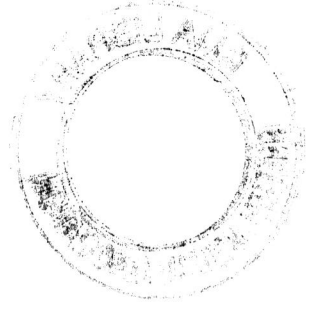

ROBBOY'S
PATHOLOGY
of the **FEMALE REPRODUCTIVE TRACT**

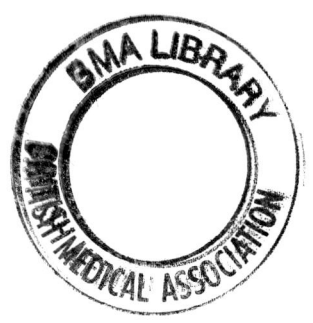

Commissioning Editor: Michael J Houston
Development Editor: Sharon Nash
Project Manager: Rory MacDonald
Design: Erik Bigland
Illustration Manager: Merlyn Harvey
Illustrator: Richard Prime
Marketing Manager(s) (UK/USA): John Canelon/Radha Mawrie

ROBBOY'S PATHOLOGY

of the FEMALE REPRODUCTIVE TRACT

SECOND EDITION

Edited by

Stanley J. Robboy MD FCAP
Professor and Vice Chairman, Department of Pathology,
Chief, Division of Diagnostic Services, Professor of Obstetrics
& Gynecology, Duke University Medical Center, Durham, NC,
USA

George L. Mutter MD FCAP
Associate Professor of Pathology, Harvard Medical School,
Department of Pathology, Brigham and Women's Hospital,
Boston, MA, USA

Jaime Prat MD PhD FRCPath
Professor and Chairman, Department of Pathology, Hospital
de la Santa Creu i Sant Pau, Autonomous University of
Barcelona, Barcelona, Spain

Rex C. Bentley MD FCAP
Associate Professor of Pathology, Department of Pathology,
Duke University Medical Center, Durham, NC, USA

Peter Russell MD FRCPA
Professor of Pathology, The University of Sydney and Director,
Department of Anatomical Pathology, Royal Prince Alfred
Hospital, Camperdown, NSW, Australia

Malcolm C. Anderson FRCPath FRCOG
Emeritus Consultant Histopathologist, Department of
Histopathology, University Hospital, Queen's Medical Centre,
Nottingham, UK

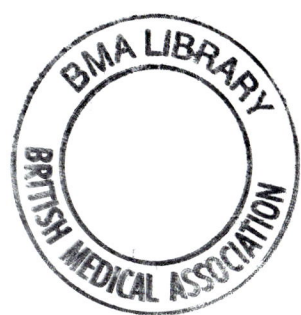

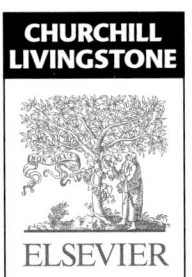

CHURCHILL
LIVINGSTONE

ELSEVIER

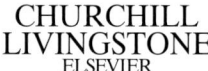

CHURCHILL LIVINGSTONE
ELSEVIER

CHURCHILL LIVINGSTONE
An imprint of Elsevier Limited.

© 2009, Elsevier Limited. All rights reserved.

First edition 2002

The right of Stanley J Robboy, George L Mutter, Jaime Prat, Rex C Bentley, Peter Russell & Malcolm C Anderson to be identified as editors of this work has been asserted by them in accordance with the Copyright, Designs and Patents Act 1988.

ISBN: 978-0-443-07477-6

British Library Cataloguing in Publication Data
A catalogue record for this book is available from the British Library

Library of Congress Cataloging in Publication Data
A catalog record for this book is available from the Library of Congress

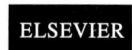

ELSEVIER
your source for books, journals and multimedia in the health sciences
www.elsevierhealth.com

Working together to grow libraries in developing countries
www.elsevier.com | www.bookaid.org | www.sabre.org

ELSEVIER   BOOK AID International   Sabre Foundation

Printed in China

The publisher's policy is to use paper manufactured from sustainable forests

Last digit is the print number: 9 8 7 6 5 4 3 2 1

Contents

CONTENTS

CHAPTER 3 VULVAR CYSTS, NEOPLASMS, AND RELATED LESIONS   59

Christopher R. Shea   Maria Angelica Selim   Stanley J. Robboy

CONTENTS

CHAPTER 4 VULVAR MESENCHYMAL NEOPLASMS AND TUMOR-LIKE CONDITIONS 95

Marisa R. Nucci   Christopher D.M. Fletcher

CHAPTER 5 VAGINA 111

Stanley J. Robboy   Peter Russell

CHAPTER 6 CERVICAL BENIGN AND NON-NEOPLASTIC CONDITIONS   141

Anais Malpica   Stanley J. Robboy

CONTENTS

CHAPTER 7 CERVIX: EPIDEMIOLOGY OF SQUAMOUS NEOPLASIA   173

Sophia S. Wang   Mark E. Sherman

CHAPTER 8 CERVICAL PRECANCER (INTRAEPITHELIAL NEOPLASIA), INCLUDING FUNCTIONAL BIOMARKERS AND COLPOSCOPY   189

Jan P.A. Baak   Mark H. Stoler   Sarah M. Bean
Malcolm C. Anderson   Stanley J. Robboy

CHAPTER 9 CERVICAL SQUAMOUS CELL CARCINOMA   227

Wenxin Zheng   Stanley J. Robboy

CHAPTER 10 CERVICAL GLANDULAR NEOPLASIA   249

*Richard C. Jaworski   Jennifer M. Roberts
Stanley J. Robboy   Peter Russell*

CONTENTS

CONTENTS

CHAPTER 15 BENIGN ENDOMETRIAL HYPERPLASIA AND EIN   367

George L. Mutter   Richard J. Zaino   Jan P.A. Baak
Rex. C. Bentley   Stanley J. Robboy

CHAPTER 16 ENDOMETRIAL ADENOCARCINOMA   393

George L. Mutter   Xavier Matias-Guiu   Sigurd F. Lax

CHAPTER 17 MESENCHYMAL UTERINE TUMORS, OTHER THAN PURE SMOOTH MUSCLE NEOPLASMS, AND ADENOMYOSIS   427

W. Glenn McCluggage   Stanley J. Robboy

CHAPTER 18 UTERINE SMOOTH MUSCLE TUMORS   457

Bradley J. Quade   Stanley J. Robboy

CHAPTER 21 NORMAL OVARIES, INFLAMMATORY AND NON-NEOPLASTIC CONDITIONS   543

Peter Russell   Stanley J. Robboy

CHAPTER 22 OVARIAN CYSTS, TUMOR-LIKE, IATROGENIC AND MISCELLANEOUS CONDITIONS 569

Peter Russell   Stanley J. Robboy

CONTENTS

CONTENTS

**CHAPTER 28 OVARIAN LYMPHOID AND
HEMATOPOIETIC NEOPLASMS 779**

Anand S. Lagoo Peter Russell Stanley J. Robboy

**CHAPTER 29 OVARIAN TUMORS:
MISCELLANEOUS AND METASTATIC 795**

Peter Russell Jennifer M. Roberts Stanley J. Robboy

CHAPTER 30 NIDATION AND PLACENTA   829

Eoghan E. Mooney   Stanley J. Robboy

CONTENTS

CHAPTER 34 DISORDERS OF SEXUAL DEVELOPMENT 945

Stanley J. Robboy   Francis Jaubert

Contributors

Malcolm C Anderson FRCOG FRCPath
Emeritus Consultant Histopathologist
University Hospital
Queen's Medical Centre
Nottingham, UK

Jan PA Baak MD PhD FRCPath FIAC(Hon)
  DrHonCausa(Antwerp)
Professor of Pathology
University of Bergen and Free University (Amsterdam);
Department of Pathology
Stavanger University Hospital
Stavanger, Norway

Sarah M Bean MD FCAP
Assistant Professor of Pathology
Department of Pathology
Duke University Medical Center
Durham, NC, USA

Rex C Bentley MD FCAP
Associate Professor of Pathology
Department of Pathology
Duke University Medical Center
Durham, NC, USA

Annie N Y Cheung MBBS MD FRCPath (UK) FHKAM(Path)
  FIAC
Professor of Pathology
Honorary Consultant
Department of Pathology
Queen Mary Hospital
The University of Hong Kong
Hong Kong, China

Rajesh Dash MD FCAP
Assistant Professor of Pathology
Department of Pathology
Duke University Medical Center
Durham, NC, USA

Emma M Doyle MB MRCOG FRCPath
Lecturer in Pathology
School of Medicine and Medical Science
University College Dublin
Dublin, Ireland

John H Eichhorn MD FASCP FIAC FCAP
Assistant Professor of Pathology
Harvard Medical School;
Department of Pathology
Massachusetts General Hospital
Boston, MA, USA

Marc Fellous MD
Faculté de Médecine Descartes
Institut Cochin
Inserm
Paris, France

Christopher D M Fletcher MD FRCPath
Professor of Pathology
Harvard Medical School;
Professor and Director of Surgical Pathology
Department of Pathology
Brigham and Women's Hospital
Boston, MA, USA

Peter Gearhart MD FACOG
Clinical Assistant Professor of Obstetrics and Gynecology
University of Pennsylvania;
Department of Obstetrics & Gynecology
Penn Hospital
Philadelphia, PA, USA

Arthur F Haney MD FACOG
Professor and Chairman
Department of Obstetrics & Gynecology
University of Chicago Medical Center
Chicago, IL, USA

Christopher B Hubbard MD
Director, Pathology Informatics
Department of Pathology
Duke University Medical Center
Durham, NC, USA

Francis Jaubert MD
Professeur Université Descartes
Praticien Hospitalier APHP
Groupe Hospitalier Necker-Enfants Malades
Paris, France

Richard C Jaworski MB BS (Hons) FRCPA
Pathologist
Douglass Hanly Moir Pathology
Macquarie Park, NSW, Australia

James V Lacey Jr MPH PhD
Investigator
Hormonal and Reproductive Epidemiology Branch
Division of Cancer Epidemiology and Genetics
National Cancer Institute
Rockville, MD, USA

Anand S Lagoo MD PhD FCAP FASCP
Associate Professor of Pathology
Director, Clinical Flow Cytometry Laboratory
Department of Pathology
Duke University Medical Center
Durham, NC, USA

Sigurd F Lax MD PhD
Associate Professor of Pathology
Medical University Graz;
Head of Department of Pathology
General Hospital Graz West
Graz, Austria

John F Madden MD
Associate Professor of Pathology
Department of Pathology
Duke University Medical Center
Durham, NC, USA

Anais Malpica MD
Professor of Pathology and Gynecologic Oncology
The University of Texas MD Anderson Cancer Center
Houston, TX, USA

Xavier Matias-Guiu MD PhD
Chairman and Professor of Pathology and Molecular
  Genetics
Department of Pathology and Molecular Genetics
Hospital Universitari Arnau de Vilanova
University of Lleida, IRBLLEIDA
Lleida, Spain

W Glenn McCluggage FRCPath
Professor of Pathology
Consultant Gynecologic Pathologist
Department of Pathology
Royal Group of Hospitals Trust
Belfast, Antrim, UK

Maria J Merino-Neumann MD
Chief, Division of Surgical Pathology
Department of Pathology
National Cancer Institute
Bethesda, MD, USA

Eoghan E Mooney MD FRCPath
Consultant Histopathologist
Department of Pathology
National Maternity Hospital
Dublin, Ireland

George L Mutter MD
Associate Professor of Pathology
Harvard Medical School;
Department of Pathology
Division of Women's and Perinatal Pathology
Brigham and Women's Hospital
Boston, MA, USA

Marisa R Nucci MD
Associate Professor of Pathology
Harvard Medical School;
Associate Pathologist
Department of Pathology
Division of Women's and Perinatal Pathology
Brigham and Women's Hospital
Boston, MA, USA

Jaime Prat MD FRCPath
Professor and Chairman
Department of Pathology
Hospital de la Santa Creu i Sant Pau
Autonomous University of Barcelona
Barcelona, Spain

Bradley J Quade MD PhD
Associate Professor of Pathology
Harvard Medical School;
Department of Pathology
Division of Women's and Perinatal Pathology
Brigham and Women's Hospital
Boston, MA, USA

Stanley J Robboy MD FCAP
Professor and Vice Chairman of Pathology
Professor of Obstetrics and Gynecology
Department of Pathology
Duke University Medical Center
Durham, NC, USA

Jennifer M Roberts MBBS (Hons) FRCPA
Senior Gynecological Pathologist
Mayne Health Laverty Pathology
North Ryde, NSW, Australia

Peter Russell MD FRCPA FRANZCOG (Hon)
Professor in Pathology
The University of Sydney;
Department of Anatomical Pathology
Royal Prince Alfred Hospital
Camperdown, NSW, Australia

Maria Angelica Selim MD FCAP
Associate Professor of Pathology and Medicine
  (Dermatology)
Director of Dermatopathology
Department of Pathology
Duke University Medical Center
Durham, NC, USA

Ruthy Shaco-Levy MD
Senior Gynecological Pathologist
Department of Pathology
Soroka Medical Center
Faculty of Health Sciences
Ben-Gurion University
Beer-Sheva, Israel

Christopher R Shea MD
Professor and Chief
Section of Dermatology;
Professor of Medicine
University of Chicago Medical Center
Chicago, IL, USA

Mark E Sherman MD
Cancer Expert
Hormonal and Reproductive Epidemiology Branch
Division of Cancer Epidemiology and Genetics
National Cancer Institute, NIH
Rockville, MD, USA

Bruce Smoller MD FCAP
Professor and Chair
Department of Pathology
University of Arkansas Medical Sciences
Little Rock, AR, USA

Mark H Stoler MD FASCP FCAP
Professor of Pathology and Clinical Gynecology;
Associate Director of Surgical Pathology and Cytopathology
Department of Pathology
University of Virginia Health System
Charlottesville, VA, USA

Sophia S Wang PhD
Investigator
Division of Cancer Epidemiology and Genetics
Environmental Epidemiology Branch
National Cancer Institute, NIH
Rockville, MD, USA

Richard J Zaino MD FCAP
Professor of Pathology
Department of Pathology
Penn State University/Milton S. Hershey Medical Center
Hershey, PA, USA

Wenxin Zheng MD FCAP
Professor of Pathology and Gynecology
Director of Gynecologic Pathology and Molecular Pathology
Department of Pathology
University of Arizona College of Medicine
Tucson, AZ, USA

Foreword

It is a privilege to have the opportunity to write the foreword for this excellent and much needed textbook. The field of gynecological pathology has continued to grow with new developments that have changed methods of diagnosis and therapy. The first edition of this textbook did much to outline the underlying principals of this field and at the same time discuss both the current state of our knowledge and practice. This second edition carries the mission further with a wider number of authors and subjects.

The text is organized in the classical manner. Beginning with embrology then proceeding with organ site discussions of benign and malignant conditions. The list of authors are from the most knowledgeable individuals in the field of female reproductive tract pathology with Dr. Robboy participating in the majority of the contributions, giving the text a smoothness not usually seen in multi-author text books.

New developments over the last decade have been carefully presented. Especially where our knowledge has exploded: such as the relationship of the human papillomavirus (HPV) and the pathogenesis of genital tract neoplasia. The references have been carefully selected to be the most comprehensive and current sources of further knowledge should the reader seek such.

Most importantly the text is very readable and is designed to assist the practitioner. Theoretical situations are minimized and have given way to practical explanations and methodologies for management of diseases that afflict the female reproductive tract. The textbook will be an essential ingredient for the library of every physician who participates in the management of these problems.

Philip J. DiSaia, MD
The Dorothy J. Marsh Chair in Reproductive Biology
Director, Division of Gynecologic Oncology
Professor, Department of Obstetrics and Gynecology
University of California, Irvine College of Medicine
Orange, California, USA

Preface

Pathology of the Female Reproductive Tract, by design, is dynamic, comprehensive and thorough, but pithy and easy to read. A decision we made when planning the 1st edition was to give the book multi-continental flavor. This was to acknowledge the reality that a common medicine is today practiced on an international scale and that the standard of care is no longer local, but global. The many advances discussed throughout the book emanate from many different countries. In this newest edition, 41 authors have been invited to participate, again representing many of the leading institutions throughout the world. As with the 1st edition, we have tried to make the text appear seamless as if prepared by a single author, yet retaining the flavor and indeed the differences that a multitude of authors and editors bring when viewing the same area. The positive response from our readers has reaffirmed the value of this approach.

To add further functionality, the authors have drawn upon their extensive personal experience, queries of trainees and junior colleagues, and discussions with senior colleagues to identify those problems and questions which are commonly encountered in practice. Unanswerable questions, today's puzzling conundrums and provocations stimulate those insights that will become tomorrow's advances. In both incorporating and filtering the ever increasing recent literature, the authors have consciously presented only those theories and explanations that we have considered hold merit.

Several aspects of the second edition are new. By involving many new authors, perspectives on presentation for individual organs by necessity have differed. In some instances, this is because medicine has evolved. Emerging new concepts about the pathogenesis of endometrial carcinoma have led to an entire new body of work on separating those lesions that are precancerous, now called endometrial intraepithelial neoplasia, from those that have histologic appearances of hyperplasia, but are biologically benign (Chapter 15). Knowledge has also exploded in our understanding of the relation between human papilloma virus (HPV) and the pathogenesis of cervical neoplasia, with new understanding about the biology of those precancerous lesions that themselves might regress spontaneously (Chapters 7 and 8). We see the beginning of major insights being made in endometrial cancer and ovarian cancer. To the extent possible, these insights are incorporated into this edition, although we anticipate a plethora of new findings in the next decade. The development of reliable immunohistochemical techniques, some borrowing from molecular diagnostics, have

provided pathologists with new tools to explore what until recently was considered classical pathology. Both Chapters 1 (embryology) and 34 (disorders of sexual development, also abnormal sexual development or intersex) heavily explore the histochemical, biochemical and genetic changes that take place over time.

A goal of this book, although never explicitly stated in the first edition, is that all of the concepts and findings presented could be used today in everyday practice. The book was not written to discuss theory, but rather what could be put into practice today. Hence, many pearls are included that we use in our daily practices. Further, a new chapter (Chapter 36) was added that systematically details the many immunohistochemical markers useful in gynecologic pathology. We hope this proves a useful reference.

If there is one area in which the editors have strayed into the future, it regards the importance of both synoptic reporting and coding, both of which make the reports rendered useful to the clinicians and managers of the electronic record in which the reports appear. Since publication of the first edition of this book, the College of American Pathologists (CAP) has entered into two key agreements that are having a major impact on all of medicine. The College has authorized the American College of Surgeons (ACS) to utilize CAP derived standardized data elements and synoptic report formats. In turn, the American College of Surgeons now requires that for an institutional tumor registry to be ACS certified, all pathology reports must incorporate pathology reporting elements deemed critical by the CAP. Synoptic reports ensure that all relevant information is included in the diagnosis rendered, allowing for better treatment of patients and easier comparison of findings across institutions. The elements of synoptic reporting are covered in Appendix C. The second major event occurred in 2005 when the coding system the CAP developed (SNOMED, or Systematized Nomenclature of Medicine) which also incorporated the United Kingdom's Clinical Terms Version 3) was adopted by the US National Library of Medicine as the major language of healthcare. The importance of this language and its role as a critical element of electronic healthcare is described in Appendix D.

To keep the volume current and manageable for the reader, the authors have emphasized inclusion of references published since 2000. To the extent feasible, earlier articles have been pruned as they are now general knowledge and easily accessible from various databases. Further, current review articles have been given preference rather than the original older articles.

The review articles often provide new insights and advances not present in the original.

Finally, during the intense multiyear endeavor required to prepare both the prior and this edition, your editors have enjoyed a buoyant spirit and have tried to portray this in the various chapters. Except where deemed outrageous by either the editors from Elsevier or our wives, we have left several purposeful elements of humor embedded in the text. Like the children's series, "Where's Elmo", we challenge the reader to find these inclusions.

We truly hope that within the year, your book will be ragged and ravaged from use.

Stanley J. Robboy
George L. Mutter
Jaime Prat
Rex C. Bentley
Peter Russell
Malcolm C. Anderson

Dedication

To our wives — Marion, Patty, Serena, Genie, Gail & Christine — the loves of our lives.

Acknowledgements

Many dedicated people, too numerous to list provided invaluable insight and contributions that have made this edition of Pathology of the Female Reproductive Tract possible. We wish especially to thank the managing and editorial staff at Elsevier without whose help this volume would have been impossible.

The editors also acknowledge the contributions made by our colleagues who participated in previous editions.

Katharine Dalziel
Harold Fox
Janice M. Lage
Anne Morse
James Padfield
Alan Stevens

Embryology

Francis Jaubert Stanley J. Robboy George L. Mutter Marc Fellous

INTRODUCTION

Understanding normal development of the embryonic genital tract gives insight into many disorders encountered in the female. These can range from relatively simple arrests of development or malformation (described by organ) to more complex abnormalities of sexual development that result from dysembryogenesis (see Chapter 34), and in some cases, to help understand the origin of some tumors, particularly sex cord-stromal and germ cell tumors of the ovary. Most early insights have come from understanding human mutations. During more recent years, targeted mutations using mouse models have disclosed key roles for genes that had not been anticipated previously. Many of these regulators modulating gonadal development involve an array of receptors, signal transduction pathways, transcription factors, extracellular ligands, and even crosstalk among intracellular signaling pathways mediating downstream transcriptional responses. Recently published references[3,16,19,26,30,41,42] provide extensive reviews and, to some degree, competing theories.

Most of the female genital tract is of mesodermal origin. Germ cells are of endodermal origin. The vulva and the epithelial lining of the vagina are ectoderm. The chronology and sequence of events that underlie the development of the female genital tract are summarized in Figures 1.1 and 1.2, and in Table 1.1. Table 1.2 lists specific genes involved in the initial steps of sexual development.

In the broadest view, sex determination takes place in three sequential steps.[37] The first is chromosomal sex determination, which occurs as a result of fertilization. Gonadal sex determination, the second critical event, results when the potential gonads actually transform into ovaries or testes in accord with the available chromosomal information. Thirdly, the secondary sex characteristics develop along female or male lines as determined by the preponderant estrogenic or androgenic hormonal milieu present systemically. Sexual identity, not to be discussed here, includes a person's sense of self (gender identity) and his/her attraction to others.

GONADAL DEVELOPMENT

Prior to the period when sex determination begins, the indifferent gonad arises from the gonadal ridge that, with the mesonephros, lies longitudinally on the dorsal aspect of the celomic cavity. At this time, the indifferent gonad is 'unisex' or, more properly, 'bipotential' due to its ability to develop into a testis or an ovary depending upon the embryo's genetic makeup.

In humans and other mammals, the karyotype 'XY' genetically defines the sex as male, whereas 'XX' defines the female sex. Sex is determined by the presence or absence of a signal from the substance initially called the testis determining factor (TDF) and now recognized as the gene called *SRY* (*Sex* determining *Region Y*) in the human, and Sry in the mouse. The gene is found on the Y chromosome. Testes are formed if this gene is expressed by the embryo before the urogenital ridge differentiates. Further male development occurs under the influence of hormones secreted later by the testes. Without *SRY*, the gonads differentiate as ovaries and the embryo develops as a female. The timely expression of *SRY* is critical to the development of male sex. In its absence, the embryo develops a female phenotype, regardless of genetic sex.[11] Although for years believed to occur by default, a gene has been identified in women (R-spondin1, RSPO1)[4a] critical for development of the ovary through signaling pathways.[4b]

The *SRY* gene is located in the region just central to the pseudoautosomal pairing region at the distal end of the short arm of the Y chromosome.[4] (The pseudoautosomal pairing region (PAR) is named for the two limited regions at the distal ends of the short and long arms of the Y chromosome where sequence identity with the X chromosome permits pairing and recombination during male meiosis.[23]) The gene, which has a strongly conserved motif,[11] encodes for a DNA binding protein, which is the binding activity product (transcriptional switch) that orchestrates the action of other genes. It does so by initiating a cascade of gene expressions that regulate the development of the testis, not all of which are known or understood.

Several lines of evidence support this thesis. These include:

- the *SRY* gene is absent from the normal X chromosome and somatic chromosomes;
- the *SRY* gene is present on the X chromosome of 'sex-reversed' XX human males;
- the homologous gene in the mouse is initially expressed just before sexual differentiation begins (the genital ridge initially swells);
- the *SRY* gene acts in the absence of germ cells;
- the *SRY* gene in the chromosomally female embryo causes it to develop as a male.[14]

Rare examples have also been identified where single basepair point mutations in the *SRY* gene or in promoter regions essential for gene expression render an XY patient as a phenotypic female with a streak gonad.[25]

Early on, *SRY* initiates induction of somatic cell migration from the mesonephros into the gonad[40] and induces indifferent cells in the genital ridge to differentiate into Sertoli cells. This is the first type of cell required to form in the embryonic testis.[39] With monoclonal antibodies, an SRY protein has been found in the nuclei of Sertoli cells and germ cells.[35] Several other genes

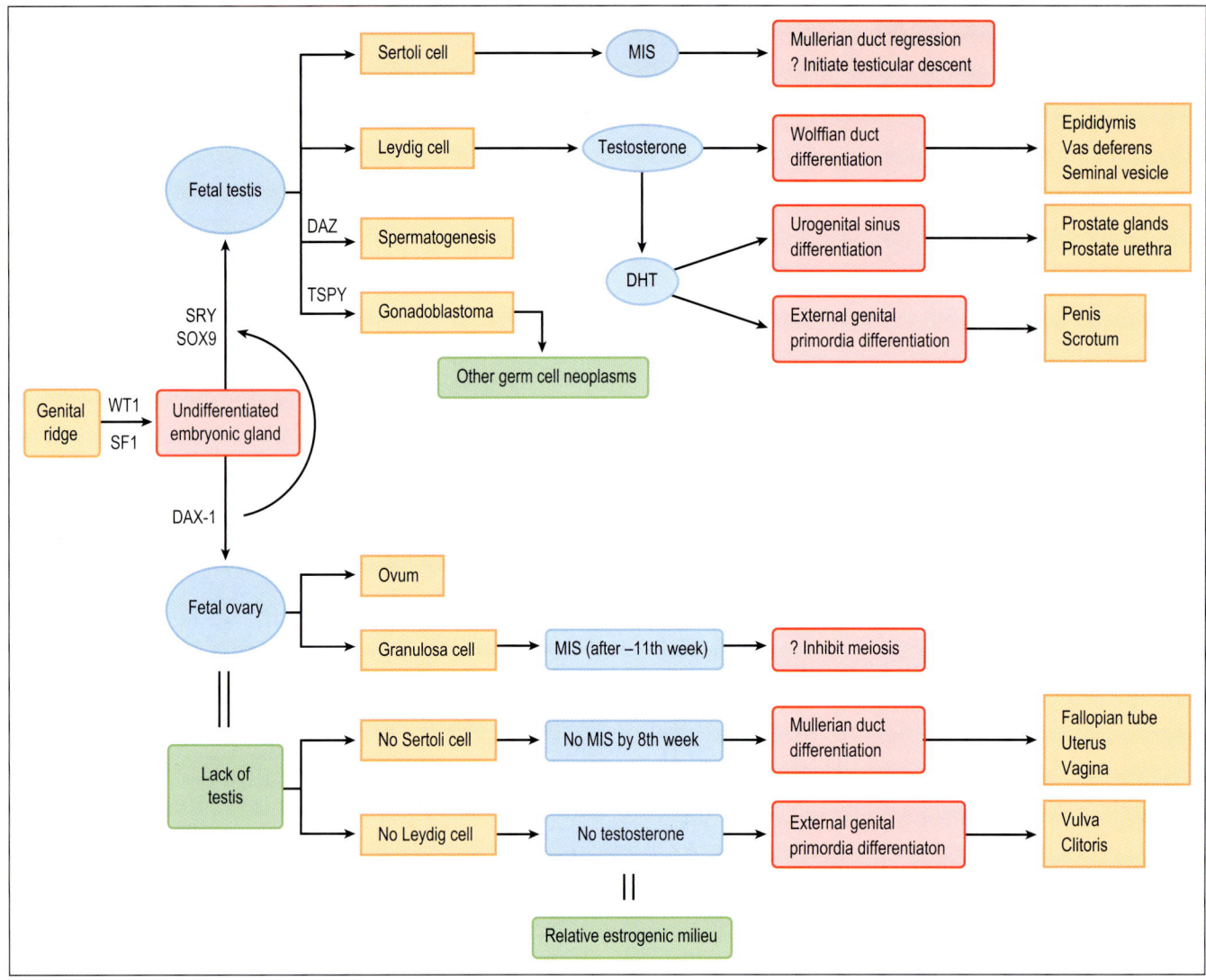

Fig. 1.1 Pathophysiology of genital tract development and neoplasia.

are thought to be important in Sertoli cell function. *SOX9*, which is named for it being an *SRY*-related HMG (high motility gene) box group, in the mouse is active in pre-Sertoli cells[27] and results in XY human females when mutations inactivate the gene. *SF1*, which *SOX9* helps regulate, is another important gene that is an orphan nuclear receptor expressed in the gonadal ridge in precursor cells of Sertoli and stromal cells. It appears as a master regulator of the reproductive system because it regulates the expression of numerous genes required for gland development and hormone synthesis.[31,32,36] Mutations in this gene in humans have been responsible for adrenal insufficiency associated with gonadal dysgenesis.[22] The gene, *DAX1*, which is required at several points in embryonic testis development,[24] also plays a key role in sex determination. Overexpression causes varying degrees of gonadal dysgenesis, and at high doses in the mouse, male-to-female sex reversal occurs. Additional references[11,23,36,37] describe in greater detail the genes involved in the rapidly evolving science of male sex determination.

In the event that the embryo does not express *SRY* on a time-sensitive basis as a transcription factor, and therefore

does not develop a testis, then other genes that are responsible for the development of the ovary activate later. In the goat, studies on XX sex reversal in polled (horned) goats have led to the discovery of a female-specific locus critical for ovarian differentiation (see discussion about *FOXL2* below).

During the development of both male and female human embryos, but before the gonads develop, the primordial germ cells migrate from the yolk sac to the urogenital ridges via the caudal part of the hindgut approximately 3 weeks after fertilization (Figure 1.3). The yolk sac, which is of considerable size, is easily recognized by its reactivity to α-fetoprotein (Figures 1.4–1.6). This migratory event is independent of eventual sex. The germ cells are large and prominent, and have clear cytoplasm and vesicular nuclei. Once they synthesize glycogen and alkaline phosphatase, they are easily identified histochemically by their demonstration of placental-like alkaline phosphatase (PLAP) and CD117 (c-kit) (Figure 1.7).

At about this time, the mesothelium on the medial surface of the urogenital ridge, which itself is located ventral to the mesonephric rudiments, begins to proliferate. By the fifth week, while still in the indifferent stage, the parenchyma is a thin

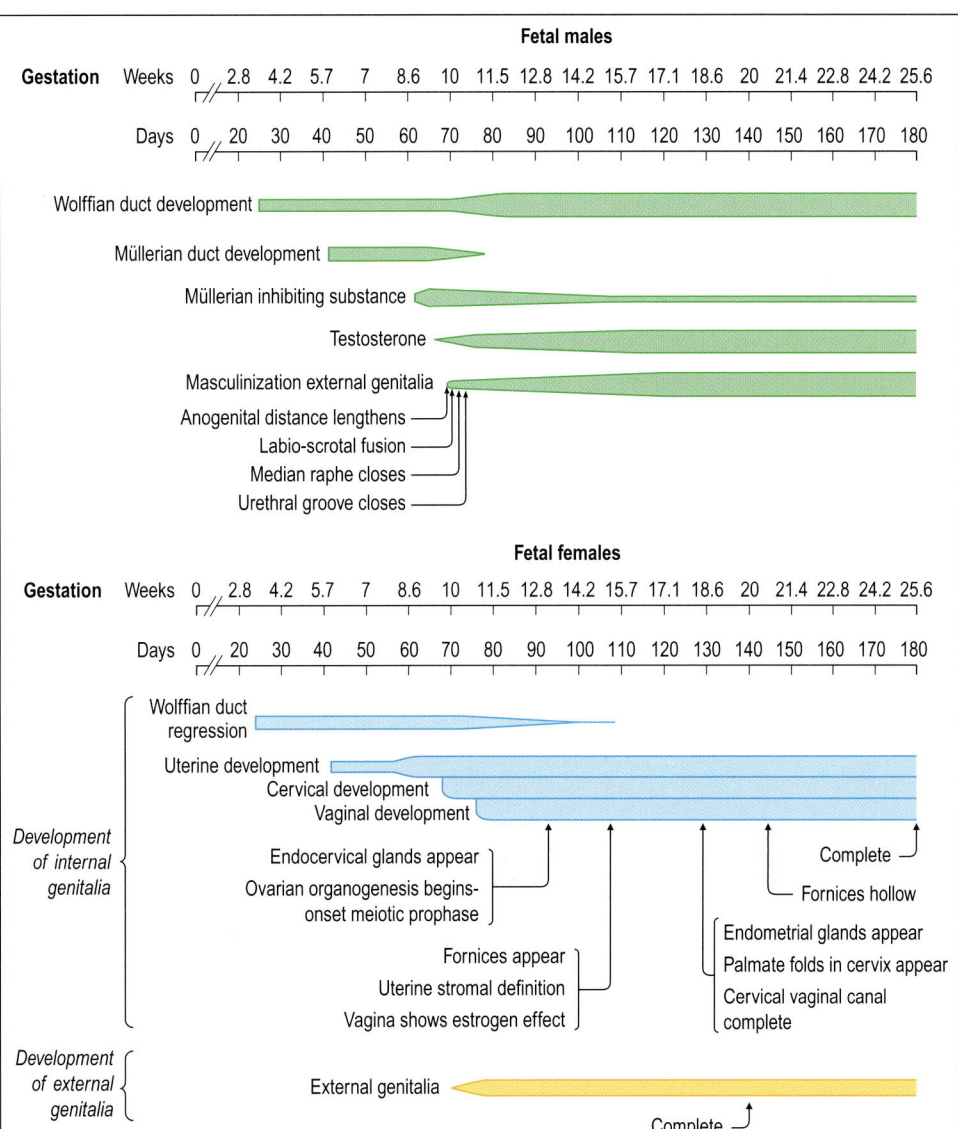

Fig. 1.2 Normal sexual development. Embryologic development is determined by several factors, all of which are time specific during embryogenesis.

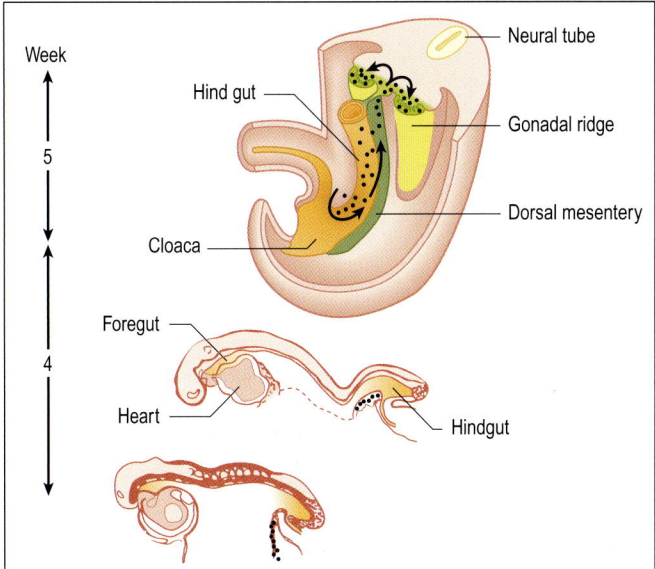

Fig. 1.3 Migration of germ cells in the human embryo. At the end of the third week, epiblast-derived cells present in the yolk sac near the allantoic base have differentiated into primordial germ cells, the latter having migrated by the fifth week along the dorsal mesentery of the hind gut to the gonadal ridges.

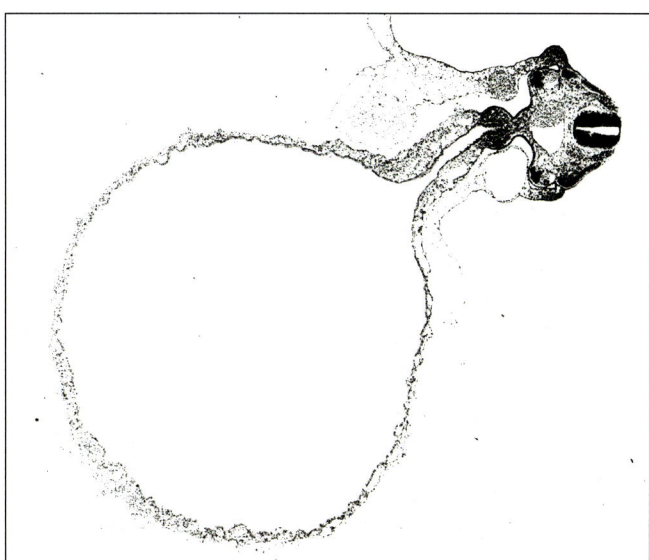

Fig. 1.4 Yolk sac with germ cell migration. Day 28.

Table 1.1 Synopsis of stages of normal embryologic development

Crown–rump (CR) (mm)	Week after ovulation	CR length, day postovulation	Carnegie stage	Description of event
		2.5 mm		Pronephric tubules form; pronephric (mesonephric) duct arises and grows caudad as solid cord.
		21 days	10	Primordial germ cells first discernable in yolk sac near caudal part of embryo.
3 mm	3.3 weeks			
		3–5 mm	12	Pronephros degenerated, but mesonephric duct reaches cloaca.
		27 days	12	Primordial germ cells discernable in hindgut.
7 mm	4 weeks			
		5 mm	13	Primordial germ cells discernable in mesonephric ridges.
		7 mm	14	Primordial germ cells discernable in gonadal ridge, which itself at this time is a thin mesodermal proliferation.
		7–9 mm		Cloaca divides into rectum and urogenital sinus.
		33 days		
12 mm	5 weeks			
		8–11 mm	16	Müllerian ducts appear as funnel-shaped opening of celomic epithelium.
		37 days		Indifferent gonad bulges into celom.
				Primitive sex cords appear.
18 mm	6 weeks			
		17 mm/48 days		Müllerian ducts about half distance to urogenital sinus.
		20+ mm	18	Testis anatomically distinct with seminiferous tubules.
23 mm	7 weeks			
			20	Ovaries initially identified by absence of distinct seminiferous tubules.
		51 days +		Müllerian ducts elongate and near urogenital sinus.
		51 days	22	Ducts approach each other.
		23–28 mm 54 days		Ducts in apposition; sinusal tubercle appears.
		27–31 mm ≥56 days		Ducts fuse and in contact with urogenital sinus.
29 mm	8 weeks			
		30? mm		So-called 'ambisexual' stage ends; experimental data for dating müllerian duct regression unclear.
		56? days		Experimentally, müllerian duct is sensitive to MIS through ≥25 mm CR size; ducts in older embryos not sensitive. Clinically, embryos 31–35 mm before effect observed; regression completed by 43–55 mm.
				Leydig cells appear.
43 mm	9 weeks			
		50? mm		Testes and ovaries acquire capacity to secrete characteristic hormones at same stage of development; testosterone coincides with histologic development of Leydig cells and immediately precedes virilization of genital tract; ovary not yet differentiated; rate-limiting step is appearance of 3 β-hydroxysteroid dehydrogenase, which is 50-fold more abundant in testis than ovary; ovary converts testosterone to estradiol, which testis cannot do; later regulation shifted to pituitary–placenta gonadotrophins where testosterone → estradiol controlled by conversion of cholesterol to pregnenolone.
		56 mm		Müllerian ducts completely fused (entire septum gone); caudal aspect proliferates; epithelium lining canal stratifies (2–3 cells layers thick).
		70 days		Anogenital distance lengthens.
60 mm	10 weeks			
		71 days		Testosterone synthesis sufficient to induce development of mesonephric duct into definitive structures (epididymis, vas deferens and seminal vesicle). Subsequently, testosterone converted peripherally into 5 α-dihydrotestosterone which causes the following transformations: Urogenital sinus → prostate Genital tubercle → glans penis Genital folds → penis (only 3.5 mm long) Genital swelling → scrotum

Table 1.1 Continued

Crown–rump (CR) (mm)	Week after ovulation	CR length, day postovulation	Carnegie stage	Description of event
		72–74 days		Fusion of labioscrotal folds.
				Closure of median raphe.
				Closure of urethral groove.
				Phallus in both sexes 3 mm long; thereafter grows in males 0.72 mm/week and females 0.20 mm/week.
		75 days		Mesonephric ducts regress if not stimulated by testosterone.
		≥60 mm		Vaginal plate first seen distinctly (complete at 140 mm; week 17). Initially, upper uterovaginal canal is large and oval in cross-section, mostly lined by pseudostratified columnar epithelium. Extensive growth begins caudally; cells stratify.
		68 mm		Uterovaginal canal occluded caudally, progresses cranially.
71 mm	11 weeks			
				Primordial follicles appear.
				Seminal vesicle develop.
				Testis at inguinal ring.
		77 mm		Extensive uterovaginal growth continues caudally.
93 mm	12 weeks			
		100–120 mm		Cervical glands appear; wavy, but undifferentiated.
		105 mm		Vaginal rudiment approaches vestibule.
				True ovarian organogenesis begins with onset of meiotic prophase.
105 mm	13 weeks			
				Male urethral organogenesis complete.
116 mm	14 weeks			
		126 mm		Primary folds of mucosa give uterine lumen W-shaped appearance on cross-section.
		130 mm		1. Vaginal rudiment reaches level of vestibular glands; uterovaginal canal (15 mm total length) divisible into vagina (one-half), cervix (one-third), and corpus (one-sixth); boundaries ill-defined.
				2. Isthmus readily distinguishable.
				3. Stromal layers of uterus begin definition.
				4. Solid epithelial anlage of anterior and posterior fornices appear.
				5. Vagina begins to show slight estrogen effect.
130 mm	15 weeks			
		139 mm		Fallopian tube begins active growth phase, begins to coil.
		140 mm		Vaginal plate completed; lower end reaches vestibule; upper end extends into endocervical canal.
				Female urogenital sinus becomes shallow vestibule.
				Primary follicles of ovary appear.
142 mm	16 weeks			
		151 mm		Vaginal plate longest and begins to canalize.
				Corpus glands appear as slight outpouchings.
153 mm	17 weeks			
		160 mm		Palmate folds of cervix appear (forerunner adult cervix).
		162 mm		Mucoid development of cervix begins.
				Smooth muscle of uterus appears.
				Estrogen effect apparent throughout vagina.
				Cavitation of vaginal canal completed.
164 mm	18 weeks			
		170 mm		Fornices hollow.
177 mm	19 weeks			
		185 mm		Dramatic increase in growth and coiling of fallopian tube (about 3 mm/week to week 34).
186 mm	20 weeks			
197 mm	21 weeks			
208 mm	22 weeks			
		210 mm		Differentiation of muscular layer of uterus complete.
		227 mm		Fundus well marked; uterus assumes adult form.
				Graafian follicles appear.

Table 1.1 Continued

Crown–rump (CR) (mm)	Week after ovulation	CR length, day postovulation	Carnegie stage	Description of event
230 mm	24 weeks			
250 mm	26 weeks			
270 mm	28 weeks			
290 mm	30 weeks			
328 mm	34 weeks			
362 mm	38 weeks	266 days		Birth.

Table 1.2 Genes involved in sex determination

Gene	Origin of name	Localization	Expressed by	Function	Phenotype if abnormal
Testis determining					
SRY = NR5A1	Sex determining Region Y (Nuclear receptor subfamily 5, Group A, Member 1)	Yp11	Genital ridge and Sertoli cells	Transcription factor	XY gonadal dysgenesis
SOX9	Srybox	17q24	Sertoli cells	Transcription factor	Campomelic dysplasia with XY gonadal dysgenesis
SF1	Steroidogenic factor-1	9q33	Ovary, adrenal gland and Sertoli cells	Transcription factor	Gonadal and adrenal agenesis in mouse
WT1	Wilms tumor suppressor gene	11p13	Primordial gonad and kidney	Transcription factor	Denys–Drash and Frasier syndromes
DAX1 = NR0B1	DAX1 = DSS-AHC on the X chromosome, where DSS = dosage sensitive sex reversal gene AHC = adrenal hypoplasia congenita gene (Nuclear receptor subfamily 0, Group B, Member 1)	Xp21.3	Genital ridge	Transcription factor	XY gonadal dysgenesis
DMRT1, DMRT2	Double sex and mab-3 related transcription factor 1	9p24.3	Testis	High and low expression, respectively, required for testis and ovarian differentiation	XY sex reversal
Ovary determining					
FOXL2	Forkhead box L2	3q23	Genital ridge, ovarian follicular cells	Forkhead transcription factor	Premature ovarian failure
WNT4	Wingless-related integration site 4 (Wingless-type MMTV integration site family, Member 4)	1p35	Leydig cells	Signaling molecule for pattern formation	Rokitansky–Kuster–Hauser syndrome
Phenotype determining					
AMH (MIS)	Antimüllerian hormone (Müllerian inhibiting substance, type 1)	19q13	Sertoli cells and in secondary follicle granulosa cells	Causes regression of fetal müllerian ducts, inhibits Leydig cells	Persistent müllerian duct syndrome
AMHR2 MISR II	Antimüllerian hormone type 2 receptor Müllerian inhibiting substance II	12q12–13	Primary sex cords; and müllerian duct	Serine threonine kinase receptor	Persistent müllerian duct syndrome

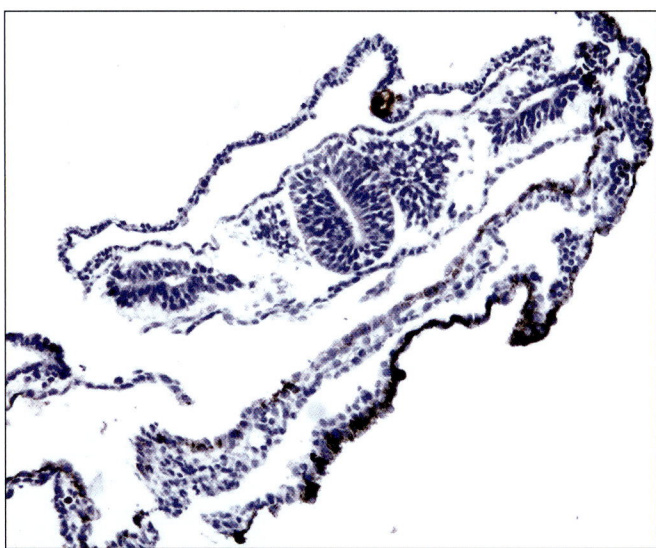

Fig. 1.5 Embryonal disk (Carnegie stage 10, about 21 days). The yolk sac is diffusely reactive for alpha-fetoprotein.

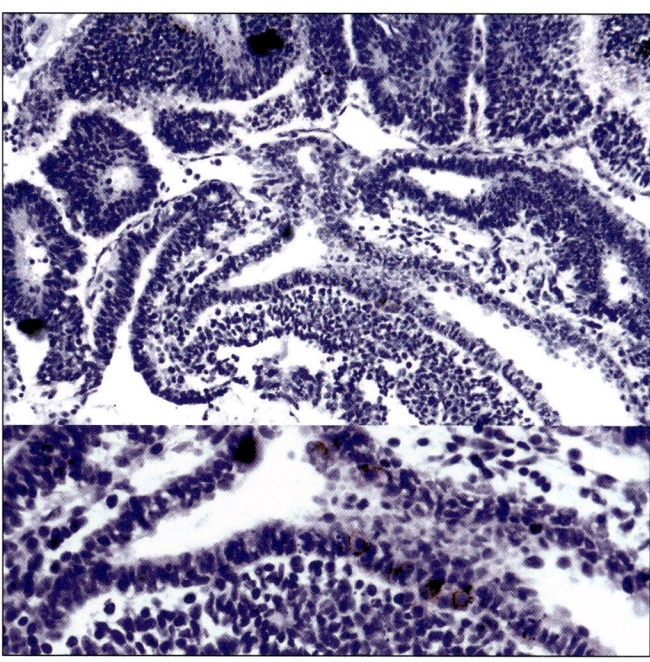

Fig. 1.7 Embryo with c-kit reactive germ cells in hindgut wall (Carnegie stage 12, about 27 days). The lower half shows the c-kit positive cells in detail (Brown).

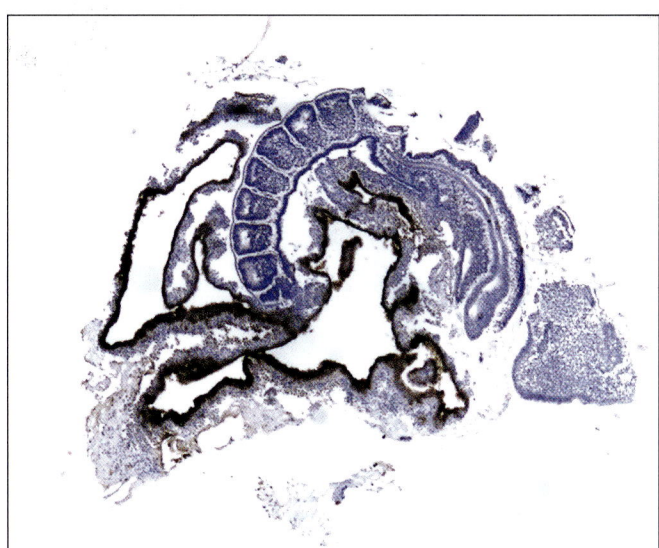

Fig. 1.6 Embryo (Carnegie stage 12, about 27 days). The yolk sac is diffusely reactive for alpha-fetoprotein.

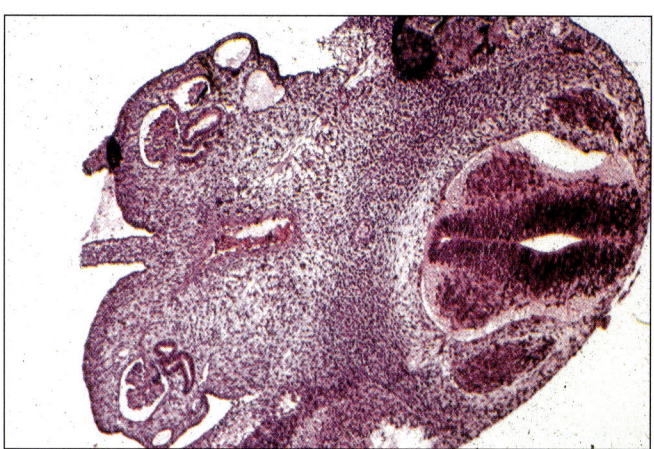

Fig. 1.8 The gonadal ridge in the 7 mm embryo (5 weeks) is much thinner than the width of the mesonephros.

wisp, measuring less than 1 mm thickness and several millimeters in width (Figures 1.8–1.10). Several transcription factors, including Wilms' tumor 1 (*WT1*) (Figure 1.11) and steroidogenic factor 1 (*SF1*), are involved in the earliest processes of gonad formation, regardless of the direction to which the gonad differentiates. These transcription factors act on the somatic cells in the gonadal primordia, but do not affect the germ cells themselves, which are still easily identifiable by their reactivity for PLAP and c-kit (Figure 1.12). Over the next several weeks the ridge develops into a recognizable, but undifferentiated, gonad (Figures 1.13 and 1.14).

During the initial stages of both testicular and ovarian development, the gonads develop independent of whether the primordial germ cells are present or absent or have proliferated abnormally. An early manifestation of the normally developing gonad is the appearance in the gonad of primary sex cords, which are temporary branched structures containing the proliferating germ cells and support cells (Figures 1.15–1.17). This process begins during the fifth week. The sex cords, the exact embryologic derivation of which is uncertain but seemingly dependent on the migration of mesonephric interstitial cells, lack a basement membrane and basal myoid cells. In a manner not yet understood, in the presence of *SRY* and with the participation of the rete and mesonephric apparatus, the sex cords transform into the tubules, which become cords of epithelial-like cells that extend from the rete in the hilus of the gonad into the medulla. The level of the connection is less important than the field effect of induction of epithelial–mesenchymal differentiation.

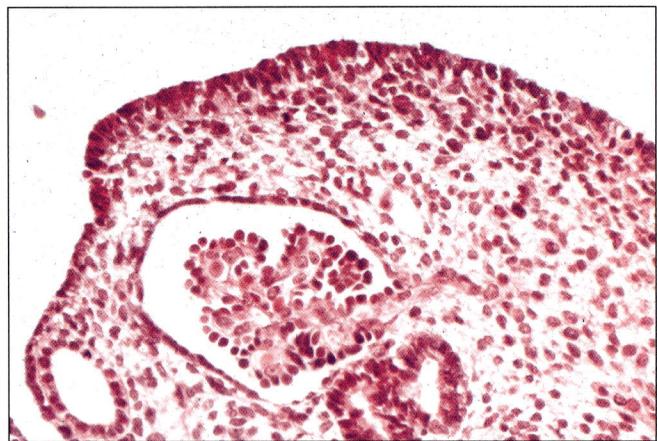

Fig. 1.9 Detail of mesonephros and gonadal ridge, 7 mm embryo.

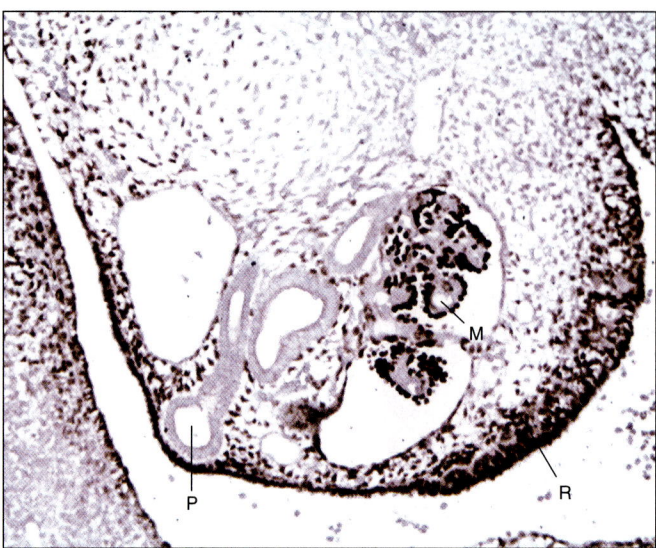

Fig. 1.11 *WT1* is expressed in the mesonephros (M) and the genital ridge (R) (Carnegie stage 13, about day 33). The residual pronephric ducts (P) do not react.

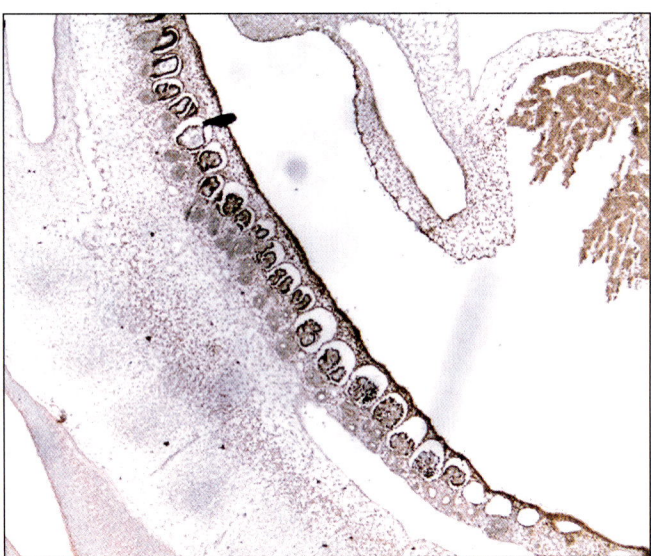

Fig. 1.10 The mesonephros, cut longitudinally, is still a predominant feature at this early stage when the gonadal ridge is forming (Carnegie stage 14, about 33 days). The gonadal ridge and underlying mesonephros are diffusely reactive for *WT1*.

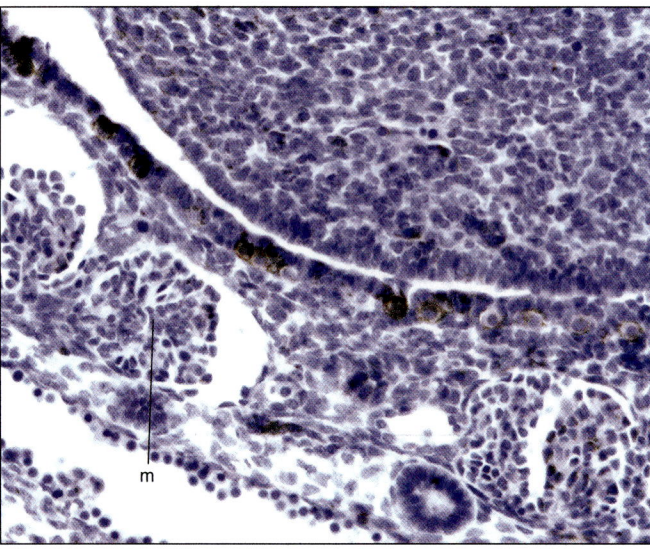

Fig. 1.12 C-kit reactive germ cells (Brown) in the genital ridge (Carnegie stage 14, about 33 days). Mesonephros (m).

In males, the testis is anatomically distinct with early tubular formation and immature Sertoli cells by postovulation day 44. (In this chapter, all dates given are postovulation.) In females, germ cells continue to increase in number (Figures 1.18 and 1.19) until ovarian differentiation is apparent some 5 weeks later, as shown by the emergence of primordial follicles. In the male, subsequently, a capsule (tunica albuginea) develops and separates the epithelial cords from the surface. The cords become the testicular tubules as the epithelial cells differentiate into the tall, clear, flask-shaped Sertoli cells of the testis (Figures 1.20–1.22) and myoid (peritubular contractile) cells appear just outside the basement membrane. The gonadal stromal cells become the interstitial or Leydig cells (Figure 1.23). In normal development, the germ cells are initially located in the lumen and move eventually between the Sertoli cells to lie on the basement membrane at the base of the tubules. The primordial germ cells preferentially colonize the medullary region of the presumptive gonads (Figures 1.24 and 1.25).[14] Even in the absence of germ cells, the somatic tissues of the undifferentiated embryonic gonad are capable of developing into a testis, albeit lacking spermatogonia and spermatogenesis.[38]

At some later time, another gene of the Y chromosome comes into play and activates the process for the development of normal spermatogenesis. The gene, called *DAZ* (Deleted in *AZ*oospermia), is less well characterized than the *SRY* gene.[10] In the absence of *DAZ*, or at least if not detectable by current methods, sperm will still develop, although defective and few in number, but capable of successful fertility.[28] *DAZ* mutation

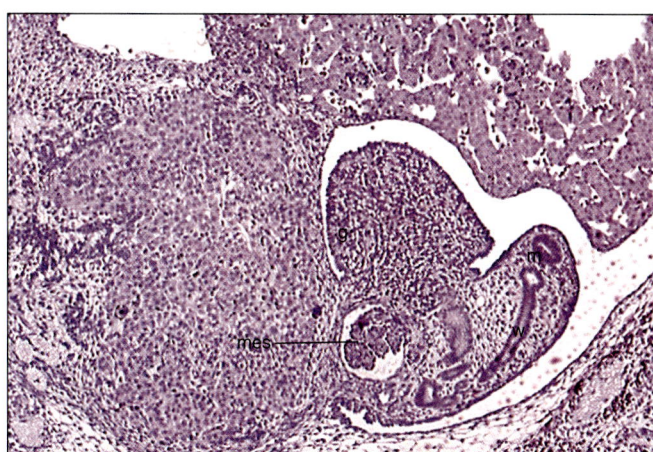

Fig. 1.13 Undifferentiated gonad (g) with wolffian (w) and müllerian (m) canals and adjacent mesonephros (mes) (Carnegie stage 16, about 37 days).

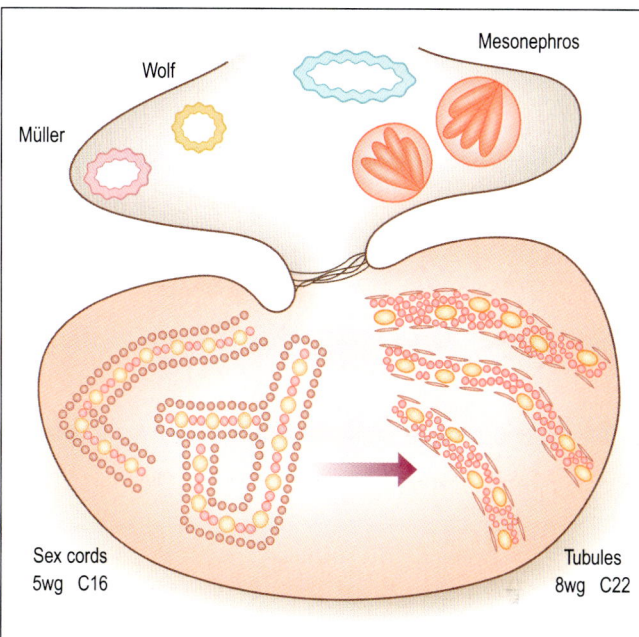

Fig. 1.15 Testicular development in male embryo from Carnegie stage 16 to 22 (~week of gestation (wg) 6–8). Within the bean-like gonad the primary sex cords develop under the influence of migrating mesonephric cells, which induce a mesenchymal to epithelial switch of differentiation similar to that happening in the metanephros under the action of *WT1*. The conversion of the sex cords to tubules is induced by the rete, which are under *SRY* control, and connected to the tubules. The primary sex cords (left) are composed of primary germ cells (pink) and stromal cells that have acquired epithelial features. Tubular differentiation (right) features acquisition of myoid cells and a peripheral basement membrane and more centrally located Sertoli and germ cells (pink).

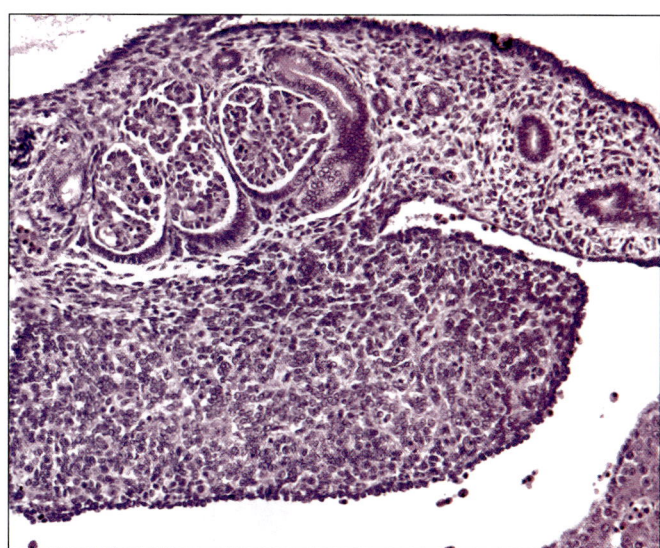

Fig. 1.14 Undifferentiated gonad with histologic suggestion of early sex cord formation (Carnegie stage 18, about 46 days).

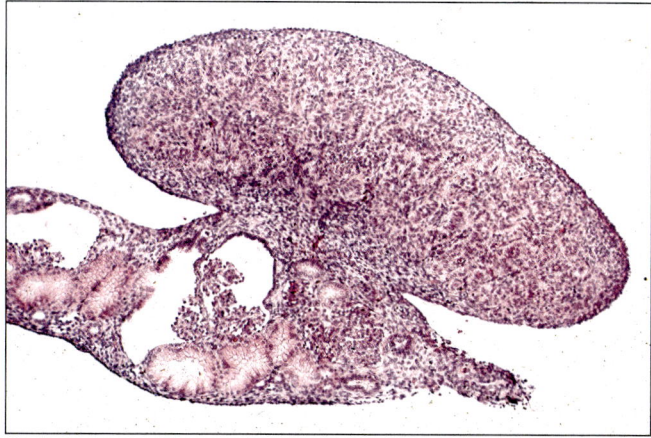

Fig. 1.16 Undifferentiated gonad at 6.5 weeks. Note enlarged size compared to mesonephros.

results in loss of the Y chromosome during mitosis, which leads to the creation of both XO and XY cell lines.

If functional *SRY* is absent (i.e., normal 46,XX females), genes associated with ovarian development activate.[5] *WNT4*, the first signaling molecule identified in the study of sex determination in mice, regulates female sexual development.[11] Part of its function is to repress male sexual differentiation. Patients with defective *WNT4* present with a Mayer–Rokitansky–Hauser-like syndrome with absence of müllerian-structures, unilateral renal agenesis, and clinical signs of androgen excess.[2] *FOXL2* is demonstrable in the genital ridge before there is any clear structural organization of the gonads.[1,7,9] Recent studies in mice have shown a robust female genetic program that activates at the onset of ovarian development.[29]

In the absence of male determining factors, the dividing germ cells are incorporated into a proliferating mass of surface epithelial cells, which results in a thickened cortex that presages the organization of the adult ovary without the development of a separating tunica (Figures 1.26–1.28). From the second to the early third trimester, this thickened cortical mass of proliferating epithelial and germ cells divides into small groups demarcated by strands of stromal tissue extending from the medulla to the cortex (Figures 1.29 and 1.30). The small groups of germ cells and epithelial cells further subdivide into

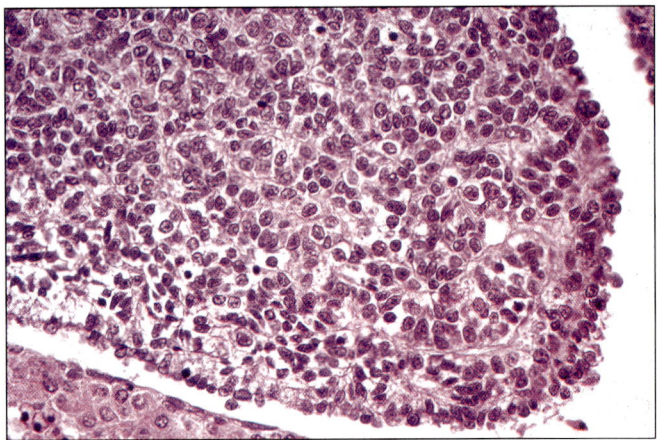

Fig. 1.17 Undifferentiated gonad at 6.5 weeks with numerous germ cells.

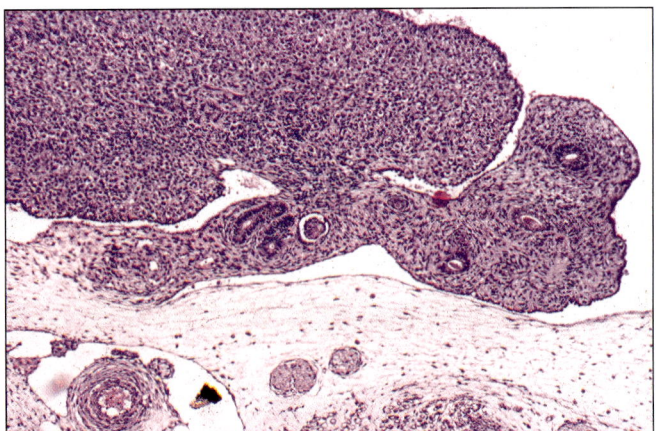

Fig. 1.18 Ovarian volume is greater than in prior weeks, 10 week fetus.

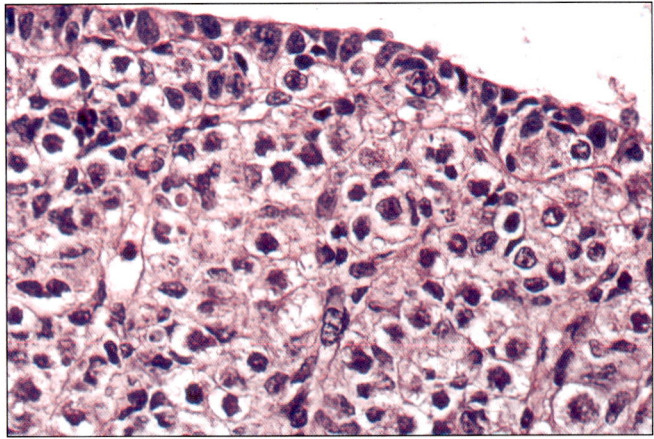

Fig. 1.19 Ovary with numerous oogonia before primordial follicles develop, 10 week fetus.

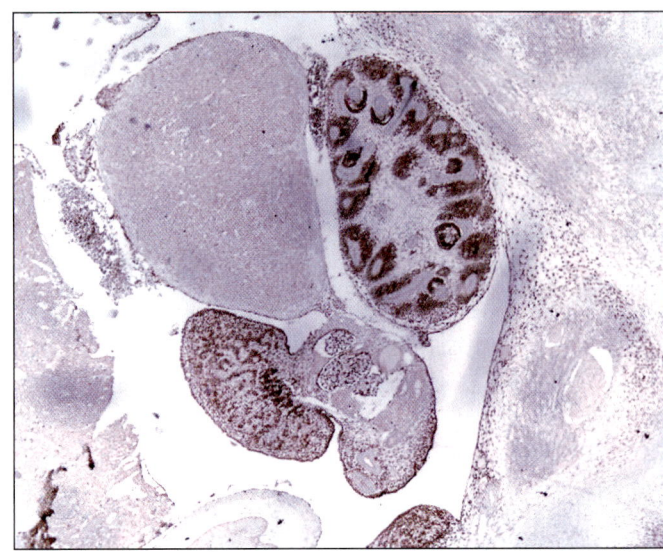

Fig. 1.20 Testis. The sex cords exhibit *WT1* reactivity (Carnegie stage 19, about 49 days).

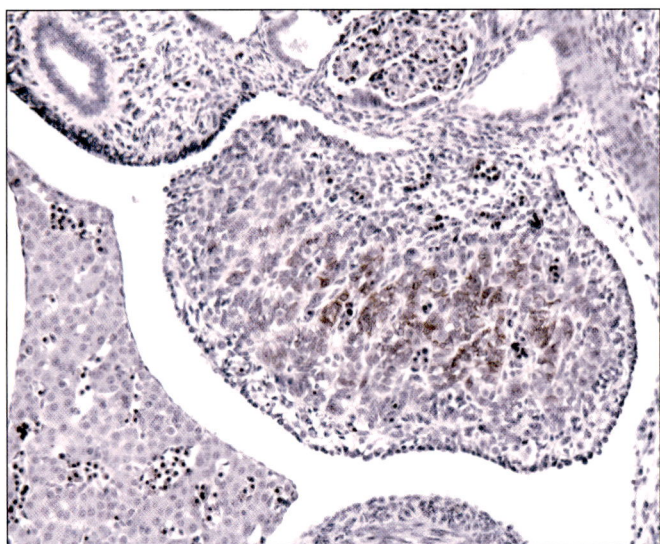

Fig. 1.21 Testis. The sex cords exhibit AMH reactivity in the cytoplasm of the Sertoli cells (Carnegie stage 19, about 49 days).

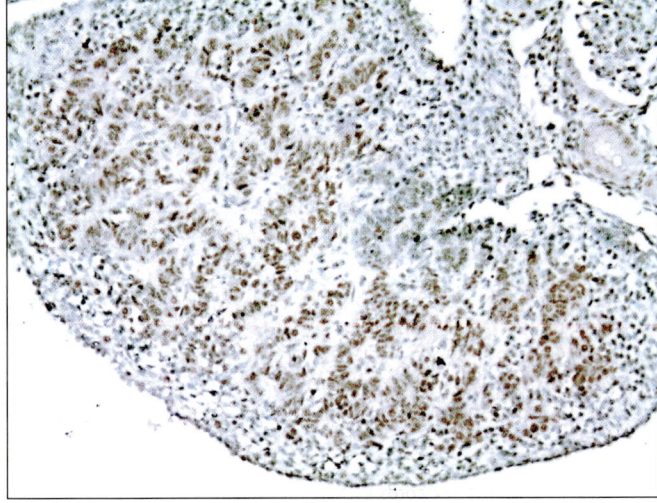

Fig. 1.22 Testis. The sex cords exhibit nuclear *SRY* reactivity (Carnegie stage 22, about 51 days).

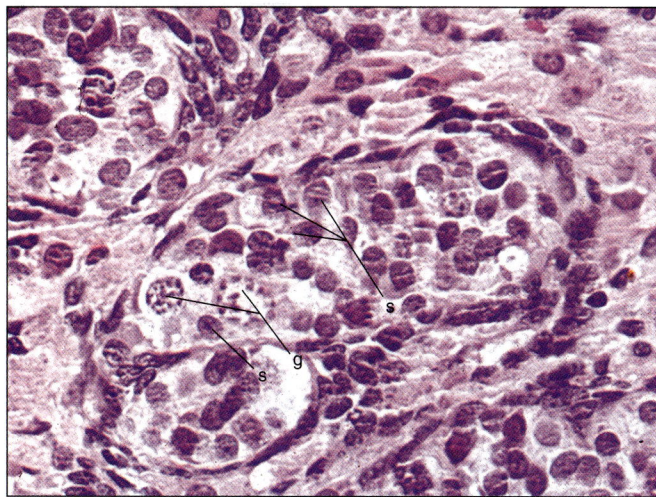

Fig. 1.23 Testis with seminiferous tubules and intratubal germ cells, 19 week fetus. g, germ cell; l, leydig cell; s, sertoli cell.

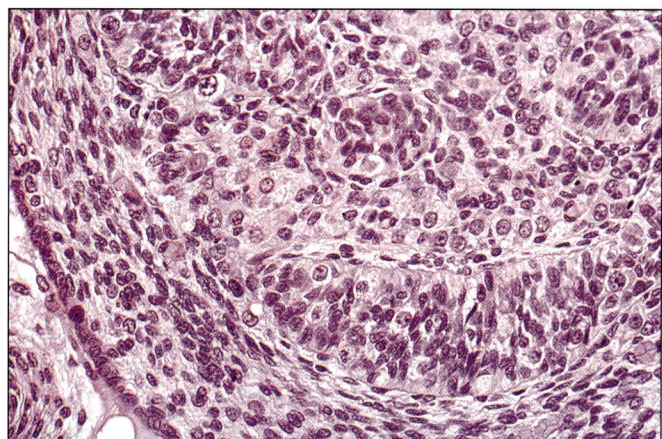

Fig. 1.24 Testis with seminiferous tubules and intratubal germ cells, 11 week fetus.

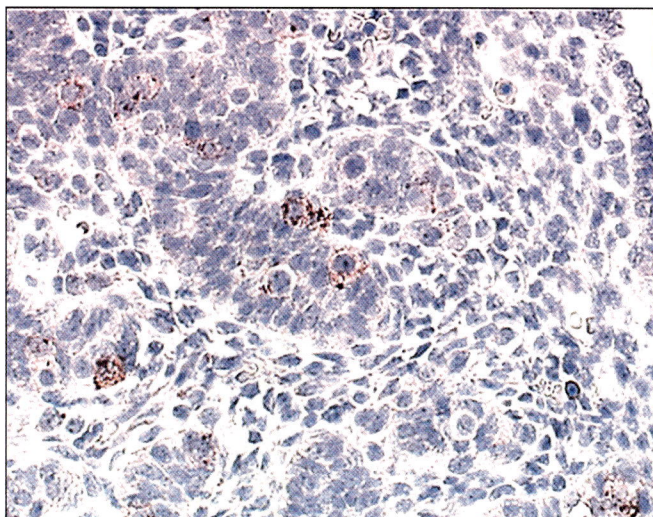

Fig. 1.25 Testis. The sex cords exhibit PLAP reactive germ cells, most of which are located superficially. At a later stage, they will become basal in location (Carnegie stage 22, about 51 days).

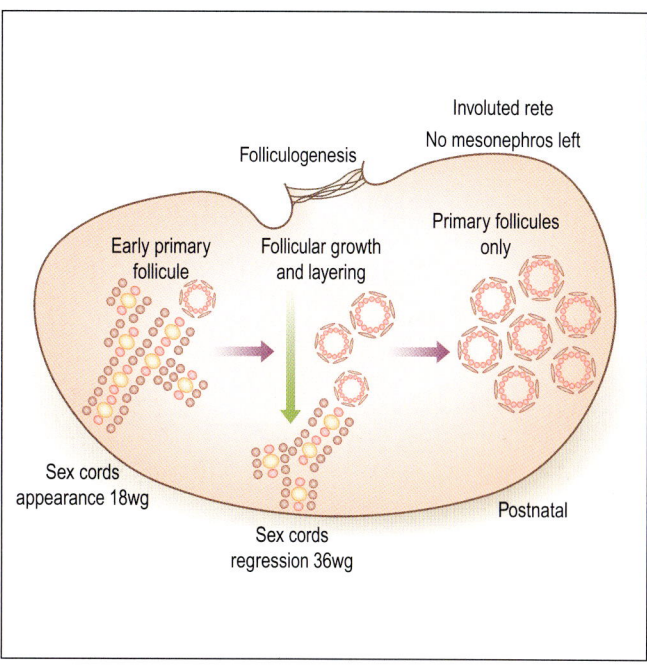

Fig. 1.26 Ovarian development from 18 weeks through birth. Until the 18th week of gestation (wg) the ovary is an undifferentiated gonad with a streak-like pattern. The primary sex cords begin their development under the influence of mesonephric cells that had migrated earlier and then remained inactive. The mesenchymal to epithelial switch of differentiation starts deeply in the parenchyma as does early primary follicular differentiation, as shown by immunohistochemical demonstration of *FOXL2* nuclear reactivity and the appearance of primary follicles of small size. The folliculogenetic process repeats itself a deeper to more superficial direction with the progressive disappearance of the primary sex cords around 36 weeks' gestation. The growth in follicles occurs under the influence of *WT1* like that of metanephric glomeruli in the kidney. Simultaneously, the primary sex cords regress by apoptotic death of the remaining cells. By birth, only primary follicles remain. Primary sex cords (left) are composed of primary germ cells (pink) and stromal cells acquiring epithelial features. Follicles (left, middle and right) disclose a central oogonium (pink) surrounded by follicular (granulosa) cells. A peripheral basement membrane envelopes each follicle.

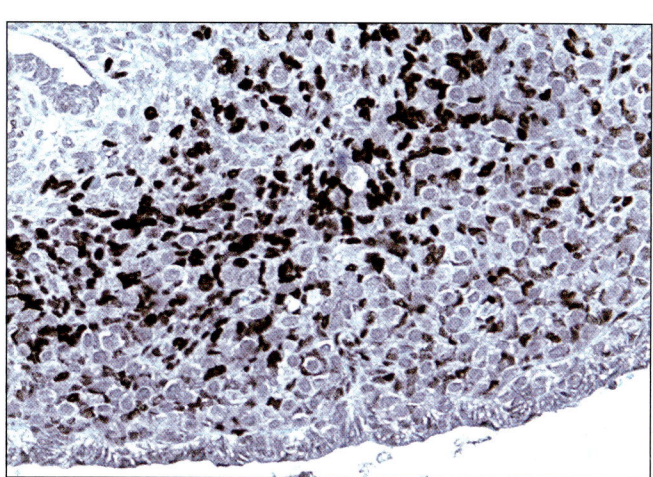

Fig. 1.27 Ovary at 10 weeks' gestation showing a mixture of germ cells (non reactive) and of stromal cells (brown reactive) (*FOXL2*).

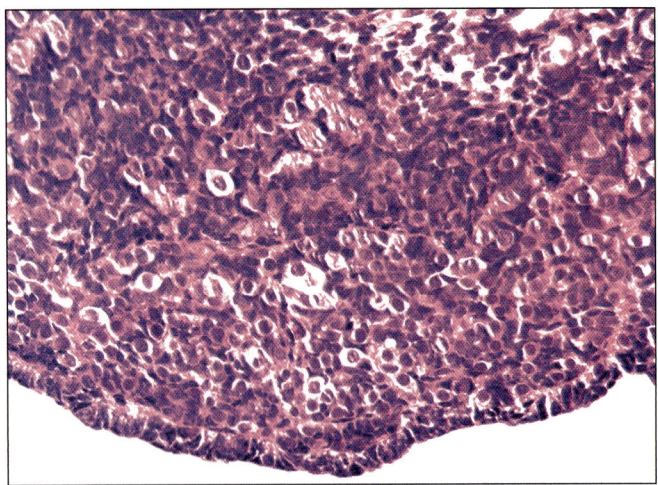

Fig. 1.28 Ovary at 10 weeks' gestation showing a mixture of germ cells and of stromal cells (H&E).

primordial follicles composed of single germ cells surrounded by a layer of epithelial cells, the primitive granulosa cells (Figure 1.31). In normal development, each germ cell is characteristically encapsulated in its own (primordial) follicle. Oogonia, not so enveloped, undergo spontaneous apoptosis. This is associated with entry into meiosis and cessation of further proliferation. By puberty, while most of the ovary shows variable concentrations of oocytes, some have developed into the antral stage and may become future ovulatory sites (Figures 1.32 and 1.33).

Until about the 15th week, the ovary is an undifferentiated gonad with a streak-like pattern. The primary sex cords begin their development under the influence of mesonephric cells that had migrated earlier and then remained inactive. The mesenchymal to epithelial switch of differentiation starts deeply in the parenchyma as does early primary follicular differentiation,

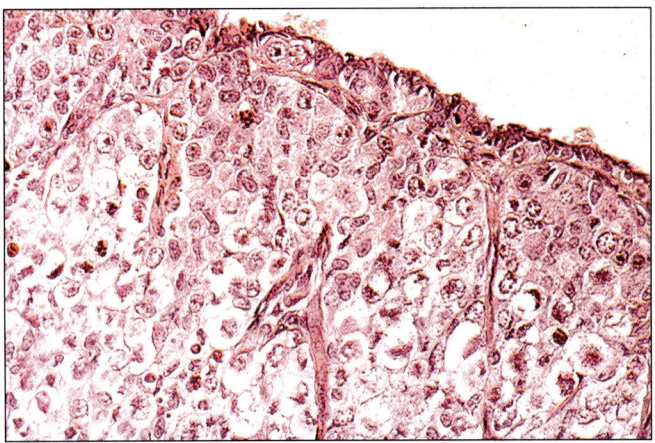

Fig. 1.29 Ovary with numerous oogonia, 17.5 week fetus.

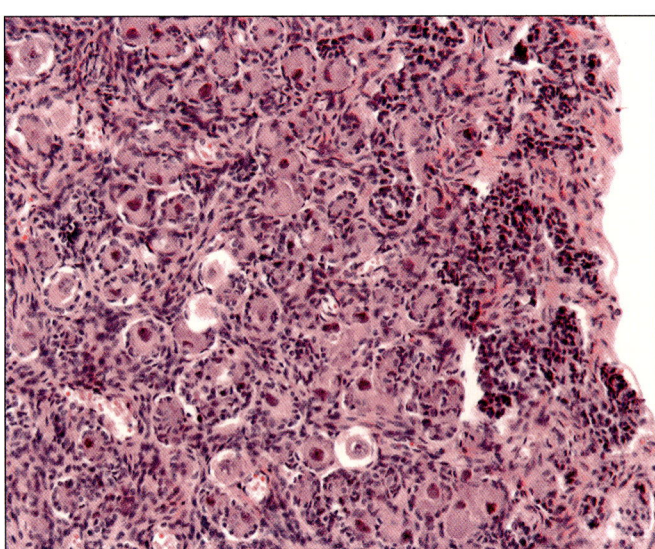

Fig. 1.30 Ovary at 36 weeks' gestation showing primary sex cords.

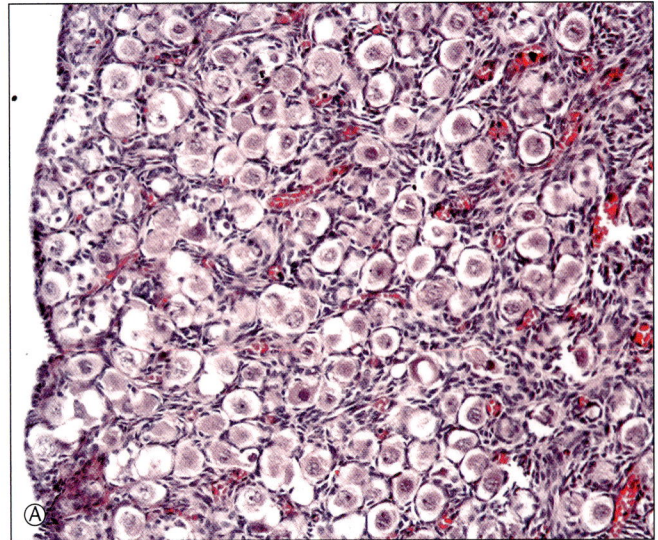

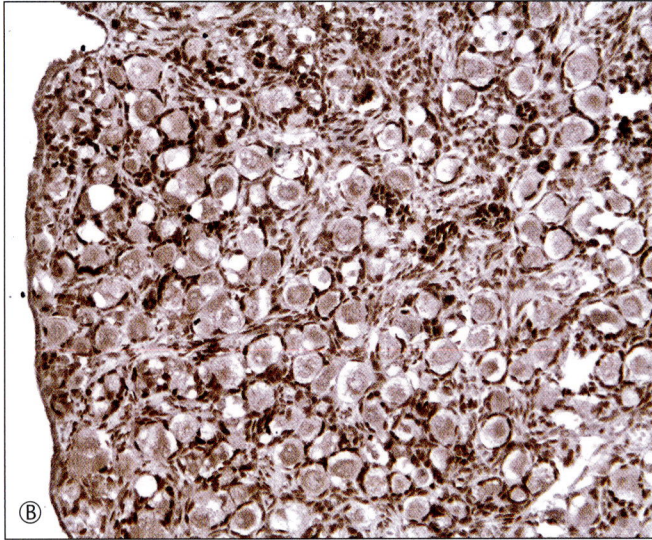

Fig. 1.31 Ovary at birth showing numerous primary follicles (A) with *FOXL2* reactivity in follicular cells (B).

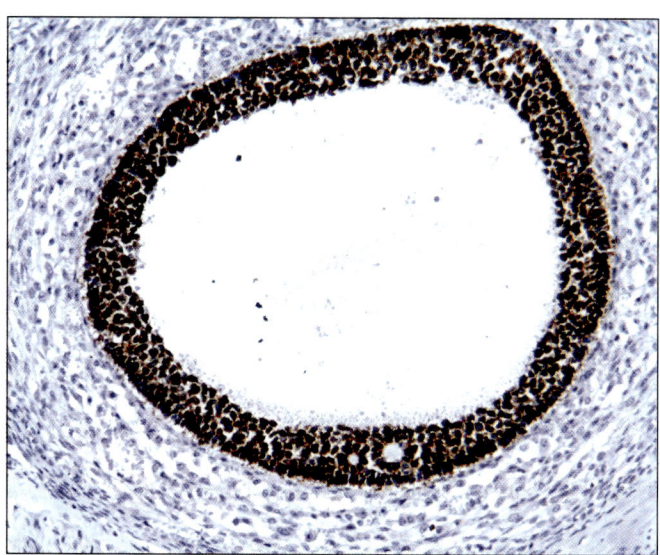

Fig. 1.32 Ovary of a 13-year-old child in which the follicular cells in follicles with an antrum are secreting AMH. This pattern is opposite of that seen prenatally.

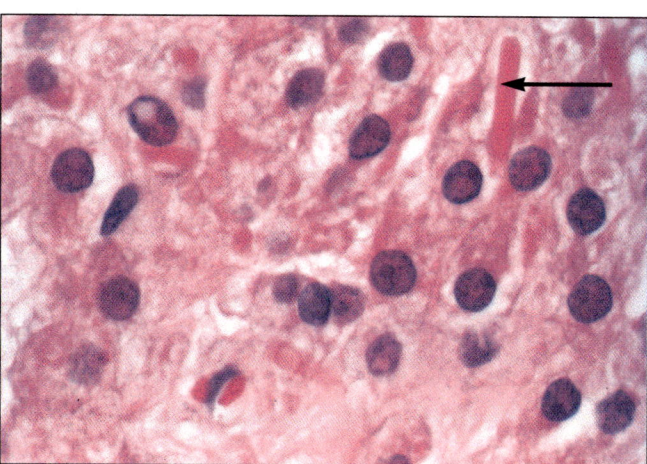

Fig. 1.34 Hilus cells with crystalloids of Reinke (arrow) surround a nerve. The crystalloids appear as proteinaceous rods.

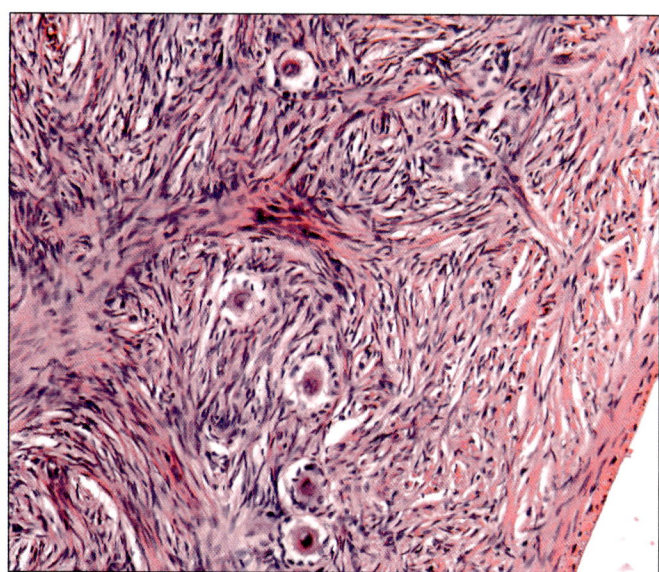

Fig. 1.33 Ovary of a 13-year-old child. The primary follicles are widely spaced (H&E).

as shown by immunohistochemical demonstration of *FOXL2* nuclear reactivity and the appearance of primary follicles of small size. The folliculogenetic process repeats itself from the deeper to the more superficial with the progressive disappearance of the primary sex cords around 36 weeks' gestation. The growth in follicles occurs under the influence of *WT1*, similar to that for metanephric glomeruli in the kidney. Simultaneously, the primary sex cords regress by apoptotic death of the remaining cells. By birth, only primary follicles remain.

If the normal male genetic constitution (46,XY) is present, some of the early epithelial proliferation contributes to the connection between the sex cords and the mesonephric tubules (rete testis). Where gonads are destined to become ovary, early epithelial proliferation degenerates in the ovarian hilus, leaving a few tubules, the rete ovarii. It is these primordial mesonephric cells that are believed to develop and envelop the individual germ cells and eventually become the follicular granulosa cells. Interstitial (Leydig) cells develop extensively in the stromal tissue of the second trimester female gonad, but degenerate in most cases by term. The few interstitial cells found in the hilus of the adult ovary are called hilus cells (Figure 1.34). Thus, the gonad develops primarily from mesodermal tissues, with the exception of the germ cells, which are endodermal in origin.

ROLE OF GERM CELLS

The primordial germ cells, which migrate to the primitive gonad, are not undifferentiated cells. By the time of their migration from the yolk sac to the gonadal ridge, they have attained some developmental potency. Occasionally, germ cells stray during migration and reach ectopic sites. If they do not die, they still may be capable of differentiation, but remarkably, always differentiate as oocytes regardless of their genetic sex. Even if the cells are in males, they differentiate as XX germ cells would normally in the ovary. It is thought that the absence of Sertoli cell differentiation is important, and the suggestion remains that all germ cells should be viewed potentially as female, regardless of the genetic sex of the patient. Follicular cells also appear important: in their absence, germ cells in ectopic sites usually degenerate and disappear. Thus, the ability of primordial germ cells to develop into oocytes or spermatogenic cells seems to reflect the tissue environment in which they grow rather than their own native chromosomal constitution. The development of the germ cells follows the somatic sex of the gonadal tissue, and not the genetic sex of the germ cells themselves.[13] In the mouse there is evidence that c-kit reactive stem cells present in bone marrow become ovarian-type germ cells.[17]

MÜLLERIAN AND WOLFFIAN DUCT DEVELOPMENT

THE MÜLLERIAN DUCT TO WEEK 8

Regardless of genetic sex, the celomic epithelium in both females and males invaginates at several points on the lateral surface of the paired urogenital ridges at the beginning of week 5 of embryonic life (Figure 1.35). They coalesce to form the paired tubes termed the müllerian (paramesonephric) ducts (Figures 1.36 and 1.37). Each of the paired ducts extends caudally in the urogenital ridge immediately lateral to and using the wolffian (mesonephric) duct as a guidewire. For proper müllerian duct migration to occur, it is essential that the wolffian duct be present. Spatially lateral to the cephalad aspect of the wolffian ducts, the müllerian ducts then cross over caudally to lie medial to them as they enter the pelvis (Figures 1.38– 1.40). By the end of week 8 of embryonic life, the müllerian ducts between the two wolffian ducts fuse to form a single structure, which is the anlage of the common uterovaginal canal (Figures 1.41 and 1.42). The tip of the müllerian duct abuts upon the posterior wall of the urogenital sinus immediately between the two orifices of the wolffian ducts (Figures

1.43–1.47). The embryologic significance of where the tip of the now fused müllerian duct abuts on the posterior wall of the urogenital sinus is controversial, in particular whether it defines the site of what will become the junction of the uterus and upper vagina,[21] or the future vaginal introitus, i.e., the hymenal membrane.

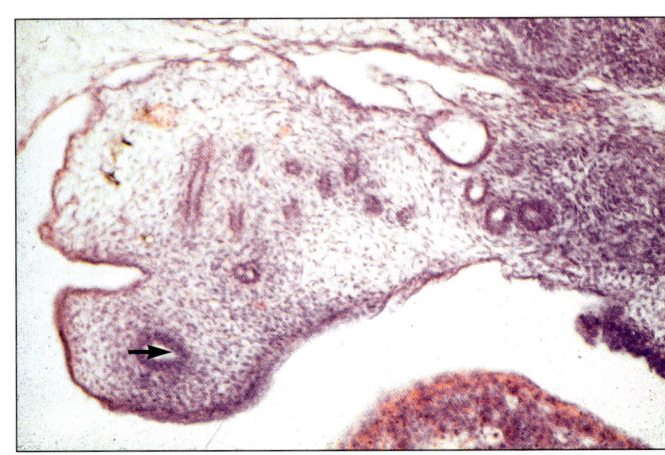

Fig. 1.37 Embryonic fallopian tube (arrow) shown further caudal to two prior figures (3 of 3).

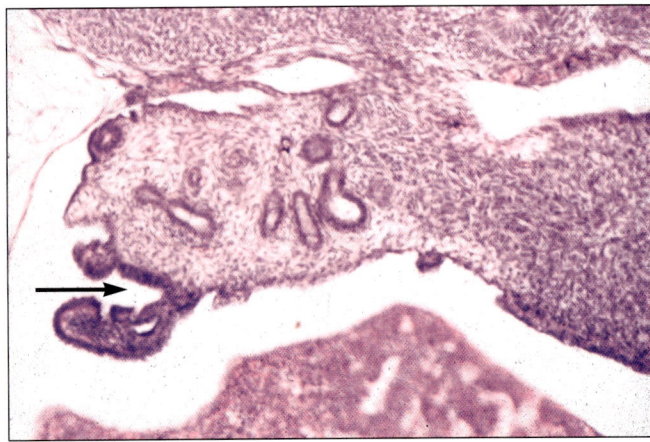

Fig. 1.35 Formation of embryonic fallopian tube with invagination of celomic epithelium (arrow), 6 week embryo (1 of 3).

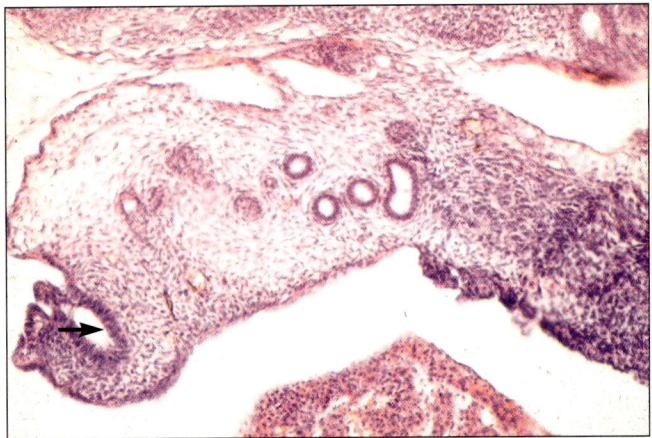

Fig. 1.36 Invagination of celomic epithelium (arrow) slightly more caudal to preceding illustration, 6 week embryo (2 of 3).

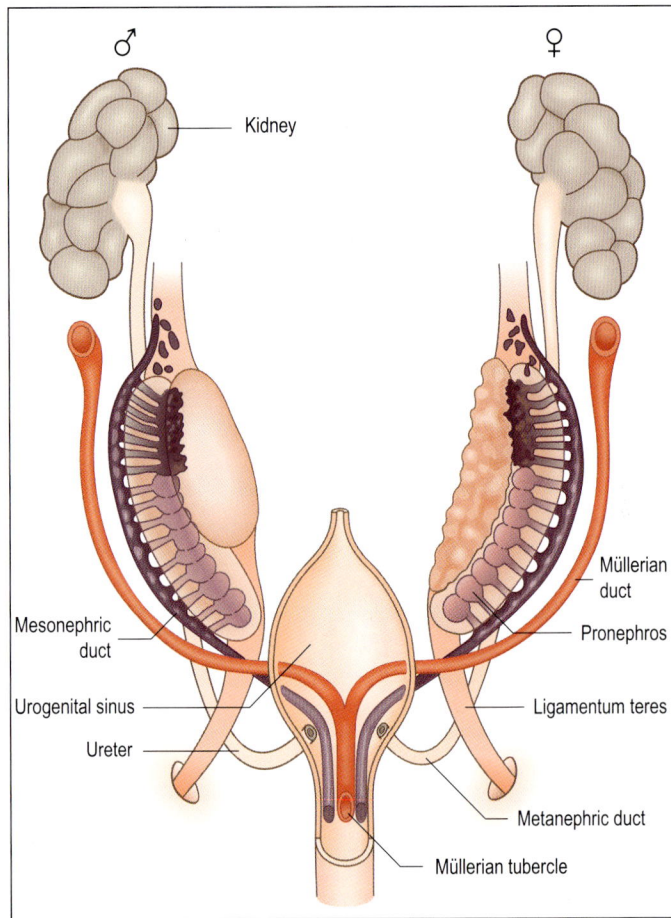

Fig. 1.38 The anlage of the genital organs in the indifferent, bisexual stage. The müllerian derivatives are red and the wolffian derivatives are blue.

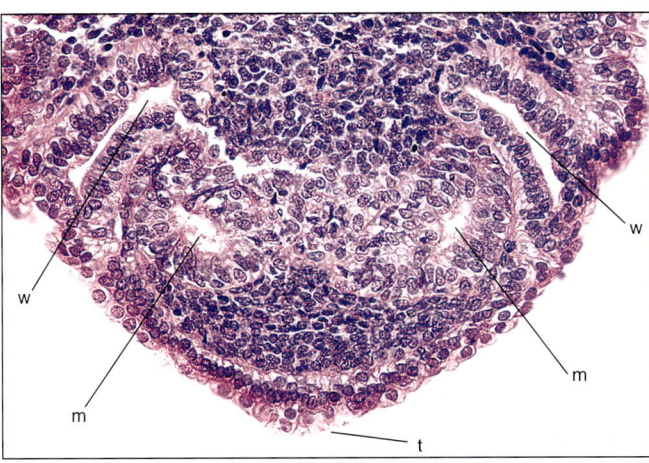

Fig. 1.39 The two müllerian ducts (m) lie between the two wolffian ducts (w). Section from urogenital sinus at level of the müllerian tubercle (t).

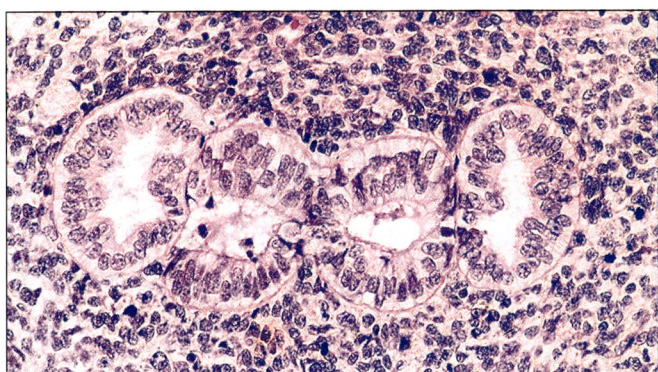

Fig. 1.40 The two müllerian ducts lie between the two wolffian ducts. The section is proximal to the urogenital sinus tubercle.

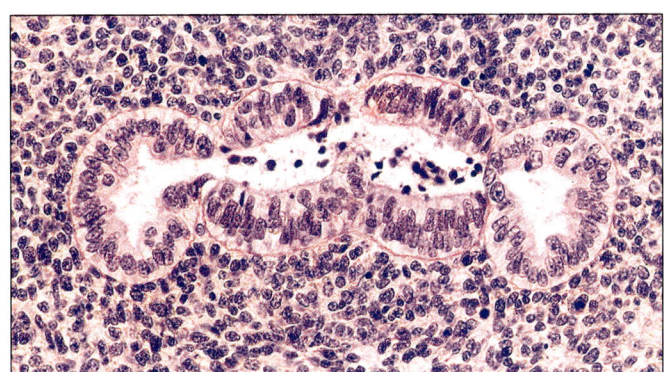

Fig. 1.41 The two müllerian ducts beginning to fuse. They lie between the two wolffian ducts.

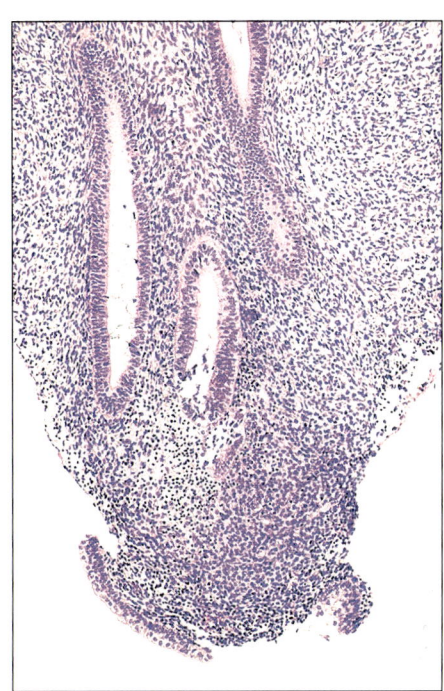

Fig. 1.42 Central single müllerian duct flanked by two wolffian ducts.

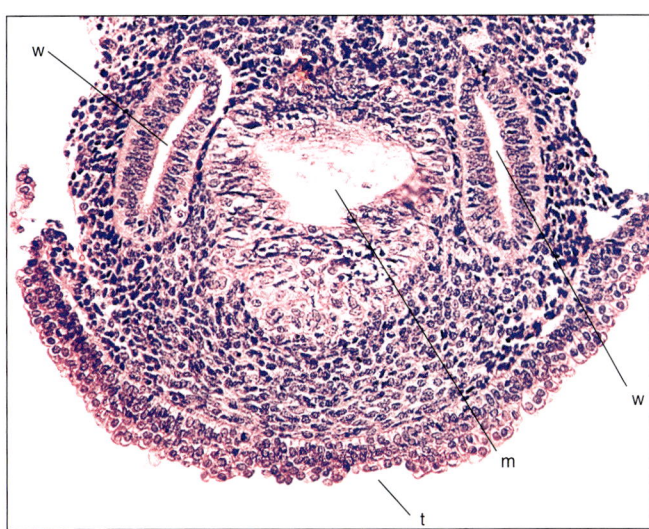

Fig. 1.43 Single müllerian duct (m) flanked by two wolffian ducts (w). Section from urogenital sinus at level of the müllerian tubercle (t).

EXTERNAL INFLUENCE ON THE DEVELOPING EMBRYONIC GENITAL TRACT DUCTS

All of the above occur in both female and male fetuses and are completed before the testis, if the embryo is male, begins to secrete antimüllerian hormone (AMH), also known as müllerian inhibiting substance (MIS). In the presence of AMH, the müllerian tissues regress, remaining only as rudimentary structures in the maturing male urogenital system.

Once the male pathway of development has begun, two hormones produced by the fetal testis then control the differentiation of the male phenotype. The first is AMH, which the Sertoli cells produce early during fetal life.[18,33] The primary function of AMH is to cause regression of the müllerian (paramesonephric) ducts in the male fetus, which it does by its effects on the mesenchyme surrounding the duct.

AMH is first secreted in effective amounts 56–62 days after fertilization, and the process of müllerian regression is normally completed by about day 77, after which the müllerian

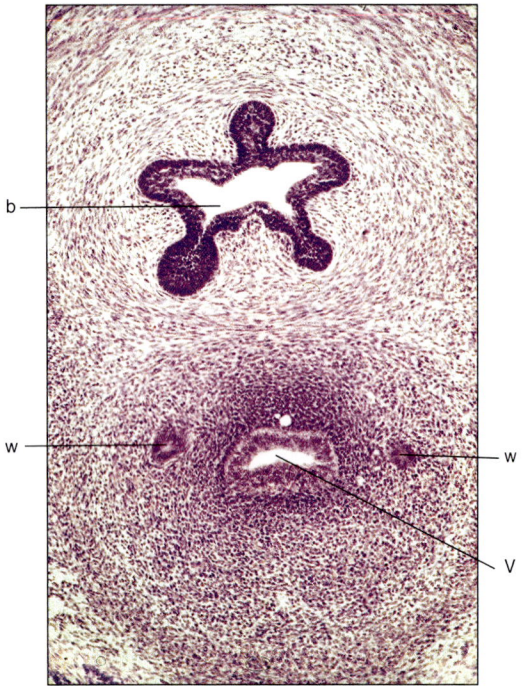

Fig. 1.44 Distal vagina (v) (12 weeks). The two wolffian tubes (w) are lateral and the bladder (b) is anterior.

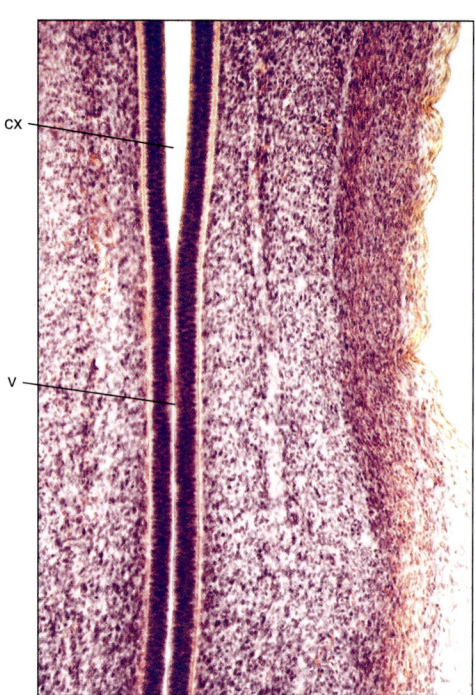

Fig. 1.46 Uterovaginal canal. The cervical canal (cx) is open and vaginal canal (v) is closed. At this stage (12 weeks), the fornix has not yet developed.

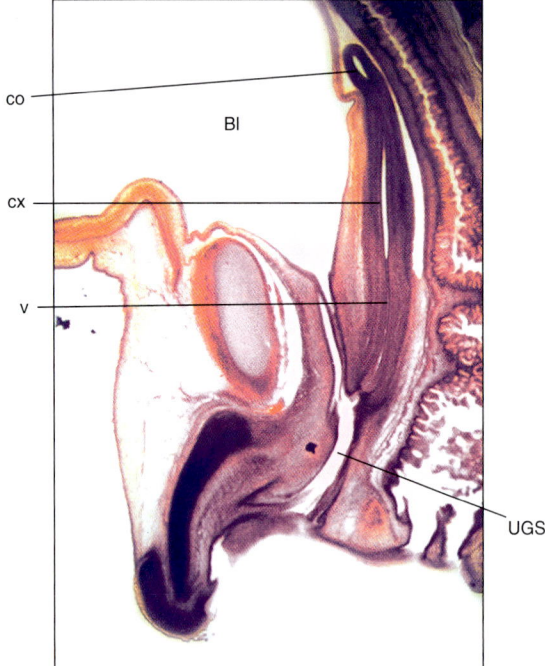

Fig. 1.45 Sagittal section of female genitalia (12 weeks). The uterine corpus (co) is small in comparison to both the elongate cervix (cx) and closed vagina (v). Other structures include urogenital sinus (UGS) and bladder (Bl).

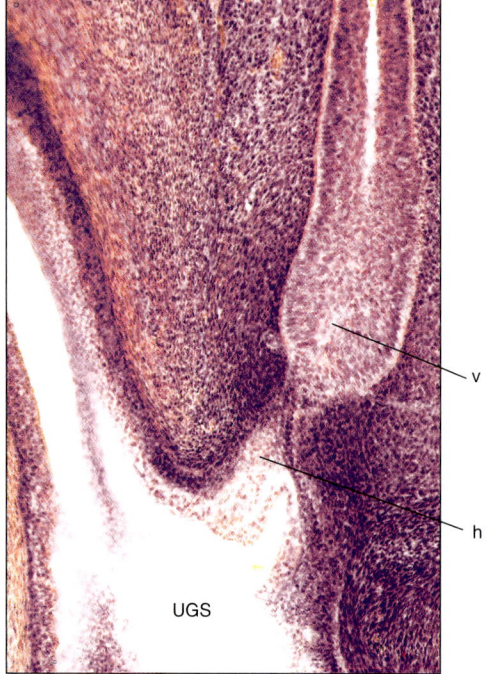

Fig. 1.47 Junction of terminal vagina (v) and urogenital sinus (UGS) (12 weeks). This junction is the anlage of the future hymen (h).

tissue is no longer sensitive to AMH. During this critical period, even relatively small amounts of AMH given over a short period of time can cause irreversible damage to the embryonic müllerian tract.[15] In the female, AMH is produced in insignificant amounts during fetal life (as there are no Sertoli cells) and the müllerian ducts develop passively to form the fallopian tubes, uterus, and vaginal wall. Other functions of AMH, secreted later in fetal life, are discussed below.

AMH has a local action, and inhibits development of the ipsilateral fallopian tube. To prevent development of both the uterus and vagina, both testes must secrete adequate amounts of AMH. Thus, a patient with a testis and a contralateral streak, ovary or ovotestis generally has a uterus and vagina and a single fallopian tube on the side with the streak or ovary. AMH immunoreactivity can be observed in Sertoli cell cytoplasm from roughly week 8 of fetal life until puberty. It is detected in the Sertoli cells in the premeiotic seminal pretubules but disappears in older tubules that have shown meiotic development.[33]

Additional functions of AMH have recently been discovered or postulated. In the female, ovarian granulosa cells begin producing AMH only after the müllerian-derived tissues (fallopian tubes, uterus, and vagina) are well developed and no longer susceptible to the regressive effects of AMH. Serum AMH levels in girls rise slowly after birth from nearly undetectable levels until reaching a plateau after 10 years of life. It is then equivalent to the adult male serum concentration. In contrast, the male serum AMH concentration is relatively high at birth, peaks at 4–12 months of age, and then falls progressively to a baseline low adult level by about 10 years of age. A major action of AMH in the young female may be to inhibit oocyte meiosis in the developing follicle. Dramatically high levels of AMH have been found in women with ovarian sex-cord tumors, thus serving potentially as a diagnostic marker or method to evaluate the effectiveness of therapy.[20] Another important action of AMH in males may be to initiate testicular descent, principally by its postulated regulatory control over the gubernaculum testis.[6] Anti-AMH is a excellent biomarker for gonadal-stromal tumor in which there is a Sertoli or granulosa cell component.[34]

The second hormone that the fetal testis secretes is testosterone. This androgenic steroid, which is critical for male development, is required for the wolffian (mesonephric) duct to differentiate into the epididymis, vas deferens, and seminal vesicle. Leydig cells appear in the testis around day 54–64 and shortly thereafter begin to produce testosterone (see Huhtaniemi[12] for a fuller analysis of the fetal testis and how it differs significantly from the adult testis). Leydig cell activity is probably stimulated by increased production of chorionic gonadotrophin by the placenta at that time. Testosterone acts locally on the ipsilateral wolffian duct by binding to a specific high affinity intracellular receptor protein. This receptor hormone complex binds DNA to regulate transcription of specific genes that govern further development. In the absence of a testis or inability of a testis to produce testosterone in adequate amounts by 10–12 weeks, or insensitivity of the wolffian duct anlage to testosterone, the epididymis, vas deferens, and seminal vesicle fail to differentiate. Only rarely are abnormally elevated testosterone levels reached sufficiently early during embryogenesis in a female fetus to cause the wolffian duct to differentiate into definitive male organs (androgen administration to the mother during pregnancy, congenital adrenogenital

syndrome, and some androgen-secreting ovarian tumors; see Chapter 34).

The development of the stromal component of the genital canal is little studied, but is clearly of major importance.[8] In addition to its role in the development of the walls of the tubular muscular organs (i.e., the vagina, cervix, uterine corpus, and fallopian tubes), there is extensive experimental evidence to indicate that the stroma also directs epithelial development. Thus, the entire structure of the female genital tract is determined by stromal–epithelial interaction.

THE MÜLLERIAN DUCT AFTER WEEK 8

If the embryo is female, or in the case of male intersex in which embryonic müllerian ducts have not been completely inhibited by the AMH that the testis secretes, the ducts continue to grow unimpeded. Cranially, the fallopian tubes are distinct (Figure 1.48) and enter into the corpus (Figure 1.49), where after a short distance, they fuse. Caudally, the urogenital sinus epithelium proliferates, growing up the embryonic müllerian ducts to replace the native embryonic glandular epithelium. A column of squamotransitional epithelial cells is formed, termed the 'vaginal plate' (Figures 1.50–1.53), which comes to occupy the entire region of the vagina and exocervix. At that time the uterovaginal canal is a straight tube without evidence of a fornix. The vaginal plate is solid. By early in the second trimester, the vaginal plate begins to degenerate, and thus the vagina shows early signs of patency. The epithelium of the vaginal plate gives rise to the epithelium that ultimately lines the vagina and exocervix.

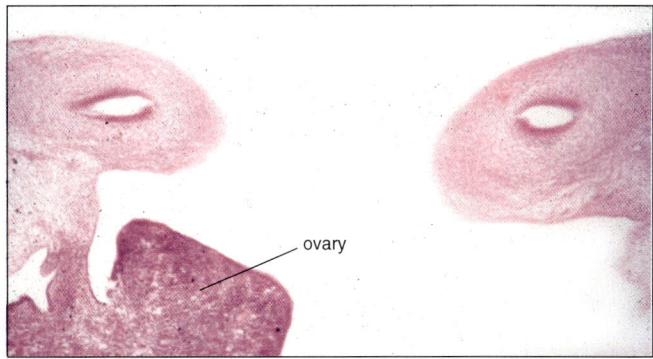

Fig. 1.48 Fallopian tubes at 12 weeks is shown attached to the ovary.

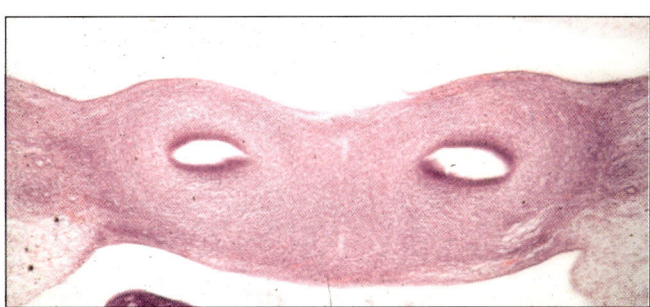

Fig. 1.49 Proximal uterine corpus with bilateral müllerian ducts (12 weeks).

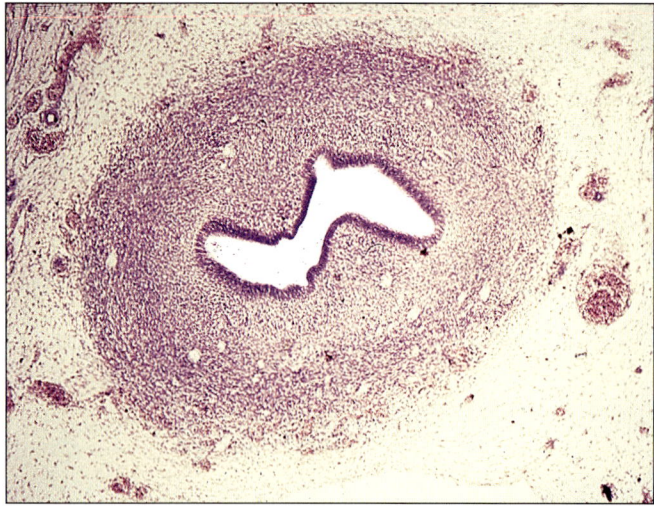

Fig. 1.50 Uterine corpus, cross-section (14 weeks).

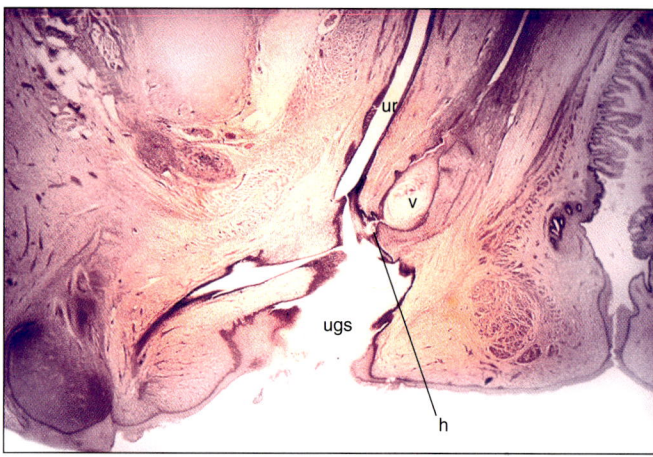

Fig. 1.53 Sagittal section of lower genital tract (16 weeks). The sinovaginal bulb is solid (v). The caudal-most covering is the region of future hymen (h). Other structures/areas include the urethra (ur) and urogenital sinus (ugs).

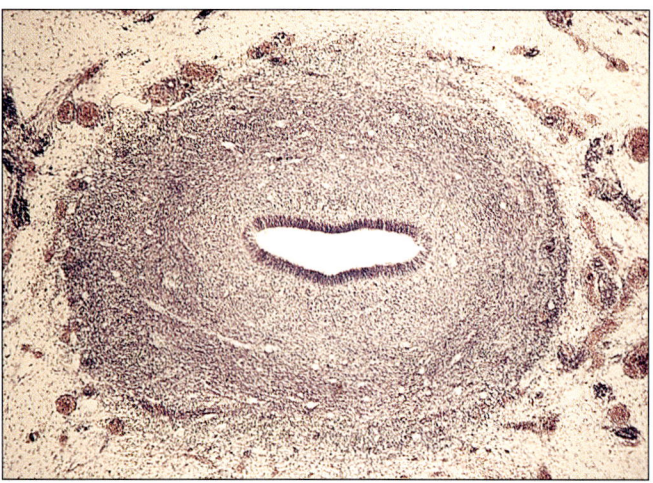

Fig. 1.51 Cervix, cross-section (14 weeks).

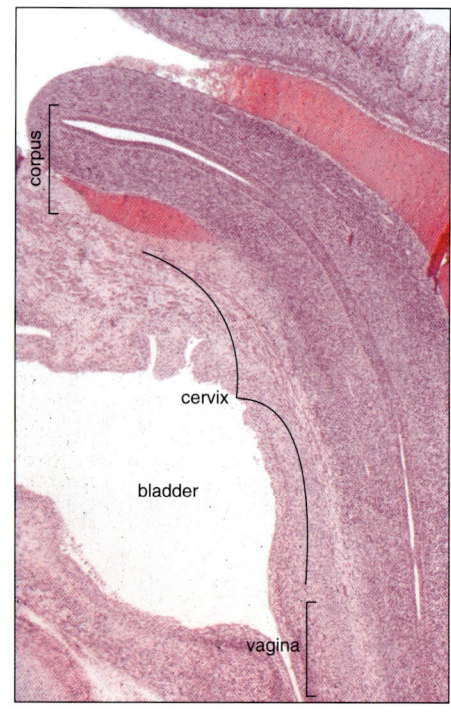

Fig. 1.54 Uterus at a stage before endometrial glands develop. The corpus is small; the cervix and vagina are much larger at this stage (14 weeks).

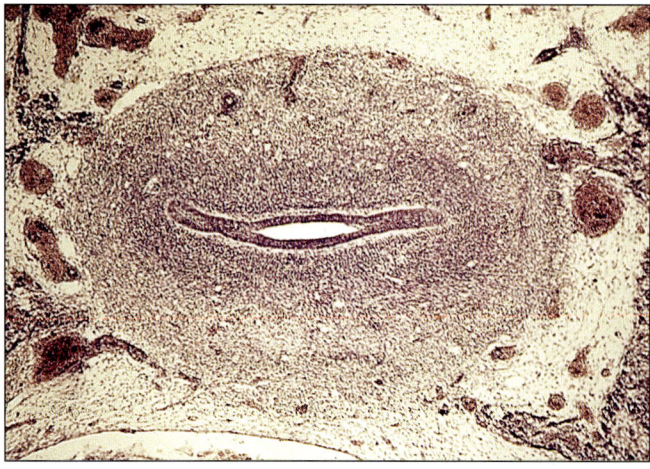

Fig. 1.52 Vagina, cross-section (14 weeks). The vaginal plate is solid in the lateral wings, and is partially opened centrally.

THE MÜLLERIAN DUCT DURING THE SECOND TRIMESTER

Smooth muscle appears in the walls of the genital tract between 18 and 20 weeks, although stromal aggregates into circular and longitudinal layers appear earlier (Figures 1.54 and 1.55). By approximately 24 weeks, the muscular portion is well developed. Vaginal, uterine, and tubal muscular walls develop around the müllerian duct alone, thus excluding the wolffian duct remnants, which are external to the true wall of the canal.

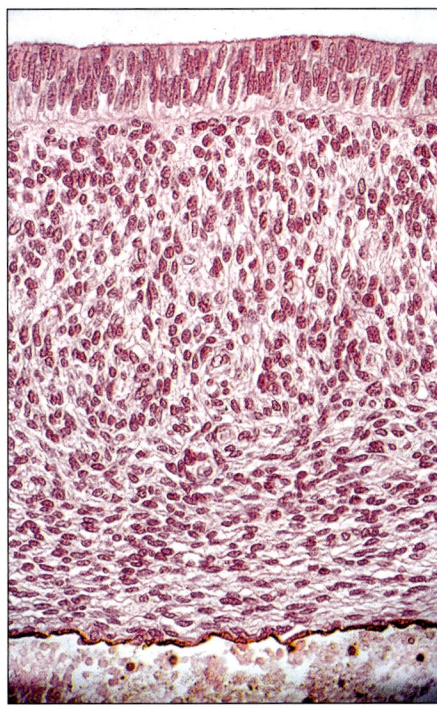

Fig. 1.55 Cross-section of wall of uterine corpus. The stroma shows presumptive longitudinal and circular aggregates (14 weeks).

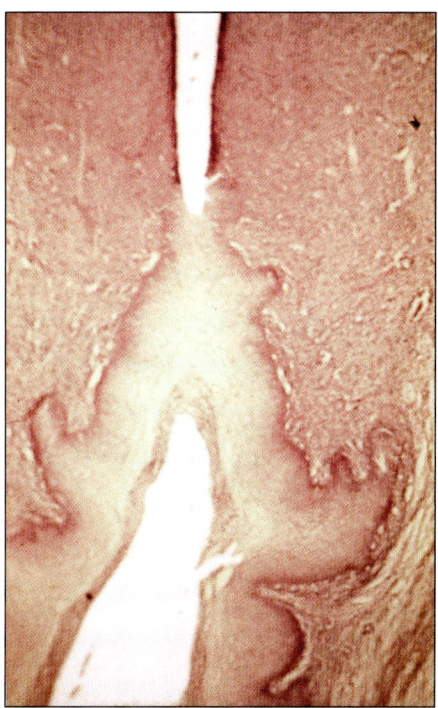

Fig. 1.57 Lower cervix and upper vagina (19 weeks). The squamous epithelium is highly glycogenated in both the vagina and cervix, presumably due to the high levels of maternal estrogens. The endocervix is a glandular tube. The earliest formation of the fornix is suggested by lateral flares of squamous epithelium.

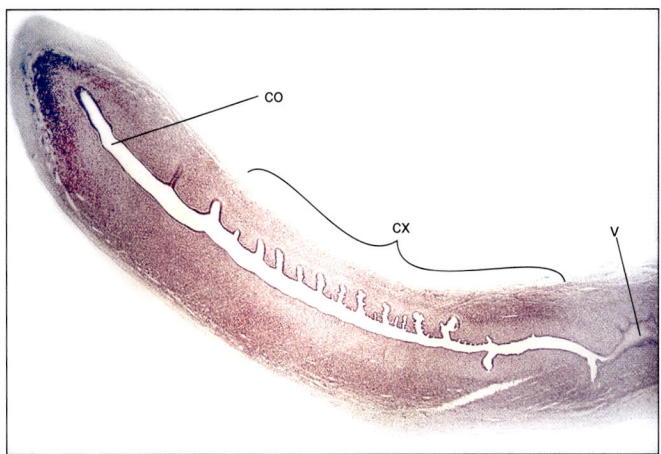

Fig. 1.56 Uterus (19 weeks). The corpus (co), which has a tube-like lumen, is one-third the size of the cervix, which shows numerous endocervical folds (cx). Only the top of the vagina (v) is present in this photograph.

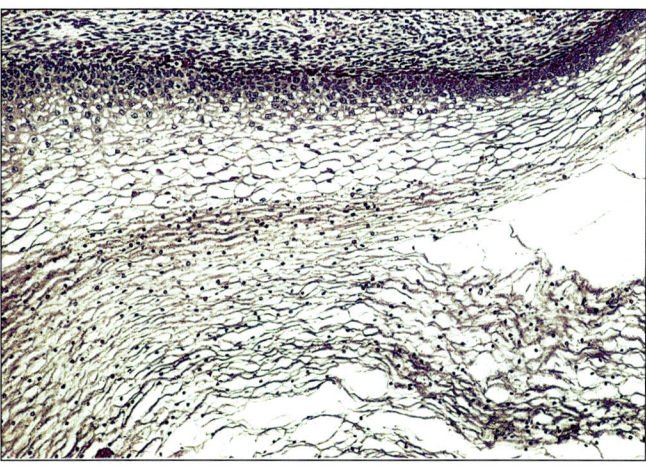

Fig. 1.58 Embryonic vaginal epithelium during continuous exposure to the estrogen, diethylstilbestrol.

Cervical glands appear at about 15 weeks. Rudimentary endometrial glands are present by 19 weeks, but the endometrium is not well developed even at term in most infants (Figure 1.56).

After about 20 weeks, at the time when estrogen levels have risen in the mother, the squamous epithelium comprising the vaginal plate of the fetus begins to show signs of intracytoplasmic glycogen accumulation (Figures 1.57 and 1.58). Eventually, there is cellular dissolution and the formation of the fully patent vagina.

EXTERNAL GENITALIA

The appearance of the external genitalia is influenced by the systemic hormonal milieu found in the developing fetus beginning somewhere about week 15. It becomes masculine when exposed to an excess of androgens and female if there is a deficiency of androgens, i.e., a relative excess of estrogens. Androgens have a positive influence on the appearance of the external genitalia. Maternal or inappropriate fetal androgens will virilize a female fetus, while high levels of circulating estrogens in pregnancy have no effect on the male fetus.

Dihydrotestosterone, the active androgen that derives from testosterone, is ultimately responsible for initiating masculinization of the external genitalia and differentiation of the prostate. 5-α reductase, found in the tissues of the external genitalia and urogenital sinus, converts testosterone to dihydrotestosterone which causes:

- the genital tubercle to enlarge and form the glans penis;
- the genital folds to enlarge and fuse to form the penile shaft with migration of the urethral orifice along the lower border of the shaft to the tip of the glans;
- the genital swellings to fuse and form a scrotum;
- the urogenital sinus tissues to differentiate into the prostate; and
- the utricle to regress.

Failure of the external genitalia to develop in males in the presence of testes may be due to a lack of adequate testosterone secretion into the systemic circulation, deficient enzyme (5-α reductase, type II) at the end-organ level to convert testosterone to dihydrotestosterone, or complete end-organ insensitivity (androgen receptor insensitivity). Lesser degrees of deficiency or end-organ insensitivity may result in partial male development characterized by a small penis, hypospadias, deficient formation of the scrotum, or a persistent urogenital sinus (vaginal opening into urethra). The effects of dihydrotestosterone begin about day 70, with fusion of the labioscrotal folds and closure of the median raphe, and continue at day 74 with closure of the urethral groove. External genital development is complete by day 120–140 (week 18–20).

The urogenital sinus, into which the vagina opens, enlarges as the embryo grows, so that it becomes the vestibule of the adult external genitalia. Consequently, the vestibule is lined, except for a variable portion anterior to the urethral orifice, by the endodermal epithelium of the urogenital sinus. This is clinically important as the endodermal-derived epithelium differs not only morphologically from the mesodermal- and ectodermal-derived epithelium, but also responds differently to a variety of stimuli, notably sex steroids.

The form of the external genitalia results from events that begin during embryonic week 4 in the mesodermal stroma immediately lateral and ventral to the cloacal plate. Just ventral to the plate, the stroma produces paired elevations of the ectoderm, which fuse to form the genital tubercle. Immediately lateral to the cloacal plate on each side, two parallel folds develop by the same mechanism: the more medial urogenital fold is destined to become the labium minor; the more lateral labioscrotal fold becomes the labium major.

The labioscrotal fold extends cranially around the genital tubercle and fuses with its partner on the other side, becoming the mons pubis. At the end of week 6, the urorectal septum fuses with the cloacal plate, thus dividing this structure into the anal membrane posteriorly and the urogenital membrane ventrally. The lateral folds are distributed primarily in relation to the urogenital membrane. In both the male and female, the lateral folds fuse across the midline in front of the anus. In the male, the fusion moves ventrally in zipper-like fashion. The urogenital folds fuse to form a portion of the wall of the penile urethra, and the labioscrotal folds fuse to form the scrotum. As female differentiation reflects the absence of this fusion, it may be difficult to detect, although by the end of the first trimester, significant fusion should have occurred in a male fetus.

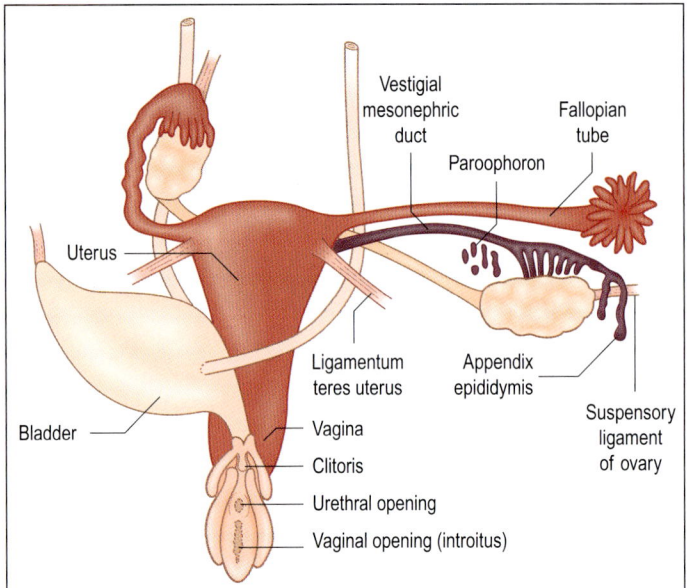

Fig. 1.59 Female differentiation of the genital organs.

In summary, female internal organs and external genitalia develop in the absence of hormones secreted by the fetal ovary, and differentiate even when gonads are absent. Unless interrupted by the regressive influence of AMH, differentiation of the müllerian ducts proceeds caudally to form fallopian tubes, a uterus, and a vagina (Figure 1.59). In the absence of the masculinizing effect of dihydrotestosterone, the undifferentiated external genital anlage develops into the vulva. The genital tubercle develops into the clitoris, the genital folds into the labia minora, and the genital swellings into the labia majora. Thus, the infant with ovaries or streak gonads has female internal and external genitalia at birth. Only if the female fetus has systematically elevated levels of androgens before week 10–12 of gestation does any degree of internal male development occur. In such cases, the external genitalia may appear ambiguous or may resemble that of a normal phenotypic male; the vagina in these instances opens into the membranous portion of the urethra. If the androgens are not elevated until after week 20, by which time the external genitalia have fully formed, the only virilizing effect is an enlarged clitoris.

REFERENCES

1. Beysen D, Vandesompele J, Messiaen L, De Paepe A, De Baere E. The human FOXL2 mutation database. Hum Mutat 2004;24:189–93.
2. Biason-Lauber A, Konrad D, Navratil F, Schoenle EJ. A WNT4 mutation associated with Mullerian-duct regression and virilization in a 46,XX woman. N Engl J Med 2004;351:792–8.
3. Brennan J, Capel B. One tissue, two fates: molecular genetic events that underlie testis versus ovary development. Nat Rev Genet 2004;5:509–21.
4. Brennan J, Karl J, Martineau J, et al. Sry and the testis: Molecular pathways of organogenesis. J Exp Zool 1998;281:494–500.
4a. Capel B: R-spondin 1 tips the balance in sex determination. *Nature Genet*, 2006;38:1304–9.
4b. Chassot AA, Ranc F, Gregoire EP, et al. Activation of β-catenin signalling by Rspol controls differentiation of the mammalian ovary. Hum Molec Genet 2008;17:1264–77.
5. Choi Y, Rajkovic A. Genetics of early mammalian folliculogenesis. Cell Mol Life Sci 2006;63:579–90.
6. Clarnette TD, Sugita Y, Hutson JM. Genital anomalies in human and animal models reveal the mechanisms and hormones governing testicular descent. Br J Urol 1997;79:99–112.

7. Cocquet J, Pailhoux E, Jaubert F, et al. Evolution and expression of FOXL2. J Med Genet 2002;39:916–21.
8. Cunha GR, Boutin EL, Turner T, Donjacour AA. Role of mesenchyme in the development of the urogenital tract. J Clean Technol Environ Toxicol Occ Med 1998;7:179–94.
9. De Baere E, Copelli S, Caburet S, et al. Premature ovarian failure and forkhead transcription factor FOXL2: blepharophimosis–ptosis–epicanthus inversus syndrome and ovarian dysfunction. Pediatr Endocrinol Rev 2005;2:653–60.
10. de Kretser DM, Burger HG. The Y chromosome and spermatogenesis. N Engl J Med 1997;336:576–8.
11. Fleming A, Vilain E. The endless quest for sex determination genes. Clin Genet 2005;67:15.
12. Huhtaniemi I. Fetal testis – a very special endocrine organ. Eur J Endocrinol 1994;130:25–31.
13. Hunter RHF. Differentiation of the gonads. In: Hunter RHF, ed. Sex Determination, Differentiation and Intersexuality in Placental Mammals. Cambridge: Cambridge University Press; 1995:69–106.
14. Hunter RHF. Mechanisms of sex determination. In: Hunter RHF, ed. Sex Determination, Differentiation and Intersexuality in Placental Mammals. Cambridge: Cambridge University Press; 1995:22–68.
15. Hunter RHF. Differentiation of the genital duct system. In: Hunter RHF, ed. Sex Determination, Differentiation and Intersexuality in Placental Mammals. Cambridge: Cambridge University Press; 1995:107–38.
16. Iyer AK, McCabe ER. Molecular mechanisms of DAX1 action. Mol Genet Metab 2004;83:60–73.
17. Johnson J, Bagley J, Skaznik-Wikiel M, et al. Oocyte generation in adult mammalian ovaries by putative germ cells in bone marrow and peripheral blood. Cell 2005;122:303–15.
18. Josso N, Racine C, di Clemente N, Rey R, Xavier F. The role of anti-Mullerian hormone in gonadal development. Mol Cell Endocrinol 1998;145:3–7.
19. Kanai Y, Hiramatsu R, Matoba S, Kidokoro T. From SRY to SOX9: mammalian testis differentiation. J Biochem (Tokyo) 2005;138:13–19.
20. Lane AH, Lee MM. Clinical applications of Mullerian inhibiting substance in patients with gonadal disorders. Endocrinologist 1999;9:208–15.
21. Ludwig KS. The Mayer–Rokitansky–Kuster syndrome. An analysis of its morphology and embryology. Part II: Embryology. Arch Gynecol Obstet 1998;262:27–42.
22. Mallet D, Bretones P, Michel-Calemard L, Dijoud F, David M, Morel Y. Gonadal dysgenesis without adrenal insufficiency in a 46,XY patient heterozygous for the nonsense C16X mutation: a case of SF1 haploinsufficiency. J Clin Endocrinol Metab 2004;89:4829–32.
23. McElreavey K, Quintana-Murci L. Y chromosome haplogroups: a correlation with testicular dysgenesis syndrome? APMIS 2003;111:106–14.
24. Meeks JJ, Weiss J, Jameson JL. Dax1 is required for testis determination. Nature Genet 2003;34:32–3.
25. Mendes JRT, Strufaldi MWL, Delcelo R, et al. Y-chromosome identification by PCR and gonadal histopathology in Turner's syndrome without overt Y-mosaicism. Clin Endocrinol 1999;50:19–26.
26. Mittwoch U. The elusive action of sex-determining genes: mitochondria to the rescue? J Theor Biol 2004;228:359–65.
27. Moreno-Mendoza N, Harley V, Merchant-Larios H. Cell aggregation precedes the onset of Sox9-expressing preSertoli cells in the genital ridge of mouse. Cytogenet Genome Res 2003;101:219–23.
28. Mulhall JP, Reijo R, Alagappan R, et al. Azoospermic men with deletion of the DAZ gene cluster are capable of completing spermatogenesis: fertilization, normal embryonic development and pregnancy occur when retrieved testicular spermatozoa are used for intracytoplasmic sperm injection. Human Reprod 1997;12:503–8.
29. Nef S, Schaad O, Stallings NR, et al. Gene expression during sex determination reveals a robust female genetic program at the onset of ovarian development. Dev Biol 2005;287:361–77.
30. Park SY, Jameson JL. Minireview: transcriptional regulation of gonadal development and differentiation. Endocrinol 2005;146:1035–42.
31. Park SY, Meeks JJ, Raverot G, et al. Nuclear receptors Sf1 and Dax1 function cooperatively to mediate somatic cell differentiation during testis development. Development 2005;132:2415–23.
32. Parker KL, Rice DA, Lala DS, et al. Steroidogenic factor 1: an essential mediator of endocrine development. Recent Prog Horm Res 2002;57:19–36.
33. Rey R, al-Attar L, Louis F, et al. Testicular dysgenesis does not affect expression of anti-mullerian hormone by Sertoli cells in premeiotic seminiferous tubules. Am J Pathol 1996;148:1689–98.
34. Rey R, Sabourin JC, Venara M, et al. Anti-Mullerian hormone is a specific marker of sertoli- and granulosa-cell origin in gonadal tumors. Hum Pathol 2000;31:1202–8.
35. Salas-Cortes L, Jaubert F, Barbaux S, et al. The human SRY protein is present in fetal and adult Sertoli cells and germ cells. Int J Dev Biol 1999;43:135–40.
36. Sekido R, Bar I, Narvaez V, Penny G, Lovell-Badge R. SOX9 is up-regulated by the transient expression of SRY specifically in Sertoli cell precursors. Dev Biol 2004;274:271–9.
37. Shimada K. Sex determination and sex differentiation. Avian Poultry Biol Rev 2002;13:1–14.
38. Short RV. Difference between a testis and an ovary. J Exp Zool 1998;281:359–61.
39. Swain A, Lovell-Badge R. A molecular approach to sex determination in mammals. Acta Paediatr 1997;86(Suppl 3):46–9.
40. Tilmann C, Capel B. Mesonephric cell migration induces testis cord formation and Sertoli cell differentiation in the mammalian gonad. Development 1999;126:2883–90.
41. Viger RS, Silversides DW, Tremblay JJ. New insights into the regulation of mammalian sex determination and male sex differentiation. Vitam Horm 2005;70:387–413.
42. Yao HH. The pathway to femaleness: current knowledge on embryonic development of the ovary. Mol Cell Endocrinol 2005;230:87–93.

Vulvar dermatoses and infections

2

Maria Angelica Selim   Bruce R. Smoller   Christopher R. Shea   Stanley J. Robboy

INTRODUCTION

The term 'vulva' derives from the Latin world for 'covering', and was originally used to refer to the uterus. Although generic references to vulvar lesions are found in ancient texts like the Talmud, the Bible, and Egyptian papyri from the second millennium BC, it was Avicenna in the eleventh century who gave one of the first detailed descriptions of vulvar disorders. Nowadays, urogenital complaints are among the most frequent problems faced by the gynecologist, family practitioner,[37,60] and dermatologist.

When a patient with a vulvar disease visits the healthcare system, three intersecting elements increase the complexity of the encounter:

1. The patient's social and cultural background affects how she perceives the problem, often leading to self-treatment and delay in seeking professional attention. Both factors can change the clinical presentation of the disease, increasing the degree of diagnostic difficulty. This problem can be exponentially increased in sexually transmitted diseases, where the patient's sexual partner is also at risk.
2. The disease can exhibit a clinical presentation different from its extragenital counterpart, because the vulva is a modified skin particularly subject to the effects of moisture and friction.[31] In addition, the vulva's anatomic location exposes it to urine, increasing maceration and predisposing it to trauma, burning, itching, and infections. The itchiness in turn can produce secondary changes, obscuring the original disease for the clinician and pathologist.
3. The most common diseases affecting the vulva are dermatologic,[2,35,37,58,69,87,96] but the clinicians caring for these complaints are usually gynecologists or family practitioners who may lack sophisticated diagnostic and therapeutic skills in skin diseases. Conversely, dermatologists may only take interest themselves with certain diseases in this organ. In summary, no single specialist is generally well trained to care for the full spectrum of vulvar disease. Multidisciplinary clinics, to which different specialists bring their expertise, are often the best forum to efficiently diagnose and treat acute or chronic vulvar diseases.[118,119]

In response to the complexity of vulvar disorders, the International Society for the Study of Vulvovaginal Disease (ISVVD) was founded with one objective being to facilitate clear communication between clinicians and pathologists caring for patients with neoplastic and non-neoplastic vulvar diseases. Accordingly, it discarded its 1987 classification, replacing it in 2006 (Table 2.1) with an entirely different classification based on microscopic morphology (generalized or localized).[75,76]

This chapter utilizes a multidisciplinary approach. The diseases are organized in order of frequency and classified with a clinical perspective using the type of lesion (patch, papule, nodule, etc.) and the symptoms produced (itch etc.), combined with the histopathologic pattern of inflammation (Figure 2.1). Both vulvar and extravulvar manifestations are covered. Not uncommonly, the latter features are the key to a correct diagnosis.

The brief glossary presented in Appendix 2.1 defines some of the more commonly used terms in dermatology and dermatopathology. To further enhance this chapter, the common dermatopathologic terms used throughout this chapter are defined in Appendix 2.2. They are divided into terms that apply to the three main layers: the surface keratin layer, the epidermis, and the dermis.

COMMON DERMATOSES AFFECTING THE VULVA

ACUTE AND CHRONIC SPONGIOTIC DERMATITIS (ECZEMAS)

Eczema or spongiotic dermatitis encompasses a variety of diseases with *spongiosis* as a common histologic finding at some stage. The spongiotic tissue reaction shows intracellular and intercellular edema leading to expanded spaces between keratinocytes. Eczema is the leading cause of chronic genital itching. All forms of endogenous and exogenous spongiotic dermatitis can affect the vulva, where they may present acutely or chronically. The location, pattern, and extent of the lesions help to define the different types of eczema.

GENERAL CLINICAL AND PATHOLOGIC FEATURES OF SPONGIOTIC DERMATITIS

Acute spongiotic dermatitis

The term 'eczema' derives from the Greek *ekzein*, 'to boil over', reflecting the clinical appearance of acute lesions. Clinically, it exhibits erythematous macules, papules, and plaques (Figure 2.2). With increasing degrees of spongiosis, lesions become vesicular or bullous and begin to weep or to ooze. The vesicles frequently progress to rupture, and their contents dry to form

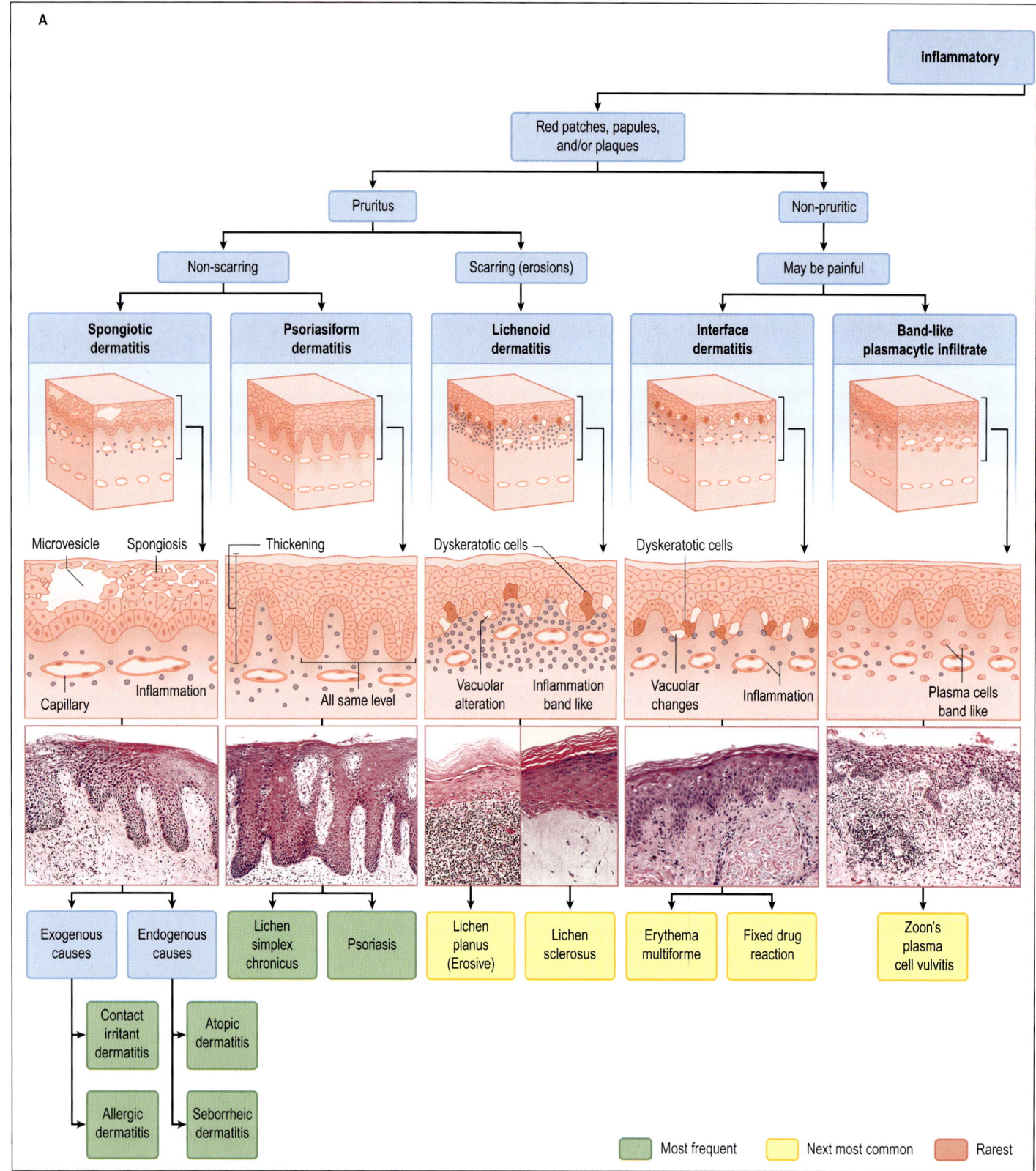

Fig. 2.1 Differential diagnoses of vulvar dermatoses. **(A)** Non-infectious inflammatory conditions. **(B)** Ulcers. **(C)** Erosions.

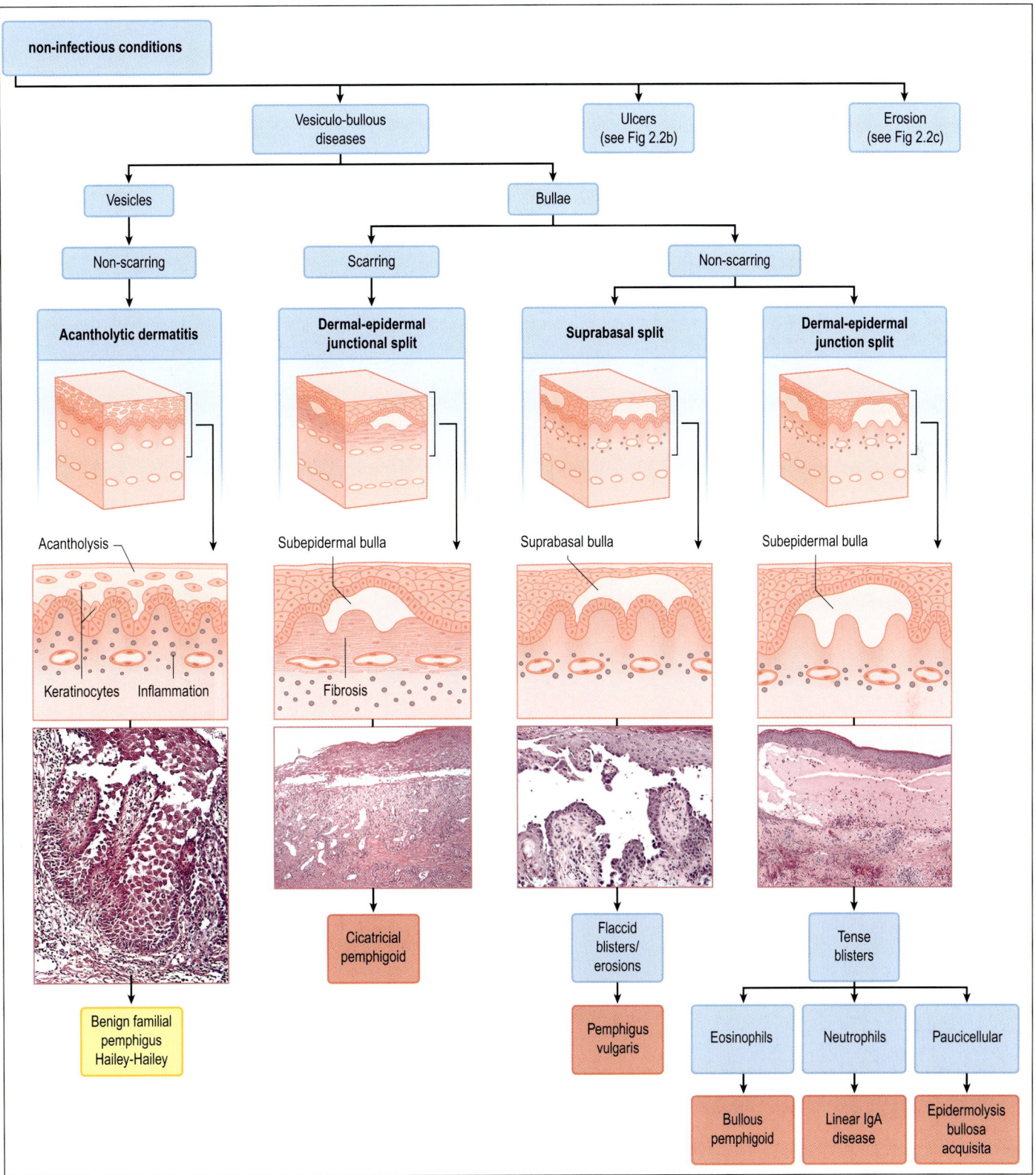

Fig. 2.1 *Continued.*

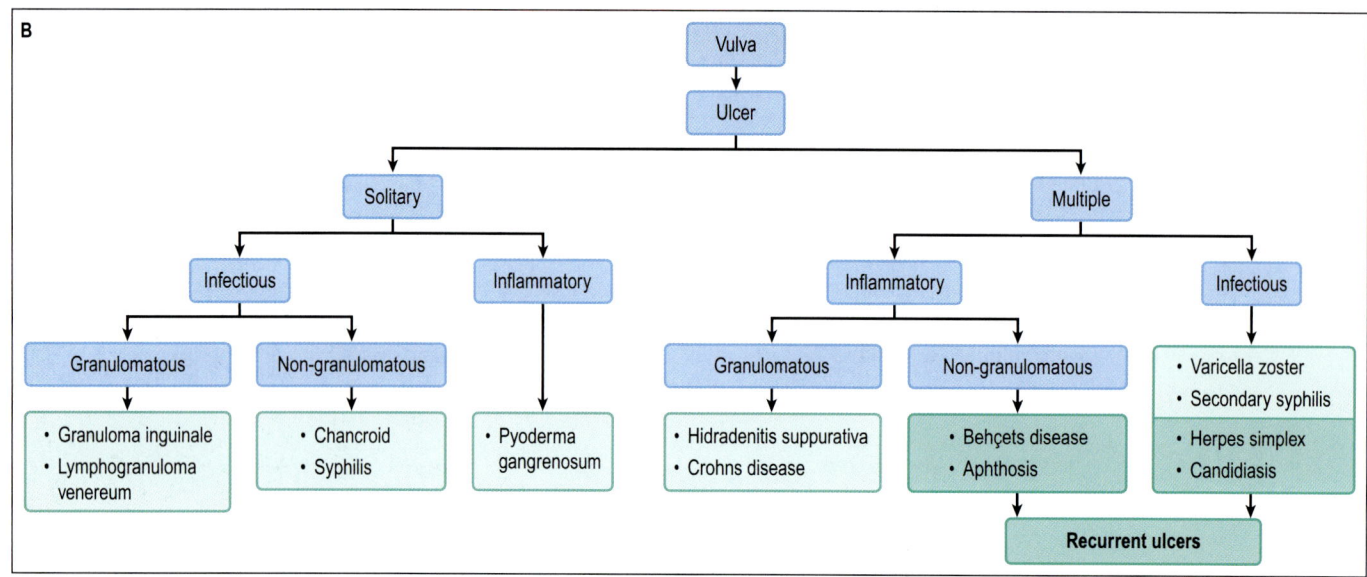

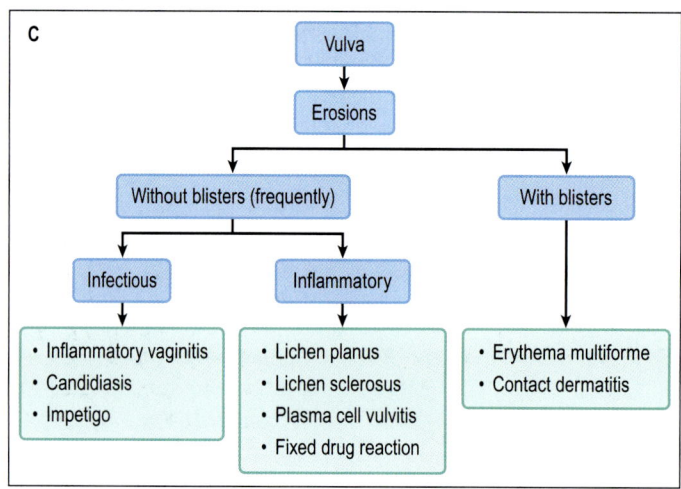

Fig. 2.1 *Continued.*

a surface crust. In the biopsy specimen the epidermis shows a variable amount of spongiosis, hyper- and parakeratosis, and exocytosis of inflammatory cells. If the spongiosis is considerable, the fluid will collect in intraepidermal vesicles that may contain lymphocytes, neutrophils, eosinophils, and Langerhans cells. Mild papillary dermal edema leading to separation of collagen fibers can be seen in association with telangiectatic vessels. The superficial vascular plexus shows a perivascular mixed inflammatory infiltrate consisting of lymphocytes, neutrophils, and eosinophils. This basic pattern of acute spongiotic dermatitis is altered by scratching or superimposed infections (impetiginization): the former produces excoriations or lichen simplex chronicus (see below); the latter is associated with neutrophils in the stratum corneum. Acute inflammation in the stratum corneum should prompt the pathologist to request special stains for bacterial (Brown–Brenn) and fungal forms (periodic acid-Schiff (PAS) and Gomori methenamine silver (GMS)).

Chronic spongiotic dermatitis

Clinically the skin exhibits a leathery appearance with accentuation of skin markings (*lichenification*). The skin also changes from red (characteristic of acute spongiotic dermatitis) to brown or hyperpigmented, particularly in racially dark individuals. Scratching from intense pruritus produces excoriations where the surface has been traumatized. Histologically there is variable hyperplasia of the epidermis (acanthosis) with overlying hyper- and parakeratosis. The elongated rete ridges are separated by a papillary dermis with prominent capillaries and thick collagen fibers arranged perpendicular to the surface. Lymphocytes are found predominantly around upper dermal vessels. In certain biopsy specimens, in the previously described background of chronic dermatitis, there are features associated with acute inflammation, specifically a notable degree of spongiosis. This coexistence of acute and chronic histologic findings is called *subacute spongiotic dermatitis* (Figure 2.3).

Table 2.1 2006 ISSVD classification of vulvar dermatoses:[75,76] pathologic subsets and their clinical correlates

Spongiotic pattern
  Atopic dermatitis
  Allergic contact dermatitis
  Irritant contact dermatitis

Acanthotic pattern (formerly squamous cell hyperplasia)
  Psoriasis
  Lichen simplex chronicus
    Primary (idiopathic)
    Secondary (superimposed on lichen sclerosus, lichen planus or other vulvar disease)

Lichenoid pattern
  Lichen sclerosus
  Lichen planus

Dermal homogenization/sclerosis pattern
  Lichen sclerosus

Vesiculobullous pattern
  Pemphigoid, cicatricial type
  Linear IgA disease

Acantholytic pattern
  Hailey–Hailey disease
  Dariers disease
  Papular genitocrural acantholysis

Granulomatous pattern
  Crohns disease
  Melkersson–Rosenthal syndrome

Vasculopathic pattern
  Aphthous ulcers
  Behçets disease
  Plasma cell vulvitis

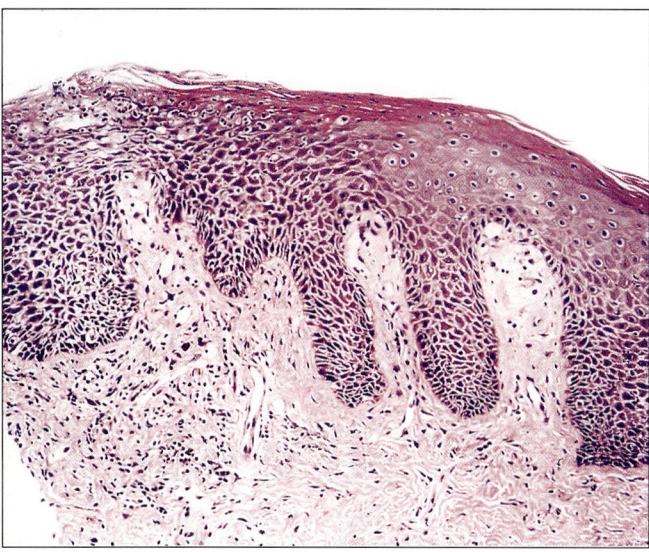

Fig. 2.3 Subacute vulvar dermatitis. The epidermis shows both active focal spongiosis (acute dermatitic change) and rete ridge elongation with collagenization in dermal papillae (chronic dermatitic change).

CLINICAL PATTERNS OF VULVAR SPONGIOTIC DERMATITIS

Endogenous vulvar spongiotic dermatitis

The two most common endogenous dermatidites are *atopic dermatitis* and *seborrheic dermatitis*. Both diseases can show the entire spectrum of eczematous lesions ranging from erythematous scaly areas to oozing to vesicle formation, and ending in lichenification. Few physicians see the acute phase. Most patients seek medical attention only during the subacute to chronic phase. Commonly, the correct diagnosis depends on identifying more distinctive extragenital lesions.

Atopic dermatitis Atopic dermatitis is a chronic, pruritic inflammation of the skin that affects individuals with a personal or family history of atopic diathesis (atopic eczema, asthma, allergic seasonal rhinitis). It typically begins in childhood with periodic flares that occur throughout life but tend to decrease in frequency with age. Spontaneous remission can be seen in adult life. Major and minor criteria are needed for diagnosis. Among the major diagnostic criteria are presence of pruritus, chronicity, history of atopy, and lesions with typical morphology such as flexural distribution. Lesions that sometimes occur during infancy and early childhood are erythematous papulovesicles involving the face and extensor surfaces of extremities. Lesions in older children are more often scaly, lichenified plaques involving mainly the popliteal and antecubital fossae. Minor diagnostic criteria include xerosis, elevated serum levels of IgE, interleukin-2 receptor, eosinophil cationic protein, E-selectin and IgG_4, increased colonization of the skin with *Staphylococcus aureus*, increased risk of viral and fungal infections, rippled hyperpigmentation, and keratosis pilaris, among others. Although the etiology and pathogenesis are still unknown, IgE-mediated late phase responses, cytokine imbalances, and cell-mediated reactions may all play important roles. Genetic factors also appear involved. One candidate gene is located on chromosome 11q13 (note that the gene for the beta subunit of the FcγRI, the high-affinity receptor for

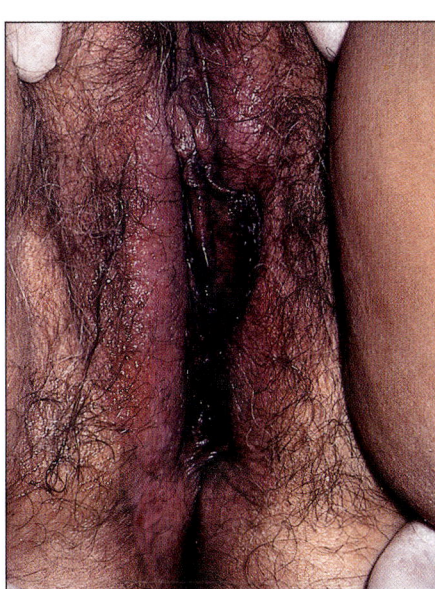

Fig. 2.2 Vulvar acute dermatitis (eczema). Erythema and edema are present, with linear excoriations due to scratching.

IgE, is localized to chromosome 11q12–q13) and another on chromosome 16q11–p13 (associated with the *IL4R* gene).

Patients with atopic dermatitis experience pruritus rather than soreness or irritation when suffering from inflamed skin. The rubbing and scratching that elicit this overpowering itchy sensation act as stimulation to perpetuate the itch and create the so called 'itch-search cycle'. Girls suffering from atopic dermatitis uncommonly show direct vulvar involvement (although as part of the atopic diathesis they have an increased propensity to experience irritant dermatitis or diaper dermatitis). On the other hand, adult women are more prone to experience genital eczema in the form of red to hyperpigmented areas, often with subtle changes of excoriation and scale due to the moisture of the area. Because vulvar involvement is part of a more general presentation of atopic dermatitis (Figure 2.2), the diagnosis is reached by the combination of a history of itching with intense relief from rubbing, morphology of cutaneous lesions, and the exclusion of infection. Therefore, biopsies are rarely necessary. The diagnosis is confirmed by the excellent response to therapy, mainly corticosteroid medications. As with children, selection of the treatment must consider the increased susceptibility these patients have to develop secondary chronic irritant dermatitis.

Seborrheic dermatitis Seborrheic dermatitis is a chronic and recurrent dermatitis that manifests as minimally symptomatic, thin, reddish plaques with greasy yellowish scale involving areas of increased sebum production. Scale and erythema involving the scalp, ears, central face, upper trunk, and flexures are the most common signs. Immunosuppressed patients may have extensive, red plaques and heavy, dry scaling. Genital lesions frequently occur in association with lesions localized in seborrheic areas with skin fold involvement, especially axillae. *Pityrosporum ovale*, the causative organism of pityriasis versicolor, may be identified by potassium hydroxide preparations of lesional scale; this yeast sometimes plays a role in seborrheic dermatitis by inducing an allergic reaction. In infants, seborrheic dermatitis spreads from the scalp (also called in this location 'cradle cap') to the face, trunk, and genitalia. The sequential spread of this chronic dermatitis occurs more frequently in infants than in adults. Seborrheic dermatitis of the external genitalia is prominent in the skin folds. It affects the hair-bearing skin of the labia majora and perineum. A classic but non-specific feature of genital seborrheic dermatitis is a glazed, shiny texture of the involved skin. The diagnosis is reached by identifying red scaling plaques on the scalp, central face, and skin folds, and the absence of *Candida* in cultures of skin scrapings. As with atopic dermatitis, the response to therapy confirms the diagnosis.

Exogenous vulvar spongiotic dermatitis
The two most common forms of spongiotic dermatitis with an exogenous cause are irritant contact dermatitis and allergic contact dermatitis.[5,21,28,52,82,84] The acute clinical presentations of allergic and irritant contact dermatitis have significant overlap and with time both evolve to a chronic lichen simplex chronicus.

Irritant contact dermatitis Irritant contact dermatitis occurs when damage to the cutaneous barrier function exceeds the skin's repair mechanisms. This dermatitis is an inflammatory reaction to direct toxic effects of a chemical, physical or

Table 2.2 Common causes of vulvar contact irritant dermatitis
Water (overwashing)
Soap (overwashing)
Detergents in shower gels and bubble baths
Antiseptic lotions, creams, etc.
Wet-wipes
Deodorant sprays
Cosmetic constituents such as perfumes or preservatives

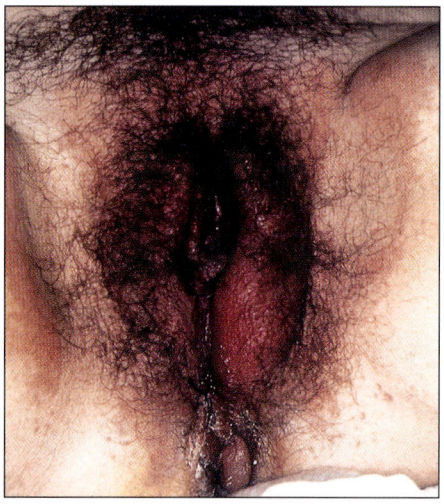

Fig. 2.4 Acute contact dermatitis to chlorhexidine. Edema and erythema are present in areas where the antiseptic chlorhexidine solution was applied during an episiotomy.

mechanical agent. Irritants may remove surface lipids and water-holding substances, damage cell membranes, denature keratins, exert direct cytotoxic effects, liberate cytokines, etc. Irritant contact dermatitis of the vulva occurs most commonly in the form of diaper dermatitis due to urine; this can also occur in adult women experiencing stress incontinence. The most common contact irritants causing vulvar dermatitis are listed in Table 2.2. Repetitive exposures are usually necessary to develop this type of dermatitis. Because the symptoms and signs occur gradually, the patient and physician often have difficulty isolating the culprit. Contact irritant dermatitis clinically presents with sharply demarcated, erythematous papules and plaques that may be weeping (Figure 2.4) and eroded if acute, or lichenified in chronic cases (see lichen simplex chronicus below). The resulting sensations of soreness and irritation, rather than itchiness, help to differentiate irritant contact dermatitis from other forms. The diagnosis involves correlation of symptoms and signs with a clinical history of potential exposures. The diagnosis is confirmed when the culprit is eliminated and the rash disappears.

Allergic contact dermatitis Allergic contact dermatitis is a cell-mediated type IV delayed hypersensitivity reaction. The rash develops 48–72 hours after exposure to the allergen. After sensitization, the patient develops allergic contact dermatitis upon each subsequent exposure. Although one exposure may be sufficient to develop the initial dermatitis, most frequently clinical reactivity becomes manifest only after repetitive exposures. The dermatitis lasts for about 2–3 weeks. The rash occurs in exposed areas. However, it may become generalized if autoeczematization (id reaction) occurs. As a general rule, infants under 5 years of age and elderly persons are less liable to develop allergic contact dermatitis as their immune systems tend not to develop type IV hypersensitivity reactions to antigens. If episodes are continuous, a patch test may be useful to study the reactants. Sometimes the offender can be the same medication given to the patient to treat this disorder (e.g., corticosteroid). A suspected substance can also be assayed by a use test, i.e., applying it under a bandage to the forearm for 48 hours. Table 2.3 lists the common causes of vulvar allergic dermatitis.

HINTS ON HISTOPATHOLOGIC INTERPRETATION OF VULVAR SPONGIOTIC DERMATITIS

Biopsy is rarely obtained on acute lesions of either irritant or allergic contact dermatitis. In such cases, the pathologist's main contribution is to confirm the clinical suspicion of spongiotic dermatitis and to rule out any other underlying dermatoses such as candidiasis or psoriasis. Performance of fungal stains for vulvar dermatitis can virtually always be justified. Rarely can the histopathologist distinguish the exogenous from the endogenous types with certainty. The cause is more likely to be identified after a detailed clinical history and an expert dermatologic examination. However, certain histologic features may point toward a particular entity:

- *Keratin changes*. Parakeratosis, particularly when also containing the nuclear remnants of neutrophils, should suggest psoriasis, seborrheic dermatitis, or a fungal infection. The location of parakeratosis around the follicular ostia, and spongiosis accentuated in the epithelium of the follicular infundibula, point toward seborrheic dermatitis.
- *Keratinocytes*. Focal keratinocyte ballooning and apoptosis suggests irritant contact dermatitis. Extensive keratinocyte necrosis, however, suggests erythema multiforme, fixed drug eruption, or dermatitis artefacta.
- *Spongiosis*. Exocytosis of eosinophils into the epidermis suggests fungal infection, allergic contact dermatitis, atopic dermatitis, or drug reaction (or more rarely, cicatricial pemphigoid or pemphigus vegetans). Neutrophils suggest fungal infection or psoriasis.

Increased numbers of Langerhans cells suggest allergic contact dermatitis.
- *Dermal infiltrate*. Eosinophils suggest allergic contact dermatitis. Marked dermal edema and dilatation of lymphatics suggest an urticarial reaction to systemic or topical drugs.

CHRONIC DERMATIDITES

LICHEN SIMPLEX CHRONICUS

Clinical features

Lichen simplex chronicus manifests as thick, scaly plaques arising after multiple cycles of rubbing and scratching in response to pruritus. The areas most frequently affected are the mons pubis and labia majora. These cutaneous changes may be the endpoint of various types of eczematous dermatitis (allergic contact dermatitis, seborrheic dermatitis, atopic dermatitis, etc.), or be superimposed upon other inflammatory processes (lichen planus, psoriasis, lichen sclerosus, etc.). Sometimes the original process that started the chronic itch–scratch cycle, perpetuating the lichen simplex chronicus changes, may have resolved by the time of the biopsy (i.e., an episode of allergic contact dermatitis, an infection with *Candida*, etc.). Clinically, the presence of thick skin with enhanced cutaneous markings (Figure 2.5) is encompassed by the term 'lichenification', referring to the rough surface of lichen overgrowing smooth-surfaced rocks.

Postinflammatory hyper- and hypopigmentation may accompany lichen simplex chronicus. Excoriations and secondary infections may result from the scratching. When thick epidermis is moist, i.e., inner surface of the labia majora, the hydrated keratin produces a white surface. Keratinocytes in these lesions have a reduced transit time through the epidermis and an increase in their mitochondrial enzymes, reflecting increased cell proliferation as well as an increase in melanocyte density. The pathogenesis of this disorder, however, remains incompletely understood. The term prurigo nodularis denotes clinical lesions with nodular growth.

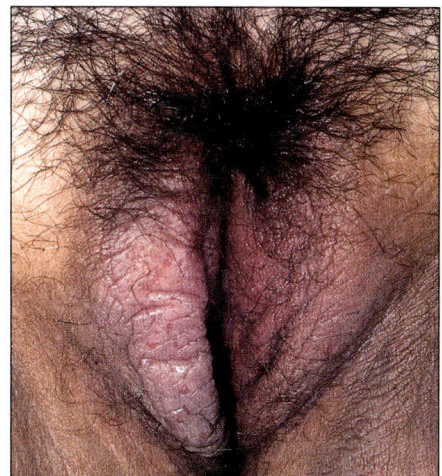

Fig. 2.5 Lichen simplex chronicus of the right labium majus. There is thickening and accentuation of skin markings, with surface excoriation due to recent scratching.

Table 2.3 Common agents causing vulvar contact allergic dermatitis
Perfumes
Preservatives in creams
Topical local anesthetics (such as benzocaine)
Topical antibiotics and antiseptics
Nail varnish
Rubber chemicals in contraceptive devices

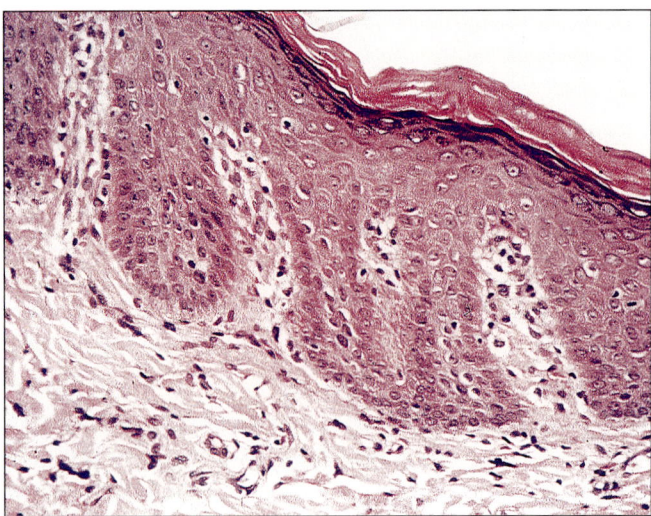

Fig. 2.6 Lichen simplex chronicus. The epidermis shows thickening of rete ridges, thickening of the granular layer, and overlying hyperkeratosis.

Microscopic features

The histologic features that characterize lichen simplex chronicus include (Figure 2.6):

- Marked orthohyperkeratosis (i.e., thickened stratum corneum devoid of keratinocyte nuclei). Parakeratosis is usually focal and may merely reflect a greater intensity of trauma or picking; the parakeratosis is less confluent than that seen in psoriasis.
- Hypergranulosis (thickened stratum granulosum).
- Acanthosis (thickened stratum spinosum). The thicker rete ridges are of less even length than those seen in psoriasis. Focal excoriation may be seen. When inflammatory exocytosis is marked, special stains for fungal forms (PAS and GMS) or bacteria (Brown–Brenn) are particularly recommended.
- Papillary dermal fibrosis. The dermal collagen bundles are thickened and tend to be vertically oriented.
- Superficial perivascular infiltrates of lymphocytes, macrophages, and sometimes eosinophils.

In prurigo nodularis the epidermis has a similar appearance but a more exaggerated acanthosis.

PSORIASIS[26]

Psoriasis (psoriasis vulgaris) is a common, multifactorial, chronic, relapsing, inflammatory dermatosis affecting 1–2% of the American population. It is diagnosed in about 5% of women presenting to a dermatologist with chronic vulvar symptoms. The most typical clinical presentation is as well-demarcated, red to salmon-colored plaques with loosely adherent, silver scales affecting the extensor surfaces of the extremities (elbows and knees), sacral region, scalp, and nails. Four main genetic loci appear associated with this disease (on chromosomes 17q, 4q, 1q, and 6p). There is a major susceptibility region for psoriasis on chromosome 5p21.3 near HLA-C. Psoriasis is associated with HLA-Cw6, B13, and B17.

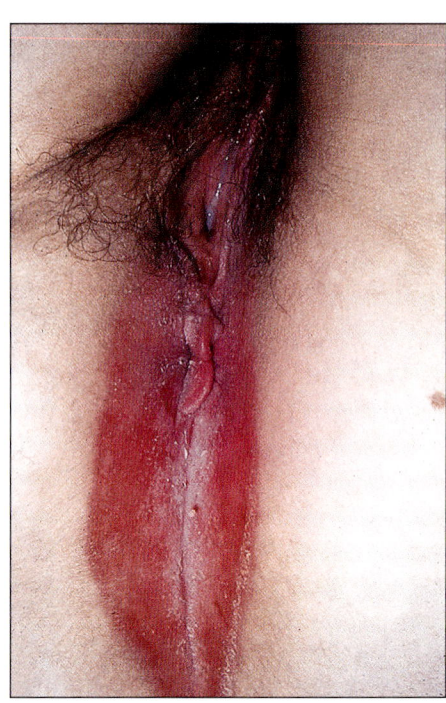

Fig. 2.7 Psoriasis of perineum and vulva. Flexural psoriasis often lacks the typical parakeratotic scale of psoriasis on other body sites. Painful erosion of the natal cleft is common.

Clinical features

The vulva and perineum are involved frequently in combination with typical lesions elsewhere on the body. Psoriasis is infrequently confined solely to the vulva. A fifth of patients develop lesions initially in areas of irritation or trauma, the so-called isomorphic or Koebner phenomenon. Genital involvement may in part reflect that this anatomic location is commonly subject to friction. Not only trauma can trigger psoriasis, but also infections and drugs. This disease affects hair-bearing areas (mons pubis and labia majora), whereas the labia minora are spared. In the anogenital region and flexural sites (inframammary fold, groin, etc.) the silvery scale can be lost, and the lesions will then present as well-demarcated, thin, intensely erythematous plaques (Figure 2.7). The intense erythema and the well-demarcated borders help to separate psoriasis from eczema. Lesions in the mons pubis usually preserve the more typical silvery scale. Persistent, painful intergluteal and perianal fissuring can be a serious complication.

Often the diagnosis is established with certainty after typical lesions develop elsewhere on the body. Nail changes in particular are seen in 30% of patients and show pitting, 'oil drop spots' (brownish-red discolorations of the nail plate), and onycholysis (lifting of the nail plate due to psoriasis in the nail bed). The flexural presentation of psoriasis with involvement of axillae, inframammary folds, retroauricular areas, and perineum can be a diagnostic challenge. Not only does this clinical presentation fail to demonstrate the classic thick-scaled lesions, but it also must be differentiated from severe seborrheic dermatitis. Cases with overlapping features of both diseases are sometimes called 'sebopsoriasis'.

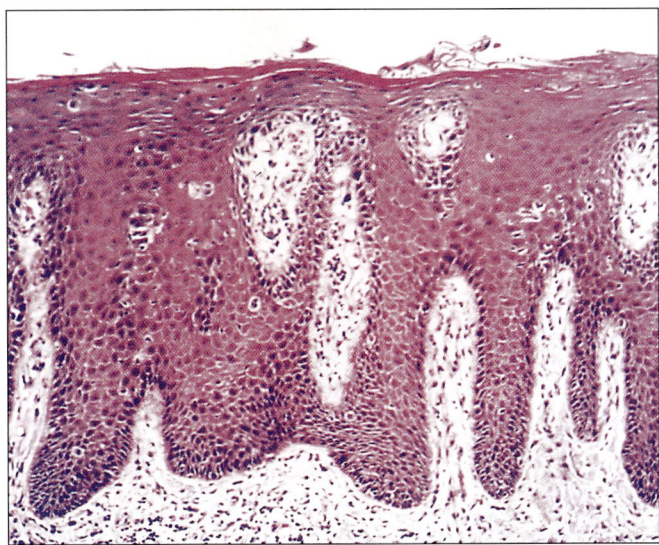

Fig. 2.8 Psoriasis. There is psoriasiform hyperplasia of rete ridges with papillary dermal edema and telangiectasia. The parakeratotic scale on the skin surface is not prominent in vulvar psoriasis.

Microscopic features

Histologically, features that characterize a classic plaque of psoriasis are:

- Stratum corneum with parakeratosis and collections of neutrophils and other inflammatory cell nuclear debris (Munros microabscesses).
- Epidermis showing psoriasiform hyperplasia with evenly elongated rete ridges, hypogranulosis, and thinned suprapapillary plates. Neutrophils migrate to the summits of the parakeratotic mounds. Collections of neutrophils in the epidermis are called spongiform pustules of Kogoj. Mitotic figures are found at different levels of the epidermis.
- Papillary dermis edema with tortuous, irregularly dilated vessels with a perivascular lymphocytic infiltrate with scattered neutrophils.

Lesions in the genital area have reduced parakeratotic surface keratin compared to classic psoriasis (Figure 2.8). Psoriasis occurring in genital regions may show more spongiosis than in other body parts. Coexistence of staphylococcal infection, repeated scratching, trauma, and chronicity, as well as partial treatment with topical steroids and a coexisting contact dermatitis (associated with the application of creams, disinfectants, etc.) can affect the histologic features. Lesions that histologically resemble pustular psoriasis may be seen in Reiters syndrome, but this rarely affects the vulva.

LESS COMMON DERMATOSES THAT FREQUENTLY INVOLVE THE VULVA

The two most common conditions in this category are lichen sclerosus and lichen planus.

LICHENOID DERMATOSES

LICHEN SCLEROSUS[2,10,11,14,32,52,59,66,83,99–101,112,115]

Lichen sclerosus, one of the most common chronic anogenital dermatoses, manifests as thickened and sclerotic dermal collagen. Most patients are middle-aged and elderly women. Sometimes it is familial.[39] Childhood presentation is uncommon, but it is important to remember it does occur lest it be confused with signs of sexual abuse.[53] Lichen sclerosus is associated with autoimmune disorders such as vitiligo, pernicious anemia, thyroid disease, etc.[13,39,86,89,102,111] Individual HLA types (DQ7, DQ8, and DQ9) have been detected more frequently in patients suffering from lichen sclerosus. One-fifth of patients show extragenital involvement as hypopigmented wrinkled patches (upper part of the trunk, the neck, the upper part of the arms, the flexor surfaces of the wrists, and the forehead). Extragenital lesions as a rule do not undergo malignant degeneration. On the other hand, genital lesions may coexist with or subsequently develop squamous cell carcinoma. In the vulva the frequency with which squamous cell carcinoma is associated with long-standing lesions of lichen sclerosus is 3–4%,[54] compared with 5.8% in penile lesions, most of them associated with human papillomavirus (HPV) infection.[93]

Although the etiology of lichen sclerosus is still unknown, infection may play a potential role, an argument based on the detection of lesional *Borrelia burgdorferi* in European countries, and the presence of CD8+ and CD57+ lymphocytic infiltrates, a profile usually associated with viral diseases, malignancies, and autoimmune disorders. The relation between lichen sclerosus and morphea is controversial. Some believe lichen sclerosus is a superficial variant of morphea, but this concept is not universally accepted.

Clinical features

The clinical presentation of lichen sclerosus is protean. The initial lesions consist of flat, ivory to white papules that coalesce to form plaques of varying sizes and shapes, with areas of telangiectasia and sometimes purpura (Figure 2.9). The early erythematous lesions with an edematous center impart a white color, and with time transform to the classic sclerotic lesions. The 'cigarette paper' atrophy in these lesions refers to the progressively wrinkled, flat or slightly depressed surface (Figure 2.10). Follicular plugging and formation of a central dell can occur. The symmetrically involved vulva and anus form the classic 'figure-of-eight' or 'hourglass'. In the vulva, lichen sclerosus extends to Harts line in the vestibule, the vaginal mucosa being uninvolved. Vulvar lesions may combine atrophic and hypertrophic areas, or may develop lichenification secondary to pruritus-related scratching. Damage to the dermoepidermal junction caused by inflammation may lead to bullae formation, sometimes blood filled due to damaged superficial telangiectatic vessels. The sclerotic background of the bullae is a clue to the diagnosis. Lichen sclerosus is a relentless and progressive disease when presenting in most adults, but not uncommonly spontaneously regresses in girls once they reach menarche.

Lichen sclerosus usually causes severe, intractable itch, to the point that some women are literally suicidal due to the intensity of the pruritus and soreness. In children, the pain experienced during micturition and defecation can lead to urinary retention or fecal impaction.[8,72] Occasionally, the condition is asymptomatic and discovered incidentally during a

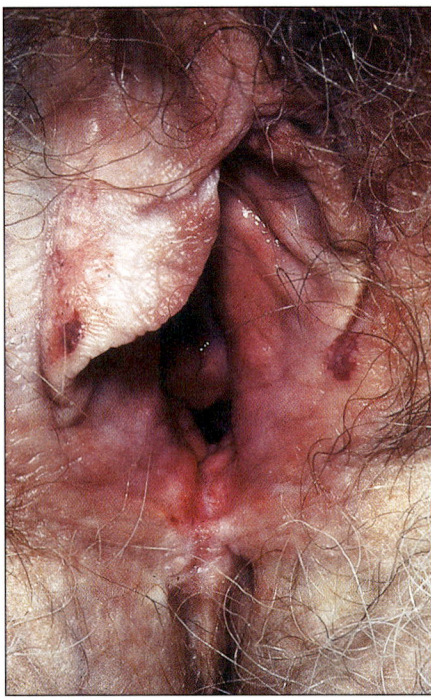

Fig. 2.9 Lichen sclerosus. Classic white areas with purpura are present on the labia majora.

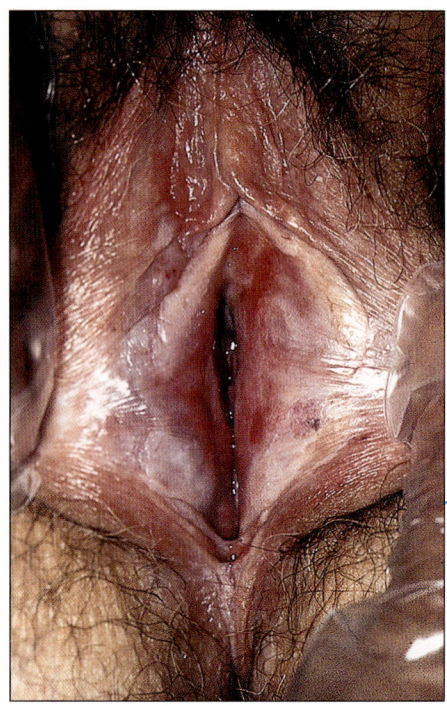

Fig. 2.11 Lichen sclerosus. The entity can scar, and resorption of the labia minora is common.

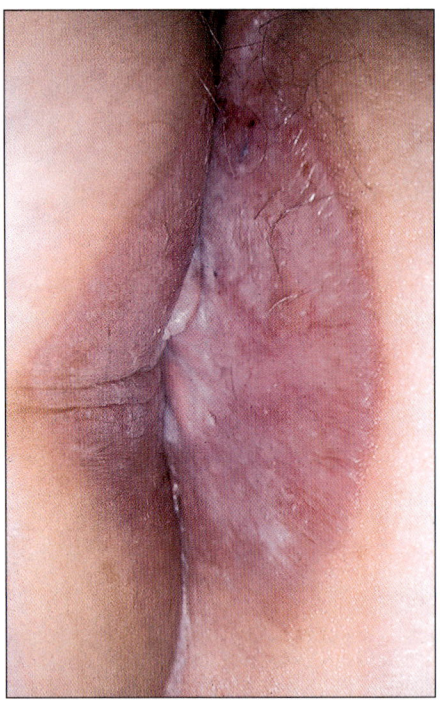

Fig. 2.10 Perianal lichen sclerosus with typical 'cigarette paper' atrophy. The skin is white and shows several purpura.

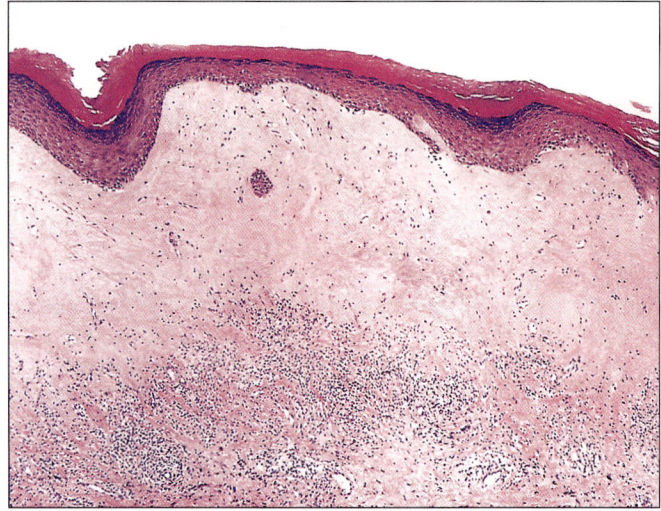

Fig. 2.12 Lichen sclerosus. There is a broad band of hyalinized collagen beneath the epidermis, and a band of lymphocytic infiltrate beneath the hyalinization. The characteristic hyalinized band may be very narrow.

routine pelvic examination. Over time, variable degrees of scarring occur at an unpredictable pace and extent. Often the labia minora partially resorb (Figure 2.11). In severe cases, vulvar stenosis, effaced anatomy, and clitoral phimosis occur. Dyspareunia is common, sometimes accompanied by frank bleeding when intercourse is attempted.

Early diagnosis and adequate treatment can prevent the distressing symptoms and severe vulvar deformities. Close surveillance facilitates early detection of squamous cell carcinoma.[45,124] Biopsy has a double role, first to confirm the diagnosis and second to help exclude a malignancy.

Microscopic features
Lichen sclerosus affects the epidermis and upper dermis (Figures 2.12 and 2.13). The variable clinical presentation parallels the diversity of histopathologic features seen at the different stages of the disease.

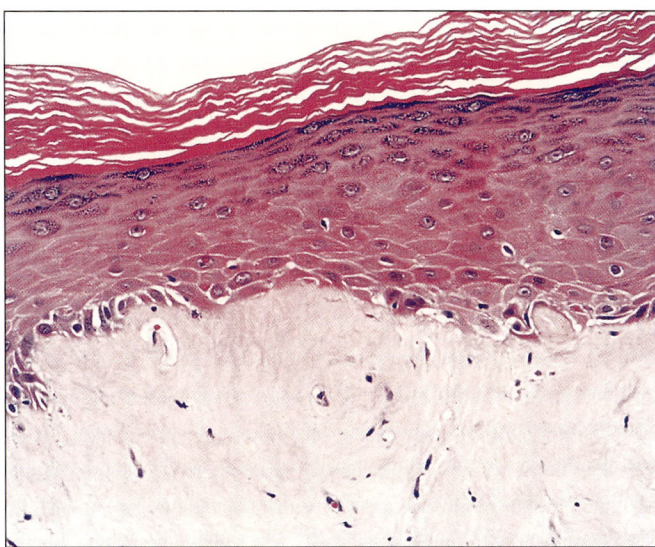

Fig. 2.13 Lichen sclerosus. A characteristic feature of lichen sclerosus is irregular damage to the basal layer of the epidermis.

Early lesion of lichen sclerosus
- Stratum corneum with compact orthokeratosis.
- Thin epidermis with vacuolar alteration of the dermoepidermal junction.
- Focal perivascular and patchy lichenoid or band-like lymphocytic infiltrate, partially effacing the dermoepidermal junction.
- Papillary dermal edema of a variable extent imparts a light and pale quality to the papillary dermal collagen. The elastic fibers are pushed downwards.

Established lesion of lichen sclerosus
- Stratum corneum with compact orthokeratosis.
- The epidermis is generally thin, but this can alternate with areas of hyperplasia (malignant transformation has been reported in hyperplastic areas). Lichen simplex chronicus, if superimposed, shows acanthosis with notable hypergranulosis. The dermoepidermal junction may show focal vacuolar alteration with a sprinkling of lymphocytes. The basement membrane may fragment, leading to the formation of PAS-positive clumps in the subjacent dermis.
- Plugs widen the ostia of eccrine glands (acrosyringia) and hair follicles (acrotrichia).
- The papillary dermis and upper reticular dermis display homogenized, thick, sclerotic, deeply eosinophilic collagen bundles. The elastic fibers are destroyed in the upper dermis. The dilated vessels embedded in the sclerosis correspond to the telangiectasias seen clinically. Melanin-laden macrophages are easily found.
- Moderately dense perivascular lymphocytic infiltrate admixed with some plasma cells and histiocytes involve the superficial vascular plexus. These vessels appear 'pushed down' by the sclerosis, displacing the inflammation to deep within the dermis.

Old lesion of lichen sclerosus
- These lesions show the sclerotic changes of an established lesion, namely a thin epidermis and absence of adnexae. In addition, the active inflammatory component is nearly

always absent. Changes of lichen simplex chronicus (acanthosis, hypergranulosis, extravasated red cells, and excoriations) may be prominent.

A biopsy taken after treatment or at an advanced stage with prominent secondary changes can be a diagnostic challenge. Examination of the slide at multiple levels, however, often reveals focal lichenoid inflammation or alteration of the collagen fibers pointing to the correct diagnosis. Elastic tissue stains may show destruction of fibers in the upper dermis, thus providing additional diagnostic information.

Pigmented lesions evolving in a background of lichen sclerosus can present alarming histologic features. It is important to remember that these changes are not associated with aggressive biologic behavior to avoid unnecessary surgical procedures.[12]

LICHEN PLANUS[2,20,23,27,38,52,64,68,70,80]

Lichen planus is a relatively common, chronic, inflammatory disease of skin and mucous membranes. Cell-mediated immune reactions to an altered antigen in basal keratinocytes, triggered by a virus, drug or allogeneic cell, may play an important role in its development. Like other lichenous disease, the clinical presentation is quite variable. Clinical variants include atrophic, hypertrophic, erosive, actinic, linear, zosteriform, and bullous types. The skin lesions resolve in most cases within 1–2 years, but mucosal lesions may persist longer. Hyperpigmentation is a common sequela after resolution, especially in darker skinned patients. Lichen planus has been associated with immunodeficiency states, internal malignancy, primary biliary cirrhosis, peptic ulcer, chronic hepatitis C infection, hepatitis B vaccination, and ulcerative colitis among other conditions. Whereas lichen sclerosus does not affect the vagina, lichen planus can manifest as desquamative vaginitis.

Clinical features
Half of the women and one-fourth of the men with cutaneous lichen planus have genital involvement. Unfortunately, it is frequently missed, for several reasons. Clinically, vulvar lichen planus can take many forms and most of them are not easy to recognize. Being a mucocutaneous interface, the vulva can be affected by cutaneous, mucosal, or combined patterns, with four clinical appearances predominating.

Cutaneous-pattern lichen planus
The cutaneous pattern shows two clinical variants, one with genital lesions similar to those seen in other cutaneous sites, and the second with hypertrophic lesions. The first group shows genital involvement as part of generalized cutaneous lichen planus: the lesions are well-defined, erythematous to violaceous, flat-topped papules and plaques without scale involving the labia minora and majora or the mons pubis (Figure 2.14). Surface changes may include fine white lines (Wickhams striae) (Figure 2.15). This type of genital lichen planus does not lead to scar formation. The hyperkeratotic white plaques of hypertrophic lichen planus are an infrequent expression of genital lichen planus. This variant can mimic malignancy and predilectorily involves the perineum and perianal region. Cutaneous lichen planus is usually very itchy; therefore, excoriations and superimposed secondary changes of lichen simplex chronicus may mask the clinical and histopathologic diagnostic features.

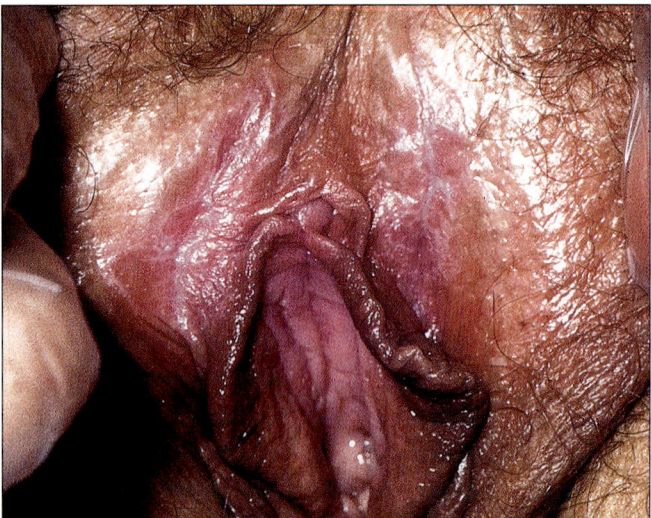

Fig. 2.14 Lichen planus of cutaneous pattern affecting the labia. There is a subtle purplish rash, which clinically is very itchy.

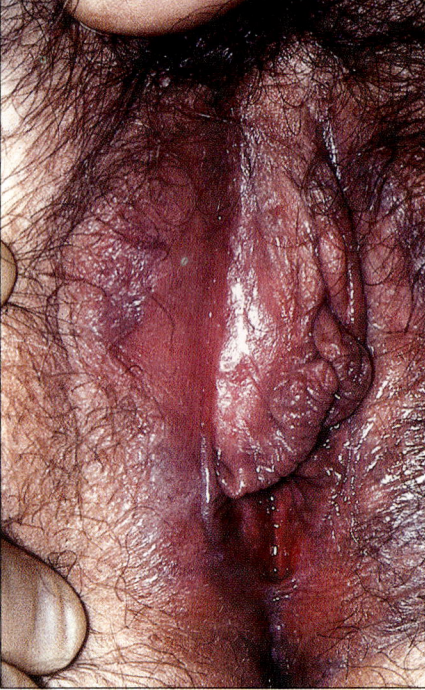

Fig. 2.15 Lichen planus in the interlabial creases. Fine white striae and erosions are present.

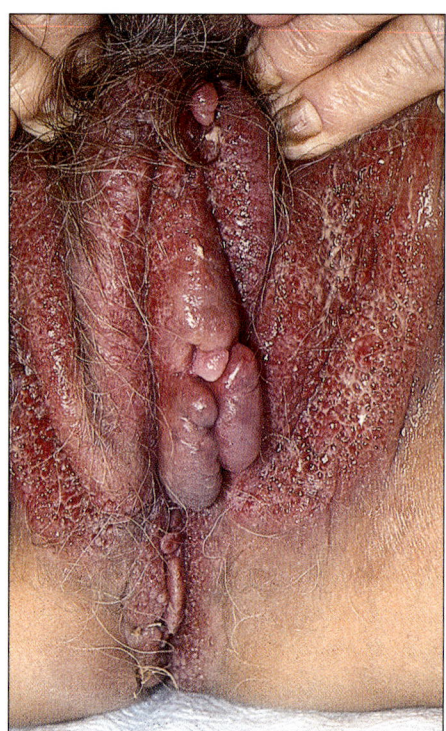

Fig. 2.16 Reticulate-pattern lichen planus. Identical changes are commonly seen on buccal mucosa.

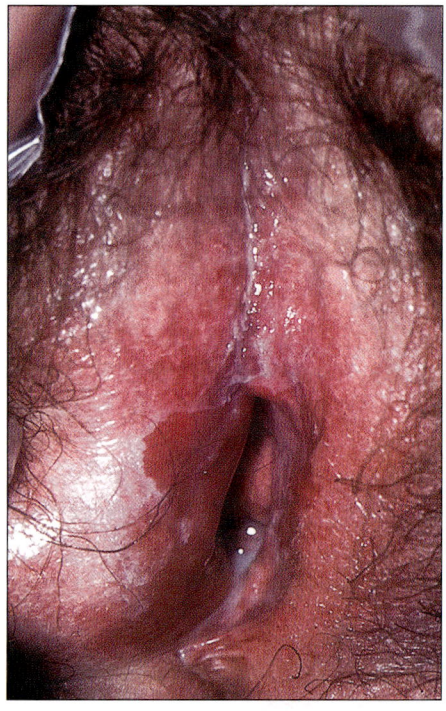

Fig. 2.17 Erosive lichen planus. Bright patches of eroded epithelium with a shaggy white edge are present at the vulvar vestibule. Vaginal disease may be present.

Mucosal lichen planus

This can be of two types: reticulate and erosive lichen planus.

Reticulate lichen planus Reticulate lichen planus manifests clinically as fine white lines running across an erythematous surface in the non-hair-bearing labial surface (Figure 2.16). The findings resemble those of lichen planus involving the oral mucosa. As in other types of lichen planus, itching leads to superimposed excoriations.

Erosive lichen planus Erosive lichen planus[25,73,80,98,103] presents with eroded, bright red, thin epithelium surrounded by reticu-

lated white lacy plaques (Figure 2.17). These lesions produce soreness, dyspareunia, postcoital bleeding, and dysuria. With time, scarring occurs that leads to labial atrophy, clitoral phimosis, and narrowing of the introitus due to adhesions. Vaginal erosive lichen planus manifests as pain and contact bleeding, and produces shortening or narrowing of the vagina. Oral lesions can be diagnostically helpful when mucosal lesions in the genital tract are not specific. The buccal mucosa shows tender erosions and ulcerations surrounded by interlacing white striae. The presence of erosive lichen planus involving the oral–vaginal–vulvar mucosae, recognized only two decades ago, is now known as the vulvovaginal–gingival syndrome. The anal mucosa may be involved, alone or together with other sites, by lesions similar to those seen in the vulva. Over time, untreated erosive lichen planus can destroy the normal anatomy of the vulva, making the introduction of a speculum for clinical examination impossible.

Mixed cutaneous and mucosal pattern lichen planus

This pattern shows cutaneous features on the labia majora and most of the labia minora, together with reticulate or erosive changes in the labia minora and vulvar vestibule, and extending variably into the vagina. These patients may experience desquamative inflammatory vaginitis due to vaginal involvement in a background of vulvar papules.

Pathology

The histopathologic diagnosis of vulvar lichen planus is often difficult. First, the appearance often differs from that of classic cutaneous lichen planus. Second, lichen simplex chronicus frequently coexists, and sometimes there is also associated lichen sclerosus. Finally, the erosive pattern, where the epithelium is lost, may be extremely difficult to diagnose due to sampling problems, secondary infection, and inflammation from topical applications. Several critical features (Figures 2.18–2.21), however, permit confident histologic diagnosis:

- Basal layer hydropic degeneration with Civatte body formation.
- Lichenoid (band-like) infiltrate in the upper dermis. Plasma cells are noted in mucosal lesions.
- Pigment incontinence (macrophages containing phagocytosed melanin) in the upper dermis.

These features may be patchy, and step sections may be required for their identification (Figure 2.21). The fully developed epidermal changes usually seen in classic cutaneous lichen

planus (saw-tooth pattern, hypergranulosis, orthokeratosis, etc.) are rarely present in vulvar lesions. Accurate diagnosis is important since the erosive form may require immunosuppressive therapy. Also, the presence of chronic lichen planus in the vulva is a risk factor for squamous cell carcinoma.[124] The differential diagnosis includes lichenoid drug reactions, which should be suspected if eosinophils are present.

IMMUNOBULLOUS DISORDERS

These vesiculobullous disorders result from congenital or acquired formation of antibodies against components involved in the adhesion of keratinocytes. Many of the blistering dis-

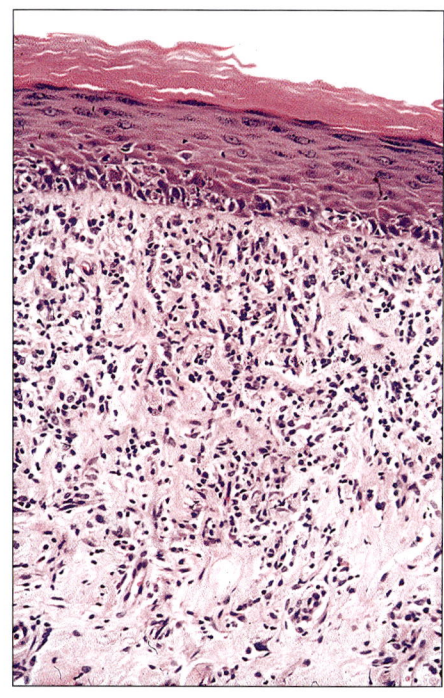

Fig. 2.19 Lichen planus. The lichenoid infiltrate may be sparse, but basal layer damage and hyperkeratosis enable the diagnosis to be made.

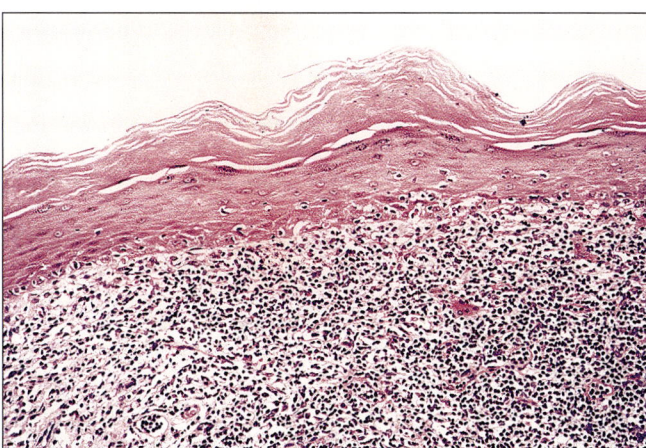

Fig. 2.18 Lichen planus. The epidermis shows hyperkeratosis, extensive basal layer destruction and a dense lichenoid infiltrate at the dermoepidermal junction. In the vulva, the histologic changes are not always as florid and classic as shown here.

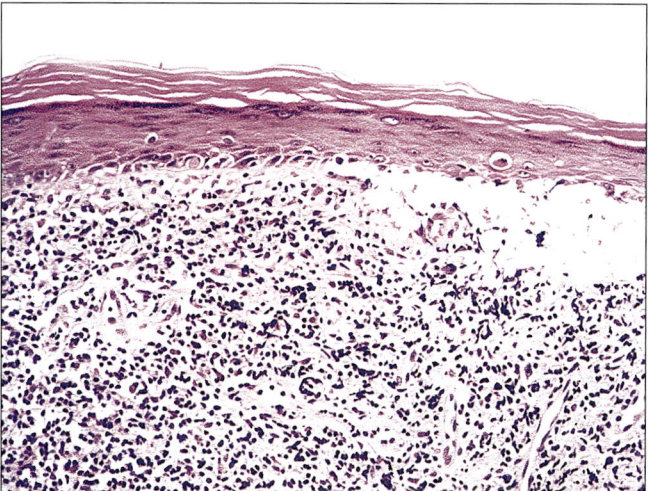

Fig. 2.20 Lichen planus. Taken from the edge of an erosion, this slide shows early basal separation occurring in lichen planus.

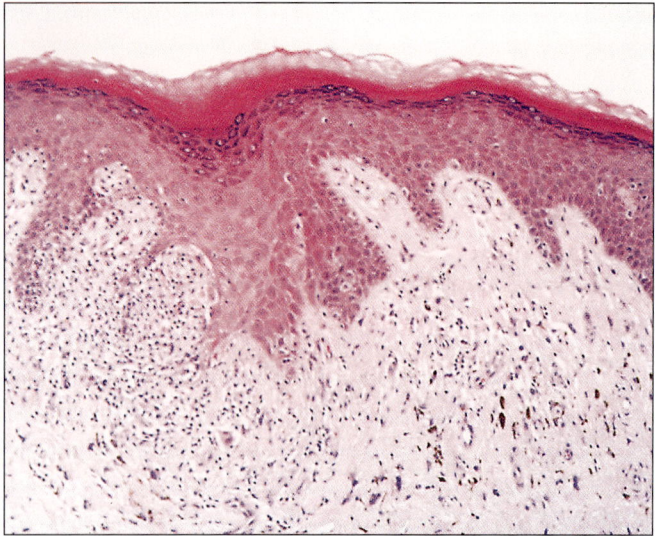

Fig. 2.21 Lichen planus. In the vulva lichen planus changes may be very focal, and show superimposed lichen simplex chronicus due to repeated scratching.

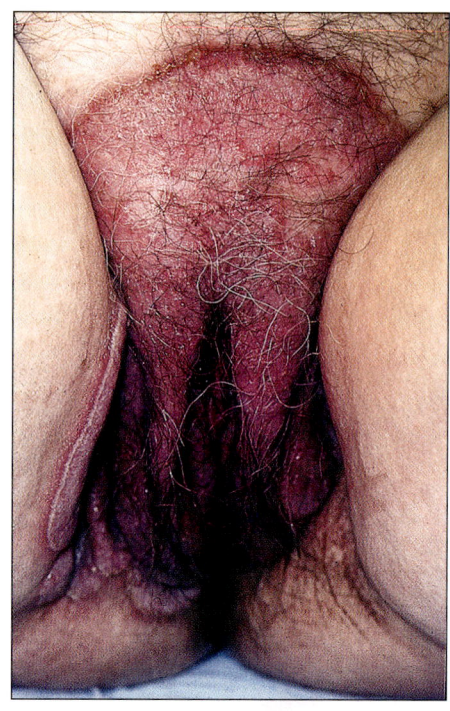

Fig. 2.22 Pemphigus vegetans. This disease preferentially involves the genital area and presents with exuberant ('vegetating'), weeping, blistering plaques.

eases that affect the skin also involve mucosal sites. In the vulva, friction and trauma foster the development of the blistering disorders, which typically present clinically as soggy, weeping, or erosive to ulcerative lesions. Clinical suspicion needs to be high in patients with erosions. Besides a detailed clinical history and careful physical examination, biopsies of the lesion for light microscopy plus perilesional skin for direct immunofluorescence are important. The most significant primary bullous skin diseases affecting the vulva are:

- Pemphigus vulgaris, and its variant pemphigus vegetans
- Cicatricial pemphigoid
- Linear IgA disease, particularly in children.

PEMPHIGUS VULGARIS[52,78,126]

Pemphigus vulgaris is an acquired, autoimmune blistering disease representing 80% of all pemphigus cases. Autoantibodies develop against the desmosomal protein, desmoglein 3, at intercellular sites among keratinocytes, leading to acantholytic blisters that break easily and form erosions.

Clinical features

Most patients have oral blisters that precede cutaneous involvement by weeks to months. Other mucosal sites affected include the conjunctiva, larynx, anorectum, vulva, vagina, and cervix. The vulvar lesions consist of erythematous, moist, eroded plaques, at the edge of which intact blisters may briefly be seen. The classic skin lesions consist of flaccid blisters on a normal or erythematous base. The blisters break easily leading to eroded and crusted areas. Trunk, groins, axillae, scalp, and face are frequently involved. These lesions extend if pressure is applied to the top of the bullae (positive Nikolsky sign). They heal without scarring. The disease activity can be follow by ELISA titers of circulating antibody to desmoglein 3. A positive direct immunofluorescence test in a patient in clinical remission often heralds a relapse. The principal cause of death is infection secondary to corticosteroid treatment. The mortality rate is 5–15%.

Microscopic features

Cutaneous and mucosal lesions are similar microscopically. The squamous epithelium shows suprabasal bullae which contain a few degenerative acantholytic cells. Scattered neutrophils and eosinophils can be seen in the bullae. Because the disease targets an adhesion protein joining keratinocytes, but not between keratinocytes and basement membrane, the basal keratinocytes remain attached to the dermis, imparting a 'tombstone appearance'. Dermal changes are non-specific. Unfortunately, the separated upper layers of the epidermis frequently fall off during the biopsy process and all that remains is the dermis with the single layer of intact basal keratinocytes. In this situation, a useful histologic clue is the presence of clefts extending deep into adnexal structures. A biopsy that includes the edge of the blister increases the chances to find early histologic findings. Careful study often demonstrates some surviving acantholytic keratinocytes. Biopsies of old lesions may exhibit a different level of clefting due to re-epithelialization, the process by which epidermis regenerates at the base of the bullae. Direct immunofluorescence usually shows IgG, especially IgG$_1$ and IgG$_4$, in the intercellular spaces. C3, IgM, and IgA are less frequently detected.

PEMPHIGUS VEGETANS

Clinical features

This rare variant of pemphigus shows well-demarcated, warty erythematous plaques with a moist, ulcerated surface that preferentially involves the pubic, perineal, and perianal areas (Figures 2.22 and 2.23). Rarely, blisters are found at the edges of the plaque. As with pemphigus vulgaris, oral lesions are invariably present, and frequently the presenting feature. Other

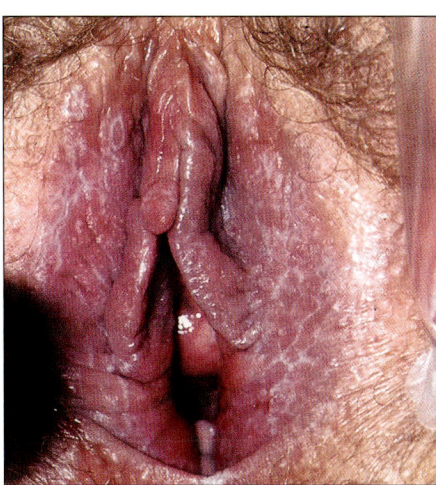

Fig. 2.23 Pemphigus vegetans. The weeping blistering nature of the lesion is shown in great detail.

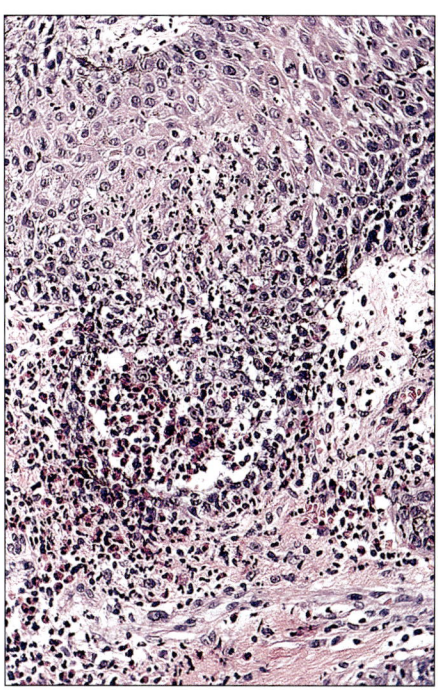

Fig. 2.25 Pemphigus vegetans. At an early stage, intraepidermal accumulations of eosinophils are a useful diagnostic picture.

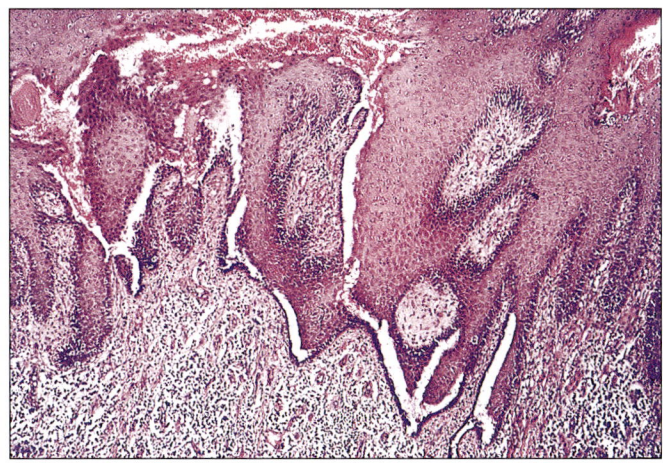

Fig. 2.24 Pemphigus vegetans. Acantholytic separation of the hyperplastic epidermis just above the basal layer is characteristic of pemphigus vegetans. There is frequently a chronic inflammatory dermal infiltrate with some inflammatory cells in the epidermis.

sites include the flexures, scalp, or face. 'Vegetans' alludes to the warty appearance of these lesions that may mislead the clinician to diagnose condyloma acuminatum or even squamous cell carcinoma. Although the warty stage is the most characteristic clinical presentation, two early stages can be detected in this disease, one with lesions similar to patients with pemphigus vulgaris (*Neumann type*) and the other with pustular lesions (*Hallopeau type*).

Microscopic features

The histologic features of pemphigus vegetans can be florid, depending on the stage at which the lesion is biopsied. The early pustular lesions of the Hallopeau type show spongiotic intraepidermal microvesicles and eosinophilic microabscesses. Acantholysis with suprabasal clefting predominates in early vesicular lesions of the Neumann type. The late warty lesions of both types show extreme acanthosis, sometimes to the point of pseudocarcinomatous hyperplasia, with prominent papillomatosis, and overlying foci of suprabasal acantholysis (Figure 2.24). Epidermal lacunae are filled with eosinophils (Figure

2.25) and dermal collections of mainly lymphocytes admixed with eosinophils. This florid inflammation may obscure the presence of focal acantholysis in the epidermis. As in pemphigus vulgaris, direct immunofluorescence shows intercellular deposits of IgG (occasionally IgM) and C3. Circulating antibodies of the IgG_2 and IgG_4 subclasses, with strong complement fixation, are commonly present in pemphigus vegetans.

BULLOUS PEMPHIGOID AND CICATRICIAL PEMPHIGOID[33,36,40,44,47,85,105,120]

Bullous pemphigoid is a chronic, subepidermal, acquired, autoimmune blistering disease. Multiple, tense blisters typically occur on itchy, urticarial, erythematous plaques or normal skin in elderly patients. Bullous pemphigoid encompasses 80% of the subepidermal bullae, with a reported incidence of 7 cases per 1 000 000.[7] These patients develop autoantibodies that target the basal cells' basement membrane attachment plaque (hemidesmosome). A 230 kDa antigenic protein (BP 230) is a member of the plakin family of proteins restricted to the intracellular hemidesmosomal plaque. A second 180 kDa antigen (BP 180) is a transmembrane protein located between the hemidesmosome and the lamina lucida. Bullous pemphigoid usually develops spontaneously, but it may also arise with specific drugs, such as furosemide, penicillins, psoralens, ibuprofen, and angiotensin-converting enzyme (ACE) inhibitors.

Cicatricial pemphigoid or benign mucous membrane pemphigoid is a chronic bullous disease that affects predominantly oral and ocular membranes, resulting in scar formation. Autoantibodies target laminin 5 and BP180, albeit in a different domain from bullous pemphigoid. Patients with autoantibodies against laminin 5 have a more recalcitrant disease, and there is a more frequent association with solid tumors.

Clinical features

Bullous pemphigoid clinically manifests with a wide range of presentations and, although less often than with pemphigus vulgaris, mucosal involvement occurs. In classic bullous pemphigoid, multiple, large, tense bullae frequently affect the vulva in the setting of widespread skin involvement. These bullae do not rupture easily and if uncomplicated, heal without scarring. Commonly, lesions appear on the thighs, flexor surfaces of the forearms, axillae, groins, and lower abdomen. Two years is the average time until the patient experiences remission.

In cicatricial pemphigoid, mucosal and squamomucosal junction areas are prominent. Even though the most frequent sites affected are the mouth, conjunctivae, and nasal mucosa, anogenital region involvement occurs in 20% of patients. Half will have eye involvement that, left untreated, can evolve to blindness. Only one-third of patients with cicatricial pemphigoid have skin involvement. Clinically the lesions affect both labia majora and minora, but particularly affect the non-hair-bearing surfaces such as the interlabial folds, labia minora, and vestibule. Blisters, if seen, are short lived, and then only when erosions are found. Patients complain of vulvar pain and soreness. The clinical appearances in the vulva (as in the mouth) may resemble erosive lichen planus. Routine histologic plus immunofluorescence tests are important. Dermal scarring is a grave sequela and may lead to destruction and fusion of the labia minora (Figure 2.26)[25,84] and urethral stenosis, the latter requiring therapeutic dilatation. This disease tends not to remit. Cicatricial pemphigoid can occur in young girls.[33,47,67,105] Some reports of isolated vulvar pemphigoid in young girls probably represent limited expressions of cicatricial pemphigoid.

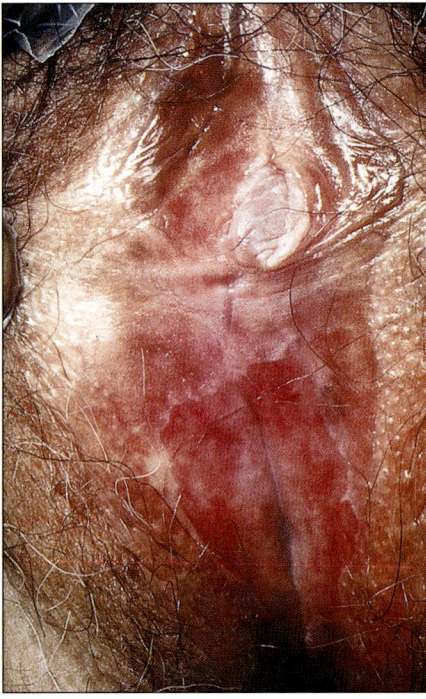

Fig. 2.26 Cicatricial pemphigoid. There is extensive scarring and loss of normal vulvar anatomy, which clinically can be indistinguishable from erosive lichen planus.

Microscopic features

In the vulva, bullous pemphigoid discloses unilocular, subepidermal blisters containing a fluid rich in eosinophils. Some neutrophils are admixed, and these increase in number with the lesion's age. As in bullae elsewhere in the body, eosinophils and neutrophils are found in the upper dermis. If the biopsy is taken from urticarial or prodromal lesions, the key findings are eosinophilic spongiosis (epidermal spongiosis with eosinophils), accumulation of clusters of eosinophils in the papillary dermis abutting the epidermal–dermal basement membrane, and papillary dermal edema.

Histologically, cicatricial pemphigoid, like bullous pemphigoid, shows subepidermal blisters, but the infiltrate and dermal changes help to separate the two entities. The inflammatory reaction in cicatricial pemphigoid changes with the age of the lesion. In those less than 48 hours old, neutrophilic collections appear in the papillary dermis. With time, eosinophils increase in number. Old lesions show variable numbers of lymphocytes and plasma cells but eosinophils remain conspicuous. As the name of the disease implies, the lesions evolve to scars. Although the scar is a characteristic of older lesions, scars can also be seen in new lesions because blisters have a tendency to recur in the same anatomic site. Polarized light is useful to highlight the new collagen in the scar. In the vulva, these fibers lie parallel to the epidermis in contrast to the haphazard arrangement of normal collagen. However, these characteristic features are rarely seen. Most biopsies show less specific changes of denuded, inflamed mucosa or a scar with re-epithelialization.

Perilesional direct immunofluorescence in both bullous and cicatricial pemphigoid usually shows a linear band of IgG with or without C3 at the dermoepidermal junction. Sometimes immunoglobulins are found, as with IgA in 20% of cases. In cicatricial pemphigoid, the diagnostic yield is highest in oral mucosal biopsy specimens. In bullous pemphigoid, levels of circulating IgG antibodies (found in 60–80% of the patients)[57] do not reflect disease activity, whereas in cicatricial pemphigoid, serial titers of IgG and IgA antibodies correlate with disease activity. In salt-split skin, the reactants are localized on the epidermal side of the lesion in bullous pemphigoid and in those cicatricial pemphigoid patients with BP180 antibodies, while cicatricial pemphigoid patients with antilaminin 5 antibodies exhibit reactivity on the dermal site of the split.

CHRONIC BULLOUS DERMATOSIS OF CHILDHOOD AND ADULT LINEAR IGA BULLOUS DERMATOSIS

Clinical features

These are rare, immunobullous disorders of unknown etiology in which linear deposits of IgA are detected in subepidermal blisters. Two clinical variants are commonly regarded as different expressions of the same entity, i.e., chronic bullous dermatosis of childhood and adult linear IgA bullous dermatosis. In both disorders, antibodies form against components of the lamina lucida. The genital area, buttocks, thighs, neck, and face are frequently involved. In the first years of life, chronic bullous dermatosis presents with the abrupt onset of large, tense bullae that have a propensity for perioral and perigenital areas, but extend to thighs and lower abdomen. The 'cluster of jewels' sign refers to an annular or polycyclic grouping, with bullae located at the margin. Initially the blisters fill with clear fluid, but secondary infection results in pustules (Figure 2.27).

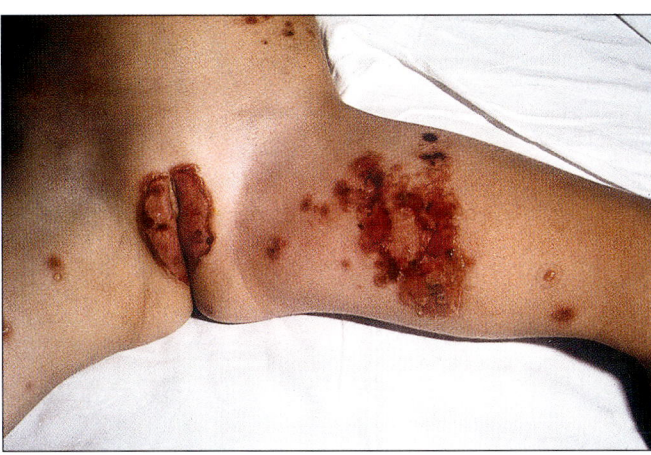

Fig. 2.27 Chronic bullous disease of childhood. The disease presents with groups of itchy blisters and erosions. The genital region is often involved.

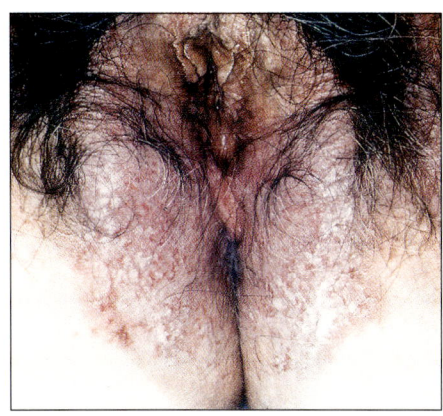

Fig. 2.28 Hailey–Hailey disease. This dyskeratotic genodermatosis presented with irritable superficially eroded plaques in flexural sites.

Commonly, this disease resolves in several months. In adults, the clinical presentation is protean and mimics other bullous disorders. Usually the lesions involve the trunk and limbs. Perineal lesions, in contrast, are less frequent. Amiodarone, vancomycin, lithium, and non-steroidal anti-inflammatory drugs (NSAIDs) can induce this immunobullous disorder.

Microscopic features

Histologically, the classic appearance is that of a subepidermal blister with neutrophilic microabscesses in the papillary dermis, a finding indistinguishable from that seen in dermatitis herpetiformis. Fibrin with leukocytolysis in the tip of the papilla favors dermatitis herpetiformis, while the presence of neutrophils parallel to the dermoepidermal junction points towards linear IgA dermatosis. However, only immunofluorescence definitively separates these two diseases. In other cases, the major inflammatory cell present is the eosinophil and the changes may resemble bullous pemphigoid, with numerous eosinophils in the subepidermal blister and dermal papillary eosinophil microabscesses. These different histologic presentations may reflect changes in lesions of different ages. In early, non-blistering areas, only an increase in eosinophils may be present in the upper dermis, with some eosinophils migrating into the focally spongiotic epidermis and discharging their granules (eosinophilic spongiosis).

INHERITED DERMATOSES

HAILEY–HAILEY DISEASE[65,122]

Clinical features

Hailey–Hailey disease is an autosomal dominant, acantholytic dermatosis involving flexural areas in which friction and sweating are frequent. It usually starts in the late teens, followed by periods of exacerbation and remission that usually improve, but do not completely resolve after puberty. Patients suffer from recurrent, erythematous, well-circumscribed, vesicular plaques that evolve into small flaccid bullae that rupture, leaving crusted, erythematous erosions. Lesions are frequently pruritic and malodorous, especially when involving the axillae,

inframammary folds, perineal area, and groin (Figure 2.28). When patients complain of increasing redness and exudation it is often a sign of secondary infection, usually bacterial in origin. The presentation of erythematous plaques with expanding, scaly, eroded borders may mimic fungal infection. The disease, when occurring in the perineal region, frequently extends to the vulva. Unusual cases are restricted to the vulva.[30,55] Some may spread to involve the vagina.[121] The responsible gene for this disease is *ATP2CL*, mapped to chromosome 3q21–q24. This gene encodes a Ca^{2+} pump of the Golgi system that interferes with intracellular Ca^{2+} signaling. Normal concentration of Ca^{2+} in the Golgi apparatus is necessary to produce adhesion proteins such as E-cadherin. High cytoplasmic Ca^{2+} may alter gene expression or, through activation of protein kinase C, lead to phosphorylation of adhesion molecules (e.g., desmoplakin) leading to disruption of desmosomes.

Microscopic features

Early lesions start with suprabasal clefting. Acantholytic cells may border the cleft or lie free in the cavity. With time, the acantholysis involves the entire epidermis, producing the characteristic image of a 'crumbling, dilapidated brick wall' (Figure 2.29). Neutrophils make up part of the parakeratotic crust, and chronic inflammatory cells are present in the superficial perivascular region. The broad lesion and degree of inflammation help to distinguish Hailey–Hailey disease from other acantholytic dermatoses. Immunofluorescence tests in difficult cases help separate it from pemphigus vulgaris. Isolated cases of squamous cell carcinoma have arisen on a background of Hailey–Hailey.[15,61]

EPIDERMOLYSIS BULLOSA

This mechanobullous disease rarely affects the vulva, except in the setting of generalized cutaneous involvement by the severe junctional and dystrophic types.

DARIERS DISEASE[4,16,104]

Clinical features

Also known as 'keratosis follicularis', this chronic acantholytic dermatosis is a genodermatosis inherited as an autosomal dom-

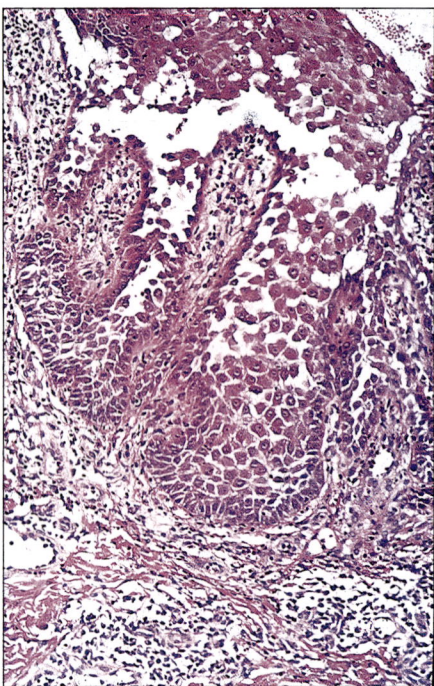

Fig. 2.29 Hailey–Hailey disease. The pattern of epidermal acantholysis in Hailey–Hailey disease is characteristic, said to resemble a crumbling brick wall. Compare this pattern of acantholysis with that seen in pemphigus vegetans.

inant disorder. It usually appears initially in adolescence with greasy, yellow to brown, crusted papules that affect the seborrheic areas of the head, neck, and trunk. These papules can coalesce to produce plaques that may occasionally have papillomatous surfaces. Verruciform lesions on the hands, like acrokeratosis verruciformis, afflict more than half of patients. Additional findings include punctate keratoses on palms and soles, longitudinal striations of the nails with distal breaks and V-shaped notches, ocular disorders, bone cysts, and mental deficiency. Although it exhibits no consistent immunologic abnormalities, Dariers disease has a predisposition to bacterial, fungal, and viral infections. Infection is more prominent in flexures like groins and causes flares of the disease as well as malodor. Involvement of the vulva is usually associated with cutaneous involvement of the groin. Because the lesions located on skin folds can be difficult to diagnose due to secondary infection, classic lesions in the seborrheic areas of the body, acral punctate keratoses, and nail changes will serve as clues to the correct diagnosis.

Acantholysis in Dariers disease reflects abnormalities in the tonofilament–desmosome complexes and adhesion complexes. Desmoplakin I and II and plakoglobin from the desmosomal attachment plaque are affected. The *ATP2A2* gene located on chromosome 12q23–q24.1 encodes the sarco/endoplasmic reticulum Ca^{2+}-ATPase type 2 isoform (SERCA2) and is the gene responsible for the acantholysis and apoptosis (dyskeratosis) seen in Dariers disease.

Papular acantholytic dyskeratosis of the vulva presents as skin-colored to white papular lesions. Previously, it was an atypical or localized form of Dariers disease or Hailey–Hailey disease, but the absence of family history or extragenital lesions separates it from both disorders.[6,106]

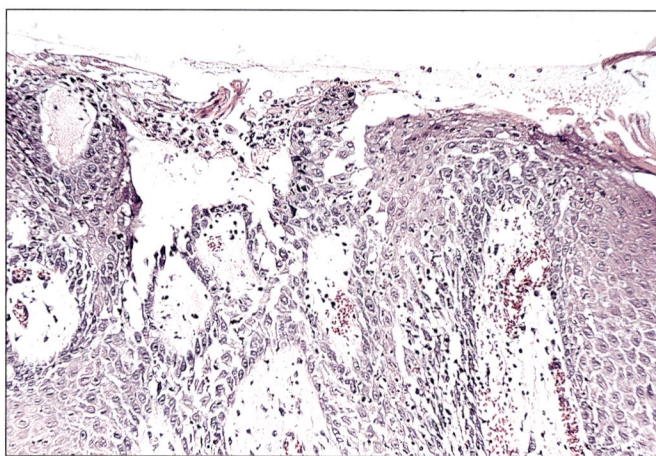

Fig. 2.30 Dariers disease with suprabasal acantholysis.

Microscopic features

Keratotic papules disclose acantholysis that involves rete ridges in which a cleft or lacuna forms (Figure 2.30). The papillary dermis typically protrudes into the lacuna that is lined by a single layer of basal cells (forming so-called 'villi'). Overlying these changes is a thick area of orthokeratosis with focal parakeratosis. Accompanying these features are dyskeratotic cells in the form of 'corp ronds' and 'grains'. Corp ronds are cells located in the upper malpighian layer and stratum corneum with a small pyknotic nucleus, clear perinuclear halo, and bright eosinophilic cytoplasm. The dense and bright peripheral rim of cytoplasm represents aggregates of tonofilaments and keratohyaline granules. Grains are small cells with elongated nuclei and a small amount of cytoplasm; electron microscopy demonstrates premature aggregation of tonofilaments. The synthesis of keratohyaline in association with clumped tonofilaments demonstrated by electron microscopy is distinctive of Dariers disease and can separate it from Hailey–Hailey disease.

OTHER INFLAMMATORY DISEASES AFFECTING THE VULVA

ZOONS VULVITIS (PLASMACYTOSIS MUCOSAE)[63,71,95,107,109,123]

A chronic inflammatory disorder of unknown etiology, Zoons vulvitis exhibits extensive plasma cells in the mucosa. Besides the vulva, it can affect the prepuce, glans penis, and oral mucosa (lips, gums, or tongue). The term 'plasmacytosis mucosae' has been proposed because of its versatility for all mucosal sites and its simplicity in conveying the concept of inflammatory cell processes.

Clinical features

The clinical presentation is similar in all locations. Usually patients after middle age present with a solitary, chronic, sore, orange-red, glistening 1–3 cm lesion on the vestibular mucosa (Figure 2.31). White edges are absent, but the clinical appearance otherwise simulates erosive lichen planus. The lesions resolve slowly, leaving behind a rusty stain from resolved microhemorrhages. Recurrences are common.

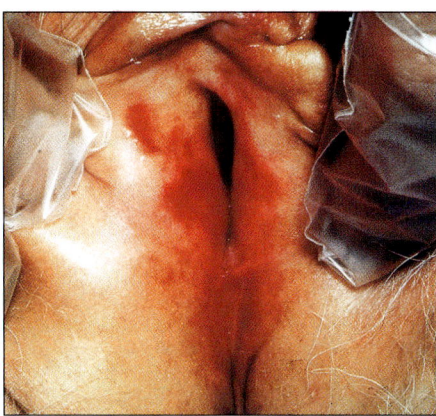

Fig. 2.31 Zoons plasma cell vulvitis. Typical orangey-red patches are present on the vestibular mucosa. These are very sore to touch.

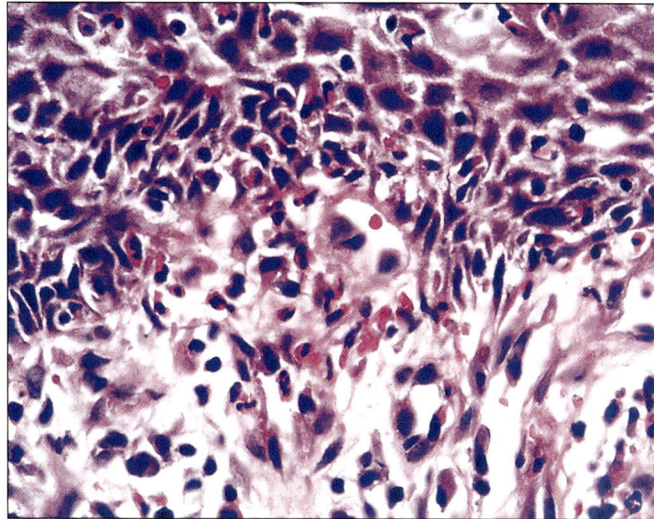

Fig. 2.33 Zoons vulvitis. Another important characteristic feature is the presence of focal red cell extravasation in upper dermis. In old lesions, there may be hemosiderin deposition.

ERYTHEMA MULTIFORME

Erythema multiforme is a self-limited, cytotoxic reaction triggered by agents such as drugs (antibiotics, oral contraceptives, NSAIDs, etc.) and infections (especially mycoplasma and viral infections, particularly herpes simplex). This disease presents at any age, but is distinctly uncommon in childhood. The characteristic reaction consists of a targetoid lesion (central zone of necrosis, blister, or erosion surrounded by erythema and edema) most frequently affecting the extremities in a symmetrical distribution. As the name implies, numerous types of lesion (macules, papules and plaques, and vesicles and bullae) can be seen in a single patient. In the genital region, it frequently presents as a bullous eruption. Most episodes are recurrent, lasting on average 2 weeks without sequelae. When more than two mucosal sites are involved, Stevens–Johnson syndrome, a variant or extreme spectrum of erythema multiforme, needs to be considered (see below). This severe variant presents with painful ulcers of the mouth and genitalia in association with the skin rash. Drugs are the most frequent etiologic culprit. Other mucosal sites affected are eyes, pharynx, esophagus, and anus.

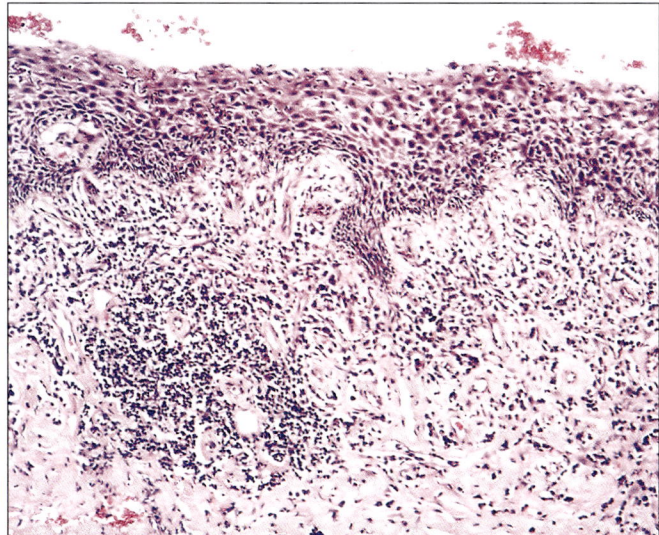

Fig. 2.32 Zoons vulvitis. Characteristic histologic features include 'lozenge-shaped' keratinocytes, epidermal atrophy (not seen in this early lesion), and a variable but usually heavy lymphoplasmacytic infiltrate in upper dermis.

Microscopic features

As the name implies, a dense, band-like mucosal infiltrate of plasma cells is admixed with lymphocytes (Figures 2.32 and 2.33). Occasional mast cells and eosinophils may also be seen. The density of plasma cells increases in parallel with the age of the lesion. The epidermis eventually becomes atrophic, with loss of the surface keratin and of the stratum granulosum. The stratum spinosum frequently exhibits flattened, lozenge-shaped keratinocytes separated by mild spongiosis. The basal layer is often irregular and may exhibit exocytosis of lymphocytes and contain occasional apoptotic basal cells. Frank ulceration occurs in but a minority of cases. The dermis shows increased numbers of dilated, thin-walled vessels, often with red cell extravasation. Scattered hemosiderin deposits reflect previous hemorrhagic episodes. Accumulated hemosiderin occurs only in genital lesions. Immunohistochemistry for light chain restriction helps exclude plasmacytoma if suspected.

Microscopic features

In erythematous patches, scattered apoptotic keratinocytes are present in the epithelium, often associated with vacuolar alteration of the basal layer, upper dermal edema and a perivascular lymphocytic infiltrate. The presence of increased numbers of eosinophils in the dermal infiltrate suggests a drug etiology. Erythema multiforme is a clinical diagnosis that usually rests on the clinical history and appearance, and the presence of other lesions outside the vulva.

BEHÇETS DISEASE[50,62,77,79]

Behçets disease is a chronic systemic disease classically defined by the triad of recurrent oral ulcers, genital ulcers, and ocular inflammation. In 1990, the International Study Group for Behçet's Disease provided diagnostic criteria for this disorder[1]

Table 2.4 International Study Group criteria for the diagnosis of Behçets disease

Criterion	Required features
Recurrent oral ulceration	Aphthous (idiopathic) oral ulceration observed by physician or patient, recurring at least three times in a 12-month period
Plus any two of the following:	
Recurrent genital ulceration	Aphthous genital ulceration or scarring observed by physician or patient
Eye lesions	Anterior or posterior uveitis; cells in the vitreous by slit lamp examination; or retinal vasculitis observed by ophthalmologist
Cutaneous lesions	Erythema nodosum-like lesions observed by physician or patient; papulopustular lesions or pseudofolliculitis; or characteristic acneiform nodules observed by physician in post-adolescent patient not on corticosteroids
Pathergy test	Interpreted at 24–48 h by physician

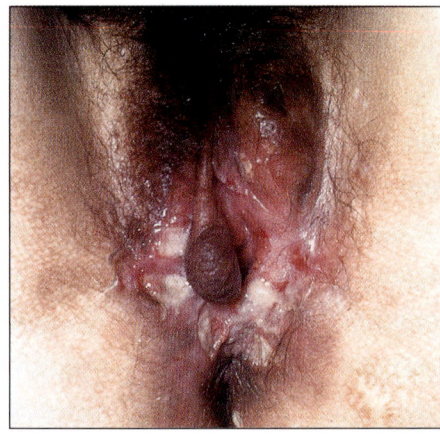

Fig. 2.34 Behçets disease. Recurrent deep painful ulcers have developed in the genital and oral epithelium.

(Table 2.4). The pathogenesis is unknown, but proposed mechanisms involve vascular damage and autoimmune responses. Turkey has the highest frequency of this disease (>80 cases per 100 000 people) whereas in the UK and US it is quite low (<2 per 100 000 people). Behçets disease typically afflicts patients in their second to third decade, with periods of flare-ups and remissions. This syndrome can cause deep ulcerations in the vulva that may lead to labial fenestration and gangrene. Complex aphthosis or aphtha major, lesions involving only genitalia and oral mucosa, is believed to be a forme fruste of Behçets disease.

Clinical features
Aphthous (small ulcers) stomatitis is the initial manifestation of Behçets disease in two-thirds of patients, and may precede other manifestations by several years. Aphthae usually affect only mucosa not fixed to bone (buccal mucosa, lip, and tongue). The patients suffer for about 10 days with erythematous-based, circular, painful, non-scarring ulcers that have a white fibrinous base. Genital and perianal aphthae are in general larger, deeper, and more painful than oral lesions (Figure 2.34). Vulvar lesions are usually multiple, sharply demarcated ulcers on an erythematous base. Among cutaneous lesions that can coexist with mucosal ulcers are sterile vesiculopustules, Sweets syndrome-like lesions, purpuric papules secondary to vasculitis, erythema nodosum, and pyoderma gangrenosum. Pathergy (i.e., lesions occurring in areas of trauma) is a diagnostic criterion for Behçets disease. Ocular involvement, ranging from the characteristic posterior uveitis to anterior uveitis, secondary glaucoma, and cataracts, is the leading cause of morbidity. Serologic titers of interleukin-8 (IL-8) correlate with disease activity. Other manifestations reflecting the multisystemic involvement of Behçets disease include arthritis, gastrointestinal signs and symptoms similar to inflammatory bowel disease, and vascular disease that varies from occlusive arterial disease to venous thrombosis and even aneurysms. Neurologic manifestations (acute meningitis, meningoencephalitis, nerve palsies, etc.) usually appear in advanced stages and are associated with poor prognosis.

Microscopic features
The histologic features are frequently non-specific, and clinical–pathologic correlation is necessary for diagnosis. Early lesions exhibit a shallow ulcer with a superficial neutrophil-rich acute inflammatory slough. The dermis contains numerous neutrophils, and there may be a lymphocytic or neutrophilic vasculitis affecting upper dermal venules, often with fibrinoid necrosis, and sometimes with thrombotic occlusion of small vessels. In the presence of ulceration, however, it is difficult to determine whether these vasculitic changes are primary or secondary. The significance of these vasculitic lesions is greater when they are found in a non-ulcerated, erythematous area away from the ulcer.

Other manifestations in the skin include erythema nodosum-like lesions, perivascular infiltrates of lymphocytes and mononuclear cells affecting vessels in the deep dermis and septa of the subcutis. Lymphocytic vasculitis may be seen in the subcutaneous tissue. Unlike erythema nodosum, this entity lacks histiocytic granulomas. In pathergic lesions, the vessels show marked neutrophilic infiltrates without the fibrinoid changes noted in the vascular wall or leukocytoclasis. This constellation of findings has been named 'pustular vasculitis' or 'Sweet-like vasculitis'.

CROHNS DISEASE[34,48,108]

Crohns disease is a granulomatous inflammation, most commonly involving the small bowel, but sometimes the large bowel, that leads to thickening and stricture formation. It affects the skin in 10–20% of patients, especially those suffering from colonic rather than ileal disease. The cutaneous changes can both precede the gastrointestinal involvement and lack any correlation in severity between cutaneous and gastrointestinal manifestations. Extraintestinal findings precede the gastrointestinal involvement in one-fourth of cases. Cutaneous lesions include continuous perianal Crohns disease, distant (metastatic) Crohns disease, oral lesions (i.e., granulomatous cheilitis), reactive skin findings (i.e., pyoderma gangrenosum, pathergy, and erythema nodosum), and nutritional skin changes. Genital Crohns disease is more frequent in children than in adults.

Clinical features
The clinical appearance of vulvar Crohns disease is variable. When associated with local colonic disease, perianal, perineal

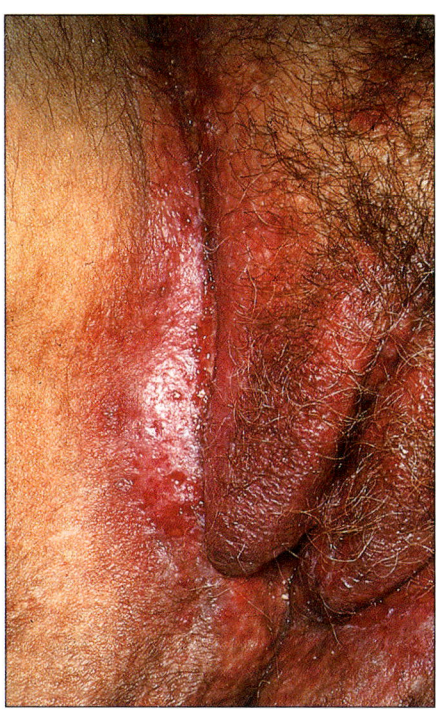

Fig. 2.35 Cutaneous Crohns disease of the perineum. The disease has infiltrated eroding plaques of the vulva and perianal skin.

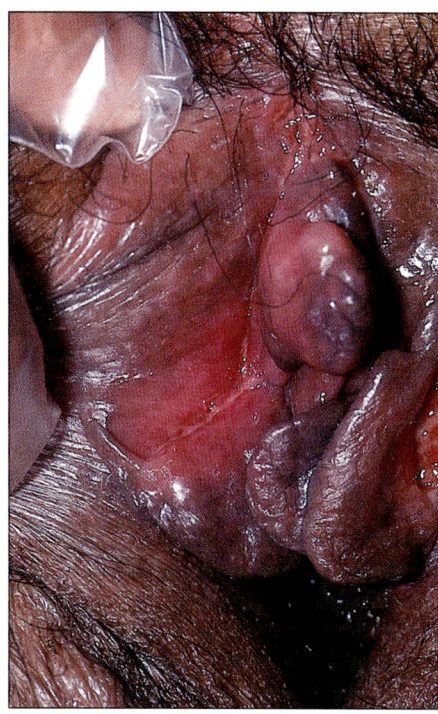

Fig. 2.36 Vulvar Crohns disease. The disease presented as painful ulceration in the interlabial creases.

ulcers and large, edematous skin tags are characteristic.[108] Sometimes fistulae extend from the affected bowel into perineal and even vulvar skin or Bartholins glands, resulting in indurated, tender, inflamed areas that drain pus. Vulvar Crohns disease may also occur when the local bowel disease is comparatively inactive, as moist, firm, erythematous plaques (Figure 2.35) on the labia majora and pubic skin. Unilateral, firm, chronic red edema leading to elephantiasis has been described. Occasionally, vulvar Crohns disease may present as chronic sloughing ulcers on the mucosal surfaces of the labia, and in the interlabial creases (Figure 2.36). The latter ulcerations are typically deep, with a knife-like, linear appearance. Occasional cases may present with a foul discharge and be due to mucinous carcinoma arising from the fistula.[90]

Microscopic features
The pathologic changes include massive dermal and subcutaneous edema, and markedly dilated lymphatics. Non-caseating sarcoidal granulomas are diagnostic, but often ill-formed aggregates of histiocytes with variable numbers of lymphocytes are seen instead. Ulcerated or fistulous lesions often show a predominance of secondary features such as fibrosis, chronic inflammation, suppuration, and granulation tissue.

HIDRADENITIS SUPPURATIVA

Hidradenitis suppurativa, a chronic suppurative folliculitis of apocrine sweat-gland-bearing skin, affects one or more flexural sites rich in apocrine glands including the axillae, pubis, groins, and perineum. This follicular occlusive disorder involving hair follicles is part of a deep scarring folliculitis triad that also includes dissecting cellulitis of the scalp and acne conglobata. The etiology is unknown, although androgens appear to play

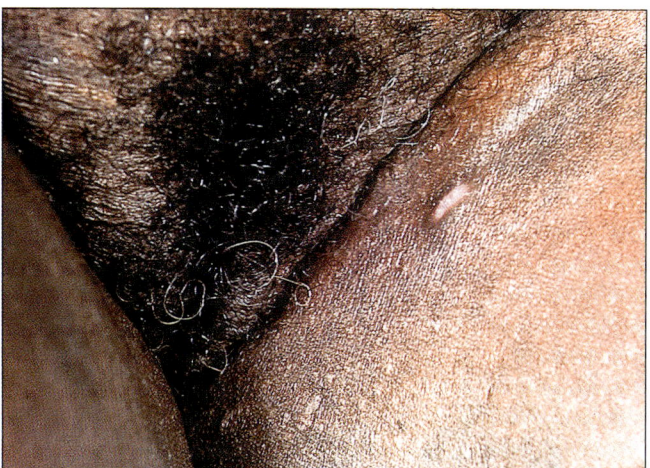

Fig. 2.37 Hidradenitis suppurativa. Discharging pustular nodules and sinuses are present in the groin creases.

a role, a notion supported by the absence of this disorder in prepubertal individuals, and the improvement of this disease with antiandrogenic drugs. It also has an inherited component, most likely as an autosomal dominant pattern. The clinical course is unclear, but common components are keratotic occlusion of dilated hair follicles (comedones), folliculitis, marked apocrine adenitis leading to apocrine gland destruction, and varying degrees of inflammation, suppuration, and formation of discharging sinus tracts. All of these changes produce substantial morbidity.

Patients usually present with recurrent painful subcutaneous abscesses, followed by sinuses from which foul pus may drain (Figure 2.37).[43] The suppuration results from secondary infection by a wide range of bacteria, including anaerobes. Squamous cell carcinoma is a rare complication, and has been reported in long-standing lesions.[110]

Hidradenitis suppurativa may be difficult to distinguish clinically and histologically from severe cutaneous involvement by Crohns disease. However, the latter usually does not affect axillae and, in contrast to hidradenitis suppurativa, affects areas lacking apocrine glands such as the inner aspects of the labia minora and vestibule. Moreover, cutaneous Crohns disease is not painful, and patients frequently have gastrointestinal manifestations. Hidradenitis suppurativa must also be distinguished from Fox–Fordyce disease, with which it sometimes coexists. Fox–Fordyce disease (apocrine miliaria) may present at puberty with pruritic papules of the axillae, vulva, and perianal regions.

VULVAR PAIN SYNDROMES

VULVAR VESTIBULITIS[41,42,46,81,125]

Clinical features
The vulvar vestibule is the ring of epithelium proximal to Harts line (see Appendix 2.1), which is in continuity with the hymen and contains the minor vestibular glands and the openings of the ducts of Bartholins and Skenes glands. Vestibulitis is a complex of introital dyspareunia and severe tenderness on light pressure (e.g., with the tip of a cotton swab).

Most women present in their twenties and thirties with dyspareunia. They often find it too painful to have intercourse or to insert tampons. Most have had normal pain-free sexual intercourse previously. Some patients give a history of severe *Candida* infection or a gynecologic procedure. Examination may show punctuate erythema (but this is not always present and may also be seen in asymptomatic women) and these areas are likely to be biopsied. The vulva is otherwise normal. Light pressure causes severe discomfort, especially over the ductal openings. *Candida* may be a contributory factor but is not the sole cause and there are no consistent microbiologic findings. Early proposals implicating papillomavirus infections have not been validated. Biopsies show peripheral nerve hyperplasia in the vestibule, without significant inflammation.[51]

Vestibulitis is more common in women with migraine, irritable bowel syndrome, and/or myalgic encephalopathy syndrome. Treatment with low-dose tricyclic antidepressant drugs often brings at least some relief. Surgical excision of the entire vestibular epithelium with advancement of vaginal mucosa is sometimes performed, but results are no different from medical and psychological management.

Microscopic features
Vestibulitis is rarely biopsied, and the histologic changes are non-specific, subtle, and of dubious significance. A sparse lymphocytic infiltrate may surround the necks of the minor vestibular glands.

DYSESTHETIC VULVODYNIA[17,24,49,114]

Clinically, a severe burning sensation affects the entire vulva, often extending onto the perineal skin, upper thighs, and abdominal wall. The pain may be worse on walking or sitting and often improves with recumbency. Dysesthetic vulvodynia tends to affect older women with a history of lumbar disc disease, constipation, or previous gynecologic surgery. Physical examination reveals only vulvar atrophic change, without tenderness to palpation. There may be altered sensitivity to light touch over the lower abdomen, pubis and thighs. A thorough neurologic examination is required to exclude cauda equina lesions or neuralgia of the pudendal nerve. Treatment with low-dose tricyclic antidepressants is often successful.

PIGMENTARY ALTERATIONS

These disorders can be divided by whether the pigmentation is increased (hyperpigmentation) or decreased (hypopigmentation). Before discussing these entities, it is useful to understand physiologic hyperpigmentation. Skin and mucosa in various body sites have different densities of melanocytes. Melanocyte concentration and melanin density are greater in genital skin, particularly in dark-skinned patients. Hormones also affect the level of pigmentation, and pregnancy increases melanogenesis, accentuating physiologic hyperpigmentation. The physiologic hyperpigmentation is most notable in the labia majora, tips of the labia minora, and posterior modified mucous membranes. Examination discloses bilateral, symmetric, brown coloration without alteration of skin thickness.

HYPERPIGMENTED VULVA

Pigmented lesions on the genitalia are found in about 10% of women. Increased pigmentation in the vulvar skin may be due to:

- Increased melanin deposition in the epidermis or dermis
- Increased thickness of the keratin layer in a verruciform or papillomatous pattern
- Increased hemosiderin deposition in the upper dermis.

Hyperpigmentation due to melanin in vulvar skin
Pigmented melanocytic nevi and melanoma are described in Chapter 3.

Idiopathic acquired pigmentation (of Laugier)/ vulvar melanosis[3,19,29]
Clinical features
Marked, macular hyperpigmentation appears on the vulva, vagina, and cervix, without a preceding history of trauma or inflammation. Lesions can reach several centimeters in diameter. Areas are often multiple (Figure 2.38). The etiology is unknown.

Microscopic features
Lesions show increased melanin deposition in the basal layer of keratinocytes and occasionally some dermal melanophages. The ideal specimen should include the edge of the lesion so that the pigmented area can be compared with normal adjacent skin. The Masson–Fontana stain serves to emphasize the increased melanin. Immunocytochemical stains show absence of increased numbers of melanocytes in the pigmented area. Lesions with melanocytic hyperplasia are best termed *lentigines*. Although vulvar melanosis shares some histologic features with lentigines, they are clinically distinct. Benign lentigo (lentigo simplex) presents as evenly pigmented macules a few

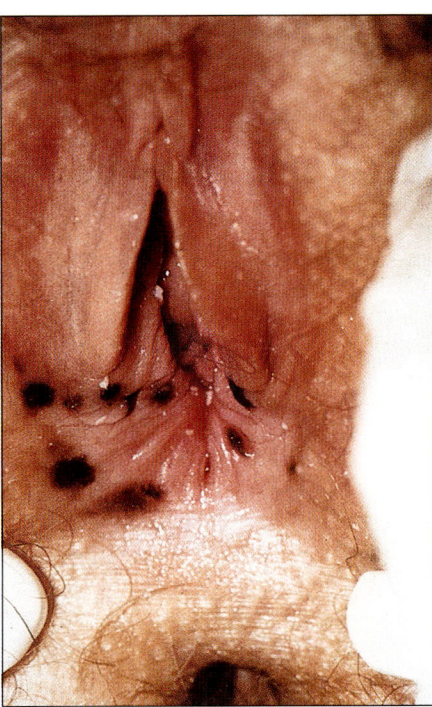

Fig. 2.38 Vulvar melanosis (of Laugier). This benign condition of young adults must be distinguished from pigmented vulvar intraepithelial neoplasia and melanoma by histology.

millimeters in diameter. Junctional nesting of nevus cells is not seen.

Postinflammatory hyperpigmentation Postinflammatory hyperpigmentation is the most common type of hyperpigmentation and usually results from increased melanin deposition in macrophages in the upper dermis following prolonged damage to epidermal keratinocytes. Sometimes, there is also stimulation of epidermal melanogenesis. Hyperpigmentation is particularly characteristic of lichen planus and fixed drug eruptions. A complete clinical history, focusing on possible previous trauma, treatment, dermatosis, or symptoms such as burning or pruritus, renders useful information in these patients.

Biopsy can help define the cause. Any hyperpigmentation with variegated color, atypical shape, or asymmetry should be biopsied. The histopathologist helps to:

- Exclude a melanocytic proliferation
- Exclude hyperpigmentation due to thick keratin
- Confirm the location of the pigment in the upper dermis
- Identify the pigment as melanin (Masson–Fontana positive) or hemosiderin (Perl positive)
- Identify the nature of the preceding inflammatory dermatosis. Examination of many levels may be necessary to find active basal layer damage, Civatte bodies, or focal lichenoid infiltrate.

Hyperpigmentation due to increased keratin in stratum corneum

Compact orthohyperkeratosis, when arranged flat, gives a pale gross appearance. It appears brown when thrown up into papillary folds. The two most common lesions affecting the vulva are acanthosis nigricans and seborrheic keratoses.

Acanthosis nigricans
Clinical features
Symmetrical, pigmented, hyperkeratotic plaques in flexural sites, particularly the axillae, neck folds, anogenital region, and groins, characterize this disorder. Mucosal involvement, particularly oral mucosa (lip and tongue), occurs in 25% of cases. The surface is papilliferous, imparting a velvety appearance, sometimes combined with larger verruciform growths on the surface. Acanthosis nigricans is an abnormal epidermal growth in response to various factors with expression of unusual keratins (e.g., 18 and 19) in basal keratinocytes. It is important to recognize acanthosis nigricans because of its potential association with the following underlying disorders.

- Multiple benign disorders, including obesity, all of which show tissue resistance to insulin and hyperinsulinemia. The effect of high insulin levels on insulin-like growth factor 1 (IGF-1) receptors on keratinocytes is believed to produce the skin changes. Stimulation of the same receptor on ovarian tissue can lead to hyperandrogenism, which also occurs in some of these syndromes.
- Benign familial acanthosis nigricans is inherited as an autosomal dominant condition and is not linked to insulin resistance. Onset of this disease is in childhood, with accentuated manifestations during puberty.
- Drug-induced forms occasionally occur with various agents including oral contraceptives, nicotinic acid, and the folate acid antagonist triazinate.
- Malignancy-associated acanthosis nigricans is a rare disorder usually seen with adenocarcinoma of the stomach or some other part of the gastrointestinal tract. Tumors in kidney, bladder, lung, and cervix, together with lymphoma, have also been sporadically associated to acanthosis nigricans. Usually the acanthosis nigricans and the neoplasm are diagnosed simultaneously. Sometimes, the cutaneous manifestation precedes or follows the tumor. Epidermal growth factor (EGF) and transforming growth factor alpha (TGF-α) are potential factors produced by these tumors and can lead to the abnormal proliferation found in acanthosis nigricans. The skin changes sometimes remit if the primary tumor can be excised before it has metastasized.
- Nevoid acanthosis nigricans localized to a single site is extremely rare.

Microscopic features
The lesions show papillomatosis with upwardly projected dermal papillae covered by thinned epidermis. Between the projections, the epidermis shows mild acanthosis with hyperkeratosis. The basal layer is mildly hyperpigmented. Sometimes, mucosal lesions show marked acanthosis and mild chronic inflammation in the submucosa. These lesions can be confused with condyloma acuminatum.

HYPOPIGMENTATION

Postinflammatory hypopigmentation
As with hyperpigmentation, hypopigmentation can follow inflammation. A possible mechanism is blockage of the transfer of melanosomes from the melanocytes to the keratinocytes. Destruction of melanocytes is also postulated in lichenoid

inflammation. Fungal and yeast infections may cause patchy mild hypopigmentation, particularly in pityriasis versicolor, which appears as pale macules. A PAS stain for fungi may be helpful in evaluating a vulvar biopsy of an irregular hypopigmented area. An important disease showing hypopigmentation is lichen sclerosus. The 'porcelain white' appearance is often the first clinical manifestation in this disease. Intraepithelial neoplasia (vulvar intraepithelial neoplasia) may also present as a white plaque. Histologically, the number of melanocytes is normal, but the melanin content is reduced in the basal layer. Melanin-laden macrophages are occasionally seen in the upper dermis, especially in patients with darker skin. Features of active or resolving inflammatory dermatosis may be noted.

Vitiligo
Clinical features
Vitiligo, an acquired leukoderma in which melanocytes are destroyed in the involved areas, affects up to 2% of the population worldwide. Locations frequently affected are face, back of the hands, axillae, groins, umbilicus, and genitalia – in other words, areas that are physiologically hyperpigmented. Vitiligo, which is usually symmetrical, often involves the perineum (Figure 2.39). Onset occurs at any age, but half appear before the age of 20 years. The depigmentation, if segmental or dermatomal, is classified as type B; generalized cases are type A. Type B is most frequent in children. It is most resistant to treatment and rarely undergoes repigmentation. One-fourth of affected individuals also have various immune abnormalities, such as an association with other autoimmune disorders and organ-specific antibodies.[94] The presence of antimelanocyte antibodies supports the immune theory as an effector of melanocytic destruction. Clinically, vitiligo appears as an insidious, progressive disease, sometimes with some repigmentation that is frequently incomplete and ephemeral. Ivory-white patches of skin with erythematous borders herald the initial stages. Of importance, textural changes, scaling, crusting, and elevation are absent. Melanocytes sometimes remain around hair follicles, showing a tiny rim of normally pigmented or hyperpigmented skin. It is from the perifollicular melanocytes that the repigmentation occurs. The pigment loss is highlighted with Woods lamp examination. Depigmented areas are brightly

white in comparison to the subtle lightening of the pigmented areas. In cases of depigmentation, it may be difficult to differentiate vitiligo from lichen sclerosus. Both are in the same group of inherited autoimmune disorders and sometimes coexist in the same patient. However, vitiligo is a purely macular lesion, lacking the atrophy or sclerosis of lichen sclerosus.

Microscopic features
Vulvar skin affected by end-stage vitiligo is completely devoid of melanin within the basal keratinocytes, and melanocytes are entirely absent in the basal layer. The ideal biopsy is taken through the edge of a lesion so that the vitiligo patch can be compared with adjacent normal skin. The edge of the vitiligo lesion may show a narrow zone of degenerating basal melanocytes and a lymphocytic infiltrate in underlying papillary dermis and lower epidermis. The Masson–Fontana stain for melanin and immunohistochemical methods for melanocytes help highlight the differences between normal and abnormal.

DRUGS

The role that topical applications play in the pathogenesis of contact dermatitis in the vulva has already been discussed. Systemically taken drugs may also elicit various types of skin reaction affecting the vulva. Such reactions are not confined to prescription-only agents. In taking a drug history, many patients will deny drug ingestion unless specifically asked about over-the-counter agents such as aspirin, acetaminophen (paracetamol), alternative or herbal remedies with unknown constituents, and food materials containing dyes or preservatives, any of which can induce skin lesions.

STEVENS–JOHNSON SYNDROME VARIANT OF ERYTHEMA MULTIFORME

Stevens–Johnson syndrome, a variant at the extreme spectrum of erythema multiforme, is considered to be an immune-mediated reaction. Known drug triggers include antibiotics (particularly sulfonamides), oral contraceptives, and many others. The severe mucosal variant of Stevens–Johnson syndrome can severely affect the vulva. Painful erythema is quickly followed by blisters that become painful, enlarging ulcers. Histologically, there is destruction of the epidermal basal layer with separation of epidermis from dermis, often augmented by severe edema of papillary dermis. Ballooning and reticular degeneration of epidermal keratinocytes is followed by extensive keratinocyte necrosis, associated with intraepidermal fluid accumulation. Eventually the keratinocytes forming the roof of the blister become completely necrotic and shed, leaving a shallow ulcer. The vulva may also be involved in the most severe (and often fatal) form of this pathologic process, *toxic epidermal necrolysis*.[88] Widespread epidermal necrosis and shedding involve much of the skin surface and the orificial–mucosal areas. This severe disease is almost always associated with drug ingestion.

FIXED DRUG ERUPTIONS

Clinical features
Fixed drug eruption is an infrequent, but recurrent reaction that occurs each time an individual is exposed to a triggering

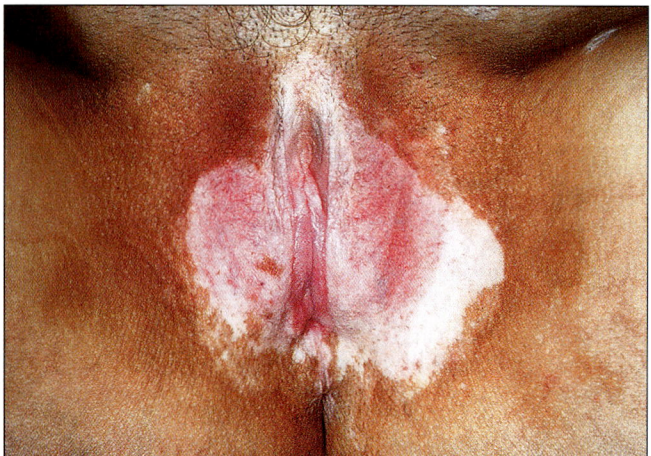

Fig. 2.39 Vitiligo with symmetrical complete loss of pigmentation.

drug. The classic presentation is that of a single, well-defined, erythematous, round to oval plaque with a dusky center and possible bulla formation leading to erosion. This lesion develops 1–2 weeks after a first exposure, reducing to 24 hours in subsequent exposures. Sites of predilection are the face, lips, buttocks, and genitalia. With recurrent episodes new locations can be involved and additional lesions can occur. Generalized fixed drug reaction can be difficult to distinguish from erythema multiforme. The reaction remits with the withdrawal of the offending drug, leaving intense hyperpigmented macules. With repeated flares followed by quiescent periods, progressive darkening occurs. Hypopigmentation sometimes occurs in patients of dark skin tone. The resolving stage is often the period when the clinician will see the eruption. Careful history taking is essential, since hypersensitivity to the drug is lifelong and the cure is to avoid the drug. More than 100 drugs are known triggering agents, the most frequent being sulfonamides, tetracyclines, tranquilizers, quinine, phenolphthalein (formerly used in laxatives), and analgesics. Some drugs may affect specific anatomic locations, such as the glans penis with tetracycline, and the lips with pyrazolones. Because many of these drugs can be purchased over the counter, the exercise of asking the patient to write a list of drugs acquired without prescription often helps identify the offending culprit.

Microscopic features

Established lesions of fixed drug eruption show a lichenoid inflammatory reaction with basal layer vacuolization and Civatte bodies associated with a heavy, superficial and deep dermal lymphocytic infiltrate. The infiltrate sometimes contains a few neutrophils and eosinophils. Macrophages are often numerous in late stages. The inflammatory infiltrate obscures the dermoepidermal junction and extends to the upper layers of the epidermis, leading to the death of keratinocytes located above the basal layer. Damage to the epidermal basal layer leads to release of melanin, which macrophages in the upper dermis capture. While these findings resemble those of erythema multiforme, fixed drug eruption also shows the presence of a mid to deep dermal inflammatory reaction, neutrophils, and prominent melanin incontinence. Occasionally, a central subepidermal bulla results from basal layer damage and keratinocyte necrosis. Extensive resolution follows removal of the drug but a flat hyperpigmented patch may remain due to the melanin pigment incontinence, which persists in the dermis.

VULVAR INFECTIONS AND INFESTATIONS

Vaginal infections may cause vulvar symptoms either by extension or by the irritant effects of vaginal discharge. Most infections are diagnosed clinically and confirmed on microbiologic identification and culture. Few are biopsied unless there are complicating factors. For example, Candida or streptococcal infection can cause a sudden and severe flare of lichen sclerosus, which might lead the clinician to perform a biopsy.

BACTERIAL INFECTIONS

Bacterial, vaginal, and cervical infections often cause vulvar symptoms, partly by the production of an irritant discharge.

Bacterial vaginosis

Bacterial vaginosis results from an overgrowth of commensal bacterial (*Gardnerella vaginalis*) and anaerobic organisms (e.g., *Morbiluncus* or *Bacteroides*) producing an increased volume of vaginal secretions. The characteristic unpleasant fishy odor is the product of bacterial amines released after exposure to an alkaline substance such as potassium hydroxide or semen. Although bacterial vaginosis lacks symptomatic manifestations (e.g., burning, itchiness, or erythema) and vulvitis is uncommon, it carries an increased risk of preterm labor in pregnant women. Rarely is a biopsy performed. The diagnosis is made with the presence of profuse milky vaginal discharge, with fishy odor when exposed to 10–20% potassium hydroxide (positive whiff test), and the presence of clue cells (squamous epithelial cells covered by coccobacilli producing a ground-glass appearance of the cytoplasm and obscuring the cell borders) on vaginal smear.

Staphylococcal infections

Like any hair-bearing skin, the labia majora or mons pubis may be the site of a superficial staphylococcal folliculitis and deep folliculitis producing furunculosis (boils). Occlusion, intertrigo, and depilated pubic hair (particularly by shaving) are important predisposing factors. Other organisms producing similar changes are *Pseudomonas*, *Malassezia furfur*, and dermatophyte fungi. The histologic appearances are identical to superficial and deep folliculitis elsewhere on the body. The exfoliative toxin produced by *S. aureus* can induce flaccid blisters or pustules in the genitalia and thighs. The warmth and moisture of the vulva provide the ideal environment for this infection. Clinical inspection reveals yellow crust and residual superficial erosions immediately after superficial fragile blisters rupture. Diagnosis is made by culture. Focal disease requires only local treatment. Oral antibiotics are the therapy of choice for extensive disease.

Streptococcal infections
Clinical features

Streptococcal infection affecting the genital area has a range of clinical presentations varying from superficial cutaneous infection to necrotizing fasciitis, a rapidly progressive necrosis of skin and subcutaneous tissue. The superficial bacterial infection, common in children between 3 and 5 years, has a predominant perianal distribution that can extend to the vulva and vagina. Adult presentation, which is uncommon, can occur alone or complicating another skin disorder.[116] Worsening of symptoms in patients with lichen sclerosus or other dermatoses sometimes heralds a secondary streptococcal infection and appropriate swabs should be taken. Streptococcal vulvitis and perianal dermatitis can produce tender, well-demarcated red skin with or without scale. The vagina shows erythematous mucosa and purulent discharge. Occasionally, anal fistulas with mucoid discharge and vulvar fissures develop. Most lesions show excoriations and lichenification secondary to scratching and rubbing. Swabs grow group A or C hemolytic streptococci, and systemic antibiotics are required to clear the infection. Cultures of the throat often yield the same organism, suggesting spread of the organism by contaminated hands.

Group A streptococci are among the organisms responsible for *necrotizing fasciitis*, which has increased in frequency over the past decade. Although single-agent necrotizing fasciitis does occur, polymicrobial infection with anaerobic and aerobic bacteria like streptococci, *Staphylococcus aureus*, *Escherichia coli*, *Bacteroides*, and *Clostridium* spp. is more common. This rare and distinct form of rapidly progressive necrosis of subcutaneous tissue and fascia can be fatal if not recognized early and aggressive therapeutic intervention pursued. The vulva is one of the sites affected, with extension of the cutaneous changes to the perineum and abdominal wall. It usually occurs in diabetics, particularly when complicated by obesity, hypertension, and peripheral vascular disease, or in the immunocompromised host. The infection's origin can be a surgical incision (e.g., episiotomy) or a local abscess of skin or Bartholins gland. The patient presents with a hot, exquisitely tender, erythematous, swollen area resistant to antibiotic treatment. At an alarming rate the skin changes from red to dusky gray-blue with bulla formation and necrosis. The soft tissue frequently feels indurated and wooden to palpation. The patient shows signs of toxicity with fever, chills, malaise, shock, and tachycardia. Patients with diabetes are often ketoacidotic.

Surgical debridement with extensive reconstructive surgery is the mainstay of treatment. Surgery typically discloses extensive subcutaneous necrosis, often spreading beyond the clinically obvious margins. The disease involves all tissue layers down to and including muscle, the deep fascia being covered with a grayish-black exudate. All necrotic tissue must be excised or the process proceeds inexorably. Antimicrobial therapy is designed to cover the results of the initial Gram stain. Mortality is high, upwards of 40%, especially when diagnosis and debridement have been delayed or invasive group A streptococcus is involved.

Microscopic features
Widespread necrosis extends from the epidermis, to subcutaneous tissue, to fascia, and sometimes to muscle. Numerous polymorphonuclear leukocytes and mononuclear cells infiltrate the tissue and necrotizing vasculitis with thrombi is apparent. Large numbers of bacterial colonies pervade the upper dermis.

Syphilis
Clinical features
Syphilis is a chronic, worldwide, sexually transmitted disease caused by the spirochete *Treponema pallidum*. Following a decline in incidence in developed countries, both infectious and congenital syphilis are becoming more common, especially in the USA. Coinfection with HIV is well recognized. Acquired syphilis is divided into four stages (primary, secondary, latent, and tertiary) with distinct clinical presentations separated by asymptomatic periods. The primary or initial lesion is the chancre, an indurated, painless, shallow ulcer with well-defined borders that occurs at the site of inoculation. Multiple lesions occur, especially in immunocompromised patients. The serum exudate from the chancre contains numerous spirochetes, which can be identified by dark-field microscopy, permitting prompt diagnosis. The primary site in women is often on the vulva or perineum; other sites include the cervix, urethra, lip, or tonsillar fossae. After healing a small discrete stellate scar develops. Regional painless lymphadenopathy occurs.

Between 4 and 8 weeks after the chancre, untreated patients develop constitutional symptoms and mucocutaneous lesions as part of secondary syphilis. Fever, lymphadenitis, and hepatitis occur in association with an erythematous exanthem of the trunk, genital area, flexor aspect of limbs, and, characteristically, the palms and soles. Atypical presentations may occur in patients with concurrent HIV infection. Pregnant women can infect the fetus via transplacental passage of the spirochete. Some cases of secondary syphilis show large, flat, fleshy, moist papules or *condylomata lata* in the labia and perineum. Condylomata lata are among the most infectious lesions in syphilis; dark-field examination shows numerous treponemes. Such lesions also occur on other mucocutaneous borders. After 3–8 weeks lesions disappear spontaneously. Diagnostic tools in secondary stage include serologic tests that measure antibodies to cardiolipin by rapid plasma reagin (RPR) or venereal disease research laboratory (VDRL) assay. Other methods detect antibodies to surface proteins of *T. pallidum* by *T. pallidum* hemabsorption (TPHA) test or microhemagglutination assay for antibodies to *T. pallidum* (MHA-TP). Latency, the period between healing of the clinical lesions and appearance of late manifestations, can last for many years. The gumma, the classic lesion of tertiary syphilis, is rarely seen on the vulva.

Microscopic features
If the diagnosis of primary syphilis is suspected clinically, identification of spirochetes by dark-field microscopy is the diagnostic tool *par excellence*. Serologic tests to confirm the diagnosis are essential. A biopsy may be necessary when the chancre has an atypical appearance or it is located in an unusual, non-genital site. Acanthosis of the epidermis is common at the edges of the ulcer, the base of which shows an infiltrate of lymphocytes and plasma cells. Blood vessels show prominent endothelial swelling.

The Warthin–Starry stain or other silver impregnation techniques may demonstrate the spirochetes; nowadays, however, more sensitive immunohistochemical stains are beginning to replace this capricious method. In primary syphilis spirochetes are usually identified at the dermoepidermal junction and within and around superficial dermal blood vessels.

Histologically, secondary syphilis exhibits variable degrees of plasmacytic infiltrate and vascular endothelial swelling. The epidermal changes range from normal to hyperplastic with spongiosis. The perivascular lymphoplasmacytic infiltrate usually involves the superficial and deep vascular plexus. Plasma cells are less prominent in macular lesions. The lymphocytic infiltrate can be so exuberant as to simulate lymphoma, but its mixed nature would be rare in such a neoplasm. Early lesions exhibit a neutrophilic vascular reaction that can sometimes simulate Sweets disease (acute febrile neutrophilic dermatosis). Neutrophilic microabscesses in the outer root sheath of the hair follicle or even follicular pustules can be identified. In late syphilitic lesions granulomas of the palisading type may simulate granuloma annulare or less frequently sarcoidal-type granulomas. Although secondary syphilis occasionally mimics other skin diseases, and may have lichenoid or psoriasiform features, the predominance of plasma cells in the infiltrate is a valuable hint that the lesion is syphilitic. Condylomata lata have epidermal hyperplasia with hyperkeratosis and patchy parakeratosis. The latter is associated with a superficial and mid-dermal perivascular lymphoplasmacytic infiltrate. Patchy alopecia of body hair with peribulbar lymphocytic infiltrate can also occur.

Gonorrhea

Neisseria gonorrhoeae is a Gram-negative diplococcus. Infection primarily affects the urethra but may spread to the vagina and cervix. Rectal and oral infections also occur. The paraurethral and Bartholins glands may be infected; in the latter, an acute abscess may ensue. Abscesses forming in the periurethral and Bartholins glands may become secondarily infected with *Staphylococcus aureus* and may be responsible for ensuing symptoms and signs. Gonococcal vulvitis is rare in adult women but is a common feature of infection in prepubertal children. Many patients are asymptomatic, which is why contact tracing is so important. Microbiologic culture is important diagnostically. Histologic examination plays no part in diagnosis.

Chancroid

This sexually transmitted infection due to the bacterium *Haemophilus ducreyi* is more prevalent in the tropics, but occurs on rare occasions in northern climates. Painful ulcers develop on the labia and perineum, and are usually multiple and contiguous, giving the appearance of a large erosion with a granulomatous base. Half of the cases present with enlarged inguinal lymph nodes. The skin lesions and nodes are rarely biopsied since the histologic changes are non-specific, inflammatory, and bear no pathognomonic features. Smears of the lesions can show the Gram-negative rods in parallel chains ('school of fish'). Selective agars that facilitate the rapid growth of this bacillus, but the low sensitivity of culture, make polymerase chain reaction (PCR) the identification test of choice.

Chlamydial infection

Chlamydia trachomatis (serotypes L1, L2, and L3) is the obligatory intracellular microorganism responsible for the sexually transmitted lymphogranuloma venereum. This infection is prevalent in tropical climates like Africa, India, and Southeast Asia, parts of the Caribbean, and Central and South America. Women are commonly asymptomatic carriers. The initial lesion is a small, painless papule or vesicle that frequently erodes, healing within several days without residual scar. Subsequently, the infection disseminates and manifests as enlarged painful inguinal and/or femoral lymph nodes. The lymph nodes can evolve to bubo formation, leading to spontaneous rupture and sinus tract formation. The groove sign reflects matted lymph nodes that have formed a mass above and below the inguinal ligament. Without treatment, extensive necrosis and scarring result in lymphedema. Esthiomene, a rare late manifestation of lymphogranuloma venereum, is a primary infection affecting the lymphatics of scrotum, penis, or vulva, and can evolve to elephantiasis of the genitalia. Progressive enlargement of the inguinal nodes follows. The primary vulvar lesions have no specific histologic features, and heal rapidly, often being no longer evident when the inguinal lymphadenopathy becomes marked. Lymph nodes are occasionally excised for histologic diagnosis, and show serpiginous or stellate abscesses with necrotic tissue and neutrophils surrounded by a macrophage and giant-cell granulomatous reaction ('suppurating granulomas'). Only one-third of cases reveal positive cultures. Therefore, the main diagnostic tools are serologic. A complement fixation titer of more than 1:64, in concert with the clinical findings previously described, is diagnostic of lymphogranuloma venereum.

Granuloma inguinale (donovanosis)

This is a mildly contagious, sexually transmitted disease caused by the bacterium *Calymmatobacterium granulomatis*, endemic in tropical and subtropical areas. The lesions present as small, ulcerated papules on the labia or vaginal introitus, which merge to create hypertrophic, velvety, beefy-red granulation tissue. This is the most frequent ulcerovegetative form. Papules can also enlarge to become nodules that may become confluent. Extensive matted ulcerations are slow to heal. This slowly progressive, destructive disease leaves disfiguring fibrous scars that, in the absence of treatment, cause extensive genital mutilation. Smears of the lesions show parasitized macrophages. The organisms (Donovan bodies) measure 1–2 micrometers, with a bipolar staining pattern in silver preparations (Warthin–Starry) giving an appearance of small safety pins.

FUNGAL INFECTIONS

Candidiasis[22,113]
Clinical features

Candidiasis is one of the most frequent infections of the genital and anal region. *Candida albicans*, the most frequent *Candida* species involved in human infection, is a normal inhabitant of the gastrointestinal tract and is found in the mouth of approximately half of normal individuals. Pregnancy, immunologic and endocrine dysfunction, immunosuppression, high-dose estrogen, antibiotic or systemic corticosteroid therapy, and debilitating states all predispose to clinical infection. Recurrent *Candida* infections, more than three episodes per year, and severe infections involving the skin should suggest underlying disorders such as diabetes or immunosuppression.

In the genital area, moisture and heat also play a role in the development of this yeast infection. *Candida* can also cause intertrigo in the groins or in folds of a pendulous abdomen. Sore red eroded patches occur in the flexures with small satellite pustules beyond their margins. Between 15 and 30% of asymptomatic women are carriers of *Candida*. Vulvovaginal candidiasis presents with vaginal and vulvar itching and burning, accompanied by vaginal discharge. Although only a fourth of all vaginitides are caused by *Candida*, it has the most prominent vulvar involvement. Therefore, a vaginitis that presents with vulvitis should initially be suspected as candidal in origin. Women of childbearing years are predominantly affected. A characteristic white curd (*Candida* comes from the Latin, *candidus* or dazzling white) appears on the vaginal walls. Erythema, edema, and fissuring of the vulva may occur.

Diagnosis is confirmed on culture of a high vaginal swab or by finding hyphae and spores on a Gram-stained film from the vaginal discharge. *C. albicans* is the culprit in most cases, but other *Candida* species such as *C. glabrata* and *C. tropicalis* are responsible in a minority and can be more resistant to conventional treatments.

Microscopic features

The diagnosis of vulvar candidiasis is frequently missed because a wide range of non-specific inflammatory changes with different degrees of severity and chronicity may accompany this infection. Diagnosis is usually quickly evident once a special stain for fungi is used (Figure 2.40). The following features should direct the pathologist to request a stain for fungi (PAS or GMS):

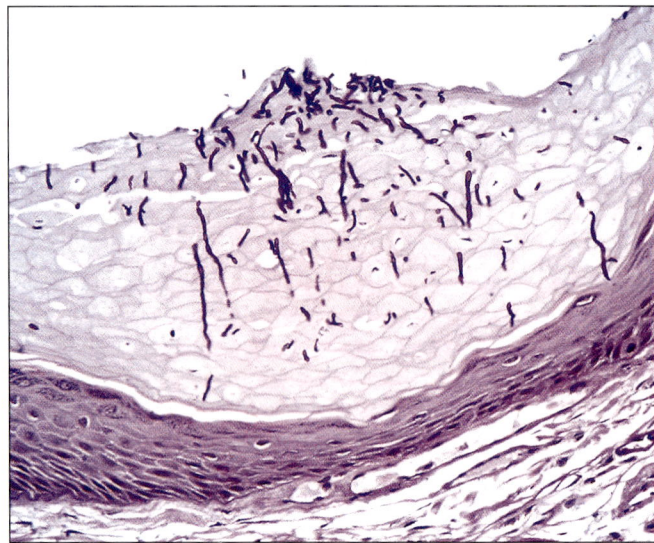

Fig. 2.40 *Candida* infection. Candidal hyphae and yeasts are present in the thickened keratin layer (D-PAS stain). In this case, there is minimal dermal inflammation.

- Parakeratosis disproportionate to the degree of epidermal spongiosis
- Parakeratosis with neutrophils
- Parakeratosis with proteinaceous scale-crust
- Epidermal spongiosis with occasional neutrophils or eosinophils
- Dermal edema with associated epidermal spongiosis.

Pityriasis versicolor

Pityriasis versicolor (tinea versicolor) is a common, non-contagious, superficial fungal infection. Clinically, it presents as chronic and recurrent scaly macules that vary in color from red-brown to white. *Malassezia globosa* in its mycelial phase is the causative agent. It occasionally involves the labia majora, producing hypopigmented or hyperpigmented patches. Hyperpigmentation may result from large melanosomes, vascular erythema or orthokeratosis, while hypopigmentation is due to azelaic acid, a tyrosinase inhibitor the organisms produce. Examination with Woods lamp accentuates the lesion, producing a dull green fluorescence. These findings differentiate this infection from erythrasma, a *Corynebacterium minutissimum* infection producing a bright, coral-red fluorescence under Woods light. The characteristic histologic finding of 'spaghetti and meatballs' is the presence in the stratum corneum of numerous round budding yeasts (blastoconidia) and short septate hyphae (pseudomycelia).

Tinea cruris
Clinical features

This superficial dermatophyte infection involves the inner upper thighs and crural folds. *Trichophyton rubrum,* the most frequent causative agent, produces a chronic infection with frequent extension to the buttocks and waist. Characteristic lesions are sharply demarcated, itchy, red patches with erythematous, scaly, advancing borders. Pustules or vesicles may occur at the edge. The vulva is rarely involved. Heat, sweating, and friction predispose to infection. When topical steroids are inadvertently applied, the appearance can change dramatically and become non-diagnostic, creating the so-called 'tinea incognita'. Although some of the erythema and scaling is initially masked by steroid use, the infection ultimately becomes more extensive and inflammatory, with papules and pustules. The annular configuration may be a clue in these cases. The unusual clinical picture may lead to a biopsy being taken, but unless the clinician is familiar with this clinical problem, a PAS stain may inadvertently not be requested. Diagnosis rests on cultures of scrapes taken from a scale at the rash's leading edge.

Microscopic features
The dermal and epidermal changes are usually minimal and non-specific. Mild epidermal acanthosis with focal spongiosis and perivascular chronic inflammation is commonly seen. A constant feature is parakeratosis overlying the epidermal changes. The hyphae in the stratum corneum are frequently scanty, but more easily visible with special stains for fungus.

VIRAL INFECTIONS

Herpes virus infections[74,91,97]
Herpes simplex virus (HSV)
Clinical features
Herpes simplex viruses, ubiquitous type 1 and type 2 DNA viruses, produce primary infection, latency, and recurrent orolabial and genital disease. Genital herpes, the most frequent sexually transmitted disease worldwide, is generally associated with HSV type 2 (70–90%) with a recent increase being noted for type 1 (10–30%).[92] In the last two decades, the seroprevalence of HSV-2 has increased in the United States by 30%, or with one million new primary genital infections yearly. Previous infection with HSV-1 (e.g., cold sore) gives some protection from HSV-2, either reducing the severity of the primary attack or preventing it altogether. Viral transmission occurs during symptomatic and asymptomatic periods of viral shedding. The virus replicates at the site of infection, then travels to the dorsal root ganglia through retrograde axonal flow and remains in a latent phase, with recurrent reactivations occurring spontaneously or following stimuli such as fever, stress, ultraviolet radiation, or immunosuppression.

Clinically, the manifestations depend on the degree of immunity present and whether it is a primary versus recurrent infection. The first episode of primary infection occurs 3–7 days after exposure, with a prodrome of general malaise associated with non-specific genital findings. The systemic manifestations include fever, myalgias, headache, and back pain coexisting with painful erythema and vulvar swelling. In time, the classic lesions develop, which are vesicles on an erythematous base arranged in clusters that evolve to pustules and/or erosions (Figure 2.41). These lesions are excruciatingly painful. Accompanying regional lymphadenopathy may last for more than a week. The vesicles heal without scarring unless there is secondary infection. Vaginal discharge can occur. Extension of the lesions, systemic complaints and complications are more frequent in women than in men with genital herpes. Lesions can spread to involve the cervix, buttock, and perineum. About 10% of patients develop urinary retention and aseptic meningitis. The severe local manifestations, marked regional lymphadenopathy, and systemic manifestations separate primary infection from recurrent disease.

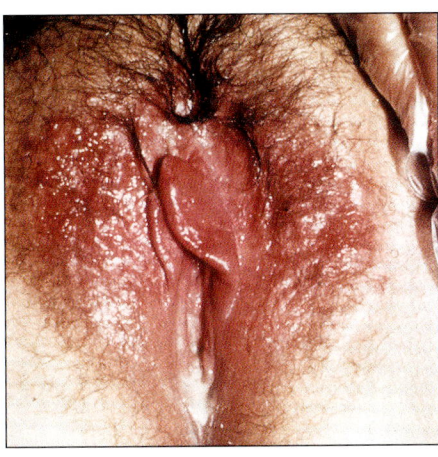

Fig. 2.41 Acute herpes simplex infection. The vulva, which shows edema, erythema, and multiple vesicles, is excruciatingly painful.

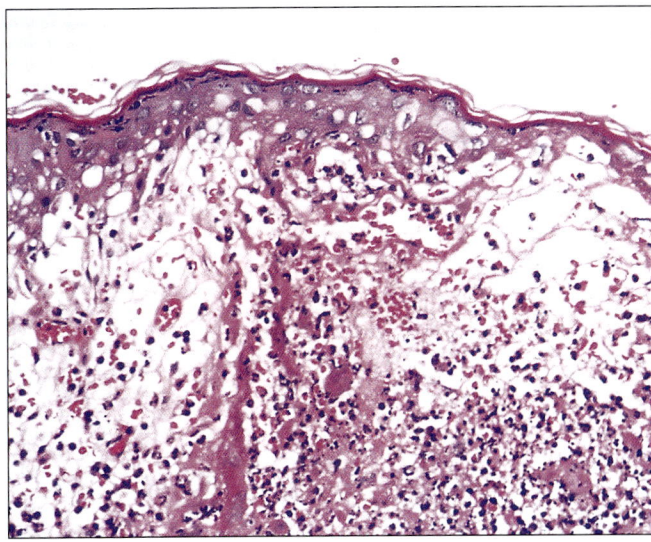

Fig. 2.42 Herpes simplex infection. There is extensive destruction of the epidermis at the edge of a blister. The reticular degeneration pattern of epidermal destruction is characteristic of acute herpes/varicella infections of skin but can also be seen in Stevens–Johnson variant of erythema multiforme.

Recurrent genital infection is in general milder and even subclinical. Usually after dysesthesia, the patients develop three to five vesicles on the genitalia for a period of 1 week. Complications are uncommon. Although variable, the average infected individual has four to seven outbreaks per year.

Genital HSV infection is more severe and protracted in immunosuppressed individuals, who have a tendency to produce pseudoepitheliomatous hyperplasia in chronic clinical cases, simulating verrucous lesions. Recurrence of previous infection is common after transplant surgery. HSV infections in HIV patients can be extensive with severe, non-healing, painful ulcers. Candidal and bacterial secondary infections are common.

The diagnosis is usually apparent clinically and may be confirmed through serologic tests, tissue culture, direct immunofluorescence, or molecular techniques. Reliable and rapid identification can be made using smears of vesicles and monoclonal immunofluorescence antibodies. The gold standard is Western blot with 99% specificity and sensitivity. PCR is the preferred test to diagnose HSV in cases of systemic spread such as encephalitis. A high percentage of cultures will be positive when taken from vesicular, pustular, and ulcerated lesions. Other infectious diseases such as *Chlamydia* and syphilis will only occasionally be in the differential diagnosis and are excluded by culture and serologic tests. Stevens–Johnson syndrome can cause acute vulvar ulceration but the skin and mouth are normally involved as well. Both Behçets and Crohns disease can cause painful ulceration, but tend to have a more chronic and less periodic history.

Microscopic features

The earliest changes appear in the nucleus of infected keratinocytes, with peripheral clumping of chromatin, homogenous ground-glass appearance, and ballooning. These early changes start at the basal layer. However, most biopsies include an established intraepidermal vesicle resulting from infected cell swelling and losing attachment (ballooning degeneration), and progressive hydropic swelling of cells transforming in large and clear keratinocytes (reticular degeneration) (Figure 2.42). Ballooning changes are specific for viral infection and the cells can be multinucleated, with eosinophilic intranuclear inclusions and/or dense eosinophilic cytoplasm. Ballooning degeneration

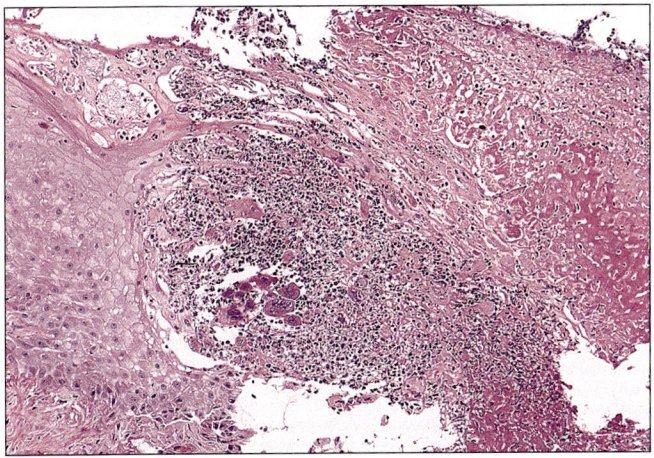

Fig. 2.43 Herpes simplex. In herpes simplex there is often severe necrosis of skin appendages and upper dermis. Viral inclusions, while prominent in this slide, may be difficult to see, and electron microscopy may be necessary to identify the viral particles.

is found mainly at the vesicular base and reticular degeneration in the superficial aspect and edges. Ulceration occurs, at the edges of which large, infected keratinocytes with intranuclear inclusions or multinucleated cells are often usually easily identified (Figures 2.43 and 2.44).

In late stages, ghost cells remain, which are infected keratinocytes where the intranuclear inclusions have turned from eosinophilic to a slate gray color. Perivascular lymphocytic and neutrophilic inflammation is seen in the upper dermis. Follicles are more often involved in recurrent lesions. If the latter is the predominant finding, the diagnosis of herpes folliculitis can be rendered. Other adnexal structures can be affected, as in herpes syringitis. Eccrine ducts and glands show changes of the viral infection. The nerves in the biopsy specimen can show inflammation, Schwann cell hypertrophy, and viral cytopathic

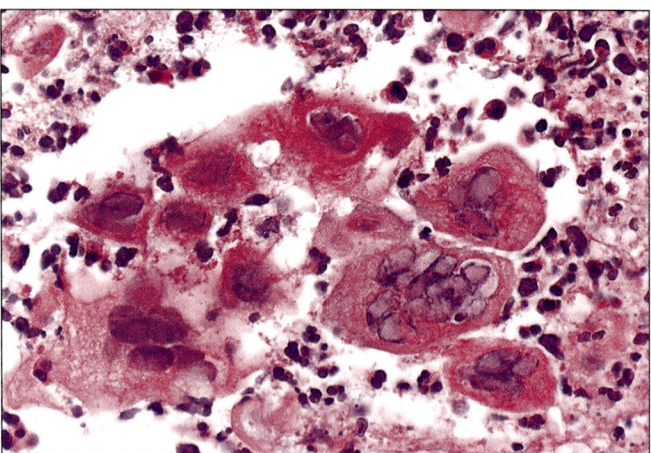

Fig. 2.44 Herpes simplex with prominent viral inclusions.

changes, demonstrating that nerves are not only a conduit for this virus but also a target of infection.

Varicella zoster virus infection
Clinical features
Varicella zoster virus is the etiology of both varicella (chickenpox) and herpes zoster (shingles). Ninety per cent of children in the United States under the age of 10 years have suffered varicella. Subsequently, the virus can remain latent in nerve ganglia until it is reactivated in 20% of immunocompetent hosts and half of immunosuppressed individuals. Reactivation may occur spontaneously or secondary to fever, stress, tissue damage, immunosuppression, etc. Herpes zoster is usually a disease of patients over 50 years, only affecting younger patients who suffered varicella during the first year of life. The incidence is increasing in immunocompromised patients, especially those infected with HIV.

In most patients herpes zoster starts with a prodrome of pain, pruritus, tingling, or tenderness in a dermatomal distribution. A painful eruption of clustered papules follows, which, in a short period of time, transform to vesicles on an erythematous base (Figures 2.45 and 2.46). The eruption usually involves one dermatome and rarely crosses the midline. Lesions similar to those seen in chickenpox can coexist with classic shingles. After several days the vesicles rupture and form adherent crusts. In the genital area, because of the moisture, friction, and thin epidermis, erosions predominate. Mucosal surfaces in proximity to the cutaneous eruption will be affected, leading especially to urinary retention. The severity of the eruption, pain, and complications increases with the patient's age or degree of immunosuppression. Complications range from postherpetic neuralgia, to ophthalmic zoster, to meningoencephalitis or motor paralysis, among others. Early recognition and treatment reduce the severity of the eruption and its sequelae. The distribution of the rash is a strong diagnostic clue. Confirmation comes from direct fluorescence antibodies or PCR viral detection. Early stages may be mistaken for other inflammatory dermatoses such as acute contact dermatitis, and a biopsy might be performed.

Microscopic features
The changes overlap with those seen in herpes simplex infections (Figure 2.42). Immunoperoxidase stains can be useful in separating herpes simplex from varicella zoster.

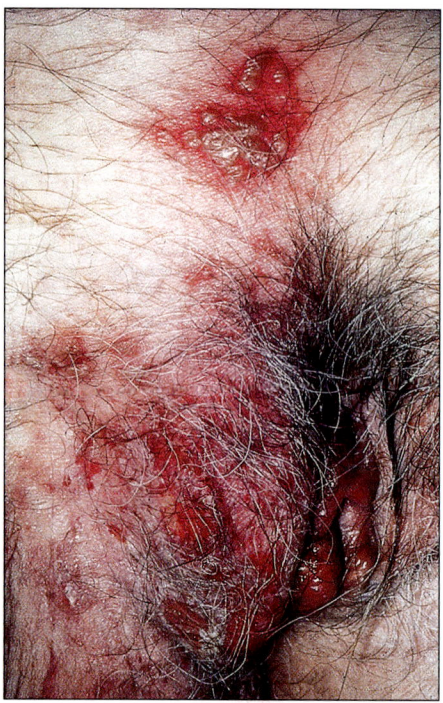

Fig. 2.45 Varicella zoster of the vulva and pubis. Unilateral groups of vesicles and pustules have an erythematous base.

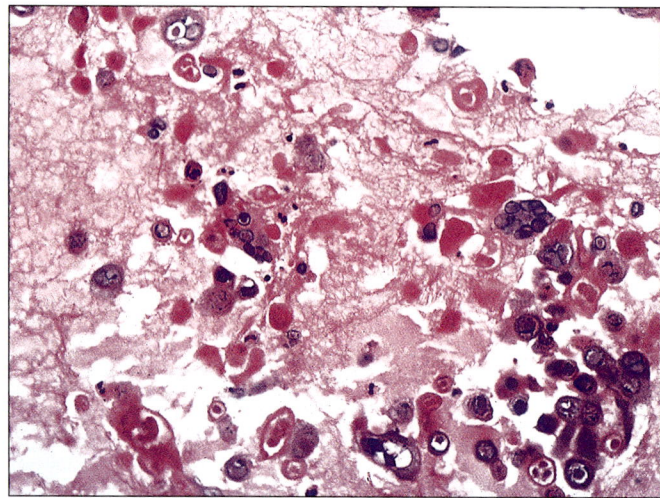

Fig. 2.46 Varicella zoster. In an early vesicular lesion the viral inclusion bodies are usually easily seen in the necrotic epithelial cells in blister content.

Other virus infections
Molluscum contagiosum
Clinical features
Molluscum contagiosum is a poxvirus infection exhibiting single or multiple, 2–8 mm dome-shaped papules with a central umbilicated core of white material. This infection predominantly affects children and adolescents. Commonly, spontaneous regression occurs. Molluscum contagiosum is usually contracted during childhood when lesions can occur anywhere in the body. In adults it occurs principally as a sexually transmitted disease involving the vulvar and perianal regions.

There may be diagnostic confusion with viral warts or occasionally with inflammatory dermatoses such as lichen planus. Primary or recurrent molluscum contagiosum often complicates HIV disease, and lesions may have very atypical appearances including giant forms or confluent lesions requiring biopsy.

Microscopic features

The histologic features of molluscum contagiosum are pathognomonic. An endophytic growth of squamous epithelium arranged as lobules is seen at low power. Eosinophilic inclusion bodies fill the cytoplasm of infected cells above the basal layer. The inclusions can acquire large dimensions and compress the nucleus of the infected keratinocytes to the periphery (Figures 2.47 and 2.48). In a fully evolved lesion, the epidermis ruptures under the pressure of the underlying proliferation almost entirely occupied by viral inclusion, and produces the charac-teristic small white core. The viral inclusion bodies become more basophilic as they enlarge.

Human papillomavirus (HPV) infections[9,18,56,117]
Clinical features

Papillomaviruses are a large group exceeding 100 genotypes of DNA viruses that infect skin and mucosae, producing warts, intraepithelial neoplasia, or invasive squamous carcinoma. Genital HPV is a common, sexually transmitted disease affecting predominantly young adults. The vulva, vagina, cervix, and anus are frequent areas of infection. All patients presenting with genital warts need to be screened for other sexually transmitted diseases. Transmission of this virus can occur from direct contact with individuals who harbor clinical or subclinical HPV lesions. Autoinoculation is a frequent event in digital and anogenital warts. The lesions are in most cases transient, but the virus may recur, persist, or enter a latent phase. Genital warts are by far the most common manifestation and the majority of infections are with HPV types which, in the normal host, carry a low risk of neoplastic change. In immunocompromised patients, HPV infections often persist and increase the risk of developing neoplasms. HPV infections affecting the genital tract can be categorized as follows:

- Those that produce warts on fully keratinized skin, i.e., common and plantar warts.
- Those that cause warts, dysplasia, and squamous cell cancer in the immunosuppressed or in patients with the rare inherited disorder, epidermodysplasia verruciformis.
- Those that infect the nasopharyngeal, conjunctival, and anogenital mucosal surfaces. These can be subdivided into low-, intermediate-, and high-risk types for the development of intraepithelial dysplasia and squamous cell cancer. As on the cervix, HPV types 16 and 18 are most definitely linked to vulvar and anal intraepithelial neoplasia and squamous cell carcinoma. However, the risk of cancerous change on the vulva and anal mucosa seems much less than on the cervix.

The clinical presentation will depend on the HPV type, the anatomic location, and the host's immune status. The following are the most frequent clinical presentations:

- Condylomata acuminata (singular: condyloma acuminatum) or anogenital warts occur on the non-hair-bearing, partially keratinized skin of the vulva (labia minora), the perineum, perianal region adjacent to the skin–mucosal interface, or in adjacent areas such as inguinal folds and mons pubis. They are discrete, skin-colored to brown, exophytic papillomas. They acquire a whitish surface when macerated in moist areas. The lesions range from several millimeters to being large and broad-based, several centimeters in size, and forming confluent plaques that may extend into the vagina, urethra, or anal canal. One-third of these cases recur. Although malignant transformation is infrequent, the chances are higher than with other types of wart. The most frequent oncogenic HPV types are HPV 16, 18, 31, 33, and 35; the most frequent HPV types associated with the benign lesions are HPV 6 and 11 (see Chapter 7).
- Papular and keratotic warts tend to occur on fully keratinized and hair-bearing skin (e.g., labia majora).
- Flat warts can be found in all situations.

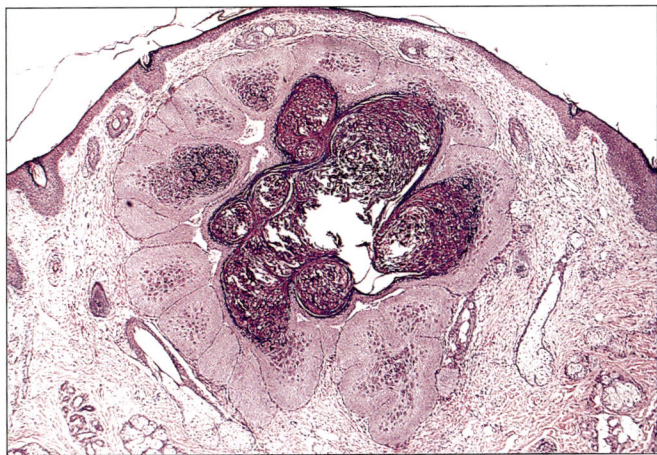

Fig. 2.47 Molluscum contagiosum. A well-defined sac encloses the virion colony. The histologic appearances of molluscum contagiosum are pathognomonic and esthetically appealing.

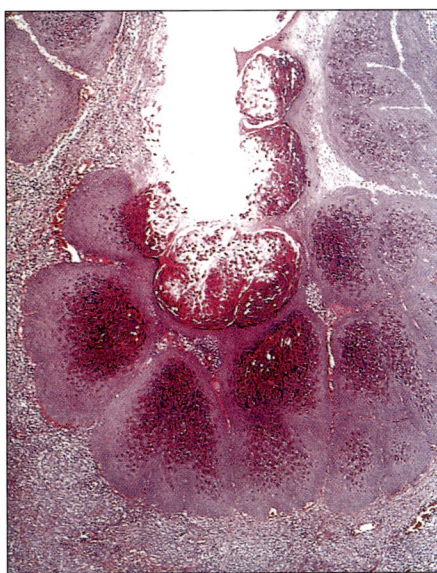

Fig. 2.48 Molluscum contagiosum. Each inverted nodule of hyperplastic squamous cells expands into the underlying dermis.

PCR has identified HPV DNA in skin with no clearly defined lesions. Dilute acetic acid will turn these abnormal areas white, albeit the acetowhite coloring only reflects thickening of the squamous epithelium and is not diagnostic of HPV infection (e.g., acetowhite coloring can be seen in *Candida* infection, psoriasis, lichen planus, or eczema). HPV can be detected not only in subclinical lesions but also in normal-appearing skin. Furthermore, the virus is resistant to heat and desiccation. This explains the high recurrence rate of lesions (e.g., 20–50% for genital warts) and supports the consideration that treatment may not prevent transmission of HPV. Genital warts are of concern to the healthcare provider when they occur in prepubertal individuals. Although transmission during delivery, from other body sites, by fomites, or from close family contact are potential explanations for this infection, the possibility that these lesions are the product of sexual abuse needs to be carefully considered.

The clinical differential diagnosis includes molluscum contagiosum, seborrheic keratoses, vulvar intraepithelial neoplasia, and papular inflammatory dermatoses such as lichen planus. Genital warts should be biopsied when there is concern about dysplastic or neoplastic change or when there is diagnostic uncertainty. Presently, no specific antiviral therapy is available. Only therapeutic measurements towards local destruction, removal, or induction of an immunologic response against the lesion are therapeutic considerations. Recently, a recombinant DNA vaccine has been developed that may change how we see HPV infection in the future.

Microscopic features

The common wart shows papillomatosis with hyperkeratosis and parakeratosis, the latter especially located in the tips of the papillae. The elongated rete ridges often show an inward orientation at the lesion's edge. Hypergranulosis with large clumps of basophilic keratohyaline material lie in the valley of the papillomatosis. Koilocytes, which are large vacuolated cells with small pyknotic single or multiple nuclei, are located in the superficial malpighian layer. The dermis shows dilated superficial vessels that may bleed into the stratum corneum, especially in areas of parakeratosis. Mild superficial perivascular chronic inflammation can also be seen.

In flat warts koilocytes present as a more or less continuous line in the upper epidermis. Condylomata acuminata show marked epidermal acanthosis with hyperkeratosis and parakeratosis, and a minor component of papillomatosis with only a few vacuolated koilocytes in the upper malpighian layers (Figure 2.49). Papillomatosis is more rounded at the base than in common warts, and koilocytes are less frequently seen than in other variants of warts and are usually present beneath the areas of parakeratosis (Figures 2.50 and 2.51). Coarse keratohyaline granules are commonly present. Changes of lichen simplex chronicus may be superimposed due to trauma to the lesion.

The histopathologist needs to know whether the warts have been treated before biopsy. Podophyllin paints and gels are still a common treatment and if applied within 48 hours of biopsy, the squamous cells may show severe nuclear and cytoplasmic atypia and large numbers of mitotic figures due to metaphase arrest. These changes can persist long after treatment has stopped and may be a pitfall in the diagnosis of intraepidermal malignancy.

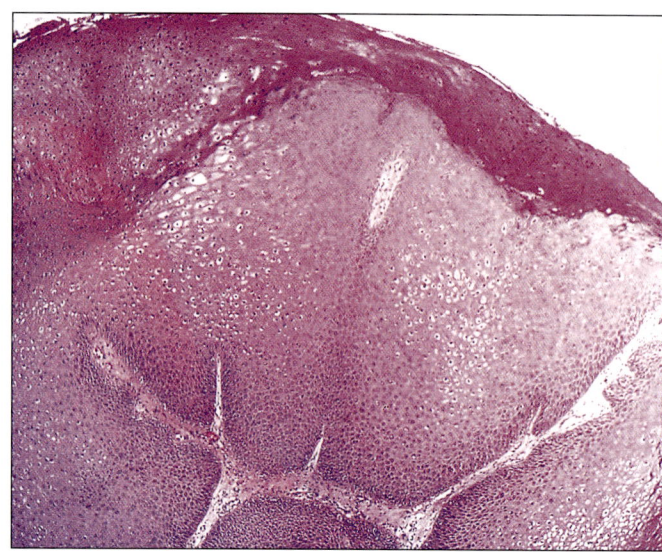

Fig. 2.49 Condyloma acuminatum. Hyperplastic thickening of epidermis with characteristic HPV koilocytosis of many of the epidermal cells.

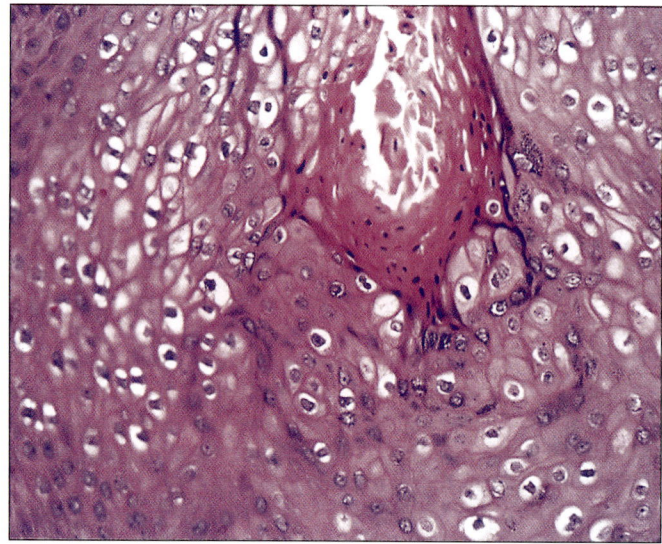

Fig. 2.50 Condyloma acuminatum. The koilocytic changes are obvious in most epidermal cells near the surface and are producing parakeratotic keratin.

PROTOZOAL INFECTIONS

Trichomoniasis

Trichomonas vaginalis, the causative organism, elicits an acute vaginitis, particularly symptomatic when there is a coexisting bacterial vaginitis, as often occurs. The profuse, offensive vaginal discharge is associated with dysuria, dyspareunia, and vulvovaginal soreness. The vulva is acutely inflamed, with marked reddening, and the vaginal wall is similarly reddened, likened to the appearance of a strawberry. Diagnosis is made by demonstrating the presence of the motile, flagellate organisms in a fresh wet saline preparation of the discharge.

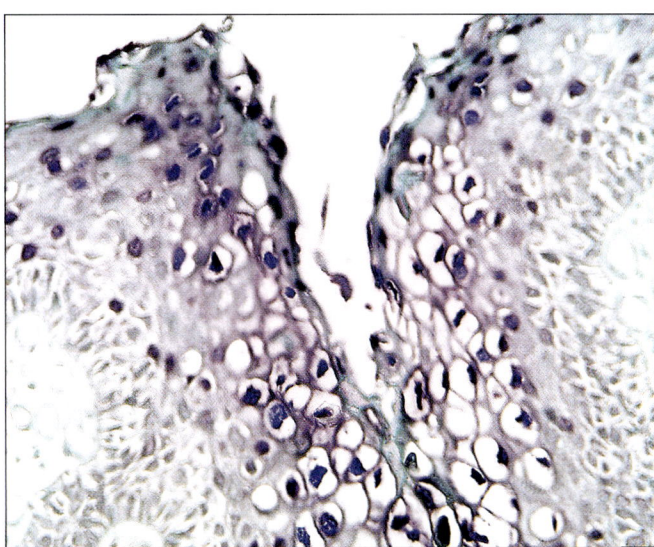

Fig. 2.51 Condyloma acuminatum. Positive reaction in the nuclei of koilocytes confirms the presence of HPV (*in situ* hybridization method for HPV).

INFESTATIONS

Scabies

Clinical features

The female mite, *Sarcoptes scabiei* var. *hominis*, infests the epidermis. The primary means of transmission is direct close contact. Factors that favor the spread of this mite include overcrowded places (especially after natural disasters, wars or economic depression), poor personal hygiene, lack of public awareness, and delayed treatment. The female mite lives out her 30-day life cycle in burrows in the epidermis where she lays her eggs, causing an allergic reaction to the mite protein. It takes 2–6 weeks after the first infestation for the host to become sensitized and develop pruritus. This period diminishes to 1–2 days with subsequent infestations.

Three clinical types have been described: papulovesicular lesions, persistent nodules, and crusted scabies. The combination of severe nocturnal itching with the finding of papules/vesicles and visible epidermal burrows in finger webs, nipples, and buttocks are clues to the diagnosis. Secondary bacterial infection is common. In women, the areola, nipples, and genitals are frequently affected. Persistent nodules affecting lower trunk, genitalia, and thighs occur in 7% of patients due to a delayed hypersensitivity reaction to the infestation.

Crusted scabies, also known as Norwegian scabies, affects immunocompromised patients (elderly individuals, HIV or transplanted patients) or patients suffering from sensory dysfunction (those infected with leprosy or paraplegia). Mites number in the millions in crusted scabies. However, allergic symptoms like itch are not so pronounced. Clinical confirmation follows by examining skin scrapings with a light microscope and mineral oil to recognize adult mites, eggs, and/or fecal pellets. Epiluminescence microscopy is also useful to see mites and eggs.

Microscopic features

Eggs, larvae, mites, and excreta are located beneath the stratum corneum when the biopsy includes a burrow. The epidermis shows spongiosis with exocytosis of eosinophils and occasionally neutrophils. There is a superficial and deep perivascular lymphocytic infiltrate with abundant eosinophils, a reaction similar to that seen with other arthropod infestations or assault. If the eosinophilic infiltrate is exuberant, flame figures (eosinophilic granules lining the collagen fibers) may be seen. Scabetic feces (scybala) or eggs are seen more often than the mite itself in vulvar biopsies.

The lesions of persistent nodular scabies have a heavy superficial and deep inflammatory infiltrate including lymphocytes, macrophages, plasma cells, eosinophils, and occasionally atypical mononuclear cells; mites are rarely found. Norwegian scabies shows massive hyperkeratosis and parakeratosis containing numerous mites and psoriasiform epidermal hyperplasia. The dermal changes resemble those of the papulovesicular variant of scabies.

Pubic (crab) lice (Phthirus pubis)

The pubic louse typically affects the axillae and pubis, but any area dense in hair follicles on the trunk or even eyelashes can be colonized. These arthropods feed at night from the patient's blood and cement their eggs to the hair, forming minute gritty projections called nits. The pruritus associated with feeding bites leads to excoriation and secondary bacterial folliculitis. Multiple bluish spots can be seen in the trunk of individuals with pubic lice (maculae ceruleae). The immune status of these patients appears to affect the infestation. Hairs can be extracted and examined under the microscope in the search for eggs. Vulvar biopsy is not required.

REFERENCES

1. Criteria for diagnosis of Behçet's disease. International Study Group for Behçet's Disease. Lancet 1990;335:1078–80.
2. Ball SB, Wojnarowska F. Vulvar dermatoses: lichen sclerosus, lichen planus, and vulval dermatitis/lichen simplex chronicus. Semin Cutan Med Surg 1998;17:182–8.
3. Barnhill RL, Albert LS, Shama SK, Goldenhersh MA, Rhodes AR, Sober AJ. Genital lentiginosis: a clinical and histopathologic study. J Am Acad Dermatol 1990;22:453–60.
4. Barrett JF, Murray LA, MacDonald HN. Darier's disease localized to the vulva. Case report. Br J Obstet Gynaecol 1989;96:997–9.
5. Bauer A, Rodiger C, Greif C, Kaatz M, Elsner P. Vulvar dermatoses – irritant and allergic contact dermatitis of the vulva. Dermatology 2005;210:143–9.
6. Bell HK, Farrar CW, Curley RK. Papular acantholytic dyskeratosis of the vulva. Clin Exp Dermatol 2001;26:386–8.
7. Bernard P, Vaillant L, Labeille B, et al. Incidence and distribution of subepidermal autoimmune bullous skin diseases in three French regions. Bullous Diseases French Study Group. Arch Dermatol 1995;131:48–52.
8. Berth-Jones J, Graham-Brown RA, Burns DA. Lichen sclerosus et atrophicus – a review of 15 cases in young girls. Clin Exp Dermatol 1991;16:14–17.
9. Beutner KR. Human papilloma virus infection of the vulva. Semin Dermatol 1996;15:2–7.
10. Carlson JA, Lamb P, Malfetano J, Ambros RA, Mihm MC, Jr. Clinicopathologic comparison of vulvar and extragenital lichen sclerosus: histologic variants, evolving lesions, and etiology of 141 cases. Mod Pathol 1998;11:844–54.
11. Carlson JA, Ambros R, Malfetano J, et al. Vulvar lichen sclerosus and squamous cell carcinoma: a cohort, case control, and investigational study with historical perspective; implications for chronic inflammation and sclerosis in the development of neoplasia. Hum Pathol 1998;29:932–48.
12. Carlson JA, Mu XC, Slominski A, et al. Melanocytic proliferations associated with lichen sclerosus. Arch Dermatol 2002;138:77–87.
13. Cattaneo A, Bracco GL, Maestrini G, et al. Lichen sclerosus and squamous hyperplasia of the vulva. A clinical study of medical treatment. J Reprod Med 1991;36:301–5.
14. Chiesa-Vottero A, Dvoretsky PM, Hart WR. Histopathologic study of thin vulvar squamous cell carcinomas and associated cutaneous lesions: a correlative study of 48 tumors in 44 patients with analysis of adjacent vulvar

intraepithelial neoplasia types and lichen sclerosus. Am J Surg Pathol 2006;30:310–8.

15. Cockayne SE, Rassl DM, Thomas SE. Squamous cell carcinoma arising in Hailey–Hailey disease of the vulva. Br J Dermatol 2000;142:540–2.
16. Craddock N, Dawson E, Burge S, et al. The gene for Darier's disease maps to chromosome 12q23–q24.1. Hum Mol Genet 1993;2:1941–3.
17. Davis GD, Hutchison CV. Clinical management of vulvodynia. Clin Obstet Gynecol 1999;42:221–33.
18. Dupin N. Genital warts. Clin Dermatol 2004;22:481–6.
19. Dupre A, Viraben R. Laugier's disease. Dermatologica 1990;181:183–6.
20. Dwyer CM, Kerr RE, Millan DW. Squamous carcinoma following lichen planus of the vulva. Clin Exp Dermatol 1995;20:171–2.
21. Eason EL, Feldman P. Contact dermatitis associated with the use of Always sanitary napkins. CMAJ 1996;154:1173–6.
22. Eckert LO, Hawes SE, Stevens CE, Koutsky LA, Eschenbach DA, Holmes KK. Vulvovaginal candidiasis: clinical manifestations, risk factors, management algorithm. Obstet Gynecol 1998;92:757–65.
23. Edwards L. Vulvar lichen planus. Arch Dermatol 1989;125:1677–80.
24. Edwards L. New concepts in vulvodynia. Am J Obstet Gynecol 2003;189(3 Suppl):S24–30.
25. Edwards L, Hays S. Vulvar cicatricial pemphigoid as a lichen sclerosus imitator. A case report. J Reprod Med 1992;37:561–4.
26. Edwards L, Hansen RC. Reiter's syndrome of the vulva. The psoriasis spectrum. Arch Dermatol 1992;128:811–4.
27. Eisen D. The vulvovaginal–gingival syndrome of lichen planus. The clinical characteristics of 22 patients. Arch Dermatol 1994;130:1379–82.
28. Elsner P, Wilhelm D, Maibach HI. Multiple parameter assessment of vulvar irritant contact dermatitis. Contact Dermatitis 1990;23:20–6.
29. Estrada R, Kaufman R. Benign vulvar melanosis. J Reprod Med 1993;38:5–8.
30. Evron S, Leviatan A, Okon E. Familial benign chronic pemphigus appearing as leukoplakia of the vulva. Int J Dermatol 1984;23:556–7.
31. Farage M, Maibach HI. The vulvar epithelium differs from the skin: implications for cutaneous testing to address topical vulvar exposures. Contact Dermatitis 2004;51:201–9.
32. Farrell AM, Dean D, Millard PR, Charnock FM, Wojnarowska F. Cytokine alterations in lichen sclerosus: an immunohistochemical study. Br J Dermatol 2006;155:931–40.
33. Farrell AM, Kirtschig G, Dalziel KL, et al. Childhood vulval pemphigoid: a clinical and immunopathological study of five patients. Br J Dermatol 1999;140:308–12.
34. Fenniche S, Mokni M, Haouet S, Ben Osman A. Vulvar Crohn disease: 3 cases. Ann Dermatol Venereol 1997;124:629–32.
35. Fischer G, Spurrett B, Fischer A. The chronically symptomatic vulva: aetiology and management. Br J Obstet Gynaecol 1995;102:773–9.
36. Fisler RE, Saeb M, Liang MG, Howard RM, McKee PH. Childhood bullous pemphigoid: a clinicopathologic study and review of the literature. Am J Dermatopathol 2003;25:183–9.
37. Foster DC. Vulvar disease. Obstet Gynecol 2002;100:145–63.
38. Franck JM, Young AW, Jr. Squamous cell carcinoma in situ arising within lichen planus of the vulva. Dermatol Surg 1995;21:890–4.
39. Friedrich EG, Jr, MacLaren NK. Genetic aspects of vulvar lichen sclerosus. Am J Obstet Gynecol 1984;150:161–6.
40. Frith P, Charnock M, Wojnarowska F. Cicatricial pemphigoid diagnosed from ocular features in recurrent severe vulval scarring. Two case reports. Br J Obstet Gynaecol 1991;98:482–4.
41. Furlonge CB, Thin RN, Evans BE, McKee PH. Vulvar vestibulitis syndrome: a clinico-pathological study. Br J Obstet Gynaecol 1991;98:703–6.
42. Gardella C. Vulvar vestibulitis syndrome. Curr Infect Dis Rep 2006;8:473–80.
43. Goldberg JM, Buchler DA, Dibbell DG. Advanced hidradenitis suppurativa presenting with bilateral vulvar masses. Gynecol Oncol 1996;60:494–7.
44. Goldstein AT, Anhalt GJ, Klingman D, Burrows LJ. Mucous membrane pemphigoid of the vulva. Obstet Gynecol 2005;105(5 Pt 2):1188–90.
45. Gomez Rueda N, Garcia A, Vighi S, Belardi MG, Cardinal L, di Paola G. Epithelial alterations adjacent to invasive squamous carcinoma of the vulva. J Reprod Med 1994;39:526–30.
46. Graziottin A, Brotto LA. Vulvar vestibulitis syndrome: a clinical approach. J Sex Marital Ther 2004;30:125–39.
47. Guenther LC, Shum D. Localized childhood vulvar pemphigoid. J Am Acad Dermatol 1990;22(5 Pt 1):762–4.
48. Gunthert AR, Hinney B, Nesselhut K, Hanf V, Emons G. Vulvitis granulomatosa and unilateral hypertrophy of the vulva related to Crohn's disease: a case report. Am J Obstet Gynecol 2004;191:1719–20.
49. Haefner HK, Collins ME, Davis GD, et al. The vulvodynia guideline. J Low Genit Tract Dis 2005;9:40–51.
50. Haidopoulos D, Rodolakis A, Stefanidis K, Blachos G, Sotiropoulou M, Diakomanolis E. Behçet's disease: part of the differential diagnosis of the ulcerative vulva. Clin Exp Obstet Gynecol 2002;29:219–21.
51. Halperin R, Zehavi S, Vaknin Z, Ben-Ami I, Pansky M, Schneider D. The major histopathologic characteristics in the vulvar vestibulitis syndrome. Gynecol Obstet Invest 2005;59:75–9.
52. Hammock LA, Barrett TL. Inflammatory dermatoses of the vulva. J Cutan Pathol 2005;32:604–11.
53. Handfield-Jones SE, Hinde FR, Kennedy CT. Lichen sclerosus et atrophicus in children misdiagnosed as sexual abuse. Br Med J (Clin Res Ed) 1987;294:1404–5.

54. Hart WR, Norris HJ, Helwig EB. Relation of lichen sclerosus et atrophicus of the vulva to development of carcinoma. Obstet Gynecol 1975;45:369–77.
55. Hazelrigg DE, Stoller LJ. Isolated familial benign chronic pemphigus. Arch Dermatol 1977;113:1302.
56. Heard I, Palefsky JM, Kazatchkine MD. The impact of HIV antiviral therapy on human papillomavirus (HPV) infections and HPV-related diseases. Antivir Ther 2004;9:13–22.
57. Helander SD, Rogers RS, 3rd. The sensitivity and specificity of direct immunofluorescence testing in disorders of mucous membranes. J Am Acad Dermatol 1994;30:65–75.
58. Heller DS, Randolph P, Young A, Tancer ML, Fromer D. The cutaneous-vulvar clinic revisited: a 5-year experience of the Columbia Presbyterian Medical Center Cutaneous-Vulvar Service. Dermatology 1997;195:26–9.
59. Hewitt J. Histologic criteria for lichen sclerosus of the vulva. J Reprod Med 1986;31:781–7.
60. Hodgson TA, Cohen AJ. Medical expenditures for major diseases, 1995. Health Care Financ Rev 1999;21:119–64.
61. Holst VA, Fair KP, Wilson BB, Patterson JW. Squamous cell carcinoma arising in Hailey–Hailey disease. J Am Acad Dermatol 2000;43(2 Pt 2):368–71.
62. Jorizzo JL, Abernethy JL, White WL, et al. Mucocutaneous criteria for the diagnosis of Behçet's disease: an analysis of clinicopathologic data from multiple international centers. J Am Acad Dermatol 1995;32:968–76.
63. Kavanagh GM, Burton PA, Kennedy CT. Vulvitis chronica plasmacellularis (Zoon's vulvitis). Br J Dermatol 1993;129:92–3.
64. Kirtschig G, Wakelin SH, Wojnarowska F. Mucosal vulval lichen planus: outcome, clinical and laboratory features. J Eur Acad Dermatol Venereol 2005;19:301–7.
65. Langenberg A, Berger TG, Cardelli M, Rodman OG, Estes S, Barron DR. Genital benign chronic pemphigus (Hailey–Hailey disease) presenting as condylomas. J Am Acad Dermatol 1992;26:951–5.
66. Leibowitch M. Lichen sclerosus. Semin Dermatol 1996;15:42–6.
67. Levine V, Sanchez M, Nestor M. Localized vulvar pemphigoid in a child misdiagnosed as sexual abuse. Arch Dermatol 1992;128:804–6.
68. Lewis FM. Vulval lichen planus. Br J Dermatol 1998;138:569–75.
69. Lewis FM. Vulval disease from the 1800s to the new millennium. J Cutan Med Surg 2002;6:340–4.
70. Lewis FM, Shah M, Harrington CI. Vulval involvement in lichen planus: a study of 37 women. Br J Dermatol 1996;135:89–91.
71. Li Q, Leopold K, Carlson JA. Chronic vulvar purpura: persistent pigmented purpuric dermatitis (lichen aureus) of the vulva or plasma cell (Zoon's) vulvitis? J Cutan Pathol 2003;30:572–6.
72. Loening-Baucke V. Lichen sclerosus et atrophicus in children. Am J Dis Child 1991;145:1058–61.
73. Lotery HE, Galask RP. Erosive lichen planus of the vulva and vagina. Obstet Gynecol 2003;101(5 Pt 2):1121–5.
74. Lowhagen GB, Bonde E, Forsgren-Brusk U, Runeman B, Tunback P. The microenvironment of vulvar skin in women with symptomatic and asymptomatic herpes simplex virus type 2 (HSV-2) infection. J Eur Acad Dermatol Venereol 2006;20:1086–9.
75. Lynch PJ. 2006 International Society for the Study of Vulvovaginal Disease classification of vulvar dermatoses: a synopsis. J Low Genit Tract Dis 2007;11:1–2.
76. Lynch PJ, Moyal-Barrocco M, Bogliatto F, Micheletti L, Scurry J. 2006 ISSVD classification of vulvar dermatoses: pathologic subsets and their clinical correlates. J Reprod Med 2007;52:3–9.
77. Magro CM, Crowson AN. Cutaneous manifestations of Behçet's disease. Int J Dermatol 1995;34:159–65.
78. Malik M, Ahmed AR. Involvement of the female genital tract in pemphigus vulgaris. Obstet Gynecol 2005;106(5 Pt 1):1005–12.
79. Mangelsdorf HC, White WL, Jorizzo JL. Behçet's disease. Report of twenty-five patients from the United States with prominent mucocutaneous involvement. J Am Acad Dermatol 1996;34(5 Pt 1):745–50.
80. Mann MS, Kaufman RH. Erosive lichen planus of the vulva. Clin Obstet Gynecol 1991;34:605–13.
81. Marinoff SC, Turner ML. Vulvar vestibulitis syndrome. Dermatol Clin 1992;10:435–44.
82. Marren P, Wojnarowska F, Powell S. Allergic contact dermatitis and vulvar dermatoses. Br J Dermatol 1992;126:52–6.
83. Marren P, Millard P, Chia Y, Wojnarowska F. Mucosal lichen sclerosus/lichen planus overlap syndromes. Br J Dermatol 1994;131:118–23.
84. Marren P, Walkden V, Mallon E, Wojnarowska F. Vulval cicatricial pemphigoid may mimic lichen sclerosus. Br J Dermatol 1996;134:522–4.
85. Marren P, Wojnarowska F, Venning V, Wilson C, Nayar M. Vulvar involvement in autoimmune bullous diseases. J Reprod Med 1993;38:101–7.
86. Marren P, Yell J, Charnock FM, Bunce M, Welsh K, Wojnarowska F. The association between lichen sclerosus and antigens of the HLA system. Br J Dermatol 1995;132:197–203.
87. McKay M. Vulvar dermatoses: common problems in dermatological and gynaecological practice. Br J Clin Pract Suppl 1990;71:5–10.
88. Meneux E, Wolkenstein P, Haddad B, Roujeau JC, Revuz J, Paniel BJ. Vulvovaginal involvement in toxic epidermal necrolysis: a retrospective study of 40 cases. Obstet Gynecol 1998;91:283–7.

89. Meyrick Thomas RH, Ridley CM, McGibbon DH, Black MM. Lichen sclerosus et atrophicus and autoimmunity – a study of 350 women. Br J Dermatol 1988;118:41–6.
90. Moore-Maxwell CA, Robboy SJ. Mucinous adenocarcinoma arising in rectovaginal fistulas associated with Crohn's disease. Gynecol Oncol 2004;93:266–8.
91. Nader SN, Prober CG. Herpesvirus infections of the vulva. Semin Dermatol 1996;15:8–16.
92. Nahmias AJ, Lee FK, Beckman-Nahmias S. Sero-epidemiological and - sociological patterns of herpes simplex virus infection in the world. Scand J Infect Dis Suppl 1990;69:19–36.
93. Nasca MR, Innocenzi D, Micali G. Penile cancer among patients with genital lichen sclerosus. J Am Acad Dermatol 1999;41:911–4.
94. Naughton GK, Reggiardo D, Bystryn JC. Correlation between vitiligo antibodies and extent of depigmentation in vitiligo. J Am Acad Dermatol 1986;15(5 Pt 1):978–81.
95. Neri I, Patrizi A, Marzaduri S, Marini R, Negosanti M. Vulvitis plasmacellularis: two new cases. Genitourin Med 1995;71:311–3.
96. O'Keefe RJ, Scurry JP, Dennerstein G, Sfameni S, Brenan J. Audit of 114 non-neoplastic vulvar biopsies. Br J Obstet Gynaecol 1995;102:780–6.
97. Palamaras I, Richardson D, Healy V, Lyons D, Byrne M, Lamba H. An atypical herpetic vulval ulcer in an African woman: an important lesson. Int J STD AIDS 2006;17:427–8.
98. Pelisse M. Erosive vulvar lichen planus and desquamative vaginitis. Semin Dermatol 1996;15:47–50.
99. Pelisse M. [Vulvar lichen sclerosus]. Rev Prat 1997;47:1674–7.
100. Pinto AP, Lin MC, Sheets EE, Muto MG, Sun D, Crum CP. Allelic imbalance in lichen sclerosus, hyperplasia, and intraepithelial neoplasia of the vulva. Gynecol Oncol 2000;77:171–6.
101. Powell JJ, Wojnarowska F. Lichen sclerosus. Lancet 1999;353:1777–83.
102. Purcell KG, Spencer LV, Simpson PM, Helman SW, Oldfather JW, Fowler JF, Jr. HLA antigens in lichen sclerosus et atrophicus. Arch Dermatol 1990;126:1043–5.
103. Ridley CM. Chronic erosive vulval disease. Clin Exp Dermatol 1990;15:245–52.
104. Ridley CM, Buckley CH. Darier's disease localized to the vulva. Br J Obstet Gynaecol 1991;98:112.
105. Saad RW, Domloge-Hultsch N, Yancey KB, Benson PM, James WD. Childhood localized vulvar pemphigoid is a true variant of bullous pemphigoid. Arch Dermatol 1992;128:807–10.
106. Saenz AM, Cirocco A, Avendano M, Gonzalez F, Sardi JR. Papular acantholytic dyskeratosis of the vulva. Pediatr Dermatol 2005;22:237–9.
107. Salopek TG, Siminoski K. Vulvitis circumscripta plasmacellularis (Zoon's vulvitis) associated with autoimmune polyglandular endocrine failure. Br J Dermatol 1996;135:991–4.
108. Schrodt BJ, Callen JP. Metastatic Crohn's disease presenting as chronic perivulvar and perirectal ulcerations in an adolescent patient. Pediatrics 1999;103:500–2.
109. Scurry J, Dennerstein G, Brenan J, Ostor A, Mason G, Dorevitch A. Vulvitis circumscripta plasmacellularis. A clinicopathologic entity? J Reprod Med 1993;38:14–18.
110. Short KA, Kalu G, Mortimer PS, Higgins EM. Vulval squamous cell carcinoma arising in chronic hidradenitis suppurativa. Clin Exp Dermatol 2005;30:481–3.
111. Sideri M, Rognoni M, Rizzolo L, et al. Antigens of the HLA system in women with vulvar lichen sclerosus. Association with HLA-B21. J Reprod Med 1988;33:551–4.
112. Smith YR, Haefner HK. Vulvar lichen sclerosus: pathophysiology and treatment. Am J Clin Dermatol 2004;5:105–25.
113. Sobel JD. Candida vulvovaginitis. Semin Dermatol 1996;15:17–28.
114. Sonnendecker EW, Sonnendecker HE, Wright CA, Simon GB. Recalcitrant vulvodynia. A clinicopathological study. S Afr Med J 1993;83:730–3.
115. Soufir N, Queille S, Liboutet M, et al. Inactivation of the CDKN2A and the p53 tumour suppressor genes in external genital carcinomas and their precursors. Br J Dermatol 2007;156:448–53.
116. Souillet AL, Truchot F, Jullien D, et al. [Perianal streptococcal dermatitis]. Arch Pediatr 2000;7:1194–6.
117. Srodon M, Stoler MH, Baber GB, Kurman RJ. The distribution of low- and high-risk HPV types in vulvar and vaginal intraepithelial neoplasia (VIN and VaIN). Am J Surg Pathol 2006;30:1513–8.
118. Sullivan AK, Straughair GJ, Marwood RP, Staughton RC, Barton SE. A multidisciplinary vulva clinic: the role of genito-urinary medicine. J Eur Acad Dermatol Venereol 1999;13:36–40.
119. Tan AL, Jones R, McPherson G, Rowan D. Audit of a multidisciplinary vulvar clinic in a gynecologic hospital. J Reprod Med 2000;45:655–8.
120. Urano S. Localized bullous pemphigoid of the vulva. J Dermatol 1996;23:580–2.
121. Vaclavinkova V, Neumann E. Vaginal involvement in familial benign chronic pemphigus (Morbus Hailey–Hailey). Acta Derm Venereol 1982;62:80–1.
122. Wieselthier JS, Pincus SH. Hailey–Hailey disease of the vulva. Arch Dermatol 1993;129:1344–5.
123. Yoganathan S, Bohl TG, Mason G. Plasma cell balanitis and vulvitis (of Zoon). A study of 10 cases. J Reprod Med 1994;39:939–44.
124. Zaki I, Dalziel KL, Solomonsz FA, Stevens A. The under-reporting of skin disease in association with squamous cell carcinoma of the vulva. Clin Exp Dermatol 1996;21:334–7.
125. Zolnoun D, Hartmann K, Lamvu G, As-Sanie S, Maixner W, Steege J. A conceptual model for the pathophysiology of vulvar vestibulitis syndrome. Obstet Gynecol Surv 2006;61:395–401; quiz 23.
126. Zosmer A, Kogan S, Frumkin A, Dgani R, Lifschitz-Mercer B. Unsuspected involvement of the female genitalia in pemphigus vulgaris. Eur J Obstet Gynecol Reprod Biol 1992;47:260–3.

APPENDIX 2.1   COMMON CLINICAL DERMATOLOGIC TERMS

Atopy (adj. **atopic**)   Inherited predisposition to hypersensitivity reactions when exposed to certain allergens. Atopic disorders include asthma, allergic rhinitis, atopic eczema, and urticaria.

Dermatosis (pl. **dermatoses**)   A non-specific term used to denote a cutaneous eruption but generally excluding solitary or multiple benign or malignant skin lesions.

Eczematous   A pattern of inflammatory skin changes characterized in the acute stages by erythema and exudation, and in the chronic form by dry, scaling, fissured skin.

Erythema   Redness of the skin due to vasodilatation of cutaneous blood vessels. This may result from inflammation or from physiologic or pathologic changes in cutaneous vasculature.

Hart's line   A visible line on the inner surface of the labia minora indicating the change from vestibular epithelium (endoderm-derived) to skin (ectoderm-derived).

Lichenification   Changes seen in skin after long-standing itching and scratching. The skin becomes thickened with exaggeration of normal skin markings. Hyperpigmentation is often a feature.

Lichenoid   Rashes sharing clinical features (of shiny purple-red papules and plaques) with lichen planus. Examples include certain drug eruptions and photosensitive disorders.

Psoriasiform   A pattern of skin inflammation in which scaling plaques are reminiscent of psoriasis. Certain drug eruptions and forms of cutaneous T-cell lymphoma are examples of psoriasiform rashes.

Vulval vestibule   That part of the vulva lying between Hart's line and the hymen. Contains the openings of the major and minor vestibular glands.

APPENDIX 2.2   COMMON DERMATOPATHOLOGIC TERMS

TERMS APPLIED TO THE SURFACE KERATIN LAYER

Hyperkeratosis   Describes thickening of the keratin layer inappropriate to the site. The thickness of the keratin layer varies according to site, for example it is normally very thin on the trunk, but very thick on the soles and palms. Hyperkeratosis may be **orthokeratotic** (in which the keratin is devoid of nuclear remnants) or **parakeratotic** (in which the keratin layer contains the remnants of nuclei from the underlying epidermis). As a general rule, orthokeratotic hyperkeratosis is associated with a thickening of the granular layer of the epidermis (**hypergranulosis**) and parakeratotic hyperkeratosis is associated with diminution of the granular layer. Parakeratosis is almost always indicative of an active abnormality in the underlying epidermis, which should be sought when parakeratosis is seen. Orthokeratotic hyperkeratosis with hypergranulosis is seen in lichen simplex chronicus (see Figure 1.6). Parakeratosis may be seen in active acute dermatitis (see Figure 1.3) and may be marked in psoriasis (see Figure 1.8).

TERMS APPLIED TO THE EPIDERMIS

Acantholysis The name given to a process in which there is loss of adhesion and contact between adjacent epidermal keratinocytes such that the cells separate one from the other with breakdown of their linking desmosomal junctions, leading to an increase in the intercellular space. Eventually the intercellular spaces become large and fluid-filled, the separated acantholytic cells tending to become rounded off and floating singly or in small clumps within a variably sized bulla. Acantholysis in the vulva is most commonly seen in Hailey–Hailey disease (see Figure 1.29) and in pemphigus vegetans (see Figure 1.30).

Acanthosis The term used to describe inappropriate thickening of the epidermal layer. The thickness of the epidermal layer varies according to site, being thin on the trunk and proximal limbs, and thick in areas such as the palms and soles where the skin is exposed to regular frictional forces. Normally thin epidermis frequently undergoes thickening in response to increased frictional forces; in the vulva this is usually due to repeated scratching (see lichen simplex chronicus). There are particular patterns of acanthosis which may assist in histologic diagnosis.

Basal layer hydropic degeneration A particular pattern of vacuolation and swelling of the cytoplasm of the basal cells of the epidermis due to the intracellular accumulation of water. This is followed by the death of the affected basal cells, some of which appear as eosinophilic spherical bodies in the basal layer or just beneath, called **colloid** or **Civatte bodies**. In the vulva, the combination of basal layer hydropic degeneration and the presence of colloid/Civatte bodies is most frequently seen in the various patterns of lichen planus (see Figure 1.19), but is also seen elsewhere in the body in systemic lupus erythematosus and dermatomyositis.

Bullae (sing. **bulla**) A bulla is another form of blister which is larger than a vesicle (a vesicle is less than 5 mm in diameter and a bulla greater than 5 mm in diameter). Although most vesicles arise within the epidermis, bullae can arise either within the epidermis or beneath the dermoepidermal junction.

Civatte body See **Basal layer hydropic degeneration**.

Exocytosis Term used to describe an invasion of the epidermis by chronic inflammatory cells (mainly lymphocytes) in associa-

tion with spongiosis and vesiculation. It is a common histologic feature of inflammatory skin disease of many types.

Papillomatosis Term used to describe the histologic appearance of marked exaggeration of the dermal papillae by elongation of rete ridges on the dermoepidermal junction and the throwing up into exaggerated folds of the surface epidermis. In the vulva, papillomatosis of epidermis is most frequently seen in condylomata acuminata and papular and keratotic warts.

Psoriasiform acanthosis In this pattern, the surface of the epidermis is mainly flat but the thickening is due to marked downward elongation of the rete ridges. The epidermis is therefore not uniformly thickened, the areas between rete ridges often showing marked thinning of the epidermis. This is the pattern of epidermal thickening seen most obviously in active psoriasis, hence its name.

Pustule A pustule is a vesicle which contains inflammatory cells in large numbers, usually neutrophil polymorphs. The presence of the cells renders the vesicle fluid thick and creamy, and the clinically visible vesicle appears white. Pustules may be seen in the vulva in bacterial infections (particularly staphylococcal and streptococcal) and in some forms of psoriasis.

Spongiosis The name given to focal intercellular edema of the epidermis leading to partial separation of the epidermal cells by edema fluid, particularly in the prickle cell layer. Accumulation of fluid between epidermal cells causes spaces to appear which may coalesce to form fluid-filled vesicles.

Vesicles Small discrete accumulations of fluid within the epidermis to form a tiny blister, which may be apparent clinically. Vesicle formation usually follows spongiosis (see above).

TERMS APPLIED TO THE DERMIS

Lichenoid infiltrate An infiltrate of chronic inflammatory cells (predominantly lymphocytes) which occupies a band-like zone in the upper dermis immediately beneath the dermoepidermal junction. It is a characteristic feature of lichen planus and the very early stages of lichen sclerosus.

Urticaria Histologically manifested by dermal edema. This may be difficult to detect histologically, but useful clues are the presence in the upper dermis of dilated small lymphatics, and the presence of a distinct pale zone of edema around upper dermal blood vessels. In acute urticaria (rarely biopsied) upper dermal capillaries and venules show margination of neutrophils; in persistent chronic urticaria there is often a scanty perivascular lymphocytic infiltrate in which special stains (e.g., chloroacetate esterase) reveal increased numbers of mast cells. Urticaria of the vulva is an important cause of itchiness, and the histologic diagnosis is frequently missed because the changes are so subtle.

Vulvar cysts, neoplasms, and related lesions

Christopher R. Shea   Maria Angelica Selim   Stanley J. Robboy

CYSTS

FOLLICULAR (EPIDERMOID) CYST

Definition
Follicular cyst is a cystic dilatation of the hair follicle epithelium.

Clinical features
The follicular cyst generally presents as a solitary, creamy-white or yellowish lesion on the labium majus (Figure 3.1). It is generally asymptomatic, but rupture may induce inflammation presenting as enlargement, tenderness, erythema, and induration. The follicular cyst usually occurs spontaneously and after age 30. Onset at an early age or occurrence in great numbers should prompt consideration of Gardner syndrome. The term 'epidermal inclusion cyst' is a misnomer when used to refer to the follicular cyst. True epidermal inclusion cysts, secondary to traumatic entrapment of epidermis beneath the surface, do occasionally occur, e.g., in old episiotomy scars or in some cases of female genital mutilation.[91,154] Likewise, 'sebaceous cyst' is an incorrect term for follicular cyst. The milium, a variant of the follicular cyst, occurs as a 1–2 mm, white, asymptomatic papule on the labium minus; some milia may alternatively represent cystically dilated eccrine ducts. Open comedones (follicular ostia dilated by keratinous plugs) can occur on the hair-bearing vulvar skin in the elderly. Idiopathic calcinosis occurs commonly in the scrotum but is rare in the vulva, where it usually presents as solitary or multiple hard nodules in the labia majora of young girls. Some cases may represent calcification of follicular cysts.

Microscopic features
Most vulvar follicular cysts represent dilatations of the most distal portion of the follicle, the infundibulum, being composed of a thin, flat, squamous epithelium lacking rete ridges, containing a granular layer, and filled with loose-packed keratin. In contrast, cysts of the more proximal follicular isthmus lack a granular layer and contain dense-packed keratin; such isthmic–catagen cysts (also designated as 'pilar' or 'tricholemmal') occur commonly on the scalp but are rare on the vulva. Hybrid cysts with combined infundibular/isthmic features, or cysts exhibiting elements of the follicular matrix, are highly characteristic of Gardner syndrome. Idiopathic vulvar calcinosis discloses small calcific nodules in the dermis. Rupture of a follicular cyst may lead to leakage of keratin, exciting a florid acute and chronic inflammatory foreign-body reaction.

STEATOCYSTOMA MULTIPLEX

Definition
Widespread, multiple, thin-walled cysts of the skin, lined by *squamous epithelium*, and including lobules of *sebaceous* cells.

Clinical features
Steatocystoma multiplex is the dominantly inherited occurrence of numerous cysts exhibiting sebaceous ductal differentiation, from adolescence onwards. Solitary steatocystoma may also occur as an isolated finding. Rarely, cases first present as multiple cysts localized to the vulva at an older age.[119] The small, creamy-colored cysts mainly occur on the presternum, axillae, and abdomen, but can also affect the genital area, specifically the labia majora (Figure 3.2). They can be diagnosed clinically by incision, leading to drainage of an oily liquid.

Microscopic features
Steatocystomas are composed of an intricately folded, thin layer of stratified squamous epithelium lined internally by a corrugated, thin, compact, and strongly eosinophilic cuticle, and lacking a granular layer. The cyst wall and surrounding dermis usually contain small sebaceous glands (Figure 3.3). This finding raises the differential diagnosis of dermoid cyst, but the latter usually occurs near the orbit and is extremely rare in the vulva, and moreover has miniaturized hair follicles as well as sebaceous glands inserting into its wall.

BARTHOLIN CYST[89]

Definition
Bartholin cyst is the cystic dilatation of a major vestibular (Bartholin) gland or its duct.

Clinical features
Bartholin cyst is the most common form of vulvar cyst, being the presenting complaint for 2% of women during their annual gynecologic visit. The Bartholin glands (Figure 3.4) are located behind the labia minora and their ducts open into the posterior lateral vestibules, just anterior to the hymeneal tegmentum. Bartholin cysts result from blockage of the drainage duct and resultant retention of secretions, perhaps following infection. Bartholin cysts are most common in the reproductive years. If large, the cyst may partially obstruct the introitus. Bartholin cysts usually present as smooth-domed nodules, generally 1–10 cm in diameter. If brown or blue, they may be mistaken clinically for melanocytic nevi. The cysts contain watery, mucoid fluid or thicker mucus. They may recur after incision

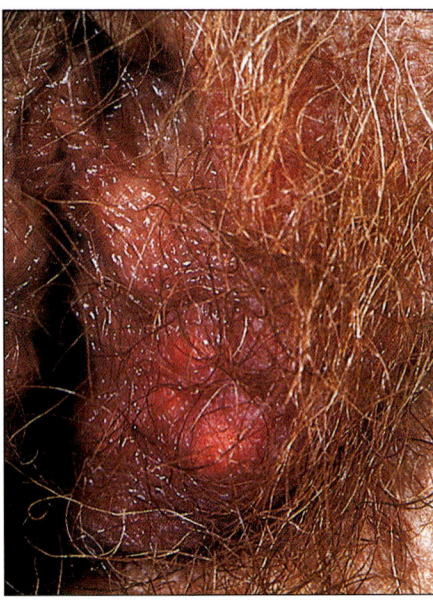

Fig. 3.1 Follicular cysts ('epidermal inclusion cysts'). Ruptured cysts become inflamed as a result of foreign body giant cell reaction to keratin leakage.

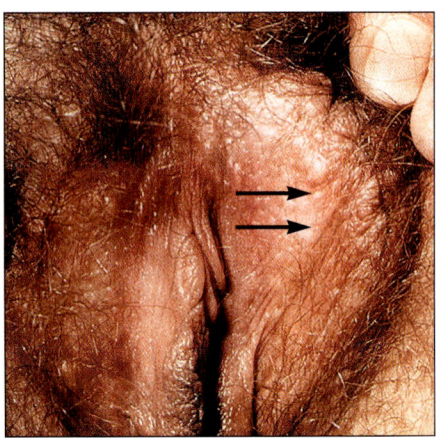

Fig. 3.2 Steatocystoma multiplex. This inherited disorder, sometimes involving the genitalia, shows multiple creamy-colored cysts (arrow).

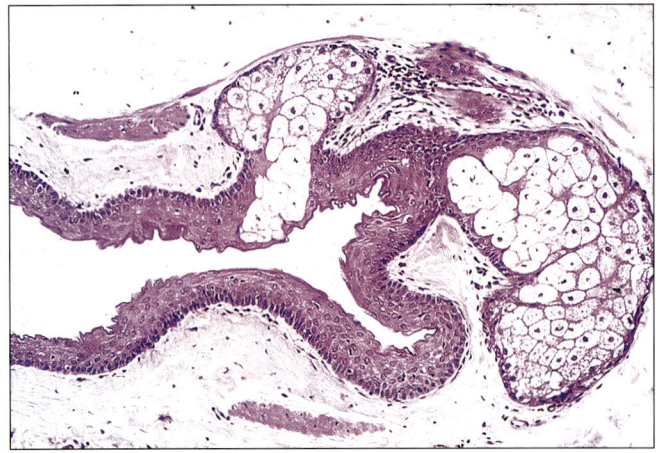

Fig. 3.3 Steatocystoma multiplex. Characteristic features include an apparently collapsed cyst with sebaceous units in the wall and a densely eosinophilic thin lining cuticle.

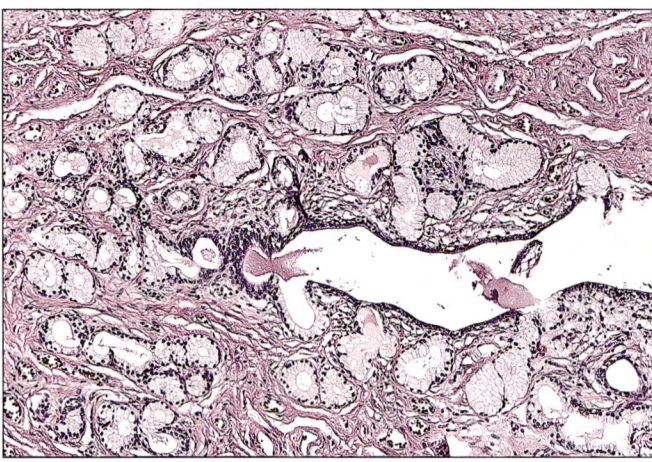

Fig. 3.4 Normal Bartholin gland. Simple tubuloalveolar glands with mucin-producing alveoli drain eventually into a central duct lined by transitional epithelium.

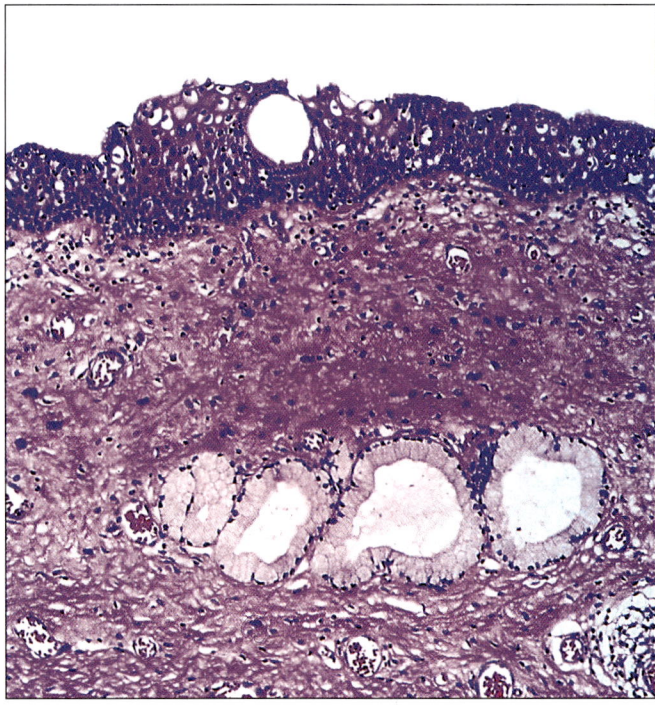

Fig. 3.5 Bartholin cyst. A thick transitional epithelium with focal squamous metaplasia lines the cyst wall (top). Normal mucus glands are frequently seen in the wall.

and drainage, and may then require surgical excision for control.

Microscopic features

Bartholin cysts show a lining of transitional epithelium, frequently exhibiting focal squamous metaplasia (Figure 3.5). Smaller mucus-filled cysts may show some remnant of the original mucus-secreting glandular epithelium, but it may be flattened or cuboidal. Normal remnants of mucus glands may be present adjacent to the cyst.

MUCINOUS CYST

Definition
Mucinous cyst is the cystic dilatation of a minor vestibular gland or its duct.

Clinical features
True mucinous cysts most commonly occur in the vulvar vestibule, including the medial labium minus and near the Bartholin glands. Onset is typically between puberty and the fourth decade, usually in parous women or those exposed to oral contraceptives. Mucinous cysts are 2 mm to 3 cm in diameter and are usually solitary. They may cause pain or urinary complaints. Excision is curative. They presumably are due to obstruction.

Microscopic features
These cysts are lined almost entirely by columnar or cuboidal mucus-secreting epithelium like that of endocervical glands (Figure 3.6). Foci of squamous metaplasia are sometimes present; they are considered to be of urogenital sinus origin.[118]

CILIATED CYST

Definition
A ciliated cyst is a cyst (most often of mucinous or Bartholin type) exhibiting ciliary differentiation.

The occasional cyst lined partially by ciliated columnar epithelium (Figure 3.7) usually represents a non-specific metaplastic change. Although sometimes associated with pregnancy or exogenous progesterone, inflammation of the vulvar vestibules (as in atopic dermatitis) may also contribute to the pathogenesis of the ciliated cyst.[55]

PARAURETHRAL (SKENE) GLAND CYST

Definition
Paraurethral gland cyst is the cystic dilatation of the paraurethral (Skene) gland or its duct.

Clinical features
The paired paraurethral glands (the female homologue of the male prostate gland) are located on either side of the urethral meatus. Ductal occlusion, probably a consequence of infection (e.g., gonococcal), leads to formation of a retention cyst, generally less than 2 cm in size, located in the upper lateral introitus. Paraurethral gland cysts occur in 1 per 2000–7000 women[19] and may be asymptomatic or lead to complaints of urinary obstruction or dyspareunia. Surgical excision should be performed only after medical therapy for any underlying infection.

Microscopic features
Paraurethral gland cysts are probably derived from the duct rather than the acini, being lined by transitional or stratified squamous epithelium upon a basement membrane, with only rare luminal cells containing intracytoplasmic mucin. Rarely, they contain calculi.

MESONEPHRIC-LIKE CYST

Definition
Mesonephric-like cyst is a thin-walled cystic space lined by a cuboidal or low columnar epithelium and encased by a small amount of smooth muscle.

Clinical features
These cysts occur in the lateral walls of the vulva as superficial, single, domed, blue or red cysts with clear, watery contents. They resemble mesonephric ducts but their embryologic basis is unclear.

CYST OF THE CANAL OF NUCK

Definition
Cyst of the canal of Nuck is a cystic remnant of the processus vaginalis peritonei.

Clinical features
These cysts are most common in the inguinal canal, where they must be differentiated from hernias. They also occur in the mons pubis and in the superior, outer region of the labium majus. Ultrasonography or magnetic resonance imaging may be helpful for definitive clinical diagnosis.[103,134] They are homol-

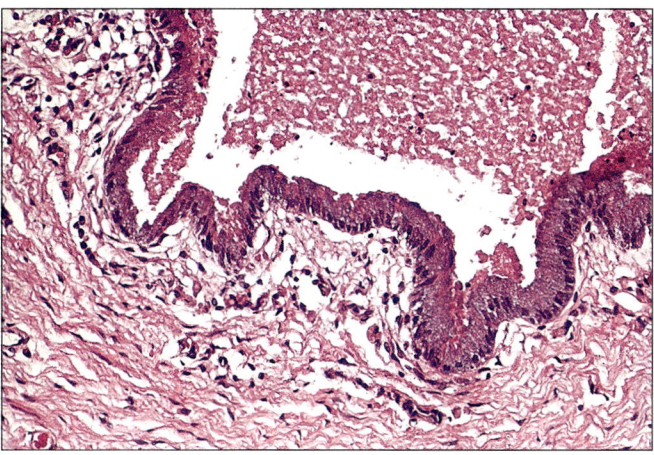

Fig. 3.6 Mucus (mucinous) cyst. Mucus-secreting columnar epithelium lines the cyst wall. Generally, the larger the cyst, the more flattened is the lining epithelium.

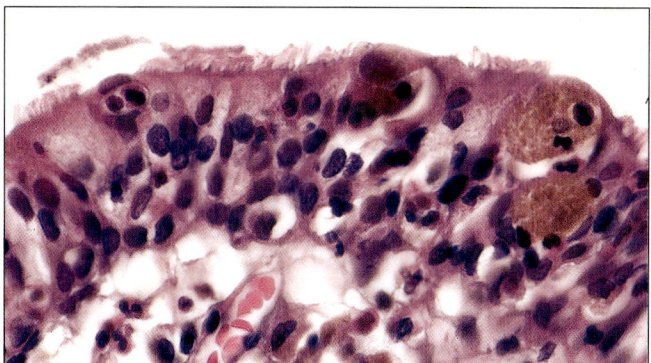

Fig. 3.7 Ciliated cells in a Bartholins gland cyst.

ogous to hydroceles in males. The processus vaginalis peritonei (canal of Nuck) is a rudimentary sac of peritoneal mesothelium carried down by the round ligament as it passes through the inguinal canal and inserts into the labium majus. Failure of this structure to obliterate normally during fetal development leads to blockage and cystic dilatation. While these cysts are usually solitary, more than one may arise if obstruction occurs at multiple sites. Generally asymptomatic, they may become tender to pressure, and may then require a procedure similar to herniorrhaphy.

Microscopic features
In their pristine state, these are thin-walled and lined by flattened mesothelium. By the time they present clinically, repeated external trauma has usually induced fibrosis of their walls, reduced or destroyed their mesothelial lining, and caused hemosiderin staining from old hemorrhage.

BENIGN KERATINOCYTIC NEOPLASMS

SEBORRHEIC KERATOSIS (VERRUCA SEBORRHEICA, BASAL CELL PAPILLOMA)

Definition
Seborrheic keratosis is a common, superficial, benign, flat, wart-like, often pigmented proliferation of keratinocytes in which keratin cysts are encased. In the vulva, as opposed to similar lesions in non-genital skin, seborrheic keratoses are believed related to human papillomavirus (HPV) infection.[4]

Clinical features
In the vulva it occurs after age 30 as a keratotic papule or plaque, often with a waxy or friable surface on the mons pubis, inguinal folds, and lateral labia majora. Occasionally, giant lesions up to several centimeters in diameter occur. The lesion characteristically appears to be 'stuck-on' to the surface of the skin. They are usually flesh-toned or tan, but sometimes appear black, simulating a melanocytic neoplasm. In such cases, specialized clinical study by skin-surface microscopy (dermatoscopy) can be helpful to exclude melanoma.[31] The characteristic horn pseudocysts can be seen clinically with the aid of a hand lens, as minute patulous depressions at the surface. Seborrheic keratoses may become irritated, traumatized, or inflamed, and may then exhibit secondary changes such as erythema or crusting.

Microscopic features
Seborrheic keratoses are raised above the surrounding skin, often have a smooth, flat base, and show surface hyperkeratosis, acanthosis, and horn pseudocysts, representing superficial invaginations from the epidermis (Figures 3.8 and 3.9). Melanin pigment is variable in amount. Cytologically they consist of bland, basaloid cells lacking significant nuclear atypia or mitotic figures. The papillary dermis is often sclerotic.

They may become irritated,[104] a phenomenon inducible experimentally by application of phorbol esters, and in clinical practice probably due to local mild trauma. Irritated seborrheic keratoses share many histologic features with inverted follicular keratoses, which tend, however, to be endophytic

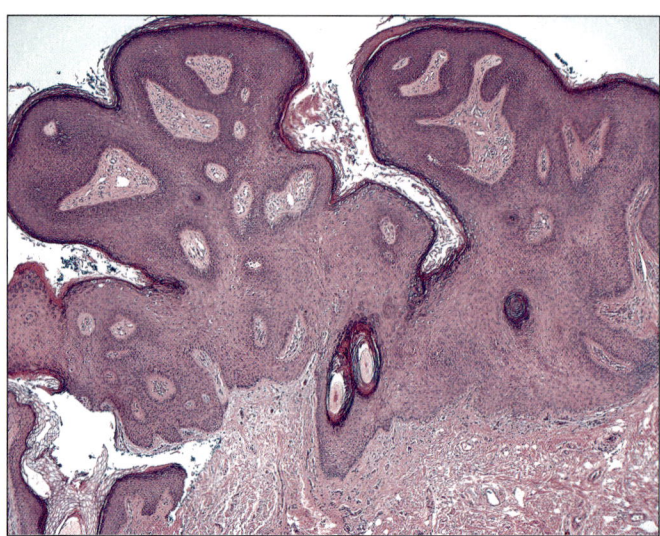

Fig. 3.8 Seborrheic keratosis. Invaginations lead to keratin-filled cysts.

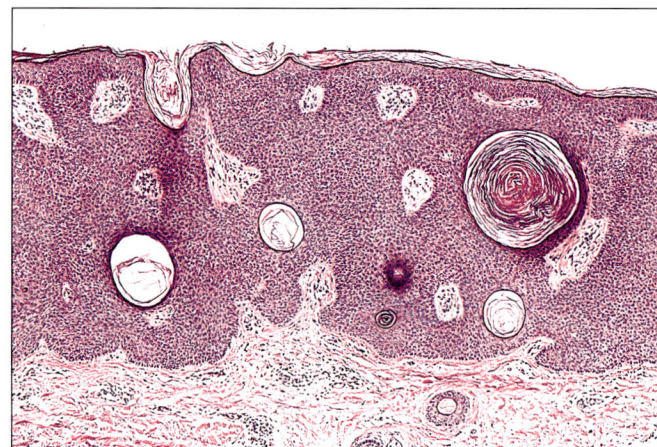

Fig. 3.9 Seborrheic keratosis. Like similar lesions on the non-genital skin, these are composed of small dark-staining basaloid cells and often contain horn cysts.

rather than exophytic. In either lesion, a variety of histologic alterations occur including inflammation, mitotic figures, dyskeratosis, parakeratosis, spongiosis, and formation of 'squamous eddies', i.e., whorled, rounded aggregates of cells resembling eddy currents in a stream. When prominent, these changes are sometimes overinterpreted as squamous cell carcinoma.[120] The key features pointing to the correct, benign diagnosis are the lack of significant cytologic atypia or of a frankly invasive growth pattern into the dermis. Occasionally moderate nuclear atypia is seen in the context of trauma or inflammation. When in doubt, it is prudent to diagnose such lesions as seborrheic keratoses with atypia, and to recommend close clinical follow-up or conservative re-excision.

KERATOACANTHOMA

Definition
Keratoacanthoma is a rapidly growing keratinocytic neoplasm that may be umbilicated and invades the dermis but rarely

metastasizes. It usually resolves spontaneously, even in the immunocompetent host. While increasingly accepted as a biologically low-grade variant of squamous cell carcinoma, some still consider it as a benign tumor *sui generis*.

Clinical features

Keratoacanthoma most often occurs on sun-exposed skin and is relatively rare on the vulva (being largely confined to the labia majora of elderly women).[22,50,99] However, its recognition is important because of its clinical and histologic similarity to conventional, invasive squamous cell carcinoma. The typical history is of sudden, rapid growth of a raised nodule having a central crater filled with compact keratin. Left alone, the crater widens but becomes shallower over a period of 3–6 months, ultimately followed by slow, spontaneous, complete regression. Most are solitary but crops of eruptive keratoacanthomas occur in the Ferguson Smith and Gryzbowski variants. Some patients also have multiple keratoacanthomas as a part of the Muir–Torre syndrome, comprising sebaceous neoplasms (benign and malignant) and colonic adenocarcinoma among other visceral tumors.[127]

Microscopic features

Keratoacanthoma consists of well-differentiated squamous epithelium with a central orthokeratotic mass opening onto the skin surface. Architecturally, it shows a well-circumscribed, symmetrical, umbilicated or crateriform, relatively superficially invaginated epithelium, rather than deeply infiltrating or irregular tongues of tumor (Figure 3.10). Notably, there is generally no high-grade atypia (VIN 3) of the surface epidermis. The tumor cells have abundant, glassy cytoplasm, and generally mild to moderate nuclear atypia (Figure 3.11). Several other histologic features said to discriminate between keratoacanthoma and conventional squamous cell carcinoma (e.g., presence of neutrophilic abscesses and intraepithelial elastic fibers in keratoacanthoma and predominance of eosinophils in the inflammatory infiltrate of keratoacanthoma versus plasma cells in conventional squamous cell carcinoma) are unreliable. Keratoacanthoma in the course of involution exhibits prominent thinning of the endophytic component and dermal fibrosis at the base.

Some pathologists dispute the concept of keratoacanthoma, except as a subset of squamous cell carcinoma.[61] However, the term can be useful when applied strictly to tumors that have many histologic features of conventional squamous cell carcinoma, but that may nevertheless undergo spontaneous resolution and therefore may not require radical extirpation. For this reason and with only the greatest of caution, should the diagnosis of keratoacanthoma be made in immunocompromised patients, who may not mount a host response adequate to induce regression. Moreover, atypical features such as extensive parakeratosis, acantholysis, high-grade atypia, focal infiltrative growth pattern, necrosis, or atypical mitotic figures mandate strong diagnostic consideration of conventional squamous cell carcinoma.

PREMALIGNANT KERATINOCYTIC NEOPLASMS

VULVAR INTRAEPITHELIAL NEOPLASIA (VIN)

Definition

VIN is a spectrum of intraepidermal pathology of the vulvar skin or mucosa, ranging from mild atypia (dysplasia) to severe cytologic and architectural abnormality equivalent to squamous cell carcinoma *in situ*.[73]

Clinical features

When symptomatic, the patient usually complains of irritation and soreness. The clinical appearances of VIN are extremely variable and may involve the skin, mucosa, or both. The range of appearances varies from banal erythematous patches, through variably verruciform plaques, to deeply pigmented macules or plaques (Figures 3.12 and 3.13). There is no absolute correlation between the pathologic grade and the clinical appearances, but grossly thickened plaques are more likely to show high-grade histopathologic changes (VIN 3). VIN may extend widely onto the perineum. Even mutilating surgical excision holds no guarantee of cure since local recurrence is frequent.[80] The strongest factor predicting recurrence is the presence of tumor at the resection margin.[71] Patients with VIN 3 require close examination of the vagina, cervix, perineum, and anal canal since these sites may harbor similar changes.[63] Staining the vulva with a 1% solution of toluidine blue is one

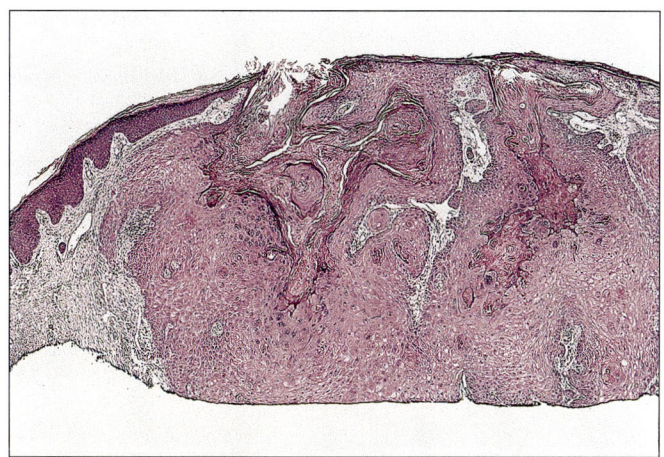

Fig. 3.10 Keratoacanthoma.

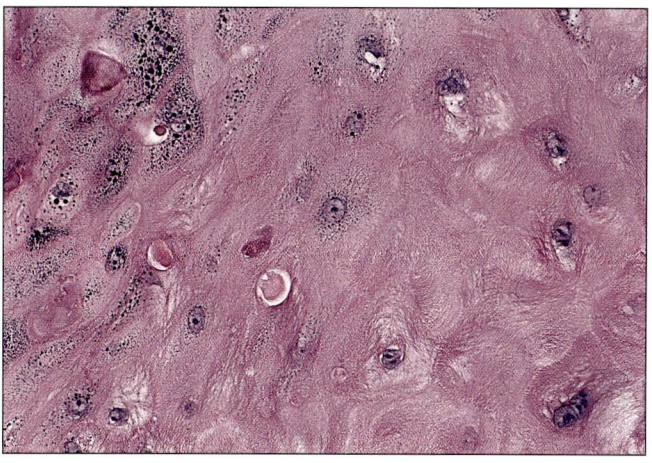

Fig. 3.11 Keratoacanthoma: detail of squamous cells.

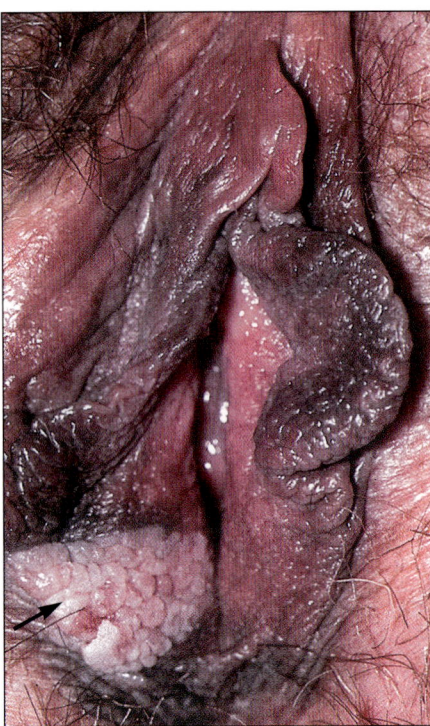

Fig. 3.12 Plaque of warty VIN 3 (arrow). The young woman also had cervical dysplasia.

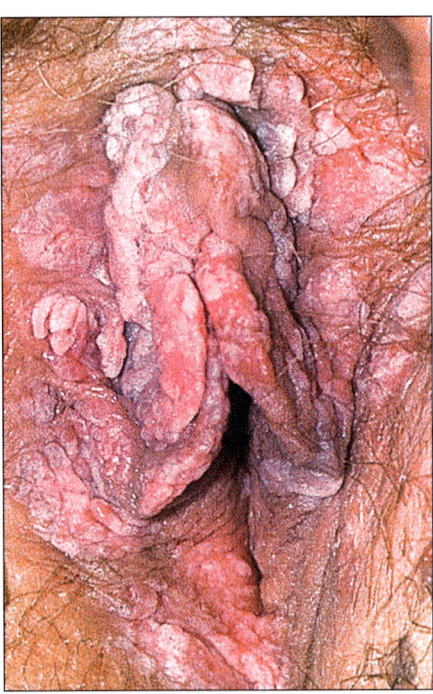

Fig. 3.13 Extensive warty VIN 3. This young lady had similar lesions in the perianal skin.

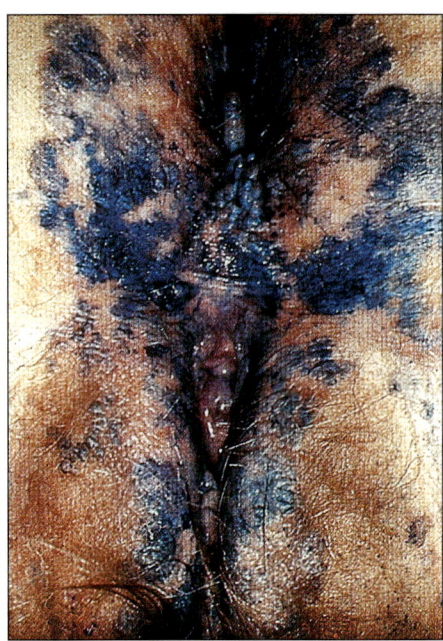

Fig. 3.14 Vulva stained with toluidine blue. Toluidine blue stains the lesion, reflecting the enormous quantity of nuclear material in the involved areas, and the minimal cytoplasm present.

virus is also commonly found (42%), but HPV 16 is rare (6%). While HPV 16 is the type most commonly associated with development of VIN-related squamous cell carcinoma, comparison of the HPV distribution in both the vagina and vulva suggests that vaginal intraepithelial neoplasia (VaIN) is more closely related to CIN than to VIN.[132]

Microscopic features

VIN is divided into grades 1–3, by analogy to CIN. The histologic criteria are:

- VIN 1 (Figure 3.15): dysplastic keratinocytes at all levels of the epithelium, with the most atypical cells confined to the lower one-third
- VIN 2 (Figure 3.16): dysplastic keratinocytes at all levels of the epithelium, with the most atypical cells confined to the lower two-thirds
- VIN 3/squamous cell carcinoma *in situ* (Figure 3.17): dysplastic keratinocytes occupying the full-thickness of the epithelium, with loss of stratification of the upper layers.

As with CIN, the grading is more reproducible for more severely atypical lesions. Considerable discordance among pathologists exists at lower grades.[110] Because this lesion is so poorly reproducible, uncommon, and is thought by some to represent only reactive change or HPV effect, the International Society for the Study of Vulvovaginal Disease (ISSVD) omits the term altogether in its new terminology.

In turn, the ISSVD now divides VIN into warty, basaloid, and mixed patterns,[57a] but we have not found the distinction easy to apply in daily practice, and do not describe the subtypes in our institutional pathology reports. The more common 'warty' pattern of VIN (Figure 3.18) shows severe atypia throughout all epidermal layers, with nuclear and cytoplasmic pleomorphism, multinucleate cells, many mitotic figures (including suprabasal and abnormal forms), and koilocytosis.

effective method to identify VIN clinically (Figure 3.14).[69] As with cervical intraepithelial neoplasia (CIN)/squamous intraepithelial lesion (SIL), virtually all cases of VIN 3 are associated with high-risk HPV, type 16 being found in over 90% of cases.[132] In VIN 1 cases, low-risk virus is found in two-thirds of cases, with HPV type 6/11 accounting for more than 40%. High-risk

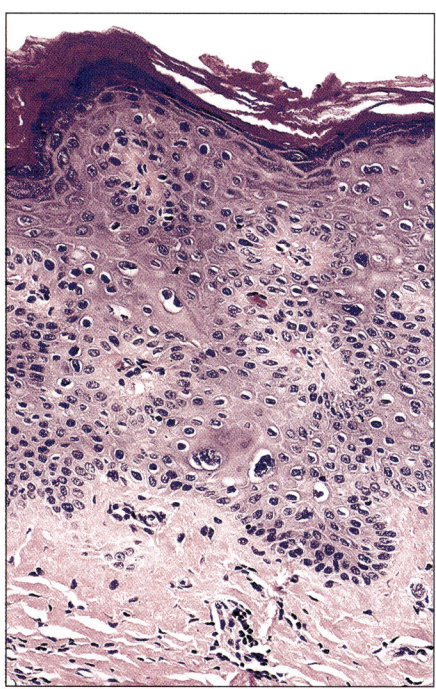

Fig. 3.15 VIN 1.

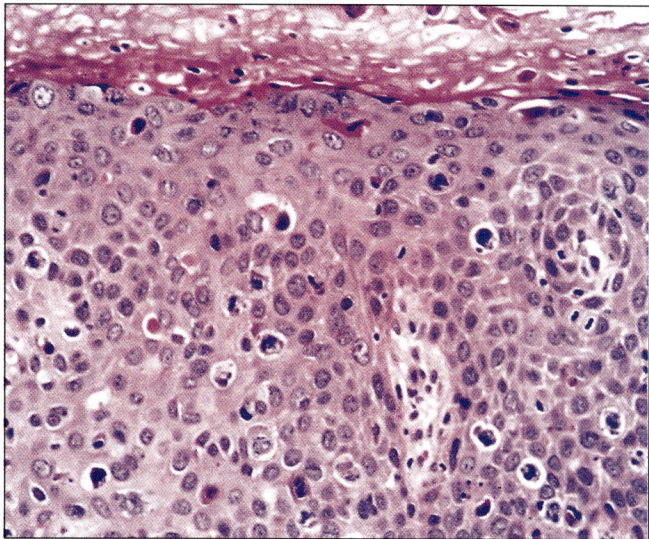

Fig. 3.17 VIN 3.

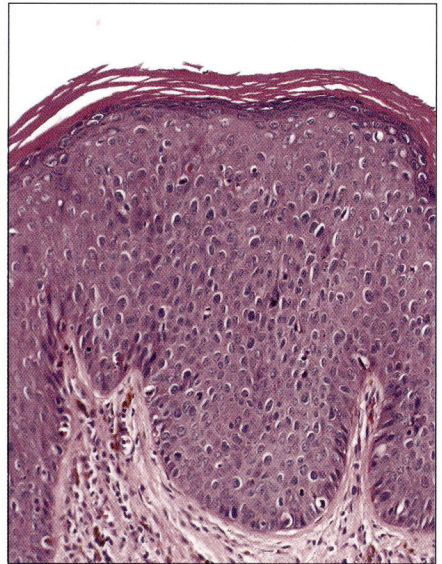

Fig. 3.16 VIN 2.

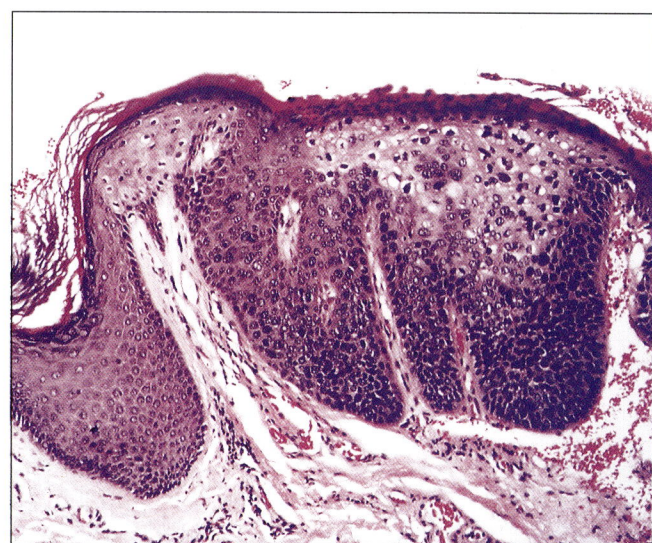

Fig. 3.18 Warty VIN 3. Koilocytic change is present near the surface.

The less common 'basaloid' pattern (Figure 3.19) is composed of smaller, more compact, atypical basaloid cells that extend from the basal layer to the surface. This variant usually displays much less pleomorphism, and atypical mitotic figures and koilocytes are rare.

As with CIN, the patterns of growth of high-grade VIN can be deceptively complex and yet still be *in situ*. The smooth borders are indicative that the tumor is not yet invasive (Figures 3.20 and 3.21).

The pathogenetic significance of VIN 1 and VIN 2 is not clearly defined. In particular, there is considerable debate about the risk of progression from VIN 1 and VIN 2 to VIN 3. More-

over, since epithelial changes similar to VIN 1 and sometimes VIN 2 occur in various forms of dermatitis having increased turnover of epithelial cells, mild vulvar atypia when taken out of context cannot necessarily be equated with VIN 1 or VIN 2. On the other hand, foci of VIN 1 and VIN 2 frequently occur in proximity to indisputable VIN 3, reinforcing the likely pathogenetic link among these categories. VIN is monoclonal in origin.[138]

The term 'VIN' reinforces currently accepted concepts of the multistep progression of tumors, and may reduce reliance on dichotomous and oversimplistic classification of lesions as either wholly benign or frankly malignant. However, the term has been criticized as overly broad, since a wide variety of neoplasms outside the dysplasia-to-carcinoma sequence (e.g., extramammary Pagets disease or even seborrheic keratosis) could also strictly be labeled as forms of intraepithelial neoplasia. Another concern is that this term may artificially divorce the early ('premalignant') changes from fully evolved carci-

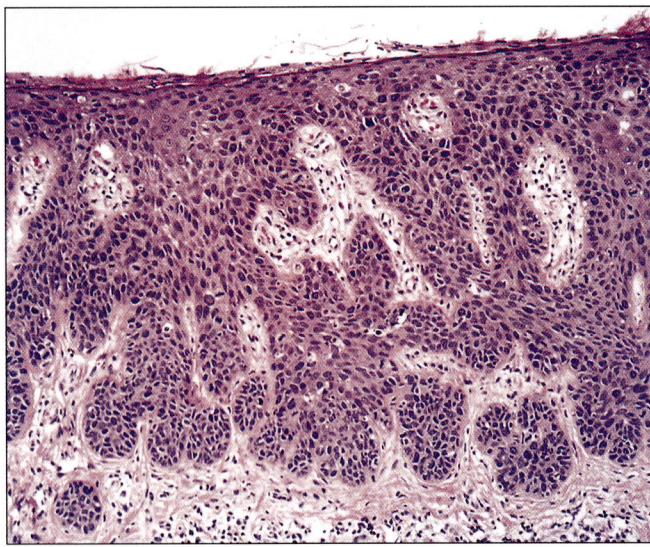

Fig. 3.19 Basaloid VIN 3. The neoplastic changes appear more uniform throughout the epidermal thickness than in warty VIN 3. The smooth borders indicate the tumor is *in situ* and not invasive.

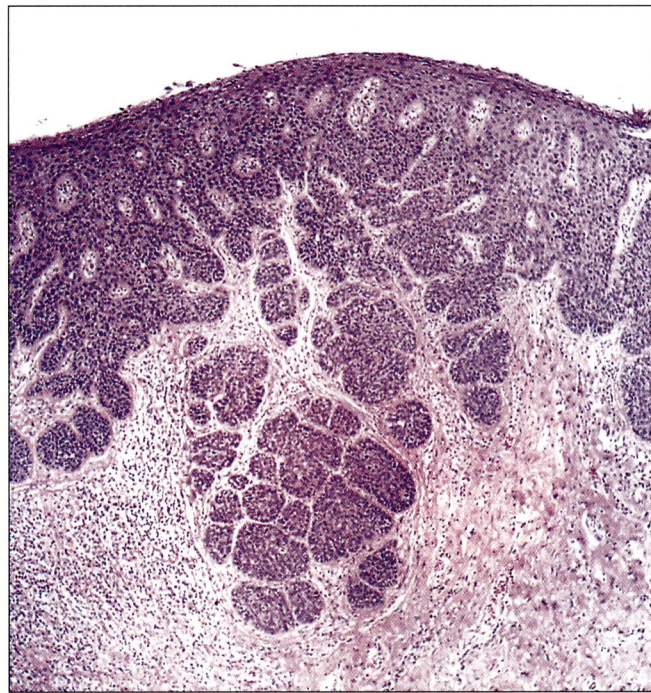

Fig. 3.21 Basaloid VIN 3 simulating microinvasive carcinoma.

Clinical features

Lesions are multiple, discrete, pigmented, warty papules that may coalesce into plaques. The distinction between bowenoid papulosis (usually VIN 1 or 2) and Bowen disease (i.e., VIN 3/squamous cell carcinoma *in situ*) was originally promulgated by dermatologists in order to obviate unnecessarily aggressive surgical therapy, since bowenoid papulosis often resolves spontaneously or with conservative therapy. Bowenoid papulosis reflects the early, infectious stages of HPV infection, which explains why it occurs commonly in women in their twenties and thirties.

Microscopic features

Severely atypical keratinocytes are seen at all levels of the epidermis, together with suprabasal mitotic figures and increased numbers of apoptotic cells. Most pathologists have abandoned the term 'bowenoid papulosis' for VIN, subtyped based on the disease's severity.

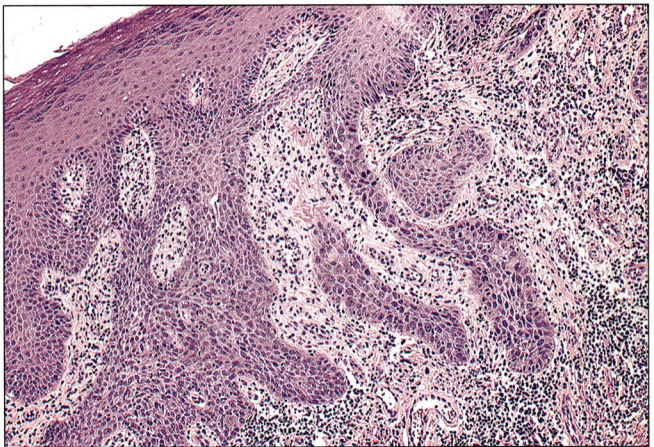

Fig. 3.20 VIN 3. The smooth borders suggest the tumor is *in situ* and not invasive. Compare with microinvasive carcinoma where the invasive tumor has sharply angulated borders.

noma. However, the term is firmly established and seems acceptable, with the firm understanding that VIN and invasive squamous cell carcinoma exist on a morphologic continuum and share a close pathogenetic relationship. By any name, the reported incidence of VIN has increased markedly in the last three decades, presumably due to increased infection by HPV.[67,68] Most pathologists prefer the term 'VIN 3/squamous cell carcinoma *in situ*' to 'Bowen disease', which is used primarily by dermatologists.

BOWENOID PAPULOSIS

Definition

Bowenoid papulosis is the occurrence, due to HPV infection, of genital or perineal papules exhibiting high-grade keratinocytic atypia.

MALIGNANT KERATINOCYTIC NEOPLASMS

MICROINVASIVE SQUAMOUS CELL CARCINOMA

Microinvasive squamous cell carcinoma is a keratinocytic neoplasm derived from the squamous mucosa in which the malignancy is less than 1 mm invasive when measured from the nearest epidermal–stromal junction of the overlying skin. Its epidemiology and pathogenesis are described in the sections on VIN (see above) and invasive squamous cell carcinoma (see below). Its gross appearance is no different from high-grade VIN (Figure 3.22).

In the earlier literature, the definition of microinvasive carcinoma was patterned after that of the cervix, the maximal invasive limit being 5 mm. This definition was abandoned as these lesions were quite commonly associated with metastases. Lesions less than 1 mm invasive generally have little if any metastatic potential,[87] although there are some reports associated with biologic malignancy.[129,147] The finding of microinvasive disease is most commonly discovered in specimens of VIN 3 removed by wide local excision or simple vulvectomies.[136]

A difficulty commonly encountered is differentiating between VIN 3 (carcinoma *in situ*) and early invasive disease (Figure 3.23). Like 'early stromal invasion' in the cervix, the earliest microinvasion may appear as an irregular tongue of cells jutting out irregularly from a bulbous tip (Figure 3.24A). Useful features when slightly more advanced are that the inva-

sive cells have increased and more eosinophilic cytoplasm when compared to neighboring basal cells, the small nests of tumor cells have irregularly irregular shapes, and the stroma is desmoplastic (Figure 3.24B,C). Not all of these features are always present. Commonly, the basal-most portions of the overlying squamous mucosa appear as bulbous tips where the basal-most cells have lost their normally ordered palisaded arrangement and the epithelial–stromal junction is blurred by a lymphocytic infiltrate. These latter features are worrisome, but by themselves are not diagnostic of microinvasion.

When the dysplastic epithelium has an increased thickness and the histologic sections are cut so as to be oblique, islands of tumor cells may seem detached within the dermis, deceptively simulating free invasion. Invasion should be diagnosed only when the clusters of squamous cells are irregular in size and outline, often with angulated borders.[58] In contrast, in VIN 3/squamous cell carcinoma *in situ*, the gland outlines are smoother and may be bulbous, and a desmoplastic stromal response absent (Figures 3.20 and 3.21). Paradoxical differentiation is also useful, when present. This is seen when there is haphazard differentiation or when the cells appear enlarged at the advancing edge of the irregular 'tongue' of squamous epithelium, in contrast to the more orderly differentiation of smaller 'basal' cells at the basement membrane to larger and more eosinophilic cells inwards and towards the epidermal surface.

INVASIVE SQUAMOUS CELL CARCINOMA

Definition
Squamous cell carcinoma (SCC) is a malignant keratinocytic neoplasm derived from epidermis or squamous mucosa and exhibiting variable degrees of atypia, invasiveness, and risk of metastasis.

Clinical features
SCC is the most common malignant tumor of the vulva, with an incidence of about 1.2 new cases/100 000 patient years.[83] SCC usually occurs in one of two clinical settings: (1) SCC associated with VIN; and (2) SCC associated with inflammatory disorders.[141,143] The former occurs almost exclusively in women under the age of 60.[68,81,105,123] There is a high incidence

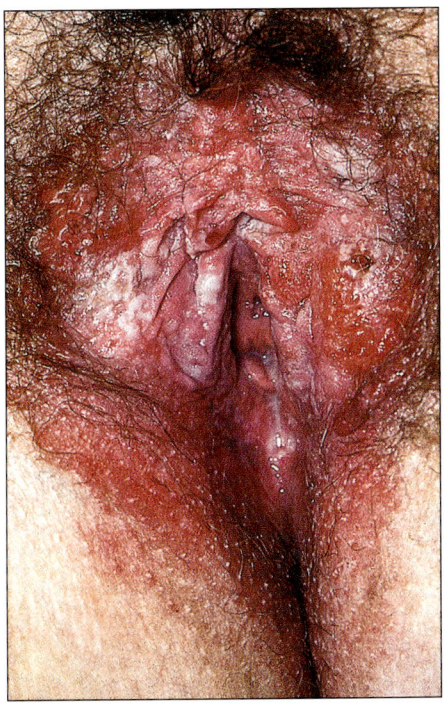

Fig. 3.22 Focal microinvasive squamous cell carcinoma arising in VIN 3. The inappropriate use of topical steroids resulted in the vulva's appearance.

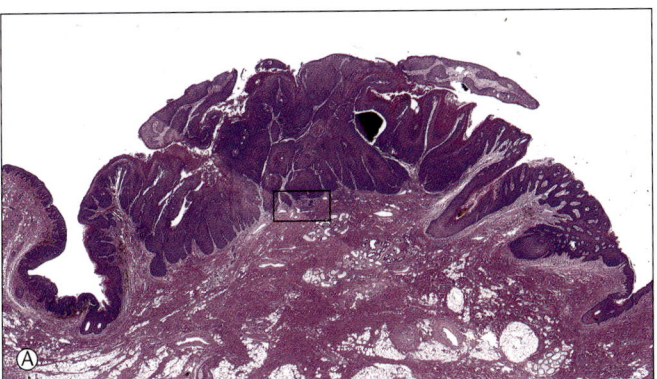 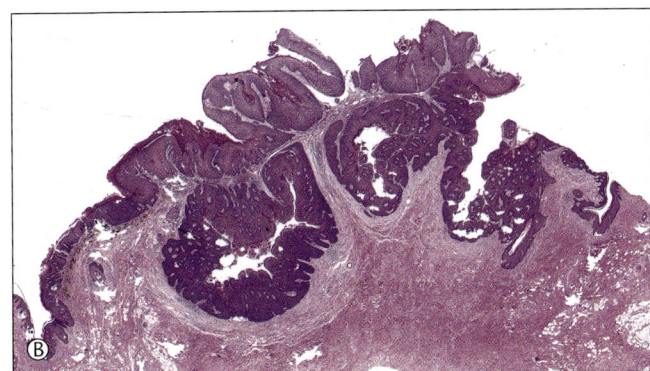

Fig. 3.23 Focal microinvasive squamous cell carcinoma arising in VIN 3. Both sections appear similar macroscopically with a large central region of squamous carcinoma *in situ*. **(A)** Small focus of sharply edged microinvasive tumor (box) arise from the most basal portion of the epidermis. **(B)** No such focus is found in the lower specimen, which is VIN 3.

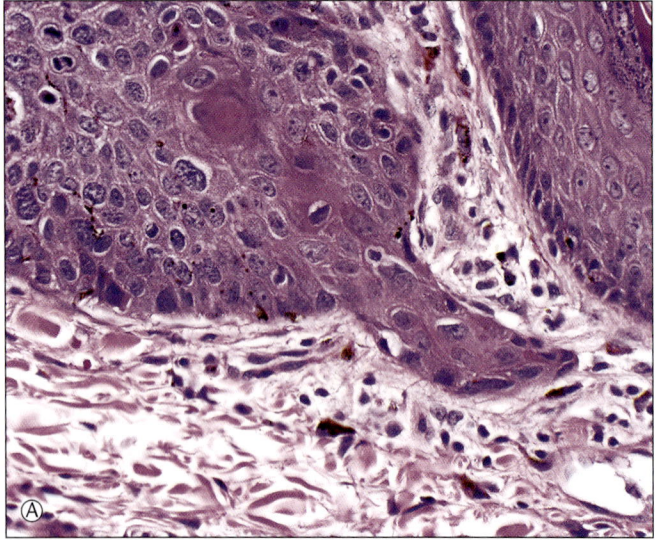

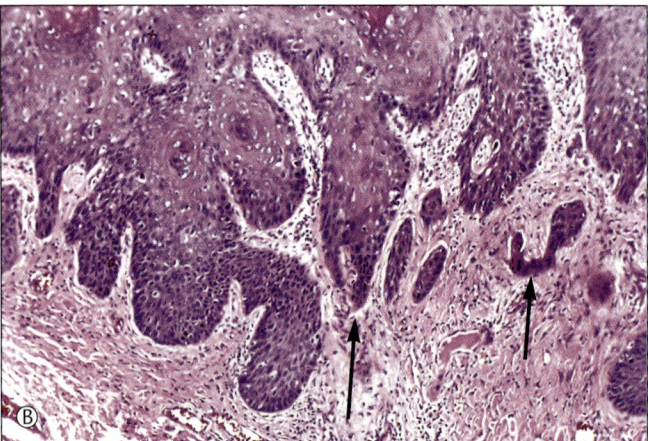

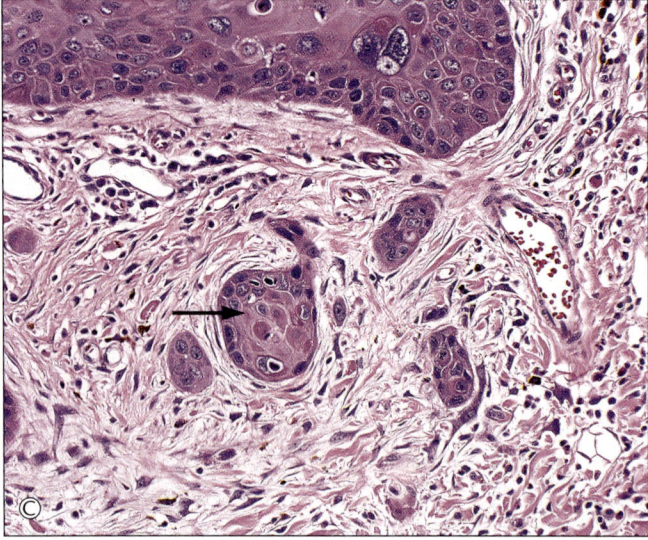

Fig. 3.24 Microinvasive squamous cell cancer. **(A)** Early stromal invasion with a tiny tongue of tumor protruding from the basal most epithelium. **(B)** The small nests of tumor cells are distinctly separate from the overlying epidermis, sometimes have irregularly irregular shapes, lie in a desmoplastic stroma and sometimes exhibit invasive cells with increased and more eosinophilic cytoplasm when compared to neighboring basal cells. The microinvasive component is easy to recognize (arrow). **(C)** Some foci are easily recognized as microinvasive (arrows), whereas the bulbous tips of the overlying epidermis that are composed of small basal cells are considered as VIN 3.

of associated lower genital tract neoplasia, particularly CIN and invasive cervical carcinoma.[63] In contrast, SCC associated with inflammatory dermatoses usually occurs in women aged 70 years or older. Many have a background disease of lichen sclerosus[15,17] or, to a lesser extent, chronic lichen planus.[44] Women with symptomatic lichen sclerosus reportedly have more than a 15% chance of later developing SCC.[15,16] This form of SCC is usually not associated with HPV infection, since *in situ* hybridization and polymerase chain reaction (PCR) methods usually fail to show evidence of the virus.

Clinically the tumor presents as an eroded plaque or ulcer (Figures 3.25 and 3.26) or nodule (Figure 3.27). The patient may complain of pruritus, pain, discharge, or bleeding, and these symptoms may be due to the antecedent chronic background vulvar disorder.

Regardless of the clinical setting in which it arises, SCC has a tendency to spread locally to infiltrate the vagina and distal urethra. The latter pattern is particularly common in the small proportion of tumors apparently originating in the clitoral region. Lymphatic spread initially takes tumor cells to the ipsi-

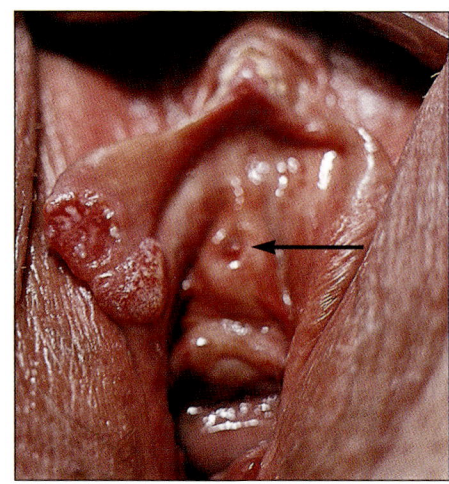

Fig. 3.25 Squamous cell carcinoma with ulceration (arrow). This elderly woman had no apparent predisposing disease.

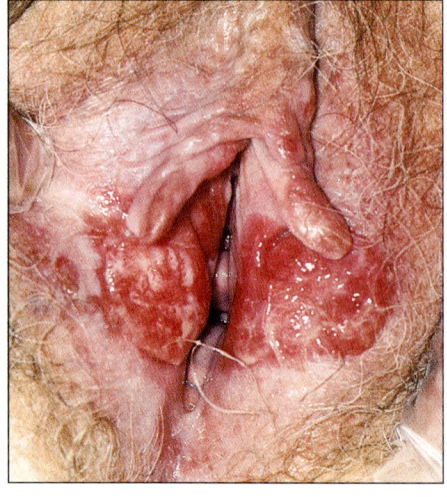

Fig. 3.26 Bilateral squamous cell carcinoma ('kissing cancers'). The tumor arose on a background of lichen sclerosus.

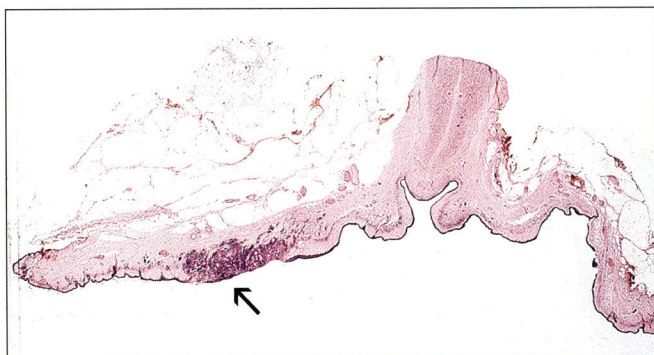

Fig. 3.27 Stage 1 squamous cell carcinoma. The tumor (arrow) is 1.8 cm in diameter. The specimen showing the tumor in the outer right side of the labium majus is a giant section through the clitoris, flanking labia minora and majora, and both the right and left sides of the vulva.

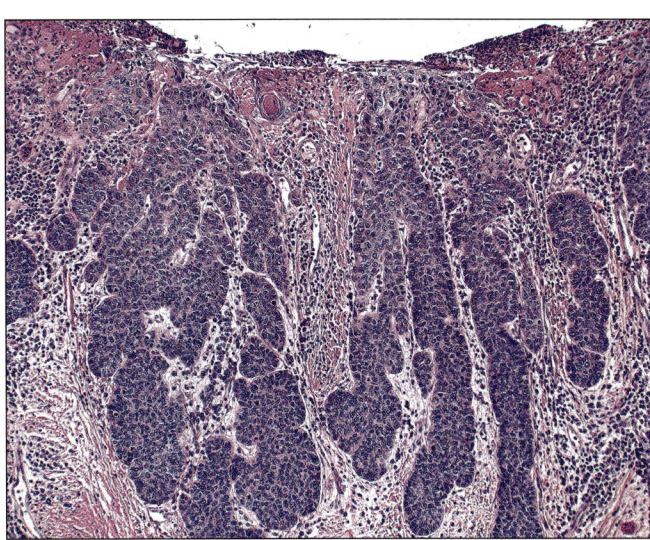

Fig. 3.28 Basaloid squamous cell carcinoma. Compare the jagged borders with basaloid VIN (Figure 3.21).

lateral inguinal lymph nodes, but more extensive lymphatic spread can encompass the contralateral inguinal nodes and the deep pelvic nodes around the iliofemoral vessels. If the superficial inguinal nodes are tumor-free, the deep pelvic nodes are unlikely to be involved. However, if the superficial inguinal nodes contain metastatic tumor, there is a 25% chance that tumor has also spread to the deep pelvic nodes, usually the medial external iliac nodes. Sentinel lymph node biopsy can also detect metastases.[30] Advanced, neglected SCC may locally invade the perirectal connective tissues, bladder, and even the pelvic bones. Such locally aggressive tumors usually have extensive inguinal and pelvic lymph node involvement, and there may also be evidence of blood-borne metastasis, e.g., to lungs and liver.

Microscopic features

Basaloid and warty variants of SCC can occur as with VIN. We have not found the distinction between the two types to be useful and do not specify the types in our reports. Basaloid carcinoma is composed of smaller, round to ovoid, basaloid cells, having a regular nucleus with limited pleomorphism (Figure 3.28), and usually arises in an area of basaloid-pattern VIN 3.

Warty SCC is a different entity from verrucous carcinoma, which, as discussed below, is a less aggressive tumor with pushing borders and bland cytology. Warty carcinoma is a conventional SCC composed of large squamous cells exhibiting marked pleomorphism including hyperchromatic nuclei, with an infiltrative growth pattern often composed of narrow, elongated strands of tumor. The term 'warty' refers both to this tumor's frequently exophytic profile and to the presence of koilocytosis.

Both basaloid and warty types of SCC associated with VIN often contain HPV 16 (75%), as does the VIN from which they arise. p16 is diffusely found in all of these HPV-positive cases.[125] Where there is associated CIN, the same HPV types can also be demonstrated in the cervix. In general, SCC associated with VIN tends to exhibit considerable nuclear pleomorphism, mitotic activity, and koilocytic change.

In contrast, most SCCs arising in the background of a vulvar dermatosis are well differentiated, with foci of keratinization, and tend to lack the high degree of atypia characteristic of VIN-associated SCC (Figure 3.29). A small percentage of dermatosis-associated SCCs are less well differentiated (Figure 3.30) or show an unusual histologic pattern such as spindle-cell (sarcomatoid) carcinoma (Figure 3.31) or acantholysis such that they may mimic adenocarcinomas. Clinicians treating vulvar carcinomas may miss the background inflammatory diseases. It is therefore important for the pathologist to examine the vulvar skin around and away from the tumor (particularly the margins of excisions) for evidence of these dermatoses (see Chapter 2).

Patients with disease-free resection margins greater than 8 mm do not experience local recurrences.[21] Histopathologic features associated with poor prognosis include large tumor size, extensive local invasion at time of first diagnosis, and involved regional lymph nodes.[95,98,109,117] A prominent stromal response, consisting of an admixture of myxoid change and immature collagen with fibroblasts at the tumor–stromal junction, is associated with more extensive lymph node metastases and a poorer survival rate.[2] Tumors exhibiting this prominent fibromyxoid response are typically flat or elevated, ulcerative lesions involving the clitoris, whereas tumors lacking this response are more commonly exophytic. Patients with four or more positive nodes, especially when associated with extracapsular extension, are nearly 6 times more likely to die from cancer and 10 times more likely to have recurrence than patients without metastases. The tumor's HPV status appears not to be prognostically important.[107]

One of the most common and difficult problems in the histopathology of SCC is to distinguish microinvasive tumor from VIN 3/SCC *in situ*. This is covered more fully above (see 'Microinvasive squamous cell carcinoma').

Natural history

The various factors are encompassed in the FIGO staging of vulvar SCC (Appendix A1). Approximate rates for 5-year survival are: Stage 1, 95%; Stage 2, 90%; Stage 3, 70%; Stage 4A, 20%; and Stage 4B, <10%. The overall 5-year survival rate is about 70%.

Treatment of vulvar SCC remains predominantly surgical, and there is a historical trend towards performance of less

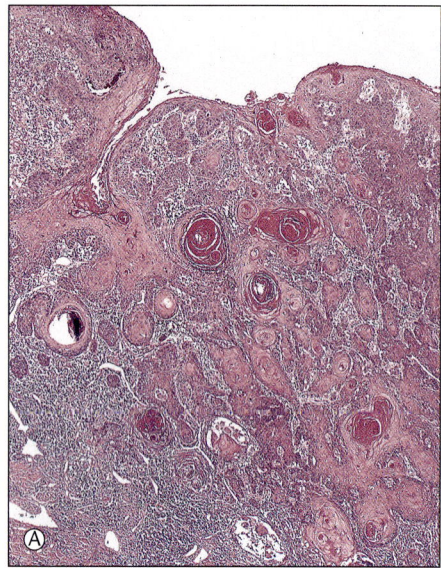

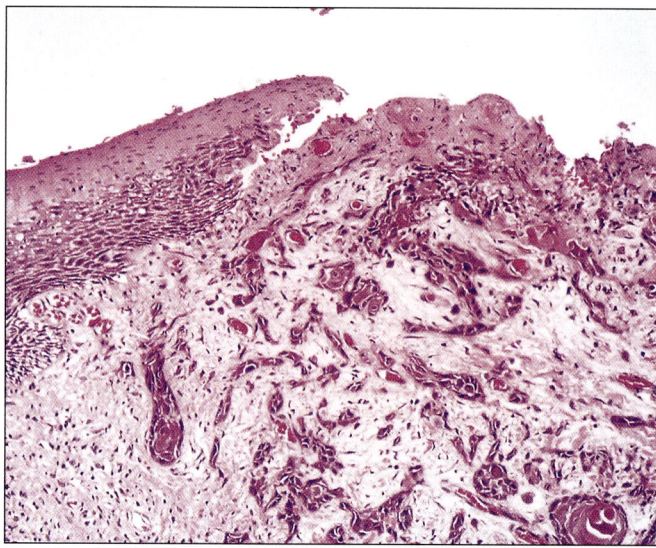

Fig. 3.30 Moderately differentiated invasive squamous cell carcinoma with some keratinization. This tumor was not associated with VIN. Adjacent vulvar skin should be carefully examined for evidence of lichen sclerosus and lichen planus in such cases.

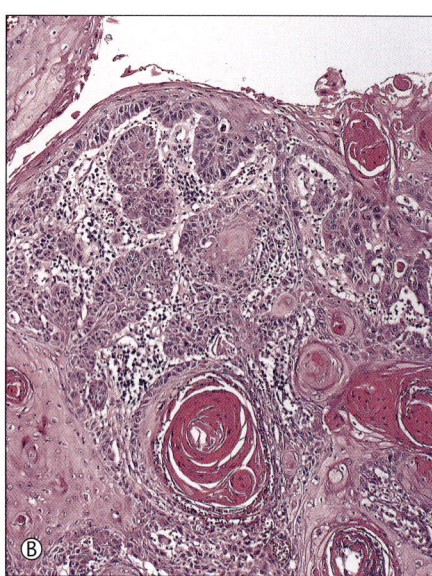

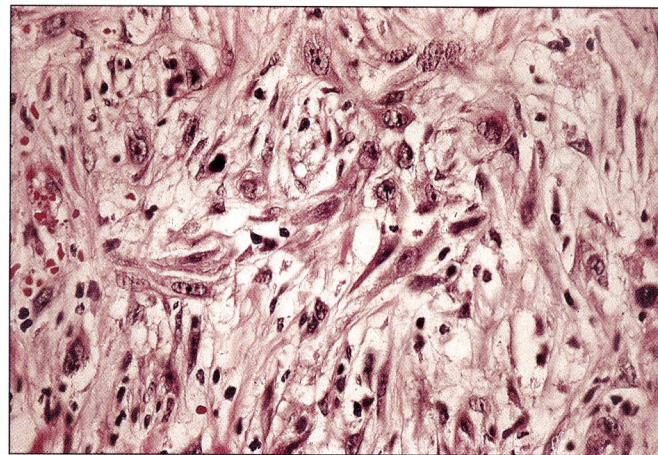

Fig. 3.29 **(A)** Invasive keratinizing squamous cell carcinoma. **(B)** Detail, keratin pearls.

Fig. 3.31 Squamous cell carcinoma, spindle cell variant (sarcomatoid).

radical surgery.[45] However, identification of tumor present or absent in the superficial ipsilateral regional inguinal nodes is crucial for staging.[28] Stage 0 is treated by wide local excision. Stage 1 tumors with a depth of invasion of 1 mm or less are currently treated with wide local excision without superficial node excision. Larger stage 1 tumors and stages 2 to 4A are treated by radical vulvectomy and bilateral inguinal/femoral lymph node removal, possibly followed by radiotherapy to pelvic nodes if the superficial nodes are involved by metastatic disease.

VERRUCOUS CARCINOMA[54,94]

Definition
Verrucous carcinoma is an exophytic, well-differentiated, indolent variant of SCC.

Clinical features
Verrucous carcinoma typically develops slowly into an exophytic mass that may eventually obscure the vulvar architecture. Its prognosis is nonetheless excellent as it does not metastasize to regional lymph nodes. However, disfiguring surgery is often necessary to achieve complete excision, and local slow regrowth may occur.

Pathology
Verrucous carcinomas typically are slow-growing lesions that develop as exophytic masses (Figure 3.32). On section, the tumor may have pushing borders into the underlying dermis, but does not show frank, destructive invasion (Figure 3.33). There is a characteristic verruciform architecture, with overlying hyperkeratosis and marked acanthosis (Figure 3.34). The rete ridges may be elongated and extend deeply into the dermis, but characteristically have a bulbous contour. Keratin pearl formation may be found even in the lesion's deepest extent. Nuclei generally show little or no cytologic atypia. The most

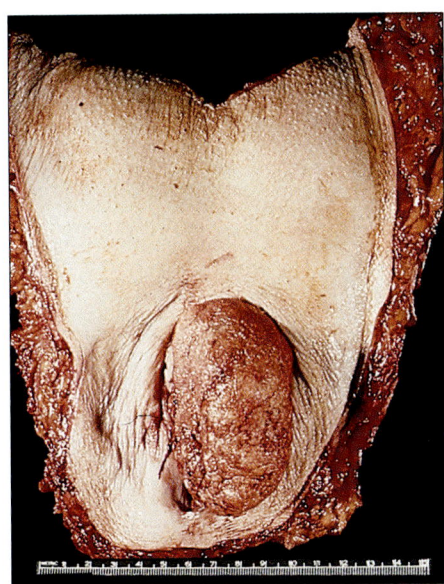

Fig. 3.32 Verrucous carcinoma. The mass is large, exophytic, and fungating.

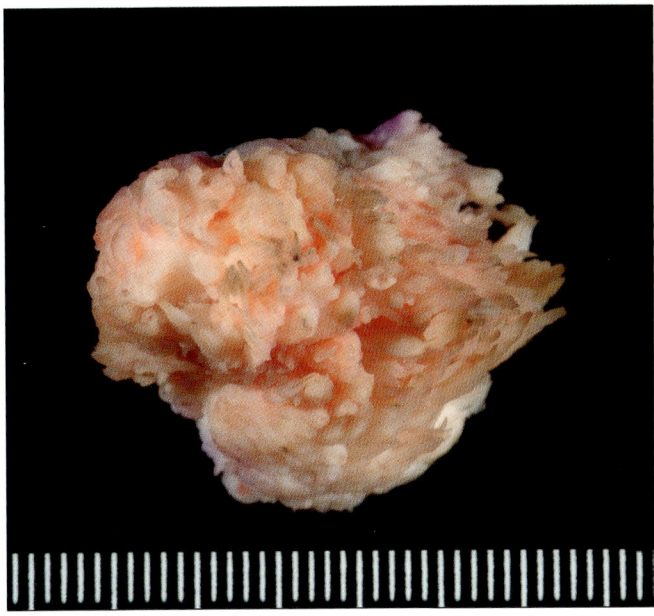

Fig. 3.35 Large condyloma acuminatum with numerous asperities. On cross section the dermoepidermal junction discloses no invasion.

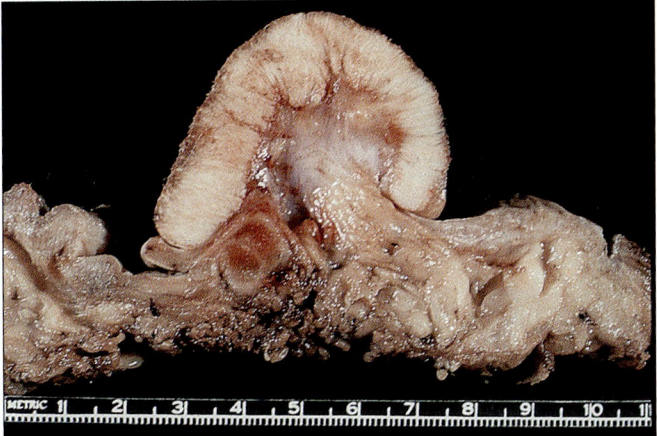

Fig. 3.33 Verrucous carcinoma. On section, the tumor is superficial without gross invasion, which microscopic examination confirmed.

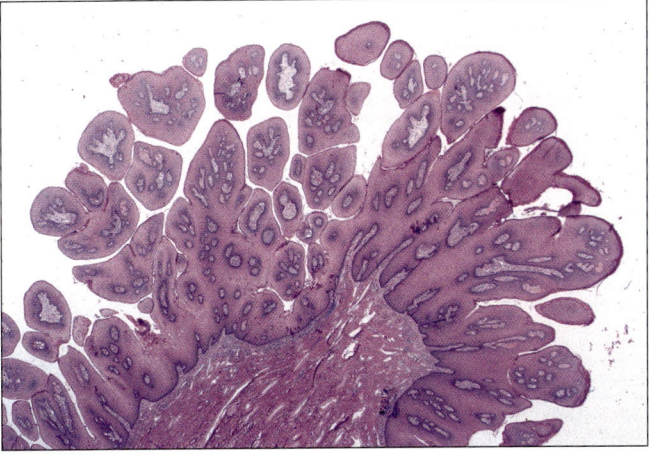

Fig. 3.36 Large condyloma acuminatum. The specimen is large, solitary, exophytic, and polypoid with a convoluted tan surface.

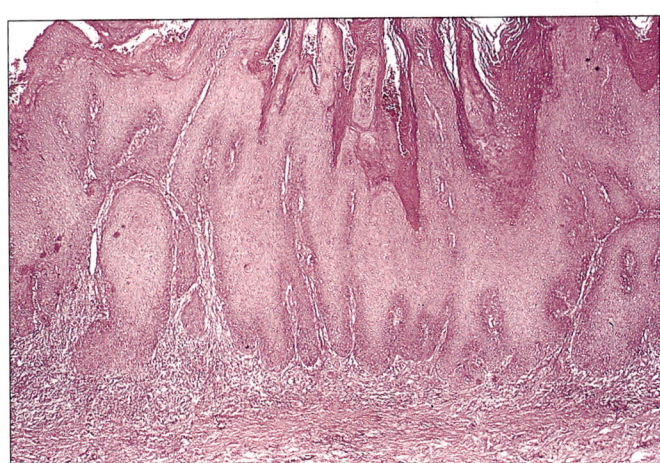

Fig. 3.34 Verrucous carcinoma. The extremely well-differentiated tumor, which is composed of large nests of squamous cells with abundant cytoplasm and relatively small, bland nuclei, has a basal border that pushes, but does not destructively invade into the dermis.

atypical cells, if any, are confined to the basal layers, the remainder being large cells with pale, eosinophilic cytoplasm. Apoptotic (dyskeratotic) cells may be prominent, but mitotic figures are sparse and usually noted mainly along the basal layer of the tongue-like downward protrusions of squamous epithelium. Atypical mitotic figures are rarely identified. HPV types 1, 2, 6, 11, 16, and 18 have been demonstrated in some cases.

Differential diagnosis

Verrucous carcinoma has considerable similarities to condyloma acuminatum when the latter enlarges and appears tumor-like (Figures 3.35 and 3.36). In this state, the lesions exhibit crusting, deep penetration, bulbous contours of down-growing

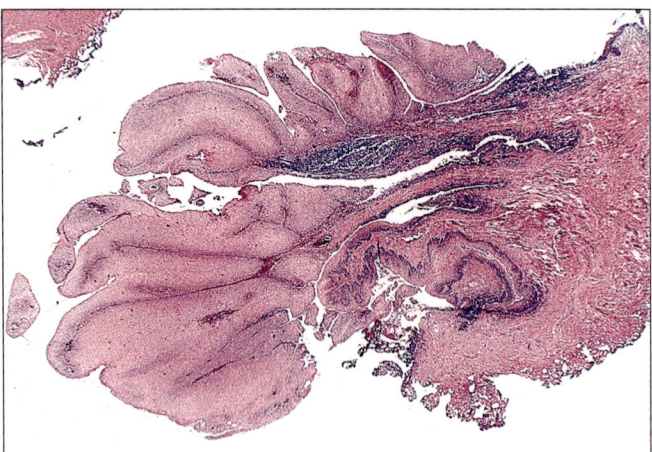

Fig. 3.37 Large condyloma acuminatum. Microscopically, the findings are typical of an ordinary condyloma, namely an acanthotic squamous proliferation lining thin fibrovascular stalks, and an absence of invasion.

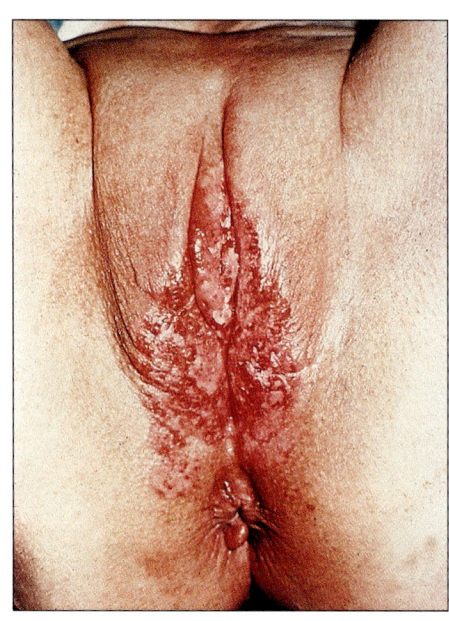

Fig. 3.38 Pagets disease, which extends to involve the perianal region.

epithelium (Figure 3.37), leading to the problematic differential diagnosis of verrucous carcinoma. 'Giant condyloma of Buschke–Lowenstein' is an obsolete and misleading eponym for verrucous carcinoma of the anogenital region. Histologically similar verrucous carcinomas also occur in other anatomic sites such as the sole of the foot (carcinoma cuniculatum), larynx, esophagus, and mouth (florid oral papillomatosis). Because verrucous carcinoma can only be diagnosed when its deep extent is available for study, it is appropriate to recommend an adequately deep biopsy whenever this diagnosis is suspected clinically or pathologically.

EXTRAMAMMARY PAGET DISEASE[40,90]

Definition
Extramammary Paget disease is a form of *in situ* adenocarcinoma of the squamous mucosa. Recent evidence that is somewhat controversial and yet to be confirmed suggests an origin from a Toker-like cell, a cell found in the breast with clear cytoplasm that reacts with cytokeratin 7 (CK7)[8,79,86,151] and thought to derive from the ostia of the mammary-like glands found in the vulva, perineum, and perianal skin.

Clinical features
The vulva is the most common site of extramammary Paget disease, accounting for about 5% of all vulvar neoplasms. It usually presents in older women as a moist, red, eroded or eczematous-appearing plaque on the anogenital region. One or both sides of the vulva can be involved, often with spread to the perianal skin (Figure 3.38). The plaques are usually irritated and sore, and may be clinically misinterpreted as an inflammatory skin disease. Indeed, since similar erosive changes may also be seen in intertrigo, fungal infections, immunobullous disorders, chronic benign familial pemphigus (Hailey–Hailey disease), etc., the clinical diagnosis usually requires biopsy confirmation.

Treatment is difficult because the disease usually extends well beyond the clinically apparent margins. In one series,[42] both frozen section analysis and visual judgment were each misleading in over a third of cases. Indeed, in our experience,

frozen section examination of resection margins is more likely than not to be inaccurate and to the point of being counterproductive. Moreover, even margin status was not particularly helpful in predicting recurrence, as about a third of patients each experienced recurrence regardless of whether the margins after initial surgery were positive or negative. The extent of the operation (wide local excision, simple vulvectomy or modified radical vulvectomy) during the initial treatment also poorly correlated with disease recurrence.[42] Mohs micrographic surgery, topical chemotherapy, and photodynamic therapy may play a role in selected cases. HER-2/neu expression has been demonstrated by some[13] but not all[11] in Paget disease of the vulva, thus hampering the proposal that trastuzumab (Herceptin), a recombinant monoclonal antibody against HER-2/neu, might be useful for patients with recurrent disease.

Microscopic features
Histologically, the epidermis contains pale-staining cells that are larger than adjacent keratinocytes, arranged singly or in small to massive nests in the epidermis (Figure 3.39). When the cells are single or few in number, they appear to be mainly within the basal layer or individually migrate into the upper epidermal layers (Figure 3.40). When massive, they may replace much of the epidermis (Figure 3.41), and in fact make the epidermis appear swollen and greatly thickened. In these instances tumor may even be found growing down hair follicles (Figure 3.42) as well as eccrine glands (Figure 3.43). On occasion, small numbers of similar cells may be seen in the underlying dermis (Figure 3.44), indicative of invasion. While upwards of 50% of patients are reported to show invasion in some series,[27] this is a distinctly unusual happening in our experience. Likewise, we find that metastases to lymph nodes are exceedingly rare.

The pale cytoplasm of the Paget cell is usually finely granular, and the nuclei are usually central and round to oval. Mitotic figures may occasionally be found. On routine staining, Paget disease may be confused with malignant melanoma *in situ*. However, the Paget cells at the basal layer are usually discrete, characteristically compress and displace the normal keratino-

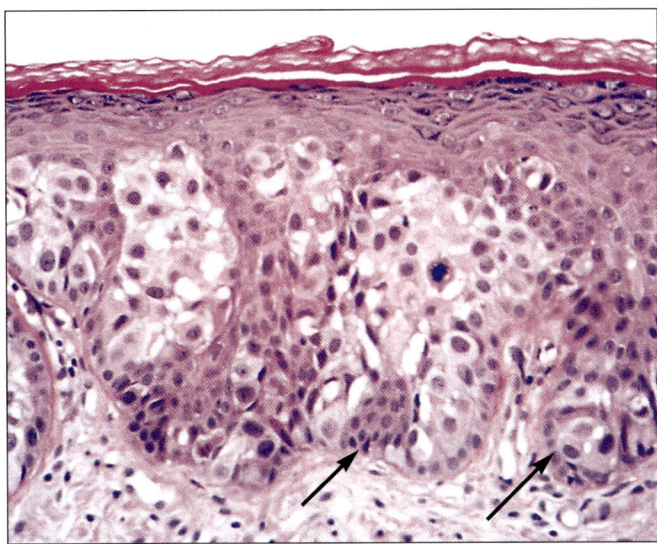

Fig. 3.39 Paget disease. Clonal nests of pale-staining dysplastic cells are located within the epidermis, including the upper layers. The tumor cells also compress the normal basal layer of squamous cells in the epidermis (arrow).

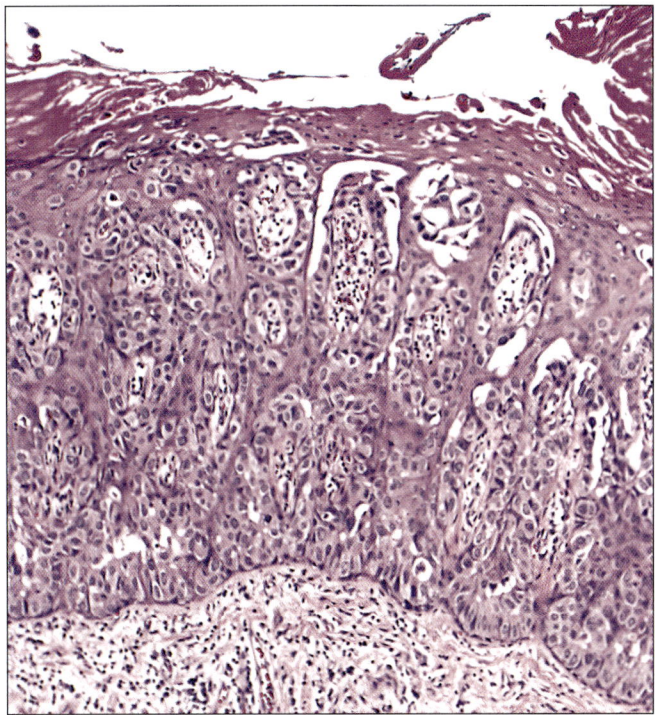

Fig. 3.41 Massive *in situ* Paget disease in which virtually the entire epidermis has been replaced.

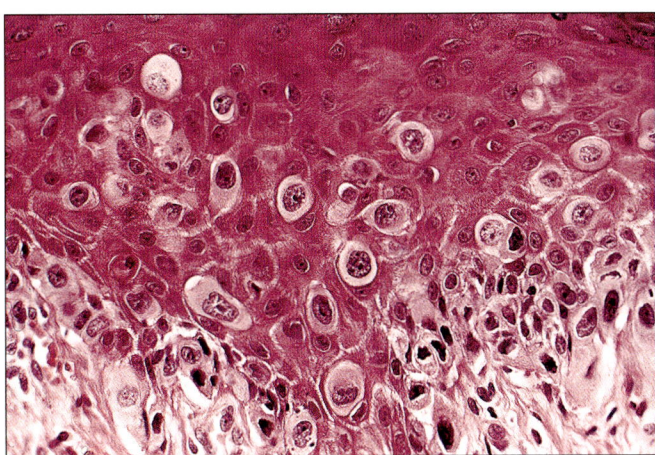

Fig. 3.40 Paget cell. These intraepithelial tumor cells have copious, pale cytoplasm occurring singly or in small clusters and appearing slightly larger than the neighboring squamous cells. Mucin stains are positive.

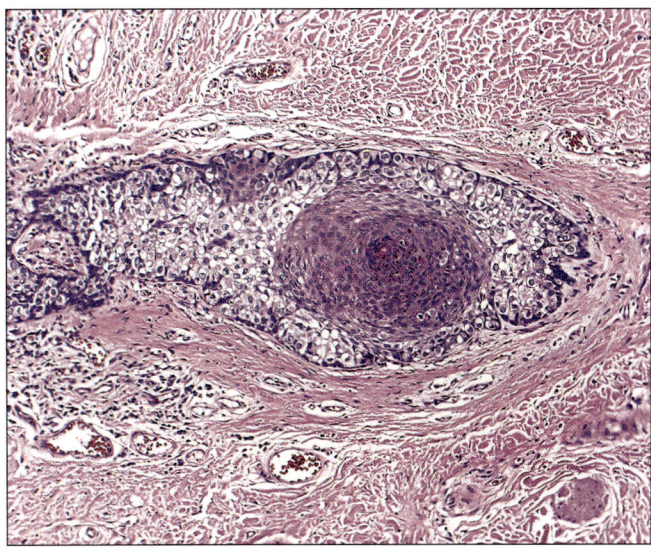

Fig. 3.42 Paget disease involving hair follicles.

cytes, whereas melanoma cells generally form a continuous proliferation.

Paget cells usually contain intracytoplasmic mucin (neutral and acidic). Periodic acid-Schiff, Alcian blue, colloidal iron, and mucicarmine stains help in the main differential diagnostic considerations. In problematic cases, immunocytochemical studies are also useful, with Paget cells selectively expressing CAM 5.2, CK7, MUC5AC, carcinoembryonic antigen (CEA), epithelial membrane antigen (EMA), and gross cystic disease fluid protein-15 (BRST-2). S-100 protein is also sometimes expressed. Such cases may require study for more specific melanocytic markers (MART-1/Melan-A, HMB45, etc.). Androgen (but not estrogen or progesterone) receptors can be detected in some cases. It can be a salutary lesson to perform occasional immunostains to observe the distressingly widespread scattering of single Paget cells beyond the field in which they are

obvious in routine H&E sections, particularly at or near surgical resections margins.

The origin of extramammary Paget disease is controversial. Some believe it represents an epidermotropic adenocarcinoma, but unlike mammary cases (in which an underlying ductal carcinoma is almost invariably present), underlying vulvar carcinoma is only rarely detected. Other postulated origins include a pluripotential stem cell within the epidermis or *in situ* malignant transformation of cells in the cutaneous sweat ducts as they insert into the epidermis. The most recent works point to the 'Toker' cell, which in the breast is an intraepidermal clear

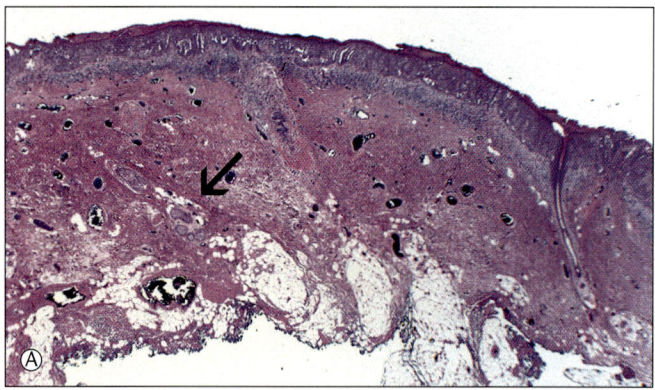

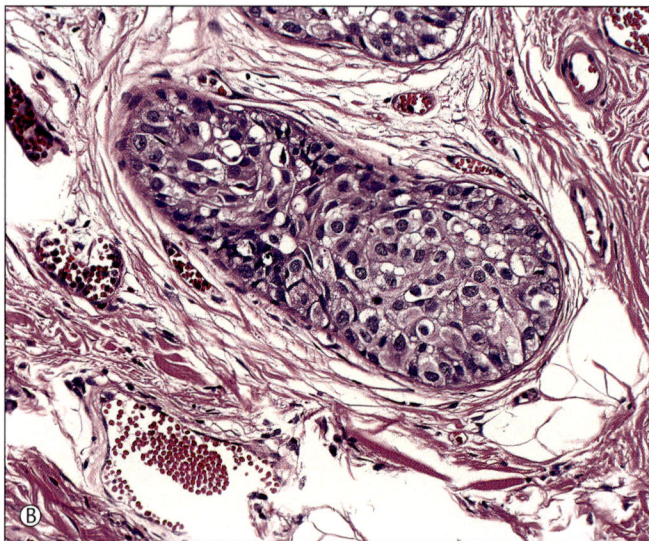

Fig. 3.43 Paget disease involving sweat glands. **(A)** Low power section of skin in which the involved gland (arrow) extends nearly to the cutaneous fat. **(B)** Detail of gland cut in cross-section.

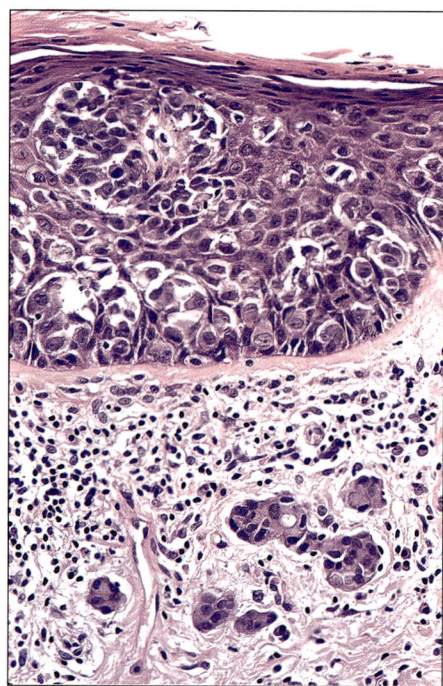

Fig. 3.44 Invasive Paget disease.

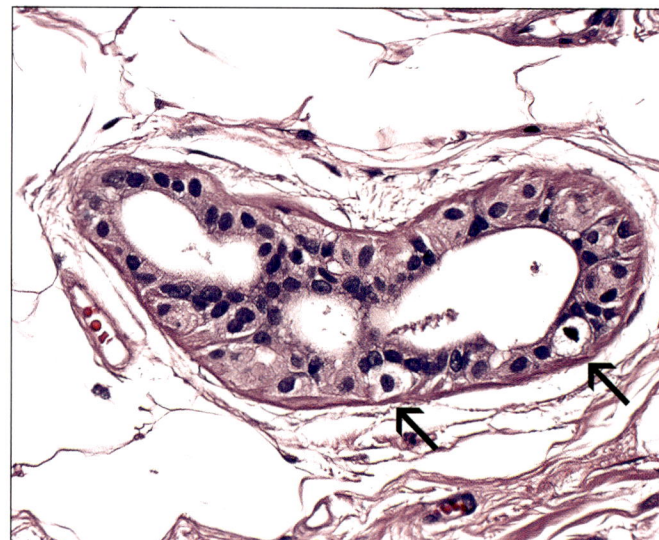

Fig. 3.45 Possible Toker cells (arrows) with copious clear cytoplasm in an isolated eccrine gland in the vulva.

cell with bland nuclear features[8,79,151] that is reactive for CK7 but not CK20.[86] It is suggested but not yet conclusive that this cell exists in the vulva (Figure 3.45). In the vulva, about a fifth of Paget cases are reactive for CK20.[27,53,79] Further, the apomucins MUC1, MUC2, and MUC5AC seem to be expressed differently in Paget disease of the vulva (MUC1+, MUC2–, MUC5AC+), the rare case of Paget disease with an underlying apocrine carcinoma (MUC1+, MUC2–, MUC5AC–), and the not much more common Paget disease in the perianal region with associated rectal adenocarcinoma (MUC1+, MUC2+, MUC5AC+). The immunoprofile of Paget disease of the breast, its underlying ductal carcinoma, and Toker cells found in 10% of nipples without breast carcinoma is MUC1+, MUC2–, MUC5AC–. Only the Bartholin gland expressed a mucin phenotype identical to that of vulvar Paget disease.

The several conclusions that might be drawn at this time are that vulvar Paget disease may arise from ectopic MUC5AC+ cells originating from Bartholin or some other unidentified glands, and that the unique expression of MUC2 in perianal Paget disease indicates that its origin from colorectal mucosa differs from that in the vulva. Cytogenetic findings suggest that at least some cases of Paget disease arise multicentrically within the epidermis from pluripotent stem cells,[139] and have a molecular basis differing from other vulvar carcinomas.[137]

BASAL CELL CARCINOMA[9,48,93,108]

Definition
Basal cell carcinoma (BCC) is a slow-growing, malignant neoplasm recapitulating hair follicular differentiation and with a propensity for local invasion and destruction but a very low risk of metastasis.

Clinical features
BCC is the most common malignant neoplasm in humans, with an annual US incidence of over 700 000 cases. Although most

BCCs occur in chronically sun-exposed skin and are a consequence of cumulative ultraviolet radiation exposure, some arise in covered sites such as the vulva and perineum. BCC represents 2–4% of all vulvar cancers. Most cases occur in patients over age 70 and present as well-circumscribed, skin-colored papules with superficial telangiectases. Pigmented variants may be mistaken for melanoma clinically. Superficial BCCs present as erythematous plaques, often with a raised, rolled, opalescent border. A less common, fibrosing or morpheiform variant presents as an indurated plaque, simulating localized scleroderma (morphea). Large, neglected BCCs (Figure 3.46) can present as fungating masses or chronic ('rodent') ulcers. Some BCCs grow to formidable sizes.

Microscopic features

A prototypical BCC consists of basaloid cells arranged in a peripheral palisade, with separation of tumor cells away from a myxoid stroma (Figure 3.47). These aspects are generally present in superficial carcinomas (those predominantly budding down from the epidermis into the papillary dermis) and the nodular variant (with rounded masses of tumor present deeper in the dermis). The less common morpheiform variant consists of jagged islands or strands of tumor cells within a desmoplastic stroma, and may be deeply infiltrative. All these patterns may occur in various combinations.

In BCC of any type mitotic figures can usually be identified, and apoptotic bodies are often numerous. Melanin pigment and amyloid are variable features. Features warranting mention in the pathology report include presence of perineural spread (a risk factor for local recurrence) and aggressive histologic types, e.g., morpheiform, micronodular, and squamous differentiation when extensive.

BASOSQUAMOUS CARCINOMA[77]

Definition

Basosquamous carcinoma is a biphasic malignant neoplasm comprising an extensive mixture of both basaloid and squamous elements.

Clinical features

The clinical appearance is not specific, but most often presents as a nodule, often with an ulcerated surface.

Microscopic features

Histopathologically one sees mixed features of BCC and SCC as described above (Figures 3.48 and 3.49). This rare occurrence may represent a 'collision' between two independent primaries, and the natural history is probably in keeping with the more aggressive SCC component. On the other hand, focal squamous differentiation within a conventional BCC is a common finding, especially when near an ulcer or surface erosion, and does not necessarily portend a worse outcome than the usual indolent BCC. The term 'metatypical' carcinoma refers to a poorly differentiated neoplasm that cannot be reliably diagnosed as either a BCC or an SCC. Such lesions have been considered to have a more aggressive potential than conventional BCC.

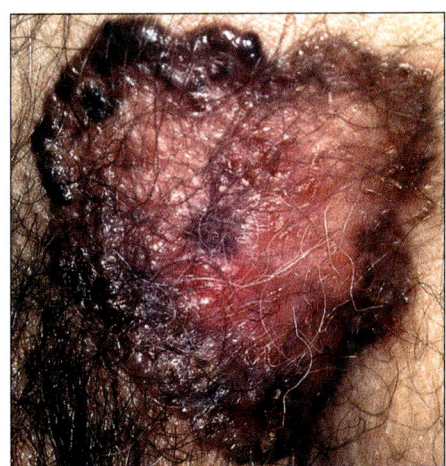

Fig. 3.46 Basal cell carcinoma of the pubis. This is an unusually large and neglected basal cell carcinoma, with pigmentation. The pearly edge can be clearly seen.

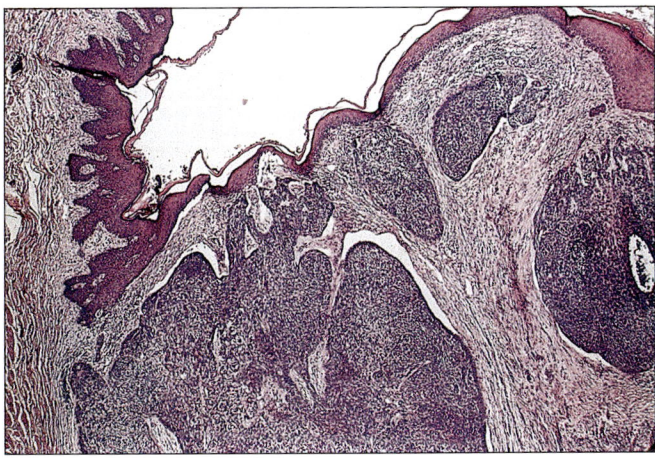

Fig. 3.47 Basal cell carcinoma. Note the artifactual separation ('clefting') of tumor cells away from the myxoid stroma.

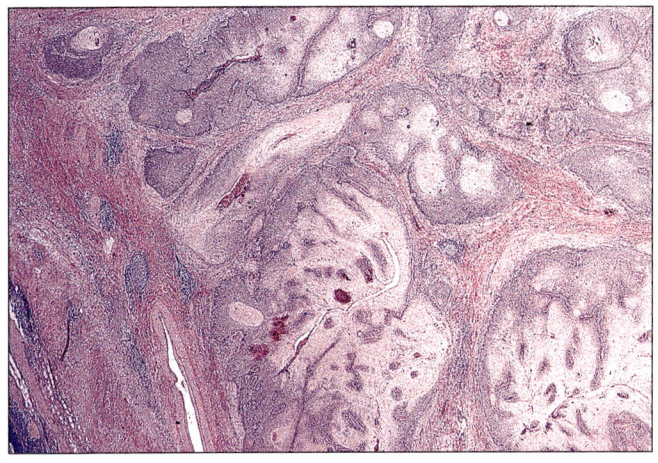

Fig. 3.48 Basosquamous carcinoma.

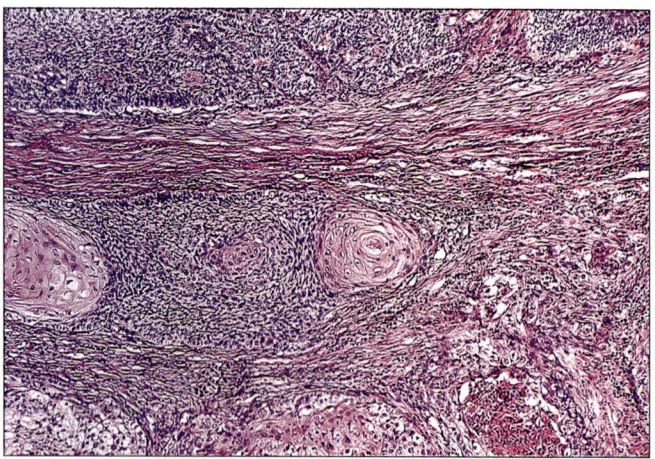

Fig. 3.49 Basosquamous carcinoma. The tumor consists largely of basal cells in which nests of squamous cells are interspersed.

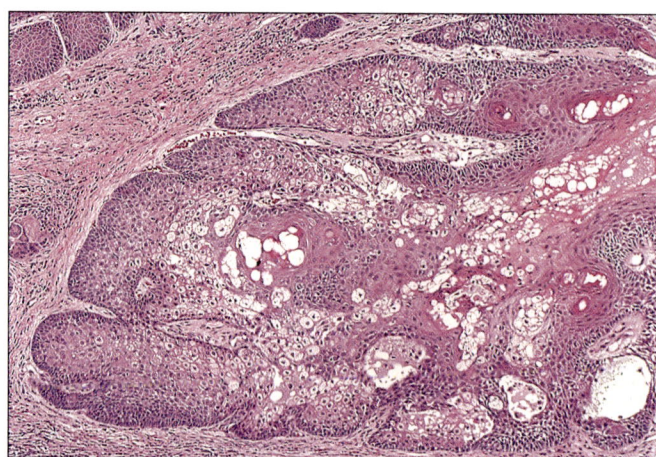

Fig. 3.50 Sebaceous carcinoma.

SEBACEOUS CARCINOMA[39,74]

Definition
Sebaceous carcinoma is a rare, aggressive, malignant neoplasm exhibiting sebaceous differentiation.

Clinical features
Most cases occur on the eyelid but vulvar examples are described, as nodules with variable ulceration. Patients with any sebaceous neoplasm, particularly if multiple, should be screened for the Muir–Torre syndrome.

Microscopic features
Atypical cells, including a number with scalloped nuclei and finely vacuolated, clear cytoplasm, are seen in the dermis (Figure 3.50). An involved epidermis in a pagetoid pattern may raise consideration of extramammary Paget disease or melanoma. In problematic cases, immunohistochemistry (e.g., positive expression of epithelial membrane antigen) may be helpful. Distinction from sebaceous adenoma/epithelioma relies on the presence of large size, ulceration, pagetoid spread, pleomorphism, and atypical mitotic figures in sebaceous carcinoma.

MELANOCYTIC LESIONS

LENTIGO[6]

Definition
A lentigo is a circumscribed macule of increased pigmentation, generally 5 mm or less in diameter, and persisting even in the absence of sun exposure.

Clinical features
Lentigines are common on the labia majora or minora. They are often deeply pigmented but usually have uniform color, sharp circumscription, and regular borders. Although some authors use the term 'lentigo' and its derivatives to describe certain forms of melanoma (e.g., lentigo maligna and mucosal–lentiginous melanoma), we discourage this usage as it conflates

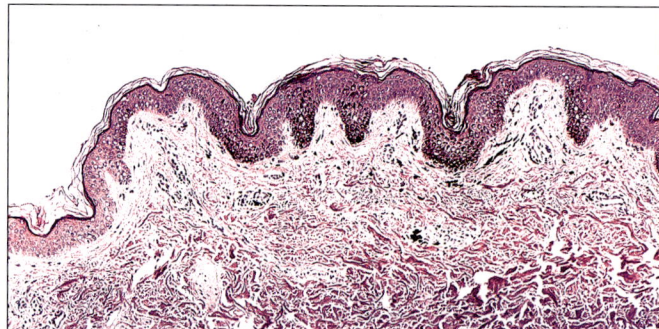

Fig. 3.51 Lentigo.

a benign with a malignant process, and also refers to a disparate variety of histologic features. Lentigines proper are not precursors of melanoma. Vulvar lentigines represent examples of lentigo simplex. The solar lentigo is a different entity caused by chronic ultraviolet radiation exposure.

Microscopic features
The epidermis of a lentigo has elongated rete ridges and increased melanin deposition in the keratinocytes (Figure 3.51). There may be increased numbers of basal melanocytes in lentigines, but the increase may be quite subtle, requiring specialized techniques (e.g., immunohistochemistry or enzyme histochemistry using DOPA as substrate) for detection. Basal layer melanocytes lack cytologic atypia. The term 'nevoid lentigo' is sometimes used for lesions having a definite increase in melanocyte number as viewed by routine light microscopy, but lacking well-formed nests as expected in a nevus proper. The term 'lentiginous nevus' is sometimes used as a synonym for atypical nevus (see below).

COMMON ACQUIRED MELANOCYTIC NEVUS

Definition
A melanocytic nevus is a benign neoplasm composed of cells exhibiting melanocytic differentiation.

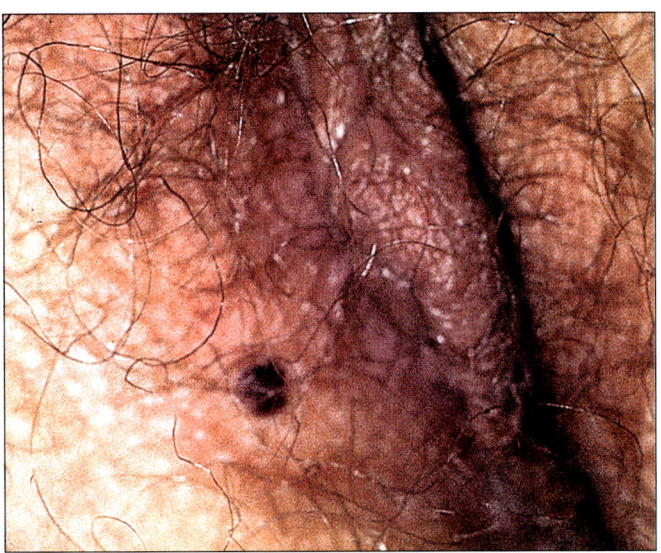

Fig. 3.52   Flat junctional melanocytic nevus. The dark color and slight irregularity of outline and pigmentation intensity in this woman of 52 years is a worrying feature and merits complete excision.

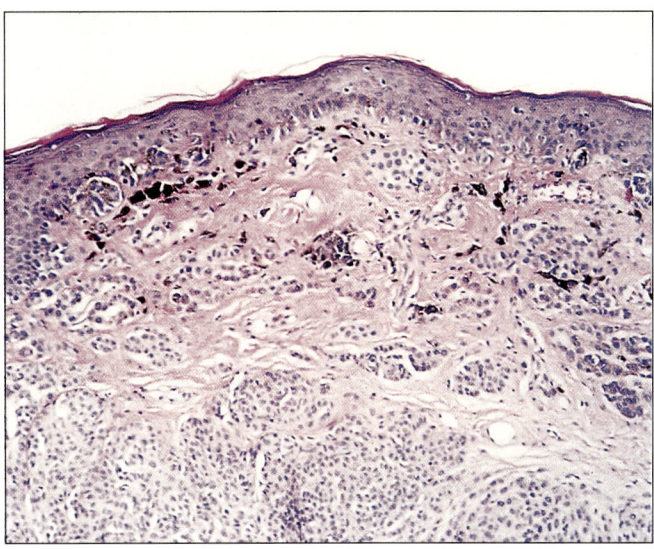

Fig. 3.53   Compound nevus. This nevus contains a mature intradermal component but with some persisting highly pigmented junctional nests.

Clinical features

Melanocytic nevi are the most common neoplasms to occur in humans. An average white adult has 10 or more. Nevi occur with some frequency on the vulva, usually on the labia majora (Figure 3.52). According to the most accepted notion of pathogenesis, nevi originate at the dermoepidermal junction, and over time progressively descend deeper into the dermis. The age-dependent stratification of nevus types supports this concept. Thus, junctional nevi (flat, deeply pigmented lesions located at the dermoepidermal junction) predominate in childhood. Later in life, the dome-shaped, brown compound nevi (with both junctional and intradermal components) are more numerous, whereas the paler, dome-shaped purely intradermal nevi are most common in later adult life. In old age, many nevi involute entirely, possibly being replaced by fat, fibrous tissue, or mucin.

An alternative concept is that nevi originate in dermal melanocytes or their precursors, and subsequently populate the epidermis. Melanocytes may have their origin in pluripotential cells in the nerve sheath precursor stage of the melanocytic differentiation pathway. Thus, maturation to a dendritic morphologic stage may produce a lentigo. Maturation to various migratory stages may produce junctional or intradermal nevi, and failure to mature may result in nevi with neuroid characteristics.[26]

Microscopic features

In purely junctional nevi, small round nests of benign-appearing regular melanocytes are present in the basal epidermis, sometimes associated with increased numbers of individual melanocytes. There may be a few melanophages in the papillary dermis, but prominent host response in the form of coarse fibrosis or notable inflammatory infiltrates should be absent (see discussion of atypical nevi, below).

In compound and dermal nevi, the relative proportion of dermal cells increases (Figure 3.53). A key element in assessing the benignity of a melanocytic lesion is to determine the presence of so-called maturation, i.e., the tendency to undergo a morphologic shift with progressive depth in the dermis. Thus,

the superficial dermal type A nevus cells frequently produce melanin, contain abundant melanosomes, and express the melanin-synthetic enzyme tyrosinase and related antigens. In their deeper dermal component, nevi consist of rounder, smaller, type B cells with a less pronounced melanogenic phenotype.[33,62] Histologically, the deepest type C nevus cells may appear neuroid and lack immunohistochemical expression of MART-1, an antigen usually expressed diffusely in type A and B cells,[14,70,72] and conversely have some immunophenotypic characteristics of Schwann cells.[111,116] Another hallmark of benignity is a tendency for quiescence in the deeper component, with reduced numbers of proliferating cells in the deeper dermis.[121] Usually there is a complete absence of mitotic figures. In contrast, most malignant melanomas consist of large, pleomorphic cells throughout and exhibit notable numbers of mitotic figures in their deep component. However, an unusual subset of melanomas exhibits a paradoxical pattern of maturation simulating that of nevi.[122]

Some nevi have considerable surface hyperkeratosis and acanthosis, resembling a seborrheic keratosis. These keratotic nevi are commonly biopsied, probably because such lesions are often clinically atypical, in contrast to their benign histologic appearance. The epidermal hyperplasia on top of a keratotic melanocytic nevus appears to result from increased cellular proliferation, in the context of adequately regulated apoptosis.[64,133]

Pigmented nevi arising in a background of lichen sclerosus may exhibit histologic features associated with malignant melanoma. This is believed to be a stromal-induced change. Awareness can prevent unnecessarily aggressive surgical procedures.[18,37]

ATYPICAL MELANOCYTIC NEVUS OF THE GENITAL TYPE[24]

Definition

A subset of nevi occurring on the vulva, perineum, or mons pubis that exhibits particular stromal changes. It differs from the atypical (dysplastic, Clark) nevus, a second form of nevus, also associated with the Clark eponym, which can be found anywhere, occurs in the more usual age spectrum, and lacks the particular stromal changes often seen in the atypical 'dysplastic' nevus.

Clinical features
Atypical nevi of the genital type are more common on the labia minora or the mucosa of the clitoral region than on the labia majora. They have also been seen in the axillae and uncommonly on male genitalia. They occur at a much younger age (median, 25 years) than vulvar melanoma.

Microscopic features
These nevi show confluent and enlarged nests of nevus cells that vary in size, shape, and position at the dermoepidermal junction. The nevus cells themselves exhibit diminished cohesion. Finally, the stromal pattern at the dermoepidermal junction is often inconspicuous and nondescript in comparison to the concentric eosinophilic fibroplasia or lamellar fibroplasia seen in the usual atypical (dysplastic) nevus (see below).

ATYPICAL (DYSPLASTIC, CLARK) NEVUS

Definition
Atypical nevi are benign melanocytic neoplasms that somewhat resemble melanoma both clinically and histologically.

Clinical features
Both atypical nevi and melanomas customarily are relatively large (>5 mm), poorly circumscribed, and asymmetric, with an irregular border and in a range of colors. Newer *in vivo* diagnostic techniques, such as viewing through a magnifying lens directly applied to the surface (dermatoscopy),[3] telespectrophotometry to assess color variation,[12] ultrasonic imaging,[130] and macroscopic spectral imaging,[152] may help clinicians make the crucial distinction between atypical nevi and melanoma, and thereby avoid unnecessary excisions.

Atypical nevi were initially described in the setting of families with a tendency to develop melanoma (dysplastic nevus syndrome). Later such nevi were recognized to occur sporadically, with an estimated prevalence in unselected white populations of about 2–9%. Atypical nevi represent a strong, independent risk factor for development of melanoma,[144] whether occurring sporadically or in the context of a familial melanoma diathesis. Moreover, there is a strong dose–response relationship, with melanoma risk rising proportionately with the number of atypical nevi present. Apart from this role as a simple marker of melanoma risk, atypical nevi on occasion may be precursor lesions to melanoma.

Microscopic features
The histopathologic features include abnormal architecture, host response, and cytology. In general, there is a high degree of consensus on the defining architectural features of atypical nevi,[57] which include peripheral extension of the junctional component (shoulder) (Figure 3.54), confluence of single melanocytes or via bridging of adjacent rete ridges, and irregular disposition, size, and shape of junctional nests (Figure 3.55). In contrast, the status of cytologic atypia as a criterion is controversial.[5] Most nevi exhibit both architectural disorder and

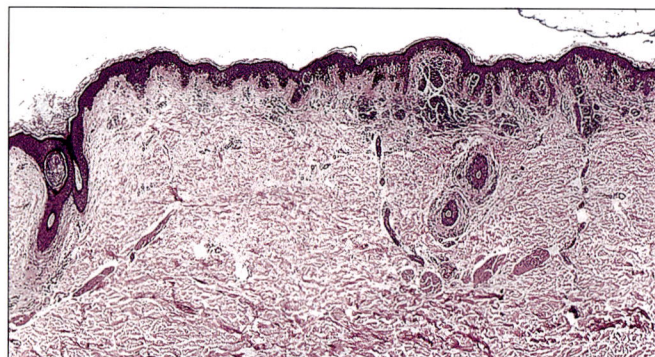

Fig. 3.54 Atypical nevus.

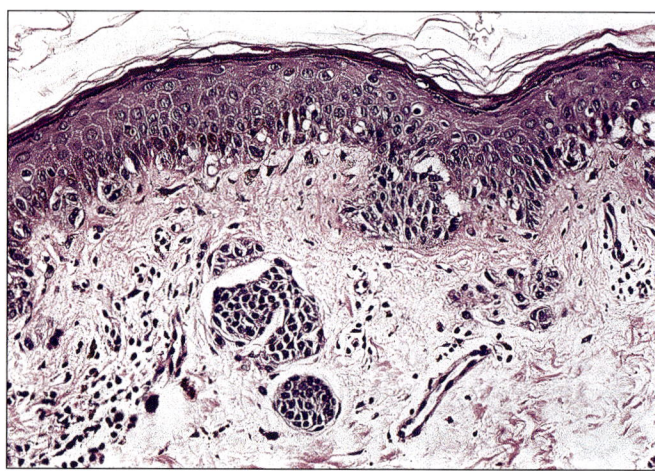

Fig. 3.55 Atypical nevus: detail of nevus cells.

at least low-grade cytologic atypia. In one series of 166 consecutive atypical nevi, 15% were highly atypical, with features suggesting (but still falling short of the full diagnostic criteria for) melanoma.[128] Of note, the degree of cytologic atypia and the extent of architectural disorder are strongly correlated.

BLUE NEVUS (DERMAL MELANOCYTOMA)

Definition
The blue nevus is a benign melanocytic neoplasm consisting of dermal cells having prominent melanin pigment.

Clinical features
Blue nevus is uncommon in the vulva but occurs frequently on the buttock. These nevi are small, blue-black, well-circumscribed skin lesions, sometimes slightly raised. The blue color occurs because the shorter (blue) wavelengths of visible light are scattered back out of the tissue, whereas the longer wavelengths, which penetrate more deeply into the skin, are absorbed by the dermal melanin and thereby subtracted from the optical signal that ultimately reaches the eye as the incident light is scattered and reflected back out of the tissue.

Microscopic features
The dermis has collections of spindle-shaped or dendritic cells containing delicate melanin pigment, intersecting with fibrotic

collagen fibers (Figures 3.56 and 3.57). Melanophages containing coarse, clumped melanin pigment are also numerous. In the cellular variant, the nevus cells are more densely packed, often forming a dumbbell-shaped nodule that may extend into the subcutis. Malignant change in blue nevi is extremely rare,[131] but atypical forms[142] warrant conservative excision.

MALIGNANT MELANOMA[35,101,113–115,133,135,148,149]

Definition
Melanoma is a malignant neoplasm that frequently metastasizes and is composed of cells exhibiting melanocytic differentiation.

Clinical features
Vulvar melanoma occurs in the labia majora and minora. It affects mainly older women, and only rarely younger women and girls.[36] Local recurrences are frequent and the overall 5-year survival rates vary from 37%[113] to 54%,[34] even when the tumor appears localized at initial presentation. As with melanoma of other sites, the pathologic features most important for prognosis are Breslow thickness and presence or absence of ulceration. Non-diploidy by flow cytometry is also a strong

independent risk factor for death.[126] Melanomas of the labia minora that involve the urethra and vagina have a particularly poor prognosis, mainly because it is difficult to achieve complete surgical excision. The overall poor prognosis of vulvar melanoma is undoubtedly due to its tendency for diagnosis after it is already deeply invasive. Therefore, early surveillance and biopsy by clinicians are crucial. Dermatoscopy by a trained examiner is of value.[31,32]

Except in the rare amelanotic[145] variant, the clinical morphology of melanoma is characteristic. There is usually marked gross asymmetry, border irregularity, and color variegation, sometimes including a play of brown, black, blue, and red (Figures 3.58 and 3.59). A white color suggests regression. Most melanomas have a prominent *in situ* (intraepidermal) component, which presents as a hyperpigmented macule. Elevation to form a plaque or nodule indicates dermal invasion, and is an ominous sign. Ulceration is a strongly negative prognostic factor. Development of satellite lesions is a form of local metastasis and carries a grave import.

Surgical treatment is based on complete local excision, with margins based on the Breslow thickness of the tumor (see

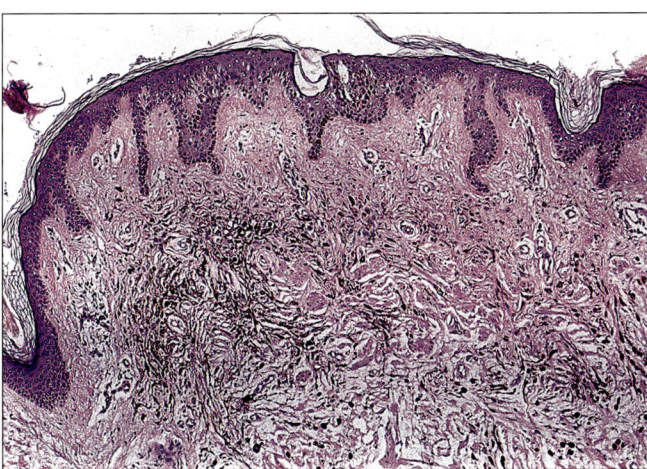

Fig. 3.56 Blue nevus.

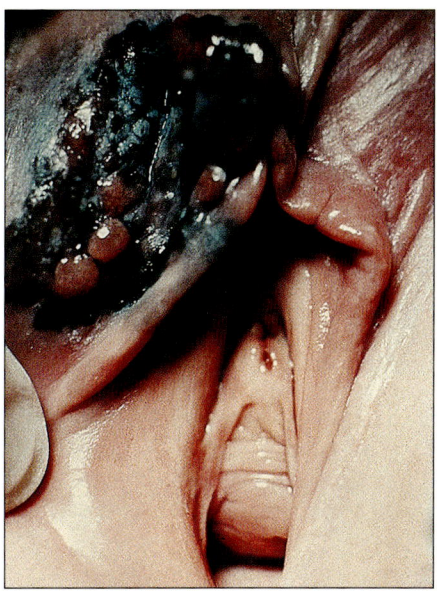

Fig. 3.58 Malignant melanoma. The tumor is darkly pigmented, elevated, and nodular.

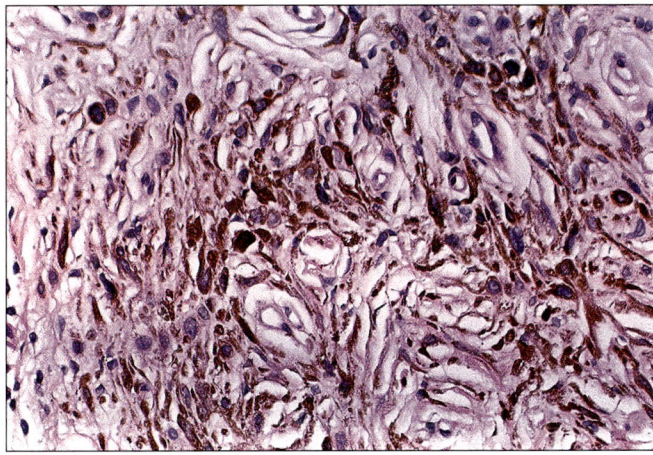

Fig. 3.57 Blue nevus: detail of nevus cells.

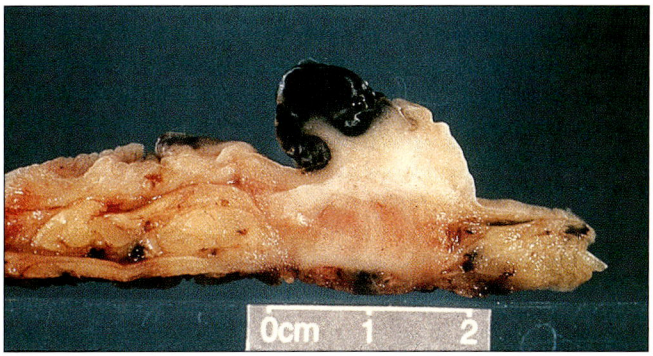

Fig. 3.59 Malignant melanoma. Cross-section shows the pigmented tumor's invasive nature.

below). Currently, melanoma *in situ* is usually treated with complete excision of the gross lesion, the full thickness of the underlying dermis, and a 5 mm rim of normal tissue. Invasive melanoma less than 1 mm thick is similarly managed, but with a 1 cm margin. Debate remains about the appropriate margins for deeper melanomas,[106] but many surgeons will remove a 2 or 3 cm margin in thick tumors. Rarely, radical vulvectomy with lymph node removal is necessary in large, neglected melanomas or those with urethral, clitoral, or lower vaginal involvement. Complete elective lymphadenectomy is now uncommonly performed for clinically non-palpable nodes, but sentinel lymph node investigation is often performed for tumors 1 mm or greater in thickness, or those attaining Clark level IV or deeper (see below). Completion lymphadenectomy is indicated in any case with gross or microscopic metastatic tumor in the sentinel node(s).[52]

Microscopic features

Melanoma historically has been classified into various histogenetic subtypes, including superficial spreading, nodular, acral–lentiginous, mucosal–lentiginous, verrucous, and lentigo maligna melanoma. This traditional terminology, while still widely used, may be misleading, e.g., 'superficial' spreading melanoma may be of any thickness, and any of these subsets of melanoma may become grossly 'nodular' if sufficiently thick. Moreover, this system largely classifies melanoma by its *in situ* component. Thus, superficial spreading melanoma is defined by the presence of an *in situ* lesion extending at least three rete ridges peripheral to the dermal component, in contrast to nodular melanoma, which lacks this lateral spread. However, it is the invasive dermal component that is most significant biologically. The various subsets based on the *in situ* component lack independent prognostic information. It is difficult to apply this classification consistently, and consensus as to classification is even poorer. Finally, more recently described forms of melanoma, such as the desmoplastic type, do not have a place in this older classification. However, the traditional classification still has some didactic utility by reinforcing the broad morphologic spectrum of melanoma, and may provide pathogenetic insights, e.g., the occurrence of the slow-growing lentigo maligna form in the context of chronic sun exposure.

Histologically, malignant melanoma *in situ* is generally composed of atypical melanocytes arranged both singly and in nests (Figure 3.60). Single cells often predominate over nests, and confluence may be extensive. Particularly in superficial spreading melanoma, the tumor cells generally exhibit high-grade cytologic atypia (large, pleomorphic nuclei with large nucleoli), as well as marked architectural disorder including pagetoid spread through the upper epidermal layers (Figure 3.61). The so-called 'lentiginous' variants usually show less pagetoid spread and often have less abundant cytoplasm, being composed of relatively small but densely hyperchromatic melanocytes, with a marked tendency to extend along the basal layer of the epidermis and adnexal epithelium.

The Breslow thickness measures the distance from the top of the granular layer of the overlying epidermis to the deepest melanoma cells in the dermis or subcutis. If the tumor is thickest in an area of ulceration (therefore lacking a granular layer), the floor of the ulcer should be used as the starting point for measurement. Periappendageal tumor cells should not be used for measurement of the Breslow thickness.

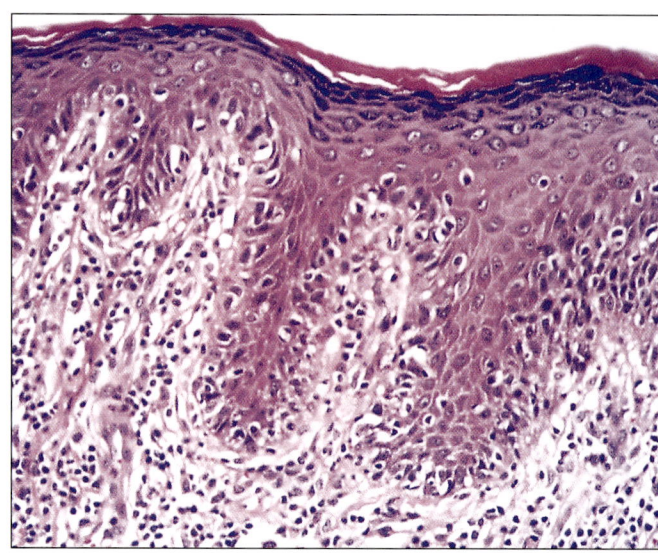

Fig. 3.60 Mucosal lentiginous melanoma. The lower levels of the epidermis contain an almost continuous line of atypical melanocytes, somewhat resembling one pattern of Paget disease.

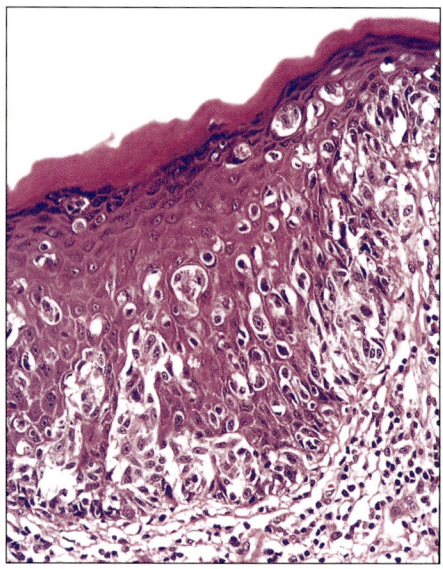

Fig. 3.61 Malignant melanoma. Atypical melanocytes, singly and in clumps, appear to migrate into the upper layers of the epidermis ('pagetoid change'), but there is no dermal invasion.

The Clark level concerns an anatomic structure, and not a thickness measurement:

- Level I: tumor confined to epidermis (or adnexal epithelium).
- Level II: tumor present in the papillary dermis but not filling or expanding it.
- Level III: tumor fills and expands the papillary dermis, but does not extend into deeper levels.
- Level IV: tumor present in the reticular dermis.
- Level V: tumor in the subcutaneous fat.

The Clark level is inapplicable to mucosal melanoma, and it is difficult to determine even on melanoma of the vulvar skin, since the anatomic boundary between the papillary and reticular dermis is difficult to delineate on the genitalia. Other problems with the Clark level concept include its low reproducibility and low predictive power. Therefore, while the Clark level is conceptually interesting and historically important, it is not always reported in present practice. The main value of the Clark level is in a subset of melanomas. The presence of reticular dermal invasion (level IV) is a negative risk factor for melanomas under 1 mm thick, which would otherwise be expected to have a relatively favorable outcome.

The concept of Clark level is tied to that of growth phase. By definition, all melanomas *in situ* (Clark level I) and some microinvasive melanomas (Clark level II) are considered to be in radial growth phase. Beyond this point, melanoma may undergo a qualitative change to tumorigenic phenotype (vertical growth phase) (Figures 3.62 and 3.63)[38] if it meets one or both of the following criteria: (1) dermal nest(s) larger than the largest intraepidermal nest of tumor; and/or (2) the presence of any dermal mitotic figures.

Melanoma is also noteworthy for its occasional spontaneous regression,[102] indicated by absence of melanoma in *situ* of the overlying epidermis, dermal fibrosis, increased vascularity, lymphocytic infiltrates, and melanophages. While regression intuitively would seem to be favorable, it actually represents a negative prognostic factor. The likely explanation is that regressed lesions may previously have attained a greater thickness, and so the measured Breslow thickness may underestimate the tumor's metastatic potential.

The main histologic features correlating with worse prognosis in melanomas are higher Breslow thickness, or the presence of ulceration, vertical growth phase, regression, intralymphatic spread, or satellitosis (melanoma cells clearly separated from the main lesion). Therefore, these data should be included in pathology reports, together with a statement regarding margins.

SKIN APPENDAGE NEOPLASMS

The vulvar skin contains hair follicles, eccrine sweat glands, apocrine glands, and sebaceous glands. In the labia majora the sebaceous glands open into the hair follicles (pilosebaceous unit) but in the labia minora they are small and superficial, opening directly onto the mucosal surface. Despite the high concentration of skin appendages in the vulva, tumors derived from them are uncommon.

HIDRADENOMA PAPILLIFERUM (PAPILLARY HIDRADENOMA)

Definition
Hidradenoma papilliferum is a benign neoplasm with cystic and papillary features, and composed of epithelium exhibiting apocrine differentiation.

Clinical features
Hidradenoma papilliferum is the only adnexal neoplasm seen frequently on the vulva. It occurs mainly in middle-aged women on the labia majora and the outer lateral surfaces of the labia minora, but may also arise in the perineum. It typically

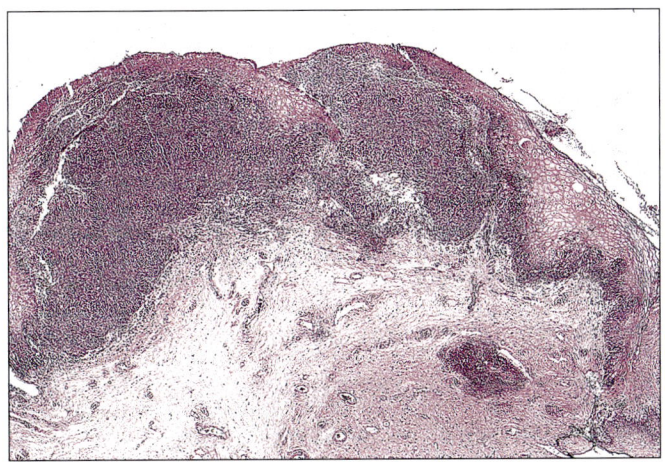

Fig. 3.62 Malignant melanoma. Vertical growth phase.

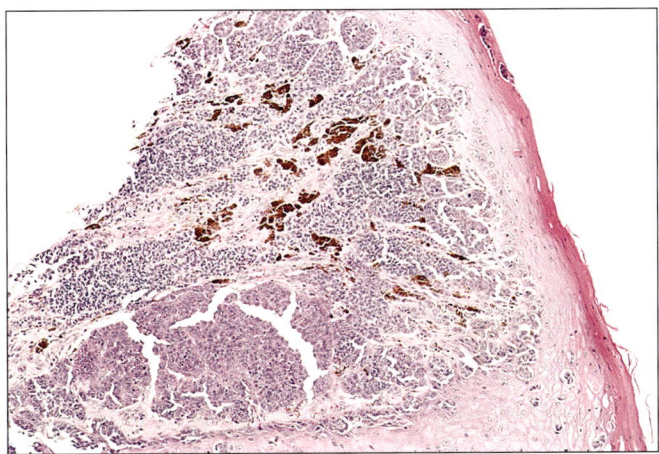

Fig. 3.63 Malignant melanoma.

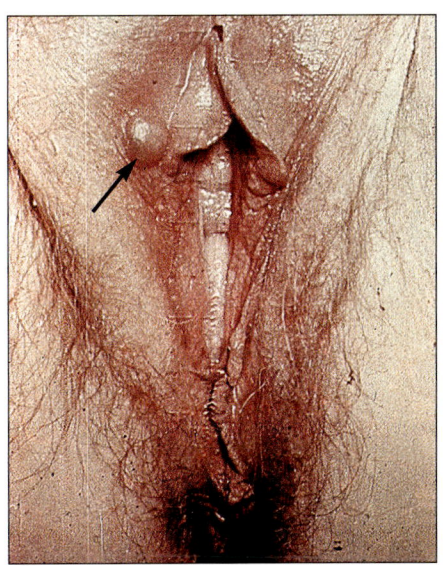

Fig. 3.64 Papillary hidradenoma (arrow).

presents as a solitary, round, firm, dome-shaped, occasionally tender nodule, 1–2 cm in diameter (Figure 3.64). Neglected, large lesions may ulcerate and bleed. Malignant change is very rare.

Microscopic features

These tumors are usually purely intradermal and are roughly spherical. Within a collagenous stroma are epithelial cells in a complex, folded, papillary pattern (Figure 3.65). Each branching papilla has a fibrovascular core and a double-layered epithelium (Figure 3.66) consisting of small, dark-staining myoepithelial cells and an inner layer of columnar or cuboidal cells, some of which are PAS positive.

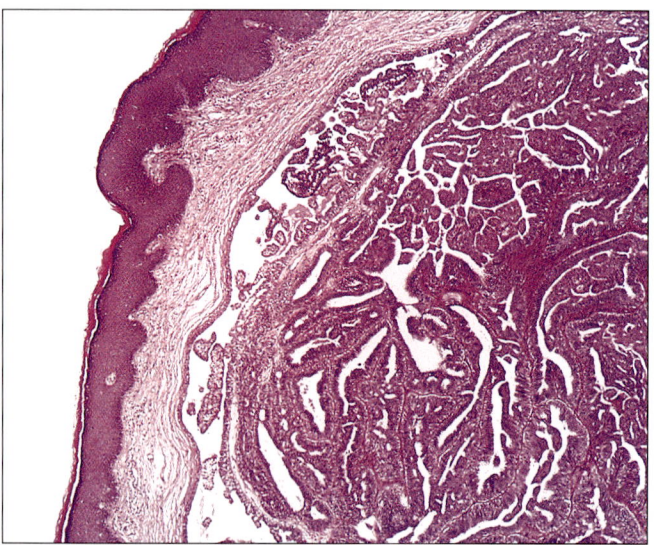

Fig. 3.65 Hidradenoma papilliferum. The complex papillary pattern of this dermal sweat gland tumor is characteristic.

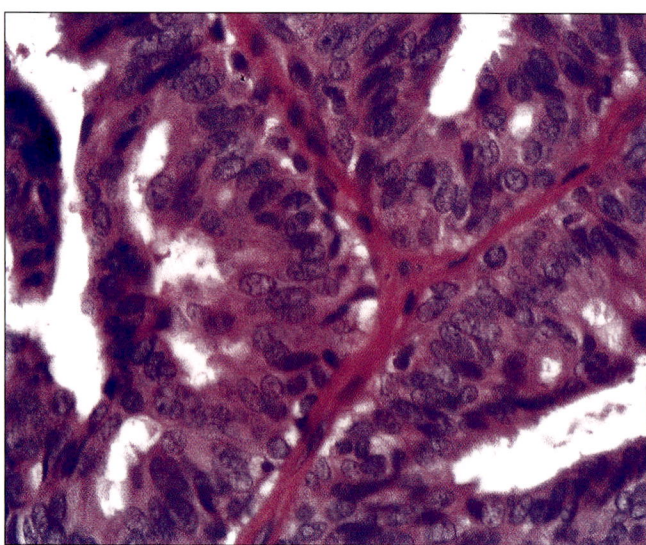

Fig. 3.66 Hidradenoma papilliferum. The papillae have a fine stromal core and focally a definite double layer, a discontinuous basal layer of myoepithelial cells beneath the tall columnar epithelial cells.

SYRINGOMA

Definition

Syringoma is a benign, microcystic neoplasm exhibiting differentiation toward eccrine ducts.

Clinical features

Syringoma most often occurs on the eyelid, often as multiple lesions. Labial syringomas may occur in the setting of eruptive syringomatosis. Syringomas are flesh-colored, dermal papules, rarely more than 3 mm in diameter, most commonly seen in young women. Malignant change is extremely rare.[46] The lesions usually remain small and treatment is rarely necessary. However, vulvar pruritus can occur and be aggravated during menses or pregnancy.[47,65]

Microscopic features

Histologically, syringomas comprise clusters of minute cystic ductal structures exhibiting a double layer of compressed epithelium, often with curved epithelial extensions attached to some of the microcysts (tadpole or frying-pan appearance) (Figure 3.67). The epithelium may undergo clear cell change due to abundance of cytoplasmic glycogen. The lumen of the microcysts often contains pink-staining, PAS-positive, proteinaceous material. Usually the stroma surrounding the glandular proliferation is fibrotic. In the chondroid syringoma (benign mixed tumor of skin), the stroma is cartilaginous. This lesion is histologically identical to the pleomorphic adenoma of the salivary gland.

TRICHOEPITHELIOMA (EPITHELIOMA ADENOIDES CYSTICUM, SUPERFICIAL TRICHOBLASTOMA)

Definition

Trichoepithelioma is a benign neoplasm exhibiting trichogenic differentiation.

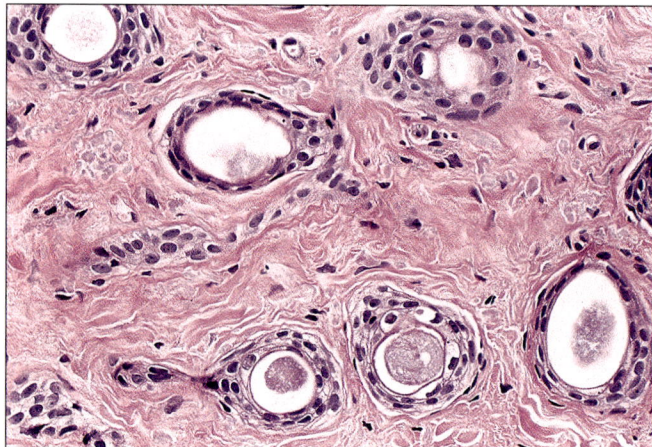

Fig. 3.67 Syringoma.

Clinical features

Trichoepithelioma occurs most often on the head and neck as a flesh-colored papule or nodule 2–8 mm in diameter, but may occur on the vulva. It is usually a solitary, sporadic lesion with onset in childhood or early adulthood. In the less common autosomal dominant form (Brooke–Spiegler syndrome), multiple lesions present in childhood on the nasolabial folds, and gradually increase in size; in this setting, trichoepithelioma may be associated with other cutaneous neoplasms such as cylindroma. Either form may be managed by conservative treatment such as shave biopsy or curettage, sometimes combined with electrodesiccation or cryotherapy.

Microscopic features

In the classic form, trichoepithelioma consists of basaloid cells that closely recapitulate follicular differentiation, especially in formation of papillary mesenchymal bodies (fibroblastic aggregates resembling abortive follicular papillae) and horn pseudocysts (resembling follicular infundibula) (Figure 3.68). The main histologic differential diagnosis is with basal cell carcinoma. In problematic cases, the presence of mitotic and apoptotic figures, myxoid stroma, and retraction of neoplastic cells from the stroma suggests basal cell carcinoma, whereas well-formed papillary–mesenchymal bodies and a more fibrous stroma suggest trichoepithelioma.[10] In the desmoplastic variant, follicular differentiation is less well developed; aggregates of neoplastic cells, usually including some keratinizing cysts, extend diffusely within a fibrous stroma, and may simulate the morpheiform pattern of basal cell carcinoma or microcystic adnexal carcinoma.

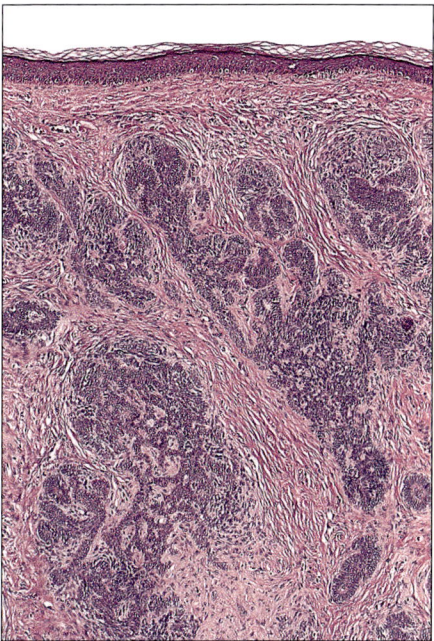

Fig. 3.68 Trichoepithelioma.

VASCULAR LESIONS

INFANTILE HEMANGIOMA (STRAWBERRY HEMANGIOMA, JUVENILE HEMANGIOENDOTHELIOMA)

Definition

Infantile hemangioma is a benign vascular neoplasm with onset in infancy and having a tendency for rapid growth followed by spontaneous regression.

Clinical features

These lesions have a predilection for the head and neck, but may also occur on the vulva and perianal skin. They are the most common vascular neoplasm of infancy, affecting 1% of newborns. Patients presenting with large, multiple, or visceral hemangiomas are at risk for high-output cardiac failure. Most lesions arise as a pink macule in the third to fifth week of postnatal life, grow rapidly into a bright-red nodule or plaque from one to several centimeters in diameter, and after about 1 year spontaneously resolve, partially or completely, leaving a scar. Lesions clinically presenting with telangiectatic vessels and peripheral pallor tend to involute more rapidly. Larger caliber hemangiomas with fast flow, in contrast, usually require therapy.[88] Moreover, ulceration and bleeding are common, particularly in larger lesions, and are further indications for treatment. As an alternative to surgical excision, laser therapy may be useful in selected cases, as may therapy with interferon and vinblastine.

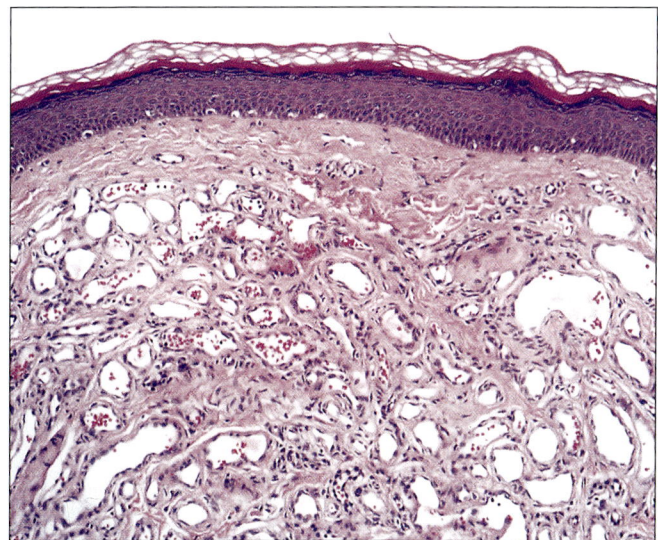

Fig. 3.69 Capillary hemangioma. This small dermal angioma is largely composed of capillary-sized channels. It is identical to those seen elsewhere in the skin.

Microscopic features

Lobular collections of small blood vessels are present in the dermis (Figure 3.69). During the early stages of the life cycle, these lesions are hypercellular and composed of numerous capillary-type vessels. In mature lesions, the vessels may become widely dilated. Regressed lesions are fibrotic and usually contain only a few dilated vessels. GLUT-1 (an antigen originally described in placenta) is a specific and sensitive marker for infantile hemangiomas, and can aid in their distinction from vascular malformations. Similarly, expression of the Wilms tumor 1 gene can distinguish proliferative vascular lesions from malformations.[82]

VENOUS MALFORMATION (CAVERNOUS HEMANGIOMA)

Definition
Venous malformation is a benign vascular lesion presenting at birth or shortly thereafter as widely dilated dermal blood vessels.

Clinical features
This lesion occurs predominantly in infants, on the head and neck area. It rarely regresses spontaneously. Use of the term 'cavernous hemangioma' is discouraged as these lesions do not represent a proliferative neoplasm as that name implies.

Microscopic features
Large blood vessels lined by a thin layer of endothelial cells are present in the dermis and subcutaneous tissue. Fibrin and red cells are numerous, and focal calcification may be seen.[25]

DEEP LYMPHATIC MALFORMATION (CAVERNOUS LYMPHANGIOMA)

Definition
Deep lymphatic malformation is a benign lesion presenting as widely dilated dermal or subcutaneous lymphatic vessels.

Clinical features
This lesion may involve the whole lower limb and extend onto the vulva. In addition to surface changes similar to those seen in superficial lymphatic malformation, there is often hypertrophy and lymphedema of the affected area. Lymphangiosarcoma is a rare complication.

Microscopic features
The dermis or deeper soft tissue contains a mass of anomalous, widely dilated lymphatics, occasionally containing scattered red cells and lined by flat endothelium (Figure 3.70). Lymphoid tissue is usually present at the periphery.

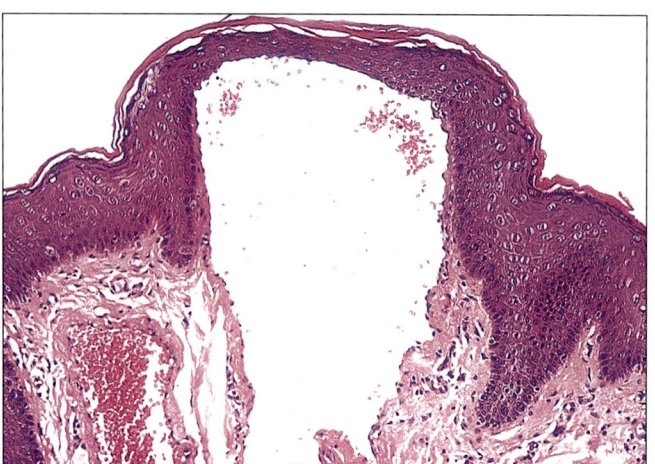

Fig. 3.70 *Cavernous lymphangioma.*

ACROCHORDON (FIBROEPITHELIAL POLYP, SKIN TAG, SQUAMOUS PAPILLOMA)

Definition
Acrochordon is a soft, skin-colored or pigmented polyp, ranging from a millimeter to a centimeter in diameter, and arising from a narrow stalk.

Clinical features
The humble acrochordon is thought to result from chronic intertriginous rubbing and therefore occurs most commonly in the inguinal folds. Other sites include the mons pubis and labia majora. Acrochordons are more common in obese, middle-aged and elderly women, and are often familial.

Microscopic features
Acrochordons are composed of a loose fibrovascular stroma covered by epidermis (Figures 3.71 and 3.72). Skin appendages are generally absent. Larger lesions may contain adipose tissue

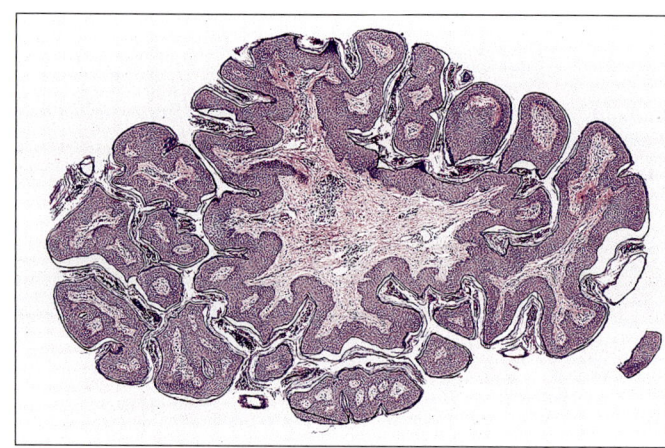

Fig. 3.71 Acrochordon.

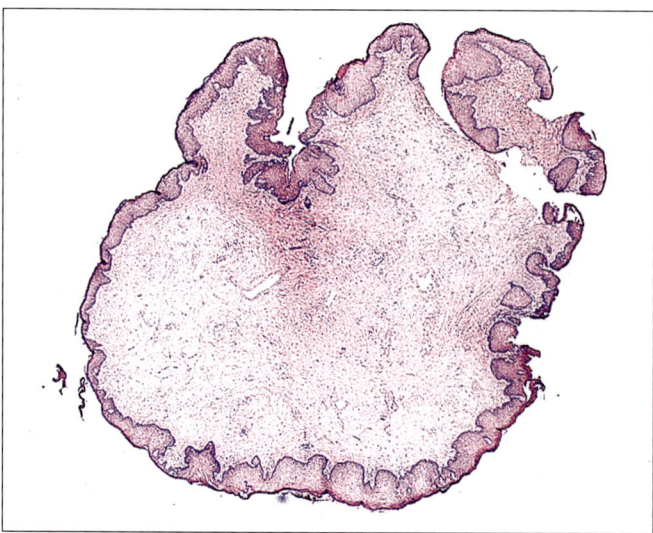

Fig. 3.72 Acrochordon.

in the stromal core, and are then designated as dermatolipomas or, if occurring in a dermatomal distribution, as nevus lipomatosus superficialis. Some dermatolipomas are associated with diabetes mellitus or hyperlipidemia.

ENDOMETRIOSIS (ENDOMETRIAL IMPLANT)

Definition
Endometriosis is the ectopic occurrence of endometrial tissue, often forming hemorrhagic cysts.

Clinical features
Implants of endometrial tissue into the vulva can occur during uterine curettage or episiotomy. Areas of endometriosis appear as purplish-blue nodules, and may cause pain or bleeding during menstruation. Please see Chapter 20.

Microscopic features
Within a fibrotic dermis are endometrial stroma and glands, sometimes exhibiting cyclic changes or decidualization. Hemosiderin deposition is common. CD10 reactivity is useful for confirming the presence of endometrial stroma.

HETEROTOPIC BREAST

Definition
Heterotopic breast is the ectopic localization of histologically normal mammary tissue.

Clinical features
A rare finding in the vulva, it most commonly presents as a small, asymptomatic, solitary, mobile nodule not fixed to the overlying skin. It may swell in late pregnancy.

Microscopic features
Terminal ducts and lobular units typical of benign breast tissue are seen (Figure 3.73). An inner columnar epithelium lines an outer myoepithelial layer (Figure 3.74). After childbirth it may show changes of lactation (Figure 3.75). Complex racemose growth (Figure 3.76), sclerosing adenosis (Figure 3.77), intraductal papilloma (Figure 3.78) or even breast carcinoma (Figure 3.79) may supervene rarely.[1,43,85]

RARE TUMORS AND TUMOR-LIKE CONDITIONS

Several tumors and tumor-like conditions encountered rarely in the vulva are described in greater detail in organs where they occur at greater frequencies.

- *Juvenile colonic polyp* arising in the vulva is exceedingly rare, being located just below the urethra and composed of radiating, occasionally dilated, tubuloacinar mucinous glands of intestinal type, set in fibrous stroma (Figures 3.80 and 3.81).[84]

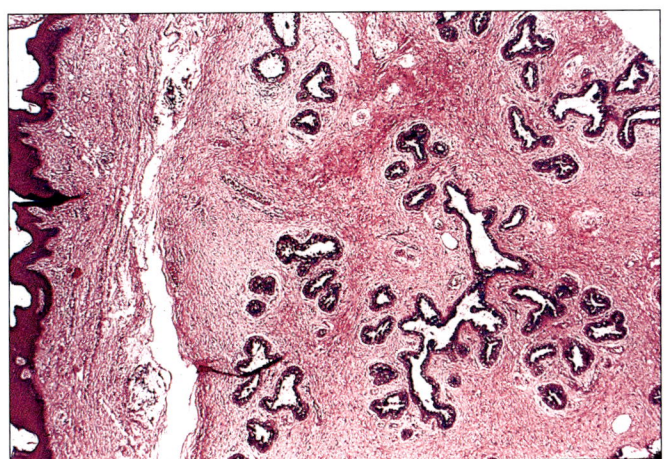

Fig. 3.73 Heterotopic breast.

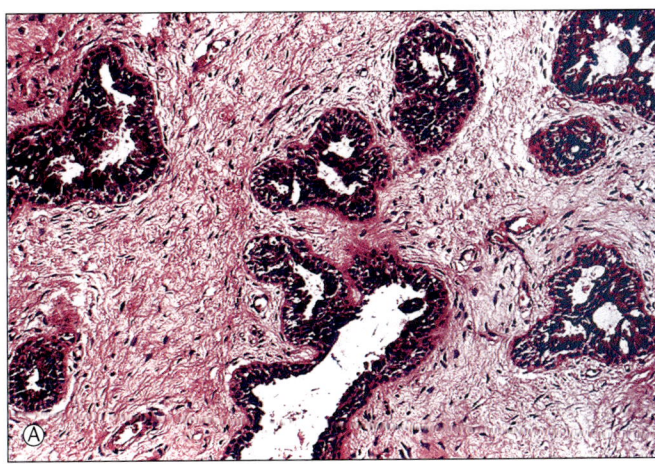
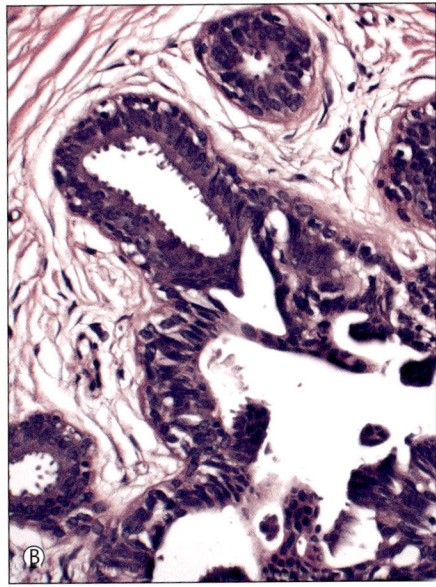

Fig. 3.74 **(A)** Heterotopic breast. **(B)** Detail of (basal) myoepithelial layer.

- *Primary yolk sac tumor* very rarely occurs in the vulvas in younger women.[7,76]
- *Neurofibromas* occur in the vulva of women with neurofibromatosis, where they can be multiple and disfiguring.
- *Solitary neurofibroma*, not part of a neurofibromatosis syndrome, usually presents as soft, raised, sometimes polypoid, tumors in the labium majus or clitoris.
- *Schwannoma* very rarely occurs in the labium majus.
- *Lipoma* derived from the subcutaneous fat of the labium majus may occur at any age. Smaller lipomas are round, lobulated, and well circumscribed, but larger tumors may become markedly protuberant and even polypoid. Histologically they are composed of mature adipocytes; *angiolipoma* is a painful variant having prominent, thin-walled vessels containing fibrin thrombi.

Please also see Chapter 4 for discussion of other mesenchymal tumors.

LANGERHANS CELL HISTIOCYTOSIS (HISTIOCYTOSIS X)[41,60,66,92,112,146]

Definition
Langerhans cell histiocytosis (LCH) is a localized or systemic accumulation of pathologic Langerhans cells.

Clinical features
LCH is a spectrum of disease characterized by proliferation of specialized, bone-marrow-derived Langerhans cells and mature eosinophils. The infiltrate of LCH is monoclonal, supporting its neoplastic nature.[150] Abnormalities of suppressor cell number and function also play a pathogenetic role, creating a permissive immunosurveillance system. Among proposed etiologic factors are viruses, defective intercellular communica-

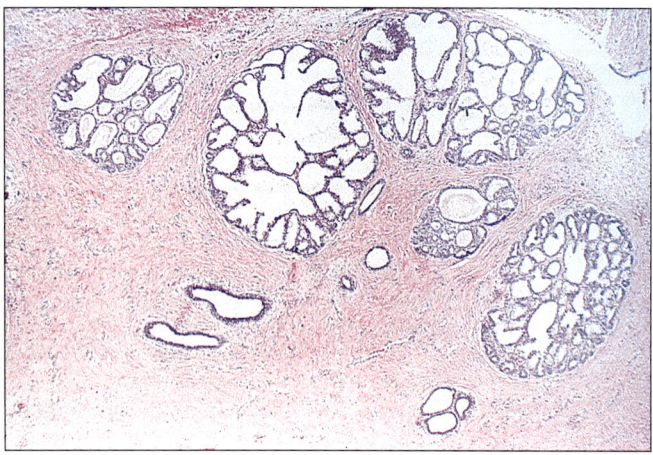

Fig. 3.75 Lactating heterotopic breast.

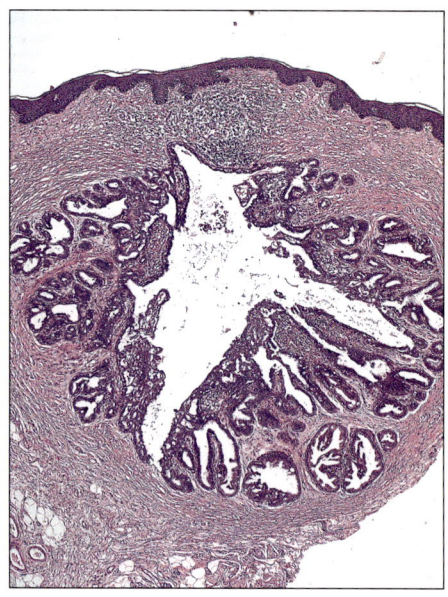

Fig. 3.76 Heterotopic breast with complex racemose glandular growth.

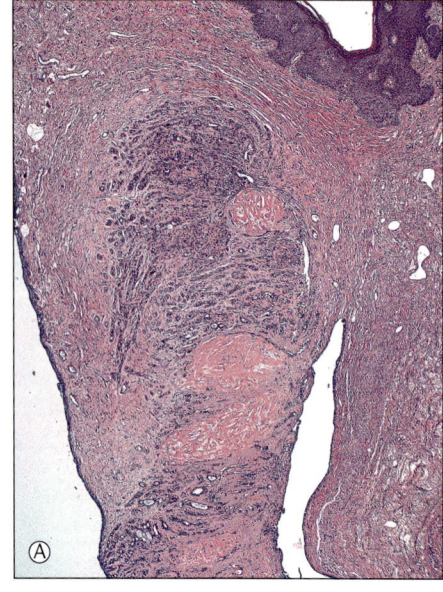

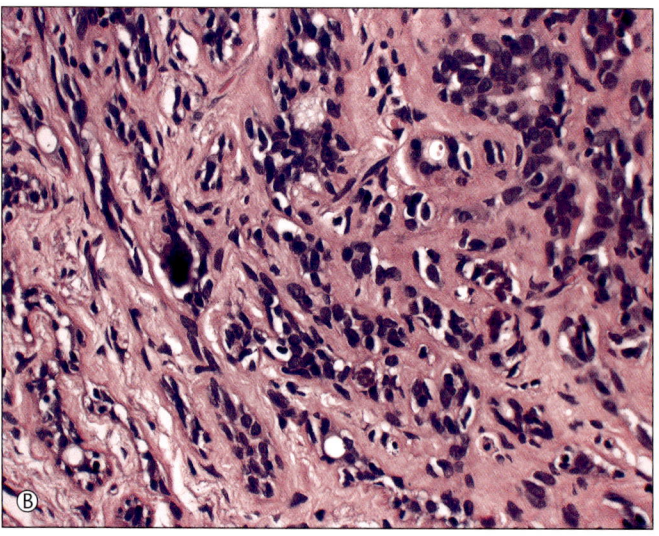

Fig. 3.77 **(A)** Sclerosing adenosis in ectopic breast. **(B)** Detail.

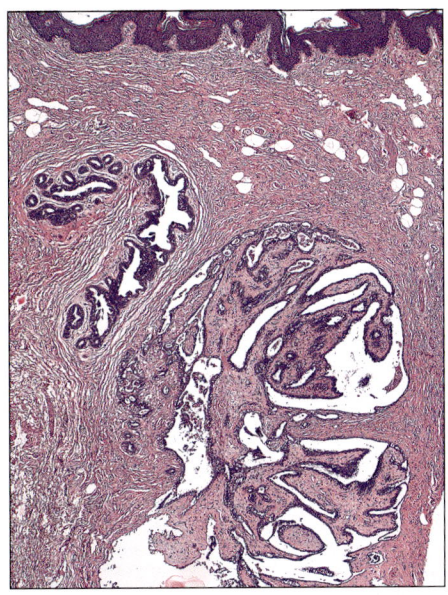

Fig. 3.78 Intraductal papilloma.

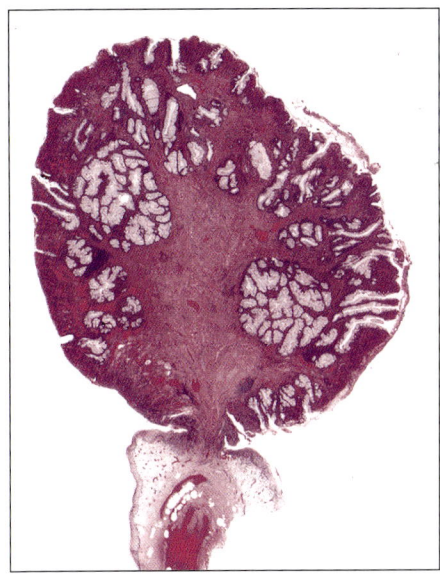

Fig. 3.80 Juvenile colonic polyp.

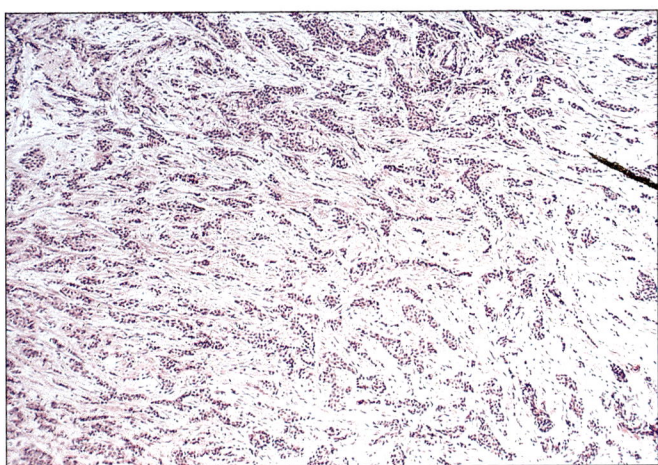

Fig. 3.79 Adenocarcinoma arising in ectopic breast.

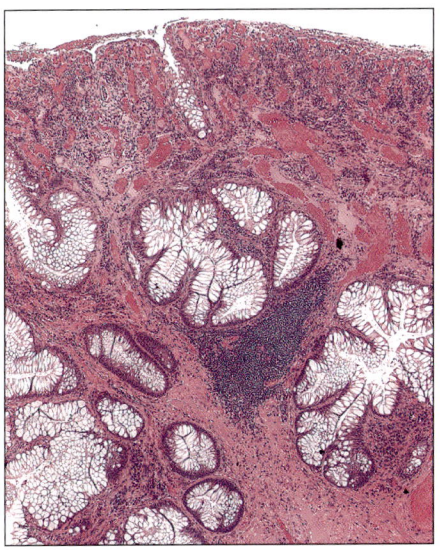

Fig. 3.81 Juvenile colonic polyp. Detail of bland but complex mucin-secreting glands.

tion (e.g., T cell–macrophage interaction), and cytokine imbalance.

In the United States the incidence is about 1200 new cases per year. LCH spans a clinical spectrum ranging from an acute, fulminant, disseminated disease of childhood (Letterer–Siwe disease) to solitary or few, indolent, chronic lesions of bone or other organs (eosinophilic granuloma). An intermediate form, showing multifocal, chronic involvement, classically presents as the triad of diabetes insipidus, proptosis, and lytic bone lesions (Hand–Schüller–Christian disease). Unifocal LCH is generally self-limited, as are multifocal, chronic cases (with the exception of infants with extrapulmonary involvement). In contrast, more than half of LCH patients under the age of 2 years with disseminated disease and organ dysfunction will die of this malady. Approximately one-third of cases of apparently isolated vulvar LCH subsequently evolve to a disseminated form, most commonly involving bones.[100]

Eosinophilic granulomas are often asymptomatic, incidental findings discovered during investigation for unrelated disorders, or they may present with bone pain or as a soft-tissue mass. They occur classically as solitary calvarial lesions in young adults. Other involved sites include vertebra, rib, mandible, femur, ilium, and scapula. One-third of patients have mucocutaneous lesions, usually infiltrated nodules and ulcerated plaques, in the mouth, axillae, oral, perineal, vulvar, or retroauricular regions (Figure 3.82). Eighty per cent of patients with the acute, disseminated Letterer–Siwe form of the disease have cutaneous lesions, frequently as the first sign, consisting of petechiae and yellow-brown, scaly and crusted papules. Eventually the lesions coalesce and evolve into an erythematous, weeping eruption mimicking spongiotic dermatitis. This

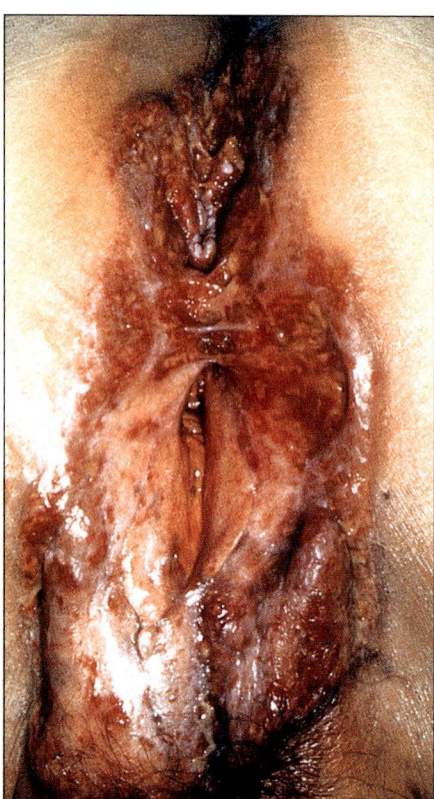

Fig. 3.82 Langerhans cell histiocytosis with affected flexural areas. This elderly woman presented with eroding plaques in the perineum and jaundice secondary to liver involvement by the tumor.

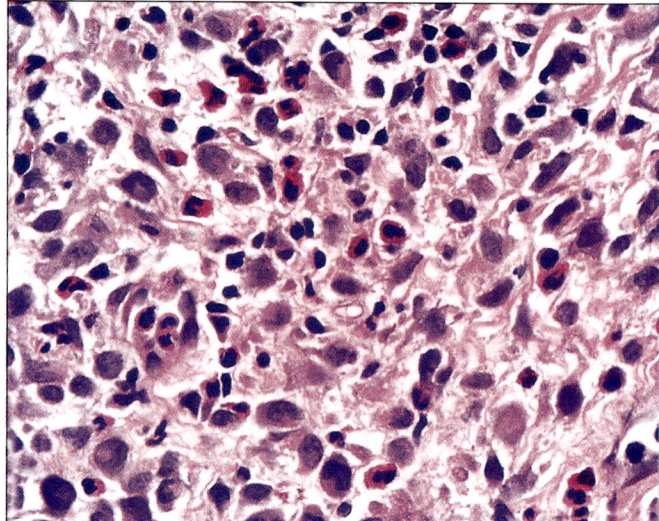

Fig. 3.83 Langerhans cell histiocytosis. The tumor infiltrate is a mixture of pleomorphic Langerhans cells, eosinophils and lymphocytes. In very young children, the infiltrate is composed almost entirely of Langerhans cells alone ('Letterer–Siwe disease').

type of eruption may be extensive, involving particularly the scalp, face, trunk, and buttocks as well as flexural areas including the vulva. The intertriginous lesions may develop secondary infections and ulceration. Patients with Letterer–Siwe syndrome commonly also experience fever, anemia, thrombocytopenia, lymphadenopathy, hepatosplenomegaly, and pulmonary infiltrates.

Microscopic features

The dermis contains infiltrates of pathologic LCH cells admixed with eosinophils and a lesser number of neutrophils, plasma cells, and lymphocytes (Figure 3.83). The LCH cell is a non-dendritic, ovoid, mononuclear cell, 15–25 μm in diameter, with a folded or reniform nucleus, central nucleolus, and a moderate amount of slightly eosinophilic, homogeneous cytoplasm.

Immunohistochemistry can be helpful for definitive diagnosis. The pathologic LCH cells strongly express S-100 protein in a cytoplasmic pattern, and also the more specific markers CD1a and langerin (CD207).[23] Notably, the pathologic LCH cells generally lack expression of several macrophage markers including the MAC-387 antigen, lysozyme, and α_1-antitrypsin, but often express CD68. Electron microscopy demonstrates the diagnostic Birbeck granule: a short, rod-like intracytoplasmic organelle, 33 nm wide and 190–360 nm long, with a midline, intermembranous, zipper-like line, and a terminal vesicular expansion imparting a 'racquet' appearance.

MERKEL CELL CARCINOMA (TRABECULAR CARCINOMA, SMALL CELL CARCINOMA OF THE SKIN, PRIMARY CUTANEOUS NEUROENDOCRINE CARCINOMA)[59]

Definition

Merkel cell carcinoma is a malignant primary neoplasm of the skin exhibiting neuroendocrine differentiation.

Clinical features

This highly aggressive tumor has a similar incidence in men and women, but women tend to survive longer. Mean age at diagnosis is about 75 years, and only 5% of cases occur before 50 years. They occur much more commonly in the skin of the head and upper trunk in the elderly, but may originate in the skin of the labia majora. Most present as a solitary, dome-shaped nodule or firm plaque, usually over 2 cm in greatest dimension. They are typically red, violaceous, or purple, with a shiny epidermal surface and telangiectases suggesting atrophy. Ulceration occurs occasionally. The tumors metastasize early and extensively via lymphatics and the bloodstream. Overall 2-year survival is 50–70%. A few cases of Merkel cell carcinoma arising from the Bartholin gland have been described. These have a poor outcome, with dissemination to regional lymph nodes or lung at the time of tumor detection or shortly thereafter.[75]

Microscopic features

This carcinoma exhibits neuroendocrine differentiation.[49] Proposed cells of origin include the epidermal Merkel cell, a dermal Merkel cell equivalent, a neural-crest-derived cell of the amine precursor uptake and decarboxylation system, and a residual epidermal stem cell. Merkel cell carcinoma is usually located predominantly within the dermis. An intraepidermal component may be present, but purely *in situ* cases are rare. Frequently the epidermis is hyperplastic. Merkel cell carcinoma has several architectural patterns. The trabecular pattern consists of interconnecting strands of dermal tumor cells with

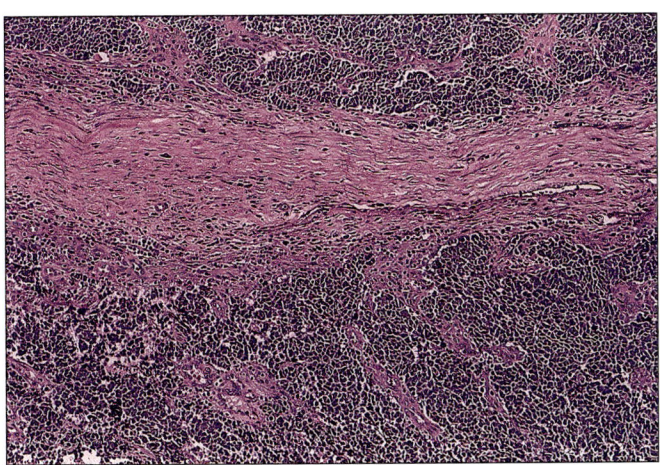

Fig. 3.84 Merkel cell tumor, trabecular pattern.

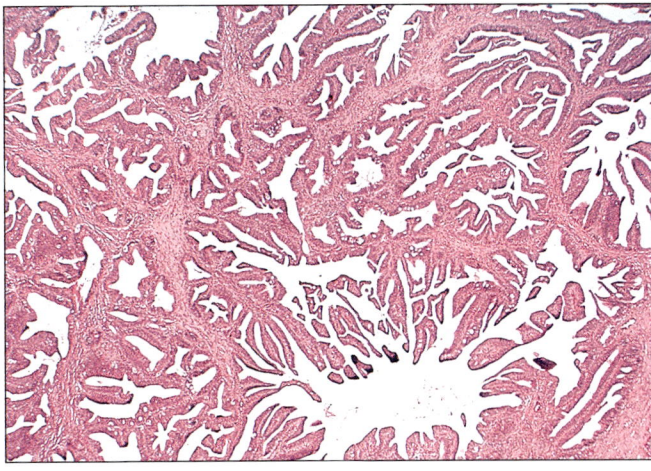

Fig. 3.86 Papillary adenocarcinoma of Bartholins gland.

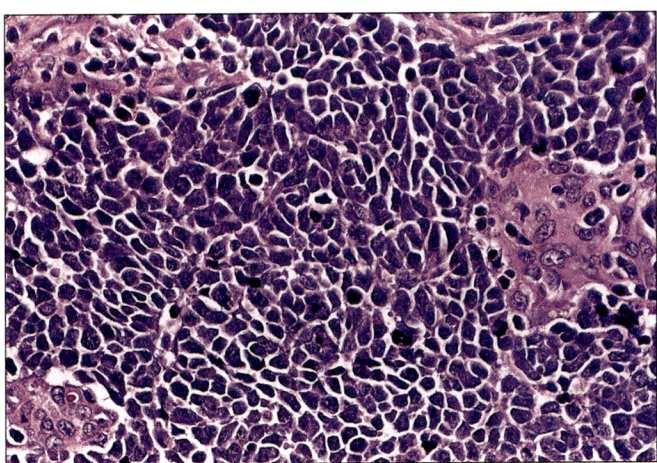

Fig. 3.85 Merkel cell carcinoma.

of primary Merkel cell carcinoma of the skin over metastatic neuroendocrine carcinoma (e.g., from a pulmonary primary), but clinical investigation is necessary in all cases.

Electron microscopy reveals a lobulated nucleus that may contain rodlets. The electron-lucent cytoplasm contains a prominent Golgi apparatus and many ribosomes. Intermediate filaments are numerous and often assume a parallel or whorled arrangement near the nucleus, accounting for the dot-like pattern of cytokeratin distribution visualized by immunohistochemistry. Desmosomes may be present. Most diagnostic is the dense core granule, 80–120 nm in diameter, the source and locus of the neuroendocrine peptides.

METASTATIC TUMORS

The most common primary sites of origin for vulvar metastases are the uterine cervix and endometrium,[51] ovary, breast, lung, kidney, and large bowel. About half of the primary tumors are of gynecologic origin.[96] The labium majus is site most frequently involved.

MISCELLANEOUS LESIONS OF AFFILIATED STRUCTURES

BARTHOLIN GLAND

Other than cysts, diseases of Bartholin gland, including hyperplasia, adenoma,[78] and carcinoma, are rare. The latter are usually adenocarcinomas of various types (papillary, Figure 3.86; mucinous, Figure 3.87; colloid, Figure 3.88) or squamous cell carcinomas,[97] but about 10–20% are adenoid cystic carcinomas (Figures 3.89 and 3.90),[153] which are histologically similar to those of the salivary glands. Nodular hyperplasia,[124] adenoma or carcinoma of Bartholin glands may present as a nodule resembling the much more common Bartholin gland cyst. At presentation, about one-fourth of all Bartholin gland carcinomas have metastasized to the superficial inguinal–femoral nodes. Wide local excision or vulvectomy with excision

formation of pseudorosettes and pseudoglands (Figure 3.84). The intermediate pattern comprises large, solid nests of neoplastic cells. In the diffuse pattern, tumor cells infiltrate among dermal collagen bundles without forming distinctive organoid aggregates. A particular Merkel cell carcinoma may contain elements of all these patterns.

The neoplastic cells are round, small, and dark, with inconspicuous nucleoli, central euchromatin, and peripheral heterochromatin (Figure 3.85). Mitotic figures and apoptotic bodies are numerous. Vascular or lymphatic invasion is not uncommon. Several histologic variants of Merkel cell carcinoma include a pagetoid type resembling extramammary Paget disease or melanoma,[56] as well as tumors with focal glandular or squamous differentiation mimicking adenocarcinoma or squamous cell carcinoma. Immunohistochemistry is helpful for definitive diagnosis. CK20 is expressed in a dot-like paranuclear pattern.[20] Other antibodies against low molecular weight cytokeratins (e.g., CAM 5.2, MNF116), while less specific, also show a similar pattern. In addition, neurofilament protein is also expressed in most cases. These findings favor the diagnosis

of inguinal nodes on both sides is the standard treatment. With adenocarcinoma, 5-year survival rates of about 50% can be expected, but this falls to about 20% when nodal metastases exist. Survival rates for SCC are rather worse, and for adenoid-cystic carcinoma, slightly better.

PARAURETHRAL (SKENE) GLAND

The Skene glands are located on both sides of the urethra and their ducts open onto either side of the urethral meatus. The duct is lined by transitional epithelium whereas the glandular structures are mucinous. Skene glands also encompass the mucinous periurethral glands that line the wall of the female urethra. Skene glands can give rise to lesions ranging from mucinous cysts to mucinous adenocarcinoma (Figure 3.91).

URETHRA

URETHRAL CARUNCLE

Definition
The urethral caruncle is a small, fleshy, sometimes painful protrusion of the mucous membrane at the meatus of the female urethra.

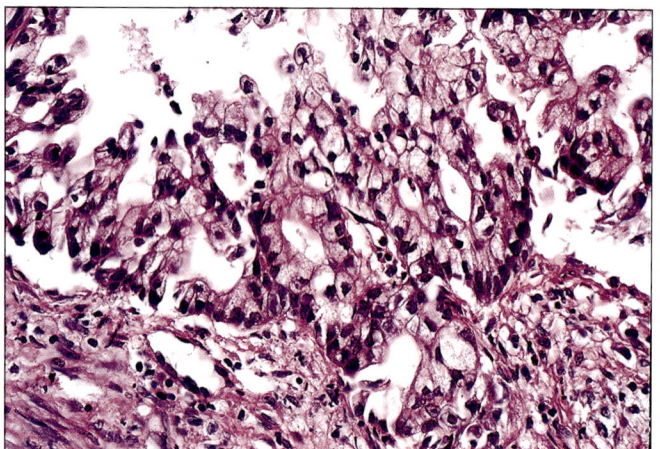

Fig. 3.87 Mucinous adenocarcinoma of Bartholin gland.

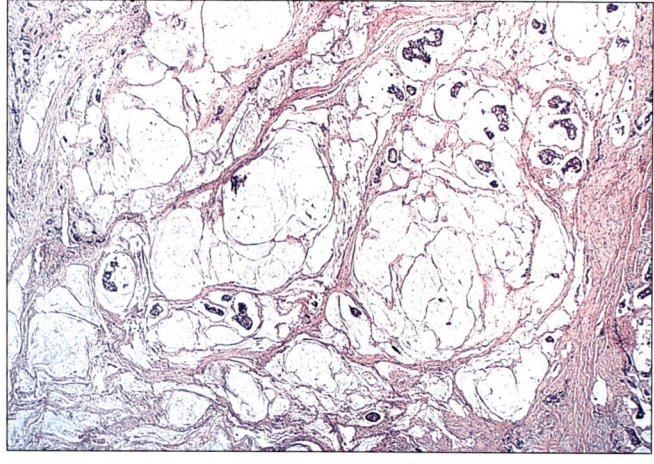

Fig. 3.88 Colloid adenocarcinoma of Bartholin gland.

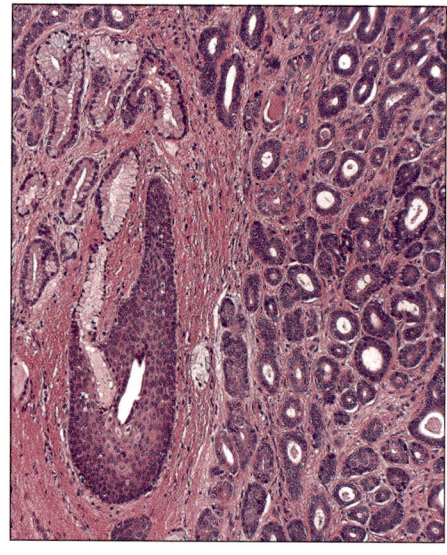

Fig. 3.90 Cystically dilated glands in a carcinoma arising from Bartholin gland.

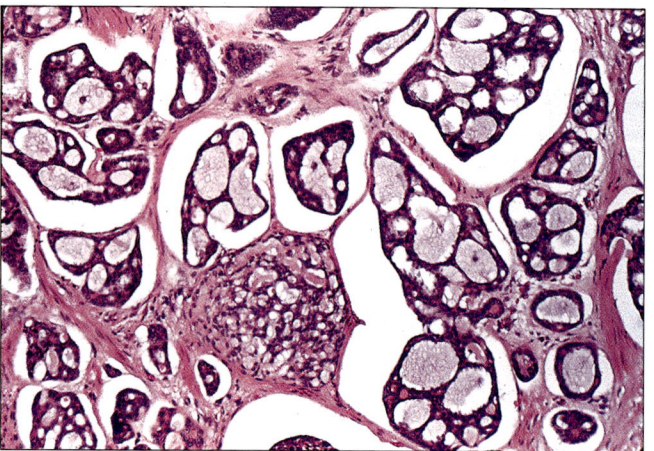

Fig. 3.89 Adenoid cystic carcinoma of Bartholin gland.

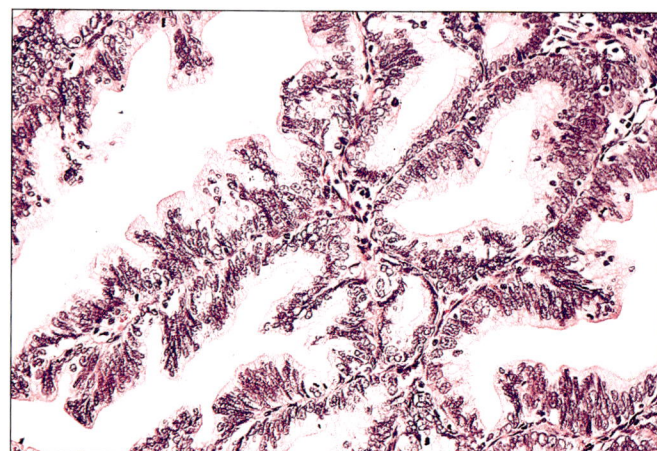

Fig. 3.91 Mucinous adenocarcinoma of Skene gland.

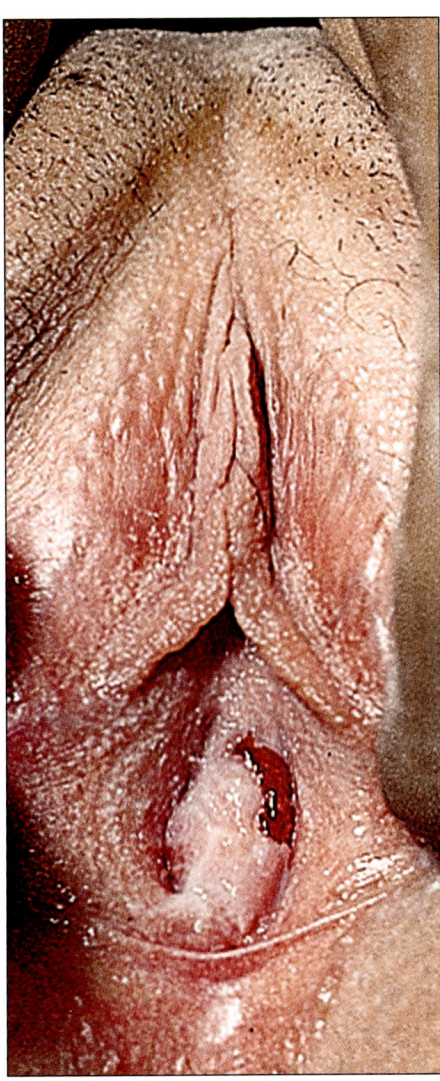

Fig. 3.92 Urethral caruncle.

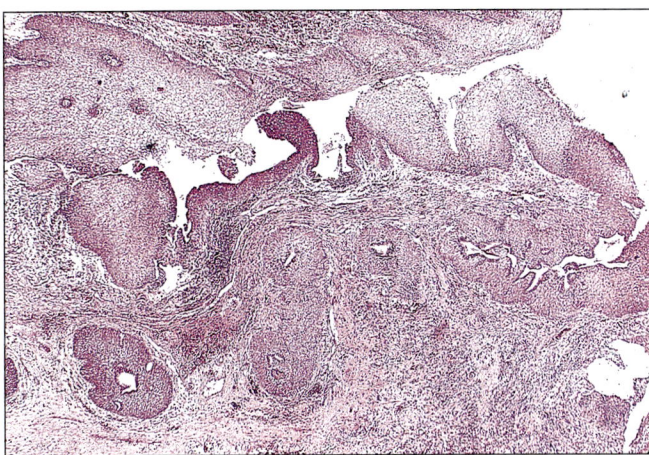

Fig. 3.93 Urethral caruncle with stroma containing a dense, chronic inflammatory cell infiltrate.

Clinical features

The caruncle may be telangiectatic, papillomatous, or composed of granulation tissue (Figure 3.92). It is common, usually after the menopause, and is often asymptomatic, although it may be painful. Caruncles can be difficult to distinguish clinically from the early stage of the much rarer urethral carcinoma. The cancer, though, tends to bleed readily and is indurated to palpation.

Microscopic features

Urethral caruncles are protuberant, polypoid masses of urethral stroma containing a dense, chronic inflammatory cell infiltrate, admixed with neutrophils if the surface is ulcerated (Figure 3.93). Sometimes, vascular proliferation is so prominent that a capillary hemangioma or pyogenic granuloma may be suspected. Islands or cords of urethral epithelium are present, distinguishing the caruncle from urethral prolapse, in which the stroma is edematous, with only a scanty inflammatory infiltrate and no included epithelium.

URETHRAL CARCINOMA[29]

Definition

Urethral carcinoma is a malignant neoplasm of urethral epithelium.

Clinical features

These rare tumors usually present in elderly women with dysuria, frequency, urgency, and hematuria. In early stages, urethral carcinoma resembles a caruncle or prolapse, but is characteristically firm to palpation, and may be friable and bleed.

Microscopic features

Almost all primary tumors of the urethra proper are SCCs arising from the squamous epithelium of the anterior third of the urethra. In advanced cases the urethral origin may be hard to identify, and such lesions may resemble an ordinary vulvar SCC. Small foci of transitional epithelium may be seen, but pure transitional cell carcinoma is extremely rare. Adenocarcinomas of the urethral region are usually derived from the paraurethral glands. The usual squamous or mixed squamous/transitional carcinoma is most often solid, but there may be papillary areas. Spread is by local invasion to the bladder neck, the rest of the vulva, and occasionally the vagina. Lymphatic spread may occur to the superficial inguinal nodes and later the deeper pelvic nodes. The 5-year survival rate is 30–40%, despite surgery and radiotherapy. Large tumors with extensive local involvement and lymph node spread have a much worse prognosis.[140]

REFERENCES

1. Abbott JJ, Ahmed I. Adenocarcinoma of mammary-like glands of the vulva: report of a case and review of the literature. Am J Dermatopathol 2006;28:127–33.
2. Ambros RA, Malfetano JH, Mihm MC. Clinicopathologic features of vulvar squamous cell carcinomas exhibiting prominent fibromyxoid stromal response. Int J Gynecol Pathol 1996;15:137–45.
3. Andreassi L, Perotti R, Rubegni P, et al. Digital dermoscopy analysis for the differentiation of atypical nevi and early melanoma: a new quantitative semiology. Arch Dermatol 1999;135:1459–65.
4. Bai H, Cviko A, Granter S, Yuan L, Betensky RA, Crum CP. Immunophenotypic and viral (human papillomavirus) correlates of vulvar seborrheic keratosis. Hum Pathol 2003;34:559–64.

5. Barnhill RL, Roush GC, Duray PH. Correlation of histologic architectural and cytoplasmic features with nuclear atypia in atypical (dysplastic) nevomelanocytic nevi. Hum Pathol 1990;21:51–8.

6. Barnhill RL, Albert LS, Shama SK, Goldenhersh MA, Rhodes AR, Sober AJ. Genital lentiginosis: a clinical and histopathologic study. J Am Acad Dermatol 1990;22:453–60.

7. Basgul A, Gokaslan H, Kavak ZN, Eren FT, Bozkurt N. Primary yolk sac tumor (endodermal sinus tumor) of the vulva: case report and review of the literature. Eur J Gynaecol Oncol 2006;27:395–8.

8. Belousova IE, Kazakov DV, Michal M, Suster S. Vulvar Toker cells: the long-awaited missing link: a proposal for an origin-based histogenetic classification of extramammary Paget disease. Am J Dermatopathol 2006;28:84–6.

9. Benedet JL, Miller DM, Ehlen TG, Bertrand MA. Basal cell carcinoma of the vulva: clinical features and treatment results in 28 patients. Obstet Gynecol 1997;90:765–8.

10. Bettencourt MS, Prieto VG, Shea CR. Trichoepithelioma: a 19-year clinicopathologic re-evaluation. J Cutan Pathol 1999;26:398–404.

11. Bianco MK, Vasef MA. HER-2 gene amplification in Paget disease of the nipple and extramammary site: a chromogenic in situ hybridization study. Diagn Mol Pathol 2006;15:131–5.

12. Bono A, Tomatis S, Bartoli C, et al. The ABCD system of melanoma detection: a spectrophotometric analysis of the Asymmetry, Border, Color, and Dimension. Cancer 1999;85:72–7.

13. Brummer O, Stegner HE, Bohmer G, Kuhnle H, Petry KU. HER-2/neu expression in Paget disease of the vulva and the female breast. Gynecol Oncol 2004;95:336–40.

14. Busam KJ, Chen YT, Old LJ, et al. Expression of melan-A (MART1) in benign melanocytic nevi and primary cutaneous malignant melanoma. Am J Surg Pathol 1998;22:976–82.

15. Carli P, Cattaneo A, De Magnis A, Biggeri A, Taddei G, Giannotti B. Squamous cell carcinoma arising in vulval lichen sclerosus: a longitudinal cohort study. Eur J Cancer Prev 1995;4:491–5.

16. Carlson JA, Lamb P, Malfetano J, Ambros RA, Mihm MC. Clinicopathologic comparison of vulvar and extragenital lichen sclerosus: histologic variants, evolving lesions, and etiology of 141 cases. Mod Pathol 1998;11:844–54.

17. Carlson JA, Ambros R, Malfetano J, et al. Vulvar lichen sclerosus and squamous cell carcinoma: a cohort, case control, and investigational study with historical perspective; implications for chronic inflammation and sclerosis in the development of neoplasia. Hum Pathol 1998;29:932–48.

18. Carlson JA, Mu XC, Slominski A, et al. Melanocytic proliferations associated with lichen sclerosus. Arch Dermatol 2002;138:77–87.

19. Ceylan H, Ozokutan BH, Karakok M, Buyukbese S. Paraurethral cyst: is conservative management always appropriate? Eur J Pediatr Surg 2002;12:212–4.

20. Chan JK, Suster S, Wenig BM, Tsang WY, Chan JB, Lau AL. Cytokeratin 20 immunoreactivity distinguishes Merkel cell (primary cutaneous neuroendocrine) carcinomas and salivary gland small cell carcinomas from small cell carcinomas of various sites. Am J Surg Pathol 1997;21:226–34.

21. Chan JK, Sugiyama V, Pham H, et al. Margin distance and other clinico-pathologic prognostic factors in vulvar carcinoma: a multivariate analysis. Gynecol Oncol 2007;104:636–41.

22. Chen W, Koenig C. Vulvar keratoacanthoma: a report of two cases. Int J Gynecol Pathol 2004;23:284–6.

23. Chikwava K, Jaffe R. Langerin (CD207) staining in normal pediatric tissues, reactive lymph nodes, and childhood histiocytic disorders. Pediatr Dev Pathol 2004;7:607–14.

24. Clark WH, Jr, Hood AF, Tucker MA, Jampel RM. Atypical melanocytic nevi of the genital type with a discussion of reciprocal parenchymal–stromal interactions in the biology of neoplasia. Hum Pathol 1998;29(1 Suppl 1):S1–24.

25. Coffin CM, Dehner LP. Vascular tumors in children and adolescents: a clinicopathologic study of 228 tumors in 222 patients. Pathol Annu 1993;28(Pt 1):97–120.

26. Cramer SF. The histogenesis of acquired melanocytic nevi. Based on a new concept of melanocytic differentiation. Am J Dermatopathol 1984;6(Suppl):289–98.

27. Crawford D, Nimmo M, Clement PB, et al. Prognostic factors in Paget's disease of the vulva: a study of 21 cases. Int J Gynecol Pathol 1999;18:351–9.

28. Creasman WT, Phillips JL, Menck HR. The National Cancer Data Base report on early stage invasive vulvar carcinoma. The American College of Surgeons Commission on Cancer and the American Cancer Society. Cancer 1997;80:505–13.

29. Dalbagni G, Zhang ZF, Lacombe L, Herr HW. Female urethral carcinoma: an analysis of treatment outcome and a plea for a standardized management strategy. Br J Urol 1998;82:835–41.

30. De Cicco C, Sideri M, Bartolomei M, et al. Sentinel node biopsy in early vulvar cancer. Br J Cancer 2000;82:295–9.

31. de Giorgi V, Massi D, Salvini C, Mannone F, Carli P. Pigmented seborrheic keratoses of the vulva clinically mimicking a malignant melanoma: a clinical, dermoscopic–pathologic case study. Clin Exp Dermatol 2005;30:17–19.

32. de Giorgi V, Massi D, Salvini C, Mannone F, Cattaneo A, Carli P. Thin melanoma of the vulva: a clinical, dermoscopic–pathologic case study. Arch Dermatol 2005;141:1046–7.

33. de Vries TJ, Fourkour A, Wobbes T, Verkroost G, Ruiter DJ, van Muijen GN. Heterogeneous expression of immunotherapy candidate proteins gp100, MART-1, and tyrosinase in human melanoma cell lines and in human melanocytic lesions. Cancer Res 1997;57:3223–9.

34. DeMatos P, Tyler D, Seigler HF. Mucosal melanoma of the female genitalia: a clinicopathologic study of forty-three cases at Duke University Medical Center. Surgery 1998;124:38–48.

35. Dunton CJ, Berd D. Vulvar melanoma, biologically different from other cutaneous melanomas. Lancet 1999;354:2013–4.

36. Egan CA, Bradley RR, Logsdon VK, Summers BK, Hunter GR, Vanderhooft SL. Vulvar melanoma in childhood. Arch Dermatol 1997;133:345–8.

37. El Shabrawi-Caelen L, Soyer HP, Schaeppi H, et al. Genital lentigines and melanocytic nevi with superimposed lichen sclerosus: a diagnostic challenge. J Am Acad Dermatol 2004;50:690–4.

38. Elder DE, Guerry Dt, Epstein MN, et al. Invasive malignant melanomas lacking competence for metastasis. Am J Dermatopathol 1984;6(Suppl):55–61.

39. Escalonilla P, Grilli R, Canamero M, et al. Sebaceous carcinoma of the vulva. Am J Dermatopathol 1999;21:468–72.

40. Fanning J, Lambert HC, Hale TM, Morris PC, Schuerch C. Paget's disease of the vulva: prevalence of associated vulvar adenocarcinoma, invasive Paget's disease, and recurrence after surgical excision. Am J Obstet Gynecol 1999;180(1 Pt 1):24–7.

41. Fernandez Flores A, Mallo S. Langerhans cell histiocytosis of vulva. Dermatol Online J 2006;12:15.

42. Fishman DA, Chambers SK, Schwartz PE, Kohorn EI, Chambers JT. Extramammary Paget's disease of the vulva. Gynecol Oncol 1995;56:266–70.

43. Fracchioli S, Puopolo M, De La Longrais IA, et al. Primary 'breast-like' cancer of the vulva: a case report and critical review of the literature. Int J Gynecol Cancer 2006;16(Suppl 1):423–8.

44. Franck JM, Young AW. Squamous cell carcinoma in situ arising within lichen planus of the vulva. Dermatol Surg 1995;21:890–4.

45. Gadducci A, Cionini L, Romanini A, Fanucchi A, Genazzani AR. Old and new perspectives in the management of high-risk, locally advanced or recurrent, and metastatic vulvar cancer. Crit Rev Oncol Hematol 2006;60:227–41.

46. Gemer O, Piura B, Segal S, Inbar IY. Adenocarcinoma arising in a chondroid syringoma of vulva. Int J Gynecol Pathol 2003;22:398–400.

47. Gerdsen R, Wenzel J, Uerlich M, Bieber T, Petrow W. Periodic genital pruritus caused by syringoma of the vulva. Acta Obstet Gynecol Scand 2002;81:369–70.

48. Gibson GE, Ahmed I. Perianal and genital basal cell carcinoma: a clinicopathologic review of 51 cases. J Am Acad Dermatol 2001;45:68–71.

49. Gil-Moreno A, Garcia-Jimenez A, Gonzalez-Bosquet J, et al. Merkel cell carcinoma of the vulva. Gynecol Oncol 1997;64:526–32.

50. Gilbey S, Moore DH, Look KY, Sutton GP. Vulvar keratoacanthoma. Obstet Gynecol 1997;89:848–50.

51. Giordano G, Gnetti L, Melpignano M. Endometrial carcinoma metastatic to the vulva: a case report and review of the literature. Path Prac Res 2005;201:751–6.

52. Glass FL, Cottam JA, Reintgen DS, Fenske NA. Lymphatic mapping and sentinel node biopsy in the management of high-risk melanoma. J Am Acad Dermatol 1998;39(4 Pt 1):603–10.

53. Goldblum JR, Hart WR. Vulvar Paget's disease: a clinicopathologic and immunohistochemical study of 19 cases. Am J Surg Pathol 1997;21:1178–87.

54. Gualco M, Bonin S, Foglia G, et al. Morphologic and biologic studies on ten cases of verrucous carcinoma of the vulva supporting the theory of a discrete clinico-pathologic entity. Int J Gynecol Cancer 2003;13:317–24.

55. Hamada M, Kiryu H, Ohta T, Furue M. Ciliated cyst of the vulva. Eur J Dermatol 2004;14:347–9.

56. Hashimoto K, Lee MW, D'Annunzio DR, Balle MR, Narisawa Y. Pagetoid Merkel cell carcinoma: epidermal origin of the tumor. J Cutan Pathol 1998;25:572–9.

57. Hastrup N, Clemmensen OJ, Spaun E, Sondergaard K. Dysplastic naevus: histological criteria and their inter-observer reproducibility. Histopathology 1994;24:503–9.

57a. Heller DS. Report of a new ISSVD classification of VIN. J Low Gen Tract Dis 2007;11:46–7.

58. Herod JJ, Shafi MI, Rollason TP, Jordan JA, Luesley DM. Vulvar intraepithelial neoplasia with superficially invasive carcinoma of the vulva. Br J Obstet Gynaecol 1996;103:453–6.

59. Hierro I, Blanes A, Matilla A, Munoz S, Vicioso L, Nogales FF. Merkel cell (neuroendocrine) carcinoma of the vulva. A case report with immunohistochemical and ultrastructural findings and review of the literature. Pathol Res Pract 2000;196:503–9.

60. Hoang MP, Owen SA, Haisley-Royster C, Allen MH, Shea CR, Selim MA. Papular eruption of the scalp accompanied by axillary and vulvar ulcerations – Langerhans cell histiocytosis (LCH) in an adult. Arch Dermatol 2001;137:1241–4.

61. Hodak E, Jones RE, Ackerman AB. Solitary keratoacanthoma is a squamous-cell carcinoma: three examples with metastases. Am J Dermatopathol 1993;15:332–42; discussion 43–52.

62. Hofbauer GF, Kamarashev J, Geertsen R, Boni R, Dummer R. Tyrosinase immunoreactivity in formalin-fixed, paraffin-embedded primary and metastatic melanoma: frequency and distribution. J Cutan Pathol 1998;25:204–9.

63. Hording U, Daugaard S, Junge J, Lundvall F. Human papillomaviruses and multifocal genital neoplasia. Int J Gynecol Pathol 1996;15:230–4.

64. Horenstein MG, Prieto VG, Burchette JL, Jr, Shea CR. Keratotic melanocytic nevus: a clinicopathologic and immunohistochemical study. J Cutan Pathol 2000;27:344–50.

65. Huang YH, Chuang YH, Kuo TT, Yang LC, Hong HS. Vulvar syringoma: a clinicopathologic and immunohistologic study of 18 patients and results of treatment. J Am Acad Dermatol 2003;48:735–9.

66. Ishigaki H, Hatta N, Yamada M, Orito H, Takehara K. Localised vulva Langerhans cell histiocytosis. Eur J Dermatol 2004;14:412–4.

67. Iversen T, Tretli S. Intraepithelial and invasive squamous cell neoplasia of the vulva: trends in incidence, recurrence, and survival rate in Norway. Obstet Gynecol 1998;91:969–72.

68. Jones RW, Baranyai J, Stables S. Trends in squamous cell carcinoma of the vulva: the influence of vulvar intraepithelial neoplasia. Obstet Gynecol 1997;90:448–52.

69. Joura EA, Zeisler H, Losch A, Sator MO, Mullauer-Ertl S. Differentiating vulvar intraepithelial neoplasia from nonneoplastic epithelial disorders. The toluidine blue test. J Reprod Med 1998;43:671–4.

70. Jungbluth AA, Busam KJ, Gerald WL, et al. A103: an anti-melan-a monoclonal antibody for the detection of malignant melanoma in paraffin-embedded tissues. Am J Surg Pathol 1998;22:595–602.

71. Junge J, Poulsen H, Horn T, Hording U, Lundvall F. Prognosis of vulvar dysplasia and carcinoma in situ with special reference to histology and types of human papillomavirus (HPV). APMIS 1997;105:963–71.

72. Kageshita T, Kawakami Y, Hirai S, Ono T. Differential expression of MART-1 in primary and metastatic melanoma lesions. J Immunother 1997;20:460–5.

73. Kaufman RH. Intraepithelial neoplasia of the vulva. Gynecol Oncol 1995;56:8–21.

74. Khan Z, Misra G, Fiander AN, Dallimore NS. Sebaceous carcinoma of the vulva. BJOG 2003;110:227–8.

75. Khoury-Collado F, Elliott KS, Lee YC, Chen PC, Abulafia O. Merkel cell carcinoma of the Bartholin's gland. Gynecol Oncol 2005;97:928–31.

76. Khunamornpong S, Siriaunkgul S, Suprasert P, Chitapanarux I. Yolk sac tumor of the vulva: a case report with long-term disease-free survival. Gynecol Oncol 2005;97:238–42.

77. Kimball KJ, Straughn JM, Conner MG, Kirby TO. Recurrent basosquamous cell carcinoma of the vulva. Gynecol Oncol 2006;102:400–2.

78. Koenig C, Tavassoli FA. Nodular hyperplasia, adenoma, and adenomyoma of Bartholin's gland. Int J Gynecol Pathol 1998;17:289–94.

79. Kuan SF, Montag AG, Hart J, Krausz T, Recant W. Differential expression of mucin genes in mammary and extramammary Paget's disease. Am J Surg Pathol 2001;25:1469–77.

80. Kuppers V, Stiller M, Somville T, Bender HG. Risk factors for recurrent VIN: role of multifocality and grade of disease. J Reprod Med 1997;42:140–4.

81. Kurman RJ, Toki T, Schiffman MH. Basaloid and warty carcinomas of the vulva. Distinctive types of squamous cell carcinoma frequently associated with human papillomaviruses. Am J Surg Pathol 1993;17:133–45.

82. Lawley LP, Cerimele F, Weiss SW, et al. Expression of Wilms tumor 1 gene distinguishes vascular malformations from proliferative endothelial lesions. Arch Dermatol 2005;141:1297–300.

83. Levi F, Randimbison L, La Vecchia C. Descriptive epidemiology of vulvar and vaginal cancers in Vaud, Switzerland, 1974–1994. Ann Oncol 1998;9:1229–32.

84. Lim C, Brewer J, Russell P. Juvenile colonic polyp occurring in the vulva. Pathology 2007;39:448–50.

85. Lopes G, DeCesare T, Ghurani G, et al. Primary ectopic breast cancer presenting as a vulvar mass. Clin Breast Cancer 2006;7:278–9.

86. Lundquist K, Kohler S, Rouse RV. Intraepidermal cytokeratin 7 expression is not restricted to Paget cells but is also seen in Toker cells and Merkel cells. Am J Surg Pathol 1999;23:212–9.

87. Magrina JF, Gonzalez-Bosquet J, Weaver AL, et al. Squamous cell carcinoma of the vulva stage IA: long-term results. Gynecol Oncol 2000;76:24–7.

88. Martinez-Perez D, Fein NA, Boon LM, Mulliken JB. Not all hemangiomas look like strawberries: uncommon presentations of the most common tumor of infancy. Pediatr Dermatol 1995;12:1–6.

89. Marzano DA, Haefner HK. The Bartholin gland cyst: past, present, and future. J Low Genit Tract Dis 2004;8:195–204.

90. Molinie V, Paniel BJ, Lessana-Leibowitch M, Moyal-Barracco M, Pelisse M, Escande JP. Paget disease of the vulva. 36 cases. Ann Dermatol Venereol 1993;120:522–7.

91. Moreira PM, Moreira IV, Faye EH, Cisse L, Mendes V, Diadhiou F. Three cases of vulvar epidermal cysts after female genital mutilation. Gynecol Obstet Fertil 2002;30:958–60.

92. Mottl H, Rob L, Stary J, Kodet R, Drahokoupilova E. Langerhans cell histiocytosis of vulva in adolescent. Int J Gynecol Cancer 2007;17:520–4.

93. Mulayim N, Foster Silver D, Tolgay Ocal I, Babalola E. Vulvar basal cell carcinoma: two unusual presentations and review of the literature. Gynecol Oncol 2002;85:532–7.

94. Nascimento AF, Granter SR, Cviko A, Yuan L, Hecht JL, Crum CP. Vulvar acanthosis with altered differentiation: a precursor to verrucous carcinoma? Am J Surg Pathol 2004;28:638–43.

95. Ndubisi B, Kaminski PF, Olt G, et al. Staging and recurrence of disease in squamous cell carcinoma of the vulva. Gynecol Oncol 1995;59:34–7.

96. Neto AG, Deavers MT, Silva EG, Malpica A. Metastatic tumors of the vulva – a clinicopathologic study of 66 cases. Am J Surg Pathol 2003;27:799–804.

97. Obermair A, Koller S, Crandon AJ, Perrin L, Nicklin JL. Primary Bartholin gland carcinoma: a report of seven cases. Aust N Z J Obstet Gynaecol 2001;41:78–81.

98. Origoni M, Dindelli M, Ferrari D, Frigerio L, Rossi M, Ferrari A. Surgical staging of invasive squamous cell carcinoma of the vulva. Analysis of treatment and survival. Int Surg 1996;81:67–70.

99. Ozkan F, Bilgic R, Cesur S. Vulvar keratoacanthoma. APMIS 2006;114:562–5.

100. Padula A, Medeiros LJ, Silva EG, Deavers MT. Isolated vulvar Langerhans cell histiocytosis: report of two cases. Int J Gynecol Pathol 2004;23: 278–83.

101. Panizzon RG. Vulvar melanoma. Semin Dermatol 1996;15:67–70.

102. Papac RJ. Spontaneous regression of cancer. Cancer Treat Rev 1996;22:395–423.

103. Park SJ, Lee HK, Hong HS, et al. Hydrocele of the canal of Nuck in a girl: ultrasound and MR appearance. Br J Radiol 2004;77:243–4.

104. Pesce C, Scalora S. Apoptosis in the areas of squamous differentiation of irritated seborrheic keratosis. J Cutan Pathol 2000;27:121–3.

105. Petry KU, Kochel H, Bode U, et al. Human papillomavirus is associated with the frequent detection of warty and basaloid high-grade neoplasia of the vulva and cervical neoplasia among immunocompromised women. Gynecol Oncol 1996;60:30–4.

106. Piepkorn M, Barnhill RL. A factual, not arbitrary, basis for choice of resection margins in melanoma. Arch Dermatol 1996;132:811–4.

107. Pinto AP, Schlecht NF, Pintos J, et al. Prognostic significance of lymph node variables and human papillomavirus DNA in invasive vulvar carcinoma. Gynecol Oncol 2004;92:856–65.

108. Pisani C, Poggiali S, De Padova L, Andreassi A, Bilenchi R. Basal cell carcinoma of the vulva. J Eur Acad Dermatol Venereol 2006;20:446–8.

109. Piura B, Rabinovich A, Cohen Y, Friger M, Glezerman M. Squamous cell carcinoma of the vulva in the south of Israel: a study of 50 cases. J Surg Oncol 1998;67:174–81.

110. Preti M, Mezzetti M, Robertson C, Sideri M. Inter-observer variation in histopathological diagnosis and grading of vulvar intraepithelial neoplasia: results of a European collaborative study. BJOG 2000;107:594–9.

111. Prieto VG, McNutt NS, Lugo J, Reed JA. The intermediate filament peripherin is expressed in cutaneous melanocytic lesions. J Cutan Pathol 1997;24:145–50.

112. Prignano F, Domenici L, Carli P, Pimpinelli N, Romagnoli P. Langerhans cell histiocytosis of the vulva: an ultrastructural study. Ultrastruct Pathol 1999;23:127–32.

113. Raber G, Mempel V, Jackisch C, et al. Malignant melanoma of the vulva. Report of 89 patients. Cancer 1996;78:2353–8.

114. Ragnarsson-Olding BK, Nilsson BR, Kanter-Lewensohn LR, Lagerlof B, Ringborg UK. Malignant melanoma of the vulva in a nationwide, 25-year study of 219 Swedish females: predictors of survival. Cancer 1999;86:1285–93.

115. Ragnarsson-Olding BK, Kanter-Lewensohn LR, Lagerlof B, Nilsson BR, Ringborg UK. Malignant melanoma of the vulva in a nationwide, 25-year study of 219 Swedish females: clinical observations and histopathologic features. Cancer 1999;86:1273–84.

116. Reed JA, Finnerty B, Albino AP. Divergent cellular differentiation pathways during the invasive stage of cutaneous malignant melanoma progression. Am J Pathol 1999;155:549–55.

117. Rhodes CA, Cummins C, Shafi MI. The management of squamous cell vulval cancer: a population based retrospective study of 411 cases. Br J Obstet Gynecol 1998;105:200–5.

118. Robboy SJ, Ross JS, Prat J, Keh PC, Welch WR. Urogenital sinus origin of mucinous and ciliated cysts of the vulva. Obstet Gynecol 1978;51:347–51.

119. Rongioletti F, Cattarini G, Romanelli P. Late onset vulvar steatocystoma multiplex. Clin Exp Dermatol 2002;27:445–7.

120. Roth LM, Look KY. Inverted follicular keratosis of the vulvar skin: a lesion that can be confused with squamous cell carcinoma. Int J Gynecol Pathol 2000;19:369–73.

121. Rudolph P, Schubert C, Schubert B, Parwaresch R. Proliferation marker Ki-S5 as a diagnostic tool in melanocytic lesions. J Am Acad Dermatol 1997;37(2 Pt 1):169–78.

122. Ruhoy SM, Prieto VG, Eliason SL, Grichnik JM, Burchette JL, Jr, Shea CR. Malignant melanoma with paradoxical maturation. Am J Surg Pathol 2000;24:1600–14.

123. Sagerman PM, Choi YJ, Hu Y, Niedt GW. Human papilloma virus, vulvar dystrophy, and vulvar carcinoma: differential expression of human papillomavirus and vulvar dystrophy in the presence and absence of squamous cell carcinoma of the vulva. Gynecol Oncol 1996;61:328–32.

124. Santos LD, Kennerson AR, Killingsworth MC. Nodular hyperplasia of Bartholin's gland. Pathology 2006;38:223–8.

125. Santos M, Landolfi S, Olivella A, et al. p16 overexpression identifies HPV-positive vulvar squamous cell carcinomas. Am J Surg Pathol 2006;30:1347–56.

126. Scheistroen M, Trope C, Koern J, Pettersen EO, Abeler VM, Kristensen GB. Malignant melanoma of the vulva: evaluation of prognostic factors with emphasis on DNA ploidy in 75 patients. Cancer 1995;75:72–80.

127. Schwartz RA, Torre DP. The Muir–Torre syndrome: a 25-year retrospect. J Am Acad Dermatol 1995;33:90–104.

128. Shea CR, Vollmer RT, Prieto VG. Correlating architectural disorder and cytologic atypia in Clark (dysplastic) melanocytic nevi. Hum Pathol 1999;30:500–5.

129. Sidor J, Diallo-Danebrock R, Eltze E, Lelle RJ. Challenging the concept of microinvasive carcinoma of the vulva: report of a case with regional lymph node recurrence and review of the literature. BMC Cancer 2006;6:157.

130. Solivetti FM, Thorel MF, Di Luca Sidozzi A, Bucher S, Donati P, Panichelli V. Role of high-definition and high frequency ultrasonography in determining tumor thickness in cutaneous malignant melanoma. Radiol Med (Torino) 1998;96:558–61.

131. Spatz A, Zimmermann U, Bachollet B, Pautier P, Michel G, Duvillard P. Malignant blue nevus of the vulva with late ovarian metastasis. Am J Dermatopathol 1998;20:408–12.

132. Srodon M, Stoler MH, Baber GB, Kurman RJ. The distribution of low and high-risk HPV types in culvar and vaginal intraepithelial neoplasia (VIN and VaIN). Am J Surg Pathol 2006;30:1513–8.

133. Stang A, Streller B, Eisinger B, Jockel KH. Population-based incidence rates of malignant melanoma of the vulva in Germany. Gynecol Oncol 2005;96:216–21.

134. Stickel WH, Manner M. Female hydrocele (cyst of the canal of Nuck): sonographic appearance of a rare and little-known disorder. J Ultrasound Med 2004;23:429–32.

135. Sugiyama VE, Shin JY, Olsen K, Kapp D, Berek J, Chan JK. Large series of 359 vulvar melanoma patients – a multivariate analysis. Obstet Gynecol 2007;109(4 Suppl):121S.

136. Sykes P, Smith N, McCormick P, Frizelle FA. High-grade vulval intraepithelial neoplasia (VIN 3): a retrospective analysis of patient characteristics, management, outcome and relationship to squamous cell carcinoma of the vulva 1989–1999. Aust N Z J Obstet Gynaecol 2002;42:69–74.

137. Takata M, Hatta N, Takehara K. Tumour cells of extramammary Paget's disease do not show either p53 mutation or allelic loss at several selected loci implicated in other cancers. Br J Cancer 1997;76:904–8.

138. Tate JE, Mutter GL, Boynton KA, Crum CP. Monoclonal origin of vulvar intraepithelial neoplasia and some vulvar hyperplasias. Am J Pathol 1997;150:315–22.

139. Teixeira MR, Kristensen GB, Abeler VM, Heim S. Karyotypic findings in tumors of the vulva and vagina. Cancer Genet Cytogenet 1999;111:87–91.

140. Thyavihally YB, Wuntkal R, Bakshi G, Uppin S, Tongaonkar HB. Primary carcinoma of the female urethra: single center experience of 18 cases. Jpn J Clin Oncol 2005;35:84–7.

141. Toki T, Kurman RJ, Park JS, Kessis T, Daniel RW, Shah KV. Probable nonpapillomavirus etiology of squamous cell carcinoma of the vulva in older women: a clinicopathologic study using in situ hybridization and polymerase chain reaction. Int J Gynecol Pathol 1991;10:107–25.

142. Tran TA, Carlson JA, Basaca PC, Mihm MC. Cellular blue nevus with atypia (atypical cellular blue nevus): a clinicopathologic study of nine cases. J Cutan Pathol 1998;25:252–8.

143. Trimble CL, Hildesheim A, Brinton LA, Shah KV, Kurman RJ. Heterogeneous etiology of squamous carcinoma of the vulva. Obstet Gynecol 1996;87:59–64.

144. Tucker MA, Halpern A, Holly EA, et al. Clinically recognized dysplastic nevi. A central risk factor for cutaneous melanoma. JAMA 1997;277:1439–44.

145. Ulmer A, Dietl J, Schaumburg-Lever G, Fierlbeck G. Amelanotic malignant melanoma of the vulva. Case report and review of the literature. Arch Gynecol Obstet 1996;259:45–50.

146. Venizelos ID, Mandala E, Tatsiou ZA, Acholos V, Goutzioulis M. Primary Langerhans cell histiocytosis of the vulva. Int J Gynecol Pathol 2006;25:48–51.

147. Vernooij F, Sie-Go DMDS, Heintz APM. Lymph node recurrence following stage IA vulvar carcinoma: two cases and a short overview of literature. Int J Gynecol Cancer 2007;17:517–20.

148. Verschraegen CF, Benjapibal M, Supakarapongkul W, et al. Vulvar melanoma at the M.D. Anderson Cancer Center: 25 years later. Int J Gynecol Cancer 2001;11:359–64.

149. Wechter ME, Gruber SB, Haefner HK, et al. Vulvar melanoma: a report of 20 cases and review of the literature. J Am Acad Dermatol 2004;50:554–62.

150. Willman CL, McClain KL. An update on clonality, cytokines, and viral etiology in Langerhans cell histiocytosis. Hematol Oncol Clin North Am 1998;12:407–16.

151. Willman JH, Golitz LE, Fitzpatrick JE. Vulvar clear cells of Toker: precursors of extramammary Paget's disease. Am J Dermatopathol 2005;27:185–8.

152. Yang P, Farkas DL, Kirkwood JM, Abernethy JL, Edington HD, Becker D. Macroscopic spectral imaging and gene expression analysis of the early stages of melanoma. Mol Med 1999;5:785–94.

153. Yang SYV, Lee JW, Kim WS, et al. Adenoid cystic carcinoma of the Bartholin's gland: report of two cases and review of the literature. Gynecol Oncol 2006;100:422–5.

154. Yoong WC, Shakya R, Sanders BT, Lind J. Clitoral inclusion cyst: a complication of type I female genital mutilation. J Obstet Gynaecol 2004;24:98–9.

Vulvar mesenchymal neoplasms and tumor-like conditions

4

Marisa R. Nucci   Christopher D.M. Fletcher

FIBROEPITHELIAL–STROMAL POLYP (PSEUDOSARCOMA BOTRYOIDES)[7,12,20,39,59,64,67,75,76,81,82,84]

Definition
A benign polypoid growth that arises from the distinctive sub-epithelial stroma of the distal female genital tract.

Clinical features
Fibroepithelial–stromal polyps, which are hormonally sensitive, most commonly occur in the vulvovaginal region of repro-ductive-aged women, quite often during pregnancy. They may, however, also occur in postmenopausal women on hormonal replacement therapy. Often, the polyps are incidental findings discovered during routine gynecologic examination. Symptoms, when present, may include bleeding, discharge or the sensation of a mass. These lesions are characteristically polyp-oid or pedunculated, varying in size but usually less than 5 cm, and are typically solitary, although multiple polyps may occur and are usually associated with pregnancy. Evidence support-ing that these lesions are hormonally driven, benign reactive proliferations include: (1) their occurrence during pregnancy, during which they can be multiple and after which they can spontaneously regress; (2) their association with hormonal replacement therapy in postmenopausal women; and (3) expres-sion of estrogen and progesterone receptors by the constituent stromal cells. Incomplete excision or continued hormonal stim-ulation (e.g., pregnancy) may be associated with recurrence.

Pathology
Gross examination typically reveals a polypoid mass with a central fibrovascular core covered by glistening squamous mucosa or skin (Figure 4.1). On occasion, multiple finger-like projections, which may clinically mimic a condyloma, are present. Histologically, these lesions exhibit: (1) a variably cel-lular stroma throughout which, but particularly located near the epithelial–stromal interface, are stellate and multinucleate stromal cells; (2) a central fibrovascular core; and (3) overlying squamous epithelium or skin, which may exhibit varying degrees of hyperplasia (Figures 4.2 and 4.3).

The stromal component has no clearly defined margin and extends right up to the epithelial–submucosal interface. Similar to non-neoplastic vulvar stroma, the stromal cells of these polyps may be reactive for desmin, actin, vimentin, and estro-gen and progesterone receptors. The most variable component of these lesions is the stroma, which may exhibit a significant degree of cellularity, nuclear pleomorphism, and mitotic activ-ity, thereby mimicking a malignant process (Figure 4.4). These worrisome histologic features are particularly, but not invari-ably, present in polyps that occur during pregnancy (and account for the historical term 'pseudosarcoma botryoides').

Differential diagnosis
Pseudosarcomatous stromal polyps can be distinguished from a malignant process by the presence of stellate and multinucle-ate stromal cells near the epithelial–stromal interface, which are characteristically present in these polyps even in the most floridly pseudosarcomatous examples, and lack of an identifi-able lesional margin. Fibroepithelial–stromal polyps are also readily distinguished from botryoid embryonal rhabdomyosar-coma as they are rare before puberty and lack both the characteristic hypercellular subepithelial (cambium) layer of sarcoma botryoides and the specific markers of skeletal muscle differentiation.

NODULAR FASCIITIS[28,57,88]

Definition
A benign, reactive myofibroblastic proliferation characterized by rapid growth and spontaneous regression.

Clinical features
Nodular fasciitis typically occurs as a rapidly growing, painful or tender subcutaneous mass in young adults. It most com-monly involves the upper limbs, particularly the forearm; however, it occasionally occurs in the vulva. These lesions are benign and local marginal excision is adequate; if left untreated they will spontaneously regress over a period of months.

Pathology
Similar to its counterparts elsewhere, nodular fasciitis involv-ing the vulva is usually a well-circumscribed, unencapsulated mass that typically measures less than 3 cm in size. Histologi-cally, it is a relatively well-circumscribed cellular proliferation of loosely arranged spindle cells set within a variably edema-tous or myxoid matrix that may exhibit microcystic change (Figure 4.5). The spindle cells, which are typically arranged in short interconnecting fascicles, have bipolar eosinophilic cyto-plasmic processes with indistinct borders and ovoid nuclei with occasional nucleoli, imparting an overall appearance to the cells that has been likened to tissue culture fibroblasts. Scat-tered inflammatory cells, particularly lymphocytes, and extrav-asated red blood cells are commonly present. Osteoclast-like giant cells are also quite common. Immunohistochemically, the

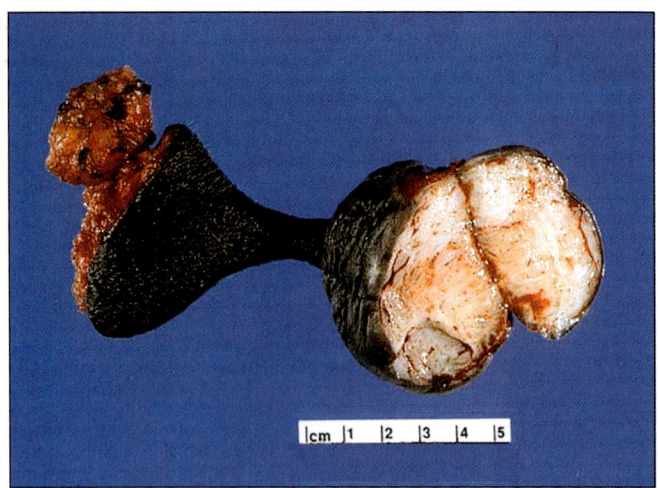

Fig. 4.1 Fibroepithelial–stromal polyp. Lesions are typically a polypoid/pedunculated mass. Courtesy of Dr J R Lewin, Jackson, MS.

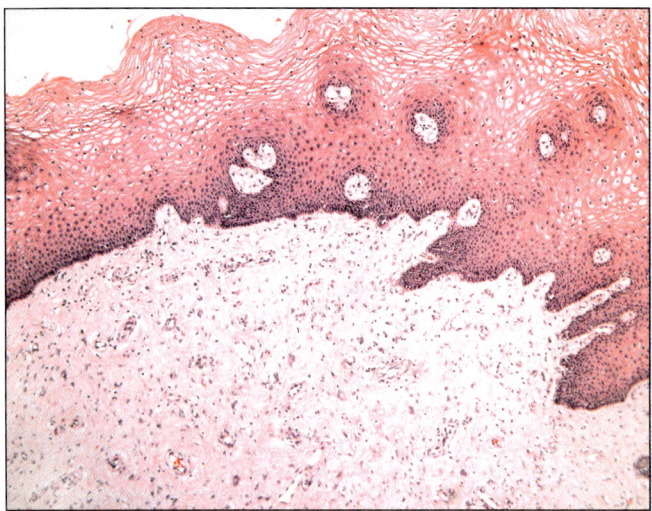

Fig. 4.2 Fibroepithelial–stromal polyp. The lesion extends up to the epithelial interface without a clearly definable margin.

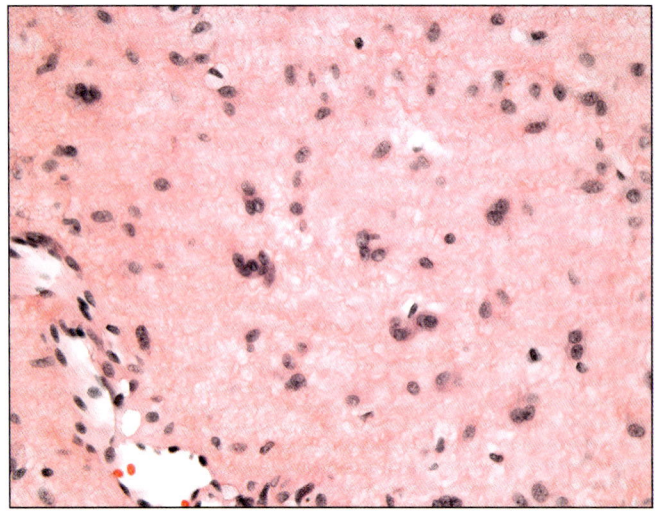

Fig. 4.3 Fibroepithelial–stromal polyp. Characteristic appearance of the stellate and multinucleate stomal cells.

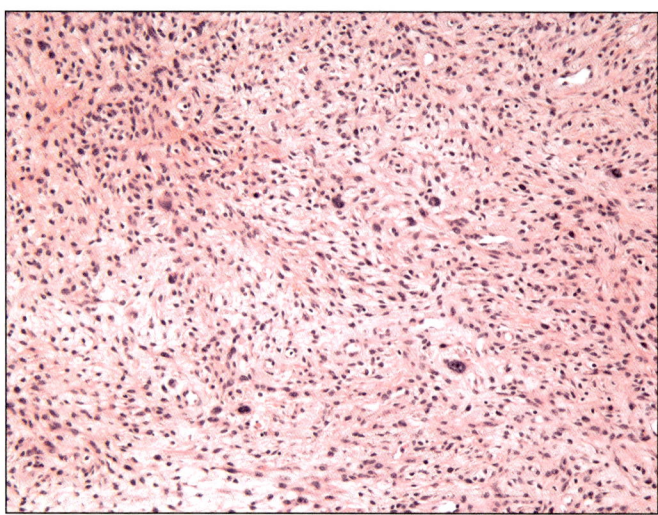

Fig. 4.4 Fibroepithelial–stromal polyp, pseudosarcomatous appearance. The stroma is hypercellular and contains cells with enlarged, pleomorphic nuclei.

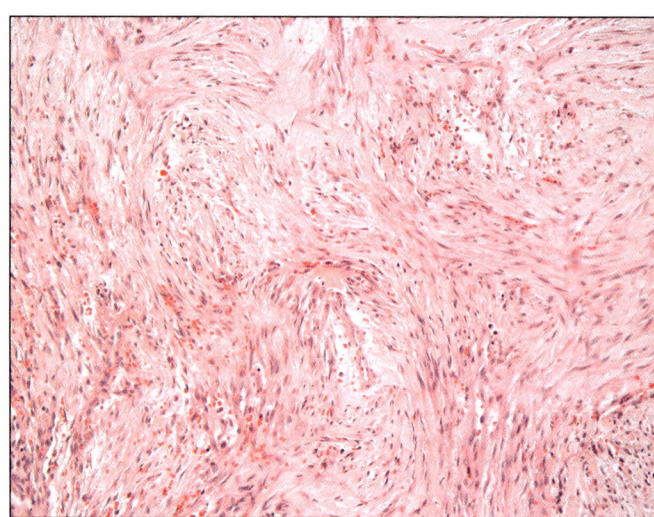

Fig. 4.5 Nodular fasciitis. Somewhat fascicular proliferation of spindle cells within an edematous matrix containing extravasated red blood cells.

spindle cells are typically reactive for smooth muscle actin and negative for desmin. Nodular fasciitis is distinguished from a sarcoma, particularly leiomyosarcoma at this site, by: (1) its lack of nuclear hyperchromasia or pleomorphism; (2) its lack of necrosis; and (3) its characteristic reactive 'tissue culture'-like myofibroblastic growth pattern.

BENIGN NEOPLASMS

ANGIOMYOFIBROBLASTOMA[25,27,40,54,71,73,83]

Definition
A benign, non-recurring tumor composed of myofibroblasts and thin-walled capillaries, which principally occurs in vulvo-vaginal soft tissue.

Clinical features

Angiomyofibroblastoma is an uncommon tumor that occurs almost exclusively in the vulvovaginal region of reproductive-aged women; however, similar tumors also occur rarely in men in the inguinoscrotal region. Clinically, it is often mistaken for a cyst on examination, in particular a Bartholin gland cyst. Local excision is typically adequate treatment, as these tumors do not recur. Exceptionally, they undergo sarcomatous transformation. Rarely they may have areas indistinguishable from aggressive angiomyxoma, suggesting that these two tumors may be related. In either of these unusual settings, excision with clear margins is essential.

Pathology

Tumors are typically small (usually < 5 cm), well-demarcated, tan/white and may have a rubbery consistency (Figure 4.6). They are composed of plump, round to ovoid or spindle-shaped cells, set within a variably edematous to collagenous matrix with alternating zones of cellularity (Figure 4.7). These cells, which have moderate amounts of eosinophilic cytoplasm and round nuclei with fine chromatin and inconspicuous nucleoli, characteristically cluster around the prominent vascular component, which is composed of numerous delicate, thin-walled capillaries (Figure 4.8). Tumor cells may be binucleate or appear somewhat epithelioid. Mitotic activity is typically sparse and occasional cases may have an adipocytic component. The spindle cells are typically reactive for desmin and negative for actin.

Differential diagnosis

Angiomyofibroblastoma is distinguished from aggressive angiomyxoma by its well-circumscribed margin, its prominent vascular component (which is typically composed of smaller caliber vessels), and its alternating zones of cellularity. As both tumors share a similar immunophenotype, distinction is based on morphologic differences.

CELLULAR ANGIOFIBROMA[45,53,62,79]

Definition

A benign tumor of vulval mesenchyme composed of a prominent vascular component admixed with a bland component of spindle cells.

Clinical features

Cellular angiofibroma is a rare benign stromal tumor that predominantly occurs in the vulva or perineum of middle-aged women (mean 54 years). Although initially described to occur exclusively at this site, they also occur in the inguinoscrotal region in men (so-called angiomyofibroblastoma-like tumor) and occasionally in extragenital sites (e.g., retroperitoneum). In the vulva, they most commonly present as a relatively small (mean 2.7 cm) subcutaneous mass that is well circumscribed and painless. Although uncommon, which limits information regarding outcome, cellular angiofibroma, if completely excised, behaves in a benign fashion with no recurrent potential. Incomplete excision may lead to regrowth of tumor;

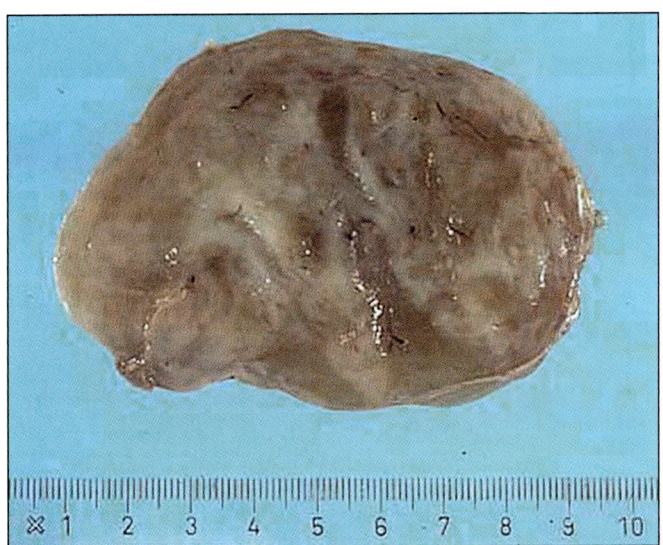

Fig. 4.6 Angiomyofibroblastoma. Well-demarcated, tan/white mass. Courtesy of Professor P P Saint-Maur, Paris, France.

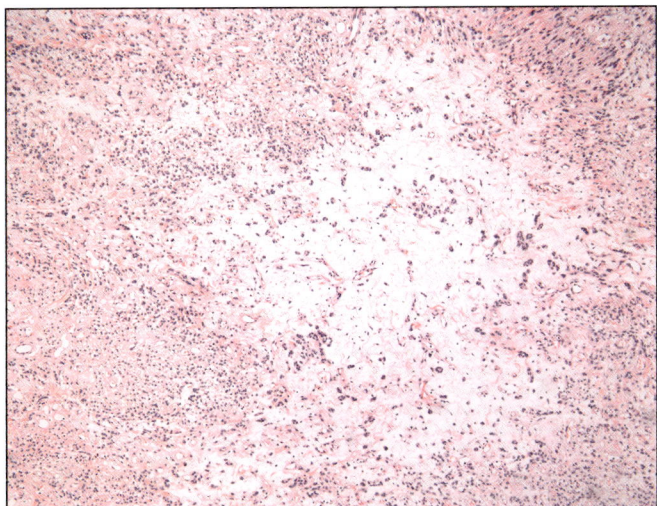

Fig. 4.7 Angiomyofibroblastoma. Alternating zones of cellularity are characteristic.

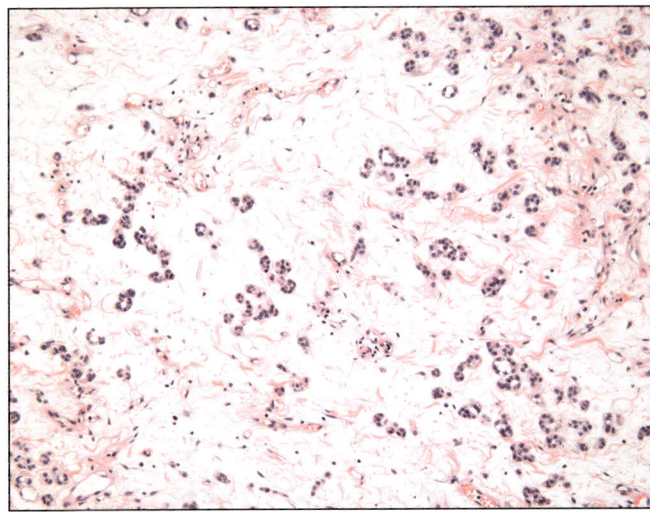

Fig. 4.8 Angiomyofibroblastoma. Numerous, thin-walled capillaries are surrounded by clusters of epithelioid and spindle cells.

therefore, local excision with negative margins is adequate treatment. Very rare cases show sarcomatous transformation.

Pathology

On gross examination, cellular angiofibroma typically is gray-white and has a firm, rubbery consistency (Figure 4.9). Histologically, it is usually well circumscribed; however, focal infiltration into surrounding soft tissue may be present. These tumors are characteristically cellular, being composed of: (1) short, intersecting fascicles of bland, spindle-shaped cells with ovoid nuclei and scant palely eosinophilic cytoplasm; (2) numerous small to medium sized, thick-walled and often hyalinized blood vessels; and (3) admixed wispy collagen bundles (Figure 4.10). In approximately 25% of cases, a usually minor component of adipose tissue is present. Mitotic activity, although brisk in some cases, is usually infrequent while necrosis and nuclear pleomorphism are typically absent. This tumor is reactive for CD34 in 60% of cases, and less commonly reactive for smooth muscle actin (20%) and desmin (8%). Half of

cases show reactivity for estrogen and progesterone receptors. Keratin, epithelial membrane antigen, and S-100 protein are negative.

Differential diagnosis

Cellular angiofibroma is distinguished from a smooth muscle tumor by its more prominent vascular component, its shorter fascicular growth pattern, and relative lack of eosinophilic cytoplasm. Its distinction from angiomyofibroblastoma is by its uniform cellularity, its larger, thick-walled and hyalinized blood vessels, and its spindle cell morphology arranged in short intersecting fascicles.

PREPUBERTAL VULVAL FIBROMA[46]

Definition

A poorly marginated, hypocellular tumor composed of bland spindle cells within a variably edematous, myxoid or collagenous matrix that occurs in prepubertal girls.

Clinical features

This vulvar tumor, which most commonly involves the labia majora of prepubertal girls, usually presents as a painless, gradual vulvar swelling or enlargement. Lesions typically are under 5 cm in size, unilateral and ill-defined submucosal or subcutaneous masses. Although only a limited number of cases have been studied, the tumors appear to be benign, except for quite frequent local recurrence when incompletely excised.

Pathology

Histologically, these tumors, which are located in submucosal or subcutaneous tissue, are poorly marginated with infiltration into surrounding tissue, including around adnexal structures and nerves, and into adipose tissue (Figure 4.11). In addition, there is no clear interface with the overlying epithelium. The lesion is hypocellular and composed of a patternless proliferation of bland, uniform spindle cells with ovoid nuclei and palely amphophilic cytoplasm set within a variably myxoid, edematous or collagenous matrix (Figure 4.12). Small to

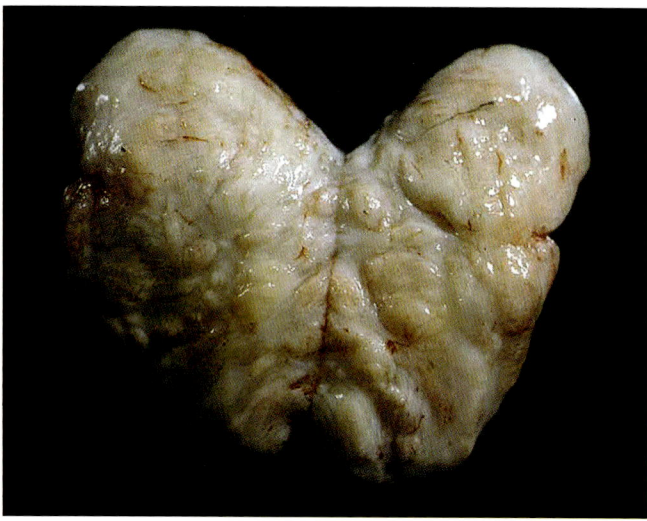

Fig. 4.9 Cellular angiofibroma. Well-demarcated, white/tan mass.

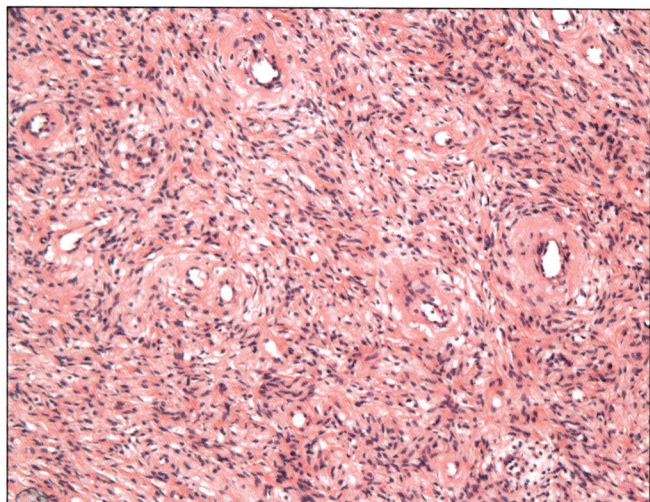

Fig. 4.10 Cellular angiofibroma. Numerous medium-sized, thick-walled vessels are surrounded by short intersecting fascicles of bland spindle cells.

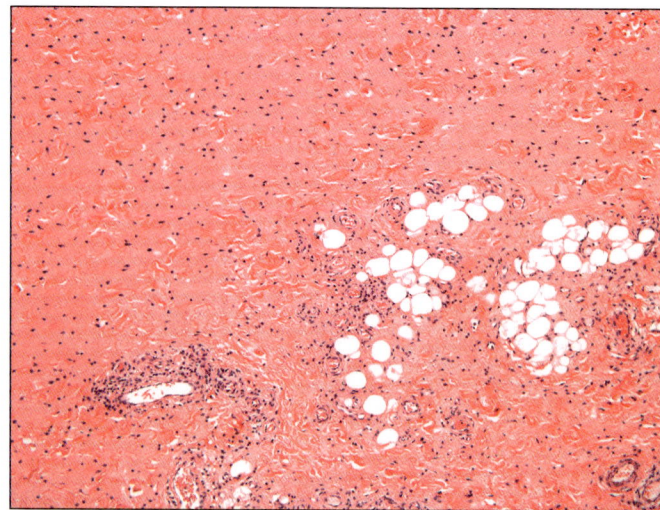

Fig. 4.11 Prepubertal fibroma. The lesion is typically poorly marginated with infiltration into adipose tissue.

medium sized vessels, some with mural thickening, are present. Mitotic activity is sparse and nuclear pleomorphism is absent. Lesional spindle cells are typically reactive for CD34 but are negative for smooth muscle actin, desmin, and S-100 protein.

DERMATOFIBROMA (FIBROUS HISTIOCYTOMA)[1,8,10,14,26,33,47,48,87,91,99]

Definition
A benign tumor of dermal connective tissue exhibiting a storiform growth pattern.

Clinical features
Most commonly occurring on the limbs or trunk of adults, dermatofibroma occasionally involves vulvar skin. Although the clinical appearance is variable, most present as a flesh-colored papule, nodule or plaque; however, some may be pigmented. The diagnosis may be suspected clinically by the presence of the so-called 'dimpling' sign – pinching of the tumor results in an inward dimpling of the lesion. Complete excision is usually not necessary unless the tumor shows unusual morphologic features (e.g., cellular, aneurysmal, plexiform, deeply infiltrative or atypical variants) as these subtypes have locally recurrent potential. Following re-excision, very rare cases of these subtypes have been associated with regional lymph node or metastatic deposits in the lung; however, there were no morphologic indicators in the primary that would predict this biologic potential.

Pathology
Dermatofibroma exhibits a storiform proliferation of bland spindle cells with varying degrees of hyalinization of the dermal collagen, which is birefringent under polarized light (Figure 4.13). The tumor is relatively well circumscribed; however, entrapment of hyalinized bundles of dermal collagen by the spindle cells at the periphery of the tumor imparts a characteristic pseudoinfiltrative pattern (Figure 4.14). Another characteristic feature is the presence of overlying epidermal hyperplasia, which is common. A number of histologic variants are recog-

nized (although these occur principally outside of the vulva) and include hemosiderotic, lipidized, aneurysmal (angiomatoid), atypical, epithelioid, plexiform, cellular, and deeply penetrating types. The spindle cells are often focally reactive for smooth muscle actin and negative for CD34, although the cellular variant may be reactive for CD34 at the periphery of the tumor. These lesions are often factor XIIIa positive, but most staining is in reactive dermal dendritic cells towards the lesional periphery.

Differential diagnosis
Dermatofibroma can be distinguished from dermatofibrosarcoma protuberans, its main differential diagnostic consideration, by: (1) its general lack of infiltration of adipose tissue (although this may be seen in the deeply penetrating variant); (2) the presence of birefringent collagen under polarized light; (3) the presence of overlying epidermal hyperplasia; (4) its

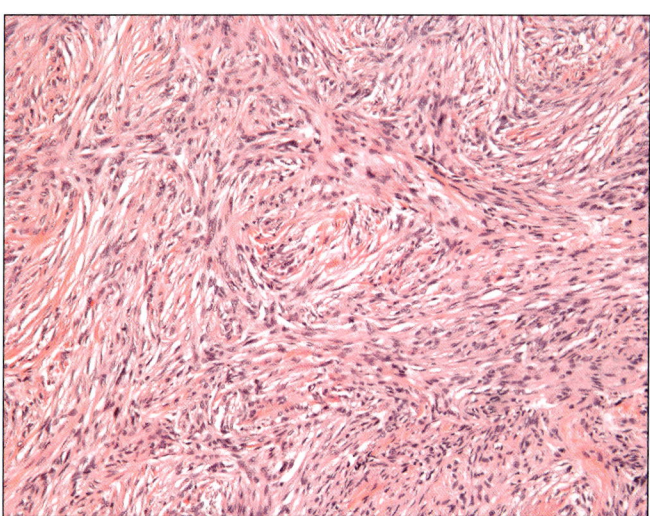

Fig. 4.13 Dermatofibroma. Characteristic storiform proliferation of bland spindle cells.

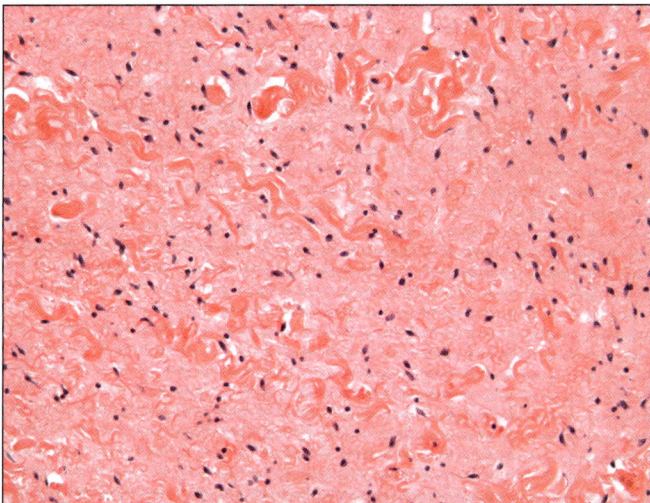

Fig. 4.12 Prepubertal fibroma. Hypocellular proliferation of bland spindle cells set within a collagenous matrix.

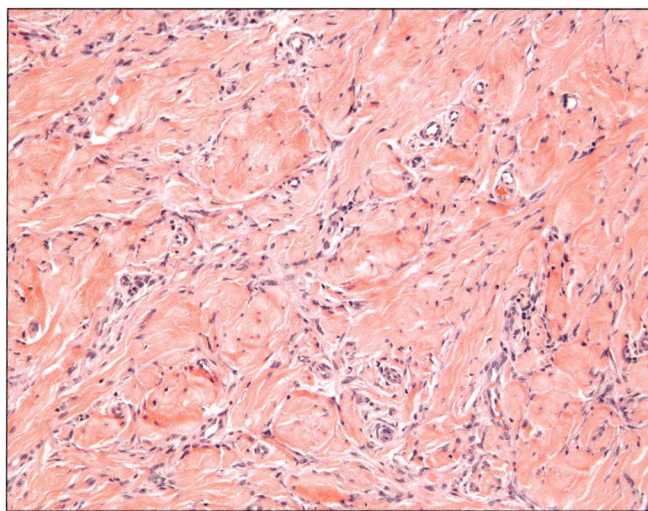

Fig. 4.14 Dermatofibroma. At the periphery of the tumor, the neoplastic spindle cells infiltrate around hyalinized collagen bundles in a characteristic pattern.

tendency not to infiltrate around adnexal structures; and (5) its lack of diffuse reactivity for CD34.

GRANULAR CELL TUMOR[36,41,51,60,89]

Definition
A tumor of neuroectodermal origin composed of cells that contain distinctive granular cytoplasm due to the accumulation of lysosomes.

Clinical features
Granular cell tumor is an uncommon neoplasm that typically arises in the skin and subcutaneous tissue of middle-aged adults with a slightly increased frequency in women. Tumors typically involve the head, neck, and trunk region, but may occasionally occur in the vulva, most often the labium majus. Patients typically present with a solitary, slowly growing, asymptomatic nodule that is usually discovered incidentally on clinical examination. If present, symptoms may include pain, increased growth, and pruritus. Complete excision with clear margins is standard treatment, although these tumors seldom recur, even if incompletely excised. Malignant examples are rare.

Pathology
Granular cell tumors are composed of strands and nests of polygonal cells with abundant eosinophilic granular cytoplasm and small, centrally placed, hyperchromatic nuclei separated by thin fibrous septa (Figure 4.15). Although distinctive, the characteristic granular cytoplasmic change, which is due to the accumulation of lysosomes, is not specific for this tumor type and may be seen in other types of neoplasms, such as smooth muscle tumors. Although many granular cell tumors are relatively well circumscribed, nearly half may show poorly defined or infiltrative margins. Nests of tumor cells adjacent to or surrounding small nerves are common. In addition, the tumor is often associated with overlying pseudoepitheliomatous hyperplasia, which may be mistaken for a squamous neoplasm if the underlying granular cell tumor is overlooked. Granular cell tumors are reactive for S-100 protein, neuron-specific enolase, CD68, and NKI-C3.

Differential diagnosis
The granular cell tumor is distinctive and few pose diagnostic difficulty. Exclusion of a smooth muscle tumor with granular cell change is the most likely differential diagnostic consideration, which can be accomplished by recognition of areas with typical smooth muscle morphology and architecture as well as coexpression of desmin, caldesmon, and smooth muscle actin.

LEIOMYOMA[69,70,78,94]

Definition
A benign tumor of smooth muscle exhibiting intersecting fascicles of spindle cells with eosinophilic cytoplasm.

Clinical features
Although genital smooth muscle tumors were initially considered within the category of superficial smooth muscle tumors, which includes pilar leiomyoma and angioleiomyoma, they are now classified separately based upon their differing clinical behavior, histologic features, and criteria for malignancy. Smooth muscle tumors of the distal female genitalia, unlike those of the uterus, are uncommon. They occur over a wide age range but are most common in the fourth and fifth decades and typically present as a painless, well-circumscribed mass usually under 3 cm in size. Not uncommonly, the clinical impression is that of a cyst. Local excision for typical leiomyomas is adequate treatment. For tumors with unusual histologic features associated with recurrent potential (see below), a margin of excision of at least 1 cm is recommended whenever possible, with close, long-term follow-up.

Pathology
Similar to uterine smooth muscle tumors, vulvar leiomyomas usually exhibit the characteristic gross appearance of benign smooth muscle tumors of the myometrium but on occasion may have a more homogeneous appearance with less obvious whorling (Figure 4.16). In most instances, they are composed of intersecting fascicles of spindle-shaped cells with moderate amounts of eosinophilic cytoplasm and elongated, blunt-ended nuclei. However, an unusual morphologic pattern, which is

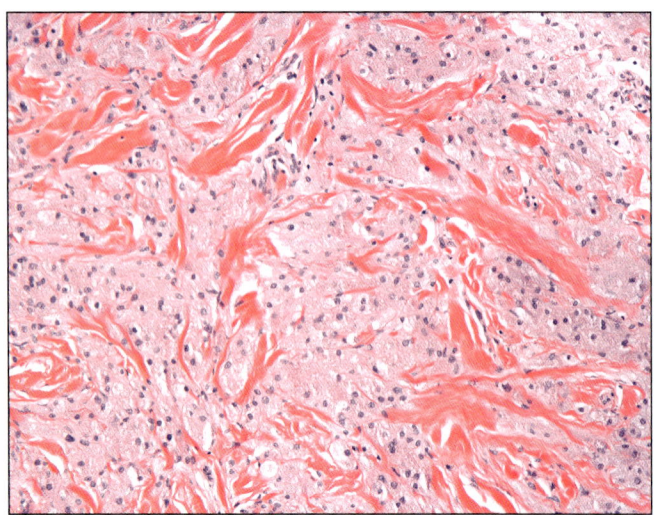

Fig. 4.15 Granular cell tumor. Nests and cords of polygonal cells with abundant eosinophilic granular cytoplasm.

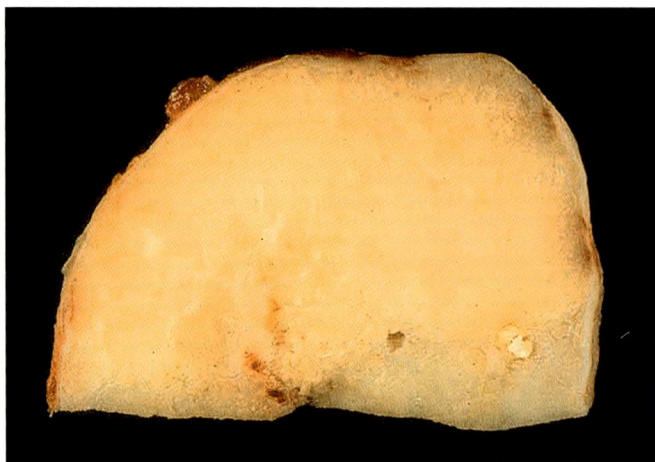

Fig. 4.16 Leiomyoma. Well-circumscribed, tan/yellow mass with a homogeneous, glistening cut surface.

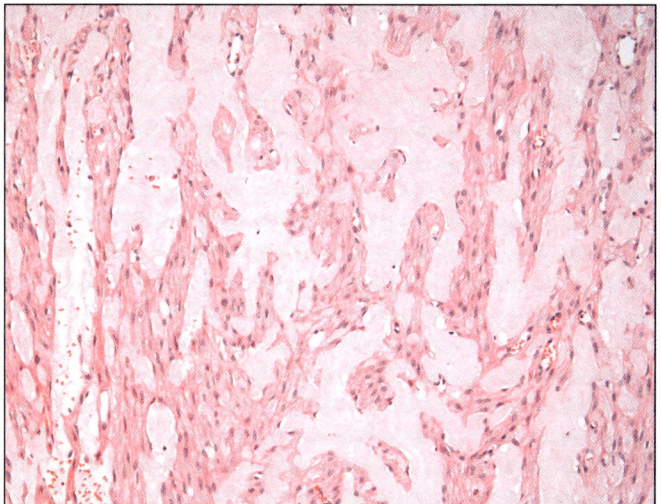

Fig. 4.17 Leiomyoma. Abundant myxohyaline matrix deposition is common in benign vulvar smooth muscle tumors.

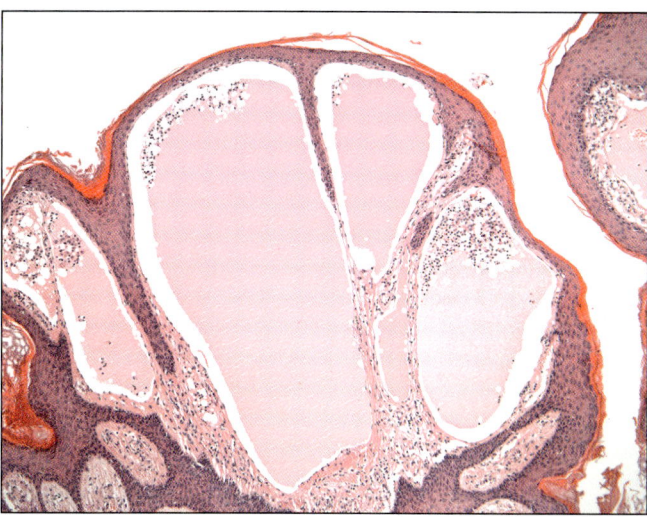

Fig. 4.18 Lymphangioma circumscriptum. Numerous dilated lymphatic channels located within the papillary dermis are closely apposed to the overlying epithelium. Note the epidermal hyperplasia and dermal lymphocytic infiltrate.

commonly present in vulvar smooth muscle tumors, is the variable deposition of myxohyaline matrix, which imparts a plexiform or lacy appearance (Figure 4.17).

Due to the relative infrequency of vulvar smooth muscle tumors in combination with few published series with long-term follow-up, there is continued difficulty in reliably predicting which tumors are benign and which have recurrent potential. While a combination of size, circumscription, nuclear atypia, and mitotic thresholds have been proposed to identify those tumors with recurrent potential, in our experience any mitotic activity, nuclear pleomorphism or infiltration of surrounding tissue may be associated with local recurrence, sometimes years after the initial excision. These observations suggest that smooth muscle tumors of the vagina and vulva fall along a biologic continuum with regard to their behavior and resist being rigidly classified into benign and malignant categories by currently definable histopathologic criteria.

From a practical standpoint, we advocate use of the term 'atypical smooth muscle tumor' for those cases having any of the following features: (1) mitotic activity; (2) nuclear pleomorphism; or (3) an infiltrative margin. Although published series have not included necrosis as a histologic criterion, leiomyosarcoma should be seriously considered in any smooth muscle neoplasm with coagulative tumor cell necrosis.

LYMPHANGIOMA CIRCUMSCRIPTUM[24,85,86,98]

Definition
An abnormality of dermal lymphatic channels exhibiting numerous dilated and cystic lymphatic spaces.

Clinical features
Lymphangioma circumscriptum may be congenital, occurring during infancy and commonly associated with other lymphatic abnormalities such as cystic hygroma or cavernous lymphangioma, or it may be acquired, which most commonly occurs in adults and is associated with secondary lymphatic damage such

as that associated with radiotherapy or chronic lymphedema. It most commonly affects the skin and subcutaneous tissue of the trunk, thighs, and buttocks, but occasionally involves the vulva. Clinically, numerous small vesicles filled with clear fluid characterize this lesion. Symptoms typically include swelling, pain, and superimposed infection secondary to excoriation. Management of congenital lesions is local excision, including removal of any large feeding lymphatic channel, which may be deep seated, as incomplete removal is commonly associated with recurrence.

Pathology
Numerous dilated and cystic lymphatic channels are present, primarily within the papillary dermis, but also within the dermis and subcutaneous tissue. Those located in the papillary dermis are closely apposed to the overlying epithelium, which results in the clinical impression of a vesicle (Figure 4.18). Associated epidermal hyperplasia and a dermal lymphocytic infiltrate are common.

ANGIOKERATOMA[13]

Definition
A lesion composed of superficial ectatic vascular channels associated with epidermal hyperplasia.

Clinical features
Angiokeratoma involving the vulva occurs over a wide age range, but typically presents before the sixth decade as an asymptomatic, red to purple, papular lesion under 1 cm in size. It often has a warty appearance due to associated epidermal changes. When present, symptoms include bleeding, pain or pruritus. The lesion may be solitary or multiple, and if multiple should raise the possibility of Fabrys disease, a rare X-linked chromosomal disorder of lipid metabolism in which there is a deficiency of lysosomal α-galactosidase.

Pathology

Angiokeratoma exhibits closely apposed, dilated, blood-filled vascular spaces within the papillary dermis, partially surrounded by the overlying epithelium (Figure 4.19). The epithelium typically shows acanthosis, hyperkeratosis, and occasionally papillomatosis, resulting in the clinical impression of a warty lesion.

OTHER RARE TUMORS

Vulvar leiomyomatosis[21,65,78] is a rare condition in which patients have numerous, ill-defined, multinodular proliferations of smooth muscle involving the vulvar submucosa. Not uncommonly, similar lesions may involve the esophagus (esophageal leiomyomatosis), which may occur either synchronously or metachronously with the vulvar lesions. Altered hormonal responsiveness by the native vulvar smooth muscle and familial factors may play a role in the pathogenesis of this disease. There is also an association with Alports syndrome, which involves defects in type IV collagen, a major component in all basement membranes, including those of smooth muscle cells. Different subtypes of type IV collagen are present in different tissue types; mutations/deletions of *COL4A6* in smooth muscle may be associated with Alports syndrome in association with vulvar leiomyomatosis.

Genital rhabdomyoma[11,38,44] most commonly involves the vagina of middle-aged women, but may occasionally occur in the vulva. Lesions are typically polypoid and patients usually present with bleeding or symptoms related to a mass. Histologically, this benign tumor exhibits a somewhat fascicular proliferation of well-differentiated rhabdomyoblasts within the submucosa (Figure 4.20). Cross-striations are usually easily identifiable (Figure 4.21). Nuclear pleomorphism is absent and mitotic activity is uncommon. Genital rhabdomyoma is distinguished from rhabdomyosarcoma by: (1) its lack of nuclear atypia; (2) its lack of mitotic activity; (3) the absence of a sub-

epithelial hypercellular zone (cambium layer); and (4) its occurrence in an older age group.

Lipoblastoma-like tumor of vulva[52] is a distinctive benign mesenchymal neoplasm involving the vulva that histologically resembles lipoblastoma in infants. In contrast to the latter, which typically occurs in the trunk and extremities of young boys under 5 years of age, this tumor occurs in the vulva of young women. Histologically, the tumors are well circumscribed and composed of lobules of immature and mature adipocytes separated by thin fibrous septa (Figure 4.22). The immature adipocytic lobules contain lipoblasts and primitive mesenchymal cells set within a myxoid stroma with a prominent capillary network mimicking myxoid liposarcoma (Figure 4.23). However, nuclear atypia is absent and mitoses are infrequent.

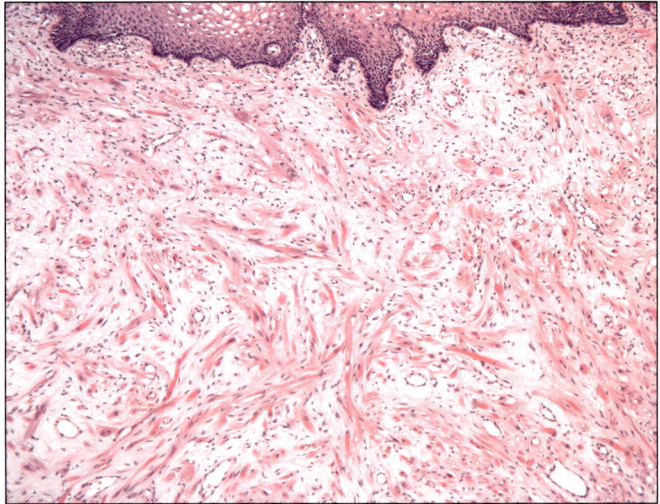

Fig. 4.20 Genital rhabdomyoma. Submucosal fascicular proliferation of well-differentiated rhabdomyoblasts.

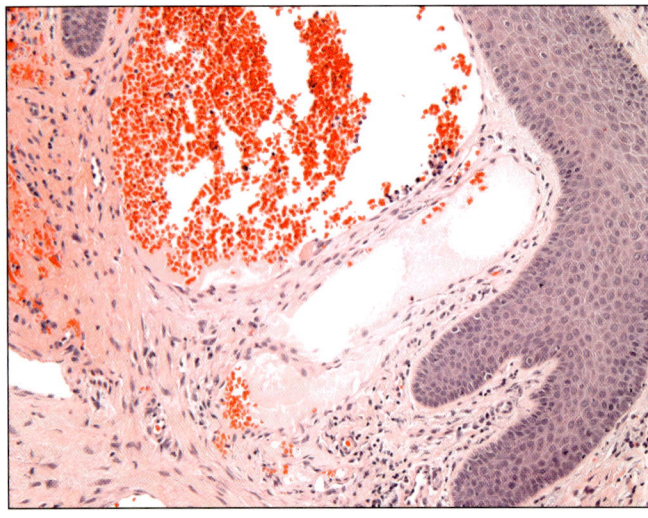

Fig. 4.19 Angiokeratoma. Dilated, blood-filled spaces within the papillary dermis are partially surrounded by epithelium.

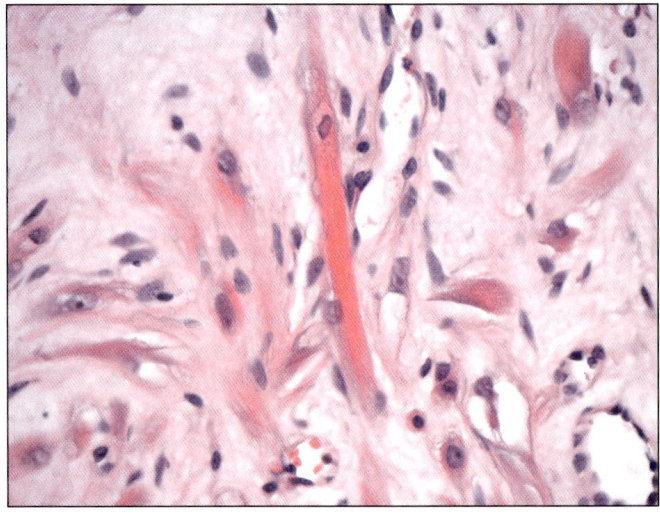

Fig. 4.21 Genital rhabdomyoma. Brightly eosinophilic cytoplasmic processes, some of which contain identifiable cross-striations.

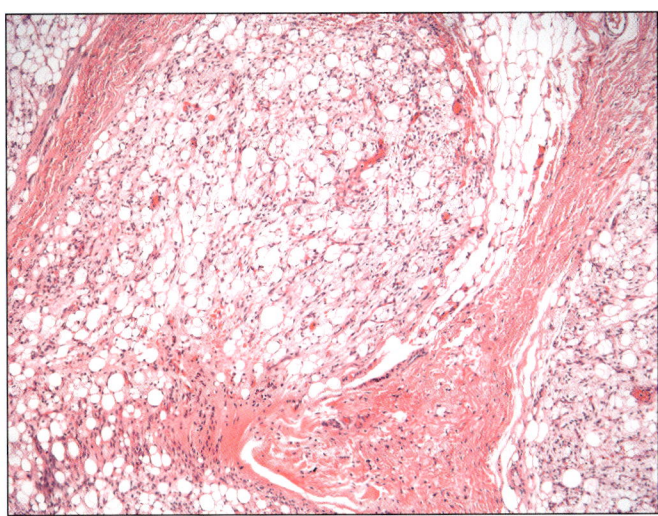

Fig. 4.22   Lipoblastoma-like tumor. Lobules of immature adipocytes within a myxoid matrix separated by thin fibrous septa.

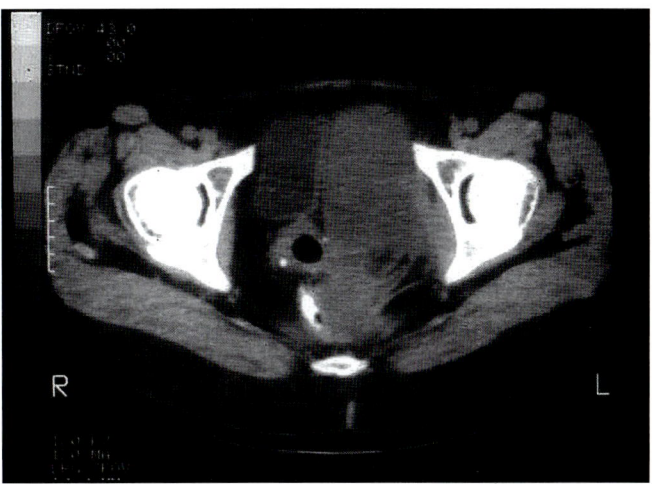

Fig. 4.24   Deep angiomyxoma. CT scan showing an infiltrative tumor mass. Courtesy of Dr R W Fortt, Newport, Wales, UK.

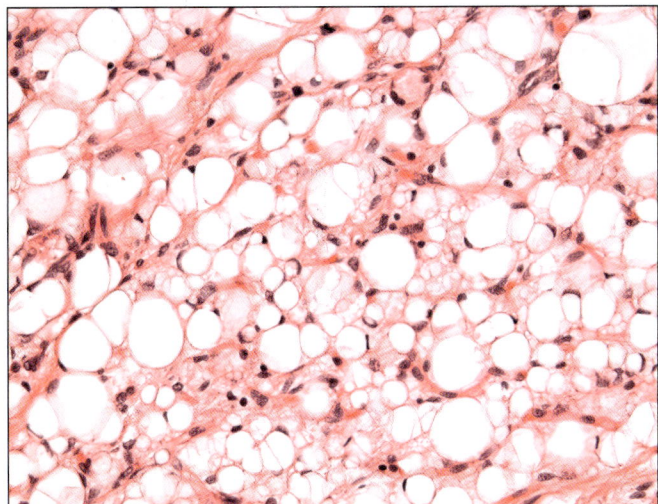

Fig. 4.23   Lipoblastoma-like tumor. Numerous lipoblasts and a delicate capillary network set within a myxoid stroma mimic myxoid liposarcoma.

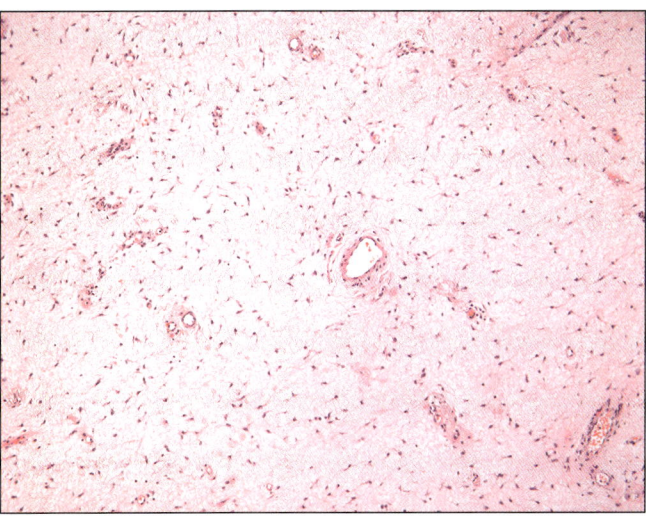

Fig. 4.25   Deep angiomyxoma. Paucicellular neoplasm punctuated by medium to large sized blood vessels.

LOCALLY RECURRENT NEOPLASMS

DEEP ANGIOMYXOMA (DEEP 'AGGRESSIVE' ANGIOMYXOMA)[4,22,34,42,50,61,80,93,95]

Definition
A locally infiltrative, non-metastasizing, hypocellular myxoid tumor of the pelvicoperineal region with the potential for local, sometimes destructive, recurrence.

Clinical features
Deep angiomyxoma occurs principally in the pelvicoperineal region of reproductive-aged women, with a median incidence in the fourth decade, but rarely also develops in the inguino-scrotal region of men, in whom the median age at presentation is in the sixth to seventh decade. Often the clinical impression is that of a labial cyst, most commonly a Bartholins gland cyst.

Tumors vary in size, but are often relatively large (>10 cm) and poorly marginated (Figure 4.24). Although there is a 30–40% risk of local, sometimes destructive recurrence, more than one recurrence is unusual and most are cured by an additional surgical excision with negative margins. Hence the currently preferred terminology is deep angiomyxoma, as these tumors are not as 'aggressive' as originally thought. Besides positive surgical margins, there are no clinical or histopathologic features that predict recurrent potential. Wide local excision with 1 cm margins is considered optimal and adequate treatment.

Pathology
Tumors typically have a gelatinous or myxoid appearance but occasionally may appear more fibrous in a recurrence, presumably due to previous surgical scar tissue. Histologically, deep angiomyxoma is a poorly marginated, paucicellular neoplasm composed of uniformly distributed bland spindle cells with round to ovoid nuclei and moderate amounts of palely eosinophilic cytoplasm, discernible as bi or multipolar cell processes (Figure 4.25). The cells are set within a copious myxoid matrix

Table 4.1 Comparison of common entities in the differential diagnosis of vulvar mesenchymal neoplasms

	Fibroepithelial stromal polyp	Angiomyofibroblastoma	Cellular angiofibroma	Superficial angiomyxoma	Deep angiomyxoma
Age at presentation	Reproductive age	Reproductive age	Reproductive age	Reproductive age	Reproductive age
Location/configuration	Typically polypoid, pedunculated	Subcutaneous	Subcutaneous	Superficial, subcutaneous, polypoid	Deep seated, not polypoid
Size	Variable	Usually <5 cm	Usually <3 cm	Usually <3 cm	Variable
Margins	Merges with normal	Well circumscribed	Usually well circumscribed; may show focal infiltration	Lobulated, well demarcated	Infiltrative, poorly demarcated
Cellularity	Variable	Alternating hyper- and hypocellular zones	Uniformly cellular	Hypocellular	Hypocellular
Vessels	Variable, usually large, thick-walled and centrally located	Numerous, capillary-sized	Abundant, small to medium sized, often thick walled and hyalinized	Delicate, elongated, thin-walled capillaries	Medium to large, thick-walled; perivascular collagen condensation and myoid bundles
Mitotic index	Variable	Typically low	Variable; may be brisk	Typically low	Rare
Clinical course	Benign, rare recurrences (e.g. during pregnancy)	Benign, no recurrent potential; rare sarcomatous transformation	Benign, no recurrent potential; rare sarcomatous transformation	30% local non-destructive recurrence	30% local, sometimes destructive, recurrence

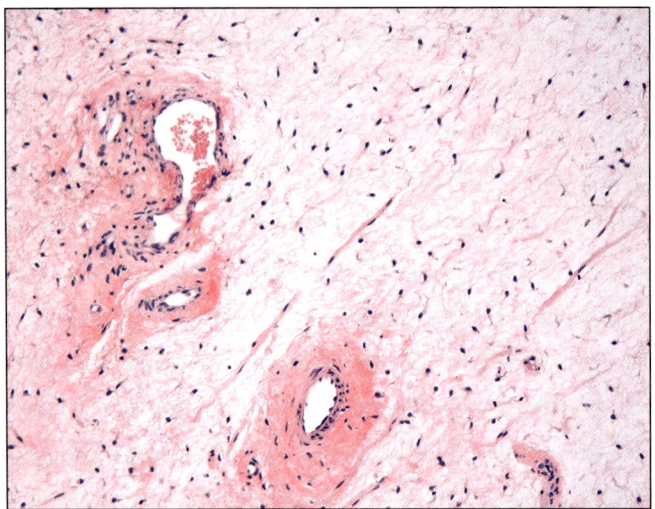

Fig. 4.26 Deep angiomyxoma. Bland spindle cells with bipolar processes within a myxoid matrix surround blood vessels with hyalinized walls. Note brightly eosinophilic smooth muscle cells.

that contains variably sized, but often medium to large, thick-walled, often hyalinized, blood vessels. Condensation of delicate fibrillary collagen around the blood vessels is characteristic, as is the presence of bundles of brightly eosinophilic smooth muscle cells (Figure 4.26). The spindle cells are typically reactive for desmin, smooth muscle actin, and estrogen and progesterone receptors, similar to normal vulval mesenchyme. Cytogenetic analysis has been performed in only a few cases but has revealed clonal chromosomal aberrations involving chromosome 12, which in one case was manifested as t(8;12)(p12;q15) that resulted in aberrant expression of the *HMGA2* gene. This gene encodes a DNA architectural factor

important in transcriptional regulation that is also rearranged in a variety of other benign mesenchymal neoplasms.

Differential diagnosis
The differential diagnosis includes superficial angiomyxoma (see below), angiomyofibroblastoma, and an edematous fibroepithelial–stromal polyp. Deep angiomyxoma is distinguished from angiomyofibroblastoma by its infiltrative margin, its vascular component (which is typically less prominent and composed of larger, thicker walled vessels), and its uniform paucicellularity. Deep angiomyxoma differs from edematous fibroepithelial–stromal polyps by its deep location, its infiltrative margin, its lack of polypoid superficial growth, and its uniformly bland cytomorphology with the lack of the characteristic stellate and multinucleate cells typical of stromal polyps.

SUPERFICIAL ANGIOMYXOMA (CUTANEOUS MYXOMA)[2,9,23]

Definition
A superficially located, multilobulated, myxoid neoplasm with a 30–40% risk of local, non-destructive recurrence.

Clinical features
Superficial angiomyxoma usually involves the head, neck, and trunk region, but does occasionally occur in the vulva. It typically occurs in the fourth decade and patients usually present with a slowly growing, painless, polypoid mass that typically measures less than 5 cm in size. Although usually solitary, multiple lesions may be associated with Carneys complex. Approximately one-third of these tumors recur locally if incompletely or marginally excised; therefore, complete excision with clear margins is recommended treatment.

Pathology

Histologically, superficial angiomyxoma is a myxoid neoplasm with a distinctive multilobulated growth pattern that is centered in the dermis and superficial subcutaneous tissue (Figure 4.27). The relatively well-demarcated myxoid nodules contain slender spindle and stellate-shaped cells, delicate thin-walled capillaries, and scattered inflammatory cells, particularly polymorphonuclear leukocytes (Figure 4.28). The presence of acute inflammatory cells is not associated with necrosis or overlying epidermal ulceration and is presumably secondary to the production of a chemotactic factor by the tumor cells. In 10–20% of cases, an epithelial component – usually in the form of a squamous epithelial-lined cyst, buds of basaloid cells or strands of squamous epithelium – is present, probably as a result of entrapped adnexal structures or stimulation of the overlying epithelium by the tumor. Immunohistochemically, the spindle cells are typically negative for actin, desmin, and S-100 protein.

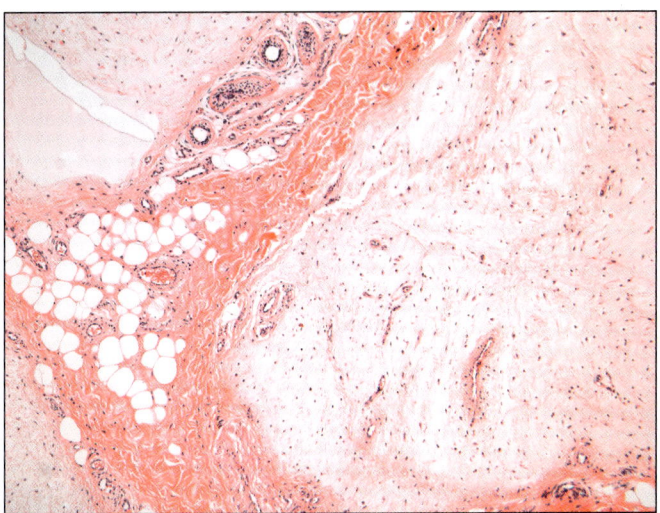

Fig. 4.27 Superficial angiomyxoma. Well-demarcated, lobulated growth pattern.

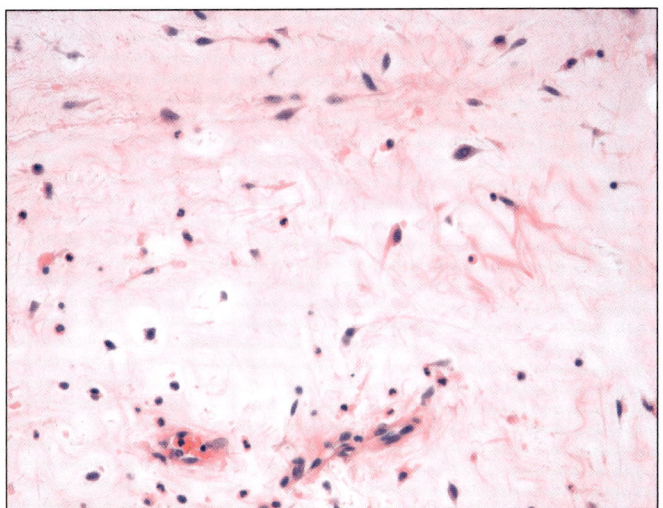

Fig. 4.28 Superficial angiomyxoma. Bland spindle- and stellate-shaped cells, delicate capillaries and a myxoid matrix are characteristic. Note the stromal acute inflammatory cells.

Differential diagnosis

Superficial angiomyxoma is distinguished from deep angiomyxoma by: (1) its superficial location; (2) its well-demarcated margins; (3) its lobulated growth pattern; (4) its lack of thick-walled blood vessels; and (5) negativity of the lesional cells for desmin.

DERMATOFIBROSARCOMA PROTUBERANS[3,5,18,30,31,55,63,66,68,92,96]

Definition

A tumor of dermal connective tissue exhibiting a monomorphic storiform proliferation of fibroblastic spindle cells and infiltration of adipose tissue.

Clinical features

Dermatofibrosarcoma protuberans most commonly occurs on the trunk, lower extremities, and groin area (although not commonly the vulva proper) of adults, principally between the third and sixth decades. Clinical presentation can vary from a flesh-colored to pigmented papule, plaque, nodule or exophytic multinodular growth. Wide local excision with clear margins is necessary to prevent recurrence; rare cases (<0.1%) have metastasized to locoregional lymph nodes, although this figure is higher (~15%) in cases that show higher grade fibrosarcomatous change.

Pathology

Histologically, the classic appearance of this tumor is that of a poorly circumscribed, storiform proliferation of uniform spindle cells involving the dermis and extending into subcutaneous adipose tissue in a characteristic lace-like or honeycomb pattern (Figure 4.29). A band of uninvolved dermis between the tumor and epidermis, which may be of normal thickness or atrophic, is typically present (Grenz zone). Entrapment of adnexal structures is common. In contrast to benign fibrous histiocytoma, polarizable collagen is typically absent. Some tumors, including ones that occur in the vulva, may exhibit

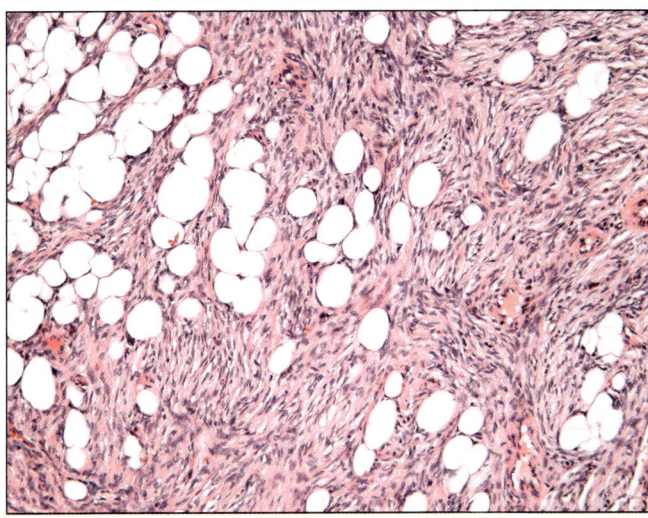

Fig. 4.29 Dermatofibrosarcoma protuberans. Storiform proliferation of spindle cells with extension into subcutaneous adipose tissue in a characteristic honeycomb pattern.

fibrosarcomatous change characterized by a herringbone, fascicular growth pattern with increased mitotic activity (Figure 4.30); tumors with this morphologic appearance have metastatic potential. Immunohistochemically, the neoplastic cells are typically diffusely reactive for CD34 and negative for factor XIIIa. Translocation between chromosomes 17 and 22, often in the form of supernumerary ring chromosomes, has been identified by cytogenetic analysis in this tumor type, including cases that have occurred in the vulva. This translocation results in the fusion of two genes, collagen type I alpha-1 (*COL1A1*) and platelet-derived growth factor β-chain (*PDGFB*).

Differential diagnosis

Dermatofibrosarcoma protuberans differs from dermatofibroma, its main differential diagnostic consideration, by: (1) its tendency to infiltrate subcutaneous adipose tissue in a characteristic honeycomb pattern (although extension into adipose tissue may be seen in the deeply penetrating variant of fibrous histiocytoma); (2) its entrapment of adnexal structures; (3) its lack of birefringent collagen under polarized light; (4) its lack of overlying epidermal hyperplasia; and (5) its diffuse reactivity for CD34.

MALIGNANT NEOPLASMS

LEIOMYOSARCOMA[17,19,69,70,74,78,94]

Definition

A rare sarcoma of vulvar soft tissue showing smooth muscle differentiation.

Clinical features

Of all sarcomas of the vulva, which as a category are rare, leiomyosarcoma represents the most common subtype. Patients are typically in their fourth or fifth decade and present with symptoms related to a mass. Tumors may be of varying size but are typically under 5 cm. Treatment varies from wide local excision to radical vulvectomy.

Pathology

Histologically, most vulvar leiomyosarcomas have a similar morphologic appearance to those that occur more commonly elsewhere in the female genital tract, being of the spindle cell type (Figure 4.31). Due to the rarity of these lesions, defining criteria to predict those tumors with metastatic potential remains problematic, yet is of paramount importance due to potential differences in clinical management. Use of the criteria proposed by Tavassoli and Norris[94] is recommended, in which tumors with three or more of the following criteria should be diagnosed as leiomyosarcoma:

- >5 cm in size;
- >5 mitoses per 10 high-power fields;
- infiltrative margin;
- moderate to severe cytologic atypia.

Although necrosis is excluded in this algorithm, its presence should strongly raise the possibility of malignancy.

PROXIMAL-TYPE EPITHELIOID SARCOMA[35,49]

Definition

Large cell variant of epithelioid sarcoma that has a predilection for the genital and perineal regions.

Clinical features

Patients typically present in the fourth decade with symptoms related to a mass lesion. Tumor size in the genital area is usually under 6 cm but tumor size in general may range up to 20 cm (median, 4 cm). Clinically, the proximal subtype acts more aggressively than the usual (distal) epithelioid sarcoma, with earlier distant metastasis following excision of the primary.

Pathology

Histologically, this tumor exhibits a diffuse and often multinodular proliferation of relatively monomorphic large cells with abundant eosinophilic cytoplasm, imparting an epithelioid appearance. Rhabdoid inclusions are frequent (Figures

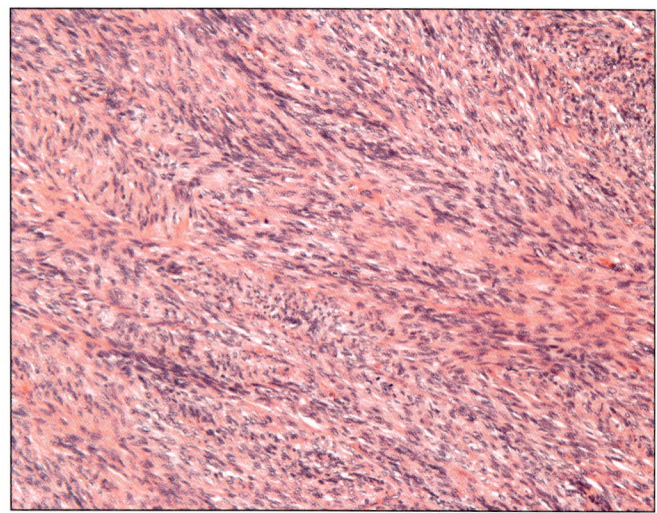

Fig. 4.30 Dermatofibrosarcoma protuberans. Fibrosarcomatous change with a fascicular growth pattern.

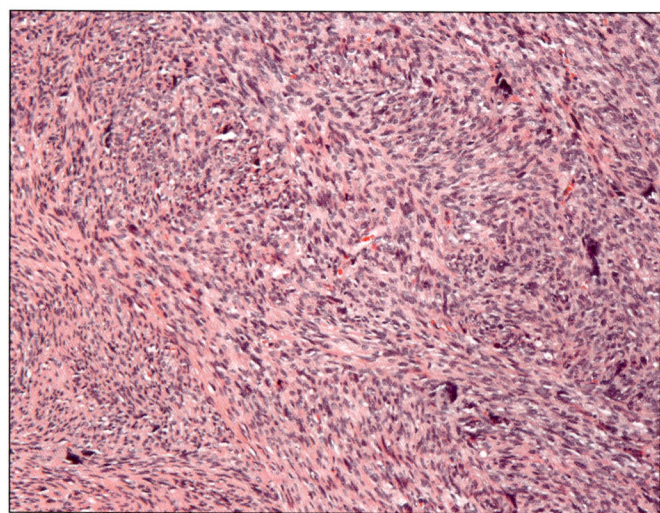

Fig. 4.31 Leiomyosarcoma, spindle cell type.

4.32 and 4.33). The tumor cells, which contain large vesicular nuclei and prominent nucleoli, commonly invade into subcutaneous or deeper soft tissue. Immunohistochemically, the tumor cells commonly react with keratin and epithelial membrane antigen. They also often express CD34 and may occasionally react for desmin and actin.

Differential diagnosis

In the genital region, the principal differential diagnosis is with carcinoma or melanoma. Proximal-type epithelioid sarcoma is distinguished from poorly differentiated carcinoma by its multinodular growth pattern, coexpression of CD34 and, occasionally, desmin, and lack of an intraepidermal *in situ* component. In addition, it differs from melanoma by the above features as well as expression of epithelial markers and lack of S-100 protein reactivity.

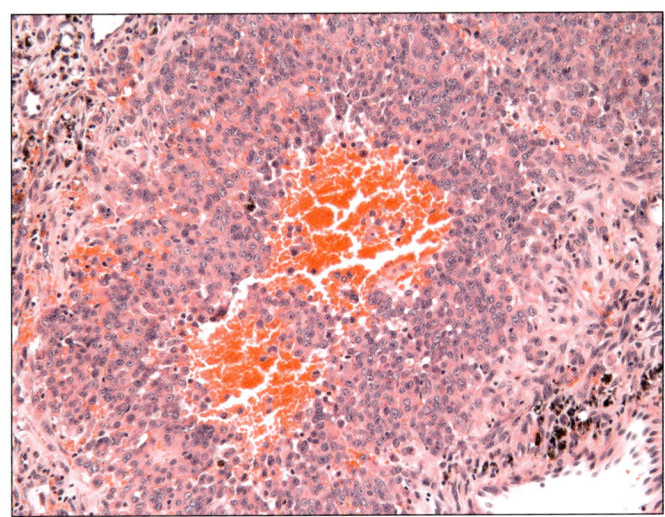

Fig. 4.32 Proximal-type epithelioid sarcoma. Multinodular, 'granulomatous' growth pattern.

LIPOSARCOMA[6,29,32,77,97]

Definition
Malignant mesenchymal neoplasm showing adipocytic differentiation.

Clinical features
Liposarcoma usually arises in the limbs, trunks, and abdominal cavity, but uncommonly also in the vulva. It occurs predominantly in middle-aged women (median 52 years) on the labia majora and is of varying size but typically is under 8 cm. Many are thought clinically to represent a lipoma. Most are of the well-differentiated subtype and have a similar clinical behavior to those that occur outside the abdominal cavity, i.e. complete excision with a clear margin is curative.

Pathology
Histologically, most tumors have the usual morphologic appearance of well-differentiated liposarcoma/atypical lipomatous tumor with variation in adipocyte size, adipocytic nuclear atypia, cellular fibrous septa (often with scattered hyperchromatic stromal cells), and occasional lipoblasts. Some, however, may have an unusual morphology that is unique to tumors that arise at this site. These tumors show an admixture of neoplastic bland spindle and round cells, variably sized adipocytes, and numerous bivacuolated lipoblasts (Figure 4.34). This unusual morphology is not associated with any difference in behavior.

OTHER RARE SARCOMAS

Other sarcomas may rarely occur in the vulva and include rhabdomyosarcoma (embryonal, alveolar, and pleomorphic subtypes),[15,16,43] alveolar soft part sarcoma,[90] extraskeletal myxoid chondrosarcoma,[56] synovial sarcoma,[72] angiosarcoma,[17,74] and Kaposi sarcoma,[37,58] among others.

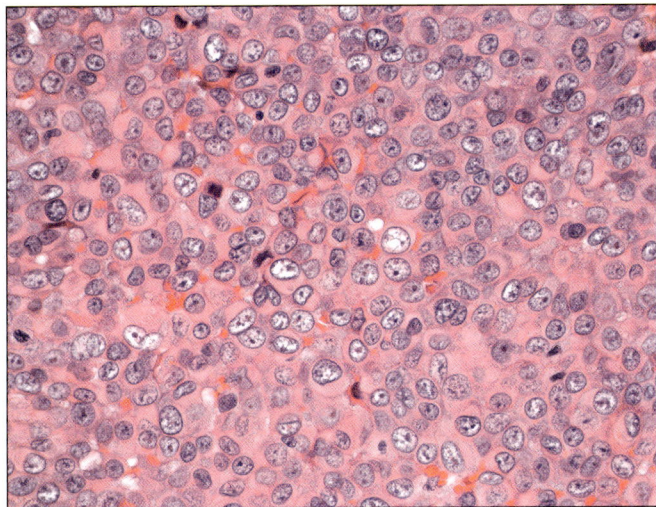

Fig. 4.33 Proximal-type epithelioid sarcoma. Tumor cells have abundant eosinophilic cytoplasm and vesicular nuclei. Note rhabdoid appearance of some cells.

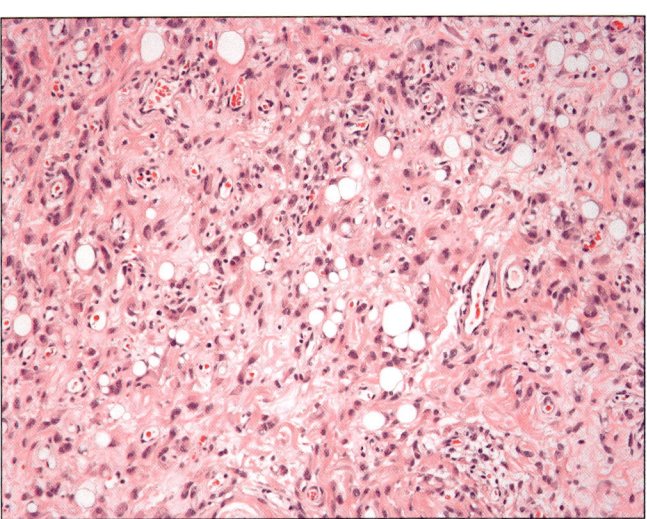

Fig. 4.34 Liposarcoma, unusual vulvar variant. Admixture of bland spindle and round cells with numerous bivacuolated lipoblasts.

REFERENCES

1. Abenoza P, Lillemoe T. CD34 and factor XIIIa in the differential diagnosis of dermatofibroma and dermatofibrosarcoma protuberans. Am J Dermatopathol 1993;15:429–34.
2. Allen PW, Dymock RB, MacCormac LB. Superficial angiomyxomas with and without epithelial components. Report of 30 tumors in 28 patients. Am J Surg Pathol 1988;12:519–30.
3. Barnhill DR, Boling R, Nobles W, Crooks L, Burke T. Vulvar dermatofibrosarcoma protuberans. Gynecol Oncol 1988;30:149–52.
4. Begin LR, Clement PB, Kirk ME, et al. Aggressive angiomyxoma of pelvic soft parts: a clinicopathologic study of nine cases. Hum Pathol 1985;16:621–8.
5. Bock JE, Andreasson B, Thorn A, Holck S. Dermatofibrosarcoma protuberans of the vulva. Gynecol Oncol 1985;20:129–35.
6. Brooks JJ, LiVolsi VA. Liposarcoma presenting on the vulva. Am J Obstet Gynecol 1987;156:73–5.
7. Burt RL, Prichard RW, Kim BS. Fibroepithelial polyp of the vagina. A report of five cases. Obstet Gynecol 1976;47:52S–54S.
8. Calonje E, Fletcher CD. Aneurysmal benign fibrous histiocytoma: clinicopathological analysis of 40 cases of a tumour frequently misdiagnosed as a vascular neoplasm. Histopathology 1995;26:323–31.
9. Calonje E, Guerin D, McCormick D, Fletcher CD. Superficial angiomyxoma: clinicopathologic analysis of a series of distinctive but poorly recognized cutaneous tumors with tendency for recurrence. Am J Surg Pathol 1999;23:910–17.
10. Calonje E, Mentzel T, Fletcher CD. Cellular benign fibrous histiocytoma. Clinicopathologic analysis of 74 cases of a distinctive variant of cutaneous fibrous histiocytoma with frequent recurrence. Am J Surg Pathol 1994;18:668–76.
11. Chabrel CM, Beilby JO. Vaginal rhabdomyoma. Histopathology 1980;4:645–51.
12. Chirayil SJ, Tobon H. Polyps of the vagina: a clinicopathologic study of 18 cases. Cancer 1981;47:2904–7.
13. Cohen PR, Young AW, Jr, Tovell HM. Angiokeratoma of the vulva: diagnosis and review of the literature. Obstet Gynecol Surv 1989;44:339–46.
14. Colome-Grimmer MI, Evans HL. Metastasizing cellular dermatofibroma. A report of two cases. Am J Surg Pathol 1996;20:1361–7.
15. Copeland LJ, Gershenson DM, Saul PB, et al. Sarcoma botryoides of the female genital tract. Obstet Gynecol 1985;66:262–6.
16. Copeland LJ, Sneige N, Stringer CA, et al. Alveolar rhabdomyosarcoma of the female genitalia. Cancer 1985;56:849–55.
17. Curtin JP, Saigo P, Slucher B, et al. Soft-tissue sarcoma of the vagina and vulva: a clinicopathologic study. Obstet Gynecol 1995;86:269–72.
18. Davos I, Abell MR. Soft tissue sarcomas of vulva. Gynecol Oncol 1976;4:70–86.
19. DiSaia PJ, Rutledge F, Smith JP. Sarcoma of the vulva. Report of 12 patients. Obstet Gynecol 1971;38:180–4.
20. Elliott GB, Reynolds HA, Fidler HK. Pseudo-sarcoma botryoides of cervix and vagina in pregnancy. J Obstet Gynaecol Br Commonw 1967;74:728–33.
21. Faber K, Jones MA, Spratt D, Tarraza HM, Jr. Vulvar leiomyomatosis in a patient with esophagogastric leiomyomatosis: review of the syndrome. Gynecol Oncol 1991;41:92–4.
22. Fetsch JF, Laskin WB, Lefkowitz M, Kindblom LG, Meis-Kindblom JM. Aggressive angiomyxoma: a clinicopathologic study of 29 female patients. Cancer 1996;78:79–90.
23. Fetsch JF, Laskin WB, Tavassoli FA. Superficial angiomyxoma (cutaneous myxoma): a clinicopathologic study of 17 cases arising in the genital region. Int J Gynecol Pathol 1997;16:325–34.
24. Flanagan BP, Helwig EB. Cutaneous lymphangioma. Arch Dermatol 1977;113:24–30.
25. Fletcher CD, Tsang WY, Fisher C, Lee KC, Chan JK. Angiomyofibroblastoma of the vulva. A benign neoplasm distinct from aggressive angiomyxoma. Am J Surg Pathol 1992;16:373–82.
26. Franquemont DW, Cooper PH, Shmookler BM, Wick MR. Benign fibrous histiocytoma of the skin with potential for local recurrence: a tumor to be distinguished from dermatofibroma. Mod Pathol 1990;3:158–63.
27. Fukunaga M, Nomura K, Matsumoto K, et al. Vulval angiomyofibroblastoma. Clinicopathologic analysis of six cases. Am J Clin Pathol 1997;107:45–51.
28. Gaffney EF, Majmudar B, Bryan JA. Nodular fasciitis (pseudosarcomatous fasciitis) of the vulva. Int J Gynecol Pathol 1982;1:307–12.
29. Genton CY, Maroni ES. Vulval liposarcoma. Arch Gynecol 1987;240:63–6.
30. Ghorbani RP, Malpica A, Ayala AG. Dermatofibrosarcoma protuberans of the vulva: clinicopathologic and immunohistochemical analysis of four cases, one with fibrosarcomatous change, and review of the literature. Int J Gynecol Pathol 1999;18:366–73.
31. Gokden N, Dehner LP, Zhu X, Pfeifer JD. Dermatofibrosarcoma protuberans of the vulva and groin: detection of COL1A1–PDGFB fusion transcripts by RT-PCR. J Cutan Pathol 2003;30:190–5.
32. Gondos B, Casey MJ. Liposarcoma of the perineum. Gynecol Oncol 1982;14:133–40.
33. Gonzalez S, Duarte I. Benign fibrous histiocytoma of the skin. A morphologic study of 290 cases. Pathol Res Pract 1982;174:379–91.
34. Granter SR, Nucci MR, Fletcher CD. Aggressive angiomyxoma: reappraisal of its relationship to angiomyofibroblastoma in a series of 16 cases. Histopathology 1997;30:3–10.
35. Guillou L, Wadden C, Coindre JM, Krausz T, Fletcher CD. 'Proximal-type' epithelioid sarcoma, a distinctive aggressive neoplasm showing rhabdoid features. Clinicopathologic, immunohistochemical, and ultrastructural study of a series. Am J Surg Pathol 1997;21:130–46.
36. Haley JC, Mirowski GW, Hood AF. Benign vulvar tumors. Semin Cutan Med Surg 1998;17:196–204.
37. Hall DJ, Burns JC, Goplerud DR. Kaposi's sarcoma of the vulva: a case report and brief review. Obstet Gynecol 1979;54:478–83.
38. Hanski W, Hagel-Lewicka E, Daniszewski K. Rhabdomyomas of female genital tract. Report on two cases. Zentralbl Pathol 1991;137:439–42.
39. Hartmann CA, Sperling M, Stein H. So-called fibroepithelial polyps of the vagina exhibiting an unusual but uniform antigen profile characterized by expression of desmin and steroid hormone receptors but no muscle-specific actin or macrophage markers. Am J Clin Pathol 1990;93:604–8.
40. Hisaoka M, Kouho H, Aoki T, Daimaru Y, Hashimoto H. Angiomyofibroblastoma of the vulva: a clinicopathologic study of seven cases. Pathol Int 1995;45:487–92.
41. Horowitz IR, Copas P, Majmudar B. Granular cell tumors of the vulva. Am J Obstet Gynecol 1995;173:1710–13.
42. Iezzoni JC, Fechner RE, Wong LS, Rosai J. Aggressive angiomyxoma in males. A report of four cases. Am J Clin Pathol 1995;104:391–6.
43. Imachi M, Tsukamoto N, Kamura T, et al. Alveolar rhabdomyosarcoma of the vulva. Report of two cases. Acta Cytol 1991;35:345–9.
44. Iversen UM. Two cases of benign vaginal rhabdomyoma. Case reports. APMIS 1996;104:575–8.
45. Iwasa Y, Fletcher CD. Cellular angiofibroma: clinicopathologic and immunohistochemical analysis of 51 cases. Am J Surg Pathol 2004;28:1426–35.
46. Iwasa Y, Fletcher CD. Distinctive prepubertal vulval fibroma: a hitherto unrecognized mesenchymal tumor of prepubertal girls: analysis of 11 cases. Am J Surg Pathol 2004;28:1601–8.
47. Iwata J, Fletcher CD. Lipidized fibrous histiocytoma: clinicopathologic analysis of 22 cases. Am J Dermatopathol 2000;22:126–34.
48. Kaddu S, McMenamin ME, Fletcher CD. Atypical fibrous histiocytoma of the skin: clinicopathologic analysis of 59 cases with evidence of infrequent metastasis. Am J Surg Pathol 2002;26:35–46.
49. Kasamatsu T, Hasegawa T, Tsuda H, et al. Primary epithelioid sarcoma of the vulva. Int J Gynecol Cancer 2001;11:316–20.
50. Kazmierczak B, Wanschura S, Meyer-Bolte K, et al. Cytogenic and molecular analysis of an aggressive angiomyxoma. Am J Pathol 1995;147:580–5.
51. Lack EE, Worsham GF, Callihan MD, et al. Granular cell tumor: a clinicopathologic study of 110 patients. J Surg Oncol 1980;13:301–16.
52. Lae ME, Pereira PF, Keeney GL, Nascimento AG. Lipoblastoma-like tumour of the vulva: report of three cases of a distinctive mesenchymal neoplasm of adipocytic differentiation. Histopathology 2002;40:505–9.
53. Laskin WB, Fetsch JF, Mostofi FK. Angiomyofibroblastoma-like tumor of the male genital tract: analysis of 11 cases with comparison to female angiomyofibroblastoma and spindle cell lipoma. Am J Surg Pathol 1998;22:6–16.
54. Laskin WB, Fetsch JF, Tavassoli FA. Angiomyofibroblastoma of the female genital tract: analysis of 17 cases including a lipomatous variant. Hum Pathol 1997;28:1046–55.
55. Leake JF, Buscema J, Cho KR, Currie JL. Dermatofibrosarcoma protuberans of the vulva. Gynecol Oncol 1991;41:245–9.
56. Lin J, Yip KM, Maffulli N, Chow LT. Extraskeletal mesenchymal chondrosarcoma of the labium majus. Gynecol Oncol 1996;60:492–3.
57. LiVolsi VA, Brooks JJ. Nodular fasciitis of the vulva: a report of two cases. Obstet Gynecol 1987;69:513–16.
58. Macasaet MA, Duerr A, Thelmo W, Vernon SD, Unger ER. Kaposi sarcoma presenting as a vulvar mass. Obstet Gynecol 1995;86:695–7.
59. Maenpaa J, Soderstrom KO, Salmi T, Ekblad U. Large atypical polyps of the vagina during pregnancy with concomitant human papilloma virus infection. Eur J Obstet Gynecol Reprod Biol 1988;27:65–9.
60. Majmudar B, Castellano PZ, Wilson RW, Siegel RJ. Granular cell tumors of the vulva. J Reprod Med 1990;35:1008–14.
61. McCluggage WG, Patterson A, Maxwell P. Aggressive angiomyxoma of pelvic parts exhibits oestrogen and progesterone receptor positivity. J Clin Pathol 2000;53:603–5.
62. McCluggage WG, Perenyei M, Irwin ST. Recurrent cellular angiofibroma of the vulva. J Clin Pathol 2002;55:477–9.
63. Mentzel T, Beham A, Katenkamp D, Dei Tos AP, Fletcher CD. Fibrosarcomatous ('high-grade') dermatofibrosarcoma protuberans: clinicopathologic and immunohistochemical study of a series of 41 cases with emphasis on prognostic significance. Am J Surg Pathol 1998;22:576–87.
64. Miettinen M, Wahlstrom T, Vesterinen E, Saksela E. Vaginal polyps with pseudosarcomatous features. A clinicopathologic study of seven cases. Cancer 1983;51:1148–51.
65. Miner JH. Alport syndrome with diffuse leiomyomatosis. When and when not? Am J Pathol 1999;154:1633–5.
66. Moodley M, Moodley J. Dermatofibrosarcoma protuberans of the vulva: a case report and review of the literature. Gynecol Oncol 2000;78:74–5.

67. Mucitelli DR, Charles EZ, Kraus FT. Vulvovaginal polyps. Histologic appearance, ultrastructure, immunocytochemical characteristics, and clinicopathologic correlations. Int J Gynecol Pathol 1990;9:20–40.

68. Naeem R, Lux ML, Huang SF, et al. Ring chromosomes in dermatofibrosarcoma protuberans are composed of interspersed sequences from chromosomes 17 and 22. Am J Pathol 1995;147:1553–8.

69. Newman PL, Fletcher CD. Smooth muscle tumours of the external genitalia: clinicopathological analysis of a series. Histopathology 1991;18:523–9.

70. Nielsen GP, Rosenberg AE, Koerner FC, Young RH, Scully RE. Smooth-muscle tumors of the vulva. A clinicopathological study of 25 cases and review of the literature. Am J Surg Pathol 1996;20:779–93.

71. Nielsen GP, Young RH, et al. Angiomyofibroblastoma of the vulva and vagina. Mod Pathol 1996;9:284–91.

72. Nielsen GP, Shaw PA, Rosenberg AE, et al. Synovial sarcoma of the vulva: a report of two cases. Mod Pathol 1996;9:970–4.

73. Nielsen GP, Young RII, Dickersin GR, Rosenberg AE. Angiomyofibroblastoma of the vulva with sarcomatous transformation ('angiomyofibrosarcoma'). Am J Surg Pathol 1997;21:1104–8.

74. Nirenberg A, Ostor AG, Slavin J, Riley CB, Rome RM. Primary vulvar sarcomas. Int J Gynecol Pathol 1995;14:55–62.

75. Norris HJ, Taylor HB. Polyps of the vagina. A benign lesion resembling sarcoma botryoides. Cancer 1966;19:227–32.

76. Nucci MR, Fletcher CD. Fibroepithelial stromal polyps of vulvovaginal tissue: from the banal to the bizarre. Pathology Case Reviews 1998;3:151–7.

77. Nucci MR, Fletcher CD. Liposarcoma (atypical lipomatous tumors) of the vulva: a clinicopathologic study of six cases. Int J Gynecol Pathol 1998;17:17–23.

78. Nucci MR, Fletcher CD. Vulvovaginal soft tissue tumours: update and review. Histopathology 2000;36:97–108.

79. Nucci MR, Granter SR, Fletcher CD. Cellular angiofibroma: a benign neoplasm distinct from angiomyofibroblastoma and spindle cell lipoma. Am J Surg Pathol 1997;21:636–44.

80. Nucci MR, Weremowicz S, Neskey DM, et al. Chromosomal translocation t(8;12) induces aberrant HMGIC expression in aggressive angiomyxoma of the vulva. Genes Chromosomes Cancer 2001;32:172–6.

81. Nucci MR, Young RH, Fletcher CD. Cellular pseudosarcomatous fibroepithelial stromal polyps of the lower female genital tract: an underrecognized lesion often misdiagnosed as sarcoma. Am J Surg Pathol 2000;24:231–40.

82. O'Quinn AG, Edwards CL, Gallager HS. Pseudosarcoma botryoides of the vagina in pregnancy. Gynecol Oncol 1982;13:237–41.

83. Ockner DM, Sayadi H, Swanson PE, Ritter JH, Wick MR. Genital angiomyofibroblastoma. Comparison with aggressive angiomyxoma and other myxoid neoplasms of skin and soft tissue. Am J Clin Pathol 1997;107:36–44.

84. Ostor AG, Fortune DW, Riley CB. Fibroepithelial polyps with atypical stromal cells (pseudosarcoma botryoides) of vulva and vagina. A report of 13 cases. Int J Gynecol Pathol 1988;7:351–60.

85. Peachey RD, Lim CC, Whimster IW. Lymphangioma of skin. A review of 65 cases. Br J Dermatol 1970;83:519–27.

86. Prioleau PG, Santa Cruz DJ. Lymphangioma circumscriptum following radical mastectomy and radiation therapy. Cancer 1978;42:1989–91.

87. Requena L, Aguilar A, Lopez Redondo MJ, Schoendorff C, Sanchez YE. Multinodular hemosiderotic dermatofibroma. Dermatologica 1990;181:320–3.

88. Roberts TA, Daly JW. Pseudosarcomatous fasciitis of the vulva. Gynecol Oncol 1981;11:383–6.

89. Robertson AJ, McIntosh W, Lamont P, Guthrie W. Malignant granular cell tumour (myoblastoma) of the vulva: report of a case and review of the literature. Histopathology 1981;5:69–79.

90. Shen JT, D'ablaing G, Morrow CP. Alveolar soft part sarcoma of the vulva: report of first case and review of literature. Gynecol Oncol 1982;13:120–8.

91. Singh GC, Calonje E, Fletcher CD. Epithelioid benign fibrous histiocytoma of skin: clinico-pathological analysis of 20 cases of a poorly known variant. Histopathology 1994;24:123–9.

92. Soergel TM, Doering DL, O'Connor D. Metastatic dermatofibrosarcoma protuberans of the vulva. Gynecol Oncol 1998;71:320–4.

93. Steeper TA, Rosai J. Aggressive angiomyxoma of the female pelvis and perineum. Report of nine cases of a distinctive type of gynecologic soft-tissue neoplasm. Am J Surg Pathol 1983;7:463–75.

94. Tavassoli FA, Norris HJ. Smooth muscle tumors of the vulva. Obstet Gynecol 1979;53:213–17.

95. Tsang WY, Chan JK, Lee KC, Fisher C, Fletcher CD. Aggressive angiomyxoma. A report of four cases occurring in men. Am J Surg Pathol 1992;16:1059–65.

96. Vanni R, Faa G, Dettori T, et al. A case of dermatofibrosarcoma protuberans of the vulva with a COL1A1/PDGFB fusion identical to a case of giant cell fibroblastoma. Virchows Arch 2000;437:95–100.

97. Vecchione A, Palazzetti P. [Anatomoclinical considerations on a case of liposarcoma with vulvar localization]. Riv Anat Patol Oncol 1967;31:177–93.

98. Vlastos AT, Malpica A, Follen M. Lymphangioma circumscriptum of the vulva: a review of the literature. Obstet Gynecol 2003;101:946–54.

99. Zelger B, Sidoroff A, Stanzl U, et al. Deep penetrating dermatofibroma versus dermatofibrosarcoma protuberans. A clinicopathologic comparison. Am J Surg Pathol 1994;18:677–86.

Vagina

5

Stanley J. Robboy   Peter Russell

NORMAL STRUCTURE

The vagina, from the Latin 'sheath', extends from the vestibule of the vulva to the uterus, lying posterior (dorsal) to the urinary bladder and anterior (ventral) to the rectum. Its axis averages 30° with the vertical and usually more than 90° with the uterus. The ventral wall is shorter than the dorsal wall, but overall the mean vaginal length is 6.2 cm.[7] It surrounds the exocervix and forms vault-like fornices between its cervical attachment and the lateral wall. In the adult, the anterior and posterior walls are slack and remain in contact with each other, whereas the lateral walls remain fairly rigid and separated. This gives an H-shaped appearance to the vaginal canal on cross-section. The vagina opens into the vestibule formed from the urogenital sinus. The vestibule lies beneath the urethra and between the inner margins of the labia minora. The vagina, urethra, and ducts of Bartholins glands open into the vestibule.

The vaginal wall consists of three principal layers: mucosa (epithelial and submucosal stroma), muscle, and adventitia. The epithelium is about 0.4 mm thick and, on gross examination, exhibits a characteristic pattern of folds or rugae separated by furrows of variable depth. The rugal pattern of the vaginal mucosa produces an undulating appearance on microscopic examination in contrast to the flat surface of the cervix. The luminal surface is lined with non-keratinized squamous epithelium, similar to cervical epithelium. The normal vaginal mucosa lacks glands. Its surface is lubricated both by fluids that pass directly through the mucosa and by cervical mucus.

The epithelial mucosa rests on a submucosa, or lamina propria, which contains elastic fibers and a rich venous and lymphatic network. Sometimes the superficial lamina propria discloses a band-like zone of loose connective tissue that contains atypical polygonal to stellate stromal cells with scant cytoplasm. Many cells are multinucleated or have multilobulated hyperchromatic nuclei. Few are mononucleate. Mitoses are not observed. These atypical stromal cells are thought to give rise to fibroepithelial polyps and have been observed within the cervix, vagina, and vulva. They are myofibroblastic in nature.[136]

The vaginal wall is an unlayered zone of smooth muscle, which is continuous with that of the uterus. The adventitia is a thin coat of dense connective tissue adjoining the muscularis. The connective tissue of the adventitia merges with the stroma, connecting the vagina to the adjacent structures. This layer contains many veins, lymphatics, nerve bundles, and small groups of nerve cells.

The surface of the vagina is moistened by a thin transudate: this fluid is acid (pH 4–5) owing to the presence of lactic acid, which is produced from the metabolism of epithelial glycogen by *Lactobacillus acidophilus*, the bacillus observed originally by Döderlein in vaginal secretions. The acidity of the vaginal fluid accounts for its considerable bacteriostatic capacity: the degree of acidity is much reduced by the presence of pus and by menstrual blood, and also by the absence of estrogens. Before puberty and, to a lesser extent, after the menopause, the vaginal mucosa is thinner and less resistant to infection than during reproductive life.

Typical of squamous epithelia elsewhere in the body, the mature, stratified squamous epithelium subdivides into the deep, intermediate, and superficial zones (Figure 5.1). The deep zone contains the basal cell layer and above this the parabasal layer. Both are the active proliferative compartments or germinal beds, as shown by the nuclear proliferation markers (the Ki-67 antigen, which is demonstrable during late G_1, G_2, and M phases of the cell cycle) (Figure 5.2). The basal cell layer consists of a single layer of columnar-like cells, approximately 10 μm thick, the long axis of which is vertically arranged. The cells have a basophilic cytoplasm and relatively large oval nuclei. Mitoses may be present. Occasional melanocytes are also found. The parabasal layer is poorly demarcated from the overlying cell layers. It consists usually of about two layers of small polygonal cells, having a total 14 μm thickness, often with intercellular bridges. The cells have basophilic cytoplasm, relatively large, centrally placed, round nuclei, and occasional mitoses.

The intermediate cell layer is of variable thickness. The cells have prominent intercellular bridges, a naviculate configuration, and a long cell axis parallel to the surface. The cytoplasm is basophilic, although some glycogen may be present. The nuclei are round, oval, or irregular, with finely granular chromatin. This layer of cells has about 10 rows of cells of about 100 μm thickness.

The superficial layer is also of variable thickness. The cells are polygonal when viewed from above and flattened when viewed in cross-section. The cytoplasm is acidophilic, and the nuclei are centrally located, small, round, and pyknotic. Keratohyalin granules are sometimes seen in the cytoplasm. This layer also contains about 10 rows of squamous cells.

Relatively little is known about the normal components of the epithelium itself. The submucosa contains various mononuclear cells demonstrable by immunocytochemical methods. The dendritic processes of Langerhans cells, about 4 per high-power field (HPF), are distributed throughout the mucosa.[98] They are found largely in the deeper layers but can extend into the superficial fields (Figure 5.3). T8 and, to a lesser degree, T4 lymphocytes are also frequently found, whereas macrophages and B lymphocytes are relatively uncommon.

111

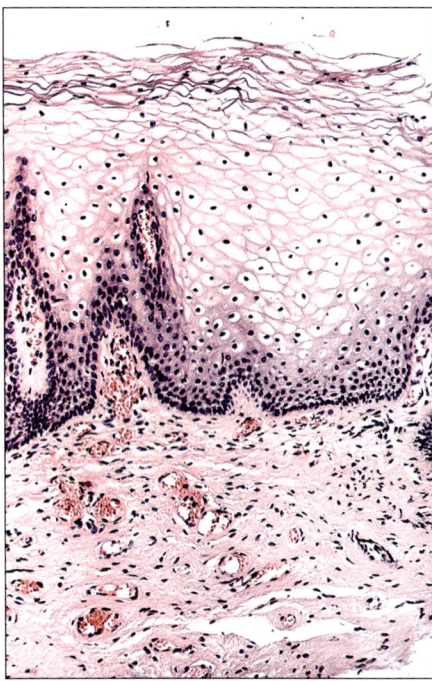

Fig. 5.1 Normal vaginal epithelium. The epithelium consists of a single layer of basal cells, several layers of parabasal cells, and thick intermediate and superficial layers of highly glycogenated cells.

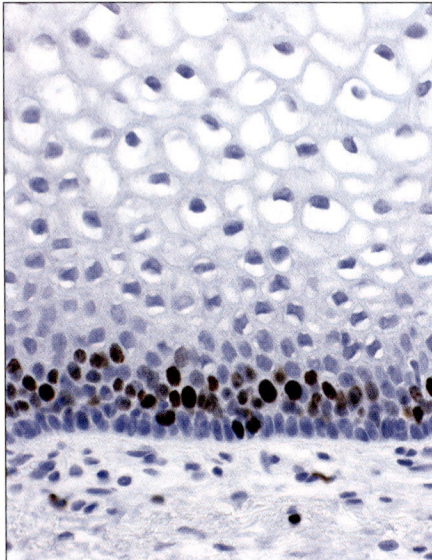

Fig. 5.2 Normal vagina. KI-67 antigen, demonstrable during the late G_1, G_2 and M phases of the cell cycle in the parabasal and basal layer of the normal vaginal mucosa.

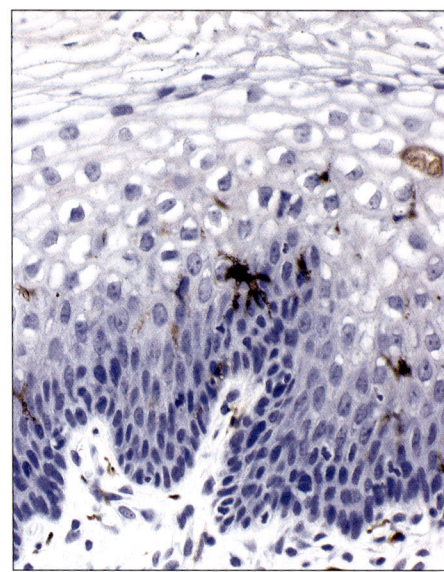

Fig. 5.3 Vagina. The dendritic processes of Langerhans cells.

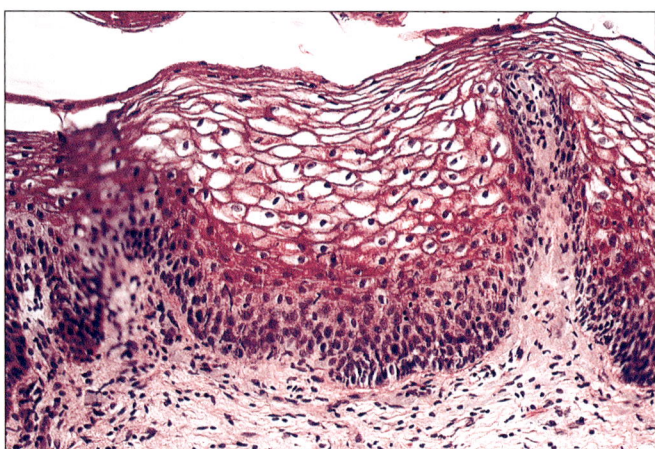

Fig. 5.4 Normal vaginal epithelium. Extensive glycogen (red) is present in the thick layers of intermediate and superficial cells (PAS stain).

Cyclic changes occur in the vaginal epithelium. Proliferation of the basal layers and general thickening of the epithelium are seen in the first half of the cycle. Estrogens stimulate maturation of the epithelium, as evidenced by increased numbers of intermediate cells and then superficial cells (Figure 5.1). A sign of maturation is the significant accumulation of glycogen in the epithelium (Figure 5.4). Full maturation to superficial cells does not occur when the estrogenic action is opposed by progesterone. Thus, in the second half of the cycle, after ovulation has taken place, maturation ceases at the level of the intermediate cells. This change is of use clinically; the number of superficial cells in a smear taken from the lateral vaginal wall (and, to a lesser extent, from the ectocervix) compared with the number of intermediate and parabasal cells gives a rough indication of the hormonal status of the woman. Variously calculated, although now considered archaic, this relationship gives the maturation index, the cornification index or the karyopyknotic index (KPI). A high KPI therefore means that the epithelium has been stimulated by unopposed estrogen. Without hormonal stimulation, the cells atrophy (Figure 5.5).

MESONEPHRIC DUCTS

The wolffian ducts, known otherwise as 'mesonephric ducts' or 'Gartners ducts', are vestigial in the adult female (Figure 5.6). They begin to irreversibly regress if not stimulated to develop by testosterone before week 13 postconception. These paired

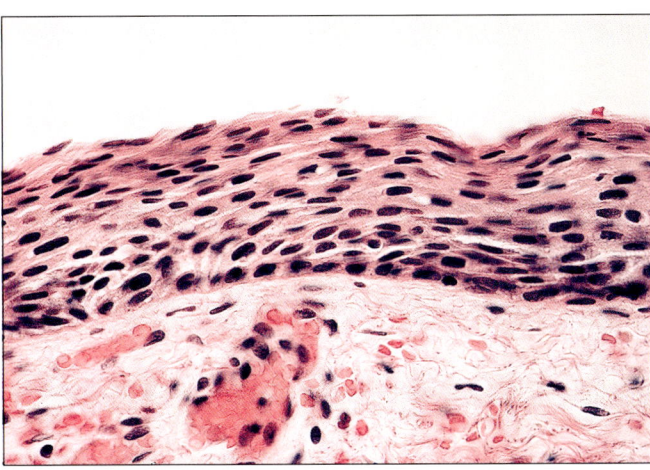

Fig. 5.5 Atrophy. In the absence of estrogenic stimulation, the number of cell layers decreases, and virtually all cells are basal and parabasal with minimal cytoplasm.

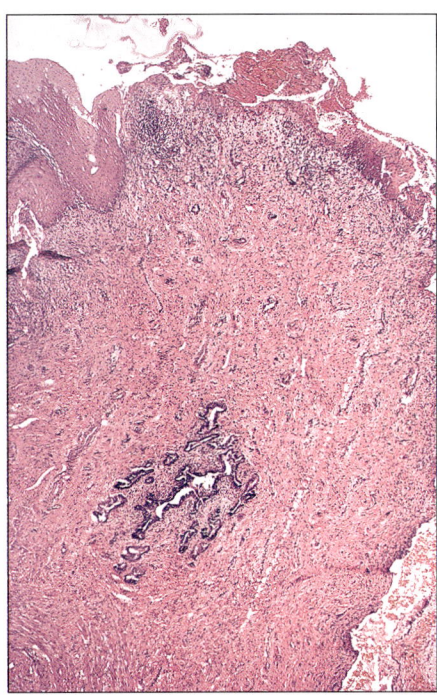

Fig. 5.7 Mesonephric duct. The mother duct, located deep in the wall of the vagina, is surrounded by smaller arborized offshoots.

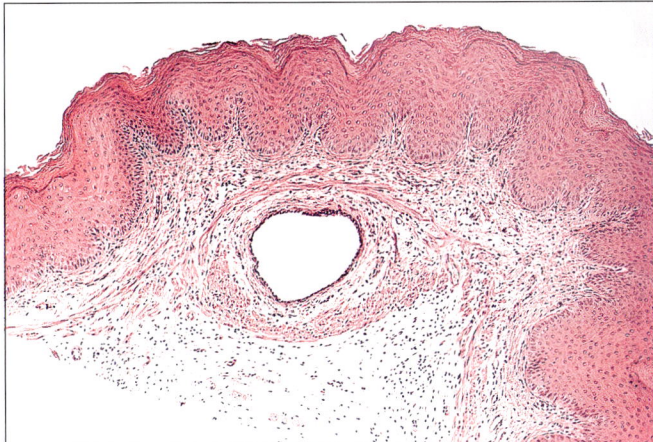

Fig. 5.6 Normal mesonephric duct. On cross-section it is a single duct in the submucosa surrounded by clusters of smooth muscle bands.

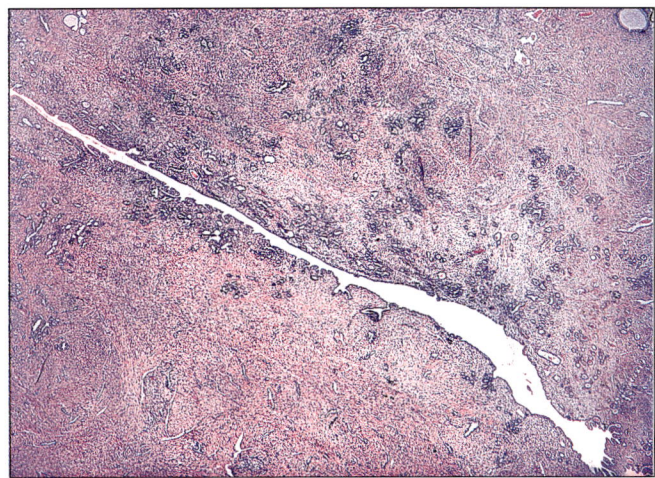

Fig. 5.8 Elongated mesonephric duct.

ducts are most commonly seen in the lateral vaginal walls, although we have encountered them in all areas. Where encountered by chance in a radical vaginectomy specimen, the ducts are virtually always invisible grossly. Usually the ducts are seen on end in tissue section, occasionally with hypertrophied smooth muscle surrounding them (Figure 5.7). They may also appear as central ducts about which are arborized glands on the periphery. Occasionally, the ducts appear as elongated tubes (Figure 5.8), also with peripheral arborized glands (Figure 5.9). The lumens are filled frequently with a deeply eosinophilic, hyalinized secretion (Figure 5.10). The single layer of cells lining the ducts is predominantly composed of nuclei. The cytoplasm is scant, relatively translucent, and lacks cilia. The nuclei frequently overlap. The chromatin is strikingly bland. Mitoses are absent. On a clinical basis individual ducts occasionally become cystic and macroscopically visible. In the cervix, these ducts may on a rare occasion appear diffusely throughout the wall and appear as mesonephric hyperplasia or even adenoma. We have also seen rare cases where the neoplasm present appeared to be a true wolffian duct carcinoma.

DEVELOPMENTAL DISORDERS

Congenital malformations of uterus and vagina result from failure of development, failure of fusion or septal reabsorption of the müllerian ducts. The spectrum of findings ranges from agenesis to duplications. They are important clinically because of their association with menstrual disorders and impaired fertility. Furthermore, women with müllerian duct anomalies have a significant risk of obstetric complications such as spontaneous abortion, stillbirth, and preterm delivery.

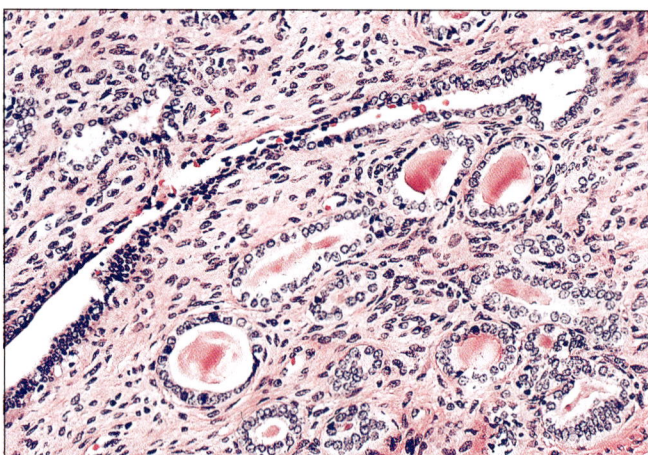

Fig. 5.9 Mesonephric duct. Smaller arborized offshoots surround the main duct.

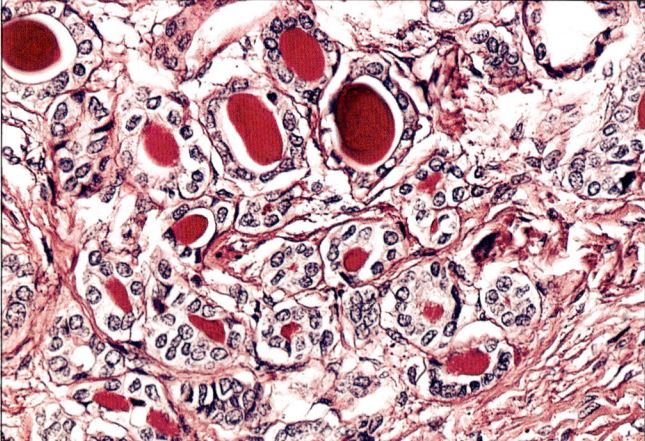

Fig. 5.10 Mesonephric duct. Detail of budding mesonephric ductules with eosinophilic secretions in the lumen.

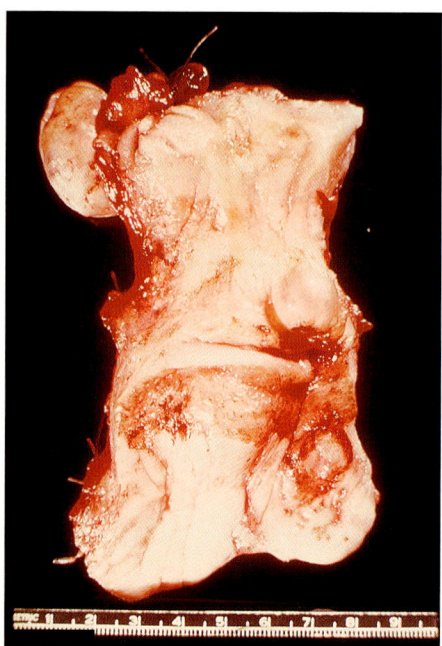

Fig. 5.11 Transverse septum.

all respects (Figure 5.4), since, embryologically, it derives from the urogenital sinus. The defect is often associated with an absent uterus and fallopian tubes (müllerian agenesis or Mayer–Rokitansky–Kuster–Hauser syndrome), and with anomalies of the urinary tract.[40,68,100] This syndrome provides insight into embryologic development and demonstrates that an intact mesonephric duct is required for the growth and caudal lengthening of the müllerian duct during fetal life. The gonads, not being of müllerian origin, are usually normal. About 25% of women with vaginal agenesis have a uterus and they may have complications from retrograde menstruation (such as an increased risk of pelvic endometriosis).

IMPERFORATE HYMEN

Imperforate hymen is the most common congenital anomaly of significance to occur in the vagina, with a frequency of 0.05%. The presence of a thick mucoid secretion that distends the vagina may provide a clue to diagnosis in the neonate, but often an imperforate hymen is not recognized until puberty, when there is retention of menstrual detritus.[69,150] If not corrected promptly, infertility may result from endometriosis and pelvic adhesions associated with retrograde menstruation.

VAGINAL AGENESIS

Vaginal agenesis refers to the absence or failure of large portions of the vagina to develop. Complete vaginal agenesis is rare, occurring in about 1 of 6000 live female births.[82] As an isolated defect, it results from incomplete caudal development and fusion of the lower part of the müllerian ducts (müllerian dysgenesis). The external genitalia usually appear normal, except for the introitus, where a short blind pouch may be present. The epithelium is highly glycogenated and normal in

TRANSVERSE VAGINAL SEPTUM

A transverse vaginal septum is uncommon,[68] occurring anywhere within the vagina (Figure 5.11). Some may be related to prenatal diethylstilbestrol exposure. A complete septum results in obstructive symptoms similar to an imperforate hymen, whereas a partial septum may allow passage of menstrual flow, but cause dyspareunia or laceration during childbirth. The microscopic appearance of the septum is typically that of a fibrovascular stroma covered on two surfaces by epithelium. The caudal surface is covered by a stratified squamous epithelium of urogenital origin, whereas the cranial aspect shows a glandular müllerian epithelium that has never transformed (Figure 5.12), as predicted from the arrested embryologic development.

MISCELLANEOUS CONGENITAL DISORDERS

Complete duplication of the vagina with a septum including muscularis extending to the introitus is rare,[38] and typically accompanies cervical and uterine duplication. Longitudinal septa that lack a muscular layer are more common. They often

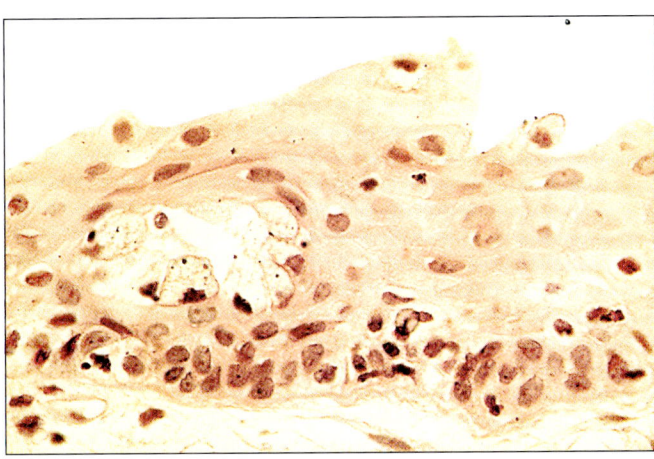

Fig. 5.12 Mucinous adenosis in transverse vaginal septum. Residual mucinous glands are embedded in metaplastic squamous epithelium on the cervical side of the transverse septum. This picture is also typical of any mucinous glands undergoing healing by the process of squamous metaplasia, whether congenital or not, or whether DES exposed or not.

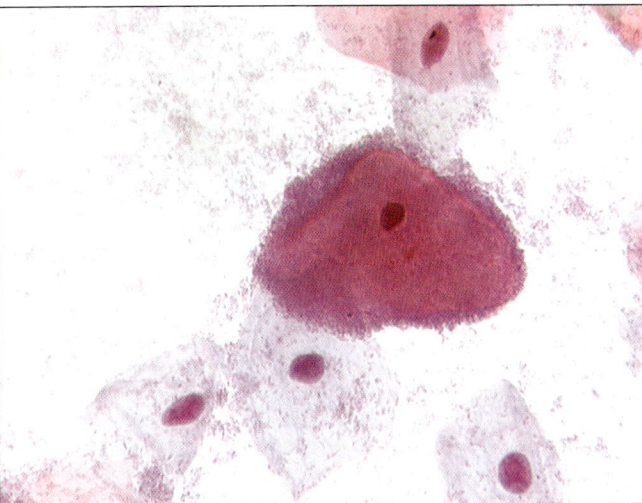

Fig. 5.13 Clue cell. Bacteria cover the cells.

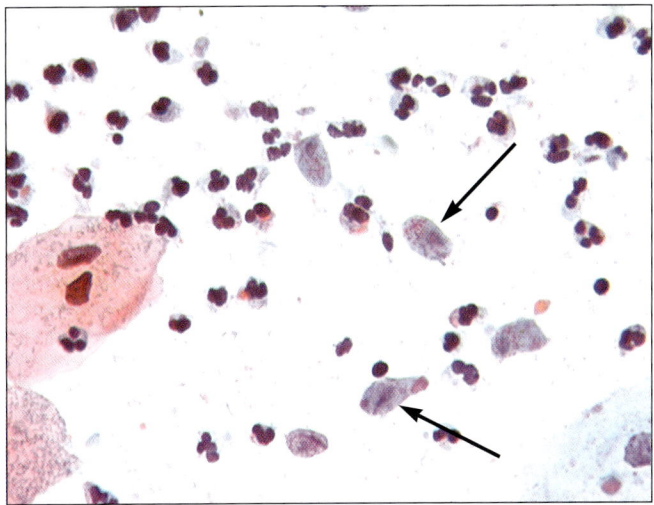

Fig. 5.14 *Trichomonas vaginalis*. The organisms appear as small bodies that stain blue and have elongated nuclei (arrows).

are clinically asymptomatic. Congenital rectovaginal fistulas are often associated with an imperforate anus. Typically, the anus opens into the posterior caudal portion of the vagina, near the fourchette.

INFLAMMATORY DISORDERS

VAGINITIS

'Vaginitis,' a generic term, refers to infection in the vagina from any cause, be it yeast, parasite, or bacterial. Vaginitis is one of the most common maladies in clinical medicine, and the reason most often cited for visits to the gynecologist. The three main categories of vaginitis are related to *Trichomonas vaginalis* infection, *Candida* vaginitis, and bacterial vaginosis.[63,130]

Bacterial vaginosis is the most common form of vaginitis, accounting for nearly 50% of all cases. The term, 'vaginosis', was introduced to indicate that, unlike the specific vaginitides, there is an increased discharge without significant inflammation, as indicated by a relative absence of polymorphonuclear leukocytes.[35] Overgrowth of facultative and anaerobic bacterial flora is the most frequent cause. This occurs most often when the pH of the vagina is no longer acid, as for example when semen is present or *Lactobacillus* species absent. *Gardnerella vaginalis*, a small Gram-variable bacillus, is responsible, at least in part, for many of the cases in women of reproductive age.[77] One study reported a crude odds ratio of nearly 75 when *G. vaginalis*, *Mycoplasma hominis*, and anaerobic bacteria were present in combination and *Lactobacillus* was absent, indicating that these organisms constitute the pathologic core of bacterial vaginosis and operate synergistically[138] in forming a biofilm.[135] The most important diagnostic finding is squamous cells covered with coccobacilli ('clue cells') (Figure 5.13).[139]

The most common cause of vaginitis throughout the reproductive period is *Trichomonas vaginalis*, a flagellate, ovoid protozoon.[9] In fresh, wet, microscopic preparations, the trichomonad is seen as a motile organism with several flagella; in dry,

fixed films it appears as a small, eosinophilic, shield-shaped object, with poorly defined cytoplasmic and nuclear outlines (Figure 5.14). Biopsies are unusual, but show a non-specific appearance of a chronic inflammatory infiltrate in the submucosa.[39] Scanning and transmission electron micrography show the organisms ingest erythrocytes, leukocytes, bacilli, and even vaginal epithelial cells.[104] The average disease is long lasting (3–5 years).[14] *Candida* infection, often as *C. albicans*, is found in a high proportion of women with vaginal discharge. It produces a characteristically cheesy discharge and its presence can be confirmed by culture and by its recognition in Papanicolaou-stained cervicovaginal smears (Figure 5.15).[32] In both conditions, a biopsy specimen is usually normal, because the organisms normally do not penetrate the mucosa nor elicit an inflammatory reaction. Both trichomoniasis and candidiasis may be very resistant to treatment, particularly if the male partner is not treated at the same time. Coital reinfection is very likely.

Actinomyces-like organisms are identified in the cervico-vaginal smears of a small percentage of women who have non-copper-containing intrauterine contraceptive devices in position (Figure 5.16). Although this finding may occasionally be associated with a real inflammatory process in the genital tract, it is probable that, in the great majority of cases, the organism is a commensal and its presence therefore is of no clinical significance.

Atrophic vaginitis, sometimes called 'senile vaginitis', occurs usually after the menopause. The lack of estrogenic stimulus to the epithelium results in a thin epithelium that is composed throughout its thickness by parabasal cells. This epithelium is much less resistant to infection than is the thick, well-estrogenized epithelium of a younger woman. The condition may present as postmenopausal bleeding; it responds well to treatment with estrogen.

Emphysematous vaginitis is a rare self-limiting disease in which multiple gas-filled cysts are present in the submucosa of the upper vagina and sometimes extending to the ectocervix.[123] It is associated with gas-forming organisms and is typically seen in pregnancy and the puerperium. Histologically, histiocytic giant cells line gas-filled cysts (Figure 5.17) and the sur-rounding vaginal wall discloses scattered and a rather inconspicuous inflammatory infiltrate, rendering a picture similar to colitis cystica profunda.

MALACOPLAKIA

Malacoplakia is an uncommon chronic granulomatous process that most commonly affects the urinary tract, but may also affect the vagina.[37,115] It results from defective macrophage function, manifesting as an inability to destroy ingested bacteria. Within a mass of polymorphonuclear leukocytes, lymphocytes, and plasma cells are histiocytes that contain small laminated bodies (Michaelis–Gutmann bodies) (Figure 5.18). These basophilic structures are nuclear-sized, sometimes with a bull's eye appearance, and contain stainable iron and calcium. Ultrastructurally, they are electron dense with a variable core of lysosome-like material. The macrophages also exhibit numerous secondary lysosomes that contain partially digested bacteria and neutrophils.

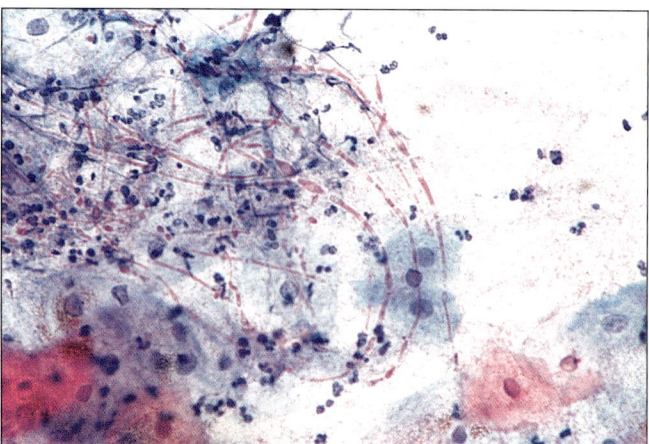

Fig. 5.15 *Candida* with pink-staining, spore-bearing hyphae.

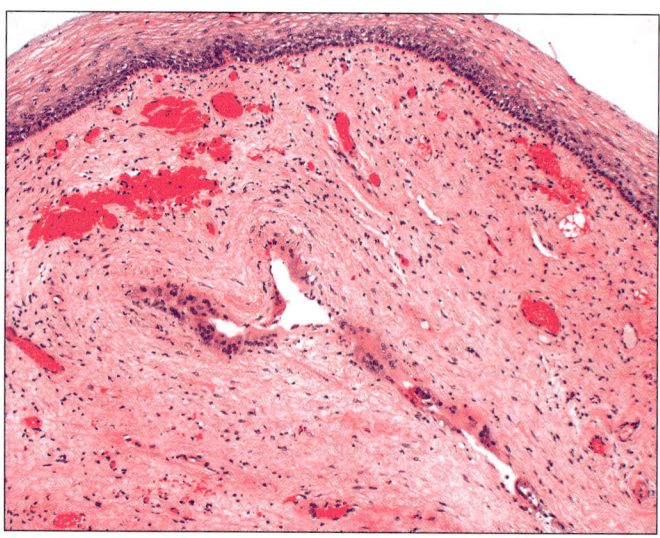

Fig. 5.17 Emphysematous vaginitis. Histiocytic giant cells line gas-filled cysts.

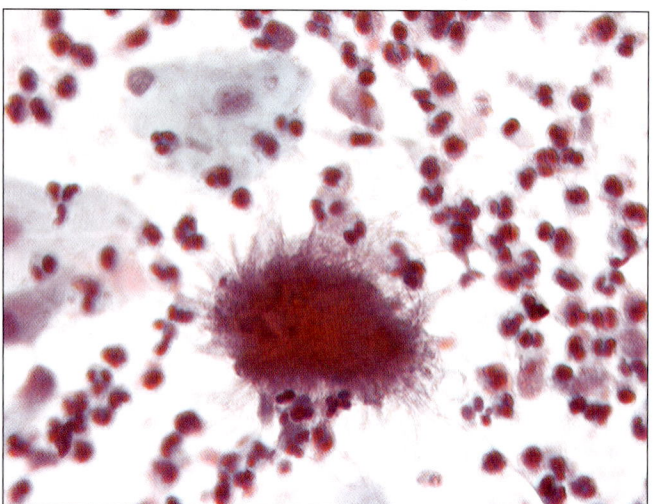

Fig. 5.16 *Actinomyces* with characteristic club-like projections.

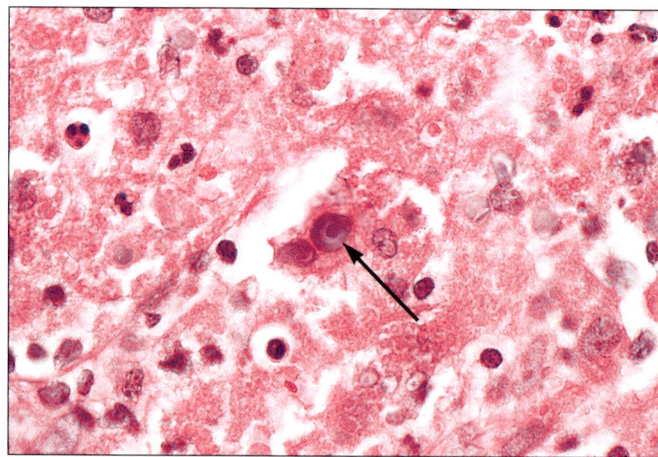

Fig. 5.18 Malacoplakia. Michaelis–Gutmann bodies (arrow).

TAMPON-RELATED LESIONS AND TOXIC SHOCK SYNDROME

Vaginal tampons may produce various lesions in the vaginal mucosa.[105] Some are grossly visible as shallow ulcers with smooth edges, but more subtle changes require colposcopy for their detection. Very early lesions appear as exfoliated small sheets of superficial squamous epithelial cells ('epithelial peeling'). Minute ulcers develop when this process reaches the underlying stroma. Tampon lesions are transient, and quickly disappear when tampon use is discontinued. Vaginal ulcerations in tampon users have been considered a portal of entry for *Staphylococcus aureus* and its toxic products in patients with toxic shock syndrome. Fever, a diffuse erythematous rash, and hypotension characterize the syndrome. It is caused by the release into the circulation of the staphylococcal toxin toxic shock syndrome toxin-1.[26] Although initially associated with tampon use, postoperative cases are being reported increasingly and the syndrome apparently may occur with any staphylococcal infection. Autopsy findings include perivasculitis, predominantly in the skin, lungs, kidneys, vagina, and other mucous membranes. The vaginal mucosa shows edema and ulceration in addition.

VAGINAL CYSTS

Vaginal cysts are uncommon and may be of paramesonephric, mesonephric, traumatic (squamous) or urogenital (usually Bartholins gland) origin. Most cysts are asymptomatic. Only when a cyst enlarges to more than 2–3 cm in diameter, usually due to infection or inspissated secretions, does the patient become aware of it. Cysts of the first two varieties are more commonly found in the upper part of the vagina. The latter two are usually encountered in the distal vagina. Except for traumatic cysts, which are usually squamous, most cysts have an embryologic basis.

Cysts derived from müllerian epithelium arise from patches of vaginal adenosis and are lined by tuboendometrial- or mucinous-type epithelia, sometimes with metaplastic squamous epithelium. They are seen most frequently in young women who were exposed prenatally to diethylstilbestrol (see below), but occur rarely in older women. Cysts of mesonephric (Gartners) duct origin are typically found in the lateral walls. Clinically apparent cysts are up to several centimeters in size, and occasionally may cause dyspareunia or other symptoms. Frequently, the mesonephric cyst has smooth muscle in its wall. The cells lining the cysts are cuboidal to columnar. The nuclei, which are large, pale, and have bland chromatin, often overlap. The cytoplasm is mucicarmine negative. Eosinophilic and mucicarmine-positive secretions are frequently present in the lumen. Occasionally, atrophic mesonephric ducts are found adjacent to the cysts, providing an additional clue to their origin.

Cysts lined by stratified squamous epithelium are nearly always traumatic inclusions of the normal vaginal mucosa (Figure 5.19). The cysts are usually single and have been reported in all areas of the vagina, although most are at the caudal end. Posterior cysts often result from epithelium trapped during episiotomy. The cause at other sites is less obvious, perhaps from trauma to the vagina during curettage. Urothelial cysts are uncommon and are lined by transitional epithe-

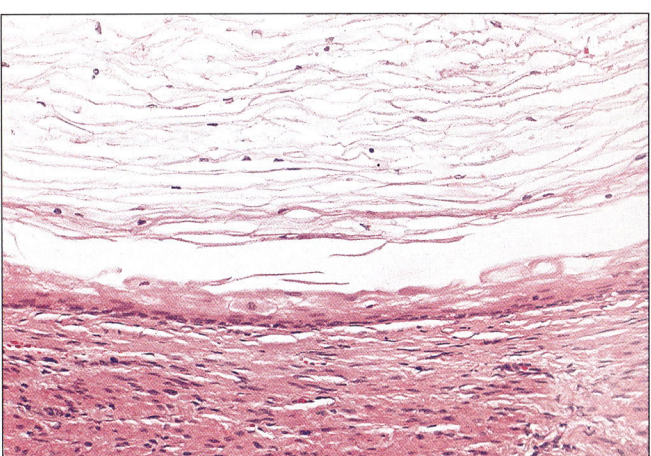

Fig. 5.19 Cyst lined by stratified squamous epithelium.

lium or a mixture of stratified columnar, stratified cuboidal, and columnar epithelium. As these cysts are derived from the urogenital sinus, they are usually situated low in the vagina, close to the urethra.

Rarely, cysts in the upper vagina are inflammatory in nature (see emphysematous vaginitis above). We have seen isolated examples of inflammatory pseudocysts of rectal origin presenting as posterior vaginal wall cysts – a trap more for the clinician than for the pathologist.

CYSTS OF THE INTROITUS

Bartholin duct cysts and mucinous cysts of vulvar origin are often misinterpreted as being of vaginal origin. Bartholin duct cysts, which are common, are recognized by ducts lined by transitional epithelium adjacent to arborized acini lined by mucin-rich cells. The occasional presence of ciliated cells in some Bartholin cysts has been responsible for a misdiagnosis of vaginal adenosis, and hence the erroneous impression that the patient has been exposed prenatally to diethylstilbestrol. Mucinous cysts (also sometimes referred to as mucous or dysontogenetic cysts) of the vulvar vestibule likely arise from mucinous glands that are normally present in this site.

BENIGN EFFECTS OF DIETHYLSTILBESTROL ON THE VAGINA

Diethylstilbestrol (DES), a synthetic, non-steroidal estrogen first synthesized in 1937 and by the mid 1940s and 1950s promoted for the treatment of habitual abortion and threatened abortion, profoundly affects the development of the vagina, and indeed the genital tract. The pathology associated with the *in utero* exposure of this class of drugs has led to many insights into embryology, anatomy, physiology, and neoplasia, and their interrelations. In 1971 its use became linked to the extremely rare development of clear cell adenocarcinoma in the vagina and cervix of offspring exposed *in utero*. By that time, estimates suggest that upwards of 3 million daughters had been so exposed.[54,97]

A variety of non-neoplastic as well as neoplastic changes occur in DES-exposed offspring. Deformities found in the upper reproductive tract include a T-shaped uterine cavity, constrictions of the uterine cavity, and hypoplasia of the uterine cavity and uterine corpus.[62] Approximately one-fifth of exposed women demonstrate gross structural changes in the cervix or vagina.[3,59] Descriptive designations include coxcomb (hood) (Figure 5.20), collar (rim), pseudopolyp (Figures 5.20 and 5.21), and ridge (Figure 5.11). The coxcomb is a protuberant ridge of tissue, usually on the anterior lip of the cervix, which is covered by squamous epithelium and contains cervical stroma. The collar is a low constricting band about a portion of the cervix. The pseudopolyp appears as a polyp due to the presence of a circumferential constricting groove, but in fact is a portion of cervix in which there is a central endocervical canal. Gross abnormalities are less common in the vagina than in the cervix. The most common is a transverse partial vaginal septum, which may make examination of the cervix by the naked eye and by colposcopy very difficult or impossible. These conditions also occur in approximately 2–4% of women who have no prenatal drug history. Over time, many structural changes disappear as the cervix remodels with age. As many as two-thirds disappear after pregnancy.[59]

VAGINAL ADENOSIS

Most women exposed prenatally to DES have some form of microscopic change in the inner half of exocervix; a substantial percentage also have changes in the vagina. The presence of glandular tissue in the vagina is called 'adenosis'. Squamous metaplasia, which when present in the vagina together with adenosis, collectively is designated 'vaginal epithelial changes'. From a mechanistic viewpoint, the metaplastic squamous epithelium represents the normal healing process by which adenosis transforms and heals. Ultimately the vaginal epithelial changes, when completely healed, appear as normal squamous epithelium.

Adenosis, in its adult microscopic form, should be suspected clinically when the vaginal mucosa contains red granular spots or patches (Figure 5.22) and fails to stain with an iodine solution (Figure 5.23). On colposcopy, adenosis appears as glandular or metaplastic epithelium that has replaced the native squamous epithelium of the vaginal mucosa. Usually, adenosis is asymptomatic, although some women have vaginal discharge or postcoital bleeding.

Adenosis, with or without squamous metaplasia, involves the upper third of the vagina in 34% of DES-exposed women. The anterior wall is involved more frequently than the posterior wall. These changes extend into the middle third of the vagina in 9% and the lower third in 2% of exposed women. In unexposed women, adenosis of the adult type is rare, but when present, is identical to that which occurs in exposed women.[109,127] An embryonic form of adenosis is also encountered on occasion;[107] it occurs naturally in tiny foci and has been found during late fetal life and childhood, and even in adults.

There are two adult (or differentiated) forms of adenosis – mucinous and tuboendometrial. Mucinous columnar cells, which by light and electron microscopy resemble those of the normal endocervical mucosa (Figures 5.12 and 5.24), comprise

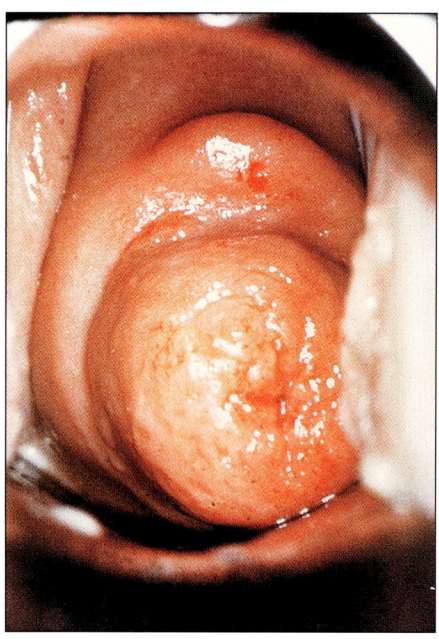

Fig. 5.20 DES-associated cervical abnormalities. A coxcomb (upper) and pseudopolyp (middle) are present.

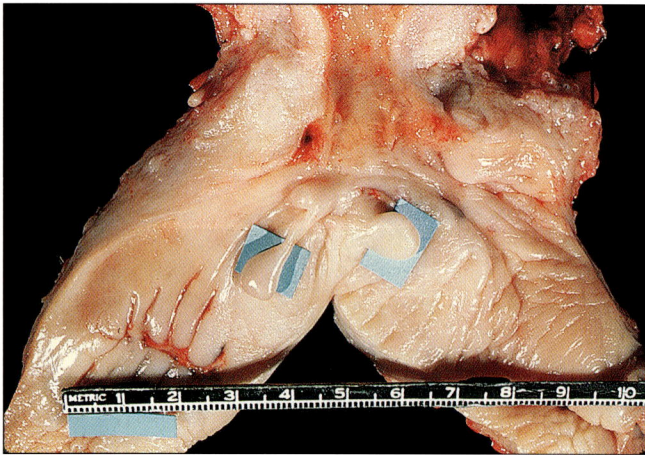

Fig. 5.21 DES-associated cervical abnormalities. The entire remains of the upper vagina and exocervix appear as several tiny tags. The cervix is hypoplastic and the fornices are obliterated.

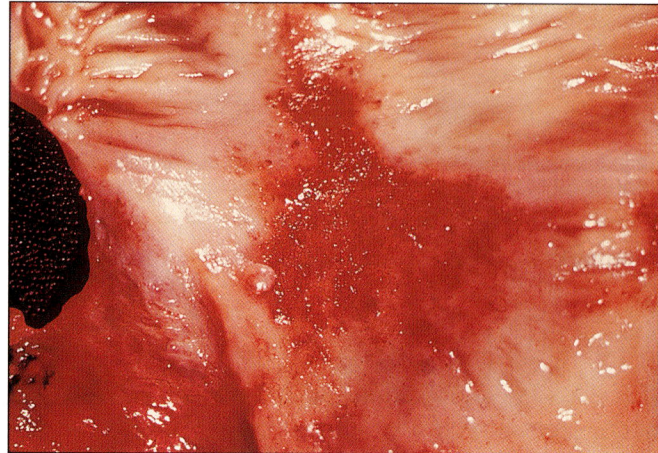

Fig. 5.22 Vaginal adenosis.

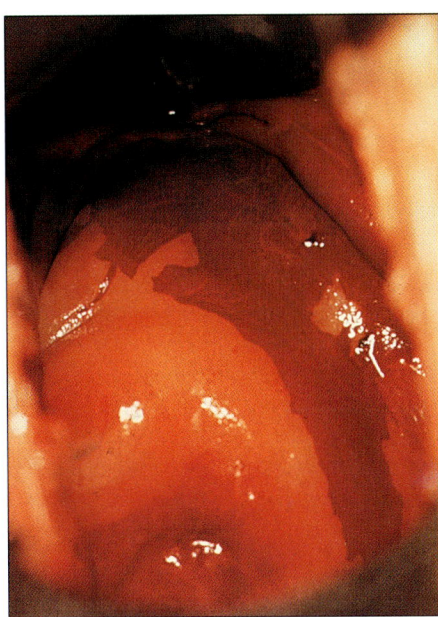

Fig. 5.23 Iodine stain of the lower genital tract. Both the cervix and portions of the vagina fail to take up the stain, indicative of a lack of glycogenated squamous epithelium.

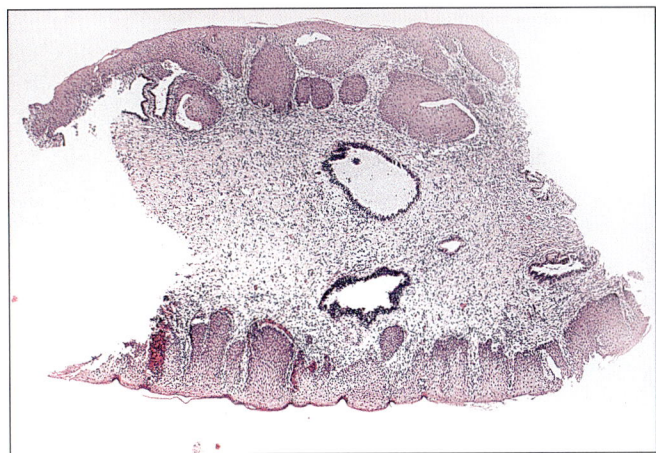

Fig. 5.25 Adenosis, tuboendometrial type.

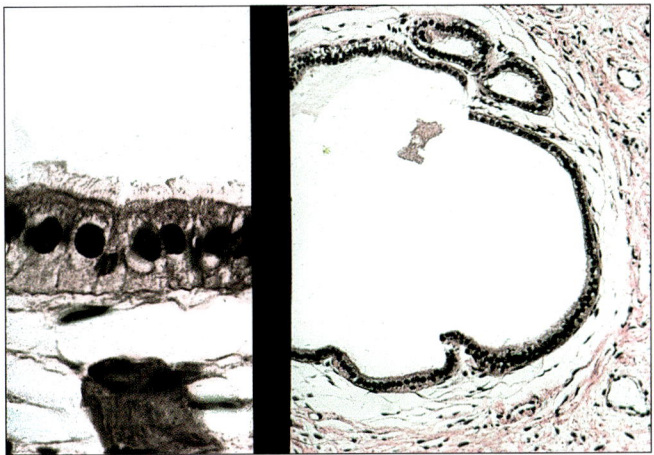

Fig. 5.26 Adenosis, tuboendometrial type. Detail of ciliated serous-type cells.

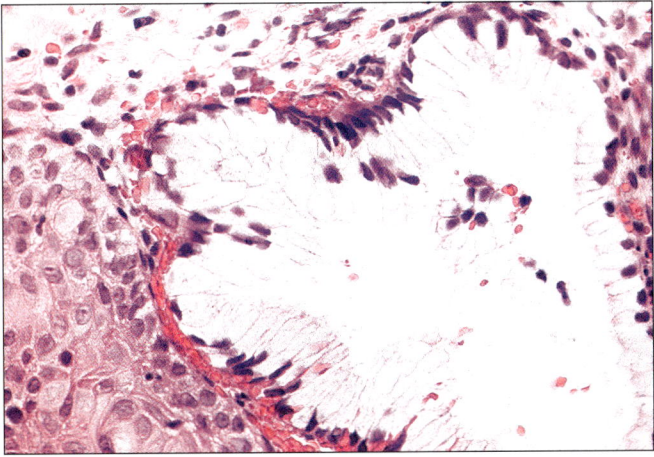

Fig. 5.24 Adenosis, mucinous type.

the glandular epithelium most frequently encountered in adenosis (62% of biopsy specimens with vaginal adenosis). As this epithelium frequently lines the surface of the vagina, it is the type of glandular epithelium most commonly seen by colposcopy, and seemingly the type also found lining the exocervix and upper vagina in stillbirths exposed *in utero* to DES. Commonly, the mucinous columnar cells also line glands within the lamina propria itself.

Tuboendometrial cells, which are often ciliated and resemble the cells lining the fallopian tube and endometrium (Figures 5.25 and 5.26), are found in 21% of specimens with adenosis. These cells are usually found in glands in the lamina propria and not on the surface of the vagina. Although adenosis is uncommon in the middle vagina and even more rare in the lower vagina, the percentage of biopsy specimens with adenosis that exhibit tuboendometrial cells in comparison to mucinous

cells increases proportionally. Mucinous and tuboendometrial cells are found together only occasionally in biopsy material.

The third type of cell found in adenosis is embryonic, i.e. a fetal form of adenosis (Figure 5.27). It is the putative precursor from which the adult form of adenosis develops postpubertally. It is this form of adenosis that is found in up to 15% of fetuses and stillbirths and occasionally in the vagina of adult women regardless of DES history,[109] and finally experimentally in human embryonic vagina grown in an athymic mouse host in a DES milieu.[108]

In most biopsy specimens, metaplastic squamous cells are found replacing adenosis to some degree, indicating the manner by which adenosis regresses. Squamous metaplasia is a normal reactive and physiologic process that occurs at one time or another in all women regardless of whether or not there was a history of prenatal exposure. It is believed to be the process by which the body heals itself of the presence of glandular tissue anywhere on the ectocervix or in the vagina (adenosis). It is unclear whether the metaplastic epithelium in a DES-exposed child is more (or less) susceptible to other disease processes than a truly uninvolved vaginal epithelium.

Remnants of columnar cells, which may be surrounded by metaplastic squamous cells or as intracellular droplets of mucin in metaplastic squamous cells, constitute the evidence for

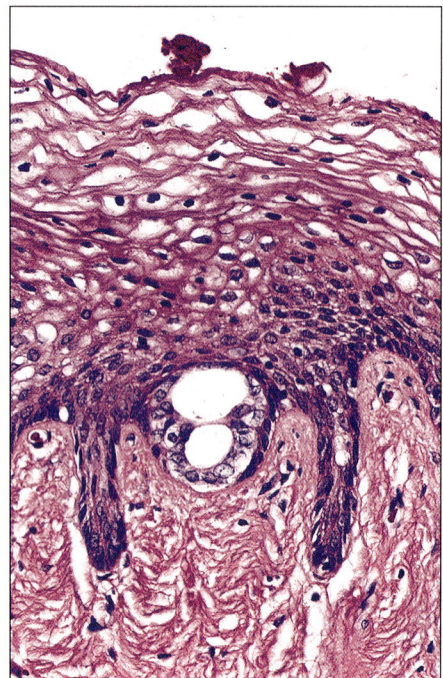

Fig. 5.27   Adenosis, fetal (embryonic) type.

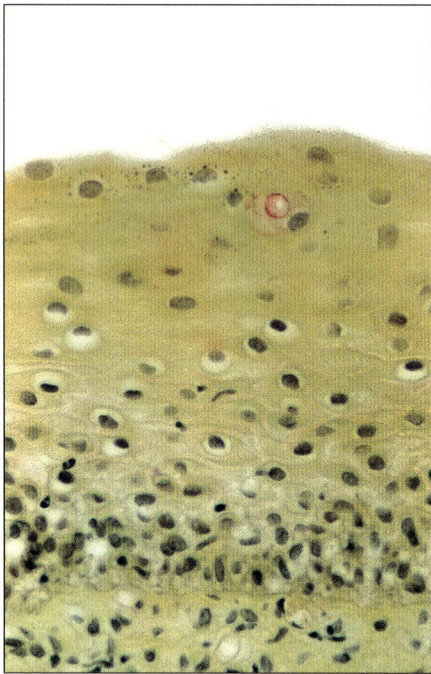

Fig. 5.28   Adenosis, intracellular droplet of mucin.

cally, the reparative process manifests as increased relative proportions of metaplastic squamous cells to mucinous columnar cells.

DES-exposed women often have abnormal colposcopic findings, i.e. mosaicism and punctation, which are often misinterpreted clinically as dysplasia. The paucity or total lack of glycogen in the early stages of squamous metaplasia accounts for the failure of the epithelium to stain with iodine. The increased vascularity, the slightly tortuous arrangement of the vessels surrounding the pegs in the lamina propria, the chronic inflammatory infiltrate, and the tile-like patterns are responsible for the atypical colposcopic motifs.[91] Hyperkeratosis accounts for the colposcopic findings of leukoplakia. Eventual maturation of the metaplastic squamous epithelium with acquisition of glycogen makes it indistinguishable from the normal (native) squamous epithelium.

Vaginal adenosis must be distinguished in a biopsy from endometriosis, which is also uncommon in the vagina. Apart from the presence of endometrial stroma, which should be considered diagnostic but is often not convincingly demonstrable, the glands of endometriosis much more closely resemble those of normal endometrium than do those of adenosis. This difference is at its most obvious during the secretory phase of the cycle. The issue may be clouded, however, by the presence of an inflammatory infiltrate around the glands of adenosis, a feature easily mistaken for endometrial stroma. Another useful point in the differential diagnosis is if the glandular epithelium contains any mucinous component. This is virtually never seen in endometriosis.

The mechanisms that operate to induce the changes seen in DES-exposed progeny may be explained in part by the changes that occur normally in the embryologic development of the lower genital tract. Both the müllerian ducts and the urogenital sinus are believed to be required for the normal vagina to develop. The primitive uterovaginal canal that is formed early in embryonic life has a muscular wall lined by columnar (müllerian) epithelium. At about week 10 of gestation, the normal transitional squamous epithelium that lines the urogenital sinus grows upwards into the vagina to replace the embryonic columnar (müllerian) epithelium. The squamous epithelium grows to extend as far as what becomes the external cervical os. If the process arrests before the external os is reached, then that area where replacement has not occurred, i.e. usually the upper vagina, retains its original columnar (müllerian) lining. This explains in part what happens as vaginal adenosis develops, although it does not explain why glandular epithelium in some cases lies only in the submucosa and not on the surface. This, possibly, may be answered by another observation. In serial sections of the normal cervix, a layer of tuboendometrial-type cells are often present deep to the normal mucinous endocervix. This same layer may persist in the DES-exposed individual and extend into the vagina.

TUMOR-LIKE CONDITIONS

FIBROEPITHELIAL POLYPS

Vaginal fibroepithelial polyps are benign growths that likely arise from a stromal layer of hormone-sensitive fibroblastic or myofibroblastic cells. Cells with a similar histologic appearance

adenosis in 48% of biopsy specimens with adenosis. Squamous metaplasia begins as reserve cell proliferation, and then progresses through immature to mature stages. The glandular epithelium gradually disappears (Figure 5.12) and intercellular pools of mucin and intracellular droplets (Figure 5.28) remain as the final vestiges of adenosis. When completely replaced by squamous epithelium, obliterated glands appear in the lamina propria as squamous pegs that are continuous with the metaplastic squamous epithelium covering the surface. Cytologi-

have been described in a band-like subepithelial–stromal zone extending from the endocervix to the vulva of normal females, and may represent the origin of these atypical cells. They commonly develop in the lower vagina of women who are pregnant or on hormone therapy,[94,99] thus implicating hormonal stimulation as a causative factor. A rare example has developed in a newborn.[21] Grossly, the polyps are single and solid (Figure 5.29), but occasionally villiform with finger-like projections (Figure 5.30), rubbery, and up to 3 cm in size. Their surface is smooth and covered by squamous epithelium. The stroma, which is composed of loose fibroconnective tissue, may contain large atypical stromal cells with delicate, pointed cytoplasmic processes, hyperchromatic, pleomorphic, irregular nuclei, and occasionally prominent nucleoli (Figures 5.31 and 5.32). Mitotic figures are uncommon, but do occur, even with atypical forms. The cells frequently express vimentin, desmin, and receptors for estrogen and progesterone.[45] In the absence of cross-striations, the stromal cells should not be called rhabdomyomatous cells. Ultrastructurally, the stromal cells resemble both fibroblasts and myofibroblasts. Fibroepithelial polyps, which are effectively treated with simple excision, should not be mistaken for a malignant growth, especially embryonal rhabdomyosarcoma, which has a cambium layer, hypercellular stroma, and strap cells, often with cross-striations. Also, the embryonal rhabdomyosarcoma usually occurs in children under the age of 4 years. The fibroepithelial polyp has sometimes been called pseudosarcoma botryoides because of the bizarre stromal cells and its potential for confusion with embryonal rhabdomyosarcoma.

PROLAPSED FALLOPIAN TUBE

Prolapse of the fallopian tube into the vagina occurs in about 0.25% of patients following vaginal hysterectomy.[27] On clinical examination, a nodule simulating granulation tissue is typically visible at the vaginal apex usually within a few weeks of the operation, but sometimes not for months later, and is usually not recognized clinically prior to biopsy. Biopsy shows glandular epithelium, often with a villous pattern suggestive of tubal

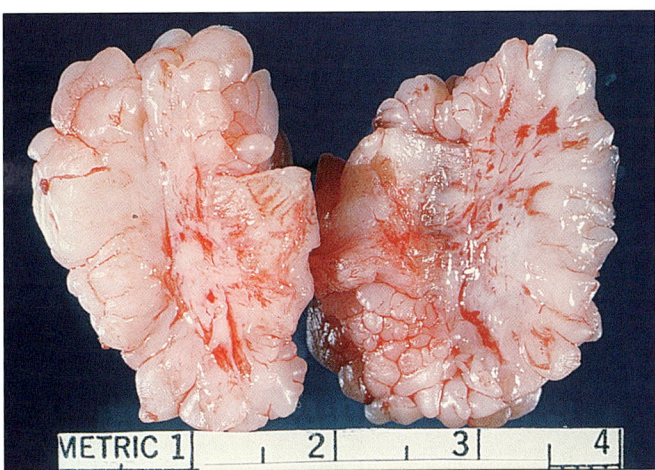

Fig. 5.29 Fibroepithelial polyp, solid.

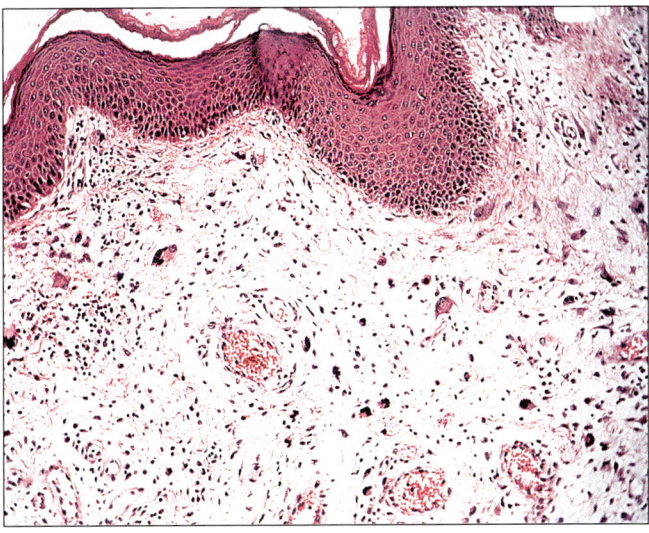

Fig. 5.31 Fibroepithelial polyp. Large atypical stromal cells with delicate, pointed cytoplasmic processes are conspicuous.

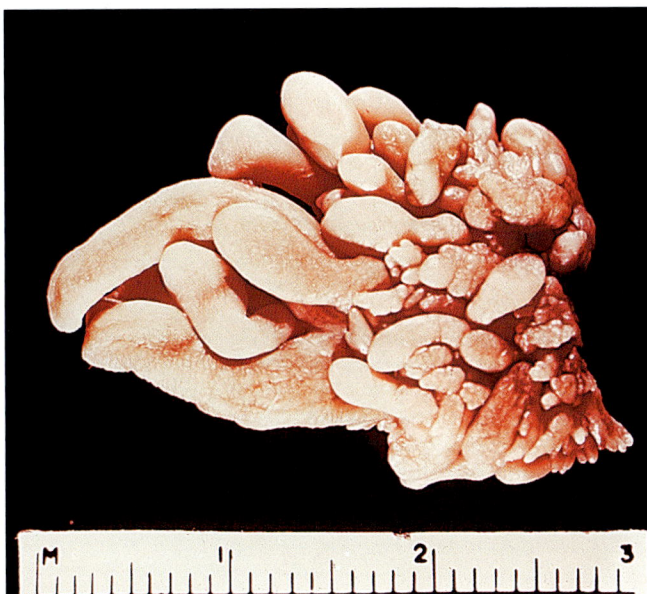

Fig. 5.30 Fibroepithelial polyp, villiform. The tumor has numerous finger-like projections.

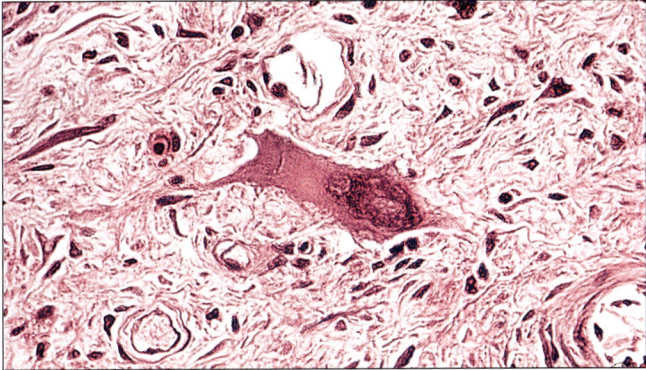

Fig. 5.32 Fibroepithelial polyp. Detail of large atypical stromal cells with delicate, pointed cytoplasmic processes.

plicae, with an intense inflammatory cell infiltrate (Figure 5.33). Nuclear crowding and stratification are common, but ciliated or secretory columnar cells may be difficult to identify. The presence of smooth muscle organized as tubal muscularis sometimes aids in the correct diagnosis. Prolapsed fallopian tube may masquerade as a simple vault granulation tissue polyp or as adenocarcinoma, a diagnosis suggested by the architecturally abnormal tubal plicae, reactive stroma, and inflammatory cytologic atypia. Florid reactive stromal proliferations arising at the stoma may also masquerade as a vaginal mesenchymal neoplasm.[79] Anecdotally, it is a rare cause of ectopic pregnancy following hysterectomy[17] and of true glandular cells in a posthysterectomy vaginal vault Papanicolaou smear.

GRANULATION TISSUE NODULE

Nodules of granulation tissue in the vaginal vault commonly develop following total abdominal hysterectomy. Nearly one-sixth of women will develop nodules over 5 mm in size, one-fifth of which are symptomatic.[117] Grossly, the nodules are red, soft, and sometimes friable. Microscopically, they are composed of usually quite immature granulation tissue with extensive numbers of plasma cells. Only about two-thirds of the nodules disappear spontaneously. These lesions are biopsied most often to exclude implanted malignancies, the most common being adenocarcinoma of the endometrium.

POSTOPERATIVE SPINDLE CELL NODULE

Spindle cell nodules resembling sarcomas develop occasionally in the genitourinary tract after surgical procedures.[41,102] Clinically, the polypoid nodules, which may be several centimeters in greatest dimension and bleed easily, have been found in or about operative sites in the vagina, endocervix, endometrium, prostate, and bladder. Microscopically, they are highly cellular and composed of an unusual proliferation of spindle cells, identified as myofibroblasts. The spindle cells have oval, elongated nuclei with evenly dispersed chromatin and abundant eosinophilic cytoplasm. The vascularity may be pronounced, disclosing a delicate network of small blood vessels, sometimes

accompanied by extravasated blood or hemosiderin (Figure 5.34). Although the mitotic rate is often high, abnormal mitoses and cytologic atypia are absent, features facilitating its differentiation from a spindle cell sarcoma, such as leiomyosarcoma. Negative immunostaining for cytokeratins also distinguishes these lesions from the rare spindle cell squamous cell carcinomas of the cervix or vagina. Local recurrence has not been reported, even after incomplete resection.

MICROGLANDULAR HYPERPLASIA

Microglandular hyperplasia, a condition defined by the presence of microglands lacking intervening stroma, is a benign condition found on occasion in the cervix. Usually associated with the use of oral contraceptives or occasionally with pregnancy, it is rarely observed in their absence. It is extremely rare in the vagina, arising in foci of the mucinous form of vaginal adenosis. Almost all of these young women were both exposed to DES *in utero* and, at the time the lesion developed, were pregnant or using oral contraceptives. Grossly, the lesion is soft, granular, tan-yellow, and usually flat. Occasionally, it may be cauliflower-like and multicentric (Figure 5.35). Micro-

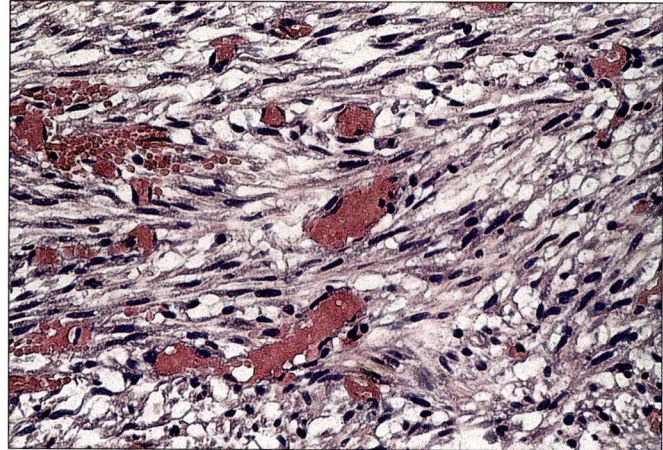

Fig. 5.34 Postoperative spindle cell nodule.

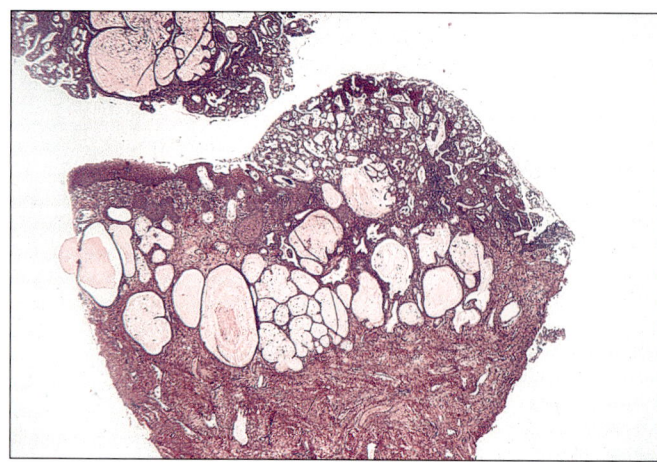

Fig. 5.35 Microglandular hyperplasia of vagina. The nodule of microglandular hyperplasia (top) has arisen on a background of mucinous adenosis (larger cysts beneath).

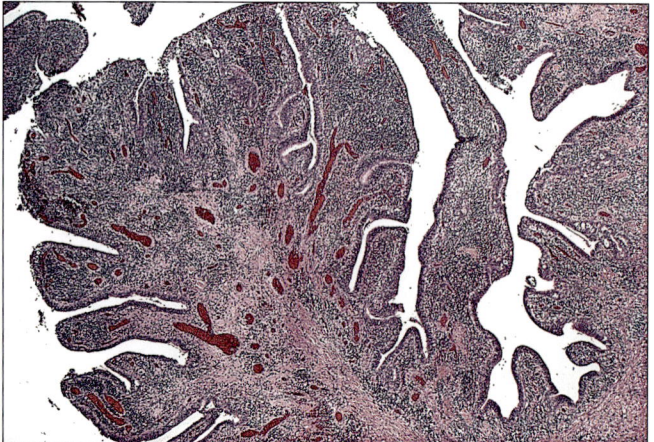

Fig. 5.33 Prolapsed fallopian tube into vagina.

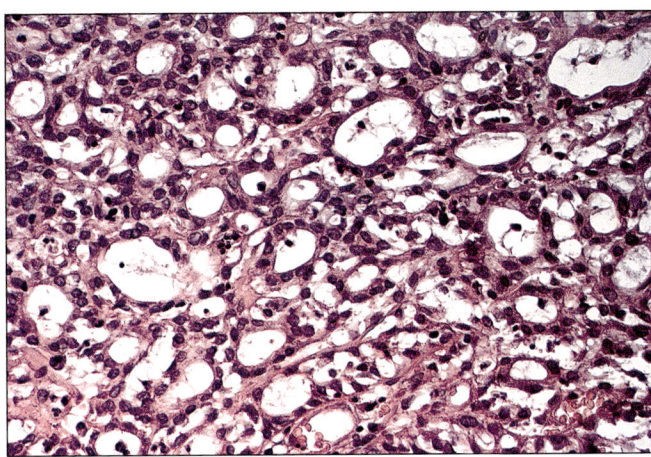

Fig. 5.36 Microglandular hyperplasia of vagina. The closely packed glands lack intervening stroma.

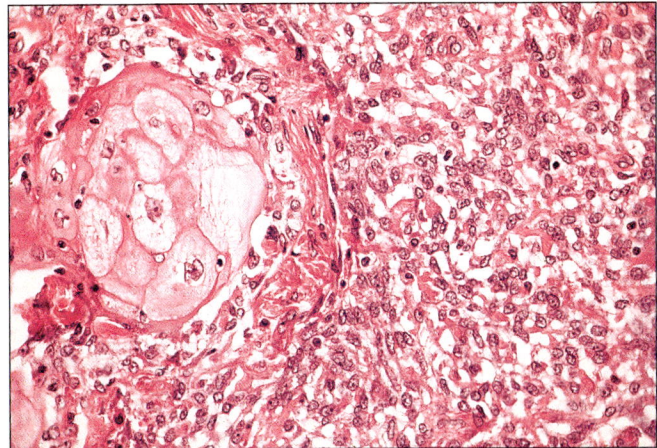

Fig. 5.37 Benign mixed tumor.

scopic examination demonstrates many small, closely packed microglands devoid of intervening stroma (Figure 5.36).

The presence of extensive nests of metaplastic squamous cells with pale eosinophilic cytoplasm may make the lesion difficult to distinguish from the solid pattern of clear cell adenocarcinoma. A clue to the diagnosis is the presence of clefts lined by mucinous epithelium that course through the metaplastic squamous epithelium. That the microglands are continuous with the clefts suggests that the microglands result from budding and arborization of the mucinous epithelium. Microglandular hyperplasia has not been shown to arise from the tuboendometrial type of adenosis. The lesion generally regresses when administration of the oral contraceptive is discontinued. Microglandular hyperplasia can be mistaken for adenocarcinoma. Microglandular hyperplasia with extensive squamous metaplasia is easily mistaken for clear cell adenocarcinoma.

ENDOMETRIOSIS

Endometriosis is rare in the vaginal wall or squamous mucosa,[103] although less rare in the deep pelvic tissues of the rectovaginal septum (see Chapter 20).

BENIGN TUMORS

Benign epithelial tumors of the vagina are uncommon. It is debatable whether genuine benign squamous papillomas, as distinct from the virus-induced condyloma acuminatum, really exist.

BENIGN MIXED TUMOR

The benign mixed tumor, a rare lesion, is composed of biphasic stromal and epithelial components. The neoplasm usually presents as a painless, slowly growing mass up to 5 cm in diameter, most frequently near the hymen. The origin is uncertain, but the immunoprofile (reactivity of the stromal component with CD10, bcl-2, and estrogen and progesterone receptors) favors

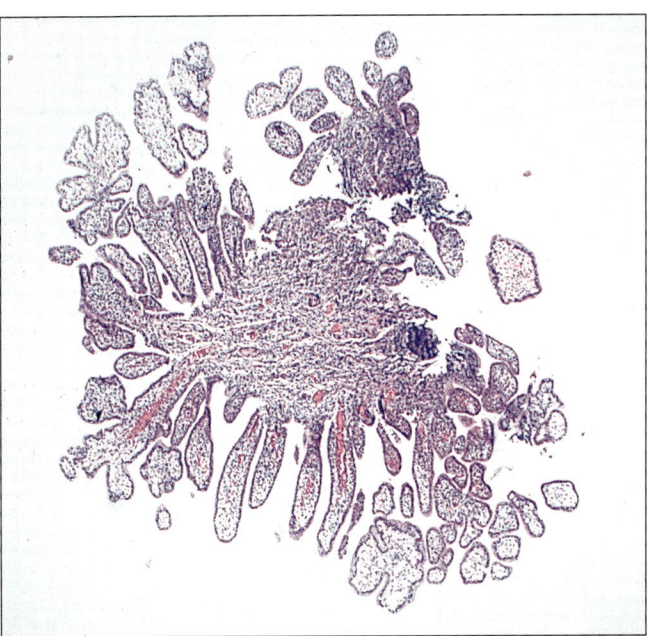

Fig. 5.38 Müllerian papilloma of infancy.

a müllerian rather than a urothelial origin.[85] The mean age at diagnosis is 30 years. The tumors are well circumscribed but non-encapsulated within the submucosa, and often are misdiagnosed preoperatively as a polyp or cyst. Microscopically, the epithelial component appears as small, but striking, nests of highly glycogenated, bland squamous cells (Figure 5.37). Glands are sometimes present. The spindle cells are sometimes arranged in loosely intersecting fascicles. In addition to reactivity with vimentin, they are sometimes reactive with cytokeratin, and show tonofilaments and desmosomes, consistent with epithelial differentiation.[16] Only a rare recurrence has been reported.[152]

MÜLLERIAN PAPILLOMA

The müllerian papilloma is a rare tumor composed of a complex arborizing fibrovascular core (Figure 5.38) lined by a mantle of bland glandular epithelium one to two cells thick (Figure 5.39). It occurs in the upper vagina of infants and young children. It has a polypoid appearance, and should not be confused with the embryonal rhabdomyosarcoma in which embryonal rhabdomyoblasts are present in the stroma. Almost all are benign, although rare local recurrences have been reported, and a solitary case after many recurrences progressed to malignancy.[1]

LEIOMYOMA

Of the mesenchymal tumors, benign smooth muscle tumors are the most common and most pedestrian. Leiomyoma, which occurs most commonly in women about 40 years of age but has a wide range, has an average size of 3 cm (range <1–15 cm in diameter). Small tumors are usually asymptomatic, whereas the larger tumors may produce pain, hemorrhage, dystocia or dyspareunia. Nearly all are well circumscribed and are treated by local excision.[114,116] An occasional tumor, especially if large, may recur.[29] The same criteria for malignancy are applied as for smooth muscle tumors elsewhere in the female genital tract. Tumors with 5 or more mitoses per 10 HPFs, especially if atypia is present, should be considered malignant. Those having between 1 and 4 mitoses per 10 HPFs are best considered potentially malignant. Leiomyomas have been reported to appear during pregnancy where there has been increased mitotic activity, minimal atypia, and an absence of aggressive behavior. Rare cases of bizarre leiomyoma have also been reported.[11]

RHABDOMYOMA

A rare, but interesting tumor is the genital rhabdomyoma, a benign neoplasm that displays a high degree of skeletal muscle differentiation and which has a predilection for the vagina. The average age at diagnosis is about 42 years (range 25–55 years).[58] The tumor presents as a solitary, polypoid to nodular mass resembling a polyp, usually less than 3 cm in diameter, although some reach 11 cm across. The overlying squamous mucosa is usually intact since the tumor arises from the wall. The texture is rubbery, and the tumor has a gray, glassy cut surface. Microscopy discloses bland, interlacing, broad strap-like or round

striated muscle cells with abundant eosinophilic cytoplasm with distinct cross-striations (Figure 5.40). Although arranged rather haphazardly and showing variation in size and shape, the cells are easily recognizable as benign, differentiated striated muscle of fetal and adult types with an immunoprofile including muscle specific actin, myoglobin, and desmin, but not smooth muscle actin. Mitoses are absent. The background connective tissue framework is a loose, collagenous to myxoid stroma with fibroblasts, and mast cells. Recurrence has not been reported following wide local excision. The differential diagnoses are embryonal rhabdomyosarcoma, which occurs in the very young, and both carcinosarcoma (malignant mixed müllerian tumor) and metastatic tumors, which occur in older women.[147]

ANGIOMYOFIBROBLASTOMA

Angiomyofibroblastoma of the vagina is a well-circumscribed myofibroblastic neoplasm that is composed of ovoid-to-round myoid tumor cells with scattered multinucleated cells (Figure 5.41). It is a distinctive benign tumor that has a diverse histo-

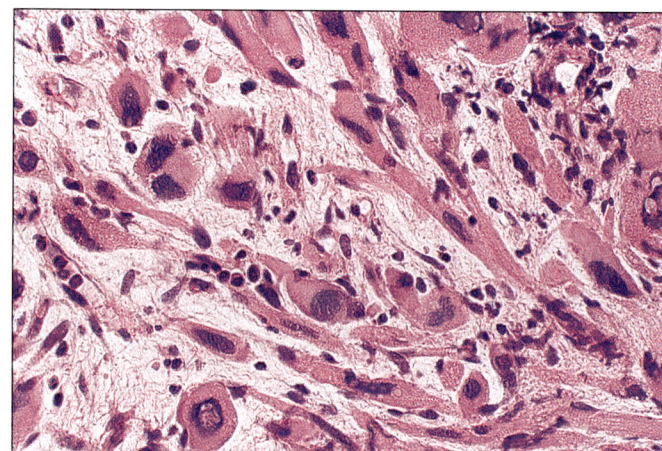

Fig. 5.40 Rhabdomyoma.

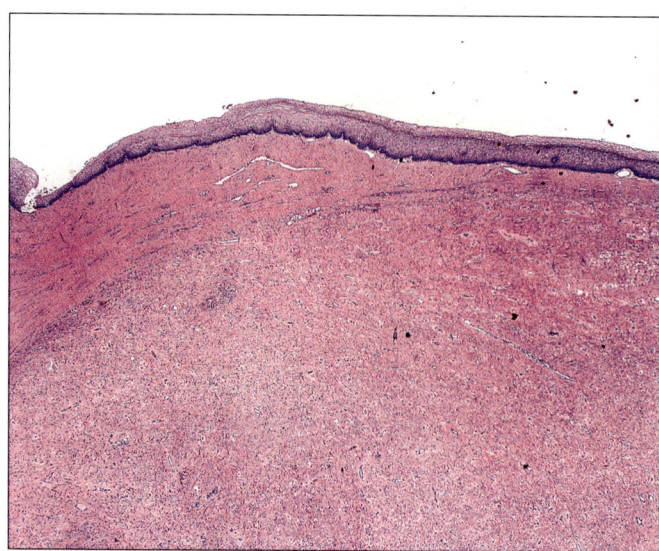

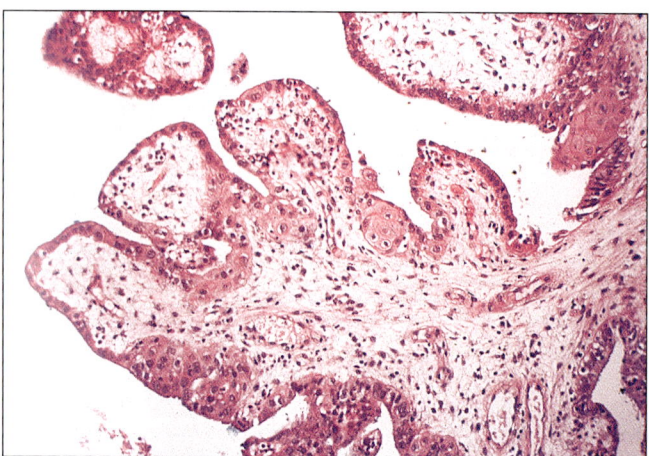

Fig. 5.39 Müllerian papilloma of infancy.

Fig. 5.41 Vaginal angiomyofibroblastoma with circumscribed borders.

logic and immunohistochemical profile. The patients are 23–71 years of age (mean 46 years). The average tumor size is 7 cm.[92] Microscopically, the neoplastic cells are spindle-shaped, plasmacytoid or epithelioid (Figure 5.42). There is minimal nuclear atypia and no more than a rare mitosis. The tumors contain small- to medium-sized blood vessels, which are thin walled, and, occasionally, ectatic and branching. Almost all are immunoreactive for vimentin and desmin, and some for smooth muscle actin (Figure 5.43) and CD34. None have recurred. This tumor forms a continuous morphologic spectrum with the clinically more aggressive angiomyxoma (see Chapter 4).[75,76]

MISCELLANEOUS BENIGN TUMORS

Several benign tumors – such as Brenner tumor,[8] paraganglioma,[46] schwannoma,[137] benign mesenchymoma,[72] and mature cystic teratoma dermoid cyst[128] – have been described with gross and microscopic findings similar to those occurring elsewhere.

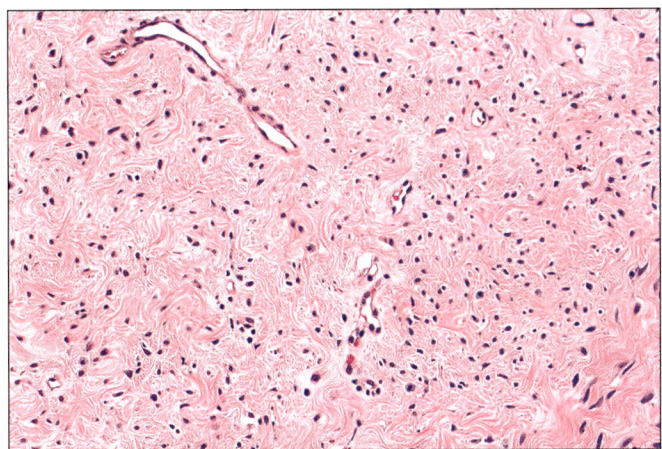

Fig. 5.42 Vaginal angiomyofibroblastoma with circumscribed borders.

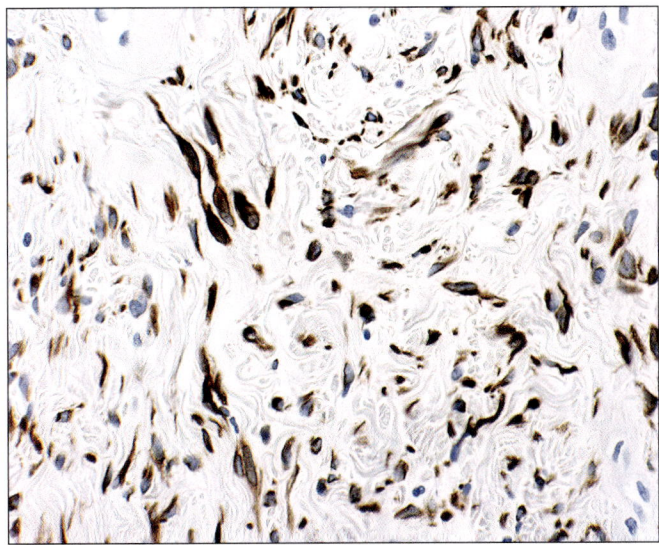

Fig. 5.43 Vaginal angiomyofibroblastoma (desmin).

SQUAMOUS NEOPLASIA

HUMAN PAPILLOMAVIRUS (HPV) INFECTION

The vaginal mucosa is frequently the site of genital papillomavirus infections, hosting approximately one-fourth of genital condylomata. The lesions may be flat, slightly raised, or verrucous with stromal papillae (asperities). While frequently small and virtually invisible without colposcopic visualization, they usually become more easily identified following application of 3% acetic acid.[51] Biopsy usually discloses cells with a characteristic perinuclear halo (koilocyte). Condylomata acuminata are predominantly HPV 6 or 11 positive[6] and they are self-limiting. Premalignant changes, which often occur, are reflected by greater degrees of cytologic atypia.[129] HPV DNA can be found in about 60% of these lesions, usually in the form of type 16. In one study of 71 patients with premalignant changes, 15 different HPV DNA types were found (HPV 16, 18, 30, 31, 35, 40, 42, 43, 51, 52, 53, 54, 56, 58 and 66).[134]

VAGINAL INTRAEPITHELIAL NEOPLASIA (VaIN)

Definition
VaIN, encompassing related terms such as dysplasia and carcinoma *in situ*, is a premalignant lesion and a forerunner of squamous cell carcinoma of the vagina.

Clinical features
VaIN is far less frequently encountered than the analogous precancerous changes in the cervix. It gives rise, however, to nearly one-fourth of all vaginal malignancies.[23] The annual incidence of VaIN 3 (see below) is 0.3/100 000 women, which compares to 38/100 000 for cervical intraepithelial neoplasia (CIN 3) and 1/100 000 for vulvar intraepithelial neoplasia (VIN 3). The ages of women with VaIN range widely, with a mean of 50 years.[5]

VaIN occurs most frequently in association with CIN, either in continuity with it or, more usually, in the vaginal vault after hysterectomy for CIN, when the line of excision has been insufficiently wide to remove an unsuspected vaginal extension of the CIN. Less frequently, VaIN may be found in the vagina at a site distant from the cervix, which may itself be entirely normal. Multifocal lower genital tract neoplasia occurs and will be dealt with in more detail below. Asynchronous intraepithelial neoplasia may develop in cervix and vagina. Approximately 4% of women who have had a hysterectomy for CIN may be found many years later to have a newly developed VaIN at the vaginal vault.[61] In one series, two-thirds of 94 women with VaIN had a prior or concurrent history of cervical neoplasia;[126] 45% of them had CIN, nearly half of whom had been treated for it on the average of 6 years earlier. Another 21% of women with VaIN had carcinoma of the cervix, 85% of whom had been treated for it on the average of 8 years earlier. This new disease may represent a further response to the carcinogenic stimulus that caused the cervical disease in the first place. Possibly, the recurrent disease may signify that tissue adjacent to that initially excised already had the potential to transform into intraepithelial neoplasia, perhaps because of initiating changes that affected a field greater than was at first apparent. The initial diagnosis is nearly always made by cytology and confirmed by colposcopy.

The histogenesis of squamous neoplasia of the vagina, both intraepithelial and invasive, is far from clear. If the squamous epithelium of the cervix, vagina, and vulva form a common field, it might be argued that they should be equally at risk for developing neoplasia when exposed to the same carcinogenic agent. Yet, the actual cellular changes that occur in the vagina (and vulva) may well differ from those in the cervix. CIN usually develops from the transformation zone. The tissue that is originally columnar in type undergoes squamous change at the very beginning of its premalignant phase. It is rare for a squamous cell carcinoma of the cervix to arise from the original squamous epithelium. However, no such transformation zone exists in the vagina, so that neoplasia must develop directly from the squamous epithelium. For the field change theory to be accepted, it is necessary to propose that the carcinogens act on the immature metaplastic cells of the cervix and on the original squamous cells of the vagina (and vulva) to produce the same end result of intraepithelial neoplasia.

Several recent investigations have studied the epidemiology of VaIN. Risk factors in common with cervical cancer include lower socioeconomic status and a history of genital warts. Every patient had demonstrable HPV (more than 1000 viral copies per cell) by blot hybridization, and 80% by immunohistochemistry.[134] Further study is necessary to determine whether there is an increased risk for vaginal neoplastic disorders in women infected with HIV, and whether this may be due in part to the woman's altered immunologic status. Patients with VaIN often report cancer 5–15 years earlier in other genital organs, most commonly as preinvasive or invasive carcinoma of the uterine cervix.[65,132]

Like intraepithelial neoplasia occurring in the cervix (CIN) and vulva (VIN), the preponderance of VaIN 1 lesions is associated with high-risk HPV types.[131] Surprisingly, HPV type 16 is found only in a rare case. VaIN 3 lesions, in contrast, are commonly (50%) associated with HPV type 16, as well as other high-risk types. While both low- and high-grade vaginal lesions may contain multiple HPV types, additional testing for viral messenger RNA has shown that in any individual lesion only one viral type is transcriptionally active. This indicates that despite the presence of more than one virus being present in any given lesion, only one is responsible for causing the intraepithelial lesion.[133]

VaIN affects the upper third of the vagina in over 90% of cases and is multifocal in half of the patients. Although usually asymptomatic, it may be suspected on vaginal smear, colposcopic examination or biopsy. Approximately half of the cases are VaIN 1, 20% VaIN 2, and 30% VaIN 3.[5] Patients with VaIN 1 to VaIN 2 are generally 15 years younger than patients with VaIN 3 (45 versus 61 years). The involved epithelium is nearly twice the thickness of normal epithelium (0.5 versus 0.3 mm).[10] Therapies have included 5-fluorouracil, CO_2 laser,[5] and partial colpectomy.[25]

Pathology

VaIN is not recognizable by gross examination. Its histologic features resemble those of CIN with all the possible variants (see Chapter 8), such as the changes seen with wart virus infection. One important difference is the absence of gland crypts in the vagina, a feature that is of significance when planning local destructive treatment for VaIN. Like CIN in the cervix, the p16 and Ki-67 are useful in helping to determine that a dysplastic process is present (Figures 5.44 and 5.45).

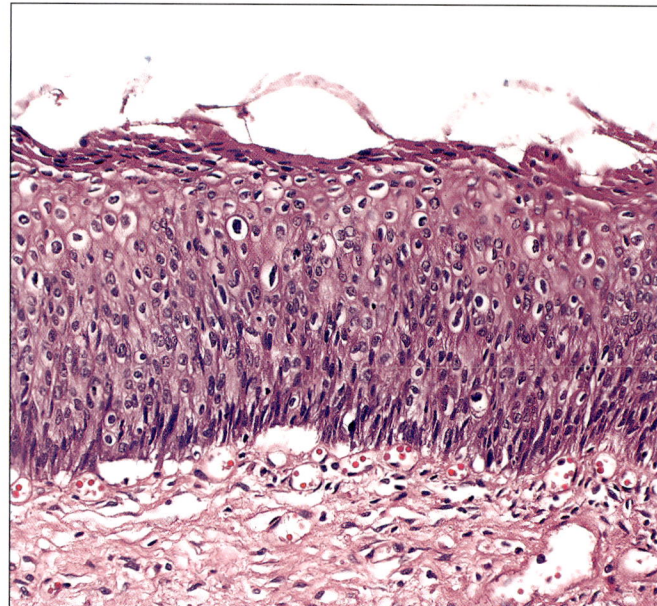

Fig. 5.44 VaIN 2.

MICROINVASIVE SQUAMOUS CELL CARCINOMA

Attempts have been made to define a microinvasive stage of vaginal carcinoma in order to spare patients at low risk for metastases from radical operations. When microinvasion is defined as tumor that penetrates less than 2.5 mm, there are no survival advantages for such patients over those with stage 1 squamous cell cancer.[33] Since the vaginal wall is only 5 mm thick, a lesion that penetrates 2.5 mm has already invaded half the wall's thickness and a new definition of microinvasion is obviously required.

INVASIVE SQUAMOUS CELL CARCINOMA

Definition

An invasive cancer composed entirely of malignant squamous cells.

Clinical features

Squamous cell carcinoma originating in the vagina is infrequent, accounting for only 1% of all gynecologic malignancies. The age-adjusted incidence is 0.6/100 000 white women in the USA. In fact, the vagina is more commonly involved by secondary spread of tumors from elsewhere than it is by primary cancer. While generally a disease of older women,[22] approximately 10% of women are less than 40 years of age; even teenagers are occasionally affected.[118] The few epidemiologic studies of vaginal carcinoma suggest that the pathogenesis is environmentally related. Additionally, skin grafts taken from extragenital sites or grafts fashioned from human amnion and used to form a neovagina sometimes assume the appearance of normal vagina,[88] and later give rise to diseases that would normally affect the vagina.[60] In one case, the neovagina had been constructed by a simple cleavage technique without tissue transplantation, suggesting that even the mechanical irritation from a prosthesis may be a potential cancer risk factor.[12] Occa-

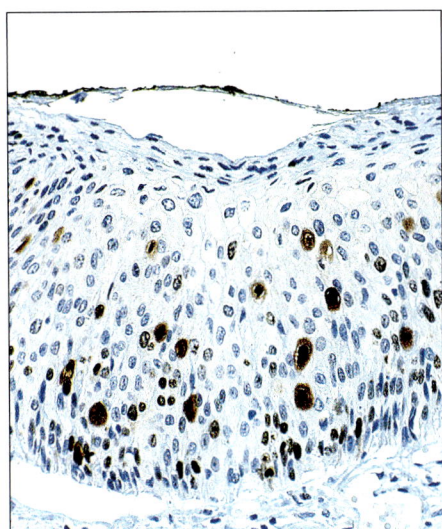 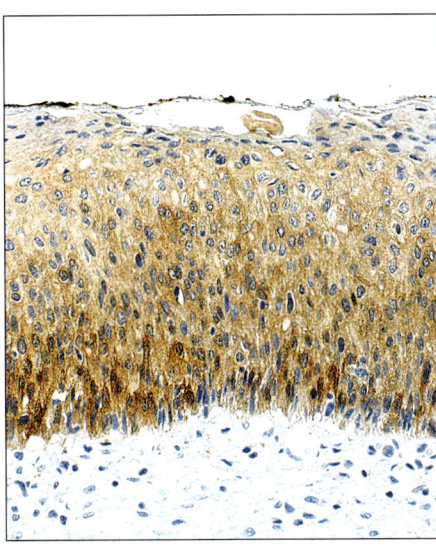

Fig. 5.45 VaIN, Ki-67 left; p16 right.

sionally the tumor that forms is more typical of those that arise in the original grafted tissue.[56] A history of prior hysterectomy is common, quite often for CIN or cervical carcinoma. Between one-fifth and three-fifths of invasive vaginal cancers have demonstrable HPV DNA, usually type 16, confirming the potential role of this virus in vaginal oncogenesis. This is more common in younger than in older patients.[53]

Pathology

As with VaIN, most lesions involve the upper vagina,[95] probably because of a topographical association with CIN. The histologic appearances of vaginal squamous cell carcinoma are those of squamous cell carcinoma in general, ranging from the keratinizing to the poorly differentiated and, in individual cases, are not distinguishable from analogous carcinomas of the vulva or cervix.

Spread and natural history

The route of lymphatic spread depends upon the anatomic location of the carcinoma. Cancers situated in the upper third of the vagina tend to spread, like those of the cervix, to the internal pelvic nodes. There is too little experience to date to determine the value of seeking and biopsying sentinel nodes.[144] Those at the lower end of the vagina spread to the inguinal nodes, as do tumors of the vulva. The outcome after treatment is poor, with 5-year survival rates of about of 33%.[31] The prognosis depends, predictably, on the stage of disease. Early stage tumors (FIGO 1–2A) tend to recur locally in the vagina, in the immediate paravaginal tissues or inguinal nodes.[154] Diagnosis in the preinvasive stage is associated with the best prognosis, emphasizing the importance of continued cytologic surveillance by vault smears in women who have had a hysterectomy for CIN.

SQUAMOUS CELL NEOPLASIA AND EXPOSURE TO DIETHYLSTILBESTROL

Despite dire early warnings, the increased risk for DES-exposed offspring over the general population of developing cervical and vaginal dysplasia and cancer has remained small. In the largest controlled study, the DES-unexposed women, in fact, had higher rates (4.0%) than the DES-exposed women (1.9%).[112] Complicating factors included morphologic criteria (or their

application) used to diagnose dysplasia (some investigators overcalled the severity of lesions), bias in patient selection (women referred because of known exposure have much higher rates than women randomly picked for evaluation), and discord between biopsy and cytologic findings. In some studies, the colposcopic appearance of squamous metaplasia had been erroneously interpreted as dysplasia. Small uniform tiles of squamous epithelium that are surrounded by vessels of small caliber, now called 'pseudomosaicism', are benign, although in the past they were often interpreted as true tiles, indicative of dysplasia. In subsequent years incidence rates were found to be slightly higher in exposed women both in the short term[111] and after more than 15 years.[47,48] Reports of invasive squamous cell cancer have been exceedingly rare[13,36,101] and a fraction of what would be expected by chance alone.

VERRUCOUS CARCINOMA

The term verrucous carcinoma is applied to a rare vaginal tumor that is exophytic with a coarsely granular or undulating surface (Figure 5.46), cells that microscopically are uniformly well differentiated and bland, and a deep margin that is usually non-invasive. Invasion, if present, is pushing rather than destructive (Figures 5.47 and 5.48). Not uncommonly, the carcinomas display koilocytosis or surface papillae with central fibrovascular cores, typical of condylomata. On microscopic examination, the tumor is extremely well differentiated, so much so that the bland cytologic features in the extensive acanthosis cannot be distinguished from normal. Definitionally, the epithelium at the stromal interface consists of broad bulbous masses of squamous cells. If jagged or irregular, the tumor is best regarded as ordinary squamous cell carcinoma. Verrucous carcinomas display a relatively indolent growth potential, with frequent local recurrence after incomplete excision. Lymph node metastasis occurs rarely. Treatment is usually wide local excision since the neoplasm is resistant to therapeutic radiation. Radiotherapy may in fact transform it to conventional squamous carcinoma. Verrucous carcinoma is also commonly misdiagnosed as giant condyloma, although we are not sure that the two are different. Tumors with a mixed pattern of both verrucous and conventional squamous carcinoma behave with

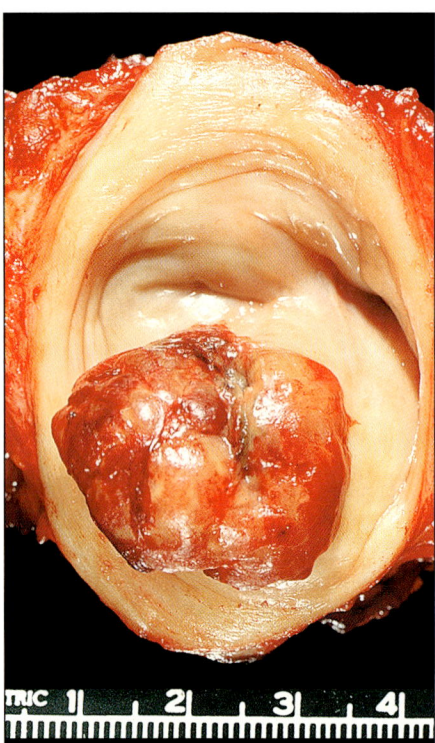

Fig. 5.46 Verrucous carcinoma.

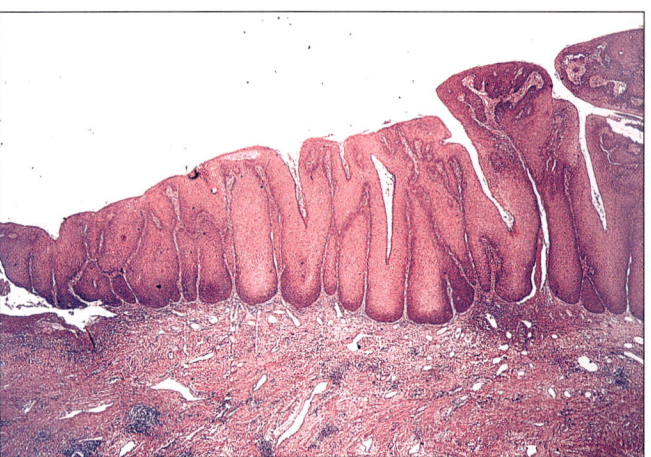

Fig. 5.47 Verrucous carcinoma. The deep margin discloses no invasion.

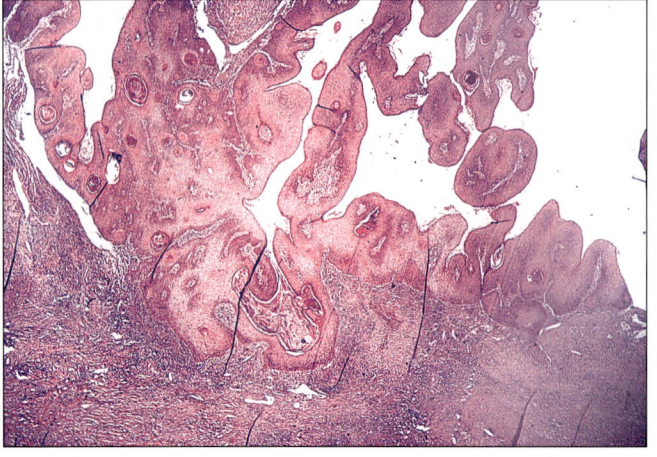

Fig. 5.48 Verrucous carcinoma. The deep margin discloses no invasion.

the aggressiveness of typical squamous cancer, and should be classified as such.

WARTY CARCINOMA

Warty carcinoma in the vagina is a homolog of the more commonly encountered warty variant of squamous cell carcinoma in the vulva. The microscopy shows marked nuclear abnormalities, perinuclear cytoplasmic cavitation (koilocytosis) in cells with little cytoplasm, and multinucleated cells. The tumor is infiltrative at the stromal interface. Preliminary data from similar tumors in the vulva indicate that they may behave in a low-grade malignant fashion.

SMALL CELL CARCINOMA

'Small cell carcinoma' is a term applied ambiguously to two separate lesions. These include: (1) anaplastic variants of squamous cell carcinoma composed of cells with small nuclei and scanty cytoplasm and resembling the cells of high-grade VaIN; and (2) carcinomas similar to the small (oat cell) neuroendocrine carcinomas of the cervix and other sites, with dense core neurosecretory granules. These tumors have also been called 'carcinoid tumors', 'argyrophil cell carcinomas', 'small cell tumors with neuroepithelial features', 'oat cell carcinoma', and 'endocrine cell carcinoma'. The tumors occur in older women as masses usually several centimeters across. Most neoplasms have spread beyond the vagina at the time of diagnosis.[52] In addition to the light microscopic findings of a small cell neoplasm, the tumor shows reactivity for chromogranin and non-specific enolase, and electron microscopy reveals features consistent with neuroendocrine cells, which include cytoplasmic- and neurosecretory-type granules, and cytoplasmic processes.[81] The small cell carcinoma needs to be differentiated from lymphoma, which may be difficult to diagnose in a small biopsy with squeeze artifact, because of different prognostic and therapeutic implications, and from small cell squamous carcinomas (by negative immunostaining for p63, which is regularly and diffusely positive in squamous carcinomas).

GLANDULAR LESIONS

ATYPICAL ADENOSIS

Atypical adenosis, characterized by glands with cellular stratification, nuclear pleomorphism, hyperchromasia, and prominent nucleoli (Figure 5.49), appears near the periphery of most clear cell carcinomas in which the excised vagina has been serially blocked for microscopic examination.[110] Atypical cells with large, irregular nuclei have also been identified in approximately 0.5% of cervical and vaginal smears from women exposed to DES antenatally. The frequent finding of tuboendometrial-type cells adjacent to the cancers (Figure 5.50), but the rarity of mucinous cells in this location, suggests that the clear cell adenocarcinoma, if it is linked to atypical adenosis, is most likely from the tuboendometrial type. At this time, this relation is considered as a hypothesis as no cases are yet known where, over time, microscopically proven atypical adenosis has progressed to carcinoma.

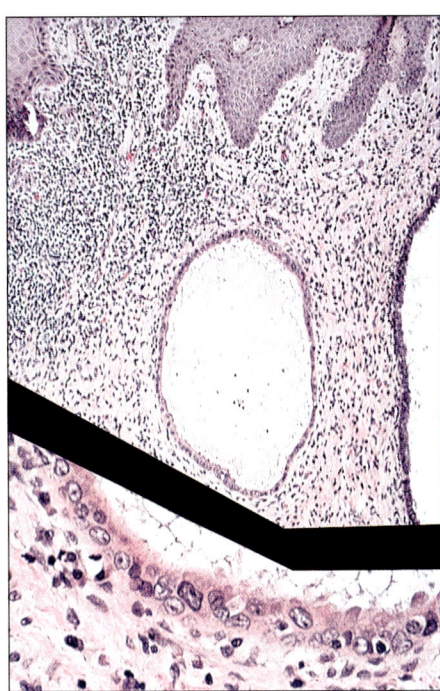

Fig. 5.49 Atypical adenosis.

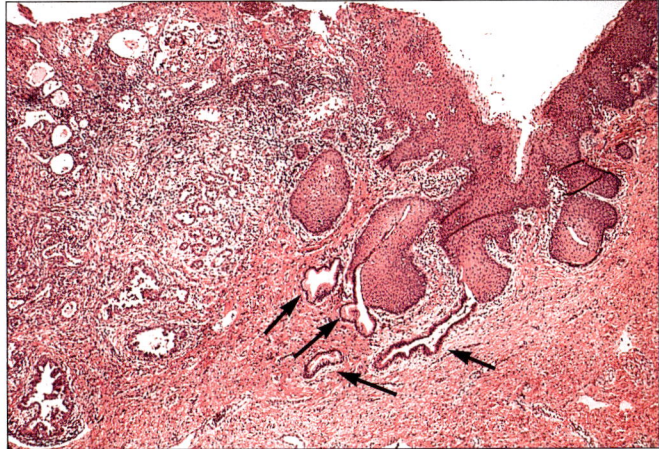

Fig. 5.50 Tuboendometrial adenosis. The adenosis (arrows) lies at the edge of the clear cell adenocarcinoma.

CLEAR CELL ADENOCARCINOMA

Clinical features

More than 750 cases of clear cell adenocarcinoma of the vagina and cervix diagnosed in females born after 1940 have been recorded, with estimates that about 25–50 new cases develop each year.[43,141] Most are from the United States, but some women with documented histories of exposure have been born in Canada, Mexico, Europe, Australia, or Africa. About three-fifths of patients reveal some evidence suggesting exposure *in utero* to DES, hexestrol or dienestrol. A few women had been exposed to steroidal estrogens or progesterone alone. While the relative risk of a vaginal cancer being associated with stilbestrol usage is high (about 40),[78,120,143] many women lack a history of drug exposure (12–22%),[122,148] confirming that this tumor occurs spontaneously. For cervical tumors alone, the majority of cases have no drug history (54% negative histories[122]), a finding in

accord with clear cell adenocarcinoma of the cervix in young women being a well-recognized entity long prior to the DES era. Clear cell adenocarcinoma of the vagina in women under the age of 20 years was known before the synthesis and use of DES in pregnancy, but less frequently. To date, even with long-term follow-up, no other tumor type has developed in association with DES exposure.[49]

The mode age at diagnosis is 19 years, which has remained remarkably uniform regardless of the patient cohort's year of birth. Although a rare patient has been as young as 7 years of age, only after the age of 14 years does the age–incidence curve rise sharply, which strongly suggests a pathogenesis related in part to puberty. It plateaus between ages 17 and 22 years and then declines rapidly,[143] with few women developing this form of cancer in their thirties or forties. Despite the strong association between drug and tumor, clear cell adenocarcinoma develops only rarely in exposed women with a cumulative incidence to date of 0.02% (1/5000),[50] a rarity confirmed by numerous other studies.[54,90,142] The greatest number of DES-exposed patients with these tumors were born in 1951–1953, the years when the drug appears to have been prescribed most frequently for pregnancy support. The final incidence will very likely prove to be slightly greater than registry estimates (but still less than its upper estimate of 0.1%) as cases are known to have been misclassified and therefore not reported,[57] and because some new tumors are still being discovered in DES-exposed women.[34] Epidemiologic studies indicate that the risk of tumor development is higher when the drug was started early in pregnancy or there has been a history of prior miscarriage.[44,54]

The risk is also increased in women who were taller or more obese than their contemporaries at age 14–15 years,[121] findings of interest since height and body mass are risk factors for endometrial cancer, the most common glandular cancer of the female reproductive tract. Rare reports of tumor formation in only one of two monozygotic twins underscore that many factors, including perhaps unidentified environmental ones, operate in carcinogenesis.

The drug only appears to have an effect if administered before week 18 of pregnancy; indeed, most of those affected were exposed in the first trimester.

Gross pathology

The tumor may involve any portion of the vagina (Figures 5.51 and 5.52) and/or cervix (Figure 5.53). Most vaginal tumors arise on the anterior wall, usually in the upper third, corresponding to the most frequent site of adenosis. The lateral and posterior walls and, occasionally, the middle and lower third of the vagina are also involved. On occasion, multicentric tumors have been demonstrated. In many cases, the areas of grossly visible tumor seem discrete, but microscopic examination usually discloses its continuity in the submucosa. Tumors have also been found on the wall opposite the main tumor, presumably as a result of implantation ('kissing lesion').

The tumors have varied in size from microscopic to large. In the years during which the entity was first being recognized, many were of substantial size, reflecting the infrequency of pelvic examinations in asymptomatic and sometimes even symptomatic young women. Most of the larger cancers were polypoid and nodular. Some were flat or ulcerated, having a granular or indurated surface. With increasing awareness that periodic examinations in exposed women should begin early in the teenage period, the tumors subsequently were discovered more often when they were small. While usually palpable, they

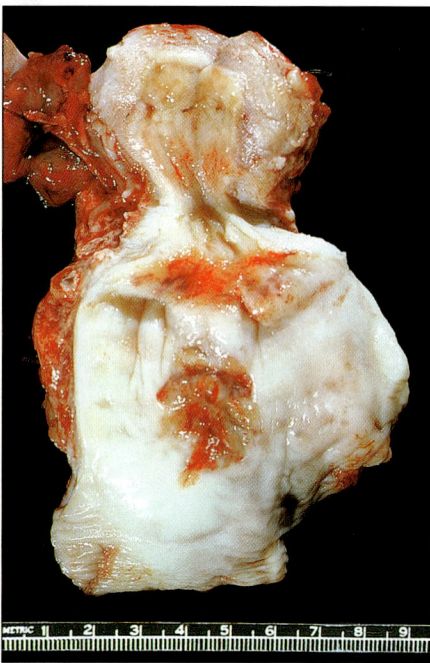

Fig. 5.51 Clear cell adenocarcinoma of vagina.

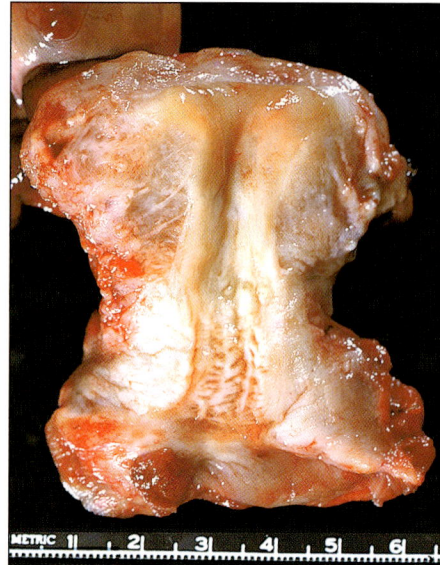

Fig. 5.53 Clear cell adenocarcinoma of exocervix.

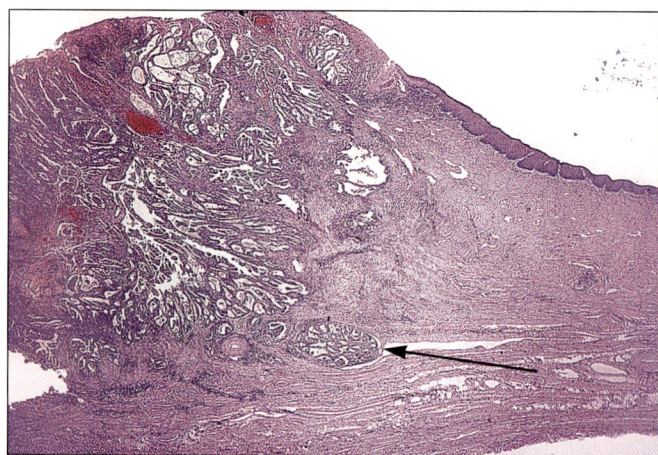

Fig. 5.54 Clear cell adenocarcinoma. The large tumor penetrates deeply into the wall and invades a major blood vessel (arrow).

Microscopic pathology

The clear cell adenocarcinomas of both vagina and cervix are identical to the müllerian clear cell adenocarcinomas of the ovary and endometrium, the latter two occurring sporadically in older women. Several histologic patterns may be observed either alone or in combination. A characteristic pattern, for which the tumor is named, consists of solid sheets of clear cells (Figure 5.55), the clear appearance of the cytoplasm being caused by the dissolution of glycogen when the specimen is processed for microscopic examination. A second pattern, the tubulocystic pattern, exhibits tubules and cysts lined by hobnail cells (Figures 5.56–5.58), by flat cells (Figures 5.59 and 5.60) or by cells that resemble müllerian-type epithelium to varying degrees. The hobnail cell displays a bulbous nucleus that protrudes into the lumen beyond the apparent cytoplasmic limits of the cell. Flat cells often appear innocuous. When only this latter epithelium is present in a small biopsy, it may be difficult to differentiate tumor from adenosis. Less common appearances include a papillary pattern, a tubular pattern resembling endometrial carcinoma, and a pattern composed of cords of cells with eosinophilic cytoplasm. Mitoses are typically infre-

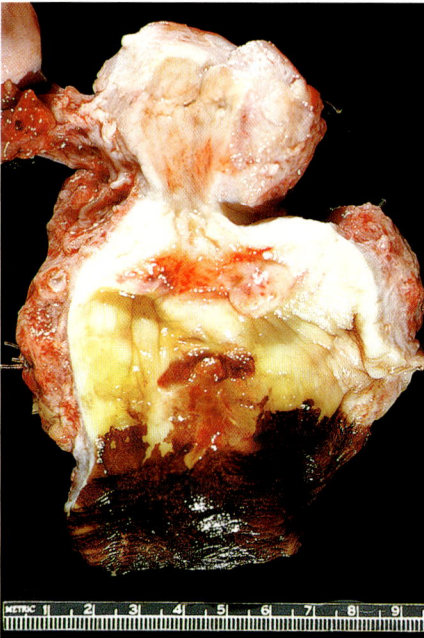

Fig. 5.52 Clear cell adenocarcinoma of vagina (Lugols iodine). The tumor has arisen at the junction of the glycogen-poor, metaplastic squamous epithelium and the glycogen-rich, original squamous epithelium (mahogany color).

may still be invisible on colposcopic examination if confined to the lamina propria and if covered by intact, normal or metaplastic squamous epithelium. Although most cancers are superficial and invade only a few millimeters into the vaginal or cervical wall, some penetrate far more deeply (Figure 5.54) or extend more centrifugally than might be anticipated on gross examination.

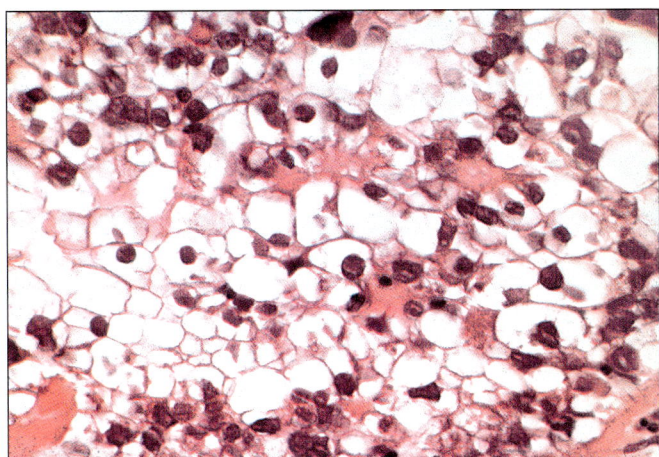

Fig. 5.55 Clear cell adenocarcinoma, clear cells.

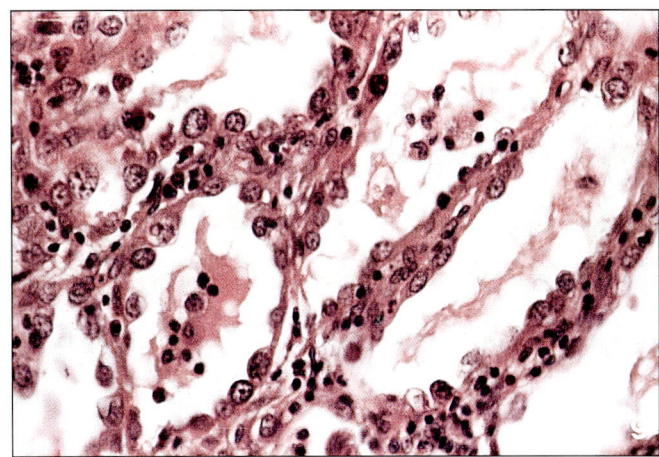

Fig. 5.58 Clear cell adenocarcinoma. The hobnail cells are slightly flattened.

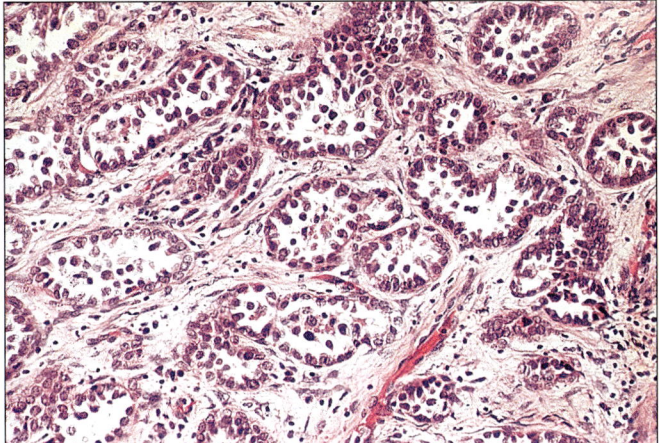

Fig. 5.56 Clear cell adenocarcinoma, hobnail cells.

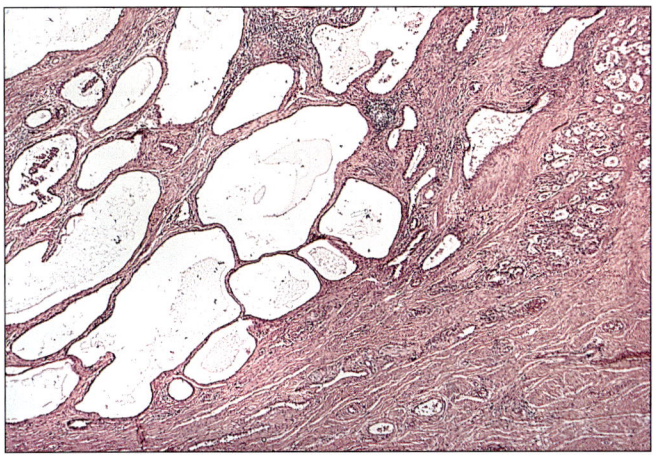

Fig. 5.59 Clear cell adenocarcinoma. Flat cells line the cysts.

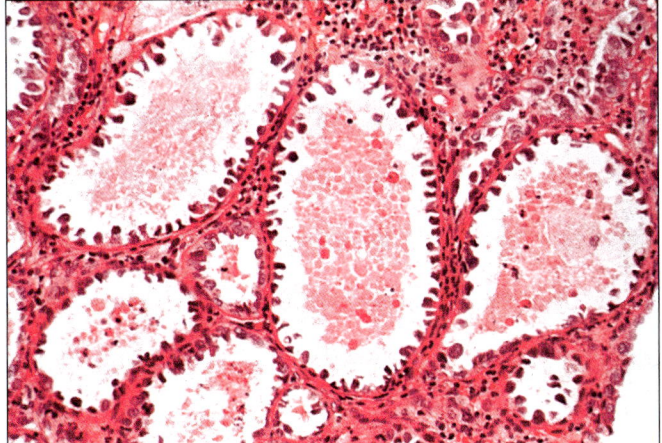

Fig. 5.57 Clear cell adenocarcinoma, hobnail cells.

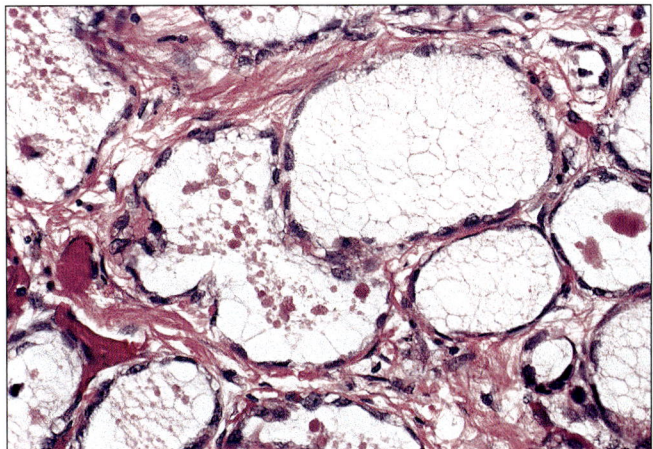

Fig. 5.60 Clear cell adenocarcinoma. Detail of flat cells lining the cysts. The perimeters of some cysts are sharply angulated.

quent. In any of these patterns, the lumina may contain mucin, but the cytoplasm is mucin free.

Clear cell adenocarcinoma is often detected cytologically, especially in the cervix (80% detection rate in the cervix versus a 33% rate in the vagina).[44] Occasionally, a suspicious or positive smear may be the first indication in an asymptomatic woman. The cancerous cells often resemble large endocervical cells or non-specific adenocarcinoma cells, but vary greatly and may appear even as undifferentiated carcinoma.

Natural history
The tumor spreads locally and metastasizes via both lymphatics and blood vessels. Approximately one-sixth of tumors

confined clinically to the lower genital tract (stage 1) will have metastasized to the pelvic lymph nodes on exploration. The frequency of nodal involvement reaches 50% when clinical stage 2 tumors are considered. Clear cell adenocarcinoma extends outside the abdominal cavity more frequently than does squamous cell carcinoma of the vagina or cervix. More than one-third of initial recurrences are in the lung or supraclavicular lymph nodes, in contrast to less than 10% for squamous cell carcinomas.

The actuarial survival rate for all patients with clear cell adenocarcinoma is high. It is about 93% at 5 years and 87% at 10 years when the tumor is stage 1. If the patient is asymptomatic at diagnosis, survival with appropriate therapy approaches 100%. Other factors associated with a better prognosis are an older age (19 years or older) at the time of diagnosis and a tubulocystic microscopic pattern.[55] Large size and/or deep invasion into the wall are associated with a poorer prognosis, but small or superficial tumors also may recur or metastasize. While nuclear aneuploidy has no effect on prognosis, nuclear atypia may be associated with a worse prognosis.[44] Pregnancy at the time of diagnosis does not affect outcome adversely.[119] Recurrences develop most often within 3 years after primary therapy, but have been found after nearly two decades. After treatment of the recurrence, approximately one-fifth of the patients survive an additional 3 years or more.

Pathogenesis

Unlike squamous cell carcinoma of the genital tract in which the etiology is generally considered established and linked to HPV,[96] no such viral associations have been found with clear cell adenocarcinoma.[149] HPV type 31, an oncogenic HPV type, occurs in one-fourth of the clear cell cancers, but in none of its metastases. Two-thirds display altered expression of the tumor suppressor protein p53, but no case has been found where mutated *p53* and the HPV virus have been found in combination. Other oncogenes that have not mutated include the K- and H-*ras* proto-oncogenes, the Wilms tumor (*WT1*) tumor suppressor gene, and the estrogen receptor gene.[15] Recent studies suggest abnormalities may exist in progesterone receptor genes. Extensive genetic instability, manifest as somatic mutation of microsatellite repeats, has been found in all DES-associated tumors examined, and in smaller quantity in half of the cancers in women who were not DES exposed.

Differential diagnosis

Several conditions are easily confused with clear cell adenocarcinoma. Two of the conditions are non-neoplastic. Microglandular hyperplasia has been described above. The Arias-Stella reaction, although usually encountered in the endometrium of pregnant women, is found occasionally in the endocervix and even in vaginal adenosis of the tuboendometrioid type. Characteristically, the Arias-Stella reaction discloses hypersecretory glands where the cells lining the glands have markedly enlarged nuclei and resemble hobnail cells. However, in clear cell adenocarcinoma, the presence of sheets of clear cells or prominent papillae should enable the two lesions to be distinguished. In addition, the hobnail-like nuclei in the Arias-Stella reaction are commonly smudged and appear as degenerative. The Arias-Stella reaction predictably shows low rates of Ki-67 nuclear reactivity and does not overexpress *p53*, both features of which are markedly different in clear cell carcinomas.[145]

Several forms of carcinoma need to be distinguished from clear cell adenocarcinoma. Tumors developing in the distal vagina may resemble transitional cell carcinomas that arise in the urogenital sinus. Renal cell carcinoma (from the left kidney) in which the metastases display clear cells may also prove extremely difficult to diagnose properly without pertinent history.[73,140] Metastatic serous carcinoma of ovarian or other origin may recapitulate the papillary pattern of clear cell carcinoma and the tumor cells resemble the hobnail cells of the latter.

ADENOCARCINOMA, NON-CLEAR CELL

The mucin-secreting adenocarcinoma is a rare tumor that contains glands resembling intestinal epithelium.[153] Most occur in older women and often involve the lower vagina (Figure 5.61). One form is low grade, even to the point of resembling a borderline mucinous tumor, and has arisen in the fistulous tracts of women with Crohns disease (Figure 5.62).[83] Also, Pagets disease of vulvar origin can spread to the vagina, occasionally

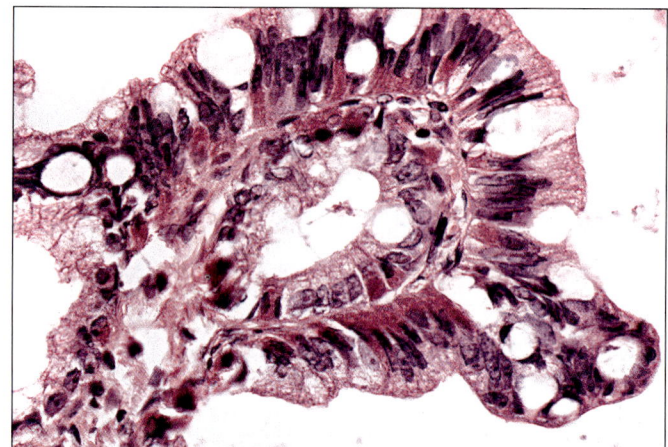

Fig. 5.61 Adenocarcinoma, intestinal type. Argentaffin cells are present.

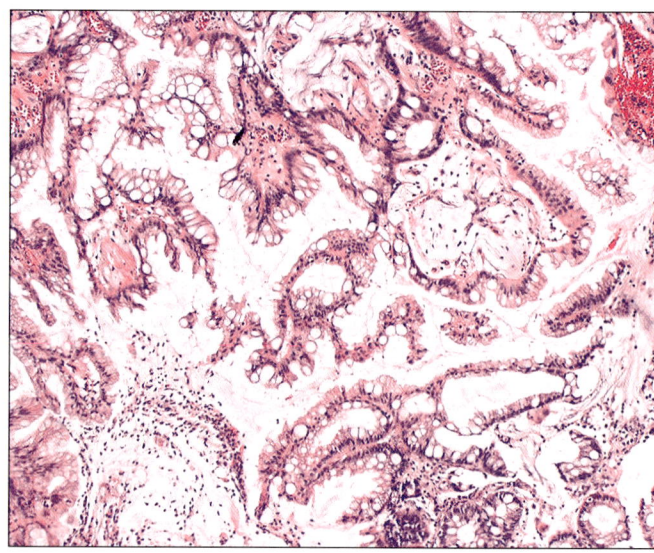

Fig. 5.62 Mucinous adenocarcinoma, well differentiated, arising in a vaginal fistulous tract in a patient with Crohns disease.

even to the cervix,[70] even though we have not encountered this.

OTHER PRIMARY MALIGNANT TUMORS OF THE VAGINA

MALIGNANT MELANOMA

Malignant melanoma is a rare primary tumor in the vagina (incidence 0.03/100 000 per year). Based on a national cancer database,[19] 1.6% of melanomas are genital, of which about one-fifth are vaginal, seven-tenths vulvar and one-tenth cervical. Most appear in women older than 50 years,[28] usually with symptoms such as bleeding or a mass lesion. Some are grossly pigmented. Some show convincing junctional activity in or adjacent to the lesion. Microscopically, most tumors disclose sheets of cells that vary from banal in appearance (Figure 5.63) to markedly irregular, but are not readily specific for any common type of primary tumor arising in the vagina. Occasionally, the tumor cells may infiltrate in the submucosa (Figure 5.64) and be extremely difficult to distinguish from inflammatory cells. An occasional tumor may be amelanotic, but recur as a pigmented melanoma.[93] While there is some debate about adverse prognostic features, complete surgical excision[80] and tumors less than 3 cm in greatest dimension[18] have been treated with some success. Regional lymph nodes are only infrequently involved. Overall, the median survival is 20 months,[80] with the 5-year survival under 20%.

LEIOMYOSARCOMA

Leiomyosarcoma of the vagina is extremely rare, even though it is the most common form of sarcoma that occurs.[24] As discussed under leiomyoma (see above), there is less certainty about the criteria distinguishing benign from malignant lesions than for such lesions in the uterus. Tumors greater than 3 cm diameter, with 5 or more mitoses per 10 HPFs or substantial cytologic atypia, or especially when infiltration is present, are best considered as malignant.

The tumor occurs over a wide age range (25–86 years) and usually presents with vaginal bleeding. The microscopic fea-

tures resemble those of uterine leiomyosarcoma. The prognosis generally is mediocre (35% 5-year survival). The most difficult aspect of therapy is to achieve adequate surgical clearance.

MISCELLANEOUS TUMORS

Most carcinomas reported as arising from mesonephric duct remnants and diagnosed as 'mesonephric carcinoma' actually have been clear cell adenocarcinomas of müllerian type upon review. Most well-documented mesonephric carcinomas have arisen in the cervix. There are exceedingly few documented in the vagina (Figure 5.65).

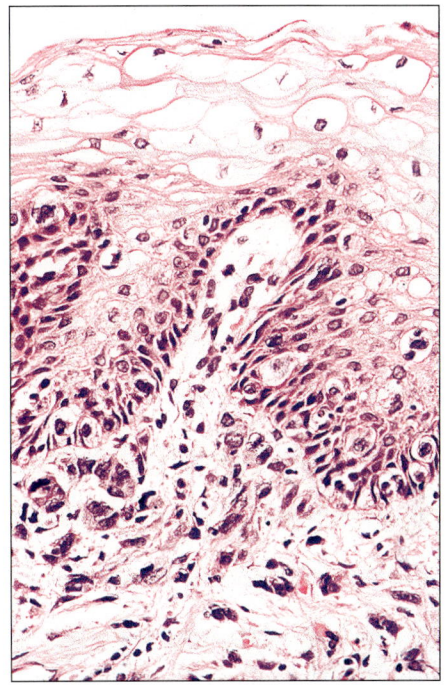

Fig. 5.64 Malignant melanoma. The tumor cells in the submucosa are extremely difficult to distinguish from inflammatory cells on medium power or lower.

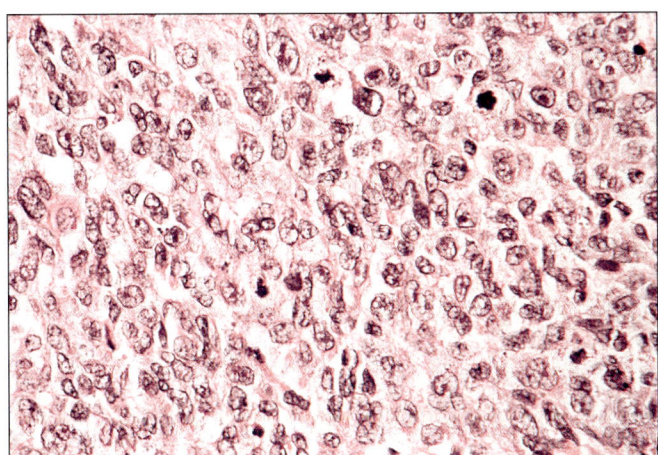

Fig. 5.63 Malignant melanoma.

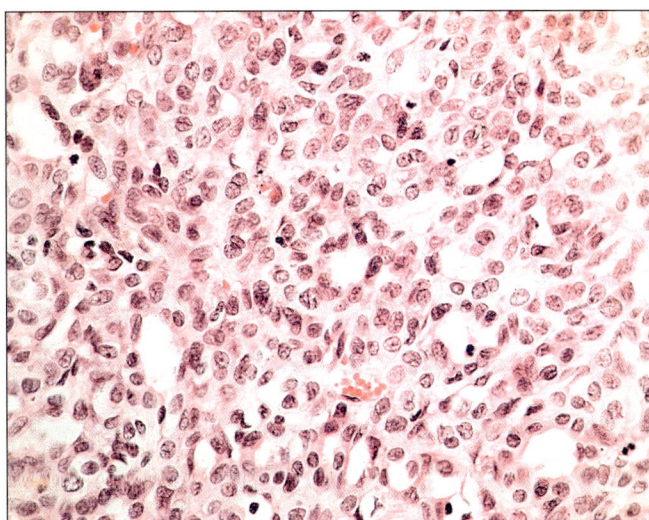

Fig. 5.65 Mesonephric duct carcinoma.

Other rare malignant primary tumors include transitional cell carcinoma (sometimes also called 'cloacogenic carcinoma'), lymphoepithelioma,[30] adenoid basal cell carcinoma,[84] basal cell carcinoma-like tumor, basaloid squamous cell carcinoma,[67] angiosarcoma,[74] papillary squamotransitional cell carcinoma,[113] serous adenocarcinoma,[106] aggressive angiomyxoma,[2] alveolar soft part sarcoma (Figure 5.66),[20,89] carcinosarcoma,[124] and other sarcomas.[87]

MALIGNANT VAGINAL TUMORS IN CHILDHOOD

EMBRYONAL RHABDOMYOSARCOMA

Embryonal rhabdomyosarcoma is a tumor composed of embryonal rhabdomyoblasts, the origin of which is the stromal mesenchyme in the lamina propria. Its former name, 'sarcoma botryoides', reflects the neoplasm's gross appearance as multiple 'grape-like' polyps. While rare in absolute numbers, the tumor is the most common vaginal neoplasm in infants and young children. The mean age at diagnosis is 2 years. Almost all occur in children under the age of 5 years,[151] although occurrences at older ages are known.

The most common symptom is vaginal bleeding, which in infants is often detected because of intermittent bloody discharge on the diaper. If large, the tumor may distend the lumen of the vagina and protrude through the introitus as soft, polypoid, grape-like masses (Figure 5.67).

Pathology

Grossly, the tumor appears as a diffusely thickened submucosa or a soft, polypoid submucosa with an overlying intact squamous epithelium. On cut section, the tumor is edematous since it diffusely involves extensively the lamina propria of the vagina (Figure 5.68). Its color is soft gray to tan. In the vagina, most tumors are polypoid and of the botryoid subtype; this type discloses a loose, myxoid hypocellular center, and just beneath the normal surface squamous epithelium, a condensed layer of neoplastic stromal cells called the 'cambium layer' (Figure 5.69), a botanical term referring to the active growth layer just underneath the bark of trees. At low-power magnification only

a minority are diffusely and evenly hypercellular (Figure 5.70), even though the International Rhabdomyosarcoma Classification considers this pattern as classic embryonal rhabdomyosarcoma.[66,86] Very few vaginal rhabdomyosarcomas are of the spindle type or the alveolar cell type.

Regardless of the tumor variant, the characteristic finding is variable numbers of stellate cells or cells with elongate tails of eosinophilic cytoplasm (Figure 5.71), some of which may contain cross-striations. Immunostains for muscle-specific actin, desmin, and myogenin, but not smooth muscle actin, are

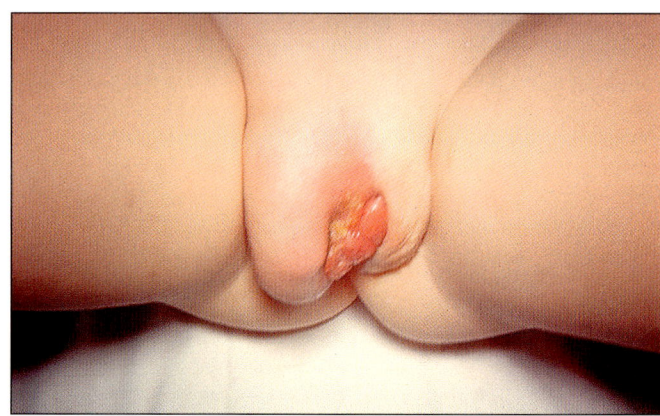

Fig. 5.67 Embryonal rhabdomyosarcoma. The tumor protrudes through the introitus as soft, polypoid, grape-like masses.

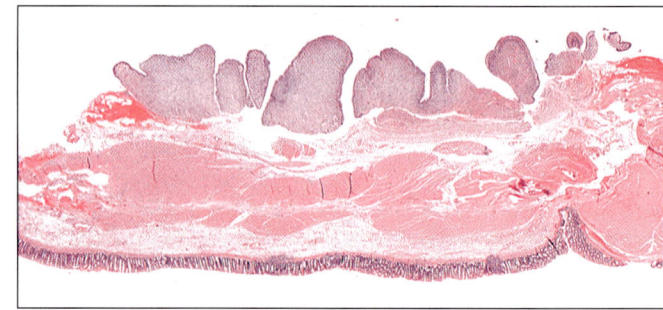

Fig. 5.68 Embryonal rhabdomyosarcoma. A cross-section through the rectovaginal septum shows that the entire vaginal submucosa is involved. The colonic musculature and mucosa are unremarkable.

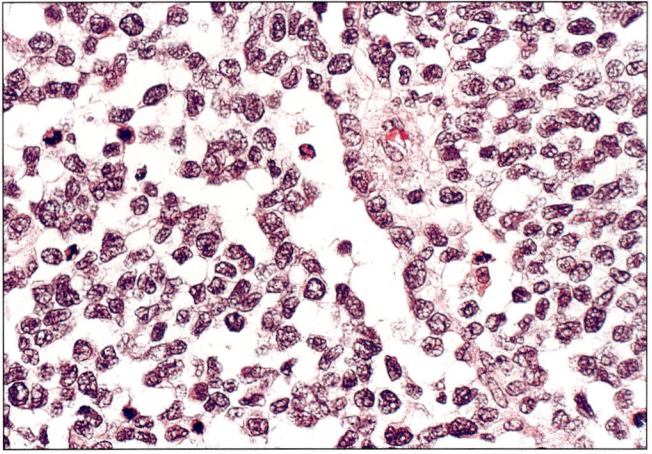

Fig. 5.66 Alveolar soft part sarcoma.

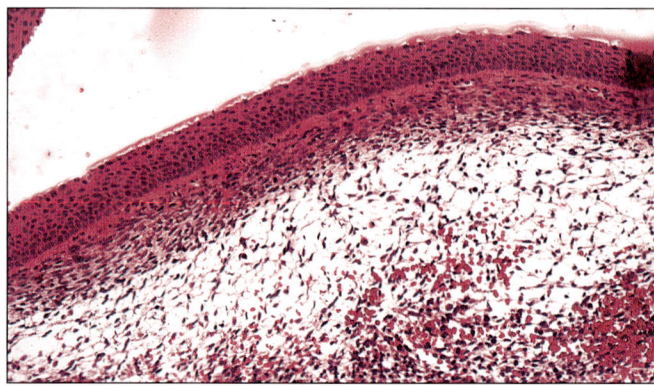

Fig. 5.69 Embryonal rhabdomyosarcoma. The cambium layer, characteristic of the tumor, is a dense zone of rhabdomyoblasts found beneath the surface epithelium.

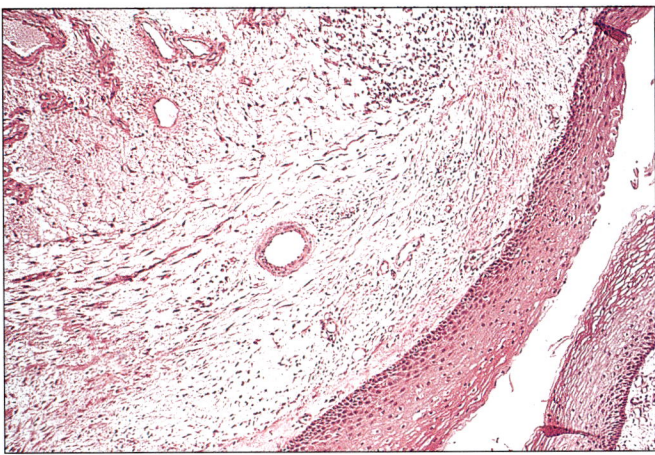

Fig. 5.70 Embryonal rhabdomyosarcoma lacking a cambium layer.

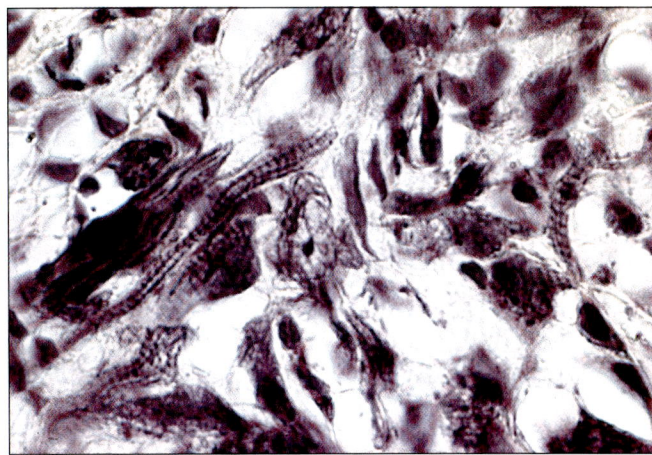

Fig. 5.72 Embryonal rhabdomyoblasts. Prominent cytoplasmic cross-striations (PTAH stain) are present.

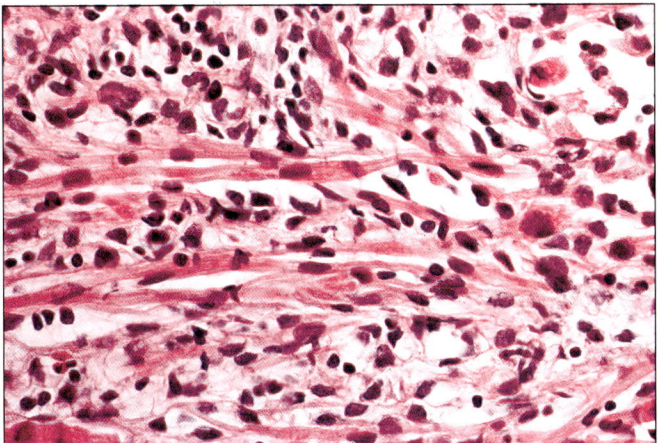

Fig. 5.71 Embryonal rhabdomyosarcoma. Rhabdomyogenic differentiation is prominent as elongate spindle cells with eosinophilic, fibrillary cytoplasm.

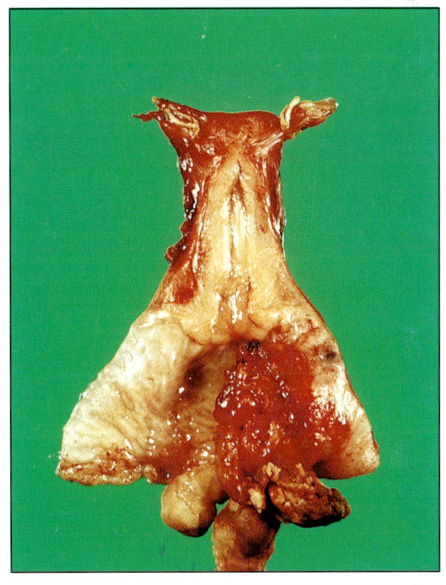

Fig. 5.73 Yolk sac carcinoma.

useful in demonstrating the skeletal muscle nature of the cells (Figure 5.72).

Natural history

The prognosis has improved greatly since the introduction of multiagent chemotherapy, especially if the tumor is stage 1.[4,125] Within stage 1 tumors, the tumor's growth pattern rather than histologic differentiation appears to be the most important prognostic discriminant. Patients with a polypoid (exophytic) intraluminal tumor, regardless whether of the botryoid type with superficially condensed tumor cells or with more evenly distributed cells, survived longer (92% 10-year survival in patients) than if the tumor grew diffusely into the wall (68% 10-year survival). Of surprise, recurrences often display a histologic pattern better than the primary. In one large series, the mitotic count dropped from 8 in the primary to 1.8 per 10 HPFs in the recurrence; the Ki-67 reactivity showed a comparable decrease.[66] To date, there is no convincing evidence that chemotherapy-induced maturation of the tumor cells influences prognosis.

YOLK SAC TUMOR

Yolk sac tumors of the vagina are germ cell tumors, equivalent to those in the ovary. Virtually all reports of this very rare tumor involve infants and children under the age of 4 years;[71] an occasional one occurs much later. Like yolk sac tumors of the ovary, they have been called 'endodermal sinus tumor' in the recent past, and before that 'mesonephroma'. The theoretical origin of these tumors is postulated to be of germ cell origin, a concept that is difficult to relate to the infant vagina. While aberrant germ cells are believed to have somehow found their way to the vagina, this theory does not account for the lack of other tumors of germ cell origin occurring in the vagina.

The tumors present with vaginal bleeding. They are polypoid, soft, and tan to white, and usually fill the vaginal lumen (Figure 5.73). The most common microscopic pattern is the reticular (honeycomb) pattern (Figure 5.74). Occasionally some may be focally solid or slightly papillary (Figure 5.75).

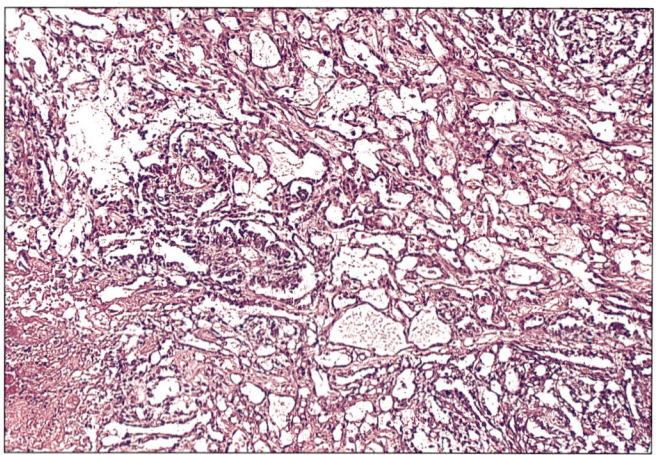

Fig. 5.74 Yolk sac carcinoma, reticular pattern.

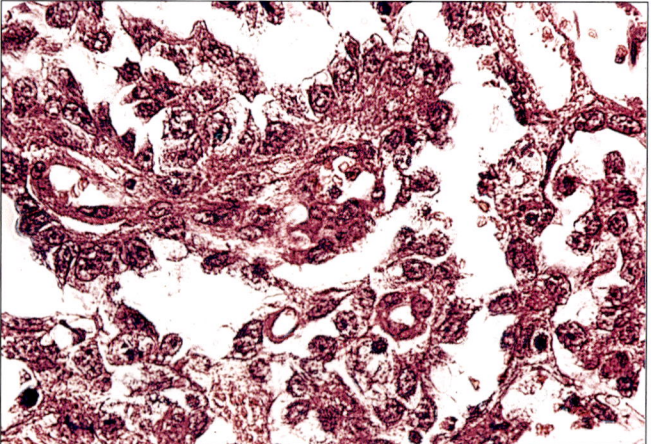

Fig. 5.75 Yolk sac carcinoma, papillary pattern.

Schiller–Duval bodies and the polyvesicular pattern are rare. The most difficult differential diagnosis is the clear cell adenocarcinoma since at times some yolk sac cells may have clear cytoplasm. Immunostains for α-fetoprotein and α_1-antitrypsin confirm the diagnosis of yolk sac tumor.

With the advent of adjuvant chemotherapy, survival rates have improved remarkably.[42] Where the condition was once considered as routinely fatal, long-term survival is now common. New forms of combination chemotherapy and partial but conservative surgery may also permit preservation of fertility.

LYMPHOMA

Vaginal lymphomas, like lymphomas throughout the genital tract, are most commonly secondary to a more generalized spread. About one-fourth[64] to one-half[146] of cases are low stage, and presumably many of these are primary. Lymphomas occur, in general, in women in their forties or older and produce an ill-defined, but very firm thickening of more than one wall and extend towards rectum, bladder or pelvic walls. At presentation, contiguous structures and/or regional lymph nodes are commonly involved.

Like elsewhere in both the upper and lower genital tract, there is a wide range in histologic types. Most are diffuse, large B-cell lymphomas irrespective of the stage at presentation, but several have been follicular lymphomas and small lymphocytic lymphomas. In diffuse, large B-cell lymphoma the sheets of neoplastic cells infiltrate deeply in the stroma, producing a dense sclerosis. The lymphoma cells lack tropism for the overlying epithelium and lymphoepithelial lesions are not seen. Rare cases of nasal-type natural killer (NK)/T cell lymphoma, plasmacytoma, and Hodgkin lymphoma have been described. Because the vagina is one of the mucosa-associated lymphoid tissues (MALT), MALT lymphoma, though rare, must be included in the differential diagnosis of vaginal neoplasms.[155]

The differential diagnosis includes inflammatory conditions, carcinoma, malignant mixed müllerian tumor, endometrial stromal sarcoma, melanoma, and primitive neuroectodermal tumor, a fact underscored by a large consultative practice where only slightly more than half of cases have been submitted correctly diagnosed by the referring pathologists.

With the wider availability and routine application of immunoperoxidase staining to paraffin sections, the distinction between these different entities is not difficult. However, the diagnosis of lymphoma must be considered first by the pathologist and appropriate special studies performed. Overdiagnosis of lymphoma is a danger in the so-called 'lymphoma-like lesions', a term signifying inflammatory lesions mimicking lymphoma.

SECONDARY TUMORS OF THE VAGINA

Secondary tumors of the vagina are four times more common than primary tumors. Most common is direct extension from tumors of adjacent organs, particularly cervix (32%) and endometrium (18%), but metastases from distant organs such as breast (Figure 5.76), bowel (Figures 5.77 and 5.78), and left

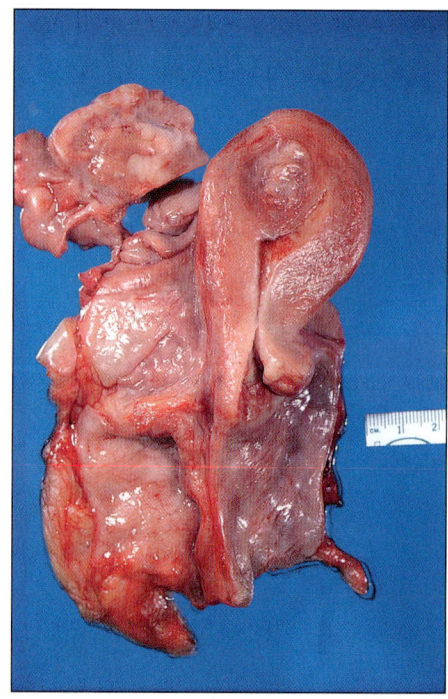

Fig. 5.76 Adenocarcinoma of breast, metastatic to vagina.

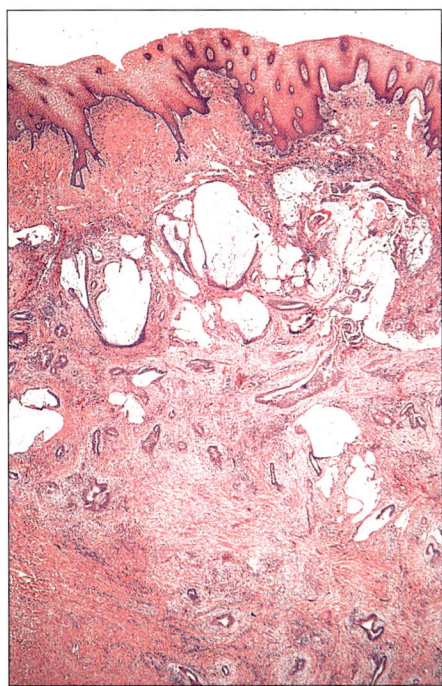

Fig. 5.77 Adenocarcinoma of colon, metastatic to vagina.

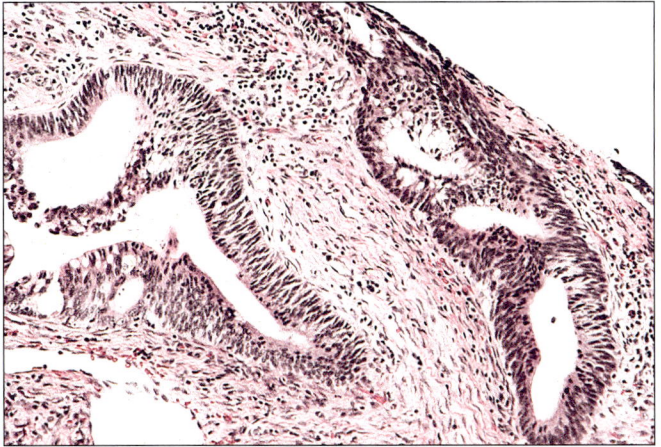

Fig. 5.78 Adenocarcinoma of colon. Detail of metastasis to vagina.

kidney[140] can also be seen. The spread may occur by direct extension, lymphatic spread or implantation at the time of hysterectomy.

REFERENCES

1. Abu J, Nunns D, Ireland D, Brown L. Malignant progression through borderline changes in recurrent Mullerian papilloma of the vagina. Histopathology 2003;42:510–11.
2. Amr SS, Elmallah KO. Aggressive angiomyxoma of the vagina. Int J Obstet Gynecol 1995;48:207–10.
3. Anderson M, Jordan J, Morse A, Sharp F. Diethylstilbestrol exposure. In: A Text and Atlas of Integrated Colposcopy, 2nd edn. London: Chapman and Hall Medical, 1996.240–2.
4. Andrassy RJ, Wiener ES, Raney RB, et al. Progress in the surgical management of vaginal rhabdomyosarcoma: a 25-year review from the Intergroup Rhabdomyosarcoma Study Group. J Pediatr Surg 1999;34:731–4.
5. Audet LP, Body G, Vauclair R, Drouin P, Ayoub J. Vaginal intraepithelial neoplasia. Gynecol Oncol 1990;36:232–9.
6. Aziz DC, Ferre F, Robitaille J, Ferenczy A. Human papillomavirus testing in the clinical laboratory 1: squamous lesions of the cervix. J Gynecol Surg 1993;9:1–7.
7. Barnhart KT, Izquierdo A, Pretorius ES, Shera DM, Shabbout M, Shaunik A. Baseline dimensions of the human vagina. Hum Reprod 2006;21:1618–22.
8. Ben-Izhak O, Munichor M, Malkin L, Kerner H. Brenner tumor of the vagina. Int J Gynecol Pathol 1998;17:79–82.
9. Benchimol M. Trichomonads under microscopy. Microscopy Microanal 2004;10:528–50.
10. Benedet JL, Wilson PS, Matisic JP. Epidermal thickness measurements in vaginal intraepithelial neoplasia – a basis for optimal CO2 laser vaporization. J Reprod Med 1992;37:809–12.
11. Biankin SA, O'Toole VE, Fung C, Russell P. Bizarre leiomyoma of the vagina: report of a case. Int J Gynecol Pathol 2000;19:186–7.
12. Bobin JY, Zinzindohoue C, Naba T, Isaac S, Mage G. Primary squamous cell carcinoma in a patient with vaginal agenesis. Gynecol Oncol 1999;74:293–7.
13. Bornstein J, Adam E, AdlerStorthz K, Kaufman RH. Development of cervical and vaginal squamous cell neoplasia as a late consequence of in utero exposure to diethylstilbestrol. Obstet Gynecol Surv 1988;43:15–21.
14. Bowden FJ, Garnett GP. Trichomonas vaginalis epidemiology: parameterising and analysing a model of treatment interventions. Sex Transm Dis 2000;76:248–56.
15. Boyd J, Takahashi H, Waggoner SE, et al. Molecular genetic analysis of clear cell adenocarcinomas of the vagina and cervix associated and unassociated with diethylstilbestrol exposure in utero. Cancer 1996;77:507–13.
16. Branton PA, Tavassoli FA. Spindle cell epithelioma, the so-called mixed tumor of the vagina. A clinicopathologic, immunohistochemical, and ultrastructural analysis of 28 cases. Am J Surg Pathol 1993;17:509–15.
17. Brown WD, Burrows L, Todd CS. Ectopic pregnancy after cesarean hysterectomy. Obstet Gynecol 2002;99(5 Pt 2):933–4.
18. Buchanan DJ, Schlaerth J, Kurosaki T. Primary vaginal melanoma: thirteen-year disease-free survival after wide local excision and review of recent literature. Am J Obstet Gynecol 1998;178:1177–83.
19. Chang AE, Karnell LH, Menck HR. The National Cancer Database report on cutaneous and noncutaneous melanoma: a summary of 84 836 cases from the past decade. The American College of Surgeons Commission on Cancer and the American Cancer Society. Cancer 1998;83:1664–78.
20. Chang HC, Hsueh S, Ho YS, Chang MY, Soong YK. Alveolar soft part sarcoma of the vagina – a case report. J Reprod Med 1994;39:121–5.
21. Colton T, Greenberg ER, Noller K, et al. Breast cancer in mothers prescribed diethylstilbestrol in pregnancy: Further follow-up. JAMA 1993;269:2096–100.
22. Creasman WT. Vaginal cancers. Curr Opin Obstet Gynecol 2005;17:71–6.
23. Creasman WT, Phillips JL, Menck HR. The National Cancer Database report on cancer of the vagina. Cancer 1998;83:1033–40.
24. Curtin JP, Saigo P, Slucher B, Venkatraman ES, Mychalczak B, Hoskins WJ. Soft-tissue sarcoma of the vagina and vulva: a clinicopathologic study. Obstet Gynecol 1995;86:269–72.
25. Curtis P, Shepherd JH, Lowe DG, Jobling T. The role of partial colpectomy in the management of persistent vaginal neoplasia after primary treatment. Br J Obstet Gynaecol 1992;99:587–9.
26. Davis CC, Kremer MJ, Schlievert PM, Squier CA. Penetration of toxic shock syndrome toxin-1 across porcine vaginal mucosa ex vivo: permeability characteristics, toxin distribution, and tissue damage. Am J Obstet Gynecol 2003;189:1785–91.
27. de Kroon CD, Bergman I, Westenberg S, van Eyk H, Thurkow AL. Prolapse of the uterine tube after subtotal hysterectomy. Br J Obstet Gynaecol 2003;110:333–4.
28. DeMatos P, Tyler D, Seigler HF. Mucosal melanoma of the female genitalia: a clinicopathologic study of forty-three cases at Duke University Medical Center. Surgery 1998;124:38–48.
29. Dhaliwal LK, Das I, Gopalan S. Recurrent leiomyoma of the vagina. Int J Gynaecol Obstet 1992;37:281–3.
30. Dietl J, Horny HP, Kaiserling E. Lymphoepithelioma-like carcinoma of the vagina – a case report with special reference to the immunophenotype of the tumor cells and tumor-infiltrating lymphoreticular cells. Int J Gynecol Pathol 1994;13:186–9.
31. Dixit S, Singhal S, Baboo HA. Squamous cell carcinoma of the vagina – a review of 70 cases. Gynecol Oncol 1993;48:80–7.
32. Eckert LO, Hawes SE, Stevens CE. Vulvovaginal candidiasis: clinical manifestations, risk factors, management algorithm. Obstet Gynecol 1998;92:757–65.
33. Eddy GL, Singh KP, Gansler TS. Superficially invasive carcinoma of the vagina following treatment for cervical cancer: a report of six cases. Gynecol Oncol 1990;36:376–9.
34. Emens JM. Continuing problems with diethylstilboestrol. Br J Obstet Gynaecol 1994;101:748–50.
35. Eschenbach DA. History and review of bacterial vaginosis. Am J Obstet Gynecol 1993;169:441–5.
36. Faber K, Jones M, Tarraza HJ. Invasive squamous cell carcinoma of the vagina in a diethylstilbestrol-exposed woman. Gynecol Oncol 1990;37:125–8.
37. Fishman A, Ortega E, Girtanner RE, Kaplan AL. Malacoplakia of the vagina presenting as a pelvic mass. Gynecol Oncol 1993;49:380–2.

38. Gastol P, Baka-Jakubiak M, Skobejko-Wlodarska L, Szymkiewicz C. Complete duplication of the bladder, urethra, vagina, and uterus in girls. Urology 2000;55:578–81.

39. Graves A, Gardner WA, Jr. Pathogenicity of Trichomonas vaginalis. Clin Obstet Gynecol 1993;36:145–52.

40. Guerrier D, Mouchel T, Pasquier L, Pellerin I. The Mayer–Rokitansky–Kuster–Hauser syndrome (congenital absence of uterus and vagina) – phenotypic manifestations and genetic approaches. J Negat Results Biomed 2006;5:1.

41. Guillou L, Gloor E, De Grandi P, Costa J. Post-operative pseudosarcoma of the vagina. A case report. Pathol Res Pract 1989;185:245–8.

42. Handel LN, Scott SM, Giller RH, Greffe BS, Lovell MA, Koyle MA. New perspectives on therapy for vaginal endodermal sinus tumors. J Urol 2002;168:687–90.

43. Hanselaar A, Boos E, Shirango H, De Wilde P, Bernheim J. Report of the Netherlands Registry of Clear Cell Adenocarcinoma: preliminary data of the 1999 update. In: DES research update 1999: Current knowledge, future directions. Bethesda, Maryland: National Institutes of Health; 1999:5.

44. Hanselaar AG, Van LN, De WP, Vooijs GP. Clear cell adenocarcinoma of the vagina and cervix. A report of the Central Netherlands Registry with emphasis on early detection and prognosis. Cancer 1991;67:1971–8.

45. Hartmann CA, Sperling M, Stein H. So-called fibroepithelial polyps of the vagina exhibiting an unusual but uniform antigen profile characterized by expression of desmin and steroid hormone receptors but no muscle-specific actin or macrophage markers. Am J Clin Pathol 1990;93:604–8.

46. Hassan A, Bennet A, Bhalla S, Ylagan LR, Mutch D, Dehner LP. Paraganglioma of the vagina: report of a case, including immunohistochemical and ultrastructural findings. Int J Gynecol Pathol 2003;22:404–6.

47. Hatch EE, Hoover RN, Herbst AL, et al. Incidence of cervical dysplasia in DES-exposed daughters: update and long-term follow-up of the DESAD cohort. In: DES research update 1999: Current knowledge, future directions. Bethesda, Maryland: National Institutes of Health; 1999:8.

48. Hatch EE, Herbst AL, Hoover RN, et al. Incidence of squamous neoplasia of the cervix and vagina in women exposed prenatally to diethylstilbestrol (United States). Cancer Causes Control 2001;12:837–45.

49. Hatch EE, Palmer JR, TitusErnstoff L, et al. Cancer risk in women exposed to diethylstilbestrol in utero. JAMA 1998;280:630–4.

50. Hatch EE, Palmer JR, TitusErnstoff L, et al. Cancer risk in women exposed to diethylstilbestrol in utero. In: DES research update 1999: Current knowledge, future directions. Bethesda, Maryland: National Institutes of Health; 1999:7.

51. Hatch K. Colposcopy of vaginal and vulvar human papillomavirus and adjacent sites. Obstet Gynecol Clin North Am 1993;20:203–15.

52. Hayashi M, Mori Y, Takagi Y, Hoshimoto K, Ohkura T. Primary small cell neuroendocrine carcinoma of the vagina – marked effect of combination chemotherapy. A case report. Oncology 2000;58:300–4.

53. Hellman K, Silfversward C, Nilsson B, Hellstrom AC, Frankendal B, Pettersson F. Primary carcinoma of the vagina: factors influencing the age at diagnosis. The Radiumhemmet series 1956–96. Int J Gynecol Cancer 2004;14:491–501.

54. Herbst A. Problems of prenatal DES exposure. In: Herbst A, Mishell D, Stenchever M, Droegmuller W, eds. Comprehensive Gynecology. St Louis: Mosby-Year Book; 1992:409–23.

55. Herbst AL, Anderson S, Hubby MM, et al. Risk factors for the development of diethylstilbestrol-associated clear cell adenocarcinoma: a case-control study. Am J Obstet Gynecol 1986;154:814–22.

56. Hiroi H, Yasugi T, Matsumoto K, et al. Mucinous adenocarcinoma arising in a neovagina using the sigmoid colon thirty years after operation: a case report. J Surg Oncol 2001;77(1):61–4.

57. Horwitz RI, Viscoli CM, Merino M, Brennan TA, Flannery JT, Robboy SJ. Clear cell adenocarcinoma of the vagina and cervix: incidence, undetected disease, and diethylstilbestrol. J Clin Epidemiol 1988;41:593–7.

58. Iversen UM. Two cases of benign vaginal rhabdomyoma. APMIS 1996;104:575–8.

59. Jefferies JA, Robboy SJ, O'Brien PC, et al. Structural anomalies of the cervix and vagina in women enrolled in the Diethylstilbestrol Adenosis (DESAD) Project. Am J Obstet Gynecol 1984;148:59–66.

60. Jobling TW, Shepherd JH, Lowe DG. Squamous cell carcinoma arising in a human amnion neovagina. J Gynecol Surg 1993;9:53–7.

61. Kalogirou D, Antoniou G, Karakitsos P, Botsis D, Papadimitriou A, Giannikos L. Vaginal intraepithelial neoplasia (VAIN) following hysterectomy in patients treated for carcinoma in situ of the cervix. Eur J Gynaecol Oncol 1997;18:188–91.

62. Kaufman RH, Adam E, Noller K, Irwin JF, Gray M. Upper genital tract changes and infertility in diethylstilbestrol-exposed women. Am J Obstet Gynecol 1986;154:1312–18.

63. Kent HL. Epidemiology of vaginitis. Am J Obstet Gynecol 1991;165:1168–76.

64. Lagoo AS, Robboy SJ. Lymphoma of the female genital tract: current status. Int J Gynecol Pathol 2006;25(1):1–21.

65. Leminen A, Forss M, Lehtvirta P. Therapeutic and prognostic considerations in primary carcinoma of the vagina. Acta Obstet Gynecol Scand 1995;74:379–83.

66. Leuschner I, Harms D, Mattke A, Koscielniak E, Treuner J. Rhabdomyosarcoma of the urinary bladder and vagina: a clinicopathologic study with emphasis on recurrent disease: a report from the Kiel Pediatric Tumor Registry and the German CWS Study. Am J Surg Pathol 2001;25:856–64.

67. Li H, Heller DS, Sama J, Bolanowski PJ, Anderson J. Basaloid squamous cell carcinoma of the vagina metastasizing to the lung – a case report. J Reprod Med 2000;45:841–3.

68. Li SY, Qayyum A, Coakley FV, Hricak H. Association of renal agenesis and mullerian duct anomalies. J Comput Assist Technol 2000;24:829–34.

69. Liang CC, Chang SD, Soong YK. Long-term follow-up of women who underwent surgical correction for imperforate hymen. Arch Gynecol Obstet 2003;269:5–8.

70. Lloyd J, Evans DJ, Flanagan AM. Extension of extramammary Paget disease of the vulva to the cervix. J Clin Pathol 1999;52:538–40.

71. Lopes LF, Chazan R, Sredni ST, deCamargo B. Endodermal sinus tumor of the vagina in children. Med Ped Oncol 1999;32:377–80.

72. Mann S, Russell P, Wills EJ, Watson GF, Atkinson K. Benign vaginal mesenchymoma showing mature skeletal muscle, smooth muscle and fatty differentiation. Report of a case. Int J Surg Pathol 1996;4:49–54.

73. MatiasGuiu X, Lerma E, Prat J. Clear cell tumors of the female genital tract. Semin Diagn Pathol 1997;14:233–9.

74. McAdam JA, Stewart F, Reid R. Vaginal epithelioid angiosarcoma. J Clin Pathol 1998;51:928–30.

75. McCluggage WG. A review and update of morphologically bland vulvovaginal mesenchymal lesions. Int J Gynecol Pathol 2005;24:26–38.

76. McCluggage WG, White RG. Angiomyofibroblastoma of the vagina. J Clin Pathol 2000;53:803–6.

77. McGregor JA, French JI. Bacterial vaginosis in pregnancy. Obstet Gynecol Surv 2000;55(5 Suppl):S1–S19.

78. McNall RY, Nowicki PD, Miller B, Billups CA, Liu T, Daw NC. Adenocarcinoma of the cervix and vagina in pediatric patients. Pediatr Blood Cancer 2004;43:289–94.

79. Michal M, Rokyta Z, Mejchar B, Pelikan K, Kummel M, Mukensnabl P. Prolapse of the fallopian tube after hysterectomy associated with exuberant angiomyofibroblastic stroma response: a diagnostic pitfall. Virchows Arch 2000;437:436–9.

80. Miner TJ, Delgado R, Zeisler J, et al. Primary vaginal melanoma: a critical analysis of therapy. Ann Surg Oncol 2004;11:34–9.

81. Mirhashemi R, Kratz A, Weir MM, Molpus KL, Goodman AK. Vaginal small cell carcinoma mimicking a Bartholin's gland abscess: a case report. Gynecol Oncol 1998;68:297–300.

82. Mizia K, Bennett MJ, Dudley J, Morrisey J. Mullerian dysgenesis: a review of recent outcomes at Royal Hospital for Women. Aust N Z J Obstet Gynecol 2006;46:29–31.

83. Moore-Maxwell CA, Robboy SJ. Mucinous adenocarcinoma arising in rectovaginal fistulas associated with Crohn's disease. Gynecol Oncol 2004;93:266–8.

84. Moore DH, Michael H, Furlin JJ, VonStein A. Adenoid basal carcinoma of the vagina. Int J Gynaecol Cancer 1998;8:261–3.

85. Murdoch F, Sharma R, Al-Nafussi A. Benign mixed tumor of the vagina: case report with expanded immunohistochemical profile. Int J Gynaecol Cancer 2003;13:543–7.

86. Newton WA, Jr, Gehan EA, Webber BL, et al. Classification of rhabdomyosarcomas and related sarcomas. Pathologic aspects and proposal for a new classification – an Intergroup Rhabdomyosarcoma Study. Cancer 1995;76:1073–85.

87. Ngan HYS, Fisher C, Blake P, Shepherd JH. Vaginal sarcoma – the Royal Marsden experience. Int J Gynaecol Cancer 1994;4:337–41.

88. Nielsen AL, Lassen M, Nielsen IM, Medgyesi S. The fate of the split thickness skin graft in neovaginas. A pathologic study of 21 cases and a review of the literature. Int J Gynaecol Pathol 1988;7:173–81.

89. Nielsen GP, Oliva E, Young RH, Rosenberg AE, Dickersin GR, Scully RE. Alveolar soft-part sarcoma of the female genital tract: a report of nine cases and review of the literature. Int J Gynaecol Pathol 1995;14:283–92.

90. Noller KL. Cancer in DES-exposed offspring. In: NIH Workshop Long term effects of exposure to diethylstilbestrol (DES); 1992; Falls Church, Virginia: Department of Health and Human Services, USA; 1992:10–11.

91. Noller KL. Role of colposcopy in the examination of diethylstilbestrol-exposed women. Obstet Gynecol Clin North Am 1993;20:165–76.

92. Ockner DM, Sayadi H, Swanson PE, Ritter JH, Wick MR. Genital angiomyofibroblastoma: comparison with aggressive angiomyxoma and other myxoid neoplasms of skin and soft tissue. Am J Clin Pathol 1997;107:36–44.

93. Oguri H, Izumiya C, Maeda N, Fukaya T, Moriki T. A primary amelanotic melanoma of the vagina, diagnosed by immunohistochemical staining with HMB-45, which recurred as a pigmented melanoma. J Clin Pathol 2004;57:986–8.

94. Ostor AG, Fortune DW, Riley CB. Fibroepithelial polyps with atypical stromal cells (pseudosarcoma botryoides) of vulva and vagina: a report of 13 cases. Int J Gynaecol Pathol 1988;7:351–60.

95. Otton GR, Nicklin JL, Dickie GJ, et al. Early-stage vaginal carcinoma – an analysis of 70 patients. Int J Gynecol Cancer 2004;14:304–10.

96. Palefsky JM, Holly EA. Molecular virology and epidemiology of human papillomavirus and cervical cancer. Cancer Epidemiol Biomarkers Prev 1995;4:415–28.

97. Palmlund I, Apfel R, Buitendijk S, Cabau A, Forsberg J. Effects of diethylstilbestrol (DES) medication during pregnancy: report from a

symposium at the 10th international congress of ISPOG. J Psychosomat Obstet Gynecol 1993;14:71–89.

98. Patton DL, Thwin SS, Meier A, Hooton TM, Stapleton AE, Eschenbach DA. Epithelial cell layer thickness and immune cell populations in the normal human vagina at different stages of the menstrual cycle. Am J Obstet Gynecol 2000;183:967–73.

99. Pearl ML, Crombleholme WR, Green JR, Bottles K. Fibroepithelial polyps of the vagina in pregnancy. Am J Perinatol 1991;8:236–8.

100. Pittock ST, Babovic-Vuksanovic D, Lteif A. Mayer–Rokitansky–Kuster–Hauser anomaly and its associated malformations. Am J Med Genet A 2005;135:314–16.

101. Piver MS, Lele SB, Baker TR, Sandecki A. Cervical and vaginal cancer detection at a regional diethylstilbestrol (DES) screening clinic. Cancer Detect Prev 1988;11:197–202.

102. Proppe KH, Scully RE, Rosai J. Postoperative spindle cell nodules of genitourinary tract resembling sarcomas. A report of eight cases. Am J Surg Pathol 1984;8:101–8.

103. Rabinerson D, Avrech O, Kaplan B, Braslavsky D, Goldman GA, Neri A. Endometrioma of the vagina in menopause. Acta Obstet Gynecol Scand 1996;75:506–7.

104. Rendon-Maldonado JG, Espinosa-Cantellano M, Gonzalez-Robles A, Martinez-Palomo A. Trichomonas vaginalis: in vitro phagocytosis of lactobacilli, vaginal epithelial cells, leukocytes, and erythrocytes. Exp Parasitol 1998;89:241–50.

105. Resnick SD. Toxic shock syndrome: recent developments in pathogenesis. J Pediatr 1990;116:321–8.

106. Riva C, Fabbri A, Facco C, Tibiletti MG, Guglielmin P, Capella C. Primary serous papillary adenocarcinoma of the vagina: a case report. Int J Gynaecol Pathol 1997;16:286–90.

107. Robboy SJ. A hypothetic mechanism of diethylstilbestrol (DES)-induced anomalies in exposed progeny. Hum Pathol 1983;14:831–3.

108. Robboy SJ, Taguchi O, Cunha GR. Normal development of the human female reproductive tract and alterations resulting from experimental exposure to diethylstilbestrol. Hum Pathol 1982;13:190–8.

109. Robboy SJ, Hill EC, Sandberg EC, Czernobilsky B. Vaginal adenosis in women born prior to the diethylstilbestrol era. Hum Pathol 1986;17:488–92.

110. Robboy SJ, Young RH, Welch WR, et al. Atypical vaginal adenosis and cervical ectropion. Association with clear cell adenocarcinoma in diethylstilbestrol-exposed offspring. Cancer 1984;54:869–75.

111. Robboy SJ, Noller KL, O'Brien P, et al. Increased incidence of cervical and vaginal dysplasia in 3980 diethylstilbestrol-exposed young women. Experience of the National Collaborative Diethylstilbestrol Adenosis Project. JAMA 1984;252:2979–83.

112. Robboy SJ, Szyfelbein WM, Goellner JR, et al. Dysplasia and cytologic findings in 4589 young women enrolled in diethylstilbestrol-adenosis (DESAD) project. Am J Obstet Gynecol 1981;140:579–86.

113. Rose PG, Stoler MH, AbdulKarim FW. Papillary squamotransitional cell carcinoma of the vagina. Int J Gynaecol Pathol 1998;17:372–5.

114. Ruggieri AM, Brody JM, Curhan RP. Vaginal leiomyoma – a case report with imaging findings. J Reprod Med 1996;41:875–7.

115. Saad AJ, Donovan TM, Truong LD. Malakoplakia of the vagina diagnosed by fine-needle aspiration cytology. Diagn Cytopathol 1993;9:559–61.

116. Sangwan K, Khosla AH, Hazra PC. Leiomyoma of the vagina. Aust N Z J Obstet Gynecol 1996;36:494–5.

117. Saropala N, Ingsirorat C. Conservative treatment of vaginal vault granulation tissue following total abdominal hysterectomy. Int J Gynaecol Obstet 1998;62:55–8.

118. Schrager LK, Friedland GH, Maude D, et al. Cervical and vaginal squamous cell abnormalities in women infected with human immunodeficiency virus. J Acquir Immune Defic Syndr Hum Retrovirol 1989;2:570–5.

119. Senekjian EK, Hubby M, Bell DA, et al. Clear cell adenocarcinoma (CCA) of the vagina and cervix in association with pregnancy. Gynecol Oncol 1986;24:207–19.

120. Sharp GB, Cole P. Vaginal bleeding and diethylstilbestrol exposure during pregnancy: relationship to genital tract clear cell adenocarcinoma and vaginal adenosis in daughters. Am J Obstet Gynecol 1990;162:994–1001.

121. Sharp GB, Cole P. Identification of risk factors for diethylstilbestrol-associated clear cell adenocarcinoma of the vagina: similarities to endometrial cancer. Am J Epidemiol 1991;134:1316–24.

122. Sharp GB, Cole P, Anderson D, Herbst AL. Clear cell adenocarcinoma of the lower genital tract. Correlation of mother's recall of diethylstilbestrol history with obstetrical records. Cancer 1990;66:2215–20.

123. Sherer DM, Hellmann M, Gorelick C, et al. Transvaginal sonographic findings associated with emphysematous vaginitis at 32 weeks' gestation. J Ultrasound Med 2006;25:515–17.

124. Shibata R, Umezawa A, Takehara K, Aoki D, Nozawa S, Hata J. Primary carcinosarcoma of the vagina. Pathol Int 2003;53:106–10.

125. Shochat S, Andrassy RJ, Ransley P. Progress in the surgical management of vaginal rhabdomyosarcoma: a 25-year review from the Intergroup Rhabdomyosarcoma Study Group – Discussion. J Pediatr Surg 1999;34:734–5.

126. Sillman FH, Fruchter RG, Chen YS, Camilien L, Sedlis A, McTigue E. Vaginal intraepithelial neoplasia: risk factors for persistence, recurrence, and invasion and its management. Am J Obstet Gynecol 1997;176:93–9.

127. Singer A, Mansell ME, Neill S. Symptomatic vaginal adenosis. Br J Obstet Gynaecol 1994;101:633–5.

128. Siu SSN, Tam WH, To KF, Yuen PM. Is vaginal dermoid cyst a rare occurrence or a misnomer? A case report and review of the literature. Ultrasound Obstet Gynecol 2003;21:404–6.

129. Smotkin D. Human papillomavirus infection of the vagina. Clin Obstet Gynecol 1993;36:188–94.

130. Sobel JD. Vaginitis. N Engl J Med 1997;337:1896–903.

131. Srodon M, Stoler MH, Baber GB, Kurman RJ. The distribution of low and high-risk HPV types in vulvar and vaginal intraepithelial neoplasia (VIN and VaIN). Am J Surg Pathol 2006;30:1513–18.

132. Stock RG, Chen ASJ, Seski J. A 30-year experience in the management of primary carcinoma of the vagina: analysis of prognostic factors and treatment modalities. Gynecol Oncol 1995;56:45–52.

133. Stoler MH, Srodon M, Baber GB, Kurman RJ. The frequency and biology of multiple HPV infection in vulvar neoplasia. Mod Pathol 2005;18(Suppl):205A.

134. Sugase M, Matsukura T. Distinct manifestations of human papillomaviruses in the vagina. Int J Cancer 1997;72:412–15.

135. Swidsinski A, Mendling W, Loening-Baucke V, et al. Adherent biofilms in bacterial vaginosis. Obstet Gynecol 2005;106(5 Pt 1):1013–23.

136. Tai LH, Tavassoli FA. Endometrial polyps with atypical (bizarre) stromal cells. Am J Surg Pathol 2002;26:505–9.

137. Terada S, Suzuki N, Tomimatsu N, Akasofu K. Vaginal schwannoma. Arch Gynecol Obstet 1992;251:203–6.

138. Thorsen P, Jensen IP, Jeune B, et al. Few microorganisms associated with bacterial vaginosis may constitute the pathologic core: a population-based microbiologic study among 3596 pregnant women. Am J Obstet Gynecol 1998;178:580–7.

139. Tokyol C, Aktepe OC, Cevrioglu AS, Altindis M, Dilek FH. Bacterial vaginosis: comparison of Pap smear and microbiological test results. Mod Pathol 2004;17:857–60.

140. Torne A, Pahisa J, Castelo BC, Fabregues F, Mallofre C, Iglesias X. Solitary vaginal metastasis as a presenting form of unsuspected renal adenocarcinoma. Gynecol Oncol 1994;52:260–3.

141. Trimble EL. The NIH consensus conference on ovarian cancer: screening, treatment, and follow-up. Gynecol Oncol 1994;55(3 Part 2):S1–S3.

142. Trimble EL, Rubinstein LV, Menck HR, Hankey BF, Kosary C, Giusti RM. Vaginal clear cell adenocarcinoma in the United States. Gynecol Oncol 1996;61:113–15.

143. Troisi R, Hatch EE, Titus-Ernstoff L, et al. Cancer risk in women prenatally exposed to diethylstilbestrol. Int J Cancer 2007;121:356–60.

144. van Dam P, Sonnemans H, van Dam PJ, Verkinderen L, Dirix LY. Sentinel node detection in patients with vaginal carcinoma. Gynecol Oncol 2004;92:89–92.

145. Vang R, Barner R, Wheeler DT, Strauss BL. Immunohistochemical staining for Ki-67 and p53 helps distinguish endometrial Arias-Stella reaction from high-grade carcinoma, including clear cell carcinoma. Int J Gynecol Pathol 2004;23:223–33.

146. Vang R, Medeiros LJ, Silva EG, Gershenson DM, Deavers M. Non-Hodgkin's lymphoma involving the vagina – a clinicopathologic analysis of 14 patients. Am J Surg Pathol 2000;24:719–24.

147. Varela CL, Delariva ML, Pelea CL. Vaginal rhabdomyomas. Int J Gynelcol Obstet 1994;47:169–70.

148. Waggoner SE, Mittendorf R, Biney N, Anderson D, Herbst AL. Influence of in utero diethylstilbestrol exposure on the prognosis and biologic behavior of vaginal clear-cell adenocarcinoma. Gynecol Oncol 1994;55:238–44.

149. Waggoner SE, Anderson SM, Vaneyck S, Fuller J, Luce MC, Herbst AL. Human papillomavirus detection and p53 expression in clear-cell adenocarcinoma of the vagina and cervix. Obstet Gynecol 1994;84:404–8.

150. Wall EM, Stone B, Klein BL. Imperforate hymen: a not-so-hidden diagnosis. Am J Emerg Med 2003;21:249–50.

151. Wierrani F, Zoubek A, Grin W, et al. Botryoid sarcoma of the infant vagina – a soft tissue sarcoma with a high probability of cure. Geburt Frauenheilk 1996;56:441–2.

152. Wright RG, Buntine DW, Forbes KL. Recurrent benign mixed tumor of the vagina. Gynecol Oncol 1991;40:84–6.

153. Yaghsezian H, Palazzo JP, Finkel GC, Carlson JA, Talerman A. Primary vaginal adenocarcinoma of the intestinal type associated with adenosis. Gynecol Oncol 1992;45:62–5.

154. Yeh AM, Marcus RBJ, Amdur RJ, Morgan LS, Million RR. Patterns of failure in squamous cell carcinoma of the vagina treated with definitive radiotherapy alone: What is the appropriate treatment volume? Int J Cancer 2001;96(Suppl):109–16.

155. Yoshinaga K, Akahira JI, Niikura H, et al. A case of primary mucosa-associated lymphoid tissue lymphoma of the vagina. Hum Pathol 2004;35:1164–6.

Cervical benign and non-neoplastic conditions

Anais Malpica   Stanley J. Robboy

6

NORMAL STRUCTURE

ANATOMY

The cervix is the lower part of the uterus. A fibromuscular junction, usually referred to as the internal cervical os, marks the junction between the muscular corpus and the predominantly fibrous cervix. The cervix projects into the vagina at the vaginal vault and has supravaginal and vaginal portions of approximately equal lengths. The vaginal mucosa is continuous with that of the cervix and the folds formed by the reflections of this mucosa at the front, back and sides of the cervix are known as the vaginal fornices. The cervix is roughly cylindrical and is about 3 cm long and 2.5 cm in diameter, although the exact dimensions and shape vary considerably, depending largely on the parity of the woman. The multiparous cervix is larger and more bulbous than the nulliparous and has an external os, which is transverse and slit-like, rather than circular, changes that are the result of the increase in size and the ectropion that occurs in pregnancy and the lacerations that happen during vaginal delivery.

The cervical canal connects the uterine cavity to the vagina and it is flattened from front to back. The external os is a rather imprecise landmark, indicating the point at which the cervical canal opens into the vagina. Tissue that lies outside the external os, on the vaginal portion of the cervix, is referred to as ecto-cervix or exocervix. That located above the external os, within the canal, is endocervix (Figures 6.1 and 6.2). While strictly incorrect, many histopathologists use these terms to describe the type of tissue found rather than its position. Thus, a biopsy consisting of stroma, glandular surface epithelium and crypts may be described as endocervical, even though the material may come from a position on the vaginal portion of the cervix, well outside the external os. Loose terminology, though often sanctioned through usage, may be misleading to the clinician. It is important that the underlying anatomic relationships are understood.

The epithelium covering the cervix is initially of two types that are laid down during embryologic development:

- original (or native) squamous epithelium
- columnar epithelium.

ORIGINAL (NATIVE) SQUAMOUS EPITHELIUM

The squamous epithelium is stratified and non-keratinizing. It is under the influence of ovarian hormones just as is the vaginal epithelium, although the changes in response to hormonal stimuli are less marked than those encountered in the vagina. The normal appearance in a woman of reproductive age is shown in Figure 6.3.

There is a more or less well defined layer of basal cells, which have a relatively high nuclear:cytoplasmic ratio, and is usually only one cell thick. The nuclei are slightly oval and oriented vertically, giving a so-called 'picket-fence' appearance; this is an important histologic marker of 'normality' in the squamous epithelium. Lying above this is a layer, four or five cells thick, of parabasal cells, also with large nuclei and sparse, dense cytoplasm. Maturation progresses to form the intermediate zone, in which the cells begin to flatten out. The nuclei of these cells are smaller and darker than those of the parabasal layer, with considerably more cytoplasm. Glycogen, demonstrable in the cytoplasm of the intermediate cells, may take on a characteristic pattern described as 'basket-weave' (Figure 6.4). The superficial cells have pyknotic nuclei, from which all nuclear detail is lost. The cytoplasm appears, in sections, as a narrow, compressed band of slightly eosinophilic material.

In describing both normal and abnormal squamous epithelium, the terms 'differentiation', 'maturation' and 'stratification' are frequently used. These terms are closely interrelated in meaning, but are not quite synonymous.

Terminology

Differentiation   Differentiation, in this context, refers to the process in which the squamous cells become fully functional as a flattened, protective layer. In the skin, which is exposed to the external environment, full differentiation involves keratinization by way of a granular layer, but in the normal cervix, where the surroundings are moist, differentiation does not involve keratinization. The epithelium is said to be 'cornified' and no granular layer is present. In normal epithelium, maturation and differentiation are virtually synonymous, i.e., the cells differentiate as they mature. In abnormal epithelium, in common with other premalignant and malignant states, the term 'differentiation' relates to the degree of morphologic and functional similarity between abnormal and normal cells at all stages of maturation. Therefore, the equivalence of 'differentiation' with 'maturation' diminishes as the epithelium becomes more abnormal.

Maturation   Maturation is closely related to differentiation in meaning, and characterizes the changes seen in cells as they reach the surface of normal squamous epithelium. Thus, a squamous cell that is mature is also well differentiated. An immature squamous cell should also show some degree of differentiation that enables it to be recognized as squamous in type.

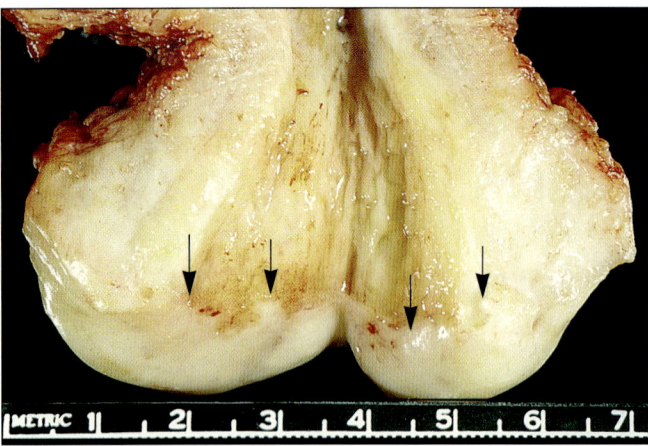

Fig. 6.1 Normal cervix. The specimen has been opened to show the rough appearance of the cervical canal in contrast to the smoothness of the ectocervix. The squamocolumnar junction (arrows) is clearly visible.

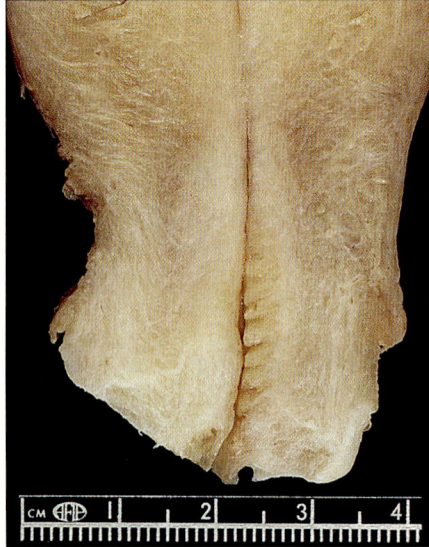

Fig. 6.2 Normal cervix. On cross-section, the normal cervix has serrated papillary folds that form the plicae of the endocervical canal.

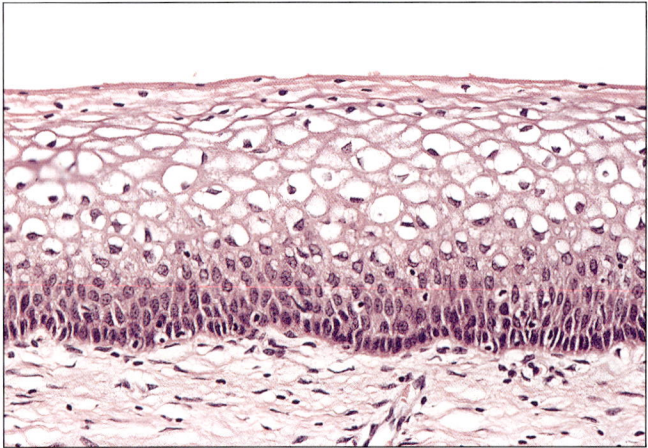

Fig. 6.3 Original squamous epithelium in a woman of reproductive age. Maturation of the squamous epithelium is obvious. The basal layer, parabasal zone, intermediate zone, and superficial layer can be clearly distinguished.

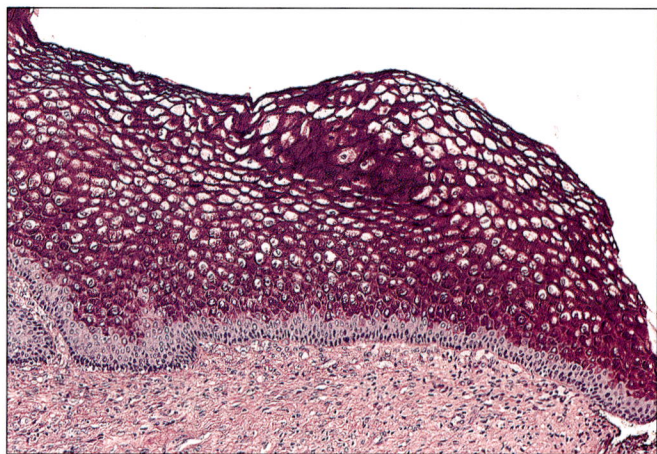

Fig. 6.4 Normal squamous epithelium. Staining with PAS shows the glycogen content of the mature and maturing epithelial cells. The 'basket-weave' pattern is clearly shown.

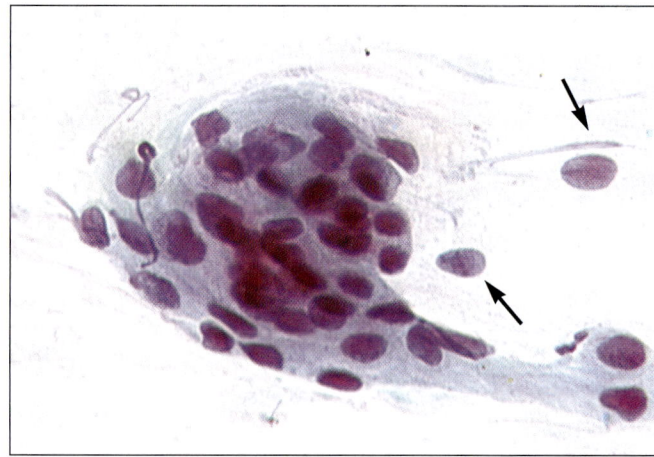

Fig. 6.5 Parabasal squamous cells in cervical smear. Cells with large nuclei with evenly distributed chromatin. Free nuclei (arrows) are present.

Stratification In squamous epithelium, stratification is a necessary and definitional consequence of maturation and differentiation. It refers to the way in which the epithelium is divided into layers of progressively more mature and flattened cells as the surface is reached.

Cytologic correlation

Parabasal squamous cells Parabasal cells exhibit a round shape and dense, green/blue cytoplasm. The large nucleus, which approximates 80–90% of the total cell size, is darkly stained with evenly distributed chromatin. Since these cells are immature squamous cells, they are generally seen in smears from postmenopausal women (Figure 6.5) or postpartum.

Intermediate squamous cells As the squamous epithelium responds to hormonal stimuli, the individual cells mature and the intermediate squamous cells reflect this change, both with an increase in the amount of cytoplasm in relation to the nucleus and in terms of total cell size. The cytoplasm becomes more transparent and tends to stain pale blue. Occasionally an area around the nucleus stains yellow, denoting the presence of glycogen. The nucleus is round with pale-staining, finely granular chromatin (Figure 6.6).

Superficial squamous cells With progressing maturation the superficial squamous cells predominate. The cells are large and polyhedral with angled edges. The pink-staining cytoplasm is virtually transparent, and the pyknotic nuclei are small and densely stained with little or no apparent chromatin structure (Figure 6.7). Keratinization does not occur normally in the cervix, although it is associated with several pathologic conditions.

HORMONAL INFLUENCES ON SQUAMOUS EPITHELIUM

After ovulation, when circulating progesterone counteracts the effect of estrogen on the epithelium, the cervical-vaginal smear shows a predominance of intermediate cells and a decreased number of superficial cells. However, this epithelium is often difficult to appreciate in histologic sections. After the menopause, when there is a deficiency of ovarian hormones, the squamous epithelium becomes much thinner, there being no maturation beyond the parabasal level. The thin epithelium is therefore composed entirely of parabasal cells and may appear quite uniform on section (Figure 6.8). The lack of a mature epithelium, coupled with the high nuclear:cytoplasmic ratio that the parabasal cells exhibit, can make the distinction from cervical intraepithelial neoplasia (CIN) difficult (see Chapter 8). However, the regular nuclear contour, the uniform chromatin pattern, and lack of conspicuous mitotic activity point to the correct diagnosis. The appearances before puberty are similar (Figure 6.9).

Cytologic correlation

The proportion of superficial to intermediate squamous cells varies throughout the menstrual cycle. Following menstruation and under the influence of estrogen, the superficial squamous cells predominate. At midcycle the smear may show very few intermediate squamous cells. The background shows few neutrophils and the cells are well separated and clearly displayed.

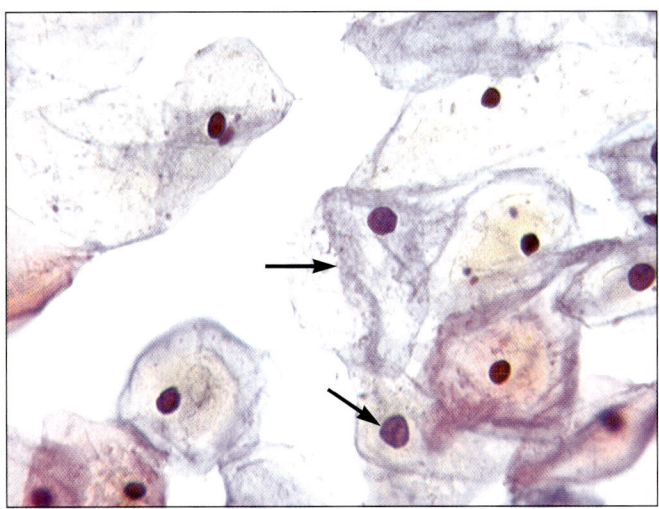

Fig. 6.6 Intermediate squamous cells. Cervical smear. Cells show larger nuclei (arrows) than the ones seen in the superficial cells.

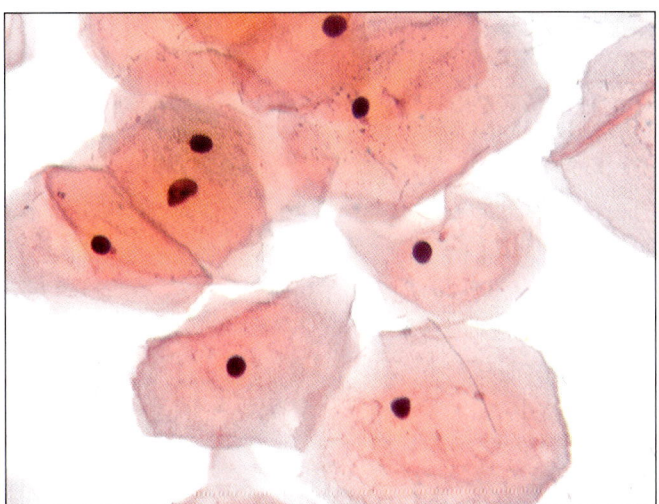

Fig. 6.7 Superficial squamous cells in cervical smear. Large cells with small pyknotic nuclei.

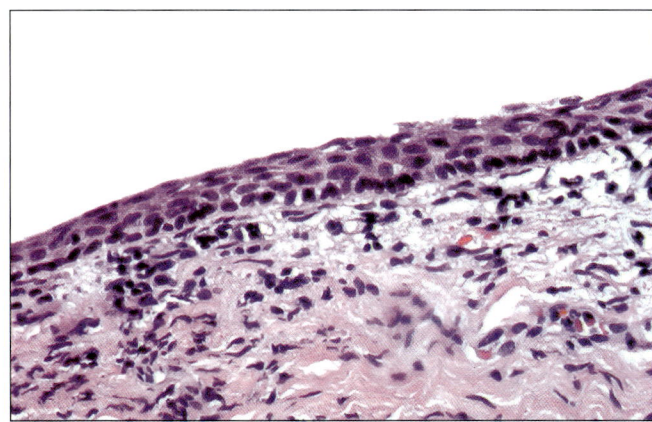

Fig. 6.8 Atrophic squamous epithelium. In a postmenopausal woman, the epithelium is thin and the cells do not mature beyond the parabasal stage.

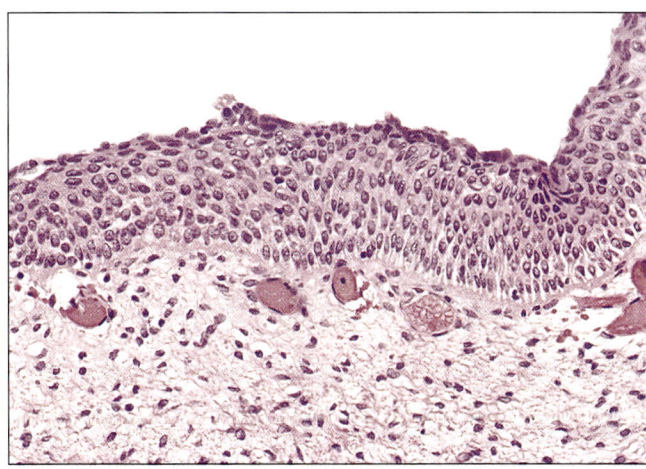

Fig. 6.9 Atrophic squamous epithelium in a 6-year-old girl.

This is the optimum time to take a cervical smear, particularly if the woman is in a cervical screening program.

Following ovulation and under the influence of progesterone, the intermediate cells dominate, forming sheets and clusters of overlapping cells with curled edges. Glycogen can be identified by the yellow staining often seen in the cytoplasm surrounding the nucleus. As this secretory phase continues, the clusters of cells become denser and more ragged looking, and there is an increase in background debris and neutrophils. Not infrequently this renders the smear inadequate for a reliable cytologic evaluation.

Postmenopausal atrophy The postmenopausal smear pattern shows a predominance of parabasal and occasional intermediate cell types with no cyclic changes (Figure 6.5). Endocervical cells are frequently not identified. Although a similar pattern is seen postpartum, squamous metaplasia and regenerative changes and endocervical cells are more frequently noted.

Endometrial cells Menstrual smears contain increased numbers of leukocytes and varying numbers of red blood cells and endometrial cells. The endometrial cells frequently are found in small darkly stained groups but can be seen in strings or as individual cells particularly in the late menstrual phase (Figure 6.10). Endometrial cells approximate the size of a neutrophil, with darkly stained coarse chromatin. The nuclei, although normally round, with darkly stained coarse chromatin often show some irregularity in shape, which may reflect degenerative change. The small amount of cytoplasm usually takes a basophilic stain. Endometrial cells should not normally be seen in a cervical smear after days 10–12 of the menstrual cycle. Not surprisingly, a menstrual smear will frequently be deemed inadequate for reliable assessment, since much cell detail can be obscured.

BASAL CELL HYPERPLASIA

In this condition the basal layer and adjacent part of the parabasal layer form an unusually well-defined stratum that is increased in thickness and conspicuous because of both nuclear enlargement and cytoplasmic basophilia (Figure 6.11). The oval basal and parabasal nuclei are usually oriented vertically and the 'picket-fence' appearance of a single layer is lost. Nuclear pleomorphism and hyperchromasia are absent. The cells above this stratum are mature and stratified. This condition is usually without import.

SQUAMOUS CELL HYPERPLASIA

The squamous epithelium of the ectocervix becomes thickened when there is uterovaginal prolapse. In these circumstances the epithelium shows acanthosis and there may be an irregularity of the epithelial–stromal junction resembling the rete ridges of the skin. Frequently, there is also (hyper) keratosis (Figure 6.12), which may or may not have a granular layer. These changes are the response to mechanical stimulation and take place in the absence of hormonal stimulation. Most prolapses are seen in women after the menopause. To further emphasize the similarity with skin, the presence of argyrophilic cells that resemble Merkel cells have been identified in the thickened, hyperkeratotic squamous epithelium associated with prolapse.

Some thickening of the squamous epithelium, often also with keratosis, is frequently seen when the cervix has healed following treatment by laser ablation, laser excision or large loop diathermy excision. These changes are usually focal and less marked than those seen with prolapse.

CERVICAL GLANDULAR EPITHELIUM

Columnar cells line the endocervical canal. The majority of these are tall, thin, mucus-secreting cells with basal nuclei,

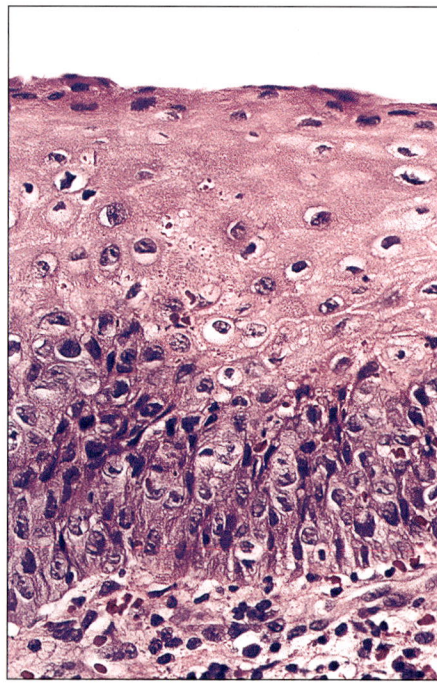

Fig. 6.11 Basal cell hyperplasia. The parabasal and basal zones are markedly expanded in an epithelium that is also somewhat thickened. The picket fence appearance of the basal layer is lost. The more superficial epithelium is glycogen-poor, but in some cases may be fully mature and exhibit abundant intracellular glycogen.

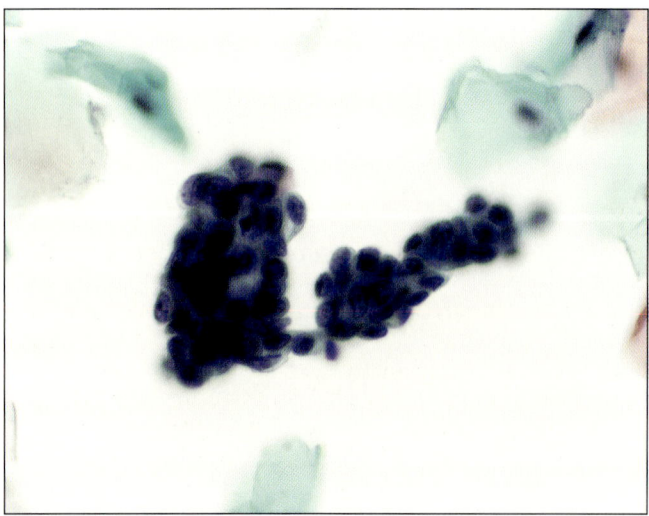

Fig. 6.10 Normal endometrial cells in cervical smear. Cells show coarse chromatin (arrows).

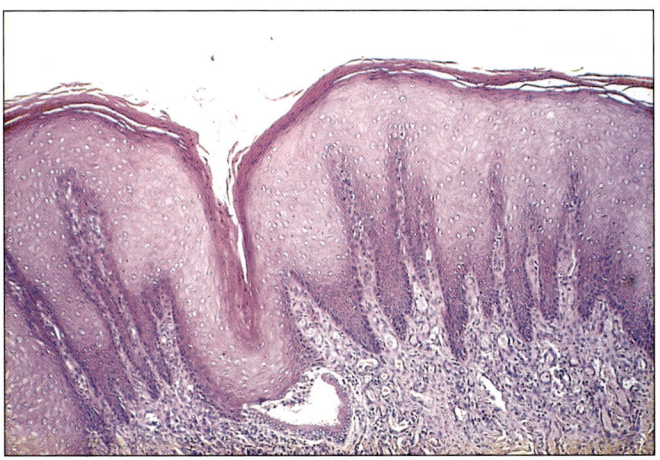

Fig. 6.12 Squamous hyperplasia. The epithelium is acanthotic with hyperkeratosis and parakeratosis.

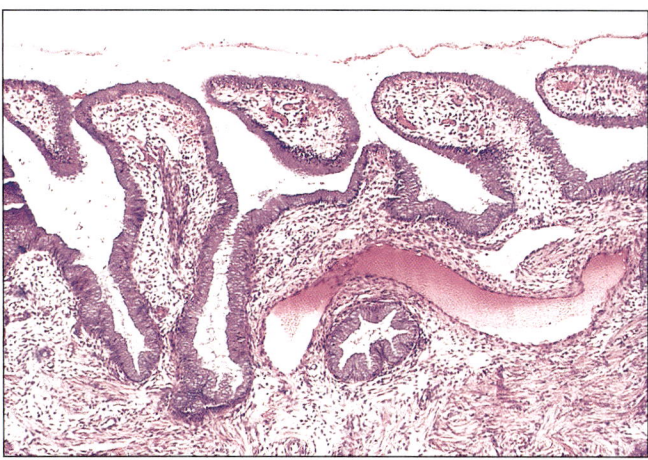

Fig. 6.14 Endocervical villi. The 'grape-like' villi seen on colposcopic examination are covered by normal columnar epithelium and contain a fibroconnective tissue core with blood vessels.

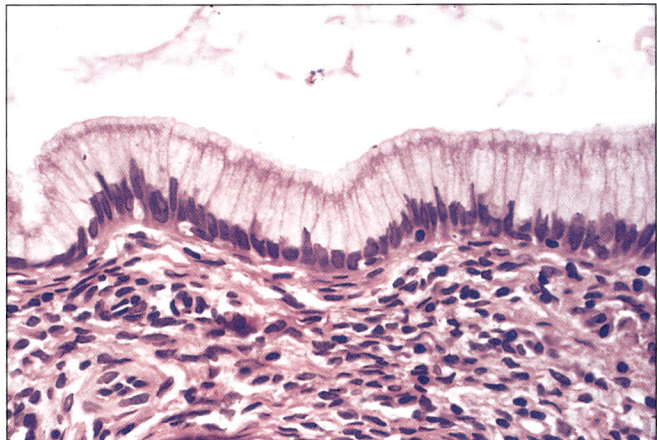

Fig. 6.13 Normal endocervical epithelium. The cells are columnar, contain mucin and the nuclei are basally located.

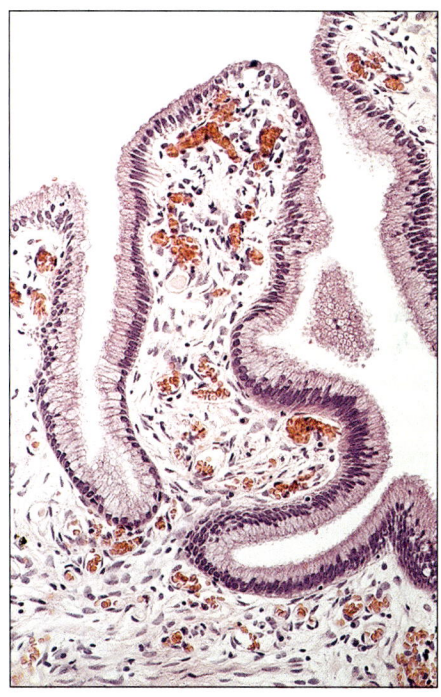

Fig. 6.15 Endocervical villi. The papillae exhibit a central fibrous core with blood vessels and a mantle of endocervical mucinous columnar cells.

presenting the familiar 'picket-fence' appearance (Figure 6.13). A minority are ciliated, a feature perhaps more readily appreciated by cytology. The epithelium takes the form of villous processes (Figures 6.14 and 6.15) that are seen most dramatically at colposcopy. Although these grape-like villi are characteristic of endocervical tissue colposcopically, they are not always easily seen, particularly in older women. They are, at all ages, more striking when adjacent to the squamocolumnar junction. A further complexity of the endocervical epithelium is the formation of crypts, which are tunnels lined by mucin-secreting epithelium passing into the substance of the cervix, usually to a depth of no more than 3 mm, but on occasion to as much as 1 cm (Figure 6.16). These structures are commonly referred to as 'glands' but as shown by serial sections they are a system of clefts that may become occluded and thereby form blind-ending tunnels. An awareness that these crypts are present is important when CIN affects the cervix (see Chapter 8). The columnar epithelium of the endocervix meets the squamous epithelium of the ectocervix at the squamocolumnar junction (Figure 6.17). The cytoplasm of the columnar cells stains with mucicarmine and alcian blue, and is reactive for various mucin antigens, e.g., MUC1, MUC4, and MUC5AC.[3]

Cytologic correlation

Frequently referred to as 'endocervical cells', glandular cells of endocervical origin are easily identified in cervical smears. They usually occur in sheets or small groups, although occasionally whole or partial fragments of villi are seen. The nuclei show a finely granular chromatin structure, sometimes with small nucleoli, and the cells have a cylindrical shape. The pale blue/gray cytoplasm is often vacuolated with poorly defined cell borders (Figure 6.18). Cilia can occasionally be seen with well-defined terminal plates (Figure 6.19). When viewed end on, the round nuclei are centrally placed within the cytoplasm and the close proximity of the cells resembles a honeycomb appearance. Endocervical cells are approximately four to five

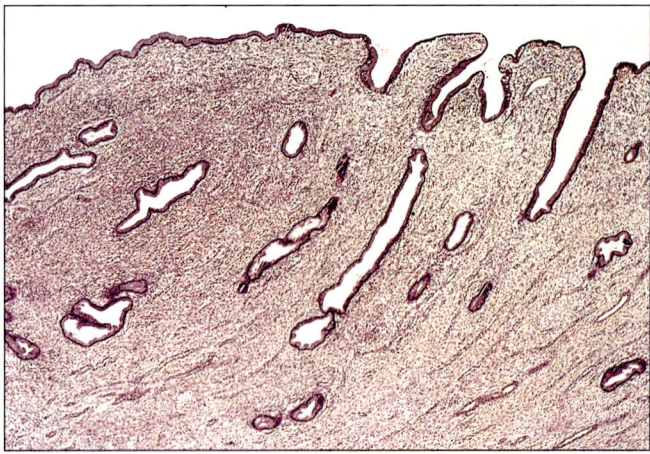

Fig. 6.16 Endocervical crypts. Tunnels that are lined by mucinous endocervical columnar epithelium penetrate into the endocervical fibromuscular stroma.

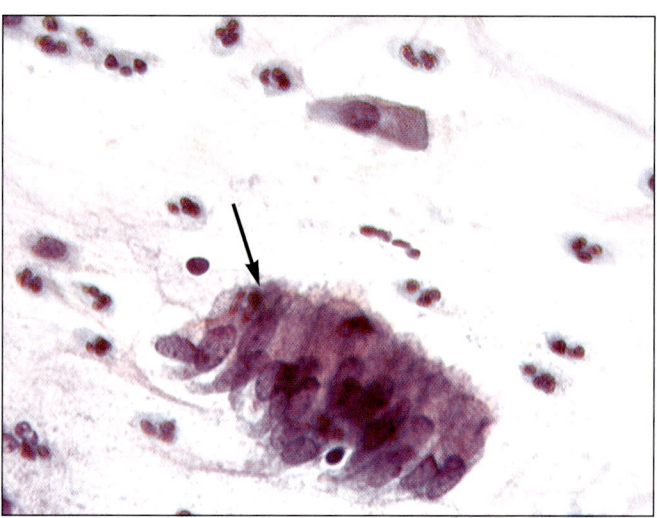

Fig. 6.19 Endocervical cells in cervical smear. Cilia are clearly seen (arrow).

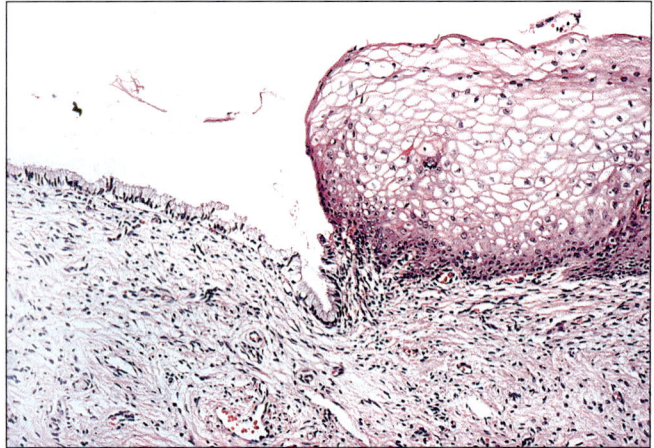

Fig. 6.17 Squamocolumnar junction. There is an abrupt transition from squamous to columnar epithelium.

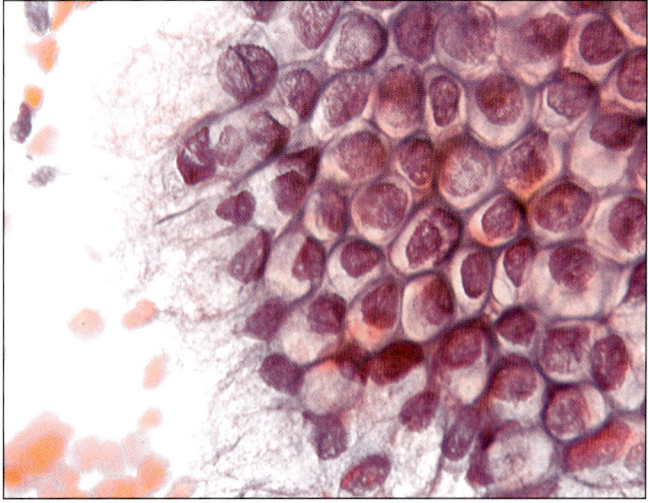

Fig. 6.18 Endocervical cells in cervical smear. Honeycomb arrangement of the cells and mucin in the cytoplasm.

times larger than endometrial cells, so misinterpretation is uncommon.

PHYSIOLOGIC CHANGES IN THE CERVIX AND THE FORMATION OF THE TRANSFORMATION ZONE

Fundamental to evolving cervical epithelial abnormalities is the formation of the transformation zone. It is in this area of the cervix that CIN and eventually invasive squamous cell carcinoma most commonly develop. The process is represented diagrammatically in Figures 6.20–6.23. Before puberty is reached, the squamocolumnar junction is situated at or near to the external cervical os (Figure 6.20). During adolescence the increasing levels of circulating ovarian hormones cause an increase in the bulk both of the body of the uterus and of the cervix, the latter growing proportionally more during this period. A consequence of this increased cervical size is its eversion outwards, rather more markedly anteriorly and posteriorly than at the sides. As a result of this change in shape, the endocervical epithelium, together with the underlying crypts and stroma, come to lie on the vaginal portion of the cervix (Figure 6.21). The 'ectopic' endocervical epithelium thus situated on the ectocervix is red and rough. It is red because the columnar epithelium is one cell layer thick and essentially transparent to the rich network of underlying blood vessels. It is rough because of the villous pattern of the endocervical tissue.

The 'transformation zone' is the area where the expected transformation to metaplastic squamous epithelium and abnormal transformation to CIN usually occurs (Figures 6.20 and 6.21). The process is a rolling outwards of the cervical stroma with its crypts and overlying epithelium. The concept of the 'healing erosion' is obsolete and should be replaced by an understanding of the formation and maturation of the transformation zone.

The process of eversion, which gives rise to the transformation zone (ectropion), occurs predominantly during adolescence. Eversion also occurs at other times, notably in the

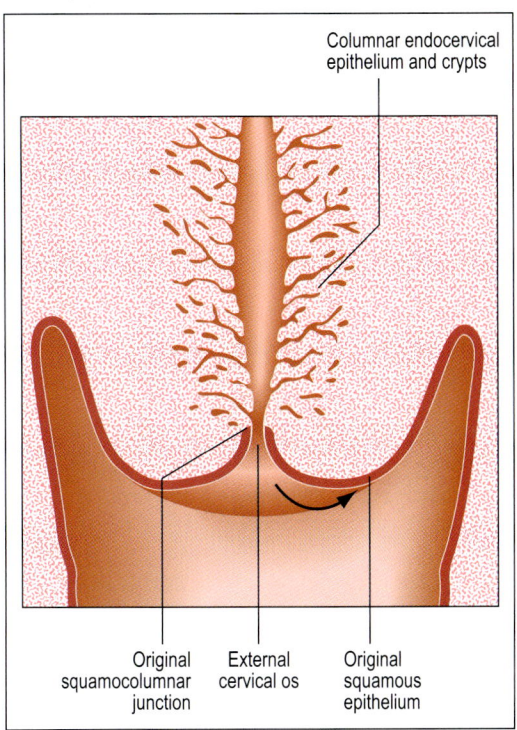

Fig. 6.20 Prepubertal cervix. The squamocolumnar junction is situated at the external cervical os. The arrow shows the direction of the movement that takes place as a result of the increase in bulk of the cervix during adolescence.

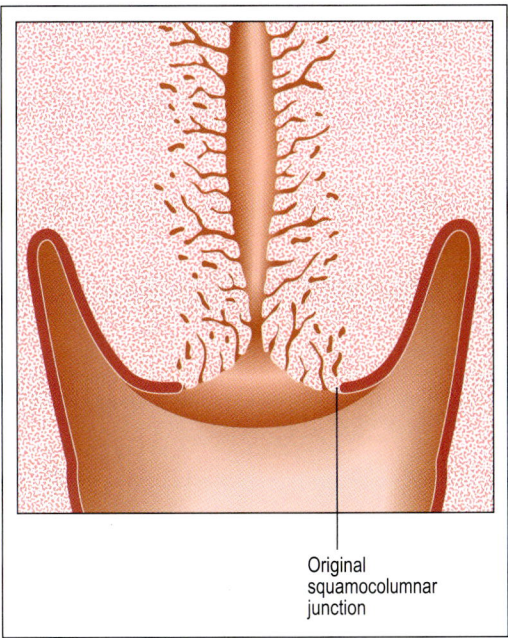

Fig. 6.21 The process of eversion. On completion, endocervical columnar tissue lies on the vaginal surface of the cervix and is exposed to the vaginal environment.

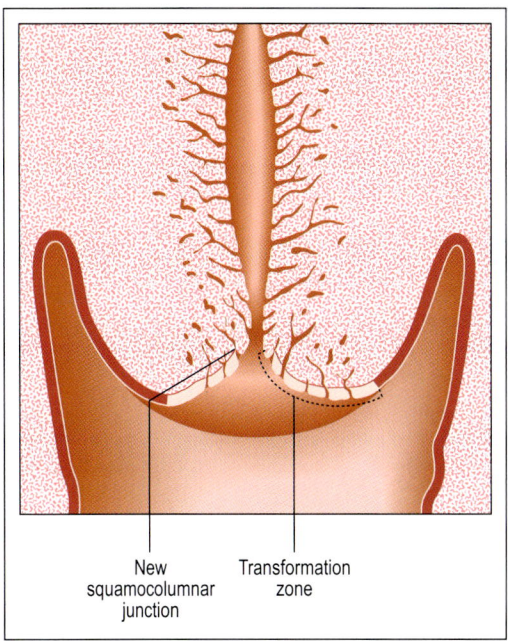

Fig. 6.22 Postadolescent cervix. The acidity of the vaginal environment is one of the factors that encourages squamous metaplastic change, replacing the exposed columnar epithelium with squamous epithelium.

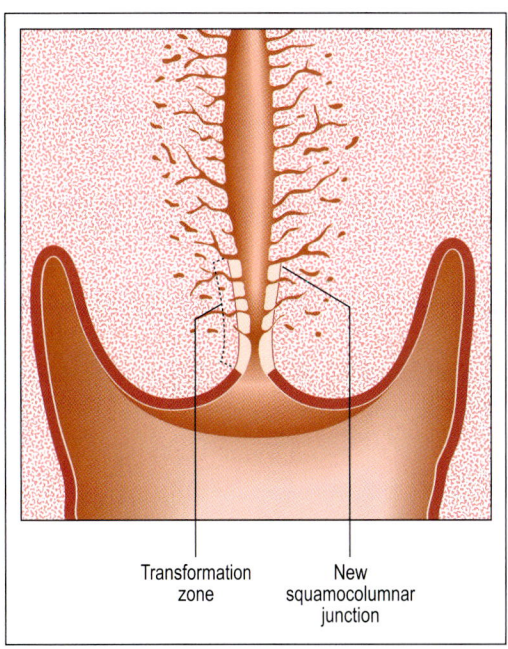

Fig. 6.23 Postmenopausal cervix. At this time, cervical inversion occurs. This phenomenon is the reverse of eversion, which was so important in adolescence. The transformation zone is now drawn into the cervical canal, often making it inaccessible to colposcopic examination.

neonatal period and with each pregnancy, after which the squamocolumnar junction regresses to approximately the same position as before that pregnancy. In addition, administration of the oral contraceptive pill contributes to the area of the transformation zone. The normal physiologic result of cervical eversion is replacement of the endocervical columnar epithelium by squamous epithelium through the process of squamous metaplasia (Figure 6.22). As the menopause approaches, this process reverses, so that the transformation zone tends to pass back into the cervical canal. This process is called 'inversion'. In the postmenopausal woman, the whole transformation zone, whether typical or atypical, may be situated inside the canal and so out of sight both to the naked eye and to colposcopy (Figure 6.23).

SQUAMOUS METAPLASIA

This mechanism of squamous metaplasia permits the much tougher and more resistant squamous epithelium to replace the highly specialized, fragile columnar cells of the endocervical epithelium normally present. There is nothing sinister about squamous metaplasia and its presence is not indicative of any increased risk for developing subsequent malignancy. The only relationship between squamous metaplasia and carcinoma is that the two conditions share the same early common path. Conditions must be right for squamous metaplasia before the precursors of squamous cell carcinoma can initiate their development in the cervix.

Squamous metaplasia is the process whereby an epithelium of squamous cells replaces the epithelium composed of mucinous columnar cells. The columnar cells do not, of course, transform into squamous cells, as mature epithelial cells of one type cannot change to differentiate and become another cell type. The stimulus to squamous metaplasia in the cervix appears to be the increased acidity of the vaginal environment compared with that of the cervical canal. Figures 6.24–6.35 show stages in the evolution of a metaplastic squamous epithe-

lium. Reserve cells are located beneath the columnar epithelial cells and they give origin to metaplastic squamous cells (Figures 6.24 and 6.25).

The origin of these reserve cells is unclear. They are normally present beneath the columnar epithelium and play an instrumental role in the replenishment of columnar cells lost by exfoliation. Studies that have analyzed cytokeratin expression in various types of cervical epithelium, including reserve cells, original squamous cells, metaplastic squamous cells, endocervical columnar cells, and neoplastic cells, have shown a close relationship in cytokeratin expression between reserve cells and endocervical columnar cells, supporting their origin from reserve cells.[52] Reserve cells first proliferate as a row of nondescript, small, round cells beneath the columnar epithelium, usually following the contour of the villi and often the more superficial crypts as well (Figure 6.26). Incomplete and immature squamous metaplasia may show columnar cells not totally replaced by squamous cells (Figure 6.27).

As the process continues, the squamous cells make up the whole thickness of the epithelium and start their differentiation to maturity, eventually rendering the metaplastic epithelium indistinguishable from normal, mature, glycogenated squamous epithelium. Metaplastic squamous epithelium may be

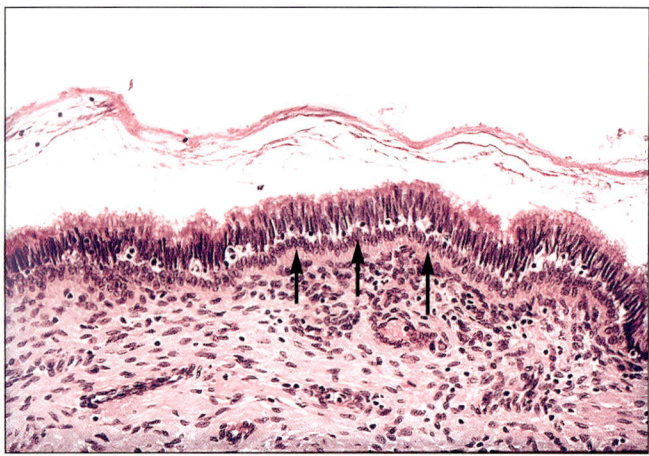

Fig. 6.24 Reserve cells. A single row of reserve cells (arrows) is present beneath the columnar epithelium.

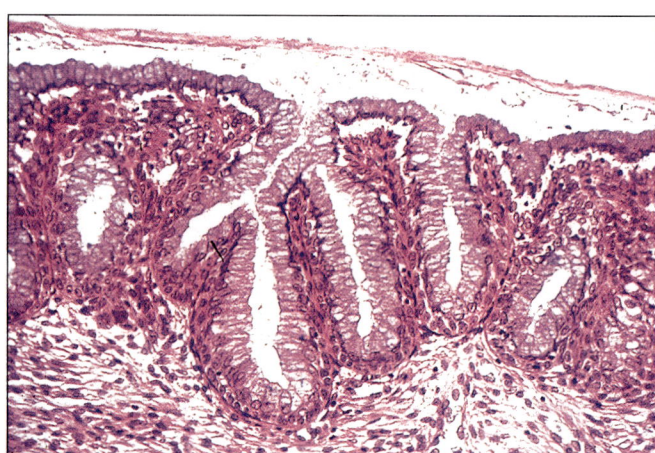

Fig. 6.26 Reserve cell proliferation. As the process continues, the reserve cells proliferate to form several layers beneath the still intact columnar epithelium. These are often sufficiently well differentiated to be recognized as squamous in nature.

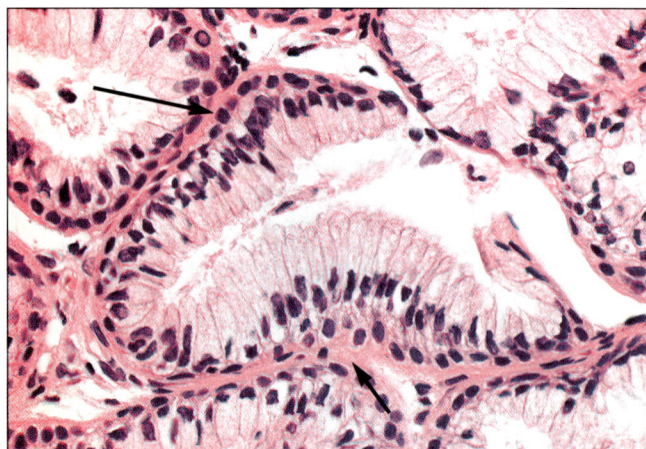

Fig. 6.25 Reserve cells. In these gland crypts, metaplastic squamous cells originate from undifferentiated reserve cells (arrows) proliferating immediately beneath mucinous columnar epithelium.

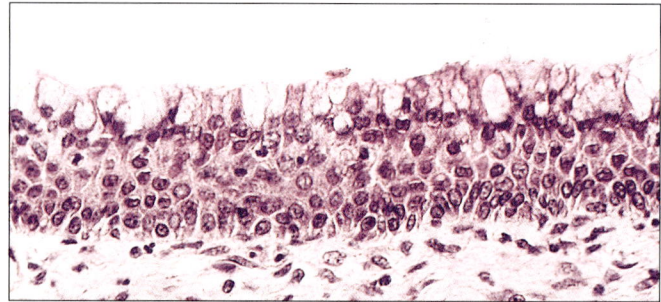

Fig. 6.27 Immature squamous metaplasia. As the process progresses, the cells acquire more abundant eosinophilic cytoplasm, stratified into multiple layers, and appear as immature squamous cells lacking intracytoplasmic glycogen. Commonly, a layer of mucinous epithelium lies superficial to the metaplastic cells.

mistaken for CIN. Figure 6.28 illustrates this dilemma. The epithelium is composed of squamous cells that are immature up to the surface of the epithelium, a feature that is often considered an important diagnostic criterion in the diagnosis of CIN regardless of grade. However, the metaplastic nuclei are regular and round or oval, each with a single, prominent nucleolus, in contrast to CIN where pleomorphism is the rule. The nuclei in metaplastic epithelium lack hyperchromasia and mitotic figures are few, confined to the basal layers, and not abnormal. In addition, normal immature squamous cells are unreactive for p16, which is a surrogate marker for integrated high-risk human papillomavirus (HPV) DNA and almost always seen in high grade CIN.[5,10,30,39]

In its final state (Figure 6.29), mature metaplastic squamous epithelium may be histologically indistinguishable from the original squamous epithelium. The only clue to its origin is the presence of underlying crypts with their mucinous epithelium (Figure 6.30). The original squamous epithelium overlaps the zone of cervical crypts very little, so that squamous epithelium found overlying crypts is almost certainly of metaplastic origin and histologically corresponding to the transformation zone.

Squamous metaplasia occurs most notably at the time of adolescence and during pregnancy but it may also be seen at other times throughout a woman's life. It is a process that may be arrested at any stage and, not uncommonly, areas of immature squamous metaplasia may be found in the cervix of women who entered the menopause long before.

Squamous metaplasia is an irreversible process so that when the transformation zone moves back into the cervical canal at the menopause, the squamous epithelium moves with it and the canal is then lined by squamous epithelium.

Although squamous metaplasia is a change that mainly involves the surface epithelium of the cervix, the crypts are also commonly affected (Figure 6.31). Sometimes the crypt

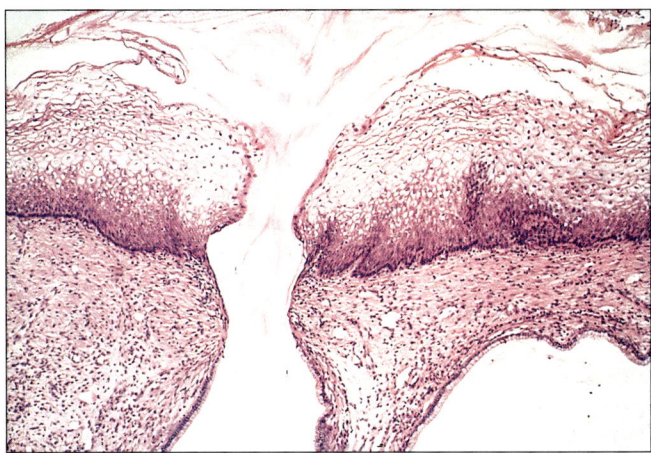

Fig. 6.30   Mature squamous metaplasia. The mature metaplastic squamous epithelium here overlies gland crypts, lined by columnar epithelium. Mucin is being discharged from a gland opening.

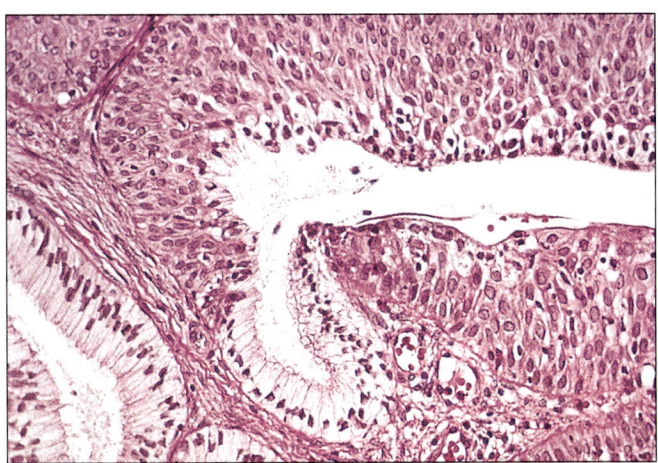

Fig. 6.28   Immature squamous metaplasia. The lack of differentiation and maturation cause confusion with intraepithelial neoplasia.

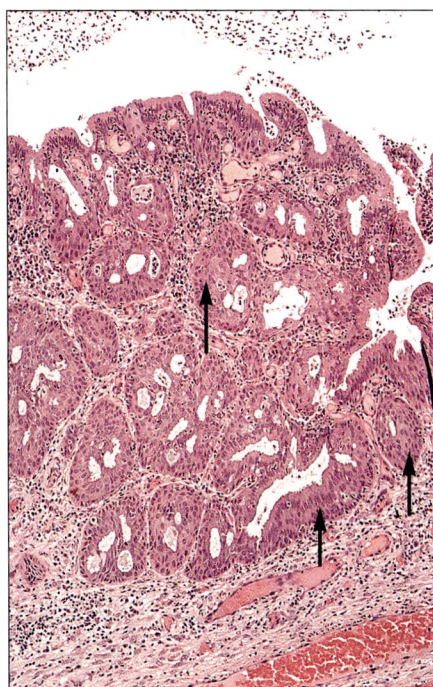

Fig. 6.31   Squamous metaplasia in an early stage exhibiting hyperplasia of the reserve cells and immature cells (arrows). At this stage, the glandular tissue is only partially replaced. As the metaplastic process continues, the amount of residual glandular tissue will decrease and then disappear.

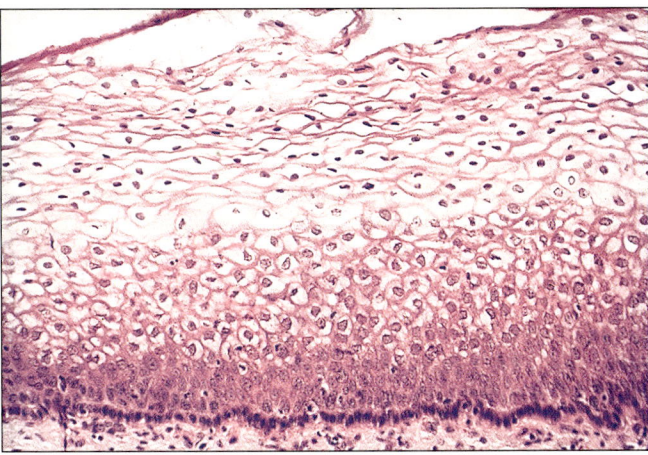

Fig. 6.29   Mature squamous metaplasia. The mature metaplastic squamous epithelium is virtually indistinguishable from original squamous epithelium.

involvement is sufficiently marked to impart an initial impression of invasive carcinoma. Attention to the cytologic appearances of the 'invasive' elements of the epithelium and the overlying epithelium should enable the distinction from carcinoma to be made without difficulty. In the cervix, the pathologist should be wary of entertaining a diagnosis of frank malignancy when there is a layer of mucinous columnar epithelium that overlies the questionably cancerous tissue.

Cytologic correlation

An important aspect associated with recognizing squamous metaplasia cytologically is that metaplastic cells exhibit a wide variety of appearances. Within a single cervical smear, both immature and mature cell types are frequently seen together with the whole spectrum of change (Figures 6.32–6.35). From a cytologic perspective, the terms 'immature' and 'mature' have a slightly different meaning from that used by histopathologists. Cells arising from a histologically mature metaplastic epithelium will be virtually indistinguishable from mature squamous cells. The term 'mature' as used by the cytologist describes cells that show some features of differentiation but still show some characteristics seen in immature metaplastic cells.

In the earliest phase of change, small round cells with a narrow rim of green-staining cytoplasm appear that closely resemble endocervical cells. The nuclei are often hyperchromatic with coarsely clumped chromatin. They are usually seen in small tight groups, a feature that makes recognition easier (Figure 6.32). The cells arising from an area of immature metaplasia are normally round in shape with large, darkly staining nuclei with a coarse chromatin pattern that may contain nucleoli or chromocenters. The cytoplasm is dense with a well-defined cell border and usually stains green (Figure 6.33 and 6.34). Differentiation from severe dysplasia should in most instances be straightforward by attention to the chromatin pattern. However, immature metaplasia remains a source of error in diagnosis.

Mature metaplasia As the metaplastic epithelium matures, the individual cells assume a squamoid appearance. The cyto-

plasm becomes more abundant and the cell appears oval or elongated. The cytoplasm may stain either blue or pink but it does not achieve the transparency of a mature squamous cell. Not infrequently the cytoplasm may be pulled out into tails and projections, the remnants of intercellular bridges. The nucleus becomes less dominant with a finer chromatin structure, but it always appears larger in comparison to the nucleus of a squamous cell (Figure 6.35).

THE CONGENITAL TRANSFORMATION ZONE

Definition

The congenital transformation zone (CTZ) is a common variant of squamous metaplasia that is found in a position peripheral to the acquired transformation zone. It appears as partially mature squamous epithelium that has an irregular, dentate junction with the stroma.

The CTZ is a variant of squamous metaplasia that exhibits incomplete maturation (Figure 6.36). The deeper layers show

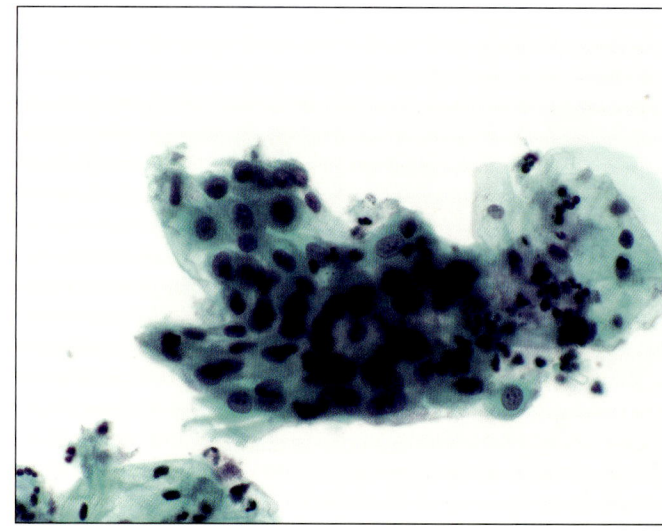

Fig. 6.33 Squamous metaplasia with darkly stained small nuclei within basophilic cytoplasm in cervical smear.

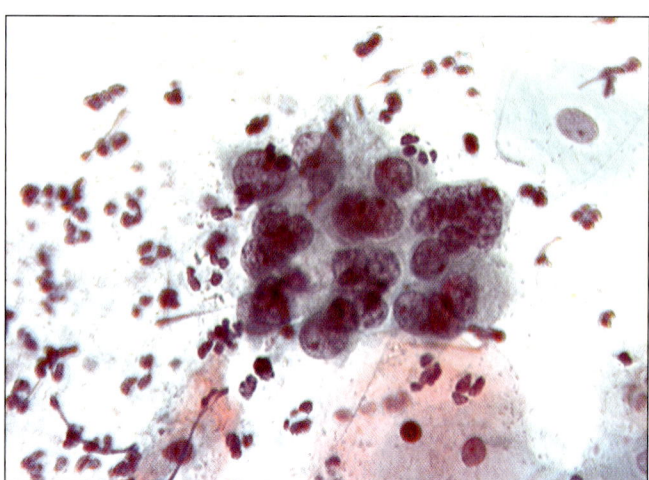

Fig. 6.32 Cervical smear. The cells, almost indistinguishable from endocervical cells, show vesicular and well-defined chromatin.

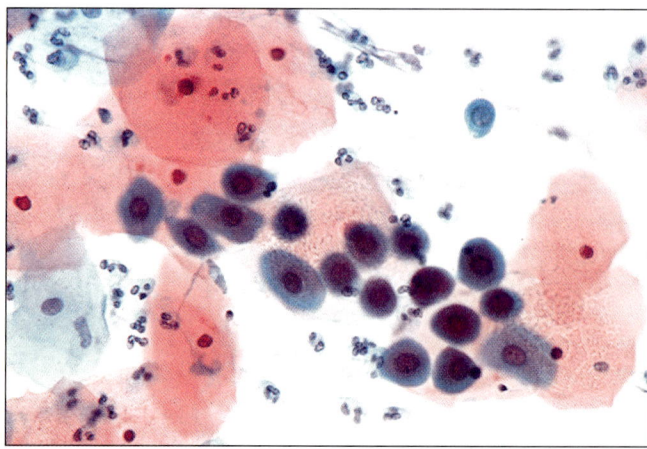

Fig. 6.34 Squamous metaplasia in cervical smear. Darkly stained, small nuclei within basophilic cytoplasm.

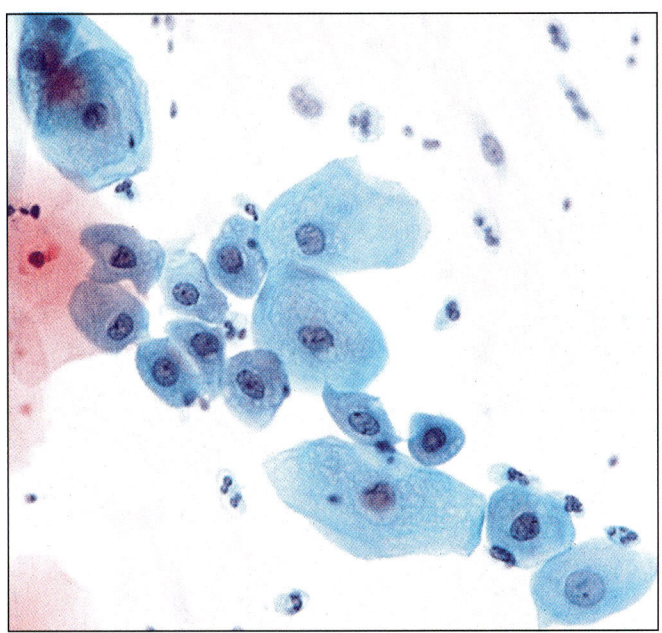

Fig. 6.35 Squamous metaplasia in cervical smear. Some cells show smaller nuclei with an increased amount of cytoplasm and a more squamoid appearance.

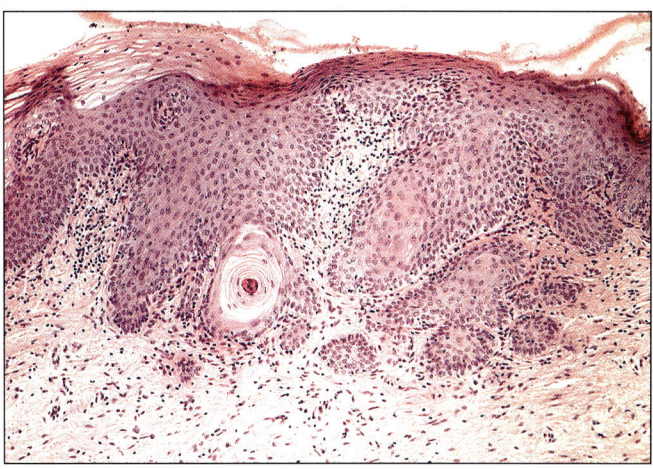

Fig. 6.37 Congenital transformation zone. An obvious keratin pearl is present deep within the epithelium.

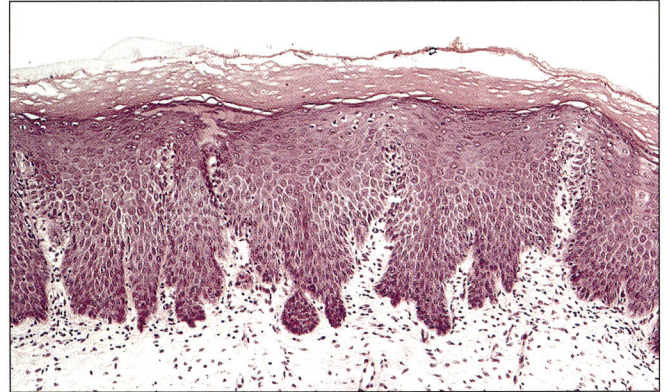

Fig. 6.36 Congenital transformation zone. The epithelium has many features of metaplastic squamous epithelium. Highly characteristic is the irregular, dentate outline of the epithelial–stromal junction.

the same features as a maturing squamous metaplasia. The nuclei are large but regular, with prominent nucleoli. There is minimal pleomorphism, and mitotic figures, which are infrequent, can usually be found with diligent searching. A layer of hyperkeratosis or parakeratosis is often present, and this layer, when thick, corresponds to the leukoplakia that is a characteristic colposcopic feature of the CTZ. One of the most striking histologic features is the pattern of its lower margin, the epithelial–stromal junction. This is always irregularly dentate, presenting an appearance akin to the rete ridges of the skin. Sometimes the tips of these epithelial incursions into the stroma appear detached from the overlying epithelium, so that they may give the impression of invasive buds. This impression may be heightened when the centers of the processes undergo differentiation, so that a whorl of keratin is seen in the center (Figure 6.37). Attention to the cytologic features will show that the CTZ is not an invasive tumor. It is unusual for there to be any stromal reaction to the CTZ. Another cardinal feature is

the absence of cytoplasmic glycogen (i.e., no 'basket-weave' pattern). This causes the epithelium to be iodine-negative on examination, further attracting the attention of the colposcopist.

HISTOGENESIS OF THE CONGENITAL TRANSFORMATION ZONE

The colposcopic and histologic appearances of the CTZ are identical to one of the appearances seen in diethylstilbestrol (DES) exposure. It is very likely that the mechanism by which the condition develops is the same. As detailed in Chapter 5, during embryogenesis transitional squamous epithelium replaces the glandular epithelium of müllerian type that originally lines the uterovaginal canal. The process starts caudally, from the urogenital sinus. In normal circumstances, this process of squamous change becomes complete, so that squamous epithelium covers the whole of the vagina and the ectocervix by the time of birth. If the cephalically directed conversion of müllerian to squamous epithelium is arrested for some reason, then some müllerian glandular epithelium remains. The müllerian epithelium, which is then known as adenosis in the vagina and ectropion on the ectocervix, most probably undergoes gradual replacement by squamous epithelium in later intrauterine life and perhaps also for some time after birth.

The product of this late squamous change is seen as the CTZ. The line of demarcation between the CTZ and the original squamous epithelium is the point at which the normal squamous development arrested. As in DES-exposed individuals, this is nearly always a single line. The process hardly ever seems to occur in a patchy fashion, which would leave areas of CTZ in the vagina.

The morphologic appearances of the CTZ through the light microscope suggest that it is more closely related to squamous metaplasia than to CIN, with minimal pleomorphism and few mitotic figures. However, the colposcopic features of the CTZ more closely resemble CIN than a benign condition, often showing an acetowhite color and mosaicism. The behavior of the CTZ, as seen in our own patients who have been followed for many years, has shown no progression towards malignancy, either to CIN or to invasive disease. The finding of a diploid chromosome content by DNA ploidy studies further negates its malignant potential. If the CTZ is the same as the similar-looking epithelial change found in DES-exposed offspring, gradual maturation over the years would be expected, finally becoming fully glycogenated and indistinguishable from mature metaplastic epithelium.

The appearances of the CTZ are often misinterpreted as being due to wart virus infection. Koilocytes may indeed be observed in an epithelium that shows the features of the CTZ, but this is a secondary phenomenon and the combination of cellular and architectural features is not the result of the virus.

Cytologic correlation

The cytologic features of cells arising from the CTZ are similar in appearance to those arising from squamous metaplasia, although on occasion there may be a predominance of cells showing cytoplasmic keratinization.

INFLAMMATORY (CERVICITIS) TO REGENERATIVE CHANGES

The term 'chronic cervicitis' often conveys differing images to the clinician, colposcopist, and pathologist. It describes the clinical appearance of a cervix that is red, inflamed and irregular on the surface. On colposcopic examination, the 'inflamed' cervix usually shows a wide transformation zone so that the changes are physiologic rather than pathologic. The transformation zone is red and rough, for the reasons described above, and the everted glandular epithelium produces excessive mucus production. The picture is further enhanced by retention cysts (nabothian cysts), which result when squamous metaplasia obliterates the outlet of cervical crypts. It is almost universal to find some degree of chronic inflammatory cell infiltrate, predominantly plasma cells with some lymphocytes, in the superficial cervical stroma, but it is only when the infiltrate becomes dense that it is justifiable to use the term 'chronic cervicitis'.

INFECTIVE CERVICITIS

The organisms most commonly responsible for active inflammation in the cervix include those that have been discussed in relation to the vagina: *Candida albicans*, *Trichomonas vaginalis*, *Neisseria gonorrhoeae*, *Gardnerella vaginalis*, and herpes simplex virus (HSV). To this list should be added *Chlamydia trachomatis*, human papillomavirus (HPV), and cytomegalovirus (CMV). Specific forms of chronic cervicitis that may be seen include tuberculous cervicitis and cervical involvement in schistosomiasis, particularly infestation by *Schistosoma hematobium*. The cervix may also be involved in syphilis, granuloma inguinale, and lymphogranuloma venereum.

A cervix that is acutely inflamed is swollen and red, often with a mucopurulent plug exuding from the external os. Histologically, acute cervicitis shows a dense infiltrate of neutrophils in the stroma. They also involve the columnar and the squamous epithelium, as well as the epithelium of the gland crypts. In severe cases, the columnar epithelium may be eroded and partially replaced by granulation tissue. These changes

result not only by infection with microorganisms but also from insults such as chemical irritation, copper-containing intrauterine contraceptive devices, inappropriate tampon use, pessaries, and the trauma of parturition or abortion.

True chronic cervicitis shows lymphocytes, histiocytes, and plasma cells in the cervical tissues. If the cells are present only in small or moderate numbers, their presence may represent the normal population of the cervix, as is seen in other organs. If the infiltrate is dense, with lymphoid follicles (Figure 6.38), particularly if there is an admixture of polymorphonuclear cells (Figure 6.39), the inflammation is active and is more likely to be pathologic. Many organisms can be isolated from cervices showing chronic cervicitis; indeed, a large number of organisms can be identified in the normal endocervix. Some histologic features

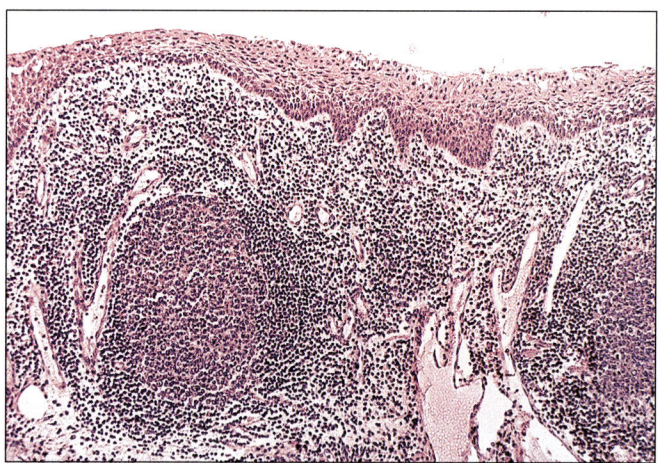

Fig. 6.38 Chronic follicular cervicitis. The cervical stroma is densely infiltrated by lymphocytes, with prominent lymphoid follicles.

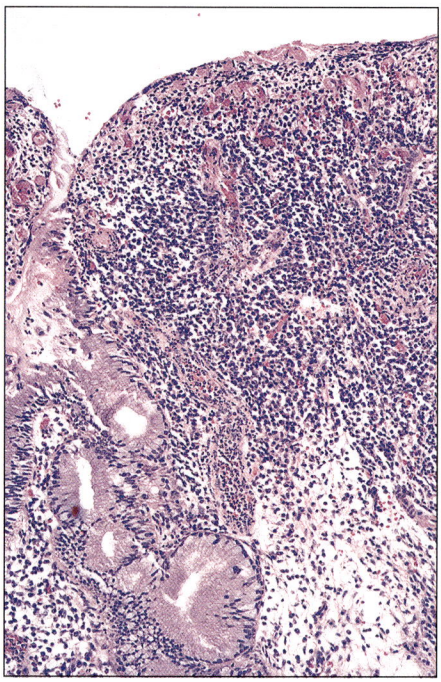

Fig. 6.39 Chronic cervicitis. There is a dense infiltrate of lymphocytes and neutrophils, with new blood vessel formation and dilated vessels packed with neutrophils.

may point to specific microorganisms being responsible for the inflammatory process.[24]

Cytologic correlation

Cervicitis is a common clinical finding and although often the result of bacterial infection (Figure 6.40) it can be due to trauma, chemical agents, viruses, and radiotherapy. On most occasions it is of little consequence cytologically or clinically. However, inflammatory changes may mask significant cellular change. The predominance of the inflammation may render dyskaryotic cells more difficult to recognize. The smear is more likely to be inadequate for a reliable assessment in the presence of marked inflammation.

The recognition of bacterial infections in cervical smears is possible and although 'clue cells' (Figure 6.41) have been linked with *Gardnerella vaginalis* (bacterial vaginosis) it is not possible to be specific cytologically and microbiologic culture is advisable.

Smears taken from an inflamed cervix may on occasion show numerous bacteria with large numbers of polymorphs. An increase in the number of polymorphs is not in itself an indication of inflammation. Increased numbers of polymorphs can be seen pre- and postmenstrually, during pregnancy, with oral contraceptive use, and in the presence of cervical ectropion. Some squamous cells may show mild nuclear enlargement (Figure 6.42) and others may show nuclear pyknosis and karyorrhexis (Figure 6.43). The cells often show eosinophilia or altered staining patterns. Nuclear enlargement of the endocervical glandular cells can occur with occasional small nucleoli and hyperchromasia and rare mitotic figures. The distinction between inflammatory changes and glandular intraepithelial neoplasia can be difficult cytologically.

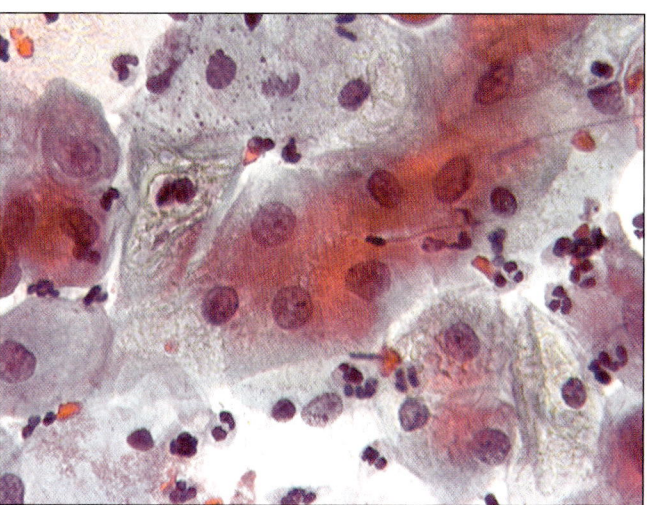

Fig. 6.42 Degenerative changes in cervical smear. General eosinophilia with mild nuclear enlargement.

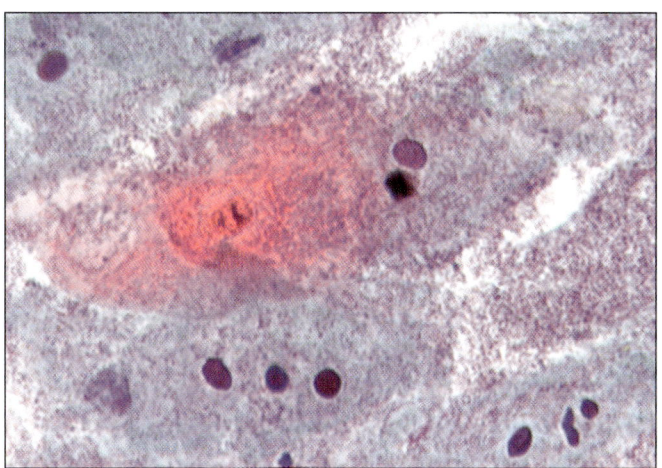

Fig. 6.40 Bacterial cervicitis in cervical smear. A heavy 'coccal' bacterial layer covers the cells and is prominent in the background.

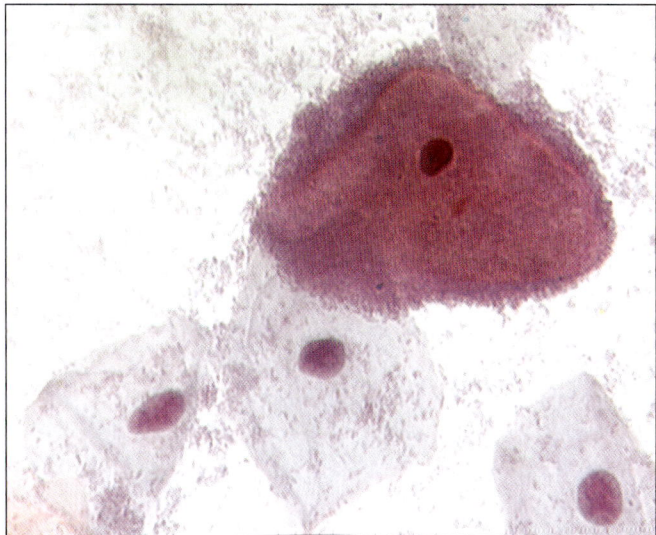

Fig. 6.41 Bacterial cervicitis in vaginal smear. 'Clue cell'. Squamous cell covered by bacteria (clue cell).

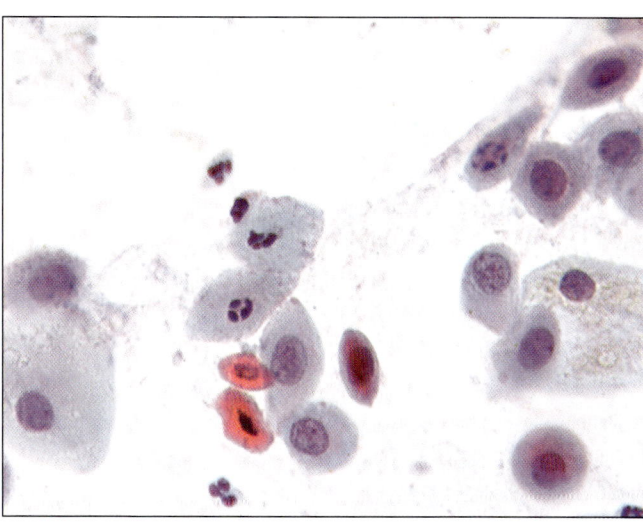

Fig. 6.43 Degenerative changes in cervical smear. Cells show pyknosis and karyorrhexis.

CHLAMYDIA TRACHOMATIS

Infection by *Chlamydia trachomatis* initially causes a polymorphonuclear infiltration of both the columnar glandular epithelium and the squamous epithelium, although the inflammation is predominantly endocervical, affecting the crypt field. There may be a focal loss of the surface columnar epithelium. A dense plasma cell infiltrate is found, particularly around the endocervical crypts (Figure 6.44). Although lymphocytes and histiocytes are always present as well, plasma cells predominate. Germinal center formation is a characteristic feature and this is usually found beneath the surface epithelium (Figure 6.38) and around the gland crypts.[24] Necrosis and destruction of underlying tissue are not features of chlamydial disease.

Cytologic correlation

The identification of the intracytoplasmic inclusions (Figure 6.45) reported by some authors is a time consuming and difficult exercise and has been challenged as a consistent and reliable indicator of the infection. In the presence of *Chlamydia* infection the cervical smear may appear to have a coccal-like background with few polymorphs, and both the squamous and glandular cells show a ragged cytoplasmic border. Because of the association between *Chlamydia* infection and follicular cervicitis, the presence of streaks of lymphocytes, some of which may be immature forms (Figure 6.46), should always raise the suggestion of *Chlamydia* infection, but the diagnosis is best made by culture or molecular diagnostic technology.

TUBERCULOSIS

Cervical tuberculosis is rare both in the United States and United Kingdom. It occurs consequent to infection from upper genital tract disease, which in turn originates from pulmonary tuberculosis. It occurs in about 8% of women with genital tuberculosis.[6,26] The clinical presentation is either as a predominantly hypertrophic lesion that clinically may be mistaken for carcinoma or predominantly ulcerative. Microscopy shows the typical epithelioid cell granulomas of tuberculosis (Figure 6.47), which may be caseating, together with hyperplasia of the epithelial elements, the latter being seen particularly in the hypertrophic variety. Langhans-type giant cells are usually

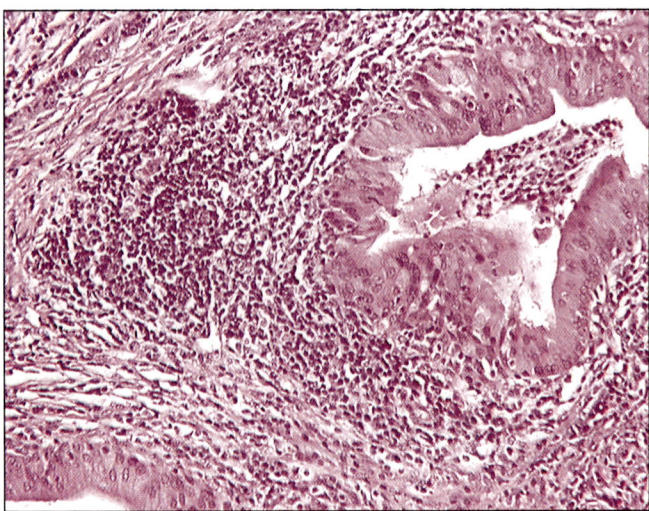

Fig. 6.44 Chlamydial cervicitis. A gland crypt surrounded by a dense infiltrate of lymphocytes and plasma cells. The infiltrate also affects the epithelium and is present in the gland lumen.

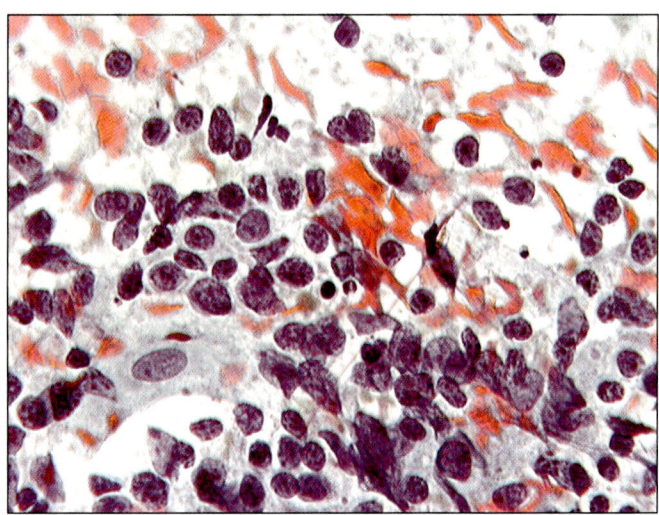

Fig. 6.46 Follicular cervicitis in cervical smear. Immature lymphocytes show variation in size and shape.

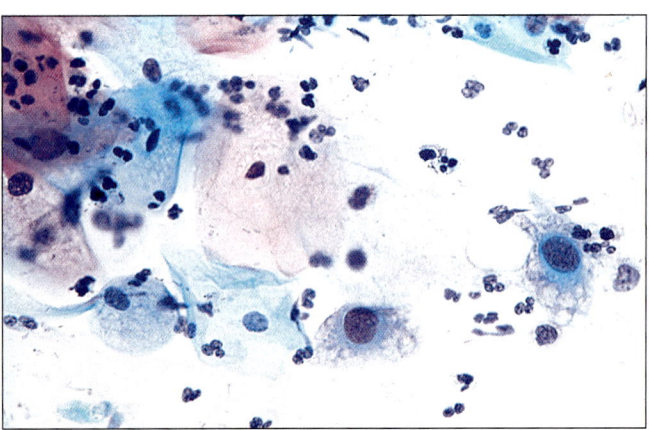

Fig. 6.45 Chlamydias infection in cervical smear. Cells show intracytoplasmic inclusions and a 'moth-eaten' appearance.

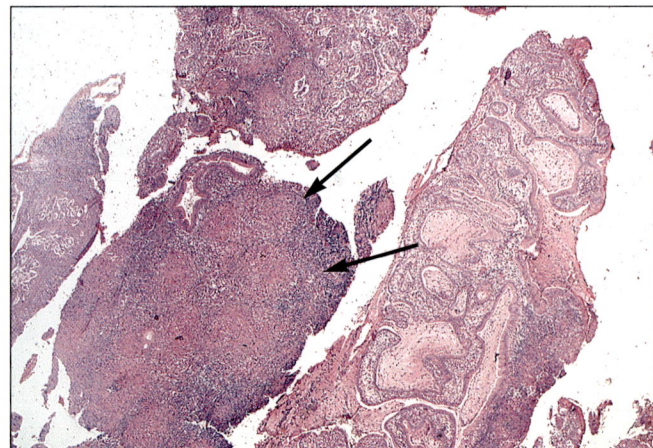

Fig. 6.47 Tuberculosis. Curetted material containing fragments of cervical tissue with prominent granulomas (arrows).

present (Figure 6.48) and the periphery of the tubercle shows a heavy infiltrate of lymphocytes and plasma cells. Acid-fast bacilli can sometimes be demonstrated.

Cytologic correlation

Large multinucleate histiocytes are occasionally seen in cervical smears where their presence cannot be regarded as specific or diagnostic. They are most frequently seen in postmenopausal smears or associated with follicular cervicitis. However, they may be seen in genital tuberculosis (Figure 6.49).

SYPHILIS

Syphilis is a chronic venereal infection caused by *Treponema pallidum*, which gains access directly through the skin and mucosa of the lower genital tract. The primary chancre is usually on the vulva but may be found on the cervix in 10–40% of women with syphilis. The cervix may be firm, nodular, and ulcerating, mimicking cervical carcinoma in some cases. The histologic features are a dense plasma cell infiltration that is most prominent beneath the epithelium (Figure 6.50). Vasculitis, exhibiting plasma cells and lymphocytes together with endothelial cell hyperplasia, is often prominent. Syphilis is one of several venereal infections that a woman may contract today.[1,9] Over one-fifth of women with human immunodeficiency virus (HIV) infection also have syphilis.[8]

HERPES SIMPLEX VIRUS (HSV)

Herpes simplex virus may give rise to an acute infection, which may be severe and necrotizing. The histologic features depend upon the stage of the disease. Even before the small, painful vesicles that are present throughout the lower genital tract appear, the parabasal cells of the squamous epithelium and the columnar endocervical epithelial cells show nuclear enlargement and cytoplasmic swelling accompanied by enlarged nucleoli. Lysis follows after about 36 hours, resulting in vacuoles within the squamous epithelium. Multinucleated giant cells are found around and beneath the vacuoles, but may also be present elsewhere in the epithelium. The multinucleated cells have pleomorphic nuclei with nuclear molding but no overlapping. The nuclear chromatin marginates to give the nuclei a ground-glass appearance (Figures 6.51 and 6.52). Rarely, a single eosinophilic intranuclear rounded inclusion (Cowdry type A inclusion) may be seen. The adjacent epithelium may show basal cell hyperplasia.

Further progression of HSV infection results in acute necrotizing cervicitis where there is extensive necrosis and destruction of stroma, glands, and vessels. These appearances are no longer diagnostic, with a dense stromal infiltrate of mixed acute and chronic inflammatory cells. The inflammation may be distinguished from infection by *Chlamydia trachomatis* because it

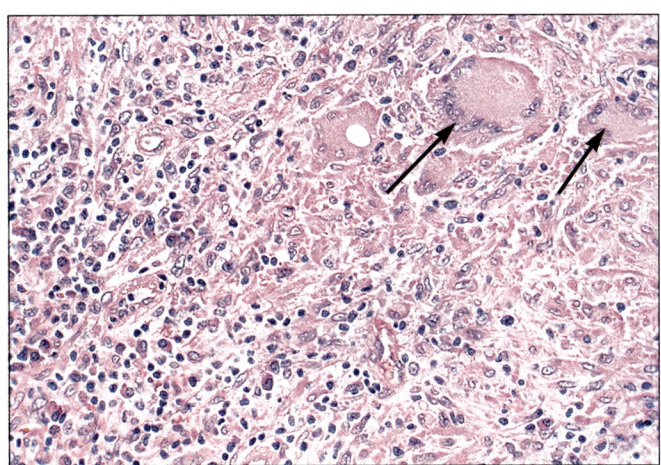

Fig. 6.48 Tuberculosis. The Langhans-type giant cells (arrows) are prominent in this poorly defined epithelioid cell granuloma.

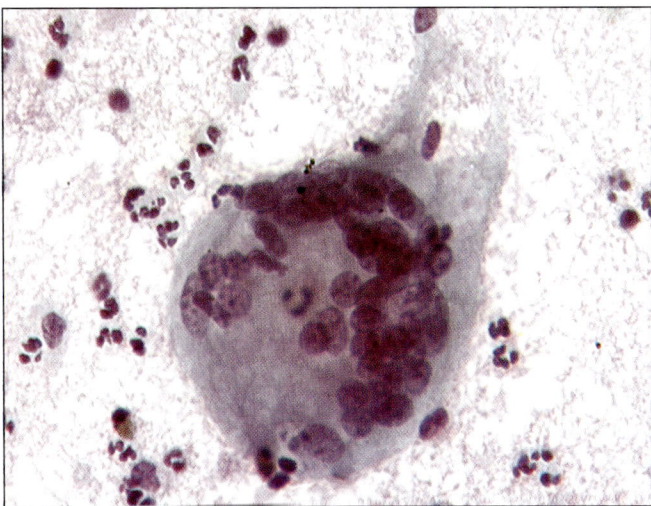

Fig. 6.49 Multinucleated histiocyte. A giant cell showing multiple small nuclei.

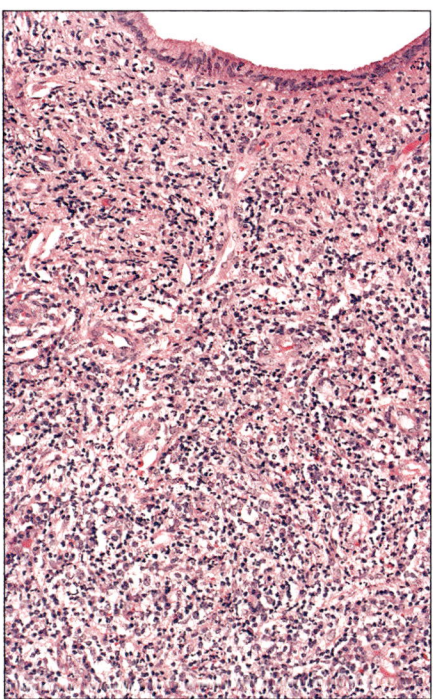

Fig. 6.50 Syphilis. A dense plasma cell infiltrate is present, with vasculitis.

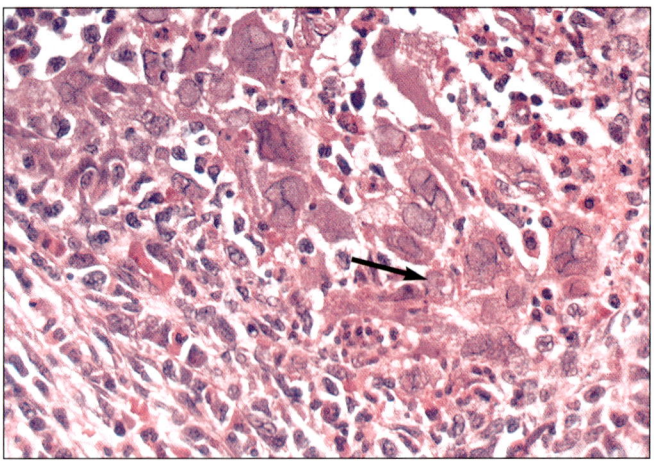

Fig. 6.51 Herpes simplex infection. There is lysis of the epithelial tissue. Multinucleated giant cells are present (arrow), showing margination of chromatin and a 'ground-glass' appearance of the nuclei.

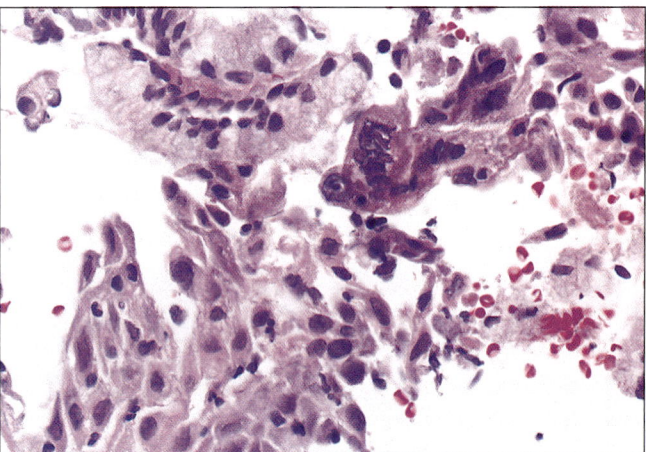

Fig. 6.52 Herpes simplex infection. Multinucleated giant cells are prominent in the disrupted epithelium.

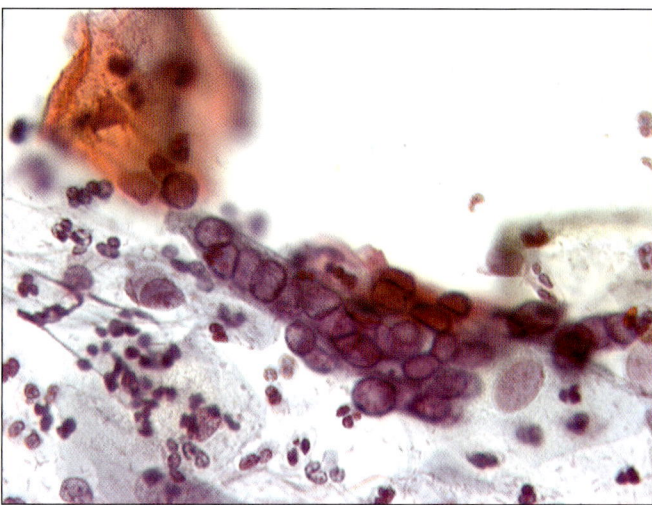

Fig. 6.53 Herpes simplex virus in cervical smear. Molded nuclei with chromatin emargination.

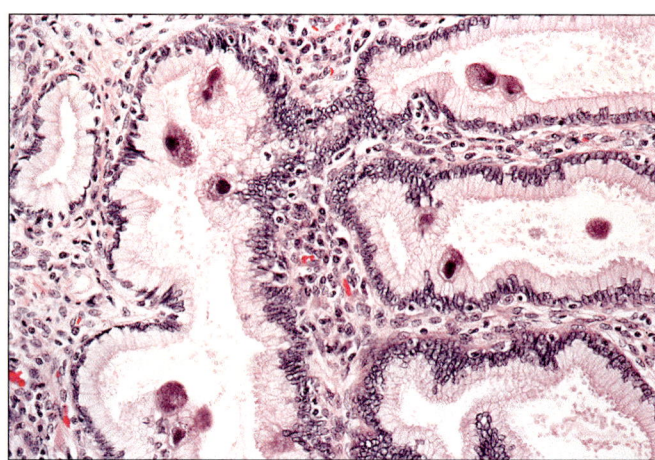

Fig. 6.54 Cytomegalovirus infection. Several endocervical cells within the crypt epithelium show large, rounded, basophilic inclusions.

is not localized to the periglandular or subepithelial zone, and extends deep into the underlying tissue, often deeper than the crypt field. Furthermore, plasma cells are not prominent and germinal centers are not encountered.

Cytologic correlation

Herpes simplex virus is primarily identified by the presence of large multinucleated cells. Multiple nuclei are present that mold one another but do not overlap. The nuclei show variation in size with margination of chromatin and a ground-glass appearance (Figure 6.53). Occasionally a single large eosinophilic or basophilic intranuclear inclusion can be identified (Cowdry type A inclusion). It is possible to recognize the features of HSV infection in cells that have only two or three nuclei. In the late stages of the infection the smear may contain only necrotic debris with few, if any, characteristic multinucleate cells. This necrotizing pattern may be misinterpreted as suggesting invasive squamous carcinoma. Conversely, the diagnosis of invasive squamous carcinoma should not be dismissed, thinking the pattern is one of necrotizing HSV infection.

CYTOMEGALOVIRUS (CMV)

Cytomegalovirus infection of the cervix may be sexually transmitted or it may occur as part of a systemic infection. The characteristic feature is the presence of large, basophilic, intranuclear inclusions, which affect only a minority of epithelial cells in the endocervical crypts (Figures 6.54–6.56) and, occasionally, in endothelial or mesenchymal cells. Associated cytoplasmic inclusions are also found. Associated morphologic features may include fibrin thrombi within small blood vessels, a dense active inflammatory infiltrate, lymphoid follicles, and vacuolated glandular epithelial cells.[33] This appearance is distinctive and the differential diagnosis from other significant lesions is not difficult. Because the abnormal nuclei are widely separated by normal cells, the distinction from high grade glandular intraepithelial neoplasia is easy.

HUMAN PAPILLOMAVIRUS (HPV)

See Chapter 8.

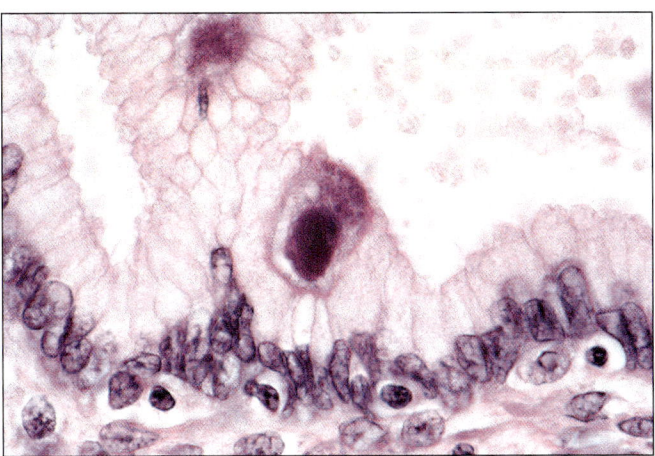

Fig. 6.55 Cytomegalovirus infection. A higher magnification of the characteristic CMV intracytoplasmic inclusion.

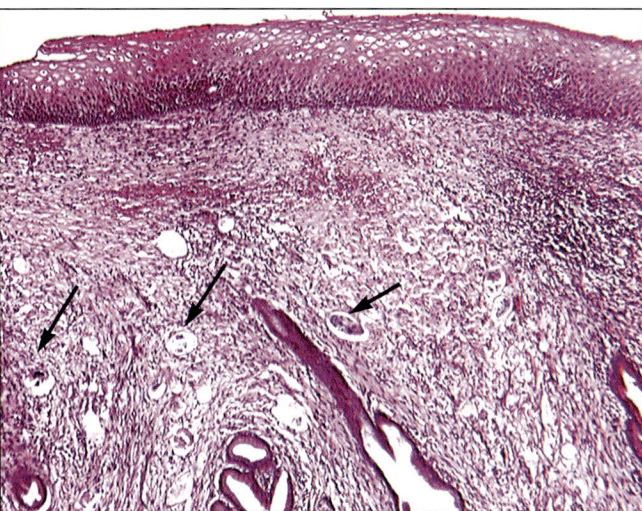

Fig. 6.57 Schistosomiasis. A patchy chronic inflammatory infiltrate surrounds ova (arrows) present in the stroma.

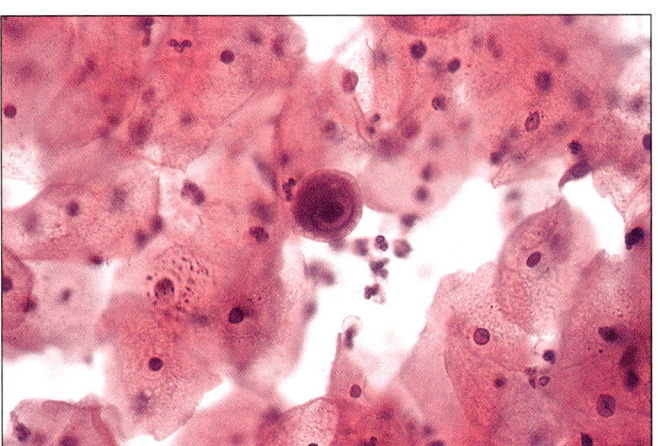

Fig. 6.56 Cytomegalovirus infection in cervical smear. A single cell shows a large central intranuclear inclusion.

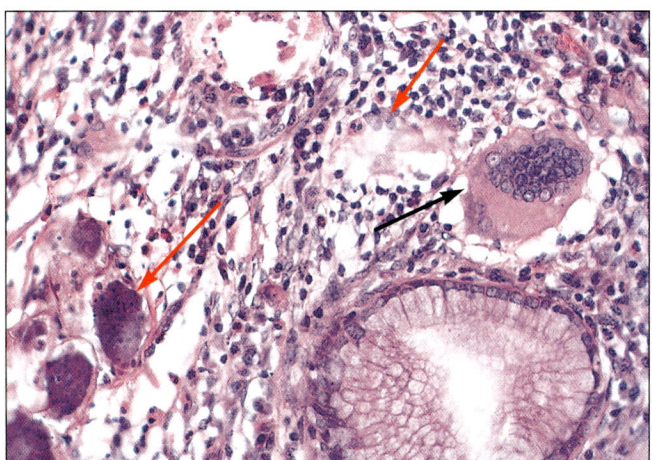

Fig. 6.58 Schistosomiasis. The tissue reaction to the ova (red arrows) includes a large, multinucleated, foreign-body giant cell (black arrow).

SCHISTOSOMIASIS

Although rare in the United States and United Kingdom, schistosomiasis is among the most important and widespread of parasitic diseases, being endemic in tropical and subtropical areas.[42] Schistosomiasis is a cause of infertility when the fallopian tube is involved. The cervical lesions are ulcerative or nodular and may present as papillomatous growths. The ova of the causative organism, *Schistosoma hematobium*, become embedded in the tissue and produce a range of tissue reactions (Figures 6.57 and 6.58). Fibrosis is commonly present and there may be multinucleated giant cells and an inflammatory exudate. The epithelial elements may be atrophic or hyperplastic. Rarely, adult worms are found in venules. The most sensitive diagnostic procedure is a bedside microscopic examination of a wet cervical biopsy crushed between two glass slides, looking for ova.[43] No studies have associated *S. hematobium* infestation with cervical cancer, although infection with the schistosomes seems to favor persistent genital HPV infection, either by traumatizing the genital epithelium and/or by local immunosuppression.[41]

Cytologic correlation

The ova of this parasite are occasionally found in cervical smears. The thick semitransparent shell can be clearly seen. The spine's location identifies the species: *S. hematobium* has a terminal spike (Figure 6.59), *S. mansoni* one that is lateral.

EPITHELIAL INFLAMMATORY CHANGES

In the presence of severe inflammatory conditions, the glandular epithelium in the cervix may show some nuclear changes, the most common being slight nuclear enlargement and pleomorphism. Although enlarged and hyperchromatic, the nuclei have an indistinct, degenerating chromatin pattern (Figures 6.60 and 6.61).[66] The cytoplasm is usually abundant and may be eosinophilic. These changes may pose serious problems in the distinction from genuine atypia but are usually mild, without mitotic activity or reduction in cytoplasm.

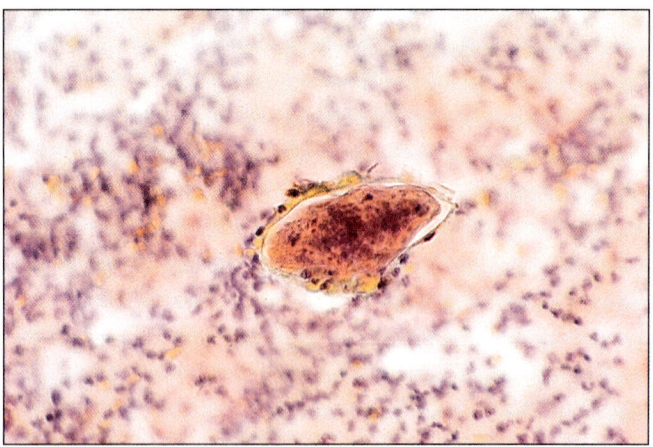

Fig. 6.59 Schistosomiasis in cervical smear. Ovum with poorly preserved terminal spike.

HEALING/REGENERATING EPITHELIUM

After portions of the cervical epithelium have been eroded from infection or treated for CIN, whether by ablation or excision, re-epithelialization may take place in several ways. In the ideal state, the surface will be recovered by a squamous epithelium that matures over the course of about 3 weeks. This is achieved by cells that migrate in from both edges of the affected area as well as from residual gland crypts. If the environment is acid, differentiation and maturation into squamous epithelium will be encouraged. Often this maturation is impaired, with the result that the healing epithelium morphologically resembles immature squamous epithelium that covers a small or large part of the treated area (Figures 6.62 and 6.63). This reparative atypia may cause the histopathologist exactly the same difficulties in differentiation from CIN as immature squamous metaplasia itself does. Clues to the diagnosis of repair are cells in which the nuclei are uniform and generally have prominent macronucleoli. The stroma is often inflamed.[64]

On the other hand, in an alkaline environment, the new epithelium that will regrow will be columnar (müllerian). This

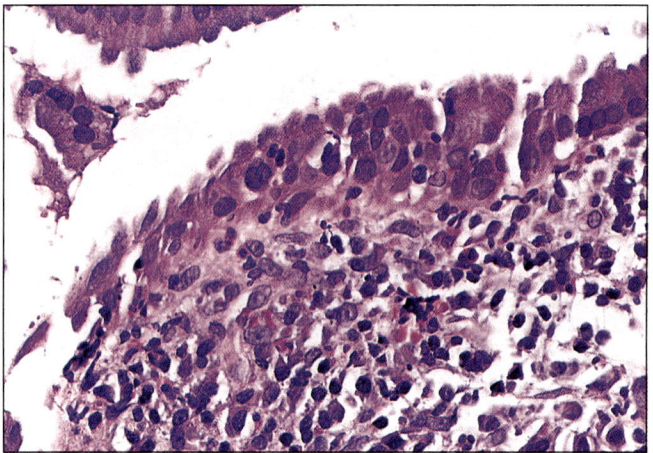

Fig. 6.60 Epithelial inflammatory changes. The nuclei are large and hyperchromatic with a degenerating chromatin pattern. There is abundant, eosinophilic cytoplasm.

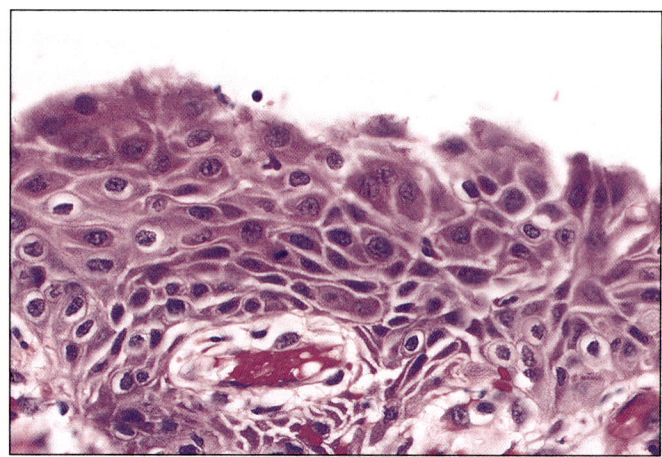

Fig. 6.62 Repair. The epithelium has regrown as poorly organized layers of immature squamous cells, lacking maturation at this stage.

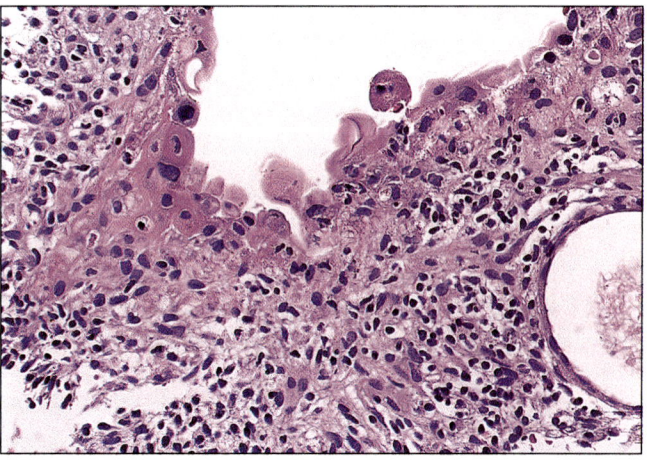

Fig. 6.61 Epithelial inflammatory changes.

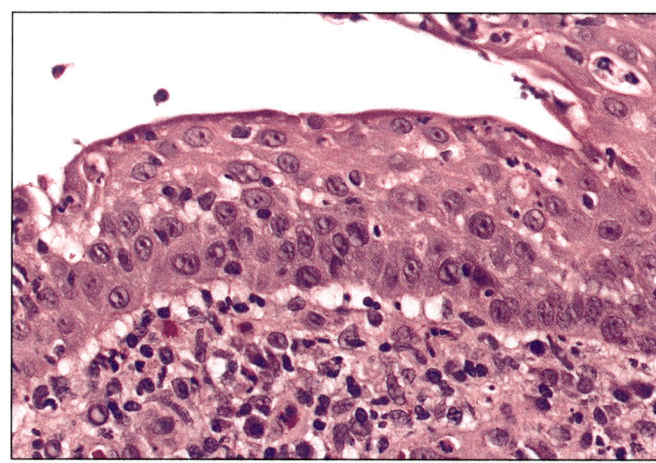

Fig. 6.63 Repair. At this stage, the repairing epithelium resembles immature squamous metaplasia.

is more likely if the area treated is large as the fluid exudate from the extensively treated surface counteracts the acidity of the vaginal environment. In this case, islands of villous, columnar, endocervical-type epithelium regenerate on the ectocervix or even in the vaginal fornices. This amounts to an iatrogenic vaginal adenosis. The biopsy will show inflamed but otherwise normal endocervical-type tissue.

Cytologic correlation

The cells from a repairing epithelium disclose large hyperchromatic nuclei with prominent chromocenters and nucleoli (Figure 6.64). Mitotic figures are not uncommon and the cytoplasm can appear eosinophilic, although green or blue staining is more likely. Not uncommonly, the cytoplasm appears pulled out in tails, the remnants of intercellular bridges (Figure 6.65). The background usually shows debris and increased numbers of polymorphs and lymphocytes. Plasma cells are rarely seen.

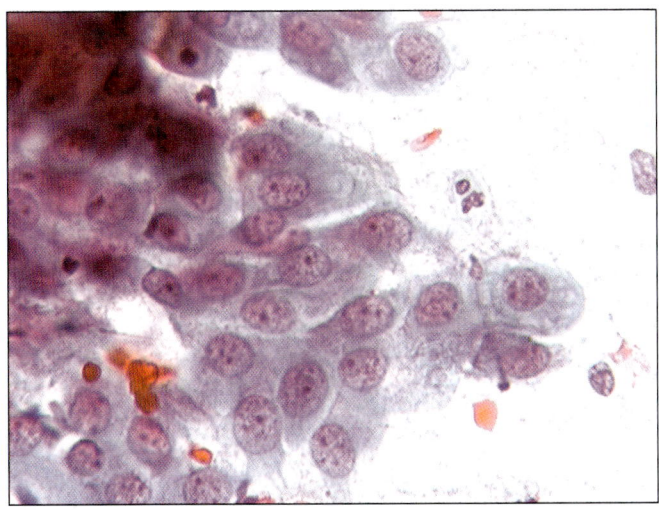

Fig. 6.64 Repair in cervical smear. Cells show prominent nuclei with evenly distributed chromatin with small nucleoli.

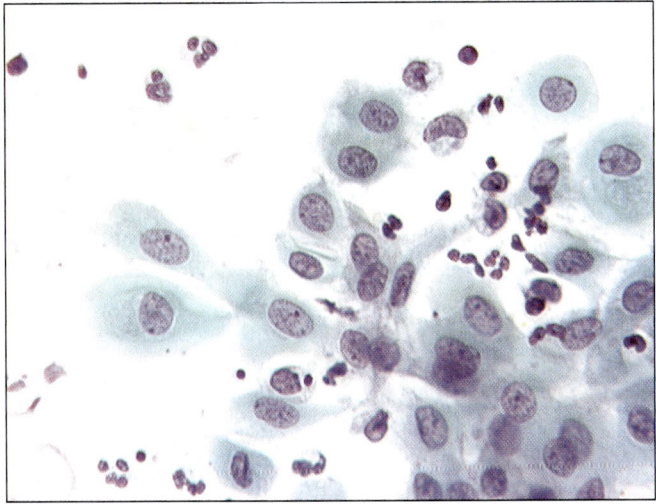

Fig. 6.65 Repair in cervical smear. Elongated cells with 'tails'.

NON-NEOPLASTIC CHANGES

MÜLLERIAN METAPLASIAS

The epithelium that lines the upper female genital tract, i.e., the fallopian tubes, endometrium, and endocervix, derives embryologically from the müllerian (paramesonephric) ducts. Although the epithelium is characteristic for each site, inappropriate müllerian epithelium may be found at any site within the tract. The typical endocervical epithelium predominantly consists of tall, columnar, mucin-secreting cells with basal nuclei, but occasional glands, or groups of glands, display ciliated (tubal) or endometrial-type cells. Similarly, ciliated cells or mucinous epithelium may be seen within the fallopian tubes. While often depicted as metaplasia, the variant epithelium should not be considered abnormal.

TUBAL, ENDOMETRIOID, AND TUBOENDOMETRIOID METAPLASIA

Although initially believed to be a reparative process after a prior cone biopsy, subsequent studies have not provided confirmation.[40] Tubal metaplasia shows tubal-type epithelium, being composed of ciliated, secretory, and intercalated (peg) cells that replace the normal endocervical epithelium composed of non-ciliated secretory and ciliated columnar cells. Its frequency ranges from 21 to 62%.[19] Tubal metaplasia is most commonly seen in premenopausal patients (mean age, 41 years) and is usually an incidental finding, but rarely is found grossly such as the presence of 'spongy mucoid tissue' or an endocervical polyp. It can also be detected on a Pap smear, especially when a cytobrush is used.

Pathology

Tubal (serous) metaplasia occurs mainly in deep glands and in the upper endocervix, but can be seen in the surface epithelium, superficial glands, and lower endocervix.[19] The involved glands are typically small or medium sized but may show variation in size and shape, including branching. The overall cell architecture may show mild atypia. Mitotic figures are rare. The adjacent stroma is often hypercellular, a finding that can be pronounced, but can also be myxoid, loose edematous, or contain focal calcifications.[40] Of interest, a few examples occurring in women exposed prenatally to DES have been extensive, involving all cervical quadrants and reaching a depth of 6.1 mm (pseudoinfiltrative endocervical tubal metaplasia).[57] In these cases, the glands showed a haphazard distribution, variability in shape and size, and were increased in number. Immunohistochemically, tubal metaplasia is unreactive for carcinoembryonic antigen (CEA),[53] and only individual cells are reactive for p16.[54]

Endometrioid metaplasia appears as an epithelium composed of columnar cells, with pseudostratified, oval nuclei. Mitotic figures can be seen. Immunohistochemically, the metaplastic endometrioid cells show reactivity for vimentin,[23] but not CEA.[63] In some cases, the metaplastic process mixes tubal and endometrioid cells, which some investigators designate as tuboendometrioid metaplasia (Figures 6.66 and 6.67). Ki-67 immunostaining shows negligible nuclear proliferation.[31]

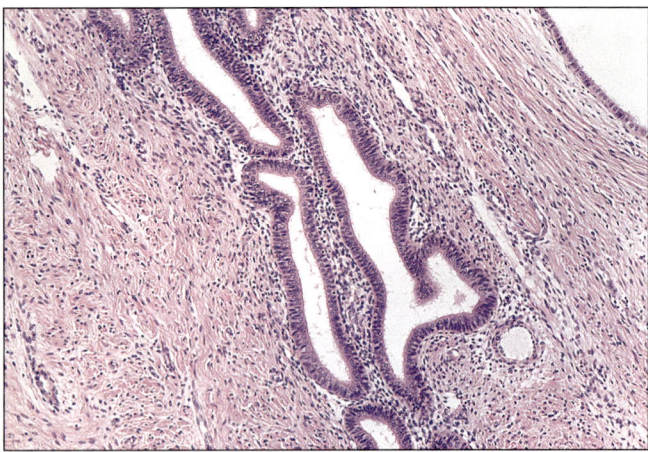

Fig. 6.66 Tuboendometrioid metaplasia. At low power, a group of glands is composed of epithelium that is darker than normal.

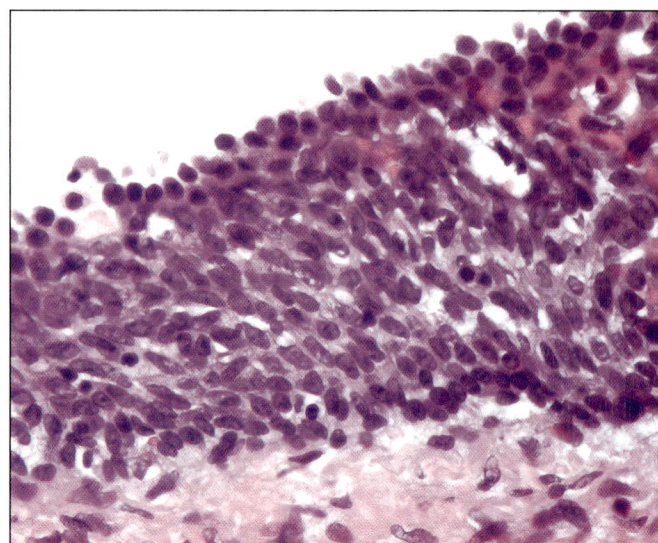

Fig. 6.68 Transitional cell metaplasia. The epithelium consists of elongated cells with nuclear grooves. There is a lack of maturation. Umbrella-like cells are in the surface of the epithelium.

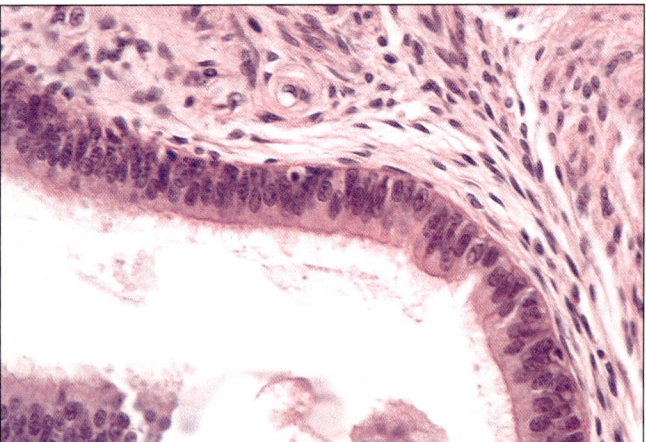

Fig. 6.67 Tuboendometrioid metaplasia. At high magnification, the epithelium can be identified as of tubal type, with cilia and a terminal bar.

Differential diagnosis

The critical differential diagnoses include adenocarcinoma *in situ* (AIS) and invasive adenocarcinoma. The former shows the presence of nuclear abnormalities such as pleomorphism, enlargement, hyperchromasia, conspicuous mitotic activity, and apoptosis. The difficulty arises when AIS arises on a background of tubal metaplasia. This form shows apical cilia in addition to the nuclear abnormalities and mitotic activity mentioned above.[46] Invasive adenocarcinoma can be recognized by the markedly irregular distribution of glands and the presence of frankly malignant cells. The presence of the stromal changes mentioned above may present a confounding factor. While the stroma about invasive adenocarcinomas is typically desmoplastic with an inflammatory infiltrate, this does not always occur. The presence of neoplastic glands in close proximity to thick-walled vessels is highly suggestive of invasive adenocarcinoma.

The cells of minimal deviation adenocarcinoma (adenoma malignum) have a bland cytology and the stroma typically lacks reactive changes. With sufficient sections, foci of marked cytologic atypia and a desmoplastic response are found, at least focally. A better clue to the correct diagnosis is its presence deep in the cervix adjacent to large muscular blood vessels, a location where normal endocervical glands are not found.[61]

Finding such diagnostic features is often not possible when examining a limited amount of cervical tissue, i.e., biopsies or loop electrosurgical excision procedure (LEEP) specimens.

TRANSITIONAL CELL METAPLASIA

Transitional cell metaplasia is a condition about which a literature has developed, but which several of the authors and editors have not convincingly encountered. It is described as forming a multilayer epithelium resembling the mucosa of the normal bladder. It is found most commonly in the cervix and vagina of peri- and postmenopausal women (mean age, 62 years; range 30–87 years).[12,58,59] This benign condition is usually an incidental finding on biopsy, but sometimes is found also in Pap smears.[11] An occasional woman has received exogenous hormones and rare cases have been found in young women who received androgens or had high androgen levels due to the adrenogenital syndrome.[23]

Pathology

In decreasing order of frequency, transitional cell metaplasia involves the transformation zone, exocervix, and endocervix. This process is usually confined to the surface epithelium, but occasionally occurs as isolated stromal nests of transitional cells, with or without lumens.[58,59] Transitional cell metaplasia exhibits a multilayered epithelium (usually >10 layers thick) composed of cells with a uniform, oval or spindled nuclei oriented vertically in the deeper epithelium and with a transition to horizontal or streaming superficially (Figure 6.68). Commonly, the superficial-most epithelial layer discloses a single layer of flattened, umbrella-like cells, much as is frequently seen with urothelium. The chromatin is delicate or smudgy, longitudinal nuclear grooves are variably seen in the non-basal cells, nucleoli are inconspicuous, and mitotic figures are absent or rare.

Immunohistochemical studies suggest that transitional cell metaplasia may represent an immature form of a transitional epithelium as there is a lack of expression of keratin 20, a marker indicative of terminal urothelial differentiation, in the presence of keratin 13, keratin 17, and keratin 18 expression. This is the same profile as seen in normal urothelium and is distinct from that of squamous or glandular cervical epithelium.[17] The superficial 'umbrella cell' is regularly p16 reactive but the rest is not.[10]

Differential diagnosis

Transitional cell metaplasia can be seen in association with various degrees of squamous dysplasia, but differs from a high-grade squamous dysplasia by the lack of marked nuclear atypia and mitotic activity. Also, Ki-67, a marker of nuclear proliferation, is seen only in rare cells of transitional cell metaplasia in contrast to its extensive reactivity in high-grade squamous dysplasia.

INTESTINAL METAPLASIA

Intestinal metaplasia is the rarest form of metaplasia in the uterine cervix, exhibiting goblet and argentaffin cells (Figure 6.69). As this process is most commonly associated with *in situ* or invasive adenocarcinomas and less commonly with adenomas, its diagnosis should be made only after careful sampling and microscopic examination to exclude any sign of malignancy (i.e., nuclear atypia, mitotic activity, or the presence of an infiltrative pattern).[66]

LESIONS OF THE ENDOCERVICAL GLANDULAR EPITHELIUM

ENDOCERVICAL TUNNEL CLUSTERS

Tunnel clusters are benign, pseudoneoplastic, glandular proliferations that are relatively common and mostly found in multigravid women over age 30.[20] There are two types, both tending to be multifocal and incidental findings: one (type A) may be small and microscopic only; the second (type B) is usually extensive and can produce marked distortion of the endocervical mucosa and underlying wall due to the presence of cysts that can penetrate up to 1.5 cm into the wall.[48] Type A is maxi-

mally 7 mm in greatest dimension and consists of a well-circumscribed, occasionally pseudoinfiltrative, proliferation of oval, round or angulated glands lined by cells that can be either cuboidal with amphophilic cytoplasm or columnar and mucus secreting (Figure 6.70). The former cells have enlarged nuclei with vesicular chromatin and conspicuous nucleoli (Figure 6.71). Nuclear hyperchromasia, if present, is of the degenerative type. Mitotic figures are absent or rare. The stroma is usually unremarkable although it can be cellular, edematous, or contain inflammatory cells. Occasionally, extravasated mucin can be seen. Localized type A tunnel clusters tend to be associated also with tunnel clusters of the more expansive type (type B), a finding suggesting the latter arises from the former due to obstruction. The expansive tunnel clusters consist of dilated glands forming distinct lobular units that contrast with the usual architectural organization of the endocervical mucosa (Figure 6.72). The cells can be cuboidal or flattened and lack mitotic activity (Figures 6.73 and 6.74). In the cystic variant,

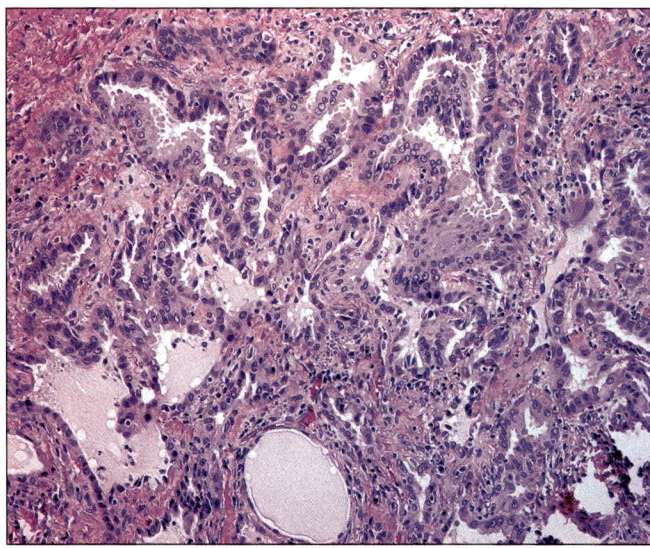

Fig. 6.70   Tunnel cluster, type A. Glands have an irregular contour.

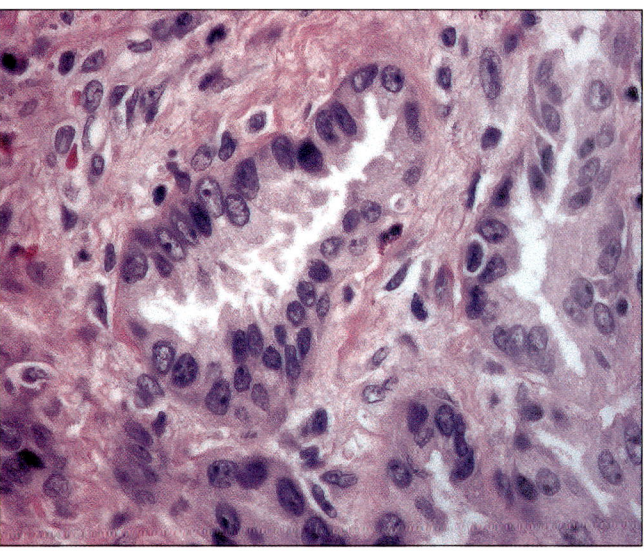

Fig. 6.71   Tunnel cluster, type A. Nuclei can be enlarged with vesicular chromatin.

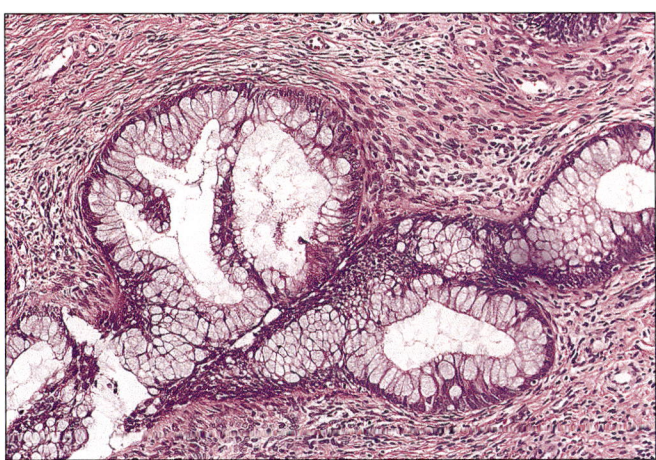

Fig. 6.69   Intestinal metaplasia. Goblet cells are prominent.

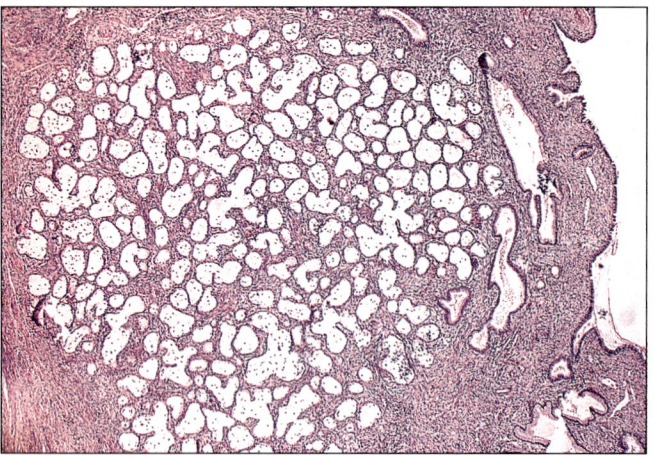

Fig. 6.72 Tunnel cluster, type B. Cystic glands in a lobular arrangement.

the individual clusters can reach up to 18 mm at greatest dimension, and penetrate up to 9 mm into the cervical wall. A rare case associated with nabothian cysts has extended through the cervical wall (1.5 cm). Tunnel clusters are negative for CEA.

Differential diagnosis

The principal concern is that tunnel cluster not be mistaken for malignancy, either as adenocarcinoma *in situ* or an endocervical adenocarcinoma, especially as the minimal deviation type (adenoma malignum) or microcystic adenocarcinoma. The absence of nuclear pseudostratification and mitotic activity allows the distinction from adenocarcinoma *in situ*. The superficial location (inner endocervical wall), and absence of symptoms, infiltrative pattern, mitoses, and overly malignant cytologic features should help to distinguish tunnel clusters from invasive adenocarcinoma.

DEEP NABOTHIAN CYSTS

Nabothian cysts, which are a normal finding in multiparous women, are mucus-filled cysts usually 2–10 mm in size located on the surface of the endocervix, corresponding in location to the normal endocervical glands. Occasionally, these cysts are found deep in the wall, almost reaching the outer surface of the uterine cervix or paracervical soft tissue. The cysts form when the duct in the gland neck becomes obstructed, leading to entrapped mucus secretions. Most women are asymptomatic, but some have had long-term chronic cervicitis.

Gross examination discloses the presence of multiple, mucin-filled cysts extending from the mucosa to the deep portion of the wall. Occasionally, the cervix is enlarged.[66] Microscopically, the cysts are either round or with slightly irregular contours (Figure 6.75). They are lined by a single layer of columnar to flattened endocervical cells without atypia or mitotic figures. Nabothian cysts differ from minimal deviation adenocarcinoma (adenoma malignum) by the lack of an obvious mass lesion, markedly irregular glands, desmoplastic response, and atypia and mitoses.

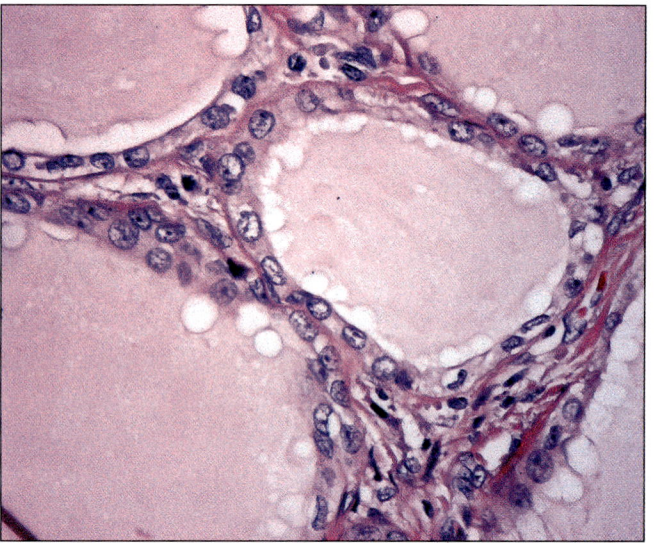

Fig. 6.73 Tunnel cluster, type B. Cuboidal epithelium.

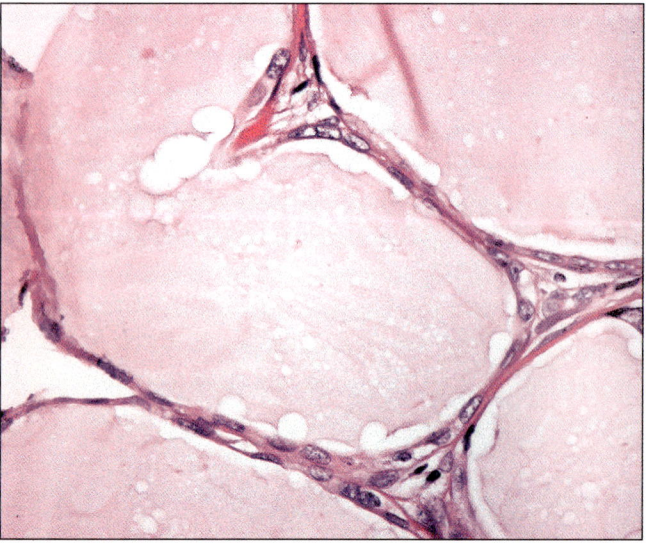

Fig. 6.74 Tunnel cluster, type B. Flattened epithelium.

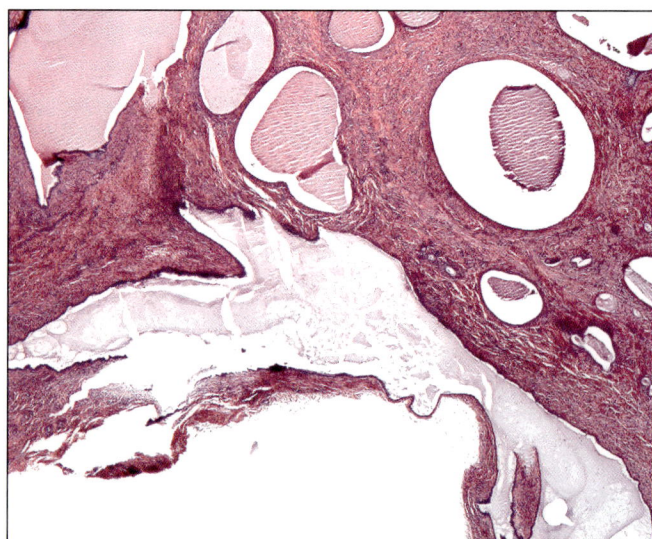

Fig. 6.75 Deep nabothian cysts.

LOBULAR ENDOCERVICAL GLANDULAR HYPERPLASIA

This uncommon pseudoneoplastic glandular proliferation, a recently described lesion, has changes suggestive of pyloric gland metaplasia. It occurs in women aged 37–71 years (mean age, 45 years), most of whom are asymptomatic. Some present with a cervical/vaginal discharge or even a cervical mass.[35,38] The cervical smear may show cells interpreted as atypical glandular cells of undetermined significance (AGUS).[25]

Pathology

Grossly, the cervix is commonly unremarkable, but sometimes there is a polypoid mass or multiple cysts within the wall. Microscopically, there is a distinct lobular proliferation of glands ranging in size from small to large and cystic (Figure 6.76). Some lobular aggregates have a centrally located dilated gland surrounded by smaller glands. The glands are mostly round, but can have undulating contours. The lining epithelium is a single layer of columnar, mucin-producing cells with bland, basal nuclei with inconspicuous nucleoli. The nuclei may be slightly enlarged with vesicular chromatin, and prominent nucleoli (Figure 6.77). In some cases, mitotic activity is even found (up to 2 mitoses per 10 HPFs). The intervening stroma may be cellular or contain inflammatory cells. The cells of endocervical lobular hyperplasia largely contain neutral mucins (periodic acid-Schiff (PAS) positive), further delineated by reactivity with HIK 1083 and MUC6, both immunomarkers for pyloric gland mucin. These findings have prompted some to designate this lesion as pyloric gland metaplasia.[25,35,36] CEA is reactive.

Pathogenesis

Recently, endocervical lobular hyperplasia has been found together with some cases of cervical minimal deviation adenocarcinomas or mucinous adenocarcinomas. As the carcinomas shared the pyloric gland immunophenotype with endocervical lobular hyperplasia, an association between these two entities has been suggested.[25,36]

DIFFUSE LAMINAR ENDOCERVICAL GLANDULAR HYPERPLASIA

This uncommon benign pseudoneoplastic glandular proliferation is seen mostly in premenopausal patients (aged 22–54 years).[21,29] In general, the lesion is an incidental finding, although some produce a watery or mucoid discharge.[13,21,29] There are no specific macroscopic findings. Microscopically, the lesion, which is clearly demarcated from the subjacent cervical stroma, exhibits a diffuse proliferation of round or abnormally shaped, small- or medium-sized glands confined to the inner endocervical wall (Figure 6.78). The glands are lined by bland, mucin-containing columnar epithelium (Figure 6.79). In the presence of inflammation, focal reactive changes may show as nuclear enlargement, chromatin clearing, and nucleoli. Mitotic figures are rare. Features helping to distinguish this lesion from minimal deviation adenocarcinoma (adenoma

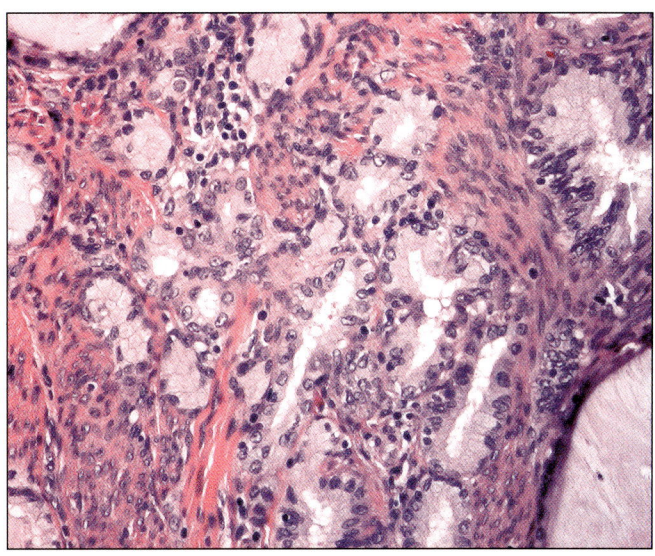

Fig. 6.77 Detail of glandular epithelium in lobular endocervical glandular hyperplasia.

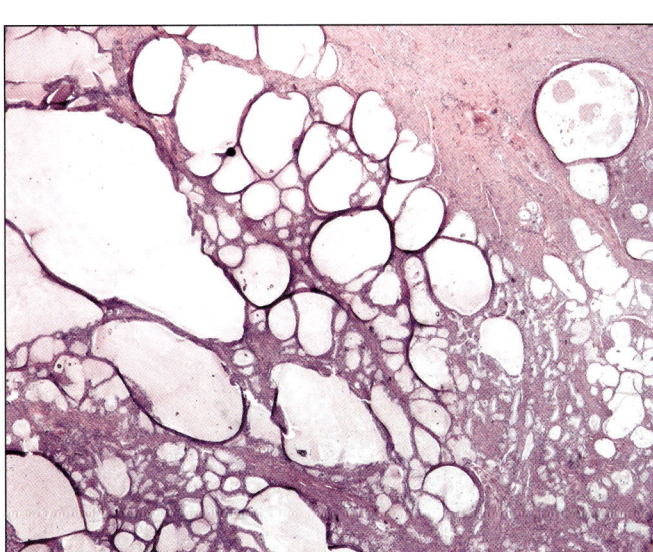

Fig. 6.76 Lobular endocervical glandular hyperplasia.

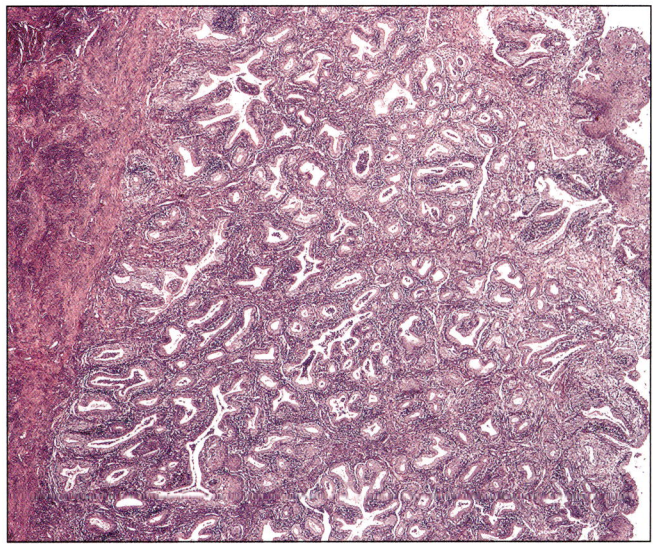

Fig. 6.78 Diffuse laminar endocervical glandular hyperplasia.

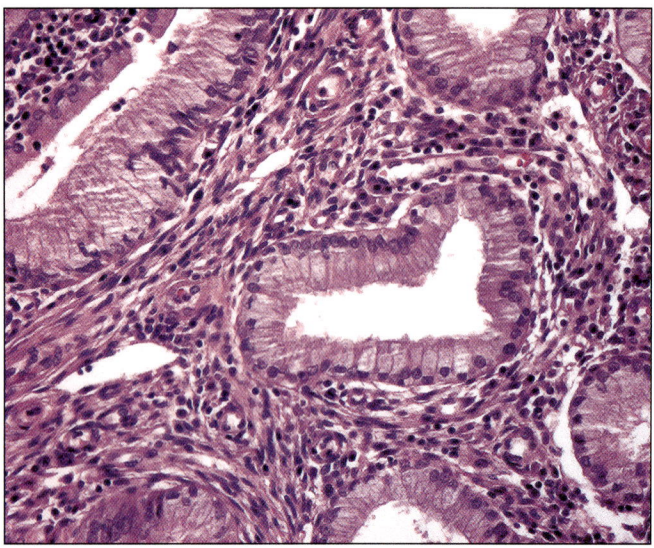

Fig. 6.79 Detail of well-differentiated glandular epithelium in diffuse laminar endocervical glandular hyperplasia.

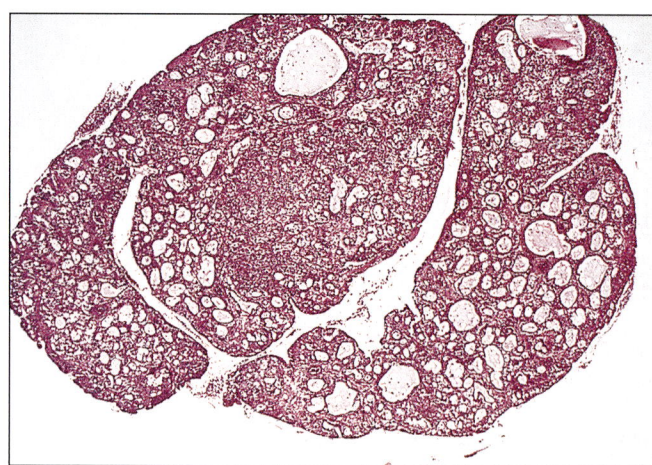

Fig. 6.80 Microglandular hyperplasia. A low-power view of microglandular hyperplasia in an endocervical polyp shows proliferation of the glandular elements.

malignum) include its superficial location and well-defined base.

LESIONS RELATED TO EXOGENOUS STIMULI

MICROGLANDULAR HYPERPLASIA

Microglandular hyperplasia refers to a particular form of glandular proliferation encountered mostly in women of reproductive age but occasionally (about 6%) in postmenopausal women. It is commonly associated with exposure to progesterone in the form of oral contraceptive therapy, Depo-Provera, or pregnancy, but in some women no hormonal background can be found. One more recent study has challenged the associations altogether.[16]

Pathology
Most occurrences are found incidentally, but some produce gross abnormalities in the forms of ectropions, polyps, or friable raised areas. Microscopically, it can be focal or multifocal. The lesion consists of closely packed glands of variable size and shape, with little intervening stroma (Figure 6.80). Acute inflammatory cells are almost always found within the gland lumens. The epithelium lining the glands is columnar or cuboidal, mucin-producing, and contains supra- or subnuclear vacuoles (Figure 6.81). The nuclei are usually uniform, but focal atypia can be encountered. Reserve cell hyperplasia and squamous metaplasia are also seen.[62] Mitotic activity is low (≤ mitoses per 10 high power fields).[37,44] Occasionally, microglandular hyperplasia can have focal areas with a solid, pseudoinfiltrative, or reticular pattern, hobnail or signet-ring cells, and stromal hyalinization.[65]

Differential diagnosis
Clinically important lesions which can be confused with microglandular hyperplasia include clear cell carcinoma and endo-

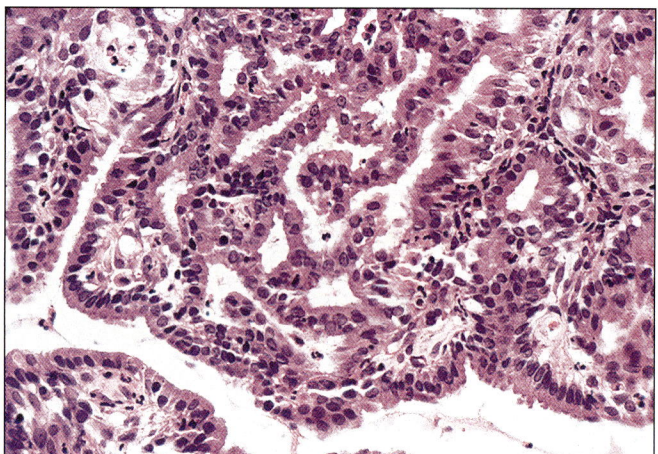

Fig. 6.81 Microglandular hyperplasia. Densely crowded small glands appear fused together without intervening stroma.

metrial adenocarcinoma with a microglandular pattern. Clear cell carcinoma is usually associated with a cervical mass, has an infiltrative pattern, and often shows several different patterns within the same tumor, including sheets of clear cells and hobnail cells within tubules. Additionally, it shows greater cytologic atypia than that seen in microglandular hyperplasia. Endometrial adenocarcinoma with a microglandular pattern can represent a true diagnostic challenge that many times cannot be resolved with only a limited tissue sample. Features that favor endometrial adenocarcinoma with a microglandular pattern include transition to other patterns of endometrial adenocarcinoma, endometrial intraepithelial neoplasia (EIN), hyperplasia or mucinous metaplasia in the background endometrium, and a lack of subnuclear vacuoles.[44,67] We have not found immunohistochemistry useful in distinguishing these lesions, although some believe vimentin reactivity favors endometrial adenocarcinoma with a microglandular pattern. CEA is unreactive in both entities.[44]

ARIAS-STELLA REACTION

The frequency with which the Arias-Stella reaction occurs in the endocervix of pregnant women ranges between 9% and 37.5%.[47] This reaction may also occur when there is a history of oral contraceptive use, but occasionally no hormonal history can be elicited.[37]

Pathology

Arias-Stella reaction in the cervix can present as involvement of an endocervical polyp or as an incidental finding in cervical tissue obtained for other reasons. It affects superficial and/or deep glands. It is most commonly seen in the upper endocervical canal but can involve glands anywhere in the endocervix.[47] Arias-Stella reaction tends to be focal, but may be extensive, producing a confluent appearance (Figure 6.82). Occasionally, the intraglandular proliferation can be striking, producing a papillary or cribriform pattern.[37] The Arias-Stella reaction exhibits large cells with clear or oxyphilic cytoplasm and large atypical nuclei demonstrating irregularity of the nuclear contour and variability of the chromatin distribution, ranging from even to dense (Figure 6.83). The nuclei typically protrude into the gland lumen, giving the cell a hobnail appearance (Figure 6.84). A rare mitotic figure can be seen as well as focally decidualized stroma. This lesion is described more fully in Chapter 14.

DECIDUAL CHANGE

Decidual change is a progestin-induced alteration of stromal tissue. Although this hormonal response is usually associated with endometrial stroma, it also affects the superficial stroma of the cervix, the lamina propria of the fallopian tube, the subcortical stroma of the ovary, and the submesothelial stroma of the peritoneum. Pathologists are more frequently encountering this lesion in the cervix as colposcopy is being used to investigate women with abnormal cervical smears. Women are being examined during pregnancy or immediately postpartum and biopsies may be taken of abnormal areas.

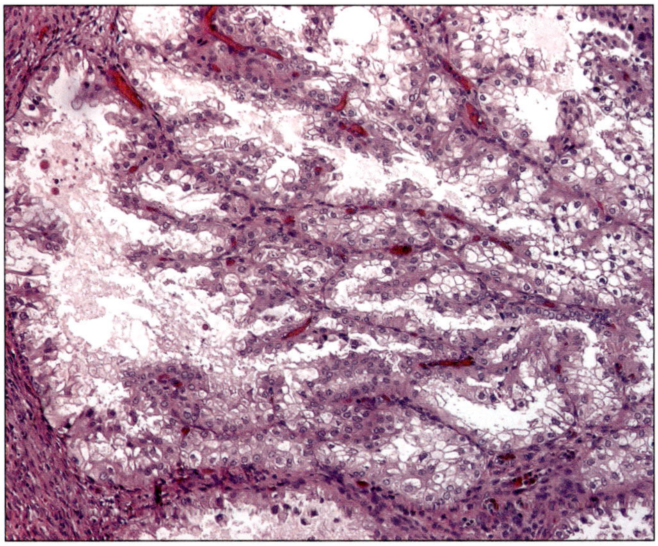

Decidual change presents to the naked eye as small, raised, vascular nodules or, less commonly, as sessile polyps. At colposcopy, the appearances can simulate those of invasive carcinoma. The affected area may have a raised, nodular, irregular contour and, in particular, prominent, often rather bizarre vessels, on the surface. Microscopy shows features that are similar to decidual change at more familiar sites (Figures 6.85 and 6.86). The cells of the superficial stroma are enlarged with copious cytoplasm. The nuclei are uniform, small and central. The change usually affects only a small area of the cervix and may be situated on both the endocervix and ectocervix. The phenomenon of decidual change in the cervix is, of course, of no consequence as it is asymptomatic and regresses soon after the pregnancy finishes.

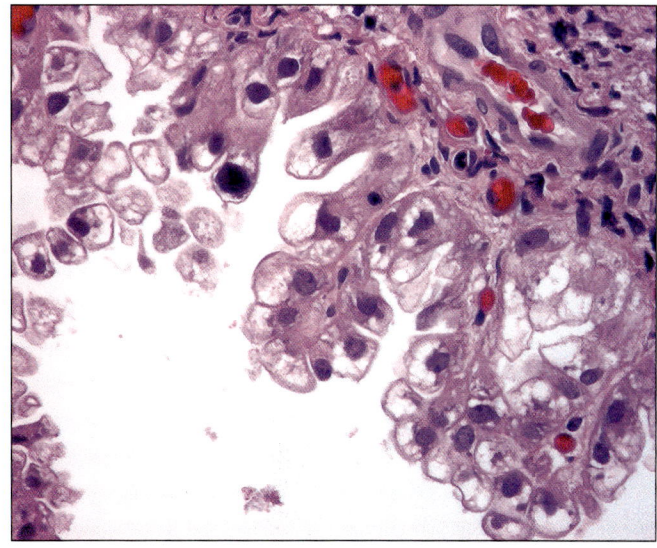

Fig. 6.83 Arias-Stella reaction in endocervix. Clear cells with enlarged, hyperchromatic nuclei.

Fig. 6.82 Arias-Stella reaction in endocervix. Unusual confluent pattern.

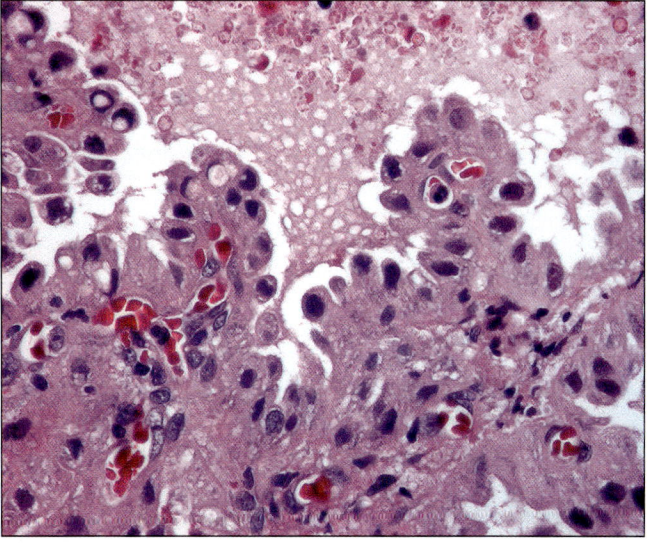

Fig. 6.84 Arias-Stella reaction in endocervix. Hobnails with eosinophilic cytoplasm.

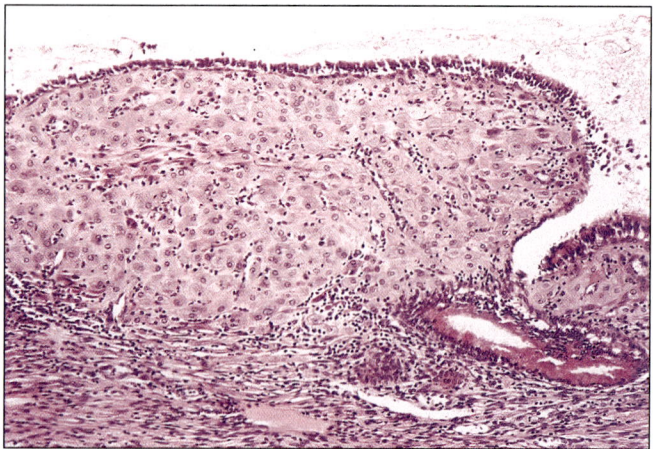

Fig. 6.85   Decidual change. A well-defined area of large, pale, decidualized stromal cells is present beneath the surface epithelium.

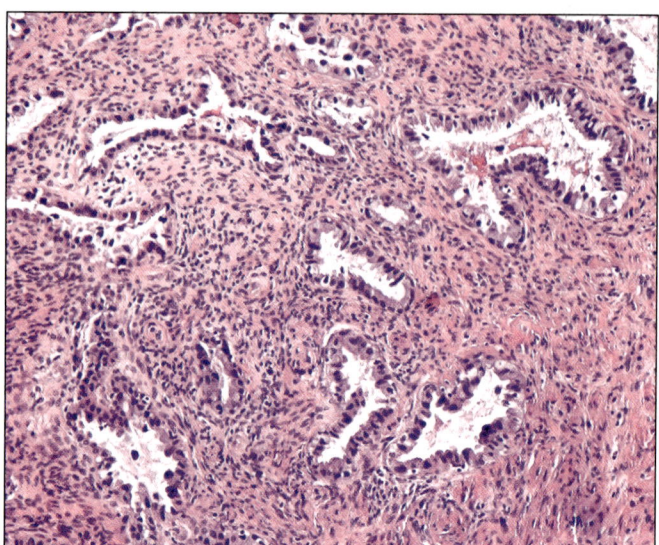

Fig. 6.87   Radiation effect. Glands of irregular size and shape.

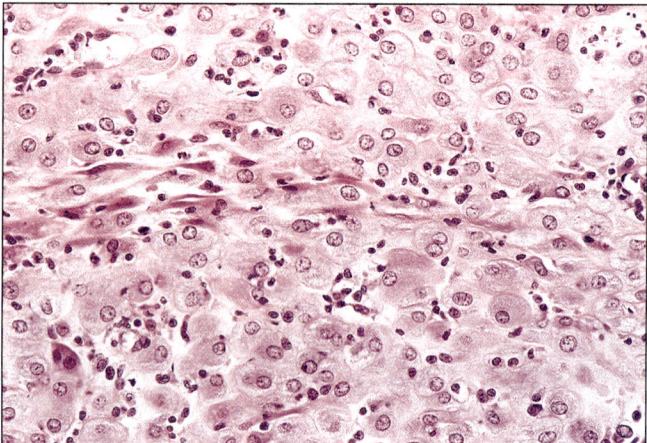

Fig. 6.86   Decidual change. At high power, the cells are identical to decidualized endometrial stromal cells.

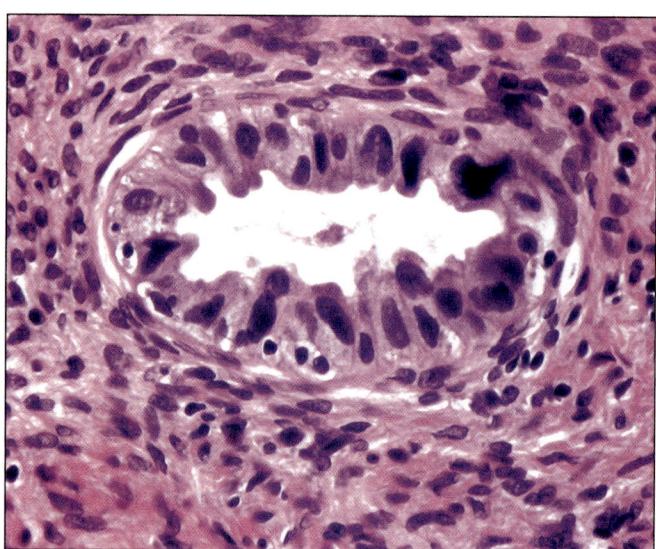

Fig. 6.88   Radiation effect with some enlarged nuclei with smudged chromatin.

RADIATION CHANGES

Radiation changes can be acute or long term. Acute changes include erosion, cytoplasmic and nuclear swelling of the squamous and endocervical cells, dilated blood vessels, and stromal changes such as necrosis, edema, and a lymphoplasmacytic infiltrate. In most patients, these acute changes gradually give way to changes associated with the long-term effects of radiation, which can persist for many years. These longer term changes include atrophy of the squamous epithelium (80% of cases), variable degrees of epithelial atypia (two-thirds of cases), and stromal changes encompassing the presence of edema, fibrosis, hyalinization, atypical fibroblasts, multinucleated cells, and focal calcification (Figures 6.87–6.91).

The blood vessels may show sclerotic changes, intimal proliferation, and atypical endothelial cells (Figure 6.90 and 6.91).[50] Additionally, the endocervical glands, which decrease in number and have either a tubular or dilated configuration (Figure 6.88), are lined by enlarged cells with eosinophilic or vacuolated cytoplasm with enlarged nuclei (Figures 6.89). These endocervical cells are usually cuboidal but can be colum-

nar or flattened. The nuclei enlarge with fine chromatin and visible nucleoli, but can also be hyperchromatic. The latter are generally scattered through the glands but occasionally are prominent and appear predominate. These epithelial changes can be focal or extensive. Mitotic figures are absent. In a rare case, multinucleated cells or eosinophilic intranuclear inclusions are present.[27]

Differential diagnosis

Adenocarcinoma *in situ* virtually always shows mitoses, a feature absent in radiation change. Clear cell adenocarcinoma may show closely packed invasive glands, mitotic figures, and a combination of architectural patterns (i.e., tubulocystic, papillary, and solid), features also absent in radiation change.

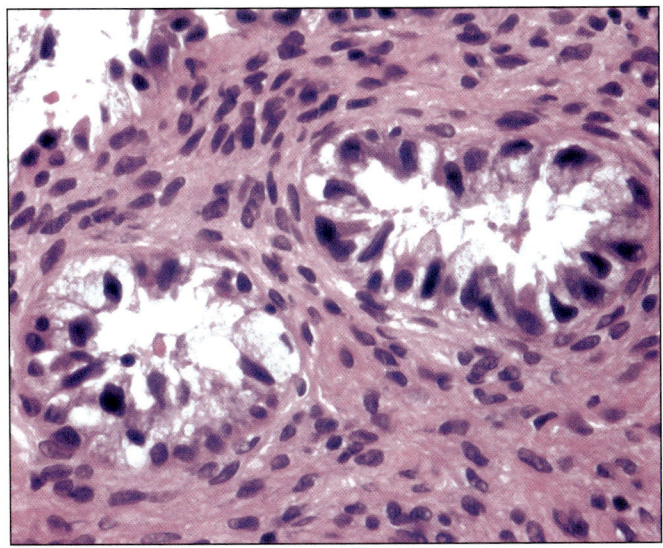

Fig. 6.89 Radiation effect. The glandular epithelium with hyperchromatic nuclei and chromatin. The cytoplasm is eosinophilic or clear.

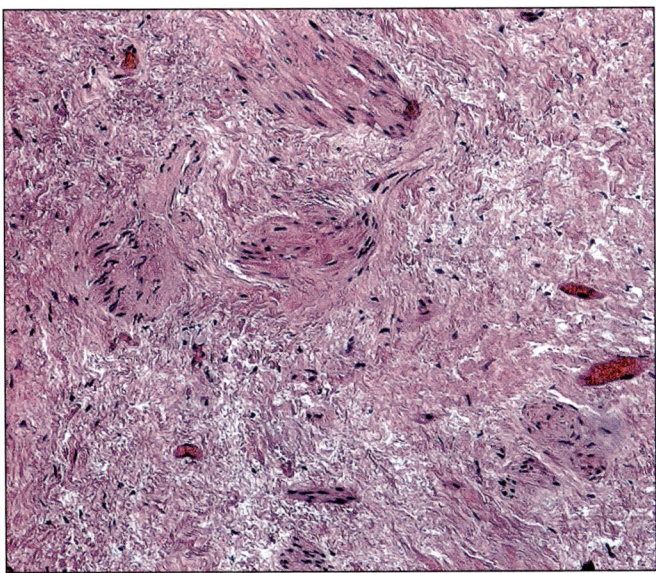

Fig. 6.90 Radiation effect, fibrotic stroma.

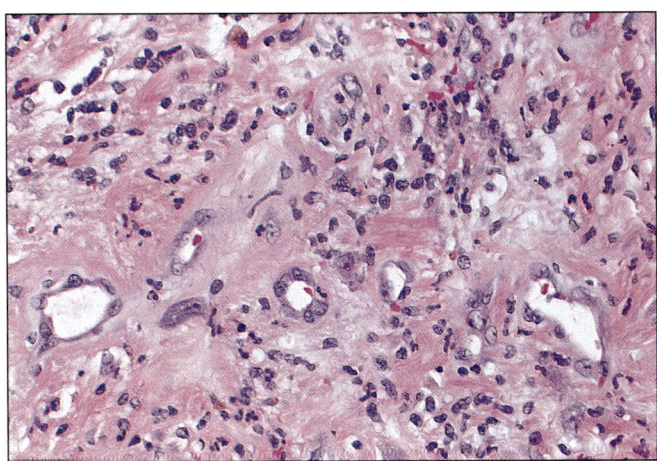

Fig. 6.91 Radiation effect. Vessels with plump endothelial cells and reactive fibroblasts in the stroma.

OTHER NON-NEOPLASTIC CONDITIONS

ENDOMETRIOSIS

Endometriosis, described in greater depth in Chapter 20, occurs in the cervix in both deep and superficial forms. The deep form is usually seen in patients with pelvic endometriosis and its recognition does not represent a diagnostic challenge. The superficial form typically consists of endometriotic glands and stroma, but in some instances the glands are sparse or absent (stromal endometriosis). It is the superficial form that can be mistaken for a number of serious diseases, including cancer, and forms the basis of the discussion to follow.

Superficial cervical endometriosis is usually seen in premenopausal patients, although the range of ages is 20–53 years.[4] It is often an incidental finding but may be detected secondary to trauma with subsequent vaginal bleeding from a surgical procedure (curettage, biopsy, loop excision or cone biopsy, and cautery). Grossly, it appears as a mucosal thickening or as nodules, blood-filled blebs or cysts (up to 2 cm in diameter). The mucosa may appear granular or hemorrhagic.[4] Microscopically, the endometriotic process tends to reside within the inner third of the cervical wall, sometimes producing ulceration. The glands are usually round to oval but occasionally are cystic (Figure 6.92). Hyperplastic or secretory changes and telescoping can be seen. The epithelial cells can show reactive atypia. The mitotic activity tends to be low, although up to three mitoses per gland can be seen. No abnormal mitotic figures are found and apoptotic bodies are rarely seen. The stroma can be focal, which, in addition to the changes listed above, complicates recognition of this lesion.[4] In difficult cases, deeper sections facilitate the recognition of this lesion since CD10 immunoreactivity is seen in endometrical stroma but also in the cervical stroma. Reactivity to CD10 cannot be seen.[32] Interestingly, in our experience, the stromal cells (rather than the glands) of implantation endometriosis in the cervix are regularly reactive for p16.

Differential diagnosis

Superficial cervical endometriosis must be distinguished from adenocarcinoma *in situ*. Confounding features rendering the correct diagnosis difficult include mitotic activity within the

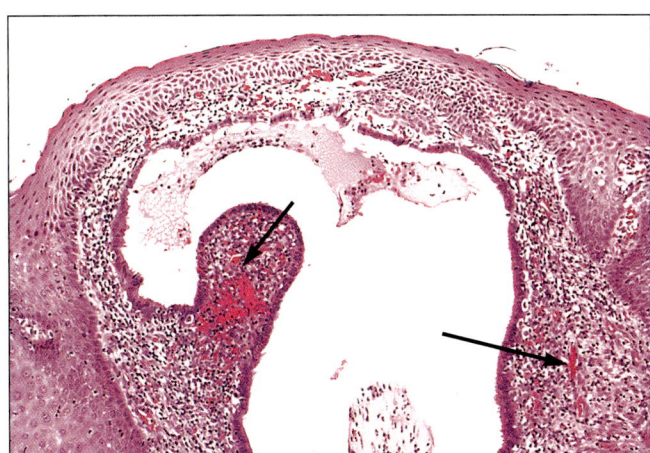

Fig. 6.92 Endometriosis. A distended glandular space, lined by endometrial-type epithelium, lies beneath the squamous epithelium of the cervix. Hemorrhagic endometrial stroma (arrows) is also present.

glandular epithelium (especially in young women), hemorrhage, inflammation, smooth muscle metaplasia, and other reactive changes within the stromal component. The absence of significant cytologic atypia, but the presence of the stromal component, which in some cases will require additional deeper sections, helps to facilitate the correct diagnosis.

Endometriosis can also be misinterpreted as atypical glandular cells of undetermined significance, high-grade squamous intraepithelial lesion, or adenocarcinoma *in situ* in cytologic smears.[28]

Rare cases of endometriosis will show exclusively the stromal component. In these instances, the lesion can simulate endometrial stromal sarcoma or Karposi's sarcoma. These latter conditions, however, usually exhibit infiltrative borders and vascular/lymphatic invasion. Karposi's sarcoma also shows spindle cells arranged in short fascicles, slit-like spaces containing red blood cells, and intra- and extracellular eosinophilic globules. Karposi's sarcoma expresses CD31 and CD34 immunoreactivity.[7,22,45]

MESONEPHRIC REMNANTS AND HYPERPLASIA

MESONEPHRIC DUCT REMNANTS

Remnants of the embryologic mesonephric duct system are common findings in hysterectomy specimens. They are also occasionally found in cone and even LEEP biopsy specimens. Remnants are found in 22% of adult cervices and in 40% of newborns and children.[49] Not uncommonly, they are detected as an abnormal cervical smear.[18,60]

Mesonephric duct remnants are most commonly found laterally, usually deep in the endocervical wall. Sometimes, they are superficial, appearing to open into an endocervical gland.[14] The usual mesonephric duct remnants appear as small groups of glands or tubules, sometimes arranged around a mother duct or a duct branch (Figure 6.93). Some appear as ducts without tubules (Figure 6.94). The lining epithelium is a single layer of cuboidal to columnar cells with scanty clear to slightly eosinophilic cytoplasm. In contrast to müllerian epithelial cells, mesonephric epithelial cells lack both mucinous secretion and cilia. The round, bland nuclei occasionally overlap. Usually there is no mitotic activity. Most of the tubular lumens contain an eosinophilic material (Figure 6.95), although occasionally it is not found.[49] There is luminal expression of CD10.[30,32] The cytoplasm lacks glycogen (PAS negative), while the luminal contents are PAS positive, diastase-resistant.[14]

MESONEPHRIC DUCT HYPERPLASIA

Three different types of hyperplasia arise from the mesonephric remnants: lobular, diffuse, and ductal.[14] The lobular type is the most common type. Its distinction from mesonephric remnants is arbitrary and based on the appearance of the lobules, which are larger, more loosely organized, and more irregularly shaped (Figure 6.96).[14,60] Lobular mesonephric hyperplasia occurs in patients with a mean age of 35 years. Usually, it is an incidental finding, but it can produce nodularity or an indurated cervix. It ranges in size from 4 to 22 mm, retains for the most part a

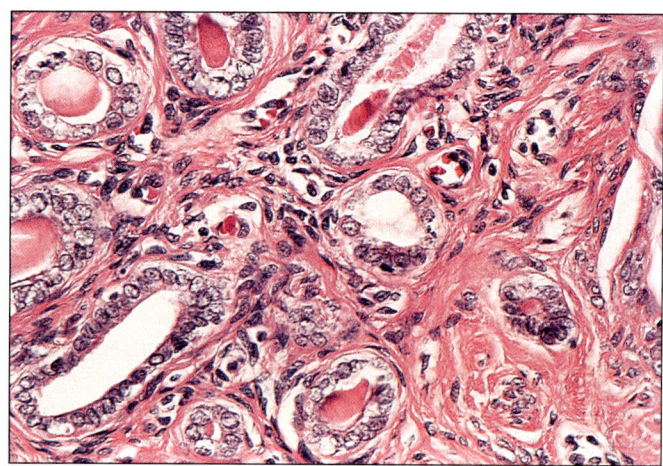

Fig. 6.94 Mesonephric remnants. The tubules consist of a single layer of low cuboidal-to-columnar epithelium. The cytoplasm lacks glycogen and is mucin negative. The cells also lack other distinguishing features, such as cilia. The nuclei are bland and large when compared to the rest of the cell, and some overlap.

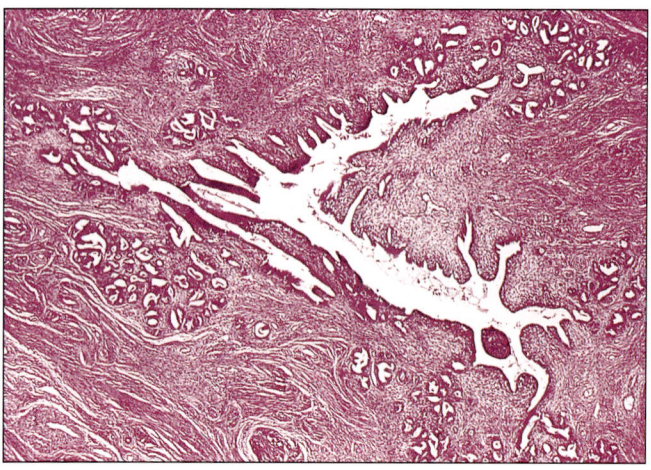

Fig. 6.93 Mesonephric remnants. Lobules of smaller tubular glands lie about a main branching duct.

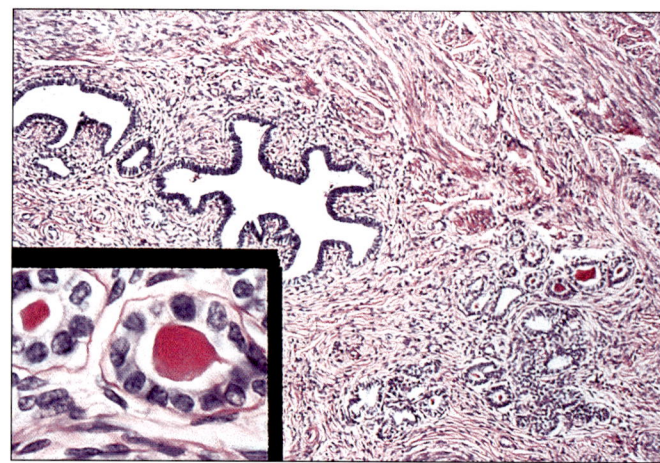

Fig. 6.95 Mesonephric remnants. In contrast to the cytoplasmic properties, the lumens nearly always contain an eosinophilic, homogeneous material that is PAS and mucicarmine positive (inset).

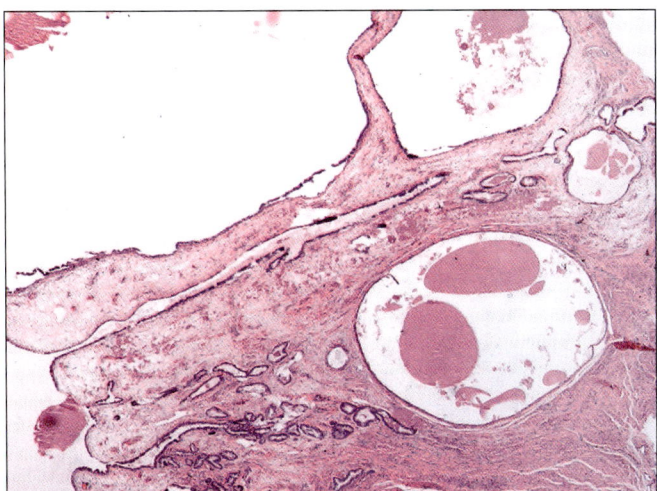

Fig. 6.96 Mesonephric hyperplasia, lobular type.

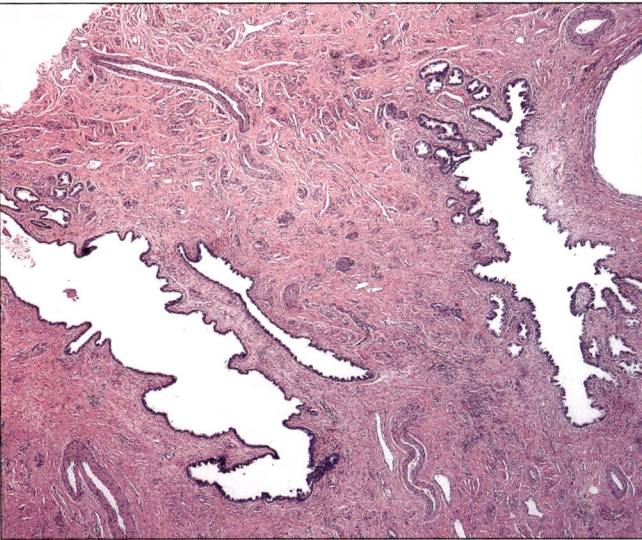

Fig. 6.98 Mesonephric hyperplasia, ductal type.

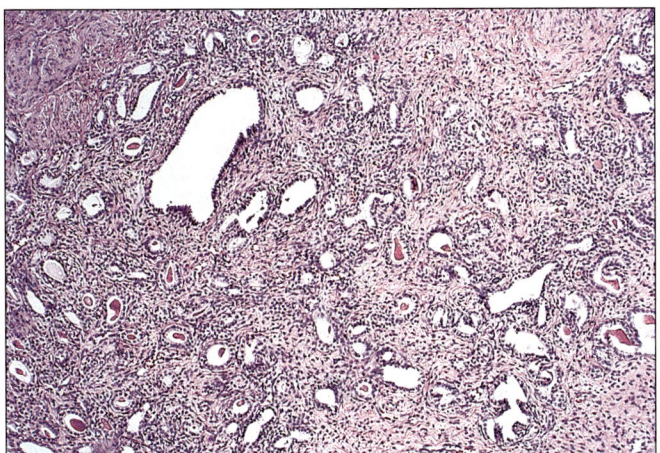

Fig. 6.97 Mesonephric duct hyperplasia, diffuse type. The central duct can still be identified but the proliferating tubules have a haphazard arrangement.

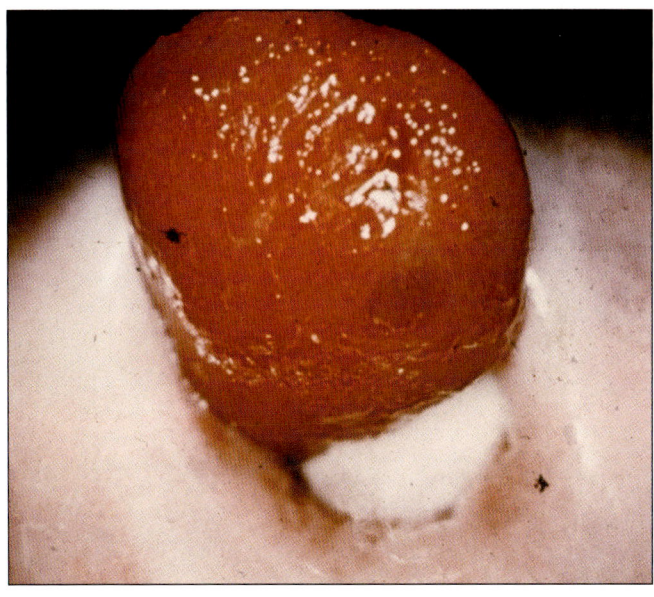

Fig. 6.99 Cervical polyp. A large polyp protrudes from the external cervical os. The surface is red and rough, covered by endocervical epithelium. Courtesy of Dr Henry J Norris, Orlando, FL.

lobular architecture, which can be lost focally, and can extend deep into the cervical wall. The cuboidal or columnar lining epithelium can form small tufts and rare mitotic figures can be found.

The second most common type of mesonephric hyperplasia is the diffuse type. The women are slightly older (mean age, 47 years) and the finding is usually incidental. Extensive disease can result in an irregular cervical shape or hypertrophy and erosion. Most lesions are 13–25 mm in size, extend deeply into the wall, and are not restricted to the lateral walls in the endocervix. Rarely, they expand into the lower uterine segment. Microscopically, there is a diffuse proliferation of mesonephric tubules, with or without ducts (Figure 6.97). A rare mitotic figure is sometimes found, but cytologic atypia is lacking.

The least common form of mesonephric hyperplasia, the ductal type (Figure 6.98), displays prominent ducts with papillary tufting, but a minimal proliferation of tubules (Figure 6.98).

Differential diagnosis

Mesonephric hyperplasias must be differentiated from mesonephric adenocarcinoma.[2,14] The latter is usually associated with symptoms and a cervical mass. In addition, the presence of nuclear atypia, conspicuous mitotic activity, vascular/lymphatic invasion, and other patterns of mesonephric adenocarcinoma, such as solid or ductal, help facilitate the correct diagnosis. Assessment of Ki-67 reactivity is helpful as about 15% of malignant cells are reactive in comparison to 1–2% of hyperplastic mesonephric cells.[51] It must also be differentiated from adenoma malignum, which also may display regular-looking glands lined by bland epithelium.

CERVICAL POLYP

Cervical polyps, which are common, are localized overgrowths of endocervical tissue (Figures 6.99–6.101). Most do not cause symptoms while others present with spotting or irregular vaginal bleeding. The polyp consists of lamina propria, with surface epithelium and underlying crypts. If the surface epithe-

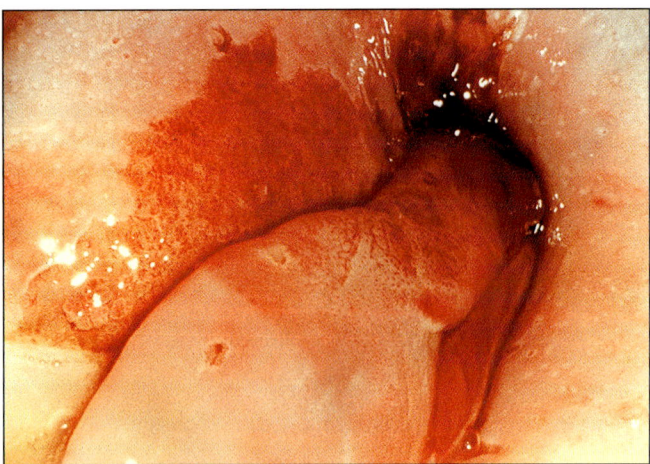

Fig. 6.100 Cervical polyp. Bleeding has been caused by mechanical friction of this polyp. The surface is smooth and has undergone squamous metaplasia.

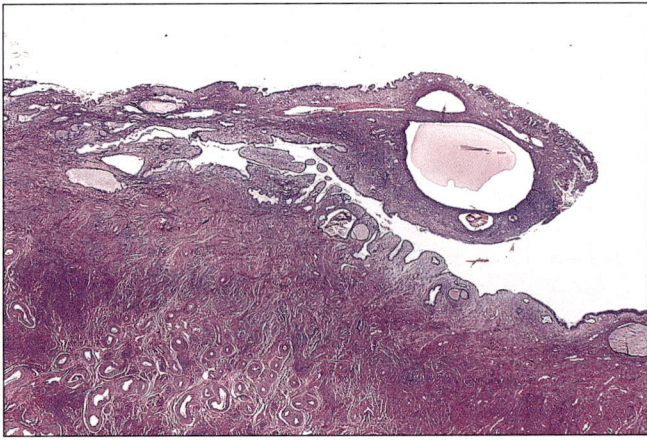

Fig. 6.101 Cervical polyp. The stroma is fibromuscular and the base contains thick-walled blood vessels. Endocervical crypts, some dilated, are present within the polyp.

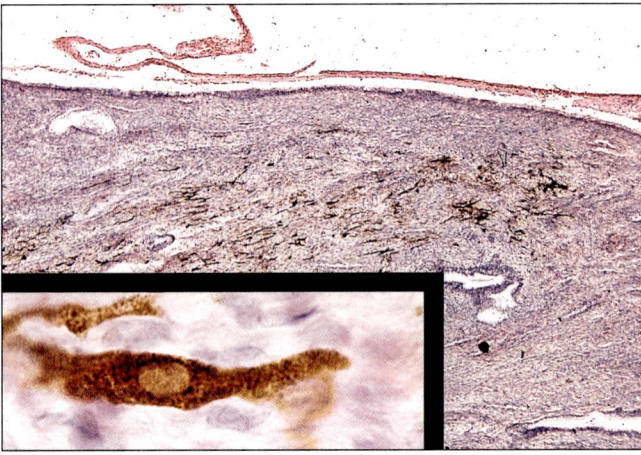

Fig. 6.102 Blue nevus. Polygonal and spindle cells filled with melanin are clustered beneath the surface epithelium in the endocervical stroma. The cytoplasm is laden with melanin granules (inset).

lium ulcerates, the underlying tissue may take on the character of granulation tissue. This is often seen with symptomatic polyps. The surface epithelium, if present, often shows squamous metaplasia of various degrees of maturity. In addition, inflammatory cells often permeate the superficial stroma with plasma cells predominating. Polyps with squamous metaplasia often contain dilated endocervical crypts. Sometimes a polyp may be composed solely of a few mucus-filled cysts covered by a layer of metaplastic squamous epithelium. Endocervical polyps must be distinguished from polyps arising in the endometrium and from leiomyomatous polyps, both of which may extend into the endocervical canal and protrude through the external os.

On occasion, the surface epithelium of a polyp can have superimposed CIN. Usually this is in association with CIN involving another area of the transformation zone, but occasionally CIN is exclusively confined to the polyp. CIN in the form of a polyp is also easy to miss; numerous mitoses are a clue to its premalignant nature. 'Cervical polyps', particularly if clinically recurrent, may be an apparently innocent presentation of embryonal rhabdomyosarcoma and attention should be given to examination of the stromal as well as to the epithelial component of the polyps.

BENIGN TUMORS

SQUAMOUS PAPILLOMA AND CONDYLOMA ACUMINATUM

Papillary lesions on the cervix are not common; the most frequently encountered is the condyloma acuminatum. Whether or not a genuine benign neoplastic papilloma of the cervix, distinct from the condyloma acuminatum, really exists is open to debate.

Histologic criteria have been suggested for distinguishing the two lesions. Squamous papillomas are reputedly solitary whereas condylomata are usually multiple. Condylomata show parakeratosis with little or no hyperkeratosis whereas the papilloma has a prominent granular layer with hyperkeratosis. We feel that such distinctions are invalid and that the two conditions, if indeed two separate conditions exist, cannot be distinguished on histologic grounds. For practical purposes, all benign, papillary squamous lesions on the cervix should be considered condylomata. (See Chapters 7 and 8 for a full discussion of condyloma acuminatum.)

LEIOMYOMA

Leiomyomas may be found in the cervix, but far less commonly than in the uterine body. Apart from their position, there are no features that distinguish them from those seen at the more usual sites (see Chapter 18). They are subject to the same histologic variants and the same forms of degeneration and may also undergo malignant change. The same criteria for malignancy are applied as in the myometrium.

A leiomyoma in the cervix causes distortion of the organ, with stretching and narrowing of the canal. Distinction must be made between a leiomyoma arising in the fibromuscular tissue of the cervix and a pedunculated leiomyoma that has arisen submucosally in the body of the uterus and has elongated sufficiently to protrude through the cervical os. Genuine cervical leiomyomas are, in our experience, rarely pedunculated.

BLUE NEVUS

This small, benign, melanocytic tumor with prominent dendrites is found in the stroma.[15] It is seen in 0.5% of uteri, but in up to 30% with step-serial sectioning.[56] The cervix is the most common non-cutaneous site for this lesion. It is asymptomatic and usually an incidental finding in biopsy, conization or hysterectomy specimens. The lesion is blue to black, flat, and usually 2–3 mm wide, although some reach 2 cm. One-fifth are multiple. Typically the lesion is in the lower endocervix and ill defined. Microscopically, blue nevi consist of polygonal and spindle cells filled with melanin (dermal melanocytes) and resemble blue nevi of the skin (Figure 6.102). Many have long dendritic processes, which may be arranged individually or appear in clusters just below and parallel to the endocervical epithelium. Macrophages usually accompany the dendritic cells in the stroma. The cytoplasm is laden with fine argentaffin- and argyrophil-positive melanin granules, but the melanin fails to react with Prussian blue and colloidal iron stains. The cells stain immunohistochemically for S-100 protein.

REFERENCES

1. Aseffa A, Ishak A, Stevens R, Fergussen E, Yohannes G, Kidan KG. Prevalence of HIV, syphilis and genital chlamydial infection among women in North-West Ethiopia. Epidemiol Infect 1998;120:171–7.
2. Bague S, Rodriguez IM, Prat J. Malignant mesonephric tumors of the female genital tract – a clinicopathologic study of 9 cases. Am J Surg Pathol 2004;28:601–7.
3. Baker AC, Eltoum I, Curry RO, et al. Mucinous expression in benign and neoplastic glandular lesions of the uterine cervix. Arch Path Lab Med 2006;130:1510–15.
4. Baker PM, Clement PB, Bell DA, Young RH. Superficial endometriosis of the uterine cervix: a report of 20 cases of a process that may be confused with endocervical glandular dysplasia or adenocarcinoma in situ. Int J Gynecol Pathol 1999;18:198–205.
5. Benevolo M, Mottolese M, Marandino F, et al. Immunohistochemical expression of p16(INK4a) is predictive of HR-HPV infection in cervical low-grade lesions. Mod Pathol 2006;19:384–91.
6. Chakraborty P, Roy A, Bhattacharya S, Addhya S, Mukherjee S. Tuberculous cervicitis: a clinicopathological and bacteriological study. J Indian Med Assoc 1995;93:167–8.
7. Cheuk W, Wong KO, Wong CS, Dinkel JE, Ben-Dor D, Chan JK. Immunostaining for human herpesvirus 8 latent nuclear antigen-1 helps distinguish Kaposi sarcoma from its mimickers. Am J Clin Pathol 2004;121:335–42.
8. Clark RA, Brandon W, Dumestre J, Pindaro C. Clinical manifestations of infection with the human immunodeficiency virus in women in Louisiana. Clin Infect Dis 1993;17:165–72.
9. Dietrich M, Hoosen AA, Moodley J, Moodley S. Urogenital tract infections in pregnancy at King Edward VIII Hospital, Durban, South Africa. Genitourin Med 1992;68:39–41.
10. Dray M, Russell P, Dalrymple C, et al. P16(INK4a) as a complementary marker of high-grade intraepithelial lesions of the uterine cervix. I: Experience with squamous lesions in 189 consecutive cervical biopsies. Pathology 2005;37:112–24.
11. Duggan MA. Cytologic and histologic diagnosis and significance of controversial squamous lesions of the uterine cervix. Mod Pathol 2000;13:252–60.
12. Egan AJM, Russell P. Transitional (urothelial) cell metaplasia of the uterine cervix: morphological assessment of 31 cases. Int J Gynecol Pathol 1997;16:89–98.
13. Farlie R, Jylling AMB, Vetner M. Diffuse laminar endocervical glandular hyperplasia – two cases presenting with excessive mucinous cervical discharge. Acta Obstet Gynecol Scand 1998;77:131–3.
14. Ferry JA, Scully RE. Mesonephric remnants, hyperplasia, and neoplasia of the uterine cervix: a study of 49 cases. Am J Surg Pathol 1990;14:1100–14.
15. Gonzalez-Campora R, Galera-Davidson H, Vazquez-Ramirez FJ, Diaz-Cano S. Blue nevus: classical types and new related entities. A differential diagnostic review. Pathol Res Pract 1994;190:627–35.
16. Greeley C, Schroeder S, Silverberg SG. Microglandular hyperplasia of the cervix: a true 'pill' lesion? Int J Gynecol Pathol 1995;14:50–4.
17. Harnden P, Kennedy W, Andrew AC, Southgate J. Immunophenotype of transitional metaplasia of the uterine cervix. Int J Gynecol Pathol 1999;18:125–9.
18. Hejmadi RK, Gearty JC, Waddell C, Ganesan R. Mesonephric hyperplasia can cause abnormal cervical smears: report of three cases with review of literature. Cytopathology 2005;16:240.
19. Jonasson JG, Wang HH, Antonioli DA, Ducatman BS. Tubal metaplasia of the uterine cervix: a prevalence study in patients with gynecologic pathologic findings. Int J Gynecol Pathol 1992;11:89–95.
20. Jones MA, Young RH. Endocervical type A (noncystic) tunnel clusters with cytologic atypia: a report of 14 cases. Am J Surg Pathol 1996;20:1312–18.
21. Jones MA, Young RH, Scully RE. Diffuse laminar endocervical glandular hyperplasia: a benign lesion often confused with adenoma malignum (minimal deviation adenocarcinoma). Am J Surg Pathol 1991;15:1123–9.
22. Katz IA, De Silva KS, Eckstein RP, Philips J. Stromal endometriosis of the cervix simulating Kaposi's sarcoma. Pathology 1997;29:426–7.
23. Kim KR, Park KH, Kim JW, Cho KJ, Ro JY. Transitional cell metaplasia and ectopic prostatic tissue in the uterine cervix and vagina in a patient with adrenogenital syndrome: report of a case suggesting a possible role of androgen in the histogenesis. Int J Gynecol Pathol 2004;23:182–7.
24. Kiviat NB, Paavonen JA, WolnerHanssen P, et al. Histopathology of endocervical infection caused by Chlamydia trachomatis, herpes simplex virus, Trichomonas vaginalis, and Neisseria gonorrhoeae. Hum Pathol 1990;21:831–7.
25. Kondo T, Hashi A, Murata S, et al. Endocervical adenocarcinomas associated with lobular endocervical glandular hyperplasia: a report of four cases with histochemical and immunohistochemical analyses. Mod Pathol 2005;18:1199–210.
26. Lamba H, Byrne M, Goldin R, Jenkins C. Tuberculosis of the cervix: case presentation and a review of the literature. Sex Transm Infect 2002;78:62–3.
27. Lesack D, Wahab I, Gilks CB. Radiation-induced atypia of endocervical epithelium: a histological, immunohistochemical and cytometric study. Int J Gynecol Pathol 1996;15:242–7.
28. Lundeen SJ, Horwitz CA, Larson CJ, Stanley MW. Abnormal cervicovaginal smears due to endometriosis: a continuing problem. Diagn Cytopathol 2002;26:35–40.
29. Maruyama R, Nagaoka S, Terao K, Honda M, Koita H. Diffuse laminar endocervical glandular hyperplasia. Pathol Int 1995;45:283–6.
30. McCluggage WG. Immunohistochemistry as a diagnostic aid in cervical pathology. Pathology 2007;39:97–111.
31. McCluggage WG, Maxwell P, McBride HA, Hamilton PW, Bharucha H. Monoclonal antibodies Ki-67 and MIB1 in the distinction of tuboendometrial metaplasia from endocervical adenocarcinoma and adenocarcinoma in situ in formalin-fixed material. Int J Gynecol Pathol 1995;14:209–16.
32. McCluggage WG, Oliva E, Herrington CS, McBride H, Young RH. CD10 and calretinin staining of endocervical glandular lesions, endocervical stroma and endometrioid adenocarcinomas of the uterine corpus: CD10 positivity is characteristic of, but not specific for, mesonephric lesions and is not specific for endometrial stroma. Histopathology 2003;43:144–50.
33. McGalie CE, McBride HA, McCluggage WG. Cytomegalovirus infection of the cervix: morphological observations in five cases of a possibly under-recognised condition. J Clin Pathol 2004;57:691–4.
34. Mikami Y, Hata S, Melamed J, Moriya M. Basement membrane material in ovarian clear cell carcinoma: correlation with growth pattern and nuclear grade. Int J Gynecol Pathol 1999;18:52–7.
35. Mikami Y, Hata S, Melamed J, Fujiwara K, Manabe T. Lobular endocervical glandular hyperplasia is a metaplastic process with a pyloric gland phenotype. Histopathology 2001;39:364–72.
36. Mikami Y, Kiyokawa T, Hata S, et al. Gastrointestinal immunophenotype in adenocarcinomas of the uterine cervix and related glandular lesions: a possible link between lobular endocervical glandular hyperplasia/pyloric gland metaplasia and 'adenoma malignum'. Mod Pathol 2004;17:962–72.
37. Nucci MR, Young RH. Arias-Stella reaction of the endocervix: a report of 18 cases with emphasis on its varied histology and differential diagnosis. Am J Surg Pathol 2004;28:608–12.
38. Nucci MR, Clement PB, Young RH. Lobular endocervical glandular hyperplasia, not otherwise specified – a clinicopathologic analysis of thirteen cases of a distinctive pseudoneoplastic lesion and comparison with fourteen cases of adenoma malignum. Am J Surg Pathol 1999;23:886–91.
39. O'Neill CJ, McCluggage WG. p16 expression in the female genital tract and its value in diagnosis. Adv Anat Pathol 2006;13:8–15.
40. Oliva E, Clement PB, Young RH. Tubal and tubo-endometrioid metaplasia of the uterine cervix: unemphasized features that may cause problems in differential diagnosis. A report of 25 cases. Amr J Clin Pathol 1995;103:618–23.
41. Petry KU, Scholz U, Hollwitz B, von Wasielewski R, Meijer CJLM. Human papillomavirus, coinfection with Schistosoma hematobium, and cervical neoplasia in rural Tanzania. Int J Gynecol Cancer 2003;13:505–9.
42. Poggensee G, Feldmeier H. Female genital schistosomiasis: facts and hypotheses. Acta Trop 2001;79:193–210.

43. Poggensee G, Sahebali S, Van Marck E, Swai B, Krantz I, Feldmeier H. Diagnosis of genital cervical schistosomiasis: comparison of cytological, histopathological and parasitological examination. Am J Trop Med Hyg 2001;65:233–6.

44. Qiu WS, Mittal K. Comparison of morphologic and immunohistochemical features of cervical microglandular hyperplasia with low-grade mucinous adenocarcinoma of the endometrium. Int J Gynecol Pathol 2003;22:261–5.

45. Robin YM, Guillou L, Michels JJ, Coindre JM. Human herpesvirus 8 immunostaining: a sensitive and specific method for diagnosing Kaposi sarcoma in paraffin-embedded sections. Am J Clin Pathol 2004;121:330–4.

46. Schlesinger C, Silverberg SG. Endocervical adenocarcinoma in situ of tubal type and its relation to atypical tubal metaplasia. Int J Gynecol Pathol 1999;18:1–4.

47. Schneider V. Arias-Stella reaction of the endocervix: frequency and location. Acta Cytol 1981;25:224–8.

48. Segal GH, Hart WR. Cystic endocervical tunnel clusters. Am J Surg Pathol 1990;14:895–903.

49. Seidman JD, Tavassoli FA. Mesonephric hyperplasia of the uterine cervix: a clinicopathologic study of 51 cases. Int J Gynecol Pathol 1995;14:293–9.

50. Shield PW. Chronic radiation effects: a correlative study of smears and biopsies from the cervix and vagina. Diagn Cytopathol 1995;13:107–19.

51. Silver SA, Devouassoux-Shisheboran M, Mezzetti TP, Tavassoli FA. Mesonephric adenocarcinomas of the uterine cervix – a study of 11 cases with immunohistochemical findings. Am J Surg Pathol 2001;25:379–87.

52. Smedts F, Ramaekers F, Leube RE, Keijser K, Link M, Vooijs P. Expression of keratin-1, keratin-6, keratin-15, keratin-16, and keratin-20 in normal cervical epithelium, squamous metaplasia, cervical intraepithelial neoplasia, and cervical carcinoma. Am J Pathol 1993;142:403–12.

53. Suh KS, Silverberg SG. Tubal metaplasia of the uterine cervix. Int J Gynecol Pathol 1990;9:122–8.

54. Tringler B, Gup CJ, Singh M, et al. Evaluation of p16INK4a and pRb expression in cervical squamous and glandular neoplasia. Hum Pathol 2004;35:689–96.

55. Tsutsumi K, Sun Q, Yasumoto S, et al. In vitro and in vivo analysis of cellular origin of cervical squamous metaplasia. Am J Pathol 1993;143:1150–8.

56. Uehara T, Takayama S, Takemura T, Kasuga T. Foci of stromal melanocytes (so-called blue naevus) of the uterine cervix in Japanese women. Virchows Archiv A, Pathol Anat Histopathol 1991;418:327–31.

57. Vang R, Vinh TN, Burks RT, Barner R, Kurman RJ, Ronnett BM. Pseudoinfiltrative tubal metaplasia of the endocervix: a potential form of in utero diethylstilbestrol exposure-related adenosis simulating minimal deviation adenocarcinoma. Int J Gynecol Pathol 2005;24:391–8.

58. Weir MM, Bell DA. Transitional cell metaplasia of the cervix: a newly described entity in cervicovaginal smears. Diagn Cytopathol 1998;18:222–6.

59. Weir MM, Bell DA, Young RH. Transitional cell metaplasia of the uterine cervix and vagina: an underrecognized lesion that may be confused with high-grade dysplasia. A report of 59 cases. Am J Surg Pathol 1997;21:510–17.

60. Welsh T, Fu YS, Chan J, Brundage HA, Rutgers JL. Mesonephric remnants of hyperplasia can cause abnormal pap smears: a study of three cases. Int J Gynecol Pathol 2003;22:121–6.

61. Wheeler DT, Kurman RJ. The relationship of glands to thick-wall blood vessels as a marker of invasion in endocervical adenocarcinoma. Int J Gynecol Pathol 2005;24:125–30.

62. Witkiewicz AK, Hecht JL, Cviko A, McKeon FD, Ince TA, Crum CP. Microglandular hyperplasia: a model for the de novo emergence and evolution of endocervical reserve cells. Hum Pathol 2005;36:154–61.

63. Yeh IT, Bronner M, Livolsi VA. Endometrial metaplasia of the uterine endocervix. Arch Pathol Lab Med 1993;117:734–5.

64. Yelverton CL, Bentley RC, Olenick S, Krigman HR, Johnston WW, Robboy SJ. Epithelial repair of the uterine cervix: assessment of morphologic features and correlations with cytologic diagnosis. Int J Gynecol Pathol 1996;15:338–44.

65. Young RH, Scully RE. Atypical forms of microglandular hyperplasia of the cervix simulating carcinoma. Am J Surg Pathol 1989;13:50–6.

66. Young RH, Clement PB. Pseudoneoplastic glandular lesions of the uterine cervix. Semin Diagn Pathol 1991;8:234–49.

67. Zaloudek C, Hayashi GM, Ryan IP, Powell CB, Miller TR. Microglandular adenocarcinoma of the endometrium: a form of mucinous adenocarcinoma that may be confused with microglandular hyperplasia of the cervix. Int J Gynecol Pathol 1997;16:52–9.

Cervix: epidemiology of squamous neoplasia

Sophia S. Wang Mark E. Sherman

From an etiologic and epidemiologic perspective, cervical cancer is among the best understood tumor of women. Experimental, clinical, and epidemiologic evidence demonstrate unequivocally that infection with one of 15 oncogenic genotypes of human papillomavirus (HPV) is required for the development of cervical cancer. However, HPV infection is extremely common, usually does not produce clinical signs, symptoms, or detectable pathology, and typically clears without treatment. Therefore, although HPV infection is a necessary cause of cervical cancer, exposure to HPV alone is insufficient for cervical carcinogenesis. It is hoped that future refinements in the multistage model of cervical carcinogenesis (Figure 7.1) will include the identification of molecular events that are both necessary and sufficient for progression of infection to neoplasia, permitting the identification of obligate cancer precursors through screening. At present, use of HPV testing as an adjunct to cytologic screening and administration of prophylactic vaccines to prevent HPV infection represent the most promising new approaches for cervical cancer prevention.

EPIDEMIOLOGY AND PUBLIC HEALTH SIGNIFICANCE

Worldwide, cervical cancer is the second most common cancer among women, accounting for 471 000 incident cases and 230 000 deaths in 2000.[149] The heaviest disease burden remains in developing countries that have high HPV prevalences and lack effective screening programs (Figure 7.2). In resource-poor regions such as East Africa, cervical cancer is the most common tumor among women, with age-standardized rates that are five times those in developed countries.[17] In contrast, in geographic regions (e.g., United States and European countries) that have had effective cytologic screening programs (Papanicolaou test) in place for a number of years, cervical cancer incidence and mortality rates have declined markedly.[13,75,196] Within these countries, most cancers arise among unscreened women. Although the success of cytologic screening in cervical cancer control is remarkable, cervical cancer rates actually began falling in the US prior to widespread screening, possibly reflecting changes in HPV cofactors (e.g., reduced childbearing) or other factors. In countries with low HPV prevalence such as China[118] and North Vietnam,[153] however, cervical cancer rates remain low, even in the absence of effective screening programs.

Squamous cell carcinomas (SCC) comprise 85% of all cervical cancers, and it is the detection of SCC precursors (cervical intraepithelial neoplasia (CIN) or squamous intraepithelial lesion (SIL)) through screening that accounts for declining cervical cancer rates in developed countries in the latter half of the twentieth century. In contrast, there is evidence that both absolute incidence rates for adenocarcinoma and relative percentages of adenocarcinoma relative to squamous cell carcinoma are increasing among young women in the US for reasons that are not well understood.[196] Historical data suggest that screening provides less protection against adenocarcinoma as compared to SCC,[132] and, in fact, many endocervical neoplasms have been identified serendipitously at the time of investigation for a concurrent squamous lesion. In recognition of this concern, improved criteria for identifying endocervical abnormalities and better terminology for reporting these findings have been introduced.[173,196]

THE ETIOLOGIC AGENT: HUMAN PAPILLOMAVIRUS (HPV)

EVIDENCE FOR CAUSALITY

Although the causal role of HPV in cervical neoplasia is now universally accepted, proving this relationship required years of research and the development of improved technologies and approaches, including accurate methods for detecting HPV DNA in exfoliative cervical specimens, improved cytologic and histologic classification of cancer precursors, and sophisticated study designs. A comprehensive summary of the evidence is presented elsewhere,[18] but summarized below.

All epidemiologic criteria for establishing causality between HPV and cervical cancer have been fulfilled:[18,88] (1) strength of the association; (2) specificity of the association; (3) consistency of the association; (4) temporality (HPV exposure precedes disease); (5) dose–response; (6) biologic plausibility; and (7) experimental evidence (e.g., viral detection in tumors). Data from an international multicenter case-control study demonstrated that HPV infection conferred a 50- to over 100-fold risk increase for cervical cancer.[139] Similar associations in case-control studies have consistently been demonstrated worldwide,[17,139,191] specifically for what are now recognized as the approximately 15 oncogenic HPV types that account for 95% of cervical cancers[140] (Table 7.1). Among oncogenic types, there are some specific disease associations such as the relatively greater role of HPV 18 in adenocarcinoma and the greater role of HPV 16 in SCC. Cohort studies have now further demonstrated that oncogenic HPV DNA detection clearly precedes development of cervical neoplasia.[119,160,205,210] Laboratory evidence has provided compelling evidence that HPV is a plausible

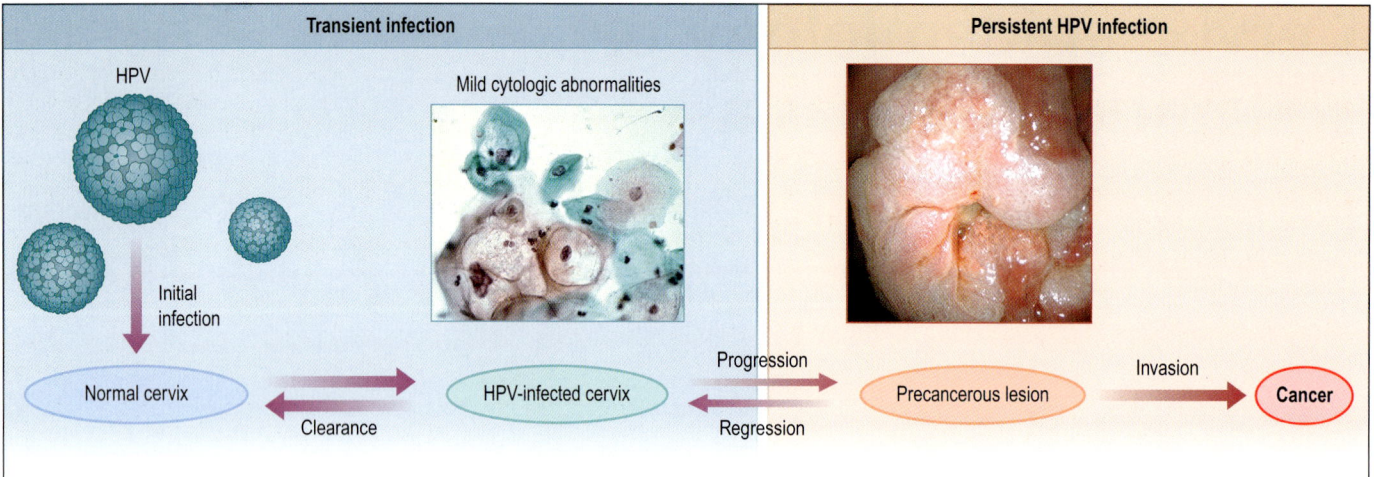

Fig. 7.1 Model of HPV-induced cervical pathogenesis, proceeding from HPV infection of the normal cervix to mild cytologic abnormalities, progression to persistent HPV infection and precancerous lesions, and finally, invasion. Of significance is the ability for precancerous lesions to regress, and the ability of most HPV-infected cervix to clear infection. Reproduced with permission from Wright and Schiffman.[207]

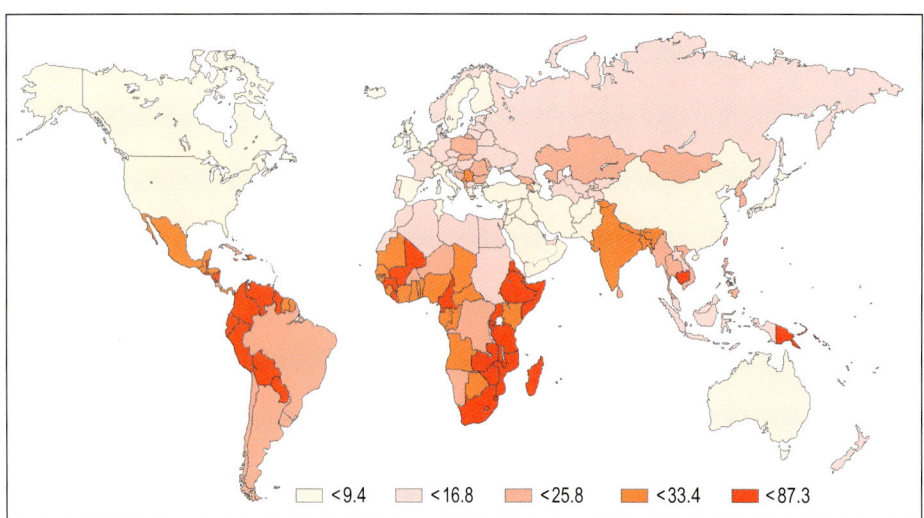

Fig. 7.2 Age-standardized incidence rate of cervix uteri per 100 000 women worldwide in the year 2002. The lowest disease burden is largely found among regions with effective screening programs (e.g., northern America) and regions where HPV prevalence is low (e.g., China). The greatest disease burden is denoted in red and is found in those countries with high HPV prevalence and without an effective screening program (e.g., East Africa). Reproduced with permission from Ferlay et al.[63]

| <9.4 | <16.8 | <25.8 | <33.4 | <87.3 |

Table 7.1 Classification of HPV types associated with genital lesions

Classification	HPV type
Oncogenic	16, 18, 31, 33, 35, 39, 45, 51, 52, 56, 58, 59, 68, 73, 82
Putatively oncogenic	26, 53, 66, 70
Non-oncogenic	6,11, 40, 42, 54, 55, 57, 84

Adapted from Munoz et al.[140]

HPV CLASSIFICATION AND PHYLOGENY

Human papillomavirus genomes consist of a single molecule of circular double-stranded DNA, measuring approximately 8000 basepairs (8 kilobases). Classification of papillomaviruses includes types, subtypes, and variants. Briefly, HPV types are delineated by a >10% difference in the nucleotide sequence of the L1 gene (described below); HPV subtypes are delineated by a 2–10% difference in this same region. HPV type variants are defined as having <2% difference in the L1 nucleotide sequence.[14] Evidence suggests that even the relatively modest genetic variations found among type variants may have biologic and clinical importance.

At present, there are over 100 HPV types identified, comprising HPV types that infect either the genital/mucosal or skin areas. Oncogenic HPV types are defined as those which are associated with cancer (cervical, anal)[213] and include HPV types 16, 18, 31, 33, 35, 39, 45, 51, 52, 56, 58, 59, 68, 73, and 82[140] (Table 7.1). Most HPV types are non-oncogenic (HPV 6, 11 are the prototypes) and their infections in the skin or mucosa result in conditions such as warts.[15,32] Among

carcinogen; the E6 and E7 genes of oncogenic HPV types immortalize and transform cervical cell lines and produce cancers in animal models (e.g., cattle, rabbits, dogs).[17,18,44] Although the concept of dose–response is not entirely applicable to HPV infection, it is accepted that clinically occult infections are associated with lower viral loads than ones that produce demonstrable pathologic lesions. More limited evidence suggests that higher loads may predict future risk of disease, especially for HPV 16.[193]

general populations (cytologically normal women), HPV type distribution varies by geographical region (Figure 7.3). HPV 16 is the most common oncogenic HPV type and possesses the highest potential for HPV persistence and progression to cervical cancer.[162] Type distribution differs by histopathologic type of cancer. Among SCCs, HPV 16 is the predominant type, followed by HPV 18, 45, 31 and 33. Among adenocarcinoma, however, HPV 18 is followed or equaled in frequency by HPV 16 and 45.[42,43]

As HPV type variants are identified, differences in their biologic behavior and clinical significance are becoming evident. Several studies have now documented an association between HPV 16 variants and the development of cervical cancer, with non-European variants conferring greater cervical cancer risk than European variants.[193,208] Although fewer data are currently available for other types, they similarly suggest that other non-European variants for HPV types 18 and 58 increase the risk for cervical cancer above that observed with European variants.[193]

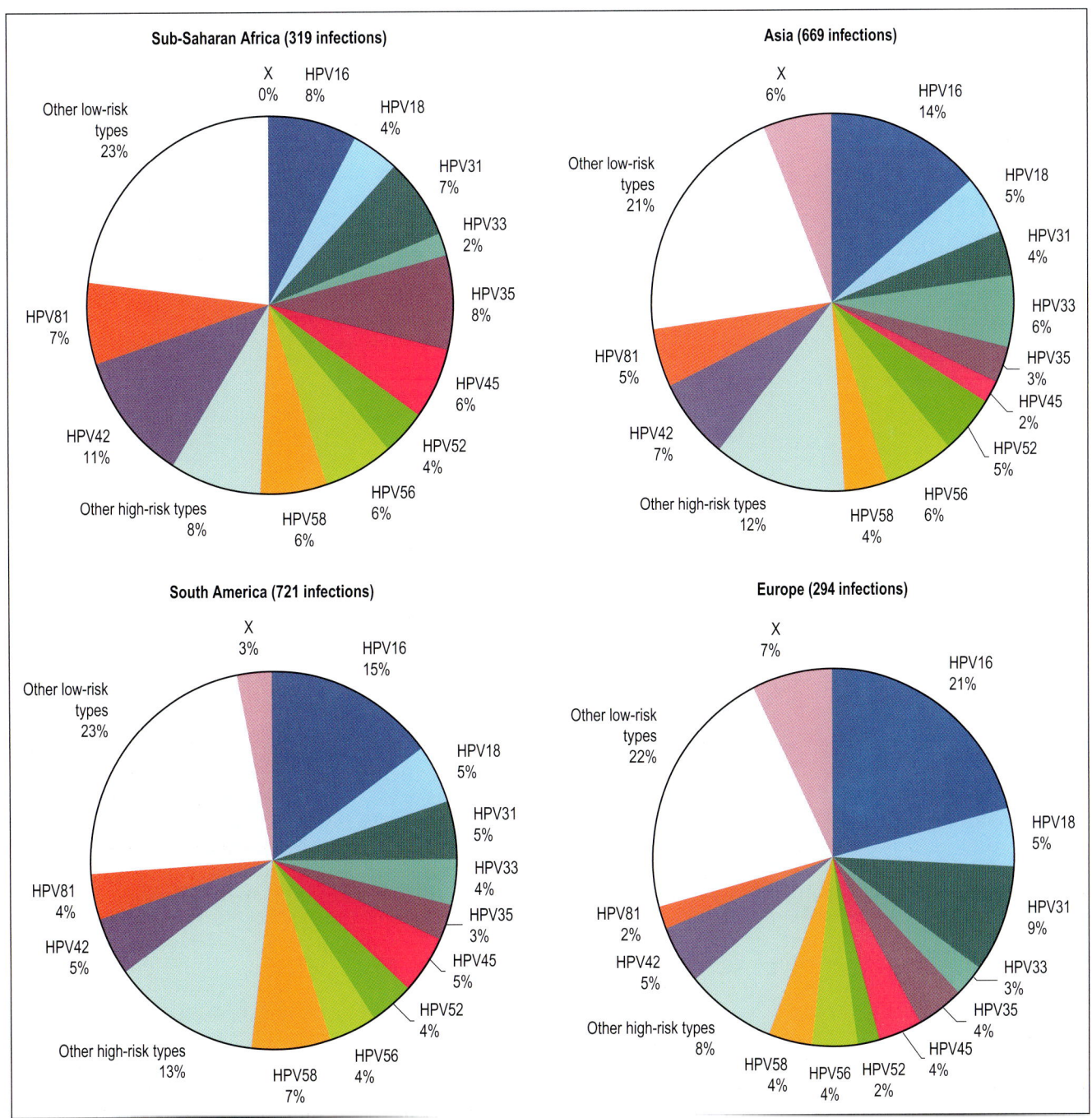

Fig. 7.3 Prevalence of HPV types in cytologically normal women worldwide, by geographic region. HPV type-specific burden varies by geography, with HPV 16 prevalence highest (21%) in Europe but HPV 18 prevalence equivalent in all regions. Reproduced with permission from Clifford et al.[41]

THE HPV GENOME

The HPV genome comprises three coding regions with eight open reading frames that are required for viral DNA replication and synthesis of the icosahedral capsids that form the protein shell of the complete non-enveloped virions (Figure 7.4).[55,62,128,137,138,213] Specifically, there are two coding regions, generally corresponding to functions required in the early (E) and late (L) periods of the viral life cycle. The six early open reading frames (ORFs) (E1, E2, E4, E5, E6, E7) regulate viral gene expression; they encode proteins that are involved in transcription, DNA replication and transformation of host cells, and recruitment of the host enzymatic machinery for these purposes. The late regions encode for two late ORFs (L1, L2) that encode the structural proteins. The third region, a small (1000 basepairs) non-coding region (NCR), also referred to as the long control region (LCR) or upstream regulatory region (URR), is responsible for RNA synthesis, modulating transcription or enhancers, and thus regulates expression of the ORFs.

EARLY GENES

E1, E2, E4, and E7 are involved in viral replication. Specifically, E1, a key regulator of viral replication and transcription, encodes the major transregulatory proteins that interact with the upstream region; the E1 protein functions as a DNA-dependent ATPase and an ATP-dependent helicase. E2 mediates the physical partitioning of episomal HPV DNA into daughter and host cells during division. Together, E1 and E2 form a protein complex that promotes the stable binding of E1 to an AT-rich sequence at the origin of viral replication. E4, which is most highly expressed in differentiated cells, encodes a protein that binds to and disrupts the cytoplasmic keratin network, contributing to the formation of cells recognized as koilocytes. E4 therefore acts late in the life cycle rather than early, as the nomenclature implies. Although the action of E4 remains incompletely understood, it seems to participate with E1 in forming a fusion protein. E4 expression is associated with the start of vegetative replication late in the viral life cycle (described below); it disrupts the cellular cytoskeleton, interfering with normal keratinocyte maturation by binding to tonofilaments. E5, which encodes a small protein that binds to a number of host membrane proteins, including growth factor receptors (e.g., platelet derived growth factor (PDGF) beta receptor), appears involved in cell transformation, although it is often lost during viral integration into the human genome (see below) and is only weakly transforming in humans.

The two remaining early genes, E6 and E7, play critical roles in HPV oncogenicity. E6 and E7 are conserved genes and are expressed in all HPV-associated neoplasia. E6 and E7 encode proteins that immortalize human keratinocytes and induce cell proliferation and transformation. Specifically, the E6 protein of oncogenic HPV types binds p53, a cell cycle regulatory protein, and leads to its destruction through a ubiquitin-dependent mechanism.[202] Therefore, E6 gene products abrogate the critical functions of the *p53* tumor suppressor gene in producing cell cycle arrest and apoptosis in response to DNA damage. E6 also inhibits *p53*-mediated apoptosis in other ways, including interfering with coactivators and interacting with Myc and Bak proteins. E7 binds to the retinoblastoma (Rb) gene product and related 'pocket proteins' (pocket protein comprises Rb, p107 and p130),[59,79] leading to dissociation of the normal E2F-Rb family complex and promoting proteolytic degradation of pocket proteins. Functionally, the inhibitory function of the Rb gene is damaged. As a result, E2F-mediated transcription of key molecules required for cell division is triggered, including DNA polymerase alpha, enzymes involved in nucleotide biosynthesis, and cyclins that control progression through S phase. Based on animal models where transgenic mice expressing E7 develop benign differentiated tumors and mice expressing E6 develop malignant neoplasms, it seems that E7 acts mainly to increase cell division, whereas E6 primarily prevents apoptosis. In summary, HPV oncogenes keep cells cycling, allowing the virus to have access to cellular machinery required for its own replication. Functionally, the HPV disrupts the normal inhibitory functions of the Rb gene and *p53* of the host cellular machinery, thereby fostering uncontrolled cell growth.

LATE GENES

The late genes, *L1* and *L2*, encode the major and minor viral capsid proteins, respectively, that form the icosahedral capsid or protein coat of the virus. In vitro, *L1* assembles into virus-like particles (VLPs), which possess morphology and antigenicity similar to whole virions, a feature exploited in vaccine development. When *L1* and *L2* are coexpressed *in vitro*, both

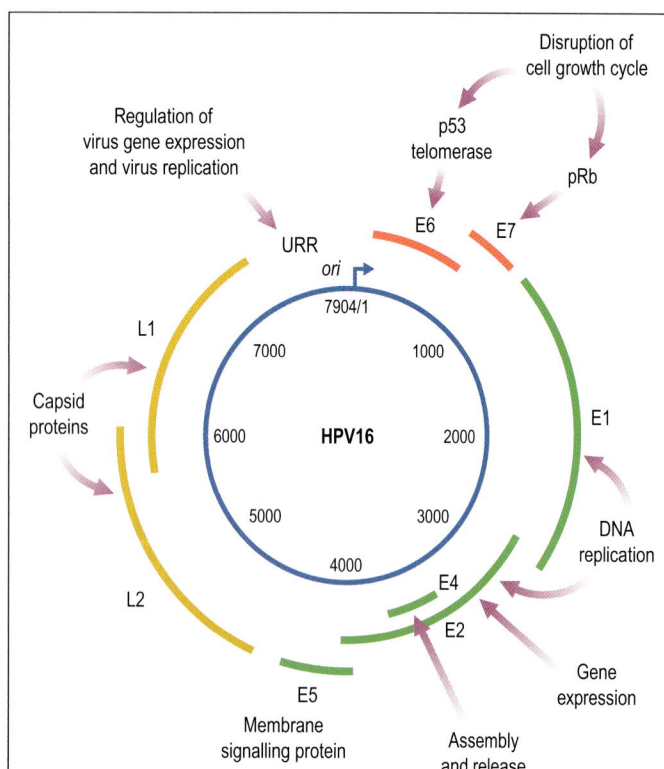

Fig. 7.4 HPV genome. Reproduced with permission from Alan Cann, University of Leicester, UK.

proteins are incorporated into VLPs. *L2* may be required for encapsidation of HPV DNA.

HPV LIFE CYCLE

The cervical transformation zone, the area between the os and the squamocolumnar junction, is the site where infection usually begins and most CIN develops.[92] At the cervical transformation zone, HPV passes through minor defects in the epithelial surface to infect the basal, reserve or stem cells. The reasons why the transformation zone is particularly susceptible to HPV infection and subsequent progression to CIN remain unknown. It has been posited that these cells express cell surface receptors that favor HPV binding and intracellular entry. It has also been suggested that the presence of replicating stem cells that do not mature provides a suitable microenvironment for infection. Immunologic or hormonal factors unique to the transformation zone might also account for this tropism. In brief, the HPV life cycle can proceed along different pathways with varied implications: (1) productive; (2) abortive; and (3) latent infections, although the existence of the last is debated.

A *productive (vegetative) infection* leads to the production of whole infectious virions. Productive infections are limited to epithelia that will undergo maturation, a process that occurs under the influence of estrogen and progesterone. In normal uninfected cervical mucosa, cell maturation proceeds as cells migrate towards the epithelial surface in conjunction with cell cycle arrest. In basal cells, HPV replication is limited by E2, a key regulator of viral replication and transcription. As cell maturation proceeds, HPV usurps the host cell's metabolic machinery by inactivating the cell cycle inhibitors p21 and p27 (see Chapter 37, showing the cell cycle machinery in HPV infection of the cervix). HPV-infected cells continue to cycle under the influence of the HPV oncoproteins E6 and E7, and the uncoupling of cell division and maturation permits viral replication and full capsid assembly. Differentiation is marked by the switch from the early to late genes where control of viral replication is no longer tightly controlled and enhanced viral replication ensues. Capsid production and virion assembly occur under the influence of E4 and L1 expression only within mature surface epithelium[180] (Figure 7.5). Morphologically, cellular maturation in uninfected epithelium exhibits cytoplasmic enlargement and nuclear condensation. In productive HPV infections, maturation proceeds but cells may display slight nuclear enlargement, sometimes double nuclei and usually cytoplasmic haloes that confer the histologic appearance of an infectious process. When there is also hyperchromatism, nuclear pleomorphism, and loss of polarity, the lesion is considered CIN 1. In smears, the presence of any degree of HPV infection or low-grade dysplasia is called low-grade squamous intraepithelial lesion (LSIL).

Under conditions that remain unexplained, productive infections switch to *abortive infections*, converting an infectious process into a neoplastic one. In abortive infections, expression of late genes and virion assembly are inhibited, permitting increased epithelial thickening that consists of immature-appearing cells expressing HPV E6 and E7 and host genes that induce markers of cell cycling (e.g., Ki-67, PCNA, minichromosome maintenance proteins). It is unclear whether some

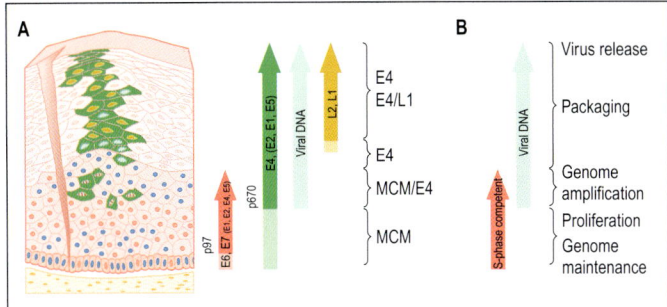

Fig. 7.5 HPV gene expression (supergroup A) during its life cycle, from HPV-infected basal cell and maturation to surface of epithelium. Upon infection, the viral genome is maintained as a low copy number episome. During epithelial differentiation, the p97 promoter directs E6 and E7 expression for S-phase entry (red) and viral replication proteins (E1, E2, E4, E5) increase in abundance (green), facilitating amplification of viral genomes (blue). E4 persists in upper epithelial layers where viral capsid proteins (L1, L2; yellow) are found. Reproduced with permission from Doorbar.[57]

HPV infections are abortive at inception, and whether those conditions account for rapid onset disease. Most cancers are preceded by type-specific HPV infections that have persisted for 10–20 years and progressed to CIN 3. In CIN 3, high levels of E6 and E7 promote continuous cell cycling and genetic instability, conditions under which additional molecular events may lead to the emergence of invasive clones. Figure 7.6 depicts the evolving HPV gene expression pattern by disease severity, from CIN 1 to CIN 3.

Understanding the factors that affect whether this process continues unabated, transforms into an abortive infection, or simply ceases is an important goal in cervical cancer research. Data suggest that early HPV infection may be a diffuse process involving the entire lower genital tract.[46] However, limited evidence also suggests that once clinically important pathology develops, HPV may become concentrated if not restricted to these focal lesions.[47] These data and the morphologic heterogeneity that can be found within an HPV-infected cervix (ranging from normal, through all grades of CIN, and cancer) demonstrate that both productive and abortive infections may be concurrent, perhaps involving cervical regions with different microenvironments that favor one or the other process. The evolving HPV gene expression during cell maturation is illustrated in Figure 7.5.

Latent infection is presently unproven, but may represent a form of persistent infection that is unassociated with active replication or transformation of the host epithelium. In this state, the virus genome could persist stably for extended periods of time, but whole virion assembly would not occur and infected host cells would remain intact. Infected cells that remain basal and do not differentiate permit low-level replication of episomal DNA with faithful partitioning of HPV DNA between parent and daughter cell.[32,145,182] Reactivation of latent HPV infection can explain the detection of multiple HPV types, including those of low prevalence, following organ transplantation and in other clinical settings in which host immunity is depressed and sexual activity is not increased. It can also account for the recurrence of laryngeal papillomas (related typically to HPV 6, 11) during childhood, when reinfection is unlikely.

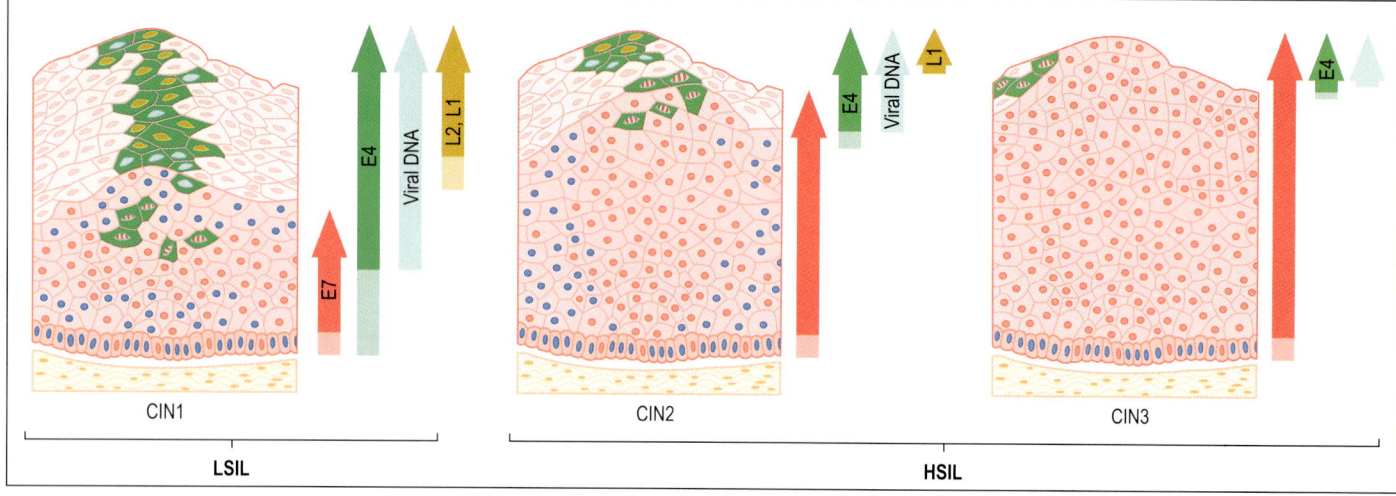

Fig. 7.6 HPV early and late gene expression from initial HPV infection through maturation, from CIN 1–CIN 3, by evolutionary HPV type. The productive cycle begins close to the basal layer and viral genome amplification begins in the parabasal cell layers. Reproduced with permission from Doorbar.[57]

HPV INTEGRATION

HPV integration into human DNA occurs in cervical carcinogenesis, but its effects differ from that of other cancer-causing viruses (e.g., hepatitis B infection and hepatocellular carcinoma). Although HPV is typically found in the episomal (nonintegrated) form in CIN, the frequency of HPV integration may increase with the degree of disease severity[106] and therefore is thought to be present as abortive infections progress and as disease progresses from CIN 1 to CIN 3 and cancer. The specific degree of integration with disease severity and specificity with HPV type, however, remains unknown. At present, there is increasing evidence that integration sites, although randomly distributed within the human genome,[193] occur principally at sites where human DNA is prone to breakage (e.g., fragile sites). Integration of HPV appears to affect only the expression of the HPV genome itself. Specifically, during integration, E1 and/or E2 are frequently disrupted and the E6 and E7 viral oncogenes are retained, ensuring constitutive expression of E6 and E7 oncogenes, a process that promotes genomic instability and carcinogenesis.

HPV MULTIPLE INFECTIONS

Infection with one HPV type does not negate the likelihood of acquiring or being protected from infection with additional HPV types.[120,187] It remains unclear whether infection resulting in seropositivity for specific HPV types also precludes reinfection.[190] This question is important with respect to the impact of HPV vaccines. Research is needed to provide added reassurance that effective prophylaxis for some types will not increase the virulence of other types. It is also important to determine if vaccination directed against specific types provides protection against additional related types. Prophylactic vaccination in animals and humans produces much higher serologic titers than natural infection, and to date vaccines seem highly protective based on limited follow-up.

HPV VIRAL LOAD

HPV viral load is defined as the amount of HPV content in samples obtained from HPV-infected women.[167,168] However, identical viral load measurements can be the result of a small number of heavily infected cells with large numbers of virions or large numbers of cells that contain few virions per cell (e.g., 1000 copies of virus in one cell or one viral copy each in 1000 cells).[166,185] For example, single koilocytes contain more viral copies than high-grade CIN cells, consistent with the understanding that the former is a marker of productive infection. Cross-sectional epidemiologic studies show that occult infections have lower loads than ones with cytologic or histologic abnormalities;[167] however, viral load values for all grades of CIN vary widely and overlap.

Complicating the measurement of HPV load is that cervical cytologic samples consist of many cell types, typically including uninfected glandular and squamous cells and variable numbers of surface cells from SILs of varying grades. Therefore, the number and size of HPV-associated lesions and the degree of surface maturation are important determinants of viral load. For example, women with focal CIN 3 may also have extensive CIN 1 and therefore, HPV load will primarily reflect the viral content per cell of the latter. The implication is that a single HPV load measurement is not useful for separating CIN 1 from higher grade lesions. Some but not all reports have found that higher HPV 16 viral loads among women with normal cytology are associated with future progression to high-grade CIN,[48,185] raising the issue about whether measuring HPV 16 load has clinical value in predicting future risk of progression.[122,211] It is also important to consider what the interpretation of 'normal cytology' actually means. As cytologists in the US generally strive for extreme sensitivity, it is possible that specimens reported as normal in some international studies would be categorized as abnormal in the US. The challenges that variable sampling and cellular heterogeneity pose with regard to measuring

HPV load may be relevant for assessment of other molecular markers.

MORPHOLOGIC FEATURES OF HPV INFECTION

HPV infection may produce a distinctive cytopathic effect that is recognizable both cytologically and histologically as a cytoplasmic halo surrounding an abnormal appearing nucleus, termed 'koilocytic atypia'.[109] Characteristically, the perinuclear haloes are large and display a sharply defined edge. Nuclei of koilocytes may show slight enlargement, irregular contours, hyperchromasia, and uneven chromatin distribution or clumping. Other findings include bi- or multinucleation, parakeratosis, and hyperkeratosis. In addition to having koilocytes in the superficial cells, tissue sections often display immature, sometimes mitotically active cells with increased ratios of nuclear to cytoplasmic area and abnormal-appearing nuclei, principally occupying the lower third of the epithelium. In all cases of CIN 1, however, some abnormal cells can be seen that will have migrated to the surface, which explains their desquamation and presence in cervical smears. The abnormal basal proliferation constitutes the findings of CIN 1 or mild dysplasia. However, studies have found that classifying individual cases as koilocytotic atypia or CIN is not reproducible and lacks clinical value, prompting a move towards using a simplified terminology, such as low-grade or high-grade squamous intraepithelial lesion (LSIL or HSIL) in cytology and corresponding terms in histology[111,173] (see Chapter 8).

Although HPV infection can be identified reliably by HPV DNA testing on cytologic specimens, microscopic recognition of HPV infections by cytology is more difficult. Many subtle changes that reflect HPV infection overlap with those found in inflammatory or reactive states. In difficult cases, cytopathologists often classify slides as atypical squamous cells when they cannot exclude a low-grade squamous intraepithelial lesion (atypical squamous cells of undetermined significance; ASCUS). HPV DNA testing can accurately identify women with ASCUS who are not HPV infected, providing reassurance that there is essentially no risk of cervical cancer for those patients at the time of testing. Therefore, HPV testing among young women identifies many infections that will spontaneously resolve.

Cells in cytologic preparations that demonstrate more profound nuclear abnormalities associated with higher ratios of nuclear to cytoplasmic areas (i.e., less maturation) are termed CIN 2 or CIN 3 (high-grade SIL or HSIL). When the majority of similar-appearing cells occupy the middle or superficial third of the epithelium in tissue sections, the lesions are termed histologic CIN 2 or CIN 3, respectively. Although far less common than findings of ASCUS, some cytologic smears will contain metaplastic, reactive or reparative cells where distinction from CIN 2 or CIN 3 is difficult, prompting a report of atypical squamous cells – cannot exclude high-grade squamous intraepithelial lesion (ASC-H). These women have a risk of underlying CIN 2 or CIN 3 that is considerably higher than women with ASCUS, but lower than women with cytology classified definitively as HSIL. A high percentage of women under age 30 years with cytology of ASCUS test positive for HPV DNA; among older women, the percentage is much lower.

IMMUNE RESPONSE TO HPV INFECTION

A major feature of HPV is its ability to evade the host immune system, a characteristic that largely accounts for its success as a human pathogen. Importantly, HPV infection does not result in cell lysis or in viremia, which minimizes exposure of host immune cells to viral antigens and limits the immune response. Sequestration of HPV within keratinocyte nuclei for much of its life cycle also shields the virus from host immune cells. In addition to physical evasion from the host immune response, HPV itself also exerts immunomodulatory effects, including downregulation of major histocompatibility complex (MHC) Class II antigens and inhibition of interferon (IFN) production. In cell lines, E6 and E7 reduce IFN-α production in natural killer cells. E6 may also downregulate interleukin (IL)-18 expression, a purportedly important molecule for cytolytic T cell responses. E5 may diminish antigen processing and presentation via acidification of endosomes.

The host immune response to infection can be considered on several levels. First, keratinocytes provide a physical barrier to infection.[179] In addition, squamous epithelium expresses MHC Class I and adhesion molecules required for immune responses. In recognition of viral pathogens, both innate and adaptive immune responses are triggered, resulting in production of interferons, cytokines, and microbicidal peptides. Interferon production promotes apoptosis of virally infected cells whereas cytokines recruit and activate macrophages, natural killer cells, and lymphocytes. The innate immunity is considered non-specific while the adaptive immune response is considered specific to the pathogen and provides immunologic memory. Because human leukocyte antigen (HLA) Class I and Class II molecules are only weakly expressed, antigen presentation of HPV seems to not result in an effective immune response.

Development of immune memory requires: (1) initial recognition of the foreign antigen by immature dendritic cells; (2) uptake of antigen by endocytosis or macropinocytosis; and (3) antigen processing for presentation in conjunction with HLA Class I and Class II molecules on the surface of cytotoxic T cells. Cytokine expression is triggered and can direct the resulting immune cascade: Th1 cytokines such as IL-2, IL-12, and IFN-γ tend to promote cytotoxic T cell and natural killer responses; Th2 cytokines, including IL-4, IL-5, IL-6, IL-10, and IL-13, favor B-cell mediated humoral responses. It is thought that a Th1 immune response is a more effective response to HPV infection and protects against CIN and cancer. Specifically, IL-2 expression is reduced in HSIL when compared to adjacent normal tissue[3] and the density of IL-4 and IL-6 staining cells is increased in SIL compared to adjacent normal tissue. Further, numbers of HLA-DR expressing cells are higher in high-grade as compared to low-grade CIN. Langerhans cells derived from SILs or the transformation zone similarly produced less IL-2 and more IL-10 than those derived from the exocervix when stimulated *in vitro*.[68] Although antibodies directed against proteins such as L1 and L2 might effectively prevent infection, it is commonly accepted that antibodies are not important effectors of regression of established HPV infections and related cervical lesions. Rather, effective humoral immunity may play a role in preventing HPV infection while an effective cellular immune response is important for eliminating an existing infection.[108,125,206]

MODEL OF HPV-INDUCED CERVICAL PATHOGENESIS

Remarkable strides have been made during the past decade in understanding how HPV induces the process of carcinogenesis. Although infection with HPV among young women is common, not all women will develop clinical manifestations of HPV infection. Of those who do, however, only 10% will develop the cervical precancer, CIN 3. Even fewer of the CIN 3 lesions will ever progress to cancer.[7] The present model of HPV-induced cervical pathogenesis (Figure 7.1) illustrates the necessity for HPV infection and most notably HPV persistence in pathogenesis. Importantly, the model illustrates the transient nature of most HPV infections among college-aged women: 70% of prevalent infections resolve within 1 year and about 90% within 2 years.[90,103,136,143,155,192,209]

The course of HPV infection depends on multiple factors. Largely it reflects viral (e.g., type, variant) characteristics, the host (e.g., immune, genetic) characteristics, and the microenvironment under which infection occurs. Epidemiologic approaches to understanding the causal nature of HPV and cervical cancer have moved beyond HPV and cervical cancer outcomes. With the current carcinogenic model, refined outcomes that include HPV persistence and progression are currently of highest scientific interest and will likely yield important clues regarding factors important for disease progression. Identification of epidemiologic and biologic factors associated with HPV persistence and progression to disease, however, has proved challenging for many reasons. First, a scientific consensus for defining HPV persistence has not yet been reached. Second, it may take approximately 15 years on average for HPV infections to progress to cancer. Because CIN 3 is both detectable and curable, it would be unethical to allow women to progress to invasion, yet CIN 3 is an imperfect surrogate for cancer. In addition, following cohorts for lengthy periods is extremely difficult and expensive. Even conducting studies based on CIN 3 endpoints requires large study populations, lengthy follow-up, and performance of repeat measurements of relevant exposures. Despite these challenges, critical clues are emerging from epidemiologic studies. Notably, HPV type 16 is unique in its tendency to persist, resulting in increased risks for progression to CIN 3.[86,90,143,162,164] Clearly, further delineation of oncogenic HPV types and their variants as they relate to HPV persistence and progression will likely yield important clues to understanding the viral influences and specific interactions with the host and its environment that are necessary for progression to CIN 3 and cancer.

HPV: ROUTES OF TRANSMISSION

HPV is sexually transmitted. Women who have not had sexual intercourse/penetration nearly always test negative for both HPV DNA and its antibodies.[5,60,100] In all women, HPV detection is closely linked to sexual behavior and the number of sexual partners.[11,65,117,135,152,203]

The absence of HPV among virgins is also considered evidence against vertical transmission. Although some report that perinatal transmission is common and children may repeatedly test positive for several years,[156] others argue that persistent detection of HPV DNA among young children results from sample contamination and that persistently positive serology may reflect detection of maternal antibodies or cross-reacting immunologic response to non-genital types.

SEXUAL BEHAVIOR AND HPV

Both case-control and cohort studies have long established that sexual behavior is the main risk factor for HPV infection, with studies reporting that approximately 39–55% of young women test positive within 24–36 months of sexual initiation.[65,89,203] The disease is more frequent in women who have had multiple partners[26] or whose husbands have had multiple partners, and among women who initiate sex earlier in life. Conversely, low rates are found among celibate women while women who have never had intercourse do not have dysplasia.[158] Although sexual behavior can be measured in a number of ways, including cumulative, new or recent sexual partners, all represent similar markers of risk for HPV infection. Today, with DNA testing of cytologic samples, estimates of HPV infection can now be more accurately determined. Although sexual behavior influences the risk of HPV acquisition, it does not determine the natural history of the infection once the HPV has been acquired.

NUMBER OF PARTNERS

Among teenagers, each new partner per month adds a 10-fold risk of incident HPV detection.[135] Among women with frequent sexual activity, such as patients in sexually transmitted disease clinics and prostitutes, risk for HPV detection plateaus, suggesting that frequent intercourse does not predict HPV persistence.[102] Although there are clear increases in risk between lifetime number of partners and cervical cancer in the population as a whole, among HPV-infected women, there is no association. Therefore, sexual activity is an important determinant of HPV exposure, but it is unrelated to outcomes among infected women.

FREQUENCY OF COITUS

At present, the frequency of intercourse or number of sexual acts is not considered an important part in the development of cervical cancer. Although there is some evidence that suggests recent intercourse is associated with testing positive for HPV, these associations are likely to reflect detection rather than true infection.

PROSTITUTION

The rates of all sexually transmitted infections are much higher in prostitutes. The characteristics among prostitutes associated with risk for cervical cancer are increased numbers of partners and early age at first intercourse. The measures of sexual activity among prostitutes, like numbers of partners, are now considered a surrogate for HPV infection.

MALE FACTORS: CONDOM USE, PROMISCUITY, AND CIRCUMCISION

Despite challenges in performing HPV tests on specimens obtained from men,[64] 'male factors' and specifically sexual behavior of men, are important determinants of cervical cancer risk among their women partners.[20] Recent studies measuring HPV infection among partners of infected men have demonstrated that their partners are more likely to become infected.[37] Increased risk of cervical cancer among partners of men with penile cancer,[35,78,171] and higher rates of cervical cancer among women whose partners travel frequently (suggesting extramarital sexual activities), suggest that a man's sexual behavior affects his partner's cervical cancer risk. This aspect of the male factor and the concept of the 'high risk male' were developed in a study of the second wives of men whose first wives had known cervical cancer. Cervical cancer and CIN were detected nearly twice as frequently in the second wives.[94] Wives of men previously married to cervical cancer patients are at increased risk for cervical neoplasia compared to the second wives where the first wife was free of this cancer.[94]

Worldwide, cervical cancer incidence rates correlate significantly with the average number of lifetime sexual partners of the men residing in a country.[19] In Spain, where cervical cancer rates are low and women typically have few sexual contacts, the risk of cervical cancer is higher[30,101] if the male partner had multiple lifetime partners, contacts with prostitutes, initiated intercourse at a young age, smoked, or had positive serology for *Chlamydia trachomatis* or a history of oral or anal sex. Detection of oncogenic HPV DNA among male partners conferred a seven-fold risk of cervical cancer among their partners; risks for monogamous women were similar to those for all women.

CONDOM USE

A meta-analysis suggests that condom use may provide modest protection against external warts and possibly other cervical lesions.[127] However, among the six studies included, only one documented lower rates of HPV DNA detection among the female partner. Given that condom users may have sporadic unprotected contacts and that condoms cannot fully cover all areas of infected genital skin and mucosal areas, such equivocal data are not surprising.

CIRCUMCISION

Circumcision of men is commonly thought to protect women from developing cervical cancer. Specifically, circumcision has been reported to be associated with reduced risk of HPV detection in penile samples and to result in lower risk of cervical cancer among women whose circumcised partners had multiple other contacts.[37]

HPV COFACTORS

HPV, although a potent carcinogen, remains insufficient for neoplastic development. Clearly, cofactors are required for

Table 7.2 Summary of evaluated HPV cofactors for squamous cell carcinoma and adenocarcinoma of the cervix

HPV cofactor	Squamous cell carcinoma	Adenocarcinoma
Smoking	↑↑	No association
Parity	↑↑	No association
Oral contraceptives/hormones	↑↑	↑
Chlamydia	↑ Evidence not sufficient	No association
HSV 2	↑ Evidence not sufficient	No association
Antioxidants	↓ Evidence not sufficient	Evidence not sufficient
Obesity	No association	↑

cervical carcinogenesis (summarized in Table 7.2). At present, multiparity, smoking behavior, and oral contraceptive use are regarded as HPV cofactors for squamous cell carcinoma[36] and thought to act as cofactors in about 75% of cervical cancers.[22] Nutrition, coinfection with other sexually transmitted diseases, genetic variation, and other exposures may act as cofactors in the remaining cases. In addition, psychosocial stress and depression-related immunosuppression have gained recent attention.[45,195] Note that HPV cofactors for SCC and cervical adenocarcinomas differ.

SMOKING

A geographic correlation between rates of smoking-related cancers such as lung cancer among men and cervical cancer among women suggested the initial links between smoking and cervical neoplasia.[204] Over 50 studies conducted to date show a two-fold increase in risk for cervical SCC in smokers compared to non-smokers.[31,112,151] These findings are consistent in both case-control and cohort studies where elevated risk among smokers persists among women infected with oncogenic HPV infections,[38,39,52,84] even after adjustment for age at first intercourse and lifetime number of sexual partners. Smoking status, intensity, and duration are all associated with cervical cancer, with current and heavy smokers possessing the highest risks. Further, cervical lesions regress in women who either quit or markedly reduce their smoking for 6 months compared to women who do not alter their habits.[186]

Biologic evidence strongly supports smoking's carcinogenic effects for SCC. The identification of tobacco-related carcinogens such as nicotine and its metabolites (e.g., cotinine) in cervical secretions of women who smoke further support the notion that smoking damages DNA (genotoxicity). Smoking, it is believed, increases free radical production and depletes antioxidants, enhancing a genotoxic-prone milieu. Smoking may also depress local and systemic immune function, possibly increasing risk for HPV persistence,[10] a prerequisite for carcinogenesis.[33] Although substantial epidemiologic and biologic evidence now associates smoking and cervical SCC, no such equivalent association with cervical adenocarcinoma has been found.

PARITY

Multiparous women are at increased risk for cervical cancer and precancer compared to nulliparous women, with a progressive elevation in risk with increasing number of live births.[25,28,38,100,141] However, cervical cancer is not associated with other reproductive factors such as age at menarche, menstrual characteristics, history of miscarriages or abortions, or age at menopause.[25,84,141] In a large multicentric case-control study, seven or more full-term pregnancies were associated with a nearly four-fold increase in squamous cell carcinoma, but not adenocarcinoma.[141] Increased exposure of the transformation zone to toxic agents at birth might account for the parity association.[9] Other studies suggest that cervical trauma during parturition might increase the risk, an explanation compatible with the observation that women who have undergone cesarean sections have a reduced risk for cervical cancer.[21] Additional biologic mechanisms that could explain the increased risk associated with parity thus include hormonal changes during pregnancy or pregnancy-related immunosuppression.[51]

METHOD OF CONTRACEPTION: ORAL CONTRACEPTIVES AND OTHERS

Relationships between contraceptive practices and risk for cervical neoplasia are difficult to study, as shown by inconsistent findings. Specifically, it is challenging to separate effects of oral contraceptive use, duration of HPV infection, and screening behavior.[12,27,29,38,133,170] A recent meta-analysis of 19 cervical cancer studies found that HPV-infected women were at increased risk for cervical cancer only after using oral contraceptives for more than 10 years.[38,74,113,170] Although similar increases in risk are reported for cervical adenocarcinoma, the association remains tentative at present.[114]

As with multiparity, long-term oral contraceptive pill usage is thought to increase risk for cervical cancer through elevated levels of circulating hormones in a woman's body. The progesterone content of the pill possibly induces an ectropion that could result in increased HPV exposure or 'mechanical trauma'. Use of the pill also potentially increases risk for cervical cancer by enhancing HPV carcinogenicity. Regulatory regions of the HPV genome contain 'hormone-recognition elements' and in vitro studies have shown that hormones further enhance transformation of HPV-infected cells.[51]

Concerns regarding hormone replacement therapy and long-acting steroid preparation such as depot-medroxyprogesterone acetate (DMPA) have also been raised. In both laboratory and animal studies, estrogen and progesterone upregulate HPV transcription. In transgenic mice that constitutively express HPV oncogenes, cervical tumors develop only after chronic administration of estradiol. However, to date, few studies have evaluated this specific question and results are currently inconclusive.[84,178] Studies attempting to evaluate relationships of endogenous hormones (e.g., estradiol, estrone, estrone-sulfate, progesterone, sex hormone-binding globulin, and dehydroepiandrosterone sulfate) with cervical precancer among pre- and postmenopausal women have been limited.

Barrier methods of contraception (diaphragm and condom) possibly protect the cervical epithelium from sexually transmitted agents like HPV in the semen, but these findings, which suggest reduced cervical cancer risk, were reported long before valid HPV tests were developed. Both HPV DNA and RNA can be found in seminal plasma and in sperm cells.[115,144,157] Although spermicides are thought to possess antiviral properties, no anti-HPV activity has been proven in vitro.[82] Thus evidence that use of intrauterine contraceptive devices reduces risk of cervical neoplasia is not compelling.

RACIAL AND NATIONALITY FACTORS/RELIGION

Race, nationality, and religious factors by themselves are not important biologic factors in the development of cervical cancer.[148] However, these factors do reflect social practices and/or inequities. In the US, secular trends among black and white women reveal similar patterns for increased detection of in situ carcinoma of the cervix, and decreased detection of invasive cervical cancer, particularly higher stages, supporting the success of screening programs. The higher cervical cancer rates among black women probably reflect inadequate screening and treatment rather than biologic differences between races.

Historically, Jewish, Mormon, and Amish women and Catholic nuns have had low incidence rates of cervical cancer, presumably reflecting limited number of sexual partners or abstinence, resulting in reduced exposure to HPV infection.[24] Specifically, Mormon women who adhered to religious proscriptions against smoking and extramarital sexual relations had lower cervical cancer risk than non-Mormons.[67] Low rates among Jewish women may reflect the practice of circumcising boys, which is supported by the reported lower rates of penile HPV infection,[36] but these data remain inconclusive.

SOCIOECONOMIC STATUS

It has long been reported that women with low socioeconomic status possess a two-fold increase in risk for invasive cervical cancer when compared to women with high socioeconomic status as commonly defined by income and education.[24] This association appears similar across race[54] and likely reflects a combination of an environmental disposition for HPV infection, where prevalence is generally higher in women with low socioeconomic status,[83,95,181] and where it is coupled with poor access to screening and treatment. Though unproven, concurrent genital infections and nutritional deficiencies may also contribute to some of the risk differences. In particular, it is unknown whether severe malnutrition such as that found in some areas of the world with the highest cancer rates may represent a contributory factor.

AGE

Although the prevalence of oncogenic HPV infection is highest among young women, the risk of HPV persistence is highest among older women. Similarly, cancer rates are low in young women and increase with age.[91,130] Rates begin increasing in women around age 25 years, presumably some years after HPV acquisition during adolescence and early adulthood. Unlike most cancers, cervical cancer rates plateau in women aged 40–50 years. It is notable that detection of CIN 3 peaks among women in the mid to late thirties, whereas invasive carcinoma peaks (decades) later. This suggests that the slowest process in carcinogenesis may be progression of CIN 3 to invasive carcinoma, whereas the steps required for progression of HPV infection to CIN 3 may occur more quickly. In summary, data suggest that CIN 3 is neither an obligate cancer precursor nor an imminent one in most instances, providing further impetus for molecular characterization of HPV-related lesions to identify lesions that will inevitably progress without treatment.

INFECTIOUS AGENTS: SEXUALLY TRANSMITTED INFECTIONS AND OTHERS

Women with cervical cancer have a higher frequency of other sexually transmitted diseases (e.g., syphilis, gonorrhea, trichomoniasis, genital herpes, *Chlamydia*) compared to women without cervical cancer. Some studies have found that the seroprevalence of herpes simplex virus 2 (HSV 2) and *Chlamydia trachomatis* is higher among women with cervical cancer than among controls, but these associations are inconsistent and could reflect inadequate adjustment for HPV infection. Other sexually transmitted infections (STIs) have not been associated with cervical cancer risk. In one view, STIs act non-specifically to promote cervical carcinogenesis by increasing cervical inflammation.

Once thought to be the etiologic agent for cervical cancer, HSV 2[8] remains a potential HPV cofactor. Recent studies indicate that women infected with HPV and also seropositive for HSV 2 and *Chlamydia* are at greater risk for cervical cancer than similar HPV-infected seronegative women.[50] Possibly, HSV may foster HPV integration and amplification in host cells. Additional studies of STIs as HPV cofactors are needed.[50]

NUTRIENTS, ANTIOXIDANTS

The evidence for poor nutritional status and increased cervical cancer risk is sparse.[69,154] Studies have either reported protective effects or no association of high antioxidant levels such as beta-carotene, lycopene, and vitamin E (tocopherol). Low folate levels have also been implicated in poor DNA repair capacity and linked to increased cervical cancer risk,[200,201] with topical administration of retinoic acid leading to lesion regression.[174] Recent Phase III chemoprevention trials, however, have shown no significant improvement of HPV lesions and precancers with folic acid or beta-carotene treatment.

IMMUNOSUPPRESSION (HIV/AIDS)

Women with impaired cellular immunity due to HIV infection,[134,145] organ transplantation (e.g., renal transplant recipients) or use of immunosuppressive drugs have increased risks of developing cervical neoplasia. They also have increased risks for HPV infection, persistence, warts, and anogenital precancer.[16,61,145,147,150,183] The prevalence of HPV infection is highest among the most severely immunosuppressed individuals possessing the lowest CD4 counts (e.g., below $200/mm^3$).[145,183] Sixty three percent of HIV-positive women have detectable HPV DNA compared to 30% in HIV-negative women. Although a similar range of HPV types were identified among HIV-infected and HIV-negative women, multiple infections were three times more common among HIV-infected women. In addition, HIV-positive women are also at greater risk for HPV persistence than HIV-negative women.[183] Women with AIDS have a 4.6-fold increased risk for CIN 3,[126] with higher risks occurring with longer times since HIV seroconversion;[66] risks were similar for invasive cancers. The US Centers for Disease Control and Prevention has designated cervical cancer among HIV-infected women as an AIDS-defining illness. However, unlike many AIDS-defining illnesses, the incidences of which have declined since the introduction of highly active antiretroviral therapy, the improved CD4 levels conferred by this therapy have only been inconsistently observed. The incidence of cervical cancer has not dropped in these women.[77,131,146,188] Thus, although impaired cellular immunity is an important risk factor for HPV infection and precursor lesions, its role in the progression to invasive cancers may be minimal.[145]

FAMILIAL AGGREGATION AND HOST GENETICS

No major gene has been found to increase risk for HPV infection or cervical cancer. However, women with affected relatives have a two-fold increase in cervical cancer risk, reflecting either shared environmental exposures or genetic predisposition.[2,70,80,81,121,124] In general, the findings have been more consistent with cervical precancer than invasive cancers. While the risk is similar for monozygotic and dizygotic twins in some studies,[2] a large Swedish study showed increased risk for precancer among monozygotic twins but not dizygotic twins. In a larger combined analysis of Scandinavian countries, familial aggregation was largely ascribed to environmental factors[2,121] and associated behaviors.

Immune status and host genetics are key factors influencing all aspects of HPV (infection, persistence) and its associated outcomes (precancer, invasion). To date, the most studied is protein expression and allelic variation of the MHC human leukocyte antigens (HLAs). HLAs present viruses and other foreign antigens to the host immune system and immune effector cells and may thus influence both recognition of HPV infection and its associated outcomes.[87] HLA Class II molecules present foreign antigens to T lymphocytes and thus play a major role in regulating immune function. HLA DRB1*13 and/or DQB1*603 appear protective against cervical cancer,[193] a protection consistently observed in multiple studies conducted in diverse populations. Enhancing this finding is the type specificity restricted to HPV 16. Increased risks associated with polymorphic variants of Class II molecules, including the DRB1*1501-DQB1*0602 haplotype and DQB1*03 alleles are less consistent,[6,199] but many of these studies lack sufficient sample sizes to detect an association.

Initial reports of the polymorphic HLA Class I antigens have identified associations, further implicating innate immunity. A few studies have reported increased risk for cervical cancer and its precursors with the HLA Class I B7 allele, but this has been inconsistent.[85,198] Decreased expression of HLA Class I molecules has long been recognized in cervical cancers and specific downregulation of HLA B7 has been associated with worse survival in cancer patients. More recently, HLA Class I molecules that bind to killer immunoglobulin receptors have been implicated in cervical cancer risk.[34] A study demonstrating reduced risk for cervical cancer and its precursors in women who possessed the HLA Class I C*0202 allele[194] prompted investigation of innate immunity, the non-specific inflammatory immune response to foreign pathogens. Because the KIR-HLA complex is believed to regulate natural killer (NK) cell-mediated innate immunity, specific inhibitory KIR-HLA ligand pairs were evaluated and demonstrated to decrease risk for cervical cancer. In contrast, the presence of the activating receptor KIR3DS1 increased risk, especially when the protective inhibitory combinations were missing. It is thus hypothesized that there may be a continuum of resistance conferred by NK cell inhibition for cervical cancer susceptibility that involves NK cell activation.

Additional immune genes investigated to date include TAP1, TAP2, and IFNA17; most recently, polymorphisms within the tumor necrosis factor (TNF) gene have been associated with increased cervical cancer risk.[53] Other non-immune-related genetic polymorphisms have not yielded consistent associations.[40,72,73,97,98,159,169] For cervical cancer, genetic involvement will probably consist of many alleles conferring modest levels of risk. The ability to evaluate multiple genes with robust intermediate outcomes (e.g., HPV persistence, CIN 3/cancer) now allows for refined analyses for understanding susceptibility in progression to cervical cancer.

SOMATIC EVENTS

To identify the molecular changes that occur at critical transitions in the natural history of HPV infection (e.g., progression from infection to persistence and then to development of cancer precursors and cancer) may provide avenues for developing improved prevention strategies. In considering the multistage carcinogenic pathway to cervical cancer, the abrogation of the tumor suppressor genes p53 and Rb by the HPV oncogenes E6 and E7, respectively, could be considered the 'first hit'.[107] Much research is therefore focused on identifying the necessary 'second hit' required for disease progression and invasion.[193] If identified, these event(s) could be translated into biomarkers of risk for early detection of cervical cancer. To date, candidate tumor suppressor genes and oncogenes have been intensively examined[116] and identified by genomic studies, including identification of chromosomal loss of heterozygosity (LOH) and comparative genetic hybridization assays. Loss of chromosomes 3p, 6, 11, 13, 16, 17, and 19 have been identified as well as chromosomal gains at 3q.[93,123,129] Identification of target genes (oncogenes/tumor suppressor genes) affected in these chromosomal regions has not yet been proven, although genes of interest (e.g., c-myc, ras, and telomerase/hTERT) have been identified. Continued investigations include biomarkers such as p16[INK4a], telomerase, aneuploidy,[58,212] and epigenetic events

such as methylation. Extensive evaluation of p16[INK4a] as an immunohistochemical biomarker consistently shows increased expression with increasing disease severity.[1,104,105,197] Translation of this marker to cytology specimens via detection through ELISA or EIA (enzyme immunoassay) might increase the utility and ease with which these markers could be applied. More importantly, prospective data on this biomarker's utility for predicting disease prior to diagnosis are needed. Another area of intense research is in identifying methylation patterns in cervical cancer. As with p16[INK4a], several groups have found methylation in cervical cancers and precancers and even in cytology specimens, but a cervix-specific methylation panel and its utility in predicting disease in prospective data have not yet been proven.[56,142,177] Recent reviews summarize the findings in this rapidly evolving area.[49,172]

PREVENTION OF CERVICAL CANCER

EARLY DETECTION OF CERVICAL CANCER

Cervical cancer is now considered a preventable disease. With advances in vaccine development and widespread administration, cervical cancer may possibly be eliminated, although clearly this goal will take many years to accomplish. Early detection of cervical cancer therefore remains of high scientific importance. Cytologic screening with the Papanicolaou smear has proven effective in reducing incidence and mortality from cervical cancer, and the identification of HPV as the etiologic agent for cervical cancer has resulted in its incorporation into screening and triage programs. Among cytology-based screening programs, HPV DNA testing is also being incorporated for clinical management of women with equivocal cytology – atypical squamous cells of undetermined significance (ASCUS). Use of combined cytologic and virologic screening among women aged 30 years and older to lengthen the screening interval to 3 years has been endorsed by the American Cancer Society and the American College of Obstetrics and Gynecology[4,96,161] (but not the College of American Pathologists). In underdeveloped countries where cytologic screening has been too difficult to implement, HPV testing may offer an alternative method for screening.

PRIMARY PREVENTION: VACCINES

Primary prevention of cervical cancer is now foreseeable as large-scale Phase III vaccine trials demonstrate the effectiveness of first generation prophylactic vaccines,[189] particularly in conferring complete protection against not only infection but also persistent HPV 16 infection and CIN.[110] Briefly, present vaccines are constructed based on virus-like particles (VLPs) for select HPV types. VLPs recapitulate the configuration of the L1 viral capsid but do not contain any viral DNA, and are thus neither infectious nor carcinogenic.[163] Cow, rabbit, and dog animal models of VLP-based papillomavirus vaccines have shown vaccine efficacy[23,99,184] and human Phase I trials have demonstrated the safety and immunogenicity of HPV 16 VLP vaccines.[76] Efficacy trials of a quadrivalent vaccine for HPV types 6, 11, 16 and 18, and a bivalent vaccine for HPV types 16 and 18 have recently been reported and approved for use by the US Food and Drug Administration (FDA).

Unlike prophylactic vaccines that are designed for administration to uninfected individuals, therapeutic vaccines for administration to infected individuals are also currently being developed. Therapeutic vaccines are designed to specifically target and destroy HPV-infected cells and thereby prevent persistent infection and progression to precancer and cancer.[175,176] Current candidates include but are not limited to a therapeutic vaccine where E7 is fused with the heat shock protein Hsp65 as an adjuvant, and an HPV 16 E7-based encapsulated plasmid DNA vaccine, both of which are currently under evaluation in animals and humans.[71,165]

CONCLUSION

Ongoing research will likely permit a clearer understanding of factors associated with HPV persistence, and those required for progression to cancer. We are also gaining a better understanding of the various host characteristics most likely relevant for eliciting an effective immune response. With advancing technology, we may soon clarify the tumor microenvironment conducive for cervical pathogenesis. Coupled with our present understanding of its natural history, cervical cancer provides a unique opportunity for researchers to identify new biomarkers that will delineate the small number of women at the highest risk for progression to cervical cancer from the large number of HPV-infected women expected to clear the infection. Until these and other newly identified biomarkers are validated, however, cytology-based screening, where used, continues to be an effective screening tool while the utility of HPV DNA testing as an adjunct to cytology evaluations offers improved management of at-risk women. In addition, numerous other technologies based on computer-assisted imaging, improved visualization, and other techniques that can be applied at the bedside are being explored. Ultimately, it is successful implementation of HPV vaccines that will reduce the burden of disease, particularly in resource-poor developing countries.

ACKNOWLEDGMENT

We thank Joseph Carreon and Patricia Madigan for their careful reviews of this manuscript.

REFERENCES

1. Agoff SN, Lin P, Morihara J, Mao C, Kiviat NB, Koutsky LA. p16(INK4a) expression correlates with degree of cervical neoplasia: a comparison with Ki-67 expression and detection of high-risk HPV types. Mod Pathol 2003;16:665–73.
2. Ahlbom A, Lichtenstein P, Malmstrom H, Feychting M, Hemminki K, Pedersen NL. Cancer in twins: genetic and nongenetic familial risk factors. J Natl Cancer Inst 1997;89:287–93.
3. al Saleh W, Giannini SL, Jacobs N, et al. Correlation of T-helper secretory differentiation and types of antigen-presenting cells in squamous intraepithelial lesions of the uterine cervix. J Pathol 1998;184:283–90.
4. American College of Obstetricians and Gynecologists. ACOG practice bulletin: clinical management guidelines for obstetrician-gynecologists. Cervical cytology screening (replaces Committee Opinion 152, March 1995). Obstet Gynecol 2003;102:417–27.
5. Andersson-Ellstrom A, Dillner J, Hagmar B, et al. Comparison of development of serum antibodies to HPV16 and HPV33 and acquisition of cervical HPV DNA among sexually experienced and virginal young girls. A longitudinal cohort study. Sex Transm Dis 1996;23:234–8.
6. Apple RJ, Erlich HA, Klitz W, Manos MM, Becker TM, Wheeler CM. HLA DR-DQ associations with cervical carcinoma show papillomavirus-type specificity. Nat Genet 1994;6:157–62.
7. ASCUS-LSIL Triage Study (ALTS) Group. Results of a randomized trial on the management of cytology interpretations of atypical squamous cells of undetermined significance. Am J Obstet Gynecol 2003;188:1383–92.
8. Aurelian L. Viruses and carcinoma of the cervix. Contrib Gynecol Obstet 1991;18:54–70.
9. Autier P, Coibion M, Huet F, Grivegnee AR. Transformation zone location and intraepithelial neoplasia of the cervix uteri. Br J Cancer 1996;74:488–90.
10. Barton SE, Maddox PH, Jenkins D, Edwards R, Cuzick J, Singer A. Effect of cigarette smoking on cervical epithelial immunity: a mechanism for neoplastic change? Lancet 1988;2:652–4.
11. Bauer HM, Ting Y, Greer CE, et al. Genital human papillomavirus infection in female university students as determined by a PCR-based method. JAMA 1991;265:472–7.
12. Beral V, Hannaford P, Kay C. Oral contraceptive use and malignancies of the genital tract. Results from the Royal College of General Practitioners' Oral Contraception Study. Lancet 1988;2:1331–5.
13. Beral V, Hermon C, Munoz N, Devesa SS. Cervical cancer. Cancer Surv 1994;19–20:265–85.
14. Bernard HU, Chan SY, Manos MM, et al. Identification and assessment of known and novel human papillomaviruses by polymerase chain reaction amplification, restriction fragment length polymorphisms, nucleotide sequence, and phylogenetic algorithms. J Infect Dis 1994;170:1077–85.
15. Beutner KR. Nongenital human papillomavirus infections. Clin Lab Med 2000;20:423–30.
16. Birkeland SA, Storm HH, Lamm LU, et al. Cancer risk after renal transplantation in the Nordic countries, 1964–1986. Int J Cancer 1995;60:183–9.
17. Bosch FX, de Sanjose S. Human papillomavirus and cervical cancer-burden and assessment of causality. J Natl Cancer Inst Monogr 2003;3–13.
18. Bosch FX, Lorincz A, Munoz N, Meijer CJ, Shah KV. The causal relation between human papillomavirus and cervical cancer. J Clin Pathol 2002;55:244–65.
19. Bosch FX, Munoz N, de Sanjose S. Human papillomavirus and other risk factors for cervical cancer. Biomed Pharmacother 1997;51:268–75.
20. Bosch FX, Munoz N, de Sanjose S, et al. Cervical carcinoma and human papillomavirus: on the road to preventing a major human cancer. J Natl Cancer Inst 2001;93:1349–50.
21. Bosch FX, Munoz N, Shah KV, Meheus A. Second International Workshop on the Epidemiology of Cervical Cancer and Human Papillomaviruses. Int J Cancer 1992;52:171–3.
22. Bosch FX, Rohan T, Schneider A, et al. Papillomavirus research update: highlights of the Barcelona HPV 2000 International Papillomavirus Conference. J Clin Pathol 2001;54:163–75.
23. Breitburd F, Kirnbauer R, Hubbert NL, et al. Immunization with virus-like particles from cottontail rabbit papillomavirus (CRPV) can protect against experimental CRPV infection. J Virol 1995;69:3959–63.
24. Brinton LA, Fraumeni JF, Jr. Epidemiology of uterine cervical cancer. J Chronic Dis 1986;39:1051–65.
25. Brinton LA, Hamman RF, Huggins GR, et al. Sexual and reproductive risk factors for invasive squamous cell cervical cancer. J Natl Cancer Inst 1987;79:23–30.
26. Brinton LA, Herrero R, Reeves WC, de Britton RC, Gaitan E, Tenorio F. Risk factors for cervical cancer by histology. Gynecol Oncol 1993;51:301–6.
27. Brinton LA, Huggins GR, Lehman HF, et al. Long-term use of oral contraceptives and risk of invasive cervical cancer. Int J Cancer 1986;38:339–44.
28. Brinton LA, Reeves WC, Brenes MM, et al. Parity as a risk factor for cervical cancer. Am J Epidemiol 1989;130:486–96.
29. Brinton LA, Reeves WC, Brenes MM, et al. Oral contraceptive use and risk of invasive cervical cancer. Int J Epidemiol 1990;19:4–11.
30. Brinton LA, Reeves WC, Brenes MM, et al. The male factor in the etiology of cervical cancer among sexually monogamous women. Int J Cancer 1989;44:199–203.
31. Brinton LA, Schairer C, Haenszel W, et al. Cigarette smoking and invasive cervical cancer. JAMA 1986;255:3265–9.
32. Broker TR, Jin G, Croom-Rivers A, et al. Viral latency: the papillomavirus model. Dev Biol (Basel) 2001;106:443–51.
33. Burger MP, Hollema H, Gouw AS, Pieters WJ, Quint WG. Cigarette smoking and human papillomavirus in patients with reported cervical cytological abnormality. BMJ 1993;306:749–52.
34. Carrington M, Wang S, Martin MP, et al. Hierarchy of resistance to cervical neoplasia mediated by combinations of killer immunoglobulin-like receptor and human leukocyte antigen loci. J Exp Med 2005;201:1069–75.
35. Cartwright RA, Sinson JD. Carcinoma of penis and cervix. Lancet 1980;1:97.
36. Castellsague X, Bosch FX, Munoz N. Environmental co-factors in HPV carcinogenesis. Virus Res 2002;89:191–9.
37. Castellsague X, Bosch FX, Munoz N, et al. Male circumcision, penile human papillomavirus infection, and cervical cancer in female partners. N Engl J Med 2002;346:1105–12.

38. Castellsague X, Munoz N. Cofactors in human papillomavirus carcinogenesis – role of parity, oral contraceptives, and tobacco smoking. J Natl Cancer Inst Monogr 2003;20–8.

39. Castle PE, Wacholder S, Lorincz AT, et al. A prospective study of high-grade cervical neoplasia risk among human papillomavirus-infected women. J Natl Cancer Inst 2002;94:1406–14.

40. Chen C, Madeleine MM, Weiss NS, Daling JR. Glutathione S-transferase M1 genotypes and the risk of vulvar cancer: a population-based case-control study. Am J Epidemiol 1999;150:437–42.

41. Clifford GM, Gallus S, Herrero R, et al. Worldwide distribution of human papillomavirus types in cytologically normal women in the International Agency for Research on Cancer HPV prevalence surveys: a pooled analysis. Lancet 2005;366:991–8.

42. Clifford GM, Smith JS, Aguado T, Franceschi S. Comparison of HPV type distribution in high-grade cervical lesions and cervical cancer: a meta-analysis. Br J Cancer 2003;89:101–5.

43. Clifford GM, Smith JS, Plummer M, Munoz N, Franceschi S. Human papillomavirus types in invasive cervical cancer worldwide: a meta-analysis. Br J Cancer 2003;88:63–73.

44. Cogliano V, Baan R, Straif K, Grosse Y, Secretan B, El Ghissassi F. Carcinogenicity of human papillomaviruses. Lancet Oncol 2005;6:204.

45. Coker AL, Bond S, Madeleine MM, Luchok K, Pirisi L. Psychosocial stress and cervical neoplasia risk. Psychosom Med 2003;65:644–51.

46. Crum CP, Nagai N, Levine RU, Silverstein S. In situ hybridization analysis of HPV 16 DNA sequences in early cervical neoplasia. Am J Pathol 1986;123:174–82.

47. Crum CP, Symbula M, Ward BE. Topography of early HPV 16 transcription in high-grade genital precancers. Am J Pathol 1989;134:1183–8.

48. Cuzick J, Terry G, Ho L, Hollingworth T, Anderson M. Type-specific human papillomavirus DNA in abnormal smears as a predictor of high-grade cervical intraepithelial neoplasia. Br J Cancer 1994;69:167–71.

49. Dallenbach-Hellweg G, Trunk MJ, von Knebel DM. Traditional and new molecular methods for early detection of cervical cancer. Arkh Patol 2004;66:35–9.

50. de Sanjose S, Munoz N, Bosch FX, et al. Sexually transmitted agents and cervical neoplasia in Colombia and Spain. Int J Cancer 1994;56:358–63.

51. de Villiers EM. Relationship between steroid hormone contraceptives and HPV, cervical intraepithelial neoplasia and cervical carcinoma. Int J Cancer 2003;103:705–8.

52. Deacon JM, Evans CD, Yule R, et al. Sexual behaviour and smoking as determinants of cervical HPV infection and of CIN3 among those infected: a case-control study nested within the Manchester cohort. Br J Cancer 2000;83:1565–72.

53. Deshpande A, Nolan JP, White PS, et al. TNF-alpha promoter polymorphisms and susceptibility to human papillomavirus 16-associated cervical cancer. J Infect Dis 2005;191:969–76.

54. Devesa SS, Diamond EL. Association of breast cancer and cervical cancer incidence with income and education among whites and blacks. J Natl Cancer Inst 1980;65:515–28.

55. DiMaio D, Mattoon D. Mechanisms of cell transformation by papillomavirus E5 proteins. Oncogene 2001;20:7866–73.

56. Dong SM, Kim HS, Rha SH, Sidransky D. Promoter hypermethylation of multiple genes in carcinoma of the uterine cervix. Clin Cancer Res 2001;7:1982–6.

57. Doorbar J. The papillomavirus life cycle. J Clin Virol 2005;32(Suppl 1):S7–15.

58. Duensing S, Munger K. Centrosomes, genomic instability, and cervical carcinogenesis. Crit Rev Eukaryot Gene Expr 2003;13:9–23.

59. Dyson N, Howley PM, Munger K, Harlow E. The human papilloma virus-16 E7 oncoprotein is able to bind to the retinoblastoma gene product. Science 1989;243:934–7.

60. Fairley CK, Chen S, Tabrizi SN, Leeton K, Quinn MA, Garland SM. The absence of genital human papillomavirus DNA in virginal women. Int J STD AIDS 1992;3:414–17.

61. Fairley CK, Chen S, Tabrizi SN, et al. Prevalence of HPV DNA in cervical specimens in women with renal transplants: a comparison with dialysis-dependent patients and patients with renal impairment. Nephrol Dial Transplant 1994;9:416–20.

62. Favre M, Ramoz N, Orth G. Human papillomaviruses: general features. Clin Dermatol 1997;15:181–98.

63. Ferlay J, Bray FG, Pisani P, Parkin DM. GLOBOCAN 2000: Cancer incidence, mortality and prevalence worldwide. 2006;IARC CancerBase No. 5

64. Franceschi S, Castellsague X, Dal Maso L, et al. Prevalence and determinants of human papillomavirus genital infection in men. Br J Cancer 2002;86:705–11.

65. Franco EL, Villa LL, Ruiz A, Costa MC. Transmission of cervical human papillomavirus infection by sexual activity: differences between low and high oncogenic risk types. J Infect Dis 1995;172:756–63.

66. Frisch M, Biggar RJ, Goedert JJ. Human papillomavirus-associated cancers in patients with human immunodeficiency virus infection and acquired immunodeficiency syndrome. J Natl Cancer Inst 2000;92:1500–10.

67. Gardner JW, Sanborn JS, Slattery ML. Behavioral factors explaining the low risk for cervical carcinoma in Utah Mormon women. Epidemiology 1995;6:187–9.

68. Giannini SL, Hubert P, Doyen J, Boniver J, Delvenne P. Influence of the mucosal epithelium microenvironment on Langerhans cells: mplications for the development of squamous intraepithelial lesions of the cervix. Int J Cancer 2002;97:654–9.

69. Giuliano AR. The role of nutrients in the prevention of cervical dysplasia and cancer. Nutrition 2000;16:570–3.

70. Goldgar DE, Easton DF, Cannon-lbright LA, Skolnick MH. Systematic population-based assessment of cancer risk in first-degree relatives of cancer probands. J Natl Cancer Inst 1994;86:1600–8.

71. Goldstone SE, Palefsky JM, Winnett MT, Neefe JR. Activity of HspE7, a novel immunotherapy, in patients with anogenital warts. Dis Colon Rectum 2002;45:502–7.

72. Goodman MT, McDuffie K, Hernandez B, et al. CYP1A1, GSTM1, and GSTT1 polymorphisms and the risk of cervical squamous intraepithelial lesions in a multi-ethnic population. Gynecol Oncol 2001;81:263–9.

73. Gostout BS, Poland GA, Calhoun ES, et al. TAP1, TAP2, and HLA-DR2 alleles are predictors of cervical cancer risk. Gynecol Oncol 2003;88:326–32.

74. Green J, Berrington de Gonzalez A, Smith JS, et al. Human papillomavirus infection and use of oral contraceptives. Br J Cancer 2003;88:1713–20.

75. Gustafsson L, Ponten J, Bergstrom R, Adami HO. International incidence rates of invasive cervical cancer before cytological screening. Int J Cancer 1997;71:159–65.

76. Harro CD, Pang YY, Roden RB, et al. Safety and immunogenicity trial in adult volunteers of a human papillomavirus 16 L1 virus-like particle vaccine. J Natl Cancer Inst 2001;93:284–92.

77. Heard I, Tassie JM, Kazatchkine MD, Orth G. Highly active antiretroviral therapy enhances regression of cervical intraepithelial neoplasia in HIV-seropositive women. AIDS 2002;16:1799–802.

78. Hellberg D, Nilsson S. Genital cancer among wives of men with penile cancer. A study between 1958 and 1982. Br J Obstet Gynaecol 1989;96:221–5.

79. Helt AM, Galloway DA. Mechanisms by which DNA tumor virus oncoproteins target the Rb family of pocket proteins. Carcinogenesis 2003;24:159–69.

80. Hemminki K, Li X, Mutanen P. Familial risks in invasive and in situ cervical cancer by histological type. Eur J Cancer Prev 2001;10:83–9.

81. Hemminki K, Vaittinen P. Familial cancers in a nationwide family cancer database: age distribution and prevalence. Eur J Cancer 1999;35:1109–17.

82. Hermonat PL, Daniel RW, Shah KV. The spermicide nonoxynol-9 does not inactivate papillomavirus. Sex Transm Dis 1992;19:203–5.

83. Hildesheim A, Gravitt P, Schiffman MH, et al. Determinants of genital human papillomavirus infection in low-income women in Washington, D.C. Sex Transm Dis 1993;20:279–85.

84. Hildesheim A, Herrero R, Castle PE, et al. HPV co-factors related to the development of cervical cancer: results from a population-based study in Costa Rica. Br J Cancer 2001;84:1219–26.

85. Hildesheim A, Schiffman M, Scott DR, et al. Human leukocyte antigen class I/II alleles and development of human papillomavirus-related cervical neoplasia: results from a case-control study conducted in the United States. Cancer Epidemiol Biomarkers Prev 1998;7:1035–41.

86. Hildesheim A, Schiffman MH, Gravitt PE, et al. Persistence of type-specific human papillomavirus infection among cytologically normal women. J Infect Dis 1994;169:235–40.

87. Hildesheim A, Wang SS. Host and viral genetics and risk of cervical cancer: a review. Virus Res 2002;89:229–40.

88. Hill AB. The environment and disease: association or causation? Proc R Soc Med 1965;58:295–300.

89. Ho GY, Bierman R, Beardsley L, Chang CJ, Burk RD. Natural history of cervicovaginal papillomavirus infection in young women. N Engl J Med 1998;338:423–8.

90. Ho GY, Burk RD, Klein S, et al. Persistent genital human papillomavirus infection as a risk factor for persistent cervical dysplasia. J Natl Cancer Inst 1995;87:1365–71.

91. Jacobs MV, Walboomers JM, Snijders PJ, et al. Distribution of 37 mucosotropic HPV types in women with cytologically normal cervical smears: the age-related patterns for high-risk and low-risk types. Int J Cancer 2000;87:221–7.

92. Jacobson DL, Peralta L, Farmer M, Graham NM, Wright TC, Zenilman J. Cervical ectopy and the transformation zone measured by computerized planimetry in adolescents. Int J Gynaecol Obstet 1999;66:7–17.

93. Kersemaekers AM, Van de Vijver MJ, Kenter GG, Fleuren GJ. Genetic alterations during the progression of squamous cell carcinomas of the uterine cervix. Genes Chromosomes Cancer 1999;26:346–54.

94. Kessler II. Venereal factors in human cervical cancer: evidence from marital clusters. Cancer 1977;39:1912–19.

95. Khan MJ, Partridge EE, Wang SS, Schiffman M. Socioeconomic status and the risk of cervical intraepithelial neoplasia grade 3 among oncogenic human papillomavirus DNA-positive women with equivocal or mildly abnormal cytology. Cancer 2005;104:61–70.

96. Kim JJ, Wright TC, Goldie SJ. Cost-effectiveness of alternative triage strategies for atypical squamous cells of undetermined significance. JAMA 2002;287:2382–90.

97. Kim JW, Lee CG, Park YG, et al. Combined analysis of germline polymorphisms of p53, GSTM1, GSTT1, CYP1A1, and CYP2E1: relation to the incidence rate of cervical carcinoma. Cancer 2000;88:2082–91.

98. Kim JW, Roh JW, Park NH, Song YS, Kang SB, Lee HP. Interferon, alpha 17 (IFNA17) Ile184Arg polymorphism and cervical cancer risk. Cancer Lett 2003;189:183–8.
99. Kirnbauer R, Chandrachud LM, O'Neil BW, et al. Virus-like particles of bovine papillomavirus type 4 in prophylactic and therapeutic immunization. Virology 1996;219:37–44.
100. Kjaer SK, Dahl C, Engholm G, Bock JE, Lynge E, Jensen OM. Case-control study of risk factors for cervical neoplasia in Denmark. II: Role of sexual activity, reproductive factors, and venereal infections. Cancer Causes Control 1992;3:339–44.
101. Kjaer SK, de Villiers EM, Dahl C, et al. Case-control study of risk factors for cervical neoplasia in Denmark. I: Role of the 'male factor' in women with one lifetime sexual partner. Int J Cancer 1991;48:39–44.
102. Kjaer SK, Svare EI, Worm AM, Walboomers JM, Meijer CJ, van den Brule AJ. Human papillomavirus infection in Danish female sex workers. Decreasing prevalence with age despite continuously high sexual activity. Sex Transm Dis 2000;27:438–45.
103. Kjaer SK, van den Brule AJ, Paull G, et al. Type specific persistence of high risk human papillomavirus (HPV) as indicator of high grade cervical squamous intraepithelial lesions in young women: population based prospective follow up study. BMJ 2002;325:572.
104. Klaes R, Benner A, Friedrich T, et al. p16INK4a immunohistochemistry improves interobserver agreement in the diagnosis of cervical intraepithelial neoplasia. Am J Surg Pathol 2002;26:1389–99.
105. Klaes R, Friedrich T, Spitkovsky D, et al. Overexpression of p16(INK4A) as a specific marker for dysplastic and neoplastic epithelial cells of the cervix uteri. Int J Cancer 2001;92:276–84.
106. Klaes R, Woerner SM, Ridder R, et al. Detection of high-risk cervical intraepithelial neoplasia and cervical cancer by amplification of transcripts derived from integrated papillomavirus oncogenes. Cancer Res 1999;59:6132–6.
107. Knudson AG. Hereditary cancer: two hits revisited. J Cancer Res Clin Oncol 1996;122:135–40.
108. Konya J, Dillner J. Immunity to oncogenic human papillomaviruses. Adv Cancer Res 2001;82:205–38.
109. Koss LG, Durfee GR. Unusual patterns of squamous epithelium of the uterine cervix: cytologic and pathologic study of koilocytotic atypia. Ann N Y Acad Sci 1956;63:1245–61.
110. Koutsky LA, Ault KA, Wheeler CM, et al. A controlled trial of a human papillomavirus type 16 vaccine. N Engl J Med 2002;347:1645–51.
111. Kurman RJ, Malkasian GD, Jr, Sedlis A, Solomon D. From Papanicolaou to Bethesda: the rationale for a new cervical cytologic classification. Obstet Gynecol 1991;77:779–82.
112. La Vecchia C, Franceschi S, Decarli A, Fasoli M, Gentile A, Tognoni G. Cigarette smoking and the risk of cervical neoplasia. Am J Epidemiol 1986;123:22–9.
113. La Vecchia C, Tavani A, Franceschi S, Parazzini F. Oral contraceptives and cancer. A review of the evidence. Drug Saf 1996;14:260–72.
114. Lacey JV, Jr, Brinton LA, Abbas FM, et al. Oral contraceptives as risk factors for cervical adenocarcinomas and squamous cell carcinomas. Cancer Epidemiol Biomarkers Prev 1999;8:1079–85.
115. Lai YM, Yang FP, Pao CC. Human papillomavirus deoxyribonucleic acid and ribonucleic acid in seminal plasma and sperm cells. Fertil Steril 1996;65:1026–30.
116. Lazo PA. The molecular genetics of cervical carcinoma. Br J Cancer 1999;80:2008–18.
117. Ley C, Bauer HM, Reingold A, et al. Determinants of genital human papillomavirus infection in young women. J Natl Cancer Inst 1991;83:997–1003.
118. Li H, Jin S, Xu H, Thomas DB. The decline in the mortality rates of cervical cancer and a plausible explanation in Shandong, China. Int J Epidemiol 2000;29:398–404.
119. Liaw KL, Glass AG, Manos MM, et al. Detection of human papillomavirus DNA in cytologically normal women and subsequent cervical squamous intraepithelial lesions. J Natl Cancer Inst 1999;91:954–60.
120. Liaw KL, Hildesheim A, Burk RD, et al. A prospective study of human papillomavirus (HPV) type 16 DNA detection by polymerase chain reaction and its association with acquisition and persistence of other HPV types. J Infect Dis 2001;183:8–15.
121. Lichtenstein P, Holm NV, Verkasalo PK, et al. Environmental and heritable factors in the causation of cancer – analyses of cohorts of twins from Sweden, Denmark, and Finland. N Engl J Med 2000;343:78–85.
122. Lorincz AT, Castle PE, Sherman ME, et al. Viral load of human papillomavirus and risk of CIN3 or cervical cancer. Lancet 2002;360:228–9.
123. Luft F, Gebert J, Schneider A, Melsheimer P, von Knebel DM. Frequent allelic imbalance of tumor suppressor gene loci in cervical dysplasia. Int J Gynecol Pathol 1999;18:374–80.
124. Magnusson PK, Sparen P, Gyllensten UB. Genetic link to cervical tumours. Nature 1999;400:29–30.
125. Man S, Fiander A. Immunology of human papillomavirus infection in lower genital tract neoplasia. Best Pract Res Clin Obstet Gynaecol 2001;15:701–14.
126. Mandelblatt JS, Kanetsky P, Eggert L, Gold K. Is HIV infection a cofactor for cervical squamous cell neoplasia? Cancer Epidemiol Biomarkers Prev 1999;8:97–106.
127. Manhart LE, Koutsky LA. Do condoms prevent genital HPV infection, external genital warts, or cervical neoplasia? A meta-analysis. Sex Transm Dis 2002;29:725–35.
128. Mantovani F, Banks L. The human papillomavirus E6 protein and its contribution to malignant progression. Oncogene 2001;20:7874–87.
129. Matthews CP, Shera KA, McDougall JK. Genomic changes and HPV type in cervical carcinoma. Proc Soc Exp Biol Med 2000;223:316–21.
130. Melkert PW, Hopman E, van den Brule AJ, et al. Prevalence of HPV in cytomorphologically normal cervical smears, as determined by the polymerase chain reaction, is age-dependent. Int J Cancer 1993;53:919–23.
131. Minkoff H, Ahdieh L, Massad LS, et al. The effect of highly active antiretroviral therapy on cervical cytologic changes associated with oncogenic HPV among HIV-infected women. AIDS 2001;15:2157–64.
132. Mitchell H, Medley G, Gordon I, Giles G. Cervical cytology reported as negative and risk of adenocarcinoma of the cervix: no strong evidence of benefit. Br J Cancer 1995;71:894–7.
133. Moreno V, Bosch FX, Munoz N, et al. Effect of oral contraceptives on risk of cervical cancer in women with human papillomavirus infection: the IARC multi-centric case-control study. Lancet 2002;359:1085–92.
134. Moscicki AB, Ellenberg JH, Vermund SH, et al. Prevalence of and risks for cervical human papillomavirus infection and squamous intraepithelial lesions in adolescent girls: impact of infection with human immunodeficiency virus. Arch Pediatr Adolesc Med 2000;154:127–34.
135. Moscicki AB, Hills N, Shiboski S, et al. Risks for incident human papillomavirus infection and low-grade squamous intraepithelial lesion development in young females. JAMA 2001;285:2995–3002.
136. Moscicki AB, Shiboski S, Broering J, et al. The natural history of human papillomavirus infection as measured by repeated DNA testing in adolescent and young women. J Pediatr 1998;132:277–84.
137. Munger K, Basile JR, Duensing S, et al. Biological activities and molecular targets of the human papillomavirus E7 oncoprotein. Oncogene 2001;20:7888–98.
138. Munger K, Howley PM. Human papillomavirus immortalization and transformation functions. Virus Res 2002;89:213–28.
139. Munoz N. Human papillomavirus and cancer: the epidemiological evidence. J Clin Virol 2000;19:1–5.
140. Munoz N, Bosch FX, de Sanjose S, et al. Epidemiologic classification of human papillomavirus types associated with cervical cancer. N Engl J Med 2003;348:518–27.
141. Munoz N, Franceschi S, Bosetti C, et al. Role of parity and human papillomavirus in cervical cancer: the IARC multi-centric case-control study. Lancet 2002;359:1093–101.
142. Narayan G, Arias-Pulido H, Koul S, et al. Frequent promoter methylation of CDH1, DAPK, RARB, and HIC1 genes in carcinoma of cervix uteri: its relationship to clinical outcome. Mol Cancer 2003;2:24.
143. Nobbenhuis MA, Walboomers JM, Helmerhorst TJ, et al. Relation of human papillomavirus status to cervical lesions and consequences for cervical-cancer screening: a prospective study. Lancet 1999;354:20–5.
144. Olatunbosun O, Deneer H, Pierson R. Human papillomavirus DNA detection in sperm using polymerase chain reaction. Obstet Gynecol 2001;97:357–60.
145. Palefsky JM, Holly EA. Immunosuppression and co-infection with HIV. J Natl Cancer Inst Monogr 2003;41–6.
146. Palefsky JM, Holly EA, Ralston ML, et al. Effect of highly active antiretroviral therapy on the natural history of anal squamous intraepithelial lesions and anal human papillomavirus infection. J Acquir Immune Defic Syndr 2001;28:422–8.
147. Palefsky JM, Minkoff H, Kalish LA, et al. Cervicovaginal human papillomavirus infection in human immunodeficiency virus-1 (HIV)-positive and high-risk HIV-negative women. J Natl Cancer Inst 1999;91:226–36.
148. Parham GP, Hicks ML. Race as a factor in the outcome of patients with cervical cancer: lift the veil to find the wounded spirit. Gynecol Oncol 1998;71:149–50.
149. Parkin DM, Bray FI, Devesa SS. Cancer burden in the year 2000. The global picture. Eur J Cancer 2001;37(Suppl 8):S4–66.
150. Penn I. Cancer in the immunosuppressed organ recipient. Transplant Proc 1991;23:1771–2.
151. Peters RK, Thomas D, Hagan DG, Mack TM, Henderson BE. Risk factors for invasive cervical cancer among Latinas and non-Latinas in Los Angeles County. J Natl Cancer Inst 1986;77:1063–77.
152. Peyton CL, Gravitt PE, Hunt WC, et al. Determinants of genital human papillomavirus detection in a US population. J Infect Dis 2001;183:1554–64.
153. Pham TH, Nguyen TH, Herrero R, et al. Human papillomavirus infection among women in South and North Vietnam. Int J Cancer 2003;104:213–20.
154. Potischman N. Nutritional epidemiology of cervical neoplasia. J Nutr 1993;123:424–9.
155. Remmink AJ, Walboomers JM, Helmerhorst TJ, et al. The presence of persistent high-risk HPV genotypes in dysplastic cervical lesions is associated with progressive disease: natural history up to 36 months. Int J Cancer 1995;61:306–11.
156. Rice PS, Cason J, Best JM, Banatvala JE. High risk genital papillomavirus infections are spread vertically. Rev Med Virol 1999;9:15–21.
157. Rintala MA, Grenman SE, Pollanen PP, Suominen JJ, Syrjanen SM. Detection of high-risk HPV DNA in semen and its association with the quality of semen. Int J STD AIDS 2004;15:740–3.

158. Robboy SJ, Szyfelbein WM, Goellner JR, et al. Dysplasia and cytologic findings in 4589 young women enrolled in diethylstilbestrol-adenosis (DESAD) project. Am J Obstet Gynecol 1981;140:579–86.

159. Roh J, Kim M, Kim J, et al. Polymorphisms in codon 31 of p21 and cervical cancer susceptibility in Korean women. Cancer Lett 2001;165:59–62.

160. Rozendaal L, Walboomers JM, van der Linden JC, et al. PCR-based high-risk HPV test in cervical cancer screening gives objective risk assessment of women with cytomorphologically normal cervical smears. Int J Cancer 1996;68:766–9.

161. Saslow D, Runowicz CD, Solomon D, et al. American Cancer Society guideline for the early detection of cervical neoplasia and cancer. CA Cancer J Clin 2002;52:342–62.

162. Schiffman M, Herrero R, Desalle R, et al. The carcinogenicity of human papillomavirus types reflects viral evolution. Virology 2005;337:76–84.

163. Schiller JT, Lowy DR. Papillomavirus-like particle vaccines. J Natl Cancer Inst Monogr 2001;50–4.

164. Schlecht NF, Kulaga S, Robitaille J, et al. Persistent human papillomavirus infection as a predictor of cervical intraepithelial neoplasia. JAMA 2001;286:3106–14.

165. Sheets EE, Urban RG, Crum CP, et al. Immunotherapy of human cervical high-grade cervical intraepithelial neoplasia with microparticle-delivered human papillomavirus 16 E7 plasmid DNA. Am J Obstet Gynecol 2003;188:916–26.

166. Sherman ME, Lorincz AT, Scott DR, et al. Baseline cytology, human papillomavirus testing, and risk for cervical neoplasia: a 10-year cohort analysis. J Natl Cancer Inst 2003;95:46–52.

167. Sherman ME, Schiffman M, Cox JT. Effects of age and human papilloma viral load on colposcopy triage: data from the randomized Atypical Squamous Cells of Undetermined Significance/Low-Grade Squamous Intraepithelial Lesion Triage Study (ALTS). J Natl Cancer Inst 2002;94:102–7.

168. Sherman ME, Wang SS, Wheeler CM, et al. Determinants of human papillomavirus load among women with histological cervical intraepithelial neoplasia 3: dominant impact of surrounding low-grade lesions. Cancer Epidemiol Biomarkers Prev 2003;12:1038–44.

169. Sierra-Torres CH, Au WW, Arrastia CD, et al. Polymorphisms for chemical metabolizing genes and risk for cervical neoplasia. Environ Mol Mutagen 2003;41:69–76.

170. Smith JS, Green J, Berrington de G, et al. Cervical cancer and use of hormonal contraceptives: a systematic review. Lancet 2003;361:1159–67.

171. Smith PG, Kinlen LJ, White GC, Adelstein AM, Fox AJ. Mortality of wives of men dying with cancer of the penis. Br J Cancer 1980;41:422–8.

172. Snijders PJ, Steenbergen RD, Heideman DA, Meijer CJ. HPV-mediated cervical carcinogenesis: concepts and clinical implications. J Pathol 2006;208:152–64.

173. Solomon D, Davey D, Kurman R, et al. The 2001 Bethesda System: terminology for reporting results of cervical cytology. JAMA 2002;287:2114–19.

174. Sporn MB, Roberts AB. Cervical dysplasia regression induced by all-trans-retinoic acid. J Natl Cancer Inst 1994;86:476–7.

175. Stanley MA. Human papillomavirus vaccines. Curr Opin Mol Ther 2002;4:15–22.

176. Stanley MA. Human papillomavirus (HPV) vaccines: prospects for eradicating cervical cancer. J Fam Plann Reprod Health Care 2004;30:213–15.

177. Steenbergen RD, Kramer D, Braakhuis BJ, et al. TSLC1 gene silencing in cervical cancer cell lines and cervical neoplasia. J Natl Cancer Inst 2004;96:294–305.

178. Stein WD, Stein AD. Testing and characterizing the two-stage model of carcinogenesis for a wide range of human cancers. J Theor Biol 1990;145:95–122.

179. Stern PL, Brown M, Stacey SN, et al. Natural HPV immunity and vaccination strategies. J Clin Virol 2000;19:57–66.

180. Stoler MH. A brief synopsis of the role of human papillomaviruses in cervical carcinogenesis. Am J Obstet Gynecol 1996;175:1091–8.

181. Stone KM, Karem KL, Sternberg MR, et al. Seroprevalence of human papillomavirus type 16 infection in the United States. J Infect Dis 2002;186:1396–402.

182. Stubenrauch F, Laimins LA. Human papillomavirus life cycle: active and latent phases. Semin Cancer Biol 1999;9:379–86.

183. Sun XW, Kuhn L, Ellerbrock TV, Chiasson MA, Bush TJ, Wright TC, Jr. Human papillomavirus infection in women infected with the human immunodeficiency virus. N Engl J Med 1997;337:1343–9.

184. Suzich JA, Ghim SJ, Palmer-Hill FJ, et al. Systemic immunization with papillomavirus L1 protein completely prevents the development of viral mucosal papillomas. Proc Natl Acad Sci U S A 1995;92:11553–7.

185. Swan DC, Tucker RA, Tortolero-Luna G, et al. Human papillomavirus (HPV) DNA copy number is dependent on grade of cervical disease and HPV type. J Clin Microbiol 1999;37:1030–4.

186. Szarewski A, Jarvis MJ, Sasieni P, et al. Effect of smoking cessation on cervical lesion size. Lancet 1996;347:941–3.

187. Thomas KK, Hughes JP, Kuypers JM, et al. Concurrent and sequential acquisition of different genital human papillomavirus types. J Infect Dis 2000;182:1097–102.

188. Viikki M, Pukkala E, Hakama M. Bleeding symptoms and subsequent risk of gynecological and other cancers. Acta Obstet Gynecol Scand 1998;77:564–9.

189. Villa LL, Costa RL, Petta CA, et al. Prophylactic quadrivalent human papillomavirus (types 6, 11, 16, and 18) L1 virus-like particle vaccine in young women: a randomised double-blind placebo-controlled multi-centre phase II efficacy trial. Lancet Oncol 2005;6:271–8.

190. Viscidi RP, Schiffman M, Hildesheim A, et al. Seroreactivity to human papillomavirus (HPV) types 16, 18, or 31 and risk of subsequent HPV infection: results from a population-based study in Costa Rica. Cancer Epidemiol Biomarkers Prev 2004;13:324–7.

191. Walboomers JM, Jacobs MV, Manos MM, et al. Human papillomavirus is a necessary cause of invasive cervical cancer worldwide. J Pathol 1999;189:12–19.

192. Wallin KL, Wiklund F, Angstrom T, et al. Type-specific persistence of human papillomavirus DNA before the development of invasive cervical cancer. N Engl J Med 1999;341:1633–8.

193. Wang SS, Hildesheim A. Viral and host factors in human papillomavirus persistence and progression. J Natl Cancer Inst Monogr 2003;35–40.

194. Wang SS, Hildesheim A, Gao X, et al. Comprehensive analysis of human leukocyte antigen class I alleles and cervical neoplasia in 3 epidemiologic studies. J Infect Dis 2002;186:598–605.

195. Wang SS, Schiffman M. Medication use, medical conditions, and the risk of human papillomavirus infection and subsequent cervical intraepithelial neoplasia 3 among women with mild cytologic abnormalities. Cancer Epidemiol Biomarkers Prev 2005;14:542–5.

196. Wang SS, Sherman ME, Hildesheim A, Lacey JV, Jr, Devesa S. Cervical adenocarcinoma and squamous cell carcinoma incidence trends among white women and black women in the United States for 1976–2000. Cancer 2004;100:1035–44.

197. Wang SS, Trunk M, Schiffman M, et al. Validation of p16INK4a as a marker of oncogenic human papillomavirus infection in cervical biopsies from a population-based cohort in Costa Rica. Cancer Epidemiol Biomarkers Prev 2004;13:1355–60.

198. Wang SS, Wheeler CM, Hildesheim A, et al. Human leukocyte antigen class I and II alleles and risk of cervical neoplasia: results from a population-based study in Costa Rica. J Infect Dis 2001;184:1310–14.

199. Wank R, Thomssen C. High risk of squamous cell carcinoma of the cervix for women with HLA-DQw3. Nature 1991;352:723–5.

200. Weinstein SJ, Ziegler RG, Frongillo EA, Jr, et al. Low serum and red blood cell folate are moderately, but nonsignificantly associated with increased risk of invasive cervical cancer in U.S. women. J Nutr 2001;131:2040–8.

201. Weinstein SJ, Ziegler RG, Selhub J, et al. Elevated serum homocysteine levels and increased risk of invasive cervical cancer in US women. Cancer Causes Control 2001;12:317–24.

202. Werness BA, Levine AJ, Howley PM. Association of human papillomavirus types 16 and 18 E6 proteins with p53. Science 1990;248:76–9.

203. Winer RL, Lee SK, Hughes JP, Adam DE, Kiviat NB, Koutsky LA. Genital human papillomavirus infection: incidence and risk factors in a cohort of female university students. Am J Epidemiol 2003;157:218–26.

204. Winkelstein W, Jr. Smoking and cervical cancer – current status: a review. Am J Epidemiol 1990;131:945–57.

205. Woodman CB, Collins S, Winter H, et al. Natural history of cervical human papillomavirus infection in young women: a longitudinal cohort study. Lancet 2001;357:1831–6.

206. Woodworth CD. HPV innate immunity. Front Biosci 2002;7:d2058–d2071.

207. Wright TC, Jr, Schiffman M. Adding a test for human papillomavirus DNA to cervical-cancer screening. N Engl J Med 2003;348:489–90.

208. Xi LF, Koutsky LA, Galloway DA, et al. Genomic variation of human papillomavirus type 16 and risk for high grade cervical intraepithelial neoplasia. J Natl Cancer Inst 1997;89:796–802.

209. Ylitalo N, Josefsson A, Melbye M, et al. A prospective study showing long-term infection with human papillomavirus 16 before the development of cervical carcinoma in situ. Cancer Res 2000;60:6027–32.

210. Ylitalo N, Josefsson A, Melbye M, et al. A prospective study showing long-term infection with human papillomavirus 16 before the development of cervical carcinoma in situ. Cancer Res 2000;60:6027–32.

211. Ylitalo N, Sorensen P, Josefsson AM, et al. Consistent high viral load of human papillomavirus 16 and risk of cervical carcinoma in situ: a nested case-control study. Lancet 2000;355:2194–8.

212. Zhang A, Zheng C, Hou M, et al. Amplification of the telomerase reverse transcriptase (hTERT) gene in cervical carcinomas. Genes Chromosomes Cancer 2002;34:269–75.

213. zur Hausen H, de Villiers EM. Human papillomaviruses. Annu Rev Microbiol 1994;48:427–47.

Cervical precancer (intraepithelial neoplasia), including functional biomarkers and colposcopy

8

Jan P.A. Baak   Mark H. Stoler   Sarah M. Bean   Malcolm C. Anderson   Stanley J. Robboy

INTRODUCTION

The traditional view of squamous carcinogenesis in the cervix has dramatically changed during the last two decades.[8,85,90,91] A clear understanding of how human papillomavirus (HPV) infection affects epithelial biology has altered long-standing concepts based purely on descriptive correlation of histology with clinical behavior. Thus older terms like dysplasia/carcinoma in situ (a four-grade system) or cervical intraepithelial neoplasia (a three-grade system) have given way or been equated with the biologic understanding that the entire spectrum of cervical neoplasia is due to HPV and that there are fundamentally only two states between normal or reactive non-neoplastic processes and cancer. The first and overwhelmingly most common is a low-grade (or even better, low risk) lesion that is the biologic manifestation of productive HPV infection. All HPVs generate this type of morphology as this type of cellular differentiation is required to make virions. These infections and their cytohistologic manifestations are almost always transient, resolving on average in about a year. Much less commonly, but significantly, HPV oncogenes, particularly from the high-risk types of HPV, are expressed in cells that are still replication competent. This produces a clonal expansion of rapidly proliferating cells that is morphologically manifest as a high-grade lesion, ultimately as a CIN 3, carcinoma in situ (CIS), or severe dysplasia (all essentially synonymous terms). These cells, the proven precursors of invasive cancer, are virologically non-infectious as no virus is made, but the viral genes drive the human (host) cells to proliferate.

Of the more than 150 HPV types known to exist, only about 30–40 affect the genital tract and, of these, probably less than 15 or so are clinically important. Most of these are oncogenic, the most common and notorious being HPV type 16 and its related viruses, like types 31, 33, 35, 56, etc. from the alpha 9 clade (a taxonomic group of organisms comprising a single common ancestor and all the descendants of that ancestor), and type 18 with its close relations such as type 45 (Table 8.1). They are called high risk or oncogenic because they are the types found in cancers. Paradoxically, while the high-risk types are the most common types affecting the cervix, most high-risk HPV infections result in only low-grade lesions. The less aggressive and generally 'benign' or low-risk forms are prototypically HPV types 6 and 11 whose biology is one of productive transient infection with only extremely rare carcinogenic examples. The low-risk group constitutes only a tenth or so of cervical infection (Table 8.2).

As pathologists have come to better understand the biology of neoplastic development, so too have they and colposcopists been humbled by the data-driven realization that morphology is subjective and limited by issues of incomplete sampling and interpretive variability. Thus, a patient may have CIN 3, but the Papanicolaou smear is negative because the cells were not collected, likewise with the biopsy. Cytology was always viewed as a screening test and tissue pathology somewhat inappropriately as the reference standard. Now we know that both are equally variable and may give the correct information on disease severity (or not at all) as the patient is put through the diagnostic process. Indeed, colposcopic biopsy was assumed by many to be an accurate assessment of the worst prevalent cervical pathology, i.e., a gold standard, even though early warnings from meticulous studies showed the standard was tarnished,[100] but understanding now affords an opportunity to compensate for these proven limitations. Despite imperfections, criteria-based approaches to diagnosis remain the best way to minimize interpretive variation and achieve practice at a standard of care level.[93]

CERVICAL INTRAEPITHELIAL NEOPLASIA (CIN): AN EVOLVING CONCEPT

NOMENCLATURE

The nomenclature used to describe the precursor conditions of invasive squamous cell carcinoma continues to be a subject of some debate. The term 'dysplasia', when introduced in the 1950s into the field of gynecologic pathology, equated the condition to an atypical hyperplasia of the cervical epithelium and, later, to a lesion less than carcinoma in situ (CIS) in which the squamous mucosa is replaced throughout its entire thickness by undifferentiated (and much later understood to be clonally proliferating) cells. The subdivision of severe dysplasia from CIS was later appreciated to have little validity on either biologic or clinical grounds, due in part to both imprecision in definitions and variability in interpretations. The latter is emphasized in numerous studies demonstrating poor inter- and intraobserver reproducibility (kappa) scores among pathologists when reviewing the same slides, and where the same pathologist has inconsistently diagnosed the findings in the same slide at different times.[70,93]

The appreciation that CIS is no more serious a condition than a high-grade dysplasia, and that CIS and dysplasia represent the same disease process, led to a simplified classification and more uniform treatment. Prior to this realization, some women with CIS were overtreated and some women with dysplasia undertreated or not even treated at all. The unity of dysplasia/CIS was supported by the tools of the times from various modalities, including light and electron microscopy,

Table 8.1 Classification of HPV types associated with genital lesions[101]

Most common types

6, 11	Condyloma acuminatum, low-grade SIL (CIN)
16	All grades SIL, squamous cell carcinoma, and more rarely other cancer types
18	All grades SIL, adenocarcinoma, squamous cell carcinoma, and small cell cancer

Less common types

30, 40, 58, 69	All grades SIL
31, 33, 35, 39, 45, 51, 52, 56	All grades SIL, squamous cell carcinoma
42, 43, 44	Low-grade SIL (CIN)
53	Normal cervical epithelium, CW1 + 2
54	Condyloma acuminatum
55	Bowenoid papulosis
59	Vulvar intraepithelial neoplasia
61, 62, 64, 67	Vaginal intraepithelial neoplasia
66	Squamous cell carcinoma
70	Vulvar papilloma

Table 8.2 Comparison of HPV frequency detected by laboratory techniques[84]

	DNA hybridization (%)	Koilocytosis (%)	1 Immunocytochemistry (%)
Condyloma	100	80	80
CIN 1	100	89	61
CIN 2	86	57	29
CIN 3 (severe dysplasia)	100	33	17
CIN 3 (carcinoma in situ)	100	20	0

image analysis, autoradiography, microspectrophotometry, and later in the 1980s molecular biologic techniques, all showing that the cells of high-grade dysplasia and CIS are virtually identical and that there are no grounds for perpetuating two diagnostic categories. What emerged was a concept of a spectrum of cervical epithelial abnormalities called cervical intraepithelial neoplasia (CIN). To the extent that the concept of a continuum is useful, it is also incompatible with rigid subdivisions into grades, although such subdivisions are helpful as a guide to management. This continuum of dysplastic changes was divided into grades where CIN 1 corresponds to mild dysplasia, CIN 2 to moderate dysplasia, and CIN 3 embraces both severe dysplasia and CIS.

The knowledge about the role of HPV (see Chapter 7),[8,85,91] and more specifically the roles of individual HPV types, suggests another division into the type of disease produced by the low-risk HPV types like HPV 6 and 11 usually resulting in low-grade dysplasia (CIN 1 and sometimes misclassified as CIN 2) and the high-risk HPV types, most commonly HPV 16 and 18 usually resulting in the full range of dysplasias, but rarely high-grade ones (CIN 2 and CIN 3/CIS).

Yet the morphologic concept of a continuum and progression or regression through grades of CIN is at odds with our current concepts of HPV epithelial biology. It implies a linearity and certainty that is not well supported by the best available data. Indeed, progression is very difficult to define in an individual due to the infrequent and incomplete sampling by cytology or small biopsy. The latter is further confounded by the previously noted diagnostic variability and the fact that the process is dynamic and constant. Since the late 1980s, the Bethesda system, the classification scheme introduced for use in reporting cervical cytology smears, has incorporated the finding of HPV as a preneoplastic condition. HPV lesions not previously considered dysplastic, including condylomatous lesions, are now grouped with CIN 1 (mild dysplasia) into a single category, low-grade squamous intraepithelial lesion (low-grade SIL, or LGSIL or LSIL). These low-grade lesions have a low-growth fraction, koilocytotic atypia (also called 'HPV cytopathic effect') and are the morphologic manifestation of productive HPV infection. These low-grade lesions might perhaps be better called 'low risk for predicting the development of high-grade precancer or cancer'. All HPV types functionally produce LSILs. In contrast, high-grade lesions are called high-grade SIL (HGSIL or HSIL), and parallel lesions are known as CIN 2 and CIN 3 (moderate dysplasia, severe dysplasia, and CIS). The relation among these various terms is shown in Figure 8.1 (see also Chapters 7 and 10).

A strength of the Bethesda system is the implication that SIL, devised initially for use in cytology, is easily transposed for use in and to describe histologic lesions (i.e., CIN 1, 2, or 3). Although this has occurred in some locales, some histopathologists would disagree with their terminologic convergence on the basis that the Bethesda system incorporates lesions that, while having the capability of becoming preneoplastic, are not yet and most likely will never become so. Because the cells from a condylomatous lesion and mild dysplasia on a smear often look identical, the former is included in the diagnosis of cytologic SIL because there is no way to differentiate the two. Yet it has now been proven that these two lesions are the same both biologically and on the basis of non-reproducibility in both tissue and Papanicolaou smears.[93] Kappa values, even among experts, are poor (~0.2, signifying poor interobserver agreement). While the histopathologist considers the features of the whole tissue, the relationships among cells within the tissue, and cellular detail, recent data show that histopathology is no more accurate or reproducible than cytopathology, and both suffer from issues of incomplete sampling. Few low-grade lesions progress, and some clinicians have long misunderstood the risk of progression, treating mild dysplasia/CIN 1 as if it had a different risk than lesions previously termed flat condyloma. As suggested above, when practitioners today think about the concept of progression, they are advised to take a probabilistic view, which incorporates assessing independently the results of cytology and biopsy, together with HPV testing. These composite results then allow derivation of an overall risk that the patient has (or soon will have) demonstrable true precancer, i.e., CIN 3. These probabilities can then be arrayed into

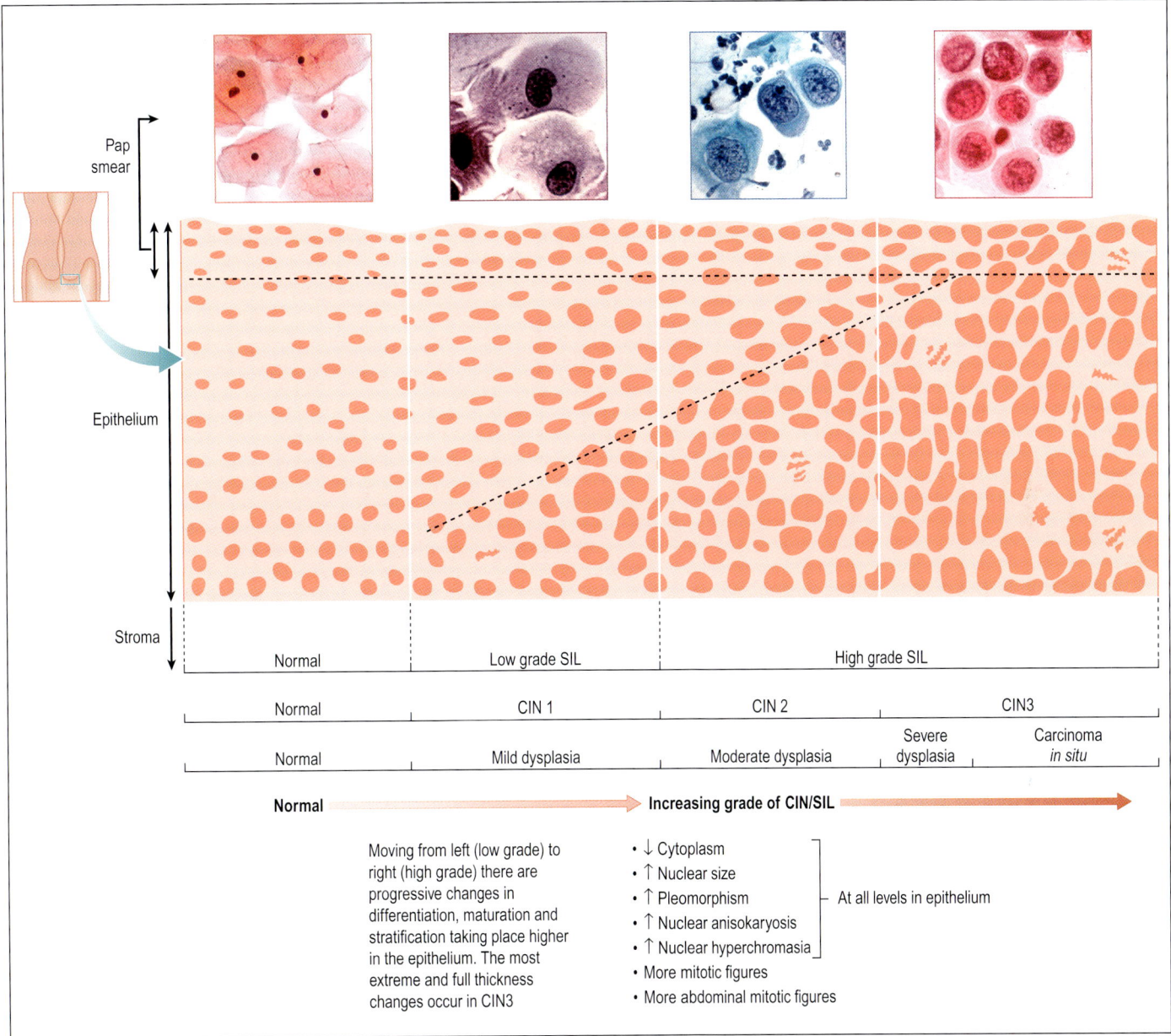

Fig. 8.1 Interrelations of naming systems in preneoplastic cervical disease. This complex chart integrates multiple aspects of the disease complex. It lists the qualitative and quantitative features that become increasingly more abnormal as the preneoplastic disease advances in severity. It also pictorially illustrates the changes in progressively more abnormal disease states and provides translation nomenclature for the dysplasia/CIS system, CIN system and Bethesda system. Finally, the scheme illustrates the corresponding cytologic smear resulting from exfoliation of the superficial-most cells, indicating that even in the most mild disease state, abnormal cells reach the surface and are shed. SIL, squamous intraepithelial lesion.

action thresholds for appropriate treatment or conservative management of the individual based on risk.[20,92]

It is true that the cytologist, in contrast to the histopathologist, can only examine cells that have been exfoliated, which by definition are the superficial-most cells in the mucosa. Yet, in some ways, the cytologic sample may be more representative of the spectrum of pathology in the cervix because of its ability to sample a much larger surface area compared to the punch biopsy. The appearance of the cytology is directly related to the underlying imagined histopathology. The fact that smear and biopsy findings from samples obtained during the same patient examination show high degrees of correlation supports the concept that CIN, even when low-grade, affects *all* layers of the epithelium. This challenges the often mistaken dogma that CIN 1 involves only the lower third of the epithelium and CIN 2 the lower and middle thirds. What seems closer to the truth is that subtleties exist in all layers, and that all are useful in differentiating the various grades of CIN. Of import, various investigators, including those of this chapter, place differing degrees of emphasis on single or combinations of findings. Yet the features are highly complementary, as in practice, colleagues easily agree about the final diagnosis, even though the features evaluated and emphasized may differ. The sections that follow, therefore, emphasize the quantitative and qualitative changes that occur throughout the epithelium in the various degrees of CIN.

FEATURES

The histopathologic assessment of a cervical biopsy must determine if CIN is present in a sample of epithelium and, if so, the grade of CIN (Figure 8.2). Both of these decisions may be difficult to make: the former because benign and physiologic changes may be mistaken for CIN; the latter because the features used for interpretation must be evaluated simultaneously in both quantitative and qualitative ways.

Cervical intraepithelial neoplasia is often divided into grades as a prognostic aid, implying that the disease evolves through a gradual progression of continuous derangements, eventually culminating in a tumor capable of invasion.[56] It is believed that the severity of the histologic abnormality helps predict the prognosis, as reported by a large meta-analysis[67] and therefore can be used as a guide in managing the patient. As a result, criteria that are purely morphologic are used to predict the clinical behavior of the abnormal epithelium. This principle is, of course, widely practiced throughout histopathology, but the correlation between appearance and behavior may not always be consistent, which in part may reflect difficulties in reproducibly using the CIN grade classification. In the cervix, this position is made all the more difficult to validate because the aim of treatment of CIN is to eradicate the disease before it becomes invasive. As a consequence, there are few reliable and substantive data available to correlate the histology of CIN with its real progression to invasive carcinoma. In other words, there is no way of knowing whether our beliefs regarding a continuum in the histologic progression of CIN to invasive cancer are correct, unless a prospective observational trial albeit ethically difficult could be conducted in which the interval between a punch biopsy and cone excision would be much longer. The fact that the average age of patients with CIN 2–3 and invasive cancer is around 35 and 50 years, respectively, indicates that most CIN 2–3 lesions require more than 15 years to develop into invasive cancer, making the hasty cone excision procedure highly debatable.

The diagnostic histopathologic criteria of CIN are shown in Table 8.3.

NUCLEAR ABNORMALITIES

The defining hallmarks of CIN are its nuclear abnormalities. These include nuclei that are enlarged, pleomorphic (irregular in size and shape), and often have a wrinkled nuclear membrane. The chromatin is increased in amount (hyperchromasia) and irregularly clumped, often along the inside of the nuclear membrane. Collectively, this constellation of features is described as 'nuclear atypia'. Neoplastic atypia is distinguished from reactive changes by the heterogeneity of the nuclear changes in CIN, contrasting with the relatively homogeneous changes in reactive atypia. Nucleoli are rare in preinvasive lesions, especially in smears. These changes may reflect the polyploidy and/or aneuploid DNA content of the cells induced by the action of HPV E6 and E7 on the host DNA synthesis system and are important for the diagnosis of CIN and for determination of its grade.

Often, there is a close correlation between the nuclear abnormality and the amount of differentiation seen. The greater the nuclear abnormality, the lesser is the differentiation observed. If a particular epithelium is extremely thin and lacks this correlation, then the severity of the nuclear changes is viewed as a more reliable indicator of the grade of the CIN than the proportion of the epithelial thickness showing maturation.

MITOTIC ACTIVITY

Mitotic activity is the histologic hallmark of cell proliferation. The conceptual distinction between normal and low-grade as well as low-grade versus high-grade CIN has much to do with the frequency, distribution, and type of mitotic activity. High-grade CIN has a proliferative phenotype as opposed to low-grade CIN, which, while slightly more proliferative in a controlled manner compared to normal, does not express the same kind of viral oncogene-driven proliferation as high-grade CIN/HSIL.

The normal squamous epithelium of the cervix has minimal if any mitotic activity, with the mitotic figures being confined to the parabasal layers. In normal or reactive changes, mitotic figures are rare and always restricted to the parabasal cells. In contrast, CIN shows an increased number of mitoses, and they may be present at any level in the epithelium. The frequency of mitoses in the epithelium increases along the continuum from normal epithelium to the most severe forms of CIN. Moreover, the number of mitotic figures in the superficial third

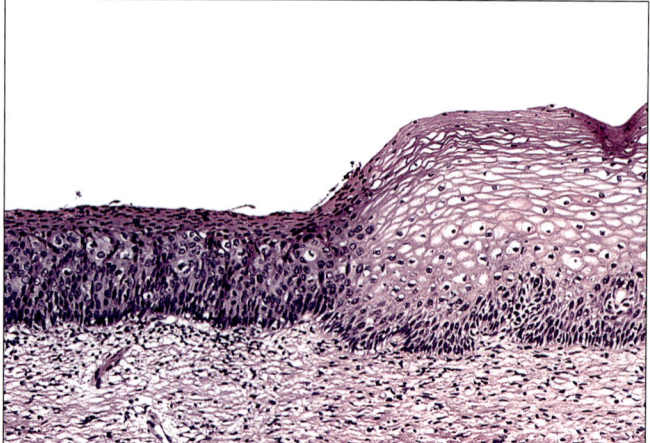

Fig. 8.2 Normal adjacent to high-grade CIN with sharp border in between.

Table 8.3 Histopathologic features of CIN (with progressively more abnormal degrees)

1. Nuclear abnormalities
   A. Nuclear:cytoplasmic ratio (↑)
   B. Hyperchromasia (↑)
   C. Nuclear pleomorphism and anisokaryosis (↑)
   D. Nuclear polarity (↑ irregular)
   E. Wrinkling of nuclear membrane (↑)

2. Mitotic activity
   A. Number of mitotic figures (↑)
   B. Height in epithelium (relation to surface) (↑)
   C. Abnormal configurations (↑)

3. Differentiation (maturation, stratification)
   A. Present or absent (↓ differentiation)
   B. Proportion of epithelium showing differentiation (↓)
   C. Proportion of unit area occupied by nuclei (↑)

of the epithelium increases as the severity of the CIN increases, demonstrating that the vertical position in the epithelium at which mitotic figures are found is a useful diagnostic indicator useful when contemplating the degree of CIN. Not all CIN lesions show mitoses above the parabasal layer, but these may be pathognomonic for CIN if they do occur.

Abnormal mitotic configurations, which are thought to reflect aneuploidy, are common in CIN, accounting for between 15% and 30% of total mitoses. CIN associated with HPV type 16 infection has the highest number of mitoses and the most abnormal forms.[21,59] The most common of these abnormal configurations is the lag-type mitosis, which is defined as a metaphase with non-attached chromatin in the area of the mitotic figure. The 'three-group metaphase' (Figure 8.3), which is where the main mass of the chromatin aligns along the equatorial plate and the non-attached condensed chromatin remains laterally at the two polar sites, has been found in 6% of CIN

1–2, 56% of CIN 3, and 93% of the high-grade CIN lesions just adjacent to microinvasive carcinoma.[60,99] Two-group metaphases (displaced chromatin at only one polar site) may also be seen (Figure 8.4). Less common than either of these forms is the multipolar mitotic figure, either as a triaster (tripolar) (Figure 8.5) or a more bizarre multipolar figure (Figure 8.6). In recognition of this volume, which has had its origin in Nottingham, UK, an occasional form has been found that appears as, and is thus named for, the famed Robin Hood of Sherwood Forest lore (Figures 8.7 and 8.8).

DIFFERENTIATION, MATURATION, AND STRATIFICATION

'Differentiation' and 'maturation' are terms that, while having slightly different meanings, are often used synonymously and interchangeably in the cervix. The definition of CIS requires

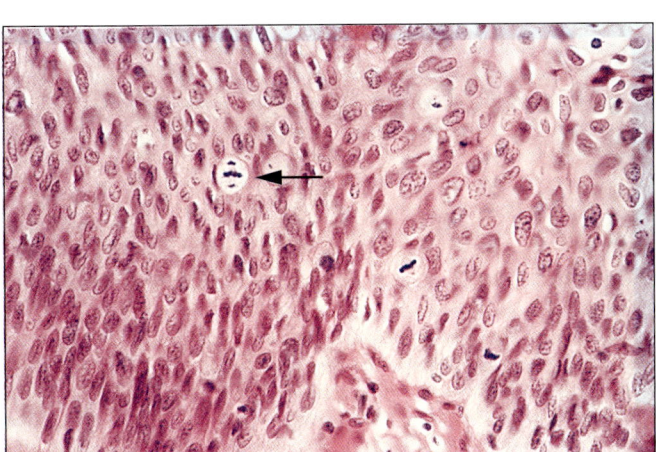

Fig. 8.3 Three-group metaphase mitosis (arrow) in CIN 3.

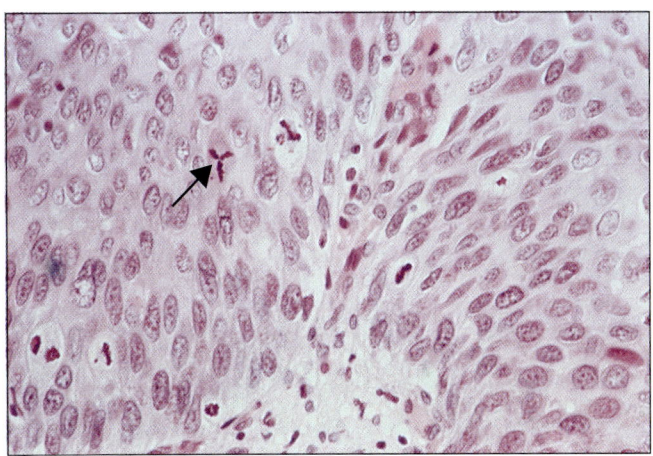

Fig. 8.5 Triaster (tripolar) mitosis (arrow) in CIN 3.

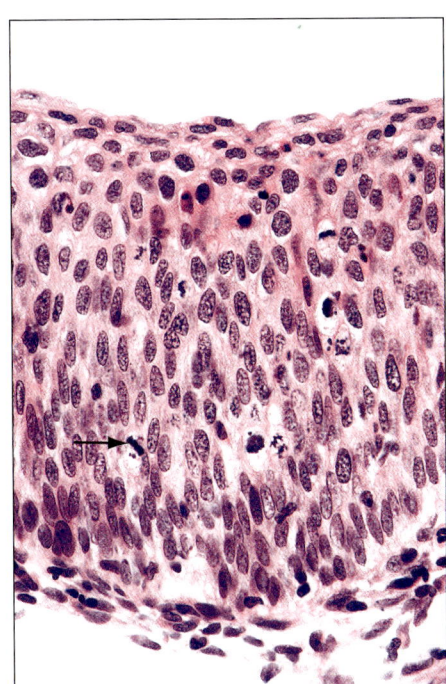

Fig. 8.4 Two-group mitosis (arrow) in CIN 3.

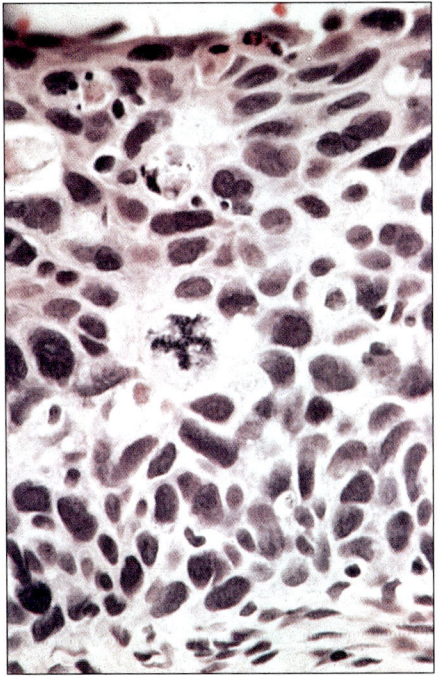

Fig. 8.6 Multipolar mitosis in CIN 3.

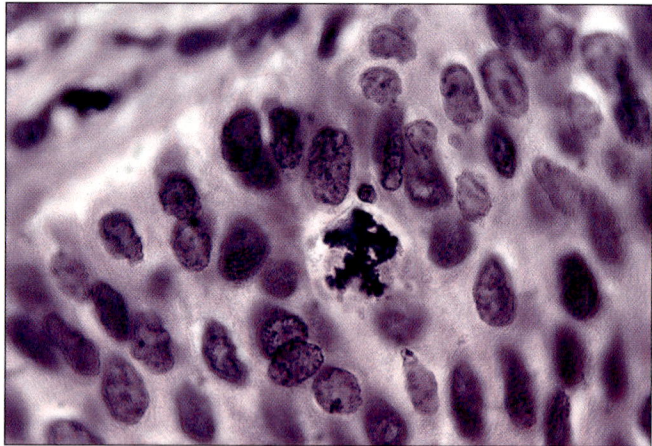

Fig. 8.7 'Robin Hood' (multipolar) mitosis in CIN 3.

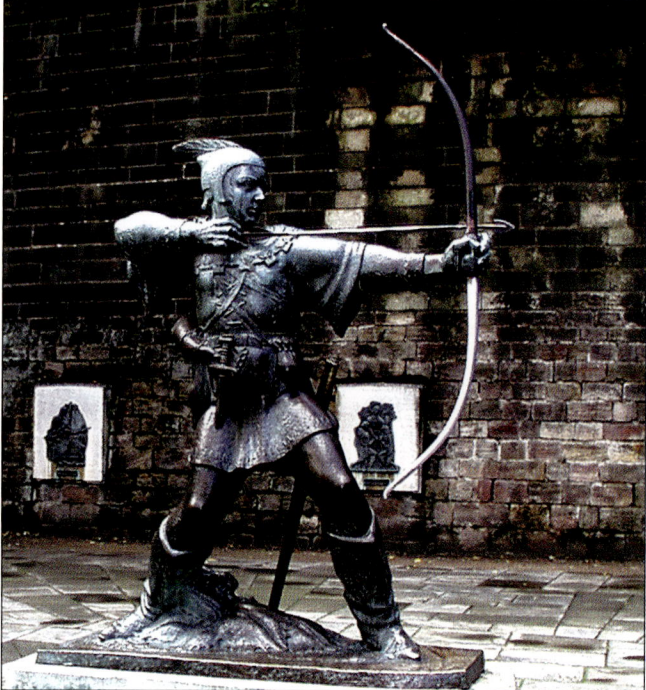

Fig. 8.8 Robin Hood statue outside Nottingham Castle, England.

that the surface epithelium lacks all differentiation, so that immature and undifferentiated cells occupy the entire thickness of the epithelium. On the other hand, some differentiation is expected in dysplasia, although this may be difficult to detect in some of the most severe forms. The presence of surface differentiation is the only way of distinguishing between CIS and severe dysplasia but, with the adoption of the CIN terminology and the term 'CIN 3', the distinction becomes irrelevant on clinical and biologic grounds. Further blurring the distinction between severe dysplasia and CIS is the common finding that some flattening of the superficial-most cells is most likely due to desiccative artifact from exposure to the atmosphere. This flattening should not be mistaken for differentiation.

The proportion of epithelial cells showing differentiation is a more useful indicator of the grade of CIN, although it must not be taken as the only criterion. For example, while CIN develops by a dysplastic process and may show little if any

differentiation, it may be difficult to distinguish from an immature, but non-dysplastic metaplastic squamous epithelium that also lacks any substantial degree of cytoplasmic differentiation. In this case, the distinguishing feature is the lack of nuclear atypia in the metaplastic process as well as much less evidence of mitotic activity. Nonetheless, distinction between the two conditions can be difficult, especially as immature metaplasia is felt by some to be a mixed bag. Many cases are in fact CIN based on the finding of high-risk HPV types, high Ki-67 proliferation indices, and follow-up studies.[32]

As normal cells differentiate and mature and migrate towards the surface, stratification is observed. One means of assessing maturation is to look for a decreasing percentage of nuclear area to overall epithelial area, reflecting a decreasing nuclear:cytoplasmic ratio at increasingly more superficial levels of epithelium. In smears, this change in ratio is quite dramatic. In normal smears, the nucleus has undergone pyknosis by the time the cell reaches the surface, so that in the smear the nuclear:cytoplasmic ratio is quite low. With increasing degrees of CIN, the individual cells have matured less so that the amount of cytoplasm present, as well as its differentiation, is less. Thus, mildly dyskaryotic (a synonym of dysplasia) cells have ample cytoplasm with a well-defined polygonal squamous shape, and moderately dyskaryotic cells show less cytoplasm and a less well-defined oval or elliptical squamous shape, whereas in CIN 3 the rim of cytoplasm that encircles the nucleus is indeed small. In CIN, the proportionally decreasing quantity of cytoplasm accounts for the changing nuclear:cytoplasmic ratio far more than the changes in nuclear size that are encountered.

In smears, the Papanicolaou stain accentuates states of maturation. The color of staining, which results in either acidophilic (pink) or basophilic (blue-green) cytoplasm, usually corresponds to normal superficial and intermediate cell types. Although this helps to distinguish the various grades of CIN, it is not a reliable criterion, being quite contingent on stain quality control factors.

DISEASE STATES

Despite the above critical comments made about reproducibility, application of qualitative features with attention to quantitative levels allows for grading of CIN.

In cervical epithelia, all productive HPV infections commonly manifest themselves both cytologically and histologically with a distinctive cytopathic effect. The cell in which this is found has been termed the 'koilocyte' (Figure 8.9). This feature, first recognized more than 50 years ago, was given the term 'koilocytotic atypia' (some use koilocytic) as these cells histologically resembled those in skin warts. Some 20 years later it was recognized that this same cell type occurred in genital warts and cervical flat condylomata and was associated with both HPV and CIN.

The 'koilocyte' is an intermediate cell that has a prominent cytoplasmic space around an atypical nucleus (Table 8.4; Figures 8.10–8.14). Due to an extensively marginated cytoplasm, the halo has a sharp edge. The cytoplasmic change is thought to be due to the abundant expression of the HPV E4 protein which binds with cytoplasmic keratin. Even in the state where the nuclei are not overtly dysplastic by size criteria, they are still, nonetheless,

Table 8.4 Koilocytic change: diagnostic criteria

Well-defined and exaggerated perinuclear halo

Condensation of the ectocytoplasm

Nuclear area two to three times a normal intermediate cell nucleus, or more

Increased nuclear:cytoplasmic ratio

Usually mild nuclear hyperchromasia

Wrinkled nuclear membrane

Sometimes degenerative nuclear changes

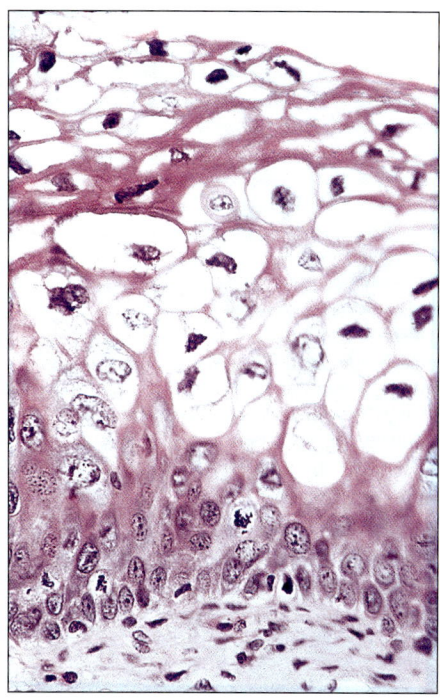

Fig. 8.11 Flat condyloma/LSIL with slight nuclear atypia. The basal layer is slightly thickened. Koilocytes are prominent.

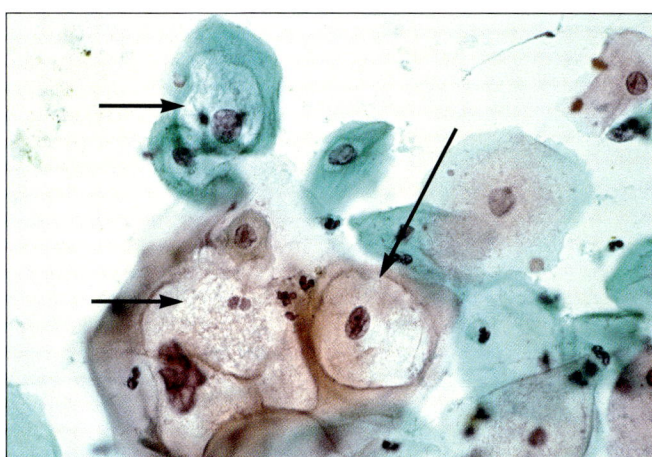

Fig. 8.9 Koilocyte (arrows) in a cervical smear.

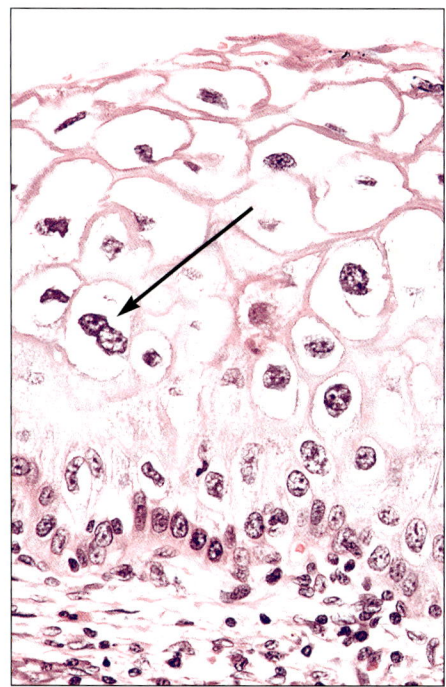

Fig. 8.10 Flat condyloma with koilocytes. The cells in the intermediate layers are ballooned with copious clear cytoplasm. One cell is binucleate (arrow).

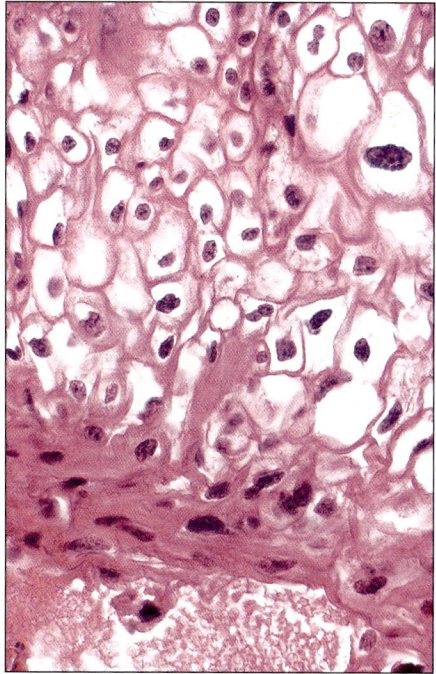

Fig. 8.12 Koilocytes in CIN 1. Several of the koilocytes show sufficient nuclear atypia to warrant the diagnosis of early CIN; but in reality 8.10–8.12 are all low-grade viral lesions.

irregular, hyperchromatic, and if near the surface may show a wrinkled nuclear membrane. The nuclei, which lack nucleoli, are usually two to four times larger in nuclear area than those of the adjacent, non-ballooned cells. Koilocytotic atypia, which under the Bethesda classification is considered a low-grade SIL, is the most common definite abnormality in cyto-

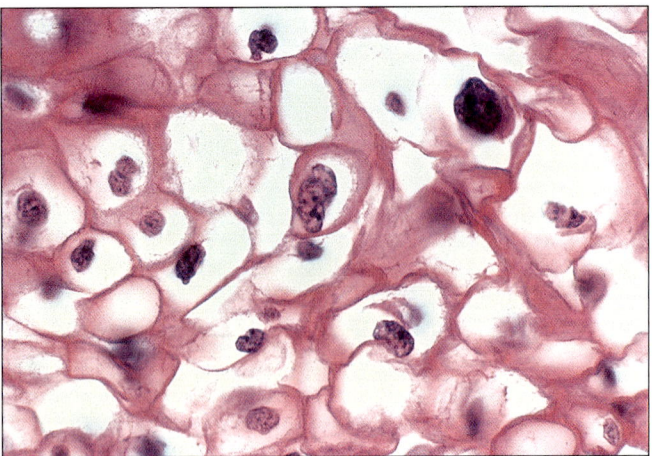

Fig. 8.13 High-power magnification of koilocytes. The nuclei are wrinkled and enlarged but show neither mitotic activity nor nucleoli.

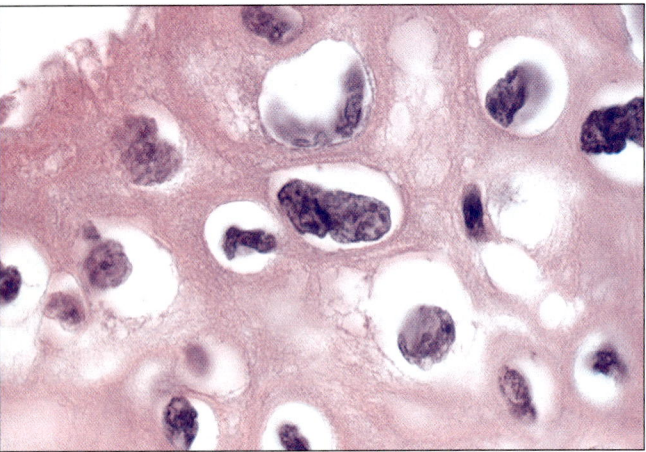

Fig. 8.14 High-power magnification of koilocytes. The nuclei are wrinkled but show neither mitotic activity nor nucleoli.

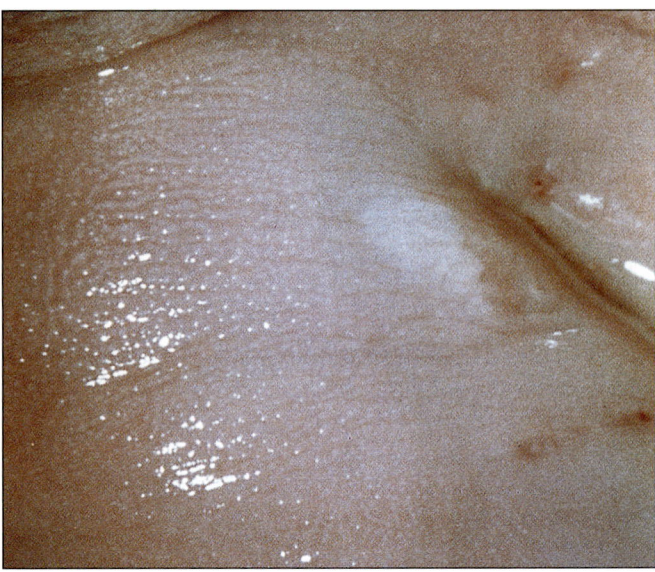

Fig. 8.15 Small condyloma acuminatum. The condyloma is exophytic but very small in size. It turned white when 3% acetic acid was applied.

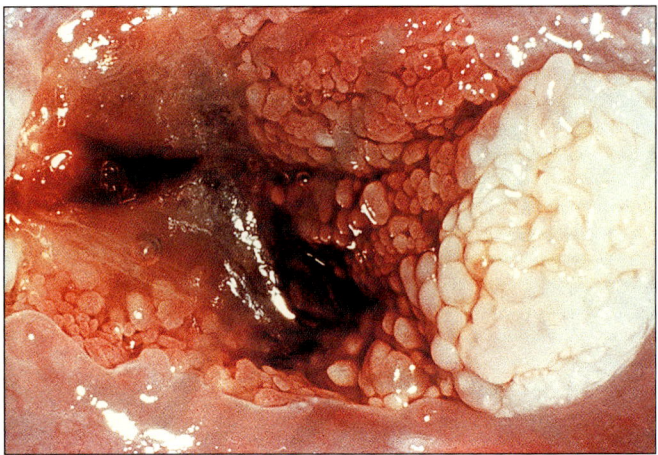

Fig. 8.16 Condyloma acuminatum. This condyloma is large and cauliflower-like.

logically screened women today, being found in up to 4% of all cervical smears.

While the term 'koilocyte' is often described as pathognomonic for HPV infection, perinuclear halos that mimic koilocytotic atypia may be caused by other infectious diseases and at times may be due to artifact. Epstein–Barr virus, when present in the cervix, may be associated with koilocytic change[96] (although this may also be due to coinfection with HPV). Likewise, when the cytoplasmic halo is less than morphologically perfect, i.e., when the borders are smooth or where the nuclei have smooth borders, and the HPV immunostains are commonly negative, trichomoniasis may be a consideration. It is therefore important that the presence of a cytoplasmic halo not be overinterpreted as being due to HPV disease. Rather it is the combination of a well-defined halo plus definite nuclear atypia as defined above that confer specificity to the morphologic findings. Other features associated with HPV infection include binucleation and meganuclei. Both are found in the mid to superficial levels. Some investigators have suggested that the latter feature or more severely pleomorphic koilocytes are more associated with high-risk HPV types. However, since over 85% of cervical HPV infections are from the high-risk group, the validity of this idea is lacking. One cannot reliably genotype a lesion by morphology.

CONDYLOMA ACUMINATUM (Figures 8.15–8.20)

In the past, condylomata acuminata of the cervix were believed to be rare. However, in the past few decades, particularly with the increasing use of colposcopy (Figure 8.15), they are now recognized with some frequency, although they are still not regarded as common. This fact is consistent with the knowledge that the acuminate architecture is somewhat more frequently associated with HPV types 6 and 11 and some other low-risk types, and that these make up only 10–15% of cervical infections. Yet HPV 6/11 account for ~95% of genital condylomata. Larger condylomata can be seen with the naked eye, and they may initially be mistaken for carcinoma (Figure 8.16).

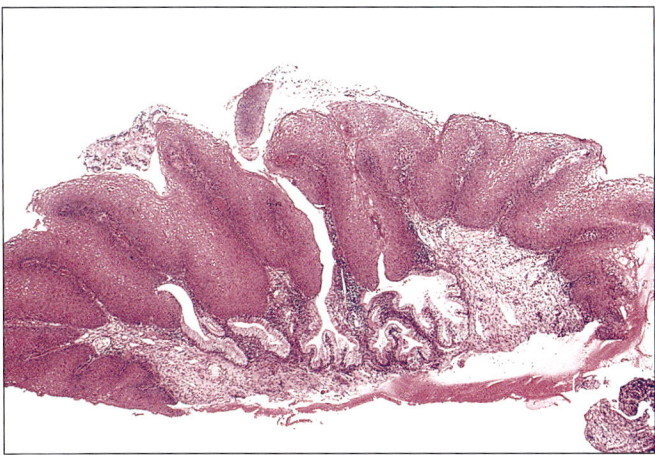

Fig. 8.17 Condyloma acuminatum that is sessile and broad.

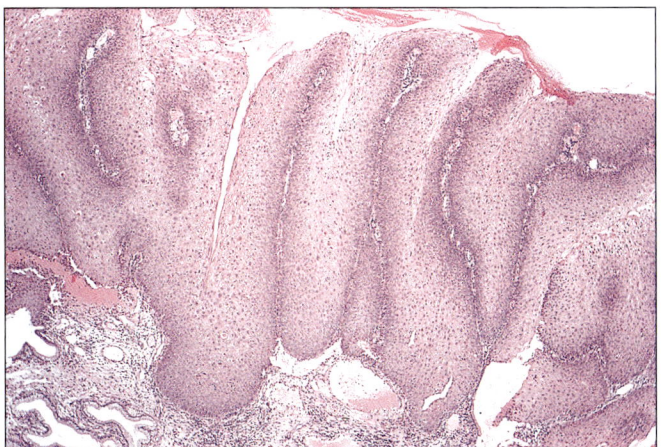

Fig. 8.18 Condyloma acuminatum. Medium magnification of sessile and broad condyloma.

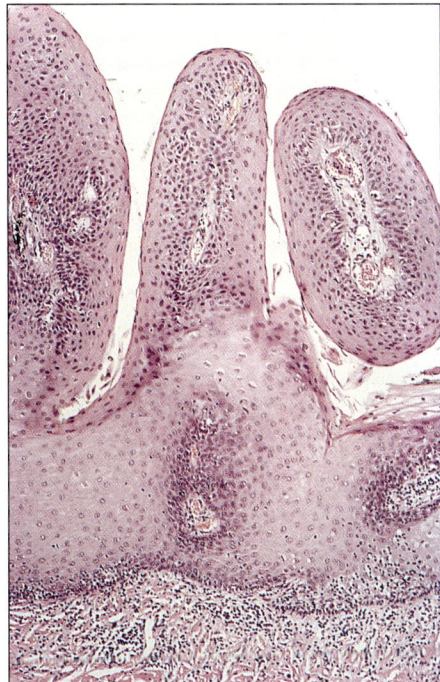

Fig. 8.19 Condyloma acuminatum with asperities.

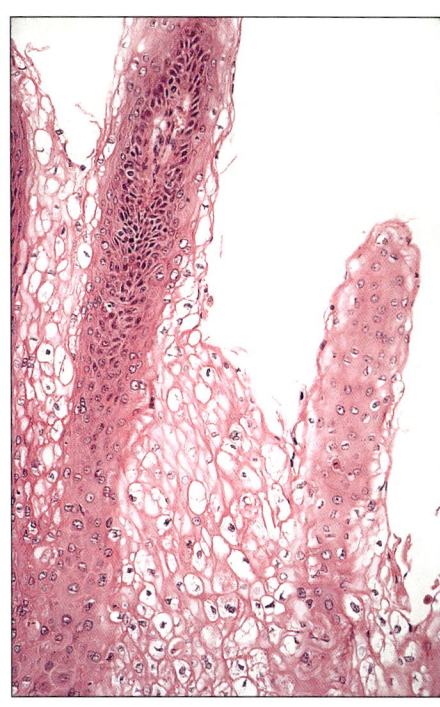

Fig. 8.20 Condyloma acuminatum with asperities. High magnification of asperity showing both koilocytes and central fibrovascular core with a central blood vessel.

Colposcopy and tissue sections reveal the true nature of the lesions, which are seen ranging from exophytic, somewhat sessile elevations (Figures 8.17 and 8.18) to tiny papillary asperities (Figures 8.19 and 8.20). The latter changes (asperities) when in the vagina are often not HPV associated, but rather are mimics or normal variation. They may be situated both in the transformation zone and on the original squamous epithelium, although the former is far more common. Characteristically, condylomata are multiple so that examination will show further lesions, perhaps very small ones, on the cervix, vagina or vulva. As colposcopic appearances of large lesions overlap with those of invasive carcinoma, biopsy is essential.

The histology of cervical condyloma shows papillomatosis, acanthosis, parakeratosis, and hyperkeratosis. At higher magnification, each asperity, i.e., each papillary frond, has a tiny blood vessel at its core. Koilocytotic atypia is usually a prominent feature, with individual cell keratinization (dyskeratosis) and multinucleation. There is often a chronic inflammatory infiltrate in the underlying cervical stroma.

If left untreated, most condylomata regress but laser vaporization or diathermy also easily eradicates them, although recurrence is common. Condylomata are frequently associated with CIN (as multitype HPV infection is common in over 40% of patients), occurring either at the same time or subsequently, so the patient with a cervical wart must have continued cytologic surveillance. Furthermore, histologic examination of the condyloma should, of course, include an assessment of atypia in the lesion itself as well as in the surrounding epithelium. It is not uncommon for a condyloma to contain cells that have sufficient atypia to warrant a diagnosis of even higher-grade CIN.

CIN 1/LSIL/MILD DYSPLASIA/FLAT CONDYLOMA (SUBCLINICAL PAPILLOMA INFECTION)
(Figures 8.21–8.35)

The flat lesions are recognizable colposcopically, cytologically, and histologically but cannot usually be seen with the naked eye (not to be confused with condyloma lata or flat warts of secondary syphilis which are external genital lesions). The colposcopic features are fully described below, but they are not altogether diagnostic. It is not usually possible to distinguish subclinical papillomavirus infection from CIN at colposcopy (because they are one and the same). Based on histology, several features in addition to the presence of koilocytes are

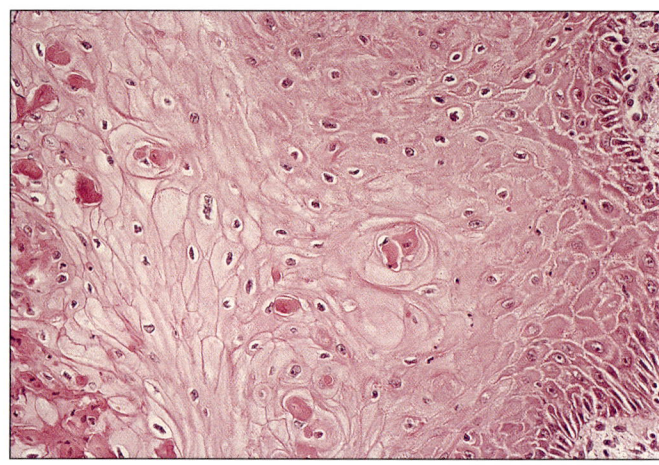

Fig. 8.23 Focal individual cell dyskaryosis in LSIL.

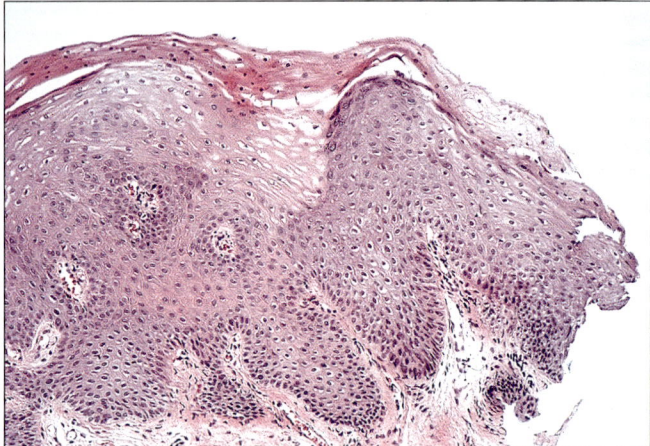

Fig. 8.21 Non-specific features commonly seen in HPV infected squamous epithelium. There is a sharp demarcation of the epithelium on the left where there is a slight loss of glycogen compared with that on the right where the glycogen loss is marked. Hyperkeratosis is present.

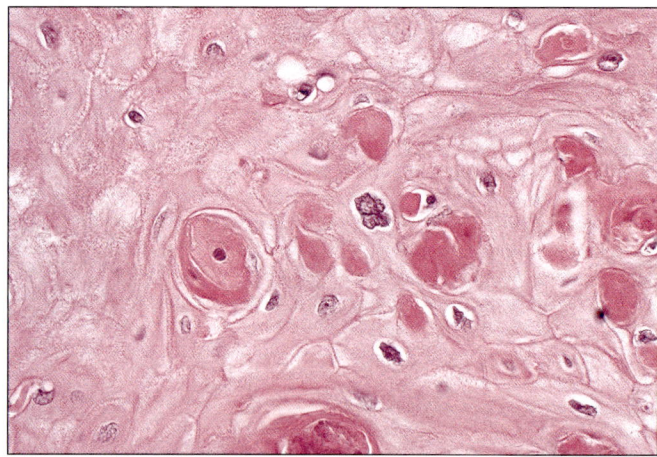

Fig. 8.24 Focal individual cell dyskaryosis in LSIL, detail.

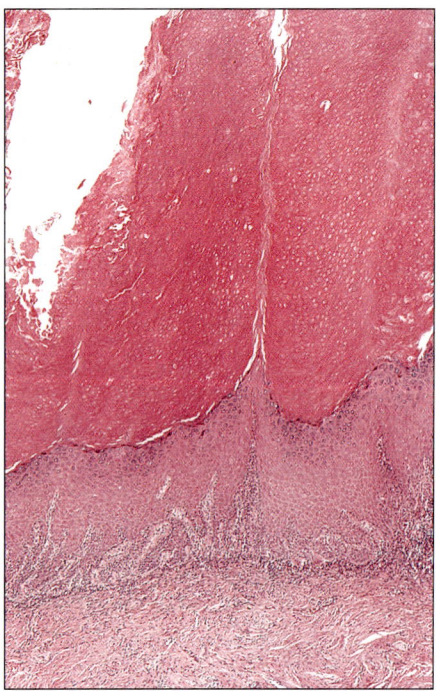

Fig. 8.22 Flat condyloma/LSIL with marked hyperkeratosis. The lesion grossly has the appearance of a cutaneous horn.

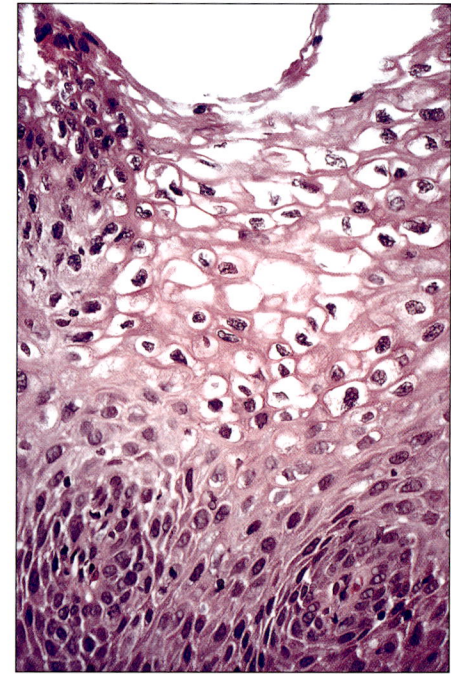

Fig. 8.25 Flat condyloma/LSIL/CIN-1.

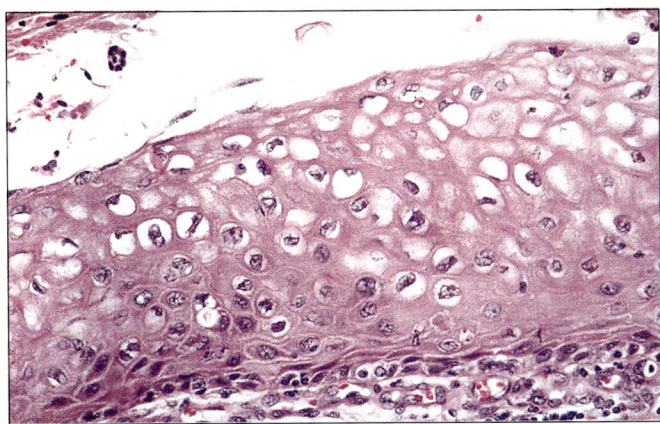

Fig. 8.26 Flat condyloma/LSIL with minimal parabasal hyperplasia.

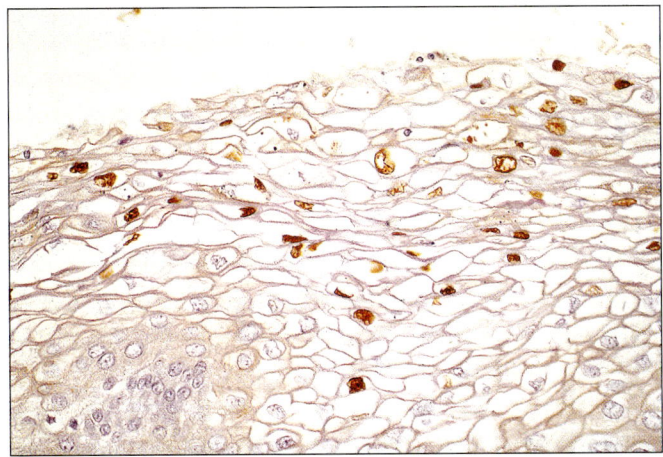

Fig. 8.27 Flat condyloma/LSIL. Immunocytochemical reactions disclose viral capsid protein in koilocytes.

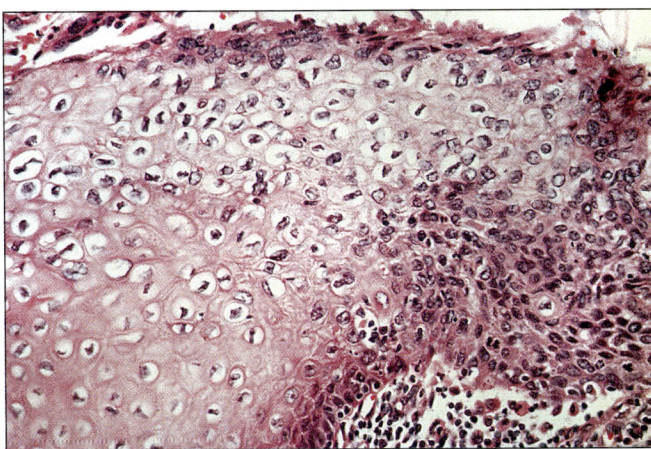

Fig. 8.28 Flat condyloma (left) adjacent to an invasive squamous cell carcinoma (not shown in picture).

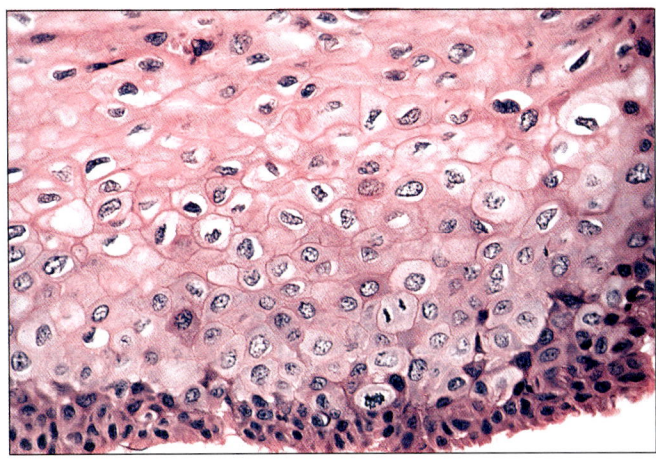

Fig. 8.29 CIN 1/LSIL. The superficial-most epithelial cells display some variation in nuclear size and shape, despite the marked cytoplasmic maturation.

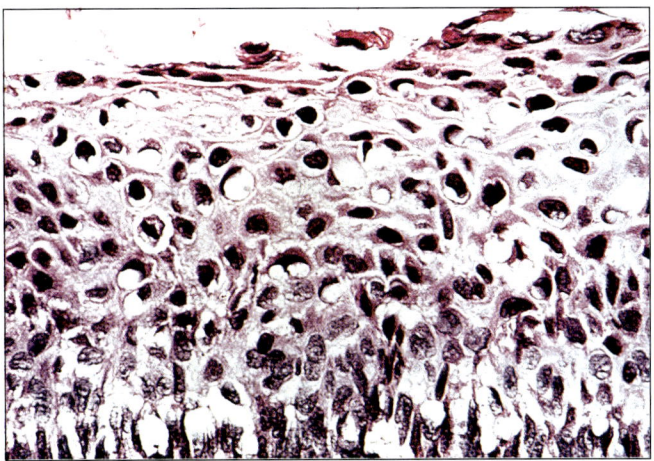

Fig. 8.30 CIN 1, called CIN 2 by some, with variable nuclear pleomorphism and substantial cytoplasmic maturation.

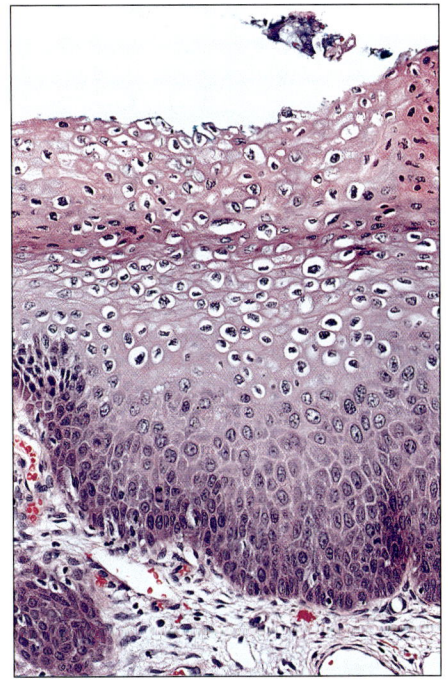

Fig. 8.31 LSIL/CIN 1 with a condylomata power architecture.

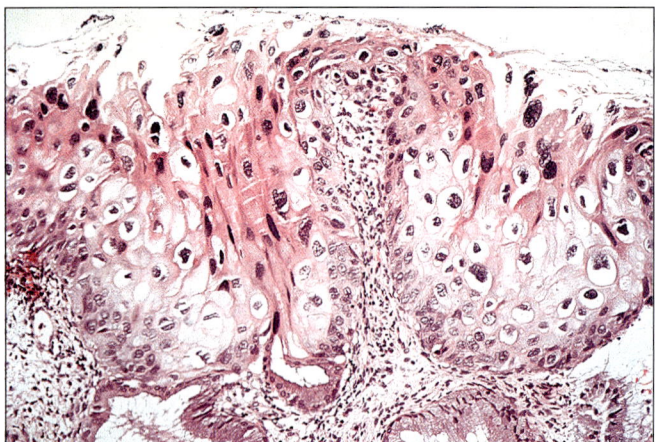

Fig. 8.32 CIN 1, with substantial nuclear pleomorphism in cells with extensive cytoplasmic maturation.

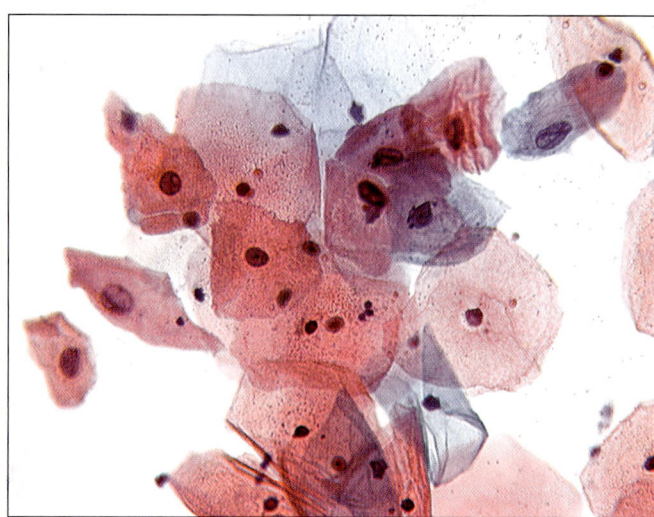

Fig. 8.35 CIN 1. Cells show dyskaryotic nuclei with abundant cytoplasm.

Table 8.5 Histologic features of condylomatous infection

Koilocytic change
Multinucleation (usually binucleation)
Individual cell keratinization
Parakeratosis
Acanthosis
Papillomatosis (in condyloma acuminatum infection only)

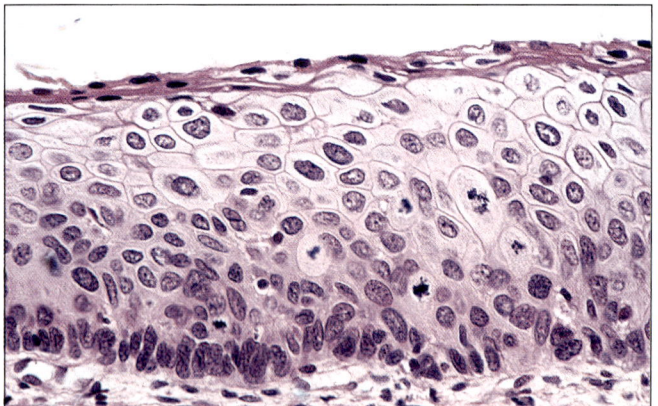

Fig. 8.33 CIN 1 with features of CIN 2 (several atypical mitoses). Such a lesion may not be reproducibly called low grade.

useful in the detection of HPV infection (Table 8.5). On low-power magnification, large areas may be composed of squamous epithelial cells lacking glycogen. While suggestive, this feature is non-specific (Figure 8.21). The cytoplasm from the basal-most cells to the surface is eosinophilic. Commonly a sharp boundary demarcates the epithelium that is glycogen rich (normal) and glycogen poor (HPV). In addition, the superficial cells in the glycogen-poor zones commonly show acanthosis, parakeratosis, and sometimes even hyperkeratosis. The last, rarely, may be quite striking (Figure 8.22).

Several other features are found with low grade lesions. Nuclei that are binucleate (Figure 8.10), or even sometimes multinucleate, are found in 95% of HPV infection.[75] These hypernucleated cells are rarely larger than other affected cells and typically are not obvious. Occasional cells may show individual cell keratinization (dyskeratosis) (Figures 8.23 and 8.24). In smears, the anucleate and nucleate keratinized cells are commonly present in sheets or plaques with poorly defined cell borders. In the vulva, but uncommonly in the cervix, prominent rete pegs and blood vessels may be surrounded by scant stroma that extends close to the surface. By themselves, these features are non-specific.

On a cellular basis, the koilocyte in histologic specimens is usually distinctive although the number of cells with koilocytic change may be few to many (Figure 8.25). Typically, the nucleus is 3–4 times enlarged in areas compared to a normal intermediate cell, uniform in size and shape, and has a halo with smooth outer borders. Typing with HPV immunostains has shown that typical koilocytes usually react with

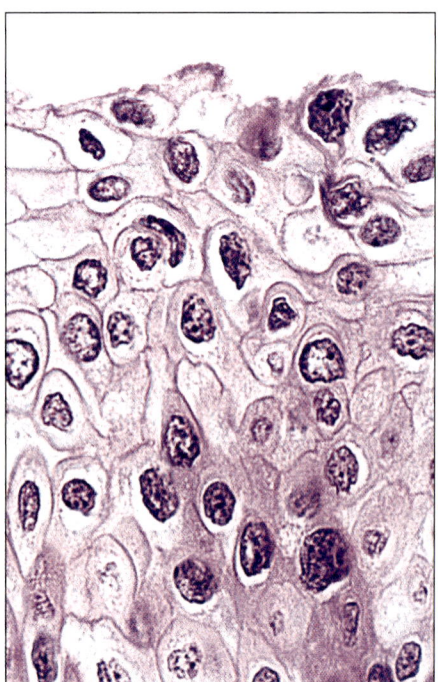

Fig. 8.34 CIN between CIN 1 and CIN 2.

antibodies in the reaction mixture which is composed of antibodies to the HPV L1 group-specific capsid protein (Figures 8.26 and 8.27). Since capsid/virion production is a temporally controlled phenomenon linked to both differentiation and lesional age, not all cells containing HPV will necessarily stain. Cells less typical for koilocytes are less likely to stain. Because of the potential social stigma often attached to a smear or biopsy specimen that is diagnosed as harboring HPV prudence dictates that no specimen should be diagnosed with the words HPV, koilocyte, or condyloma unless the overall microscopic picture is distinctive.

Koilocytes are usually found in condylomata and CIN 1 lesions unified under the LSIL nomenclature. They are uncommon in CIN 2 and 3 for reasons discussed below. Flat condylomata, on occasion, may lie adjacent to high-grade lesions, or occasionally even adjacent to carcinomas.

In all low-grade lesions histologically diagnosed as CIN 1, the upper two-thirds of the epithelium usually shows substantial to extensive differentiation, although abnormal nuclei persist throughout the full thickness of the epithelium (if this were not so, a diagnosis by cytologic smear would not be possible; see above) (Figures 8.29–8.34). In CIN 1 the diagnostic features are concentrated in the lower portion of the epithelium, with nuclear abnormalities being most obvious in the basal third of the epithelium. Mitotic figures, if present, are few in number and confined to the basal third of the epithelium. Abnormal forms are uncommon, but highly prejudicial to the diagnosis of CIN.

The dysplastic features in the upper portion of the epithelium include individual nuclei with a minor degree of pleomorphism in relation to neighboring nuclei, loss of polarity to varying (but usually small) degrees, wrinkled nuclear membrane, and various degrees of hyperchromasia. Usually, the nuclei remain slightly to moderately enlarged as they migrate towards the surface; however, not infrequently, they also increase slightly to moderately in size, a byproduct of unscheduled host DNA synthesis as HPV replicates its own genome. Regardless, the overall percentage of nuclear area to total epithelial area in the upper half of the squamous mucosa is usually 20–40%, but under 50%. Most specimens will also disclose concomitant features of HPV infection, especially in the form of koilocytes as described. In smears, the mildly dyskaryotic cells have ample cytoplasm with a well-defined squamous shape (*vida supra*) (Figure 8.35).

CIN 2 INCLUDING MODERATE DYSPLASIA AND PART OF HSIL (Figures 8.36–8.42)

In CIN 2, the upper half of the epithelium shows some differentiation and maturation, with, as in CIN 1, nuclear atypia persisting to the surface. Nuclear abnormalities are more marked than in CIN 1, and more nuclei with greater degrees of abnormality are found high in the epithelium. Mitotic figures, which may be abnormal, are present in the basal two-thirds of the epithelium. If attention is focused upon the findings in the upper portion of the epithelium, the changes would be similar qualitatively, but more advanced quantitatively in comparison to CIN 1. More nuclei are pleomorphic in relation to neighboring nuclei, lack polarity to various degrees, have wrinkled nuclear membranes, and show various degrees of hyperchromasia. Using the point counting method, overall, the percentage of nuclear area to total epithelial area is roughly

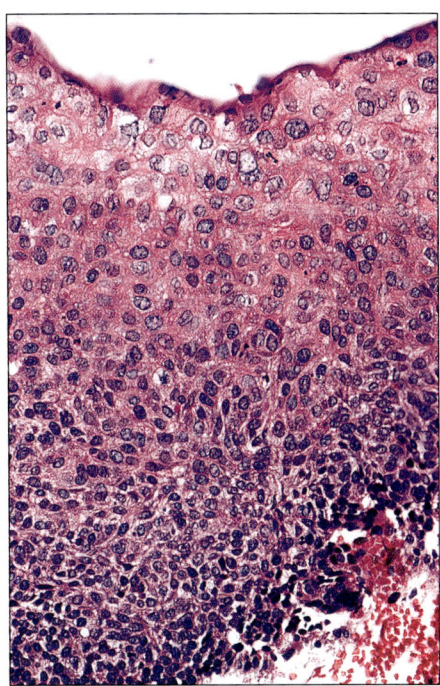

Fig. 8.36 CIN 2. The cytoplasmic maturation is less than that seen in CIN 1 and largely confined to the upper third of the epithelium.

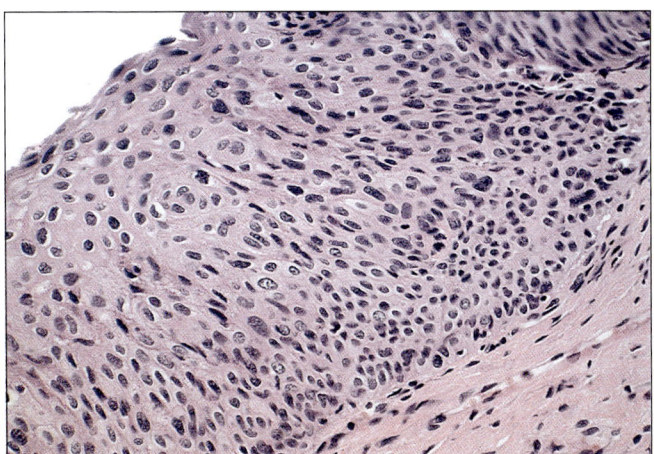

Fig. 8.37 CIN 2 (left) merging with CIN 3 (right).

40–60% in the upper half of the epithelium. The diagnosis of CIN 2 is the least reproducible form of CIN. It is an equivocal biologic state and probably represents a mixture of true CIN 1/LSIL (approximately one-third) and true precancer/CIN 3/HSIL (approximately two-thirds).[19]

CIN 3 (Figures 8.43–8.47)

In CIN 3 any maturation, if present, is confined to the superficial third of the epithelium. Generally, it is minimal to completely absent. Nuclear abnormalities are marked throughout the whole thickness of the epithelium. Similarly, mitotic figures are found at all levels of the epithelium and may be numerous, with many abnormal configurations. The findings in the upper

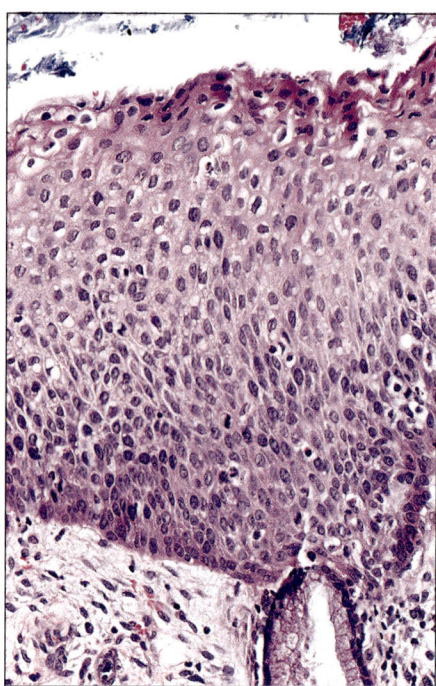

Fig. 8.38   CIN 2. Many of the abnormal nuclei in the upper epithelium are larger than that seen in the basal epithelium.

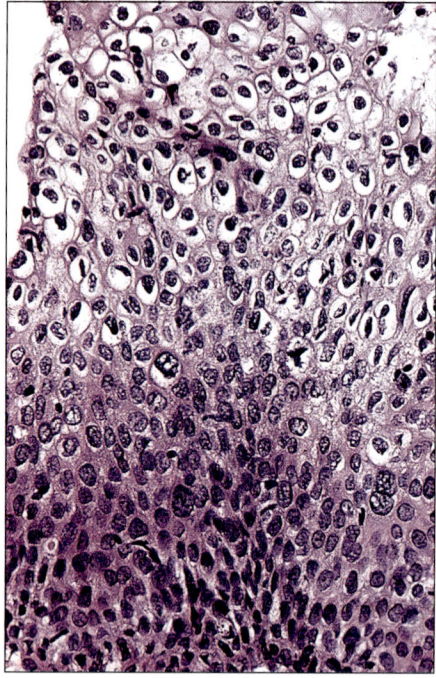

Fig. 8.39   CIN 2.

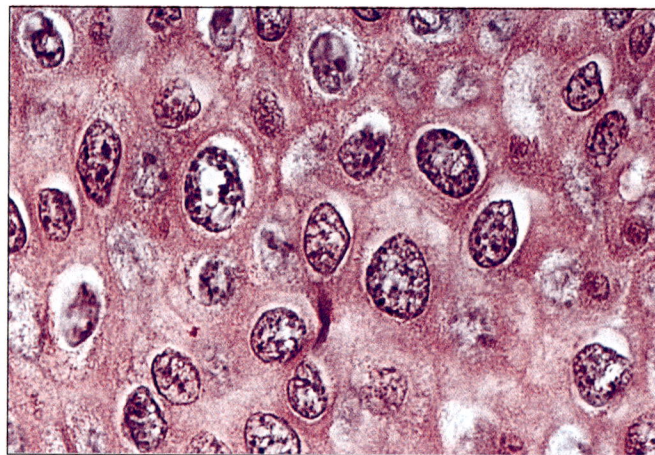

Fig. 8.40   CIN 2. The section, although cut tangentially, shows some cytoplasmic maturation towards the surface.

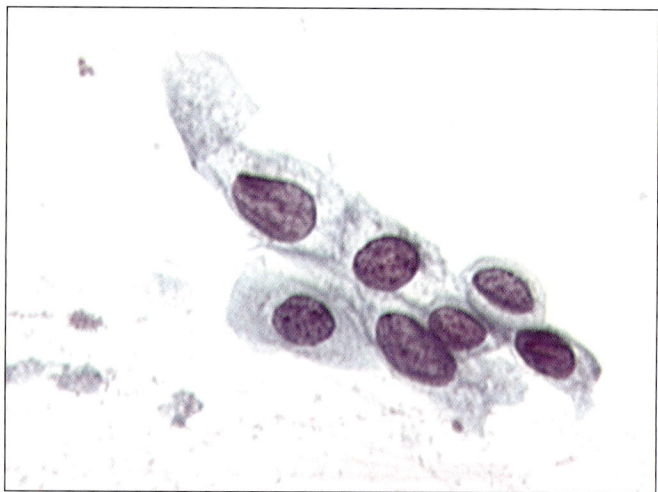

Fig. 8.41   CIN 2. The nuclei are large, occupying more than half the total cell size.

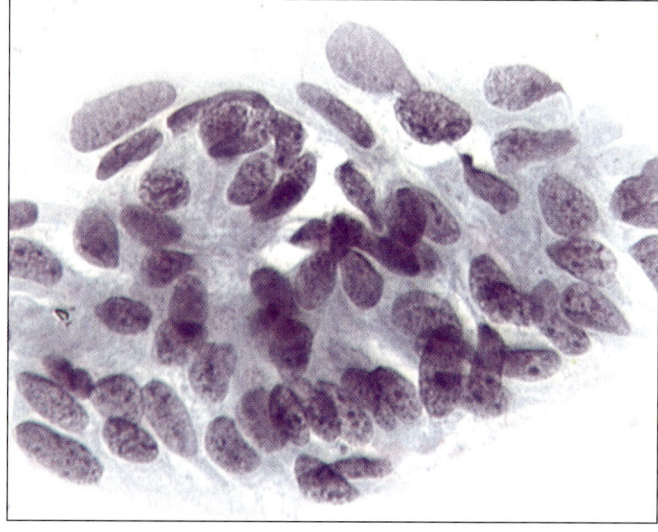

Fig. 8.42   CIN 2. A sheet of cells with dyskaryotic nuclei and reduced amounts of cytoplasm shows some differentiation.

portion of the epithelium include more extensive nuclear changes. Using the point counting method, in general, the percentage of area consisting of nuclear material can exceed 60% in the upper half of the epithelium. In smears, the rim of cytoplasm is quite thin, and the nucleus occupies virtually the entire cell (Figure 8.43).

The above should be used as a general guide to the central features of the distinct grades of CIN, since examples of the

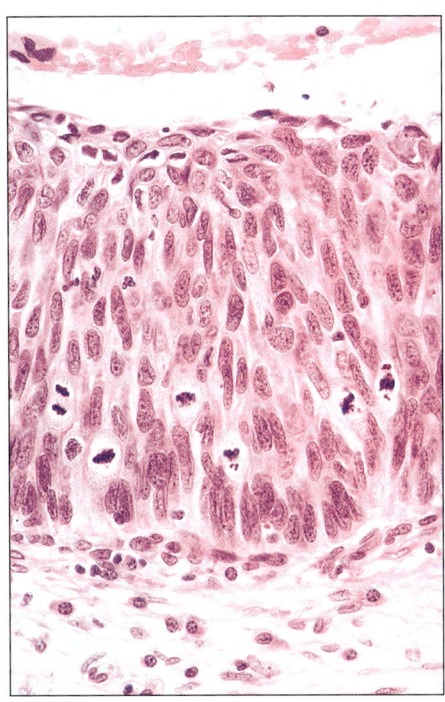

Fig. 8.43 CIN 3.

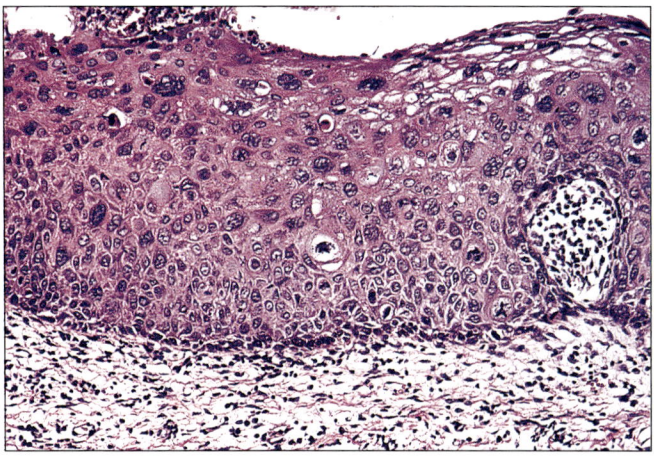

Fig. 8.46 CIN 3. The superficial nuclei are markedly enlarged and bizarre in shape.

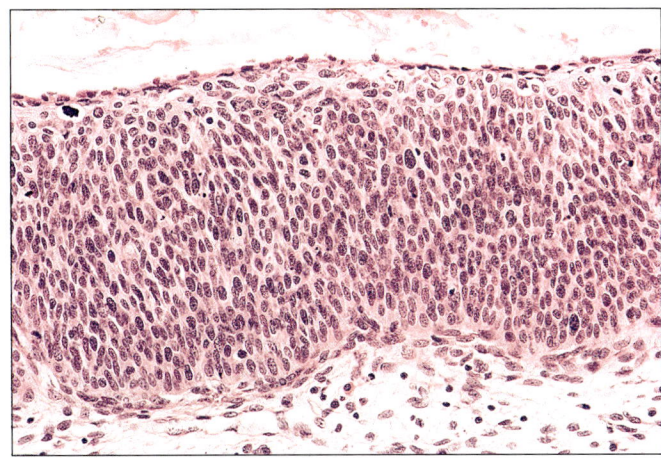

Fig. 8.44 CIN 3. Maturation is lacking throughout the entire thickness of the epithelium.

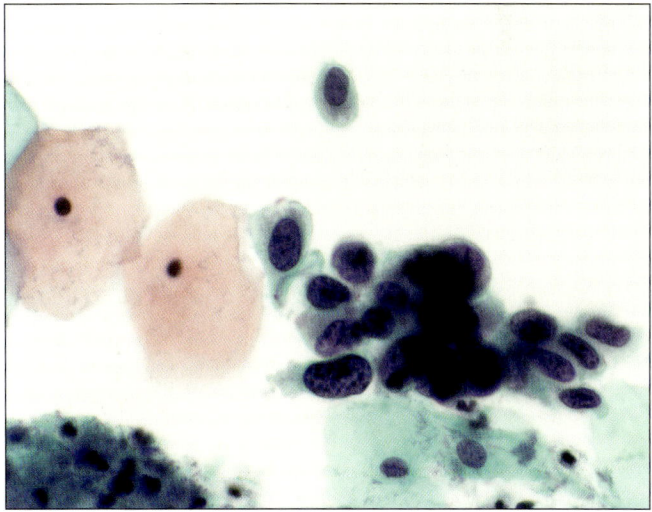

Fig. 8.47 Cervical intraepithelial neoplasia, high grade. Cervical smear.

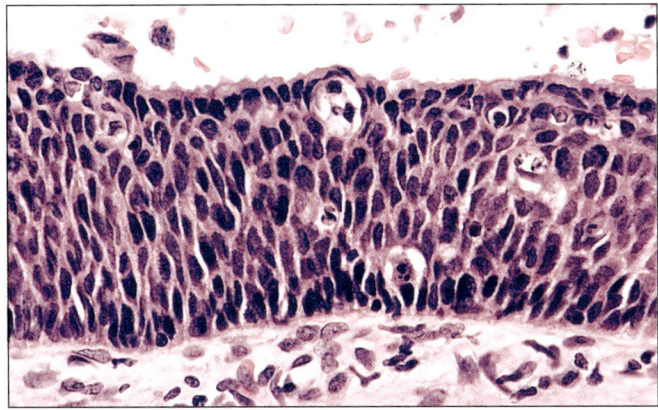

Fig. 8.45 CIN 3 in which a thin residual layer of mucinous columnar cells resides atop the CIN. More commonly, CIN 3 overgrows the glandular cells.

same CIN grade may have varying appearances. For example, one specimen may emphasize a lack of differentiation and stratification throughout (Figure 8.44), whereas others may show more prominent mitoses, some being abnormal (Figure 8.45), or bizarre nuclei located in superficial levels (Figure 8.46). Many of the histologic features used in the grading of CIN may vary independently of each other, so it is obvious that the emphasis put on each of these criteria may vary from one specimen to another. All of this variation contributes to a lack of reproducibility in diagnosis.

Like histology, assignment of an overall grade of CIN to a smear is as subjective as the assessment-based examination of the individual cells. The cervical smear will frequently contain cells showing all degrees of CIN, and it is the most severe cell type that determines the grade (Figure 8.47). A smear containing only a few dysplastic cells but all showing a marked degree of abnormality, almost certainly reflects CIN 3. Likewise, a smear containing a majority of dysplastic cells of moderate degree with only occasional severely dysplastic cells, while seemingly suggestive of CIN 2, will often disclose CIN 3 on conization.

AREAS OF DIAGNOSTIC DIFFICULTY

THE SCANT ENDOCERVICAL CURETTAGE

Absent any generally accepted criteria for what constitutes either an adequate or scant specimen, a problem pathologists frequently encounter is the language to use when reporting a curettage specimen where the diagnostic tissue is less than adequate. This is true also for endometrium, where only endocervical tissue is present. Many specimens, even with copious amounts of material, consist largely of mucus, which itself is not of diagnostic value. Often the only diagnostic cellular component present consists of little more than a few small strips of mucinous columnar epithelium devoid of any underlying stroma. To diagnose a specimen as 'unsatisfactory' would generally require that the clinician repeat a painful procedure for which there have been no published studies analyzing sensitivity and specificity or the utility for evaluating what condition is actually present in the endocervical canal. We diagnose endocervical curettages descriptively (mucus, mucinous columnar cells, fragment of endocervix, fragments of exocervix) and when necessary with the qualifiers 'scant, rare, miniscule quantities of, etc.' A typical example is 'scant mucus and mucinous columnar epithelium.' When the specimen consists of just a few exfoliated mucinous cells, some of us diagnose 'rare exfoliated mucinous cells, inadequate for further diagnosis,' which serves as a trigger for the clinician to rethink the issue. We distinguish between strips of mucinous columnar cells and rare isolated exfoliated mucinous cells as the former reflects the curettage while the latter may represent little more cells already exfoliated into the mucus. Although the endocervical curettage is primarily used to assess the extent of squamous neoplasia, it also helps in evaluating the present or absence of glandular tumors and precancers that may involve the endocervix.

SQUAMOUS EPITHELIUM WITH SLIGHTLY ENLARGED NUCLEI AND EPITHELIAL CHANGES OF UNCERTAIN SIGNIFICANCE

The entity 'squamous epithelium with slightly enlarged nuclei (SEN)' defines a condition diagnosed principally to provide correspondence with the cytologic diagnosis of ASCUS (atypical squamous cell of undetermined significance) or NCBD (nuclear changes bordering on dyskaryosis) (Figure 8.48). Since ASCUS is a cytologic equivocation and a risk assessment rather than a biologic entity, SEN should be used at a minimum if at all.

The term 'SEN', while not standard in the literature, portrays a concept that has been advocated and named 'borderline' in the UK and Europe.[1,24] Quite commonly, when the cytologic smear indicates a very slight degree of abnormality, the gynecologist is forced to ponder what follow-up testing is needed when the biopsy findings are reported as normal (e.g., no pathologic diagnosis, or no diagnostic abnormality recognized) for lack of a more precise terminology. In reality, many such biopsies disclose nuclei that are enlarged, yet are uniform in size and shape in an epithelium that shows substantial differentiation (Figures 8.49 and 8.50). Mitoses, if present, are not atypical. These findings are insufficient for a diagnosis of dysplasia. In one study, all cases of CIN 1 were reviewed using uniform and strict criteria, resulting in a reclassification of 12% to borderline.[1] Recorrelation with the cytologic smears indicated the borderline group had negative smears in 76% of cases and borderline (ASCUS) smears in the remaining 24%. No smear was dysplastic. Based on a prospective 4-year review at one of our institutions (SJR), squamous epithelium with slightly enlarged nuclei correlates with cytologic smears as follows: normal, 9%; reactive, 35%; ASCUS, 22%; CIN 1, 31%; and CIN 2, 3% (unpublished data). Another way of viewing this entity is that it does not really exist based on the above correlations.

The UK National Health Service Cervical Screening Programme National Coordinating Network has considered this

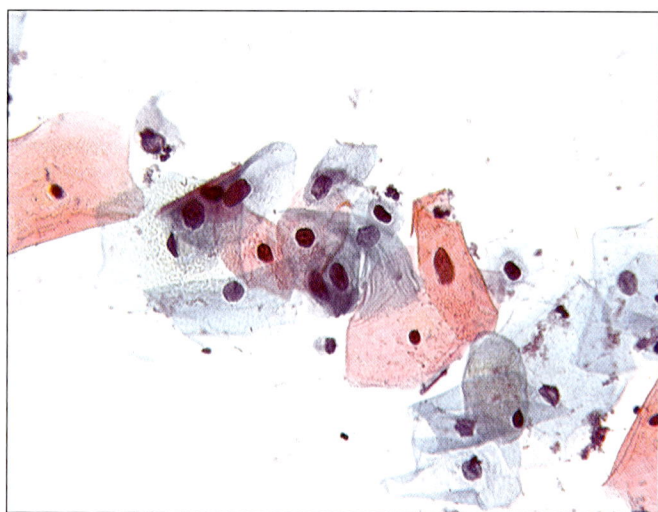

Fig. 8.48 Borderline nuclear change. The nuclear changes are insufficient for an unequivocal diagnosis of CIN. Such changes are termed ASCUS (atypical squamous cell of undetermined significance) or sometimes as NCBD (nuclear changes bordering on dyskaryosis).

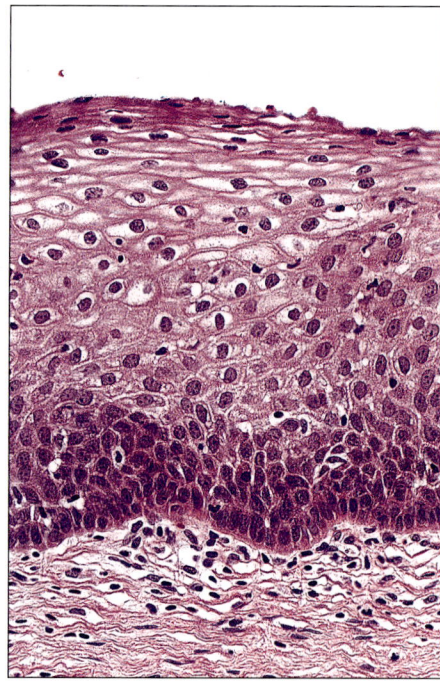

Fig. 8.49 Slightly enlarged nuclei. The basal layers are thickened. The nuclei in the superficial half of the epithelium are also slightly enlarged, but essentially normal.

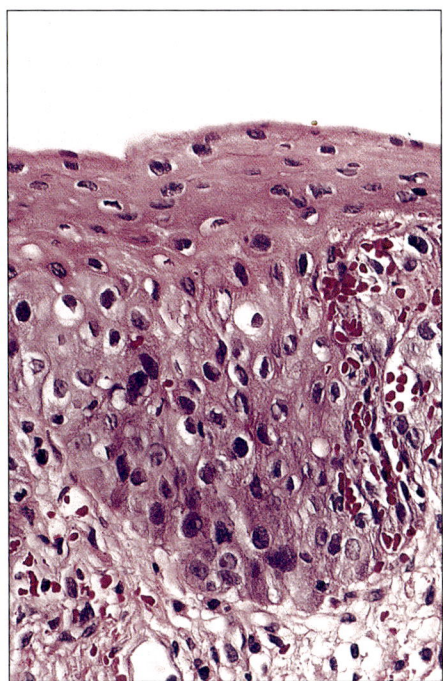

Fig. 8.50 Squamous epithelium with superficially located, slightly enlarged nuclei. The basal layers are also slightly increased in number.

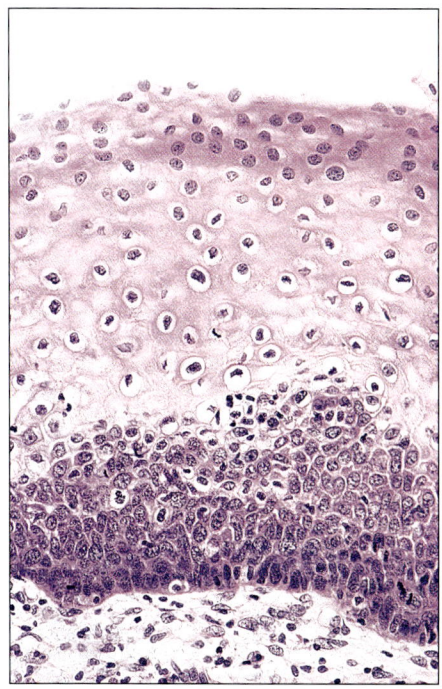

Fig. 8.51 Excessive differentiation. The basal and parabasal epithelium are remarkably abnormal, consistent with a high-grade dysplasia, and yet the upper epithelium is normal. The quandary exists whether such a case should be categorized as CIN or as basal cell hyperplasia.

issue and recommended the term 'epithelial changes of uncertain significance' for an essentially similar condition. The Working Party felt a need for a category to encompass those lesions where the pathologist was uncertain as to whether there was CIN 1 or not. The features it states that can be found in these circumstances include:

- nuclear enlargement
- a minor degree of nuclear pleomorphism
- normal mitoses
- koilocytosis-associated features.

These criteria disclose overlap with some of those used to diagnose CIN 1. In the US the concept would be split between CIN 1 and normal/reactive states. In our consultation practice, as more than half of community-diagnosed CIN 1 is called down to normal, HPV testing would be helpful to adjudicate these judgments just as in cytology. In other words, HPV-negative SEN is of no consequence, whereas HPV-positive SEN is really like CIN 1.

BASAL CELL HYPERPLASIA

Basal cell hyperplasia shows regular replication of basal layers with nuclear enlargement. However, nuclear pleomorphism and hyperchromasia are absent. Differentiation is relatively normal in the upper half of the epithelium. While the significance of basal cell hyperplasia and its long-term implications are unknown, it may reflect the early stages of dysplasia occurring in the 'original' (native) squamous epithelium.

In some cases, the distinction between basal cell hyperplasia and high-grade CIN can be difficult, if not impossible, to make, and much depends upon the belief of the pathologist. Such cases exist where the basal and parabasal cells are remarkably abnormal, and yet the upper two-thirds of the epithelium is relatively normal (Figures 8.51 and 8.52). Emphasis on the

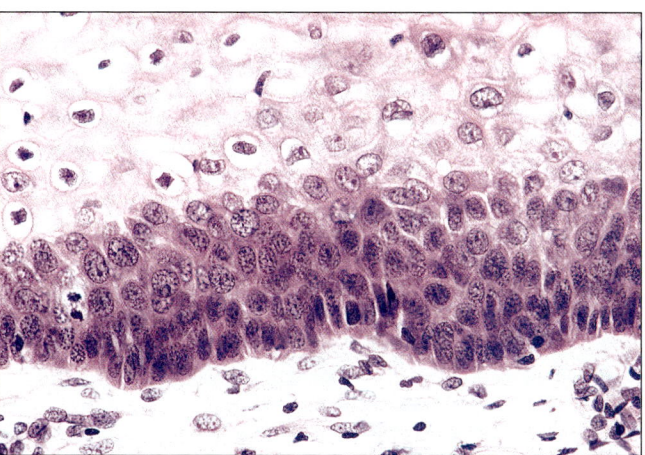

Fig. 8.52 High magnification of excessive differentiation.

upper layers leads to a diagnosis of basal cell hyperplasia, whereas emphasis on the basal layers leads to a diagnosis of high-grade CIN. Ki-67 and p16 immunohistochemistry can be helpful in making the distinction.

IMMATURE SQUAMOUS METAPLASIA AND ATYPICAL SQUAMOUS METAPLASIA

Squamous metaplasia is a physiologic process characterized by reserve cell hyperplasia, early squamous differentiation, variable polarity, and nuclear enlargement, any part of which may sometimes be quite exaggerated (see Chapter 6). Nuclear pleomorphism and hyperchromasia are absent, thus rendering to the epithelium an appearance of somewhat bland nuclei of uniform size and shape (the nuclei are remarkably round). During the time when metaplastic squamous cells develop, they may undermine and replace endocervical columnar cells. At times the nuclei can be enlarged and yet be relatively uniform, which elicits differences in diagnoses among pathologists as to whether the lesion is an immature squamous metaplasia or CIN, especially when columnar cells are present on the surface (Figure 8.53). HPV-associated features are rarely seen in immature metaplastic squamous epithelium.

It can be difficult to distinguish immature squamous metaplasia with minimal nuclear changes from CIN (Table 8.6). Typically, immature metaplastic squamous cells have abundant cytoplasm and homogeneous round nuclei with fine speckled chromatin and a small nucleolus. The frequency of MIB1 (Ki-67) reactive nuclei is low and the staining intensity minimal.[47] Cylindrical cells can occur intermingled with, or at the surface of, the immature cells and then are a strong diagnostic criterion, but are not always present. Whenever substantial nuclear pleomorphism is found, CIN should be diagnosed even if columnar cells are present on the surface (Figure 8.54). MIB1 staining is a useful differential diagnostic feature, as it typically is unremarkable in immature squamous metaplasia but appears strongly and diffusely throughout the epithelium in CIN.

REPAIR (REACTIVE EPITHELIAL CHANGES)

Repair of the squamous epithelium is a condition that commonly mimics the features of mild dysplasia.[102] Unlike dyspla-

sia, the stroma in repair is virtually always chronically and often floridly inflamed. The nuclei are uniform, with no or minimal pleomorphism. The chromatin is bland and evenly distributed. Nucleoli of 'bull's eye' or macronucleolar appearance are often easily found (Figure 8.55). Mildly dysplastic epithelium, in contrast, is infrequently associated with an intensely inflamed stroma, but has nuclei that are pleomorphic and commonly display coarse chromatin and mitoses.

LOW ESTROGEN STATES AND ATROPHY

In low estrogen states, i.e., after the menopause and in women taking low estrogen oral contraceptives, the cervical squamous epithelium is usually thin and may be composed entirely of parabasal cells. While mild nuclear hyperchromasia is often seen, the nuclei are uniform in size and shape and a constant amount of cytoplasm surrounds most nuclei. Nuclear pleomorphism is absent. In some postmenopausal women, the cervix may exhibit a spectrum of epithelial alterations, including prominent perinuclear halos, nuclear hyperchromasia, some variation in nuclear size, and multinucleation. In one study, all cases showing these changes were negative for HPV by PCR analysis.[37] Several features help to distinguish this

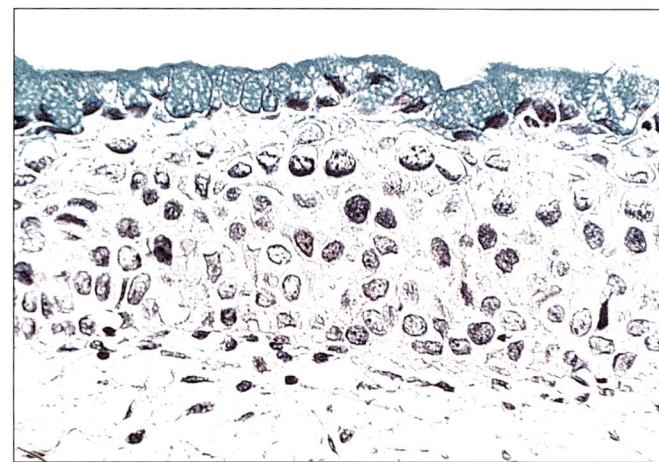

Fig. 8.54 CIN with pleomorphic nuclei beneath the surface columnar mucinous epithelium.

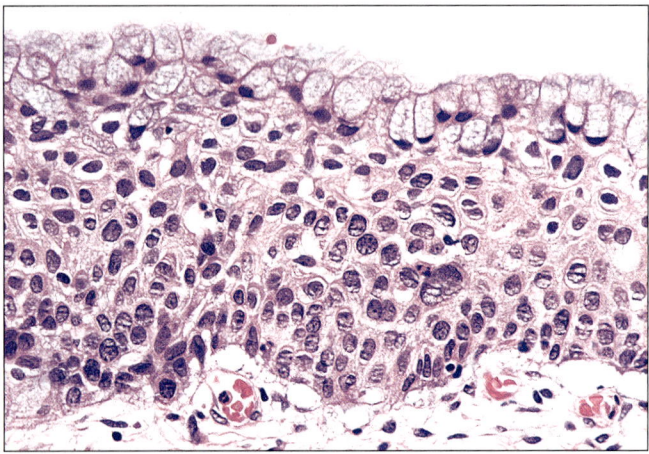

Fig. 8.53 Immature squamous metaplasia versus CIN 2, with surface columnar epithelium.

Table 8.6 Differential diagnostic features of immature squamous metaplasia and CIN		
Feature	Immature squamous metaplasia	CIN
Nuclei	Round	Variable
Chromatin	Homogeneous	Course, clumped
Nucleolus	Single, small	Often large and multiple
Cylindrical cells	Strong argument when present, but often absent	Absent
MIB1 (Ki-67)	Small, dot-like	Often abundant

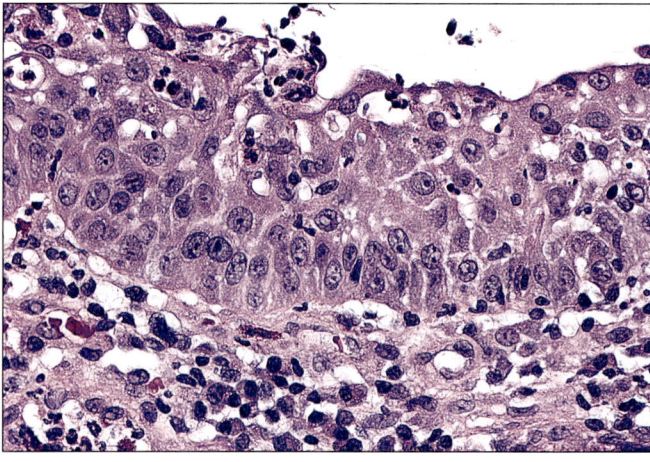

Fig. 8.55 Repair. The nuclei lack pleomorphism and often disclose prominent nucleoli.

change, named 'postmenopausal squamous atypia', from HPV-associated low-grade squamous intraepithelial lesions. They include less variation in nuclear size and staining intensity, more finely and evenly distributed nuclear chromatin, and greater uniformity of perinuclear halos in the former. MIB1 expression can also be useful, as positive nuclei are typically limited to the lower layers, but must be interpreted with care as very thin epithelium may lack superficial cells. The latter can mimic CIN. However, caution is warranted. Correlation with HPV testing is important as many studies demonstrate a 'bump' in HPV prevalence in the postmenopausal age group.

THIN EPITHELIUM

In an epithelium that has only a few layers of cells, it is commonly impossible to confidently diagnose the presence of CIN. There is often the concern that the epithelium is not naturally thin, and that some artifactual process is responsible for the removal of multiple superficial layers. In the absence of severe inflammation, CIN should usually be diagnosed (Figure 8.56). Sometimes, the number of cell layers present is sufficient to diagnose CIN, or even probable high-grade CIN, but further definition is precluded (Figure 8.57).

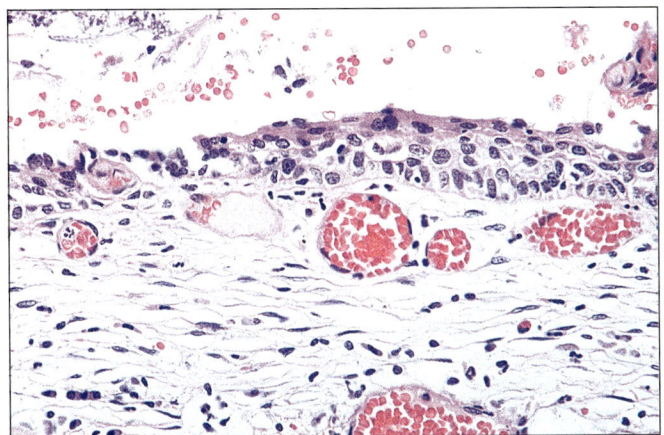

Fig. 8.56 Thin epithelium, probably CIN. The nuclei are clearly atypical.

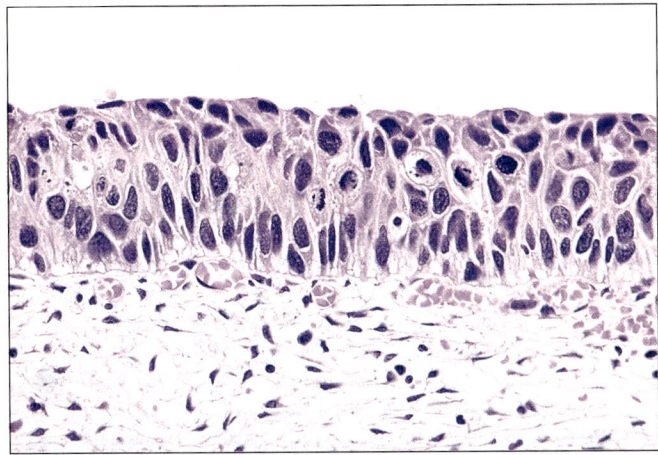

Fig. 8.57 Thin epithelium with high-grade CIN. The number of cell layers present is sufficient to diagnose high-grade CIN, but further definition is precluded.

INVASIVE SQUAMOUS CELL CARCINOMA

Not uncommonly, one of the most difficult diseases to distinguish from CIN 3 is invasive squamous cell carcinoma. This occurs most commonly if the biopsy is superficial and is devoid of an obvious stromal component. In such examples, the epithelium appears as sheets of irregularly folded tumor lying on a thin basement membrane. The most appropriate diagnosis is that of 'at least CIN 3 (or squamous cell CIS), cannot exclude invasion'. In one study testing for cellular features that distinguish the two diseases, several histologic features found in the cone biopsy specimens were preferentially associated with invasive tumor.[54] These included giant bizarre cells that were irregular, hyperchromatic, and up to five times the size of a basal cell (67% vs 6%), large keratinized cells with distinct cell borders (87% vs 0%), keratin pearls (41% vs 0%), necrosis, often comedo-like (80% vs 8%), and neovascularized tumor cells close to the endothelial lining and lacking intervening connective tissue (57% vs 0%). In 74% of the invasive cancer cases, a component of CIN 3 was present, of which 35% showed large keratinized cells or keratin pearls in the *in situ* components. This suggested that the presence of either feature in biopsy specimens showing CIN 3 might signify the presence of invasive lesions elsewhere in the cervical mucosa.

A not unusual situation is where the diagnosis of CIN is correct, but the results of hysterectomy show the disease process to be more extensive than expected. Occasionally, the surface and the endocervical glands are involved only with CIN, as suggested by a history of only CIN on smears (even when reviewed retrospectively) and the absence of any abnormality clinically. However, the hysterectomy specimen shows that the wall harbors a small cancer or on occasion is permeated by a quite large carcinoma (see Chapter 9).

ARTIFACT

Fragmentation and thermal artifact in cone and loop electrosurgical excision procedure (LEEP) biopsy specimens are major problems affecting correct diagnosis.[22,34] When specimens are fragmented into multiple small pieces, it is difficult, if not impossible, to evaluate margins. Thermal artifact, which is often caused by low-voltage techniques, results in an epithelium that appears smudged and unreadable. Cellular and nuclear details are lost (Figure 8.58). In a LEEP biopsy correctly done, the thermal artifact produces a very thin rim, usually a fraction of a millimeter wide, at the periphery of the specimen. The outermost layer, the carbonization zone, is usually quite thin. The coagulation zone is deeper and is significantly larger and more readily apparent. Unacceptable thermal artifact occurs when the coagulation zone is wide (Figure 8.59), resulting in extensive loss of cellular detail. A recent randomized control trial that evaluated pure cut versus traditional blending settings in large loop excisions of the transformation zone found no significant differences in thermal artifact. In the deep stroma, however, the blended setting had a thicker thermal artifact band (0.382 mm) than the pure cut setting (0.325 mm).[63]

MISCELLANEOUS CONDITIONS

One of the more bizarre situations rarely encountered is where the cervix is treated for CIN, but the results of hysterectomy

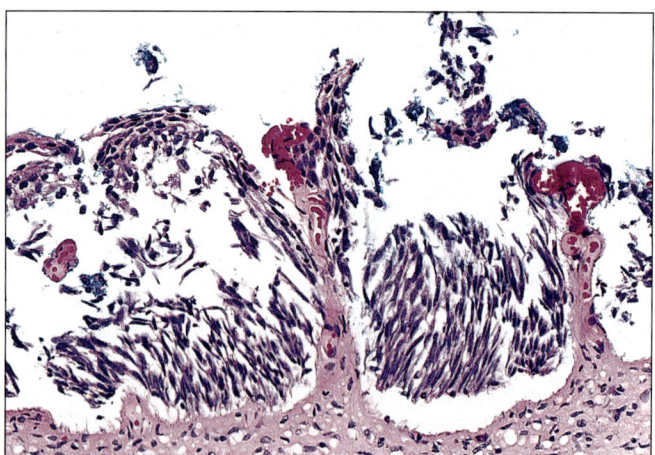

Fig. 8.58 Thermal artifact with LEEP biopsy. The epithelium has lost all cellular detail.

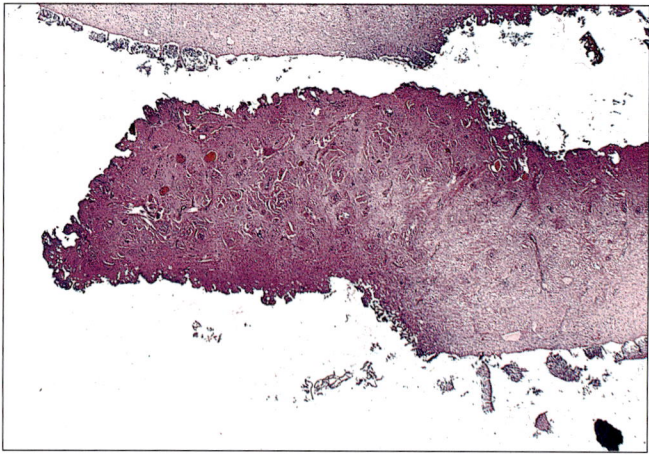

Fig. 8.59 Thermal artifact with LEEP biopsy. The stroma shows extensive coagulative changes.

show the CIN process involves more than the cervix. There are the rare reported cases where hysterectomy and bilateral salpingo-oophorectomy performed to treat the CIN disclosed that the disease had extended to the endometrium and fallopian tubes, and there extensively replaced the normal glandular mucosa.[73,83]

BIOMARKERS

WHY ARE DEEP EPITHELIAL LAYER BIOMARKERS PROGNOSTIC?

The microscopic image of a cervical epithelium is a snapshot (a 'photo') of a dynamic process (a 'film') that normally would consist of many images if taken over time. The question why measurement of biomarkers in the deep epithelium helps predict CIN behavior pulls together the different dynamic biologic aspects discussed above.

The cervical epithelium is a dynamic tissue of socially and orderly upward-moving cells with tightly balanced and controlled proliferation and differentiation. HPV infection disturbs this process. Through oncoproteins E6 and E7, HPV

immobilizes/degrades, thereby reducing and finally annihilating pRb and p53 in the cells found in the lower half of the epithelium, which otherwise would be available for their usual function of slowing the normal maturation process. The result of the metabolic 'take-over' is a high (abnormal) proliferation of cells even reaching up into the superficial layers (mitoses or Ki-67 positive cells and abnormal chromatin patterns) and altered differentiation markers, which historically is seen as a high-grade lesion. Once the virally transformed cells are cleared by the host's immune system, pRb and p53 functions in the deep layers restart. This is so far the earliest sign of cure and normalization of epithelial cell metabolism.

Thereafter, perhaps by some weeks, proliferation as reflected by the number of Ki-67 reactive cells falls, initially in the deep layer. These newly 'cured' normal cells (now mostly Ki-67 negative) will move up, mature, and reach the epithelial surface in several weeks. Quite some time after pRb and p53 have normalized, signs of abnormal proliferation and differentiation in the superficial layers (diagnostic for CIN 3) also disappear and return to normal. Thus, assessing pRb and p53 in the deep epithelial cell layers predicts the future events that would have taken place in the superficial epithelium some weeks from when the biopsy was taken. It may be that the clearance and cure process expressed by the biomarkers is not always that it simply just slowly disappears – it may be that, depending on the balance between the host's defense system on the one hand, and the aggression of HPV on the other, a CIN 3 lesion regresses to CIN 2, hangs there for some time, increases back to CIN 3, and only then totally regresses or even persists ('hanging' of cells at CIN 2 is perhaps the only explanation why pathologists ever see a CIN 2). Quantifying biomarkers therefore can change the pathologist's role from reporting static morphology to the much more exciting possibility of dynamically interpreting and forecasting future events taking place in the tissue.

In this context it is of the utmost importance that biomarker analysis be performed using specified geographical areas of the epithelium. Average measurements – ignoring whether taken from the basal, deep or superficial layers – obviate the dynamic nature of the cervical epithelium, obscuring important prognostic information. It is the strength of pathologists with their familiarity of the biology and dynamics of tissues that allows them to extract the biologically relevant information correctly. Not considering this important facet of tissue, i.e., geographical location, means losing important information.

Ki-67 CELL CLUSTERS

The development and behavior of CIN correlate with proliferation. In paraffin sections, the MIB1 antibody is equivalent to Ki-67, a widely used biomarker correlated with proliferation, and its immunohistochemical staining pattern is stable, robust, and contrast rich. In evaluating Ki-67 reactive cell clusters as a diagnostic adjunct in distinguishing CIN from normal or benign reactive cervical squamoepithelial lesions, it is important to prevent overdiagnosis, and Ki-67 reactive to tangentially cut parabasal cells, inflammatory cells, and immature metaplasia must be carefully excluded.

Ki-67 immunoquantitation is an important diagnostic adjunct for grading of CIN,[45,51] and its diagnostic import is best understood when expressed numerically as the 90th percentile stratification index, or Stratification Index-90 (SI90) (Figure 8.60). Cells are identified equidistant along the basement membrane, and then the location of the uppermost Ki-67 reactive cell recorded as a percentage of the distance to the mucosal surface. The 90th out of 100 recordings is considered

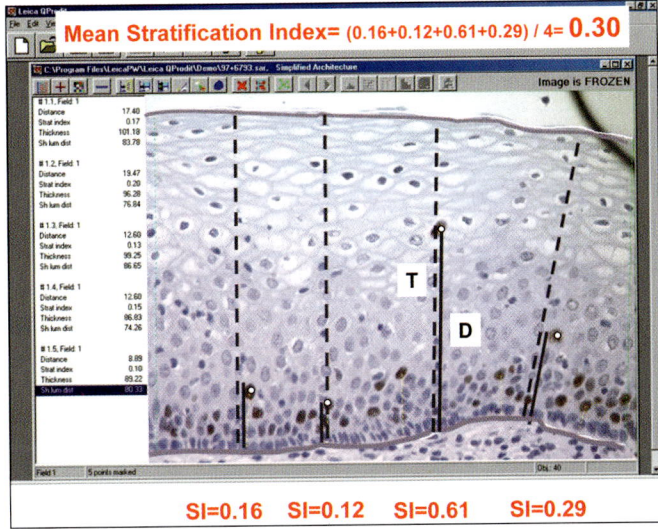

Mean Stratification Index= (0.16+0.12+0.61+0.29) / 4= **0.30**

SI=0.16   SI=0.12   SI=0.61   SI=0.29

Fig. 8.60 Ki-67 and quantitative image analysis method. After the operator clicks the mouse on all Ki-67 reactive nuclei, the system automatically draws a perpendicular line from that point to the basal membrane plus a dotted line at that point over the full thickness of the epithelium. The system then calculates thickness (T) of the epithelium at that point, distance (D) of the point to the basal membrane, the stratification index (SI = D/T) and others, examples of which are on the left. The SIs for the four nuclei measures are 0.16, 0.12, 0.61 and 0.29, respectively. The program automatically calculates many quantitative features per sample, e.g., the mean SI of the four measurements = (0.16 + 0.12 + 0.61 + 0.29)/4 = 0.30. With multivariate analysis, the 90th percentile (SI90) of all individual SI measurements per case is the strongest factor (more significant than the mean SI) for grade description and also to predict progression. The number of Ki-67 reactive nuclei per 100 μm basal membrane is the next strongest discriminator for grade, while the percentage of Ki-67 positive nuclei in the middle third of the epithelium (MIDTHIRD) is the only factor that adds to the prognostic value of SI90. Reproduced with permission from Baak et al.[8]

the SI90. This number is an excellent proxy of the degree of dysplasia.

In normal epithelium, MIB1 reactivity is limited to the parabasal region and maximally to the lower one-third of the epithelium in CIN 1, whereas in high-grade CIN, MIB1 reactive nuclei are also found in higher epithelial cells. Typically, in CIN 3, MIB1 reactive nuclei are also present under the surface. The SI quantifies the MIB1 localization. The distance from a nucleus to the basal membrane is measured, and divided by the epithelial thickness where the nucleus is found. Thus, the SI of nuclei close to the basal membrane is low, e.g., 0.1, whereas it is closer to 1.0 the higher the nuclei in the superficial layer.

The SI90 (as opposed to other indices such as SI50) is highly sensitive diagnostically and has the best correlation with CIN assessments by examination with H&E alone. Another aspect of quantifying the SI90 is to take into account the 'Ki-67 crowding'. From experience, the number of Ki-67 reactive nuclei along the basement is much higher in CIN 3 than in CIN 1. An important objective measure is the relative number of Ki-67 reactive nuclei per 100 μm basal membrane (increased numbers of Ki-67 reactive nuclei correlate with higher grade). In performing the SI90, cell columns should be chosen for measurement that are equidistant from each other along the basement membrane. Use of these features forms a highly discriminating method to distinguish the three CIN grades, achieving 97% levels of agreement among experts, with equally good sensitivity, specificity, and positive and negative predictive values. Ki-67 immunoquantitative parameters also correlate well with the presence of *hr*HPV in CIN lesions.[51]

p16

The cyclin-dependent kinase 2A inhibitor, p16[INK4], hereafter p16, helps distinguish CIN from reactive lesions.[39] Since a retinoblastoma protein (Rb)-dependent negative feedback loop regulates p16 expression, continuous inactivation of Rb by *hr*HPV E7 results in increased p16 levels. Hence, increased p16 levels may reflect HPV-induced dysplasia with deregulated E7 expression.[87] Marked overexpression of p16 protein, i.e., diffuse and strong immunostaining (Figure 8.61A), is

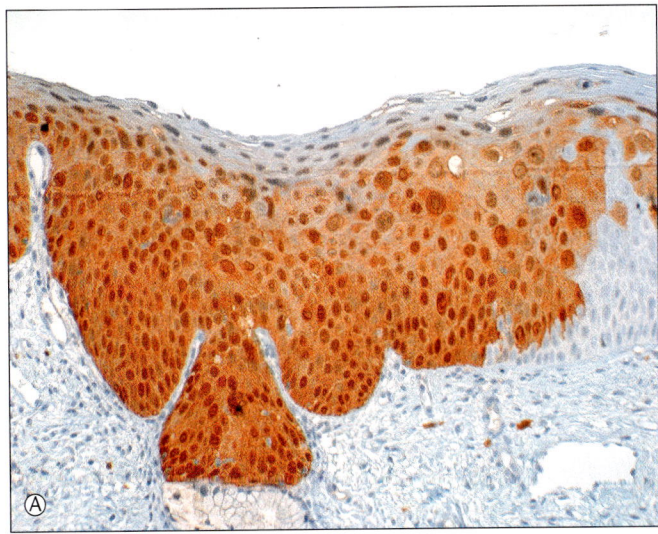

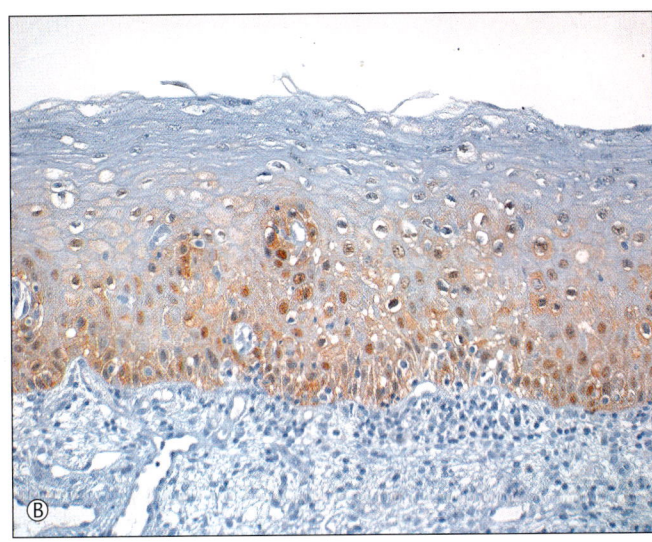

Fig. 8.61 p16 reactivity in CIN. **(A)** CIN 3, with strong p16 reactivity. **(B)** CIN 1, with weak p16 reactivity.

present in virtually all cervical cancers and high-grade preneo-plastic lesions infected by high- and intermediate-risk HPVs, i.e., subtypes 16, 18, 31, 33, 52, and 58, in contrast to the weak/focal staining (Figure 8.61B) in HPV 6/11 or similar low-grade infected lesions.[82] p16 overexpression is sensitive (84%) and specific (98%) in detection of *hr*HPV.[15] At low magnification, p16 staining facilitates finding a dysplastic area, especially if the epithelium is heavily infested with leukocytes, as often occurs in CIN lesions.[42] In addition, overexpressed p16 helps identify individual dyskaryotic cells in fluid-based cytologic smears.[62]

NATURAL HISTORY OF CIN, USING MOLECULAR MARKERS TO ASSESS RISK

A potential shortcoming of the microscopic pathology grade is that it assesses *epithelial* features exclusively and usually only those visible with the standard H&E stain, thereby not taking into account other possibly valuable information. Another serious disadvantage is that the three distinct grades used in CIN (or two in SIL) can easily give a faulty static impression of a *solidified sculpture*, as if CIN/SIL were a static event whereas, in reality, a CIN lesion is a dynamic process (a balance) that can progress and persist but also regress. This emphasizes the need to interpret the actual morphologic impression of a CIN lesion in *dynamic terms*, rather than in *static morphologic grades*. Such adjunctive methods are also important, not only for better distinction of CIN from non-neoplastic lesions, but also the ability to predict the risk of

progression of low-grade and regression of high-grade CIN lesions much more accurately. A caveat in this concept of predictive ability is the confounding caused by sampling by biopsy not being totally accurate of the entire range of potential dysplasia present.

Inasmuch as CIN involves progressive dysfunction of proliferation and differentiation of cervical epithelial cells, many studies have focused on evaluating the merits of proliferation and differentiation-related features.[7,10,44–51] Without doubt, p16 and Ki-67 (MIB1) are the most widely available, robust, stable, and strongest diagnostic and predictive biomarkers currently available for the handling of CIN lesions. Others, such as the retinoblastoma protein (pRb), p53, cytokeratins 13 (CK13) and 14 (CK14), etc. add substantial insight.[39,66]

HPV infection often results in nothing more than minimal reactive epithelial cell changes with some leukocytic infiltrate, or a low-grade lesion, lesions that are destined to regress in 80–90% of cases (Figure 8.62). About 10–20% of those infected with *hr*HPV develop a real precancer or high-grade CIN lesion.[12] Clearance of the virally infected cells by the immune system is followed by regression of cervical lesions. Altered transcriptional regulation of the viral oncogenes E6 and E7, especially in the oncogenic types, results in a topographical shift of E6/E7 expression from the differentiated layers to the proliferating (para) basal cell layers. When overexpressed in proliferating cells, E6 and E7 interfere with the cell cycle control that p53 and pRb regulate, respectively.[89] These morphologically abnormal cells proliferate and expand towards the surface (just as normal cells do) but without normal maturation. The degree of abnormal maturation is expressed as a high-grade

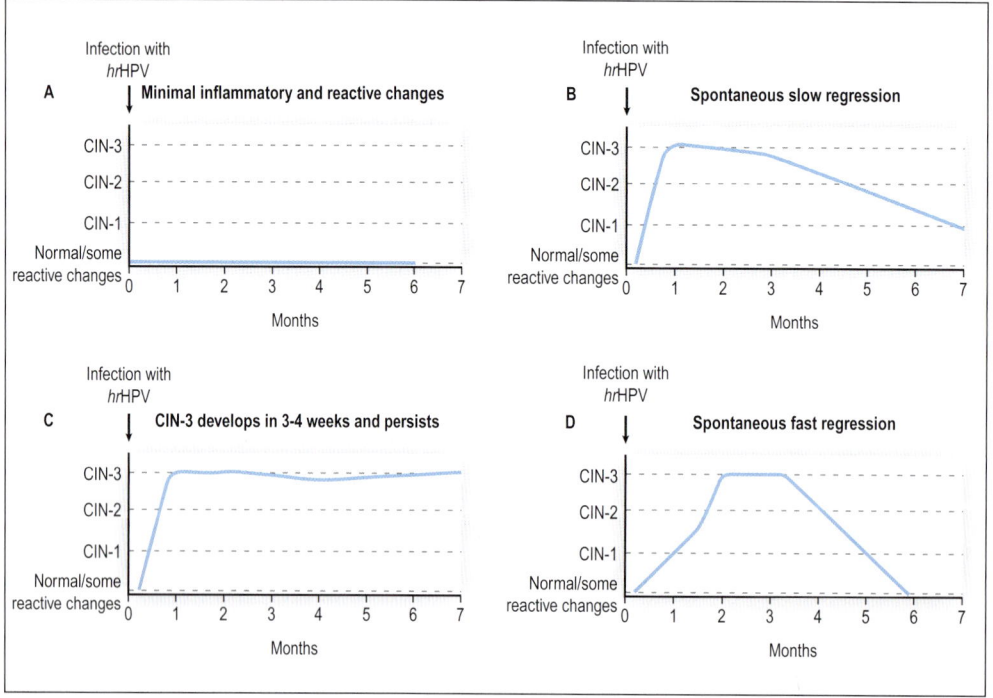

Fig. 8.62 Hypothetical courses after *hr*HPV infection. **(A)** 80% of cases after infection with *hr*HPV show no neoplasia, just minimal reactive epithelial and inflammatory changes, which disappear once the infection has cleared. This may take several months. **(B)** Development of CIN 3 after several days or weeks. The neoplastic cells develop in the parabasal cell layers (CIN 1) and, in the days after, move to the middle layer where they are visible as CIN 2. After 2–4 weeks, sometimes earlier and sometimes later, CIN 3 is present. This may then persist. **(C, D)** Examples of slow and fast regression. The initial full-blown CIN 3 persists for 1.5–2 months and then slowly clears. The first change indicative of healing is increased nuclear pRb expression in the deep epithelial cell layers. After some weeks, MIB1 positive nuclei start to disappear and epithelial CIN 2 and CIN 1 patterns replace the original CIN 3. Finally, minimal epithelial and reactive changes remain, often accompanied by transepithelial CK14 and CK13 changes as late (fading) signs of HPV infection.

CIN. The dysplastic cells are estimated to arrive at the surface within one to several weeks and then desquamate, so a full-blown CIN 3 may develop in a few weeks, although many, mostly low-grade CINs regress spontaneously, usually over 8–14 months. In contrast, regression of CIN 3 is harder to prove but yet likely.[61,98]

BIOMARKERS AND BIOLOGIC AGGRESSION OF CIN LESIONS

CIN 3 with and without coexistent endocervical CGIN

Although the incidence of invasive squamous cell cancer has markedly declined over the years, the incidence of cervical adenocarcinomas has correspondingly increased.[86] A commonly given explanation is that glandular adenocarcinomas and their precursor lesions are often missed by conventional cytology. As the lesions are located higher in the cervical canal, they are less accessible to conventional brush sampling methods. Only 43% of patients with glandular lesions prior to conization of the cervix were detected by endocervical curettage (ECC).[74] Moreover, the squamous lesions are treated and eliminated, which, in long screened populations, means the relative frequency of glandular lesions will increase.

Indicators in CIN 3 for possible coexistence of a glandular lesion can alert the gynecologist to perform an extensive cone biopsy high up in the endocervix. Such a high-risk cervical glandular intraepithelial neoplasia (CGIN) indicator could also serve as a safety net against false-negative endocervical curettage. The frequency of *hr*HPV genotypes (16, 18, 31, 33, 35, 39, 45, 51, 52, 56, 58, 59, 66 and 68) differs for CIN 3 patients with and without high-grade CGIN. Despite little difference in the frequency of HPV 16 or HPV 45 between CIN 3 patients with or without high-grade CGIN, the frequency of HPV 18 is significantly higher, and the frequency of *hr*HPV genotypes other than HPV 16, 18, and 45 lower in CIN lesions coexisting with CGIN than in solitary CIN lesions. This suggests that CIN 3s, coexisting with high-grade glandular lesions, may have some etiologic differences from squamous lesions without coexisting glandular lesions.[14] CIN 3 epithelial cell cycle regulator expression may reflect these differences and thereby indicate coexistent CGIN. Indeed, in one recent study, CIN 3s with coexistent CGIN had a significantly lower percentage of pRb ($p = 0.03$) and p53 ($p = 0.03$) reactive nuclei in the lower half of the epithelium than CIN 3s without coexistent CGIN.[43]

Prognostic value of Ki-67 and other biomarkers in low-grade lesions

As discussed above, the Ki-67 SI90 is a sensitive marker for the grade of dysplasia present. In small histologic punch (marker) biopsies, the marker also better predicts progression to CIN 3 than CIN grade alone. The prognostically strongest Ki-67 features are:[48,50]

- Average Ki-67 reactive nucleus is more than 57% of the distance towards the surface.
- More than 30% of the Ki-67 reactive nuclei are located in the middle third of the epithelium.

The prognostic value of the various cell cycle regulatory proteins and markers of squamous differentiation have also been examined in various studies. Telomerase analysis has rendered variable results,[17,49,78] which is understandable as its activity

reflects a rather late step in the sequence of progress from CIN 3 to squamous cell carcinoma, thus explaining why it is not prognostic for early CIN progression.[39] The results for pRb, p53, cyclins A, E, and D, p16, p21, p27, telomerase, involucrin, CK13 and CK14 do not always agree with each other, but this too can be partly understood by inappropriate technology used in certain studies, which have not taken into account the biologic dynamics of cervical epithelium, as follows.

Epithelial cells are born in the parabasal layer, and in the normal process of maturation, migrate to the surface (where they desquamate). An average, which assesses biomarkers throughout all layers of the entire epithelial thickness rather than within specific compartments, blurs important dynamic information. Biomarkers should be viewed separately in the basal, deeper and upper half of the epithelium. Experience has shown that a high Ki-67 stratification index and reduced pRb expression in the lower squamous epithelium best predicts the progression of early CIN lesions (Figure 8.63). The reduced pRb expression indicates suppressed pRb, which translates as the brake on proliferation (like the brake on an automotive gas pedal) being removed, allowing the engine to race, which the heightened Ki-67 activity reflects. Moreover, reduced cytokeratin (CK13 and CK14) expression identifies a subgroup with an even greater risk of progression, but this additional prognostic value of CK13 and CK14 is only in the prognostically high-risk subgroup with high Ki-67 and low pRb. Loss of involucrin and CK13 expression occurs only in high-grade lesions and is therefore related to future lesion grade. Finally, loss of CK14 expression is also significantly more frequent in high-grade than in low-grade lesions.[88] Quantitation of combined Ki-67, Rb, CK13 and CK14 in early CIN lesions provides the most accurate information about their progression risk.[8,49]

Based on the above findings, a biochemical model for the development of an early CIN lesion has been developed (Figure 8.63). Central in this hypothesis is that *hr*HPV E7, when expressed during HPV infection, impairs pRb, which acts normally to reduce growth. When impaired by E7, the growth-reducing effect of Rb diminishes as shown by increased and upward proliferation (as a result, the Ki-67 SI increases and finally exceeds a critical level of 0.57). The first sign of healing and disappearance of morphologic CIN features is increased Rb in the deep layers of the epithelium (Figure 8.64). Shortly after, proliferation reduces, and the subsequent upward spread of proliferating cells is also reduced, as manifest by lowering Ki-67 reactivity. Naturally, p53 is also impaired (by E6), but the prognostic role of pRb is much stronger and overshadows the significance of p53 in predicting early CIN progression. However, in HSIL (CIN 2–3) lesions, p53 has some additional value to pRb in identifying CIN 3 lesions that will regress (see below).

PREDICTION OF CIN 2 AND 3 BEHAVIOR WITH BIOMARKER PATTERNS

Biomarker patterns may also be prognostic in CIN 2–3, which has important implications. Left untreated, many cervical biopsies continue to show persistent disease (CIN 2–3 endures in follow-up biopsies). Consequently, many physicians now ablate all CIN 2–3s, even though, without treatment, about 15–43% will spontaneously regress (i.e., no CIN 2–3 detected on follow-up) (Table 8.7). Based on the populations examined, the average age of patients with CIN 2–3 is around 29–40 years,

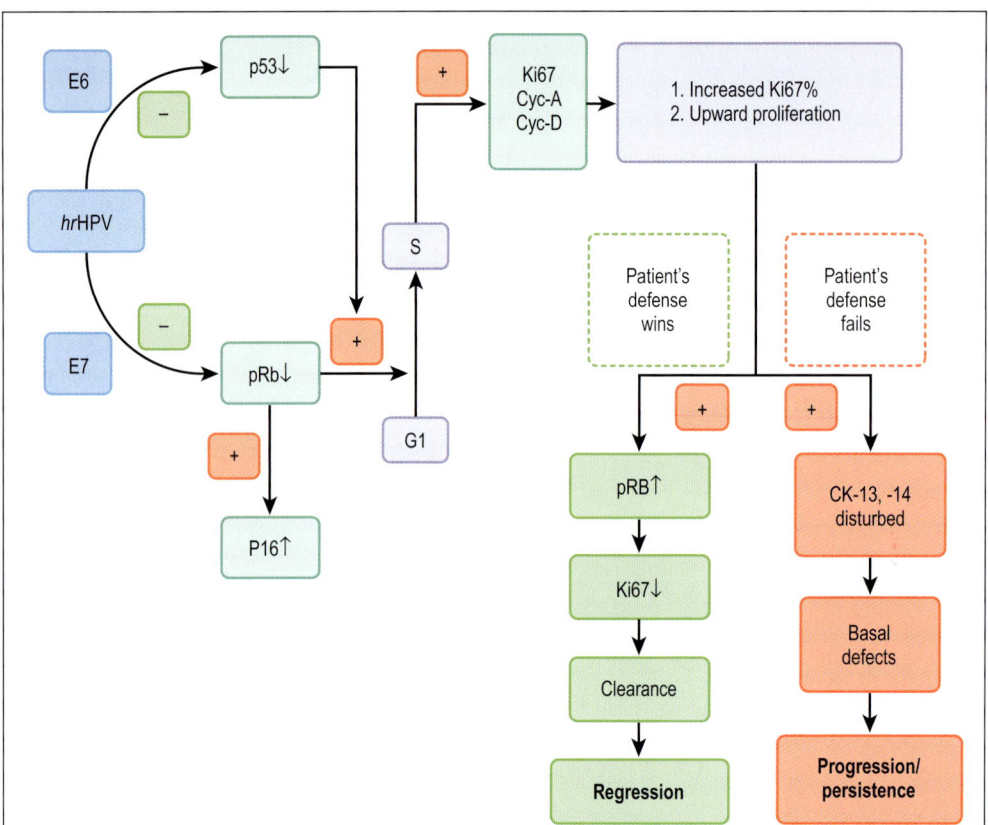

Fig. 8.63 HPV and the development of an early CIN lesion. Reproduced with permission from Baak et al.[8]

Table 8.7 Natural history of CIN: a meta-analysis[66,67,94]

	Regress (%)	Persist (%)	Progress to CIS (CIN 3) (%)	Progress to invasion (%)
HPV lacking CIN	80	15	5	0
CIN 1	57	32	11	1
CIN 2	43	35	22	5
CIN 3	32	<56	–	>12

whereas patients with microinvasive cancer are on average 5–10 years older. Stage 1 cancers occur in the late forties to fifties (Figure 8.65) (Of course, exceptions occur, (micro-)invasive cancers can also occur at much younger ages). Complicating the decision as to whether or not to treat CIN 2–3 is the reality that excision, with either cold-knife/laser cone or diathermic loop method, is a considerable medical procedure, with potentially serious complications, cervical insufficiency being the most clinically important. Because many patients treated for CIN 2–3 will at some later time become pregnant, cervical insufficiency becomes a major concern and not uncommonly leads to immature birth,[81] demanding preventive cervical cerclage under general anesthesia at 16–20 weeks' gestation. Obviously, today's goal of clinical value is to prevent unnecessary cone and LEEP treatment. The ideal remedy would be to identify those CIN 2–3s that would regress spontaneously.

In one study, in order to identify factors related to histologically proven persistence or regression in CIN 2–3, small histologic colposcopically directed (punch) biopsies were analyzed for HPV genotypes and different immunoquantitative proliferation, cell cycle regulation, and differentiation markers.[9]

Special attention was paid to p53 and pRb in biopsies as potential markers for *hr*HPV E6 and E7 function.[103] An interval of at least 100 days for all cases separated the initial marker and subsequent LEEP/cone biopsy, thus mitigating the effects of the initial punch biopsy procedure, which causes considerable damage, and, consequently, a local inflammatory and repair response in the first 3–6 weeks after biopsy. Healing is generally complete within 100 days, lessening the chance that the follow-up specimen would be over-read due to regenerative changes. All lesions were reactive for both p16 and *hr*HPV; 63% were reactive for HPV 16 or HPV 16 admixtures, while 37% had other *hr*HPV types.

Forty-three per cent of lesions had histologically regressed, similar to reports of regression seen by others.[98] The initial punch (marker) biopsies of the persistent CIN 2–3s compared to specimens with regressive CIN 2–3 had significantly decreased pRb and p53 detected in the deep half of the epithelium than non-persistent HSILs. The degree of reactivity to p16, Ki-67, and cyclin D1, lesion extent in the punch (marker) biopsy, and patient age were all unrelated to persistence or regression as later found in follow-up cone biopsies. HPV 16-positive CIN 2–3 lesions had a lower regression percentage of pRb and p53 than those with other HPV types. While statistically not significant, HPV 16-containing lesions tended to persist more frequently.[9] However, the percentages of pRb and p53 reactive nuclei in the deep half of the epithelium of a histologic punch cervical biopsy were much stronger predictors of CIN 3 regression than HPV genotype, a finding of prospective observational cohort studies.

Some studies also suggest that interactions among HPV and human leukocyte antigen (HLA) types support a role for

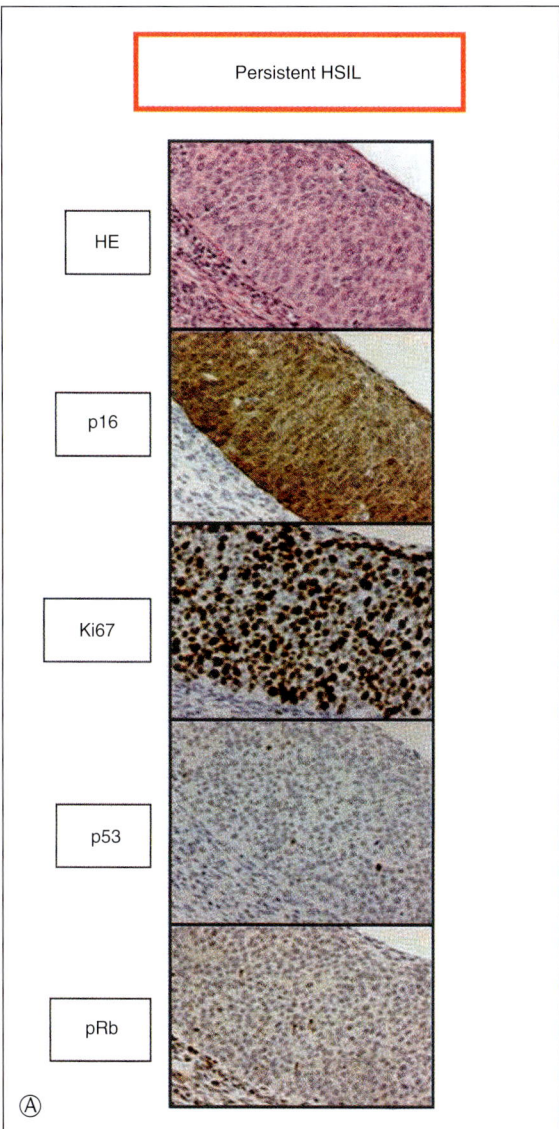

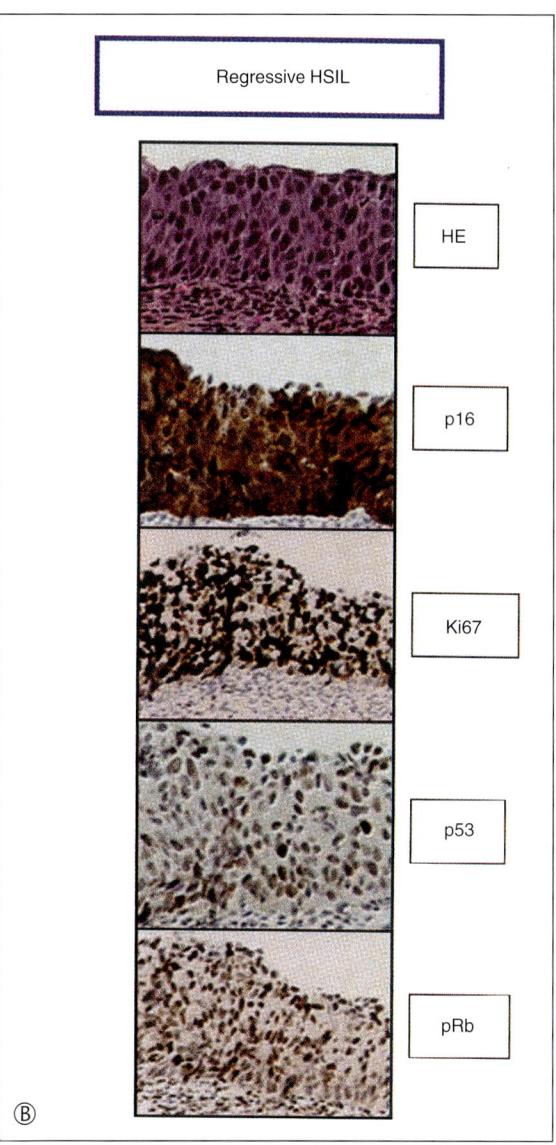

Fig. 8.64 (A, B) Immunocytochemical findings in persistent and regressing CIN 3.

HLA-restricted HPV-specific immune responses in determining disease outcome.[98] It seems that the interaction (balance) between a patient's immune response and HPV factors results in a prognostically important epithelial cell reaction measured by epithelial pRb and p53. Additionally, recent studies show that CIN 2–3 with and without coexistent CGIN can also be distinguished by combined pRb and p53 in the lower half of the epithelium. Those with CGIN had both low pRb and p53, whereas those without CGIN had high values of either pRb or p53 in the deep epithelium.[43] However, these studies are confounded by the failure to control for lesion size and the potential therapeutic effect of biopsy and postbiopsy inflammation. Hence they are still preliminary and cannot yet be viewed as robust enough for individual patient management.

INTERPRETING DYNAMIC BIOMARKER PATTERNS

The following is a hypothetical approach for handling a cervical punch biopsy in the surgical pathology laboratory when behavioral predictions are desired (Figure 8.66). In presenting it, the reader must always be cognizant of sampling confounding, recognizing that the punch biopsy does not always accurately reflect the worst disease present, and in up to half of instances may miss the worst pathology and in addition to the *sampling considerations*, the cost effectiveness of doing multiple stains in multiple biopsies should be considered.

Analysis of early CIN lesions
- Analyze the diagnostic H&E-stained section for routine evaluation.
- Scan a serial section, stained for p16, to identify diffusely reactive squamous areas. These are nearly always dysplastic (false-positive p16 reactivity is rare and easily recognized).
- Evaluate the next serial section with Ki-67. Ki-67-positive cell clusters further support a diagnosis of CIN.
- Perform quantitative Ki-67 image analysis for objective grading support and progression risk indication in case of

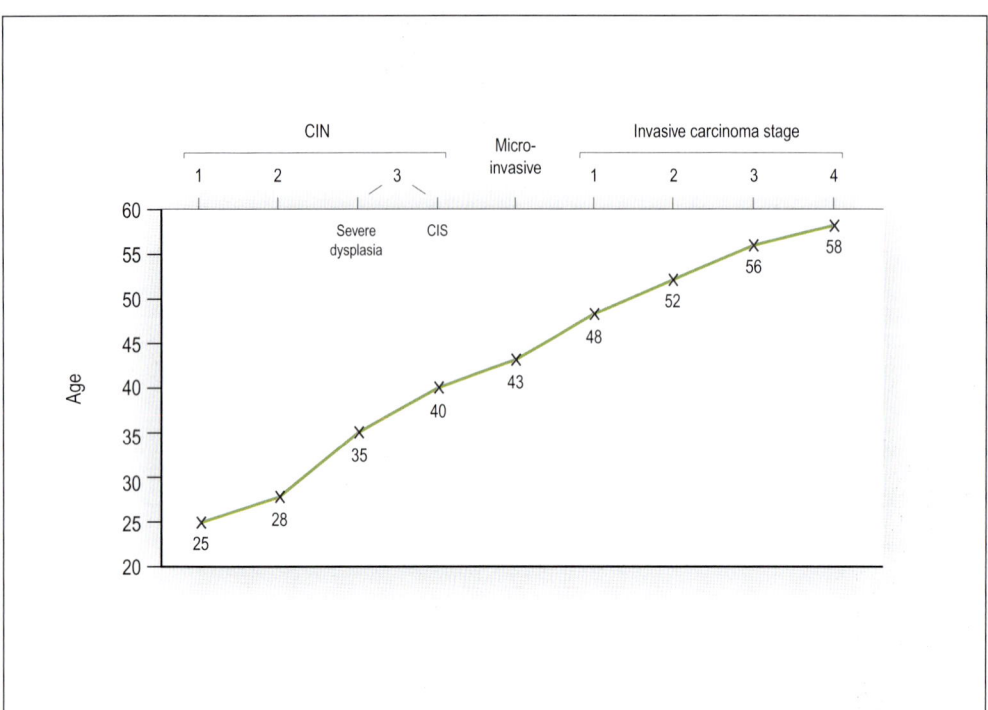

Fig. 8.65 Ages of occurrence of squamous cell carcinoma of the cervix and its precursor states. Mean ages are presented for each category.

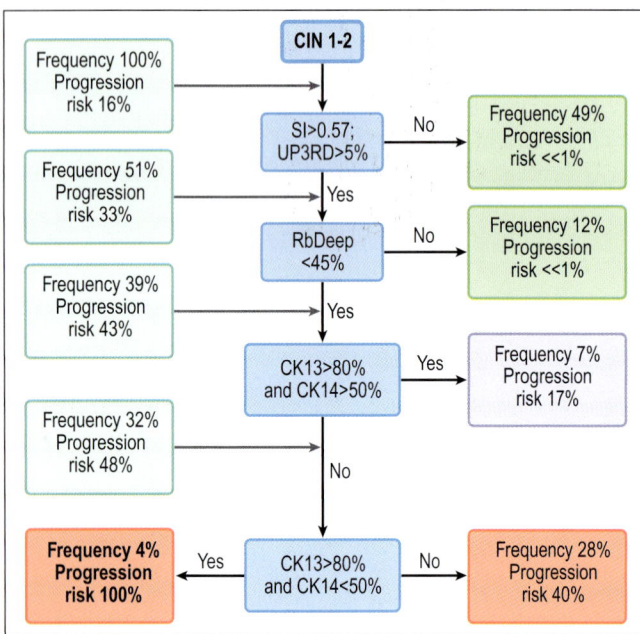

Fig. 8.66 Prognostic biomarker-based decision scheme of an early CIN lesion. Reproduced with permission from Baak et al.[8]

CIN 1 and CIN 2. If the Ki-67 SI90 exceeds 0.57 and/or the percentage of Ki-67-positive nuclei in the middle third layer of the epithelium exceeds 30%, the likelihood of progression to CIN 3 in the follow-up is high (about 30%).

- In the subsequent section, analyze the percentage of pRb-positive nuclei in the lower half of the epithelium.
- Interpret the results as follows. If the combination of Ki-67/SI90 > 0.57 occurs together with Rb < 40%,

progression risk in early CIN to CIN 3 is high (about 50%). The progression risk in the remaining patients is near zero. Moreover, in the subgroup at high risk according to Ki-67 and Rb, a combination of CK13 < 80% and CK14 < 50% epithelial cells identifies patients with an excessively high progression risk. In the other patients, the cytokeratins are not informative.

Analysis of late CIN lesions

- The results for CIN 2 and 3 are promising, but have not been validated to the same degree as for low-grade CIN.
- Evaluate the percentage of pRb and p53 reactive nuclei in the deep half of the epithelium.
- If the percentage of pRb nuclei exceeds 40%, or the percentage of p53 nuclei exceeds 15%, the likelihood of regression is high.
- All other CIN 2–3 lesions will probably persist or even progress.
- Moreover, if the pRb and p53 are low, the likelihood of concurrent high-grade CGIN is much higher than if either the pRb or p53 is low.

OTHER HISTOLOGIC FINDINGS AFFECTING MANAGEMENT AND PROGNOSIS

When contemplating management, it is vital to remember that CIN affects gland crypts in addition to the surface epithelium (Figures 8.67–8.69). The greater the grade, the greater are the number and depth of involved crypts. In CIN 3 cone biopsy specimens, nearly 90% have involved crypts.[5] The mean depth of involvement is 1.2 mm, but 5% extend deeper than 3 mm and some even reach a depth of over 5.2 mm.[95] We have seen cases even greater than 6 mm deep.

Extreme care must be taken not to mistake crypt involvement for invasive cancer. When the CIN involves only a portion

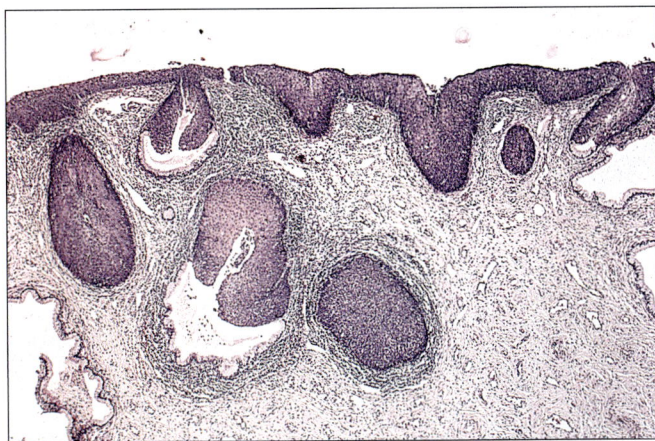

Fig. 8.67 CIN 3 with endocervical crypt involvement. Several crypts are only partially replaced; the endocervical mucosa remains intact. Where the CIN 3 has replaced in entirety the crypt, the smooth perimeter indicates that the lesion is *in situ* and has not invaded into the stromal wall of the cervix.

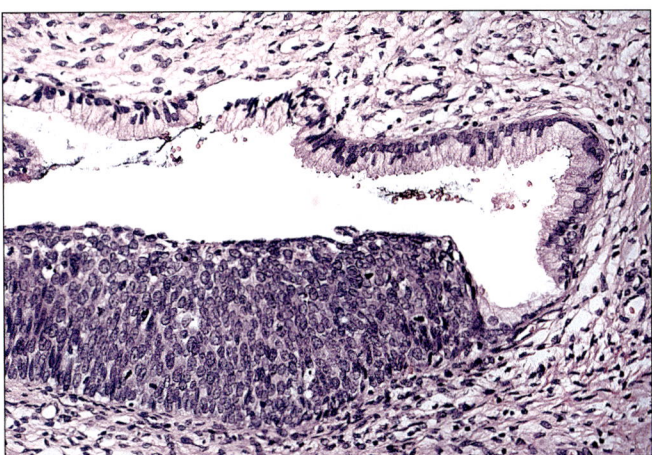

Fig. 8.69 CIN 3 with endocervical crypt involvement.

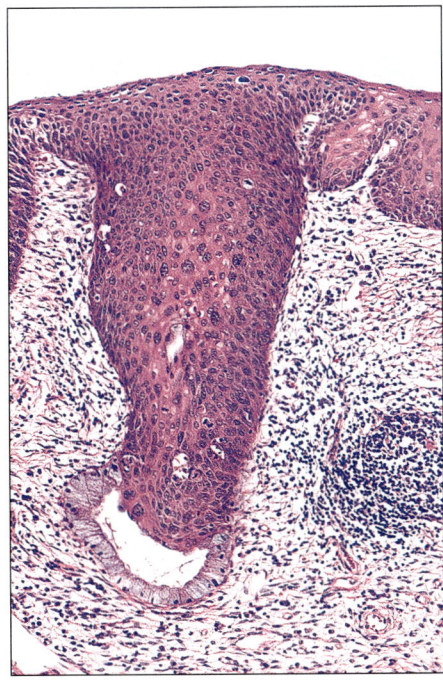

Fig. 8.68 CIN 3 with endocervical crypt involvement. The perimeter is smooth, indicative that the CIN is replacing the gland crypt rather than invading into the underlying stroma.

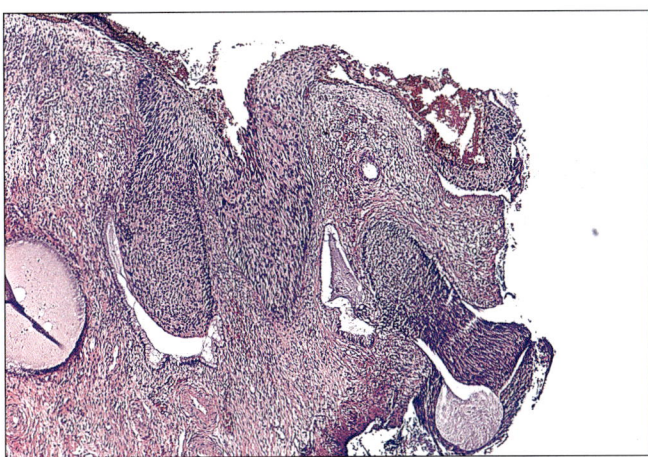

Fig. 8.70 CIN 3 involving resection margin.

of the crypt, thus exposing some of the lining composed of mucinous columnar cells, the correct diagnosis is usually obvious. Difficulties arise when the CIN replaces the crypts in their entirety, especially in a biopsy specimen. In this instance the clue that the disease process is not invasive cancer, but CIN that involves a crypt, lies with its shape. Crypts that are involved have perimeters that are round to oblong and smooth, reflecting that the normal crypt lining has been replaced. Sometimes the crypt diameter may be expanded slightly. The stroma about the crypt is normal. Tumor that is invasive usually has irregular and sharply angulated borders. It is difficult to give precise guidelines regarding stroma that surrounds the tumor when it

is slightly desmoplastic or even heavily inflamed. While always disconcerting for invasion, we have seen many examples of CIN 3 where there is a markedly edematous stroma and inflammatory reaction about the glands without any concrete sign of invasion.

Not infrequently, cone biopsy specimens disclose CIN 3 either reaching to the resection margins or involving the endocervical crypts (Figure 8.70), both of which may confer an increased risk of residual disease. Residual squamous dysplasia is detected in 8–85% of women with positive margins on cone biopsy and in 0–55% of women with negative margins.[35] In a study of 782 women treated for CIN with large loop excision, 9% of margins were involved, but within 2 years, the treatment failure rate was 30%.[69] With uninvolved margins, 5% of these patients proved to still have residual disease. Endocervical glandular involvement, age exceeding 40 years, and the presence of satellite lesions were all identified as independent risk factors for the appearance of a subsequent lesion. Among a cohort of 390 patients, 22% had recurrent CIN 3 or developed invasive carcinoma after cold knife conization with positive margins. Persistent or recurrent disease was more common in women with both ectocervical and endocervical margin involvement as opposed to singular ectocervical or endocervical positive margins.[64,79] Because of this, we generally remark in our

215

reports if the dysplasia comes with 0.1–0.5 mm of the resection margin, the number varying by institution.

If an endocervical curettage was positive for CIN, 54% had high-grade CIN with cone biopsy.[57] A retrospective study of 152 women who underwent ECC at the time of conization concluded that only the endocervical margin status predicted residual disease (and not ECC).[77a]

In one study where hysterectomy was performed soon after the cone biopsy, 61% of patients who had both involved margins and involved crypts had residual CIN (29% of women with uninvolved margins and crypts also had residual CIN in the hysterectomy specimen).[21a] In a second phase of the same investigation, women treated with cone biopsy alone were followed over a long period. Of women with both involved margins and involved crypts, 23% developed a subsequent recurrence, which compared to only 8% of women in whom both the margins and crypts were initially normal. The average time to the first recurrence was 2.2 years. In predicting recurrence, positive margins and involved crypts were each found to be independent prognostic factors with equal predictive value.

With knowledge that the status of the endocervical margin can have a substantial effect on immediate therapy and later disease progression, a lively debate has ensued over the years about the wisdom of using frozen sections to examine cone biopsy specimens.[11] The consensus has been that complete examination of specimens by frozen section is less thorough than if the specimen is first fixed in formalin and then carefully blocked. It is the common experience that cone specimens cut into 12 or more pieces not infrequently show only a small focus of high-grade CIN which would easily have been missed by frozen section examination. In the example shown, the entire focus of CIN 3 was under 1 mm in total size (Figure 8.71). Frozen-section examination of large specimens is also tedious in effort and expense. However, in those institutions where frozen-section evaluation of the endocervical margins is performed routinely, the overall experience has been highly satisfactory.[13] A number of institutions also report excellent correlation between the frozen sections and permanent sections in cases of CIN 3[27] and microinvasive cancer.[25] Yet the artifacts and tissue loss at frozen section can compromise the evaluation of early invasion. Furthermore, rarely will the astute gynecologist need to alter the approach based on the finding of micro-

invasion. Hence, frozen-section evaluation of conization is generally discouraged.

An obvious concern in the management of CIN is to ensure that the therapy is not excessive for the degree of abnormality present. Conversely, it is important not to treat lesions inadequately and miss an occult carcinoma as a result. In a meta-analysis examining the use of various diagnostic techniques, both punch biopsy and cone biopsy with or without colposcopy missed significant numbers of invasive cancers (Table 8.8).[95]

In one of the largest case series, 2.7% of 600 patients with CIN 3 had invasive carcinomas detected in a subsequent cone biopsy specimen.[53] Another 1% had microinvasive carcinomas. The major features identified in CIN 3 associated with the latter were:[2]

- extensive involvement of surface epithelium, often with multiquadrant disease
- deep involvement of endocervical crypts by expansile CIN 3
- luminal necrosis.

One study has shown that the mean size of CIN 3 lesions exhibiting microinvasion is seven times greater than if invasion were absent and 100-fold greater than with CIN 1.[97] Several studies have shown that care must also be exercised to remove the entire lesion when locally destructive methods are used in the treatment of high-grade CIN. In a multicenter retrospective study, the British Society for Colposcopy and Cervical Pathology identified 49 women who subsequently developed invasive carcinoma following therapy with laser vaporization, cold coagulator, diathermy or cryosurgery.[4] Most of these tumors were ascribed to failure to recognize the early invasive disease at the time the patients were initially assessed. Fortunately, radical reoperation has been performed in these patients with low morbidity and excellent cure rates.[6]

REGRESSION AND PROGRESSION TO INVASIVE CARCINOMA

Regression Practical data are difficult to find regarding the transit times from dysplasia to invasive carcinoma. In one of the better older studies,[80] the median transit times for progression from mild (CIN 1), moderate (CIN 2), and severe (CIN 3) dysplasia to CIS (CIN 3) were 5 years (58 months), 3 years (38 months), and 1 year (12 months), respectively. The regression rate for the high-grade abnormality reverting to normal

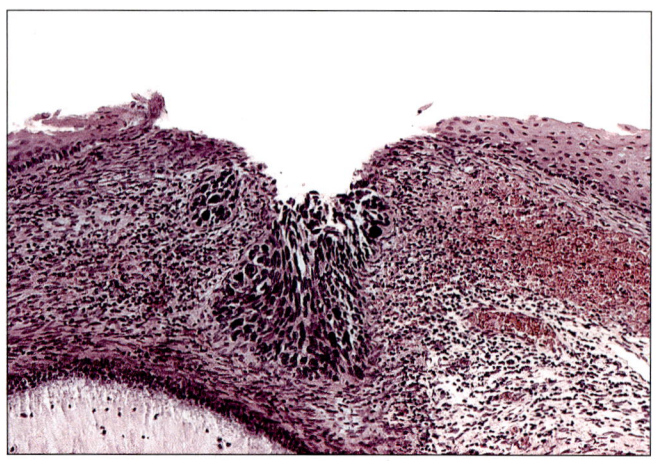

Fig. 8.71 Focus of CIN 3 under 1 mm in total size.

Table 8.8 Occult invasive cancer as an unexpected finding after biopsy or conization[95]

Procedure	Total patients (*n*)	Patients with more severe lesion on subsequent surgical specimen (%)	Invasive lesions missed (%)
Punch biopsy	4334	16.7	6.0
Colposcopically directed biopsy	1930	4.0	0.8
Cone biopsy without invasive cancer	1734	?	2.1

was 6%, a lower number than anticipated, attributed to the fact that biopsies were not taken. It was believed that removing even a small piece of tissue from a field of CIN materially altered the disease's natural history. In contrast, others found higher regression rates:[36] 50% of patients followed by cytology and biopsy experienced regression during the next 10 years. In the same interval, only 1.4% of all patients with dysplasia showed progression to CIS. In part the rates of progression and regression are related to the initial severity of the CIN, as shown by a meta-analysis of all papers published since 1950[67] (Table 8.7).

In a more recent study based on a historical cohort of women whose Papanicolaou smear histories were recorded continuously between 1962 and 1980, and during which time CIN was managed conservatively, both CIN 1 and CIN 2 were more likely to regress (usually within 2 years) than to progress. The risk of progression from CIN 1 to CIN 3 or worse was only 1% per year, but the risk of progression from CIN 2 was 16% within 2 years and 25% within 5 years, in agreement with meta-analyses.[67] Most of the excess risk for carcinomas developing from CIN 2 or 3 occurred within the first 2 years after the initial cervical abnormality was identified.[31]

Two decades ago, it was generally assumed that the progression through CIN grades occurred incrementally, starting as CIN 1 and over many years progressing through CIN 2 to CIN 3 before becoming invasive. However, this is not based on actual observations, and with the current state of technologies is also impossible to prove. The biopsies necessary to confirm the diagnoses on each occasion would destroy the tissue under study and colposcopic observations are insufficiently reliable to diagnostically render such a claim. Moreover, there are very rare reports of cases in which CIN 2 and even CIN 1 have apparently developed directly into invasive carcinoma, without reaching the stage of CIN 3. It is possible that a small, very aggressive, newly formed clone of abnormal cells appearing in the deeper epithelium becomes genetically changed, driving the daughter cells into an invasive behavior so that these lesions immediately invade, bypassing CIN 3. On the basis of such observations, some have argued for treating all patients who have CIN, irrespective of its degree, but this would mean enormous overtreatment and has not been widely adopted. Also, it has never been fully excluded that the lesions were adequately sampled.

Progression   In the natural history of CIN, the relationship of CIN to invasive carcinoma is also important. The two assumptions that (1) a significant proportion of women with CIN would eventually develop invasive carcinoma if not treated, and (2) most invasive squamous cell carcinomas are preceded by a demonstrable intraepithelial phase, have been the basis of cervical screening programs to detect CIN by cytology and allow treatment during the preinvasive phase. Clearly, the goal of early treatment is to eradicate squamous cell carcinoma in a preinvasive state. Despite cervical screening being the most effective cancer preventive program currently available, total eradication has not been obtained. There are numerous reasons why this hope has not been fully realized, including poor coverage by the screening programs of the population most at risk, poor quality of the screening, and the possibility that some invasive carcinomas may not be preceded by a demonstrable preinvasive phase. Even so, a woman who has had even one screening during her lifetime will have nearly a six-fold lower incidence rate of cervical cancer (decreasing from about 34 to 4.2/100 000 women-years).[23]

Several works provided some of the earlier insights into the relationship between CIN and invasive carcinoma. One highly quoted study showed that 14% of 59 women whose CIS (now CIN 3) remained untreated developed invasive carcinoma. It was later admitted that many of the original diagnoses were incorrect and that only 14 of the patients had acceptable CIS. Thus the percentage rose to 57%, i.e., 8 of 14 women developed invasive carcinoma over a period of 10 years. Later still, it was reported that 31 of these women had been followed for at least 12 years and that 22 (71%) of them had developed invasive disease.[41] Other reports from that time were similar.[72] Of 127 women with 'epithelial atypia', 26% ultimately developed invasive carcinoma. In a fuller account of the same patients, it was admitted that only 67 had a recognizable abnormality still present at the end of the first year of follow-up. Of the 67 who remained in the series, two-thirds eventually developed invasive carcinoma. While the more recent amended rates are rarely quoted, they may well provide a more reliable indication of the malignant potential of CIN than their earlier and more widely quoted figures. Most investigations have found that the time for progression from CIN 3 to occult invasive cancer takes between 5 and 25 years, with most series reporting times of over 10 years. Estimates of transit time from CIN to microinvasive/subclinical carcinoma are about 10 years with another 4–5 years elapsing until the tumor causes symptoms.[30]

These estimates are in accord with the average ages when women develop CIN (25–40 years), microinvasive carcinoma (43 years), stage 1 squamous cell carcinoma (48 years), and stage 4 squamous cell carcinoma (58 years) (Figure 8.65).

A common issue in evaluating the natural progression of CIN is the effect introduced by both biopsy and conization. The former can theoretically affect the diseased tissues that remain in place, while conization certainly can ablate all tissues, removing the entire lesion. To overcome the difficulty that the method of diagnosis may interfere with the natural history of the disease, 52 women were traced who had positive smears diagnosed at least 2 years previously but had had neither biopsies nor any treatment.[38] Ten of these women (19%) developed invasive carcinoma, including some preclinical invasive carcinomas.

A notable study involved 948 women who had CIS (CIN 3) diagnosed by histology, most of whom had cone biopsies.[58,71] Of this group, 131 continued to have abnormal cytology, indicative of residual disease. No further treatment was given to these patients but they were followed closely. After 10 years, 18% had developed invasive carcinoma and after 20 years, the number had risen to 36%. Of those whose cytology was normal after the initial treatment, 1.5% developed invasive carcinoma and 0.8% developed recurrent CIS. One explanation of the latter figures is that the propensity to develop new disease may remain where there is some residual infection or other promoting factors (relative risk of 3.2). A recent retrospective study of 33 women revealed that the invasive cancer was in 67% and 94% of women within 5 and 10 years, respectively, after their CIN/CGIN was treated.[26]

The figures quoted for the progression from CIN to invasive carcinoma thus vary widely, from 0.17 to 71%. Several difficulties exist in characterizing this relationship. First, all reliable methods for diagnosing CIN involve the removal of tissue with the associated risk of interfering with the disease's natural progression. Second and more importantly is an ethical consideration. Once it becomes apparent that there is a substantial risk of a woman developing invasive carcinoma from unattended CIN, it is unthinkable not to provide treatment. Because currently available methods to assess follow-up are destructive (biopsy), progression to cancer cannot be observed and therefore precise rates of progression from CIN to invasive carcinoma are now virtually impossible to determine. Another factor to consider when evaluating follow-up studies, making certain conclusions difficult, is that the invasive or higher grade lesions may be unrelated to the original lesion, but caused by reinfection.

In examining the natural history of CIN following conization, caution must be exercised in attributing the reappearance of an abnormality to the development of new disease. In one large study, 672 women were treated with conization for CIS and had resection margins free of tumor.[53] Of this group, 4% had abnormal smears detected within 3 months and 5% within 1 year, suggesting that the original tumor had never been fully resected. Another 2.5% developed abnormal smears during the ensuing 2–6 years. In general, the recurrence rate and time of recurrence were strongly correlated with the presence or absence of initial disease in the resection margins (Table 8.9).

During the past several decades disquieting new trends have developed. Since the 1960s and the era of the 'sexual revolution' in the United States and elsewhere, the average age of CIN development has begun falling progressively, such that the averages for CIN 1, CIN 2, and CIN 3 fell to between 25 and 30 years of age and more recently even further. There is concern that the age when invasive carcinoma will develop will drop also. The second issue involves reports of young women developing invasive carcinoma of the cervix after recent prior negative cytology.[16,76] Some of these lesions have been called rapidly progressive cancer, a condition discussed elsewhere (see Chapter 9).

There are several explanations for these findings. Some of the smears were probably false negatives that would have been found to contain malignant cells or at least dysplastic cells on review. Others may have been genuine false negatives, in which either the cytologic sample was inadequate, the tumor was located high in the endocervical canal, or the tumor did not exfoliate cells and none were present in the smears (discussed above).[33] However, it is impossible to escape the conclusion that at least some of these women had true progression from a normal histology to invasive carcinoma. This has occurred in a short period between the collection of the smear and the diagnosis of the carcinoma, sometimes in less than a year. It seems reasonable to speculate that, although the mean time interval for the progression through CIN to invasive carcinoma

may be 10–15 years, a few women will fall at the two extremes of the distribution curve of the length of natural history. Some may have such a long natural history that progression to invasion will never occur in the course of their lifetime; these women would be categorized as non-progressive. On the other hand, there may be those women at the other extreme, in whom the natural history of the disease runs a very rapid course, measured in months rather than years. These may be the patients described in the above reports. Indeed, very rarely do women under age 20 develop rapidly lethal invasive cancer. This hypothesis presumes that one disease process is occurring and that the difference in the behavior in different women is the result of extreme variations in the length of the natural history of the same disease. Another suggestion for which there are only preliminary data is that certain HPV types associated with cervical cancer intrinsically foster short transit time. This may correlate with the finding that HPV type 18 is rarely detected in cases of high-grade CIN, but commonly in cervical cancers that have metastasized.[52]

COLPOSCOPY, A TECHNIQUE (SOMEWHAT) USEFUL FOR DETECTION OF CIN

CORRELATION BETWEEN CYTOLOGY AND HISTOLOGY

Since the publication in 1987 by the *Wall Street Journal* about incorrectly read cytology smears, there has been increased awareness of quality and liability issues associated with the Papanicolaou smear. A substantial literature has accumulated since that time, as exemplified by a symposium in 1997 on that subject by the College of American Pathologists.[40] One common theme was the question of what constitutes an error or false-negative smear. While most false-negative rates were between 2% and 28%,[65] the issue often is far more subtle. In evaluating these rates, it is important to understand what components are truly being measured. If a patient has cancer but the smear truly contains no abnormal cells, is this a false negative? Equally perplexing is the question whether to include or exclude consideration of cells considered ASCUS or those cells showing signs of HPV infection, or even low-grade CIN itself.

A theme implicit in most articles is that histologic findings are always correct and that therefore histology is the gold standard. While it is beyond the scope of this chapter to examine this subject in detail, several studies have shown convincingly that the findings in tissue biopsies and cervical smears are complementary.[93] An abnormal finding by either modality should not be dismissed as artifact when not confirmed by the other. In a prospective examination of 3404 paired biopsies and cytologic smears, 481 paired cases (14%) had discordant diagnoses, defined as differing by more than one degree of CIN or as CIN or carcinoma identified by only one modality.[33] Eighteen initial diagnostic differences arose from cytologic screening errors, 16 from interpretive errors by staff pathologists, and one from superficial initial histologic sections. Of these, 33 involved lesions with CIN 1. Only two involved high-grade CIN (0.06%); both smears initially interpreted as atrophy were in fact examples of CIN 3. (Perhaps even this could have been prevented by routinely using additional biomarkers, such as MIB1 and p16, in case of 'atrophic' smears.) The remaining examples of discordance resulted from sampling differences.

Table 8.9 Reappearance of disease after conization[53]			
Results of follow-up	Free margins	Ambiguous margins	Involved margins
Women treated by conization for CIS (n)	672	40	6
Abnormal <3 months	3.6%	20%	100%
Abnormal 4 months–1 year	1.3%	12.5%	–
Abnormal >1.1 year	2.5%	0%	–

The cytologic smear contained the diagnostic lesion in 40% of the cases and the surgical biopsy detected the remainder, emphasizing the utility of pairing these sampling techniques in patients at risk for CIN. Not infrequently, the discordant, but verified finding of an abnormality on cytopathology alone led to re-examination of the patient and discovery of a preneoplastic lesion somewhere in the endocervical canal. Clearly, if cytologic and histologic diagnoses are discordant but valid independently, then the diagnosis of the more advanced disease state should be favored for purposes of patient safety.

DISTRIBUTION AND SITE OF ORIGIN OF CIN

Cervical neoplasia is thought in most cases to arise within the transformation zone, a term used in colposcopy to define the area between the original and new (current) squamocolumnar junction. The 'original' squamocolumnar junction is the border demarcating the native embryologic squamous epithelium found on the ectocervix and the mucinous columnar epithelium lining the endocervix. In most women, over time, some of the columnar epithelium is replaced by metaplastic squamous epithelium, so that a 'new' squamocolumnar junction forms between it and the residual (original) mucinous endocervical columnar epithelium (see Chapter 5). Since light microscopy cannot be used reliably to distinguish between original squamous epithelium and mature, glycogenated but metaplastic squamous epithelium, the concept of the 'last cervical gland' was devised.[18] The last cervical gland indicates the most distal (outer, vaginal or caudal) extent of the original endocervical-type columnar epithelium and thus is the most useful clue to the location of the original squamocolumnar junction. It is postulated that abnormalities present in the squamous epithelium distal to the last gland have arisen in squamous epithelium that was 'original' (native), while those that are proximal have arisen in the metaplastic squamous epithelium that transformed from the original glandular epithelium.

Measurements have shown that most CIN occurs proximal to the last gland. In half of the cases, the most proximal (cranial) boundary of the CIN is before the last endocervical gland and one-third end at the last gland. Only one-sixth appear to be located entirely distal to the last gland.[18] In virtually all of the latter, their proximal borders end at the last gland. This observation has been put forward to support the concept that the last gland divides two embryologically distinct epithelia, a concept yet to be verified. It is suggested that each field acts independently, and each differs concerning the histologic types of intraepithelial neoplasia that usually develop. CIN that arises in the transformation zone or the endocervix is mostly non-keratinizing (usually large cell type). It is proposed that these intraepithelial neoplasias originate in the basal cells of the transformation zone or the endocervical reserve cells, and reflect where immature squamous metaplasia and reserve cell hyperplasia occur. The carcinomas found distal to the last gland more often are keratinizing, suggesting that these neoplasias have arisen from the basal layer of the original (native) squamous epithelium. Under 10% of invasive squamous cell carcinomas arise from the original squamous epithelium.[68] Similarly, 11% of microinvasive squamous cell carcinomas arise from the original squamous epithelium.

Most studies have shown that CIN lesions are small, but increase in size with the severity of the disease. CIN 3 lesions average 2.5 mm with an average linear extent of 6.3 mm. Sixty-five per cent of CIN 3 lesions involve two or more quadrants. Approximately 10–25% of lesions that arise in the transformation zone extend more than 1 cm into the endocervical canal. An occasional case may exceed 4 cm. In one study, nearly all lesions involved the anterior or posterior lips (94%), and fewer the lateral edges (38%),[29] which affects how biopsies are taken.[3] Other more recent studies have shown CIN 2–3 to be randomly distributed,[55] or slightly more common posteriorly than anteriorly, but equally laterally right and left lateral edges.[77] Based on results from the ALTS (ASCUS/LSIL Triage Study for Cervical Cancer) studies, CIN occurred more commonly on the anterior and posterior lips, but the data were confounded by the tendency for these areas to be more often acetowhite in the absence of CIN.[28] Of course patient age and presenting morphology bias all of these measurements.

Colposcopic paradigm With this background, epithelial abnormalities of the cervix are initially recognized by exfoliative cytology, further evaluated by colposcopy and definitively diagnosed by histology. The indication for referral for colposcopy in nearly all cases is an abnormal cervical smear. This section presents a broad outline of the principles involved and discusses briefly the important part that the colposcopic examination plays in the management of women with preclinical neoplasia of the cervix.

Colposcopy is a technique for examining the cervix using relatively low, stereoscopic magnification and bright illumination. All colposcopes have a movable base, adjustable supporting arm, bright light source and variable magnification. The colposcopic examination is usually carried out as an outpatient procedure. The cervix is exposed using a speculum and, after being gently cleaned with saline on a cotton wall ball, is examined with the colposcope. Topography, vascular pattern, color, and surface contour are all observed, both before and after the application of acetic acid. Lugols iodine is often applied at the end of the colposcopic examination to identify glycogenated and non-glycogenated epithelium.

Using these features a colposcopist can assess the degree of CIN abnormality and identify an early invasive carcinoma, at the same time selecting the most appropriate sites for punch biopsy so that a precise histologic diagnosis may be made. Colposcopy also enables the lesional extent to be determined accurately. An atypical transformation zone may extend off the cervix into the vaginal fornices or even, very occasionally, some way down the vaginal walls.

The uses of colposcopy can be summarized as:

- To determine the extent and distribution of the lesion.
- To select the sites for directed biopsy.
- To confirm the cytologic findings.
- To rule out invasive carcinoma.

COLPOSCOPIC APPEARANCES

NORMAL COLPOSCOPIC FINDINGS

The normal colposcopic findings are: the original squamous epithelium, the original columnar epithelium, and squamous metaplasia (the typical transformation zone).

ORIGINAL SQUAMOUS EPITHELIUM

Normal original squamous epithelium presents a uniform, relatively featureless appearance with a smooth surface contour, which does not become white after the application of acetic acid (Figures 8.72 and 8.73). The vessels are usually inconspicuous and are mostly of hairpin type, showing one ascending and one descending branch of very fine caliber, forming a small loop. If the surface epithelium is thin, it is sometimes possible to observe the whole loop by colposcopy. Generally only the tip of the loop is visible, so that these hairpin capillaries are usually seen as regularly and densely arranged small dots.

COLUMNAR EPITHELIUM

Normal columnar epithelium is easily recognized by its characteristic grape-like or villous appearance. Before application of acetic acid, the colposcopist will see that each columnar epithelial villus contains a fine capillary. As the villus is covered by no more than a single layer of columnar cells, the blood in the capillary gives columnar epithelium its typically red appearance. Following application of acetic acid, the villi often appear white and swollen and are more easily recognizable (Figure 8.74).

SQUAMOUS METAPLASIA

The transformation zone in the cervix lies between the external os and the current squamocolumnar junction. It is usually covered at least in part by mature normal squamous metaplasia, but, at some earlier time, was covered by columnar epithelium. The new epithelium results from transformation of columnar to squamous epithelium, through the process of squamous metaplasia.

Mature metaplasia

Fully mature, squamous epithelium of metaplastic origin exhibits gland openings and typical branching vessels (Figure 8.75). The surface contour resembles that of original squamous epithelium so that, in the absence of prominent branching vessels, gland openings or retention cysts, distinction from original squamous epithelium may be impossible.

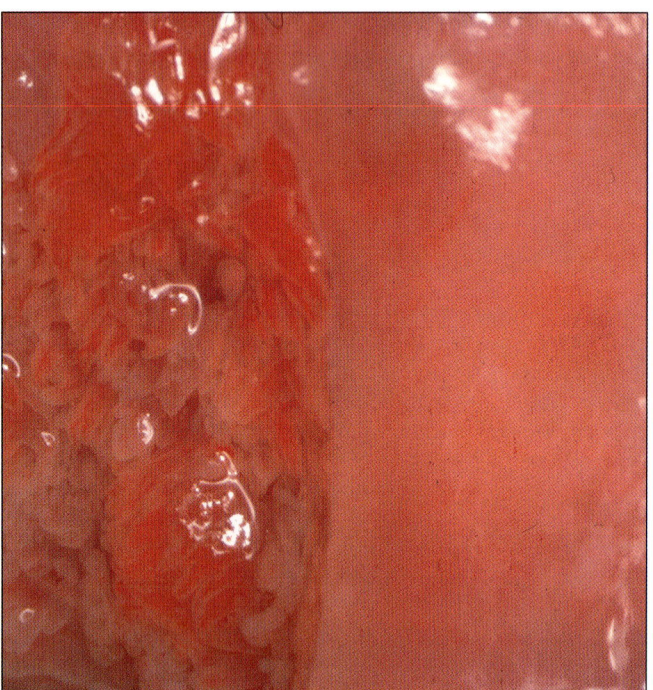

Fig. 8.72 Original squamous epithelium. On the right, the original squamous epithelium is smooth, shiny and featureless. Very fine vessels can just be discerned. The sharp squamocolumnar junction separates the squamous epithelium from the villous endocervix.

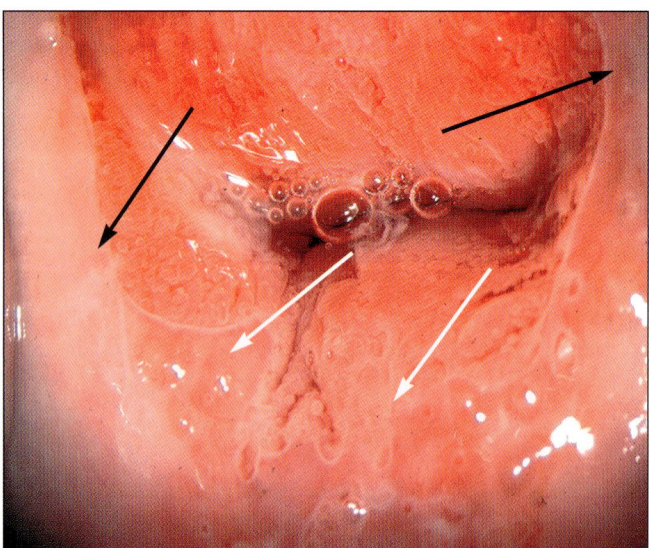

Fig. 8.73 Normal cervix. Original squamous epithelium is seen at the two lateral aspects of the cervix (black arrows). Patchy squamous metaplasia is present on the posterior lip (white arrows).

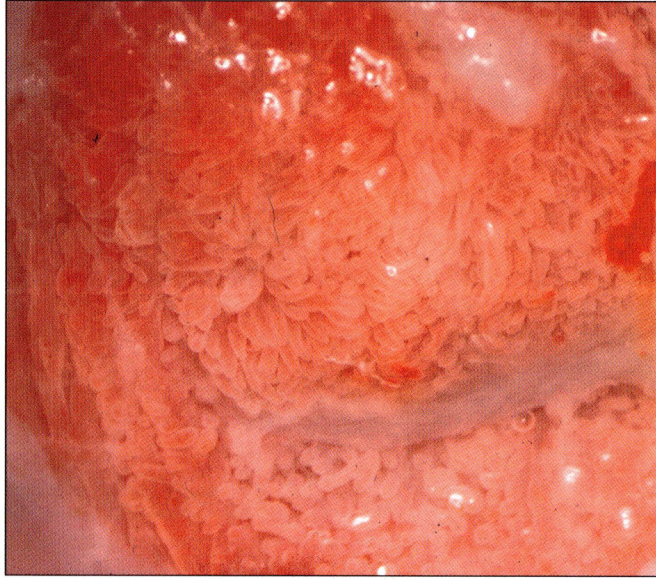

Fig. 8.74 Columnar epithelium. After application of acetic acid, the endocervical villi separate, become prominent and slightly white. Compare with Figure 6.14.

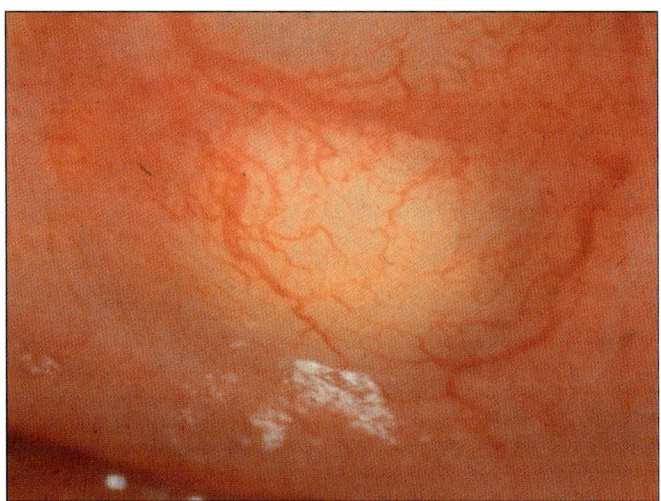

Fig. 8.75 Mature squamous metaplasia. The surface is smooth with pale retention cysts beneath it. Branched vessels are prominent.

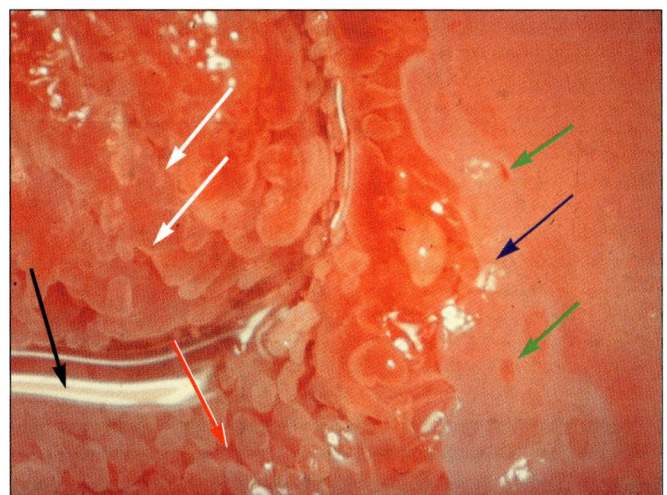

Fig. 8.76 Squamous metaplasia. Original squamous epithelium is present on the right and the transverse, slit-like external os (black arrow) is seen on the left. Normal endocervical villi are present on the posterior lip (red arrow). There is an irregular crescent of maturing squamous metaplasia adjacent to the squamocolumnar junction (blue arrow), which is slightly acetowhite and shows gland openings (green arrows). On the anterior lip are diagonal columns of very immature metaplasia (white arrows) where the endocervical villi are fused (compare this appearance with its histologic counterpart, Figure 6.26).

Immature metaplasia

Recognition of immature or active metaplasia, which is epithelium that is in the process of being transformed from columnar to squamous, is difficult to fully evaluate (Figure 8.76). The epithelium is often acetowhite and is easily confused with abnormal epithelium. Indeed, it is often difficult to differentiate between immature metaplasia and cervical intraepithelial neoplasia, especially in some conditions such as young women who were exposed to diethylstilbestrol (DES) (see Chapter 5).

The process of squamous metaplasia occurs in a patchy fashion. Cervical columnar epithelium often appears as a series of ridges and clefts. If this is the case, the epithelium along the surface of the ridges is usually the first to undergo metaplasia.

Table 8.10 Abnormal colposcopic findings

Table 8.10 Abnormal colposcopic findings

- Atypical transformation zone
  Mosaic
  Punctation
  Acetowhite epithelium
  Leukoplakia
  Atypical vessels

- Suspect frank invasive carcinoma

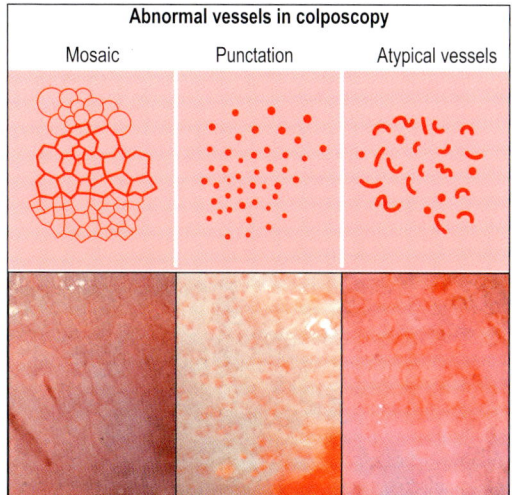

Fig. 8.77 Abnormal vessels in colposcopy.

ABNORMAL COLPOSCOPIC FINDINGS

In CIN, one or more features of the atypical transformation zone would be expected (Table 8.10). Some of these features may also occur with entities other than CIN, e.g., immature squamous metaplasia, the congenital transformation zone, and HPV infection.

MOSAIC AND PUNCTATION

These are both patterns of the small blood vessels that arise in the stromal plexus beneath the epithelium and pass into the epithelium surrounded by a very sparse stromal core (Figure 8.77). If the vessels branch and anastomose, forming a basket-like pattern around epithelial blocks, a mosaic pattern results (Figures 8.78 and 8.79). On the other hand, if the vessel travels towards the surface and then turns back again without branching, a punctation pattern will be seen (Figures 8.80 and 8.81). The two patterns often coexist on the same cervix. The degree of histologic abnormality that the epithelium shows may be roughly predicted by the intercapillary distance, the coarseness of the vessels and the regularity of the pattern. The greater the intercapillary distance, the coarser the vessels and more irregular the pattern, the more severe the histologic grade of CIN is likely to be. However, it is wrong to believe that colposcopy itself is capable of making a precise histologic diagnosis of an epithelial abnormality.[100] An experienced colposcopist can often predict the degree of abnormality present but this will not always be reliable. The final diagnosis must always be histologic.

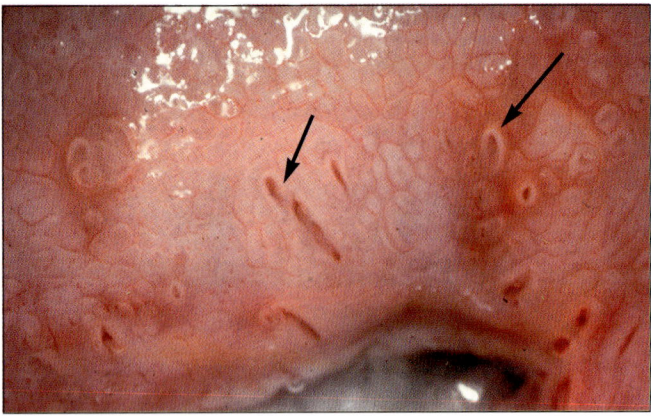

Fig. 8.78 Mosaic. The epithelium is acetowhite and there is a prominent abnormal vascular pattern of intercommunicating horizontal vessels just beneath the surface, giving rise to the mosaic appearance. Gland openings (arrows) are obvious. Biopsy showed CIN 3.

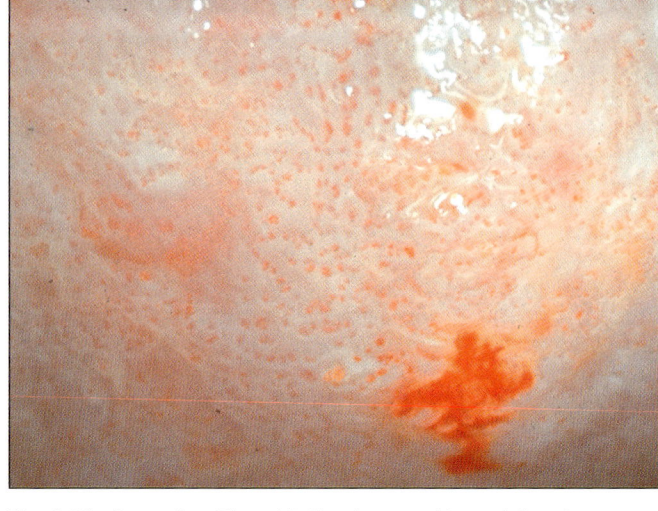

Fig. 8.81 Punctation. The epithelium is acetowhite and there is a prominent 'stippling' of vessels that do not intercommunicate. Biopsy showed CIN 3.

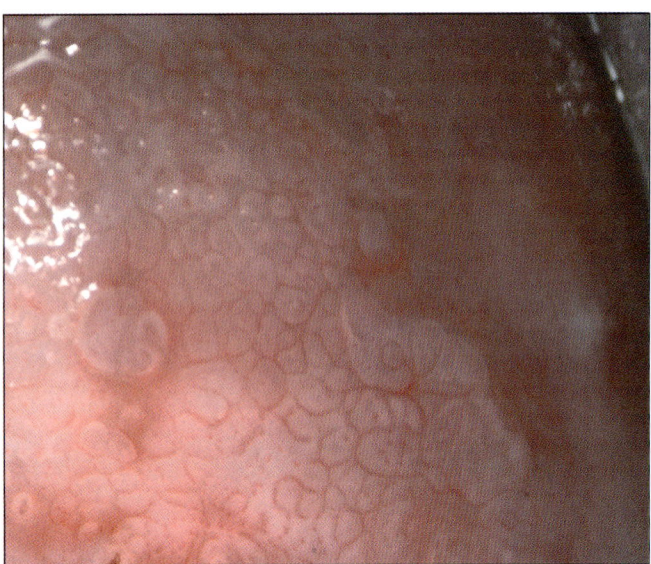

Fig. 8.79 Mosaic. Biopsy showed CIN 3.

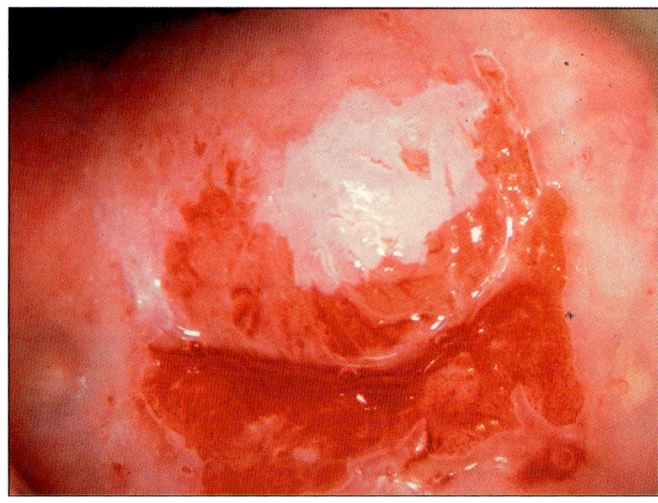

Fig. 8.82 Acetowhite epithelium. A small area of abnormal epithelium is sharply defined after the application of acetic acid. Biopsy showed CIN 3.

ACETOWHITE EPITHELIUM

Application of aqueous acetic acid (3–5%) to the cervix causes a color change when CIN (or some of the other changes listed above) are present. The acetic acid has the effect of making the abnormal epithelium appear white and opaque, whiter than it was before the application of the acetic acid and whiter than the normal epithelium after the application of acetic acid (Figures 8.82 and 8.83). The whiteness, usually referred to as 'acetowhite epithelium', is related to the amount of nuclear material present.

LEUKOPLAKIA

Leukoplakia appears as a well-defined white area, often slightly raised and with a 'waxy', shiny surface (Figure 8.84). It differs from acetowhite epithelium as it is white before acetic acid application and the acetic acid has no effect on its whiteness.

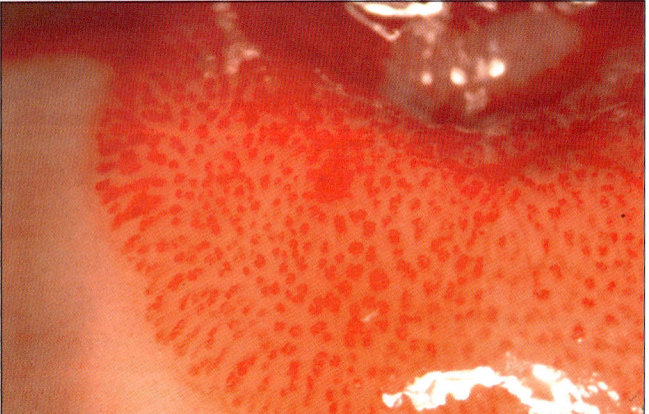

Fig. 8.80 Punctation. A sharply defined area of marked punctation is occupying the transformation zone of the posterior lip. Acetic acid has not been applied. Biopsy showed CIN 3.

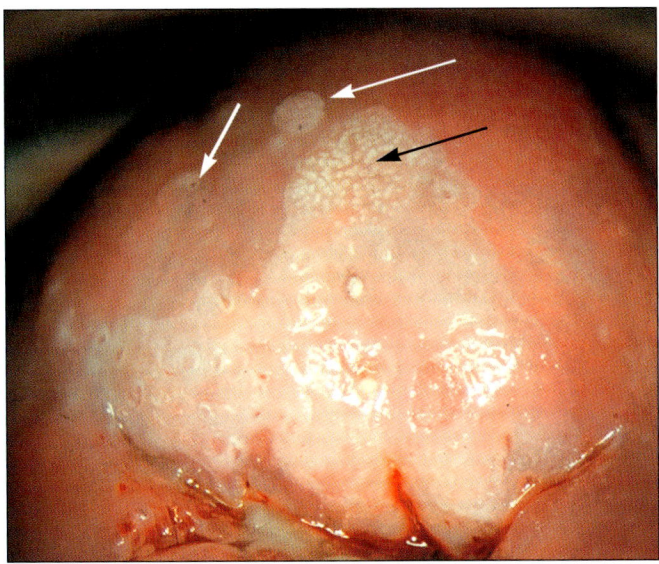

Fig. 8.83 Acetowhite epithelium. The abnormal epithelium is apparently confined to the anterior lip. One area shows white, raised 'asperities' (black arrow) and 'satellite' lesions are present (white arrows). Both these features suggest that HPV infection is present. Biopsy showed CIN 3 and HPV changes.

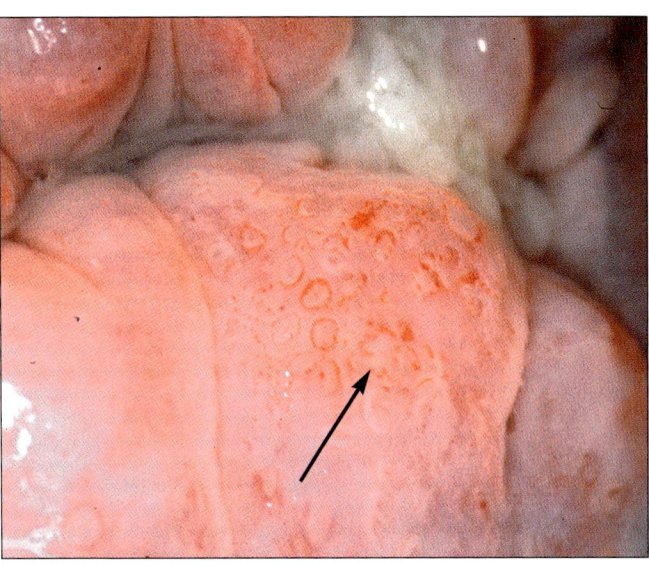

Fig. 8.85 Atypical vessels. This extensive atypical transformation zone is markedly acetowhite and shows a vascular pattern on the posterior lip that is basically a mosaic. In places (arrow) the mosaic pattern has broken and there are small, irregular, comma-shaped vessels running parallel to the surface. The surface contour is slightly nodular. These features suggest that the lesion may be more advanced than CIN. Biopsy showed microinvasive squamous carcinoma.

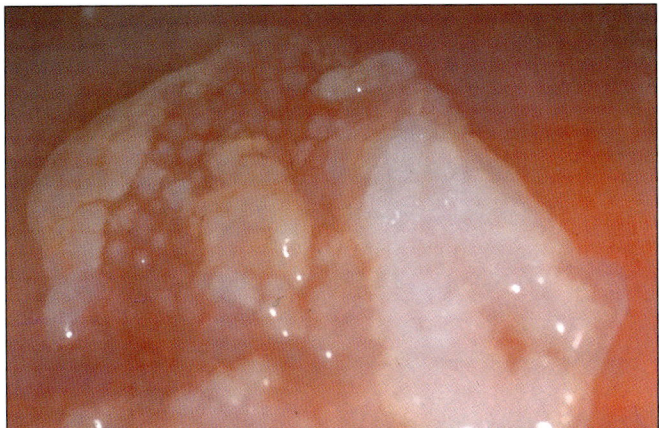

Fig. 8.84 Leukoplakia. Raised plaques that are white before the application of acetic acid are present on the anterior lip. Biopsy showed CIN 2 with keratosis.

While the finding of leukoplakia indicates keratinized epithelium, the underlying features that enable the degree of abnormality to be assessed are masked by the keratin, so that biopsy is essential.

ATYPICAL VESSELS

Atypical vessels indicate the possibility of a more advanced abnormality, perhaps early invasive carcinoma. These atypical vessels are basically punctate or mosaic patterns, but turn and run a short way parallel to the surface of the epithelium, forming commas, spirals, and irregular shapes (Figures 8.77 and 8.85).

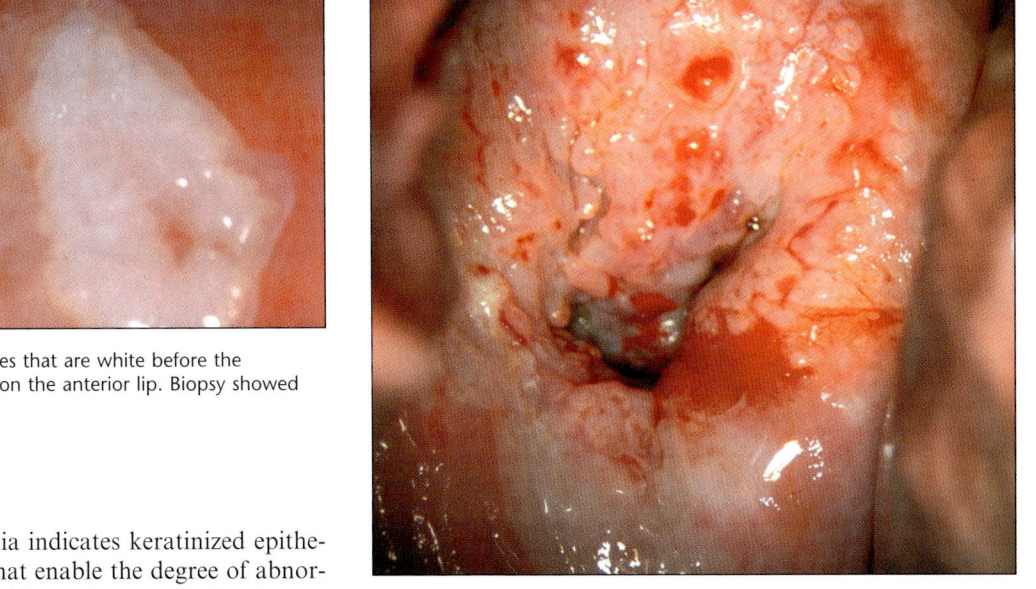

Fig. 8.86 Invasive squamous cell carcinoma. The surface is densely acetowhite and nodular, with bizarre vessels and areas of hemorrhage.

SUSPECT FRANK INVASIVE CARCINOMA

This term refers to cases where a preclinical invasive carcinoma is present, usually larger than microinvasive carcinoma. The surface contour is irregular and nodular. There is intense acetowhiteness and coarse, bizarre, and irregular vessels (Figure 8.86).

CONGENITAL TRANSFORMATION ZONE

While most areas of columnar epithelium undergoing squamous metaplasia fully mature into glycogenated squamous epithelium, showing the features described above, in some patients metaplastic change results in a persistently acetowhite epithelium that is non-glycogenated. These changes are primarily confined to the cervix, but in 4% of women they extend to involve the vagina, usually anteriorly and posteriorly.

This type of transformation zone may develop during intrauterine life, or later but prior to sexual activity, and is not associated with an increased risk of neoplastic change. It is colposcopically significant as it shares some features with CIN. The epithelium is acetowhite, has a fine mosaic pattern, and is either non-glycogenated or patchily and partially glycogenated.

OTHER COLPOSCOPIC FINDINGS

Wart virus infection

Colposcopy can identify condylomata acuminata (Figure 8.87), which need to be distinguished from invasive carcinoma, because both show nodularity of the surface contour and prominent vasculature. Biopsy of suspected condylomata is mandatory for this reason.

Non-condylomatous wart virus infection (subclinical papillomavirus infection, HPV changes) is frequently identified colposcopically. Acetowhiteness is the rule and satellite lesions are common, a feature distinguishing it from CIN. In addition, the more marked lesions show changes in surface contour, such as a cerebriform pattern (Figure 8.88) or asperities. It is often the case, however, that colposcopy alone cannot differentiate between CIN and HPV infection when all that is seen is an area of otherwise featureless acetowhite epithelium.

Glandular lesions

Cervical glandular intraepithelial neoplasia and invasive adenocarcinoma may show colposcopic abnormalities (Figure 8.89), but distinction from squamous lesions is not usually possible.

Vagina

Vaginal intraepithelial neoplasia generally shows the same colposcopic features that have been described for CIN. Acetowhiteness and punctation are often present, but a mosaic pattern is rare. Because of the area involved and the folded nature of the mucosa, full colposcopic examination of the vagina is a lengthy procedure.

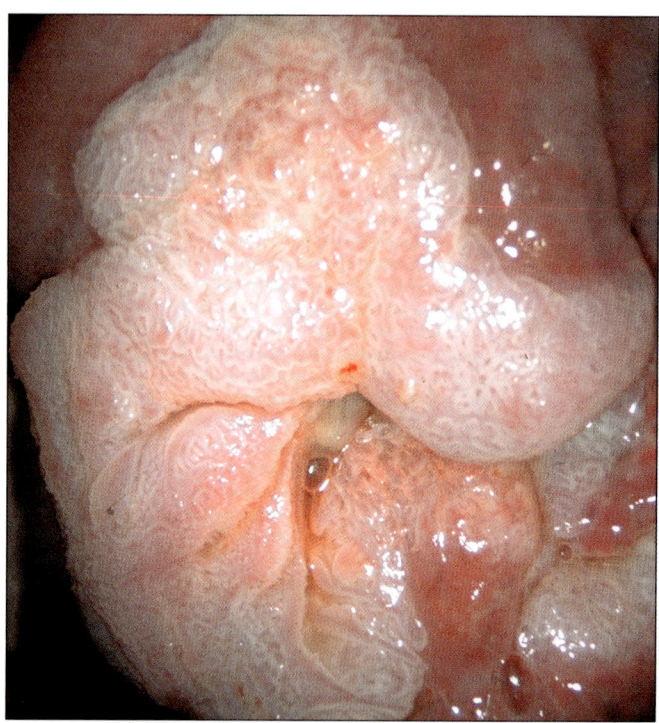

Fig. 8.88 Wart virus infection. There is an extensive raised area of acetowhite epithelium, with prominent vessels. The surface contour has been likened to the gyri of the brain, hence the term 'cerebriform'.

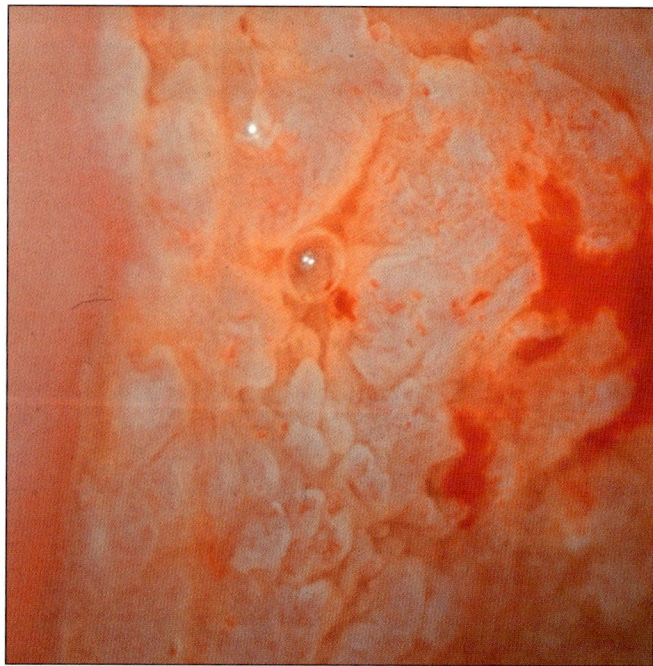

Fig. 8.89 Invasive adenocarcinoma. This example shows large, irregular villi that are acetowhite. The tissue is fragile and hemorrhage has occurred.

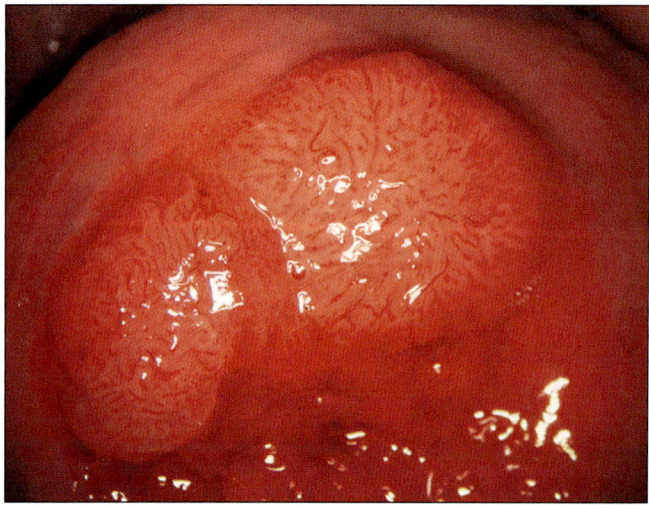

Fig. 8.87 Condyloma. Two viral warts are present on the anterior lip. They are composed of delicate, finger-like fronds, each with a central vessel.

REFERENCES

1. Al-Nafussi AI, Colguhoun MK. Mild cervical intraepithelial neoplasia (CIN 1): a histological overdiagnosis. Histopathology 1990;17:557–61.
2. Al-Nafussi AI, Hughes DE. Histological features of CIN3 and their value in predicting invasive microinvasive squamous carcinoma. J Clin Pathol 1994;47:799–804.
3. Allard JE, Rodriguez M, Rocca M, Parker MF. Biopsy site selection during colposcopy and distribution of cervical intraepithelial neoplasia. J Low Genit Tract Dis 2005;9:36–9.
4. Anderson MC. Invasive carcinoma of the cervix following local destructive treatment for cervical intraepithelial neoplasia. Br J Obstet Gynaecol 1993;100:657–63.
5. Anderson MC, Hartley RB. Cervical crypt involvement by intraepithelial neoplasia. Obstet Gynecol 1980;55:546–50.
6. Ayhan A, Otegen U, Guven S, Kucukali T. Radical reoperation for invasive cervical cancer found in simple hysterectomy. J Surg Oncol 2006;94:28–34.
7. Baak JP, Kruse AJ. Use of biomarkers in the evaluation of CIN grade and progression of early CIN. Methods Mol Med 2005;119:85–99.
8. Baak JP, Kruse AJ, Robboy SJ, Janssen EA, van Diermen B, Skaland I. Dynamic behavioural interpretation of cervical intraepithelial neoplasia with molecular biomarkers. J Clin Pathol 2006;59:1017–28.
9. Baak JP, Kruse AJ, Garland SM, et al. Combined p53 and retinoblastoma protein detection identifies persistent and regressive cervical high-grade squamous intraepithelial lesions. Am J Surg Pathol 2005;29:1062–6.
10. Baak JPA, Kruse AJ, Janssen E, van Diermen B. Ki67 predicts progression in early CIN: validation of a multivariate progression-risk model. Cell Oncol 2005;27:357.
11. Baker P, Oliva E. A practical approach to intraoperative consultation in gynecologic pathology. Int J Gynecol Pathol 2008; in press.
12. Baseman JG, Koutsky LA. The epidemiology of human papillomavirus infections. J Clin Virol 2005;32(Suppl):S16.
13. Behtash N, Karimi Zarchi M, Hamedi B, Azmoode Ardalan F, Tehranian A. The value of frozen sectioning for the evaluation of resection margins in cases of conization. Arch Gynecol Obstet 2007;276:529–32.
14. Bekkers RLM, Bulten J, Wiersma-van Tilburg A, et al. Coexisting high-grade glandular and squamous cervical lesions and human papillomavirus infections. Br J Cancer 2003;89:886–90.
15. Benevolo M, Mottolese M, Marandino F, et al. Immunohistochemical expression of p16(INK4a) is predictive of HR-HPV infection in cervical low-grade lesions. Mod Pathol 2006;19:384–91.
16. Berkeley AS, LiVolsi VA, Schwartz PE. Advanced squamous cell carcinoma of the cervix with recent normal Papanicolaou tests. Lancet 1980;ii:375–6.
17. Bravaccini S, Sanchini MA, Amadori A, et al. Potential of telomerase expression and activity in cervical specimens as a diagnostic tool. J Clin Pathol 2005;58:911–14.
18. Burghardt E, Ostor AG. Site and origin of squamous cervical cancer: a histomorphologic study. Obstet Gynecol 1983;62:117–27.
19. Castle PE, Stoler MH, Solomon D, Schiffman M. The relationship of community biopsy-diagnosed cervical intraepithelial neoplasia grade 2 to the quality control pathology-reviewed diagnoses: an ALTS report. Am J Clin Pathol 2007;127:805–15.
20. Castle PE, Sideri M, Jeronimo J, Solomon D, Schiffman M. Risk assessment to guide the prevention of cervical cancer. Am J Obstet Gynecol 2007;197:356. e1–6.
21. Crum CP, Ikenberg H, Richart RM, Gissman L. Human papillomavirus type 16 and early cervical neoplasia. N Engl J Med 1984;310:880–3.
21a. Demopoulos RI, Horowitz LF, Vamvakas EC. Endocervical gland involvement by cervical intraepithelial neoplasia grade III: predictive values for residual and/or recurrent disease. Cancer 1991;68:1932–6.
22. dos Santos L, Odunsi K, Lele S. Clinicopathologic outcomes of laser conization for high-grade cervical dysplasia. Eur J Gynaecol Oncol 2004;25:305–7.
23. Fidler HK, Boyes DA, Worth AJ. Cervical cancer detection in British Columbia. J Obstet Gynaecol Br Commonwealth 1968;75:392–404.
24. Fox H, Buckley CH. Current problems in the pathology of intra-epithelial lesions of the uterine cervix. Histopathology 1990;17:1–6.
25. Giuntoli RL, 2nd, Winburn KA, Silverman MB, Keeney GL, Cliby WA. Frozen section evaluation of cervical cold knife cone specimens is accurate in the diagnosis of microinvasive squamous cell carcinoma. Gynecol Oncol 2003;91:280–4.
26. Gornall RJ, Boyd IE, Manolitsas T, Herbert A. Interval cervical cancer following treatment for cervical intraepithelial neoplasia. Int J Gynecol Cancer 2000;10:198–202.
27. Gu M, Lin F. Efficacy of cone biopsy of the uterine cervix during frozen section for the evaluation of cervical intraepithelial neoplasia grade 3. Am J Clin Pathol 2004;122:383–8.
28. Guido RS, Jeronimo J, Schiffman M, Solomon D. The distribution of neoplasia arising on the cervix: results from the ALTS trial. Am J Obstet Gynecol 2005;193:1331–7.
29. Heatley M. Distribution of cervical intraepithelial neoplasia: are hysterectomy specimens sampled appropriately? J Clin Pathol 1995;48:323–4.
30. Herrero R, Munoz N. Human papillomavirus and cancer. Cancer Surveys 1999;33:75–98.
31. Holowaty P, Miller AB, Rohan T, To T. Natural history of dysplasia of the uterine cervix. J Nat Cancer Inst 1999;91:252–8.
32. Iaconis L, Hyjek E, Ellenson LH, Pirog EC. p16 and Ki-67 immunostaining in atypical immature squamous metaplasia of the uterine cervix: correlation with human papillomavirus detection. Arch Pathol Lab Med 2007;131:1343–9.
33. Ibrahim SN, Krigman HR, Coogan AC, et al. Prospective correlation of cervicovaginal cytologic and histologic specimens. Am J Clin Pathol 1996;106:319–24.
34. Ioffe OB, Brooks SE, DeRezende RB, Silverberg SG. Artifact in cervical LLETZ specimens: correlation with follow-up. Int J Gynecol Pathol 1999;18:115–21.
35. Jakus S, Edmonds P, Dunton C, King SA. Margin status and excision of cervical intraepithelial neoplasia: a review. Obstet Gynecol Surv 2000;55:520–7.
36. Johnson LD, Nickerson RJ, Easterday CL, Stuart RS, Hertig AT. Epidemiological evidence for the spectrum of change from dysplasia through carcinoma in situ to invasive cancer. Cancer 1968;22:901–14.
37. Jovanovic AS, Mclachlin CM, Shen LH, Welch WR, Crum CP. Postmenopausal squamous atypia: a spectrum including 'pseudo-koilocytosis'. Mod Pathol 1995;8:408–12.
38. Kinlen LJ, Spriggs AI. Women with positive cervical smears but without surgical intervention. Lancet 1978;ii:463–5.
39. Klaes R, Benner A, Friedrich T, et al. p16(INK4a) immunohistochemistry improves interobserver agreement in the diagnosis of cervical intraepithelial neoplasia. Am J Surg Pathol 2002;26:1389–99.
40. Kline TS. The Papanicolaou smear – a brief historical perspective and where we are today. Arch Pathol Lab Med 1997;121:205–9.
41. Kottmeier HL. Evolution et traitement des epitheliomas. Rev Fr Gynecol Obstet 1961;56:821–6.
42. Kruse AJ. Quantitative biomarkers to identify low- and high-risk early CIN lesions. Amsterdam: Vrije Universiteit; 2003.
43. Kruse AJ, Skaland I, Munk AC, Janssen E, Gudlaugsson E, Baak JP. Low p53 and retinoblastoma protein expression in cervical intraepithelial neoplasia grade 3 lesions is associated with coexistent adenocarcinoma in situ. Hum Pathol 2008;39(4):573–8.
44. Kruse AJ, Buhr-Wildhagen S, Janssen EA, Baak JP. The relationship between syntactic structure analysis features, histological grade and high-risk HPV DNA in cervical intraepithelial neoplasia. Cell Oncol 2004;26:135–41.
45. Kruse AJ, Baak JP, de Bruin PC, van de Goot FR, Kurten N. Relationship between the presence of oncogenic HPV DNA assessed by polymerase chain reaction and Ki-67 immunoquantitative features in cervical intraepithelial neoplasia. J Pathol 2001;195:557–62.
46. Kruse AJ, Baak JP, Helliesen T, Kjellevold KH, Robboy SJ. Prognostic value and reproducibility of koilocytosis in cervical intraepithelial neoplasia. Int J Gynecol Pathol 2003;22:236–9.
47. Kruse AJ, Baak JP, Helliesen T, Kjellevold KH, Bol MG, Janssen EA. Evaluation of MIB-1-positive cell clusters as a diagnostic marker for cervical intraepithelial neoplasia. Am J Surg Pathol 2002;26:1501–7.
48. Kruse AJ, Gudlaugsson E, Helliesen T, et al. Evaluation of prospective, routine application of Ki-67 immunoquantitation in early CIN for assessment of short-term progression risk. Anal Quant Cytol Histol 2004;26:134–40.
49. Kruse AJ, Skaland I, Janssen EA, et al. Quantitative molecular parameters to identify low-risk and high-risk early CIN lesions: role of markers of proliferative activity and differentiation and Rb availability. Int J Gynecol Pathol 2004;23:100–9.
50. Kruse AJ, Baak JP, Janssen EA, et al. Ki67 predicts progression in early CIN: validation of a multivariate progression-risk model. Cell Oncol 2004;26:13–20.
51. Kruse AJ, Baak JP, de Bruin PC, et al. Ki-67 immunoquantitation in cervical intraepithelial neoplasia (CIN): a sensitive marker for grading. J Pathol 2001;193:48–54.
52. Kurman RJ, Schiffman MH, Lancaster WD, et al. Analysis of individual human papillomavirus types in cervical neoplasia: a possible role for type 18 in rapid progression. Am J Obstet Gynecol 1988;159:293–6.
53. Larsson G. Conization for cervical dysplasia and carcinoma in situ: long term follow-up of 1013 women. Ann Chir Gynecol 1981;70:79–85.
54. Leung KM, Chan WY, Hui PK. Invasive squamous cell carcinoma and cervical intraepithelial neoplasia III of uterine cervix – morphologic differences other than stromal invasion. Am J Clin Pathol 1994;101:508–13.
55. Lurie S, Eliaz M, Boaz M, Levy T, Golan A, Sadan O. Distribution of cervical intraepithelial neoplasia across the cervix is random. Am J Obstet Gynecol 2007;196:125.e1–3.
56. Mariuzzi GM, Montironi R, Di Loreto C, Sisti S. Multiparametric quantitation of the progression of cervix preneoplasia towards neoplasia. Pathol Res Pract 1989;185:606–11.
57. Massad LS, Chronopoulos FT, Cejtin HE. Correlating cone biopsy histology with operative indications. Gynecol Oncol 1997;65:286–90.
58. McIndoe WA, McLean MA, Jones RW, Mullins PR. The invasive potential of carcinoma in situ of the cervix. Obstet Gynecol 1984;64:451–4.
59. Mittal K, Demopoulos RI, Tata M. A comparison of proliferative activity and atypical mitoses in cervical condylomas with various HPV types. Int J Gynecol Pathol 1998;17:24–8.
60. Mourits MJE, Pieters WJLM, Hollema H, Burger MPM. 3-Group metaphase as a morphologic criterion of progressive cervical intraepithelial neoplasia. Am J Obstet Gynecol 1992;167:591–5.

61. Munk AC, Kruse AJ, Van Diermen B, et al. Cervical intraepithelial neoplasia grade 3 (CIN-3) lesions can regress. AMPIS 2008: in press.

62. Murphy N, Ring M, Killalea AG, et al. p16INK4A as a marker for cervical dyskaryosis: CIN and cGIN in cervical biopsies and ThinPrep smears. J Clin Pathol 2003;56:56–63.

63. Nagar HA, Dobbs SP, McClelland HR, Price JH, McClean G, McCluggage WG. The large loop excision of the transformation zone cut or blend thermal artefact study: a randomized controlled trial. Int J Gynecol Cancer 2004;14:1108–11.

64. Narducci F, Occelli B, Boman F, Vinatier D, Leroy JL. Positive margins after conization and risk of persistent lesion. Gynecol Oncol 2000;76:311–14.

65. Naryshkin S. The false-negative fraction for Papanicolaou smears: how often are 'abnormal' smears not detected by a 'standard' screening cytologist? Arch Pathol Lab Med 1997;121:270–2.

66. Nucci MR, Castrillon DH, Bai H, et al. Biomarkers in diagnostic obstetric and gynecologic pathology: a review. Adv Anat Pathol 2003;10:55–68.

67. Ostor AG. Natural history of cervical intraepithelial neoplasia – a critical review. Int J Gynecol Pathol 1993;12:186–92.

68. Ostor AG. Studies on 200 cases of early squamous cell carcinoma of the cervix. Int J Gynecol Pathol 1993;12:193–207.

69. Paraskevaidis E, Lolis ED, Koliopoulos G, Alamanos Y, Fotiou S, Kitchener HC. Cervical intraepithelial neoplasia outcomes after large loop excision with clear margins. Obstet Gynecol 2000;95(6 Pt 1):828–31.

70. Parker MF, Zahn CM, Vogel KM, Olsen CH, Miyazawa K, O'Connor DM. Discrepancy in the interpretation of cervical histology by gynecologic pathologists. Obstet Gynecol 2002;100:277–80.

71. Paul C. The New Zealand cervical cancer study: could it happen again? Br Med J 1988;297:533–9.

72. Petersen O. Spontaneous course of cervical precancerous conditions. Am J Obstet Gynecol 1956;72:1063–71.

73. Pins MR, Young RH, Crum CP, Leach IH, Scully RE. Cervical squamous cell carcinoma in situ with intraepithelial extension to the upper genital tract and invasion of tubes and ovaries: report of a case with human papilloma virus analysis. Int J Gynecol Pathol 1997;16:272–8.

74. Poynor EA, Barakat RR, Hoskins WJ. Management and follow-up of patients with adenocarcinoma in situ of the uterine cervix. Gynecol Oncol 1995;57:158–64.

75. Prasad CJ, Sheets E, Selig AM, Mcarthur MC, Crum CP. The binucleate squamous cell – histologic spectrum and relationship to low-grade squamous intraepithelial lesions. Mod Pathol 1993;6:313–17.

76. Prendiville W, Guillebaud J, Bamford P, Beilby J, Steele SJ. Carcinoma of the cervix with recent normal Papanicolaou tests. Lancet 1980;ii:835–54.

77. Pretorius RG, Zhang X, Belinson JL, et al. Distribution of cervical intraepithelial neoplasia 2, 3 and cancer on the uterine cervix. J Low Genit Tract Dis 2006;10:45–50.

77a. Ramchandani SM, Houck KL, Hernandez E, Gaughan JP. Predicting persistent/recurrent disease in the cervix after excisional biopsy. MedGenMed 2007;9:24.

78. Reesink-Peters N, Helder MN, Wisman GBA, et al. Detection of telomerase, its components, and human papillomavirus in cervical scrapings as a tool for triage in women with cervical dysplasia. J Clin Pathol 2003;56:31–5.

79. Reich O, Lahousen M, Pickel H, Tamussino K, Winter R. Cervical intraepithelial neoplasia III: long-term follow-up after cold-knife conization with involved margins. Obstet Gynecol 2002;99:193–6.

80. Richart RM, Barron BA. A follow-up study of patients with cervical dysplasia. Am J Obstet Gynecol 1969;105:386–93.

81. Sadler L, Saftlas A, Wang W, Exeter M, Whittaker J, McCowan L. Treatment for cervical intraepithelial neoplasia and risk of preterm delivery. JAMA 2004;291:2100–6.

82. Sano T, Oyama T, Kashiwabara K, Fukuda T, Nakajima T. Expression status of p16 protein is associated with human papillomavirus oncogenic potential in cervical and genital lesions. Am J Pathol 1998;153:1741–8.

83. Sasa H, Imai K, Kudo K, Kita T, Aida S, Furuya K. A case of uterine cervical carcinoma in situ with replacement of the entire corpus endometrium. J Low Genit Tract Dis 2007;11:279–80.

84. Sato S, Okagaki T, Clark BA, Twiggs LB. Sensitivity of koilocytosis, immunocytochemistry and electron microscopy as compared to DNA hybridization in detecting human papillomavirus in cervical and vaginal condyloma and intraepithelial neoplasia. Int J Gynecol Pathol 1986;5:297–307.

85. Schiffman M, Castle PE, Jeronimo J, Rodriguez AC, Wacholder S. Human papillomavirus and cervical cancer. Lancet 2007;370:890–907.

86. Smith HO, Tiffany MF, Qualls CR, Key CR. The rising incidence of adenocarcinoma relative to squamous cell carcinoma of the uterine cervix in the United States – a 24-year population-based study. Gynecol Oncol 2000;78:97–105.

87. Snijders PJ, Steenbergen RD, Heideman DA, Meijer CJ. HPV-mediated cervical carcinogenesis: concepts and clinical implications. J Pathol 2006;208:152–64.

88. Southern SA, McDicken IW, Herrington CS. Loss of cytokeratin 14 expression is related to human papillomavirus type and lesion grade in squamous intraepithelial lesions of the cervix. Hum Pathol 2001;32:1351–5.

89. Steenbergen RDM, de Wilde J, Wilting SM, Brink AATP, Snijders PJF, Meijer CJLM. HPV-mediated transformation of the anogenital tract. J Clin Virol 2005;32(Suppl):S25–33.

90. Stoler M. The impact of human papillomavirus biology on the clinical practice of cervical pathology. Pathol Case Rev 2005;10:119–27.

91. Stoler MH. Human papillomaviruses and cervical neoplasia: a model for carcinogenesis. Int J Gynecol Pathol 2000;19:16–28.

92. Stoler MH. ASC, TBS, and the power of ALTS. Am J Clin Pathol 2007;127:489–91.

93. Stoler MH, Schiffman M. Interobserver reproducibility of cervical cytologic and histologic interpretations: realistic estimates from the ASCUS-LSIL Triage Study. JAMA 2001;285:1500–5.

94. Syrjanen KJ. Condyloma acuminatum and other HPV-related squamous cell tumors of the genitoanal area. In: Gross G, Vonkrogh G, eds. Human Papillomavirus Infections in Dermatovenereology. 2000 Corporate Blvd NW/Boca Raton/FL 33431: CRC Press; 1997:151–80.

95. Sze EHM, Rosenzweig BA, Birenbaum DL, Silverman RK, Baggish MS. Excisional conization of the cervix uteri. J Gynecol Surg 1989;5:235–68.

96. Szkaradkiewicz A, Wal M, Kuch A, Pieta P. Human papillomavirus (HPV) and Epstein–Barr virus (EBV) cervical infections in women with normal and abnormal cytology. Pol J Microbiol 2004;53:95–9.

97. Tidbury P, Singer A, Jenkins D. CIN-3 – the role of lesion size in invasion. Br J Obstet Gynaecol 1992;99:583–6.

98. Trimble CL, Piantadosi S, Gravitt P, et al. Spontaneous regression of high-grade cervical dysplasia: effects of human papillomavirus type and HLA phenotype. Clin Cancer Res 2005;11:4717–23.

99. Van Leeuwen AM, Pieters WJ, Hollema H, Burger MP. Atypical mitotic figures and the mitotic index in cervical intraepithelial neoplasia. Virchows Arch 1995;427:139–44.

100. Welch WR, Robboy SJ, Kaufman RH, et al. Pathology of colposcopic findings in 2635 diethylstilbestrol-exposed young women. Gynecol Oncol 1985;21:277–86.

101. Wright TC, Park TW. Cervical cancer and its precursors – an introduction. In: Langdon SP, Miller WR, Berchuk A, eds. Biology of Female Cancer. 2000 Corporate Blvd NW/Boca Raton/FL 33431: CRC Press; 1997:221–43.

102. Yelverton CL, Bentley RC, Olenick S, Krigman HR, Johnston WW, Robboy SJ. Epithelial repair of the uterine cervix: assessment of morphologic features and correlations with cytologic diagnosis. Int J Gynecol Pathol 1996;15:338–44.

103. Zielinski GD, Snijders PJF, Rozendaal L, et al. The presence of high-risk HPV combined with specific p53 and p16(INK4a) expression patterns points to high-risk HPV as the main causative agent for adenocarcinoma in situ and adenocarcinoma of the cervix. J Pathol 2003;201:535–43.

Cervical squamous cell carcinoma

9

Wenxin Zheng   Stanley J. Robboy

MICROINVASIVE CARCINOMA

Microinvasive carcinoma, a concept introduced over 50 years ago, refers to cancer of the cervix that is in its earliest state of invasion, and as such has a prognosis much better than the rest of stage 1 carcinomas. The difference in prognosis between microinvasive and deeply invasive cancers is central to our thinking about early carcinoma of the cervix. It raises the question of whether very early invasive carcinoma can be treated with less than a radical operation without jeopardizing the patient's chance for curative resection. If so, is it possible to define by histology the point in the growth of the tumor at which radical treatment becomes necessary? The ideal definitions of microinvasive carcinoma (stage 1A) and early clinical invasive carcinoma (stage 1B) ought to reflect this possible difference in therapeutic approach. A diagnosis of microinvasive carcinoma should indicate a tumor which, although locally invasive, has negligible, if any, potential for metastasizing. This is important since the incidence of this disease entity has risen substantially over the past 25 years. Presumably this is related to greater accessibility to and improved methods of cytologic screening, for this condition is now most often diagnosed after women present with abnormal smears interpreted as high-grade cervical intraepithelial neoplasia (CIN).

Treatment failure of early cervical cancer is of two types: local recurrence due to incomplete removal of the initial neoplasm or 'new disease' at the site, and recurrence due to metastatic disease. Both types have to be factored into decisions about therapy since they determine the surgical modes of treatment recommended, be it cone biopsy, simple hysterectomy, extrafascial hysterectomy, or radical hysterectomy with or without lymph node dissection. While this text does not explore the types of surgical approach in detail, they are introduced here for the very practical reason that the various histologic parameters are assessed in each.

STAGING

Definition

In 1994 the International Federation of Gynecologists and Obstetricians (FIGO) revised its staging system for carcinoma of the cervix (Appendix A3). Microinvasion was defined with the following two requirements:

- The tumor must be identified only by microscopic examination. Any lesion visible macroscopically on clinical examination, regardless of size, must be upstaged to at least stage 1B.
- The tumor, by direct measurement of the glass tissue slide, may invade to a maximum depth of 5 mm and a maximum width of 7 mm. Any lesion that is larger must be upstaged to at least stage 1B.

Nevertheless, the diagnostic parameters of microinvasive carcinoma remain ill defined and even in institutions where there is extensive experience in this disease, review of cases from earlier years required that about a fourth to half had to be excluded from analyses because of inadequate diagnostic criteria.[9]

History and controversy

The search for a definition of microinvasive carcinoma is the quest for histologic criteria that reliably identify the maximum extent of disease that can safely be treated in a conservative fashion. In 1937 when FIGO introduced its first clinical staging system for cervical cancer, stage 1 was defined as carcinoma strictly confined to the cervix. No further subdivisions were made. In 1964, stage 1 was divided into cases with early stromal invasion (stage 1A) and all other cases (stage 1B). In 1973, stage 1A was more narrowly defined. It was a cancer that could be diagnosed only by histologic examination. It was divided into those showing early stromal invasion (minute invasive foci), the remainder being termed 'occult' cancer.

Two central themes predominated in the controversy about microinvasive cancer:

- The biology of early cancer and the histopathologic features critical for a correct diagnosis. Recognition of confounding histopathologic features is also important, i.e., features that if present should cause the lesion to be upstaged.
- The purpose underlying the design of the classification schemes. Is the scheme designed for statistical analysis (e.g., FIGO staging) or as a guide to treatment (e.g., SGO staging)?

The FIGO classification scheme as conceived permits institutions across the world to compare the results of treatment statistically on a stage-by-stage basis. The thrust of the classification is to divide tumors into several groups, all of which are associated with statistically significant differing probabilities of survival. As such, the system is primarily an epidemiologic tool. It has never been designed to recommend treatment. More specifically, the classification should not give rise to the unrealistic expectation that the definition will guarantee the safety

227

of conservative therapy[57] and major differences in survival of patients are to be expected for each stage. Thus, larger FIGO stage 1A tumors are associated with a substantial rate of nodal metastases, documented to be about 7–8%, while for even small tumors with only 2–3 mm of invasion, it is about 2%.[6]

In contrast to FIGO, the scheme devised by the Society of Gynecologic Oncologists (SGO) is treatment oriented and forms the basis of therapy in most institutions in the United States. As such, the SGO has striven to develop criteria for lower stage cancers that are of such constraint that the prescribed treatment should minimize, if not eliminate, treatment failures. The ultimate goal has been to define criteria that will reduce the likelihood of treatment failure to as close as practicable to zero, while maximizing benefits of local (conservative) therapy. This has led to examination of the following histopathologic features: early stromal invasion, 'spray bud' pattern of invasion (used differently by various investigators – to be defined subsequently), 'tongues' of invasive tumor, confluence of tumor growth, lymphatic channel invasion, point from which depth of tumor invasion should be measured, maximal horizontal spread of tumor, and finally, surgical margins that are involved with tumor.

In 1973, the SGO implemented its first treatment-oriented definition. The key points are:

- Stromal invasion is 3 mm or less.
- Lymphovascular involvement is absent.

A microinvasive lesion is one in which the neoplastic epithelium invades the stroma in one or more places to a depth of 3 mm or less below the base of the epithelium, and in which lymphatic or blood vessel involvement is not demonstrated.[68]

In 1994 FIGO, responding to wishes of many American gynecologic oncologists, modified its classification scheme so that substage 1A1 now approximates the 1973 original SGO definition of microinvasion. However, areas of contention still persist, especially since the FIGO definition of this substage eliminated from its definition any reference to histology.[8] These issues are discussed below and the implications summarized in Table 9.1.

MORPHOLOGIC FEATURES

Patterns of growth

The earliest stage at which invasion can be recognized is where a well-defined, tiny bud of invasive cells emanates from the base of CIN on the surface of the cervix or in endocervical glands (Figure 9.1). The bud projects into the stroma, clearly having disrupted the adjacent smooth basement membrane (Figure 9.2). In one large series a single bud accounted for one-third of all the microinvasive cancers.[58] Not uncommonly, multiple small buds are present that extend into the stroma (Figures 9.3 and 9.4). Sometimes, the invasive buds of cells may be better differentiated (i.e., the cytoplasm is more copious and eosinophilic) than the adjacent CIN. In these earliest phases of growth, the tumor has been called 'early stromal invasion', which is the original definition of the FIGO substage 1A1 in its 1985 classification. Generally, early stromal invasion is best described as invasive buds that are present either in continuity with an *in situ* lesion, or tumor cells separated by not more than

Table 9.1 Comparison of FIGO and SGO criteria of microinvasive cancer

	FIGO stage	SGO equivalency
≤3 mm depth	IA1	IA
≤5 mm depth	IA2	1B
≤7 mm width	IA1 or IA2	–
≥7 mm width	IB	–
Lymphatics positive	–	IB
Confluence	–	?IB
Early stromal invasion	–	–

– not a criterion.

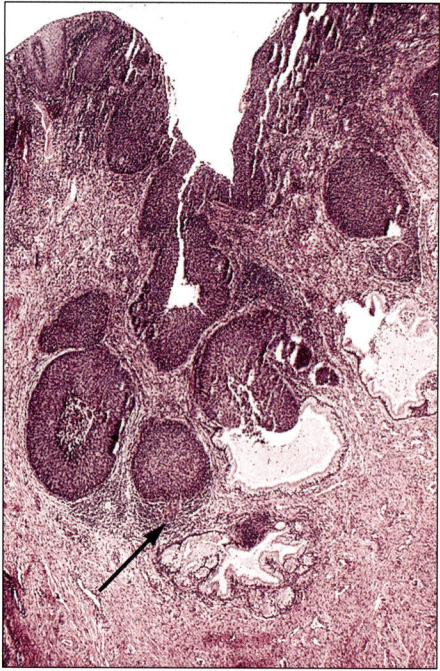

Fig. 9.1 Microinvasive carcinoma (early stromal invasion). A tiny focus of early stromal invasion (arrow) that is barely perceptible arises from extensive CIN 3 that fills endocervical glands.

1 mm from the nearest involved surface or glandular basement membrane. By definition, early stromal invasion can only be identified microscopically. Early stromal invasion is a distinct histologic entity with a distinctly favorable prognosis.

Microinvasive cancers that appear as tiny nests of cells extending into the stroma and separate from the overlying surface have been named 'spray bud' (Figures 9.5 and 9.6). The spray bud pattern of growth is usually less than 1–2 mm deep and rarely found to a depth of 3 mm in the stroma. Many tumors with the spray bud pattern also show concomitant 'early stromal invasion', suggesting that the spray buds may reflect an emerging time sequence in the natural progression of the disease (Figures 9.5–9.8).

As the lesions enlarge, the growths become broader and longer and have been known as 'tongues' of growth, although this term is now rarely used. Finally, as the tumor becomes

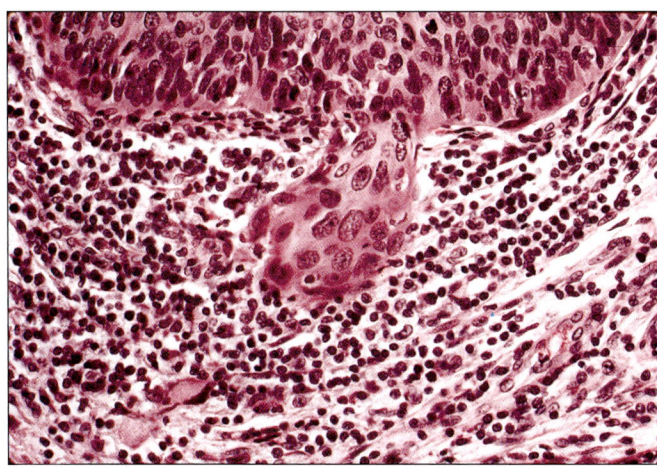

Fig. 9.2 Microinvasive carcinoma (early stromal invasion). At high magnification, an extensive inflammatory infiltrate surrounds the small cluster of tumor cells that have broken through the basement membrane to invade the stroma.

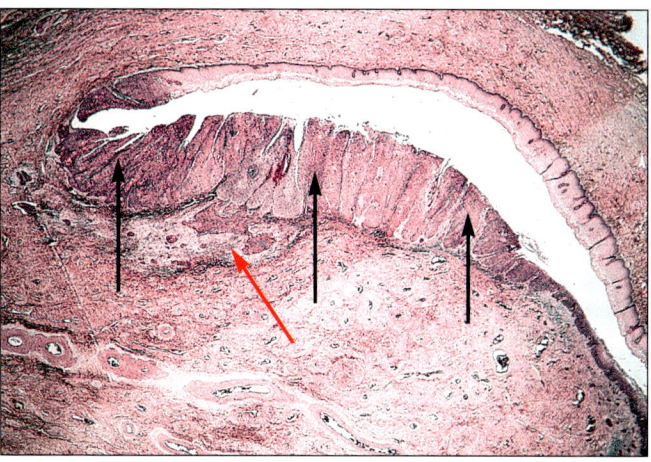

Fig. 9.5 Microinvasive carcinoma. The ectocervix near the fornix discloses extensive CIN 3 (black arrows). A focus of microinvasive tumor is at the base (red arrow).

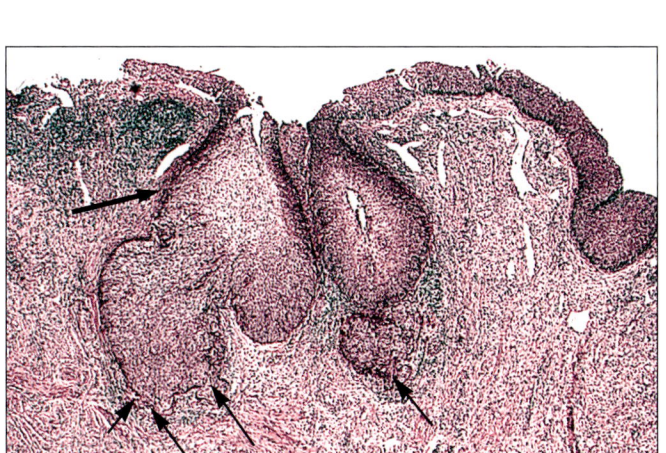

Fig. 9.3 Microinvasive carcinoma (early stromal invasion). Several foci of tumor (thin arrows) arise at the base of endocervical glands replaced by CIN 3 (thick arrow).

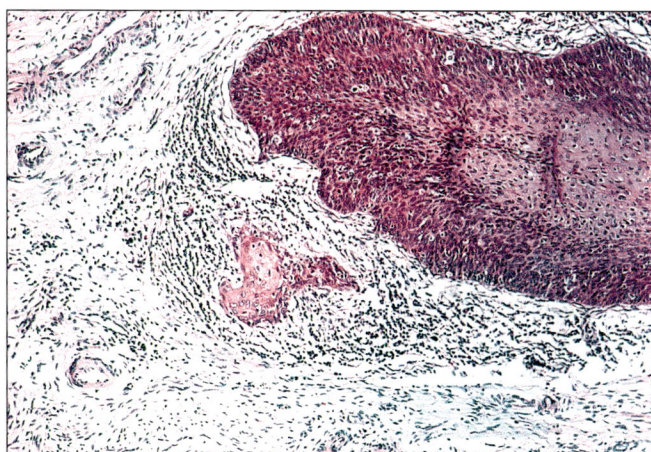

Fig. 9.6 Microinvasive carcinoma. A small nodule of invasive tumor, which appears well differentiated, is close to the base of an endocervical gland replaced by CIN 3.

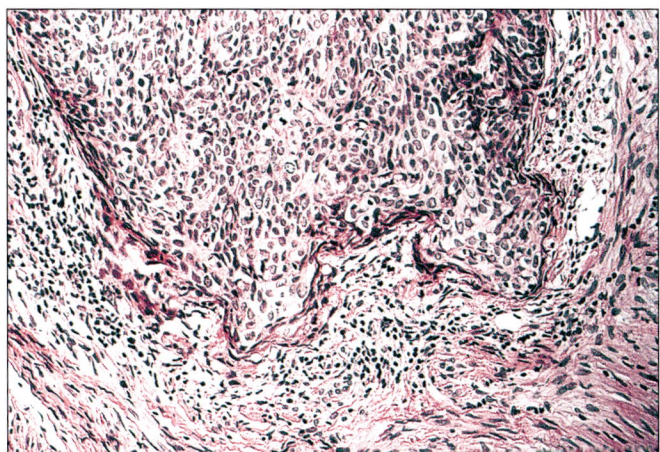

Fig. 9.4 Microinvasive carcinoma (early stromal invasion). The minute invasive foci show irregular contour.

more advanced, this pattern usually changes to produce a confluent growth pattern (Figures 9.9–9.11). While there has been some ambiguity in the literature as to the definition of confluence, it is generally felt to represent the following situations:

- solid growth of tumor cells more than 1 mm diameter in size; and
- intertwined cords of tumor, much like thick tangled roots of a tree.

In general, the appearance of a so-called 'confluent growth pattern' is related to tumor size; the larger microinvasive carcinomas nearly always present a confluent pattern. These lesions, while invisible clinically, can usually be appreciated macroscopically when looking at an H&E slide, and thus form the basis of what was given the substage of 1A2 under the 1985 FIGO classification. While there has been some controversy about treatment of lesions that have a confluent pattern of growth and yet 1–3 mm invasive, reports where there have been recurrences almost always show original tumors with the same finding of confluence.

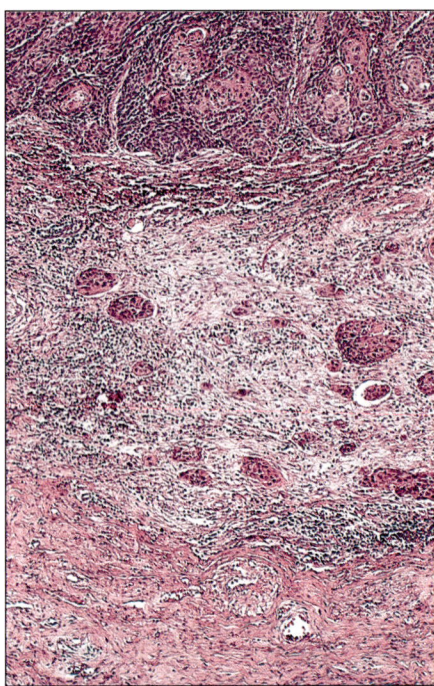

Fig. 9.7 Microinvasive carcinoma, spray bud pattern. At high magnification, numerous clusters composed of small numbers of tumor cells are present in a desmoplastic stroma with a mild inflammatory infiltrate. Stromal retraction secondary to processing artifact creates the false impression of lymphovascular space invasion.

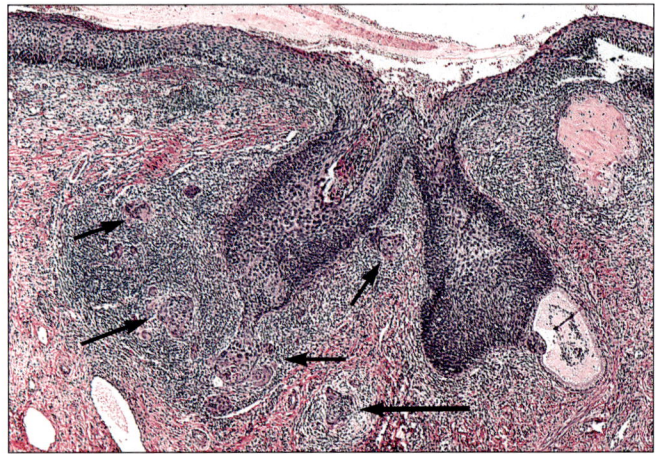

Fig. 9.8 Microinvasive carcinoma. Multiple small foci of tumor (short arrows) arise from CIN 3 that has replaced an endocervical gland. Some invasive foci are larger than others, and one is detached altogether (longer arrow). The endocervical gland on the right is only partially replaced by CIN 3.

Other morphologic features become apparent as the invasion advances. There is frequently a pronounced stromal reaction to the infiltrating carcinoma, which may be expressed as a localized lymphocytic reaction or a loosening of the stroma. Sometimes both of these features are seen together. Some feel this may represent an immunologic reaction that keeps the incipient invasion in check or may destroy it altogether. These features are of help to the pathologist in deciding whether invasion has occurred or not. As the invasion becomes more advanced, other histologic changes have to be taken into

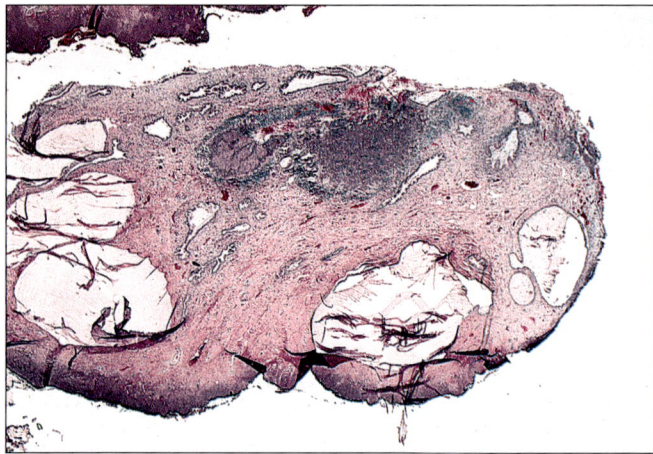

Fig. 9.9 Microinvasive carcinoma, confluent pattern. The absence of an intact overlying surface epithelium makes it difficult to determine from where the invasion should be measured.

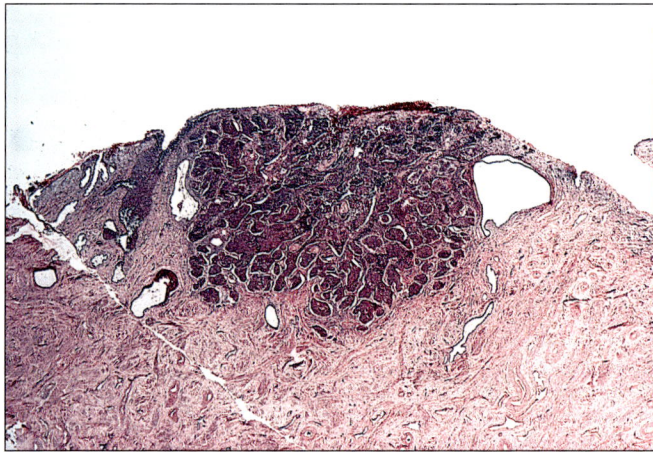

Fig. 9.10 Microinvasive carcinoma, confluent pattern. The depth of invasion being slightly greater than 3 mm stages this tumor as 1A2 by FIGO rules, but 1B by SGO rules.

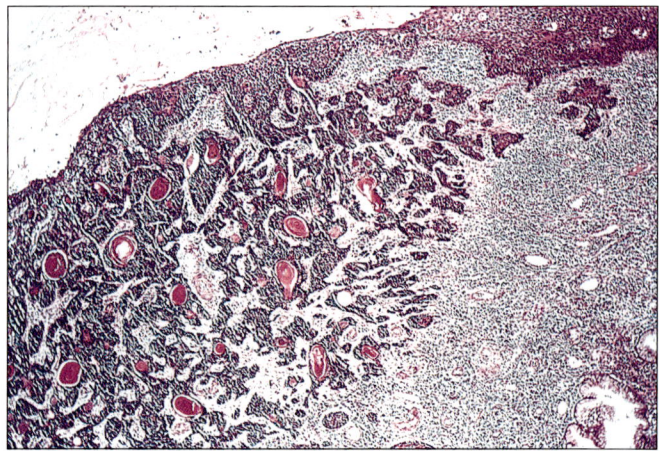

Fig. 9.11 Microinvasive carcinoma. The tumor, which shows a confluent pattern of growth, invades slightly less than 5 mm deep and is slightly less than 7 mm wide. This tumor is stage 1A2 by FIGO rules, but 1B by SGO rules.

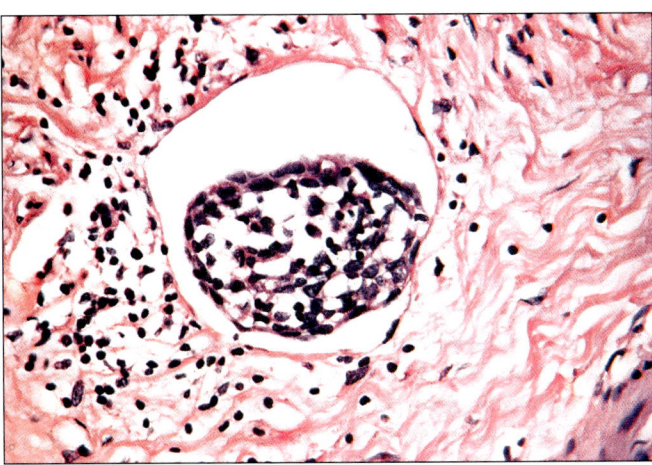

Fig. 9.12 Lymphovascular involvement in microinvasive carcinoma. Sparse endothelial cells line the channel.

account. These are lymphovascular involvement and the dimensions of the tumor.

Lymphovascular space involvement (LVSI)

The presence of tumor in endothelium-lined spaces, either lymphatics or blood vessels, should always be sought in invasive carcinomas (Figure 9.12). Until recently when the antibody D2-40 was introduced that was reactive to lymphatic vessels, it was impractical to tell the difference between lymphatic and blood vessels under the microscope. It would seem reasonable to argue that a tumor that has LVSI is more likely to have lymph node metastases. This would imply a worse prognosis and the need for more radical treatment. The evidence on this point is, unfortunately, conflicting. Step-serial sections from some studies were examined from 30 cervices diagnosed as microinvasive carcinoma. The maximum invasion was between 2 and 5 mm from the surface epithelium. Thirty per cent of the women had 'capillary-like space' involvement based on the first cut of tissue from the blocks, a number that increased to 57% with serial sections. Although these women had all been treated with radical hysterectomy and pelvic lymphadenectomy, no metastasis was found in the lymph nodes. This study concluded that the presence of tumor in lymphatic spaces was of no value by itself in predicting which patients are likely to have lymph node metastases. However, others report that the presence of lymphatic channel involvement is an important indication of increased risk of metastases.[6,48] In our own experience LVSI and lymph node metastases have never been seen with the spray bud pattern of tumor invasion.

Further problems relate to pathologist experience in deciding whether lymphatic channel involvement is truly present or simply an artifact of tissue processing. It is well documented that the stroma in which the invasive buds lie can retract during preparation of the tissue sections for microscopic examination. A clear space can easily be mistaken for an LVSI. The diagnosis should be made only if the nuclei of the endothelial cells can be recognized, which itself is not always easy to determine with confidence.

Finally, there is a serious dilemma in recommendations for treatment. If it is believed that the presence of lymphatic channel involvement indicates an increased risk of lymph node metastasis, then radical treatment would seem necessary, even though the depth of invasion is very slight. This problem has not yet been resolved. A perplexing aspect regarding the goals of the FIGO and SGO staging systems is exemplified by the issue posed by the finding of LVSI. The FIGO classification scheme, which is primarily for epidemiologic analyses, permits such invasion in substage 1A1. In contrast, in the treatment-oriented SGO scheme, the presence of LVSI requires the tumor as a whole to be upstaged which then requires more extensive and aggressive treatment.[11] From a practical point of view, it is recommended to record if LVSI is present in microinvasive carcinoma cases, even though the management may be individualized.

Tumor dimensions

There is substantial disagreement over the maximum depth of invasion that should be permitted in the definition of microinvasive carcinoma. Even so, it is generally accepted that the deeper the invasion, the worse the prognosis and the greater the need for radical treatment. Tumor volume predicts the prognosis more reliably than measurements in only one or even two dimensions. The volume is assessed by examining step-serial sections. When the distance between the sections is known, a third dimension can be calculated. With this method, no metastases were seen with a tumor volume of up to 500 mm^3, i.e., dimensions of $5 \times 10 \times 10$ mm, provided that no LVSI was seen. With current maximum measurements of $5 \times 7 \times 7$ mm, the total volume is about 250 mm^3 or one half that originally proposed. As this method of assessment is not practicable in most laboratories, the ensuing recommendation has been that the measurement of tumor size should be made in two dimensions, depth and width.

Extent of spread

As microinvasive carcinoma is most commonly detected as an unexpected finding in a cone biopsy specimen from a patient whose earlier biopsy specimen disclosed only CIN, it is usually impossible to make detailed planometric measurements for correlative studies. It is important, therefore, to determine whether any other simple measurements can be made that will correlate with other prognostic variables. One suggestion has been to examine the number of quadrants involved. In one study, 2% of patients had lymph nodes metastases if only one quadrant was involved, a number which increased to 11% if two quadrants were involved, and 13% if three or four quadrants were involved. No classification scheme takes the number of quadrants involved into consideration for staging nor does any classification scheme take into account the 12% of cases that have multifocal microinvasive carcinoma.[63]

The maximum extent of horizontal spread when reporting stage 1A lesions is another issue of controversy about which little agreement exists, either from philosophy or actual data. (Other equivalent terms used include lateral spread, superficial spread or 'radial growth', as opposed to 'vertical growth'.) Several earlier studies suggested that 10 mm should be the maximum horizontal spread allowable for inclusion of a tumor within the category of microinvasive carcinoma. The FIGO compromised and settled in its 1985 classification scheme at 7 mm on the premise that a tumor of $7 \times 10 \times 5$ mm (width, length, depth) would have a maximum volume of 350 mm^3 and thus would be a tumor still under 500 mm^3. The 1995 FIGO compromise keeps the maximum width at 7 mm. The American SGO ignored the measurement altogether. Overall, the percentage of lymph node metastases increased significantly if the lesion was more than 3 mm invasive; it was 3.4% if the lesion were less than 7 mm wide and 9.1% if it were wider.

Depth of invasion

Of all variables evaluated for the assessment of microinvasion, depth of invasion is the one that is universally considered the easiest to measure, the most objective, and certainly the one most commonly appraised by all pathologists during the routine examination of this disease. That is not to say it is the best. The interobserver variability is also the lowest among the various features considered. The current FIGO staging method recommends that measurement be made from the base of epithelium where invasion occurs to the deepest point of carcinoma in a vertical line. In most microinvasive squamous carcinomas, invasion occurs either from the base of the surface squamous epithelium or originates from both the surface epithelium and endocervical glands simultaneously. In such cases, measurement should be made from the base of surface epithelium involved by high-grade CIN. In some cases invasion is limited to the periphery of a few endocervical glands without surface involvement. In such cases, measurement is made from the base of the glands to the deepest point. The deepest measurement counts when multiple foci of microinvasion are present.

Among the many literature reports on microinvasion, whether presenting the findings of an individual series of patients or meta-analyses of all published articles, there is a general uniform agreement that lesions 3–5 mm invasive are associated with lymph node metastases in about 4–8% of cases. Even in one recent study examining lesions invasive <3 mm, the recurrence rate was 6% during the 10-year follow-up period.[61] Radical hysterectomy is usually the treatment of choice in tumors invading 3–5 mm.

There is also widespread agreement that tumors that invade less than 1 mm into the underlying stroma are virtually never associated with lymph node metastases, although there are some reports describing this phenomenon.[41] However, substantial controversy exists about the frequency of lymph node metastases if a lesion is 2–3 mm invasive. If the frequency of lymph node metastases at this depth was rare, then the appropriate method to achieve a cure would be extrafascial hysterectomy, or if fertility were of issue, possibly large conization biopsy. On the other hand, multiple analyses have shown that lesions 2–3 mm invasive are associated with a 2% or higher rate of lymph node metastases. While a less aggressive approach is favored by many, these results would argue that the decision about therapy must be individualized, and in some cases, especially if the tumor pattern is confluent or if there is LVSI, then radical hysterectomy might be considered the prudent, conservative, and optimal therapy.

An important aspect of the controversy regarding depth of invasion may well hark back to the histologic pattern of tumor present. Almost all analyses on the subject of microinvasive cancer report that the frequency of metastases associated with disease less than 3 mm invasive is extremely low, being about 1–2%.[6] However, as this includes the two-thirds of cases that are spray bud and early stromal invasion type[8] and do not metastasize, then it becomes apparent that the average 2% rate is, in fact, a composite, the other one-third being larger, i.e., 2–3 mm, and carrying a significantly worse prognosis. If each of the articles cited in the meta-analysis was re-reviewed

(assuming sufficient data were available about the cases), by simple mathematics, the frequency of involved lymph nodes might be expected to rise to 5% (two-thirds at 0% and one-third at 5% equals an average of 1–2%), a figure that approaches that of lesions 3–5 mm in depth. One meta-analysis indicates that six times as many patients will die of their disease with invasion of 1–3 mm (1995 FIGO definition) as will die if the microinvasion is only of early stromal invasion (1985 FIGO definition).[8]

> If the goal of the changes in the new staging definitions was to achieve better prognostication in patients with stage 1A disease, then this aim has not been achieved; instead by eliminating an extremely low-risk subcategory, it has resulted in a loss of diagnostic accuracy.[8]

In essence, the now current FIGO classification scheme dilutes the utility of stage 1A1 since a large percentage of cases consist of early stromal invasion that makes treatment results highly favorable. If cases of early stromal invasion are removed from the category of neoplasms invading up to a depth of 3 mm, then the percentage of patients who die from these cancers will approach the rate of those patients with cancers 35 mm invasive.

Diagnosis

Overdiagnosis of microinvasive carcinoma is frequently encountered in daily practice. This is mainly caused by misinterpreting tangential cuts of glandular involvement by high-grade CIN. Solid nests of high-grade CIN appear to extend into the stroma, but the peripheries of these solid nests are usually smooth, which is helpful for the diagnosis of non-invasive lesions. Sometimes irregular, tongue-like processes with surrounding fibrosis seem to invade the stroma. In such instances, deeper cuts usually confirm the glandular extension. In the event of true stromal invasion, isolated single tumor cells or irregular tumor islands can be found in the stroma. Stromal edema and chronic inflammation beneath the benign squamous mucosa or CIN often obscures the basement membrane and simulates microinvasion. It is our experience that examination for the presence or absence of basement membrane seldom yields conclusive information. We recommend searching for cellular anaplasia and stromal fibrosis, which are expected in the area of true microinvasion. Occasionally, entrapped atypical cells in the stroma may result from previous procedures, such as biopsy or conization. Understanding the potential cause of artifacts may be helpful to avoid overdiagnosis of microinvasion.

Although microinvasion can be identified in cervical biopsy specimens, the depth of invasion may not represent the maximal depth. The true depth of invasion is best determined by a comprehensive microscopic examination of the entire specimen obtained from loop electrosurgical excision procedure (LEEP), conization, trachelectomy, or hysterectomy. It is important to assess the depth of invasion and surgical resection margin accurately. We recommend the method of sectioning along the long axis of the cervical canal in a clockwise fashion and try best to avoid tangential sections, which invariably result in inaccurate measurement of the depth of invasion. LEEP specimens require no inking since a thermal artifact is universally present in the resection margin. However, a cold knife cone requires differential ink with one color at the endocervical margin and the other color on the peripheral or deep margin. According to previous experience, if the surgical margins of cone specimen were clear of microinvasive carcinoma, the chance of finding residual invasive carcinoma in the subsequent hysterectomy specimen is 4%.[11] There is a significant risk factor for tumor recurrence even when only high-grade CIN was positive on resection margins.

Cytologic findings

The cytology of microinvasive carcinoma is controversial, as some cytologists believe that the distinction between CIN 3 and the earliest stages of invasion cannot be made on cell appearances alone. It is certainly true that no features are sufficiently robust to permit the diagnosis of microinvasion with certainty. On the other hand, subtle features, when recognized, can suggest that early invasion should be strongly considered.

A striking feature is the unusually greater degree of cytoplasmic differentiation. The cytoplasm increases in quantity and frequently stains pale pink. Occasionally, the nucleus in this type of cell is dyskaryotic. The cell itself is more elongate than usual and has poorly defined cell borders. This is sometimes referred to as 'soft differentiation' (Figure 9.13).

Other features include odd cytoplasmic shapes with club-like cytoplasmic projections (Figure 9.14). The cells may form loosely associated sheets rather that the tight groups of cells or strings of discrete cells that are more often seen in CIN 3. The nuclei often show finely clumped chromatin, sometimes with nuclear clearing. If nucleoli are seen, then invasive cancer should be suspected.

It must be emphasized that the current FIGO and SGO classifications are only provisional and while constantly improving, are still interim working definitions. These provisional definitions should therefore not be taken as dictates to specific treatment.[5]

In summary, microinvasive carcinoma, as described above, is a diagnosis based almost wholly on microscopic examination. A summary of the various histologic appearances and putative growth phases are shown in Figure 9.15. It is a condition, also, that is easily misdiagnosed. Upwards of 25% of cases are either cases of carcinoma *in situ* that have been overcalled or cases of invasive carcinoma that have been missed.[37] The mean ages of occurrence in several series were from the high thirties to low forties. In one population-based study where the mean age was slightly less, the patients were on the average 9 years older than those with only CIN 3 and 8 years younger than those with stage 1B cancer. Although some cases can be suspected by cytologic smear, the more common presentation is as an incidental finding during a workup for high-grade dysplasia. The treatment for patients with substage 1A2 (3–

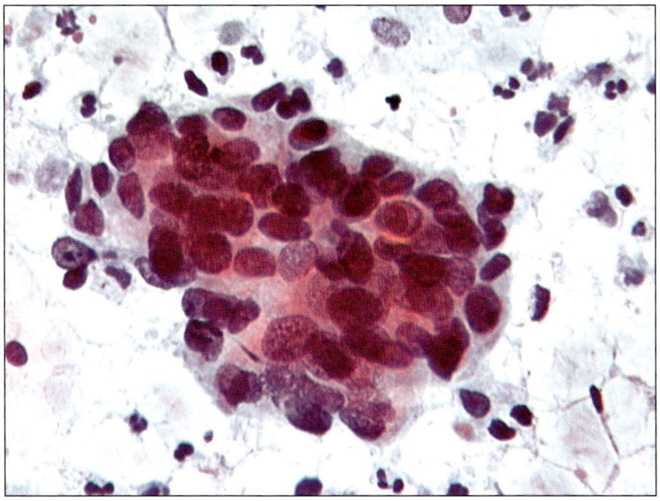

Fig. 9.13 Microinvasive carcinoma. Pink-staining cytoplasm suggests 'soft differentiation'.

Fig. 9.14 Microinvasive carcinoma. Pleomorphic nuclei with indistinct pink-staining cytoplasm.

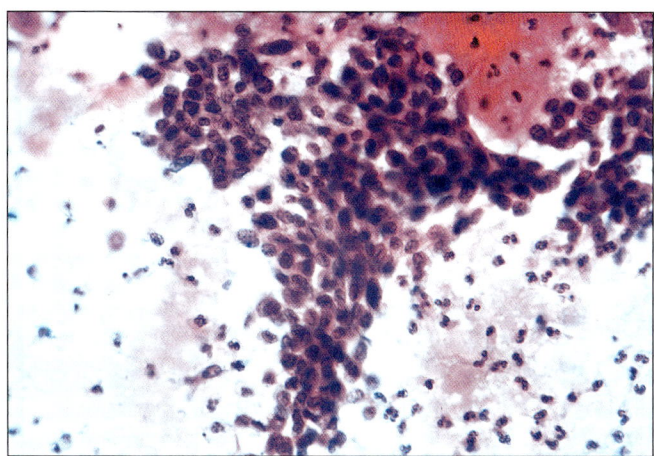

Fig. 9.15 Comparison of microinvasive carcinomas.

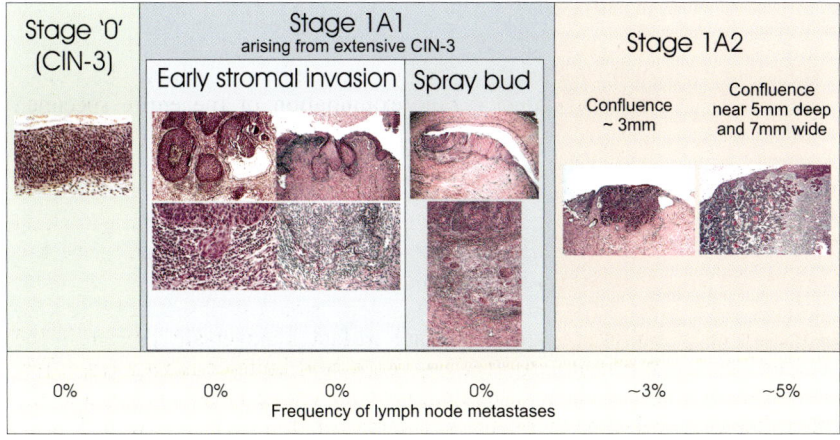

5 mm depth invasion) is usually radical hysterectomy. The treatment for substage 1A1 where the lesion invades < 1 mm is usually cone biopsy or sometimes simple hysterectomy. Tumors of a size in between can be treated on occasion by radical hysterectomy, although the emerging trend is to treat such lesions more conservatively. If the tumor is to be removed by loop conization, care must be taken to ensure that the specimen is removed in one piece so that accurate measurements of tumor size can be made. Clearly, any recommendation must be modified in the individual patient who is concerned about fertility conservation.[69] Recurrence is rare, but has been recorded in 1–2% of cases where treatment has been 'conservative'.

INVASIVE CARCINOMA

Cancer of the cervix is the second most common cancer in women worldwide after cancer of the breast. It is the single most common female genital cancer in developing countries. Each year worldwide, more than 370 000 new cases are diagnosed (about 10% of all new cases of cancer found in women worldwide and about 4% in the United States).[59] In the United States, cervical cancer is a distant third most common neoplasm of the female genital tract (9710 cases, or about 13% of all genital cancers), after endometrium (41 200 cases) and ovary (20 180 cases).[34] Breast cancer, by comparison, is 22 times more common (214 000 cases in the United States).

The lifetime risk of a woman developing cervical cancer is 3% worldwide and 1.1% in the United States. In terms of incidence the rates for cervical cancer show a wide geographic variation, which are partially explained by differences in health-care systems, intensity of screening programs, and exposure to major risk factors. A nearly 10-fold difference exists between the lowest rate (4.9/100 000 Chinese women) and the highest rate (45/100 000 women in Central America).[59] The incidence rate in the United States is 7.3/100 000 for Caucasian women and 11.7/100 000 for Afro-American women.[50]

Cervical cancer causes about 3700 deaths each year in the United States (2.0 deaths/100 000 women). It is responsible for 1.4% of all deaths from neoplasia and 13% of all deaths from genital tract cancer. This compares with 409 00 deaths annually from breast cancer, 15 300 from ovarian cancer, and 7350 from cancer of the uterine corpus.[34]

During the past 50 years, both the incidence and the mortality rates for cervical cancer have declined precipitously in most developed countries. In the United States, the incidence has declined nearly 75% (from 34/100 000 in 1947) while the mortality rate has declined by more than 60%. The single most important factor in this decline is the success from intensive screening with cytology smears. In an early study from British Columbia, a seven-fold reduction was found even with only a single smear taken during reproductive years (29 versus 4.5 cancers/100 000 women years in unscreened versus screened populations, respectively). Repeated studies have shown the single most common factor associated with the development of cervical cancer is the history of never having had a cytologic smear taken.[2] Marked variations for various populations relate to environmental, socioeconomic, and cultural factors as well as access to screening programs.

Squamous cell carcinoma (SCC) is by far the most common tumor of the cervix. While SCCs accounted for upwards of

90% of primary neoplasms several decades ago, the overall frequency has dropped to about 60–80%. The various patterns of adenocarcinoma comprise much of the rest. The remaining primary malignancies of the cervix include sarcomas, lymphomas, and melanomas. Endometrial tumors not uncommonly spread to the cervix. It is unusual to find other tumors metastasizing to the cervix.

SQUAMOUS CELL CARCINOMA

Definition
A malignant neoplasm composed of squamous cells. While generally derived from stratified squamous epithelium, it may occur in sites, such as the endocervix, where columnar epithelium is normally present.

Gross features
Early invasive carcinoma of the cervix may appear quite striking colposcopically, but to the unaided eye the diagnosis is not always easy to make as the features are not characteristic. The tumor may present as a rough, raised, red granular area that bleeds on manipulation. Often, it is difficult macroscopically to distinguish an early invasive carcinoma from ectropion, which is where endocervical-type epithelium lines the ectocervix.

The gross features of a more advanced tumor depend upon its site of origin, the pattern of growth, and the rate of necrosis. Most squamous cell carcinomas, by the time they become clinically apparent, involve the external os and are visible on speculum examination (Figures 9.16 and 9.17). However, there are some patients who recently have had a speculum examination that showed no grossly observable tumor, but clearly had tumor diffusely present in the wall at the time of the examination (Figures 9.18 and 9.19). Not until the superficial normal epithelium sloughed did the underlying tumor become grossly apparent. A few cervical cancers remain entirely within the canal so that they are not seen, and are classified clinically as squamous cell carcinomas arising in the endocervix. These may expand the endocervix to produce a 'barrel-shaped' cervix (defined as a diameter greater than 4 cm) (Figure 9.20). Thus, the growth pattern of an SCC may be either predominantly exophytic, in which case it grows out from the surface, often

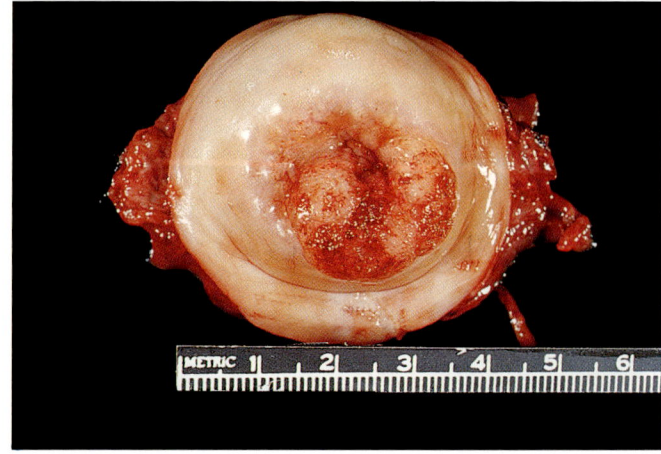

Fig. 9.16 Squamous cell carcinoma. Tumor protrudes through the external os and involves the exocervix.

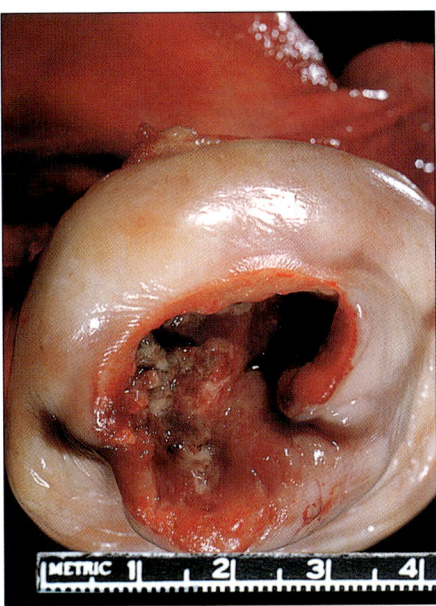

Fig. 9.17 Ulcerated squamous cell carcinoma of cervix.

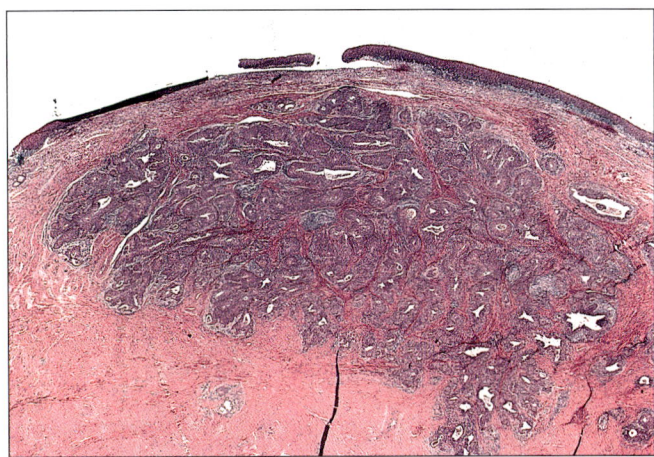

Fig. 9.19 Macroscopically invisible 'occult' squamous cell carcinoma. The tumor diffusely involves the wall. The overlying epithelium is relatively normal. The tumor in this instance was not obvious to the clinician, who noted at the time of examination only that the cervix might be slightly more firm than normal.

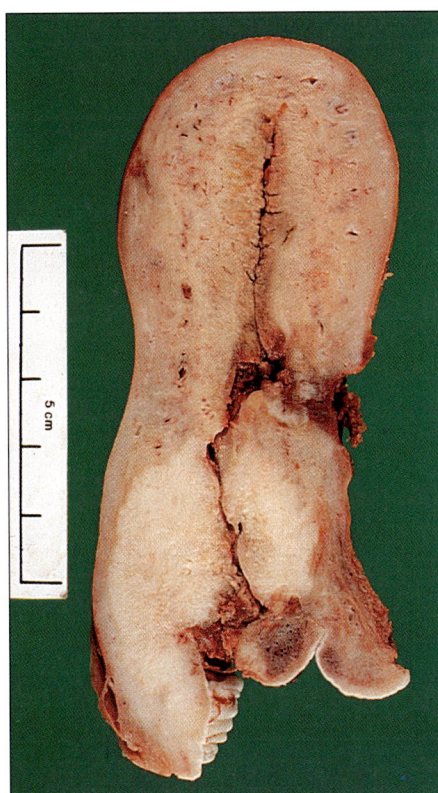

Fig. 9.18 Squamous cell carcinoma. The uterus, cut in cross-section, discloses an extensive tumor infiltrating throughout the wall of the endocervix (white).

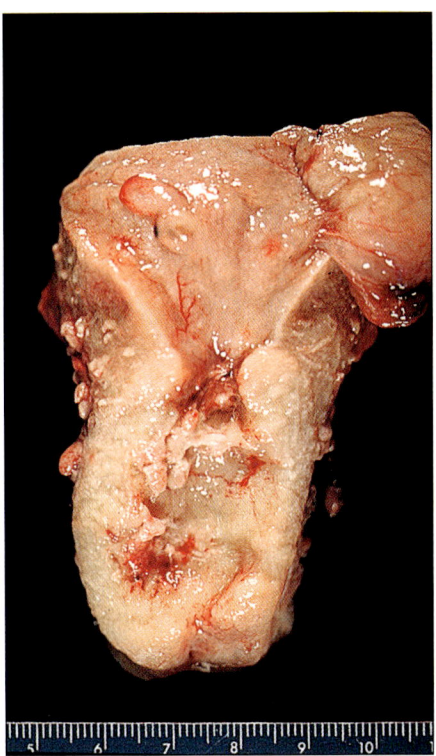

Fig. 9.20 'Barrel-shaped' cervix.

as a polypoid excrescence (Figure 9.21), or mainly endophytic so that it infiltrates into the surrounding structures, without much surface growth. Infiltrative lesions that extensively permeate the stroma often result in hard lesions with minimal surface change. If necrosis is marked, ulceration occurs. Ulcer-

ative examples usually involve the ectocervix and sometimes the upper vaginal vault. Giant cross-sections through the operative specimens are effective in identifying the extent of spread in these tumors (Figures 9.22 and 9.23).

Microscopic features used in classification

No classification system currently in use for invasive SCC faithfully provides reliable prognostic correlations. In general, the systems emphasize type and degree of differentiation of the predominant cell. One of the more common classifications

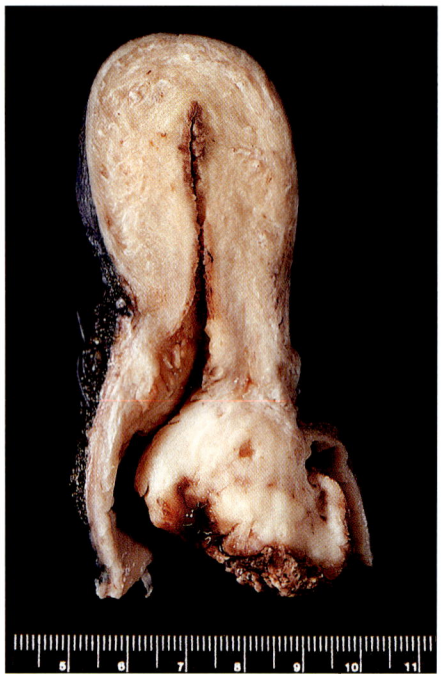

Fig. 9.21 Squamous cell carcinoma. The tumor replaces the entire posterior wall of the cervix.

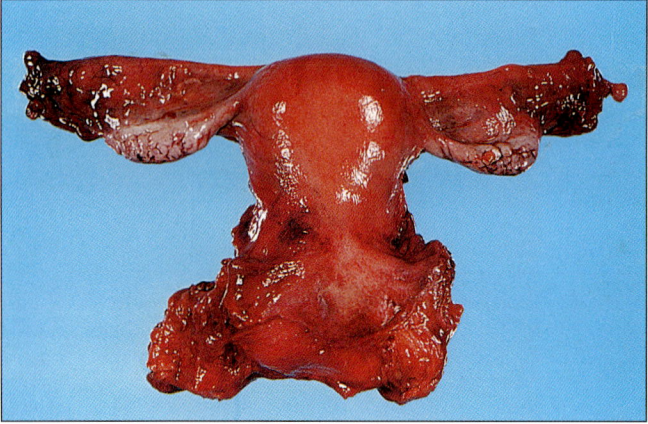

Fig. 9.22 Radical hysterectomy specimen. The cervix has been removed with attached extrafascial tissues (paracervical/parametrial).

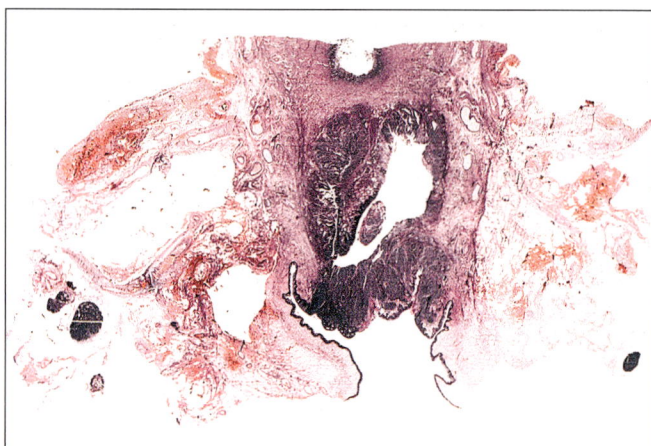

Fig. 9.23 Frontal giant section of a radical hysterectomy specimen. The tumor diffusely involves the entire cervix. Both parametria contain lymph nodes.

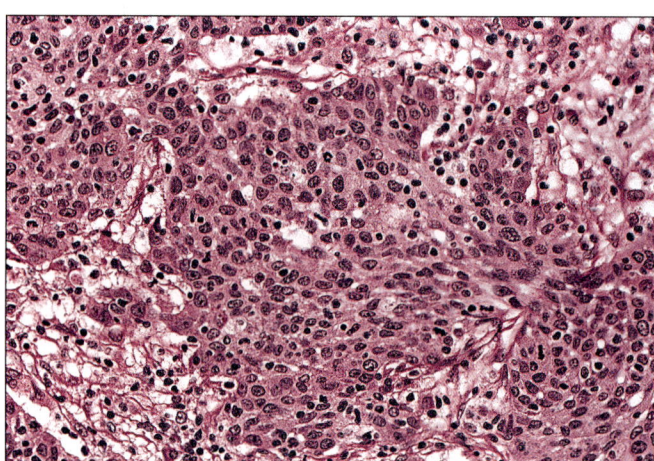

Fig. 9.24 Squamous cell carcinoma, large cell, non-keratinizing type.

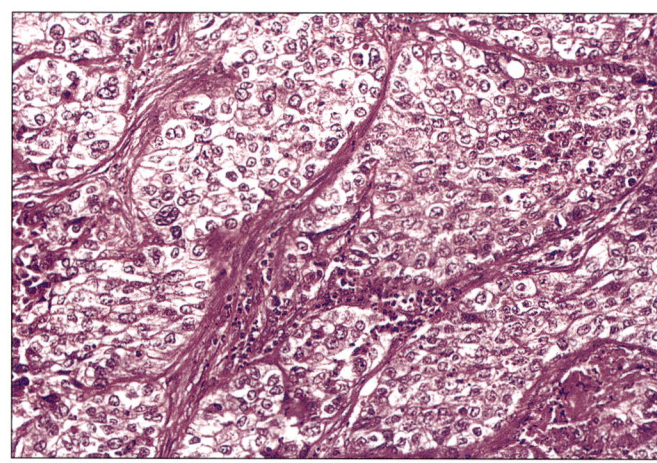

Fig. 9.25 Squamous cell carcinoma, large cell, non-keratinizing type. The nuclei are highly pleomorphic, suggesting the tumor is poorly differentiated.

(that of Reagan and coworkers) divides pure squamous cell lesions into the following:

1. *Large-cell, non-keratinizing carcinomas* (Figure 9.24), which account for two-thirds of cases, contain cells that are generally recognizable as squamous from their polygonal shape. There may be individual cell keratinization, but keratin pearls are not seen. Cellular and nuclear pleomorphism may be minimal or extensive (Figure 9.25) and mitotic figures may be quite numerous. Cell borders may be distinct, sometimes with intercellular bridges. An occasional tumor may focally show differentiation as if it were mimicking the normal squamous lining of the exocervix (Figure 9.26). The more poorly differentiated cells involve deeper stromal areas of tumor while the more superficial portions show

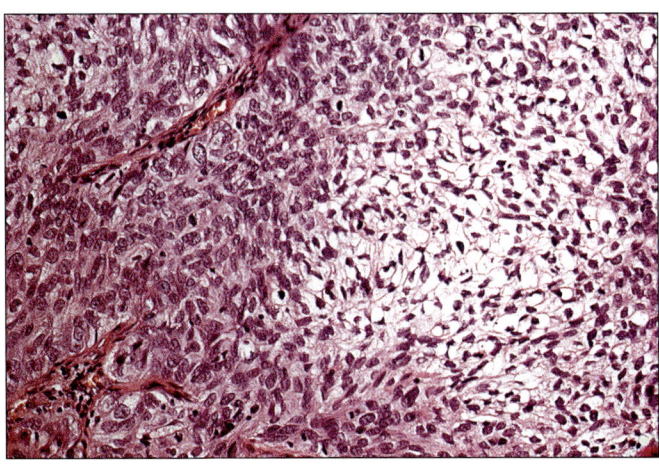

Fig. 9.26 Glycogen-rich squamous cell carcinoma, large cell, non-keratinizing type. Much of the tumor shows cellular differentiation with glycogen accumulation, reminiscent of the maturation that occurs in the normal squamous epithelium of the cervix.

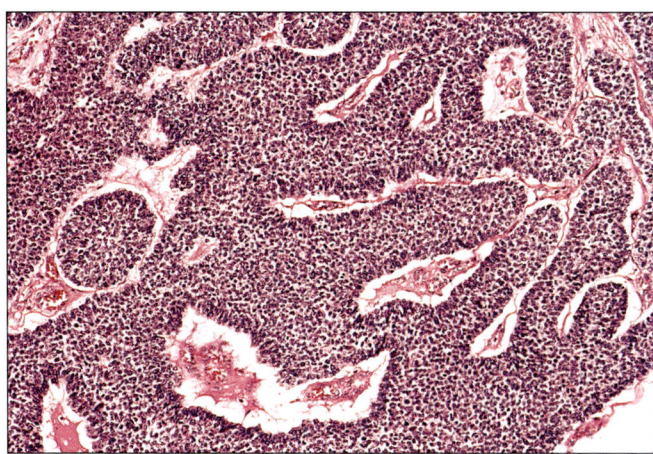

Fig. 9.28 Basaloid (small cell) squamous cell carcinoma. The cells contain minimal cytoplasm.

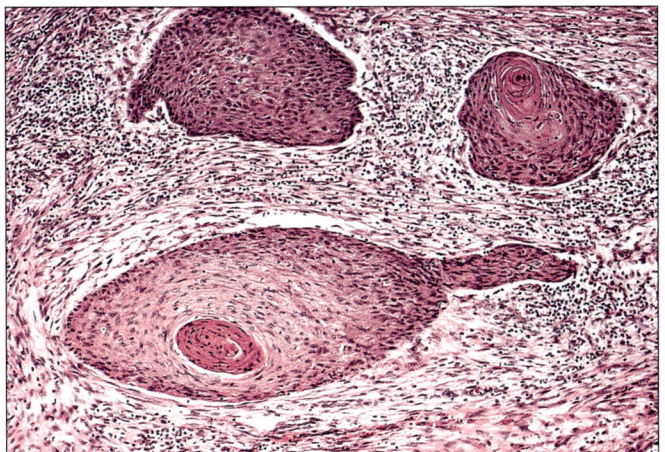

Fig. 9.27 Squamous cell carcinoma, large cell, keratinizing type. Keratin pearls are present. The irregular angulations that protrude from the tumor nests into the stroma are indicative of invasion.

cytoplasmic differentiation with accumulation of extensive intracytoplasmic glycogen (not to be confused with clear cell adenocarcinoma, where the tumor is uniform throughout).

2. *Keratinizing carcinomas* (Figure 9.27), which account for one-sixth of cases, by definition require the presence of keratin pearl formation. This diagnosis can be made even if only one pearl is found. Keratin pearls are circular whorls of squamous epithelium with central nests of acellular keratin. Usually, the tumor cells appear mature and are organized in nests or cords. Individual squamous cells are large and usually show abundant eosinophilic cytoplasm. The cells are tightly adherent and may show prominent intercellular bridges. The nuclei may be enlarged or pyknotic. Mitotic activity is relatively sparse compared with the other tumor types. While many cells commonly display individual cell keratinization (dyskeratosis), this feature, i.e., in the absence of squamous pearls, is insufficient by itself to establish the diagnosis of the keratinizing subtype.

3. *Basaloid squamous cell carcinomas* (previously called small-cell, non-keratinizing carcinoma) (Figure 9.28), which account for the remaining one-sixth of cases, describe a pattern consisting of small, oval-shaped basaloid cells with scant cytoplasm (resembling the cells commonly seen in CIN 3 lesions) that grow in masses and nests. The nuclei are usually fairly uniform, hyperchromatic, small, and display abundant mitotic activity. Necrosis is frequently observed. While foci of squamous differentiation and keratinization may sometimes be present, keratin pearls are absent. These tumors resemble the vaginal and vulvar tumors designated as basaloid carcinoma, and by definition, lack the characteristic argyrophilic, immunohistochemical, and ultrastructural features of endocrine carcinomas, also often called 'small cell carcinoma'. Except for their size and growth pattern, there is little to characterize these latter tumors as squamous cell. Many cases reported as small cell are argyrophilic, with a small cell pattern resembling the small cell, anaplastic ('oat cell') carcinoma of the bronchus. Tumors of this type in the cervix have been associated with a particularly poor prognosis and are described below as endocrine tumors.

Many reports inconsistently group lesions primarily by cell size (large and small) and secondarily by keratinization (present or absent). Some are the opposite. This is related in part to the revision in 1973 of the 1959 classification scheme where the small cell carcinoma form of squamous cell carcinoma was changed to small cell, non-keratinizing type. In reality, nearly all keratinizing tumors are of the large cell type. There is no small-cell, keratinizing carcinoma.

The modified Broder system, which has poor clinical correlation, is rarely used today. It includes:

1. Well-differentiated (grade 1; mature squamous cells with abundant keratin, pearl formation, and sometimes intercellular bridges).
2. Moderately differentiated (grade 2; less abundant cytoplasm, cell borders less distinct, nuclei with greater pleomorphism, and high mitotic activity).
3. Poorly differentiated (grade 3; masses and nests of small, primitive-appearing oval cells with scant cytoplasm and

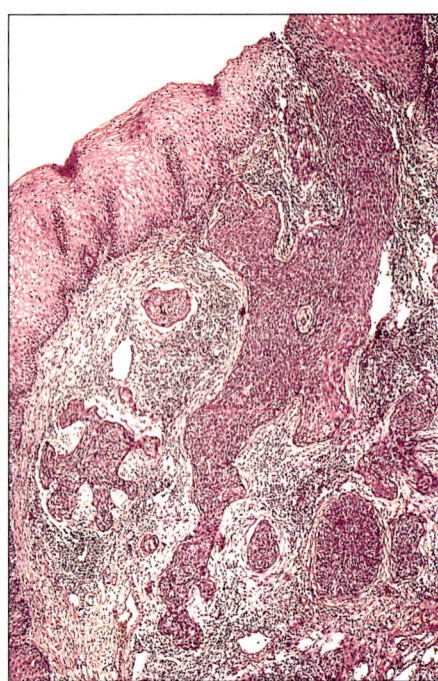

Fig. 9.29 Invasive squamous cell carcinoma. The tumor displays highly angular protrusions diagnostic of invasion, while the stroma about the invasive tumor displays a marked desmoplastic response.

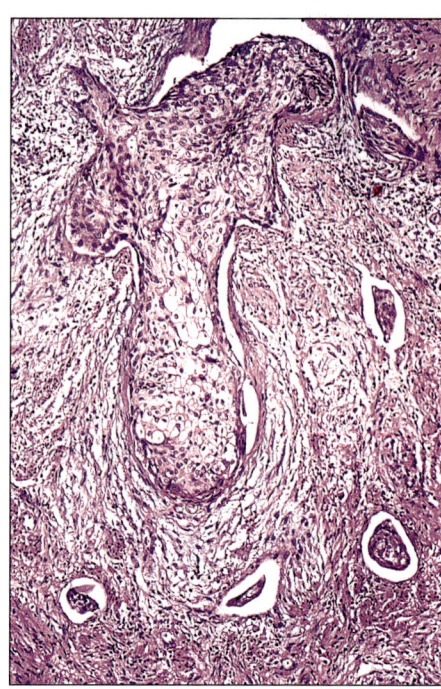

Fig. 9.30 Squamous cell carcinoma, invasive. The angulated tumor buds are diagnostic of invasion. Tumor is also present in four lymphatic channels.

hyperchromatic, and spindle-shaped nuclei with high mitotic activity).

Additional microscopic features   Tumors classified as SCCs of the cervix often show extensive variation in patterns of growth, cell types, and degrees of cellular differentiation. Most carcinomas infiltrate as networks of anastomosing bands with intervening stroma that on section appear as irregular islands, some rounded and some angular and spiked. Often, particularly in the early tumors, CIN may be found on the surface and at the edge of the invasive tumor. Occasionally it may be difficult to distinguish between invasive nests of tumor in the stroma and CIN in the gland crypts. Useful clues of invasive cancer are an irregular outer perimeter (Figure 9.24), the presence of a desmoplastic stromal response (Figures 9.29 and 9.30) or sharp angulations of the tumor (Figures 9.27, 9.29 and 9.30) suggesting invasive growth through stromal planes.

Invasive SCC displays considerable morphologic heterogeneity among cases. Most exhibit compact masses and nests of neoplastic squamous epithelium, often with keratinization of individual cells and/or central necrosis of the nests. Sometimes the necrosis is of the comedo type, i.e., centrally filled with keratin and necrotic debris, which most likely indicates a high tumor load in relation to the blood supply. Other tumors display large masses of squamous cells with little intervening stroma. Some invade as cords and individual cells, with considerable variation in size, shape, and degree of keratinization. Unlike CIN, the new growth of capillary-like vascular structures (neovascularization) shows tumor cells close to the endothelial lining without intervening connective tissue.

Immunostains   Cytokeratins are the principal immunostains that help identify squamous cells, but they are rarely needed to diagnose a tumor that is a pure squamous cell carcinoma. Low- and high-molecular-weight cytokeratins, with differing patterns of distribution, are found in poorly differentiated and non-keratinizing carcinomas. High-molecular-weight cytokeratins are present in well-differentiated keratinizing carcinomas. Involucrin – a protein present in cells of stratified squamous epithelium that have differentiated beyond the basal stage, and is thus a marker for squamous differentiation distinct from keratin – is present in some invasive SCCs depending on their degree of cellular differentiation. Involucrin is found within the most differentiated areas.[30]

Carcinoembryonic antigen (CEA) and a subfraction, called TA-4 (tumor-associated antigen), of squamous cell carcinoma antigen (SCCA) can be found in squamous cell carcinomas, but are not routinely used. SCCA has the greatest utility as a serum tumor marker as it is elevated in 60% of cases, but rarely elevated with adenocarcinoma. CEA levels reflect stage and have no value in screening. Overexpression of p21 in large cell keratinizing and non-keratinizing tumors has been associated with a poor prognosis. *p53* mutations are rare in cervical carcinoma. Human papillomavirus (HPV), as discussed elsewhere, is present in virtually all tumors. Together with p16, a surrogate marker for HPV infection, HPV help differentiate primary cervical carcinoma from metastasis.[18]

Cytology   The cytologic features associated with invasive squamous carcinoma are well described although it is accepted that invasive carcinoma is underrecognized cytologically. One reason for this is the preconceived impression that many have, based on textbook pictures of bizarre keratinizing cells. The true pattern associated with most cases is that of poorly preserved cells in a background of cell necrosis including inflammatory changes (Figure 9.31). Often the background is as

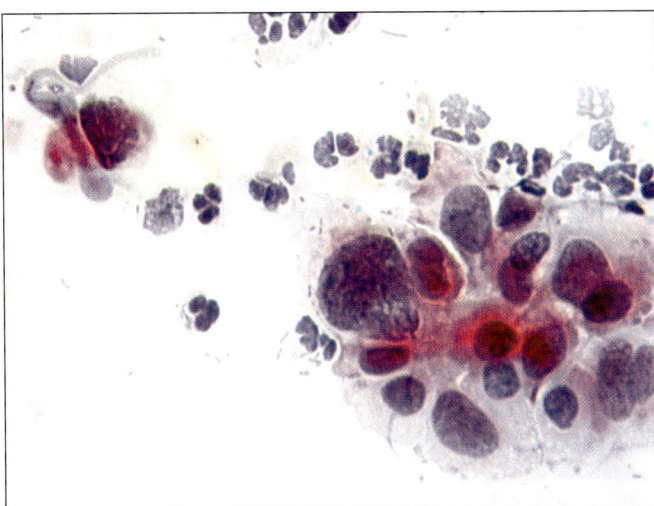

Fig. 9.31 Squamous cell carcinoma, large cell, non-keratinizing type. Pale-staining pleomorphic nuclei.

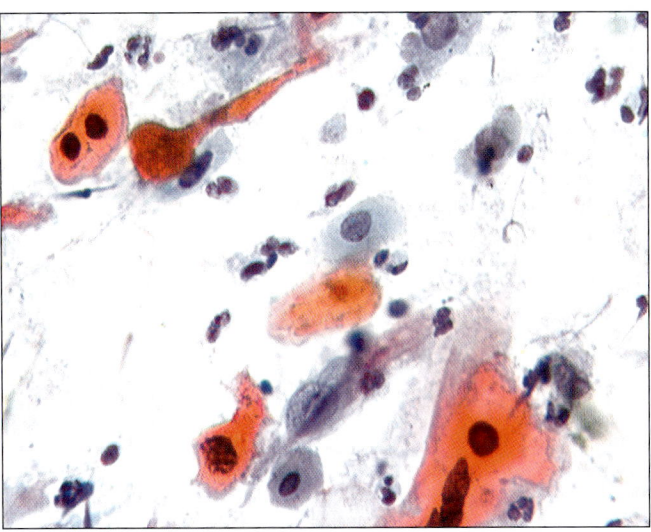

Fig. 9.33 Squamous cell carcinoma, large cell, keratinizing type. Bizarre keratinized cells with necrosis.

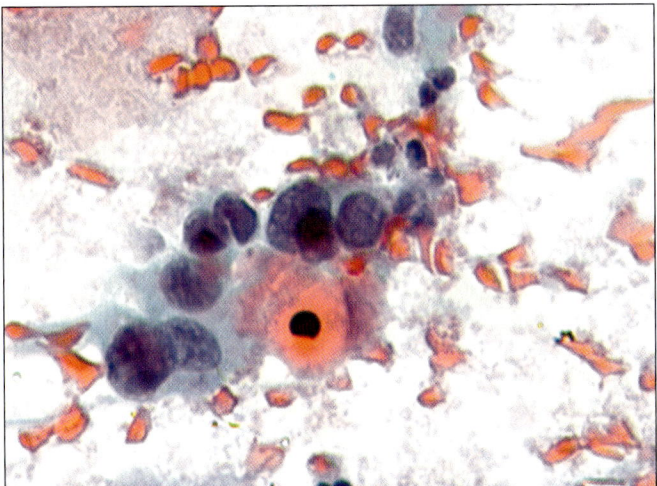

Fig. 9.32 Squamous cell carcinoma, large cell, non-keratinizing type. Large, pale, pleomorphic nuclei.

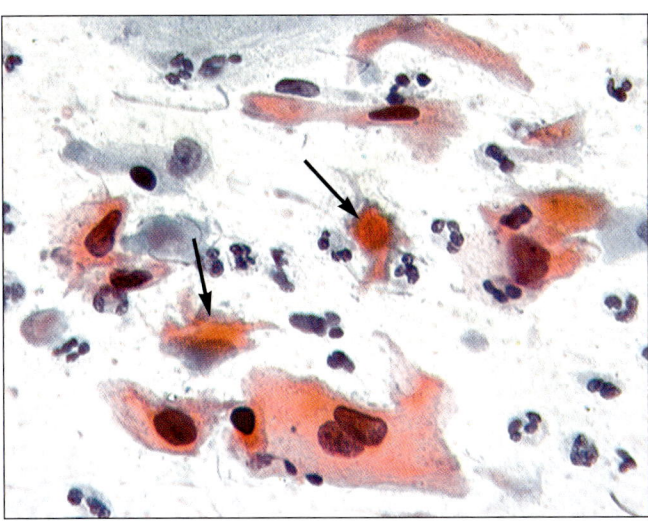

Fig. 9.34 Squamous cell carcinoma, large cell, keratinizing type. Bizarre keratinization and some anucleate forms (arrows).

important as the cytology of the cells. Small, highly keratinized cells or cells showing a wide variation in size and shape are important to recognize. Some cells may show hyperchromasia but others appear pale and insignificant (Figure 9.32). Careful evaluation of all these features is essential.

Large cell keratinizing carcinoma may show bizarre, elongated, and 'tadpole' forms (Figure 9.33), often associated with excessive keratinization (Figure 9.34), but well-differentiated carcinoma cells may be confused with regenerative tissue cells or squamous metaplasia. When few cells are present, screening becomes more challenging and subtle cytologic detail more important.

Ultrastructure Electron microscopy is rarely helpful in the examination of squamous cell cancer. Intracytoplasmic tono-filaments, desmosome–tonofilament complexes, and inter-cellular microvilli are present in well-differentiated tumors, but disappear with decreasing differentiation. Neurosecretory (dense core) granules are absent.

Clinicopathologic correlation

Cervical cancer has several modes of presentation, each of which reflects the extent of tumor spread. Depending upon the level of routine medical care received, the majority of patients present initially with an abnormal Pap smear. The survival of stage 1 patients is greater than 95%. About 60% of patients present with intermittent painless vaginal bleeding, which is usually postmenopausal, but is sometimes postcoital.

With more advanced disease, bleeding may become continuous and accompanied by a malodorous discharge. As the endo-pelvic fascia envelops the cervix in an anterior–posterior fashion and therefore serves as a natural barrier, cervical cancer preferentially grows within the parametria and involves the ureters before it infiltrates the bladder or rectum.[54] Ureteral obstruction and death from renal failure mark the natural course of untreated cervical cancer. Pain, present in under 10% of cases, frequently refers to the flank or leg, indicating that tumor may have invaded the pelvic wall or lumbosacral nerve

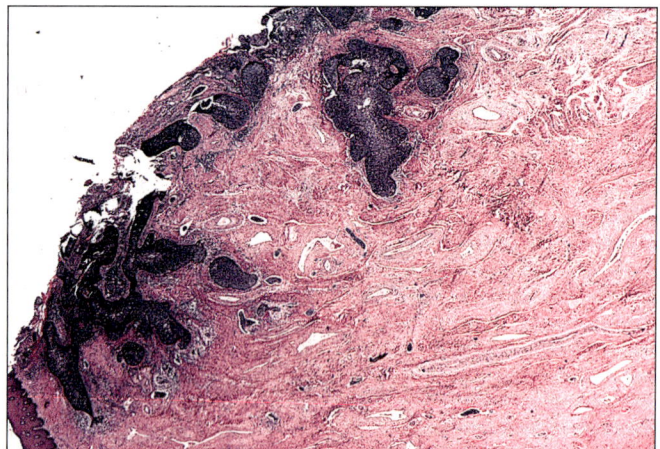

Fig. 9.35 Squamous cell carcinoma in lymphovascular channels.

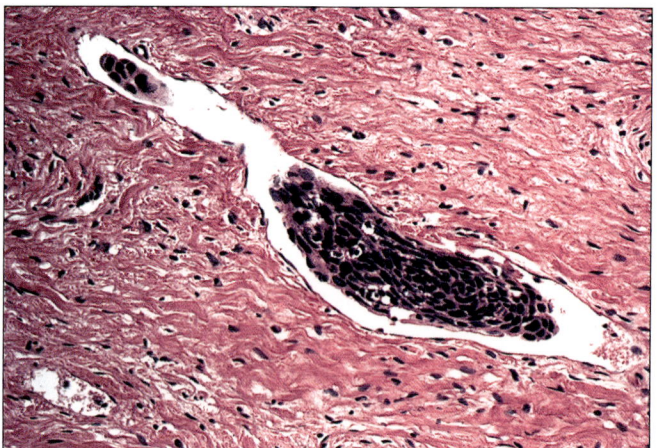

Fig. 9.36 Lymphovascular channel with tumor. Endothelial cells line the vessel.

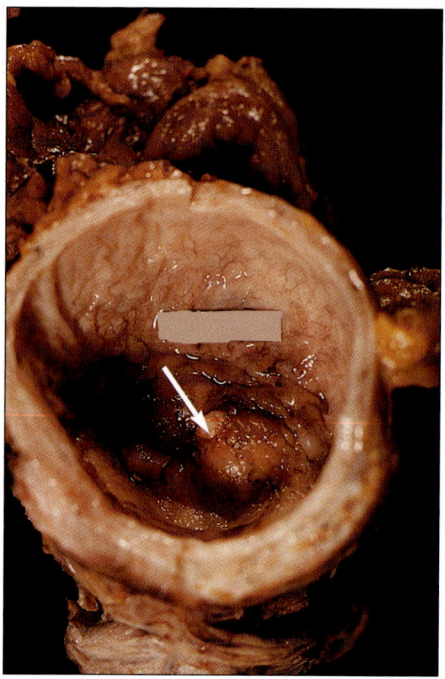

Fig. 9.37 Squamous cell carcinoma (arrow) involving bladder mucosa.

roots. Edematous lower extremities signify involved lymphatics. During the latest stages in the evolution of the cancer, dysuria, hematuria, rectal bleeding, or constipation may herald bladder or rectal involvement.

The age in a woman's life when cancer appears has lowered in recent decades. Earlier, the average age of patients with stage 1 tumor was 48 years, and 50–60 years for stages 2–3. During the past two decades, tumors have occurred in progressively younger women. Currently, 25% of stage 1B tumors occur in women under 40 years of age; 5% occur in women 30 years of age or younger.

Clinical behavior

Squamous cell carcinomas spread primarily by local extension and lymphatic invasion (Figures 9.30, 9.35 and 9.36). Local extension includes adjacent vaginal mucosa, parametrial soft tissue and pelvic wall, corpus uteri, bladder (Figure 9.37) and rectum. Spread into the peritoneum is uncommon, and when grossly absent, the peritoneal cytologic wash is almost always negative (98.3%).[76] Lymphatic spread mutually involves parametrial, paracervical, obturator, hypogastric, external iliac, and sacral lymph nodes and secondarily, common iliac, inguinal, and para-aortic nodes. A close correlation exists among stage, frequency, and location of lymph node metastasis. Thus, tumor is found in pelvic lymph nodes in 15%, 30% and 40% of patients with stage 1, 2 and 3/4 disease, respectively. Para-aortic lymph nodes are involved in 0%, 15% and 20%, correspondingly. About one-third of patients with para-aortic node involvement have metastases to the scalene nodes.

Large and small cell tumor types differ in their modes and speed of invasion and spread: large cell tumors show early root-like stromal infiltration with rapid lymphatic invasion and extrauterine spread; small cell types are often bulky, but also spread early.

Most recurrences are local (Figure 9.38) and occur within 3 years of the initial diagnosis.

Prognostic features

Numerous prognostic factors have been studied in patients with cervical carcinoma. In general, the more important features relate to the physical size of the tumor. Some prognostic features, also considered below, are determined by microscopic examination of the tumor.

Correlations with tumor size Stage, which relates to the anatomic extent of the disease and is largely a function of tumor size, is generally considered to be the single most important determinant of outcome[23] (Table 9.2).

In most studies, size has been defined using the diameter of the tumor, which is based on two-dimensional measurements.[42] When used as a continuous variable, it is a good predictor of survival.[21,28] In some studies, size has also been measured in terms of volume, and this has been found to be a key prognostic index.[40,60,70] Tumors with a volume <2 cm³ had 5-year survival rates of about 90% in contrast to those with volumes >30 cm³ (~65% survival). (If recalculated to the theoretical shape of a sphere, although not correct as cervical tumors may assume any three-dimensional shape, volumes of 2 cm³ and

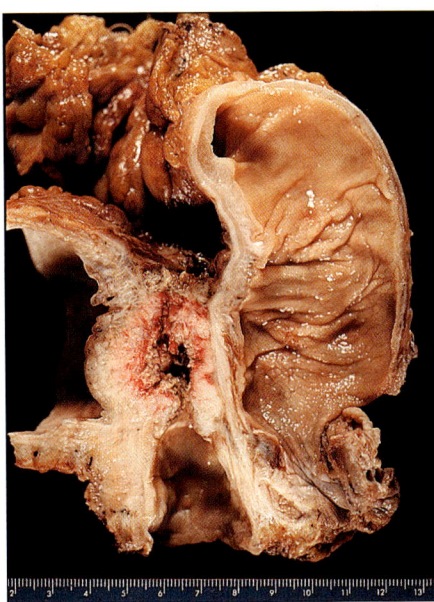

Fig. 9.38 Squamous cell carcinoma, recurrent. Hysterectomy has been previously performed. The local recurrence at the site of the removed cervix indents the rectum posteriorly and bladder wall anteriorly.

Table 9.2 FIGO stage and survival

FIGO stage	Five-year survival (%)
IA1	98–100*
IA2	97
IB	84
IIA	73
IIB	65
III	36
IV	13

* Related to definition used. Early stromal invasion and spray bud pattern are associated with rates of essentially 100%. Definitions including invasion up to 3 mm and/or confluence have rates closer to 98%.

Table 9.3 Depth of invasion in stage 1 tumors

Depth of invasion (mm)	Vascular invasion (%)	Positive lymph node (%)	Five-year survival (%)
< 3	3	3	99
4–5	11	5	96
6–10	21	6	91
11–15	65	31	72
> 19	69	47	63

30 cm^3 equal diameters of 1.6 cm and 3.8 cm, respectively.) With the availability of MRI techniques, precise volumetric measurement has now become a routine possibility in recent years, regardless of whether the patient is treated with radical surgery or radiotherapy. The measurement can be made without excising the tumor.

Depth of invasion, a feature easily obtained in a surgically removed specimen, is proportional to the volume of tumor present. In stage 1 tumors, it is a reasonably reliable indicator of survival (Table 9.3).

The finding of LVSI by tumor has long been recognized as an adverse prognostic sign.[14,22] However, the critical question is whether this feature is of independent import, or simply related to overall tumor size and therefore of secondary import. Some other factor such as the quantity of positive LVSI might be a more important predictor.[65] While it has been reported that the survival of patients with and without LVSI is not significantly different, a high degree of correlation exists between the presence of tumor in lymphatic channels and lymph node metastases, even when corrected for size of clinical tumor. The frequency of lymph node metastases was approximately 25% higher if the lymphatic channels were involved than not.

The primary lymphatic drainage of the cervix is to the paracervical and parametrial lymph nodes and then to the obturator nodes, the external iliac nodes, and the internal iliac (hypogastric) nodes. From these sites, progressive involvement is of the common iliac nodes and subsequently the para-aortic nodes. The sacral nodes may occasionally be involved, perhaps by retrograde spread from the inguinal nodes. Even the supraclavicular nodes may, on occasion, be involved.

It is generally agreed that features of prognostic significance are the presence and number of lymph node metastases, the number of nodal groups involved,[36] and the size of the metastases themselves. While these features may reflect the size of the primary cervical tumor, some report that the presence of nodal metastases is in itself an independent prognostic factor.[21] Survival rates decrease with increasing numbers of involved nodes.[32] One series of low stage tumors reported a 90% survival rate with no involved nodes, 70% with one to three involved nodes, and 38% with over four involved nodes.[60] For patients with positive nodes, survival was better if the cervical tumor was small rather than large (82% versus 48%). Lymph node metastases smaller than 2 mm were associated with much higher survival rates than if the metastases exceeded 2 cm (85% versus 38%, respectively).[13,60]

Correlations with microscopic findings In comparison to the physical size of the primary tumor, prognostic features related to histology, although still of statistical significance, have proven to be of lesser import. Important features include mitotic activity, type of growth (endophytic or exophytic), grading, and histologic type.

Some believe that the tumor's histologic type may influence survival. Certain tumors with a pattern other than pure squamous cell, such as adenosquamous carcinoma and neuroendocrine carcinoma (small cell carcinoma, non-squamous type), may have slightly worse prognoses; this is covered below for respective tumor types. For the variants of pure squamous cell carcinoma, it seems doubtful that there is any intrinsic prognostic adversity associated with any specific histologic type. Several articles, with somewhat differing findings, have addressed features associated with recurrence in women whose lymph nodes showed no histologic tumor at radical hysterectomy. In one study a high nuclear grade and small cell histology were the major adverse factors, lymphatic permeation, age less than 36 years, tumor size > 28 mm or surgical clearance < 5 mm also being significant.[75]

There is frequently an inflammatory cell infiltrate in the stromal tissue between the invasive islands of the tumor, composed mainly of lymphocytes and plasma cells. It must be assumed that these cells represent the host's immune response against the tumor antigens. Some series have shown that patients whose carcinomas were associated with a marked lymphocytic and plasma cell reaction of the stroma had a better prognosis with a lower incidence of nodal metastases than patients who showed little or no stromal reaction. Occasionally eosinophilic polymorphs may be the most prominent cell type. Sometimes a foreign body reaction is seen, presumably against keratin-containing cells, and this may indicate a better prognosis. As an important aside, a stromal inflammatory response should not be confused with a desmoplastic response or used to define a tumor as invasive.

The relation of new vessel formation in cervical cancers has also been explored. Even though there is some evidence for increased density of newly formed vessels in both preinvasive[12,17,55,74] and invasive lesions, reports conflict as to whether increased vessel density may[16,56] or may not be independent factors predicting both lymph node metastasis and disease-free survival. We have not found this evaluation to be practical in daily use.

Molecular biology and prognosis-related biomarkers Various attempts have been made to identify features reflective through immunostains and other molecular biologic studies that have prognostic significance. While the HPV types present in tumors from older and younger women are similar,[26] there is some evidence that type 18 is more common in small cell types and adenosquamous carcinomas. In one study, the 5-year disease-free survival rate was reported as 100% for patients with intermediate-risk HPV-associated tumors, 58% for patients with HPV 16-positive tumors, and 38% for patients with HPV 18-positive tumors. In multivariate analysis, patients with HPV 18-associated tumors had a relative risk of death 2.4 times greater than that for patients with HPV 16, and 4.4 times greater than that for patients with a tumor associated with a viral type different from HPV 16/18.[47]

Specifically, abrogations of the functions of p53 and retinoblastoma tumor suppressor gene proteins are believed to occur via interaction with the HPV E6 and E7 viral proteins, respectively. Numerous recent investigations have examined various genetic alterations associated with cervical cancer, including oncogene and tumor suppressor gene expression,[4,7,39,44,51,53] cell cycle protein expression,[25,73] tumor proliferation markers,[77] cell adhesion molecules,[20,78] loss of heterogeneity,[33,38] and microsatellite instability.[64,73] Some of these studies have attempted to discern the changes important in pathogenesis from those that may reflect progression of the cancer. In general, the findings are insufficiently mature to help assess the prognosis in any individual case and thus affect a patient's treatment plan.

Differential diagnosis

Clear cell adenocarcinoma The cells of squamous cell cancer may diffusely contain extensive intracytoplasmic glycogen (Figure 9.26). Unlike clear cell adenocarcinomas where the change is uniform throughout, the glycogenated elements are confined only to superficial portions of the epithelium. Clear cell adenocarcinoma, in addition to solid areas, usually has a papillary portion or tubulocystic areas with hobnail cells.

Small cell cancer of the neurosecretory (endocrine) type Neurosecretory granules are the hallmark feature. Most neu-

rosecretory cancers have a distinctive growth pattern. Small nests and typically individual cells diffusely infiltrate the stroma. Sometimes they differentiate towards rosettes, trabeculae, and ribbons. The cytoplasm is scant. The round to spindle-shaped nuclei lack prominent nucleoli and are intensely hyperchromatic. The smudged chromatin obscures nuclear and nucleolar details. A characteristic crush artifact is frequently present. Electron microscopy frequently discloses the presence of dense core (neurosecretory) granules, while immunostains exhibit reactivity for chromogranin, synaptophysin, neuron-specific enolase, and S-100 protein. In contrast, squamous cell carcinomas composed of small cells have oval-shaped nuclei and granular chromatin arranged in cohesive nests; squamous differentiation is found occasionally in the centers of some nests.

Epithelioid trophoblastic tumor (ETT) ETT describes an unusual trophoblastic tumor with features resembling a carcinoma that is distinct from placental site trophoblastic tumor and choriocarcinoma (see Chapter 32).[71] ETT frequently involves the endocervix and lower uterine segment.[19] ETT displays a nodular proliferation of monomorphic population of intermediate-sized epithelioid trophoblasts with eosinophilic or clear cytoplasm, forming nests and cords. The center of tumor nests often displays an area of hyalinization or eosinophilic debris, resembling keratinous material in a squamous cell carcinoma. Occasionally, ETT shows focal replacement of the surface and/or glandular epithelium with stratified neoplastic cells, simulating high-grade CIN. A high index of suspicion, a clinical presentation in a young woman having a relatively low, but definitely elevated level of serum human chorionic gonadotrophin (hCG; <2500 mIU ml), and/or an intrauterine mass identified by ultrasound help to make a correct diagnosis. Histologically, the absence of a definite squamous intraepithelial lesion, the presence of decidualized stromal cells in the neighborhood, reactivity for α-inhibin, human placental lactogen (hPL), and cytokeratin 18 (CK18) help to confirm the diagnosis of ETT. Anti-HLA-G, a recently introduced antibody specific to intermediate trophoblastic cells, has a great value in this differential diagnosis.

SPECIAL CONSIDERATIONS

Pregnancy

The incidence of invasive carcinoma during pregnancy is approximately one in every 2000 pregnancies to more recently about one per 10 000 pregnancies.[80] In most recent large series, nearly all of the patients had microinvasive carcinoma (stage 1A) or carcinomas still confined to the cervix (stage 1B). The pathologic features are not statistically different from cancers in patients who were not pregnant. As modern neonatal intensive care units now report close to a 100% survival for 7-month fetuses, a delay in therapy between the time of diagnosis earlier in pregnancy and definitive therapy several months later does not appear to adversely affect the mother.[80]

Cervical stump carcinoma

While supracervical hysterectomy has become increasingly rare, there are still many women with a retained cervical stump. The cancers that occur in the stump, nevertheless, account for about 5% of all cervical cancers. The proportion of squamous cell carcinoma to adenocarcinoma, and other clinical pathologic features resemble that of cervical carcinoma in general.[29]

Effects of radiotherapy on cervical carcinoma

Biopsies are often taken during and after a course of radiotherapy to assess the response of the tumor to the treatment.

The initial gross change is a decrease in tumor size. The rapidity of this change is quite variable, although most tumors will have regressed within 3 months of the cessation of treatment. During this period of regression, the tumor is initially hyperemic, then becomes necrotic. The necrotic slough separates and contraction of the underlying tissue ensues because of fibrosis.

Microscopically, the effect on cell division that radiation induces is reflected in reduced numbers of mitotic figures. Those that remain often appear even more abnormal than before the radiation was instituted. At the same time, the same cells tend to exhibit better differentiation, with more abundant cytoplasm that may appear keratinized. Degenerative changes are superimposed, with hyperchromatic nuclei that are sometimes pyknotic and sometimes enlarged and bizarre in shape (Figure 9.39). Vacuolization is seen, both in the cytoplasm and in the nuclei. The stroma shows a variable inflammatory infiltrate composed of both acute and chronic inflammatory cells, with fibrosis. Endothelial proliferation may be prominent and is often seen to progress to complete obliteration of the lumen of many arterioles. Areas of necrosis are almost universal; sometimes the biopsies consist entirely of necrotic material. Assessment should, of course, be made on the least degenerated areas.

Micrometastasis

Current methods of detecting lymph node metastasis in cervical cancer are limited to routine histopathologic analysis. Although immunohistochemical analysis is currently used for the detection of breast cancer micrometastasis in sentinel lymph nodes and this procedure is being actively investigated in staging procedures for cervical cancer, the incidence and significance of micrometastases detected by immunohistochemical methods in cervical cancer are largely undefined. The term 'micrometastasis' is used to describe small foci of metastases, found only microscopically. While there is no universally agreed upon definition of a micrometastasis, in breast cancer staging, for example, the division is at 2 mm. No dimension has yet been proposed for the cervix.

Immunohistochemical analyses for cervical cancer use markers for keratin, a protein found in cervical epithelial cells but not normally found in lymph node tissue. In a study of keratin expression in primary tumors and lymph nodes in stages 1A2 through 1B2 cervical cancer, 50% of 32 patients with cervical cancer and 44% of 150 histologically uninvolved lymph nodes showed cytokeratin 19 transcription. The highest levels of transcription were found in lymph nodes from patients with poorly differentiated tumors or where there was LVSI. The amount of cytokeratin 19 expression related to the presence of other adverse prognostic features.[79] In two studies immunohistochemical analyses identified 8–15% of patients with lymph node micrometastasis not initially identified by H&E analysis.[35,45] The number of positive lymph nodes was less than 1%. The data were conflicting as to whether the patients with micrometastases did or did not have a statistically significant probability of having other high-risk factors, including LVSI. Overall, it is too early to draw definitive conclusions concerning the clinical implications of immunohistochemically detected lymph node micrometastasis in cervical cancer.

'Mucin-secreting' carcinoma

Approximately 25–35% of carcinomas lacking definitive glandular structures have intracellular mucin demonstrable with the use of mucin stains. Some have named this as 'mucin-secreting squamous cell carcinoma', or sometimes 'mucoepidermoid carcinoma' (Figure 9.40). Others suggest that these tumors are slightly more aggressive than the typical squamous cell carcinoma, but this has not been borne out uniformly.[15,66] In the absence of any substantial information indicating that these tumors have a significantly different clinical pathologic behavior from the typical squamous carcinoma, we see no reason to regard this as a distinct entity. For the same reason, we see no value in the routine staining for mucin in all invasive squamous cell carcinomas to identify these tumors.

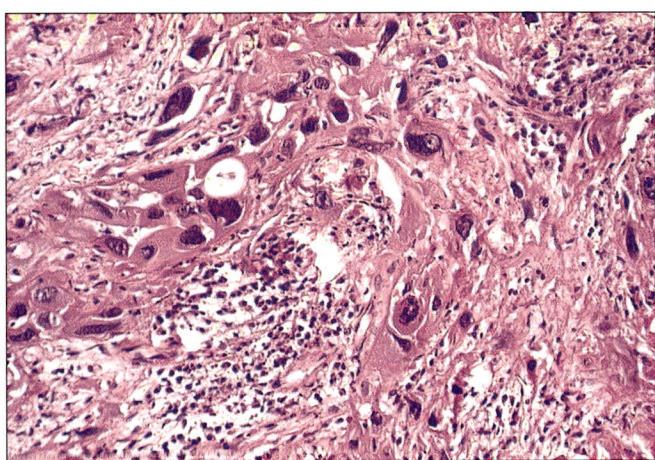

Fig. 9.39 Squamous cell carcinoma with radiation change. The nuclei are enlarged, pleomorphic, and have smudged chromatin.

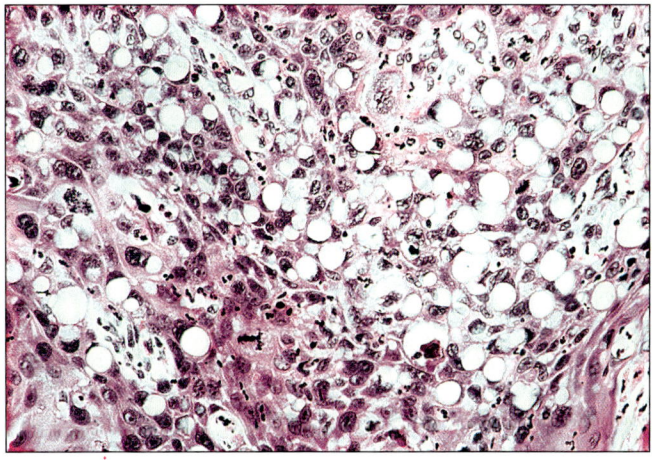

Fig. 9.40 Squamous cell carcinoma with intracellular mucin. Most tumors display less mucin.

VERRUCOUS CARCINOMA

Verrucous carcinoma is usually regarded as a variant of squamous cell carcinoma. It is usually large, bulky, and exophytic but sometimes warty, fungating or even ulcerated, and usually associated with HPV 6 infection. Its deceptively benign cytologic features distinguish it from the more common form of invasive squamous cell carcinoma. It is rare, occurs preferentially in older women, and is found anywhere throughout the lower genital tract or perivulvar regions. It grows slowly in size, encroaching on adjoining structures. On sectioning, the sessile tumor commonly invades into the stroma at its base, but the deep margin characteristically is broad and sharply circumscribed. As the tumor invades along a wide front in a 'pushing' fashion, it keeps a well-defined deep margin.

The high degree of differentiation of verrucous carcinoma is striking on both low- and high-power microscopic examination. Other than for its immense bulk and the fact that it can recur, the cells are so well differentiated that they often appear benign, or at most only slightly atypical (Figure 9.41). Not infrequently, it is misdiagnosed initially as a wart, hence the name 'verrucous'. The atypia is also minimal at the basal layers adjacent to the basement membrane. The tumor invades by pushing into the underlying stroma, even if the neoplasm appears as bulbous pegs. Isolated groups of invasive cells typical of squamous cell carcinoma are absent. Laminated keratin whorls are sometimes present within the epithelium. If irregular prongs of squamous epithelium and small clusters of neoplastic squamous cells infiltrate at the base, then it must be suspected that squamous cell carcinoma has supervened. Mitotic activity is low, and then is usually confined to the basal cells. Koilocytosis is minimal and sometimes absent. An intense inflammatory infiltrate has been associated with verrucous carcinoma of the cervix but is, in itself, non-specific.

An accurate diagnosis can only be made if the biopsy is sufficiently large to include the rete ridge pattern at the base of the lesion as well as the more superficial, well-differentiated, keratotic areas. The correct diagnosis is impossible if only the surface layers are examined. Moreover, the pathologist should always be made aware of the gross appearance of the tumor. Correct diagnosis is important, because treatment requires wide local excision. While the tumor rarely metastasizes, obviating the need for lymphadenectomy, local recurrences are common. Occasionally, verrucous carcinoma pursues a relentless course manifested by uncontrolled local recurrence. Radiotherapy has no effect on the tumor.

Condylomata that are exophytic may occasionally enlarge dramatically, particularly during pregnancy, and may regress spontaneously. Microscopically, the exophytic asperities of condylomata are rounded or pointed papillary projections with central and often prominent fibrovascular cores, a feature lacking in verrucous carcinoma. Both condylomata and verrucous carcinomas are superficial, but the former is usually small compared to the verrucous carcinoma, which is usually large and broad based.

Verrucous carcinoma must also be differentiated from several other malignant conditions. Squamous cell carcinomas of any variety may be extremely well differentiated. The presence of small groups of invasive, anaplastic cells in the underlying stroma excludes verrucous carcinoma. In situ squamous carcinoma is also distinguished by a greater degree of nuclear atypicality and the fact that it is not grossly appreciated as a large exophytic mass.

LYMPHOEPITHELIOMA

Lymphoepithelial carcinoma exhibits malignant squamous cells enveloped in an intense stromal chronic inflammatory infiltrate (Figure 9.42). The cells have moderate cytoplasm, and often vesicular nuclei with prominent nucleoli.[62] The epithelial nature of the tumor is obvious when the cells are aggregated into nests or examined for cytokeratin filaments (Figure 9.43), but when scattered in small clusters or even individual cells, differentiation from lymphoma can be difficult. This tumor is rare in Caucasian women, but has been described more commonly in Japanese women. The Epstein–Barr virus, which is common in this tumor when in the nasopharynx, has not been identified in the cervix.[49] The frequency of nodal metastasis is low and the prognosis is generally favorable.[72]

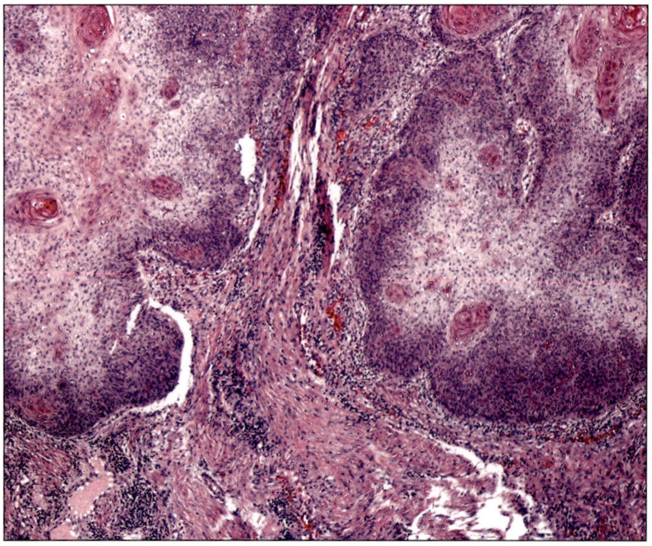

Fig. 9.41 Verrucous carcinoma.

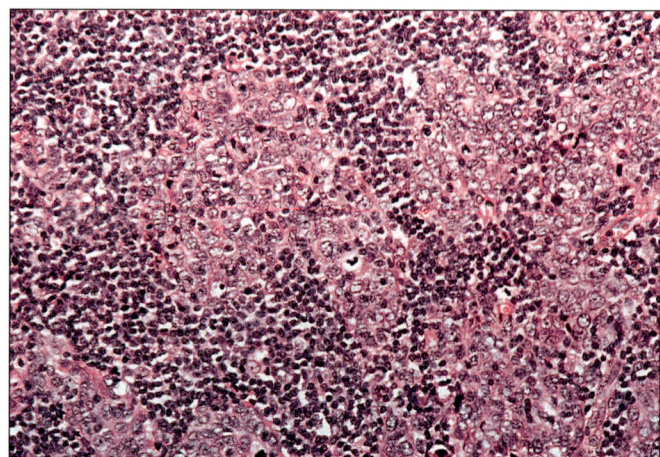
Fig. 9.42 Lymphoepithelioma.

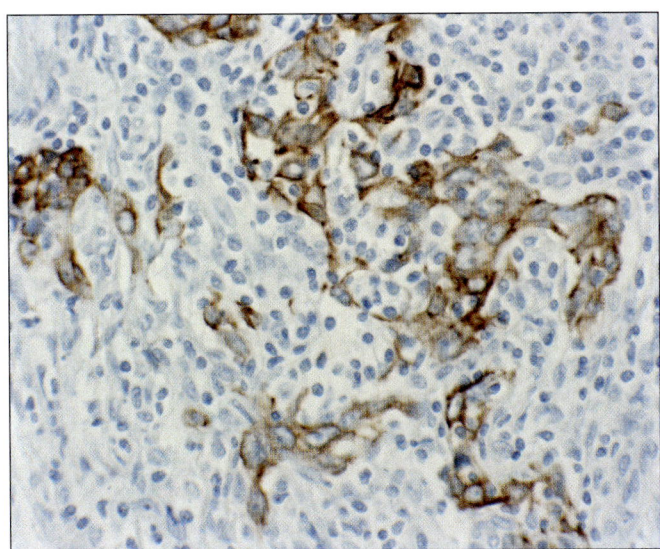

Fig. 9.43 Lymphoepithelioma. The squamous component reacts with the cytokeratin.

RAPIDLY PROGRESSIVE CARCINOMA

On an anecdotal basis, virtually every physician has experienced the patient who has been followed closely with one or more smears, and yet has experienced the explosive growth of a new tumor that seems to have suddenly appeared from nowhere over a very short period. This phenomenon, which has been named 'rapidly progressive cervical cancer' or sometimes as an 'interval cancer', is defined as a cervical cancer that has been diagnosed within 3 years of a last true-negative Papanicolaou smear.[67] This time period has been selected because of the recommendation by the American Cancer Society that the time interval between screenings should be 3 years for women who are at low risk for the development of cervical cancer and who in the past have had negative smears.

While this concept of rapidly progressive cervical cancer has had a long history, it seems unlikely, even today, that this phenomenon truly exists as a specific entity based on any particular histology.[67] In general, most studies on cervical cancer report that upwards of three-fourths of patients who develop cervical cancer have never previously had a cytologic smear, had the prior screening at excessively long intervals (>5 years) or had a known prior abnormal smear that was never followed up.

At best, the category of rapidly progressive cancers where the prior smears were correctly read and showed no evidence of tumor, applies to only a small percentage of women who develop cervical cancer. In one large series, adenocarcinomas (and adenosquamous carcinomas) were found more frequently (37%) than in most series of squamous cancer.[67] The women were also younger (mean age, 42 years). Most of the tumors were small (stage 1B) and symptomatic (with bleeding, discharge, or pain). It was questioned in some of these cases whether the endocervical component had been adequately screened. Some authorities believe that there are essentially no cases of rapid onset when the cases are confirmed as having an adequate and correctly read negative smear.

We have seen rare cases in which the squamous cancer proved to be extensive and diffusely invaded the wall of the cervix or, as vaginal intraepithelial neoplasia (VaIN), involved the entire length of the vagina. On clinical examination the cervix was thought to be normal or at most slightly firm, but without suspicion of cancer. The endocervix and the squamous epithelium in the ectocervix were normal both by cytologic examination and in a few instances by colposcopy. Only when the tumor became of sufficient size that the overlying surface was necrotic did the true nature of the cancer become apparent. This is most likely the explanation for many cases of rapidly progressive cervical cancer. While there is no way to determine the entire incubation period, it is likely that the tumor began in endocervical glands, taking many years to percolate and grow to sufficient size to involve the exocervix surface.

On the other hand, there may well be a specific small category that is not yet well understood.[24] An occasional patient who is in her twenties to very early thirties and white will develop the explosive growth of a carcinoma. Often it is an adenocarcinoma or adenosquamous carcinoma. Within incredibly short periods of times, sometimes in less than 1–2 years, it becomes a tumor that is stage 3 or 4.[31] These tumors appear quite anaplastic on microscopic examination. Occasionally, such cases may be in association with HIV infection. HPV 18, while having a relative risk of 1.6 in these women compared to normal-onset carcinomas, seems an inadequate explanation for the phenomenon. These types of cases are indeed rare.

PAPILLARY SQUAMOTRANSITIONAL CELL CARCINOMA

A rare form of cervical cancer has been described in which the tumor is papillary and has transitional or squamous differentiation that resembles transitional cell carcinoma of the urinary tract.[1,52] Like most squamous cell carcinomas of the cervix, patients with papillary tumors show a wide range in age (mean, 50 years). The tumors are discovered because of abnormal bleeding or an abnormal Papanicolaou smear. Nearly all are HPV 16 positive.[46] Grossly, the tumor size may range from 0.7 to 6 cm, and the clinical stages may range from intraepithelial to 3B. Microscopically, the prominent features are a papillary architecture with fibrovascular cores lined by a multilayered, atypical epithelium that is predominantly squamous, mixed squamous, and transitional, or predominantly transitional, and resembles a high-grade squamous intraepithelial lesion of the cervix. Nearly all tumors are immunoreactive for cytokeratin 7. About one-tenth are reactive for cytokeratin 20. These potentially aggressive malignant tumors need to be distinguished from the far more common and benign papillary lesions of the cervix. An additional consideration in the differential diagnosis of such neoplasms includes villoglandular carcinomas of the cervix. However, unlike papillary squamotransitional cell carcinomas, villoglandular lesions, as the name implies, are stratified columnar adenocarcinomas without any squamous features.

REFERENCES

1. Al-Nafussi AI, Al-Yusif R. Papillary squamotransitional cell carcinoma of the uterine cervix: an advanced stage disease despite superficial location: report of two cases and review of the literature. Eur J Gynaecol Oncol 1998;19:455–7.

2. Amadori A, Gentilini P, Bucchi L, et al. A registry-based study of follow-up failures in the screening experience of cervical cancer patients. Int J Gynecol Cancer 1998;8:251–6.

3. Averette HE, Austin JMJ, Boronow RC, et al. SGO Clinical Practice Guidelines. Chicago: Society of Gynecologic Oncologists; 1996.

4. Baykal C, Ayhan A, Al A, Yuce K, Ayhan A. Overexpression of the c-Met/HGF receptor and its prognostic significance in uterine cervix carcinomas. Gynecol Oncol 2003;88:123–9.

5. Benedet JL. Cervical cancer staging systems: the endless debate. Gynecol Oncol 1997;65:6–7.

6. Benedet JL, Anderson GH. Stage IA carcinoma of the cervix revisited. Obstet Gynecol 1996;87:1052–9.

7. Biesterfeld S, Schuh S, Muys L, Rath W, Mittermayer C, Schroder W. Absence of epidermal growth factor receptor expression in squamous cell carcinoma of the uterine cervix is an indicator of limited tumor disease. Oncol Rep 1999;6:205–9.

8. Burghardt E, Ostor A, Fox H. The new FIGO definition of cervical cancer stage IA: a critique. Gynecol Oncol 1997;65:1–5.

9. Copeland LJ. Microinvasive cervical cancer: the problem of studying a disease with an excellent prognosis. Gynecol Oncol 1996;63:1–3.

10. Cote RJ, Peterson HF, Chaiwun B, et al. Role of immunohistochemical detection of lymph-node metastases in management of breast cancer. International Breast Cancer Study Group. Lancet 1999;354:896–900.

11. Creasman WT. Stage IA cancer of the cervix: finally some resolution of definition and treatment? Gynecol Oncol 1999;74:163–4.

12. Davidson B, Goldberg I, Kopolovic J. Angiogenesis in uterine cervical intraepithelial neoplasia and squamous cell carcinoma: an immunohistochemical study. Int J Gynecol Pathol 1997;16:335–8.

13. Dawlatly B, Lavie O, Cross PA, et al. Prognostic factors in surgically treated stage IB–IIB squamous cell carcinoma of the cervix with positive lymph nodes. Int J Gynecol Cancer 1998;8:467–70.

14. Delgado G. Lymphovascular space involvement in cervical cancer: an independent risk factor. Gynecol Oncol 1998;68:219.

15. Dilek FH, Kucukali T. Mucin production in carcinomas of the uterine cervix. Eur J Obstet Gynecol Reprod Biol 1998;79:149–51.

16. DiLeo S, Caschetto S, Garozzo G et al. Angiogenesis as a prognostic factor in cervical carcinoma. Eur J Gynaecol Oncol 1998;19:158–62.

17. Dobbs SP, Hewett PW, Johnson IR, Carmichael J, Murray JC. Angiogenesis is associated with vascular endothelial growth factor expression in cervical intraepithelial neoplasia. Br J Cancer 1997;76:1410–5.

18. Elishaev E, Gilks CB, Miller D, et al. Synchronous and metachronous endocervical and ovarian neoplasms: evidence supporting interpretation of the ovarian neoplasms as metastatic endocervical adenocarcinomas simulating primary ovarian surface epithelial neoplasms. Am J Surg Pathol 2005;29:281–94.

19. Fadare O, Parkash V, Carcangiu ML, Hui PH. Epithelioid trophoblastic tumor: clinicopathologic features with an emphasis on uterine cervical involvement. Mod Pathol 2006;19:75–82.

20. Fadare O, Reddy H, Wang J, Hileeto D, Schwartz PE, Zheng W. E-Cadherin and beta-catenin expression in early stage cervical carcinoma: a tissue microarray study of 147 cases. World J Surg Oncol 2005;3:38.

21. Finan MA, DeCesare S, Fiorica JV, et al. Radical hysterectomy for stage IB1 vs IB2 carcinoma of the cervix: does the new staging system predict morbidity and survival? Gynecol Oncol 1996;62:139–47.

22. Francke P, Maruyama Y, Van Nagell J, DePriest P. Lymphovascular invasion in stage IB cervical carcinoma: prognostic significance and role of adjuvant radiotherapy. Int J Gynecol Cancer 1996;6:208–12.

23. Fyles AW, Pintilie M, Kirkbride P, Levin W, Manchul LA, Rawlings GA. Prognostic factors in patients with cervix cancer treated by radiation therapy: results of a multiple regression analysis. Radiother Oncol 1995;35:107–17.

24. Gallup DC, Nolan TE, Hanly MG, Otken LB, Gallup DG, Maier RC. Characteristics of patients with rapidly growing cervical cancer. South Med J 1997;90:611–5.

25. Goff BA, Sallin J, Garcia R, VanBlaricom A, Paley PJ, Muntz HG. Evaluation of p27 in preinvasive and invasive malignancies of the cervix. Gynecol Oncol 2003;88:40–4.

26. Gostout BS, Podratz KC, McGovern RM, Persing DH. Cervical cancer in older women: a molecular analysis of human papillomavirus types, HLA types, and p53 mutations. Am J Obstet Gynecol 1998;179:56–61.

27. Greene FL. American Joint Committee on Cancer and American Cancer Society. AJCC Cancer Staging Manual, 6th edn. New York: Springer; 2002.

28. Grigsby PW. Stage IB1 vs IB2 carcinoma of the cervix: should the new FIGO staging system define therapy? Gynecol Oncol 1996;62:135–6.

29. HannounLevi JM, Peiffert D, Hoffstetter S, et al. Carcinoma of the cervical stump: retrospective analysis of 77 cases. Radiother Oncol 1997;43:147–53.

30. Heatley MK, Cork K. Involucrin and cytokeratin intermediate filament protein expression in cervical carcinoma. Int J Gynecol Cancer 1998;8:37–40.

31. Hildesheim A, Hadjimichael O, Schwartz PE, et al. Risk factors for rapid-onset cervical cancer. Am J Obstet Gynecol 1999;180(3 Pt 1):571–7.

32. Hopkins MP, Lavin JP. Cervical cancer in pregnancy. Gynecol Oncol 1996;63:293.

33. Huettner PC, Gerhard DS, Li L, et al. Loss of heterozygosity in clinical stage IB cervical carcinoma: relationship with clinical and histopathologic features. Hum Pathol 1998;29:364–70.

34. Jemal A, Siegel R, Ward E, Murray T, Xu J, Thun MJ. Cancer statistics – 2006. CA Cancer J Clin 2006;56:106–30.

35. Juretzka MM, Jensen KC, Longacre TA, Teng NN, Husain A. Detection of pelvic lymph node micrometastasis in stage IA2–IB2 cervical cancer by immunohistochemical analysis. Gynecol Oncol 2004;93:107–11.

36. Kamura T, Shigematsu T, Kaku T, et al. Histopathological factors influencing pelvic lymph node metastases in two or more sites in patients with cervical carcinoma undergoing radical hysterectomy. Acta Obstet Gynecol Scand 1999;78:452–7.

37. Kavanagh AM, Brown R, Fortune D, et al. Misclassification of microinvasive cervical cancer and carcinoma-in-situ of the cervix. Int J Gynecol Cancer 1998;8:46–50.

38. Kersemaekers AM, Hermans J, Fleuren GJ, van de Vijver MJ. Loss of heterozygosity for defined regions on chromosomes 3, 11 and 17 in carcinomas of the uterine cervix. Br J Cancer 1998;77:192–200.

39. Kim YT, Park SW, Kim JW. Correlation between expression of EGFR and the prognosis of patients with cervical carcinoma. Gynecol Oncol 2002;87:84–9.

40. Kinney WK, Hodge DO, Egorshin EV, Ballard DJ, Podratz KC. Identification of a low-risk subset of patients with stage IB invasive squamous cancer of the cervix possibly suited to less radical surgical treatment. Gynecol Oncol 1995;57:3–6.

41. Kohlberger P, Edwards L, Hacker NF. Microinvasive squamous cell carcinoma of the cervix: immunohistochemically detected prognostic factors in a case with poor clinical outcome. Gynecol Oncol 2003;90:443–5.

42. Lambin P, Kramar A, Haie-Meder C, et al. Tumour size in cancer of the cervix. Acta Oncol 1998;37:729–34.

43. Lecuru F, Neji K, Robin F, et al. Microinvasive carcinoma of the cervix. Which approach in 1998? Bull Cancer 1998;85:319–27.

44. Lee JS, Kim HS, Jung JJ, Lee MC, Park CS. Expression of vascular endothelial growth factor in cervical carcinoma and its relation to angiogenesis and p53 and c-erbB-2 protein expression. Gynecol Oncol 2002;85:469–75.

45. Lentz SE, Muderspach LI, Felix JC, Ye W, Groshen S, Amezcua CA. Identification of micrometastases in histologically negative lymph nodes of early-stage cervical cancer patients. Obstet Gynecol 2004;103:1204–10.

46. Lininger RA, Wistuba I, Gazdar A, Koenig C, Tavassoli FA, Albores-Saavedra J. Human papillomavirus type 16 is detected in transitional cell carcinomas and squamotransitional cell carcinomas of the cervix and endometrium. Cancer 1998;83:521–7.

47. Lombard I, Vincent Salomon A, Validire P, et al. Human papillomavirus genotype as a major determinant of the course of cervical cancer. J Clin Oncol 1998;16:2613–9.

48. Marana HRC, de Andrade JM, Matthes ADD, Spina LAR, Carrara HHA, Bighetti S. Microinvasive carcinoma of the cervix. Analysis of prognostic factors. Eur J Gynaecol Oncol 2001;22:64–6.

49. Martorell MA, Julian JM, Calabuig C, Garcia-Garcia JA, Perez-Valles A. Lymphoepithelioma-like carcinoma of the uterine cervix – a clinicopathologic study of 4 cases not associated with Epstein–Barr virus, human papillomavirus, or simian virus 40. Arch Pathol Lab Med 2002;126:1501–5.

50. Morris M, Tortolero-Luna G, Malpica A, et al. Cervical intraepithelial neoplasia and cervical cancer. Obstet Gynecol Clin North Am 1996;23:347–410.

51. Nakagawa S, Yoshikawa H, Kimura M, et al. A possible involvement of aberrant expression of the FHIT gene in the carcinogenesis of squamous cell carcinoma of the uterine cervix. Br J Cancer 1999;79:589–94.

52. Nakamura E, Shimizu M, Fujiwara K, et al. Papillary squamous cell carcinoma of the uterine cervix: diagnostic pitfalls. APMIS 1998;106:975–8.

53. Nevin J, Laing D, Kaye P, et al. The significance of Erb-b2 immunostaining in cervical cancer. Gynecol Oncol 1999;73:354–8.

54. Nguyen HN, Averette HE. Biology of cervical carcinoma. Semin Surg Oncol 1999;16:212–6.

55. Obermair A, Bancher-Todesca D, Bilgi S, et al. Correlation of vascular endothelial growth factor expression and microvessel density in cervical intraepithelial neoplasia. J Natl Cancer Inst 1997;89:1212–7.

56. Obermair A, Wanner C, Bilgi S, et al. Tumor angiogenesis in stage IB cervical cancer: correlation of microvessel density with survival. Am J Obstet Gynecol 1998;178:314–9.

57. Ostor AG. Pandora's box or Ariadne's thread? Definition and prognostic significance of microinvasion in the uterine cervix. Squamous lesions In: Rosen PR, Fechner RE, eds. Pathology Annual 1995, Vol 30, Part 2 Stamford, CT: Appleton and Lange; 1996.

58. Ostor AG, Rome RM. Micro–invasive squamous cell carcinoma of the cervix – a clinico–pathologic study of 200 cases with long–term follow-up. Int J Gynecol Cancer 1994;4:257–64.

59. Parkin DM, Pisani P, Ferlay J. Estimates of the worldwide incidence of 25 major cancers in 1990. Int J Cancer 1999;80(6):827–41.

60. Pickel H, Haas J, Lahousen M. Prognostic factors in cervical cancer. Eur J Obstet Gynecol Reprod Biol 1997;71:209–13.

61. Raspagliesi F, Ditto A, Quattrone P, et al. Prognostic factors in microinvasive cervical squamous cell cancer: long-term results. Int J Gynecol Cancer 2005;15:88–93.

62. Reich O, Pickel H, Purstner P. Exfoliative cytology of a lymphoepithelioma-like carcinoma in a cervical smear. A case report. Acta Cytol 1999;43:285–8.

63. Reich O, Pickel H, Tamussino K, Winter R. Microinvasive carcinoma of the cervix: site of first focus of invasion. Obstet Gynecol 2001;97:890–2.

64. Rodriguez JA, Barros F, Carracedo A, Mugica-van Herckenrode CM. Low incidence of microsatellite instability in patients with cervical carcinomas. Diagn Mol Pathol 1998;7:276–82.

65. Roman LD, Felix JC, Muderspach LI, et al. Influence of quantity of lymph-vascular space invasion on the risk of nodal metastases in women with early-stage squamous cancer of the cervix. Gynecol Oncol 1998;68:220–5.

66. Samlal RA, Ten Kate FJ, Hart AA, Lammes FB. Do mucin-secreting squamous cell carcinomas of the uterine cervix metastasize more frequently to pelvic lymph nodes? A case-control study. Int J Gynecol Pathol 1998;17:201–4.

67. Schwartz PE, Hadjimichael O, Lowell DM, Merino MJ, Janerich D. Rapidly progressive cervical cancer: the Connecticut experience. Am J Obstet Gynecol 1996;175(4 Pt 2):1105–9.

68. Sevin B, Jones HI. Carcinoma of the cervix uteri, 2nd edn. Chicago: Society of Gynecologic Oncologists; 1997.

69. Sevin BU. Management of microinvasive cervical cancers. Semin Surg Oncol 1999;16:228–31.

70. Sevin BU, Nadji M, Lampe B, et al. Prognostic factors of early stage cervical cancer treated by radical hysterectomy. Cancer 1995;76(10 Suppl):1978–86.

71. Shih IM, Kurman RJ. Epithelioid trophoblastic tumor: a neoplasm distinct from choriocarcinoma and placental site trophoblastic tumor simulating carcinoma. Am J Surg Pathol 1998;22:1393–403.

72. Skinner EN, Horowitz IR, Majmudar B. Lymphoepithelioma-like carcinoma of the uterine cervix. Southern Med J 2000;93:1024–7.

73. Skomedal H, Kristensen GB, Lie AK, Holm R. Aberrant expression of the cell cycle associated proteins TP53, MDM2, p21, p27, cdk4, cyclin D1, RB, and EGFR in cervical carcinomas. Gynecol Oncol 1999;73:223–8.

74. Smith McCune K, Zhu YH, Hanahan D, Arbeit J. Cross-species comparison of angiogenesis during the premalignant stages of squamous carcinogenesis in the human cervix and K14-HPV16 transgenic mice. Cancer Res 1997;57:1294–300.

75. Stockler M, Russell P, McGahan S, et al. Prognosis and prognostic factors in node-negative cervix cancer. Int J Gynecol Cancer 1996;6:477–82.

76. Takeshima N, Katase K, Hirai Y, Yamawaki T, Yamauchi K, Hasumi K. Prognostic value of peritoneal cytology in patients with carcinoma of the uterine cervix. Gynecol Oncol 1997;64:136–40.

77. Tsang RW, Fyles AW, Li Y, et al. Tumor proliferation and apoptosis in human uterine cervix carcinoma I: correlations between variables. Radiother Oncol 1999;50:85–92.

78. Van de Putte G, Kristensen GB, Baekelandt M, Lie AK, Holm R. E-cadherin and catenins in early squamous cervical carcinoma. Gynecol Oncol 2004;94:521–7.

79. Van Trappen PO, Gyselman VG, Lowe DG, et al. Molecular quantification and mapping of lymph-node micrometastases in cervical cancer. Lancet 2001;357:15–20.

80. van Vliet W, van Loon AJ, ten Hoor KA, Boonstra H. Cervical carcinoma during pregnancy: outcome of planned delay in treatment. Eur J Obstet Gynecol Reprod Biol 1998;79:153–7.

Cervical glandular neoplasia

Richard C. Jaworski   Jennifer M. Roberts   Stanley J. Robboy   Peter Russell

10

CERVICAL GLANDULAR INTRAEPITHELIAL NEOPLASIA

Definition

Cervical glandular intraepithelial neoplasia (CGIN) is a range of dysplastic changes in the glandular epithelium of the uterine cervix presumed to be precursors of adenocarcinoma.

Terminology

Precursor lesions of invasive adenocarcinoma of the uterine cervix have had various names historically, which reflects the belief that a spectrum exists from very mild changes to severe abnormalities. These include cervical glandular atypia, glandular dysplasia, endocervical dysplasia, columnar cell dysplasia, cervical intraepithelial glandular neoplasia, cervical glandular intraepithelial neoplasia, and adenocarcinoma *in situ* (AIS). We refer to this entire spectrum as 'cervical glandular intraepithelial neoplasia'.

Earlier investigators recognized three grades of CGIN[60] in keeping with the terminology used for squamous CIN, but this has proven unrealistic. Squamous CIN is graded partly on separate architectural criteria that, while simple, are more numerous than those available in grading glandular lesions. Three grades, with only subtle differences among them, are not reproducible, and far less so than for corresponding squamous lesions. Two recent systems use three grades with terms such as glandular atypia, glandular dysplasia and atypical hyperplasia, but we find these difficult to define with precision.[117,232] To be practical, a grading system must be within the capability of the non-specialist pathologist to apply reproducibly. Even squamous intraepithelial lesions, in the Bethesda System, for example, are grouped into two categories for this reason. A more practical approach is to divide the spectrum of glandular changes into two grades, an approach we advocate. These are variously referred to as low-grade CGIN (LCGIN) and high-grade CGIN (HCGIN), or endocervical glandular dysplasia and AIS.[92,116,202]

Clinical features

In the past CGIN was a relatively uncommon lesion; however, with the increasing proportion of cervical neoplasms representing adenocarcinomas, more precursor lesions are being seen.[74,116] Compared to high-grade squamous intraepithelial lesions (HSIL), HCGIN is much less common, with reported ratios varying from 1:26 to 1:237. In one Australian cytology registry the incidence per 1000 screened women of histologically confirmed HCGIN was 0.06 in 1990 compared to 1.98 for squamous carcinoma *in situ*. By 2002 the respective reported incidences were 0.12 and 2.89. In that study, the incidence of squamous cell carcinoma *in situ* was in the order of 20–30 times higher than HCGIN.[149]

On average, coexistence of squamous CIN or carcinoma with HCGIN is seen in approximately 50% of cases.[250] In one study, 63% of cases of HCGIN showed associated CIN, with 8% having an associated microinvasive or frankly invasive squamous cell carcinoma.[93]

HCGIN may be present for some years before an invasive adenocarcinoma supersedes it. Supporting evidence is that patients with HCGIN are, on average, 35–46 years of age, or 5–11 years younger than women with invasive adenocarcinoma.[32,126,128,149] In one study, the mean ages were 39, 43, 43, and 48 years for LCGIN, HCGIN, microinvasive adenocarcinoma, and invasive adenocarcinoma, respectively.[116] In another series, unrecognized HCGIN was found in cervical biopsies 3–7 years before invasive adenocarcinoma was found in 5 of 18 women.[23] In another study, nearly half the women with invasive adenocarcinoma had unrecognized atypical endocervical cells in the smears at least 2–8 years before, indicating a long evolution of the disease.[21] Similarly, patients treated for HCGIN over similar periods have had lesions that progressed into invasive adenocarcinoma.[80]

Like squamous CIN, most patients with CGIN are asymptomatic. Occasionally, abnormal vaginal bleeding is noted. The lesion is usually found because of abnormalities in cervical smears taken as part of routine screening or as an unanticipated finding in a cervical biopsy performed for a suspected squamous lesion.

Pathogenesis/etiology

Epidemiologic risk factors for cervical adenocarcinoma include low socioeconomic status, multiple sexual partners (particularly before the age of 20), weight gain, and oral contraceptive use (long term).[219] More recent data have implicated human papilloma virus (HPV).[77,255] Both HPV DNA and HPV mRNA have been identified in HCGIN, with HPV types 16 and 18 being found in the majority of cases.[53,123,255] HPV 18 is the more common form in CGIN (43% of cases) and HPV 16 the next most common (23% of cases).[48]

Diagnosis

CGIN is a microscopic diagnosis. CGIN, whether low or high grade, lacks a distinctive gross appearance. Furthermore, most colposcopists believe CGIN has no specific colposcopic features. As the abnormal glandular epithelium is only slightly thicker than normal, it is difficult to appreciate colposcopically, even when it involves the surface mucosa of the transformation zone.

HCGIN (high-grade cervical glandular intraepithelial neoplasia)

HCGIN has three main histologic subtypes: endocervical HCGIN, endometrioid HCGIN, and intestinal HCGIN.[92,93] Endocervical HCGIN, either alone or in combination with other types, is the most frequent variety.[93] Other less common types of HCGIN described include clear cell, serous, adenosquamous, villoglandular, and ciliated (tubal) HCGIN.[68,97,99,197,213]

Endocervical HCGIN shows glands with nuclear atypia, nuclear pseudostratification, small to moderate amounts of juxtaluminal cytoplasm containing mucin, scattered juxtaluminal mitoses (normal and/or abnormal), and apoptotic bodies (Figures 10.1–10.6).[3,20,92,93,99] Endometrioid HCGIN as originally described exhibits marked nuclear pseudostratification and absent cytoplasmic mucin or mucin staining confined to the luminal border.[93] In many ways, this distinction between endocervical and endometrioid HCGIN is artificial as the endometrioid features represent endocervical-type cells that have lost their intracytoplasmic mucin. Intestinal-type HCGIN,

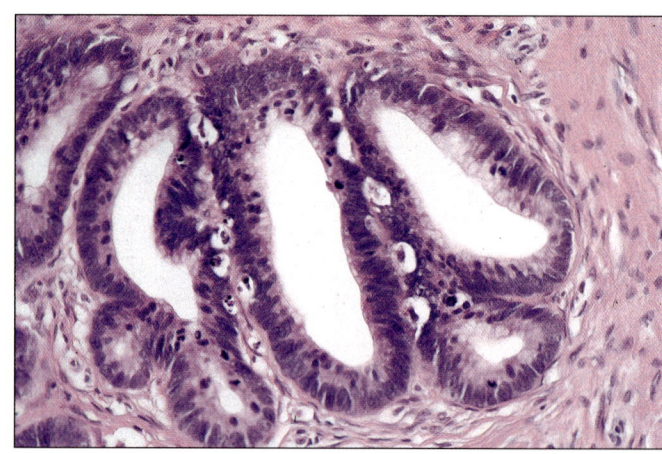

Fig. 10.1 HCGIN endocervical subtype.

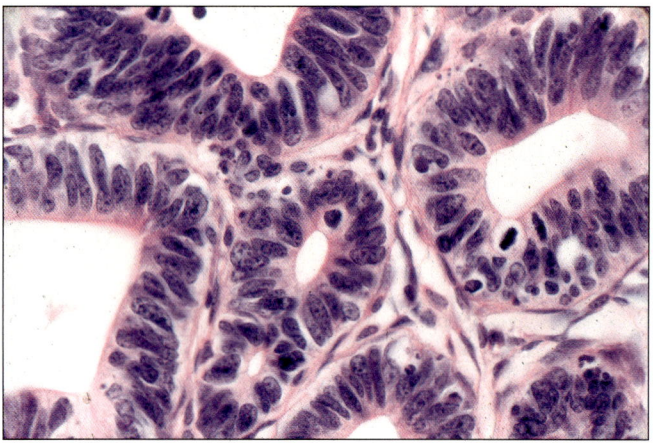

Fig. 10.2 HCGIN. The nuclei are abnormal and show stratification.

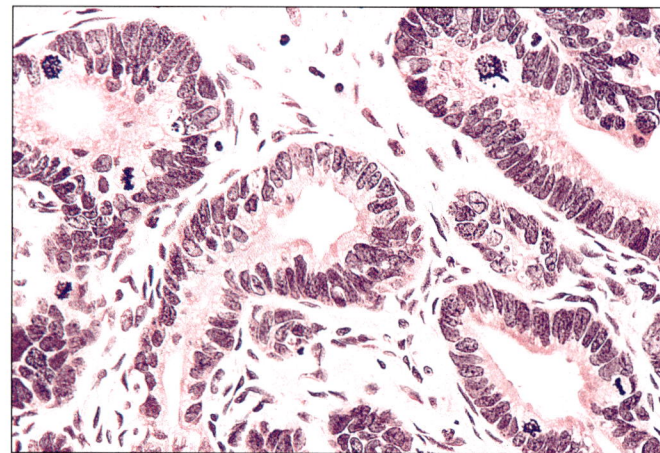

Fig. 10.3 HCGIN. Numerous abnormal mitoses are present.

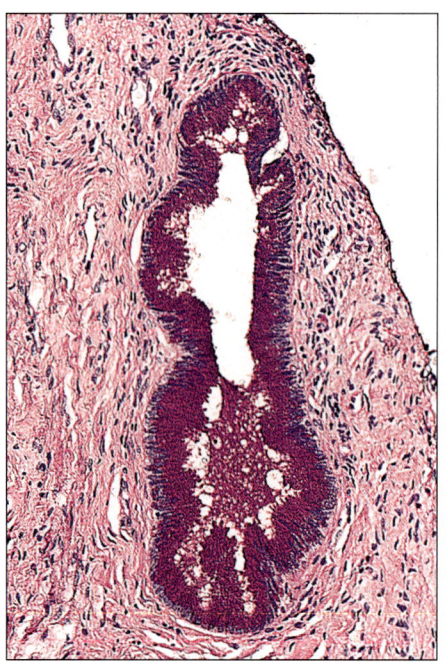

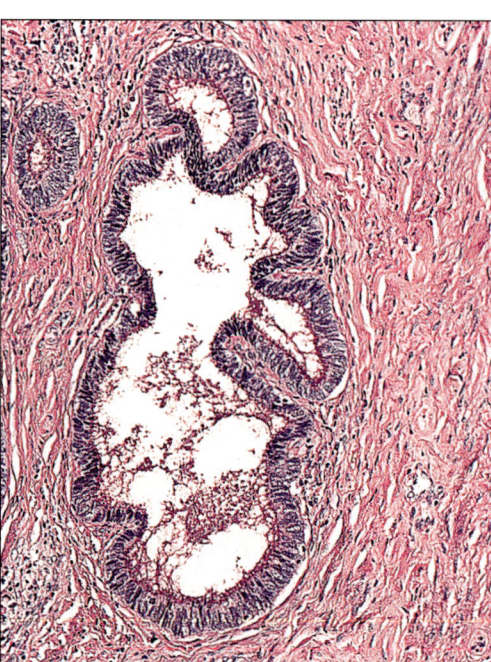

Fig. 10.4 HCGIN compared with a normal gland. The abnormal gland (right) shows little mucin in comparison to extensive mucin in the normal endocervical gland (left). (PAS stain after diastase digestion.)

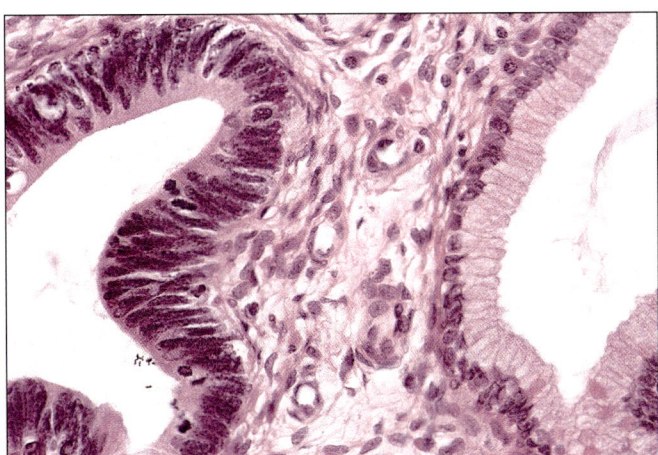

Fig. 10.5 HCGIN compared with normal gland.

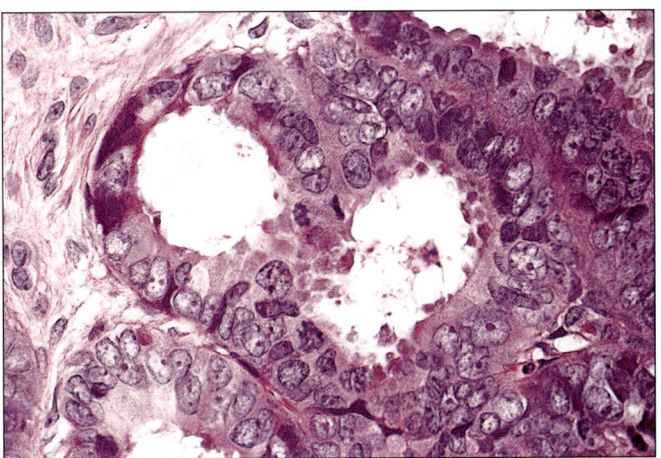

Fig. 10.6 HCGIN. The nuclei are abnormal and show some stratification.

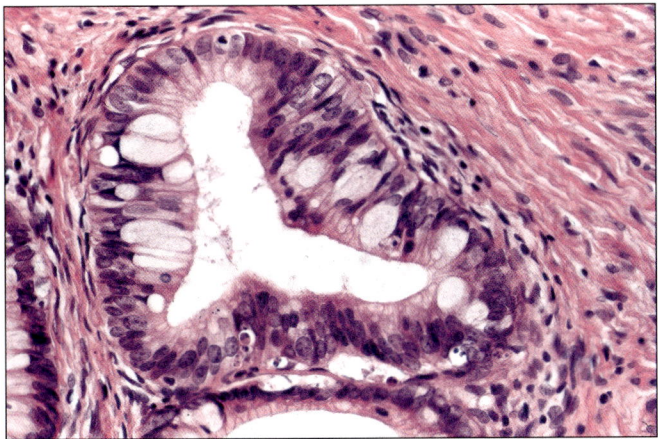

Fig. 10.7 HCGIN, intestinal subtype with goblet cells.

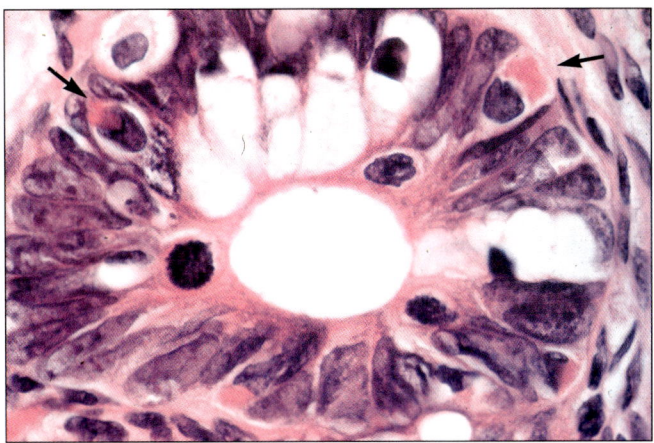

Fig. 10.8 HCGIN, intestinal subtype with neuroendocrine cells. Neuroendocrine cells (arrows) show basal granular cytoplasm and are argentaffin positive.

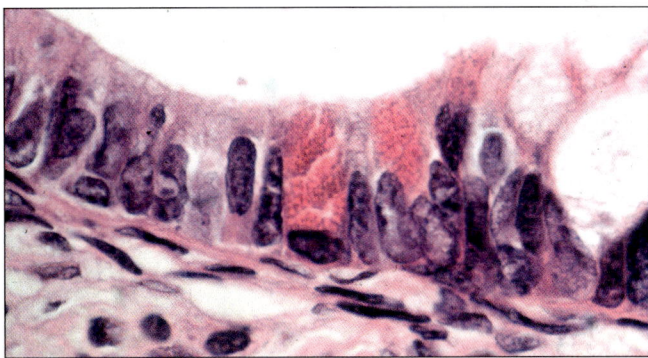

Fig. 10.9 HCGIN, intestinal subtype with Paneth cells.

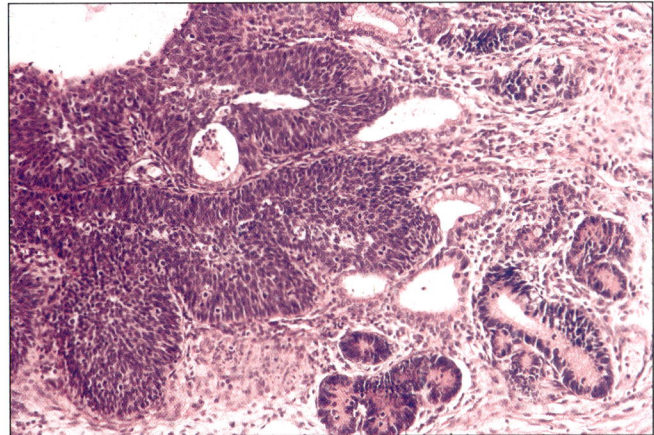

Fig. 10.10 HCGIN with numerous mitoses in endocervical glands at edge of CIN 3 growing into the glands.

a form of intestinal metaplasia, exhibits goblet cells (Figure 10.7). Occasionally, neuroendocrine cells (Figure 10.8), which are argentaffin positive, and even Paneth cells (Figure 10.9) may be seen.[93] Pure intestinal metaplasia without CGIN is rare.

HCGIN involves the transformation zone in over two-thirds of cases. It can be found at the edge of squamous CIN (Figure 10.10), invasive squamous cell carcinoma, or an invasive adenocarcinoma. It often affects the surface epithelium and the superficial (Figure 10.11) and deep regions of the endocervical crypts.[92,93] It is also commonly found alone in glands beneath normal metaplastic squamous epithelium or CIN (Figure 10.12). The lesions may be focal or diffuse (Figures 10.13 and 10.14), and extensive sectioning may be necessary both for their

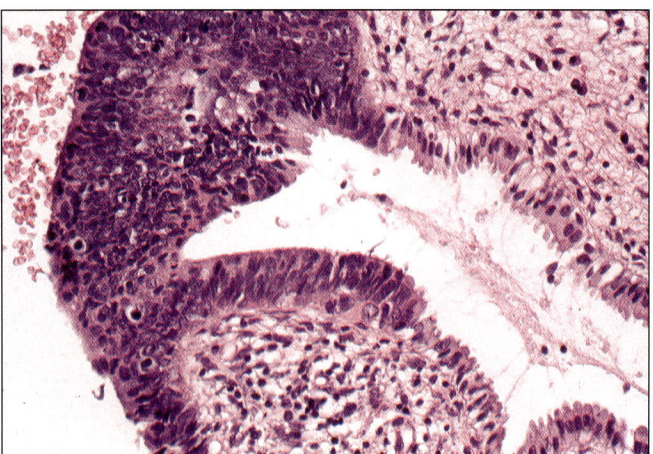

Fig. 10.11 HCGIN involving the surface epithelium and neck of an endocervical crypt.

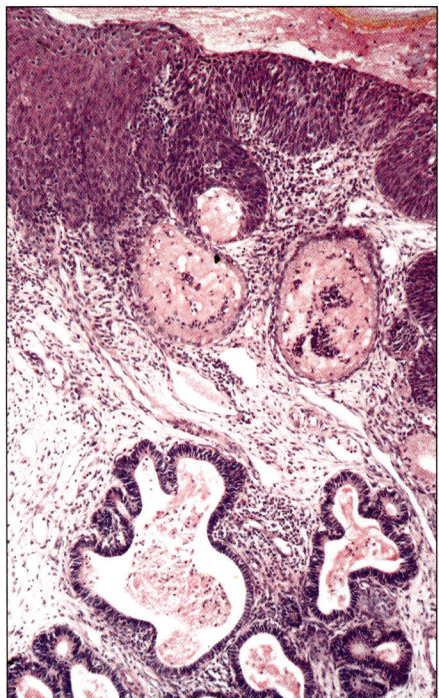

Fig. 10.12 HCGIN located deep to the surface epithelium that shows CIN 3.

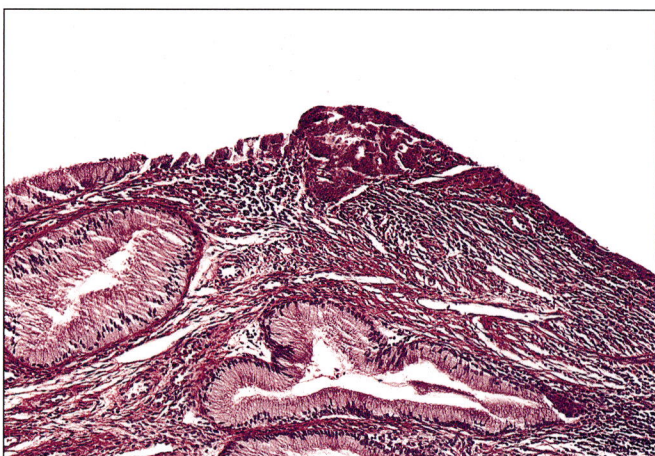

Fig. 10.13 HCGIN. The abnormality is present as a single focus near the squamocolumnar junction. More than 20 sections were required to identify this single focus in the hysterectomy specimen.

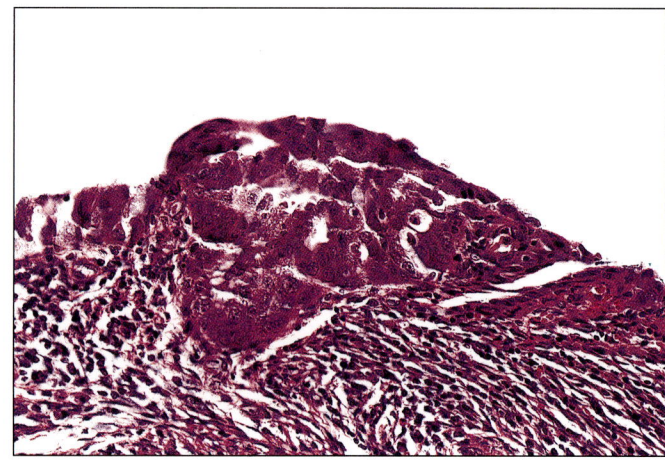

Fig. 10.14 HCGIN. Detail of single focus.

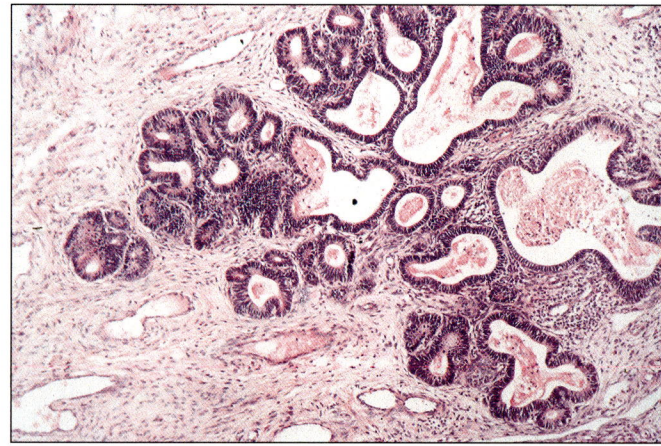

Fig. 10.15 HCGIN simulating tunnel cluster formation.

detection and to exclude invasive adenocarcinoma.[92,93] HCGIN also extends up the endocervical canal for a variable distance (up to 30 mm).[19] In patients younger than 36 years, HCGIN is less likely to show prominent extension up the endocervical canal.[159] If not directly adjacent to the squamous CIN, the CGIN may be located high in the endocervical canal. In 14% of cases, CGIN is multifocal.[19,159,170,204,250] True skip lesions, where foci of HCGIN are separated by several millimeters of normal glands, are rare.[250]

The glands involved by HCGIN may show various architectural patterns, simulating tunnel clusters (Figure 10.15), villoglandular papillae (Figure 10.16), and budding (Figures 10.17–10.19). Serous HCGIN, which is rare, shows micropapillae where the tumor cells appear as a 'pile-of-stones' and the papillae lack fibrovascular stromal cores (Figure 10.20). The

presence of a prominent cribriform pattern is usually indicative of adenocarcinoma. An abrupt transition commonly separates HCGIN from normal endocervical glandular epithelium.[93,250] The glands of HCGIN are usually surrounded by a compact stroma.[92,93] In addition, the microscopic architecture of the

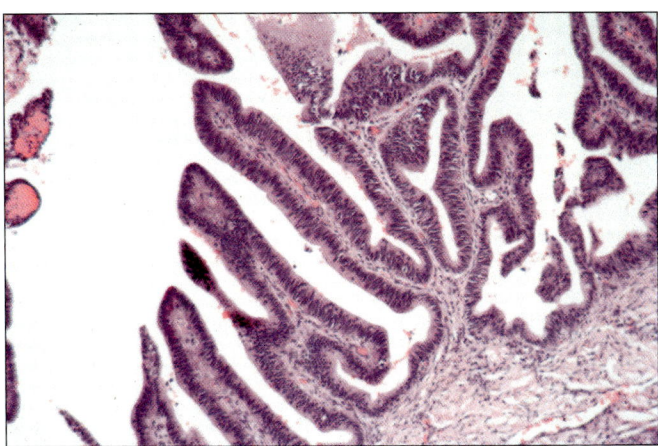

Fig. 10.16 Villoglandular HCGIN.

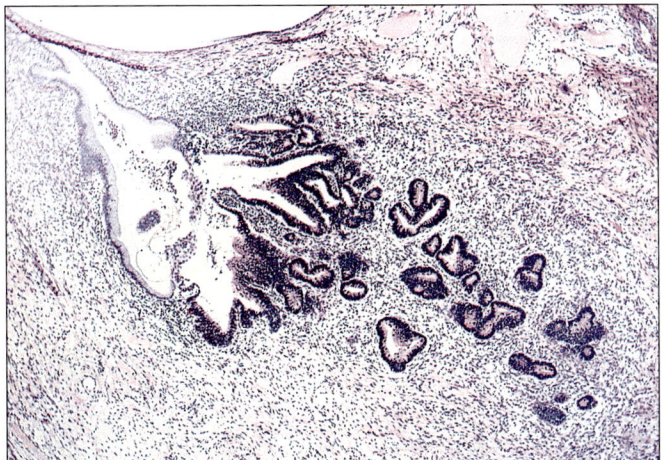

Fig. 10.17 HCGIN. Small abnormal clusters of buds have evolved from a normal endocervical gland.

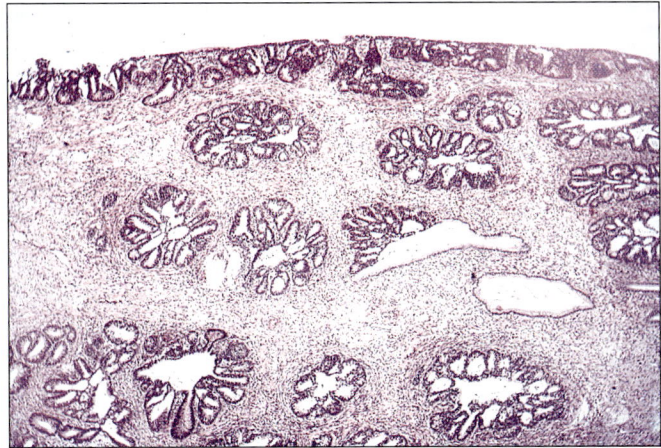

Fig. 10.18 HCGIN. There is an abnormal proliferation of glands, but none with a cribriform pattern.

endocervix is usually not disturbed by the presence of CGIN (Figure 10.21).

As with squamous CIN, CGIN lesions can be small, focal, and difficult to locate. Not uncommonly, a smear may be abnormal in the face of repeated normal biopsies and even

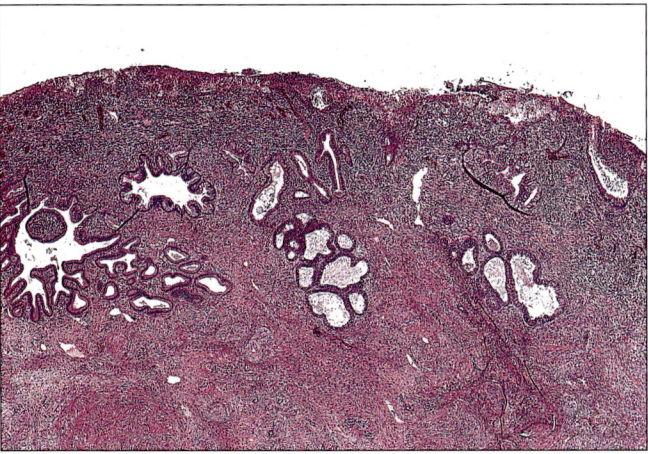

Fig. 10.19 HCGIN. The glands in the superficial cervical stroma are closely packed, suggestive of abnormal budding and growth.

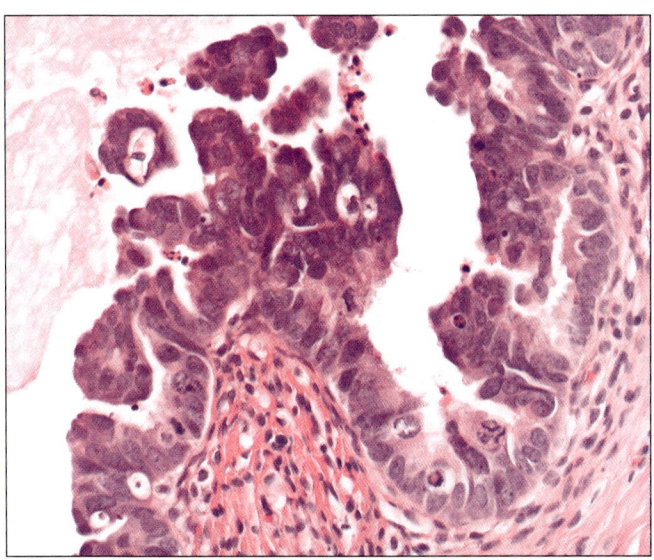

Fig. 10.20 HCGIN, papillary serous subtype.

conization. Extensive sectioning of the hysterectomy specimen may be required to locate the single abnormal focus.

LCGIN (low-grade cervical glandular intraepithelial neoplasia)

The issue of the existence of LCGIN (endocervical glandular dysplasia) is currently one of the most controversial areas in cervical glandular pathology with supporters and detractors.[62,87,92,116,128,249,250] That glandular lesions exist with morphologic features resembling, but falling short of, HCGIN (AIS) is in no doubt. The issues are what we call them and, more importantly, their biologic significance. We reserve the term LCGIN for glandular abnormalities displaying some (Figure 10.22) but not all the features of HCGIN and not associated with inflammation or reparative changes.

The features of LCGIN are qualitatively less severe than those of HCGIN (Table 10.1) and, as such, form part of a morphologic spectrum. A recently described scoring system improves reproducibility. Each feature, nuclear atypia, stratification, and the sum of mitoses/apoptosis (counted in the

253

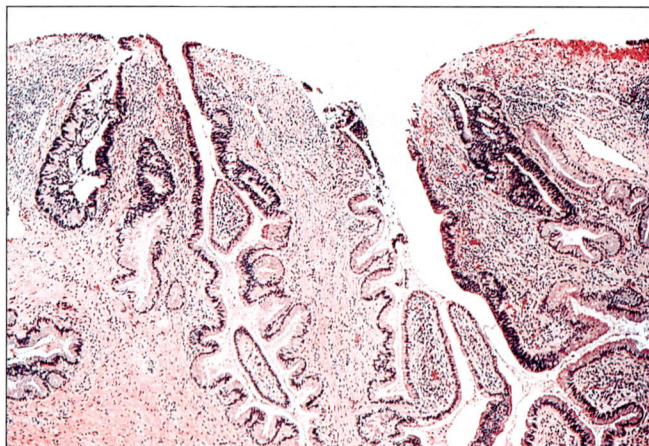

Fig. 10.21 HCGIN. The architecture of the endocervix is not altered by the glandular abnormalities.

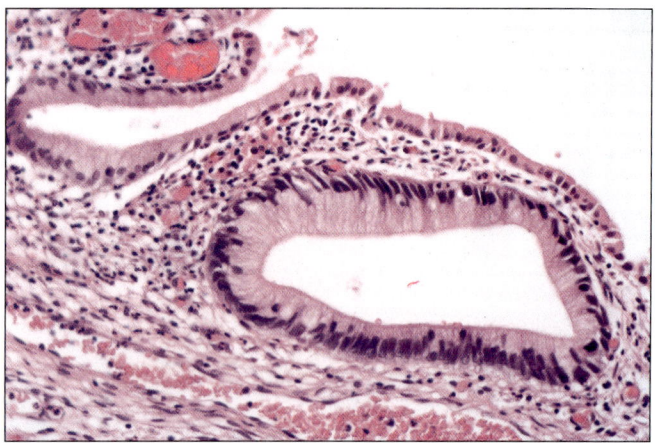

Fig. 10.22 LCGIN. The nuclei are larger than normal and hyperchromatic, they occupy more of the cell with some occupying part of the luminal half, and a very rare mitosis can sometimes be seen. Contrast to the normal glandular tissue above.

Table 10.1 Features of CGIN

Feature.	Normal	Low-grade CGIN	High-grade CGIN
Intracellular mucin	Easily observed	Some loss	Moderate to absent
Nuclear : cytoplasmic ratio	Low	Moderate	Moderate to high
Mitoses	None to occasional	None to few	Few to frequent
Apoptosis	None	None to few	Few to frequent
Nuclear size	Small	Enlarged	Enlarged
Nuclear pleomorphism	None	Slight to none	Slight to marked
Hyperchromasia	None to slight	Slight to moderate	Slight to marked
Nuclear polarity	High	High to slight loss	Usually disorganized

two most active glands and the average number used) is scored 0–3. The sum of the three scores is interpreted as 0–3 = benign, 4–5 = LCGIN (endocervical glandular dysplasia), and 6–9 = HCGIN (AIS).[87]

LCGIN can be found in association with HCGIN or invasive adenocarcinoma (up to 77% of cases) and squamous abnormalities (CIN in 57% of cases).[32,77] Unlike squamous CIN, most series dealing with HCGIN report fewer cases of LCGIN than HCGIN.[86,116,249] Possibly, LCGIN could be underdiagnosed in cases with squamous abnormalities, the appearance of the latter being more likely to attract the pathologist's attention. In a similar manner, the presence of LCGIN could also be overlooked in cases of HCGIN. However, in our experience, when specifically sought, cases of pure LCGIN prove uncommon. This view is supported by one series, where only 30 cases were identified in 1220 cone biopsies, most having more than 50 slides prepared per cone.[32]

The precise relationship between LCGIN and HCGIN and invasive adenocarcinoma remains to be defined. We believe that LCGIN and HCGIN form a morphologic spectrum that stratifies using a two-tiered grading system. That LCGIN is closely related to HCGIN finds support in aneuploidy being

found in 33% of cases, its association with c-*myc* oncogene expression, younger age of patients compared to those with HCGIN and invasive adenocarcinoma, frequency of HPV with LCGIN in some reports and its location adjacent to, and in some cases in continuity with, HCGIN.[77,79] In addition, some lesions termed 'superficial (early)' AIS, but which we would regard as fulfilling the criteria of LCGIN, also show positive immunostaining for p16^{INK4A} and have high rates of MIB1 expression.[239] Thus, it may be that the cells of LCGIN may prove to have similar or identical molecular changes to those of HCGIN. However, there appear to be clinical and biologic differences between the two as LCGIN occurs at an earlier age than HCGIN and, in our experience, invasive adenocarcinoma arises directly from areas of HCGIN and not from LCGIN.

In practice, the important issue is to recognize that a particular glandular lesion falls into the spectrum of CGIN. Strong morphologic clues include nuclear hyperchromasia and atypia, nuclear pseudostratification, and mitotic and apoptotic activity. In problematic cases, ancillary stains for p16^{INK4A} and MIB1(Ki-67) may be useful.[239]

Immunohistochemistry

In the past, immunohistochemistry played a minor role in the diagnosis of HCGIN. Carcinoembryonic antigen (CEA) reactivity occurs in 63–78% of cases.[137,157] CA125 is found in the normal luminal surface and secretory products of the endocervical crypts, but in HCGIN it is absent or localized to the perinuclear region of the cytoplasm as an accumulation of atypical coarse granules.[157] P53 is expressed focally in 20% of cases.[139] MIB1, a biomarker for increased nuclear proliferative activity, exhibits reactivity in more than 10% of cells in 86% of cases of CGIN.[30] Cdc6, another marker for cellular proliferation, also shows reactivity in 79% of cases.[22] Epithelial specific antigen (ESA) is normally expressed by the basolateral membrane of endocervical cells in the normal endocervix. Progression to diffuse cytoplasmic membrane staining has been reported in cases of LCGIN (80%) and HCGIN (84%).[136] The stromal cells surrounding glands showing HCGIN are estrogen receptor (ER) positive and alpha-smooth muscle actin negative

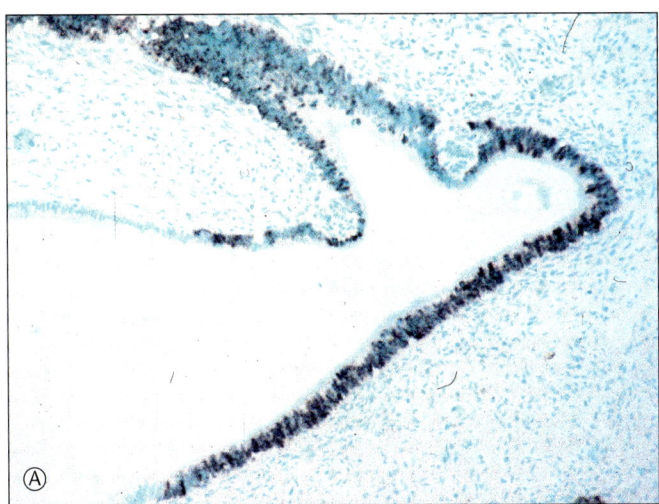

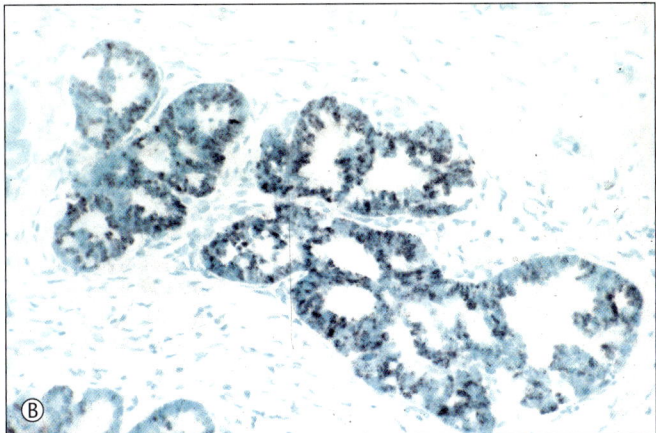

Fig. 10.23 HCGIN. *In situ* hybridization for HPV 18 (A) and HPV 16 (B) from separate cases.

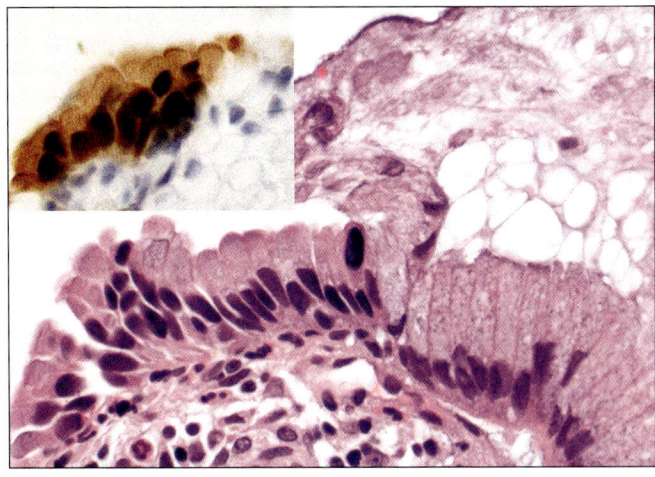

Fig. 10.24 Surface LCGIN and adjacent normal endocervical glandular epithelium. Note the nuclear enlargement, hyperchromasia and mild stratification. Apoptotic bodies are absent. Inset: LCGIN showing p16 reactivity.

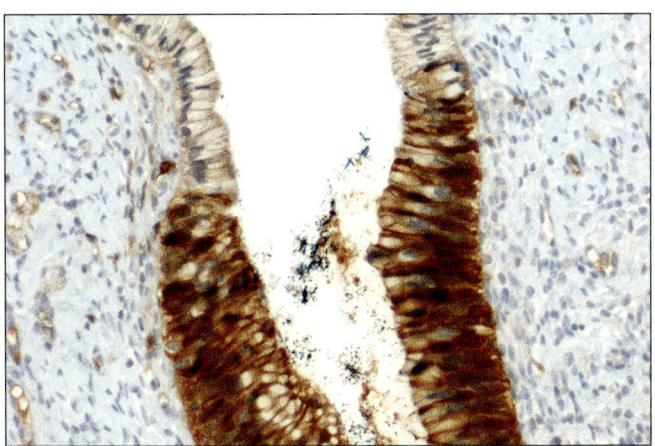

Fig. 10.25 HCGIN. Strong reactivity for p16.

in contrast to the stromal cells associated with invasive adenocarcinoma.[145]

While HPV DNA is demonstrated frequently by *in situ* hybridization in CGIN (Figure 10.23), this technology is expensive and not conducive to routine practice.[123] Recently, p16[INK4A] has emerged as a potentially useful marker for diagnosing CGIN (Figures 10.24 and 10.25). The cyclin dependent kinase 4 inhibitor, also known as p16[INK4A], is the product of the CDKN2A gene located on chromosome 9p21 and specifically binds to cyclin D-cyclin dependent kinase 4/6 complexes to control the cell cycle at the G_1–S interphase.[141,155,218]

Overexpression of p16[INK4A] is induced when high-risk HPV DNA integrates into the cell genome. In one series, all 26 cases of adenocarcinoma showed reactivity, including where there was associated *in situ* carcinoma. LCGIN showed some focal reactivity and normal endocervix, no reactivity.[158] The distinction between HCGIN and benign lesions requires attention to methodologic detail as p16[INK4A] is focally expressed in tuboendometrioid metaplasia and is diffusely expressed in proliferative endometrium (see below).[187] Possibly, MIB1, p16[INK4A] and bcl-2 may serve as a diagnostic panel.[141] HCGIN is typically diffusely reactive for p16[INK4A], shows a high proliferation index with MIB1, and is bcl-2 negative or at most focally positive.[30,141] Accurate application of such markers may clarify whether

LCGIN is a neoplastic condition and a precursor to endocervical glandular malignancy. Moreover, while these ancillary tests are useful, the mainstay of diagnosis should be careful morphologic examination.[141]

Cytology and cytologic–pathologic correlations
Terminology
Uniform terminology for the cytologic prediction of CGIN has yet to be achieved. Endocervical AIS/HCGIN was omitted as a separate entity in the 1991 Bethesda System (TBS) but included within the umbrella term 'Atypical glandular cells of undetermined significance' (AGUS). In the 2001 Bethesda System 'AIS' became a separate category.[211] Cases showing some features suggestive of, but not diagnostic of AIS, are 'Atypical endocervical cells, favor neoplastic'. The lowest reporting category for abnormal endocervical cells is 'Atypical endocervical cells, NOS'. The Australian Modified Bethesda System 2004 has similar categories, namely 'AIS', 'Possible AIS' and 'Atypical endocervical cells of undetermined significance'.[65] The UK reports only two categories, '?Glandular neoplasia', which also includes predictions of invasive and endometrial disease, and 'Borderline nuclear change in endo-

Table 10.2 Comparison of cytologic reporting systems for endocervical glandular abnormalities

The Bethesda System	Australian system	British terminology
Adenocarcinoma *in situ*	Adenocarcinoma *in situ*	?Glandular neoplasia
Atypical endocervical cells, favor neoplastic	Possible AIS	
Atypical endocervical cells, NOS	Atypical endocervical cells of undetermined significance	Borderline nuclear change in endocervical cells

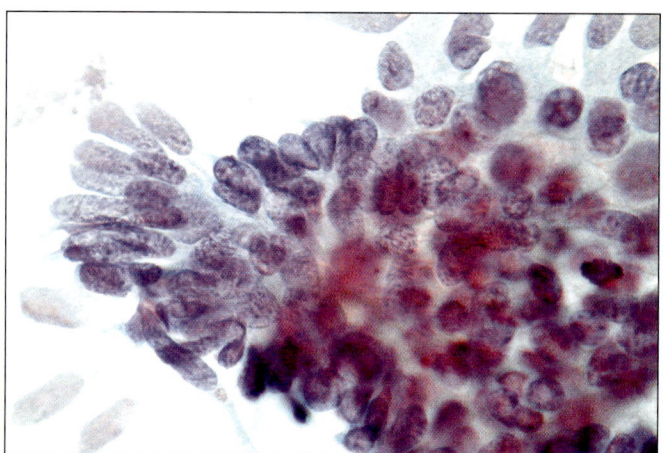

Fig. 10.26 AIS (HCGIN), endocervical subtype (Pap smear). A crowded sheet with ragged edges. Hyperchromatic elongated nuclei show palisading and feathering at the edges of the sheet. Note the mitotic figure in the sheet.

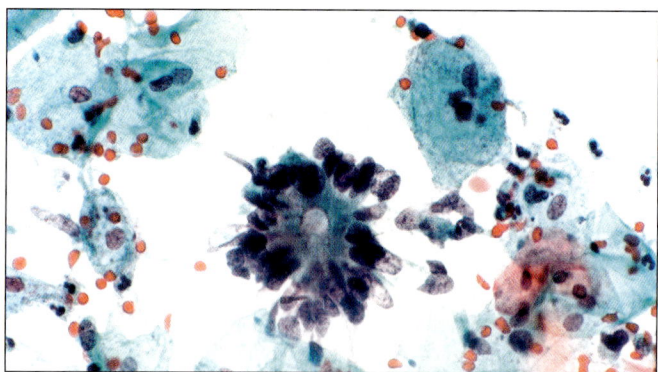

Fig. 10.27 AIS (HCGIN), endocervical subtype (Pap smear). A rosette displays a central lumen and a ragged periphery.

cervical cells'.[75] Some have further subdivided '?Glandular neoplasia' into 'Severe endocervical dyskaryosis/AIS' and 'Endocervical dyskaryosis'.[138] These categories probably do not correlate exactly with the Bethesda System or the Australian system (Table 10.2)

AIS is predicted in approximately 0.002–0.03% of all cervical smear reports and 'Possible AIS' in a similar proportion.[138,148,188,190,212] This variation probably reflects different disease incidence (these populations also vary in frequency of reporting of squamous abnormalities), different positive predictive values (see below), and varying expertise in recognition of AIS.

The historical view that the Papanicolaou smear has low sensitivity for AIS is changing.[149,209] While relevant studies are few, emerging evidence indicates that the sensitivity of the cervical smear for detecting AIS is in the order of 40–69%.[127,187a,199,205] This compares favorably with sensitivity for CIN 3, which has been reported as ranging between 43% and 75%.[7,187a,199] False-negative reports result from either sampling error or laboratory error, which can be in screening or in interpretation by senior staff. In a study of smears taken up to 3 years preceding histologic AIS, sampling error accounted for 77% of false-negative reports, while only 23% were due to laboratory error.[192] A College of American Pathologists' (CAP) *Interlaboratory Comparison Program in Cervicovaginal Cytology* showed the laboratory false-negative rate for AIS was significantly greater than that for HSIL and squamous cell carcinoma.[185,186] Problematically, unless the true prevalence of AIS in the population can be determined, the true sensitivity of the Papanicolaou test will remain unknown.

In studies of the accuracy of a cytologic prediction of AIS, positive predictive values (PPVs) ranged from 63 to 100% for any histologic high-grade lesion (HSIL, AIS or carcinoma) and from 49 to 94% for a histologic high-grade glandular lesion (AIS or adenocarcinoma).[138,148,188,190,203,238] When the cytologic report was 'Possible AIS', PPVs ranged from 42 to 75% for any histologic high-grade lesion and from 44 to 72% for a histologic high-grade glandular lesion.[148,188,190,203] Accurate prediction of AIS may be confounded by the presence of coexisting HSIL.[108,121,187a,199,223] Also, nearly one-fifth of cases predicted as AIS prove to be invasive on histology,[188,190,211] suggesting a morphologic overlap between intraepithelial and invasive endocervical glandular lesions.

Cytologic morphology

The endocervical subtype is the most common variant of the three well-differentiated AIS subtypes. Typical architectural features include crowded sheets of columnar cells with palisading and feathering of nuclei at group edges, pseudostratification, small strip-off sheets and gland openings within the sheets (Figure 10.26).[25] In addition, short strips are typical, also displaying palisading and pseudostratification. Rosettes are also a feature (Figure 10.27). The nuclei, while typically enlarged and oval in shape with coarse granular chromatin, show a wide variation in chromasia and chromatin structure. Mitoses and apoptosis are helpful features if seen. While the presence of ciliated cells is usually associated with benign findings such as tubal metaplasia, rare cases of ciliated tubal-type AIS and adenocarcinoma have, however, been described.[165,197]

Endometrioid AIS is less common and more difficult to recognize, presenting as small glandular cells in compact crowded groups.[125] The architectural features of the endocervical type are absent or subtle, with little evidence of feathering or ragged group edges.[25] Clues include pseudostratified strips and part-bare nuclei at the edges of sheets and strips (Figure 10.28). Component cells have small round nuclei and little cytoplasm. Nuclei can vary in size and chromasia. Apoptosis and mitoses are seen. Endometrioid AIS may resemble the glandular component of directly sampled lower uterine segment/endometriosis, but lacks the accompanying population of endometrial stromal cells (Figure 10.29).[25,129]

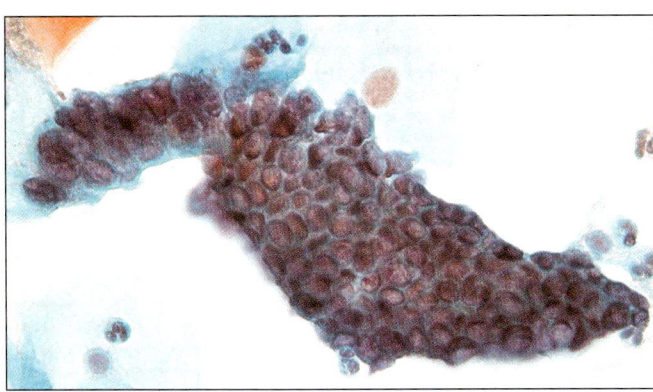

Fig. 10.28 AIS (HCGIN), endometrioid subtype (Pap smear). A compact crowded sheet lacking ragged edges. Clues to the diagnosis are nuclear variability and the 'strip-off sheet' at the top, showing pseudostratification.

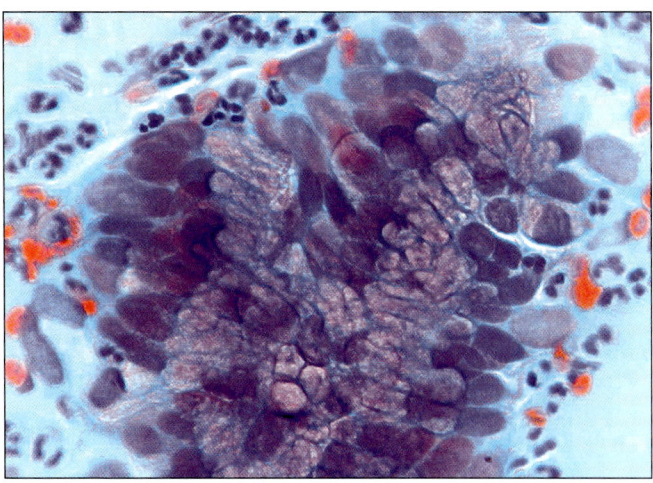

Fig. 10.30 AIS (HCGIN), intestinal subtype (Pap smear) with goblet cells in a partly air-dried crowded sheet.

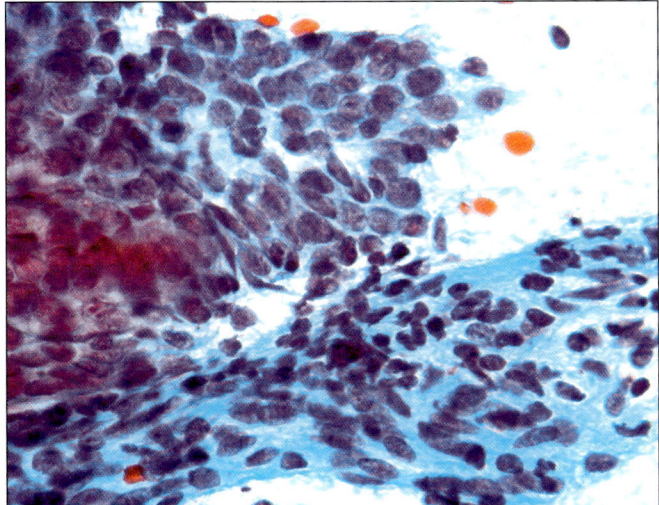

Fig. 10.29 Directly sampled endometrium (Pap smear) is a source of diagnostic confusion with endometrioid AIS. The presence of attached endometrial stroma below the epithelial sheet suggests benignancy.

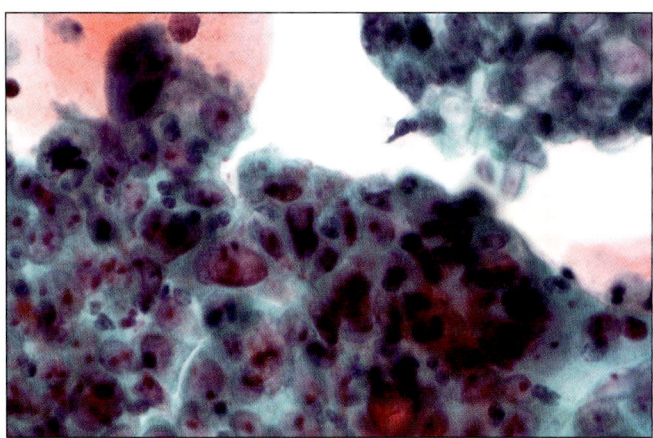

Fig. 10.31 AIS (HCGIN), poorly differentiated subtype (Pap smear). A disorganized sheet with variably enlarged nuclei, displaying prominent nucleoli and fine chromatin. Note the mitosis in the upper left corner.

Intestinal AIS is also less common and sometimes accompanies other subtypes. Again, the characteristic feature is crowded sheets, with many goblet cells containing large mucous vacuoles that tend to distort the nuclei. AIS architecture may be present but disarranged somewhat by the presence of abundant vacuoles (Figure 10.30).[25]

Poorly differentiated AIS is difficult to recognize on cytology and may resemble reactive change/repair. Loosely packed sheets may lack pseudostratification. Nuclear enlargement is prominent, with oval to round shapes, prominent nucleoli, and finely granular chromatin (Figure 10.31). Features that suggest abnormality rather than repair include cells with fragile disintegrating cytoplasm and the presence of rosette or acinus-like structures (Figure 10.32). Often the diagnosis must be based on the presence of better differentiated groups within the same smear.[25]

Microglandular hyperplasia has been reported to occasionally mimic AIS, but can usually be recognized by the admixture of glandular and immature metaplastic cells with microlumina and fenestrations and no significant nuclear atypia.[4,31]

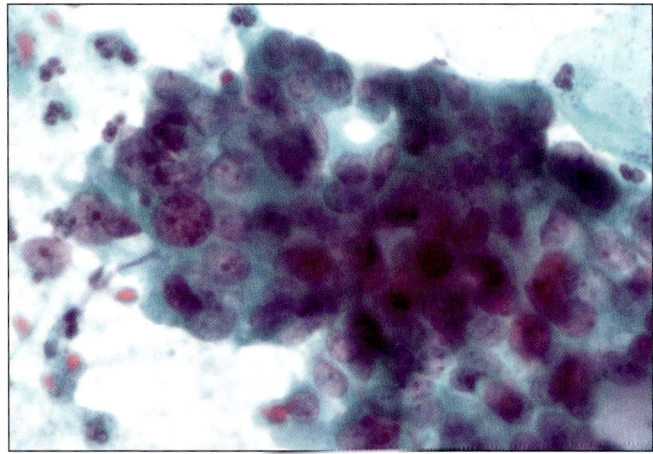

Fig. 10.32 AIS (HCGIN), poorly differentiated subtype (Pap smear). High nuclear : cytoplasmic ratios, bare nuclei at the edge and an acinus (top) provide evidence of the neoplastic nature of the sheet.

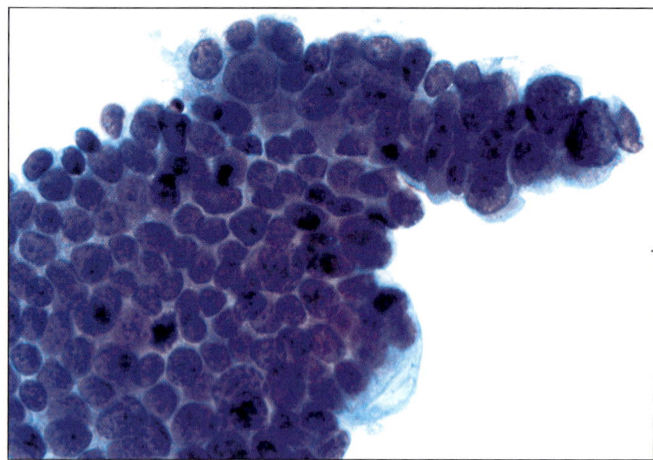

Fig. 10.33 AIS (HCGIN) (ThinPrep). Pseudostratified strips can be very helpful in liquid-based preparations.

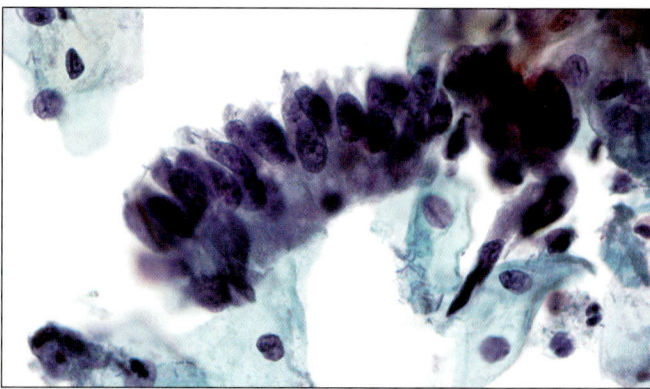

Fig. 10.35 AIS (HCGIN) (ThinPrep). A crowded smooth-edged sheet with pleomorphic nuclei and a 'strip-off sheet' at the top with pseudostratified nuclei. Nuclear detail is excellent, feathering is absent.

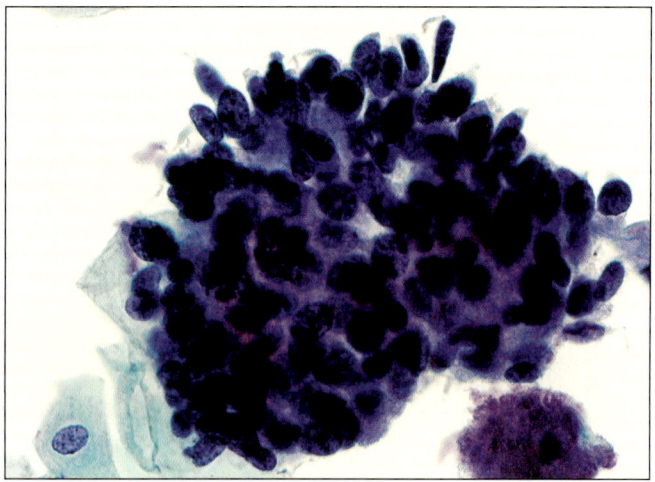

Fig. 10.34 AIS (HCGIN) (ThinPrep). A crowded hyperchromatic sheet with mitoses, nuclear variability, and some subtle feathering at the top.

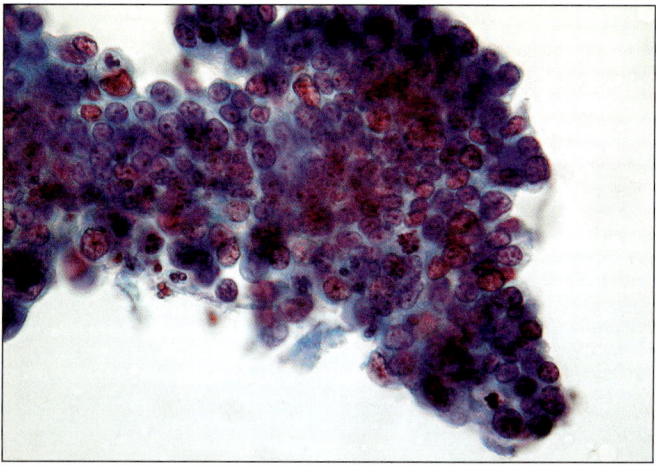

Fig. 10.36 AIS (HCGIN) (ThinPrep). A crowded sheet with subtle glandular features and no feathering.

The increased use of liquid-based cytology (LBC) for cervical screening has resulted in a need to learn somewhat different appearances of endocervical neoplasia. Glandular groups with this methodology are more three-dimensional than with the usual cervical smear and show diminution of several typical architectural features of AIS, in particular the shearing of cells at the edge of groups that contributes to the appearance of feathering in conventional smears, although this is not universally agreed.[16a,94,171,189] Nuclear features are better preserved in samples collected in fluid medium (Figures 10.33–10.36).[94,171,189] Data are still conflicting as to whether or not liquid-based specimens enable detection of AIS with greater efficacy than the cervical smear.[8,13,72,151,182,187,189,200,230,237] An advantage of this new methodology is the opportunity to perform immunohistochemical stains, such as p16[INK4A] and P-cadherin, on the original cytology samples.[134,156,158]

With the recent development and use of interactive computer-assisted screening of LBC slides, it will be important to determine the accuracy of these systems in highlighting abnormal glandular groups for human review. In our trial we found that use of the ThinPrep Imaging System (TIS) had a similar sensitivity for detection of AIS as manual screening of Thin-

Prep slides[191]. However, in subsequent routine use over three years, we have found that the current TIS algorithm favors the selection of single cells over diagnostic large sheets, which presents a problem in the recognition of AIS, particularly the endometrioid subtype.

Prediction of low-grade CGIN

Considerable controversy exists regarding the prediction of LCGIN on cervical cytology. Neither the Bethesda System 2001 nor the Australian reporting system recognizes an ability to accurately predict LCGIN on Papanicolaou tests. This view is further supported by the outcome data for the reporting categories 'less than' AIS (see Table 10.1). Rather than predicting a lesion of lower histologic grade than AIS, these categories predict a lesser probability of histologic AIS.[46,148,188,190,203] In a British study in which a histologic diagnosis of LCGIN was expected following a cytologic prediction of 'endocervical dyskaryosis', only 16% had LCGIN, 18% had a high-grade glandular lesion (HCGIN or carcinoma), while the remainder showed no glandular abnormality, a metaplastic process or non-neoplastic atypia.[138] In contrast, some investigators claim an ability to grade the severity of CGIN on a Papanicolaou smear, using specific architectural, cellular, and nuclear char-

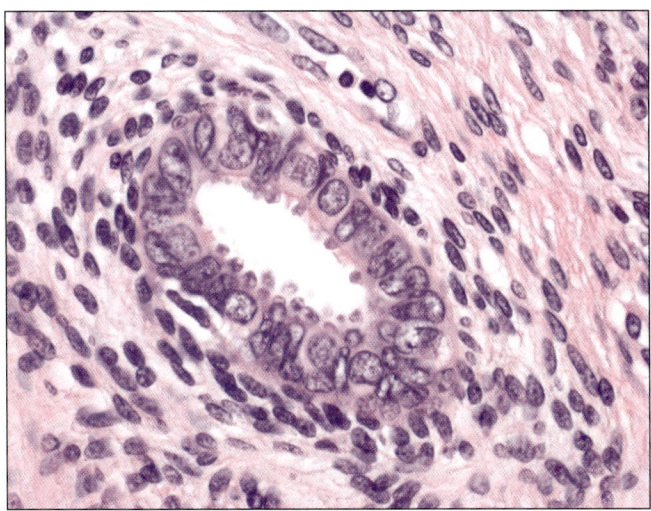

Fig. 10.37 Tuboendometrioid metaplasia.

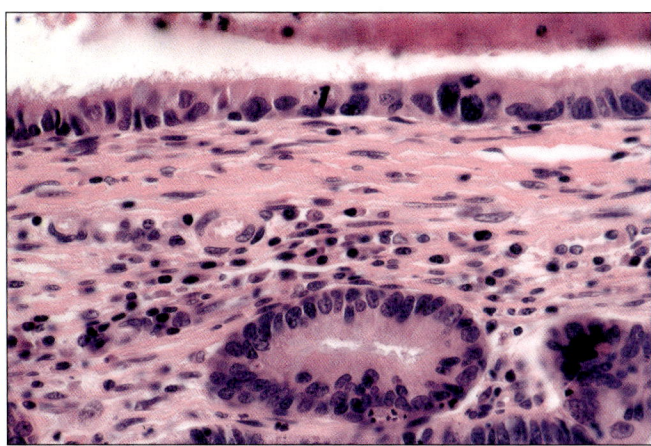

Fig. 10.38 Ciliated HCGIN.

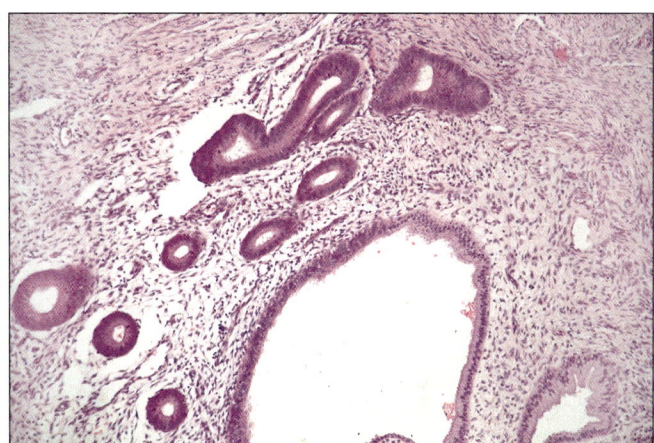

Fig. 10.39 Superficial cervical endometriosis.

acteristics, and to successfully correlate this with histologic findings.[224–226]

Management of cytologic predictions

A Papanicolaou test prediction of 'AIS' or 'Atypical endocervical cells, favor neoplasia'/'Possible AIS' requires histologic confirmation.[241a] Colposcopy should be performed to exclude clinically overt invasive carcinoma and to determine whether there is coexistent squamous disease. However, colposcopy is usually negative in cases of uncomplicated AIS. The lesion may be confined to the canal and even when it is not, there are usually no colposcopically diagnostic features.[241] Diagnostic conization is recommended after a negative colposcopy.[241] Management of reports of 'Atypical endocervical cells' with its much reduced predictive outcome, is more problematic and has been extensively discussed.[65,241] Colposcopy is uniformly recommended. While a negative colposcopy does not exclude a significant glandular lesion, it does exclude overtly invasive carcinoma and does help determine the extent of any squamous disease present. Squamous disease alone is a not infrequent outcome when 'Atypical endocervical cells' are reported.[194,241] HPV testing may prove useful in this group[45,115,194] and the American Society for Colposcopy and Cervical Pathology has recently incorporated testing for high-risk HPV DNA into its management guidelines for these women.

Differential diagnosis/problematic issues

Several benign glandular lesions simulate CGIN. The most common is tubal metaplasia, which displays in varying proportions a mixture of ciliated, secretory, and resting (intercalary or peg) cells, even within a single case (Figure 10.37). Glands exhibiting tubal metaplasia lack nuclear atypia and mitoses are seen only occasionally. Apoptotic bodies are inconspicuous. The glands may be associated with endometrioid-type stroma. Endometrioid metaplasia also shows bland nuclei that lack significant mitotic activity. CD10-positive endometrioid stroma may also be present. Immunohistochemically, tuboendometrioid metaplasia shows a low MIB1 staining rate and strong widespread positive staining for bcl-2. It also exhibits p16^{INK4A} in 62% of cases, but unlike HCGIN, the reactivity is only focal.[30] Tuboendometrioid metaplasia may show reactivity for

CEA in 39% of cases but unlike HCGIN expresses vimentin.[137] The presence of cilia usually implies a benign process, but of note, ciliated CGIN also occurs (Figure 10.38).[197]

Superficial cervical endometriosis (Figure 10.39) may be confused with CGIN histologically.[14] The latter may be particularly problematic in patients followed with cytologic smears after cone biopsy. The endometriotic foci are usually confined to the inner third of the cervical wall. The endometrioid glands are typically evenly spaced, show bland cytologic features, and are surrounded, at least focally, by endometrial-type stroma, which may show focal hemosiderin deposition. Inflammation and hemorrhage may obscure the stromal cells. Mitotic figures are seen in 37% of cases.[14]

Endocervical glands may show a variety of architectural and cytologic changes in response to inflammation. This may lead to a suspicion of CGIN. In inflammatory/reparative changes, the nuclei become enlarged and show chromatin clearing and prominent nucleoli. Nuclear pleomorphism may occur, but the chromatin is often smudged (Figure 10.40). Pseudostratification and mitotic activity are minimal. Apoptotic bodies are generally absent. Our experience is that endocervical glands in some patients may also show mild morphologic changes during the menstrual cycle. Occasionally, a normal-appearing mitosis can be found in normal endocervical glands and should not raise concern (Figure 10.41).

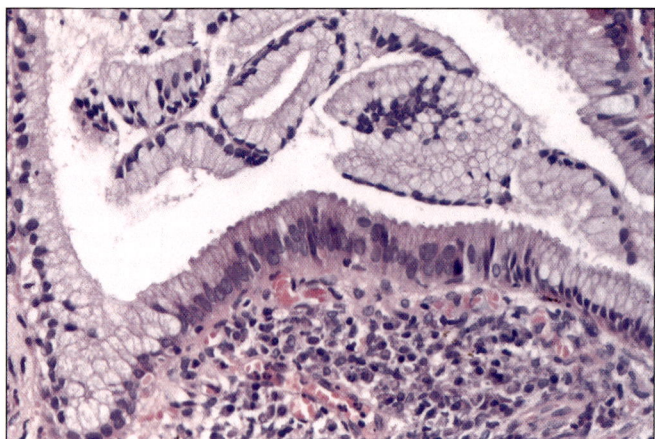

Fig. 10.40 Endocervical gland showing inflammatory changes.

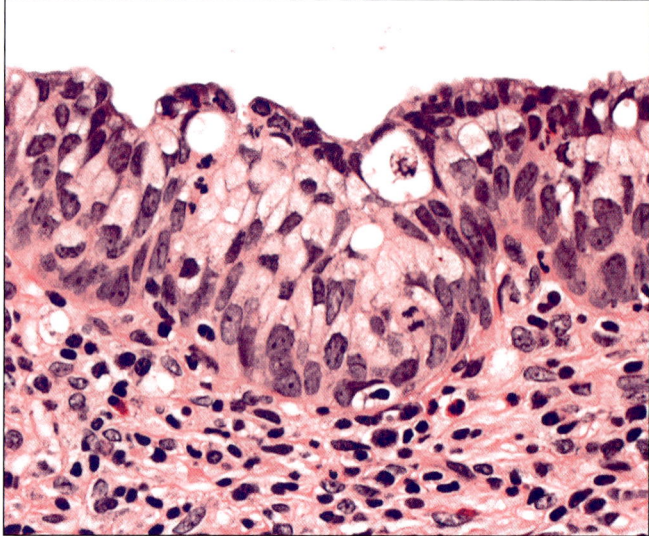

Fig. 10.42 Stratified mucin-producing intraepithelial lesion (SMILE) in a case also with HCGIN and CIN 3 elsewhere in the cervix.

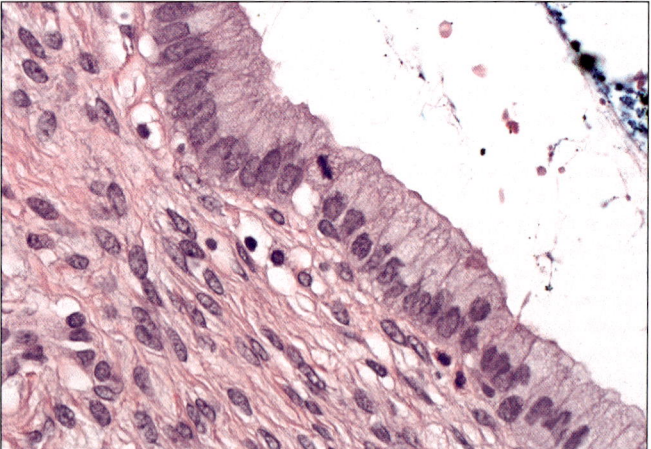

Fig. 10.41 Normal endocervical gland showing a mitotic figure.

Radiation therapy results in widely spaced glands that are often tubular or dilated and lined by flattened to cuboidal large cells with at most a slight increase in nuclear : cytoplasmic ratio. The cytoplasm is finely vacuolated or eosinophilic. There is often loss of nuclear polarity and the nuclei show dispersed chromatin and one or two prominent eosinophilic nucleoli. Focal cytoplasmic CEA reactivity occurs and does not distinguish it from CGIN.[130]

The Arias-Stella reaction involves the endocervical glands in 10% of gravid uteri (Figure 14.66). Superficial glands are more commonly involved than deep. The involved glands typically have a single layer of enlarged hyperchromatic pleomorphic nuclei that protrude into the lumen producing a 'hobnail' appearance. The glandular cells may also show intranuclear cytoplasmic inclusions as well as optically clear nuclei. Mitoses are exceedingly rare or absent.[162,163]

CGIN may occasionally involve areas of microglandular hyperplasia within the cervix. In such cases, the presence of residual microglandular hyperplasia not involved by CGIN is the key to establishing the diagnosis. Similarly, CGIN may also involve other benign endocervical glandular lesions, such as tunnel clusters.[141]

A stratified mucin-producing intraepithelial lesion (SMILE) exhibits stratified epithelium resembling CIN in which there is conspicuous mucin production (Figure 10.42). Mucin is present throughout the epithelium, varying from indistinct cytoplasmic clearing to discrete vacuoles. The lesion shows a rounded or lobulated contour at the epithelial–stromal interface and a high MIB1 index. SMILE is an unusual cervical intraepithelial lesion best regarded as a variant of cervical columnar cell neoplasia based on phenotype. SMILE is usually associated with CIN, CGIN or invasive carcinoma.[173]

Clinical behavior/management

Unlike squamous CIN where complete excision with a cone biopsy is usually sufficient for cure, the optimal treatment for HCGIN remains debatable. In a meta-analysis, 27% of patients treated with conization where the margins were free of abnormality had residual HCGIN in the subsequent hysterectomy specimen. This figure reached 59% if the margins on cone biopsy were positive.[11,61,82,169,204,250] Some believe that the disease-free endocervical margin in a cone biopsy must be at least 10 mm to consider the lesion completely excised.[61] Except where preservation of fertility is desired, hysterectomy may be the prudent definitive therapy for HCGIN.[82] If a lesser procedure is performed, cold-knife or laser cone biopsy is more effective than loop electrosurgical excision, especially for the endocervical margin.[2,107,234] Furthermore, patients with HCGIN and positive margins on cone biopsy are at moderate risk of harboring an occult invasive endocervical adenocarcinoma that has already developed.[154] The optimal management of LCGIN is even more controversial, with treatment options including cytologic follow-up or management along the lines of HCGIN.

PRECLINICAL CARCINOMA

MICROINVASIVE (EARLY INVASIVE) ADENOCARCINOMA

Definition

Microinvasive adenocarcinoma refers to the earliest form of invasive adenocarcinoma and is classified generally in a manner similar to microinvasive squamous cell carcinoma.

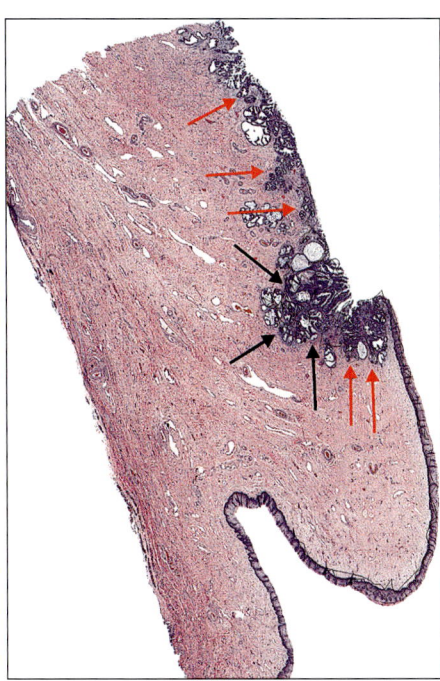

Fig. 10.43 Microinvasive adenocarcinoma. A giant section through the cervix shows a microinvasive carcinoma arising adjacent to the squamocolumnar junction. CGIN is present from that point to the cranial-most resection margin.

Pathology

Microinvasive adenocarcinoma of the cervix (Figure 10.43) is an entity, the existence of which has been controversial until recently.[167] One problem in the debate has been the lack of agreement on the histologic criteria that identify the earliest stages of invasion and distinguish it from CGIN. A second problem has been whether adopting such a category helps in determining management.

Identifying the first steps of invasion in squamous lesions is usually straightforward. This is a function of the relative simplicity, morphologically, of the epithelial–stromal interface – the boundary between CIN and the underlying supporting stroma. The finger-like processes of early stromal invasion breaking through the basement membrane are easily identified. With CGIN, by contrast, this interface is far more complex and difficult to assess.

To identify early invasion requires an ability to recognize which glandular structures represent CGIN involving pre-existing crypts and which are truly invasive. Several characteristic growth patterns of microinvasive adenocarcinoma occur singly or in combination.[168]

- Small, finger-like processes extend into the stroma from the base of the epithelium or detached cellular clusters are found lying free in the stroma. The individual cells are larger than those of HCGIN with more abundant eosinophilic cytoplasm (Figures 10.44–10.46). This pattern of invasion is, in our experience, uncommon.
- Tentacular invasion with variably shaped and sized neoplastic glands (Figure 10.47) associated with a stromal reaction.
- Prominent cribriform pattern (Figure 10.48) or prominent intraglandular papillae.

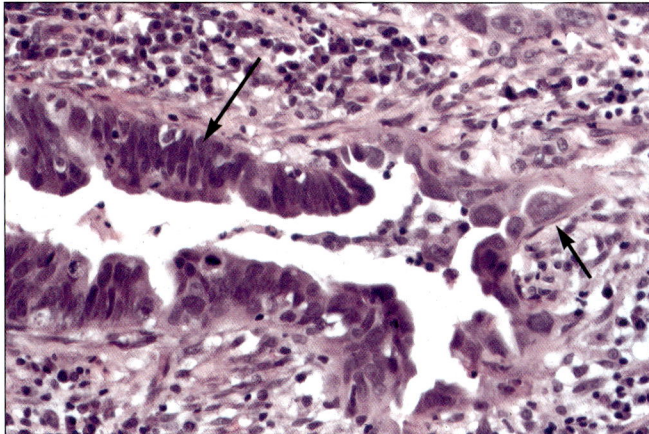

Fig. 10.44 HCGIN and microinvasive adenocarcinoma. The architecture and cytology change substantially at the junction of the *in situ* (long arrow) and invasive disease (short arrow).

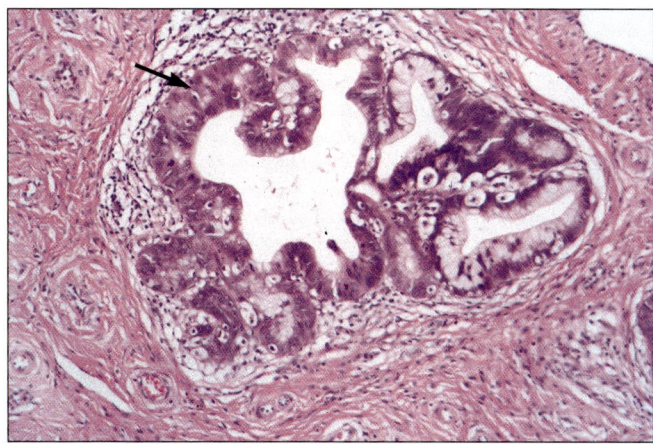

Fig. 10.45 Microinvasive adenocarcinoma arising in HCGIN. While the perimeter of some of the major gland is smooth (arrow), definite breaks and foci of invasion indicate early stromal invasion.

- Some cases invade on a broad front, similar to their squamous counterpart, with relatively discrete demarcation from the underlying stroma (Figure 10.49).
- Rarely, there is solid growth with only a minor, well-formed glandular component (Figure 10.50). Spread of invasive tumor between the normal crypts near the surface may also occur.
- Extension of glands beyond the normal crypt field is another marker for invasion (Figure 10.48). However, this often proves difficult to recognize if all crypts in one section are involved so that there are no normal crypts for reference.
- Close proximity of glands to thick-walled blood vessels (distance from the closest gland to a thick-walled vessel less than or equal to the thickness of the vessel wall) appears to be a useful feature in the diagnosis of invasive endocervical adenocarcinoma.[233]
- Perhaps the most difficult pattern to diagnose occurs where well-differentiated glands are found singly or in

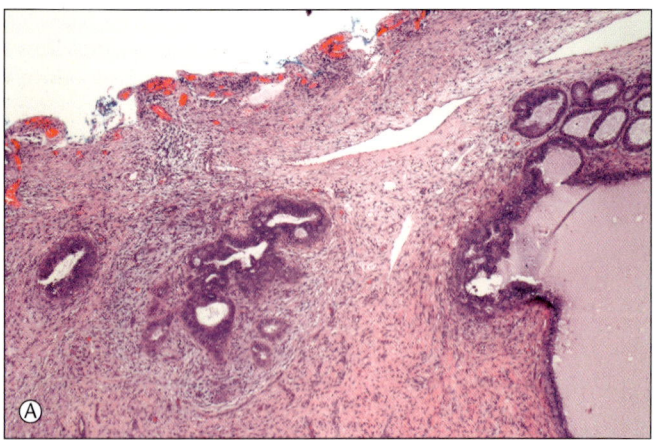

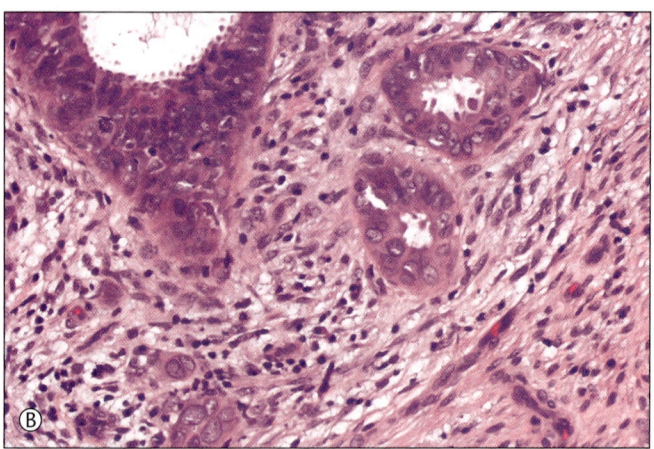

Fig. 10.46 (A, B) Microinvasive adenocarcinoma.

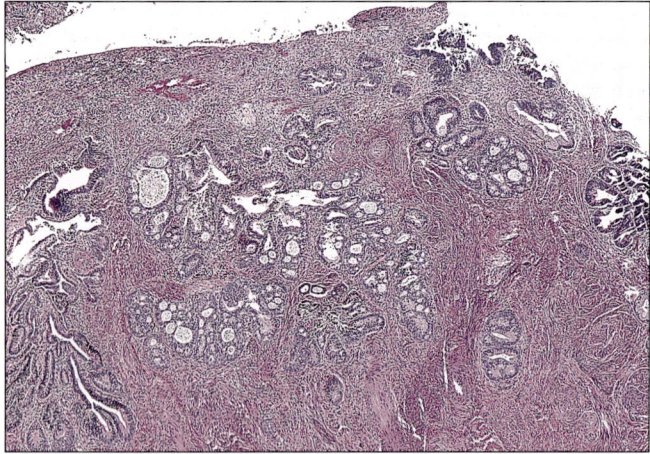

Fig. 10.47 Microinvasive adenocarcinoma. Numerous glands are present. The irregular growth pattern, the presence in some of a cribriform pattern, and irregular outlines are indicative of early invasive carcinoma.

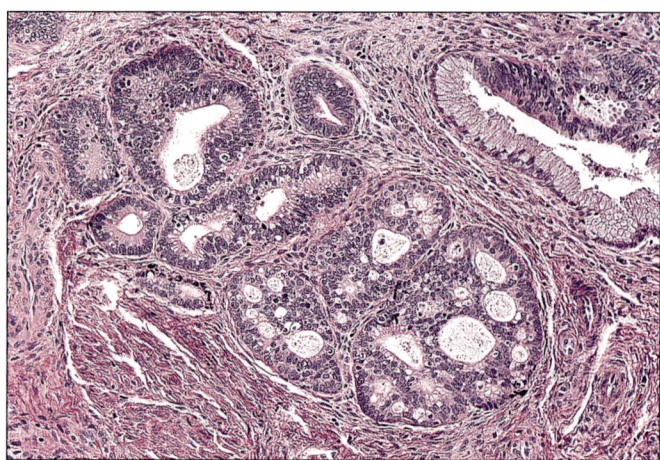

Fig. 10.48 Microinvasive adenocarcinoma. Several glands with a cribriform pattern and adjacent glands with HCGIN are located just beneath the normal crypt field (not shown in photograph).

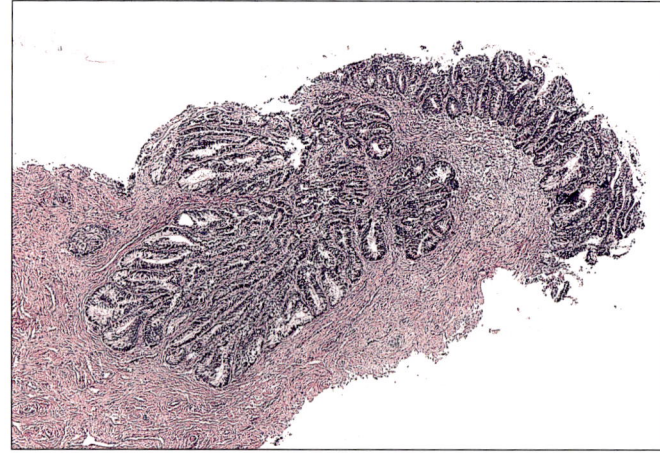

Fig. 10.49 Microinvasive adenocarcinoma. The tumor is 2 mm in greatest dimension and composed of thickly packed glands.

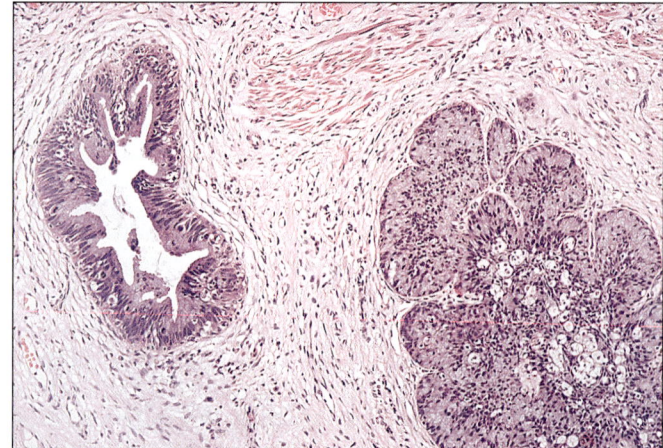

Fig. 10.50 Microinvasive adenocarcinoma. On the right is a large, complex gland that is solid and has a highly irregular outline with blunt extensions into the stroma.

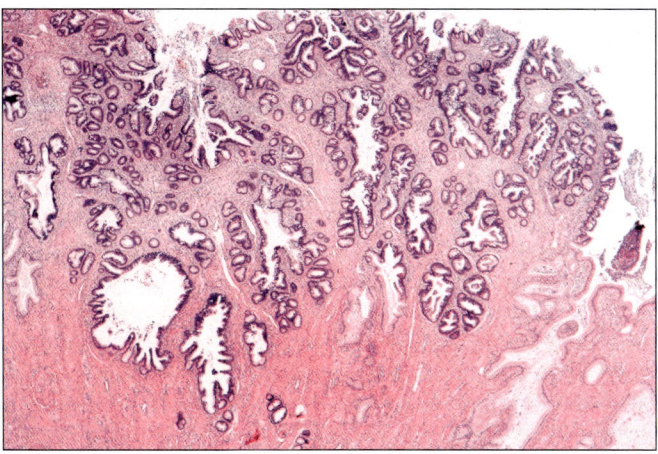

Fig. 10.51 In some cases it may be difficult to distinguish HCGIN from invasive tumor when extensive changes are present. The deeply invasive glands suggest this case is invasive.

groups, well beyond the deepest normal crypt in the absence of any stromal reaction. This pattern closely mimics some cases of diffusely invasive endometrioid adenocarcinoma of the corpus.

While the above description of features describing microinvasive adenocarcinoma may appear straightforward, in practice it often proves difficult and subjective when employed in any individual case (Figure 10.51). Indeed, the identification of early invasion in cervical glandular lesions may not always be possible, and in approximately 10–15% of patients the pathologist may be uncertain.[141] The inevitable result is errors of over- and underdiagnosis.

The FIGO system (1995) for staging carcinoma of the cervix makes no distinction between squamous and glandular lesions. Stage 1A1 defines invasion to less than 3 mm in depth and less than 7 mm in width; stage 1A2 defines invasion between 3 and 5 mm in depth and less than 7 mm in width. Vascular space invasion does not alter the stage. While invasion should be measured ideally from the point of origin from the adjacent *in situ* component, this is rarely practical with glandular neoplasia. Most pathologists measure the depth of penetration from the surface of the lesion and in most cases this measurement corresponds to tumor thickness.[167] An alternative and rarely used method is to define microinvasion on the basis of tumor volume of <500 mm.[3,28]

Microinvasive adenocarcinoma and microinvasive adenosquamous carcinoma comprise approximately 12% of microinvasive cervical tumors.[49] The distribution is similar to that of HCGIN. Most (78%) have the midpoint of the invasive focus in the region of the squamocolumnar junction or transformation zone.[126] Moreover, multiple invasive foci were seen in only 10% of cases in one study. In a substantive study where microinvasion was defined as depth of invasion or tumor thickness of at most 5 mm, the length of microinvasive adenocarcinomas ranged from 0.8 to 21 mm and the tumor volume ranged between 3 and 1000 mm³. The tumors were multicentric in 21 of 77 cases (interpreted as most commonly involving both cervical lips without continuity at 3 o'clock and 9 o'clock). 'Skip' lesions – defined as separation of more than 3 mm between discrete microinvasive adenocarcinomas in the same lip – were not found.[167]

Cytologic correlation

Microinvasive adenocarcinoma can sometimes be predicted cytologically. Features include those of AIS, which are always present. Syncytia of glandular cells, small cells in supercrowded sheets, papillary groupings, and dissociated cells are suggestive of the diagnosis. Nuclear features include pleomorphism with irregular chromatin and nucleoli. Tumor diathesis may also be present. Collectively, these criteria help predict microinvasion in over two-fifths of cases.[9,152] In practical terms, microinvasion can be accurately defined only histologically. The major role of cytology in this circumstance is identifying the existence of high-grade neoplasia of endocervical columnar cell origin.

Clinical behavior/management

There is no doubt that pathologists can recognize some glandular lesions that are invasive but apparently still early in their natural history. What is uncertain is the maximum size where less than radical treatment is safe. Whether a diagnosis of microinvasive adenocarcinoma has the same clinical value as microinvasive squamous cell carcinoma is undecided, although there is mounting evidence supporting their similar clinical behavior.

When early invasive adenocarcinoma is defined by a 5 mm depth of invasion or less, no patient treated by radical hysterectomy had parametrial involvement.[168] No adnexal tumors were found in patients in whom one or both ovaries were removed. Two per cent of patients had pelvic lymph node metastases, a figure that in reality may be lower as some cases in the meta-analysis lacked pertinent information. Of these patients, 3.4% developed recurrences and 1.4% died. The relationship of capillary–lymphatic space involvement, lymph node metastasis, and recurrence remains uncertain. Fifty per cent of patients with positive margins had residual disease in the subsequent hysterectomy specimen. As no patient treated with conization suffered a recurrence, early invasive adenocarcinoma seems to behave like its squamous counterpart. In addition, cone biopsy is considered acceptable treatment only if the specimen has been adequately sampled and the margins free.[168] In a Surveillance, Epidemiology and End Results (SEER) database review of 301 cases of microinvasive adenocarcinoma of which 131 were FIGO stage 1A1 and 170 were stage 1A2, only one of 140 women who had lymphadenectomy had a single positive lymph node. This patient had stage 1A2 disease. Moreover, of four women with tumor-related deaths, three were stage 1A2. Overall, the prognosis for microinvasive adenocarcinoma is excellent and in 96 cases, simple hysterectomy alone proved adequate.[231] In a more recent study evaluating depth of invasion, none of 48 patients with tumor under 5 mm invasive had involved parametria or nodes, whereas 8 of the 36 with invasion greater than 5 mm had nodal metastases. None of the former developed a recurrence whereas one-sixth of the latter developed recurrent disease. These data argue that for patients with tumor less than 5 mm effective invasion and negative margins, pelvic lymphadenectomy may be omitted.[15] Similarly, in a study of 32 patients with FIGO stage 1A1 and 1A2 adenocarcinomas of the cervix where invasion was strictly defined, the method of measurement was standardized, and villoglandular, papillary serous, and clear cell carcinomas were excluded, no recurrences have been reported to date. No patients had lymph node metastasis. One patient died of metastatic ovarian carcinoma 82 months after her diagnosis of cervical carcinoma. Two of 27 (7%) patients have chronic leg edema secondary to lymph node dissection. The authors concluded that, given the excellent prognosis, the absence of lymph node metastases, and a lymph node dissection complication rate of 7%, less radical surgery should be considered in this low-risk patient population.[34]

Tumor volume in one, but not another, study was more predictive than depth of invasion in foretelling lymph node metastasis and/or recurrence.[101,106]

Unlike squamous carcinoma where large numbers of cases have been studied, insufficient information exists about the natural history of early cervical adenocarcinoma to allow firm conclusions regarding treatment to be drawn. Radical therapy will undoubtedly be used in some cases. Clearly, some young women with early invasive adenocarcinomas might best be served by treating the tumor in the same way as microinvasive squamous cell carcinoma.

INVASIVE ADENOCARCINOMA

ENDOCERVICAL-TYPE ADENOCARCINOMA (INCLUDING FEATURES OF ADENOCARCINOMA IN GENERAL)

Definition
Carcinomas of the glandular epithelium form a substantial group of invasive cervical cancers. In the last five decades the proportion of cervical carcinomas of glandular origin has risen in comparison to those of squamous type, from about 6% in the 1950s and 1960s to 12.6% in the 1990s, with current estimates in the range of 10–20%.[92,206,210,215,227,228,248] Part of this apparent increase is due to the effects of the screening programs that are now so widespread. They detect many precursor lesions, especially those of squamous cell carcinoma, with a subsequent reduction of that tumor type. However, as many glandular lesions are more difficult to diagnose in the precursor stages, many remain undetected until they present as clinical carcinoma, thereby increasing the proportion of clinical carcinomas that are of glandular type.[127,180] As well as a relative increase in the incidence of cervical adenocarcinoma, there is some evidence for an absolute increase in incidence in both the United States and Northern Europe, particularly in women under the age of 35 years.[27,132,172,176]

Clinical features
The mean age of patients with adenocarcinoma of the cervix is about 55 years, and on a per-stage basis this is about the same (stage 1, 47 years; stage 2, 55 years; stage 3, 59 years) as for patients with squamous cell carcinoma. There is some suggestion that the mean age of patients with stage 1 tumor has fallen (in one series from 58 to 44 years), but this does not seem greatly different from squamous cell cancers where the same phenomenon has been observed.[6] Most patients complain of vaginal bleeding or discharge. A third of patients are asymptomatic. At the time of diagnosis, 67.8% of patients are found to be FIGO stage 1, 23.8% stage 2, 7.4% stage 3, and 1% are stage 4. The older the age group, the higher the proportion of cases with a more advanced FIGO stage.[36]

Pathogenesis/etiology
Some evidence indicates that cervical adenocarcinoma shares some epidemiologic risk factors with squamous cell carcinoma

and is a sexually transmitted disease, linked to HPV exposure.[18,219] In contrast to squamous cell carcinoma in which HPV genotype 16 is most common, multiple studies have shown that both HPV types 16 and 18 are common. While some, but not all, studies suggest HPV type 18 is more common in adenocarcinoma,[84,240] it is unclear how this is influenced by specific histologic cell types[5] or even HPV type variants.[29,43] The HPV status, however, is not predictive of disease outcome. Interestingly, *PTEN* mutation is frequently detected in HPV-negative adenocarcinomas of the cervix and is seen most commonly in the endometrioid subtype.[147] Cofactors that show significant positive associations with adenocarcinoma overall and among HPV-positive women include poor hygiene, low levels of formal education, high parity, and HSV 2 seropositivity.[33]

Most adenocarcinomas and squamous cell carcinomas are thought to arise from the transformation zone from subcolumnar reserve cells. In some studies adenocarcinomas have been associated with use of oral contraceptives (particularly use > 10 years and with preparations containing a more potent progestational agent), especially in women under the age of 35 years.[26,33,216,219] However, other studies have found no such increased risk after accounting for HPV infection, sexual history, and cytologic screening.[83,119] Also, it appears that oral contraceptives do not modulate the expression of cervical neoplasia in favor of adenocarcinoma.[81] On the other hand, use of hormone replacement therapy, especially unopposed estrogens, in older women may be associated with an increased risk of cervical adenocarcinoma.[118] Yet other reports indicate that adenocarcinomas share some epidemiologic associations with endometrial carcinoma, including a slight tendency toward patient obesity, hypertension, and nulligravidity.[112,219]

Patients with the Peutz–Jeghers syndrome have a genetic predisposition to the development of adenoma malignum (minimal deviation adenocarcinoma, mucinous type).[58] A link between cervical and ovarian glandular neoplasms exists as occasional women with mucinous cervical adenocarcinoma develop primary ovarian mucinous neoplasms including adenocarcinoma. This association is seen in both the presence and absence of the Peutz–Jeghers syndrome.[58,133]

Classification and pathology
One current classification scheme orders the pure invasive glandular cancers in descending frequency.[248] For simplicity of presentation, the pure endocervical type will be presented as the paradigm and will include generalized discussions about pathology, biology, and clinical treatment. This will be followed by variants with specific items covered.

Grossly, half of cervical adenocarcinomas are exophytic, usually as a polypoid or papillary mass (Figure 10.52). Some may be nodular, with diffuse enlargement or ulceration. About one-sixth are small and not visible, usually because of their location within the endocervical canal. Even in the absence of visible signs or symptoms, the tumor may infiltrate deeply into the wall (Figure 10.53). Generally, the gross appearance is not helpful in predicting the histologic appearance.[244]

The endocervical tumor type accounts for at least 80% of cervical adenocarcinomas. Whilst cervical adenocarcinoma is often referred to as mucinous adenocarcinoma, it is not always overtly mucinous. Commonly it is mucin-poor due to less than a high degree of differentiation and instead is composed of cells with eosinophilic cytoplasm. The tumor also has readily found

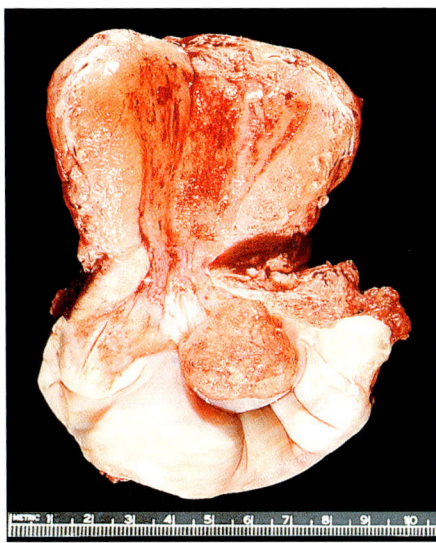

Fig. 10.52 Adenocarcinoma. The tumor appears as a polypoid mass at the squamocolumnar junction.

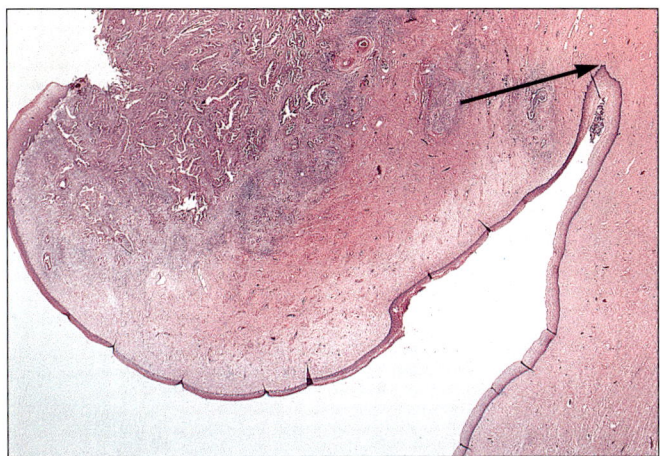

Fig. 10.53 Adenocarcinoma. The tumor diffusely involves the inner half of the endocervical wall. It also involves focally the outermost wall of the ectocervix, penetrating to almost involve the fornix (arrow).

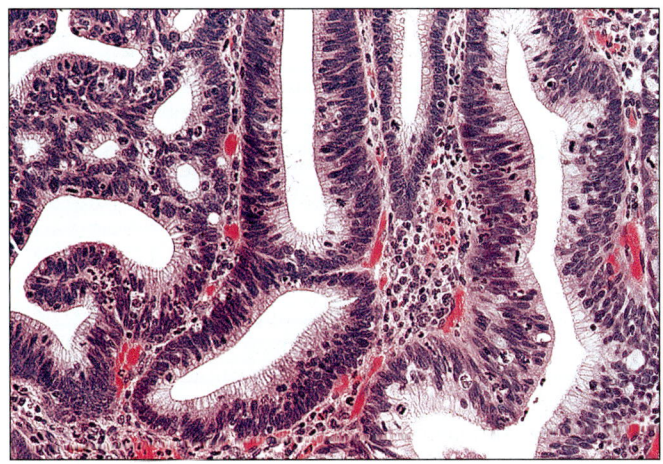

Fig. 10.54 Endocervical pattern of adenocarcinoma.

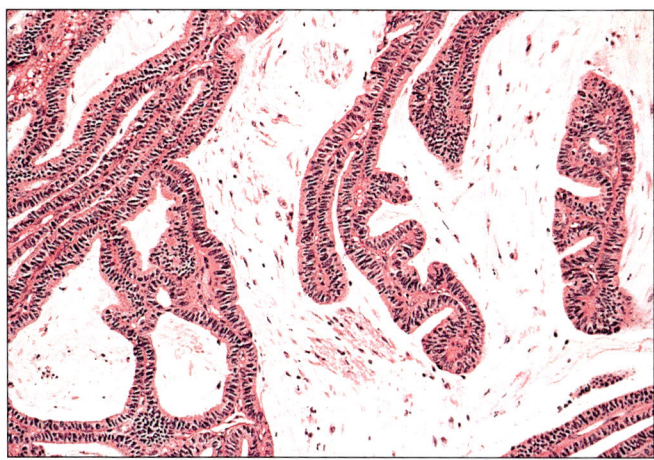

Fig. 10.55 Papillary pattern in endocervical adenocarcinoma. Extracellular mucin is present.

mitoses and commonly seen apoptotic bodies (Figure 10.54). Mucin stains show a spectrum of staining with a subset showing prominent intracytoplasmic mucin whilst others show little or no mucin. This has led to confusion, with these latter tumors being regarded as endometrioid. Cervical adenocarcinoma also shows marked variability in mucin expression which includes mucins of pyloric gland and intestinal type.[252] These tumors show a range of architectural differentiation, with some composed of well-formed glands and others that show solid areas. Gland size may vary from small to cystic, and the glands may be widely spaced or closely packed, often with a cribriform pattern. Papillary projections may be seen within the glandular lumina (Figure 10.55). The tumors often, at least focally, elicit a desmoplastic stromal response; however, in some cases no stromal reaction is seen. Some tumors show prominent numbers of acute inflammatory cells within both the stroma and the gland lumens.

Grading of the tumors follows the general FIGO system for glandular tumors as described elsewhere for endometrium and ovary. Grade 1 tumors (well-differentiated tumors) grow in glandular formations with less than 5% of areas being solid. Grade 3 tumors (poorly differentiated tumors) are more than 50% composed of solid tumor nests; the cells may show pseudorosette formation or palisading of nuclei and little intracytoplasmic mucin.

Immunohistochemistry

Typical endocervical adenocarcinomas are often, but not always, cytoplasmic CEA positive and are negative for vimentin. Estrogen receptor (ER) is usually negative; however, focal weak reactivity may be present. In contrast, primary endometrial adenocarcinomas of endometrioid type are strongly vimentin and ER positive and negative for CEA. However, some cases may be focally positive for CEA with strong staining usually seen in benign squamous elements. The situation with mucinous adenocarcinoma of the endometrium and endometrioid adenocarcinoma of the cervix is less clear. A recent study found that ER reactivity was more dependent on the site of origin, being more common in endometrial than cervical tumors. Moreover, vimentin reactivity was more dependent on differentiation, being more commonly expressed in endometrioid than in mucinous tumors. It appears that tumors that show strong positive

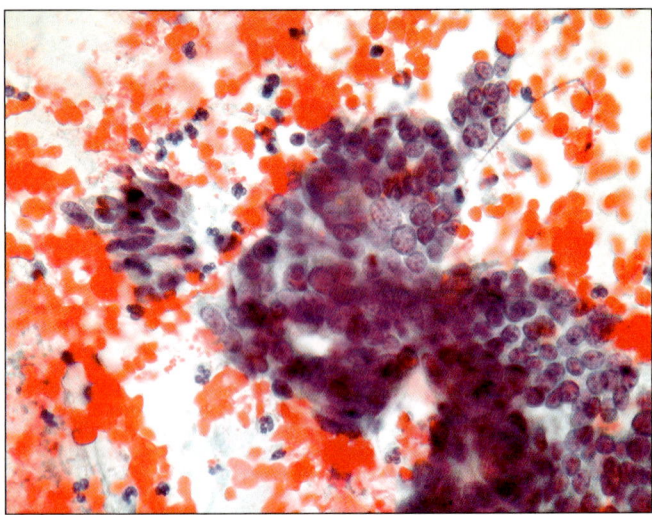

Fig. 10.56 Endocervical adenocarcinoma (Pap smear) exhibiting a crowded sheet with gland openings, a strip of pseudostratified nuclei, a small three-dimensional group of cells, and heavy background blood staining.

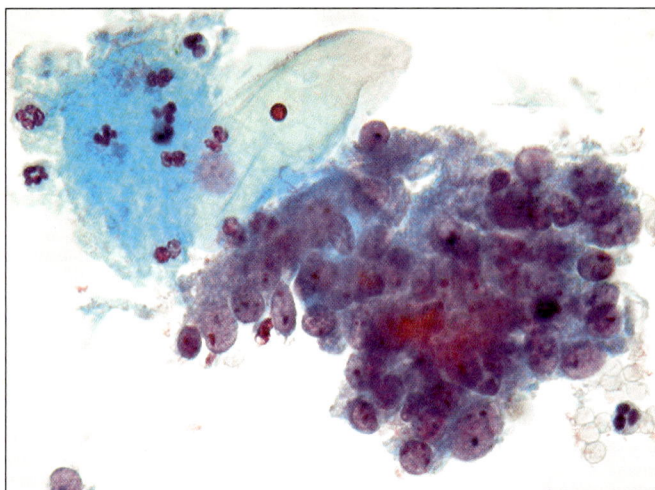

Fig. 10.57 Adenocarcinoma (ThinPrep) showing a group of malignant glandular cells with lysed blood in the background.

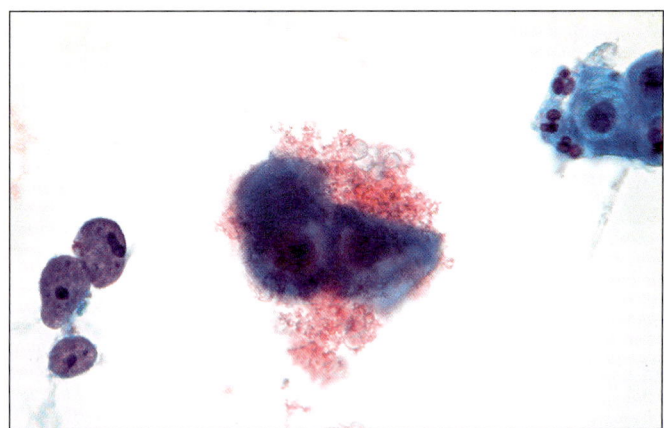

Fig. 10.58 Adenocarcinoma (ThinPrep) with bare malignant nuclei.

staining for vimentin and ER are almost invariably of endometrial origin.[105,140,141]

Cytology and cytologic correlation

Invasive cervical adenocarcinoma is reported rarely in cervical smears, with a frequency of about 0.0025%.[212] The sensitivity of the Papanicolaou smear for cervical adenocarcinoma is 45–76%, a figure comparable to AIS.[114,198] About half the false-negative reports can be accounted for by sampling error while the other half are due to laboratory error (screening or interpretative errors). However, one study reported that laboratory errors outnumber sampling errors by nearly 3:1.[50]

The specificity of a cytologic prediction of endocervical adenocarcinoma is high, with Positive Predictive Values (PPVs) (albeit based on small numbers) in the order of 90–100% if all high-grade histologic outcomes are included.[111,138,203]

Morphologically, invasive endocervical adenocarcinoma shares many features with AIS. Features helpful in correctly predicting histologic invasion include: heavy blood staining, abundant abnormal glandular epithelium, supercrowding of sheets, small three-dimensional groups, papillary clusters, tumor diathesis, single malignant cells with nuclear pleomorphism and macronucleoli, and mitotic figures (Figure 10.56).[24,25,47,198] While invasive squamous cell carcinoma is sometimes predicted on the basis of appearances of a small number of cells, with respect to adenocarcinoma, reliance on the presence of a few classic malignant criteria, which may be subtle in any particular case, can easily lead to false-negative reports.[25] There may be morphologic clues to the histologic subtype of the tumor; these are discussed with the appropriate histology descriptions.

Liquid based cytology may be more sensitive than conventional cytology in the detection of cervical adenocarcinoma.[8,200] The reduction in screening false negatives has been attributed to enhanced cytologic detail and the elimination of obscuring elements such as blood.[94,200] The three-dimensionality of cell groups may render visualization of individual nuclei within groups more difficult.[41] A background of lysed blood and inflammatory debris may be maintained, providing a clue to the presence of invasion (Figures 10.57 and 10.58).[94] A 'clinging' diathesis has been described,[41,171] as has also been noted with squamous cell carcinoma.[235] As with *in situ* disease, establishing the efficacy of computer-assisted interactive screening of thin-layer slides for recognition of cervical adenocarcinoma is important.[55a]

Differential diagnosis

The histologic differential diagnosis of cervical adenocarcinoma includes benign glandular lesions (see Chapter 6) including tunnel clusters (types A and B), microglandular hyperplasia, lobular endocervical glandular hyperplasia, diffuse laminar endocervical glandular hyperplasia, and deep nabothian cysts, as well as secondary adenocarcinoma metastatic to the cervix. In general, when faced with a problematic endocervical glandular lesion, features that favor a benign lesion include: (1) superficial location and lack of deep infiltration; (2) lobulation; (3) well-defined margins; (4) bland nuclear features; (5) inconspicuous mitotic and apoptotic activity; and (6) absence of a stromal reaction. Whilst exceptions to the above can be seen in some benign lesions, assessment of the overall cytologic and architectural features usually allows the correct diagnosis to be achieved.[248] A caveat is that benign glandular lesions may coexist with adenocarcinoma as highlighted by a recent report of endocervical adenocarcinoma occurring in association with, and possibly arising from, lobular endocervical glandular hyperplasia.[113]

On the basis of cytologic smears alone, it is not always easy to distinguish between endometrial and endocervical adenocarcinoma, as all of the various subtypes of adenocarcinoma can occur in both sites. While endometrial carcinoma is described as presenting with fewer, smaller cells which form balls rather than sheets, many of the cytologic differences between endometrial and endocervical carcinoma can be explained in terms of the sampling method, i.e., directly sampled cells (the usual case in endocervical carcinoma) versus shed cells (the usual case in endometrial carcinoma).[57] In addition, endometrial carcinoma is typically accompanied by a watery, granular diathesis, rather than a necrotic one.

Adenocarcinoma cells from a site other than the uterus can also cause diagnostic difficulties in Papanicolaou tests. Tumors arising from elsewhere in the female genital tract (e.g., fallopian tube, ovary, peritoneum) generally have a clean background and tumor cells may show degenerative changes. Papillary clusters and psammoma bodies suggest an ovarian origin.[41] Metastatic carcinomas involving the cervix arise most commonly from gastrointestinal tract, ovary, and breast, and are said to be characterized by a clean background.[214] In contrast, bowel and bladder carcinoma which directly invade the female genital tract often have a necroinflammatory diathesis due to fistula formation.

Benign conditions can mimic adenocarcinoma, leading to false-positive reports. Inflammatory/reactive groups of cells may show enlarged nuclei, varying in size and chromatin pattern and often with prominent variable nucleoli. In such cases, features not usually associated with reactive change should be searched for, such as high nuclear : cytoplasmic ratio, fragile cytoplasm, syncytial appearance of cells within a sheet, loose cohesion at the edge of sheets, single cells, apoptosis and mitoses, and disordered polarity.[25] Another rare differential diagnosis is the Arias-Stella reaction which may produce markedly pleomorphic cells with large abnormal nuclei, prominent nucleoli, and pale, vacuolated cytoplasm (Figure 10.59).[17,153,178] Knowledge of the patient's pregnant status is very important to prevent a false-positive prediction of adenocarcinoma.

Clinical behavior/management

Collectively, the prognosis for adenocarcinoma is essentially that of squamous carcinoma or slightly worse.[10,36,175,184,229] Differences in survival rates for squamous cell carcinoma and adenocarcinoma in stage 1 and 2 disease may be due to the relative ineffectiveness of radiotherapy as a primary treatment in cases of adenocarcinoma.[12,36] The features that influence prognosis are similar to those for squamous cell carcinoma, largely grade, tumor size, lymphatic–capillary space invasion, stage, and lymph node status.[6,12,37,63,144,160] In addition, the ratio of mitotic index to apoptotic index is also of prognostic significance.[131] On a per-stage basis, the 5-year survival for adenocarcinoma is: stage 1A1, 100%; stage 1A2, 93%; stage 1B, 83%; stage 2, 37–62.9%; stage 3, 13–31%; and stage 4, 0–6%.[12,36,175] Longest survival is seen in patients with early stage disease, younger patients, and those treated with primary surgery.[12]

VILLOGLANDULAR ADENOCARCINOMA

Definition, clinical history and pathogenesis

Villoglandular adenocarcinoma, an uncommon variant of endocervical cell carcinoma described only recently, shows villoglandular fronds similar to that seen in villoglandular adenoma of the colon (Figure 10.60). It occurs most commonly in young women (average age, 35–45 years) but has been described in women ranging from 22 to 69 years.[39,97,98] A link with oral contraceptive use has been suggested.[97] These tumors are associated with HPV (type 16 more commonly than type 18) and do not manifest K-ras-2 and p53 gene point mutational damage.[5,98] Immunohistochemically, they overexpress Ki-67 (MIB1), and show no reactivity for p53 and estrogen and progesterone receptors.[179]

Pathology

The tumor presents as a polypoid mass that is papillary and friable, arising in the endocervical canal. Microscopically, it shows by a surface papillary component of variable thickness. The papillae are long and slender, occasionally short

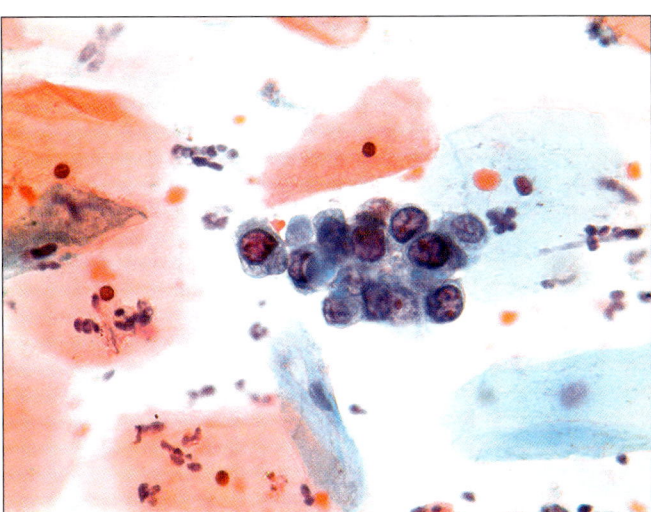

Fig. 10.59 Arias-Stella reaction (Pap smear) showing a cluster of atypical pleomorphic cells with glandular features. The patient was 5 days post termination of pregnancy. Follow-up examinations were negative.

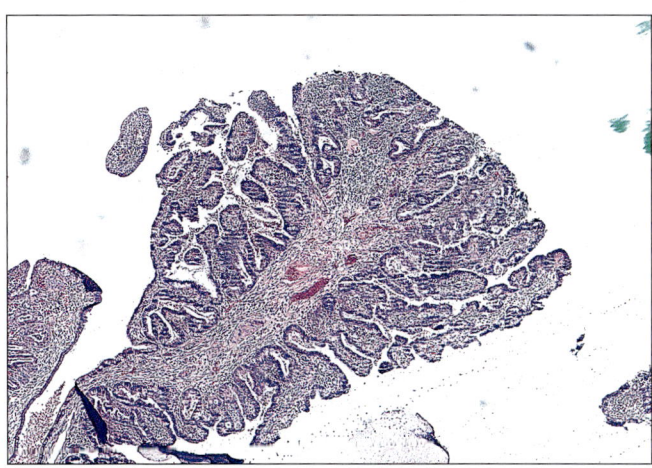

Fig. 10.60 Villoglandular adenocarcinoma. The tumor resembles a villous adenoma of colon.

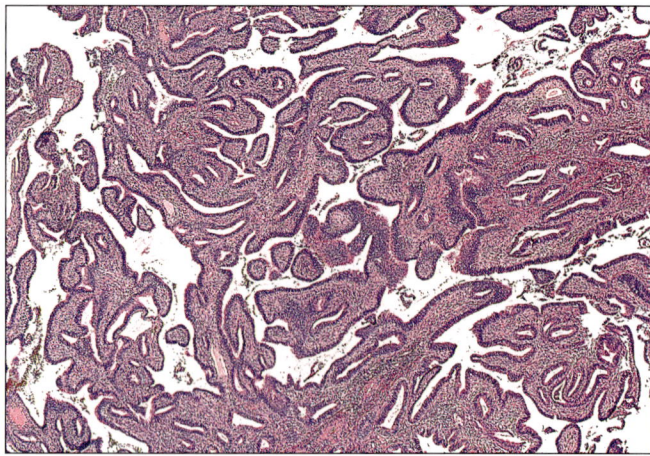

Fig. 10.61 Villoglandular adenocarcinoma. The villi have a substantial stromal core.

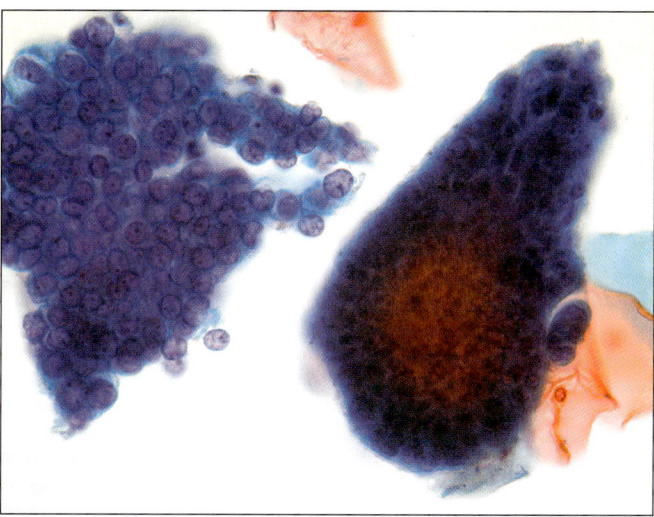

Fig. 10.63 Villoglandular adenocarcinoma (ThinPrep) showing a papillary structure on the right with a smooth palisaded edge and stromal core. Nuclear detail is better seen in the sheet on the left, where nuclei are crowded but not pleomorphic.

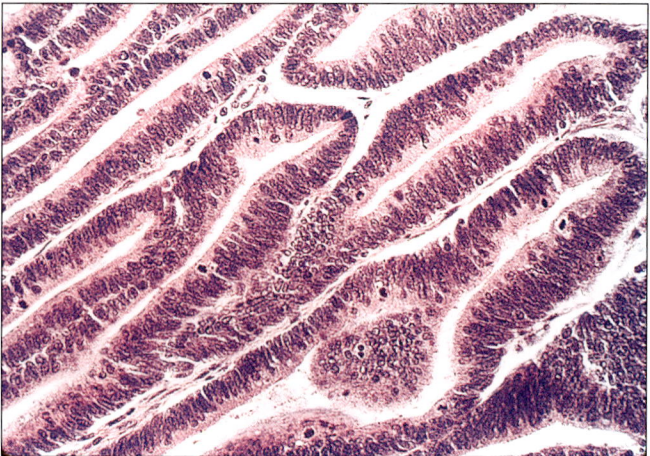

Fig. 10.62 Villoglandular adenocarcinoma. The villi have a negligible stromal core.

and broad, and covered by epithelium with at most mild to moderate cytologic atypia. The amount of stroma in the villi may be substantial (Figure 10.61) or minimal (Figure 10.62). The epithelium may be pseudostratified, but lacks tufting and solid areas. In the majority of cases, the epithelium is of endocervical type but endometrioid and intestinal epithelium may also be seen.[208] The invasive portion of the tumor, if present, is composed of elongated branching glands separated by a fibrous stroma like that seen in the stroma of the papillae but sometimes it may be myxoid or desmoplastic. Most tumors are either entirely exophytic or show only superficial invasion, confined to the inner third of the cervical wall. Grossly, they are usually well circumscribed. Those tumors that lack invasion may be regarded as villoglandular variants of CGIN. A tumor should not be placed in this group if any adverse prognostic feature (e.g., presence of coexisting papillary serous adenocarcinoma or small cell carcinoma) is present.[102,248] As a cautionary note, we have also seen cases where the superficial tumor, seen on biopsy, was villoglandular, but where the deeper tumor found in the subsequent hysterectomy specimen was more of a typical invasive adenocarcinoma.

Villoglandular adenocarcinoma has distinct cytologic appearances.[1,16,35,109,161] Smears contain many large cohesive sheets, with crowded nuclei and loss of the normal honeycomb structure. Most characteristic are true papillary structures with stromal cores covered by palisaded columnar cells with intact cytoplasm. Both the sheets and the papillae have smooth edges, which contrasts with the feathered edges typically seen in AIS. Rosettes and strips of pseudostratified cells may also be seen. Nuclei are small, moderately hyperchromatic, and round to oval with minimal pleomorphism and small or absent nucleoli (Figure 10.63). The nuclear features are not clearly malignant and if close attention is not paid to the architectural features, the diagnosis may be missed. In fact, in five papers describing cytologic appearances of villoglandular carcinoma, of a total of 24 retrospectively diagnostic cervical smears, only six were recognized as showing glandular neoplasia prior to biopsy.[1,16,35,109,161]

The differential diagnosis of villoglandular adenocarcinoma includes papillary endocervicitis, müllerian papilloma, müllerian adenofibroma, and müllerian adenosarcoma.[248]

Clinical behavior/management

Because of the good prognosis initially reported with pure forms of this tumor, routine management by radical hysterectomy has been questioned. Indeed, in some early reports, patients treated by cone biopsy or simple hysterectomy suffered no recurrences. However, in some more recent reports some cases have pursued an aggressive clinical course. Six cases have been documented where there has been pelvic nodal spread (one with bulky nodes), and in the majority of these cases lymphatic invasion was present in the primary tumors.[56,102,110,220,221] One patient had recurrence 30 months after initial treatment and died of disease after 46 months.[221] In addition, one case has been reported in a 28-year-old pregnant patient with a 2.5 cm polypoid cervical tumor who subsequently developed recurrent pelvic masses and died 5 years after diagnosis secondary to complications associated with recurrent tumor.[44] Recurrence of villoglandular adenocarcinoma in an episiotomy scar has also been reported.[76] Conservative management (cone biopsy and colposcopic and cytologic follow-up) should probably be reserved only for tumors that are purely villoglandular, *in situ* or minimally invasive, without lymphatic capillary space invasion and that have been completely excised. Moreover, we and others believe that the diagnosis should not be rendered unequivocally on a small biopsy as other components may be present and the patient may be undertreated.[51]

ADENOMA MALIGNUM (MINIMAL DEVIATION ADENOCARCINOMA, MUCINOUS TYPE)

Definition

Adenoma malignum is a rare form of adenocarcinoma in which the tumor is exceedingly well-differentiated microscopically, even to the point where the mucin-rich glands lack any cytologic feature of malignancy.[58,67] The distinction of adenoma malignum from other forms of cervical adenocarcinoma was proposed because of the deceptively innocent histologic appearance that often led to an initial diagnosis of a benign lesion.[143] Today, the term 'minimal deviation adenocarcinoma' is often used synonymously with 'adenoma malignum'.[207] Complicating the understanding of its usage has been its designation to include an extremely well-differentiated form of endometrioid cervical adenocarcinoma.[120,135,246] If the term minimal deviation adenocarcinoma is used, the specific histologic subtype should be designated.

Clinical features

Adenoma malignum accounts for about 1% of all cervical adenocarcinomas.[78] The age range of patients with adenoma malignum is 25–72 years (mean age, 42 years).[58] Patients with the Peutz–Jeghers syndrome have an increased risk of developing adenoma malignum.[58,142,245] Synchronous or metachronous ovarian mucinous neoplasms with histologic features resembling cystadenoma, proliferating (borderline) tumor, and well-differentiated adenocarcinoma may also occur and have been interpreted as representing independent primary ovarian tumors or metastases.[58] Mucinous epithelium, often with nuclear atypia, may be seen in the endometrium and fallopian tubes, most likely due to direct extension from the endocervical mucinous tumor. The genetic locus of Peutz–Jeghers syndrome has been mapped to the telomeric region of chromosome 19p. In the sporadic form of adenoma malignum, a putative tumor suppressor gene is located at D19S216 on chromosomal band 19p13.3 and plays an important role in adenoma malignum tumor genesis.[124] The most common presenting sign of the cervical tumor, as with most cervical carcinomas of any bulk, is abnormal vaginal bleeding. A mucoid, watery or purulent vaginal discharge may be present.

Pathology

Grossly, adenoma malignum resembles and is indistinguishable from other types of endocervical adenocarcinoma. It may be polypoid or ulcerative and the cervical wall is typically firm or indurated. In early lesions, the cervix may even look normal. The mucosa is usually hemorrhagic, friable or mucoid. On section, the cervix usually shows thickening by yellow or tan-white tumor tissue and mucin-filled cysts are occasionally prominent (Figures 10.64 and 10.65).[58]

A histologic diagnosis of adenoma malignum may be impossible in small superficial biopsies. Multiple biopsies, cone

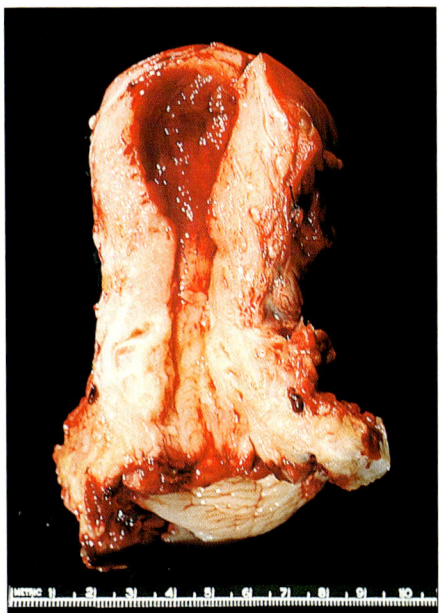

Fig. 10.64 ('Minimal deviation adenocarcinoma') ('Adenoma malignum'). The tumor diffusely pervades the entire thickness of the endocervical wall.

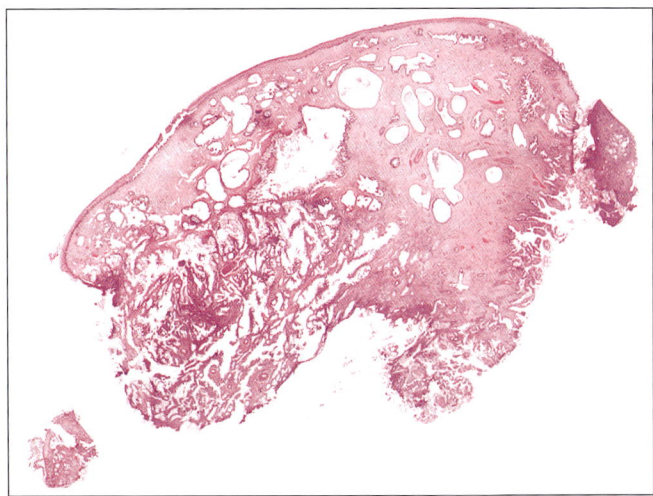

Fig. 10.65 ('Minimal deviation adenocarcinoma') ('Adenoma malignum'). Cross-section of wall showing tumor throughout.

biopsy or examination of the hysterectomy specimen may be required to make the diagnosis. Several features are key and include glands that are unusually deeply invasive (more than 8 mm into the wall) (Figure 10.66) and present where they should not be (adjacent to deep blood vessels) (Figure 10.67), as well as the presence of vascular invasion and less commonly perineural space invasion. The presence of major blood vessels deep in the tumor is a useful clue, particularly when examining a frozen section. Other features include endocervical glands with complex outlines that vary in size and range from small and regular to large, irregularly shaped, and excessively convoluted with papillary projections into the lumina. A stromal response (whether desmoplastic or loose and edematous) to the neoplastic glands is a useful diagnostic aid and is more commonly encountered in the deeper aspect of the tumor. Unfor-

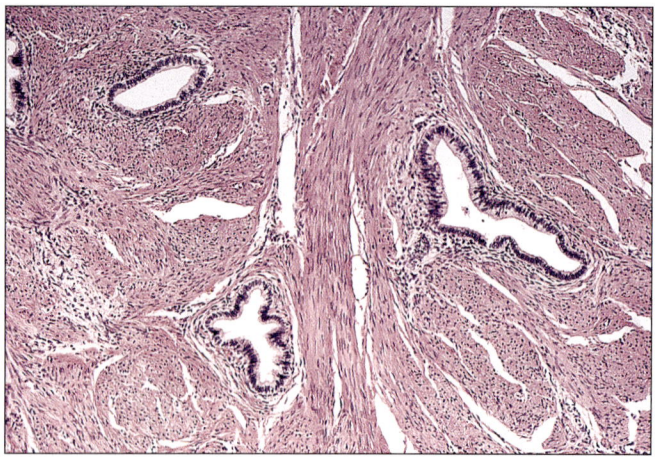

Fig. 10.66 Well-differentiated glands of (minimal deviation adenocarcinoma) ('adenoma malignum'). The glands are present deep in the muscular wall of the endocervix.

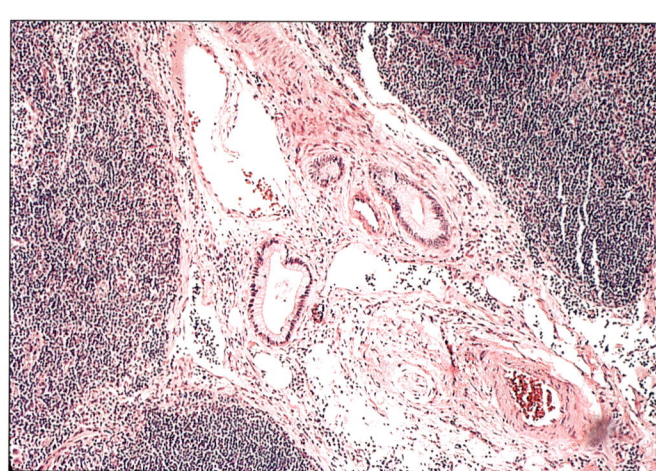

Fig. 10.68 Lymph node with metastatic (minimal deviation adenocarcinoma) ('adenoma malignum'). The glands are so well differentiated that they appear microscopically normal.

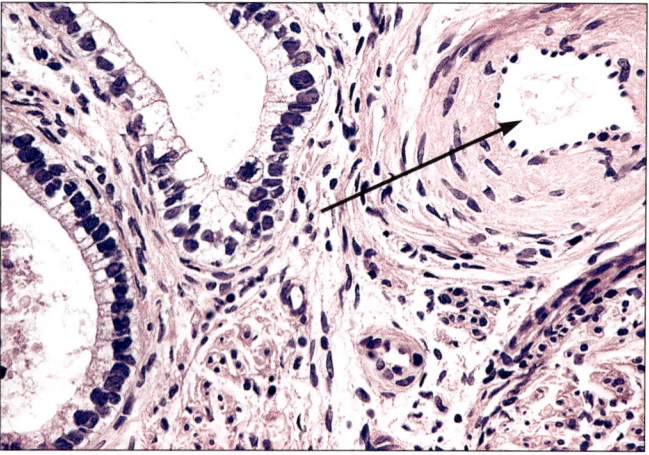

Fig. 10.67 (Minimal deviation adenocarcinoma) ('Adenoma malignum'). Extremely well-differentiated glands deep in the wall adjacent to a major blood vessel (arrow).

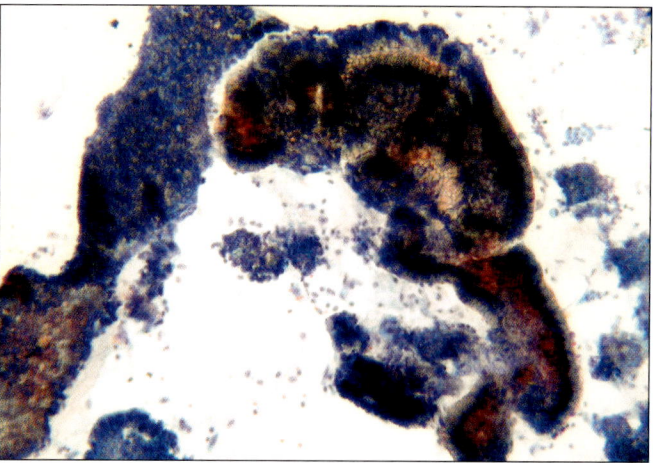

Fig. 10.69 Adenoma malignum (Pap smear). The abundant complex crowded sheets have smooth edges and yellowish cytoplasmic mucus.

tunately, this change is not seen around every neoplastic gland and may not be seen at all in small biopsy specimens. Mitotic figures are rare (fewer than one per 10 high-power fields). Cellular abnormalities range from entirely normal to mildly atypical (common) to foci that are frankly malignant. The glands are usually lined by a single layer of columnar, mucin-producing cells resembling endocervical gland cells that appear normal except for size and shape. The nuclei are basally located and have inconspicuous nucleoli. However, closer inspection often discloses glands with slight loss of polarity of the lining cells with enlarged atypical hyperchromatic nuclei. Not uncommonly, whilst most of the tumor is extremely well differentiated, there will be several foci somewhere that are clearly diagnostic of carcinoma. Lymph node metastases often show mucinous glands that are extremely well differentiated (Figure 10.68).

Cytologic prediction of adenoma malignum is challenging.[64] Smears display many large branching sheets of enlarged glandular cells with retention of the honeycomb pattern and peripheral palisading. Nuclei can be enlarged but are uniform, with smooth nuclear membranes, occasional irregularities in shape, and fine chromatin. Small nucleoli may be present.[64,78] Cytoplasm is abundant and vacuolated or lacy and this cytoplasmic mucus has been reported to stain a golden-yellow color with the Papanicolaou method (Figure 10.69).[70,91] Golden-yellow mucus can also be seen in abundance in the background. This staining reflects gastric metaplasia, which is not unique to adenoma malignum but can also be seen in pyloric gland metaplasia, which may accompany endocervical glandular hyperplasia.[70] The presence of more usual-type adenocarcinoma cells with increased nuclear atypia and pleomorphism may provide a useful clue to the nature of the abundant bland endocervical material seen on cervical smears in adenoma malignum.[64,78]

Differential diagnosis

Great care must be taken not to mistake adenoma malignum for 'look-alikes'. These include diffuse laminar endocervical glandular hyperplasia, deep nabothian cysts, adenomyoma of endocervical type, endocervical glandular tunnel clusters, lobular endocervical glandular hyperplasia, and endocervicosis. Diffuse laminar endocervical glandular hyperplasia is an incidental finding in hysterectomy or cone biopsy specimens.[96]

Moderate-sized, evenly spaced, extremely well-differentiated endocervical glands are present within the inner one-third of the cervical wall and are sharply demarcated from the underlying cervical stroma. A marked inflammatory response is often present. On occasion, entirely normal endocervical glands can be found deep in the wall as an incidental finding. Usually the glands are few in number, but occasionally they may be florid.[42]

Another condition easily confused with adenoma malignum is a benign endocervical adenomyoma where extremely well-differentiated glands lined by endocervical mucinous epithelium are admixed with smooth muscle.[59] A further condition that may be confused with adenoma malignum is endocervical tunnel clusters (type A), in which a benign lobulated proliferation of small-caliber, non-dilated, closely packed glands is found virtually always as an incidental finding. While most glands are arranged around a central primary or secondary endocervical cleft and as a group are well circumscribed, occasionally the borders may be irregular and have a pseudoinvasive appearance. Occasionally, some areas may show cytologic atypia.[95]

Lobular endocervical glandular hyperplasia, like adenoma malignum, may produce a gross abnormality of the cervix. The lobular proliferation of benign-appearing endocervical glands, the hallmark of the condition, is usually confined to the inner cervical wall. The intervening cervical stroma is unremarkable.[146,164]

Endocervicosis, a condition that usually involves the urinary bladder, but may also involve the deep cervix, is of unknown pathogenesis. In the few cases described, the lesion grossly consisted of firm rubbery masses 1–2.5 cm in size, and was located in the outer half of the anterior cervical wall and separate from the normal endocervical glands lining the endocervix. Microscopically, the mucinous glands are of variable size and shape, and exhibit endocervical-type glands with bland cytologic features. Desmoplasia is absent.[247]

Histochemistry using a combined Alcian blue (pH 2.5)–periodic acid Schiff (PAS) stain may be useful. Normal endocervical glands with their high content of acid and neutral mucins stain a purple to violet color, whereas the glands of cervical adenoma malignum (and conventional adenocarcinomas) stain red because of the almost exclusive presence of neutral mucin.[71,141] Reticulin stains in the tumor show disruption of the basement membrane.

Immunohistochemistry may be useful in distinguishing probable tumor and a benign lesion, with elevated Ki-67 and more extensive diffuse cytoplasmic staining with CEA suggestive of malignancy.[38,58,217] Moreover, in a recent study, both adenoma malignum and well-differentiated adenocarcinoma of usual type could be distinguished from endocervical glandular hyperplasia by identifying surrounding alpha-smooth muscle actin-positive stromal cells and by the absence or decreased number of ER-positive stromal cells in the malignant tumors.[145]

In adenoma malignum the typical well-differentiated glands are negative for *p53*; however, the less well-differentiated areas may exhibit focal positive staining.[85] DNA measurements of the glands of adenoma malignum disclose patterns similar to those of normal endocervical glands except for the presence of 4c to 6c aneuploid cells.[100] Reports of HPV identification strongly suggest HPV is involved in only a minority of cases.[5,54,55,177,236,242]

Some studies have shown that adenoma malignum, as it is well differentiated, reacts with HIK-1083 (M-GGMC-1), an antibody sensitive to pyloric gland-type mucin, in the majority of cases.[89,91,195,222,243] Some cases of lobular endocervical glandular hyperplasia are also HIK-1083 reactive,[146] suggesting that gastric metaplasia may play a role in the development of adenoma malignum minimal deviation adenocarcinoma and some other cervical adenocarcinomas.[88,90,222] Despite some literature assertions, we believe lobular endocervical glandular hyperplasia is a clinically and histopathologically benign process.[146,162]

Clinical behavior/management

Despite its histologically bland appearance, adenoma malignum invades deeply and commonly metastasizes to lymph nodes. Hematogenous dissemination of tumor is exceptional and tumor recurrence is most commonly in the abdominopelvic region.[58] Studies concerning prognosis report inconsistent findings compared to other well-differentiated cervical adenocarcinomas.[58,78,100,104,143,207] In a literature review of tumors that were clinically staged before treatment, 50% of patients with stage 1 tumors and 80% of patients with stage 2 tumors died of recurrent tumor despite radical treatment in most cases.[58]

INTESTINAL-TYPE ADENOCARCINOMA (INCLUDING SIGNET-RING CELL AND COLLOID ADENOCARCINOMA)

Intestinal-type adenocarcinoma is composed of cells similar to those seen in colorectal adenocarcinomas, the most prominent and characteristic feature being the presence of goblet cells (Figure 10.70). The intestinal type of adenocarcinoma usually has a glandular pattern, but may have papillary areas. Neuroendocrine cells and occasionally Paneth cells may be present. Intestinal-type change may be found diffusely or only focally within a mucinous carcinoma. Cytologically, the intestinal subtype may show prominent cytoplasmic goblet-like mucous vacuoles, which indent the nucleus. It is presumed, but not documented in the literature, that these tumors arise from intestinal-type CGIN.[196,208] The main differential diagnosis is with metastatic intestinal adenocarcinoma. Primary cervical intestinal-type adenocarcinoma is generally reactive with cytokeratin 7 and unreactive with cytokeratin 20 and *Cdx2*.[183]

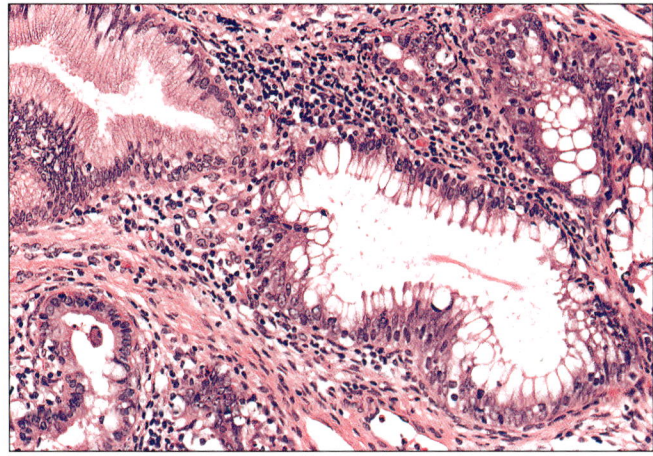

Fig. 10.70 Intestinal (goblet cell) pattern of adenocarcinoma.

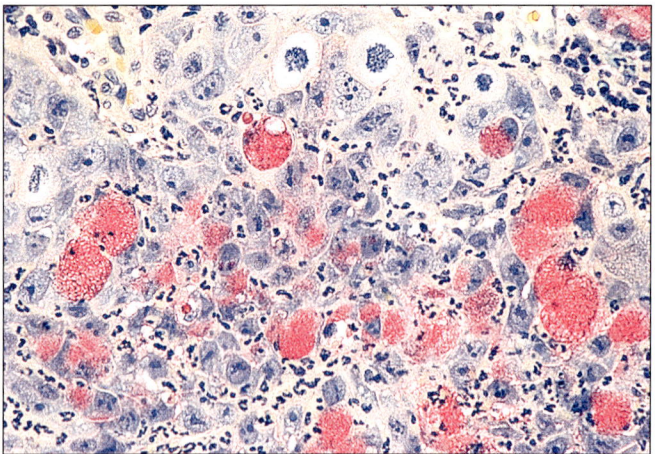

Fig. 10.71 Signet-ring cells in intestinal pattern of adenocarcinoma.

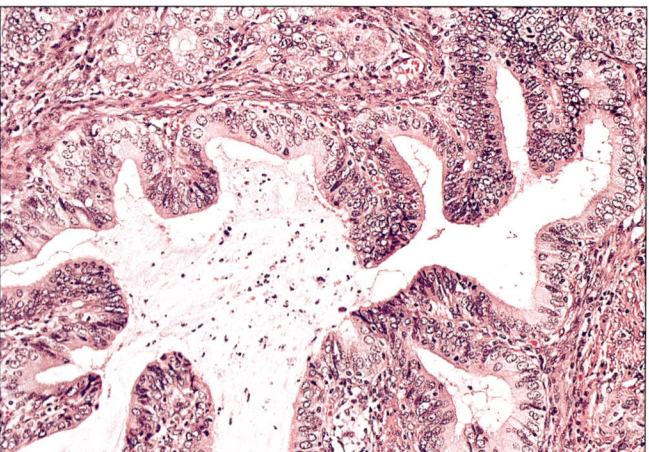

Fig. 10.72 Endometrioid pattern of adenocarcinoma.

Signet ring carcinomas occurring either in a pure form or, more usually, as part of an endocervical or intestinal carcinoma are uncommon.[69,150] Characteristically, cells with eccentric nuclei and pale, mucin-filled cytoplasm growing singly, in clusters, nests or in columns are present (Figure 10.71). Colloid carcinomas are rare and show lakes of mucin containing neoplastic glands and occasionally signet-ring cells.

ENDOMETRIOID ADENOCARCINOMA

The reported frequency of endometrioid adenocarcinoma ranges discrepantly from 7 to 50%[201,251] and is related to whether mucin-poor tumors are included within the classification of the typical endocervical adenocarcinoma or as the specific 'endometrioid' variant.[141,201] Typical endometrioid adenocarcinoma should have tubular glands and sometimes villous papillae as seen in typical and villoglandular endometrioid adenocarcinoma of the uterine corpus (Figure 10.72). Ciliated cells are occasionally present. Cytologically, endometrioid carcinoma may resemble endometrioid AIS, with clusters of small glandular cells with crowded, hyperchromatic, coarsely textured nuclei, which may be mistaken for lower uterine segment.[114] Rare endometrioid adenocarcinomas have arisen in endome-

triosis. CEA is positive in 75% of mucinous carcinomas, but is negative or only focally positive in endometrioid types.[181] The diagnosis can only be made if the endometrium itself is normal; because of the lack of precision that usually accompanies endocervical curettage, the diagnosis is best made on the complete hysterectomy specimen.

MINIMAL DEVIATION ADENOCARCINOMA, ENDOMETRIOID TYPE

Minimal deviation adenocarcinoma of the endometrioid type is an entity acceded by some because it refers to the occasional endometrioid adenocarcinoma of the cervix that has a deceptively benign histologic appearance.[248] This definition expands upon the original description of adenoma malignum that was confined to the mucinous tumor that resembles normal endocervical epithelium. In these cases the architecture and distribution of the glands and the presence of at least low-grade nuclear atypia help achieve the correct diagnosis. Cilia and/or apical snouts are commonly seen in these tumors.[246] Rarely, an endometrial adenocarcinoma arising from the corpus may invade into the cervical stroma without eliciting a stromal reaction and exhibit maturation, thus causing confusion with tuboendometrioid metaplasia.[248] A recent report of three cases with cervical cytology indicates that Papanicolaou smear appearances of this tumor may mimic those of AIS, although a diathesis may be present.[166]

ADENOSQUAMOUS CARCINOMA

Definition
Adenosquamous carcinoma is defined as a tumor having both glandular and squamous cell differentiation, with each component plainly visible on H&E-stained slides without special histochemical stains. The most recent World Health Organization classification places adenosquamous carcinoma into the group of 'uncommon carcinomas and neuroendocrine tumors'.[232] The occurrence of scattered mucin-producing cells in an otherwise typical-appearing squamous cell carcinoma has been referred to as mucoepidermoid carcinoma, an unnecessary term. There is no convincing evidence that such tumors behave differently.

Clinical features
Adenosquamous carcinoma accounts for approximately 4% of all cervical cancer.[206] Like both squamous cell carcinoma and adenocarcinoma, the mean age when the tumor develops is 57 years, although in individual cases it may occur in young women. There appears to be a slight association with pregnancy. When the tumor is still in an *in situ* stage, the mean age of the patient is 35 years. The risk factors closely resemble those of squamous cell carcinoma, e.g., multiple sexual partners. HPV types 16 and 18 are frequently identified. The reserve cell is generally regarded as the cell of origin of adenosquamous carcinoma, as it gives rise independently to both adenocarcinoma and squamous cell carcinoma.

Pathology
The tumor may be polypoid, ulcerated or nodular, and grossly indistinguishable from adenocarcinoma and squamous cell

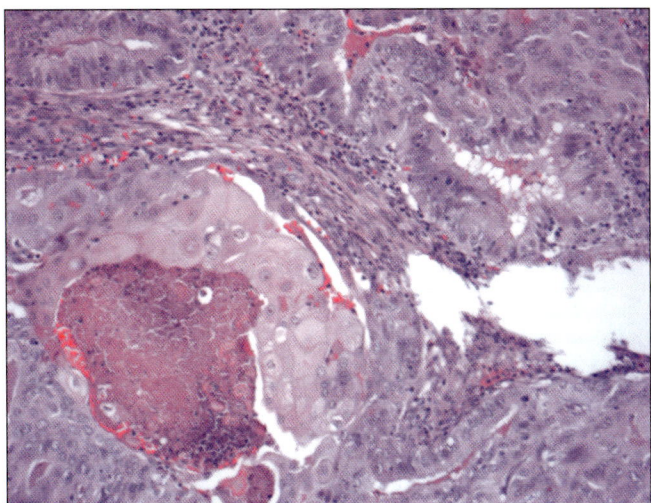

Fig. 10.73 Adenosquamous carcinoma.

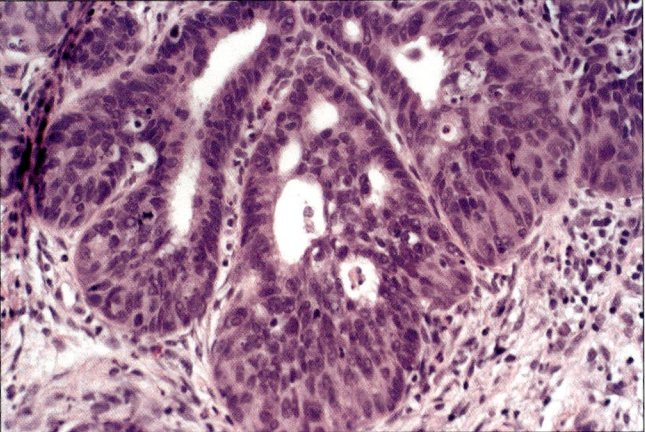

Fig. 10.74 Endocervical glandular component of adenosquamous carcinoma.

carcinoma of the endocervix. On microscopic examination, adenosquamous carcinomas are composed of various amounts of glands and squamous epithelium, which are intimately admixed (Figure 10.73). The glandular component is usually of endocervical type (Figure 10.74), but may be mucinous, including signet-ring type. Tumors with an endometrioid appearance and bland (non-malignant) appearing squamous differentiation should be classified as endometrioid adenocarcinomas of the cervix with squamous differentiation. In practice, most tumors are poorly differentiated and the presence of either component, but especially the glandular component, may not be readily apparent with a superficial glance. Although mucin stains may be helpful to highlight the poorly formed glands or intracellular mucin, glandular differentiation should also be evident on H&E slides alone. In some tumors the squamous component may show prominent cytoplasmic glycogen accumulation. A gradient from basal cells that are glycogen poor to more superficial cells that are progressively more glycogen rich helps distinguish it from clear cell carcinoma where the glycogen content is uniform throughout. Adenosquamous carcinoma is usually easy to distinguish from adenoid basal carcinoma as the latter cells are uniform, with generally bland nuclear features, exhibit peripheral palisading and have scant cytoplasm. Cytologically, adenosquamous carcinoma demon-

strates a variable admixture of malignant squamous and glandular elements. When one component predominates, the other may not be appreciated and the true nature of the neoplasm may not be established until biopsy.

Clinical behavior/management

The belief that adenosquamous carcinoma has a poorer prognosis than squamous cell carcinoma or adenocarcinoma[40,52,122] has been repeatedly challenged.[6,73,206,229] In one large series,[206] patients with adenocarcinoma, squamous cell carcinoma, and adenosquamous carcinoma had no significant difference in 5-year survival in any clinical stage except American Joint Committee on Cancer stage II, where squamous cell carcinoma had a better survival. Of interest, patients with adenosquamous carcinoma and positive lymph nodes had the highest 5-year survival rate, whereas women with adenocarcinoma and positive nodes had a sharply reduced survival rate. Recent data suggest that patients with adenosquamous carcinoma have a better prognosis than endocervical adenocarcinoma in patients who are stage 1, and sometimes stage 2.[37,52,206] Regardless, adenosquamous histology, like most cancers, predicts a poor outcome for patients with advanced-stage disease.[52]

CLEAR CELL ADENOCARCINOMA

Definition

Clear cell adenocarcinoma, a tumor named for its common histologic appearance of sheets of cells with clear cytoplasm, accounts for only 2–4% of cervical adenocarcinomas. While this tumor occurs in young women who were exposed to diethylstilbestrol (DES) *in utero* (see Chapter 5), it occurs at all ages in other women (with a bimodal age distribution), and is most commonly seen in postmenopausal women.[66] The 10-year survival rate for patients with cervical clear cell carcinoma is 57%.[103]

Pathology

Grossly, tumors may be endocervical or ectocervical. Histologically, clear cell adenocarcinoma of the cervix shows the same variety of patterns seen elsewhere in the female genital tract (endometrium, ovary, and vagina). These include solid areas with clear cells, as well as tubules and cysts lined by clear cells or by cells showing nuclei that may be enlarged, pleomorphic and protrude into the lumen, imparting a hobnail appearance. The tumor cells (clear and hobnail) may also be arranged in papillae, which often have hyalinized fibrovascular cores. Tumor nuclear grade is usually 2 or 3 and mitoses are infrequent. The clear cells contain abundant intracytoplasmic glycogen. Intraluminal but not intracytoplasmic mucin may be present.

On Papanicolaou smear, clear cell adenocarcinoma may display large nuclei with prominent single nucleoli and variable hyperchromasia. Cytoplasm is abundant but wispy and may disintegrate to create a pattern of large bare nuclei (Figure 10.75).[57] Psammoma bodies have been reported in a cervical smear showing clear cell carcinoma of the cervix.[174]

Differential diagnosis

Clear cell carcinoma may be confused with the Arias-Stella reaction, microglandular hyperplasia, mesonephric hyperplasia, and, in children, cervical yolk sac tumor. The Arias-Stella

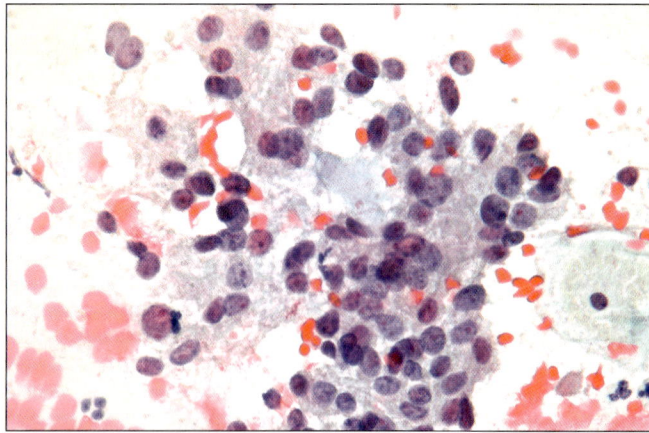

Fig. 10.75 Clear cell adenocarcinoma (Pap smear) showing pleomorphic malignant cells with prominent nucleoli and wispy, disintegrating cytoplasm.

reaction is seen in about 10% of gravid uteri. Although typically involving only a few glands, it may occasionally be more diffuse. Distinction from clear cell carcinoma rests on the lack of a mass, stromal invasion, and the absence of cells arranged in a solid sheet. Some cases of microglandular hyperplasia may show markedly dilated tubules that at low power may resemble the tubulocystic pattern of clear cell carcinoma, but typically glands contain small numbers of neutrophil polymorphs in the lumens. Additionally, the cells are bland with fine nuclear chromatin and show cytoplasmic mucin.

SEROUS ADENOCARCINOMA

Definition

This very rare tumor is histologically identical to the common serous adenocarcinoma of the ovary, endometrium, and peritoneum. It accounts for 3% of cervical adenocarcinomas (in either pure form or mixed with another type of adenocarcinoma) and has a bimodal age distribution, with one peak occurring before the age of 40 years and the second after the age of 65.[254] Serous carcinoma usually presents with abnormal vaginal bleeding, an abnormal cervical smear or a watery vaginal discharge.

Pathology

Grossly it resembles other types of cervical adenocarcinoma and microscopically shows a complex pattern of papillae with cellular budding, nuclei with grade 2 or 3 cytologic features, and sometimes psammoma bodies. An *in situ* component may be present. Nearly half of cases exhibit a second admixed pattern, most commonly low-grade villoglandular adenocarcinoma but endocervical, clear cell and endometrioid adenocarcinoma may be admixed.[254] Spread to the cervix from serous adenocarcinoma of the ovary, endometrium, and peritoneum should be excluded before a diagnosis of a primary cervical tumor is made. A helpful point is that serous adenocarcinoma of the cervix is frequently CEA positive in contrast to this tumor when arising in other sites.

Cytologically, serous carcinoma can, as expected from the histology, show pseudopapillary clusters and balls of atypical cells, as well as single cells displaying extreme cytologic atypia with enlarged irregular nuclei and large nucleoli. Interestingly,

however, the superficial portion of the tumor may be better differentiated than the deeper portions, so that the predominant cytologic appearance may be of branching, monolayered sheets with smooth edges and only mild to moderate nuclear pleomorphism.[253] While these sheets may be mistaken for reactive glandular atypia, if seen in combination with dissociated, more pleomorphic cells, bare nuclei, and tumor diathesis, the appearances are readily interpreted as malignant.[35,253]

Clinical behavior/management

Forty per cent of patients die of extensive metastases within 5 years of diagnosis.[254] Patients with stage 1 tumors have a similar outcome to those with usual-type cervical adenocarcinoma, while those with advanced stage disease have a poor prognosis.[254] While most metastases are to pelvic and para-aortic lymph nodes, other sites involved are lung, peritoneum (with production of ascites), liver, and skin. Features associated with a poor prognosis include age <65 years, stage 2 and higher tumors, tumor size >2 cm, depth of tumor invasion >10 mm, lymph node metastases, and elevated serum CA125. Tumor grade or composition (pure or mixed) does not appear to correlate with outcome.

REFERENCES

1. Ajit D, Dighe S, Gujral S. Cytologic features of villoglandular adenocarcinoma of the cervix. Acta Cytol 2004;48:288–9.
2. Akiba Y, Kubushiro K, Fukuchi T, et al. Is laser conization adequate for therapeutic excision of adenocarcinoma in situ of the uterine cervix? J Obstet Gynaecol Res 2005;31:252–6.
3. Ali-Fehmi R, Qureshi F, Lawrence WD, Jacques SM. Apoptosis, proliferation, and expression of p53 and bcl-2 in endocervical glandular intraepithelial lesions and invasive endocervical adenocarcinoma. Int J Gynecol Pathol 2004;23:1–6.
4. Alvarez–Santin C, Sica A, Rodriguez M, Feijo A, Garrido G. Microglandular hyperplasia of the uterine cervix. Cytologic diagnosis in cervical smears. Acta Cytol 1999;43:110–3.
5. An HJ, Kim KR, Kim IS, et al. Prevalence of human papillomavirus DNA in various histological subtypes of cervical adenocarcinoma: a population-based study. Mod Pathol 2005;18:528–34.
6. Angel C, DuBeshter B, Lin JY. Clinical presentation and management of stage I cervical adenocarcinoma: a 25 year experience. Gynecol Oncol 1992;44:71–8.
7. Anon. Performance Measures for Australian Laboratories reporting Cervical Cytology 2005. Royal College of Pathologists of Australasia Cytopathology Quality Assurance Program 2005. Surry Hills, NSW: RCPA; 2005.
8. Ashfaq R, Gibbons D, Vela C, Saboorian MH, Iliya F. ThinPrep Pap Test. Accuracy for glandular disease. Acta Cytol 1999;43:81–5.
9. Ayer B, Pacey F, Greenberg M. The cytologic diagnosis of adenocarcinoma in situ of the cervix uteri and related lesions. II. Microinvasive adenocarcinoma. Acta Cytol 1988;32:318–24.
10. Ayhan A, Al RA, Baykal C, Demirtas E, Yuce K, Ayhan A. A comparison of prognoses of FIGO stage IB adenocarcinoma and squamous cell carcinoma. Int J Gynecol Cancer 2004;14:279–85.
11. Azodi M, Chambers SK, Rutherford TJ, Kohorn EI, Schwartz PE, Chambers JT. Adenocarcinoma in situ of the cervix: management and outcome. Gynecol Oncol 1999;73:348–53.
12. Baalbergen A, Ewing-Graham PC, Hop WC, Struijk P, Helmerhorst TJ. Prognostic factors in adenocarcinoma of the uterine cervix. Gynecol Oncol 2004;92:262–7.
13. Bai H, Sung CJ, Steinhoff MM. ThinPrep Pap Test promotes detection of glandular lesions of the endocervix. Diagn Cytopathol 2000;23:19–22.
14. Baker PM, Clement PB, Bell DA, Young RH. Superficial endometriosis of the uterine cervix: a report of 20 cases of a process that may be confused with endocervical glandular dysplasia or adenocarcinoma in situ. Int J Gynecol Pathol 1999;18:198–205.
15. Balega J, Michael H, Hurteau J, et al. The risk of nodal metastasis in early adenocarcinoma of the uterine cervix. Int J Gynecol Cancer 2004;14:104–9.
16. Ballo MS, Silverberg SG, Sidawy MK. Cytologic features of well-differentiated villoglandular adenocarcinoma of the cervix. Acta Cytol 1996;40:536–40.
16a. Belsley NA, Tambouret RH, Misdraji J, Muzikansky A, Russell DK, Wilbur DC. Cytologic features of endocervical glandular lesions: Comparison of

SurePath, ThinPrep, and conventional smear specimen preparations. Diagn Cytopathol 2008;36(4):232–7.

17. Benoit JL, Kini SR. 'Arias-Stella reaction'-like changes in endocervical glandular epithelium in cervical smears during pregnancy and postpartum states – a potential diagnostic pitfall. Diagn Cytopathol 1996;14:349–55.

18. Berrington de Gonzalez A, Sweetland S, Green J. Comparison of risk factors for squamous cell and adenocarcinomas of the cervix: a meta-analysis. British J Cancer 2004;90:1787–91.

19. Bertrand M, Lickrish GM, Colgan TJ. The anatomic distribution of cervical adenocarcinoma in situ: implications for treatment. Am J Obstet Gynecol 1987;157:21–5.

20. Biscotti CV, Hart WR. Apoptotic bodies: a consistent morphologic feature of endocervical adenocarcinoma in situ. Am J Surg Pathol 1998;22:434–9.

21. Boddington MM, Spriggs AI, Cowdell RH. Adenocarcinoma of the uterine cervix: cytological evidence of a long preclinical evolution. Br J Obstet Gynaecol 1976;83:900–3.

22. Bonds L, Baker P, Gup C, Shroyer KR. Immunohistochemical localization of cdc6 in squamous and glandular neoplasia of the uterine cervix. Arch Pathol Lab Med 2002;126:1164–8.

23. Boon ME, Baak JP, Kurver PJ, Overdiep SH, Verdonk GW. Adenocarcinoma in situ of the cervix: an underdiagnosed lesion. Cancer 1981;48:768–73.

24. Boon ME, Ouwerkerk-Noordam E, van Leeuwen AW, Kok LP, van Haaften-Day C. How to improve cytologic screening for endocervical adenocarcinoma? Eur J Gynaecol Oncol 2002;23:481–5.

25. Bowditch R. Specific high risk patterns. In: Bowditch R, ed. Challenges in Cytology Confronting Difficult High Grade Lesions. Sydney: NSW Cervical Screening Program; 2002:27–101.

26. Brinton LA, Herrero R, Reeves WC, de Britton RC, Gaitan E, Tenorio F. Risk factors for cervical cancer by histology. Gynecol Oncol 1993;51: 301–6.

27. Bulk S, Visser O, Rozendaal L, Verheijen RH, Meijer CJ. Cervical cancer in the Netherlands 1989–1998: decrease of squamous cell carcinoma in older women, increase of adenocarcinoma in younger women. Int J Cancer 2005;113:1005–9.

28. Burghardt E. Microinvasive carcinoma in gynaecological pathology. Clin Obstet Gynaecol 1984;11:239–57.

29. Burk RD, Terai M, Gravitt PE, et al. Distribution of human papillomavirus types 16 and 18 variants in squamous cell carcinomas and adenocarcinomas of the cervix. Cancer Res 2003;63:7215–20.

30. Cameron RI, Maxwell P, Jenkins D, McCluggage WG. Immunohistochemical staining with MIB1, bcl2 and p16 assists in the distinction of cervical glandular intraepithelial neoplasia from tubo-endometrial metaplasia, endometriosis and microglandular hyperplasia. Histopathology 2002;41:313–21.

31. Cangiarella JF, Chhieng DC. Atypical glandular cells – an update. Diagn Cytopathol 2003;29:271–9.

32. Casper GR, Ostor AG, Quinn MA. A clinicopathologic study of glandular dysplasia of the cervix. Gynecol Oncol 1997;64:166–70.

33. Castellsague X, Diaz M, de Sanjose S, et al. Worldwide human papillomavirus etiology of cervical adenocarcinoma and its cofactors: implications for screening and prevention. J Natl Cancer Inst 2006;98: 303–15.

34. Ceballos KM, Shaw D, Daya D. Microinvasive cervical adenocarcinoma (FIGO Stage 1A Tumors): Results of surgical staging and outcome analysis. Am J Surg Pathol 2006;30:370–4.

35. Chang WC, Matisic JP, Zhou C, Thomson T, Clement PB, Hayes MM. Cytologic features of villoglandular adenocarcinoma of the uterine cervix: comparison with typical endocervical adenocarcinoma with a villoglandular component and papillary serous carcinoma. Cancer 1999;87:5–11.

36. Chen RJ, Lin YH, Chen CA, Huang SC, Chow SN, Hsieh CY. Influence of histologic type and age on survival rates for invasive cervical carcinoma in Taiwan. Gynecol Oncol 1999;73:184–90.

37. Chen RJ, Chang DY, Yen ML, et al. Prognostic factors of primary adenocarcinoma of the uterine cervix. Gynecol Oncol 1998;69:157–64.

38. Cina SJ, Richardson MS, Austin RM, Kurman RJ. Immunohistochemical staining for Ki-67 antigen, carcinoembryonic antigen, and p53 in the differential diagnosis of glandular lesions of the cervix. Mod Pathol 1997;10:176–80.

39. Collinet P, Prolongeau JF, Vaneecloo S. Villoglandular papillary adenocarcinoma of the uterine cervix. Eur J Obstet Gynecol Reprod Biol 1999;86:101–3.

40. Costa MJ, McIlnay KR, Trelford J. Cervical carcinoma with glandular differentiation: histological evaluation predicts disease recurrence in clinical stage I or II patients. Hum Pathol 1995;26:829–37.

41. Covell JL, Wilbur DC, Guidos B, Lee KR, Chhieng DC, Mody DR. Epithelial abnormalities: glandular. In: Solomon D, Nayar R, eds. The Bethesda System for Reporting Cervical Cytology. New York: Springer-Verlag; 2004:123–56.

42. Daya D, Young RH. Florid deep glands of the uterine cervix. Another mimic of adenoma malignum. Am J Clin Pathol 1995;103:614–7.

43. De Boer MA, Peters LAW, Aziz MF, et al. Human papillomavirus type 18 variants: histopathology and E6/E7 polymorphisms in three countries. Int J Cancer 2005;114:422–5.

44. Dede M, Deveci G, Deveci MS, et al. Villoglandular papillary adenocarcinoma of the uterine cervix in a pregnant woman: a case report and review of literature. Tohoku J Exp Med 2004;202:305–10.

45. Derchain SF, Rabelo-Santos SH, Sarian LO, et al. Human papillomavirus DNA detection and histological findings in women referred for atypical glandular cells or adenocarcinoma in situ in their Pap smears. Gynecol Oncol 2004;95:618–23.

46. DeSimone CP, Day ME, Tovar MM, Dietrich CS, 3rd, Eastham ML, Modesitt SC. Rate of pathology from atypical glandular cell Pap tests classified by the Bethesda 2001 nomenclature. Obstet Gynecol 2006;107:1285–91.

47. DiTomasso JP, Ramzy I, Mody DR. Glandular lesions of the cervix. Validity of cytologic criteria used to differentiate reactive changes, glandular intraepithelial lesions and adenocarcinoma. Acta Cytol 1996;40:1127–35.

48. Duggan MA, Benoit JL, McGregor SE, Inoue M, Nation JG, Stuart GC. Adenocarcinoma in situ of the endocervix: human papillomavirus determination by dot blot hybridization and polymerase chain reaction amplification. Int J Gynecol Pathol 1994;13:143–9.

49. Elliott P, Coppleson M, Russell P, et al. Early invasive (FIGO stage IA) carcinoma of the cervix: a clinico-pathologic study of 476 cases. Int J Gynecol Cancer 2000;10:42–52.

50. Erzen M, Mozina A, Bertole J, Syrjanen K. Factors predicting disease outcome in early stage adenocarcinoma of the uterine cervix. Eur J Obstet Gynecol Reprod Biol 2002;101:185–91.

51. Fadare O, Zheng W. Well-differentiated papillary villoglandular adenocarcinoma of the uterine cervix with a focal high-grade component: is there a need for reassessment? Virchows Arch 2005;447:883–7.

52. Farley JH, Hickey KW, Carlson JW, Rose GS, Kost ER, Harrison TA. Adenosquamous histology predicts a poor outcome for patients with advanced-stage, but not early-stage, cervical carcinoma. Cancer 2003;97:2196–202.

53. Farnsworth A, Laverty C, Stoler MH. Human papillomavirus messenger RNA expression in adenocarcinoma in situ of the uterine cervix. Int J Gynecol Pathol 1989;8:321–30.

54. Ferguson AW, Svoboda-Newman SM, Frank TS. Analysis of human papillomavirus infection and molecular alterations in adenocarcinoma of the cervix. Mod Pathol 1998;11:11–18.

55. Fukushima M, Shimano S, Yamakawa Y, et al. The detection of human papillomavirus (HPV) in a case of minimal deviation adenocarcinoma of the uterine cervix (adenoma malignum) using in situ hybridization. Jpn J Clin Oncol 1990;20:407–12.

55a. Friedlander MA, Rudomina D, Lin O. Effectiveness of the Thin Prep Imaging System in the detection of adenocarcinoma of the gynecologic system. Cancer 2008;114(1):7–12.

56. Garcea A, Nunns D, Ireland D, Brown L. A case of villoglandular papillary adenocarcinoma of the cervix with lymph node metastasis. BJOG 2003;110:627–9.

57. Geisinger KR, Stanley MW, Raab SS, Silverman JF, Abati A. Invasive glandular malignancies of the gynecologic tract. In: Geisinger KR, Stanley MW, Raab SS, Silverman JF, Abati A, eds. Modern Cytopathology. Philadelphia: Churchill Livingstone; 2004:167–96.

58. Gilks CB, Young RH, Aguirre P, DeLellis RA, Scully RE. Adenoma malignum (minimal deviation adenocarcinoma) of the uterine cervix. A clinicopathological and immunohistochemical analysis of 26 cases. Am J Surg Pathol 1989;13:717–29.

59. Gilks CB, Young RH, Clement PB, Hart WR, Scully RE. Adenomyomas of the uterine cervix of endocervical type: a report of ten cases of a benign cervical tumor that may be confused with adenoma malignum. Mod Pathol 1996;9:220–4.

60. Gloor E, Hurlimann J. Cervical intraepithelial glandular neoplasia (adenocarcinoma in situ and glandular dysplasia). A correlative study of 23 cases with histologic grading, histochemical analysis of mucins, and immunohistochemical determination of the affinity for four lectins. Cancer 1986;58:1272–80.

61. Goldstein NS, Mani A. The status and distance of cone biopsy margins as a predictor of excision adequacy for endocervical adenocarcinoma in situ. Am J Clin Pathol 1998;109:727–32.

62. Goldstein NS, Ahmad E, Hussain M, Hankin RC, Perez-Reyes N. Endocervical glandular atypia: does a preneoplastic lesion of adenocarcinoma in situ exist? Am J Clin Pathol 1998;110:200–9.

63. Goodman HM, Buttlar CA, Niloff JM, et al. Adenocarcinoma of the uterine cervix: prognostic factors and patterns of recurrence. Gynecol Oncol 1989;33:241–7.

64. Granter SR, Lee KR. Cytologic findings in minimal deviation adenocarcinoma (adenoma malignum) of the cervix. A report of seven cases. Am J Clin Pathol 1996;105:327–33.

65. Screening to prevent cervical cancer. Guidelines for the management of asymptomatic women with screen-detected abnormalities. NHMRC, 2005. Online. Available: www.csp.nsw.gov.au/nhmrc/index.php.

66. Hanselaar A, van Loosbroek M, Schuurbiers O, Helmerhorst T, Bulten J, Bernhelm I. Clear cell adenocarcinoma of the vagina and cervix. An update of the central Netherlands registry showing twin age incidence peaks. Cancer 1997;79:2229–36.

67. Hart WR. Symposium part II: special types of adenocarcinoma of the uterine cervix. Int J Gynecol Pathol 2002;21:327–46.

68. Hasumi K, Ehrmann RL. Clear cell carcinoma of the uterine endocervix with an in situ component. Cancer 1978;42:2435–8.
69. Haswani P, Arseneau J, Ferenczy A. Primary signet ring cell carcinoma of the uterine cervix: a clinicopathologic study of two cases with review of the literature. Int J Gynecol Cancer 1998;8:374–9.
70. Hata S, Mikami Y, Manabe T. Diagnostic significance of endocervical glandular cells with 'golden-yellow' mucin on pap smear. Diagn Cytopathol 2002;27:80–4.
71. Hayashi I, Tsuda H, Shimoda T. Reappraisal of orthodox histochemistry for the diagnosis of minimal deviation adenocarcinoma of the cervix. Am J Surg Pathol 2000;24:559–62.
72. Hecht JL, Sheets EE, Lee KR. Atypical glandular cells of undetermined significance in conventional cervical/vaginal smears and thin-layer preparations. Cancer 2002;96:1–4.
73. Helm CW, Kinney WK, Keeney G, et al. A matched study of surgically treated stage IB adenosquamous carcinoma and adenocarcinoma of the uterine cervix. Int J Gynecol Cancer 1993;3:245–9.
74. Hemminki K, Li X, Vaittinen P. Time trends in the incidence of cervical and other genital squamous cell carcinomas and adenocarcinomas in Sweden, 1958–1996. Eur J Obstet Gynecol Reprod Biol 2002;101:64–9.
75. Herbert A. BSCC terminology for cervical cytology: two or three tiers? Why not five, seven or even 14? Cytopathology 2004;15:245–51.
76. Heron DE, Axtel A, Gerszten K, et al. Villoglandular adenocarcinoma of the cervix recurrent in an episiotomy scar: a case report in a 32-year-old female. Int J Gynecol Cancer 2005;15:366–71.
77. Higgins GD, Phillips GE, Smith LA, Uzelin DM, Burrell CJ. High prevalence of human papillomavirus transcripts in all grades of cervical intraepithelial glandular neoplasia. Cancer 1992;70:136–46.
78. Hirai Y, Takeshima N, Haga A, Arai Y, Akiyama F, Hasumi K. A clinicocytopathologic study of adenoma malignum of the uterine cervix. Gynecol Oncol 1998;70:219–23.
79. Hlupic L, Jukic S, Svagelj D, Kos M. Malignant potential of dysplastic endocervical epithelium assessed by ploidy status, S-phase fraction and C-myc expression. Coll Antropol 2003;27:247–57.
80. Hocking GR, Hayman JA, Ostor AG. Adenocarcinoma in situ of the uterine cervix progressing to invasive adenocarcinoma. Aust N Z J Obstet Gynaecol 1996;36:218–20.
81. Honore LH, Koch M, Brown LB. Comparison of oral contraceptive use in women with adenocarcinoma and squamous cell carcinoma of the uterine cervix. Gynecol Obstet Invest 1991;32:98–101.
82. Hopkins MP. Adenocarcinoma in situ of the cervix – the margins must be clear. Gynecol Oncol 2000;79:4–5.
83. Hopkins MP, Morley GW. A comparison of adenocarcinoma and squamous cell carcinoma of the cervix. Obstet Gynecol 1991;77:912–7.
84. Huang LW, Chao SL, Chen PH, Chou HP. Multiple HPV genotypes in cervical carcinomas: improved DNA detection and typing in archival tissues. J Clin Virol 2004;29:271–6.
85. Ichimura T, Koizumi T, Tateiwa H, et al. Immunohistochemical expression of gastric mucin and p53 in minimal deviation adenocarcinoma of the uterine cervix. Int J Gynecol Pathol 2001;20:220–6.
86. Ioffe OB, Sagae S, Moritani S, Dahmoush L, Chen TT, Silverberg SG. Symposium part 3: Should pathologists diagnose endocervical preneoplastic lesions 'less than' adenocarcinoma in situ?: Point. Int J Gynecol Pathol 2003;22:18–21.
87. Ioffe OB, Sagae S, Moritani S, Dahmoush L, Chen TT, Silverberg SG. Proposal of a new scoring scheme for the diagnosis of noninvasive endocervical glandular lesions. Am J Surg Pathol 2003;27:452–60.
88. Ishii K, Ota H, Katsuyama T. Lobular endocervical glandular hyperplasia represents pyloric gland metaplasia? Am J Surg Pathol 2000;24:325; author reply 325–6.
89. Ishii K, Hidaka E, Katsuyama T, Ota H, Shiozawa T, Tsuchiya S. Ultrastructural features of adenoma malignum of the uterine cervix: demonstration of gastric phenotypes. Ultrastruct Pathol 1999;23:375–81.
90. Ishii K, Hosaka N, Toki T, et al. A new view of the so-called adenoma malignum of the uterine cervix. Virchows Arch 1998;432:315–22.
91. Ishii K, Katsuyama T, Ota H, et al. Cytologic and cytochemical features of adenoma malignum of the uterine cervix. Cancer 1999;87:245–53.
92. Jaworski RC. Endocervical glandular dysplasia, adenocarcinoma in situ, and early invasive (microinvasive) adenocarcinoma of the uterine cervix. Semin Diagn Pathol 1990;7:190–204.
93. Jaworski RC, Pacey NF, Greenberg ML, Osborn RA. The histologic diagnosis of adenocarcinoma in situ and related lesions of the cervix uteri. Adenocarcinoma in situ. Cancer 1988;61:1171–81.
94. Johnson JE, Rahemtulla A. Endocervical glandular neoplasia and its mimics in ThinPrep Pap tests. A descriptive study. Acta Cytol 1999;43:369–75.
95. Jones MA, Young RH. Endocervical type A (noncystic) tunnel clusters with cytologic atypia. A report of 14 cases. Am J Surg Pathol 1996;20:1312–8.
96. Jones MA, Young RH, Scully RE. Diffuse laminar endocervical glandular hyperplasia. A benign lesion often confused with adenoma malignum (minimal deviation adenocarcinoma). Am J Surg Pathol 1991;15:1123–9.
97. Jones MW, Silverberg SG, Kurman RJ. Well-differentiated villoglandular adenocarcinoma of the uterine cervix: a clinicopathological study of 24 cases. Int J Gynecol Pathol 1993;12:1–7.
98. Jones MW, Kounelis S, Papadaki H, et al. Well-differentiated villoglandular adenocarcinoma of the uterine cervix: oncogene/tumor suppressor gene alterations and human papillomavirus genotyping. Int J Gynecol Pathol 2000;19:110–7.
99. Jordan LB, Abdul-Kader M, Al-Nafussi A. Uterine serous papillary carcinoma: histopathologic changes within the female genital tract. Int J Gynecol Cancer 2001;11:283–9.
100. Kaku T, Enjoji M. Extremely well-differentiated adenocarcinoma ('adenoma malignum') of the cervix. Int J Gynecol Pathol 1983;2:28–41.
101. Kaku T, Kamura T, Sakai K, et al. Early adenocarcinoma of the uterine cervix. Gynecol Oncol 1997;65:281–5.
102. Kaku T, Kamura T, Shigematsu T, et al. Adenocarcinoma of the uterine cervix with predominantly villoglandular papillary growth pattern. Gynecol Oncol 1997;64:147–52.
103. Kaminski PF, Maier RC. Clear cell adenocarcinoma of the cervix unrelated to diethylstilbestrol exposure. Obstet Gynecol 1983;62:720–7.
104. Kaminski PF, Norris HJ. Minimal deviation carcinoma (adenoma malignum) of the cervix. Int J Gynecol Pathol 1983;2:141–52.
105. Kamoi S, AlJuboury MI, Akin MR, Silverberg SG. Immunohistochemical staining in the distinction between primary endometrial and endocervical adenocarcinomas: another viewpoint. Int J Gynecol Pathol 2002;21:217–23.
106. Kaspar HG, Dinh TV, Doherty MG, Hannigan EV, Kumar D. Clinical implications of tumor volume measurement in stage I adenocarcinoma of the cervix. Obstet Gynecol 1993;81:296–300.
107. Kennedy AW, Biscotti CV. Further study of the management of cervical adenocarcinoma in situ. Gynecol Oncol 2002;86:361–4.
108. Keyhani-Rofagha S, Brewer J, Prokorym P. Comparative cytologic findings of in situ and invasive adenocarcinoma of the uterine cervix. Diagn Cytopathol 1995;12:120–5.
109. Khunamornpong S, Siriaunkgul S, Suprasert P. Well-differentiated villoglandular adenocarcinoma of the uterine cervix: cytomorphologic observation of five cases. Diagn Cytopathol 2002;26:10–14.
110. Khunamornpong S, Maleemonkol S, Siriaunkgul S, Pantusart A. Well-differentiated villoglandular adenocarcinoma of the uterine cervix: a report of 15 cases including two with lymph node metastasis. J Med Assoc Thai 2001;84:882–8.
111. Kirwan JM, Herrington CS, Smith PA, Turnbull LS, Herod JJ. A retrospective clinical audit of cervical smears reported as 'glandular neoplasia'. Cytopathology 2004;15:188–94.
112. Kjaer SK, Brinton LA. Adenocarcinomas of the uterine cervix: the epidemiology of an increasing problem. Epidemiol Rev 1993;15:486–98.
113. Kondo T, Hashi A, Murata SI, et al. Endocervical adenocarcinomas associated with lobular endocervical glandular hyperplasia: a report of four cases with histochemical and immunohistochemical analyses. Mod Pathol 2005;18:1199–210.
114. Krane JF, Granter SR, Trask CE, Hogan CL, Lee KR. Papanicolaou smear sensitivity for the detection of adenocarcinoma of the cervix: a study of 49 cases. Cancer 2001;93:8–15.
115. Krane JF, Lee KR, Sun D, Yuan L, Crum CP. Atypical glandular cells of undetermined significance. Outcome predictions based on human papillomavirus testing. Am J Clin Pathol 2004;121:87–92.
116. Kurian K, al-Nafussi A. Relation of cervical glandular intraepithelial neoplasia to microinvasive and invasive adenocarcinoma of the uterine cervix: a study of 121 cases. J Clin Pathol 1999;52:112–7.
117. Kurman RJ, Norris HJ, Wilkinson EJ. Tumors of the cervix. In: Tumors of the cervix, vagina, and vulva. Washington: Armed Forces Institute of Pathology; 1992:37–139.
118. Lacey JV, Jr, Brinton LA, Barnes WA, et al. Use of hormone replacement therapy and adenocarcinomas and squamous cell carcinomas of the uterine cervix. Gynecol Oncol 2000;77:149–54.
119. Lacey JV, Jr, Brinton LA, Abbas FM, et al. Oral contraceptives as risk factors for cervical adenocarcinomas and squamous cell carcinomas. Cancer Epidemiol Biomarkers Prev 1999;8:1079–85.
120. Landry D, Mai KT, Senterman MK, et al. Endometrioid adenocarcinoma of the uterus with a minimal deviation invasive pattern. Histopathology 2003;42:77–82.
121. Laverty C. Can the Pap smear diagnose adenocarcinoma precursors? The reliability and clinical significance of a cytological prediction of adenocarcinoma in situ. In: Chanen W, Atkinson K, eds. Current Status: Future Directions. 9th World Congress of Cervical Pathology and Colposcopy. Bologna: Monduzzi Editore; 1991:121–26.
122. Lea JS, Coleman RL, Garner EO, Duska LR, Miller DS, Schorge JO. Adenosquamous histology predicts poor outcome in low-risk stage IB1 cervical adenocarcinoma. Gynecol Oncol 2003;91:558–62.
123. Leary J, Jaworski R, Houghton R. In situ hybridization using biotinylated DNA probes to human papillomavirus in adenocarcinoma-in situ and endocervical glandular dysplasia of the uterine cervix. Pathology 1991;23:85–9.
124. Lee JY, Dong SM, Kim HS, et al. A distinct region of chromosome 19p13.3 associated with the sporadic form of adenoma malignum of the uterine cervix. Cancer Res 1998;58:1140–3.
125. Lee KR. Adenocarcinoma in situ with a small cell (endometrioid) pattern in cervical smears: a test of the distinction from benign mimics using specific criteria. Cancer 1999;87:254–8.
126. Lee KR, Flynn CE. Early invasive adenocarcinoma of the cervix. Cancer 2000;89:1048–55.

127. Lee KR, Minter LJ, Granter SR. Papanicolaou smear sensitivity for adenocarcinoma in situ of the cervix. A study of 34 cases. Am J Clin Pathol 1997;107:30–5.
128. Lee KR, Sun D, Crum CP. Endocervical intraepithelial glandular atypia (dysplasia): a histopathologic, human papillomavirus, and MIB-1 analysis of 25 cases. Hum Pathol 2000;31:656–64.
129. Lee KR, Genest DR, Minter LJ, Granter SR, Cibas ES. Adenocarcinoma in situ in cervical smears with a small cell (endometrioid) pattern: distinction from cells directly sampled from the upper endocervical canal or lower segment of the endometrium. Am J Clin Pathol 1998;109:738–42.
130. Lesack D, Wahab I, Gilks CB. Radiation-induced atypia of endocervical epithelium: a histological, immunohistochemical and cytometric study. Int J Gynecol Pathol 1996;15:242–7.
131. Leung TW, Xue WC, Cheung AN, Khoo US, Ngan HY. Proliferation to apoptosis ratio as a prognostic marker in adenocarcinoma of uterine cervix. Gynecol Oncol 2004;92:866–72.
132. Liu S, Semenciw R, Mao Y. Cervical cancer: the increasing incidence of adenocarcinoma and adenosquamous carcinoma in younger women. Can Med Assoc J 2001;164:1151–2.
133. LiVolsi VA, Merino MJ, Schwartz PE. Coexistent endocervical adenocarcinoma and mucinous adenocarcinoma of ovary: a clinicopathologic study of four cases. Int J Gynecol Pathol 1983;1:391–402.
134. Longatto Filho A, Albergaria A, Paredes J, Moreira MA, Milanezi F, Schmitt FC. P-cadherin expression in glandular lesions of the uterine cervix detected by liquid-based cytology. Cytopathology 2005;16:88–93.
135. Mai KT, Perkins DG, Yazdi HM, Thomas J. Endometrioid carcinoma of the endometrium with an invasive component of minimal deviation carcinoma. Hum Pathol 2002;33:856–8.
136. Markaki S, Lazaris D, Papaspirou I, Paulou V. The expression of epithelial specific antigen in cervical intraepithelial neoplasia and adenocarcinoma. Eur J Gynaecol Oncol 2004;25:101–3.
137. Marques T, Andrade LA, Vassallo J. Endocervical tubal metaplasia and adenocarcinoma in situ: role of immunohistochemistry for carcinoembryonic antigen and vimentin in differential diagnosis. Histopathology 1996;28:549–50.
138. Mathers ME, Johnson SJ, Wadehra V. How predictive is a cervical smear suggesting glandular neoplasia? Cytopathology 2002;13:83–91.
139. McCluggage G, McBride H, Maxwell P, Bharucha H. Immunohistochemical detection of p53 and bcl-2 proteins in neoplastic and non-neoplastic endocervical glandular lesions. Int J Gynecol Pathol 1997;16:22–7.
140. McCluggage WG. Recent advances in immunohistochemistry in gynaecological pathology. Histopathology 2002;40:309–26.
141. McCluggage WG. Endocervical glandular lesions: controversial aspects and ancillary techniques. J Clin Pathol 2003;56:164–73.
142. McGarrity TJ, Kulin HE, Zaino RJ. Peutz–Jeghers syndrome. Am J Gastroenterol 2000;95:596–604.
143. McKelvey J, Goodlin R. Adenoma malignum of the cervix. Cancer 1963;16:549–57.
144. McLellan R, Dillon MB, Woodruff JD, Heatley GJ, Fields AL, Rosenshein NB. Long-term follow-up of stage I cervical adenocarcinoma treated by radical surgery. Gynecol Oncol 1994;52:253–9.
145. Mikami Y, Kiyokawa T, Moriya T, Sasano H. Immunophenotypic alteration of the stromal component in minimal deviation adenocarcinoma ('adenoma malignum') and endocervical glandular hyperplasia: a study using oestrogen receptor and alpha-smooth muscle actin double immunostaining. Histopathology 2005;46:130–6.
146. Mikami Y, Hata S, Fujiwara K, Imajo Y, Kohno I, Manabe T. Florid endocervical glandular hyperplasia with intestinal and pyloric gland metaplasia: worrisome benign mimic of 'adenoma malignum'. Gynecol Oncol 1999;74:504–11.
147. Minaguchi T, Yoshikawa H, Nakagawa S, et al. Association of PTEN mutation with HPV-negative adenocarcinoma of the uterine cervix. Cancer Lett 2004;210:57–62.
148. Mitchell H. Outcome after a cytological prediction of glandular abnormality. Aust N Z J Obstet Gynaecol 2004;44:436–40.
149. Mitchell H, Hocking J, Saville M. Cervical cytology screening history of women diagnosed with adenocarcinoma in situ of the cervix: a case-control study. Acta Cytol 2004;48:595–600.
150. Moritani S, Ichihara S, Kushima R, Sugiura F, Mushika M, Silverberg SG. Combined signet ring cell and glassy cell carcinoma of the uterine cervix arising in a young Japanese woman: a case report with immunohistochemical and histochemical analyses. Pathol Int 2004;54:787–92.
151. Moss SM, Gray A, Legood R, Henstock E. Evaluation of HPV/LBC. Cervical Screening Pilot Studies, 2002. Online. Available: www.cancerscreening.nhs.uk/cervical/lbc-pilot-evaluation.pdf
152. Mulvany N, Ostor A. Microinvasive adenocarcinoma of the cervix: a cytohistopathologic study of 40 cases. Diagn Cytopathol 1997;16:430–6.
153. Mulvany NJ, Khan A, Ostor A. Arias-Stella reaction associated with cervical pregnancy. Report of a case with a cytologic presentation. Acta Cytol 1994;38:218–22.
154. Muntz HG, Bell DA, Lage JM, Goff BA, Feldman S, Rice LW. Adenocarcinoma in situ of the uterine cervix. Obstet Gynecol 1992;80:935–9.
155. Murphy N, Heffron CC, King B, et al. P16(INK4A) positivity in benign, premalignant and malignant cervical glandular lesions: a potential diagnostic problem. Virchows Arch 2004;445:610–15.
156. Murphy N, Ring M, Killalea AG, et al. p16INK4A as a marker for cervical dyskaryosis: CIN and cGIN in cervical biopsies and ThinPrep smears. J Clin Pathol 2003;56:56–63.
157. Nanbu Y, Fujii S, Konishi I, Nonogaki H, Mori T. Immunohistochemical localizations of CA 125, carcinoembryonic antigen, and CA 19-9 in normal and neoplastic glandular cells of the uterine cervix. Cancer 1988;62:2580–8.
158. Negri G, Egarter-Vigl E, Kasal A, Romano F, Haitel A, Mian C. p16INK4a is a useful marker for the diagnosis of adenocarcinoma of the cervix uteri and its precursors: an immunohistochemical study with immunocytochemical correlations. Am J Surg Pathol 2003;27:187–93.
159. Nicklin JL, Wright RG, Bell JR, Samaratunga H, Cox NC, Ward BG. A clinicopathological study of adenocarcinoma in situ of the cervix. The influence of cervical HPV infection and other factors, and the role of conservative surgery. Aust N Z J Obstet Gynaecol 1991;31:179–83.
160. Nola M, Tomicic I, Dotlic S, Morovic A, Petrovecki M, Jukic S. Adenocarcinoma of uterine cervix – prognostic significance of clinicopathologic parameters. Croat Med J 2005;46:397–403.
161. Novotny DB, Ferlisi P. Villoglandular adenocarcinoma of the cervix: cytologic presentation. Diagn Cytopathol 1997;17:383–7.
162. Nucci MR. Symposium part III: tumor-like glandular lesions of the uterine cervix. Int J Gynecol Pathol 2002;21:347–59.
163. Nucci MR, Young RH. Arias-Stella reaction of the endocervix: a report of 18 cases with emphasis on its varied histology and differential diagnosis. Am J Surg Pathol 2004;28:608–12.
164. Nucci MR, Clement PB, Young RH. Lobular endocervical glandular hyperplasia, not otherwise specified: a clinicopathologic analysis of thirteen cases of a distinctive pseudoneoplastic lesion and comparison with fourteen cases of adenoma malignum. Am J Surg Pathol 1999;23:886–91.
165. O'Connell F, Cibas ES. Cytologic features of ciliated adenocarcinoma of the cervix: a case report. Acta Cytol 2005;49:187–90.
166. Odashiro AN, Odashiro DN, Nguyen GK. Minimal deviation endometrioid adenocarcinoma of the cervix: report of three cases with exfoliative cytology. Diagn Cytopathol 2006;34:119–23.
167. Ostor A, Rome R, Quinn M. Microinvasive adenocarcinoma of the cervix: a clinicopathologic study of 77 women. Obstet Gynecol 1997;89:88–93.
168. Ostor AG. Early invasive adenocarcinoma of the uterine cervix. Int J Gynecol Pathol 2000;19:29–38.
169. Ostor AG, Duncan A, Quinn M, Rome R. Adenocarcinoma in situ of the uterine cervix: an experience with 100 cases. Gynecol Oncol 2000;79:207–10.
170. Ostor AG, Pagano R, Davoren RA, Fortune DW, Chanen W, Rome R. Adenocarcinoma in situ of the cervix. Int J Gynecol Pathol 1984;3:179–90.
171. Ozkan F, Ramzy I, Mody DR. Glandular lesions of the cervix on thin-layer Pap tests. Validity of cytologic criteria used in identifying significant lesions. Acta Cytol 2004;48:372–9.
172. Parazzini F, La Vecchia C. Epidemiology of adenocarcinoma of the cervix. Gynecol Oncol 1990;39:40–6.
173. Park JJ, Sun D, Quade BJ, et al. Stratified mucin-producing intraepithelial lesions of the cervix: adenosquamous or columnar cell neoplasia? Am J Surg Pathol 2000;24:1414–9.
174. Parkash V, Chacho MS. Psammoma bodies in cervicovaginal smears: incidence and significance. Diagn Cytopathol 2002;26:81–6.
175. Pecorelli S. Annual report on the results of treatment in gynecological cancer. Int J Gynecol Obstet 2003;25(Suppl 1):1–211.
176. Peters RK, Chao A, Mack TM, Thomas D, Bernstein L, Henderson BE. Increased frequency of adenocarcinoma of the uterine cervix in young women in Los Angeles County. J Natl Cancer Inst 1986;76:423–8.
177. Pirog EC, Kleter B, Olgac S, et al. Prevalence of human papillomavirus DNA in different histological subtypes of cervical adenocarcinoma. Am J Pathol 2000;157:1055–62.
178. Pisharodi LR, Jovanoska S. Spectrum of cytologic changes in pregnancy. A review of 100 abnormal cervicovaginal smears, with emphasis on diagnostic pitfalls. Acta Cytol 1995;39:905–8.
179. Polat A, Dusmez D, Pata O, Aydin O, Egilmez R. Villoglandular papillary adenocarcinoma of the uterine cervix with immunohistochemical characteristics. J Exp Clin Cancer Res 2002;21:425–7.
180. Raab SS, Snider TE, Potts SA, et al. Atypical glandular cells of undetermined significance. Diagnostic accuracy and interobserver variability using select cytologic criteria. Am J Clin Pathol 1997;107:299–307.
181. Rahilly MA, Williams AR, al-Nafussi A. Minimal deviation endometrioid adenocarcinoma of cervix: a clinicopathological and immunohistochemical study of two cases. Histopathology 1992;20:351–4.
182. Ramsaroop R, Chu I. Accuracy of diagnosis of atypical glandular cells – conventional and ThinPrep. Diagn Cytopathol 2006;34:614–9.
183. Raspollini MR, Baroni G, Taddei A, Taddei GL. Primary cervical adenocarcinoma with intestinal differentiation and colonic carcinoma metastatic to cervix: an investigation using Cdx-2 and a limited immunohistochemical panel. Arch Pathol Lab Med 2003;127:1586–90.
184. Recoules-Arche A, Rouzier R, Rey A, et al. [Does adenocarcinoma of uterine cervix have a worse prognosis than squamous carcinoma?] Gynecol Obstet Fertil 2004;32:116–21.
185. Renshaw AA. Making the cut: what can be regularly and reliably identified in gynecologic cytology? Diagn Cytopathol 2006;34:181–3.

186. Renshaw AA, Mody DR, Lozano RL, et al. Detection of adenocarcinoma in situ of the cervix in Papanicolaou tests: comparison of diagnostic accuracy with other high-grade lesions. Arch Pathol Lab Med 2004;128:153–7.
187. Riethdorf L, Riethdorf S, Lee KR, Cviko A, Loning T, Crum CP. Human papillomaviruses, expression of p16, and early endocervical glandular neoplasia. Hum Pathol 2002;33:899–904.
187a. Roberts JM, Thurloe JK. Comparative sensitivities of ThinPrep and Papanicolaou smear for adenocarcinoma in situ (AIS) and combined AIS/high-grade squamous intraepithelial lesion (HSIL): comparison with HSIL. Cancer 2007;111(6):482–6.
188. Roberts JM, Thurloe JK, Bowditch RC, Laverty CR. Subdividing atypical glandular cells of undetermined significance according to the Australian modified Bethesda system: analysis of outcomes. Cancer 2000;90:87–95.
189. Roberts JM, Thurloe JK, Bowditch RC, Humcevic J, Laverty CR. Comparison of ThinPrep and Pap smear in relation to prediction of adenocarcinoma in situ. Acta Cytol 1999;43:74–80.
190. Roberts JM, Thurloe JK, Biro C, Hyne SG, Williams KE, Bowditch RC. Follow up of cytologic predictions of endocervical glandular abnormalities: histologic outcomes in 123 cases. J Lower Genit Tract Dis 2005;9:71–7.
191. Roberts JM, Thurloe JK, Bowditch RC, et al. A three-armed trial of the ThinPrep Imaging System. Diagn Cytopathol 2007;35:96–102.
192. Ruba S, Schoolland M, Allpress S, Sterrett G. Adenocarcinoma in situ of the uterine cervix: screening and diagnostic errors in Papanicolaou smears. Cancer 2004;102:280–7.
193. Sabo D, Shorie J, Biscotti C. Detection of adenocarcinoma using the ThinPrep Imaging System. Cancer Cytopathol 2005;105:374A.
194. Saqi A, Gupta PK, Erroll M, et al. High-risk human papillomavirus DNA testing: a marker for atypical glandular cells. Diagn Cytopathol 2006;34:235–9.
195. Sato S, Ito K, Konno R, Okamoto S, Yajima A. Adenoma malignum. Report of a case with cytologic and colposcopic findings and immunohistochemical staining with antimucin monoclonal antibody HIK–1083. Acta Cytol 2000;44:389–92.
196. Savargaonkar PR, Hale RJ, Pope R, Fox H, Buckley CH. Enteric differentiation in cervical adenocarcinomas and its prognostic significance. Histopathology 1993;23:275–7.
197. Schlesinger C, Silverberg SG. Endocervical adenocarcinoma in situ of tubal type and its relation to atypical tubal metaplasia. Int J Gynecol Pathol 1999;18:1–4.
198. Schoolland M, Allpress S, Sterrett GF. Adenocarcinoma of the cervix. Cancer 2002;96:5–13.
199. Schoolland M, Segal A, Allpress S, Miranda A, Frost FA, Sterrett GF. Adenocarcinoma in situ of the cervix. Cancer 2002;96:330–7.
200. Schorge JO, Hossein Saboorian M, Hynan L, Ashfaq R. ThinPrep detection of cervical and endometrial adenocarcinoma: a retrospective cohort study. Cancer 2002;96:338–43.
201. Schorge JO, Lee KR, Flynn CE, Goodman A, Sheets EE. Stage IA1 cervical adenocarcinoma: definition and treatment. Obstet Gynecol 1999;93:219–22.
202. Scully RE, Bonfiglio TA, Kurman RJ, Silverberg SG, Wilkinson EJ. Histological typing of female genital tract tumours. In: World Health Organization International Histological Classification of Tumours, 2nd edn. Berlin: Springer-Verlag; 1994:13–15.
203. Segal A, Frost FA, Miranda A, Fletcher C, Sterrett GF. Predictive value of diagnoses of endocervical glandular abnormalities in cervical smears. Pathology 2003;35:198–203.
204. Shin CH, Schorge JO, Lee KR, Sheets EE. Conservative management of adenocarcinoma in situ of the cervix. Gynecol Oncol 2000;79:6–10.
205. Shin CH, Schorge JO, Lee KR, Sheets EE. Cytologic and biopsy findings leading to conization in adenocarcinoma in situ of the cervix. Obstet Gynecol 2002;100:271–6.
206. Shingleton HM, Bell MC, Fremgen A, et al. Is there really a difference in survival of women with squamous cell carcinoma, adenocarcinoma, and adenosquamous cell carcinoma of the cervix? Cancer 1995;76(10 Suppl):1948–55.
207. Silverberg SG, Hurt WG. Minimal deviation adenocarcinoma ('adenoma malignum') of the cervix: a reappraisal. Am J Obstet Gynecol 1975;121:971–5.
208. Skopelitou A, Hadjiyannakis M. Enteric type villoglandular papillary adenocarcinoma of the uterine cervix associated with in situ squamous cell carcinoma. Case report and review of the literature. Eur J Gynaecol Oncol 1996;17:309–14.
209. Smith HO, Padilla LA. Adenocarcinoma in situ of the cervix: sensitivity of detection by cervical smear: will cytologic screening for adenocarcinoma in situ reduce incidence rates for adenocarcinoma? Cancer 2002;96:319–22.
210. Smith HO, Tiffany MF, Qualls CR, Key CR. The rising incidence of adenocarcinoma relative to squamous cell carcinoma of the uterine cervix in the United States – a 24-year population-based study. Gynecol Oncol 2000;78:97–105.
211. Solomon D, Davey D, Kurman R, et al. The 2001 Bethesda System: terminology for reporting results of cervical cytology. JAMA 2002;287:2114–9.
212. Sparkes J, Schoolland M, Barrett P, Kurinczuk JJ, Mitchell KM, Sterrett GF. Trends in the frequency and predictive value of reporting high grade abnormalities in cervical smears. Cancer 2000;90:215–21.
213. Steiner G, Friedell GH. Adenosquamous carcinoma in situ of the cervix. Cancer 1965;18:807–10.
214. Tabbara SO, Covell JL. Other malignant neoplasms. In: Solomon D, Nayar R, eds. The Bethesda System for Reporting Cervical Cytology. New York: Springer-Verlag; 2004:157–67.
215. Tamimi HK, Figge DC. Adenocarcinoma of the uterine cervix. Gynecol Oncol 1982;13:335–44.
216. Thomas DB, Ray RM. Oral contraceptives and invasive adenocarcinomas and adenosquamous carcinomas of the uterine cervix. The World Health Organization Collaborative Study of Neoplasia and Steroid Contraceptives. Am J Epidemiol 1996;144:281–9.
217. Toki T, Shiozawa T, Hosaka N, Ishii K, Nikaido T, Fujii S. Minimal deviation adenocarcinoma of the uterine cervix has abnormal expression of sex steroid receptors, CA125, and gastric mucin. Int J Gynecol Pathol 1997;16:111–6.
218. Tringler B, Gup CJ, Singh M, et al. Evaluation of p16INK4a and pRb expression in cervical squamous and glandular neoplasia. Hum Pathol 2004;35:689–96.
219. Ursin G, Pike MC, Preston-Martin S, d'Ablaing G, 3rd, Peters RK. Sexual, reproductive, and other risk factors for adenocarcinoma of the cervix: results from a population-based case-control study (California, United States). Cancer Causes Control 1996;7:391–401.
220. Utsugi K, Shimizu Y, Akiyama F, Hasumi K. Villoglandular papillary adenocarcinoma of the uterine cervix with bulky lymph node metastases. Eur J Obstet Gynecol Reprod Biol 2002;105:186–8.
221. Utsugi K, Shimizu Y, Akiyama F, Umezawa S, Hasumi K. Clinicopathologic features of villoglandular papillary adenocarcinoma of the uterine cervix. Gynecol Oncol 2004;92:64–70.
222. Utsugi K, Hirai Y, Takeshima N, Akiyama F, Sakurai S, Hasumi K. Utility of the monoclonal antibody HIK1083 in the diagnosis of adenoma malignum of the uterine cervix. Gynecol Oncol 1999;75:345–8.
223. van Aspert-van Erp AJ, Smedts FM, Vooijs GP. Severe cervical glandular cell lesions with coexisting squamous cell lesions. Cancer 2004;102:218–27.
224. van Aspert-van Erp AJ, van't HofGrootenboer AB, Brugal G, Vooijs GP. Endocervical columnar cell intraepithelial neoplasia. II. Grades of expression of cytomorphologic criteria. Acta Cytol 1995;39:1216–32.
225. van Aspert-van Erp AJ, van't HofGrootenboer AB, Brugal G, Vooijs GP. Endocervical columnar cell intraepithelial neoplasia. I. Discriminating cytomorphologic criteria. Acta Cytol 1995;39:1199–215.
226. van Aspert-van Erp AJ, van't HofGrootenboer AB, Brugal G, Vooijs GP. Endocervical columnar cell intraepithelial neoplasia (ECCIN). 3. Interobserver variability in feature use. Anal Cell Pathol 1996;10:115–35.
227. Vesterinen E, Forss M, Nieminen U. Increase of cervical adenocarcinoma: a report of 520 cases of cervical carcinoma including 112 tumors with glandular elements. Gynecol Oncol 1989;33:49–53.
228. Visioli CB, Zappa M, Ciatto S, Iossa A, Crocetti E. Increasing trends of cervical adenocarcinoma incidence in Central Italy despite Extensive Screening Programme, 1985–2000. Cancer Detect Prev 2004;28:461–4.
229. Waldenstrom AC, Horvath G. Survival of patients with adenocarcinoma of the uterine cervix in western Sweden. Int J Gynecol Cancer 1999;9:18–23.
230. Wang N, Emancipator SN, Rose P, Rodriguez M, Abdul-Karim FW. Histologic follow-up of atypical endocervical cells. Liquid-based, thin-layer preparation vs. conventional Pap smear. Acta Cytol 2002;46:453–7.
231. Webb JC, Key CR, Qualls CR, Smith HO. Population-based study of microinvasive adenocarcinoma of the uterine cervix. Obstet Gynecol 2001;97(5 Pt 1):701–6.
232. Wells M, Ostor AG, Crum CP, et al. Pathology and genetics tumors of the breast and female genital organs. In: Tavassoli FA, Devilee P, eds. World Health Organization Classification of Tumors. Lyon: IARC Press; 2003:275–6.
233. Wheeler DT, Kurman RJ. The relationship of glands to thick-wall blood vessels as a marker of invasion in endocervical adenocarcinoma. Int J Gynecol Pathol 2005;24:125–30.
234. Widrich T, Kennedy AW, Myers TM, Hart WR, Wirth S. Adenocarcinoma in situ of the uterine cervix: management and outcome. Gynecol Oncol 1996;61:304–8.
235. Wilbur DC, Dubeshter B, Angel C, Atkison KM. Use of thin-layer preparations for gynecologic smears with emphasis on the cytomorphology of high-grade intraepithelial lesions and carcinomas. Diagn Cytopathol 1996;14:201–11.
236. Wilczynski SP, Walker J, Liao SY, Bergen S, Berman M. Adenocarcinoma of the cervix associated with human papillomavirus. Cancer 1988;62:1331–6.
237. Williams AR. Liquid-based cytology and conventional smears compared over two 12-month periods. Cytopathology 2006;17:82–5.
238. Wilson C, Jones H. An audit of cervical smears reported to contain atypical glandular cells. Cytopathology 2004;15:181–7.
239. Witkiewicz A, Lee KR, Brodsky G, Cviko A, Brodsky J, Crum CP. Superficial (early) endocervical adenocarcinoma in situ: a study of 12 cases and comparison to conventional AIS. Am J Surg Pathol 2005;29:1609–14.
240. Woodman CBJ, Collins S, Rollason TP, et al. Human papillomavirus type 18 and rapidly progressing cervical intraepithelial neoplasia. Lancet 2003;361:40–3.
241. Wright TC, Jr, Cox JT, Massad LS, Twiggs LB, Wilkinson EJ. 2001 Consensus guidelines for the management of women with cervical cytological abnormalities. JAMA 2002;287:2120–9.

241a. Wright TC, Jr., Massad LS, Dunton CJ, Spitzer M, Wilkinson EJ, Solomon D. 2006 consensus guidelines for the management of women with abnormal cervical cancer screening tests. Am J Obstet Gynecol 2007;197(4):346–55.

242. Xu JY, Hashi A, Kondo T, et al. Absence of human papillomavirus infection in minimal deviation adenocarcinoma and lobular endocervical glandular hyperplasia. Int J Gynecol Pathol 2005;24:296–302.

243. Yamashita S, Nagai N, Oshita T, et al. Clinicocytopathological and immunohistochemical study of adenoma malignum of the uterine cervix. Hiroshima J Med Sci 2000;49:167–73.

244. Yeh IT, LiVolsi VA, Noumoff JS. Endocervical carcinoma. Pathol Res Pract 1991;187:129–44.

245. Young RH. Sex cord-stromal tumors of the ovary and testis: their similarities and differences with consideration of selected problems. Mod Pathol 2005;18(Suppl):S81.

246. Young RH, Scully RE. Minimal-deviation endometrioid adenocarcinoma of the uterine cervix. A report of five cases of a distinctive neoplasm that may be misinterpreted as benign. Am J Surg Pathol 1993;17:660–5.

247. Young RH, Clement PB. Endocervicosis involving the uterine cervix: a report of four cases of a benign process that may be confused with deeply invasive endocervical adenocarcinoma. Int J Gynecol Pathol 2000;19:322–8.

248. Young RH, Clement PB. Endocervical adenocarcinoma and its variants: their morphology and differential diagnosis. Histopathology 2002;41:185–207.

249. Zaino RJ. Glandular lesions of the uterine cervix. Mod Pathol 2000;13:261–74.

250. Zaino RJ. Symposium part I: adenocarcinoma in situ, glandular dysplasia, and early invasive adenocarcinoma of the uterine cervix. Int J Gynecol Pathol 2002;21:314–26.

251. Zaino RJ. The fruits of our labors: distinguishing endometrial from endocervical adenocarcinoma. Int J Gynecol Pathol 2002;21:1–3.

252. Zhao S, Hayasaka T, Osakabe M, et al. Mucin expression in nonneoplastic and neoplastic glandular epithelia of the uterine cervix. Int J Gynecol Pathol 2003;22:393–7.

253. Zhou C, Matisic JP, Clement PB, Hayes MM. Cytologic features of papillary serous adenocarcinoma of the uterine cervix. Cancer 1997;81:98–104.

254. Zhou C, Gilks CB, Hayes M, Clement PB. Papillary serous carcinoma of the uterine cervix: a clinicopathologic study of 17 cases. Am J Surg Pathol 1998;22:113–20.

255. Zielinski GD, Snijders PJ, Rozendaal L, et al. The presence of high-risk HPV combined with specific p53 and p16INK4a expression patterns points to high-risk HPV as the main causative agent for adenocarcinoma in situ and adenocarcinoma of the cervix. J Pathol 2003;201:535–43.

Miscellaneous cervical neoplasms

11

Anais Malpica   Stanley J. Robboy

EPITHELIAL TUMORS

GLASSY CELL CARCINOMA

Definition
Glassy cell carcinomas are poorly differentiated malignant neoplasms exhibiting cells with abundant, granular, lightly eosinophilic cytoplasm imparting a so-called ground-glass appearance.

General features
These tumors, which account for only 1–5% of all cervical carcinomas,[35] are commonly associated with human papillomavirus (HPV) 18 and occasionally with HPV 16.[50,51,61,71]

Pathogenesis
The tumors strongly express high and low molecular weight cytokeratins, as do the squamous components of adenosquamous carcinomas. They also express MUC1 (a membrane-bound mucin core protein) and MUC2 (a secretory-type mucin core protein), like the glandular (adeno) component of adenosquamous carcinomas. Within the World Health Organization classification of tumors of the uterine cervix they are therefore considered poorly differentiated variants of adenosquamous carcinoma.[50,90] Some believe they originate from multipotent stem or reserve cells with the capacity for both glandular and squamous differentiation.[50]

Clinical features
Glassy cell carcinomas occur in younger women (mean age, 44 years).[44,65] Initially, they were believed to arise in association with pregnancy, but recent studies have not confirmed this.[35,44] Patients most frequently present with uterine bleeding. An occasional asymptomatic case may be detected in a routine Pap smear.

Pathology
Tumors are usually bulky, exophytic masses, the sizes of which usually range from 3 to 7 cm. Invasion is frequently shallower than suspected from the size of the protuberant mass. These tumors disclose nests and sheets of large cells with abundant eosinophilic or amphophilic, ground-glass or finely granular cytoplasm, and large nuclei and macronucleoli (Figure 11.1). The mitotic index is high and cell borders are distinct (Figures 11.2 and 11.3). There is frequently a marked inflammatory infiltrate. Rare foci of obvious squamous or glandular differentiation and intracellular mucin may be seen. While no preinvasive lesion has been identified, a small pro-

portion of cases show associated squamous cell carcinoma *in situ.*

The tumors are reactive for low and high molecular weight cytokeratins, MUC1 and MUC2,[50] but not estrogen or progesterone receptors.[7]

Ultrastructural features
The glassy cell appearance is due to the presence of extensive abundant polyribosomes and rough endoplasmic reticulum in the cytoplasm of the neoplastic cells. Abortive gland formation, well-developed tonofilaments, desmosomal complexes, interdigitating microvilli, and cytoplasmic microfilaments provide further evidence that the neoplasms are adenosquamous in type,[23] even though it is unclear whether they are still more primitive in evolution than poorly differentiated, nonkeratinizing squamous cell carcinomas.

Differential diagnosis
Tumors with more than a minor degree of squamous differentiation should be considered as poorly differentiated squamous cell carcinoma.

Prognosis
Although the earliest studies of glassy cell carcinomas considered these tumors to be aggressive with a uniformly poor survival rate, subsequent studies have demonstrated that survival is related to stage of the disease at diagnosis.[44,79,92]

MALIGNANT MESONEPHRIC TUMOR, INCLUDING MESONEPHRIC ADENOCARCINOMA

Definition
These are malignant tumors derived from the remnants of the mesonephric ducts. They include mesonephric adenocarcinomas and the very rare malignant mixed mesonephric tumors (not to be confused with carcinosarcomas, also known as malignant mixed müllerian tumors). The malignant mixed mesonephric tumors disclose a sarcomatous component, either homologous or heterologous, in addition to adenocarcinoma.[9]

General features
These tumors are rare, with fewer than 40 cases reported. The mean age at presentation is in the low 40 s, but the range is wide (24–72 years). Most patients present with uterine bleeding and a visible cervical lesion; however, some are found incidentally.[9,18,27,80] They arise from mesonephric remnants, which are normally found in about one-fifth of uterine cervices. Areas of

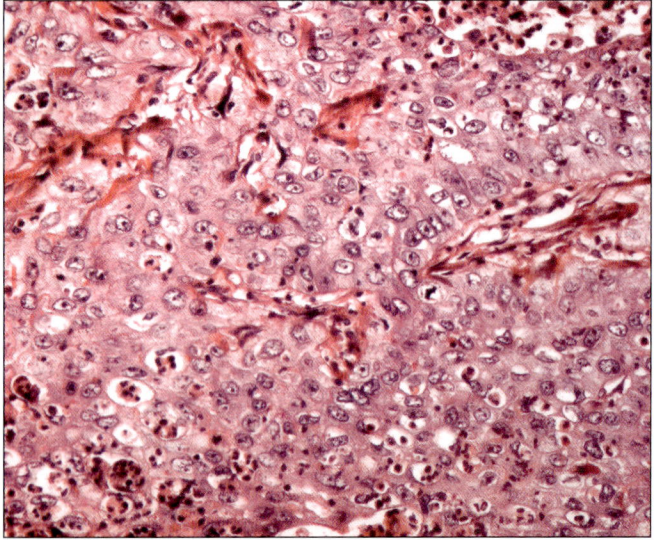

Fig. 11.1 Glassy cell carcinoma.

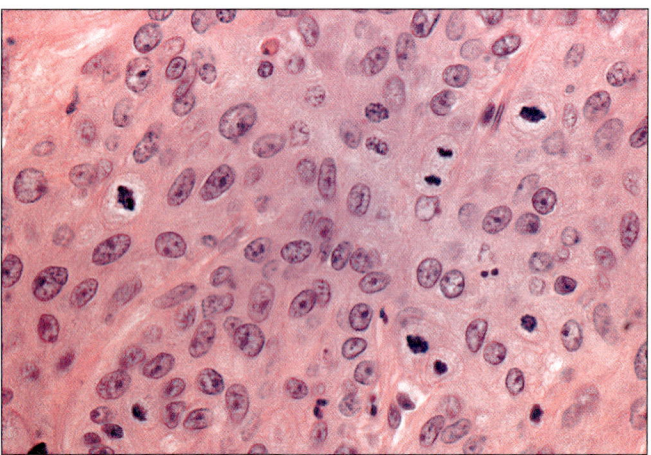

Fig. 11.2 Glassy cell carcinoma. Prominent features at high power include cytoplasm with a ground-glass appearance and nuclei with a prominent macronucleous, and many mitotic figures.

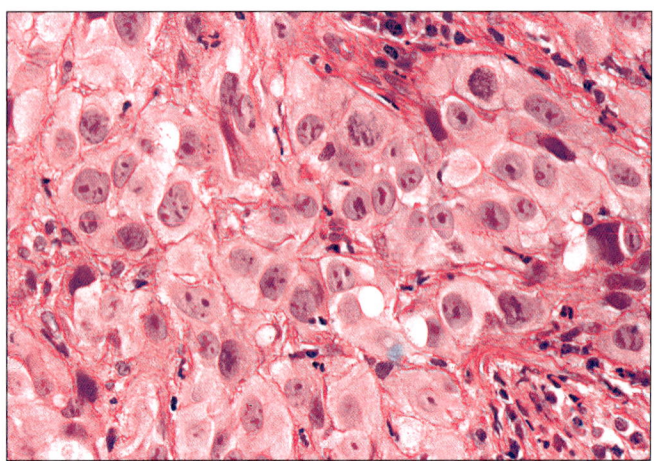

Fig. 11.3 Glassy cell carcinoma disclosing cells with prominent cell borders.

mesonephric remnants or hyperplasia have been identified in the majority of cases.[9,18,80]

Pathology

The tumors range in size from 1 to 8.5 cm,[9,18,80] commonly enlarge the cervical wall or are polypoid. Less frequently, they produce no gross alterations. Microscopically, most are pure mesonephric adenocarcinomas (Figure 11.4). They may exhibit ductal (glandular), tubular, retiform, solid, or sex-cord like patterns. The ductal and tubular patterns are the most common. The cells are columnar or cuboidal, with mild to moderate pleomorphism, and variable mitotic activity. They lack the intracellular mucin found in the usual endocervical adenocarcinoma, and the glycogen found in the usual clear cell adenocarcinoma. As in non-neoplastic mesonephric tubules, at least some of the luminal spaces of this type of carcinoma contain a dense eosinophilic material (Figure 11.5). Rare cases are biphasic with a sarcomatoid component. The tumors usually display a non-specific malignant spindle cell component; however, heterologous elements such as osteosarcoma, rhabdomyosarcoma, and atypical cartilage may be found.[9,18]

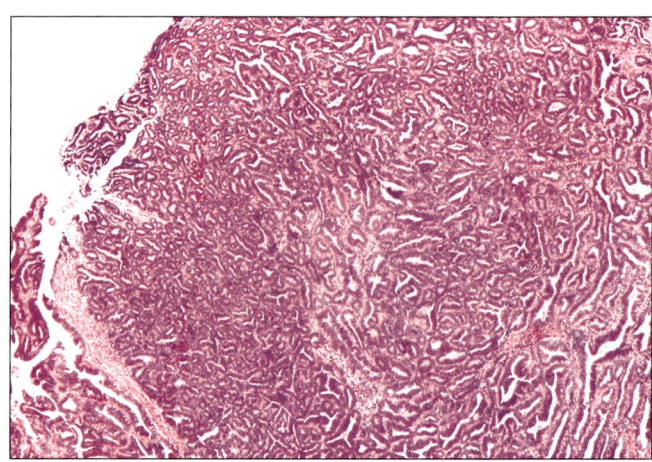

Fig. 11.4 Mesonephric adenocarcinoma with oval and irregularly shaped glands.

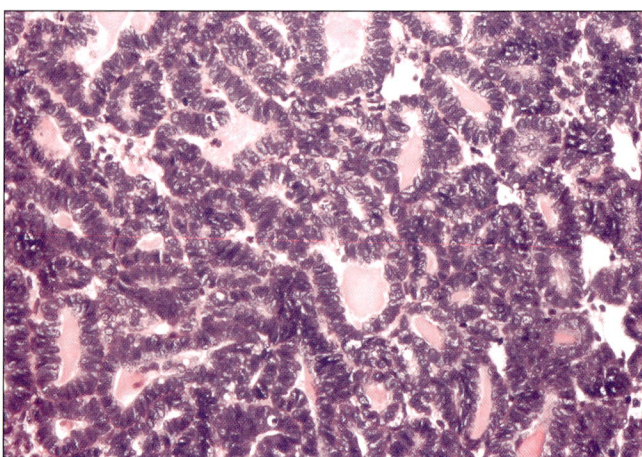

Fig. 11.5 Mesonephric adenocarcinoma with intraluminal eosinophilic material.

Immunohistochemical studies

These tumors are universally reactive for epithelial markers, including pancytokeratin, cytokeratin 7 (CK7), low molecular weight keratin (CAM 5.2), and epithelial membrane antigen (EMA). Mesonephric adenocarcinomas are usually reactive for calretinin and vimentin (Figure 11.6) and unreactive for estrogen and progesterone receptors, cytokeratin 20 (CK20), and monoclonal carcinoembryonic antigen (mCEA).[80] In addition, reactivity to CD10 or CALLA (common acute lymphoblastic leukemia antigen) is variable.[9,68] In the rare cases in which there was focal reactivity for CEA, the antibody used was polyclonal.[9] Androgen receptors are expressed in approximately 33% of cases.[80]

Differential diagnosis

Diffuse mesonephric hyperplasia lacks a back-to-back glandular pattern. Mild to moderate atypia, more than an occasional mitosis, and the presence of vascular or perineural invasion support the diagnosis of mesonephric adenocarcinoma.

The presence of background mesonephric hyperplasia, the presence of intraluminal dense eosinophilic material and the expression of calretinin differentiate mesonephric adenocarcinoma from primary cervical adenocarcinoma of endometrioid type.

Similarly, endometrial adenocarcinoma of various types (i.e., endometrioid, clear cell, and serous) may be differentiated from mesonephric adenocarcinoma by these same features. Also, atypical endometrial hyperplasia commonly accompanies endometrial adenocarcinoma of endometrioid type. Serous carcinomas of the endometrium disclose marked cytologic atypia, p53 reactivity, and lack reactivity with calretinin and CD10 as frequently seen in mesonephric adenocarcinomas. Clear cell carcinomas of endometrial but also cervical origin have histologic features that are usually easy to identify (i.e., the presence of clear cells and hobnail cells arranged in a combination of patterns including tubulocystic, papillary, and solid); attention to the cytologic and histologic features will facilitate the correct diagnosis.

Endometrial stromal sarcoma may be suggested by the sarcomatous component of a biphasic mesonephric tumor.

Although these tumors may exhibit focal glandular differentiation, they typically show nests or sheets of oval/round uniform cells in association with a distinct meshwork of fine vascular spaces that mimics the arterioles of proliferative phase endometrium. These features are all absent in mesonephric tumors of the biphasic type.

Carcinosarcoma may be suggested by the biphasic type of mesonephric tumors. However, the recognition of the features considered typical of mesonephric adenocarcinoma in the epithelial component and the use of immunohistochemical studies, as mentioned above, facilitate the distinction.

Uterine tumors resembling ovarian sex-cord tumors rarely occur in the cervix, usually have a well-circumscribed/pushing border, and lack the eosinophilic intraluminal material, as well as areas of mesonephric hyperplasia in the vicinity as seen in mesonephric tumors.

Prognosis

Mesonephric adenocarcinomas often present in an early stage and have a better prognosis than their müllerian counterparts, whereas malignant mixed mesonephric tumors may present in advanced stage and behave in aggressive fashion similar to the malignant mixed müllerian tumors.[9]

ADENOID BASAL CARCINOMA

Definition

Adenoid basal carcinomas are composed of uniform, bland, basaloid cells arranged in nests with peripheral palisading. They may show focal glandular or squamous differentiation.[13] Because they have an excellent prognosis when showing only the typical features throughout, some have proposed changing their name to 'adenoid basal epitheliomas'.[43]

General features

Adenoid basal carcinomas are rare, accounting for less than 1% of cervical cancers. They usually develop in postmenopausal women, mostly 55–75 years of age (range, 19–91 years).[13,43] Almost all women are asymptomatic, but the disease

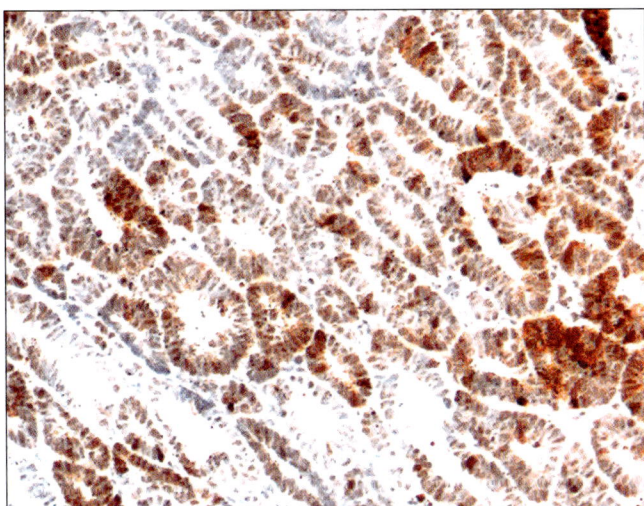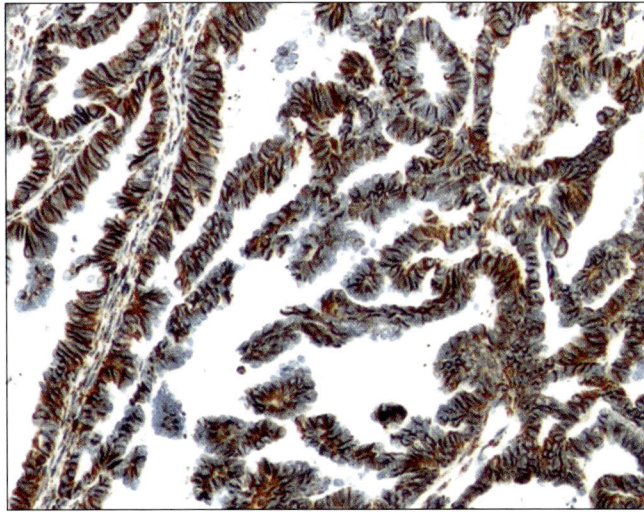

Fig. 11.6 Mesonephric adenocarcinoma, reactive for calretinin (left) and vimentin (right).

is usually detected during evaluation of an abnormal Pap smear that proves to be an associated cervical intraepithelial neoplasia (CIN). The tumors appear to originate from pluripotent reserve cells[40] and most are associated with HPV 16.[61,70]

Pathology

They usually show no grossly visible tumor. Induration, erosion, ulceration, and slight abnormalities of the cervical mucosa have been described in rare cases.[13]

Adenoid basal carcinomas or 'epitheliomas' exhibit multiple, small, well-defined, round or oval nests of epithelial cells haphazardly distributed in the cervical stroma without eliciting a desmoplastic response (Figures 11.7 and 11.8). The lesions typically do not reach the endocervical canal surface, although occasionally they may originate from an overlying dysplastic squamous epithelium.[28] Tumor cells are small, uniform, cuboidal, oval or spindle, with palisading towards the periphery of the nests (Figure 11.9). Nuclei are bland and uniform, and

mitotic activity tends to be low although variable: 0–9 mitoses per 10 high-power fields (HPFs).[13,28] The cytoplasm, if clear, results from accumulated intracytoplasmic glycogen.[40] Areas of glandular differentiation or squamous metaplasia may sometimes be seen within the epithelial nests (Figures 11.10 and 11.11). The presence of squamous metaplasia may be marked, producing expansion of the nests to where the lesion mimics a squamous cell tumor. In these cases, a rim of basaloid cells still persists at the periphery of the nests. There is no necrosis. The cervical mucosa and endocervical glands usually show CIN. These tumors show no vascular or perineural invasion and usually elicit no stromal response. In rare cases some edema and a mild chronic inflammatory infiltrate may be seen around the tumor nests. While most cases are accompanied by high-grade CIN or squamous carcinoma *in situ*, rare cases are found with superficially invasive or frankly invasive squamous carcinoma, adenoid cystic carcinoma, adenosquamous carcinoma, clear cell carcinoma, and neuroendocrine carcinoma. Adenoid

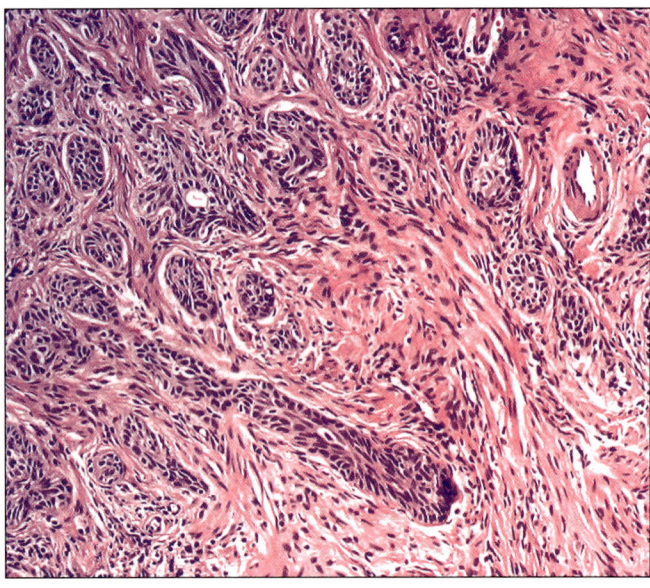

Fig. 11.7 Adenoid basal carcinoma (epithelioma) composed of round, oval or slightly distorted nests.

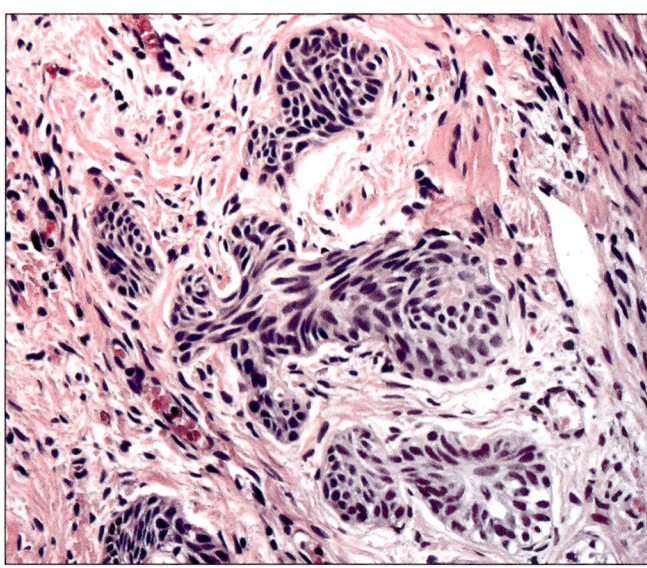

Fig. 11.9 Adenoid basal carcinoma (epithelioma) with bland cytology and peripheral palisading.

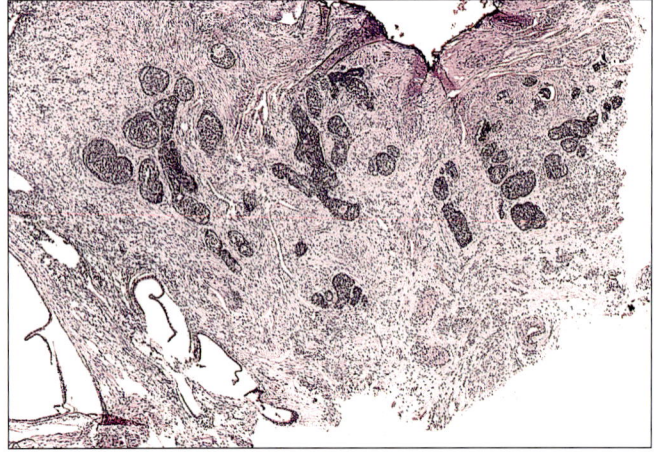

Fig. 11.8 Adenoid basal carcinoma (epithelioma) infiltrating deep in the cervical stroma.

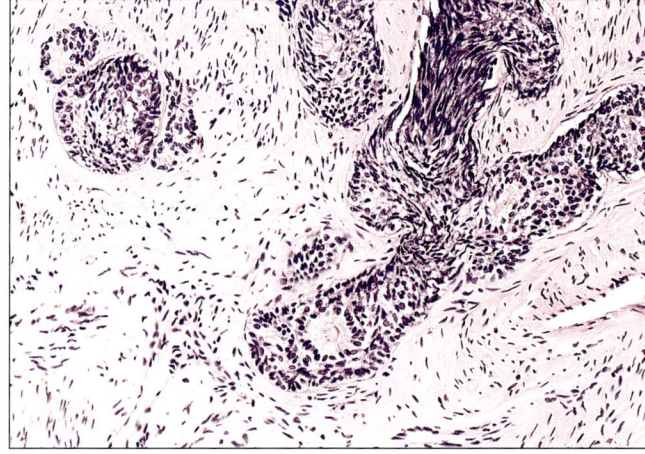

Fig. 11.10 Adenoid basal carcinoma (epithelioma) with focal glandular formation.

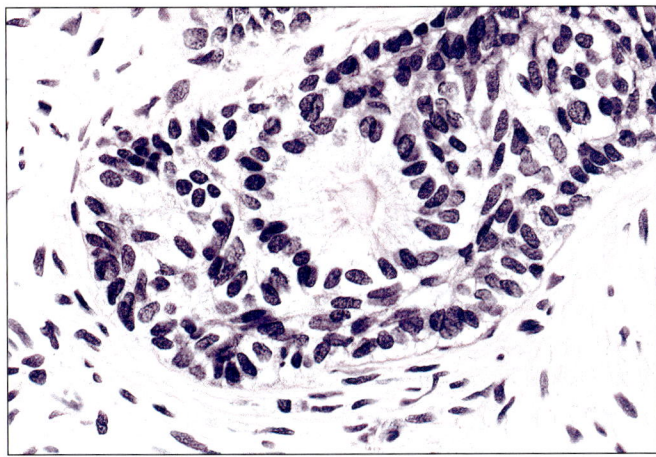

Fig. 11.11 Adenoid basal carcinoma. Detail of glandular formation.

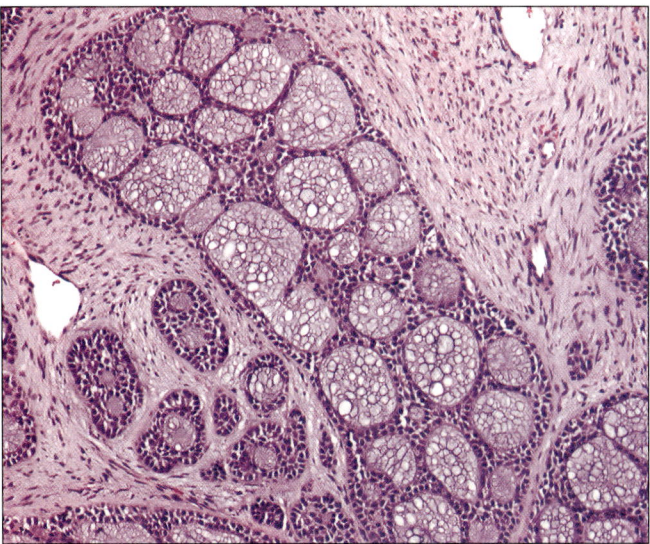

Fig. 11.12 Adenoid cystic carcinoma.

basal carcinomas have even been found near malignant mixed müllerian tumors of the cervix.[28,40,43,70]

Immunohistochemical features

Adenoid basal carcinomas react consistently for CAM 5.2, CK7, EMA, and CEA, and inconsistently for S-100 protein.[40,43] The use of CAM 5.2 has been advocated for distinguishing adenoid basal carcinomas from invasive squamous carcinomas since it enhances the basaloid cells present in the former.[43]

Prognosis

Typical cases of adenoid basal carcinoma behave in a benign fashion without metastases to lymph nodes or other sites, local recurrences or deaths.[43] Based on published photographs, we believe that the rare cases reported to behave aggressively[28] have abnormally large cells compared with those usually seen in adenoid basal carcinomas, are arranged in cords, and have elicited a striking myxoid stromal response, indicative of high-grade invasive carcinomas.

Differential diagnosis

Adenoid basal hyperplasia is a superficial lesion with epithelial nests smaller than those seen in adenoid basal carcinomas. The epithelial nests reside within 0.5 mm of the basement membrane of the overlying or adjacent epithelium and are connected to it.

Adenoid cystic carcinomas tend to produce gross lesions. Microscopically, the nodules are larger than the tumor nests seen in adenoid basal carcinomas and display a cribriform pattern and hyaline cylinders. Necrosis is present. Vascular invasion is commonly seen.

Basaloid squamous carcinomas, like their counterparts at other sites, exhibit larger islands of small, intermediate, or large neoplastic cells with peripheral palisading and numerous mitoses. Their behavior in the uterine cervix is unknown.[36]

ADENOID CYSTIC CARCINOMA

Definition

Adenoid cystic carcinomas of the cervix have histologic features mimicking those of similar tumors of salivary glands and upper respiratory tract.

General features

These tumors are rare and mostly seen in postmenopausal women (mean age, 72 years),[28] but occasionally in women under age 40.[54] Uterine bleeding is the most common presentation with a rare case detected incidentally.[28] Similar to adenoid basal carcinomas, these tumors appear to originate from reserve cells. In some cases, HPV 16 has been detected.[39]

Pathology

These tumors have a variable appearance from small polypoid lesions to large exophytic, friable masses to deeply invasive endophytic tumors.[28] Microscopically, tumors are composed of cords, nests, sheets, and trabeculae of small, relatively uniform basaloid cells. Clear cell changes may be present.[40] A distinct cribriform pattern containing either an amorphous hyaline eosinophilic basement membrane-like material or basophilic mucin or eosinophilic secretion is seen (Figure 11.12). Mitotic activity is variable, ranging from scanty to very high.[28,40] Necrosis is often present and extensive. Stromal changes are typically prominent, ranging from hyalinization to myxoid or fibroblastic. The solid variant lacks the typical cribriform pattern, but the tumor is recognized in these cases by the presence of abundant periodic acid-Schiff (PAS)-positive basement membrane material around the tumor cells that grow in solid nests, cords, and trabeculae.[2] Small foci may show squamous differentiation. The tumors may also be associated with adenoid basal carcinoma, *in situ* or invasive squamous carcinoma, or adenocarcinoma.[28,40] The tumors have a tendency to involve vascular spaces and to have lymph node metastases at an early stage.[54]

Immunohistochemical studies

Tumor cells are reactive for broad spectrum cytokeratin (MNF116), CAM 5.2, CK7, and EMA. CEA may also be expressed. S-100 protein reactivity occurs in some cases[40] while others are unreactive or just focally and weakly reactive.[2,28]

Prognosis

These tumors exhibit an aggressive behavior. Nearly half of the patients will die of locally recurrent or metastatic disease within 8 months to 8 years of diagnosis.[28]

NEUROENDOCRINE TUMORS

Neuroendocrine tumors of the uterine cervix are rare.[63] According to the approach proposed in 1997 by a workshop sponsored by the College of American Pathologists and the National Cancer Institute, they are best classified as: typical (classic) carcinoid tumors, atypical carcinoid tumors, small cell neuroendocrine carcinomas, and large cell neuroendocrine carcinomas.[4] These tumors may originate from the cells containing neuroendocrine granules seen in 20% of normal cervices or from cervical reserve or stem cells.[34,59,81] Additionally, association with HPV 16 or 18 has been described in atypical carcinoids, small cell neuroendocrine carcinomas, and large cell neuroendocrine carcinomas.[1,6,38,59,81,91]

TYPICAL (CLASSIC) CARCINOID TUMOR

The least common of the neuroendocrine tumors[59,63] exhibit the typical carcinoid features seen elsewhere in the body. Cytologic atypia is non-existent or minimal, mitotic figures are not found or rare, and there is no necrosis (Figure 11.13).[4]

ATYPICAL CARCINOID

The second least common of the neuroendocrine tumors[59,63] exhibits mild to moderate cytologic atypia, up to 10 mitotic figures per 10 HPFs, and focal necrosis[4] (Figures 11.4 and 11.15).

SMALL CELL NEUROENDOCRINE CARCINOMA

The most common neuroendocrine tumors account for 0.5–1% of all cervical carcinomas.[22,59,63] Their diagnostic features include small cells with minimal cytoplasm, nuclei with finely granular chromatin, absence of nucleoli, numerous mitotic figures, and extensive necrosis.

General features

Patients range from 22 to 87 years of age (mean age, fifth decade).[1,33,87] Most patients present with vaginal bleeding. Occasionally, the tumors are detected in an abnormal Pap smear. In rare cases, there is clinical and biochemical evidence of hormone production, such as Cushing's syndrome (due to corticotrophin production), syndrome of inappropriate antidiuretic hormone production (due to vasopressin production), carcinoid syndrome (due to serotonin production), and hypoglycemia (due to insulin production).[1,46,77] The tumors in most patients are FIGO stage 1 or 2.[5,22,63,82,87]

Pathology

The tumors range in size from 1 to 10 cm.[87] Microscopically, they are composed of oval or spindle cells with scanty cytoplasm and hyperchromatic nuclei with finely granular chromatin and no nucleoli. The cells are arranged in nests, trabeculae or sheets (Figures 11.16 and 11.17). There are numerous mitoses and apoptotic bodies. Molding of the nuclei and necrosis are common. Vascular/lymphatic involvement is usually promi-

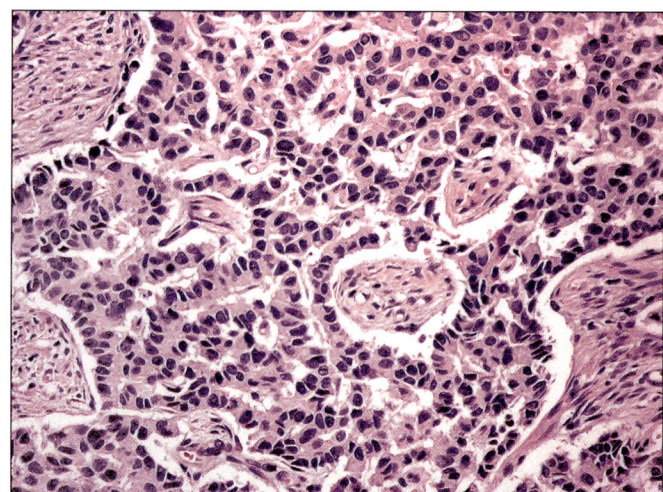

Fig. 11.14 Atypical carcinoid with trabecular pattern.

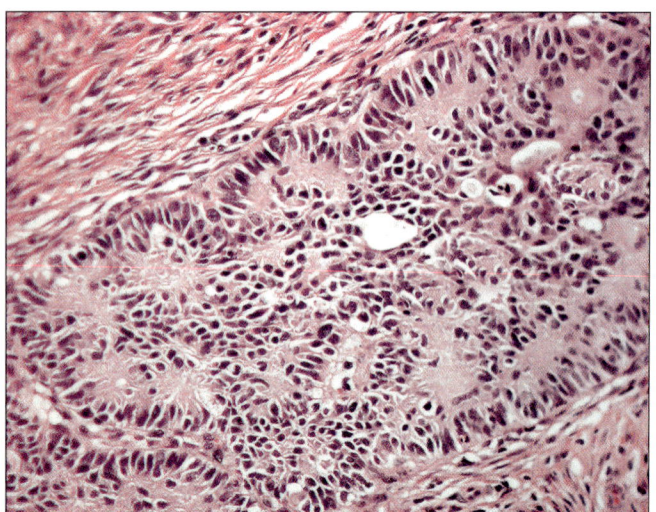

Fig. 11.13 Typical (classic) carcinoid.

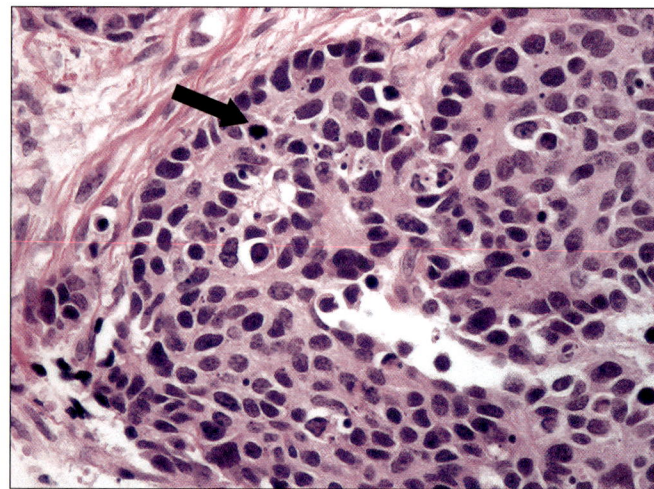

Fig. 11.15 Atypical carcinoid with mitotic arrow (arrow).

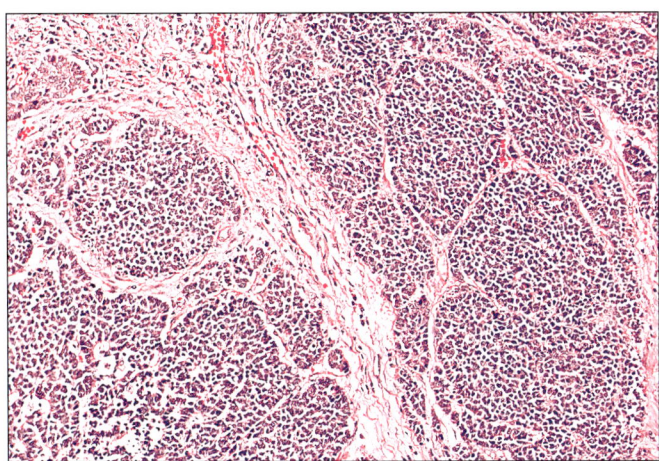

Fig. 11.16 Neuroendocrine carcinoma, small cell type. Nests and trabeculae of tumor cells.

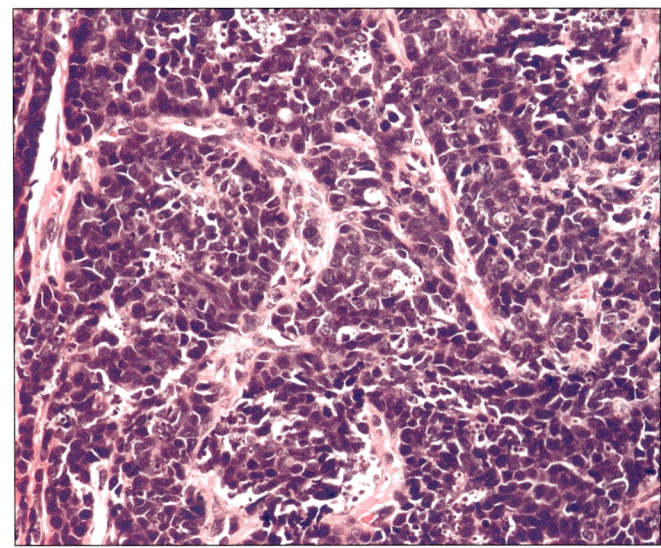

Fig. 11.17 Neuroendocrine carcinoma, small cell type.

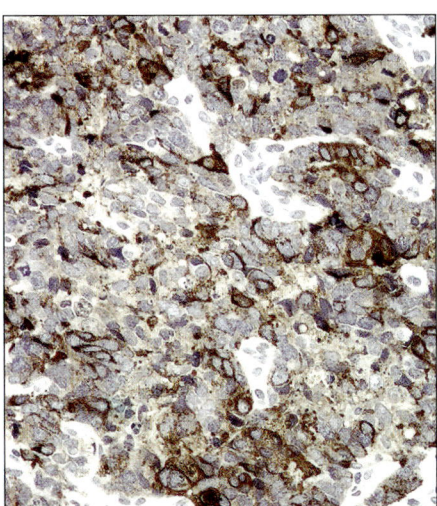
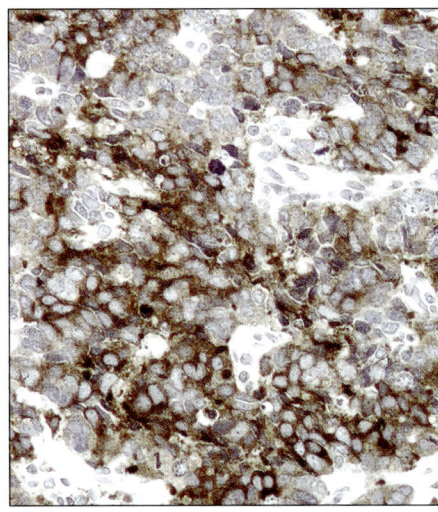

Fig. 11.18 Neuroendocrine carcinoma small cell type, reactive for chromogranin (left) and synaptophysin (right).

nent. An associated large cell neuroendocrine carcinoma, *in situ* or invasive squamous or adenocarcinoma may be found.[22,47]

Immunohistochemical studies

Although the tumor cells react with keratin, chromogranin, synaptophysin, neuron-specific enolase (NSE), and CD56 (neural cell adhesion molecule, NCAM) (Figure 11.18), the percentage of cases reactive with each varies according to different studies. Keratin reactivity may be absent[6] or present in 100% of the cases.[22] Chromogranin reactivity has been found in 32%, 50%, and 76% of the cells in three different studies.[3,82,87] Synaptophysin reactivity ranges from 50 to 90%.[82,87] NSE expression occurs in up to 75% of cases[82] and CD56 expression has been seen in 71–88% of the cases.[3,87] The latter is thought to be the most sensitive marker for the diagnosis of small cell carcinoma of the uterine cervix.[3] Of interest, one study showed that half of cases failed to express chromogranin and synaptophysin, while other studies have shown that at least one neuroendocrine marker is expressed in 88% and 95% of the

cases.[82,87] Thyroid transcription factor-1 (TTF-1) reactivity is variable in contrast to the reactivity shown in cases of small cell carcinoma arising in the lung.[47] C-kit reactivity is infrequent in small cell carcinoma of the cervix.[88]

Prognosis

Small cell carcinomas are highly aggressive neoplasms with an overall survival rate of 29–33% at 5 years.[5,87]

Differential diagnosis

Poorly differentiated squamous carcinomas are occasionally composed of small cells, but they have more cytoplasm than those of a small cell carcinoma, are usually arranged in cohesive sheets, and they have nucleoli. In difficult cases, reactivity for CD56, chromogranin, and synaptophysin may be useful in establishing the neuroendocrine nature of a tumor, and p63 in identifying squamous differentiation.[62a]

Lymphomas and melanomas are equally rare but require only standard immunohistochemical studies to differentiate them from small cell neuroendocrine carcinomas.

LARGE CELL NEUROENDOCRINE CARCINOMA

Definition

The second most common neuroendocrine tumors of the cervix, which account for 0.6% of the invasive cervical carcinomas,[59,63,76] exhibit an insular or trabecular pattern, at least focally, and high-grade neoplastic cells with abundant or moderate amounts of cytoplasm.

Clinical features

The mean age of the women is 34 years, but the range is wide (21–62 years).[34] The most common presentation is vaginal bleeding, but some tumors are detected due to an abnormal Pap smear. The tumors are usually FIGO stage 1 or 2.[34,56,74,76]

Pathology

The tumors often are polypoid and exophytic, although they may be ill defined and not even grossly visible. Some are up to 6 cm in size and with a variable cut surface, ranging from tan-brown to yellow-gray or white, with areas of hemorrhage and necrosis.[34,76] Microscopically, the tumor cells are relatively uniform (Figure 11.19), showing moderate or abundant cytoplasm and nuclei with vesicular chromatin and nucleoli. The mitotic index is high (>10 mitoses per 10 HPFs). Geographic necrosis is commonly seen (Figure 11.20). The neoplastic cells

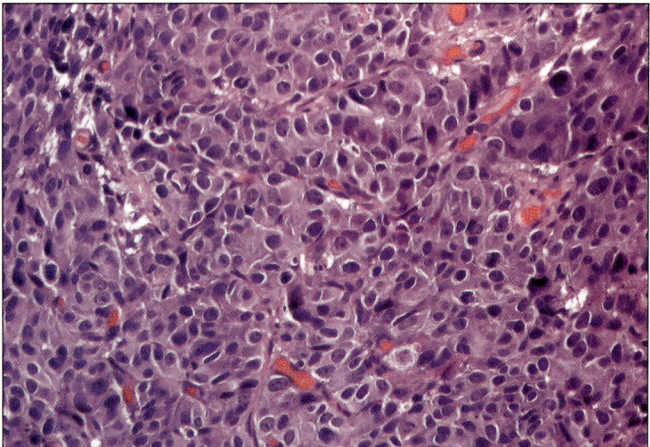

Fig. 11.19 Neuroendocrine carcinoma, large cell type.

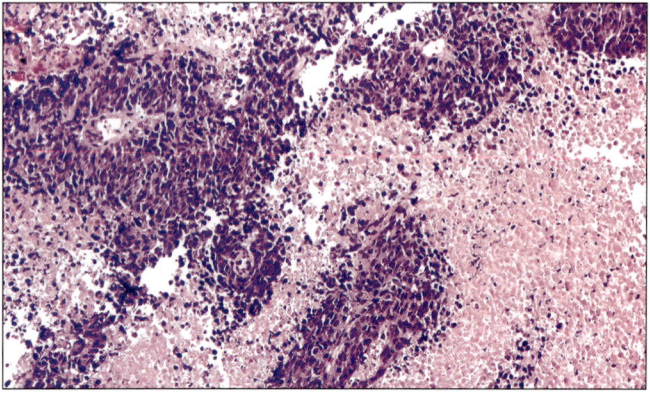

Fig. 11.20 Neuroendocrine carcinoma, large cell type, showing geographic necrosis.

are arranged, at least focally, in an insular or trabecular pattern, and in solid sheets. Vascular invasion is usually present and prominent. Focal glandular differentiation may be noted. In addition, the tumors may be associated with adenocarcinoma *in situ*, CIN, invasive adenocarcinoma (mucinous or endometrioid), or small cell carcinoma.[34,59,76,93]

Immunohistochemical studies

The neoplastic cells express chromogranin, although only 25% do so. They are also reactive for synaptophysin, although the expression of this marker is less reliable than the former.[34,56,76]

Prognosis

The outcome for patients with large cell neuroendocrine carcinomas is poor, 65% dying typically within 3 years of diagnosis despite the administration of adjuvant therapy. Intra-abdominal/intrapelvic and extra-abdominal metastases, including liver, kidney, adrenal gland, lymph nodes, lung, and brain, are usually seen.[34,76]

Differential diagnosis

Small cell carcinomas exhibit cells with scanty cytoplasm, hyperchromatic nuclei, and no nucleoli.

Adenocarcinoma may be erroneously suggested by the presence of focal glandular differentiation within a large cell neuroendocrine carcinoma, or the association with either an adenocarcinoma *in situ* or invasive adenocarcinoma. Attention to the cytologic and histologic features typically seen in large cell neuroendocrine carcinomas (i.e., an insular or trabecular pattern and the relative uniformity of the tumor cells), as well as the use of neuroendocrine markers, will assist in making this distinction. It is important to remember that focal expression of neuroendocrine markers sometimes occurs in otherwise typical adenocarcinomas or adenosquamous carcinomas of the cervix.[34]

Poorly differentiated squamous carcinomas should have at least focal evidence of keratin production or intercellular bridges. The absence of these two features in addition to the presence of high-grade nuclei, macronucleoli, numerous mitotic figures and apoptotic bodies, geographic necrosis, and prominent vascular invasion should raise the possibility of large cell neuroendocrine carcinoma.

Malignant melanomas may show a combination of junctional activity, melanin, and reactivity for S-100 protein and/or HMB45 to allow their distinction from large cell neuroendocrine carcinomas.

SARCOMAS OR TUMORS WITH A SARCOMATOUS COMPONENT

Sarcomas of the uterine cervix are rare, accounting for approximately 0.5% of the malignant tumors at this site.[15] The most common is embryonal rhabdomyosarcoma (sarcoma botryoides), followed by leiomyosarcoma. Other rarities include endometrial stromal sarcoma, alveolar soft part sarcoma, malignant peripheral sheath tumor, angiosarcoma, alveolar rhabdomyosarcoma, liposarcoma, osteosarcoma, so-called PEComa (perivascular epithelioid cell tumor), and malignant fibrous histiocytoma.[12,15,16,25,26,29,67,75,83]

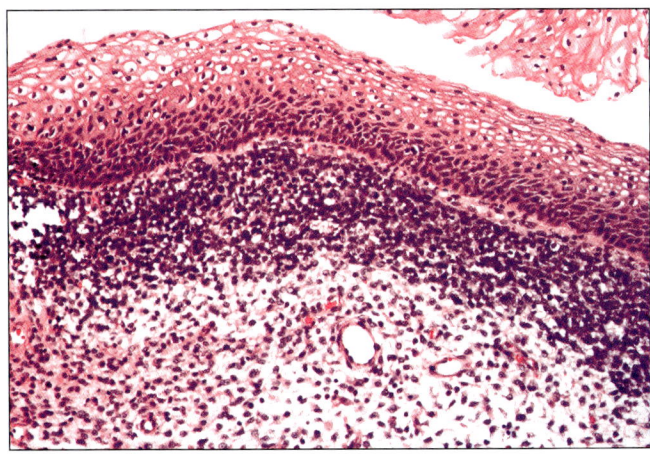

Fig. 11.21 Embryonal rhabdomyosarcoma, with prominent cambium layer.

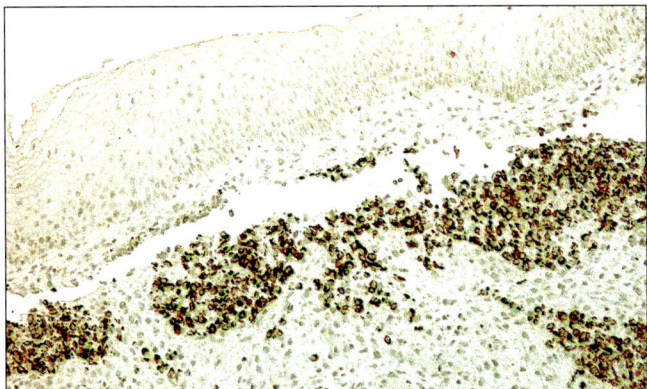

Fig. 11.22 Embryonal rhabdomyosarcoma, cambium layer reactive for desmin.

EMBRYONAL RHABDOMYOSARCOMA

Primary embryonal rhabdomyosarcomas (sarcoma botryoides) arising from the uterine cervix are rare.[66] They mostly affect young women aged 12–26 years (average, 18 years). Exceptional cases in women of up to 45 years are known. The most common symptom is vaginal bleeding. In some cases, a mass protrudes through the introitus or the tumor is detected during a routine gynecologic examination. The tumors are polypoid and 2–10 cm in size. Microscopically, they have a 'cambium layer' represented by a subepithelial condensation of tumor cells (Figure 11.21). The neoplastic cells vary in appearance, ranging from small cells to cells with definitive rhabdomyoblastic differentiation.[89] The neoplastic cells are reactive for desmin, myo-D1, and myogenin (Figure 11.22). With treatment, the overall survival rate nears 80%.[10]

LEIOMYOSARCOMA

These equally rare tumors tend to occur in perimenopausal patients, with an average age of 46 years; the most common presenting symptom is vaginal bleeding.[45] In addition to the spindle cell type, epithelioid, myxoid, and xanthomatous variants have been described.[30,37,45,84] The diagnostic criteria are identical to those for the uterine body. Two of the three following features must be present to make such diagnosis: diffuse moderate to severe atypia (i.e., readily appreciable at low power), coagulative tumor cell necrosis, and a mitotic rate of at least 10 mitoses per 10 HPFs.[11]

PECOMA

A few cases of perivascular epithelioid cell neoplasm (PEComa), a mesenchymal tumor composed of perivascular epithelioid cells that coexpress melanocytic and muscle markers, have been reported in the cervix. The typical histologic features of these tumors include the presence of epithelioid cells intermixed or not with spindled cells, arranged in a fascicular, nested or sheet-like pattern, and a prominent intrinsic vasculature that ranges from delicate, arborizing capillaries to thick, small arteries. The nuclear grade is variable. The mitotic index is low (<1 mitosis per 50 HPFs). The patients are aged 28–48 years, and the tumors generally are 2–3 cm in size. One of the three reported cases has been related to the tuberous sclerosis complex. In this case, aggregates of HBM-45 reactive perivascular epithelioid cells were also present in the myometrium, small bowel, and ovarian hilus. Immunohistochemically these tumors react for smooth muscle actin and at least one melanocytic marker, HMB45 being the most sensitive marker. Melan-A and Mitf (microphthalmia-associated transcription factor) are the next most sensitive markers. The patients showed no evidence of recurrent disease after 3 years of follow-up.[26,29]

ADENOSARCOMA

Definition

Tumors characterized by a benign neoplastic epithelial component and a malignant mesenchymal component.

General features

Adenosarcomas of the uterine cervix are less common than their counterparts in the uterine corpus.[19,49] The patients are aged 11–67 years (mean age, 36 years) and usually present with abnormal bleeding.[49,52]

Pathology

Tumors are 1.5–20 cm in size and have a polypoid configuration. They are usually solitary but may be multiple.[49,52] Typically, they show relatively bland, occasionally atypical, glandular elements that are intermixed with a low-grade homologous sarcoma. A leaf-like pattern due to growth of the stromal component into dilated glandular spaces and/or the tumor surface is characteristic. Most cases show a distinctive band of stromal hypercellularity immediately subjacent to the epithelium (periglandular cuffing). Features differentiating adenosarcomas from their notionally benign counterparts (adenofibromas) include one or more of the following: a stromal mitotic count of 2 or more mitoses per 10 HPFs, marked stromal cellularity (usually as periglandular cuffing), and more than mild nuclear atypia of the stromal cells.[19] In reality, most diagnostic cases display at least two of these features (Figures 11.23 and 11.24). Usually, the epithelial component is endocervical type with focal squamous metaplasia, although endometrioid or tubal-type epithelia may be seen. In nearly all cases,

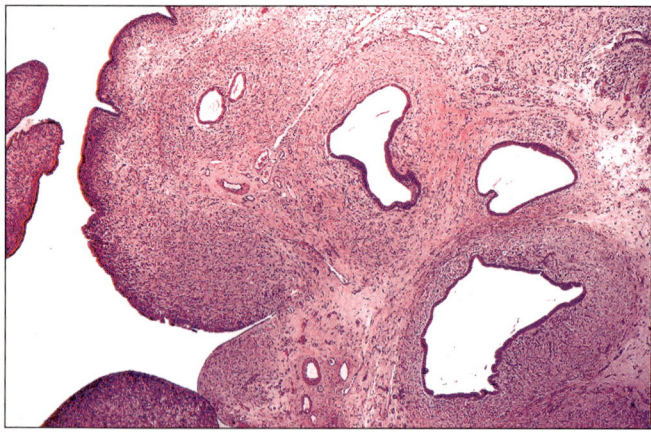

Fig. 11.23 Adenosarcoma with prominent periglandular cuffing.

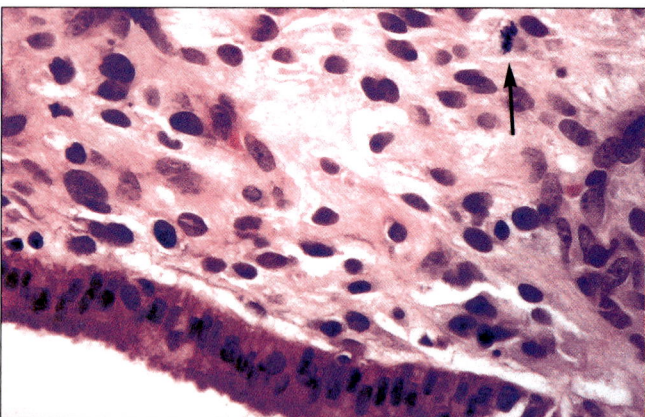

Fig. 11.24 Adenosarcoma with stromal cell atypia and a rare mitotic figure (arrow).

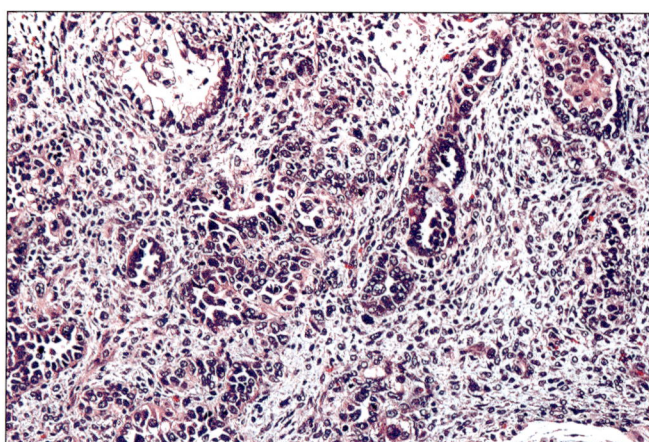

Fig. 11.25 Carcinosarcoma (malignant mixed müllerian tumor).

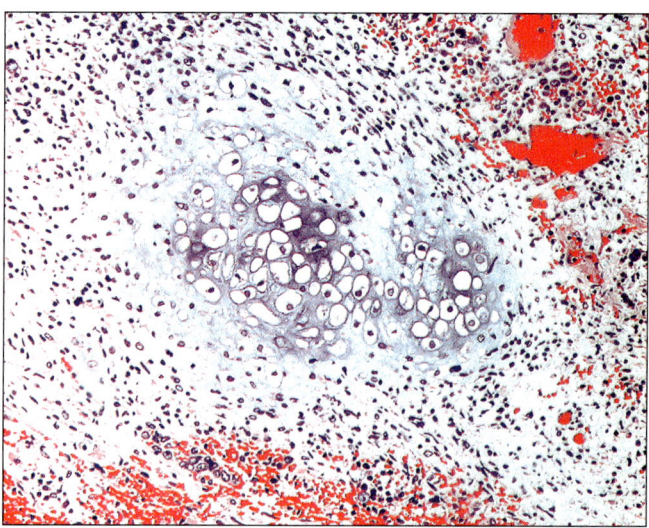

Fig. 11.26 Carcinosarcoma with cartilaginous differentiation.

focal epithelial atypia will be present, showing copious eosinophilic cytoplasm, enlarged nuclei, and irregularly shaped cells. By definition, these features are insufficient to diagnose a malignant epithelial component. The sarcomatous component occasionally will show heterologous elements in the form of striated muscle, cartilage, lipoblasts or bone.[49,52,73] At times, the tumors will show 'sarcomatous overgrowth', defined as exceeding 25% of the tumor volume[19] or having a high-grade as well as low-grade sarcoma.[69]

Differential diagnosis

Adenofibromas are composed of benign epithelium and benign stroma, and lack the stromal cytologic atypia, hypercellularity or requisite mitotic activity in the stroma. As discussed in Chapter 17, many pathologists, including some of the editors, doubt adenofibromas exist or can be diagnosed, because some adenosarcomas may appear histologically so well differentiated, and yet may act clinically aggressively. We recommend a very low threshold for adenosarcomas when any pathologic doubt exists or there is a clinical history of 'recurrent polyps'.

Endocervical polyps usually lack the leaf-like pattern and the microscopic features that allow the diagnosis of adenosarcoma.

Malignant mixed müllerian tumors have a malignant epithelial component in addition to the sarcomatous component.

Embryonal rhabdomyosarcomas have a characteristic hypercellular layer of tumor cells beneath the covering epithelium (so-called cambium layer), not dissimilar to adenosarcomas, but this fades quickly into looser mesenchyme containing small, dark, mitotically active cells with focally demonstrable cross-striations, and lack the distinct leaf-like pattern so commonly seen in adenosarcomas. Reactivity with myxoid markers (myogenin and Myo-D1) is universal.

Prognosis

In general, the prognosis for adenosarcomas is good, with a low incidence of recurrences and metastases.[49] Tumors with sarcomatous overgrowth have a more aggressive course.[69]

CARCINOSARCOMA (MALIGNANT MIXED MÜLLERIAN TUMOR)

These tumors, by definition, consist of malignant epithelial and malignant stromal components (Figures 11.25 and 11.26) and occur infrequently in the uterine cervix.[41] Most patients are elderly (mean age, 60 years),[20,41,78] but the tumor may be seen in children and the very old.[78] HPV 16 has been found in a few cases.[41] The most common symptoms at presentation are vaginal bleeding or spotting, with an occasional asymptomatic case being detected by a cervical smear. Tumors generally are polypoid and range in size from 1 to 10 cm. Microscopically, the epithelial component may be an endometrioid adenocarcinoma, squamous carcinoma, basaloid squamous carcinoma, adenoid cystic carcinoma or adenoid basal carcinoma, while the mesenchymal component may be homologous (fibrosarcoma, endometrial stromal sarcoma, high-grade spindle cell sarcoma) or heterologous (rhabdomyosarcoma, chondrosarcoma). The differential diagnosis includes adenosarcoma, as discussed above, and sarcomatoid carcinoma. Most cases present with FIGO stage 1 disease.[20,78] Although the experience with cervical carcinosarcomas is limited, the prognosis seems better than that for the counterparts arising in the uterine corpus.[20,78]

MALIGNANT MELANOMA

Malignant melanomas arising in the cervix are exceptionally rare.[24] While the age range is wide (19–78 years), most women are postmenopausal.[17] The most common symptom is vaginal bleeding. Occasional tumors are detected during routine clinical examination by a cervical smear or the discovery of a distant metastasis.[14,17]

Pathology
The tumors are usually polypoid and red, brown, gray, black or blue. Frequently, they are ulcerated. About 25% of cases are amelanotic. The neoplastic cells are routinely epithelioid or spindle (Figure 11.27). Intranuclear inclusions and multinucleated tumor giant cells may be seen. Occasional variants include desmoplastic melanoma[48] and a clear cell type with polygonal cells containing glycogen and mimicking clear cell carcinoma.[31]

Immunohistochemically, the neoplastic cells are always reactive for either S-100 protein or HMB45, and usually for both.[17,48,55] Criteria that substantiate the primary origin in the cervix include the presence of a junctional component (Figure 11.28), the presence of melanosis in the squamous or glandular epithelium, and the absence of a primary or regressed mela-

noma elsewhere, especially the skin, uveal tract, and other mucosal sites.[17] Most cases of melanoma present with FIGO stage 1 or 2 disease. These tumors are aggressive; the 5-year survival rates for stage 1, 2, and 3/4 cases are 25%, 14%, and 0%, respectively. The overall mean survival rate for all cervical melanomas is 2.4 years.[17]

LYMPHOMA AND LEUKEMIA

Definition
These are malignant lymphoproliferative or hematopoietic tumors that arise in the cervix or are metastatic to it.

GENERAL FEATURES

Most cases of lymphoma or leukemia involving the uterine cervix represent a manifestation of widespread disease. Most lymphomas primary in the cervix are of the diffuse large B-cell type; the next most common type is follicular lymphoma.[8,53,86] Much more rare are cases of mantle cell lymphoma, Burkitt lymphoma, natural killer (NK)/T-cell lymphoma of the nasal type, peripheral T-cell lymphoma and Hodgkin lymphoma.[53,57,64,72,86] Although occurring over a wide age range (20–80 years), cervical lymphomas are predominantly seen in premenopausal women (median age, 41 years). Bleeding is the most common symptom, although occasionally atypical lymphoid cells on a routine cervical smear have led to detection.[57]

Macroscopic features
The cervix is typically diffusely enlarged and barrel shaped[57] (Figure 11.29), and often appears as a polyp or cervical mass. Only rarely is the mucosa abnormal due to tumor ulceration. The tumor cut surface is usually fleshy, rubbery or firm, and homogeneous or white to tan (Figure 11.30). Focal necrosis or hemorrhage may be seen. Granulocytic sarcomas may give a green color when freshly cut, giving rise to the term 'chloroma'.

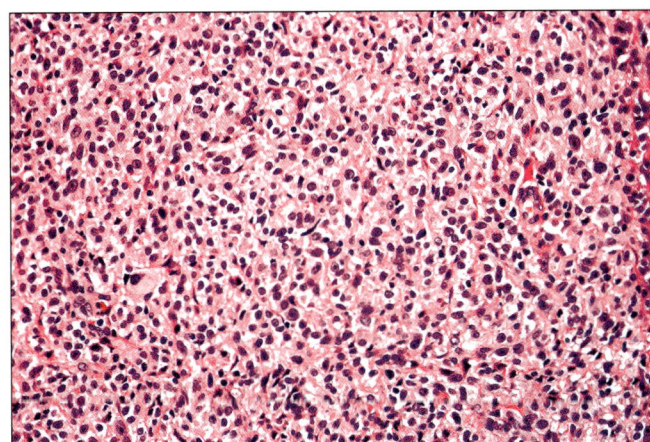

Fig. 11.27 Malignant melanoma, epithelioid cells.

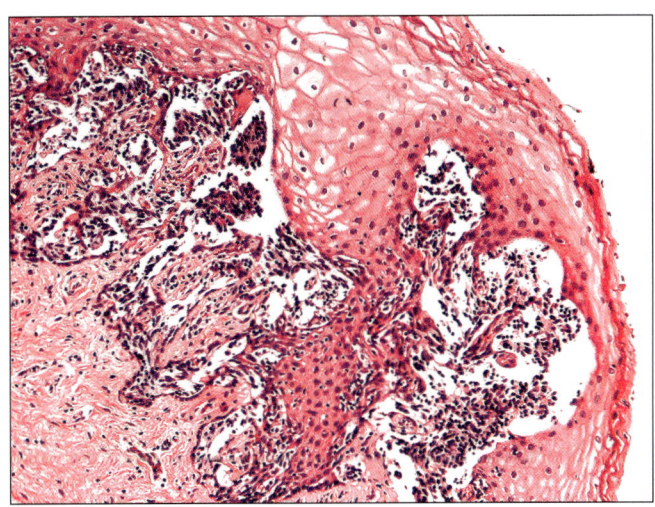

Fig. 11.28 Malignant melanoma, junctional component.

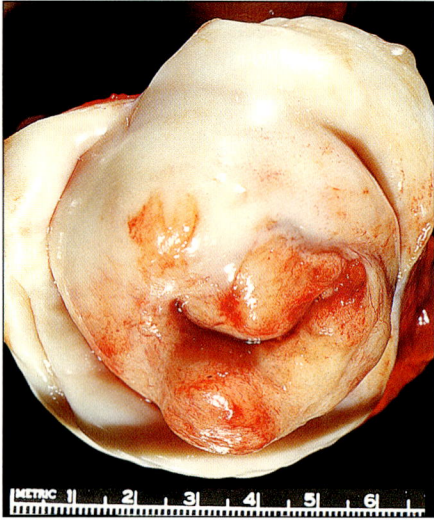

Fig. 11.29 Lymphoma. A rubbery, fleshy mass diffusely enlarges the cervix.

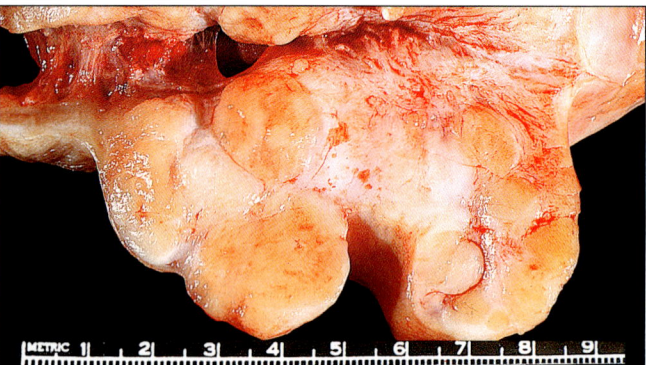

Fig. 11.30 Lymphoma. The tumor, cut in cross-section, is fleshy and rubbery without necrosis.

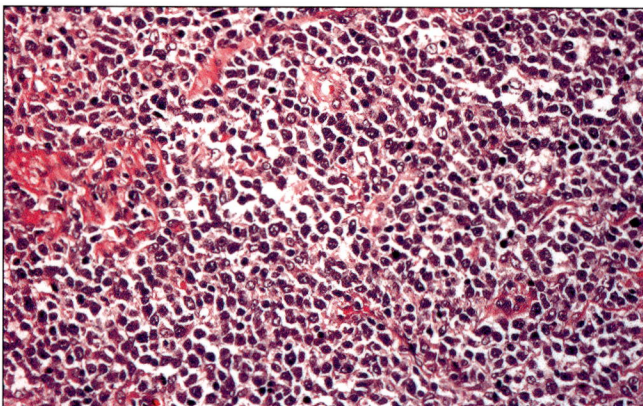

Fig. 11.31 Diffuse large B-cell lymphoma.

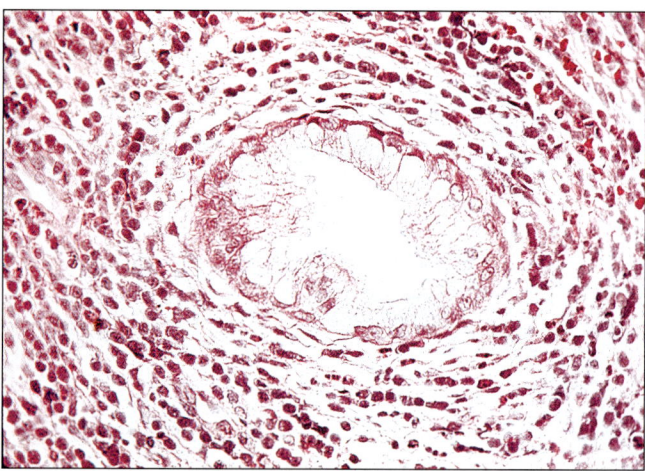

Fig. 11.32 Lymphoma. The tumor infiltrates about, but does not replace or destroy the endocervical glands.

Microscopic features

Most cases extend deep into the wall. In diffuse large B-cell lymphomas, neoplastic cells separate or surround endocervical glands without destroying the endocervical or squamous epithelium. Often, collagenous stroma separates the tumor from the ectocervical epithelium. The neoplastic cells are moderate to large, mostly rounded, with slightly pleomorphic nuclei, with vesicular chromatin, small nucleoli, and numerous mitoses (Figures 11.31 and 11.32). Follicular lymphomas tend to infiltrate along the blood vessels walls at the periphery of the tumor.[57]

Immunohistochemical studies

- A screening panel consisting of CD3, CD20, CD45, and keratin is useful to ascertain whether the tumor is a B-cell lymphoma (CD20+) (Figure 11.33), T-cell lymphoma (CD3+), granulocytic sarcoma (only CD45+), or carcinoma (keratin+).
- In lymphomas composed of small cells, a panel consisting of CD5, CD10, cyclin D1, CD23, bcl-2, and bcl-6 helps to differentiate between a follicular lymphoma (CD10+, bcl-6+, bcl-2+) and follicular hyperplasia (bcl-2−), or chronic lymphocytic leukemia/small lymphocytic lymphoma (CD5+, CD23−, cyclin D1+).

- For B-cell proliferations with large or intermediate cells or blasts, reactivity for CD10, CD79a, cyclin D1, bcl-6, Ki-67, T-cell lymphoblastic lymphoma (TdT), Epstein–Barr virus–latent membrane protein (EBV–LMP), and EBNA2 suggests precursor B-acute lymphoblastic lymphoma (CD79a+, CD10±, TdT±), diffuse large B-cell lymphoma (CD10±, bcl-6±, Ki-67 reactivity in <90% of nuclei), blastic variant of mantle cell lymphoma (cyclin D1+), and Burkitts lymphoma (CD10+, TdT−, Ki-67 reactivity in >99% of nuclei).
- CD15 and CD30 are necessary to confirm the diagnosis of classic Hodgkins lymphoma and CD57 for the lymphocyte-predominant variant.
- The uncommon NK/T-cell neoplasms are better defined with antibodies to CD30 and ALK1 (anaplastic large cell lymphoma), CD1a and TdT, and TIA-1 and EBV antigens (cytotoxic T-cells and nasal-type NK cell tumors).
- To diagnose granulocytic sarcoma, testing with myeloperoxidase, CD4, CD68, and CD117 is required.[57]

Prognosis

The 5-year survival for patients with primary diffuse large B-cell lymphoma of the uterine cervix generally falls in a range of 67–100%.[86] In one series, the 5-year survival was zero.[86]

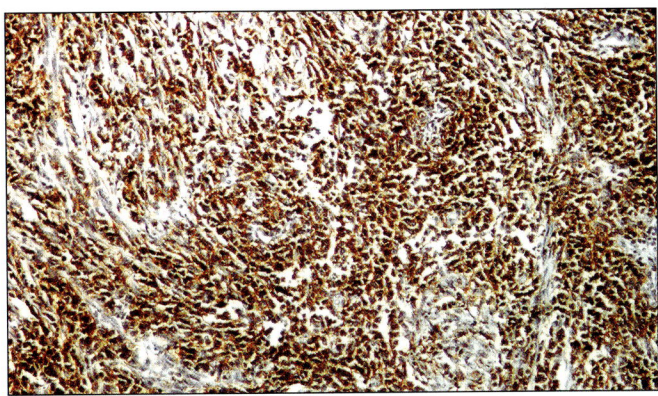

Fig. 11.33 Diffuse large B-cell lymphoma, reactive for CD20.

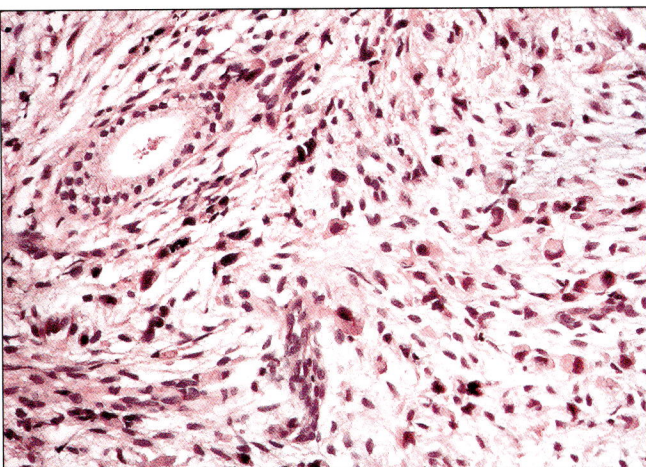

Fig. 11.34 Metastatic gastric carcinoma with signet-ring cell features.

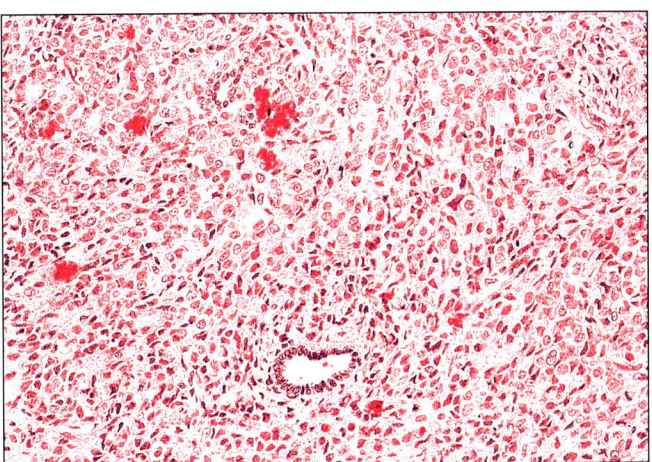

Fig. 11.35 Metastatic gastric carcinoma, tumor diffusely permeates the wall and insinuates about and among endocervical glands without displacing or destroying the glands.

Differential diagnosis

Patients with a lymphoma-like lesion tend to be in the fourth decade of life, and experience bleeding and pelvic pain. Although a cervical mass is usually absent, erosion, erythema, bleeding at touch, nodularity, or a friable exophytic growth may be seen. Some patients have had the Epstein–Barr virus.[42] Commonly, the infiltrate is superficial, rarely extending deeper than the endocervical glands. The infiltrate may be diffuse or nodular and contains a mixture of mature lymphocytes, polyclonal plasma cells, and polymorphonuclear cells with numerous mitoses. Immunohistochemically, B-cells predominate and the plasma cells exhibit polyclonality. Rare cases have monoclonal B-cells by polymerase chain reaction. Since it is necessary to demonstrate the presence of deep invasion, a cervical cone may be required for diagnosis.[57]

Poorly differentiated carcinomas and neuroendocrine carcinomas are differentiated from lymphomas and leukemias by reactivity for keratin and neuroendocrine markers such as CD56, synaptophysin, and chromogranin.

Primitive neuroectodermal tumors (PNET) may cause diagnostic difficulties and attention to features such as the presence of fibrillary material and rosettes, as well as the use of immunomarkers such as synaptophysin and neurofilaments help facilitate the diagnosis. CD99 is not specific for PNET as it may often be detected in lymphoblastic lymphomas.[57]

METASTATIC TUMORS TO THE CERVIX

Secondary involvement of the uterine cervix is commonly seen as a result of contiguous spread from carcinoma arising in the endometrium.[21] Metastases to the uterine cervix are infrequent, representing 1.5% of the cases in a large series of metastatic tumors to the female genital tract.[58,62] In decreasing order of frequency, the primary sites of these metastatic tumors are: ovaries, large bowel, stomach, breasts, and kidneys.[58] Occasionally, tumors arising in the lungs, pancreaticobiliary tract, and fallopian tubes, as well as appendiceal carcinoids or melanomas may metastasize to the cervix.[32,58] Bizarrely, peritoneal mesothelioma may also secondarily involve the cervix.[21]

Metastases to the cervix are usually detected after the primary tumor has been diagnosed; however, they may represent the initial presentation of disease. In certain cases, the disease is discovered after an abnormal Pap smear.[58,60,85] Histologic and cytologic features that raise the possibility of a metastatic tumor include extensive signet-ring cell formation (Figure 11.34), a permeative growth pattern (Figure 11.35), the presence of an 'Indian single cell file' arrangement, a lack of an associated *in situ* component, an unusually prominent lymphovascular involvement, multifocality and, in specific instances, the presence of a papillary serous carcinoma pattern.[21,60] In addition, reactivity for CK7, CEA, gross cystic disease fluid protein-15 (GCDFP-15), and TTF-1, and non-reactivity for p16, support the diagnosis of metastatic disease.

REFERENCES

1. Abeler VM, Holm R, Nesland JM, Kjorstad KE. Small cell carcinoma of the cervix. A clinicopathologic study of 26 patients. Cancer 1994;73:672–7.
2. Albores-Saavedra J, Manivel C, Mora A, et al. The solid variant of adenoid cystic carcinoma of the cervix. Int J Gynecol Pathol 1992;11:2–10.
3. Albores-Saavedra J, Latif S, Carrick KS, et al. CD56 reactivity in small-cell carcinoma of the uterine cervix. Int J Gynecol Pathol 2005;24:113–17.

4. Albores-Saavedra J, Gersell D, Gilks GB, et al. Terminology of endocrine tumors of the uterine cervix: results of a workshop sponsored by the College of American Pathologists and the National Cancer Institute. Arch Pathol Lab Med 1997;121:34–9.

5. Alfsen GC, Kristensen GB, Skovlund E, et al. Histologic subtype has minor importance for overall survival in patients with adenocarcinoma of the uterine cervix: a population-based study of prognostic factors in 505 patients with non-squamous cell carcinomas of the cervix. Cancer 2001;92:2471–83.

6. Ambros RA, Park JS, Shah KV, Kurman RJ. Evaluation of histologic, morphometric, and immunohistochemical criteria in the differential diagnosis of small-cell carcinomas of the cervix with particular reference to human papillomavirus types 16 and 18. Mod Pathol 1991;4:586–93. Erratum in Mod Pathol 5:40.

7. Atlas I, Gajewski W, Falkenberry S, et al. Absence of estrogen and progesterone receptors in glassy cell carcinoma of the cervix. Obstet Gynecol 1988;91:136–8.

8. Au WY, Chan BCP, Chung LP, Choy C. Primary B-cell lymphoma and lymphoma-like lesions of the uterine cervix. Am J Hematol 2003;73:176–9.

9. Bagué S, Rodríguez IM, Prat J. Malignant mesonephric tumors of the female genital tract. A clinicopathologic study of 9 cases. Am J Surg Pathol 2004;28:601–7.

10. Behtash N, Mousavi A, Tehranian A, et al. Embryonal rhabdomyosarcoma of the uterine cervix: case report and review of the literature. Gynecol Oncol 2003;91:452–5.

11. Bell SW, Kempson RL, Hendrickson MR. Problematic uterine smooth muscle neoplasms: a clinicopathologic study of 213 cases. Am J Surg Pathol 1994;18:535–58.

12. Boarman CH, Webb MJ, Jefferies JA. Low grade endometrial stromal sarcoma of the ectocervix after therapy for breast cancer. Gynecol Oncol 2000;79:120–3.

13. Brainard JA, Hart WR. Adenoid basal epitheliomas of the uterine cervix. A reevaluation of distinctive cervical basaloid lesions currently classified as adenoid basal cell carcinoma and adenoid basal cell hyperplasia. Am J Surg Pathol 1998;22:965–75.

14. Cantuaria G, Angioli R, Nahmias J, et al. Primary malignant melanoma of the uterine cervix. Gynecol Oncol 1999;75:170–4.

15. Carcangiu ML. Tumours of the uterine cervix. Mesenchymal tumours. In: Tavassoli FA, Devilee P, eds. World Health Organization Classification of Tumours: Tumours of the Breast and Female Genital Organs. Lyon: IARC Press; 2003:280–3.

16. Chang KL, Crabtree GS, Lim-Tan SK, et al. Primary uterine endometrial stromal neoplasms. A clinicopathologic study of 117 cases. Am J Surg Pathol 1990;14:415–38.

17. Clark K, Butz WR, Hapke MR. Primary malignant melanoma of the uterine cervix: a case report with world literature. Int J Gynecol Pathol 1999;18:265–73.

18. Clement PB, Young RH, Keh P, et al. Malignant mesonephric neoplasms of the uterine cervix: a report of eight cases, including four with a malignant spindle cell component. Am J Surg Pathol 1995;19:1158–71.

19. Clement PB, Scully RE. Mullerian adenosarcoma of the uterus: a clinicopathologic analysis of 100 cases with a review of the literature. Hum Pathol 1990;21:363–81.

20. Clement PB, Zubovits JT, Young RH, Scully RE. Malignant mullerian tumors of the uterine cervix: a report of nine cases of a neoplasm with morphology often different from its counterpart in the corpus. Int J Gynecol Pathol 1998;17:211–22.

21. Clement PB. Miscellaneous primary tumors and metastatic tumors of the uterine cervix. Semin Diagn Pathol 1990;7:228–48.

22. Conner MG, Richter H, Moran CA, et al. Small cell carcinoma of the cervix: a clinicopathologic and immunohistochemical study of 23 cases. Ann Diagn Pathol 2002;6:345–8.

23. Costa MJ, Kenny MB, Hewan-Lowe K, Judd R. Glassy cell features in adenosquamous carcinoma of the uterine cervix. Histologic, ultrastructural, immunohistochemical, and clinical findings. Am J Clin Pathol 1991;96:520–8.

24. De Matos P, Tyler D, Seigler HE. Mucosal melanoma of the female genitalia: a clinicopathologic study of forty-three cases at Duke University Medical Center. Surgery 1998;124:38–48.

25. Emerich J, Senkus E, Konefka T. Alveolar rhabdomyosarcoma of the uterine cervix. A case report. Gynecol Oncol 1996;63:398–403.

26. Fadare O, Parkash V, Yilmaz Y, et al. Perivascular epithelioid cell tumor (PEComa) of the uterine cervix associated with intraabdominal 'PEComatosis': a clinicopathologic study with comparative genomic hybridization analysis. World J Surg Oncol 2004;2:35.

27. Ferry JA, Scully RE. Mesonephric remnants, hyperplasia, and neoplasia in the uterine cervix: a study of 49 cases. Am J Surg Pathol 1990;14:1100–11.

28. Ferry JA, Scully RE. 'Adenoid cystic' carcinoma and adenoid basal carcinoma of the uterine cervix. A study of 28 cases. Am J Surg Pathol 1988;12:134–44.

29. Folpe AL, Mentzel T, Lehr HA, et al. Perivascular epithelioid cell neoplasms of soft tissue and gynecological origin. A clinicopathologic study of 26 cases and review of the literature. Am J Surg Pathol 2005;29:1558–75.

30. Fraga M, Prieto O, Garcia-Caballero T, et al. Myxoid leiomyosarcoma of the uterine cervix. Histopathology 1994;25:381–4.

31. Furuya M, Shimizu M, Nishihara H, et al. Clear cell variant of malignant melanoma of the uterine cervix: a case report and review of the literature. Gynecol Oncol 2001;80:409–12.

32. Gerolymatos A, Yannacou N, Bontis N, et al. Primary fallopian tube adenocarcinoma with metastasis to the uterine cervix. A case report. Eur J Gynaec Oncol 1993;6:469–78.

33. Gersell DJ, Mazoujian G, Mutch DG, Rudloff MA. Small-cell undifferentiated carcinoma of the cervix. A clinicopathologic, ultrastructural, and immunocytochemical study of 15 cases. Am J Surg Pathol 1988;12:684–98.

34. Gilks CB, Young RH, Gersell DJ, Clement PB. Large-cell carcinoma of the uterine cervix: a clinicopathologic study of 12 cases. Am J Surg Pathol 1997;21:905–14.

35. Gray HJ, Garcia R, Tamimi HK, et al. Glassy cell carcinoma of the cervix revisited. Gynecol Oncol 2002;85:274–7.

36. Grayson W, Cooper K. A reappraisal of 'basaloid carcinoma' of the cervix, and the differential diagnosis of basaloid cervical neoplasms. Adv Anat Pathol 2002;9:290–300.

37. Grayson W, Fourie J, Tiltman AJ. Xanthomatous leiomyosarcoma of the uterine cervix 1998. Int J Gynecol Pathol 1998;17:89–90.

38. Grayson W, Rhemtula H, Taylor LF, et al. Detection of human papillomavirus in large-cell neuroendocrine carcinoma of the uterine cervix: a study of 12 cases. J Clin Pathol 2002;55:108–14.

39. Grayson W, Taylor L, Cooper K. Detection of integrated high-risk human papilloma virus in adenoid cystic carcinoma of the uterine cervix. J Clin Pathol 1996;49:805–9.

40. Grayson W, Taylor LF, Cooper K. Adenoid cystic and adenoid basal carcinoma of the uterine cervix. Comparative morphologic, mucin, and immunohistochemical profile of two rare neoplasms of putative 'reserve cell origin'. Am J Surg Pathol 1999;23:448–58.

41. Grayson W, Taylor LF, Cooper K. Carcinosarcoma of the uterine cervix. A report of eight cases with immunohistochemical analysis and evaluation of human papillomavirus status. Am J Surg Pathol 2001;25:338–47.

42. Hachisuga T, Ookuma Y, Fukuda K, et al. Detection of Epstein–Barr virus DNA from a lymphoma-like lesion of the uterine cervix. Gynecol Oncol 1992;46:289–99.

43. Hart WR. Special types of adenocarcinoma of the uterine cervix. Int J Gynecol Pathol 2002;21:327–46.

44. Hopkins MP, Morley GW. Glassy cell carcinoma of the uterine cervix. Am J Obstet Gynecol 2004;190:67–70.

45. Irvin W, Presley A, Andersen W, Taylor P, Rice L. Leiomyosarcoma of the cervix. Gynecol Oncol 2003;91:636–42.

46. Ishibashi-Ueda H, Imakita M, Yutani C, et al. Small-cell carcinoma of the uterine cervix with syndrome of inappropriate anti-diuretic hormone secretion. Mod Pathol 1996;9:397–400.

47. Ishida GM, Kato N, Hayasaka T, et al. Small-cell neuroendocrine carcinomas of the uterine cervix: a histological, immunohistochemical, and molecular genetic study. Int J Gynecol Pathol 2004;23:366–72.

48. Ishikura H, Kojo T, Ichimura H, Yoshiki T. Desmoplastic malignant melanoma of the uterine cervix. Histopathology 1998;33:93–4.

49. Jones MW, Lefkowitz M. Adenosarcoma of the uterine cervix: a clinicopathologic study of 12 cases. Int J Gynecol Pathol 1995;14:223–9.

50. Kato N, Katayama Y, Kaimori M, Motoyama T. Glassy cell carcinoma of the uterine cervix: histochemical, immunohistochemical, and molecular genetic observations. Int J Gynecol Pathol 2002;21:134–40.

51. Kenny MB, Unger ER, Chenggis ML, et al. In situ hybridization for human papillomavirus DNA in uterine adenosquamous carcinoma with glassy cell features ('glassy cell carcinoma'). Am J Clin Pathol 1992;98:180–7.

52. Kerner H, Lichtig C. Mullerian adenosarcoma presenting as cervical polyps: a report of seven cases and review of the literature. Obstet Gynecol 1993;81:655–9.

53. Kosari F, Daneshbod Y, Parwaresch R, et al. Lymphoma of the female genital tract. A study of 186 cases and review of the literature. Am J Surg Pathol 2005;29:1512–20.

54. Koyfman SA, Abidi A, Ravichandran P, et al. Adenoid cystic carcinoma of the cervix. Gynecol Oncol 2005;99:477–80.

55. Kristiansen SB, Anderson R, Cohen DM. Primary malignant melanoma of the cervix and review of the literature. Gynecol Oncol 1992;47:398–403.

56. Krivak TC, McBroom JW, Sundborg MJ, et al. Large-cell neuroendocrine carcinoma: a report of two cases and review of the literature. Gynecol Oncol 2001;82:187–91.

57. Lagoo AS, Robboy SJ. Lymphoma of the genital tract. Int J Gynecol Pathol 2006;25:1–21.

58. Lemoine NR, Hall PA. Epithelial tumors metastatic to the uterine cervix. A study of 33 cases and review of the literature. Cancer 1986;57:2002–5.

59. Mannion C, Park WS, Man YG, et al. Endocrine tumors of the cervix. Morphologic assessment, expression of human papilloma virus, and evaluation for loss of heterozygosity on 1p, 3p, 11q, and 17p. Cancer 1998;83:1391–400.

60. Martinez-Roman S, Frumovitz M, Deavers MT, Ramirez P. Metastatic carcinoma of the gallbladder mimicking advanced cervical carcinoma. Gynecol Oncol 2005;97:942–5.

61. Matthews-Greer J, Dominguez-Malagon H, Herrera GA, et al. Human papillomavirus typing of rare cervical carcinomas. Arch Pathol Lab Med 2004;128:554–6.

62. Mazur MT, Hsueh S, Gersell DJ. Metastases to the female genital tract: analysis of 325 cases. Cancer 1984;63:593–6.

62a. McCluggage WG. Immunohistochemistry as a diagnostic aid in cervical pathology. Pathology 2007;39:97–111.

63. McCusker ME, Cote TR, Clegg LX, Tavassoli FA. Endocrine tumors of the uterine cervix: incidence, demographics, and survival with comparison to squamous cell carcinoma. Gynecol Oncol 2003;88:333–9.

64. Mhawech P, Medeiros LJ, Bueso-Ramos C, et al. Natural killer-cell lymphoma involving the gynecologic tract. Arch Pathol Lab Med 2000;124:1510–13.

65. Mikami M, Ezawa S, Sakaiya N, et al. Response of glassy-cell carcinoma of the cervix to cisplatin, epirubicin, and mitomycin C. Lancet 2000;355:1159–60.

66. Miyamoto T, Shiozawa T, Nakamura T, Konishi I. Sarcoma botryoides of the uterine cervix in a 46-year-old woman: case report and review of the literature. Int J Gynecol Pathol 2003;23:78–82.

67. Neilsen GP, Oliva E, Young RH, et al. Alveolar soft-part sarcoma of the female genital tract: a report of nine cases and review of the literature. Int J Gynecol Pathol 1995;14:283–92.

68. Ordi J, Romagosa C, Tavassoli FA, et al. CD10 expression in epithelial tissues and tumors of the gynecological tract: a useful marker in the diagnosis of mesonephric, trophoblastic, and clear cell tumors. Am J Surg Pathol 2001;27:178–86.

69. Park HM, Park MH, Kim YJ, et al. Mullerian adenosarcoma with sarcomatous overgrowth of the cervix presenting as a cervical polyp: a case report and review of the literature. Int J Gynecol Cancer 2004;14:1024–9.

70. Parwani AV, Smith Sehdev AE, Kurman RJ, et al. Cervical adenoid basal tumors comprised of adenoid basal epithelioma associated with various types of invasive carcinoma: clinicopathologic features, human papillomavirus DNA detection, and p16 expression. Hum Pathol 2005;36:82–90.

71. Pirog EC, Kleter B, Olgac S, et al. Prevalence of human papillomavirus DNA in different histological subtypes of cervical adenocarcinoma. Am J Pathol 2000;157:1055–62.

72. Pomares Arias E, Payeras Mas M, Conchillo A, et al. Linfoma difuso de células T de cervix uterino: una localización inusual de un tumor poco frecuente. An Med Interna 2000;17:432–3.

73. Ramos P, Ruiz A, Carabias E, et al. Mullerian adenosarcoma of the cervix with heterologous elements: report of a case and review of the literature. Gynecol Oncol 2002;84:161–6.

74. Rhemtula H, Grayson W, van Iddekingen B, Tiltman A. Large-cell neuroendocrine carcinoma of the uterine cervix. A clinicopathological study of five cases. S Afr Med J 2001;91:525–8.

75. Rodriguez AO, Truskinovsky AM, Kasrazadeh M, Leiserowitz GS. Malignant peripheral nerve sheath tumor of the uterine cervix treated with radical vaginal trachelectomy. Gynecol Oncol 2006;100:201–4.

76. Sato Y, Shimamoto T, Amada S, et al. Large-cell neuroendocrine carcinoma of the uterine cervix: a clinicopathological study of six cases. Int J Gynecol Pathol 2003;22:226–30.

77. Seckl MJ, Mulholland PJ, Bishop AE, et al. Hypoglycemia due to an insulin-secreting small-cell-carcinoma of the cervix. N Engl J Med 1999;341:733–6.

78. Sharma NK, Sorosky JI, Bender D, et al. Malignant mixed mullerian tumor (MMMT) of the cervix. Gynecol Oncol 2005;97:442–5.

79. Shingleton HM, Bell MC, Fregmen A, et al. Is there really a difference in survival of women with squamous cell carcinoma, adenocarcinoma, and adenosquamous carcinoma? Cancer 1995;76:1948–55.

80. Silver SA, Devouassoux-Shisheboran M, Mezzeti TP, Tavassoli FA. Mesonephric adenocarcinomas of the uterine cervix: a study of 11 cases with immunohistochemical findings. Am J Surg Pathol 2001;25:379–87.

81. Stoler MH, Mills SE, Gersell DJ, Walker AN. Small-cell neuroendocrine carcinoma of the cervix. A human papillomavirus type 18 associated cancer. Am J Surg Pathol 1991;5:28–32.

82. Straughn JM, Richter HE, Conner MG, et al. Predictors of outcome in small-cell carcinoma of the cervix – a case series. Gynecol Oncol 2001;83:216–20.

83. Takecuchi K, Murata K, Funaki K, et al. Liposarcoma of the uterine cervix: case report. Eur J Gynaecol Oncol 2000;21:290–1.

84. Toyoshima M, Okamura C, Nikura H, et al. Epithelioid leiomyosarcoma of the uterine cervix: a case report and review of the literature. Gynecol Oncol 2005;97:957–60.

85. Treszezamsky A, Altuna S, Diaz L, et al. Metastases to the uterine cervix from a gastric carcinoma presenting with obstructive renal failure. Int J Gynecol Cancer 2003;13:555–7.

86. Vang R, Medeiros LJ, Ha CS, Deavers M. Non-Hodgkin's lymphoma involving the uterus: a clinicopathologic analysis of 26 cases. Mod Pathol 2000;13:19–28.

87. Viswanathan AN, Deavers MT, Jhingran A, et al. Small-cell neuroendocrine carcinoma of the cervix: outcome and patterns of recurrence. Gynecol Oncol 2004;93:27–33.

88. Wang HL, Lu DW. Over-expression of c-kit protein is an infrequent event in small-cell carcinomas of the uterine cervix. Mod Pathol 2004;17:732–8.

89. Weiss SW, Goldblum JR. Rhabdomyosarcoma. In: Weiss SW, Goldblum JR, eds. Enzinger and Weiss's Soft Tissue Tumors, 4th edn. St Louis: Mosby; 2001:875–35.

90. Wells M, Ostor AG, Crum CP, et al. Tumours of the uterine cervix. Epithelial tumours. In: Tavassoli FA, Devilee P, eds. World Health Organization Classification of Tumours: Tumours of the Breast and Female Genital Organs. Lyon: IARC Press; 2003:260–89.

91. Wistuba II, Thomas B, Behrens C, et al. Molecular abnormalities associated with endocrine tumors of the uterine cervix. Gynecol Oncol 1999;72:3–9.

92. Yazigi R, Sanstad J, Munoz AK, et al. Adenosquamous carcinoma of the cervix: prognosis in stage IB. Obstet Gynecol 1990;75:1012–15.

93. Yun K, Cho NP, Glassford GN. Large-cell neuroendocrine carcinoma of the uterine cervix: a case report of a case with coexisting cervical intraepithelial neoplasia and human papillomavirus 16. Pathology 1999;31:158–61.

The normal endometrium

Rex C. Bentley   George L. Mutter   Stanley J. Robboy

12

NORMAL STRUCTURE OF THE UTERUS

The mature, non-gravid uterus is pear-shaped and about 8–9 cm in length. The cervix accounts for about one-third of its length. The myometrium consists of discrete bundles of smooth muscle fibers, arranged in a basket-weave pattern that is more compact near the endometrium than toward the serosa. The use of magnetic resonance imaging (MRI) has shown the presence of a specialized zone of myometrium situated immediately beneath the endometrium, referred to as the 'junctional zone', which structurally and functionally differs from the outer myometrium.[3] At the level of the internal os, the size and number of the muscle cells diminish, and fibrocollagenous tissue forms a correspondingly larger component of the uterine wall. The outer zone of the corporeal musculature is continuous over the outer cervix and muscular layer of the vagina. The collagenous tissue of the body (corpus uteri) and cervix (cervix uteri) softens during pregnancy, largely by separation of the bundles of fibers into their constituent fibrils. This effect is reproducible in laboratory animals by administering relaxin, a polypeptide obtained from the corpus luteum of pregnancy.

The cavity of the uterine body is flattened anteroposteriorly and shield-shaped when viewed from the front (Figure 12.1). It narrows toward its lower end, the isthmus (also known as the 'lower uterine segment'). The isthmus grows rapidly in the early stages of pregnancy and produces most of the lower segment of the pregnant uterus.

The uterine blood supply comes predominantly from the uterine branch of the internal iliac artery on each side. Each uterine artery anastomoses with the ovarian artery above and with the vaginal artery below. These anastomoses form a sinuous arterial channel along each lateral wall of the uterus within the broad ligament. Branches of this channel penetrate the outer third of the uterine wall and then divide to form the circulus vasculosus at this depth. Arteries radiate inward from this ring to supply the inner myometrium and the endometrium. The veins follow a similar course but are straighter. They are poorly developed in the dense inner third of the myometrium. The arterial vascular plexus in the myometrium can be a very useful anatomic landmark when assessing depth of invasion of endometrial carcinomas. Invasion into the region of the plexus almost always indicates invasion into the outer half of the myometrium.[35]

COMPONENTS OF THE NORMAL ENDOMETRIUM

The mucosal lining of the uterus consists of glands, stroma, and blood vessels. Glandular changes are most easily observed in the common and significant pathologic conditions in the uterus and it is the glands that are viewed, in the main, to determine the activity of the endometrium and its response to the hormonal environment. Much is made, both morphologically and biochemically, of what the glandular epithelial cells secrete. However, if the function of the endometrium, which is to form a receptive site for nidation, is considered, then it becomes apparent that the influence of the glands and their secretions is short lived, having a nutrient effect on the blastocyst only during the 24 hours or so when it is in the uterine cavity before implantation takes place (on or about day 7 postovulation). Once nidation has occurred, the relationship between the conceptus and its mother is the interface between the trophoblast and the decidualized endometrial stroma. Glandular activity plays no further part, and the functional importance of the stroma should not be underestimated.

The endometrium merges with the mucosa of the fallopian tube at its upper extreme and with the endocervical epithelium at its lower end. The junction with the fallopian tube epithelium is usually abrupt, although the exact position may vary considerably. Uncommonly, endometrium may line the tube some centimeters lateral to the cornu (a condition referred to as 'endometrialization' and to be distinguished from endometriosis – see Chapter 20). At the junction of the endometrium with the endocervical epithelium, however, there is a gradual transition from one type of mucosa to the other, sometimes over a distance of as much as 1 cm. This is the lower uterine segment, which contains the isthmic endometrium consisting of glands with features between those of the endometrium proper and the endocervix (Figures 12.2 and 12.3). Not uncommonly endometrial glands will be found deep to the endocervical lining, at this point appearing like a cuff providing an outer lining about an inner shell. Glands of the lower uterine segment show practically none of the morphologic effects that hormonal stimulation elicits in the fundus so that the isthmic component in curettings does not give any indication of hormonal activity. An appreciation of this becomes important when the curettings consist of isthmic endometrium only. Care must be taken to recognize this tissue for what it is, so that the inactivity in these pieces is not taken to mean that the

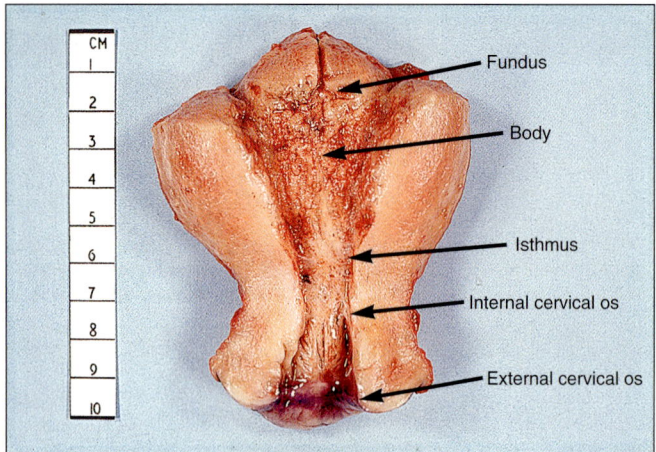

Fig. 12.1 Opened uterus. The landmarks are indicated.

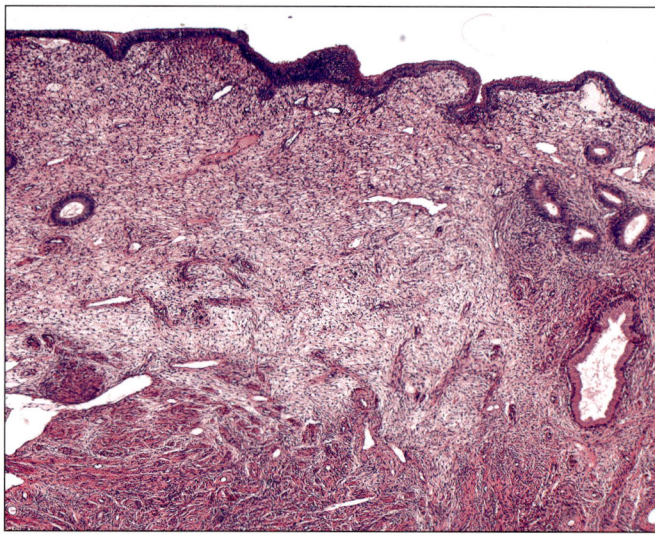

Fig. 12.3 Isthmic endometrium. In a hysterectomy specimen, the isthmic endometrium is seen as a zone of poorly developed glands in fibrous stroma.

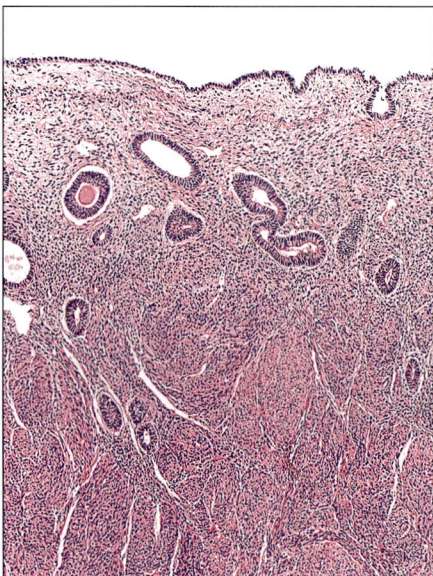

Fig. 12.2 Isthmic endometrium. Appearances in a hysterectomy specimen.

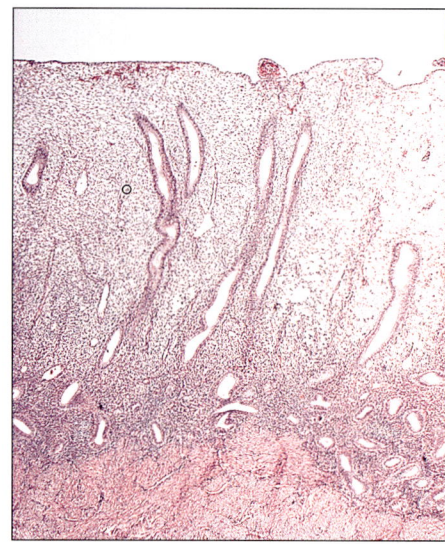

Fig. 12.4 Normal endometrium, low power.

endometrium as a whole is not being stimulated or is not responding. Glands in this area are prone to be partly lined by epithelium containing a mixture of undistinguished columnar cells admixed with ciliated cells – arguably either a form of tubal metaplasia or persistence of the primitive or archetypal tubal epithelium in this region of the uterus. The stroma of the lower uterine segment differs from that of the endometrium proper in being rather more fibrous and displaying cells that are generally more spindled. The glands are typically flattened and slit-like, and the epithelial cells lack mucosubstances.

The endometrium from the uterine body and fundus is generally fairly uniform, with little variation in appearance from one area to another. There is variation, however, depending on the position of the tissue in relation to the surface epithelium and the endometrial–myometrial junction (Figure 12.4). In other words, the functional endometrium is stratified into layers, a stratification that becomes more pronounced as the menstrual cycle progresses (Figure 12.5).

The basal layer (stratum basalis) is adjacent to the myometrium, and consists of tubular glands, occasionally branching, lined by simple to pseudostratified epithelium in a more basophilic, compact stroma (Figures 12.6 and 12.7). The glandular epithelium shows no evidence of secretory activity whatever the phase of the cycle, and there is no or minimal mitotic activity in either glands or stroma. As the overall volume of glands is small compared with that in the functional layer, the stroma is relatively more prominent. The stromal cells also appear more prominent as they are composed of largely spindled nuclei and have inapparent cytoplasm.

The remaining endometrium is the functional zone (stratum functionalis), which is further subdivided into the superficial compact layer (stratum compactum) and the deeper spongy layer (stratum spongiosum). This distinction only becomes striking in the late secretory (postovulatory or luteal) phase (Figure 12.8). At that time the spongy layer consists of glands

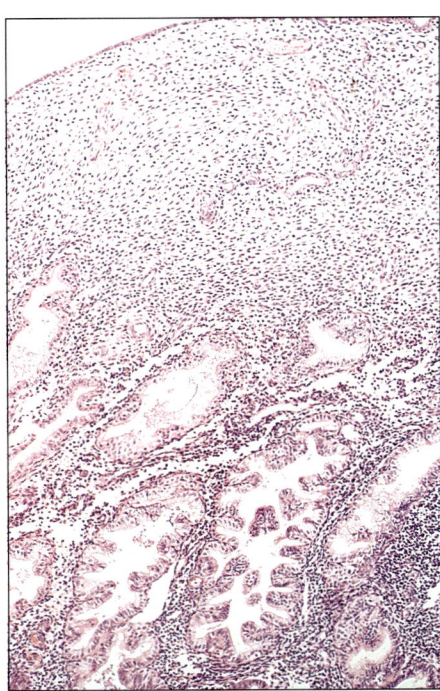

Fig. 12.5   Late secretory phase endometrium (day 28).

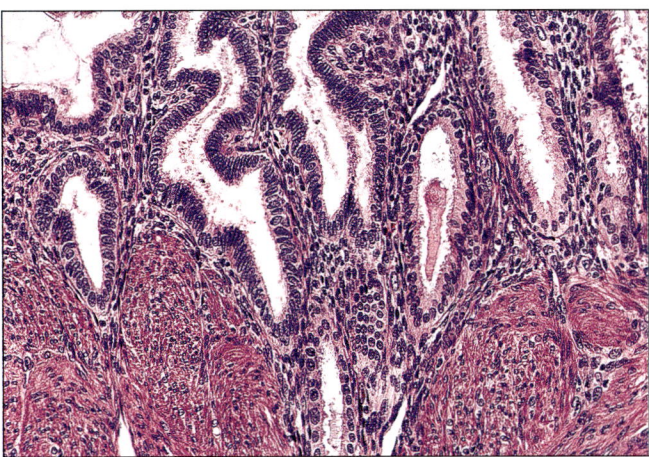

Fig. 12.7   Normal endometrium. Basal zone.

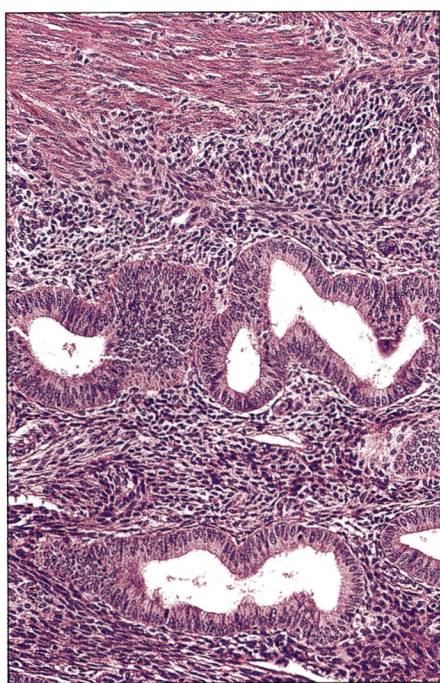

Fig. 12.6   Normal endometrium. Basal zone.

showing maximal secretory activity but a relatively unresponsive stroma that does not develop a good predecidual response apart from the immediate vicinity of the spiral arterioles. Stroma in the more superficial compact layer, on the other hand, responds remarkably to hormonal stimulation with a prominent predecidual reaction and numerous granulated lymphocytes (see below). Glands in this zone are stretched thin by the expanding stroma, and demonstrate less secretory activity. It is apparent therefore that the morphology of the

endometrial stromal and glandular cells is a function not only of the systemic hormonal environment, but also of position in the corpus or lower uterine segment, and vertical location within the endometrial layers. As material from all of these layers routinely appears in curettings, the pathologist must be aware of characteristic appearances at all sites throughout the menstrual cycle.

SURFACE EPITHELIUM

The surface epithelium of the endometrium is continuous with the glandular epithelium and is generally similar (Figure 12.9). However, the constituent cells show less marked cyclic variation than the cells in the glands, responding relatively weakly to circulating sex steroids, and are frequently ciliated. Although subnuclear vacuolation and mitotic activity are seen, these features do not always accurately reflect the time of the cycle. There is usually no problem in identifying surface epithelium in curettings, but the few small epithelial strips that may constitute an entire aspiration sample can be difficult if not impossible to characterize with any degree of certainty.

GLANDULAR CELLS

The endometrial glandular cells are of three types: the secretory cell (Figure 12.10), the ciliated cell (Figure 12.11), and the clear cell (Figure 12.12).

- The secretory cells are by far the most abundant and their morphology varies with the time of the menstrual cycle. The various appearances will be covered when the phases of the cycle are described.
- The ciliated cells are more frequent near the cornua and towards the endocervix as well as being quite common in the surface epithelium. Although a normal constituent of the endometrium, the ciliated cells are particularly under the influence of estrogens and become more prominent in conditions of estrogen excess (e.g. anovulatory cycles). They are usually obvious in estrogen-primed tissue with hyperplasia. As ciliated cells are found so commonly, they must be considered as normal and not as 'ciliated metaplasia' as described elsewhere in the literature.

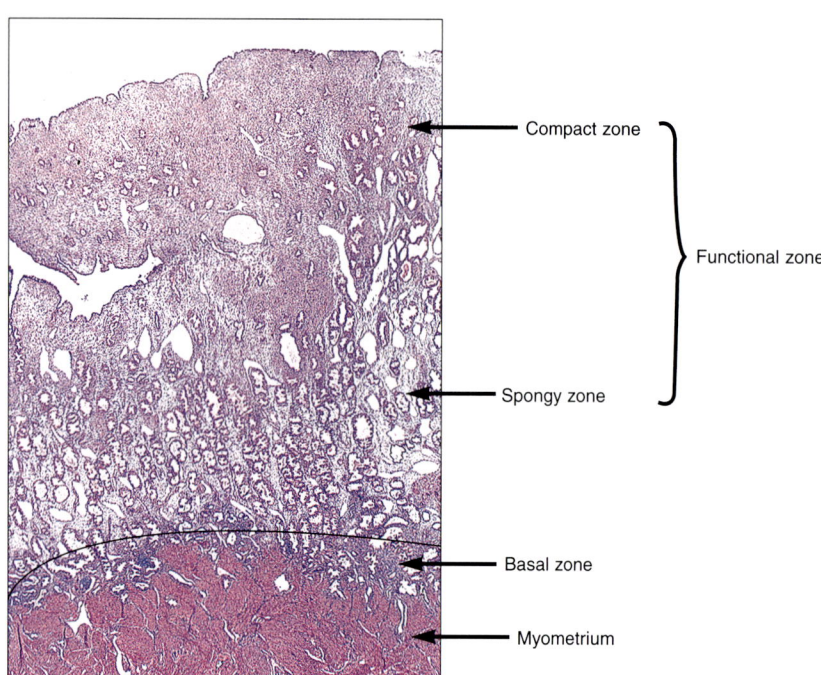

Compact zone

Functional zone

Spongy zone

Basal zone

Myometrium

Fig. 12.8 Late secretory phase endometrium (day 27). The stratification is demonstrated.

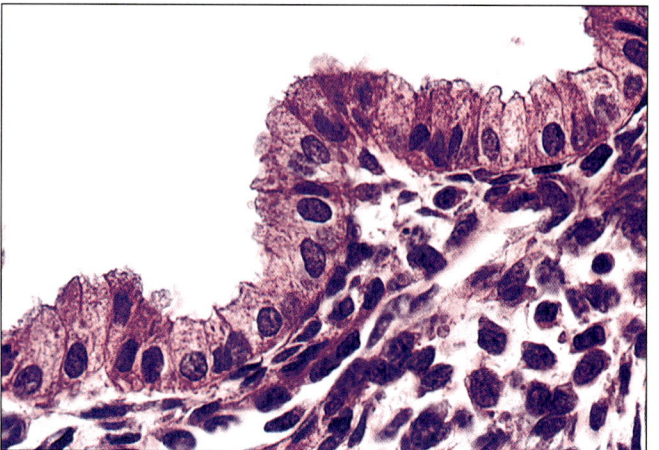

Fig. 12.9 Surface epithelium.

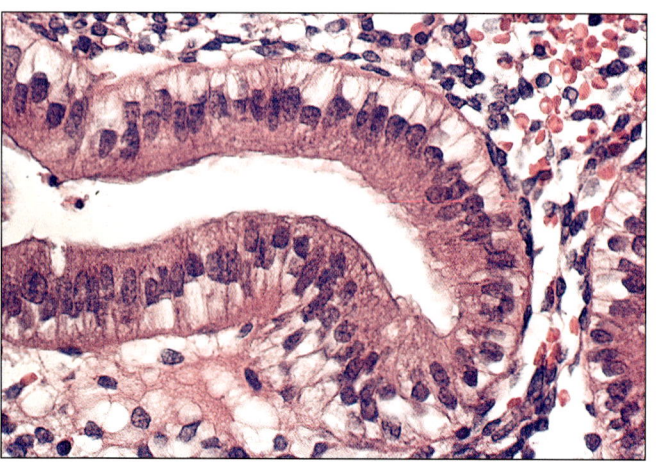

Fig. 12.10 Early secretory phase endometrium (day 17).

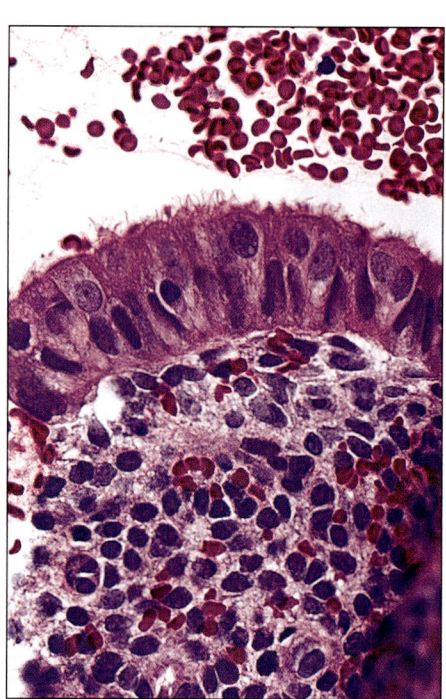

Fig. 12.11 Ciliated epithelium.

Furthermore, in specimens, especially aspirates, where only strips of cells are produced, the presence of cilia is useful to suspect that an estrogenic milieu is present, whether from endogenous or exogenous sources, and that the specimen is not atrophic.

- The clear cells are much less common and are thought to be precursors of the ciliated cells. They are most frequently seen in the proliferative phase and in cystic (benign forms of) hyperplasia.

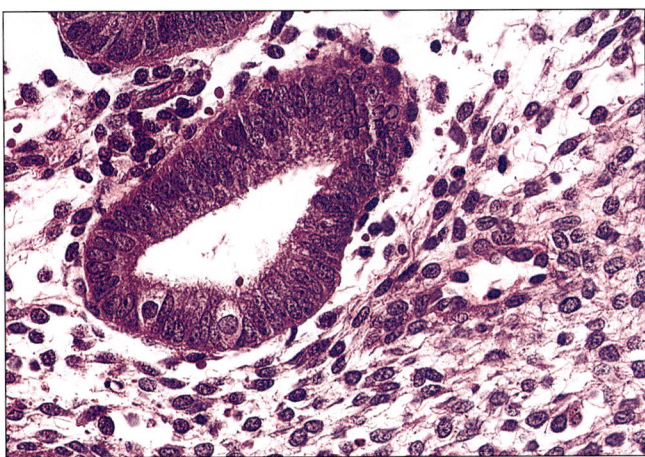

Fig. 12.12 Clear cells in glandular epithelium.

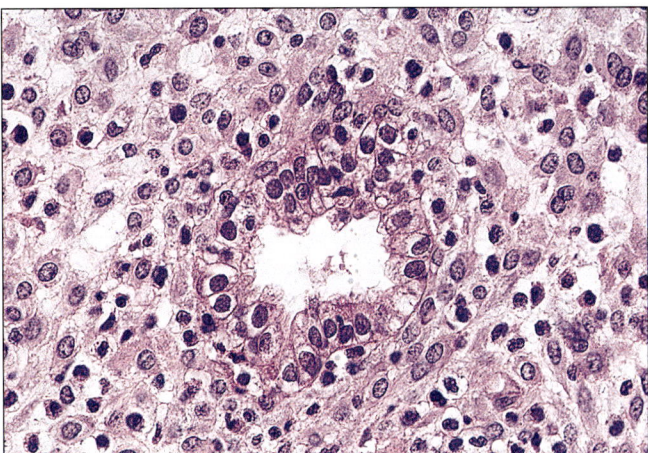

Fig. 12.14 Endometrial stroma. Late secretory phase (day 27), compact layer. The stromal cells show decidual change and have abundant cytoplasm. Granulated lymphocytes are present.

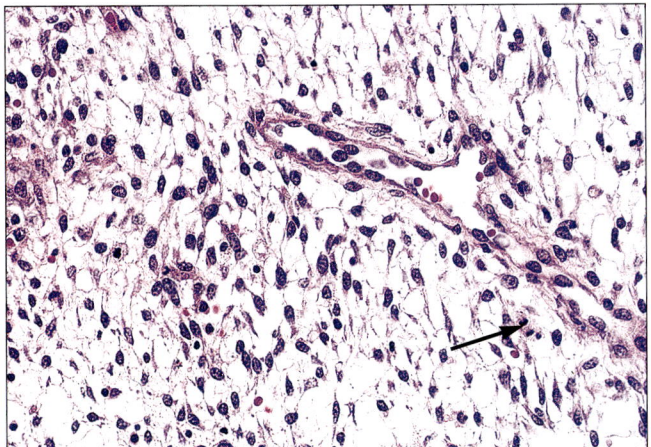

Fig. 12.13 Endometrial stroma. Proliferative phase. Stromal mitotic activity (arrow) is seen. Part of a spiral arteriole is present.

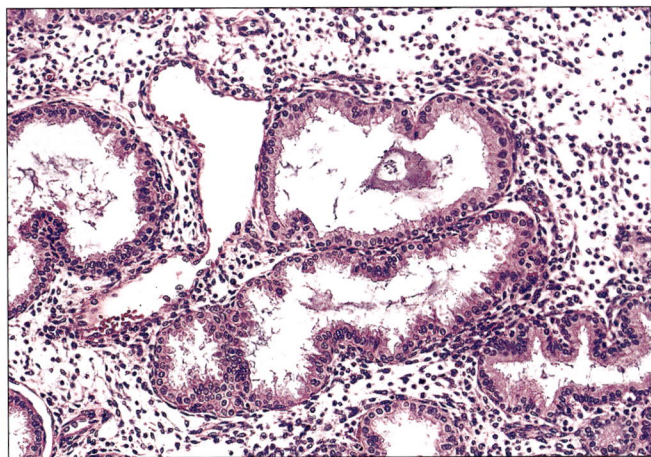

Fig. 12.15 Endometrial stroma. Late secretory phase (day 27), spongy layer. The glands are active but the stromal cells are small with no decidual change.

STROMAL CELLS

The morphology of the endometrial stromal cells varies dramatically throughout the menstrual cycle. During the proliferative phase, the stromal cells are small and mostly compact, with oval, hyperchromatic nuclei and inapparent cytoplasm. In the mid-proliferative phase, at the preovulatory peak of serum estrogen levels, stromal cells are separated by increased intercellular edema. At the end of the proliferative phase the nuclei become slightly larger and their chromatin a little less dense (Figure 12.13). The stroma again becomes edematous in the middle of the secretory phase, reaching a peak at about day 22 of a normalized 28-day cycle (again due to an estrogen peak), after which the cells of the compact zone progressively undergo predecidual change, developing into polygonal cells with vesicular nuclei and abundant, pale cytoplasm with well-defined cell borders (Figure 12.14). The terms 'predecidua' and 'pseudodecidua' are often used to describe this change in the morphology of the stromal cells as a response to endogenous progesterone before implantation and stromal changes that exogenous hormones induce in native endometrium (or at ectopic sites, e.g., peritoneum or fallopian tubes), respectively. The term 'decidua' is reserved for the change seen in pregnancy.

While the semantic value of this distinction is arguable from a medical point of view, the social consequences can be substantial if the change is ascribed to pregnancy when it is not. While the morphologic changes in the cells are qualitatively the same whether they have been brought about by physiologic levels of the hormone in the second half of the cycle or in pregnancy or by synthetic progestins, as in oral contraceptives, there is usually a quantitative difference in both the amount of cytoplasm present in any given cell and in the proportion of stromal cells with the change. In general, decidual change is extensive and uniform in pregnancy and in patients receiving exogenous progestins, whereas in premenstrual endometrium a significant proportion of the cells are only minimally or partially affected. Decidual change is first apparent adjacent to the spiral arterioles; however, towards the end of the secretory phase and in pregnancy the change becomes diffuse. The stromal cells that are situated deeper in the endometrium, lying between the active glands of the spongy layer, show little, if any, decidual change and remain fairly nondescript (Figure 12.15). Occasionally, small bundles of smooth muscle may be found in the endometrial stroma (Figure 12.16). The decidual cells of the endometrial stroma, together with an exponential increase in granulated lymphocytes and natural killer (NK) cells, and the synthesis of a variety of extracellular matrix proteins including laminin and fibronectin, play a central role in the process of nidation (see Chapter 30).[9] Interleukin-1 has also been implicated in the induction of pinopodes and decidual integrins, which also seem to play an important role in successful implantation.[4]

ENDOMETRIAL LYMPHOCYTES

Several subpopulations of T-lymphocytes reside in the normal endometrium. CD4+ and CD8+ T-cells are randomly scattered throughout the functional layer (Figure 12.17) and, in the absence of an inflammatory process, show only a modest variation in density throughout the menstrual cycle, increasing towards menstruation.[42] In any form of endometritis, they aggregate near and around glands and can be seen within the gland lumens (Figure 12.18), along with CD68+ or CD163+ macrophages (Figures 12.19 and 12.20). Macrophages are normally found in all areas of the functional and basal zones.[1]

By contrast, small, rounded cells with hyperchromatic nuclei that are usually kidney-shaped or segmented increase in number in the endometrial stroma in the second half of the cycle (Figures 12.21 and 12.22). These cells are known as endometrial granulocytes, endometrial granular cells, or K-cells. The cytoplasm contains eosinophilic granules of variable size, so that the cells are also often mistaken for infiltrating polymorphonuclear leukocytes, particularly in the presence of early or imminent menstrual fragmentation (neutrophils are not seen in a normal endometrium until menstruation is well established and their presence at other times of the cycle indicates inflammation). These cells are large granulated lymphocytes that, on flow cytometric analysis, exhibit the unusual T-cell phenotype CD56+, CD3−, CD16− and also have a natural killer function.[11] They derive from the peripheral

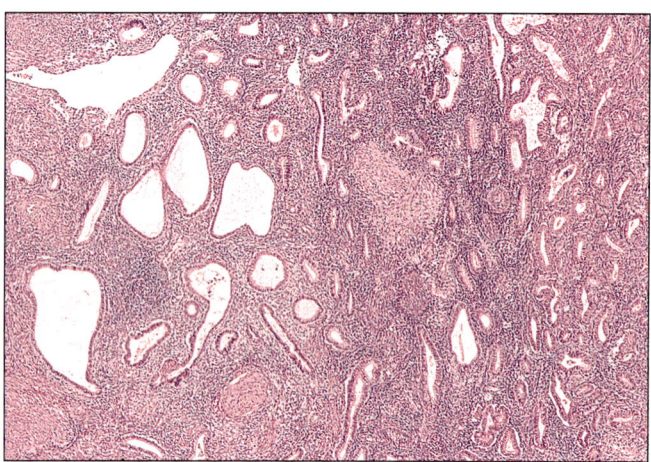

Fig. 12.16   Smooth muscle in endometrial stroma.

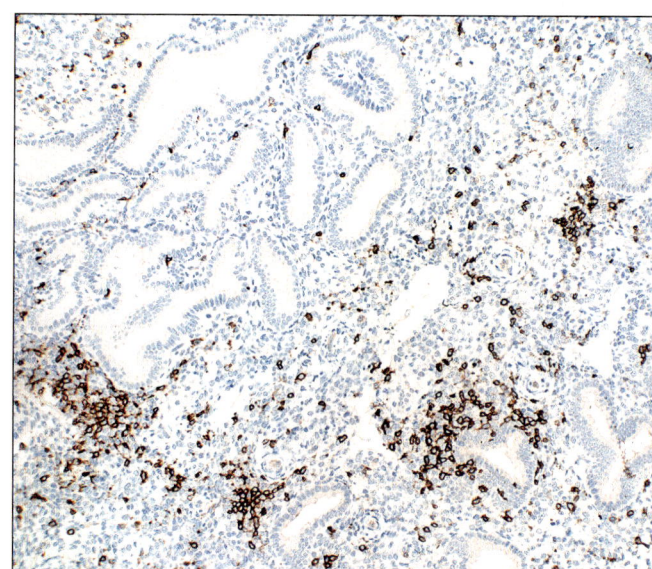

Fig. 12.18   Chronic endometritis with CD8 reactive T-cells aggregated about glands.

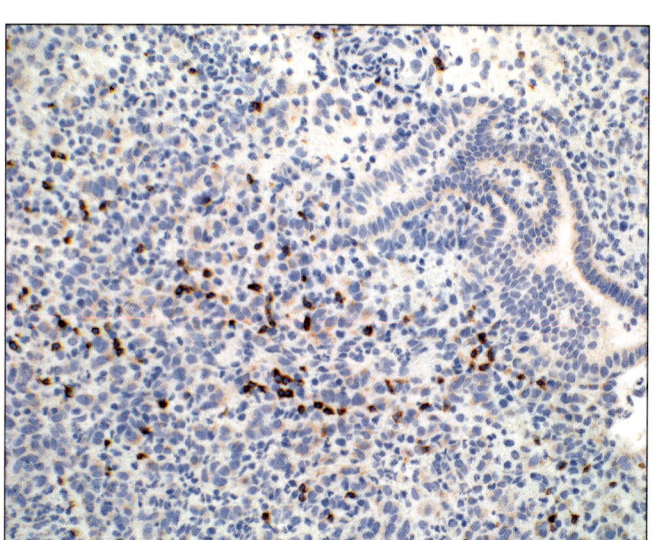

Fig. 12.17   Normal late secretory endometrium with CD8 reactive T-cells randomly scattered throughout the stroma.

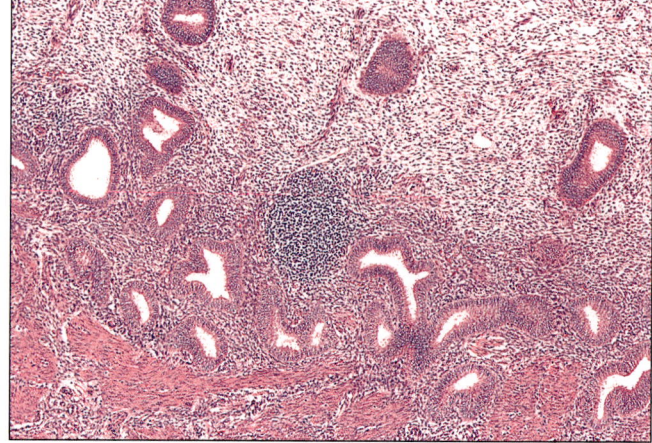

Fig. 12.19   Normal endometrium. Focal collection of lymphocytes.

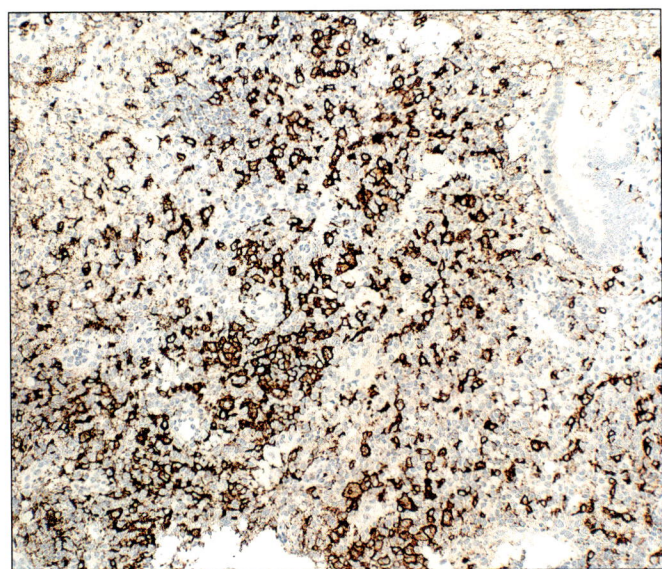

Fig. 12.20 Chronic endometritis with CD163 reactive macrophages aggregated about glands.

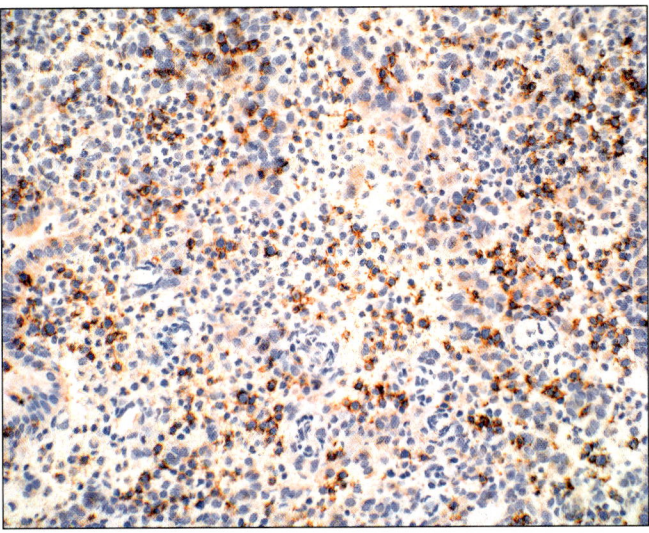

Fig. 12.23 CD56 reactive large granulated lymphocytes with a natural killer cell phenotype in normal late secretory endometrium.

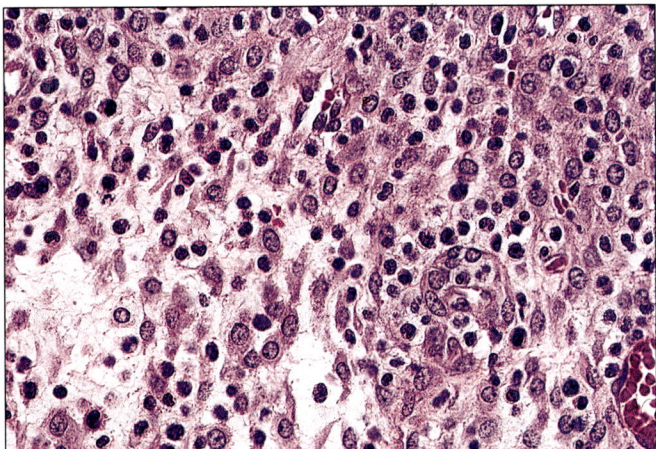

Fig. 12.21 Endometrial lymphocytes. The cells have hyperchromatic, kidney-shaped nuclei and eosinophilic granules in the cytoplasm.

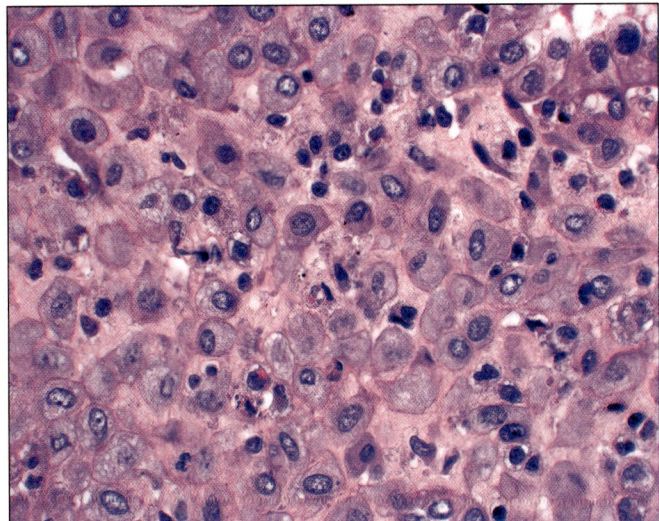

Fig. 12.22 Large granular lymphocytes in stroma of normal late secretory endometrium.

blood, colonize the endometrium, and may be specific to the uterus.[11,38] Endometrial granulated lymphocytes increase in number dramatically in the late secretory phase of the menstrual cycle (Figures 12.18 and 12.23), sometimes reaching a population density exceeding 25% of all stromal cells. If conception and implantation occur, they continue to increase in number and make up about 70% of the stromal lymphocytes in the first trimester of pregnancy.[11,30] Despite this dramatic cyclic variation, these cells lack progesterone and estrogen receptors. It is probable that steroid hormones influence the population indirectly by means of products made by endometrial stromal or epithelial cells, which themselves express steroid hormone receptors.[30] These uterine NK cells are in close association with extravillous trophoblast in early pregnancy.[13] Furthermore, the decidual NK cells have receptors for trophoblast human leukocyte antigen (HLA) Class I molecules, suggesting a possible role in the maternal–fetal interaction, perhaps more specifically in the control of trophoblast invasion and migration.[12,14] They may also function in angiogenesis.[32]

BLOOD VESSELS

The arterial supply of the endometrium is from the radial arteries that arise from the arcuate arteries in the myometrium. The radial arteries branch near the endometrial–myometrial interface, forming the basal arteries. As these ascend through the functionalis to the endometrial surface, they become the spiral arterioles (Figure 12.24). The spiral arterioles respond to the varying levels of ovarian hormones and become prominent in the second half of the secretory phase, under the influence of progesterone. Coiling becomes most pronounced when the stromal edema is reabsorbed prior to menstruation. In the proliferative phase, the arterioles show little coiling and are confined to the deeper levels of the functionalis. There is an irregular network of venous channels with the veins frequently intersecting, forming venous lakes.

ENDOMETRIUM DURING THE NORMAL MENSTRUAL CYCLE

Only a brief account is presented here of the changes that are seen in the endometrium as the menstrual cycle progresses. Fuller accounts are available in numerous monographs.[8,22,39] The main features throughout the cycle are summarized and illustrated in Figure 12.25. The endometrial cycle is customarily divided into two main phases, the proliferative (preovulatory) phase and the secretory (postovulatory or luteal) phase, to which can be added the menstrual phase and the interval phase. This division of the cycle is related, of course, to the hormones stimulating it, estrogen predominating in the proliferative phase and progesterone in the secretory phase. The idealized 28-day endometrial cycle begins on the first day of menses with ovulation on day 14. Normal cycling endometrium is usually diagnosed by reference to that cycle day that best fits the histologic appearance (e.g., secretory endometrium, day 24).

PROLIFERATIVE PHASE (Figures 12.4 and 12.26–12.30)

This part of the cycle generally lasts for 2 weeks but its length may vary over quite a wide range, this being largely responsible for the patient-to-patient variation in the length of the menstrual cycle. Remembering that menstrual dating starts from the first day of clinical bleeding, proliferative activity commences before menstrual bleeding from the previous cycle has finished and, at this early phase of the cycle, the endometrium is thin with sparse, small, straight glands and a loose stroma of spindled cells. At 8–10 days, the endometrial thickness increases, mainly as a result of stromal edema induced by estrogen, which reaches a peak at about day 10. With the preovulatory serum levels of estrogen then subsiding and with it stromal edema, the continued growth of the glands overtakes that of the stroma, so that they become slightly tortuous (Figures 12.4 and 12.26). This process becomes more exaggerated close to the time of ovulation (Figures 12.27 and 12.28). Glandular epithelium takes on a 'pseudostratified' appearance, with nuclei staggered at various heights in the cell, although most are in the basal half. The epithelial cells have smooth sharp luminal borders and basophilic or amphophilic cytoplasm (Figure 12.29). Mitoses are frequent in both glands and stroma, and are a direct result of stimulation by estrogen. Using these morphologic criteria, the proliferative endometrium may be dated as early, mid or late proliferative but this degree of 'accuracy' is rarely possible or, indeed, necessary.

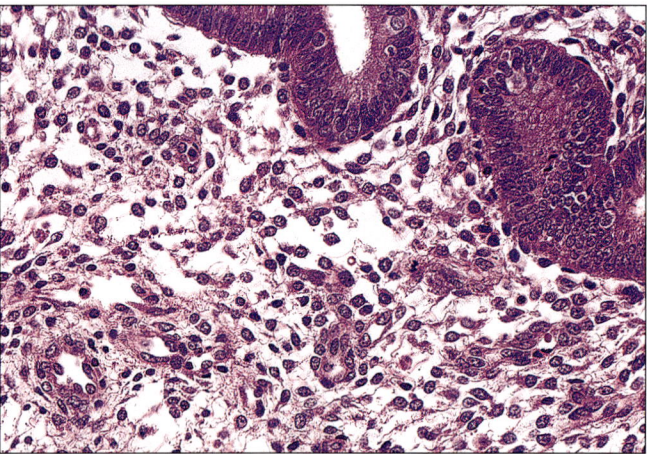

Fig. 12.24 Spiral arterioles in the proliferative phase.

Day of Cycle		Before 14	15-16	17	18	19-22	23	24-25	26-27	28+
Post-ovulatory day		-	1-2	3	4	5-8	9	10-11	12-13	14+
Cycle phases		Proliferative	'Interval'	Early secretory		Mid-secretory			Late secretory	Menstrual
Key feature		Mitoses	Mitoses and subnuclear vacuoles	Maximum subnuclear vacuoles	Subnuclear vacuoles present	Stromal edema	Focal decidua around spiral arteries	Patchy decidua	Extensive decidua	Stromal crumbling
Microscopic features of functional zone	Stroma	Loose stroma. Mitoses	Same as proliferative	Loose stroma, scanty mitoses	Loose stroma	Stromal edema	Focal decidua around spiral arteries. Edema prominent	Decidua throughout stroma. Some edema	Extensive decidua. Prominent granulated lymphocytes	Stromal crumbling. Hemorrhage
	Glands	Straight to tightly coiled tubules. Mitoses	Some subnuclear vacuoles, otherwise as proliferative	Extensive subnuclear vacuoles	Dilated glands. Some subnuclear vacuoles	Dilated glands with irregular outline. Luminal secretion		'Saw tooth' glands	Prominent 'saw tooth' glands	Disrupted glands. Secretory exhaustion. Regenerating epithelium
Appearances		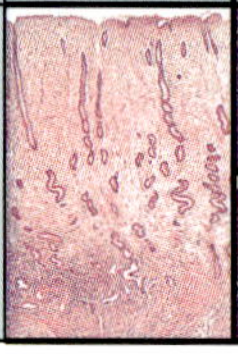	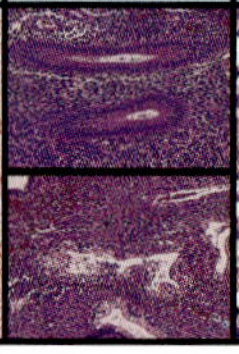	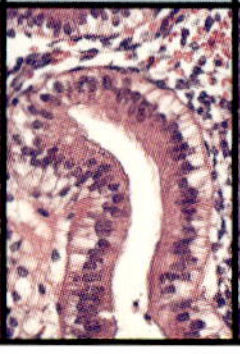	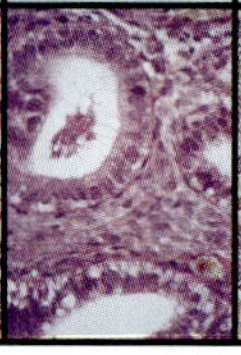	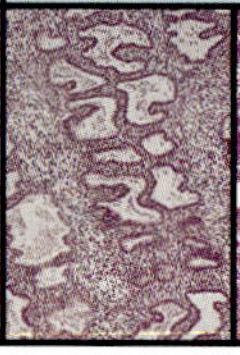	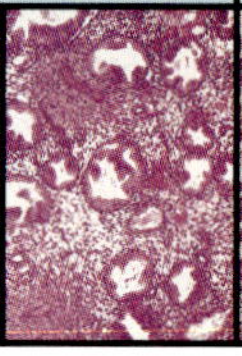	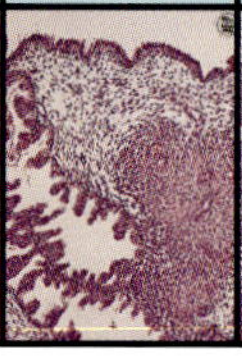	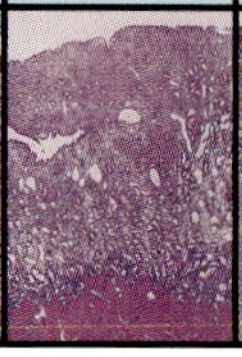	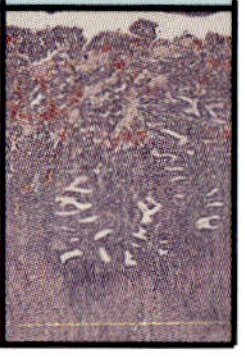

Fig. 12.25 Main histologic features of the menstrual cycle.

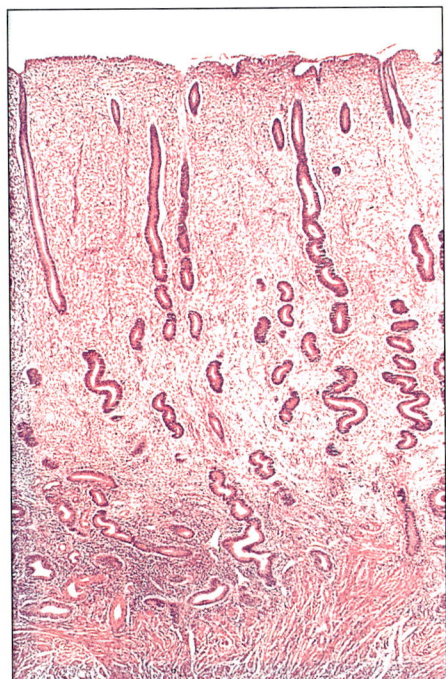

Fig. 12.26 Proliferative endometrium. Low power.

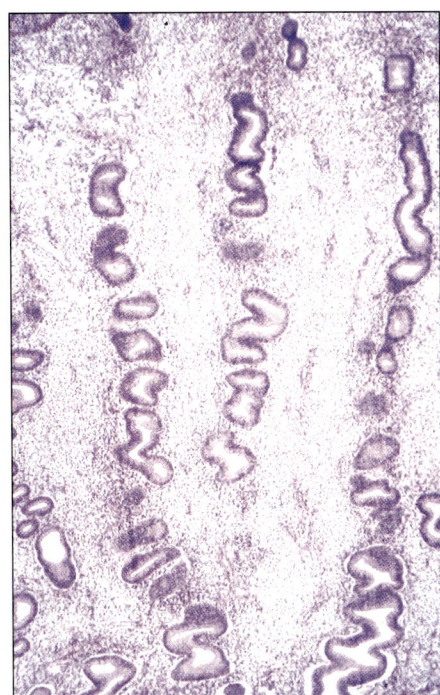

Fig. 12.28 Proliferative endometrium with tortuous coiled glands just prior to ovulation.

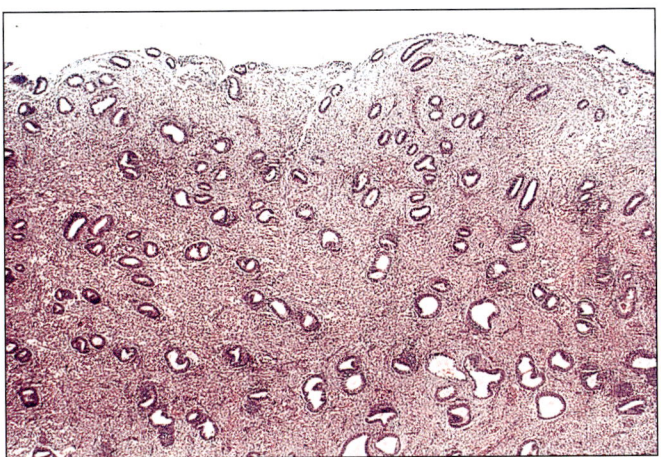

Fig. 12.27 Proliferative phase endometrium.

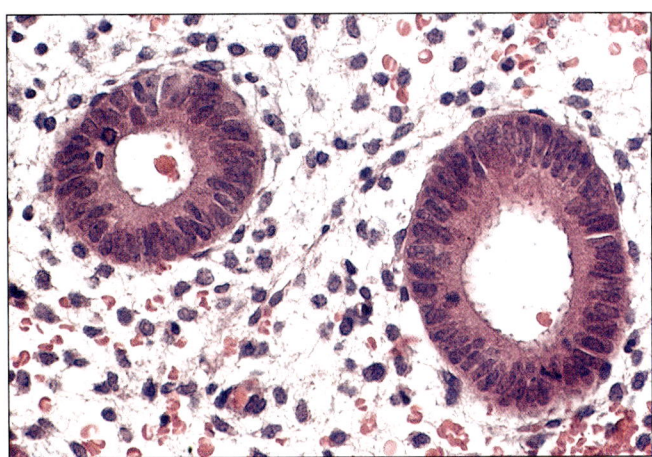

Fig. 12.29 Proliferative phase endometrium.

INTERVAL PHASE (Figure 12.31)

The short period of no more than 48 hours between ovulation and the appearance of the first secretory changes in the endometrium, induced by rising serum progesterone levels, is termed the 'interval phase'. It can only be inferred from clear biochemical evidence of a luteinizing hormone peak and an absence of conspicuous subnuclear vacuolation in the endometrial glandular epithelial cells (see below).

Morphologic changes in the endometrium are not apparent until 36–48 hours after ovulation has occurred, so that the earliest evidence of secretory activity develops on the second postovulatory day (i.e., the second half of day 16 of a 'normalized' 28-day cycle, assuming ovulation at the end of day 14). At this stage, there is an overlap of proliferative and secretory activity. The endometrial glands show both mitotic activity and

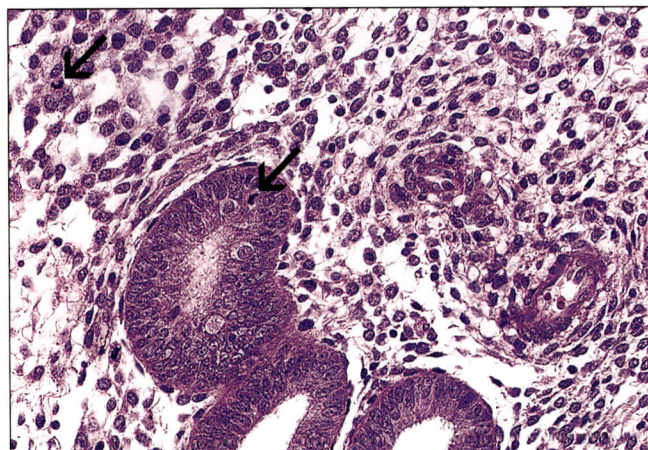

Fig. 12.30 Proliferative phase endometrium. Mitotic figures are present in the glandular epithelium and in the stroma (arrows). A spiral arteriole is prominent.

305

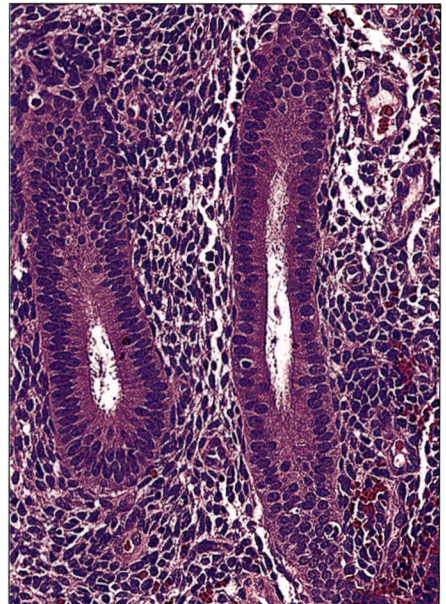
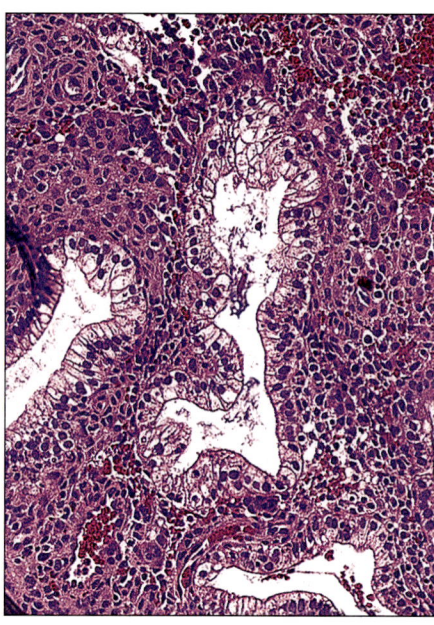

Fig. 12.31 'Interval phase' endometrium. At the very beginning of the secretory phase, there is an overlap of proliferative and secretory activity, so that mitotic figures and secretory vacuoles are present in the glandular epithelium at the same time. The right side appears more like a later secretory pattern, thus a mixed pattern.

a hint of early secretory activity, so that the endometrium is referred to as being in transition from the proliferative phase. This period of overlap is also known as the 'interval phase' (Figure 12.31). The first morphologic sign of secretion in the endometrium is the presence of subnuclear vacuolation, a clear zone that forms between the nucleus and the basement membrane of the cell. This appears initially at day 16 in individual cells but is not yet pathognomonic of ovulation.

SECRETORY PHASE (Figures 12.32–12.54)

After ovulation the development and involution of the corpus luteum is controlled in a very precise way (see Chapter 21). The response of the endometrium to the changing levels of both estrogen and progesterone follows a predictable pattern so that the appearances seen in the secretory phase of the cycle allow accurate dating. The average interval between ovulation and the onset of menstruation is 14 days but it may normally vary from 11 to 17 days.[41] The secretory phase is often divided into early, mid, and late phases, but these phases are variably (and arbitrarily) defined by different authorities.

Morphologically, the earliest the change is sufficient to unequivocally document ovulation is day 17, or 3 days after ovulation. These subnuclear vacuoles reflect the presence of glycogen that has been leached from the cell during tissue processing. Nonetheless, periodic acid-Schiff (PAS) stains will demonstrate the small amount that remains (Figure 12.32). It seems odd that secretory vacuoles first appear in a basal position, when the secretion has eventually to be discharged into the lumen. At any time in the cycle, it is normal for a few cells to display poorly formed subnuclear vacuoles, so the presence of a few such cells should not be regarded as proof of ovulation.

EARLY SECRETORY PHASE (Figures 12.32–12.35)

The appearance of the subnuclear vacuolation heralds the onset of the early secretory phase, which lasts from the first to

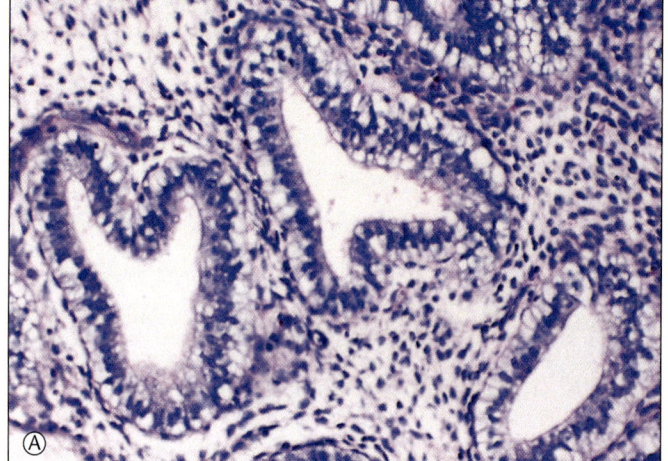

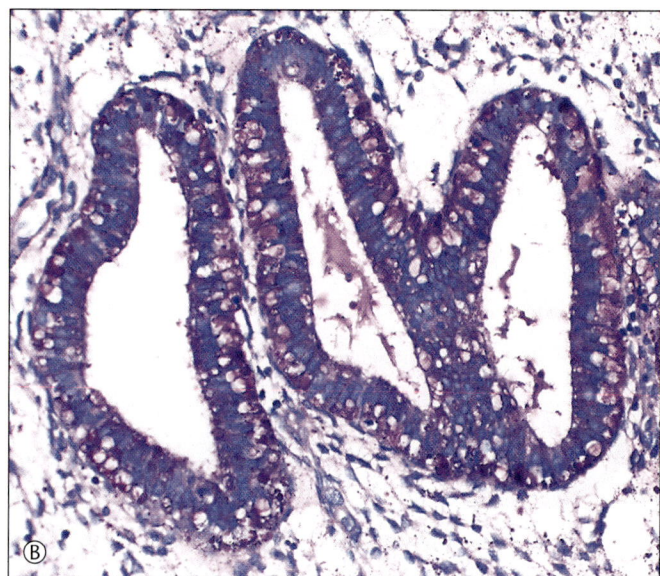

Fig. 12.32 Early secretory phase endometrium (day 17) with prominent subnuclear vacuoles. **(A)** Diastase digestion removes the glycogen granules seen clearly **(B)** with the native PAS stain.

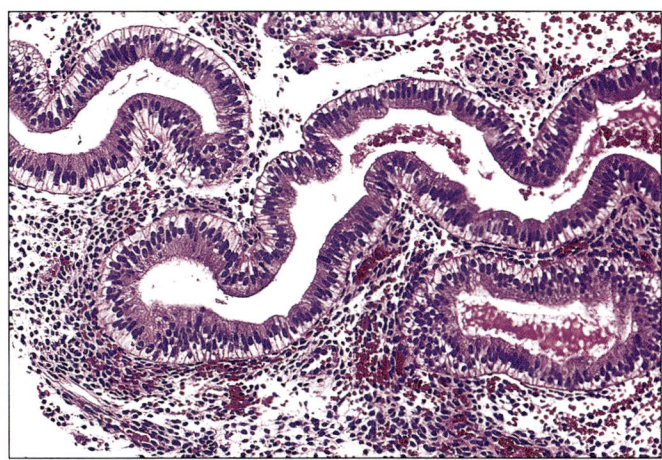

Fig. 12.33 Early secretory phase endometrium (day 17). The glands are becoming tortuous and subnuclear vacuolation is prominent.

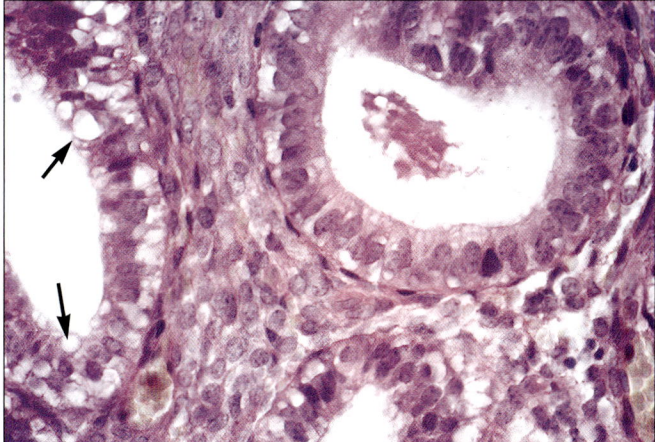

Fig. 12.34 Early secretory phase endometrium (day 18). The subnuclear vacuolation is less prominent and less regular. Secretory vacuoles are also seen on the luminal side of the nucleus (arrows).

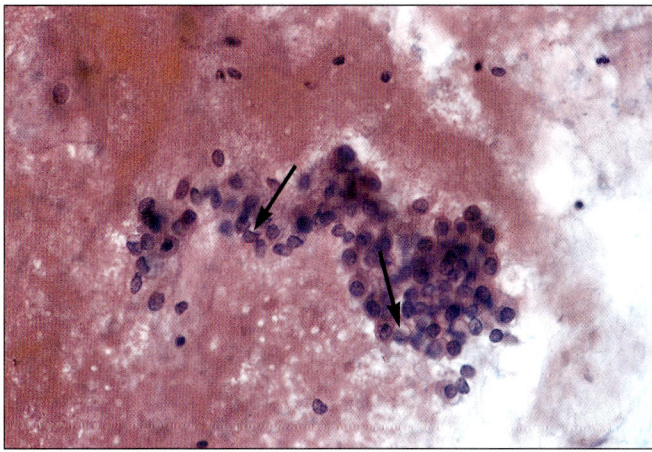

Fig. 12.35 Cytology. Early secretory phase. Some cells show a subnuclear vacuole (arrows).

the fifth postovulatory day (cycle days 15–19). On day 3 after ovulation (day 17) the basal vacuoles are at their most prominent. Uniformly sized vacuoles push the nuclei into alignment (loss of nuclear pseudostratification) in the middle of the cell (Figures 12.10 and 12.33). The combination of clear basal vacuoles and aligned dark nuclei resemble a row of 'piano keys'. The glands become more tortuous during this part of the cycle and, although the epithelial cells are no longer dividing, the surface area of the glands increases. By day 18, the subnuclear vacuoles are less regular and similar secretory vacuoles are additionally present in the cytoplasm on the luminal side of the nucleus (Figure 12.34). Both 16- and 18-day endometrium have pseudostratified nuclei and variably sized basal vacuoles, but can readily be distinguished by the paucity of mitoses at day 18. Occasionally, the vacuoles can be seen on cytologic preparations (Tao Brush technique) (Figure 12.35).

MID-SECRETORY PHASE (Figures 12.36–12.46)

The mid-secretory phase lasts from cycle days 19 to 25, when histologic dating is primarily based upon the sequential appearance of specific progesterone-induced stromal changes, rather than detailed examination of the glands. The distribution of stromal changes within different zones of the endometrial thickness is important to be aware of, particularly in disrupted curettage material. The care taken to identify the endometrial surface of randomly oriented tissue fragments and dating the changes in these areas is rewarded by accuracy and reproducibility.

Stromal changes, in response to ovulation and rising serum progesterone levels, begin with edema within the functional zone on day 19. Edema is greatest at days 20–22 (Figure 12.36), coinciding with the second estrogen peak in the menstrual cycle. Dating within this window is particularly difficult, both because the histologic appearance of edema may be modified by artifact, and paucity of confirmatory discrete glandular benchmarks. By the end of this period the stromal edema highlights the thin-walled spiral arterioles and their immediately adjacent stromal cells, which appear 'naked' and suspended within the functional layer of the endometrium. At the same time, and partly as a result of this change, the endometrial layers become more apparent (Figures 12.37 and 12.46). The basal layer is now clearly distinguished from the functional endometrium.

At day 23, the edema starts to regress and at the same time the stromal cells commence decidualization. This change is first appreciated in the immediate vicinity of the spiral arterioles and beneath the surface epithelium (Figures 12.41, 12.43, 12.44, and 12.46). The previously 'naked' spiral arterioles are now cuffed by predecidua (decidualized stromal cells), but still suspended in the otherwise loose, edematous stroma. At 24 days predecidua extends to bridge vascular elements (Figures 12.44 and 12.46). The stromal edema is progressively reabsorbed as predecidua forms focally under the surface lining at 25 days. Somewhat paradoxically, mitoses are frequently seen in the stromal cells of mid-secretory endometrium, peaking at day 23.

Several changes occur in the character of the glands (Figures 12.36–12.40). In cross-section, the outlines of the glands become markedly irregular, in striking contrast to the round or oval pattern seen in the proliferative phase (Figures 12.41–12.43). This is due to the glands widening in their diameter, which

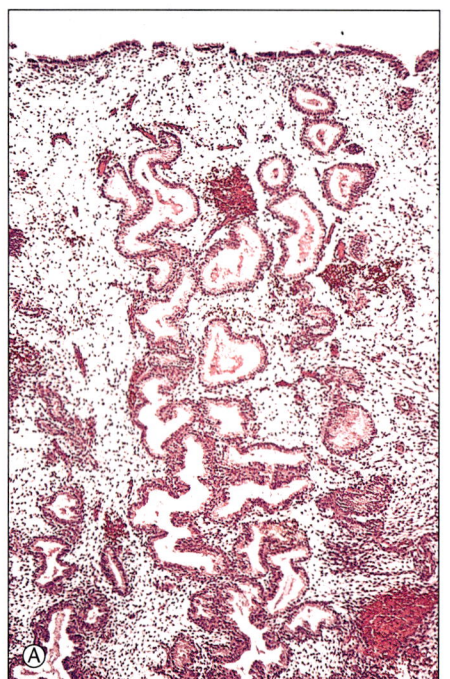

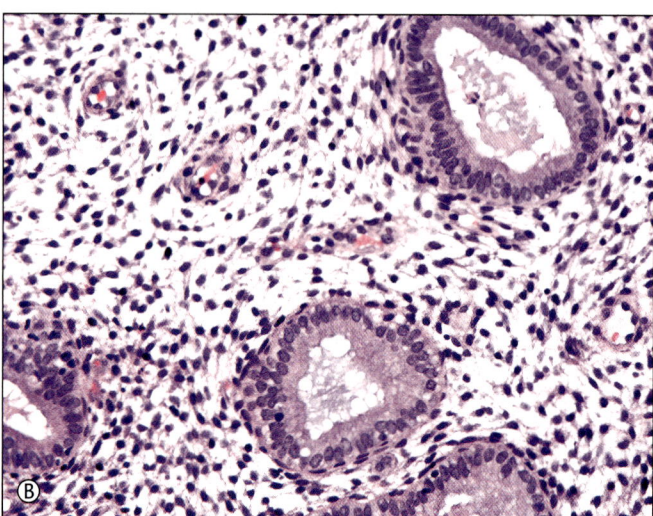

Fig. 12.36 **(A)** Mid-secretory phase endometrium (days 20–22) with loose, edematous stroma. **(B)** Detail.

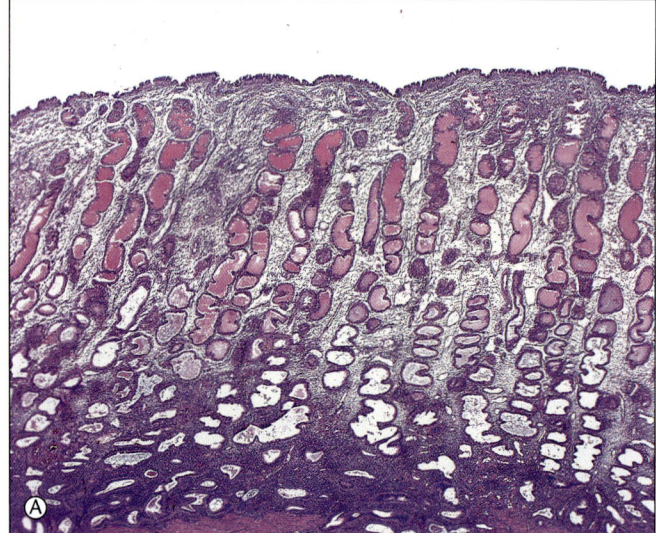

Fig. 12.37 Mid-secretory phase endometrium (days 20–22). **(A)** Peak of intraluminal secretion in compactum layer. **(B)** Detail.

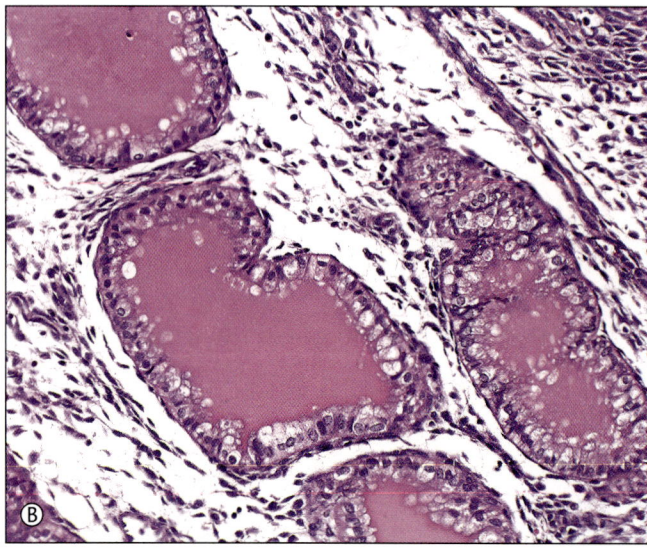

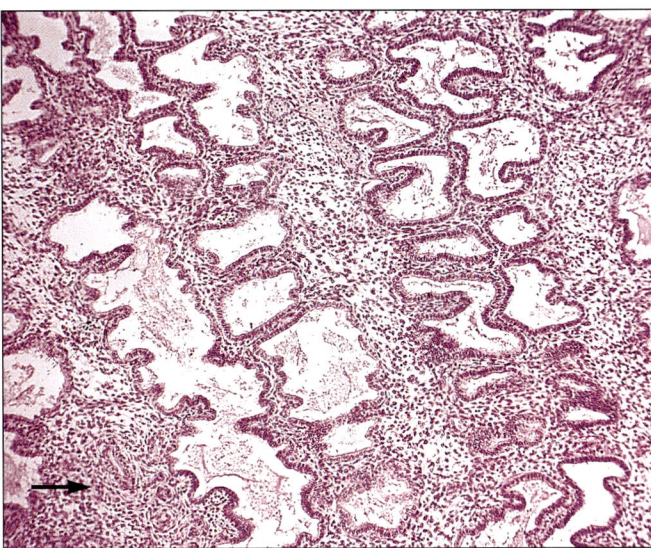

Fig. 12.38 Mid-secretory phase endometrium (days 20–22). The stroma cells about the spiral arteries (arrows) have not developed into predecidua.

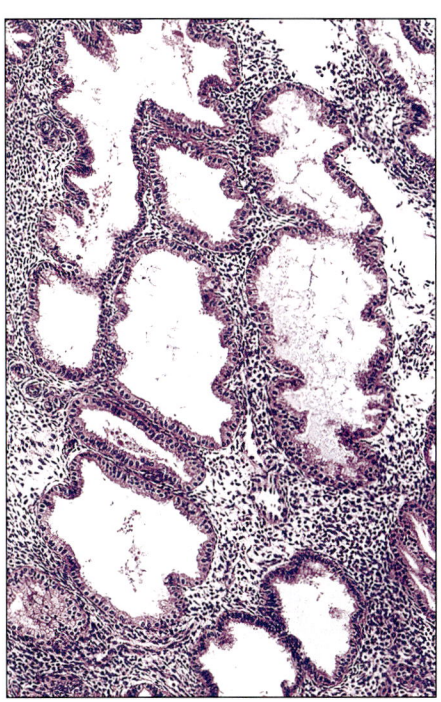

Fig. 12.40 Mid-secretory phase endometrium (days 20–22). The glands are irregular with minimal serration and the stromal cells about the spiral arteries lack cytoplasm development consistent with predecidua.

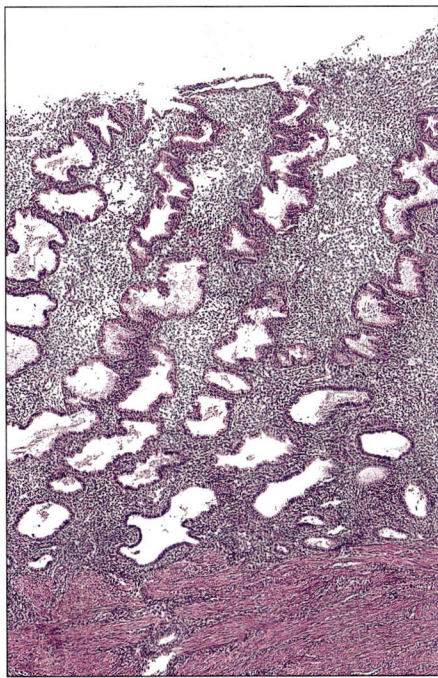

Fig. 12.39 Mid-secretory phase endometrium (days 20–22).

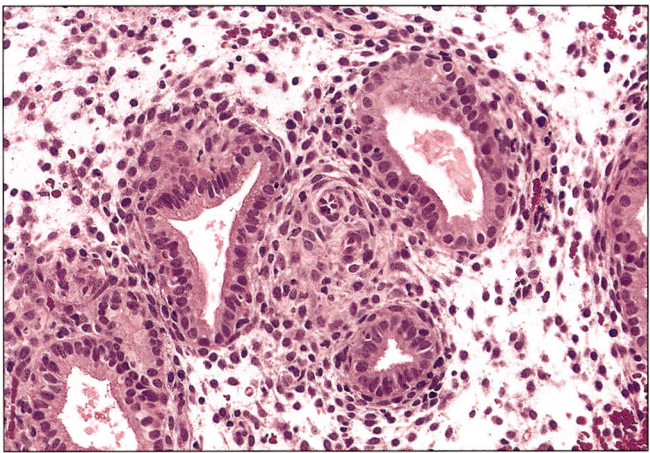

Fig. 12.41 Mid-secretory phase endometrium (day 23). The stroma about the spiral arteries shows the earliest predecidual development.

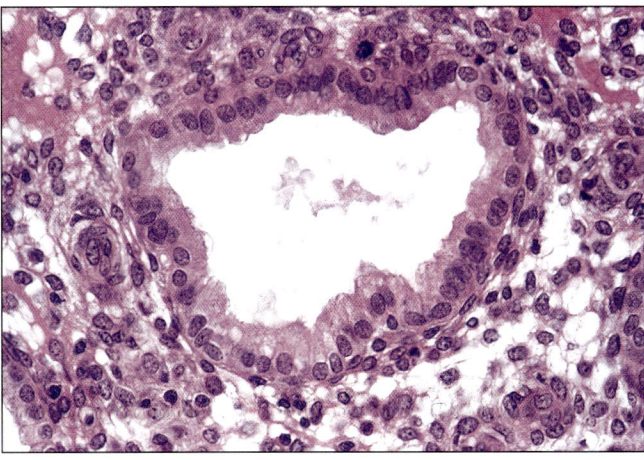

reflects a change from glands that are tightly coiled in the proliferative phase. The lining epithelium also changes character and begins to develop slight papillary infoldings. This progresses, together with the dilated outline, to give the so-called 'saw-toothed pattern' (Figure 12.44). Finally, there is no longer the pseudostratified appearance of the nuclei that typifies the late proliferative phase, and mitoses cease to be apparent.

The secretory vacuoles have by now all moved to the luminal pole of the cell, and are in the process of being discharged into the lumen. The apical surface of the cell is rough and indistinct ('fluffy') because it has been broken by the process

Fig. 12.42 Mid-secretory phase endometrium (day 23).

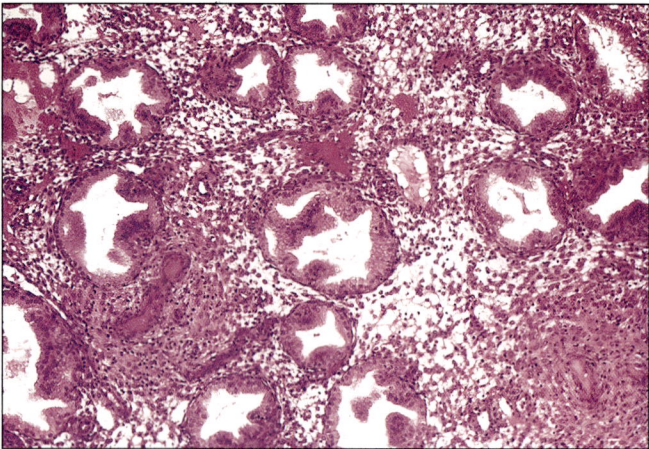

Fig. 12.43 Mid-secretory phase endometrium (day 23) with predecidua about spiral arteries.

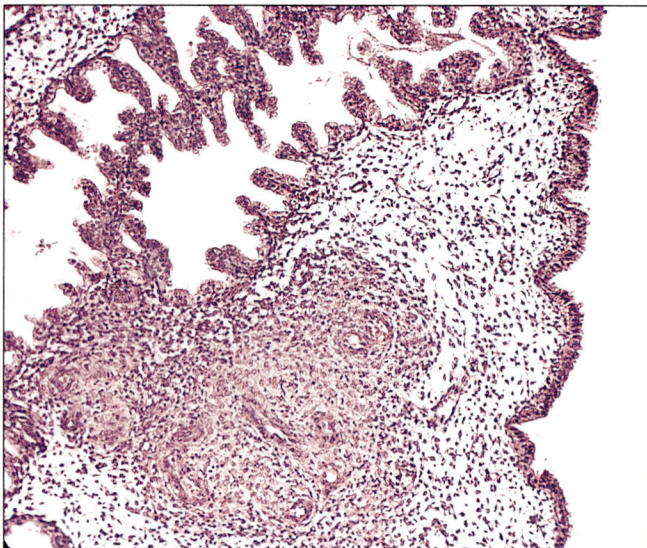

Fig. 12.44 Mid-secretory phase endometrium (day 24). The glands are serrated and the predecidua has begun to bridge among spiral arteries.

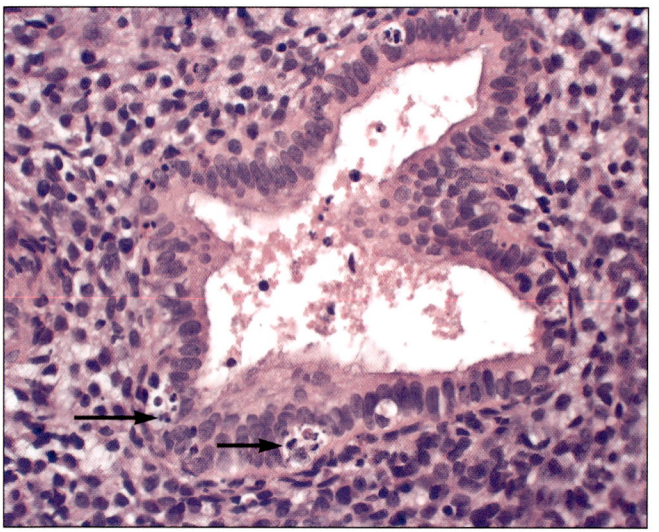

Fig. 12.45 Apoptotic bodies (arrows) in mid-secretory phase endometrium.

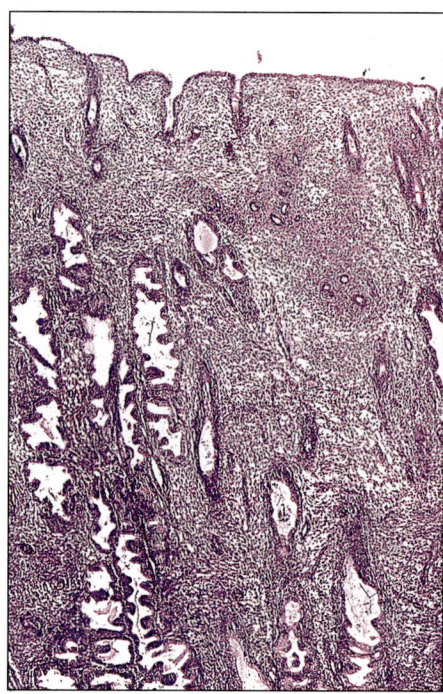

Fig. 12.46 Mid-secretory phase endometrium (days 24–25). The glands are serrated and the predecidua has begun to bridge among many spiral arteries.

of apocrine secretion and vacuoles are seen in the cell's luminal cytoplasm. Pale staining fragments of cell cytoplasm may be found within the gland lumens. The nuclei are basal, round, vesicular and pale staining. It is during this period, the so-called 'peak' of intraluminal secretions, at which time the endometrium is optimally structured for implantation around day 21, that the luminal content can become intensely eosinophilic (Figure 12.37). Apoptotic bodies normally appear in the glandular epithelium in response to progesterone's downregulation of the proto-oncogene *bcl-2* (Figure 12.45).[28] These apoptotic bodies should not be misinterpreted as infiltrating neutrophils.

LATE SECRETORY PHASE (Figures 12.47–12.54)

The late secretory phase (days 26–28) shows further extension of predecidual change from the surface lining downwards. At day 26, the stroma just under the endometrial lining epithelium shows a band of continuous predecidual change, and projects more deeply to include all of the stratum compactum by day 27, when numerous granulated lymphocytes are evident (Figures 12.14 and 12.47). The stroma in the deeper spongy zone appears featureless and undifferentiated (Figures 12.49 and 12.50). The glands also show differences according to their position relative to the surface. In the central, spongy part of the endometrium the glands have a characteristic 'saw-toothed' appearance (Figures 12.50 and 12.51). The epithelial cells are now full of secretion and are of a moderately tall, columnar type. The glands of the stratum compactum, on the other hand, appear to be fewer in number (an illusion, as each gland in the spongy layer must have an opening onto the surface) and are lined by flat to cuboidal cells with some luminal membrane breakdown (the beginning of 'secretory exhaustion') (Figures 12.52 and

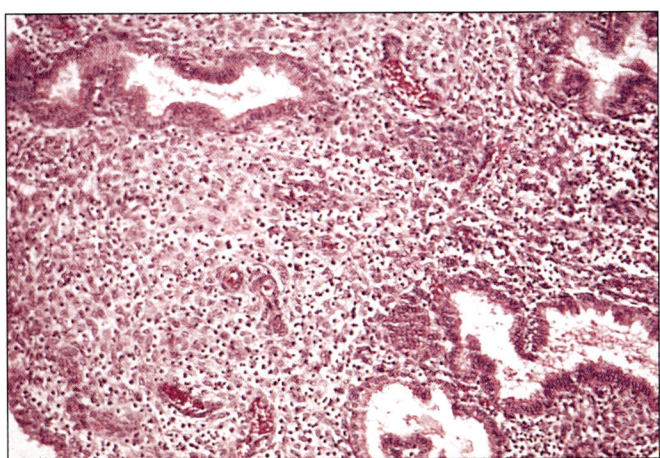

Fig. 12.47   Late phase endometrium (day 26).

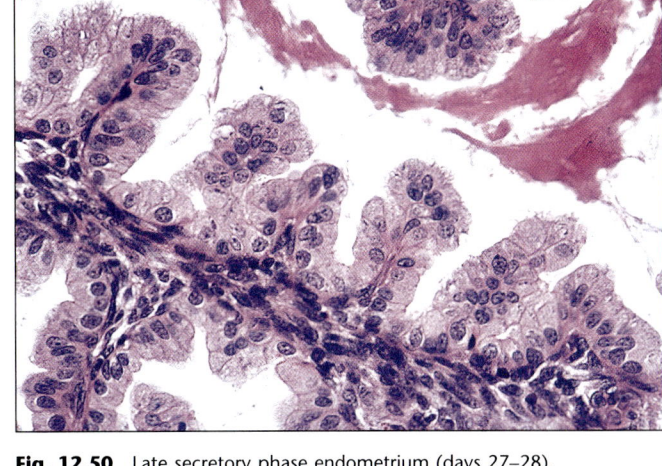

Fig. 12.50   Late secretory phase endometrium (days 27–28).

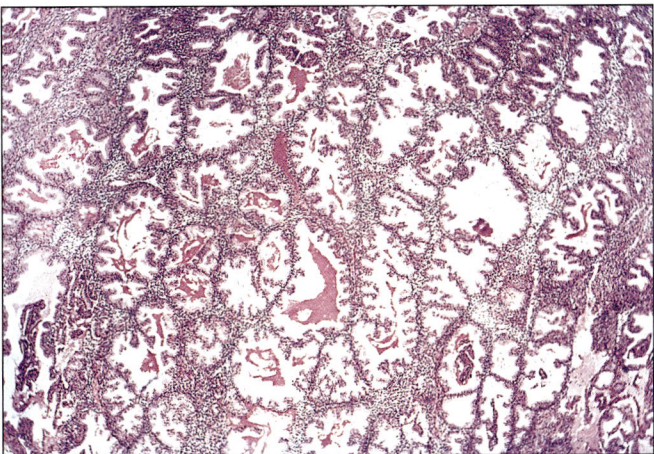

Fig. 12.48   Late secretory phase endometrium (days 27–28).

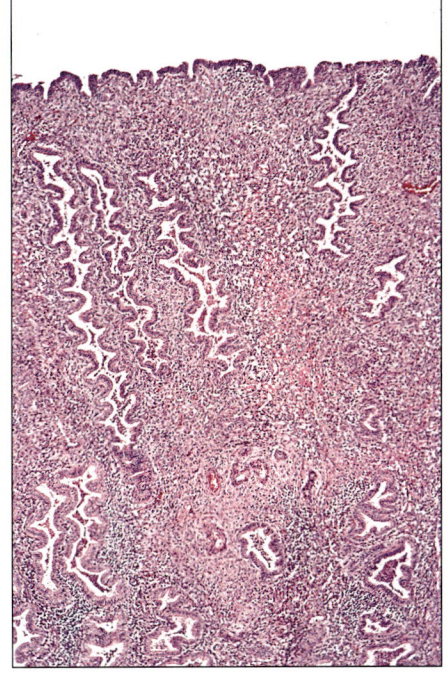

Fig. 12.51   Late secretory phase endometrium (days 27–28).

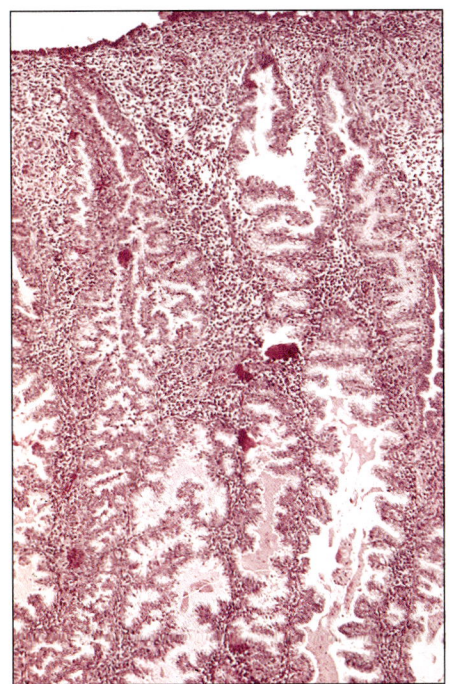

Fig. 12.49   Late secretory phase endometrium (day 27).

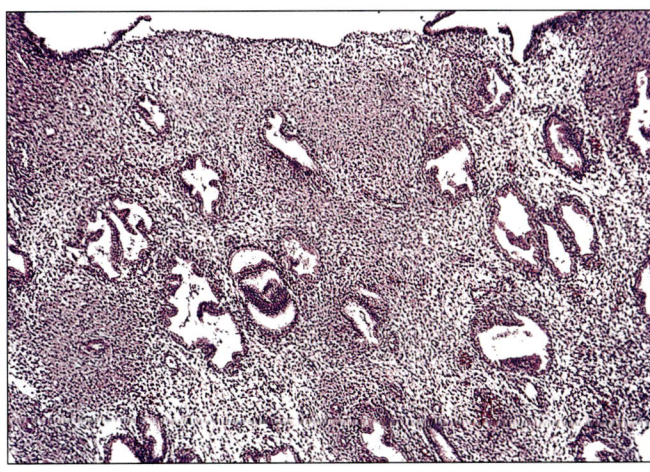

Fig. 12.52   Late secretory phase endometrium (day 27).

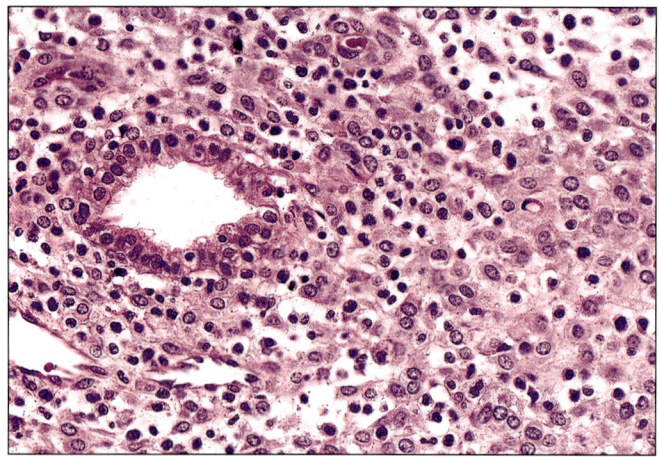

Fig. 12.53 Late secretory phase endometrium (day 27). The glandular epithelium shows 'secretory exhaustion'.

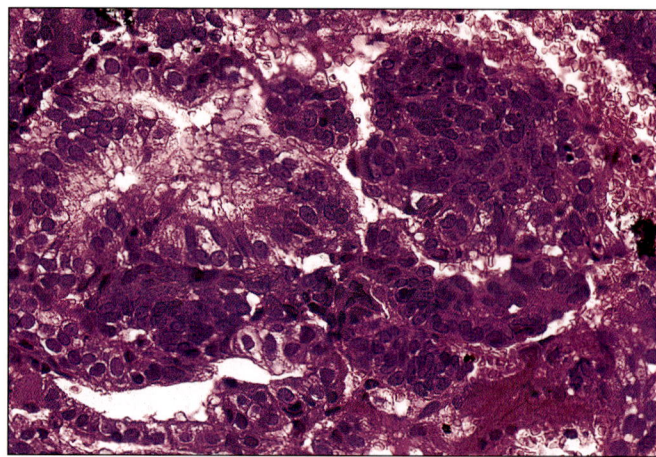

Fig. 12.55 Menstrual phase endometrium. The stroma is crumbling and the glands are breaking up and show 'secretory exhaustion'.

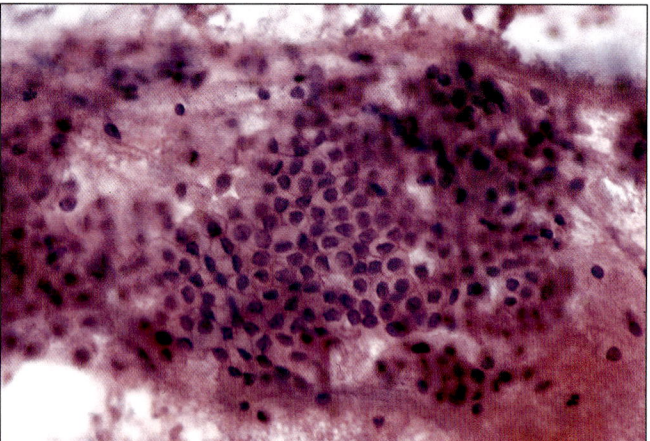

Fig. 12.54 Cytology. Late secretory phase. Cells show diffuse cytoplasmic vacuolation, with hazy appearance.

12.53). The cytoplasm in these cells is extensive, but appears bubbly and largely empty of contents (Figure 12.54).

MENSTRUAL PHASE (Figures 12.55–12.62)

If conception and implantation have not occurred by day 24 (postovulatory day 10), leading to an absence of human chorionic gonadotrophin (hCG) stimulation, the corpus luteum fails in its ability to maintain itself ('corpus luteum involution'), leading to a marked fall in progesterone output. The late secretory phase then leads inevitably to the menstrual phase, normally starting on day 28. This is recognized histologically by very fine crumbling or fragmentation of the stroma and glandular collapse. Two very characteristic changes, especially when seen in combination, are compact balls of stromal cells which, with hematoxylin, have an unusually deep blue color, and overlying epithelial cells, which appear degenerative. A third change, often seen, is the presence of plump epithelial glandular cells displaying secretory exhaustion. These tissue fragments are separated by red blood cells and neutrophils.

The appearances of menstrual endometrium can confuse inexperienced pathologists because the stromal crumbling

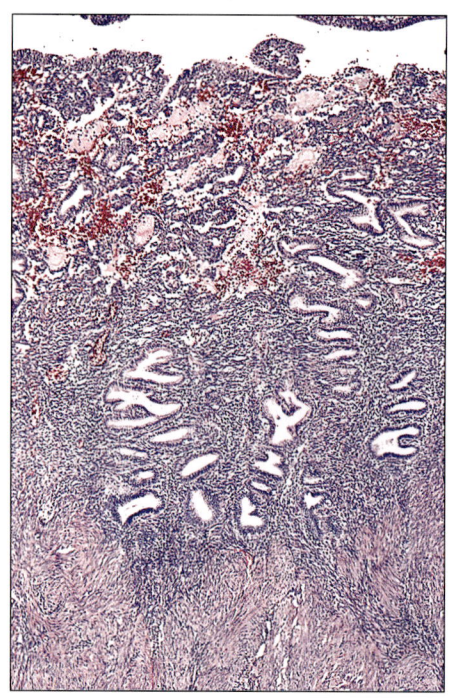

Fig. 12.56 Menstrual phase endometrium.

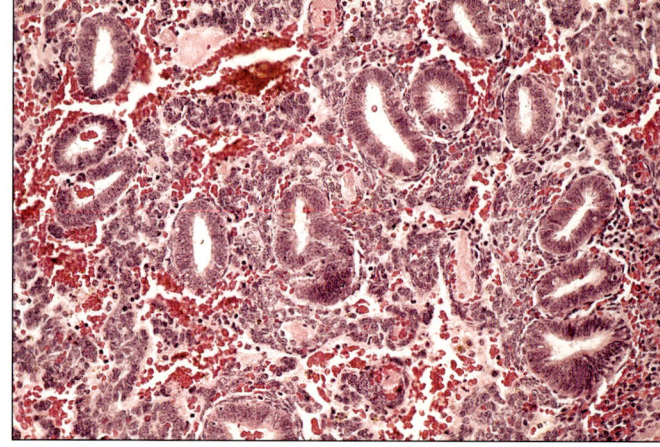

Fig. 12.57 Menstrual phase endometrium. Stromal crumbling and glandular collapse are well established, giving a false impression of glandular crowding.

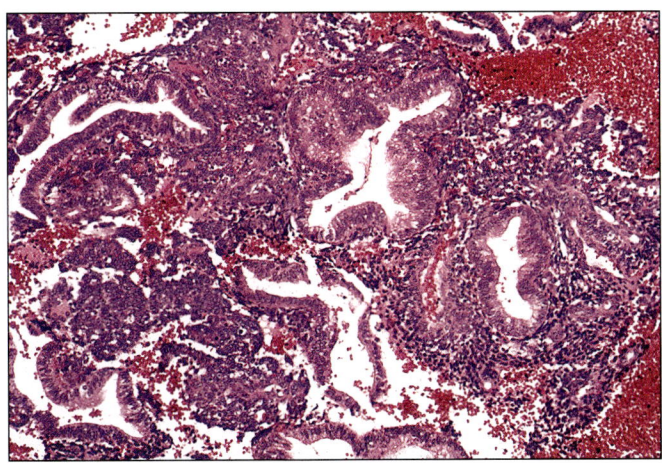

Fig. 12.58 Menstrual phase endometrium.

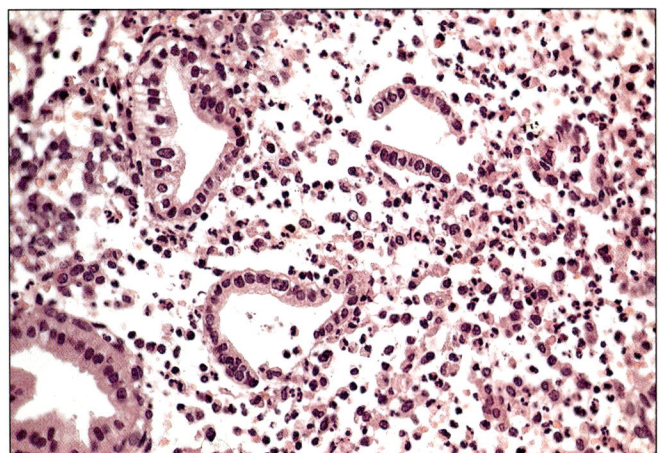

Fig. 12.61 Late menstrual phase endometrium. Inflammation is present in the background and the endometrial glands are extensively fragmented.

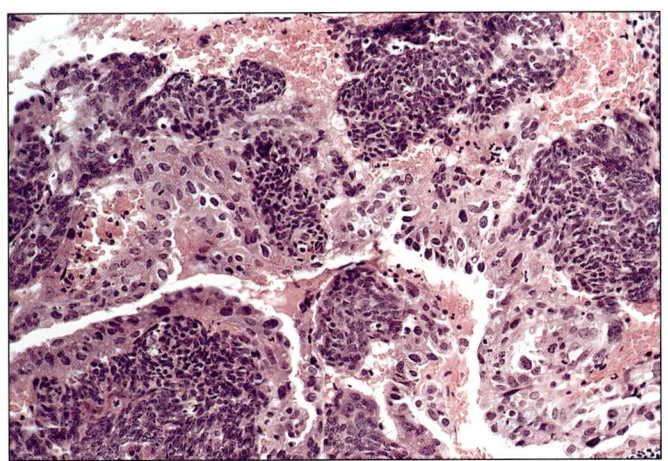

Fig. 12.59 Menstrual phase endometrium. The nodules of collapsed, condensed stroma have colloquially been called 'blue balls'.

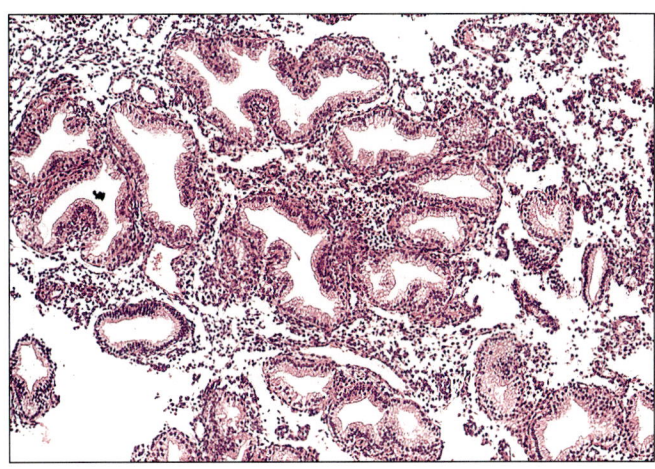

Fig. 12.62 Early menstrual phase endometrium. Stromal crumbling is present but the glands still show some secretory activity.

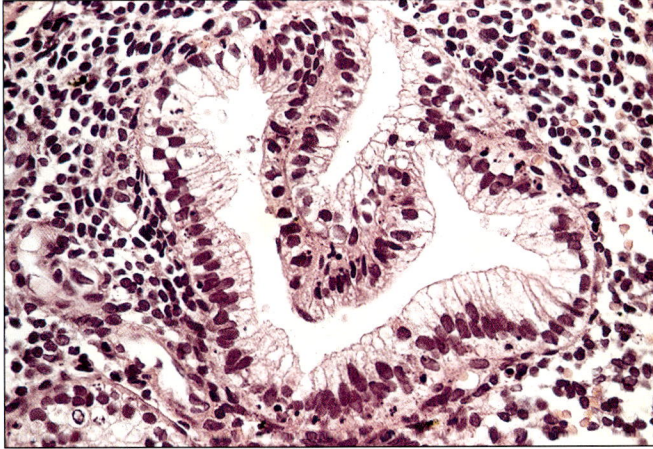

Fig. 12.60 Menstrual phase endometrium. The gland shows 'secretory exhaustion'.

results in irregular, collapsing glands, often coming together to give a 'back-to-back' pattern that may be misinterpreted as hyperplasia or even malignancy. Attention to the rest of the material on the slide will show the remains of secretory glands and, perhaps, some areas where the stroma remains intact and shows decidual change. In addition, the highly cellular stromal balls are occasionally misinterpreted as small cell carcinoma of either endometrium or cervix due to the very high nuclear to cytoplasmic ratios and prominent nuclear molding and apoptosis.

Histologic examination of curettings taken during menstruation is usually uninformative, as fragmenting tissue obscures the architecture at the same time as the degenerative changes that take place very rapidly once menstruation commences blur the true epithelial morphology. From the configuration of the larger intact fragments plus the appearances of the glandular cells, especially by the presence of secretory change, it is often possible to indicate whether the cycle just finishing has been ovulatory or anovulatory. Actual secretory activity and mitotic figures are not seen at the time of menstruation. These cell activities cease quickly once the blood supply to the cells is compromised. In general, if the curettage is being undertaken to diagnose a suspected underlying hormonal abnormality or cause of infertility, it is best performed when intact tissue can be obtained, outside of menses. On the other hand, for the workup of abnormal bleeding, curettage can be done at any time, even while the bleeding occurs.

There is insufficient space here to discuss fully the complex process of menstruation which, suffice to say, involves unique modulations of all the hemostatic mechanisms with which we are familiar. Very briefly, the process follows a chain of events that begins with involution of the corpus luteum. Falling levels of estradiol and progesterone have direct effects upon vascular, stromal, and glandular elements, which then develop a secondary cascade of dynamic interactions. Stromal breakdown, the pathognomonic histologic feature of menstruation, is initiated by the progesterone drop, which forces stromal cells into apoptosis.[15] At the same time, a sequence of vascular effects is initiated as follows:

1. Falling levels of estradiol reduce the intracapillary and intravenular hydrostatic pressure.
2. This drop in pressure in the vessels allows reabsorption of stromal edema fluid.
3. Loss of edema fluid from the stroma rapidly causes a decrease in endometrial thickness.
4. The spiral arterioles, which are structured as irregular spirals, collapse and kink.
5. Obstruction of blood flow in the spiral arterioles caused by kinking results in ischemia of the overlying endometrial tissue.
6. About 20 hours after menstruation starts, intense prostaglandin-induced vasoconstriction controls the blood loss.[10,18]

It follows from this outline that true menstruation cannot occur in the absence of ovulation. The complete process depends on falling levels of both estrogen and progesterone. From a morphologic point of view, the absence of fragments of endometrial epithelium showing changes of secretory exhaustion is one clue that the process is anovulatory. A second clue that the breakdown is anovulatory in type is the presence of fibrin thrombi, not normally seen in a true menstrual phase endometrium. The level in the endometrium at which the tissue remains rather than is shed is thus determined by the level at which the dependence on the spiral arteriole blood supply ceases. Usually, the basal layer remains, with a variable, narrow band of the spongy zone. The remaining tissue is then ready to begin proliferating again at the start of the next cycle. In fact, it is usually possible to appreciate an overlap between the menstrual breakdown and beginning proliferation; curettings taken after menstruation is well established will often contain crumbling tissue, intact basal endometrium, and early proliferating endometrium. A further feature of the endometrium at menstruation is the presence of a neutrophil polymorph infiltrate, which is seen as a response to necrotic tissue and does not indicate acute infection.

ENDOMETRIUM AFTER THE MENOPAUSE

Once the ovaries cease their cyclic production of estrogen and progesterone, the endometrium is no longer subject to its normal stimulation and undergoes atrophy. The endometrium

after the menopause is usually thin and inactive, although varying somewhat in thickness (Figures 12.63–12.65), and becoming quite atrophic in the elderly. The glands are typically small and sparse, and are often not evenly distributed throughout the tissue. They exhibit an epithelium composed of cuboidal or flattened cells (Figure 12.66). The stroma becomes fibrous and the stromal cells lose virtually all their cytoplasm, with the result that the stroma of the postmenopausal endometrium may appear remarkably cellular. Commonly, the endometrium is so thin and meager in amount that biopsy specimens yield only strips of atrophic surface endometrial epithelium (Figures 12.67–12.69). Exposure to low levels of estrogen, either exogenous or endogenous, can result in a mildly expanded endometrium in which rare mitoses can be seen. This is quaintly referred to as 'weakly proliferative' endometrium.

Some common variants of the pattern just described should be mentioned, in particular the so-called 'cystic atrophy' pattern. The endometrium in this state has glands that are distended, often only slightly (Figure 12.70), but sometimes

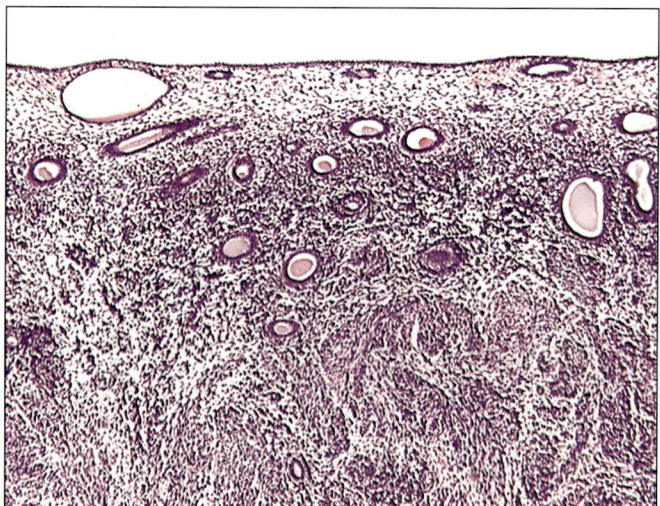

Fig. 12.63 Atrophic postmenopausal endometrium.

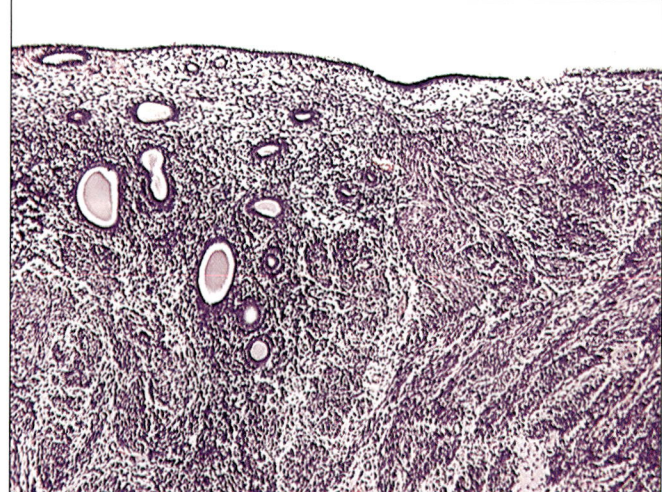

Fig. 12.64 Atrophic postmenopausal endometrium. In some areas, the endometrium is entirely absent.

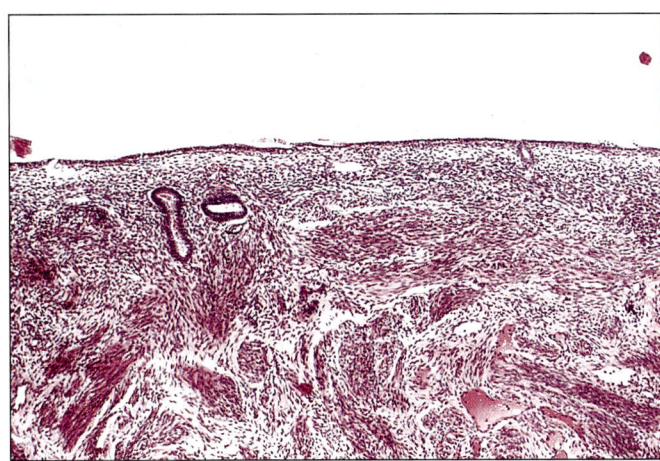

Fig. 12.65 Atrophic postmenopausal endometrium that is thin with rare atrophic glands and minimal stroma.

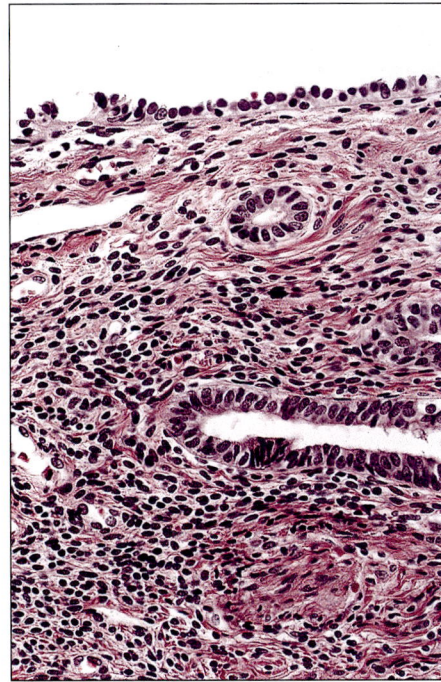

Fig. 12.66 Atrophic postmenopausal endometrium with a slightly fibrous stroma.

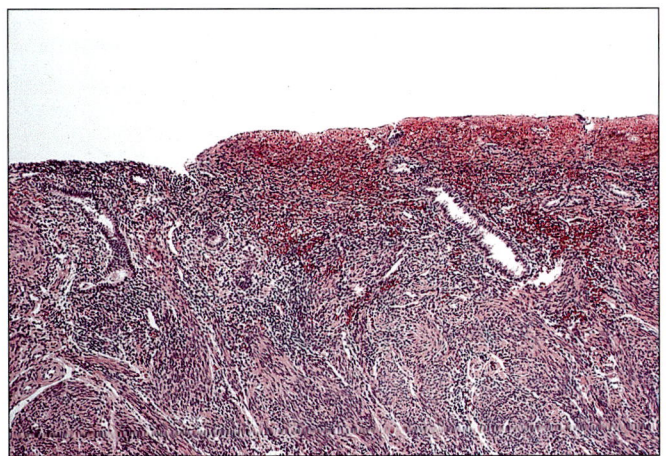

Fig. 12.67 Atrophic postmenopausal endometrium. Appearances in hysterectomy specimen following curettage.

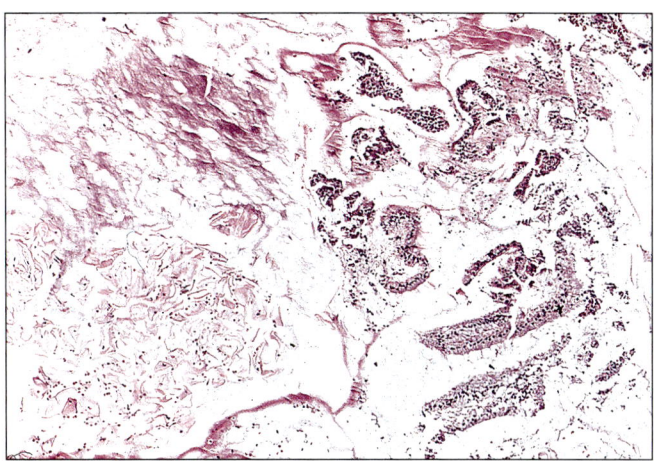

Fig. 12.68 Atrophic postmenopausal endometrium. Scanty endometrial curettage specimen, with tiny broken epithelial fragments, mucus and blood.

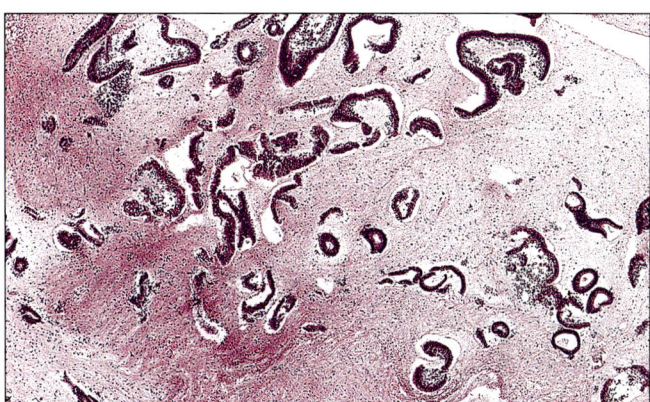

Fig. 12.69 Atrophic postmenopausal endometrium. Scanty curettage specimen.

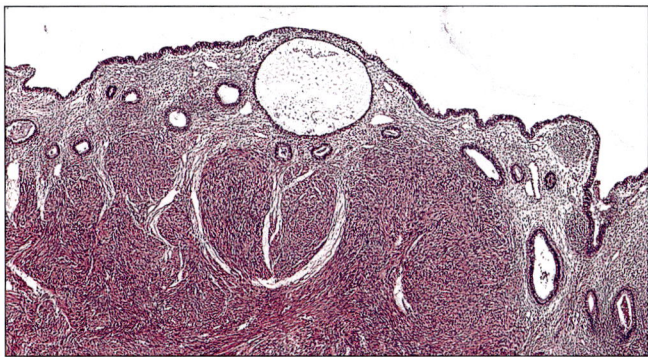

Fig. 12.70 Atrophic postmenopausal endometrium, with some cystic dilatation.

strikingly so (Figure 12.71). The epithelium lining the distended glands is flattened and inactive and the lumens contain material that is partly non-specific secretion and partly transudate. This change may occasionally be so marked and widespread as to be apparent to the naked eye on opening the uterus (so-called 'Swiss cheese endometrium'). This condition may arise in two ways: (1) as a result of benign hyperplasia present at the time

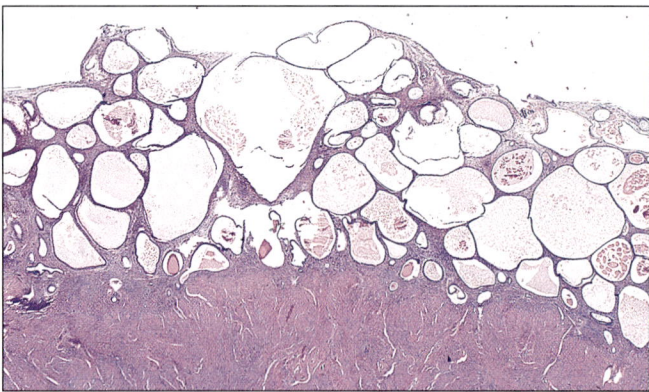

Fig. 12.71 Cystic atrophic postmenopausal endometrium.

of the menopause regressing as its hormonal support diminishes, with the architectural cystic pattern remaining without the accompanying cellular activity; and (2) as a simple obstruction of the endometrial gland ostia by the stromal fibrosis that occurs after the menopause. It must be remembered that the epithelium of the endometrium secretes not only in response to progesterone but also produces a non-specific, seromucinous secretion at other times: before puberty, after the menopause, and in the first half of the menstrual cycle. Obstruction of the glands will therefore always produce an accumulation of this secretion in the lumens, resulting in distension.

It is, of course, paramount to distinguish cystic atrophy from postmenopausal hyperplasia: the atrophic appearance of the epithelium and the lack of mitotic figures in glands and stroma of the former condition distinguish the two. The presence of a proliferative endometrium in a woman past the age of 60 years is abnormal and, in the absence of a history of exogenous estrogen usage, is regarded by many as hyperplasia.

METHODS OF ENDOMETRIAL SAMPLING

DILATATION AND CURETTAGE (D&C)

For decades, diagnostic curettage has been the most common operation performed on women,[40] and all histopathologists, however inexperienced, will have had some experience of endometrial curettings. The procedure is not without its limitations. Hemorrhage, infection, and uterine perforation may occur and, because cervical dilatation is painful, the risks associated with the necessary general anesthetic are also present. Furthermore, although a carefully performed curettage should involve removing essentially all the endometrium from the uterine cavity, this ideal is rarely achieved. Consequently, as many as 5% of hyperplasias or carcinomas remain without detection in curettage immediately preceding hysterectomy.[33] Most specimens are adequate for a reliable histologic assessment.

ENDOMETRIAL BIOPSY

Removal of a single strip of endometrium may be undertaken as an outpatient procedure, without cervical dilatation or general anesthetic. A sharp curette that is considerably smaller than that used for conventional curettage is used but nevertheless the procedure may cause moderate pain. This technique is rarely used.

VABRA ASPIRATOR

This is a suction curette device composed of a 3–4 mm diameter steel cannula that has an opening on one side of its bent tip. The endometrial tissue is obtained by suction with an attached syringe. The amount of material this procedure captures varies from specimens that are as abundant as a curettage, usually in women of reproductive age, to blood and minute fragments, often in a postmenopausal woman, which may not be adequate for histologic assessment.

PIPELLE BIOPSY

This is probably the most widely used outpatient method used today in the United States and Europe to sample the endometrial cavity. The device is a flexible plastic tube, 3.1 mm in diameter, with a solid tip and a side port. A vacuum is created by the withdrawal of a piston from the cannula and, as the device is gently rotated and moved from side to side as it is withdrawn from the uterus, endometrial tissue is sucked into the cannula by the slight negative pressure. This procedure is quick and while causing significantly less pain than the Novak curette or Vabra aspirator, it is nonetheless uncomfortable, especially if the cervix must be dilated. Although it produces less tissue, the diagnostic accuracy of the Pipelle biopsy is similar to that of the Vabra aspirator.[20] It is no less reliable than other techniques for identifying endometrial carcinoma,[7,27] although some studies have suggested a poor pick-up rate for early, low-volume tumors.[6,31]

CYTOLOGIC EVALUATION OF THE ENDOMETRIUM

Cervical smears, while generally inadequate and unreliable for the recognition of endometrial adenocarcinoma, let alone subtly assessing endometrial status, may on occasion disclose the presence of malignant endometrial cells [5,24] The presence of normal endometrial cells up to days 10–12 of the menstrual cycle is within normal limits and cytologists rarely report them. It is good cytologic practice to report morphologically normal endometrial cells seen beyond days 10–12 or in postmenopausal women. Identifying endometrial intraepithelial neoplasia (EIN) and differentiating it from proliferative and secretory endometrial cells are unrealistic possibilities using conventional cervical smears.

DIRECT ENDOMETRIAL CYTOLOGIC SAMPLING

The study of cytologic samples obtained by direct sampling is a challenging yet rewarding area for the cytologist.[25,26] In Japan, there is a significant literature supporting its use. In recent years, in the United States, there has also been a resurgent interest using the Tao Brush technique in combination with liquid-based cytology.[19,36,37] The Tao Brush, a highly optimized device for collecting endometrial cytology specimens, allows for sampling without excessive manipulation of a substantial (3 cm) portion of the endometrial cavity. The brush's outer sheath minimizes endocervical and vaginal cell contamination. The smooth, rounded end minimizes the chances of uterine wall injury or inadvertent myometrial perforation. The flexible wire core allows the device's sampling portion to glide over uterine cavity irregularities. It is also constructed so that the outer sheath can be precisely retracted to the level of the cervical internal os. Of import, the technique is relatively painless.

In practice, the sheathed Tao Brush is inserted to the level of the uterine fundus. The overlying sheath is then retracted, exposing the brush's bristles to the endometrium lining the uterine cavity. Because the brush's bristles are arrayed in the fashion of an augur, the brush is rotated about four or five times in one direction, using an action similar to that used in winding a wrist watch. The sheath is replaced over the brush bristles in order to entrap the collected material *in utero*. After the closed assembly is safely removed from the uterus, the brush is pushed out of its cannula and exposed to fixative; the brush is then cut off into liquid fixative.

In the experience with over 2000 cytobrush specimens to date,[19] endometrial cytology has proven to be an effective technique for the discovery and diagnosis of malignant and premalignant states. An important facet is that the brush often returns small fragments of endometrium, similar to a mini-biopsy. In brushings from 656 hysterectomy specimens, cell blocks advanced the 'exact' diagnostic agreement of cytology slides to source tissue slides from 80 to 93% (Figures 12.72–12.74).

HYSTEROSCOPY

In recent years, hysteroscopy has become a valuable additional method for assessing the uterine cavity.[34] Hysteroscopy,[21] accompanied where necessary by biopsy or Pipelle aspiration, is rapidly replacing curettage in the investigation of menstrual disorders, with significant cost-benefits. The hysteroscope is a rigid optical instrument 4 mm in diameter with a distal lens. Its widespread use became practical with the development of

high-powered fiberoptic light sources, together with the refinement of methods for distending the uterine cavity. During hysteroscopic examination, the instrument is introduced through the cervix, with 0.9% saline or carbon dioxide gas as the most commonly used distension medium. Exposure to the hypotonic saline solution can create significant histologic artifact if the tissue is not rapidly fixed.

ENDOMETRIAL RESECTION (ABLATION)

The advent of hysteroscopy as a reliable method of assessing the uterine cavity, in conjunction with directed biopsy or other forms of endometrial sampling, has led the way to conservative methods of treating abnormal uterine bleeding. If certain qualifying criteria are met, including biopsy-proven absence of hyperplasia or malignancy, the patient may be treated by endometrial ablation rather than hysterectomy.[17] Although most

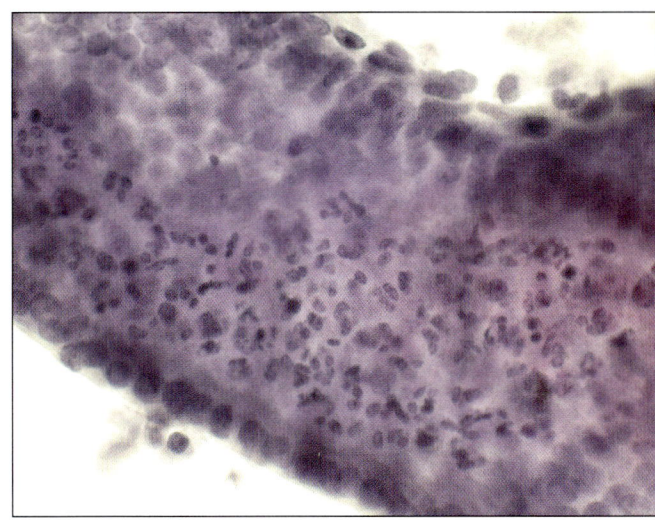

Fig. 12.73 Endometrial smear with breakdown and neutrophilic infiltrate. Tao Brush technique. (Courtesy of Dr John Maksem.)

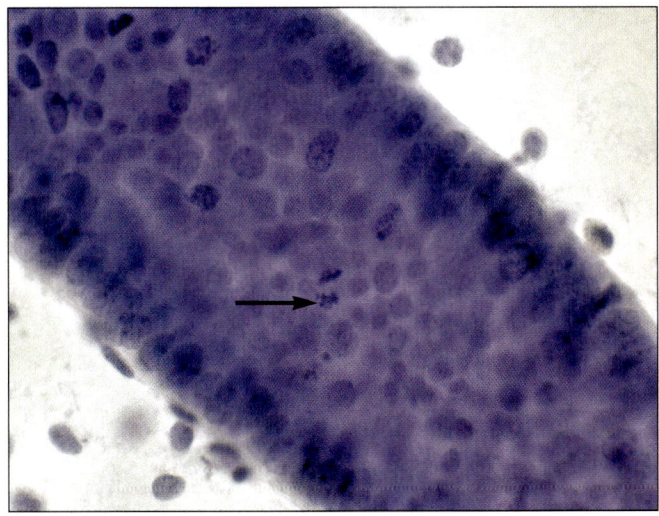

Fig. 12.72 Endometrial smear with mitosis (arrow) in proliferative endometrium. Tao Brush technique. (Courtesy of Dr John Maksem.)

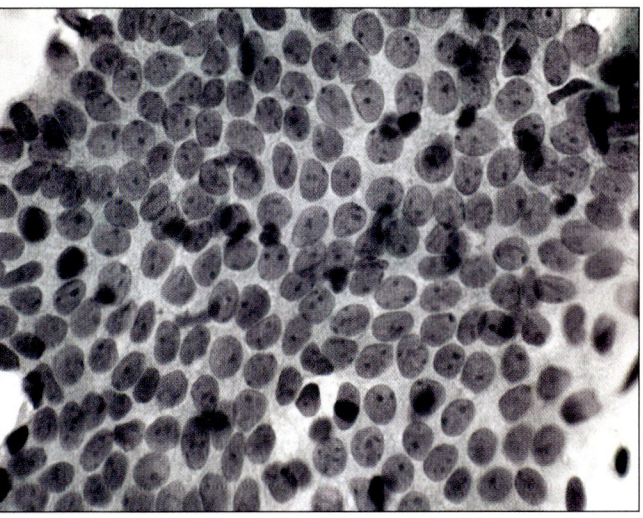

Fig. 12.74 Atrophic endometrial smear with small bland stromal cells. Tao Brush technique. (Courtesy of Dr John Maksem.)

centers treating patients by endometrial ablation employ hysteroscopy, this is not an absolute prerequisite. The techniques aim to remove the entire endometrium, including the basal layer, thereby preventing regrowth, and inducing a therapeutic Ashermans syndrome, where synechiae form and the anterior and posterior walls become adherent. Many different methods have been used in the past and several are still available. The most widely used are laser ablation, endometrial resection, and rollerball ablation.[29] In recent years, numerous different technologies have become available, including thermal balloon (ThermaChoice), circulated hot fluid (Hydro ThermAblator), cryotherapy (HerOption), radiofrequency electrosurgery (NovaSure), and microwave energy (MEA). All are effective if properly applied. Endometrial resection is the only method of special interest to the histopathologist because it produces a specimen. The procedure uses the cutting loop of a resecting hysteroscope. The depth of cut with a resection loop is 3–4 mm. Because the endometrial thickness varies from 3 to 12 mm during the menstrual cycle, the endometrium is usually first suppressed with either danazol or gonadotrophin-releasing hormone analogues. This hormonal manipulation must be taken into account by the histopathologist interpreting the resected material.

Endometrial resection produces a specimen that looks rather like bulky endometrial curettings but as it consists largely of myometrium, the tissue is firmer than curettings in the fixed state (Figure 12.75). Microscopic examination confirms that the tissue is composed predominantly of myometrium, most pieces being covered by thin, inactive endometrium if the patient has been properly prepared (e.g., with danazol). Endocervical tissue is often present. Diathermy artifact frequently hinders histologic interpretation, particularly at the edges of the fragments. It is important to look for hyperplasia and carcinoma, although these should both have been excluded before the procedure was undertaken.[17] The presence of adenomyosis correlates with a poor outcome following endometrial ablation[23] due to the superficial adenomyotic islands regenerating into pockets of functioning endometrium. Whether this diagnosis can be made with any confidence in the resected material

is debatable, because of random orientation of the pieces of tissue and the normal irregularity of the endometrial–myometrial junction. Even in cases where endometrial resection has failed to control uterine bleeding and the patient has subsequently undergone a hysterectomy that has shown adenomyosis histologically, we have been unable to identify adenomyosis retrospectively with confidence in the resection specimen. Despite these mitigating factors, a histologic suspicion of adenomyosis in the endomyometrial strips should be communicated to the surgeon in the ultimate interests of managing patient expectations.

Several reports describe large series of patients who have undergone endometrial resection.[16] Over 80% of patients have been satisfied with the procedure.[2,34] In unsatisfactory cases, a repeat procedure can sometimes be performed without resorting to hysterectomy. Women in whom the procedure fails to cure the symptoms may then be treated by hysterectomy. If performed within weeks of ablation, often there is a foreign-body giant cell reaction and carbonaceous debris affecting the lining of the cavity. This debris is cleared over the course of ensuing months, when gross examination of the uterus usually shows a narrow cavity, often with patches of endometrium visible. Microscopy shows residual endometrium, often poorly organized, and a zone of fibrosis in the underlying myometrium (Figure 12.76).

PROBLEMS IN INTERPRETATION OF ENDOMETRIAL SPECIMENS

The endometrium is a composite tissue. Glands, stroma, blood vessels, and lymphocytes all contribute to the physiologic and non-physiologic changes that together enable a histologic diagnosis to be made. If any of these components is lacking, or if the relations among them are disrupted, the validity of a histologic diagnosis is compromised. To definitively identify the phase of the menstrual cycle requires intact endometrial functionalis capable of being oriented. Problems therefore arise in interpreting the endometrial tissue if the specimen is scanty, broken, or traumatized during its collection.

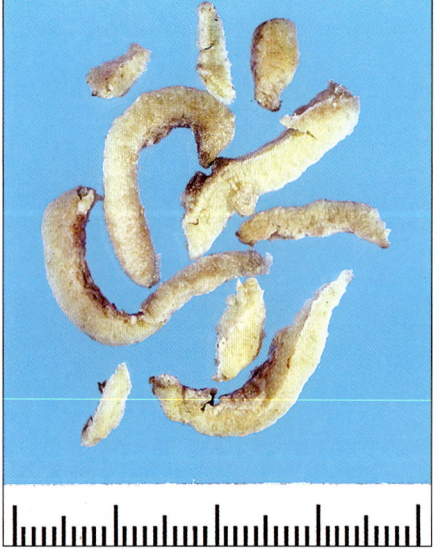

Fig. 12.75 Endometrial resection specimen.

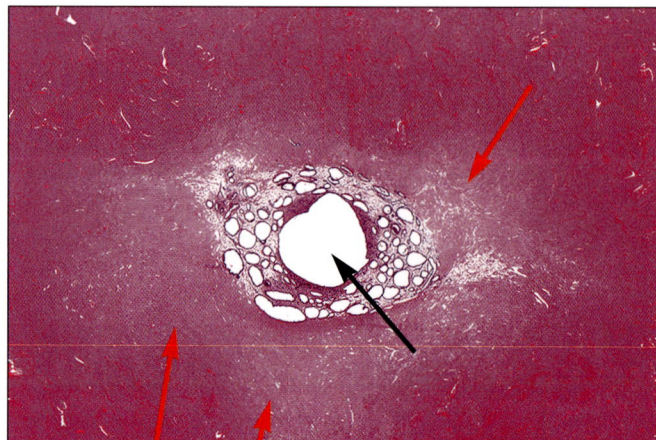

Fig. 12.76 Failed endometrial ablation. A narrow uterine cavity is present (black arrow) with somewhat disorganized residual endometrium. Deep to this is a zone of fibrosis (red arrows) in the central myometrium.

ADEQUACY

A very scanty specimen may be a problem with any method of collection of an endometrial sample, but seems to be more frequently encountered with material obtained by outpatient methods, such as the Pipelle biopsy. If the endometrium is abundant, as it is during the late proliferative and secretory phase of a normal cycle, as well as in many cases where there is hyperplasia or carcinoma, an adequate diagnostic sample is likely to be obtained, irrespective of the method of sampling.

If little endometrial tissue is present in the uterus, as in postmenopausal atrophy, a very scanty specimen usually results irrespective of the method of collection. The scanty specimen may consist of mucus and blood with tiny broken strips of surface and glandular epithelium, sometimes with a little stroma attached, but often with no stroma at all (Figures 12.68, 12.69 and 12.77), and frequently cervical tissue removed *en passant*.

In these circumstances, it is tempting simply to dismiss the specimen as inadequate and unsuitable for diagnosis. Certainly, these specimens are not suitable for a definitive diagnosis or exclusion of pathology, but, nevertheless, some comment can usually be made that may help the gynecologist. The epithelium may be classified as inactive if it is cuboidal or columnar without evidence of mitotic figures or secretory vacuoles, or proliferative if even only one mitotic figure is seen. If secretory vacuoles are present, either subnuclear or supranuclear, the epithelium may be designated as secretory in type (Figure 12.78). For specimens taken in the course of monitoring women on hormone replacement therapy (HRT), for example, comments such as these can be helpful. It is important to avoid the statement that the specimen is 'inadequate for histologic assessment', since the expected result in an atrophic endometrium is a scant specimen. The statement of inadequacy may force the gynecologist in this instance to unnecessarily repeat the procedure.

In postmenopausal women, 'inadequate' should be reserved for those specimens where there is literally no endometrial tissue at all. We find it useful in these cases simply to report the tissue components that are present and note that the material is 'unsuitable for further useful comment', allowing the individual gynecologist to decide what other diagnostic workup, if any, is indicated. This approach is particularly pertinent in the not uncommon scenario of a postmenopausal patient having a D&C for 'thickened endometrium seen on ultrasound'. At the same time, however, both the pathologist and the gynecologist must be aware that these very scanty specimens cannot guarantee that no pathology is present in the endometrium. It is false to believe that if hyperplasia or carcinoma is present, then there is ample tissue in the uterus to provide a specimen containing the abnormality, but experience warns us that this is not necessarily so. We have all come across cases where the biopsy (or even curettings) has been scanty and apparently negative and a subsequent hysterectomy has revealed carcinoma.

DISSOCIATION ARTIFACT

If the stroma separating endometrial glands is disrupted or lost, then the relations of the glands to each other become disturbed. This usually means that the glands lie closer together than normal (Figures 12.79 and 12.80) but sometimes they are widely separated by mucus or clear space. This false crowding may be sufficiently marked to give a back-to-back appearance and an erroneous impression of hyperplasia or even carcinoma. The most commonly encountered situation in which this phenomenon occurs is in menstrual endometrium, when due allowance can usually be made because the phase of the cycle is obvious (Figure 12.81). Dissociation artifact is more of a problem when traumatic sampling damages the stroma at other times in the cycle. The changes are usually focal, so that at least some of the endometrium appears normal but groups of glands are crowded, without intervening stroma. Careful examination will show that the stroma between and around these glands has been disrupted, so that the abnormal architectural pattern can be disregarded. Additionally, there is rarely if ever any significant complexity to the crowded glandular structures (multiple lumens, irregular outlines, etc.) that are common in neoplasia and their precursors. Sometimes, however, even careful examination may fail to resolve the dilemma (Figures 12.82 and 12.83).

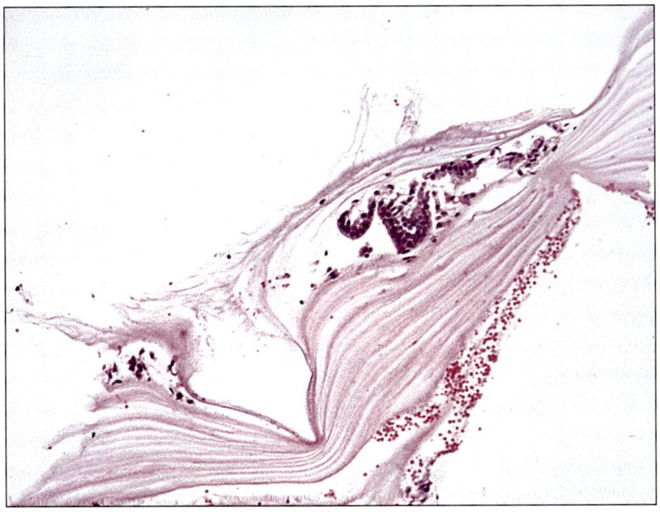

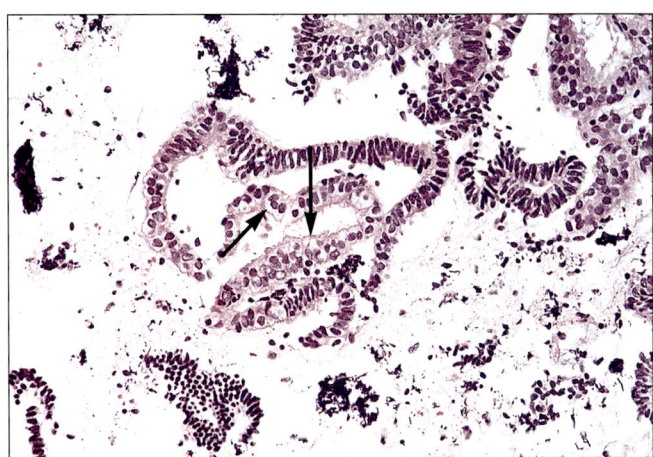

Fig. 12.77 Pipelle aspiration specimen. A single strip of epithelium is present amongst the mucus.

Fig. 12.78 Pipelle aspiration specimen. A very scanty specimen in which a little secretory activity is discernible (arrows).

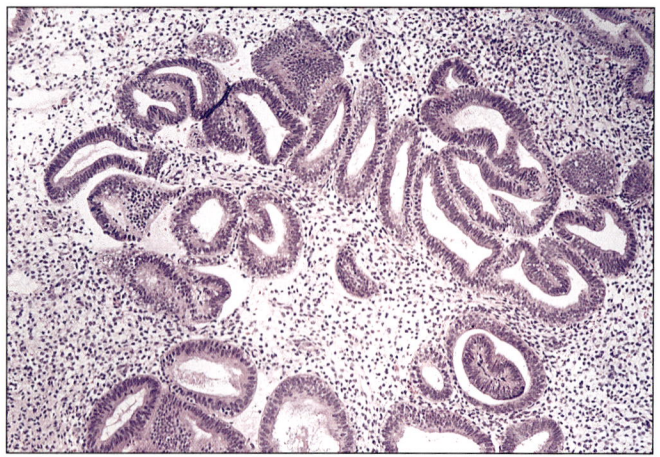

Fig. 12.79 Endometrial curettings. The glands are artifactually crowded because of traumatic breaking of the stroma.

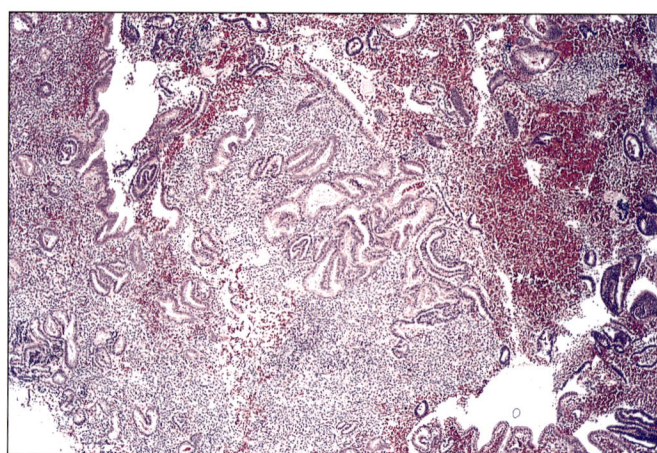

Fig. 12.82 Endometrial curettings. The stroma is broken and the crowding of the glands may be artifactual as a result of this.

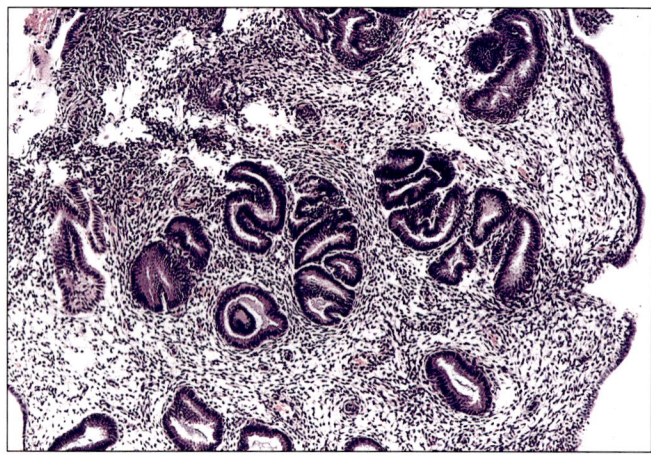

Fig. 12.80 Endometrial curettings. The glands are artifactually crowded because of traumatic fragmentation of the stroma. These appearances must not be mistaken for complex hyperplasia.

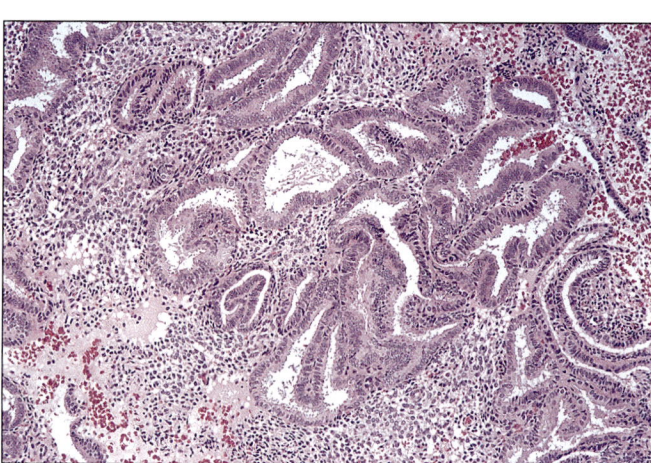

Fig. 12.83 Endometrial curettings (higher power of Figure 12.82). Although there is some stromal break-up, this does not seem enough to account for the degree of crowding. Experts disagreed as to whether what is shown here is complex hyperplasia or not.

TELESCOPING ARTIFACT

This is another effect of trauma on the endometrium brought about at the time of sampling, whereby the glands undergo intussusception, producing a gland-within-gland appearance. The result is what appears, at first sight, to be a complex glandular pattern at low magnification (Figure 12.84). An erroneous diagnosis of hyperplasia or even carcinoma may be made. Closer examination shows that each of these apparently complex glandular structures is completely surrounded by a circle of epithelium representing the original gland outline (Figures 12.85–12.87) and it is this feature that enables true hyperplasia to be excluded. This differential diagnosis is a genuine one only for those inexperienced in proliferative phase endometrium, where a non-secretory epithelial phenotype and mitotic activity complicate the picture.

Other patterns may be encountered, such as apparent focal reduplication of glands, which is also most probably artifactual (Figure 12.88).

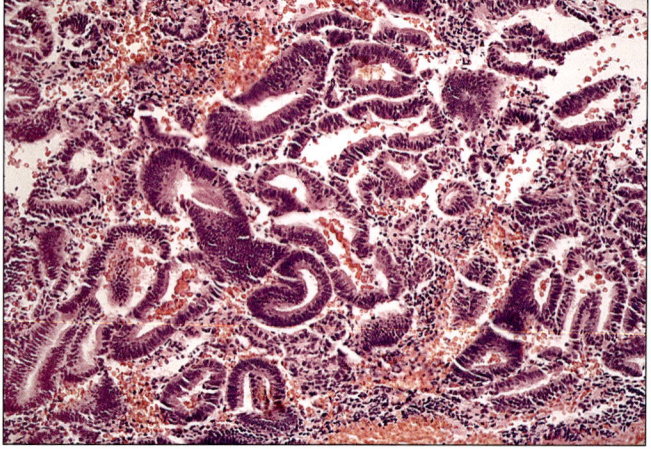

Fig. 12.81 Endometrial curettings. The glands are artifactually crowded because of menstrual breakdown of the stroma.

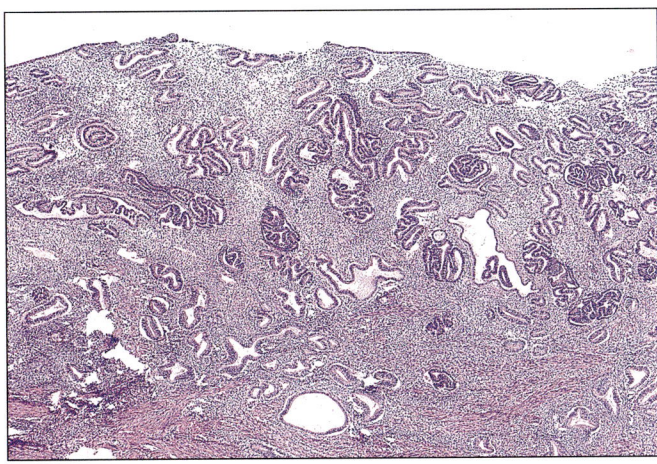

Fig. 12.84 Endometrial curettings. Telescoping artifact. Low power.

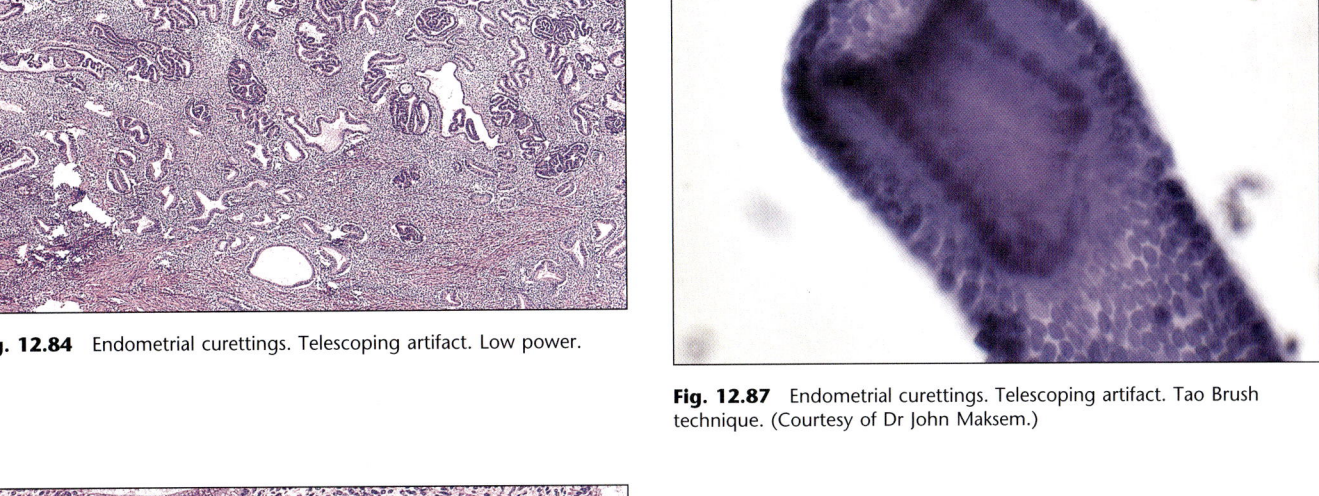

Fig. 12.87 Endometrial curettings. Telescoping artifact. Tao Brush technique. (Courtesy of Dr John Maksem.)

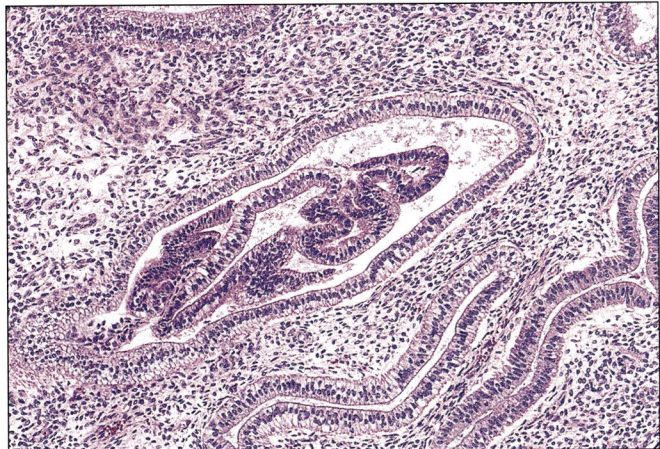

Fig. 12.85 Endometrial curettings. Telescoping artifact.

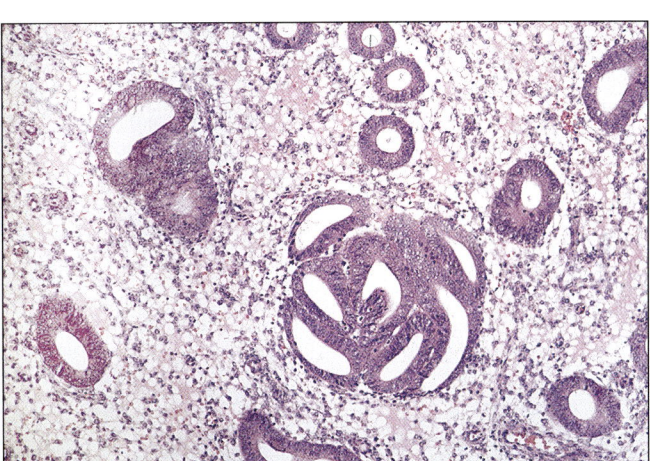

Fig. 12.88 Endometrial curettings. Artifact. This appearance, where there seems to be reduplication of one glandular unit, is distinct from telescoping as there is no surrounding epithelial rim. No stromal damage is apparent, so the process is different from the artifactual crowding resulting from that. Although previously categorized as 'focal adenomatous hyperplasia', this feature is likely to be an artifact.

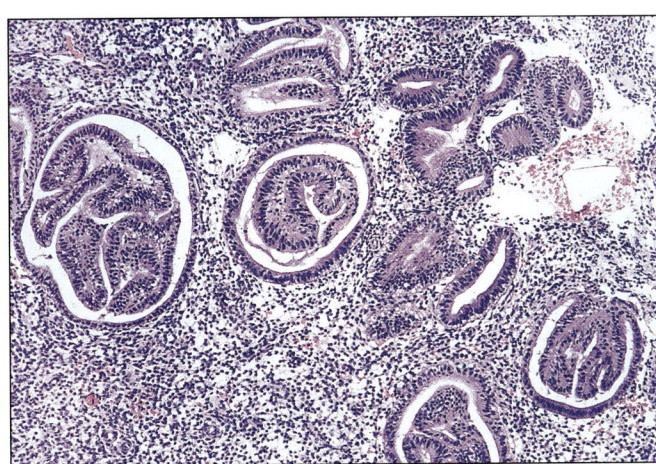

Fig. 12.86 Endometrial curettings. Telescoping artifact. This apparently complicated pattern is most probably the result of glandular epithelium intussuscepting as the curettage is performed. The presence of a complete epithelial circle surrounding the unit allows hyperplasia to be excluded.

FIXATION ARTIFACT

If fixation of the endometrial specimen is poor or delayed, the stroma may retract away from the glands, leaving an artifactual clear space around the glands. At low magnification, this may give a false impression of subnuclear vacuolation and so compromise accurate dating of the sample (Figure 12.89). Careful examination under high power allows this artifact to be recognized. Endometrium autolyzes rapidly and timely exposure to fixative is important in hysterectomy specimens so as to avoid a major 'laboratory' error from which no recovery is possible. Many pathology services recommend the surgeon open the uterus before placing it in adequate fixative.

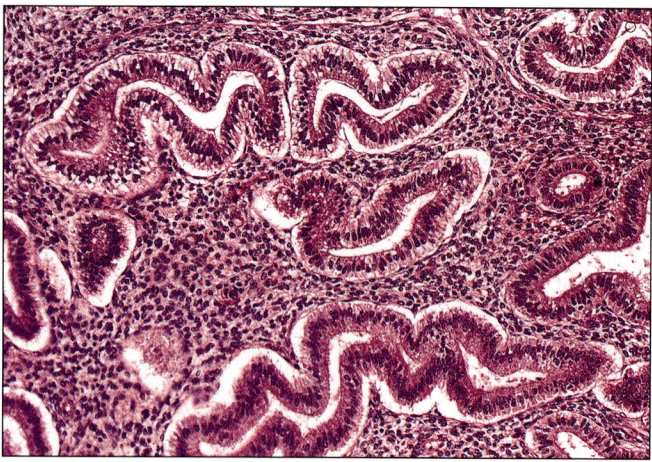

Fig. 12.89 Endometrium. Fixation artifact.

LEGITIMATE TISSUE CONTAMINANTS

Non-endometrial components are frequently and legitimately found in curettings. Endocervical tissue is common; it is nearly always easy to identify and should not cause any problems. Microglandular hyperplasia, however, is not always easily recognizable and care must be taken not to mistake it for endometrial pathology because of its superficial resemblance to hyperplasia or carcinoma. Endocervical stroma containing plasma cells can, if not correctly identified, mislead the pathologist to diagnose endometritis, particularly if the clinical notes indicate 'removal of intrauterine contraceptive device' or some such. Stratified squamous epithelium from the ectocervix or vagina is also seen quite often. Occasionally, but of great import, the diagnosis of cervical intraepithelial neoplasia (CIN) is first made as a result of cervical contamination of endometrial curettings.

Fragments of smooth muscle may represent normal myometrium or a submucous leiomyoma, a distinction that it is not always possible to make from the pattern of the muscle bundles. The presence of adipose tissue in endometrial curettings means that the uterus has likely been perforated, although a rare uterine tumor such as lipoleiomyoma can contain fat. This information should immediately be communicated to the clinician (although, in our experiences, clinicians often already know that perforation has happened or report that the patient is not having any detectable adverse effects). Fetal tissues (bone, cartilage, neural tissue) may be found unexpectedly, without clinical reference to a recent miscarriage.

REFERENCES

1. Booker SS, Jayanetti C, Karalak S, Hsiu JG, Archer DF. The effect of progesterone on the accumulation of leukocytes in the human endometrium. Am J Obstet Gynecol 1994;171:139–42.
2. Broadbent JAM, Magos AL. Endometrial resection follow up: late onset of pain and the effect of depot medroxyprogesterone acetate. Br J Obstet Gynaecol 1995;102:673.
3. Brosens JJ, Desouza NM, Barker FG. Uterine junctional zone: function and disease. Lancet 1995;346:558–60.
4. Bulletti C, de Ziegler D. Uterine contractility and embryo implantation. Curr Opin Obstet Gynecol 2006;18:473–84.
5. DuBeshter B. Endometrial cancer: predictive value of cervical cytology. Gynecol Oncol 1999;72:271–2.
6. Ferry J, Farnsworth A, Webster M, Wren B. The efficacy of the pipelle endometrial biopsy in detecting endometrial carcinoma. Aust N Z J Obstet Gynaecol 1993;33:76–8.
7. Guido RS, Kanbourshakir A, Rulin MC, Christopherson WA. Pipelle endometrial sampling: sensitivity in the detection of endometrial cancer. J Reprod Med 1995;40:553–5.
8. Heller DS. The normal endometrium. New York: Igaku–Shoin Medical; 1994.
9. Hoozemans DA, Schats R, Lambalk CB, Homburg R, Hompes PG. Human embryo implantation: current knowledge and clinical implications in assisted reproductive technology. Reprod Biomed Online 2004;9:692–715.
10. Jabbour HN, Sales KJ. Prostaglandin receptor signalling and function in human endometrial pathology. Trends Endocrinol Metab 2004;15:398–404.
11. Kammerer U, Marzusch K, Krober S, Ruck P, Handgretinger R, Dietl J. A subset of CD56+ large granular lymphocytes in first-trimester human decidua are proliferating cells. Fertil Steril 1999;71:74–9.
12. King A, Burrows T, Loke YW. Human uterine natural killer cells. Nat Immun 1996;15:41–52.
13. King A, Burrows T, Verma S, Hiby S, Loke YW. Human uterine lymphocytes. Hum Reprod Update 1998;4:480–5.
14. King A, Hiby SE, Verma S, Burrows T, Gardner L, Loke YW. Uterine NK cells and trophoblast HLA class I molecules. Am J Reprod Immunol 1997;37:459–62.
15. Labied S, Kajihara T, Madureira PA, et al. Progestins regulate the expression and activity of the forkhead transcription factor FOXO1 in differentiating human endometrium. Mol Endocrinol 2006;20:35–44.
16. Lethaby A, Hickey M, Garry R. Endometrial destruction techniques for heavy menstrual bleeding. Cochrane Database Syst Rev 2005:CD001501.
17. Lewis BV. Guidelines for endometrial ablation. Br J Obstet Gynaecol 1994;101:470–3.
18. Lumsden M, Norman J. Menstruation and menstrual abnormality. In: Shaw RW, Soutter WP, Stanton SL, eds. Gynaecology, 2nd edn. New York: Churchill Livingstone; 1997:421–40.
19. Maksem JA, Meiers I, Robboy SJ. A primer of endometrial cytology with histological correlation. Diag Cytopathol 2007;35:817–44.
20. Manganiello PD, Burrows LJ, Dain BJ, Gonzalez J. Vabra aspirator and pipelle endometrial suction curette – a comparison. J Reprod Med 1998;43:889–92.
21. Marsh F, Duffy S. The technique and overview of flexible hysteroscopy. Obstet Gynecol Clin North Am 2004;31:655–68, xi.
22. Mazur MT, Kurman RJ. Normal endometrium and infertility evaluation. New York: Springer; 1995.
23. McCausland V, McCausland A. The response of adenomyosis to endometrial ablation/resection. Hum Reprod Update 1998;4:350–9.
24. Mitchell H, Giles G, Medley G. Accuracy and survival benefit of cytological prediction of endometrial carcinoma on routine cervical smears. Int J Gynecol Pathol 1993;12:34–40.
25. Morse A, Beard RW. Endometrial cytology [editorial]. J Roy Soc Med 1984;77:997–8.
26. Morse AR, Ellice RM, Anderson MC, Beard RW. Reliability of endometrial aspiration cytology in the assessment of endometrial status. Obstet Gynecol 1982;59:513–8.
27. Ong S, Duffy T, Lenehan P, Murphy J. Endometrial pipelle biopsy compared to conventional dilatation and curettage. Irish J Med Sci 1997;166:47–9.
28. Otsuki Y, Misaki O, Sugimoto O, Ito Y, Tsujimoto Y, Akao Y. Cyclic bcl-2 gene expression in human uterine endometrium during menstrual cycle. Lancet 1994;344:28–9.
29. Solnik JM, Guido RS, Sanfilippo JS, Krohn MA. The impact of endometrial ablation technique at a large university women's hospital. Am J Obstet Gynecol 2005;193:98–102.
30. Stewart JA, Bulmer JN, Murdoch AP. Endometrial leucocytes: expression of steroid hormone receptors. J Clin Pathol 1998;51:121–6.
31. Tanriverdi HA, Barut A, Gun BD, Kaya E. Is pipelle biopsy really adequate for diagnosing endometrial disease? Med Sci Monit 2004;10:CR271–4.
32. van den Heuvel MJ, Xie X, Tayade C, et al. A review of trafficking and activation of uterine natural killer cells. Am J Reprod Immunol 2005;54:322–31.
33. Vorgias G, Lekka J, Katsoulis M, Varhalama E, Kalinoglou N, Akrivos T. Diagnostic accuracy of prehysterectomy curettage in determining tumor type and grade in patients with endometrial cancer. MedScape General Med 2003;5:7.
34. Waller KG, Lewis BV. Hysteroscopy. In: Shaw RW, Soutter WP, Stanton SL, eds. Gynaecology, 2nd edn. New York: Churchill Livingstone; 1997:41–52.
35. Williams JW, Hirschowitz L. Assessment of uterine wall thickness and position of the vascular plexus in the deep myometrium: implications for the measurement of depth of myometrial invasion of endometrial carcinomas. Int J Gynecol Pathol 2006;25:59–64.
36. Wu HH, Casto BD, Elsheikh TM. Endometrial brush biopsy. An accurate outpatient method of detecting endometrial malignancy. J Reprod Med 2003;48:41–5.
37. Wu HH, Harshbarger KE, Berner HW, Elsheikh TM. Endometrial brush biopsy (Tao brush). Histologic diagnosis of 200 cases with complementary cytology: an accurate sampling technique for the detection of endometrial abnormalities. Am J Clin Pathol 2000;114:412–8.
38. Yamaguchi T, Kitaya K, Daikoku N, Yasuo T, Fushiki S, Honjo H. Potential selectin L ligands involved in selective recruitment of peripheral blood

CD16(–) natural killer cells into human endometrium. Biol Reprod 2006;74:35–40.

39. Zaino RJ. The logical patterns of the normal endometrial cycle. Interpretation of endometrial biopsies and curettings. In: Silverberg SG, ed. Biopsy Interpretation Series. Philadelphia: Lippincott-Raven; 1996:53–99.

40. Zaino RJ. Indications and methods for sampling the endometrium. Interpretation of endometrial biopsies and curettings. In: Silverberg

SG, ed. Biopsy Interpretation Series.Philadelphia: Lippincott-Raven; 1996:1–10.

41. Zaino RJ. The physiology of the menstrual cycle. Interpretation of endometrial biopsies and curettings. In: Silverberg SG, ed. Biopsy Interpretation Series. Philadelphia: Lippincott-Raven; 1996:11–21.

42. Zaino RJ. Interpretation of endometrial biopsies and curettings. In: Silverberg SG, ed. Biopsy Interpretation Series. New York: Lippincott-Raven; 1996.

Exogenous hormones and their effects on the endometrium

13

Rex C. Bentley   Stanley J. Robboy

INTRODUCTION

Exogenous hormonal agents represent one of the most commonly prescribed medications in women. Hormonal therapies are used for a wide range of indications, including birth control, postmenopausal hormone replacement, dysfunctional uterine bleeding, endometriosis, infertility, and the treatment of neoplastic and preneoplastic lesions of the endometrium and breast. These drugs can be administered by many methods, including oral, parenteral, transdermal, transvaginal, vaginal rings, and subcutaneous or intrauterine implants. Consequently, a significant proportion of endometrial specimens that the surgical pathologist evaluates show the effects of these exogenous hormonal agents. At first glance, the spectrum of changes seen with hormone therapy appears unwieldy broad, and it is certainly true that nearly any endometrial appearance can be attributed to therapy with hormones. With a basic understanding of the effects of estrogens and progestins on the normal endometrium, however, substantial order emerges for this confusing pathologic array. Essentially, it is possible to predict the common appearances of hormone therapy based on the known effects of the endogenous steroid hormones on normal endometrium.

ESTROGENS

The basic effect of estrogens on the endometrium is to induce proliferation of the endometrial glands and stroma, including vascular endothelium. The degree of proliferation can vary in proportion to the estrogenic stimulus. Very low levels of estrogen or a very weak estrogen will lead to an inactive or atrophic endometrium. Higher levels lead to weakly proliferative and, finally, to normally or excessively (hyperplastic) proliferative endometrium with the highest levels (Figure 13.1). The degree of proliferative activity can usually be assessed by the mitotic activity in both the glandular epithelium and the stroma. Women who are many years postmenopause may have little response to estrogen, presumably due in part to profound endometrial atrophy (Figure 13.2). A number of estrogenic drugs on the market are listed in Table 13.1.

Persistent exposure to a significant estrogenic stimulus, such as occurs in anovulation, leads to a pattern of continued, unrelieved proliferation. The endometrium cannot support such continued growth. Whether the estrogen source is endogenous or exogenous, the histologic consequence is the same: a combination of proliferative endometrium with episodic coexisting stromal breakdown, or shedding, which accounts for the clinical presentation of irregular bleeding (Figure 13.3). This pattern is also called 'anovulatory bleeding' or 'anovulatory shedding'. Because the endometrial vessels become abnormally large, bleeding can also be quite severe. Some pathologists mistakenly refer to the shedding endometrium as 'menstrual', but it is important to distinguish this appearance from the appearance of menstrual endometrium occurring at the end of a normal cycle. In normal endometrium, the endometrial glands transform soon after ovulation to a secretory pattern and by the time menstrual bleeding begins will still show some residual changes, most commonly secretory exhaustion (see Chapter 12). This change is absent in anovulatory-type bleeding or where the drug administered is progestin-poor. Another common difference is the presence of large fibrin thrombi in the vessels of anovulatory shedding endometrium (Figure 13.4). They are absent from menstrual endometrium because of the marked fibrinolytic activity typical of normal menstruation.

With more prolonged estrogen exposure, the proliferating glands tend to lose their uniformity of size, shape, and distribution, leading to so-called disordered proliferative endometrium. Cystic dilatation of glands and 'tubal' metaplasia are commonly present. With continued, longer term, unopposed estrogen exposure, a high proportion of patients will ultimately develop benign endometrial hyperplasia. A small number will also go on to develop endometrial intraepithelial neoplasia (EIN), formerly called 'atypical hyperplasia' or even adenocarcinoma (see Chapters 15 and 16).

PROGESTINS

The effect of progestins on the endometrium depends on 'priming' by estrogen, which induces progesterone receptors in the endometrial cells. One important feature of progestins is that they act to downregulate estrogen and progesterone receptors; in other words, they reduce the sensitivity of the endometrium to both of these hormones. Prolonged exposure to progestins can thus lead to a histologic picture that is paradoxically similar to the atrophy seen in a postmenopausal or hormone-suppressed patient. Some commonly used progestins are shown in Table 13.2.

In the short term, however, progestins induce secretory differentiation in endometrial glands and decidual-type change in the stroma, i.e., the classic changes of a normal secretory endometrium (Figure 13.5) and over approximately the same time scale. The glands develop large glycogen vacuoles that are then secreted into the increasingly complex gland lumina (Figure

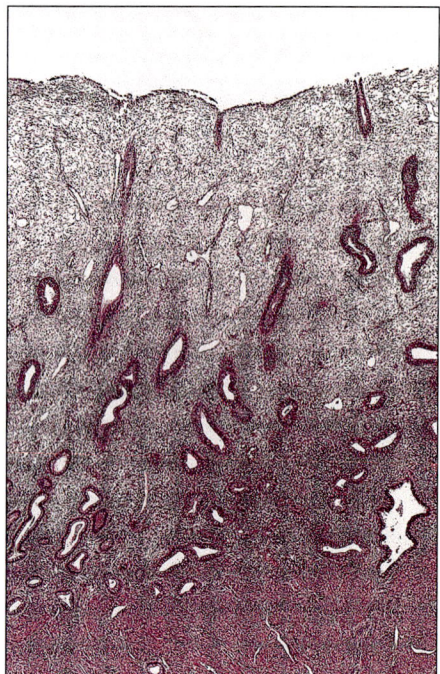

Fig. 13.1 Normal proliferative endometrium (normal estrogen effect).

Table 13.1 Representative estrogenic agents available in the USA

Generic name	US brand name
Estradiol	Estrace
Estradiol valerate	Delestrogen, Gynogen, Valergen
Estradiol (transdermal)	Estraderm, Climara, Fempatch
Diethylstilbesterol	
Conjugated equine estrogens	Premarin
Synthetic conjugated estrogens	Cenestin
Mestranol	
Ethinyl estradiol	Estinyl

From Cada.[13]

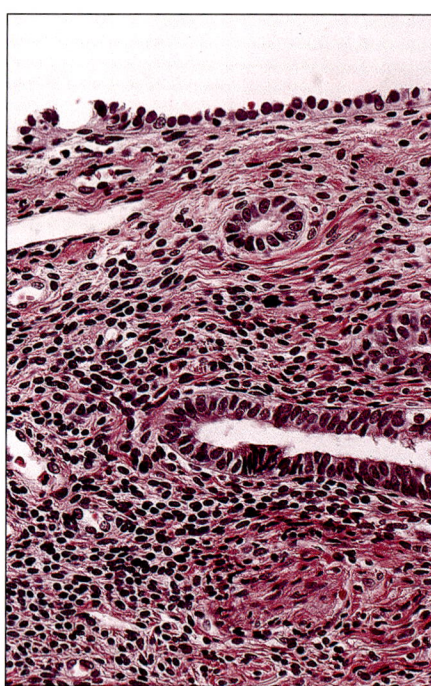

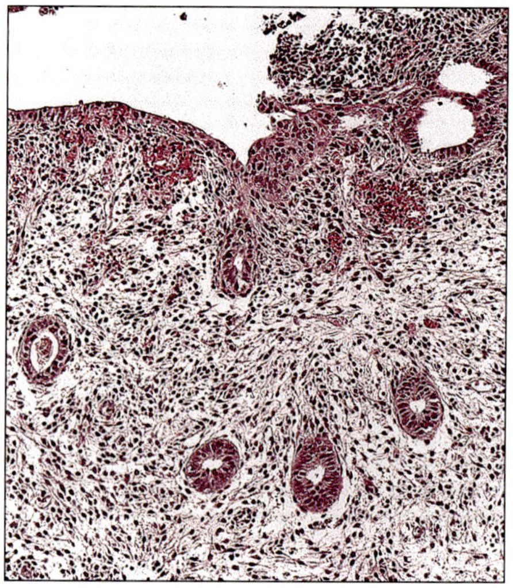

Fig. 13.2 Atrophic endometrium. The few glands present have minimal cytoplasm and small nuclei. The endometrial stroma is dense.

13.6). At the same time, the stromal cells enlarge strikingly, with abundant granular cytoplasm, and appear relatively cohesive, regardless of whether the endometrium is normal (Figure 13.7) or harbors an abnormality, such as a polyp (Figure 13.8).

With continued exposure or repeated cycles, the receptor downregulation causes the glands to lose their sensitivity to estrogens and they develop progressively less secretory change

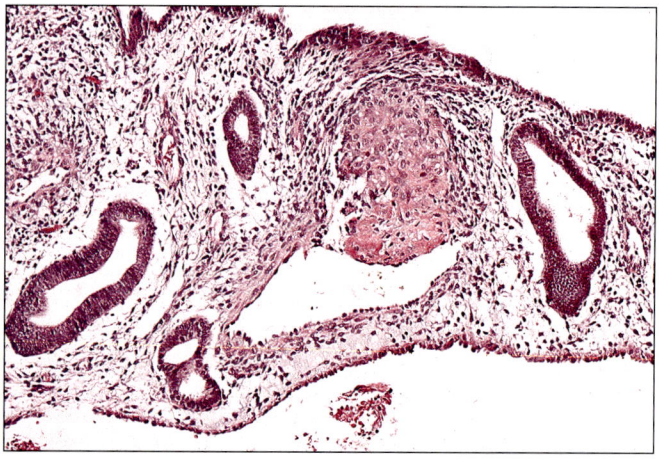

Fig. 13.3 Unopposed estrogen, HRT, proliferative endometrium with breakdown. Present are proliferative endometrium (left) and menstrual type endometrium with stromal balls and eosinophilic epithelial cells (right). This pattern is identical to anovulation in the premenopausal patient.

Fig. 13.4 Fibrin thrombi in endometrium with anovulatory bleeding. The patient had been on tamoxifen.

Table 13.2 Representative progestational agents available in the USA

Generic name	US brand name
Progesterone	Prometrium, Crinone
Hydroxyprogesterone	Hylutin
Medroxyprogesterone	Provera, Depo-Provera, Cycrin, Amen, Curretab
Megesterol acetate	Megace
Norgestrel	
Drospirenone	
Levonorgestrel	Norplant
Norethindrone	Aygestin
Norethynodrel	
Desogestrel	
Norgestimate	

From Cada.[13]

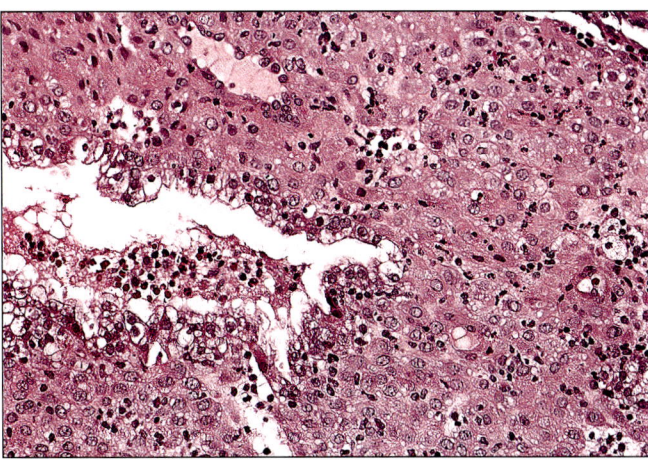

Fig. 13.6 Secretory glands with decidualized endometrium (on progesterone).

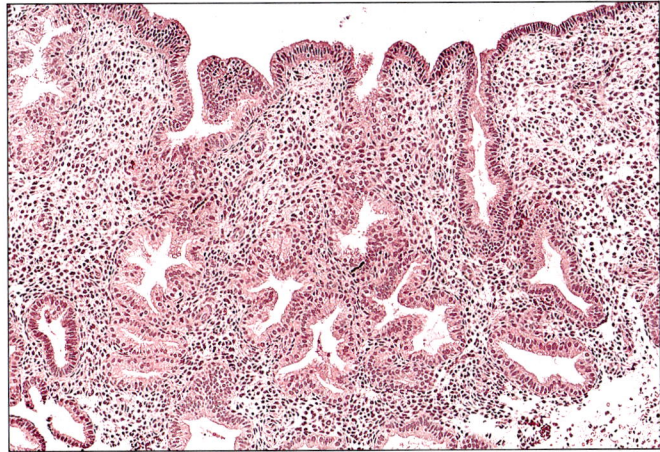

Fig. 13.5 Early secretory endometrium (normal progesterone effect). The woman, who was older, had received progesterone for 20 days.

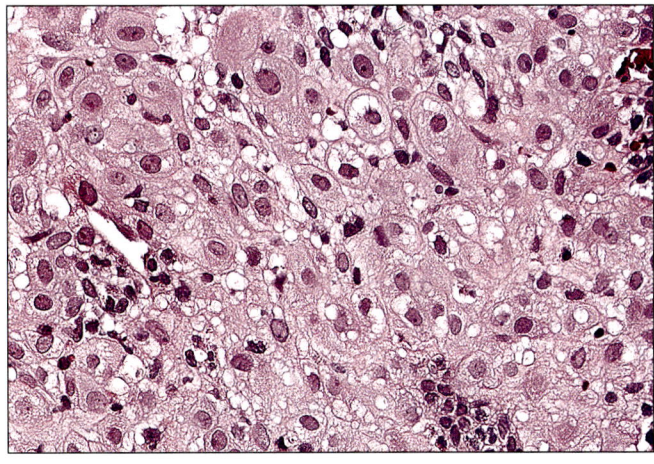

Fig. 13.7 Decidualized endometrium (on progesterone).

('secretory exhaustion'), such that they ultimately appear atrophic. At this stage, which only occurs after prolonged exposure or multiple cycles, the appearance is that of decidualized stroma with widely dispersed atrophic glands, often referred to as a 'pill' endometrium (Figure 13.9). More slowly, the stroma also begins to be suppressed by the receptor downregulation, and over months to years will also become attenuated and atrophic, ultimately losing most of its decidual features. At this point, the appearances resemble endometrial atrophy due to menopause or hormone suppression.

Exposure to high-dose progestins (often given for dysfunctional uterine bleeding and usually with a good initial response) can, paradoxically, cause secondary necrosis of the superficial endometrium, often in the form of wedge-shaped infarcts, and renewed bleeding. The hysteroscopic appearances are often alarming. Both the continued bleeding and the hysteroscopic findings lead the clinician to perform a dilatation and curettage (D&C) to exclude hyperplasia or malignancy and yielding abundant, macroscopically suspicious tissue fragments.

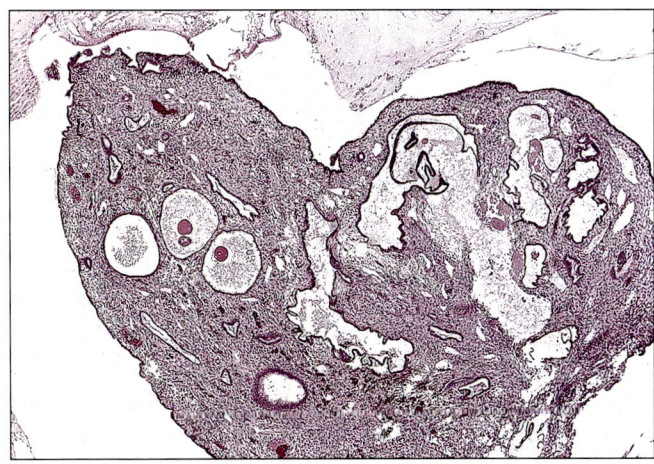

Fig. 13.8 Decidual response of stroma in polyp (on Megace).

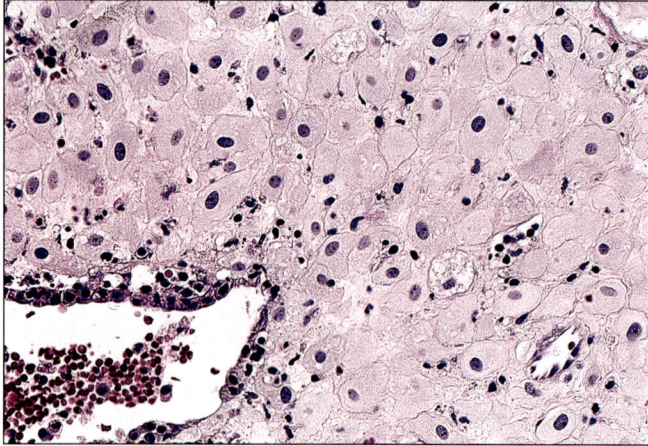

Fig. 13.9 'Pill' endometrium. Atrophic gland in decidualized stroma in woman receiving progesterone.

Occasionally, patients will spontaneously pass large intact sheets of decidualized endometrium ('decidual casts').

ORAL CONTRACEPTIVES

Oral contraceptives (OCs) are one of the most widely used medications in the developed world. They are used as treatment for several common medical problems in addition to contraception, including dysfunctional uterine bleeding and endometriosis. Most OCs are based on a combination of an estrogen and a progestin, given over 21 consecutive days of the cycle, followed by 7 days of placebo tablets yielding a withdrawal week. A variety of types have been developed (Table 13.3). Sequential OCs contain estrogen during the first half of the cycle, with progestin added during the second half. Because of the increased risk of endometrial cancer with some sequential formulations,[91] combined OCs and progestin-only formulations are now the most commonly used types. Combined pills can be monophasic, in which there is a fixed dose of estrogen and a progestin in combination for the 21 days of each cycle, or they can be biphasic or triphasic, depending on whether the progestin dose is altered once or twice during the cycle. In contrast to some sequential OCs and estrogen-only hormone-replacement regimens, which increase the risk of endometrial carcinoma, combined OCs are protective, with the degree of protection increasing with the length of therapy. Patients with 10 years of OC use have about a 75% reduction in endometrial carcinoma.[72,88,93] OC use is also associated with a 30–50% decrease in the risk of ovarian carcinoma, and this lowered risk persists for at least 20 years after cessation of their use.[51,87]

COMBINED ORAL CONTRACEPTIVES

The histologic appearance of the endometrium in a patient on combined OCs is extremely variable, but is dominated by the progestin effects. It depends on various factors, some poorly understood, including the type of pill, the duration of therapy, precise dose of the individual pill, levels of compliance with the regimen, and endogenous hormone synthesis and metabo-

Table 13.3 Composition of representative oral contraceptives available in the USA

Generic name	US brand name
Combination monophasic	
Ethinyl estradiol/norethindrone	Loestrin 1/20, Loestrin 1.5/30, Junel, Brevicon, Nortrel, Modicon Genora 0.5/35, Necon, Norinyl 1+35, Ortho-Novum 1/35, Ovcon-35
Ethinyl estradiol/levonorgestrel	Levlen, Nordette, Alesse, Aviane, Lessina, Levlite
Ethinyl estradiol/norgestrel	Lo/Ovral, Ovral, Cryselle
Ethinyl estradiol/ethynodiol diacetate	Demulen 1/35, Demulen 1/50, Zovia 1/50, Mestranol/norethindrone, Norinyl 1+50, Ortho-Novum 1/50, Norethin 1/50M, Genora 1/50, Nelova 1/50M
Ethinyl estradiol/desogestrel	Desogen, Ortho-Cept
Ethinyl estradiol/norgestimate	Ortho-Cyclen, Sprintec
Ethinyl estradiol/drospirenone	Yasmin, Yaz
Biphasic	
Ethinyl estradiol/norethindrone	Ortho-Novum 10/11, Jenest-28, Necon 10/11
Ethinyl estradiol/desogestrel	Mircette, Kariva
Triphasic	
Ethinyl estradiol/norethindrone	Ortho-Novum 7/7/7, Tri-Norinyl, Estrostep, Aranelle
Ethinyl estradiol/norgestimate	Ortho Tri-Cyclen
Ethinyl estradiol/levonorgestrel	Tri-Levlen, Triphasil-21, Trivora-28, Enpresse
Progestin-only (mini-pill)	
Norethindrone	Micronor, Nor-QD
Norgestrel	Ovrette

From Cada.[13]

lism.[27,45,58] Certain generalizations are possible, however. Within the first several cycles of a combined OC, there is a mixture of proliferative and secretory features seen in the endometrium ('asynchronous' or 'discordant' endometrium). The glands tend to remain relatively straight and narrow, resembling proliferative endometrial glands but with cuboidal rather than columnar epithelium, and with very minimal mitotic activity. Subnuclear vacuoles may be seen, especially with the first 2 weeks of the cycle. Decidual change can be seen early but is usually more evident after several cycles have been completed. Despite the stromal changes, spiral arterioles do not develop normally.[27,92] With prolonged therapy over many cycles the glands develop secretory exhaustion (Figures 13.10 and 13.11) and become increasingly small, inactive, and ultimately atrophic (Figures 13.12–13.14). As this occurs, the stromal decidual changes become increasingly well developed, until the endome-

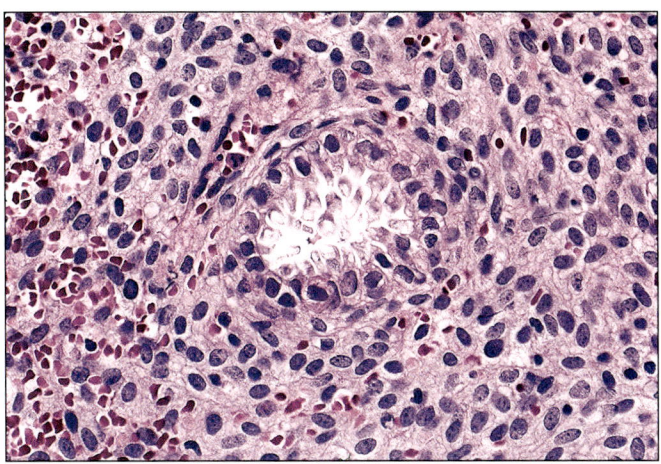

Fig. 13.10 Combined oral contraceptive, secretory exhaustion. The glands are small and show only rudimentary evidence of secretory activity in the form of apical snouts.

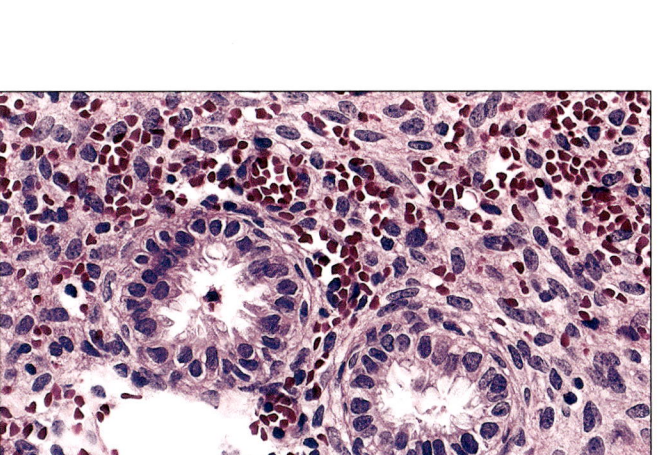

Fig. 13.11 Combined oral contraceptive, secretory exhaustion. The glands are small and show only rudimentary evidence of secretory activity in the form of apical snouts.

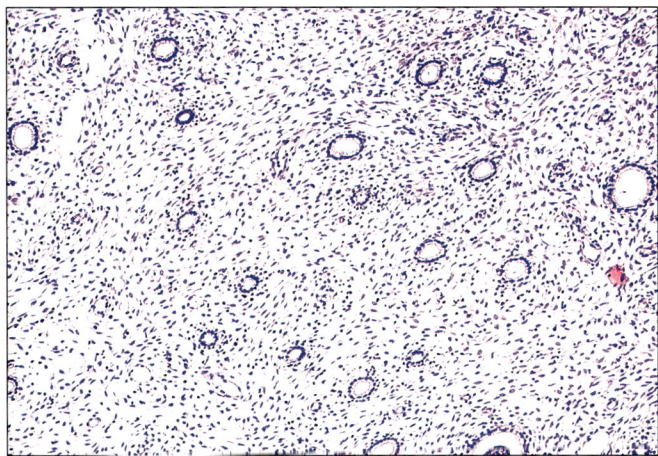

Fig. 13.12 Gland atrophy with combined oral contraceptive. The stromal decidual response is minimal.

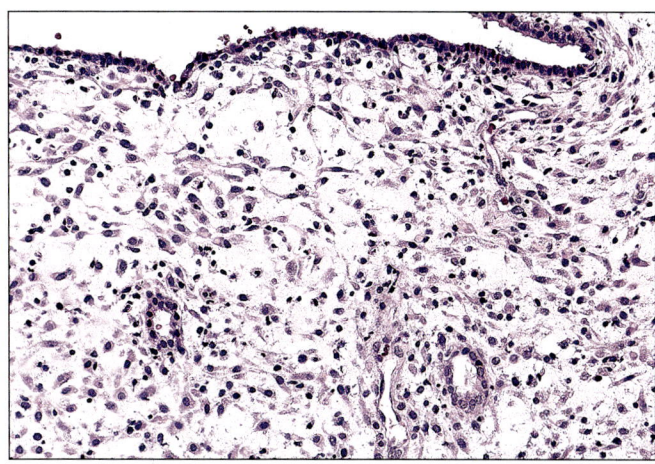

Fig. 13.13 Gland atrophy with combined oral contraceptive. The stromal decidual response is minimal (Ortho-Cyclen).

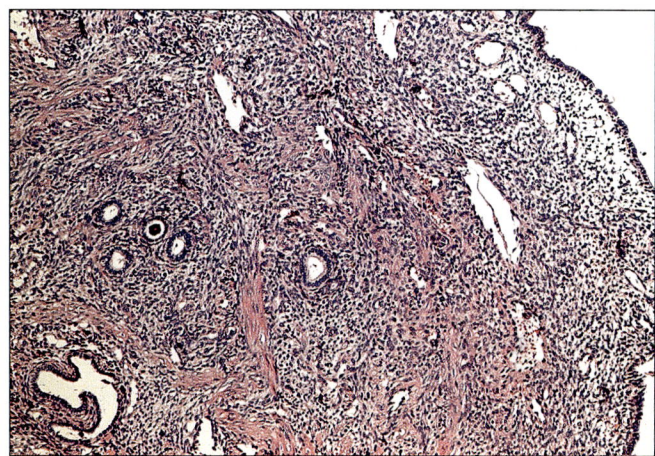

Fig. 13.14 Gland atrophy with combined oral contraceptive (Ortho-Novum).

trium is uniformly decidualized, with only rare, atrophic-appearing glands. This is the classic appearance of the so-called 'pill' endometrium (Figures 13.15–13.17). Prominent ectatic thin-walled veins are also seen, which often contain thromboses in patients having breakthrough bleeding (Figures 13.18 and 13.19). The classic 'pill' endometrium is not seen in all patients, and there is a spectrum from well-developed stromal changes to complete atrophy, with only a very thin endometrium showing little or no identifiable decidual change. The atrophic changes are seen more frequently with some of the lower dose regimens.[45]

Formulations that include short estrogen-only periods have been used in an attempt to lower the overall dose of hormones. Mircette, for example, has 21 days of combination treatment followed by a 2-day, hormone-free interval and 5 days of unopposed estrogen. Technically, this is a sequential OC, but to date it has not had the safety issues associated with the older, higher dose sequential therapies. This formulation has a distinctly different histologic pattern than the combined OCs. Biopsies taken during the estrogen-only portion of the cycle show proliferative endometrium while biopsies taken during the combined portion of the cycle show secretory endometrium.

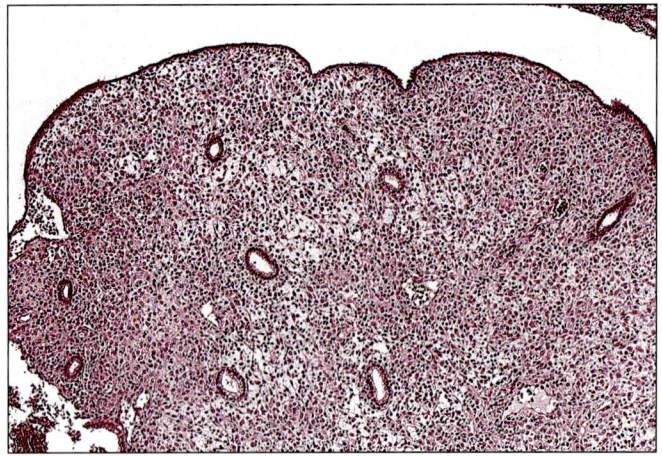

Fig. 13.15 Prominent stroma decidual response with combined oral contraceptive. The glands are atrophic (Ortho-Cyclen).

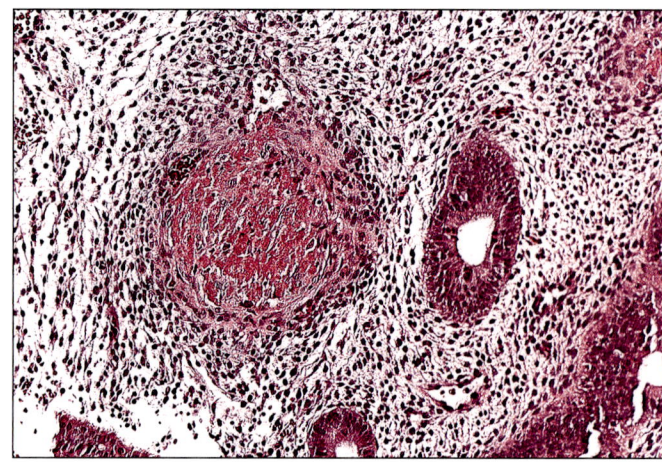

Fig. 13.18 Thrombi occluding a thin-walled vein (combined oral contraceptive).

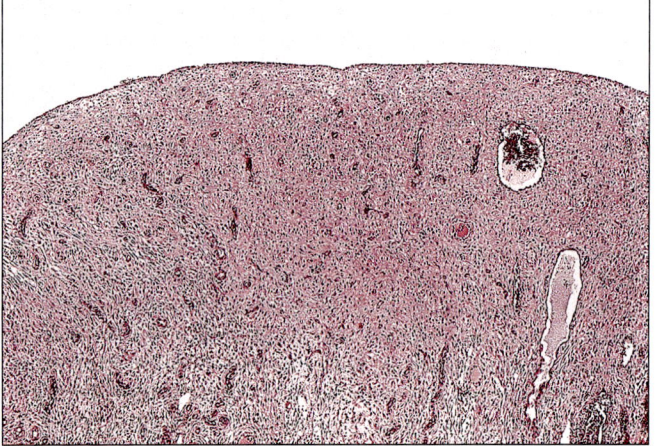

Fig. 13.16 Combined oral contraceptive (Loestrin), with classic 'pill' endometrium. The stroma is massively decidualized and contains widely scattered, atrophic glands.

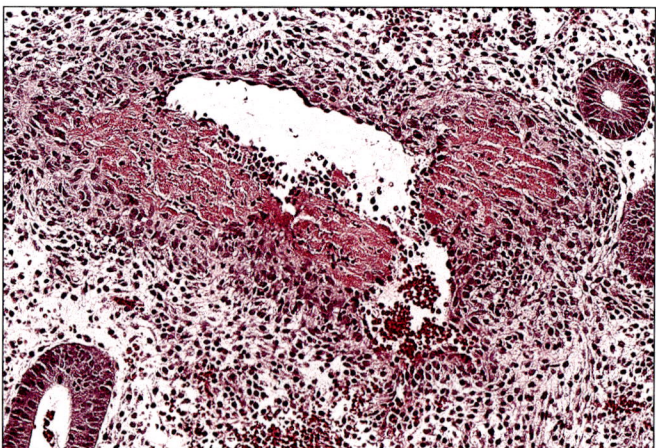

Fig. 13.19 Thrombi in prominent ectatic thin-walled veins (combined oral contraceptive).

PURE PROGESTIN ORAL CONTRACEPTIVES ('MINI-PILL')

In contrast to the combined OCs, the pure progestin OC (the 'mini-pill', 300 mcg norethisterone) is taken daily without interruption during the cycle. The mechanism of contraception differs from combined OCs in that ovulation is not consistently suppressed. Instead, contraception is due to the production of relatively thick cervical mucus that is impermeable to sperm, and to the atrophic endometrium that will not support implantation. The endometrial changes seen with the mini-pill are not distinctly different from those seen with combined OCs, but marked atrophy is more common and biopsy frequently yields only scanty material. In addition, proliferative endometrium is not infrequently seen, and this correlates with abnormal bleeding.[49]

LONG-TERM, PROGESTIN-ONLY CONTRACEPTION

Several systems have been developed for long-term, progestin-only contraception. Medroxyprogesterone acetate micro-

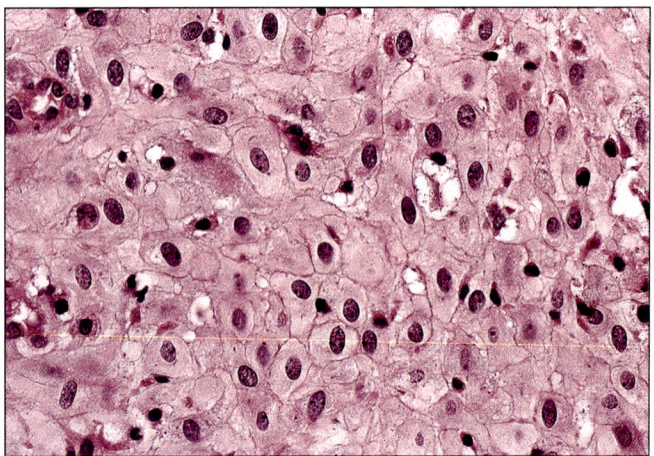

Fig. 13.17 Combined oral contraceptive (Loestrin) with well-developed decidual change (high magnification).

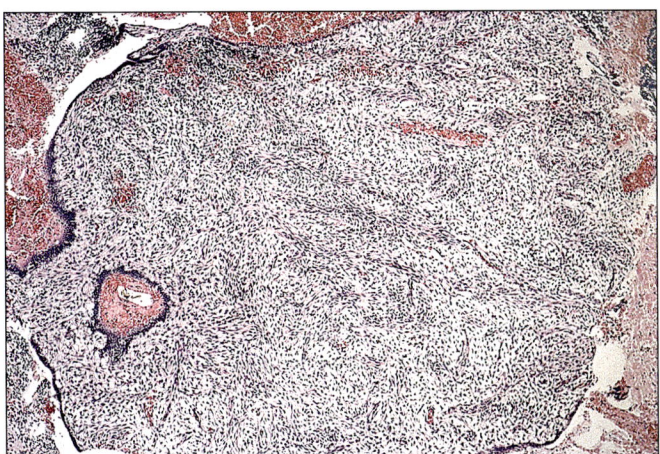

Fig. 13.20 Decidualized endometrium with long-term Depo-Provera use.

crystals in an aqueous solution (Depo-Provera) are used as an intramuscular injection. The slow dissolution of the crystals maintains effective progestin levels for several months, allowing for an injection schedule of every 3 months. Levels of progestin are typically higher than with the mini-pill. Early after injection, some women develop exaggerated hypersecretory changes that resemble gestational endometrium, including the presence of Arias-Stella reaction. By 3–6 months these changes have resolved and stromal decidual changes develop, resembling those seen with combined OCs as described above. Long-term treatment can result in atrophy or pure decidua-like change (Figure 13.20), just as with combined OCs.[45,70]

The Norplant system consists of several silastic tubes containing levonorgestrel. The tubes are slightly permeable to steroids, and the progestin is slowly released for a period of 3–5 years. As in other progestin-only regimens, ovulation occurs in about one-third of cycles, and contraception is by production of thick cervical mucus and an endometrium inimical to implantation. There are relatively few studies on the histologic findings with Norplant,[41,42] but the findings seem to be similar to other progestin-only regimens, with atrophy being the most common finding. Proliferative endometrium can also be seen, and correlates with irregular bleeding patterns.[69]

Devices that supply progestins directly to the endometrium are also used. The most common of these uses a slow-release formulation of levonorgestrel in combination with an intrauterine device (Mirena). Although physically located within the endometrium, absorption is systemic and they can be used for treatment of extrauterine disease such as endometriosis.[1,11] Histologically, the endometrium shows extensive decidualization.[46]

HORMONE-REPLACEMENT THERAPY (HRT)

COMMON TYPES OF HRT

Three general types of HRT have been used clinically: unopposed estrogen, cyclic estrogen and progestin, and combined estrogen and progestin formulations. Because of the markedly increased risk of endometrial cancer with unopposed estrogen,

only the latter two are in common use today. A common variation in Australia is continuous estrogen with either cyclic or continuous progestin. While the exact agents used and their dosage can vary, within each of these groups the histologic findings tend to be similar, and thus they will be discussed as categories.

The number of patients receiving long-term (>5 years) HRT dropped precipitously after two large studies showed an increase in cardiovascular risk rather than the predicted protective effects.[2,4] In the US, the number of prescriptions for HRT in the national Medicaid program fell by 57% between 2002 and 2004.[84] Nonetheless, HRT continues to be commonly used as short-term therapy for symptoms related to menopause.

UNOPPOSED ESTROGEN

Historically, estrogen alone was given as hormone replacement for postmenopausal women, and the beneficial effects of this therapy in preventing osteoporosis and cardiovascular disease have been well documented. Then a series of case control studies subsequently demonstrated a markedly increased risk of endometrial adenocarcinoma in women using long-term estrogens unopposed by progestins. Patients receiving unopposed estrogens for 5 years or more have an approximately six-fold increase in endometrial carcinoma. With the addition of progestins, the risk of endometrial carcinoma fell to near control levels.[3,65,66,90] The risk of endometrial carcinoma is dose related, but even low-dose estrogens (0.3 mg conjugated estrogens or equivalent) are associated with a risk of carcinoma if not combined with a progestin.[24,32,33] Estrogens applied as vaginal creams do not appear to have significant risk.[89] Although current practice is treatment with combined therapy, occasional patients are still treated with estrogen alone.

The endometrium from a woman being treated with unopposed estrogens will most commonly appear proliferative, and may in fact be indistinguishable from a normal proliferative endometrium in a premenopausal patient. This is especially likely if the patient is younger or immediately postmenopausal. There may also be a lesser degree of proliferation that is described as weakly proliferative, especially if the estrogen dose is low.[29] If the patient is bleeding, the endometrium will often have associated stromal breakdown with proliferative glands (Figure 13.3), a feature that specifically suggests unopposed estrogen exposure. Unfortunately, conventional microscopy cannot distinguish these changes due to exogenous estrogens from the effects of endogenous estrogen, as in anovulatory bleeding, or from the effects of other agents that may act as estrogenic agents in the endometrium. These include tamoxifen, various drugs and pharmaceutical agents such as digitalis or phenothiazines, and herbal preparations such as ginseng.

Long-term estrogen exposure can lead to a full spectrum of appearances, ranging from disordered proliferative changes to benign endometrial hyperplasia, EIN, or even adenocarcinoma.[27] Disordered proliferative endometrium shows a basic pattern of proliferative endometrium, with the addition of irregularly dilated and focally branched glands. This condition is most commonly seen in women not on therapy during the perimenopause and is not felt to be preneoplastic (see Chapter 15). Tubal metaplasia is common. The hallmark of benign endometrial hyperplasia is the development of endometrial compartment-wide irregular gland shape and distribution, which in many areas has glandular crowding to more than a

1:1 gland:stroma ratio. EIN may emerge from benign endometrial hyperplasia as a localized lesion with discrete cytology.[62]

Even with low-dosage administration, after long-term use the risk of developing benign endometrial hyperplasia or EIN is substantially increased.[89] Adenocarcinomas exhibit severe glandular crowding, usually with a cribriform or papillary architecture, and at least mild nuclear atypia (see Chapter 16). As is the case for those carcinomas associated with prolonged exposure to endogenous estrogens, the tumors developing where the exogenous estrogens are unopposed are usually low grade and minimally invasive, and the long-term survival rates are extremely high. Patients who develop adenocarcinomas usually have a minimum of 2–3 years of unopposed estrogen use. The risk does increase over time, with the highest risk in patients who have taken estrogens for 10 or more years.[58] Of note, some reports indicate that unopposed estrogens are also associated with an increased risk of endometrioid and clear cell ovarian carcinomas, perhaps reflecting the involvement of endometriosis in the pathogenesis of these particular tumor types.[68]

CYCLIC ESTROGEN–PROGESTERONE

Because unopposed estrogens elevate the risk of endometrial adenocarcinoma, HRT today nearly always includes a progestin (if the patient has a uterus). The most commonly used agents are conjugated equine estrogen (Premarin) in combination with medroxyprogesterone acetate (Provera). Cyclic or sequential HRT uses daily estrogen for the first 21–25 days of the month with daily progestin added for the last 10–13 days.[63] Consistent reduction of mitotic rates in glandular epithelium is found after generally only 9 or more days of progesterone administration in each cycle.[60,61] This regimen mimics to some degree the normal progression of these hormones during a menstrual cycle and typically results in a withdrawal bleed at the end of each cycle. Longer cycle lengths (i.e., 12 weeks instead of 4 weeks) have shown a decrease in the protective effect of the progestin and are not generally recommended.[9]

The pathologic findings in the endometrium are somewhat but not entirely predictable based on our understanding of normal endometrial cycles. Not surprisingly, biopsies taken from the estrogen-only portion of the cycle typically have a proliferative or weakly proliferative appearance, and may be histologically identical to a normal proliferative endometrium (Figures 13.21–13.23). Biopsies taken after the initiation of the progestin are more variable. Most show some degree of secretory change, beginning about 3 days after the beginning of the progestin therapy, but the changes lack the well-ordered daily progression seen in normal secretory endometrium and cannot be 'dated' in the same fashion (see Chapter 12).[14,38,86] Frequently, the glandular component develops no further than an early secretory appearance, with variably developed glycogen vacuoles persisting even late into the artificial cycle. The stroma shows a variable response to the progestin, and may develop a spotty decidual response by day 10 after progestin initiation. This is often described in pathology reports as gland–stromal asynchrony, and can be due to various other factors, including intrauterine devices (IUDs), oral contraceptives, underlying mass lesions such as leiomyomas or polyps, chronic endometritis, and other types of hormone such as mifepristone, clomiphene, and gonadotrophins. Although this sequence of

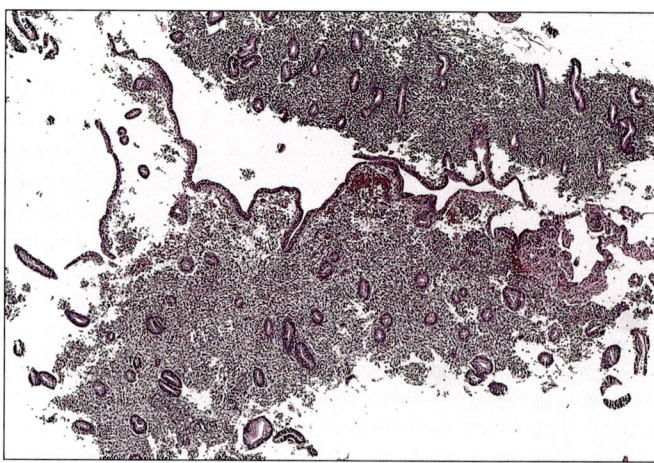

Fig. 13.21   Cyclic HRT, weakly proliferative pattern.

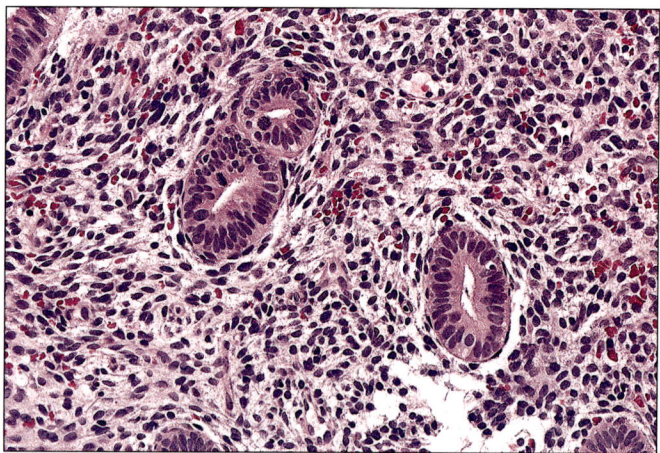

Fig. 13.22   Cyclic HRT, weakly proliferative pattern (high magnification).

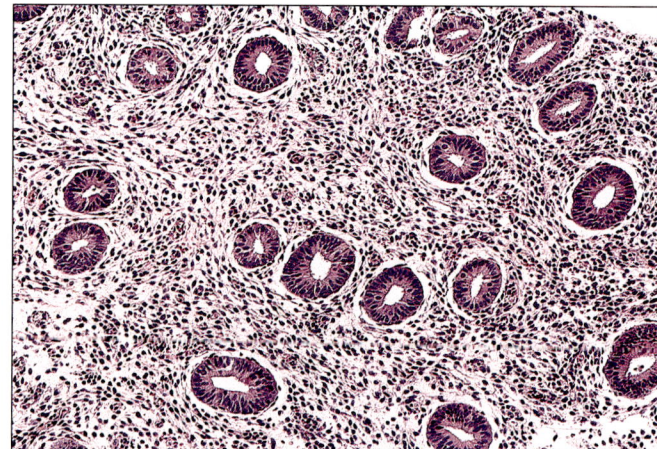

Fig. 13.23   Proliferative endometrium with cyclic HRT.

incomplete cycling is the most common picture with cyclic HRT, other patterns are not infrequent. Some patients will have normal menstrual changes (Figure 13.24) impossible to distinguish from women who have never taken HRT. Up to a fifth of patients will have quiescent endometrium, a picture of

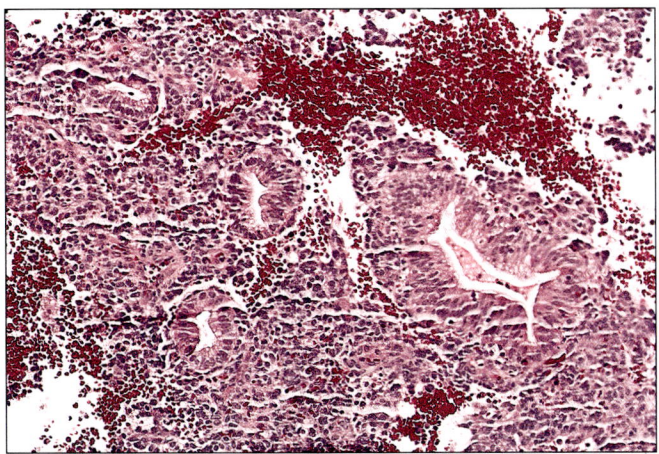

Fig. 13.24 Normal menstrual endometrium with focal secretory changes in woman receiving HRT.

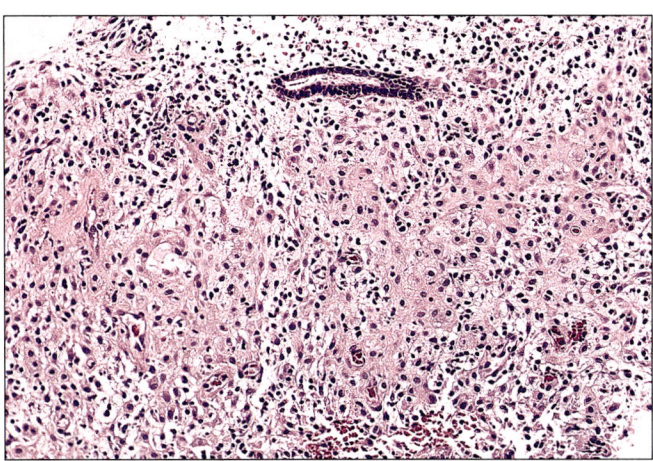

Fig. 13.25 Combined HRT (Prempro), extensive stromal decidual change. The stroma shows a well-developed decidual change, with inactive glands. This pattern can mimic the 'pill' endometrium.

an endometrium with some growth, but without the active signs of proliferation and development seen in a normal proliferative or secretory pattern. This group of patients generally does not experience monthly withdrawal bleeds.

Other patterns are seen less frequently, but can sometimes be helpful in managing patients. For example, if biopsies show a marked decidual change in the stroma, even during the estrogen portion of the cycle, it suggests that the progestin is overwhelming the estrogen, and the relative doses may need to be adjusted. Likewise, if biopsies taken from the latter portion of the progestin phase of the cycle show a well-developed proliferative pattern, then the progestin dose may be too low. Finally, if the biopsies show changes consistent with atrophy, then the endometrium is not responding at all to the hormones, and atrophy is causing the bleeding. This information can be helpful in trying to manage irregular bleeding in patients on cyclic HRT.

Our understanding of precisely why the endometrium responds so variably to cyclic HRT is poor, but presumably reflects multiple host factors (age, years postmenopause, level of endogenous hormones) and medication-specific factors (precise drug, dose, and duration).

COMBINED ESTROGEN–PROGESTERONE

Continuous combined estrogen–progestin HRT protects against the carcinogenic effects of unopposed estrogen. These regimens generally have a relatively predictable and uniform effect on the endometrium. As described above, the continuous long-term use of progesterone leads to downregulation of both estrogen and progesterone receptors, diminishing the responsiveness of the endometrium. This leads to the most common appearance, namely an atrophic or inactive endometrium.[45,67] There may be weak, poorly developed decidual change in the stromal cells, and the glandular component may show a few glycogen vacuoles suggesting progestin effect in the glands, but these findings are variable. Least commonly, there is a well-developed stromal decidual change, similar to that seen with oral contraceptives (Figure 13.25). Metaplastic changes such as tubal metaplasia, eosinophilic metaplasia, squamous metaplasia, and papillary syncytial metaplasia are more common with combined continuous HRT.[27]

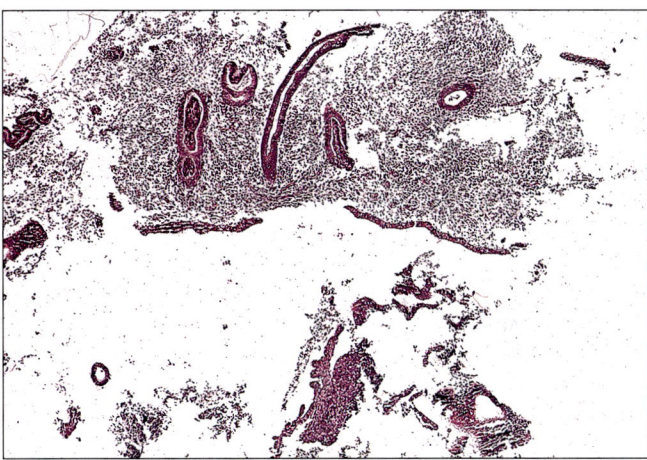

Fig. 13.26 Combined HRT (Prempro), proliferative with breakdown. This unusual pattern is identical to that seen with anovulation in the premenopausal patient. It indicates continuous estrogen stimulation to the endometrium with an insufficient opposing level of progestin.

As with the cyclic regimens, variations from these expected findings are frequent and can sometimes be helpful in managing patients. For example, a clearly proliferative pattern in the endometrium would suggest an inadequate dose of the progestational agent, especially if there is ongoing breakdown (i.e., an anovulatory-like pattern) (Figures 13.26–13.28).

OTHER HORMONAL AGENTS

TAMOXIFEN

Tamoxifen has been widely used in the treatment and now the prevention of breast cancer, where it functions as an antiestrogen.[47] In the endometrium, tamoxifen is a weak estrogen agonist, i.e., a compound with estrogenic properties that competes for the estrogen receptor. In the presence of high estrogen levels, as found in premenopausal women, it competes for receptor and thus blocks the effects of estrogen. In the presence

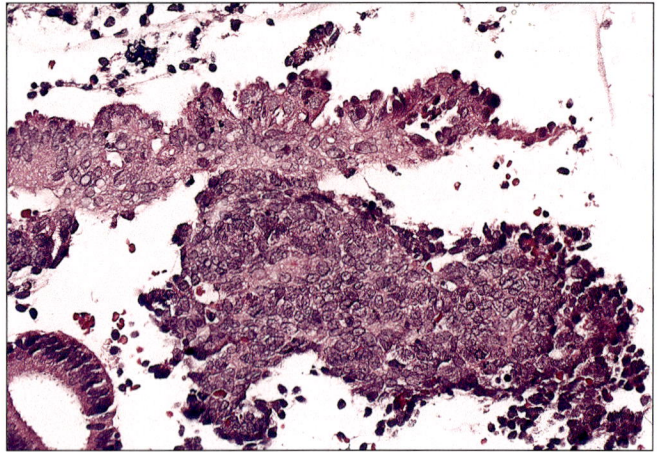

Fig. 13.27 Detail of stromal breakdown with combined HRT (Prempro).

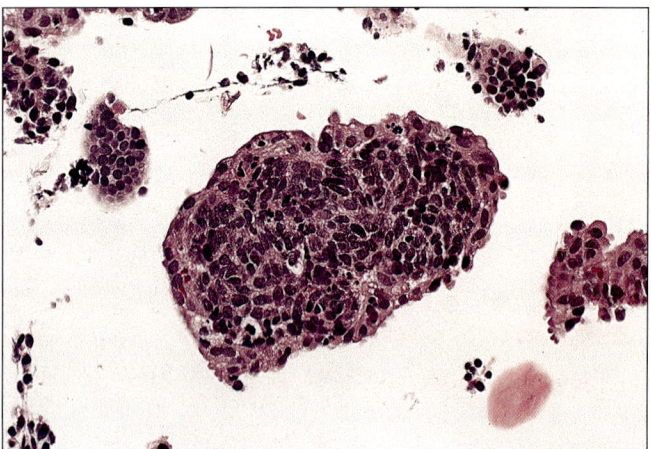

Fig. 13.28 Detail of stromal breakdown with combined HRT (Prempro).

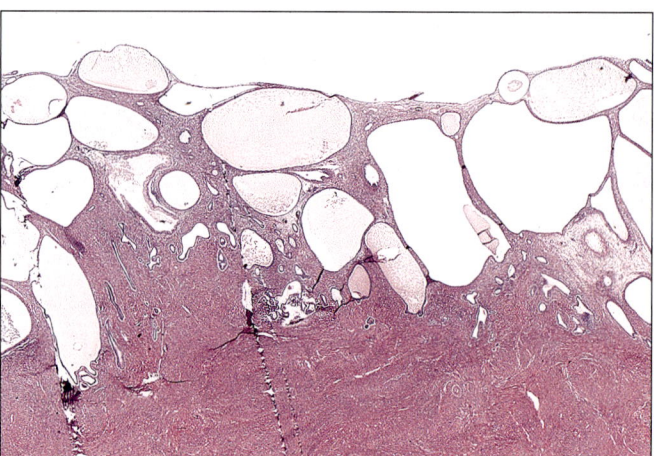

Fig. 13.29 Tamoxifen, cystic atrophy. Large cystic glands are present in the endometrium. Courtesy of H. Krigman, Missouri Baptist Hospital.

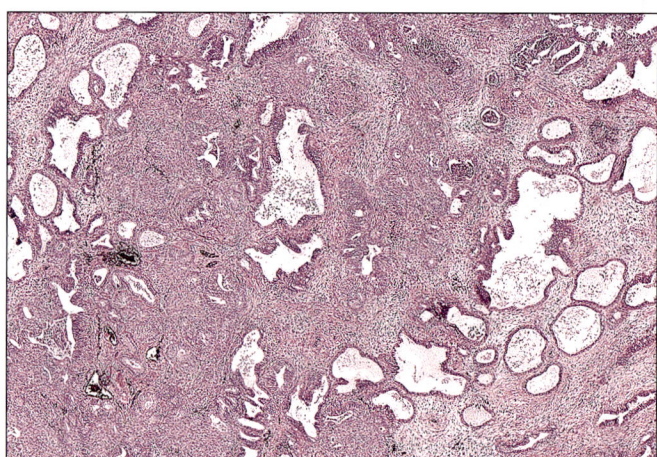

Fig. 13.30 Tamoxifen, polyp. This polyp also showed extensive squamous metaplasia, a not uncommon finding.

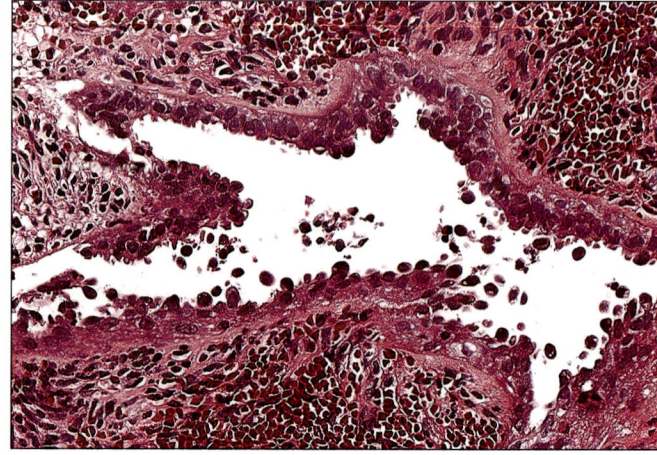

Fig. 13.31 Tamoxifen, serous epithelial atypia. This finding has also been reported in association with polyps in tamoxifen users. (Courtesy of Dr Hannah Krigman.)

of very low estrogen levels, i.e., in the postmenopausal patient, weak estrogenic activity is seen in the endometrium.[20] While most postmenopausal women will continue to have atrophic or (regular or cystic) inactive endometrium (Figure 13.29), a few will develop the pathologic changes associated with chronic unopposed estrogen stimulation.[80] As might be expected, women receiving tamoxifen who are symptomatic have far greater frequencies of endometrial pathologies than women who are asymptomatic (93% vs 25%).[19,74]

Multiple reports have described unusual-appearing endometrial polyps in tamoxifen-treated patients, with cystically dilated glands sometimes containing luminal secretions, a variety of metaplasias, massive fibrosis and, more rarely, decidualized stroma (Figures 13.30 and 13.31).[48,71] Some of these changes may be dose related.[21] Many of the polyps are 20 mm or more in size, which is larger than seen with any other form of HRT. No studies have yet indicated why this drug alone has such a peculiar effect on the endometrial stroma.[21] Malignancies are occasionally found in polyps associated with tamoxifen therapy and at rates much higher than in healthy non-users (3% vs 0.5%).[17]

Endometrial carcinomas arise at approximately the same rate as with unopposed estrogen at far greater rates than women not receiving HRT. The risk is related to the duration of therapy, and is increased approximately four-fold in patients exposed to tamoxifen for more than 5 years.[8] Some initial anecdotal reports and small series suggested that tamoxifen-induced carcinomas might be more frequently high grade, but larger subsequent series including results from the NSABP B-14 study have shown a similar proportion of high-grade tumors to those arising sporadically.[75,82] Most cancers are low-grade, low-stage endometrioid adenocarcinomas.[18,73] Uterine sarcomas also occur rarely in association with tamoxifen therapy,[5] but most of these examples are carcinosarcomas and one should be careful, given the current body of opinion that places such neoplasms into the category of 'metaplastic carcinomas' (see Chapter 20), not to view this as either unusual or unexpected.

RALOXIFENE

For many years it was thought that there was only one receptor for estrogen, and that the endometrial side effects of estrogens were thus inextricably linked to the desirable effects on bone and cardiovascular system. It is now known that there are at least two estrogen receptors, which modulate different effects. This has led to the development of selective estrogen receptor modulators (SERMs), designed for relatively tissue-specific effects.[52] The first of these to come into wide use was raloxifene.

Raloxifene, an antiestrogen designed initially for breast cancer treatment, has been investigated extensively for its selective beneficial effects on bone and cardiovascular systems. In animal studies, it lacks the weak estrogenic activity seen in endometrium with tamoxifen, and thus might be expected to lack any association with endometrial hyperplasia and carcinoma. Endometrial biopsies from postmenopausal women taking raloxifene show atrophy or inactive endometrium,[10] confirming (at least histologically) that there is essentially no estrogenic effect. Other studies have shown no increase in endometrial thickness as measured by ultrasound.[26] To date, there has been no demonstrated increase in endometrial hyperplasia or carcinoma in these patients when sampled histologically,[34] although in a very small percentage of women (3.3% vs 1.5% placebo) the endometrial thickness has increased by more than 5 mm during the treatment period as measured by ultrasound.[22] Long-term follow-up studies now confirm that patients receiving raloxifene have neither increased endometrial hyperplasia nor carcinoma when compared to control groups, although there has been an increase in endometrial polyps.[35,57]

AROMATASE INHIBITORS

Aromatase inhibitors, a new class of endocrine agents, block the peripheral conversion of steroid into estradiol by inhibiting the aromatase enzyme. Letrozole, anastrozole, and exemestane are the three mostly thoroughly studied members of this drug class. These drugs are used primarily to treat estrogen-receptor-positive breast cancers in postmenopausal women (in this situation they are highly effective)[54,77,78] and, more recently, endometriosis.[11] Because they reduce circulating estrogen levels to near zero, the primary effect on the endometrium is atrophy, and the rate of endometrial carcinoma is lower than in

tamoxifen-treated patients.[12,16] As measured by transvaginal ultrasound, aromatase inhibitors do not increase endometrial thickness. Some preliminary evidence suggests that aromatase inhibitors could even help treat pre-existing endometrial hyperplasias.[31] Although aromatase inhibitors effectively shut down endometrial proliferation, endometrial polyps continue to develop, an observation that contradicts current dogma that endometrial polyps are estrogen induced.[28]

PHYTOESTROGENS AND OTHER DIETARY AGENTS

Dietary and herbal remedies are widely used worldwide for relief of menopausal symptoms. Commonly used herbs include black cohosh (*Cimicifuga racemosa*), chaste tree berry (*Vitex agnus-castus*), dong quai (*Angelica sinensis*), ginseng (*Panax ginseng* and other *Panax* species), evening primrose oil (*Oenothera biennis*), motherwort (*Leonurus cardiaca*), red clover (*Trifolium pratense*), and licorice (*Glycyrrhiza glabra*). In many cases the active ingredients of these herbal preparations have not been clearly identified.[50]

Phytoestrogens, new forms of SERM still being evaluated, are plant estrogens that occur naturally as constituents of many plants, most notably beans and a variety of grains and seeds. Soybeans and flaxseed are commonly cited in the lay literature as sources of phytoestrogens,[39,50] which have a weak estrogen-like effect in the body. One tantalizing observation is that Asian women, who are known to have a much lower incidence of endometrial carcinoma than Western women, consume much higher amounts of phytoestrogen-rich foods, such as soy and tofu. Human studies suggest that a diet high in phytoestrogens may protect against endometrial adenocarcinoma and provide benefits in bone density.[53] Nationwide population-based studies, while not specifically evaluating phytoestrogens, suggest that a diet with a low fruit and vegetable intake is associated with higher rates of endometrial cancer.[81]

The most common types of phytoestrogen in plants and foods are the 'isoflavones'. The richest sources in nature are the leaves of the subterranean red clover with levels of up to 5 g per 100 g dry weight, and soybeans with levels up to 300 mg per 100 g dry weight. The most commonly studied phytoestrogens within this group are genistein and daidzein.

The initial data available on the effects on the endometrium itself suggest that phytoestrogens likely function as weak estrogen agonists. Long-term exposure to high doses may increase the risk of endometrial hyperplasia in postmenopausal women,[6,85] but most evidence suggests that short-term exposure to lower doses has no discernable histologic effect on endometrium.[64] In premenopausal women, the endometrium appears to cycle normally (Figure 13.32).

Wild yam preparations contain diosgenin, which can be converted to progesterone in a laboratory but not in the human body. Whether dietary supplementation with wild yams has any histologic effects on the endometrium is unknown.[50]

CLOMIPHENE/OVULATION INDUCTION THERAPY

Clomiphene citrate (Clomid) is an agent with strong affinity for the estrogen receptor. It binds essentially irreversibly to the

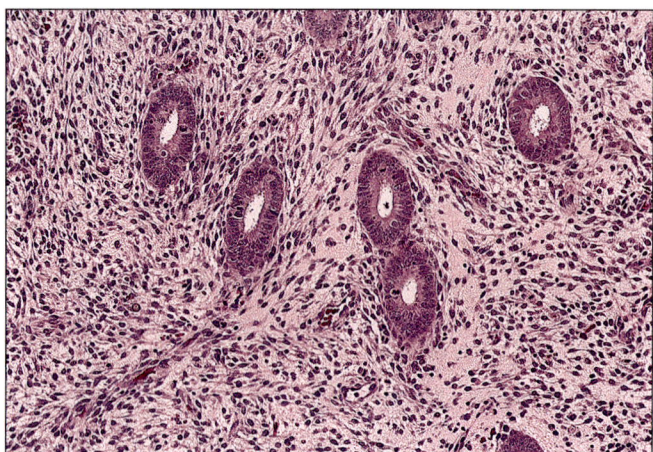

Fig. 13.32 Phytoestrogen, with well-developed proliferative endometrium.

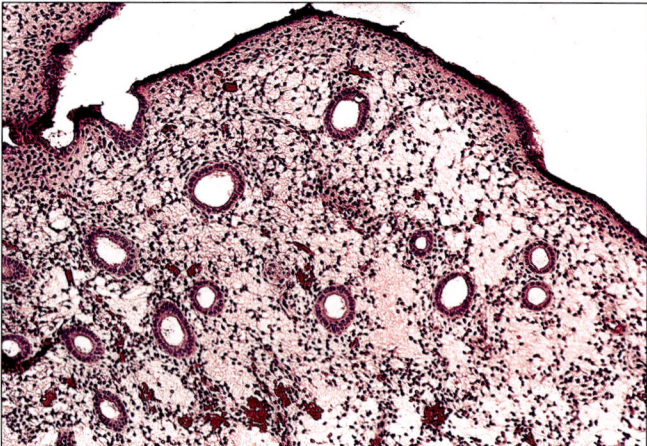

Fig. 13.33 Markedly edematous stroma (clomiphene). Courtesy of Dr Karen Ireland, Liberty Lake, WA.

receptor, reducing turnover. Its clinical usefulness stems from its effects on the hypothalamus, which interprets this activity as a low level of estrogen, causing increased gonadotrophin-releasing hormone (GnRH) stimulation of the pituitary, and hence increased follicle-stimulating hormone (FSH) production. This increases ovarian estrogen production, which then feeds back to the pituitary and causes a luteinizing hormone (LH) surge, followed by ovulation.[45] This drug, used to induce ovulation, is usually given on cycle days 5–10, with ovulation occurring 5–10 days after its administration. The increased stimulation of the dominant follicle results in higher serum estrogen and progesterone levels during the resulting secretory phase.

The effects of clomiphene on the endometrium are relatively subtle.[7,43] In a clomiphene-induced secretory phase, the glandular development is delayed relative to the time of ovulation (Figure 13.33). Although delayed, the early secretory changes are unusually well developed, with large, uniform subnuclear glycogen vacuoles that persist longer than in a normal cycle. Later in the cycle, decidual changes in the stroma are less prominent, and a coiled glandular architecture persists. These findings probably represent the antiestrogenic effects of clomi-

phene in combination with the high circulating levels of estrogen and progesterone.[7]

Experimental studies suggest that clomiphene may affect the developing lower genital tract in fetuses similar to the drug, diethylstilbestrol (DES) (see Chapter 5).[23] Care should be exercised that women who receive this drug for infertility are not already inadvertently in the early months of pregnancy.

In more recent years, ovulation induction has involved more complex regimens, generally involving administration of GnRH agonists, antagonists, FSH, and human chorionic gonadotrophin (hCG). Studies on the endometrial morphology are understandable few, and it is difficult to extrapolate the results to different regimens, but at least some studies suggest a relative delay in secretory phase maturation, similar to that seen with clomiphene. Other studies show in phase or even advanced date endometrium.[76,83] Although difficult to study, the endometrial alterations may be clinically significant as the alterations in endometrial histology may be responsible for the reduced rate of successful implantation seen in some patients.

MIFEPRISTONE ('MORNING-AFTER' PILL)

The progestin antagonist mifepristone (RU486) has received wide publicity as an agent of early abortion, but also has potential applications as a contraceptive. Mifepristone competes for the progesterone receptors. It may also have a second mechanism of action, which is antagonizing estrogen-dependent endometrial growth by stimulation of the androgen receptor.[63] In postmenopausal women, it acts as a weak progestin. As a postcoital agent to induce early abortion, it is given in large doses (200 mg) and effectively appears to block secretory development of the endometrium. It also shows promise as an oral contraceptive agent in low doses (2.5 or 5 mg) given daily, where it blocks normal secretory development while allowing ovulation to occur. It has also been used successfully in the treatment of uterine leiomyomas.[15]

In controlled studies with monkeys, the stromal cells are targeted, with resultant inhibition of edema and endometrial growth.[36] Treatment with mifepristone alone shows a strikingly compact stroma, indicating that mifepristone antagonizes the development of estrogen-dependent stromal edema, an effect that is reversed by progesterone. In glands, mifepristone is antiprogestogenic, but not antiestrogenic. Its strong inhibitory effect on glands is shown by a scarcity of cells containing vacuoles, again nullified in progesterone-treated animals.

Biopsies of patients receiving mifepristone as an abortifacient often show significantly delayed maturation relative to the clinical dates, similar to a luteal phase defect. The changes of long-term treatment with mifepristone are notable for a marked increase in endometrial hyperplasias, similar to expectations when receiving unopposed estrogens.[63] The hyperplasia risk may be dose dependent, and lower doses of long-term mifepristone may not be associated with increased risks of endometrial hyperplasia.[30]

Mifepristone is the first of a large family of progesterone receptor antagonists to come into clinical use. Numerous progesterone receptor modulators are in development, with potential use in a wide variety of gynecologic conditions. Undoubtedly, some will come into clinical use in the future.[79]

GONADOTROPHIN-RELEASING HORMONE AGONISTS

Pulsatile release of GnRH from the hypothalamus is the normal stimulus to the pituitary to secrete FSH and LH. Paradoxically, chronic non-pulsatile treatment has the opposite effect, after an initial surge of inhibiting FSH and LH secretion, apparently via downregulation of the GnRH receptors in the pituitary. Several GnRH agonists make use of this pathway to suppress pituitary gonadotrophin secretion, including leuprolide acetate, buserelin acetate, and goserelin acetate. Administering these agents blocks ovarian follicle development and induces a marked reduction in estrogen and progesterone levels, comparable to a postmenopausal state. Indeed, long-term treatment with these agents is limited due to the side effects of marked hypoestrogenemia, including profound bone density loss.

Currently, GnRH agonists are used to reduce the size of uterine leiomyomas and endometrial stromal sarcomas. They are also used in the diagnosis and treatment of endometriosis, and in the suppression of ovulation during oocyte harvest for *in vitro* fertilization. Histologically, it is not surprising that the endometrium from patients treated chronically with GnRH shows profound atrophy.[40]

GONADOTROPHINS

Gonadotrophins are used primarily to treat infertility. Human menopausal gonadotrophins, LH and FSH, are extracted from the urine of postmenopausal women. Human chorionic gonadotrophin is closely related to LH, and can be used to simulate the mid-cycle LH surge in ovulation induction. The effects of these agents on the endometrium are not clear. Various conflicting findings report delayed, normal, or advanced histologic maturation relative to the clinical dates, as well as hypersecretory changes similar to Arias-Stella reactions.[25,45,58]

CORTICOSTEROIDS

High doses of corticosteroids can have a progestational effect on the endometrium. Presumably, this is due to a weak affinity for the progestin receptor. The histologic appearance is similar to other progestational agents. Chronic lower dose therapy will eventually result in endometrial atrophy.

DANAZOL

Danazol is a weak androgen that is structurally related to testosterone and is used to treat endometriosis and endometrial hyperplasia. The endometrial changes resemble those seen with other progestational agents. As with other progestins, long-term therapy usually leads to atrophy[37,56] or reduction in severity of hyperplasia.[55]

TREATMENT OF HYPERPLASIA, EIN, AND CARCINOMA

Hormonal therapy, primarily high-dose progestin therapy, has long been used to treat endometrial hyperplasia, and is increas-

ingly being used as therapy for EIN and even well-differentiated adenocarcinomas in women who are poor surgical candidates. This includes young women who wish to preserve fertility. Relatively high doses of progestins are used, typically 20–40 mg/day oral medroxyprogesterone acetate (Provera), 80 mg/day megestrol (Megace), or intramuscular depo-medroxyprogesterone acetate (Depo-Provera). Repeat biopsy is usually obtained (typically at around 3 months) to evaluate response to therapy. The histologic response to this therapy requires progesterone receptors within lesional tissue, a condition met in almost all benign endometrial hyperplasias and EIN, and many adenocarcinomas.[27]

In those patients who respond, the endometrium shows typical secretory changes in the first weeks of therapy (Figure 13.34). By 3 months, the endometrium shows diffuse and profound decidualization, with widely scattered atrophic-appearing glands similar to the decidua seen in pregnancy (Figure 13.35). Although this pattern strongly correlates with a long-term response to therapy, it does not guarantee that the lesion

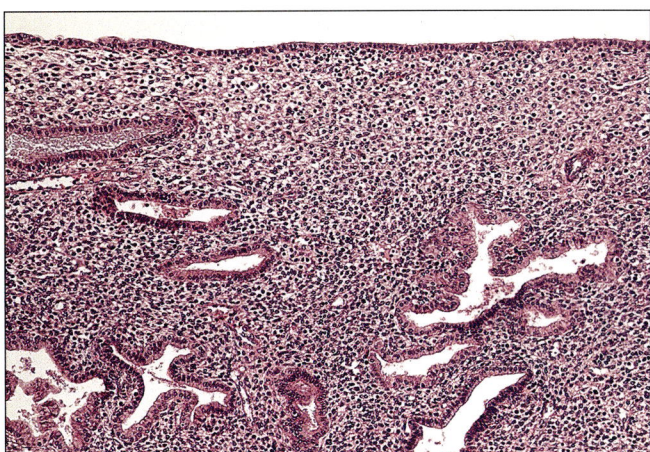

Fig. 13.34 Changes in an endometrium treated with progesterone for simple hyperplasia. This woman had initially used high-dose Premarin over a long period. After a short period of receiving Depo-Provera, some of the endometrial glands show secretory changes. The stroma has become decidualized.

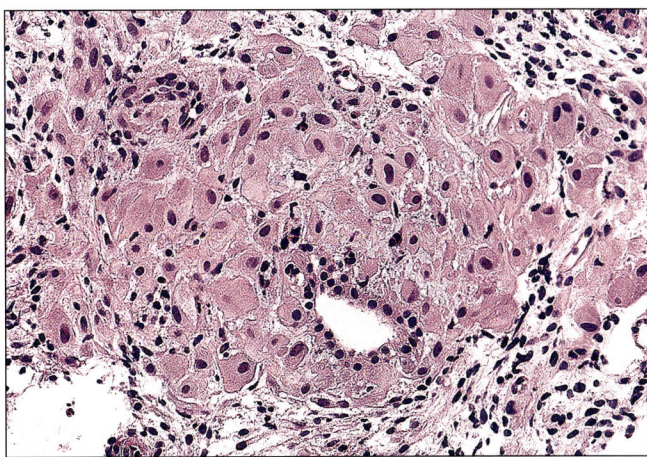

Fig. 13.35 Stroma decidual changes, similar to 'pill' endometrium with Megace. Long-term treatment of a patient with endometrial cancer has, in some areas, resulted in atrophic glands in a decidualized stroma.

will regress. Progestin-altered glands of persistent premalignant EIN lesions and adenocarcinoma may become widely separated by an expanded decidualized stroma, and acquire a bland nuclear cytology. This can make persistent disease difficult to recognize in biopsies taken while the patient is still receiving hormonal therapy. Close follow-up is always warranted.

A rare patient will show little or no response to therapy with progestins. The decidual response will be minimal or absent altogether, and there may be no histologic evidence at all that the tumor has been treated with progestins. More problematic are those patients who show a marked decidual response punctuated by clusters of glands with a cytology different from the background (Figures 13.36–13.38). If the pathologist reviews the slide without knowing the history of hyperplasia, it is difficult, if not impossible, to correctly interpret the biopsy as showing a partial response to progestin therapy. The degree of gland crowding often does not reach the degree seen in untreated

hyperplasia, but more glands are present than would be expected in an entirely decidualized endometrium. When faced with such a biopsy, it is critically important to obtain a full history, and if possible, to review the initial biopsies for comparison.

Progestin therapy has also been associated with the development of squamous metaplasia in hyperplasias or carcinomas.[59] When present, the metaplasia can be profound (Figures 13.39–13.41). If the history is not known, the extensive squamous differentiation can cause diagnostic confusion with other entities (adenoacanthoma, squamous cell carcinoma, etc.).

Progestin-treated hyperplasias and well-differentiated endometrioid carcinomas can also be mistaken for various different neoplastic processes, especially in the absence of a complete clinical history (see Table 13.4). The most common confusion is with secretory adenocarcinoma, which is the variant of endometrioid carcinoma showing features of early secretory differentiation (see Chapter 16). The large basal intracytoplasmic

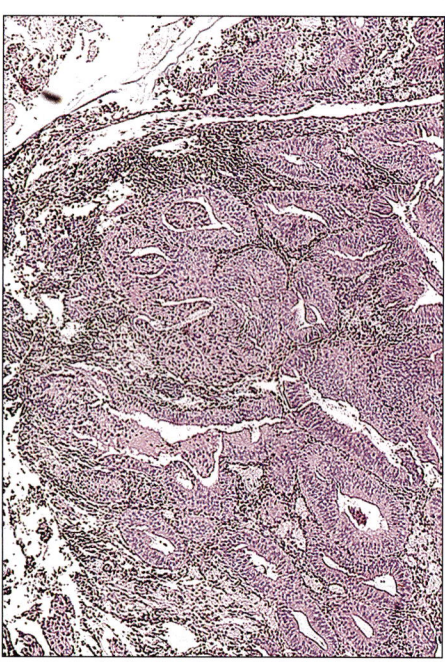

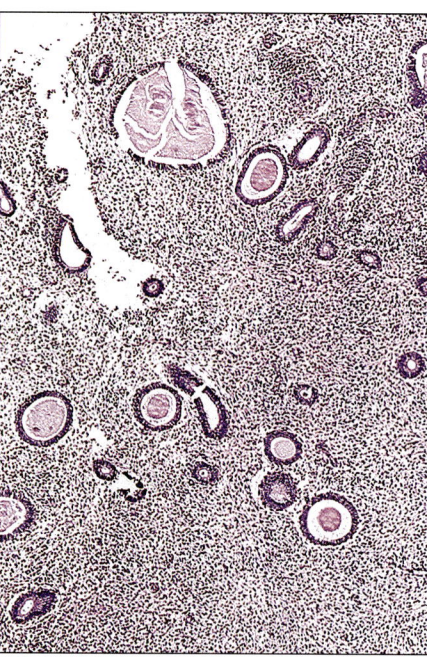

Fig. 13.36 Endometrial carcinoma, re-biopsy after 3 months of high-dose progestin therapy (Megace), partial response. The right side shows a marked stromal decidual change with an increased number of glands compared to the complete response seen in Figure 13.35. Without history, definitive recognition as partially treated hyperplasia or carcinoma would not be possible. The left side shows the original adenocarcinoma for comparison.

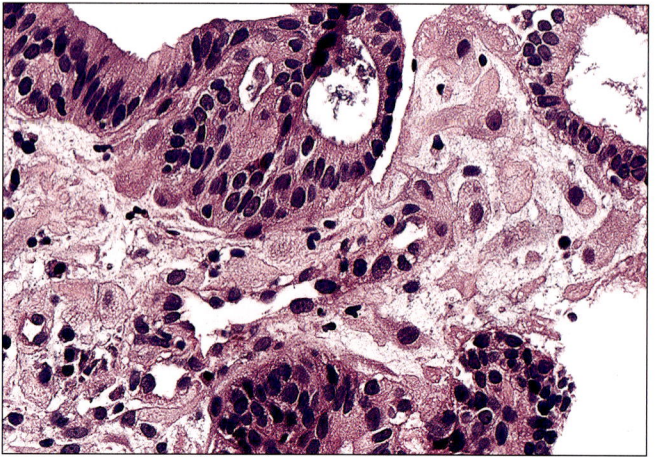

Fig. 13.37 Extensive decidua with partial response of cancer to Megace.

Fig. 13.38 Decidua with partial response of cancer to Megace.

Table 13.4 Progestin treatment. Effect on endometrial hyperplasia and carcinoma: differential diagnosis

	Sheets of epithelium	High-grade nuclei	Subnuclear vacuoles	Intracellular mucin	Decidualized stroma
Progestin effect	+/–	+/–	+/–	–	+++
Secretory carcinoma	–	–	+++	–	–
Clear cell carcinoma	+++/–	+++/–	–	–	–
Mucinous carcinoma	+/–	+/–	–	+++	–
Secretory endometrium	–	–	+++/–	–	+++/–

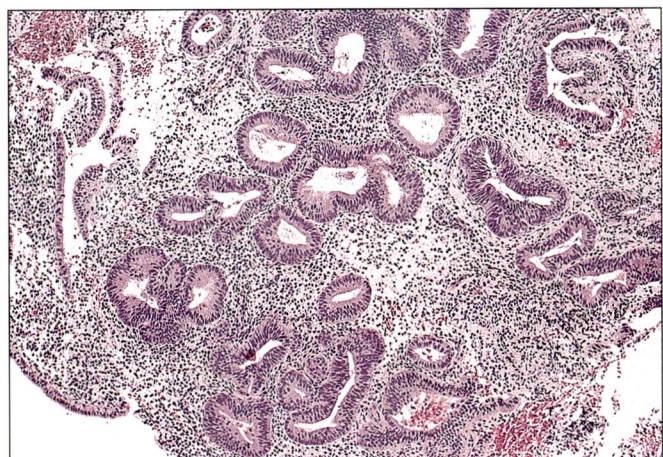

Fig. 13.39 Simple endometrial hyperplasia, prior to treatment with progesterone.

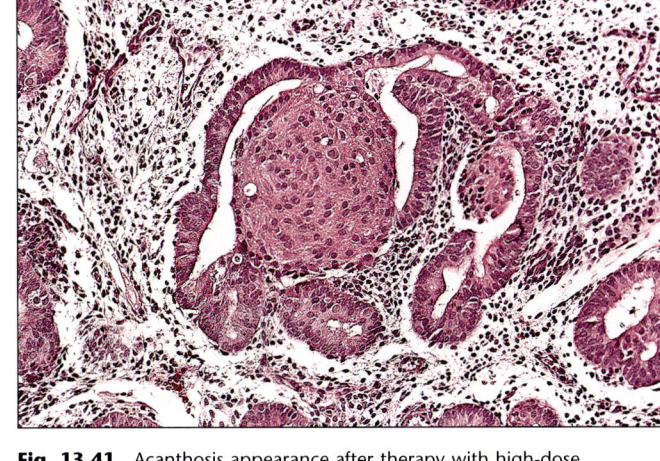

Fig. 13.41 Acanthosis appearance after therapy with high-dose progestins (Megace).

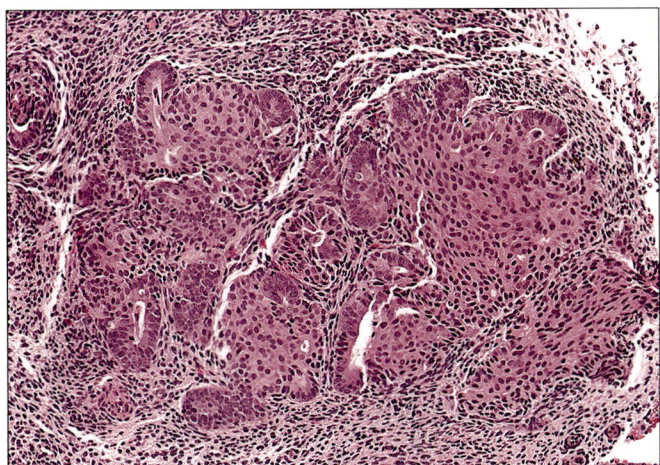

Fig. 13.40 Three months of treatment with high-dose progestins (Megace). Extensive squamous metaplasia is now present, giving a much more complex-appearing pattern than was present in the pretreatment biopsy.

glycogen vacuoles are striking. A key distinguishing feature is the absence of stromal decidual change in true spontaneous secretory carcinomas, while progestin-treated carcinomas typically will develop stromal changes, at least focally. If the biopsy is performed early after the initiation of progestin therapy, however, it may be impossible to distinguish these stromal changes on histologic grounds alone.

Cytoplasmic vacuolization can also suggest mucinous adenocarcinoma. However, unlike the mucinous carcinoma where the mucin casts a foamy appearance throughout the luminal half of the cell and has an amphophilic color, the cytoplasmic vacuoles associated with progestin therapy are clear. Moreover, mucin stains will show only small amounts of apical mucin associated with progestin therapy, in contrast to the large cytoplasmic mucin vacuoles seen in mucinous adenocarcinoma.

The presence of clear cytoplasm may cause confusion with a clear cell adenocarcinoma. Attention to the high-grade nuclear atypia and solid or hobnail architectural patterns will distinguish this from a progestin-treated adenocarcinoma, which will lack these features.

Finally, the normal secretory endometrium should not be overinterpreted as neoplastic. The glandular architecture during the secretory phase is normally more crowded and complex than during the proliferative phase. True 'secretory hyperplasia' or 'secretory endometrial intraepithelial neoplasia' is rare, and is generally recognized by transitions to areas with a more typical morphology. Secretory carcinomas can be recognized by the presence of architectural features of adenocarcinoma, such as cribriform architecture, and also will often show transitions to more typical endometrioid adenocarcinoma. One helpful feature is that when the endometrium fits into a defined histologic cycle date, it is unlikely to represent a neoplastic process.

REFERENCES

1. Abou-Setta AM, Al-Inany HG, Farquhar CM. Levonorgestrel-releasing intrauterine device (LNG-IUD) for symptomatic endometriosis following surgery. Cochrane Database Syst Rev 2006:CD005072.
2. Anderson GL, Limacher M, Assaf AR, et al. Effects of conjugated equine estrogen in postmenopausal women with hysterectomy: the Women's Health Initiative randomized controlled trial. JAMA 2004;291:1701–12.
3. Anonymous. Effects of hormone replacement therapy on endometrial histology in postmenopausal women. The Postmenopausal Estrogen/Progestin Interventions (PEPI) Trial. JAMA 1996;275:370–5.
4. Archer DF, Viniegrasibal A, Hsiu JG, Seltman HJ, Muesing R, Ross B. Endometrial histology, uterine bleeding, and metabolic changes in postmenopausal women using a progesterone-releasing intrauterine device and oral conjugated estrogens for hormone replacement therapy. Menopause 1994;1:109–16.
5. Arenas M, Rovirosa A, Hernandez V, et al. Uterine sarcomas in breast cancer patients treated with tamoxifen. Int J Gynecol Cancer 2006;16:861–5.
6. Arici A, Bukulmez O. Phyto-oestrogens and the endometrium. Lancet 2004;364:2081–2.
7. Benda JA. Clomiphene's effect on endometrium in infertility. Int J Gynecol Pathol 1992;11:273–82.
8. Bernstein L, Deapen D, Cerhan JR, et al. Tamoxifen therapy for breast cancer and endometrial cancer risk. J Natl Cancer Inst 1999;91:1654–62.
9. Bjarnason K, Cerin A, Lindgren R, Weber T. Adverse endometrial effects during long cycle hormone replacement therapy. Maturitas 1999;32:161–70.
10. Boss SM, Huster WJ, Neild JA, Glant MD, Eisenhut CC, Draper MW. Effects of raloxifene hydrochloride on the endometrium of postmenopausal women. Am J Obstet Gynecol 1997;177:1458–64.
11. Brown PM, Farquhar CM, Lethaby A, Sadler LC, Johnson NP. Cost-effectiveness analysis of levonorgestrel intrauterine system and thermal balloon ablation for heavy menstrual bleeding. BJOG 2006;113:797–803.
12. Buzdar A, Howell A, Cuzick J, et al. Comprehensive side-effect profile of anastrozole and tamoxifen as adjuvant treatment for early-stage breast cancer: long-term safety analysis of the ATAC trial. Lancet Oncol 2006;7:633–43.
13. Cada DJ, ed. Facts and comparisons. In: Drug Facts and Comparisons 2000. St Louis: Mosby; 1999:217–44.
14. Carranza Lira S, Martinez Chequer JC, Santa Rita MT, Ortiz de la Pena A, Perez Y, Fernandez RL. Endometrial changes according to hormone replacement therapy schedule. Menopause 1998;5:86–9.
15. Chabbert-Buffet N, Meduri G, Bouchard P, Spitz IM. Selective progesterone receptor modulators and progesterone antagonists: mechanisms of action and clinical applications. Hum Reprod Update 2005;11:293–307.
16. Coates AS, Keshaviah A, Thurlimann B, et al. Five years of letrozole compared with tamoxifen as initial adjuvant therapy for postmenopausal women with endocrine-responsive early breast cancer: update of study BIG 1–98. J Clin Oncol 2007;25:486–92.
17. Cohen I, Bernheim J, Azaria R, Tepper R, Sharony R, Beyth Y. Malignant endometrial polyps in postmenopausal breast cancer tamoxifen-treated patients. Gynecol Oncol 1999;75:136–41.
18. Cohen I, Azaria R, Fishman A, Tepper R, Shapira J, Beyth Y. Endometrial cancers in postmenopausal breast cancer patients with tamoxifen treatment. Int J Gynecol Pathol 1999;18:304–9.
19. Cohen I, Perel E, Flex D, et al. Endometrial pathology in postmenopausal tamoxifen treatment: comparison between gynaecologically symptomatic and asymptomatic breast cancer patients. J Clin Pathol 1999;52:278–82.
20. Cohen I, Altaras MM, Beyth Y, et al. Estrogen and progesterone receptors in the endometrium of postmenopausal breast cancer patients treated with tamoxifen and progestogens. Gynecol Oncol 1997;65:83–8.
21. Cohen I, Perel E, Tepper R, et al. Dose-dependent effect of tamoxifen therapy on endometrial pathologies in postmenopausal breast cancer patients. Breast Cancer Res Treat 1999;53:255–62.
22. Cummings SR, Eckert S, Krueger KA, et al. The effect of raloxifene on risk of breast cancer in postmenopausal women: results from the MORE randomized trial. Multiple Outcomes of Raloxifene Evaluation. JAMA 1999;281:2189–97.
23. Cunha GR, Taguchi O, Namikawa R, Nishizuka Y, Robboy SJ. Teratogenic effects of clomiphene, tamoxifen, and diethylstilbestrol on the developing human female genital tract. Hum Pathol 1987;18:1132–43.
24. Cushing KL, Weiss NS, Voigt LF, McKnight B, Beresford SAA. Risk of endometrial cancer in relation to use of low-dose, unopposed estrogens. Obstet Gynecol 1998;91:35–9.
25. Dallenbach-Hellweg G, Poulsen H, eds. Iatrogenic changes. In: Atlas of Endometrial Histopathology, 2nd edn. Berlin: Springer; 1996:105–28.
26. Davies GC, Huster WJ, Shen W, et al. Endometrial response to raloxifene compared with placebo, cyclical hormone replacement therapy, and unopposed estrogen in postmenopausal women. Menopause 1999;6:188–95.
27. Deligdisch L. Hormonal pathology of the endometrium. Mod Pathol 2000;13:285–94.
28. Duffy S, Jackson TL, Lansdown M, et al. The ATAC ('Arimidex', Tamoxifen, Alone or in Combination) adjuvant breast cancer trial: first results of the endometrial sub-protocol following 2 years of treatment. Hum Reprod 2006;21:545–53.
29. Ettinger B, Bainton L, Upmalis DH, Citron JT, VanGessel A. Comparison of endometrial growth produced by unopposed conjugated estrogens or by micronized estradiol in postmenopausal women. Am J Obstet Gynecol 1997;176:112–7.
30. Fiscella K, Eisinger SH, Meldrum S, Feng C, Fisher SG, Guzick DS. Effect of mifepristone for symptomatic leiomyomata on quality of life and uterine size: a randomized controlled trial. Obstet Gynecol 2006;108:1381–7.
31. Garuti G, Cellani F, Centinaio G, Montanari G, Nalli G, Luerti M. Prospective endometrial assessment of breast cancer patients treated with third generation aromatase inhibitors. Gynecol Oncol 2006;103:599–603.
32. Grady D, Ernster VL. Hormone replacement therapy and endometrial cancer: are current regimens safe? J Natl Cancer Inst 1997;89:1088–9.
33. Grady D, Gebretsadik T, Kerlikowske K, Ernster V, Petitti D. Hormone replacement therapy and endometrial cancer risk: a meta-analysis. Obstet Gynecol 1995;85:304–13.
34. Grady D, Ettinger B, Moscarelli E, et al. Safety and adverse effects associated with raloxifene: multiple outcomes of raloxifene evaluation. Obstet Gynecol 2004;104:837–44.
35. Grady D, Herrington D, Bittner V, et al. Cardiovascular disease outcomes during 6.8 years of hormone therapy: Heart and Estrogen/progestin Replacement Study follow-up (HERS II). JAMA 2002;288:49–57.
36. Greb RR, Kiesel L, Selbmann AK, et al. Disparate actions of mifepristone (RU 486) on glands and stroma in the primate endometrium. Hum Reprod 1999;14:198–206.
37. Grio R, Piacentino R, Marchino GL, Bocci A, Navone R. Danazol in the treatment of endometrial hyperplasia. Panminerva Med 1993;35:231–3.
38. Habiba MA, Bell SC, Al-Azzawi F. Endometrial responses to hormone replacement therapy: histological features compared with those of late luteal phase endometrium. Hum Reprod 1998;13:1674–82.
39. Hale GE, Hughes CL, Robboy SJ, Agarwal SK, Bievre M. A double-blind randomized study on the effects of red clover isoflavones on the endometrium. Menopause 2001;8:338–46.
40. Heller DS. Hormonal effects on the endometrium – dysfunctional uterine bleeding, iatrogenic hormonal effects, and luteal phase defects. New York: Igaku-Shoin; 1994.
41. Hickey M, Simbar M, Young L, Markham R, Russell P, Fraser IS. A longitudinal study of changes in endometrial microvascular density in Norplant implant users. Contraception 1999;59:123–9.
42. Hickey M, Simbar M, Markham R, et al. Changes in vascular basement membrane in the endometrium of Norplant users. Hum Reprod 1999;14:716–21.
43. Homburg R, Pap H, Brandes M, Huirne J, Hompes P, Lambalk CB. Endometrial biopsy during induction of ovulation with clomiphene citrate in polycystic ovary syndrome. Gynecol Endocrinol 2006;22:506–10.
44. Hompes PG, Mijatovic V. Endometriosis: the way forward. Gynecol Endocrinol 2007;23:5–12.
45. Ireland K, Zaino RJ. Iatrogenic patterns: what hath the physician wrought? In: Zaino RJ, ed. Interpretation of Endometrial Biopsies and Curettings. New York: Lippincott-Raven; 1996:143–73.
46. Jones RL, Critchley HO. Morphological and functional changes in human endometrium following intrauterine levonorgestrel delivery. Hum Reprod 2000;15(Suppl 3):162–72.
47. Jordan VC, Brodie AM. Development and evolution of therapies targeted to the estrogen receptor for the treatment and prevention of breast cancer. Steroids 2007;72:7–25.
48. Kennedy MM, Baigrie CF, Manek S. Tamoxifen and the endometrium: review of 102 cases and comparison with HRT-related and non-HRT-related endometrial pathology. Int J Gynecol Pathol 1999;18:130–7.
49. Kim-Bjorklund T, Landgren BM, Johannisson E. Morphometric studies of the endometrium, the fallopian tube and the corpus luteum during contraception with the 300 micrograms (NET) minipill. Contraception 1991;43:459–74.
50. Kronenberg F, Fugh-Berman A. Complementary and alternative medicine for menopausal symptoms: a review of randomized, controlled trials. Ann Intern Med 2002;137:805–13.
51. La Vecchia C. Oral contraceptives and ovarian cancer: an update, 1998–2004. Eur J Cancer Prev 2006;15:117–24.
52. Lewis JS, Jordan VC. Selective estrogen receptor modulators (SERMs): mechanisms of anticarcinogenesis and drug resistance. Mutation Res, Fundamental Mol Mech Mutagen 2005;591:247–63.
53. Lof M, Weiderpass E. Epidemiologic evidence suggests that dietary phytoestrogen intake is associated with reduced risk of breast, endometrial, and prostate cancers. Nutr Res 2006;26:609–19.
54. Lonning PE. Adjuvant endocrine treatment of early breast cancer. Hematol Oncol Clin North Am 2007;21:223–38.
55. Mais V, Cossu E, Angioni S, Piras B, Floris L, Melis GB. Abnormal uterine bleeding: medical treatment with vaginal danazol and five-year follow-up. J Am Assoc Gynecol Laparosc 2004;11:340.
56. Marchini M, Fedele L, Bianchi S, Dinoa G, Nava S, Vercellini P. Endometrial patterns during therapy with danazol or gestrinone for endometriosis – structural and ultrastructural study. Hum Pathol 1992;23:51–6.
57. Martino S, Disch D, Dowsett SA, Keech CA, Mershon JL. Safety assessment of raloxifene over eight years in a clinical trial setting. Curr Med Res Opin 2005;21:1441–52.
58. Mazur M, Kurman RJ, eds. Effects of hormones. In: Diagnosis of Endometrial Biopsies and Curettings: A Practical Approach. New York: Springer; 2004:121–40.

59. Miranda MC, Mazur MT. Endometrial squamous metaplasia: an unusual response to progestin therapy of hyperplasia. Arch Pathol Lab Med 1995;119:458–60.

60. Moyer DL, Felix JC. The effects of progesterone and progestins on endometrial proliferation. Contraception 1998;57:399–403.

61. Moyer DL, Delignieres B, Driguez P, Pez JP. Prevention of endometrial hyperplasia by progesterone during long-term estradiol replacement – influence of bleeding pattern and secretory changes. Fertil Steril 1993;59:992–7.

62. Mutter GL, Zaino RJ, Baak JPA, Bentley RC, Robboy SJ. The benign endometrial hyperplasia sequence and endometrial intraepithelial neoplasia (EIN). Int J Gynecol Pathol 2007;26:103–14.

63. Narvekar N, Cameron S, Critchley HO, Lin S, Cheng L, Baird DT. Low-dose mifepristone inhibits endometrial proliferation and up-regulates androgen receptor. J Clin Endocrinol Metab 2004;89:2491–7.

64. Nikander E, Rutanen EM, Nieminen P, Wahlstrom T, Ylikorkala O, Tiitinen A. Lack of effect of isoflavonoids on the vagina and endometrium in postmenopausal women. Fertil Steril 2005;83:137–42.

65. Persson I. Cancer risk in women receiving estrogen–progestin replacement therapy. Maturitas 1996;23:S37–S45.

66. Persson I, Weiderpass E, Bergkvist L, Bergstrom R, Schairer C. Risks of breast and endometrial cancer after estrogen and estrogen–progestin replacement. Cancer Causes Control 1999;10:253–60.

67. Piegsa K, Calder A, Davis JA, McKay Hart D, Wells M, Bryden F. Endometrial status in post-menopausal women on long-term continuous combined hormone replacement therapy (Kliofem(R)): a comparative study of endometrial biopsy, outpatient hysteroscopy and transvaginal ultrasound. Eur J Obstet Gynecol Reprod Biol 1997;72:175–80.

68. Purdie DM, Bain CJ, Siskind V, et al. Hormone replacement therapy and risk of epithelial ovarian cancer. Br J Cancer 1999;81:559–63.

69. Rhoton-Vlasak A, Chegini N, Hardt N, Williams RS. Histological characteristics and altered expression of interleukins (IL) IL-13 and IL-15 in endometria of levonorgestrel users with different uterine bleeding patterns. Fertil Steril 2005;83:659–65.

70. Rivera R, Yacobson I, Grimes D. The mechanism of action of hormonal contraceptives and intrauterine contraceptive devices. Am J Obstet Gynecol 1999;181(5 Pt 1):1263–9.

71. Schlesinger C, Kamoi S, Ascher SM, Kendell M, Lage JM, Silverberg SG. Endometrial polyps: a comparison study of patients receiving tamoxifen with two control groups. Int J Gynecol Pathol 1998;17:302–11.

72. Schlesselman JJ. Risk of endometrial cancer in relation to use of combined oral contraceptives. A practitioner's guide to meta-analysis. Hum Reprod 1997;12:1851–63.

73. Seidman JD, Kurman RJ. Tamoxifen and the endometrium. Int J Gynecol Pathol 1999;18:293–6.

74. Seoud M, Shamseddine A, Khalil A, et al. Tamoxifen and endometrial pathologies: a prospective study. Gynecol Oncol 1999;75:15–19.

75. Silva EG, Tornos CS, Follenmitchell M. Malignant neoplasms of the uterine corpus in patients treated for breast carcinoma – the effects of tamoxifen. Int J Gynecol Pathol 1994;13:248–58.

76. Simon C, Oberye J, Bellver J, et al. Similar endometrial development in oocyte donors treated with either high- or standard-dose GnRH antagonist compared to treatment with a GnRH agonist or in natural cycles. Hum Reprod 2005;20:3318–27.

77. Smith IE, Dowsett M. Aromatase inhibitors in breast cancer. N Engl J Med 2003;348:2431–42.

78. Smith IE, Dowsett M, Ebbs SR, et al. Neoadjuvant treatment of postmenopausal breast cancer with anastrozole, tamoxifen, or both in combination: the Immediate Preoperative Anastrozole, Tamoxifen, or Combined with Tamoxifen (IMPACT) multicenter double-blind randomized trial. J Clin Oncol 2005;23:5108–16.

79. Spitz IM. Progesterone receptor antagonists. Curr Opin Investig Drugs 2006;7:882–90.

80. Suh-Burgmann EJ, Goodman A. Surveillance for endometrial cancer in women receiving tamoxifen. Ann Intern Med 1999;131:127–35.

81. Terry P, Baron JA, Weiderpass E, Yuen J, Lichtenstein P, Nyren O. Lifestyle and endometrial cancer risk: a cohort study from the Swedish Twin Registry. Br J Cancer 1999;82:38–42.

82. Treilleux I, Mignotte H, Clement-Chassagne C, Guastalla P, Bailly C. Tamoxifen and malignant epithelial–nonepithelial tumours of the endometrium: report of six cases and review of the literature. Eur J Surg Oncol 1999;25:477–82.

83. Tropea A, Miceli F, Minici F, et al. Endometrial evaluation in superovulation programs: relationship with successful outcome. Ann N Y Acad Sci 2004;1034:211–8.

84. Udell JA, Fischer MA, Brookhart MA, Solomon DH, Choudhry NK. Effect of the women's health initiative on osteoporosis therapy and expenditure in Medicaid. J Bone Mineral Res 2006;21:765–71.

85. Unfer V, Casini ML, Costabile L, Mignosa M, Gerli S, Di Renzo GC. Endometrial effects of long-term treatment with phytoestrogens: a randomized, double-blind, placebo-controlled study. Fertil Steril 2004;82:145–8, quiz 265.

86. Vandermooren MJ, Hanselaar AGJM, Borm GF, Rolland R. Changes in the withdrawal bleeding pattern and endometrial histology during 17 beta-estradiol–dydrogesterone therapy in postmenopausal women: a 2 year prospective study. Maturitas 1994;20:175–80.

87. Vessey M, Painter R. Oral contraceptive use and cancer. Findings in a large cohort study, 1968–2004. Br J Cancer 2006;95:385–9.

88. Weiderpass E, Adami HO, Baron JA, Magnusson C, Lindgren A, Persson I. Use of oral contraceptives and endometrial cancer risk (Sweden). Cancer Causes Control 1999;10:277–84.

89. Weiderpass E, Baron JA, Adami HO, et al. Low-potency oestrogen and risk of endometrial cancer: a case-control study. Lancet 1999;353:1824–8.

90. Weiderpass E, Adami HO, Baron JA, et al. Risk of endometrial cancer following estrogen replacement with and without progestins. J Natl Cancer Inst 1999;91:1131–7.

91. Weiss NS, Sayvetz TA. Incidence of endometrial cancer in relation to the use of oral contraceptives. N Engl J Med 1980;302:551–4.

92. Wynants P, Ide P. Endometrial morphology during a normophasic and a triphasic regimen: a comparison. Contraception 1986;33:149–57.

93. Ziel HK, Finkle WD, Greenland S. Decline in incidence of endometrial cancer following increase in prescriptions for opposed conjugated estrogens in a prepaid health plan. Gynecol Oncol 1998;68:253–5.

Endometritis, metaplasias, polyps, and miscellaneous changes

14

George L. Mutter   Marisa R. Nucci   Stanley J. Robboy

INFLAMMATORY AND INFECTIOUS PROCESSES

In the United States, pelvic inflammatory disease (PID) affects 10% of women during the reproductive years, 25% of whom experience serious sequelae, including infertility, ectopic pregnancy or chronic pelvic pain.[41] Many will require hospital admission and surgery. The medical costs of managing the disease are enormous. Although most interest in PID centers on the fallopian tubes, the disease is defined as an infection of the whole upper genital tract, including the endometrium. Endometritis should therefore be viewed not as a localized discrete entity, but as part of a widespread inflammatory disorder, usually considered as acute endometritis and chronic endometritis according to the inflammatory cell infiltrate present. Some microorganisms that infect the endometrium produce a recognizable constellation of inflammatory changes so that it is often possible from the histologic appearances to suggest what organism is causing the endometritis in a particular woman. More often the features are insufficiently characteristic to attribute the inflammation to a specific microorganism, even if a precipitating cause such as abortion can be identified. Our classification of endometritis incorporates the specific histology linked to infective organisms or related to other etiologic factors where known (Table 14.1).

Endometrial inflammation is recognized, as in other organs, primarily by the presence of inflammatory cells. However, as the endometrium may normally contain inflammatory cells, the diagnosis of endometritis is often not straightforward. Lymphocytes are a normal constituent and their presence does not necessarily indicate endometritis. Even the presence of focal collections of lymphocytes, which are usually perivascular, should not be considered abnormal. When arranged in follicles with transformed lymphocytes forming a germinal center, endometritis is likely.[26] As plasma cells are seldom found in a normal endometrium, their presence is indicative of chronic endometritis. Neutrophil polymorphonuclear leukocytes may also be found in the normal cycle, especially in appreciable numbers once menstruation is well established. Granulated lymphocytes, or CD56+ uterine natural killer (NK) cells, present in the stroma during the second half of the cycle, and especially in predecidua, are easily mistaken for neutrophils.[18,55] Macrophages are always present in the normal endometrium, but in their usual appearance resembles endometrial stromal cells, rendering separation difficult.

ENDOMETRITIS

Patients with endometritis often present with the clinical features of PID. They will have a history of fever and lower abdominal pain, with leukocytosis and bilateral adnexal or cervical motion tenderness on bimanual pelvic examination. If the infecting organism is less virulent or if the disease is early in its natural history, the symptoms, such as menstrual abnormalities, pelvic pain or infertility, may not initially indicate the clinical diagnosis of endometritis. Although most cases of acute salpingitis are accompanied by endometritis, it is not known how often endometritis occurs in isolation without involving the fallopian tubes. The diagnosis of endometritis is therefore often a histologic one that, particularly in the case of non-specific endometritis, is not associated with a specific clinical presentation or cause.

NON-SPECIFIC ENDOMETRITIS

The histologic diagnosis of acute endometritis is made when significant numbers of neutrophils are present in the endometrial stroma at a time other than the menstrual phase of the cycle (Figure 14.1). Isolated or rare neutrophils are insufficient for a diagnosis of acute endometritis. The usual pattern is that of patchy distribution, with or without microabscesses. In most instances, it is relatively straightforward to distinguish between menstrual endometrium and acutely inflamed, non-menstrual endometrium, particularly if other histologic features of inflammation or repair, including edema, hemorrhage, venule ectasia, collections of lymphocytes or inflamed glands, are present (Figure 14.2). If the neutrophils are present because of menstruation, other features of menstruation will be present, such as secretory vacuoles in the glandular epithelium and predecidual change of the stroma with diffuse breakdown. The diagnosis of acute endometritis during menstruation is difficult because there is some overlap between menstrual and inflammatory histologic features. Although it may seem important to distinguish between those features that are the results of physiologic, cyclic changes and those that are pathologic, it may not always be possible to do so.

The acute inflammatory process in acute endometritis most often involves only the upper functional layer of the endometrium, so that when menstruation occurs, the inflamed tissue is shed and, assuming that the precipitating cause of the inflammation is no longer present, a new functional layer develops

343

Table 14.1 Classification of endometritis

Specific microorganism
  Neisseria
  Tuberculosis
  Chlamydia
  Mycoplasma
  Cytomegalovirus
  Herpes simplex virus

No specific microorganism
  Associated with intrauterine contraceptive device
  Granulomatous (excluding tuberculosis)
  Histiocytic
  Postpartum
  Postabortal
  Pyometra
  Not otherwise specified (chronic non-specific)

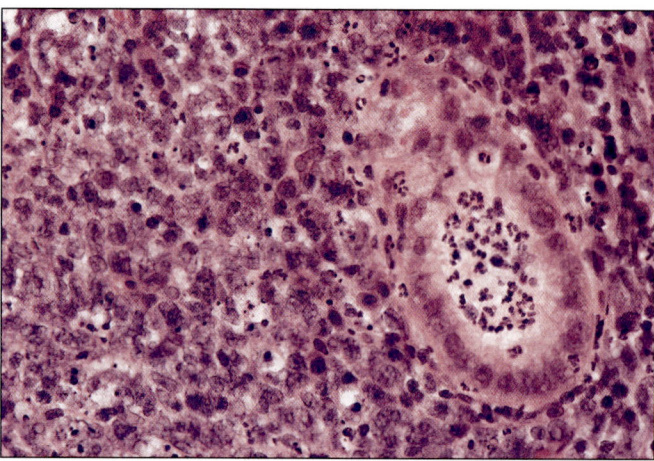

Fig. 14.2 Acute endometritis. Polymorphs are present throughout the stroma and in the gland lumina.

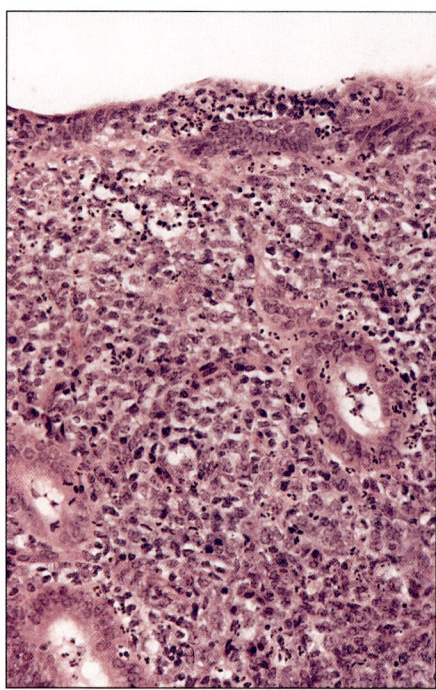

Fig. 14.1 Acute endometritis. Polymorphs are present in the surface epithelium and throughout the stroma.

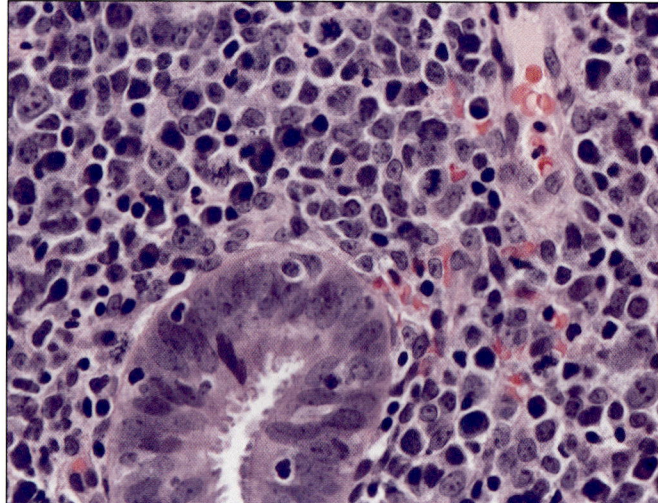

Fig. 14.3 Chronic endometritis. Plasma cells are prominent in the stroma. Detail: Plasma cells.

from the healthy regenerating basal layer. In more severe examples, the inflammation may persist, eventually progressing to chronic endometritis.

If plasma cells are present, often together with the changes described above, then a diagnosis of chronic endometritis is made (Figure 14.3). A clear distinction between acute endometritis and chronic endometritis is artificial, however, as the two phases of inflammation often merge and coexist. Frequently the plasma cells of chronic endometritis accompany lymphocytes and there can be no doubt that, in these circumstances, the lymphocytes contribute to the inflammatory process. Indeed, lymphocytes may predominate in the infiltrate, contributing significantly to the increased stromal cellularity. However, lymphocytes in isolation are not diagnostic of chronic endometritis. The density of the plasma cell infiltrate naturally

varies depending upon the severity of the inflammation. Furthermore, the infiltrate may be superficial, as seen with an intrauterine contraceptive device, or may involve all layers of the endometrium.

A not uncommon problem occurs when only a rare plasma cell is identified or it is a minor component of the infiltrate. If on a low-power magnification the endometrium looks 'dirty' with numerous lymphocytes (Figure 14.4), a careful search under higher magnification often shows scattered plasma cells that justify a diagnosis of chronic endometritis. Areas worthy of particular attention include stroma adjacent to luminal breakdown or glands engorged with inflammatory cells. As plasma cells may be a normal component within the stroma of an endometrial polyp, care must be taken to ensure that only the functionalis is assessed and not fragments of polyp.

As a diagnosis of chronic endometritis depends upon the presence of plasma cells, it is important that these are identified with maximum accuracy. Plasma cells are generally easy to recognize if they are present in reasonable numbers, but we have found that in the endometrium, as opposed to any other

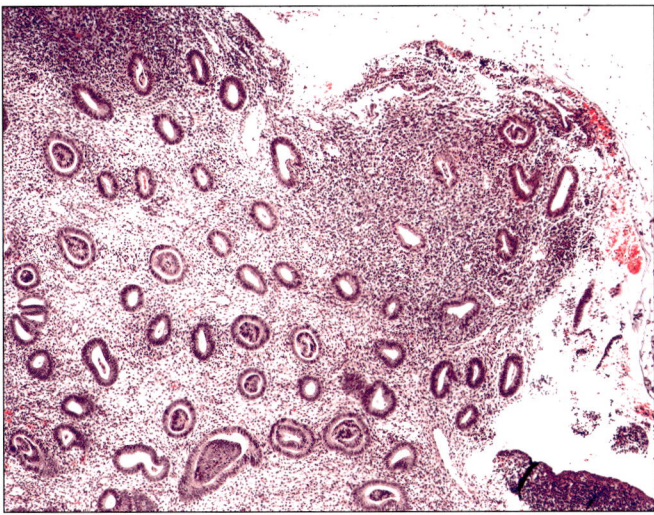

Fig. 14.4 Chronic endometritis. At low magnification, the presence of a patchy infiltrate of inflammatory cells makes the stroma appear dirty. At high magnification, a rare plasma cell can be found.

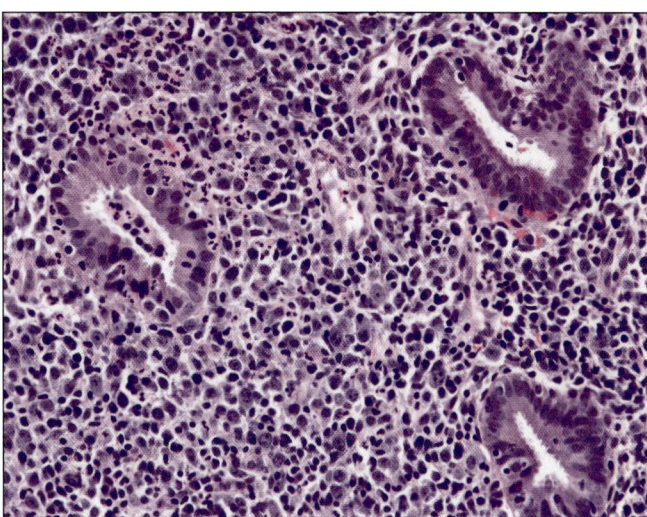

Fig. 14.5 Chronic endometritis. The glands show neither secretory nor proliferative activity. Numerous plasma cells are present in the stroma and there is pus in gland lumina.

organ, they can appear smudged or are easily overlooked if sparse. In these cases, a methyl green-pyronin stain or reactivity with syndecan-1 (CD-138)[3] assists in their identification. However, the clinical significance of sparse plasma cell infiltration identified by these methods is not clear.

A final problem in the diagnosis occurs when the endometrium shows a diffuse infiltrate of lymphocytes ('dirty' endometrium) but no plasma cells. This finding should be described in the report with the suggestion that it may represent chronic endometritis. A related observation appears to be particularly relevant in patients being investigated for recurrent miscarriage. In such cases, a frequently observed pattern is aggregation of a mixture of CD8+ T-cells and CD56+ NK cells adjacent to glands, in the absence of clinical signs of infection.

The glands may be involved in the inflammatory process[48a] in two ways. There may be an infiltrate of inflammatory cells, predominantly neutrophils, affecting the epithelium of the glands and the lumina may contain pus. In addition, as the process becomes more advanced, the glandular response to hormonal stimulation becomes impaired, the glands appearing inactive, with neither proliferation nor secretion (Figure 14.5). Once an endometrium shows signs of endometritis, precise dating is not possible. It is probably not even reliable to categorize the endometrium as either proliferative or secretory. Dating is unnecessary in a patient who has significant endometritis. The histologic features of endometritis are summarized in Table 14.2.

SPECIFIC FORMS OF ENDOMETRITIS

CHLAMYDIA TRACHOMATIS AND *NEISSERIA GONORRHOEAE*

Many upper genital tract infections result from the sexually transmitted organisms *Chlamydia trachomatis* and *Neisseria gonorrhoeae*.[26,46] Infection by the former exhibits tiny, supranuclear, intracytoplasmic vacuoles containing inclusions, but as these are not readily apparent by microscopic examination, immunohistologic or molecular methods are usually required

Table 14.2 Histologic features of endometritis
Neutrophil infiltrate
Plasma cell infiltrate
Lymphocyte infiltrate – focal collections with germinal centers
Edema
Vascular ectasia
Necrosis and fragmentation of stroma
Suppression of glandular hormonal response

for confirmation of this infection. Polymerase chain reaction (PCR) identifies *C. trachomatis* in one-fourth of plasma cell endometritis specimens, and these can also be cultured.[32,45] Endometritis due to either *Chlamydia* or *Neisseria* has large numbers of plasma cells in the endometrial stroma, neutrophils in the endometrial surface epithelium (five or more per high-power field) and lymphoid aggregates with transformed lymphocytes,[27] thus providing clues to the diagnosis. Intraluminal neutrophils and subepithelial hemorrhages are also usually present, but these findings are less specific. Histopathology alone can suggest, but not reliably distinguish between, these organisms. Prominent lymphoid follicles with transformed lymphocytes point more to chlamydial infection while extensive stromal fragmentation favors gonococcal infection.[26]

MYCOPLASMA

Infection with the mycoplasma *Ureaplasma urealyticum* produces subtle but distinctive changes that may be easily missed. The changes are focal, composed of lymphocytic clusters with histiocytes and occasional neutrophils. Plasma cells are not prominent. These focal collections often lie beneath the surface epithelium, around glands and surrounding spiral arterioles. The changes are best seen when the endometrial stroma is most edematous, from day 20 to day 23, a time when the looseness of the stroma allows the small collections of cells to be spotted more easily. In many of these patients, *U. urealyticum* has also been cultured from the uterine cervix, suggesting an ascending infection.

CYTOMEGALOVIRUS

Cytomegalovirus (CMV) infection of the endometrium has been reported rarely and may be associated with pregnancy and immunosuppression as well as being found in women with no known underlying disorder. The infection discloses the characteristic viral cytopathic effects in epithelial and sometimes endothelial cells. The affected cells are grossly enlarged and each usually contains a single large, basophilic intranuclear inclusion that is surrounded by a narrow clear space separating it from the nuclear membrane (Figure 14.6). Immunocompetent patients often also show an accompanying dense inflammatory infiltrate, with plasma cells, lymphocytes, and eosinophils.

HERPES SIMPLEX VIRUS

Like CMV infection, herpes simplex virus (HSV) infection of the endometrium is rare. It may occur as an ascending process associated with cervical infection or result from disseminated virus in immunosuppressed patients. It may cause postpartum endometritis in cases where neonates have died from disseminated HSV infection.[26] Infection of the endometrium produces changes similar to those associated with HSV elsewhere, namely extensive acute inflammation with necrosis. Cowdry type A inclusions and, occasionally, multinucleated giant cells with ground-glass nuclei may be identified in glandular epithelium or in the stroma.

TUBERCULOUS ENDOMETRITIS

Although tuberculosis is now infrequent in many countries, occasional examples in the female genital tract are still encountered, and more may be seen in the future resulting from the emergence of drug-resistant strains of *Mycobacterium tuberculosis* and the immunosuppression of AIDS. Tuberculosis of the female genital tract is virtually always secondary to disease of the lungs or gastrointestinal tract, which often occurred many

years previously. About three-fourths of women with tuberculosis of the genital tract have endometrial involvement. The fallopian tubes are almost always involved and the endometrium is affected secondarily by passage of the bacteria down the tube into the uterine cavity.

The disease may present without gynecologic symptoms or it may be associated with infertility, irregular bleeding or amenorrhea. The principal histologic feature is epithelioid cell granulomas. These may be sparse, so that a thorough search of the material is required if tuberculosis is suspected clinically. The granulomas are usually small and central caseation is unusual, especially in women who have normal, or near normal, menstrual cycles (Figure 14.7). Caseation is found only when there is amenorrhea or after the menopause, for it is only when the endometrium no longer periodically sheds that there exists sufficient time for the granulomas to develop *de novo* and then caseate. The disease process affects all layers of the endometrium.

The epithelioid cell granuloma of tuberculous endometritis contains a central collection of epithelioid cells with both Langhans and foreign body type giant cells (Figure 14.8). There is usually a peripheral collar of lymphocytes. Because caseation is absent, the granulomas more closely resemble those of sar-

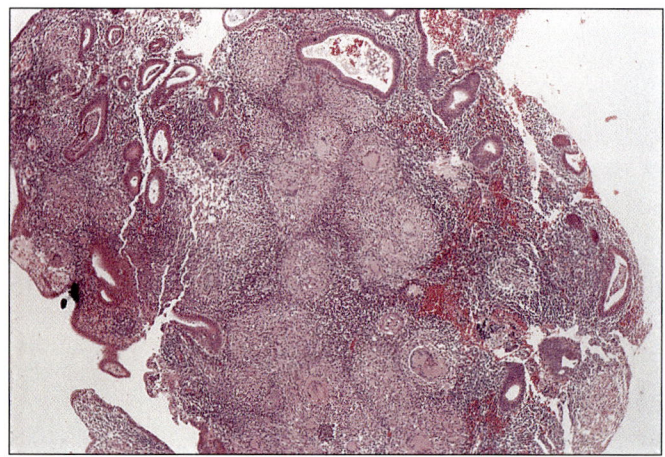

Fig. 14.7 Tuberculous endometritis.

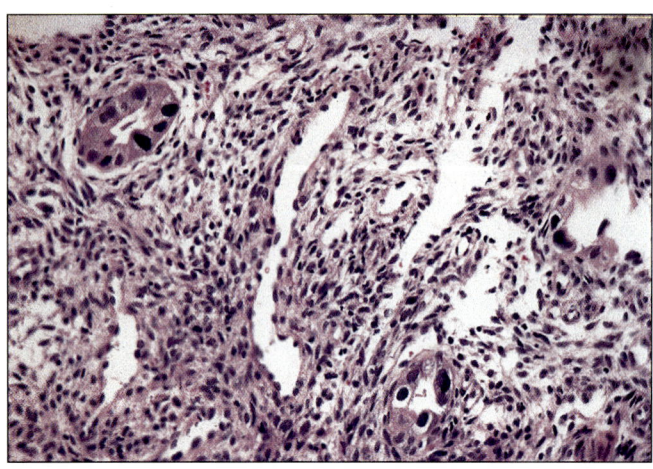

Fig. 14.6 Cytomegalovirus infection. Cells with grossly enlarged nuclei are present in small glands.

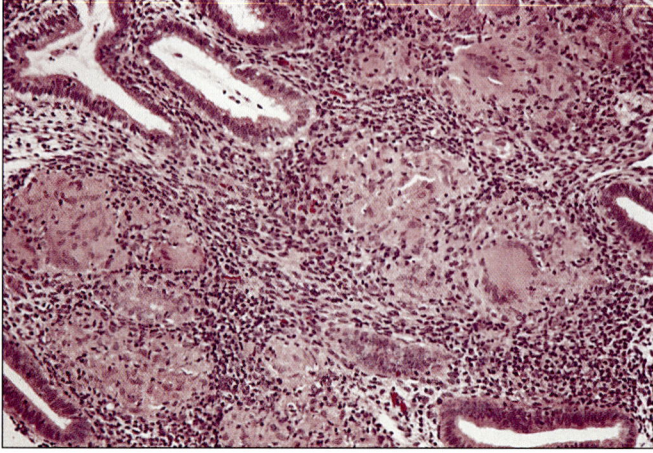

Fig. 14.8 Tuberculous endometritis. Non-caseating epithelioid cell granulomas are distributed throughout the stroma.

coidosis, a feature reinforced by their being well circumscribed. Uterine sarcoidosis rarely presents without proven sarcoidosis elsewhere in the body.

Culture of the endometrial tissue best confirms the diagnosis. In a 30-year-old classic study that has not been repeated, acid-fast bacilli were demonstrated in less than 2% of 1134 women with culture-proven organisms.[42] Treatment results in the granulomas being replaced either by fibrous tissue or by becoming transient lymphoid follicles that eventually disappear completely, the lymphocytic infiltrate remaining in the endometrium for many years.

ACTINOMYCES ISRAELI

Infection by *Actinomyces israeli* has long been associated with intrauterine contraceptive device (IUD) usage. This organism is a slow-growing, filamentous, Gram-positive anaerobe that is not normally found in the lower genital tract (Figure 14.9). When found in cervical smears or curettings, half the women lack symptoms. Microscopic examination of the curettings shows densely matted filaments of the Gram-positive organisms (Figure 14.10). Gomori methenamine silver stain is positive in *Actinomyces*, which is a useful means of identifying

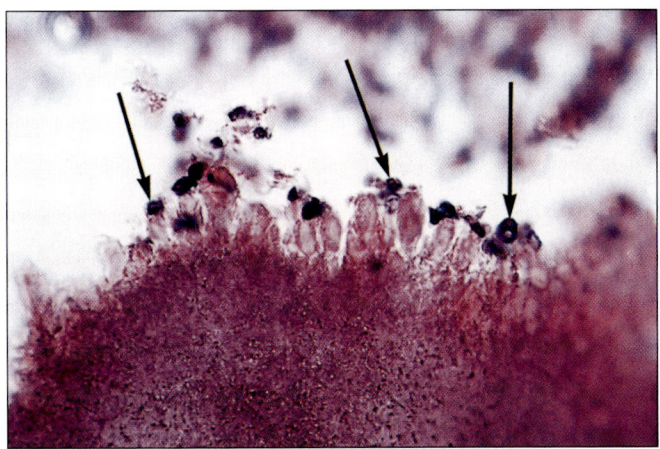

Fig. 14.9 *Actinomyces.* Sulfur granule with clubs (arrows) of a patient with an intrauterine device.

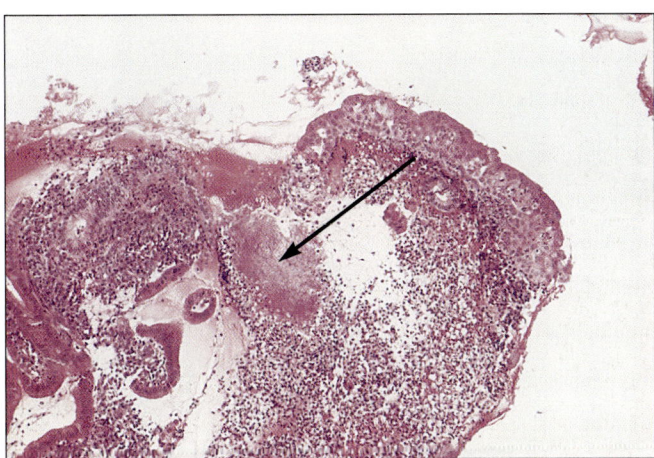

Fig. 14.10 Intrauterine contraceptive device. *Actinomyces*-like organisms (arrow) in curettings of a women with an intrauterine device.

non-infectious pseudoactinomycotic radiate granules (negatively staining) that are even more common than actual organisms in women with an IUD.[43] There is usually some degree of associated endometritis, with a dense infiltrate of neutrophils. Sulfur granules, if present, appear in sinus tracks bathed in pus (Figure 14.11). The infection may progress to pelvic actinomycosis.[48] The risk of infection by *A. israeli* relates less to the type of IUD in use than the length of time it has been in place in the uterine cavity, 85% of cases occurring when the IUD has been worn for 3 or more years.

OTHER FORMS OF ENDOMETRITIS

GRANULOMATOUS ENDOMETRITIS

Granulomas may be found in the endometrium as an expression of a wide variety of diseases, both local and systemic. Although tuberculous endometritis comes first to mind, it is probably no longer the most common form. Sarcoidosis is associated with well-formed, clearly demarcated epithelioid cell granulomas lacking central necrosis. It occurs usually, but not always, in women with known systemic disease. However, as necrosis is unusual in tuberculous endometritis, endometrial sarcoid should only be diagnosed if the disease is present elsewhere in the body. Other causes of granulomatous endometritis include postablation repair, foreign bodies, fungal infection, parasites, and the specific infections described above, particularly *Ureaplasma*. An effort should be made to identify a treatable, infective cause if it is present. Fungi may be identified using periodic acid-Schiff (PAS) or Grocott stains but it is questionable whether a time-consuming search for acid-fast bacilli is worth undertaking, because of the very low chance of identifying the organism, even in culture-proven cases.[33] The identification of pigment or birefringence under polarized light points to a foreign body reaction. A clinical history may also be useful in coming to a conclusion.

HISTIOCYTIC ENDOMETRITIS

On rare occasions, the endometrium discloses a massive infiltrate of histiocytes that contain abundant lipid, together with

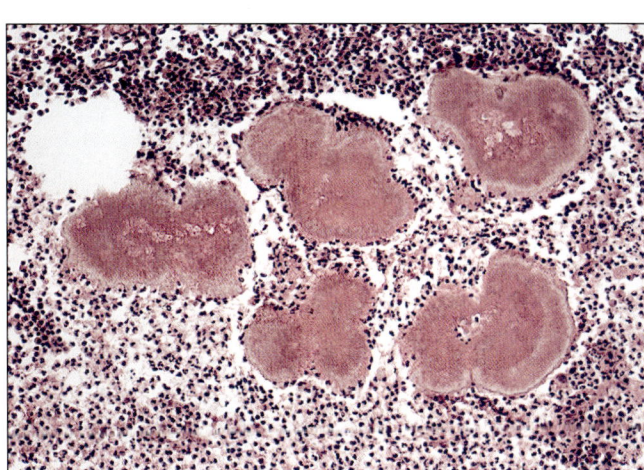

Fig. 14.11 *Actinomyces.* Sulfur granules surrounded by pus.

multinucleated giant cells, hemosiderin, cholesterol clefts, plasma cells, lymphocytes, and occasional neutrophils. This may occur in association with pyometra, due to postmenopausal cervical stenosis, or as the result of cervical carcinoma. The terms 'pseudoxanthoma' and 'xanthogranuloma' have also been used but the term 'histiocytic endometritis' is preferred. The condition bears no relation to the focal clusters of foamy macrophages sometimes found in the stroma of endometrial hyperplasias and carcinomas. Appearances similar to histiocytic endometritis may be seen in the fallopian tube. Malacoplakia is a rare variant of histiocytic endometritis. The appearances are generally similar to those already described but in addition Michaelis–Gutmann bodies are present. These are small, round, laminated calcospherules that may be found both in the histiocyte cytoplasm and extracellularly.

POSTPARTUM AND POSTABORTAL ENDOMETRITIS

Endometritis occurs in 2–5% of women following vaginal delivery, 20–55% of women following cesarean section, and 1–8% of women having termination of pregnancy in a hospital setting. Plasma cell infiltrates are characteristic of postpartum chronic endometritis (Figure 14.12). Microbiologic examination shows that the infection is caused most frequently by cultured being *U. urealyticum* and *Gardnerella vaginalis*. The latter is most commonly associated with bacterial vaginosis and clinical evidence of bacterial vaginosis is associated with a six-fold increase in the risk of postcesarean endometritis.[43] Furthermore, recent studies have shown that bacterial vaginosis is associated with a higher risk of endometritis[62] and upper genital tract infection[27] in the non-pregnant state. Pyometra has also been reported postpartum.[47]

Following spontaneous abortion, the infective organisms are more likely to be the usual pathogens, *Escherichia coli*, *Staphylococcus aureus*, *Neisseria gonorrhoeae* and *Streptococcus viridans*.

The histopathologic features of the endometrium in these forms of endometritis are usually those of an acute infection, with prominence of neutrophils and tissue necrosis. Organisms are often identified by Gram stain.

PYOMETRA

Inflammation of the endometrium is most dramatic when pyometra, pus filling the uterine cavity, develops. This is often due to a blocked cervical canal in conditions such as cervical carcinoma or, more frequently, postmenopausal stenosis. Introduction of foreign material through fistulous tracts is another common cause. As the term implies, the cavity of the distended uterus is filled with pus and the endometrium usually shows the features of severe acute and chronic inflammation (Figure 14.13). In some cases, where the distension is considerable, pressure markedly thins the endometrium, such that it becomes merely an attenuated layer of stroma covered by surface epithelium. An acute and chronic inflammatory infiltrate permeates the stroma, and may also extend into the superficial myometrium (Figure 14.14). Squamous metaplasia may develop in the surface epithelium and glands, and at its most extreme is known as ichthyosis uteri. Squamous cell carcinoma, rarely, may also occur.

ENDOMETRIAL METAPLASIAS

Endometrial metaplasia is a change in cellular differentiation to a type that is not present in the normal endometrium. Metaplastic cells have an altered cytoplasmic appearance and variable nuclear changes that may or may not be associated with an altered architecture. Metaplasia in the endometrium most commonly affects the epithelial element, but occasionally involves the stromal component. Because altered differentiation may be seen in benign, premalignant, or malignant endometria, a simple diagnosis of endometrial metaplasia is rarely

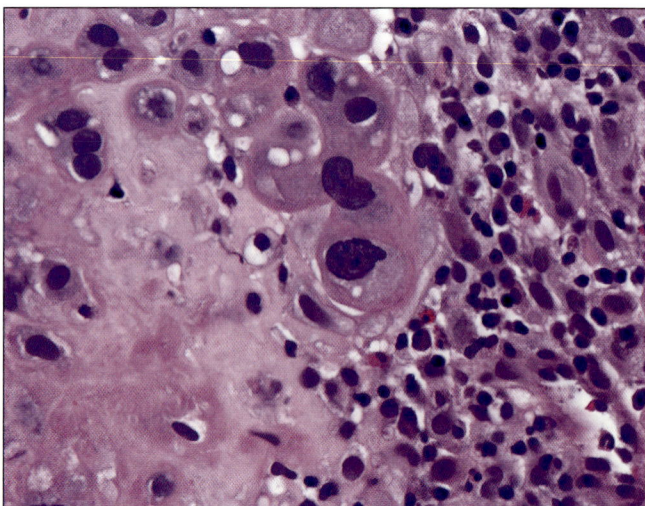

Fig. 14.12 Postabortal chronic endometritis. Plasma cells are adjacent to a recent nodular implantation site.

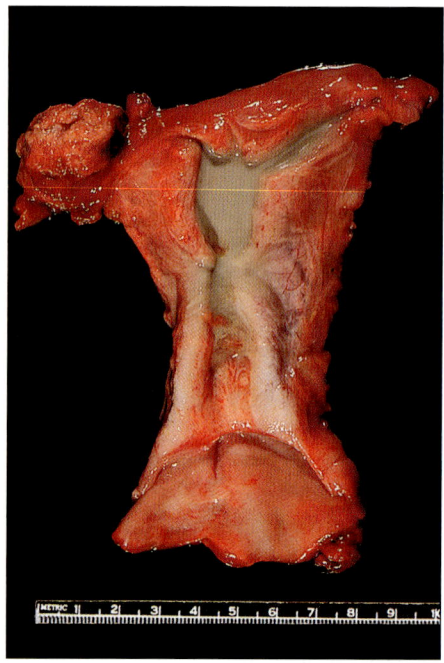

Fig. 14.13 Pyometra.

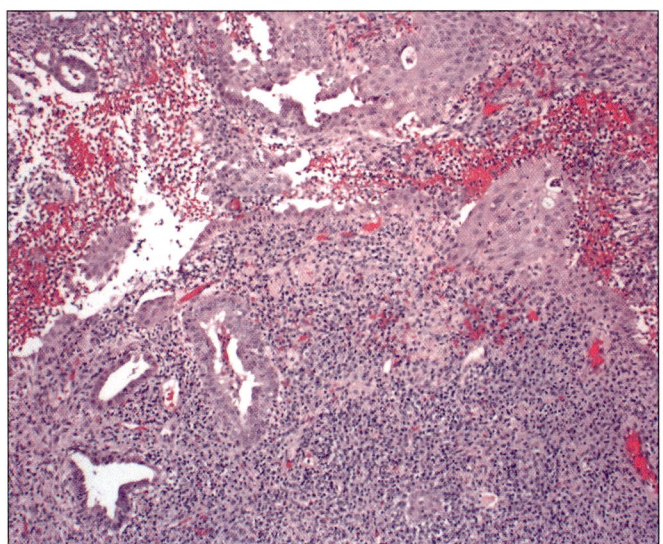

Fig. 14.14 Acute inflammatory infiltrate and severe epithelial reactive change in pyometra.

Table 14.3 Major classes of endometrial epithelial metaplasia

	Degenerative/Repair	Hormonal	Neoplastic
Topography	Focal/Multifocal	Regularly irregular	Local and expansive
Mechanism	Stromal breakdown, surface repair	Hormonal stimulation	Monoclonal expansion of muted cell
Examples	Papillary syncytial metaplasia	Disordered proliferative endometrium with tubal metaplasia	EIN, adenocarcinoma

sufficient to fully convey the lesion's clinical significance. Whenever possible, endometrial metaplasia should be clearly placed within the broader diagnostic context of a reactive, hormonal, or neoplastic process.

EPITHELIAL METAPLASIAS

The epithelium of the upper female genital tract, whether endocervical, endometrial or tubal, is all of common paramesonephric (müllerian) origin, but each area shows its own characteristic cell type: mucus-secreting in the cervix, ciliated in the fallopian tube, and columnar with secretory potential in the endometrium. The most common forms of endometrial metaplasia are those in which endometrial glands assume a morphology resembling that seen elsewhere along the müllerian duct, such as serous, mucinous, or squamous. Müllerian-derived structures thus maintain an element of plasticity in which any of a number of pathogenetic mechanisms may incite differentiation inappropriate for the particular anatomic location. The resultant metaplasia is accompanied by the appearance of differentiated structures and protein expression patterns usually associated with a specific non-endometrial cell type, such as intracellular mucin in mucinous metaplasia, cilia in tubal metaplasia, or keratin in squamous metaplasia. In practice, use of the term 'metaplasia' is not constrained to a change in differentiation, having been extended as a descriptive label for some non-specific degenerative changes.

Endometrial metaplasias are best considered a spectrum of altered differentiation states in which the pathologist should attempt to determine the underlying mechanism, and use terminology that clearly communicates clinical significance to the referring physician. This is rarely accomplished by a freestanding diagnosis of 'metaplasia', which simply declares a lesion to be non-endometrioid in appearance without specifying it as benign, premalignant, or malignant.

Etiology and natural history
The term 'metaplasia' applies to a broad range of cytologic appearances caused by degenerative, hormonal, or neoplastic processes (Table 14.3). The overall low magnification topography of metaplastic changes within the endometrial compartment, combined with the local histologic context, are extremely useful in ascertaining a likely cause.[36,37] Degenerative changes can be localized to areas of inflammation, stromal breakdown, or recent surface repair. Hormonally induced changes tend to be diffusely and randomly scattered throughout the upper endometrial compartment (functionalis), whereas premalignant and malignant processes are monoclonal expansions that begin as localizing lesions offset by the normal background.

ARIAS-STELLA REACTION

The Arias-Stella reaction, also called phenomenon, change and effect, refers to hypersecretory glands in the gestational endometrium, the hallmark of which is cells with nuclear atypia exhibiting enlargement, hyperchromasia and irregularity. The importance of this change is the difficulty that often occurs in distinguishing it from hyperplasia, or indeed from adenocarcinoma. The Arias-Stella change is due to increased gonadotropin stimulation and may be seen in both normal or ectopic pregnancy.

Pathology
The diagnosis is exclusively microscopical (Figure 14.15). No gross changes are seen. Characteristically, nuclei in the hypersecretory glands bulge into the gland lumina beyond the apparent cell limits and resemble, but should not be mistaken for, the hobnail cells of clear cell carcinoma. It is our impression that the nucleus usually appears degenerative and smudged and chromatin is not apparent. Atypical mitotic figures have been reported, but we have never even seen normal mitotic figures in this condition. Although not obligatory for the diagnosis of the Arias-Stella phenomenon, most examples show exaggerated secretory activity that is very often associated with architectural complexity, with prominent infoldings. The curetted

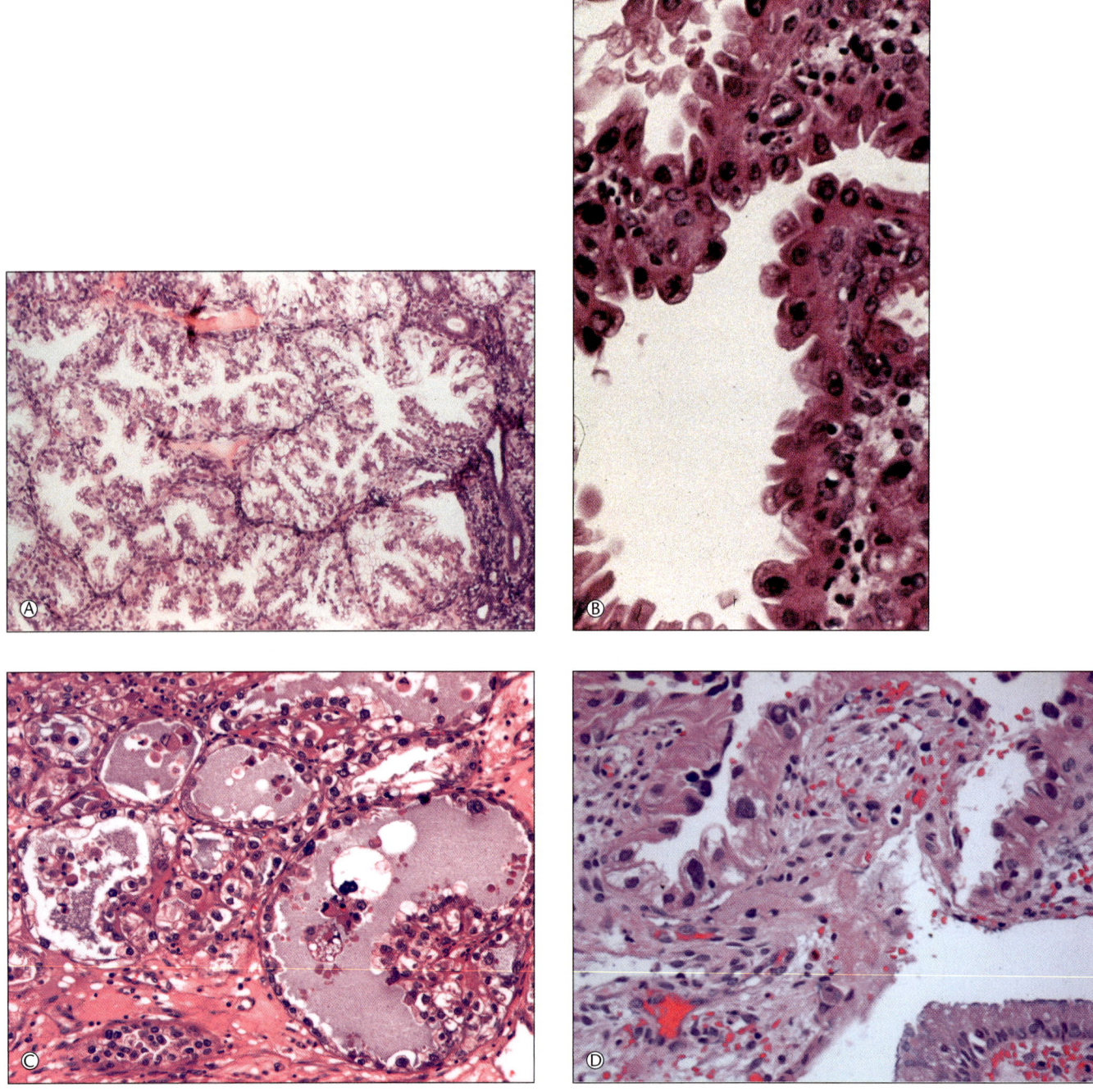

Fig. 14.15 Arias-Stella reaction. **(A)** Hypersecretory change in endometrium in which a rare nucleus is enlarged. **(B)** The hobnail cell change with bulbous nuclei protruding beyond their cytoplasmic limits is so pronounced as to mimic the hobnail pattern in the papillary form of clear cell adenocarcinoma. **(C)** Hobnail cell of Arias-Stella reaction change mimicking the hobnail pattern in the tubulocystic form of clear cell adenocarcinoma. **(D)** Arias-Stella reaction in endocervix.

material in such circumstances will often show other features associated with gestation, such as decidual change, although these changes may be seen in the absence of pregnancy. In addition, the Arias-Stella phenomenon generally occurs in a younger age group than hyperplasias do and the clinical features may aid the diagnosis.

The genetic underpinnings of müllerian metaplasia are just now emerging. Genetic mediators of müllerian differentiation include members of the homeobox gene superfamily, HOX, where coordinate expression of HOX genes determines differentiation state.[17] Altered HOX gene expression, through hormonal[38,53] or epigenetic mechanisms,[7,58] is capable of re-determining differentiation state. For example, HOXA11 expression can be induced by progestins and in müllerian epithelium is associated with acquisition of mucinous differentiation.[63]

Many instances of degenerative 'metaplasia' will show an underlying cause, such as physical irritation due to an intrauterine mass lesion (submucous fibroid, polyp), inflammatory conditions (endometritis), or breakdown of endometrial stroma. Most are not true metaplasias demonstrating features of specialized altered differentiation, but rather histologic mimics where use of the term descriptively augments a more specific diagnosis of endometritis or breakdown. An example is 'papillary syncytial metaplasia', which exhibits papillary fronds of epithelium that have lost nuclear polarity and can be seen in association with breakdown of supporting stroma, irritation of the uterine lining epithelium, or as part of a reparative process.

Hormonally induced metaplasias are common and not always abnormal, particularly in the case of estrogen-induced tubal change. Estrogens may induce tubal metaplasia of endometrial glands in a random interspersed pattern throughout the entire endometrial compartment at a density depending on dose and duration of exposure. Estrogen-induced tubal metaplasia is most frequently seen in women around the time of the menopause and just afterwards, and is associated with abnormal uterine bleeding and often with a history of recent estrogen therapy. It is important to realize that ciliated cells are normally sporadically present in the endometrium, particularly the lining epithelium, and may not indicate a hormonally induced change.

A particular pitfall in dealing with endometrial neoplasms with altered (metaplastic) differentiation is the incorrect assumption that metaplasia and neoplasia are mutually exclusive processes. Tight homogeneous clusters of metaplastic glands offset by a background of glands with contrasting cytology raises the possibility of endometrial intraepithelial neoplasia (EIN) or even adenocarcinoma.[34] Squamous, mucinous, tubal, or secretory differentiation may be acquired features intrinsic to a premalignant (EIN) or malignant (adenocarcinoma) neoplastic clone.[11,23,59] In these instances, altered differentiation is best noted descriptively appended to a primary diagnosis of EIN or adenocarcinoma (Table 14.4). Individual examples of EIN or adenocarcinoma can demonstrate quite unstable differentiation states in which admixed cytologies line individual glands or populate different regions of the neoplastic field.[23,34,35] In the case of premalignant lesions, all the usual EIN criteria must be met (see Chapter 15),[57] and the observed change in cellular differentiation may be a part of the characteristic altered cytology. Overtly malignant processes, espe-

cially mucinous and secretory adenocarcinomas, may have unusually bland nuclei as part of their altered differentiation state.

METAPLASIAS TO A TUBAL EPITHELIUM

Tubal differentiation is the most commonly encountered form of endometrial metaplasia, accounting for 60% of examples of metaplasia in the endometrium. Cilia are the most distinctive manifestation, but changes evident even at low magnification are increased cytoplasmic volume and eosinophilic staining properties. Interspersed between cuboidal ciliated cells are occasional round secretory cells in a pattern resembling that of the normal fallopian tube. The density of cilia varies greatly, and even a cilia-poor epithelium that demonstrates characteristic cytoplasmic properties of admixed round and columnar cells may be considered serous-like ('seroid') or tubal in character (Figure 14.16). Some cilia-depleted tubal metaplasias display such prominent micropapillary or eosinophilic features that they may be considered mixed-type metaplasias (Figure 14.17). Tubal differentiation may be induced by estrogen exposure or be a manifestation of a neoplastic clone.

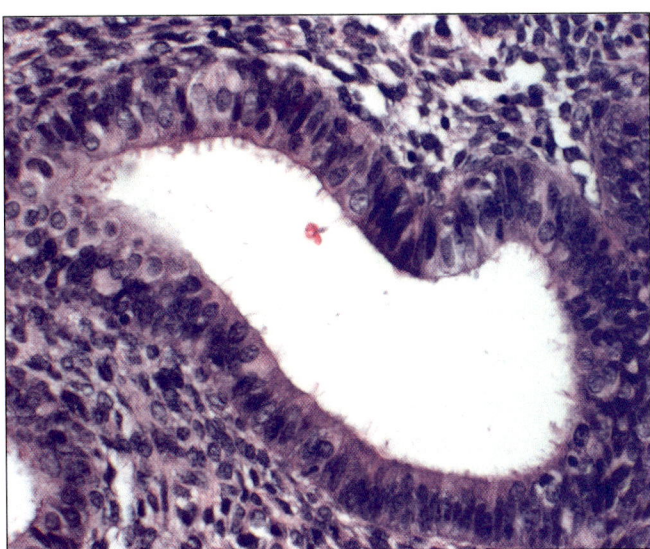

Fig. 14.16 Tubal (ciliated cell) metaplasia.

Table 14.4 Diagnostic terminology of benign, premalignant, and malignant endometrial epithelial metaplasias

Differentiation	Benign	Premalignant	Malignant
Tubal	Normal proliferative endometrium with tubal metaplasia Disordered proliferative endometrium with tubal metaplasia Benign endometrial hyperplasia with tubal metaplasia	EIN with tubal differentiation	Endometrial adenocarcinoma, endometrioid type, with tubal differentiation
Squamous	Chronic endometritis with squamous differentiation (ichthyosis uteri) Isolated squamous morules (requires follow-up)	EIN with morular squamous differentiation	Endometrial adenocarcinoma, endometrioid type, with squamous (morular, non-morular) differentiation
Mucinous	Mucinous degenerative changes Polyp, mixed endometrial and endocervical type Benign mucinous differentiation	EIN with mucinous differentiation	Endometrial adenocarcinoma, endometrioid type, with mucinous differentiation
Secretory	Secretory endometrium, mixed type Hypersecretory endometrium (includes Arias-Stella)	EIN with secretory differentiation	Endometrial adenocarcinoma, endometrioid type, with secretory differentiation

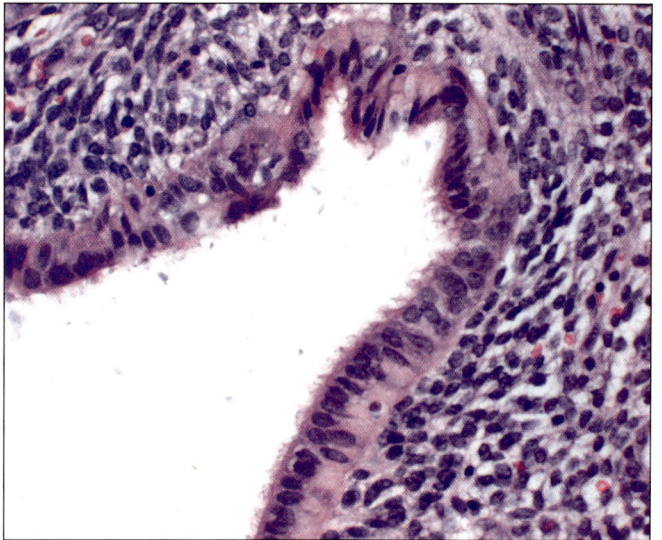

Fig. 14.17 Tubal metaplasia with eosinophilic cytoplasm.

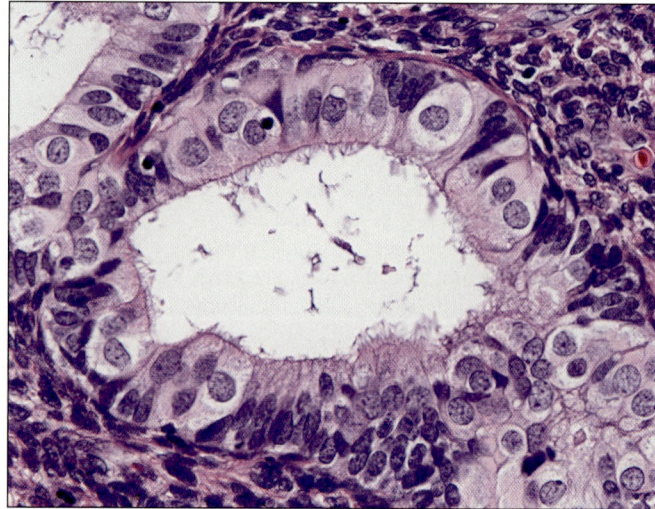

Fig. 14.19 EIN with ciliated tubal differentiation.

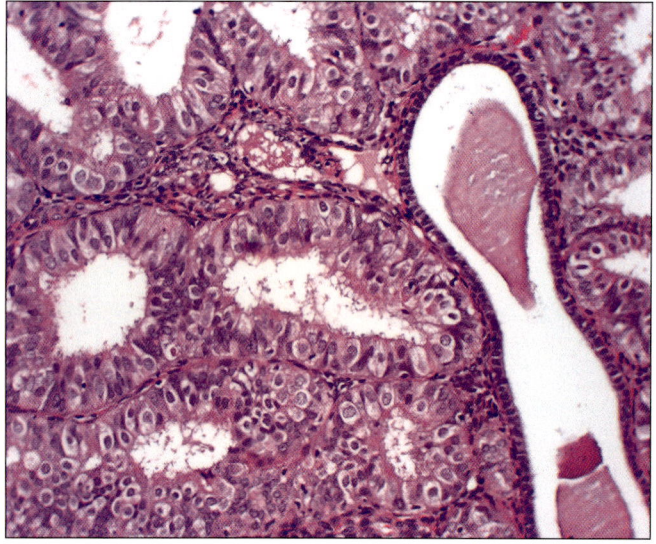

Fig. 14.18 EIN with ciliated tubal differentiation.

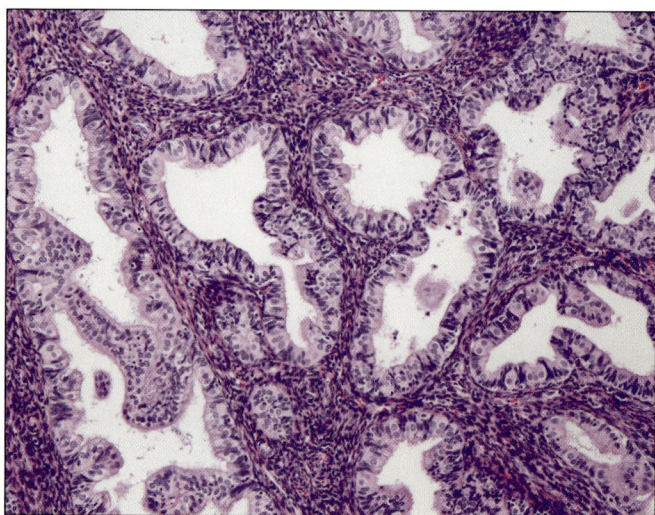

Fig. 14.20 EIN with tubal differentiation. Tubal–micropapillary changes.

A difficult, but practical problem is the significance that should be given to the finding of tubal metaplasia. It is frequent in the normal proliferative endometrium, suggesting that this can be a normal physiologic finding of little clinical import, other than indicative of a background estrogenic milieu. It also occurs in half of endometrial adenocarcinomas.[23] Precancerous EIN lesions with localized clonal architecture (Figure 14.18) may also demonstrate tubal differentiation within affected neoplastic glands (Figure 14.19).[24] In some cases tubal differentiation is a homogeneous cytologic change delimiting an EIN clone. More commonly, tubal glands within the EIN lesion have variable cilia formation, and are admixed with micropapillary or endometrioid cytologies (Figure 14.20) in flanking glands. Many EIN lesions arise from an endometrial field altered by unopposed estrogens. Background glands may also demonstrate tubal metaplasia characteristic of an estrogen effect, but these appear scattered amongst the cysts and irregularly spaced glands rather than in clusters. Some EIN lesions with tubal differentiation occur within an inactive or even atrophic background, implying that estrogens, while common, are not essential for tubal differentiation within neoplastic clones.

METAPLASIAS TO A SQUAMOUS EPITHELIUM

Squamous metaplasia may be seen as a stratified epithelium lining the uterine cavity, or as expansile round morules within individual glands. When an isolated finding, the former typically results from chronic irritation or infection. Squamous metaplasia of the morular type, however, is most common in a neoplastic setting. Squamous differentiation within endometrial glands occurs in many premalignant EIN[23] lesions and approximately 25% of adenocarcinomas.[35,57] Not uncommonly, a single or several foci of squamous morules is found isolated in a small biopsy specimen, but prove to be located at the periphery of an EIN or malignant lesion. This has prompted the clinical recommendation that a dilatation and curettage (D&C) should be performed when such unexplained lesions are found.

Even though morules may be an intimate component of a premalignant EIN lesion, it is the glandular element that has biologic potential to progress to carcinoma.[64] Conserved molecular markers such as β-catenin mutation in both the squamous and glandular elements of EIN, as well as the adenocarcinoma, suggest all are derived from a common clone.[13] Loss of estrogen and progesterone receptors, and reduced mitotic activity occur specifically in the squamous but not glandular elements,[10,52] suggesting that squamous differentiation confers a terminal differentiation state with behavior and biologic potential quite different from that of the accompanying glands.

Figure 14.21 summarizes a model in which precancerous endometrioid lesions develop and eventually cast off squamous morules. Intraglandular morules arise as a transdifferentiation event within a clonal population of premalignant endometrial glands. In contrast to mitotically quiescent and hormone receptor-depleted morules (Figures 14.22–14.24, asterisks), accompanying glandular elements (Figures 14.22–14.24, arrows) are mitotically active and retain competence to respond to the cancer-promoting effects of estrogens or the involuting effects of progestins. Resulting cancers are derived from the glandular elements, and primarily have a glandular phenotype. If the lesion is treated with progestins, or exposed to progestins during natural menstrual cycles, the glandular components may involute, leaving residual isolated squamous morules with little or no accompanying glandular lesion (Figures 14.25 and 14.26).

Squamous morules in EIN lesions may be particularly striking, displaying what amounts to a rosette pattern of glands, the glands encircling and seeming to grow out of the central morule. This particular pattern in premenopausal women has sometimes been called 'adenoacanthosis', and must not be overinterpreted as a cribriform pattern diagnostic of adenocarcinoma.[28,41] In general, individual glands, even when many, surrounding a single squamous morule are considered as acanthosis. In contrast, confluence of non-morular squamous elements into large

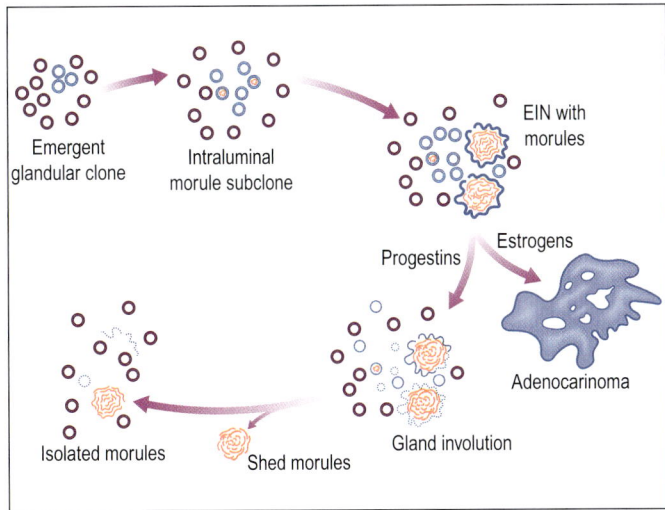

Fig. 14.21   Natural history of endometrial morules.

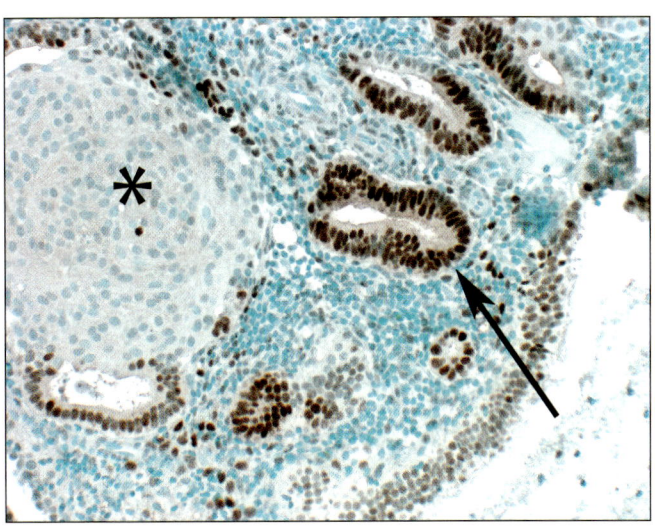

Fig. 14.23   Squamous morules in EIN lose estrogen responsiveness. Immunohistochemistry showing estrogen receptors in glands (arrow) but not in squamous morules (asterisk).

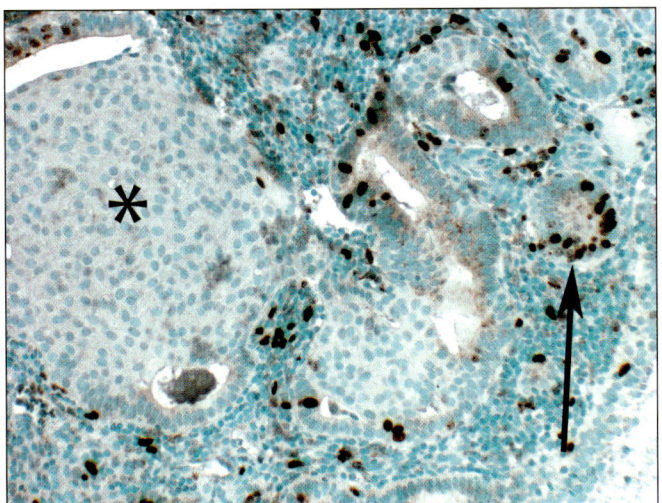

Fig. 14.22   Squamous morules in EIN are mitotically quiescent. Mitotic activity shown by Ki-67 (MIB1) immunohistochemistry is high in glands (arrow) but not in squamous morules (asterisk).

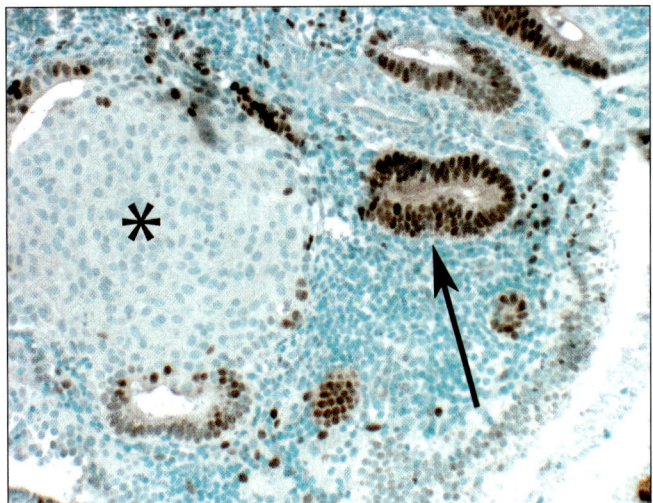

Fig. 14.24   Squamous morules in EIN lose progesterone responsiveness. Immunohistochemistry showing progesterone receptors in glands (arrow) but not in squamous morules (asterisk).

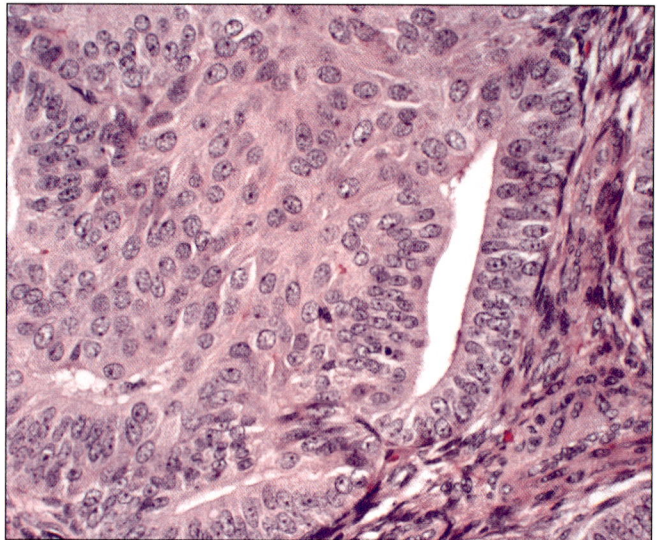

Fig. 14.25 EIN with squamous morules, before progestin therapy.

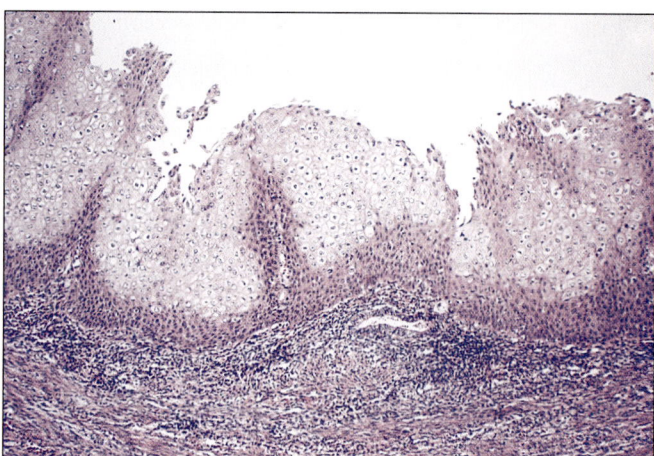

Fig. 14.27 Ichthyosis uteri, in which the surface of the endometrium is replaced by stratified squamous epithelium.

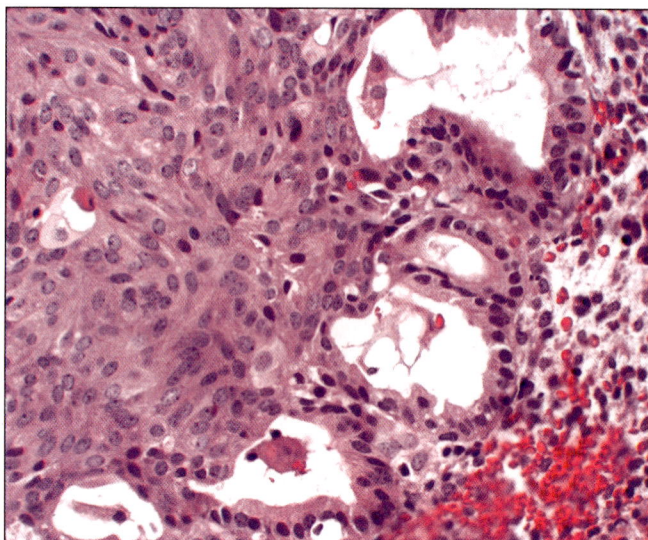

Fig. 14.26 Rebiopsy after 4 months' therapy with progestins. The squamous components are unchanged, but cells of the glandular epithelium demonstrate reduction of epithelial thickness and nuclear size.

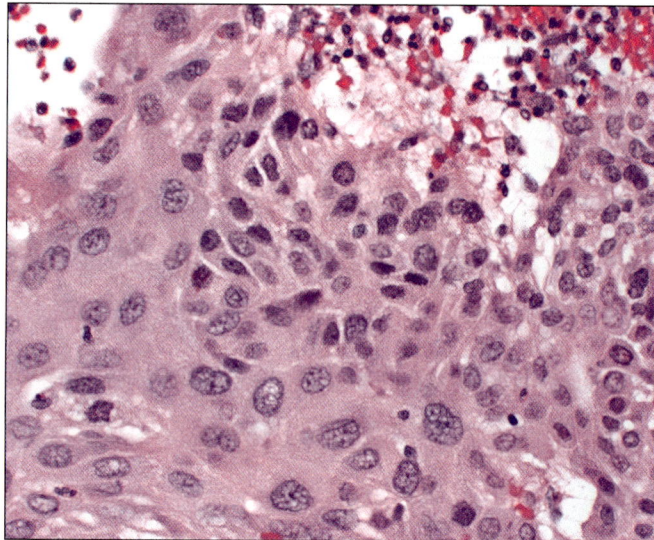

Fig. 14.28 Well-differentiated squamous cells in chronic endometritis.

irregular expanses without intervening glands should raise concern of a squamous cell carcinoma of the endometrium.

ICHTHYOSIS UTERI

Ichthyosis uteri defines a stratified squamous uterine lining epithelium (Figure 14.27) that extends downwards to individual glands and demonstrates intercellular bridges and even keratin pearls.[6,14] Chronic endometritis, over protracted intervals of several years, almost always is the antecedent condition (Figure 14.28). Much more common in the pre-antibiotic era, ichthyosis uteri is now rare and most commonly encountered in women with anatomic abnormalities favoring recurrent infection, such as fistulous tracts into the uterine cavity. We have encountered cases in which primary squamous cell carcinoma of the endometrium has been associated with ichthyosis uteri of the adjacent, non-malignant endometrium, although there is no evidence that ichthyosis itself is premalignant.

ISOLATED SQUAMOUS MORULES

Not uncommonly, the presence of isolated squamous morules is the only clue that something more serious may be present elsewhere in the endometrium (Figure 14.29). The endometrium may be proliferative or secretory, the glands small and uniform with little nuclear atypia and a low mitotic count. In one study neither of the two women that came to hysterectomy had evidence of more severe disease and three treated conservatively were subsequently found to have normal endometrium.[44] In contrast, several patients we have seen treated with D&C or hysterectomy showed EIN or cancer nearby. Possible mechanisms for presentation of isolated squamous morules in an otherwise unremarkable endometrial biopsy include morule persistence following involution of a previous glandular lesion (Figure 14.20), or morule shedding (Figure 14.30) from a coexisting glandular lesion missed due to sampling error. Isolated morules should always be clearly described, with diagnosis of the underlying glandular pattern and careful clinical correlation or follow-up. On rare occasions, persistent trophoblastic nodules have been confused with squamous morules.

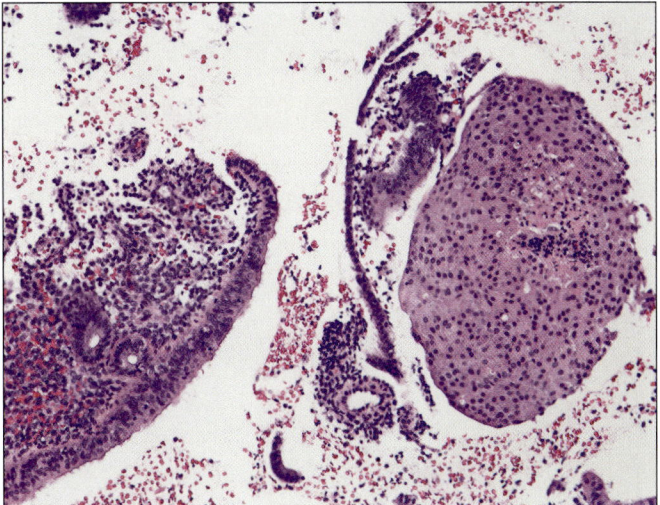

Fig. 14.29 Isolated squamous morule.

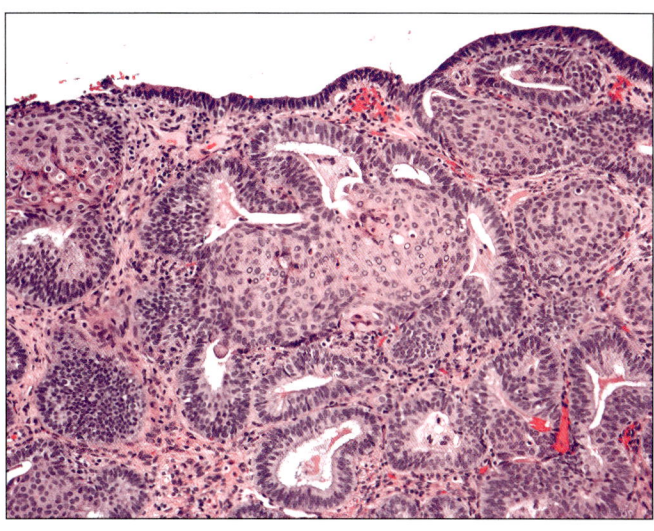

Fig. 14.31 Squamous morules in EIN.

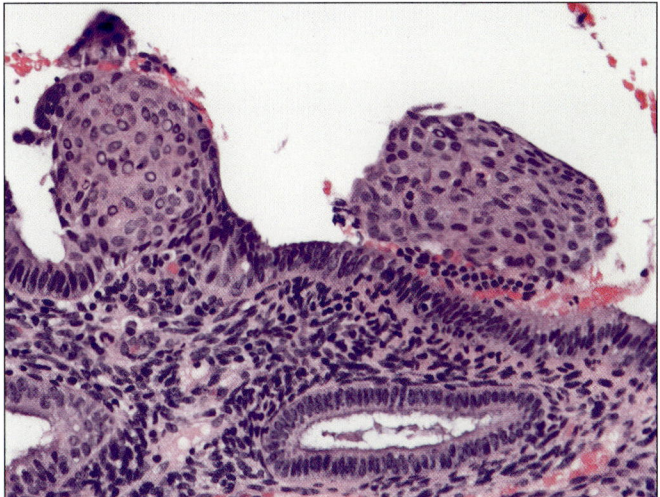

Fig. 14.30 Squamous morules shedding from the luminal surface.

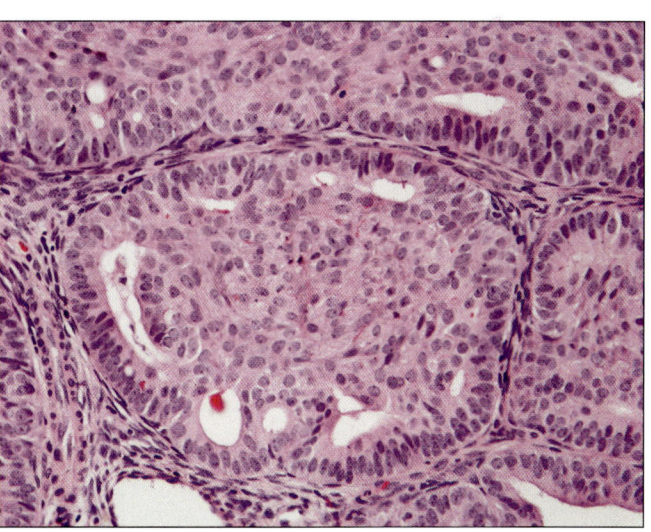

Fig. 14.32 Squamous morules with marginal glands, mimicking cribriform adenocarcinoma.

EIN WITH SQUAMOUS MORULES

Squamous morules within the gland tracts of EIN lesions are not always easily recognizable as well-differentiated squamous cells. The morules form central rounded epithelial aggregates that are usually continuous at the periphery with the endometrial glandular epithelium (Figure 14.31). The morules may appear to enlarge into sheets with multiple glands arranged radially around the periphery. These should not be confused with cribriform adenocarcinoma, which it may resemble (Figure 14.32). Key features are peripheral glands displaced by an expansile solid central component, and transition from glandular to squamous cytology within individual lumens. Central comedo necrosis of squamous morules is common (Figure 14.33) in the context of EIN, but of no clinical significance.

A diagnosis of EIN is made exclusively by careful evaluation of the glandular cytology and architecture, which must meet all criteria specified in the following chapter on EIN, including size greater than 1 mm, cytologic change, and area of glands exceeding that of stroma. Intermingled morules, which are hormonally unresponsive and lack mitotic activity

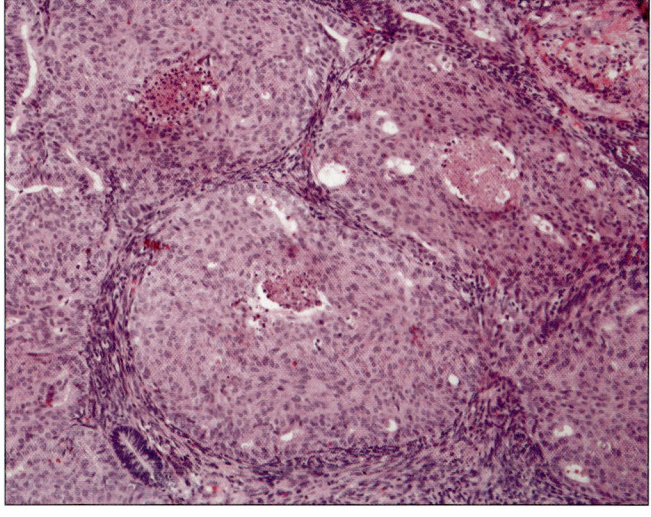

Fig. 14.33 Central necrosis in a squamous morule.

(Figures 14.22–14.24), should not be incorporated into the size and area estimates. This can be accomplished either by focusing upon a morule-depleted area of the glandular lesion or by mentally subtracting the interposed squamous areas.

METAPLASIAS TO A MUCINOUS EPITHELIUM

Mucinous metaplasia of the endometrium is not uncommon, and may range from isolated pockets of extracellular mucin to prominent cytoplasmic mucin droplets in endocervical-like epithelium. Specialized stains are typically unnecessary to evaluate these metaplasias, as the amphophilic bubbly to foamy appearance of mucin on routine H&E-stained sections is characteristic. In general, degenerative processes demonstrate extracellular mucin or disorganized variably sized cytoplasmic droplets, and it is the cases with prominent or regimented intracellular mucinous vacuoles that are most problematic. These are separated into different clinical outcome and thus diagnostic categories based upon architecture.[44,60] Papillary mucinous change is a special case of complex architecture that may be either premalignant or malignant, depending on the location, extent, and type of papillary change.

Resemblance of some endometrial mucinous metaplasias to normal endocervical epithelium and the bland cytology of many endometrial mucinous neoplasms create diagnostic challenges for the pathologist. This is particularly so when scanty amounts of mucinous epithelium, especially those with prominent aligned cytoplasmic vacuoles, are too fragmented to evaluate the underlying architecture. General familiarity with the varied appearances of normal endocervical epithelium is most helpful in these circumstances, and fractional D&C may assist in discriminating between an endometrial and an endocervical site of origin. Not uncommonly, a layer of basal reserve cells exhibiting cytoplasmic eosinophilia identifies the tissue as normal endocervix transformation zone. Tissue from the lower uterine segment or fragments of mixed endometrial–endocervical polyps are banal examples of mucinous epithelium presenting in association with endometrial stroma within an endometrial sample. Aside from these obviously benign contexts, the presence of well-differentiated mucinous epithelium within endometrial tissue fragments is a significant abnormality that requires explanation.

MUCINOUS DEGENERATIVE CHANGES

Mucin droplets may be seen in association with degenerative changes or syncytial repair associated with stromal breakdown. In these cases, there are disorganized cellular aggregates of cuboidal to columnar eosinophilic cells that may also show focal tubal and mucinous differentiation, the latter most often in the form of intracytoplasmic and extracellular mucin droplets (Figure 14.34). A minor degree of architectural complexity as evidenced by multilayering of the cells and irregular slit-like spaces can be seen in association with reparative changes and should be distinguished from the more worrisome architectural features associated with mucinous metaplasia as outlined below.

BENIGN MUCINOUS DIFFERENTIATION

Benign tubular glands or flat uterine lining surface sometimes show mucinous epithelium with a simple architecture. These

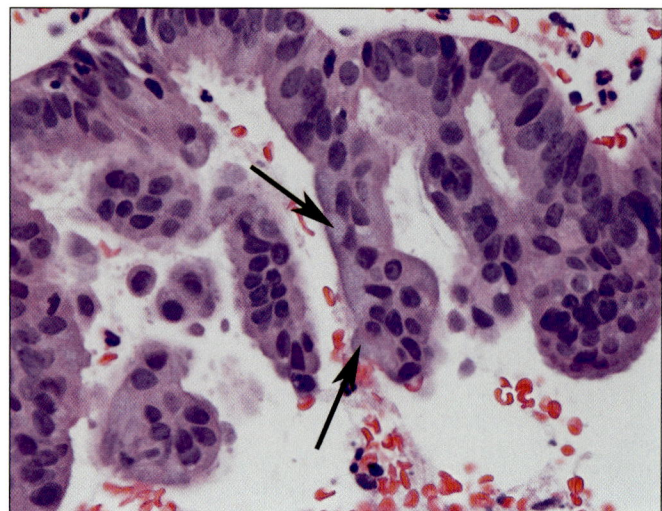

Fig. 14.34 Degenerative mucinous change. Cytoplasmic droplets (arrows).

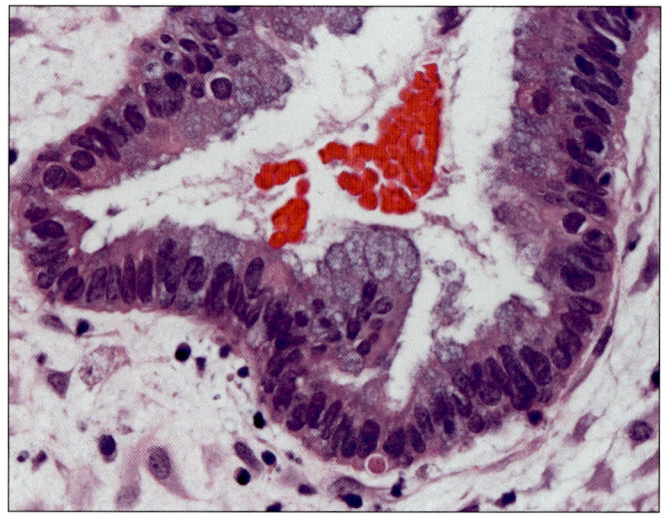

Fig. 14.35 Benign mucinous metaplasia of endometrium in pregnancy.

may be single layers of columnar epithelium with either focal cytoplasmic mucin droplets or, less commonly, rows of tall columnar cells that are identical to those seen in the endocervix with basally located nuclei and abundant vacuolated, mucin-rich cytoplasm (Figure 14.35). Goblet cells may also occasionally be seen. The presence of endometrial-type stroma between the glands enables differentiation from endocervical contaminants. Some examples are fragments of partly sampled or unrecognized mixed endometrial–endocervical polyps, but others involve glands within the native endometrium. The presence of focal cytoplasmic mucin droplets is often seen in curettings from patients on hormone replacement therapy and is also often present in close association with tubal-type change. Lack of glandular crowding and absence of a complex exophytic architecture are key elements in discrimination from a neoplastic process.

EIN AND ADENOCARCINOMA WITH MUCINOUS DIFFERENTIATION

EIN may demonstrate mucinous metaplasia within the crowded glands that define the lesion (Figure 14.36). Extent of mucinous differentiation varies between adjacent, and even within individual, EIN glands. Intermediate extents of vacuole formation are common, phasing in and out between areas of mucinous and endometrioid differentiation (Figure 14.37). When gland lining epithelium is simple, and architecture restricted to tubular or slightly branching forms, these are unlikely to be confused with carcinoma. Papillary proliferation, confined to redundant folds within individual endometrial glands ('intraglandular'), may also be seen in EIN.

Very well-differentiated endometrial adenocarcinomas with mucinous differentiation are most readily distinguished from EIN by the presence of a conspicuous exophytic surface papillary, or microglandular cribriform architectural component.[4]

Cytology may be bland, and alternating endometrioid and mucinous differentiation within individual surfaces is a clue to its non-endocervical origin. The papillary fronds of well-differentiated adenocarcinoma are supported by a complicated delicate branching stromal support network, and may appear in a biopsy or curettage as detached 'free-floating' filiform fragments (Figure 14.38), often admixed with a microglandular component. These microglandular mucinous proliferations show small glands with rigid, 'punched out' lumens superficially resembling microglandular hyperplasia of the endocervix (Figure 14.39). Very small or highly fragmented pieces of tissue with this appearance may or may not represent a well-differentiated mucinous adenocarcinoma of the endometrium, the diagnosis of which depends on the amount of tissue, its preservation, and fragmentation. In scanty specimens, we diagnose a 'complex mucinous epithelial proliferation' and advise a follow-up endometrial sampling.

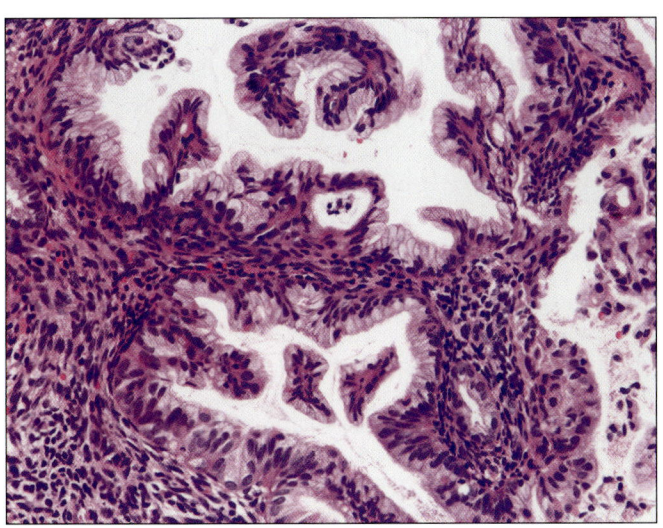

Fig. 14.36 EIN with mucinous differentiation.

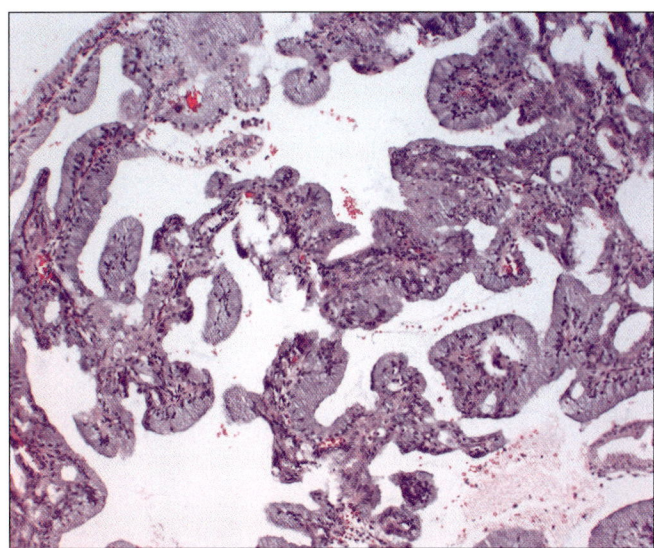

Fig. 14.38 Well-differentiated endometrial adenocarcinoma, endometrioid type, with mucinous differentiation. Filiform pattern.

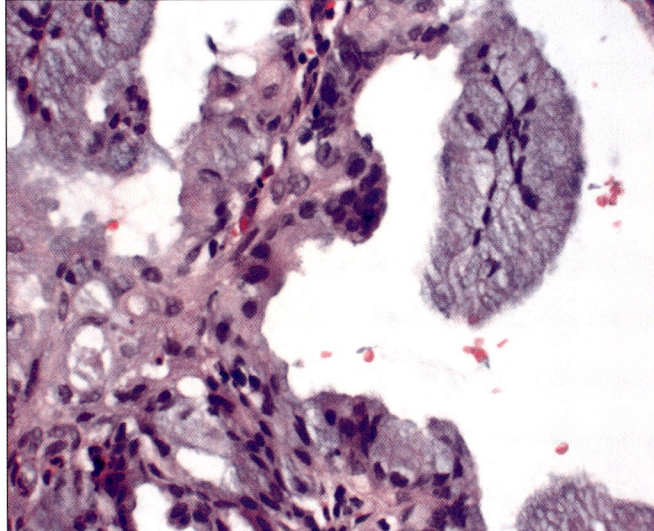

Fig. 14.37 Detail of mucinous epithelium in filiform mucinous adenocarcinoma, showing alternating mucinous and non-mucinous differentiation.

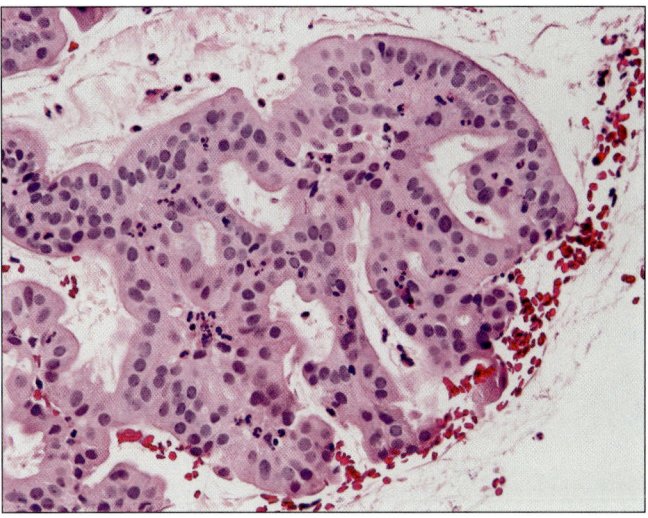

Fig. 14.39 Well-differentiated endometrial adenocarcinoma, endometrioid type, with mucinous differentiation. Microglandular pattern.

METAPLASIAS TO A SECRETORY EPITHELIUM

Normal secretory change, a normal response of endometrial glands to circulating progestins, is also accompanied by a characteristic change in the stromal cells to a cell resembling decidua. These changes, strictly speaking, are physiologic and not metaplastic. Neoplastic glands of EIN and adenocarcinoma may be capable of mounting a secretory response to progestins, and this may appear as subnuclear vacuoles in patients who have recently ovulated or received hormonal therapy (Figures 14.40 and 14.41). Not all secretory changes, however, are caused by progestational stimulation. A subset of neoplastic lesions develops prominent cytoplasmic secretory vacuoles as an integral feature of their neoplastic growth, independent of ambient progestational exposure (Figure 14.42). In those instances of EIN and adenocarcinoma with secretory changes in the absence of progestin exposure, the stroma is free of pseudodecidual changes, and secretory change is confined

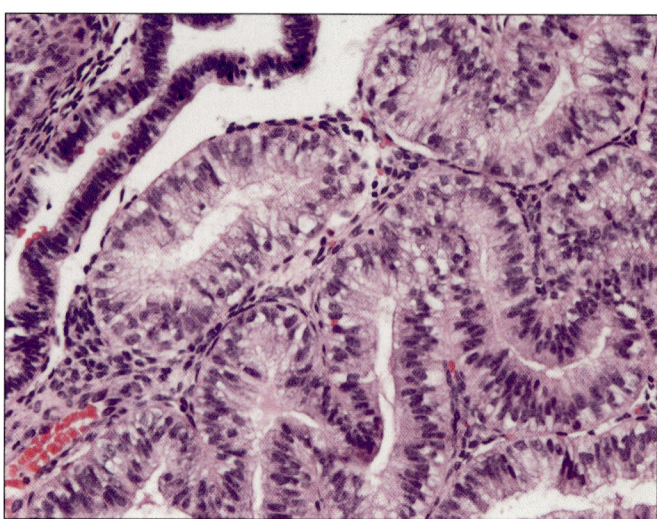

Fig. 14.42 EIN glands with secretory differentiation, occurring without progestin exposure. Comparison background gland in upper left.

to architecturally and cytologically abnormal glands. These can be diagnosed as EIN or adenocarcinoma with secretory differentiation.

'METAPLASIAS' TO NON-SPECIFIC CELL TYPES

Some changes in endometrial epithelial appearance do not resemble any particular differentiated müllerian cell type, and thus cannot be properly considered metaplasias. Nonetheless, the term 'metaplasia' is sometimes loosely applied to these processes to indicate their unusual appearance, but they are usually best diagnosed using more specific terminology.

EOSINOPHILIC METAPLASIA

An eosinophilic change can be associated with a variety of endometrial alterations such as ciliated cell metaplasia (Figure 14.16), squamous metaplasia, papillary metaplasia, and adenocarcinoma; as such, it is fair to question its status as a true metaplasia. Many eosinophilic metaplasias contain features overlapping with other altered differentiation states, such as mucin expression (85% of cases)[65] or micropapillary architecture. The metaplasia can take several forms. When isolated and associated with a simple lining epithelium, the change is always benign. This change is most commonly encountered within endometrial polyps, but occurs within the endometrial glands of the functionalis, usually in an inflammatory setting.

More commonly, the term 'eosinophilic metaplasia' refers to a change that is also known as oxyphil or oncocytic metaplasia. The cells showing eosinophilic metaplasia, which may be either on the surface or in the glands, are of tall columnar type with abundant eosinophilic cytoplasm that ranges from homogeneous to granular and a bulging surface membrane similar to the oncocytes seen in other organs such as the salivary glands, pancreas, thyroid, and kidney. The nuclei are centrally placed, large and round to oval, with a delicate chromatin pattern. The eosinophilia corresponds to myriads of mitochondria as shown by electron microscopy.[29] Like most other metaplasias, this change can be associated with a spec-

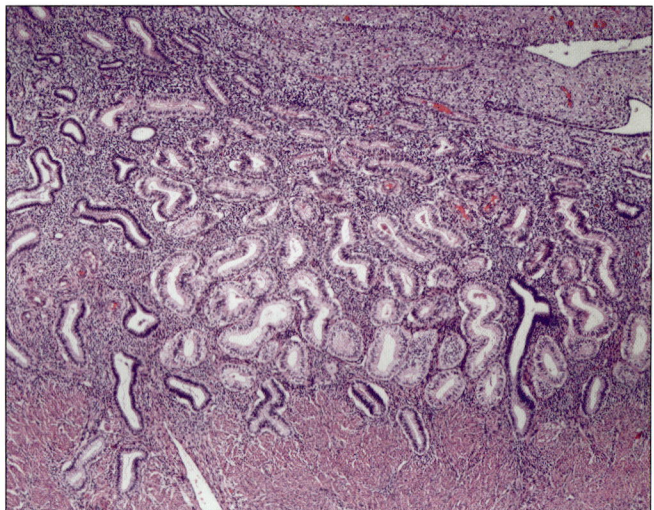

Fig. 14.40 Residual EIN with secretory differentiation, in basalis following progestin therapy.

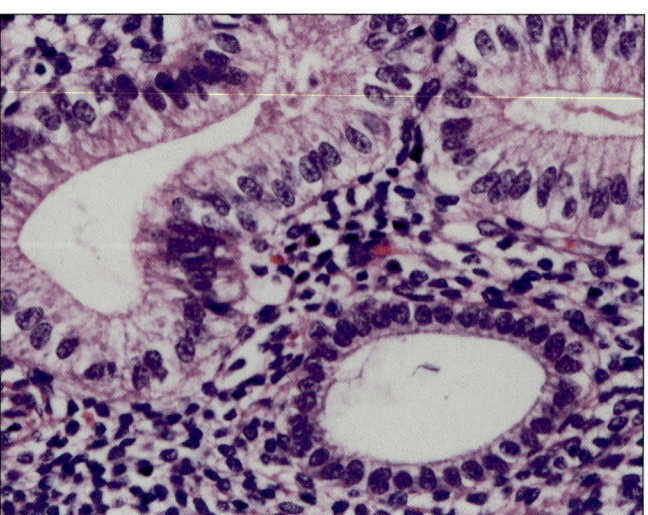

Fig. 14.41 Residual EIN glands with secretory changes (top) following withdrawal of progestin therapy. An overrun background gland is present in the lower right.

trum of endometrial changes ranging from benign to malignant.

As with other types of metaplasia, eosinophilic change is worrisome when associated with architectural complexity. In particular, intraglandular papillary proliferations exhibiting eosinophilic change can be associated with EIN (Figure 14.43). Similar to other types of metaplasia, eosinophilic change may be the alteration in differentiation associated with premalignant change.

PAPILLARY METAPLASIA

Papillary metaplasia is a descriptive term without any specific cellular basis. It involves glandular tissue thrown into papillae and is principally used to reflect degenerative processes that may involve endometrial glands and epithelial surfaces[44] in addition to a tufted pattern of intraglandular differentiation in EIN (Figure 14.44) and adenocarcinoma. It lacks the pleomorphic nuclear cytology and coarse chromatin seen in serous adenocarcinomas, which also show papillary tufting. It is of

practical diagnostic significance because endometria with this histologic feature may present an unusually broad differential diagnosis, including degenerative, reactive, and neoplastic processes.

EIN lesions may show micropapillary differentiation where a crowded focus of glands is distinguished by small intraluminal tufts protruding from a flat simple epithelium (Figure 14.45). These can be confused with adenocarcinoma when tufting defines a complicated luminal architecture mimicking a maze-like or cribriform architecture (Figure 14.46). Tangential sectioning artifacts of the papillary areas create numerous clefts communicating to the central lumen, and redundant 'saw-toothed' folds contained within the boundaries of an encasing basement membrane. Nuclear cytology is round and bland or monomorphic, unlike the highly atypical exfoliative nuclei characteristic of the papillary branching typifying an adenocarcinoma as serous. Micropapillary areas are often admixed with, or blend into, other EIN glands with tubal or endometrioid differentiation.

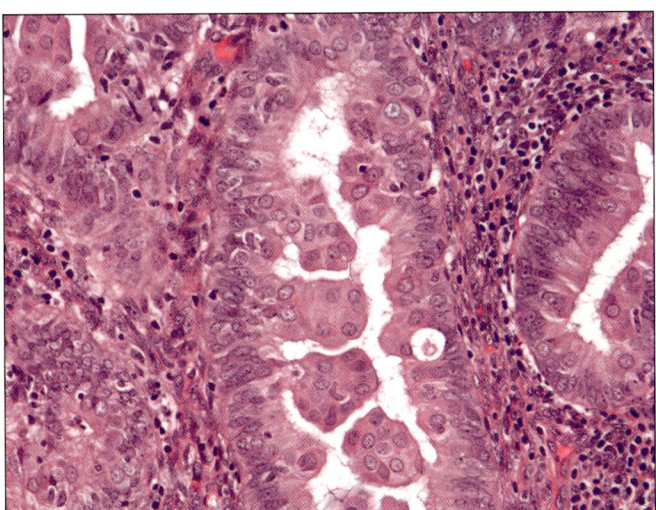

Fig. 14.43 EIN with eosinophilic differentiation.

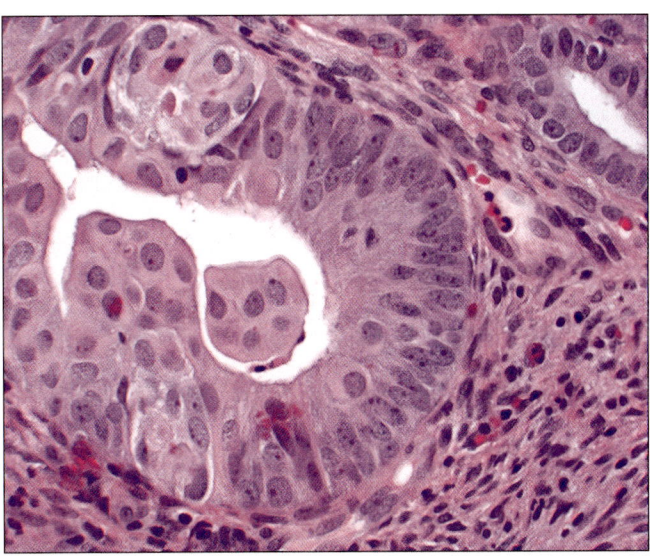

Fig. 14.45 EIN with micropapillary differentiation.

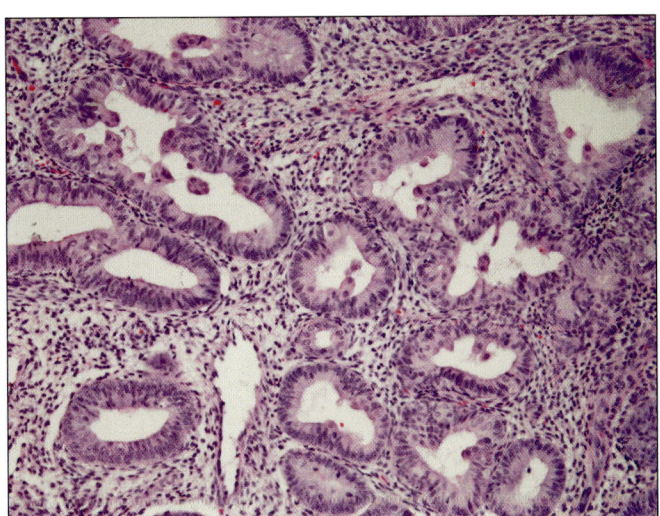

Fig. 14.44 EIN with micropapillary differentiation.

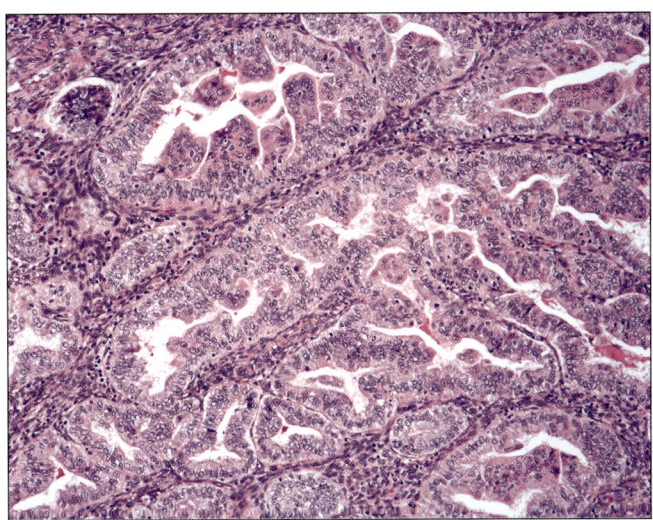

Fig. 14.46 EIN with micropapillary differentiation. Complex intraglandular redundant folds.

PAPILLARY SYNCYTIAL METAPLASIA

Papillary syncytial metaplasia is a degenerative process in which collapsed sheets of epithelium with abundant pink cytoplasm resemble squamous cells, but lack true squamous differentiation (Figure 14.47). This has also been called 'surface syncytial change' and 'eosinophilic syncytial metaplasia'. It is found in nearly one-fifth of curettage specimens and appears as syncytial aggregates of eosinophilic, cuboidal to spindly epithelial cells.[65] The underlying stroma is nondescript to tight balls, indicative of menstruation or anovulatory bleeding (Figure 14.48). True papillae, with a fibrovascular core, are not seen (Figure 14.49). The women in whom these appearances are seen are usually premenopausal, with an average age of 38 years, and have presented with abnormal uterine bleeding caused by conditions where there is non-menstrual endometrial shedding. Papillary syncytial metaplasia is not a true 'metaplasia' but a degenerative change caused by endometrial breakdown.[31]

MICROPAPILLARY 'HOBNAIL' METAPLASIA

This form of metaplasia is rare, and likely represents a variety of etiologies including exfoliation artifact, degenerative changes associated with underlying necrosis, Arias-Stella-like changes, and changes associated with endometrial polyps. On morphologic grounds, hobnail cell metaplasia exhibits glandular cells with rounded, apical nuclear protrusions beyond the apparent cytoplasmic borders into the gland lumina (Figure 14.50). Clear cell metaplasia shows cells with abundant, clear cytoplasm. Before considering the diagnosis of metaplasia, the diagnosis of clear cell adenocarcinoma and the Arias-Stella phenomenon of pregnancy need to be excluded.

MESENCHYMAL METAPLASIAS

OSSEOUS METAPLASIA

Osseous tissue in the endometrial stroma is a rarely encountered condition that is often associated with a previous history

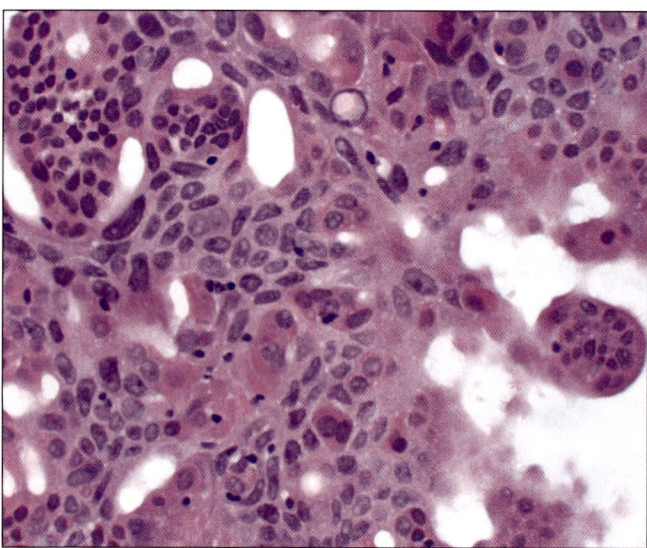

Fig. 14.47 Papillary syncytial metaplasia, a mimic for squamous differentiation.

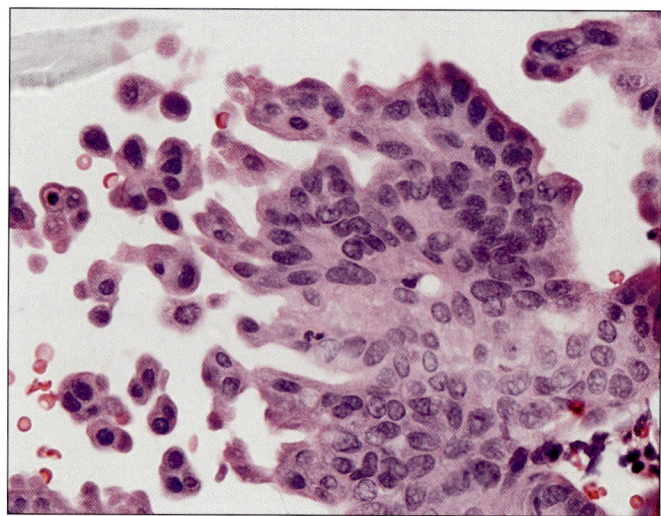

Fig. 14.49 Papillary syncytial metaplasia, exophytic. Fibrovascular cores are absent.

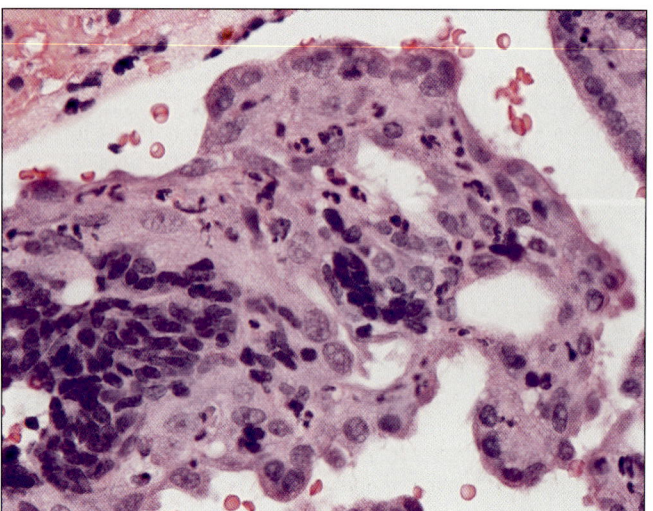

Fig. 14.48 Papillary syncytial metaplasia overlying stromal breakdown.

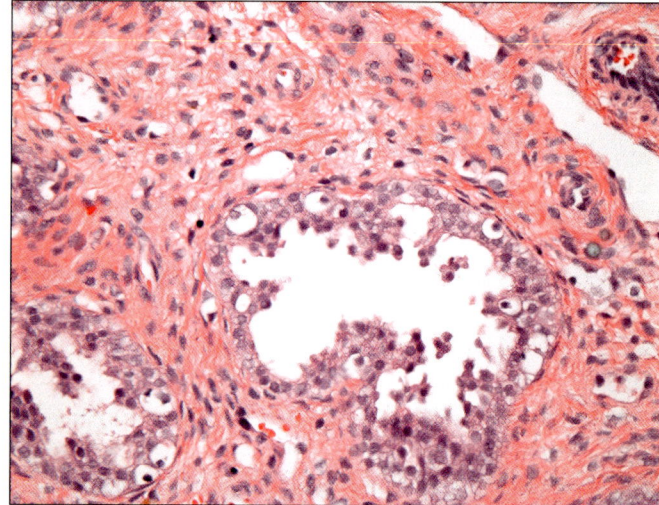

Fig. 14.50 Micropapillary ('hobnail') metaplasia.

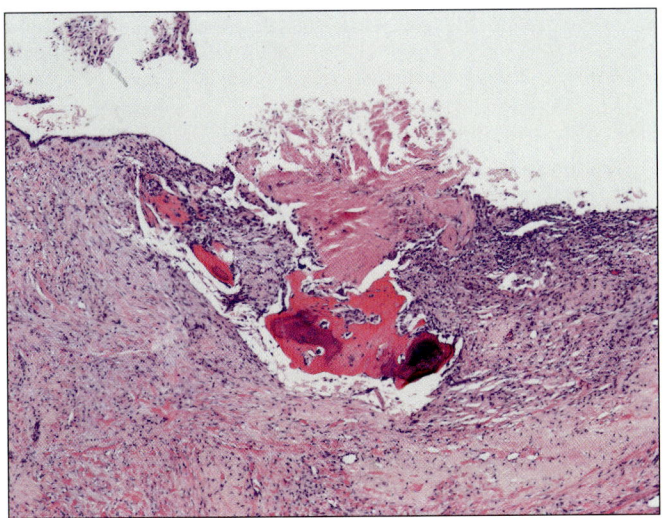

Fig. 14.51 Osseous metaplasia following endometrial ablation.

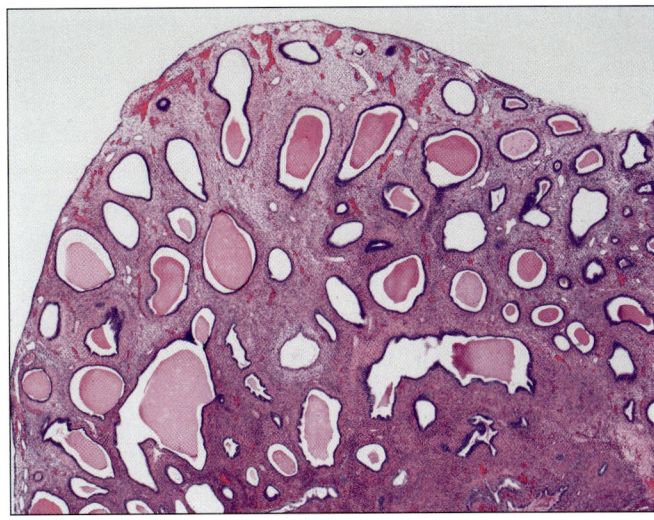

Fig. 14.52 Endometrial polyp with fibrous stroma and irregular cystic glands.

of abortion or instrumentation (Figure 14.51). Some may be residual fetal bone incorporated into the endometrium. Others are doubtless genuine metaplasia, albeit sometimes induced by the retention of fetal bones.[2,9] Most cases occur in women between 20 and 40 years and are associated with infertility.[1] It occurs also in postmenopausal women.[56]

ENDOMETRIAL EXTRAMEDULLARY HEMOPOIESIS

Extramedullary hemopoiesis is a rare finding associated with hematologic disease, and thus not strictly a metaplastic condition. The finding of endometrial extramedullary hemopoiesis may herald the presence of an underlying hematologic abnormality.[12]

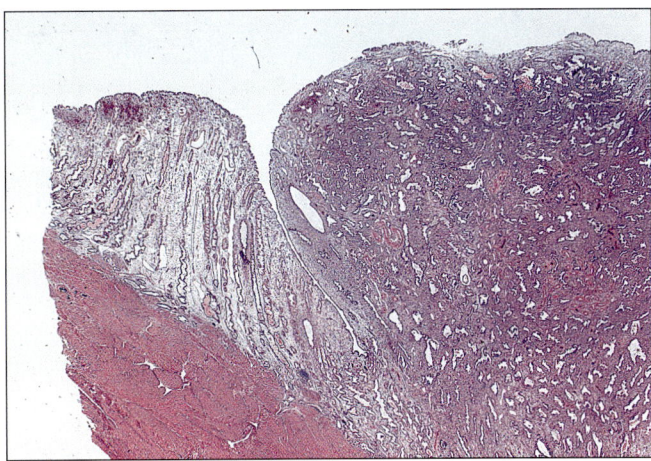

Fig. 14.53 Endometrial polyp. The polyp is composed of inactive endometrium with slightly irregular glands and compact stroma. The adjacent endometrium is in the secretory phase and the stroma is edematous.

ENDOMETRIAL POLYPS

Definition
Endometrial polyps, which by definition protrude into the uterine cavity, are biphasic growths of endometrial glands and stroma with blood vessels. Smooth muscle is also sometimes present.

Etiology and natural history
Polyps arise as monoclonal overgrowths of genetically altered endometrial stromal cells with secondary induction of polyclonal benign glands through as yet undefined stromal–epithelial interactive mechanisms.[20] Chromosomal analysis of polyp stroma shows in the majority of cases clonal translocations, involving 6p21–22, 12q13–15, or 7q22 regions.[15] One breakpoint gene, the HMGIC gene at 12q15, is also rearranged in uterine leiomyomas, lipomas, pleomorphic adenomas, and pulmonary chondroid hamartomas.[8]

Endometrial polyps variably respond to circulating estrogens and progesterone. Most commonly the polyp is nonfunctional, lacking those normal cyclic changes seen in the adjacent normal endometrium. The glands are frequently entirely inactive, showing neither proliferative nor secretory activity. Some or many of the glands may be dilated, slightly branching, or irregularly distributed. An irregular gland pattern

is common and should not give cause for concern or be separately diagnosed as an endometrial hyperplasia, especially when it is uniformly distributed throughout the entire polyp (Figure 14.52).

Functioning polyps are less common than those already described and are composed of glands that show secretory activity during the secretory phase. The glands in the polyp may sometimes be indistinguishable from those in the rest of the endometrium but this is unusual. More often, the glands in the polyp are out of step with non-polyp endometrial glands. Secretory activity in the polyp either lags behind or the secretory changes are less well developed, and not all polyp glands are in synchrony (Figure 14.53).

In recent years, there have been numerous reports of endometrial polyps occurring in women treated with tamoxifen for breast cancer.[16,39,49,54,61] It is clear that women on tamoxifen have a higher incidence of endometrial polyps than the rest of the population and that their polyps are likely to be much larger, more fibrotic, more likely to show mucinous metaplasia, and more likely to contain hyperplasia or carcinoma than women not on tamoxifen treatment.[5,21]

Clinical features

Endometrial polyps may be found at any age, but are most frequent around and shortly after the menopause. They are present in about 13–17% of women.[25]

From a practical viewpoint, is the recognition of a polyp in curettings of any importance? If the patient is complaining of abnormal bleeding, the diagnosis of an endometrial polyp may indicate the cause for those symptoms, particularly if hemorrhage or necrosis can be demonstrated. If EIN or adenocarcinoma is found in what is thought to be a polyp at curettage, the patient should be managed in exactly the same way as would have been done had the changes been in a non-polypoid area. The mass effect of a polyp can obstruct access of flexible devices such as the Pipelle to areas of the uterine cavity, making them less accessible for sampling. Use of a rigid curette to completely shear away the polyp, or sampling through a carefully positioned hysteroscope, decreases the effective 'blind spots'.

Gross features

Endometrial polyps range in size from a slightly rounded protuberance to a large, broad-based or pedunculated, oval structure filling the uterine cavity. They may also expand the cervical canal and present at the external cervical os. Pedunculated polyps are the easiest to recognize and often attract the most attention (Figure 14.54). Many polyps are sessile and have a broad base of attachment to the internal surface of the uterus. Some sessile polyps are only slightly raised and are easy to miss on gross examination. About 20% of polyps are multiple. The surface may be smooth and shiny and there is often hemorrhage, particularly at the tip. Small cysts may be observed beneath the surface (Figure 14.55). Necrosis is sometimes present, although this is uncommon in benign polyps. The cut surface may be uniform or it may show cysts, hemorrhage, and necrosis.

Microscopic features

The diagnosis of a polyp in a curetting depends upon the finding of at least two of three particular histologic features and exclusion of mimics. These are: (1) irregularly shaped and positioned glands; (2) stroma altered by fibrosis or excessive collagen; and (3) thick-walled blood vessels (Figures 14.56 and 14.57). In addition, as polyps elongate, the glands often get stretched such that parallel glands with intervening fibrous stroma becomes a useful clue to the diagnosis (Figure 14.58).[50] Lower uterine segment and deep endometrial basalis are normal tissues that can closely resemble and be confused with polyps. Requiring at least one polyp fragment to contain luminal surface epithelium from uterine cavity lining excludes basalis. Lower uterine segment may be recognized by a relatively low density of glands, collagenous stroma devoid of endometrial character, and intermediate mucinous differentiation. It may perhaps be thought that a piece of endometrium in curettings that is covered on three sides by surface epithelium should be considered a polyp, but this is not always necessarily so. Sheets of normal endometrium when folded and distorted by fixation can be sectioned in such a way that it is completely covered by surface epithelium in the plane of section. Correspondingly, fragments of polyps commonly only have epithelium covering a fraction of the surface.

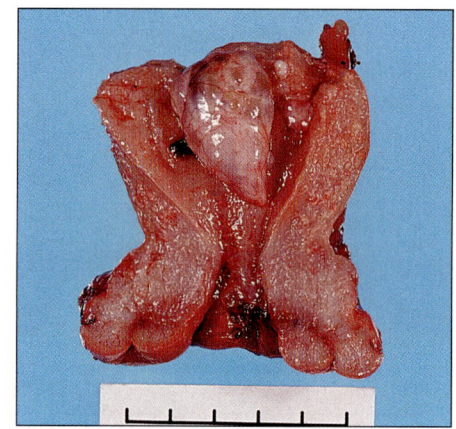

Fig. 14.55 Endometrial polyp. Cystic glands are discernible.

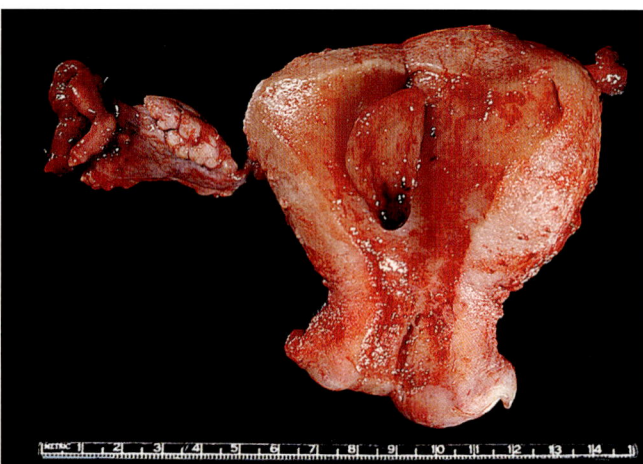

Fig. 14.54 Endometrial polyp. The polyp arises on a narrow pedicle at one cornu and has a hemorrhagic tip.

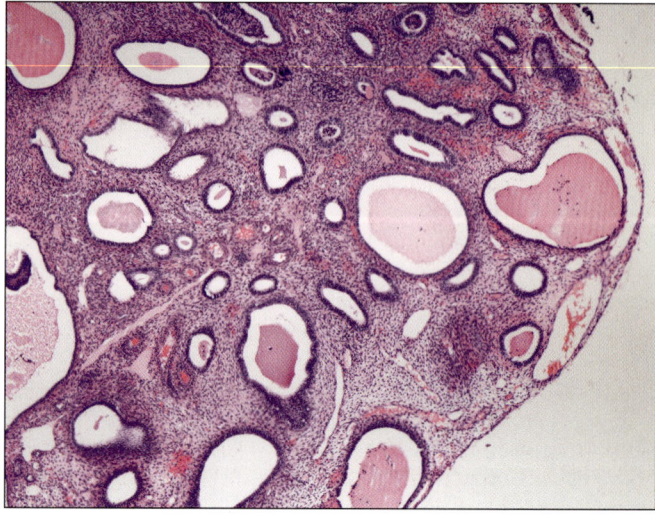

Fig. 14.56 Endometrial polyp. Irregular bland glands with cysts and fibrous stroma.

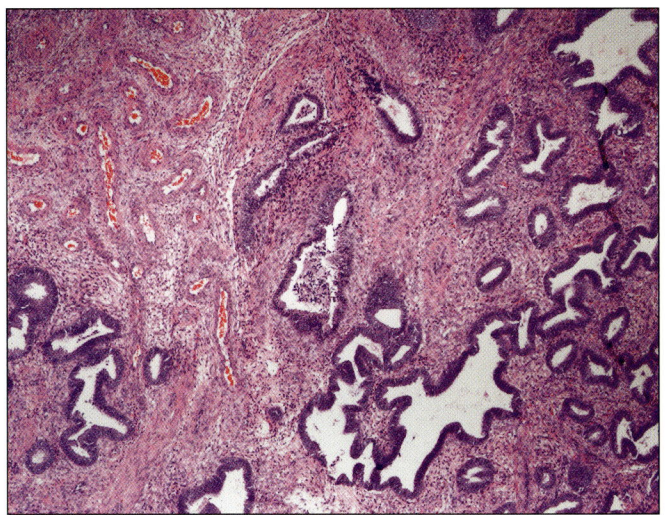

Fig. 14.57 Endometrial polyp. Fibrous stroma with prominent vessels.

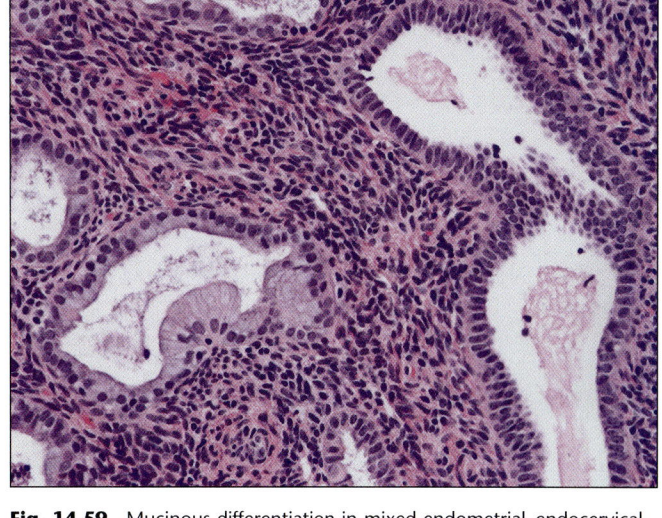

Fig. 14.59 Mucinous differentiation in mixed endometrial–endocervical type polyp.

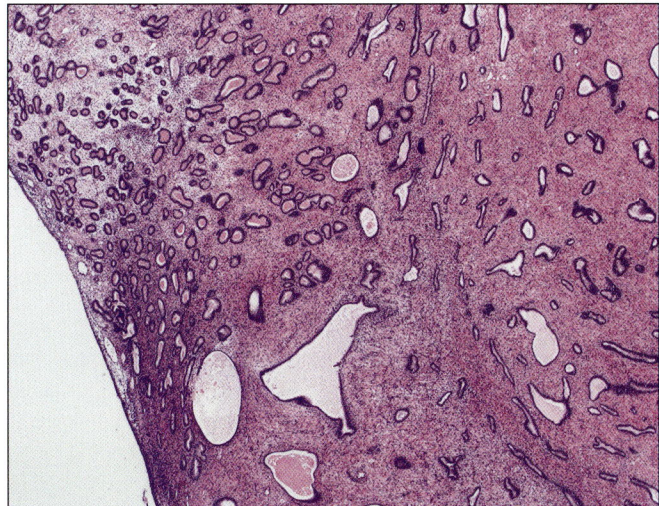

Fig. 14.58 Endometrial polyp. Gland density may be irregular within the polyp and at the interface with adjacent endometrium. Some compressed glands are parallel to the polyp-normal interface.

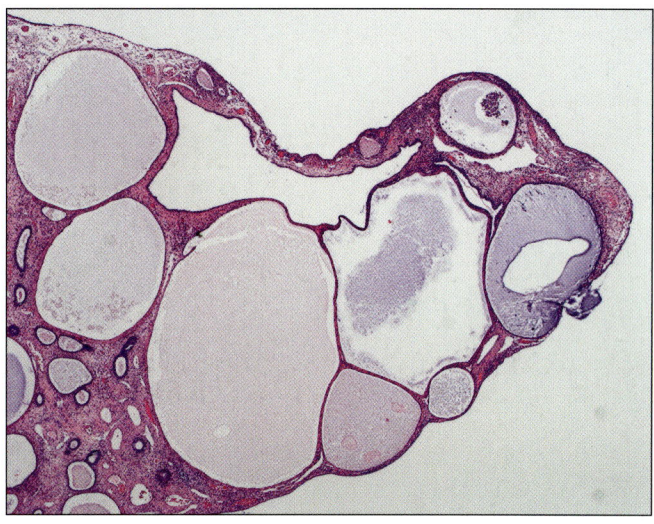

Fig. 14.60 Endometrial polyp, senile type. The glands are cystic with flaccid walls.

Admixtures of mucinous and endometrial-type glands can be seen within endometrial polyps (Figure 14.59). The mucinous component demonstrates cytoplasmic mucin resembling that of the normal endocervix. When mucinous glands are prominent, occasional interspersed endometrial glands, commingled endometrial stroma, and lack of overlying squamous metaplasia are useful in distinguishing them from cervical polyps.

In postmenopausal women, the polyps are usually composed of exaggerated glands lined by atrophic epithelium (Figure 14.60). Those with dilated glands lined by thin, atrophic epithelium surrounded by pale, fibrous stroma (Figure 14.61) are often called senile polyps. These are clearly a remnant of the time when the endometrium was active, and the pattern described represents a regressed state following a period of growth, perhaps many years previously.

EIN, when seen in polyps, may be recognized as a discrete geographic focus of crowded glands with a cohesive cytology

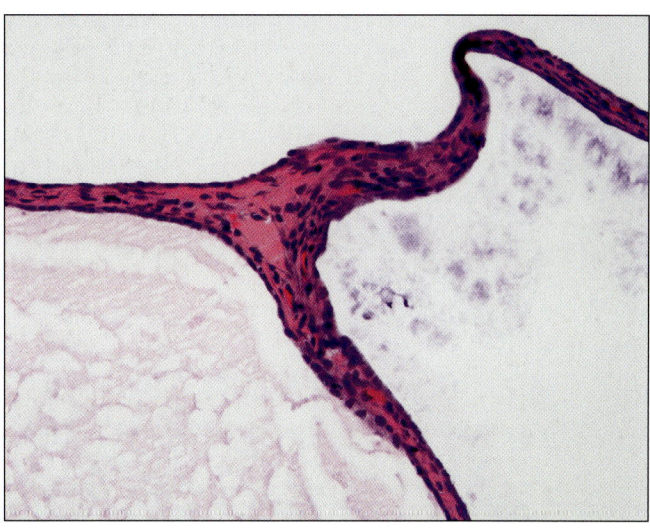

Fig. 14.61 Endometrial polyp, senile type. Cystic glands are lined by flattened epithelium.

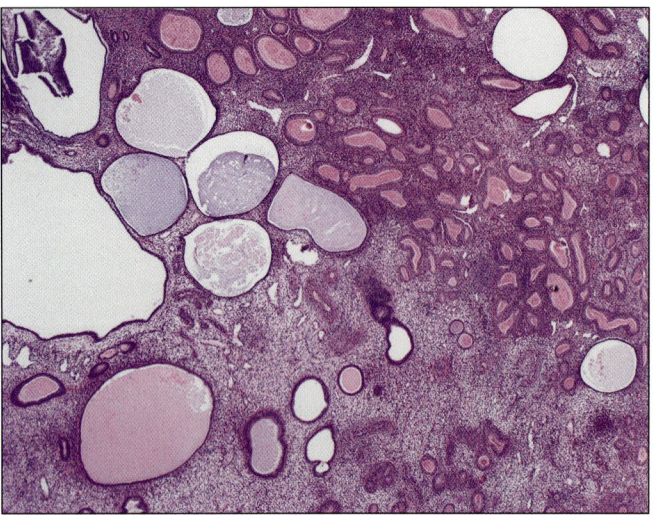

Fig. 14.62 EIN in endometrial polyp. Increased gland density and cytologic change are seen within the EIN focus (upper right).

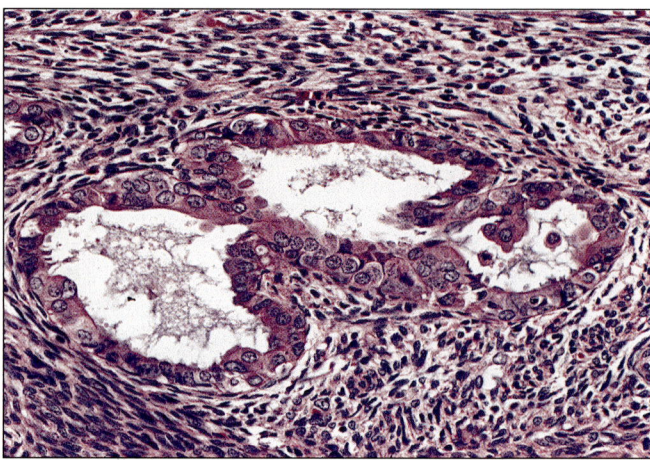

Fig. 14.63 Radiation changes.

that differs from the background polyp (Figure 14.62). Polyps with EIN need to be distinguished from a carcinoma arising in a pre-existing polyp and a polypoid carcinoma, which depends on finding a benign fibrous stalk or benign glandular elements in the polypoid mass.

ATYPICAL POLYPOID ADENOMYOMA

See Chapter 17.

MISCELLANEOUS CONDITIONS

ASHERMANS SYNDROME

Ashermans syndrome, defined as synechiae within the endometrial cavity, often causes menstrual disorders and infertility (62% and 43% of patients, respectively).[19] The most common causes are curettage after a missed abortion or during the puerperium. Genital tuberculosis, in countries where this disease is still common, is a principal causative factor. Hysterosalpingography and hysteroscopy are the usual methods of definitive diagnosis.

There are no gross features as the specimens usually consist of fragments of fibrous tissue with varying amounts of entrapped residual endometrial glands. The rare hysterectomy specimen discloses massive fibrosis of the residual 'endometrium'.

Treatment usually consists of lysing the adhesions followed by immediate insertion of an intrauterine device, together with a course of estrogens. The usual measure of successful treatment is with regard to the ability to achieve a term delivery.[30,51] Placenta accreta is not an uncommon complication during the subsequent pregnancy, usually because the endometrium is absent and the placental villi have implanted directly into the myometrium.

RADIATION EFFECT

Radiation delivered for therapy of cervical or other pelvic malignancies may alter the histology of what initially was normal endometrium. Grossly, no changes are seen, unless the absence of lush endometrium 2–3 mm thick is considered abnormal. The endometrium is usually paper thin, and more akin to an atrophic endometrium. The chief microscopic features are glands in which the nuclei are irregular in size and shape, but in which the chromatin is usually smudged (Figure 14.63). Mitoses are absent. The glands are either normal or slightly irregular in shape, but lack any evidence of any usual features of carcinoma with which it is commonly mistaken. Normal glands affected by radiotherapy lack signs of invasion or a cribriform arrangement of the cells. The glands are also usually spaced as normal glands.

THE EFFECTS OF THE INTRAUTERINE CONTRACEPTIVE DEVICE ON THE ENDOMETRIUM

Often, the IUD appears to have no demonstrable effect on the endometrium, although subtle, local changes are almost invariable. Focally compressed endometrium may be seen at the site of contact (Figure 14.64), which may vary between a slight indentation of the surface to deep implantation almost through the endometrium or even into the myometrium (Figure 14.65). Rarely, an IUD may penetrate the uterine wall and even lie in the peritoneal cavity. Commonly, near the point where the IUD is in contact with the endometrium, a fibroblastic overgrowth will develop to ensheath the IUD as if it were a foreign body. The surface epithelium at the point of contact with the IUD may also show atypical features, with loss of cellular polarity and nuclear enlargement and pleomorphism. Squamous metaplasia of the surface epithelium has been seen on occasion. The stroma may exhibit focal edema and dilated blood vessels. Small foci of an exaggerated decidual-like response to progesterone may also be evident.

Inflammation is the most important complication of an IUD in the endometrium, particularly with the non-copper-containing types. It is common to observe a sparse, focal scattering of neutrophils in the superficial stroma close to the

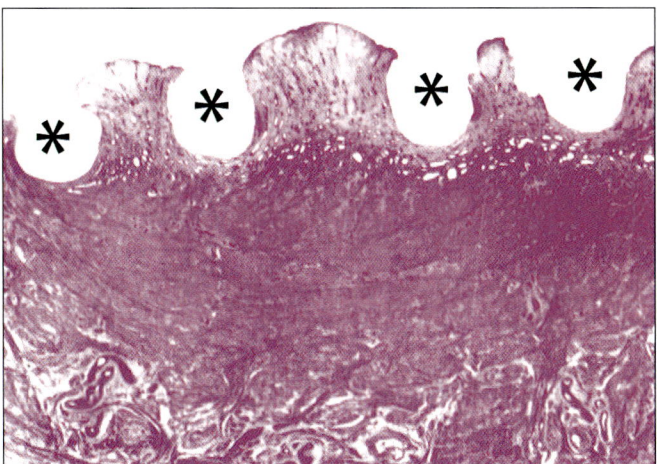

Fig. 14.64 Intrauterine contraceptive device. Imprint of a Lippes loop in the endometrium. The endometrium is normal between the depressions (asterisks) caused by the IUD itself.

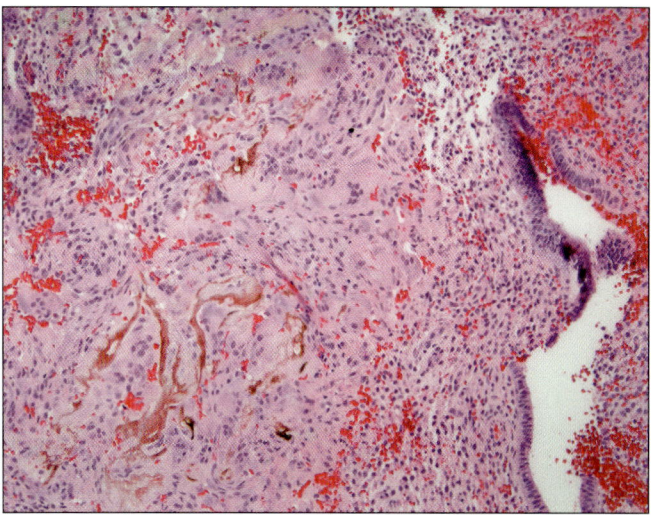

Fig. 14.66 Re-epithelized surface with underlying coagulative debris and giant cells 2 years after endometrial ablation.

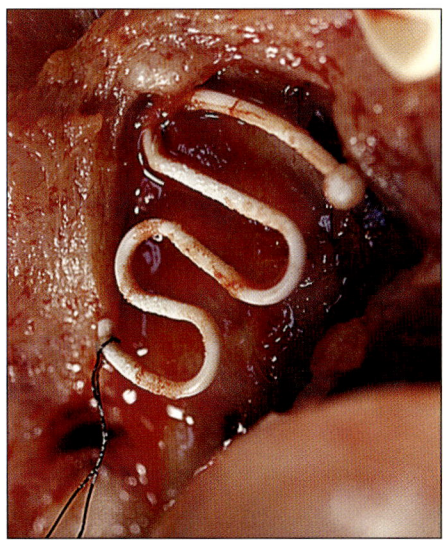

Fig. 14.65 Intrauterine contraceptive device. A Lippes loop in position in an opened uterus. Adhesions are attached to the loop.

contact point with the device, as well as neutrophils and nuclear debris in gland lumina. These minor local inflammatory changes are thought to result more often from irritation rather than from infection, as the uterine cavity becomes sterile again within 48 hours after the device has been inserted. Even so, some organisms are probably introduced with it. More widespread and severe inflammatory changes, however, result from infection. In these circumstances, the full picture of acute or chronic endometritis may be seen with a stromal infiltrate of neutrophils, plasma cells and lymphocytes, pus in the gland lumina, and suppression of the glandular hormonal cyclic response.

ENDOMETRIAL ABLATION

Procedures for endometrial ablation have grown in popularity as a method to treat benign symptomatic disease. Diffuse coagulative necrosis lacking any granulomatous component domi-

nates the histologic picture for the first few weeks. It closely resembles the artifact commonly seen on the periphery of surgical specimens obtained by cauterizing sampling devices, but is more extensive and uniform. As collagen replaces the necrotic tissue, the appearance varies from well-formed, non-caseating granulomas that are difficult to distinguish from those of infective origin to foreign-body giant cells surrounding debris (Figure 14.66). Not all endometrial epithelium is destroyed during ablation, and residual glands that regrow may be inaccessible to future biopsy attempts because of obscuring adhesions. For this reason endometrial ablation is not advised for treatment of premalignant disease, where complete sampling during follow-up surveillance biopsies is desired.

REFERENCES

1. Bahceci M, Demirel LC. Osseous metaplasia of the endometrium: a rare cause of infertility and its hysteroscopic management. Hum Reprod 1996;11:2537–9.
2. Basu M, Mammen C, Owen E. Bony fragments in the uterus: an association with secondary subfertility. Ultrasound Obstet Gynecol 2003;22:402–6.
3. Bayer-Garner IB, Nickell JA, Korourian S. Routine syndecan-1 immunohistochemistry aids in the diagnosis of chronic endometritis. Arch Pathol Lab Med 2004;128:1000–3.
4. Bergeron C, Ferenczy A. Oncocytic metaplasia in endometrial hyperplasia and carcinoma. Int J Gynecol Pathol 1988;7:93–5.
5. Berliere M, Radikov G, Galant C, Piette P, Marbaix E, Donnez J. Identification of women at high risk of developing endometrial cancer on tamoxifen. Eur J Cancer 2000;36:S35–S36.
6. Bewtra C, Xie QM, Hunter WJ, Jurgensen W. Ichthyosis uteri: a case report and review of the literature. Arch Pathol Lab Med 2005;129:e124–e125.
7. Block K, Kardana A, Igarashi P, Taylor HS. In utero diethylstilbestrol (DES) exposure alters Hox gene expression in the developing mullerian system. FASEB J 2000;14:1101–8.
8. Bol S, Wanschura S, Thode B, et al. An endometrial polyp with a rearrangement of HMGI-C underlying a complex cytogenetic rearrangement involving chromosomes 2 and 12. Cancer Genet Cytogenet 1996;90:88–90.
9. Bolaji I, Saridogan E, Hasan N, Baithun S, Djahanbakhch O. Prolonged retention of fetal bones with osseous metaplasia of the endometrium. Int J Gynaecol Obstet 1995;50:65–6.
10. Brachtel EF, Sanchez-Estevez C, Moreno-Bueno G, Prat J, Palacios J, Oliva E. Distinct molecular alterations in complex endometrial hyperplasia (CEH) with and without immature squamous metaplasia (squamous morules). Am J Surg Pathol 2005;29:1322–9.
11. Cheng W, Liu J, Yoshida H, Rosen D, Naora H. Lineage infidelity of epithelial ovarian cancers is controlled by HOX genes that specify regional identity in the reproductive tract. Nat Med 2005;11:531–7.
12. Creagh TM, Bain BJ, Evans DJ, Reid CD, Young RH, Flanagan AM. Endometrial extramedullary haemopoiesis. J Pathol 1995;176:99–104.

13. Crum CP, Lomo L, Lin MC, Nucci MR, Mutter GL. Morular metaplasia of the endometrium revisited: a followup study. Lab Invest 2004;84(Suppl 1):195A.

14. Crum CP, Richart RM, Fenoglio CM. Adenoacanthosis of endometrium: a clinicopathologic study in premenopausal women. Am J Surg Pathol 1981;5:15–20.

15. Dal Cin P, Vanni R, Marras S, et al. Four cytogenetic subgroups can be identified in endometrial polyps. Cancer Res 1995;55:1565–8.

16. Deligdisch L, Kalir T, Cohen CJ, de Latour M, Le Bouedec G, Penault-Llorca F. Endometrial histopathology in 700 patients treated with tamoxifen for breast cancer. Gynecol Oncol 2000;78:181–6.

17. Deutchman ME, Hartman KJ. Postpartum pyometra: a case report. J Fam Pract 1993;36:449–52.

18. Disep B, Innes BA, Cochrane HR, Tijani S, Bulmer JN. Immunohistochemical characterization of endometrial leucocytes in endometritis. Histopathology 2004;45:625–32.

19. Fernandez H, Al-Najjar F, Chauveaud-Lambling A, Frydman R, Gervaise A. Fertility after treatment of Asherman's syndrome stage 3 and 4. J Minim Invasive Gynecol 2006;13:398–402.

20. Fletcher J, Pinkus J, Lage J, Morton C, Pinkus G. Clonal 6p21 rearrangement is restricted to the mesenchymal component of an endometrial polyp. Genes Chrom Cancer 1992;5:260–3.

21. Goldstein SR, Zeltser I, Horan CK, Snyder JR, Schwartz LB. Ultrasonography-based triage for postmenopausal patients with uterine bleeding. Am J Obstet Gynecol 1997;177:102–8.

22. Hollier LM, Scott LL, Murphree SS, Wendel GD, Jr. Postpartum endometritis caused by herpes simplex virus. Obstet Gynecol 1997;89:836–8.

23. Jovanovic AS, Boynton KA, Mutter GL. Uteri of women with endometrial carcinoma contain a histopathologic spectrum of monoclonal putative precancers, some with microsatellite instability. Cancer Res 1996;56:1917–21.

24. Kaku T, Silverberg SG, Tsukamoto N, et al. Association of endometrial epithelial metaplasias with endometrial carcinoma and hyperplasia in Japanese and American women. Int J Gynecol Pathol 1993;12:297–300.

25. Kim KR, Peng R, Ro JY, Robboy SJ. A diagnostically useful histopathologic feature of endometrial polyp: the long axis of endometrial glands arranged parallel to surface epithelium. Am J Surg Pathol 2004;28:1057–62.

26. Kiviat NB, Wolner-Hanssen P, Eschenbach DA, et al. Endometrial histopathology in patients with culture-proved upper genital tract infection and laparoscopically diagnosed acute salpingitis. Am J Surg Pathol 1990;14:167–75.

27. Korn AP, Bolan G, Padian N, Ohm-Smith M, Schachter J, Landers DV. Plasma cell endometritis in women with symptomatic bacterial vaginosis. Obstet Gynecol 1995;85:387–90.

28. Lax SF, Pizer ES, Ronnett BM, Kurman RJ. Comparison of estrogen and progesterone receptor, Ki-67, and p53 immunoreactivity in uterine endometrioid carcinoma and endometrioid carcinoma with squamous, mucinous, secretory, and ciliated cell differentiation. Hum Pathol 1998;29:924–31.

29. Lehman MB, Hart WR. Simple and complex hyperplastic papillary proliferations of the endometrium – a clinicopathologic study of nine cases of apparently localized papillary lesions with fibrovascular stromal cores and epithelial metaplasia. Am J Surg Pathol 2001;25:1347–54.

30. Mencaglia L, Tonellotto D. Endometrial ablation: a review. In: Blanc B, Marty R, DeMontgolfier R, eds. Office and Operative Hysteroscopy. Paris: Springer-Verlag France; 2002:197–202.

31. Moritani S, Kushima R, Ichihara S, et al. Eosinophilic cell change of the endometrium: a possible relationship to mucinous differentiation. Mod Pathol 2005;18:1243–8.

32. Mount S, Mead P, Cooper K. Chlamydia trachomatis in the endometrium: can surgical pathologists identify plasma cells? Adv Anat Pathol 2001;8:327–9.

33. Muller-Holzner E, Ruth NR, Abfalter E, et al. IUD-associated pelvic actinomycosis: a report of five cases. Int J Gynecol Pathol 1995;14:70–4.

34. Mutter GL. Histopathology of genetically defined endometrial precancers. Int J Gynecol Pathol 2000;19:301–9.

35. Mutter GL. Diagnosis of premalignant endometrial disease. J Clin Pathol 2002;55:326–31.

36. Mutter GL. Endometrial carcinogenesis: an integrated molecular, histologic, and functional model of a dualistic disease. In: Giordano A, Bovicelli A, Kurman R, eds. Molecular Pathology of Gynecologic Cancer. Totowa, NJ: Humana; 2007:73–90.

37. Mutter GL, Ince TA. Molecular pathogenesis of endometrial cancer. In: Fuller A, Seiden MV, Young R, eds. Uterine Cancer: American Cancer Society Atlas of Clinical Oncology. Hamilton, Ontario, Canada: Decker; 2004:10–21.

38. Naora H. Developmental patterning in the wrong context: the paradox of epithelial ovarian cancers. Cell Cycle 2005;4:1033–5.

39. Neven P, De Muylder X, Van Belle Y. Tamoxifen-induced endometrial polyp. N Engl J Med 1997;336:1389; author reply 1389–90.

40. Newkirk GR. Pelvic inflammatory disease: a contemporary approach. Am Fam Physician 1996;53:1127–35.

41. Nielsen AL, Nyholm HC. Endometrial adenocarcinoma of endometrioid subtype with squamous differentiation: an immunohistochemical study of MIB-1 (Ki-67 paraffin), cathepsin D, and c-erbB-2 protein (p185). Int J Gynecol Pathol 1995;14:230–4.

42. Nogales-Ortiz F, Ildefonso T, Nogales F. The pathology of female genital tuberculosis. Obstet Gynec 1979;53:422–8.

43. Nogales-Ortiz F, Tarancon I, Nogales FF, Jr. The pathology of female genital tuberculosis. A 31-year study of 1436 cases. Obstet Gynecol 1979;53:422–8.

44. Nucci M, Crum CP, Prasad C, Mutter GL. Mucinous endometrial epithelial proliferations: a morphologic spectrum of changes with diverse clinical significance. Mod Pathol 2000;12:1137–42.

45. Paukku M, Puolakkainen M, Paavonen T, Paavonen J. Plasma cell endometritis is associated with Chlamydia trachomatis infection. Am J Clin Pathol 1999;112:211–15.

46. Peeling RW, Brunham RC. Chlamydiae as pathogens: new species and new issues. Emerg Infect Dis 1996;2:307–19.

47. Peipert JF, Montagno AB, Cooper AS, Sung CJ. Bacterial vaginosis as a risk factor for upper genital tract infection. Am J Obstet Gynecol 1997;177:1184–7.

48. Pritt B, Mount SL, Cooper K, Blaszyk H. Pseudoactinomycotic radiate granules of the gynaecological tract: review of a diagnostic pitfall. J Clin Pathol 2006;59:17–20.

48a. Quenby S, Bates M, Doig T, et al. Pre-implantation endometrial leukocytes in women with recurrent miscarriage. Hum Reprod 1999;14:2386–91.

49. Ramondetta LM, Sherwood JB, Dunton CJ, Palazzo JP. Endometrial cancer in polyps associated with tamoxifen use. Am J Obstet Gynecol 1999;180:340–1.

50. Reslova T, Tosner J, Resl M, Kugler R, Vavrova I. Endometrial polyps. A clinical study of 245 cases. Arch Gynecol Obstet 1999;262:133–9.

51. Roy KH, Mattox JH. Advances in endometrial ablation. Obstet Gynecol Surv 2002;57:789–802.

52. Saegusa M, Okayasu I. Frequent nuclear beta-catenin accumulation and associated mutations in endometrioid-type endometrial and ovarian carcinomas with squamous differentiation. J Pathol 2001;194:59–67.

53. Samuel S, Naora H. Homeobox gene expression in cancer: insights from developmental regulation and deregulation. Eur J Cancer 2005;41:2428–37.

54. Schlesinger C, Kamoi S, Ascher SM, Kendell M, Lage JM, Silverberg SG. Endometrial polyps: a comparison study of patients receiving tamoxifen with two control groups. Int J Gynecol Pathol 1998;17:302–11.

55. Searle RF, Jones RK, Bulmer JN. Phenotypic analysis and proliferative responses of human endometrial granulated lymphocytes during the menstrual cycle. Biol Reprod 1999;60:871–8.

56. Shimizu M, Nakayama M. Endometrial ossification in a postmenopausal woman. J Clin Pathol 1997;50:171–2.

57. Silverberg SG, Mutter GL, Kurman RJ, Kubik-Huch RA, Nogales F, Tavassoli FA. Tumors of the uterine corpus: epithelial tumors and related lesions. In: Tavassoli FA, Stratton MR, eds. WHO Classification of Tumours: Pathology and Genetics of Tumours of the Breast and Female Genital Organs. Lyon: IARC Press; 2003:221–32.

58. Taylor HS, Arici A, Olive D, Igarashi P. HOXA10 is expressed in response to sex steroids at the time of implantation in the human endometrium. J Clin Invest 1998;101:1379–84.

59. Taylor HS, Igarashi P, Olive DL, Arici A. Sex steroids mediate HOXA11 expression in the human peri-implantation endometrium. J Clin Endocrinol Metab 1999;84:1129–35.

60. Vang R, Tavassoli FA. Proliferative mucinous lesions of the endometrium: analysis of existing criteria for diagnosing carcinoma in biopsies and curettings. Int J Surg Pathol 2003;11:261–70.

61. Vosse M, Renard F, Coibion M, Neven P, Nogaret JM, Hertens D. Endometrial disorders in 406 breast cancer patients on tamoxifen: the case for less intensive monitoring. Eur J Obstet Gynecol Reprod Biol 2002;101:58–63.

62. Watts DH, Krohn MA, Hillier SL, Eschenbach DA. Bacterial vaginosis as a risk factor for post-cesarean endometritis. Obstet Gynecol 1990;75:52–8.

63. Yoshida H, Broaddus R, Cheng W, Xie S, Naora H. Deregulation of the HOXA10 homeobox gene in endometrial carcinoma: role in epithelial-mesenchymal transition. Cancer Res 2006;66:889–97.

64. Zaino RJ, Kurman RJ. Squamous differentiation in carcinoma of the endometrium: a critical appraisal of adenoacanthoma and adenosquamous carcinoma. Semin Diagn Pathol 1988;5:154–71.

65. Zaman SS, Mazur MT. Endometrial papillary syncytial change. A nonspecific alteration associated with active breakdown. Am J Clin Pathol 1993;99:741–5.

Benign endometrial hyperplasia and EIN

George L. Mutter   Richard J. Zaino   Jan P.A. Baak   Rex. C. Bentley   Stanley J. Robboy

INTRODUCTION AND TERMINOLOGY

Prolonged estrogen exposure unmitigated by opposing progestins and the appearance of an abnormal endometrial histology have long been associated with an increased risk for endometrioid (type I) endometrial adenocarcinoma. The risk, which is 2–10-fold increased with unopposed estrogen exposure in a dose- and duration-dependent manner,[40,44,59] has been calculated from large epidemiologic studies of cancer outcomes in women of known hormonal exposure. Pathologic confirmation of the presence of endometrial changes secondary to unopposed estrogen exposure helps to establish that there is an abnormal hormonal state, but is of little value in determining which specific patients are most likely to get cancer and which specific histologic changes are an immediate precursor to cancer.

An integrated picture of endometrial carcinogenesis incorporating hormonal, genetic, histopathologic, and clinical outcome parameters underlies the diagnostic strategies outlined in this chapter. The process of carcinogenesis is driven by a continuous and ongoing complex interaction between genetic and non-genetic factors over long periods of time. As early as the 1950s, it was recognized that intervals exceeding 15 years were common between the last normal endometrial biopsy and endometrioid adenocarcinoma. Contrary to long-standing assumption, the change to malignancy is not accompanied by a gradual morphologic progression in which a continuous histologic spectrum of changes is related to a progressively increased endometrial cancer risk. Rather, it is the precipitous emergence of endometrial intraepithelial neoplasia (EIN) which heralds heightened cancer risk.

In the past, both generalized hormonal responses and localized premalignant lesions have been lumped under the term 'endometrial hyperplasia', subdivided by architectural complexity and cytologic atypia.[43] Although this practice has been widespread, it fails to optimally stratify patients according to those pathologic mechanisms and cancer risks necessary for appropriate therapeutic triaging. Diagnoses are poorly reproducible.[57] Recent molecular studies have provided evidence that the use of the term 'hyperplasia' is conceptually correct for some but not all of these lesions. For these reasons we have chosen to present a practically oriented disease classification in which the hormonal effects of unopposed estrogens (benign hyperplasia) and emergent neoplastic precancerous lesions (EIN) are separately diagnosed using non-overlapping terminology and discrete criteria (Table 15.1).[3]

It must be acknowledged that the use of the term 'hyperplasia' is problematic, given its complex history and varied diagnostic application. However, the subset of largely polyclonal proliferations that result from a physiologic response of the endometrium to an abnormal estrogenic stimulus precisely fits the general definition of hyperplasia, and rightly should be labeled such. In contrast, the clonal subset has the characteristics of a non-invasive neoplasm, and should be diagnosed as such (EIN). Compelling genetic, biologic, and histologic evidence supports the use of these two diagnostic terms in a new way.

DISORDERED PROLIFERATIVE TO BENIGN ENDOMETRIAL HYPERPLASIA SEQUENCE

DEFINITION

Benign endometrial hyperplasia is a functional class of diffuse estrogen-induced lesions characterized by irregular remodeling of glands, and variably accompanied by vascular thrombi, stromal breakdown, and randomly scattered cytologic changes. It is preceded by disordered proliferative endometrium, an intermediate step between normal proliferative and benign hyperplastic endometrium. The combination and severity of features progressively increases with duration of exposure and may be retained even if the estrogen level declines or is quenched by addition of progestins (benign hyperplasia with superimposed progestin effect). They are best construed as a sequence of changes, whereby the appearance at any single timepoint is uniquely dependent on the preceding combination and duration of hormonal exposures. Benign hyperplasia of the endometrium has also been referred to as disordered proliferative, proliferative with architectural changes of unopposed estrogens, and non-atypical hyperplasia.

CLINICAL FEATURES

Benign endometrial hyperplasia is encountered most frequently around the time of the menopause or postmenopause, when the normal cycle of sequentially regulated estrogen and progesterone is perturbed in tempo and amount. It can also occur, however, in young women and teenagers, in whom anovulatory cycles are also the norm. In a woman of childbearing age, there is characteristically prolonged or excessive bleeding at intervals that are initially longer than normal. As the endometrial bulk increases through proliferation, the bleeding may become more frequent and almost continuous. The causes of excessive bleeding are multiple. Dilated and delicate superficial blood vessels undergo thrombosis, which contributes to intermittent bleeding. As the condition depends upon estrogen

Table 15.1 Endometrial diagnostic terminology

Nomenclature	Topography	Functional category	Treatment
Benign hyperplasia	Diffuse	Prolonged estrogen effect	Hormonal therapy, symptomatic
Endometrial intraepithelial neoplasia	Focal progressing to diffuse	Precancerous	Hormonal or surgical
Endometrial adenocarcinoma, endometrioid type, well differentiated	Focal progressing to diffuse	Malignant	Surgical stage-based

stimulation for its development, the fluctuation of estrogenic support results in irregular episodes of extensive apoptotic endometrial stromal cell death and breakdown of the tissue.

Persistent estrogen production may be associated with ovarian abnormalities such as granulosa cell tumors, thecomas, polycystic ovary disease or exogenous administration of estrogens. Most patients eventually become symptomatic and present with abnormal vaginal bleeding. An unknown proportion have no symptoms and the abnormality only becomes apparent when baseline biopsies are taken for hormone replacement therapy.

ETIOLOGY

The administration of estrogen unopposed by progestin for postmenopausal hormone replacement therapy is known to cause the development of a persistent proliferative state with resultant disseminated architectural abnormalities throughout the endometrial field.[7] This category of changes referable to unopposed estrogens encompasses individual examples of such diverse histopathology that it is tempting to finely subdivide them by their morphologic appearance, but this is of little clinical significance. The primary pathology in all these cases is a systemic hormonal imbalance, albeit one in which the endometrium is secondarily altered and a frequent source of symptomatic bleeding.

In the first half of a normal cycle, unopposed estrogen brings about proliferation, with mitotic activity of both glands and stroma. Ovulation occurs 14 days after onset of menses, followed by secretion of progesterone, the effect of which is to stimulate secretory activity in the endometrium and, at the same time, to inhibit proliferation through downregulation of estrogen receptors. If ovulation does not occur until much later than day 14, or does not happen at all, the estrogen remains unopposed and proliferation continues. This prolonged proliferation as a result of anovulation first gives rise to disordered proliferative endometrium after a period of about 3 weeks. The serum level of estrogen is not necessarily raised, although in some circumstances it may be.

Longer intervals of estrogen stimulation cause an even greater exaggeration of the proliferative phase, with an increasingly irregular distribution of individually variable endometrial glands which are known as benign hyperplasia. Looked at in this way, disordered proliferative endometrium and benign endometrial hyperplasia may be regarded as a physiologic response of a normal endometrium to prolonged and unopposed estrogen stimulation.

Microinfarcts and estrogen withdrawal are responsible for symptomatic bleeding.[14,48] Both mechanisms may be effective at different times in patients with benign hyperplasia. Patchy stromal breakdown secondary to estrogen-induced micro-

thrombi can produce intermittent spotting. A relative reduction in the prolonged estrogen stimulation causes apoptosis of the endometrial glands and stroma of the hypertrophied functionalis, and resultant heavy shedding. Occasionally, decline in estrogen levels is sufficiently gradual that generalized apoptosis and shedding fail to take place.

Superimposition of progesterone upon a benign endometrial hyperplasia occurs in women with delayed ovulation, idiosyncratic corpus luteum development in the perimenopausal years, or therapeutic administration of progestins following an extended follicular phase. Downregulation of estrogen receptors by progestins leads to a dominant progestational effect, regardless of the presence or absence of continued estrogen production. In this environment menstrual shedding is delayed, as progestins have the capacity to directly support the endometrium. Progesterone-related stromal and secretory glandular changes develop within the setting of irregular glands previously developed under the influence of estrogens. Thus, although the causal event in benign hyperplasia is unopposed estrogen, the histologic appearance at diagnosis may be heavily modified by intermittent or accompanying progestins.

GROSS FEATURES

Initial changes, seen after only 3 weeks of unopposed estrogens (1 week beyond expected ovulation date), are subtle. The endometrium may be moderately but uniformly thickened with a smooth surface lining. Scattered microcysts, although often present, are not apparent on gross examination. With further estrogen exposure, the uterus may enlarge and the endometrium often is irregularly thickened, pale to tan, with a nodular surface (Figure 15.1). Foci of hemorrhage may be present in the areas of breakdown. Ultrasound may help identify the thickened endometrium.[45]

MICROSCOPIC FEATURES

Endometrial curettage in a woman who has benign endometrial hyperplasia is likely to generate abundant curettings that require two or more cassettes for adequate processing. The morphologic features are characteristically diffuse and widespread, as would be expected for a tissue responding uniformly to an underlying systemic hormonal cause. This contrasts with the initially focal distribution of EIN. Although many histologic changes have been described, few specimens demonstrate them all.

The histologic changes of disordered proliferative and benign endometrial hyperplasia are conceptually and morphologically well represented as a unified disease spectrum, separate and discontinuous from EIN. Disordered proliferative

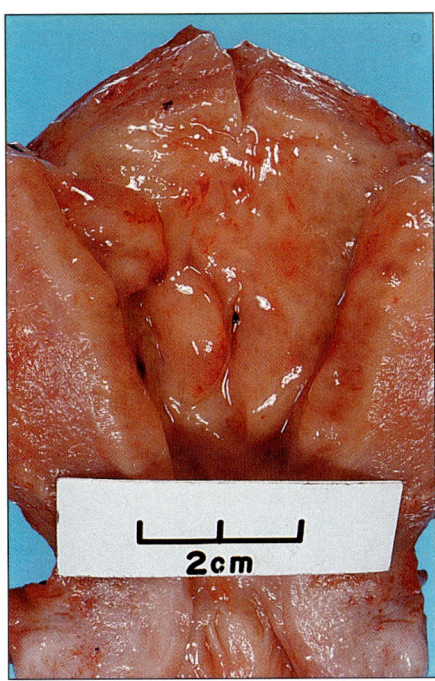

Fig. 15.1 Benign endometrial hyperplasia. The endometrium is diffusely thickened with a nodular surface but no overt polyp formation. Microscopy showed benign endometrial hyperplasia with multiple cysts.

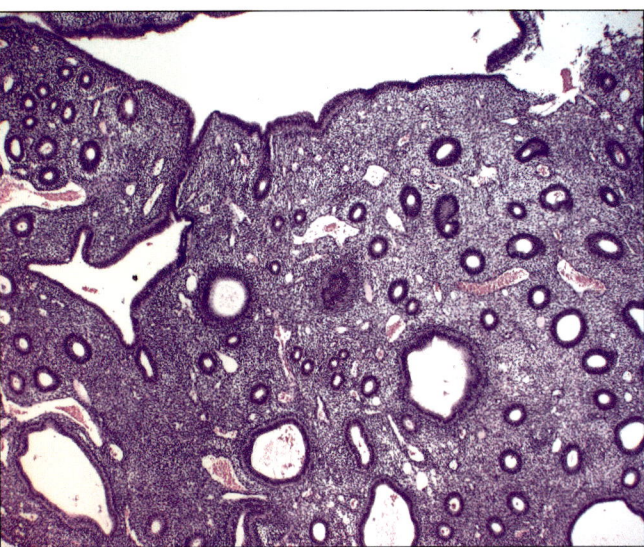

Fig. 15.2 Disordered proliferative endometrium demonstrating glands at low density with scattered cyst formation. Placement of glands is quite regular, and branching is slight, indicating a minimal extent of remodeling.

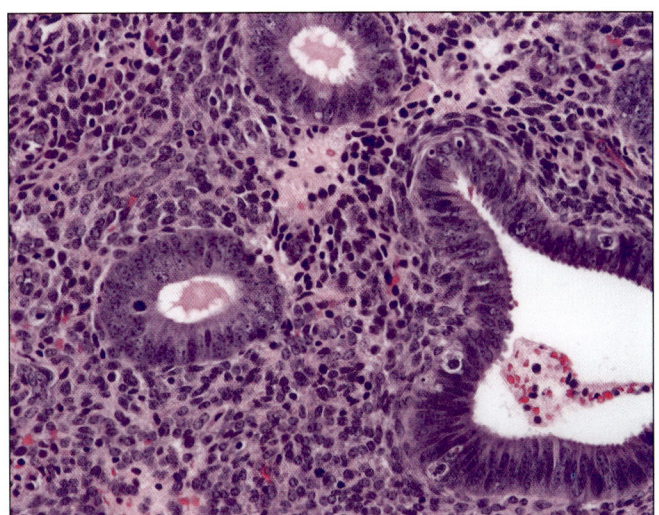

Fig. 15.3 Cytology of disordered proliferative glands resembles that of normal proliferative endometrium, surrounded by a dense stroma.

endometrium and the earliest phases of benign hyperplasia of the endometrium thus share a common pathogenesis, and present a continuous spectrum of overlapping histopathologic features (Table 15.2) rather than sharply different appearances. Precise discrimination is somewhat arbitrary and of little immediate clinical importance. Early effects of unopposed estrogen are scattered cysts in an otherwise normal-appearing proliferative endometrium, known as disordered proliferative endometrium. These are usually considered deviations from the normal endometrial cycle, and are rarely confused with premalignant (EIN) lesions. Continued exposure causes a progressive spectrum of histopathologic change including increasing irregularity of gland density and shape, scattered alterations of cytologic appearance known as benign hyperplasia. Established benign hyperplasias demonstrate a high degree of remodeling between glands and stroma of the expanded, hyperplastic, endometrial compartment. Stromal breakdown and associated reactive epithelial changes commonly develop, and must be carefully distinguished from neoplastic processes.

Cessation or progesterone inhibition of estrogenic stimulation may occur at any time, at which point benign hyperplasias lose their mitotic activity and the endometrium is no longer proliferative. Architectural changes of the estrogen-driven interval are retained, so that a diagnosis of benign hyperplasia can provide indirect evidence of the prior hormonal state of unopposed estrogens.

DISORDERED PROLIFERATIVE ENDOMETRIUM (CYSTS AND TUBAL METAPLASIA)

Disordered proliferative endometrium is an exaggeration of the normal proliferative phase and, as such, much of the tissue is similar to that seen in normal proliferative endometrium. The pathognomonic feature of persistent estrogen stimulation is architectural changes of individual glands distributed randomly throughout the entire hormonally responsive region of the endometrium (superficial functionalis). The overall ratio of glands to stroma is not significantly increased from that of a normal proliferative phase. The changes involve the entire endometrial compartment, and are evident at low magnification as sacculated dilatations (microcysts) randomly scattered amongst tubular glands; it is this feature that commonly draws attention to the condition (Figure 15.2). The mitotically active glands are similar to those seen in the proliferative phase, composed of a simple but often pseudostratified epithelium. Nuclear shape is oval to elongated (Figure 15.3). The stroma is usually dense, cellular, and abundant, thus separating the glands. Gland density is low. Some background tubular glands are slightly irregular, and minimal budding and branching are commonly seen.

Table 15.2 Histological features of benign endometrial hyperplasia (not all are present in every case)

Feature	Comment	Disordered proliferative	Benign hyperplasia[a] Active phase	Exhausted phase	Benign hyperplasia with superimposed progestin effect	Shedding following benign hyperplasia[b]	Appearance
Mitotic activity	Similar to normal proliferation	+	+				
Scattered cysts	Within functionalis, random placement	+	+	+	+		
Tubal metaplasia	Randomly involves scattered tubular or cystic glands ± cilia	+	+	+	+		
Variable gland density	'Regularly irregular' secondary to gland proliferation and remodeling		+	+	+		
Bulky specimen	Reflects prolonged proliferative activity		+	+	+		
Fibrin thrombi	Often separate or displaced		+	+	+	+	
Microinfarcts with epithelial change	Randomly placed, multifocal, with intervening intact		+	+	+		

Table 15.2 Continued

Feature	Comment	Disordered proliferative	Benign hyperplasia[a] Active phase	Exhausted phase	Benign hyperplasia with superimposed progestin effect	Shedding following benign hyperplasia[b]	Appearance
Low or absent mitoses	Reflects decline in estrogen			+	+	+	
Secretory change	Variable extent depending on exposure				+	+	
Stromal predecidualization	May be patchy or lacking, depending on progestin exposure				+	+	
Global breakdown	Architectural clues obscured, cytology degenerative					+	

[a]Diagnosis is 'benign endometrial hyperplasia'. Subphases need not be specified.
[b]Indistinguishable from menstrual endometrium, with or without confirmation of ovulation. If present, fibrin thrombi can be described as a feature consistent with a hormonally abnormal antecedant cycle.

Ciliated cell change (tubal metaplasia) of endometrial glandular cells is common, reflecting estrogen's pivotal role in the process (Figure 15.4). The estrogen-primed cell often has substantial cytoplasm. Characteristically, glands affected by tubal differentiation are randomly interspersed amongst proliferative glands, and they may demonstrate tubular, branching, or cystic architecture.

BENIGN ENDOMETRIAL HYPERPLASIA (REMODELING, FIBRIN THROMBI, AND MICROINFARCTS)

Benign endometrial hyperplasia develops from disordered proliferative endometrium under the continued influence of unopposed estrogens. The entire endometrial compartment contains variable gland densities caused by remodeling of stroma and glands to the extent that in some areas the gland to stroma ratio exceeds 1 (Figure 15.5). It is the change in gland density that offsets benign hyperplasia from disordered proliferative endometrium. Individual glands may be tubular, cystic, or branching, and these forms are commingled throughout (Figures 15.6 and 15.7). On a large scale the endometrium appears uniformly affected; however, at medium magnification local admixtures of individually variable glands present quite differing appearances between separate microscopic fields. This combination of low magnification uniformity, made up of variable medium magnification fields, can be described as 'regularly irregular'.

The cytology of benign endometrial hyperplasia does not change between architecturally crowded and uncrowded areas. This reflects the systemic hormonal etiology of the process which similarly exposes the entire endometrium, and allows its distinction from EIN. Absolute cytologic presentation may change over time with the evolving hormonal state of the patient, and superimposition of local factors such as breakdown and repair. During the established phase of active estrogen exposure glands are proliferative and interposed tubal metaplasia is common.

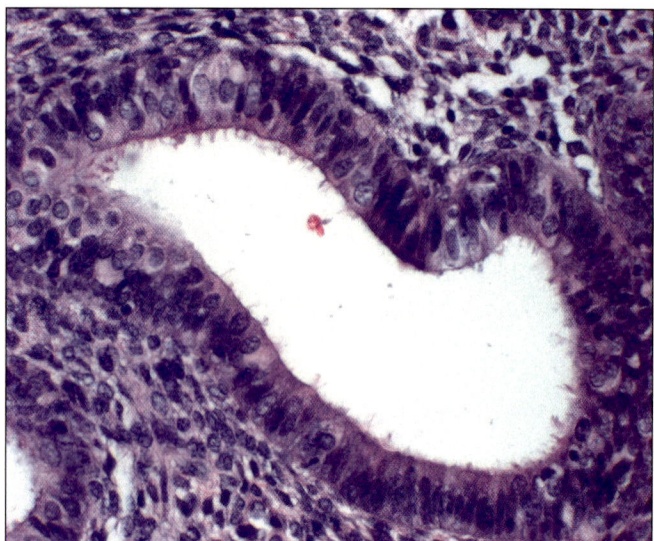

Fig. 15.4 Tubal differentiation with cilia formation, interposed round epithelial cells, and eosinophilic cytoplasm is a common estrogen effect in disordered proliferative endometrium and benign endometrial hyperplasia.

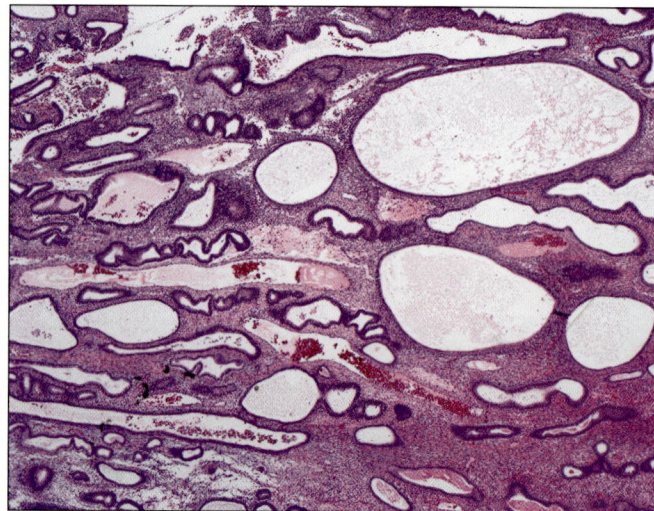

Fig. 15.6 Benign endometrial hyperplasia with randomly interspersed cystic and tubular glands. The entire endometrial compartment is involved, but local remodeling of glands with stroma creates regional heterogeneity of gland density.

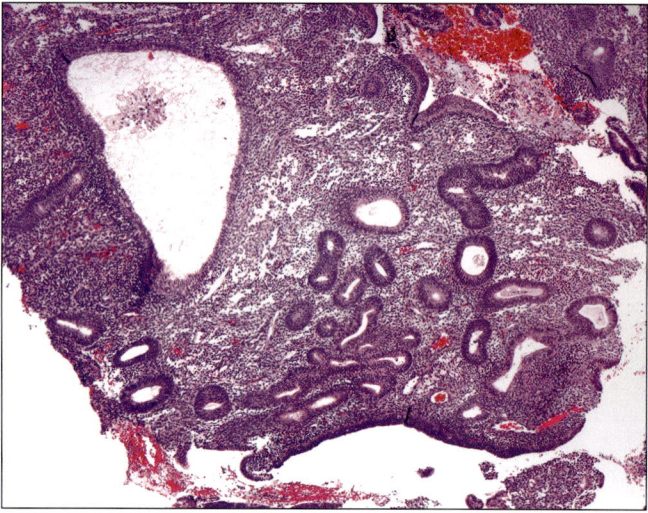

Fig. 15.5 Benign endometrial hyperplasia with a focal collection of crowded glands. Even though the overall distribution of glands is random, some may by chance collect in close proximity. In benign hyperplasias the cytology of glands in the crowded focus is similar to that of uncrowded areas, and may include interspersed tubal differentiation.

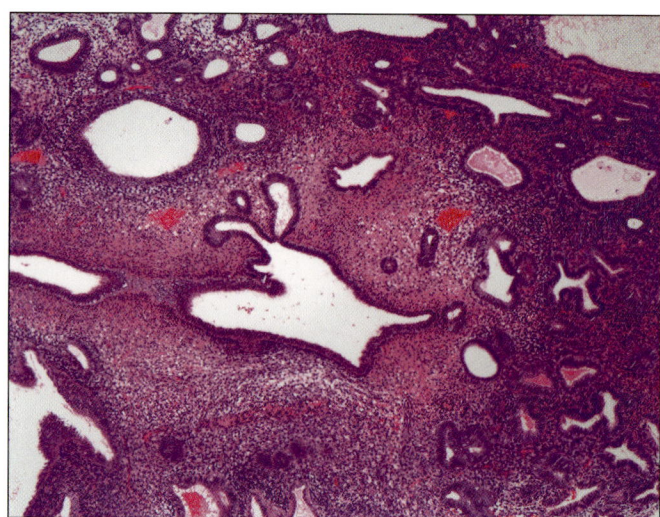

Fig. 15.7 Benign endometrial hyperplasia with variable gland density composed of tubular, cystic, and branching glands.

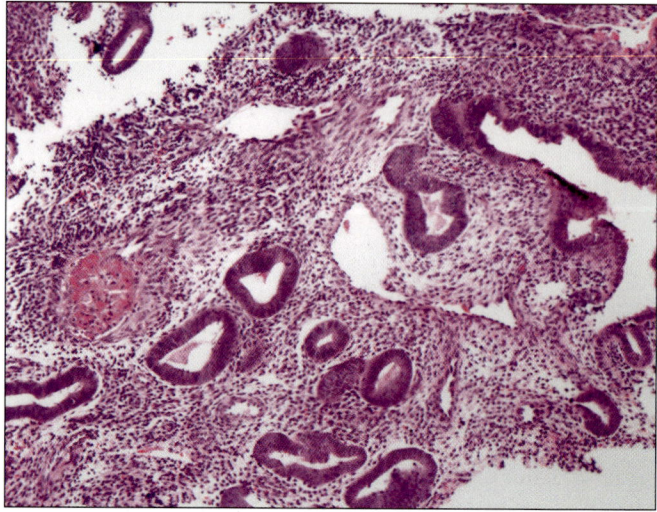

Fig. 15.8 Vascular ectasia and fibrin thrombi are commonly seen in superficial blood vessels of benign endometrial hyperplasia.

Some time after initiation of cystic gland dilatation, the endothelial lining of ectatic superficial endometrial vessels may be damaged and occlusive luminal fibrin thrombi form (Figure 15.8). Unopposed estrogen states such as those related to benign endometrial hyperplasia are the most common setting in which fibrin thrombi are seen in the intact endometrial functionalis.[14] Fibrin thrombi are rarely seen in architecturally normal late secretory endometrium, and there is no evidence that vascular thrombosis is a primary mechanism of cyclic synchronized menstrual shedding. They accumulate in increasing numbers under the continued influence of unopposed estrogens. Thrombi are often intimately associated with discrete areas of surrounding stromal breakdown, which has been interpreted either as a cause or effect of the vascular lesion (Figure 15.9). Whatever the sequence and mechanism of events, the

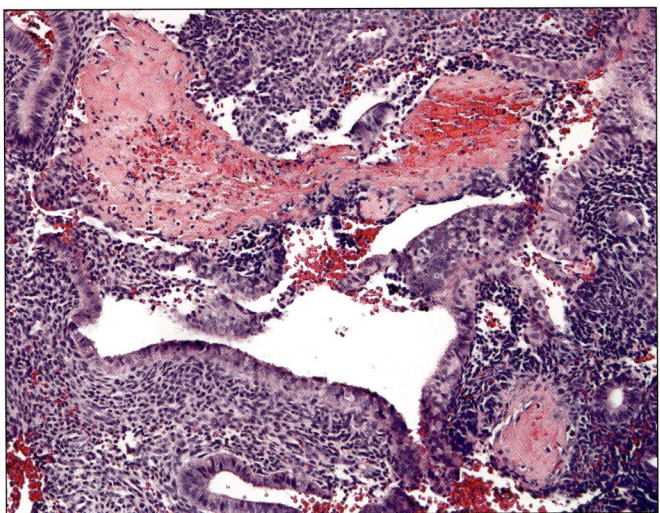

Fig. 15.9 Stromal breakdown associated with fibrin vascular thrombi in benign endometrial hyperplasia. The majority of thrombi seen in benign hyperplasia are dislodged as separate fragments.

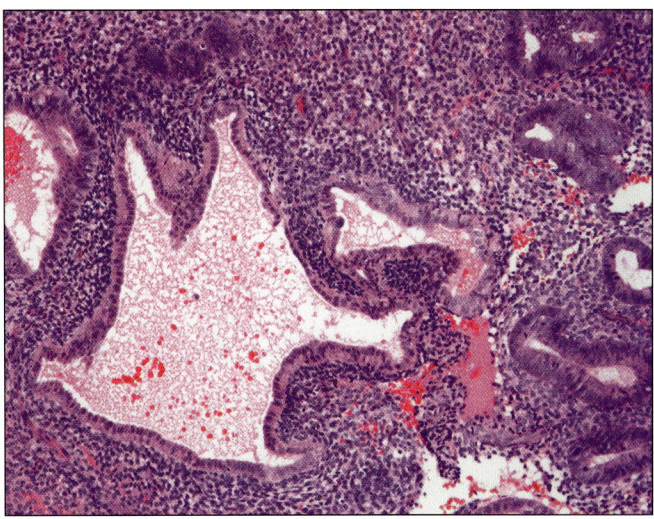

Fig. 15.10 Stromal breakdown in benign endometrial hyperplasia alters cytology of the adjacent epithelium, and may lead to gland displacement.

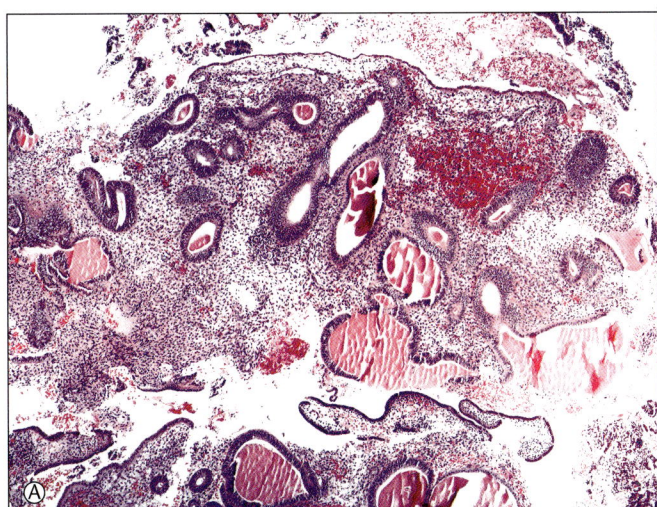

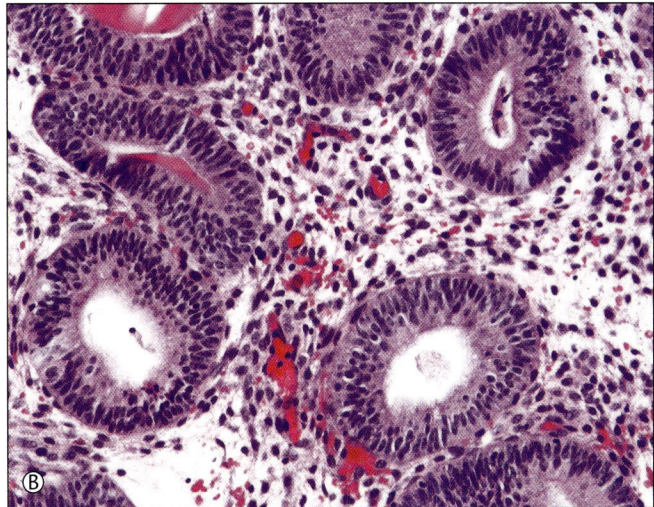

Fig. 15.11 **(A, B)** Benign endometrial hyperplasia, exhausted phase. Quiescent, inactive-appearing glands with scattered cysts caused by a decline in estrogen following a prolonged period of stimulation.

two are linked in benign hyperplasias, and are responsible for patchy non-synchronous endometrial breakdown and resultant symptoms of spotting and intermenstrual bleeding. Collapse of intervening broken-down stroma may lead to close apposition of endometrial glands, degenerative epithelial changes (Figure 15.10), and dislodgement of vascular thrombi from their tissue context. It is the close association of these epithelial changes with stromal breakdown that permits their distinction from EIN.

Estrogen production from persistent follicles or by peripheral conversion following the menopause is inconstant. When the estrogen level declines slowly, massive breakdown does not occur and the glands lose mitotic activity. These endometria retain the architectural features of a bulky endometrium with altered gland architecture and any pre-existing fibrin thrombi, but the glands demonstrate an inactive appearance and may be karyorrhectic (Figure 15.11). With prolonged low estrogen levels, endometrial bulk declines towards an atrophic pattern, sometimes with cysts.

BENIGN ENDOMETRIAL HYPERPLASIA WITH SUPERIMPOSED PROGESTIN EFFECT

Superimposition of endogenous or exogenous progestins upon benign endometrial hyperplasia shuts down mitotic activity, and may initiate secretory change with or without subsequent stromal predecidualization (Figure 15.12). The most common endogenous progesterone source is delayed ovulation in a perimenopausal woman, where the corpus luteum is typically unable to elaborate normal quantities and duration of progesterone. Similar effects can be seen in women having benign hyperplasia treated by low dose or intermittent progestins, such as are seen in many oral contraceptive formulations.

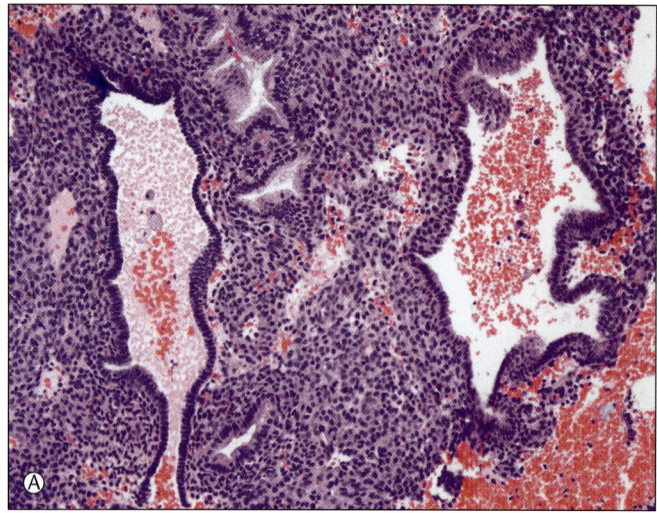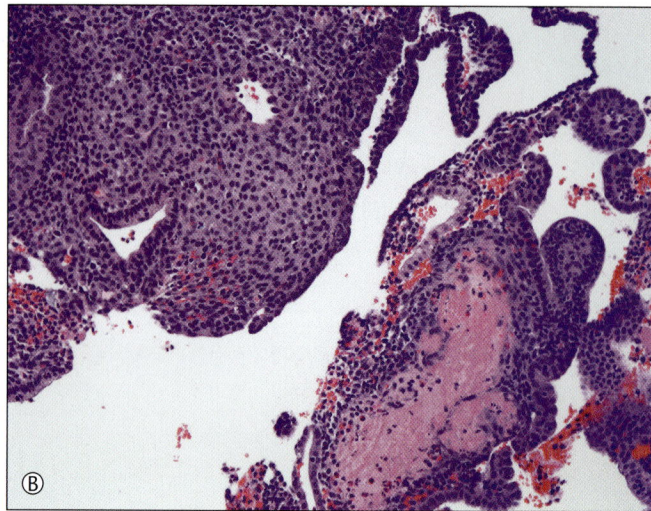

Fig. 15.12 (A, B) Delayed ovulation following protracted estrogen stimulation superimposes secretory change and stromal predecidualization upon pre-existing cysts and thrombi of a benign endometrial hyperplasia.

This group of non-mitotic, architecturally altered, endometria has frequently been described as 'non-atypical' hyperplasia, especially when there is insufficient progesterone to cause stromal predecidualization. The process is widespread throughout the endometrial compartment, although the secretory response of glands may be patchy or irregular when progestin levels are subphysiologic.

WITHDRAWAL SHEDDING FOLLOWING BENIGN HYPERPLASIA

Cessation of estrogenic stimulation, such as occurs systemically upon shutdown or exhaustion of the persistently active ovarian follicle, leads to rapid endometrial-wide stromal breakdown and heavy menses. This occurs through a direct apoptotic effect upon endometrial stromal and epithelial cells, rather than thrombosis-initiated infarction responsible for breakdown during the estrogen-rich period. Evidence of secretory and predecidual change may or may not be present, depending on whether delayed ovulation occurred and the extent of tissue preservation. Architectural features of cysts and irregular gland distribution are increasingly obscured by stromal collapse, eventually yielding a nondescript collection of individual glands with extensive reactive changes. For these reasons, it can be difficult to confirm in the late stages of shedding whether the preceding cycle was normal or abnormal, or whether a benign hyperplasia was present or not. Fibrin thrombi, which are durable sequelae of many benign hyperplasias, remain identifiable despite extensive stromal breakdown (Figure 15.13).

DIFFERENTIAL DIAGNOSIS

It is necessary to distinguish benign endometrial hyperplasia from a variety of conditions, both physiologic and pathologic. These include changes induced by artifacts during the gathering of the specimen, misinterpretation of a variety of normal appearances, endometrial epithelial metaplasias and other pathologic states.

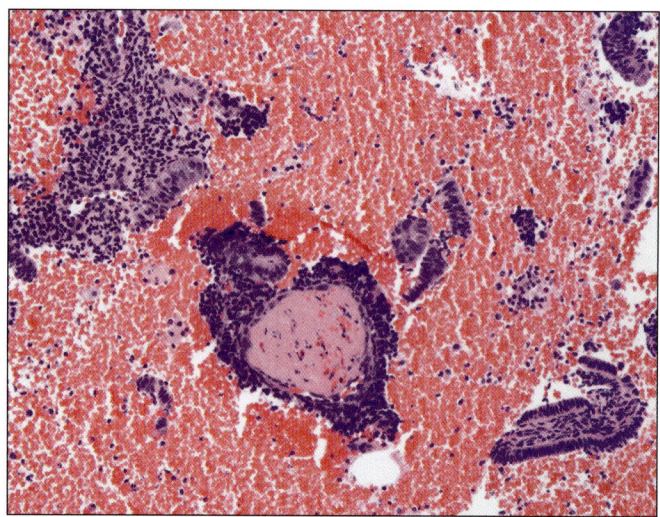

Fig. 15.13 Withdrawal shedding of benign hyperplasia is caused by rapid decline of supportive sex hormones. Fibrin thrombi scattered amongst nondescript stromal aggregates may be the only identifiable residua, as more specific diagnostic features are obscured or 'erased' by massive breakdown.

NORMAL ENDOMETRIUM

Immediately following menses and at the beginning of the proliferative phase, the endometrial functionalis is thin, with endometrial basalis comprising the majority of the tissue seen. Irregularly spaced and occasionally branching glands of the basalis must be distinguished from benign hyperplasia. The glands of basal endometrium are dark and irregular and may be cystic but they are localized to the endomyometrial junction (Figure 15.14). The basal stroma is dense and cellular. Endometrium sampled between cessation of menses and onset of proliferation is much scantier than that of benign hyperplasias, and there is usually evidence of recent repair along the luminal surface.

Just before ovulation occurs, the endometrium of the normal late proliferative phase may be quite thick and the glands may

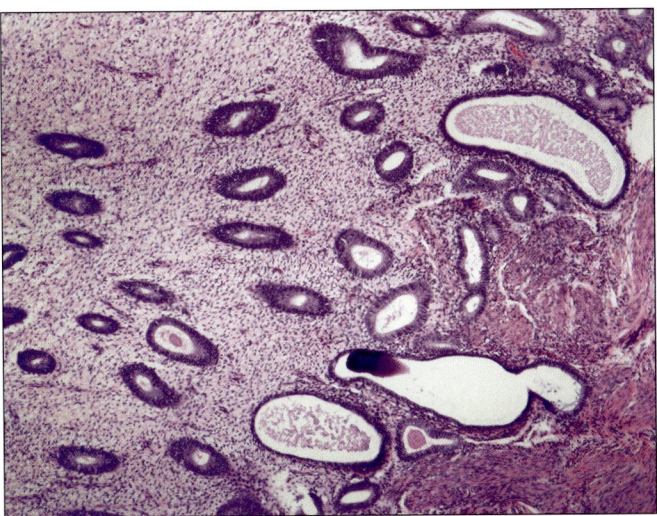

Fig. 15.14 The glands of normal basal endometrium may be cystic but they are localized to the endomyometrial junction.

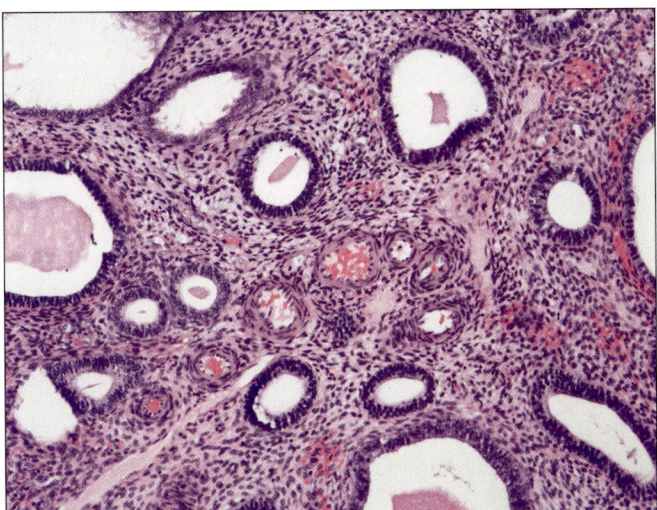

Fig. 15.15 Endometrial polyps may have cysts resembling the pattern of benign endometrial hyperplasia, but they have a denser, more fibrous, stroma and thick-walled blood vessels.

appear numerous. A slight variation in size and shape of the glands may be apparent but the pattern is uniform throughout the curetted material, cysts are rare, and there is no branching.

DISORDERED PROLIFERATIVE ENDOMETRIUM

Disordered proliferative endometrium, as discussed above, has scattered cystic or branching glands which individually may resemble those of benign hyperplasia. It is distinguished from benign hyperplasia by its uniformly low gland density and regular distribution of mitotically active glands which closely resemble those of the normal proliferative endometrium.

ENDOMETRIAL POLYPS

Endometrial polyps, especially when fragmented, are commonly misdiagnosed. Within individual polyp fragments, the irregularly distributed and occasionally branching glands with occasional cysts bear some resemblance to benign endometrial

hyperplasia (Figure 15.15). Epithelial coverage along three fragment surfaces is a frequently discussed, but rarely seen and non-specific feature. The majority of polyps are fractured internally during sampling so they may have one or no surfaces covered by epithelium. Large warped sheets of thickened benign endometrial hyperplasia, on the other hand, may present as fragments extensively or entirely covered by surface endometrium in the plane of sectioning. Thick-walled blood vessels and fibrous stroma commonly seen in polyps are lacking in benign endometrial hyperplasia. Further clues are provided by careful examination of all available fragments. Because polyps are localizing lesions, specimens obtained by undirected biopsy or curettage typically contain commingled native endometrium with a completely different histologic pattern. This is not the case with benign endometrial hyperplasia where the entire functionalis is affected.

POSTMENOPAUSAL CYSTIC ATROPHY

A commonly encountered pattern that may be mistaken for the exhausted phase of benign endometrial hyperplasia is seen during the perimenopausal and postmenopausal periods and is composed of prominent cystically dilated glands in scant, often septated, fibrous stroma. In the past this was one of two patterns often called 'Swiss cheese endometrium'. The terms 'cystic atrophy' or 'cystic atrophic endometrium' currently describe these appearances and show cuboidal or flattened and inactive cells lining the distended glands. In contrast, the epithelium of benign endometrial hyperplasia is thicker and may be pseudostratified. Furthermore, the glands in cystic atrophy lack budding and infoldings.

ENDOMETRIAL INTRAEPITHELIAL NEOPLASIA (EIN)

Distinction of benign endometrial hyperplasia from EIN is critical because the former will result in symptomatic hormonal management and the latter aggressive attempts at lesion ablation by surgery or high dose progestin therapy. This is discussed later in this chapter. Benign hyperplasia is a diffuse condition in which the cytology of regions of crowded glands resembles that of uncrowded areas. Locally random admixtures of tubal or reactive (adjacent to stromal breakdown) glands are common in benign endometrial hyperplasia. In contrast, EIN lesions demonstrate coordinated changes in cytology within crowded areas of glands that offset them from the background.

TREATMENT

The underlying mechanism for elaboration of unopposed estrogens in a patient with benign endometrial hyperplasia will commonly determine appropriate clinical management. Endogenous causes of benign endometrial hyperplasia in the young and perimenopausal patient include failed or delayed ovulation. Anovulatory women of reproductive age should be evaluated by a reproductive endocrinologist to determine whether there is a primary endocrine abnormality, or if anovulation is secondary to other treatable factors such as stress or low body weight. Resultant infertility can be treated by hormonal induction of ovulation or through a variety of assisted reproductive techniques. Most women experience occasional anovulatory or delayed ovulatory menstrual cycles during the perimenopausal window with onset of erratic ovarian responsiveness to gonadotrophins. The symptom of irregular bleeding in these patients can to a certain extent be treated by progestins, which, when withdrawn, cause shedding of the overstimulated endometrium. A benign endometrial hyperplasia in the postmenopausal woman without a history of exogenous (pharmacologic) estrogen use requires explanation. Elaboration of estrogenic compounds by hormonally active ovarian tumors should be considered especially in this group, but may also occur in the younger patient.

Clinical evaluation of the risk for cancer will determine the appropriate follow-up and need for endometrial biopsy following a diagnosis of benign endometrial hyperplasia. Women with intractable chronic anovulation, such as that caused by polycystic ovarian syndrome or associated with obesity, may be exposed to unopposed estrogen for years and thus have 5–10-fold increased endometrial cancer risk.

ENDOMETRIAL INTRAEPITHELIAL NEOPLASIA (EIN)

DEFINITION

EIN is the histopathologic presentation of a monoclonal endometrial premalignant glandular lesion prone to malignant transformation into endometrioid (type I) endometrial adenocarcinoma.

EIN fulfills all levels of evidence[31] required to define a precancerous lesion according to consensus standards established in 2004 by the National Cancer Institute (USA)[6] (Table 15.3).

Table 15.3 Expected features of premalignant lesions which are met by EIN

Evidence type	Precancer feature	EIN evidence
Natural history	A precancer must be different from the normal tissue from which it arises	EIN is monoclonal EIN genotype diverges from normal
Natural history	The resulting cancer must arise from cells within the precancer	EIN to cancer lineage continuity May share PTEN mutations May share K-ras mutations May share MLH1 changes Both EIN and cancer are monoclonal
Natural history	A precancer must be different from the cancer into which it develops	EIN to cancer lineage hierarchy Increasing burden of PTEN and microsatellite changes
Clinical utility	There must be a method by which the precancer can be diagnosed	Subjective diagnostic criteria Histomorphometry reference standard (D-Score)
Clinical utility	The precancer is associated with an increased risk of cancer	39% concurrent cancer rate 45-fold increased future cancer risk

Based on data from Mutter.[31]

This definition of a precancerous lesion provides a set of expected features generalizable to a wide variety of organ sites and epithelial types.

The precancerous properties of EIN are ones previously ascribed to atypical endometrial hyperplasia, a common ground which is the basis for managing EIN lesions in a manner similar to that of atypical endometrial hyperplasia. Clinical management parallels aside, the pathology of EIN lesions is sufficiently distinctive to prevent them from being cleanly equated to any previous hyperplasia subgroup (see Figure 15.36, 'Where have all the hyperplasias gone?'). Other terms that have been applied to suspected premalignant endometrial lesions, using a variety of diagnostic criteria, include 'adenomatous hyperplasia', 'marked adenomatous hyperplasia', 'atypical hyperplasia types II and III', 'anaplasia', and 'glandular hyperplasia with atypical epithelial proliferation'.[57] None of these previously described entities includes all of the diagnostic elements used today for EIN diagnosis.

CLINICAL FEATURES

Because there are no systematic endometrial screening programs, and the PAP smear is ineffective for screening, EIN is detected almost always within the context of an endometrial biopsy performed in response to patient symptoms, incidental to workup of an unrelated disorder, or when monitoring women receiving hormone replacement therapy. Postmenopausal bleeding or vaginal bleeding or irregular menses in the perimenopausal period are the most common signs. Especially in perimenopausal women, a coexisting condition such as benign endometrial hyperplasia or adenocarcinoma, but not the EIN itself, may lead to the bleeding. The postmenopausal patient with a non-cycling atrophic endometrium may experience symptomatic bleeding directly from an EIN lesion.

The average age of women with EIN is 52 years, which is about 8 years earlier than the average age of 60 for endometrioid endometrial adenocarcinoma in the same patient population.[3] The interval for progression from EIN to adenocarcinoma can be more directly estimated in individual patients who undergo protracted surveillance following an EIN diagnosis. Once patients with concurrent adenocarcinoma are excluded (defined as cancer found within the first year of follow-up), the average interval to diagnosis of adenocarcinoma is 4 years.[3]

CANCER OUTCOMES IN WOMEN WITH EIN

Untreated EIN, whether diagnosed objectively by histomorphometry, or subjectively using criteria from Table 15.4, has a high likelihood of progression to adenocarcinoma. EIN lesions that do not progress to cancer may involute, or stably persist for protracted periods of time. Absence of an EIN lesion in an initial representative biopsy, including those with only benign hyperplasia, confers very high (99%) negative predictive value for concomitant or future adenocarcinoma.[3]

Morphometric EIN diagnosis using computerized image analysis incorporates three variables (see D-Score in 'Biomarkers' section below) to generate a 'D-Score', which is interpreted as an EIN when the value is less than 1. A clinical outcome study incorporating 477 endometrial 'hyperplasia' patients who had no concomitant cancer with the first year of follow-up and restratified by histomorphometry into EIN (D-Score <1)

Table 15.4 Diagnostic features of EIN (all must be met)

EIN criterion	Comments
Architecture	Area of glands exceeds that of stroma (glands/stroma >1)
	Lesion composed of individual glands which may branch slightly and vary in shape.
Cytology	Nuclear and/or cytoplasmic features of epithelial cells differ between architecturally abnormal glands and normal background glands
	May include change in nuclear polarity, nuclear pleomorphism, or altered cytoplasmic differentiation state
	If no normal glands present, highly abnormal cytology
Size	Maximum linear dimension exceeds 1 mm
Exclude mimics	Benign conditions with overlapping criteria: disordered proliferative, basalis, secretory, polyps, repair, etc.
Exclude cancer	Carcinoma if maze-like glands, solid areas, or significant cribriforming

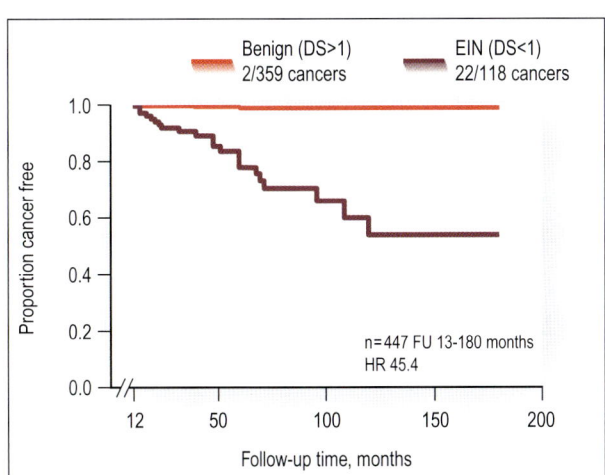

Fig. 15.16 Forty-five-fold elevated prospective cancer risk in women with EIN at endometrial biopsy (red) compared to women with benign, non-EIN endometria (blue).

and benign (D-Score > 1) categories showed that the EIN group had an overall 45-fold increased frequency of endometrial cancer (Figure 15.16).[3] EIN has proven to discriminate better between benign and premalignant conditions than the WHO classification scheme in general usage since 1994. In the latter, a diagnosis of atypical hyperplasia vs non-atypical hyperplasia in the same patient population predicts only a seven-fold cancer risk.

Of import, 39% of patients with EIN had cancer diagnosed within the first year, in contrast to 0% of patients where the morphometric score was benign (not EIN). This explains the historical observation that cancer is very often present in a hysterectomy performed shortly after a diagnostic biopsy showing only premalignant findings. Sampling error is a major deficiency in detection of concurrent carcinoma in the initial biopsy.

Subjective (non-morphometric) EIN diagnosis from H&E-stained slides at a standard microscope without specialized equipment, using guidelines shown in Table 15.4, also has a high level of clinical outcome predictive value.[31,46] In a hospital-based clinical outcome study, 84 successive endometrial hyperplasias of all types with known clinical outcomes were reclassified according to subjective and histomorphometric EIN schema.[17] All subjective EIN diagnoses had a D-Score <1, confirming that subjective implementation of the EIN criteria conforms well with that achieved by formal morphometry. All eight cancer occurrences during follow-up were captured in the high-risk subjective EIN (8/25) and morphometric EIN (D-Score <1, 8/38) groups.

MOLECULAR ETIOLOGY AND NATURAL HISTORY

EIN IS A MONOCLONAL NEOPLASM

EIN lesions begin as localized monoclonal outgrowths of mutated endometrial cells with a changed cytology and architecture that enables their recognition when compared to the background source polyclonal field.[32] Monoclonal growth is a generalizable feature of premalignant epithelial lesions, also being present in precancers originating at other sites such as vulva,[52] cervix,[11] oral mucosa,[8] and esophagus.[61] It is the clonal origin of EIN that determines its localized emergence and expansile growth properties over time. The clonal nature of EIN lesions has been demonstrated by various markers such as non-random X chromosome inactivation and clonal propagation of altered microsatellites.[22,32,34] The non-random X chromosome inactivation and altered DNA microsatellites used to score clonality do not necessarily reflect a causal role for those specific marker genes in endometrial carcinogenesis. Rather, monoclonal outgrowth shown by non-random X inactivation is the non-specific functional consequence of a cell that has acquired a growth advantage relative to its neighbors. Clonally altered microsatellites, seen in approximately 20% of EIN lesions and endometrial adenocarcinomas, are merely a symptom of a form of sporadic DNA instability that also accelerates mutation rates at other, non-microsatellite, genetic loci.[41]

Insights into how endometrial precancers behave have been facilitated by application of molecular markers to paraffin-embedded human materials. Precancerous endometrial lesions identified through molecular analysis have an identical microscopic appearance to that seen in patients developing cancer during clinical follow-up. Histomorphometric analysis of premalignant endometrial lesions identified by monoclonal growth and lineage continuity with actual carcinomas that developed in the same patients showed that virtually all precancers have a histomorphometric D-Score <1, a feature noted in clinical outcome studies to confer elevated cancer risk.[3]

GENETIC CHANGES IN EIN

Each EIN lesion is the end result of multiple mutations that occur in varying permutations and order of invocation between patients. Within individual patients, those exact genetic alterations present in an EIN lesion are carried forward to the cancer, establishing them as physical progenitors of carcinoma.[32,33] The clone which comprises an EIN lesion may acquire additional mutations during subsequent clonal expansion, a key element of progression to carcinoma and development of intratumoral heterogeneity.[33,36] Comparison of the extent and range of genomic damage between premalignant and malignant phases indicates a greater cumulative mutational load in cancers, a feature that must contribute to their differing morphology and behavior. For example, while 55% of EIN lesions have demonstrable inactivating events (mutation and/or deletion)[13] of the *PTEN* tumor suppressor gene, the proportion rises to 83% in those cancers which follow an EIN lesion.[36] Similarly, for those lesions with microsatellite instability, the burden of altered microsatellite alleles increases between EIN and carcinoma.[32,33]

Inactivation of the *PTEN* tumor suppressor gene is the most frequent genetic change in endometrioid-type endometrial adenocarcinoma, occurring in approximately 42% of all reported cases,[30] increasing to 83%[36] in cancers preceded by an EIN lesion. Because *PTEN* inactivation occurs early in carcinogenesis, it is an informative marker for exploring the premalignant phases of disease. Sixty-three per cent of EIN lesions lack immunohistochemically detectable PTEN protein in a clonal distribution.[35] Despite this very strong association, and the fact that experimental *PTEN* inactivation in mice leads to a high incidence of endometrial cancer,[49] additional genetic changes must occur before affected cells acquire histopathologic features diagnostic of EIN, and an elevated endometrial cancer risk.

Several other genes known to be structurally altered in endometrial carcinomas are already abnormal in EIN lesions. Most are somatically acquired rather than inherited defects, as they are intact in the background endometrial tissues. Activating mutations of the KRAS2 cellular oncogene are clonally present in the cells of 16% of EIN lesions.[10,12,38] Microsatellite instability caused by defective DNA mismatch repair is seen in 20–25% of EIN lesions. β-catenin mutations involve 25–30%[25] of endometrial cancers and their premalignant counterparts. Conservation of particular genetic changes between the EIN and carcinoma phases within individual patients is concrete evidence that the cells of EIN are the physical progenitors of carcinoma.

Defective DNA mismatch repair and resultant microsatellite instability, usually secondary to epigenetic inactivation of the MLH1 gene,[13] is present in 15–20% of sporadic endometrioid endometrial cancers[4,16] and a similar proportion of EIN lesions.[32] When present, it produces a hypermutable state within affected cells that extends to non-microsatellite areas of the genome, thereby accelerating the rate of accumulation of a critical mutational burden necessary for malignant transformation.[41] Defective DNA mismatch repair also occurs in a familial setting, where patients with hereditary non-polyposis colorectal cancer (HNPCC) syndrome have a 22–43% lifetime endometrial cancer risk.[27] HNPCC-associated endometrial cancers are usually of the endometrioid type, and may include a premalignant phase.[51]

The threshold between EIN and adenocarcinoma is experimentally less documented than the benign–EIN interface. Well-differentiated endometrioid adenocarcinoma has no uniquely present markers different from those seen in EIN. Rather, adenocarcinomas tend to have a higher density of genetic damage involving a broader repertoire of genes, some of which were already abnormal in the premalignant phase. Changes in *PTEN*, K-*ras*, microsatellite instability, and β-catenin may all be present in either.

THE ROLE OF ESTROGENS AND PROGESTINS

Hormonal risk factors for EIN are the same as those previously described for atypical endometrial hyperplasia, with estrogens acting as promoters and progestins as protectors. In the Postmenopausal Estrogen/Progestin Interventions (PEPI) Trial, 12% of women receiving unopposed estrogens developed atypical hyperplasia over the 3-year surveillance period compared to 0% of placebo controls.[56] Estrogen risks are obviated by addition of progestins such as medroxyprogesterone acetate, which protects against development of endometrial hyperplasia,[55,56] and when administered in a combined low dose oral contraceptive formulation may reduce endometrial cancer risk below that of the population background.[50,54]

Hormonal and genetic mechanisms are linked in the very earliest stages of endometrial carcinogenesis through the selective effects of hormones upon genetically defective compared to intact endometrial cells. Hormones act upon 'latent' precancers, which are somatically mutated, histologically unremarkable, endometrial glands detectable only with specialized biomarkers. This is a preclinical phase of disease properly described as 'latent' in that additional changes in the affected cells are required before they develop any histologic phenotype, or even clinically measurable increased cancer risk. They are not an entity appropriate for clinical diagnosis or patient management, but are key in understanding the link between genetic and hormonal carcinogenesis mechanisms.

De novo somatic mutation of endometrial glandular cells occurs in most women as a random event during monthly regeneration, a process that generates kilograms of new endometrial tissue throughout the reproductive years. The *PTEN* tumor suppressor gene is a useful biomarker for the earliest stages of carcinogenesis, as it inactivates well before established disease develops. Forty-three per cent of normal premenopausal naturally cycling women have small numbers of immunohistochemically detected *PTEN*-deficient endometrial glands, which when microdissected bear acquired mutations and deletions of the *PTEN* gene itself.[35] Progression from this stage to carcinoma must be extremely inefficient, as the lifetime risk of endometrial cancer is only 2.6%.[42] These first events of endometrial carcinogenesis occur with sufficient frequency that they can be considered a feature of 'normal' endometrial biology rather than part of a pathologic state.

PTEN-defective latent precancers, as well as established EIN lesions, maintain high levels of nuclear estrogen and progesterone receptors.[35] Physiologic expression of endometrial gland PTEN protein is greatest in a mitotic, estrogen-rich environment, when its tumor suppressor functions are required to control the rate of cell division.[37] Under estrogen stimulation *PTEN* mutant cells would thus be expected to have a selective proliferative advantage that is lost upon progesterone exposure when genetically intact glands shut down *PTEN* expression.

Under conditions of a normal monthly menstrual cycle, progesterone exposures are insufficient to ablate latent precancers, only 17% of which disappear a year later.[35] If the dose and duration of progestins are increased to therapeutic levels, *PTEN* mutant latent precancers undergo a 90% rate of involution, thereby resetting the carcinogenesis 'clock'.[60] These events are all inapparent at the level of routine histology.

Two major conclusions can be drawn from these data. First, although inactivation of genes like *PTEN* is a frequent element of endometrial carcinogenesis, loss of *PTEN* function in histologically unremarkable glands cannot, and should not, be construed as evidence for heightened clinical cancer risk. It is simply too early an event to place in any meaningful clinical management context. Second, inactivated cells may persist for intervals of several years,[35] providing a genetically predisposed cell population that is a target for, and effector of, prospective hormonal risk modulation. Longitudinal studies of the fate of latent endometrial precancers under differing hormonal and clinical circumstances are required before their clinical implications can be fully understood.

GROSS FEATURES

Most EIN lesions are themselves grossly inapparent. They expand by interactively remodeling the stroma relative to the neoplastic glands. This makes the boundaries difficult to distinguish grossly, as they are unaccompanied by gross distortion or compression of the flanking normal tissues. One circumstance in which EIN may be grossly evident is when a thin atrophic background endometrium lacks the bulk necessary to contain the expanding EIN lesion without distortion. For this reason, some EIN lesions in postmenopausal patients are visible as local thickenings.

The background endometrium which contains an EIN lesion, however, is often itself grossly abnormal. Many EIN lesions are focally distributed against a background of benign endometrial hyperplasia, which can have a thickened and multicystic appearance. EIN may present within otherwise grossly unremarkable sessile or pedunculated endometrial polyps. The pathologist should sample grossly visible lesions, while keeping in mind that EIN is a disease that is most often detected by random sampling of undistinguished regions of the endometrium. Thoroughness of sampling is therefore a key element in successful detection of EIN lesions, especially those that are physically small and localized at the time of diagnosis.

MICROSCOPIC FEATURES OF EIN

Focal origin of EIN lesions explains why most are represented in only some of the many tissue fragments that comprise a typical endometrial biopsy or curettage specimen. The first step in diagnosis is thus low magnification scanning of all tissue fragments in search of architecturally crowded patterns that visually punctuate a more uniform background (Figure 15.17). Closer examination will show a change in cytology of the crowded focus relative to the background endometrium, in addition to all other features listed in Table 15.4 and discussed in detail below.

Large-scale topography has been greatly underestimated as a useful feature in endometrial precancer diagnosis. This is due to previous overemphasis on cytology, with the false expectation that problematic differential diagnoses can be resolved with higher magnification. This is rarely the case with EIN for two reasons. First, many EIN lesions arise from a pathologic endometrial field such as a benign endometrial hyperplasia, where cytology of individual scattered glands is already abnormal and altered by tubal metaplasia or regional breakdown. It is the geographic aggregation of similarly altered endometrial glands, a reflection of clonal growth, which is seen in EIN but not benign endometrial hyperplasia. Secondly, the cytologic

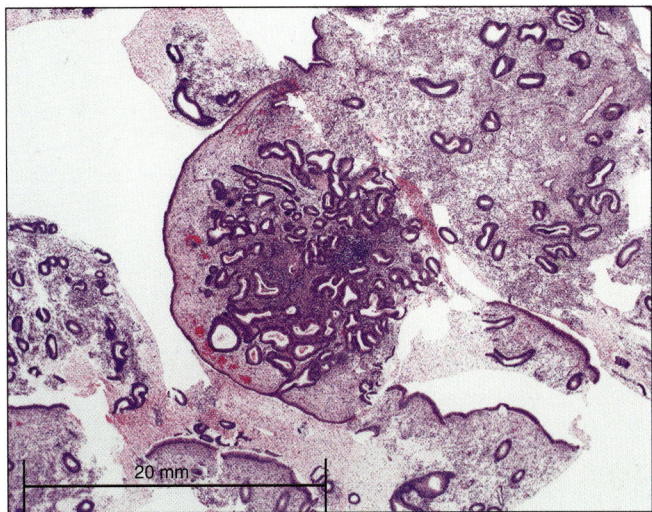

Fig. 15.17 This discrete EIN lesion is readily visible under low magnification as a 1.5 mm diameter region of crowded glands against a regular background of proliferative endometrium. Only one tissue fragment was involved. The patient was diagnosed with endometrioid endometrial adenocarcinoma 2 years later.

changes of EIN can most reliably be recognized when comparing the lesion's epicenter with the adjacent or background endometrium. This requires awareness, on a large scale, of which fragments and regions should be compared.

EIN DIAGNOSTIC CRITERIA

EIN diagnostic criteria include shared features conserved amongst all lesions (the first three items of Table 15.4), and exclusion of benign mimics and carcinoma. It is the latter that requires experience to recognize, as familiarity with a broad range of benign entities that share some features with EIN is a prerequisite to avoid misdiagnosis.

All five EIN diagnostic criteria must be met in every case to maintain a high level of diagnostic specificity and clinical predictive value. The demonstrably strong outcome predictive value of an individual parameter such as crowded gland architecture should not be taken as evidence that other features such as lesion cytology are of lesser value. It is the combined application of multiple diagnostic features that confers robustness to an EIN diagnosis.

1. Architecture: Area of glands exceeds that of stroma

EIN lesions are composed of aggregates of individual tubular or slightly branching glands, in which the surface area of glands is greater than that of the stroma which contains them (Figure 15.18). The 'crowded' appearance of these clusters is what makes localizing EIN lesions so readily visible under low magnification. Expanses of obviously benign cysts, commonly encountered in the atrophic endometrium of the postmenopausal patient, or within the benign endometrial hyperplasia from which an EIN has arisen, should be avoided in this assessment.

Growing EIN lesions have an 'epicenter' with maximal concentration of neoplastic glands that may become less densely distributed towards the periphery. Margins with adjacent

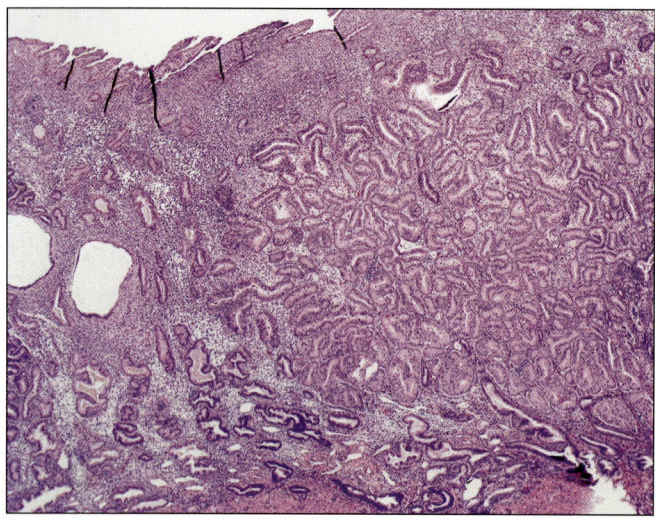

Fig. 15.18 EIN lesions are composed of aggregates of individually tubular or slightly branching glands, in which the surface area of the glands is greater than that of the stroma which contains them.

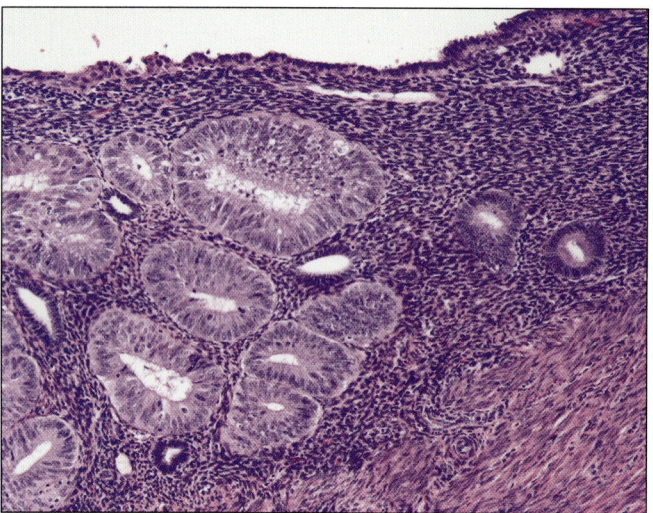

Fig. 15.19 Growth of EIN lesions occurs through percolation of affected peripheral glands between and amongst overrun normal glands. Extension is lateral rather than exophytic, preserving a smooth uterine cavity surface lining which obscures recognition of EIN at gross examination.

normal tissues tend to be expansive rather than compressive, with a peripheral spray of EIN glands projecting between, and amongst, overrun normal glands (Figure 15.19). Non-invasive dynamic remodeling between glands and stroma, rather than invasion, is probably responsible for changes in gland density.[20,39] The stroma intervening between glands of EIN will have an appearance dependent on the regional and hormonal context, ranging from the lush stroma of the functionalis, to more fibrous non-cycling stroma within the basalis or a polyp. Attempts to interpret endometrial stroma as 'desmoplastic' or altered in response to 'invasion' are of no diagnostic benefit because of the irreproducible[5] nature of that determination.

The endometrial compartment can be thought of as glands (combined epithelium and internal lumina) distributed within supportive stroma. The size of glands and distances between them codetermine the amount of intervening stroma, which

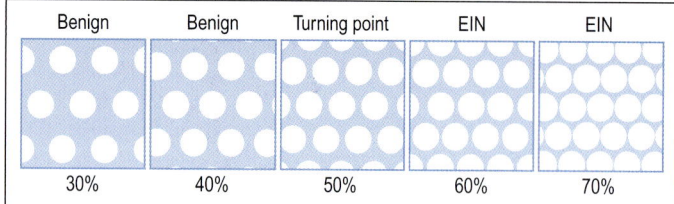

Fig. 15.20 Appearance of glands (white) packed at different densities within endometrial stroma (gray). Gland area as percentage of tissue area.

may be expressed as the percentage of the endometrial compartment occupied by stroma, or volume percentage stroma (Figure 15.20). Because gland and stromal areas together add up to 100%, decreases in stroma are proportionally accompanied by increases in glands. When the gland area exceeds that of stroma (volume percentage stroma <55%), the lesion is likely to be a monoclonal precancer, and the patient has an increased risk for development of carcinoma during clinical follow-up. Fortunately for the pathologist, this can intuitively be translated to 'gland area exceeds stromal area'.

When evaluating extent of gland crowding (training can be done against reference images (Figure 15.20, online photomicrographs at www.endometrium.org) or through use of simple ocular counting grids), the area for analysis should be free of displacement artifact. A conscious awareness of an intact stromal compartment will prevent misinterpretation of sheared or disrupted specimens. Inexpensive ocular grids with 50–100 regularly placed points indicated by intersecting lines are easy to use, and allow rapid calculation of volume percentage stroma (number of points over stroma/number of points over glands and stroma) within any selected microscopic field. More formal computerized histomorphometry is discussed below in the 'Biomarkers' section.

2. Cytology: The cytology of EIN changes relative to the background endometrium from which it has arisen

Altered cytology within the same glands that demonstrate the architectural features of EIN is an important criterion for diagnosis that must be judged independently in each patient by comparison with the native background endometrium. There is no single cytologic appearance across all EIN lesions, which may differ dramatically between patients, and even change over time in individual patients as the hormonal environment fluctuates.

The nature of cytologic change can include nuclear and/or cytoplasmic components. EIN lesions may have round non-stratified, or elongated pseudostratified nuclei (Figure 15.21). Classic cytologic 'atypia', defined as a round non-polarized nuclear morphology with prominent nucleoli, although often present, is not required for EIN diagnosis. The cytoplasm may retain endometrioid differentiation or acquire non-endometrioid differentiation of tubal, mucinous, secretory, or eosinophilic epithelium. The latter are discussed in detail in Chapter 14 on endometrial 'metaplasias', a subset of which are premalignant EIN lesions. A comparison of background with EIN cytology makes it possible to recognize a changed cytology at the contrasting interface despite a variable appearance between EIN lesions. The term 'cytologic demarcation' is a

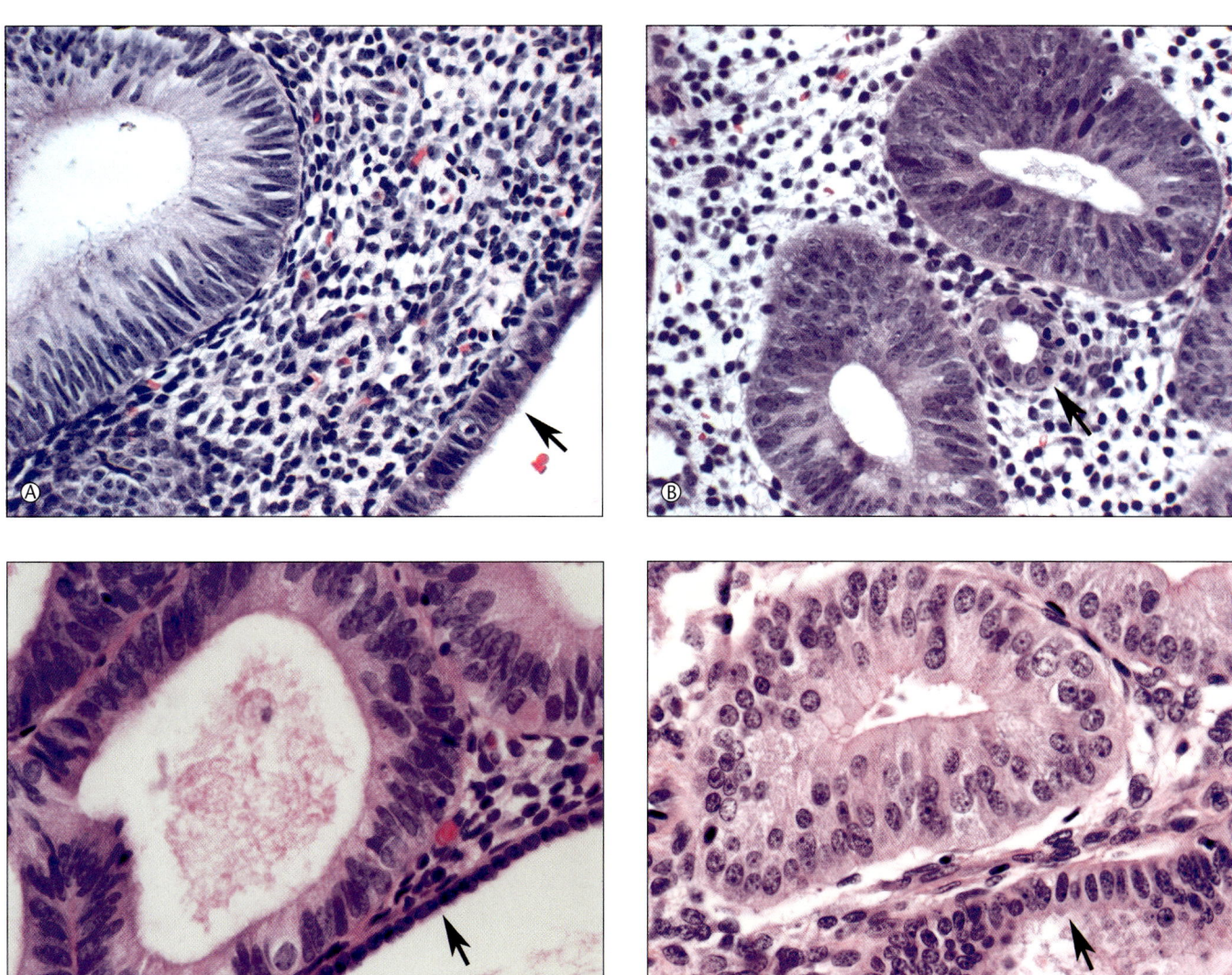

Fig. 15.21 The cytologic appearance of EIN glands varies between examples, but in each case there is a distinctive change in cytology in comparison with matched background glands (arrowheads) of the same patient. Images A–D illustrate differing extents of nuclear polarization, and ratio of nuclei to cytoplasm.

good description of this feature, where cytology as well as architecture demarcates the perimeter of the lesion. For lesions that are no longer localized, or which do not have readily identifiable perimeters, individually overrun normal glands may be available for comparison (Figure 15.21). This is discussed further in the 'Common EIN diagnostic problems' section that follows.

EIN, like endometrioid adenocarcinoma, generally lacks the markedly pleomorphic hobnailed nuclei seen in serous or clear cell adenocarcinoma of the endometrium (non-endometrioid type II tumors). In the presence of such cytology, a non-endometrioid neoplasm or surface spread from an adjacent high-grade carcinoma should be considered. When in their early stage of development, serous or clear cell adenocarcinomas may spread along the uterine surface lining or overtake the spaces of pre-existing glands, and may lack their otherwise distinctive complicated architecture. P53 immunohistochemistry, usually positively staining in serous endometrial adenocarcinomas, may help in recognizing this process.

3. Size: The lesion must be at least 1 mm in dimension

The perimeter of an EIN lesion used for measurement should be drawn at the margin of a suitably dense arrangement of cytologically altered glands, a position often located internal to the outermost distribution of individual neoplastic glands, which become rarified on the periphery (Figure 15.22). The 1 mm size needs to be present in only one linear measurement. Elongated or irregularly shaped lesions may have a width of lesser extent. Separate foci cannot be added to achieve this minimum size – it must be met in a single focus.

The minimum size requirement confers clinical outcome predictive value to an EIN diagnosis while reducing the risk of overdiagnosis. Cancer outcome prediction is dependent on the ability to reliably measure extent of gland crowding, a difficult task unless a critical mass of representative glands is included in the assessment. There are many processes, such as estrogen-induced tubal metaplasia, and local reactive changes, where tiny clusters of three or four glands may demonstrate an altered

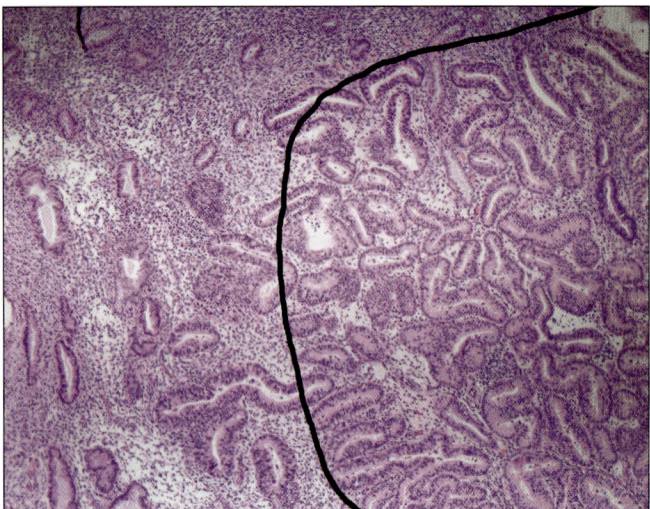

Fig. 15.22 The perimeter of an EIN lesion used to measure maximum linear extent should be drawn at the margin of a suitably dense (gland greater than stromal area) arrangement of cytologically altered glands, a position that is often internal to the outermost distribution of individual neoplastic glands which become rarified on the periphery. The epicenter of this EIN lesion is to the right.

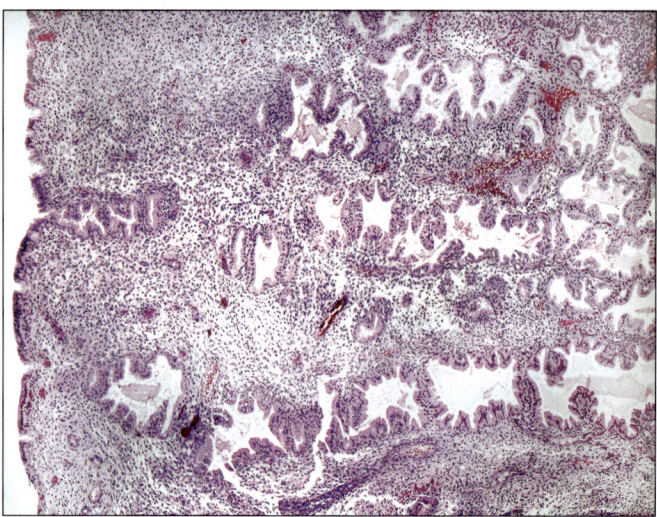

Fig. 15.24 Density of secretory endometrial glands in this 27-day normal endometrium is very high in the deep functionalis (right) where there is less predecidual change than towards the luminal surface (left). Gradual transition and recognition of the sawtooth configuration of lumens assists in discrimination from EIN.

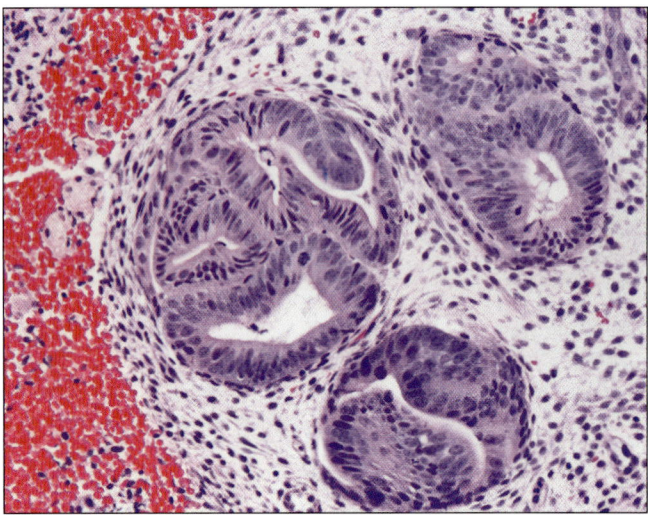

Fig. 15.23 Glands artifactually pushed together or telescoped into a crowded discrete focus will lack the cytologic change of EIN.

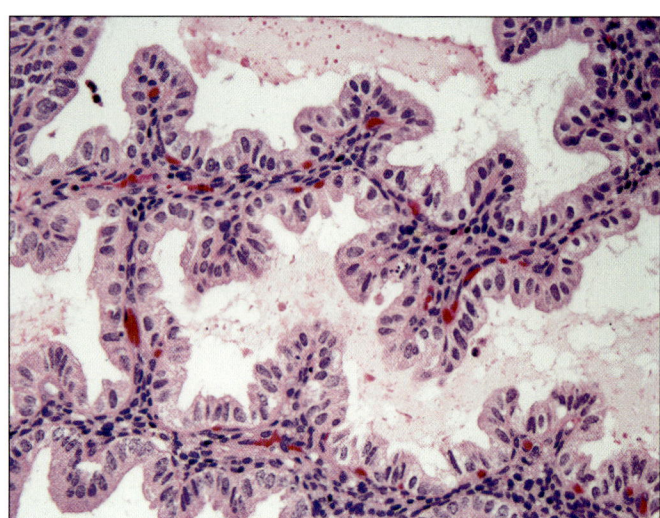

Fig. 15.25 Detail of normal 27-day secretory glands showing round nuclei, complex luminal contours, and scant stroma. This appearance of irregular glands that are not separated by stroma must not be misinterpreted as EIN.

cytology unrelated to premalignant change. The minimum size reduces considerably the likelihood of overreacting to these processes. Lesions smaller than 1 mm, or excessively fragmented specimens with few or no individual fragments 1 mm in dimension, represent a class of endometria subdiagnostic for EIN that are discussed below.

4. Exclusion of benign mimics
Normal tissues that can be mistaken for EIN
Glands artifactually pushed together or telescoped into a crowded discrete focus may have angular contours due to extrinsic compression, and will lack the cytologic change of EIN (Figure 15.23). Normal tissues with irregularly placed glands such as lower uterine segment or uterine basalis can usually be identified by their more fibrous stromal context and

usually quiescent epithelium. The gland density of late secretory endometrium may be very high in the deep functionalis where the predecidual change may be minimal (Figure 15.24). When the endometrium breaks down, either in the normal menstrual phase of the cycle or as a result of estrogen withdrawal, the glands collapse and the stroma crumbles. This frequently results in irregular glands lacking much stromal separation and there is a real danger of misinterpretation as EIN (Figure 15.25). When an EIN-like area is focal, it is important that the surrounding stroma is intact and the cytology of the localizing lesion differs distinctly from the background.

Benign processes that can be mistaken for EIN
Fragments of polyps are commonly overdiagnosed as 'hyperplasia', and the combination of irregularly placed glands and

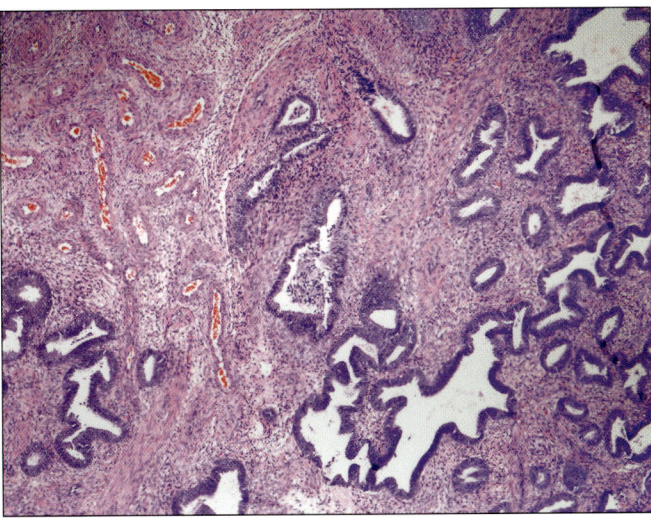

Fig. 15.26 Polyps may have regions of high gland density, but the cytology of these areas is usually similar to that seen elsewhere in the polyp. Polyps can be recognized by their altered stroma, thick vessels, and random irregular glands.

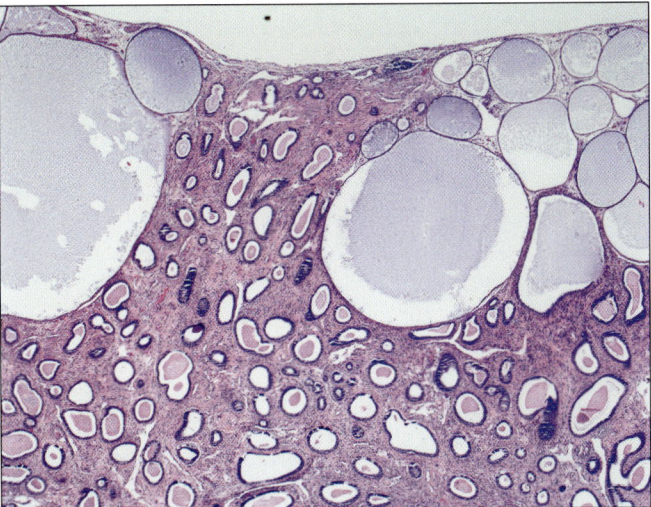

Fig. 15.27 Collections of bland endometrial cysts may be seen in atrophic endometria or senile polyps, and these will have a very low stromal density and lining epithelium with a more attenuated cytology than uninvolved areas.

variable cytology makes them prone to misdiagnosis as EIN. EIN lesions may be one component of an otherwise benign endometrial polyp, as discussed below. Polyps usually exhibit altered stroma, thick vessels, and random irregular glands (Figure 15.26). EIN lesions within polyps usually stand out as a discrete focus in comparison to the remaining polyp.

Benign endometrial hyperplasia should not be confused with EIN, although EIN lesions often arise in that background. Benign hyperplasia changes involve the entire endometrial compartment, and have an irregular random pattern of architectural and cytologic alterations unlike the localizing and expansile features of EIN.

Collections of bland endometrial cysts may be seen in atrophic endometria or senile polyps, and these will have a very low stromal density and lining epithelium with a more attenu-

ated cytology than uninvolved areas (Figure 15.27). They have a sufficiently distinctive appearance unlikely to be confused with EIN, but which may otherwise meet the formal architectural and size criteria for EIN.

5. Exclusion of carcinoma

Distinction between EIN and adenocarcinoma is of clinical importance. Not uncommonly, foci of adenocarcinoma will appear to have developed from the EIN, in which case both entities should be included in the final diagnosis. Also, coexistence of adenocarcinoma with EIN occurs frequently, as shown by the high percentage of patients with EIN diagnosed with carcinoma within the first year if hysterectomy is performed.[3]

EIN lesions are composed of clusters of individually recognizable glands with a simple lining epithelium, whereas adenocarcinomas may have one or more specific patterns not seen in EIN, such as solid, cribriform, or complex interlacing maze-like growth (Figure 15.28). These architectural changes of endometrial cancer reflect loss of basement membrane contact dependence of epithelial cells (loss of contact dependent growth) or promiscuous growth as folded sheets rather than tubular glands. These features specifically apply to EIN lesions which maintain endometrioid differentiation. EIN lesions with non-endometrioid differentiation, especially those with squamous morular or micropapillary change, may have epithelial stratification in the absence of malignant behavior. Precise criteria for defining the precancer–cancer threshold are thus dependent on differentiation state (see Chapter 14).

EIN lesions with tightly packed glands may be difficult to distinguish from adenocarcinoma (Figure 15.29). Lesions composed of confluent glands separated by thread-like strands of intervening connective tissue, with abutting glands having a polygonal appearance resembling fitted elements of a mosaic, are candidates for a diagnosis of adenocarcinoma. Caution must be exercised, however, to avoid overinterpretation of artifactually compressed or displaced EIN glands as adenocarcinoma.

In those instances where myometrium is included, presence of myoinvasion is diagnostic of carcinoma. The absence of myometrial invasion does not, however, preclude a diagnosis of carcinoma as up to 30% of carcinomas may be confined to the endometrium, and myoinvasion usually is not represented in a superficial biopsy. EIN may occasionally affect endometrial glandular elements in foci of adenomyosis within the myometrium, so that abnormal, non-malignant glands are present deep in the myometrium (Figure 15.30). Stromal response to invasion, desmoplasia, is a useful diagnostic feature, if present, in cases of myoinvasion (Figure 15.31), but of no benefit in distinction between EIN and carcinoma within the endometrial compartment itself. Commonly, even extensive myoinvasion shows no desmoplastic reaction.

COMMON EIN DIAGNOSTIC PROBLEMS

Some specimens defy diagnosis. The condition of the specimen may be suboptimal, confounding factors present, or the specimen may have an unusual presentation new to the diagnostician. Most important in these cases is to clearly convey to the clinician the non-diagnostic nature of the case, while specifically identifying the particular problem. Strategies for dealing with specific diagnostic difficulties are presented below.

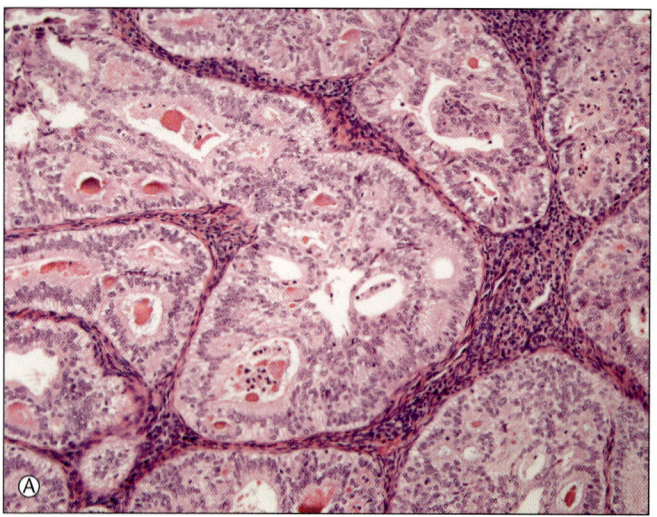

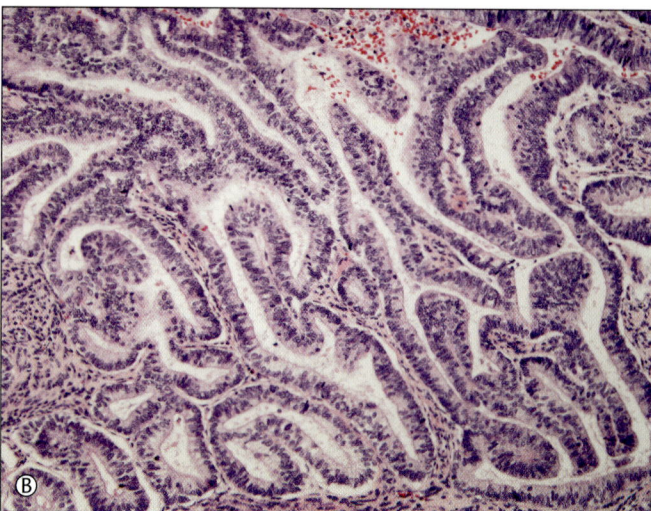

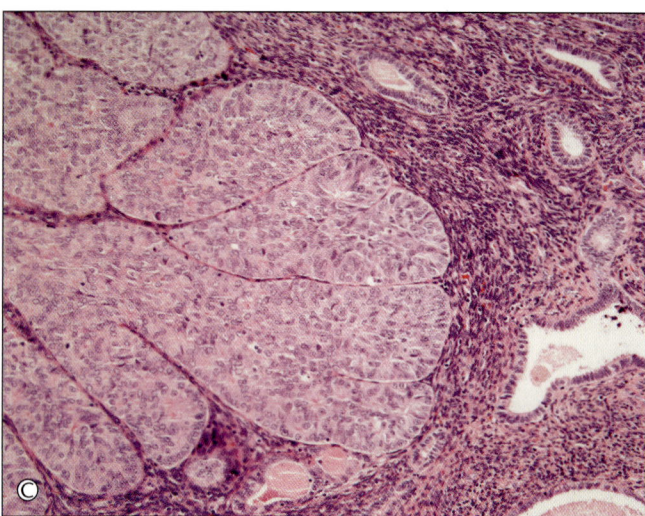

Fig. 15.28 Well-differentiated adenocarcinoma should be diagnosed whenever a cribriform **(A)**, complex maze-like **(B)**, or solid **(C)** pattern of epithelial growth is present.

Non-localizing (widespread) EIN

One-fifth of EIN lesions are diffuse and non-localizing by the time of initial presentation. This is not an indication of malignancy, as even when widespread, EIN may remain confined to the endometrial compartment for prolonged periods or even undergo complete involution in response to progestin therapy. Complicating the diagnosis is that these fragments lack clear interfaces of lesion and background for interpreting the cytologic change. It is usually possible to recognize the EIN either by: (1) reference to interspersed 'overrun' normal glands suitable for confirmation of cytologic change between EIN and background glands (Figure 15.32b); or (2) an obviously complicated architecture and greatly abnormal cytology that easily excludes a benign process, but rather focuses attention upon distinction between EIN and well-differentiated adenocarcinoma.

EIN within an endometrial polyp

For the third of EIN cases that occur within an endometrial polyp, the usual diagnostic criteria apply. The reference point for recognition of cytologic change must be the uninvolved areas of polyp, rather than comparison to non-polypoid endometrial surface. Almost all EIN lesions within polyps are recognized under low magnification as a defined focus (Figure 15.33). A dense, fibrous stroma within the polyp may influence the pattern by which the neoplastic glands grow outward. EIN foci within polyps are usually sharply delimited from the fibrous background. Sometimes, however, EIN glands channeled by the grain of dense collagen into a loose spray may be difficult to distinguish from invasive carcinoma. The presence of cribriform or maze-like lumens favors a diagnosis of adenocarcinoma.

Localizing lesions subdiagnostic for EIN

Occasionally, large fragments of endometrial tissue contain discrete dense clusters of cytologically altered endometrial glands that are subdiagnostic of EIN either because of a focus size less than 1 mm or a density of glands that is less than required (Figure 15.34). Some represent an early phase of EIN development in which the disease burden has not yet achieved a sufficient level to appear in fully diagnostic form. Others are tangentially sectioned regions of peripheral aspects of a lesion.

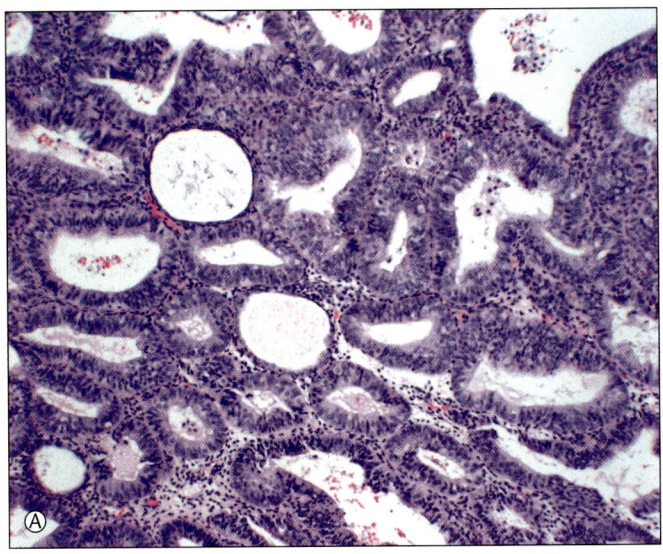

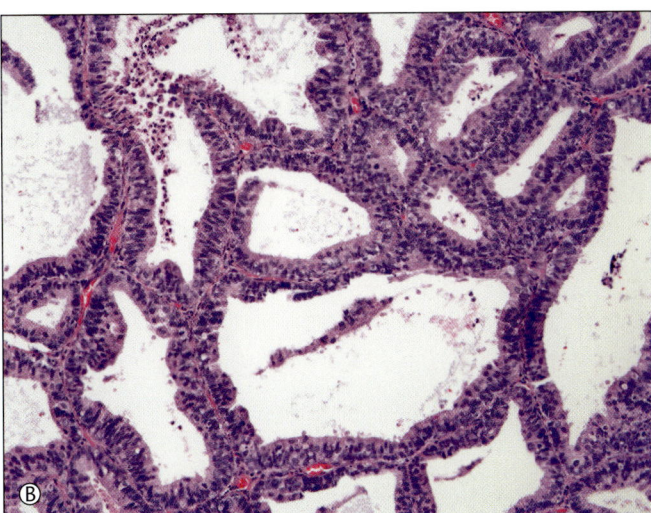

Fig. 15.29 Compact growth of individual glands in EIN **(A)** can be difficult to distinguish from the confluent glands of well-differentiated adenocarcinoma **(B)**. EIN lesions are composed of clusters of individually recognizable glands with a simple lining epithelium, which even when closely packed maintain their integrity as individual elements with some interposed stroma. Disappearance of intervening stroma, except for a threadlike vascular core, with a polygonal or 'mosaic' architecture is more characteristic of adenocarcinoma.

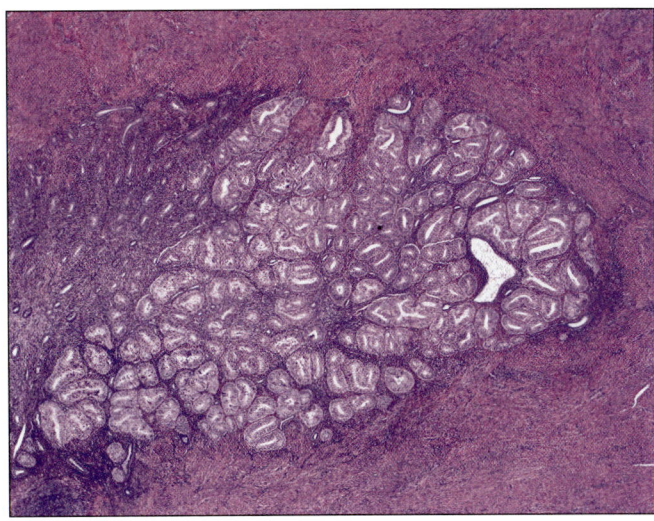

Fig. 15.30 EIN extending into an area of adenomyosis. Within the myometrium, the area is surrounded by endometrial stroma and normal glands remain.

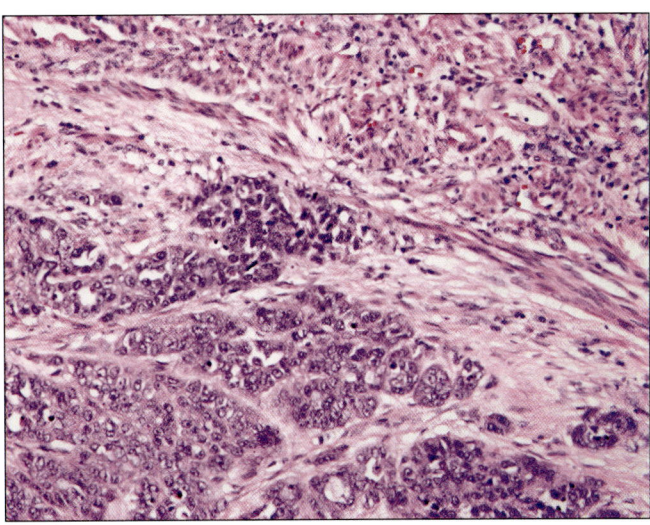

Fig. 15.31 Endometrial adenocarcinoma, desmoplastic myometrial reaction. Connective tissue adjacent to the invasive epithelial nests has a loose appearance with an increased collagen content and spindly reactive cells.

Deeper sections (levels) of the tissue block infrequently resolve these possibilities. A descriptive diagnosis of 'microscopic focus of crowded, cytologically altered endometrial glands suspicious for EIN' is appropriate. Lesions suspicious for EIN occur at about one-sixth the frequency of readily diagnosable EINs. Until more studies become available, careful clinical correlation and follow-up biopsies are recommended.

Excessively fragmented tissue

Definitive diagnosis of highly fragmented tissue is always difficult. The problem is greatest when multiple small tissue fragments contain neoplastic glands from edge to edge. In some cases the aggregate tissue is sufficiently abundant so as not to be confused with a benign process, but insufficient to discriminate between EIN and well-differentiated adenocarcinoma.

The latter may be suspected if very high grade nuclei, or cribriform or solid neoplastic epithelium are present.

Non-endometrioid EIN

Not all EIN lesions maintain endometrioid differentiation, with some displaying complete, or more often partial, mucinous, squamous morular, tubal, eosinophilic, or micropapillary differentiation (Figure 15.35). A rule of thumb is that the usual EIN diagnostic criteria apply, and that the altered differentiation state is only one of the many ways in which lesion cytology can be offset from the background. The change in cytology may involve the cytoplasm primarily, with a variable degree of nuclear change. To some extent, the specific type of altered differentiation dictates additional elements that must be incorporated into the diagnosis. For example, the morular

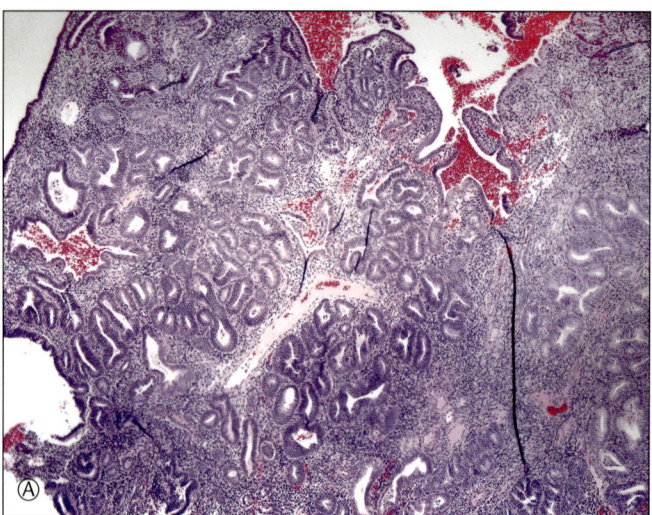
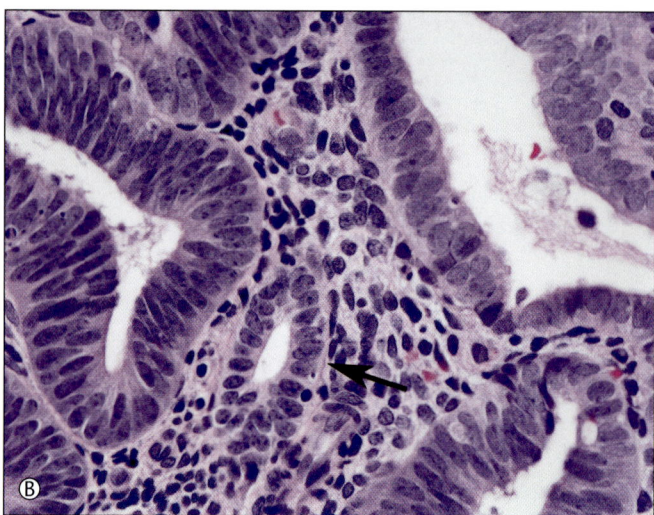

Fig. 15.32 (A, B) EIN lesion occupying the entire endometrial compartment which is difficult to diagnose because it lacks boundaries with areas of normal endometrium. It can be recognized as an EIN by the high gland density and evidence of cytologic change when compared to interspersed 'overrun' normal glands (arrowhead). This 47-year-old patient was diagnosed at hysterectomy 8 months later with well-differentiated adenocarcinoma.

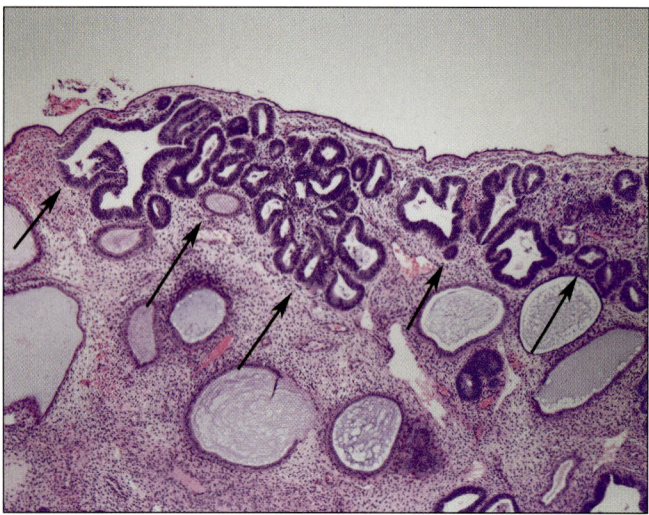
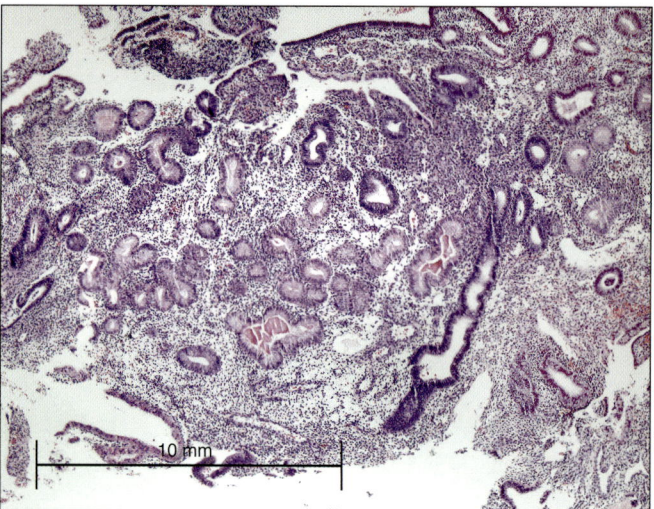

Fig. 15.33 EIN lesion within an endometrial polyp. There is a tight cluster of cytologically altered glands (arrowheads) when compared to those elsewhere in the polyp.

Fig. 15.34 Small, non-compact cluster of cytologically altered glands subdiagnostic of EIN. This should not be diagnosed as EIN because the affected glands in center field are too loosely arranged, and fail to meet the criterion of gland area exceeding stromal area. These can be diagnosed descriptively.

component of EIN with squamous morules should be ignored in calculating the ratio of glands to stroma. Morules are functionally inert, and it is the abundance of glandular elements relative to stroma that determines cancer risk. Morules surrounded by glands present a cribriform-like appearance that should not be confused with adenocarcinoma. Guidelines for separation of EIN from carcinoma may be modified in non-endometrioid lesions. These are discussed and illustrated in detail, for each differentiation state, in Chapter 14.

Hormonally treated EIN

There are no accepted criteria for assessing premalignant endometrial lesions while under the influence of progestins. Administration of high dose progestins such as Megace is an increasingly common clinical intervention that greatly alters the appearance of the EIN itself, often making it non-diagnostic. The extent of stromal pseudodecidual change is often the only clue to the presence of this confounding factor. Glands are pushed apart by stromal pseudodecidualization, and nuclei become smaller and less mitotically active (Figure 15.36). Combined, these changes dramatically alter the appearance of a post-therapy EIN lesion compared to its pre-therapy appearance. 'Improvement' in cytology or lessening of gland crowding cannot be viewed as evidence of clearance of an EIN lesion when the follow-up biopsy is taken in the presence of active progestational agent. Furthermore, rebiopsy of a hormonally treated EIN while still on progestins may be a premature endpoint to assess lesion involution, as the patient has not yet had the benefit of withdrawal shedding, a significant component of the ablative process.

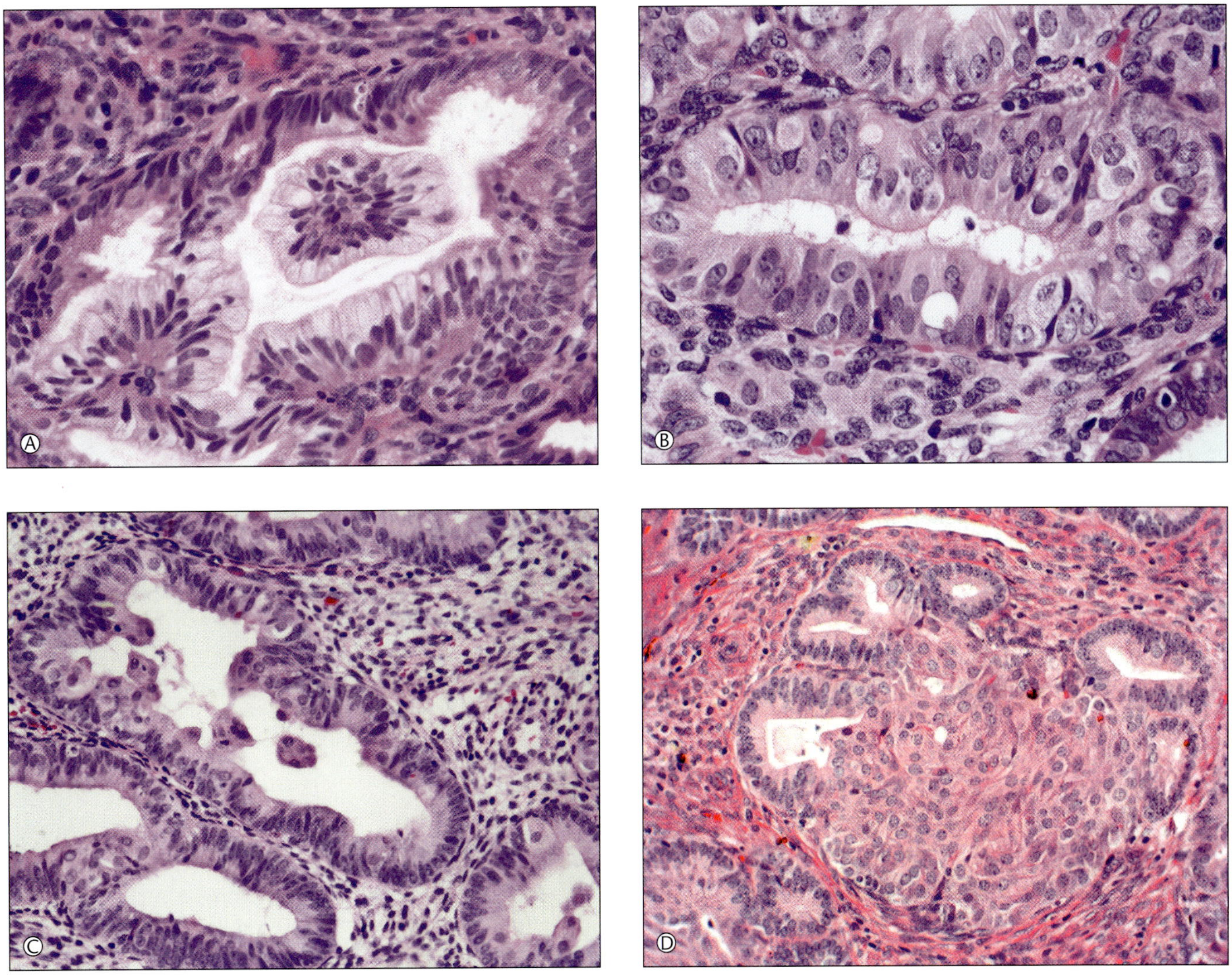

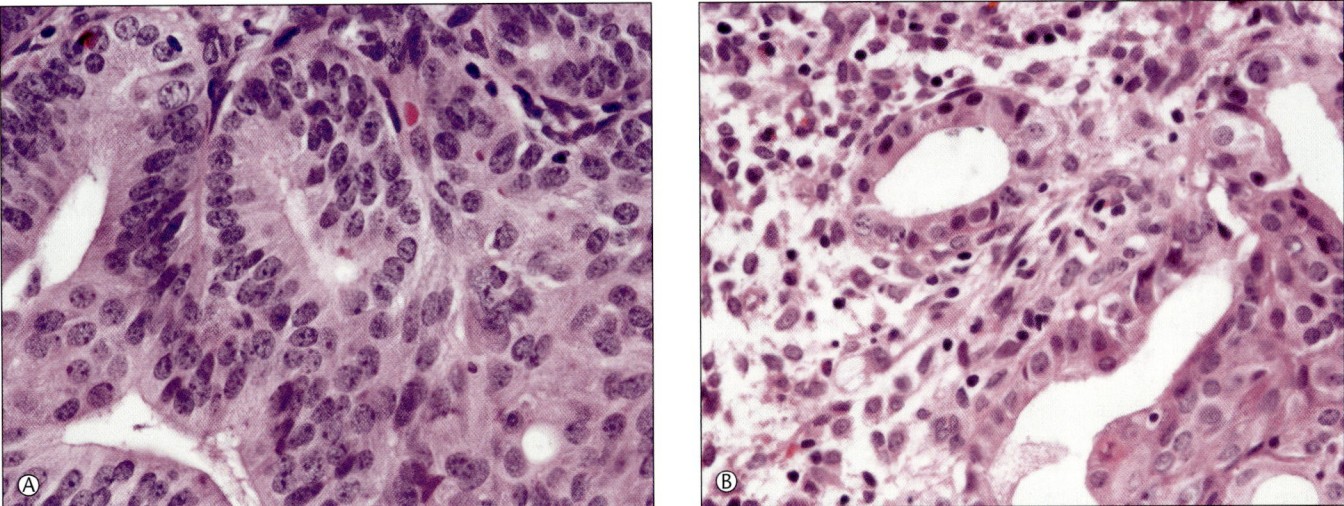

Fig. 15.35 Cytology of non-endometrioid EIN lesions may include complete, or more often partial, mucinous **(A)**, tubal **(B)**, micropapillary **(C)**, or squamous morular **(D)** differentiation. Altered differentiation, primarily a cytoplasmic feature, is the nature of the cytologic change that characterizes these EIN lesions. Non-endometrioid lesions present specific interpretive difficulties. Squamous morules surrounded by glands have a cribriform-like appearance that should not be confused with adenocarcinoma.

Fig. 15.36 EIN cytology altered by 3 months of high dose progestin (Megace) therapy. Pre-therapy glands **(A)** have plump nuclei and a moderately thick epithelium. After therapy **(B)**, persistent EIN glands are pushed apart by stromal pseudodecidualization, and nuclei become smaller and less mitotically active.

The confounding effects of ongoing progestin therapy create a problem for the clinician who wants to know if the patient has been adequately treated as of the time of the biopsy. There are a few useful strategies compatible with appropriate management of the patient:

1. If either adenocarcinoma or (criteria-meeting) EIN is present, it should be diagnosed with a mention of the noted progestational effects.
2. If there are any architecturally localizing, cytologically distinctive glandular lesions, they should be described and a comment made that although subdiagnostic, EIN cannot be excluded while the patient is under active progestin therapy.
3. If the entire endometrium is decidualized with a very low density of secretorily exhausted, uniformly appearing glands, a diagnosis of 'endometrium with stromal and glandular changes of progestin therapy' can be made.

The best way to resolve any diagnostic uncertainty introduced by hormonal therapy is to rebiopsy 2–4 weeks following a withdrawal bleed. The hormonal effects will no longer be present, thereby permitting accurate assessment of the presence or absence of residual EIN. The clinical context and the intent of the managing physician must be understood before invoking this option. Withdrawal may not be feasible in women with subcutaneous or intrauterine devices impregnated with hormone. Often treatment plans do not have lesion ablation as a primary objective, but rather lesion stabilization by indefinite and continuous progestin therapy.

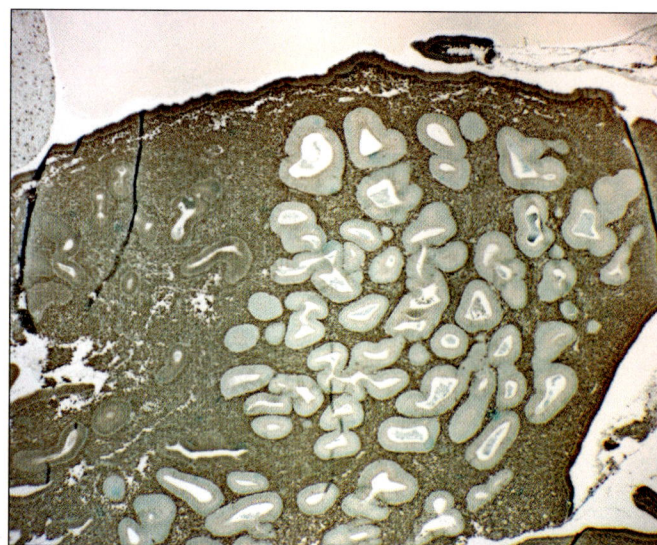

Fig. 15.37 Localized EIN lesion highlighted by *PTEN* immunohistochemistry showing loss of signal within the lesion, in contrast to background proliferative glands and stroma. Sixty-three per cent of EIN lesions lack PTEN tumor suppressor protein in a monoclonal distribution, usually through a combination of genomic deletion and mutation.

BIOMARKERS

Specialized biomarkers have played a crucial role in defining the entity of EIN, and provide valuable tools for training and prospective diagnostic standardization. DNA-based assays of clonality or genetic mutations are expensive, generally unavailable, and unnecessary for diagnostic purposes. There are no serum biomarkers of EIN that have value as an early detection system, and cytology-based approaches lack sensitivity. Most importantly, for a biomarker to be of practical benefit it must offer information which complements or exceeds at reasonable cost that already available by routine microscopy. This last standard is met in limited fashion by two different marker systems.

PTEN IMMUNOHISTOCHEMISTRY

PTEN tumor suppressor inactivation permits visual delineation of affected EIN lesions by routine immunohistochemistry. Two-thirds of EIN lesions are null for this protein, (Figure 15.37). One-third of EIN lesions express normal levels of the PTEN protein, making it relatively insensitive to render decisions regarding individual patients. Of equal concern, frequent inactivation of this marker at a preclinical stage means that demonstration of isolated *PTEN*-null glands in the absence of otherwise diagnostic EIN cannot be considered a high cancer risk state.[35] It may, however, have some value when localizing lesions are found to be *PTEN* null, and thus likely EIN, in otherwise difficult or equivocal diagnostic situations such as within endometrial polyps[19] or secretory endometrium. Lesions that express the PTEN protein, the normal state for endome-

trial tissues, are non-informative. It is a somewhat difficult assay to perform, requiring use of reagents that have been validated in paraffin sections against mutational data (antibody 6h2.1), applied to freshly cut sections following antigen retrieval.[35]

QUANTITATIVE HISTOMORPHOMETRY

The D-Score as measured by an interactive computerized morphometric workstation from H&E-stained slides has provided a discovery platform to define EIN diagnostic criteria, and a stable reference tool for objective EIN diagnosis. Variables of volume percentage stroma, gland outer surface density, and standard deviation of shortest nuclear axis are algorithmically combined to generate the D-Score,[2] a threshold function diagnostic of EIN at a value of less than 1. Workstations are composed of an autofocusing microscope with automated stage and videocamera attached to a computer. Morphometry is only performed on a selected area, usually within a single fragment, chosen by a pathologist. Field selection remains a subjective component of morphometry, as does recognition of those confounding conditions likely to give erroneous results (normal secretory endometrium, endometrial polyps). The high clinical outcome predictive value (Figure 15.14), reproducibility (>95% between laboratories), and commercial availability of analytical systems (QProdit system, Leica, Cambridge, UK) have enabled its clinical use in locations (primarily Europe) where centralized triaging to high volume specialized laboratories is common. Sets of morphometry-annotated histologic sections offer standardized materials for pathologists to train against or perform quality control checks of subjective diagnoses.[29]

TREATMENT

The negative cancer predictive value of a representative endometrial biopsy which lacks EIN is very high, at 99%.[3] If the clinician is confident of sampling adequacy, and the pathologist has not indicated some particular problem in interpretation of the specimen, observational follow-up with symptom management can be justified. Not all cases are so straightforward, however, as there will be individual cases where there is lingering concern of sampling adequacy, discordance between the clinical presentation and pathologic diagnosis rendered, or interpretive uncertainty by the pathologist. In these instances the diagnostic process may be considered incomplete, and repeat sampling indicated.

EXCLUSION OF COEXISTING ADENOCARCINOMA

Thirty-nine per cent of EIN lesions coexist with well-differentiated adenocarcinoma that may not be evident on the initial biopsy.[3] Tissue sampling devices that access the endometrium via the uterine lumen cannot obtain access to blind luminal pockets, and have a tendency to underrepresent tissues deep to the surface lining. Myoinvasive cancers are easily missed if the bulk of tumor is below the endometrial–myometrial interface. Women with abnormally configured luminal cavities or extensive intrauterine adhesions can be difficult to sample adequately.

HYSTERECTOMY

Management of women with a diagnosis of EIN centers on two objectives: (1) exclusion of a coexisting carcinoma, management of which would supersede that of the EIN itself; and (2) ablation of EIN as a cancer preventative strategy. Hysterectomy fulfills both goals by simultaneously removing the EIN lesion itself while providing a definitive pathology specimen for exclusion of adenocarcinoma. Although hysterectomy is the most common therapy for EIN, not all patients are good surgical risks, and young women with isolated EIN may desire uterus-sparing therapy to maintain reproductive potential. Topical endometrial ablation by thermal or cautery-mediated devices applied directly to the endometrial lining are not recommended as a treatment option because they may leave residual islands of lesional tissue behind, and create intrauterine adhesions which hinder post-treatment surveillance by rebiopsy.

HORMONAL THERAPY OF EIN TO REDUCE ENDOMETRIAL CANCER RISK

Although current practice favors hysterectomy for EIN in women past childbearing age, there is an active interest in developing uterus-sparing alternatives for younger women and those who present unfavorable surgical risks. Progestin-based hormonal therapies capable of ablating EIN lesions offer the best alternative to surgery, but the optimal regimens, expected clinical response, and attendant risks remain to be defined. Essentially, all EIN lesions are hormonally competent, with detectable progesterone receptors.[35] Endometrial gland apoptosis can be initiated by progestins,[9,26] and those that bear abnormalities of the *PTEN* gene are particularly susceptible to involution following progestin therapy.[60]

There are two schools of thought regarding the therapeutic intent of progestin therapy for premalignant endometrial disease. For both, close follow-up is mandatory and repeated sampling strongly recommended.

The first concept is that circulating progestins can stabilize a premalignant lesion, preventing its progression to adenocarcinoma as long as the hormonal exposure is maintained. In this model, continuous uninterrupted high dose delivery to the endometrium for an indefinite period is desired. Side effects of long-term systemic progestin therapy make this impractical for most women. Progestin-impregnated intrauterine devices capable of locally delivering supraphysiologic quantities of hormone at low systemic levels effectively control over half of well-differentiated endometrial cancers,[28] and by extrapolation are likely to have a similar effect on EIN. More studies are needed to define long-term outcomes.

A different therapeutic objective is permanent ablation of premalignant lesions following progestin therapy during a time-delimited therapeutic window. As previously shown for atypical endometrial hyperplasia,[15,21] EIN lesions may regress completely under the influence of high dose progestins, although it is not possible to predict individual case response in advance. *In vitro* data, which shows that progestins induce apoptotic cell death of neoplastic endometrial cells, support this objective.[1] Continuously administered progestins are followed in a few days by a gradual decline in the apoptotic rate as the effect extinguishes, but withdrawal after a period of high dose exposure dramatically increases the apoptotic rate 10-fold.[53] This provides one rationale for interrupted, rather than continuous, progestin therapy for ablation. In this scenario, the maximal therapeutic effect of apoptosis, and synchronized shedding of lesion-bearing endometrial tissues occurs through repeated cyclic withdrawal of hormone following a priming interval. The Gynecologic Oncology Group is just now launching a clinical trial of interrupted vs continuous progesterone therapy for women with EIN.

PRIOR CLASSIFICATION

The hyperplasia nomenclature for endometrial cancer precursors has been confusing, reflecting repeated reclassification into varying numbers of component entities using overlapping terminology and inconsistent criteria. Some of the more common terms and systems used over the past three decades included: simple vs complex hyperplasia; atypical vs non-atypical hyperplasia; cystic atrophy vs hyperplasia; disordered proliferative vs simple hyperplasia; mild, moderate, and marked hyperplasia with/without atypia; adenomatous hyperplasia, anaplasia and carcinoma *in situ*. Typically the range of entities was determined by the number of possible permuted combinations of particular morphologic features rather than insight into the nature of underlying biologic groups, or even range of available clinical management options.

The most widely used classification of the past decade, adopted by the World Health Organization (WHO) in 1994[43] divides endometrial hyperplasia into four groups according to atypical or non-atypical cytology and simple or complex architecture. The presence of cytologic atypia, recognized as nuclear enlargement, the presence of nucleoli, or a change from an elongated to more ovoid or round nucleus, has been viewed as the predominant feature which increases risk for adenocarcinoma, observed to be of the order of a 14-fold elevation.[24] The definitions of architectural complexity and nuclear atypia that are used in this classification rest on a multitude of features that are inconsistently present across all instances of a single diagnostic category.[23] Concern about the reliability of pathologists to apply multiple criteria to distinguish among these forms of hyperplasia led to several reproducibility studies, disclosing only moderate to poor interobserver reproducibility.[5,23,47]

The Gynecologic Oncology Group (GOG) recently completed a study of the reproducibility of the community-based diagnosis of atypical hyperplasia in about 300 women.[58] The panel agreed with the diagnosis of atypical hyperplasia in only 39% of cases, interpreting about one-fourth of cases as a less significant process and about one-fourth of cases as adenocarcinoma. Even the GOG expert pathologists had a very low order of agreement among themselves. Interobserver reproducibility was lowest for the diagnosis of atypical hyperplasia, with interobserver overall kappas of 0.29, compared with 0.54–0.62 for EIN.[17] Hysterectomy subsequently performed within 12 weeks of initial diagnosis revealed the presence of coexisting adenocarcinoma in the uterus in 43% of cases. These disturbing results raised serious questions about the ability of pathologists to use the WHO hyperplasia system to recognize and distinguish endometrial precancers from otherwise benign, and malignant, endometrial conditions.

WHERE HAVE ALL THE HYPERPLASIAS GONE?

All lesions need to be individually reassigned using criteria described in this chapter. New diagnostic criteria such as lesion size and manner of cytology interpretation cut across previous hyperplasia categories (complex/non-complex, atypical/non-atypical). As a result, there is no direct or absolute concordance between WHO hyperplasia and EIN schema diagnosis (Figure 15.38). Seventy-nine per cent of atypical hyperplasia, 44% of complex non-atypical hyperplasias, and 5% of simple non-

atypical hyperplasias are classifiable as premalignant EIN lesions. After removing EIN lesions, remaining lesions are reassigned largely into specific categories such as endometrial polyp, disordered proliferative endometrium, benign endometrial hyperplasia, and a variety of normal structures such as endometrial basalis and lower uterine segment. Of import, in long-term follow-up studies only about 0.6% of these women will subsequently develop carcinoma over the next decade.

REFERENCES

1. Amezcua CA, Lu JJ, Felix JC, Stanczyk FZ, Zheng W. Apoptosis may be an early event of progestin therapy for endometrial hyperplasia. Gynecol Oncol 2000;79:169–76.
2. Baak JP, Mutter GL. EIN and WHO94. J Clin Pathol 2005;58:1–6.
3. Baak JP, Mutter GL, Robboy S, et al. The molecular genetics and morphometry-based endometrial intraepithelial neoplasia classification system predicts disease progression in endometrial hyperplasia more accurately than the 1994 World Health Organization classification system. Cancer 2005;103:2304–12.
4. Basil JB, Goodfellow PJ, Rader JS, Mutch DG, Herzog TJ. Clinical significance of microsatellite instability in endometrial carcinoma. Cancer 2000;89:1758–64.
5. Bergeron C, Nogales F, Masseroli M, et al. A multicentric European study testing the reproducibility of the WHO classification of endometrial hyperplasia with a proposal of a simplified working classification for biopsy and curettage specimens. Am J Surg Pathol 1999;23:1102–8.
6. Berman JJ, Bores-Saavedra J, Bostwick D, et al. Precancer: a conceptual working definition. Results of a Consensus Conference. Cancer Detect Prev 2006;30:387–94.
7. Boerrigter PJ, van de Weijer PH, Baak JP, Fox H, Haspels AA, Kenemans P. Endometrial response in estrogen replacement therapy quarterly combined with a progestogen. Maturitas 1996;24:63–71.
8. Califano J, Van der Riet P, Westra W, et al. Genetic progression model for head and neck cancer: implications for field cancerization. Cancer Res 1996;56:2488–92.
9. Dahmoun M, Boman K, Cajander S, Westin P, Backstrom T. Apoptosis, proliferation, and sex hormone receptors in superficial parts of human endometrium at the end of the secretory phase. J Clin Endocrinol Metab 1999;84:1737–43.
10. Duggan BD, Felix JC, Muderspach LI, Tsao J-L, Shibata DK. Early mutational activation of the c-Ki-ras oncogene in endometrial carcinoma. Cancer Res 1994;54:1604–7.
11. Enomoto T, Haba T, Fujita M, et al. Clonal analysis of high-grade squamous intra-epithelial lesions of the uterine cervix. Int J Cancer 1997;73:339–44.
12. Enomoto T, Inoue M, Perantoni A, et al. K-ras activation in premalignant and malignant epithelial lesions of the human uterus. Cancer Res 1991;51:5304–14.
13. Esteller M, Catasus L, Matias-Guiu X, et al. hMLH1 promoter hypermethylation is an early event in human endometrial tumorigenesis. Am J Pathol 1999;155:1767–72.
14. Ferenczy A. Pathophysiology of endometrial bleeding. Maturitas 2003;45: 1–14.
15. Ferenczy A, Gelfand M. The biologic significance of cytologic atypia in progestogen-treated endometrial hyperplasia. Am J Obstet Gynecol 1989;160:126–31.
16. Goodfellow PJ, Buttin BM, Herzog TJ, et al. Prevalence of defective DNA mismatch repair and MSH6 mutation in an unselected series of endometrial cancers. Proc Natl Acad Sci U S A 2003;100:5908–13.
17. Hecht JL, Ince TA, Baak JP, Baker HE, Ogden MW, Mutter GL. Prediction of endometrial carcinoma by subjective endometrial intraepithelial neoplasia diagnosis. Mod Pathol 2005;18:324–30.
18. Hecht JL, Ince TA, Baker HE, Mutter GL. Concordance of WHO hyperplasia and EIN classification of endometrial precancers. Lab Invest 2003;83:191A.
19. Hecht JL, Pinkus JL, Pinkus GS. Enhanced detection of atypical hyperplasia in endometrial polyps by PTEN expression. Appl Immunohistochem Mol Morphol 2004;12:36–9.
20. Hopfer H, Rinehart CA, Jr, Vollmer G, Kaufman DG. In vitro interactions of endometrial stromal and epithelial cells in Matrigel: reorganization of the extracellular matrix. Pathobiology 1994;62:104–8.
21. Horn LC, Schnurrbusch U, Bilek K, Einenkel J. Endometrial hyperplasia: the risk of progression to carcinoma in a series of 538 cases. Geburtshilfe Frauenheilkd 2001;61:501–6.
22. Jovanovic AS, Boynton KA, Mutter GL. Uteri of women with endometrial carcinoma contain a histopathologic spectrum of monoclonal putative precancers, some with microsatellite instability. Cancer Res 1996;56:1917–21.
23. Kendall BS, Ronnett BM, Isacson C, et al. Reproducibility of the diagnosis of endometrial hyperplasia, atypical hyperplasia, and well-differentiated carcinoma. Am J Surg Pathol 1998;22:1012–19.

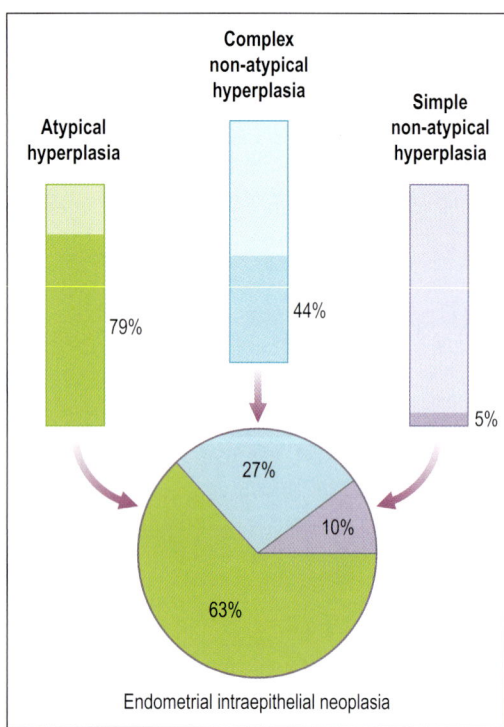

Fig. 15.38 Percentage of WHO hyperplasias rediagnosed as EIN (bars), and proportional sources of all EINs (pie).

24. Kurman R, Kaminski P, Norris H. The behavior of endometrial hyperplasia: a long term study of 'untreated' hyperplasia in 170 patients. Cancer 1985;56:403–12.
25. Matias-Guiu X, Catasus L, Bussaglia E, et al. Molecular pathology of endometrial hyperplasia and carcinoma. Hum Pathol 2001;32:569–77.
26. Mertens HJ, Heineman MJ, Evers JL. The expression of apoptosis-related proteins Bcl-2 and Ki67 in endometrium of ovulatory menstrual cycles. Gynecol Obstet Invest 2002;53:224–30.
27. Millar AL, Pal T, Madlensky L, et al. Mismatch repair gene defects contribute to the genetic basis of double primary cancers of the colorectum and endometrium. Hum Mol Genet 1999;8:823–9.
28. Montz FJ, Bristow RE, Bovicelli A, Tomacruz R, Kurman RJ. Intrauterine progesterone treatment of early endometrial cancer. Am J Obstet Gynecol 2002;186:651–1.
29. Mutter GL. Endometrial precancer type collection. Online. Available: http://www.endometrium.org
30. Mutter GL. PTEN, a protean tumor suppressor. Am J Pathol 2001;158:1895–8.
31. Mutter GL. Diagnosis of premalignant endometrial disease. J Clin Pathol 2002;55:326–31.
32. Mutter GL, Baak JPA, Crum CP, Richart RM, Ferenczy A, Faquin WC. Endometrial precancer diagnosis by histopathology, clonal analysis, and computerized morphometry. J Pathol 2000;190:462–9.
33. Mutter GL, Boynton KA, Faquin WC, Ruiz RE, Jovanovic AS. Allelotype mapping of unstable microsatellites establishes direct lineage continuity between endometrial precancers and cancer. Cancer Res 1996;56:4483–6.
34. Mutter GL, Chaponot M, Fletcher J. A PCR assay for non-random X chromosome inactivation identifies monoclonal endometrial cancers and precancers. Am J Pathol 1995;146:501–8.
35. Mutter GL, Ince TA, Baak JPA, Kust G, Zhou X, Eng C. Molecular identification of latent precancers in histologically normal endometrium. Cancer Res 2001;61:4311–14.
36. Mutter GL, Lin MC, Fitzgerald JT, et al. Altered PTEN expression as a diagnostic marker for the earliest endometrial precancers. J Natl Cancer Inst 2000;92:924–30.
37. Mutter GL, Lin MC, Fitzgerald JT, Kum JB, Ziebold U, Eng C. Changes in endometrial PTEN expression throughout the human menstrual cycle. J Clin Endocrinol Metab 2000;85:2334–8.
38. Mutter GL, Wada H, Faquin W, Enomoto T. K-ras mutations appear in the premalignant phase of both microsatellite stable and unstable endometrial carcinogenesis. Mol Pathol 1999;52:257–62.
39. Osteen KG, Rodgers WH, Gaire M, Hargrove JT, Gorstein F, Matrisian LM. Stromal-epithelial interaction mediates steroidal regulation of metalloproteinase expression in human endometrium. Proc Natl Acad Sci U S A 1994;91:10129–33.
40. Parazzini F, La Vecchia C, Bocciolone L, Franceschi S. The epidemiology of endometrial cancer. Gynecol Oncol 1991;41:1–16.
41. Parsons R, Li G, Longley M, et al. Hypermutability and mismatch repair deficiency in RER+ tumor cells. Cell 1993;75:1227–36.
42. Ries LAG, Eisner MP, Kosary CL, et al. SEER cancer statistics review, 1975–2002. Bethesda, MD: National Cancer Institute. Online. Available: http://seer.cancer.gov/csr/1975_2002.
43. Scully RE, Bonfiglio TA, Kurman RJ, Silverberg SG, Wilkinson EJ. Uterine Corpus. Histological Typing of Female Genital Tract Tumors. New York: Springer-Verlag; 1994:13–31.
44. Shapiro S, Kelly JP, Rosenberg L, et al. Risk of localized and widespread endometrial cancer in relation to recent and discontinued use of conjugated estrogens. N Engl J Med 1985;313:969–72.
45. Shipley CF, III, Simmons CL, Nelson GH. Comparison of transvaginal sonography with endometrial biopsy in asymptomatic postmenopausal women. J Ultrasound Med 1994;13:99–104.
46. Silverberg SG, Mutter GL, Kurman RJ, Kubik-Huch RA, Nogales F, Tavassoli FA. Tumors of the uterine corpus: epithelial tumors and related lesions. In: Tavassoli FA, Stratton MR, eds. WHO Classification of Tumours: Pathology and Genetics of Tumours of the Breast and Female Genital Organs. Lyon: IARC Press; 2003:221–32.
47. Skov BG, Broholm H, Engel U, et al. Comparison of the reproducibility of the WHO classifications of 1975 and 1994 of endometrial hyperplasia. Int J Gynecol Pathol 1997;16:33–7.
48. Song J, Rutherford T, Naftolin F, Brown S, Mori G. Hormonal regulation of apoptosis and the Fas and Fas ligand system in human endometrial cells. Mol Hum Reprod 2002;8:447–55.
49. Stambolic V, Tsao MS, Macpherson D, Suzuki A, Chapman WB, Mak TW. High incidence of breast and endometrial neoplasia resembling human Cowden syndrome in pten+/– mice. Cancer Res 2000;60:3605–11.
50. Stanford JL, Brinton LA, Berman ML, et al. Oral contraceptives and endometrial cancer: do other risk factors modify the association? Int J Cancer 1993;54:243–8.
51. Sutter C, Lenbach-Hellweg G, Schmidt D, et al. Molecular analysis of endometrial hyperplasia in HNPCC-suspicious patients may predict progression to endometrial carcinoma. Int J Gynecol Pathol 2004;23:18–25.
52. Tate JE, Mutter GL, Boynton KA, Crum CP. Monoclonal origin of vulvar intraepithelial neoplasia and some vulvar hyperplasias. Am J Pathol 1997;150:315–22.
53. Wang S, Pudney J, Song J, Schwartz PE, Zheng W. Mechanisms involved in the evolution of progestin resistance in human endometrial hyperplasia – precursor of endometrial cancer. Gynecol Oncol 2003;88:108–17.
54. Weiderpass E, Adami HO, Baron JA, Magnusson C, Lindgren A, Persson I. Use of oral contraceptives and endometrial cancer risk (Sweden). Cancer Causes Control 1999;10:277–84.
55. Woodruff JD, Pickar JH. Incidence of endometrial hyperplasia in postmenopausal women taking conjugated estrogens (Premarin) with medroxyprogesterone acetate or conjugated estrogens alone. Am J Obstet Gynecol 1994;170:1213–23.
56. Writing Group for the PEPI Trial. Effects of hormone replacement therapy on endometrial histology in postmenopausal women. The Postmenopausal Estrogen/Progestin Interventions (PEPI) Trial. JAMA 1996;275:370–5.
57. Zaino RJ. Endometrial hyperplasia: is it time for a quantum leap to a new classification? Int J Gynecol Pathol 2000;19:314–21.
58. Zaino R, Trimble C, Silverberg S, Kauderer J, Curtin J. Reproducibility of the diagnosis of atypical endometrial hyperplasia (AEH): a Gynecologic Oncology Group (GOG) study. Cancer 2006;106:804–11.
59. Zeleniuch-Jacquotte A, Akhmedkhanov A, Kato I, et al. Postmenopausal endogenous oestrogens and risk of endometrial cancer: results of a prospective study. Br J Cancer 2001;84:975–81.
60. Zheng W, Baker HE, Mutter GL. Involution of PTEN-null endometrial glands with progestin therapy. Gynecol Oncol 2004;92:1008–13.
61. Zhuang Z, Vortmeyer AO, Mark EJ, et al. Barrett's esophagus: metaplastic cells with loss of heterozygosity at the APC gene locus are clonal precursors to invasive adenocarcinoma. Cancer Res 1996;56:1961–4.

Endometrial adenocarcinoma

George L. Mutter   Xavier Matias-Guiu   Sigurd F. Lax

INTRODUCTION AND TERMINOLOGY

Carcinoma of the endometrium is increasing in frequency compared with carcinoma of the cervix, although the degree of the change in this relationship varies from country to country. It is now the most common gynecologic cancer in the United States, with a lifetime risk of 2.5%.[144] It is most common in postmenopausal women. The median age at presentation is 63 years. Ninety per cent of cases are found in women past the menopause and only 1% are under age 40 years.[144] However, these figures should not color the pathologist's opinion on curettings from young women for there is a danger that a well-differentiated carcinoma may be incorrectly diagnosed as premalignant (endometrial intraepithelial neoplasia (EIN), Chapter 15) for no reason other than that carcinomas are so rare in those under age 40 years.

MAJOR TYPES OF ENDOMETRIAL ADENOCARCINOMA

Extensive epidemiologic, molecular, and behavioral information suggests that there are two distinct forms of endometrial carcinoma, commonly referred to as type I and type II, which correspond to endometrioid and non-endometrioid histotypes, respectively (Table 16.1).[101] The histologic recognition of the subtypes is an important factor in predicting the outcome and is of help in planning the most appropriate treatment. A histologic classification of endometrial carcinomas is given in Table 16.2.

The two main types of endometrial carcinoma exhibit different molecular alterations, consistent with a dualistic model of endometrial tumorigenesis.[103] According to this model, the estrogen-related type I tumors frequently demonstrate one or more of the following: microsatellite instability, inactivated *PTEN* tumor suppressor gene, *K-ras* mutations, and abnormalities in the β-catenin gene (*CTNNB-1*) associated with β-catenin nuclear accumulation.[114] In contrast, the estrogen-independent type II tumors show loss of heterozygosity at different loci, altered *p53*, and abnormalities in genes regulating mitotic checkpoints.[160] Studies using cDNA microarrays confirm that these two classes of tumor have distinctively different gene expression profiles.[124]

ENDOMETRIAL ADENOCARCINOMA, ENDOMETRIOID TYPE (TYPE I)

Endometrioid tumors account for the majority of sporadic endometrial carcinomas (70–80%). They occur in younger, pre- and perimenopausal women, in association with the estrogen-related risk factors described below. The tumors usually have an indolent course, and frequently are preceded by EIN. In comparison with other tumors, they are better differentiated, more likely to have diploid DNA content, show less myometrial invasion, low potential for lymphatic spread, frequently maintain estrogen and progesterone receptors, and carry a generally favorable prognosis.

ENDOMETRIAL ADENOCARCINOMA, NON-ENDOMETRIOID TYPE (TYPE II)

In contrast, non-endometrioid tumors occur in older, postmenopausal women, and account for 10–20% of endometrial carcinomas. They are not associated with clinical evidence of estrogen stimulation, and typically arise from atrophic endometrium, frequently in the setting of endometrial polyps. The tumors most often have serous or clear cell cytologies, or the very poorly differentiated phenotype of carcinosarcoma or undifferentiated carcinoma. They have rapid courses, a high degree of nuclear pleomorphism, frequent aneuploid DNA content, deeper myometrial invasion, a higher risk of lymphatic spread, low sensitivity to progestin, and a poor prognosis.

UNIQUE AND HYBRID TYPES OF CARCINOMA

Although the dualistic model is applicable to a high proportion of endometrial carcinomas, not all tumors fit in. In fact, a gray zone exists between the two broad types, with a significant number of tumors showing overlapping clinical, morphologic, and molecular features. Moreover, there is an ongoing debate about whether a histologic subset of endometrioid carcinomas (those that are poorly differentiated or have high nuclear grade) should be assigned to the type II group. Furthermore, it is now accepted that a non-endometrioid component may emerge from a pre-existing endometrioid carcinoma. The probable mechanism for this is development of genetic heterogeneity within elements of a type I tumor, and progressive expansion

Table 16.1 Differences between endometrioid and non-endometrioid endometrial adenocarcinomas

	Endometrioid (Type I)	Non-endometrioid (Type II)	References
Histologic patterns	Endometrioid, mucinous, adenosquamous, secretory	Serous, clear cell	165
Grade	1–3	Not applicable	
Behavior	Indolent	Aggressive	
Average age (years)	59	66	50
Risk factors	Endocrine (unopposed estrogen)	Unknown	
Precursor lesion	EIN	?EGD, ?serous EIC	10, 127, 195
p53 mutation	5–10%	80–90%	20, 160
PTEN inactivation	55%	11%	126
K-ras inactivation	13–26%	0–10%	20, 94, 114
β-Catenin mutation	25–38%	Rare	114
MLH1 inactivation	17%	5%	60, 61
Loss of estrogen and progesterone receptors	27–30%	76–81%	94

EGD, endocervical glandular dysplasia; EIC, endometrial intraepithelial carcinoma; EIN, endometrial intraepithelial neoplasia.

Table 16.2 Histopathologic classification of endometrial carcinoma

Endometrioid adenocarcinoma
  Variants
  Endometrioid adenocarcinoma with squamous differentiation
  Villoglandular adenocarcinoma
  Secretory adenocarcinoma
  Ciliated cell adenocarcinoma

Serous adenocarcinoma

Clear cell adenocarcinoma

Mucinous adenocarcinoma

Squamous cell carcinoma

Mixed carcinoma

Undifferentiated carcinoma

of a particularly aggressive tumor subclone with genetic and behavioral features resembling that of type II tumors.[114] Some unique tumor types, such as carcinosarcomas, demonstrate clinical and molecular features that do not fit cleanly into either of the prototype endometrioid and non-endometrioid categories.[165]

HEREDITARY ENDOMETRIAL CARCINOMA

Women with an inherited predisposition for endometrial neoplasia have a distinctive clinical presentation of endometrioid endometrial adenocarcinomas.[18] They tend to develop disease 15 years earlier than sporadic occurrences and the prognosis is favorable. Most have the hereditary non-polyposis colorectal carcinoma syndrome (HNPCC), a rare heritable genetic condition affecting about 1% of the population.[138] In addition to a high incidence of colorectal cancer, the lifetime risk of endometrial adenocarcinoma is 70% in these women.[184] Their tumors show many of the histopathologic and genetic features of type

I carcinomas, including transit through a premalignant hyperplasia phase,[82,143] endometrioid histopathology of resultant carcinomas,[171] and genetic alterations in mismatch repair genes (mainly *MSH-2*, *MSH-6*, and *MLH-1*)[81,138] and *PTEN*.[196]

RISK FACTORS IN ENDOMETRIAL CARCINOMA

ESTROGENS

The overriding stimulus behind the development of both endometrial hyperplasia and endometrial carcinoma is the effect of estrogens, both endogenous and exogenous. From 1940 and for the next three decades, the incidence of endometrial cancer in the United States was fairly constant. Beginning in 1969, a notable rise in the number of cancer registrations occurred, which coincided with a four-fold increase in the use of estrogens for the alleviation of peri- and postmenopausal symptoms. Since then, numerous case control studies covering many thousands of patients have examined the relation between endometrial cancer and estrogen use.

Despite methodologic criticisms, particularly with regard to the choice of controls and the accuracy of the histologic diagnosis (most of the estrogen-induced tumors were very well-differentiated and many may have been EIN), it is apparent that the relative risk of developing endometrial carcinoma in women taking unopposed estrogens is elevated three- to six-fold,[28,29] rising to 9.5-fold if unopposed estrogen has been used for 10 years or longer.[72] The increased risk persists for several years after the estrogen is discontinued.[73] The risk is roughly similar whether the estrogens are taken continuously or cyclically.

The additional administration of progestins for several days of each month reduces the risk of carcinoma to baseline population levels. Although progestins are usually prescribed for either 7 or 10 days per month in women taking estrogen-replacement therapy, the protection from endometrial cancer is much greater if progestins are used for at least

10 days or given continuously as combined estrogen–progestin therapy.[140]

TAMOXIFEN

The antiestrogen tamoxifen is widely used as an adjuvant therapy for women with breast cancer. Tamoxifen is a non-steroidal compound that competes with estrogen for estrogen receptors. In women of childbearing age it antagonizes endogenous estrogens and induces endometrial inactivity or atrophy, but in postmenopausal women, who are normally hypoestrogenic, it may have a weak estrogenic effect. Thus in some women it behaves as an agonist, in that it has combined with a receptor on the endometrial cell to produce a reaction similar to that of naturally occurring estrogen.

Tamoxifen administration is associated with an overall slightly increased risk (two to three times) of endometrial adenocarcinoma.[40] Carcinoma occurrences are mainly of early stage and low grade, but a small subset of aggressive carcinosarcomas – malignant mixed müllerian tumors (MMMT) – are disproportionately increased, at four times expected.[44] There is conflicting evidence about the level of risk related to length of treatment. Most studies have found that the risk increases with longer duration of tamoxifen administration[134,182] whereas others have found no such relationship.[87] Not surprisingly perhaps, women in whom pretreatment screening showed endometrial lesions, including polyps and hyperplasia, were at a higher risk of developing carcinoma during tamoxifen treatment, which has been put forward as an argument for gynecologic screening of women before starting this therapy, especially when symptomatic.[21,109]

The assumption that tamoxifen-mediated endometrial carcinogenesis involves estrogenic pathways has been challenged following the finding that estrogen receptor reactivity is equally random amongst tamoxifen-treated and non-tamoxifen-treated endometrial carcinomas in breast cancer patients and because tamoxifen may induce DNA adduct formation in endometrial tissues.[93,95,96] In addition to the increased risk of endometrial carcinoma, women treated with tamoxifen are particularly prone to developing endometrial polyps, especially ones of gigantic size[40] (see Chapter 14).

ENDOGENOUS RISK FACTORS

Endogenous estrogen as an etiologic factor in endometrial carcinoma has been understood for many years as these women are known to have a number of constitutional stigmata. Later menopause and low parity are both factors relating to an increased overall lifetime estrogen exposure. Infertility has been linked with anovulation, while obesity, hypertension, and diabetes are noted as common risk factors for endometrial carcinoma. Uncommon pathologic sources of endogenous estrogen include ovarian thecoma and granulosa cell tumors.

POLYCYSTIC OVARY SYNDROME (PCOS)

PCOS is a constellation of endocrine disorders expressing at least two of the following features: anovulation or infrequent ovulation, androgen excess, and polycystic ovaries.[149] The patients are usually infertile, have elevated estrogen levels, and associated insulin resistance may cause type 2 diabetes.[54] When present, characteristic theca–lutein cysts exhibit a luteinized theca interna, but not luteinized granulosa cells of affected ovarian follicles. Endometrial carcinoma occurs in less than 5% of those women with polycystic ovaries[156] but, as the women are all young, this number comprises a significant proportion of endometrial carcinomas in women under age 45 years.

The broad entity of PCOS functionally integrates many features previously shown to individually increase endometrial cancer risk.[88] Primary endocrine defects in PCOS are peripheral insulin resistance and excess ovarian production of androgens. In young women, these factors increase endometrial cancer risk by inducing anovulation and reducing progesterone levels. In older patients, bioavailable estrogens are increased through peripheral conversion of circulating androgens and a reduced level of sex hormone binding globulin (thereby liberating free estradiol).[22,175]

OBESITY

Numerous studies firmly link obesity as a highly significant risk factor in women developing endometrial cancer,[67,133] a sevenfold increased risk associated with a weight of 200 pounds compared with less than 125 pounds.[27] The exact role that obesity plays, however, is far from clear and appears to be quite complicated. The association in women past the menopause is commonly explained in terms of increased aromatization of androgens to estrogens (estrone and estradiol) in adipose tissue, this being the major source of estrogens in women of this age group. The level of serum sex hormone binding globulin (SHBG) in the blood is inversely proportional to the degree of obesity. Women with endometrial carcinoma have lower levels of SHBG than controls, but the difference disappears when corrected for obesity.

DIABETES

The work relating diabetes to the risk of endometrial carcinoma has produced conflicting results. One problem encountered is definitional as some authors refer to clinical diabetes while others use an abnormal glucose tolerance test as the criterion for diagnosis – for example, 3–17% of women with endometrial carcinoma have clinical diabetes and 17–64% have an abnormal glucose tolerance test. One recent case control study found a relative risk of developing endometrial carcinoma of 2.8 when corrected for obesity, suggesting the relationship is probably real.[98]

OVARIAN LESIONS

Ovarian lesions are associated with prolonged, excessive, and unopposed estrogen production that sometimes cause benign endometrial hyperplasia, EIN, and endometrioid adenocarcinoma that is almost always low grade and early stage. The most common lesions include granulosa cell tumor, thecoma, polycystic ovary disease, and hyperthecosis.

SEX CORD-STROMAL TUMORS

Granulosa cell tumor is a relatively uncommon tumor that mainly affects women shortly after the menopause. Most tumors produce increased estrogens and about half the women affected present with postmenopausal bleeding, one-third having proliferative endometrium. Endometrial carcinomas occur in 9–13% of women with granulosa cell tumors.[111] Thecomas occur in women of any age although mainly over 40 years. Most patients present with menstrual irregularities or postmenopausal bleeding as manifestations of estrogen production.[19] One-fifth of thecomas are associated with endometrial carcinoma.[23]

NON-NEOPLASTIC LESIONS

Women with diffuse ovarian stromal hyperthecosis demonstrate luteinized cells, either singly or in groups, dispersed throughout the ovarian stroma, which is typically hyperplastic. When accompanied by hyperandrogenism, as is frequently the case, the clinical presentation may be that of PCOS. Endometrial carcinoma is found in over one-third of women with diffuse hyperthecosis.[151]

Stromal hyperplasia is an abnormal proliferation of ovarian stromal cells without the presence of luteinized cells or prominent cystic follicles. The condition is found mainly during and shortly after the menopause. A mild or moderate degree of stromal hyperplasia is a common histologic finding and it is impossible to state the percentage of women with stromal hyperplasia of the ovary who develop endometrial carcinoma. However, examination of hysterectomy specimens from women with endometrial carcinoma frequently shows some degree of ovarian stromal hyperplasia.

REPRODUCTIVE FACTORS

Nulliparity is a strong independent risk factor for endometrial carcinoma.[27,118,135] Women with endometrial carcinoma are less likely to have had children than normal controls and, if they are parous, they will have had fewer children. Infertility, particularly that associated with anovulation and progesterone insufficiency, is also associated with the risk of developing endometrial carcinoma.[27,57] Nulliparity is significant only when the endometrial carcinoma develops before the menopause and not after.[97] This suggests very strongly that the estrogenic hormonal disturbances that prevent conception also encourage malignant change in the endometrium. The protective effect of pregnancy applies only to full-term pregnancy. Induced and spontaneous abortions are not associated with reduced risk,[27] particularly if the spontaneous abortion occurs late in reproductive life and is not followed by a subsequent full-term pregnancy.[118]

Most studies have shown an association between early age at menarche, late age at natural menopause, and total length of ovulation span,[118] although these findings are not universal. The use of oral contraceptives reduces the risk of endometrial cancer, in some studies by half.[86,119,153]

It is further apparent that the risk for developing endometrial carcinoma is greater when there are multiple risk factors. This means that a woman who is obese and nulliparous is at even higher risk if she is given unopposed estrogen hormone replacement therapy. It is not clear, however, whether the factors combine to give an additive or multiplicative effect.

CIGARETTE SMOKING

Cigarette smoking reduces the risk of endometrial carcinoma. The effect is limited primarily to women whose disease is detected after the menopause and, among these women, current smokers show the greatest reduction in risk, former smokers being less affected.[15,26,185] Smoking does not appear to reduce the risk of endometrial carcinoma before the menopause. Indeed, there may even be increased risk.[185] In the postmenopausal group, smoking appears to reduce the risk to the greatest extent in subjects who are multiparous, obese, or have not used exogenous hormones.[26]

The mechanism whereby cigarette smoking reduces risk is not clear. One study has shown that serum estrogen levels were unaffected but that androstenedione levels were slightly higher in smokers.[15] Paradoxically, women with advanced stage endometrial carcinoma (stages 2–4) were more likely to be smokers than women with early stage disease (stages 0–1).[47]

ENDOMETRIOID ADENOCARCINOMA

Definition

A cancer in which the glandular pattern, when well-differentiated, has cytologic features most like a normal proliferative endometrium.

Clinical features

The most common subtype of endometrial cancer is endometrioid, its pure form constituting about 60% of all endometrial carcinomas. Most neoplasms develop slowly in the setting of hyperestrogenism against a background of benign endometrial hyperplasia and EIN, although some arise in atrophic endometrium.[127] Endometrioid carcinoma is predominantly a disease of the sixth and seventh decades and 75% of cases occur after the menopause. Only 5% occur in women less than 40 years old. They are low grade, non-myoinvasive, associated with a good prognosis, and often develop after a long history of anovulatory cycles or estrogen therapy. Endometrial carcinoma rarely occurs in pregnancy.[62,154]

Women with endometrioid carcinoma most often present with abnormal vaginal bleeding, which means in the majority of cases postmenopausal bleeding. The fact that they bleed, however, simply means that the tumor is often large or advanced. Smaller carcinomas may be asymptomatic. Surprisingly frequently, asymptomatic tumor is documented in women who have an endometrial biopsy before instituting hormone-replacement therapy, or had the tumor discovered initially at autopsy.[79] Patients with advanced disease may complain of pelvic pain, which reflects the tumor spread.

Until recent years, the diagnosis has been made by endometrial biopsy or curettage but imaging techniques now play a part and hysteroscopy with directed endometrial biopsy is being used more often. Outpatient endometrial sampling techniques generally have a good diagnostic rate for endometrial carcinoma, but may need to be followed by confirmatory curettage.[52]

Gross features

Endometrioid carcinoma can present variously to the naked eye when the uterus is opened. The uterus may be slightly or grossly enlarged but it may be of normal size or even small and atrophic, particularly in a postmenopausal woman. Most tumors arise in the corpus but some originate in the lower uterine segment. The tumor may present as a single mass, two or three separate masses (Figure 16.1), or a diffuse thickening of the endometrium. Carcinomas are situated more frequently on the posterior than the anterior wall. The most common appearance is of a raised, rough, perhaps papillary area of the endometrium with a shaggy surface and ulceration, frequently occupying at least half of the surface area of the endometrium (Figure 16.2).

Sometimes the tumor is polypoid, with a fairly narrow base. When this is the case, its surface may be smooth and hemorrhagic and the uterine cavity distended, with concomitant thinning of the uterine wall. When the tumor is polypoid, the remaining endometrium usually appears thin. Myometrial invasion may be obvious to the naked eye (Figure 16.3), with either pushing or infiltrating borders (Figure 16.4), but frequently it is difficult to appreciate the degree of myometrial invasion grossly. There seems to be no correlation between the degree of exophytic growth of the tumor within the uterine cavity and the presence of myometrial invasion.[112] However, a tumor diameter of more than 2 cm generally is associated with a poorer prognosis and a higher frequency of distant failure.

Microscopic features

The glandular pattern and cellular features generally resemble that of the proliferative phase endometrium, although showing a more complicated architecture that may include solid growth, maze-like interconnected lumens, villoglandular appearance, or cribriform growth (Figures 16.5–16.7). Multilayered epithelial cells are nearly always seen. Occasionally cribriform fragments have a microglandular appearance easily confused with a cervical lesion (Figure 16.8). Solid growth may vary widely

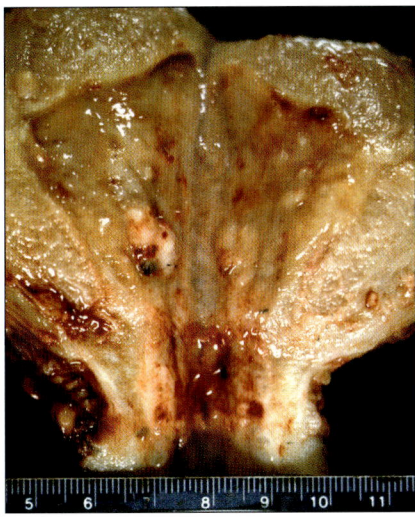

Fig. 16.1 Endometrial adenocarcinoma. The tumor involves only part of the endometrium and appears as apparently separate foci.

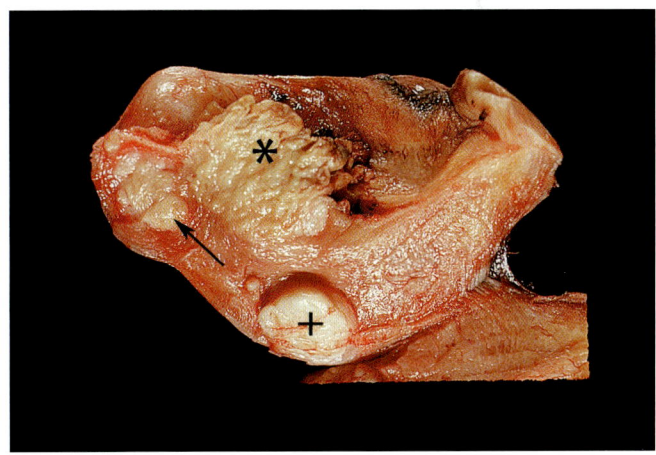

Fig. 16.3 Endometrial adenocarcinoma. A section through the wall of a uterus shows carcinoma protruding into the lumen (*) and invading deeply into the myometrium (black arrow). A leiomyoma is also present (+).

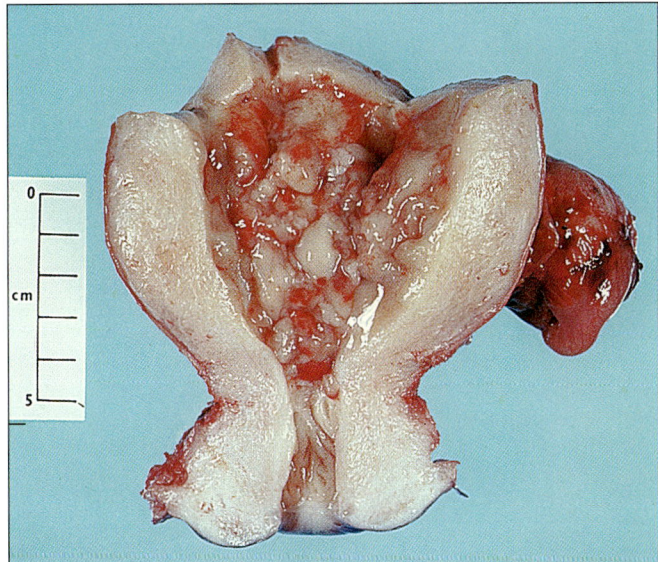

Fig. 16.2 Endometrial adenocarcinoma. The tumor involves most of the endometrium.

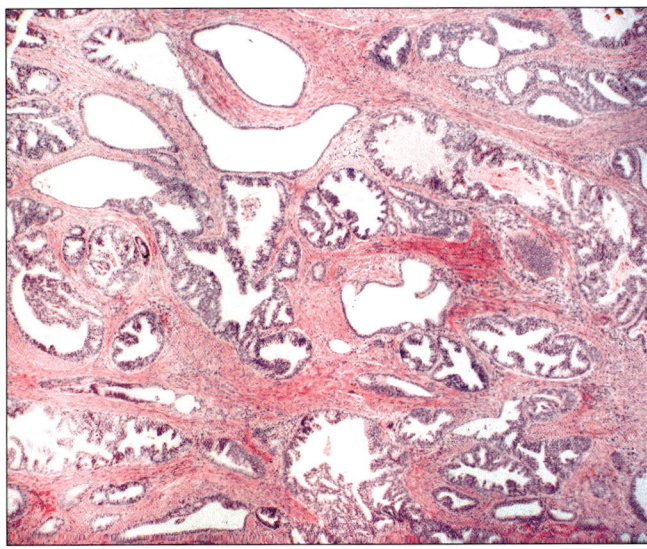

Fig. 16.4 Endometrial adenocarcinoma, endometrioid pattern. Well-differentiated (grade 1) tumor, invading the myometrium.

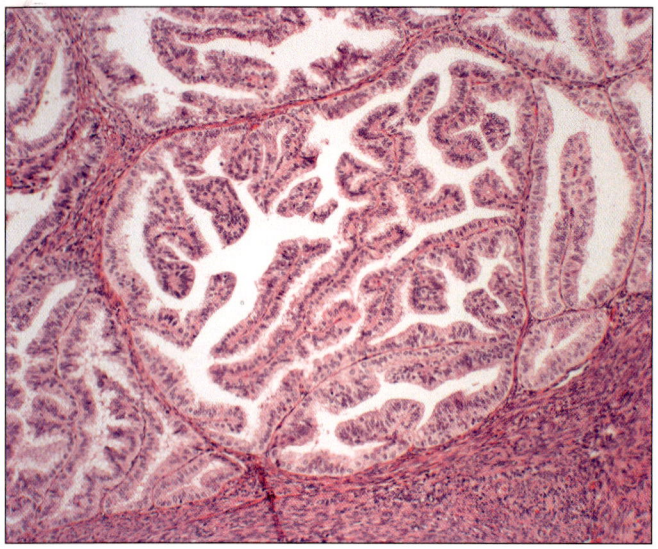

Fig. 16.5 Endometrial adenocarcinoma, endometrioid pattern. Well-differentiated (grade 1) tumor with maze-like gland arrangement.

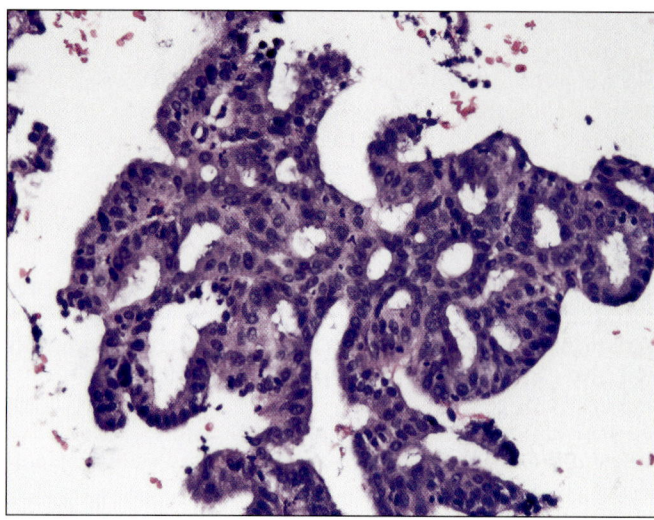

Fig. 16.8 Endometrial adenocarcinoma, endometrioid type, with microglandular cribriform architecture. These delicate lesions tend to be exophytic, and may appear highly fragmented in biopsy specimens.

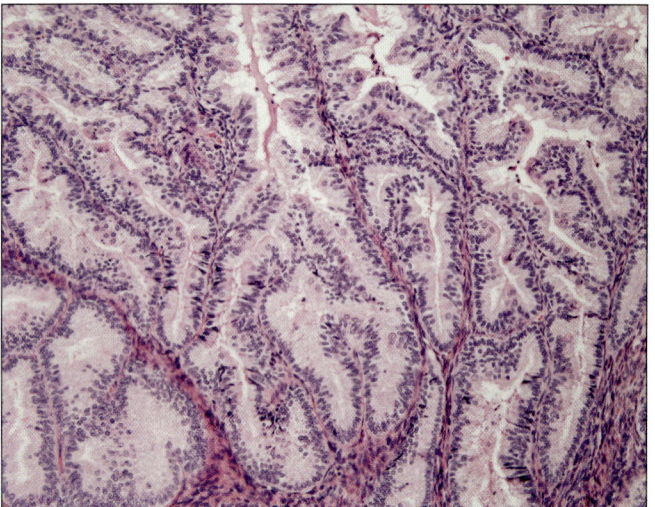

Fig. 16.6 Endometrial adenocarcinoma, intraendometrial. The branching glands with maze-like lumens indicate an architecture of folded sheets of neoplastic epithelium, rather than dense packing of tubular structures.

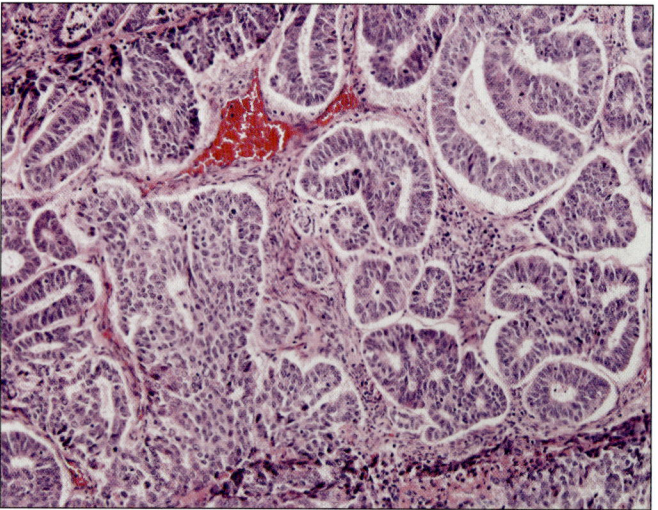

Fig. 16.9 Endometrial adenocarcinoma, endometrioid pattern. Moderately differentiated (grade 2) tumor with admixed solid and glandular areas.

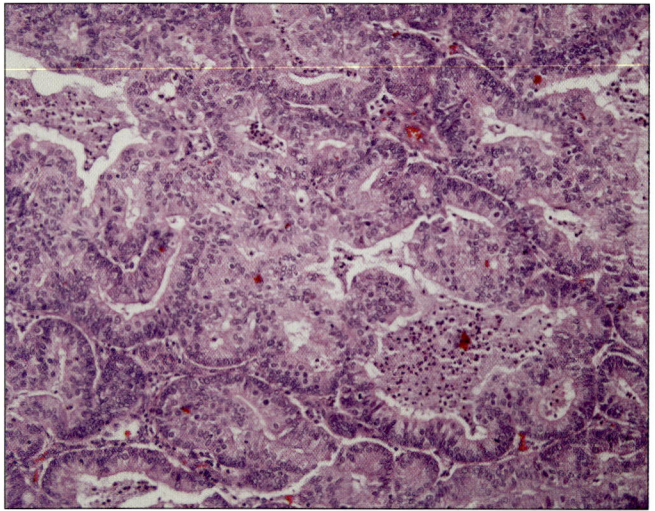

Fig. 16.7 Endometrial adenocarcinoma, endometrioid pattern. Extensive cribriform areas.

in extent, a feature of importance in tumor grading (Figures 16.9–16.11). Glands that are confluent without intervening stroma demonstrate varying degrees of modeling, sometimes assuming polygonal (mosaic-like) shapes (Figure 16.12).

The individual epithelial cells are larger than would be expected in the proliferative phase. Compared with the normal endometrium, the carcinoma cells have a distinctly altered cytology that varies between patients and even within areas of a single tumor, but may include rounded nuclei, clumped chromatin, and prominent nucleoli. Individual tumors frequently demonstrate patchy changes in differentiation to mucinous, squamous, tubal, or other cytologies, and in these cases cytoplasmic as well as nuclear features stand out from the normal background. Some endometrioid adenocarcinomas secrete abundant extracellular mucin but lack much intracytoplasmic mucin (Figure 16.13), a feature that distinguishes them from mucinous adenocarcinoma.

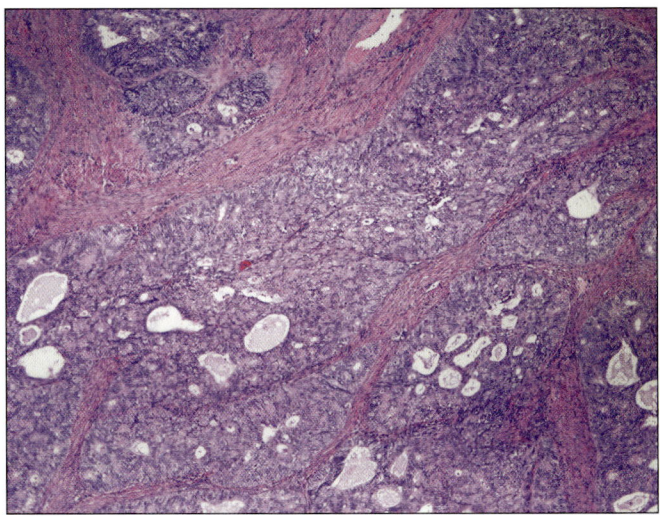

Fig. 16.10 Endometrial adenocarcinoma, endometrioid pattern. Poorly differentiated (grade 3) tumor. Although gland lumina are apparent, more than 50% of the tumor is solid.

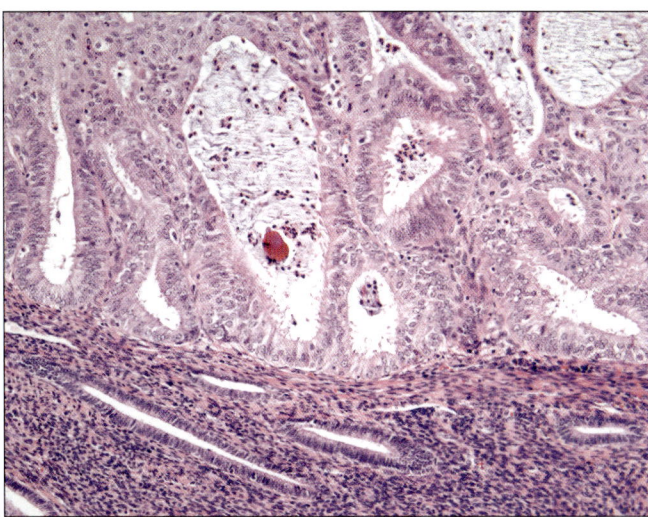

Fig. 16.13 Endometrial adenocarcinoma, endometrioid pattern. There is abundant mucin production, but no intracytoplasmic mucin.

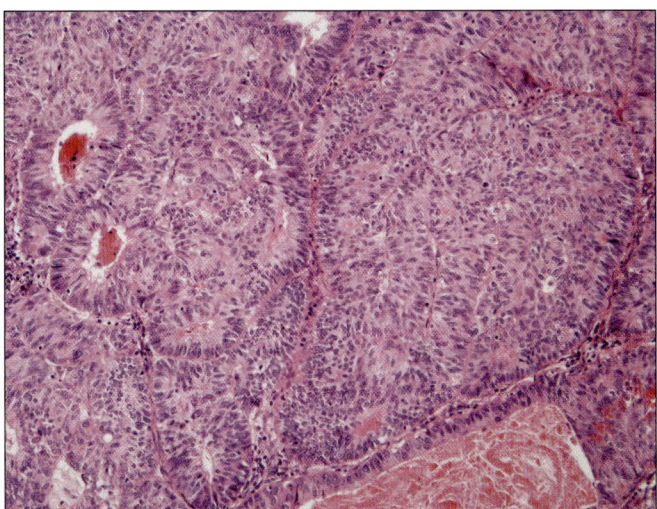

Fig. 16.11 Endometrial adenocarcinoma, endometrioid pattern. Poorly differentiated (grade 3) tumor.

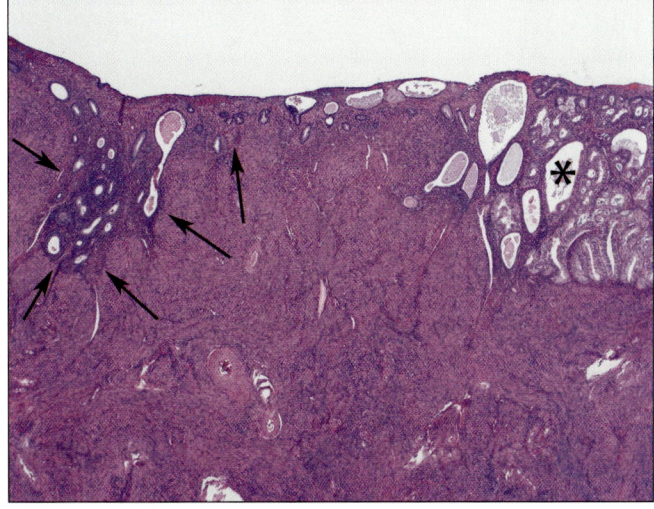

Fig. 16.14 Endometrial adenocarcinoma, intraendometrial. Well-differentiated (grade 1) tumor, confined to the endometrium (*). The endometrial–myometrial junction is non-linear (arrows).

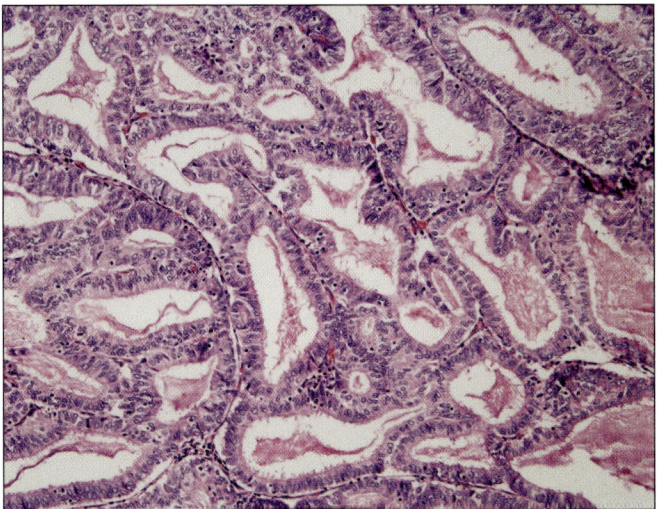

Fig. 16.12 Endometrial adenocarcinoma, endometrioid pattern. Well-differentiated (grade 1) tumor with confluent glands and cribriform areas.

Mitotic figures are usually present but may be scanty in well-differentiated tumors.

Endometrial adenocarcinomas, like their precursor EIN lesions, spread within the endometrial compartment by extension of newly formed, well-differentiated neoplastic glands into the adjacent stroma (centrifugal growth) (Figures 16.14 and 16.15). In turn, the adjacent endometrial stroma responds by remodeling, rarely demonstrating a classic desmoplastic change. For this reason, qualitatively assessing the character of the endometrial stroma is non-contributory in resolving premalignant from malignant disease within the endometrial compartment itself. Carcinoma is recognized within the endometrial compartment by presence of at least one of the following: a cribriform pattern of the glands, a solid mass of glandular epithelium, meandering interconnected lumens formed by folded sheets of neoplastic epithelium, or irregular, angulated and tapering glandular contours. Several features may be present together. These points are represented in Figure 16.16.

Foamy histiocytes are commonly seen in the endometrial stromal compartment of patients with a carcinoma. Nearly a fifth of cases contain stromal cells laden with lipid (Figure 16.17) but there is no correlation between the presence of these cells and the grade of the tumor or the survival of the patient.[41] This change is simply a reactive response to tumor cells that have died. The presence of such histiocytic cells in endometrial biopsies showing EIN should always lead to further diagnostic workup for coexistent carcinoma.

The concept of invasion is often confused. Tumor, even when confined to the endometrial compartment, may be invasive into the endometrial stroma. Myoinvasive disease, often simplified to 'invasive', should be diagnosed only when malignant glands have transgressed the endometrial–myometrial junction into the underlying muscular uterine wall, but even this is not always straightforward. Because the endometrial–myometrial boundary is irregular, one clue we commonly use is whether isolated normal endometrial glands can be found at the junction and just deep to the tumor (Figure 16.18). Sometimes a desmoplastic myometrial response may be the primary diagnostic feature of superficial myoinvasion, but more often than not, tumor that is myoinvasive elicits no desmoplastic response. Accessibility of sampling devices to deeper tissues limits the ability to diagnose myoinvasive disease, even when present in the patient.

Cytologic correlation

There are no established guidelines for routine endometrial cytologic screening, but exfoliated neoplastic endometrial cells are sometimes encountered in cervical Papanicolaou smears. Unfortunately, recognition of malignant features is often hampered by the degenerative changes that follow exfoliation or the shedding of cells from the endometrium many hours before. Up to two-thirds of women with endometrial adenocarcinoma have malignant cells in their cervical cytology specimen and high-grade as well as high-stage tumors seem to be detected more frequently.[155] In cervical smears, malignant endometrial cells characteristically appear as small clusters with darkly stained nuclei (Figure 16.19) or perhaps as single discrete cells that are easily overlooked.

Transcervical cytology sampling devices have been designed to directly access the endometrium.[110] The malignant cells in an endometrial aspirate are freshly removed and rapidly fixed so the features are well preserved and can be widely variable, from large single cells to small clusters as well as large sheets (Figure 16.20). The cellular features can be quite subtle, suggesting a well-differentiated adenocarcinoma, or pleomorphic and bizarre, suggesting a poorly differentiated adenocarcinoma. Advances in the design of the Tao Brush, together with liquid-based cytologic techniques, now promise much higher yields and even clusters of cells equivalent to a microbiopsy.[110]

The key cytoarchitectural features of endometrioid glandular neoplasia are shown in Figure 16.20. EIN and well-differentiated adenocarcinomas may present as tufted epithelial structures similar to those seen with syncytial metaplasia with small and often distorted acini or bridging epithelial structures

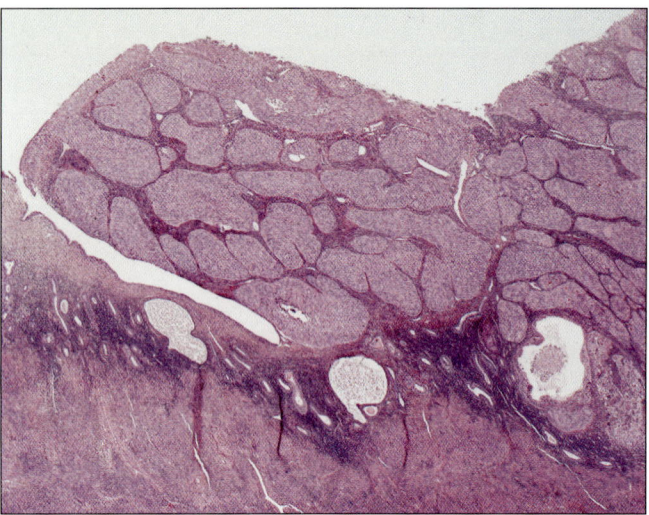

Fig. 16.15 Endometrial adenocarcinoma, intraendometrial. The tumor is exophytic and entirely intraendometrial, its deep margin following the line of the endometrial-myometrial junction.

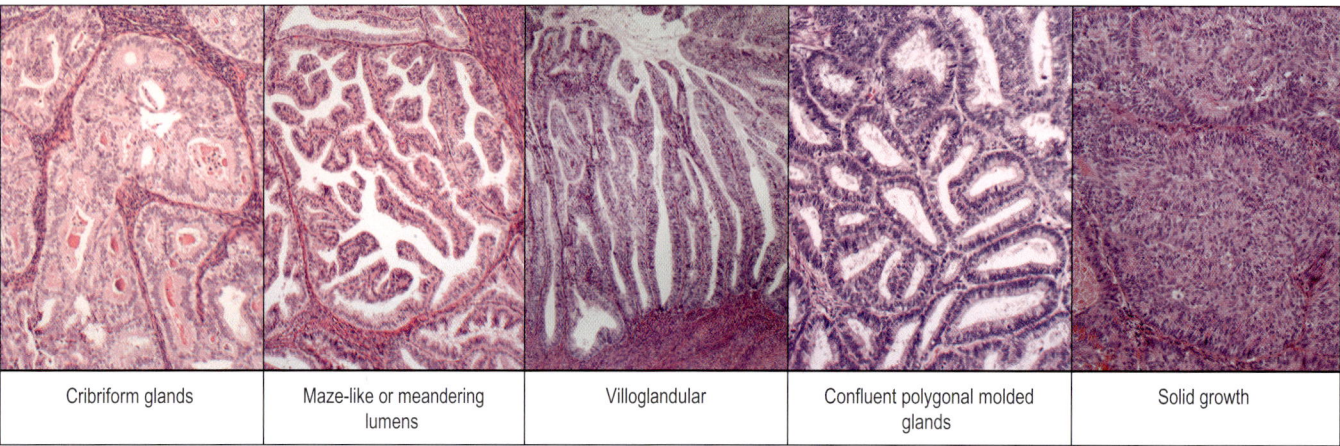

| Cribriform glands | Maze-like or meandering lumens | Villoglandular | Confluent polygonal molded glands | Solid growth |

Fig. 16.16 Intraendometrial adenocarcinoma. Glandular architectural patterns that may be seen in non-myoinvasive areas.

that lack stromal support. Small sheet-like to cup-like aggregates of cells with highly pseudostratified nuclei are another appearance. Changes diagnostic of overt adenocarcinoma include cribriform structures (comprising solid aggregates of cells punctuated by lumens), expanded mucin-filled vacuoles in aggregates of cells with or without polymorphonuclear neutrophilic emperipolesis, elongated villoglandular structures, solid cell aggregates, and abundant and widely scattered dyshesive anaplastic cells in a necroinflammatory background. These smears are also easily used for immunocytochemical studies. Since the final classification rests with the histologic pattern based on glandular features as well as cellular appearance, a diagnosis of adenocarcinoma is sufficient for the cytologist.

On rare occasions following the recognition of malignant glandular cells in an endometrial aspirate the curettage may be negative. In this eventuality the possibility of an ovarian lesion should be considered and eliminated. This occurs rarely, but more often than generally believed. We have seen several of these cases where an endometrial lesion was also present. An experienced cytologist is unlikely to mistake malignant adenocarcinoma cells.

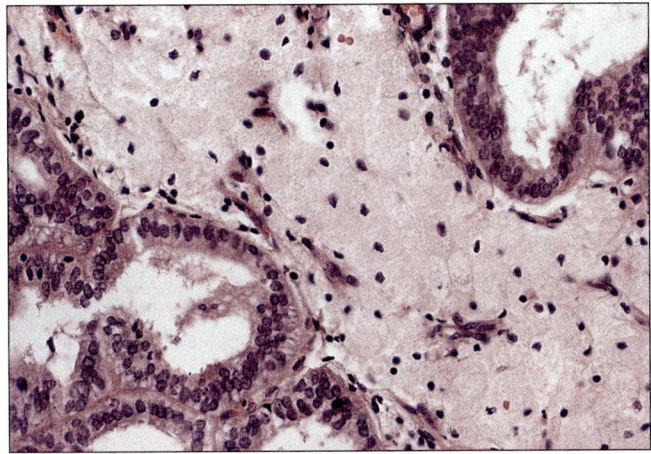

Fig. 16.17 Endometrial adenocarcinoma. Foam cells in the stroma.

OTHER VARIANTS OF ENDOMETRIOID ADENOCARCINOMA

Four histologic variants of endometrioid adenocarcinoma are recognized.[165] All show a particular type of cellular differentiation related to cyclic or hyperplastic endometrium, or peculiar architecture.

Endometrial adenocarcinoma, endometrioid type, with squamous differentiation   One-fourth of endometrial adenocarcinomas display focal squamous differentiation (Figures 16.21 and 16.22). In the late 1960s the distinction was made between tumors where the squamous component was well or poorly differentiated. The former tumors were called 'adenoacanthoma' and the latter 'adenosquamous carcinoma'. Numerous studies have confirmed the significantly better prognosis associated with adenoacanthoma and endometrial carcinoma without squamous differentiation (about 90% survival at 5 years) as compared to adenosquamous carcinoma (65%), a distinction related largely to the grade of the glandular component. Well differentiated squamous components, often reported as being 'benign' or even as 'squamous metaplasia', are, in reality, neoplastic and metaplastic at the same time, as shown by conservation of β-catenin mutations between squamous and glandular elements.[150] The squamous elements may be described as being 'terminally differentiated' and 'hormonally incompetent', an integral part of the tumor incapable of estrogen stimulation and independent growth.

Most studies are hampered by the poor reproducibility in the current classification of these tumors. Usable criteria are needed for the recognition of squamous differentiation, so that a solid focus of adenocarcinoma in endometrial carcinoma will not be mistaken for squamous differentiation. The International Society of Gynecological Pathologists (ISGP) has suggested criteria in response to this need (Table 16.3).[164] In large studies where the glandular and squamous components were graded independently, differentiation of the squamous component was shown to parallel that of the glandular component closely. Thus, the prognosis can be predicted by the glandular

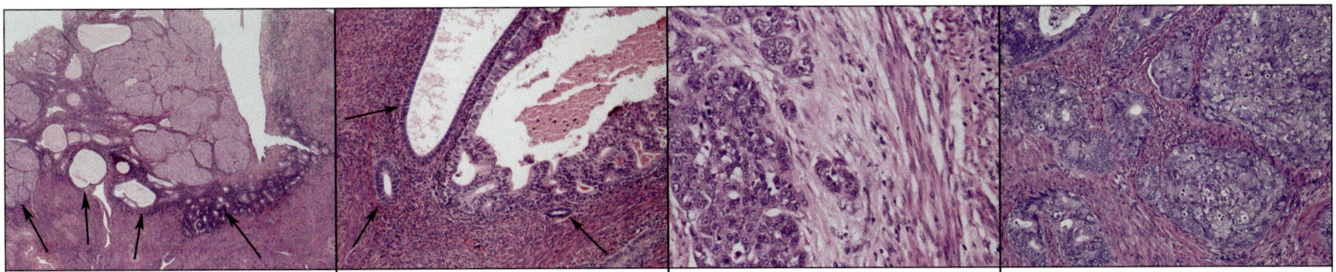

NO	NO	YES	YES
This tumor is entirely intraendometrial, but the irregular junction between the endometrium and myometrium imparts a false impression of myoinvasion. Endometrial stroma (arrows) surrounds the tumor.	Tumor extending into islands of adenomyosis can be recognized by a surrounding mantle of endometrial stroma and/or benign adenomyotic glands (arrows).	Invasion into the myometrium by malignant glands which have incited a desmoplastic stromal response.	Invasion into the myometrium by malignant glands that have minimal desmoplastic response. These have penetrated almost to the serosa.

Fig. 16.18 Myoinvasion in endometrial adenocarcinoma.

grade alone. The utility of the terms 'adenoacanthoma' and 'adenosquamous carcinoma' is that they are short, and reflect tumors where both the glandular and squamous components are well or poorly differentiated, respectively. In other words, adenoacanthoma usually has a low-grade glandular compo-nent, while adenosquamous carcinoma usually has a high-grade glandular component. The glandular component is much easier to grade in a reproducible fashion. Grading of the glan-dular component is also superior in predicting lymph node metastasis and 5-year survival. Furthermore, proportional hazard models indicate that the grade of the squamous com-ponent is not an independent prognostic variable.[189]

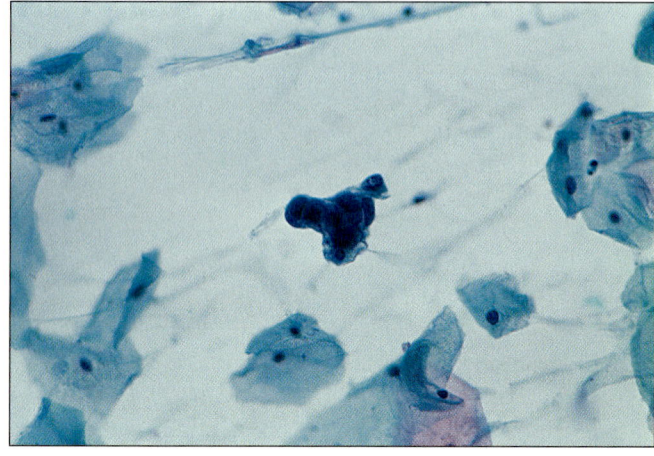

Fig. 16.19 Endometrial adenocarcinoma, cytology. Malignant glandular cells in a cervical smear.

Table 16.3 Criteria for identifying squamous differentiation in endometrioid adenocarcinoma[164]

Squamous differentiation is suggested by the presence of any of the following:
 	
• Keratin or keratin pearls demonstrated without special stains
• Intercellular bridges
• At least three of the following:
  – sheet-like growth without gland formation or palisading
  – distinct cell margins
  – deeply eosinophilic or 'glassy' cytoplasm
  – a decreased nuclear:cytoplasmic ratio compared with the rest of the tumor

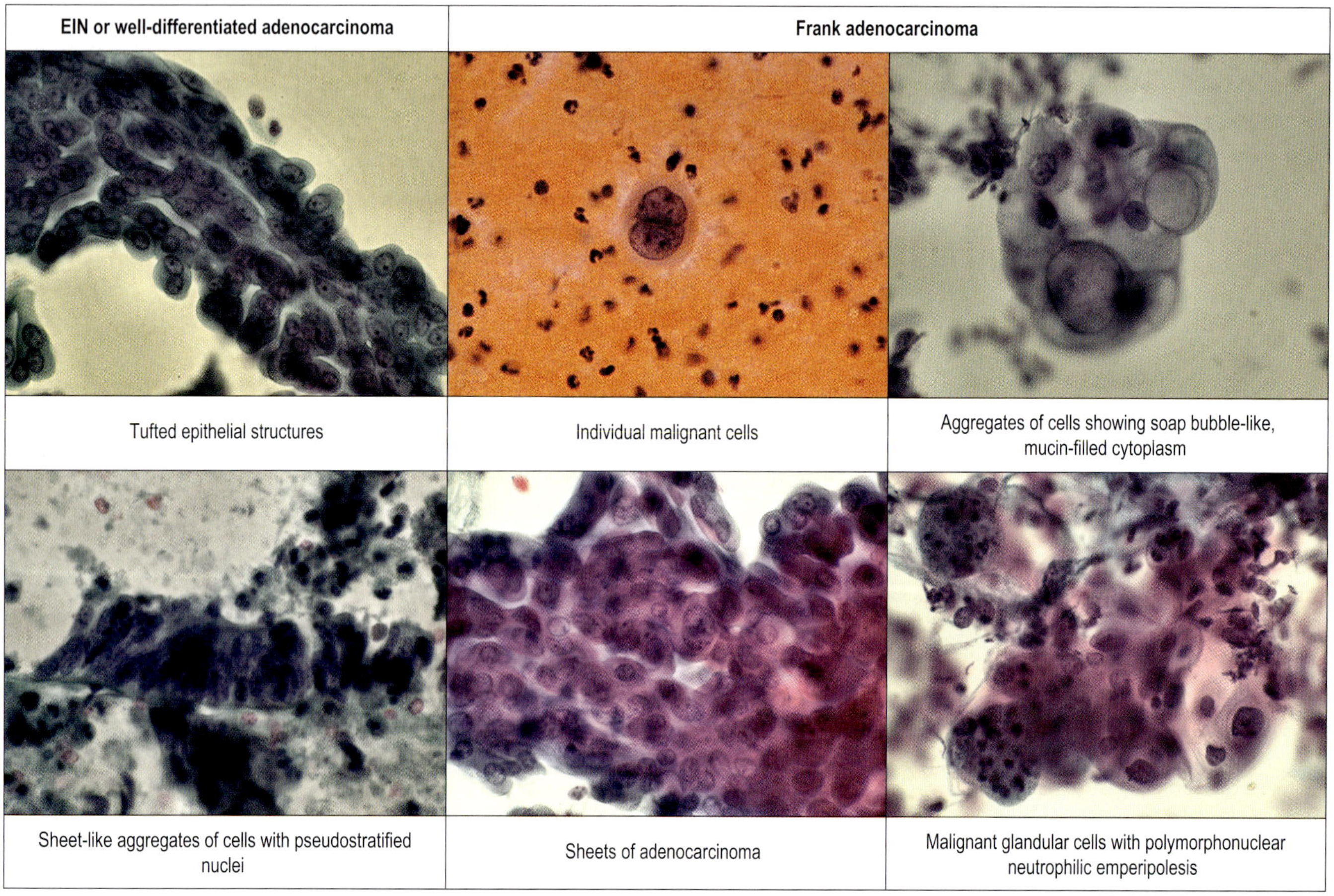

EIN or well-differentiated adenocarcinoma	Frank adenocarcinoma	
Tufted epithelial structures	Individual malignant cells	Aggregates of cells showing soap bubble-like, mucin-filled cytoplasm
Sheet-like aggregates of cells with pseudostratified nuclei	Sheets of adenocarcinoma	Malignant glandular cells with polymorphonuclear neutrophilic emperipolesis

Fig. 16.20 Brush cytology of endometrioid endometrial glandular neoplasia. (Courtesy of John Maksem, MD, Orlando, FL.)

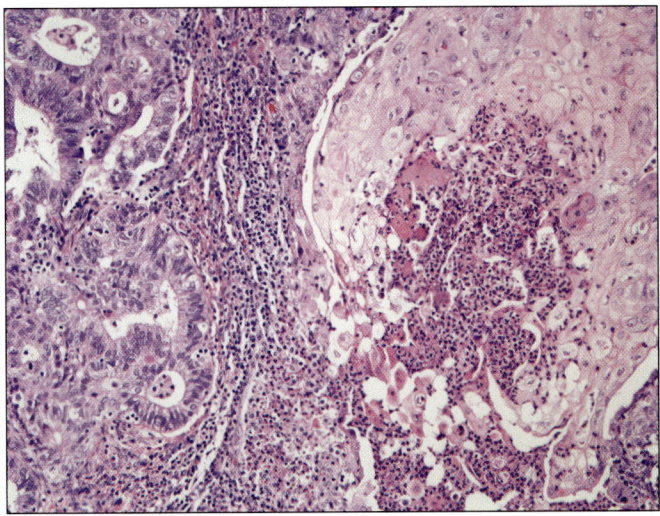

Fig. 16.21 Endometrial adenocarcinoma, endometrioid type, with squamous change.

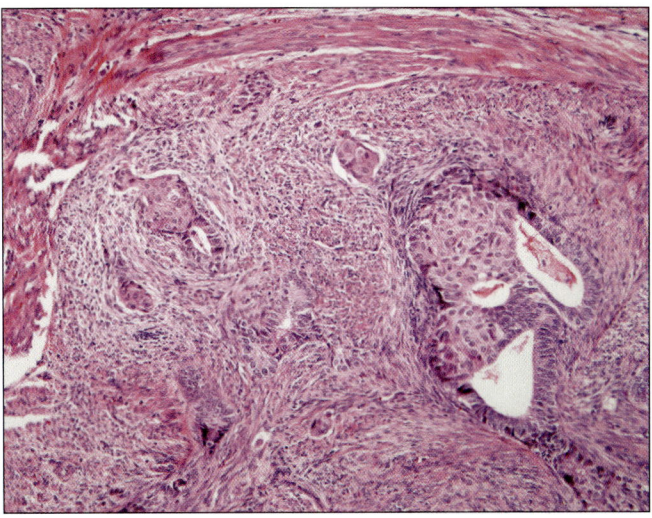

Fig. 16.24 Endometrial adenocarcinoma, endometrioid type, myoinvasive with squamous change.

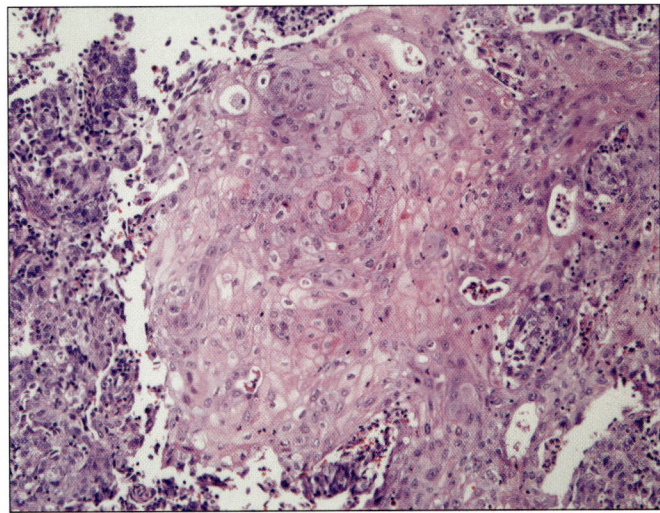

Fig. 16.22 Endometrial adenocarcinoma, endometrioid type, with squamous change. Squamous (right) and glandular (left) components in a moderately differentiated (grade 2) tumor.

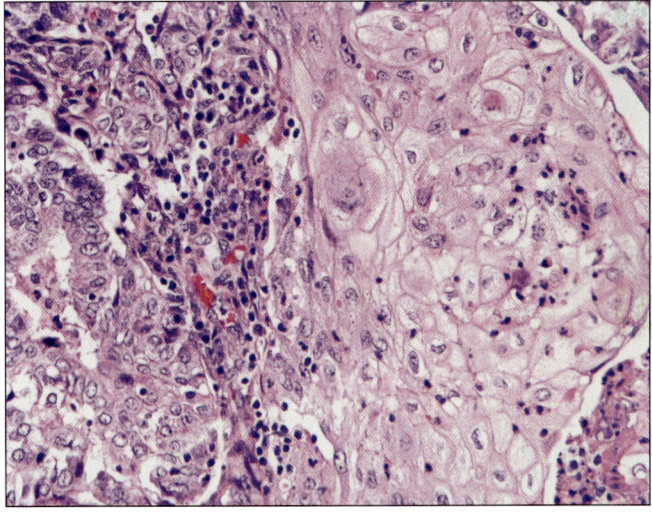

Fig. 16.25 Endometrial adenocarcinoma, endometrioid type, with squamous change.

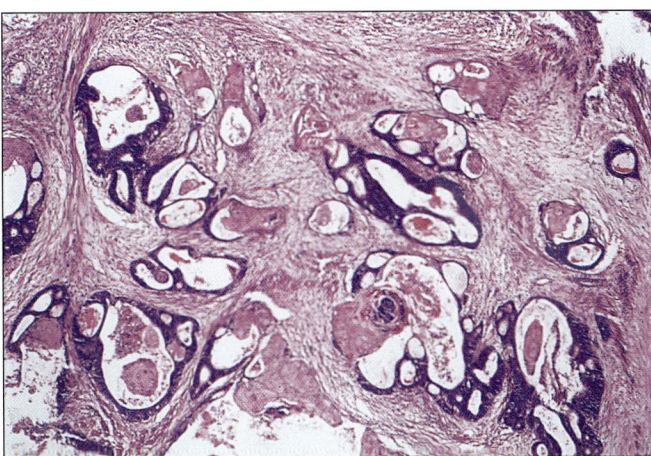

Fig. 16.23 Endometrial adenocarcinoma, endometrioid type, with squamous change.

As a result of comparative studies and the difficulties in classifying lesions as adenoacanthoma and adenosquamous carcinoma, the ISGP/WHO recommends that the term 'adenocarcinoma with squamous differentiation' replace 'adenoacanthoma' and 'adenosquamous carcinoma'. Grading is to be based solely on the glandular component. We believe that if the term 'adenosquamous carcinoma' is used, it should be reserved for those tumors in which the squamous component shows unequivocal cytologic malignancy, mitotic activity or destructive stromal infiltration (Figures 16.23 and 16.24).[164] In the same vein, 'adenoacanthoma' should be reserved for tumors in which the squamous component is uniformly well differentiated throughout, in small nests, and without mitotic activity or destructive stromal infiltration. The cytologic appearances associated with adenocarcinoma with squamous change are mainly those of the adenocarcinoma element and are therefore similar to the features already described (Figure 16.25). In addition, cells are present that are clearly identifiable as squamous in type, having enlarged nuclei with aberrant chromatin distribution and pleomorphism (Figure 16.26).

Endometrial adenocarcinoma, endometrioid type, with secretory differentiation 'Secretory adenocarcinomas' are an uncommon variant of endometrioid adenocarcinoma composed of well-differentiated glands resembling those of early or mid-secretory endometrium (Figure 16.27).[39] The most common changes are subnuclear and/or supranuclear vacuolation. In addition, there may be solid areas consisting of small polygonal cells with clear cytoplasm. Unlike clear cell carcinoma, the nuclei are only mildly to moderately polygonal and hobnail features are absent. The tumor may consist entirely of secretory glands, although usually the changes are focally distributed. Secretory adenocarcinomas are associated with a good prognosis.[164] There are two types of secretory carcinoma: those in which the secretory change is induced by circulating progestins,

and those in which secretory differentiation is an intrinsic feature of the neoplasm independent of background hormonal state. The presence or absence of progestin-induced stromal change and the menopausal status of the patient distinguish these etiologies.[176] The tumor's general architecture and the cells' intrinsic columnar shapes are not altered by progestin induction of secretory change, thus distinguishing these tumors from clear cell adenocarcinomas (see below). It is not uncommon where a woman has had both a biopsy and hysterectomy to have one show secretory adenocarcinoma and the other only typical non-secretory adenocarcinoma, an indication that the secretory change is a manifestation of the ovulatory cycle.

Endometrial adenocarcinoma, endometrioid type, with ciliated cell differentiation 'Ciliated cell carcinoma' is rare.[105,164] Ciliated cells are uncommon in adenocarcinomas of the endometrium but occasionally individual ciliated cells can be found with diligent searching. More rarely, extensive ciliated differentiation is present throughout (Figures 16.28 and 16.29). Only

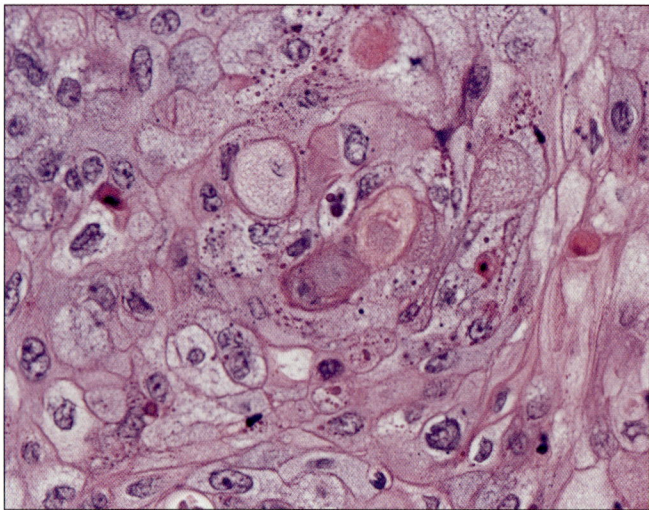

Fig. 16.26 Endometrial adenocarcinoma, endometrioid type, with squamous change. High power view of squamous component of same case as in Figure 16.24.

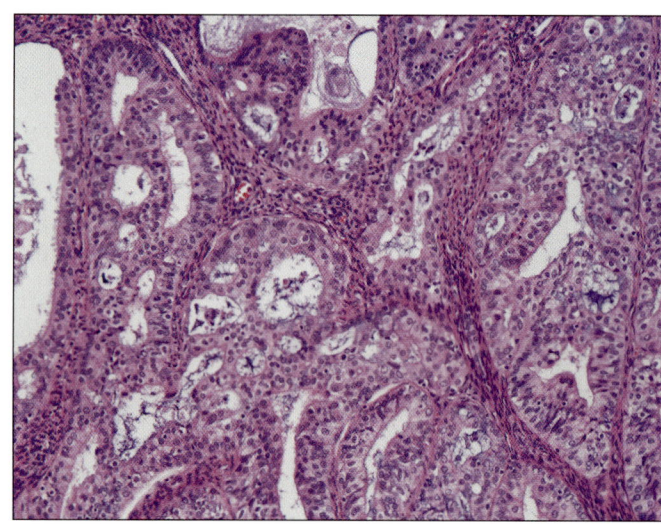

Fig. 16.28 Endometrial adenocarcinoma, ciliated type.

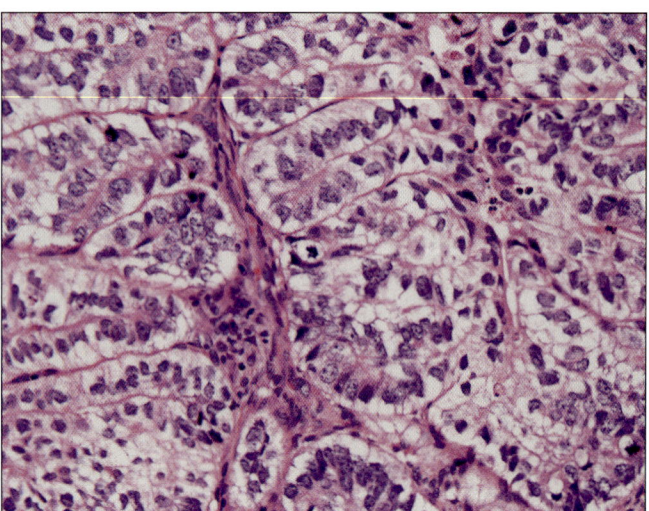

Fig. 16.27 Endometrial adenocarcinoma, endometrioid type, with secretory differentiation. This tumor resembles a day 17 secretory endometrium with characteristic and prominent subnuclear vacuoles.

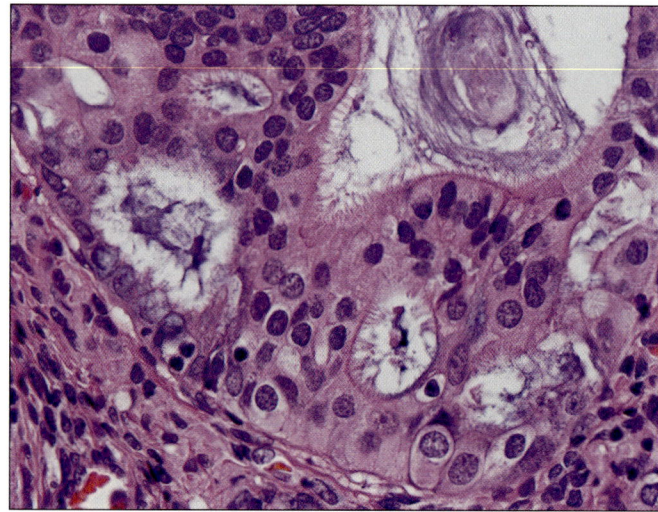

Fig. 16.29 Endometrial adenocarcinoma, ciliated type, high magnification view of cilia.

if at least 75% of the tumor cells are ciliated should the tumor be termed a 'ciliated cell carcinoma'.[77] Some well-differentiated ciliated tumors may be difficult to distinguish from premalignant EIN lesions. Thus the diagnosis of ciliated cell carcinoma should be made with great caution. In some cases only the presence of myometrial or lymphatic invasion establishes the diagnosis. Endometrioid carcinomas with ciliated cell differentiation have a good prognosis.[77]

Endometrial adenocarcinoma, endometrioid type, villoglandular variant This variant consists of slender, long, delicate papillae in well-differentiated neoplasms that may be predominantly of typical endometrioid type or entirely papillary (Figure 16.30).[190] This tumor is similar to villoglandular adenocarcinoma arising in the endocervix, where it occurs in younger women and is often associated with a better prognosis. Psammoma bodies may rarely be encountered.[137] They are a more consistent feature of serous carcinomas. The cytologic features are the same as those of typical endometrioid carcinoma, with nuclei usually having grade 1 features. Because these tumors are well differentiated, they are usually associated with a favorable outcome.[59] However, tumors in which the invasive elements are of villoglandular papillary pattern may be associated with a poorer prognosis.[9] Some of the editors avoid the term villoglandular adenocarcinoma as the villoglandular portion is usually exophytic where the tumor can be expansive, whereas the portion invasive into the wall shows a more typical adenocarcinoma.

Villoglandular adenocarcinomas need to be distinguished from serous carcinomas, as the latter have a poorer prognosis. The term 'papillary carcinoma' is imprecise and should not be used for endometrial tumors. Papillary, without further designation, could refer to the villoglandular variant, endometrioid carcinoma itself, or serous carcinoma. Clear cell adenocarcinomas and mucinous adenocarcinomas may have papillary areas but they are usually sufficiently different in overall appearance for confusion to be avoided.

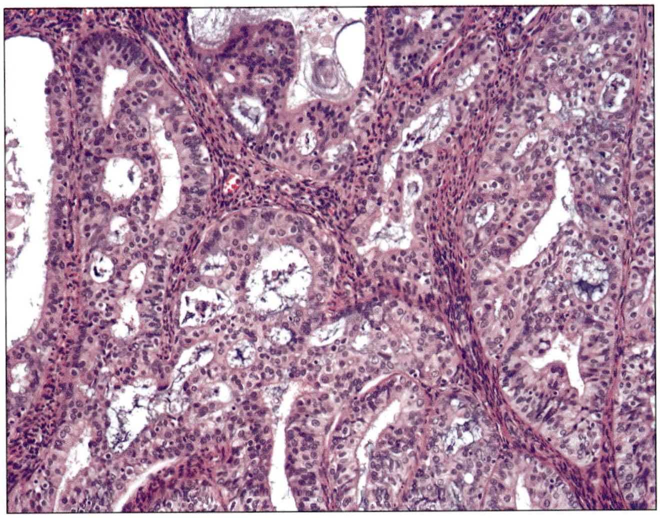

Differential diagnosis

Well-differentiated endometrioid adenocarcinoma may be difficult to distinguish from EIN, which is the most frequent differential diagnosis in curettings. This problem has been discussed in detail in Chapter 15. EIN consists of individual lumen-bearing glands grouped together, whereas a cribriform pattern, solid growth, meandering interconnected lumens, or villoglandular architecture generally are diagnostic of adenocarcinoma (Figures 16.31 and 16.32). Myoinvasion clearly points towards a diagnosis of carcinoma, but biopsy and curettage devices rarely sample the myometrial wall. Unfortunately, the picture is further clouded by some invasive carcinomas showing few, if any, of these features; Figure 16.33 shows an example of an adenocarcinoma that has invaded almost to the serosa, but both the architectural and nuclear differentiation are so good that the tumor appears to satisfy none of the cri-

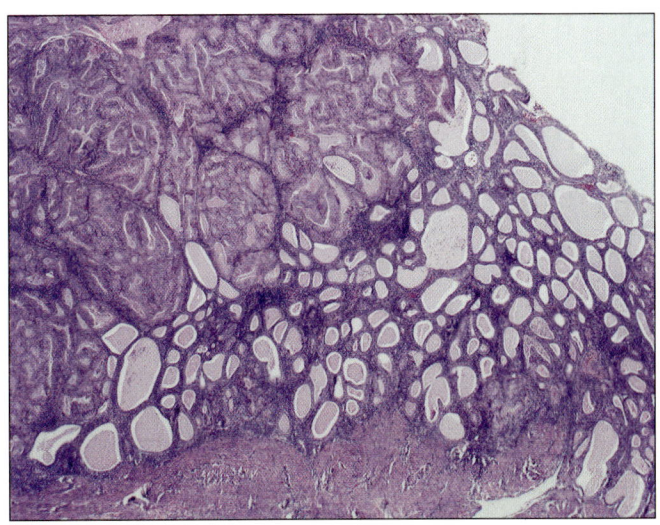

Fig. 16.31 Endometrial adenocarcinoma, intraendometrial (left). The endometrium on the right is a premalignant EIN composed of packed round glands.

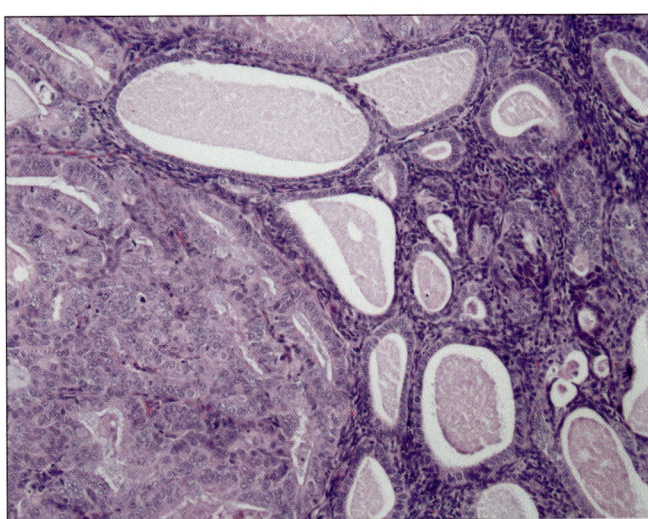

Fig. 16.32 Endometrial adenocarcinoma, intraendometrial. Individual tubular glands of EIN are present on the right and adenocarcinoma, with cribriform glands, on the left.

Fig. 16.30 Endometrial adenocarcinoma, endometrioid type, with villoglandular architecture.

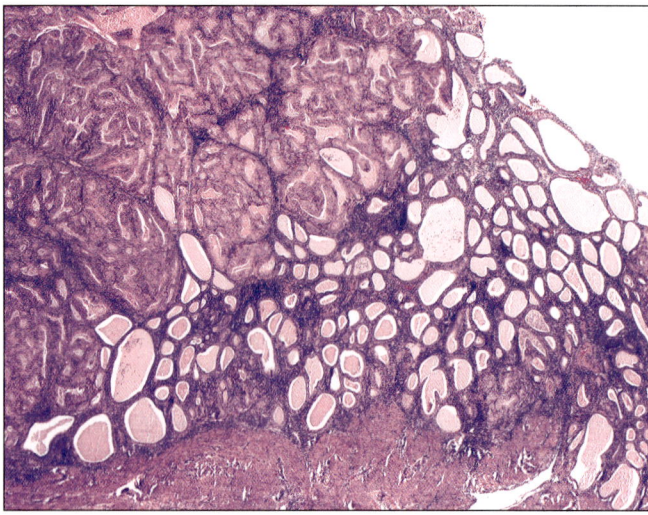

Fig. 16.33 Endometrial adenocarcinoma, endometrioid type, well differentiated, with myoinvasion. Individual glands are simple and lined by cytologically bland epithelium, unusual features of deeply myoinvasive disease.

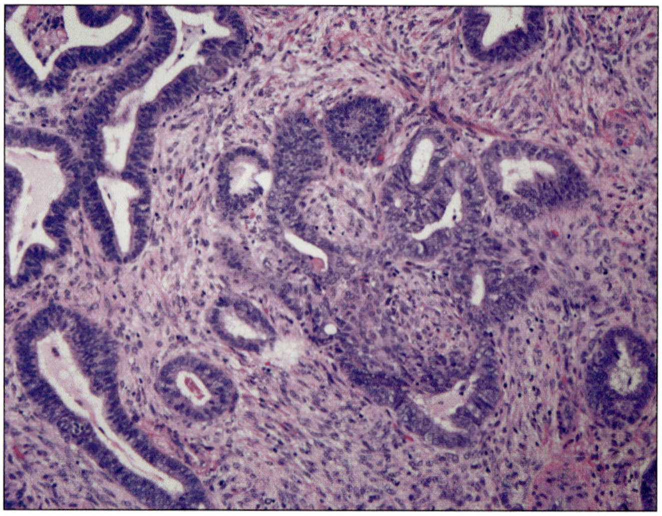

Fig. 16.34 Atypical polypoid adenomyoma. Neoplastic glands with squamous morules are offset by a densely muscular stroma.

teria for a diagnosis of carcinoma. Myometrial invasion is, of course, diagnostic, but is a criterion only available in hysterectomy specimens and therefore only of use in establishing the final diagnosis. The features discussed in Chapter 15 are those that are of value in curettings, when the decision needs to be made whether to proceed to hysterectomy or not.

Several groups have systematically examined endometrial biopsy material in women with and without myoinvasive adenocarcinoma to discover features predictive of myoinvasion. In one study that visually scored many discrete histologic features, paired endometrial samplings and hysterectomy specimens were examined in a training set of 306 cases and then tested with a challenge of 214 cases.[108] The training set enabled the identification of one significant predictive architectural feature (glandular complexity) and two cytologic features (nuclear pleomorphism and prominence of nucleoli) that achieved a 99.5% sensitivity and 57% specificity of myoinvasion detection in the challenge set. The complicated architectural patterns that are illustrated are quite varied and include a cribriform pattern, although many of the profiles appear to vary only in degree from those seen in EIN. Another study used objective computerized morphometry applied to a similar training set of biopsies with and without accompanying myoinvasive disease.[16] Parameters of gland outer surface density (outer gland perimeter), volume percentage epithelium (volume of glands including lumens relative to the entire specimen), epithelial thickness, and nuclear shape variation were combined in a 4-Class Rule to yield probability estimates of myoinvasion likelihood.

Ability of the 4-Class Rule to predict deep myoinvasion was confirmed in a recent Gynecologic Oncology Group study.[128] Biopsy classification into one of the two highest grade categories captured 92% of the deep myoinvasive cancer outcomes. Biopsy classification in one of the two lower grade categories had excellent negative predictive value for deep myoinvasion (99%). Larger scale architectural parameters measuring epithelial abundance (volume percentage epithelium, outer surface density, epithelial thickness) were most associated with presence or absence of myoinvasion at any depth. Variation in nuclear size (anisokaryosis, measured as standard deviation of nuclear diameter) emerged as the single variable most associated with deep myoinvasion. These morphometric data confirm an earlier observation which showed that the presence of extreme nuclear pleomorphism worsens clinical outcome relative to that expected by architectural features alone.[191]

In biopsy specimens, extremely well-differentiated carcinomas that arise in the region of the junction between the lower uterine segment and the upper endocervix and that contain some mucin can be extremely difficult to distinguish from endocervical squamous metaplasia with mucin. Both show cells with moderate eosinophilia, occasional cells with intracytoplasmic mucin, and, of concern, small foci with a cribriform pattern. At times the distinction cannot be made, and in these cases the pathologist should clearly communicate to the gynecologist that further evaluation is necessary. Sometimes, hysterectomy must be performed to adequately document the presence of the tumor.

Well-differentiated endometrioid adenocarcinoma with myometrial invasion may be difficult to distinguish from *atypical polypoid adenomyoma* as both contain glands with architectural atypia, separated by tissue that is predominantly smooth muscle. The squamous morules that are characteristic of atypical polypoid adenomyoma may be mistaken for squamous change in endometrial adenocarcinoma (Figure 16.34). Women with atypical polypoid adenomyoma are generally younger than those with classic endometrioid carcinomas, but these are not necessarily mutually exclusive entities. Many atypical polypoid adenomyomas recur, and many will have obvious cancer at hysterectomy.

Poorly differentiated carcinomas composed of extensive solid tumor may show spindled cells and give a 'pseudosarcomatous' appearance. Just because there are recognizable glands does not mean the tumor is biphasic and may lead to an erroneous diagnosis of *carcinosarcoma*. Conversely, it is also apparent that the mesenchymal and epithelial elements of carcinosarcomas may both show reactivity with cytokeratins and vimentin.[7,49,116] Thus, cytokeratin reactivity in the stromal element does not necessarily mean that carcinoma is present in a sarcoma. In some cases a distinction is impossible to make.

The interpretation of *menstrual endometrium* or endometrium with glandular and stromal breakdown in curettings may give rise to difficulties, especially in differentiation with adenocarcinoma. The absence of stroma between the glandular elements may give the impression of confluent glands or in some cases even of solid epithelial growth. The piled up epithelium may lose nuclear polarity and acquire prominent nucleoli. However, the coarse chromatin and nuclear pleomorphism of malignancy are lacking and a genuine cribriform pattern and invasion are never present. Mitoses are lacking. Furthermore, the glands of menstrual endometrium regularly exhibit some residual secretory change and a careful search will identify typical areas of stromal fragmentation as opposed to areas of coagulative necrosis (see Chapter 12).

The *metaplastic changes* described in Chapter 14 may be difficult to distinguish from carcinoma, particularly when associated with EIN. Hormonally induced metaplasias, such as tubal metaplasia resulting from estrogen stimulation, have a distinctive topography in which metaplastic glands are diffusely interspersed amongst non-metaplastic glands. This differs from the expanding geographic foci of premalignant and malignant neoplastic processes. While careful attention to cytologic features, the architectural pattern, and lack of invasion should enable the correct diagnosis to be made, the presence of metaplastic changes, not infrequently, is associated with cancer.

The distinction between endometrial adenocarcinoma and *endocervical adenocarcinoma* may be difficult, if not impossible, to make in curettings. Fractional curettage assists in delimiting sites of involvement, but surface extension along the lower uterine segment may lead to a distribution at diagnosis well beyond the original site of origin. Even though most endometrial carcinomas are of endometrioid type and most endocervical carcinomas are of mucinous type, endometrioid carcinomas may arise in the cervix and mucinous adenocarcinomas not uncommonly arise in the endometrium. Further, tumors involving the endocervix, lower uterine segment, and corpus may show progressive changes in the extent of mucinous differentiation, thus further hindering assignment of the area of origin by biopsy alone.

An immunostain panel of three markers can help in the differential diagnosis. Estrogen receptor and vimentin are more likely to be expressed in endometrial than cervical adenocarcinomas, whereas cervical adenocarcinomas more frequently express carcinoembryonic antigen (CEA).[7,116] Recently, p16 immunohistochemistry has proven useful in the distinction, particularly when combined with other markers such as estrogen receptor, vimentin, and CEA.[132] In particular, strong immunoreactivity for p16 in all tumor cells is more frequently found in endocervical than in endometrial adenocarcinoma.[13] Reactivity for integrated human papillomavirus (HPV) in DNA isolated from tumor tissue strongly supports a cervical origin, as it is present in 80–90% of cervical and essentially no endometrial adenocarcinomas.[123,141] Tissue processing and HPV polymerase chain reaction testing for this purpose are not generally available, however. The type of stroma may also be diagnostic. Clearly the presence of endometrial-type stroma supports an endometrial, rather than endocervical, origin.

A distinction has to be made among *papillary carcinomas* of the endometrium. The villoglandular variant of endometrioid adenocarcinoma, serous adenocarcinoma, clear cell adenocarcinoma, and mucinous adenocarcinoma may all have a papillary architecture. Villoglandular endometrioid adenocarcinoma consists of cells characteristic of the endometrioid type. Columnar and darkly staining, they are well differentiated, usually with little nuclear atypia. The epithelial cells of serous carcinoma tend to be small and cuboidal rather than columnar, and nuclear atypia is often marked. Indeed, an immediately obvious discrepancy between high-grade nuclear changes in an apparently well-differentiated adenocarcinoma (irrespective of growth pattern) should alert the pathologist to the possibility of a serous carcinoma. Clear cell adenocarcinomas rarely only show papillary areas. Usually solid areas of clear cells and tubulocystic areas with a 'hobnail' pattern of the epithelium are also present. The morphology of the epithelial cells in mucinous adenocarcinoma, with regular, basal nuclei and abundant, mucin-rich cytoplasm allows the distinction from other papillary carcinomas of the endometrium to be made easily.

Behavior and treatment

Endometrioid adenocarcinoma and its variants present early, mainly because the predominant symptom is postmenopausal bleeding, which is both obvious and alarming. What is rarely acknowledged, even in gynecology texts, is that many endometrial carcinomas are asymptomatic. Eighty per cent of patients present with clinical stage 1 disease, although some are found to have more advanced disease at surgery. Five-year survival rates are currently 96% for stage 1 disease, 67% for stage 2, and 23% for stage 3.[144] The behavior of the variants is the same, grade for grade, as that of typical endometrioid adenocarcinoma.[161]

The standard treatment is surgical, consisting of hysterectomy with bilateral salpingo-oophorectomy, with or without adjuvant radiotherapy. Practices vary regarding pelvic and para-aortic lymph node dissection. These additional procedures are rarely undertaken in the United Kingdom but may be carried out in the United States and other parts of the world, particularly central Europe, if frozen section of the hysterectomy specimen demonstrates deep myometrial invasion, cervical involvement, or a non-endometrioid type. Local delivery of high-dose progestins by hormone-impregnated intrauterine devices may be effective in controlling local disease with a low rate of systemic complications.[121] Systemic treatment with progestins may be beneficial but, as the tumors that respond are those with estrogen and progesterone receptors that are of early stage and low grade with a favorable outcome anyway, practical use of these agents is limited.[56,142] Chemotherapy and adjunctive radiotherapy are still being evaluated for advanced and recurrent disease.[14,158,180]

Appearances following radiation

Curetted specimens may be received following radiation therapy for endometrial carcinoma. Occasionally the radiation may be given preoperatively. The tumor's histologic response to radiation is variable and sometimes no changes can be detected. It is usual for changes to be seen in both neoplastic and non-neoplastic epithelial cells. Most prominent among these are nuclear enlargement, pleomorphism, and hyperchromasia, often resulting in markedly bizarre forms (Figure 16.35). As these alterations are seen in both benign and malignant cells, identifying residual carcinoma can be difficult.

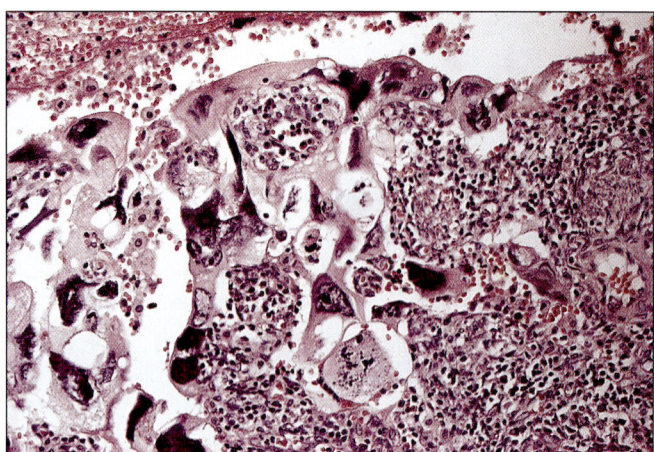

Fig. 16.35 Endometrial adenocarcinoma. Appearances following radiation.

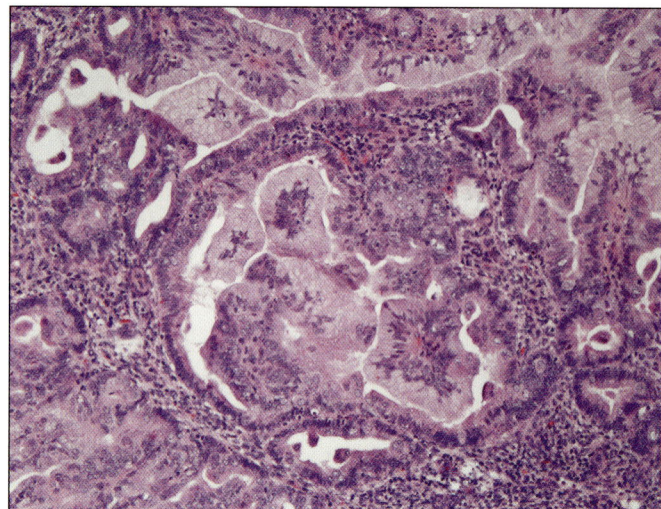

Fig. 16.36 Endometrial adenocarcinoma, endometrioid type, with mucinous differentiation. An area of mucinous carcinoma is present in the center.

MUCINOUS ADENOCARCINOMA

Definition
An endometrial carcinoma composed predominantly of cells containing prominent intracytoplasmic mucin, resembling the mucinous tumors found in the endocervix. Mucinous adenocarcinoma comprises 1–9% of all endometrial adenocarcinomas.[120,148] Mucinous endometrial adenocarcinomas usually arise in conjunction with an endometrioid component, and thus can be considered within the endometrioid class of endometrial carcinomas.

Clinical features
The clinical features and presentation of women with mucinous adenocarcinoma of the endometrium are similar to those with endometrioid adenocarcinoma. A higher frequency of mucinous adenocarcinomas is reported in patients receiving tamoxifen and synthetic progestogens,[37,45] suggesting that there might be a different histogenetic mechanism for this tumor, namely, progestogens encouraging mucinous metaplasia.[37,45]

Gross features
No macroscopic features distinguish mucinous from endometrioid adenocarcinoma, apart from the infrequent prominence of the secreted tenacious mucus.

Microscopic features
Mucinous adenocarcinoma of the endometrium resembles mucinous tumors found in the endocervix. While many endometrial carcinomas contain focal mucin, the mucinous component in a mucinous adenocarcinoma should involve at least half the cells.[161] The involved cells are tall with basal nuclei and prominent intracytoplasmic mucin (Figures 16.36 and 16.37). Mucicarmine, periodic acid-Schiff (PAS) and Alcian blue are all useful to amplify the staining. Most tumors are well differentiated (grade 1) but grade 2 and grade 3 tumors are occasionally described.[120] More likely than not, poorly differentiated tumors lose their ability to produce mucin. Lymph node metastases may be extremely well differentiated. Mucinous adenocarcinoma differs from benign and premalignant mucinous metaplasia by the usual criterion of malignancy.[148]

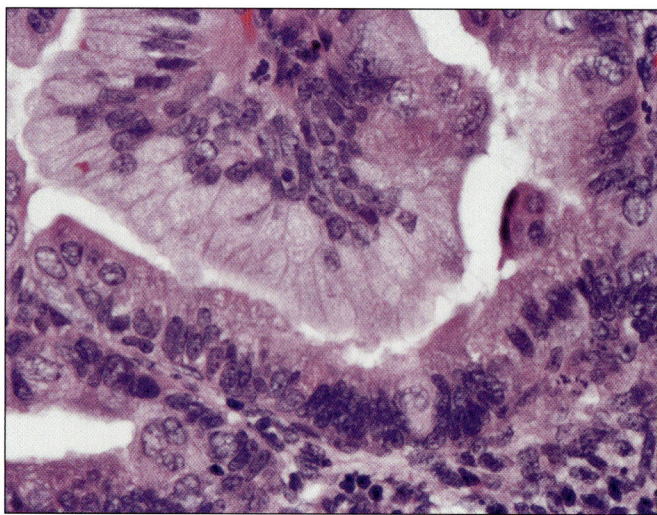

Fig. 16.37 Endometrial adenocarcinoma, endometrioid type, with mucinous differentiation. Detail of columnar cells with cytoplasmic mucin.

In some cases exophytic complex filiform papillary fragments of mucinous endometrial adenocarcinoma are encountered in biopsy specimens. An extremely bland cytology, rare mitoses, and a tendency to break apart into small fragments make these tumors extremely difficult to recognize, as they resemble endocervical epithelium. The abundance of mucinous epithelium, delicate supportive stroma, and alternating mucinous and non-mucinous differentiation (Figure 16.38), often coexisting with a microglandular component (Figure 16.39),[187,192] are typical.[131] At hysterectomy, non-exophytic regions of tumor are commonly seen, and these may or may not retain the extensive mucinous differentiation of the papillary surface tumor (Figure 16.40).

Behavior and treatment
The behavior of mucinous adenocarcinoma is that of endometrioid carcinomas. As most are well differentiated, the prognosis is generally favorable.[164] Treatment is primarily surgical.

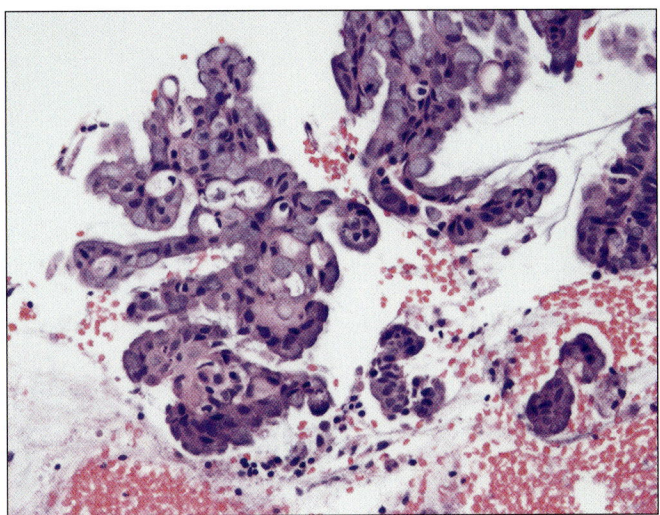

Fig. 16.38 Endometrial adenocarcinoma, endometrioid type, with mucinous differentiation. Exophytic fronds of branching mucinous epithelium contain microcribriform structures.

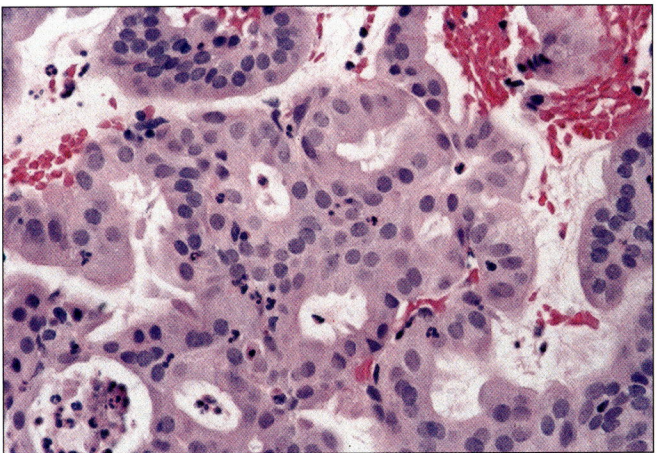

Fig. 16.39 Microglandular cribriform architecture in an endometrial adenocarcinoma, endometrioid type, with mucinous differentiation.

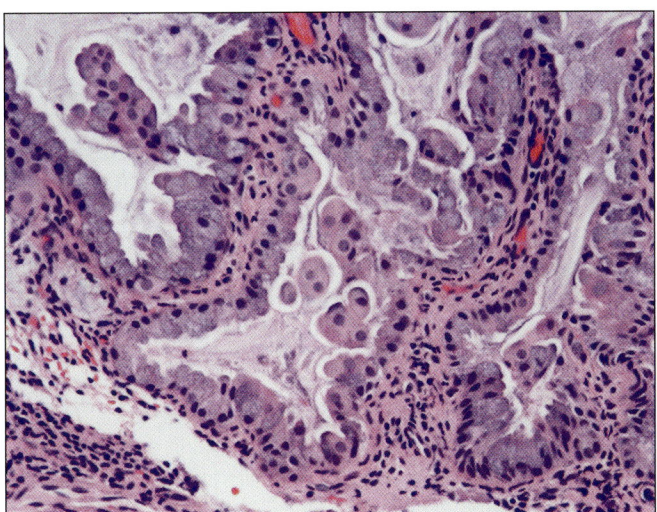

Fig. 16.40 Endometrial adenocarcinoma, endometrioid type, with mucinous differentiation. Non-exophytic component of same tumor as Figure 16.38 showing a greater degree of endometrioid differentiation and scattered intracytoplasmic mucin.

SQUAMOUS CELL CARCINOMA

Definition
An endometrial carcinoma composed entirely of malignant squamous epithelium, similar to squamous cell carcinomas found elsewhere.

Clinical features
Squamous cell carcinoma of the endometrium is rare. The median age of patients is 61 years, similar to that of endometrioid adenocarcinoma.[91] Earlier reports included a high proportion of women who had endometritis and pyometra but this has been less apparent for the last four decades.[91] Many cases are associated with benign squamous metaplasia of the endometrium (ichthyosis uteri), a condition encountered only in older women, often in association with intrauterine infection. The clinical presentation is no different from that of endometrioid carcinoma.

Gross features
There are no gross features that distinguish squamous cell carcinoma from endometrioid adenocarcinoma.

Microscopic features
The tumor's microscopic appearance resembles that of squamous cell carcinomas found in other sites (Figures 16.41–16.43). It has long been believed that the diagnosis should be made only if there is no evidence of coexistent adenocarcinoma and if careful examination of the cervix excludes a primary tumor in that organ. Where squamous cell carcinoma is present synchronously in both the uterine body and cervix, the assumption has been that the tumor originated in the cervix and spread upwards. More recent views suggest that sometimes the opposite may be true, namely, that some fraction start in the endometrium and spread to the cervix.[46] Another alternative is that some squamous cell carcinomas are overgrowths of adenosquamous carcinomas.

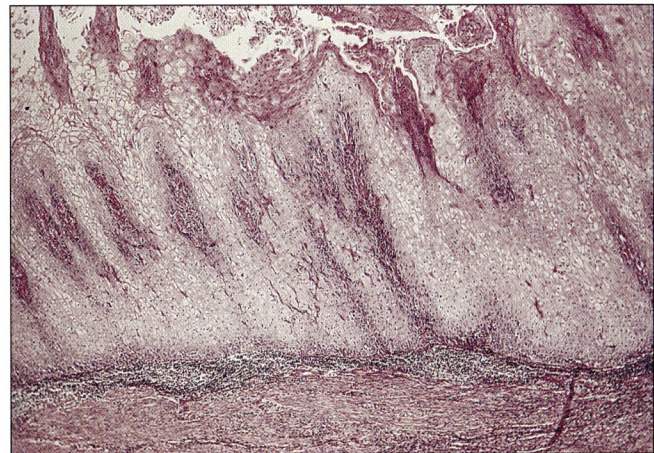

Fig. 16.41 Icthyosis uteri. The entire endometrium, with the exception of a little basal stroma, is replaced by stratified squamous epithelium. Squamous cell carcinoma was present adjacent to this field (see Figure 16.44) but it is difficult to decide whether the appearances shown here amount to carcinoma or not.

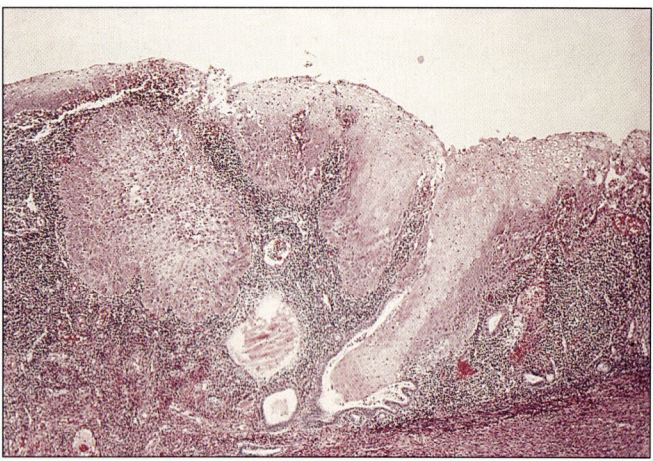

Fig. 16.42 Squamous cell carcinoma, arising in a field of squamous metaplasia ('ichthyosis uteri').

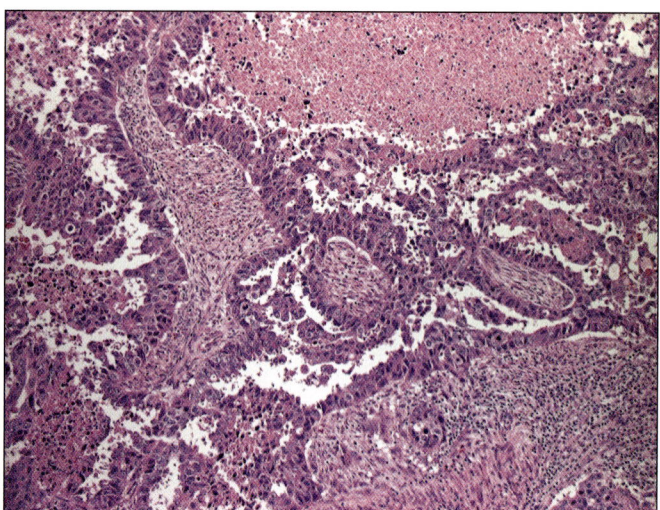

Fig. 16.44 Endometrial adenocarcinoma, serous type.

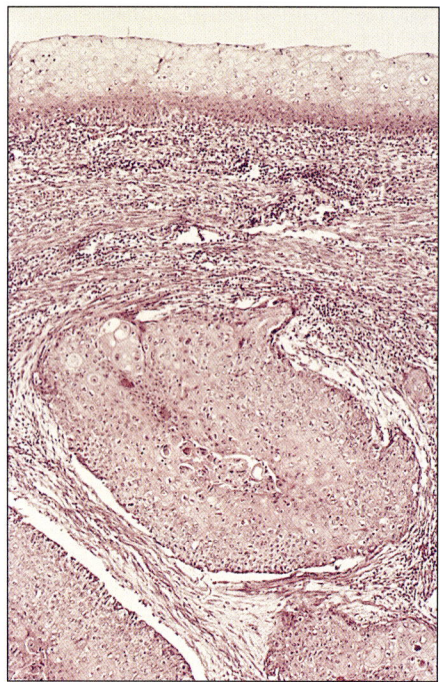

Fig. 16.43 Squamous cell carcinoma. Apparently benign squamous metaplasia is also present, replacing the overlying endometrium.

Behavior and treatment

The prognosis is exceedingly poor,[164] with 26% of reported cases surviving only a median of 9 months after diagnosis.[91] Treatment is primarily by surgery. Adjunctive radiotherapy does not improve survival. The addition of cisplatin-based chemotherapy to postoperative radiotherapy may prolong survival in some patients.[91,168]

SEROUS ADENOCARCINOMA

Definition

Serous adenocarcinoma is an aggressive form of endometrial cancer exhibiting a predominantly papillary architecture com-

posed of exfoliative bulbous hobnail-like cells with marked nuclear atypia. Although 'serous adenocarcinoma' is the tumor's official name, the term 'papillary serous carcinoma' is more commonly used synonymously in the literature.

Clinical features

Serous adenocarcinoma is a poor prognostic form of endometrial cancer.[76,159] It accounts for 1–10% of all endometrial cancers. It is lower in population-based studies but higher in reports from gynecologic oncology centers.[1,159] The patients are generally about 4–10 years older than women with endometrioid carcinomas, rarely have received exogenous estrogen therapy, and lack previous or concurrent EIN or hyperplasia.[78] Most women are parous (90%). Few are obese (10%) or have diabetes.[70] Typically they have normal serum estrogen levels.[162]

Gross features

Serous carcinomas generally have the same gross features as endometrioid carcinomas, although many appear as bulky, necrotic masses.[160] The uterus is more frequently atrophic as compared with endometrioid carcinomas.

Microscopic features

Histologically, serous adenocarcinomas closely resemble the more common ovarian serous carcinomas in their many guises (see Chapter 24). They typically have complex, branching papillae with usually broad, thick fibrovascular cores, but occasionally thin to delicate cores (Figure 16.44). The papillae are covered by a stratified epithelium with a prominent and very characteristic tufting or budding pattern, with many groups of detached cells lying free between the papillae (Figure 16.45). This pattern notwithstanding, serous adenocarcinoma may also show a glandular or solid pattern. Unlike endometrioid adenocarcinoma, the glandular structures are irregularly shaped and often lined by polygonal rather than columnar cells.[159] The nuclei are usually high grade, with marked pleomorphism and large macronucleoli along with occasional bizarre and hyperchromatic giant nuclei. Psammoma bodies are found in about 25% of cases (Figure 16.46).[51] A high percentage of cases exhibit striking lymphovascular invasion

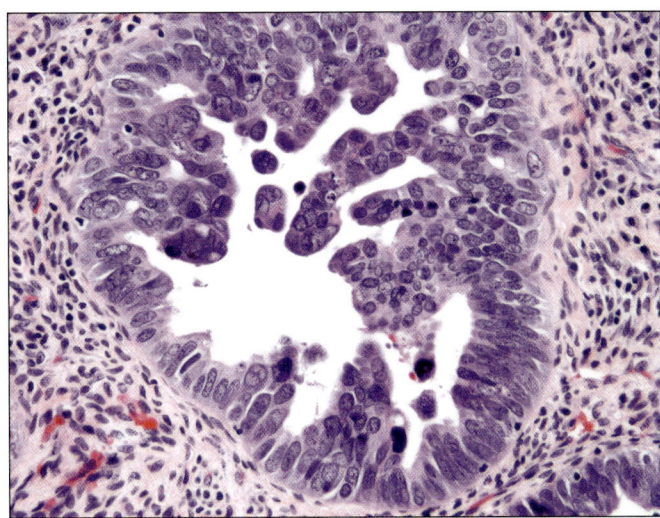

Fig. 16.45 Endometrial adenocarcinoma, serous type. High-grade nuclei with exfoliation in a 'hobnail' pattern.

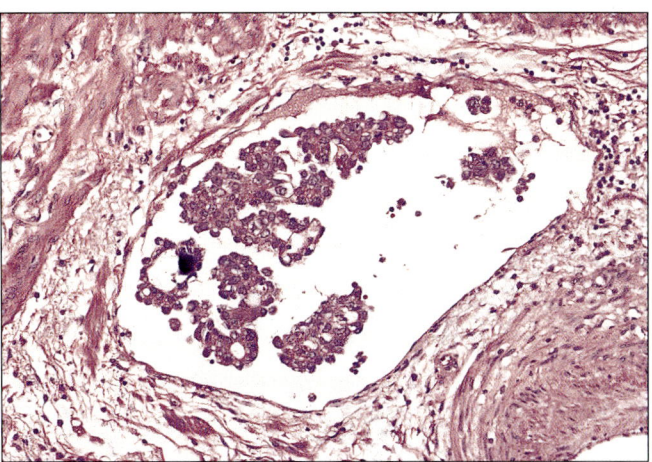

Fig. 16.47 Endometrial adenocarcinoma, serous papillary pattern. Tumor in a myometrial lymphatic.

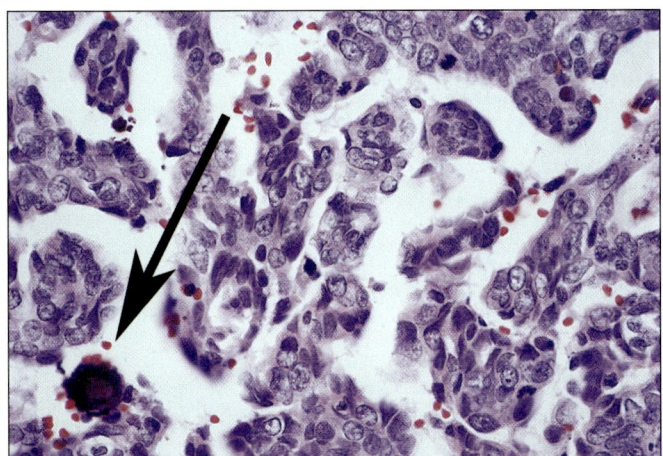

Fig. 16.46 Endometrial adenocarcinoma, serous type. A psammoma body (arrow) is present.

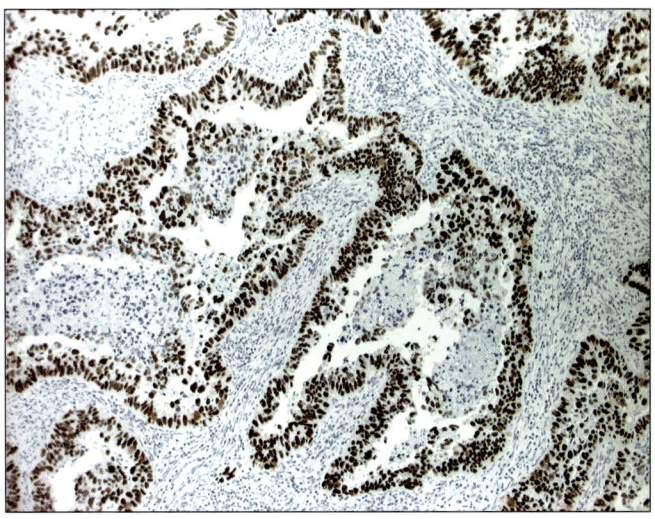

Fig. 16.48 Endometrial adenocarcinoma, serous type. Intense nuclear p53 staining of almost all tumor cells indicates clonal *p53* mutation.

(Figure 16.47) and deep myometrial invasion.[76] Serous endometrial carcinomas also have a higher incidence of cervical and lower uterine segment involvement.[108]

Serous adenocarcinoma of the endometrium may occur in a pure form or associated with other types of endometrial carcinoma, such as endometrioid or clear cell adenocarcinoma, or it may be found in endometrial polyps.[160,163] These mixed tumors have the same poor prognosis as pure serous carcinomas and should be treated as serous carcinomas if at least one-fourth of the tumor has features of serous differentiation.[159] Unlike its ovarian counterpart, serous adenocarcinoma of the endometrium is not graded but considered high grade by definition.[173]

Immunohistochemistry

The molecular changes of *p53* mutation in 80–90% of serous carcinomas is reflected in *p53* immunohistochemistry, which typically shows a diffuse and intense nuclear staining pattern involving almost all tumor cells (Figure 16.48).[102,160] Less frequently, *p53* frameshift mutations lead to a truncated protein that is not detected by the antibodies.[102] Ki-67 immunohistochemistry shows a high labeling index (about 40%) in serous carcinoma, and estrogen and progesterone receptors are absent or only weakly expressed in most tumors.[104] The *PTEN* gene is intact, and expressed in normal levels in most serous carcinomas.[48]

PRECURSOR LESIONS

SEROUS ENDOMETRIAL INTRAEPITHELIAL CARCINOMA (SEROUS EIC)

Recently, serous EIC has been described and hypothesized as the immediate precursor of serous adenocarcinoma.[10,160] Serous EIC exhibits single or multiple layers of malignant cells that

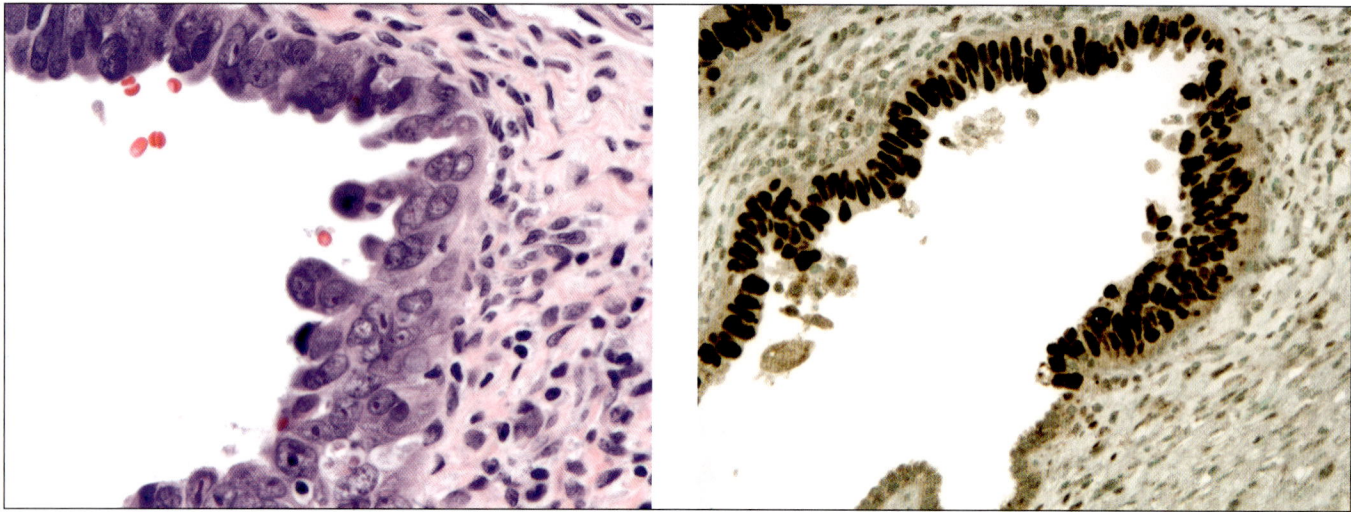

Fig. 16.49 Serous EIC spreading over endometrial surfaces. Hobnail pattern with highly atypical nuclei that are reactive with p53.

replace the endometrial surface epithelium or glands. The cells have pleomorphic nuclei and frequent mitotic figures, resembling the cells of high-grade tumor. Immunoreactivity resembles that seen in uterine serous adenocarcinomas (Figure 16.49), including intense nuclear staining for p53, high Ki-67 index, and loss of estrogen (Figure 16.50) and progesterone receptors.[160]

Serous EIC is frequently and specifically associated with concurrent serous adenocarcinoma of the endometrium but may be observed in association with clear cell adenocarcinoma.[10,104] Isolated serous EIC, a very rare lesion,[194] demonstrates intrinsically malignant behavior, as it has the capacity for peritoneal metastasis to abdominal sites.[17,186] In one study the endocervix was involved by serous EIC in 22% of women with uterine serous carcinoma, the fallopian tube in 5% of cases, the ovary in 10%, and the peritoneal surfaces or omentum in 25% of cases.[159] Extensive serous EIC may cover most of the surface and the glands of the endometrium and, thus, can hardly be distinguished from minimally invasive serous carcinoma.

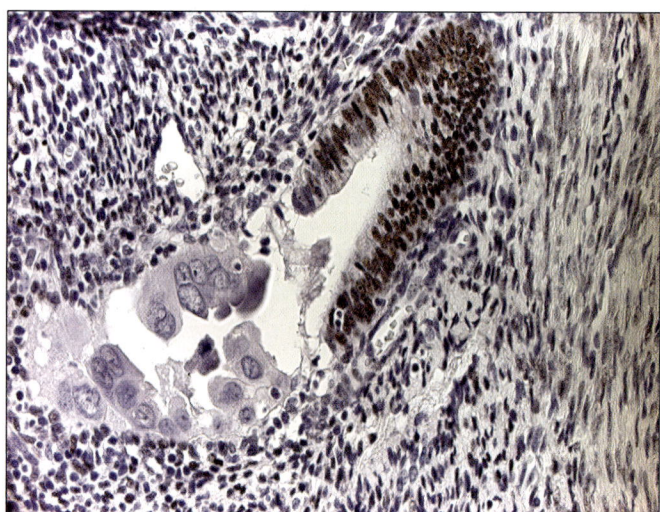

Fig. 16.50 Serous EIC extending into a pre-existing endometrial gland. Atypical malignant cells have lost estrogen receptor. ER immunohistochemistry.

ENDOMETRIAL GLANDULAR DYSPLASIA (EMGD)

Recently, an atypical glandular lesion of endometrium has been described and designated endometrial glandular dysplasia (EmGD) (Figure 16.51).[186a,195] It has been proposed as a putative precursor of serous EIC[106] based on histologic similarities, molecular p53 staining, and loss of heterozygosity patterns. A new cytoplasmic marker for serous endometrial cancer, which is called insulin-like growth factor II mRNA binding protein 3 (IMP3) and serves in an oncofetal protein function, has an increased level of expression from EmGD (14%) to serous EIC (89%) to serous adenocarcinoma (94%). At this time, the nature, biology, and clinical importance of this lesion is still in debate and controversial. In particular, its frequency in endometrium without cancer is unknown and its clinical impact has not been validated. Finally, EmGD might be confused with reactive changes.

Endometrial glandular dysplasia usually involves single glands or small groups of glands mostly under 1 mm in size but may occasionally reach 2 mm in maximum diameter. The nuclei are either hyperchromatic or vesicular with clumped chromatin but never show the severe degree of nuclear atypia of serous EIC and serous adenocarcinoma. Endometrial glandular dysplasia is frequently found associated with serous EIC (75%) and more frequently with serous compared to endometrioid adenocarcinoma (53% vs 2%).

Differential diagnosis

Serous adenocarcinoma must be distinguished from its papillary endometrioid counterpart, villoglandular adenocarcinoma.[190] Architecturally, villoglandular adenocarcinoma

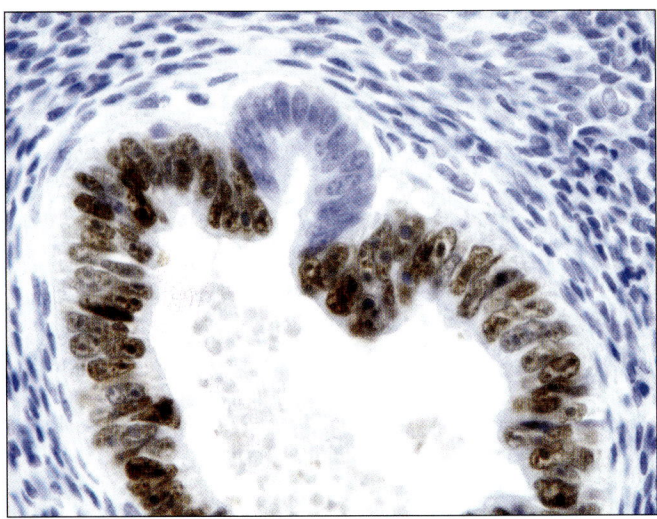

Fig. 16.51 Endometrial glandular dysplasia (EmGD). Pseudostratified moderately atypical glandular cells with patchy p53 staining are characteristic of EmGD. p53 immunohistochemistry.

exhibits long delicate papillae usually covered by columnar epithelium with pseudostratified nuclei, whereas serous carcinoma shows plump papillae with tufting. On a cellular basis, nuclear atypia is only mild to moderate in villoglandular carcinoma compared to the marked nuclear atypia in serous carcinoma. Serous carcinomas with a predominant glandular pattern should not be confused with endometrioid adenocarcinomas since the latter usually reveal more regularly shaped glands and less nuclear atypia.

Overlap of cellular features exists between serous and clear cell carcinomas.[159] In particular, hobnail-shaped cells, which are characteristic of clear cell carcinoma, may also occur in serous carcinoma but they are usually larger. In contrast to clear cell carcinomas, serous carcinomas lack a tubulocystic or a solid pattern as well as stromal hyalinization, and lack a considerable amount of cells with clear cytoplasm. Compared to clear cell carcinomas, serous carcinomas may also show substantial nuclear polymorphism and frequent mitoses.

Behavior and treatment

The most striking feature of endometrial serous adenocarcinoma is its aggressive behavior leading to a poor overall prognosis (14% 10-year survival). This poor outcome particularly relates to frequent extrauterine disease at the time of diagnosis; 72% of patients whose disease preoperatively appears confined to the uterus already have extrauterine disease found at operation.[70] Even minimal myometrial invasion is frequently associated with widespread disease.[33]

Early clinical studies have shown poor outcome for stage 1 cases, but this may be due in part to incomplete staging procedures.[69] Cancer death may even occur in stage 1A disease.[34] Grade and depth of myometrial invasion are not significant predictors for peritoneal spread of disease.[70] Most likely, this reflects spread via tubal reflux and subsequent peritoneal carcinomatosis,[166] which is unusual for other forms of endometrial cancer. There is no evidence that endometrial serous carcinoma is a component of a multifocal disease process

arising independently in the endometrium, and pelvic and abdominal serosa. On the other hand, spread of serous adenocarcinoma originating from the fallopian tube[43] or ovaries into the uterine cavity through the fallopian tubes cannot be ruled out as a potential source for the uterine tumor, and certainly has been seen in our practices on occasion. Not surprisingly, a disproportionately large fraction of patients with relapsed endometrial carcinomas have serous adenocarcinoma. Whereas serous adenocarcinomas comprise less than 10% of endometrial carcinomas, they account for about 50% of treatment failures.[76]

First-line treatment for women with endometrial serous carcinoma is surgery: total abdominal hysterectomy with bilateral salpingo-oophorectomy with or without pelvic and para-aortic node dissection. Because this tumor is aggressive, some form of adjunctive therapy is desirable but it is not yet clear which type is most effective. The platinum-based chemotherapeutic agents that are widely used for ovarian serous carcinoma appear to be of limited value and the results of trials using various protocols of irradiation are awaited.[78] Patients with early-stage disease have a survival advantage, underlining the need for precise staging procedures.[90]

CLEAR CELL ADENOCARCINOMA

Definition

An endometrial adenocarcinoma exhibiting clear or sometimes eosinophilic cells and 'hobnail'-shaped cells arranged in a papillary, tubulocystic or solid pattern, similar to the clear cell adenocarcinomas that occur in the vagina, cervix, and ovary.

Clinical features

Clear cell adenocarcinomas account for 1–6% of endometrial carcinomas and occur at an older age (mean age 65–69 years) than endometrioid adenocarcinoma.[2,33,164] The women generally are less often obese, less often have diabetes mellitus, and less frequently have taken hormone-replacement therapy.[38,89] Like all other forms of endometrial cancer, bleeding is the most common initial clinical manifestation.

Gross features

There are no gross features that distinguish clear cell adenocarcinoma from other varieties of endometrial carcinoma but, like serous carcinoma, it occurs more frequently on a background of an atrophic endometrium.

Microscopic features

Clear cell adenocarcinomas occur in the vagina, cervix, and ovary as well as the endometrium. The histologic appearances are the same at all sites and are striking and unmistakable, both because of the variety of patterns presented and the characteristic nature of the patterns themselves. In order of decreasing frequency the most common patterns are papillary (Figure 16.52), glandular, solid (Figure 16.53), and tubulocystic (Figure 16.54). Most clear cell adenocarcinomas have a mixture of at least two of these patterns. The epithelial cells lining the cysts in the tubulocystic areas frequently contain very little cytoplasm, so that the enlarged and pleomorphic nuclei appear to protrude into the lumens, presenting a 'hobnail' appearance

(Figure 16.55). However, the most prominent diagnostic feature of the clear cell adenocarcinoma is clear cytoplasm in many cells (although not necessarily the majority). Nothing in the cytoplasm stains with H&E since the glycogen that is present is leached out during normal fixation and processing. Mucin, if present, is found only in the lumens of the glands formed by the clear cells. None is intracytoplasmic. The stroma may be dense and hyalinized, particularly in tubulocystic areas. Nuclear pleomorphism is often marked and the tumors are of a high nuclear grade. The frequency of mitotic figures is variable. Architectural grading is difficult, because the tumor is not structurally related to a normal tissue with which it can be compared. Nuclear grade may be used,[164] but the recent WHO classification considers clear cell adenocarcinomas as high grade by definition.[173]

Differential diagnosis

Clear cell adenocarcinoma has to be separated particularly from secretory and serous endometrial carcinoma as well as from yolk sac tumor. Secretory carcinoma, a variant of endo-

metrioid adenocarcinoma, usually shows a glandular pattern with well-formed glands but it may become solid and, subsequently, be difficult to distinguish from clear cell carcinoma. Usually, nuclear atypia and polymorphism are less pronounced in secretory compared to clear cell carcinoma. The cells of secretory carcinoma are typically columnar with rectangular subnuclear vesicles imitating early secretory endometrium and not hobnail shaped. In addition, secretory carcinoma is rarely papillary or cystic, whereas these features are characteristic for many clear cell carcinomas.

Clear cell and serous carcinomas may at times have areas that are indistinguishable. However, both tumors have a range of patterns where there are differences. Serous carcinoma is rarely solid and does not show a tubulocystic pattern. It also lacks more than a few cells with clear cytoplasm. In some cases,

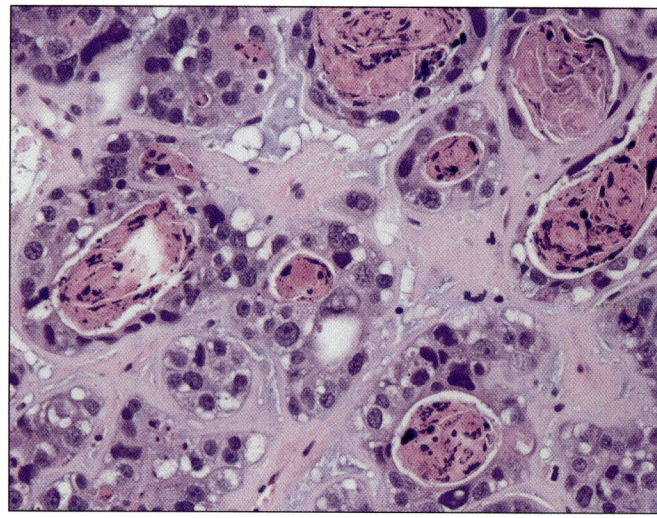

Fig. 16.54 Clear cell adenocarcinoma of endometrium, tubulocystic pattern.

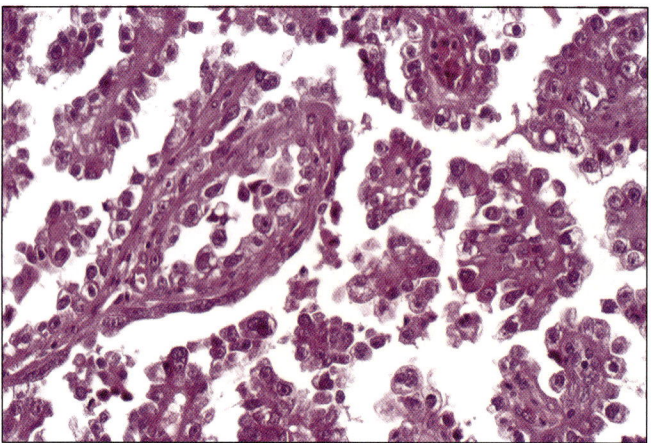

Fig. 16.52 Endometrial adenocarcinoma, clear cell type. A papillary area in a clear cell adenocarcinoma.

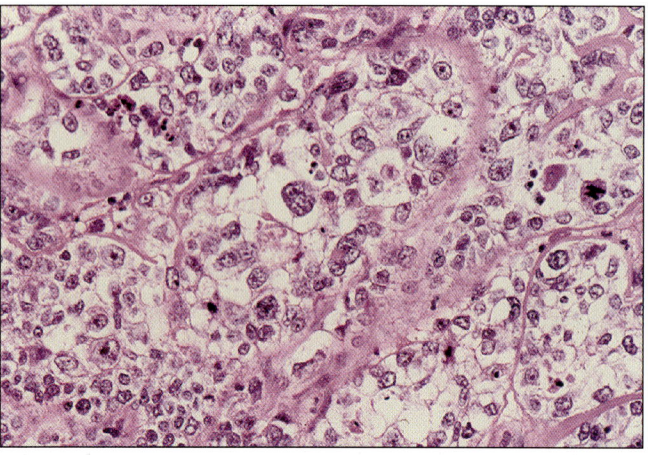

Fig. 16.53 Endometrial adenocarcinoma, clear cell type, solid growth.

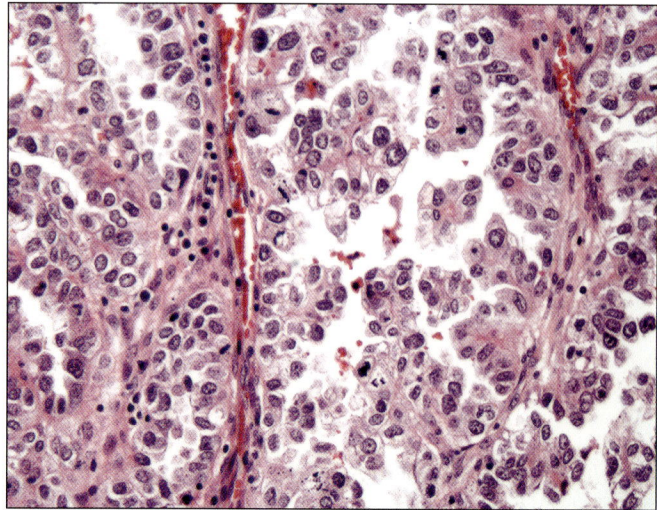

Fig. 16.55 Endometrial adenocarcinoma, clear cell pattern. An area of 'hobnailing'.

particularly in mixed serous and clear cell carcinomas, there may be an overlap of histologic features. There is evidence that p53 immunostaining is less pronounced in clear cell compared to serous carcinoma.[104] Due to similar clinical behaviors, the distinction between serous and clear cell carcinomas is far less important than the separation of secretory from clear cell carcinomas.

Yolk sac tumors, particularly with clear cytology, are rare in the uterus and exceedingly rare in the endometrium.[169] In contrast to clear cell carcinoma which typically occurs in the postmenopause, the patients are young, in the third or fourth decade. As Schiller–Duval bodies are seen in only a small minority of yolk sac tumors, detection of α-fetoprotein (AFP) or $α_1$-antitrypsin by immunohistochemistry as well as elevated serum AFP are helpful diagnostic tools.

Clear cell adenocarcinomas may at times be exceedingly difficult to distinguish from Arias-Stella change in the endometrium (Figure 16.56), but the differential is critical as therapy differs in diametrically opposed ways. While both show bulbous nuclear enlargement, pleomorphism, and hyperchromasia, the nuclear chromatin is virtually always smudged in Arias-Stella change, whereas the chromatin material in at least some areas in clear cell adenocarcinoma should be crisp. Other signs are often useful. Arias-Stella change is often associated with decidua and in women who are usually young, whereas clear cell adenocarcinoma may show solid areas composed of clear cells and the patients are invariably past the menopause.

Behavior and treatment

The prognosis for women with endometrial clear cell adenocarcinoma is poorer than for endometrioid carcinoma, with 5- and 10-year disease-free survival rates reported as 43–68% and 39%, respectively.[4,33] Two-thirds of patients suffer relapses outside the pelvis. Pathologic stage and age are the two most important prognostic factors.[4] Stage 1 tumors, particularly if confined to an endometrial polyp, are associated with a better prognosis.[33] Treatment is primarily surgical.

MIXED CARCINOMA

Although it is common to find small areas of one histologic type in a tumor that is predominantly of another type, it is uncommon where the mixture exceeds 10%. Such tumors are referred to as 'mixed carcinomas'. If 25% of an endometrial carcinoma is composed of serous carcinoma, the prognosis is that associated with serous carcinoma.[159] However, how the presence of 10–25% of tumor elements of an unfavorable histologic type affects prognosis is not clear.

UNDIFFERENTIATED CARCINOMA

This term, while semantically incorrect, is applied, by common usage, to those neoplasms that are demonstrably epithelial in nature but not otherwise differentiated. Less than 2% of endometrial tumors are classified as undifferentiated carcinomas.[3,161] Some of these are of large cell type and may show some attempt at gland formation. These are therefore probably the most

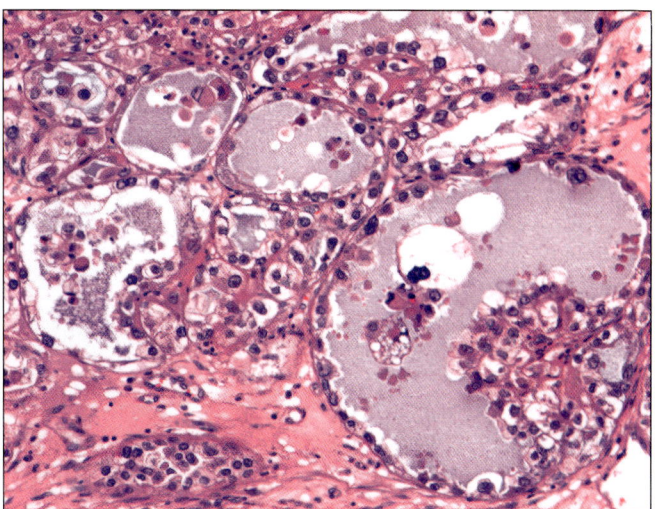

Fig. 16.56 Focus of exaggerated Arias-Stella phenomenon where the cells have pleomorphic, enlarged, and hyperchromatic nuclei that protrude into the glandular lumen, resulting in a 'hobnail' appearance. At times, this change is difficult to distinguish from clear cell adenocarcinoma. We have not encountered mitioses, but they have been reported to occur.

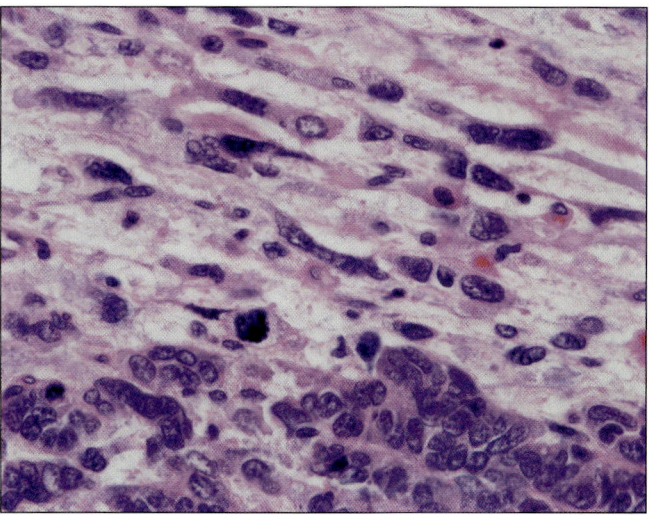

Fig. 16.57 Endometrial carcinosarcoma. Nests of high-grade epithelial carcinoma (bottom) are admixed with malignant cells that have undergone sarcomatous transformation (top).

anaplastic examples of the tumors described above. Other tumors described as undifferentiated carcinoma are of small cell type and a few have positive neuroendocrine markers. We classify these separately, even though no difference in survival has been shown between large cell and small cell types.[3] The prognosis is poor.

CARCINOSARCOMA

Endometrial carcinosarcomas are epithelial malignancies with a malignant mesenchymal component that may include homologous or heterologous sarcomatous elements (Figures 16.57

and 16.58). Long known as malignant mixed müllerian tumors (MMMT) or sometimes as malignant mixed mesodermal tumors, they were redesignated as endometrial carcinosarcomas by the WHO in 2003 to reflect current understanding that they are primarily epithelial tumors that have developed a mesenchymal component.[63,165]

Evidence suggests that carcinosarcomas share some molecular and epidemiologic risk factors with endometrioid-type endometrial carcinoma, including *PTEN* mutation,[8] microsatellite instability,[174] obesity, use of exogenous hormones, and nulliparity.[84,193] Carcinosarcomas, however, may demonstrate an expression profile independent of other forms of endometrial cancer,[115] and have a worse prognosis than other high-grade endometrial carcinomas.[179] Carcinosarcoma is sufficiently distinctive that it should be a separate entity of its own rather than considered as a subset of another endometrial tumor type. This tumor is discussed in greater detail in Chapter 17.

OTHER TYPES OF ENDOMETRIAL CARCINOMA

Small cell carcinomas (Figures 16.59 and 16.60), both with[181] and without[80] positive neuroendocrine markers, have been reported, some associated with paraneoplastic syndromes.[32,157] *Signet-ring cell carcinoma*,[122] *transitional cell carcinoma*,[66,107,170] *glassy cell carcinoma* (Figure 16.61),[74] *mucinous adenocarcinoma of intestinal* type,[117,192] and *lymphoepithelioma-like carcinoma*[183] have also been reported.

Endometrioid carcinomas with sertoliform differentiation[55,113,178] are tumors with areas composed of glands resembling sex cord-stromal tumors. The glands are in the form of closely packed tubules or trabeculae with basally oriented nuclei and clear to fibrillary cytoplasm (Figures 16.62 and 16.63). The non-sertoliform areas of the tumors consist of typical endometrioid adenocarcinoma (see also Chapter 17).

Another rare variant is *endometrial adenocarcinoma with trophoblastic differentiation*.[24,25,139,177] These tumors are poorly differentiated endometrial adenocarcinomas containing syncytiotrophoblast-like giant cells that are reactive for the beta

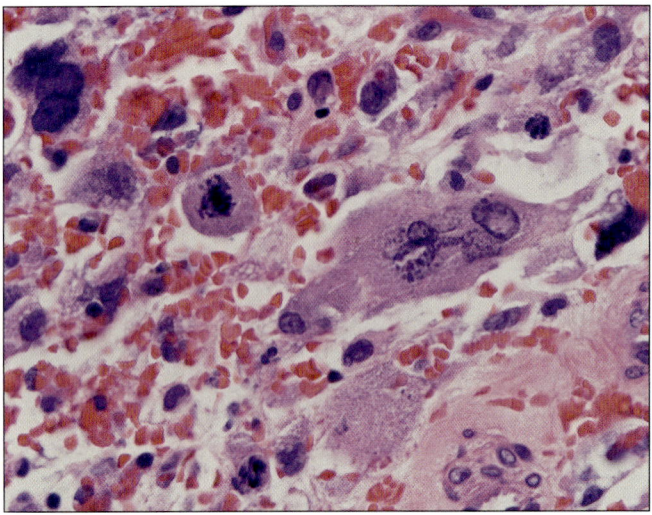

Fig. 16.58 Endometrial carcinosarcoma. Sarcomatous elements within endometrial carcinosarcoma demonstrating rhabdoid differentiation.

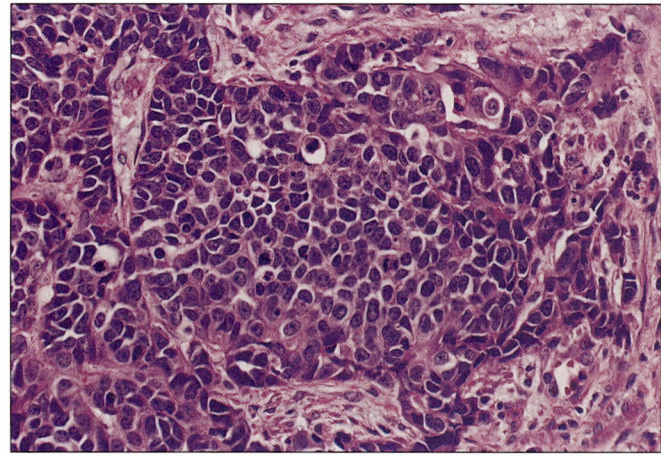

Fig. 16.60 Detail of small cell carcinoma.

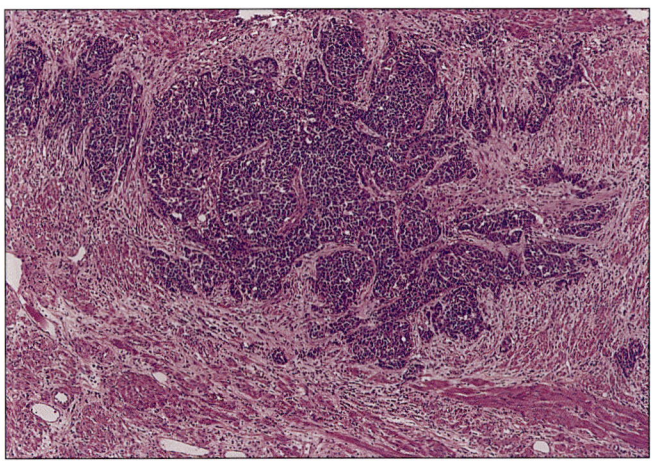

Fig. 16.59 Small cell carcinoma.

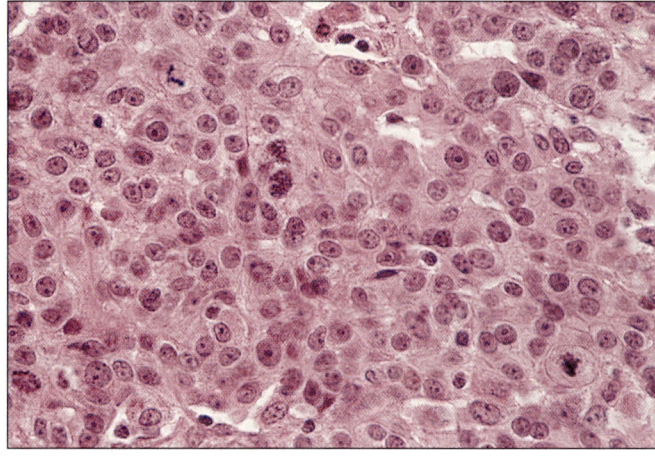

Fig. 16.61 Glassy cell carcinoma.

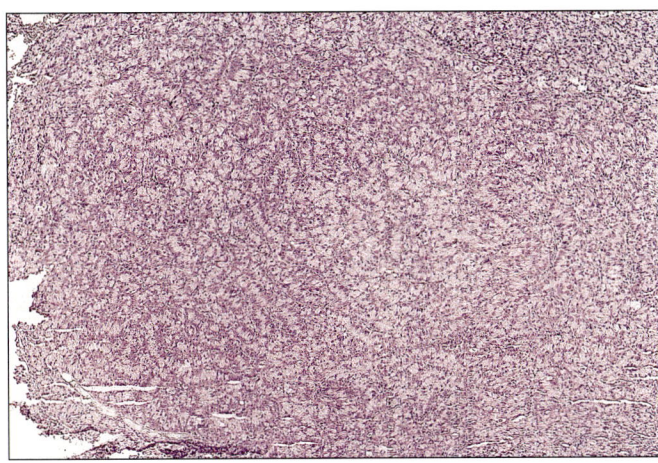

Fig. 16.62 Endometrial adenocarcinoma, sertoliform pattern.

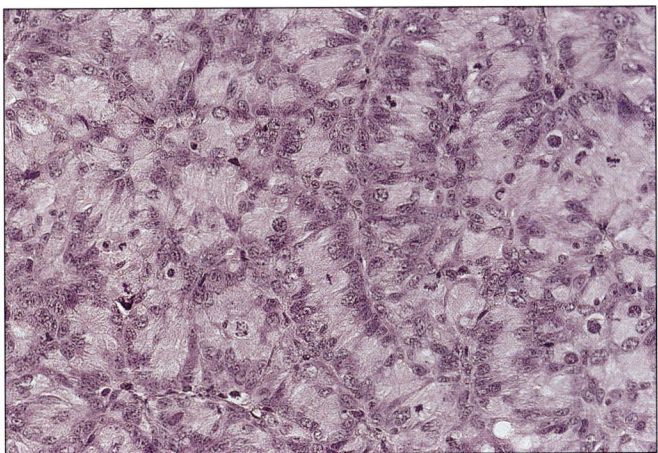

Fig. 16.63 Endometrial adenocarcinoma, detail of sertoliform pattern.

subunit of human chorionic gonadotrophin (hCG). Some patients also having raised levels of serum β-hCG.[25] Their clinical behavior is aggressive.

SYNCHRONOUS ENDOMETRIAL AND OVARIAN CARCINOMA

A perplexing problem encountered all too often by the practicing pathologist is to determine whether a tumor involving the endometrium and one or both ovaries has arisen in one organ and metastasized to the other(s), or whether the tumors are truly independent, but synchronous primaries.[188] This distinction can be very difficult when the histologies are similar but not exact, or if the tumor in the second organ occurs at a subsequent time. This distinction, however, is of great clinical importance, due to the significantly better prognosis of patients with synchronous primary tumors.

Several histologic features help distinguish primary from metastatic tumors in the endometrium and ovaries.[146] The presence of a precancerous process is strong evidence of *in situ* genesis. If the cancer is endometrioid, this would include EIN. Serous carcinomas do not have such a definitive counterpart for this purpose, because the presumed precursor lesion (serous EIC) is closely mimicked by secondary surface spread outwards from a main tumor mass. Potentially precancerous processes in the ovary, such as endometriosis or a pre-existing benign or borderline tumor of similar histologic type, suggest de novo development of the cancer in the ovary. Disparate histologic types (but not grade) of synchronous endometrial and ovarian tumors are also good evidence of independent primaries. On the other hand, similar histology cannot be taken as evidence of metastasis from one organ to the other. About 15–25% of ovarian tumors with endometrioid histology are associated with a histologically similar lesion in the endometrium. These lesions are usually regarded as well-differentiated independent neoplasms due to their high survival rates.

Multinodular implants on the surface of both ovaries favors metastatic disease rather than an ovarian primary. Synchronous tumors that are regarded as metastases are usually of high histologic grade, e.g., poorly differentiated endometrioid carcinomas, carcinosarcomas, and non-endometrioid carcinomas (serous and clear cell). Metastases from the ovary to the endometrium also occur, and most of these are surface spread of serous cancer via the fallopian tube. In these cases the uterus shows small tumor nodules perched on the superficial endometrium as might be expected of an implant. Such lesions are rare.

While many molecular tests are useful, most lack the specificity needed to be the magic bullet that distinguishes primary tumors from metastases. Conservation of highly specific molecular changes between tumors at different sites supports metastasis of a unicentric process.[85] There are, however, two fundamental barriers in applying this in practice: (1) independent tumors may share genetic alterations that are common players on the path to tumor formation; and (2) the most commonly performed tests (immunohistochemistry) examine nonspecific protein endpoints without characterizing more specific underlying genetic changes. An excellent example is p53 immunohistochemistry of synchronous ovarian and endometrial serous carcinomas. Irrespective of origin, most of these will abnormally accumulate p53 protein in their nuclei. DNA sequencing to characterize underlying mutations as shared or different is required to resolve them as unicentric versus multicentric processes. Such specialized, and expensive, sequence confirmation of mutations that serve as clonal 'markers' is not routine practice in most pathology departments today. Furthermore, there is the additional complication that metastases may acquire additional changes, making them genetically different from the primary tumor.

To help distinguish synchronous primary tumors from metastatic disease, several groups have tried to identify immunohistochemical changes that can serve as a diagnostic adjunct to histologic evaluation. Intranuclear accumulation of the developmental transcription factor WT1 is rarely (<10%) seen in serous carcinomas of endometrial origin,[5,53] in contrast to over 90% of extrauterine serous carcinomas (ovary, fallopian tube, peritoneum).[71,75] A practical limitation of using WT1 as a marker is a high frequency of randomly distributed staining heterogeneity. This makes many tumors

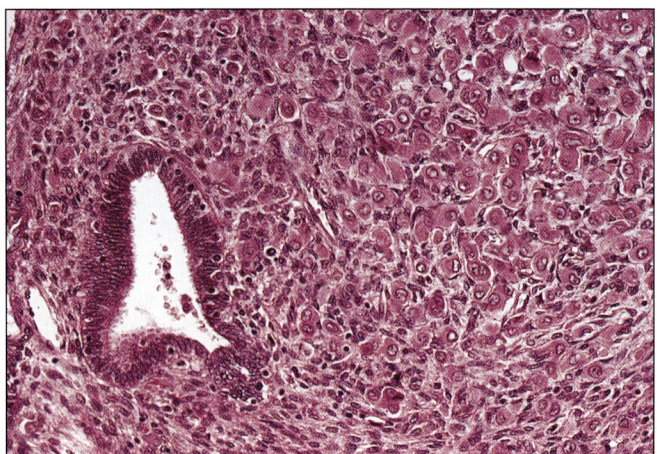

Fig. 16.64 Metastatic carcinoma. The metastatic carcinoma cells have copious cytoplasm and nondescript nuclei. The tumor cells diffusely permeate the stroma.

Table 16.4 Grading of endometrioid endometrial carcinoma*

Grade 1	5% or less of non-squamous solid growth
Grade 2	6–50% of non-squamous solid growth
Grade 3	More than 50% of non-squamous growth

*Serous, clear cell, and carcinosarcoma tumors are not graded.
Notable nuclear atypia inappropriately severe for the architectural grade of the tumor raises the grade by one (to a maximum of grade 3). In tumors with squamous differentiation, grading is based on the glandular component.

difficult to simply report as positive or negative, and leads to the expectation of some degree of staining discordance between primary tumor and its metastasis. Surprisingly, there is little literature exploring the utility of the well-established ovarian cancer marker CA125 in diagnosing synchronous primary tumors.

TUMORS METASTATIC TO THE ENDOMETRIUM

The most common tumors that metastasize to the endometrium are those that arise in the pelvis, cervical and ovarian carcinoma being the most frequent. Metastasis to the uterus from extrapelvic sites are distinctly uncommon and only a minority of these affect the endometrium, most being confined to the myometrium. Carcinomas of the breast (particularly lobular carcinoma), colon, stomach, and pancreas are the most frequent tumors to metastasize to the uterus but less common metastases have been reported from kidney, bladder, gall bladder, thyroid, and cutaneous malignant melanoma.

The metastatic tumor in the endometrium frequently has a characteristic appearance that enables the primary tumor to be identified. For instance, lobular carcinoma from the breast often presents a characteristic 'Indian-file' pattern. Metastatic signet-ring cell carcinomas of stomach or colon are equally characteristic. More often, however, the metastatic tumor cells have no diagnostic features and are diffusely distributed through the stroma, showing copious cytoplasm and nondescript nuclei (Figure 16.64).

PROGNOSTIC FACTORS IN ENDOMETRIAL CARCINOMA

The prognosis in a patient with endometrial carcinoma depends on multiple factors, including histologic type and grade, depth of myometrial invasion, vascular channel involvement, age at diagnosis and, of course, the tumor stage. Other factors, such as steroid hormone receptor status and genetic and molecular changes, are currently being examined in detail.

TUMOR TYPE

It is clear from the above descriptions that some histologic types are associated with a better prognosis than others. Endometrioid adenocarcinoma, including its variants of villoglandular adenocarcinoma, secretory carcinoma, mucinous adenocarcinoma, ciliated cell carcinoma, and endometrioid adenocarcinoma with squamous differentiation are associated with a relatively good prognosis. On the other hand, all non-endometrioid carcinomas, including serous carcinoma, clear cell adenocarcinoma, carcinosarcoma, and undifferentiated carcinoma, have unfavorable outcomes. Pure squamous cell carcinoma of the endometrium also bears a poor prognosis.

HISTOLOGIC GRADE

Histologic grading is clinically prognostic and thus required for all varieties of endometrioid endometrial carcinomas. In contrast, virtually all non-endometrioid endometrial adenocarcinomas (including serous, clear cell, and carcinosarcoma subtypes) demonstrate aggressive behavior regardless of stratification by grade. For this reason, all non-endometrioid endometrial adenocarcinomas are considered high grade, and specification of a grade in the diagnosis provides no further information on prognosis.

The most commonly used grading system is that of the International Federation of Gynecology and Obstetrics (FIGO) and is recommended by the World Health Organization (Table 16.4).[165] This three-tired grading system is applied to endometrioid and mucinous adenocarcinomas and classifies carcinomas as well differentiated (grade 1), moderately differentiated (grade 2), and poorly differentiated (grade 3). The grading procedure is based on the amount of solid non-squamous areas in a tumor. Grade 1 tumors (Figures 16.65 and 16.66) are composed of cells and glands that closely resemble those of normal endometrium, with a well-preserved glandular pattern, scanty stroma, and some lack of uniformity of the epithelial cells. Less than 5% of the tumor, exclusive of any squamous component, shows a solid growth pattern. Often there is no solid tumor at all. Grade 2 tumors (Figures 16.67) show a less well-defined glandular pattern, although this is still easily discernible. The cells are more irregular, with multilayering and large, pleomorphic nuclei. From 6 to 50% of the tumor, exclusive of the squamous component, is solid. More than 50% of a grade 3 tumor (Figures 16.68) is composed of non-squamous solid growth and often the glandular pattern may be hardly recognizable, the cells being arranged in solid sheets and cords.

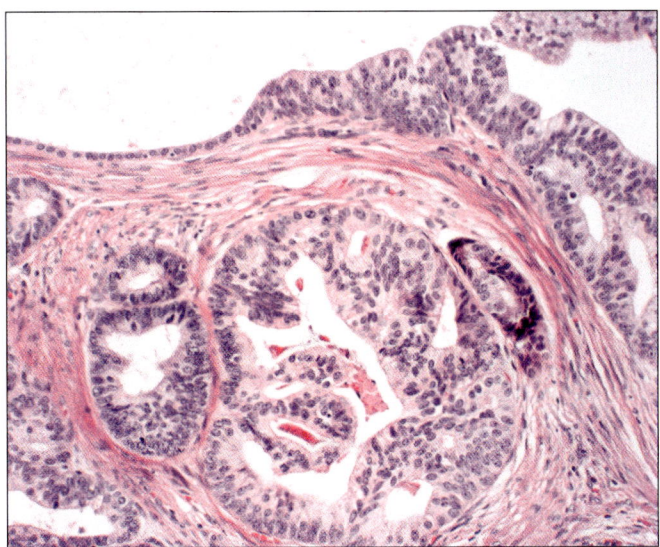

Fig. 16.65 Endometrial adenocarcinoma, endometrioid type. Well-differentiated (grade 1) tumor. Less than 5% of the tumor is solid and the cells show very little cytologic change.

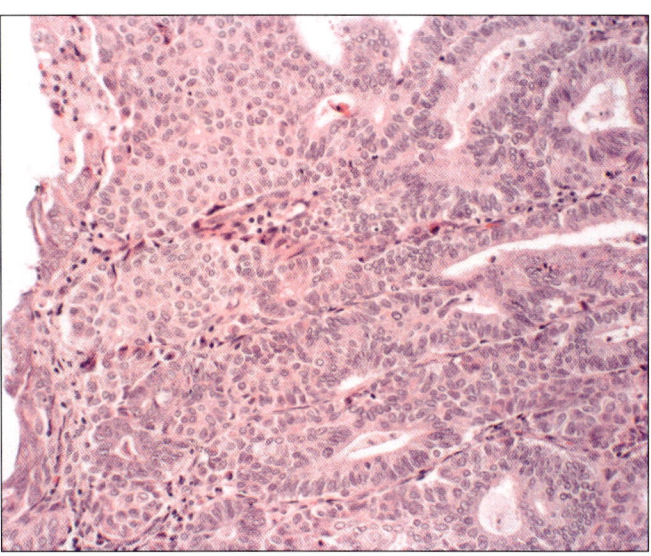

Fig. 16.67 Endometrial adenocarcinoma, endometrioid type. Moderately differentiated (grade 2) tumor. Between 5% and 50% of the tumor is solid.

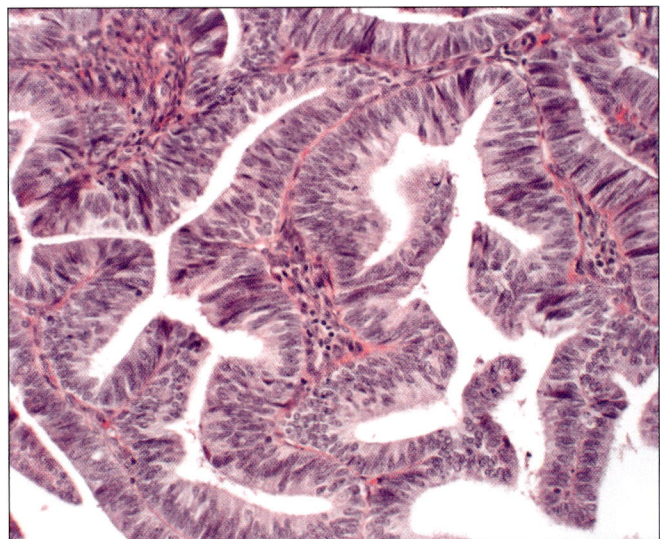

Fig. 16.66 Endometrial adenocarcinoma, endometrioid pattern. Well-differentiated (grade 1) tumor.

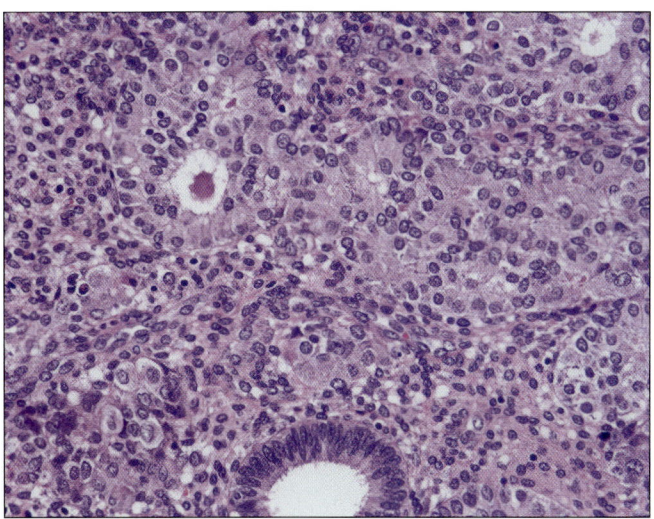

Fig. 16.68 Endometrial adenocarcinoma, endometrioid pattern. Poorly differentiated (grade 3) tumor. More than 50% of the tumor is solid.

Nuclear pleomorphism may be marked, often with prominent, enlarged, and irregular nucleoli. Mitotic activity is not a primary feature of tumor grading, but in general mitotic activity and likelihood of finding abnormal mitotic figures increases with grade.

This FIGO system of endometrioid endometrial carcinoma grading relies first and foremost on the architectural pattern of the glands, but the histologic grade should be raised by one level in those cases which demonstrate severe cytologic atypia.[191] The features taken into account in nuclear grading (Table 16.5)[41,130,167] are graphically represented in Figure 16.69. Nuclear atypia, which justifies elevating histologic grade by one unit, is defined in Table 16.5 as 'high grade'.[191] Usually the architectural and nuclear grades correspond, but when at

Table 16.5 Nuclear grading of endometrial carcinoma

Low grade	High grade (severe atypia)
Little variation in shape	→ Marked variation in shape
Little variation in size	→ Marked variation in size (some markedly enlarged)
Hypochromasia	→ Marked hyperchromasia (may be focal)
No variation in staining intensity	→ Marked variation in staining intensity
Evenly distributed chromatin	→ Coarsely clumped chromatin
Nucleoli not prominent	→ Prominent nucleoli
Sparse mitoses	→ Frequent mitoses with abnormal forms

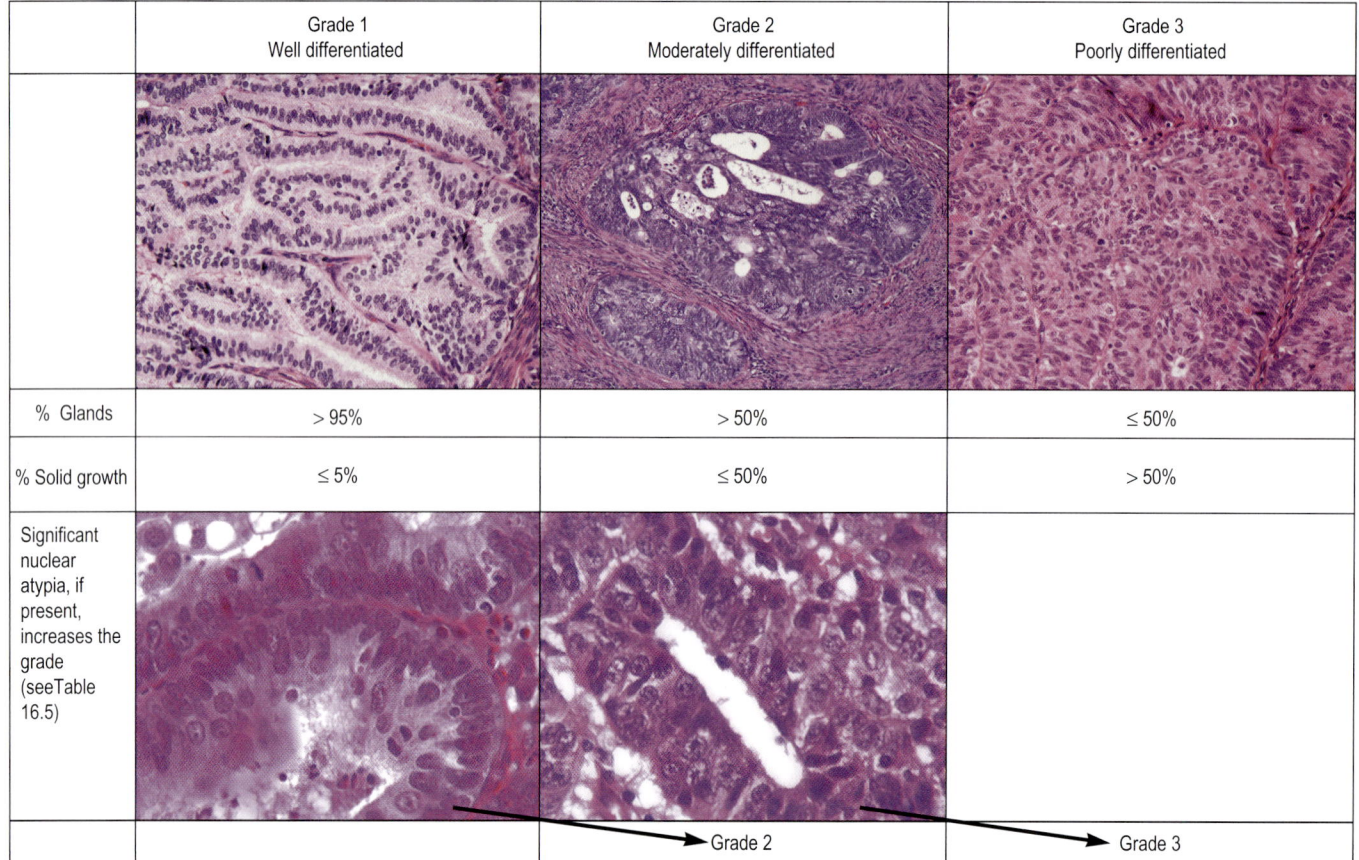

	Grade 1 Well differentiated	Grade 2 Moderately differentiated	Grade 3 Poorly differentiated
% Glands	> 95%	> 50%	≤ 50%
% Solid growth	≤ 5%	≤ 50%	> 50%
Significant nuclear atypia, if present, increases the grade (seeTable 16.5)		Grade 2	Grade 3

Fig. 16.69 Grading of endometrial adenocarcinoma, endometrioid type. The grade depends primarily on the architectural pattern, but significant nuclear atypia changes a grade 1 tumor to grade 2, and a grade 2 tumor to grade 3.

variance, the nuclear grade is often the more reliable indicator of prognosis.[130,167] When the final grade is elevated due to severe cytologic atypia, a note should appear in the report so that the clinician is alerted that the patient falls into this special category.

STAGE AND DEPTH OF MYOMETRIAL INVASION

A critical determinant in the outcome of a woman with endometrial carcinoma is the stage of the tumor at the time of diagnosis. This is true for all tumor types. The staging system most widely used is that recommended by FIGO, which the International Union Against Cancer (UICC) has also adopted[11,42] (see Appendix A). Precise histologic assessment of myometrial invasion and cervical involvement is crucial for the staging of early disease.

Patients with more than 50% myometrial thickness invasion are at increased risk for extrauterine metastases, including pelvic and para-aortic lymph node metastases. These patients often require more aggressive surgical staging,[100] which may include pelvic and para-aortic lymphadenectomy, as well as postoperative adjunctive therapy. Maximum depth of myoinvasion is measured in millimeters from the endometrial–myometrial junction, and expressed as a percentage of the total myometrial thickness. Problems arise, however, in assessing the depth of invasion, the most important of which is accurately identifying the endometrial–myometrial junction. It may be quite difficult when the boundary is distorted by the tumor itself or other lesions such as fibroids. Residual areas of normal endometrium (Figure 16.18) or overrun normal glands are informative benchmarks, when available. Bulky exophytic tumors can be difficult to orient against recognizable landmarks in a single histologic section. Assessment of the endometrial–myometrial boundary location at the site of deepest invasion requires a combination of gross and histologic evaluation.

Endometrial carcinoma extending into foci of adenomyosis should not be considered invasive unless tumor cells extend outwards into the myometrium itself.[6] In that case, depth of invasion is measured not from the point of adenomyotic transgression, but from the endometrial–myometrial junction underling the surface endometrium.

VASCULAR INVASION

Vascular and lymphatic channel invasion are seen in approximately one-fifth of endometrial carcinomas and the finding correlates significantly with the extension of the primary tumor, depth of myometrial invasion, and histologic grade.[83] Patients with lymph node metastasis have a significantly higher incidence of vascular invasion than those without. The presence of vascular invasion has been shown to be a powerful independent indicator for increased risk of recurrence[125] and diminished survival in patients with clinical stage 1 endometrial adenocarcinoma.[34,68] Women with stage 1 endometrial adenocarcinoma who have vascular invasion should therefore be considered for adjunctive therapy.[68]

Care must be exercised in determining what is true vascular invasion. Quite commonly, especially if the invasion is limited to a single focus and is superficial, the chances are substantial that only separation artifact is being observed. We prefer to see several unequivocal foci before diagnosing lymphatic invasion as being present.

AGE

The patient's age at the time of diagnosis is often a critical factor in determining the prognosis of a patient with endometrial carcinoma.[3] Generally, endometrial carcinoma in younger women, particularly before the menopause, is associated with a 5-year survival approaching 100%. One study found a 5-year survival of 96% for women aged 40–49 years compared with only 53% for women of 70–79 years.[41] Increasing age is associated with a higher grade and stage of endometrioid tumors and the likelihood of a non-endometrioid-type tumor, but this accounts for only part of the difference in survival. An additional factor may be that a relative lack of immunocompetence is more prevalent in older patients.

STEROID HORMONE RECEPTORS

The endometrium is a hormone target tissue and hormones obviously play an important part in the origin of endometrial carcinoma. This is especially true of the endometrioid class of tumors, but of diminished relevance in non-endometrioid tumors. Unlike the former, the latter have not been associated with estrogen-mediated carcinogenesis, and often lack estrogen (ER) and progesterone receptors (PR).

Hormone receptor evaluation by immunohistochemical methods, using monoclonal antibodies specific for human ER and PR, can be done on very small pieces of tissue, and scored specifically within tumor cells. Essentially, all endometrioid carcinomas are reactive for ER, whereas PR levels depend on the histologic grade of the tumor, well-differentiated carcinomas generally having higher PR concentrations compared with poorly differentiated tumors.[152] There is some evidence that immunohistochemical determination of PR may be an independent predictor of clinical course in patients with endometrioid carcinoma,[65,92] and receptor studies may prove to be of some value to help determine which patients might or might not be suitable for hormonal therapy. A multitude of recently described ER and PR subtypes has increased the complexity of possible hormonal responses beyond a simple one-hormone, one-receptor model. Relevance of receptor subtypes to disease course and management is not yet completely understood, and is a subject of ongoing investigation.

MOLECULAR PATHOLOGY

As mentioned before, two different molecular pathways have been proposed for endometrioid and non-endometrioid types of endometrial carcinoma.[101,114]

Endometrioid carcinomas usually show one or more of the following alterations: (1) microsatellite instability; (2) alterations of *PTEN*; (3) *K-ras* mutations; and (4) alterations in *CTNNB-1*.

Microsatellite instability reflects a widespread alteration in the length of short, tandem repeat microsatellite DNA sequences in tumor tissue.[30,35] It occurs in the endometrial carcinomas that develop in the setting of the hereditary non-polyposis colorectal cancer (HNPCC) syndrome as a result of the presence of inherited mutations in mismatch repair genes (*MSH-2*, *MLH-1*, *MSH-6*).[136] However, it also occurs in 20–40% of sporadic endometrioid carcinomas. In these cases, microsatellite instability is caused by mismatch repair deficiency due to inactivation of *MLH-1* by promoter methylation.[60] *MLH-1* promoter hypermethylation and microsatellite instability are early events in the process of endometrial tumorigenesis, occurring in the premalignant phases.[58] Endometrial carcinomas with microsatellite instability show 'secondary' mutations in genes that contain microsatellites in their coding sequence. Mutations in these genes, such as the proapoptotic tumor suppressor gene *BAX*, may be responsible for tumor progression.[36]

The most frequent altered gene in endometrioid carcinoma is *PTEN*, a tumor suppressor gene located on chromosome 10. Mutations in *PTEN* occur in 35–80% of endometrioid carcinomas, and this is visible as loss of PTEN protein by immunohistochemistry (Figures 16.70 and 16.71).[172] Alterations in *PTEN* cause activation of the PI3K-AKT signaling pathway, which is involved in the regulation of cell survival and proliferation. *PTEN* alterations are early events in endometrial carcinogenesis. Isolated PTEN protein null endometrial glands exhibiting *PTEN* mutations but retaining steroid hormone

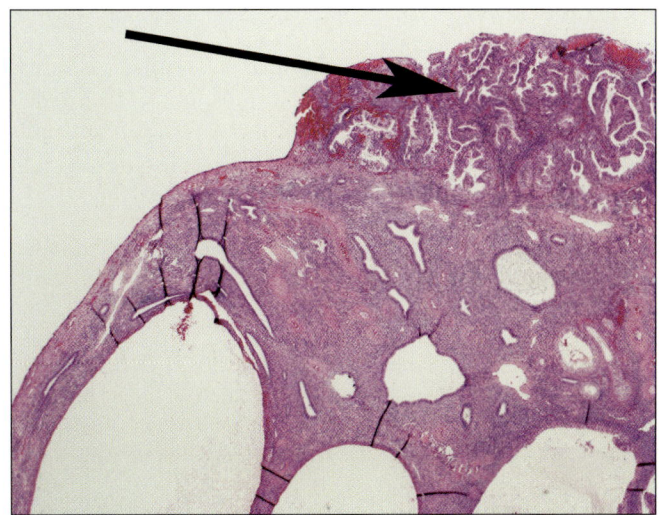

Fig. 16.70 Endometrial adenocarcinoma (black arrow), arising in a polyp.

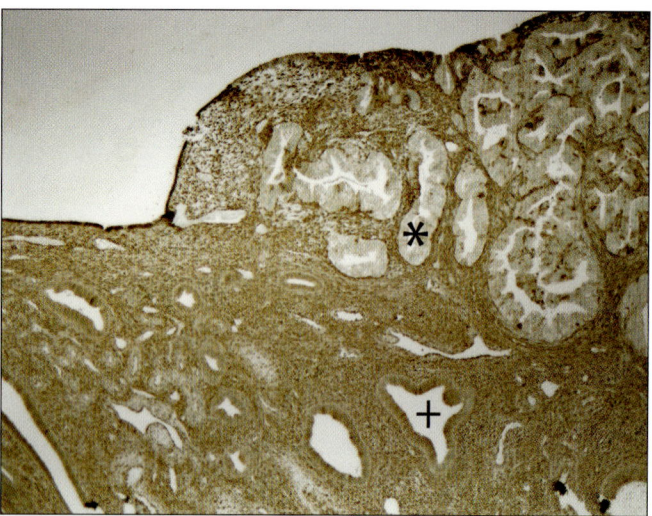

Fig. 16.71 Endometrial adenocarcinoma immunohistochemistry with PTEN. Same case as Figure 16.70. The malignant glands are lacking in the PTEN tumor suppressor protein (*) in contrast to background polyp glands (+).

THE SPREAD OF ENDOMETRIAL CARCINOMA

Endometrial carcinoma spreads initially by invading the myometrium and cervix. Advanced tumors may penetrate the myometrium fully and spread to the adnexa. They may further infiltrate adherent small bowel. Infiltration of the broad ligament, such as in cervical carcinoma, also happens occasionally. Lymphatic spread is to the external iliac and internal iliac (hypogastric) lymph nodes and thence to the common iliac and para-aortic groups. If the tumor extends to involve the cervix, the lymphatic spread will be to the internal iliac and obturator lymph nodes as well. It is important for the pathologist to examine the cervix and determine whether or not it is involved by the tumor. A diagnosis of involvement limited to the endocervical mucosa (stage 2A) can only be made by the pathologist. A common area of difficulty is when the tumor involves the entire lower uterine segment, stopping just at the junction of the upper endocervix. For purposes of staging, we regard this as not involving the endocervix. Involvement of the underlying endocervical stroma upstages the tumor to at least stage 2B. The most common route of spread, especially for endometrioid tumors, is by direct extension, although sometimes lymphatic spread, especially with serous tumors, is observed.

A further route of tumor dissemination is by loose carcinoma cells passing along the fallopian tube and gaining access to the peritoneal cavity, especially common in serous carcinomas where intra-abdominal spread may occur without any myoinvasion at the primary endometrial site.[166] The ovary is involved in 10–15% of advanced cases of endometrial carcinoma. When the ovary contains an appreciable amount of tumor of endometrial pattern, the possibility of a coexistent but separate primary ovarian tumor of endometrioid type must be borne in mind.

receptors may be seen in normal cycling endometrium and persistent proliferative endometrium.[129] The alteration of *PTEN* could render these endometrial cells more sensitive to stimulation by estrogen. As these cells proliferate they undergo further mutation. Clonal clusters of cytologically abnormal glands regarded as the earliest form of endometrial precancer are known as endometrial intraepithelial neoplasia (EIN, Chapter 15). Several studies have reported a significant association between *PTEN* mutations and microsatellite instability.[31] Some controversy exists with regard to the prognostic significance of alterations in *PTEN*, but one study has shown a favorable prognosis for tumors exhibiting *PTEN* mutations.[145]

k-RAS is mutated in 10–30% of endometrial carcinomas, and also in endometrial precancers, suggesting a role in early steps of tumorigenesis.[99]

Mutations in the β-catenin gene (*CTNNB-1*) occur in 25–40% of endometrioid carcinomas.[64] β-Catenin is a normal component of the cell membrane, and is involved in cell-to-cell adhesion. Mutated *CTNNB-1* results in stabilization of β-catenin, cytoplasmic and nuclear accumulation, and participation in transcriptional activation of genes involved in cell cycle machinery, apoptosis, and signaling. Some studies indicate that *CTNNB-1* may be involved in the development of endometrioid carcinomas with squamous differentiation.[150]

In contrast to endometrioid carcinomas, the non-endometrioid carcinomas show altered *p53*,[160] and loss of heterozygosity at multiple loci, reflecting the phenomenon of chromosomal instability. They also show higher frequency of c-erb B2 amplification.[147] *P53* mutations occur in up to 90% of serous carcinoma, and also occur in serous endometrial intraepithelial carcinoma (serous EIC), its putative precursor. In fact, *p53* immunostaining can be a useful tool that helps in identifying both lesions. *P53* mutations are also frequently detected in grade 3 endometrioid carcinomas and clear cell carcinomas but significantly less frequently compared to serous carcinomas.[12,102]

REFERENCES

1. Abeler VM, Kjorstad KE. Serous papillary carcinoma of the endometrium: a histopathological study of 22 cases. Gynecol Oncol 1990;39:266–71.
2. Abeler VM, Kjorstad KE. Clear cell carcinoma of the endometrium: a histopathological and clinical study of 97 cases. Gynecol Oncol 1991;40:207–17.
3. Abeler VM, Kjorstad KE. Endometrial adenocarcinoma in Norway. A study of a total population. Cancer 1991;67:3093–103.
4. Abeler VM, Vergote IB, Kjorstad KE, Trope CG. Clear cell carcinoma of the endometrium. Prognosis and metastatic pattern. Cancer 1996;78:1740–7.
5. Al-Hussaini M, Stockman A, Foster H, McCluggage WG. WT-1 assists in distinguishing ovarian from uterine serous carcinoma and in distinguishing between serous and endometrioid ovarian carcinoma. Histopathology 2004;44:109–15.
6. Ali A, Black D, Soslow RA. Difficulties in assessing the depth of myometrial invasion in endometrial carcinoma. Am J Pathol 2007;26:115–23.
7. Alkushi A, Irving J, Hsu F, et al. Immunoprofile of cervical and endometrial adenocarcinomas using a tissue microarray. Virchows Arch 2003;442:271–7.
8. Amant F, de la RM, Dorfling CM, et al. PTEN mutations in uterine sarcomas. Gynecol Oncol 2002;85:165–9.
9. Ambros RA, Ballouk F, Malfetano JH, Ross JS. Significance of papillary (villoglandular) differentiation in endometrioid carcinoma of the uterus. Am J Surg Pathol 1994;18:569–75.
10. Ambros RA, Sherman ME, Zahn CM, Bitterman P, Kurman RJ. Endometrial intraepithelial carcinoma: a distinctive lesion specifically associated with tumors displaying serous differentiation. Hum Pathol 1995;26:1260–7.
11. American Joint Committee on Cancer. Corpus uteri. AJCC Cancer Staging Manual. New York: Springer; 2002:267–73.
12. An HJ, Logani S, Isacson C, Ellenson LH. Molecular characterization of uterine clear cell carcinoma. Mod Pathol 2004;17:530–7.
13. Ansari-Lari MA, Staebler A, Zaino RJ, Shah KV, Ronnett BM. Distinction of endocervical and endometrial adenocarcinomas – immunohistochemical

p16 expression correlated with human papillomavirus (HPV) DNA detection. Am J Surg Pathol 2004;28:160–7.

14. Aoki Y, Watanabe M, Amikura T, et al. Adjuvant chemotherapy as treatment of high-risk stage I and II endometrial cancer. Gynecol Oncol 2004;94:333–9.

15. Austin H, Drews C, Partridge EE. A case-control study of endometrial cancer in relation to cigarette smoking, serum estrogen levels, and alcohol use. Am J Obstet Gynecol 1993;169:1086–91.

16. Baak JPA. Manual of Quantitative Pathology in Cancer Diagnosis and Prognosis. New York: Springer; 1991.

17. Baergen RN, Warren CD, Isacson C, Ellenson LH. Early uterine serous carcinoma: clonal origin of extrauterine disease. Am J Pathol 2001;20: 214–19.

18. Bandera CA, Boyd J. The molecular genetics of endometrial carcinoma. Prog Clin Biol Res 1997;396:185–203.

19. Barrenetxea G, Schneider J, Centeno MM, et al. Pure theca cell tumors. A clinicopathologic study of 29 cases. Eur J Gynaecol Oncol 1990;11:429–32.

20. Berchuck A, Boyd J. Molecular basis of endometrial cancer. Cancer 1995;76(Suppl):2034–40.

21. Berliere M, Charles A, Galant C, Donnez J. Uterine side effects of tamoxifen: a need for systematic pretreatment screening. Obstet Gynecol 1998;91: 40–4.

22. Bernasconi D, Del Monte P, Meozzi M, et al. The impact of obesity on hormonal parameters in hirsute and nonhirsute women. Metabolism 1996;45:72–5.

23. Bjorkholm E, Silfversward C. Theca-cell tumors. Clinical features and prognosis. Acta Radiol Oncol 1980;19:241–4.

24. Black K, Sykes P, Ostor AG. Trophoblastic differentiation in an endometrial carcinoma. Aust N Z J Obstet Gynaecol 1998;38:472–3.

25. Bradley CS, Benjamin I, Wheeler JE, Rubin SC. Endometrial adenocarcinoma with trophoblastic differentiation. Gynecol Oncol 1998;69:74–7.

26. Brinton LA, Barrett RJ, Berman ML, Mortel R, Twiggs LB, Wilbanks GD. Cigarette smoking and the risk of endometrial cancer. Am J Epidemiol 1993;137:281–91.

27. Brinton LA, Berman ML, Mortel R, et al. Reproductive, menstrual, and medical risk factors for endometrial cancer: results from a case-control study. Am J Obstet Gynecol 1992;167:1317–25.

28. Brinton LA, Hoover RN. Estrogen replacement therapy and endometrial cancer risk: unresolved issues. The Endometrial Cancer Collaborative Group. Obstet Gynecol 1993;81:265–71.

29. British Gynaecological Cancer Group. Oestrogen replacement and endometrial cancer. A statement by the British Gynaecological Cancer Group. Lancet 1981;1:1359–60.

30. Burks RT, Kessis TD, Cho KR, Hedrick L. Microsatellite instability in endometrial carcinoma. Oncogene 1994;9:1163–66.

31. Bussaglia E, del Rio E, Matias-Guiu X, Prat J. PTEN mutations in endometrial carcinomas: a molecular and clinicopathologic analysis of 38 cases. Hum Pathol 2000;31:312–17.

32. Campo E, Brunier MN, Merino MJ. Small cell carcinoma of the endometrium with associated ocular paraneoplastic syndrome. Cancer 1992;69:2283–8.

33. Carcangiu ML, Chambers JT. Early pathologic stage clear cell carcinoma and uterine papillary serous carcinoma of the endometrium: comparison of clinicopathologic features and survival. Int J Gynecol Pathol 1995;14:30–8.

34. Carcangiu ML, Tan LK, Chambers JT. Stage IA uterine serous carcinoma: a study of 13 cases. Am J Surg Pathol 1997;21:1507–14.

35. Catasus L, Machin P, Matias-Guiu X, Prat J. Microsatellite instability in endometrial carcinomas: clinicopathologic correlations in a series of 42 cases. Hum Pathol 1998;29:1160–4.

36. Catasus L, Matias-Guiu X, Machin P, Munoz J, Prat J. BAX somatic frameshift mutations in endometrioid adenocarcinomas of the endometrium: evidence for a tumor progression role in endometrial carcinomas with microsatellite instability. Lab Invest 1998;78:1439–44.

37. Cheng W, Liu J, Yoshida H, Rosen D, Naora H. Lineage infidelity of epithelial ovarian cancers is controlled by HOX genes that specify regional identity in the reproductive tract. Nat Med 2005;11:531–7.

38. Christopherson WM, Alberhasky RC, Connelly PJ. Carcinoma of the endometrium: I. A clinicopathologic study of clear-cell carcinoma and secretory carcinoma. Cancer 1982;49:1511–23.

39. Clement PB, Young RH. Endometrioid carcinoma of the uterine corpus: a review of its pathology with emphasis on recent advances and problematic aspects. Adv Anat Pathol 2002;9:145–84.

40. Cohen I. Endometrial pathologies associated with postmenopausal tamoxifen treatment. Gynecol Oncol 2004;94:256–66.

41. Connelly PJ, Alberhasky RC, Christopherson WM. Carcinoma of the endometrium. III. Analysis of 865 cases of adenocarcinoma and adenoacanthoma. Obstet Gynecol 1982;59:569–75.

42. Creasman WT, Odicino F, Maisonneuve P, et al. Carcinoma of the corpus uteri. Int J Gynaecol Obstet 2006;95(Suppl 1):S105–S143.

43. Crum CP, Drapkin R, Miron A, et al. The distal fallopian tube: a new model for pelvic serous carcinogenesis. Curr Opin Obstet Gynecol 2007;19:3–9.

44. Curtis RE, Freedman DM, Sherman ME, Fraumeni JF, Jr. Risk of malignant mixed mullerian tumors after tamoxifen therapy for breast cancer. J Natl Cancer Inst 2004;96:70–4.

45. Dallenbach-Hellweg G, Hahn U. Mucinous and clear cell adenocarcinomas of the endometrium in patients receiving antiestrogens (tamoxifen) and gestagens. Am J Pathol 1995;14:7–15.

46. Dalrymple JC, Russell P. Squamous endometrial neoplasia – are Fluhmann's postulates still relevant? Int J Gynecol Cancer 1995;5:421–5.

47. Daniell HW. More advanced-stage tumors among smokers with endometrial cancer. Am J Clin Pathol 1993;100:439–43.

48. Darvishian F, Hummer AJ, Thaler HT, et al. Serous endometrial cancers that mimic endometrioid adenocarcinomas: a clinicopathologic and immunohistochemical study of a group of problematic cases. Am J Surg Pathol 2004;28:1568–78.

49. de Brito PA, Silverberg SG, Orenstein JM. Carcinosarcoma (malignant mixed mullerian (mesodermal) tumor) of the female genital tract: immunohistochemical and ultrastructural analysis of 28 cases. Hum Pathol 1993;24:132–42.

50. Deligdisch L, Holinka C. Endometrial carcinoma: two diseases? Cancer Detect Prev 1987;10:237–46.

51. Demopoulos RI, Genega E, Vamvakas E, Carlson E, Mittal K. Papillary carcinoma of the endometrium: morphometric predictors of survival. Am J Pathol 1996;15:110–18.

52. Dijkhuizen FP, Mol BW, Brolmann HA, Heintz AP. The accuracy of endometrial sampling in the diagnosis of patients with endometrial carcinoma and hyperplasia: a meta-analysis. Cancer 2000;89:1765–72.

53. Egan JA, Ionescu MC, Eapen E, Jones JG, Marshall DS. Differential expression of WT1 and p53 in serous and endometrioid carcinomas of the endometrium. Int J Gynecol Pathol 2004;23:119–22.

54. Ehrmann DA. Polycystic ovary syndrome. N Engl J Med 2005;352:1223–36.

55. Eichhorn JH, Young RH, Clement PB. Sertoliform endometrial adenocarcinoma: a study of four cases. Am J Pathol 1996;15:119–26.

56. Elit L, Hirte H. Current status and future innovations of hormonal agents, chemotherapy and investigational agents in endometrial cancer. Curr Opin Obstet Gynecol 2002;14:67–73.

57. Escobedo LG, Lee NC, Peterson HB, Wingo PA. Infertility-associated endometrial cancer risk may be limited to specific subgroups of infertile women. Obstet Gynecol 1991;77:124–8.

58. Esteller M, Catasus L, Matias-Guiu X, et al. hMLH1 promoter hypermethylation is an early event in human endometrial tumorigenesis. Am J Pathol 1999;155:1767–72.

59. Esteller M, Garcia A, Martinez-Palones JM, Xercavins J, Reventos J. Clinicopathologic features and genetic alterations in endometrioid carcinoma of the uterus with villoglandular differentiation. Am J Clin Pathol 1999;111:336–42.

60. Esteller M, Levine R, Baylin SB, Ellenson LH, Herman JG. MLH1 promoter hypermethylation is associated with the microsatellite instability phenotype in sporadic endometrial carcinomas. Oncogene 1998;17:2413–17.

61. Faquin WC, Fitzgerald JT, Lin MC, Boynton KA, Muto MG, Mutter GL. Sporadic microsatellite instability is specific to neoplastic and preneoplastic endometrial tissues. Am J Clin Pathol 2000;113:576–82.

62. Fine BA, Baker TR, Hempling RE, Intengan M. Pregnancy coexisting with serous papillary adenocarcinoma involving both uterus and ovary. Gynecol Oncol 1994;53:369–72.

63. Fujii H, Yoshida M, Gong ZX, et al. Frequent genetic heterogeneity in the clonal evolution of gynecological carcinosarcoma and its influence on phenotypic diversity. Cancer Res 2000;60:114–20.

64. Fukuchi T, Sakamoto M, Tsuda H, Maruyama K, Nozawa S, Hirohashi S. Beta-catenin mutation in carcinoma of the uterine endometrium. Cancer Res 1998;58:3526–8.

65. Fukuda K, Mori M, Uchiyama M, Iwai K, Iwasaka T, Sugimori H. Prognostic significance of progesterone receptor immunohistochemistry in endometrial carcinoma. Gynecol Oncol 1998;69:220–5.

66. Fukunaga M, Ushigome S. Transitional cell carcinoma of the endometrium. Histopathology 1998;32:284–6.

67. Furberg AS, Thune I. Metabolic abnormalities (hypertension, hyperglycemia and overweight), lifestyle (high energy intake and physical inactivity) and endometrial cancer risk in a Norwegian cohort. Int J Cancer 2003;104:669–76.

68. Gal D, Recio FO, Zamurovic D, Tancer ML. Lymphovascular space involvement – a prognostic indicator in endometrial adenocarcinoma. Gynecol Oncol 1991;42:142–5.

69. Gitsch G, Friedlander ML, Wain GV, Hacker NF. Uterine papillary serous carcinoma: a clinical study. Cancer 1995;75:2239–43.

70. Goff BA, Kato D, Schmidt RA, et al. Uterine papillary serous carcinoma: patterns of metastatic spread. Gynecol Oncol 1994;54:264–8.

71. Goldstein NS, Uzieblo A. WT1 immunoreactivity in uterine papillary serous carcinomas is different from ovarian serous carcinomas. Am J Clin Pathol 2002;117:541–5.

72. Grady D, Gebretsadik T, Kerlikowske K, Ernster V, Petitti D. Hormone replacement therapy and endometrial cancer risk: a meta-analysis. Obstet Gynecol 1995;85:304–13.

73. Green PK, Weiss NS, McKnight B, Voigt LF, Beresford SA. Risk of endometrial cancer following cessation of menopausal hormone use (Washington, United States). Cancer Causes Control 1996;7:575–80.

74. Hachisuga T, Sugimori H, Kaku T, Matsukuma K, Tsukamoto N, Nakano H. Glassy cell carcinoma of the endometrium. Gynecol Oncol 1990;36:134–8.

75. Hashi A, Yuminamochi T, Murata SI, Iwamoto H, Honda T, Hoshi K. Wilms tumor gene immunoreactivity in primary serous carcinomas of the fallopian tube, ovary, endometrium, and peritoneum. Int J Gynecol Pathol 2003;22:374–7.

76. Hendrickson M, Martinez A, Ross J, Kempson R, Eifel P. Uterine papillary serous carcinoma, a highly malignant form of endometrial adenocarcinoma. Am J Surg Path 1982;6:93–108.

77. Hendrickson MR, Kempson RL. Ciliated carcinoma – a variant of endometrial adenocarcinoma: a report of 10 cases. Am J Pathol 1983;2:1–12.

78. Hendrickson MR, Longacre TA, Kempson RL. Uterine papillary serous carcinoma revisited. Gynecol Oncol 1994;54:261–3.

79. Horwitz RI, Feinstein AR, Horwitz SM, Robboy SJ. Necropsy diagnosis of endometrial cancer and detection-bias in case/control studies. Lancet 1981;2:66–8.

80. Huntsman DG, Clement PB, Gilks CB, Scully RE. Small-cell carcinoma of the endometrium. A clinicopathologic study of sixteen cases. Am J Surg Pathol 1994;18:364–75.

81. Hutter P, Couturier A, Membrez V, Joris F, Sappino AP, Chappuis PO. Excess of hMLH1 germline mutations in Swiss families with hereditary non-polyposis colorectal cancer. Int J Cancer 1998;78:680–4.

82. Ichikawa Y, Tsunoda H, Takano K, Oki A, Yoshikawa H. Microsatellite instability and immunohistochemical analysis of MLH1 and MSH2 in normal endometrium, endometrial hyperplasia and endometrial cancer from a hereditary nonpolyposis colorectal cancer patient. Jpn J Clin Oncol 2002;32:110–12.

83. Inoue Y, Obata K, Abe K, et al. The prognostic significance of vascular invasion by endometrial carcinoma. Cancer 1996;78:1447–51.

84. Inthasorn P, Carter J, Valmadre S, Beale P, Russell P, Dalrymple C. Analysis of clinicopathologic factors in malignant mixed Mullerian tumors of the uterine corpus. Int J Gynecol Cancer 2002;12:348–53.

85. Irving JA, Catasus L, Gallardo A, et al. Synchronous endometrioid carcinomas of the uterine corpus and ovary: alterations in the beta-catenin (CTNNB1) pathway are associated with independent primary tumors and favorable prognosis. Hum Pathol 2005;36:605–19.

86. Jick SS, Walker AM, Jick H. Oral contraceptives and endometrial cancer. Obstet Gynecol 1993;82:931–5.

87. Jordan VC, Assikis VJ. Endometrial carcinoma and tamoxifen: clearing up a controversy. Clin Cancer Res 1995;1:467–72.

88. Kaaks R, Lukanova A, Kurzer MS. Obesity, endogenous hormones, and endometrial cancer risk: a synthetic review. Cancer Epidemiol Biomarkers Prev 2002;11:1531–43.

89. Kanbour-Shakir A, Tobon H. Primary clear cell carcinoma of the endometrium: a clinicopathologic study of 20 cases. Int J Gynecol Pathol 1991;10:67–78.

90. Kato DT, Ferry JA, Goodman A, et al. Uterine papillary serous carcinoma (UPSC): a clinicopathologic study of 30 cases. Gynecol Oncol 1995;59:384–9.

91. Kennedy AS, Demars LR, Flannagan LM, Varia MA. Primary squamous cell carcinoma of the endometrium: a first report of adjuvant chemoradiation. Gynecol Oncol 1995;59:117–23.

92. Kerner H, Sabo E, Friedman M, Beck D, Samare O, Lichtig C. An immunohistochemical study of estrogen and progesterone receptors in adenocarcinoma of the endometrium and in the adjacent mucosa. Int J Gynecol Cancer 1995;5:275–81.

93. Kim SY, Suzuki N, Laxmi YR, et al. Formation of tamoxifen-DNA adducts in human endometrial explants exposed to alpha-hydroxytamoxifen. Chem Res Toxicol 2005;18:889–95.

94. Kounelis S, Kapranos N, Kouri E, Coppola D, Papadaki H, Jones MW. Immunohistochemical profile of endometrial adenocarcinoma: a study of 61 cases and review of the literature. Mod Pathol 2000;13:379–88.

95. Kuwashima Y, Kurosumi M, Kobayashi Y, et al. Random nuclear p53 overexpression pattern in tamoxifen-mediated endometrial carcinoma. Int J Gynecol Pathol 1998;17:135–9.

96. Kuwashima Y, Kurosumi M, Kobayashi Y, et al. Tamoxifen mediated human endometrial carcinogenesis may not involve estrogenic pathways: a preliminary note. Anticancer Res 1996;16:2993–6.

97. La Vecchia C, Franceschi S, Decarli A, Gallus G, Tognoni G. Risk factors for endometrial cancer at different ages. J Natl Cancer Inst 1984;73:667–71.

98. La Vecchia C, Negri E, Franceschi S, D'Avanzo B, Boyle P. A case-control study of diabetes mellitus and cancer risk. Br J Cancer 1994;70:950–3.

99. Lagarda H, Catasus L, Arguelles R, Matias-Guiu X, Prat J. K-ras mutations in endometrial carcinomas with microsatellite instability. J Pathol 2001;193:193–9.

100. Larson DM, Connor GP, Broste SK, Krawisz BR, Johnson KK. Prognostic significance of gross myometrial invasion with endometrial cancer. Obstet Gynecol 1996;88:394–8.

101. Lax SF. Molecular genetic pathways in various types of endometrial carcinoma: from a phenotypical to a molecular-based classification. Virchows Arch 2004;444:213–23.

102. Lax SF, Kendall B, Tashiro H, Slebos RJ, Hedrick L. The frequency of p53, K-ras mutations, and microsatellite instability differs in uterine endometrioid and serous carcinoma: evidence of distinct molecular genetic pathways. Cancer 2000;88:814–24.

103. Lax SF, Kurman RJ. A dualistic model for endometrial carcinogenesis based on immunohistochemical and molecular genetic analyses. Verh Dtsch Ges Pathol 1997;81:228–32.

104. Lax SF, Pizer ES, Ronnett BM, Kurman RJ. Clear cell carcinoma of the endometrium is characterized by a distinctive profile of p53, Ki-67, estrogen, and progesterone receptor expression. Hum Pathol 1998;29:551–8.

105. Lax SF, Pizer ES, Ronnett BM, Kurman RJ. Comparison of estrogen and progesterone receptor, Ki-67, and p53 immunoreactivity in uterine endometrioid carcinoma and endometrioid carcinoma with squamous, mucinous, secretory, and ciliated cell differentiation. Hum Pathol 1998;29:924–31.

106. Liang SX, Chambers SK, Cheng L, Zhang S, Zhou Y, Zheng W. Endometrial glandular dysplasia: a putative precursor lesion of uterine papillary serous carcinoma. Part II: molecular features. Int J Surg Pathol 2004;12:319–31.

107. Lininger RA, Ashfaq R, Bores-Saavedra J, Tavassoli FA. Transitional cell carcinoma of the endometrium and endometrial carcinoma with transitional cell differentiation. Cancer 1997;79:1933–43.

108. Longacre TA, Chung MH, Jensen DN, Hendrickson MR. Proposed criteria for the diagnosis of well-differentiated endometrial carcinoma. A diagnostic test for myoinvasion. Am J Surg Pathol 1995;19:371–406.

109. Machado F, Rodriguez JR, Leon JP, Rodriguez JR, Parrilla JJ, Abad L. Tamoxifen and endometrial cancer. Is screening necessary? A review of the literature. Eur J Gynaecol Oncol 2005;26:257–65.

110. Maksem JA. Performance characteristics of the Indiana University Medical Center endometrial sampler (Tao Brush) in an outpatient office setting, first year's outcomes: recognizing histological patterns in cytology preparations of endometrial brushings. Diagn Cytopathol 2000;22:186–95.

111. Malmstrom H, Hogberg T, Risberg B, Simonsen E. Granulosa cell tumors of the ovary: prognostic factors and outcome. Gynecol Oncol 1994;52:50–5.

112. Mariani A, Webb MJ, Keeney GL, Lesnick TG, Podratz KC. Surgical stage I endometrial cancer: predictors of distant failure and death. Gynecol Oncol 2002;87:274–80.

113. Matadial L, Escoffery CT, Bowen-Chatoor JS. Sertoliform variant of endometrioid carcinoma of the ovary. West Indian Med J 1995;44:72–3.

114. Matias-Guiu X, Catasus L, Bussaglia E, et al. Molecular pathology of endometrial hyperplasia and carcinoma. Hum Pathol 2001;32:569–77.

115. Maxwell GL, Chandramouli GV, Dainty L, et al. Microarray analysis of endometrial carcinomas and mixed mullerian tumors reveals distinct gene expression profiles associated with different histologic types of uterine cancer. Clin Cancer Res 2005;11:4056–66.

116. McCluggage WG. Recent advances in immunohistochemistry in gynaecological pathology. Histopathology 2002;40:309–26.

117. McCluggage WG, Roberts N, Bharucha H. Enteric differentiation in endometrial adenocarcinomas: a mucin histochemical study. Int J Gynecol Pathol 1995;14:250–4.

118. McPherson CP, Sellers TA, Potter JD, Bostick RM, Folsom AR. Reproductive factors and risk of endometrial cancer. The Iowa Women's Health Study. Am J Epidemiol 1996;143:1195–202.

119. Medl M. [Oral contraceptives and endometrial and ovarian carcinomas]. Gynakol Geburtshilfliche Rundsch 1998;38:105–8.

120. Melhem MF, Tobon H. Mucinous adenocarcinoma of the endometrium: a clinico-pathological review of 18 cases. Am J Pathol 1987;6:347–55.

121. Montz FJ, Bristow RE, Bovicelli A, Tomacruz R, Kurman RJ. Intrauterine progesterone treatment of early endometrial cancer. Am J Obstet Gynecol 2002;186:651–7.

122. Mooney EE, Robboy SJ, Hammond CB, Berchuck A, Bentley RC. Signet-ring cell carcinoma of the endometrium: a primary tumor masquerading as a metastasis. Am J Pathol 1997;16:169–72.

123. Moreira MA, Longato-Filho A, Taromaru E, et al. Investigation of human papillomavirus by hybrid capture II in cervical carcinomas including 113 adenocarcinomas and related lesions. Int J Gynecol Cancer 2006;16:586–90.

124. Moreno-Bueno G, Sanchez-Estevez C, Cassia R, et al. Differential gene expression profile in endometrioid and nonendometrioid endometrial carcinoma: STK15 is frequently overexpressed and amplified in nonendometrioid carcinomas. Cancer Res 2003;63:5697–702.

125. Morrow CP, Bundy BN, Kurman RJ, et al. Relationship between surgical-pathological risk factors and outcome in clinical stage I and II carcinoma of the endometrium: a Gynecologic Oncology Group study. Gynecol Oncol 1991;40:55–65.

126. Mutter GL. PTEN, a protean tumor suppressor. Am J Pathol 2001;158:1895–8.

127. Mutter GL, Baak JPA, Crum CP, Richart RM, Ferenczy A, Faquin WC. Endometrial precancer diagnosis by histopathology, clonal analysis, and computerized morphometry. J Pathol 2000;190:462–9.

128. Mutter GL, Kauderer J, Baak JPA, Alberts DA. Biopsy histomorphometry predicts uterine myoinvasion by endometrial carcinoma: a Gynecologic Oncology Group study. Hum Pathol 2008;39:866–74.

129. Mutter GL, Lin MC, Fitzgerald JT, et al. Altered PTEN expression as a diagnostic marker for the earliest endometrial precancers. J Natl Cancer Inst 2000;92:924–30.

130. Nordstrom B, Strang P, Lindgren A, Bergstrom R, Tribukait B. Carcinoma of the endometrium: do the nuclear grade and DNA ploidy provide more prognostic information than do the FIGO and WHO classifications? Am J Pathol 1996;15:191–201.

131. Nucci M, Crum CP, Prasad C, Mutter GL. Mucinous endometrial epithelial proliferations: a morphologic spectrum of changes with diverse clinical significance. Mod Pathol 2000;12:1137–42.

132. O'Neill CJ, McCluggage WG. p16 expression in the female genital tract and its value in diagnosis. Adv Anat Pathol 2006;13:8–15.

133. Olson SH, Trevisan M, Marshall JR, et al. Body mass index, weight gain, and risk of endometrial cancer. Nutr Cancer 1995;23:141–9.

134. Ozsener S, Ozaran A, Itil I, Dikmen Y. Endometrial pathology of 104 postmenopausal breast cancer patients treated with tamoxifen. Eur J Gynaecol Oncol 1998;19:580–3.

135. Parazzini F, La Vecchia C, Bocciolone L, Franceschi S. The epidemiology of endometrial cancer. Gynecol Oncol 1991;41:1–16.

136. Parc YR, Halling KC, Burgart LJ, et al. Microsatellite instability and hMLH1/hMSH2 expression in young endometrial carcinoma patients: associations with family history and histopathology. Int J Cancer 2000;86:60–6.

137. Parkash V, Carcangiu ML. Endometrioid endometrial adenocarcinoma with psammoma bodies. Am J Surg Pathol 1997;21:399–406.

138. Peel DJ, Ziogas A, Fox EA, et al. Characterization of hereditary nonpolyposis colorectal cancer families from a population-based series of cases. J Natl Cancer Inst 2000;92:1517–22.

139. Pesce C, Merino MJ, Chambers JT, Nogales F. Endometrial carcinoma with trophoblastic differentiation. An aggressive form of uterine cancer. Cancer 1991;68:1799–802.

140. Pike MC, Peters RK, Cozen W, et al. Estrogen–progestin replacement therapy and endometrial cancer. J Natl Cancer Inst 1997;89:1110–16.

141. Pirog EC, Kleter B, Olgac S, et al. Prevalence of human papillomavirus DNA in different histological subtypes of cervical adenocarcinoma. Am J Pathol 2000;157:1055–62.

142. Randall TC, Kurman RJ. Progestin treatment of atypical hyperplasia and well-differentiated carcinoma of the endometrium in women under age 40. Obstet Gynecol Surv 1997;90:434–40.

143. Renkonen-Sinisalo L, Bützow R, Leminen A, Lehtovirta P, Mecklin JP, Järvinen HJ. Surveillance for endometrial cancer in hereditary nonpolyposis colorectal cancer syndrome. Int J Cancer 2007;120:821–4.

144. Ries LAG, Melbert D, Krapcho M, et al. SEER cancer statistics review, 1975–2005. Bethesda, National Cancer Institute; 2008 Online. Available: http://seercancergov/csr/1975_2005/.

145. Risinger JI, Hayes K, Maxwell GL, et al. PTEN mutation in endometrial cancers is associated with favorable clinical and pathologic characteristics. Clin Cancer Res 1998;4:3005–10.

146. Robboy SJ, Datto MB. Synchronous endometrial and ovarian tumors: metastatic disease or independent primaries? Hum Pathol 2005;36:597–9.

147. Rolitsky CD, Theil KS, McGaughy VR, Copeland LJ, Niemann TH. HER-2/neu amplification and overexpression in endometrial carcinoma. Am J Pathol 1999;18:138–43.

148. Ross JC, Eifel PJ, Cox RS, Kempson RL, Hendrickson MR. Primary mucinous adenocarcinoma of the endometrium. A clinicopathologic and histochemical study. Am J Surg Pathol 1983;7:715–29.

149. Rotterdam ESHRE/ASRM-Sponsored PCOS Consensus Workshop Group. Revised 2003 consensus on diagnostic criteria and long-term health risks related to polycystic ovary syndrome (PCOS). Hum Reprod 2004;19:41–7.

150. Saegusa M, Okayasu I. Frequent nuclear beta-catenin accumulation and associated mutations in endometrioid-type endometrial and ovarian carcinomas with squamous differentiation. J Pathol 2001;194:59–67.

151. Sasano H, Fukunaga M, Rojas M, Silverberg SG. Hyperthecosis of the ovary. Clinicopathologic study of 19 cases with immunohistochemical analysis of steroidogenic enzymes. Am J Pathol 1989;8:311–20.

152. Satyaswaroop PG, Mortel R. Sex steroid receptors in endometrial carcinoma. Gynecol Oncol 1993;50:278–80.

153. Schlesselman JJ. Risk of endometrial cancer in relation to use of combined oral contraceptives. A practitioner's guide to meta-analysis. Hum Reprod 1997;12:1851–63.

154. Schneller JA, Nicastri AD. Intrauterine pregnancy coincident with endometrial carcinoma: a case study and review of the literature. Gynecol Oncol 1994;54:87–90.

155. Schorge JO, Hossein SM, Hynan L, Ashfaq R. ThinPrep detection of cervical and endometrial adenocarcinoma: a retrospective cohort study. Cancer 2002;96:338–43.

156. Scully RE, Young RH, Clement PB. Tumor-like lesions. In: Scully RE, Young RH, Clement PB, eds. Tumors of the Ovary, Maldeveloped Gonads, Fallopian Tube, and Broad Ligament. Washington, DC: Armed Forces Institute of Pathology; 1998:409–50.

157. Sekiguchi I, Suzuki M, Sato I, Ohkawa T, Kawashima H, Tsuchida S. Rare case of small-cell carcinoma arising from the endometrium with paraneoplastic retinopathy. Gynecol Oncol 1998;71:454–57.

158. Shaeffer DT, Randall ME. Adjuvant radiotherapy in endometrial carcinoma. Oncologist 2005;10:623–31.

159. Sherman ME, Bitterman P, Rosenshein NB, Delgado G, Kurman RJ. Uterine serous carcinoma. A morphologically diverse neoplasm with unifying clinicopathologic features. Am J Surg Pathol 1992;16:600–10.

160. Sherman ME, Bur ME, Kurman RJ. p53 in endometrial cancer and its putative precursors: evidence for diverse pathways of tumorigenesis. Hum Pathol 1995;26:1268–74.

161. Sherman ME, Silverberg SG. Advances in endometrial pathology. Clin Lab Med 1995;15:517–43.

162. Sherman ME, Sturgeon S, Brinton LA, et al. Risk factors and hormone levels in patients with serous and endometrioid uterine carcinomas. Mod Pathol 1997;10:963–8.

163. Silva EG, Jenkins R. Serous carcinoma in endometrial polyps. Mod Pathol 1990;3:120–8.

164. Silverberg S, Kurman R. Endometrial Carcinoma. Tumors of the Uterine Corpus and Gestational Trophoblastic Disease. Washington, DC: Armed Forces Inst. of Pathology; 1991:47–89.

165. Silverberg SG, Mutter GL, Kurman RJ, Kubik-Huch RA, Nogales F, Tavassoli FA. Tumors of the uterine corpus: epithelial tumors and related lesions. In: Tavassoli FA, Stratton MR, eds. WHO Classification of Tumors: Pathology and Genetics of Tumors of the Breast and Female Genital Organs. Lyon: IARC Press; 2003:221–32.

166. Snyder MJ, Bentley R, Robboy SJ. Transtubal spread of serous adenocarcinoma of the endometrium: an underrecognized mechanism of metastasis. Int J Gynecol Pathol 2006;25:155–60.

167. Sorbe B, Risberg B, Frankendal B. DNA ploidy, morphometry, and nuclear grade as prognostic factors in endometrial carcinoma. Gynecol Oncol 1990;38:22–7.

168. Sorosky JI, Kaminski PF, Kreider J, Podczaski ES, Olt GJ, Zaino R. Endometrial squamous cell carcinoma following whole pelvic radiation therapy: response to carboplatin. Gynecol Oncol 1995;57:426–9.

169. Spatz A, Bouron D, Pautier P, Castaigne D, Duvillard P. Primary yolk sac tumor of the endometrium: a case report and review of the literature. Gynecol Oncol 1998;70:285–8.

170. Spiegel GW, Austin RM, Gelven PL. Transitional cell carcinoma of the endometrium. Gynecol Oncol 1996;60:325–30.

171. Sutter C, Lenbach-Hellweg G, Schmidt D, et al. Molecular analysis of endometrial hyperplasia in HNPCC-suspicious patients may predict progression to endometrial carcinoma. Am J Pathol 2004;23:18–25.

172. Tashiro H, Blazes MS, Wu R, et al. Mutations in PTEN are frequent in endometrial carcinoma but rare in other common gynecological malignancies. Cancer Res 1997;57:3935–40.

173. Tavassoli FA, Stratton MR. Tumors of the Breast and Female Genital Organs. Lyon: IARC Press; 2003.

174. Taylor NP, Zighelboim I, Huettner PC, et al. DNA mismatch repair and TP53 defects are early events in uterine carcinosarcoma tumorigenesis. Mod Pathol 2006;19:1333–8.

175. Tchernof A, Labrie F, Belanger A, Despres JP. Obesity and metabolic complications: contribution of dehydroepiandrosterone and other steroid hormones. J Endocrinol 1996;150(Suppl):S155–S164.

176. Tobon H, Watkins GJ. Secretory adenocarcinoma of the endometrium. Am J Pathol 1985;4:328–35.

177. Tunc M, Simsek T, Trak B, Uner M. Endometrium adenocarcinoma with choriocarcinomatous differentiation: a case report. Eur J Gynaecol Oncol 1998;19:489–91.

178. Usadi RS, Bentley RC. Endometrioid carcinoma of the endometrium with sertoliform differentiation. Am J Pathol 1995;14:360–4.

179. Vaidya AP, Horowitz NS, Oliva E, Halpern EF, Duska LR. Uterine malignant mixed mullerian tumors should not be included in studies of endometrial carcinoma. Gynecol Oncol 2006;103:684–7.

180. Vaidya AP, Littell R, Krasner C, Duska LR. Treatment of uterine papillary serous carcinoma with platinum-based chemotherapy and paclitaxel. Int J Gynecol Cancer 2006;16(Suppl 1):267–72.

181. van Hoeven KH, Hudock JA, Woodruff JM, Suhrland MJ. Small cell neuroendocrine carcinoma of the endometrium. Am J Pathol 1995;14:21–9.

182. Van Leeuwen FE, Benraadt J, Coebergh JWW, et al. Risk of endometrial cancer after tamoxifen treatment of breast cancer. Lancet 1994;343:448–52.

183. Vargas MP, Merino MJ. Lymphoepithelioma-like carcinoma: an unusual variant of endometrial cancer. A report of two cases. Am J Pathol 1998;17:272–6.

184. Watson P, Vasen HFA, Mecklin JP, Järvinen H, Lynch HT. The risk of endometrial cancer in hereditary nonpolyposis colorectal cancer. Am J Med 1994;96:516–20.

185. Weir HK, Sloan M, Kreiger N. The relationship between cigarette smoking and the risk of endometrial neoplasms. Int J Epidemiol 1994;23:261–6.

186. Wheeler DT, Bell KA, Kurman RJ, Sherman ME. Minimal uterine serous carcinoma: diagnosis and clinicopathologic correlation. Am J Surg Pathol 2000;24:797–806.

186a. Yi X, Zheng W. Endometrial glandular dysplasia and endometrial intraepithelial neoplasia. Curr Opin Obstet Gynecol 2008;20:20–5.

187. Young RH, Scully RE. Uterine carcinomas simulating microglandular hyperplasia. A report of six cases. Am J Surg Pathol 1992;16:1092–7.

188. Zaino R, Whitney C, Brady MF, DeGeest K, Burger RA, Buller RE. Simultaneously detected endometrial and ovarian carcinomas – a prospective clinicopathologic study of 74 cases. A Gynecologic Oncology Group study. Gynecol Oncol 2001;83:355–62.

189. Zaino RJ, Kurman R, Herbold D, et al. The significance of squamous differentiation in endometrial carcinoma. Data from a Gynecologic Oncology Group study. Cancer 1991;68:2293–302.

190. Zaino RJ, Kurman RJ, Brunetto VL, et al. Villoglandular adenocarcinoma of the endometrium: a clinicopathologic study of 61 cases. A Gynecologic Oncology Group study. Am J Surg Pathol 1998;22:1379–85.

191. Zaino RJ, Kurman RJ, Diana KL, Morrow CP. The utility of the revised International Federation of Gynecology and Obstetrics histologic grading of

endometrial adenocarcinoma using a defined nuclear grading system: a Gynecologic Oncology Group study. Cancer 1995;75:81–6.

192. Zaloudek C, Hayashi GM, Ryan IP, Powell CB, Miller TR. Microglandular adenocarcinoma of the endometrium: a form of mucinous adenocarcinoma that may be confused with microglandular hyperplasia of the cervix. Am J Pathol 1997;16:52–9.

193. Zelmanowicz A, Hildesheim A, Sherman ME, et al. Evidence for a common etiology for endometrial carcinomas and malignant mixed mullerian tumors. Gynecol Oncol 1998;69:253–7.

194. Zheng W, Khurana R, Farahmand S, Wang Y, Zhang ZF, Felix JC. p53 immunostaining as a significant adjunct diagnostic method for uterine surface

carcinoma: precursor of uterine papillary serous carcinoma. Am J Surg Pathol 1998;22:1463–73.

195. Zheng W, Liang SX, Yu H, Rutherford T, Chambers SK, Schwartz PE. Endometrial glandular dysplasia: a newly defined precursor lesion of uterine papillary serous carcinoma. Part I: morphologic features. Int J Surg Pathol 2004;12:207–23.

196. Zhou XP, Kuismanen S, Nystrom-Lahti M, Peltomaki P, Eng C. Distinct PTEN mutational spectra in hereditary non-polyposis colon cancer syndrome-related endometrial carcinomas compared to sporadic microsatellite unstable tumors. Hum Mol Genet 2002;11:445–50.

Mesenchymal uterine tumors, other than pure smooth muscle neoplasms, and adenomyosis

17

W. Glenn McCluggage   Stanley J. Robboy

INTRODUCTION

Uterine mesenchymal tumors form a large and varied group. The most common benign and malignant tumors, the leiomyoma and leiomyosarcoma, respectively, are described in Chapter 18. Considerably less common are the tumors of endometrial stromal origin, which may be benign (endometrial stromal nodule, ESN) or malignant (endometrial stromal sarcoma, ESS). Many morphologic variations exist such as the related neoplasm, uterine tumor resembling ovarian sex-cord tumor. Another variety is the mixed müllerian tumor, composed of both glandular and mesenchymal elements, each of which may be benign or malignant. Other mesenchymal tumors, both benign and malignant, are rare. Some tumors – in particular, but not exclusively, the mixed müllerian tumor – may contain tissue types not normally seen in the uterus, such as striated muscle or cartilage. These are referred to as 'heterologous elements', to distinguish them from the 'homologous elements', such as endometrial stroma and smooth muscle, which are normal uterine constituents. Malignant mesenchymal tumors of all types comprise about 2–3% of malignant tumors of the uterus. A simple classification of these tumors is given in Table 17.1 and their key features are illustrated in Figure 17.1.

ENDOMETRIAL STROMAL TUMORS

Definition

Endometrial stromal tumors are neoplasms composed of stromal cells resembling those of the normal proliferative phase endometrium. The diagnosis rests on finding uniform small cells with often scanty, nondescript, poorly recognized cytoplasm. The nuclei, which often are haphazardly oriented, may show somewhat pointed polar tails. In addition, a rich arborizing vascular pattern of small arteriolar vessels is often seen, sometimes together with hyalinized collagen and foamy macrophages in the absence of necrosis. These neoplasms have a rich reticulin meshwork that encircles the tumor cells individually.

Classification

The classification of endometrial stromal tumors has changed several times during the past two decades. Until the 1990s, the tumors were considered as benign stromal nodules if the margins were smooth and pushing, and mitoses few. 'Endolymphatic stromal myosis' described tumors composed entirely of pure endometrial stroma with irregular margins and involvement of vascular channels. These lesions were considered as low-grade neoplasms, especially if the mitotic count was fewer than 10 mitoses per 10 high-power fields (HPFs). Lesions were considered as stromal sarcoma if the mitotic count was 10 or more mitoses per 10 HPFs. Beginning in the 1970s the terminology was changed to better reflect the natural behaviors. The category of endolymphatic stromal myosis was combined into the stromal sarcomas, with the new group then divided into low-grade ESS and high-grade ESS based on mitotic count, with low-grade neoplasms having <10 mitoses per 10 HPFs and high-grade neoplasms having >10 mitoses per 10 HPFs.

Until recently, this terminology was in widespread use. The tumors regarded by many as high-grade ESS, however, are a heterogeneous collection, composed partly of tumors containing endometrial stromal cells as defined above, but also of anaplastic tumors consisting of larger cells showing marked nuclear atypia. The latter occur in women of older age than endometrial stromal tumors, have very high mitotic counts, and are associated with a much worse prognosis. Their histologic appearances are more like the mesenchymal elements of a carcinosarcoma than a classic endometrial stromal tumor. It appears more sensible, therefore, to divide these tumors into ESN, ESS, and undifferentiated endometrial or uterine sarcoma. In this classification, the terms low-grade and high-grade ESS no longer apply. This classification has been incorporated into the 2003 World Health Organization (WHO) classification and is used here.[126] Using this newest classification, some tumors previously classified as high-grade ESS are now referred to as ESS while others are now termed undifferentiated endometrial or uterine sarcoma. Most of the latter group of neoplasms bears little or no morphologic resemblance to normal endometrial stroma and there is little evidence that they are derived from endometrial stroma. Rare tumors contain areas of both ESS and undifferentiated sarcoma.

General features

A characteristic t(7;17) chromosomal translocation, which results in fusion of two zinc finger genes (JAZF1 and JJAZ1), has been found in some cases of ESS and ESN,[89] suggesting a genetic basis for tumor pathogenesis. This finding is more prevalent in endometrial stromal tumors of classic histology rather than in the variant patterns.[41]

Most endometrial stromal neoplasms react diffusely with CD10 (Figure 17.2),[74] although fibrous variants may be negative. Not uncommonly, endometrial stromal neoplasms will exhibit diffuse alpha-smooth muscle actin (α-SMA) reactivity, while desmin and h-caldesmon are generally negative or at most focally positive.[107] Some cases will show anticytokeratin

427

Table 17.1 Uterine neoplasms with a mesenchymal component other than pure smooth muscle neoplasms

Endometrial stromal nodule (and variants)

Endometrial stromal sarcoma (and variants)

Mixed endometrial stromal and smooth muscle tumor

Uterine tumor resembling ovarian sex-cord tumor (UTROSCT)

Undifferentiated uterine or endometrial sarcoma

Mixed müllerian tumors
? Adenofibroma
Adenosarcoma (including with sarcomatous overgrowth)
? Carcinofibroma
Carcinosarcoma (malignant mixed müllerian tumor) (homologous and heterologous)

Pure heterologous sarcomas

Pure benign mesenchymal lesions

Perivascular epithelioid cell tumor (PEComa)

Atypical polypoid adenomyoma

reactivity. Other markers which may be positive are WT1,[122] estrogen and progesterone receptors,[103] androgen receptor,[87] cellular retinol binding protein-1,[97] and bcl-2.[8] CD34 is negative.[8] These markers are of limited value in the diagnosis of endometrial stromal neoplasms but hormone receptor reactivity may predict those neoplasms that will respond to adjuvant therapy in the form of hormonal preparations.

Proliferating endometrial stroma in curettings

An issue common to all pathologists is the frequency of having to evaluate small amounts of tissue and yet render authoritative diagnoses. This is especially true when tissue from endometrial curettings, polypectomy specimens or ablation procedures contains cellular, proliferating endometrial stroma, a finding that may indicate the presence of an endometrial stromal nodule or sarcoma. A cellular or highly cellular leiomyoma may also enter into the differential diagnosis. The distinction between an endometrial stromal nodule and sarcoma depends on assessment of margins, which cannot be done in a fragmented specimen. A panel comprising CD10, h-caldesmon, desmin, and oxytocin receptor should help distinguish endometrial stroma from smooth muscle.[17]

In a postmenopausal woman, the presence of a cellular proliferating endometrial stromal lesion in curettings usually warrants a diagnostic hysterectomy. If the patient has not yet reached menopause and wishes to preserve reproductive function, careful investigation, including imaging of the uterus, needs to be undertaken before local excision of a well-circumscribed nodule is undertaken.

ENDOMETRIAL STROMAL NODULE

Definition

The rarest of the endometrial stromal tumors, the endometrial stromal nodule is a benign tumor composed of well-differentiated endometrial stromal cells forming a well-circumscribed nodule with largely smooth, non-infiltrative margins.

Clinical features

Endometrial stromal nodule occurs at any age during reproductive or later years. Most are incidental findings in a hysterectomy specimen while others present with abnormal uterine bleeding.

Gross features

The tumors are discrete, round lesions that are usually solitary, ranging from under 1 cm to 15 cm (Figure 17.3). A few are situated in the endometrium and some involve both endometrium and myometrium, but most are entirely within the myometrium, without any apparent connection to the endometrium. Like leiomyomas, these neoplasms may form polyps in the uterine cavity or, more rarely, project into the pelvic cavity from the serosal surface. They are soft and most have a yellowish cut surface that does not show the whorled pattern characteristic of a leiomyoma for which they may be mistaken. Cysts may be present.

Microscopic features

The principal distinguishing feature of the ESN is the expansile, non-infiltrating, smooth margin (Figures 17.4 and 17.5) that contrasts with the infiltrating, irregular margin of stromal sarcoma.[4] Occasional finger-like processes may be present at the lesion's periphery, but none should exceed 3 mm in dimension. The edge should be extensively sampled, especially when the tumor is large, to exclude areas of invasion greater than 3 mm, which would result in a diagnosis of ESS. The term 'endometrial stromal tumor with limited infiltration' has been proposed for those neoplasms with marginal irregularities >3 mm but without the typical infiltrative permeative pattern of most ESS.[28]

The cells comprising ESN resemble those of proliferative phase endometrial stroma and are of uniform size and shape without appreciable cytologic atypia (Figure 17.6). Nuclei are round to ovoid. There is usually scant cytoplasm, although occasionally it is abundant. Reactivity with Ki-67 is low.[53] Mitotic activity is also usually low, but the mitotic count is not a criterion in the diagnosis of ESN.[16] If appreciable numbers of mitotic figures in an otherwise typical ESN are found, caution is advised with careful follow-up, since there is little published by way of long-term outcome in such cases. The ESN is usually vascular with numerous small arteriole-like vessels, but blood vessel invasion is not seen, which is another indication of its benign nature. Stromal foam cells may be present, which may represent histiocytes, tumor cells or both (Figure 17.7). Sex cord-like structures and true endometrioid glands may sometimes be present, as in the other forms of stromal tumor. An occasional tumor may exhibit hyalinized fibrous tissue in the form of a 'starburst' radiating into the endometrial stroma tumor (Figure 17.8).

A smooth muscle and striated muscle component has also been reported, the latter an extremely rare phenomenon.[63,93] These variations may also be present in ESS.

Treatment and prognosis

Most women with an ESN will have been treated by hysterectomy, as the neoplasm is usually an incidental finding following the procedure. Among 60 women followed for up to 16 years there were no recurrences, even though some tumors had high mitotic counts and minor irregularities of the margin.[125] When the lesion is discovered following 'myomectomy', hysterectomy

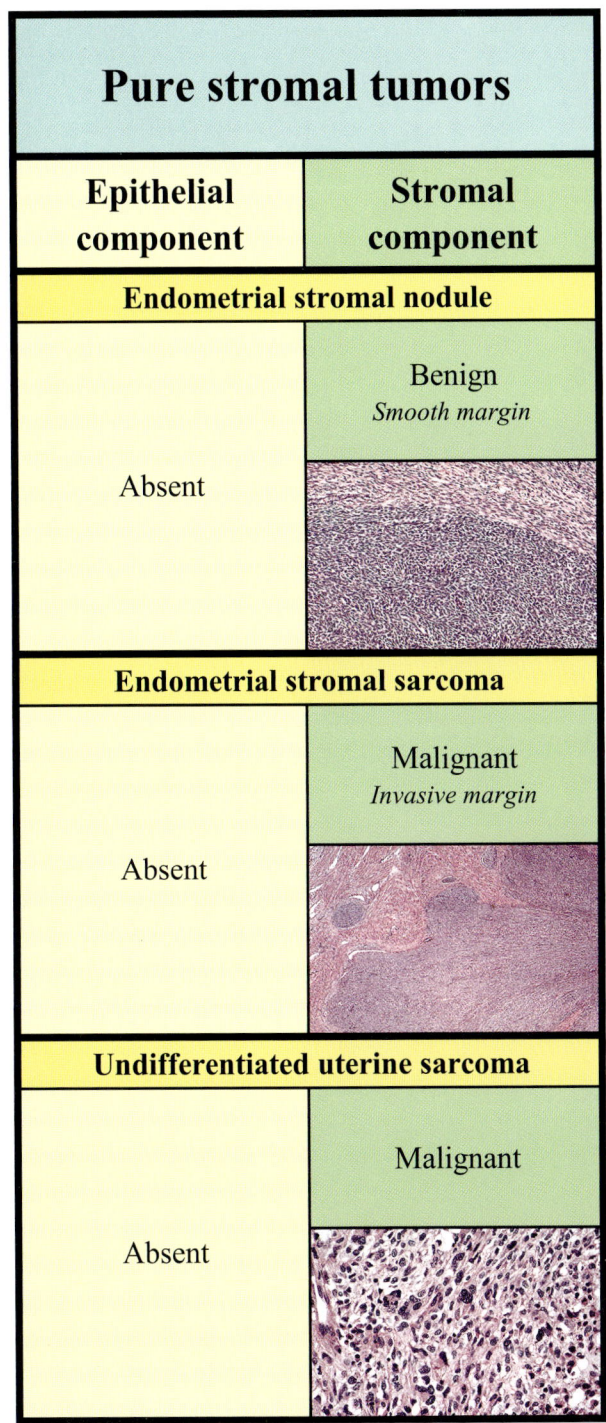

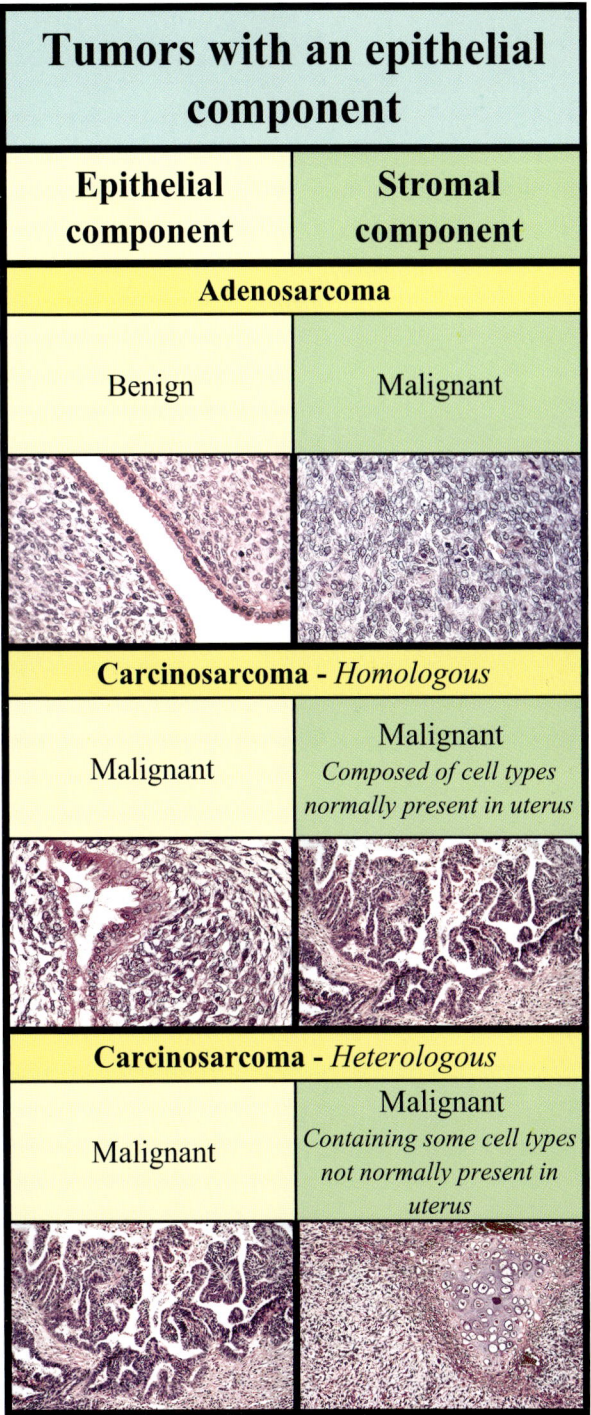

Fig. 17.1 Architectural classification of endometrial tumors with a stromal component.

is advised since an ESS cannot be excluded without examination of the margins.

Differential diagnosis

The stromal nodule differs from stromal sarcoma by its broad, smooth pushing margin in contrast to the serpiginous jagged interface between the sarcoma and the surrounding myometrium.[91] This is the main differentiating feature between the two tumors, the stromal sarcoma often also exhibiting vascular permeation. As both the stromal nodule and the ESS con-

sist of differentiated endometrial stromal cells, the cytologic appearance cannot be used to distinguish the two, although undifferentiated sarcoma can be excluded.

Cellular and highly cellular leiomyomas can be difficult to distinguish from both the ESN and the ESS. The leiomyoma has a fascicular growth pattern, contains cleft-like spaces and thick-walled muscular arteries, and may have a slightly irregular outline merging with the surrounding myometrium.[95] Leiomyomatous tumor cells frequently merge into the media of larger vessels, while those of endometrial stromal tumors are

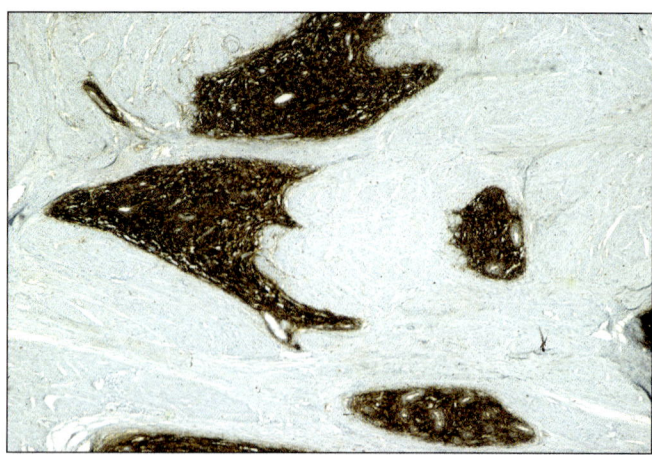

Fig. 17.2 CD10 reactivity in endometrial stromal sarcoma, but common to all tumors of endometrial stroma.

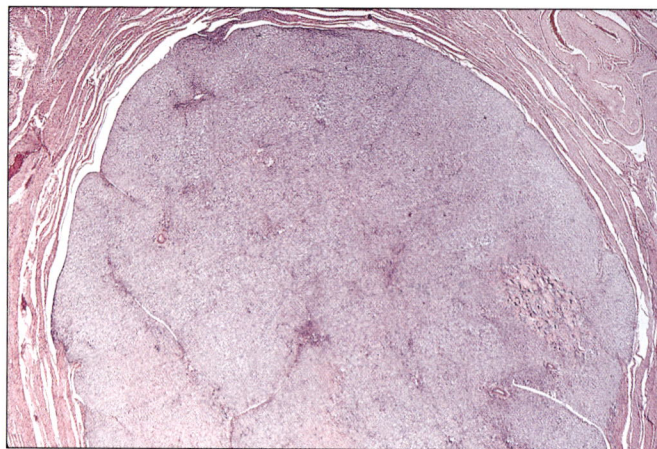

Fig. 17.5 Endometrial stromal nodule, the border of which is well demarcated.

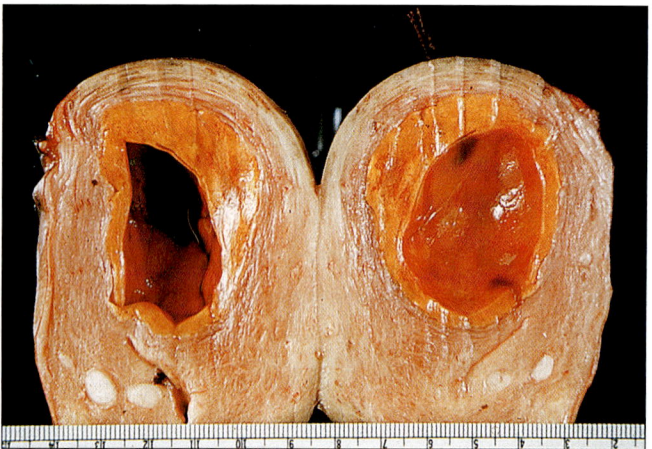

Fig. 17.3 Endometrial stromal nodule. The tumor is yellow with a cystic center and a clearly defined margin.

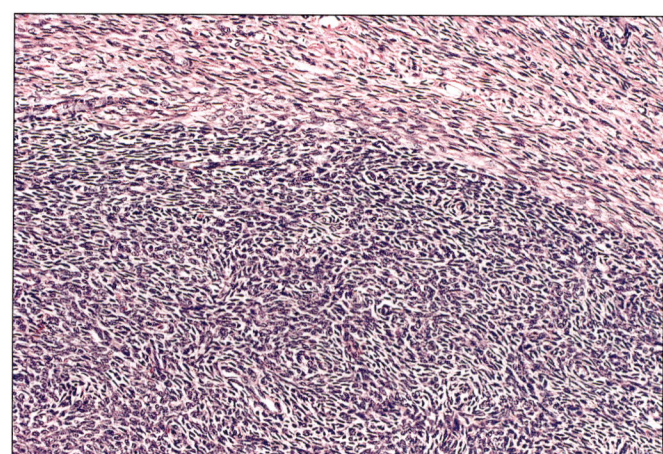

Fig. 17.6 Endometrial stromal nodule. The tumor is composed of cells resembling endometrial stromal cells.

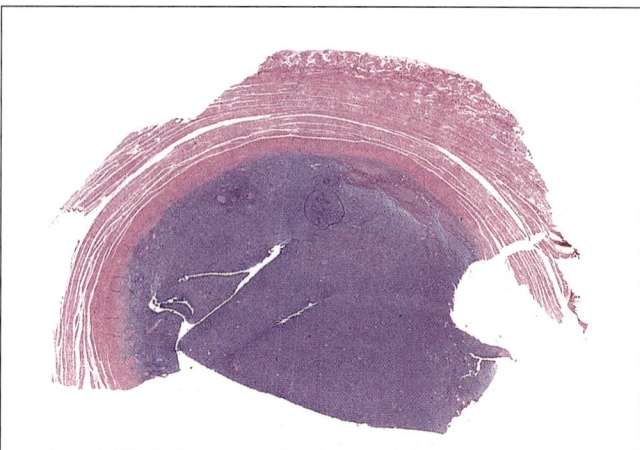

Fig. 17.4 Endometrial stromal nodule. At very low magnification, the well-defined margin is clearly seen.

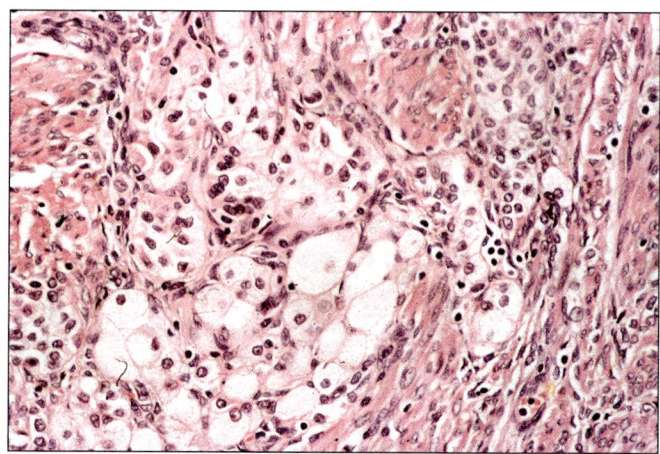

Fig. 17.7 Endometrial stromal tumor with component of foam cells.

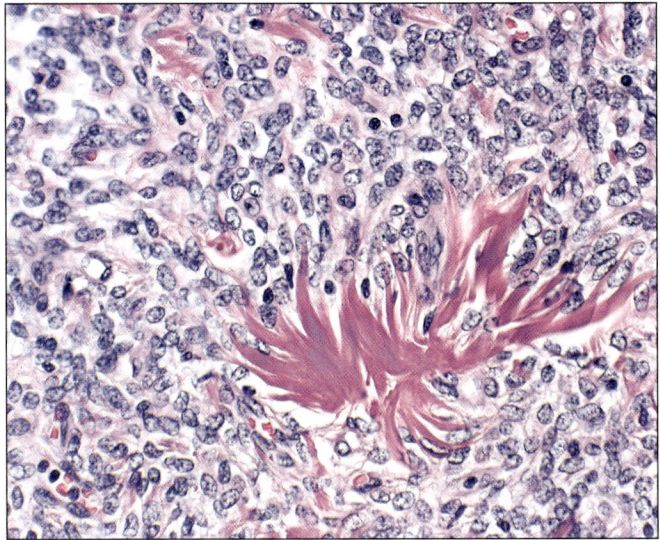

Fig. 17.8 Hyalinized stroma radiating in a 'starburst' pattern as rays penetrating into the neoplastic stromal nodule. This tumor specimen contains no smooth muscle component.

Table 17.2 Comparison of immunophenotype of endometrial stromal and cellular leiomyomatous neoplasm

	Endometrial stromal neoplasm	Cellular leiomyomatous neoplasm
CD10	Diffusely reactive	Negative; sometimes reactive (focal or diffuse)
α-SMA	Negative; sometimes reactive (focal or diffuse)	Diffusely reactive
Desmin	Negative; rarely focally reactive	Diffusely reactive
h-Caldesmon	Negative	Diffusely reactive
Oxytocin receptor	Negative	Diffusely reactive

α-SMA, alpha-smooth muscle actin.

separated from the media of these vessels by the vascular adventitia. The ESN may contain foam cells. In addition, the ESN usually exhibits a rich network of small arteriole-like vessels. As both the ESN and cellular leiomyoma are benign tumors, the distinction is of little clinical consequence in a hysterectomy specimen. However, the distinction may be important in a curette or 'myomectomy' specimen, since a hysterectomy is usually performed for an endometrial stromal lesion in order to exclude an ESS (see Chapter 18 for discussion of therapeutic considerations regarding cellular leiomyoma, leiomyoma of uncertain malignant potential – so-called 'STUMP' tumor – and leiomyosarcoma).

A panel of immunohistochemical stains, including desmin, h-caldesmon, CD10, and oxytocin receptor, helps distinguish between a smooth muscle and an endometrial stromal neoplasm,[17,76,90,107,122] although there may be considerable immunophenotypic overlap, reflecting the origin of endometrial stroma and smooth muscle from a common progenitor cell within the uterus. Table 17.2 compares the immunophenotype of an endometrial stromal and a cellular leiomyomatous neoplasm.

ENDOMETRIAL STROMAL SARCOMA

Definition
Endometrial stromal sarcoma, a malignant tumor with an infiltrating margin, is composed of cells similar to a normal proliferative phase endometrial stroma. Many show vascular invasion, either within or outside the uterus.

Clinical features
ESS usually occurs in women of middle age, but rarely occurs in teenagers.[86] Although the risk factors for endometrial carcinoma seem to play no role in the pathogenesis of ESS, sporadic examples, both within the uterus[1] and arising in pelvic endometriosis,[79] have developed after prolonged estrogen therapy. Thus, unopposed estrogens are best avoided following hysterectomy in patients with a history of endometriosis. When a

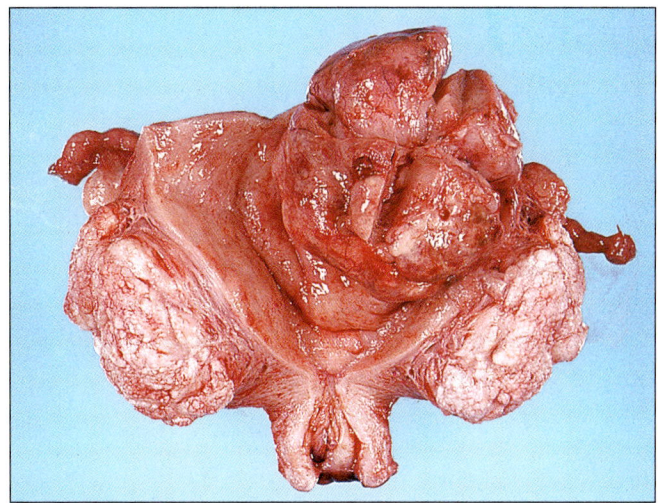

Fig. 17.9 Endometrial stromal sarcoma. The opened uterus displays the typical tumor's polypoid, smooth-surfaced appearance.

diagnosis of extrauterine ESS is made, spread from an undetected uterine primary should be excluded. Some ESSs are incidental findings in a hysterectomy specimen, but most present with abnormal vaginal bleeding.

Gross features
The gross appearance of a uterus containing an ESS varies. The uterus may be enlarged with a polypoid tumor protruding into and greatly distending the uterine cavity (Figure 17.9). When this occurs, the mass is typically round with a smooth surface, a feature that often distinguishes this tumor macroscopically from the polypoid variant of endometrial carcinoma, which usually has a rough or papillary surface. Necrosis and some cystic change may be seen grossly (Figure 17.10). Occasionally, the cystic change may be prominent (Figure 17.11). In other cases an infiltrative growth pattern is seen, producing an area where the uterine wall is thickened. If the uterus is cut across when fresh and then fixed, the cut surface may take on the appearance of the surface of a towel, as the infiltrating cords of tumor stand out from the surface, the result of differential

shrinkage after fixation. Some tumors infiltrate the myometrium with a 'worm-like' appearance.

Microscopic features

The cells of the tumor are identical to those in ESN. They are uniform and resemble the stromal cells of normal proliferative phase endometrium with usually scanty cytoplasm (Figures 17.12 and 17.13). Some contain hyalinized foci with the formation of collagen in thick bundles, with particularly prominent vascularity, the so-called 'hyaline-vascular' type (Figure 17.14). Rarely, hyalinized fibrous tissue in the form of a starburst, a non-specific finding in an endometrial stromal tumor with or without a smooth muscle component, may be found radiating into the neoplastic stromal parenchyma (Figure 17.8).[14]

A striking feature of many, although not all, ESSs and the origin of the alternative name of 'endolymphatic stromal myosis' is the nature of the infiltrating margin of the tumor. Broad, rounded bands and jagged, serpentine processes of stromal cells infiltrate extensively into the myometrium, between the muscle fibers and particularly into the lymphatic and vascular spaces (Figures 17.15–17.18). There may be extension into vessels outside the uterus. The intrinsic vascular pattern of these tumors is also distinctive, comprising small arterioles, reminiscent of the spiral arterioles of normal endometrium and thin-walled vascular channels. Nuclear atypia is usually absent or mild (Figure 17.19) and mitotic figures are generally less than 10 per 10 HPFs. However, the mitotic count is not a criterion for diagnosis.[16]

Other morphologic patterns, similar to those sometimes seen in ESN, may occur such as the presence of foam cells, sex cord-like areas, and the formation of endometrioid glands. Smooth muscle differentiation may also occur (see below). Fibrous, myxoid, and epithelioid variants of endometrial stromal tumor have been described,[94] as well as rhabdoid areas (Figure 17.20).[80] Skeletal muscle differentiation and adipose tissue have rarely been described[5] and occasionally foci of pseudocartilage (Figure 17.21) are encountered. These variant patterns may result in problems in differential diagnosis but the behavior is that of the corresponding stromal neoplasm.[134]

While accepting that undifferentiated uterine sarcoma must be separated from ESS, some have maintained that low-grade and high-grade ESS should still be distinguished from each other. In this scheme, the high-grade ESS when compared to

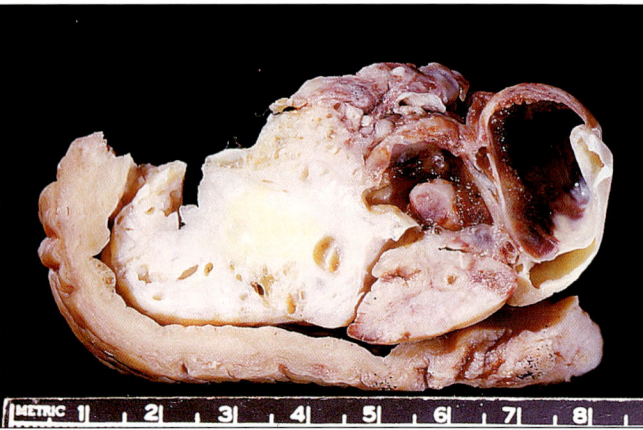

Fig. 17.10 Endometrial stromal sarcoma, with areas of cystic change.

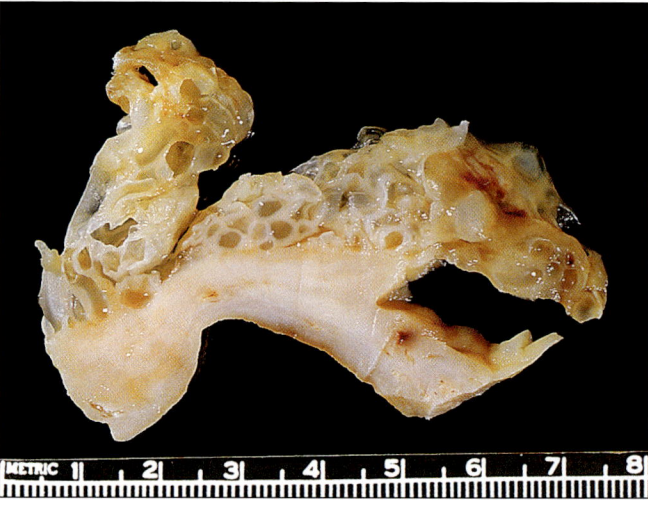

Fig. 17.11 Endometrial stromal sarcoma, with extensive cystic change.

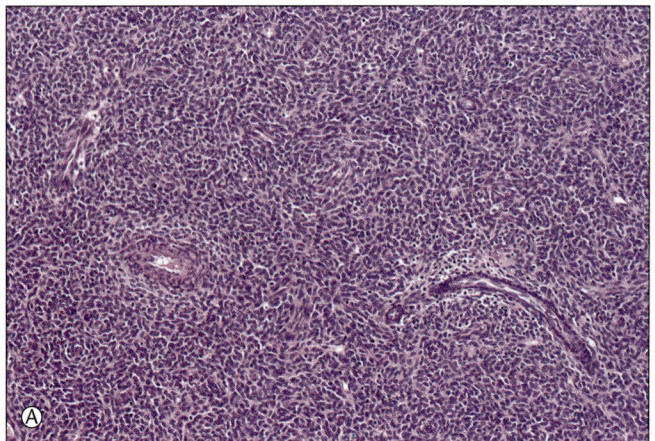

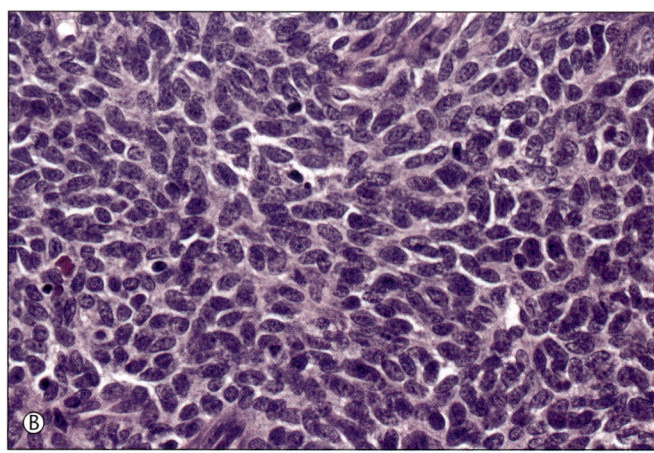

Fig. 17.12 Endometrial stromal sarcoma. **(A)** The component cells are similar to endometrial stromal cells in the proliferative phase and they are uniform. Numerous small blood vessels typify this tumor. **(B)** Detail of stromal cells.

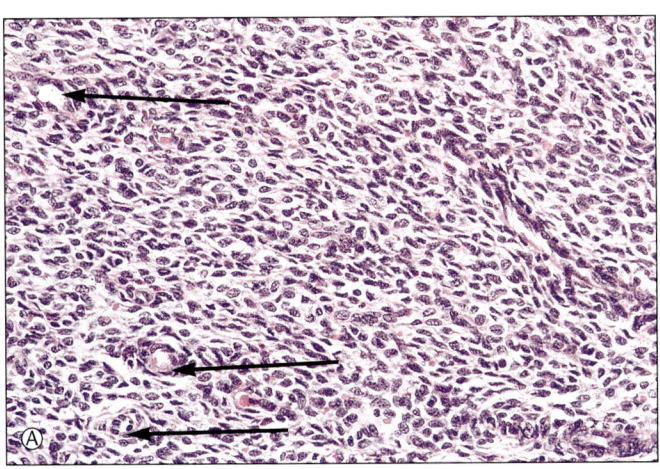
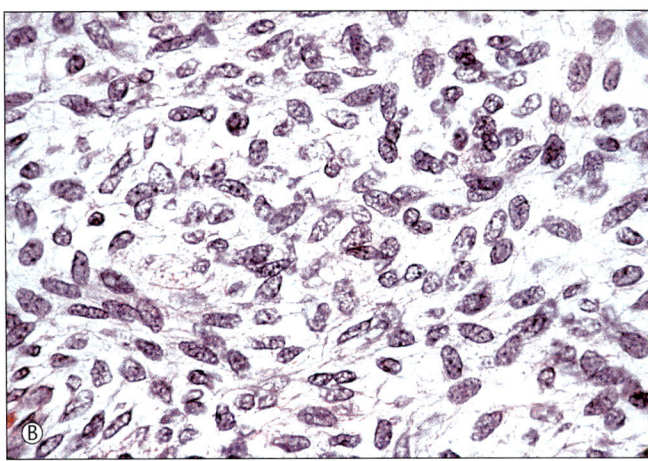

Fig. 17.13 Endometrial stromal sarcoma. The stroma in both parts is looser than in the preceding figure.

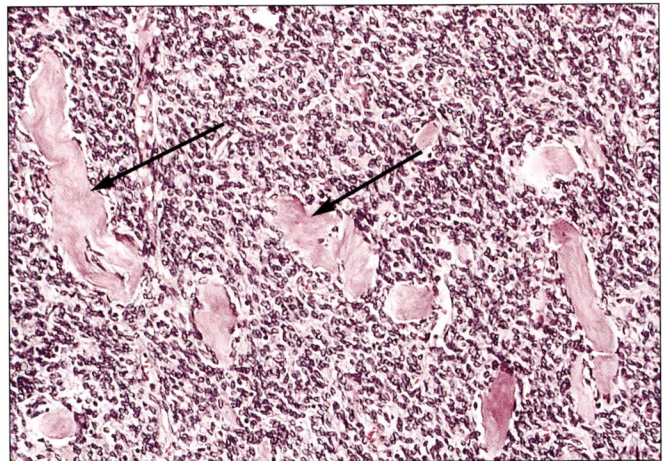

Fig. 17.14 Endometrial stromal sarcoma. Areas of collagenization (arrows) are present.

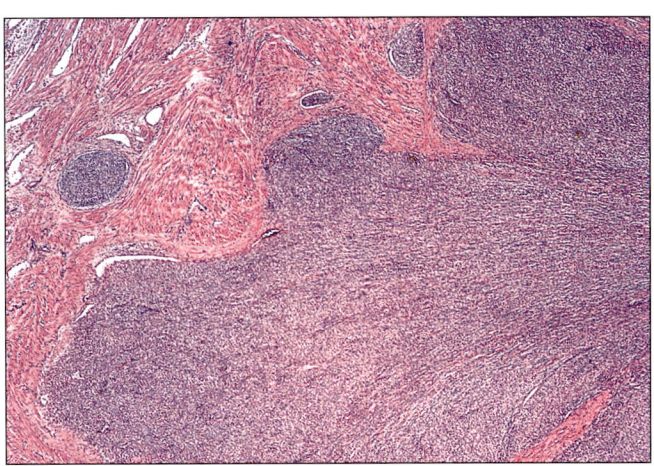

Fig. 17.15 Endometrial stromal sarcoma. The irregularly infiltrating margin distinguishes this tumor from an endometrial stromal nodule.

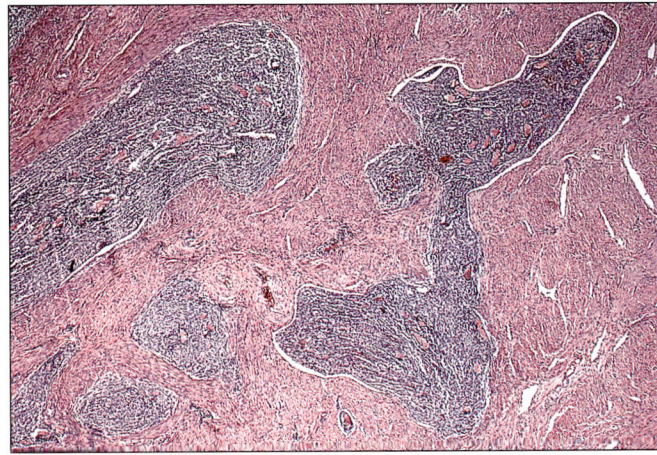

Fig. 17.16 Endometrial stromal sarcoma. The cellular tumor invades in a serpentine fashion between smooth muscle bundles and into vessels.

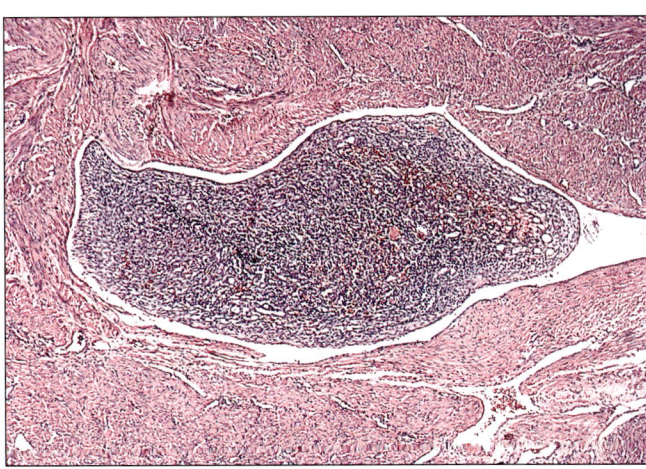

Fig. 17.17 Endometrial stromal sarcoma. Tumor is present within a vascular space.

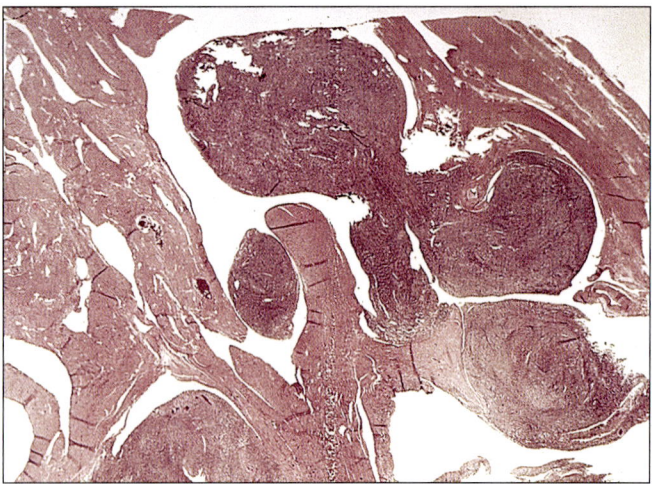

Fig. 17.18 Endometrial stromal sarcoma invading vascular channels.

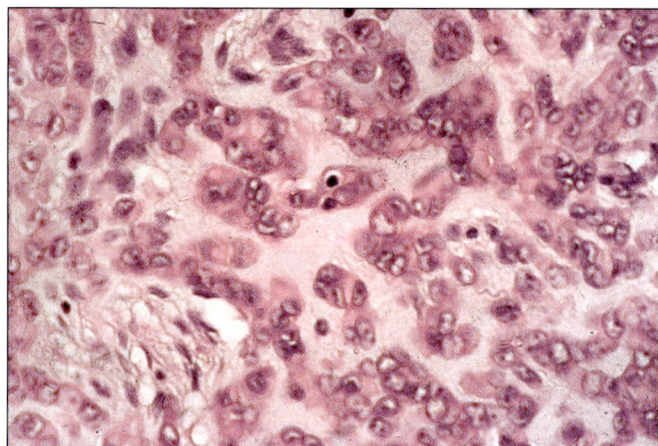

Fig. 17.20 Endometrial stromal sarcoma containing cells with rhabdoid appearance.

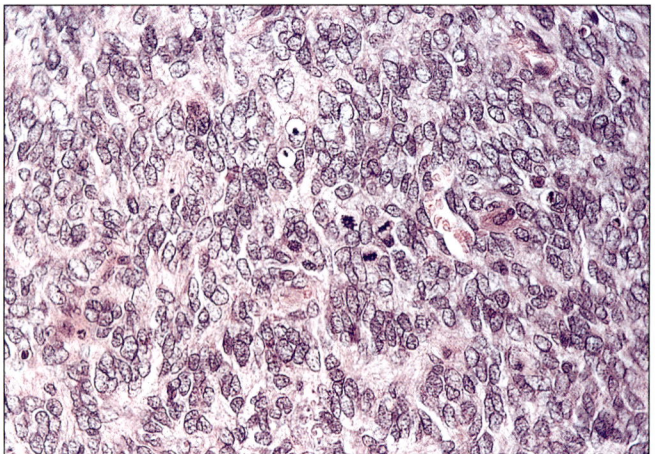

Fig. 17.19 Endometrial stromal sarcoma.

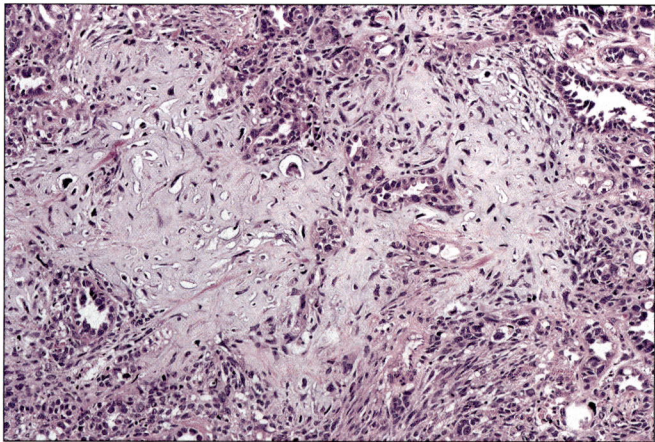

Fig. 17.21 Endometrial stromal sarcoma with focus of pseudocartilage.

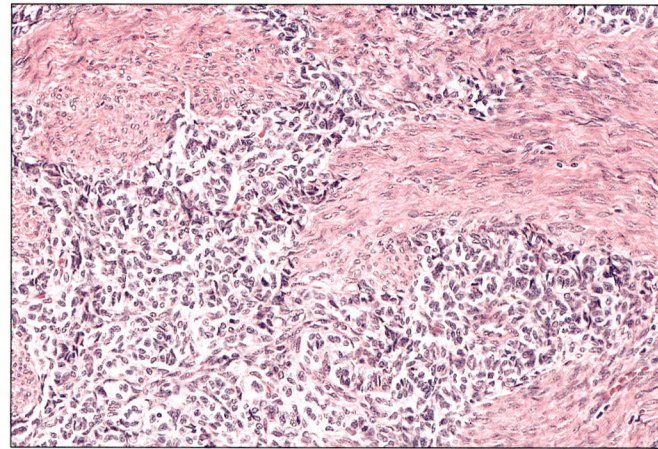

Fig. 17.22 Endometrial stromal sarcoma. Infiltrating margin.

the cells of low-grade ESS has larger, more vesicular nuclei, with more prominent chromatin clumps and nucleoli. Mitotic figures are more frequent, sometimes exceeding 20 or more per 10 HPFs. These tumors infiltrate the myometrium directly (Figure 17.22) and destructively, in contrast to the myometrial and vascular involvement typifying the low-grade ESS. What is important, however, is that both grades maintain the vascular pattern and reticulin meshwork of the endometrial stroma, albeit in an irregular pattern. Most investigators today recognize only one all-inclusive grade of ESS.

Treatment and prognosis

Treatment of ESS is predominantly surgical in the form of hysterectomy and bilateral salpingo-oophorectomy.

The outcome in patients with ESS depends largely on the extent of the tumor at the time of diagnosis. Staging, although not recognized by FIGO for stromal tumors, is in practice assessed identically as for endometrial carcinoma. A surgical stage greater than 1 is a univariate predictor of an unfavorable outcome.[83] In the case of what appears to be a large ESN, extensive sampling, especially at the periphery, is required to confidently exclude ESS. ESS generally has a good prognosis, with 5- and 10-year actuarial survival for patients with stage 1 tumors of 98% and 89%, respectively.[16] About 20% of stage 1 tumors recur, this figure being higher for stage 2–4 neoplasms. Several other features may help predict outcome. A small study has suggested that tumors with a high MIB1 proliferation index may have an increased risk of recurrence or metastasis.[101] Studies of larger numbers of cases are required to confirm this.

ESS usually contains estrogen and progesterone receptors[103] and there is evidence that progestins are of benefit in the treatment of women with this disease, particularly following recurrences after surgery and for advanced stage disease.[59] Recently aromatase inhibitors or gonadotrophin-releasing hormone agonists have been used in the treatment of recurrent or metastatic tumor.[119] Pelvic radiotherapy may be useful in treating local disease when there is extrauterine spread.

Differential diagnosis

ESS is distinguished from ESN by the nature of the interface with the surrounding myometrium. ESS is an infiltrative neoplasm while ESN is well circumscribed, although slight marginal irregularity is allowable, as described previously. Vascular invasion excludes ESN. Distinction of ESS from those cellular leiomyomas with a slightly irregular margin is by the same criteria used in the distinction between benign ESN and cellular leiomyoma. Unusual morphologic variants of ESS raise their own peculiar diagnostic considerations and are discussed below.

Adenomyosis with stromal predominance or adenomyosis with sparse glands may be misdiagnosed as ESS. Careful sampling usually demonstrates areas of more typical usual adenomyosis with glands. Additionally, in adenomyosis the constituent cells generally appear atrophic without mitotic activity, in contrast to the proliferative expansile appearance of the stromal cells in ESS where mitotic figures are usually identified, even if sparse. Usually the smooth muscle surrounding the foci of adenomyosis is hypertrophied, this feature being absent in ESS. Adenomyosis may exhibit vascular invasion but this is usually much less obvious than in ESS, which often also exhibits extrauterine vascular invasion.

ENDOMETRIAL STROMAL TUMOR VARIANTS

Both ESN and ESS may contain areas with several unusual morphologic features. These include fibrous and myxoid areas, epithelioid and rhabdoid foci.[80,92,94] The following sections describe other variants of endometrial stromal tumor, including endometrial stromal tumor with endometrioid glandular differentiation, mixed endometrial stromal–smooth muscle tumor, and endometrial stromal tumor with sex cord-like areas. These morphologic variations in endometrial stromal neoplasm result in no special clinical manifestations and have no known impact on behavior, which is that of the underlying endometrial stromal tumor.

ENDOMETRIAL STROMAL TUMOR WITH ENDOMETRIOID GLANDS

Definition

Presence of well-formed epithelial elements of endometrioid glandular type in an endometrial stromal neoplasm of either ESN or ESS type.

Pathology

These tumors show varying numbers of focally distributed, benign endometrioid glands (Figure 17.23).[23] Because of their focality, they are found often only with extensive sampling. The presence of glands, which does not affect the neoplasm's behavior, may be explained either by focal epithelial differentiation or entrapment of endometrial or adenomyotic glands. An occasional case will exhibit many epithelial elements, resulting in diagnostic dilemmas. Sometimes, the glands will vary from atypical to carcinomatous and may be present in primary uterine or extrauterine tumors or in recurrent endometrial stromal neoplasms. Endometrioid glands appear more common in extrauterine neoplasms (see discussion on aggressive endometriosis below).

Differential diagnosis

Endometrial stromal neoplasms containing focal benign endometrioid glands should be distinguished from endometrial stromal tumors with sex cord-like areas. While both can look similar, the endometrioid foci usually have areas that are more obviously epithelial and usually show well-formed tubules that are distinct from the surrounding stroma whereas the sex-cord structures often blend into the stroma. Immunohistochemistry can also be helpful, with sex cord-like foci showing reactivity against inhibin or calretinin, or even against smooth muscle antigens, whereas the endometrioid glands are reactive against cytokeratins, including cytokeratin 7[23] (sex cord-like areas may show some reactivity for cytokeratins).

This differential diagnosis is perhaps unimportant, as the endometrial stromal element determines the behavior of both these groups of tumors. The great disparity between the volume of stroma and the number of glands present, together with the appearance of the stroma as well as its propensity to extensive vascular invasion, enables ESS to be differentiated from adenomyosis. Similar features in an extrauterine tumor allow its distinction from endometriosis. Most likely, many cases reported as aggressive endometriosis represent extrauterine ESS with extensive endometrioid glandular differentiation. Adenosarcoma characteristically shows cuffing of the stromal cells around the glands (so called 'periglandular cuffing'), a feature

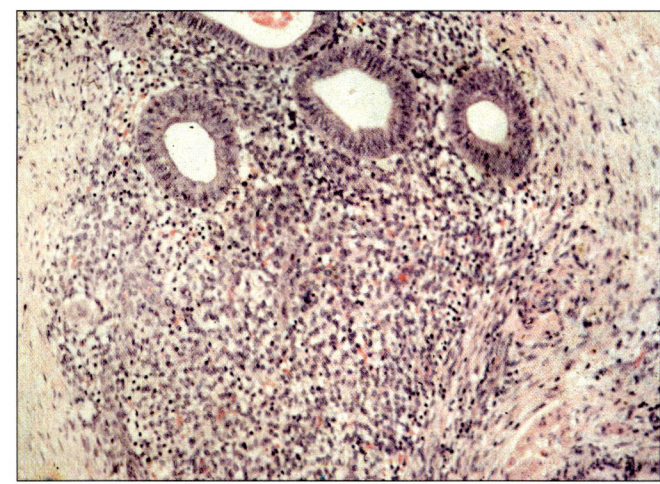

Fig. 17.23 Endometrial stromal sarcoma with focal endometrioid gland formation.

not seen in stromal neoplasms with endometrioid glands. Adenosarcoma rarely shows significant myometrial invasion unless there is sarcomatous overgrowth. If the endometrioid glands show atypia or malignant change, carcinosarcoma should be considered. The mesenchymal element of carcinosarcoma is usually composed of pleomorphic, undifferentiated cells, with or without heterologous elements, similar to those seen in undifferentiated endometrial or uterine sarcoma. Similarly, the epithelial component usually exhibits a high degree of atypia.

MIXED ENDOMETRIAL STROMAL AND SMOOTH MUSCLE TUMOR

Definition
Uterine tumors that contain prominent elements of both smooth muscle and endometrial stromal tissue.[19,51,81,91]

Pathology
The gross appearance of these tumors does not differ from that of stromal neoplasms lacking smooth muscle. On microscopic examination, these tumors not only resemble ESN and ESS but also contain areas of elongated, eosinophilic cells that morphologically resemble smooth muscle and are reactive for smooth muscle antibodies. The smooth muscle elements are usually, but not always, morphologically benign. Small areas of smooth muscle differentiation in endometrial stromal neoplasms are not unusual and the tumor should only be considered mixed if they are prominent. Some suggest the minor component should comprise at least 30% of the tumor before the diagnosis of mixed endometrial stromal–smooth muscle tumor is made, although this figure is arbitrary. The smooth muscle component sometimes has a starburst appearance with central hyalinization and blunt radiations, although this morphologic feature is not specific for a mixed endometrial stromal and smooth muscle tumor. A rare case of mixed endometrial stromal–smooth muscle tumor may even exhibit endometrioid glandular differentiation.[81]

It is important that mixed endometrial stromal–smooth muscle neoplasms be distinguished from ESS infiltrating the myometrium. Delineation requires close correlation between the gross and microscopic features with knowledge as to where tissue blocks have been taken from.

These uncommon tumors have previously been referred to as 'stromomyomas', an inappropriate term implying the neoplasm is benign. Their behavior depends on the endometrial stromal element. One of the early tumors reported metastasized 17 years later at which time study showed it was an ESS with smooth muscle elements.[52]

ENDOMETRIAL STROMAL TUMOR WITH SEX CORD-LIKE ELEMENTS

Definition
Endometrial stromal neoplasms, either ESN or ESS, containing focal sex cord-like differentiation like that found in ovarian sex-cord tumors. This tumor, sometimes given the acronym, ESTSCLE, differs from the condition 'uterine tumor resembling ovarian sex cord tumor' sometimes called UTROSCT, where the sex-cord element is extensive, involving most or all of the tumor.

Pathology
The gross appearance does not differ from the corresponding stromal neoplasm, either ESN or ESS. Microscopically, areas of the tumor exhibit cells typical of an endometrial stromal neoplasm as previously described. The sex cord-like areas, which vary in prominence, appear as anastomosing trabeculae, cords, nests, and sometimes tubular structures (Figures 17.24 and 17.25).[45] The immunophenotype of the sex cord-like foci is variable. Some are reactive for cytokeratins while others exhibit smooth muscle differentiation. Some (but not all) cases show reactivity with markers of ovarian sex-cord-stromal tumors, including inhibin, calretinin, and CD99.[45,70,73] The histogenesis of these neoplasms is discussed more fully in the following section on uterine tumors resembling ovarian sex-cord tumors.

Treatment and prognosis
Treatment is surgical. The behavior of the tumor is that of the corresponding stromal neoplasm, either ESN or ESS.

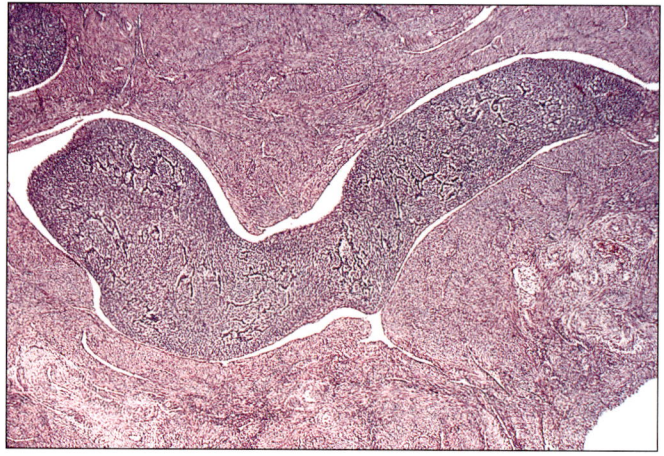

Fig. 17.24 Endometrial tumor resembling ovarian sex-cord tumor.

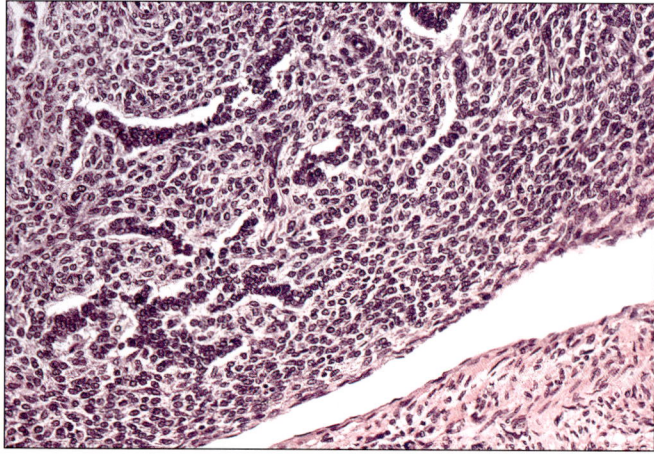

Fig. 17.25 Endometrial tumor resembling ovarian sex-cord tumor, detail.

UTERINE TUMOR RESEMBLING OVARIAN SEX-CORD TUMOR

Definition

Uterine tumors that are predominantly or entirely composed of elements resembling ovarian sex-cord tumors.

Uterine neoplasms containing elements that resemble ovarian sex-cord tumors were originally divided into two groups. One consisted of focal differentiation into sex cord-like elements in an otherwise typical endometrial stromal tumor (type 1), whereas the other was composed predominantly or even exclusively of a pattern reminiscent of an ovarian sex-cord tumor (type 2). The former are now generally termed 'endometrial stromal tumor with sex cord-like elements', reflecting the predominance of the endometrial stromal component. The latter, reflecting the predominance of the sex-cord pattern, are now called 'uterine tumor resembling ovarian sex-cord tumor' and abbreviated with the acronym UTROSCT. Occasional tumors occur within the cervix.[48]

Gross features

These tumors are generally round, well-circumscribed masses that may be submucosal, intramural or subserosal. The cut surface is gray, yellow or tan. They are soft with a uniform appearance and lack the characteristic whorled pattern of a leiomyoma.

Microscopic features

The tumors are usually well circumscribed but focally may show some irregularity with infiltration of the surrounding myometrium. The 'sex cords' that resemble those found in ovarian tumors may take several forms and appear as anastomosing trabeculae, cords, retiform areas, small nests, and sometimes well-formed tubules with lumens or combinations thereof (Figures 17.26 and 17.27).[84] Very rarely, structures resembling Call–Exner bodies are present. Sometimes the cells have eccentric nuclei and glassy eosinophilic cytoplasm, resulting in a rhabdoid appearance.[43,80] Cells with foamy cytoplasm may also be present. The sex cord-like areas are separated by stroma which may be cellular or hyalinized and hypocellular.

The sex cord-like elements have a varied and inconsistent immunophenotype and show variously reactivity with epithelial, myoid, and ovarian sex-cord-stromal markers (i.e., inhibin (Figure 17.28), CD56, and calretinin) and hormone receptors.[43,77]

Histogenesis

The origin and nature of the sex cord-like elements remain controversial. It has long been thought that the resemblance to ovarian sex-cord tumors is coincidental and that the trabecular and tubular elements are not of true sex-cord origin, but rather are derived either from endometrial stroma or myometrium. Ultrastructural and immunohistochemical studies support this view,[32,78] in some instances even suggesting smooth muscle differentiation.[106] A competing ultrastructural study has identified

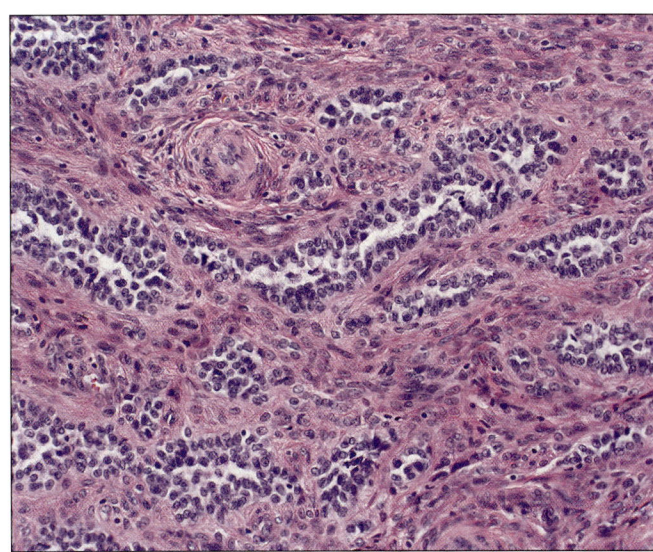

Fig. 17.27 Detail of sex cords in a uterine tumor resembling ovarian sex-cord tumor.

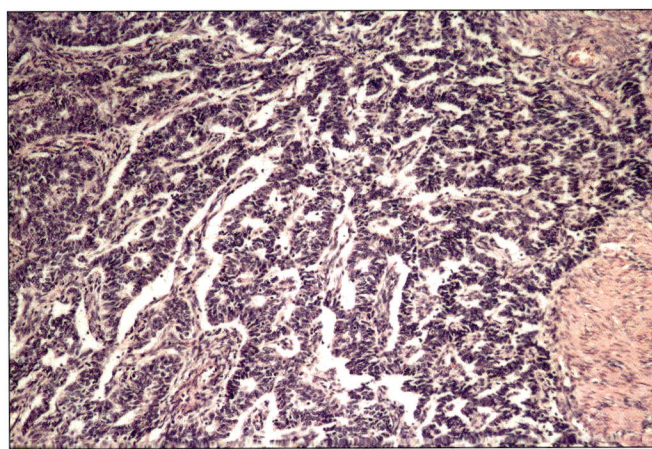

Fig. 17.26 Endometrial tumor resembling ovarian sex-cord tumor with unusually pronounced sex-cord elements.

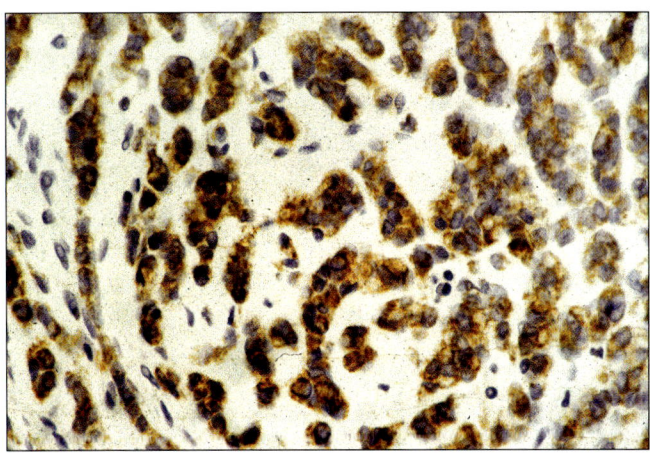

Fig. 17.28 Uterine tumor resembling ovarian sex-cord tumor exhibiting inhibin reactivity.

Charcot–Bottcher crystals, indicative of Sertoli cell differentiation.[50] Further, additional studies have shown reactivity with inhibin, calretinin, CD56 and CD99, markers of ovarian sex-cord tumors,[26,43,45] providing evidence for true sex-cord differentiation. We believe that these neoplasms are derived from multipotential uterine mesenchymal cells that have the capacity for diffrntiation along endometrial stromal, sex cord, epithelial or myoid lines.

Treatment and prognosis

Treatment is surgical. Although the behavior of UTROSCT is not well established, these tumors are generally considered neoplasms of low malignant potential with a small but definite risk of local recurrence or metastasis.

UNDIFFERENTIATED UTERINE OR ENDOMETRIAL SARCOMA

Definition

This rare malignant tumor displays pleomorphic mesenchymal cells with a high mitotic index that do not resemble the cells of the endometrial stroma and show no evidence of smooth muscle or any other specific differentiation.

Pathology

Undifferentiated sarcomas are usually bulky and polypoid, with obvious necrosis, distending the uterine cavity and even appearing at the external cervical os. Deep myometrial involvement is usually present. On microscopic examination, the cells comprising this group of tumors do not resemble endometrial stromal cells, but are generally larger. They exhibit marked variation in nuclear size and shape, with hyperchromasia (Figures 17.29–17.32). The chromatin is coarsely clumped and there are frequently large nucleoli. The cells are bizarre, rounded or simply spindle shaped, occasionally having abundant eosinophilic cytoplasm. Collagenization and vascularity are less a feature than in endometrial stromal neoplasms. Mitotic figures are numerous, almost always exceeding 10 per 10 HPFs and sometimes approaching 50 per 10 HPFs. Extensive necrosis is frequently present.

Treatment and prognosis

No reliable data are available for women with undifferentiated uterine sarcoma, because even the more recent series of endometrial stromal tumors do not make a distinction between high-grade ESS and undifferentiated uterine sarcoma. However,

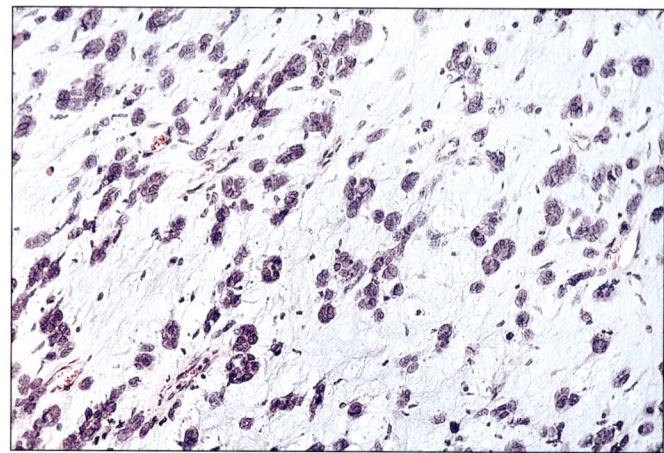

Fig. 17.30 Undifferentiated uterine sarcoma, with myxoid change.

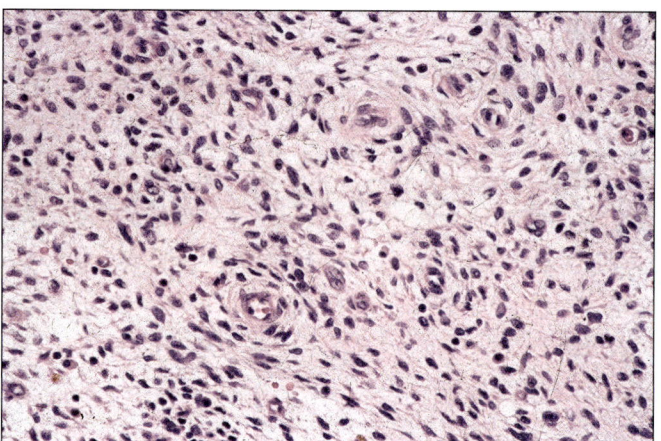

Fig. 17.31 Undifferentiated uterine sarcoma, banal pattern.

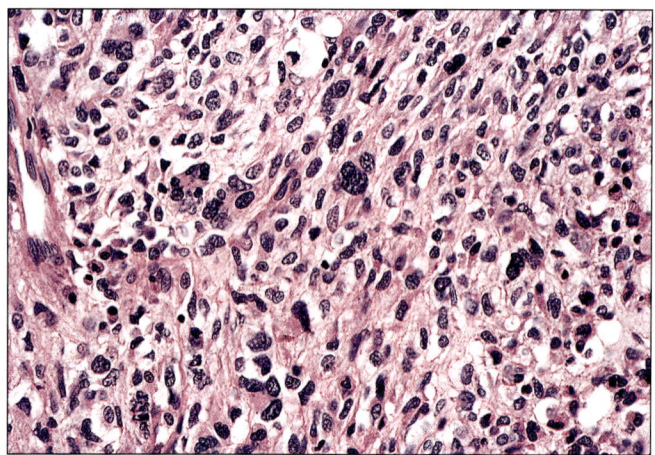

Fig. 17.29 Undifferentiated uterine sarcoma. There is marked atypia and the cells do not resemble those of endometrial stroma.

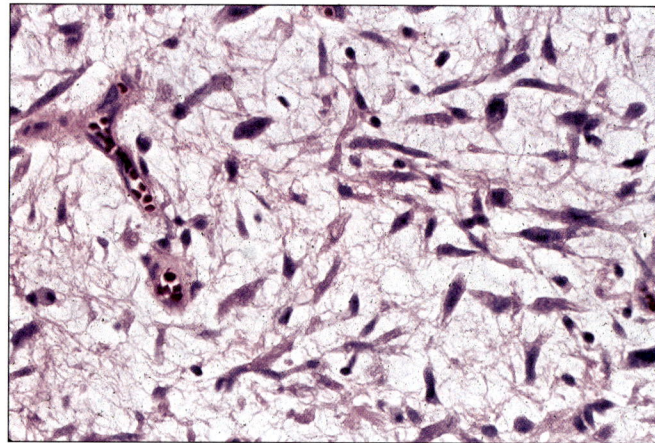

Fig. 17.32 Undifferentiated uterine sarcoma, with a past history of radiation.

it is clear that undifferentiated uterine sarcoma is a much more aggressive neoplasm than ESS. Local recurrences and distant metastases result in a high mortality within 2 years of diagnosis. Treatment is primarily surgical with or without the addition of adjuvant radiotherapy or chemotherapy. The precise value of these adjuvant modalities is largely unknown, although radiotherapy may be effective in controlling the growth of local disease.

Differential diagnosis

The undifferentiated uterine sarcoma is distinguished from ESS mainly by cellular characteristics, the former being composed of larger mesenchymal cells that are poorly differentiated. Leiomyosarcoma is excluded by the absence of smooth muscle differentiation and lack of reactivity for smooth muscle antibodies, although focal staining for α-SMA sometimes occurs. Careful sampling should be undertaken to exclude a carcinosarcoma or adenosarcoma, neoplasms in which an epithelial component is present. Other pure uterine sarcomas, such as rhabdomyosarcoma, are excluded by a combination of morphologic and immunohistochemical features.

MIXED MÜLLERIAN TUMORS

The body of the uterus, along with the fallopian tubes, the cervix, and the upper part of the vagina, develop from the primitive paramesonephric (müllerian) ducts, which in turn are derived from the mesenchyme of the urogenital ridge and the celomic lining epithelium. This anlage gives rise to all the elements of which the uterus is eventually composed: myometrial smooth muscle, endometrial stroma, and endometrial glands. Thus smooth muscle tumors of the uterus, the endometrial stromal tumors discussed above as well as endometrial carcinomas are all müllerian in origin. The term 'mixed müllerian tumor' is applied to the group of uterine tumors (these tumors may also more rarely arise in the ovary, fallopian tube or cervix) composed of both mesenchymal and epithelial elements, all components of which are of müllerian origin. These mixed neoplasms are more common in the uterus than elsewhere, probably because the epithelium and mesenchyme at this site share a common embryologic origin. The classification of these tumors (Table 17.3), which is based on combinations of whether the epithelial and mesenchymal elements are benign or malignant, is controversial as disagreement exists as

to whether several of the conditions, chiefly adenofibroma and carcinofibroma, occur with any frequency to justify a specific name.

ADENOFIBROMA

Definition

Adenofibroma, a tumor of the uterus (and rarely also of the cervix) that many, including several editors of this book, believe exists with such infrequency to hardly justify it as an entity, theoretically consists of benign epithelial and benign mesenchymal elements, both of which are an integral component of the tumor. This tumor is exceedingly rare, and must be differentiated from the far more common adenosarcoma with a subtle malignant stromal component.[135] Those who believe adenofibroma does not exist consider the lesion as an exceedingly well-differentiated form of adenosarcoma.

Clinical features

Adenofibromas are mainly tumors of postmenopausal women with a median age of around 68 years and a range from 19 to over 80 years. Like any tumor filling the endometrial cavity, the most common presenting symptom is abnormal vaginal bleeding. Occasional cases have been associated with tamoxifen therapy.[42]

Pathology

Grossly, the tumor occupies and distends the uterine cavity, arising as a broad-based polypoid mass, often lobulated or papillary (Figure 17.33). When the cervix is affected, the tumor may distend the cervical canal or present as a cervical polyp. It is soft, firm or rubbery and the cut surface may be spongy or overtly cystic.

Microscopic features

A bland epithelium that is usually of endometrioid type but which may be endocervical, ciliated or even squamous covers broad or fine papillary stromal fronds (Figures 17.34 and 17.35). Cells of fibroblastic type and more rarely endometrial

Table 17.3 Classification of mixed müllerian tumors of the uterus		
Epithelial component (neoplastic)	**Mesenchymal component (neoplastic)**	**Tumor**
Benign	Benign	Adenofibroma*
Benign	Malignant	Adenosarcoma
Malignant	Benign	Carcinofibroma*
Malignant	Malignant	Carcinosarcoma

*It is controversial whether these entities exist in sufficient numbers to warrant specific names.

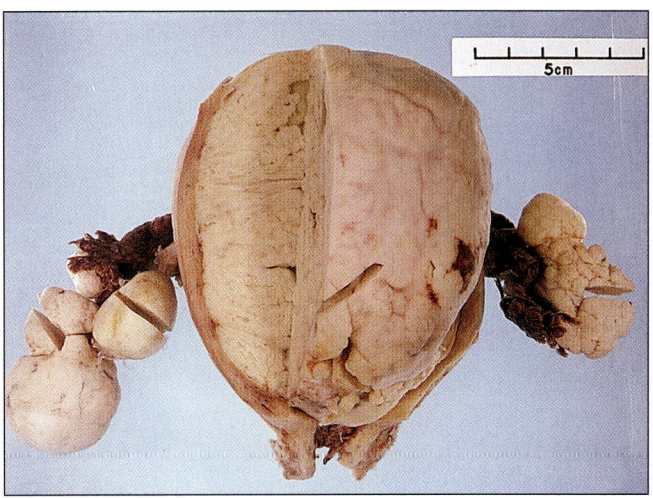

Fig. 17.33 Adenofibroma.

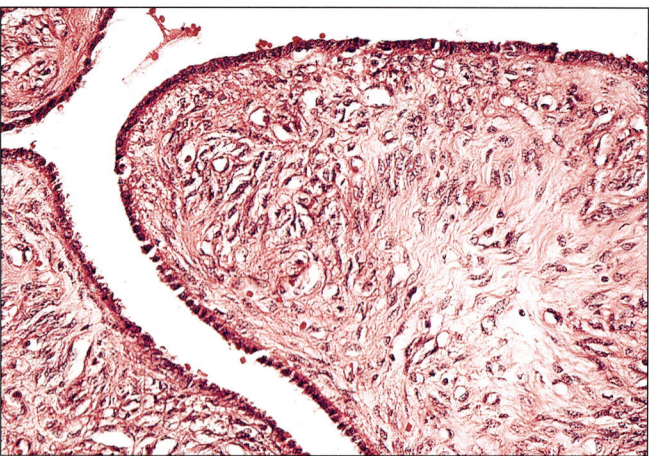

Fig. 17.34 Adenofibroma. The bland surface epithelium covers cellular and fibrous stroma.

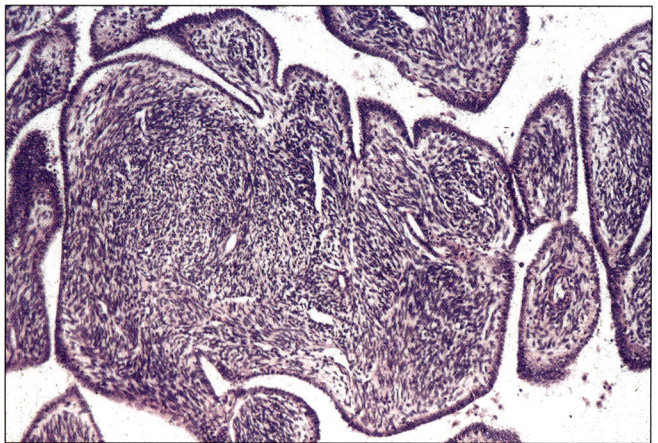

Fig. 17.35 Adenofibroma. The bland surface epithelium covers cellular and fibrous stroma.

stroma or smooth muscle make up the mesenchymal element; rarely skeletal muscle or adipose components have been reported: such lesions have been designated lipoadenofibroma or adenomyofibroma.[40,116] The stroma may be cellular or fibrous. Mitotic figures are usually absent and should not exceed 1 per 10 HPFs in the most active areas; greater mitotic activity than this number warrants a diagnosis of adenosarcoma which is much more common. Periglandular cuffing by stromal cells should result in consideration of adenosarcoma. The stromal elements are cytologically bland without nuclear pleomorphism. Occasionally, an adenocarcinoma arises within an adenofibroma but this is probably a coincidental association.[129]

Treatment and prognosis

While by definition the adenofibroma is benign, hysterectomy is the most appropriate treatment. This is mainly because adenosarcoma cannot be excluded in curettings or biopsy, as discussed later, but also because recurrence of adenofibroma treated by curettage or local excision may occur, even in the absence of mitotic activity. It is for these reasons that many consider this a lesion that does not exist, but rather is a well-differentiated form of adenosarcoma.

Differential diagnosis

At the heart of the controversy whether or not adenofibroma exists as an entity is the ability to distinguish it from adenosarcoma. The critical features are the number of mitotic figures in the stroma, morphology of the stromal cells and the presence of periglandular cuffing by stromal cells. Mitotic counts greater than 1 per 10 HPFs warrant a diagnosis of müllerian adenosarcoma, a diagnosis that should also be made if there is marked stromal cellularity, more than mild nuclear atypia or periglandular stromal cuffing.[22] Even in the absence of mitoses, we have encountered cases that have recurred. A confident diagnosis of adenofibroma cannot be made on curetted or avulsed material because adenosarcoma cannot be excluded unless the whole tumor is available for examination. Thus, a hysterectomy is required to ensure that the tissue examined was not just the most benign area of an adenosarcoma. Using these strict criteria, the diagnosis of adenofibroma is made only rarely, comprising only about 5% of one large series of adenofibromas and adenosarcomas. Cases have been reported in which repeated curettages have been carried out because the tumor was wrongly thought to be benign before a diagnosis of adenosarcoma has eventually been made.[22]

The architectural pattern of the glandular elements, with abundant intervening mesenchyme, and the benign appearance of the epithelial cells serve to separate this tumor from carcinoma. On the other hand, it is important to recognize the difference between adenofibroma and a benign endometrial (or endocervical) polyp. A benign polyp does not require further treatment. While the distinction can be difficult, the neoplastic condition should be considered if the lesion has a papillary surface pattern and a stroma that is cellular. The stroma of endometrial polyps tends to be more hyaline than that of adenofibroma.

ADENOSARCOMA

Definition

A mixed tumor composed of benign neoplastic glandular elements and sarcomatous, albeit often low-grade, stromal elements.

Clinical features

Adenosarcoma occurs in all age groups (14–89 years) but is mainly seen in women after the menopause (median age 58 years). The most common presenting symptom is abnormal vaginal bleeding but some patients present with pelvic pain or a vaginal discharge. Some patients have taken tamoxifen therapy or have had prior radiation therapy.[22,24]

Gross features

Adenosarcoma most commonly arises from the endometrium, including the lower uterine segment, but rare cases arise in the endocervix and within the myometrium, probably from adenomyosis. Some tumors form multiple polyps. The uterine cavity is filled and distended by a coarsely lobulated, soft, spongy or rubbery, polypoid and sometimes large mass (Figure 17.36). Occasionally, it may project through the cervical os. The cut surface may show variably sized cysts or clefts. There is often hemorrhage and focal necrosis. The margin of the tumor is usually clearly defined.

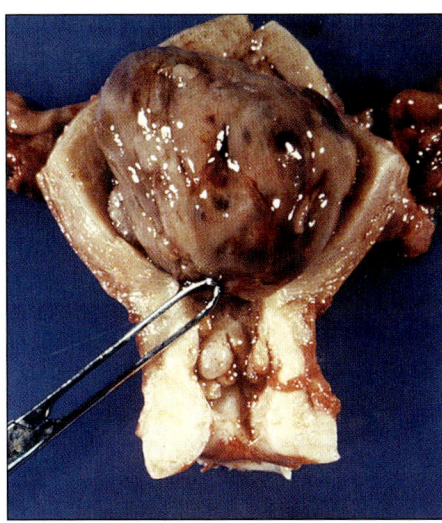

Fig. 17.36 Adenosarcoma. The tumor is large, polypoid and smooth surfaced, distending the uterine cavity.

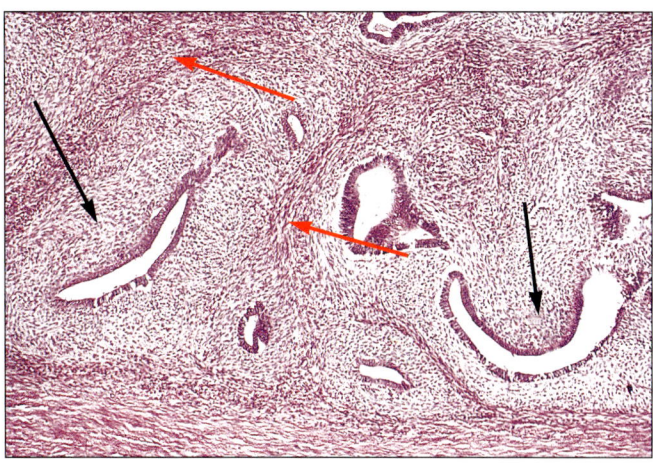

Fig. 17.38 Adenosarcoma. Cleft-like spaces and tubular glands are surrounded by cellular stroma (black arrows) with more fibrous stroma in the background (red arrows).

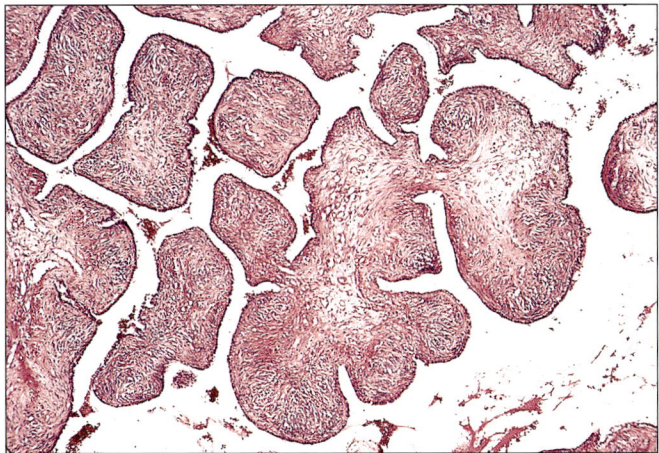

Fig. 17.37 Adenosarcoma. The cut surface shows numerous slit-like spaces. In some areas the histology is identical to that called adenofibroma. At low magnification, it also resembles a phylloides tumor of the breast.

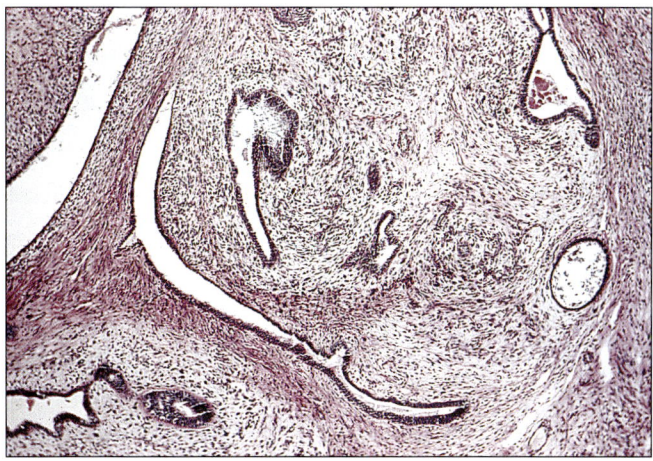

Fig. 17.39 Adenosarcoma with cleft-like glands surrounded by a cellular stroma.

Microscopic features

The mixed nature of the tumor is exemplified by the presence of both glandular and stromal elements, the latter tending to predominate. An essential feature is an epithelial lining that is well differentiated but neoplastic (described often as 'benign') and the malignant nature of the mesenchymal component, thereby placing the tumor halfway along the spectrum of mixed müllerian tumors, with adenofibroma at one end and carcinosarcoma at the other. At low power magnification the tumor often has a leaf-like pattern, resembling a phylloides tumor of the breast (Figure 17.37).

The glands are widely separated by the abundant stromal component and are usually lined by cuboidal or low columnar epithelium (Figures 17.38 and 17.39). In most cases, this epithelium resembles that of proliferative or hyperplastic endometrium, although epithelium of ciliated, endocervical, and occasionally squamous type may also be seen. Some glands are dilated while others are slit-like. Commonly, the epithelium appears active, showing mitotic activity or subnuclear vacuoles

despite the advanced age of some patients, even when the adjacent endometrium is atrophic. Focal nuclear atypia of the epithelial element is present in about one-third of cases, which may amount to severe atypical hyperplasia. Commonly, some of the epithelial cells will be cuboidal, with a large nucleolus and prominent eosinophilic cytoplasm (Figure 17.40). Rarely a carcinoma arises within a pre-existing adenosarcoma, suggesting this may be the histogenetic origin of a small number of carcinosarcomas (see discussion on histogenesis of carcinosarcomas below).

The stromal component, which is often low grade, is composed of spindled and/or round cells, the former usually arranged in whorls and the latter loosely dispersed. One of the most characteristic features of adenosarcoma is the manner in which the stromal cells concentrate about the glandular components, forming a cuff ('periglandular cuffing') or so-called 'cambium' layer (Figures 17.38 and 17.39). This cellular zone, in contrast to the more hyaline or fibrous areas away from the glands, is where the maximum nuclear atypia and mitotic activity is found (Figures 17.41 and 17.42). While a mitotic count of 1 per 10 HPFs is often found in these tumors, it may be less

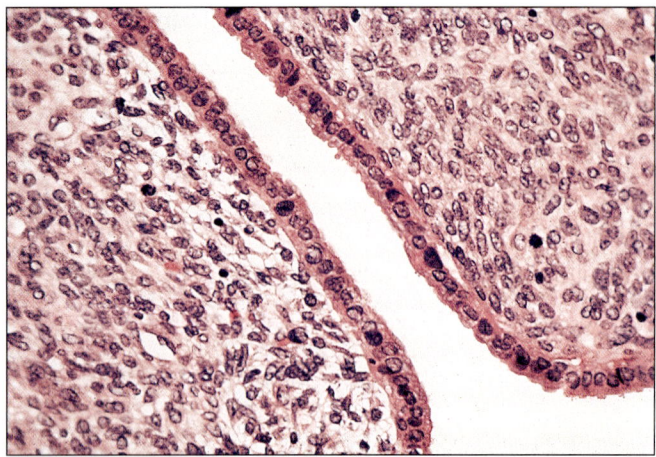

Fig. 17.40 Adenosarcoma. The cuboidal cells with markedly eosinophilic cytoplasm that line the spaces are neoplastic (and benign) but the stroma is the malignant component found in metastases.

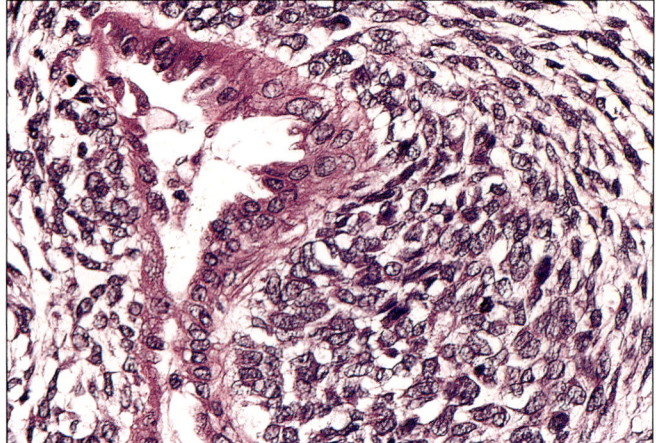

Fig. 17.41 Adenosarcoma. Increased cellularity in the stroma adjacent to glandular epithelium.

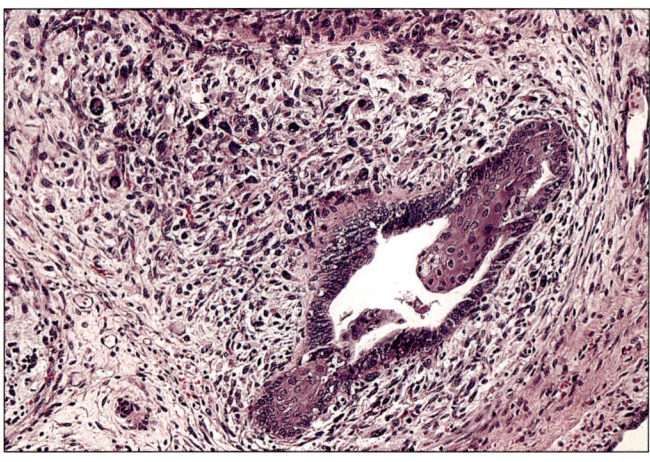

Fig. 17.42 Adenosarcoma. The periglandular stroma shows pleomorphism in addition to increased cellularity. Metaplastic squamous epithelium arises from the glandular epithelium.

in some. Also within many areas in any individual neoplasm, it is less. In practice, if the characteristic leaf-like pattern is present with periglandular cuffing, a diagnosis of adenosarcoma is made in the absence of mitotic figures. Many adenosarcomas contain exclusively homologous mesenchymal elements, composed of tissue types that are normally found in the uterus, including endometrial stromal sarcoma or undifferentiated sarcoma. About one-fourth of the tumors have heterologous elements with embryonal rhabdomyoblasts predominating, but features of chondrosarcoma and liposarcoma also occur. Sex cord-like elements (Figure 17.43), identical to those seen in endometrial stromal neoplasms, may be present within the mesenchymal component.[20]

Most adenosarcomas are confined to the endometrium. A small number invade into the inner half of the myometrium. Deep invasion is rare in the absence of sarcomatous overgrowth (see below).

Treatment and prognosis
The treatment of choice is total abdominal hysterectomy with bilateral salpingo-oophorectomy. The role of adjuvant radiotherapy and chemotherapy has not been fully evaluated but apparently benefits some patients, both with primary and recurrent tumor.[19,135]

Adenosarcoma has a relatively low malignant potential (unless associated with sarcomatous overgrowth – see below) compared with carcinosarcoma, although about 25% of patients die from their disease.[21] Recurrences are usually confined to the vagina, pelvis or abdomen. They may be late, for which reason long-term follow-up is needed, and are usually composed solely of the mesenchymal element (Figure 17.44).[124] Distant metastasis, which occurs in 5% of cases, is almost always composed of pure sarcoma.[22] Not unexpectedly, myometrial invasion is associated with an increased risk of recurrence.[22]

Differential diagnosis
Adenosarcoma is distinguished from adenofibroma by the presence of a stromal mitotic count of 1 or more per 10 HPFs (although, as discussed, this is not always present), marked stromal cellularity with periglandular cuffing, or more than mild nuclear atypia of the stromal cells. As adenosarcoma is so much more common than adenofibroma, if in doubt, diag-

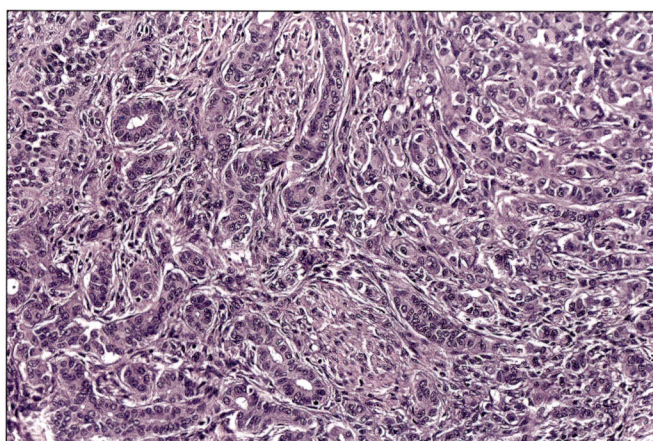

Fig. 17.43 Adenosarcoma with sex-cord elements.

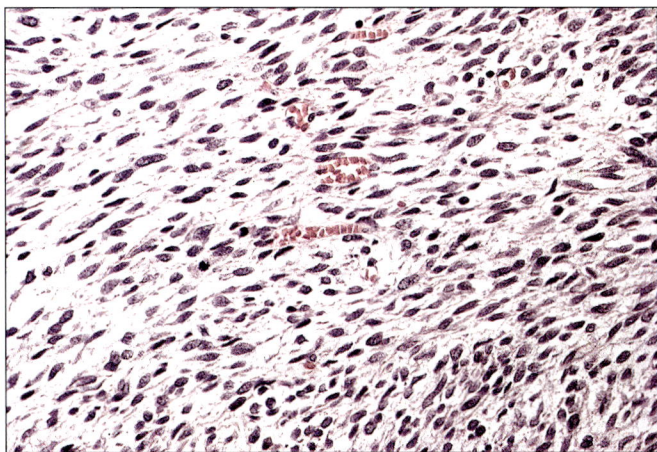

Fig. 17.44 Recurrent adenosarcoma. Recurrent and metastatic tumors are composed of the malignant stromal element only.

nose low-grade adenosarcoma to ensure optimal management, including long-term follow-up.

Carcinosarcoma is composed of clearly malignant epithelial elements, usually with a diffuse distribution, that have substantially different architectural and cytologic appearances from those seen in adenosarcoma. The stromal component of most carcinosarcomas tends to be highly pleomorphic and less well differentiated than in most adenosarcomas and lacks the periglandular cuff of increased stromal cellularity that is so characteristic of adenosarcoma. Sometimes a carcinoma may arise in a pre-existing adenosarcoma.

Benign endometrial polyps have stroma like the adjacent endometrium or the stroma may be hyaline or fibrous. The epithelial component usually resembles the adjacent endometrium with some distended glands. Multilayering and mild architectural atypia are not uncommon. If the stroma of an endometrial polyp is markedly cellular with nuclear atypia and mitotic activity, then adenosarcoma should be considered, particularly if there is periglandular cuffing and the epithelial cells differ from the adjacent endometrium.

The atypical polypoid adenomyoma, a lesion generally regarded as benign in the literature but which some of us consider as a low-grade malignancy, is composed of stroma that is predominantly cellular smooth muscle and may exhibit some mitotic activity (see below). The epithelial elements usually show greater atypia than is seen in adenosarcoma and foci of squamous differentiation (acanthotic morules), sometimes with central necrosis, are characteristic. Recurrence is not infrequent after excision.

Endometrial stromal sarcoma may have occasional trapped endometrial glands at the margin of the tumor and, rarely, endometrioid glandular differentiation may be present within the tumor. The distribution of these glands, however, differs from that in adenosarcoma and periglandular stromal cuffing is not seen. Other uterine sarcomas, such as undifferentiated sarcoma, may contain entrapped glands but these are not an integral component of the tumor.

ADENOSARCOMA WITH SARCOMATOUS OVERGROWTH

Adenosarcomas in which more than 25% of the tumor is composed of pure sarcoma are designated as 'adenosarcoma with sarcomatous overgrowth'.[18,21] The sarcomatous component is usually composed of more poorly differentiated tumor with a higher mitotic rate than in the sarcomatous element of the residual adenosarcoma. The presence of sarcomatous overgrowth in an adenosarcoma predicts a poor prognosis[18,57,131] and is often associated with deep myometrial invasion or distant metastasis.

CARCINOFIBROMA

Carcinofibroma is a tumor composed of a malignant epithelial element and a benign but neoplastic stromal component. Its existence is not agreed upon. It does not appear in the classifications of some authorities and has not been described in the literature since the 1980s. However, it is included herein since it appears in the recently updated WHO classification of tumors of the breast and female genital organs.[126] Carcinofibroma of the uterus, if it exists, is extremely rare and if the diagnosis is to be made, it should be done so with great caution, as many carcinomas of the endometrium elicit a prominent fibroblastic stromal reaction. The distinction between a non-neoplastic fibroblastic proliferation of the stroma and a true neoplastic mesenchymal element is very difficult, if not impossible, to make reliably. It is doubtful whether a diagnosis of carcinofibroma should ever be made on a biopsy specimen, a hysterectomy being required to exclude a carcinosarcoma with a focally bland mesenchymal element. The authors and editors have never diagnosed a carcinofibroma.

CARCINOSARCOMA

Definition
A mixed tumor composed of epithelial elements and mesenchyme, both of which are histologically malignant. This tumor, which is the most common of all mixed müllerian tumors, has long been recognized under a variety of different terms used throughout the years. Those containing only homologous mesenchymal elements were called 'carcinosarcoma' and those with heterologous elements were known as 'mixed mesodermal tumor' or 'malignant mixed müllerian tumor' (MMMT). With the recognition that homologous and heterologous tumors behave similarly, the terminology for all variants is now 'carcinosarcoma' with MMMT as an acceptable alternative. Note that the adjective 'mixed', both in MMMT and in the older 'mixed mesodermal tumor', refers to the mixture of epithelial and stromal elements and not the mixture of different mesenchymal cell types that are commonly encountered in these tumors.

Clinical features
Carcinosarcoma accounts for 2–5% of all malignancies of the uterine corpus.[11] It is most common in postmenopausal women (median age 66 years), but sometimes occurs in younger women and children. The most common presentation is abnormal vaginal bleeding, but a bloody or watery discharge, abdominal pain or an abdominal mass may also be the first symptoms. Gastrointestinal or urinary tract symptoms suggest extrauterine spread. Although the conventional Papanicolaou smear is insensitive (60%) for detecting carcinosarcoma, when the result is abnormal the Papanicolaou is an important stage-independent adverse prognosticator.[117]

Carcinosarcoma shares risk factors with endometrial carcinoma, but the influence of these factors is weaker than with carcinoma. A history of prior pelvic irradiation has been reported in 7–37% of cases in the earlier literature for the treatment of benign conditions such as abnormal uterine bleeding and, more recently, following treatment for cervical cancer. The time interval between radiation therapy and development of the carcinosarcoma generally is between 10 and 20 years.

Carcinosarcoma may also develop after long-term treatment with tamoxifen for breast cancer.[82] However, there is no conclusive evidence that tamoxifen has either a direct carcinogenic effect or is even involved in these tumors' genesis. Alternative explanations are that tamoxifen treatment is now so widespread that carcinosarcoma must occur spontaneously on a statistical basis of chance alone, or that women with breast cancer treated with tamoxifen are surviving longer and therefore have more opportunity to develop carcinosarcomas. On the other hand, carcinosarcoma shares some risk factors with endometrial carcinoma (and, as discussed later, most carcinosarcomas are in reality carcinomas with sarcomatous metaplasia[71]), and some possess estrogen and progesterone receptors.[3] Since tamoxifen may be implicated in the development of endometrial carcinoma, not unexpectedly some patients may develop carcinosarcoma.

Gross features

Carcinosarcomas lack a characteristic naked-eye appearance. Some arise in atrophic uteri while others develop into such enormous masses that the uterus proper cannot be identified. The tumor in these cases diffusely enlarges the uterus by infiltrating and expanding its wall. More typically, carcinosarcoma forms a broad-based polyp that fills and expands the uterine cavity (Figure 17.45), often protruding through the cervix (Figure 17.46). The cut surface may show extensive necrosis and hemorrhage, and gritty or hard areas may be present, corresponding to bone or cartilage. The surface of the tumor is often smooth, in contrast to the roughness of most adenocarcinomas. Myometrial invasion is obvious macroscopically in most cases. Occasional cases arise within and are confined to an otherwise benign endometrial polyp.

Microscopic features

The microscopic features of carcinosarcoma are striking. Both the epithelial and mesenchymal elements are malignant (Figure 17.47), the carcinomatous component corresponding to any müllerian type. Often there is a sharp demarcation between the epithelial and stromal elements. Most frequently the epithelial component is a poorly differentiated serous carcinoma (Figure 17.48), and squamous elements are not infrequently seen (Figure 17.49). Endometrioid differentiation is less common. On rare occasions, squamous cell carcinoma is the sole epithelial component. Other epithelial patterns may be encountered, such as mucinous carcinoma, clear cell carcinoma or undifferentiated carcinoma. The proportion of the tumor that is epithelial varies greatly. Sometimes the sarcomatous component predominates to such an extent that the carcinoma may be difficult to identify and extensive sampling is necessary to demonstrate this. Any uterine neoplasm composed of high-grade sarcoma, especially with heterologous elements, should be extensively sampled to exclude a carcinosarcoma. In some cases, the carcinoma predominates.

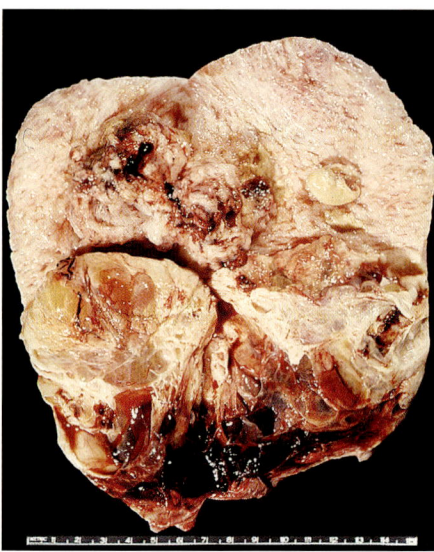

Fig. 17.45 Carcinosarcoma. A solid, partially cystic, and necrotic mass that expands the uterine cavity.

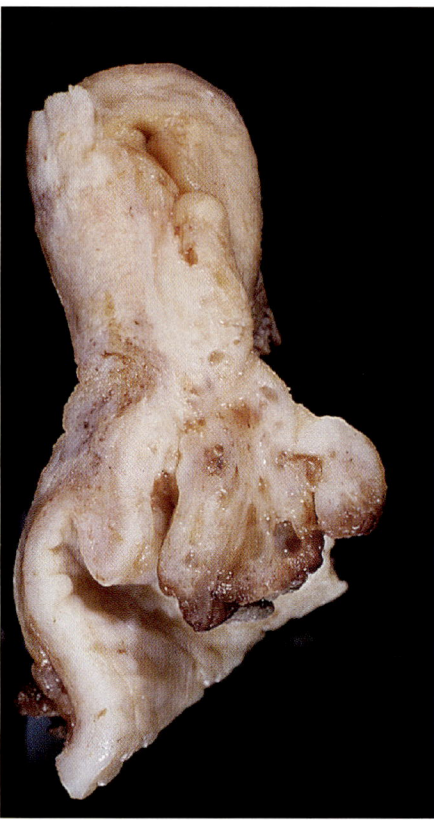

Fig. 17.46 Carcinosarcoma. This tumor presented as a pedunculated polypoid mass that extended into the cervical canal and protruded from the cervix.

The stromal element may be homologous or heterologous but usually is obviously malignant. The homologous carcinosarcoma contains a mesenchymal element that is composed of cell types that are normally found in the uterus. Endometrial stromal sarcoma, fibrosarcoma, and undifferentiated sarcoma are the most common homologous components but leiomyo-

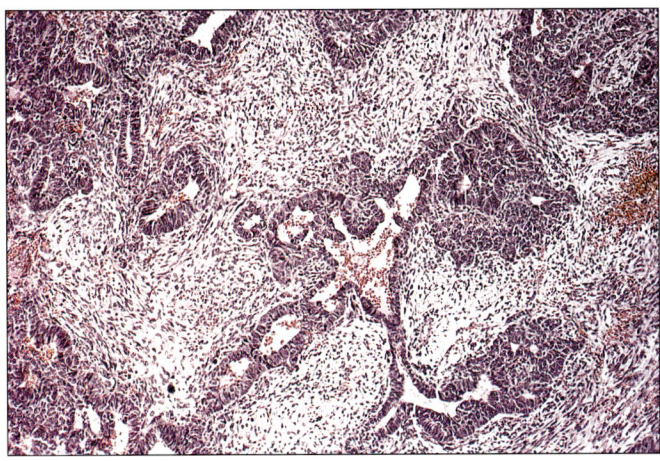

Fig. 17.47 Carcinosarcoma. A homologous tumor containing malignant stroma and malignant epithelium of types native to the uterus.

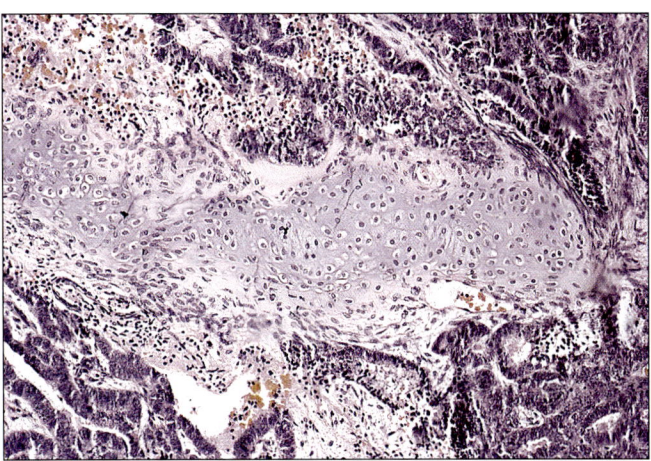

Fig. 17.50 Carcinosarcoma, heterologous. Heterologous carcinosarcomas contain components that are foreign to the normal uterus, e.g., cartilage.

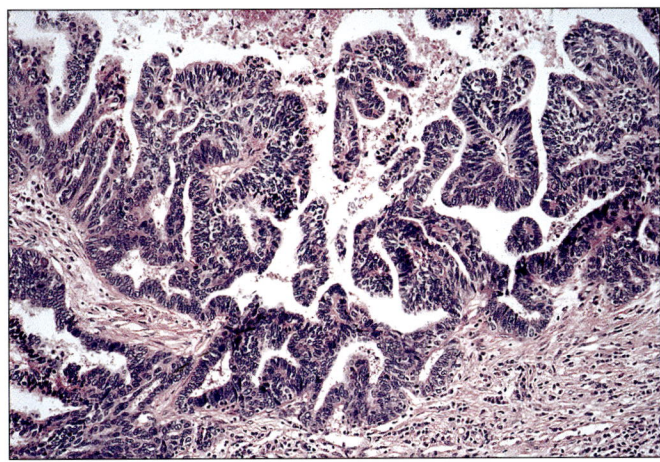

Fig. 17.48 Carcinosarcoma. The carcinomatous component is often of endometrioid pattern.

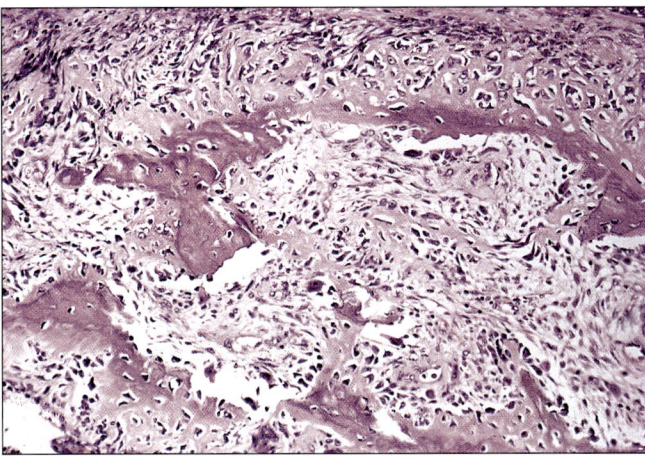

Fig. 17.51 Carcinosarcoma, heterologous. Malignant osteoid is present.

sarcoma is also seen and many tumors contain mixtures of these tissue types.

The heterologous elements most common in carcinosarcoma in order of decreasing frequency are rhabdomyosarcoma, chondrosarcoma (Figure 17.50), osteosarcoma (Figure 17.51), and liposarcoma. The most frequently encountered heterologous element is striated muscle, which is easily identified if the rhabdomyoblasts are well differentiated and have cross-striations. The cross-striations can be identified on H&E staining but recognition may be helped by staining with phosphotungstic acid hematoxylin (PTAH) or immunohistochemistry. Relatively large cells that may be strap-like, round or oval with atypical nuclei and granular eosinophilic cytoplasm (racket cells) are readily accepted as rhabdomyoblasts, even in the absence of cross-striations (Figures 17.52 and 17.53). They are more difficult to recognize if they are sparse and occur singly (Figure 17.54). Immunohistochemistry, using antibodies to myoglobin, desmin, and sarcomeric actin (Figure 17.55), helps confirm their presence. Chondrosarcoma is the next most commonly encountered heterologous element and osteosarcoma and liposarcoma (Figure 17.56) are rare. Other uncommonly reported elements include neuroectodermal tissue,[33] yolk sac

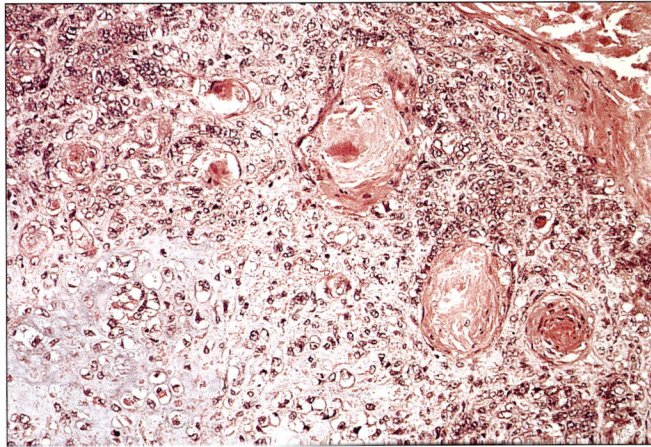

Fig. 17.49 Carcinosarcoma. A squamous epithelial component is present.

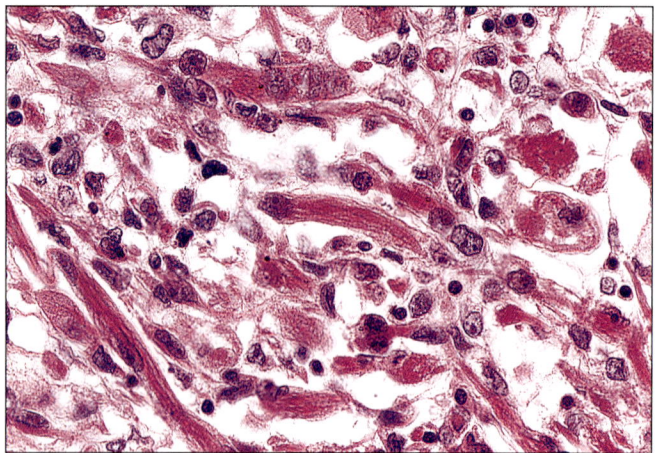

Fig. 17.52 Carcinosarcoma, heterologous. Rhabdomyoblasts appear here as elongated, strap-like cells.

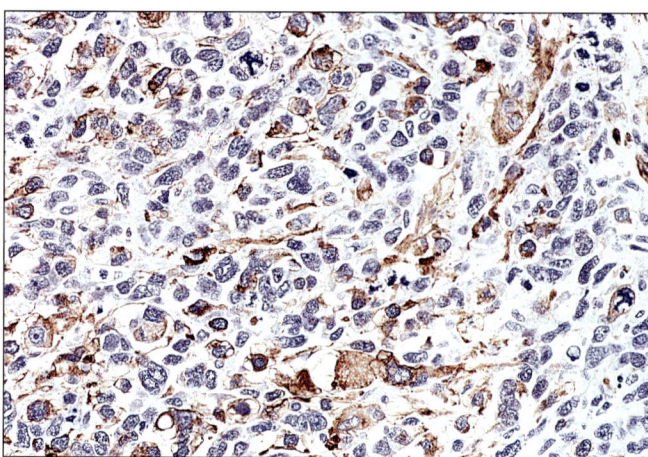

Fig. 17.55 Carcinosarcoma, heterologous. The rhabdomyoblasts are immunohistochemically positive for actin.

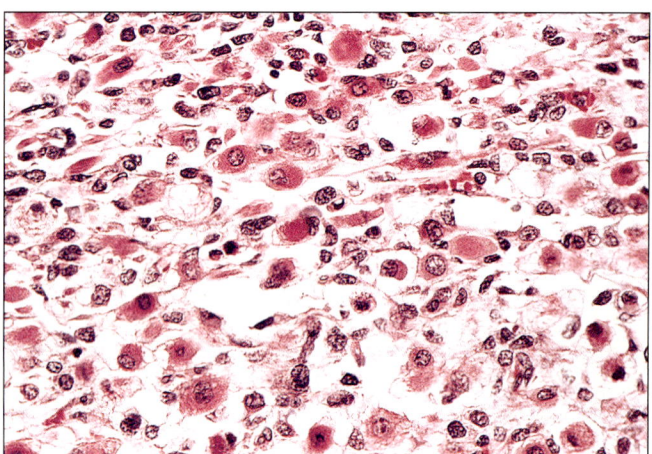

Fig. 17.53 Carcinosarcoma, heterologous. Rhabdomyoblasts are often present as pleomorphic, rounded cells with copious eosinophilic cytoplasm.

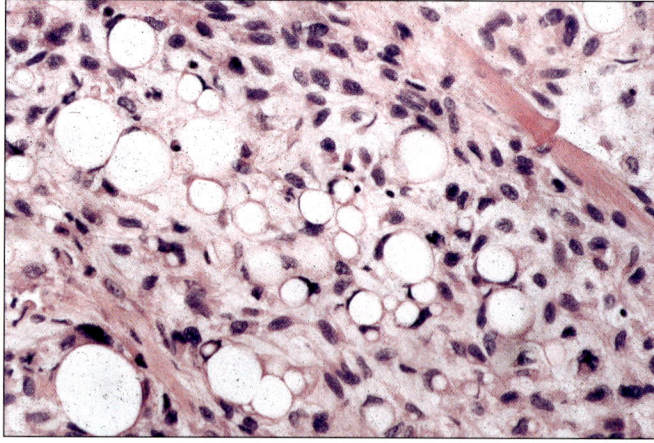

Fig. 17.56 Carcinosarcoma, heterologous with lipoblasts (liposarcoma).

tumor that may be associated with high serum levels of α-fetoprotein,[100,112] melanocytic[2] and neuroendocrine elements. Carcinosarcomas typically contain cells with a marked degree of anaplasia, with striking variations in nuclear size and shape, bizarre mitotic figures, and giant cells. This first impression of pleomorphism is often the initial pointer to the histologic diagnosis. Cells with a rhabdoid appearance may be present. There is often extensive necrosis, deep myometrial invasion, and cervical involvement with lymphovascular permeation and often extrauterine spread.

Treatment and prognosis

Carcinosarcomas, if stage 1 or 2, are usually treated by total abdominal hysterectomy and bilateral salpingo-oophorectomy. Omentectomy is often performed due to the propensity for abdominal dissemination. The role of adjuvant radiotherapy and chemotherapy is uncertain, with more recent reports expressing greater optimism than in the past.[15,62,132] The prognosis is poor, ranging from 11 to 35% 5-year survival. In the past heterologous in contradistinction to homologous stromal elements were believed to be associated with a poorer prognosis, and a rhabdomyosarcomatous component had the worst prognosis of all. Chondrosarcoma was thought to confer a

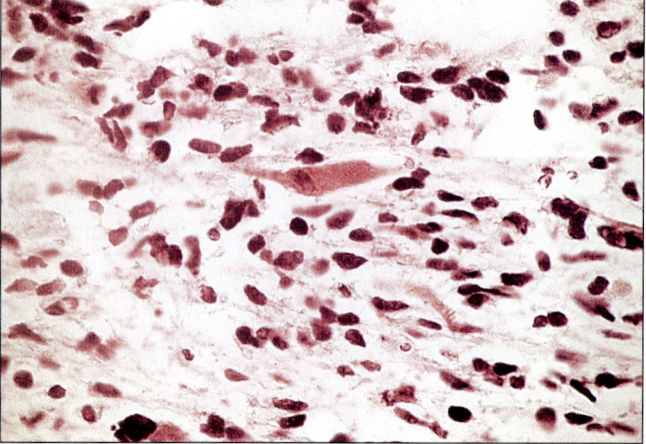

Fig. 17.54 Carcinosarcoma, heterologous. Rhabdomyoblasts may occur singly.

more favorable outcome. Recent reports refute these suspicions. Heterologous elements,[127] variations in histologic grade, and mitotic activity in the stroma have little bearing on the eventual outcome. Conversely, the epithelial elements may be prognostically significant with serous, clear cell or undifferentiated elements imparting a worse prognosis. Stage, however, is still the single most important prognostic factor. However, recurrences may occur even in those cases lacking myometrial infiltration.

Associated with a good prognosis are early stage disease, limited spread in relation to myometrial and cervical involvement, and absence of vascular invasion. Increased numbers of lymph nodes collected also correlate with longer disease-free and overall survival.[127] Five-year survival rates of 50% have been reported in women with stage 1 disease. Parity may also be a statistically independent prognostic factor. In a series of 83 patients, women with four or more children formed a subgroup of long-term survivors, even where the interval from the birth of the last child exceeded 20 years.[66]

Differential diagnosis

Not uncommonly, a definitive diagnosis of carcinosarcoma cannot be made from uterine biopsy or curettings. The specimen may be scanty, only one element may be represented, or there may be extensive hemorrhage or necrosis. Whether the specimen is from a diagnostic curettage or from a hysterectomy, carcinosarcoma may be difficult to distinguish from undifferentiated carcinoma, particularly if there are pleomorphic and poorly differentiated areas with a 'pseudosarcomatous' appearance in the latter neoplasm. In contrast to monophasic tumors (undifferentiated carcinomas and sarcomas), the epithelial and mesenchymal elements of carcinosarcoma should not merge with one another. Although immunohistochemistry has been thought useful to differentiate undifferentiated carcinoma from carcinosarcoma, both the mesenchymal and epithelial elements of carcinosarcomas may show reactivity for many epithelial and connective tissue markers.[27] Thus, cytokeratin staining of the stromal element does not mean that the tumor is a carcinoma with poorly differentiated areas. In reality this distinction may be unimportant since the critical prognostic element is the epithelial component. Similarly, as there is no evidence that homologous and heterologous carcinosarcomas behave differently, there seems little point in going to extreme lengths in order to identify heterologous elements within a carcinosarcoma, other than as an academic exercise.

Distinction from pure uterine sarcomas is made by finding obvious epithelial elements in carcinosarcoma. Adenosarcomas are distinguished by the well-differentiated 'benign' nature of the epithelium and the characteristic mesenchymal cuffing around the glands. Some low grade endometrioid carcinomas have spindle cell foci that should be differentiated from carcinosarcoma. These spindle cell elements may exhibit squamoid differentiation. In carcinosarcoma, the mesenchymal component is usually high grade with obvious anaplasia.

Histogenesis of carcinosarcomas

There are several possible ways in which carcinosarcomas may originate:

- the 'collision' theory suggests that the epithelial and mesenchymal elements have arisen independently

and collided to give the impression of a single mixed tumor
- the 'combination' theory claims that both elements arose from a stem cell that had the ability to differentiate along both lines
- the 'conversion' theory suggests that the sarcomatous element derives from the carcinoma during the tumor's evolution.

The combination and conversion theories are not mutually exclusive. There is no doubt that collision tumors do rarely occur but these are relatively easy to identify in hysterectomy specimens because there will be areas of separate carcinoma and sarcoma.[58,71,72] A small number of carcinosarcomas probably represent a carcinoma arising in a pre-existing adenosarcoma but this is rare.

The 'conversion' theory is currently widely accepted, whereby the sarcomatous component develops from the carcinoma.[71,72] Tumors arising by this mechanism should be monoclonal, in contrast to collision tumors derived from two distinct clones. Evaluation of p53 and K-ras mutations[133] as well as immunohistochemical[35] and cytogenetic[29] studies on cultured cell lines from carcinosarcomas has confirmed that most, although not all, carcinosarcomas are monoclonal, further supporting the conversion theory of histogenesis. Concordance of p53 staining between the epithelial and mesenchymal components has been interpreted as evidence for monoclonality.[67]

There is now also abundant evidence that the carcinomatous component is the 'driving force' in most uterine carcinosarcomas and, analogous to the situation in other organs such as breast and urinary bladder, these tumors are in reality 'metaplastic' carcinomas or carcinomas with sarcomatous 'metaplasia',[71,72] although the term carcinosarcoma is retained. The pattern of spread generally resembles that of high-grade endometrial carcinoma. Lymphatic and vascular invasion, when identified, usually consists exclusively of carcinoma.[120] Metastatic deposits, whether local or distant, are predominantly, but not exclusively, composed of carcinoma.[120] These findings, although not supported by all,[34] suggest that the epithelial component invades much more readily than the mesenchymal component. Furthermore, the behavior of carcinosarcoma does not depend upon the grade, mitotic index or the presence of and types of heterologous element within the stromal component but is more closely related to the features of the epithelial element.[114] High-grade endometrioid, undifferentiated, serous and clear cell carcinomatous components are associated with a high frequency of metastasis.

Because this evidence supports the premise that the epithelial elements dictate prognosis, these findings have been interpreted to indicate that carcinosarcomas are 'conversion' tumors with the sarcomatous element evolving from a carcinoma by a 'metaplastic' process. As a result, some authors now believe carcinosarcomas should be classified with endometrial adenocarcinomas rather than with sarcomas, a view with which we agree.[71,72,120] A study designed specifically to assess whether high-grade and histologically unfavorable types of endometrial adenocarcinoma behave in the same way as carcinosarcoma has, nevertheless, shown that the outcome is worse in carcinosarcomas than in grade 3 endometrioid adenocarcinomas and serous and clear cell carcinomas.[35] Based on this, some feel that carcinosarcoma should not be classified along with endometrial carcinomas but should remain separate from these.

OTHER SARCOMAS

Endometrial stromal sarcoma, undifferentiated sarcoma, and leiomyosarcoma together comprise the great majority of malignant mesenchymal tumors of the uterine body. As discussed above, most uterine carcinosarcomas are metaplastic carcinomas. Only brief mention of other very rare primary uterine sarcomas needs be made. These are the pure heterologous sarcomas and mixed sarcomas with heterologous elements ('mixed' in this context meaning a mixture of mesenchymal tissue types). These diagnoses should be made only after there has been a very thorough search for epithelial elements to exclude a carcinosarcoma or adenosarcoma (occasional residual entrapped benign endometrial glands may be present in pure uterine sarcomas). Probably, some tumors represent carcinosarcomas or adenosarcomas in which the epithelial element has not been identified or has been overgrown by the sarcomatous component. Included in the category of pure sarcoma are the pure heterologous sarcomas, rhabdomyosarcoma (embryonal, alveolar or pleomorphic),[10,60,111] malignant fibrous histiocytoma,[110] osteosarcoma,[37,55] chondrosarcoma,[56] angiosarcoma,[86] liposarcoma,[61] and alveolar soft-part sarcoma.[102] The histologies are similar to their counterparts elsewhere. Sarcomas without an epithelial component but containing a mixture of homologous and heterologous elements are exceedingly rare.

BENIGN OR BORDERLINE MESENCHYMAL TUMORS

There have been occasional reports of benign mesenchymal neoplasms arising within the uterus. These have included lipoma, rhabdomyoma, hemangioma, lymphangioma, and solitary fibrous tumor.

UTERINE PERIVASCULAR EPITHELIOID CELL TUMOR (PECOMA)

A perivascular epithelioid cell has been proposed as the cell of origin of epithelioid angiomyolipoma, lymphangioleiomyomatosis, clear cell sugar tumor, and some other rare mesenchymal neoplasms. These lesions, which may occur in patients with the tuberous sclerosis complex, typically show HMB45-positive epithelioid cells and have been designated as PEComas. They usually also react with smooth muscle markers.[96] Presently, there is some degree of uncertainty about their existence in the uterus. Although they have been documented as tumors containing HMB45 reactive epithelioid cells with clear to eosinophilic cytoplasm (Figures 17.57–17.59),[128] a second interpretation has been that neoplastic epithelioid smooth muscle clear cells express HMB45[44,113] since uterine epithelioid leiomyosarcomas are known to have clear cells that may express HMB45.[113,115] Ultrastructural examination in occasional cases has revealed melanosomes, providing compelling evidence that the entity of PEComa does exist, however. Regardless of histogenesis, uterine PEComas are neoplasms of low malignant potential with an uncertain behavior and best treated by hysterectomy.

In one small series, the patients were 30–40 years old and the tumors were 1–30 cm in size.[31] Most were stage 1. Microscopically, the tumors showed an epithelioid arrangement of

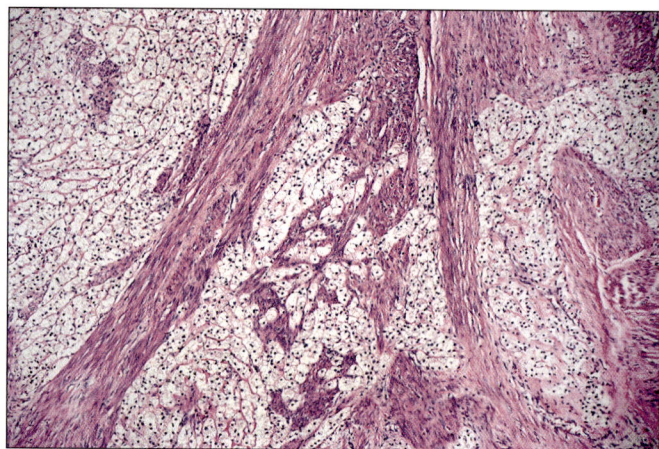

Fig. 17.57 Uterine PEComa composed of epithelioid cells with abundant clear cytoplasm.

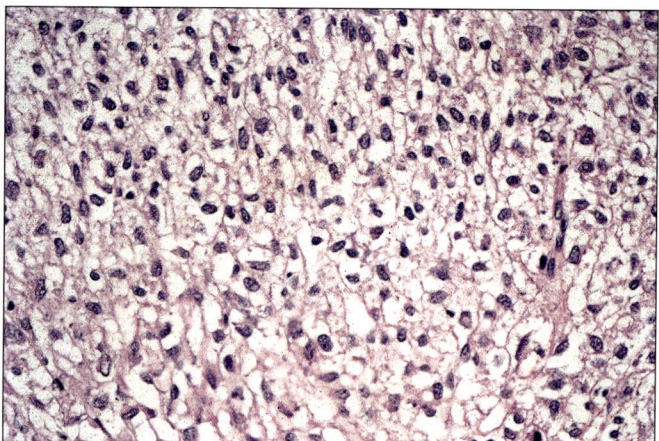

Fig. 17.58 Uterine PEComa.

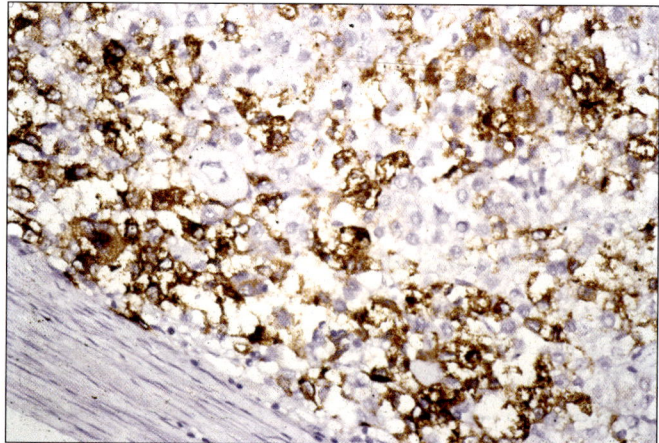

Fig. 17.59 Uterine PEComa with HMB45 reactivity.

tumor cells, with abundant clear to eosinophilic pale granular cytoplasm. Moderately atypical nuclei and coagulative necrosis were found in several cases and the mitotic figures ranged from 0 to 11 per 10 HPFs. Immunohistochemically, the tumors were uniformly reactive for vimentin, HMB45 and h-caldesmon, variably for smooth muscle actin and desmin, and unreactive for Melan-A and S-100.

ATYPICAL POLYPOID ADENOMYOMA

Definition
A rare polypoid uterine tumor consisting of architecturally complex and cytologically atypical endometrial glands in a stroma composed predominantly of smooth muscle or fibromyomatous tissue.[38]

Clinical features
These tumors occur mainly before the menopause, the median age being about 40 years.[123] Most have been associated with menstrual disturbance. Many patients are nulliparous and some have a clinical history of infertility. Occasional cases have arisen in patients with Turners syndrome who received long-term unopposed estrogen.

Gross features
Atypical polypoid adenomyomas are most often situated in the lower uterine segment and may also rarely arise in the endocervix.[9] Their average size is 2 cm in greatest dimension and they have round, bulging surfaces. Their polypoid nature is not always obvious. They may be sessile and broad based, and may be mistaken for a submucosal leiomyoma on gross examination. The cut surface may also be reminiscent of a leiomyoma because of the prominent smooth muscle component. Small cysts may sometimes be apparent.

Microscopic features
The epithelial element of atypical polypoid adenomyoma exhibits haphazardly arranged, irregular glands that may be widely separated or arranged in groups or lobules (Figures 17.60–17.62). Many glands are branched and the architectural appearance often resembles that seen in endometrial intraepithelial neoplasia. The epithelium is endometrioid but varies in appearance from cuboidal to low columnar to pseudostratified. Most cases show extensive squamous metaplasia involving the glandular elements, commonly as rounded 'morules'. Keratinization, if present, may show central necrosis. In one series, 45% of atypical polypoid adenomyomas contained glands with such architectural complexity that they were virtually indistinguishable from well-differentiated endometrioid adenocarcinoma. Of these, 20% showed superficial myometrial invasion, for which reason some investigators prefer the term 'atypical polypoid adenomyoma of low malignant potential' for this group.[64]

The stroma of atypical polypoid adenomyoma, which is an integral and characteristic part of the tumor, consists largely of smooth muscle, most cells showing strong reactivity with smooth muscle antibodies.[118] In most cases, however, fibrous tissue seen as sclerotic areas is also present. On this basis, some prefer the term 'atypical polypoid adenomyofibroma' as the preferred designation.[118] Stromal mitotic activity is generally low (<3 mitoses per 10 HPFs), although greater activity (up to 5 mitoses per 10 HPFs) may be seen focally in the more cellular areas. The margin between the tumor and the underlying myometrium is rounded, pushing, and usually well delineated.

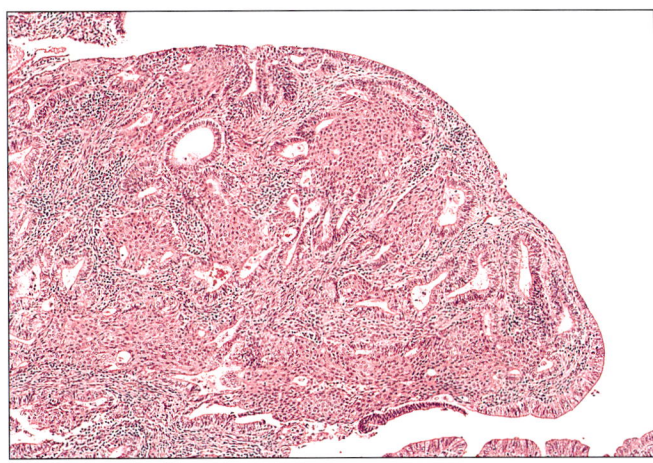

Fig. 17.60 Atypical polypoid adenomyoma. The polyp is composed of hyperplastic glands showing squamous metaplasia arranged haphazardly within smooth muscle stroma.

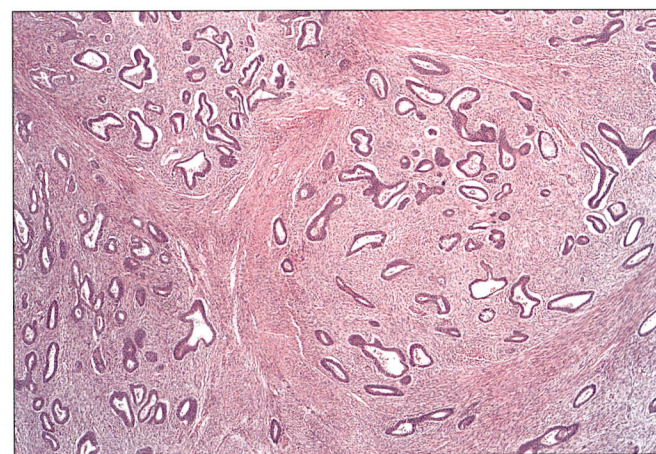

Fig. 17.61 Atypical polypoid adenomyoma composed of glands within a myomatous stroma.

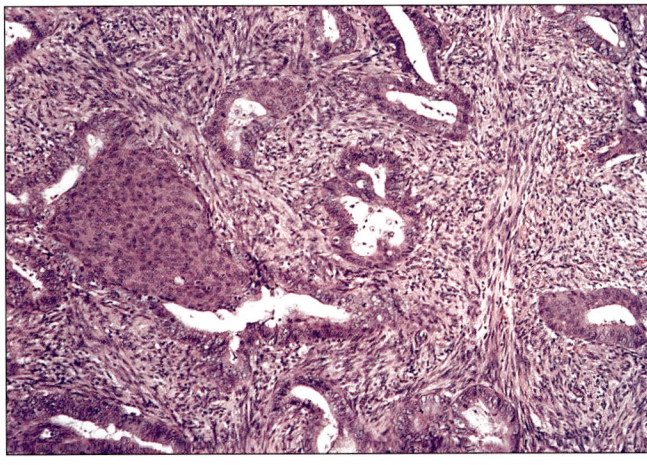

Fig. 17.62 Atypical polypoid adenomyoma. Many glands exhibit squamous metaplasia.

Transition to adenocarcinoma

Transitions from atypical polypoid adenomyoma to invasive endometrioid adenocarcinoma are well documented.[13] In contrast to the usual young age of women who have atypical polypoid adenomyoma, some developing adenocarcinoma are postmenopausal. One 40-year-old patient with Turners syndrome had a long history of estrogen administration.[121] The potential for malignant change may be realized in older women, perhaps because the lesion has been present longer, or when long-term unopposed estrogens have been administered.[121]

Treatment and prognosis

Atypical polypoid adenomyoma is generally a 'benign' tumor with a significant risk of recurrence if inadequately removed initially and a very low risk of malignant change. Many women with this tumor are treated by hysterectomy either because the diagnosis was not made preoperatively or because the curettings raised the possibility of adenocarcinoma. If a confident diagnosis of atypical polypoid adenomyoma has been made on curettings, hysterectomy is the treatment of choice. However, treatment by polypectomy or complete curettage may be undertaken, thereby preserving reproductive function, providing there is close follow-up subsequently. In one series, 45% of patients so treated experienced at least one recurrence but successful pregnancies were recorded, even after two recurrences.[64] Recurrence is more likely if the epithelial element shows severe atypia.

Differential diagnosis

The presence in biopsy or curettage material of the atypical proliferating glands of atypical polypoid adenomyoma, set in fibromuscular stroma, can be difficult to distinguish from endometrioid adenocarcinoma invading the myometrium. This distinction is important because atypical polypoid adenomyomas generally are 'benign' or of a low order degree of malignancy. They occur usually in women before the menopause, can be treated conservatively, and allow for preservation of childbearing potential. We believe, in contradistinction to others, that immunohistochemical stains for actin or desmin are not useful to separate the atypical polypoid adenomyoma and endometrial cancer. These biomarkers demonstrate the smooth muscle stromal component in atypical polypoid adenomyoma, but also the smooth muscle of the myometrium with the admixed reactive fibroblastic desmoplasia of the carcinomatous stroma. Typical features of adenocarcinoma, e.g., a cribriform pattern or marked cytologic atypia, point to a diagnosis of malignancy. Most atypical polypoid adenomyomas exhibit no more than mild or moderate cytologic atypia. It is unusual in curettings from an endometrioid carcinoma to obtain only fragments of myoinvasive tumor without free tumor fragments and with such a picture an atypical polypoid adenomyoma should be considered.

Many simple endometrial polyps contain a minor component of smooth muscle within the stroma. This does not signify an atypical polypoid adenomyoma. Typical adenomyomas may also occur within the uterus. These are composed of benign endometrial glands with minimal cytologic atypia and architectural complexity embedded in a fibromyomatous stroma. Generally, endometrial-type stroma surrounds the glandular component and the former is in turn surrounded by smooth muscle. These lesions may be associ-ated with underlying adenomyosis. The term adenomyoma has also been used for adenomyosis which forms a localized myometrial mass.

ADENOMYOSIS

Although not a neoplasm, adenomyosis is included in this chapter as, for some neoplasms already discussed, it contains both epithelial and stromal elements.

Definition

Adenomyosis is a non-neoplastic condition in which admixed endometrial stroma and glands are found within the myometrium.[6,99]

Background

In the normal uterus, the junction between the endometrium and the myometrium is not delineated by any limiting layer or membrane. Rather, endometrial glands and stroma often appear to make minor incursions into the myometrium, without being considered pathologic. Involvement of the superficial myometrium by endometrial tissue therefore occurs to varying degrees and it is normal to find irregularity of the endometrial–myometrial junction, with endometrial glands and stroma apparently invading a little distance into the muscle. A consequence of this lack of a definitive junction has been the problem in defining the term 'adenomyosis', generally stated to be 'a benign condition with the invasive growth of endometrial tissue into smooth muscle'. 'Superficial adenomyosis', a term lacking any clinical utility, has been used to describe myometrial invasion that is greater than this normal amount, but is not deep within the muscle.

The borderline that separates these degrees of endometrial penetration into the myometrium is ill defined, for which reason we find it most expedient to consider the appearances as normal or of sufficient depth to be designated as adenomyosis. A useful practical way of paraphrasing this dilemma is that superficial adenomyosis is frequently an incidental finding on histologic examination, while more deeply penetrating adenomyosis is visible to naked-eye inspection of the uterus. The distance to which the endometrium extends into the myometrium has often been expressed as the number of microscopic fields from the definable junction; one medium-power field has been suggested as the minimum needed for a diagnosis of adenomyosis (about 2–3 mm for a 10× objective). Alternatively, the depth of penetration of the endometrial tissue into the myometrium can be expressed as a proportion of the overall thickness of the myometrium. While arbitrary, 25% has been suggested (also 2–3 mm in a 1 cm thick wall).

The other criterion that is often used is an absolute measurement, but there is little overall agreement on this measurement. While 2.5 mm is widely accepted in much of the pathology literature,[109] it has no medical basis. An objective study correlating depth of adenomyosis with the severity of menorrhagia has convincingly shown that significant menorrhagia occurs even with adenomyotic foci penetrating 1 mm into the myometrium,[69] with the frequency of clinical symptoms increasing with adenomyosis at deeper levels. The presence of focal smooth muscle hypertrophy around the islands of endometrium helps in distinguishing adenomyosis from a normal extension of endometrium into the myometrium.

Clinical features

Adenomyosis occurs mostly in the late reproductive years and involves from 5 to 70% of surgically removed uteri.[7] These widely varying figures reflect differences in the diagnostic stringency. Two studies found a prevalence of 21% and 25%,[98] which is now the more generally accepted range. The symptoms are non-specific and not diagnostic, since many women suffer from menorrhagia or dysmenorrhea and do not have adenomyosis as shown by hysterectomy. Contrary to previously held beliefs, recent studies have also shown that adenomyosis is not particularly associated with other forms of uterine pathology, such as leiomyomas[39] and prolapse, although parity is associated with an increased frequency.[130] A decreased risk in women who smoke has been suggested.[98] One study has shown that the incidence of adenomyosis amongst postmenopausal breast cancer patients treated with tamoxifen is three to four times higher than the rate reported in postmenopausal women not taking tamoxifen.[25]

Using traditional clinical criteria, the correct diagnosis of adenomyosis is made in less than one-third of cases. The growing tendency to treat some gynecologic disorders, such as menorrhagia, by methods other than hysterectomy has led to a need for more precise methods for the diagnosis of adenomyosis because patients with deep adenomyosis respond poorly to endometrial ablation and other non-surgical procedures.[69] Magnetic resonance imaging (MRI),[49] vaginal ultrasound,[104,105] and myometrial needle biopsy[68] have all been investigated as a means of achieving this end.

Pathogenesis

That adenomyosis is the result of a benign, non-neoplastic infiltration of endometrial stromal and glandular elements into the myometrium has long been accepted, although why this should happen remains a mystery. A number of factors play a role in the pathogenesis of adenomyosis and the mechanisms of its development.

MRI has drawn attention to a specialized zone of myometrium situated immediately beneath the endometrium, referred to as the 'junctional zone'.[12] This zone structurally and functionally differs from the outer myometrium. There is conjecture that an abnormality of this zone, in which there is subendometrial smooth muscle hypertrophy with distortion of normal zonal architecture and loss of inner myometrial function, predisposes to secondary infiltration of the myometrium by endometrial elements.[12]

The most commonly used method to induce adenomyosis in experimental animals has been long-term estrogen therapy. Evidence suggests that prolactin also plays a key role, possibly by inducing myometrial smooth muscle cells in the junctional zone to degenerate.[88]

Immune factors may also play a part, some suggesting that impaired immune-related growth control in ectopic endometrium may be necessary for the maintenance of adenomyosis.[30] The concept that adenomyosis is the result of direct invasion into the myometrium has also been questioned. One study believes that established adenomyosis is preceded by the formation of stromal nodules that develop from the perivascular stromal cells (pericytes) to endometrial

stromal cells that subsequently proliferate and develop glandular elements.[65]

Gross features

The uterus harboring adenomyosis may be of normal size if the condition is mild. In most cases with significant clinical symptoms, however, the uterus is enlarged, either by a diffuse increase in bulk that may affect only one wall, or by more or less focal involvement that results in intramural masses that can mimic the naked-eye appearance of leiomyomas. In its most extreme form, adenomyosis results in a grossly enlarged and globular uterus. Most of the increased uterine size results from the smooth muscle hypertrophy that accompanies the invading endometrium. Little of the increased bulk results from the volume of the endometrial tissue itself. The smooth muscle hypertrophy results in a fairly characteristic gross appearance of the cut surface of an adenomyotic uterus. The affected area has a prominent trabeculated pattern, the hypertrophic swirls of smooth muscle separating duller, gray foci of endometrium that often appear as petechiae (Figure 17.63). Cystic spaces (due to cystically dilated glands) are seen in a minority of cases and occasionally blood is present in the cystic cavities. The lesion edges are poorly defined in contrast to the sharply defined edges of a leiomyoma, and the cut surface does not bulge in the manner so characteristic of leiomyomas. It is often impossible to distinguish adenomyosis from leiomyomas clinically and from gross inspection of the uterine serosa at the time of surgery.

Not uncommonly, both conditions coexist. The upshot is that attempts to remove foci of unrecognized adenomyosis in the same way that leiomyomas are shelled out by myomectomy sometimes leads to a hysterectomy being performed once uncontrollable bleeding is encountered resulting from the lack of well-defined margins with a plane of cleavage. A macroscopic variant of adenomyosis is the so-called 'adenomyoma', which is a well-defined area of adenomyosis with marked smooth muscle hypertrophy that has the gross appearance of a leiomyoma but which, on microscopy, contains islands of endometrium. This is not a combined lesion consisting of a

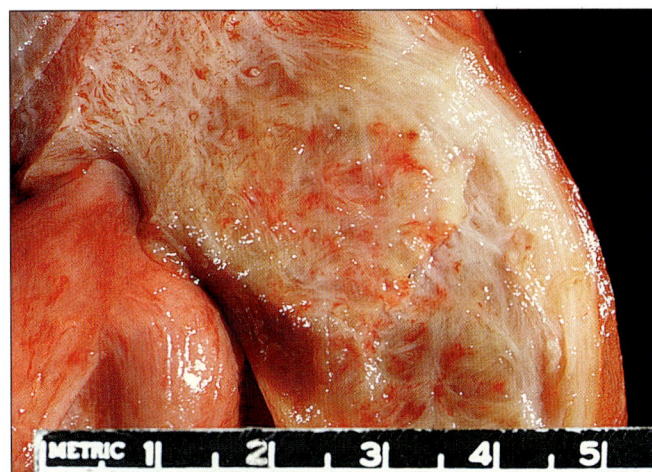

Fig. 17.63 Adenomyosis. Thickened, poorly circumscribed trabeculae about pinpoint hemorrhagic cysts distort the myometrial wall.

leiomyoma into which adenomyosis has grown. It is more correctly considered as localized adenomyosis in which the muscle hypertrophy has developed in an extreme fashion.

Microscopic features

The histologic features of adenomyosis are well known and straightforward. The infiltrating islands of endometrium usually consist of both glands and stroma (Figures 17.64 and 17.65). The glandular tissue is commonly, although not always, inactive and of basal endometrial pattern. Occasionally, secretory changes are seen in the glands in the adenomyotic foci and, in pregnancy or with exogenous hormones, decidual change may occur in the stroma. The hypertrophied myometrial smooth muscle immediately surrounding the infiltrating endometrial tissue has been alluded to above as the main reason for the increased size of the uterus in adenomyosis. These changes are also apparent microscopically, being recognized as rounded masses of smooth muscle (Figure 17.66), sometimes seeming to compress the glandular elements in the manner characteristic of the mammary intracanalicular fibroadenoma, and regularly producing triangular or 'shark's fin'-shaped islands with the stromal elements fading into the corners. Unusual changes in adenomyosis, such as glandular dilatation, epithelial metaplasias, and stromal fibrosis, have been described in association with tamoxifen.[75] It is not unusual to find adenomyotic foci in small vascular channels within the myometrium.

In most cases, endometrial glands are obvious in most of the adenomyotic foci, making the diagnosis simple. Occasionally, however, the glandular component is sparse or even absent, so that the myometrium appears infiltrated by endometrial stroma resulting in a differential diagnosis of endometrial stromal sarcoma.[36] These appearances may involve most of the adenomyotic foci or may be present only focally. Not uncommonly, small foci composed only of stroma are found at the periphery of larger areas that contain glands. Extensive sampling usually demonstrates foci of more typical adenomyosis with glandular elements. The most important features pointing to a diagnosis of adenomyosis rather than endometrial stromal sarcoma are that typical adenomyosis is present elsewhere in the uterus and that the foci are microscopic without gross evidence of tumor. In both typical adenomyosis and adenomyosis with sparse glands, stromal elements may sometimes be found within vascular and lymphatic channels,[108] again raising the concern of endometrial stromal sarcoma. However, the vascular involvement is minimal compared to that seen with sarcoma. The absence of a tumor mass and the presence of typical adenomyosis elsewhere in the uterus in these circumstances mitigate against the erroneous diagnosis of endometrial stromal sarcoma.

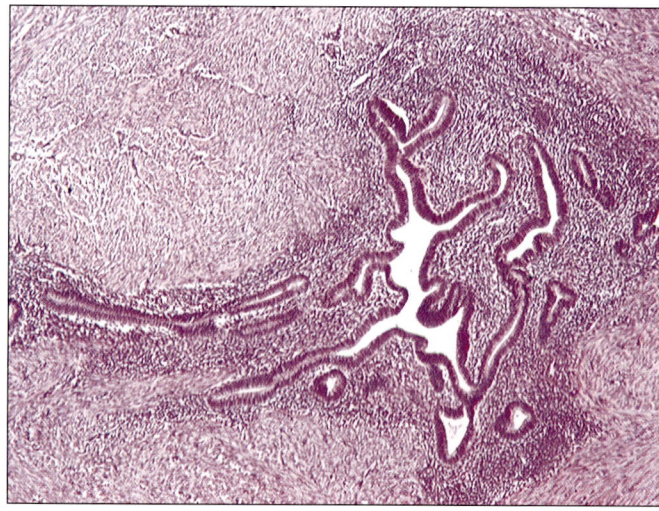

Fig. 17.65 Adenomyosis. The infiltrating islands of endometrium consist of both glands and stroma. The glands are inactive and of basal pattern.

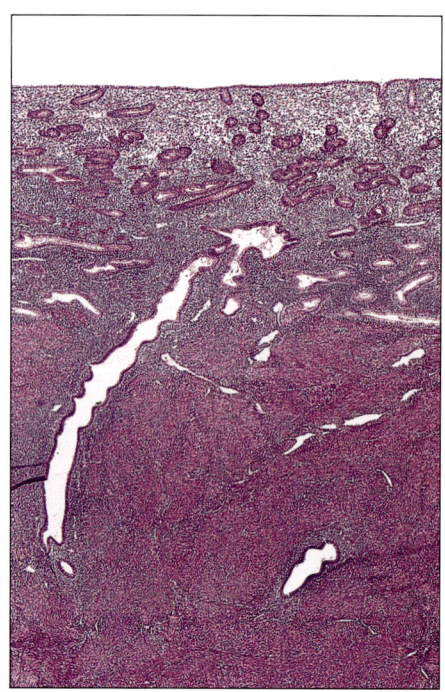

Fig. 17.64 Adenomyosis. Endometrial tissue infiltrates the myometrium.

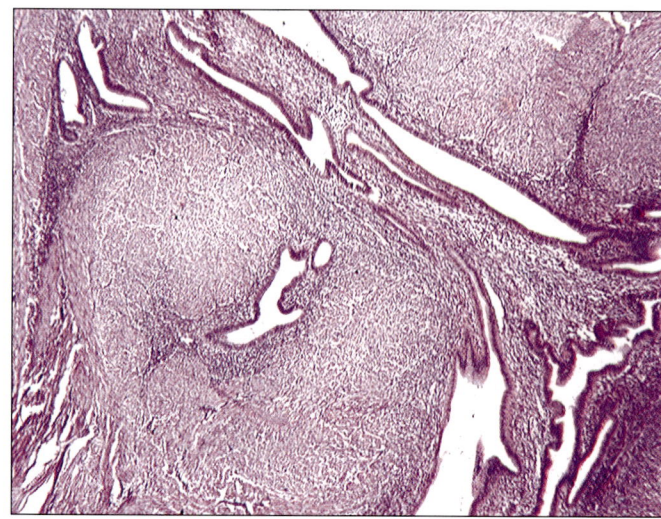

Fig. 17.66 Adenomyosis with smooth muscle proliferation. Nodules of proliferating smooth muscle are clearly seen.

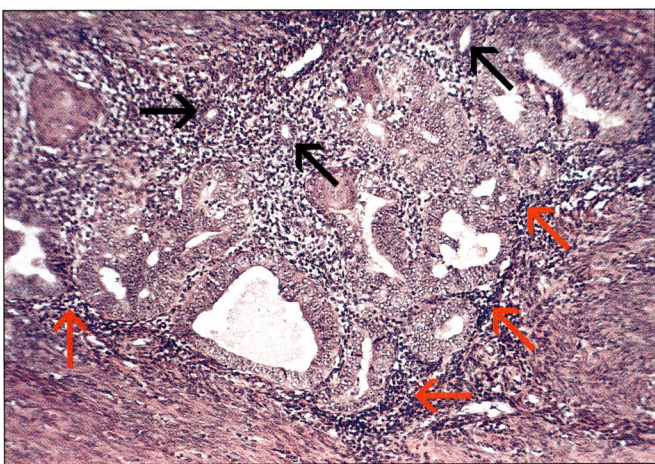

Fig. 17.67 Adenocarcinoma arising in adenomyosis. Endometrial stroma (arrows) surrounds the malignant glands, which are not invading the myometrium from this focus of adenomyosis.

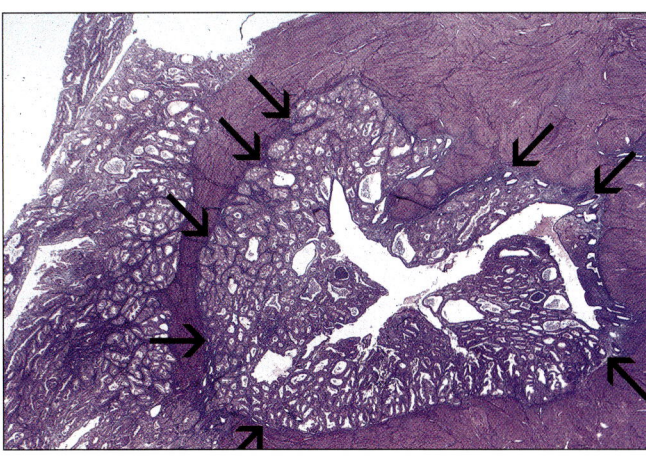

Fig. 17.68 Adenocarcinoma in which numerous foci of adenomyosis (arrows) lie at the periphery (interphase with adjacent myometrium).

In most instances, there will be no confusion regarding the benign nature of adenomyosis since the glands and stroma are arranged orderly and distinctly separate from the encompassing myometrium. Difficulty arises when small patches of adenomyosis are mistaken for early myoinvasive carcinoma in a patient with endometrial cancer, or when an endometrial adenocarcinoma is present and involves the adenomyotic foci. In addition, an intraendometrial adenocarcinoma may involve or rarely even arise in foci of adenomyosis, further increasing diagnostic interpretations.[54,85] For the diagnosis of carcinoma arising in adenomyosis to be made, benign endometrial tissue must be identified in that particular focus, with stromal cells separating some glands (Figure 17.67), so that there is a clear transition between benign and malignant tissue. Endometrial stromal cells should be seen to separate the endometrial glands, whether benign or malignant, from the surrounding myometrium. The involvement of adenomyosis by an intraendometrial adenocarcinoma (Figure 17.68), even when deep in the myometrium, is not associated with the poor prognosis that deep myometrial penetration by invasive carcinoma would confer.[85] The distinction is therefore an important one to make so that the patient is not upstaged and inappropriate adjuvant therapy administered.

In new work that was based on a large series and just published,[46,47] presaging more progress to come regarding how adenomyosis involved by cancer affects survival, comparisons were made of consecutive cases where the myometrium contained tumor within the adenomyosis or was uninvolved by adenomyosis altogether. CD10 helped determine if stroma enveloped the carcinoma or the carcinomatous component was truly myoinvasive. FIGO grade 1 endometrial endometrioid adenocarcinoma in adenomyosis was found associated with myometrial invasion in 91% of cases versus only 78% if there were no adenomyosis present, suggesting that the adenomyosis increased the potential surface area within the adjacent myometrium for myoinvasion to occur. Not uncommonly (35%), myoinvasion arose exclusively from the adenomyotic foci. Deep (outer half) myometrial invasion was also more common in the adenomyosis group (35% vs 18%). No prognostic information was available.

REFERENCES

1. Altaras MM, Jaffe R, Cohen I, Gruber A, Yanai-Inbar I, Bernheim J. Role of prolonged excessive estrogen stimulation in the pathogenesis of endometrial sarcomas: two cases and a review of the literature. Gynecol Oncol 1990;38:273–7.
2. Amant F, Moerman P, Davel GH, et al. Uterine carcinosarcoma with melanocytic differentiation. Int J Gynecol Pathol 2001;20:186–90.
3. Ansink AC, Cross PA, Scorer P, Lopes AD, Monaghan JM. The hormonal receptor status of uterine carcinosarcomas (mixed Mullerian tumours): an immunohistochemical study. J Clin Pathol 1997;50:328–31.
4. Baker P, Oliva E. Endometrial stromal tumours of the uterus: a practical approach using conventional morphology and ancillary techniques. J Clin Pathol 2007;60:235–43.
5. Baker PM, Moch H, Oliva E. Unusual morphologic features of endometrial stromal tumors – a report of 2 cases. Am J Surg Pathol 2005;29:1394–8
6. Benagiano G, Brosens I. History of adenomyosis. Best Prac Res Clin Obstet Gynecol 2006;20:449–63.
7. Bergeron C, Amant F, Ferenczy A. Pathology and physiopathology of adenomyosis. Best Prac Res Clin Obstet Gynecol 2006;20:511–21.
8. Bhargava R, Shia J, Hummer AJ, Thaler HT, Tornos C, Soslow RA. Distinction of endometrial stromal sarcomas from 'hemangiopericytomatous' tumors using a panel of immunohistochemical stains. Mod Pathol 2005;18: 40–7
9. Biscreglia M. Atypical polypoid adenomyoma. Adv Anat Pathol 2002;9: 256–60.
10. Borka K, Patai K, Rendek A, Sobel G, Paulin F. Pleomorphic rhabdomyosarcoma of the uterus in a postmenopausal patient. Path Oncol Res 2006;12:102–4.
11. Brooks BE, Zhan M, Cote T, Baquet CR. Surveillance, epidemiology, and end results analysis of 2677 cases of uterine sarcoma 1989–1999. Gynecol Obstet 2004;93:204–8.
12. Brosens JJ, Desouza NM, Barker FG. Uterine junctional zone: function and disease. Lancet 1995;346:558–60.
13. Buenerd A, Dargent D, Scoazec JY, Berger G. Carcinomatous transformation of an atypical polypoid adenomyofibroma of the uterus. Ann Pathol 2003;23:63–6.
14. Cady FM, Kuhn E, Holt JB. Images in pathology. Endometrial stromal sarcoma with hyalinizing giant rosettes and separate leiomyoma with palisading nuclei in the same uterus. Int J Surg Pathol 2006;14:326–7.
15. Callister M, Ramondetta LM, Jhingran A, Burke TW, Eifel PJ. Malignant mixed Mullerian tumors of the uterus: analysis of patterns of failure, prognostic factors, and treatment outcome. Int J Radiat Oncol Biol Phys 2004;58:786–96.
16. Chang KL, Crabtree GS, LimTan SK, Kempson RL, Hendrickson MR. Primary uterine endometrial stromal neoplasms. A clinicopathologic study of 117 cases. Am J Surg Pathol 1990;14:415–38.
17. Chu PG, Arber DA, Weiss LM, Chang KL. Utility of CD10 in distinguishing between endometrial stromal sarcoma and uterine smooth muscle tumors: an immunohistochemical comparison of 34 cases. Mod Pathol 2001;14: 465–71.
18. Clement PB. Mullerian adenosarcomas of the uterus with sarcomatous overgrowth. A clinicopathological analysis of 10 cases. Am J Surg Pathol 1989;13:28–38.

19. Clement PB. The pathology of uterine smooth muscle tumors and mixed endometrial stromal-smooth muscle tumors: a selective review with emphasis on recent advances. Int J Gynecol Pathol 2000;19:39–55.

20. Clement PB, Scully RE. Mullerian adenosarcomas of the uterus with sex cord-like elements. A clinicopathologic analysis of eight cases. Am J Clin Pathol 1989;91:664–72.

21. Clement PB, Scully RE. Müllerian adenofibroma of the uterus with invasion of myometrium and pelvic veins. Int J Gynecol Pathol 1990;9:363–71.

22. Clement PB, Scully RE. Mullerian adenosarcoma of the uterus: a clinicopathologic analysis of 100 cases with a review of the literature. Hum Pathol 1990;21:363–81.

23. Clement PB. Endometrial stromal sarcomas of the uterus with extensive endometrioid glandular differentiation: a report of three cases that caused problems in differential diagnosis. Int J Gynecol Pathol 1992;11:163–73.

24. Clement PB, Oliva E, Young RH. Mullerian adenosarcoma of the uterine corpus associated with tamoxifen therapy: a report of six cases and a review of tamoxifen-associated endometrial lesions. Int J Gynecol Pathol 1996;15:222–9.

25. Cohen I, Beyth Y, Tepper R, et al. Adenomyosis in postmenopausal breast cancer patients treated with tamoxifen: a new entity? Gynecol Oncol 1995;58:86–91.

26. Czernobilsky B, Mamet Y, Ben David M, Atlas I, Gitstein G, Lifschitz-Mercer B. Uterine retiform Sertoli–Leydig cell tumor: report of a case providing additional evidence that uterine tumors resembling ovarian sex cord tumors have a histologic and immunohistochemical phenotype of genuine sex cord tumors. Int J Gynecol Pathol 2005;24:335–40.

27. de Brito PA, Silverberg SG, Orenstein JM. Carcinosarcoma (malignant mixed mullerian (mesodermal) tumor) of the female genital tract: immunohistochemical and ultrastructural analysis of 28 cases. Hum Pathol 1993;24:132–42.

28. Dionigi A, Oliva E, Clement PB, Young RH. Endometrial stromal nodules and endometrial stromal tumors with limited infiltration: a clinicopathologic study of 50 cases. Am J Surg Pathol 2002;26:567–81.

29. Emoto M, Iwasaki H, Kikuchi M, Shirakawa K. Characteristics of cloned cells of mixed mullerian tumor of the human uterus – carcinoma cells showing myogenic differentiation in vitro. Cancer 1993;71:3065–75.

30. Ferenczy A. Pathophysiology of adenomyosis. Hum Reprod Update 1998;4:312–22.

31. Fukunaga M. Perivascular epithelioid cell tumor of the uterus: report of four cases. Int J Gynecol Pathol 2005;24:341–6.

32. Fukunaga M, Miyazawa Y, Ushigome S. Endometrial low-grade stromal sarcoma with ovarian sex cord-like differentiation: report of two cases with an immunohistochemical and flow cytometric study. Pathol Int 1997;47:412–5.

33. Fukunaga M, Nomura K, Endo Y, Ushigome S, Aizawa S. Carcinosarcoma of the uterus with extensive neuroectodermal differentiation. Histopathology 1996;29:565–70.

34. George E, Manivel JC, Dehner LP, Wick MR. Malignant mixed mullerian tumors: an immunohistochemical study of 47 cases, with histogenetic considerations and clinical correlation. Hum Pathol 1991;22:215–23.

35. George E, Lillemoe TJ, Twiggs LB, Perrone T. Malignant mixed mullerian tumor versus high-grade endometrial carcinoma and aggressive variants of endometrial carcinoma: a comparative analysis of survival. Int J Gynecol Pathol 1995;14:39–44.

36. Goldblum JR, Clement PB, Hart WR. Adenomyosis with sparse glands: a potential mimic of low-grade endometrial stromal sarcoma. Am J Clin Pathol 1995;103:218–23.

37. Hardisson D, Simon RS, Burgos E. Primary osteosarcoma of the uterine corpus: report of a case with immunohistochemical and ultrastructural study. Gynecol Oncol 2001;82:181–6.

38. Heatley MK. Atypical polypoid adenomyoma: a systematic review of the English literature. Histopathology 2006;48:609–10.

39. Hever A, Roth RB, Hevezi PA, et al. Molecular characterization of human adenomyosis. Mol Hum Reprod 2006;12:737–48.

40. Horie Y, Ikawa S, Kadowaki K, Minagawa Y, Kigawa J, Terakawa N. Lipoadenofibroma of the uterine corpus: report of a new variant of adenofibroma (benign mullerian mixed tumor). Arch Pathol Lab Med 1995;119:274–6.

41. Huang HY, Ladanyi M, Soslow RA. Molecular detection of JAZF1-JJAZ1 gene fusion in endometrial stromal neoplasms with classic and variant histology – evidence for genetic heterogeneity. Am J Surg Pathol 2004;28:224–32.

42. Huang KT, Chen CA, Cheng WF, et al. Sonographic characteristics of adenofibroma of the endometrium following tamoxifen therapy for breast cancer: two case reports. Ultrasound Obstet Gynecol 1996;7:363–6.

43. Hurrell D, McCluggage WG. Uterine tumour resembling ovarian sex cord tumour is an immunohistochemically polyphenotypic neoplasm which exhibits coexpression of epithelial, myoid and sex cord markers. J Clin Pathol 2007;60:1148–54.

44. Hurrell DP, McCluggage WG. Uterine leiomyosarcoma with HMB45+ clear cell areas: report of two cases. Histopathology 2005;47:540–2.

45. Irving JA, Carinelli S, Prat J. Uterine tumors resembling ovarian sex cord tumors are polyphenotypic neoplasms with true sex cord differentiation. Mod Pathol 2006;19:17–24.

46. Ismiil N, Rasty G, Ghorab Z, et al. Adenomyosis involved by endometrial adenocarcinoma is a significant risk factor for deep myometrial invasion. Ann Diagn Pathol 2007;11:252–7.

47. Ismiil ND, Rasty G, Ghorab Z, et al. Adenomyosis is associated with myometrial invasion by FIGO 1 endometrial adenocarcinoma. Int J Gynecol Pathol 2007;26:278–83.

48. Kabbani W, Deavers MT, Malpica A, et al. Uterine tumor resembling ovarian sex-cord tumor: report of a case mimicking cervical adenocarcinoma. Int J Gynecol Pathol 2003;22:297–302.

49. Kang S, Turner DA, Foster GS, Rapoport MI, Spencer SA, Wang JZ. Adenomyosis: specificity of 5 mm as the maximum normal uterine junctional zone thickness in MR images. Am J Roentgenol 1996;166:1145–50.

50. Kantelip B, Cloup N, Dechelotte P. Uterine tumor resembling ovarian sex cord tumors: report of a case with ultrastructural study. Hum Pathol 1986;17:91–4.

51. Kempson RL, Hendrickson MR. Smooth muscle, endometrial stromal, and mixed Mullerian tumors of the uterus. Mod Pathol 2000;13:328–42.

52. Khalifa MA, Hansen CH, Moore JL, Rusnock EJ, Lage JM. Endometrial stromal sarcoma with focal smooth muscle differentiation: recurrence after 17 years: a follow-up report with discussion of the nomenclature. Int J Gynecol Pathol 1996;15:171–6.

53. Kir G, Cetiner H, Karateke A, Gurbuz A, Bulbul D. Utility of MIB-1 and estrogen and progesterone receptor in distinguishing between endometrial stromal sarcomas and endometrial stromal nodules, highly cellular leiomyomas. Int J Gynecol Cancer 2005;15:337–42.

54. Koshiyama M, Suzuki A, Ozawa M, et al. Adenocarcinomas arising from uterine adenomyosis: a report of four cases. Int J Gynecol Pathol 2002;21:239–45.

55. Kostopoulou E, Dragoumis K, Zafrakas M, Myronidou Z, Agelidou S, Bontis I. Primary osteosarcoma of the uterus with immunohistochemical study. Acta Obstet Gynecol Scand 2002;81:678–80.

56. Kostopoulou E, Dragoumis K, Kellartzis D, Zafrakas M, Kriaka A, Leontsini M. Primary myxoid chondrosarcoma of the uterus: report of a case with immunohistochemical study. Eur J Gynaecol Oncol 2003;24:76–8.

57. Krivak TC, Seidman JD, McBroom JW, MacKoul PJ, Aye LM, Rose GS. Uterine adenosarcoma with sarcomatous overgrowth versus uterine carcinosarcoma: comparison of treatment and survival. Gynecol Obstet 2001;83:89–94.

58. Lam KY, Khoo US, Cheung A. Collision of endometrioid carcinoma and stromal sarcoma of the uterus: a report of two cases. Int J Gynecol Pathol 1999;18:77–81.

59. Larson B, Silfversward C, Nilsson B, Pettersson F. Endometrial stromal sarcoma of the uterus. A clinical and histopathological study. The Radiumhemmet series 1936–1981. Eur J Obstet Gynecol Reprod Biol 1990;35:239–49.

60. Levine PH, Mittal K. Rhabdoid epithelioid leiomyosarcoma of the uterine corpus – a case report and literature review. Int J Surg Pathol 2002;10:231–6.

61. Levine PH, Wei XJ, Gagner JP, Flax H, Mittal K, Blank SV. Pleomorphic liposarcoma of the uterus: case report and literature review. Int J Gynecol Pathol 2003;22:407–11.

62. Livi L, Paiar F, Shah N, et al. Uterine sarcoma: twenty-seven years of experience. Int J Radiat Oncol Biol Phys 2003;57:1366–73.

63. Lloreta J, Prat J. Endometrial stromal nodule with smooth and skeletal muscle components simulating stromal sarcoma. Int J Gynecol Pathol 1992;11:293–8.

64. Longacre TA, Chung MH, Rouse RV, Hendrickson MR. Atypical polypoid adenomyofibromas (atypical polypoid adenomyomas) of the uterus: a clinicopathologic study of 55 cases. Am J Surg Pathol 1996;20:1–20.

65. Mai KT, Yazdi HM, Perkins DG, Parks W. Pathogenetic role of the stromal cells in endometriosis and adenomyosis. Histopathology 1997;30:430–42.

66. Marth C, Windbichler G, Petru E, et al. Parity as an independent prognostic factor in malignant mixed mesodermal tumors of the endometrium. Gynecol Oncol 1997;64:121–5.

67. Mayall F, Rutty K, Campbell F, Goddard H. P53 immunostaining suggests that uterine carcinosarcomas are monoclonal. Histopathology 1994;24:211–4.

68. McCausland AM. Hysteroscopic myometrial biopsy: its use in diagnosing adenomyosis and its clinical application. Am J Obstet Gynecol 1992;166(6 Pt 1):1619–26; discussion 1626–8.

69. McCausland AM, McCausland VM. Depth of endometrial penetration in adenomyosis helps determine outcome of rollerball ablation. Am J Obstet Gynecol 1996;174:1786–93.

70. McCluggage WG. Uterine tumours resembling ovarian sex cord tumours: immunohistochemical evidence for true sex cord differentiation. Histopathology 1999;34:374–5.

71. McCluggage WG. Uterine carcinosarcomas (malignant mixed Mullerian tumors) are metaplastic carcinomas. Int J Gynecol Cancer 2002;12:687–90.

72. McCluggage WG. Malignant biphasic uterine tumours: carcinosarcomas or metaplastic carcinomas? J Clin Pathol 2002;55:321–5.

73. McCluggage WG. A critical appraisal of the value of immunohistochemistry in diagnosis of uterine neoplasms. Adv Anat Pathol 2004;11:162–71.

74. McCluggage WG. Immunohistochemistry as a diagnostic aid in cervical pathology. Pathology 2007;39:97–111.

75. McCluggage WG, Desai V, Manek S. Tamoxifen-associated postmenopausal adenomyosis exhibits stromal fibrosis, glandular dilatation and epithelial metaplasias. Histopathology 2000;37:340–6.

76. McCluggage WG, Sumathi VP, Maxwell P. CD10 is a sensitive and diagnostically useful immunohistochemical marker of normal endometrial stroma and of endometrial stromal neoplasms. Histopathology 2001;39: 273–8.

77. McCluggage WG, McKenna M, McBride HA. CD56 is a sensitive and diagnostically useful immunohistochemical marker of ovarian sex cord-stromal tumors. Int J Gynecol Pathol 2007;26:322–7.

78. McCluggage WG, Shah V, Walsh MY, Toner PG. Uterine tumour resembling ovarian sex cord tumour – evidence for smooth muscle differentiation. Histopathology 1993;23:83–5.

79. McCluggage WG, Bailie C, Weir P, Bharucha H. Endometrial stromal sarcoma arising in pelvic endometriosis in a patient receiving unopposed oestrogen therapy. Br J Obstet Gynaecol 1996;103:1252–4.

80. McCluggage WG, Date A, Bharucha H, Toner PG. Endometrial stromal sarcoma with sex cord-like areas and focal rhabdoid differentiation. Histopathology 1996;29:369–74.

81. McCluggage WG, Cromie AJ, Bryson C, Traub AI. Uterine endometrial stromal sarcoma with smooth muscle and glandular differentiation. J Clin Pathol 2001;54:481–3.

82. McCluggage WG, Abdulkader M, Price JH, et al. Uterine carcinosarcomas in patients receiving tamoxifen. A report of 19 cases. Int J Gynecol Cancer 2000;10:280–4.

83. Melilli GA, DiVagno G, Greco P, et al. Endometrial stromal sarcoma: a clinicopathologic study. Eur J Gynaecol Oncol 1999;20:33–4.

84. Miliaras D, Bontis J. Uterine tumor resembling sex-cord ovarian tumors: one more case of the pure type suggests a neoplasm with benign behavior. Eur J Gynaecol Oncol 1997;18:133–5.

85. Mittal KR, Barwick KW. Endometrial adenocarcinoma involving adenomyosis without true myometrial invasion is characterized by frequent preceding estrogen therapy, low histologic grades, and excellent prognosis. Gynecol Oncol 1993;49:197–201.

86. Moinfar F, Azodi M, Tavassoli FA. Uterine sarcomas. Pathology 2007;39:55–71.

87. Moinfar F, Regitnig P, Tabrizi AD, Denk H, Tavassoli FA. Expression of androgen receptors in benign and malignant endometrial stromal neoplasms. Virchows Arch 2004;444:410–4.

88. Mori T, Singtripop T, Kawashima S. Animal model of uterine adenomyosis: is prolactin a potent inducer of adenomyosis in mice? Am J Obstet Gynecol 1991;165:232–4.

89. Nucci MR, Harburger D, Koontz J, Dal Cin P, Sklar J. Molecular analysis of the JAZF1-JJAZ1 gene fusion by RT-PCR and fluorescence in situ hybridization in endometrial stromal neoplasms. Am J Surg Pathol 2007;31:65–70.

90. Nucci MR, O'Connell JT, Huettner PC, Cviko A, Sun D, Quade BJ. h-Caldesmon expression effectively distinguishes endometrial stromal tumors from uterine smooth muscle tumors. Am J Surg Pathol 2001;25:455–63.

91. Oliva E, Clement PB, Young RH. Endometrial stromal tumors: an update on a group of tumors with a protean phenotype. Adv Anat Pathol 2000;7:257–81.

92. Oliva E, Clement PB, Young RH. Epithelioid endometrial and endometrioid stromal tumors: a report of four cases emphasizing their distinction from epithelioid smooth muscle tumors and other oxyphilic uterine and extrauterine tumors. Int J Gynecol Pathol 2002;21:48–55.

93. Oliva E, Clement PB, Young RH, Scully RE. Mixed endometrial stromal and smooth muscle tumors of the uterus: a clinicopathologic study of 15 cases. Am J Surg Pathol 1998;22:997–1005.

94. Oliva E, Young RH, Clement PB, Scully RE. Myxoid and fibrous endometrial stromal tumors of the uterus: a report of 10 cases. Int J Gynecol Pathol 1999;18:310–9.

95. Oliva E, Young RH, Clement PB, Bhan AK, Scully RE. Cellular benign mesenchymal tumors of the uterus: a comparative morphologic and immunohistochemical analysis of 33 highly cellular leiomyomas and six endometrial stromal nodules, two frequently confused tumors. Am J Surg Pathol 1995;19:757–68.

96. Oliva E, Wang WL, Branton P, et al. Expression of melanocytic ('PEComa') markers in smooth muscle tumors of the uterus: an immunohistochemical analysis of 86 cases. Lab Invest 2006;86(Suppl): 191A.

97. Orlandi A, Ferlosio A, Ciucci A, et al. Cellular retinol-binding protein-1 expression in endometrial stromal cells: physiopathological and diagnostic implications. Histopathology 2004;45:511–7.

98. Parazzini F, Vercellini P, Panazza S, Chatenoud L, Oldani S, Crosignani PG. Risk factors for adenomyosis. Hum Reprod 1997;12:1275–9.

99. Parker WH. Etiology, symptomatology, and diagnosis of uterine myomas. Fertil Steril 2007;87:725–36.

100. Phillips KA, Scurry JP, Toner G. Alpha-fetoprotein production by a malignant mixed mullerian tumour of the uterus. J Clin Pathol 1996;49:349–51.

101. Popiolek D, Yee H, Levine P, Vamvakas E, Demopoulos RI. MIB1 as a possible predictor of recurrence in low-grade endometrial stromal sarcoma of the uterus. Gynecol Oncol 2003;90:353–7.

102. Radig K, Buhtz P, Roessner A. Alveolar soft part sarcoma of the uterine corpus – report of two cases and review of the literature. Pathol Res Pract 1998;194:59–63.

103. Reich O, Regauer S, Urdl W, Lahousen M, Winter R. Expression of oestrogen and progesterone receptors in low-grade endometrial stromal sarcomas. Br J Cancer 2000;82:1030–4.

104. Reinhold C, Tafazoli F, Wang L. Imaging features of adenomyosis. Hum Reprod Update 1998;4:337–49.

105. Reinhold C, Atri M, Mehio A, Zakarian R, Aldis AE, Bret PM. Diffuse uterine adenomyosis: morphologic criteria and diagnostic accuracy of endovaginal sonography. Radiology 1995;197:609–14.

106. Rollins SE, Clement PB, Young RH. Uterine tumors resembling ovarian sex cord tumors frequently have incorporated mature smooth muscle imparting a pseudoinfiltrative appearance. Lab Invest 2007;87(Suppl):212A.

107. Rush DS, Tan J, Baergen RN, Soslow RA. h-Caldesmon, a novel smooth muscle-specific antibody, distinguishes between cellular leiomyoma and endometrial stromal sarcoma. Am J Surg Pathol 2001;25:253–8.

108. Sahin AA, Silva EG, Landon G, Ordonez NG, Gershenson DM. Endometrial tissue in myometrial vessels not associated with menstruation. Int J Gynecol Pathol 1989;8:139–46.

109. Seidman JD, Kjerulff KH. Pathologic findings from the Maryland Women's Health Study: practice patterns in the diagnosis of adenomyosis. Int J Gynecol Pathol 1996;15:217–21.

110. Selvaggi L, DiVagno G, Maiorano E, et al. Giant malignant fibrous histiocytoma of the uterus. Arch Gynecol Obstet 1997;259:197–200.

111. Shintaku M, Sekiyama K. Leiomyosarcoma of the uterus with focal rhabdomyosarcomatous differentiation. Int J Gynecol Pathol 2004;23: 188–92.

112. Shokeir MO, Noel SM, Clement PB. Malignant Mullerian mixed tumor of the uterus with a prominent alpha-fetoprotein-producing component of yolk sac tumor. Mod Pathol 1996;9:647–51.

113. Silva EG, Deavers MT, Bodurka DC, Malpica A. Uterine epithelioid leiomyosarcomas with clear cells: reactivity with HMB-45 and the concept of PEComa. Am J Surg Pathol 2004;28:244–9.

114. Silverberg SG, Major FJ, Blessing JA, et al. Carcinosarcoma (malignant mixed mesodermal tumor) of the uterus. A Gynecologic Oncology Group pathologic study of 203 cases. Int J Gynecol Pathol 1990;9:1–19.

115. Sinipson KW, Albores-Saavedra J. HMB-45 reactivity in conventional uterine leiomyosarcomas. Am J Surg Pathol 2007;31:95–8.

116. Sinkre P, Miller DS, Milchgrub S, Hameed A. Adenomyofibroma of the endometrium with skeletal muscle differentiation. Int J Gynecol Pathol 2000;19:280–3.

117. Snyder MJ, Robboy SJ, Vollmer RT, Dodd LG. An abnormal cervicovaginal cytology smear in uterine carcinosarcoma is an adverse prognostic sign: analysis of 25 cases. Am J Clin Pathol 2004;122:434–9.

118. Soslow RA, Chung MH, Rouse RV, Hendrickson MR, Longacre TA. Atypical polypoid adenomyofibroma (APA) versus well-differentiated endometrial carcinoma with prominent stromal matrix: an immunohistochemical study. Int J Gynecol Pathol 1996;15: 209–16.

119. Spano JP, Soria JC, Kambouchner M, et al. Long-term survival of patients given hormonal therapy for metastatic endometrial stromal sarcoma. Med Oncol 2003;20:87–93.

120. Sreenan JJ, Hart WR. Carcinosarcomas of the female genital tract: a pathologic study of 29 metastatic tumors: further evidence for the dominant role of the epithelial component and the conversion theory of histogenesis. Am J Surg Pathol 1995;19:666–74.

121. Staros EB. Atypical polypoid adenomyoma with carcinomatous transformation: a case report. Surg Pathol 1991;4:157–66.

122. Sumathi VP, Al-Hussaini M, Connolly LE, Fullerton L, McCluggage WG. Endometrial stromal neoplasms are immunoreactive with WT-1 antibody. Int J Gynecol Pathol 2004;23:241–7.

123. Tahlan A, Nanda A, Mohan H. Uterine adenomyoma: a clinicopathologic review of 26 cases and a review of the literature. Int J Gynecol Pathol 2006;25:361–5.

124. Taskin S, Bozaci EA, Sonmezer M, Ekinci C, Ortac F. Late recurrence of uterine Mullerian adenosarcoma as heterologous sarcoma: three recurrences in 8 months increasing in number and grade of sarcomatous components. Gynecol Oncol 2006;101:179–82.

125. Tavassoli FA, Norris HJ. Mesenchymal tumours of the uterus. VII. A clinicopathological study of 60 endometrial stromal nodules. Histopathology 1981;5:1–10.

126. Tavassoli FA, Devilee P, eds. Pathology and Genetics of Tumours of the Breast and Female Genital Organs. WHO Classification of Tumours series. Lyon: IARC Press; 2003.

127. Temkin SM, Hellmann M, Lee YC, Abulafia O. Early-stage carcinosarcoma of the uterus: the significance of lymph node count. Int J Gynecol Cancer 2007;17:215–9.

128. Vang R, Kempson RL. Perivascular epithelioid cell tumor ('PEComa') of the uterus: a subset of HMB-45-positive epithelioid mesenchymal neoplasms with an uncertain relationship to pure smooth muscle tumors. Am J Surg Pathol 2002;26:1–13.

129. Venkatraman L, Elliott H, Steele EK, McClelland HR, McCluggage WG. Serous carcinoma arising in an adenofibroma of the endometrium. Int J Gynecol Pathol 2003;22:194 7.

130. Vercellini P, Parazzini F, Oldani S, Panazza S, Bramante T, Crosignani PG. Adenomyosis at hysterectomy: a study on frequency distribution and patient characteristics. Hum Reprod 1995;10:1160–2.

131. Verschraegen CF, Vasuratna A, Edwards C, et al. Clinicopathologic analysis of mullerian adenosarcoma: The M.D. Anderson Cancer Center experience. Oncol Rep 1998;5:939–44.

132. Villena-Heinsen C, Diesing D, Fischer D, et al. Carcinosarcomas – a retrospective analysis of 21 patients. Anticancer Res 2006;26: 4817–23.

133. Wada H, Enomoto T, Fujita M, et al. Molecular evidence that most but not all carcinosarcomas of the uterus are combination tumors. Cancer Res 1997;57:5379–85.

134. Yilmaz A, Rush DS, Soslow RA. Endometrial stromal sarcomas with unusual histologic features – a report of 24 primary and metastatic tumors emphasizing fibroblastic and smooth muscle differentiation. Am J Surg Pathol 2002;26:1142–50.

135. Zaloudek CJ, Norris HJ. Adenofibroma and adenosarcoma of the uterus: a clinicopathologic study of 35 cases. Cancer 1981;48:354–66.

Uterine smooth muscle tumors

18

Bradley J. Quade   Stanley J. Robboy

INTRODUCTION

The benign smooth muscle tumor, the leiomyoma, is the most common of all uterine neoplasms. Its malignant counterpart, the leiomyosarcoma, is the most common of the malignant non-epithelial tumors. A classification of smooth muscle tumors of the uterus is given in Table 18.1. The diagnostic features that enable a distinction to be made between them are discussed in detail below.

LEIOMYOMA

Definition

A benign smooth muscle tumor that most commonly affects the uterine body, but also may be found in the cervix, uterine ligaments and, rarely, the ovary or fallopian tube. The tumor also is known colloquially as 'fibroid', and although an unscientific term, its use is universal and understood by all.

Incidence

The true incidence of uterine leiomyomas, or 'fibroids' as they are colloquially known, is uncertain, even though they are the most frequent tumor found in the female genital tract. They are clinically evident in 20–30% of women over 30 years of age,[22,168] rising to more than 40% in those over 40 years old.[64] In a series of 1000 uteri that were serially examined, over 56% contained leiomyomas.[180] In other studies, 69–77% of women who underwent hysterectomy for non-cancerous conditions were found to have leiomyomas.[32,88] Many of these women presented because of the symptoms caused by their tumors, but undoubtedly a high proportion of women harbor leiomyomas completely without symptoms. Furthermore, multiple leiomyomas are found in the majority of hysterectomy specimens,[32] indicating the smooth muscle tumorigenesis in the uterus is an exceedingly frequent event. The location of symptomatic tumors often correlates, and presumably determines, the nature of symptoms.[168] Although benign, leiomyomas pose a major public health burden.[108] An estimate of the total annual cost resulting from symptomatic leiomyomas exceeds $4600 per patient.[62]

There are racial differences in the incidence of uterine leiomyomas. The Nurses' Health Study II estimated the relative risk for leiomyomas to be two to three times greater in black than in Caucasian women.[104] In one study,[88] 89% of black women and 59% of white women had leiomyomas in uteri removed at hysterectomy. The average age at diagnosis was 4 years younger in black women. They also had a higher body weight and larger number of leiomyomas. Furthermore, black women were more likely to have anemia and severe pelvic pain than their white counterparts.[88] This increased risk of uterine leiomyomas cannot be explained by a higher prevalence of risk factors such as body weight or smoking history.[105,159] Recently, a higher prevalence for genetic polymorphisms in the estrogen receptor-α and catechol-O-methyltransferase (an enzyme involved in estrogen metabolism) was observed in black women with leiomyomas, but it remains uncertain to what extent these polymorphisms account for the higher tumor incidence.[3,4] In fact, a number of nuclear receptors are differentially expressed by leiomyomas in black women compared to other ethnic groups.[195]

Like the contribution of race, familial patterns of inheritance also suggest that genetic risk factors are important in the pathobiology of leiomyomas.[56,97,102,158]

Etiology

The precise etiology of leiomyomas is unknown, but the hormonal milieu is pivotal.[46] Leiomyomas are tumors that occur during the reproductive period, a time when hormonal influences are maximal. They first become apparent after the menarche, become enlarged during pregnancy and shrink after menopause. Even so, experimental attempts to induce their development by exogenous estrogens in animals have failed to produce anything more than fibromuscular proliferations in the peritoneum. It is remarkable that the human uterine wall should be such a common site for leiomyomas in contrast to their rarity elsewhere, because smooth muscle tumors can arise in any tissue as a neoplastic change of mural smooth muscle in vessels as well as hollow viscera. Recent evidence affirms the view that estrogens and estrogen receptors are important in the pathogenesis of leiomyomas.[181] Studies comparing gene expression in leiomyomas with that in normal myometrium show that leiomyomas maintain a high level of sensitivity to estrogen during the estrogen-dominated proliferative phase of the menstrual cycle.[6] Furthermore, cultured cells from leiomyomas have a significantly higher response to estrogen than do matched cultures of myometrial cells from the same patient, particularly if the tissue is taken for culture in the proliferative phase.[7] Semi-quantitative immunohistochemistry for estrogen and progesterone receptors correlates with tumor growth rate.[75] Accelerated growth, sufficient to require hysterectomy, also occurs in women taking tamoxifen for breast cancer treatment.[12,94]

Further information on the origin of leiomyomas has come from studying their clonality. Originally, glucose-6-phosphate dehydrogenase isoforms were used as a marker for X chromosome inactivation,[98,184] but this has been supplanted by newer

Table 18.1 Classification of smooth muscle tumors

Leiomyoma
    Variants of leiomyoma
        Degenerated leiomyoma
        Atypical leiomyoma
        Mitotically active leiomyoma
        Cellular leiomyoma
        Epithelioid leiomyoma (plexiform, leiomyoblastoma, clear cell)
        Myxoid leiomyoma
        Leiomyomas with heterologous elements
    Unusual growth patterns
        Diffuse (intrauterine) leiomyomatosis
        Intravascular leiomyomatosis
        Benign metastasizing leiomyomatosis
        Disseminated peritoneal leiomyomatosis

Smooth muscle tumors of uncertain malignant potential (a term to be discouraged)

Leiomyosarcoma
    Variants of leiomyosarcoma
        Epithelioid leiomyosarcoma
        Myxoid leiomyosarcoma

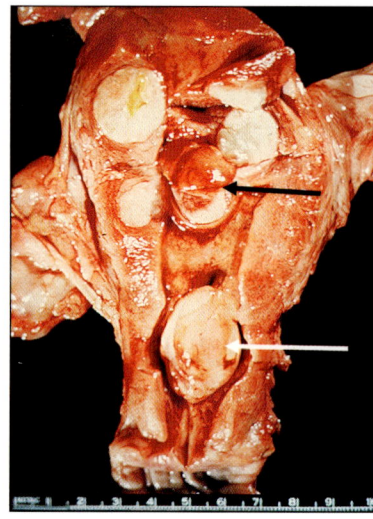

Fig. 18.1 Multiple leiomyomas. On cut section, the tumors are well circumscribed, bulging above the cut surface. These leiomyomas are intramural and one is submucosal (black arrow). A prolapsed, submucosal leiomyoma protrudes into the endocervical canal (white arrow).

molecular biologic techniques that exploit methylation differences between polymorphic loci on the active and inactive X chromosomes.[63,107,204] These methods confirm that each leiomyoma derives from a single transformation event. Interestingly, these studies also suggest that each tumor is a distinct clone, reinforcing the notion that smooth muscle tumorigenesis is an exceedingly common event.

The genetic mechanisms by which initiation and growth of leiomyomas occur so frequently are not fully understood. Cytogenetic analysis of these benign smooth muscle tumors, however, has revealed important clues.[97,156] Nearly one-half of leiomyomas have chromosomal rearrangements large enough to be seen in G-banded karyotypes. These chromosomal rearrangements are generally simple, which is in sharp contrast to the aberrations seen in leiomyosarcoma. To date, recurrent aberrations have allowed definition of seven cytogenetic subgroups: t(12;14)(q14–15;q23–24), del(7)(q22q32), rearrangements of 6p21 and 10q22, trisomy 12, and deletions of 3q and 1p.[97,170] Of these, the translocation between chromosomes 12 and 14 and the rearrangements involving chromosome 6 are perhaps the best understood. Both rearrangements involve genes for two closely related non-histone chromatin proteins: *HMGA1* at 6p21 and *HMGA2* at 12q15.[51,165,199] Rearrangements involving *HMGA1* and *HMGA2* are also associated with lipomas, endometrial polyps, vulvar aggressive angiomyxoma, and several other benign mesenchymal neoplasms.[82,175] Evidence suggests that inappropriate expression of AT-hook DNA binding domains from *HMGA2* are relevant in uterine leiomyoma.[89,144,203] Interestingly, rearranged 10q22 disrupts a gene for another class of chromatin protein, namely the histone acetyltransferase *MYST4*, which raises the possibility that chromatin regulation more broadly is important in uterine leiomyoma pathobiology.[113] Beyond such mechanistic insights, cytogenetic studies may also have some practical significance. Tumors with chromosomal rearrangements are on average larger and often within the uterine wall.[149] In addition, some aberrations are associated with specific variants of uterine leiomyomas.

An autosomal dominant syndrome, Reed syndrome[148] (Mendelian Inheritance in Man #150800 and #605839), exhibits a predisposition towards cutaneous and uterine leiomyomas as well as renal cell carcinoma. This syndrome has inactivated fumarate hydratase,[182,197] an enzyme of the Krebs cycle. Germline fumarate hydratase mutations behave like those in classical tumor suppressor genes. Some non-syndromic (i.e., typical 'garden variety') leiomyomas also have a subset, particularly those from symptomatic younger women, that may have deleted fumarate hydratase.[56,87,95]

Transcriptional profiling has been used to study uterine smooth muscle tumors.[10,143,152,163,164,186,203] Typical of this experimental approach, a seemingly large number (into the hundreds!) have been found. While lists of dysregulated genes produced by various groups overlap to some degree, and while much more study is needed to understand fully the significance of these transcriptional profiles, it seems that the transcriptional profiles for uterine leiomyomas are much closer to myometrium than to leiomyosarcoma and atypical leiomyomas, and that malignant transformation appears to coincide in downregulation of gene expression more frequently than upregulation.[143] Three potential mechanisms proposed to account for differential gene regulation in the smooth muscle transcriptome include: (1) differential expression of non-histone chromatin proteins such *HMGA2* and *MYST4*; (2) altered expression of tuberin and the glucocorticoid receptor;[194–196] and (3) abnormal regulation of micro-RNAs, which in turn might regulate *HMGA2*.[192]

Gross features

Leiomyomas occur anywhere within the myometrium. They also occur occasionally in the cervix (see Chapter 11). The most frequent location is within the myometrial wall where, if numerous or large, they can also grossly distort the uterus (Figures 18.1 and 18.2). Those situated close to the endometrium or the serosa are referred to as submucosal and subserosal (Figures 18.3 and 18.4), respectively. From each of these locations, the leiomyoma may protrude, either into the uterine cavity or into the peritoneal cavity. Submucosal leiomyomas may lead to

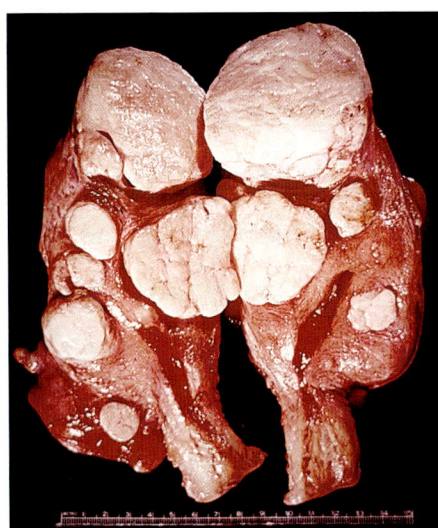

Fig. 18.2 Multiple leiomyomas. These are predominantly intramural. The bulging cut surfaces are clearly shown.

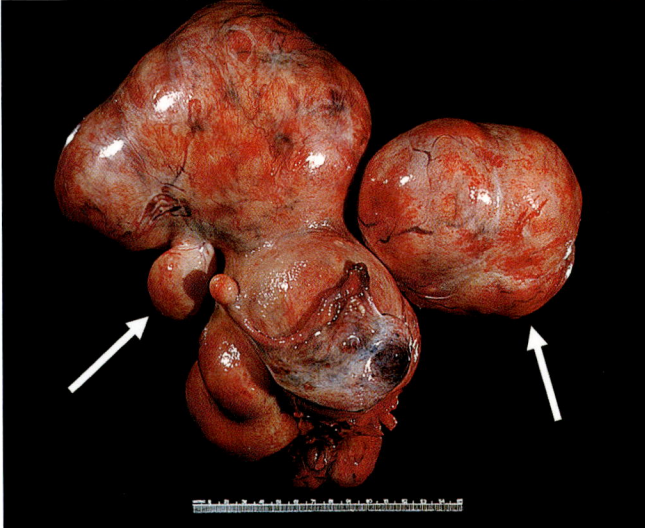

Fig. 18.3 Multiple leiomyomas. This unopened uterus is greatly distorted by leiomyomas, two of which (arrows) are subserosal and pedunculated.

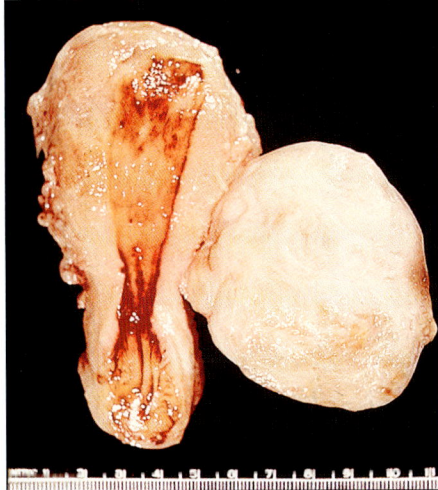

Fig. 18.4 Subserosal leiomyoma. A single large subserosal pedunculated leiomyoma is present.

atrophy or erosion of the mucosal surface and hence intermenstrual bleeding. As the muscular action of the uterus acts to expel the mass, the leiomyoma becomes pedunculated, giving rise to a fibroid polyp or a submucosal pedunculated leiomyoma (Figure 18.5). The former may be subjected to further traction by isthmic contractions and may present at the external cervical os, often with an infarcted tip (Figure 18.6). These women often report cramps not unlike the Braxton Hicks contractions seen in mid-to-late pregnancy. A subserosal, pedunculated leiomyoma may, on rare occasions, establish a blood supply from an adjacent, adherent structure, such as the omentum, bowel or peritoneum. Eventually its anchorage to

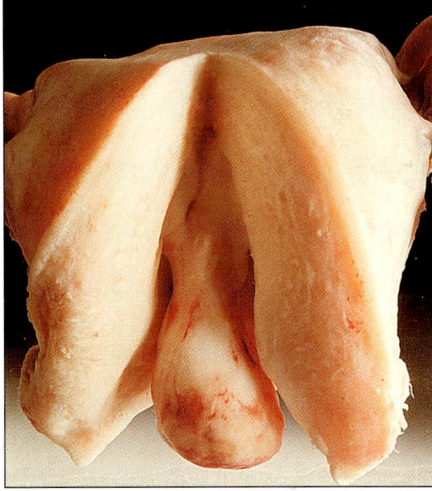

Fig. 18.5 Polypoid leiomyoma. A pedunculated submucosal leiomyoma protrudes through the external os.

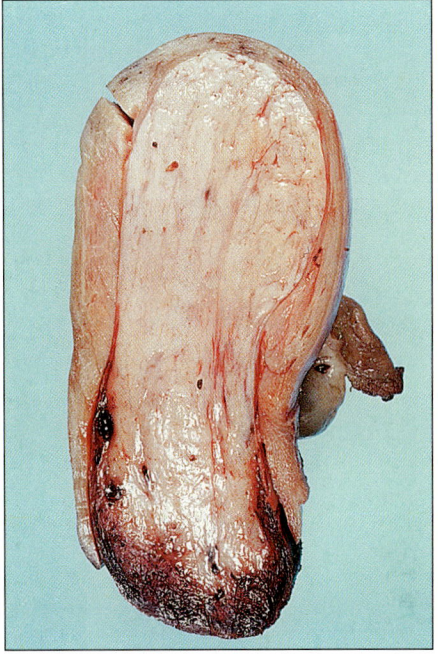

Fig. 18.6 Polypoid leiomyoma. A large, soft, submucosal prolapsed leiomyoma protrudes through the external cervical os and markedly dilates the cervical canal. The vaginal surface of the leiomyoma is hemorrhagic and the cause of bleeding.

the uterus, together with its dependence on its uterine blood supply, may sever. This is then termed a 'parasitic' leiomyoma, which must not be mistaken for a metastasis from a malignant smooth muscle tumor.

The cut surface of a leiomyoma typically shows a whorled, spiral pattern of fibers to the naked eye (Figure 18.7). The leiomyoma is firm and rubbery and its cut surface both pops up (rises above the cut surface in the unfixed state as a result of decompression) and is resistant to indentation by the examining thumb or finger, in contrast to some examples of leiomyosarcoma. It is usually paler than its surrounding myometrium. A striking feature is the very sharp demarcation between it and the surrounding normal myometrium. This forms a plane of cleavage that enables the leiomyoma to be shelled out at myomectomy. The loss of this cleavage plane is an important feature that offers the pathologist a clue that malignant change may have occurred (i.e., infiltration) or that a different diagnosis should be entertained (e.g., adenomyoma or adenomatoid tumor).

Several variations from the typical naked-eye appearance of leiomyoma may be encountered if any one of the several varieties of degeneration to which these benign tumors are commonly prone has occurred. Although these patterns are considered in more detail in subsequent sections, any deviation from the typical gross appearance requires more thorough histologic sampling, particularly at the interface between tumor and myometrium and in areas of gross necrosis, hemorrhage, softness or believed malignancy.

Microscopic features

A leiomyoma consists of interlacing bundles of smooth muscle cells. The sharp demarcation from surrounding myometrium that has been noted macroscopically is also prominent microscopically (Figure 18.8). The smooth muscle cells are markedly elongated and have eosinophilic cytoplasm and tapered, cigar-shaped nuclei. In a typical leiomyoma, the nuclei are uniform and mitotic figures absent or sparse (Figure 18.9). Abundant reticulin is present. The smooth muscle cells of a leiomyoma are usually more closely packed than those of the surrounding myometrium, so that the tumor usually appears more cellular

and the small blood vessels appear compressed and less randomly distributed. Such increased cellularity is often particularly striking in women past menopause. With estrogen withdrawal, along with the shrinkage of the uterus that occurs after the menopause, the amount of cytoplasm in the smooth muscle cells of the normal myometrium and in the leiomyoma diminishes dramatically so that the entire tissue appears darker and richer in nuclei. This change is usually more noticeable in the leiomyoma than in the surrounding muscle. Absence of mitotic activity is just one feature that enables a distinction from leiomyosarcoma to be made in these circumstances. The nuclei in a leiomyoma are generally arranged in a fascicular fashion, but occasionally there is palisading resulting in a pattern similar to that seen in a neurilemmoma (schwannoma) (Figures 18.10 and 18.11).

Marked attenuation of overlying endometrium may be seen in some mucosal leiomyomas (Figure 18.8). By extension, the presence of aglandular functionalis in curettings is a hint that dysfunctional uterine bleeding might be due to a nearby leiomyoma.

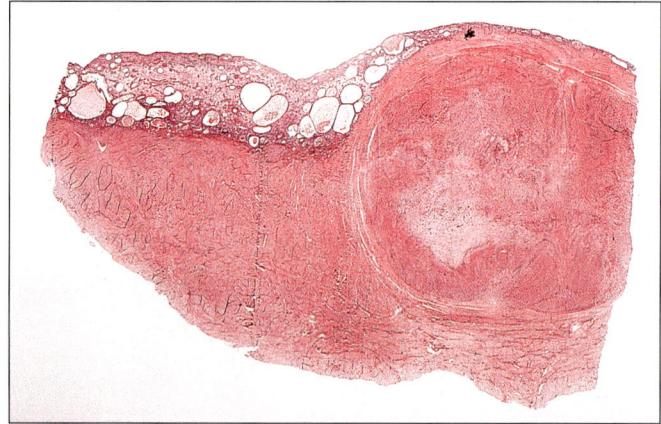

Fig. 18.8 Submucosal leiomyoma. At this low magnification the sharp line of demarcation between the leiomyoma and the surrounding myometrium is clearly shown. In this submucosal position, the overlying endometrium is compressed and atrophic.

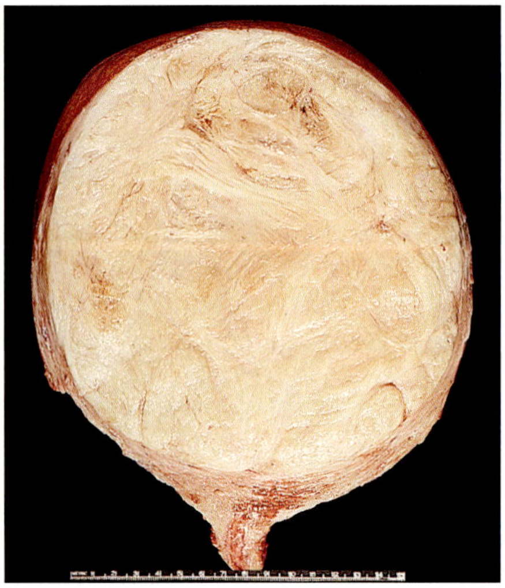

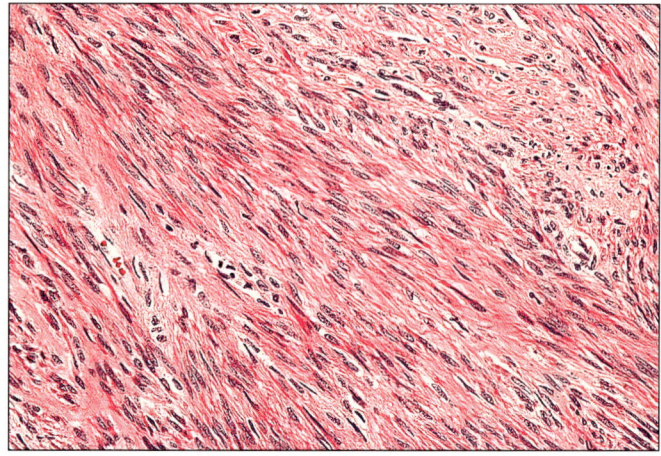

Fig. 18.9 Leiomyoma. The smooth muscle cells are markedly elongated and have eosinophilic cytoplasm and elongated, cigar-shaped nuclei. The nuclei are uniform and mitotic figures absent or sparse.

Fig. 18.7 Leiomyoma. The cut surface shows the spiral, whorled pattern of fibers in a typical tumor.

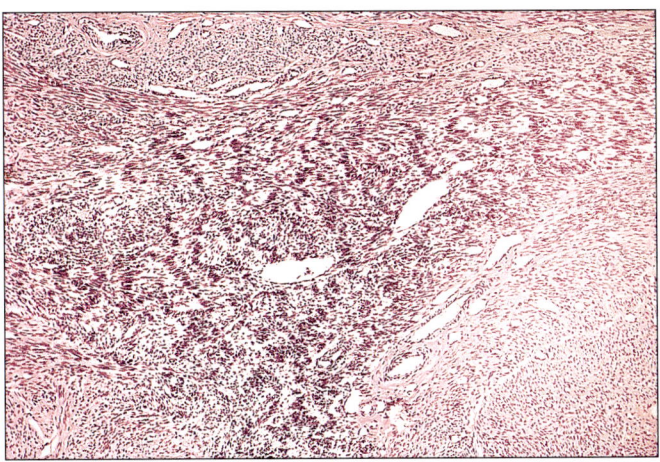

Fig. 18.10 Leiomyoma. Palisading of nuclei (plexiform tumorlet). A focal area of an otherwise typical leiomyoma shows striking nuclear palisading.

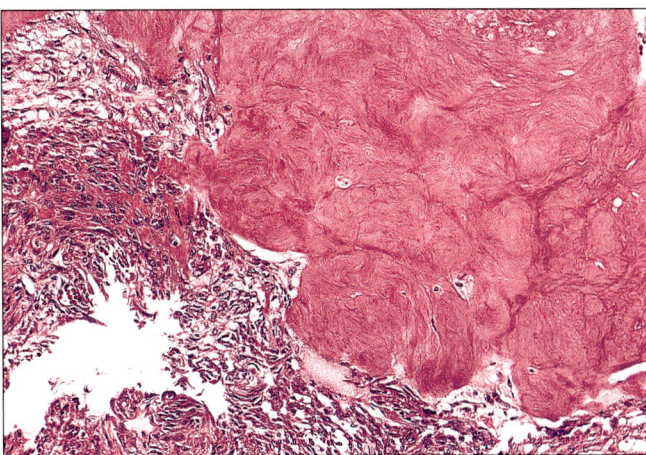

Fig. 18.12 Hyaline change. The leiomyoma has a uniform, eosinophilic, ground-glass appearance. Blood vessels are also involved.

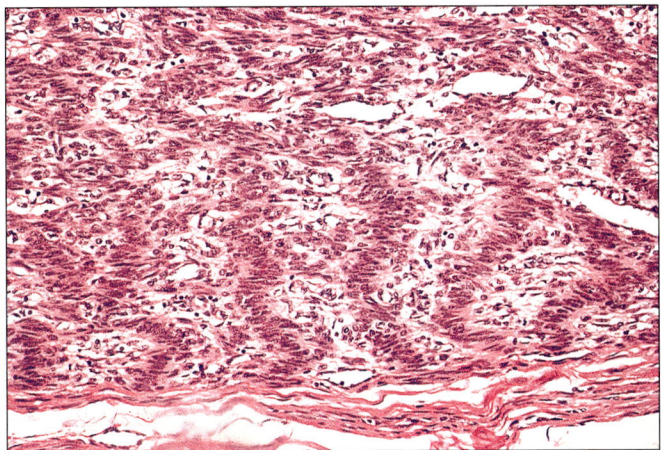

Fig. 18.11 Leiomyoma. Nuclear palisading.

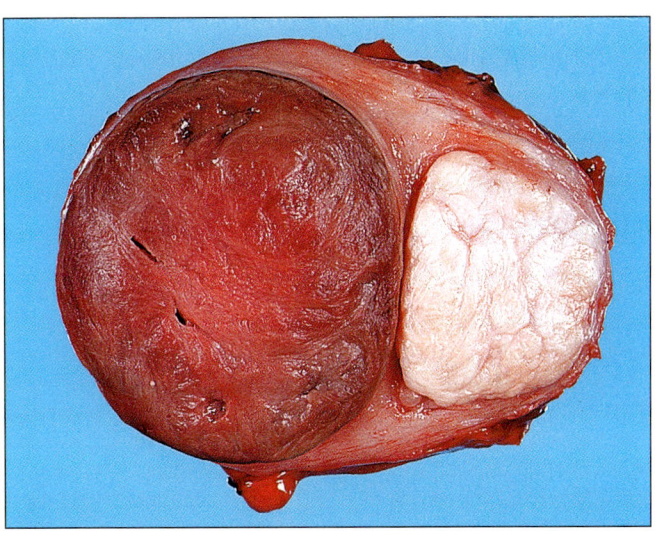

Fig. 18.13 Red degeneration (necrobiosis). The cut surface of the leiomyoma on the left is red and more homogeneous, with loss of the whorled appearance.

VARIANTS OF LEIOMYOMA

DEGENERATED LEIOMYOMA

A variety of degenerative changes can occur in leiomyomas. The larger the leiomyoma, the more likely some degenerative form will be present. Several mechanisms likely contribute to this, including ischemia and hormonal effects. More than one pattern of degeneration may be observed in the same leiomyoma.

By far the most common form of degeneration is *hyaline degeneration* whereby expanded septa have lost their fibrillary structure, assuming a uniform, pale eosinophilic, ground-glass appearance (Figure 18.12). This change may be localized or it may affect extensive areas of the tumor, occasionally even the whole of it. This form of degeneration may be accompanied by surviving muscle cells oriented into lacework patterns. The blood vessels within an area of hyaline necrosis undergo the same change and can be seen as pale outlines, a point of distinction from the coagulative tumor cell necrosis seen in leiomyosarcoma where the vessels are often spared (e.g., see Figures 18.46–18.48).[17]

Degenerated areas may liquefy, resulting in *hydropic* or *cystic degeneration*. When extreme, such a degenerated leio-

myoma may take on a peculiar multinodular appearance.[28,154] The terms *mucoid* and *myxoid degeneration* are used to describe changes that seem very little different from hyaline change, with or without cystic change. In myxoid change, the scattered nuclei are embedded in an amorphous, slightly amphophilic matrix whereas in mucoid degeneration the matrix appears to be mucinous in nature. The mucoid and myxoid forms of degeneration lack practical importance and the two terms are often used interchangeably without distinguishing between them.

Red degeneration (*necrobiosis*), on the other hand, is a form of degeneration that occurs characteristically, but not exclusively, in pregnancy and the process often causes pain and fever. Necrobiosis (red degeneration) results in the cut surface taking on a more homogeneous look, with loss of the whorled appearance. At the same time the color becomes a deeper pink or red (due to staining by fresh blood pigment) and the consistency softer (Figure 18.13). Over time, the periphery of a leiomyoma that has undergone red degeneration may become white and calcified. Unlike hyaline change, the microscopic appearance in red degeneration shows the ghosts of the muscle cells and their nuclei (Figure 18.14). Uncommonly, a leiomyoma may undergo necrosis, resulting in a soft, structureless, pale gray mass. This change is seen most often in submucous leiomyomas that protrude into the endometrial cavity.

Calcific degeneration is seen more often in women after the menopause.

Fatty degeneration, if it exists, is rare. In most circumstances fat in a myometrial mass is part of a lipoleiomyoma. In these tumors, the fat is within recognizable adipocytes; in contrast, fatty degeneration discloses the lipid in the smooth muscle cells themselves or in histiocytes.

In general, benign forms of necrosis tend to be unifocal, centrally located, rounded in shape, and relatively uniform in color and consistency of the gross cut surface. The microscopic border exhibits a gradual transition from viable to fully necrotic tumor. Inflammation, granulation, and early hyaline change may be found in these transitional areas. Atypical ghost cells should not be present. Vascular sparing within larger areas of degeneration is unusual. Not infrequently, thrombosis may be seen in the tumor. The overall impression rendered is that of an ongoing or chronic process with a corresponding host reaction. These features are important to recognize and distinguish from the pattern of necrosis found in malignant smooth muscle tumors.

LEIOMYOMA TREATED WITH GONADOTROPHIN-RELEASING HORMONE ANALOGUES

In recent years, gonadotrophin-releasing hormone (GnRH) analogues or agonists have been used to treat uterine leiomyomas. During treatment, both the uterus and its leiomyomas decrease in size, but most of the latter return to their original size once treatment is stopped or within a year even if treatment is continued. Treated leiomyomas have a significant increase in estrogen receptor content.[188] GnRH analogues are mostly used as an adjunct to surgery, reducing the need for transfusion and, perhaps, permitting vaginal hysterectomy to be performed because the uterus has shrunk in size.[172] Medical management may also be used in perimenopausal women as a temporary measure to reduce menorrhagia prior to the onset of menopause.

Gross features

If coagulative necrosis is extensive or involves the whole tumor, the leiomyoma is soft and exhibits a dusky or red color. The appearance seen more usually is of partial necrosis, when there are well-delineated, often centrally located red zones within the leiomyoma (Figure 18.15).

Microscopic features

The most striking feature that may be present is coagulative necrosis exhibiting nuclear pyknosis, karyorrhexis, karyolysis, and markedly increased cytoplasmic eosinophilia.[30] This may affect a small group of cells or extensive areas within the leiomyoma (Figure 18.16) and be surrounded by a rim of inflammatory cells. Apoptosis may be prominent.[69] Changes in cellularity generally are not significant, but both decreased[37] and increased cellularity[30] have been reported. A massive lymphocytic infiltration[14,91] and thickening of blood vessels walls with narrowing of the lumen may also be seen.[37] In our experi-

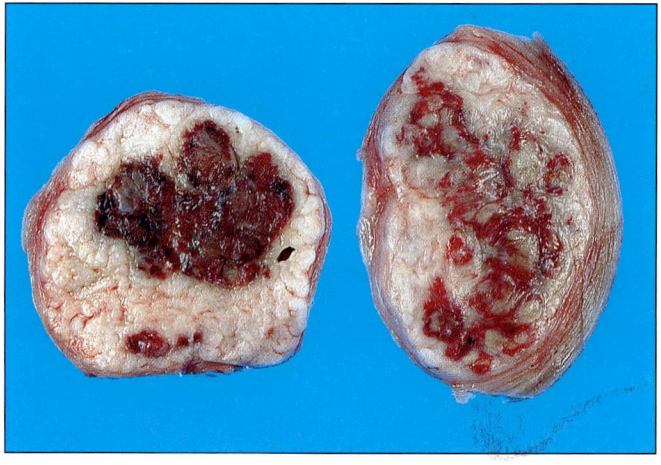

Fig. 18.15 Treatment with gonadotrophin-releasing hormone analogues. The leiomyoma shows focal areas of hemorrhagic necrosis.

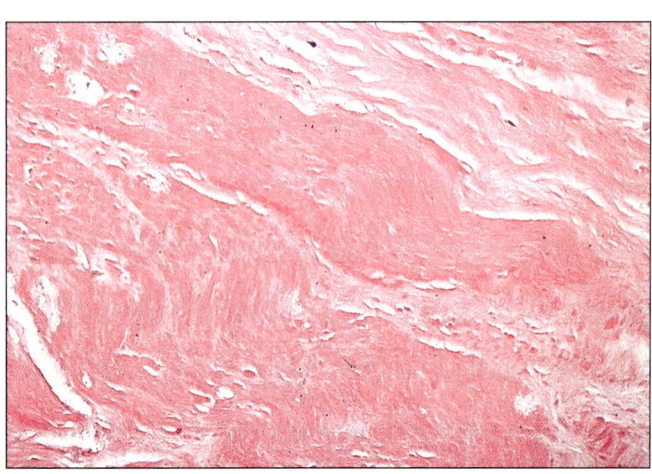

Fig. 18.14 Red degeneration (necrobiosis). The ghosts of the muscle cells and their nuclei remain.

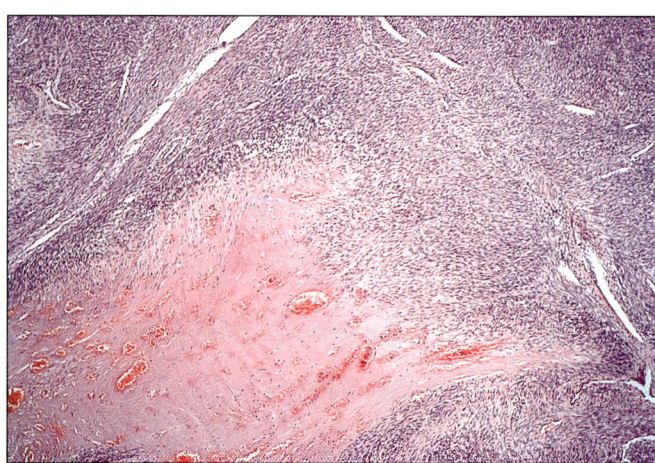

Fig. 18.16 Treatment with gonadotrophin-releasing hormone analogues. There are well-demarcated areas of coagulative necrosis with a rim of inflammatory cells.

ence, GnRH analogue therapy, however, is associated with little or no difference in histologic appearance in the majority of instances. A study of cell proliferation indices (Ki-67 and proliferating cell nuclear antigen) suggests that the reduction in size of leiomyomas treated by GnRH agonists is due to a reduction in the number of cycling cells, presumably secondary to reduced levels of estrogen and progesterone receptors.[191]

LEIOMYOMA TREATED BY INTERVENTIONAL RADIOLOGY

In addition to conservative medical management with GnRH analogues and selective estrogen receptor modulators (e.g., raloxifene) and less invasive surgical procedures such as laparoscopic or hysteroscopic myomectomy, recent advances in interventional radiology have been made for the management of uterine leiomyomas. In some cases, these techniques are unsuccessful and hysterectomy ensues. As these minimally invasive technologies become more widespread, pathologists will increasingly encounter surgical specimens from these cases and need to distinguish treatment effects from other types of degeneration, particularly the pattern of necrosis associated with malignancy.

Selective arterial embolization is one such conservative method for treating uterine leiomyomas.[146,147,160,200] The procedure is performed under local anesthesia and involves femoral artery puncture with catheterization of hypogastric and then uterine arteries. Polyvinylformaldehyde particles, 150–600 μm in diameter, are introduced until complete devascularization of the targeted tumor is achieved. The procedure is often accompanied by pelvic pain that lasts 12–18 hours. A postembolization syndrome (defined by a greater severity of ischemic pain accompanied by low-grade fever, elevated neutrophil counts, malaise, nausea, and vomiting), premature ovarian failure, sepsis, and even death are among the other complications associated with this procedure.[42,166,189] Perhaps the complication most of interest to pathologists is the delay in diagnosis of leiomyosarcoma.[53,79,132,166] In about 80–90% of women who underwent embolization, the symptoms improved sufficiently for surgical treatment to be avoided.[42,146] Gross examination of hysterectomy specimens may sometimes reveal distended small arteries occluded by small aggregates of translucent spheres that might conjure up the notion of a bizarre parasitic infection to the unaware examiner. Such vessels may be found throughout the specimen, and not necessarily in proximity to leiomyomas. Microscopically, a foreign-body giant cell reaction surrounds the amorphous spheroids after the initial period following installation.[31,198] The leiomyomas themselves may show various patterns of necrosis, including hyaline, coagulative, and suppurative types, or they may show no apparent change at all.[31,198]

Another emerging technology for the non-invasive treatment of leiomyoma is ablation by magnetic resonance (MR) guided focused ultrasound (FUS or MRgFUS).[169,171,177] Patients are placed in a specialized MR scanner that has been modified to include a large panel of ultrasound transducers. The emissions from this arrayed ultrasound transducer coordinated to constructively interfere in a small focus, resulting in very rapid tissue heating in the zone targeted by MR imaging. The resulting thermal necrosis may grossly mimic the pattern of geographic tumor necrosis seen in leiomyosarcoma because it is sharply demarcated, geometrically complex, and often associated with hemorrhage. One clue that distinguishes this treatment effect from malignant-type geographic tumor necrosis is the firmness of the tissue section. Sudden thermal ablation results in massive protein denaturation, resulting in a hard, unyielding cut surface, whereas necrosis in leiomyosarcomas produces additional softening in tissue, often compared to 'fish flesh'. Microscopic inspection of FUS treatment effect is also notable for the sharp transition from viable to non-viable tissue, at least in the short term following treatment. Interstitial hemorrhage may be prominent. In contrast to leiomyosarcoma, the necrosis following FUS is comprised of a remarkably bland eosinophilia typical of thermal denaturation.

ATYPICAL LEIOMYOMA

Definition

This variant was formally renamed in the most recent World Health Organization (WHO) Classification of Tumours monograph.[67] Symplastic leiomyoma, bizarre leiomyoma, and pleomorphic leiomyoma are older synonyms for this tumor. Of note, the word 'symplastic' is derived from a 'symplast', a multinucleated cell created either by the fusion of cells into one cytoplasmic mass, or by the division of the nucleus of a single cell. The term is more usually applied to plant cells and bacteria.

In series in which most patients were treated by hysterectomy and a minority by myomectomy, no deaths or recurrences were recorded, underscoring the benign nature of this variant.[40,41,55] Despite its good reputation, we have seen atypical leiomyomas, particularly those with diffuse atypia, recur following conservative surgical treatment for fibroids in our practices. In one instance, the atypical tumor even appeared to evolve into a leiomyosarcoma with geographic tumor necrosis and extremely high proliferative activity. In addition, recent cytogenetic and molecular studies, described below, suggest that there may be greater similarity between atypical leiomyoma and leiomyosarcoma than just the morphologic atypia. These observations and the need to exclude malignancy make this variant of uterine smooth muscle tumors clinically relevant.

Consequently, we take a much more cautious approach to the management of atypical leiomyoma following myomectomy, especially when the atypia is diffuse or the tumor is large (i.e., >5 cm), by recommending follow-up with non-invasive imaging to exclude regrowth in the first several years. When an atypical leiomyoma recurs, we also believe that hysterectomy should be given due consideration. In contrast, once thorough histologic sampling of a hysterectomy specimen has established the diagnosis of atypical leiomyoma, no further management is required.

Gross features

There often is nothing that distinguishes an atypical leiomyoma from the usual type of leiomyoma to the naked eye. Some tumors may be more yellow or tan than usual, or have areas of hemorrhage, softening, cavitation or myxoid change.[40] When such gross findings are present, greater scrutiny of the tumor by histology is prudent.

Microscopic features

Bizarre, pleomorphic tumor cells with atypical nuclei characterize this tumor (Figures 18.17–18.19). Many of the bizarre

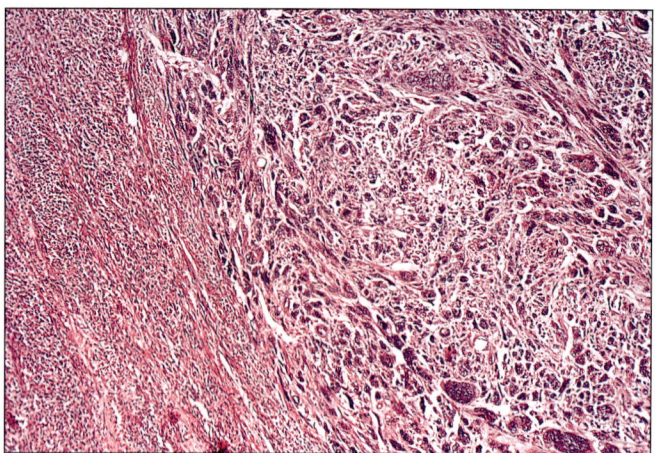

Fig. 18.17 Atypical leiomyoma. An area of this leiomyoma shows markedly pleomorphic and enlarged nuclei, some of which are multilobed.

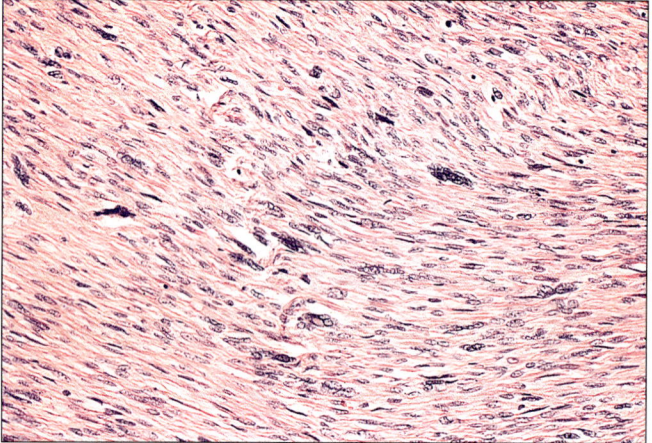

Fig. 18.18 Atypical leiomyoma. Scattered enlarged and multilobed nuclei are seen.

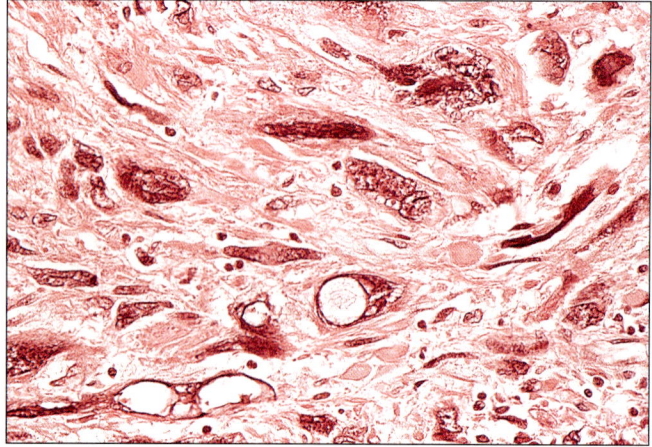

Fig. 18.19 Atypical leiomyoma. Clusters of bizarre, hyperchromatic, often multinucleated smooth muscle cells are present within an otherwise typical leiomyoma. Intranuclear vacuolation is present.

cells are multinucleated or have multilobed nuclei, but greatly enlarged, hyperchromatic mononuclear cells also are common. Some of the nuclear features are degenerative, with smudged chromatin, vacuolation, karyorrhexis, and pyknosis. Most tumors, however, also contain some cells that have nuclear features that are more disquieting, where the chromatin is coarsely clumped or granular, with areas of clearing and enlarged nucleoli.[40] In practical terms, the nuclear atypia should be appreciated easily at lower magnification (i.e., with 4 or 10× objectives) in the vast majority of cases. In contrast, mild nuclear hyperchromasia or enlargement noticed only at the highest magnification (i.e., with 40× objectives) should not prompt the diagnosis of an atypical leiomyoma. The exception to this latter rule is when such minimal nuclear changes are present consistently in every tumor cell, emphasizing their monoclonal phenotype. Although the cell-to-cell variation is minimal in this subset, their nuclear atypia should stand out clearly when compared to smooth muscle cells of the adjacent myometrium. More commonly, multinucleated cells may be found focally, multifocally or diffusely, and occupy more than 25% of the tumor in most cases.[40] In one study of 24 cases, 50% had the multinucleated cells evenly distributed throughout the tumor.[41] The cellularity of the mononuclear component varies, but tends to be higher than usual.

As atypical leiomyomas by definition are smooth muscle tumors that show cellular atypia and may sometimes have increased mitotic rates, it is important that they be correctly distinguished from leiomyosarcomas. Proliferative activity in atypical smooth muscle tumors classified as being benign is often low, but mitotic figures up to 7 per 10 high-power fields (HPFs) using the highest count method have been reported.[40,41,139] Of note, these more mitotically active tumors tend to be smaller and the increased proliferation is typically focal. The mitotic figures are only rarely atypical (e.g., multipolarity, extreme polyploidy, or lagging chromosomes during the later stages of mitosis). If atypical smooth muscle cells are present in a multifocal or diffuse distribution in association with an elevated mitotic activity, a diagnosis of sarcoma must be considered. Furthermore, these tumors may show degeneration, edema, and hyaline change, with the symplastic cells seemingly associated with the edge of the degenerating areas. Geographic coagulative tumor cell necrosis, sometimes a prominent feature of malignant leiomyosarcomas (see below), however, must not be present.

Cytogenetic and molecular features
Nearly half of atypical leiomyomas show loss of heterozygosity for loci on the short arm of chromosome 1, suggesting that they might harbor a tumor suppressor gene for atypical smooth muscle tumors on 1p.[25] Interestingly, the expression profiles of atypical leiomyomas with 1p– resemble more closely that of leiomyosarcomas than the profiles of myometrium and leiomyomas of the usual histologic type.[25]

MITOTICALLY ACTIVE LEIOMYOMA

Definition
A benign smooth muscle tumor, usually of a size under 8 cm with an increased mitotic rate.[38,125,139] Increased proliferative rates have been associated with increased progestin levels, such those seen during the secretory phase.[201]

Microscopic features

These leiomyomas have from 5 to 14 mitotic figures per 10 HPFs when counted in the most active area. This increased proliferative rate is frequently, but not always, diffusely distributed. If focal increases in proliferation are appreciated, one should consider the possibility that the proliferation is being stimulated by some local factor such as nearby ischemic necrosis or mucosal inflammation and ulceration in a polypoid submucosal tumor. Atypical mitotic figures are not characteristic of mitotically active leiomyomas and should prompt a more thorough examination of the tumor. By definition, geographic tumor necrosis and atypia must not be present, otherwise the tumor would be classified as a leiomyosarcoma or atypical leiomyoma. Of note, tumors in series classified as mitotically active leiomyomas are usually small (2–3 cm) and nearly all are smaller than 8 cm. Consequently, larger smooth muscle tumors with increased proliferative activity should be scrutinized for other features of malignancy.

In general, we reserve the diagnosis of mitotically active leiomyoma for tumors in which the increased proliferation is widespread, if not diffuse. This requirement recognizes the intrinsic biologic feature of this variant. In our opinion, reactive proliferation does not reflect the same pathobiology. Consequently, we will not classify a tumor as being of the mitotically active variant when a mitogenic stimulus can be identified.

Although very uncommon, smooth muscle tumors with mitotic counts higher than 14 mitotic figures per 10 HPFs are highly suspicious for malignancy, even in the absence of necrosis and atypia.

CELLULAR LEIOMYOMA

Definition

A benign smooth muscle tumor that has a markedly increased number of cells per unit area when compared with the surrounding myometrium and the vast majority of other leiomyomas. While there is no specific quantitative definition for this benign variant, practical considerations with regard to the gross and microscopic features of cellular leiomyoma, as well as its distinction from other malignant tumors, justify its recognition in clinical practice.

Gross features

A leiomyoma that is cellular may appear to the naked eye very much like an ordinary leiomyoma or it may be subtly different. It is a pale, round tumor that is sharply demarcated from the surrounding myometrium. The whorled pattern characteristic of a leiomyoma may be lacking and the color tends to be tan or creamy-yellow rather than pinkish-white. The most striking difference between a cellular leiomyoma and the usual leiomyoma is that the former is characteristically soft, a feature that this tumor has in common with some leiomyosarcomas. Soft 'fibroids' must always be sampled extensively and, as with all unusual smooth muscle tumors, tissue from the perimeter and any variegated areas should be sampled.

Microscopic features

The cells comprising this variant are similar to those seen in an ordinary leiomyoma and range from spindle shaped to round, depending on the angle at which they are sectioned. They have scanty cytoplasm and are closely packed so that the section is dark blue with little or no magnification (Figure

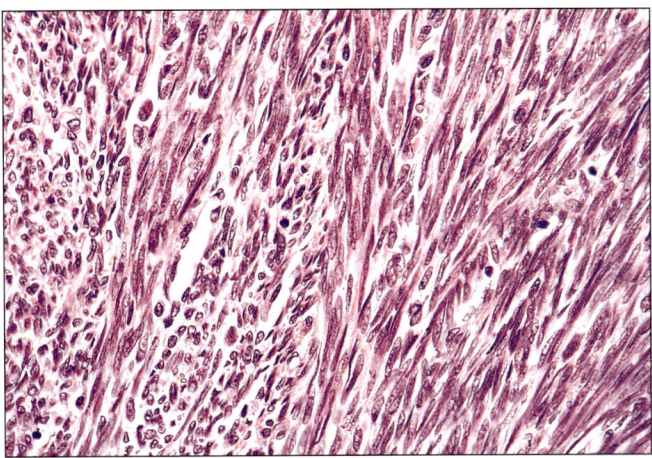

Fig. 18.20 Cellular leiomyoma. The nuclear features are the same as those of a typical leiomyoma, but the nuclei are more closely packed.

18.20). In fact, recognizing this basophilia without or at very low magnification is one practical test for determining if the cellularity of a particular tumor is beyond the spectrum of typical leiomyomas. A fascicular pattern is present in some areas. The blood vessels are typically large with thick muscular walls and cleft-like spaces are often seen, possibly representing compressed vessels or edema.[131] Unlike the usual leiomyoma, cellular leiomyomas often show focal extensions into and appear to merge with the adjacent myometrium. The mitotic count is variable, but usually low. Nuclear atypia is absent. As noted earlier, such microscopic features may also be seen in a minority of leiomyomas removed from postmenopausal patients.

Differential diagnosis

The cellular leiomyoma must be distinguished from leiomyosarcoma and an endometrial stromal neoplasm. The cellular leiomyoma lacks the coagulative tumor cell necrosis, nuclear atypia, and mitotic activity that is characteristic of leiomyosarcoma. The distinction from an endometrial stromal nodule may be more difficult. The microscopic features that favor a diagnosis of cellular leiomyoma rather than endometrial stromal tumor are: a fascicular growth pattern; large caliber, thick-walled vessels; merging or slight interdigitation with the adjacent myometrial fascicles; the presence of cleft-like spaces and the absence of foamy histiocytes, which are often present in endometrial stromal tumors.[131] Further help is given by immunocytochemistry. Most cellular leiomyomas strongly and uniformly express h-caldesmon, desmin, and smooth muscle actin, and some may express CD10, often in a less intense and less uniform fashion than the markers of smooth muscle differentiation. The prototypical endometrial stromal neoplasm (both benign nodules and sarcomas) uniformly expresses CD10, but lacks cytoskeletal proteins found in smooth muscle differentiation.[70,109,124,130] Both cellular leiomyomas and endometrial stromal nodules are benign. The differentiation between them is of little practical importance in a hysterectomy specimen, but can be problematic in endometrial curetting and myomectomy specimens since a low-grade endometrial sarcoma enters in the differential diagnosis.

Cytogenetic features

The cellular variant may be associated with two chromosomal aberrations: deletion of 1p and rearranged 10q22.[25,113] Whether all cellular leiomyomas have these or related chromosomal aberrations remains to be determined.

HEMORRHAGIC CELLULAR LEIOMYOMA

Definition

This variant, also sometimes referred to as 'apoplectic leiomyoma', occurs in pregnancy and during oral contraceptive treatment, and exhibits hemorrhage and cystic change.[117,122] There is some overlap with the changes of GnRH analogue therapy (see above).

Pathology

One or more leiomyomas show areas of hemorrhage with cystic change. Microscopically, the smooth muscle is densely cellular, surrounding stellate zones of hemorrhage. Mitotic activity may be increased (up to 8 mitotic figures per 10 HPFs), but there is no atypia. Vascular changes may also be prominent.

EPITHELIOID LEIOMYOMA

Definition

A smooth muscle tumor composed predominantly of rounded cells rather than the more usual spindle-shaped cells of a common leiomyoma. Three subtypes are usually recognized:

- leiomyoblastoma;
- clear cell leiomyoma; and
- plexiform tumor.

Gross features

On naked-eye inspection of the uterus, this variant is often not appreciably different from the ordinary leiomyoma. The tumors are well circumscribed and may be softer and more yellow than the ordinary non-epithelioid type. Most are found in the company of ordinary leiomyomas in the uterus and, when this is the case, there is typically only one epithelioid leiomyoma among several ordinary ones.

Microscopic features

The cells are usually arranged in a clustered, cord-like or network fashion and contain rounded nuclei with finely stippled chromatin and a single nucleolus. The *leiomyoblastoma* consists of rounded cells with eosinophilic cytoplasm and an usually slight degree of cytoplasmic vacuolation (Figures 18.21 and 18.22). (Some pathologists disdain the term 'leiomyoblastoma' for these tumors because it implies the malignancy consists of primitive cells, analogous to neuroblastoma.[26]) The *clear cell leiomyoma* shows, in addition to the features of epithelioid leiomyoma described above, conspicuous cytoplasmic vacuoles that contain glycogen, lipid or both (Figure 18.23). The third subtype is the *plexiform tumor*, with cells arranged in a more prominent pattern of interwoven islands or cord of rounded cells. The cells are smaller and darker than those of the other epithelioid leiomyomas, and are often separated by septa of extracellular matrix. Sometimes these tumors appear as multiple, microscopic foci, which have been referred to as 'plexiform tumorlets'. The histologic phenotype of plexiform tumors may be more a result of abundant elabora-

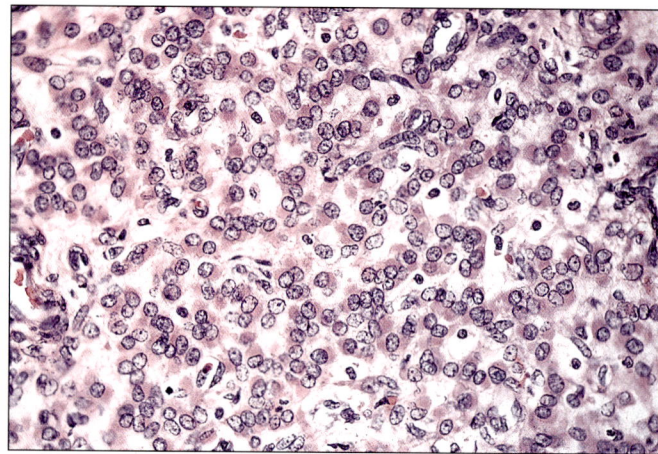

Fig. 18.21 Epithelioid leiomyoma, leiomyoblastoma type. The tumor is composed of uniform, round cells with eosinophilic cytoplasm.

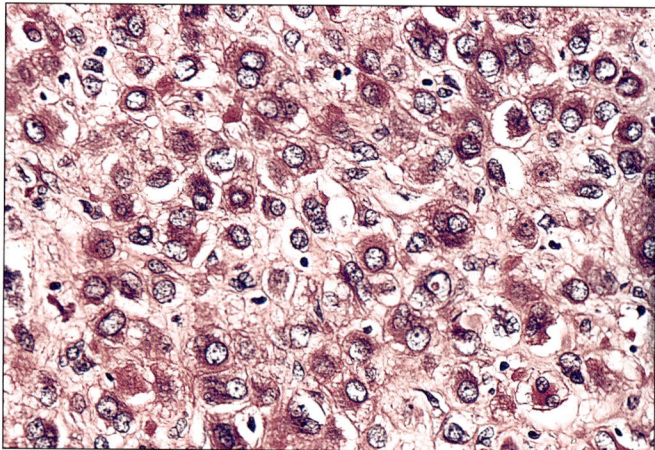

Fig. 18.22 Epithelioid leiomyoma, leiomyoblastoma type.

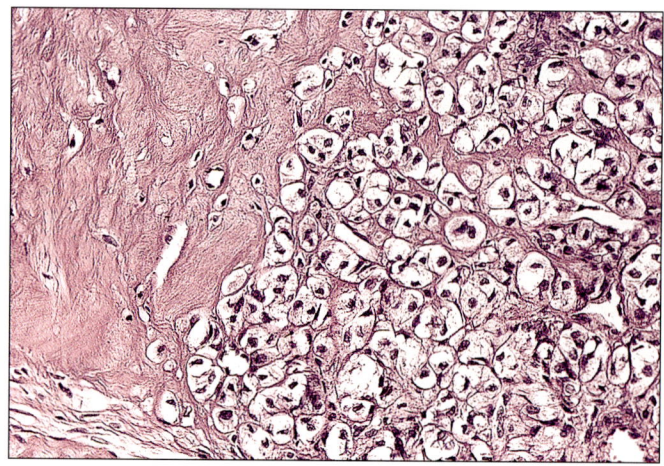

Fig. 18.23 Epithelioid leiomyoma, clear cell leiomyomatous type. Conspicuous cytoplasmic vacuolation is present, in addition to the other features of epithelioid leiomyoma.

tion of extracellular matrix material than of epithelioid differentiation.

The true nature of these variants as smooth muscle tumors is confirmed by all of these types having been seen in continuity with ordinary leiomyomas, a direct transition being recognized in at least half the tumors. Immunohistochemical and electron microscopic studies of leiomyoblastoma and plexiform tumor have confirmed their smooth muscle origin.[13,74] The malignant potential of epithelioid leiomyomas is discussed below.

MYXOID LEIOMYOMA

Definition

A benign smooth muscle tumor with extensive myxoid change.

Microscopic features

Myxoid change occurs in clinically benign smooth muscle tumors, but this phenomenon must be distinguished from myxoid leiomyosarcoma. Myxoid leiomyosarcomas show infiltrative growth, extensive myxoid change, and some degree of nuclear enlargement and pleomorphism (see below). The myxoid stroma in leiomyomas arises from the myxoid degeneration of collagen surrounding nodules of smooth muscle. This connective tissue transformation tends to leave large, thick-walled vessels in its wake (Figure 18.24), a feature not found in myxoid leiomyosarcoma. When the border between a myxoid tumor and adjacent myometrium becomes infiltrated and the cells large and atypical, the odds become high that the lesion in question is malignant.

LEIOMYOMAS WITH HETEROLOGOUS ELEMENTS

The most common heterologous element in a well-circumscribed leiomyoma-like uterine mass consists of endometrial glands and stroma.[173] This is termed an *adenomyoma*, but it is not clear whether the lesion represents focal adenomyosis with reactive smooth muscle proliferation or a truly neoplastic leiomyoma with benign heterologous elements. Adenomyomas grossly may be less well circumscribed than typical leiomyoma and punctate hemorrhagic foci may be recognized by the astute examiner.[173] When this mass protrudes into the uterine cavity it is best referred to as an adenomyomatous polyp, to avoid confusion with the atypical polypoid adenomyoma (see Chapter 17).

Otherwise, typical leiomyomas may rarely contain other more exotic mature heterologous elements. Of these, the most common is the *lipoleiomyoma* (Figures 18.25–18.28).[150,161,193] In this tumor, the lipid is present within adipocytes, which distinguishes it from the very rare fatty degenerate leiomyoma where the lipid resides within the degenerating smooth muscle cells themselves or in histiocytes. The tumor should also be distinguished from the even rarer lipoma and liposarcoma of the uterus, although the latter may not occur as a primary tumor in the uterus.[65] As noted elsewhere, dysregulated *HMGA2* may be found in cutaneous lipoma and uterine leiomyoma and lipoleiomyoma.[73,135]

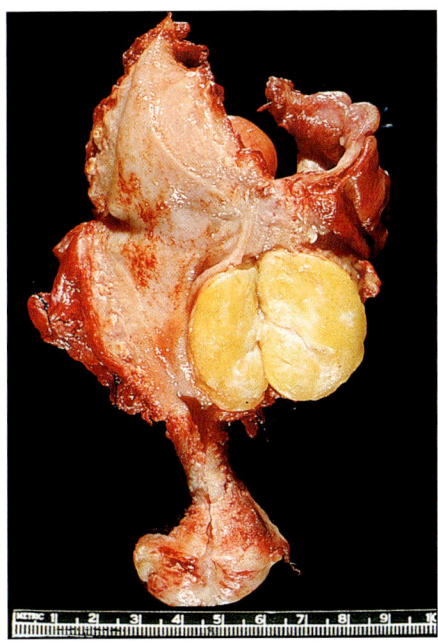

Fig. 18.25 Lipoleiomyoma. Depending on the fat content, these tumors are seen grossly as yellow, well-circumscribed, intramural masses.

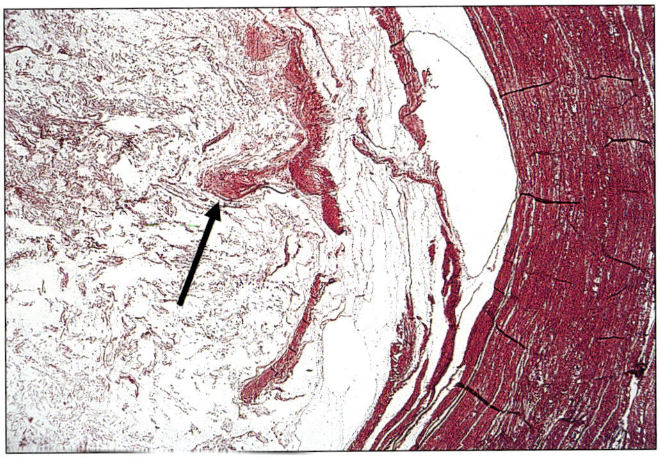

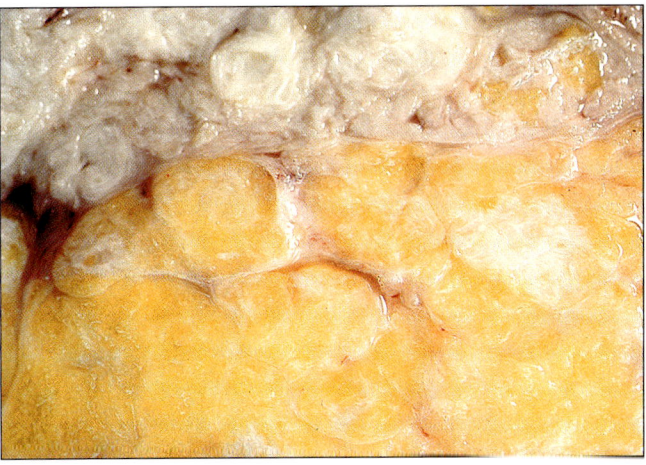

Fig. 18.24 Myxoid leiomyoma. Myxoid degeneration of collagen replaces and separates smooth muscle bundles. A preserved blood vessel (arrow) is present.

Fig. 18.26 Lipoleiomyoma. The mixture of yellow adipose tissue with white smooth muscle is apparent.

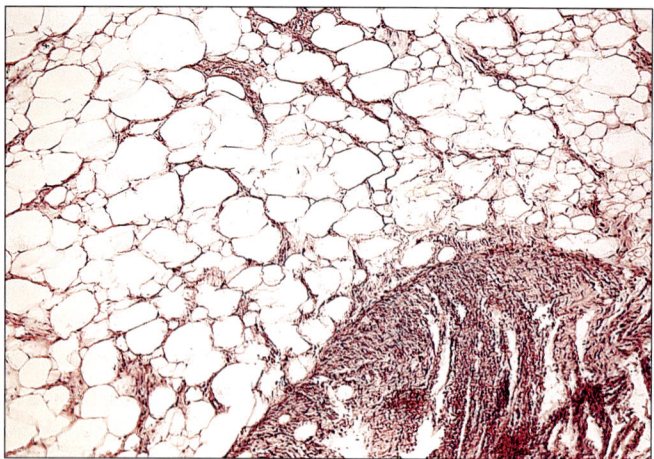

Fig. 18.27 Lipoleiomyoma. Adipocytes are predominant.

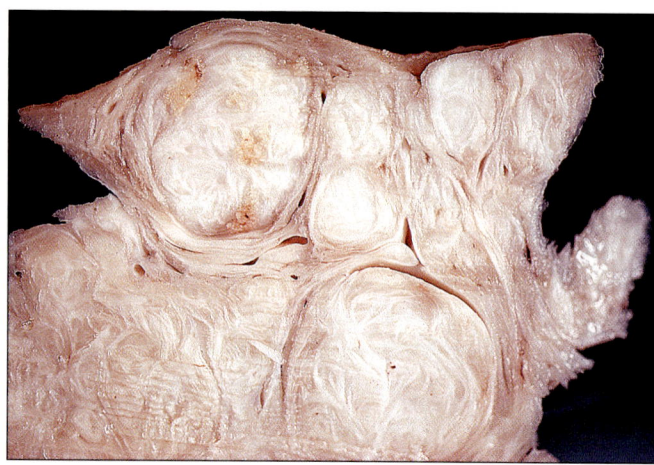

Fig. 18.29 Diffuse leiomyomatosis. The cut surface of this part of a uterine wall shows the normal myometrium virtually replaced by multiple leiomyomas, some of which are very small.

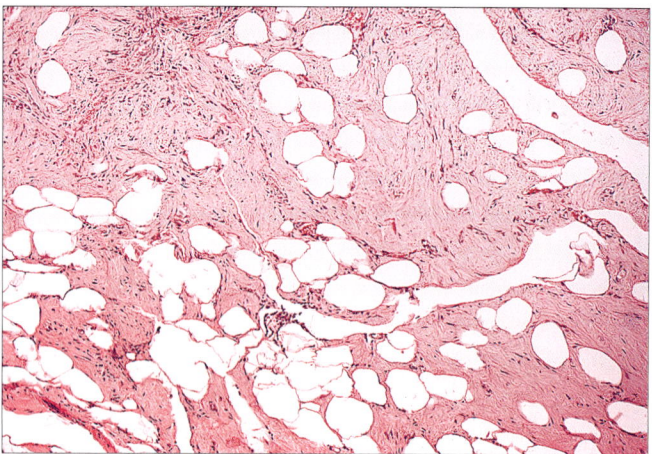

Fig. 18.28 Lipoleiomyoma. There are fewer adipocytes in this example than in Figure 18.27 and they are scattered throughout the smooth muscle.

Examples of *osseous, chondroid*[190] and *skeletal muscle*[106] *metaplasia* have also been reported. A *sex cord-like pattern* has been described in a single case of disseminated peritoneal leiomyomatosis.[103] Sex cord-like differentiation also occurs in uterine leiomyomas; however, when extensive, a variant of endometrial stromal neoplasia should be considered, i.e., the so-called 'uterine tumor resembling ovarian sex-cord tumor' (UTROSCT).[128] A *neurilemmoma-like* phenotype may be appreciated when nuclear palisading is prominent (Figures 18.10 and 18.11).[45]

UNUSUAL GROWTH PATTERNS OF LEIOMYOMAS

Leiomyomas may have a number of special and unusual growth patterns. These are diffuse leiomyomatosis, intravascular leiomyomatosis, benign metastasizing leiomyoma, and disseminated peritoneal leiomyomatosis. Although of considerable biologic interest, their rarity precludes a lengthy discussion.

DIFFUSE LEIOMYOMATOSIS

Definition

A rare condition in which there are tens to hundreds of small ill-defined leiomyomatous nodules in a symmetrically enlarged uterus.[16,26,39,115] Clonality analysis of this unusual growth pattern suggests that each nodule represents a distinct clone, implying a peculiar propensity to tumor initiation in these rare affected individuals.[15] Recently, a case of diffuse uterine leiomyomatosis complicated by uterine rupture and lytic bone metastasis during pregnancy has been reported.[179]

Gross features

The uterus is symmetrically enlarged and may reach considerable dimensions, weighing even 1 kg.[26] The serosal surface is bosselated.[115] The nodules, which range from microscopic to 2–3 cm in diameter, are paler than the surrounding myometrium and often present a whorled or trabeculated appearance that may resemble adenomyosis (Figure 18.29).[115]

Microscopic features

The nodules consist of uniform benign cellular smooth muscle bundles that are less well defined than the usual uterine leiomyomas. They tend to merge with each other and with the surrounding less cellular myometrium. Clustered capillaries may be present in the center of the nodules and are surrounded by hyalinized stroma. Mitotic figures are rare and atypia is lacking. Leiomyomas of the usual type may be present in the same uterus.

INTRAVASCULAR LEIOMYOMATOSIS

Definition

This term describes an uncommon condition in which morphologically benign smooth muscle is present within the lumens of veins. If this invasion is of microscopic proportion only and is confined to the limits of the leiomyoma, then the term 'leiomyoma with vascular invasion' is used and the condition is of no consequence. Intravenous leiomyomatosis involves extension of the intravascular element beyond the confines of the leiomyoma, 80% spreading outside the uterus into the pelvic veins and, occasionally, along the inferior vena cava and into the chambers of the heart.[111,116,167,183,187] Dysregulated *HMGA2* and simple chromosomal aberrations similar to those found in typical uterine leiomyoma have been noted, but the molecular mechanism responsible for this angioinvasive phenotype remains unclear.[34,140]

Gross features

Intravascular leiomyomatosis is usually apparent on gross examination (Figure 18.30). The uterus is enlarged and, when cut across, the intravenous elements may pop up as 'worm-like' coils of firm, rubbery tissue.

Microscopic features

Uterine leiomyomas may or may not be present. When present, continuity may sometimes be demonstrated between the extravascular and intravascular components. Some cases totally lack an extravascular component and the smooth muscle merges with the vessel wall, perhaps indicating a vascular origin.[119,126] The smooth muscle situated within the veins is usually that of an ordinary leiomyoma, although it may have increased vascularity (Figure 18.31) and show more hyaline

change (Figure 18.32). Many variants of leiomyoma have been described in intravenous leiomyomatosis and include cellular, epithelioid, symplastic, myxoid, and lipoleiomyoma.[27,92] The clinical behavior of these variants is the same as that of the usual type.

Intravenous leiomyomatosis differs from leiomyosarcoma by its lack of mitotic activity, atypia, and coagulative necrosis, and from endometrial stromal sarcoma by demonstration of its smooth muscle immunophenotype.

Clinical features and treatment

The patients present with the same symptoms as women with ordinary leiomyomas. The condition is seen most frequently in women over the age of 50 years. Treatment is by total hysterectomy and bilateral salpingo-oophorectomy, along with removal of as much of the extrauterine tumor as possible. Intravascular tumor remaining after hysterectomy may need further surgical treatment. The presence of estrogen receptors in some cases has prompted treatment by GnRH analogues or tamoxifen.[8,59,86,100] The prognosis of intravenous leiomyomatosis is largely determined by the degree of hemodynamic compromise. The only deaths reported have been associated with intracardiac involvement.

BENIGN METASTASIZING LEIOMYOMA

Definition

This is a very rare phenomenon in which histologically benign smooth muscle tumors are present at distant sites, particularly the lungs (Figure 18.33), in women who have histologically benign uterine leiomyomas.[29,133,174,202] The grossly evident, generally solitary tumor mass in benign metastasizing leiomyoma is distinct from the multifocal, bland microscopic smooth muscle proliferations associated with inactivation of the tuberous sclerosis loci in the lungs of women with lymphangioleiomyomatosis.[33,54,68] Cytogenetic analysis of five cases of benign metastasizing leiomyoma revealed deletion of 19q and 22q in all five cases; a subset of cases also showed deletions of 1p or 13q as well as 6p rearrangement.[123]

Careful and critical analysis of the published cases has shown that few can be accepted as genuine examples of 'benign' metastasis. Mitotic counts on the uterine tumors are not

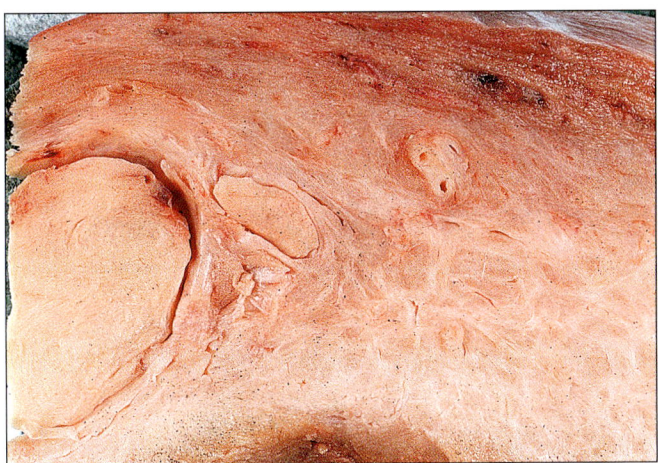

Fig. 18.30 Intravenous leiomyomatosis. Tumor masses are present within distended blood vessels.

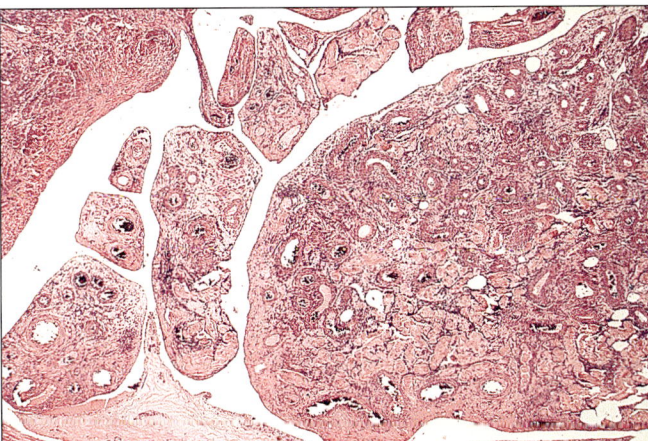

Fig. 18.31 Intravenous leiomyomatosis. Multiple nodules of vascular leiomyoma are present within a grossly distended vessel.

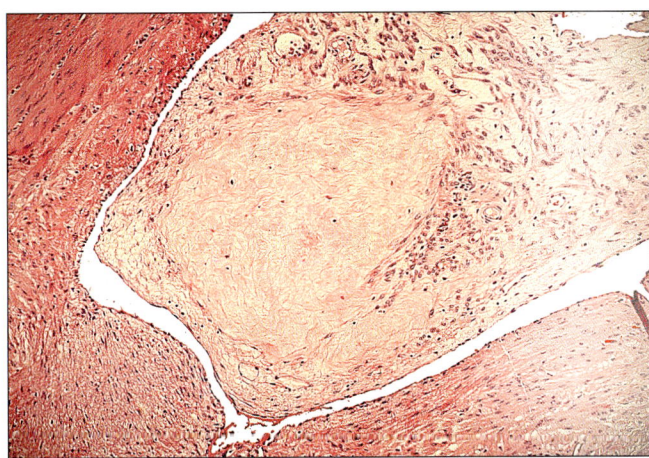

Fig. 18.32 Intravenous leiomyomatosis. This example shows hyaline degeneration of the intravascular element.

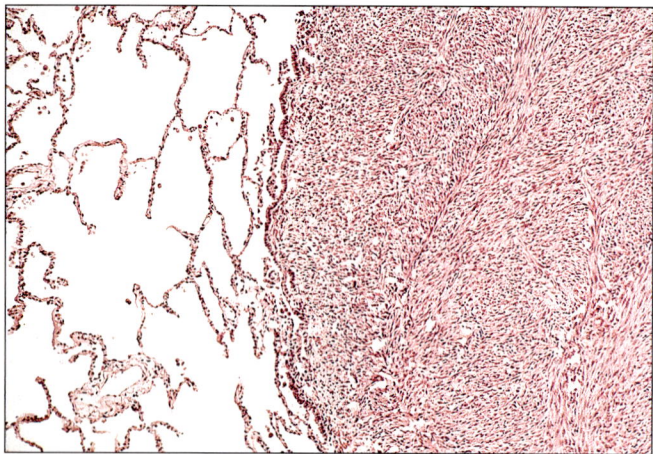

Fig. 18.33 Metastasizing leiomyoma. The section of lung (left) contains a leiomyoma (right).

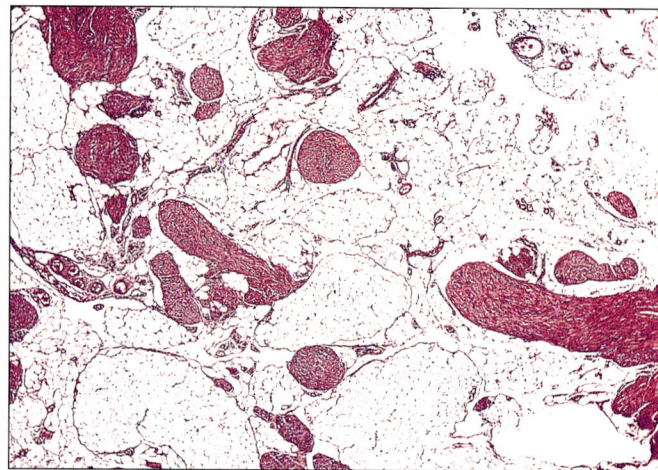

Fig. 18.34 Peritoneal leiomyomatosis. Multiple tiny nodules of smooth muscle are scattered throughout the omentum.

recorded in many reports and, where multiple uterine leiomyomas have been present, not all have been histologically sampled, factors that raise doubts over their benign nature. A high proportion of women with benign metastasizing leiomyomas, however, had a prior dilatation and curettage, myomectomy or hysterectomy, raising the possibility that surgery had predisposed to the subsequent spread. Pulmonary metastasis both before and after resection of intravenous leiomyomatosis has been reported;[9,116] this observation raises the possibility that benign metastasizing leiomyoma originates from unrecognized intravenous leiomyomatosis. It is also possible that some cases in which concomitant leiomyomas of the uterus and smooth muscle tumors in the lungs have been found represent distinct and genuine primary tumors in two sites. Evidence supporting benign metastasizing leiomyoma being a genuine phenomenon is that primary smooth muscle tumors of the lung are exceedingly rare and that estrogen receptors and a response to hormone treatment have been demonstrated in the pulmonary tumor diagnosed as benign metastasizing leiomyoma.[29,44,81] Treatment is by the removal of as much of the 'metastatic' tumor as is feasible, but hormonal treatment using progestins,[114] luteinizing hormone-releasing hormone (LHRH) analogues,[57] and raloxifene[18] has also been tried. Progression is slow.

DISSEMINATED PERITONEAL LEIOMYOMATOSIS
(see Chapter 33)

Definition
This exceedingly rare condition exhibits multiple small, nodular deposits of histologically benign smooth muscle that are found in the superficial subperitoneal tissues (Figures 18.34 and 18.35), including the serosa of the uterus, tubes and ovaries as well as the omentum.[11,60,101,141,178]

Features
The condition affects women of reproductive age and there is a strong association with hormonal stimulation, as many affected women have been pregnant, puerperal or taking oral contraceptives at the time of diagnosis. Similar appearances have been produced experimentally in animals by administra-

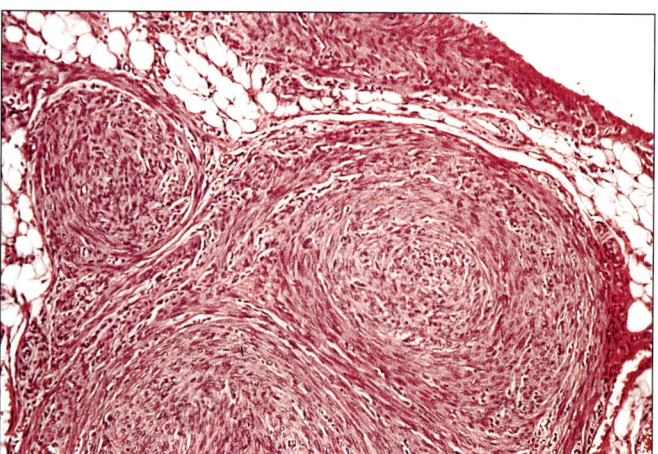

Fig. 18.35 Peritoneal leiomyomatosis. At higher magnification, the whorled nature of the smooth muscle bundles can be appreciated.

tion of estrogen alone or in combination with progestins, raising the possibility of a multicentric origin involving metaplasia of subperitoneal mesenchymal stem cells to smooth muscle, fibroblasts, myofibroblasts, and decidual cells. Specifically, the condition was thought by some to represent fibrosis and smooth muscle metaplasia of ectopic nodules of decidua found in the omentum and peritoneum during pregnancy (Figure 18.36). A study undertaking clonality analysis based on patterns of X chromosome inactivation, however, has shown that the same parental X chromosome was nonrandomly inactivated in all of the peritoneal smooth muscle tumors in each of the four patients analyzed.[141] This finding would not be expected if the condition were metaplastic, but rather is consistent with either metastasis from a single primary tumor or selection for an X-linked allele in clonal multicentric lesions.

When first encountered, the unsuspecting surgeon's or pathologist's impression may be that of ovarian serous carcinomatosis. The tumorous lesions of peritoneal leiomyomatosis may be up to 10 cm, but most tumorlets are less than 1 cm and may even be as small as microscopic collections of smooth muscle cells. Although we have seen cases in which only a small

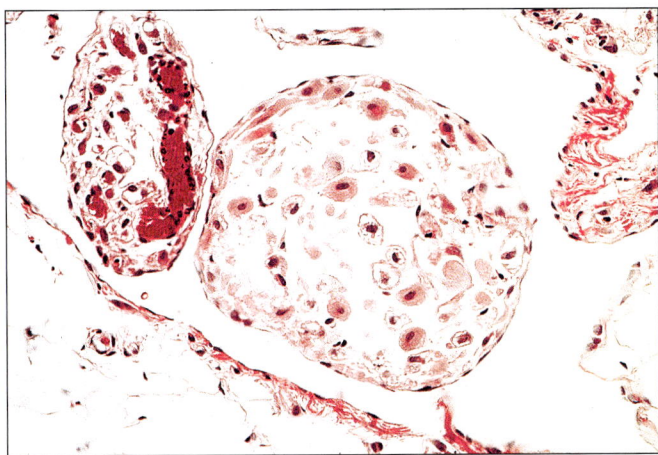

Fig. 18.36 A decidual nodule on the peritoneum of a patient with peritoneal leiomyomatosis.

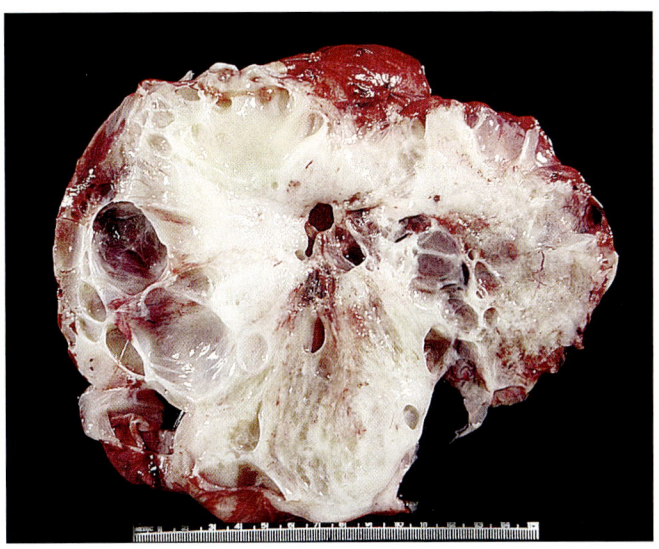

Fig. 18.37 Leiomyosarcoma. Extensive areas of cystic degeneration are present in this example.

number of tumor nodules were found, smooth muscle tumorlets too numerous to count typify this disorder. Unlike carcinomatosis, the lesions of peritoneal leiomyomatosis truly resemble diminutive 'fibroids'. They are well-circumscribed, firm nodules having the same tan to slightly pink, often whorled incised surface as their uterine counterpart. This parallel to utrine 'fibroids' extends to the microscopic level, as each tumorlet consists of histologically bland fascicles of smooth muscle. Foci of endometrial glands and stroma may occasionally be found and such an adenomyomatous appearance poses an interesting question as to their origin.

The condition is an incidental finding and nearly all reported cases have run a benign course. Nevertheless, six cases of malignancy are known to have developed in diffuse peritoneal leiomyomatosis.[1,2,48,145,153] One patient developed bony metastatic lesions and died within 2 years.[153]

LEIOMYOSARCOMA

Definition
A malignant tumor composed entirely of smooth muscle. This tumor is the malignant counterpart of the leiomyoma and is the most common pure sarcoma of the uterus.

Incidence
The incidence of leiomyosarcoma is 0.67/100 000 women years and the proportion of uterine smooth muscle tumors that are malignant ranges from 0.13 to 6%, a 50-fold variation reflecting usage of differing diagnostic criteria. Taking into account that many benign leiomyomas go unrecognized, perhaps two or three women per 1000 with smooth muscle tumors of the uterus have a leiomyosarcoma. The age of women with leiomyosarcoma is about 10 years older than those with leiomyoma, most being over 40 years of age. The tumor is more common in black than in white women, but the difference is less than that estimated for leiomyoma.[21] The incidence in women who are on tamoxifen therapy for breast cancer is increased compared to those who are not.[23,52,110]

Gross features
The gross appearance of leiomyosarcoma commonly, but not always, differs greatly from that of a leiomyoma. Most are diagnosed because the tumor irregularly pervades the adjacent myometrium. Of those presenting as a circumscribed mass, many are not diagnosed by the naked eye because of the overlap in appearance between malignant change and the various forms of degeneration. Leiomyosarcoma has a cut surface that may appear paler, and perhaps more yellow, than a leiomyoma. Areas of hemorrhage and necrosis (Figure 18.37), often irregular in shape and color, are frequently found in leiomyosarcoma. A plethora of more or less meaningless similes describe the texture and color of leiomyosarcoma, such as 'fleshy', 'luxuriant', 'brain-like', 'fish-like', 'putty-like', and 'snowy'. A valuable feature is the loss of the sharp line of demarcation (Figure 18.38), separating the tumor from the normal myometrium, which is so characteristic of a leiomyoma. This change denotes invasion and is not always so apparent in early tumors. Another herald is when the nodule does not bulge above the cut surface. Malignant tumors lack the decompressive force of benign tumors. Most leiomyosarcomas also lack the prominent whorled appearance of the cut surface that is so familiar in leiomyomas.

Consistency is another useful indicator of malignant change in a smooth muscle tumor. Leiomyomas are usually firm and rubbery when an attempt is made to indent the cut surface with a finger or thumb. Leiomyosarcomas, on the other hand, are softer and less resilient, permitting the examining thumb to push into them. These features are not diagnostic individually, but they can be used as a guide for selecting the blocks for histology in a uterus that contains many smooth muscle tumors. Every tumor must be cut across, its cut surface examined by the naked eye, and its consistency assessed. If none shows any special features, there is no need to take more than a few sections altogether, but the presence of the features in Table 18.2 is an indication that more thorough sampling must be undertaken, particularly including the interface with the adjacent myometrium or with areas of hemorrhage and necrosis. We avoid providing a rule of thumb for the number of sections

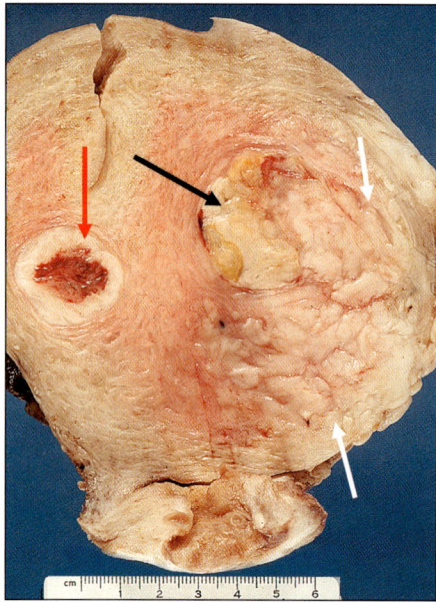

Fig. 18.38 Leiomyosarcoma. This example arises in a leiomyoma (black arrow). The tumor irregularly spreads into the wall of the uterus (white arrows). A typical leiomyoma (red arrow) is present by comparison.

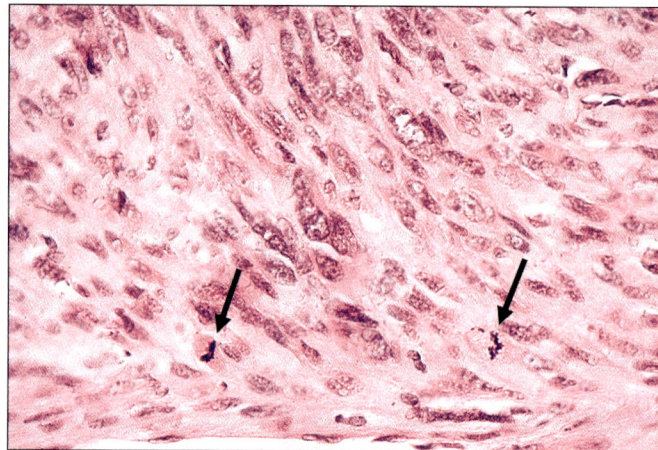

Fig. 18.39 Leiomyosarcoma. Leiomyosarcomas are hypercellullar and this example shows considerable nuclear atypia and abundant mitotic activity (arrows).

Table 18.2 Macroscopic features suspicious for malignancy in a smooth muscle tumor
Loss of whorled pattern
Heterogeneity
Margin not well defined, blurred, merging, irregular
Yellow, tan or gray color
Softer, less rubbery, less resilient
Absence of a bulging surface

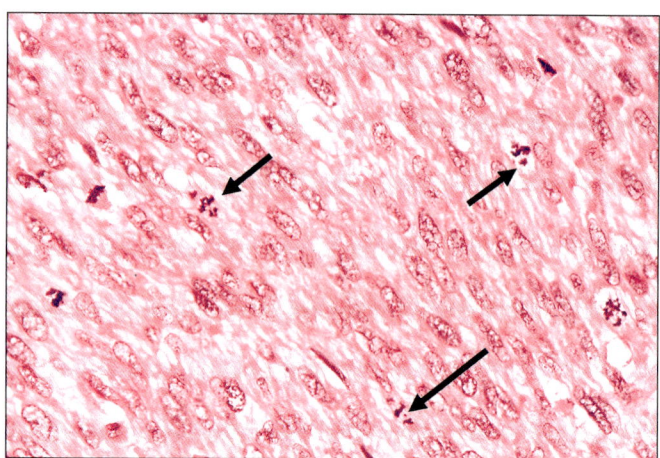

Fig. 18.40 Leiomyosarcoma. Abnormal mitotic figures (arrows) are prominent in this example.

required, such as '1 per cm' as is often stated, as this could foster a less than critical examination of the gross specimen. We have seen not infrequently where a less than critical gross examination leads to an excessive number of uninformative normal sections and sections where malignanttumor is poorly represented and eaily missed. Repeated experience has shown that typical leiomyomas need few if any sections, whereas emphasis is required on those lesions considered suspicious. Leiomyosarcomas are frequently found in uteri that contain leiomyomas, and at times can be seen to arise in one of many leiomyomas. Leiomyosarcomas are more likely to be a solitary, dominant mass than leiomyomas.

Microscopic features

Compared with leiomyomas, leiomyosarcomas are generally more densely cellular and contain frequent mitotic figures (Figures 18.39–18.44). The degree of smooth muscle differentiation is variable, both between tumors and within an individual leiomyosarcoma. Well-differentiated leiomyosarcomas consist of elongated smooth muscle cells with regular nuclei that differ little from those of leiomyoma. At the other end of the spectrum, a poorly differentiated leiomyosarcoma displays rounded and pleomorphic cells that have virtually no resem-

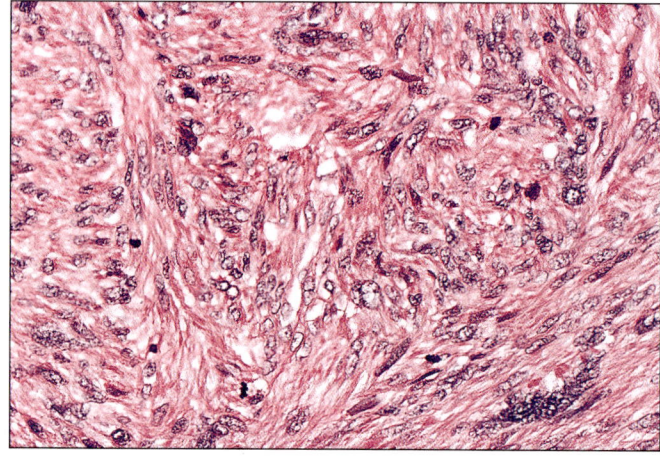

Fig. 18.41 Leiomyosarcoma. Nuclear atypia and mitotic activity.

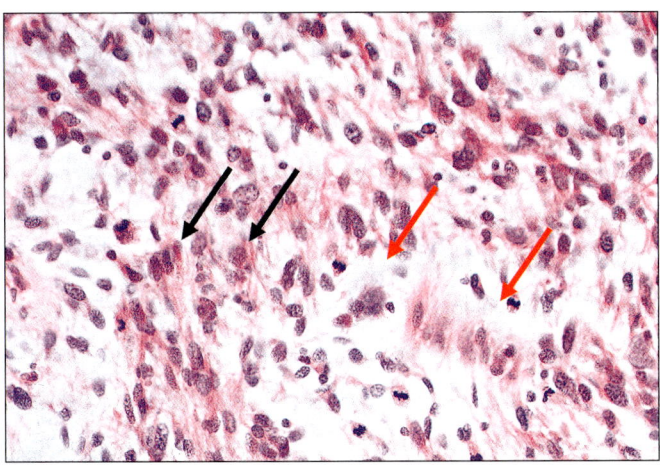

Fig. 18.42 Leiomyosarcoma. This example shows focal myxoid (red arrows) and epithelioid (black arrows) features.

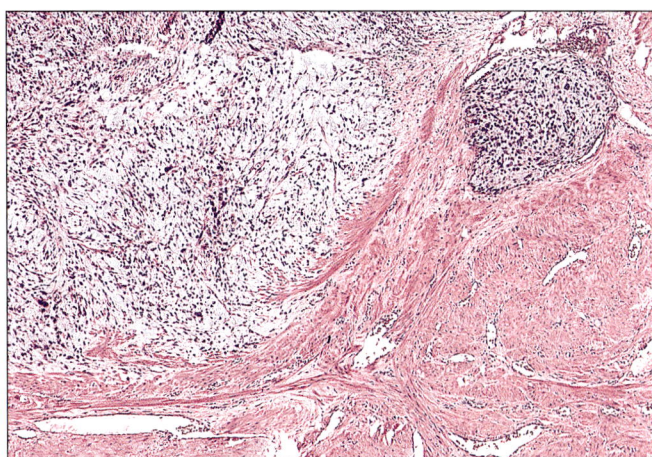

Fig. 18.45 Leiomyosarcoma. The tumor is infiltrating into the surrounding myometrium.

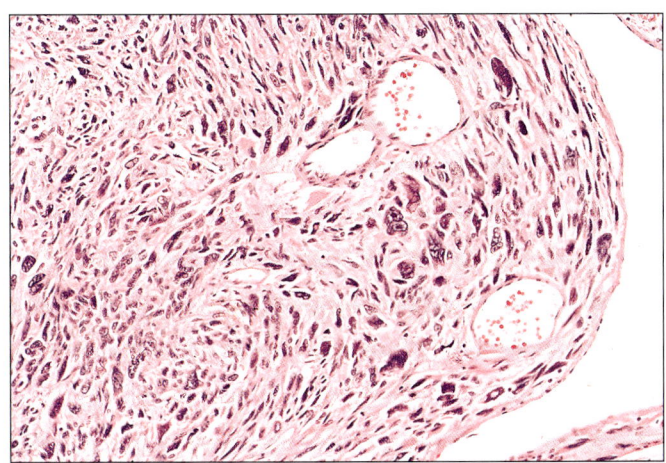

Fig. 18.43 Leiomyosarcoma. Marked nuclear pleomorphism, with some multinucleated cells, is present.

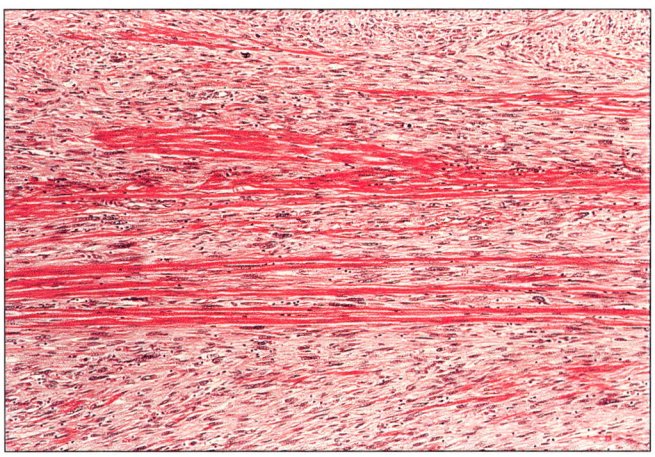

Fig. 18.46 Leiomyosarcoma. Myometrial smooth muscle fibers are separated and destroyed by infiltrating leiomyosarcoma.

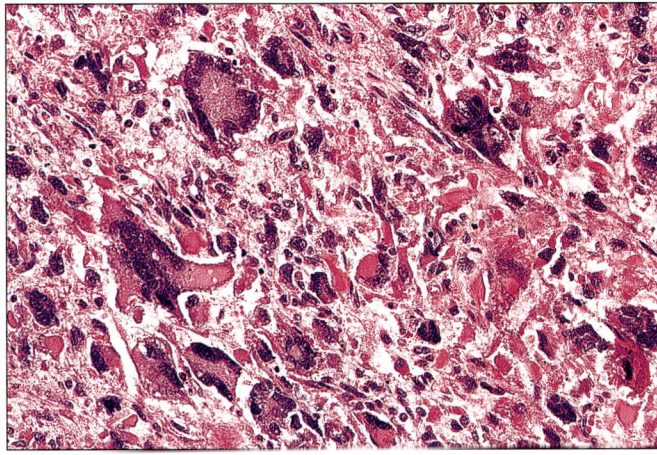

Fig. 18.44 Leiomyosarcoma. Some leiomyosarcomas contain large numbers of giant cells.

blance to normal smooth muscle cells. Nuclear as well as cellular pleomorphism, nuclear hyperchromasia, and giant cells also exemplify increasing anaplasia of the tumor. Areas of coagulative necrosis and hemorrhage, sometimes obvious macroscopically, are also seen microscopically. Commonly, leiomyosarcomas have invaded the adjacent myometrial tissue at the time of diagnosis (Figures 18.45 and 18.46), even to the extent of breaking through the serosal surface of the uterus and involving other pelvic organs. Vascular invasion also may be present.

THE APPROACH TO THE HISTOLOGIC DIAGNOSIS OF LEIOMYOSARCOMA

Much has been written about the histologic criteria for the diagnosis of leiomyosarcoma and its distinction from leiomyoma. Features that play a part in this differential diagnosis include mitotic activity, nuclear atypia, coagulative necrosis, degree of cellularity, degree of differentiation, presence of tumor giant cells, atypical mitotic figures, vascular invasion, and invasion of the surrounding myometrium. The last two are unquestionably diagnostic of malignancy (with the exception of intravenous leiomyomatosis, see above) and associated with a dismal prognosis. These two extremes are easy to diagnose. If a smooth muscle tumor is well circumscribed, composed of cells that are uniform in size and shape, has no intravascular component, cytologic atypia and necrosis are lacking, and the mitotic index is less than 5 mitotic figures per 10 HPFs, then the tumor is a leiomyoma. On the other hand, if the tumor has infiltrative margins, intravascular growth, marked cytologic atypia and coagulative tumor cell necrosis, a mitotic index greater than 10 mitotic figures per 10 HPFs, and abnormal mitotic figures, then the tumor is an overt leiomyosarcoma. It is when a smooth muscle neoplasm has features somewhere between these extremes that difficulty and controversy exists.

What specific criteria enable a histologic diagnosis of leiomyosarcoma to be made and how may the histopathologic findings be used to guide treatment in patients with tumors falling between the readily diagnosed pathologic extremes? One of the landmark papers on leiomyosarcoma emphasized the value of the mitotic count and used 10 mitotic figures per 10 HPFs as the threshold for the diagnosis of sarcoma.[176] Since then, many publications have based the diagnosis almost exclusively on mitotic count, some authors maintaining that any smooth muscle tumor having 10 or more mitotic figures per 10 HPFs is a leiomyosarcoma, regardless of the degree of atypia.[64]

As some patients with tumors containing 5–9 mitotic figures per 10 HPFs succumb, it is clear that the approach to the definitive diagnosis must be based on multiple qualitative and quantitative factors. That some of these tumors behave unpredictably has led some to introduce the concept of the 'smooth muscle tumor of uncertain malignant potential' or 'STUMP',[83] a term that can unwittingly obscure the true diagnosis when misused. This group is largely defined by mitotic activity. The evidence indicates that when account is also taken of invasiveness, nuclear atypia, necrosis, size of tumor, and age of patient, tumors can be allocated to benign or malignant categories with greater certainty and the term 'of uncertain malignancy' can be avoided in most cases (Tables 18.3 and 18.4).[151] This point is illustrated by a study that looked at 15 uterine smooth muscle tumors with the histologic features of typical leiomyomas

Table 18.3 Factors used to assess the malignancy of smooth muscle tumors

Age of patient

Tumor size

Appearance of incised surface

Invasiveness of tumor margins

Vascular invasion

Significant nuclear atypia

Geographic coagulative tumor cell necrosis

Elevated mitotic index

Atypical mitotic figures

Table 18.4 A comparison of features seen in groups of smooth muscle tumors (after Robboy et al[151])

Parameter	Leiomyoma	Atypical smooth muscle tumor[a]		Leiomyosarcoma
		Probably benign	Probably malignant	
Age (average)	30s	30s	50s	50s
Invasiveness	None	Rare	Many	All
Tumor margins	Distinct	Distinct	Variable	Indistinct
Vascular invasion	None	None	33%	33%
Size (average)	<5 cm	6 cm	5–15 cm	>10 cm
Incised surface	Bulging	Bulging	Variable	Soft, irregular
Necrosis	None	33%	All	All
Nuclear atypia	None	Mild	Marked	Marked
Mitoses – atypia absent[b]	<5	5–14	5–14	≥10
Mitoses – atypia present	<5	5–10	5–10	≥10
Abnormal mitoses	None	Rare	Occasional	Frequent
Adjunct from the literature, not to supplant histologic features				
p16[20]	10%	20%	>20%	>50%
Ki-67[112]	Low (<5%)	Intermediate (5–10%)	Intermediate (5–10%)	High (≥15%)

[a]Includes lesions variously described as atypical leiomyomas, smooth muscle tumors of uncertain malignant potential, and smooth muscle tumors of low malignant potential.
[b]Mitotic activity is expressed as the number of readily identifiable mitotic figures per 10 HPFs in the most proliferative areas. The evaluation of mitotic activity differs when nuclear atypia is present or absent. We appreciate that other authors, such as the group at Stanford University, classify tumors with minimal atypia, without necrosis, and with mitotic activity ≥15 mitotic figures per 10 HPFs as being 'mitotically active leiomyoma with limited experience'. Based on our observation of malignant behavior in some tumors with these features, we believe that a threshold for malignancy above 14 mitotic figures per 10 HPFs is too high. Consequently, we would not classify these tumors as benign. In the presence of atypia, we agree that the threshold for diagnosis of malignancy is lower and set our cut-off at 10 mitotic figures per 10 HPFs.

except for the presence of mitotic counts ranging from 5 to 15 per 10 HPFs.[139] By definition, all lacked cytologic atypia. The tumors ranged from 1.3 to 8 cm in diameter and the women were followed up for a mean of 2.5 years. No local recurrences or metastases were detected. The clinically benign nature of these tumors indicates that the term 'leiomyomas with increased mitotic activity' can be more appropriate than 'smooth muscle tumors of uncertain malignant potential'. These tumors, of note, were mostly small in size.

It has become clear over the last three decades that mitotic activity is only one of multiple histologic features that must be evaluated when assessing the potential malignancy of smooth muscle tumors and from time to time slightly different proposals for diagnosis and classification have been put forward. A recent study analyzed 213 problematic smooth muscle neoplasms, excluding epithelioid and myxoid tumors, in women who had follow-up for at least 2 years, most considerably longer.[17] From the many histologic features that were assessed, mitotic index, the degree of cytologic atypia, and the presence or absence of coagulative tumor cell necrosis emerged as the most important predictors of behavior. A diagnostic strategy was devised utilizing these three criteria. Atypia was classified as either absent to mild or moderate to severe, coagulative tumor cell necrosis was scored as either present or absent, and the mitotic index was recorded as the number of mitotic figures per 10 HPFs. These features are shown graphically in Figure 18.47, in which we have simplified the classification slightly and unified the various atypical categories (atypical leiomyoma, atypical leiomyoma with low risk of recurrence, and smooth muscle tumor of low malignant potential) into the single category of 'atypical leiomyoma'.

By employing three variables in the assessment of smooth muscle tumors, this diagnostic strategy moves away from complete dependence on mitotic count. Indeed, mitotic index is the last feature to be taken into account in this scheme and, in many tumors, a mitotic count is not needed for diagnosis. Smooth muscle tumors that show no or mild atypia and no coagulative tumor cell necrosis are leiomyomas, irrespective of mitotic count. On the other hand, tumors that show diffuse moderate or severe atypia and have coagulative tumor cell necrosis are leiomyosarcomas. Figure 18.47 shows that it is only the intermediate tumors that need a mitotic count for the determination of malignancy. In reality, the schema is not quite as foolproof as once believed, as indicated by one of the authors himself as additional experience has been gained. Tumors lacking coagulative necrosis on rare occasion will metastasize.

A slightly different approach to assessing the factors pertinent to malignancy was taken in a study that analyzed 28 leiomyosarcomas that metastasized.[78] This showed that, in addition to mitotic activity greater than 5 per 10 HPFs, significant atypia, and coagulative tumor cell necrosis, the finding of a tumor larger than 3 cm in diameter and, to a lesser extent, patient age over 50 years were factors associated with metastasis and mortality. No tumor under 3 cm metastasized.

DIAGNOSTIC CRITERIA

Mitotic activity

If it is agreed that the mitotic count plays a role in the diagnosis of leiomyosarcoma of the uterus, then it is appropriate to look in more detail at the validity and reproducibility of mitotic

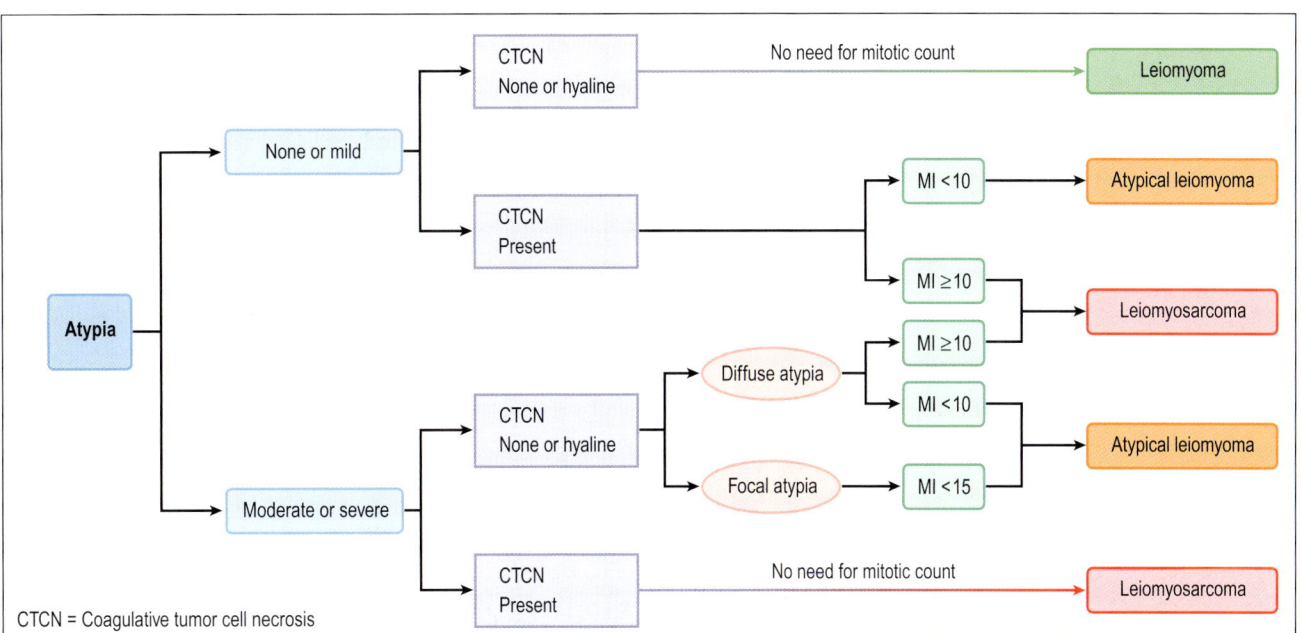

Fig. 18.47 The histologic diagnosis of leiomyosarcoma. The tumor is initially assessed at low power for atypia, a higher power being needed for confirmation and in questionable cases. Necrosis is then sought. If it is present, it is decided whether it is of coagulative type or hyaline. Cases at the two extremes can be categorized without mitotic counts. If there is no atypia and no necrosis or just hyaline necrosis, the tumor is a leiomyoma. If there is diffuse moderate or severe atypia and coagulative tumor cell necrosis is present, the tumor is a leiomyosarcoma. If there is no atypia but coagulative tumor cell necrosis is present, or if atypia is present and coagulative tumor cell necrosis is lacking, a mitotic count is required. The mitotic index determines whether the tumor is a leiomyosarcoma or an atypical leiomyoma. In cases where moderate or severe atypia is seen but there is no coagulative tumor cell necrosis, the distribution of the atypia, whether diffuse or focal, is also taken into account.

counting. In one classic study, this problem was approached by circulating the same stained slides of smooth muscle tumors of the uterus to a number of experienced practicing pathologists, asking them to record the mitotic counts for each tumor and to recommend management.[162] The results were dramatically inconsistent. For example, one slide was given a mitotic count of zero by one pathologist and 22 by another, while the count for another tumor ranged from 2 to 34 mitotic figures per 10 HPFs. The conclusion was that mitotic counting (without rigor or standardization) was not reliable or reproducible, and could not be used as a precise basis for diagnosis, prognosis or treatment.

There are many variables in mitotic counting:

- The number of sections taken from the tumor.
- The thickness of the sections.
- Failure of the pathologist to locate the most proliferative area of the tumor.
- Too few or too many fields counted.
- Mitotic figures unrecognized or mistaken for pyknotic or otherwise degenerating nuclei.
- Pyknotic and degenerating nuclei erroneously interpreted as mitotic figures.
- Different sized high-power fields used by different pathologists.
- The rapidity of fixation.

Some of these points deserve elaboration. If mitotic counting is to be of any value, then the most active part of the tumor must be assessed, as it is this area that will most greatly influence the rapidity of tumor growth. It follows that adequate and appropriate sampling must be based on careful gross examination. Perhaps the most perplexing variable is the interpretation of what should be called a mitotic figure, which is the main reason for the different results in the study quoted above.[162] Many dark, irregular nuclear structures are present in smooth muscle tumors, particularly when there is atypia, and it is important that apoptotic and degenerating nuclei not be misinterpreted as mitotic figures and vice versa. Only definite mitotic figures should be counted, while questionable cells should be ignored. The rapidity of fixation also has an effect on the number of mitotic figures that can be recognized in a section. Dividing cells that have already begun the process of mitosis when the blood circulation ceases will either continue towards completion of the mitosis in an apparently normal manner or become unrecognizable from chromatin clumping. Consequently, the mitotic count potentially may fall during the interval between when the tissue is removed from the body and fixation takes place. Studies have shown reductions in mitotic counts of 13% in soft tissue tumors and 30% in epithelial cells in the colon if fixation is delayed by 2 hours. Thus, a higher count may be found at the incised surface of a tumor than in its center and a tumor that is left for some hours before fixation may give a misleadingly low count. The size of a 'high-power field' will vary depending on the microscope's configuration and all the components in the optical path. All these factors should be specified in publications in which mitotic counts feature significantly.

Recent exposure to progestins can increase mitotic activity of smooth muscle tumors and this information should be sought from clinicians or the medical record in difficult cases. Likewise, low-grade ischemia or proximity to an inflamed or ulcerated mucosa can induce a reactive increase in mitotic count. Pedunculated submucous fibroid polyps not infrequently show focally elevated mitotic activity for this reason and 'ordinary' fibroids sometimes show mitoses near areas of hyaline necrosis.

The following rules apply for mitotic counting:

- There should be prompt, good fixation.
- Well-stained (but not overstained) sections, not more than 4–5 μm thick, must be used.
- An adequate number of sections must be examined.
- Counting must be from the most active area and the highest count must be used.
- At least four sets of 10 HPFs must be counted.
- Only definite mitotic figures should be counted.
- Avoid areas of obvious ischemic change – the periphery or growing edge is a good place to start.

Although not part of the formal criteria, atypical mitotic figures are often found in leiomyosarcomas (Figure 18.40). Examples of atypical mitotic figures include spindle poles in excess of two (i.e., tri- and tetrapolar metaphases), chromosomes lagging far behind the separating groups in later phases of division (as they may be damaged by cycles of chromosomal fusion and subsequent breakage), and extreme polyploidy (which admittedly is a subjective appraisal as accurate enumeration requires other cytogenetic or molecular techniques). Each of these forms of atypia reflects cytogenetic aberrations that characterize malignant smooth muscle tumors and a mechanism to generate genomic instability. Consequently, presence of atypical mitotic figures in a uterine smooth muscle tumor should prompt a thorough histologic evaluation in search of other parameters indicative of malignancy.

Recognizing the vagaries in counting mitoses, interest has grown in developing a more accurate and easily applied surrogate for evaluating proliferative rate in uterine smooth muscle tumors. Such a technique ideally would be insensitive to pyknotic and degenerating nuclei that mimic metaphase chromosomes. Flow cytometry has been used by some investigators,[5,19,93,137] but its general unavailability and lack of a clear advantage over mitotic counting has limited its use. In addition, immunohistochemistry for the Ki-67 and proliferating cell nuclear antigens have been tested.[5,112] Unfortunately, there is no consensus on how to score expression of these proliferation markers. Nevertheless, Ki-67 expression, as determined by MIB1 staining, may be useful on some situations. For example, as it is difficult to count mitoses in smooth muscle tumor fragments found in endometrial curettings, it may be helpful to use MIB1 staining in order to confirm one's histologic impression and prevent gross under- or overcounting.

Finally, it has to be said that, even if all these points are standardized, mitotic counting is a 'tedious, time consuming and thoroughly boring'[121] procedure and a technique that requires intuition, tuition, and practice. Even when unnecessary for diagnostic purposes, careful mitotic counting should be performed as it is the most prognostic of histologic parameters.

Atypia

Although often referred to as cellular (or cytologic) atypia, it is really only the nuclei that are assessed for atypia. Cytoplasm is not evaluated, other than to note that it is reduced in amount in proportion to an increase in the nuclear:cytoplasmic ratio and in the determination of the epithelioid phenotype. Atypia in this context embraces the features of nuclei used to distinguish between benign and malignant tumors generally (Figures 18.39, 18.43, and 18.44). Paramount is nuclear pleomorphism, with a variable increase in nuclear size, irregularities of nuclear membrane, chromatin clumping, and prominent nucleoli also being taken into account. An increase in the number of nuclei, when none of these features is present, does not constitute atypia. Crowded, normal nuclei are seen in a cellular leiomyoma. Significant atypia (moderate or severe) can be identified readily under the low power of the microscope. Mild atypia is subtler, requires evaluation under a higher power, and does not carry the same diagnostic import as do greater degrees of atypia. One difficulty in applying this approach occurs when the nuclear atypia is very uniform from tumor cell to tumor cell. The monomorphic quality of such tumors suggests that there is less intratumoral genetic heterogeneity than typical for leiomyosarcoma. This difficulty in recognizing nuclear atypia can be overcome when one compares the tumor nuclei to nuclei in the adjacent myometrium. This comparison reveals the increases in nuclear size, chromasia, and chromatin distribution in this subset of low-grade leiomyosarcomas.

Necrosis

Several types of necrosis are found in uterine smooth muscle tumors. As recognition of coagulative tumor cell necrosis is important in the diagnosis of leiomyosarcomas, it is essential to distinguish among the various forms of necrosis that occur. Hyaline necrosis is the commonest form encountered in leiomyoma, so the distinction between coagulative tumor cell necrosis and hyaline necrosis is, in practice, most important to make. The main points of distinction (Table 18.5) are that coagulative tumor cell necrosis shows an abrupt transition from viable to necrotic tissue without interposed inflammation, granulation or hyalinized tissue (Figures 18.48 and 18.49). Ghost outlines of cells may be seen within the coagulative necrosis and often there is some preservation of nuclei, enabling hyperchromasia and pleomorphism to be identified. The pre-existing vascular structures are frequently preserved (Figure 18.50), whereas they are usually involved in the process of hyaline necrosis (Figure 18.12). The contour of interface between viable and necrotic tumor is often geometrically complex, evoking comparison to islands on a map. This 'geographic' tumor necrosis is often multifocal and distributed throughout the tumor. In contrast, benign necrosis typically consists of a single, often centrally located region with a simple, rounded border. There has been criticism about using the term 'coagulative tumor cell necrosis' in this context with suggestions of alternatives.[61,66] Now that the term has been introduced and defined for this purpose, there seems little point in changing it again.

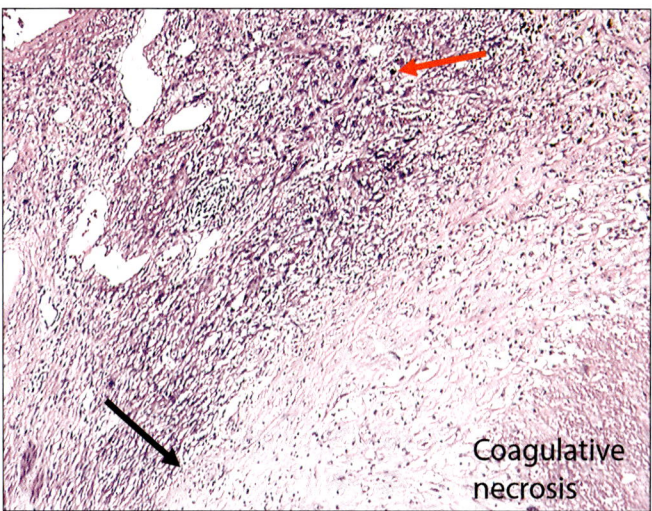

Fig. 18.48 Coagulative tumor cell necrosis. Nuclear atypia (red arrow) is present at the edge of the area of necrosis. Demarcation between the necrotic area and the healthy tissue (black arrow) is sharp. Some tumor cells with partially viable nuclei extend into the coagulum.

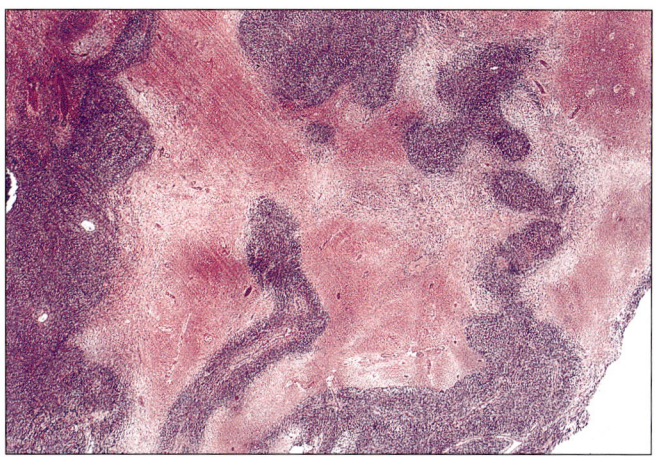

Fig. 18.49 Coagulative necrosis. There are sharp lines of demarcation between the areas of necrosis and the viable areas within the tumor.

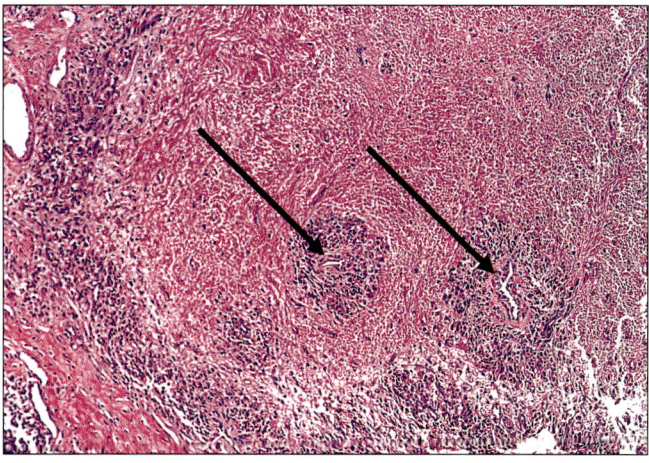

Fig. 18.50 Coagulative necrosis. The blood vessels (arrows) and cuff of surrounding tissue are spared.

Table 18.5 Smooth muscle tumors: distinction between coagulative and hyaline necrosis		
Parameter	Coagulative necrosis	Hyaline necrosis
Margin	Abrupt	Gradual
Vessels	Spared	Involved
Nuclei in necrotic zone	May be atypical	Pale and 'mummified'
Outline	Complex 'geographic'	Simple

Coagulative necrosis is also a feature of leiomyomas treated with GnRH analogues. The distinction between this type of necrosis and the coagulative tumor cell necrosis found in leiomyosarcomas may be difficult. Treatment with GnRH analogues does not result in nuclear atypia elsewhere in the tumor and thick-walled blood vessels may be prominent.[30,37] Focused ultrasound effect, used in the ablation of 'fibroids', may mimic the pattern of necrosis found in leiomyosarcoma. Macroscopic tissue hardening, as well as histologic blandness and hypereosinophilia associated with thermal denaturation, should provide the clues needed to correlate with the clinical history and arrive at the correct diagnosis.

Finally, the histologic features typical of ischemic or hormonally induced degeneration and subsequent host tissue reaction typically found in leiomyomas may also occasionally be seen in leiomyosarcoma. Consequently, the presence of such benign degenerative changes cannot be used to exclude malignancy.

Tumor invasiveness

Tumor invasiveness is useful in predicting subsequent clinical behavior.[136,151] In studies using this criterion, the invasiveness described is usually grossly obvious but, in practice, we have found that this feature can sometimes be difficult to evaluate, especially as small areas of invasion tend to be grossly overlooked. Therefore, it probably receives less weight as a criterion than is due. In many publications, mention of invasion is given only when tumor has spread beyond the confines of the uterus, which signifies that the tumor is already in an advanced stage. Little mention is made of tumors invasive into the myometrium, which represents significant tumor spread. Also, there has been remarkably little discussion about the diagnostic criteria of invasion. The problem exists, as in the endometrium, of what distinguishes an undulating border from true invasiveness. Infiltrating cells of leiomyosarcoma usually do not respect the anatomic boundary defined by myometrial fascicles, whereas the benign smooth muscle cells in leiomyoma do (Figures 18.45 and 18.46). Undulating interdigitations between myometrium and leiomyomatous masses should be regarded as pseudoinvasion. Similarly, it can be questioned whether invasion is present if there is intravascular spread within the tumor. In the majority of cases, a careful gross examination combined with thorough microscopy will determine whether or not invasion into the surrounding myometrium or vascular space has occurred.

Size

Leiomyosarcomas are often greater than 10 cm at presentation and are the largest tumor mass when multiple fibroids are present. For this reason, larger masses, particularly those 10 cm and above, should be targeted for careful gross examination. In addition, tumor size is critical in helping to determine the potential for biologic as opposed to histologic malignancy. Tumors under 5 cm in diameter are rarely associated with aggressive behavior[45,84,136] and probably none under 3 cm metastasizes.[78] This feature is key as it can help resolve the not uncommon challenging problem in management in which a small but grossly typical leiomyoma is found on microscopic examination to have a high mitotic count.[151] On the other hand, rapid tumor growth, especially during and after menopause or during leuprolide therapy, may be the first indication of malignancy in a uterine smooth muscle tumor.

Age

Malignant uterine smooth muscle tumors typically occur a decade or more later than their benign counterpart. Consequently, large dominant fibroids in perimenopausal and postmenopausal women are of much greater concern than in younger women. Age may also affect potential malignancy. Metastases may be less common in young women and most clinically malignant sarcomas of the uterus in women younger than 35 years of age have an obviously malignant microscopic appearance.[136,151]

CONCLUSIONS

The recently proposed scheme described above[17] represents a significant advance in the diagnosis of smooth muscle tumors. The authors have refined and redefined diagnostic criteria that have been in use for some years and have made an attempt to correlate these findings with the clinical outcome. The number of patients in some diagnostic groups is small and the follow-up period for many of the patients is short, so that the validity of the predictions in categories is not as certain.

Useful though this diagnostic strategy is as a means of assessing smooth muscle tumors, we feel that a broader view should be taken and that features additional to atypia, necrosis, and mitotic index must always be considered when categorizing a tumor, recommending treatment, and predicting prognosis. Other features that need to be taken into account include: age of the patient, the size of the tumor and its gross appearance, tumor's margin, and vascular invasion (Table 18.3). Table 18.4 incorporates all of these features in a strategy that separates the clearly benign from the clearly malignant tumors and gives guidance for the intermediate groups.[151] Lastly, the diagnosis of 'smooth muscle tumor of uncertain malignant potential' or 'STUMP' should be used most sparingly.

VARIANTS OF LEIOMYOSARCOMA

EPITHELIOID LEIOMYOSARCOMA

Definition

A very rare malignant smooth muscle tumor that is composed predominantly of rounded cells rather than the more usual spindle-shaped cells.

Microscopic features

It has long been believed that the presence of atypia and mitotic activity is more sinister if the tumor has an epithelioid cell morphology than in the usual type of smooth muscle tumor. For this reason, criteria for the diagnosis of leiomyosarcomas include a lower mitotic count for epithelioid tumors than for tumors of usual spindle cell type.[83] As epithelioid smooth muscle tumors are uncommon, it has been difficult to amass a series of cases sufficient to be useful. In one larger series (80 cases) features indicative of malignancy were the presence of necrosis, vascular invasion, significant nuclear pleomorphism, and a mitotic count of greater than 3 mitotic figures per 10 HPFs.[129] If none of these four features was present, the tumor behaved in a malignant fashion in under 10% of cases; however, if one, two or three features were identified, malignant behavior was observed in 42%, 56%, and 88% of patients, respectively. It is disquieting that nearly 1 in 10 epithelioid tumors that showed no necrosis, no vascular invasion, no significant nuclear pleomorphism, and mitotic counts of less than 3 per 10 HPFs still behaved in a malignant fashion. Another smaller retrospective study confirmed the importance of these features in predicting malignant behavior[138] but clearly further work on these rare tumors is still needed.

MYXOID LEIOMYOSARCOMA

Definition
A very rare smooth muscle tumor with extensive gross and microscopic myxoid stroma that, despite a low mitotic count, often demonstrates clinically malignant biologic behavior.

Gross features
Myxoid leiomyosarcomas are usually large and if confined to the uterus have a gelatinous cut surface with apparently well-circumscribed borders.[85,155]

Microscopic features
The tumors show a copious myxomatous stroma with sparse tumor cells (Figures 18.51–18.53). Identification of these as smooth muscle cells may be difficult in some areas but both light and electron microscopic examination usually shows the characteristic features of smooth muscle cells in other areas. Most of the few cases reported have had sparse mitotic figures. Of the first six tumors reported,[85] all had mitotic indices from 0 to 2 per 10 HPFs but, in subsequent cases, about 20% contained 5 or more mitoses per 10 HPFs.[134] A single example had as many as 30 abnormal mitotic figures per 10 HPFs.[90] We have seen cases that lacked mitoses, but had already spread widely into the adnexa and tissue about the uterus. The typically low mitotic count in these tumors is largely due to the separation of cells by the abundant stroma, so that there are few nuclei in each high-power field. Infiltrating margins may be apparent and vascular space involvement is frequently observed. Most cases in the literature have been defined retrospectively, after the observation of malignant biologic behavior, although some of the later cases showed some pathologic features of malignancy.

MOLECULAR BIOLOGY OF LEIOMYOSARCOMA

Clearly, difficulty may be encountered in predicting the behavior of uterine smooth muscle tumors using conventional histopathologic techniques. There is hope that the rapidly developing field of molecular biology may provide additional and perhaps more reliable criteria to help in the management of women with these enigmatic tumors.

Gene expression
Overexpression of the tumor suppressor gene *p53* is associated with malignancy and a poor prognosis in a wide variety of tumors. Several studies have looked at *p53* overexpression and mutation in uterine smooth muscle tumors.[5,35,58,118] Overexpression and mutation of *p53* is present in a significant minority of leiomyosarcomas (25–47%) but not in leiomyomas. Intermediate figures are found in atypical leiomyomas and smooth muscle tumors often referred to as 'of uncertain malignant potential'. Furthermore, there is evidence that strong overexpression of *p53* is linked to high-grade morphology[118] and a poorer prognosis.[5] It has been suggested that, because most of the mutations in *p53* are transitions, the tumors are likely to arise as a result of spontaneous errors in DNA synthesis and repair.[99]

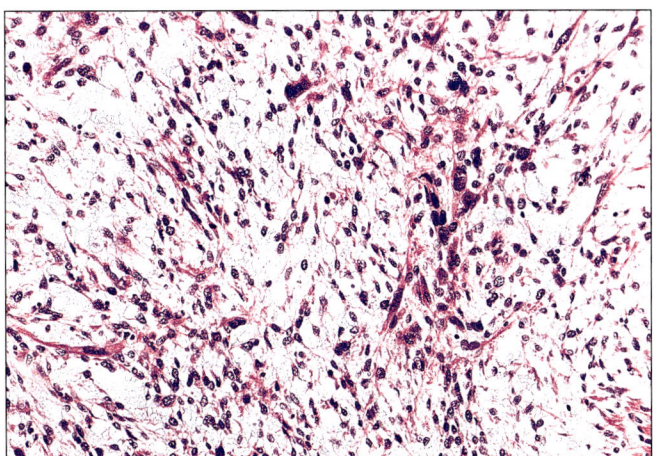

Fig. 18.52 Myxoid leiomyosarcoma. The cells are widely separated by myxoid material. Nuclear atypia is present.

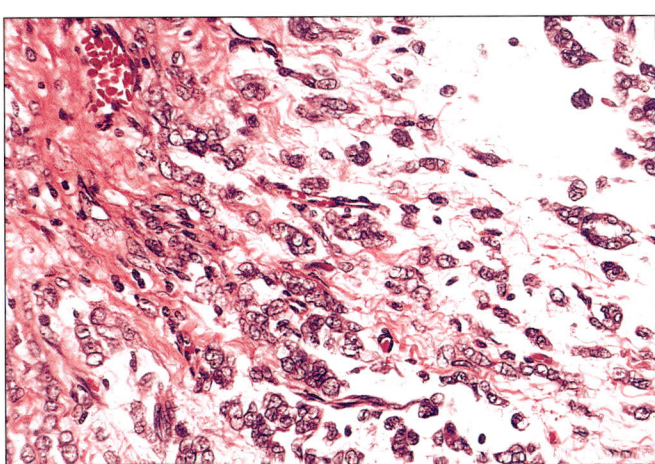

Fig. 18.51 Myxoid leiomyosarcoma. This example also has features of an epithelioid smooth muscle tumor. Mitotic figures are sparse.

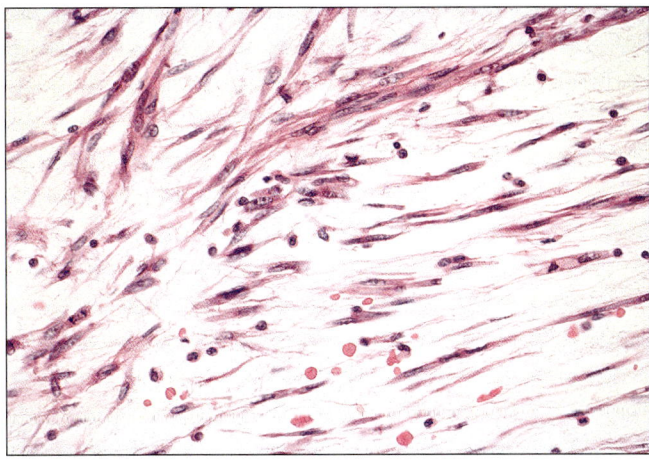

Fig. 18.53 Myxoid leiomyosarcoma.

Overexpression of the c-myc proto-oncogene occurs in about 50% of both leiomyomas and leiomyosarcomas,[77] but the pattern of staining differs, being in a perinuclear location in leiomyomas and diffuse in sarcomas. Overexpression does not correlate with survival. K-ras is overexpressed in a small minority of leiomyomas but not at all in leiomyosarcomas.[58] The MDM2 gene, in contrast, is overexpressed in some leiomyosarcomas but not in leiomyomas.[58] The lack of gamma-smooth muscle isoactin gene, in a pilot study, correlated 100% with a histologic diagnosis of leiomyosarcoma.[185] Abnormalities of the retinoblastoma–cyclin D pathway have been found in about 90% of leiomyosarcomas,[36] which is not surprising when one considers that the retinoblastinoma gene is among the genes on 13q that is deleted in about three-fourths of leiomyosarcomas.[72] These different patterns of molecular alterations in leiomyomas and leiomyosarcomas may lead to the conclusion that they are different entities.[58]

Recently, p16, also known as INK4 or cyclin-dependent kinase inhibitor 2A (CDKN2A), was shown to possibly play an important role in malignant smooth muscle tumor pathobiology.[20,80] P16 protein binds the CDK4–cyclin D complex and acts as a negative cell cycle regulator. Consequently, p16 deletion results in a loss of tumor suppression phenotype. Although p16 likely contributes to sarcomagenesis, its usefulness as a clinical tool to distinguish between benign and malignant smooth muscle tumors remains to be proven.

Proliferation markers

Proliferating cell nuclear antigen (PCNA) is a protein involved with copying DNA and therefore in cell division. It can be demonstrated immunohistochemically on fixed histologic material using the antibody PC10. The Ki-67 antigen provides a means of identifying proliferating normal and neoplastic cells in histologic sections, using the MIB1 antibody. Together these may provide a more reliable indication of cell division and proliferation than the crude mitotic index. The results of recent studies have shown statistically significant higher mean levels of PCNA and Ki-67 in uterine leiomyosarcomas compared with leiomyomas,[5,24] although it is uncertain how much additional useful information either provides beyond that given by conventional morphologic examination.[76] In one study, the percentage of MIB1-positive tumor cells helped predict prognosis and extent of tumor spread.[24] The power of MIB1-positivity as a predictor seems enhanced when linked to alpha-smooth muscle actin expression, which is lacking in leiomyosarcoma.[5]

Flow cytometry, cytogenetics, and molecular genetics

Analysis of leiomyosarcomas by flow cytometry has produced mixed results. Studies show that between about 55 and 70% of the tumors are aneuploid.[5,76] While most studies report that neither ploidy nor S-phase fraction offers additional value to clinical and histologic factors already described,[96,120] one concluded that DNA ploidy helped identify cases that might have an adverse prognosis.[76]

Cytogenetic analyses show that leiomyosarcomas have both complex numerical and structural chromosomal aberrations.[47,156,157] The large variability in aberrations found among the metaphases from the same leiomyosarcoma also suggest, in contrast to benign leiomyoma, that genomic instability is a hallmark of malignancy in uterine smooth muscle tumors.[47]

Loss of heterozygosity (LOH) analysis and comparative genomic hybridization (CGH), two different means to assess allelic imbalance, also detect complex genomic aberrations. In particular, frequent losses of 10q and 13q as well as occasional gain of 17p and losses of 2p and 16q have been observed.[72,142] Recently, scoring LOH at seven tumor suppressor loci (p16, p21, p53, VHL, XRCC23, RB1, and NM-23) was shown in a small cohort to segregate benign and malignant uterine smooth muscle tumors.[43]

At least some leiomyosarcomas have X inactivation that differs from their accompanying leiomyomas, suggesting that the benign and malignant tumors arose from independent transformations and that leiomyosarcomagenesis occurs de novo.[205] Whether malignant transformation of certain leiomyomas (e.g., atypical leiomyoma) occurs, it remains to be proven fully.

Treatment and prognosis

Treatment of leiomyosarcoma is by hysterectomy, with or without removal of the ovaries. Radiotherapy has little place, although some patients experience increased disease-free survival, especially if factors indicating a poor prognosis are present.[50,71,127] Chemotherapy has not been fully evaluated for recurrent and advanced disease. The 5-year survival is on the order of 20–30%. Recurrences develop locally in the pelvis and abdomen and the majority of fatal cases show metastasis to the chest.

Tumor stage is the strongest prognostic variable[78] but other factors that indicate poor prognosis are infiltrating margins, obvious malignancy on naked-eye inspection, blood vessel invasion, marked anaplasia, and a high mitotic rate.[49,50] Premenopausal women experience a longer disease-free survival than those past the menopause.[50] Pushing margins and apparent containment of the tumor within a leiomyoma are potentially good prognostic signs. Of the histologic parameters, mitotic count is the most predictive and should be reported in every new case.[49]

PRACTICAL CONSIDERATIONS

The final comment on the difficult subject of smooth muscle tumors should be practical. The pathologist has to examine specimens either from myomectomy or from a hysterectomy and decide on the diagnosis of the tumor, so that appropriate treatment can be instituted. Most tumors fall at the two extremes of the spectrum and are either clearly benign or malignant. It is only occasionally that a smooth muscle tumor falls into the difficult intermediate category. In a myomectomy specimen, the diagnosis of sarcoma demands treatment by hysterectomy, although there have been cases reported of leiomyosarcomas of the good prognosis group diagnosed where there was no further treatment and the patient remained disease free. Difficulty arises if an atypical leiomyoma or a smooth muscle tumor of low malignant potential is encountered, particularly if a myomectomy was done rather than a hysterectomy because of desire to preserve fertility or based on strong patient preference. In these circumstances, subsequent hysterectomy is usually preferred unless the issue of childbearing is critical and the patient understands the potential subsequent risks and the need for careful follow-up.

If the specimen is from a hysterectomy and the tumor is non-infiltrative, no further action is usually indicated, even if a diagnosis of leiomyosarcoma is reached. The exception may be in an older woman or one who has an anaplastic tumor with evidence of vascular invasion. These are features associated with a poor prognosis and, although further treatment in the form of chemotherapy or radiotherapy may be felt desirable, the outcome is unlikely to be altered.[151] Further sections and lengthy deliberations over a 'suspicious' smooth muscle tumor in a hysterectomy specimen will generally have little bearing on the subsequent management of the patient. If the tumor is a leiomyosarcoma, a smooth muscle tumor of low malignant potential or an atypical leiomyoma, then the patient should have more careful follow-up than if it is a leiomyoma, so that possible recurrences can be recognized and dealt with rapidly.

REFERENCES

1. Abulafia O, Angel C, Sherer DM, Fultz PJ, Bonfiglio TA, DuBeshter B. Computed tomography of leiomyomatosis peritonealis disseminata with malignant transformation. Am J Obstet Gynecol 1993;169:52–4.
2. Akkersdijk GJ, Flu PK, Giard RW, van Lent M, Wallenburg HC. Malignant leiomyomatosis peritonealis disseminata. Am J Obstet Gynecol 1990;163:591–3.
3. Al-Hendy A, Salama SA. Catechol-O-methyltransferase polymorphism is associated with increased uterine leiomyoma risk in different ethnic groups. J Soc Gynecol Invest 2006;13:136–44.
4. Al-Hendy A, Salama SA. Ethnic distribution of estrogen receptor-alpha polymorphism is associated with a higher prevalence of uterine leiomyomas in black Americans. Fertil Steril 2006;86:686–93.
5. Amada S, Nakano H, Tsuneyoshi M. Leiomyosarcoma versus bizarre and cellular leiomyomas of the uterus: a comparative study based on the MIB-1 and proliferating cell nuclear antigen indices, p53 expression, DNA flow cytometry, and muscle specific actins. Int J Gynecol Pathol 1995;14:134–42.
6. Andersen J, Barbieri RL. Abnormal gene expression in uterine leiomyomas. J Soc Gynecol Invest 1995;2:663–72.
7. Andersen J, DyReyes VM, Barbieri RL, Coachman DM, Miksicek RJ. Leiomyoma primary cultures have elevated transcriptional response to estrogen compared with autologous myometrial cultures. J Soc Gynecol Invest 1995;2:542–51.
8. Andrade LA, Torresan RZ, Sales JF, Jr, Vicentini R, De Souza GA. Intravenous leiomyomatosis of the uterus. A report of three cases. Pathol Oncol Res 1998;4:44–7.
9. Arif S, Ganesan R, Spooner D. Intravascular leiomyomatosis and benign metastasizing leiomyoma: an unusual case. Int J Gynecol Cancer 2006;16:1448–50.
10. Arslan AA, Gold LI, Mittal K, et al. Gene expression studies provide clues to the pathogenesis of uterine leiomyoma: new evidence and a systematic review. Hum Reprod 2005;20:852–63.
11. Aruh L, Taskin O, Demir N. Recurrent leiomyomatosis peritonealis disseminata. Int J Gynaecol Obstet 1993;43:330–1.
12. Attilakos G, Fox R. Regression of tamoxifen-stimulated massive uterine fibroid after conversion to anastrozole. J Obstet Gynaecol 2005;25:609–10.
13. Balaton AJ, Vuong PN, Vaury P, Baviera EE. Plexiform tumorlet of the uterus: immunohistological evidence for a smooth muscle origin. Histopathology 1986;10:749–54.
14. Bardsley V, Cooper P, Peat DS. Massive lymphocytic infiltration of uterine leiomyomas associated with GnRH agonist treatment. Histopathology 1998;33:80–2.
15. Baschinsky DY, Isa A, Niemann TH, Prior TW, Lucas JG, Frankel WL. Diffuse leiomyomatosis of the uterus: a case report with clonality analysis. Hum Pathol 2000;31:1429–32.
16. Beattie GJ, Williams AR, Duncan A, Smart GE. Diffuse leiomyomatosis of the uterus with local pelvic spread. Acta Obstet Gynecol Scand 1993;72:492–4.
17. Bell SW, Kempson RL, Hendrickson MR. Problematic uterine smooth muscle neoplasms. A clinicopathologic study of 213 cases. Am J Surg Pathol 1994;18:535–58.
18. Benetti-Pinto CL, Soares PM, Petta CA, De Angelo-Andrade LA. Pulmonary benign metastasizing leiomyoma: a report of 2 cases with different outcomes. J Reprod Med 2006;51:715–718.
19. Blom R, Guerrieri C, Stal O, Malmstrom H, Simonsen E. Leiomyosarcoma of the uterus: a clinicopathologic, DNA flow cytometric, p53, and mdm-2 analysis of 49 cases. Gynecol Oncol 1998;68:54–61.
20. Bodner-Adler B, Bodner K, Czerwenka K, Kimberger O, Leodolter S, Mayerhofer K. Expression of p16 protein in patients with uterine smooth muscle tumors: an immunohistochemical analysis. Gynecol Oncol 2005;96:62–6.
21. Brooks SE, Zhan M, Cote T, Baquet CR. Surveillance, epidemiology, and end results analysis of 2677 cases of uterine sarcoma 1989–1999. Gynecol Oncol 2004;93:204–8.
22. Buttram VC, Jr. Uterine leiomyomata – aetiology, symptomatology and management. Prog Clin Biol Res 1986;225:275–96.
23. Chew SB, Carmalt H, Gillett D. Leiomyosarcoma of the uterus in a woman on adjuvant tamoxifen therapy. Breast 1996;5:429–31.
24. Chou CY, Huang SC, Tsai YC, Hsu KF, Huang KE. Uterine leiomyosarcoma has deregulated cell proliferation, but not increased microvessel density compared with uterine leiomyoma. Gynecol Oncol 1997;65:225–31.
25. Christacos NC, Quade BJ, Dal CP, Morton CC. Uterine leiomyomata with deletions of 1p represent a distinct cytogenetic subgroup associated with unusual histologic features. Genes Chromosomes Cancer 2006;45:304–12.
26. Clement PB. Pure mesenchymal tumors. In: Clement PB, Young RH, eds. Tumors and tumorlike lesions of the uterine corpus and cervix. New York: Churchill Livingstone; 1993:265–328.
27. Clement PB, Young RH, Scully RE. Intravenous leiomyomatosis of the uterus. A clinicopathological analysis of 16 cases with unusual histologic features. Am J Surg Pathol 1988;12:932–45.
28. Clement PB, Young RH, Scully RE. Diffuse, perinodular, and other patterns of hydropic degeneration within and adjacent to uterine leiomyomas. Problems in differential diagnosis. Am J Surg Pathol 1992;16:26–32.
29. Cohen JD, Robins HI. Response of 'benign' metastasizing leiomyoma to progestin withdrawal. Case report. Eur J Gynaecol Oncol 1993;14:44–5.
30. Colgan TJ, Pendergast S, LeBlanc M. The histopathology of uterine leiomyomas following treatment with gonadotropin-releasing hormone analogues. Hum Pathol 1993;24:1073–7.
31. Colgan TJ, Pron G, Mocarski EJ, Bennett JD, Asch MR, Common A. Pathologic features of uteri and leiomyomas following uterine artery embolization for leiomyomas. Am J Surg Pathol 2003;27:167–77.
32. Cramer SF, Patel A. The frequency of uterine leiomyomas. Am J Clin Pathol 1990;94:435–8.
33. Crooks DM, Pacheco-Rodriguez G, DeCastro RM, et al. Molecular and genetic analysis of disseminated neoplastic cells in lymphangioleiomyomatosis. Proc Natl Acad Sci U S A 2004;101:17462–7.
34. Dal Cin P, Quade BJ, Neskey DM, Kleinman MS, Weremowicz S, Morton CC. Intravenous leiomyomatosis is characterized by a der(14)t(12;14)(q15;q24). Genes Chromosomes Cancer 2003;36:205–6.
35. de Vos S, Wilczynski SP, Fleischhacker M, Koeffler P. P53 alterations in uterine leiomyosarcomas versus leiomyomas. Gynecol Oncol 1994;54:205–8.
36. Dei Tos AP, Maestro R, Doglioni C, et al. Tumor suppressor genes and related molecules in leiomyosarcoma. Am J Pathol 1996;148:1037–45.
37. Demopoulos RI, Jones KY, Mittal KR, Vamvakas EC. Histology of leiomyomata in patients treated with leuprolide acetate. Int J Gynecol Pathol 1997;16:131–7.
38. Dgani R, Piura B, Ben Baruch G, et al. Clinical–pathological study of uterine leiomyomas with high mitotic activity. Acta Obstet Gynecol Scand 1998;77:74–7.
39. Domnitz SW, Roth JA, Corwin LJ. Diffuse leiomyomatosis of the uterus in pregnancy. A case report. J Reprod Med 1994;39:61–6.
40. Downes KA, Hart WR. Bizarre leiomyomas of the uterus: a comprehensive pathologic study of 24 cases with long-term follow-up. Am J Surg Pathol 1997;21:1261–1270.
41. Downes KA, Hart WR. Uterine bizarre ('symplastic') leiomyomas: morphology and behavior. Lab Invest 1997;76:99A.
42. Edwards RD, Moss JG, Lumsden MA, et al. Uterine-artery embolization versus surgery for symptomatic uterine fibroids. N Engl J Med 2007;356:360–70.
43. Esposito NN, Hunt JL, Bakker A, Jones MW. Analysis of allelic loss as an adjuvant tool in evaluation of malignancy in uterine smooth muscle tumors. Am J Surg Pathol 2006;30:97–103.
44. Esteban JM, Allen WM, Schaerf RH. Benign metastasizing leiomyoma of the uterus: histologic and immunohistochemical characterization of primary and metastatic lesions. Arch Pathol Lab Med 1999;123:960–2.
45. Evans HL, Chawla SP, Simpson C, Finn KP. Smooth muscle neoplasms of the uterus other than ordinary leiomyoma. A study of 46 cases, with emphasis on diagnostic criteria and prognostic factors. Cancer 1988;62:2239–47.
46. Flake GP, Andersen J, Dixon D. Etiology and pathogenesis of uterine leiomyomas: a review. Environ Health Perspect 2003;111:1037–54.
47. Fletcher JA, Morton CC, Pavelka K, Lage JM. Chromosome aberrations in uterine smooth muscle tumors: potential diagnostic relevance of cytogenetic instability. Cancer Res 1990;50:4092–7.
48. Fulcher AS, Szucs RA. Leiomyomatosis peritonealis disseminata complicated by sarcomatous transformation and ovarian torsion: presentation of two cases and review of the literature. Abdom Imaging 1998;23:640–4.
49. Gadducci A, Fabrini MG, Bonuccelli A, et al. Analysis of treatment failures in patients with early-stage uterine leiomyosarcoma. Anticancer Res 1995;15:485–8.
50. Gadducci A, Landoni F, Sartori E, et al. Uterine leiomyosarcoma: analysis of treatment failures and survival. Gynecol Oncol 1996;62:25–32.
51. Gattas GJ, Quade BJ, Nowak RA, Morton CC. HMGIC expression in human adult and fetal tissues and in uterine leiomyomata. Genes Chromosomes Cancer 1999;25:316–22.

52. Gillett D. Leiomyosarcoma of the uterus in a woman taking adjuvant tamoxifen therapy. Med J Aust 1995;163:160–1.

53. Goldberg J, Burd I, Price FV, Worthington-Kirsch R. Leiomyosarcoma in a premenopausal patient after uterine artery embolization. Am J Obstet Gynecol 2004;191:1733–5.

54. Goncharova EA, Goncharov DA, Spaits M, et al. Abnormal growth of smooth muscle-like cells in lymphangioleiomyomatosis: role for tumor suppressor TSC2. Am J Respir Cell Mol Biol 2006;34:561–72.

55. Grases PJ, Ubeda A, Grases P, Tresserra E, Labastida R. Leiomioma pleomorfico del utero. Espectro clinico-patologica en siete casos. Progresos en Obstetricia y Ginecologia 1997;40:351–6.

56. Gross KL, Panhuysen CI, Kleinman MS, et al. Involvement of fumarate hydratase in nonsyndromic uterine leiomyomas: genetic linkage analysis and FISH studies. Genes Chromosomes Cancer 2004;41:183–90.

57. Hague WM, Abdulwahid NA, Jacobs HS, Craft I. Use of LHRH analogue to obtain reversible castration in a patient with benign metastasizing leiomyoma. Br J Obstet Gynaecol 1986;93:455–60.

58. Hall KL, Teneriello MG, Taylor RR, et al. Analysis of Ki-ras, p53, and MDM2 genes in uterine leiomyomas and leiomyosarcomas. Gynecol Oncol 1997;65:330–5.

59. Hameleers JA, Zeebregts CJ, Hamerlijnck RP, Elbers JR, Hameeteman TM. Combined surgical and medical approach to intravenous leiomyomatosis with cardiac extension. Acta Chir Belg 1999;99:92–4.

60. Hardman WJ, III, Majmudar B. Leiomyomatosis peritonealis disseminata: clinicopathologic analysis of five cases. South Med J 1996;89:291–4.

61. Hart WR. Problematic uterine smooth muscle neoplasms. Am J Surg Pathol 1997;21:252–5.

62. Hartmann KE, Birnbaum H, Ben-Hamadi R, et al. Annual costs associated with diagnosis of uterine leiomyomata. Obstet Gynecol 2006;108:930–7.

63. Hashimoto K, Azuma C, Kamiura S, et al. Clonal determination of uterine leiomyomas by analyzing differential inactivation of the X-chromosome-linked phosphoglycerokinase gene. Gynecol Obstet Invest 1995;40: 204–8.

64. Hendrickson MR, Kempson RL. Smooth muscle neoplasms. In: Surgical Pathology of the Uterine Corpus. Philadelphia: Saunders; 1980:472.

65. Hendrickson MR, Kempson RL. Pure mesenchymal neoplasms of the uterine corpus. In: Fox H, Wells M, eds. Haines and Taylor Obstetrical and Gynaecological Pathology, 4th edn. New York: Churchill Livingstone; 1995:519–86.

66. Hendrickson MR, Kempson RL, Bell SW. Problematic uterine smooth muscle neoplasms – response. Am J Surg Pathol 1997;21:253–5.

67. Hendrickson MR, Tavassoli FA, Kempson RL, McCluggage WG, Haller U, Kubik-Huch RA. Mesenchymal tumours and related lesions. In: Tavassoli FA, Devilee P, eds. Pathology and Genetics of Tumours of the Breast and Female Genital Organs. Lyon: IARC Press; 2003:233–44.

68. Henske EP. Metastasis of benign tumor cells in tuberous sclerosis complex. Genes Chromosomes Cancer 2003;38:376–81.

69. Higashijima T, Kataoka A, Nishida T, Yakushiji M. Gonadotropin-releasing hormone agonist therapy induces apoptosis in uterine leiomyoma. Eur J Obstet Gynecol Reprod Biol 1996;68:169–73.

70. Hirsch MS, Huettner PC, Cviko A, Quade BJ, Nucci MR. CD10 (CALLA) positive/h-caldesmon negative immunophenotype effectively distinguishes endometrial stromal tumors from uterine smooth muscle tumors. Mod Pathol 2002;15:198A.

71. Hoffmann W, Schmandt S, Kortmann RD, Schiebe M, Dietl J, Bamberg M. Radiotherapy in the treatment of uterine sarcomas. A retrospective analysis of 54 cases. Gynecol Obstet Invest 1996;42:49–57.

72. Hu J, Khanna V, Jones M, Surti U. Genomic alterations in uterine leiomyosarcomas: potential markers for clinical diagnosis and prognosis. Genes Chromosomes Cancer 2001;31:117–24.

73. Hu J, Surti U, Tobon H. Cytogenetic analysis of a uterine lipoleiomyoma. Cancer Genet Cytogenet 1992;62:200–2.

74. Hyde KE, Geisinger KR, Marshall RB, Jones TL. The clear-cell variant of uterine epithelioid leiomyoma. An immunohistologic and ultrastructural study. Arch Pathol Lab Med 1989;113:551–3.

75. Ichimura T, Kawamura N, Ito F, et al. Correlation between the growth of uterine leiomyomata and estrogen and progesterone receptor content in needle biopsy specimens. Fertil Steril 1998;70:967–71.

76. Jeffers MD, Oakes SJ, Richmond JA, Macaulay EM. Proliferation, ploidy and prognosis in uterine smooth muscle tumours. Histopathology 1996;29:217–23.

77. Jeffers MD, Richmond JA, Macaulay EM. Overexpression of the c-myc proto-oncogene occurs frequently in uterine sarcomas. Mod Pathol 1995;8:701–4.

78. Jones MW, Norris HJ. Clinicopathologic study of 28 uterine leiomyosarcomas with metastasis. Int J Gynecol Pathol 1995;14:243–249.

79. Joyce A, Hessami S, Heller D. Leiomyosarcoma after uterine artery embolization. A case report. J Reprod Med 2001;46:278–80.

80. Kawaguchi K, Oda Y, Saito T, et al. Mechanisms of inactivation of the p16INK4a gene in leiomyosarcoma of soft tissue: decreased p16 expression correlates with promoter methylation and poor prognosis. J Pathol 2003;201:487–95.

81. Kayser K, Zink S, Schneider T, et al. Benign metastasizing leiomyoma of the uterus: documentation of clinical, immunohistochemical and lectin-histochemical data of ten cases. Virchows Arch 2000;437:284–92.

82. Kazmierczak B, Dal Cin P, Wanschura S, et al. HMGIY is the target of 6p21.3 rearrangements in various benign mesenchymal tumors. Genes Chromosomes Cancer 1998;23:279–85.

83. Kempson RL, Hendrickson MR. Pure mesenchymal neoplasms of the uterine corpus. In: Fox H, ed. Haines and Taylor Obstetrical and Gynaecological Pathology, 3rd edn. Edinburgh: Churchill Livingstone; 1987:411–56.

84. Kempson RL, Hendrickson MR. Pure mesenchymal neoplasms of the uterine corpus: selected problems. Semin Diagn Pathol 1988;5:172–98.

85. King ME, Dickersin GR, Scully RE. Myxoid leiomyosarcoma of the uterus. A report of six cases. Am J Surg Pathol 1982;6:589–98.

86. Kir G, Kir M, Gurbuz A, Karateke A, Aker F. Estrogen and progesterone expression of vessel walls with intravascular leiomyomatosis; discussion of histogenesis. Eur J Gynaecol Oncol 2004;25:362–6.

87. Kiuru M, Lehtonen R, Arola J, et al. Few FH mutations in sporadic counterparts of tumor types observed in hereditary leiomyomatosis and renal cell cancer families. Cancer Res 2002;62:4554–7.

88. Kjerulff KH, Langenberg P, Seidman JD, Stolley PD, Guzinski GM. Uterine leiomyomas. Racial differences in severity, symptoms and age at diagnosis. J Reprod Med 1996;41:483–90.

89. Klötzbucher M, Wasserfall A, Fuhrmann U. Misexpression of wild-type and truncated isoforms of the high-mobility group I proteins HMGI-C and HMGI(Y) in uterine leiomyomas. Am J Pathol 1999;155:1535–42.

90. Kunzel KE, Mills NZ, Muderspach LI, d'Ablaing G, III. Myxoid leiomyosarcoma of the uterus. Gynecol Oncol 1993;48:277–80.

91. Laforga JB, Aranda FI. Uterine leiomyomas with T-cell infiltration associated with GnRH agonist goserelin. Histopathology 1999;34:471–2.

92. Lam PM, Lo KW, Yu MM, Lau TK, Cheung TH. Intravenous leiomyomatosis with atypical histologic features: a case report. Int J Gynecol Cancer 2003;13:83–7.

93. Layfield LJ, Liu K, Dodge R, Barsky SH. Uterine smooth muscle tumors: utility of classification by proliferation, ploidy, and prognostic markers versus traditional histopathology. Arch Pathol Lab Med 2000;124:221–7.

94. Le Bouedec G, De Latour M, Dauplat J. Tamoxifen and uterine fibroids. Eur J Cancer 1998;34:S19–S21.

95. Lehtonen R, Kiuru M, Vanharanta S, et al. Biallelic inactivation of fumarate hydratase (FH) occurs in nonsyndromic uterine leiomyomas but is rare in other tumors. Am J Pathol 2004;164:17–22.

96. Lennart K, Lennart B, Ulf S, Bernard T. Flow cytometric analysis of uterine sarcomas. Gynecol Oncol 1994;55(3 Pt 1):339–42.

97. Ligon AH, Morton CC. Leiomyomata: heritability and cytogenetic studies. Hum Reprod Update 2001;7:8–14.

98. Linder D, Gartler SM. Glucose-6-phosphate dehydrogenase mosaicism: utilization as a cell marker in the study of leiomyomas. Science 1965;150:67–9.

99. Liu FS, Kohler MF, Marks JR, Bast RC, Jr, Boyd J, Berchuck A. Mutation and overexpression of the p53 tumor suppressor gene frequently occurs in uterine and ovarian sarcomas. Obstet Gynecol 1994;83:118–24.

100. Lo KW, Lau TK. Intracardiac leiomyomatosis. Case report and literature review. Arch Gynecol Obstet 2001;264:209–10.

101. Losch A, Kainz C, Gitsch G, Breitenecker G. Leiomyomatosis peritonealis disseminata – a case report. Wien Klin Wochenschr 1996;108:153–6.

102. Luoto R, Kaprio J, Rutanen EM, Taipale P, Perola M, Koskenvuo M. Heritability and risk factors of uterine fibroids – the Finnish Twin Cohort study. Maturitas 2000;37:15–26.

103. Ma KF, Chow LT. Sex cord-like pattern leiomyomatosis peritonealis disseminata: a hitherto undescribed feature. Histopathology 1992;21:389–91.

104. Marshall LM, Spiegelman D, Barbieri RL, et al. Variation in the incidence of uterine leiomyoma among premenopausal women by age and race. Obstet Gynecol 1997;90:967–73.

105. Marshall LM, Spiegelman D, Manson JE, et al. Risk of uterine leiomyomata among premenopausal women in relation to body size and cigarette smoking. Epidemiology 1998;9:511–7.

106. Martin-Reay DG, Christ ML, LaPata RE. Uterine leiomyoma with skeletal muscle differentiation. Report of a case. Am J Clin Pathol 1991;96:344–7.

107. Mashal RD, Fejzo ML, Friedman AJ, et al. Analysis of androgen receptor DNA reveals the independent clonal origins of uterine leiomyomata and the secondary nature of cytogenetic aberrations in the development of leiomyomata. Genes Chromosomes Cancer 1994;11:1–6.

108. Mauskopf J, Flynn M, Thieda P, Spalding J, DuChane J. The economic impact of uterine fibroids in the United States: a summary of published estimates. J Womens Health (Larchmt) 2005;14:692–703.

109. McCluggage WG, Sumathi VP, Maxwell P. CD10 is a sensitive and diagnostically useful immunohistochemical marker of normal endometrial stroma and of endometrial stromal neoplasms. Histopathology 2001;39: 273–8.

110. McCluggage WG, Varma M, Weir P, Bharucha H. Uterine leiomyosarcoma in patients receiving tamoxifen therapy. Acta Obstet Gynecol Scand 1996;75:593–5.

111. Miranda-Guardiola F, Josa M, Valls VV, Azqueta M, Anguera II, Pare C. A case of uterine leiomyomatosis extending into the right heart with an unusual echocardiographic appearance. Echocardiography 1997;14:149–52.

112. Mittal K, Demopoulos RI. MIB-1 (Ki-67), p53, estrogen receptor, and progesterone receptor expression in uterine smooth muscle tumors. Hum Pathol 2001;32:984–7.

113. Moore SD, Herrick SR, Ince TA, et al. Uterine leiomyomata with t(10;17) disrupt the histone acetyltransferase MORF. Cancer Res 2004;64:5570–7.

114. Motegi M, Takayanagi N, Sando Y, et al. [A case of so-called benign metastasizing leiomyoma responsive to progesterone]. Nihon Kyobu Shikkan Gakkai Zasshi 1993;31:890–5.

115. Mulvany NJ, Ostor AG, Ross I. Diffuse leiomyomatosis of the uterus. Histopathology 1995;27:175–9.

116. Mulvany NJ, Slavin JL, Ostor AG, Fortune DW. Intravenous leiomyomatosis of the uterus: a clinicopathologic study of 22 cases. Int J Gynecol Pathol 1994;13:1–9.

117. Myles JL, Hart WR. Apoplectic leiomyomas of the uterus. A clinicopathologic study of five distinctive hemorrhagic leiomyomas associated with oral contraceptive usage. Am J Surg Pathol 1985;9:798–805.

118. Niemann TH, Raab SS, Lenel JC, Rodgers JR, Robinson RA. p53 protein overexpression in smooth muscle tumors of the uterus. Hum Pathol 1995;26:375–9.

119. Nogales FF, Navarro N, Martinez de Victoria JM, et al. Uterine intravascular leiomyomatosis: an update and report of seven cases. Int J Gynecol Pathol 1987;6:331–9.

120. Nola M, Babic D, Ilic J, et al. Prognostic parameters for survival of patients with malignant mesenchymal tumors of the uterus. Cancer 1996;78:2543–50.

121. Norris HJ. Editorial: Mitosis counting – III. Hum Pathol 1976;7:483–4.

122. Norris HJ, Hilliard GD, Irey NS. Hemorrhagic cellular leiomyomas ('apoplectic leiomyoma') of the uterus associated with pregnancy and oral contraceptives. Int J Gynecol Pathol 1988;7:212–24.

123. Nucci MR, Dal Cin P, Drapkin R, Fletcher CD, Fletcher JA. Unique cytogenetic profile in so-called benign metastasizing leiomyoma: evidence of a distinct clinicopathological entity. Mod.Pathol 2003;16:202A.

124. Nucci MR, O'Connell JT, Huettner PC, Cviko A, Sun D, Quade BJ. h-Caldesmon expression effectively distinguishes endometrial stromal tumors from uterine smooth muscle tumors. Am J Surg Pathol 2001;25:455–63.

125. O'Connor DM, Norris HJ. Mitotically active leiomyomas of the uterus. Hum Pathol 1990;21:223–7.

126. Ohmori T, Uraga N, Tabei R, et al. Intravenous leiomyomatosis: a case report emphasizing the vascular component. Histopathology 1988;13:470–2.

127. Olah KS, Dunn JA, Gee H. Leiomyosarcomas have a poorer prognosis than mixed mesodermal tumours when adjusting for known prognostic factors: the result of a retrospective study of 423 cases of uterine sarcoma. Br J Obstet Gynaecol 1992;99:590–4.

128. Oliva E, Clement PB, Young RH. Endometrial stromal tumors: an update on a group of tumors with a protean phenotype. Adv Anat Pathol 2000;7:257–81.

129. Oliva E, Nielsen GP, Clement PB, Young RH, Scully RE. Epithelioid smooth muscle tumors of the uterus. A clinicopathologic analysis of 80 cases. Lab Invest 1997;76:107A.

130. Oliva E, Young RH, Amin MB, Clement PB. An immunohistochemical analysis of endometrial stromal and smooth muscle tumors of the uterus: a study of 54 cases emphasizing the importance of using a panel because of overlap in immunoreactivity for individual antibodies. Am J Surg Pathol 2002;26:403–12.

131. Oliva E, Young RH, Clement PB, Bhan AK, Scully RE. Cellular benign mesenchymal tumors of the uterus. A comparative morphologic and immunohistochemical analysis of 33 highly cellular leiomyomas and six endometrial stromal nodules, two frequently confused tumors. Am J Surg Pathol 1995;19:757–68.

132. Papadia A, Salom EM, Fulcheri E, Ragni N. Uterine sarcoma occurring in a premenopausal patient after uterine artery embolization: a case report and review of the literature. Gynecol Oncol 2007;104:260–3.

133. Parenti DJ, Morley TF, Giudice JC. Benign metastasizing leiomyoma. A case report and review of the literature. Respiration 1992;59:347–50.

134. Peacock G, Archer S. Myxoid leiomyosarcoma of the uterus: case report and review of the literature. Am J Obstet Gynecol 1989;160:1515–18.

135. Pedeutour F, Quade BJ, Sornberger K, et al. Dysregulation of HMGIC in a uterine lipoleiomyoma with a complex rearrangement including chromosomes 7, 12, and 14. Genes Chromosomes Cancer 2000;27:209–15.

136. Perrone T, Dehner LP. Prognostically favorable 'mitotically active' smooth-muscle tumors of the uterus. A clinicopathologic study of ten cases. Am J Surg Pathol 1988;12:1–8.

137. Peters WA, III, Howard DR, Andersen WA, Figge DC. Deoxyribonucleic acid analysis by flow cytometry of uterine leiomyosarcomas and smooth muscle tumors of uncertain malignant potential. Am J Obstet Gynecol 1992;166(6 Pt 1):1646–53.

138. Prayson RA, Goldblum JR, Hart WR. Epithelioid smooth-muscle tumors of the uterus: a clinicopathologic study of 18 patients. Am J Surg Pathol 1997;21:383–91.

139. Prayson RA, Hart WR. Mitotically active leiomyomas of the uterus. Am J Clin Pathol 1992;97:14–20.

140. Quade BJ, Dal Cin P, Neskey DM, Weremowicz S, Morton CC. Intravenous leiomyomatosis: molecular and cytogenetic analysis of a case. Mod Pathol 2002;15:351–6.

141. Quade BJ, McLachlin CM, Soto-Wright V, Zuckerman J, Mutter GL, Morton CC. Disseminated peritoneal leiomyomatosis. Clonality analysis by X chromosome inactivation and cytogenetics of a clinically benign smooth muscle proliferation. Am J Pathol 1997;150:2153–66.

142. Quade BJ, Pinto AP, Howard DR, Peters WA, III, Crum CP. Frequent loss of heterozygosity for chromosome 10 in uterine leiomyosarcoma in contrast to leiomyoma. Am J Pathol 1999;154:945–50.

143. Quade BJ, Wang TY, Sornberger K, Dal Cin P, Mutter GL, Morton CC. Molecular pathogenesis of uterine smooth muscle tumors from transcriptional profiling. Genes Chromosomes Cancer 2004;40:97–108.

144. Quade BJ, Weremowicz S, Neskey DM, et al. Fusion transcripts involving HMGA2 are not a common molecular mechanism in uterine leiomyomata with rearrangements in 12q15. Cancer Res 2003;63:1351–8.

145. Raspagliesi F, Quattrone P, Grosso G, Cobellis L, Di Re E. Malignant degeneration in leiomyomatosis peritonealis disseminata. Gynecol Oncol 1996;61:272–4.

146. Ravina JH, Aymard A, CiraruVigneron N, et al. Selective arterial embolization for hemorrhagic uterine leiomyomas. Presse Med 1998;27:299–303.

147. Ravina JH, Bouret JM, CiraruVigneron N, et al. Interest of particulate arterial embolization in the treatment of some uterine myoma. Bull Acad Natl Med 1997;181:233–46.

148. Reed WB, Walker R, Horowitz R. Cutaneous leiomyomata with uterine leiomyomata. Acta Derm Venereol 1973;53:409–16.

149. Rein MS, Powell WL, Walters FC, et al. Cytogenetic abnormalities in uterine myomas are associated with myoma size. Mol Hum Reprod 1998;4:83–6.

150. Resta L, Maiorano E, Piscitelli D, Botticella MA. Lipomatous tumors of the uterus. Clinico-pathological features of 10 cases with immunocytochemical study of histogenesis. Pathol Res Pract 1994;190:378–83.

151. Robboy SJ, Mehta K, Norris HJ. Malignant potential and pathology of leiomyomatous tumors of the uterus. Clin Consult Obstet Gynecol 1990;2:2–9.

152. Roth TM, Klett C, Cowan BD. Expression profile of several genes in human myometrium and uterine leiomyoma. Fertil Steril 2007;87:635–41.

153. Rubin SC, Wheeler JE, Mikuta JJ. Malignant leiomyomatosis peritonealis disseminata. Obstet Gynecol 1986;68:126–30.

154. Saeed AS, Hanaa B, Faisal AS, Najla AM. Cotyledonoid dissecting leiomyoma of the uterus: a case report of a benign uterine tumor with sarcomalike gross appearance and review of literature. Int J Gynecol Pathol 2006;25:262–7.

155. Salm R, Evans DJ. Myxoid leiomyosarcoma. Histopathology 1985;9:159–69.

156. Sandberg AA. Updates on the cytogenetics and molecular genetics of bone and soft tissue tumors: leiomyoma. Cancer Genet Cytogenet 2005;158:1–26.

157. Sandberg AA. Updates on the cytogenetics and molecular genetics of bone and soft tissue tumors: leiomyosarcoma. Cancer Genet Cytogenet 2005;161:1–19.

158. Sato F, Mori M, Nishi M, Kudo R, Miyake H. Familial aggregation of uterine myomas in Japanese women. J Epidemiol 2002;12:249–53.

159. Sato F, Nishi M, Kudo R, Miyake H. Body fat distribution and uterine leiomyomas. J Epidemiol 1998;8:176–80.

160. Scialli AR. Alternatives to hysterectomy for benign conditions. Int J Fertil Womens Med 1998;43:186–91.

161. Sieinski W. Lipomatous neometaplasia of the uterus. Report of 11 cases with discussion of histogenesis and pathogenesis. Int J Gynecol Pathol 1989;8:357–63.

162. Silverberg SG. Reproducibility of the mitosis count in the histologic diagnosis of smooth muscle tumors of the uterus. Hum Pathol 1976;7:451–54.

163. Skubitz KM, Skubitz AP. Differential gene expression in leiomyosarcoma. Cancer 2003;98:1029–38.

164. Skubitz KM, Skubitz AP. Differential gene expression in uterine leiomyoma. J Lab Clin Med 2003;141:297–308.

165. Sornberger KS, Weremowicz S, Williams AJ, et al. Expression of HMGIY in three uterine leiomyomata with complex rearrangements of chromosome 6. Cancer Genet Cytogenet 1999;114:9–16.

166. Spies JB, Spector A, Roth AR, Baker CM, Mauro L, Murphy-Skrynarz K. Complications after uterine artery embolization for leiomyomas. Obstet Gynecol 2002;100(5 Pt 1):873–80.

167. Steinmetz OK, Bedard P, Prefontaine ME, Bourke M, Barber GG. Uterine tumor in the heart: intravenous leiomyomatosis. Surgery 1996;119:226–9.

168. Stewart EA. Uterine fibroids. Lancet 2001;357:293–8.

169. Stewart EA, Gedroyc WM, Tempany CM, et al. Focused ultrasound treatment of uterine fibroid tumors: safety and feasibility of a noninvasive thermoablative technique. Am J Obstet Gynecol 2003;189:48–54.

170. Stewart EA, Morton CC. The genetics of uterine leiomyomata: what clinicians need to know. Obstet Gynecol 2006;107:917–21.

171. Stewart EA, Rabinovici J, Tempany CM, et al. Clinical outcomes of focused ultrasound surgery for the treatment of uterine fibroids. Fertil Steril 2006;85:22–9.

172. Stjernquist M. Treatment of uterine fibroids with GnRH-analogues prior to hysterectomy. Acta Obstet Gynecol Scand Suppl 1997;164:94–7.

173. Tahlan A, Nanda A, Mohan H. Uterine adenomyoma: a clinicopathologic review of 26 cases and a review of the literature. Int J Gynecol Pathol 2006;25:361–5.

174. Takemura G, Takatsu Y, Kaitani K, et al. Metastasizing uterine leiomyoma. A case with cardiac and pulmonary metastasis. Pathol Res Pract 1996;192:622–9.

175. Tallini G, Dal Cin P. HMGI(Y) and HMGI-C dysregulation: a common occurrence in human tumors. Adv Anat Pathol 1999;6:237–46.

176. Taylor HB, Norris HJ. Mesenchymal tumors of the uterus. IV. Diagnosis and prognosis of leiomyosarcomas. Arch Pathol 1966;82:40–4.

177. Tempany CM, Stewart EA, McDannold N, Quade BJ, Jolesz FA, Hynynen K. MR imaging-guided focused ultrasound surgery of uterine leiomyomas: a feasibility study. Radiology 2003;226:897–905.

178. Thejls H, Pettersson B, Nordlinder H. Leiomyomatosis peritonealis disseminata. Acta Obstet Gynecol Scand 1986;65:373–4.

179. Thomas EO, Gordon J, Smith-Thomas S, Cramer SF. Diffuse uterine leiomyomatosis with uterine rupture and benign metastatic lesions of the bone. Obstet Gynecol 2007;109:528–30.

180. Tiltman AJ. Adenomatoid tumours of the uterus. Histopathology 1980;4:437–43.

181. Tiltman AJ. Smooth muscle neoplasms of the uterus. Curr Opin Obstet Gynecol 1997;9:48–51.

182. Tomlinson IP, Alam NA, Rowan AJ, et al. Germline mutations in FH predispose to dominantly inherited uterine fibroids, skin leiomyomata and papillary renal cell cancer. Nat Genet 2002;30:406–10.

183. Topcuoglu MS, Yaliniz H, Poyrazoglu H, et al. Intravenous leiomyomatosis extending into the right ventricle after subtotal hysterectomy. Ann Thorac Surg 2004;78:330–2.

184. Townsend DE, Sparkes RS, Baluda MC, McClelland G. Unicellular histogenesis of uterine leiomyomas as determined by electrophoresis by glucose-6-phosphate dehydrogenase. Am J Obstet Gynecol 1970;107:1168–73.

185. Trzyna W, McHugh M, McCue P, McHugh KM. Molecular determination of the malignant potential of smooth muscle neoplasms. Cancer 1997;80:211–17.

186. Tsibris JC, Segars J, Coppola D, et al. Insights from gene arrays on the development and growth regulation of uterine leiomyomata. Fertil Steril 2002;78:114–21.

187. Uchida H, Hattori Y, Nakada K, Iida T. Successful one-stage radical removal of intravenous leiomyomatosis extending to the right ventricle. Obstet Gynecol 2004;103(5 Pt 2):1068–70.

188. Van d Ven J, Sprong M, Donker GH, Thijssen JH, Mak-Kregar S, Blankenstein MA. Levels of estrogen and progesterone receptors in the myometrium and leiomyoma tissue after suppression of estrogens with gonadotropin releasing hormone analogs. Gynecol Endocrinol 2001;15(Suppl 6):61–8.

189. Volkers NA, Hehenkamp WJ, Birnie E, et al. Uterine artery embolization in the treatment of symptomatic uterine fibroid tumors (EMMY trial): periprocedural results and complications. J Vasc Interv Radiol 2006;17:471–80.

190. Volpe R, Canzonieri V, Gloghini A, Carbone A. 'Lipoleiomyoma with metaplastic cartilage' (benign mesenchymoma) of the uterine cervix. Pathol Res Pract 1992;188:799–801.

191. Vu K, Greenspan DL, Wu TC, Zacur HA, Kurman RJ. Cellular proliferation, estrogen receptor, progesterone receptor, and bcl-2 expression in GnRH agonist-treated uterine leiomyomas. Hum Pathol 1998;29:359–63.

192. Wang T, Zhang X, Obijuru L, et al. A micro-RNA signature associated with race, tumor size, and target gene activity in human uterine leiomyomas. Genes Chromosomes Cancer 2007;46:336–47.

193. Wang X, Kumar D, Seidman JD. Uterine lipoleiomyomas: a clinicopathologic study of 50 cases. Int J Gynecol Pathol 2006;25:239–42.

194. Wei J, Chiriboga L, Mizuguchi M, Yee H, Mittal K. Expression profile of tuberin and some potential tumorigenic factors in 60 patients with uterine leiomyomata. Mod Pathol 2005;18:179–88.

195. Wei JJ, Chiriboga L, Arslan AA, Melamed J, Yee H, Mittal K. Ethnic differences in expression of the dysregulated proteins in uterine leiomyomata. Hum Reprod 2006;21:57–67.

196. Wei JJ, Chiriboga L, Mittal K. Expression profile of the tumorigenic factors associated with tumor size and sex steroid hormone status in uterine leiomyomata. Fertil Steril 2005;84:474–84.

197. Wei MH, Toure O, Glenn GM, et al. Novel mutations in FH and expansion of the spectrum of phenotypes expressed in families with hereditary leiomyomatosis and renal cell cancer. J Med Genet 2006;43:18–27.

198. Weichert W, Denkert C, Gauruder-Burmester A, et al. Uterine arterial embolization with tris-acryl gelatin microspheres: a histopathologic evaluation. Am J Surg Pathol 2005;29:955–61.

199. Williams AJ, Powell WL, Collins T, Morton CC. HMGI(Y) expression in human uterine leiomyomata. Involvement of another high-mobility group architectural factor in a benign neoplasm. Am J Pathol 1997;150:911–18.

200. Wood C, Maher P. Endoscopic treatment of uterine fibroids. Baillieres Clin Obstet Gynaecol 1998;12:289–316.

201. Wu X, Blanck A, Olovsson M, Moller B, Favini R, Lindblom B. Apoptosis, cellular proliferation and expression of p53 in human uterine leiomyomas and myometrium during the menstrual cycle and after menopause. Acta Obstet Gynecol Scand 2000;79:397–404.

202. Yoshitomi A, Sato A, Imokawa S, et al. [A case of so-called benign metastasizing leiomyoma]. Nihon Kyobu Shikkan Gakkai Zasshi 1994;32:373–7.

203. Zaidi MR, Okada Y, Chada KK. Misexpression of full-length HMGA2 induces benign mesenchymal tumors in mice. Cancer Res 2006;66:7453–9.

204. Zhang P, Zhang C, Hao J, et al. Use of X-chromosome inactivation pattern to determine the clonal origins of uterine leiomyoma and leiomyosarcoma. Hum Pathol 2006;37:1350–6.

Fallopian tube

Wenxin Zheng   Stanley J. Robboy

19

INTRODUCTION

As the fallopian tube is the intermediary between the ovary and the uterus, it is the seat of various interactions that culminate in a normally implanted pregnancy. Its multiple functions include conditioning of both gametes before fertilization, guiding their journeys before encounter, providing an appropriate chemical environment for fertilization, supplying nutriment to the fertilized ovum for its first few hours of life, and delivering it to the uterine cavity at the proper time for nidation. The exact processes by which these various mechanisms are accomplished are still rather poorly understood, partly because many of them vary significantly from species to species, so that the study of experimental animals does not always help to understand the situation in women.

ANATOMY, HISTOLOGY, AND FUNCTION OF THE FALLOPIAN TUBE

ANATOMY

The fallopian tubes are derived from the müllerian ducts, which begin as invaginations of the celomic lining epithelium lateral to the cranial end of the mesonephric ducts at 5 weeks of intrauterine development. The lower ends fuse to the mesonephric bodies in the 7 week embryo, after which the mesonephric ducts undergo regression. The tube is 9–12 cm long *in vivo* but, being a muscular organ, its length can vary considerably. After fixation, it appears shorter, shrinking to a serpentine form. At the medial end, the tube is attached to the uterine cornu above and in front of the ovarian ligament, and above and behind the round ligament of the uterus. A sheet of pelvic peritoneum is folded over the tube, joining beneath it to form the mesosalpinx and then, beneath the mesovarium and ovarian ligament, to become the broad ligament. On the lateral wall of the pelvis, the tube arches backward over the ovary, its ostium facing the medial aspect of the latter.

The fallopian tube is divided into four zones, which, extending laterally to medially, are the infundibulum, the ampulla, the isthmus, and the interstitial (or intramural) portions. The infundibulum is the lateral end of the tube and forms the funnel-like expansion, about 1 cm in length and diameter that ends in a variable number of irregular, fringe-like extensions, the fimbriae. Medial to the infundibulum and making up about half of the length of the tube is the ampullary portion. The ampulla is narrower than the infundibulum and runs a tortuous course. The isthmus, which is 2–3 cm in length, has a narrower lumen and more muscular wall than the ampulla. The interstitial portion of the tube has a lumen with a simple, stellate or almost circular cross-section. In this segment of the tube, the muscle of the tubal wall merges with that of the myometrium.

HISTOLOGY

The fallopian tube is composed of a mucosal lining, a muscular layer, and an outer serosa. The mucosa consists of non-stratified epithelium and a sparse underlying fibrovascular lamina propria. The epithelium (Figure 19.1) comprises four cell types: ciliated cells, secretory cells, intercalary (or peg) cells, and reserve basal (or undifferentiated) cells. The ciliated cells have a centrally placed nucleus with a perinuclear halo, a prominent terminal bar, and definable surface cilia. The nuclei of the secretory cells vary in position, depending on the stage in the menstrual cycle. The intercalary cells are secretory cells that have discharged their secretions with the result that the cell walls are collapsed around the nucleus. The ciliated component is the most prominent near the fimbrial end of the tube and the secretory cells are more numerous in the isthmus than they are in the ampulla.

The tubal epithelium shows well-defined histologic alterations in response to cyclic hormonal variations, which affect the height of the epithelial cells, rather than the number of cilia, as happens in other primates. In the proliferative phase of the cycle the estrogen predominance results in epithelial cells with increasing height whereas in the progesterone-dominated secretory phase, the cell height may be as little as half that seen in the first half of the cycle. Similarly, the height of both epithelial cell types is low in pregnancy. Oral contraceptives produce a similar appearance to those of pregnancy, the epithelial cells being relatively flat and showing a lack of secretory activity, features that doubtless play some part in the effectiveness of the medication. In the late postmenopausal state, the epithelium becomes thin and atrophic (Figure 19.2).

In cross-section, at low-power magnification, the mucosa of the tubal ampulla (Figure 19.3) forms a complicated maze-like pattern of folds (the plicae) that branch but do not join. The epithelial surfaces of the plicae are apposed to one another so that even in the widest part of the tube the traversing ovum is not floating in a spacious lumen but is at all times nurtured by the ciliated and secretory epithelium with which it is in contact on all sides. These folds become less complex as the medial end of the tube is approached, becoming stellate in the isthmus (Figure 19.4) and forming an irregular, almost rounded outline to the lumen in the interstitial part. In postmenopausal women, the plical stroma becomes fibrous and the plicae themselves

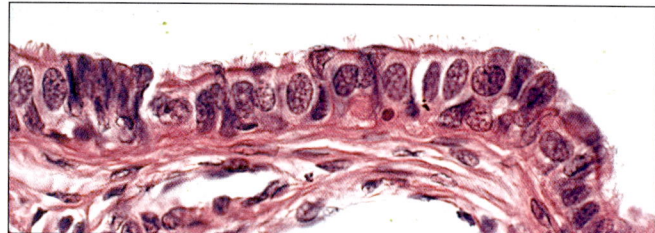

Fig. 19.1 Normal tubal epithelium. Tall ciliated cells predominate.

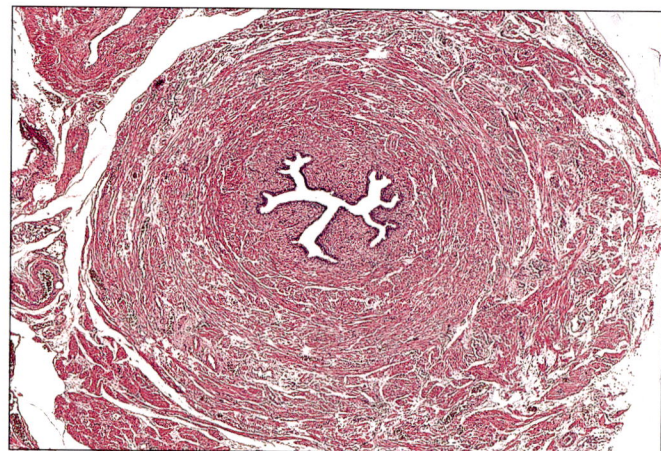

Fig. 19.4 Normal isthmus. The lumen is narrow and stellate and the wall is thick.

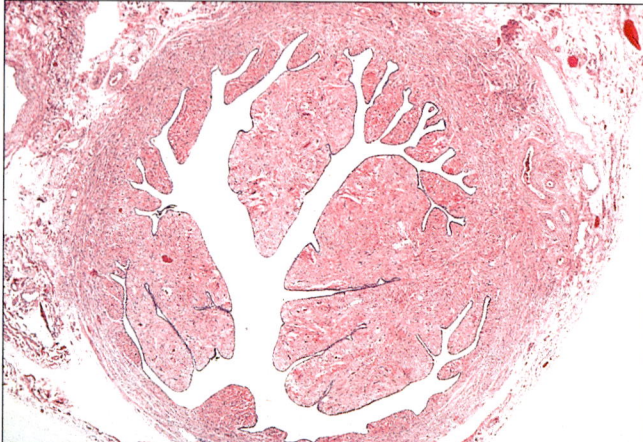

Fig. 19.2 Atrophic tubal mucosa. The epithelium is thin and atrophic and the plical lamina propria is fibrotic.

FUNCTION

The fallopian tube has three main functions in the reproductive process. First, it is responsible for transferring the ovum into its lumen when discharged from the ovary's rupturing follicle. Second, it provides an environment in which the sperm can fertilize the ovum. Third, it transfers the fertilized, cleaving embryo into the uterus after a timed interval of 3–4 days.

Sperm transport

The mechanisms of sperm transport in the tube are not known. It is apparent that there is a rapid postcoital sperm movement along the whole genital tract and that, in different segments of the tract, including the tube, a number of 'storage compartments' are established from which sperm release occurs slowly. Although reduced sperm motility is a factor in male infertility, it is accepted that sperm do not have to be motile to be transported along the female genital tract. No information is known about the active part, if any, that the tube plays in sperm transport.

Ovum transport

Ovum transport has been studied in detail, the two essential elements being muscular activity and ciliary action. It would seem that these two mechanisms play a complementary role in ovum transport. Even so, each does not always appear necessary. Reproduction can take place when the ciliary action is paralyzed and ciliary action alone will carry the ovum across the ampullary part of the tube. The muscular contractions of the tubal wall are both phasic and tonic; it can undergo transient contractions as well as alter its basal tone. Contractile activity of the muscle takes place in coordinated waves. These result in peristaltic pulses along segments of the tube, although these are propagated only along random short lengths, with junctional pauses. The positions are probably related to changes in the muscular thickness and arrangement at the ampullary–isthmic junction and the isthmic–interstitial junction. Some claim that muscular activity is not essential for transport of the oocyte along its course.

The ciliary action in the tube is towards the uterus and is under the influence of many mediators. Physiologic levels of prostaglandins $F_{2\alpha}$, E_1 and E_2 stimulate the ciliary activity as

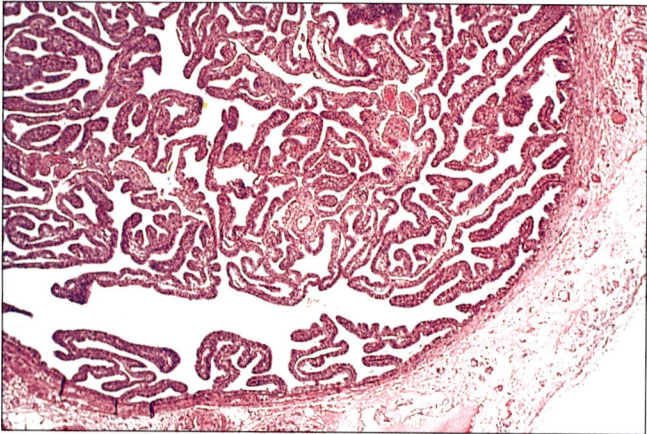

Fig. 19.3 Normal ampulla. The mucosa forms a complex maze-like pattern of folds that branch but do not join.

club shaped, an appearance that may be mistaken for one sequela of infection, and the epithelium flattened.

The tubal musculature is arranged in a basket-weave fashion. This layer is thinnest at the tube's outer end and becomes progressively thicker as the cornu is approached. A subepithelial layer of mainly longitudinal muscle appears at the isthmus and continues along the interstitial portion. At this point, the spiral muscle becomes continuous with the myometrium.

do β-adrenergic agonists, the latter effect being potentiated by estrogen and progesterone. Recent data have shown that progesterone affects the tubal ciliary beat frequency.[39] Incubation with progesterone suppresses the beat frequency by 40–50% but estradiol has no effect. Cilia from the tubal ampulla beat significantly faster than those from fimbrial segments.

INFLAMMATION OF THE FALLOPIAN TUBES

Inflammatory disease resulting from infection of the fallopian tubes and adjacent ovary is an increasing problem. The investigation and treatment of women with the disease is demanding more and more in the way of time and other resources. Identification of the disease early in its natural history is important to enable treatment to be effected before the damage becomes extensive and the consequent surgery destructive.

INFECTIVE SALPINGITIS

Infective salpingitis may be divided into the two major categories of non-granulomatous and granulomatous (or tuberculous?) salpingitis.

NON-GRANULOMATOUS SALPINGITIS

Non-granulomatous salpingitis is predominantly a disease of young, sexually active women, 70% of those with the disease being under the age of 25. Other factors that have an influence on the development of salpingitis include the method of contraception, induced abortion, and instrumentation of the cervix. Among the infective organisms responsible for salpingitis, *Chlamydia trachomatis* and *Neisseria gonorrhoeae* remain of paramount importance and are responsible for ascending salpingitis.[18] Other causative microbial agents are: the anerobic bacteria (bacteroides, clostridia and streptococci), *Mycoplasma hominis* and *Ureaplasma urealyticum*, and miscellaneous organisms such as *Haemophilus influenzae* and group A streptococci. Bacterial vaginosis is a common concurrent disorder of women with acute salpingitis, and bacterial vaginosis microorganisms are commonly isolated from the upper genital tracts of patients with pelvic inflammatory disease.[18] In practice, however, microbiologic investigations often show that the cultured material is already sterile by the time of the investigation, or else there is a combination of organisms.

The spread of etiologic organisms from the lower to the upper genital tract is canalicular, through the cervical canal and endometrial cavity and then into the fallopian tubes. Blockage of this route, either by cornual resection of the fallopian tubes or by sterilization, reduces the risk of salpingitis.[1] Salpingitis begins as a mucosal rather than a serosal infection.

Gross features
In the acute phase of the disease, the tube is swollen, edematous, and congested. The acutely inflamed tube is rarely seen histologically, as treatment of the acute phase is medical rather than surgical.

In chronic salpingitis, the tube is thickened and congested, with adhesions on the surface, often binding the tube and ovary closely together. A pyosalpinx is a grossly enlarged tube,

increased in both diameter and length, usually thick walled and containing pus. A hydrosalpinx characteristically shows a retort shape and is greatly enlarged with paper-thin walls. In both conditions, the fimbrial ends fuse, sealing the tube. Not uncommonly, the fimbriae cannot be identified.

Microscopic features
The plicae are greatly swollen and densely infiltrated by neutrophils (Figure 19.5). The epithelial cells soon lose their cilia and the epithelium is shed in severe disease. The lumen contains pus (Figure 19.6). As the disease progresses to chronic salpingitis (Figures 19.7 and 19.8), the inflammatory infiltrate consists predominantly of plasma cells and then lymphocytes. The progression from acute to chronic non-granulomatous salpingitis may take several courses. If the fimbrial end of the tube remains patent, a chronic interstitial salpingitis may ensue, in which case the tube is thickened and the plicae fuse together, this plical conglutination being the hallmark of chronic salpingitis. Widespread plical conglutination results in an appearance termed 'follicular salpingitis' (Figure 19.9) (the 'follicular' rather confusingly referring to the epithelium-lined spaces rather than lymphoid collections). The inflammatory process

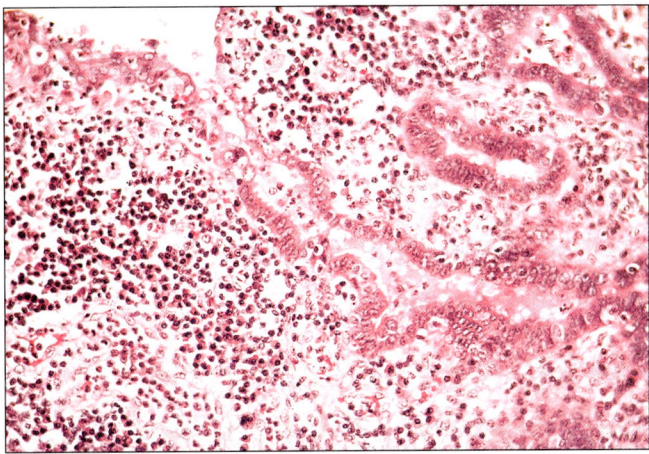

Fig. 19.5 Acute salpingitis. The plicae are edematous and infiltrated by polymorphs.

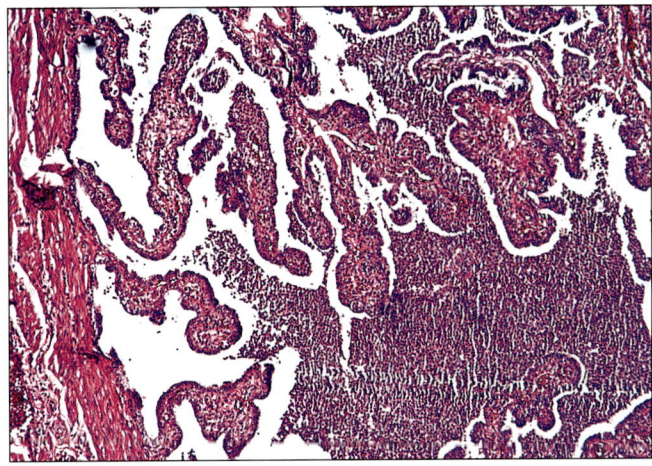

Fig. 19.6 Acute salpingitis. The lumen is filled with pus and the plicae are engorged and inflamed.

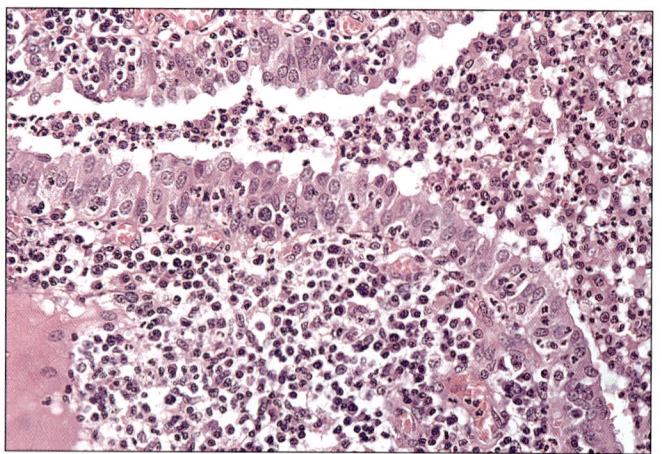

Fig. 19.7 Chronic salpingitis. In this early stage of the disease, the plicae are infiltrated by plasma cells and lymphocytes and there is pus in the lumen. The epithelium is intact, although containing inflammatory cells.

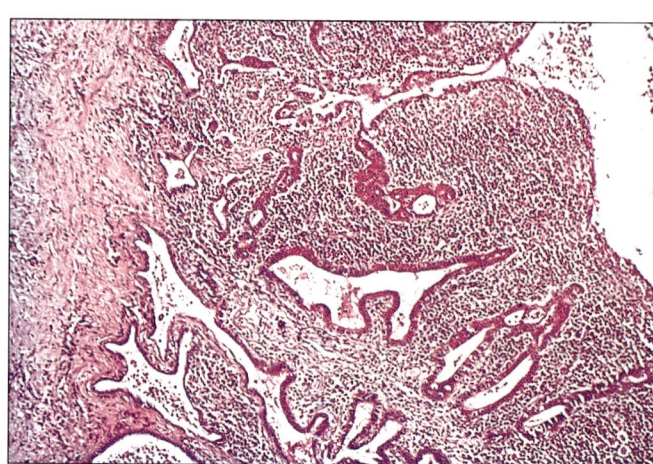

Fig. 19.9 Chronic salpingitis. The plicae are becoming fused, forming separate channels in the lumen. Inflammation is still active.

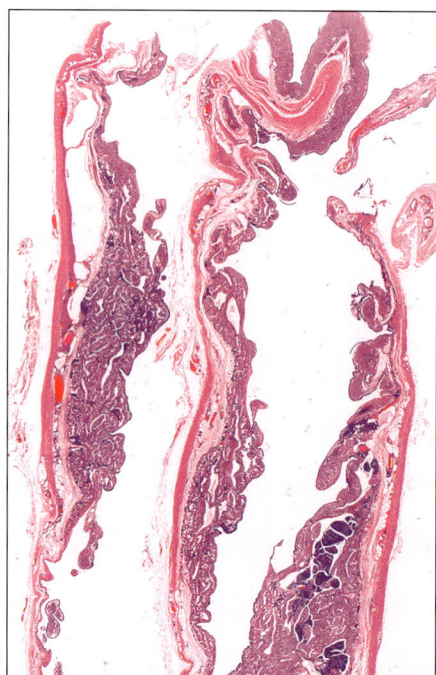

Fig. 19.8 Chronic salpingitis. The infiltrate is now predominantly lymphocytic, with germinal centers.

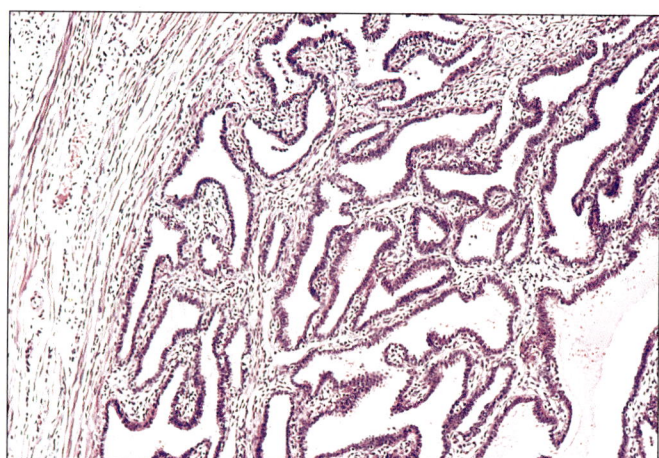

Fig. 19.10 Chronic salpingitis, healed. The inflammation has subsided and is near absent, but the plicae remain fused by fibrosis.

may eventually become quiescent, so that the architectural sequelae of chronic salpingitis may be seen without the inflammatory infiltrate that indicates current inflammatory activity (Figure 19.10). Severe inflammation in the tube may spread to the adjacent ovary, resulting in a tubo-ovarian abscess (Figure 19.11). Occlusion of the fimbrial end of the tube prevents release of the tubal contents, so that a pyosalpinx may result (Figure 19.12). As the exudate is reabsorbed into the tubal wall concurrently with the quiescence of the inflammatory process, clear fluid replaces this pus and a hydrosalpinx results (Figures 19.13 and 19.14). A small hydrosalpinx in which there is plical conglutination will have a 'honeycomb' cut surface and is termed a 'hydrosalpinx follicularis' (Figure 19.15). The

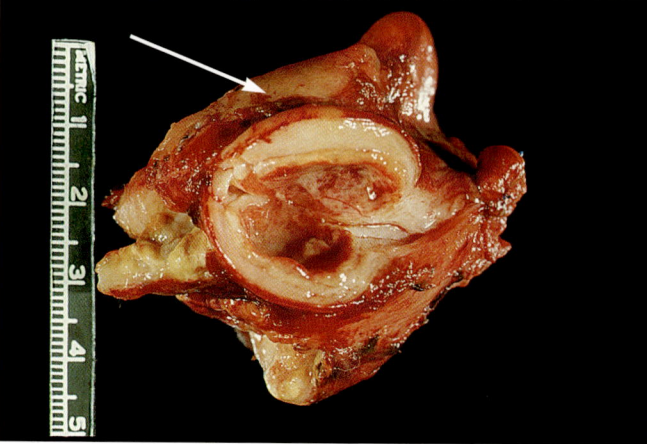

Fig. 19.11 Tubo-ovarian abscess. The central mass is the ovary, which contains an abscess. Its cavity communicates with pus in the lumen of the tube (arrow).

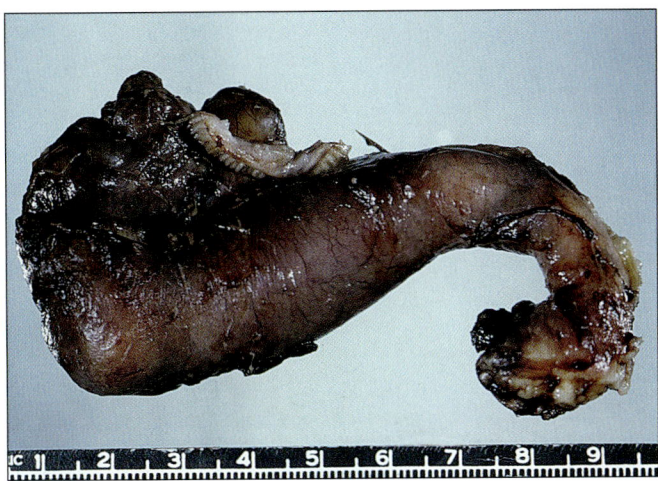

Fig. 19.12 Pyosalpinx.

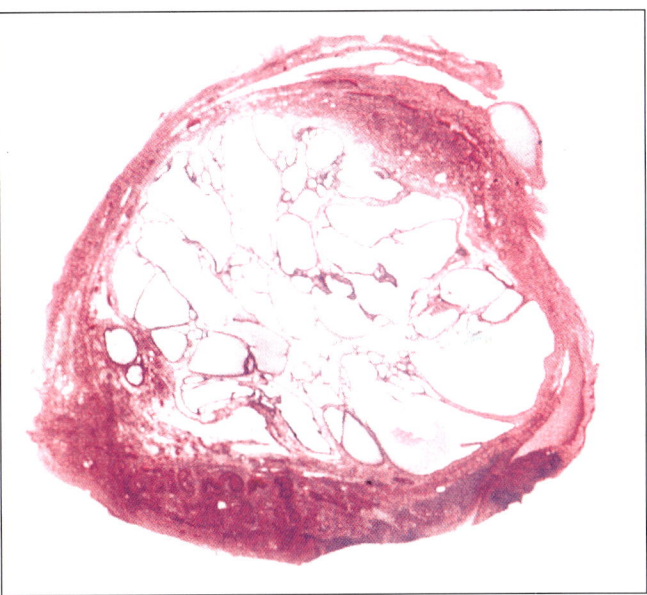

Fig. 19.15 Hydrosalpinx follicularis.

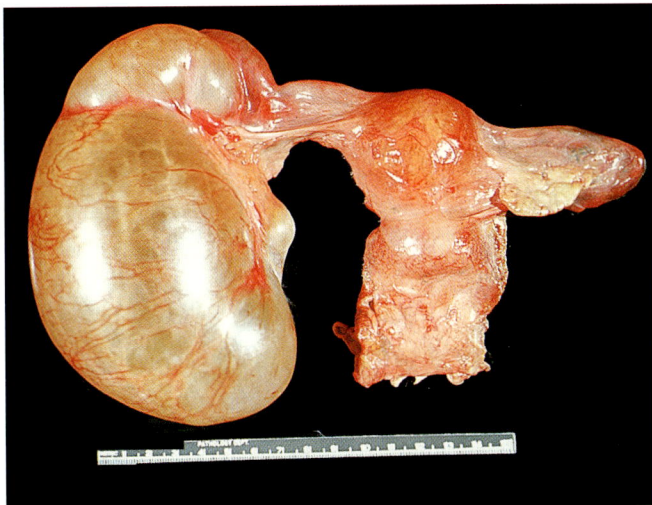

Fig. 19.13 Hydrosalpinx.

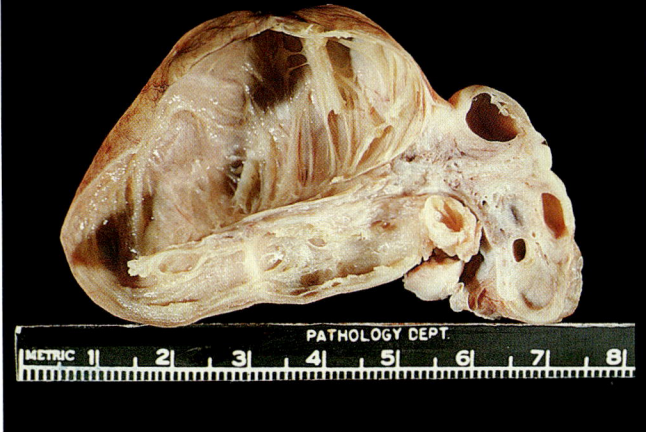

Fig. 19.14 Hydrosalpinx. The convoluted shape (often called 'retort shaped') of the tube is seen on section.

relations among these inflammatory changes are shown in Figure 19.16.

The term 'pelvic inflammatory disease' (PID) implies chronic salpingitis with involvement of the surrounding structures, including ovary and parametrium. Adhesions are present on the surface of the tube, often spreading to involve the uterine serosa. PID typically has remissions and exacerbations and is difficult to eradicate. As a result of this cycle of events, in which acute salpingitis leads to chronic salpingitis, quiescence and then an exacerbation of the acute episode again, the histologic finding of acute on chronic salpingitis is commonplace. In these circumstances, the background architectural features of chronic salpingitis are seen, but the cellular infiltrate is predominantly of neutrophils, with pus in the lumen.

Pyosalpinx   The lumen is filled with pus (Figure 19.17) and the wall is thinned, although the attenuation is commonly less marked than in hydrosalpinx. Acute and chronic inflammatory cells infiltrate the plicae and wall as evidence of the usual process of an acute exacerbation superimposed on a chronic inflammatory state.

Hydrosalpinx   In hydrosalpinx (Figures 19.13 and 19.14) and hydrosalpinx follicularis (Figure 19.15) the epithelium is generally thin and non-ciliated, although a few areas of morphologically normal cells may be seen. The wall of a hydrosalpinx is markedly thinned, with loss of smooth muscle and plicae. Usually, by this advanced stage in the disease process, there is little, if any, residual inflammatory infiltrate in the tissues of the wall. From a practical point of view, hydrosalpinx is commonly misdiagnosed as 'serous cystadenoma' since it commonly presents as an adnexal mass in the clinic. A careful microscopic examination identifying the muscular layer is diagnostic for hydrosalpinx.

GRANULOMATOUS SALPINGITIS

Granulomatous salpingitis is nearly always tuberculous in origin. All age groups may be affected but the pattern of the

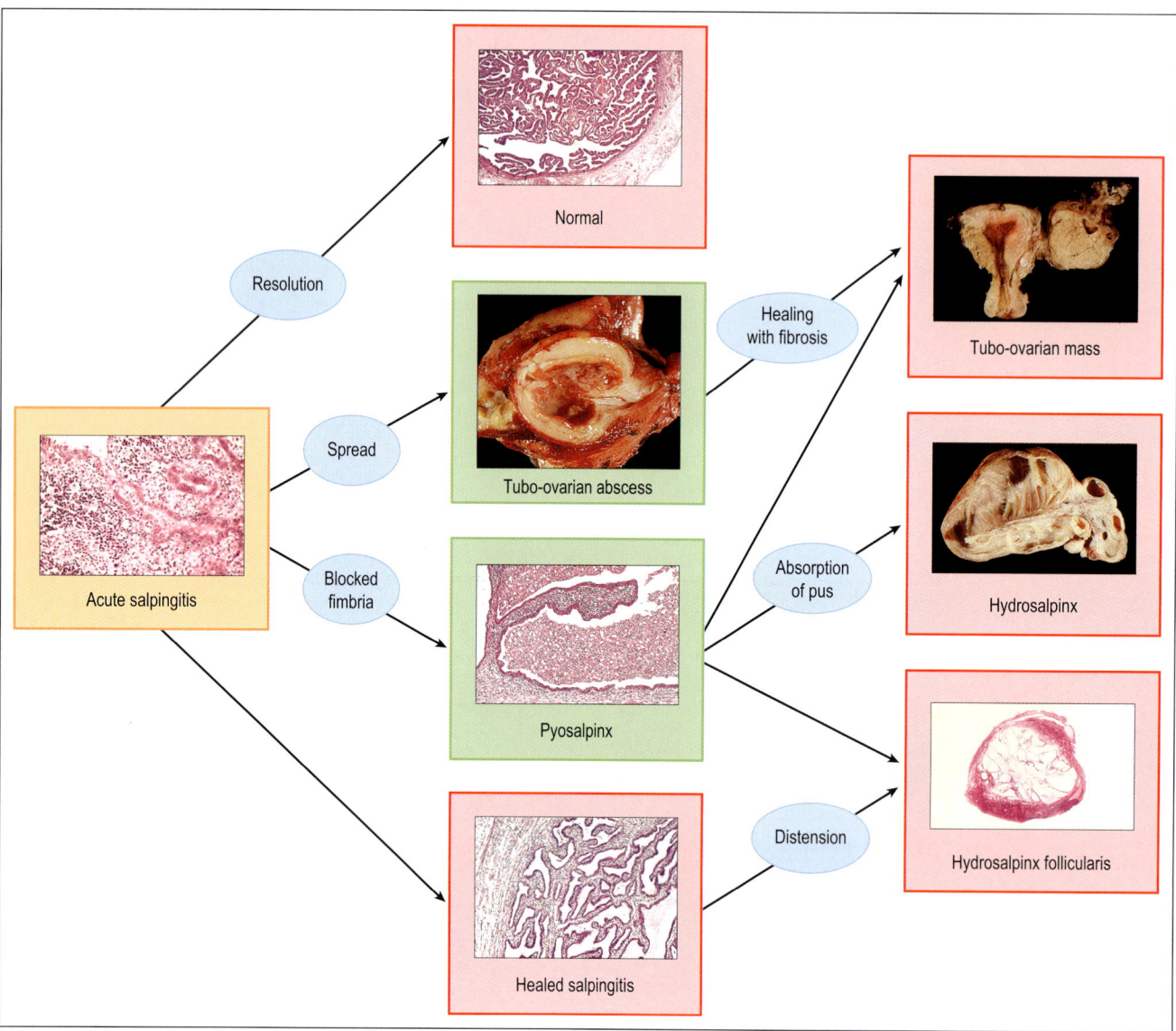

Fig. 19.16 Relations among the appearances and stages of inflammation of the fallopian tube.

disease has changed over the last few decades. Until the 1970s, tuberculosis of the female genital tract in the developed world affected mainly women of childbearing age but more recently the majority of cases are in postmenopausal women.[29] Whereas previously the main complaint of these women was infertility, tuberculosis accounting for about 40% of all cases of infertility,[49] the common symptoms are now pain and bleeding.[29] Thus, the condition should always be borne in mind as a possibility, albeit a rare one, in infertile women. When tuberculosis affects the female genital tract, the tube is affected in nearly all cases and involvement of the endometrium is always secondary to it. The pelvic disease is, in turn, secondary to primary disease in the lungs or bowel, spreading to the tubes by hematogenous and lymphatic routes, respectively.

Gross features

Tuberculous salpingitis is nearly always bilateral. The tube is thickened and congested and there are serosal adhesions. The fimbrial end of the tube is usually patent and the lumen may

contain caseous debris (Figure 19.18). The wall is thickened and foci of caseation may be recognized within the tissue of the wall.

Microscopic features

The hallmark of tuberculous salpingitis histologically is the epithelioid cell granuloma that is situated in the lamina propria of the plicae (Figures 19.19 and 19.20) and, rarely, within the muscular wall. Caseation may or may not be present, but is more often seen in older women. A surrounding, dense lymphocytic infiltrate is found, both in the plical lamina propria and in the muscle, the latter usually being more conspicuous. A frequent finding is the presence of striking epithelial proliferation of the endosalpinx, a feature that may cause confusion with carcinoma (see below). Schaumann bodies are occasionally seen in tuberculous salpingitis (Figure 19.19). Although typically associated with sarcoidosis, these rounded, concentrically laminated calcified bodies may be seen in most forms of epithelioid cell granuloma. They are

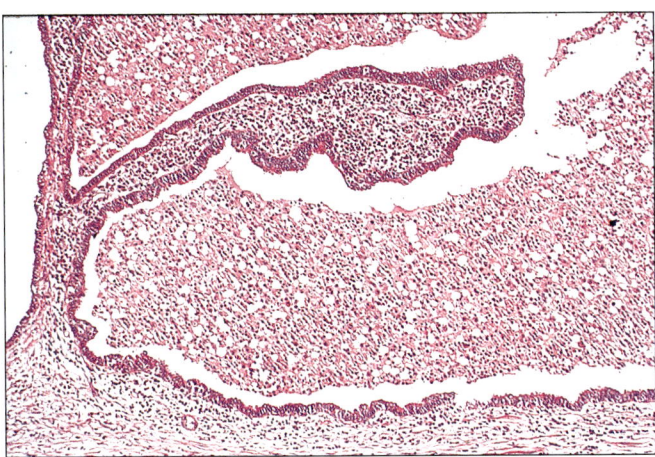

Fig. 19.17 Pyosalpinx. The lumen contains pus.

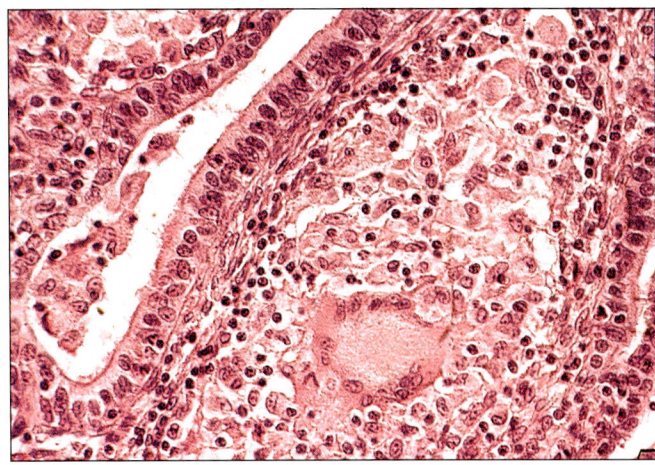

Fig. 19.20 Tuberculous salpingitis.

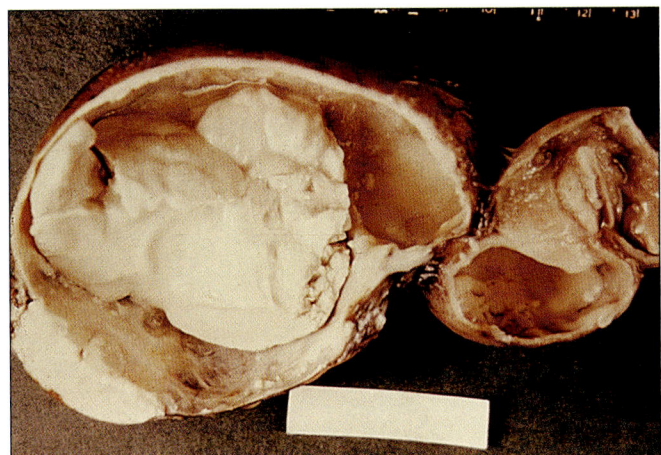

Fig. 19.18 Tuberculous salpingitis. The wall is greatly distended and thinned and the lumen contains caseous material.

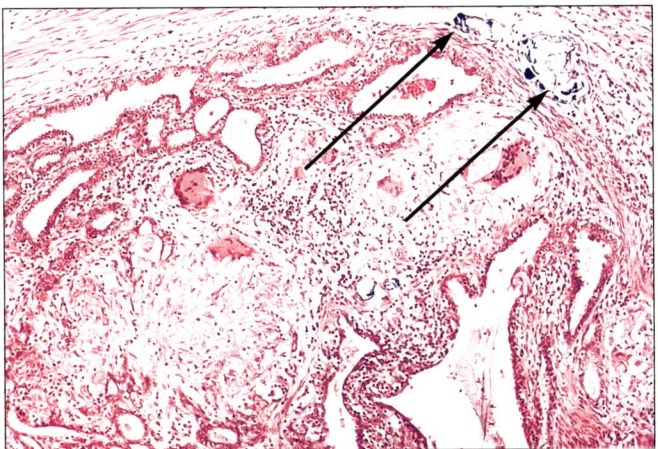

Fig. 19.19 Tuberculous salpingitis. Epithelioid cell granulomas are present with giant cells. Schaumann bodies are also seen (arrows).

rather more common in tubal tuberculosis than in tuberculosis elsewhere.

The histologic suggestion of tubal tuberculosis is confirmed if acid-fast bacilli are found in the sections but this is achieved in only 1% of cases in which the culture or guinea pig inoculation proves positive. On a practical basis, staining is not useful. With the development of molecular pathology, polymerase chain reaction (PCR)-based tuberculosis-specific bacilli DNA can be detected in 48 hours.[48] The differential diagnosis of tuberculous salpingitis in Europe is sarcoidosis, Crohns disease, and foreign-body granuloma. Worldwide, other conditions include schistosomiasis, blastomycosis, coccidioidomycosis, histoplasmosis, and enterobiasis. A positive diagnosis of tuberculosis is often not possible and the decision to treat the patient must rest on the degree of suspicion that the histologic picture raises, together with absence of other indications of sarcoid and Crohns disease. The chances of a normal pregnancy occurring after treatment for tuberculous salpingitis are low and there is an increased risk of spontaneous abortion and ectopic pregnancy.

PELVIC INFLAMMATORY DISEASE AND INTRAUTERINE CONTRACEPTIVE DEVICE USE

INTRAUTERINE CONTRACEPTIVE DEVICE

Intrauterine contraceptive devices (IUDs) have been used for centuries. During the first half of the twentieth century their use was marred by an associated high incidence of infection and they were prohibited in some countries as a result. With the advent of the new, inert plastic devices their popularity has increased again in the belief that the infective side effects would be minimal. The main effect of an IUD is to induce a local inflammatory reaction in the endometrium that spreads to involve the entire genital tract because of luminal transmission of the fluids that accumulate in the uterine lumen. As a result, fertilization of ova in the fallopian tube occurs at a much lower rate.[47] Increased numbers of inflammatory cells are present in the tubal lamina propria of women wearing an IUD.[66] From the late 1960s through to the early 1980s, the literature contained reports of serious PID from infection complicating the apparently successful use of IUDs. Recent findings, however, show the IUD is not associated with an increased risk of PID when no active infection is present, nor are they associated with increased risk of ectopic pregnancy or subsequent infertility.[8,43,62]

Of particular interest, IUD usage has been associated with infection by *Actinomyces israelii*,[6] which is very rare in the absence of an IUD. The risk of pelvic actinomycosis developing is related less to the type of IUD in use than the length of time it has been in the uterine cavity, 85% of cases occurring in women who have worn an IUD continuously for 3 or more years. Tubo-ovarian abscesses (Figure 19.21) may result and the *Actinomyces*-like organisms can be identified in the pus (Figure 19.22).

Although some organisms may be introduced at the time the IUD is being fitted, the uterine cavity is probably sterile within 48 hours and the risk of pelvic infection is only increased for about 20 days after insertion. The subsequent infection may be the result of the coil thread acting as a wick, up which organisms travel to the uterine cavity and subsequently to the tubes. The early literature strongly supported the wicking effect in the multithreaded Dalkon shield. Microscopic pits have been observed on the surface of the coil, and electron microscopy has shown that the plastic surface of the coil has become coated with cellular elements, the composition of which changes over time. Our own experience suggests that the human body sees the IUD as a foreign body, and attempts to ensheath it so as to seal it off.

SALPINGITIS ISTHMICA NODOSA

Definition

An uncommon abnormality of the fallopian tube, salpingitis isthmica nodosa (SIN) occurs in 1% of Caucasian women and 10% of black women whose mean age is 26 years. SIN consists of nodular swelling of the isthmic segment of the fallopian tube and is associated with diverticula of the lumen and smooth muscle proliferation. It has characteristic radiologic features and is significantly more common in women with ectopic pregnancy and infertility.

Pathology

SIN may be recognized grossly as a rounded, firm swelling, up to 2 cm in diameter, at the isthmic end of the tube (Figure 19.23), often merging with the cornual extremity of the uterus. The nodules are often bilateral and, occasionally, there may be more than one swelling on each tube. Most cases, however, cannot be detected macroscopically. The histologic appearances are striking and consist of a thickened wall due to hypertrophied musculature with epithelial-lined channels running between the muscle bundles and reaching close to the serosa (Figures 19.24 and 19.25). The epithelium lining these spaces is of normal, tubal type. The central lumen is always recognizable and the additional channels communicate with it and with each other, but not with the peritoneal cavity.

Histogenesis

The histogenesis of SIN remains unknown. Three alternatives are that:

- The condition is inflammatory.
- The outcome results from 'mechanical' pressure, analogous to diverticular disease of the large bowel.
- It is a condition analogous to adenomyosis in the uterus.

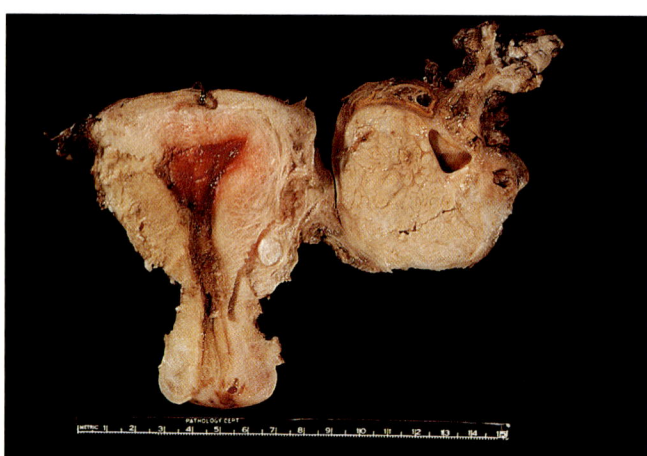

Fig. 19.21 *Actinomyces* infection causing a tubo-ovarian abscess.

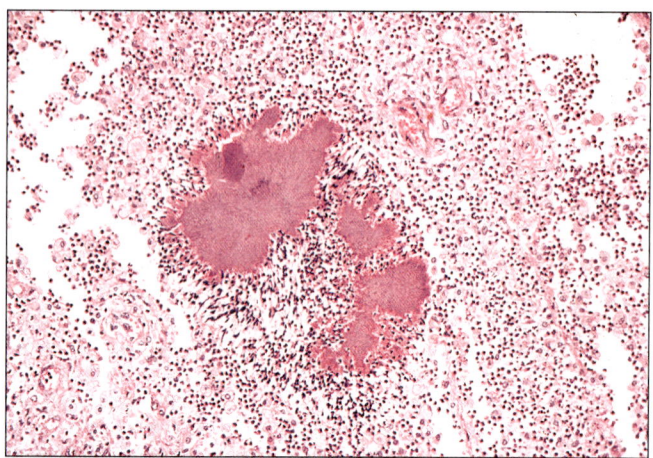

Fig. 19.22 *Actinomyces*-like organisms in pus.

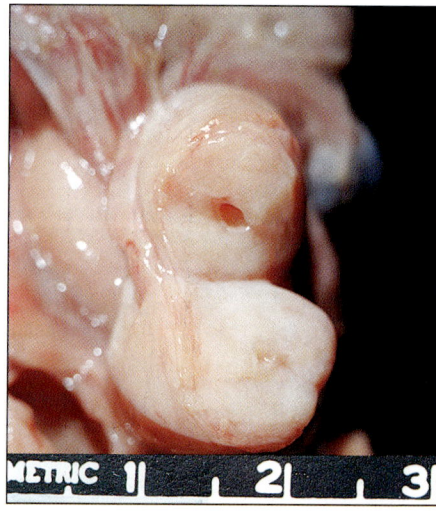

Fig. 19.23 Salpingitis isthmica nodosa. The firm, round, isthmic nodule is bisected to demonstrate the central lumen.

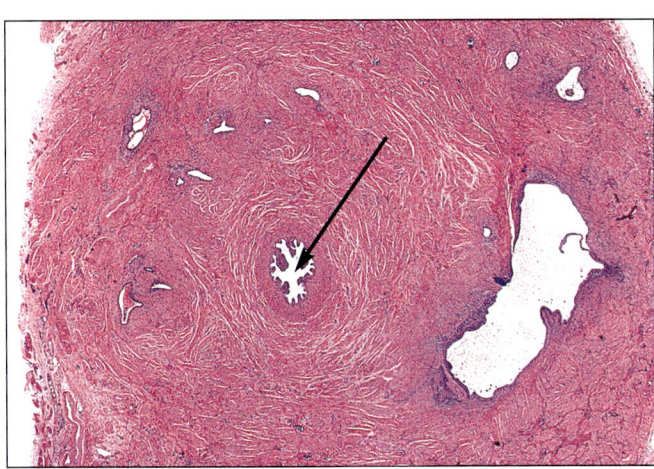

Fig. 19.24 Salpingitis isthmica nodosa. The original lumen is still discernible near the center (arrow). The wall of the tube is greatly thickened by muscular hypertrophy and separate channels are present throughout the wall.

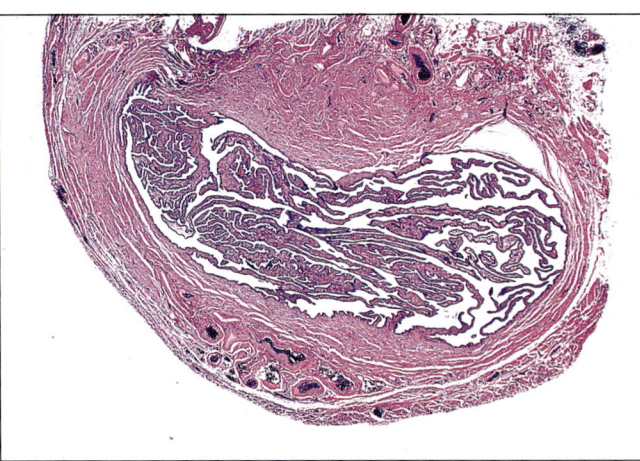

Fig. 19.26 Sterilization procedure, complete transection. This section of the tube shows the complete circumference of muscular wall surrounding the mucosa, confirming complete transection of the tube.

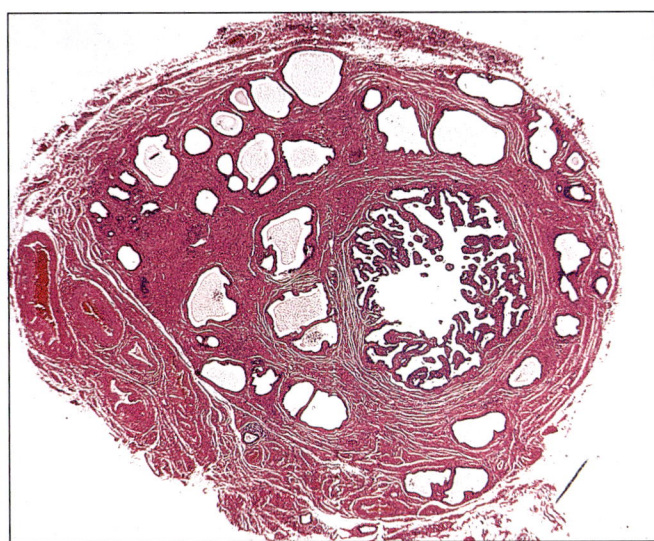

Fig. 19.25 Salpingitis isthmica nodosa.

That SIN is the result of inflammatory changes is unlikely because of its low incidence compared with salpingitis, its position in the isthmus (inflammatory changes are more often in the ampulla), and the absence of fibrosis and of a cellular infiltrate. In favor of the mechanical theory is the finding of continuity between the original lumen and the peripheral channels, as well as the demonstration of small, direct outpouchings of epithelium into the muscle, which appear to initiate the process. The analogy with diverticulosis of the sigmoid colon is strengthened by the occurrence of SIN in the most muscular segment of the tube. However, such pulsion diverticula would perhaps be simpler and more finger-like than the channels seen in SIN. The proposal that the condition is the tubal counterpart of adenomyosis seems the most plausible explanation of the findings.

Differential diagnosis

Salpingitis isthmica nodosa should be distinguished from endometriosis, chronic (infective) salpingitis, and neoplasia. A diag-

nosis of endometriosis requires the presence of endometrial-type stroma surrounding the epithelial component, the latter consisting predominantly of non-ciliated, columnar cells, although areas of ciliation may be seen. Stroma is absent in SIN, the epithelium abutting directly onto the muscle. The distinction from chronic salpingitis is made by identifying smooth muscle bundles, which usually are prominent between the multiplicity of epithelial channels in SIN. In the inflammatory condition the channels are formed by fusion of the plicae with the result that fibrous tissue only, not muscle, intervenes between the diverticula. SIN is distinguished from carcinoma by the regular distribution of widely spread glands, lack of nuclear atypia, and absence of a reactive stromal response.

TUBAL STERILIZATION

Thirty per cent of females over the age of 35 years in the UK have been sterilized.[24] Many methods are used, the most popular being the Pomeroy operation and methods incorporating the use of clips or rings. The Pomeroy operation is an open procedure in which a loop of the tubal isthmus is pulled up and ligated with an absorbable suture followed by excision of the isolated loop. Histologic examination provides evidence that the operation has been carried out properly. Clips are also widely used in the UK. The clips are placed over the isthmus, where the tube is thinnest, so that the tubal lumen is completely occluded. Falope rings, made of silastic, are placed over a loop of tube that is pulled up. The application of clips and rings is usually done as a laparoscopic procedure.

Pathology

An important aspect in the cut-up and preparation of the excised specimen for microscopic examination is that sufficient sections be made to show the complete cross-section of the tube (Figure 19.26). The details of cut-up are given (see Chapter 35). An efficient method is to cut the fallopian tube into sections no more than 1–2 mm thick so that usually a single slide contains up to six sections. In this manner, even if some sections are embedded improperly or cut on a bias, at least a few should show the complete cross-section, if in fact it is present. Any case where none of the pieces shows a complete cross-section should be reported as incomplete (Figure 19.27). The most common examples in our experience occur where the surgeon has removed arteries and fascia or only the tubal fimbria. In these cases, it commonly happens that the clinician had difficulty definitively identifying the fallopian tube, even though this information was not transmitted to the pathologist. It is most important that an incomplete ligation be clearly reported to the clinician, in part for medico-legal consideration. If the pathologist reports a complete ligation, where review of the slides reveals that only a portion of the tube is present but none where is there proof that the fallopian tube is completely transected, then the burden of negligence falls on the pathologist. In the event that a complete cross-section cannot be identified, it is also wise practice to personally communicate this fact to the clinician and document it in the report, so as to remove the pathologist from any form of contributory negligence.

Appearances following sterilization

The histopathologist frequently encounters the results of sterilization when examining hysterectomy specimens. The Pomeroy operation leaves a gap in the tube where a segment has been excised, usually 0.5–2 cm in the middle portion of the tube. Often, a clip or ring causes necrosis of the tissue that it has compressed, so that the clip or ring falls away, also leaving a defect, usually within 1 cm of the cornu. Frequently, particularly if the procedure has been carried out recently, the clip or ring is still in position on the fallopian tube, usually covered by a layer of newly formed peritoneum.

If the clip has been properly applied, microscopy of the tissue held between its jaws shows a markedly attenuated thin membrane, the consequences of pressure atrophy. It is not usually necessary, however, to separate the jaws of the clip and examine the tissue between, unless the sterilization has failed. The layer of 'neo-peritoneum' covering the clip often shows a sparse infiltrate of lymphocytes. Very occasional foreign-body giant cells may also be seen. The histologic changes associated with the presence of a clip on the tube are localized, and trans-verse sections taken a couple of millimeters to either side of the clip often show no abnormality. Frequently the narrow segment of tube between the clip and the uterine cornu shows some degree of dilatation and 'endometrial colonization'.

Examination of the fallopian tube following failed sterilization

The overall failure rate of female sterilization ranges from 2 to 10 per 1000 but as many as 45 failures per 1000 have been recorded when residents in training have applied the clips. Most failures associated with the application of clips are due to faulty technique, either because the wrong structure has been clipped (usually the round ligament) or because the tube has not been completely occluded.[24] Pregnancy may also result after tubal occlusion because of luteal-phase pregnancy or slippage of the clip.

When a failure has occurred, a further sterilization procedure will almost always be performed. This may be a repeat ligation but is more likely to be a bilateral salpingectomy or even hysterectomy. The gynecologist should be aware how important it is that the pathologist is informed that the specimen is from a failed sterilization and full details must be given on the histopathology request form. The pathologist is required to make a detailed gross examination of the specimens and issue a report that records the lengths of the specimens, the presence or absence of occlusive devices, and their exact positions. The specimens should be photographed (Figures 19.28 and 19.29). The clips are carefully examined for defects before they are removed from the specimens, which may require the dissection of the 'reperitonealized' layer from the surface. If there is a suspicion that the clip is defective, it should be removed carefully by unhooking the spring, separating the jaws and gently teasing the clip away from the included tissue, which will then allow close examination by the manufacturer if necessary. Blocks of tissue for processing are taken from the flattened portion of the tube held in the jaws of the clip. Step-serial, longitudinal sections can then be cut and examined, looking for evidence of a patent lumen and recanalization (Figure 19.30). Further transverse sections are taken from the tube on either side of the clip and randomly from the other parts of the

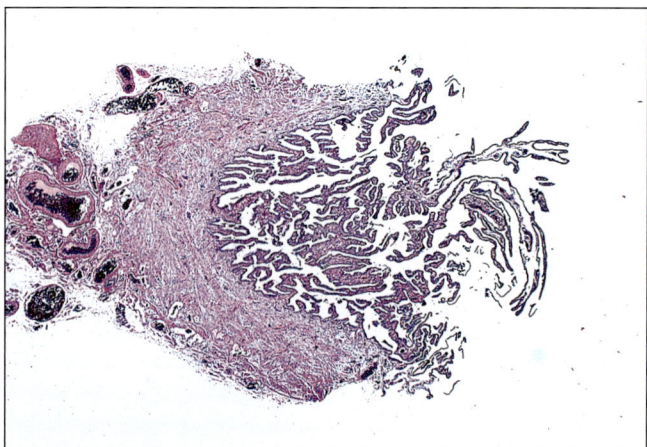

Fig. 19.27 Sterilization procedure, incomplete transection. This is one of many sections from this sterilization procedure. Although tubal mucosa and muscular wall are present, the muscle does not surround the mucosa completely so that the transection cannot be confirmed as complete.

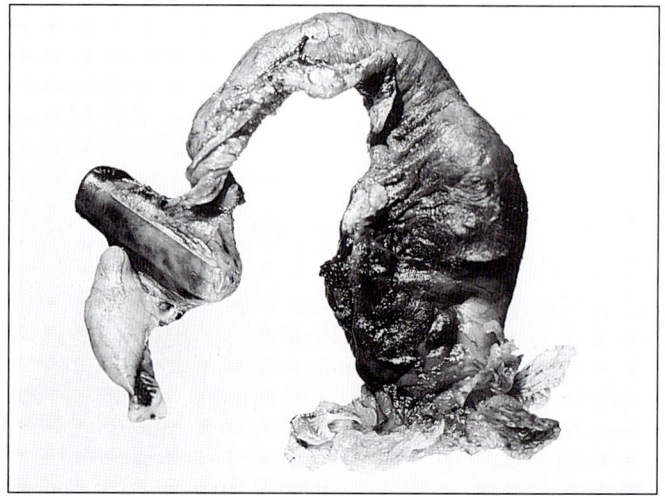

Fig. 19.28 Salpingectomy following failed sterilization. The Filshie clip appears to be correctly applied to the isthmic portion of the tube.

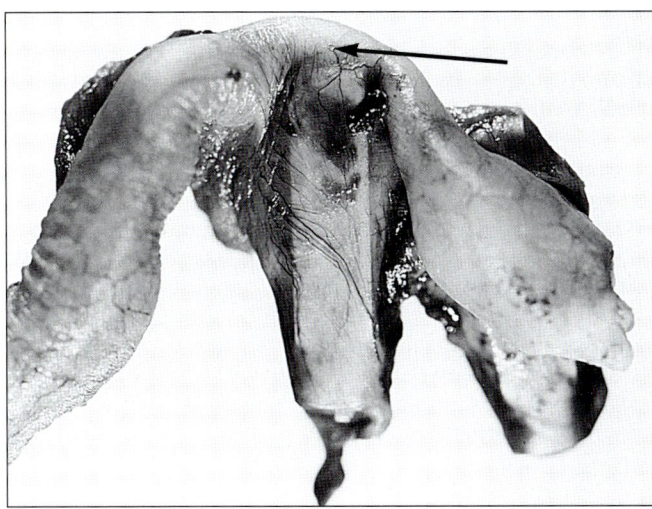

Fig. 19.29 Salpingectomy following failed sterilization. The jaws of the Filshie clip do not enclose the full diameter of the tube. A narrow portion (arrow) that contains the lumen is not compressed.

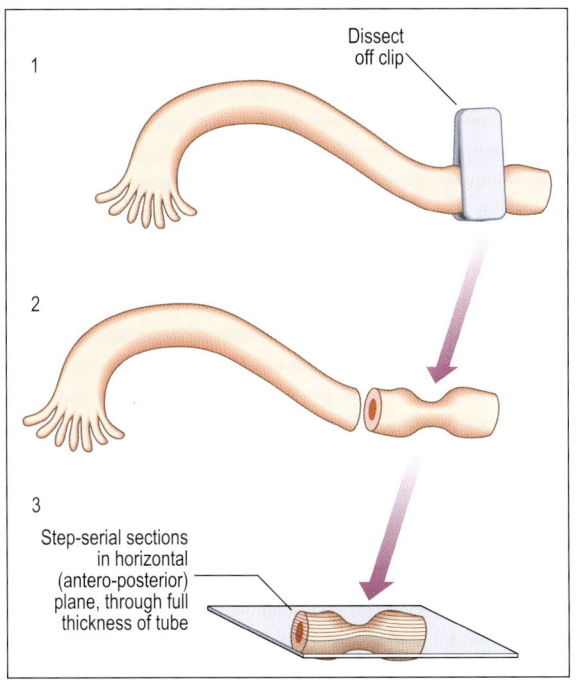

Fig. 19.30 Method of examining a salpingectomy specimen following failed sterilization if the clip appears to be correctly applied.

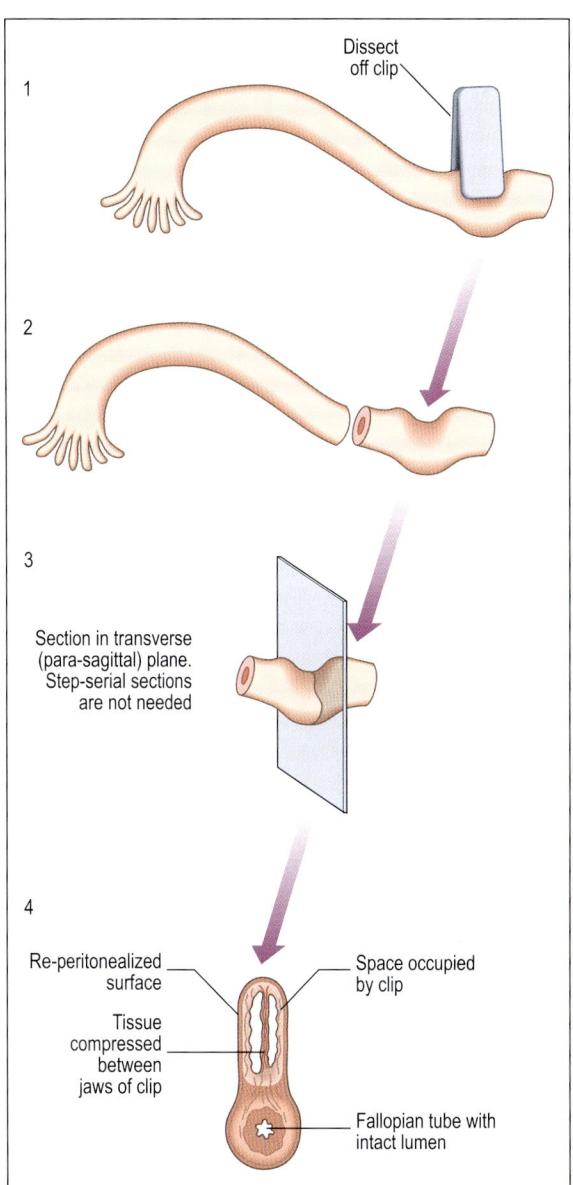

Fig. 19.31 Method of examining salpingectomy specimen following failed sterilization if the clip appears to compress only part of the diameter of the tube.

tube. If the device has been improperly applied, a section is taken in an appropriate plane to demonstrate a patent lumen running alongside the tissue defect that has been left after removal of the clip (Figure 19.31).

These methods of examination are clearly very different from those that will be carried out if the pathologist thinks that the specimen has come from a straightforward sterilization or reversal of sterilization. The specimen itself should alert the pathologist to the nature of the case because it is likely to be different from that received from either of the above procedures. However, it is the responsibility of the gynecologist to give the pathologist the necessary information, either personally or on the request form, so that the appropriate full examination is done.

TUBAL PREGNANCY

Etiology and pathogenesis

Any factor that impairs the tube's ability to transport the fertilized ovum will predispose to tubal implantation of the ovum. Hence, congenital tubal abnormalities, failed tubal sterilization, reconstructive tubal surgery, salpingitis isthmic nodosa, and, most importantly, postinflammatory tubal damage are all associated with an increased incidence of tubal pregnancies.[55]

The fertilized ovum may on occasion also implant in a normal tube. It has been argued that in these cases conception occurred during a cycle in which there was delayed ovulation and a shortened, inadequate luteal phase. The argument continues that as the corpus luteum began to decay, the conceptus had not yet reached a stage where its trophoblast was producing sufficient human chorionic gonadotropin (hCG) to prevent luteolysis. During the menstrual bleeding that then followed, the ovum was flushed back into the tube by a reflux of menstrual blood. Findings that support this hypothesis are that tubal gestation occurs only in humans and in primates that menstruate, and by the not uncommon finding that the tube with the pregnancy is on the side opposite to the corpus luteum of pregnancy. This latter phenomenon can also be due to transperitoneal or transuterine migration of the fertilized ovum into the contralateral tube where, due to its relatively advanced stage of development, it implants.

Natural history

Implantation occurs most commonly in the ampulla and may be plical, plicomural or mural. It may also occur in the isthmus and interstitial portion. The earliest stages of pregnancy usually proceed in a manner that does not differ in any significant respect from the same process in an intrauterine site. The complications of tubal abortion, hemorrhage or rupture soon supersede in all cases.

Tubal abortion   A high proportion of tubal pregnancies abort at an early stage and may be expelled from the fimbrial end of the tube. This is invariably the case if implantation has been fimbrial or plical, simply because these sites offer insufficient tissue for adequate placentation, but it is also seen with mural implantation. There is often intramural and intraluminal hemorrhage and subsequent fetal death. Following abortion, degenerating chorionic villi may be retained in the tube as so-called 'chronic ectopic pregnancy' or they may be expelled via the uterus or be gradually absorbed. Hyalinized ghost villi may be identified in the tube as an incidental finding many months later.[30]

Tubal hemorrhage   Although decidual change may be seen in the lamina propria of the fallopian tube, both at full term in segments excised for sterilization after delivery and in tubal pregnancy, the change is focal and poorly developed. In normal pregnancy in the uterine body, decidualized endometrium acts as a buffer that constrains trophoblastic invasion. In the absence of this buffering zone in a tubal pregnancy, trophoblast infiltrates destructively into the vessels and muscle of the tube wall, resulting in hemorrhage and rupture. Even if there is no rupture, hemorrhage is invariably present at the time of presentation of a tubal ectopic pregnancy. Massive hemorrhage into the uterine wall may result if the implantation is interstitial.

Tubal rupture   Tubal rupture complicates about 50% of cases of tubal pregnancy and appears to be due partly to the limited distensibility of the tube and partly to transmural trophoblastic invasion with penetration of the serosa. It is particularly likely to occur when the implantation is isthmic, because of this area's limited distensibility. Rupture is usually acute and is accompanied by intraperitoneal hemorrhage and the clinical features of an acute abdomen. Less commonly, there is a slow leakage of tubal contents and blood from the tube, which results in a gradually enlarging peritubal hematoma and causes

dense adhesions between the tube and surrounding structures such as omentum and intestines. Occasionally, the ureters obstruct as a result of involvement in this peritubal mass. Although tubal rupture usually results in fetal death, the fetus occasionally retains sufficient attachment to its blood supply to maintain its viability. The trophoblast grows out through the rupture site and forms a secondary placental site in the abdomen or broad ligament. A secondary abdominal pregnancy of this type can occasionally proceed to term. Few tubal pregnancies proceed to term without rupture of the viscus.

Pathology

Tubal changes   The fallopian tube, as received by the pathologist after salpingectomy, can show a range of appearances that vary with the site of nidation, viability of the fetus, duration of pregnancy, and presence or absence of rupture. In typical cases the tube is focally or generally distended whilst the peritoneal surface is congested and sometimes inflamed (Figure 19.32). The fimbrial ostium can be occluded by blood clot or blood may be oozing from the ostium. If rupture has occurred, blood clot and placental tissue are sometimes seen protruding through the rupture site (Figure 19.33), and blood clot may envelop the tube. On opening the tube a complete amniotic sac and fetus is occasionally seen (Figures 19.34 and 19.35). More commonly, the lumen contains only fresh and old blood clot (Figure 19.36).

Histologic examination is usually required to confirm the diagnosis of tubal gestation (Figure 19.37). A critical aspect is determination of the tissue to be submitted for microscopic examination. In nearly all cases, any tissue within the blood clot will contain chorionic villi. Occasionally, they will be attached to the tubal wall. The villi may appear fully normal, but more often show postmortem change such as fibrosis or hydropic swelling. Dysmorphic changes, associated with chromosomal anomalies or molar change (e.g. triploidy), are only rarely seen as these do not constitute the cause for the pregnancy loss. In some cases many sections of the blood clot have to be examined before placental villi are seen. In the rare case no residual villous tissue will be found, the only detectable abnormalities being the presence of inflammatory debris and non-specific granulation tissue. A reticulin stain on the 'blood

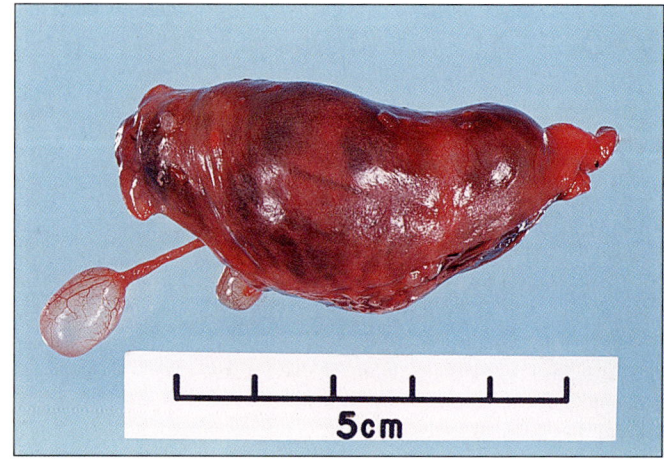

Fig. 19.32   Tubal ectopic pregnancy.

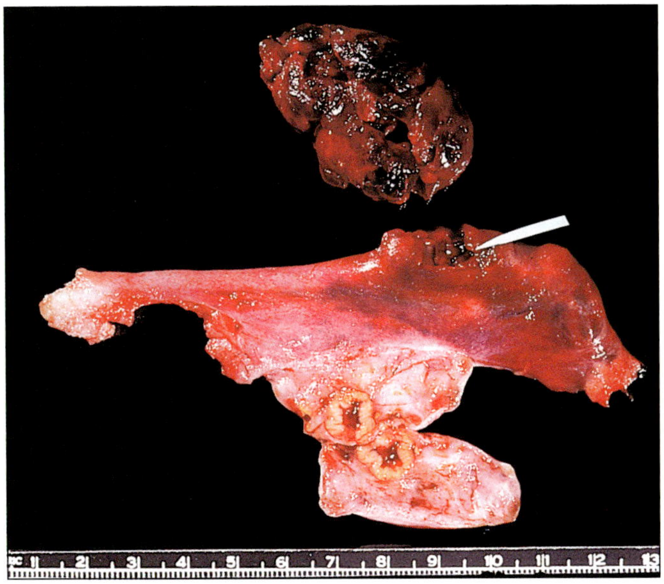

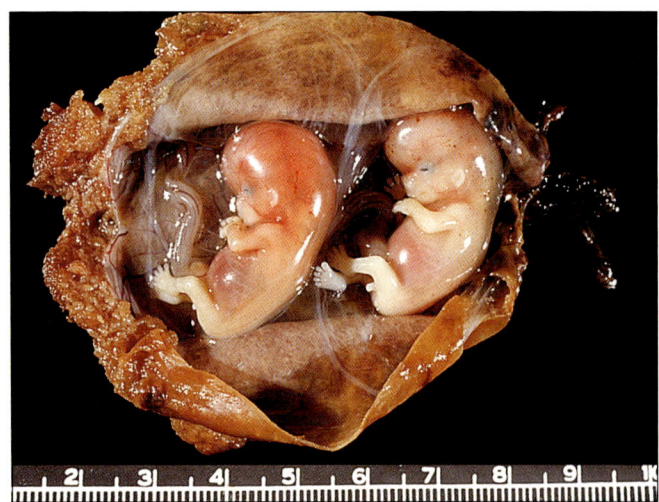

Fig. 19.35 Tubal ectopic pregnancy. Twin fetuses are present.

Fig. 19.33 Ruptured tubal ectopic pregnancy.

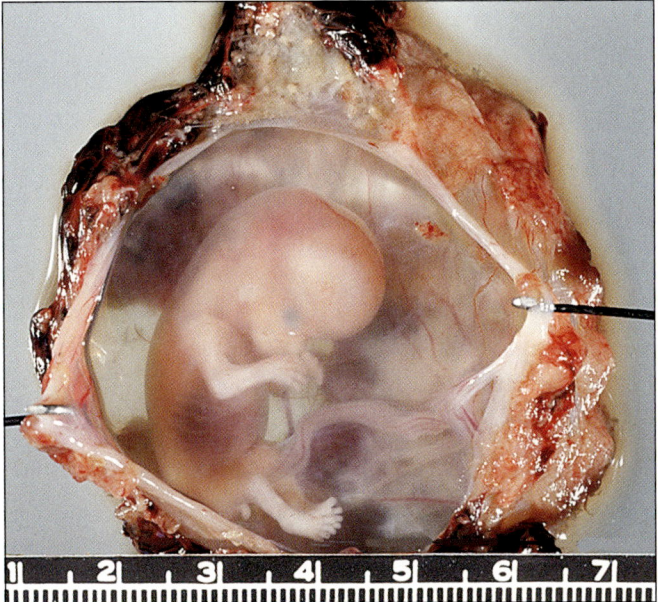

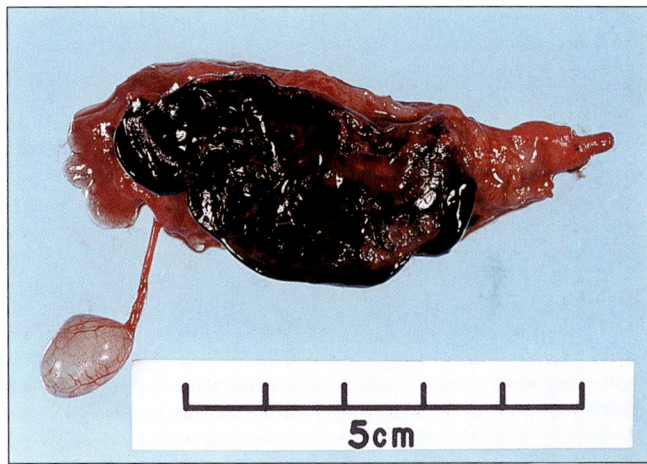

Fig. 19.36 Tubal ectopic pregnancy. Sectioning shows only blood clot.

Fig. 19.34 Tubal ectopic pregnancy. A fetus is present.

clot' is very often helpful as it highlights the outline of dead villi that are inapparent in the H&E sections. Even in such circumstances, however, an implantation site can often be identified by the presence of extra villous trophoblastic cells that have infiltrated the tubal wall and invaded the vascular spaces. Curiously, tubal tissue more than a short distance from the region of the ectopic pregnancy may show no abnormality other than a minor degree of non-specific inflammation. It is important to take a block from the fallopian tube medial to the implantation site to assess the presence or absence of pre-existing salpingitis, usually manifest as plical adhesions, as this offers not only some pointer as to a likely cause of the present ectopic, but is useful in the further management of the patient. Salpingitis is usually bilateral and a

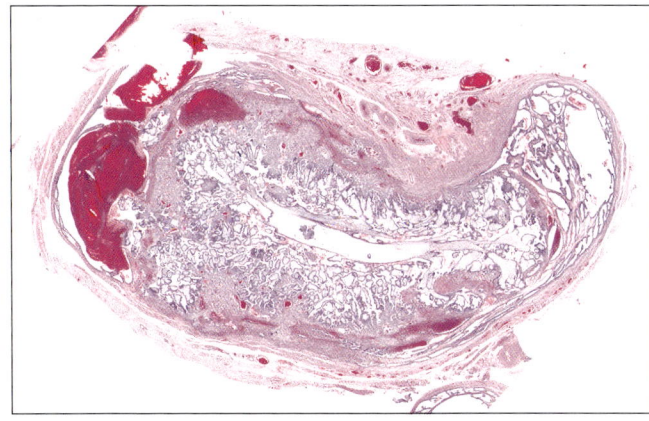

Fig. 19.37 Tubal ectopic pregnancy, showing a virtually intact gestation sac. Chorionic villi are easily identifiable. A tiny fragment of embryo is present in the gestational sac itself. The fallopian tube parenchyma (right) shows evidence of old healed salpingitis with confluent plicae.

second ectopic in the contralateral tube is more likely in such patients (who frequently end up having some form of assisted conception).

Laparoscopic salpingostomy Although salpingectomy offers almost a 100% cure, laparoscopic methods are widely used that not only prevent death but also allow rapid recovery, preserve fertility, and reduce costs.[12] Linear salpingostomy is now the standard laparoscopic operation when an ectopic pregnancy is unruptured but measures more than 4 cm by ultrasound. The products of conception are removed after an incision is made along the bulging antimesenteric border of the tube. The specimen the pathologist receives consists mainly of blood clot but frequently contains chorionic villi and trophoblastic fragments, enabling the diagnosis to be confirmed.

Uterine changes In tubal pregnancies the uterine endometrium undergoes decidual change to a degree compatible to that found in an intrauterine pregnancy in about 45% of cases.[55] The endometrial glands are hypersecretory and an Arias-Stella change is seen focally in 60–70% of cases showing gestational changes. These appearances can, however, occur in any type of pregnancy and are not a specific feature of an ectopic gestation. In contrast to intrauterine pregnancies, curetted material shows little necrosis or inflammation. Indeed, this often is an important clue to the presence of an ectopic pregnancy. Depending on the time interval between fetal demise and curettage, the endometrium may show relatively poorly formed secretory changes, be inactive or even proliferative. In evaluating a curettage or biopsy specimen as part of a clinically suspected ectopic pregnancy, we have never personally encountered the situation where there was a documented pregnancy in the fallopian tube and chorionic villi were simultaneously found in the endometrial cavity. However, the pathologist must always be aware that villi are easily dislodged during tissue processing and may be artifactually introduced as contaminants into another case. Clues as to this possibility include position of the villi relative to other tissue fragments, lack of implantation site in the maternal tissues, and discordance between villous maturity and clinically suspected ectopic gestational age.

NON-NEOPLASTIC LESIONS

METAPLASIAS

As in the cervix and endometrium, it is questionable whether the finding of a type of müllerian epithelium that is inappropriate to the site should strictly be referred to as 'metaplasia'. Nevertheless, the presence of mucinous epithelium and endometrial epithelium in the fallopian tube mucosa must be considered abnormal.

MUCINOUS METAPLASIA

This is an extremely rare finding in which mucinous epithelium, similar to that found in the normal endocervix, replaces areas of tubal epithelium (Figure 19.38). Mucinous metaplasia may occur in women with Peutz–Jeghers syndrome and may be associated with both ovarian and cervical mucinous tumors.

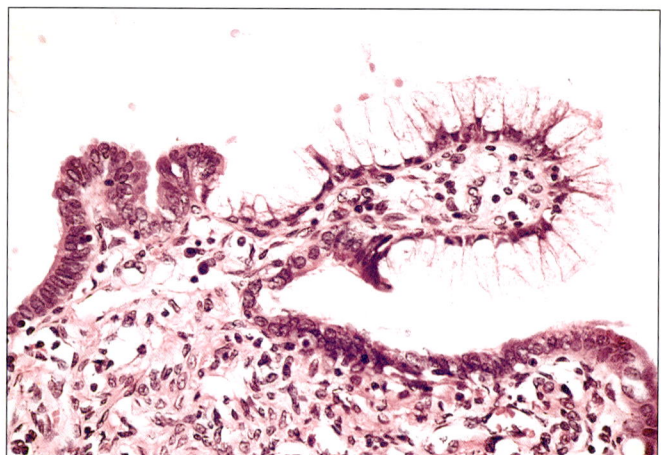

Fig. 19.38 Mucinous metaplasia.

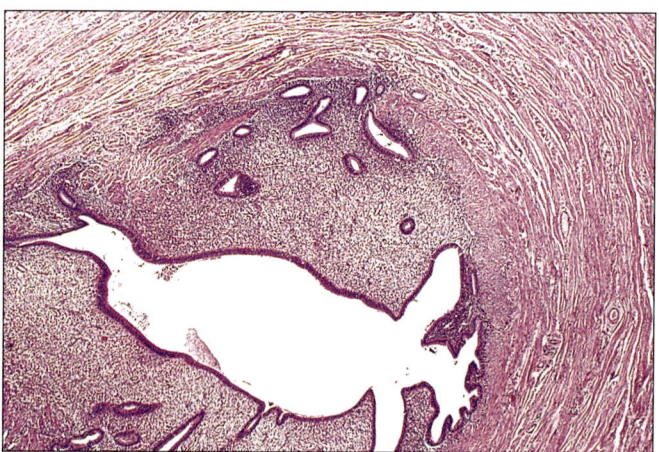

Fig. 19.39 Endometrial replacement ('endometrialization or endometrial colonization'). Endometrial glands and stroma replace the tubal mucosa in the isthmus.

These findings suggest that some tubal mucinous metaplasia may represent mucosal spread from a mucinous neoplasm elsewhere in the female genital tract.

ENDOMETRIAL REPLACEMENT AND ENDOMETRIOSIS

Uterine endometrium is sometimes found in the interstitial and isthmic segments of the fallopian tube (Figure 19.39). This change is identified both as an incidental finding in hysterectomy specimens and, more significantly, in cornual resections for infertility. The lesion represents a shift of the junction between endometrium and fallopian tube mucosa into the fallopian tube. It may be considered a normal morphologic variation even though it is often called 'endometriosis' or 'endometrial colonization'. This phenomenon, which may be related to the micro environment adaptation, is often encountered in histologic examination of the tubal proximal stump, usually 1–4 years after tubal ligation. The interstitial and isthmic segments of the fallopian tube occur in up to 25% and 10% of women, respectively.[60] Endometrial colonization can also be caused by complete occlusion of the fallopian tube. It accounts for

15–20% of cases of infertility and may be associated with tubal pregnancy.[60]

Typical or serosal tubal endometriosis is most commonly associated with endometriosis elsewhere in the pelvis. In this condition, the myosalpinx and mucosa are not usually involved. In some cases of pelvic endometriosis, with or without tubal involvement, the plicae are expanded by masses of pseudoxanthoma cells, a lesion called pseudoxanthomatous salpingitis or pseudoxanthomatous salpingiosis.

TRANSITIONAL METAPLASIA

Walthard rests are extremely common, small collections of cells, rarely more than 1 mm or so in diameter, situated immediately beneath the tubal serosa (Figures 19.40 and 19.41). The cells are of rather nondescript type but some show longitudinal grooves in the nuclear membrane, resembling the appearance seen in Brenner tumor of the ovary. There is speculation that the cells of the Walthard rest and Brenner tumor arise in the same way, by transitional cell metaplasia of the serosal mesothelium. Walthard rests are most often seen on the outer third of the tube and on the mesosalpinx and seem particularly frequent when adhesions bind the tube and ovary together. They

may be solid or cystic. Walthard rests are of no significance whatsoever, apart from the importance of being recognized grossly for what they are and not mistaken clinically for pelvic tuberculosis, endometriosis, or disseminated tumor. Grossly, Walthard rests are clear to tan-white soft nodules, usually less than 1 mm in diameter (Figure 19.42).

Compared with the very common transitional cell metaplasia of the serosa that Walthard rests represent, transitional cell metaplasia of the mucosa is extremely rare. It is likely that this is the same change that is described as 'reserve cell metaplasia' and may serve as a possible source of tubal transitional cell carcinomas.[23]

OTHER FORMS OF METAPLASIA

Squamous metaplasia and oncocytic metaplasia are both extremely rare.

DECIDUAL CHANGE

The stromal cells of the fallopian tube lamina propria readily undergo decidual change (Figure 19.43). It is seen in about one-third of salpingectomy specimens containing ectopic

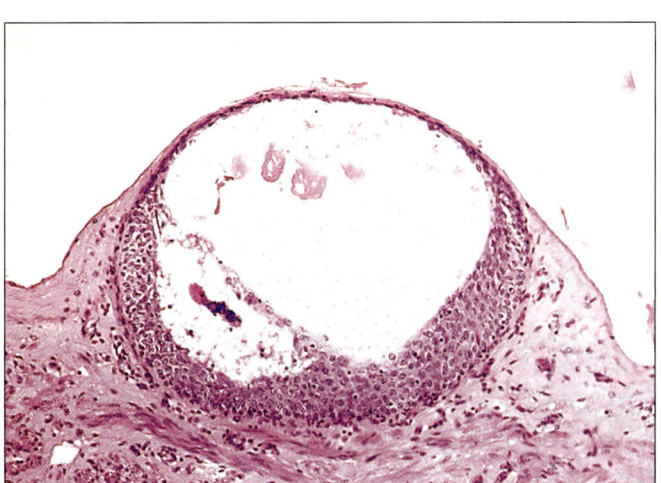

Fig. 19.40 Walthard rest.

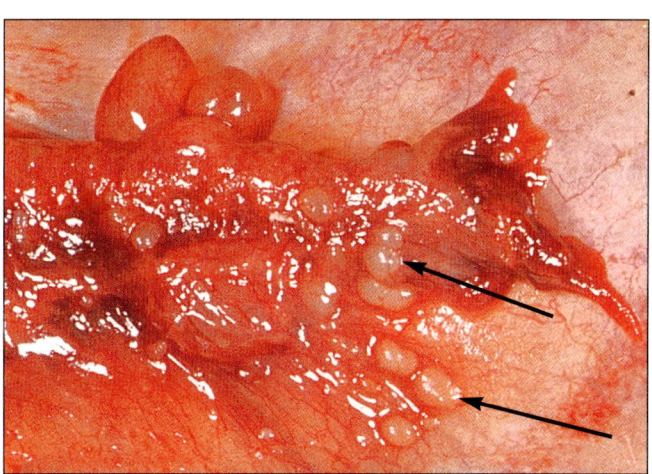

Fig. 19.42 Walthard rests. Cystic Walthard rests (arrows) are present on the surface of the tube.

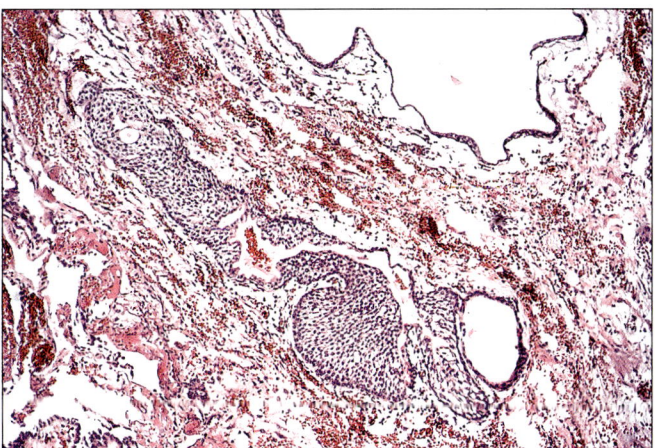

Fig. 19.41 Walthard rest.

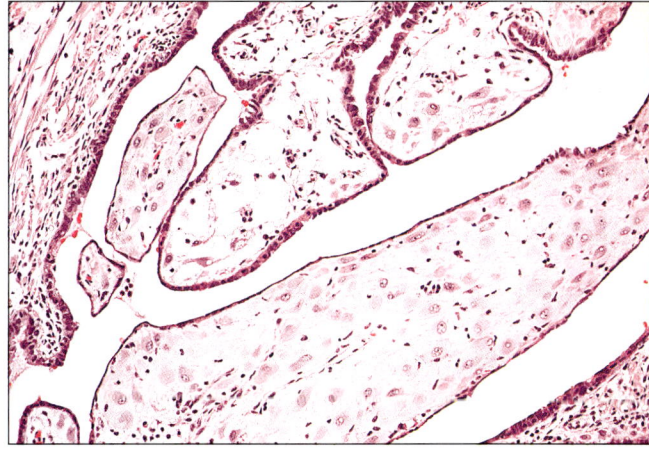

Fig. 19.43 Decidual change.

pregnancies, and in 5–8% of tubal segments excised for sterilization performed during cesarean section or in the immediate postpartum period.[60]

TORSION OF THE FALLOPIAN TUBE

The fallopian tube usually undergoes torsion with the ovary. Both become twisted together, often because the ovary is enlarged. However, torsion may affect either organ independently and the tube is particularly at risk if it is diseased, as with a hydrosalpinx. The torsed tube is swollen and dark red-blue (Figure 19.44). Microscopy shows marked congestion initially (Figure 19.45), followed by infarction.

PROLAPSE OF THE FALLOPIAN TUBE

Tubal prolapse occurs occasionally after a hysterectomy, especially with vaginal hysterectomy. On clinical examination, a lesion simulating granulation tissue is seen at the vaginal apex. A misdiagnosis of papillary adenocarcinoma may happen if the

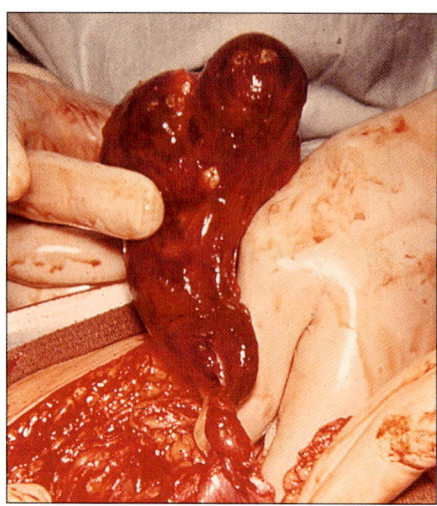

Fig. 19.44 Torsion of the tube. A hydrosalpinx is present, an abnormality that precipitated twisting.

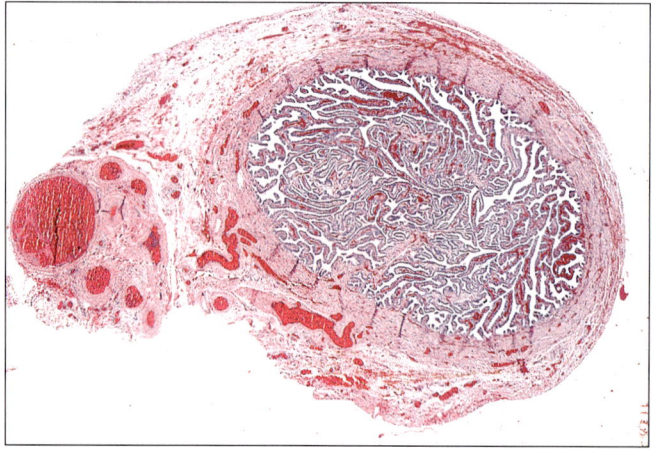

Fig. 19.45 Torsion of the tube. At this early stage there is marked congestion. Infarction may follow.

tubal plicae and their lining of bland epithelium are not correctly recognized (see Chapter 5).

MUCOSAL EPITHELIAL PROLIFERATION

Definition

Proliferation of the mucosal epithelium is a condition of the fallopian tube epithelium in which there is an increase in epithelial thickness with crowding and stratification of nuclei but lacking the histologic features of carcinoma. The change occurs in nearly one-fifth of otherwise normal tubes. This finding is often associated with unopposed estrogenic stimulation and serous borderline ovarian tumors but may occur without any known predisposing conditions.

Microscopic features

The epithelium is thickened and shows stratified nuclei, nuclear crowding, loss of polarity, nuclear atypia, and small papillary tufts, but sparse mitotic figures (Figure 19.46). The nuclear atypia appears as elongated and slightly enlarged nuclei with an increased nuclear:cytoplasmic ratio in the hyperplastic cells. The chromatin of the hyperplastic cells is finely granular. One or two small nucleoli are usually observed in each cell. The changes are seen more frequently in association with salpingitis. It is known that a mild degree of epithelial proliferation is encountered frequently and that note should therefore only be taken of a moderate or marked degree of the change, which is rarely encountered (3% of cases) in normal tubes obtained for sterilization or hysterectomy specimens. In contrast, epithelial proliferation of moderate or marked degree occurs in 25% to over 40% of tubes accompanying a wide variety of neoplastic conditions.[67] However, progression of these proliferative conditions to invasive tubal carcinoma has not been documented. The significance of this condition, therefore, cannot yet be assessed with certainty.

EPITHELIAL PROLIFERATION ASSOCIATED WITH SALPINGITIS

Definition

Reactive hyperplasia of tubal epithelium that is associated with tuberculous and non-tuberculous salpingitis. It may be

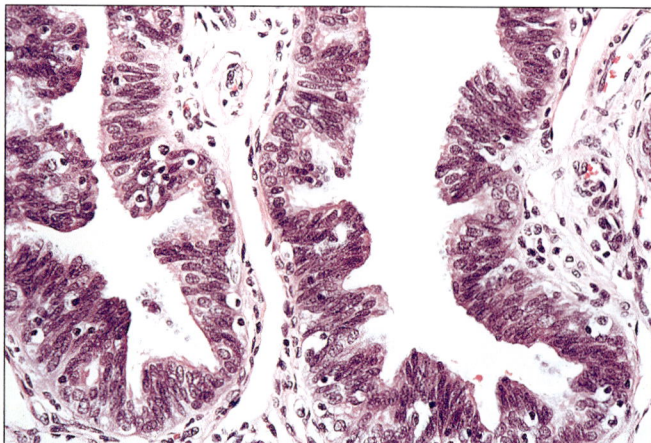

Fig. 19.46 Mucosal epithelial proliferation.

mistaken for carcinoma since the salpingitis may present as pseudocarcinomatous hyperplasia.[15]

Microscopic features

This change results in the formation of multiple small glandular structures, often arranged in a highly complex pattern, amid inflamed, often edematous tubal plicae (Figures 19.47–19.49). The complexity of the architectural pattern is compounded by the fusion of adjacent plicae, resulting in a striking back-to-back pseudoglandular pattern or a sieve-like pattern.[15] Epithelial stratification is often present and there may be loss of nuclear polarity. Nuclear atypia is of a mild-to-moderate degree only. Nucleoli are prominent in only half of the cases. Mitotic figures are rarely observed and these are normal. Moderate-to-marked chronic inflammatory changes are, of course, always present.

Reactive atypical hyperplasia may be distinguished from adenocarcinoma by the lack of solid epithelial areas, a feature nearly always seen in tubal carcinoma, the presence of only mild-to-moderate nuclear atypia and sparse, normal mitotic figures. Adenocarcinoma commonly shows moderate to severe atypia with prominent nucleoli and frequent mitotic figures.

TUMORS OF THE FALLOPIAN TUBE

Primary tubal neoplasms, most of which are malignant, are rare and uncommonly diagnosed preoperatively. Their WHO classification is shown in Table 19.1.[60] Because most tumors are so rare, only a few are covered below.

BENIGN TUMORS

ADENOMATOID TUMOR

Definition

The adenomatoid tumor, also referred to as 'benign mesothelioma', is the most common benign tumor of the fallopian tube but, nevertheless, is rare. It is always an incidental finding, usually in women who are in middle age or elderly, and is never symptomatic. Similar tumors are found in the uterus and ovary. Multiple small, slit-like or ovoid spaces lined by a single layer of flattened epithelium-like cells typify this condition.

Pathology

The adenomatoid tumor appears as a round or oval nodule, usually 1–3 cm in diameter, distending the tube (Figure 19.50). It is usually subserosal and in the outer wall, although it may be confined to the endosalpinx or spread throughout the wall. The neoplasm shows numerous slit-like, ovoid and round spaces of various sizes, separated by bands of connective tissue (Figure 19.51). The spaces are lined by a single layer of low cuboidal or flattened cells with eosinophilic cytoplasm and oval nuclei (Figures 19.52–19.54). The tumor is not encapsulated and infiltrates the muscle of the tubal wall at its margins.

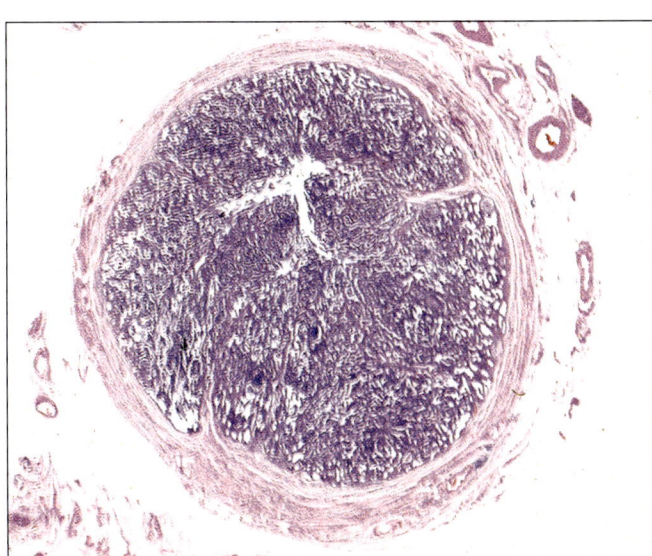

Fig. 19.47 Epithelial proliferation associated with salpingitis. The diameter of the tube is greatly increased by what appears to be solid tissue.

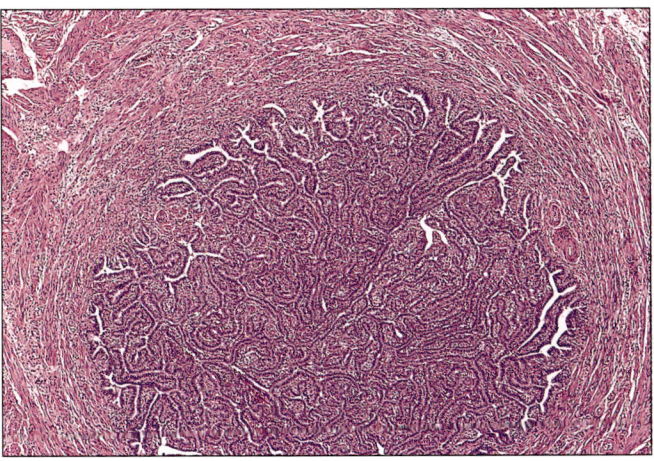

Fig. 19.48 Epithelial proliferation associated with salpingitis.

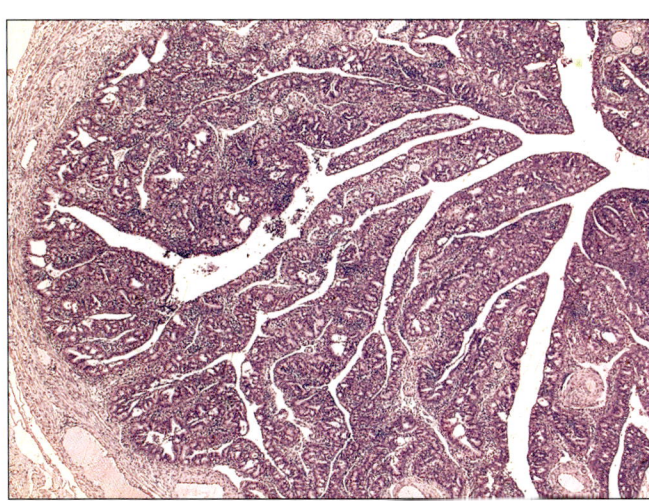

Fig. 19.49 Epithelial proliferation associated with salpingitis. At higher power, the combination of inflammatory infiltrate and epithelial proliferation is apparent.

Table 19.1 WHO classification of tumors of the fallopian tube

- *Epithelial tumors*
  Benign
      Endometrioid polyp
      Papilloma
      Metaplastic papillary tumor
  Malignant
      Adenocarcinoma *in situ*
      Serous adenocarcinoma
      Mucinous adenocarcinoma
      Endometrioid adenocarcinoma
      Clear cell adenocarcinoma
      Transitional cell carcinoma
      Squamous cell carcinoma
      Mixed carcinoma
      Undifferentiated carcinoma

- *Mixed epithelial–mesenchymal tumors*
  Malignant
      Adenosarcoma
      Carcinosarcoma

- *Soft tissue tumors*
  Benign
      Leiomyoma
      Others
  Malignant
      Leiomyosarcoma
      Others

- *Mesothelial tumors*
  Solitary mesothelioma
  Adenomatoid tumor

- *Germ cell tumors*
  Teratoma
  Mature
      Dermoid cyst
      Solid
  Immature
  Struma
  Carcinoid
  Others

- *Trophoblastic disease*
  Hydatidiform mole
  Choriocarcinoma

- *Secondary tumors*

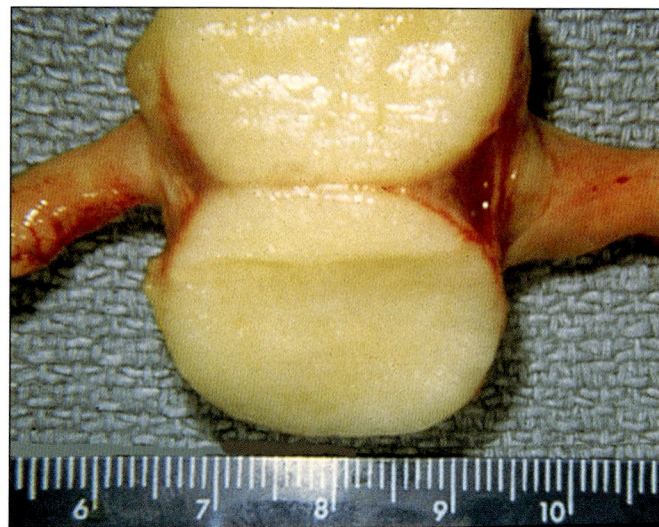

Fig. 19.50 Adenomatoid tumor.

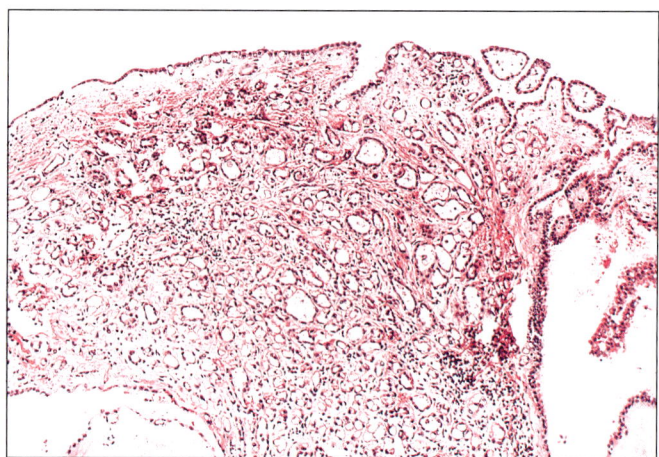

Fig. 19.51 Adenomatoid tumor, which at low-power magnification discloses numerous slit-like, ovoid, and round spaces of various sizes, separated by bands of connective tissue.

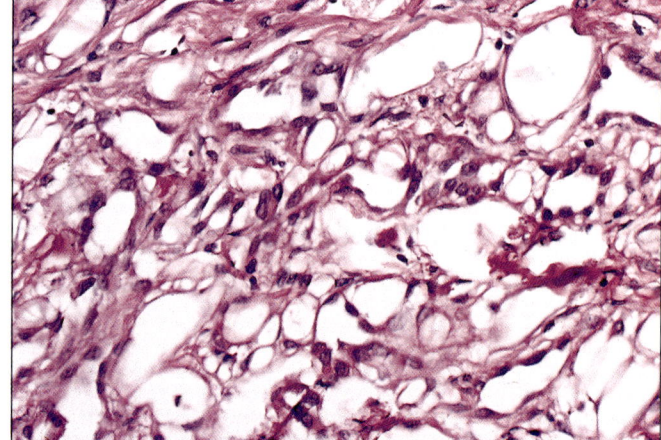

Fig. 19.52 Adenomatoid tumor disclosing slit-like, ovoid, and round spaces of various sizes.

The main interest in these clinically unimportant tumors is in their histogenesis. Suggestions of their origin include mesonephric, vascular, lymphatic, müllerian, and mesothelial derivation. Electron microscopic and, more recently, immunohistochemical studies indicate it is of mesothelial origin.

METAPLASTIC PAPILLARY TUMOR

These rare lesions have been identified as incidental findings in tubal segments excised postpartum for sterilization.[60] They are composed of papillary nests of budding, proliferating cells with abundant eosinophilic cytoplasm (Figures 19.55 and 19.56). Rare mitotic figures may be seen. Whether these are genuine

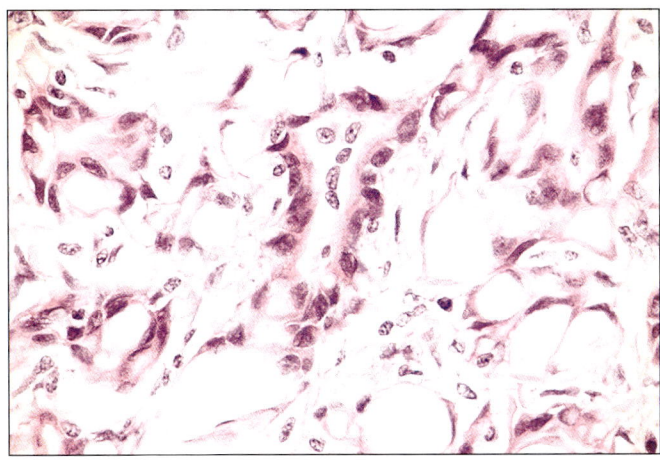

Fig. 19.53 Adenomatoid tumor with variation in appearances.

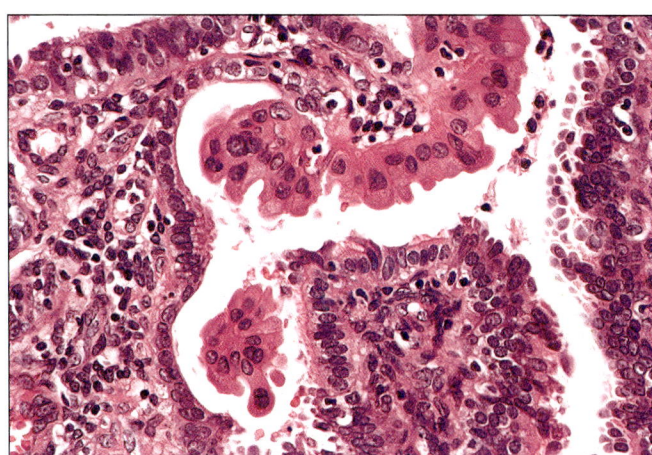

Fig. 19.56 Metaplastic papillary lesion of pregnancy.

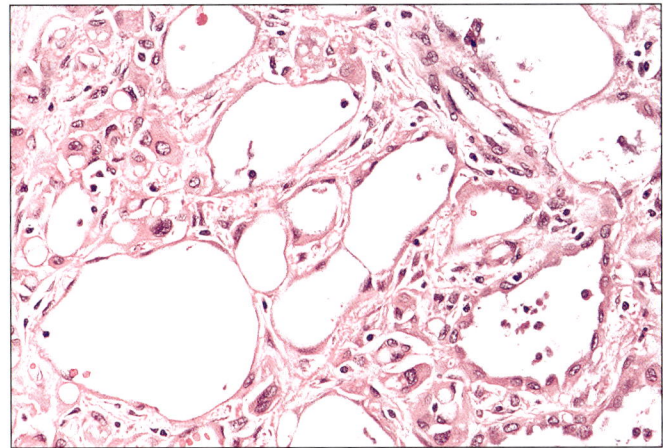

Fig. 19.54 Adenomatoid tumor with lymphatic-like channels.

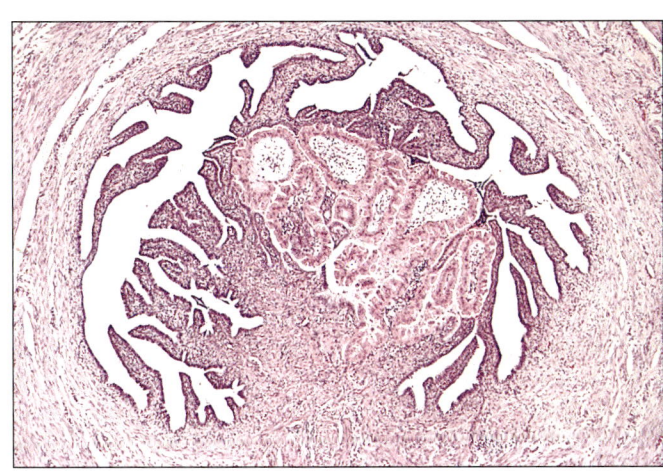

Fig. 19.55 Metaplastic papillary lesion of pregnancy.

neoplastic lesions or the result of metaplasia and proliferation occurring during pregnancy is not known.

LEIOMYOMAS

Leiomyomas are rare compared with the uterine variety and are usually small.[59]

OTHER BENIGN TUMORS

Of the rare benign tumors, about 50 mature cystic teratomas (dermoid cysts) have been reported, nearly all as incidental findings.[33] It resembles grossly and histologically the ovarian mature cystic teratoma. It is thought to arise from misplaced germ cells, in this case extragonadal.

Rare examples of placental site nodule[10,46] and placental site trophoblastic tumor[63] have also been reported in the fallopian tube. Occasional serous cystadenomas resemble their ovarian counterparts, and rare papillomas, ranging up to 3 cm in diameter, may occur in tubal lumen.

Very rare neoplasms are neurilemmoma, lipoma, chondroma, lymphangioma, ganglioneuroma, and hemangioma.[60]

BORDERLINE TUMORS

Compared with their ovarian counterparts, borderline tumors of the fallopian tube are uncommon, with limited experience about their clinical behavior. Most of the very limited number are serous and a very rare case is endometrioid.[4,32,72] Primary mucinous borderline tumor has never been reported. When such cases are encountered, secondary spread to the tube from an undetected appendiceal mucinous tumor should always be excluded first.

The serous borderline tumor of the fallopian tube shows formation of papillary projections with focally prominent epithelial stratification and atypia. None has recurred, suggesting that these extremely uncommon tumors can be managed conservatively.[72]

MALIGNANT TUMORS

ADENOCARCINOMA *IN SITU* (AIS)

Adenocarcinoma *in situ* (AIS) is commonly called carcinoma *in situ* (CIS). This lesion, invisible macroscopically, shows replacement of the normal tubal epithelium by obviously malignant cells, with nuclear atypia, prominent nucleoli, and mitotic activity similar to that of tubal carcinoma cells (Figure 19.57). The epithelium is flat or only slightly papillary. This lesion is most commonly found in women with breast cancer or in *BRCA* mutation carriers,[42,51] who today have prophylactic oophorectomy with incidental salpingectomy, performed at a time long before the lesion in the tube has had a chance to develop into an overt cancer. In older women, the diagnosis of AIS should be made with some degree of caution. Not uncommonly, we have seen cases in which what initially seems to be AIS proves not to be. With additional sections, more obvious tumor in the fallopian tube was apparent that had refluxed from a primary tumor in the endometrium. Also, AIS is not an uncommon finding in women with ovarian serous, peritoneal or endometrial carcinoma.[71] What is actually *in situ* tumor and what represents implanted cancer cluster is not always clear. How such changes should be interpreted is a function of one's view of the nature of serous neoplasia and subject to the same mindset alluded to above. One striking feature of tubal AIS is that the majority of tumor cells show diffuse strong p53 nuclear staining. This is helpful when the morphologic diagnosis is in doubt.

ADENOCARCINOMA

Definition

A malignant tumor arising from the epithelium of the fallopian tube mucosa.

General features

Primary malignant tumors of the fallopian tube are rare; secondary tumors are much more common. Of tumors arising elsewhere that can affect the tube, ovarian carcinoma is the most frequent and because of the histologic similarity between the most common of the ovarian carcinomas – the serous adenocarcinoma and primary tubal carcinoma – strict criteria must be applied before rendering a diagnosis of tubal carcinoma.[61] The bulk of the tumor must lie in the tube, its histologic appearance must reflect the features of tubal epithelium, and the ovary and uterus must be normal or contain less tumor than the tube. In addition, if intact mucosa is left, a transition from benign to malignant epithelium is helpful. Using these criteria, genuine primary carcinoma of the fallopian tube is indeed rare, comprising only 0.3% of malignant gynecologic tumors with an annual incidence rate of about 5 per million women.[28] Of course, these diagnostic criteria would necessarily exclude a tumor that has arisen in the tube and has then spread to engulf the ovary, resulting in a tumor mass that involves both organs. In these circumstances the tumor would usually be designated as of ovarian origin, a function of the currently prevailing mindset, and, in our view, not wholly valid.

Tubal carcinogenesis and the putative precursor lesions of tubal carcinomas

Because tubal carcinoma is so rare, little is known about its pathogenesis. The incidence is higher in nulliparous compared with parous women, but there is no evidence of any increased incidence in women on hormone treatment. New evidence suggests that altered *p53* and *BRCA* tumor suppressor genes may be related to the occurrence of tubal carcinoma. Altered *p53* was found in over half[71] to all[54] tubal AIS. Nearly all of the *p53* reactive cases in one series showed transitions from negative to either partial positive and then uniformly strong positive or abruptly to strong positive that corresponded at high magnification to atypical glandular epithelium consisting of cells with more hyperchromatic and larger nuclei with coarser chromatin than adjacent *p53* unreactive epithelial cells.

In an unpublished study of high-risk patients with either ovarian or breast cancer or known *BRCA* mutations, up to half of the tubal epithelium with atypical morphologic changes but

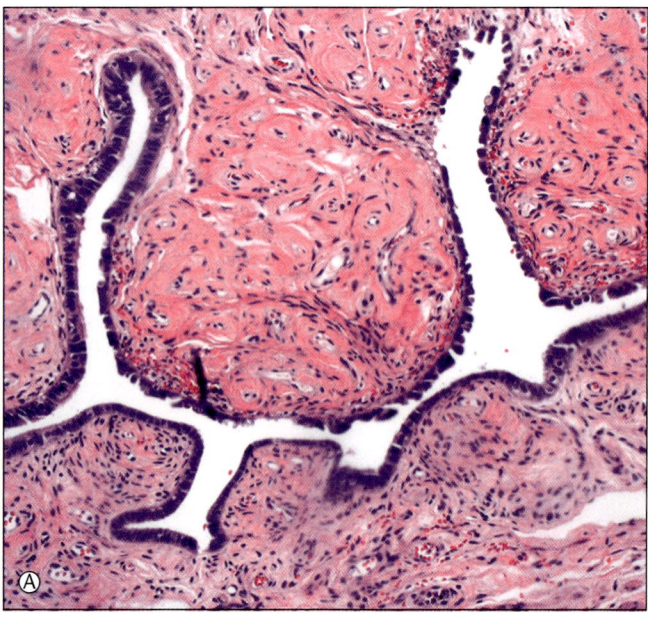

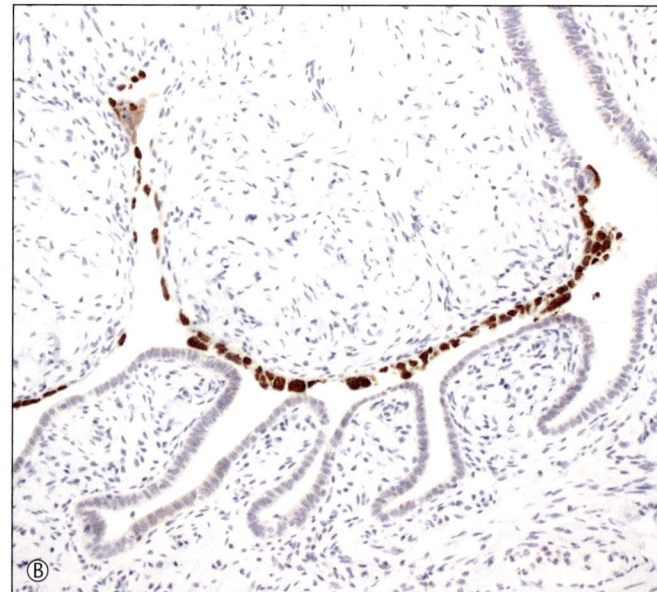

Fig. 19.57 Atypical tubal epithelium with positive *p53* nuclear reactivity.

falling short of CIS showed diffuse overexpression of *p53* (Figure 19.58). A similar finding of common *p53* alteration in dysplastic tubal epithelia and in 'normal' looking tubal epithelia has also been reported recently.[13,36,42] Among women with *BRCA1* germline mutations who underwent prophylactic salpingo-oophorectomy and whose ovaries were histologically negative for carcinoma, the frequency of proliferative and atypical lesions, including CIS, was increased.[11] Early tubal carcinomas are commonly found in *BRCA* mutation carriers.[16,36] Although no DNA sequence analysis was performed in these studies, these lines of evidence suggest that alterations of *p53* and *BRCA1* may function in the pathogenesis of tubal carcinogenesis, and that cancer develops in a step-wise fashion from benign tubal epithelium, to dysplastic changes, to CIS, and eventually invasive carcinoma.

Potential role of tubal epithelia contributing to ovarian serous carcinogenesis

Ovarian epithelial cancer, particularly ovarian serous carcinoma, is believed to arise from the ovarian surface epithelium or ovarian epithelial inclusions (see Chapter 23). In recent years, new evidence, largely circumstantial, has implicated the

fallopian tube in the pathogenesis of both ovarian and/or peritoneal carcinomas:[36,50]

* The tubal lining possesses all of the known hormone receptors including estrogen, progesterone, and gonadotropins that potentially serve as the targets for the cancer-promoting hormones.[38,68,69]
* The fallopian tube, particularly the fimbrial end, may contribute to the formation of ovarian epithelial inclusions[35] as the fimbrial end closely interacts with the ovarian surface.[2]
* Hysterectomy or salpingectomy reduces the risk of ovarian cancer.
* Ovulating hens have a high incidence of ovarian cancer and, of those with cancer, a high frequency show preinvasive disease in their oviducts.[25,57,65]
* A high incidence of tubal intraepithelial neoplastic changes, including CIS with positive *p53* overexpression, is present in women with ovarian or peritoneal cancer and in *BRCA* mutation carriers.[11,36,52,71]
* There are similarities in expression profiles between normal fallopian tube epithelium and ovarian serous carcinoma.[40]

Although the exact role that the fallopian tube plays in the pathogenesis of ovarian serous carcinoma is unknown, it is now recognized that the tubal epithelia is more prone to develop cancer than previously thought. One practical point emanating from these recent advances is the need to carefully examine the fallopian tubes by serial blocking of all submitted tissues if early neoplastic lesions are to be found. This is especially important for prophylactically removed ovaries and tubes.[42,53] Future studies of tubal epithelia and ovarian serous carcinomas by using cutting edge molecular techniques such as laser capture microdissection, cell lineage analysis, comparative genomic hybridization, and expression array analysis may reveal genes that are important in serous tubal carcinogenesis and the tubal role in contributing to ovarian carcinogenesis.

Clinical features

The mean age of patients with fallopian tube adenocarcinoma is about 60 years (age range, 26–86). Only 6% occur in women under 40 years old.[5,17] The diagnostic triad of serosanguineous vaginal discharge, pain, and pelvic mass is seen in only a minority of women with the disease while the correct preoperative diagnosis is made in only about 5% of cases.[5] The current clinical staging system for carcinoma of the fallopian tube, shown in an abbreviated fashion in Appendix A, may be too simple. A recent proposal would expand the scope of staging for non-invasive tubal carcinomas as well as fimbrial carcinomas. The tumor also appears associated with an increased frequency of ovarian and endometrial carcinomas, perhaps reflecting a field change. There is also increased incidence in women who have breast and peritoneal carcinomas.[60,71]

Gross features

Tubal carcinoma has a variable gross appearance, usually causing enlargement of the tube, the lumen being filled with tumor, with or without thickening of the wall (Figure 19.59). The tumor may protrude through the fimbrial end or the tube may be retort shaped, resembling a hydrosalpinx or a sausage. Rarely, the tube is of normal size and shape. About 20% of tubal carcinomas are bilateral.[5]

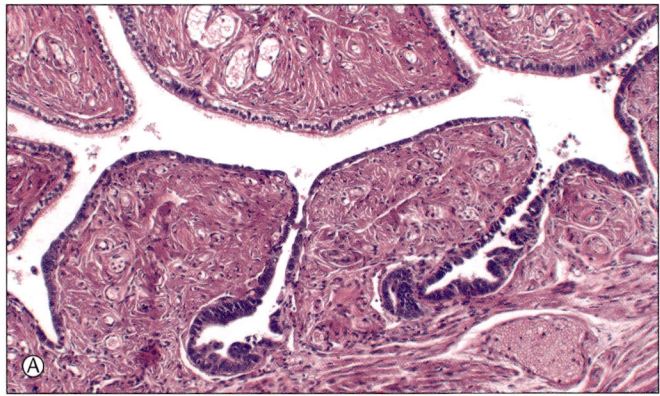
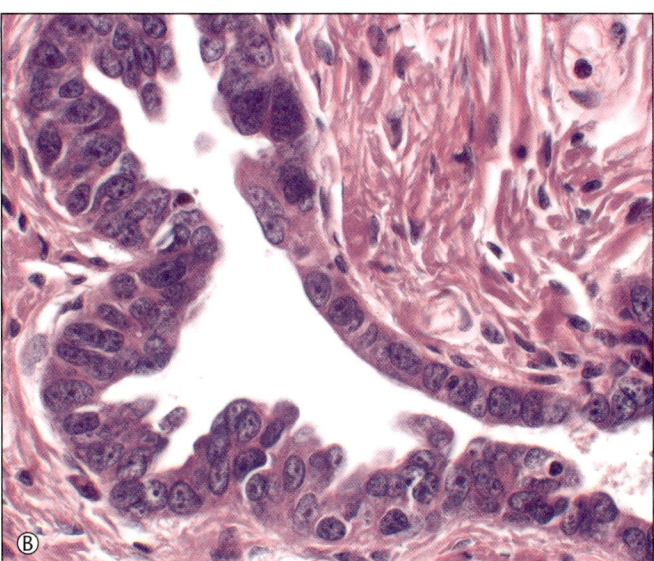

Fig. 19.58 Adenocarcinoma *in situ* with nuclear stratification and prominent macronucleoli (above); detail of nuclei (below).

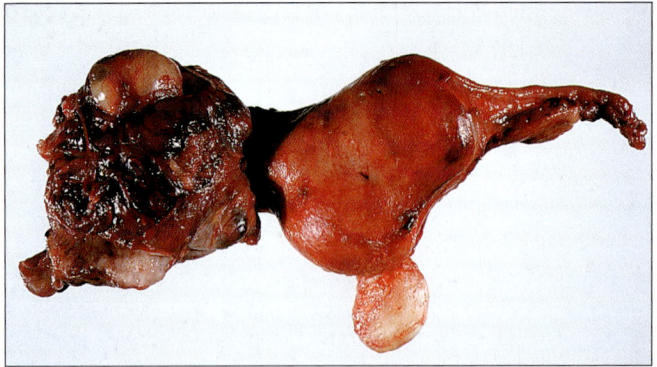

Fig. 19.59 Adenocarcinoma. The tube is enlarged, with solid, papillary, luminal growth.

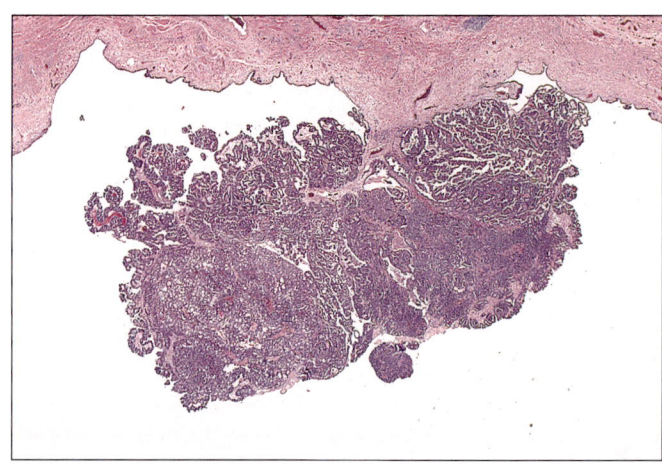

Fig. 19.61 Adenocarcinoma. The tumor is entirely mucosal and intraluminal.

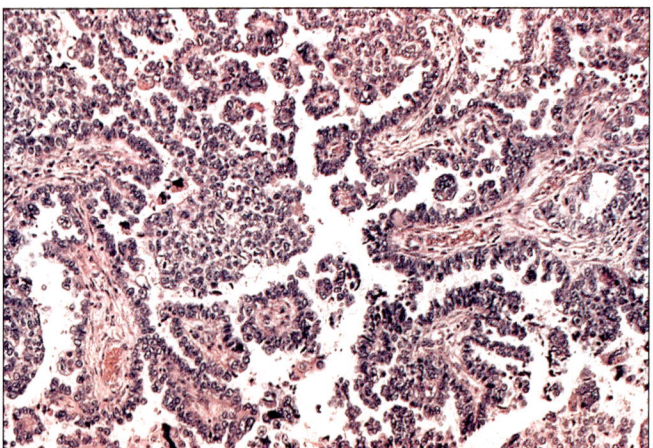

Fig. 19.60 Adenocarcinoma. A well-differentiated tumor showing a typical papillary pattern.

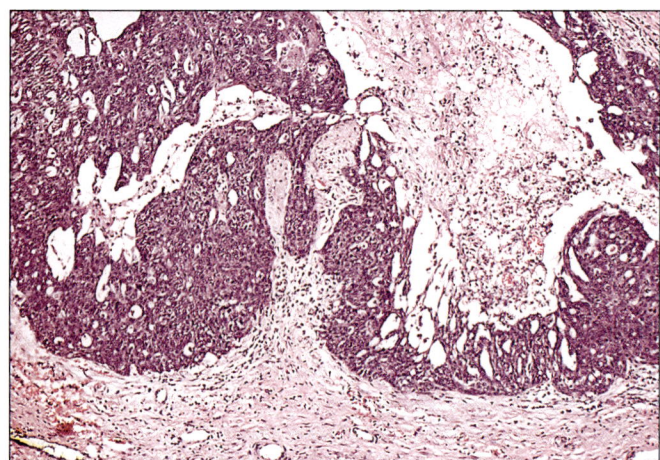

Fig. 19.62 Adenocarcinoma, grade 2.

Microscopic features

As the carcinomas arise from a müllerian epithelium, they are of serous, mucinous, endometrioid, clear cell, transitional cell, and squamous cell types. Among *BRCA*-positive cases, the tubal fimbria was the most common site for early serous carcinoma.[42]

Serous adenocarcinoma This is the most common type of fallopian tube carcinoma, comprising about half of the total cases.[5] It bears a resemblance to the serous adenocarcinoma of the ovary. The predominant pattern is papillary, with a gradation through alveolar to solid as the grade increases. Most tumors are grade 3.[5] Grade 1 tumors show an almost entirely papillary pattern, with cuboidal cells covering papillae that have delicate fibrovascular branching cores (Figures 19.60 and 19.61). A transition from benign epithelium through dysplastic changes to AIS and to malignancy may be observed. In grade 2 tumors, the papillary pattern is still obvious but irregular glands and alveolar structures are seen (Figures 19.62 and 19.63). The epithelium of the papillae is cuboidal or columnar, and nuclear atypia and the presence of nucleoli increase along with the increasing architectural grade. The poorly differentiated tumor (grade 3) is predominantly solid and composed of cells showing marked nuclear pleomorphism and a high mitotic rate (Figures 19.64 and 19.65). Necrotic foci are common but

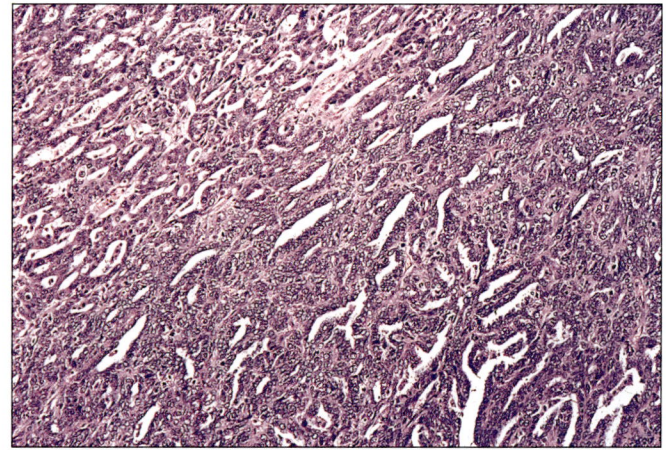

Fig. 19.63 Adenocarcinoma, grade 2.

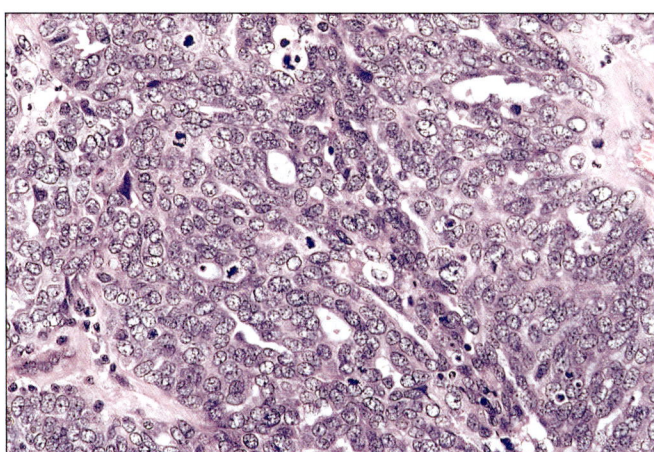

Fig. 19.64 Adenocarcinoma, grade 3.

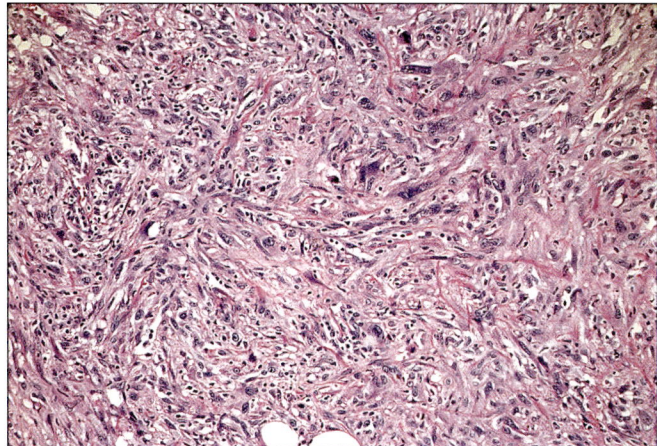

Fig. 19.65 Adenocarcinoma, grade 3.

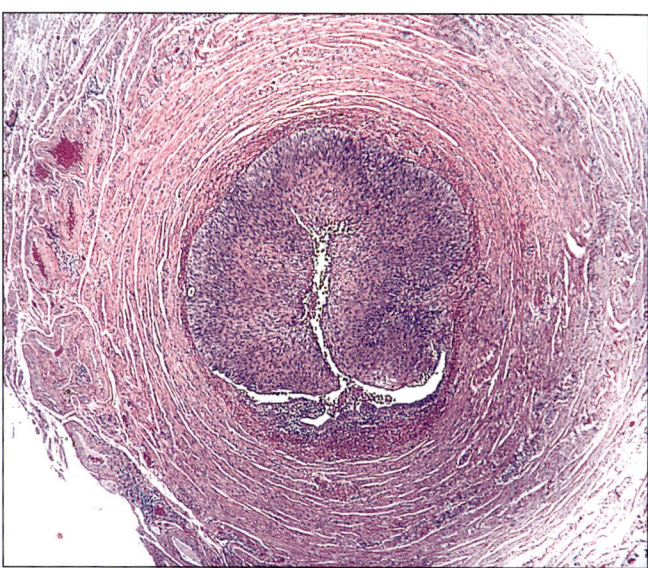

Fig. 19.66 Squamous cell carcinoma *in situ* in the tube.

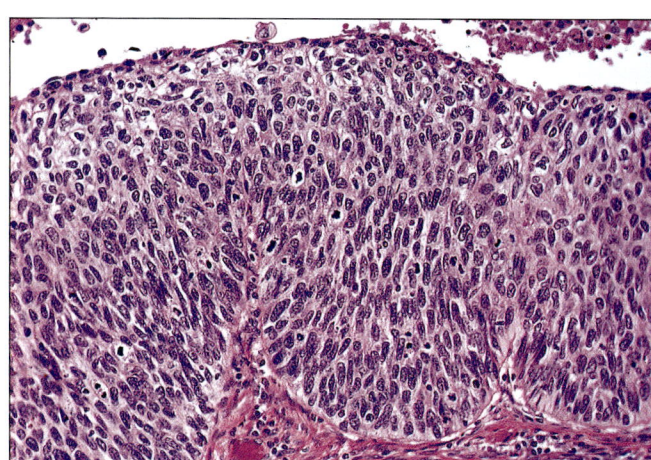

Fig. 19.67 Squamous cell carcinoma *in situ* in the tube.

even in the most poorly differentiated tumors some papillary structures are usually apparent.

Endometrioid adenocarcinoma About 12–25% of fallopian tube carcinomas are of endometrioid type.[5,26,45] Their pattern resembles that of endometrioid adenocarcinomas in the uterus and ovary and is predominantly more glandular and less papillary than serous adenocarcinomas. They are less likely to be bilateral than serous adenocarcinomas.[45] A subtype of endometrioid carcinoma may resemble the female adnexal tumor of probable wolffian origin (FATWO), and shows a mostly solid proliferation of small, oval to spindle cells punctured by small to cystic glands, many with luminal PAS-positive colloid-like secretions. Foci of typical endometrioid carcinoma are usually present but may be minor. These tumors usually are non-invasive.

Transitional cell carcinoma Transitional cell carcinoma is the third most common histologic type of carcinoma found in the fallopian tube. One recent report found that 12% of tubal carcinomas were entirely of transitional cell type[5] while another found that as many as 57% of tubal carcinomas contained a transitional cell element.[64] These tumors are arranged as solid nests that show stratification. The cells have clear cytoplasm that may be slightly eosinophilic and some nuclei show nuclear grooves, the so-called 'coffee bean' appearance.[5] In our view, many such cases are more likely to be poorly differentiated serous carcinomas with a broad papillary or pseudopapillary growth pattern than a truly transitional cell type.

Clear cell carcinoma Clear cell carcinoma of the fallopian tube is rare, comprising about 2% of tubal carcinomas.[5] The tumor has the same appearances as seen in the uterus and ovary. Solid zones of clear cells and papillary areas are present, together with a tubulocystic pattern with prominent hobnail cells.

Squamous cell carcinoma Primary squamous cell carcinoma in the fallopian tube has been reported, but is rare.[14] Most cases are thought to represent spread of intraepithelial neoplasia from the cervix through the endometrium (Figures 19.66 and 19.67).[14]

Spread, treatment and prognosis of tubal carcinoma

The spread of tubal carcinoma is generally similar to that of ovarian carcinoma. Transluminal spread into the peritoneal cavity with subsequent implantation on peritoneal surfaces is the predominant mode of spread, but direct involvement of adjacent organs, particularly ovary and uterus, is also important. Occasionally, spread may occur transluminally to involve endometrium and endocervix. Lymphatic spread from the fimbria is principally to the pelvic nodes, and to the para-aortic nodes from that portion of the tube near the uterus. In one small series, two of six patients with disease limited to the fallopian tube already had nodal metastases.[17,20]

Initial treatment is surgical, consisting of total hysterectomy with bilateral salpingo-oophorectomy and with staging procedures as for ovarian carcinoma. Postoperative radiation therapy is of some value but combination chemotherapy with cisplatin-containing agents, similar to that used for ovarian carcinoma, is most widely used.

Survival depends upon the extent of the disease at the time of diagnosis. The overall 5-year survival for stages 1 and 2 is about 50–60% and for stages 3 and 4 is about 15–20%.[56,58] The overall 5-year survival for all stages is under 40%. Histologically, grade 3 lesions have the worst outcome but a better prognosis is associated with endometrioid type[5] and an inflammatory reaction around the tumor. Many biologic markers have been tested to predict the prognosis of fallopian tube carcinoma. One study showed that *p53* overexpression is a poor prognostic marker, with a seven-fold higher relative risk compared to those carcinomas without *p53* overexpression.[71] However, controversial reports with no significant prognostic role for *p53* are also present.[34] The most import adverse prognostic factor remains as advanced stage. Other adverse factors have included increasing age, vascular space invasion, and a high volume of residual tumor.

CARCINOSARCOMA

Definition

A rare mixed tumor composed of malignant glands and malignant mesenchyme, with an annual incidence of about 0.25 cases per million women.[28] Carcinosarcoma may be found anywhere along the female genital tract and, although much more common in the endometrium and ovary, about 70 cases of this tumor have been reported in the fallopian tube.

Clinical features

The mean age at diagnosis is 59 years, with a range of 14–79 years. The majority of patients are postmenopausal although 17% are under 50 years old at diagnosis. Presentation is with non-specific abdominal symptoms of pain or distension, often with vaginal spotting or bleeding. Physical examination usually reveals a pelvic mass, although initial evaluation may be normal.

Pathology

Carcinosarcomas of the tube are often relatively small when diagnosed. Larger tumors are difficult to distinguish from ovarian primaries. They appear grossly as polypoid growths filling the lumen of the tube, often with areas of hemorrhage and necrosis (Figure 19.68).

Microscopically, carcinosarcoma discloses a malignant epithelial element which may or may not have the pattern of an

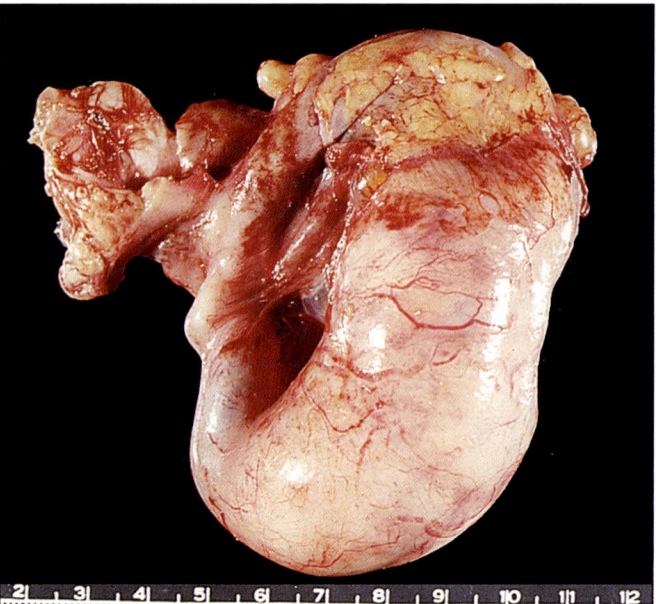

Fig. 19.68 Carcinosarcoma.

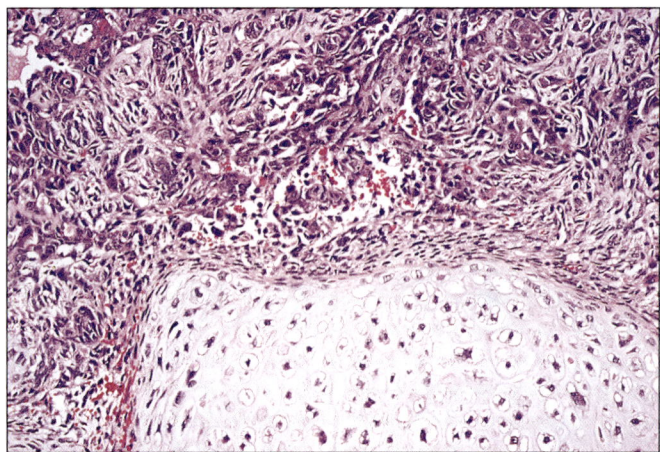

Fig. 19.69 Carcinosarcoma. A heterologous tumor containing cartilage.

endometrioid adenocarcinoma, together with a mesenchymal element. As in the endometrium and ovary, the mesenchymal element may be homologous, containing elements indigenous to the endometrium, or heterologous, containing elements foreign to the endometrium, such as cartilage (Figure 19.69) or striated muscle.

Treatment and prognosis

Recommended treatment is by surgery, followed by radiotherapy and/or chemotherapy. The prognosis is poor, the 5-year survival rate being about 15% and the mean survival only 16–20 months. Early stage disease is associated with a better prognosis,[22] and several long-term survivals are recorded.[28]

OTHER MALIGNANT TUMORS

Other rare malignant tumors that have been reported arising in the tube include leiomyosarcoma,[21] embryonal rhabdomyosarcoma,[9] immature teratoma,[37] and choriocarcinoma.[44]

TUMORS METASTATIC TO THE FALLOPIAN TUBE

Numerically, tumors metastatic to the fallopian tube (Figures 19.70–19.72) are far more significant than primaries, accounting for 80–90% of all tubal neoplasms. Most of these (60%) are suspected to have arisen from the ovary and reach the tube by direct spread.

PARATUBAL TISSUES AND BROAD LIGAMENTS

CYSTS

Cysts lying alongside the fallopian tube are referred to as perisalpingeal or parovarian cysts (Figure 19.73). Their origin is either from müllerian (paramesonephric) elements or wolffian (mesonephric) remnants.

MESONEPHRIC CYSTS

The mesonephric remnants are the epoophoron and paroophoron, which continue as vestigial tubular structures between the tube and ovary, passing medially towards the body of the uterus, to enter it at about the level of the internal cervical os and pass anterolaterally in the cervix as Gartners duct. Non-neoplastic, non-cystic mesonephric remnants are universally present between the tube and the ovary and are seen as a collection of thick-walled tubular structures lined by cuboidal epithelium with smooth muscle in their walls (Figure 19.74). These remnants may become cystic at any point along their course, so that mesonephric cysts may be found within the mesosalpinx and broad ligament or they may be pedunculated and situated just lateral to the ovary (Kobelts cyst). Typically, the mesonephric cyst is lined by a single layer of epithelium that is of low columnar or cuboidal, ciliated or non-ciliated type. Smooth muscle may be prominent in the wall of these cysts, often together with dense connective tissue and elastic fibers.

PARAMESONEPHRIC CYSTS

The paramesonephric cysts, when small, tend to be more laterally situated than those of mesonephric origin. The hydatid of Morgagni, usually seen as a cyst on a pedicle arising from the

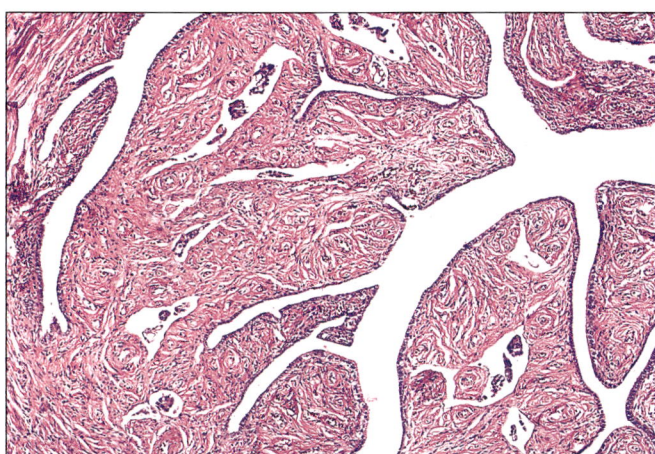

Fig. 19.70 Metastatic serous adenocarcinoma of the ovary in the fallopian tube.

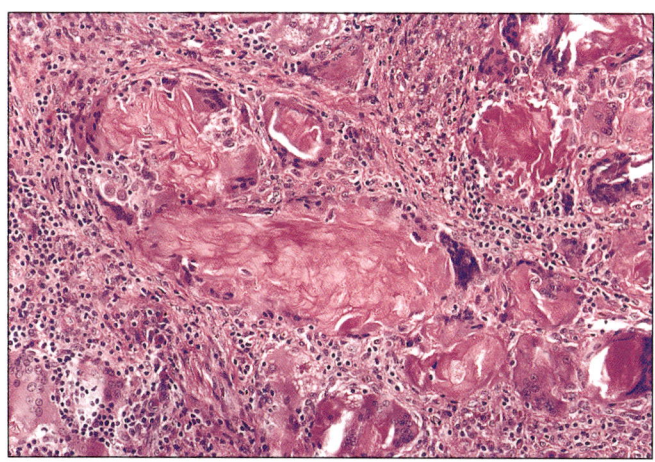

Fig. 19.72 Metastatic squamous cell carcinoma. A foreign body reaction has occurred.

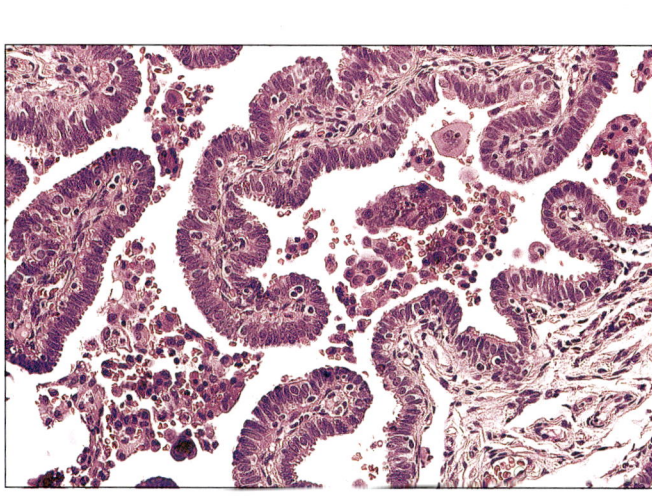

Fig. 19.71 Metastatic serous adenocarcinoma of the ovary in the fallopian tube.

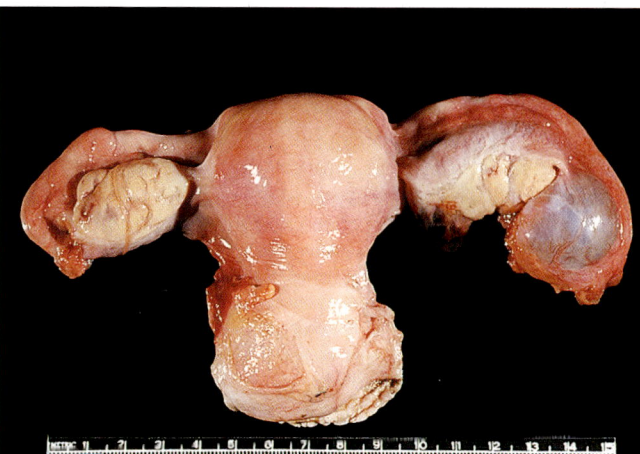

Fig. 19.73 Broad ligament cyst. This parovarian, or paratubal cyst, is thin walled and contains clear watery fluid.

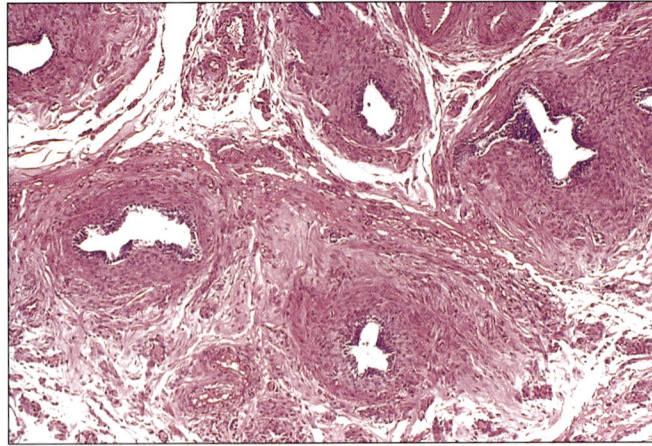

Fig. 19.74 Mesonephric remnants.

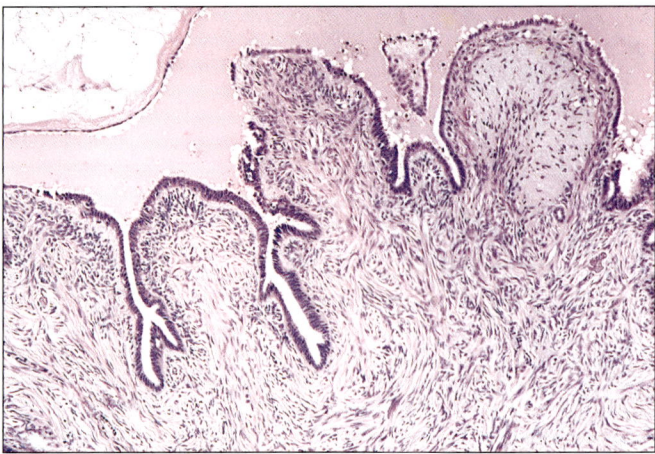

Fig. 19.76 Broad ligament cyst. Coarse, polypoid projections into the lumen may be seen.

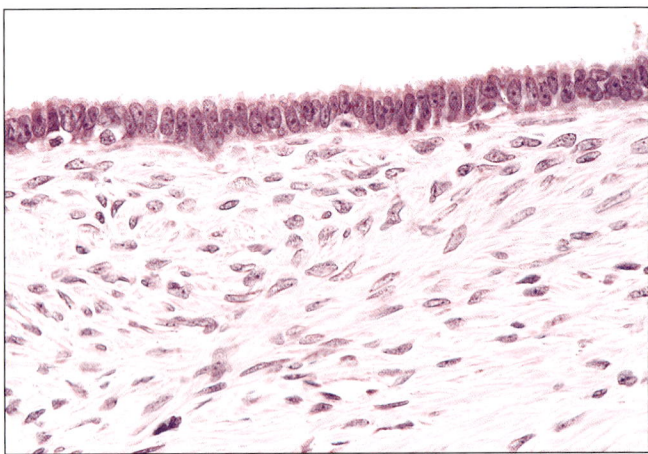

Fig. 19.75 Broad ligament cyst.

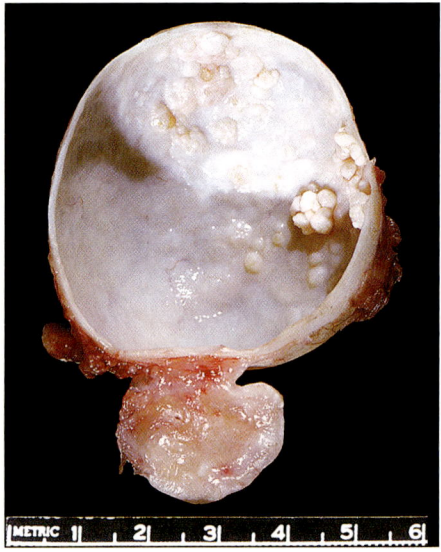

Fig. 19.77 Broad ligament cyst. A large cyst has papillary excrescences that arise from the internal surface.

fimbria, is the commonest example of a paramesonephric cyst. Others are found in close proximity to the tube or on its subserosal aspect. Paramesonephric cysts, often also termed 'broad ligament cysts', are lined by a single layer of columnar cells that may also be ciliated or non-ciliated (Figures 19.75 and 19.76). Smooth muscle is often present in their wall but is less prominent than in the mesonephric variety. Distinction between the two types of cyst is not always possible.

Larger paramesonephric cysts may have papillary excrescences arising from the internal surface (Figure 19.77). Benign, borderline, and malignant tumors of serous type have been reported in the broad ligament.[3] Although it is accepted that these are likely to be paramesonephric in origin, their histogenesis is unimportant in relation to management. Cases of endometrioid adenocarcinoma have also been reported, some arising from endometriosis.[60]

ADRENAL REST

An encapsulated collection of adrenal cortical cells is encountered as 1–3 mm yellow nodules in the broad ligament or mesosalpinx in as many as one-fourth of women (Figure 19.78).

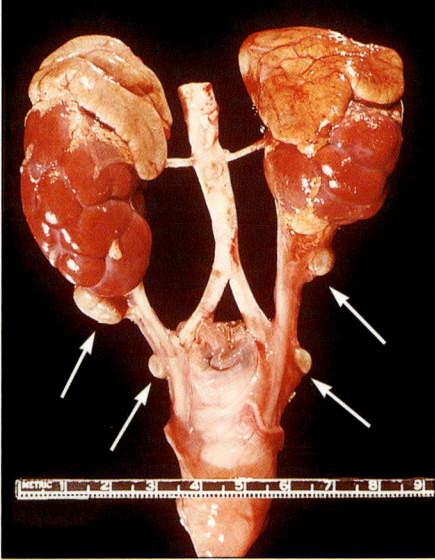

Fig. 19.78 Adrenal rests. Although no longer related to the fallopian tubes, the adrenal rests (arrows) are clearly seen in these dissected organs from an infant.

Also termed 'Marchands rest', the heterotopic adrenal cells are identical to those of the adrenal cortex and are arranged in cords mimicking the zona fascicularis of the latter (Figure 19.79). Benign and malignant tumors may arise from them.

FEMALE ADNEXAL TUMOR OF PROBABLE WOLFFIAN ORIGIN (FATWO)

Definition
A tumor of the broad ligament for which there is very strong evidence of a wolffian origin. About 40 cases have been reported.[60]

Clinical features
The patients are 15–81 years of age. The tumors are asymptomatic and usually incidental findings, although a large tumor may present as a mass.

Gross features
The tumors are unilateral, ranging from 0.5 to 18 cm in diameter, and are situated within the leaves of the broad ligament or pedunculated from it. Virtually all have bosselated, smooth outer surfaces. The cut surfaces (Figure 19.80) are gray-white to tan in color and rubbery to firm in consistency. Some are gritty, with focal areas of calcification that are sometimes sufficiently extensive to be seen on pelvic X-ray. Cystic areas are sometimes present.

Microscopic features
Three main histologic patterns are described in these tumors:

- a sieve-like pattern (Figure 19.81), in which there are hollow tubules of varying size and shape, sometimes with cyst formation;
- closely packed tubules, giving a dense, solid appearance (Figure 19.82). The tubules are winding, branching, and anastomosing, and are lined by cuboidal or columnar epithelial cells; and
- diffuse, solid sheets of cells.

The nuclei are round or oval and pale, with evenly dispersed chromatin. Most tumors have a low mitotic count. Some of those that behave in a malignant fashion contain pleomorphic

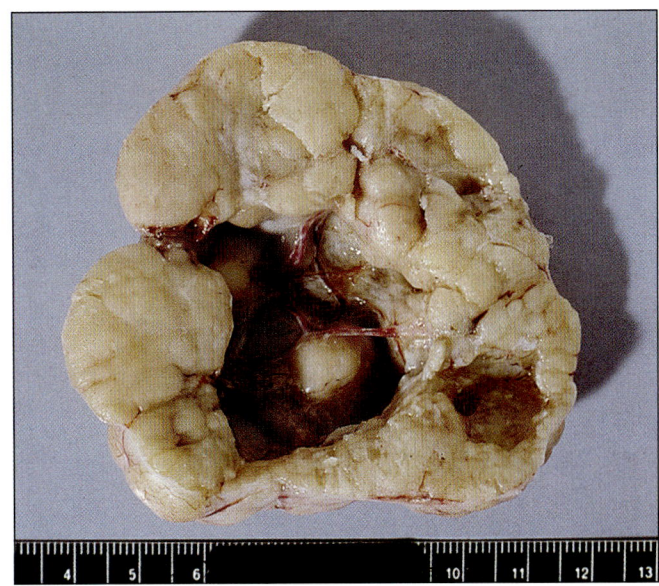

Fig. 19.80 Adnexal tumor of probable wolffian origin.

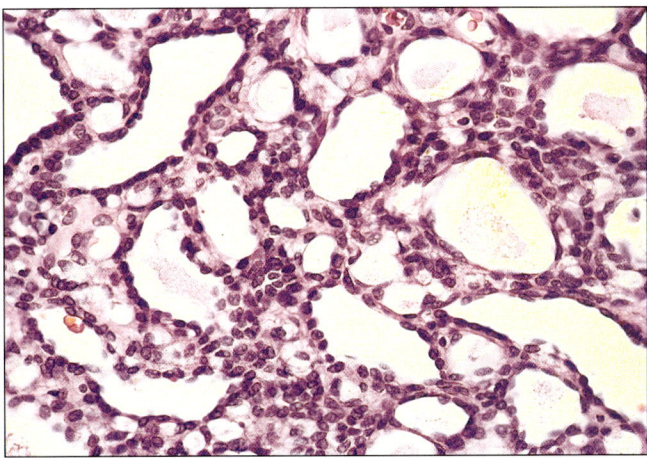

Fig. 19.81 Adnexal tumor of probable wolffian origin. Solid areas between the cysts.

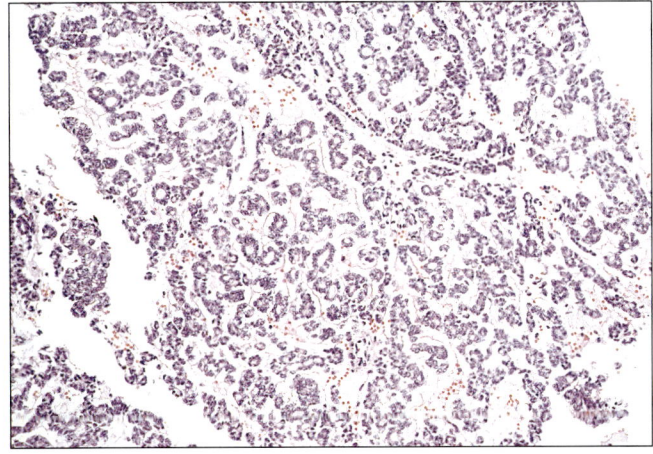

Fig. 19.82 Adnexal tumor of probable wolffian origin. Closely packed tubules.

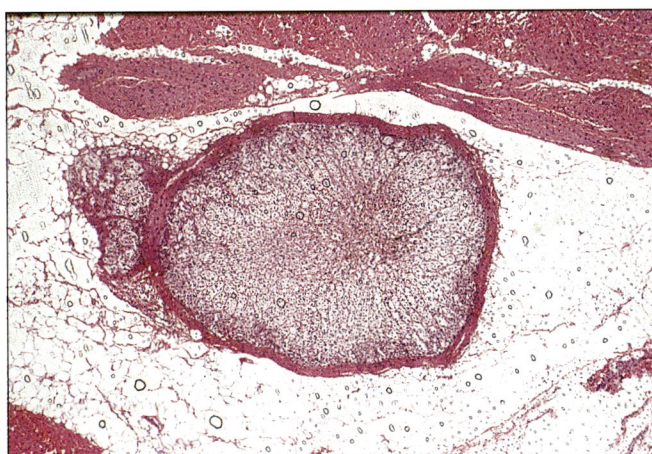

Fig. 19.79 Adrenal rest.

nuclei and numerous mitotic figures, but not all clinically malignant tumors display these features.[60]

Origin

The tumors found in the broad ligament and mesosalpinx are considered by convention to be of wolffian origin because of their occurrence in the broad ligament, which is where wolffian remnants are located. Also, they do not resemble müllerian tumors by light microscopy, electron microscopy or immuno-histochemistry.[60] However, as the majority of FATWOs share histologic features of sex cord-stromal tumors, particularly of Sertoli cell tumors or Sertoli–Leydig cell tumors, a possible extragonadal sex cord-stromal origin has been proposed.[70] It is difficult to study the tumor origin because of low incidence.

Differential diagnosis

The differential diagnosis is sex cord-stromal tumors, particularly those containing Sertoli cells. No stromal cells of Leydig type have been demonstrated, nor has any patient shown hormonal manifestations. Inhibin reactivity is not helpful to differentiate FATWOs, Sertoli cell or Sertoli–Leydig cell tumors as all of these tumors are consistently reactive.[31,41,70] In addition, although some areas of the tumors have a passing similarity to granulosa cell tumors, endometrioid adenocarcinomas, and clear cell carcinomas, these resemblances are only superficial and do not stand up to close scrutiny, although occasional confusion may occur.[27]

Prognosis

Five women have been reported with FATWOs that behaved in a malignant fashion.[7,19] All others have been benign, with follow-up ranging from a few months to 15 years.

REFERENCES

1. Abbuhl SB, Muskin EB, Shofer FS. Pelvic inflammatory disease in patients with bilateral tubal ligation. Am J Emerg Med 1997;15:271–4.
2. Ahmad-Thabet SM. The fimbrio-ovarian relation and its role on ovum picking in unexplained infertility: the fimbrio-ovarian accessibility tests. J Obstet Gynaecol Res 2000;26:65–70.
3. Altaras MM, Jaffe R, Corduba M, et al. Primary parovarian cystadenocarcinoma: clinical and management aspects and literature review. Gynecol Oncol 1990;38:268–72.
4. Alvarado-Cabrero I, Navani SS, Young RH, et al. Tumors of the fimbriated end of the fallopian tube: a clinicopathologic analysis of 20 cases, including nine carcinomas. Int J Gynecol Pathol 1997;16:189–96.
5. Alvarado-Cabrero I, Young RH, Vamvakas EC, et al. Carcinoma of the fallopian tube: a clinicopathological study of 105 cases with observations on staging and prognostic factors. Gynecol Oncol 1999;72:367–79.
6. Bazot M, Davenne C, Benzakine Y, et al. Actinomycotic tuboovarian abscess: dynamic CT findings. J Radiologie 1997;78:513–6.
7. Brescia RJ, Cardoso de Almeida PC, Fuller AF Jr, Dickersin GR, Robboy SJ. Female adnexal tumor of probable Wolffian origin with multiple recurrences over 16 years. Cancer 1985;56:1456–61.
8. Bromham DR. Intrauterine contraceptive devices – a reappraisal. Br Med Bull 1993;49:100–23.
9. Buchwalter CL, Jenison EL, Fromm M, et al. Pure embryonal rhabdomyosarcoma of the fallopian tube. Gynecol Oncol 1997;67:95–101.
10. Campello TR, Fittipaldi H, O'Valle F, Carvia RE, Nogales FF. Extrauterine (tubal) placental site nodule. Histopathology 1998;32:562–5.
11. Carcangiu ML, Radice P, Manoukian S, et al. Atypical epithelial proliferation in fallopian tubes in prophylactic salpingo-oophorectomy specimens from BRCA1 and BRCA2 germline mutation carriers. Int J Gynecol Pathol 2004;23:35–40.
12. Carson SA, Buster JE. Current concepts – ectopic pregnancy. N Engl J Med 1993;329:1174–81.
13. Cass I, Holschneider C, Datta N, et al. BRCA-mutation-associated fallopian tube carcinoma: a distinct clinical phenotype? Obstet Gynecol 2005;106:1327–34.
14. Cheung ANY, So KF, Ngan HYS, et al. Primary squamous cell carcinoma of fallopian tube. Int J Gynecol Pathol 1994;13:92–5.
15. Cheung AN, Young RH, Scully RE. Pseudocarcinomatous hyperplasia of the fallopian tube associated with salpingitis. A report of 14 cases. Am J Surg Pathol 1994;18:1125–30.
16. Colgan TJ, Murphy J, Cole DE, et al. Occult carcinoma in prophylactic oophorectomy specimens: prevalence and association with BRCA germline mutation status. Am J Surg Pathol 2001;25:1283–9.
17. Cormio G, Lissoni A, Maneo A, et al. Lymph node involvement in primary carcinoma of the fallopian tube. Int J Gynecol Cancer 1996;6:405–9.
18. Crossman SH. The challenge of pelvic inflammatory disease. Am Fam Physician 2006;73:859–64.
19. Daya D. Malignant female adnexal tumor of probable Wolffian origin with review of the literature. Arch Pathol Lab Med 1994;118:310–12.
20. di Re E, Grosso G, Raspagliesi F, et al. Fallopian tube cancer. Incidence and role of lymphatic spread. Gynecol Oncol 1996;62:199–202.
21. Ebert A, Goetze B, Herbst H, et al. Primary leiomyosarcoma of the fallopian tube. Ann Oncol 1995;6:618–9.
22. Ebert AD, Perez-Canto A, Schaller G, et al. Stage I primary malignant mixed müllerian tumor of the fallopian tube: report of a case with five-year survival after minimal surgery without adjuvant treatment. J Reprod Med 1998;43:598–600.
23. Egan AJM, Russell P. Transitional (urothelial) cell metaplasia of the fallopian tube mucosa: morphological assessment of three cases. Int J Gynecol Pathol 1996;15:72–6.
24. Filshie GM. Sterilization. In: Clements RV, ed. Safe Practice in Obstetrics and Gynaecology: A Medico-Legal Handbook. Edinburgh: Churchill Livingstone; 1994:337–43.
25. Fredrickson TN. Ovarian tumors of the hen. Environ Health Perspect 1987;73:35–51.
26. Fujiwaki R, Takahashi K, Ryuko K, et al. Primary endometrioid carcinoma of the fallopian tube. Acta Obstet Gynecol Scand 1996;75:508–10.
27. Fukunaga M, Bisceglia M, Dimitri L. Endometrioid carcinoma of the fallopian tube resembling a female adnexal tumor of probable wolffian origin. Adv Anat Pathol 2004;11:269–72.
28. Hellstrom AC, Auer G, Silfversward C, et al. Prognostic factors in malignant mixed müllerian tumor of the fallopian tube. Int J Gynecol Cancer 1996;6:467–72.
29. Honore LH. Pathology of the fallopian tube and broad ligament. In: Fox H, Wells M, eds. Haines and Taylor Obstetrical and Gynaecological Pathology, 4th edn. New York: Churchill Livingstone; 1995:623–71.
30. Jacques SM, Qureshi F, Ramirez NC, et al. Retained trophoblastic tissue in Fallopian tubes: a consequence of unsuspected ectopic pregnancies. Int J Gynecol Pathol 1997;16:219–24.
31. Kommoss F, Oliva E, Bhan AK, et al. Inhibin expression in ovarian tumors and tumor-like lesions: an immunohistochemical study. Mod Pathol 1998;11:656–64.
32. Krasevic M, Stankovic T, Petrovic O, et al. Serous borderline tumor of the fallopian tube presented as hematosalpinx: a case report. BMC Cancer 2005;5:129.
33. Kutteh WH, Albert T. Mature cystic teratoma of the fallopian tube associated with an ectopic pregnancy. Obstet Gynecol 1991;78:984–6.
34. Lacy MQ, Hartmann LC, Keeney GL, et al. c-erbB-2 and p53 expression in fallopian tube carcinoma. Cancer 1995;15:2891–6.
35. Lauchlan SC. The secondary müllerian system revisited. Int J Gynecol Pathol 1994;13:73–9.
36. Lee Y, Medeiros F, Kindelberger D, et al. Advances in the recognition of tubal intraepithelial carcinoma: applications to cancer screening and the pathogenesis of ovarian cancer. Adv Anat Pathol 2006;13:1–7.
37. Li S, Zimmerman RL, LiVolsi VA. Mixed malignant germ cell tumor of the fallopian tube. Int J Gynecol Pathol 1999;18:183–5.
38. Lu JJ, Zheng Y, Yuan J-M, et al. Decreased luteinizing hormone receptor mRNA expression in human ovarian epithelial cancer. Gynecol Oncol 2000;79:158–68.
39. Mahmood T, Saridogan E, Smutna S, et al. The effect of ovarian steroids on epithelial ciliary beat frequency in the human Fallopian tube. Hum Reprod 1998;13:2991–4.
40. Marquez RT, Baggerly KA, Patterson AP, et al. Patterns of gene expression in different histotypes of epithelial ovarian cancer correlate with those in normal fallopian tube, endometrium, and colon. Clin Cancer Res 2005;11:6116–26.
41. McCluggage WG. Value of inhibin staining in gynecological pathology. Int J Gynecol Pathol 2001;20:79–85.
42. Medeiros F, Muto MG, Lee Y, et al. The tubal fimbria is a preferred site for early adenocarcinoma in women with familial ovarian cancer syndrome. Am J Surg Pathol 2006;30:230–6.
43. Mohllajee AP, Curtis KM, Peterson HB. Does insertion and use of an intrauterine device increase the risk of pelvic inflammatory disease among women with sexually transmitted infection? A systematic review. Contraception 2006;73:145–53.
44. Muto MG, Lage JM, Berkowitz RS, et al. Gestational trophoblastic disease of the fallopian tube. J Reprod Med 1991;36:57–60.
45. Navani SS, Alvarado-Cabrero I, Young RH, et al. Endometrioid carcinoma of the fallopian tube: a clinicopathologic analysis of 26 cases. Gynecol Oncol 1996;63:371–8.

46. Nayar R, Snell J, Silverberg SG, et al. Placental site nodule occurring in a fallopian tube. Hum Pathol 1996;27:1243–5.
47. Ortiz ME, Croxatto HB, Bardin CW. Mechanisms of action of intrauterine devices. Obstet Gynecol Surv 1996;51:S42–51.
48. Ortu S, Molicotti P, Sechi LA, et al. Rapid detection and identification of Mycobacterium tuberculosis by real time PCR and Bactec 960 MIGT. New Microbiol 2006;29:75–80.
49. Parikh FR, Nadkarni SG, Kamat SA, et al. Genital tuberculosis – a major pelvic factor causing infertility in Indian women. Fertil Steril 1997;67:497–500.
50. Piek JM, Kenemans P, Verheijen RH. Intraperitoneal serous adenocarcinoma: a critical appraisal of three hypotheses on its cause. Am J Obstet Gynecol 2004;191:718–32.
51. Piek JM, Verheijen RH, Menko FH, et al. Expression of differentiation and proliferation related proteins in epithelium of prophylactically removed ovaries from women with a hereditary female adnexal cancer predisposition. Histopathology 2003;43:26–32.
52. Piek JMJ, van Diest PJ, Zweemer RP, et al. Dysplastic changes in prophylactically removed Fallopian tubes of women predisposed to developing ovarian cancer. J Pathol 2001;195:451–6.
53. Powell CB, Kenley E, Chen LM, et al. Risk-reducing salpingo-oophorectomy in BRCA mutation carriers: role of serial sectioning in the detection of occult malignancy. J Clin Oncol 2005;23:127–32.
54. Rabczynski JK, Kochman AT. Primary cancer of the fallopian tube with transitional differentiation. Clinical and pathological assessment of 6 cases. Neoplasma 1999;46:128–31.
55. Ramirez NC, Lawrence WD, Ginsburg KA. Ectopic pregnancy. A recent five-year study and review of the last 50 years' literature. J Reprod Med 1996;41:733–40.
56. Rauthe G, Vahrson HW, Burkhardt E. Primary cancer of the fallopian tube. Treatment and results of 37 cases. Eur J Gynaecol Oncol 1998;19:356–62.
57. Rodriguez-Burford C, Barnes MN, Berry W, et al. Immunohistochemical expression of molecular markers in an avian model: a potential model for preclinical evaluation of agents for ovarian cancer chemoprevention. Gynecol Oncol 2001;81:373–9.
58. Rosen AC, Ausch C, Hafner E, et al. A 15-year overview of management and prognosis in primary fallopian tube carcinoma. Austrian Cooperative Study Group for Fallopian Tube Carcinoma. Eur J Cancer 1998;34:1725–9.
59. Schust D, Stovall DW. Leiomyomas of the fallopian tube. A case report. J Reprod Med 1993;38:741–2.
60. Scully RE, Young RH, Clement RB. Tumors of the broad ligament and other uterine ligaments. Washington, DC: Armed Forces Institute of Pathology; 1998:499–511.
61. Sedlis A. Carcinoma of the fallopian tube. Surg Clin North Am 1978;58:121–9.
62. Steen R, Shapiro K. Intrauterine contraceptive devices and risk of pelvic inflammatory disease: standard of care in high STI prevalence settings. Reprod Health Matters 2004;12:136–43.
63. Su YN, Cheng WF, Chen CA, et al. Pregnancy with primary tubal placental site trophoblastic tumor: a case report and literature review. Gynecol Oncol 1999;73:322–5.
64. Uehira K, Hashimoto H, Tsuneyoshi M, et al. Transitional cell carcinoma pattern in primary carcinoma of the fallopian tube. Cancer 1993;72:2447–56.
65. Wilson JE. Adenocarcinomata in hens kept in a constant environment. Poult Sci 1958;37:1253.
66. Wollen AL, Sandvei R, Mork S, et al. In situ characterization of leukocytes in the fallopian tube in women with or without an intrauterine contraceptive device. Acta Obstet Gynecol Scand 1994;73:103–12.
67. Yanai YI, Siriaunkgul S, Silverberg SG. Mucosal epithelial proliferation of the fallopian tube: a particular association with ovarian serous tumor of low malignant potential? Int J Gynecol Pathol 1995;14:107–13.
68. Zheng W, Lu J, Luo F, et al. Ovarian epithelial tumor growth promotion by FSH and inhibition of the effect by LH. Gynecol Oncol 2000;76:80–8.
69. Zheng W, Magid MS, Kramer EE, et al. Follicle-stimulating hormone receptor is expressed in human ovarian surface epithelium and fallopian tube. Am J Pathol 1996;148:47–53.
70. Zheng W, Senturk BZ, Parkash V. Inhibin immunohistochemical staining: a practical approach for the surgical pathologist in the diagnoses of ovarian sex cord-stromal tumors. Adv Anat Pathol 2003;10:27–38.
71. Zheng W, Sung CJ, Cao P, et al. Early occurrence and prognostic significance of p53 alteration in primary carcinoma of the fallopian tube. Gynecol Oncol 1997;64:38–48.
72. Zheng W, Wolf S, Kramer EE, et al. Borderline papillary serous tumor of the fallopian tube. Am J Surg Pathol 1996;20:30–5.

Endometriosis

Stanley J. Robboy   Arthur Haney   Peter Russell

INTRODUCTION

Endometriosis is the condition in which endometrial tissue, composed of both endometrial-type glandular epithelium and stroma, is found at sites outside the uterine cavity. In the past, adenomyosis and endometriosis were linked by a common terminology, the former being referred to as 'endometriosis interna' and the latter as 'endometriosis externa'. The two conditions are distinct,[90] however, with different symptoms and different epidemiologic and etiologic patterns: adenomyosis results from invagination of the basal endometrium lining the endometrial cavity into the uterine wall (see Chapter 17); endometriosis in most cases develops from endometrium that has implanted in the peritoneal cavity after retrograde transmission from the uterus through the fallopian tube.

CLINICAL FEATURES OF ENDOMETRIOSIS

Endometriosis, a condition described in European history for over 300 years,[78] is almost exclusively a disease of women in their reproductive years. It is currently the third leading cause of gynecologic hospitalization in the United States.[99] Its true incidence is unknown, although most reports estimate that it occurs in about 4–13% of all women of reproductive age,[29,62] 25–50% of infertile women,[7,52,113] 5–25% of those admitted for pelvic pain, 50% of teenagers with intractable dysmenorrhea,[29] and up to 7% of those admitted with pelvic masses. To determine the true incidence would require use of the most sensitive diagnostic test, laparoscopy, on a population of unselected premenopausal asymptomatic women. Clearly, such a prospective trial will never be performed.

Although earlier reports indicated that the typical patient was in her late thirties or early forties, the diagnosis is nowadays more frequently made in the late twenties or early thirties, and not infrequently in adolescence.[28] This difference may stem not from a change in the disease itself, but rather, in part, from the current widespread use of laparoscopy for the investigation of infertility. Delayed childbearing, which is common today, has also had an influence. In the past, the diagnosis was made only after symptoms appeared. The condition has not been reported before puberty, which is not surprising, as the sex steroid hormones needed for endometrial growth are not present in sufficient strength. Endometriosis may also occur after the menopause, mostly in postmenopausal women who have taken hormone medication.[26] In the minority who have not, other hormonal sources that are continuous and can sustain the process of endometriosis should be sought. One example is peripheral conversion of androgens in obese women.

Racial differences in the incidence of endometriosis,[86] although once thought to be important, now appear to be inconsequential as recent studies have more adequately controlled for childbearing patterns, socioeconomic and other relevant factors. Women with endometriosis are generally of lower parity than non-sufferers. The relationship between endometriosis and infertility is almost certainly a vicious circle. The hormonal milieu in a woman who does not achieve pregnancy encourages the development of endometriosis. Once endometriosis develops, its presence contributes to the infertile state and the circle is established. Conversely, pregnancy often has a beneficial effect on the disease. The typical patient with endometriosis is said to be a strong, well-educated career woman who has postponed having a family.

Most women with endometriosis present with secondary dysmenorrhea, dyspareunia, pelvic pain or infertility. However, only about 5% have all four major symptoms. A small number of women with endometriosis develop a pelvic mass or, occasionally, ascites.[102] Many women with endometriosis are also asymptomatic. In one study two-fifths of the women in whom endometriosis was discovered during laparoscopic tubal ligation had no symptoms.[11]

For reasons that are unknown, the amount and character of the pain that the patient experiences correlate poorly with the actual extent of disease found.[63] Women with minimal disease may have marked pain. At the opposite extreme, extensive disease may be found and yet the patient is relatively asymptomatic. In one study of 618 women diagnosed by laparoscopy, the stage and severity of pelvic endometriosis were out of proportion to the pelvic pain experienced in 40% of the patients. Local biochemical and physical effects seem to be more important factors than the anatomic location and extent of the endometriosis.[149] The presence of activated and degranulating mast cells has also been suggested as participating in the pathogenesis of the pain.[9,48,138]

DISTRIBUTION OF ENDOMETRIOSIS

The sites where endometriosis is most commonly found vary among series. The frequency depends greatly on whether the diagnosis rests on clinical or histologic findings, the two varying significantly either because the biopsies may not confirm the clinical findings[156] or the clinical site was not biopsied at all. In descending order of frequency, the two most frequent sites based on clinical findings are the uterosacral ligaments and ovaries (Table 20.1).[133] In most series, these two sites are each

Table 20.1 Clinical location of endometrial implants

Location	Frequency*
Uterosacral ligaments	63%
Ovaries	
Superficial	56%
Deep (endometrioma)	20%
Ovarian fossae	33%
Anterior vesicle pouch	22%
Pouch of Douglas	19%
Intestines	5%
Fallopian tubes	5%
Uterus	5%

*Most individuals have multiple sites of involvement.
From Shaw.[133]

Table 20.2 Location of endometriosis based upon biopsy findings

Location	Frequency*
Ovary	36%
Fallopian tube	14%
Uterine serosa	12%
Cul-de-sac	6%
Cervix	3%
Colon	3%
Peritoneum	3%
Appendix	2%
Broad ligament	2%
Pelvis	2%
Uterosacral ligament	2%
Vagina	2%
Abdominal wall	1%
Bladder	1%
Fibrous tissue	1%
Parametrium	1%
Rectum	1%
Small intestine	1%
Other sites (>20)	7%

*Based on 1323 biopsies and operative specimens.
From Stern et al.[136]

affected in over 60% of instances (due to multisite involvement). Most other sites are in the pelvis and include the pouch of Douglas, pelvic peritoneum, uterine surface, and fallopian tubes. The frequency of involvement ranges from 5 to 20%.

Since the diagnosis of endometriosis is made largely on a clinical basis, biopsies are performed selectively and thus affect what the pathologist encounters. In addition, many cases of endometriosis are incidental findings in bilateral salpingo-oophorectomy specimens (with or without hysterectomy) removed for other unrelated reasons. Thus, in contrast to clinical series, the ovary is the principal tissue where the pathologist sees endometriosis (36% of specimens) (Table 20.2).[136] The fallopian tube, uterine serosa, and cul-de-sac each account for 6–14% of biopsy-proven specimens. The uterosacral ligaments are rarely biopsied, which explains why this site accounts for under 2% of biopsy-proven endometriosis.

About 5–12% of women have extrapelvic disease on a clinical basis. The intestines are the most commonly involved site, especially where there is contact with the pelvic organs. Such sites, in descending order of frequency, include the sigmoid colon (in all levels, including the lamina propria, submucosa, muscularis propria, and subserosal mesentery),[161] rectosigmoid,[47,66] appendix, and ileum.[129] Endometriosis is well known to occur, although not commonly, in operative scars,[91,115,159] inguinal region,[20] lungs,[6,22] lymph nodes,[2] pleura, skin,[163] umbilicus,[24,155] ureter,[164,165] vagina, and vulva. It is also found very rarely in some distant sites,[14] including brain,[64] bone, diaphragm,[6] heart and muscle, liver,[30] and presacral nerve.[1]

EPIDEMIOLOGY OF ENDOMETRIOSIS

Several risk factors have been identified that are associated with the development of endometriosis. Some evidence suggests that there may be a genetic basis to endometriosis as it occurs far more commonly in monozygotic than dizygotic twins.[145] The common features that appear to increase the risk of endometriosis relate to an increased exposure to menstruation, i.e. longer duration of flow or higher volumes of retrograde menstruation in states where estrogenic stimulation is maintained.[44,126] It is also frequent in women with cervical ste-

nosis. The disease is more common where there is reduced parity, which reflects delayed childbearing, and is infrequent among multiparous women.[126] The risk is reduced for women using concurrent oral contraceptive medication, but not for such non-hormonal methods as intrauterine devices or diaphragms.[153] The risk increases after the use of the oral contraception medication is discontinued.

The occurrence of endometriosis relates also to increasing age, peaking at ages 40–44 years.[153] This may reflect increased numbers of menstrual cycles that have occurred before the menopause has begun and the major source of estrogenic stimulation has ceased. Compared to women aged 25–29 years, the relative risk of endometriosis is 2.1 for women aged 30–34 years, 4.5 during the ages 35–39 years, and finally 6.1 for ages 40–44 years.

PATHOGENESIS OF ENDOMETRIOSIS

Many theories have been proffered to explain the histogenesis of endometriosis (Table 20.3). Generally, they divide into those that favor:

- *transplantation* of endometrial fragments to ectopic sites
- *metaplasia* of the multipotential celomic peritoneum
- *induction* of undifferentiated mesenchyme in ectopic sites to form endometriotic tissues after exposure to substances released from shed endometrium.

Table 20.3 Theories of histogenesis of endometriosis

Theory	Comment
Transplanted endometrium	
Retrograde menstruation	Peritoneal implantation after passage through fallopian tubes
Lymphatic dissemination	Explains lymph node deposits
Vascular dissemination	Explains pulmonary deposits
Direct invasion	No evidence endometriosis penetrates wall of uterus, except in adenomyosis
Uterotubal	No evidence endometriosis penetrates wall of fallopian tube
Metaplasia *in situ*	
Celomic metaplasia	No experimental evidence
Embryonic rests	Experience limited to equivocal case reports
Wolffian duct remnants	
Müllerian duct remnants	
Induction	May occur, but requires exfoliated endometrium, e.g., deciduosis

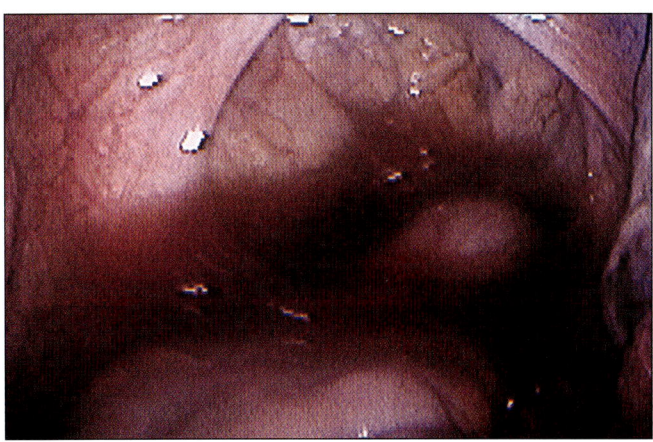

Fig. 20.1 Blood in pelvis from retrograde flow during menses.

TRANSPLANTATION

The most easily understood, scientifically supported, and widely accepted mechanism is that at menstruation, some of the menstrual products flow in a retrograde fashion through the lumen of the fallopian tubes into the pelvic peritoneal cavity.[56,57] The material drops to the pelvic floor and implants, in time regenerating into recognizable endometrium. This pathophysiology explains the most common sites of endometriosis. Abundant evidence indicates that menstrual retrograde flow does happen and, indeed, is a common phenomenon. Over 90% of women have blood in their pelvis at the time of menstruation, as identified by fluid examined at laparoscopy (Figure 20.1).

The frequency with which endometriotic implants are found in the pelvic cavity both usually and under special conditions supports an origin from transplanted menstrual products. Studies have shown that the most frequent sites are where the menstrual products flow from the fimbrial ends of the tubes. In addition to the ovary, the uterosacral ligaments are the most frequently involved area, with implants in the latter usually being located near the tubal ostium.[67] The uterine position is also of importance.[69] Disease, if exclusively located anteriorly, is found only in patients with anterior uteri. It is found significantly more commonly anteriorly in patients with severely anteflexed uteri. In contrast, when the uterus is retroflexed, anterior disease is uncommon.[57] The more frequent finding of endometriosis in the left rather than the right ovary, confirmed in several studies,[69,150] suggests that the endometrial retrograde flow is entrapped on entry by a shield (or 'microenvironment') formed in part by the sigmoid colon, which commonly leans on the left ovary and fallopian tube and is also fixed to the left pelvic brim by filmy adhesions.[150] Finally, as endometrial growth depends upon ovarian hormones and as the ovary is adjacent to the fallopian tube ostia, it is not surprising that the ovary is so commonly a site of the disease.

Further proof that menstrual material is viable has been obtained by collecting samples of menstrual products and injecting them subcutaneously into the anterior abdominal wall of animals. Excisional biopsy of the injection sites after several weeks showed lesions that resembled endometriosis in some subjects. These experiments show without doubt that endometrium shed at menstruation is viable and has the ability to implant and grow, further strengthening support for the theory that retrograde menstruation is important in the pathogenesis of endometriosis.[113]

Animal studies also support that menstrual products have the potential to implant and grow on a peritoneal surface. Early experimental studies in monkeys resulted in the development of endometriosis when the upper vagina was transected and the cervix turned into the peritoneal cavity, thereby creating an artificial uteropelvic fistula. In baboons, a species with a high rate of spontaneous endometriosis, blood-stained peritoneal fluid was 10-fold more frequent (62% vs 6%) during menses than during non-menstrual phases.[35] Retrograde menstruation was also observed more frequently in animals that had spontaneously developed endometriosis than in animals that were free of disease and had a normal pelvis. Finally, the experimental intrapelvic injection of menstrual endometrium led to the development of endometriosis much more frequently than if normal secretory endometrium was injected.[34,36] More recent work with this non-human primate model suggests that endometriosis develops in two distinct phases, the first being invasive and dependent on ovarian steroids and the second, which is the active phase of the disease, expressing endogenous estrogen biosynthesis. Following inoculation with menstrual endometrial tissues in two consecutive menstrual cycles, lesions develop similar to those seen in humans. By the first month the lesions express estrogen receptor beta, but it is only after 10 months that the lesions fully express aromatase.[46]

Experimental studies have also shown that human endometrium, when explanted onto human peritoneum, can attach and grow.[124,158] Invasion through the mesothelium by the stroma seems to occur rapidly, proof of invasion being measured by assessing the presence of the mesothelium. Over 90% of the explants grew through the cytokeratin-positive mesothelial layer, with intact mesothelium running up to the point of attachment.

Several other routes of transplantation, i.e. vascular spread, lymphatic spread, and direct implantation, have been observed. All help explain the occurrence of disease at distant or unusual sites. Endometriosis in a location such as within the parenchyma of the lung is usually accepted as vascular spread. Excised endometria from rabbits when injected into the ear veins of the individual hosts resulted in pulmonary endometriosis in 79% of the animals.[139] Fragments of endometrium may be seen in lymphatics in about 5% of women with endometriosis,[146] and occasionally in lymph nodes,[2] a phenomenon easiest explained by lymphatic spread. Finally, endometriosis in operative scars and in the cervix after cone biopsy or loop excision is easy to understand, as the endometrial tissue reaches the site by spillage at the time of operation or by direct implantation. The latter has also been experimentally documented. While all three of these mechanisms occur, their relative rarity shows that they are not the principal means by which endometriosis develops in most women.

The occurrence of endometriosis in young girls has been used as an argument that endometriosis arises by metaplasia, although the same facts can be used to argue that endometriosis is a phenomenon related in the majority of cases to retrograde menstrual flow. It does not occur much before the age of 11 years,[43] and when occurring in young women shortly after the onset of their menarche, is found associated with müllerian anomalies causing outflow tract obstruction.[139] On average, the elapsed time between the onset of menarche and the development of symptoms that require surgical intervention is 3 years if the woman has müllerian anomalies with outflow tract obstruction; it is nearly 7 years if outflow tract obstruction is present but the pelvic anatomy is normal.

METAPLASTIC THEORY

The metaplastic theory, for which there is scant data, proposes that endometriosis arises in the pelvis and elsewhere by endometrial metaplasia of the peritoneal serosa or serosa-like structures. This potential of pelvic peritoneum, invoked to explain the origin of epithelial tumors of the ovary, has fostered the concept of the so-called 'secondary müllerian system',[88] attributing to the pelvic peritoneum the ability to differentiate, if appropriately stimulated, into any of the recognized types of müllerian epithelium. A tenet of this theory is that endometriosis should be capable of development in situations where retrograde menstrual flow is impossible, such as in the prostate, bladder, and epididymides of men. In the few cases recorded, however, the men all had several years of therapy with synthetic estrogen, usually for prostatic carcinoma. The origin in these cases was thought to be the prostatic utricle, which is the vestigial remnant of the paramesonephric duct in the male. Rather than representing metaplasia, the development of endometriosis may represent simply a stimulation of the pre-existing müllerian duct epithelium.

In one study, the pelvic peritoneum and ovarian surface epithelium were examined to determine whether the epithelium adjacent to endometriosis exhibited signs of a metaplastic process.[105] Ber-EP4 antigen (a marker for epithelial differentiation) and estrogen and progesterone receptors (as markers of müllerian differentiation) were absent in normal peritoneum, but reactive in endometriosis and focally reactive in the adjacent peritoneal epithelium. Ovarian surface epithelium from normal control ovaries and ovaries adjacent to endometriotic lesions showed focal reactivity for these markers. All stromal cells uniformly lacked marker evidence of epithelial differentia-

tion. While these findings were interpreted to indicate that the mesothelium adjacent to endometriosis possibly acquires characteristics of müllerian-type epithelium, the results can just as easily be interpreted in the opposite manner. Unlike normal ovarian serosa, which is focally reactive for all three markers, the peritoneum is indeed negative. The endometriosis that implants can have microscopic extensions into the neighboring peritoneum, accounting for the spotty findings only in the region of the endometriosis. The more frequent finding of Ber-EP4 reactivity in normal ovarian surface epithelium compared to normal peritoneal mesothelium also suggests a fundamental difference in these two epithelia.

The reality of the metaplastic theory has been questioned.[111] One argument that proponents for both sides of the controversy have made concerns the development of endometriosis in women who congenitally lack a uterus (Rokitansky–Kuster–Hauser syndrome). If, by the implantation theory, endometriosis requires a source of transplanted endometrium, how can this occur in the absence of a uterus? In reality, patients with the Rokitansky–Kuster–Hauser syndrome usually have a portion of at least one fallopian tube associated with a rudimentary nubbin of uterus. One case, initially published as an example of endometriosis with an absent uterus, was later reported after new operative findings disclosed a functioning endometrium in a right rudimentary horn and retrograde menstruation through a fallopian tube with hematosalpinx.[3] In another instance, a 24-year-old woman with mosaic Turners syndrome was found to have endometrioma arising from the uterine serosa. However, as she had been receiving cyclic hormone-replacement therapy (HRT) for 5 years after laparoscopic gonadectomy and was having cyclic menstrual flow, it is likely that the endometriosis arose from retrograde menstruation.[140]

Another argument advanced in favor of the metaplastic theory is the apparent transitions sometimes observed between serosal inclusion cysts and endometriotic foci, but these findings too can be explained differently and have no experimental basis. On occasion, we have seen examples where an occasional cyst or gland lined by 'müllerian epithelium' lies adjacent to typical implants of endometriosis on the uterine serosa, peritoneum, or in the ovary. Rather than assigning the development of the endometriosis to the isolated gland, the gland might be unrelated or simply a focus of endometriosis where the stroma is absent. This would not obviate that the endometriosis developed by implantation. A second argument against the metaplastic theory concerns why men do not develop endometriosis at a high frequency, assuming the peritoneal epithelium has the potential to undergo celomic metaplasia. One answer has been the fact that the testes secrete müllerian inhibiting substance (MIS), but this acts only locally and therefore is an insufficient answer as to why men are free of endometriosis.

Another form of the metaplastic theory, development from embryonic rests, has been postulated by the finding of endometrial glands that appear to have arisen directly from some form of non-endometrial-type embryonic structure. In the embryonic ducts adjacent to the fallopian tube, allegedly wolffian ducts from the photographs in one study,[94] there was a gradual replacement of the muscular coat to a stroma that immunohistochemically resembled endometrial-type stroma. The theory put forward – namely, that the embryonic duct remnants were of celomic origin and therefore had the potential to differentiate into endometrial tissue – is generally not accepted to explain the common occurrence of endometriosis.

INDUCTION THEORY

A final theory, the induction concept, offers interesting aspects linked to the transplantation postulate. In this theory, it is not the transplanted endometrium itself that grows, but some substance within the endometrium that is secreted and induces the surrounding host tissues to generate the development of endometriotic epithelium and stroma. Experimental studies from over 30 years ago showed that when menstrual products encased in Millipore filters were implanted into the abdominal wall, some animals developed lesions that the investigators claimed to resemble endometriosis in the connective tissue adjacent to the implanted filters. In retrospect, it cannot be guaranteed that the filters remained intact. Further, the illustrations of the purported endometriosis are far from convincing and the tissue had no functional characteristics of endometrium.[57]

CATAMENIAL PNEUMOTHORAX

Catamenial pneumothorax is a condition suggested to theoretically develop on the basis of induction.[139] Catamenial pneumothorax, which differs from parenchymal pulmonary endometriosis, is a state where hemothorax and chest pain are the major symptoms of pleural and diaphragmatic endometriosis. The disease begins 2–3 days after the onset of menses. The pneumothorax is right-sided 90% of the time when associated with catamenia, but right-sided only 57% of the time when the pneumothorax is idiopathic. Recurrent pneumothorax is virtually always associated with menses. Most instances occur in parous women, but not in association with pregnancy. Most women with catamenial pneumothorax lack parenchymal pulmonary endometriosis.

A key argument for induction in association with catamenial pneumothorax is that particles over $22\,\mu m$ in size do not pass through the lacunas in the peritoneal lining of the diaphragm, which generally would eliminate fragments of endometrium, but not the inducing substances that might be liberated from degenerating endometrial cells.[139] As peritoneal fluid circulates in a clockwise direction, running down the left peritoneal gutter, across the pelvic floor, up the right peritoneal gutter, and to the right diaphragm, it is argued that substances may be introduced that then induce the formation of endometriosis in the pleural space. Problematically, many of the women with catamenial pneumothorax have evidence of diaphragmatic defects, suggesting that even in this disease state, transplantation may well be the most probable explanation. In one series of eight patients where the pneumothorax had a catamenial character by clinical history, diaphragmatic abnormalities were found as holes only (1), endometrial implants (3), and both holes and endometrial implants (4), indicative that diaphragmatic abnormalities play a fundamental role in catamenial pneumothorax.[6] With removal of the endometriotic focus in the diaphragm (or other thoracic locations), the syndrome of catamenial pneumothorax ends.[49,107,141]

In summary, the vast clinical experience and more recent experimental studies in non-human primates have shown that the etiology of endometriosis involves the transplantation of exfoliated endometrial cells. Retrograde menstruation and intraperitoneal implantation accounts for the vast majority of cases.[57] In some cases, induction by substances within the cells, even other routes of transport such as lymphatics or blood vessels, appear to be implicated. Some of the potential keys, as discussed below, are the elements that subsequently are needed to permit the endometriosis to develop into a pathologic disease process. These include the influence of the peritoneal milieu, i.e., the contents of the peritoneal fluid, and factors such as hormones, genetics, and immunologic aspects.

ETIOLOGIC FACTORS IN ENDOMETRIOSIS

GENETIC FACTORS

Heritable factors are important in the development of endometriosis.[122,154,157] In an early study of women with histologically proven endometriosis, a surprisingly large proportion of their female relatives were similarly affected (6% of sisters, 8% of mothers, and 7% of first-degree female cousins). In contrast, only 1.0% of their husbands' sisters and 0.9% of their husbands' mothers were affected. Furthermore, those women with endometriosis whose first-degree relatives were affected were more likely to have a severe form of the disease than those women whose first-degree relatives were not affected. In another study comparing 515 cases with 149 control cases (women without endometriosis determined by laparoscopy performed during sterilization), endometriosis was found in 3.9% of mothers of cases but in only 0.7% of mothers of controls. It was also found in 4.8% of sisters of cases, but only 0.6% of sisters of controls. The relative risk of endometriosis in a first-degree relative was 7.2. The manifestations of endometriosis were far more severe in women with a positive family history than in those without (26% vs 12%).[100] Recent pilot surveys also suggest that there are high concordance rates for the presence of endometriosis in monozygotic but not dizygotic twins.[54,74] Large international collaborative projects are currently being undertaken to identify the multifactorial mode of inheritance.[75]

HORMONAL ASPECTS

As the endometrium is a hormone-responsive tissue, it is not surprising that endometriosis undergoes cyclic patterns of growth and differentiation indicating that it responds to ovarian direction. The finding of endometriosis almost exclusively in the reproductive years and its association with leiomyomas and endometrial polyps also lead to the suggestion that hormonal influences may play an important part in its etiology. Multiple lines of evidence support the importance of prolonged estrogenic stimulation. Endometriosis is more common in women and primates where there are prolonged periods of unopposed estrogen exposure or in obese women who have higher levels of endogenous estrogen.[113] Conversely, it is much rarer in women who have decreased estrogen production during reproductive life. It often disappears after the menopause or, when found on histologic examination, appears in an atrophic state. It may also regress with medical suppression, but reappears once ovarian activity resumes.[45]

An important facet in the manifestations of endometriosis is therefore the ovary. Its microenvironmental steroid hormone concentrations are exceedingly high, measuring 1000-fold higher in follicles than in plasma.[80] The fluid found in the peritoneum originates mainly as an ovarian exudate, especially from around the developing follicle and corpus luteum, and has steroid hormone levels that also exceed those occurring in plasma. During the follicular phase, the concentration of estradiol in the peritoneal fluid increases progressively, rising after ovulation to a maximum of 40 000 pg/mL, which is a level 100 times that in the plasma. Progesterone levels mirror, and are also higher than, plasma levels. During the follicular phase, the levels in the peritoneal fluid are low (5–10 ng/mL), but jump abruptly after ovulation to 2000 ng/mL, decreasing slowly thereafter.

PERITONEAL ENVIRONMENT

Accumulating reports suggest that endometriosis is linked to abnormal immune function, which would explain why only some women develop the disease even though retrograde menstruation is so common.[39] In turn, the local environment of peritoneal fluid that surrounds the endometriotic implant may provide the specific microenvironment that dynamically links the reproductive and immune systems.[10,82,112,118]

In addition to the hormonal milieu established by the ovary, peritoneal fluid contains multiple types of free-floating cells, including macrophages, mesothelial cells, leukocytes, lymphocytes, eosinophils, and mast cells. Macrophages are estimated to account for over 80% of the cells in normal women.[32] In women with endometriosis, there is a pronounced increase in the number of total leukocytes, including macrophages, helper T-lymphocytes, and natural killer cells, supporting the suggestion that active immunologic processes are occurring.

Whether the changes observed are cause or effect remains unknown. The number of peritoneal macrophages is higher and many have increased expression of antigen markers. These macrophages secrete a number of factors thought to play important roles in both the growth and regulation of the endometriotic foci, especially in terms of proliferation of fibroblasts and endothelial cells that are involved in inflammation, tissue repair, and new vascular growth. Growth factors identified are epidermal growth factor, transforming growth factor, platelet-derived growth factor, and basic fibroblast growth factor. Some cytokines identified are interleukins 1, 6 and 8, tumor necrosis factor-alpha, and monocyte chemoattractant protein-1. The cytokines are also important in gamete function, fertilization and embryo development, implantation and postimplantation survival of the conceptus.

It would seem that the concentration of substances in these many secretions present in the local environment must have a substantial influence on the superficially implanted cells and could explain differences between the appearances and responsiveness of superficial endometriosis with that of the eutopic endometrium.

The differences that exist between superficial implants and those deeper (indicated in current classifications) may reflect the different local microenvironments to which each area of endometriosis is exposed. Peritoneal fluid factors probably regulate the superficial implants, whereas blood and ovarian hormonal factors regulate deep-seated endometriosis and cystic ovarian endometriosis.[80] A consequence of this theory is that the differences in deeply situated endometriosis or in the endometrium itself versus superficial endometriosis may be due more to the local environment than to any inherent differences in the tissues themselves. An extension of this theory concerns what is clinically significant endometriosis. If superficial endometriosis is considered as a natural condition that develops frequently on the basis of retrograde endometrial flow during menses, disappears spontaneously in most women, and is rarely associated with infertility or pain, it is questioned whether this form should be considered endometriosis at all. Some suggest that this should be considered normal. It might be questioned whether only endometriotic tissue that has penetrated at least 5 mm beneath the peritoneal surface, and is therefore deep, should be considered clinically significant endometriosis, which correlates with more aggressive behavior and is reflected by pelvic pain and infertility. Some have suggested that the classification should be based not on depth, but on more functional characteristics.[18]

OTHER FACTORS

ANGIOGENESIS

Excessive angiogenesis in the endometrium is a mechanism proposed to help explain the pathogenesis of endometriosis. One hypothesis tested is that the endometrium in women with endometriosis has an enhanced ability to proliferate, which in turn might lead to enhanced growth in the peritoneal cavity following implantation.[59] Proliferation of endothelial cells was measured with a monoclonal antibody against CD34 antigen, a glycoprotein expressed on the luminal surface of endothelial cells, and the proliferating cell nuclear antigen (PCNA), a nuclear protein whose expression peaks during the S phase of the cell cycle. An endothelial cell proliferation index was calculated as a percentage of proliferating endothelial cells per mm^2 divided by the total number of endothelial cells per mm^2. The endometrium of the women with endometriosis was abnormal, the proliferation index of the endometrium in the proliferative phase being many times higher (≥ 12) in women with endometriosis than controls.

Another marker of angiogenesis, integrin $\alpha_v\beta_3$,[59] is found in endothelial cells. It binds multiple ligands, including fibrinogen, von Willebrand factor, fibronectin, laminin, and thrombin. When blocked by monoclonal antibodies, it inhibits the growth of new blood vessels. The percentage of vessels in the endometrium of patients with endometriosis expressing this marker is significantly increased. In both of the above studies, it was concluded that the endometrium in patients with endometriosis had both enhanced proliferation and an increased ability to implant and survive in ectopic locations.

Under the transplantation theory, the retrograde endometrial flow must attach to and implant within the peritoneal cavity, and then establish and maintain an adequate blood supply. Growth of a new vascular bed is therefore critical if the endometriosis is to develop. Studies of vascular endothelial growth factor showed similarities in the endometrium of women without endometriosis and those with endometriosis.[41] The endometrial glandular epithelium of the latter women formed endometriotic deposits characterized as 'red' lesions, supporting the theory that the endometriosis in the study arose from the peritoneal seeding of viable endometrial cells during retrograde menstruation and that red lesions were the first stage of implantation. That there was a significantly higher growth factor present in red lesions compared with black lesions is consistent with the black lesions being older and showing changes reflecting some degrees of fibrosis and inactivation.

Other studies have shown that the vessel density in endometriosis does not differ from that of the normal endometrium nor from that found in various types of endometriotic lesions. The luminal diameter, however, was decreased in older ('black') lesions and within any individual patient. Differences were commonly observed in vessel densities, both in different types of lesion and within the same types of lesion.[95] In summary, these results do not unequivocally explain whether angiogenesis fosters the growth of endometriotic explants or simply mirrors their level of activity.

Some evidence suggests that a key to angiogenic activity may lie in the contents of the peritoneal cavity rather than in the endometriotic explant itself.[134] Potent angiogenic growth factors are increased in the peritoneal fluid in patients with this disease. The activated peritoneal fluid macrophages and infiltrating macrophages are a rich source of this angiogenic growth factor.

PROSTAGLANDINS

Prostaglandins, the origin of which is uncertain in the peritoneal fluid but which may possibly derive from peritoneal macrophages, the peritoneal lining itself, or even the retrograde menstrual endometrium, were once considered important in endometriosis.[32] The literature has remained inconsistent, as evidenced by conflicting reports that the levels are normal in some women but abnormal in others. There is even disagreement about which of the many known prostaglandins may be important.

MORPHOLOGIC FEATURES OF ENDOMETRIOSIS

GENERAL

In the most elemental terms, endometriosis can be diagnosed by finding both endometrial glands and stroma in the operative specimen. The appearances, however, can be protean and affected by topography, age of the lesion, and age of the patient. The laparoscopic appearances of the lesions are depicted in Figures 20.1–20.4.

GROSS FEATURES

The ages of the endometriotic deposits affect their gross appearances. The various colors reflect the deposit's functional states. Yellow-red surface stains, which reflect breakdown of blood products on the involved surfaces, often herald the presence of the earliest detectable lesions (Figure 20.2). Occasionally, early lesions will show vesicle formations (Figure 20.3), a state before the endometriotic foci begin to cycle and undergo tissue and blood breakdown. The red lesions also reflect an early form of

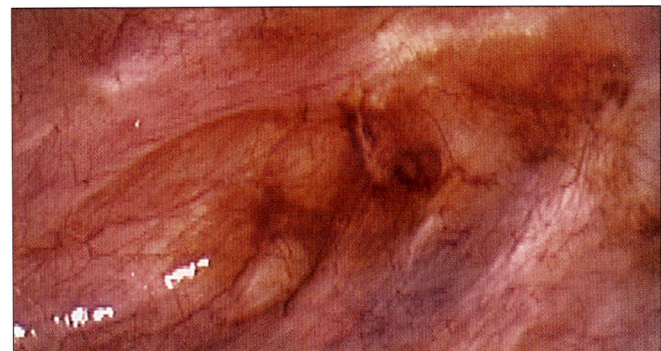

Fig. 20.2 Yellow-red stain of endometriosis. This is the earliest manifestation of endometriosis seen laparoscopically.

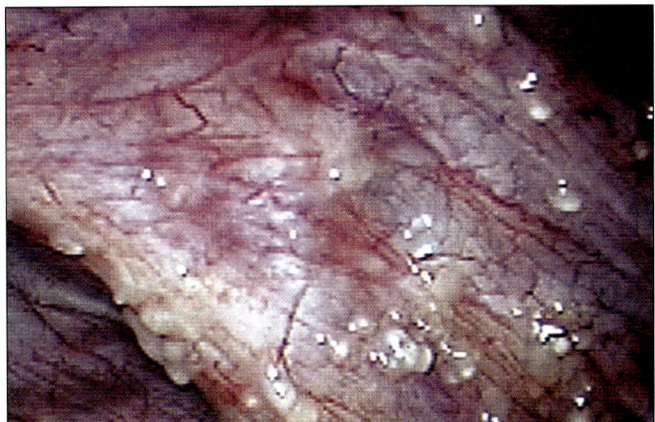

Fig. 20.3 Vesicle formation in endometriosis on broad ligament.

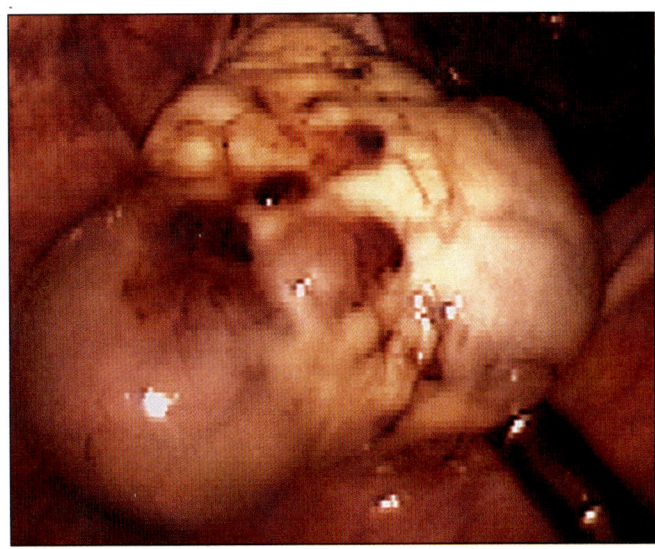

Fig. 20.4 Multiple red lesions on ovary.

the disease.[42] The endometriosis is actively growing (Figures 20.4 and 20.5). These red lesions evolve into the black (advanced) lesions in which some degree of bleeding has resolved (Figures 20.6 and 20.7). This is the most common form seen by the pathologist in operative specimens. Some

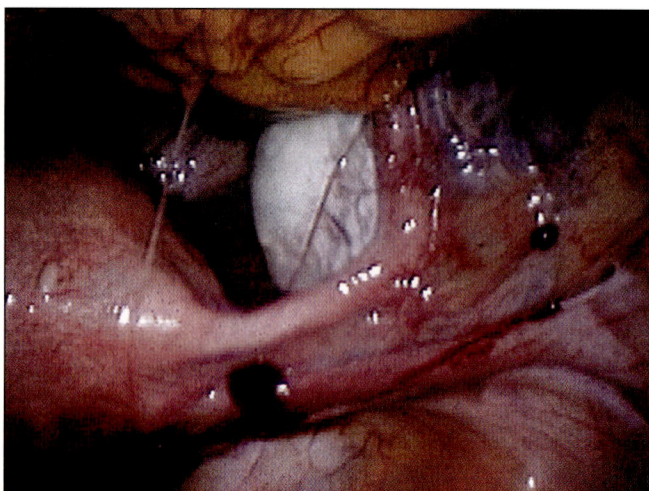

Fig. 20.5 Red lesions on broad ligament and ovary.

lesions may be brown to slightly yellow-brown, which indicates the presence of hemosiderin. These lesions are also called 'café-au-lait spots'. The oldest, or white lesions, have fibrosis and scarring and often the color reflects the advanced degree of healing (Figure 20.8). Strangely, it is the white lesion where endometriosis is most easily confirmed histologically.[137] This may relate to the complete fibrotic encapsulation of the peritoneal implant protecting the transplanted endometrial cells from destruction by tissue macrophages. As lesions begin at different times, the various foci may differ from site to site in this multifocal condition. Seldom are endometriotic lesions solitary.

The changes seen laparoscopically are also seen macroscopically in the surgical specimen. In general, the first grossly recognizable lesions are blister-like blebs, some 2–3 mm in diameter, on the surface of the target organs (Figure 20.9). They are red and represent highly vascularized implants.[17] The tiny red lesions are the exclusive form of endometriosis found in 20% of adolescents with this disease. They have yet to show

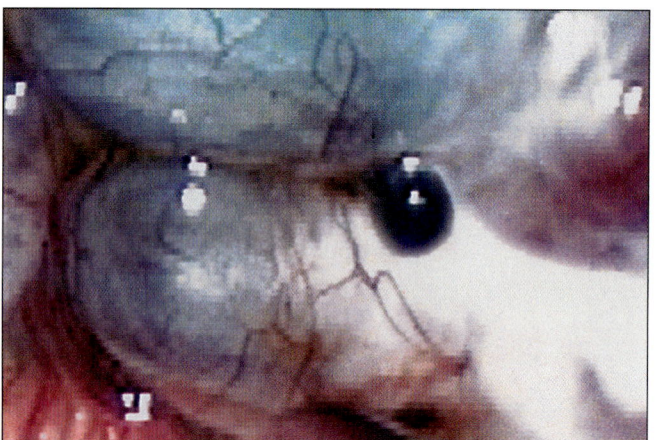

Fig. 20.6 Black lesion on ovary.

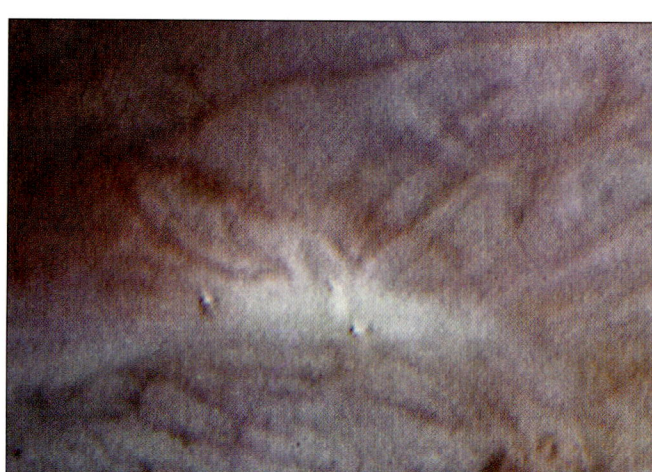

Fig. 20.8 White lesion due to extensive fibrosis.

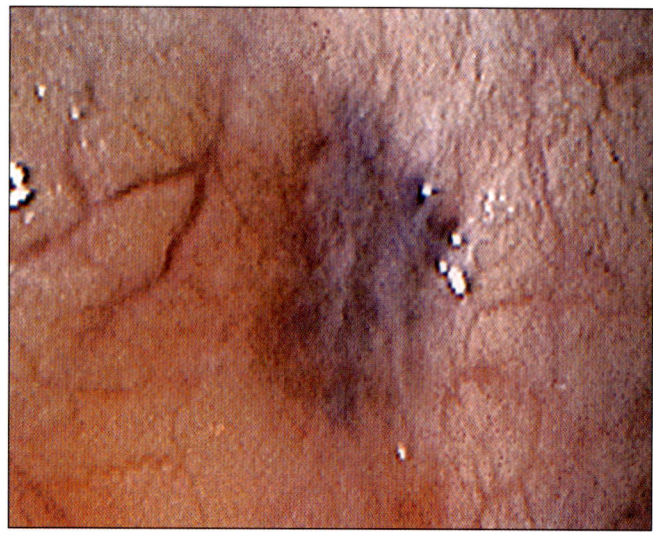

Fig. 20.7 Black lesion in endometriosis with early scarring.

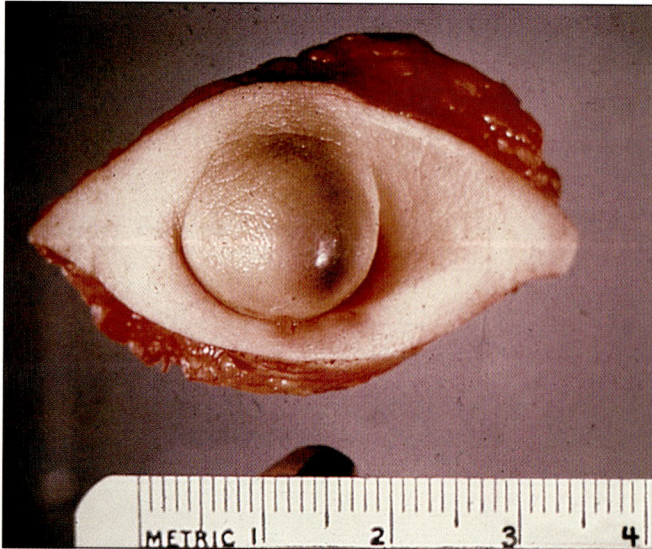

Fig. 20.9 Red, newly formed lesion of umbilical endometriosis. The 3 mm raised hemorrhagic papule appeared only recently.

signs of repeated bleeding and scarring (fibrosis). Some investigators[79] believe that many of the red lesions should not be considered as endometriosis, assuming that virtually all women have retrograde menstruation and therefore some red lesions.

As the lesions advance in age, they enlarge, reaching a size of 3 mm to sometimes over 1 cm, sometimes singly or as a collection. As they go through repeated cycles, they become pigmented and blacker, largely from intraluminal debris, old blood, hemorrhagic stroma, hemosiderin-laden macrophages, and even some scarring. These lesions may be raised, bluish-red to bluish-black, and may resemble mulberries or blueberries (Figure 20.10). If they are more extensively fibrotic and scarred, they may also appear puckered ('powder burn') (Figure 20.11).

Lesions that heal have undergone extensive fibrosis and scarring and are white. They have minimal stroma and are poorly vascularized. Black-and-white scarred lesions predominate in later years.

The disease site affects whether the endometriosis is serosal (including subserosal/subperitoneal) or whether it can be found deep within an organ (e.g., ovary). Implants of endometriosis grow poorly on the surface of the peritoneal mesothelium,[16] as scanning electronic microscopic studies have shown. Rather, mesothelium quickly grows over the implant, encapsulating it as if it were a foreign body, or the stroma grows into the wall. In the peritoneum, such nodules appear to be located subperitoneally. In the ovary, these nodules enlarge during cyclical 'menstruation', first appearing as small indentations into the cortex, and with time invaginating substantially into the ovarian substance. On cross-section, these foci of developing endometriomas show the wall and base to actually consist of the ovarian cortex/serosa, the so-called 'inverted cortex' (Figure 20.12). Sometimes, the pearl-white appearance of the ovarian cortex is still recognizable. The tissue covering the endometrioma, i.e., the peritoneal cover, is an operculum consisting of fibrous tissue and mesothelium.

At some sites, the lesions may become grossly cystic, but the cysts generally do not become large, except in the ovary. In general, the cyst wall is rarely thicker than 2 mm, and the endometriotic tissue rarely more than 1.5 mm thick.[104] The term 'chocolate cyst' is often used to describe these cystic lesions (Figures 20.13 and 20.14). The term, though, can be misleading. It is purely descriptive, referring to the chocolate-colored contents. In fact, any hemorrhagic dysfunctional cyst can have the same appearance, be it from an old hemorrhagic corpus luteum, unruptured follicular cyst, to an endometrioid adenocarcinoma with extensive hemorrhage and necrosis.

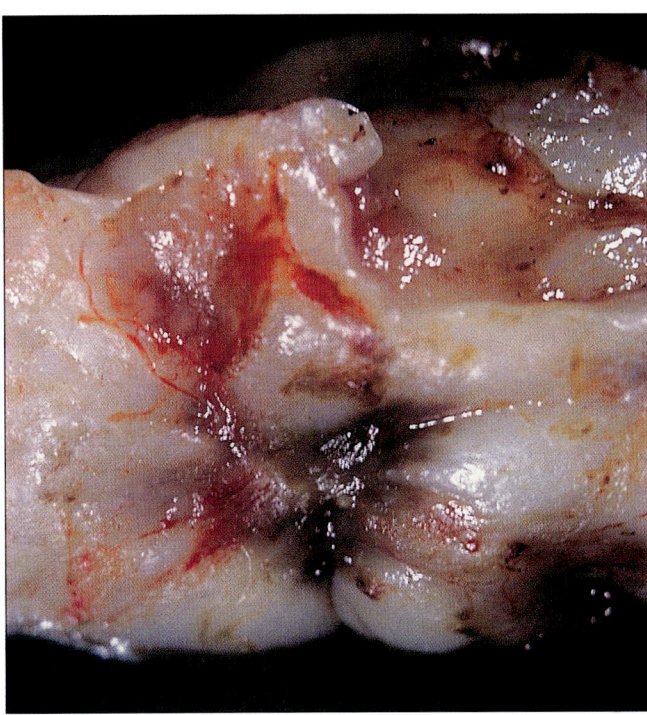

Fig. 20.11 Scarred ('powder burn') lesion of endometriosis. The consequent extensive fibrosis has resulted in a puckered surface.

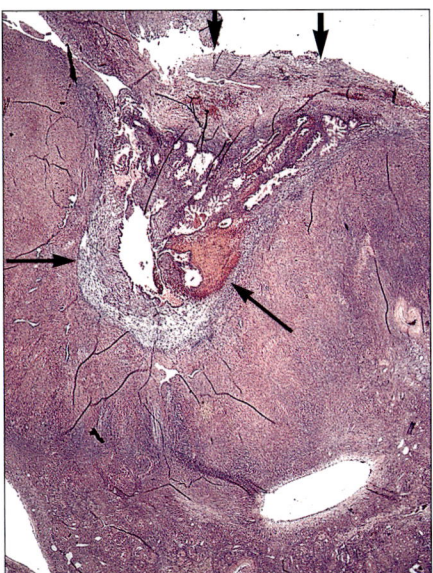

Fig. 20.12 Inverted cortex of ovarian endometrioma. The inverted ovarian cortex lies at the base (thin arrow) of the endometrioma. A fibrous operculum (thick arrow) covers the upper surface of the endometrioma.

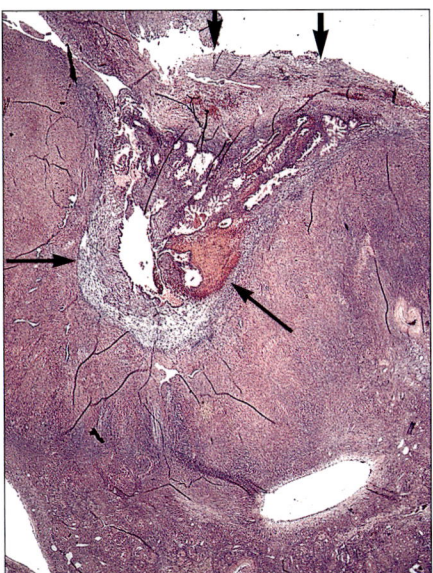

Fig. 20.10 Black ('mulberry') lesion of endometriosis.

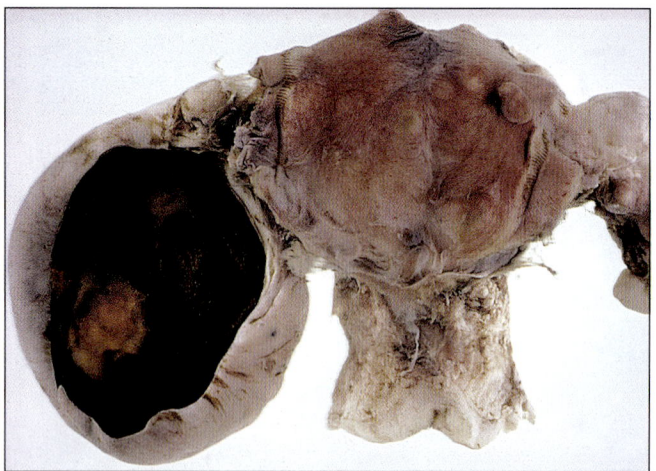

Fig. 20.13 'Chocolate cyst' of ovary. The endometrioma is large, but has not yet completely replaced the ovary.

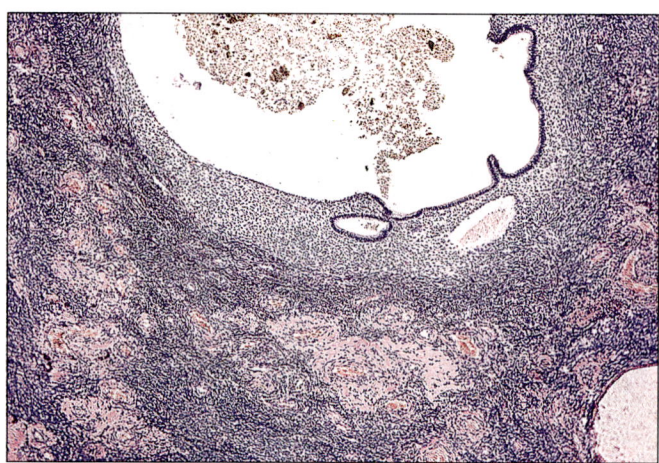

Fig. 20.15 Endometriosis of ovary. The endometrial-type epithelium is one cell thick and is sharply defined and distinct from the underlying endometrial-type stroma, which itself is also distinct from the deeper ovarian parenchyma.

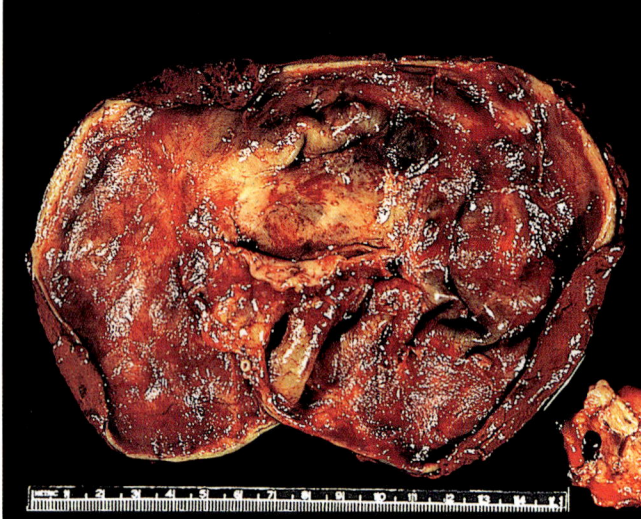

Fig. 20.14 Large endometrioma of ovary. The endometrioma has completely replaced the ovary.

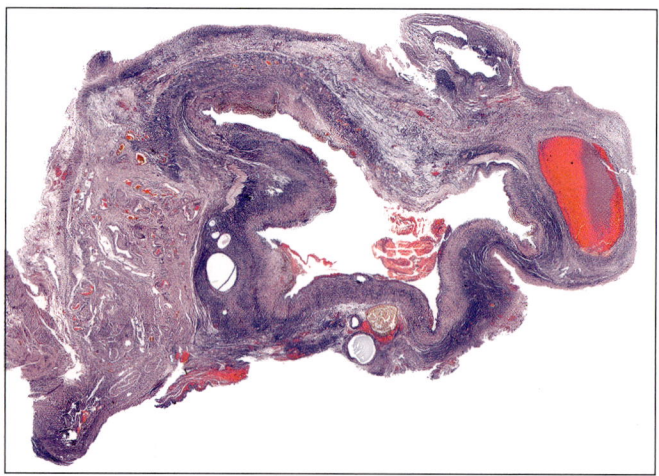

Fig. 20.16 Endometrioma of ovary. Courtesy of Dr Myron Tannenbaum, Clearwater, FL.

In some cases, an organ involved with endometriosis may be greatly distorted by extensive fibrosis and scarring. Adhesions to surrounding structures are usually present and form an important basis of staging the severity of disease present.

Another feature that affects the appearance of the endometriosis is the age of the woman. A woman who is in her reproductive years will have the typical lesions, the microscopic appearances of which are as described below. Women who are postmenopausal or who lack a source of estrogen stimulation will often have lesions marked by atrophy or near disappearance of either the epithelial or stromal component.

MICROSCOPIC FEATURES

Endometriosis consists of endometrial glands surrounded by endometrial stroma. This definition is important and both components must be more or less typical if errors in diagnosis are to be avoided. Usually the features of endometriosis are

quite easy to identify. On a low-power magnification, the epithelium appears as a thin, dark layer that is sharply delineated from the underlying, paler stroma (Figures 20.15 and 20.16). The luminal surface of the epithelium may be slightly jagged and irregular. On high-power examination, the epithelium is one cell layer thick and has the appearance of an endometrial epithelium (Figures 20.17 and 20.18). The cells are usually tall and columnar with elongate cigar-shaped nuclei showing regular vertical orientation. The cytoplasm is eosinophilic and cilia are often identified. The glands usually appear to be relatively inactive, with only sparse mitoses, but florid proliferative and secretory activity may at times be observed.

The stroma generally resembles the normal stroma found in the endometrium, and consists of small spindle-shaped cells with inconspicuous cytoplasm. A delicate reticulin network that is much finer than that of native ovarian stroma supports the cells, as silver impregnation staining reveals. The presence of reticulin is also useful in some organs to distinguish between endometriosis and stroma that normally lacks reticulin investiture, e.g., cervix.[76] Various degrees of decidualized stromal

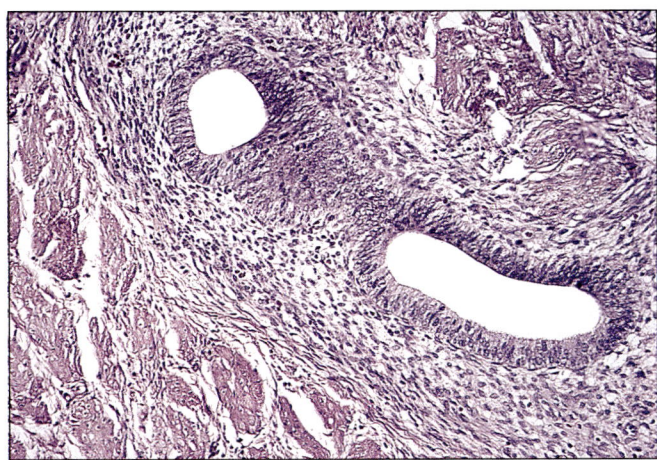

Fig. 20.17 Endometriosis in broad ligament.

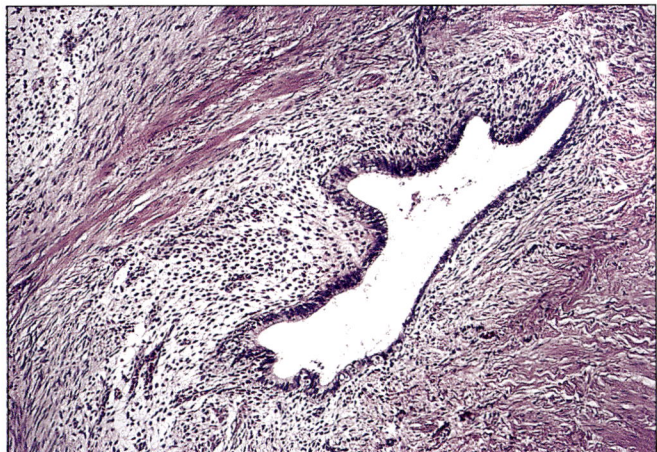

Fig. 20.18 Endometriosis in broad ligament. The epithelial layer is distinct from the underlying stroma.

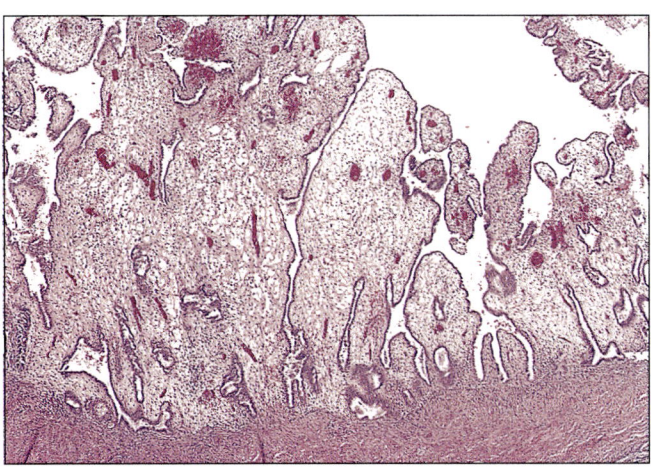

Fig. 20.19 Decidual response of endometriosis to exogenous progestins.

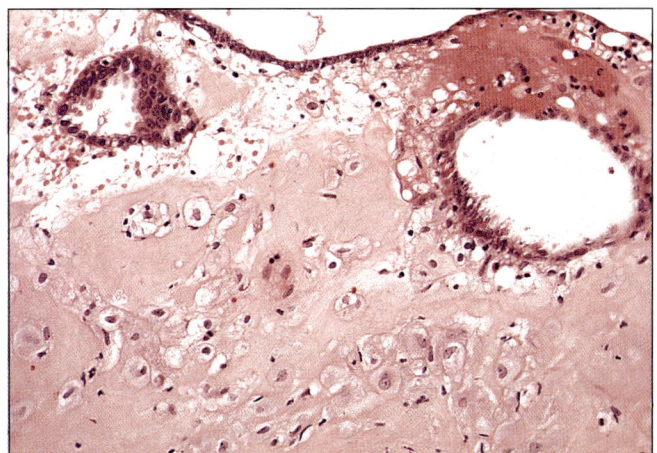

Fig. 20.20 Florid decidual response of endometriosis in pregnancy.

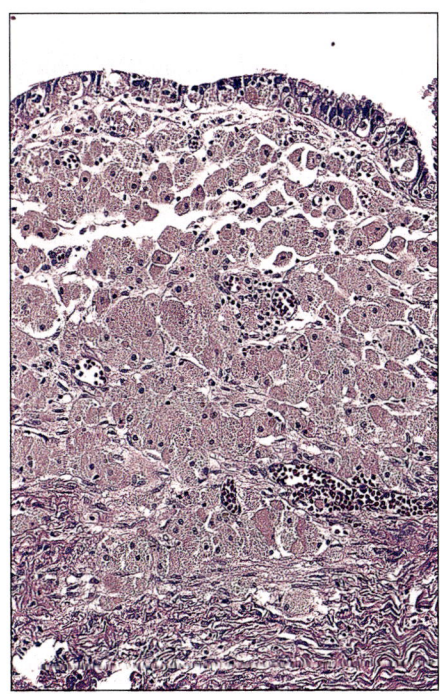

Fig. 20.21 Endometriosis with mildly pigmented, hemosiderin-laden macrophages.

cells may be seen if the endometriotic focus is cyclically functional. The cells may show a (pseudo)decidual response during the latter part of the menstrual cycle in association with exogenous administration of progestins (Figure 20.19) and during pregnancy (Figure 20.20).

Sometimes, macrophages may be present that are slightly (Figure 20.21), focally (Figure 20.22) or heavily (Figure 20.23) hemosiderin laden. Smooth muscle fibers may be associated with the stromal component of endometriotic foci, most commonly in randomly arranged small groups, but sometimes forming an incomplete sheath around chronic cysts, especially in pelvic sites.[8]

The epithelial and stromal components may not always be satisfactorily identified. This is consistent with the character of the endometrial fragments in the menstrual debris as the autolytic process of menses may yield isolated glandular or stromal cells. In cystic lesions, which are common in the ovary, the endometriosis may appear to be composed solely of stroma, or sometimes stroma with fibrosis or hemosiderin-laden macrophages; however, in the absence of epithelium, the diagnosis cannot be established conclusively. Often, the epithelium may not at first be apparent. In some cases, multiple sections are necessary to disclose the characteristic findings. Particular

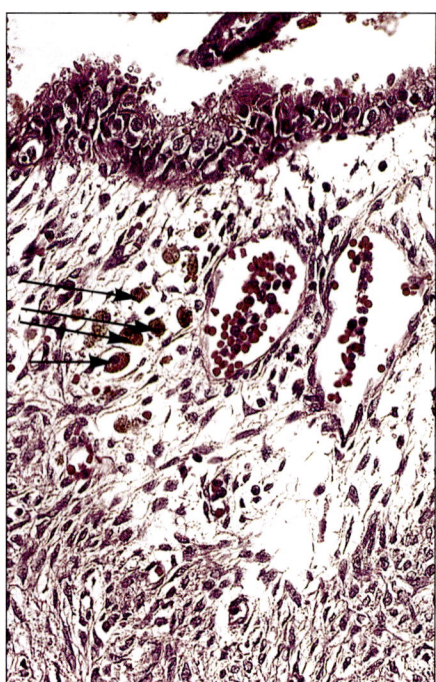

Fig. 20.22 Endometriosis with several hemosiderin-laden macrophages (arrows).

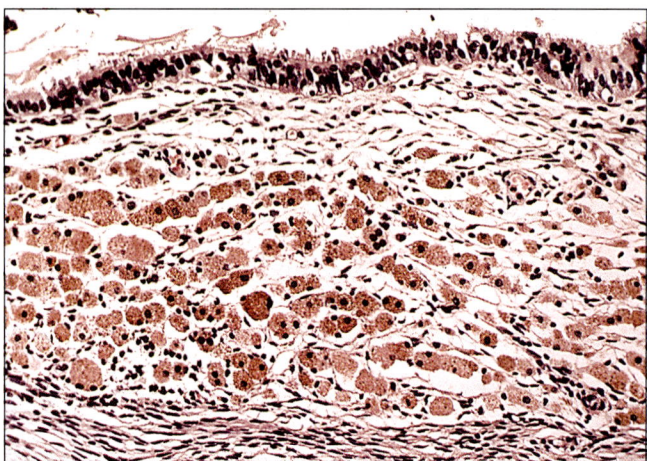

Fig. 20.23 Endometriosis with markedly pigmented, hemosiderin-laden macrophages.

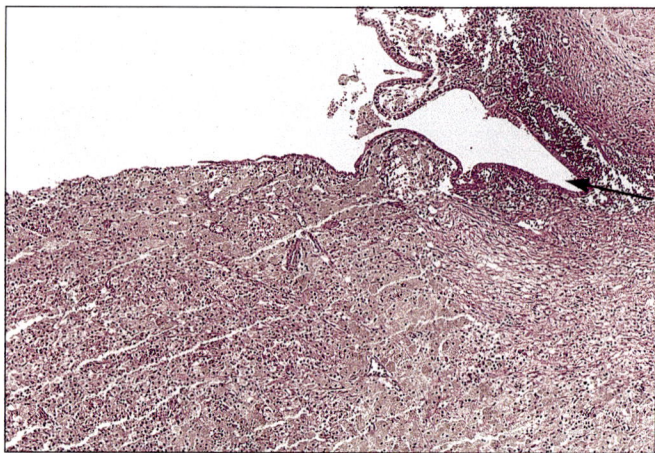

Fig. 20.24 Endometriotic epithelium in a protected crevice. Occasionally, the epithelium from an endometrioma cannot be found except in an invagination where pressure atrophy is lacking (arrow), or during specimen preparation where the epithelium has not been wiped away. The photograph shows epithelium around the protected crevice. In the extreme circumstance, only a dozen cells or so may be found in the crevice itself.

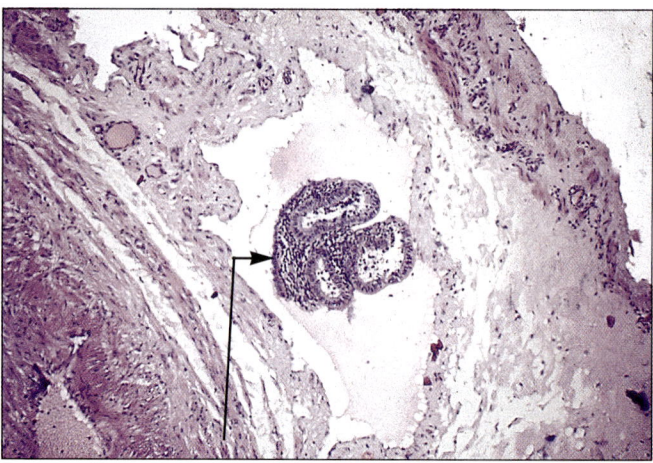

Fig. 20.25 Endometriosis in a subserosal lymphatic vessel of the uterus. The several endometrial-type glands present are invested with only a minute amount of stroma (arrow).

attention should be paid when examining the slides to small crevice-like invaginations in the stroma (Figure 20.24). These areas are commonly overlooked, but often are the only zones where the epithelium is retained. Such a zone may amount to no more than a rare microscopic focus, and is extremely easy to overlook, even when there is a conscientious effort to seek it. In one series of 77 patients with non-pigmented peritoneal lesions, 73 biopsy specimens showed both glands and stroma, 12 showed only endometrial-type stroma and 10 had neither.[68] On a practical basis, there seems to be no merit in diagnostic criteria that are so rigid that they exclude many clinically obvious cases of endometriosis. Except for ovarian endometriosis where several lesions described above are easily confused with endometriosis, a presumptive diagnosis based clinically on the laparoscopic findings, or the finding of stroma alone in the biopsy specimen is generally sufficient to diagnose endometriosis.

At times, the stromal component may not be altogether obvious. This is exemplified by several cases. In one, obvious endometrial-type glands invested with only a minute amount of stroma were located in a subserosal lymphatic vessel in the uterus of a patient with extensive pelvic endometriosis (Figure 20.25). In other cases, the stromal component may simply be absent, requiring that the diagnosis be inferred from the other disease present. For example, a small endometrial-type gland was found within a pelvic nerve in a patient who had florid endometriosis throughout the entire pelvis, the region of the bladder, and about the ureters (Figure 20.26). A third example is where a müllerian-type gland on the serosa of an organ was immediately adjacent to more typical appearing foci of endometriosis (Figure 20.27). A final type of problem occurs in

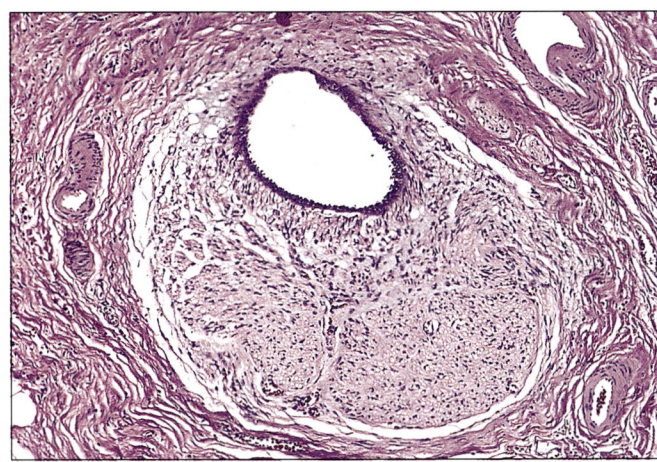

Fig. 20.26 Endometriosis within a pelvic nerve. The diagnosis is inferred in the absence of stroma as florid endometriosis was present throughout the entire pelvis, the region of the bladder, and about the ureters.

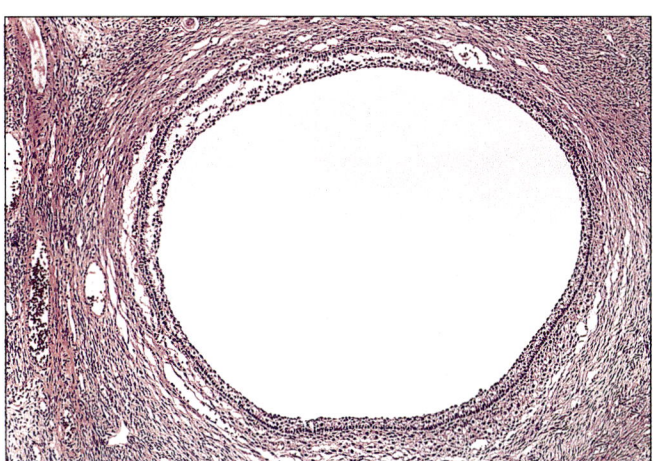

Fig. 20.28 Graafian follicle of ovary. The granulosa layer is composed of uniform cells, thus lacking the lining layer of epithelium seen in endometriosis.

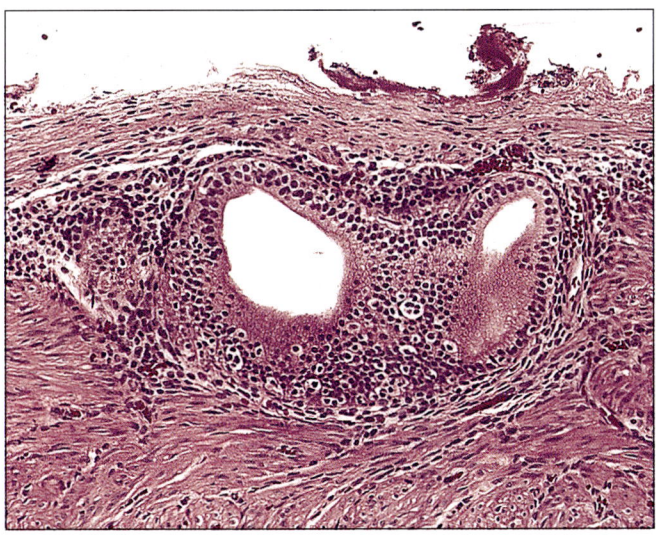

Fig. 20.27 Müllerian-type gland devoid of stroma on uterine serosa. A field nearby, but not in the photograph, showed typical endometriosis.

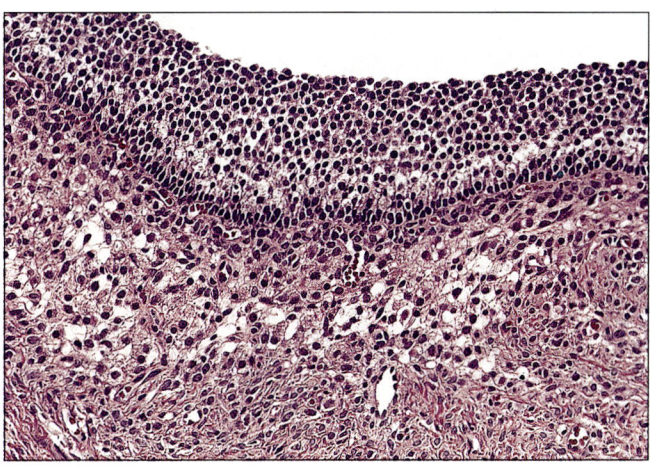

Fig. 20.29 Granulosa layer in ovarian follicle. High-power magnification discloses uniform small cells lacking a supporting vasculature. The granulosa also lacks the lining of a luminal epithelium seen in endometriosis.

postmenopausal women where the endometriotic components are atrophic and difficult to appreciate.

There are two particular, normal morphologic appearances that may be confused with endometriosis, either causing the endometriosis to be overlooked or, conversely, leading to the diagnosis of endometriosis being made improperly. The former situation where the endometriosis is missed occurs when it is confused with a normal follicle in the ovary that is in an advanced state of maturity (Figures 20.28 and 20.29). Because of the plane of section, the follicle lacks an obvious cumulus oophorus. The entire thickness of cells that line the follicle is composed of granulosa cells. All lack cytoplasmic maturation and thus appear as closely packed nuclei that are uniform. They lack any degree of pleomorphism, which is so typical of endometrial stroma. There is also a conspicuous absence of vessels in the preovulatory granulosa layer, further differentiating it from the stroma of endometriosis. Additionally, in endometriosis the innermost layer of cells consists of epithelium that

contrasts, often starkly to the practiced eye, with the underlying stromal cells (Figures 20.15 and 20.18).

The other, more common misdiagnosis where endometriosis is mistakenly identified occurs in lesions composed of hemosiderin-laden macrophages. Such lesions are often end-stage hemorrhagic follicles or resolving corpora lutea (Figure 20.30). If epithelium is present, the diagnosis of endometriosis is established. If epithelium is absent, a useful clue to the diagnosis of a follicle or corpus luteum is the finding of clusters of luteinized theca cells deep in the focus in question. These findings are often subtle.

In postmenopausal women and women receiving selective estrogen response modulators, which are predominantly estrogen antagonists, foci of endometriosis in the peritoneal structures may be particularly difficult to identify and, when suspected, may be difficult to document conclusively. The lesions in this age group are typically atrophic and either the epithelial cells or sometimes the stromal cells are absent or, at most, debatably present. The stroma may also in part be fibrotic. In circumstances where the typical appearances of

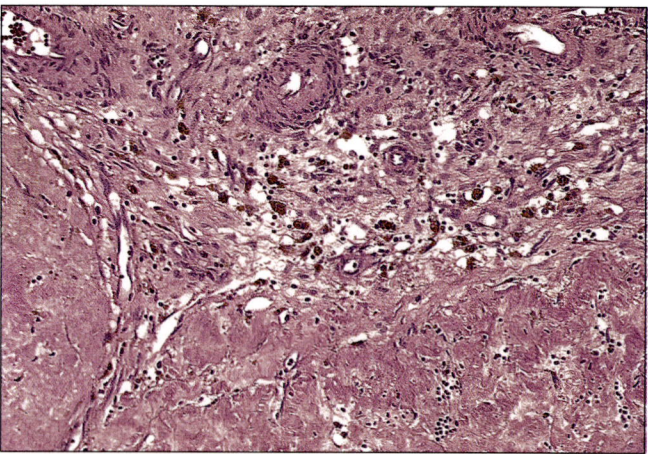

Fig. 20.30 Resolving corpus luteum with hemosiderin-laden macrophages. This appearance is easily misinterpreted as endometriosis.

endometriosis are not found, it may be impossible to make a definitive diagnosis. At times the most appropriate diagnosis concludes with the inconclusive comment that the appearance is 'compatible with, but not diagnostic of'.

Although endometriosis can be hormonally responsive, the endometriotic foci usually do not reflect the histologic appearances expected at the appropriate stages of the menstrual cycle. Indeed, they commonly lack cyclic changes. The morphologic appearance of tissue can provide some insight into which foci of endometriosis will be hormonally responsive. For example, implants with greater amounts of fibrosis show progressively less hormonal responsiveness.[98] Endometriomas are less often in phase with the corresponding endometrium than ordinary implants (22% vs 43%). Finally, implants that are functionally synchronous with the corresponding eutopic endometrium have more stroma than those that are out of phase.

These results suggest that the architectural relationships among the various cellular elements affect the endometriotic response to cyclic endogenous hormones, the classic gland–stromal interaction, critical to endocrine responsiveness. In general, the hormonal responsiveness of the implants reflects the quantity of stroma that surrounds the glands, its degree of vascularity, the degree of fibrosis, the presence of surface epithelium, characteristics of the glands themselves, and the presence of local stromal hemorrhage. The steroid receptor content is variable in the various lesions.[144]

While not generally discussed in the literature, endometriosis when present in tissue with native smooth muscle can sometimes induce marked hypertrophy. This is not unusual in endometriosis in the bowel wall, uterine ligaments, and bladder. The local muscular hypertrophy that is induced is morphologically identical to that characteristic in uterine adenomyosis.

Differential diagnosis
Several conditions that are commonly misdiagnosed as endometriosis (or vice versa) have been described above. Corpus luteum cysts are the lesions most likely to be confused microscopically with chronic endometriotic cysts, since both have a ragged hemorrhagic internal surface. Microscopically, both are lined, at least focally, by fibrous tissue, and granulation tissue in which there are clusters of pale vacuolated cells. Endometrial glands and stroma are, of course, absent.

Serosal inclusion cysts are exceedingly common superficial cortical lesions. They are lined by cuboidal cells of surface epithelial type or by cells more typically identified as serous. They are commonly associated with psammoma bodies. The lesions are distinguished from small superficial endometriotic lesions by an epithelial lining that is generally not endometrial in type, and by their lack of endometrial stroma, hemorrhage or associated adhesions.

Mesothelial cysts are superficial lesions that do not impinge on the ovarian cortex. They are lined by cuboidal cells with small round nuclei that are readily distinguished from columnar endometrial cells with their cigar-shaped nuclei. Endometrial stroma is absent. They are usually the end result of inflammatory processes involving the ovarian capsular surface, so that adhesions and chronic inflammatory cells are often present.

Rete ovarii and parovarian vestigial remnants may superficially resemble endometriotic foci. The rete have a characteristic ramifying pattern and are surrounded by condensed ovarian, rather than endometriotic stroma lacking evidence of hemorrhage. Rete tubules are lined by cuboidal or columnar cells. Paramesonephric and mesonephric remnants are lined by tubal and cuboidal epithelium, respectively, with cuffs of smooth muscle.

Mature adult cystic teratomas (see Chapter 27) should not cause confusion if there is an opportunity to examine the surgical specimen macroscopically or if multiple blocks have been sectioned. However, individual slides may show a cyst lining composed of macrophages, granulation tissue, and fibrous tissue – a picture also seen in endometriotic (and corpus luteum) cysts. Close scrutiny of the macrophage zone should reveal the pathognomonic hair fragments or squamous cells.

In the peritoneal cavity, deciduosis and disseminated leiomyomas are manifestations of müllerian tissue present in the pregnant and the non-pregnant state, respectively. The subperitoneal foci of stroma decidualize and resemble the endometriotic lesions of pregnant women or patients receiving progesterone therapy. The absence of endometrial glands excludes endometriosis.

OVARY

The best known manifestation of endometriosis in the ovary is the 'chocolate cyst' (Figure 20.13). Grossly, this is a moderately thin-walled cyst containing dark purple-brown, semisolid, sticky material that may sometimes be similar in color, although not in consistency, to chocolate. The appearance of this material is due to hemorrhage into the lumen of the cyst with the resultant degradation of blood pigments. Although the finding of a 'chocolate cyst' highly suggests endometriosis, it is not diagnostic, as a similar appearance may develop in any circumstance where there has been hemorrhage into a cyst. This may be seen with a corpus luteum cyst, a follicular cyst or even a neoplastic cyst. Other gross manifestations of endometriosis, described above, include mulberry (Figure 20.10) or blueberry-like structures, or sometimes an end-stage likened to powder burns (Figure 20.11). Today, these are all called 'black' lesions.

The microscopic features of cystic endometriosis in the ovary may present as any of a number of patterns. Commonly, the full picture of endometriosis is seen with a mucosal lining composed of easily recognizable glands and an underlying stroma readily recognized as being of endometrial type (Figure 20.15). A clear demarcation between the endometrial stroma and the surrounding ovarian stroma is also usually apparent. This pattern is easily diagnosed. Many endometriomas, if small enough, can be shown to be superficial in location. A cross-section of the ovary in these cases often discloses that the ovarian cortex lies deep to (i.e., beneath) the endometriotic stroma (Figure 20.12). The fibrous cap above the endometriosis appears more like an operculum that has grown in from the adjacent epithelial surface of the ovary to have covered the endometrial implant. It is as if the new overgrowth had acted to wall off the endometriotic implant, much like the type of reaction that occurs about a foreign body. These findings suggest that in at least some cases the endometriosis develops as endometrium that has implanted onto the ovarian serosa.

A more difficult lesion to identify is where the endometrial epithelium is reduced to a single layer of cuboidal cells that are nondescript or distorted. The epithelium, if atrophic, may resemble that of a simple cystadenoma. The cytoplasm may also be unusually eosinophilic, such that the cells resemble oxyphils, and even at first glance raise the question of neoplasia (Figure 20.31). The nuclei are generally situated in the basal half of the cell, but may even be in the center of the cell, and may show considerable pleomorphism. Distinction from the epithelium of a mucinous cystadenoma is usually easy, although there is the suggestion that some mucinous lesions may arise in endometriosis.[89] Distinction from a serous cystadenoma may be more difficult. The presence of an underlying endometrial-type stroma, even if minute in amount, is sufficient to confirm the diagnosis of endometriosis. CD10 reactivity is useful in establishing the presence of the stroma.[96,143]

The overall shape of an endometriotic cyst on microscopic section tends to be more irregular than that of common epithelial neoplastic cysts. Endometriosis nearly always gives the impression of a collapsed cyst. Just deep to the epithelium there may or may not be an easily discerned band of endometrial-type stroma, characterized by closely packed, small, dark cells. There may have been hemorrhage into this zone, with the resultant accumulation of pigment-laden macrophages.

The most extreme histologic pattern, and perhaps the most unusual, is when the epithelium lining the cyst is lost and the repeated hemorrhage into surrounding ovarian stroma has effaced any endometrial stroma, replacing the environs of the cyst with fibrous tissue (Figure 20.24). Within the fibrous layer, hemosiderin-laden macrophages are scattered in uneven aggregates. On many occasions, a cyst that is quite clearly a 'chocolate cyst' on macroscopic examination and so is purportedly of endometriotic type contains no recognizable endometrial tissue on microscopic examination. Rather it shows only the fibrotic appearances just described. This may also represent a histologic sampling error as the endometriotic cells may have an uneven distribution within the endometrioma wall. It is in these circumstances that the histopathologist can do no more than comment that the features are compatible with endometriosis.

Ovarian endometriosis may also be non-cystic and recognized as a small collection of irregular glandular structures within a field of endometrial-type stroma. It is sometimes possible to trace apparent transitions between serosal inclusion cysts and endometriotic foci. Indeed, the distinction between the two can be difficult. The ovary affected by endometriosis often has surface adhesions. The condition is frequently bilateral.

A rare feature occasionally reported in endometriosis is the presence of Liesegang rings, which are acellular, ring-like structures that may form within and around inflamed or necrotic tissue.[116] They appear as multiple eosinophilic, sharply demarcated, ring-like structures that are highly periodic acid-Schiff positive. Almost all such cases involving the female genital tract have been found in endometriomas of the ovary.

Epithelial 'metaplasias' have been described in endometriosis, but in our experience are largely so common and interspersed that we consider them more of an intrinsic component than an abnormality.[50] Serous (tubal) metaplasia as alternating groups of ciliated and secretory cells is the most frequent (found in nearly half of cases) and may be either focal or widespread. Endometriotic lesions showing a prominent tubal metaplasia have been called 'endosalpingiosis', a term we avoid as confusing. Clear cell metaplasia has been described in over a tenth of cases, but this can be difficult to distinguish from secretory changes, and particularly from the Arias-Stella reaction. Mucinous metaplasia is relatively rare and is usually focal. Squamous metaplasia has been reported to occur in long-standing endometriotic cysts.

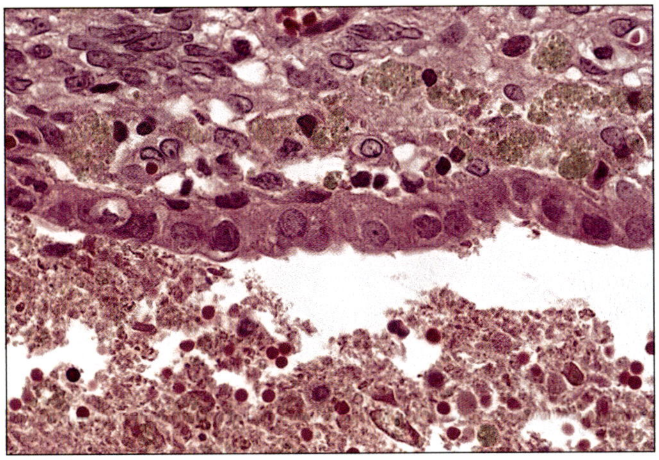

Fig. 20.31 Cuboidal, markedly eosinophilic cells of endometriosis.

FALLOPIAN TUBE

Endometriosis of the fallopian tube has several patterns of appearance. A relatively uncommon, but highly distinctive form is the presence of endometrial tissue lining the tubal lumen itself, replacing the tubal mucosa ('endometrialization'). Rather than finding the tubal plicae covered by ciliated epithelium, endometrial glands and stroma are present. The endometriosis commonly fills the entire lumen of the proximal tube's isthmic segment, but sometimes is present only as large nodules (Figure 20.32). Whether this condition should rightly be called endometriosis is a moot point, since it may represent an exceptionally high junction between endometrium and fallopian tube epithelium, a junction that is usually situated at the inner end of the isthmic portion of the tube. Regardless of histogenesis, this condition often produces complete blockage of the affected tube and is associated with infertility (see Chapter 19).

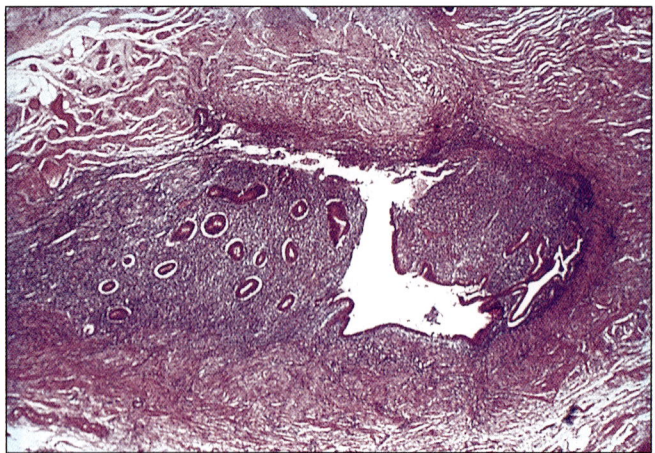

Fig. 20.32 Endometriosis of fallopian tube.

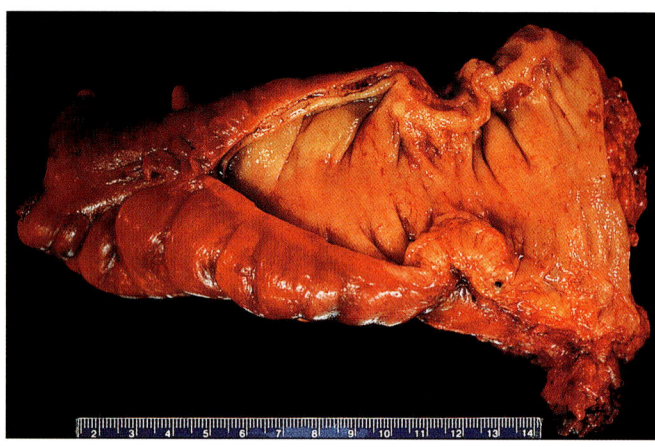

Fig. 20.33 Stricture induced by endometriosis in colonic wall.

The more common situation is to find the endometriosis as a surface phenomenon on the outer peritoneal surface of the tube, the endometrial glands and stroma being situated in the subserosal layer. As at most non-ovarian sites, endometriosis of the fallopian tube is composed of small, non-cystic glands and easily recognizable endometrial stroma. Fibrosis and signs of hemorrhage may be seen but these features are not usually prominent. Occasionally, overgrowth of the muscle may be seen, but this is exceptional and much less pronounced than in the bowel or uterine ligaments (see below).

Sometimes, the endometriosis may be found in the wall, where it must be distinguished from salpingitis isthmica nodosa, a disease thought akin to adenomyosis of the uterine myometrium. The latter is usually localized to the tubal wall, lacking other findings on the serosa. Salpingitis isthmica nodosa, grossly, often appears nodular, which microscopically is due to reactive smooth muscle hyperplasia about the glandular epithelium. Unequivocal endometrial-type stroma is not present in salpingitis isthmica nodosa. The two conditions may occur together.

Endometriosis on the tubal surface or present in the mesosalpinx or broad ligament often needs to be distinguished from small microscopic foci of serous epithelium arising in these locations or even small foci of serous borderline tumor metastatic from the ovary. The serous forms have been called 'endosalpingiosis' by many, although others prefer to classify the disease in a more histogenetic and functional form depending upon the appearance of the tissue. The authors are divided with regard to terminology. Some prefer 'serous metaplasia', 'serous adenoma of borderline malignancy' or 'müllerian inclusion cyst', depending upon the histologic appearance and whether the lesion appears to have originated there or is metastatic from another location, usually the ovary.

Regardless of the terminology preferred, the distinction between endometriosis and serous lesions can sometimes be difficult. Quite commonly, the stroma that is present is miniscule in amount and has the appearance of reactive fibroblasts. In the absence of unequivocal endometrial-type stroma, endometriosis cannot be diagnosed. Adding further difficulty to the diagnosis is the relative infrequency of hemosiderin-laden macrophages, even in well-developed foci of endometriosis in this location. Psammoma bodies are typical of serous disease and are rarely if ever seen in endometriosis. The two conditions may coexist and sometimes do.

CERVIX

Historically, endometriosis involving the cervix has been relatively infrequently seen (3% of biopsy and hysterectomy specimens). With the increased usage of loop electrosurgical excision and cone biopsy procedures, the frequency anecdotally has risen. The microscopic findings are as described above. Cervical implants may also represent transient adherence of endometrial cells shed during menses.

GASTROINTESTINAL TRACT

Extrapelvic endometriosis most commonly involves the gastrointestinal tract,[129] usually affecting those parts of the bowel that lie in proximity to the genital organs. It occurs in 5% of women with endometriosis. Symptoms, when present, depend on the site involved, and commonly are abdominal or rectal pain, or constipation.[65,147] Dysmenorrhea, dyspareunia, and infertility frequently accompany concomitant pelvic disease. Local symptoms reflect abnormal peristalsis or a distorted intestinal lumen. Constipation may occur with endometriosis in the distal colon, while patients with small intestinal lesions may have diarrhea or loose stools. Catamenial hematochezia may be a consequence of submucosal implants of endometriosis involving the bowel.

The gross appearance is usually that of a thickened bowel wall. At times, the endometriosis may simulate a colonic carcinoma if there is a circumferential stricture of the wall (Figure 20.33), but usually the endometriosis is distinctive in that there is prominent muscular hypertrophy. This thickened area of bowel wall is white and rubbery and sometimes discloses small, cystic spaces just visible to the naked eye (Figure 20.34). The wall also lacks the grittiness, scarring, and irregular tongues of invasive tumor seen with carcinomas. Usually, the mucosa is intact. Rectal bleeding, if present, is due to endometriotic tissue that swells during menstruation, resulting in mucosal tears.[47] Endometriosis may also resemble a polypoid

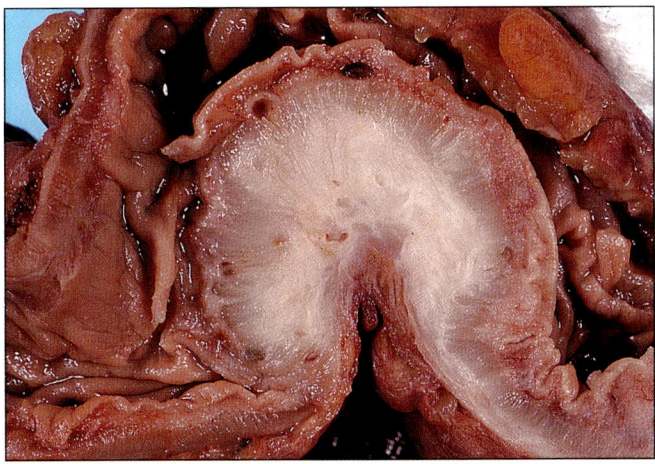

Fig. 20.34 Endometriosis in colonic wall. Extensive fibrosis and muscle hypertrophy account for the white and tan-brown color, respectively.

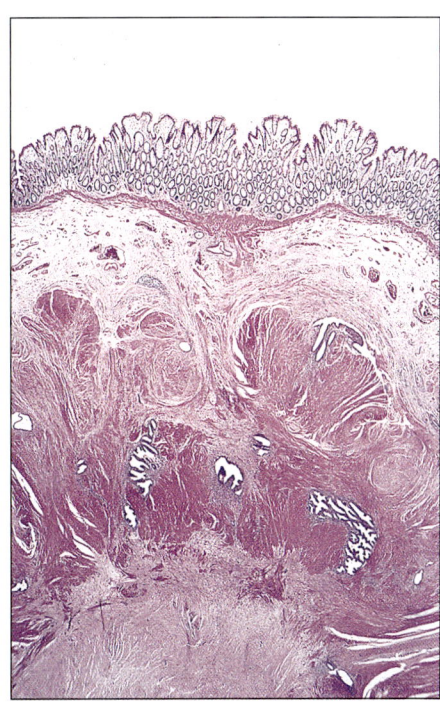

Fig. 20.36 Endometriosis in smooth muscle of colonic wall.

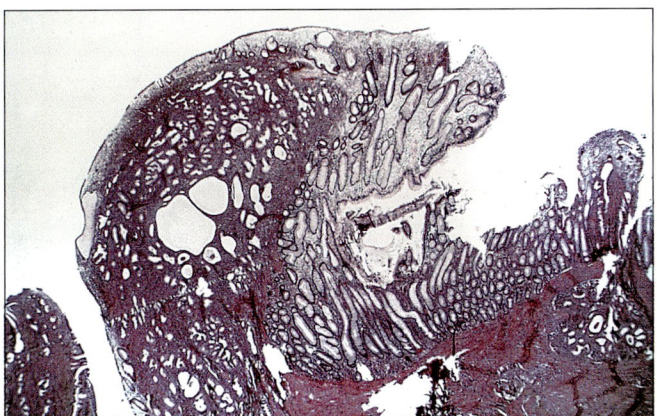

Fig. 20.35 Polypoid endometriosis in colonic wall.

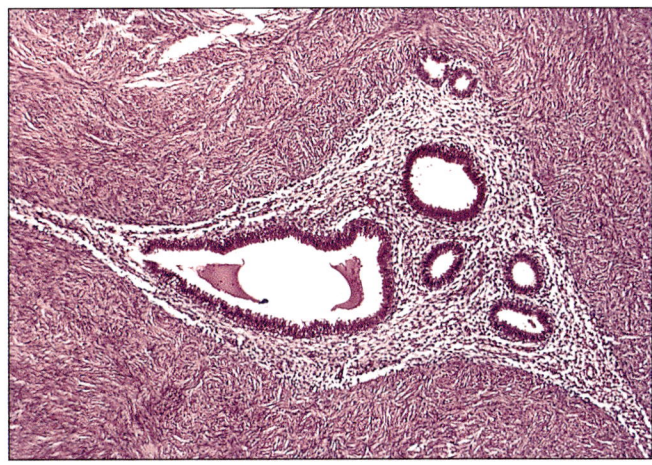

Fig. 20.37 Endometriosis in smooth muscle of colonic wall, medium power magnification.

neoplasm, which on endoscopic examination might easily be mistaken for an adenocarcinoma (Figure 20.35). Microscopically, typical foci of endometriosis are seen throughout the bowel wall (Figures 20.36 and 20.37), and sometimes may involve the submucosa (Figure 20.38). Occasionally, if endometriosis is not clinically evident and not present in the immediate zone of the biopsy, inflammatory bowel disease may be erroneously diagnosed.[87]

URINARY TRACT

The urinary tract is involved in 1.2% of women with endometriosis.[129] Of these, the bladder is most commonly affected (five-sixths of cases) and the disease is usually limited to the serosa. The wall, when involved, is usually thickened from fibrosis and muscular proliferation around the endometriotic foci. The ureter is affected less often (one-sixth of cases) and the kidney and urethra very rarely. Endometriosis can induce dramatic retroperitoneal fibrosis on occasion and if the ureter is entrapped, represents an important cause of ureteric obstruction.[60]

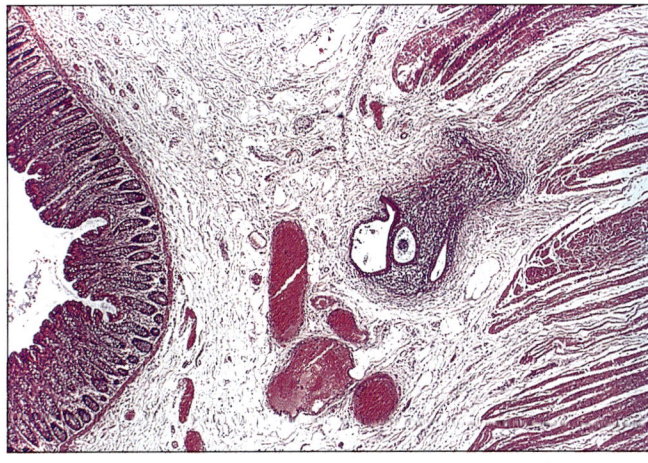

Fig. 20.38 Endometriosis in submucosa of colonic wall.

ABDOMINAL WALL

Endometriosis in abdominal wall scars is seen most frequently following hysterotomy, a procedure that was a commonly used method of mid-trimester abortion in the early 1970s. The frequency with which endometriosis has been seen subsequently in the abdominal wall of women subjected to this operation emphasizes that endometrium has the potential to implant and proliferate when spilt into a wound. Although cesarean section is a common procedure, endometriosis is rarely a sequel. Many cases reported following cesarean section appear due to direct progression of endometrium through the deficiency in the uterine wall rather than iatrogenically implanted disease and are thus more akin to adenomyosis. Endometriosis in the needle track has been reported following amniocentesis. It has also followed operations such as myomectomy or cesarean section that open the uterine cavity and thereby allow spillage of endometrium into the wound. Only rarely is it found in the scars of other operations, such as hysterectomy or appendectomy. Proponents of lymphatic spread in the pathogenesis of endometriosis have used this finding to support their beliefs, suggesting that the lymphatics are obliterated at the scar, so that endometrial tissue traveling along them becomes lodged.

LYMPH NODES

Endometriosis is only occasionally found in lymph nodes (Figure 20.39), which is surprising given extensive disease in the peritoneum and the occasional observation of endometrial cells in the myometrial lymphatics. When present in pericolic lymph nodes, it is easy to mistake the endometriosis for a metastatic adenocarcinoma of the intestines.[2,47,65] The presence in the lymph node of an endometrial-type epithelium that is associated with endometrial-type stroma should allow the diagnosis to be made with some ease. Occasionally, the stroma may be decidualized, especially if the patient is pregnant or is taking progestational-type medication.

Far more commonly, pelvic or para-aortic lymph nodes may contain glands lined by a serous or endometrioid-type epithelium. In the absence of stroma, these glands may represent müllerian inclusion cysts,[101] a lesion described elsewhere and which often appears associated with metastases from borderline serous tumors of the ovary[101] (see Chapter 33).

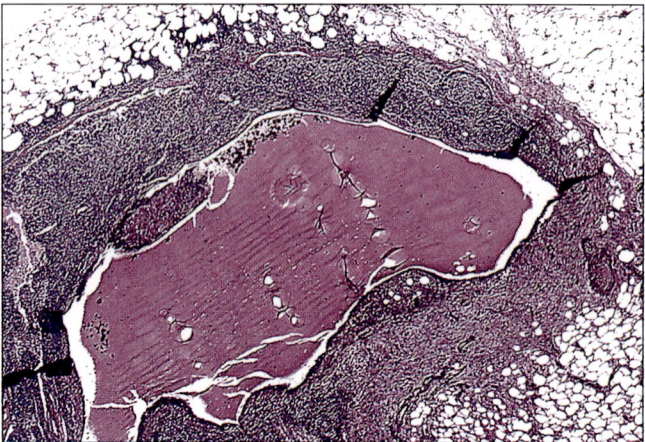

Fig. 20.39 Endometriosis in colonic lymph node.

SPECIAL CONSIDERATIONS

Endometriosis is sometimes detected on the serosa of the uterus or immediately in a subserosal location (Figure 20.40). The difficulty in diagnosis occurs when the patient has concomitant adenomyosis. In these cases, however, the adenomyosis is usually confined to the inner portion of the myometrium and there is usually a substantial portion of uninvolved myometrium between the two conditions.

Similarly, endometriosis in the vagina must be distinguished from adenosis that is of the tuboendometrial type. Adenosis usually involves the mucosa. If in a submucosal location, there is still often a connection to the mucosa. Endometrial-type stroma is also absent. Endometriosis, in contrast, is usually located deep in the wall, has endometrial-type stroma around glands, and is often separated from the vaginal mucosa by an area of uninvolved wall (Figure 20.41).

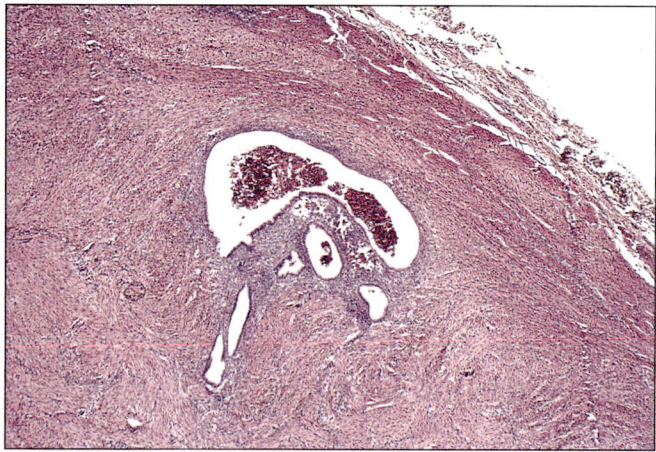

Fig. 20.40 Subserosal endometriosis in uterus.

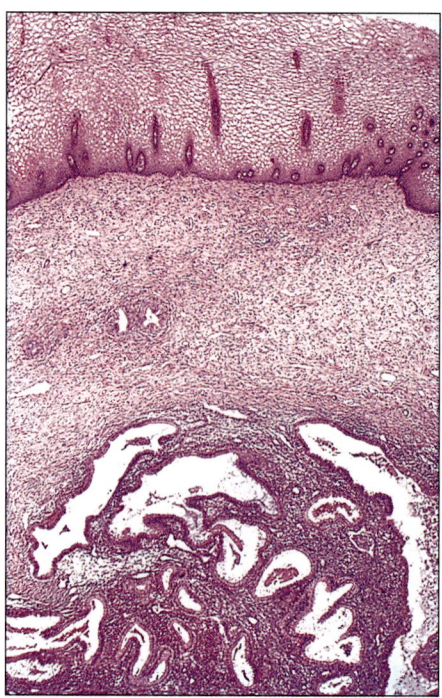

Fig. 20.41 Endometriosis separated from the vaginal mucosa by a broad zone of uninvolved wall.

In the peritoneum, small nodules of endometriosis may disclose an abundance of histiocytes filled with ceroid, a wax-like, golden to yellow-brown pigment that is probably a type of lipofuscin. These have sometimes been called 'necrotic pseudoxanthomatous nodules'.[27]

CLASSIFICATION OF ENDOMETRIOSIS

The schemes used to classify endometriosis have undergone substantial change since they were first introduced nearly 50 years ago. The various classifications introduced evolved from being based on the histology of resected specimens and those that emphasized anatomic staging, similar to contemporary systems for staging malignancies based on extent of disease.[31,61] The scheme used most commonly today is the 1996 Revised Classification of Endometriosis by the American Society for Reproductive Medicine.[21,127] The goal of the classification scheme is to predict, on the basis of disease severity, the chance of conception.

This classification stratifies endometriosis not only by the extent of disease present, emphasizing ovary, fallopian tube, peritoneum, and cul-de-sac, but also by the severity of disease found. It also assesses damage from the disease, namely pelvic adhesions. It has a weighted point score that assesses the extent of the endometriosis among organs and even within an organ, i.e., superficial (<1 mm) vs invasive (>5 mm) disease. It assesses the unilaterality of the disease, size of endometriomas, and type of adhesions (filmy vs dense). The cumulative scores result in a stage designation: Stage 1 is minimal disease (1–5 points), Stage 2 is mild disease (6–15 points), Stage 3 is moderate disease (16–40 points), and Stage 4 is extensive disease (>40 points).

Several areas have been identified where the classification scheme needs to more accurately represent the disease present:

- Predictive abilities: Virtually all schemes poorly predict pregnancy rates, which is the main goal of the system. It also poorly predicts response to treatment. Current schemes also help little in the evaluation and management of endometriosis when there is pelvic pain.[31,61,120] Possibly, a Stage 5 is needed requiring >70 points, since patients with this score or higher do not conceive. Over half of women with scores under 70 do conceive.[21]
- Limited reproducibility: Interobserver reproducibility is only fair to good.[121] When the same observer scored the endometriosis based on what was seen by two different operative methods (laparoscopy and laparotomy), the correlations were worse, especially for the disease in the ovaries and cul-de-sac. Evaluation of disease found in the peritoneum was the most consistent.[92]
- Potential for observational error: Non-pigmented lesions may be difficult to see, and are often related to the surgeon's experience and anticipation of such lesions.
- Failure to consider the morphology of the lesion: Lesions, as they age, change from red to a dark color. This relates to functional characteristics of the lesions, including production of various biochemicals.
- Better correlation is needed between extent of disease and pelvic pain[23] and also severity of pelvic symptoms.[151]

- Inclusion of all disease: Endometriosis in extrapelvic locations needs to be included in any classification scheme in order to compare findings among institutions.[129]

INFERTILITY IN ENDOMETRIOSIS

Infertility and endometriosis go hand in hand, both in humans[130] and non-human primates.[37] Although precise figures of the relationship are difficult to determine, estimates are that about 30–50% of women with endometriosis suffer from infertility and 25–50% of infertile women have endometriosis. The cause of this infertility is not clear,[58] especially if the amount of disease present is minimal. In baboons, the primate model most extensively studied experimentally, fecundity is normal if the animal has only minimal disease, but is reduced with progressively more severe disease.[34,37]

The most obvious reasons for infertility would appear to be mechanical, resulting from tubal blockage or distortion, but these factors are not obvious in most cases nor does evidence support these suggestions. Endometriosis may occasionally obliterate the tubal lumina, but this appears only in a minority of cases. Tubal scarring and fixation, with tethering of the fimbriae that would interfere with ovum pick-up, are sometimes observed. Although many women with endometriosis show what appears to be the stigma of chronic salpingitis, the incidence of these changes is no higher in infertile women than in those who conceive.

A second reason for infertility may be related to the implants themselves, although the mechanisms involved are not at all clear. The strongest evidence for a causal link between the implants and decreased cycle fecundity involved women who underwent a therapeutic donor insemination program on the basis of a severe male factor (e.g., aspermia).[68] Those women who had visible endometriosis subsequently had lower cycle fecundity after insemination when compared to women free of implants. However, even those data do not conclusively demonstrate causality and do not exclude some other underlying more important explanatory factor.[58]

More subtle causes for the association must be sought.[117] Potential mechanisms being explored include endocrine dysfunction (inadequate mid-cycle luteinizing hormone surge and inadequate corpus luteum), tubal dysfunction, luteinized unruptured follicle syndrome, altered components of follicular fluid, dysfunctional eutopic endometrium, immune dysfunction (dysfunctional T-lymphocytes, antiendometrial antibodies with specific B-lymphocyte activation, autoimmune syndrome with non-specific B-lymphocyte activation), alterations in circulating blood components (elevated levels of cytokines, direct toxic effects of serum), and peritoneal fluid inflammation.[58] In the experimental situation, there is some evidence that the intraperitoneal inflammation itself rather than the implants is responsible for the reduced fecundity, comparable to the mechanism of contraception of the intrauterine device.

MALIGNANCY IN ENDOMETRIOSIS

The exact incidences of tumor-like forms of endometriosis, endometriosis with adenomas, and malignant change in endometriosis are unknown. Tumor-like conditions take the form of nodules or even large masses that microscopically show no more than florid endometriosis. These masses can be in the pelvis (Figure 20.42), fat (Figures 20.43 and 20.44), or even located within organs (Figures 20.45 and 20.46). The endometriosis can also be seen adjacent to, but continuous with (Figure 20.47) or even within (Figure 20.48) endometrioid adenomas.

Most likely endometriosis has no greater malignant potential than the endometrium proper, but neither has it any less potential for malignant change. For any number of reasons, the frequency of endometriosis transforming to cancer has been difficult to determine. Extensive sampling may be required to find a small focus of endometriosis adjacent to a malignant tumor or a cancer may destroy the endometriotic tissue from which it arose. Often, only the frequency of concomitant endometriosis has been recorded without a specific statement of how many cancers arose from the endometriotic tissue.

In general, the criteria for establishing an origin of malignancy from endometriosis include the following:

- Both cancer and benign endometrial tissue should be seen in the same organ.

- Both should bear the same histologic relation to each other that the cancer of the uterine corpus bears to the non-malignant portion of the endometrium.
- The cancer must be shown to have arisen in this tissue and not invaded it from some other source.

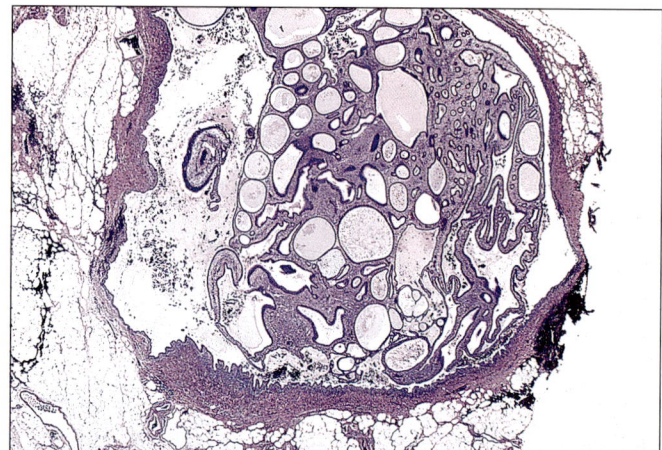

Fig. 20.44   Florid (adenoma) endometriosis in omentum.

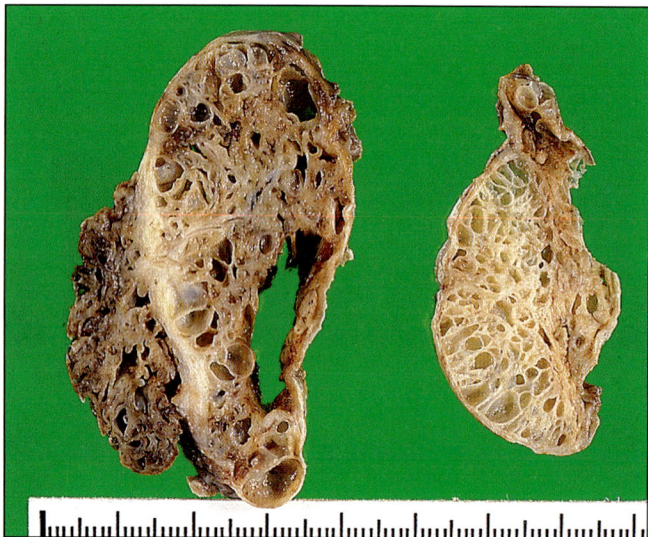

Fig. 20.42   Florid endometriosis as pelvic mass.

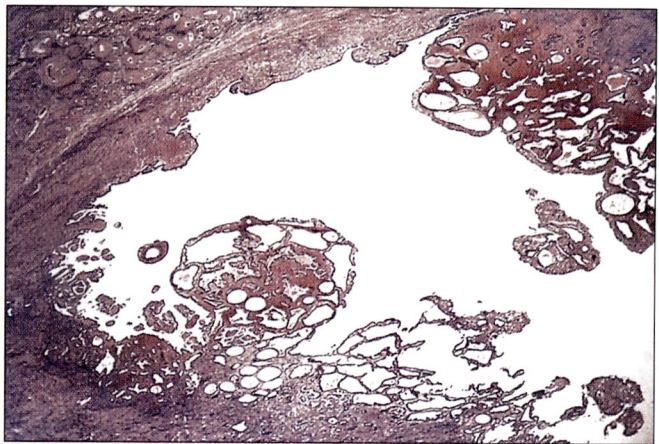

Fig. 20.45   Florid endometriosis within ovary.

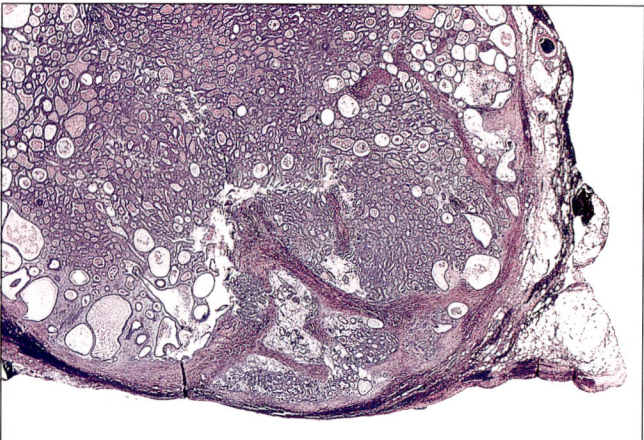

Fig. 20.43   Florid (adenoma) endometriosis in omentum.

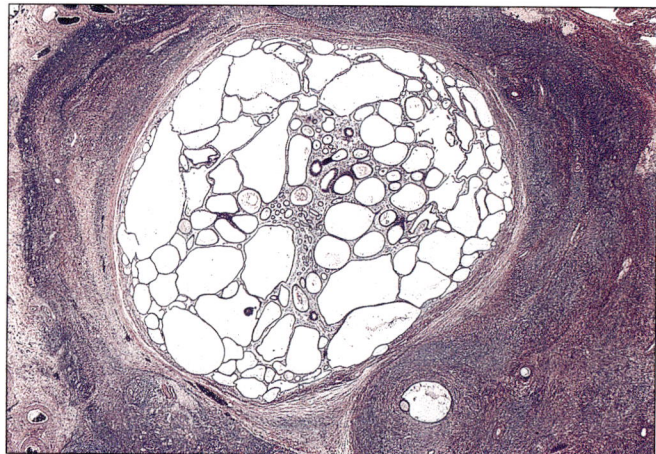

Fig. 20.46   Florid endometriosis within ovary.

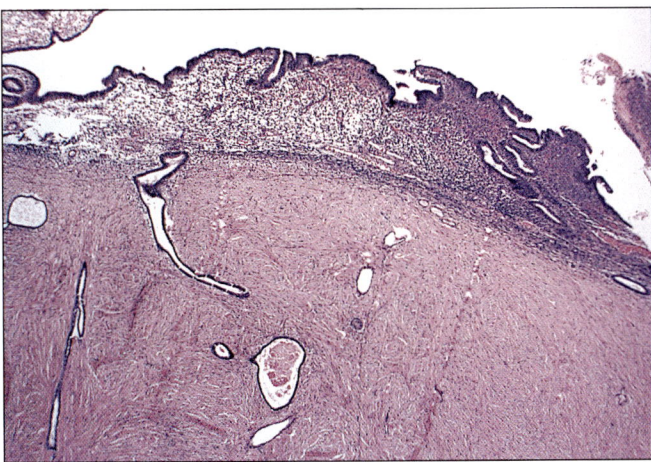

Fig. 20.47 Endometriosis in continuity with endometrioid adenofibroma of ovary.

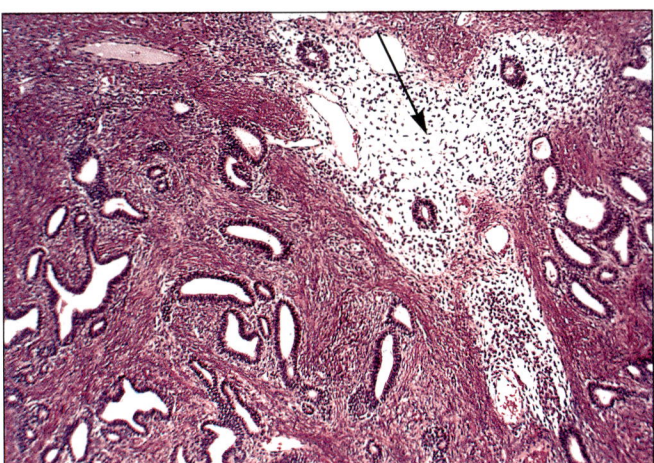

Fig. 20.48 Focus of endometriosis (arrow) within an endometrioid adenofibroma of ovary.

Table 20.4 Tumors and tumor-like conditions arising in endometriosis

Tumor-like conditions

Polyp
    Tamoxifen associated[128]

Benign tumors

Polypoid endometriosis[114]

Adenoma
    Endometrioid[53] (Figures 20.43–20.44)

Adenofibroma
    Endometrioid[110] (Figure 20.47)

Premalignancies

Atypical endometriosis[51,131] (Figures 20.49–20.52)

Borderline tumors
    Serous[51]
    Mucinous[51]

Malignant tumors

Epithelial malignancies
    Endometrioid[51,124] (Figures 20.53 and 20.54)
      Adenoacanthoma
      Adenosquamous carcinoma (Figure 20.55)
    Clear cell[51,77,124] (Figure 20.56)
    Serous (rare)
    Mucinous (rare)
    Squamous cell carcinoma[19]

Stromal malignancies
    Stromal sarcoma[119] (Figures 20.57 and 20.58)

Malignancy with mixed components
    Adenosarcoma[38,93] (Figures 20.59–20.61)
    Carcinosarcoma (malignant mixed müllerian tumor)

- The tumor should be of a histologic type known to arise in the native endometrium (Table 20.4).
- A gradual transition from benign to malignant epithelium is helpful, or at least documented atypia in the endometriosis adjacent to the malignant tumor.

These criteria are fulfilled in less than 10% of published cases. However, in nearly one-fourth of cases endometriosis can be identified in other parts of the affected organ (e.g., ovary), even though it is not in continuity with the tumor.

The changes leading to malignancy are those described for endometrium. At the earliest stage, the endometriosis is 'florid', a term that might also be considered as analogous to endometrial intraepithelial neoplasia (EIN) (hyperplasia) of the endometrium. Nuclear atypia, which can be slight (Figure 20.49) or more marked (Figure 20.50), can also be seen, and probably represents a higher degree of abnormality. As in the endometrium, cases will be seen where the endometriosis is quite atypical (Figure 20.51) or merges into endometrioid adenocarcinoma (Figure 20.52), such that it is difficult to even determine what portion is still precancerous.

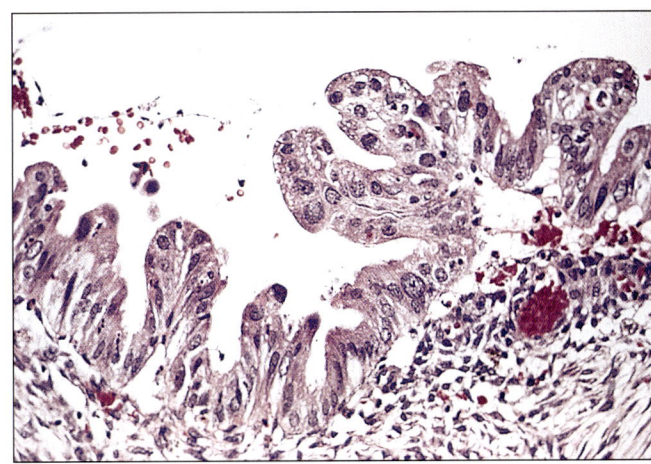

Fig. 20.49 Mild nuclear atypia in endometriosis.

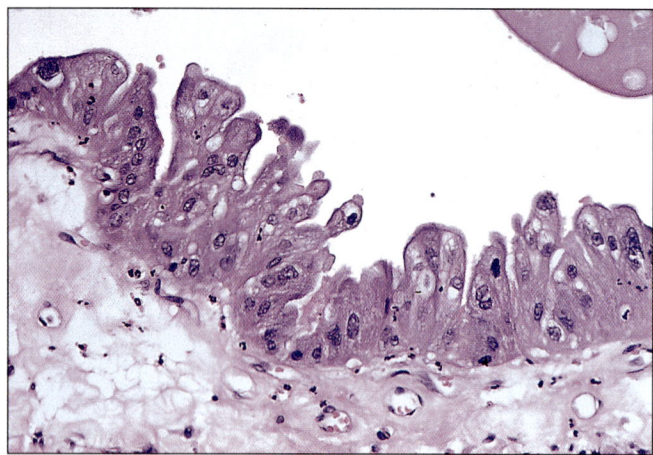

Fig. 20.50   Marked nuclear atypia in endometriosis.

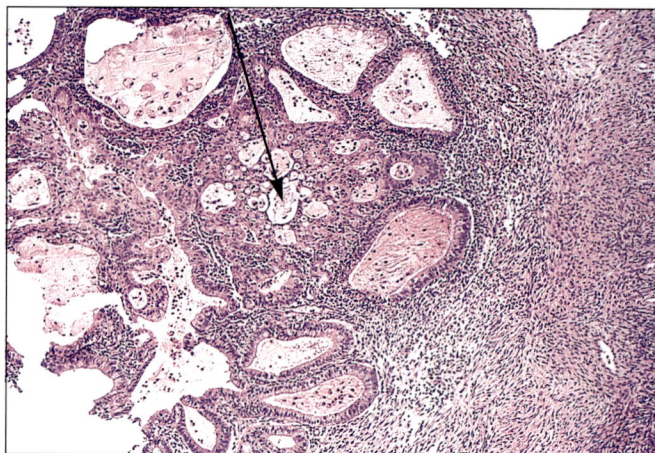

Fig. 20.53   Endometrioid adenocarcinoma (arrow) arising in atypical endometriosis.

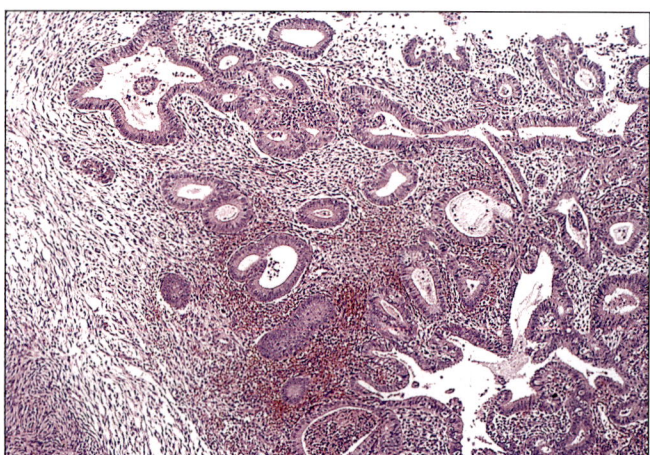

Fig. 20.51   Atypical endometriosis with focal back-to-back glands.

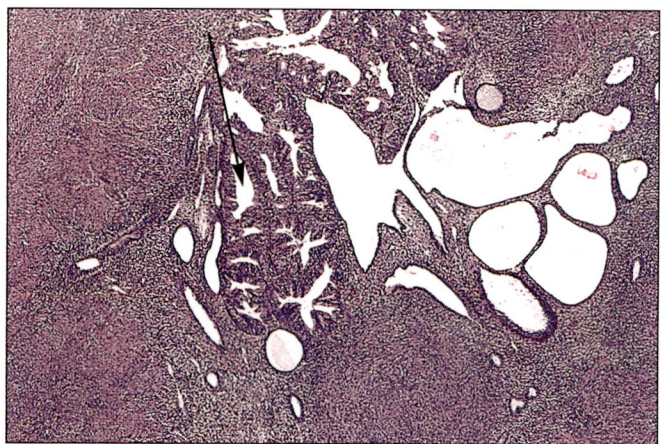

Fig. 20.54   Endometrioid adenocarcinoma arising in endometriosis. The tumor (arrow) is encompassed by endometriosis.

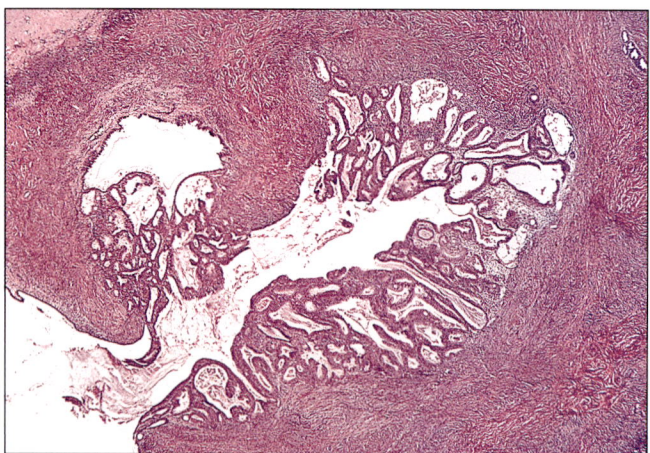

Fig. 20.52   Marked atypical endometriosis merging into endometrioid adenocarcinoma.

We have estimated the frequency of malignant transformation at 1.1–3%,[136] a level slightly greater than others.[13,40,109] The level of uncertainty relates to the sampling issues noted above. Among 1021 cases of endometriosis, malignancy was found in 56 (5.5%). However, only 11 (1.1%) were identified as arising

within endometriosis with an additional 20 (1.9%) arising in the same organ but at some measurable distance from the microscopic endometriosis. The remaining 35 malignancies arose in patients with endometriosis, but in organs where no endometriosis was observed. In a report from a population-based study from a national cancer registry involving more than 20 000 women with endometriosis followed for a mean time of over 11 years, the relative risk of subsequently developing ovarian cancer was 1.9, rising to 4.2 among those subjects with a long-standing history of ovarian endometriosis.[15] The development of ovarian cancer was also raised in a second study with long-term follow-up.[97]

The ovary is by far the most common site where malignancy arises in association with endometriosis,[106,148] accounting for about 75% of such cases. However, tumor develops at virtually every site where endometriosis is found: cul-de-sac,[85] fallopian tube, groin, large bowel,[73,160] lymph node, omentum, pleura, rectovaginal septum,[162] scars,[5,25] ureter,[125] urinary bladder, vagina,[93,132] and vulva.[135]

Endometrioid adenocarcinoma (Figures 20.53–20.55) and clear cell adenocarcinoma (Figure 20.56) are the most common malignancies found to arise in ovarian endometriosis, accounting for roughly two-thirds of all such reported cases.[103,136,142]

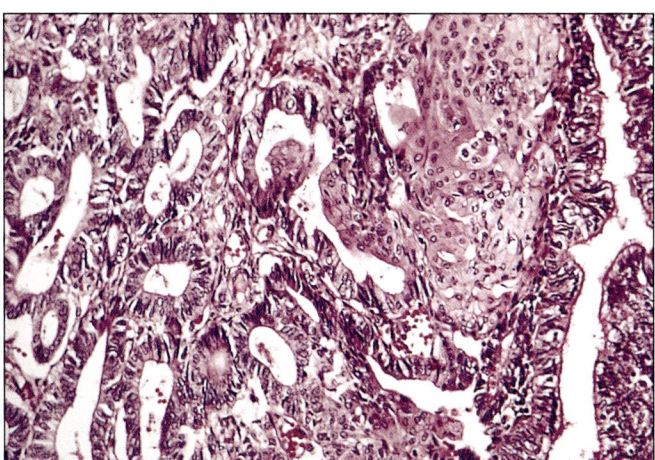

Fig. 20.55 Adenosquamous carcinoma in endometrioma of ovary.

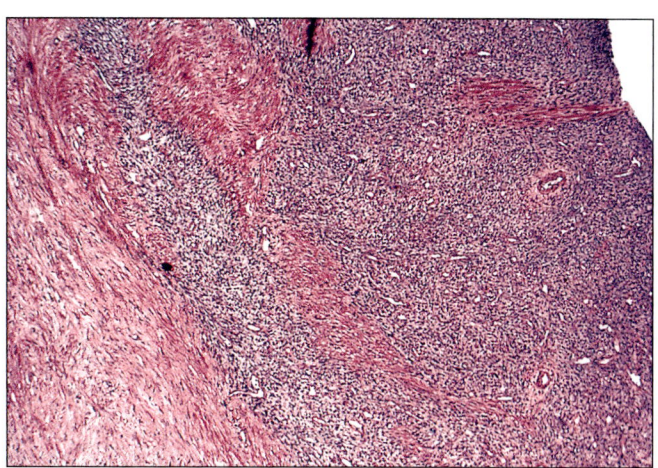

Fig. 20.57 Stromal sarcoma arising in endometriosis.

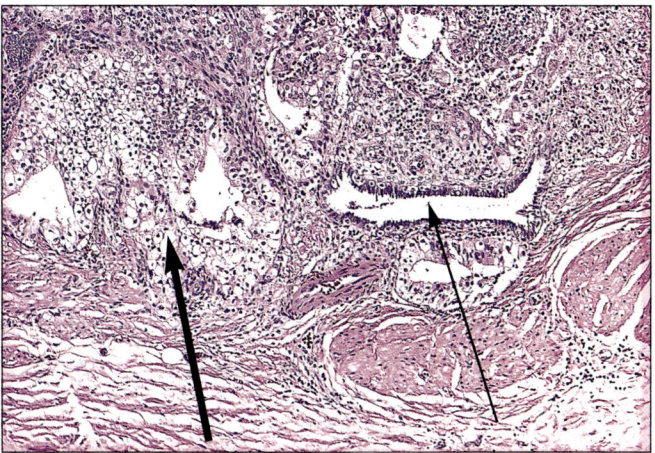

Fig. 20.56 Clear cell adenocarcinoma (thick arrow) associated with endometriosis (thin arrow).

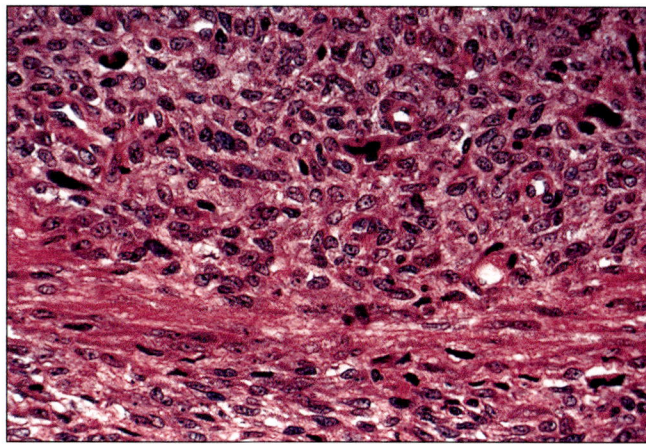

Fig. 20.58 Stromal sarcoma with marked nuclear atypicality arising in endometriosis.

While endometrioid adenocarcinoma is the more common of the two entities by a ratio between 1.3 : 1 to about 4 : 1,[152] women who have clear cell adenocarcinoma are often reported to have a much higher frequency of coexistent pelvic endometriosis. The rate of about 25–50% is much higher than for any other cell type, including endometrioid adenocarcinoma.[33,71] Mixtures of both endometrioid and clear cell adenocarcinoma are common. The association between clear cell adenocarcinoma, endometrioid adenocarcinoma, and endometriosis has been used in the past as credence that clear cell adenocarcinomas are of müllerian rather than wolffian origin. This same association has also supported the view that clear cell adenocarcinomas of the ovary should be considered a subdivision of endometrioid tumors. More direct evidence, discussed below, further supports the numerous histologic observations that endometrioid and clear cell ovarian adenocarcinomas may arise through malignant transformation of endometriotic lesions. It has also been suggested, but not proven, that clear cell carcinoma, when found in the ovary, is of endometriotic origin rather than being an ovarian tumor of 'common epithelial origin'.

Cancers of all other cell types arising in endometriosis are relatively uncommon. Endometriosis was found maximally in 8% of serous tumors in one study,[71] but in all other studies serous and all other cell types were present in under 5% of cases, regardless of whether it occurred in the ovary or extragonadally.[71,136,152] Endometrial-type stromal sarcoma (Figures 20.57 and 20.58), even though reported to be the second most common malignant neoplasm arising in extraovarian endometriosis, is nonetheless rare. The tumor we have seen with surprising frequency has been adenosarcoma arising in extrapelvic endometriosis (Figures 20.59–20.61).

A difficult association to link is between serous adenocarcinoma and endometriosis. On occasion, the cancer is intimately associated with the endometriosis and can seem to have arisen from it. In one recent study in which 13 cases of invasive serous tumor were seen in patients with endometriosis, only five involved the same ovary as the endometriosis and none was contiguous with endometriosis. We have, however, seen cases where the serous tumor is intimately involved with the endometriosis. Serous borderline tumors have also been found occasionally in association with endometriosis, possibly coincidentally.[123]

PATHOGENESIS OF MALIGNANCY

The transition from endometriosis to malignancy is thought similar to the process by which any ordinary epithelium

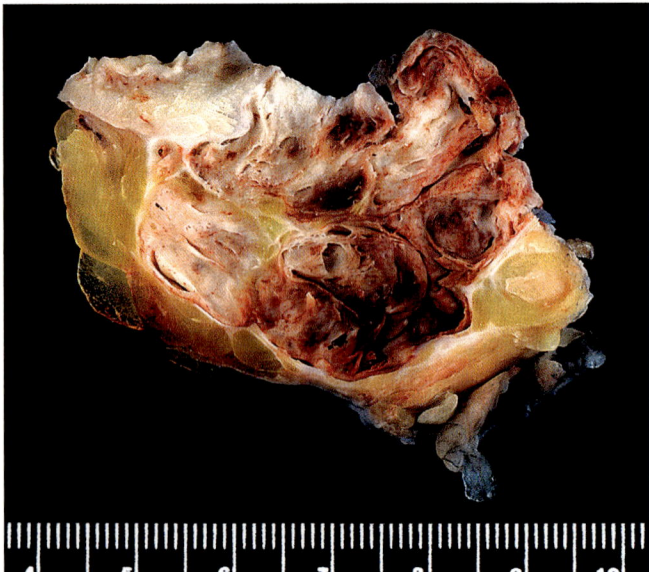

Fig. 20.59 Adenosarcoma arising in omental endometriosis. The tumor, which was bloody and of a different texture, differed from the endometriosis spread throughout the abdominal cavity that was otherwise more rubbery and had evoked a fibrous stromal reaction.

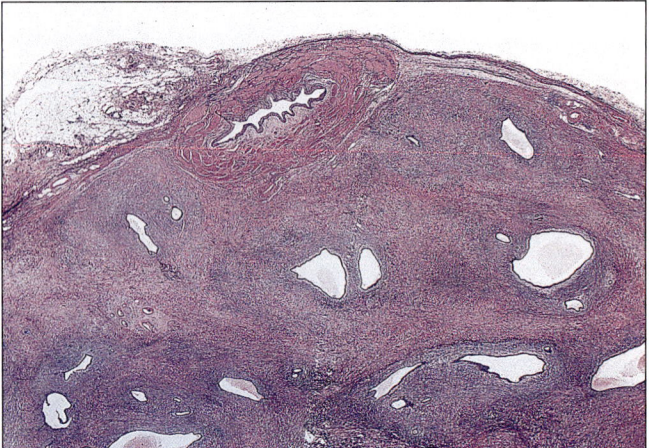

Fig. 20.60 Adenosarcoma with periglandular cuffing in extrapelvic adenosarcoma.

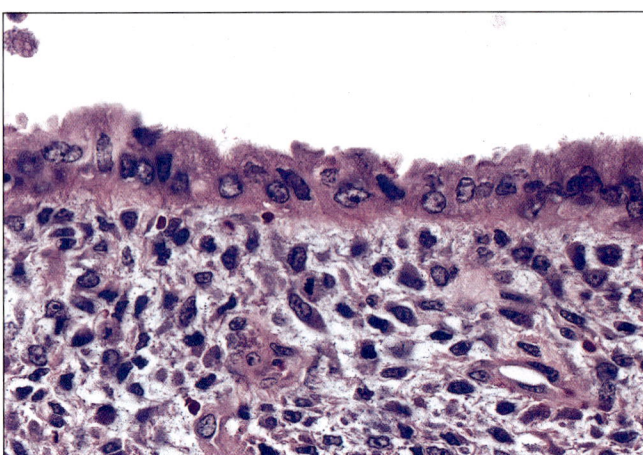

Fig. 20.61 Adenosarcoma in the intestinal wall, high magnification. The epithelium shows cuboidal cells with atypical nuclei and copious eosinophilic cytoplasm.

becomes malignant. Atypical endometriosis, akin to atypical hyperplasia in the endometrium, is considered to provide the bed, if not the transitional stage itself, from which the cancers arise.[131] Applications using molecular pathology are just beginning, but indicate that this line of reasoning may well be correct.[83] Severely atypical epithelium in half the cases of endometriosis has aneuploid DNA, whereas the normal lining epithelium of all endometriotic cysts without atypia is diploid.[12] In one study, aneuploidy of chromosome 17, a chromosome believed to be involved in the genesis of ovarian cancer, was found in 65% of endometriotic cells, but in only 25% of normal endometrial epithelium.[84] This finding suggested that a multistep pathway involving somatic genetic alterations is involved in the development of endometriosis itself and its progression, an idea others have endorsed.[81] Conversely, progressive reduction to loss in estrogen receptor alpha and progesterone receptor expression have been observed as endometriosis progresses to atypical endometriosis and then to clear cell adenocarcinoma, as might be expected.[4]

Studies of endometriotic cysts, 4–10 cm in dimension, have been conducted to determine the type of clonality present. In one series, all 11 cases showed monoclonality,[72] and in a second study, three of five cases were monoclonal.[108] These results suggested that some endometriotic cysts are probably tumors, and, possibly, should be considered as endometrioid cystadenomas. Finally, when both the cancer and its associated endometriosis were examined by various molecular biologic techniques, the malignant portions showed changes that might be expected in cancer. For example, receptor expression, positive in the endometriosis, was lost in the cancer. Proliferation rates, as measured by Ki-67, increased from low rates in the endometriosis to high rates in the cancer; *p53* oncogene was also abnormal in the cancer.[55] In another study,[70] each case where the carcinoma arose within the endometriosis and in two-thirds of cases where the carcinoma was adjacent to the endometriosis showed loss of heterozygosity on the arm of chromosome 12 or X-chromosome inactivation consistent with a common lineage. One case also showed a *p53* mutation in both the endometriosis and its adjacent carcinoma. These findings support the numerous histologic observations that endometrioid and clear cell ovarian adenocarcinomas may arise through malignant transformation of endometriotic lesions.

REFERENCES

1. Abrao MS, Podgaec S, Carvalho FM, Pinotti JA. Endometriosis in the presacral nerve. Int J Gynecol Obstet 1999;64:173–5.
2. Abrao MS, Podgaec S, Dias JA, Jr, et al. Deeply infiltrating endometriosis affecting the rectum and lymph nodes. Fertil Steril 2006;86:543–7.
3. Acien P, Lloret M, Chehab H. Endometriosis in a patient with Rokitansky–Kuster–Hauser syndrome. Gynecol Obstet Invest 1988;25:70–2.
4. Akahane T, Sekizawa A, Okuda T, Kushima M, Saito H, Okai T. Disappearance of steroid hormone dependency during malignant transformation of ovarian clear cell cancer. Int J Gynecol Pathol 2005;24:369–76.
5. Alberto VO, Lynch M, Labbei FN, Jeffers M. Primary abdominal wall clear cell carcinoma arising in a Caesarean section scar endometriosis. Irish J Med Sci 2006;175:69–71.
6. Alifano M, Roth T, Broet SC, Schussler O, Magdeleinat P, Regnard JF. Catamenial pneumothorax – a prospective study. Chest 2003;124:1004–8.
7. Allaire C. Endometriosis and infertility – a review. J Reprod Med 2006;51:164–8.
8. Anaf V, Simon P, Fayt I, Noel J. Smooth muscles are frequent components of endometriotic lesions. Hum Reprod 2000;15:767–71.
9. Anaf V, Chapron C, El Nakadi I, De Moor V, Simonart T, Noel JC. Pain, mast cells, and nerves in peritoneal, ovarian, and deep infiltrating endometriosis. Fertil Steril 2006;86:1336–43.

10. Arici A, Oral E. The peritoneal environment in endometriosis. In: Diamond MP, Osteen KG, eds. Endometrium and Endometriosis. Oxford: Blackwell Science; 1997:161–73.
11. Balasch J, Creus M, Fabregues F, et al. Visible and non-visible endometriosis at laparoscopy in fertile and infertile women and in patients with chronic pelvic pain: a prospective study. Hum Reprod 1996;11:387–91.
12. Ballouk F, Ross JS, Wolf BC. Ovarian endometriotic cysts – an analysis of cytologic atypia and DNA ploidy patterns. Am J Clin Pathol 1994;102:415–9.
13. Benoit L, Arnould L, Cheynel N, et al. Malignant extraovarian endometriosis: a review. EJSO 2006;32:6–11.
14. Bergqvist A. Different types of extragenital endometriosis – a review. Gynecol Endocrinol 1993;7:207–21.
15. Brinton LA, Gridley G, Persson I, Baron J, Bergqvist A. Cancer risk after a hospital discharge diagnosis of endometriosis. Am J Obstet Gynecol 1997;176:572–9.
16. Brosens IA. Histologic appearances of endometriosis throughout the pelvis. In: Diamond MP, Osteen KG, eds. Endometrium and Endometriosis. Oxford: Blackwell Science; 1997:27–35.
17. Brosens IA. Endometriosis – a disease because it is characterized by bleeding. Am J Obstet Gynecol 1997;176:263–7.
18. Brosens IA, Brosens JJ. Redefining endometriosis – is deep endometriosis a progressive disease? Hum Reprod 2000;15:1–3.
19. Campagnutta E, Sopracordevole F, Spolaor L, Doglioni C, Parin A, Scarabelli C. Squamous cell carcinoma in ovarian endometriosis – a case report. J Reprod Med 1994;39:557–60.
20. Candiani GB, Vercellini P, Fedele L, Vendola N, Carinelli S, Scaglione V. Inguinal endometriosis – pathogenetic and clinical implications. Obstet Gynecol 1991;78:191–4.
21. Canis M, Donnez JG, Guzick DS, et al. Revised American Society for Reproductive Medicine classification of endometriosis: 1996. Fertil Steril 1997;67:817–21.
22. Chahine B, Malbranque G, Lelong J, Ramon P, Tillie-Leblond I. Catamenial haemoptysis during hormone replacement treatment. Rev Mal Respir 2007;24(3 Pt 1):339–42.
23. Chapron C, Fauconnier A, Dubuisson JB, Barakat H, Vieira M, Breart G. Deep infiltrating endometriosis: relation between severity of dysmenorrhoea and extent of disease. Hum Reprod 2003;18:760–6.
24. Chen TH. Umbilical endometriosis. Eur J Plast Surg 1998;21:51–2.
25. Chene G, Darcha C, Dechelotte P, Mage G, Canis M. Malignant degeneration of perineal endometriosis in episiotomy scar: case report and review of the literature. Int J Gynecol Cancer 2007;17:709A–14.
26. Choi SW, Lee HN, Kang SJ, Kim HO. A case of cutaneous endometriosis developed in postmenopausal woman receiving hormonal replacement. J Am Acad Dermatol 1999;41(2 Pt 2 Suppl):327–9.
27. Clement PB. Reactive tumor-like lesions of the peritoneum. Am J Clin Pathol 1995;103:673–6.
28. Coccia ME, Rizzello F, Comparetto C, et al. Endometriosis and pain in an adolescent population. In: Proceedings of the World Meeting on Gynecologic Pelvic Pain and Endometriosis. Bolognia; 2006:101–5.
29. Cramer DW, Missmer SA. The epidemiology of endometriosis. In: Yoshinaga K, Parrott EC, eds. Endometriosis: Emerging Research and Intervention Strategies. New York: New York Academy of Sciences; 2002:11–22.
30. Cravello L, D'Ercole C, LeTreut YP, Blanc B. Hepatic endometriosis: a case report. Fertil Steril 1996;66:657–9.
31. Damario MA, Rock JA. Classification of endometriosis. Semin Reprod Endocrinol 1997;15:235–44.
32. Dawood MY. Macrophages and macrophage-derived factors in normal reproductive tissues and endometriosis. In: Diamond MP, Osteen KG, eds. Endometrium and Endometriosis. Oxford: Blackwell Science; 1997:146–51.
33. De la Cuesta RS, Eichhorn JH, Rice LW, Fuller AF, Nikrui N, Goff BA. Histologic transformation of benign endometriosis to early epithelial ovarian cancer. Gynecol Oncol 1996;60:238–44.
34. D'Hooghe TM. Clinical relevance of the baboon as a model for the study of endometriosis. Fertil Steril 1997;68:613–25.
35. D'Hooghe TM, Bambra CS, Raeymaekers BM, Koninckx PR. Increased incidence and recurrence of recent corpus luteum without ovulation stigma (luteinized unruptured follicle syndrome?) in baboons with endometriosis. J Soc Gynecol Invest 1996;3:140–4.
36. D'Hooghe TM, Bambra CS, Raeymaekers BM, Dejonge I, Lauweryns JM, Koninckx PR. Intrapelvic injection of menstrual endometrium causes endometriosis in baboons (Papio cynocephalus and Papio anubis). Am J Obstet Gynecol 1995;173:125–34.
37. D'Hooghe TM, Riday AM, Bambra CS, Suleman MA, Raeymaekers BM, Koninckx PR. The cycle pregnancy rate is normal in baboons with stage I endometriosis but decreased in primates with stage II and stage III–IV disease. Fertil Steril 1996;66:809–13.
38. Dincer AD, Timmins P, Pietrocola D, Fisher H, Ambros RA. Primary peritoneal mullerian adenosarcoma with sarcomatous overgrowth associated with endometriosis: a case report. Int J Gynecol Pathol 2002;21:65–8.
39. Dmowski WP, Braun DP. Immunologic aspects of endometriosis. In: Diamond MP, Osteen KG, eds. Endometrium and Endometriosis. Oxford: Blackwell Science; 1997:174–81.
40. Dogan S, Agic A, Eilers W, Finas D, Diedrich K, Hornung D. Endometriosis and risk of malignancy. Geburt Frauenheil 2006;66:739–44.
41. Donnez J, Smoes P, Gillerot S, Casanas-Roux F, Nisolle M. Vascular endothelial growth factor (VEGF) in endometriosis. Hum Reprod 1998;13:1686–90.
42. Donnez J, Van Langendonckt A, Casanas-Roux F, et al. Current thinking on the pathogenesis of endometriosis. Gynecol Obstet Invest 2002;54(Suppl):52–62.
43. Emmert C, Romann D, Riedel HH. Endometriosis diagnosed by laparoscopy in adolescent girls. Arch Gynecol Obstet 1998;261:89–93.
44. Eskenazi B, Warner ML. Epidemiology of endometriosis. Obstet Gynecol Clin North Am 1997;24:235–58.
45. Evers JLH, Land JA, Dunselman GAJ, vander Linden PJQ, Hamilton CJCM. 'The Flemish Giant': reflections on the defense against endometriosis, inspired by Professor Emeritus Ivo A. Brosens. Eur J Obstet Gynecol Reprod Biol 1998;81:253–8.
46. Fazleabas AT, Brudney A, Gurates B, Chai D, Bulun S. A modified baboon model for endometriosis. In: Yoshinaga K, Parrott EC, eds. Endometriosis: Emerging Research and Intervention Strategies. New York: New York Academy of Sciences; 2002:308–17.
47. Ferguson CM, Compton CC, Ryan JM, Mark EJ, Fernaneezdel Castillo C, Sategh RA. A 45-year-old woman with abdominal pain and a polypoid mass in the colon – endometriosis of the sigmoid colon. N Engl J Med 1996;335:807–12.
48. Fujiwara H, Konno R, Netsu S, et al. Localization of mast cells in endometrial cysts. Am J Reprod Immunol 2004;51:341–4.
49. Fukunaga M. Catamenial pneumothorax caused by diaphragmatic stromal endometriosis. APMIS 1999;107:685–8.
50. Fukunaga M, Ushigome S. Epithelial metaplastic changes in ovarian endometriosis. Mod Pathol 1998;11:784–8.
51. Fukushima N, Mukai K. 'Ovarian-type' stroma of pancreatic mucinous cystic tumor expresses smooth muscle phenotype. Pathol Int 1997;47:806–8.
52. Giudice LC, Tazuke SI, Swiersz L. Status of current research on endometriosis. J Reprod Med 1998;43:252–62.
53. Grouls V, Berndt R. Endometrioid adenoma (polypoid endometriosis) of the omentum maius. Pathol Res Pract 1995;191:1049–52.
54. Hadfield RM, Mardon HJ, Barlow DH, Kennedy SH. Endometriosis in monozygotic twins. Fertil Steril 1997;68:941–2.
55. Han AC, Hovenden S, Rosenblum NG, Salazar H. Adenocarcinoma arising in extragonadal endometriosis: an immunohistochemical study. Cancer 1998;83:1163–9.
56. Haney AF. Etiology and histogenesis of endometriosis. Prog Clin Biol Res 1990;323:1–14.
57. Haney AF. The pathogenesis and etiology of endometriosis. In: Thomas EJ, Rock JA, eds. Modern Approaches to Endometriosis. Boston: Kluwer; 1991.
58. Haney AF. Endometriosis-associated infertility. Reprod Med Rev 1998;6:145–61.
59. Healy DL, Rogers PAW, Hii L, Wingfield M. Angiogenesis: a new theory for endometriosis. Hum Reprod 1998;4:736–40.
60. Henkel A, Christensen B, Schindler AE. Endometriosis: a clinically malignant disease. Eur J Obstet Gynecol Reprod Biol 1999;82:209–11.
61. Hoeger KM, Guzick DS. Classification of endometriosis. Obstet Gynecol Clin North Am 1997;24:347–59.
62. Hompes PGA, Mijatovic V. Endometriosis: the way forward. Gynecol Endocrinol 2007;23:5–12.
63. Hurd WW. Criteria that indicate endometriosis is the cause of chronic pelvic pain. Obstet Gynecol 1998;92:1029–32.
64. Ichida M, Gomi A, Hiranouchi N, et al. A case of cerebral endometriosis causing catamenial epilepsy. Neurology 1993;43:2708–9.
65. Insabato L, Pettinato G. Endometriosis of the bowel with lymph node involvement. A report of three cases and review of the literature. Pathol Res Pract 1996;192:957–61; discussion 962.
66. Insabato L, Darmiento FP, Tornillo L. A rectal endometrioma producing intestinal obstruction. J Clin Gastroenterol 1994;19:82–4.
67. Ishimaru T, Masuzaki H. Peritoneal endometriosis – endometrial tissue implantation as its primary etiologic mechanism. Am J Obstet Gynecol 1991;165:210–4.
68. Jansen RP. Minimal endometriosis and reduced fecundability: prospective evidence from an artificial insemination by donor program. Fertil Steril 1986;46:141–3.
69. Jenkins S, Olive DL, Haney AF. Endometriosis: pathogenetic implications of the anatomic distribution. Obstet Gynecol 1986;67:335–8.
70. Jiang XX, Morland SJ, Hitchcock A, Thomas EJ, Campbell IG. Allelotyping of endometriosis with adjacent ovarian carcinoma reveals evidence of a common lineage. Cancer Research 1998;58:1707–12.
71. Jimbo H, Yoshikawa H, Onda T, Yasugi T, Sakamoto A, Taketani Y. Prevalence of ovarian endometriosis in epithelial ovarian cancer. Int J Gynecol Obstet 1997;59:245–50.
72. Jimbo H, Hitomi Y, Yoshikawa H, et al. Evidence for monoclonal expansion of epithelial cells in ovarian endometrial cysts. Am J Pathol 1997;150:1173–8.
73. Jones KD, Owen E, Berresford A, Sutton C. Endometrial adenocarcinoma arising from endometriosis of the rectosigmoid colon. Gynecol Oncol 2002;86:220–2.
74. Kennedy S. Is there a genetic basis to endometriosis? Semin Reprod Endocrinol 1997;15:309–18.
75. Kennedy S. The genetics of endometriosis. Eur J Obstet Gynecol Reprod Biol 1999;82:129–33.

76. Kim KR. Utility of trichrome and reticulin stains in the diagnosis of superficial endometriosis of the uterine cervix. Int J Gynecol Pathol 2001;20:173–6.

77. Klein AE, Bauer TW, Marks KE, Belinson JL. Papillary clear cell adenocarcinoma of the groin arising from endometriosis. Clin Orthop Relat Res 1999;(361):192–8.

78. Knapp VJ. How old is endometriosis? Late 17th- and 18th-century European descriptions of the disease. Fertil Steril 1999;72:10–14.

79. Koninckx PR. Biases in the endometriosis literature – illustrated by 20 years of endometriosis research in Leuven. Eur J Obstet Gynecol Reprod Biol 1998;81:259–71.

80. Koninckx PR, Kennedy SH, Barlow DH. Endometriotic disease: the role of peritoneal fluid. Hum Reprod 1998;4:741–51.

81. Koninckx PR, Barlow D, Kennedy S. Implantation versus infiltration: the Sampson versus the endometriotic disease theory. Gynecol Obstet Invest 1999;47(Suppl 1):3–10.

82. Koninckx PR, Kennedy SH, Barlow DH. Pathogenesis of endometriosis: the role of peritoneal fluid. Gynecol Obstet Invest 1999;47(Suppl 1):23–33.

83. Korner M, Burckhardt E, Mazzucchelli L. Higher frequency of chromosomal aberrations in ovarian endometriosis compared to extragonadal endometriosis: a possible link to endometrioid adenocarcinoma. Mod Pathol 2006;19:1615–23.

84. Kosugi Y, Elias S, Malinak LR, et al. Increased heterogeneity of chromosome 17 aneuploidy in endometriosis. Am J Obstet Gynecol 1999;180:792–7.

85. Kusaka M, Mikuni M, Nishiya M. A case of high-grade endometrial stromal sarcoma arising from endometriosis in the cul-de-sac. Int J Gynecol Cancer 2006;16:895–9.

86. Kyama MC, D'Hooghe TM, Debrock S, Machoki J, Chai DC, Mwenda JM. The prevalence of endometriosis among African–American and African–Indigenous women. Gynecol Obstet Invest 2004;57:40–2.

87. Langlois NEI, Park KGM, Keenan RA. Mucosal changes in the large bowel with endometriosis: a possible cause of misdiagnosis of colitis? Hum Pathol 1994;25:1030–4.

88. Lauchlan SC. The secondary mullerian system revisited. Int J Gynecol Pathol 1994;13:73–9.

89. Lee KR, Nucci MR. Ovarian mucinous and mixed epithelial carcinomas of mullerian (endocervical-like) type: a clinicopathologic analysis of four cases of an uncommon variant associated with endometriosis. Int J Gynecol Pathol 2003;22:42–51.

90. Leyendecker G, Kunz G. Endometriosis and adenomyosis. New insight into uterine (patho)physiology. Zentralbl Gynakol 2005;127:288.

91. Liang CC, Liou B, Tsai CC, Chen TC, Soong YK. Scar endometriosis. Int Surg 1998;83:69–71.

92. Lin SY, Lee RK, Hwu YM, Lin MH. Reproducibility of the revised American Fertility Society classification of endometriosis using laparoscopy or laparotomy. Int J Gynecol Obstet 1998;60:265–9.

93. Liu LT, Davidson S, Singh M. Mullerian adenosarcoma of vagina arising in persistent endometriosis: report of a case and review of the literature. Gynecol Oncol 2003;90:486–90.

94. Mai KT, Yazdi HM, Perkins DG, Parks W. Development of endometriosis from embryonic duct remnants. Hum Pathol 1998;29:319–22.

95. Matsuzaki S, Canis M, Darcha C, Dechelotte P, Pouly JL, Bruhat MA. Angiogenesis in endometriosis. Gynecol Obstet Invest 1998;46:111–5.

96. McCluggage WG, Oliva E, Herrington CS, McBride H, Young RH. CD10 and calretinin staining of endocervical glandular lesions, endocervical stroma and endometrioid adenocarcinomas of the uterine corpus: CD10 positivity is characteristic of, but not specific for, mesonephric lesions and is not specific for endometrial stroma. Histopathology 2003;43:144–50.

97. Melin A, Sparen P, Persson I, Bergqvist A. Endometriosis and the risk of cancer with special emphasis on ovarian cancer. Hum Reprod 2006;21:1237–42.

98. Metzger DA, Szpak CA, Haney AF. Histologic features associated with hormonal responsiveness of ectopic endometrium. Fertil Steril 1993;59:83–8.

99. Missmer SA, Cramer DW. The epidemiology of endometriosis. Obstet Gynecol Clin North Am 2003;30:1–19, vii.

100. Moen MH, Magnus P. The familial risk of endometriosis. Acta Obstet Gynecol Scand 1993;72:560–4.

101. Moore WF, Bentley RC, Berchuck A, Robboy SJ. Some mullerian inclusion cysts in lymph nodes may sometimes be metastases from serous borderline tumors of the ovary. Am J Surg Pathol 2000;24:710–8.

102. Muneyyirci-Delale O, Neil G, Serur E, Gordon D, Maiman M, Sedlis A. Endometriosis with massive ascites. Gynecol Oncol 1998;69:42–6.

103. Munkarah AR. Malignant transformation of endometriosis. In: Diamond MP, Osteen KG, eds. Endometrium and Endometriosis. Oxford: Blackwell Science; 1997:42–6.

104. Muzii L, Bianchi A, Bellati F, et al. Histologic analysis of endometriomas: what the surgeon needs to know. Fertil Steril 2007;87:362–6.

105. Nakayama K, Masuzawa H, Li SF, et al. Immunohistochemical analysis of the peritoneum adjacent to endometriotic lesions using antibodies for Ber-EP4 antigen, estrogen receptors, and progesterone receptors: implication of peritoneal metaplasia in the pathogenesis of endometriosis. Int J Gynecol Pathol 1994;13:348–58.

106. Ness RB. Endometriosis and ovarian cancer: thoughts on shared pathophysiology. Am J Obstet Gynecol 2003;189:280–94.

107. Nezhat C, Seidman DS, Nezhat F, Nezhat C. Laparoscopic surgical management of diaphragmatic endometriosis. Fertil Steril 1998;69:1048–55.

108. Nilbert M, Pejovic T, Mandahl N, Iosif S, Willen H, Mitelman F. Monoclonal origin of endometriotic cysts. Int J Gynecol Cancer 1995;5:61–3.

109. Nishida M, Watanabe K, Sato N, Ichikawa Y. Malignant transformation of ovarian endometriosis. Gynecol Obstet Invest 2000;50(Suppl):18–23.

110. Nuovo M, Bayani E, Gerold T, Leong M, Mir R. Endometrioid cystadenofibroma developing in juxtahepatic endometriosis: a case report. Int J Surg Pathol 1998;6:109–12.

111. Oral E, Arici A. Pathogenesis of endometriosis. Obstet Gynecol Clin North Am 1997;24:219–33.

112. Oral E, Olive DL, Arici A. The peritoneal environment in endometriosis. Hum Reprod 1996;2:385–98.

113. Osteen KG, Bruner KL, Eisenberg E. The disease endometriosis. In: Diamond MP, Osteen KG, eds. Endometrium and Endometriosis. Oxford: Blackwell Science; 1997:20–4.

114. Parker RL, Dadmanesh F, Young RH, Clement PB. Polypoid endometriosis – a clinicopathologic analysis of 24 cases and a review of the literature. Am J Surg Pathol 2004;28:285–97.

115. Patterson GK, Winburn GB. Abdominal wall endometriomas: report of eight cases. Am Surg 1999;65:36–9.

116. Perrotta PL, Ginsburg FW, Siderides CI, Parkash V. Liesegang rings and endometriosis. Int J Gynecol Pathol 1998;17:358–62.

117. Prentice A, Ingamells S. Endometriosis and infertility. Hum Reprod 1996;11:51–5.

118. Ramey JW, Archer DF. Peritoneal fluid – its relevance to the development of endometriosis. Fertil Steril 1993;60:1–14.

119. Reich O, Regauer S. Aromatase expression in low-grade endometrial stromal sarcomas: an immunohistochemical study. Mod Pathol 2004;17:104–8.

120. Roberts CP, Rock JA. The current staging system for endometriosis: does it help? Obstet Gynecol Clin North Am 2003;30:115–32.

121. Rock JA. The revised American Fertility Society classification of endometriosis: reproducibility of scoring. Zoladex Endometriosis Study Group. Fertil Steril 1995;63:1108–10.

122. Ross HL, Bischoff FZ, Elias S. Genetics of endometriosis. In: Diamond MP, Osteen KG, eds. Endometrium and Endometriosis. Oxford: Blackwell Science; 1997:70–4.

123. Rutgers JL, Scully RE. Ovarian mixed-epithelial papillary cystadenomas of borderline malignancy of mullerian type. A clinicopathologic analysis. Cancer 1988;61:546–54.

124. Sainz de la Cuesta R, Eichhorn JH, Rice LW, Fuller AF, Jr, Nikrui N, Goff BA. Histologic transformation of benign endometriosis to early epithelial ovarian cancer. Gynecol Oncol 1996;60:238–44.

125. Salerno MG, Masciullo V, Naldini A, Zannoni GF, Vellone V, Scambia G. Endometrioid adenocarcinoma with squamous differentiation arising from ureteral endometriosis in a patient with no history of gonadal endometriosis. Gynecol Oncol 2005;99:749–52.

126. Sangihaghpeykar H, Poindexter AN. Epidemiology of endometriosis among parous women. Obstet Gynecol 1995;85:983–92.

127. Schenken RS, Guzick DS. Revised endometriosis classification: 1996. Fertil Steril 1997;67:815–6.

128. Schlesinger G, Silverberg SG. Tamoxifen-associated polyps (Basalomas) arising in multiple endometriotic foci: a case report and review of the literature. Gynecol Oncol 1999;73:305–11.

129. Schwartz JL, Schwartz LB. Extrapelvic endometriosis. In: Diamond MP, Osteen KG, eds. Endometrium and Endometriosis. Oxford: Blackwell Science; 1997:247–54.

130. Seibel MM, Zilberstein M. Endometriosis: mechanisms of infertility. In: Diamond MP, Osteen KG, eds. Endometrium and Endometriosis. Oxford: Blackwell Science; 1997:182–7.

131. Seidman JD. Prognostic importance of hyperplasia and atypia in endometriosis. Int J Gynecol Pathol 1996;15:1–9.

132. Shah C, Pizer E, Veljovich DS, Drescher CW, Peters WA, III, Paley PJ. Clear cell adenocarcinoma of the vagina in a patient with vaginal endometriosis. Gynecol Oncol 2006;103:1130–2.

133. Shaw RW. An Atlas of Endometriosis. New York: Parthenon; 1993.

134. Smith SK. Angiogenesis. Semin Reprod Endocrinol 1997;15:221–7.

135. Soliman NF, Hillard TC. Hormone replacement therapy in women with past history of endometriosis. Climacteric 2006;9:325–35.

136. Stern RC, Dash R, Bentley RC, Snyder MJ, Haney AF, Robboy SJ. Malignancy in endometriosis: frequency and comparison of ovarian and extraovarian types. Int J Gynecol Pathol 2001;20:133–9.

137. Stratton P, Winkel CA, Sinaii N, Merino MJ, Zimmer C, Nieman LK. Location, color, size, depth, and volume may predict endometriosis in lesions resected at surgery. Fertil Steril 2002;78:743–9.

138. Sugamata M, Ihara T, Uchiide I. Increase of activated mast cells in human endometriosis. Am J Reprod Immunol 2005;53:120–5.

139. Suginami H. A reappraisal of the coelomic metaplasia theory by reviewing endometriosis occurring in unusual sites and instances. Am J Obstet Gynecol 1991;165:214–8.

140. Tazuke SI, Milki AA. Endometrioma of uterine serosa in a woman with mosaic Turner's syndrome receiving hormone replacement therapy. Hum Reprod 2002;17:2977–80.

141. Terada Y, Chen FS, Shoji T, Itoh H, Wada H, Hitomi S. A case of endobronchial endometriosis treated by subsegmentectomy. Chest 1999;115:1475–8.
142. Toki T, Fujii S, Silverberg SG. A clinicopathologic study on the association of endometriosis and carcinoma of the ovary using a scoring system. Int J Gynecol Cancer 1996;6:68–75.
143. Toki T, Shimizu M, Takagi Y, Ashida T, Konishi I. CD10 is a marker for normal and neoplastic endometrial stromal cells. Int J Gynecol Pathol 2002;21:41–7.
144. Toki T, Horiuchi A, Li SF, Nakayama K, Silverberg SG, Fujii S. Proliferative activity of postmenopausal endometriosis: a histopathologic and immunocytochemical study. Int J Gynecol Pathol 1996;15:45–53.
145. Treloar SA, O'Connor DT, O'Connor VM, Martin NG. Genetic influences on endometriosis in an Australian twin sample. Fertil Steril 1999;71:701–10.
146. Ueki M. Histologic study of endometriosis and examination of lymphatic drainage in and from the uterus. Am J Obstet Gynecol 1991;165:201–9.
147. Urbach DR, Reedijk M, Richard CS, Lie KI, Ross TM. Bowel resection for intestinal endometriosis. Dis Colon Rectum 1998;41:1158–64.
148. Van Gorp T, Amant F, Neven P, Vergote I, Moerman P. Endometriosis and the development of malignant tumours of the pelvis. A review of literature. Best Pract Res Clin Obstet Gynaecol 2004;18:349–71.
149. Vercellini P. Endometriosis: what a pain it is. Semin Reprod Endocrinol 1997;15:251–61.
150. Vercellini P, Aimi G, De Giorgi O, Maddalena S, Carinelli S, Crosignani PG. Is cystic ovarian endometriosis an asymmetric disease? Br J Obstet Gynaecol 1998;105:1018–21.
151. Vercellini P, Fedele L, Aimi G, Pietropaolo G, Consonni D, Crosignani PG. Association between endometriosis stage, lesion type, patient characteristics and severity of pelvic pain symptoms: a multivariate analysis of over 1000 patients. Hum Reprod 2007;22:266–71.
152. Vercellini P, Parazzini F, Bolis G, et al. Endometriosis and ovarian cancer. Am J Obstet Gynecol 1993;169:181–2.
153. Vessey MP, Villardmackintosh L, Painter R. Epidemiology of endometriosis in women attending family planning clinics. BMJ 1993;306:182–4.
154. Vigano P, Somigliana E, Vignali M, Busacca M, Di Blasio AM. Genetics of endometriosis: current status and prospects. Front Biosci 2007;12:3247–55.
155. von Stemm AM, Meigel WN, Scheidel P, Gocht A. Umbilical endometriosis. J Eur Acad Dermatol Venereol 1999;12:30–2.
156. Walter AJ, Hentz JG, Magtibay PM, Cornella JL, Magrina JF. Endometriosis: correlation between histologic and visual findings at laparoscopy. Am J Obstet Gynecol 2001;184:1407–11; discussion 11–13.
157. Wieser F, Wenzl R, Taylor RN, Diedrich K, Hornung D. Genetic basis of endometriosis. Gynakologie 2004;37:676–80.
158. Witz CA, Monotoya-Rodriguez IA, Schenken RS. Whole explants of peritoneum and endometrium: a novel model of the early endometriosis lesion. Fertil Steril 1999;71:56–60.
159. Wolf Y, Haddad R, Werbin N, Skornick Y, Kaplan O. Endometriosis in abdominal scars: a diagnostic pitfall. Am Surg 1996;62:1042–4.
160. Yantiss RK, Clement PB, Young RH. Neoplastic and pre-neoplastic changes in gastrointestinal endometriosis – a study of 17 cases. Am J Surg Pathol 2000;24:513–24.
161. Yantiss RK, Clement PB, Young RH. Endometriosis of the intestinal tract – a study of 44 cases of a disease that may cause diverse challenges in clinical and pathologic evaluation. Am J Surg Pathol 2001;25:445–54.
162. Yazbeck C, Poncelet C, Chosidow D, Madelenat P. Primary adenocarcinoma arising from endometriosis of the rectovaginal septum: a case report. Int J Gynecol Cancer 2005;15:1203–5.
163. Ying AJ, Copeland LJ, Hameed A. Myxoid change in nondecidualized cutaneous endometriosis resembling malignancy. Gynecol Oncol 1998;68:301–3.
164. Zugor V, Schott GE. Endometriosis involving the ureter – the Erlangen experience exemplified by two case reports. Akt Urol 2007;38:55–8.
165. Zugor V, Krot D, Rosch WH, Schrott KM, Schott GE. Endometriosis of the ureter and urinary bladder. Urologe 2007;46:71–8.

Normal ovaries, inflammatory and non-neoplastic conditions

21

Peter Russell Stanley J. Robboy

ANATOMY, HISTOLOGY AND FUNCTION OF THE OVARIES

ANATOMY

The ovaries are paired, almond-shaped bodies weighing 3–5 g and measuring approximately $30 \times 20 \times 10$ mm in an adult. They normally enlarge in pregnancy and shrink after the menopause. The external surface is smooth until after puberty, when it begins to become somewhat irregularly contoured in the course of maturation and rupture of the follicles.

The whole of the length of the hilum is attached to the posterior surface of the broad ligament by the loose fibromuscular mesovarium. The strongly muscular ovarian ligament attaches the medial pole to the uterine cornu just below and behind the fallopian tube. The lateral pole of the ovary attaches to the pelvic wall by the suspensory ligament (infundibulopelvic ligament), a peritoneal fold containing the principal vascular supply and lymphatic drainage of the ovary. Veins from the left ovary drain into the left renal vein. Those of the right ovary drain into the right renal vein in 10% of women and directly into the inferior vena cava in the other 90%.[80]

The cut surface of the ovary shows a narrow, white outer cortex and a grayish pink, rather less firm medulla that forms the bulk of the organ. The medulla varies in consistency because of the follicles and corpora albicantia, which are often obvious macroscopically.

HISTOLOGY

The ovary is covered by a single layer of cells, a serosal investment that originates from the celomic epithelium lining the ventromedial surface of the gonadal blastema. This is a highly specialized mesothelial layer, continuous with the mesothelium of the peritoneal cavity at the ovarian hilus. Previously referred to as the 'germinal epithelium', this layer is more appropriately called the 'surface epithelium' or simply the 'serosa'. The cells are cuboidal in young women (Figure 21.1) but flatten in later life. Immunohistochemically, the serosal cells stain for vimentin, N-cadherin, calretinin,[23] and cytokeratin-7, but generally lack staining for cytokeratin-20 and CA125. They are more active than the peritoneal mesothelial cells to which they are related and secrete or have receptors for inhibin, estrogen, progesterone, and androgens, as well as a range of growth factors and cytokines, such as epidermal growth factor, transforming growth factor-β, and tumor necrosis factor-α.[9] They form a delicate layer that is often damaged or removed completely by handling at the time of operation. It shows variation from a single, flattened layer to a pseudostratified or genuinely stratified low columnar epithelium, with the formation of solid cellular invaginations, nests and cords, crypts and inclusion cysts, as well as the formation of evaginations or surface papillations of varied size and complexity. These changes are seen to a lesser extent in the adult human, but are more obvious in fetal life. The ovarian serosa is discussed further in relation to the histogenesis of epithelial tumors in both the ovary and the peritoneum (see Chapters 23 and 33, respectively).

Beneath the ovarian serosa lies the cortex, which is roughly divisible into an outer, fibrous, relatively acellular, collagenous zone, often termed the 'tunica albuginea', and an inner, more cellular active cortex. The tunica albuginea is usually a well-defined layer in an active ovary, averaging about 0.3 mm as measured from the serosa to the most superficially placed primordial follicle, but in some conditions, notably anovulatory states such as the polycystic ovary syndrome (see below), this outer cortical zone becomes an even more obvious 'capsule', being wider and more densely collagenous. The underlying cellular part of the cortex contains the primordial, ripening, and mature follicles; its appearances vary considerably at different ages and, to some extent, during the menstrual cycle and pregnancy. The cortical stroma consists of uniform spindled cells arranged in bundles, often with a striking fine storiform pattern. From these cells arise the interstitial lutein cells and the theca that forms the outer part of the follicle.

The central portion of the ovary is the medulla and, in young women, it consists of active follicles and cellular stroma. The blood vessels, which enter at the hilum, are accompanied by a small amount of connective tissue generally poor in cells. As women approach middle age, the medulla fills with corpora albicantia and by a meshwork of blood vessels with thick, hyalinized walls that render them more prominent than formerly. The medulla now also appears more prominent than earlier in life. On transverse section, the ovary therefore has an outer, dark cortical zone and an inner, less cellular medulla. After the menopause, the cortical stroma characteristically shrinks but postmenopausal stromal hyperplasia may occur (see below).

PHYSIOLOGIC FUNCTION OF THE OVARIES

OVARIAN DEVELOPMENT

The ovary has two major functions: the release of mature ova at the time of ovulation and the secretion of steroid hormones. These are controlled by the cyclic release of pituitary

543

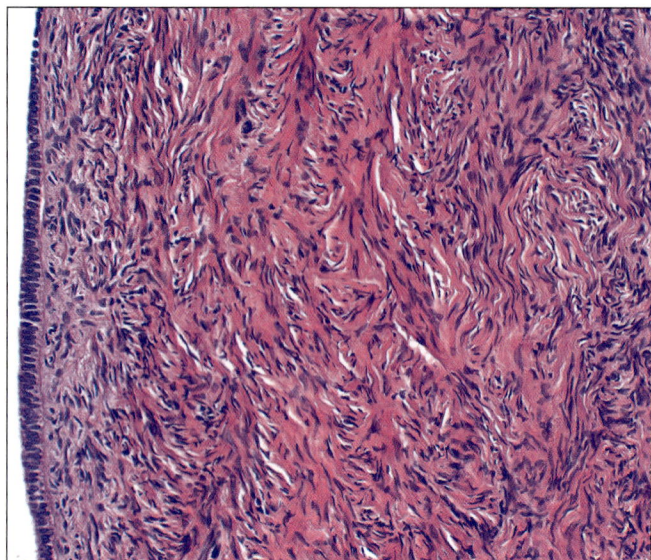

Fig. 21.1 Cuboidal surface epithelial cells covering the ovary of perimenopausal patient. They are separated from the cellular cortex by the narrow tunica albuginea.

follicle-stimulating hormone (FSH) and luteinizing hormone (LH). These hormones are, in turn, regulated by gonadotrophin-releasing hormone (GnRH), which the hypothalamus secretes into the pituitary portal circulation. The ovarian steroid hormones stimulate the growth of the reproductive organs, foster the development of secondary sexual characteristics, and help maintain the implanted blastocyst. The production of these hormones depends upon the development and ripening of the follicles and the formation of the corpus luteum.

FOLLICULOGENESIS

The primordial germ cells arise from the endoderm at the junction of the hindgut and the yolk sac and migrate by ameboid movement, via the hindgut mesentery to the gonadal ridge, the migration commencing 3 weeks after fertilization.[136] As a consequence of this migration, the gonads develop at a crown–rump length of 5.5 mm, but they remain sexually indifferent until the crown–rump length is 17 mm (about day 42). Then, in the testis, the presumptive Sertoli cells, which are non-germinal elements, outline the sex cords. In the ovary, by contrast, the proliferating germ cells comprise the dominant growth,[99] forming a finite complement of about six million ova by the sixth month of fetal life, to which there is no later addition. This proliferation is evident by the eighth week and very marked by the 13th week when the ovary consists largely of oogonial and oocytic clusters that taper proximally, with 'cords' only in the rete. Subsequent differentiation is centrifugal.[141] Pregranulosa cells enclose individual germ cells to form primordial follicles (Figure 21.2A). At the primary oocyte stage, the cells are in the prophase of the first meiotic division and DNA synthesis resumes only in the event of fertilization. At birth, the ovary consists largely of scanty, loose stroma, enclosing primordial and ripening follicles and folded around stems of vascular connective tissue. The characteristic ovarian stroma develops during the first year. The total number of germ cells at birth exhibits a considerable variation around an

approximate average of 500 000, already a significant loss from the second trimester maximum.

RIPENING OF THE FOLLICLES

Follicle ripening begins in the third trimester of intrauterine life, becoming more frequent later. The ripening of a follicle at this stage of life is followed by its atresia. The number of ripening follicles becomes considerable in the first 2 years of postnatal life, falls to a low level at 4 years and then increases again. At puberty individual follicles start to rupture and form corpora lutea, which then in turn regress.

Women, like other primates, typically develop a single dominant follicle resulting in a single ovulation in each cycle. The mechanism of selection and maturation of a dominant follicle is not well understood. The early follicular phase rise of FSH may be important in the recruitment of the dominant follicle and the transient decrease in FSH during the midfollicular phase does not allow the development of subdominant follicles. The largest follicle has more granulosa cells and therefore more FSH receptors, enabling its continued growth despite the low FSH levels.[142]

The ripening process comprises enlargement of the ovum, formation of the zona pellucida around it, proliferation of the granulosa cells, and formation of a cavity among the latter. The enlarging follicle sinks deeper into the ovary, probably because of differential theca proliferation, and then expands and ruptures. When it ruptures, about 36 hours after the onset of the midcycle LH surge, it has been developing for some 12 weeks. It is likely that several hundred primordial follicles initiate growth each month, but only 20 or so become 'precursor' follicles. These potential preovulatory follicles are capable of undergoing complete maturation and ovulating within about 2 weeks, the length of a normal follicular phase, provided they receive the appropriate gonadotrophic stimulation. At this stage, the follicle is about 2–5 mm in diameter, with a fluid-filled antrum, at least one million granulosa cells, and a single healthy oocyte. The other follicles undergo atresia at an early stage of development.

Granulosa cell proliferation begins when the ovum starts to enlarge. The cells change from flat to cuboidal and then form several layers around the ovum (Figure 21.2B). Between the granulosa cells small droplets that are periodic acid-Schiff (PAS) positive form; these condense around the ovum to form small spaces. Enlargement or fusion of these spaces produces first an arcuate crevice and then a reniform cavity, the antrum (Figure 21.2C). The granulosa cells form a palisade at the periphery of the follicle and in turn are surrounded by a pale layer of specialized ovarian stroma, the theca interna. A basal lamina separates the granulosa cells from the cells of the theca interna. The theca externa is a poorly defined zone formed by the merging of the theca interna with the surrounding ovarian stroma (Figure 21.2D). The cytoplasm of the cells of the theca interna increases in amount and becomes foamy or granular and can be shown in frozen sections to contain sudanophilic and doubly refractile lipids. The nuclei become rounded and vesicular. In the dominant preovulatory follicle, the theca cell layer is well supplied with blood vessels but the granulosa cell layer remains avascular.

The follicular fluid is a modified transudate from the theca and adjacent vessels, which are believed to become more permeable because of local liberation of histamine. The same

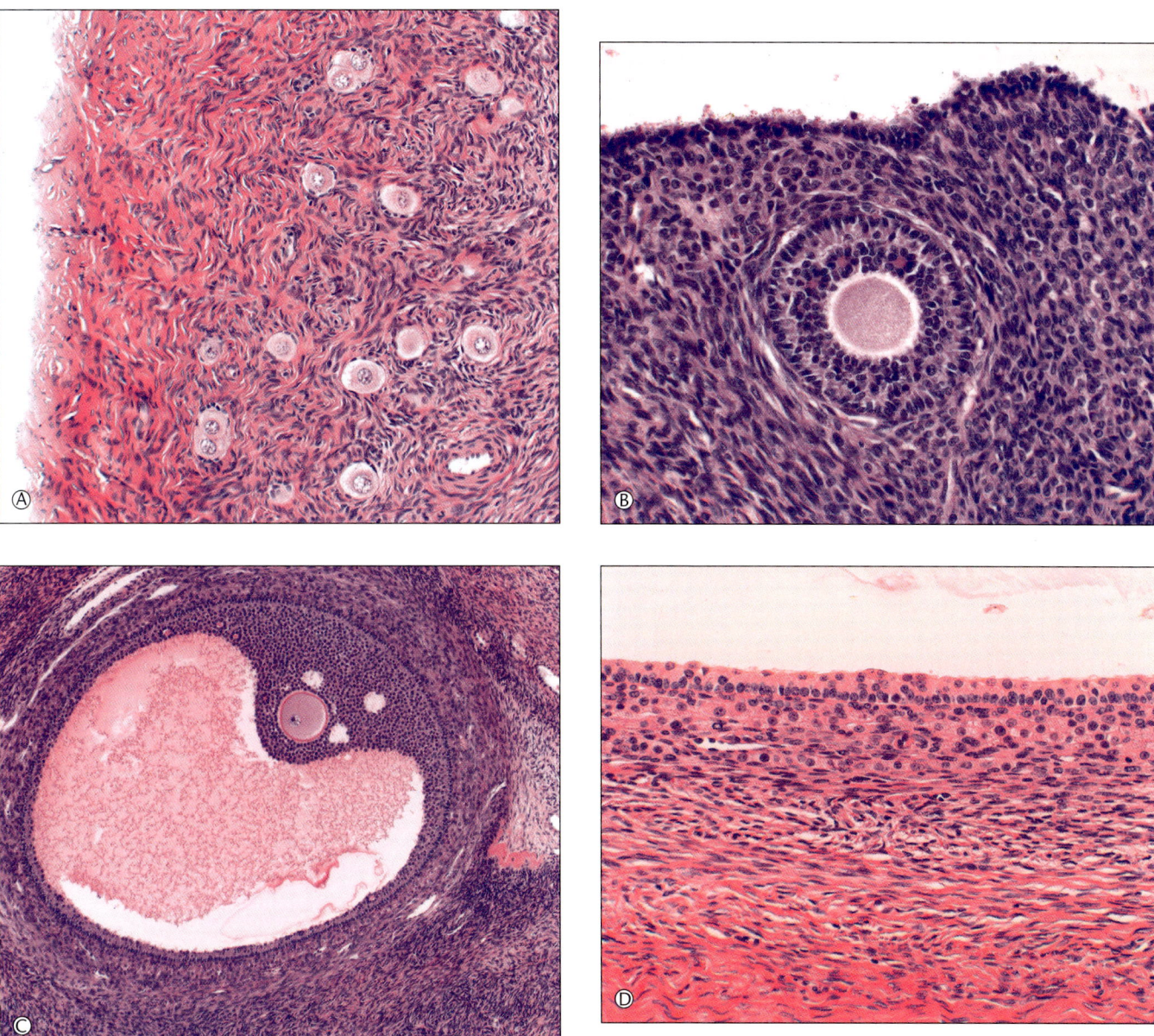

Fig. 21.2 Preovulatory follicles. **(A)** Cellular superficial cortex containing a number of primordial follicles. An unusual variation is the presence of binovular follicles. **(B)** A late primary or preantral follicle with a prominent zona pellucida surrounding the ovum and an occasional Call–Exner body within the developing granulosa cell layer (above the ovum). The spindle-shaped cells of the emerging theca are apparent. A regressing cystic follicle forms the upper margin of the field. **(C)** Secondary or Graafian follicle with an eccentric cumulus oophorus containing the oocyte. **(D)** Developing follicle showing the granulosa cell layer subtended by theca interna (plump cells) and theca externa (spindle cells) layers.

process of transudation leads to the development of a loose-textured vascular shell around the outside of the follicle, the theca externa. As the antrum enlarges, the granulosa cell layer becomes generally thinned, but persists as a mound, the cumulus oophorus, around the ovum (Figure 21.2C). Granulosa cells aspirated from the developing follicle at this stage tend to be single or in small clusters with scanty amphophilic cytoplasm (Figure 21.3). Outside the cumulus the theca interna shows a corresponding thickening, the theca cone, which has a role in loosening the coherence of the tissues. The mature, preovulatory follicle is known as a Graafian follicle. The final phase in follicular maturation is abrupt and largely mediated by the LH surge and a complex interaction of local cyto-kines.[12,70] It includes rapid accumulation of follicular fluid, loosening of the theca, and discharge of the fluid contents and

ovum with the few attendant granulosa cells that form the corona radiata. The follicle then collapses, taking on a corrugated outline that becomes exaggerated as transformation into a corpus luteum advances. Bleeding into the thecal tissues may occur at about the time of ovulation but, since the granulosa is as yet avascular, there is normally no bleeding into the follicular cavity and peritoneum.

FORMATION OF THE CORPUS LUTEUM

The formation of the corpus luteum comprises two processes: (1) blood vessels grow into the collapsed granulosa cell layer from the theca, carrying theca cells with them (some bleeding now takes place into the cavity and, because of this, the corpus luteum of the current cycle appears bluish when seen through the surface of the ovary); and (2) luteinization of the granulosa cell layer occurs (Figure 21.4), the cells becoming strikingly large and pale, and readily distinguishable from the smaller and somewhat less pale luteinized theca cells ('theca–lutein cells'). Among the theca–lutein cells are some darker, angular cells with hyperchromatic nuclei, the so-called 'K cells', which contain alkaline phosphatase and are most probably CD4+ and CD8+ T-lymphocytes in equal numbers.[17] Ultrastructural studies of the luteinized cells show abundant smooth endoplasmic reticulum with vesicular dilatations, mitochondria with tubular cristae, and numerous small lipid droplets, which are the familiar general features of the steroid-secreting cell. There is also an intracellular and intercellular canalicular system that probably conveys secretion to the perivascular spaces.

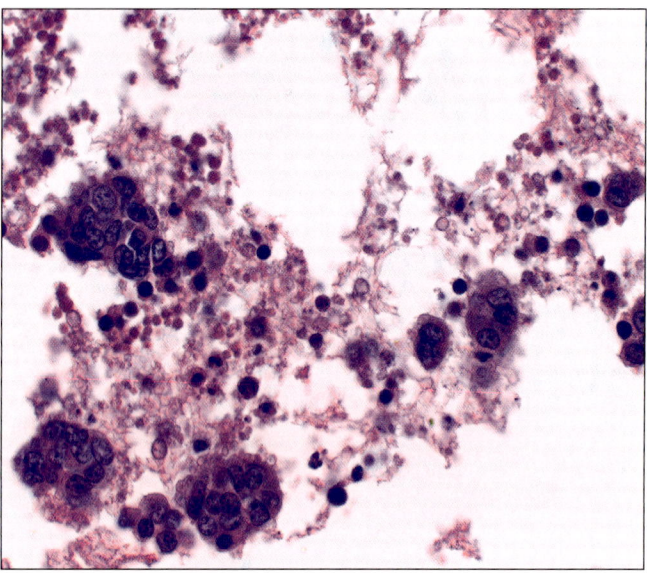

Fig. 21.3 Shed granulosa cells from a mature preovulatory follicle.

When pregnancy occurs, the corpus luteum remains unchanged for about 50 days. It then doubles in size during the following 10 days and remains thus enlarged until about day 80, when it begins to shrink as the placenta takes over progesterone production. Hyaline bodies, about 10–20 μm in size, are found sparingly among the luteinized cells only in the corpus luteum of pregnancy (Figure 21.5A). Another histologic feature that, when present, distinguishes the corpus luteum of pregnancy from that of menstruation is the organization of the central coagulum to produce mature, avascular, collagenous connective tissue over a time period not available to the corpus luteum of menstruation prior to its programmed involution (Figure 21.5B).

INVOLUTION OF THE CORPUS LUTEUM

Unless stimulated by beta-human chorionic gonadotrophin from trophoblast the fertilized zygote produces, the corpus luteum begins its programmed involution at about day 9, i.e., about day 23 of a normal 28-day cycle. The biologic mechanisms responsible for this process of elimination of the corpus luteum (structural luteolysis) are complex and centered around apoptosis.[24,96,111] Hyaline and fatty changes appear to a variable extent in the luteinized granulosa cells (Figure 21.6A), together with an increase of acid phosphatase and PAS-positive intracellular material. This apoptotic change may occur acutely, with frank necrosis (Figure 21.6B). The average corpus luteum reaches about 1.5 cm in maximum size. It has shrunk only slightly by the end of the cycle, but then rapidly gets smaller. As it does so, its wavy lemon-yellow form becomes thinner and the color deepens to a darker yellow or orange. Eventually, the luteal pigment and the cells disappear. After several months, the corpus luteum completes its transformation into a much folded, collapsed shell of white, hyaline collagen, the corpus albicans (Figure 21.6C), the size and indeed the presence of which is determined by the amount of bleeding that occurs into the mature corpus luteum.[111] Corpora albicantia persist in the medulla and are often conspicuous on the cut surface, particu-

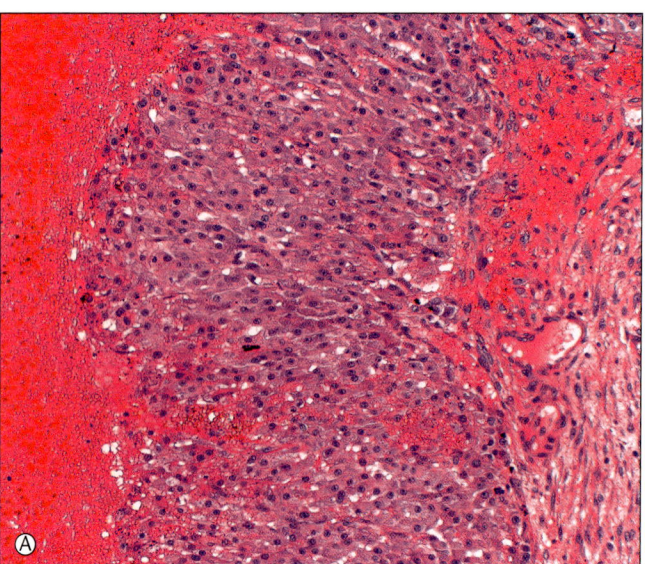

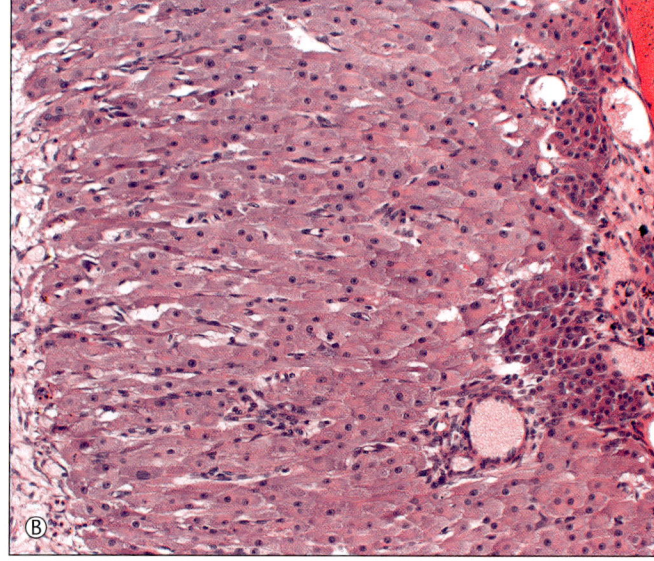

Fig. 21.4 Corpus luteum. **(A)** Early corpus luteum with antrum at the top, granulosa lutein layer in the centre and poorly formed theca at the base but no vascularization of the granulosa. **(B)** Mature corpus luteum with vascularized granulosa and immature granulation tissue organizing the central coagulum (top).

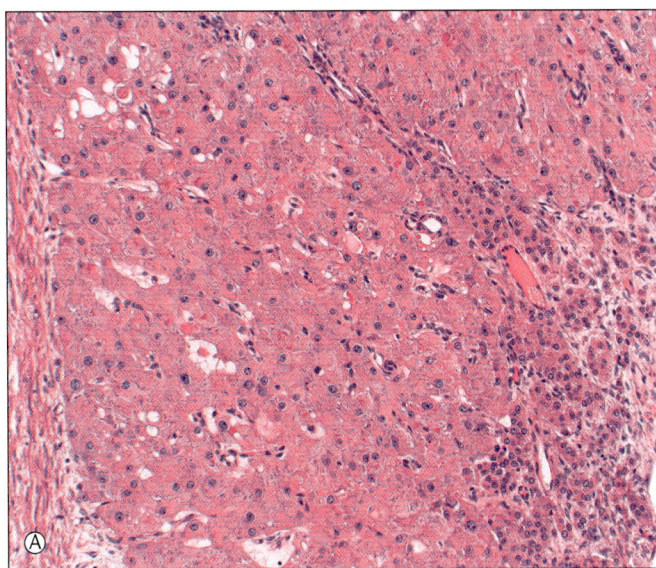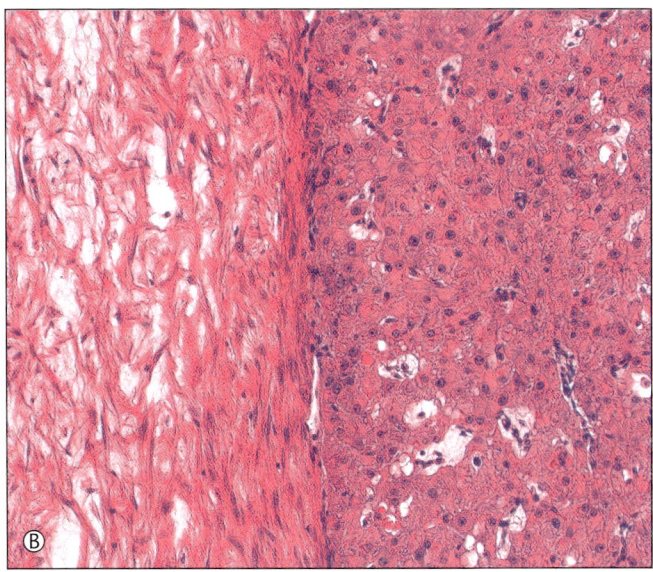

Fig. 21.5 Corpus luteum of pregnancy. **(A)** Established corpus luteum of pregnancy with organizing granulation tissue lining antrum at the top, granulosa lutein layer in the centre, containing scattered hyaline bodies, and well-formed theca at the base. **(B)** Active corpus luteum of pregnancy with avascular collagenous connective tissue of many weeks' age lining central antrum (top).

larly in later life. Regression of the corpus luteum of pregnancy is occasionally accompanied by residual microcalcispherule formation (Figure 21.6D).

FOLLICULAR ATRESIA

During each cycle many follicles start to mature but usually only one ruptures to form a corpus luteum. Occasionally, two or three synchronous corpora lutea are found (one mechanism of multiple pregnancies). The follicles that do not complete maturation become atretic. In atretic antral follicles, granulosa cells stop proliferating and become apoptotic. Atresia may start at any stage during maturation and proceeds at rates varying from follicle to follicle and in different parts of the same follicle, the region of the cumulus being the last affected.[60] The main effectors of this apoptosis are caspases, which are activated by either Fas/tumor necrosis factor-alpha (TNF-α) receptor or elements of the bcl-2 family.[112] Atresia is triggered by a lack of some essential factors supporting follicular development. Specifically, terminal follicular development is strictly dependent upon gonadotrophin supply (FSH, then LH in the final preovulatory stage). In addition, paracrine factors (growth factors, cytokines, steroids, constituents of extracellular matrix) also play important roles in amplifying gonadotrophin action in follicular cells.[110] The features of atresia include degeneration and shrinkage of the ovum, apoptosis of the granulosa cells or their transformation into connective tissue cells (Figure 21.7A), reversion of the cells of the theca interna to their original stromal form, invasion and obliteration of the shrinking cavity by stromal cells, and the formation of a hyalinized, collagenous membrane at the margin of the follicle. Eventually, the hyaline membrane alone persists to mark the site of the former follicle, which now appears as a compact white or gray nodule with a wavy outline, the corpus fibrosum (Figure 21.7B).

The commonest variations in the progress of atresia are persistent luteinization of the theca, leading to fatty change in the theca–lutein cells and persistence of granulosa cells, espe-

cially at the site of the cumulus (Figure 21.7C). Macrophages laden with lipofuscin may accumulate around corpora albicantia and corpora fibrosa and may remain there for long periods. Care should be taken not to confuse degenerating luteinized cells containing lipofuscin and old hemorrhage with endometriosis (in which the typical epithelial component might not be immediately apparent).

The residue of encircling cellular stroma left after follicular atresia contributes to production of cellular stroma that characterizes the mature ovary, and is absent at birth. The medullary stroma involutes to a varying extent in the third year of life, concurrently with the development of the larger blood vessels in the medulla. It remains prominent near the hilum. The cortical stroma forms by intrinsic proliferation of the peripheral mesenchyme, probably in response to the stretch stimulus caused by the presence of multiple centrally placed follicles, with large antra, that develop during the first year of life. Stroma formation is therefore largely dependent on follicular activity and is depressed if follicles are lacking or inactive and increased if maturation and atresia are excessive, as in the polycystic ovary syndrome. The medullary and juxta–hilar stroma thus has a direct 'follicular' ancestry, which makes it easier to understand why the tumors that may rarely arise from it are similar to those that develop in the functioning cortical stroma, tumors of sex cord-stromal type. During pregnancy, follicle maturation and atresia diminish in the first 10 weeks. They then become more active and are associated with marked theca-cell luteinization (Figure 21.7C).

THE HORMONAL BACKGROUND OF THE OVARIAN CYCLE

The first stages of follicle maturation under normal conditions are of uncertain cause, although the development of an ovarian follicle to the point of ovulation is intrinsically related to its capacity for estrogen synthesis. Ripening to the early antrum stage is under the control of pituitary FSH to which the larger follicles are more responsive. Local interaction between estro-

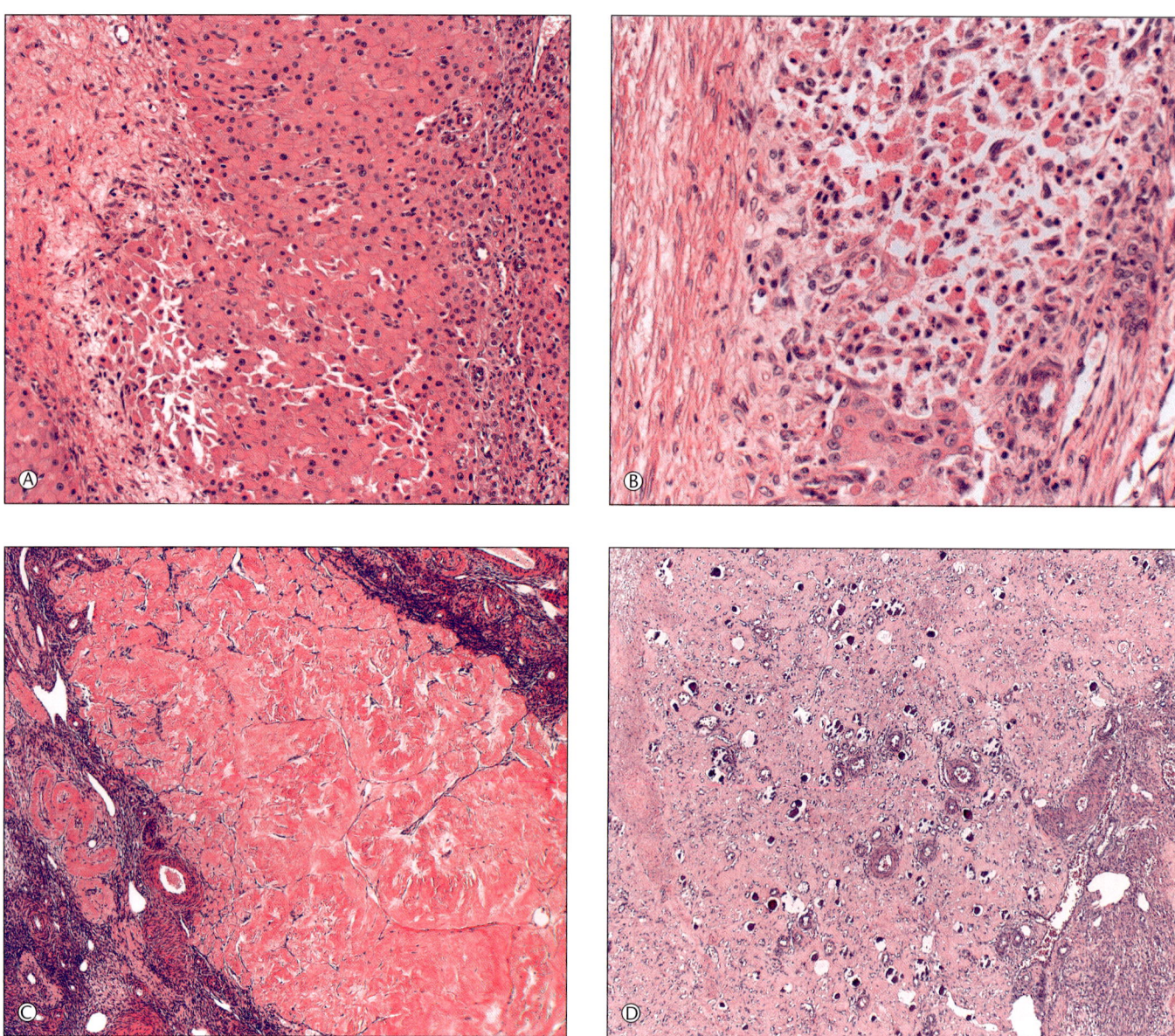

Fig. 21.6 Regression of corpus luteum. **(A)** Regressing corpus luteum, showing considerable diminution in size of luteal cells (early apoptosis) and complete vascularization of the granulosa. **(B)** Very uncommon hyperacute regression (diffuse apoptosis) of a corpus luteum, with frank necrosis. Surviving granulosa cells to left. **(C)** Corpus albicans. **(D)** Regressed corpus luteum of pregnancy with prominent microcalcispherules.

gens and gonadotrophins also helps to coordinate preovulatory follicular maturation. Follicular estrogens feeding back to the hypothalamic–pituitary axis control gonadotrophin secretion, the secretion of FSH showing peaks on about days 4 and 14. Other critical factors are:

- activin, which promotes ovarian follicular development, inhibits androgen production, and increases FSH and insulin secretion;
- follistatin, an activin-binding protein, which neutralizes activin bioactivity;[47] and
- inhibin, a gonadal peptide that selectively suppresses the secretion of FSH.

Granulosa cells within the follicle synthesize inhibin, and its initial transport from the ovary appears to be by way of the lymphatics.

Thecal development, which requires the presence of LH, enhances the production and steroidogenic use of cholesterol. In the early follicular phase, LH acts through specific receptors, constitutively present on thecal cells, for stimulating androgen production. A positive correlation has recently been established between androgen receptor expression and follicular cell proliferation.[70] Furthermore, androgens are active through a conversion to estrogens in granulosa cells. The acute follicular enlargement leading to ovulation is associated with the peak of LH secretion on day 14 of the normal 28-day cycle, triggered by estrogen secreted by the dominant follicle. If pregnancy does not ensue, the corpus luteum has a maximum lifespan of about 14 days. As mentioned above, its degeneration begins by day 23 (day 9 postovulation). Its persistence during that time is dependent on the continuous low level of LH secretion, but on no other known luteotrophic stimulus. When pregnancy

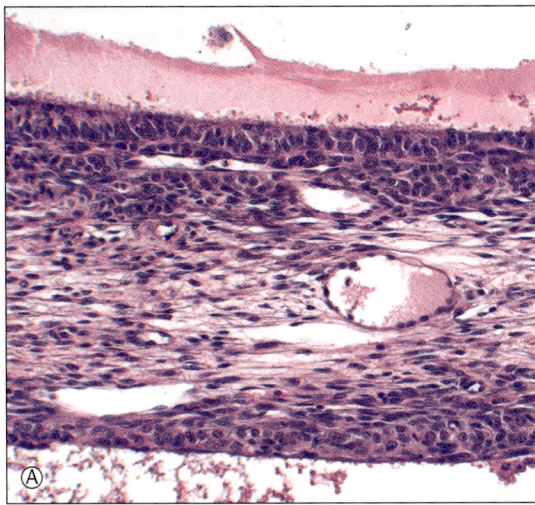

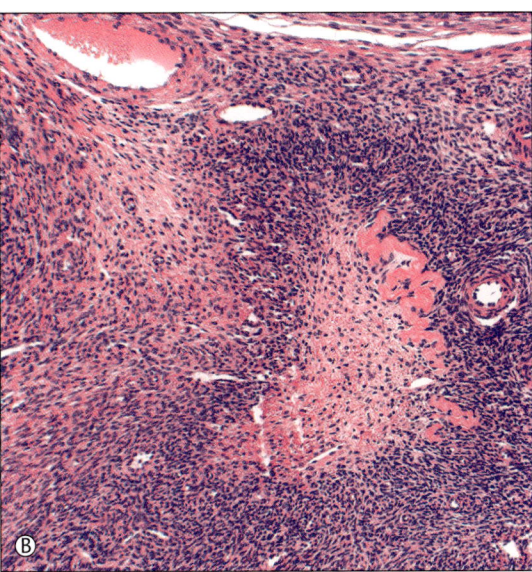

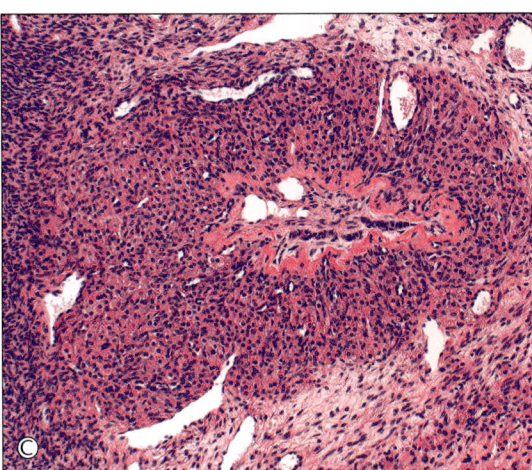

Fig. 21.7 Follicular atresia. **(A)** Adjacent cystic follicles with early atresia in the lower follicle. The granulosa is degenerate and has been partly shed into the antrum. **(B)** Small follicle showing advanced atresia with typical festooned contour and fibroblastic tissue occupying the site of the original antrum. **(C)** Atretic follicle in early pregnancy displaying partial luteinization of the theca interna layer and, interestingly, central persistence of small cords of granulosa cells.

occurs, chorionic gonadotrophin fosters maintenance of the corpus luteum.

All of the known steroidogenic sites in the ovary produce each of the main ovarian hormones from acetate by way of cholesterol. These include progesterone, androstenedione, testosterone, dihydroandrosterone, estradiol, and estrone 1, which are the main successive stages in cholesterol transformation. Each steroidogenic site, however, produces only one or a few, preferentially. The exact roles of the granulosa cells and theca cells in the preovulatory follicle are difficult to study; the complex interrelationships of the cells to each other are virtually impossible to reproduce *in vitro*. However, it is clear that the granulosa cells can synthesize pregnenolone and progesterone and convert androgens to estrogens by aromatization. Thecal tissue produces mainly androstenedione, with small amounts of estradiol. As the granulosa cell layer in the preovulatory follicle is avascular, the hormonal environment of these cells (and also that of the oocyte) is different from that of the blood. It is dependent, in part, upon the activity of the adjacent theca cells. This means that the products of the granulosa cells have to diffuse through at least some of the theca cell layer to reach the ovarian venous blood. While analysis of the follicular fluid gives only an indirect indication of the activity of the follicular cells of both types, the dominant and therefore the most active preovulatory follicle in an ovary has the highest levels of estradiol in the fluid. This dominant follicle has the highest estrogen : androgen ratio in its secreted hormones of all the follicles and its granulosa cells have the highest capacity for androgen aromatization *in vitro*. Aromatase activity in the granulosa cells falls off shortly before ovulation, and synthesis of progesterone commences just prior to ovulation in response to the LH surge.

The levels of LH, FSH, and estradiol fall after ovulation, but there is sufficient LH to maintain the sensitive luteinized granulosa cells of the corpus luteum. Together the luteinized theca cells and luteinized granulosa cells of the corpus luteum produce both estradiol and its major product progesterone. Normal corpus luteum function depends on numerous regulatory factors, such as prostaglandins, oxytocin, steroids, growth factors, cytokines, etc. Studying luteal cell interactions (steroidogenic large and small luteal cells as well as non-steroidogenic 'accessory' cells of the corpus luteum) has produced new evidence of communication within the corpus luteum that influences its function.[39] The theca cells produce primarily estrogen and the luteinized granulosa cells produce mainly progesterone, which is reflected in the high plasma progesterone level during this phase of the cycle and the high pregnanediol excretion from the time of ovulation until the day or two preceding menstruation. Both hormones reach their peak in the midsecretory phase of the cycle, when estradiol levels are similar to those of the mid-to-late follicular phase. The stromal tissue produces mainly androstenedione, which has about one-tenth the androgenic activity of testosterone and is partly converted into the latter peripherally. The effects of these hormones on the pituitary are largely mediated through the hypothalamus. Secretion of FSH is inhibited by sufficient amounts of either estrogens or progesterone; the effect of estrogens on the secretion of LH is thought to be diphasic, being stimulatory over a short length of time and inhibitory in the long term.

The ovaries are the primary source of androgens in the postmenopausal period when testosterone production in particular is maintained or even boosted, presumably due to increased stimulation of the ovarian stroma by LH.[20]

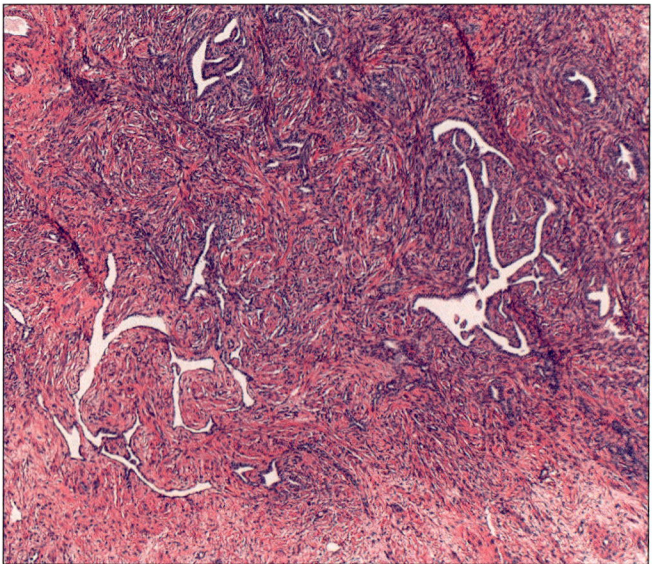

Fig. 21.8 Normal rete ovarii, with jagged branching of slit-like epithelial-lined spaces.

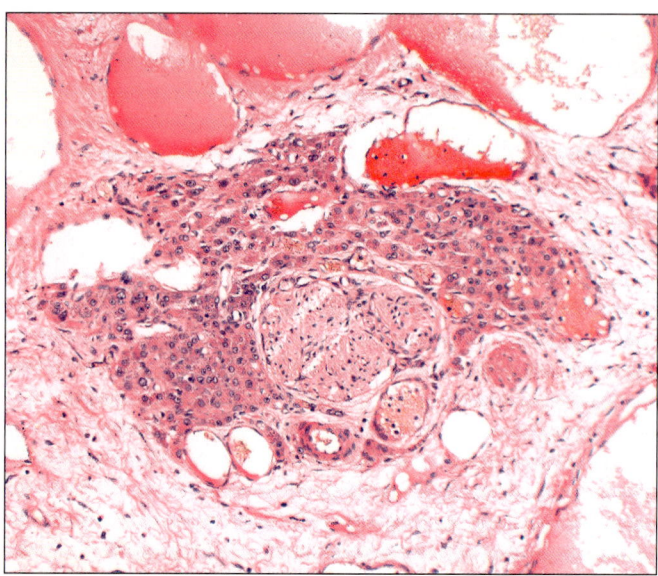

Fig. 21.9 Hilus cells. Aggregate of hilus cells in close apposition to both autonomic nerve and dilated vascular spaces.

THE OVARIAN HILUM AND ITS VICINITY

The epoophoron, the homologue of which is the efferent ducts of the wolffian duct in the male, lies in the lateral part of the mesosalpinx. It consists of a main tubule of mesonephric origin and lies parallel to the lateral end of the fallopian tube. A series of secondary tubules run at right angles from it towards the ovary (Kobelts tubes). It is formed by epithelium surrounding a narrow lumen and enclosed, as is the mesonephric duct at most sites, by a wall of smooth muscle.

The rete ovarii consists of multiple intercommunicating channels lined by deeply staining, cuboidal to flattened epithelial cells exhibiting a characteristically angular, jagged-looking cross-section (Figure 21.8). Nearer to the ovary the rete tubules are more rounded in outline and in this situation they often show traces of a muscle and connective tissue covering. The origin of the rete ovarii is disputed. It is generally considered as homologous with the straight seminiferous tubules of the testis. The relevant immunoprofile of the rete tubules includes strong positive staining for CD10[122] and negative staining for calretinin.[23]

Small groups of lutein-like cells are found in the mesovarium and in the ovarian hilum, often adjacent to nerves. These are the so-called 'ovarian hilar' (hilum or hilus) cells (Figure 21.9). It is possible that hilar cells may be derived either from luteinized ovarian stromal cells that have wandered into the hilum or from perineural fibroblasts. They resemble the interstitial cells of the testis (Leydig cells) and contain lipofuscin pigment and Reinke crystals. While they probably produce both androgens and estrogens, it is the former role that distinguishes them and is responsible for a characteristic immunoprofile. Along with theca interna cells of the normal ovarian follicles and the Leydig cell component of Sertoli–Leydig cell tumors, these cells express α-inhibin and calretinin.[23] They participate in the ovarian renin–angiotensin system, which is also linked to androgen secretion. More recently, these cells have been shown to secrete vascular endothelial growth factor, a crucial mediator in the cyclic angiogenesis of the corpus luteum.[53]

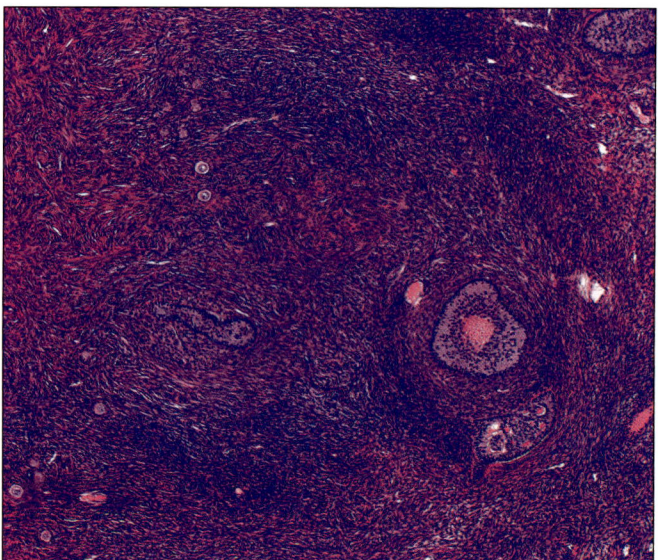

Fig. 21.10 Dysplastic follicles in partial resistant ovary syndrome. Bizarre-shaped follicles with normal primordial follicles at top left.

FOLLICULAR FAILURE

FOLLICULAR DYSGENESIS (DYSPLASIA)

Definition

Dysplastic primary (preantral) and secondary (antral) follicles are occasionally encountered in otherwise normally functioning ovaries. The term 'follicular dysgenesis' has been applied to polyovular primordial follicles (i.e., containing two or more oocytes; see Figure 21.2A). However, we believe it is most appropriately applied to developing follicles that differ morphologically from normal by disorganized proliferated granulosa, frequently without an antrum despite the follicular size, and containing multiple Call–Exner bodies (Figure 21.10). These lesions have been likened to microscopic gonadoblasto-

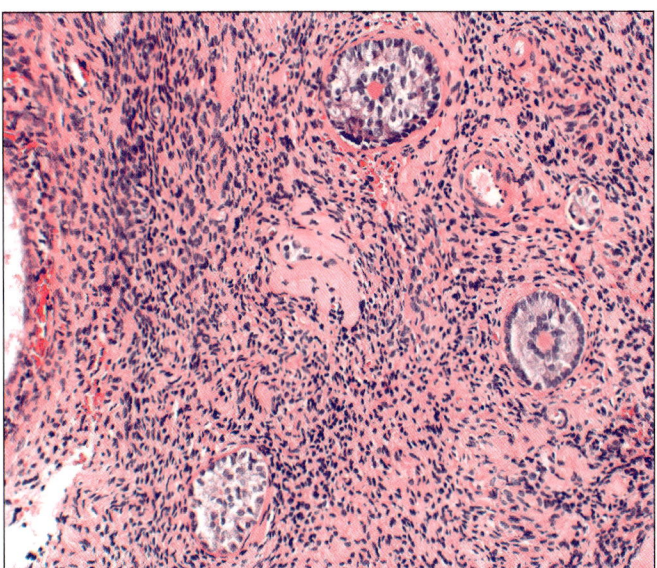

Fig. 21.11 Dysplastic follicles in partial resistant ovary syndrome. Higher power of dysplastic follicles showing superficial resemblance to structures seen in SCTAT associated with the Peutz–Jeghers syndrome.

mas. They frequently occur (25%) in the ovaries of infants and young children. A similar morphologic pattern is seen in some cases of documented hypergonadotrophic premature ovarian failure (Figures 21.10 and 21.11), but the relationship of the follicular changes to altered hypothalamic–pituitary–ovarian function remains unclear. Dysplastic follicles also occur in cases of autoimmune oophoritis and of ovarian fibromatosis (see below).

Microscopic features

The follicular outline is distorted with irregular extensions into the adjacent stroma (Figure 21.10). Sometimes follicular fragmentation produces small nests or cords of granulosa cells. Mitoses are reduced in these cells. Rarely, the cells contain cytoplasmic lipid. A prominent cuff of focally or partially luteinized theca interna cells surrounds about one-third of dysplastic follicles. Atresia of the dysplastic follicles is generally accompanied by persistent granulosa, a phenomenon only occasionally observed in normal ovaries. Occasional dysplastic follicles show convoluted and rounded deposits of hyaline PAS-positive material similar to, and continuous with, the basement membrane (glassy membrane) of the regressing follicles. These deposits are interposed between the cords of granulosa cells in a manner resembling sex-cord tumors with annular tubules (SCTAT).

OVARIAN FAILURE

Definition

Failure of the ovary to ovulate or even to produce its steroids, broadly speaking, may be caused by a multiplicity of factors, ranging from never functioning or functioning abnormally from the start, or more commonly failing at some later time in life in association with abnormal gonadotrophin levels, either elevated or depressed. *Premature ovarian failure* refers to

secondary amenorrhea (with well-developed secondary sex characteristics and a history of normal menarche) with continuously raised gonadotrophin levels, where the last menstrual period occurs prior to 40 years of age. However, premature ovarian failure should not be regarded as merely an early normal menopause.

Other terms commonly used include:

- *Hypergonadotrophic hypogonadism* (primary ovarian failure), which results from a congenital or acquired intrinsic ovarian defect, or failure of the ovaries to respond to pituitary gonadotrophins despite the presence of follicles.
- *Hypogonadotrophic hypogonadism*, which results from the pituitary gland failing to secrete gonadotrophins (FSH and LH) in amounts sufficient to stimulate the ovaries.

Both ovarian failure and hypogonadotrophic hypogonadism can present as primary or secondary amenorrhea. The median age at menopause in Western populations of women is approximately 51 years. While about 5% of women experience 'early' cessation of ovarian function at or prior to age 45, by convention, premature ovarian failure (a preferable term to premature menopause[71]) is reserved for the 1% of women who experience hypergonadotrophic amenorrhea prior to age 40 years.[139]

Whilst reproductive senescence in most species can be explained in the same general terms as physiologic senescence, in women ovarian function comes to a relatively abrupt halt at an age when the impact of somatic senescence on most other functions is minimal.[102] The human ovary is endowed at birth with a fixed number of primordial follicles, which steadily decreases throughout life due to atresia and recruitment for ovulation. A causal relationship between follicular depletion and normal menopause clearly exists and there is a gradual acceleration towards follicular wastage, commencing more than a decade before cessation of menstrual activity. This suggests that follicle dynamics rather than neuroendocrine function determines the onset of menopause, both normal and premature.

Four broad etiologic categories are known for premature ovarian failure:[138]

1. *Genetic*. Clear-cut X chromosome deletions or transpositions,[26,36,51,88,114,134] particularly those in the critical region, result in a truncated reproductive lifespan. Autosomal anomalies are less frequent causes.[144]
2. *Autoimmune*. Premature ovarian failure may accompany any autoimmune polyglandular failure syndrome, most often in linkage with antithyroid and antiadrenal antibodies.[29,65,77]
3. *Iatrogenic*. Repeated ovarian surgery, uterine vascular embolization,[83] the underlying disease that led to surgery, or chemotherapy may trigger the failure.[28,121]
4. *Environmental*. Environmental toxicants are difficult to pinpoint but, amongst others, industrial toxins[101,107] and galactose consumption[54,56] have been implicated.

The probability that one or other of these mechanisms is operative will be more or less likely depending on the woman's age at diagnosis.[100,139]

Clinical features

Ovarian failure divides into two broad clinicopathologic sub-types: (1) premature follicular depletion ('true premature menopause'), irreversible ovarian failure due to depleted follicles (afollicular ovarian failure); and (2) the much rarer resistant ovary syndrome ('gonadotrophin insensitivity syndrome'), in which primordial follicles are present but fail to respond appropriately to gonadotrophin stimulation (follicular ovarian failure). Patients with apparent ovarian failure associated with chronic (autoimmune) oophoritis fit best into the latter category on therapeutic grounds, namely the possibility, in practice very slight, that ovarian function and reproductive capability will recover. This separation into afollicular and follicular forms is somewhat artificial, since many of the former are very likely end stages of various disorders. This distinction is nonetheless critical clinically, since premature follicular depletion signifies permanent loss of reproductive function.

Although ovarian biopsy, currently by minilaparoscopic techniques through a 2 mm port,[127] is not necessary for the diagnosis of ovarian failure, it is the best means to distinguish afollicular from follicular types and is therefore useful in counseling patients desiring pregnancy.[1,52] Recent research suggests that serum antimüllerian hormone (AMH) levels can differentiate follicular from afollicular patients.[86,104] Recent developments and sporadic success with physiologic estradiol/progesterone replacement cycles in such women[87] and cryopreservation of oocytes from unstimulated follicles[69] offer promise of alternatives to oocyte donation programs. This latter also requires ovarian biopsy.

A combined pathologic and etiologic classification of ovarian failure is given in Table 21.1.

Table 21.1 Ovarian failure: pathologic and etiologic classification

Afollicular (premature follicular depletion, true premature menopause)
  Exogenous (iatrogenic)
    Surgery
    Radiation
    Chemotherapeutic and other drugs
    Environmental toxins
  Endogenous (spontaneous)
    Chromosomal, genetic, maldeveloped gonads
      Familial
      Galactosemia
      Mucopolysaccharidosis
      Blepharophimosis
      Malouf syndrome
      Perrault syndrome
      Roberts-SC phocomelia syndrome
    Autoimmune
    Infection (mumps, others)
    Hemorrhage
    Malignant infiltration
    Idiopathic
Follicular (Savage syndrome, gonadotrophin-insensitivity syndrome)
  Idiopathic resistant ovary syndrome
  Chronic (autoimmune) oophoritis
  Galactosemia
  Blepharophimosis

AFOLLICULAR OVARIAN FAILURE (PREMATURE FOLLICULAR DEPLETION, TRUE PREMATURE MENOPAUSE)

Etiology

Sometimes the cause of premature ovarian failure is obvious from the patient's history, e.g., bilateral oophorectomy for neoplastic or non-neoplastic disease, prior radiation or chemotherapy. These exogenous or iatrogenic factors are discussed later.

Genetic abnormalities more commonly present with primary rather than secondary amenorrhea, and include perturbations of the X chromosomes[36,37,51,129,134,152] as well as autosomal defects. Normal ovarian function requires two functioning X chromosomes. X monosomy as in Turners syndrome, mixed gonadal dysgenesis (Swyers syndrome; 46,XY), and so-called 'pure gonadal dysgenesis' (46,XX)[64] are well-documented causes of primary afollicular ovarian failure. Other reported associations include 47,XXX,[59,67] 48,XXXX,[135] 45,X/46,XX mosaicism,[40,42] structurally abnormal X chromosomes,[90] and balanced[13] and unbalanced[7] translocations of the X chromosome, including deletions of the distal portions of the Xq encompassing the fragile X locus.[22] The fragile X syndrome results from hyperexpansion and hypermethylation of a CGG repeat tract in the 5' untranslated region of the FMR1 gene. This methylation causes the gene to be transcriptionally silenced. Recent reports of premutation-specific phenotypes unrelated to fragile X syndrome have shown up to 20-fold increased risks for premature ovarian failure among female carriers.[3,57,106]

About 10% of patients with premature ovarian failure have a family member with the same condition and a higher percentage if presenting during their teenage years.[100] Some have a known specific genetic abnormality such as galactosemia. The mechanism of ovarian damage in galactosemia remains unknown, but appears to be independent of dietary management and most investigators favor a toxic effect of galactose or its metabolites on germ cells/follicular structures.[54,56] Ovarian failure has been documented in females with the blepharophimosis ptosis epicanthus inversus syndrome (BPES), a human disorder caused by mutations in the forkhead transcription factor gene FOXL2 of chromosome 3 and is characterized by facial dysmorphism,[94] and rarely in association with the Malouf syndrome,[117] the Perrault syndrome,[15] the Roberts-SC phocomelia syndrome,[38] the noggin mutation,[41,82] the cutis marmorata telangiectatica congenita syndrome,[143] Mulibrey nanism,[74,75] and specific types of leukodystrophy.[140]

The contribution of infections (including viral diseases) to premature ovarian failure is not known. Mumps oophoritis, although suspected clinically, has not been documented pathologically.

Although the etiology remains elusive in most cases with a normal 46,XX karyotype, several rare specific immune causes have been discovered. Clinical gonadal failure has been reported in both type I and type II autoimmune polyendocrine syndromes.[6,19,27,49] These include Addisons,[35] Graves, and Hashimotos diseases,[48,100] rheumatoid arthritis,[34] myasthenia gravis,[137] diabetes mellitus,[44] pernicious anemia,[95] hypoparathyroidism,[95,115] and systemic lupus erythematosus,[103] ranging, in some studies, up to 20–40% of patients with premature ovarian failure.

Further support lies in the demonstration of antiovarian antibodies in many premature ovarian failure patients (both

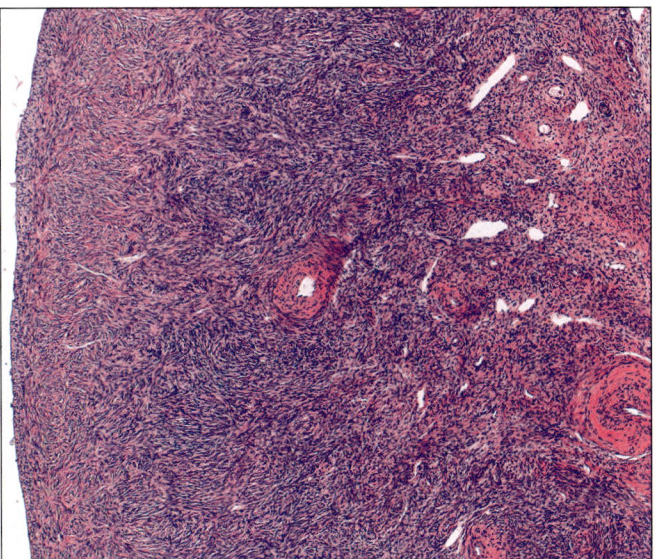

Fig. 21.12 Premature follicular depletion. Dense cortical stroma devoid of primordial or developing follicles.

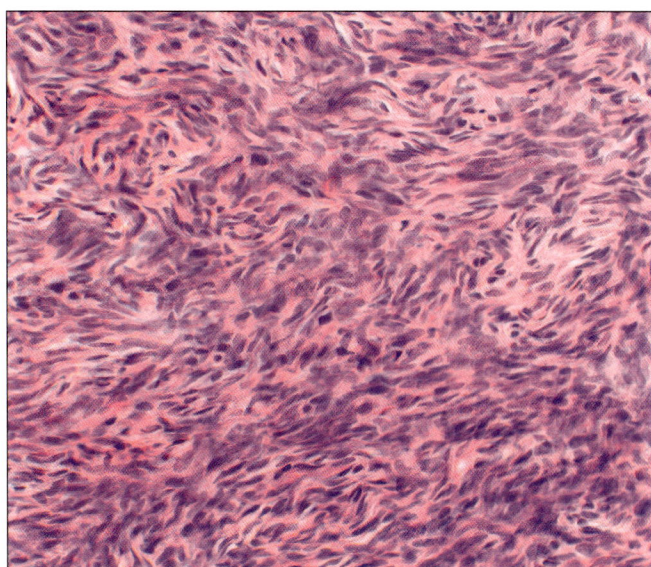

Fig. 21.13 Premature follicular depletion. Undistinguished ovarian cortical stroma that would be difficult to differentiate from that seen in streak gonads.

with and without associated autoimmune disorders), and reports of response to corticosteroid therapy. Antibodies in patients' sera have reacted against steroid-producing cells, gonadotrophins and their receptors, corpus luteum, zona pellucida, and oocytes,[55] as well as producing a cytotoxic effect on granulosa cells in culture. Because of the association with other autoimmune diseases, investigation and close follow-up are recommended in such patients with premature ovarian failure.[11,50,76] Although premature ovarian failure was once considered permanent, a substantial number of patients experience spontaneous remission.[126] Hormone replacement therapy remains the cornerstone of treatment, and the best chance of achieving a pregnancy is through oocyte donation.[4]

A minority of patients with premature follicular depletion have no etiologic factor that can be demonstrated clinically or histologically. Such unexplained cases may be due to an as yet undefined genetic defect resulting in congenitally small ovaries with reduced numbers of primordial follicles, or increased utilization of follicles or rapid follicular atresia.

Microscopic features
The cortical stroma is dense and hypercellular and notable for a complete absence of primordial and antral follicles (Figure 21.12), although a rare primordial follicle does not exclude the diagnosis. Serosal epithelial inclusions are common, and care is needed to avoid confusing the smaller ones with primordial or preantral follicles. Atretic follicles (usually at corpus fibrosum stage) may be present, which indicates previous follicular activity. The deeper cortex and medulla often show evidence of previous ovulation, most commonly in the form of corpora albicantia, but occasionally regressing corpora lutea. If there is no evidence of past or present follicular activity, nor any apparent corticomedullary differentiation (Figure 21.13), it may be difficult, especially in small laparoscopic biopsies, to confidently differentiate such an ovary from a streak (see above). Minor stromal changes may be present, such as small clusters of luteinized stromal cells or minor inflammatory foci that, in serial sections, exhibit no relationship to follicular

remnants. It is reasonable to speculate that such infiltrates represent the end result of a chronic autoimmune oophoritis.

FOLLICULAR OVARIAN FAILURE

Resistant ovary syndrome (Savage syndrome, gonadotrophin-insensitivity syndrome)
Definition This is a follicular form of premature ovarian failure in which the ovary contains numerous morphologically normal primordial follicles, but most show no evidence of development. A rare follicle may reach the preantral stage and occasional follicles will reach the antral stage. In cases of secondary amenorrhea, stigmata of previous ovulation are usually present. Continuous hypersecretion of pituitary gonadotrophins, and insensitivity of the ovaries to exogenous stimulation by human gonadotrophins, even in massive doses, are central to the diagnosis. Approximately 10% of cases of ovarian failure fall into this group.

Etiology An established association exists in general between autoimmune disease and premature ovarian failure (see above), but this has not been specifically or widely extended to resistant ovary syndrome until recent studies reported a strong association between the latter and myasthenia gravis.[30] The key appears to be via blocking antibodies to the FSH receptor or a receptor-related membrane domain, analogous to the blocking antibodies of the acetylcholine receptor of myasthenia gravis. Some patients suffer from galactosemia or BPES and the overlap between afollicular and follicular variants of premature ovarian failure only adds uncertainty to speculation as to etiology.

The history of apparently normal menstrual activity prior to the onset of symptoms and a resistance to exogenous gonadotrophins suggests that the resistant ovary syndrome is usually an acquired disorder not related to any intrinsic abnormality of FSH. Since gonadotrophin receptors are modulated by local estrogen production, an abnormality in estrogen metabolism may also be causative. It should also be noted that, in the physiologic perimenopausal period, the last remaining follicles are

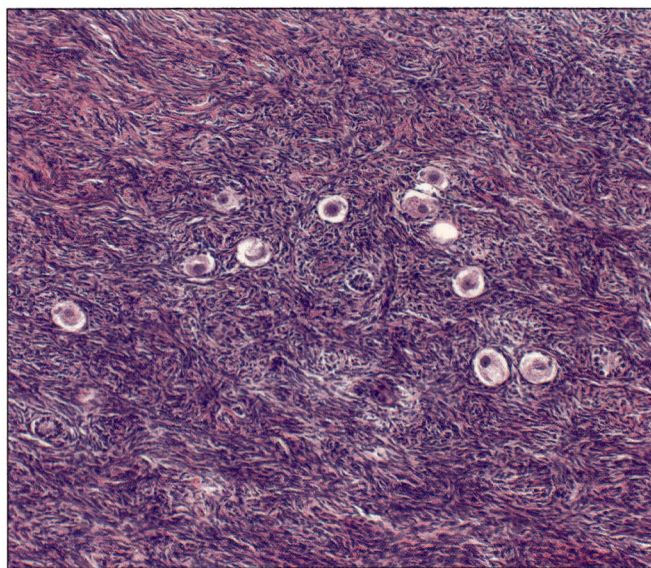

Fig. 21.14 Resistant ovary syndrome in patient with galactosemia. Cluster of primordial follicles in dense cortical stroma. No inflammatory infiltrate present.

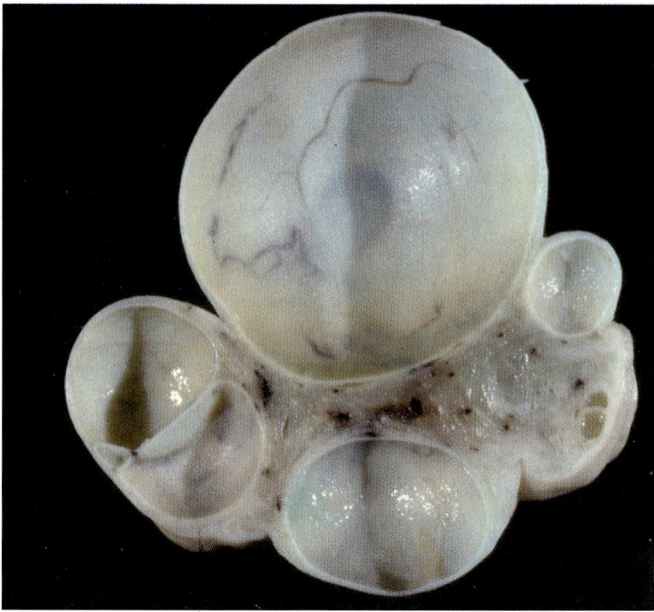

Fig. 21.15 Autoimmune oophoritis displaying multiple large cystic follicles.

relatively resistant to gonadotrophin stimulation and that, by analogy, the picture of resistant ovary syndrome in women with premature ovarian failure may merely reflect a stage of premature perimenopause preceding total follicular depletion.

Microscopic features   The cortical stroma appears uniformly dense and superficially sclerotic. Primordial follicles are variable in number and, as in normal ovaries, there is a tendency to clustering (Figure 21.14). Adequately sized biopsies and step-sectioning of these assume some importance in this context. Ova are histologically viable. In cases of partial ovarian resistance, i.e., those with some follicular development, dysplastic primary follicles are commonly observed. These are often enlarged and have rounded or irregular profiles outlined by thickened basement membranes. Call–Exner bodies may be numerous. Sometimes the granulosa cells are broken up by hyaline material forming small round nodules and ribbons in a pattern resembling that seen in SCTAT (see Chapter 26; Figure 21.11). Sometimes the hyaline material almost completely replaces the follicles. Morphologically similar follicles have been found in ovaries of stillborn fetuses, infants and children, and have been most commonly identified in fetuses of 30–41 weeks' gestational age, a period when massive physiologic reduction of oocytes normally occurs. In occasional cases, oocytes are replaced by non-laminated granular basophilic material that may or may not be calcium. Rare early antral follicles may be present and evidence of previous ovulation, e.g., corpora albicantia, is not unexpected. Follicular atresia, when present, appears to be normal, with disappearance of the granulosa.

Some biopsies show the expected complement of primordial follicles but no evidence whatsoever of developing or atretic follicles, and these cases are histologically indistinguishable from those of hypogonadotrophic hypogonadism. No inflammatory infiltrate is present. Foci of stromal luteinization are seen in about one-third of cases.

Behavior and treatment   Ovarian resistance to gonadotrophins may be relative rather than absolute. The process may be episodic, spontaneous remissions being known.[8,113] Thus, ovarian function and reproductive capacity are not necessarily irrevocably lost in such patients and, in fact, there are several reports of return of the menses and, rarely, pregnancies following a diagnosis of resistant ovary syndrome. Estrogen therapy and high dose gonadotrophin therapy sometimes overcome the ovarian 'resistance'.

Autoimmune oophoritis

Etiology   While antiovarian antibodies or the association of ovarian failure in a patient with various autoimmune type disorders are often taken as *prima facie* evidence of autoimmune oophoritis, such observations are not conclusive. In turn, some patients who fall into the clinicopathologic category of follicular ovarian failure as defined above have a florid chronic oophoritis, histologic characteristics of which leave no doubt as to its autoimmune basis, but antiovarian antibodies are rarely reported.[14] From experimental studies, it would appear that firstly there is some defect in the immune system, including reduced natural killer cell activity, that permits the development of organ-specific autoimmunity, and secondly there is some ovarian target under attack. Neither the nature of the immune defect nor the ovarian target is understood.[118] Furthermore, susceptibility in both mice and women appears to be associated with genes outside the major histocompatibility complex. Circulating antibodies to ooplasm, zona pellucida and steroid-producing cells, and the inflammatory CD4+ T-cell mechanism are critical pathogenetic pathways. Autoimmune oophoritis presents as either primary or secondary amenorrhea, preceded by progressive oligomenorrhea and hypomenorrhea.

Gross features   The ovaries are often of normal size, but many are greatly enlarged and even multicystic (Figure 21.15).

Microscopic features   All cases have shown inflammatory infiltrates specifically directed at follicular cells. The infiltrates consist of lymphocytes and plasma cells, sometimes with a

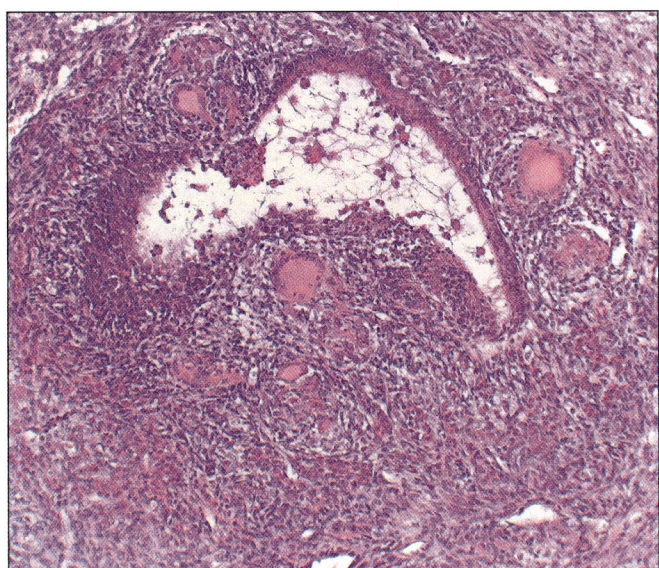

Fig. 21.16 Chronic oophoritis in an 18-year-old girl with premature ovarian failure. Perifolliculitis which includes a well-formed sarcoid-like granuloma.

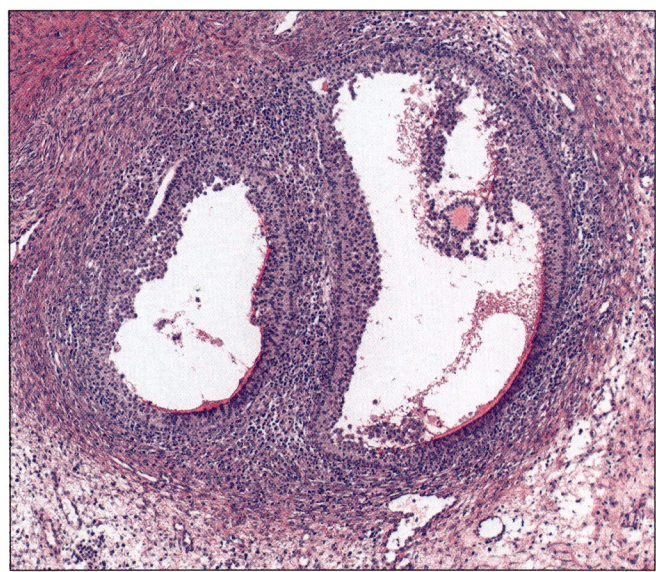

Fig. 21.18 Chronic autoimmune oophoritis. Antral follicle with heavy chronic inflammatory infiltrate in theca and lighter infiltrate in granulosa that appears degenerate, especially in region of cumulus oophorus. Follicular fluid contains fibrin and a few inflammatory cells.

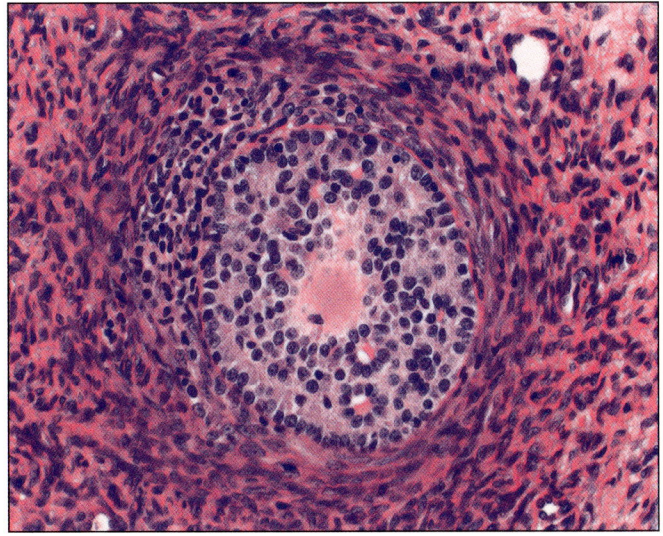

Fig. 21.17 Chronic autoimmune oophoritis. Primary follicle with partial cuffing (left side) by an inflammatory infiltrate in the theca interna. Stroma elsewhere is not infiltrated.

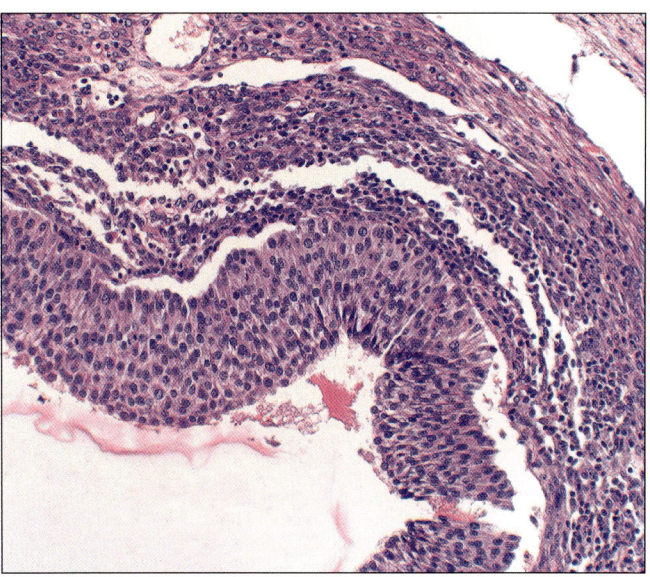

Fig. 21.19 Chronic autoimmune oophoritis. Cystic follicle with moderate chronic inflammatory cell infiltrate in theca.

granulomatous and eosinophilic reaction directed at follicular cells as well[91] (Figure 21.16). The usual histologic pattern is that of a lymphoplasmacytic infiltrate closely apposed to the theca interna of developing follicles – the more advanced the follicles, the denser the inflammatory infiltrate and the greater the preponderance of plasma cells. The granulosa of affected follicles is only focally and sparsely infiltrated by inflammatory cells, but secondary degenerative features, such as hydropic change and apoptosis, may be observed. The follicular fluid contains few, if any, inflammatory cells (Figures 21.17–21.19). Primordial follicles are apparently entirely spared. With atresia of developing follicles, the inflammatory infiltrate subsides to some extent, though rarely completely (Figures 21.20 and 21.21). Dysplastic follicles may also be seen, similar to those described in the resistant ovary syndrome (see above). If ovulation occurs, both granulosa and theca–lutein layers of the corpora lutea are heavily infiltrated by lymphocytes and plasma cells (Figures 21.22 and 21.23). Focal necrosis may be present. The infiltrate occasionally is predominantly eosinophilic (Figure 21.24).[124] The infiltrate contains a mixture of B cells (including plasma cells), T cells (both T4+ and T8+), macrophages, and a few natural killer cells. The cystic structures seen macroscopically are developing follicles or involuting corpora lutea, most likely due to elevated levels of pituitary gonadotrophins. The intervening stroma is unremarkable.

Behavior and treatment Although uncommon, autoimmune oophoritis is important to recognize as it represents a definable, potentially treatable process that leads to premature ovarian failure and also indicates that the patient is at increased risk of having or developing other endocrine or non-endocrine auto-

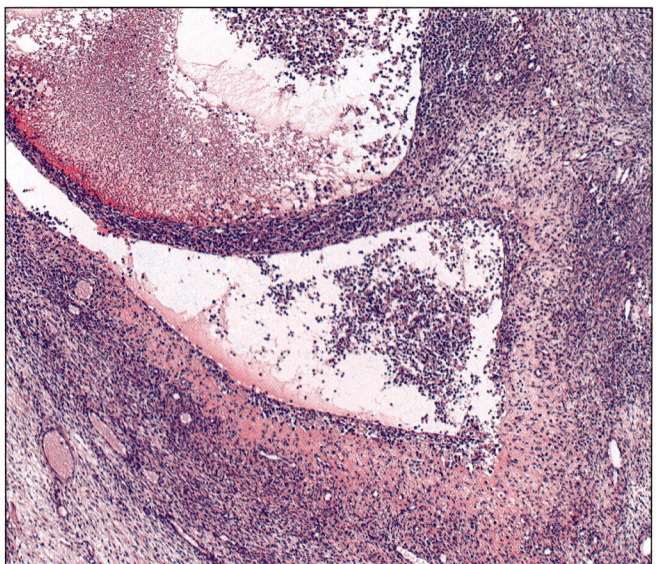

Fig. 21.20 Chronic autoimmune oophoritis. Atretic follicle, with diffuse lymphoplasmacytic infiltrate.

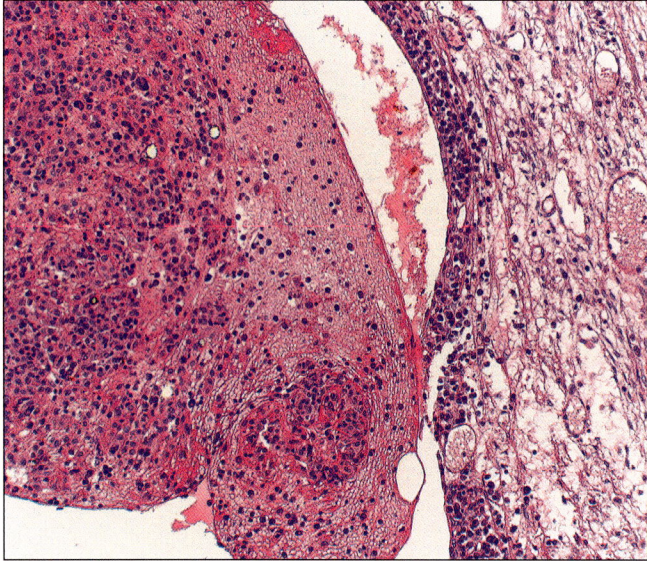

Fig. 21.21 Partially atretic cystic follicle in autoimmune oophoritis. Infiltration of the theca interna is noted to the right, while the granulosa is grossly disrupted and cells are shed into the antral fluid along with plasma and lymphoid cells.

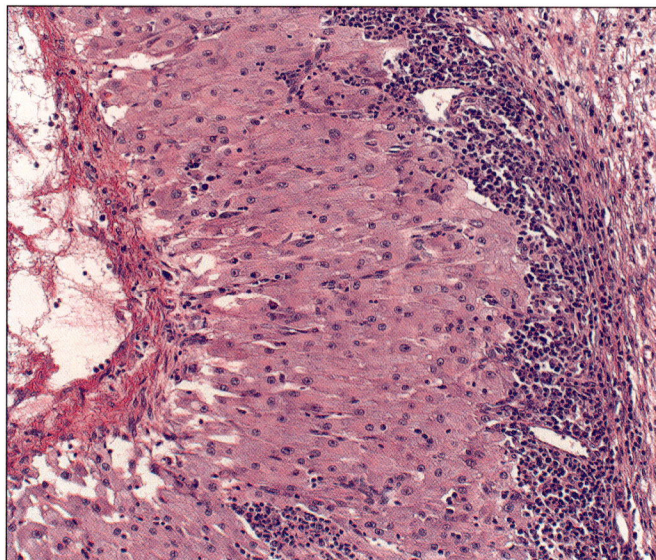

Fig. 21.22 Chronic autoimmune oophoritis. A 48-year-old woman with menorrhagia and a past history of Addison and Hashimoto disease. Fresh corpus luteum with inflammatory infiltrate involving chiefly theca-lutein layer. Only sparse inflammatory cells in central coagulum at right.

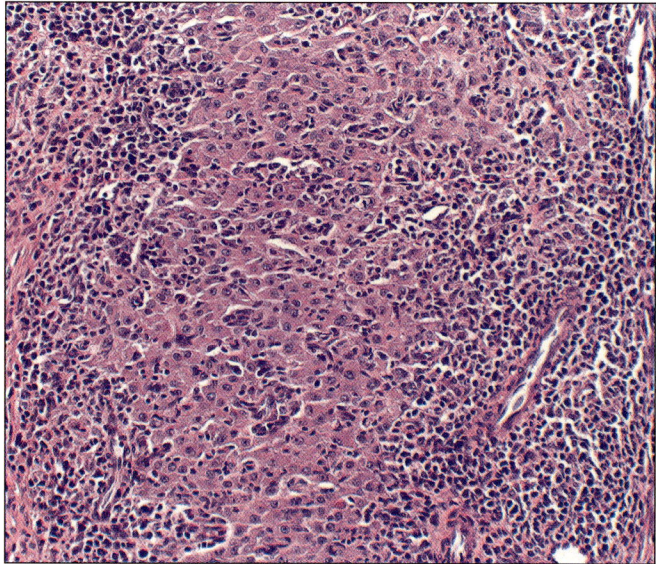

Fig. 21.23 Autoimmune oophoritis in 26-year-old woman with secondary infertility (same case as Figure 21.15). Heavy inflammatory infiltrate in wall of fresh corpus luteum with disruption of granulosa cells.

immune disease (which may develop even several years after onset of amenorrhea). Anti-adrenal antibodies may be useful predictors that adrenal failure may ensue. At present, no proven therapies are known that will improve follicular function for these women.[119]

HYPOGONADOTROPHIC HYPOGONADISM

Etiology

This syndrome results from intrinsic disorders of the hypothalamus or hypophysis, or to local anatomic alterations or infiltrations, which interfere with secretion of releasing factors or gonadotrophins.[105,148] Acquired causes are more common and include tumors,[149] infections, granulomas, anorexia nervosa, radiation, surgery, and head trauma.

Congenital or hereditary causes include dysmorphic and polyglandular syndromes, isolated gonadotrophin deficiency, and Kallmann syndrome (hypothalamic hypogonadism and anosmia).[66]

Microscopic features

Primordial follicles are plentiful, but lack follicular development. If the onset of failure occurs after the menarche, corpora fibrosa or albicantia may be evident. The cortical and medullary stroma is unremarkable and there is no inflammation. To this extent the picture may be indistinguishable from the resistant ovary syndrome (Figure 21.25).

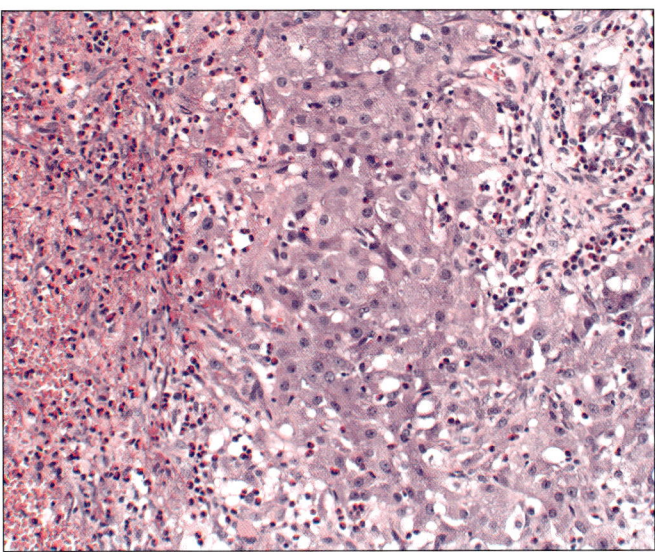

Fig. 21.24 Chronic autoimmune oophoritis. The inflammatory infiltrate concentrated at the margins of the granulosa lutein layer contains mostly eosinophils rather than plasma cells. Courtesy of Dr J Lewis, Perth, Australia.

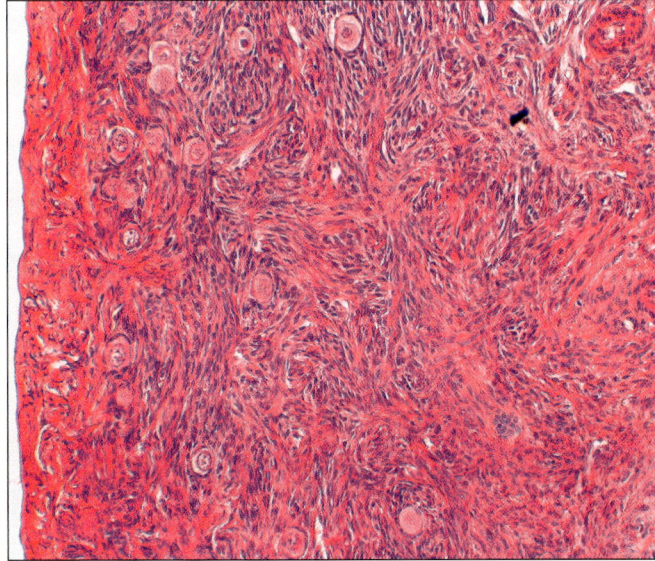

Fig. 21.25 Hypogonadotropic hypogonadism. Dense cortical ovarian stroma with many primordial follicles. No evidence of current or past follicular activity.

ANOMALIES OF OVARIAN DEVELOPMENT AND DESCENT

SUPERNUMERARY AND ACCESSORY OVARIES

Anomalies of ovarian development and descent are rarely encountered. Ectopic ovarian tissue may occur in the presence or absence of normally sited ovaries. Where this occurs in association with normally sited ovaries they can be divided into 'supernumerary' and 'accessory' ovaries. Such anomalies are either isolated or occur with other congenital genitourinary malformations (such as unicornuate or bicornuate uterus, vaginal aplasia, accessory adrenal glands, lobulated liver).[151] The additional ovarian tissue possesses functional potential.

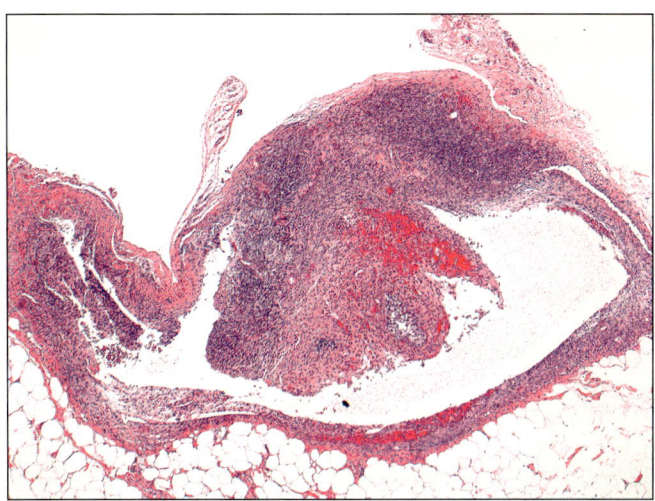

Fig. 21.26 Supernumerary ovary in 32-year-old woman occurring in omentum. No history of previous pelvic or abdominal surgery.

Supernumerary ovaries[62,93] are located at some distance from the eutopic ovary. They are found in the pelvis (in relation to the uterus, bladder or pelvic wall) and abdomen (retroperitoneum, omentum, mesentery of the colon, kidney) (Figure 21.26), and are not connected to the normal ovary. They may be single or multiple. They range in size from a few millimeters across to the dimensions of a normal ovary and may contain grossly visible follicular structures. The vast majority are incidental findings at autopsy, laparoscopy, or surgery. The documented sites of accessory and supernumerary ovarian tissue may possibly explain the origin of non-müllerian ovarian-type tumors in extraovarian sites such as broad ligament and retroperitoneum as well as accounting for persistent menstruation after bilateral oophorectomy. Exceptionally rare cases of documented pathology in supernumerary ovaries have been reported.[10,72,85]

Accessory ovarian tissue (the more common of the two variants) typically is seen as small nodules up to 1 cm across, situated near a normally placed ovary, either within or suspended from the posterior leaf of the broad ligament (Figure 21.27), and physically connected to that normal ovary.[151] These small pieces of tissue have been mistaken for lymph nodes at operation in the past and only diagnosed upon histologic examination. They are mostly solitary and rarely display pathology.[5,92]

DYSTOPIC OVARIES

One or both ovaries, structurally and functionally normal, may be found in abnormal positions due to aberrant descent into the pelvis.[150] They have been identified as high as the lower pole of the kidney, close to their embryologic site of origin, within the retroperitoneal tissues, and as low as the inguinal canal. In some instances, malposition (dystopia) or maldescent of the ovaries is associated with ipsilateral anomalies of the müllerian duct derivatives.[79,84] In some patients, displacement may be due to torsion, detachment, and parasitic attachment to the omentum or other intraperitoneal structures.

OVARIAN AGENESIS

Confusion exists concerning the terms 'agenesis' and 'dysgenesis' (see Chapter 34) and many of the reports in the early

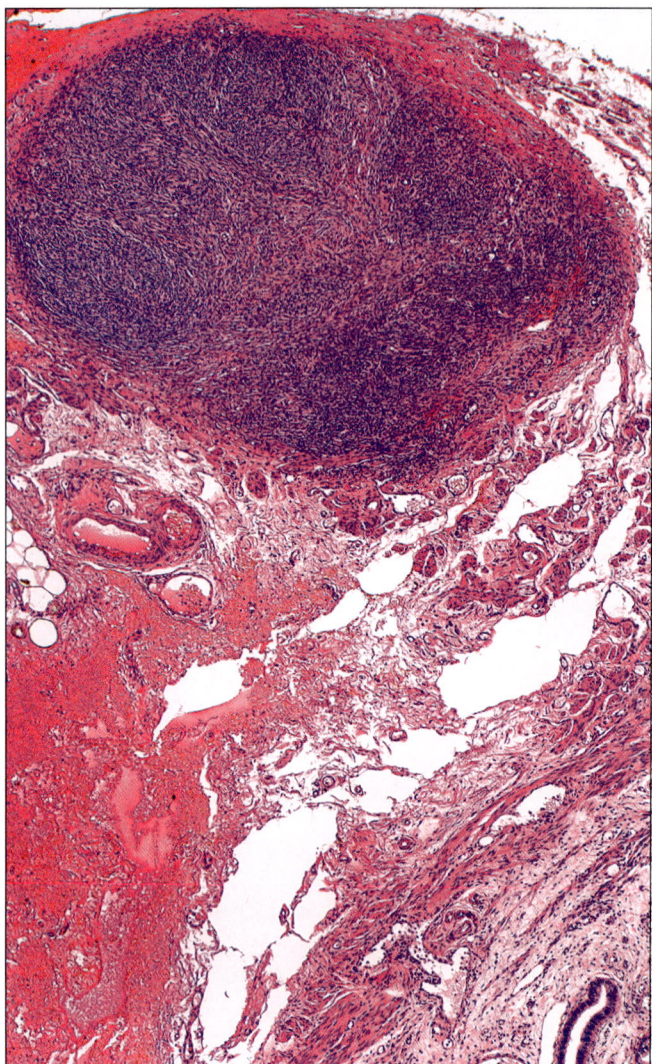

Fig. 21.27 Small nodule of ovarian cortical tissue in the posterior leaf of the broad ligament. Incidental finding in hysterectomy specimen. No history of previous pelvic or abdominal surgery. Note endosalpingiosis at lower right corner.

literature undoubtedly were examples of streak gonads rather than true agenesis.

Rarely, one ovary may be absent in an otherwise normal woman.[116] Associated findings include agenesis or malformation of the ipsilateral fallopian tube,[45] uterus, round ligament, kidney and ureter, alone or in combination.[79] However, most reported cases of absent ovaries are probably due to antenatal torsion of an otherwise normal fallopian tube and ovary with necrosis and resorption of the adnexal structures.

OVARIAN HYPOPLASIA

This 'entity' overlaps with both ovarian dysgenesis and premature ovarian failure, depending on the pathogenesis of the particular abnormality observed. Ovaries in patients with Turners syndrome (with 45,X or mosaic karyotype) may have greatly reduced numbers of primordial follicles and little evidence of follicular activity at any stage of childhood or adult life. In most adult patients with Turners syndrome, the end result of this ovarian 'hypoplasia' is a typical fibrous streak (see Chapter 34).

SPLENOGONADAL FUSION

This rare developmental abnormality, which occurs early in intrauterine development, is admixed splenic and gonadal tissues resulting in the presence of splenic tissue in proximity to the ovary and hilar ductules.[33] Splenogonadal fusion may be continuous, in which case a fibrous cord connects the splenic tissue in the pelvis with the spleen, or discontinuous, where no cord is present and nodules of splenic tissue are present along its presumed path. Many of these patients have severe congenital malformations of the extremities such as phocomelia.[18] The coexistence of these abnormalities suggests that both were induced sometime between weeks 5 and 8 of gestation, possibly by vascular disruption due to administration of drugs or by intercurrent viral disease.

'UTERUS-LIKE MASS' REPLACING OVARY

In this rare condition the ovary[108] or adjacent broad ligament[2] is replaced by a uterus-like mass with a central cavity lined by endometrial tissue and surrounded by a thick smooth muscle wall. This lesion is most likely a congenital malformation of müllerian duct origin with no normal ovarian development having taken place, an interpretation supported by the presence of congenital abnormalities of the urinary tract in several reported cases.

INFECTIOUS INFLAMMATORY DISEASES

BACTERIAL OOPHORITIS

PELVIC INFLAMMATORY DISEASE (PID)

Definition
Most examples of acute and chronic suppurative oophoritis are associated with PID, a generic term for infection of the female genital organs. PID usually begins as ascending, often recurrent, infection of the genital tract that tends to localize in the fallopian tubes but may also involve adjacent structures such as peritoneum and ovaries.

Etiology
Gonococci and chlamydiae are the bacteria most commonly isolated. Once tissue damage has occurred, secondary bacterial invaders, chiefly anaerobic, may replace the initial organisms. Acute salpingitis results in the production of inflammatory exudate, including fibrin, from the tubal serosa and ostia, leading to adhesions to adjacent pelvic and sometimes abdominal organs.

Isolated ovarian abscesses, unassociated with salpingitis, are unusual. In almost all cases there is a predisposing factor such as a recent gynecologic operation, childbirth or use of an intrauterine contraceptive device (IUD). *Escherichia coli* and *Bacteroides* spp. are the most common organisms isolated. As opposed to the insidious development of ovarian abscesses in association with PID, isolated abscesses have an acute presentation, usually with abdominal pain. Rupture is likely if surgical treatment is not prompt. Acute peritonitis and pelvic abscess are likely sequelae.

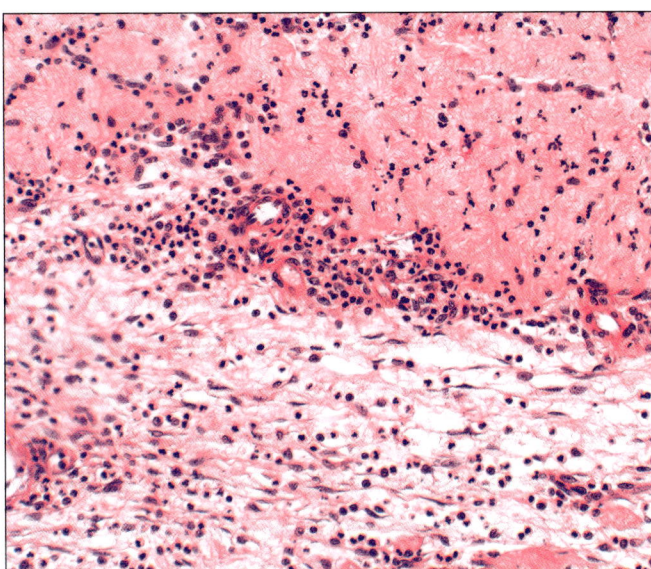

Fig. 21.28 Acute suppurative oophoritis. Edematous parenchyma with diffuse neutrophilic infiltrate which even involves a corpus fibrosum (top).

The presence of an IUD increases the risk of developing PID compared with non-users, and especially predisposes to unusual organisms such as *Actinomyces* spp. (see below). Oophoritis may complicate other pelvic and abdominal infections such as diverticulitis and appendicitis.

Secondary infection of pre-existing cysts is a recognized clinical risk. One per cent of mature cystic teratomas are said to become infected, usually by coliforms. Endometriotic cysts are also prone to secondary suppurative inflammation.

Gross features

The ovaries usually resist the invasion of pathogenic bacteria, and their involvement in PID is often limited to a peri-oophoritis, even in the presence of tubo-ovarian inflammatory masses. However, recurrent or severe PID may result in ovarian parenchymal involvement, initially as an acute diffuse oophoritis. Abscess formation, usually in continuity with a pyosalpinx (tubo-ovarian abscess) sometimes follows and this may result in permanent loss of ovarian parenchyma. In chronic PID there may be an increase in cystic follicles and follicular or corpus luteum cysts, but chronic PID does not influence growth of follicles or their ability to ovulate. An outer layer of dense fibrous tissue is usually present.

Microscopic features

Acute diffuse oophoritis shows neutrophil infiltration, edema, vascular dilatation, and focal hemorrhage. Follicular structures may be involved (Figure 21.28). Abscesses display central accumulations of necrotic debris or cavities lined by granulation tissue admixed with inflammatory cells (Figure 21.29). Large foamy lipid-laden macrophages (xanthoma cells) may be conspicuous if there has been extensive hemorrhage and necrosis. Hemosiderin and lipofuscin (ceroid) pigment may also be demonstrable.

Acute peri-oophoritis exhibits neutrophil infiltration and fibrin exudation. Groups of peritoneal macrophages adhere to the serosal surfaces. The exudate becomes organized by the ingrowth of proliferating fibroblasts and capillaries, i.e., granulation tissue. Concurrent with this reparative process is a pro-

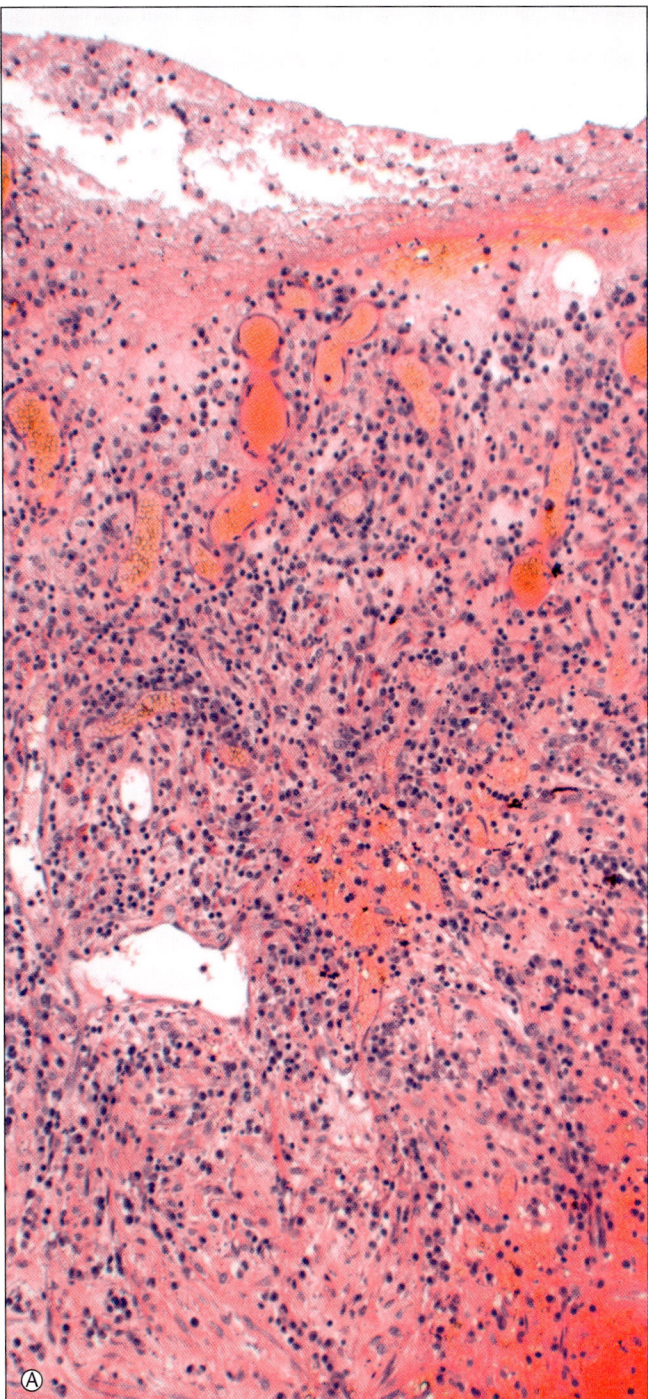

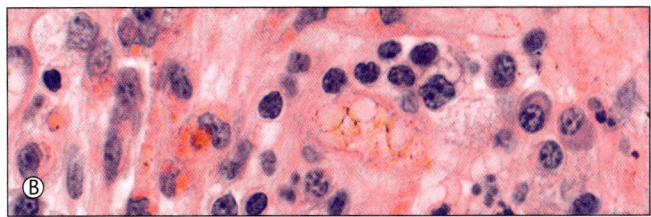

Fig. 21.29 Ovarian abscess (chronic phase). **(A)** Thick fibrous wall with shaggy lining. Heavy infiltrate of chronic inflammatory cells. **(B)** Detail of cellular infiltrate – plasma cells, lymphocytes, and foamy macrophages.

liferation of mesothelial cells, which may be quite exuberant. Peri-oophoritis resolves but leaves behind adhesions, scattered lymphocytes, and sometimes psammoma bodies as residua of the inflammatory process.

Chronic diffuse oophoritis is rarely observed in patients with PID (Figure 21.30). Focal lymphocytic infiltrates are associated with autoimmune oophoritis.

In most cases of suppurative oophoritis, the fallopian tubes are also inflamed. However, in cases of isolated ovarian abscess, endosalpingitis is absent, although there may be tubal edema and perisalpingitis.

XANTHOGRANULOMATOUS OOPHORITIS (INFLAMMATORY PSEUDOTUMOR)

This rare variant of chronic oophoritis occurs in women with a history of chronic PID.[130] *Bacteroides* spp. have been isolated from some cases. Inflammatory pseudotumors probably result from exaggerated prolonged repair reactions in cases of oophoritis that have involved an unusual degree of necrosis or hemorrhage, with consequent abundance of lipid breakdown products.

Macroscopically, pseudotumors are firm, yellow, well-circumscribed masses (4–8 cm in diameter), with foci of hemorrhage and necrosis. Stigmata of PID are generally present elsewhere. Microscopically, sheets of foamy macrophages dominate the picture, interspersed with non-vacuolated, sometimes multinucleated histiocytes and other inflammatory cells. The foamy cells contain lipid as well as PAS-positive cytoplasmic granules (lysosomes). Hemosiderin deposition and fibroblastic proliferation are usually present.

MALACOPLAKIA

This chronic inflammatory process rarely involves the female genital tract of postmenopausal women,[31] being more often identified in the renal pelvis and bladder. The lower genital tract (especially the vagina) is more commonly affected than the ovaries (see Chapter 5).

ACTINOMYCOSIS

Etiology

Pelvic actinomycosis is rare and in older reports was almost always secondary to ileocecal disease.[16] Although actinomycotic PID, associated with IUD use, has been recognized since the 1920s, the popularity of the new generation IUDs in the 1960s was followed by a spate of reports, which continue.[46] There appears to be a correlation with prolonged IUD usage[133] although rare reports have been unassociated with IUD use.[21] The organism is readily identified in cervicovaginal smears of 8–30% of IUD users, but only rarely, and in small numbers, in non-users. Up to 25% of those with positive smears develop clinical PID (not necessarily due to actinomycosis).

Culture of the organisms is successful in less than one-third of the histologically confirmed cases but other anaerobic bacteria are isolated from the abscesses in most cases. Almost all patients with actinomycotic PID have an actinomycotic endometritis. Uterine curettings and tissue adherent to a removed IUD can also be used for histologic examination and culture.

Gross features

Adnexal involvement is frequently unilateral and forms a large distorted tubo-ovarian mass. Bilateral involvement may mimic pelvic malignancy at laparotomy.[43] Sectioning shows multiple shaggy abscesses containing purulent bloodstained material separated by dense fibrous scar tissue (Figure 21.31). Sulfur granules may be evident macroscopically.

Microscopic features

The actinomycotic colonies are located in the centre of abscesses and are surrounded by polymorphs and necrotic debris (Figure 21.32). Occasional multinucleated histiocytes may be seen in close proximity to the colonies. Foamy histiocytes are often conspicuous in the adjacent granulation tissue. Plasma cells and lymphocytes are more obvious in the peripheral zone of fibrous tissue. The colonies consist of branching filaments; the central

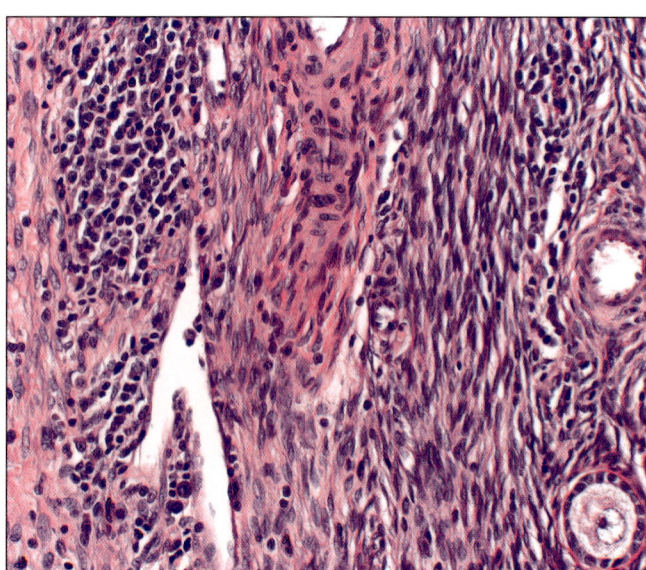

Fig. 21.30 Chronic lymphoplasmacytic oophoritis. Patchy infiltrate adjacent to a resolving abscess.

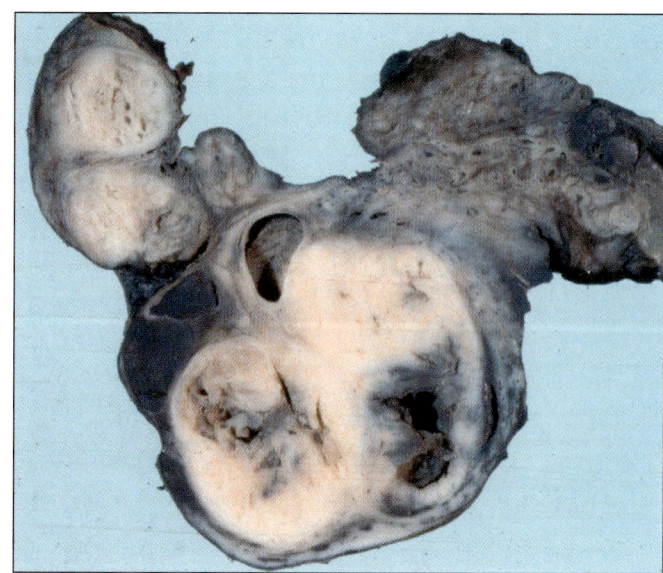

Fig. 21.31 Ovarian actinomycosis. Right adnexal mass from 43-year-old woman who had been using an IUD for 10 years. Thick-walled necrotic cavities in ovary and thickened fallopian tube. A residual cystic follicle is recognizable (center).

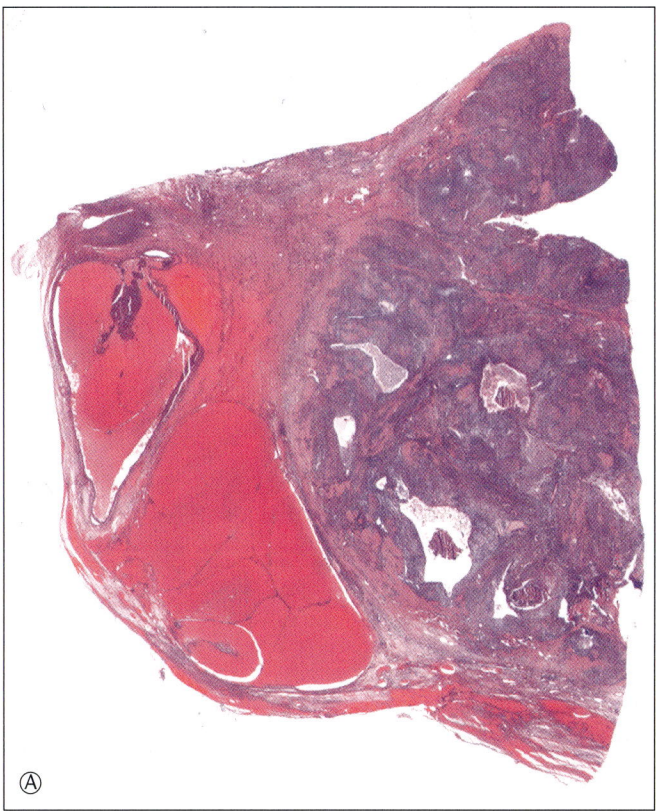

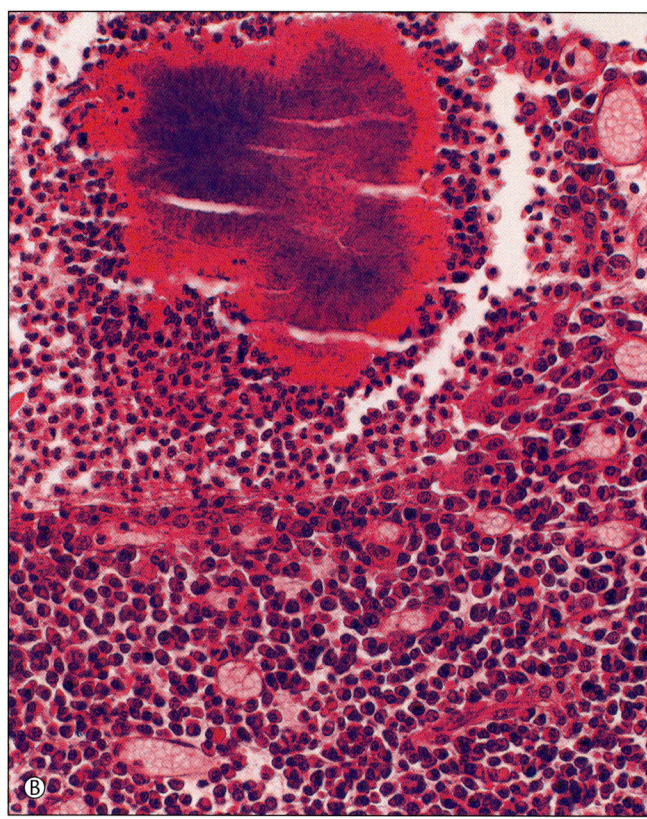

Fig. 21.32 Ovarian actinomycosis (same case as Figure 21.31). **(A)** Survey showing confluent, communicating abscess cavities, with cystic follicles to left. **(B)** Detail of cellular infiltrate composed of lymphocytes, plasma cells, neutrophils (adjacent to 'sulfur granule').

denser portion is hematoxylinophilic, but the peripheral radiating clubs are eosinophilic. The organisms are Gram positive and acid fast with certain of the modified stains (Putt stain) but not in solutions where full-strength acids are used (traditional Ziehl Neelsen stain). With these stains, the organism can often be seen as a central core through the length of the club.

TUBERCULOSIS

Etiology

Although most genital tuberculosis is thought to be bloodborne from a pulmonary focus, less than half the patients have a history of tuberculosis or an abnormal chest X-ray. Within the pelvis, tubercle bacilli preferentially lodge in the fallopian tubes, from which direct spread to the ovaries may occur. Less commonly, the infection spreads via lymphatics from a tuberculous focus in the urinary or gastrointestinal tracts. Overall, the incidence of genital tuberculosis is low and stable in most Western countries,[146] with the ovaries being involved in 20–63% of such patients (Figure 21.33). They may also be involved incidentally in tuberculous peritonitis (see Table 21.2 for a differential diagnosis of tuberculoid granulomas and Chapter 33 for further details).

VIRAL OOPHORITIS

MUMPS

Transient acute oophoritis may occur during the course of mumps and the exanthems. While orchitis is a well-known and common manifestation of mumps infection in males, the occur-

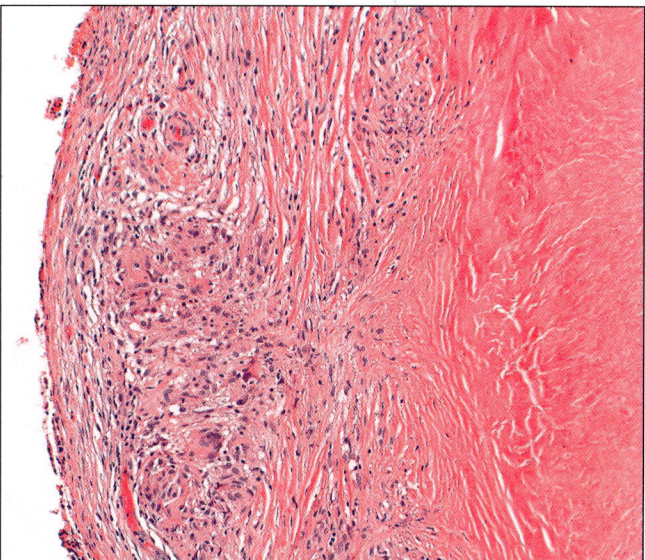

Fig. 21.33 Microbiologically confirmed peritoneal tuberculosis involving the ovarian cortex.

rence of oophoritis in infected females is less well recognized and is said to be less frequent, in the order of 5%. There are no reports in the literature of the histologic features of mumps oophoritis.

CYTOMEGALOVIRUS (CMV)

CMV infection of the female genital organs, while usually secondary to viremia, may be transmitted venereally. CMV

Table 21.2 Oophoritis: differential diagnosis by tissue reaction[a]

Acute or chronic suppuration
  Acute diffuse oophoritis associated with pelvic inflammatory disease
  Ovarian abscess associated with pelvic inflammatory disease
  Isolated ovarian abscess
  Actinomycosis
  Foreign body
  Coccidioidomycosis, blastomycosis
  Schistosomiasis[b]

Acute serositis (without parenchymal inflammation)
  Ruptured tubal ectopic gestation
  Generalized peritonitis
  Peritoneal carcinomatosis

Eosinophilic infiltration
  Foreign body reactions, especially starch[c]
  Enterobiasis[c]
  Schistosomiasis[c]
  Autoimmune oophoritis[b]
  Isolated non-infectious granulomatous oophoritis[b]

Lymphoplasmacytic infiltration
  Autoimmune oophoritis
  Resolving phases of suppurative oophoritis
  Cytomegalovirus oophoritis

Foreign-body granulomas
  Exogenous substances, e.g. sutures, talc, starch, radiographic media,
    parasites, intestinal contents
  Endogenous substances, e.g. contents of mature cystic teratomas,
    keratin from uterine adenoacanthomas, cauterized tissue

Sarcoidal granulomas
  Sarcoidosis
  Crohns disease
  Foreign-body reactions, especially starch[c]
  'Cortical granulomas'
  Autoimmune oophoritis[b]

Necrotizing granulomas
  Tuberculosis[c]
  Foreign-body reactions, especially starch[b,c], radiographic media[b,c]
  Enterobiasis[c]
  Coccidioidomycosis, blastomycosis
  Isolated non-infectious granulomatous oophoritis
  Schistosomiasis[b]

[a]Note that an etiologic agent may be associated with more than one type of reaction.
[b]Rare feature of the condition.
[c]Predominantly serosal lesions.

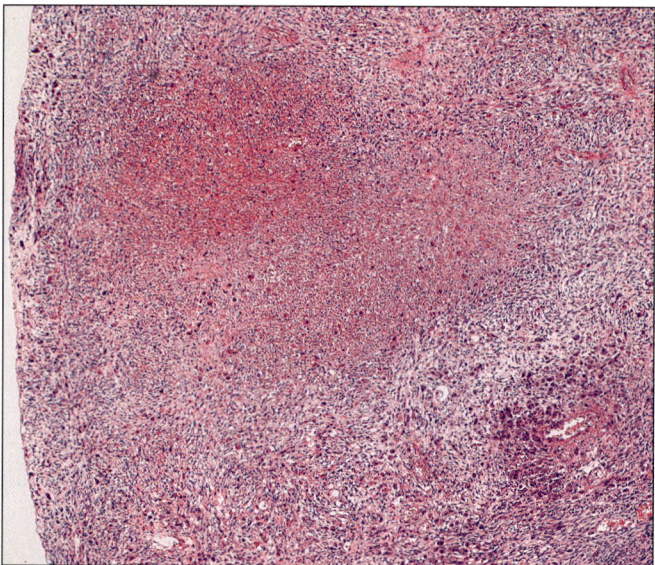

Fig. 21.34 Cytomegalovirus oophoritis from an immunosuppressed 37-year-old woman. Wedge-shaped cortical infarct.

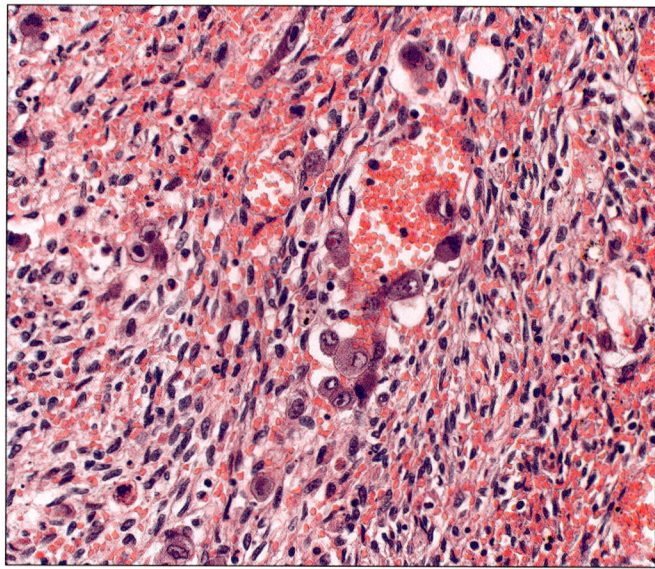

Fig. 21.35 Detail of Figure 21.34. Infected endothelial and stromal cells with intranuclear and intracytoplasmic inclusions.

PARASITIC OOPHORITIS

SCHISTOSOMIASIS (BILHARZIASIS)

Etiology

Genital schistosomiasis is rare, its incidence being partly a function of international travel to or through endemic areas,[89] and represents so-called ectopic disease, i.e., not related directly to the life cycle of the organism. Worms preferentially lodge in the mesenteric and portal (*Schistosoma mansoni* and *S. japonicum*) or vesical veins (*S. haematobium*) but may gain access to the genital tract via venous anastomoses such as those between the hemorrhoidal and hypogastric veins, and between mesenteric and ovarian veins. It is usually an incidental finding, although some patients with upper genital tract

oophoritis is rare, being reported only in immunosuppressed patients, most commonly due to HIV infection.[97,120,123]

In most cases, the ovaries show focal hemorrhagic cortical necrosis, associated with polymorph and lymphoplasmacytic infiltration (Figure 21.34). Within and bordering this area, infected stromal and endothelial cells are readily identified by their enlargement and pleomorphism. The characteristic basophilic intranuclear inclusions are easily found and intracytoplasmic inclusions may also be present (Figure 21.35). A chronic inflammatory cell infiltrate is present in the surrounding viable parenchyma.

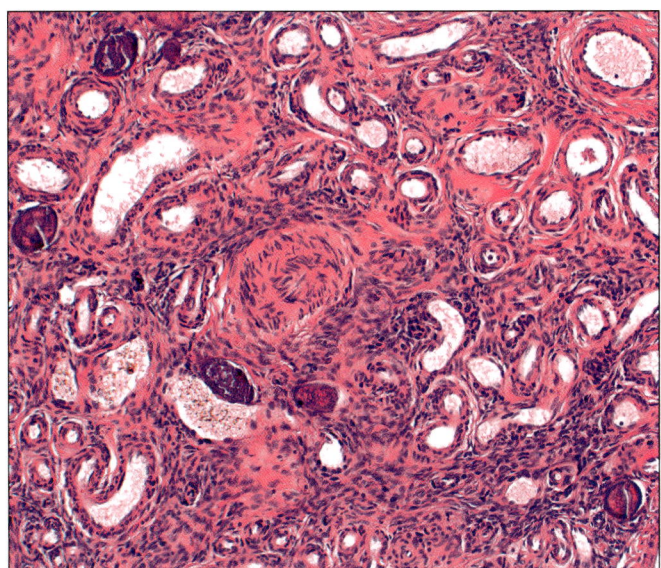

Fig. 21.36 Ovarian medulla containing degenerate, calcified, schistosomal ova. Note the complete absence of an inflammatory reaction.

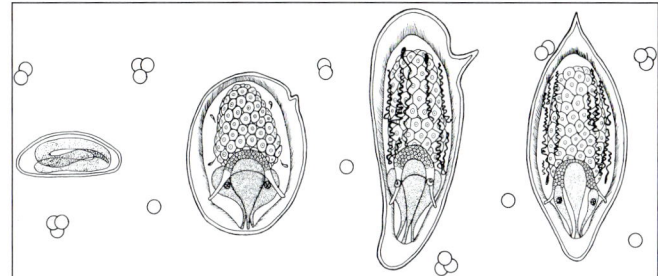

Fig. 21.37 Parasitic ova. From left to right: *S. haematobium, S. japonicum, S. mansoni, E. vermicularis*. Circles represent the size of red blood cells.

infections have symptoms suggestive of PID. The genital tract is involved more frequently in *S. haematobium* than in *S. mansoni* infection. *S. haematobium* predominantly involves the lower genital tract, while *S. mansoni* has a predilection for tubes and ovaries.

Microscopic features

If the schistosomal infection is merely an incidental finding, the ovaries are likely to be of normal size. Small white nodules are present on their surfaces, and often elsewhere on the pelvic peritoneum as well. This appearance may simulate metastatic carcinoma. In patients clinically affected, the ovaries may be enlarged up to three times their normal size. They display necrosis, abscesses, tubo-ovarian adhesions, and adhesions to other pelvic structures in most cases.

Living worms and dead ova usually provoke little tissue reaction (Figure 21.36) but dead worms and living ova, when they enter the tissues, incite a granulomatous reaction. Ova are more commonly identified than worms. The cellular infiltrate consists of epithelioid cells, foreign-body giant cells, lymphocytes, plasma cells, and eosinophils. Some granulomas appear tuberculoid. Sometimes the cellular reaction to freshly laid ova is predominantly eosinophilic, with formation of abscesses. The Splendore–Hoeppli phenomenon (radiating eosinophilic deposits around ova) may also be observed. The peripheral zone of the granulomas consists of fibrous tissue that gradually increases in amount and may replace entire lesions. Dead ova frequently calcify. These are found within the ovarian parenchyma and, more often, within veins of the outer uterine wall or broad ligament.

Schistosomal ova can be readily differentiated from each other in histologic preparations if spines are visible in the plane of section. The ova are 80–160 μm in length and 30–90 μm in width. *S. haematobium* and *S. mansoni* are elongate. *S. haematobium* has a terminal spine while *S. mansoni* has a lateral one. *S. japonicum* is round to ovoid and has a lateral spine that is less prominent than that of *S. mansoni* (Figure 21.37).

ENTEROBIASIS

Etiology

Pelvic peritoneal granulomas due to *Enterobius* (*Oxyuris*) *vermicularis* (pinworm, threadworm) are rare complications of gastrointestinal infestation and have been reported in females only. Parasites are thought to gain entry to the peritoneal cavity by ascending the genital tract after migrating to the introitus from the anus. On reaching the peritoneal cavity the worms die and their ova are released, inciting the inflammatory reaction. The granulomas are usually located in the pelvis and may involve the serosal surfaces or even the ovarian parenchyma.[68,145] If numerous, they may simulate peritoneal carcinomatosis.

Pathology

Macroscopically, ovarian granulomas are soft yellow-brown serosal nodules, up to 1 cm in diameter, sometimes associated with adhesions. Larger lesions may show central softening.

Microscopically, the granulomatous inflammation is centered on the ova, which are oval (up to 60 μm long and 30 μm wide) with double-contoured smooth shells, flattened on one side, in which embryonic structures may be identified. Degenerate worms are rarely identified. Ova (and worms) are surrounded by necrotic debris containing numerous eosinophils and, beyond this, there is a zone of granulation tissue that includes epithelioid histiocytes and lymphocytes. The granulomas show peripheral fibrosis. The ova and, indeed, entire granulomas may undergo calcification.

The finding of large necrotizing pelvic granulomas, particularly if associated with an eosinophilic infiltrate, should prompt a search for a possible causative parasite by processing additional tissue and cutting step-sections if appropriate. *Enterobius* ova can be distinguished from those of *Schistosoma* by their smaller size and lack of spines (Figure 21.37).

ECHINOCOCCOSIS

Echinococcosis is an infestation by the cestode *Echinoccocus granulosus*, which is prevalent in sheep- and cattle-raising areas of Australia, New Zealand, and South America, and also in the Middle East, Iceland, and some European countries. Genital involvement is rare and occurs in only 0.1–0.3% of infected females. The uterus is more commonly affected than the ovary. Ovarian involvement may represent primary infection (if embryos emerging from the gut pass through both liver and lungs before establishing themselves in the tissues) or secondary infection (if it follows rupture of a primary hepatic cyst, either into the vascular system or peritoneal cavity). Such ovarian involvement may present clinically and on ultrasound as ovarian cysts.[81,147]

Hydatid cysts measure up to 16 cm in diameter and show the characteristic triple-layered wall consisting of innermost germinal epithelium (with its brood capsules and scolices), hyaline-laminated membrane, and outermost adventitial fibrous tissue (of host origin). Calcification of the cyst wall, a very useful radiologic sign, is usually associated with regression of the cyst following death of the parasite.

FUNGAL OOPHORITIS

COCCIDIOIDOMYCOSIS

Etiology

This fungal disease is endemic in certain semi-arid areas of North, Central and South America and is caused by *Coccidioides immitis*. Genital infection is rare, even in cases of disseminated fatal coccidioidomycosis, which generally occurs in immunosuppressed patients. As in tuberculosis, genital involvement usually results from blood-borne spread of organisms from a pulmonary lesion that is generally radiologically inactive or apparently healed. Pelvic coccidioidomycosis is usually associated with peritonitis.

Pathology

In cases of adnexal involvement the tubes and ovaries show dense serosal adhesions and multiple small white nodules are apparent on the serosal surfaces. In addition, the ovaries may contain abscess cavities.

The inflammatory reaction is either tuberculoid granulomatous, which may progress to caseation and cavitation, or suppurative with microabscess formation. The fungal elements are seen in tissues as spherules (sporangia) measuring 20–200 µm in diameter that have thin doubly refractile walls. The enclosed endospores, 2–3 µm in diameter, are released into the tissues upon rupture of the spherules. A rapid diagnosis of pelvic coccidioidomycosis may be made by identifying the spherules in wet preparations of peritoneal fluid or purulent exudates.

BLASTOMYCOSIS

Genital tract involvement in North American blastomycosis is rare and results from venereal transmission or hematogenous spread from a pulmonary lesion. The tissue reaction to the fungus is similar to that seen in coccidioidomycosis, i.e., either suppurative or tuberculoid granulomatous inflammation. The budding, thick-walled yeast bodies, 8–20 µm diameter, are readily found in sections.

NON-INFECTIOUS INFLAMMATORY DISEASES

SARCOIDOSIS

Etiology

Sarcoidosis rarely involves the female genital tract – even in the active stage of the disease when granulomas may be widely disseminated throughout the body. The uterus is more often affected than the adnexa. Most reported cases have been in

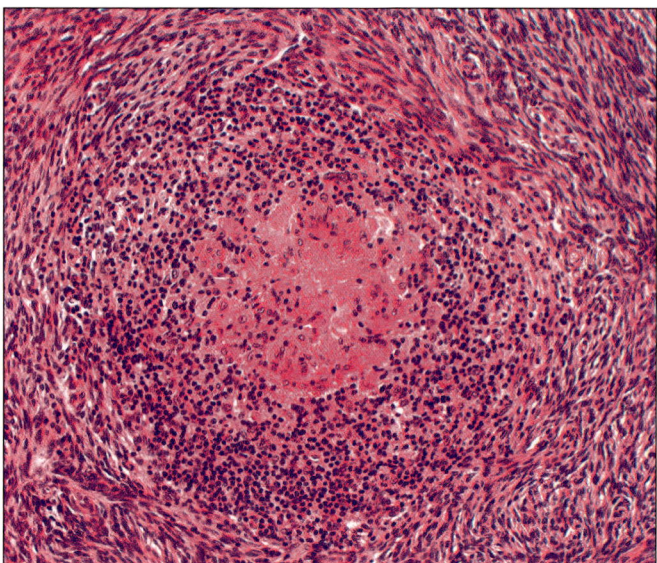

Fig. 21.38 Sarcoidosis. Typical sarcoidal granuloma in ovarian cortex, an incidental finding in a postmenopausal woman with known clinical sarcoidosis. No microorganisms or foreign bodies could be identified.

patients with current or recent evidence of pulmonary sarcoidosis.[125] An elevated serum CA125 may be present.

Microscopic features

Ovarian granulomas are distributed at random through the cortex, medulla, and hilus. As in extragenital sites, the discrete non-caseating granulomas are composed of epithelioid histiocytes with small numbers of giant cells of Langhans or foreign-body type, sometimes containing crystalloid inclusions. A diagnosis of ovarian sarcoidosis in the absence of systemic disease should be made with great caution since the histologic changes alone are not pathognomonic (Table 21.2; Figure 21.38). Tuberculosis and mycoses, especially if endemic in the patient's locality, should be excluded by the appropriate special stains and preferably culture. The sections should be screened with the aid of polarizing filters for foreign bodies, particularly starch granules and parasitic elements.

CROHNS DISEASE

The ovary is very rarely and only 'accidentally' involved in Crohns disease.[109] Ovarian involvement is the result of direct extension of the inflammatory process from the adherent segment of intestine. The right ovary, by virtue of its proximity to the terminal ileum, is more commonly affected, but left adnexal involvement has also been reported. Crohns disease may also cause ovarian vein thrombosis with consequent ovarian pain and enlargement.[32,98]

Ovarian granulomas may be restricted to the serosa and superficial cortex, or widely distributed in the parenchyma. They are sarcoidal in type and set in a background of lymphocytic infiltration. A more destructive combined suppurative and granulomatous reaction has also been described, in association with an ileo-ovarian 'fistula'. The ipsilateral fallopian tube is generally involved as well. There should be no problem in differential diagnosis once the clinical and surgical details are available. However, it is prudent to exclude infective causes of granulomatous oophoritis, such as actinomycosis or tuberculosis (Table 21.2), which may also be associated with ileocecal disease.

CORTICAL GRANULOMAS

'Cortical granulomas' are seen in 10–15% of postmenopausal ovaries and usually in association with stromal 'proliferations'. They probably represent transitional stages in involuting hyperthecosis, although other interpretations are possible. The granulomas are well circumscribed, 100–500μm in diameter and consist of loose ovarian stroma containing small numbers of lymphocytes and epithelioid cells (which may represent either luteinized stromal cells or macrophages), multinucleated giant cells, and occasional anisotropic fat crystals. The lesions are well vascularized but eventually become fibrotic and hyalinized.

ISOLATED NON-INFECTIOUS GRANULOMAS

Isolated non-infectious granulomas typically occur in premenopausal women without evidence of systemic granulomatous disease or of genital tract infection of potentially granulomatous type. In most patients the granulomas are incidental findings and there is a history of previous surgery (in the preceding several months or years) involving the now affected ovary, suggesting the possibility that the granulomas may be a reaction to traumatized or devitalized tissues.

The granulomas are multiple and may be bilateral. They are small, with an acellular hyaline core bordered by palisading histiocytes and peripheral fibrosis. The lesions resemble the necrobiotic rheumatoid-like granulomas that may be found in the cervix following cone biopsy or loop excision of transformation zone.

AUTOIMMUNE OOPHORITIS

See discussion under 'Ovarian failure' (above).

NECROTIZING ARTERITIS

Etiology
A small proportion of patients with necrotizing arteritis suffer from a systemic connective tissue disorder such as lupus erythematosus, while others give a history of drug therapy, especially penicillin, suggesting an allergic basis to the lesion. In the majority, however, no underlying cause can be identified and these appear to be cases of idiopathic isolated visceral necrotizing vasculitis. Further investigation and follow-up of asymptomatic patients with uterine and adnexal involvement are usually unrewarding in uncovering systemic disease.[128]

Microscopic features
Medium-sized arteries and arterioles are affected (Figure 21.39). The most striking feature is fibrinoid necrosis of the media with some associated disruption of the internal elastic lamina. Fibrin is often seen in the lumen, but thrombosis and tissue infarction do not occur. An inflammatory infiltrate, chiefly lymphocytic,

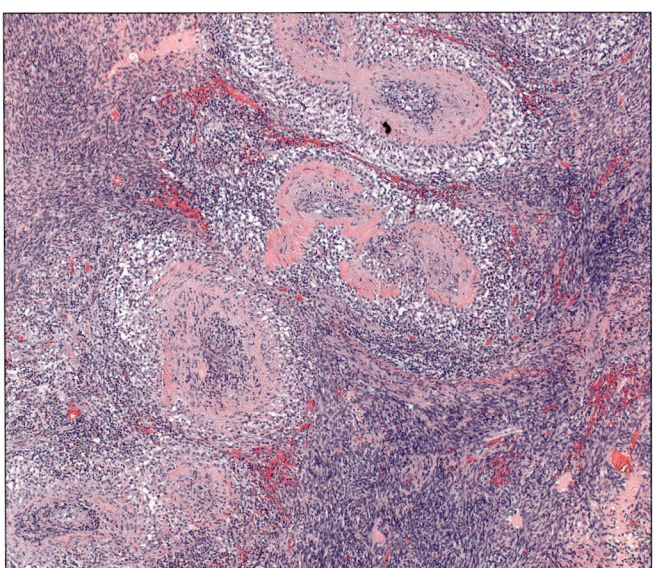

Fig. 21.39 Isolated necrotizing arteritis. Incidental finding in an ovary which also contained a small benign transitional cell tumor. No evidence of systemic vasculitis.

is present throughout the vessel wall and adventitia. Neutrophils and eosinophils, but not giant cells, may be present in small numbers. If eosinophils are prominent, the possibility of polyarteritis nodosa should be considered (see below).

GIANT CELL ARTERITIS

Classic giant cell arteritis affects large and medium-sized arteries, especially the temporal and intracranial vessels. Less commonly, giant cell arteritis affects smaller arteries and arterioles, and this variant may be either disseminated or anatomically restricted. In the latter group, the female genital organs are commonly involved, including the ovaries in about half of cases.[58] All the reported cases have been in postmenopausal women, of whom about one-half suffered from polymyalgia rheumatica. Treatment appears to be unnecessary in these asymptomatic women. By contrast, occasional cases have presented in severely ill women with an ovarian mass ('pseudotumor') and display either typical giant cell arteritis or polyarteritis nodosa on histology.[73] Such patients need to be further investigated.

Microscopic features
Small arteries and arterioles show random segmental involvement. There is intimal edema and fibrosis that result in luminal narrowing. The medium is expanded by a granulomatous inflammatory infiltrate consisting of lymphocytes and histiocytes, some epithelioid and multinucleated giant cells. There is destruction of elastic fibers, especially in the internal elastic lamina. Inflammatory cells, mainly lymphocytes, extend into the intima and adventitia. Eosinophils are conspicuous by their absence. Fibrinoid necrosis and thromboses are rarely seen.

POLYARTERITIS NODOSA

The female genital tract, including the ovaries, rarely may be involved in polyarteritis nodosa.[63,132] Radiographic demonstra-

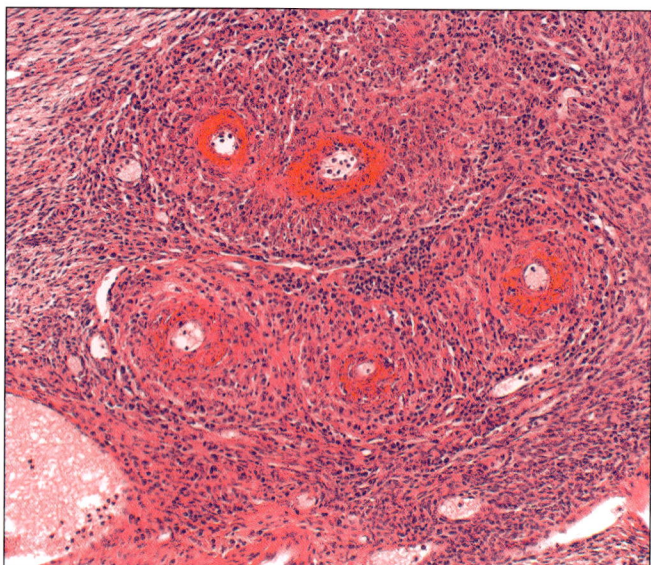

Fig. 21.40 Acute necrotizing arteritis in patient with systemic evidence of polyarteritis nodosa.

tion of microaneurysms, which have a predilection for arterial bifurcations, is important in confirming the diagnosis. It is arguable whether a 'localized' form that involves the ovaries[78] should be classified as polyarteritis nodosa or isolated necrotizing arteritis (see above).

Microscopic features

Medium-sized and small arteries are affected. They show fibrinoid necrosis and an acute, predominantly eosinophilic, inflammatory infiltrate (Figure 21.40). In older lesions, lymphocytes and plasma cells are also present. Thromboses may develop and these may result in infarction of distal tissues.

PUERPERAL OVARIAN VEIN THROMBOPHLEBITIS

Etiology

The pathologist rarely encounters puerperal ovarian vein thrombophlebitis and thrombosis, a potentially life-threatening condition, because standard management does not include oophorectomy.[25,131] The condition complicates about one in 600 deliveries, and abortions less frequently. It is part of the spectrum of pelvic thrombophlebitis but selective involvement of the ovarian veins makes the condition clinically distinct from non-puerperal cases in which the uterine and iliac veins are predominantly affected. Some consider the condition to be infective, with the primary source being the placental bed. Postpartum hypercoagulability, together with dilatation and stasis, potentiate thrombosis in the inflamed veins. Peculiarities in ovarian venous blood flow postpartum (antegrade on the right but retrograde on the left) result in preferential spread of infection to the right side.[61] The right side is involved in 90% of unilateral cases and 14% of all cases are bilateral. Venography, ultrasonography, and computer-assisted tomographic scanning have been used to facilitate non-invasive diagnosis.

Microscopic features

At laparotomy, the thrombosed ovarian veins are markedly enlarged (up to 10 mm in diameter), tortuous, tense and firm;

thrombus sometimes extends into the ovaries. The inferior vena cava, left renal vein or both may be involved in continuity. The ovaries and fallopian tubes are dark and congested, but their viability is not usually compromised and infarction rarely occurs. The ovarian veins, if available for histologic examination, show thrombophlebitis.

REFERENCES

1. Abe N, Takeuchi H, Kikuchi I, Kinoshita K. Effectiveness of microlaparoscopy in the diagnosis of premature ovarian failure. J Obstet Gynaecol Res 2006;32:224–9.
2. Ahmed AA, Swan RW, Owen A, Kraus FT, Patrick F. Uterus-like mass arising in the broad ligament: a metaplasia or mullerian duct anomaly? Int J Gynecol Pathol 1997;16:279–81.
3. Allen EG, He W, Yadav-Shah M, Sherman SL. A study of the distributional characteristics of FMR1 transcript levels in 238 individuals. Hum Genet 2004;114:439–47.
4. Anasti JN. Premature ovarian failure: an update. Fertil Steril 1998;70:1–15.
5. Andrade LA, Gentilli AL, Polli G. Sclerosing stromal tumor in an accessory ovary. Gynecol Oncol 2001;81:318–9.
6. Arif S, Varela-Calvino R, Conway GS, Peakman M. 3 beta hydroxysteroid dehydrogenase autoantibodies in patients with idiopathic premature ovarian failure target N- and C-terminal epitopes. J Clin Endocrinol Metab 2001;86:5892–7.
7. Ashraf M, Jayawickrama NS, Bowen-Simpkins P. Premature ovarian failure due to an unbalanced translocation on the X chromosome. Bjog 2001;108:230–2.
8. Aslam MF, Gilmour K, McCune GS. Spontaneous pregnancies in patients with resistant ovary syndrome while on HRT. J Obstet Gynaecol 2004;24:573–4.
9. Auersperg N, Ota T, Mitchell GW. Early events in ovarian epithelial carcinogenesis: progress and problems in experimental approaches. Int J Gynecol Cancer 2002;12:691–703.
10. Badawy SZ, Kasello DJ, Powers C, Elia G, Wojtowycz AR. Supernumerary ovary with an endometrioma and osseous metaplasia: a case report. Am J Obstet Gynecol 1995;173:1623–4.
11. Bakalov VK, Vanderhoof VH, Bondy CA, Nelson LM. Adrenal antibodies detect asymptomatic auto-immune adrenal insufficiency in young women with spontaneous premature ovarian failure. Hum Reprod 2002;17:2096–100.
12. Balasch J, Fabregues F. Pregnancy after administration of high dose recombinant human LH alone to support final stages of follicular maturation in a woman with long-standing hypogonadotrophic hypogonadism. Reprod Biomed Online 2003;6:427–31.
13. Banerjee N, Kriplani A, Takkar D, Kucheria K. Balanced X; 22 translocation in a patient with premature ovarian failure. Acta Genet Med Gemellol (Roma) 1997;46:241–4.
14. Bannatyne P, Russell P, Shearman RP. Autoimmune oophoritis: a clinicopathologic assessment of 12 cases. Int J Gynecol Pathol 1990;9:191–207.
15. Bellassoued M, Mnif M, Marouene H, et al. [Perrault's syndrome: two cases]. Ann Endocrinol (Paris) 2001;62:534–7.
16. Benkiran L, Gamra L, Lamalmi N, et al. [Pelvic actinomycosis simulating adnexal malignant tumor]. Med Trop (Mars) 2002;62:73–6.
17. Best CL, Pudney J, Welch WR, Burger N, Hill JA. Localization and characterization of white blood cell populations within the human ovary throughout the menstrual cycle and menopause. Hum Reprod 1996;11:790–7.
18. Bonneau D, Roume J, Gonzalez M, et al. Splenogonadal fusion limb defect syndrome: report of five new cases and review. Am J Med Genet 1999;86:347–58.
19. Borgaonkar MR, Morgan DG. Primary biliary cirrhosis and type II autoimmune polyglandular syndrome. Can J Gastroenterol 1999;13:767–70.
20. Burger HG, Davis SR. The role of androgen therapy. Best Pract Res Clin Obstet Gynaecol 2002;16:383–93.
21. Burlando SC, Paz LA, De Feo LG, Benchetrit G, Rimoldi D, Predari SC. [Ovarian abscess due to Actinomyces sp. in absence of an intrauterine contraceptive device]. Medicina (B Aires) 2001;61(5 Pt 1):577–80.
22. Bussani C, Papi L, Sestini R, et al. Premature ovarian failure and fragile X premutation: a study on 45 women. Eur J Obstet Gynecol Reprod Biol 2004;112:189–91.
23. Cao QJ, Jones JG, Li M. Expression of calretinin in human ovary, testis, and ovarian sex cord-stromal tumors. Int J Gynecol Pathol 2001;20:346–52.
24. Carambula SF, Pru JK, Lynch MP, et al. Prostaglandin F2alpha- and FAS-activating antibody-induced regression of the corpus luteum involves caspase-8 and is defective in caspase-3 deficient mice. Reprod Biol Endocrinol 2003;1:15.
25. Carr S, Tefera G. Surgical treatment of ovarian vein thrombosis. Vasc Endovascular Surg 2006;40:505–8.
26. Causio F, Fischetto R, Leonetti T, Schonauer LM. Ovarian stimulation in a woman with premature ovarian failure and X-autosome translocation. A case report. J Reprod Med 2000;45:235–9.

27. Cemeroglu AP, Bober E, Dundar B, Buyukgebiz A. Autoimmune polyglandular endocrinopathy and anterior hypophysitis in a 14 year-old girl presenting with delayed puberty. J Pediatr Endocrinol Metab 2001;14:909–14.
28. Chen WY, Manson JE. Premature ovarian failure in cancer survivors: new insights, looming concerns. J Natl Cancer Inst 2006;98(13):880–1.
29. Chernyshov VP, Radysh TV, Gura IV, Tatarchuk TP, Khominskaya ZB. Immune disorders in women with premature ovarian failure in initial period. Am J Reprod Immunol 2001;46:220–5.
30. Chiauzzi VA, Bussmann L, Calvo JC, Sundblad V, Charreau EH. Circulating immunoglobulins that inhibit the binding of follicle-stimulating hormone to its receptor: a putative diagnostic role in resistant ovary syndrome? Clin Endocrinol (Oxf) 2004;61:46–54.
31. Chou SC, Wang JS, Tseng HH. Malacoplakia of the ovary, fallopian tube and uterus: a case associated with diabetes mellitus. Pathol Int 2002;52:789–93.
32. Cil T, Tummon IS, House AA, et al. A tale of two syndromes: ovarian hyperstimulation and abdominal compartment. Hum Reprod 2000;15:1058–60.
33. Cualing H, Wang G, Noffsinger A, Fenoglio-Preiser C. Heterotopic ovarian splenoma: report of a first case. Arch Pathol Lab Med 2001;125:1483–5.
34. Cutolo M, Sulli A, Pizzorni C, Craviotto C, Straub RH. Hypothalamic–pituitary–adrenocortical and gonadal functions in rheumatoid arthritis. Ann N Y Acad Sci 2003;992:107–17.
35. Dal Pra C, Chen S, Furmaniak J, et al. Autoantibodies to steroidogenic enzymes in patients with premature ovarian failure with and without Addison's disease. Eur J Endocrinol 2003;148:565–70.
36. Davis CJ, Davison RM, Payne NN, Rodeck CH, Conway GS. Female sex preponderance for idiopathic familial premature ovarian failure suggests an X chromosome defect: opinion. Hum Reprod 2000;15:2418–22.
37. Davison RM, Fox M, Conway GS. Mapping of the POF1 locus and identification of putative genes for premature ovarian failure. Mol Hum Reprod 2000;6:314–8.
38. de Ravel TJ, Fryns JP, Van Driessche J, Vermeesch JR. Complex chromosome re-arrangement 45,X,t(Y;9) in a girl with sex reversal and mental retardation. Am J Med Genet 2004;124A:259–62.
39. Del Vecchio RP. The role of steroidogenic and nonsteroidogenic luteal cell interactions in regulating progesterone production. Semin Reprod Endocrinol 1997;15:409–20.
40. Devi AS, Metzger DA, Luciano AA, Benn PA. 45,X/46,XX mosaicism in patients with idiopathic premature ovarian failure. Fertil Steril 1998;70: 89–93.
41. Di Pasquale E, Beck-Peccoz P, Persani L. Hypergonadotropic ovarian failure associated with an inherited mutation of human bone morphogenetic protein-15 (BMP15) gene. Am J Hum Genet 2004;75:106–11.
42. Diao FY, Xu M, Liu JY. [Analysis of X chromosome mosaicism in patients with premature ovarian failure by fluorescent in-situ hybridization]. Zhonghua Fu Chan Ke Za Zhi 2003;38:20–3.
43. Dogan NU, Salman MC, Gultekin M, Kucukali T, Ayhan A. Bilateral actinomyces abscesses mimicking pelvic malignancy. Int J Gynaecol Obstet 2006;94:58–9.
44. Dorman JS, Steenkiste AR, Foley TP, et al. Menopause in type 1 diabetic women: is it premature? Diabetes 2001;50:1857–62.
45. Dueck A, Poenaru D, Jamieson MA, Kamal IK. Unilateral ovarian agenesis and fallopian tube maldescent. Pediatr Surg Int 2001;17(2–3):228–9.
46. Dunn TS, Cothren C, Klein L, Krammer T. Pelvic actinomycosis: a case report. J Reprod Med 2006;51:435–7.
47. Eldar-Geva T, Spitz IM, Groome NP, Margalioth EJ, Homburg R. Follistatin and activin A serum concentrations in obese and non-obese patients with polycystic ovary syndrome. Hum Reprod 2001;16:2552–6.
48. Estienne V, Duthoit C, Costanzo VD, et al. Multicenter study on TGPO autoantibody prevalence in various thyroid and non-thyroid diseases; relationships with thyroglobulin and thyroperoxidase autoantibody parameters. Eur J Endocrinol 1999;141:563–9.
49. Falorni A, Laureti S, Santeusanio F. Autoantibodies in autoimmune polyendocrine syndrome type II. Endocrinol Metab Clin North Am 2002;31:369–89, vii.
50. Falorni A, Laureti S, Candeloro P, et al. Steroid-cell autoantibodies are preferentially expressed in women with premature ovarian failure who have adrenal autoimmunity. Fertil Steril 2002;78:270–9.
51. Fassnacht W, Mempel A, Strowitzki T, Vogt PH. Premature ovarian failure (POF) syndrome: towards the molecular clinical analysis of its genetic complexity. Curr Med Chem 2006;13:1397–410.
52. Fernandes AM, Arruda Mde S, Bedone AJ. Twin gestation two years after the diagnosis of premature ovarian failure in a woman on hormone replacement therapy. A case report. J Reprod Med 2002;47:504–6.
53. Ferrara N, Frantz G, LeCouter J, et al. Differential expression of the angiogenic factor genes vascular endothelial growth factor (VEGF) and endocrine gland-derived VEGF in normal and polycystic human ovaries. Am J Pathol 2003;162:1881–93.
54. Forges T, Monnier-Barbarino P. [Premature ovarian failure in galactosaemia: pathophysiology and clinical management]. Pathol Biol (Paris) 2003;51: 47–56.
55. Forges T, Monnier-Barbarino P, Faure GC, Bene MC. Autoimmunity and antigenic targets in ovarian pathology. Hum Reprod Update 2004;10: 163–75.
56. Forges T, Monnier-Barbarino P, Leheup B, Jouvet P. Pathophysiology of impaired ovarian function in galactosaemia. Hum Reprod Update 2006;12:573–84.
57. Gersak K, Meden-Vrtovec H, Peterlin B. Fragile X premutation in women with sporadic premature ovarian failure in Slovenia. Hum Reprod 2003;18:1637–40.
58. Gil H, Chirouze C, Magy N, et al. [Giant cell arteritis of the ovary: a rare localization of Horton's disease]. Rev Med Interne 1999;20:825–6.
59. Goswami R, Goswami D, Kabra M, Gupta N, Dubey S, Dadhwal V. Prevalence of the triple X syndrome in phenotypically normal women with premature ovarian failure and its association with autoimmune thyroid disorders. Fertil Steril 2003;80:1052–4.
60. Gougeon A. Regulation of ovarian follicular development in primates: facts and hypotheses. Endocr Rev 1996;17:121–55.
61. Hadas-Halpern I, Patlas M, Fisher D. Postpartum ovarian vein thrombophlebitis: sonographic diagnosis. Abdom Imaging 2002;27:93–5.
62. Hartigan K, Pecha B, Rao G. Intrarenal supernumerary ovary excised with partial nephrectomy. Urology 2006;67:424 e11– e12.
63. Herve F, Heron F, Levesque H, Marie I. Ascites as the first manifestation of polyarteritis nodosa. Scand J Gastroenterol 2006;41:493–5.
64. Hisama FM, Zemel S, Cherniske EM, Vladutiu GD, Pober BR. 46,XX gonadal dysgenesis, short stature, and recurrent metabolic acidosis in two sisters. Am J Med Genet 2001;98:121–4.
65. Hoek A, Schoemaker J, Drexhage HA. Premature ovarian failure and ovarian autoimmunity. Endocr Rev 1997;18:107–34.
66. Hoffman B, Bradshaw KD. Delayed puberty and amenorrhea. Semin Reprod Med 2003;21:353–62.
67. Holland CM. 47,XXX in an adolescent with premature ovarian failure and autoimmune disease. J Pediatr Adolesc Gynecol 2001;14:77–80.
68. Hong ST, Choi MH, Chai JY, Kim YT, Kim MK, Kim KR. A case of ovarian enterobiasis. Korean J Parasitol 2002;40:149–51.
69. Hovatta O. Cryopreservation and culture of human primordial and primary ovarian follicles. Mol Cell Endocrinol 2000;169(1–2):95–7.
70. Hugues JN, Cedrin-Durnerin I. [Role of luteinizing hormone in follicular and corpus luteum physiology]. Gynecol Obstet Fertil 2000;28:738–44.
71. Kalantaridou SN, Nelson LM. Premature ovarian failure is not premature menopause. Ann N Y Acad Sci 2000;900:393–402.
72. Kamiyama K, Moromizato H, Toma T, Kinjo T, Iwamasa T. Two cases of supernumerary ovary: one with large fibroma with Meig's syndrome and the other with endometriosis and cystic change. Pathol Res Pract 2001;197:847–51.
73. Kariv R, Sidi Y, Gur H. Systemic vasculitis presenting as a tumorlike lesion. Four case reports and an analysis of 79 reported cases. Medicine (Baltimore) 2000;79:349–59.
74. Karlberg N, Jalanko H, Perheentupa J, Lipsanen-Nyman M. Mulibrey nanism: clinical features and diagnostic criteria. J Med Genet 2004;41:92–8.
75. Karlberg S, Tiitinen A, Lipsanen-Nyman M. Failure of sexual maturation in Mulibrey nanism. N Engl J Med 2004;351(24):2559–60.
76. Kasperlik-Zaluska AA, Czarnocka B, Czech W. Autoimmunity as the most frequent cause of idiopathic secondary adrenal insufficiency: report of 111 cases. Autoimmunity 2003;36:155–9.
77. Kauffman RP, Castracane VD. Premature ovarian failure associated with autoimmune polyglandular syndrome: pathophysiological mechanisms and future fertility. J Womens Health (Larchmt) 2003;12:513–20.
78. Kaya E, Utas C, Balkanli S, Basbug M, Onursever A. Isolated ovarian polyarteritis nodosa. Acta Obstet Gynecol Scand 1994;73:736–8.
79. Kaya H, Sezik M, Ozkaya O, Kose SA. Mayer–Rokitansky–Kuster–Hauser syndrome associated with unilateral gonadal agenesis. A case report. J Reprod Med 2003;48:902–4.
80. Koc Z, Ulusan S, Oguzkurt L. Right ovarian vein drainage variant: is there a relationship with pelvic varices? Eur J Radiol 2006;59:465–71.
81. Konar K, Ghosh S, Konar S, Bhattacharya S, Sarkar S. Bilateral ovarian hydatid disease – an unusual case. Indian J Pathol Microbiol 2001;44: 495–6.
82. Kosaki K, Sato S, Hasegawa T, Matsuo N, Suzuki T, Ogata T. Premature ovarian failure in a female with proximal symphalangism and Noggin mutation. Fertil Steril 2004;81:1137–9.
83. Kovacs P, Stangel JJ, Santoro NF, Lieman H. Successful pregnancy after transient ovarian failure following treatment of symptomatic leiomyomata. Fertil Steril 2002;77:1292–5.
84. Kriplani A, Banerjee N, Aminni AC, Kucheria K, Takkar D. Hernia uterus inguinale in a 46,XX female. A case report. J Reprod Med 2000;45:48–50.
85. Kuga T, Esato K, Takeda K, Sase M, Hoshii Y. A supernumerary ovary of the omentum with cystic change: report of two cases and review of the literature. Pathol Int 1999;49:566–70.
86. La Marca A, Pati M, Orvieto R, Stabile G, Carducci Artenisio A, Volpe A. Serum anti-mullerian hormone levels in women with secondary amenorrhea. Fertil Steril 2006;85:1547–9.
87. Laml T, Schulz-Lobmeyr I, Obruca A, Huber JC, Hartmann BW. Premature ovarian failure: etiology and prospects. Gynecol Endocrinol 2000;14:292–302.
88. Layman LC. Genetic causes of human infertility. Endocrinol Metab Clin North Am 2003;32:549–72.
89. Lee KF, Hsueh S, Tang MH. Schistosomiasis of the ovary with endometriosis and corpus hemorrhagicum: a case report. Changgeng Yi Xue Za Zhi 2000;23:438–41.

90. Leppig KA, Disteche CM. Ring X and other structural X chromosome abnormalities: X inactivation and phenotype. Semin Reprod Med 2001;19:147–57.
91. Lewis J. Eosinophilic perifolliculitis: a variant of autoimmune oophoritis? Int J Gynecol Pathol 1993;12:360–4.
92. Lim MC, Park SJ, Kim SW, et al. Two dermoid cysts developing in an accessory ovary and an eutopic ovary. J Korean Med Sci 2004;19:474–6.
93. Litos MG, Furara S, Chin K. Supernumerary ovary: A case report and literature review. J Obstet Gynaecol 2003;23:325–7.
94. Loffler KA, Zarkower D, Koopman P. Etiology of ovarian failure in blepharophimosis ptosis epicanthus inversus syndrome: FOXL2 is a conserved, early-acting gene in vertebrate ovarian development. Endocrinology 2003;144:3237–43.
95. Maclaren N, Chen QY, Kukreja A, Marker J, Zhang CH, Sun ZS. Autoimmune hypogonadism as part of an autoimmune polyglandular syndrome. J Soc Gynecol Investig 2001;8(1 Suppl Proceedings):S52–4.
96. Manase K, Endo T, Henmi H, et al. The significance of membrane type 1 metalloproteinase in structural involution of human corpora lutea. Mol Hum Reprod 2002;8:742–9.
97. Manfredi R, Alampi G, Talo S, et al. Silent oophoritis due to cytomegalovirus in a patient with advanced HIV disease. Int J STD AIDS 2000;11:410–2.
98. Marcovici I, Goldberg E. Ovarian vein thrombosis associated with Crohn's disease: a case report. Am J Obstet Gynecol 2000;182:743–4.
99. Martins da Silva SJ, Bayne RA, Cambray N, Hartley PS, McNeilly AS, Anderson RA. Expression of activin subunits and receptors in the developing human ovary: activin A promotes germ cell survival and proliferation before primordial follicle formation. Dev Biol 2004;266:334–45.
100. Massin N, Czernichow C, Thibaud E, Kuttenn F, Polak M, Touraine P. Idiopathic premature ovarian failure in 63 young women. Horm Res 2006;65:89–95.
101. Matikainen T, Perez GI, Jurisicova A, et al. Aromatic hydrocarbon receptor-driven Bax gene expression is required for premature ovarian failure caused by biohazardous environmental chemicals. Nat Genet 2001;28:355–60.
102. McDonough PG. Selected enquiries into the causation of premature ovarian failure. Hum Fertil (Camb) 2003;6:130–6.
103. Medeiros MM, Silveira VA, Menezes AP, Carvalho RC. Risk factors for ovarian failure in patients with systemic lupus erythematosus. Braz J Med Biol Res 2001;34:1561–8.
104. Meduri G, Massin N, Guibourdenche J, et al. Serum anti-Mullerian hormone expression in women with premature ovarian failure. Hum Reprod 2007;22:117–23.
105. Meysing AU, Kanasaki H, Bedecarrats GY, et al. GNRHR mutations in a woman with idiopathic hypogonadotropic hypogonadism highlight the differential sensitivity of luteinizing hormone and follicle-stimulating hormone to gonadotropin-releasing hormone. J Clin Endocrinol Metab 2004;89:3189–98.
106. Mila M, Mallolas J. [Fragile X syndrome: premature ovarian failure. Preimplantation and preconception genetic diagnosis]. Rev Neurol 2001;33 Suppl 1:S20–3.
107. Miller KP, Borgeest C, Greenfeld C, Tomic D, Flaws JA. In utero effects of chemicals on reproductive tissues in females. Toxicol Appl Pharmacol 2004;198:111–31.
108. Mitra ANAGISS. Uterus-like mass of the ovary. J Obstet Gynaecol 1997;17:94–5.
109. Monneuse O, Pilleul F, Gruner L, Barth X, Tissot E. MRI evaluation in a rare case of Crohn's disease complicated by abscess of the ovary. Gastroenterol Clin Biol 2006;30:153–4.
110. Monniaux D, Huet C, Pisselet C, Mandon-Pepin B, Monget P. [Mechanism, regulation, and manipulations of follicular atresia]. Contracept Fertil Sex 1998;26(7–8):528–35.
111. Morales C, Garcia-Pardo L, Reymundo C, Bellido C, Sanchez-Criado JE, Gaytan F. Different patterns of structural luteolysis in the human corpus luteum of menstruation. Hum Reprod 2000;15:2119–28.
112. Morita Y, Tilly JL. Oocyte apoptosis: like sand through an hourglass. Dev Biol 1999;213:1–17.
113. Mueller A, Berkholz A, Dittrich R, Wildt L. Spontaneous normalization of ovarian function and pregnancy in a patient with resistant ovary syndrome. Eur J Obstet Gynecol Reprod Biol 2003;111:210–3.
114. Murray A, Ennis S, MacSwiney F, Webb J, Morton NE. Reproductive and menstrual history of females with fragile X expansions. Eur J Hum Genet 2000;8:247–52.
115. Myhre AG, Halonen M, Eskelin P, et al. Autoimmune polyendocrine syndrome type 1 (APS I) in Norway. Clin Endocrinol (Oxf) 2001;54:211–7.
116. Mylonas I, Hansch S, Markmann S, Bolz M, Friese K. Unilateral ovarian agenesis: report of three cases and review of the literature. Arch Gynecol Obstet 2003;268:57–60.
117. Narahara K, Kamada M, Takahashi Y, et al. Case of ovarian dysgenesis and dilated cardiomyopathy supports existence of Malouf syndrome. Am J Med Genet 1992;44:369–73.
118. Nelson LM. Autoimmune ovarian failure: comparing the mouse model and the human disease. J Soc Gynecol Investig 2001;8(1 Suppl Proceedings):S55–7.
119. Nelson LM, Bakalov VK. Mechanisms of follicular dysfunction in 46,XX spontaneous premature ovarian failure. Endocrinol Metab Clin North Am 2003;32:613–37.
120. Nieto Y, Ross M, Gianani R, et al. Post-mortem incidental finding of cytomegalovirus oophoritis after an allogeneic stem cell transplant. Bone Marrow Transplant 1999;23:1323–4.
121. Oktay K, Buyuk E, Davis O, Yermakova I, Veeck L, Rosenwaks Z. Fertility preservation in breast cancer patients: IVF and embryo cryopreservation after ovarian stimulation with tamoxifen. Hum Reprod 2003;18:90–5.
122. Ordi J, Romagosa C, Tavassoli FA, et al. CD10 expression in epithelial tissues and tumors of the gynecologic tract: a useful marker in the diagnosis of mesonephric, trophoblastic, and clear cell tumors. Am J Surg Pathol 2003;27:178–86.
123. Ortiz-Rey JA, Touza F, Perez-Valcarcel J, Perez-Villanueva J. [Oophoritis due to cytomegalovirus in a female AIDS patient]. Med Clin (Barc) 1997;108:357–8.
124. Page K, Pagidas K, Derosa MC, Quddus MR. Eosinophilic perifolliculitis presenting as a painful cystic ovarian mass in a woman with fibromyalgia: a case report. J Reprod Med 2006;51:141–4.
125. Parveen AS, Elliott H, Howells R. Sarcoidosis of the ovary. J Obstet Gynaecol 2004;24:465.
126. Patel B, Haddad R, Saxena I, Gossain VV. Spontaneous long-term remission in a patient with premature ovarian failure. Endocr Pract 2003;9:380–3.
127. Pellicano M, Zullo F, Cappiello F, Di Carlo C, Cirillo D, Nappi C. Minilaparoscopic ovarian biopsy performed under conscious sedation in women with premature ovarian failure. J Reprod Med 2000;45:817–22.
128. Pilch H, Schaffer U, Gunzel S, et al. (A)symptomatic necrotizing arteritis of the female genital tract. Eur J Obstet Gynecol Reprod Biol 2000;91:191–6.
129. Prueitt RL, Chen H, Barnes RI, Zinn AR. Most X;autosome translocations associated with premature ovarian failure do not interrupt X-linked genes. Cytogenet Genome Res 2002;97(1–2):32–8.
130. Punia RS, Aggarwal R, Amanjit, Mohan H. Xanthogranulomatous oophoritis and salpingitis: late sequelae of inadequately treated staphylococcal PID. Indian J Pathol Microbiol 2003;46:80–1.
131. Quarello E, Desbriere R, Hartung O, Portier F, d'Ercole C, Boubli L. [Postpartum ovarian vein thrombophlebitis: report of 5 cases and review of the literature]. J Gynecol Obstet Biol Reprod (Paris) 2004;33:430–40.
132. Ramos-Casals M, Trejo O, Garcia-Carrasco M, et al. Triple association between hepatitis C virus infection, systemic autoimmune diseases, and B cell lymphoma. J Rheumatol 2004;31:495–9.
133. Ramos J, Torroba A, Garcia Santos J, Marin M. [A 41 year–old female with abdominal pain and fever of 24 hours.]. An Med Interna 2004;21:507–13.
134. Rizzolio F, Bione S, Sala C, et al. Chromosomal rearrangements in Xq and premature ovarian failure: mapping of 25 new cases and review of the literature. Hum Reprod 2006;21:1477–83.
135. Rooman RP, Van Driessche K, Du Caju MV. Growth and ovarian function in girls with 48,XXXX karyotype – patient report and review of the literature. J Pediatr Endocrinol Metab 2002;15:1051–5.
136. Russell P, Farnsworth A. Surgical Pathology of the Ovaries. 2 ed. New York: Churchill Livings; 1997.
137. Ryan MM, Jones HR, Jr. Myasthenia gravis and premature ovarian failure. Muscle Nerve 2004;30:231–3.
138. Santoro N. Research on the mechanisms of premature ovarian failure. J Soc Gynecol Investig 2001;8(1 Suppl Proceedings):S10–2.
139. Santoro N. Mechanisms of premature ovarian failure. Ann Endocrinol (Paris) 2003;64:87–92.
140. Schiffmann R, van der Knaap MS. The latest on leukodystrophies. Curr Opin Neurol 2004;17:187–92.
141. Sforza C, Vizzotto L, Ferrario VF, Forabosco A. Position of follicles in normal human ovary during definitive histogenesis. Early Hum Dev 2003;74:27–35.
142. Sharif K, Afnan M. Ovarian function and ovulation induction. In: Shaw RW, Soutter WP, Stanton SL, eds. Gynaecology. 2 ed. New York: Churchill Livingstone; 1997:223–36.
143. Sills ES, Harmon KE, Tucker MJ. First reported convergence of premature ovarian failure and cutis marmorata telangiectatica congenita. Fertil Steril 2002;78:1314–6.
144. Simpson JL, Rajkovic A. Ovarian differentiation and gonadal failure. Am J Med Genet 1999;89:186–200.
145. St Georgiev V. Chemotherapy of enterobiasis (oxyuriasis). Expert Opin Pharmacother 2001;2:267–75.
146. Steller J. [Ovarian tuberculosis]. Gynakol Geburtshilfliche Rundsch 2001;41:236–9.
147. Tampakoudis P, Assimakopoulos E, Zafrakas M, Tzevelekis P, Kostopoulou E, Bontis J. Pelvic echinococcus mimicking multicystic ovary. Ultrasound Obstet Gynecol 2003;22:196–8.
148. Timmreck LS, Reindollar RH. Contemporary issues in primary amenorrhea. Obstet Gynecol Clin North Am 2003;30:287–302.
149. Trimarchi CP, Russo P. Cyclic estrogen-progestin hormone therapy as a new therapeutic approach in the treatment of functional alterations of the hypothalamus–pituitary–ovary axis: case reports. Endocr Res 2002;28:155–60.
150. Trinidad C, Tardaguila F, Fernandez GC, Martinez C, Chavarri E, Rivas I. Ovarian maldescent. Eur Radiol 2004;14:805–8.
151. Vendeland LL, Shehadeh L. Incidental finding of an accessory ovary in a 16-year-old at laparoscopy. A case report. J Reprod Med 2000;45:435–8.
152. Zinn AR. The X chromosome and the ovary. J Soc Gynecol Investig 2001;8(1 Suppl Proceedings):S34–6.

Ovarian cysts, tumor-like, iatrogenic and miscellaneous conditions

22

Peter Russell   Stanley J. Robboy

DYSFUNCTIONAL CYSTS

Definition

Dysfunctional ovarian cysts are derived from the follicular apparatus either before or after ovulation and are classified as outlined in Table 22.1. They may either result from, or cause, disordered hypothalamic–pituitary–ovarian function. Although not always functional in the sense of producing steroid hormones, the cysts all have or have had the potential to do so at some stage in their development.

Ultrasound examination is used widely in the diagnosis and surveillance of these cysts, which achieve clinical importance if they exceed 3 cm and do not disappear on repeat scanning within another 2–3 weeks. Although the cysts usually resolve spontaneously, their resolution can be accelerated by transvaginal ultrasound-guided needle drainage. This procedure can be both diagnostic and therapeutic. Such management may prevent unnecessary ovarian surgery.

'Polycystic ovaries' is a term that should be reserved for the abnormal ovaries found in association with functional hyperandrogenism (the Stein–Leventhal and related clinical syndromes – see below). The ovaries commonly have thick white capsules, and display multiple cystic follicles and small, luteinized follicular cysts of atretic type, absence of stigmata of recent ovulation, and occur with a characteristic disturbance of hypothalamic–pituitary function. Ovaries displaying several cysts, but otherwise not fitting into this category, should be called 'multicystic' or 'polyfollicular' in order to avoid confusion.

Corpus luteum cysts are also derived from the follicular apparatus but show evidence of prior ovulation that distinguishes them from follicular cysts. Ovulation is indicated by convolution of the cyst lining (which results from collapse of the follicle) with the characteristic invaginations of theca-lutein (paralutein) cells into the inner zone of granulosa lutein cells. A layer of fibrous tissue lining the inner surface of the cyst, resulting from organization of the corpus luteum hematoma, also indicates that ovulation has occurred.

Features distinguishing the various types of cyst derived from the follicular apparatus are illustrated diagrammatically in Figure 22.1.

CYSTS DERIVED FROM PREOVULATORY FOLLICLES (FOLLICULAR CYSTS)

Etiology

The etiology of follicular cysts (by definition ≥3 cm in diameter) is not always obvious but in most cases reflects disordered function of the pituitary–ovarian axis. Pathologic cystic change may develop either in the follicular growth phase or during atresia. Unluteinized follicular cysts, which produce predominantly estradiol, result from excessive ovarian stimulation (either by endogenous follicle-stimulating hormone (FSH) or by ovulation-induction agents) or an abnormal response to normal stimulation.

Granulosa lutein cysts are follicular cysts with predominant luteinization of the granulosa cells (which are internal to the basal lamina – Figure 22.1B); like corpora lutea, they secrete progesterone. An unknown proportion of granulosa lutein cysts results from failure of follicular rupture at the expected time of ovulation. This circumstance is the basis of the luteinized unruptured follicle (LUF) syndrome.

Theca–lutein cysts are follicular cysts with luteinization predominantly of the theca interna (which is external to the basal lamina – Figure 22.1C). Androstenedione is the characteristic steroid product. These cysts develop when there is prolonged exposure to luteinizing hormone (LH) or beta-human chorionic gonadotropin (β-hCG), either endogenous, such as in polycystic ovary syndrome (see below) or hyperreactio luteinalis syndrome of pregnancy (multiple theca–lutein cysts), or exogenous, as in the ovarian hyperstimulation syndrome. Atretic follicular cysts are also capable of elaborating androstenedione.

Clinical features

Ovarian cysts in the fetus are more frequent than were once thought, with an estimated incidence of about one in 2500 births. They are usually diagnosed in the third trimester by ultrasound or MRI.[41,49] Therapeutic intervention is usually prompted by acute torsion in the newborn period or persistence of cysts greater than 5 cm in diameter in children beyond 6 months of age.

In prepubertal girls, follicular cysts form a significant proportion of ovarian lesions that come to surgical intervention. Common clinical presentations are pain, vomiting, diarrhea, and constipation, sometimes precipitated by ovarian torsion. A less common but well-recognized association is with isosexual pseudoprecocity, either idiopathic or associated with hypothyroidism, or the McCune–Albright syndrome (polyostotic fibrous dysplasia).[22]

During the reproductive years, unluteinized follicular cysts may produce sufficient estradiol to cause irregular or prolonged (dysfunctional) uterine bleeding. The endometrium in such cases may show disordered proliferative phase changes or hyperplasia. Granulosa lutein cysts secrete progesterone, but rarely in sufficient amounts to disturb the menstrual cycle. Atretic cysts, if numerous (as in the polycystic ovary

Table 22.1 Classification of dysfunctional ovarian cysts

Cysts derived from preovulatory follicles
    Follicular cyst – unluteinized
    Follicular cyst – luteinized
        Granulosa lutein cyst
        Theca–lutein cyst
    Follicular cyst – atretic

Cysts derived from corpus luteum
    Cystic corpus luteum
    Corpus luteum cyst
    Corpus albicans cyst

Simple cysts

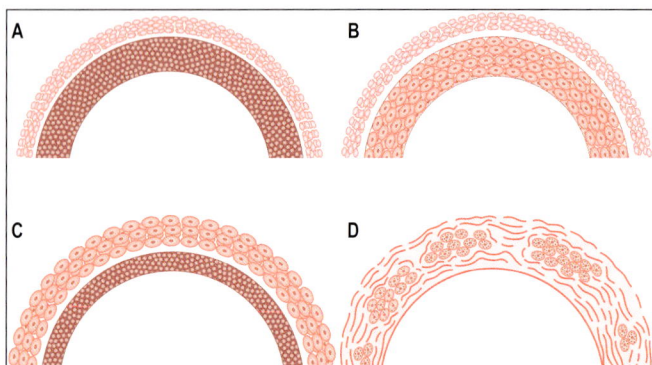
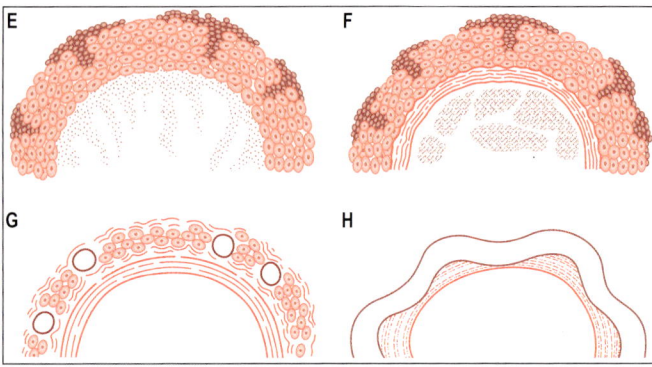

Fig. 22.1 Comparative morphology of dysfunctional cysts. **(A)** Unluteinized follicular cyst. **(B)** Granulosa lutein cyst. **(C)** Theca-lutein cyst. **(D)** Involuting follicular cyst. **(E)** Cystic corpus luteum. **(F)** Corpus luteum cyst (early). **(G)** Corpus luteum cyst (late). **(H)** Corpus albicans cyst. Microscopic features are: (a) unluteinized granulosa, (b) basal lamina, (c) unluteinized theca interna, (d) luteinized granulosa, (e) luteinized theca, (f) involuting luteinized cells, (g) granulosa lutein layer, (h) theca (para) lutein layer, (i) fibrin, (j) loose fibrous tissue, (k) blood, (l) dense fibrous tissue, (m) prominent blood vessels, (n) acellular hyalinized fibrous tissue.

syndrome), may synthesize sufficient androstenedione to produce hirsutism or virilization. Observation of these cysts shows that most regress spontaneously over a few cycles and that therapy with contraceptive agents does not accelerate this process.[29] Persistence should raise the specter of neoplasia.

During pregnancy, pre-existing follicular cysts may become luteinized. New cysts rarely develop but a notable exception is the hyperreactio luteinalis syndrome (multiple theca–lutein cysts). Large solitary luteinized follicular cysts may present as adnexal masses in the third to fourth months of pregnancy or postpartum, or are incidental findings at cesarean section.

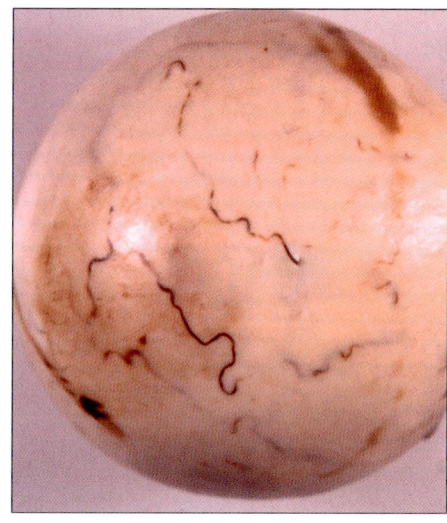

Fig. 22.2 Dysfunctional cyst. A large simple cyst with a yellowish blush showing through the thin wall and to the smooth external surface.

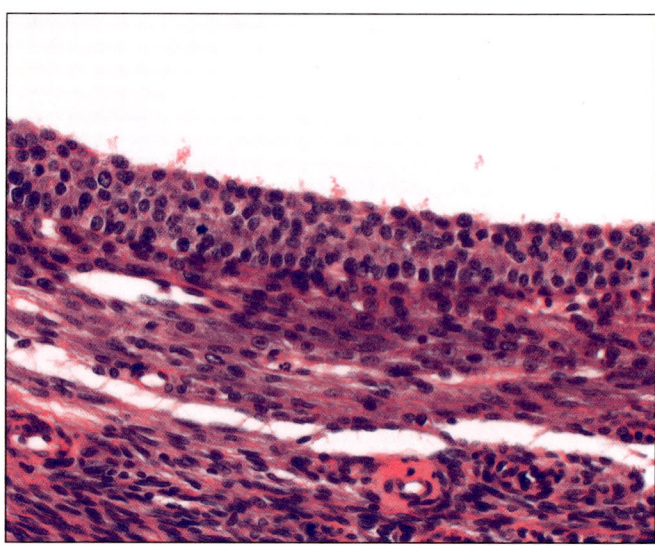

Fig. 22.3 Unluteinized follicular cyst. About four layers of uniform small granulosa cells are present above the basal lamina.

Symptomatic follicular cysts are rare after the menopause, although some sporadic follicular activity (generally without ovulation) continues in the early years.

Gross features
These are usually single and 3–10 cm in diameter (Figure 22.2). Solitary luteinized follicle cysts of pregnancy and puerperium have a median diameter of 25 cm. They are smooth-lined and contain clear proteinaceous fluid or altered blood.

Microscopic features
Unluteinized follicular cysts show the microscopic features of physiologic growing cystic follicles, with well-preserved granulosa and theca layers separated by a basal lamina (Figure 22.3). However the cumulus oophorus and oocyte are no longer present. The lining may be somewhat attenuated secondary to dilatation. There is no trace of the festooned pattern of a corpus luteum. During involution the lining is often incomplete and later appears as small clusters of lutein cells in the com-

pressed ovarian stroma, which becomes progressively fibrotic. As involution continues, distinguishing features become increasingly difficult to identify and definitive diagnosis may not be possible (Figure 22.4); in this situation the cyst is better designated 'simple' (see below).

Cytologically, unluteinized follicular cysts contain numerous granulosa cells that have been shed into the fluid and reflect the normal lining. The cells are arranged singly and in tight clusters (see Figure 21.1E). The clusters may be irregular in shape, some with papillary configurations. Granulosa cells contain round to oval nuclei and a small rim of distinct cytoplasm. The chromatin is coarsely granular. Nuclear grooves are occasionally seen. Mitoses may be identified. The cells are uniform with negligible variation from cell to cell. Degenerative changes may be present.

Luteinized follicular cysts show the general features of unluteinized follicular cysts as described above, but in addition some of the cells in the cyst wall are luteinized. The granulosa (granulosa lutein cyst – Figure 22.5) or theca layer (theca-lutein cyst – Figures 22.6, 22.22, and 22.23) luteinize, or occasionally both, although the cyst is classified according to the layer predominantly affected. Luteinization appears as enlarged cells with increased eosinophilic or finely vacuolated cytoplasm. The changes are analogous to those in a corpus luteum.

Cytologically, luteinized follicular cysts contain single and/ or clusters of granulosa cells, some or all of which are luteinized. The clusters may form papillary or spherical groups. Luteinized granulosa cells have round to oval nuclei with coarse chromatin and may have small prominent nucleoli. Cell cytoplasm is ample and foamy. Mitotic figures are not unusual in the cell clusters. The cells are predictable and without pleomorphism. Degenerative changes may be present in single cells with obvious nuclear pyknosis.

Atretic follicular cysts are lined by ovarian stroma in which there are small clusters of luteinized theca cells. They may be indistinguishable from involuting follicular cysts of other types (Figures 22.7 and 22.8).

Other histologic alterations may be seen in the ovary if follicular cysts are associated with some specific clinicopathologic syndromes. For example, 'polycystic ovaries' also show subcapsular fibrosis and focal stromal luteinization, and the ovaries in hyperreactio luteinalis and the hyperstimulation syndrome exhibit marked stromal edema and hemorrhage.

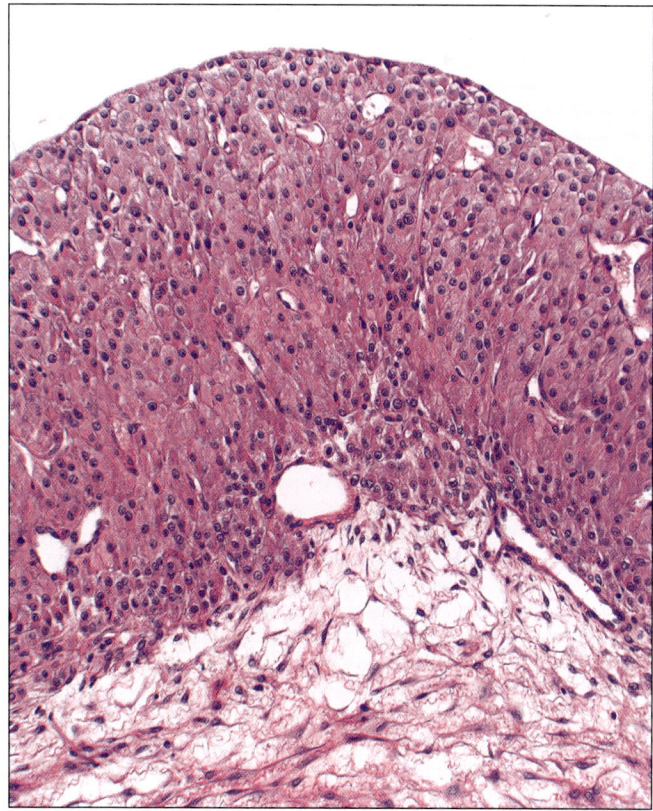

Fig. 22.5 Granulosa lutein cyst lined by large eosinophilic cells. The thecal layer is relatively inconspicuous.

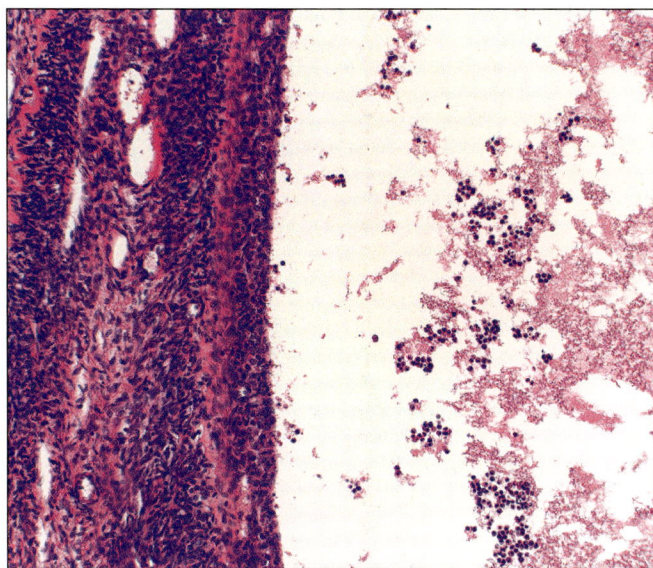

Fig. 22.4 Involuting follicular cyst. Smooth internal contour and inapparent lining cells of follicular origin. Shed granulosa cells in the lumen are a useful guide to diagnosis.

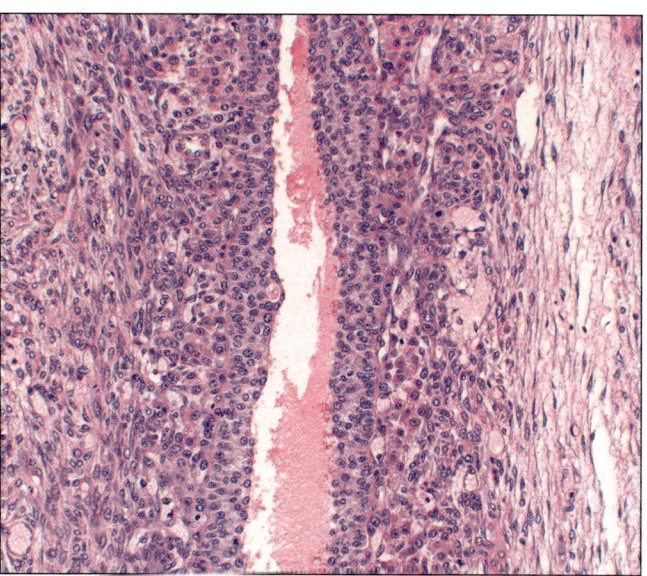

Fig. 22.6 Theca-lutein cyst. Thick lining of small granulosa cells with large luteinized theca cells beneath basal lamina (from patient with polycystic ovary syndrome).

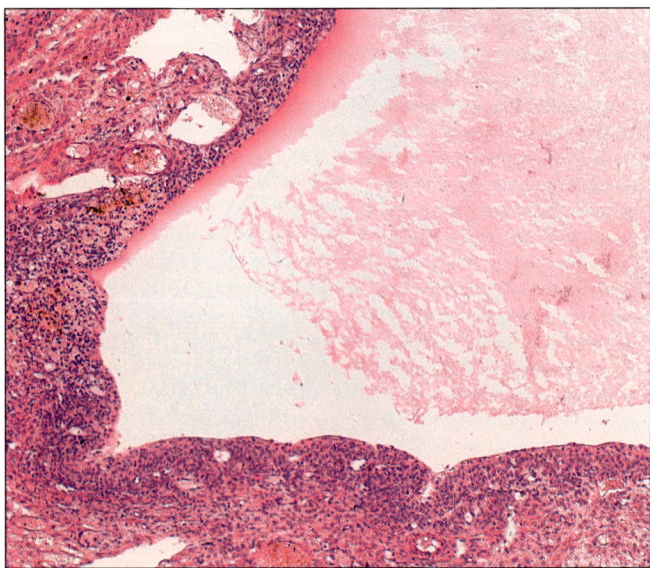

Fig. 22.7 Atretic cyst from patient with polycystic ovary syndrome. Note smooth internal contour and fibrous wall.

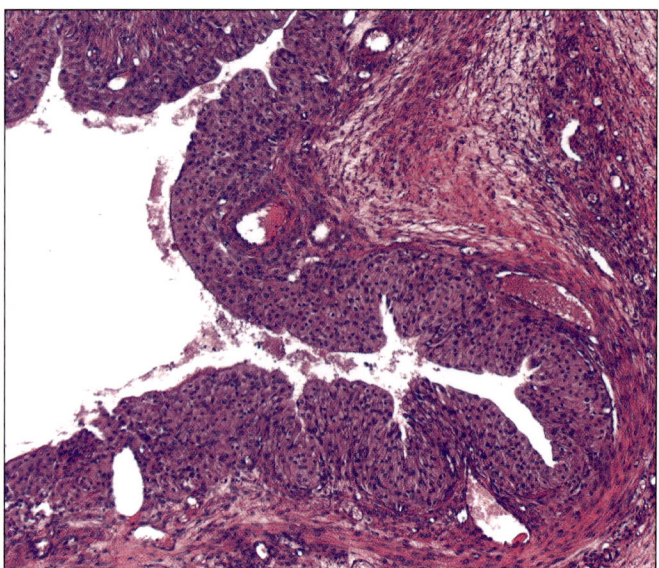

Fig. 22.9 Wall of ruptured cystic corpus luteum with early luteinization of granulosa and theca.

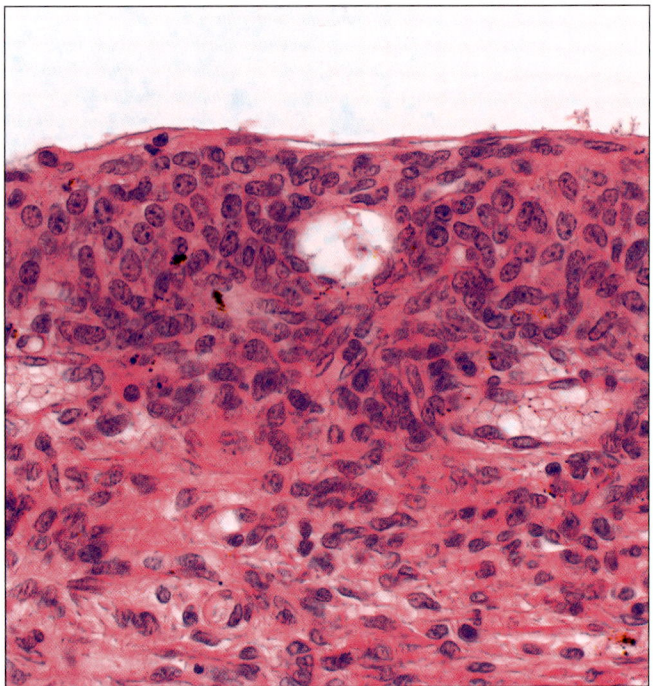

Fig. 22.8 Detail of Figure 22.7. Clusters of follicular cells of uncertain type close to cyst lumen.

Differential diagnosis

Cysts derived from a corpus luteum can be distinguished from luteinized follicular cysts by their retention, partially or focally, of their convoluted lining with invaginations of paralutein cells, and by their innermost lining of fibrous tissue (the result of organization of the central coagulum). In addition, a well-defined vascular zone may be evident.

Cystic granulosa cell tumors may be difficult to distinguish from follicular cysts. They are often considerably larger and always unilateral. The neoplastic cells lining the cysts may show prominent luteinization and may display mitotic activity. Although most granulosa cell tumors are estrogenic, 15–30%

of the cystic variants are clinically androgenic, a feature not associated with follicular cysts except in the specific clinical situations mentioned above.

CORPUS LUTEUM CYSTS

Etiology

These are cysts derived from corpora lutea of menstruation or pregnancy that result from excessive central hemorrhage. Small physiologic hemorrhages occur 2–4 days after ovulation during the stage when the corpus luteum vascularizes. They usually organize rapidly, but if the hemorrhage is excessive and the corpus luteum becomes overdistended with blood, involution is likely to be delayed.

Clinical features

Most are asymptomatic. In some non-pregnant women, this delayed involution (sometimes called 'persistent corpus luteum') and its continuing production of progesterone may result in minor menstrual disturbances (so-called 'irregular shedding').

Gross features

Corpora lutea of menstruation rarely exceed 3 cm (average size 2 cm) but may do so if there is an unusually large fluid-filled central cavity. Cystic corpora lutea of pregnancy often exceed 5 cm and may exceed 10 cm in diameter. They are not infrequently identified on routine ultrasound examination in early pregnancy. They contain clear fluid or altered blood. Rupture may be evident. They are generally smooth-lined with an incomplete band of yellow tissue in the wall.

Microscopic features

Cystic corpora lutea display the same features as their non-cystic counterparts. The distension leads to some attenuation of the convolutions but without loss of distinctive cell layers (Figure 22.9). The fibrous tissue lining contains mature collagen demonstrable with a trichrome connective tissue stain. Although hemorrhage in the cyst wall and surrounding stroma

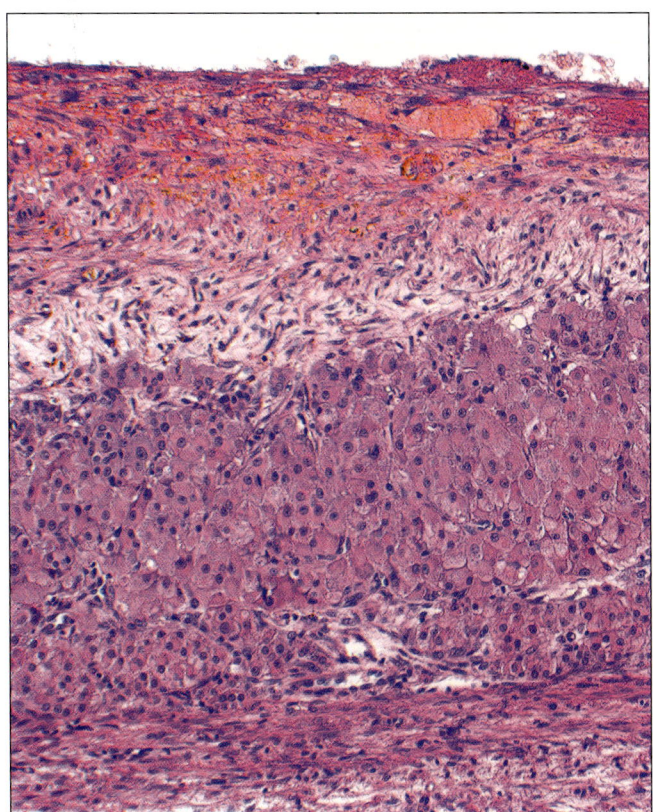

Fig. 22.10 Early corpus luteum cyst. Organizing hematoma at top and thin zone of involuting vacuolated luteinized cells below.

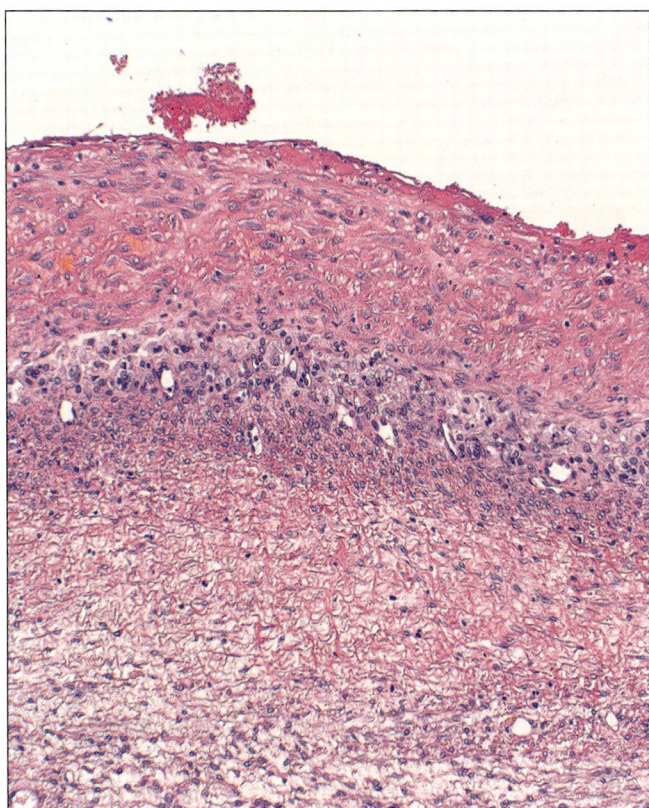

Fig. 22.11 Late corpus luteum cyst. Inner zone of fibrous tissue with involuting vacuolated luteinized cells beneath.

may partially obscure morphologic features, vestiges of the convoluted lining can be seen microscopically if carefully sought. Peripheral clusters of small paralutein (theca–lutein) cells may still be seen between larger groups of granulosa lutein cells (Figure 22.10). The granulosa and theca–lutein cells are smaller than those seen in a fresh corpus luteum. The nuclei are small, hyperchromatic, and lack mitotic activity, while the cytoplasm is usually finely vesicular. With progressive involution, fewer and smaller islands of lutein cells are found within the increasingly fibrotic wall, but a well-defined zone of small blood vessels remains to mark the phase of vascularization (Figure 22.11).

Cytologically, corpus luteum cysts contain numerous fully luteinized granulosa cells, singly and in clusters, and mixed with fresh blood and scattered hemosiderin-laden macrophages. Unlike those from follicular cysts, these cells are large, polyhedral in shape with a low nuclear:cytoplasmic ratio. Nuclei are eccentric, round to slightly oval, with finely granular chromatin and prominent nucleoli. Nuclear grooves are not present and binucleation may be apparent. Cytoplasm is ample, finely granular, and contains tiny vacuoles. Yellowish cytochrome pigment may also be present. Hemorrhagic corpus luteum cysts may be identified by these features as well as the presence of abundant fibrin and some fibroblasts in the smear background. Regressing corpora lutea may contain large luteinized cells, as well as numerous macrophages with yellow hematoidin pigment.

Differential diagnosis

Luteinized follicular cysts appear macroscopically like corpus luteum cysts but are less likely to be hemorrhagic. The micro-

scopic distinction hinges around evidence of ovulation as indicated above. Follicular cysts generally lack the zone of vascularization. Some long-standing cysts may be very difficult to classify.

Endometriotic cysts may be impossible to distinguish macroscopically from corpus luteum cysts but may be suspected if there is evidence of endometriosis elsewhere in the submitted specimens or if the diagnosis is indicated clinically. The microscopic identification of endometrial glands or stroma within the cyst quickly excludes this lesion from the differential diagnosis. When degenerate, a useful clue is the presence of organized fibrous tissue outside the layer of foamy decidualized cells of an endometriotic cyst, which contrasts with the fibrous tissue layer inside similar appearing luteinized cells of the corpus luteum cyst.

CORPUS ALBICANS CYSTS

The corpus albicans is typically a small solid hyalinized fibrous scar, but occasionally it has a central cavity containing clear fluid. The cysts are rarely more than 1 cm in diameter, and develop after corpora lutea involute. The mechanism of fluid retention or accumulation is not known.

Microscopically, the cyst wall is composed of a convoluted ribbon-like band of hyalinized acellular fibrous tissue, usually with an innermost lining of looser fibrous connective tissue with a smoother outline (Figure 22.12). The cysts are nonfunctional and are too small to produce symptomatic adnexal masses.

SIMPLE (UNCLASSIFIED) CYSTS

Definition
These are ovarian cysts or cyst-like structures that lack identifiable linings. Some produce symptomatic adnexal masses but most are incidental findings. The cysts are usually less than 10 cm in diameter, solitary, and have a smooth internal surface and a variable content of clear fluid or altered blood. Most are of follicular origin, although some arise as epithelial cysts.

Microscopic features
The lining usually consists only of a narrow band of dense fibrous tissue or compressed ovarian stroma. There may be occasional small clusters of involuting lutein cells in the cyst wall, suggesting an origin from the follicular apparatus. Sometimes there is a complete or partial lining of apparent epithelial cells that are too attenuated for their origin to be identified (Figure 22.13A) but, even here, persistent immunostaining for α-inhibin may be present (Figure 22.13B). Some cysts undoubtedly represent epithelial cystomas (Figure 22.14). Some are lined by granulation tissue or organizing hematoma. Such lesions may be endometriotic in origin but lack overall the necessary diagnostic features. There is probably no benefit in precisely categorizing 'simple' cysts. All are benign and most are non-neoplastic.

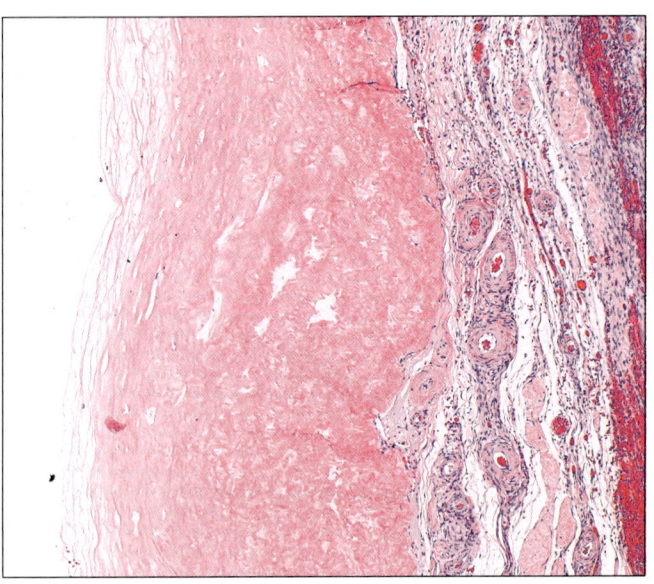

Fig. 22.12 Corpus albicans cyst. A layer of acellular hyalinized fibrous tissue, now devoid of residual granulosa cells but retaining the festooned architectural pattern, lines the cystic space.

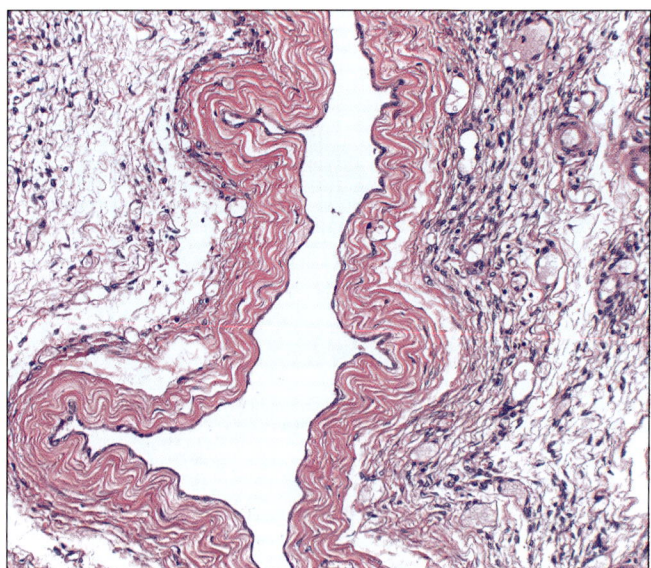

Fig. 22.14 Simple cyst. Lined by ovarian stroma and attenuated, undistinguished epithelial cells.

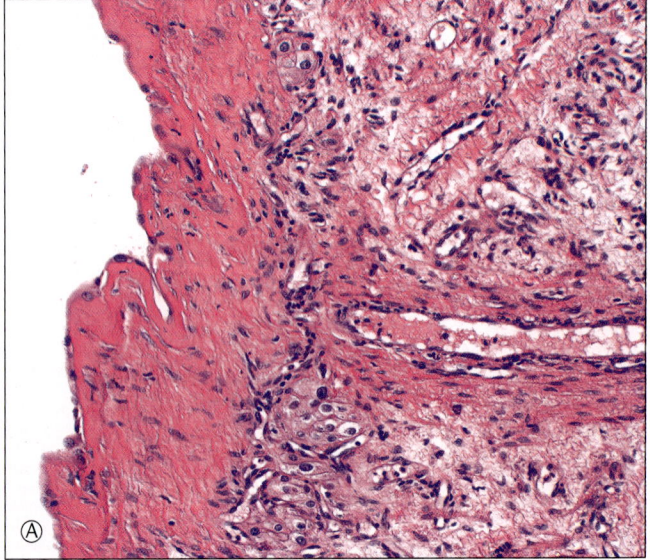

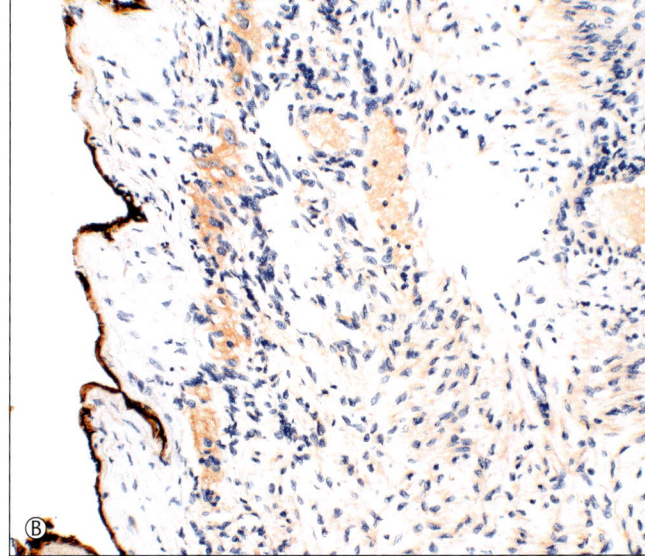

Fig. 22.13 Simple cyst. **(A)** A dense fibrous tissue wall is lined by barely perceptible 'epithelial' cells. Occasional lutein-like cells beneath this fibrous layer suggest origin from the follicular apparatus. **(B)** Persistent immunostaining of the lining cells for α-inhibin (as well as the lutein-like cells in the wall) support this interpretation.

TUMOR-LIKE LESIONS ASSOCIATED WITH PREGNANCY

Non-neoplastic ovarian lesions encountered exclusively in pregnancy or the puerperium are grouped together to emphasize the importance of their recognition by pathologists. These lesions involute spontaneously after the pregnancy ends and radical surgery is clearly inappropriate treatment. Other ovarian enlargements not necessarily exclusive to pregnancy are also seen, e.g., corpus luteum cysts, endometriotic cysts, and parovarian cysts.

LUTEOMAS OF PREGNANCY (NODULAR THECA–LUTEIN HYPERPLASIA)

Definition
These are multinodular, often multicentric or bilateral, tumor-like masses of lutein cells that develop during an otherwise normal pregnancy (presenting usually in the third trimester) and involute in the puerperium.

Clinical features
About one-fourth of patients become hirsute or virilized. Female fetuses may be born with signs of masculinization (see Chapter 34).

Etiology
The lesions most likely arise from the lutein cells found during pregnancy as isolated groups in the stroma or in the walls of atretic follicles. Some patients have a history suggestive of polycystic ovary syndrome, and luteomas in these patients possibly arise from the hyperplastic, often luteinized, stromal cells existing before the onset of pregnancy. Beta-human chorionic gonadotropin (β-hCG) is necessary for the development of luteomas but is unlikely to be the only etiologic factor since the lesions are not associated with trophoblastic disease or with early pregnancy, when β-hCG levels are at their highest. Morphologic and clinical similarities exist between luteomas and multiple theca–lutein cysts (hyperreactio luteinalis), and it is possible that they are related forms of theca–lutein cell hyperplasia. However, in contrast to luteomas, hyperreactio luteinalis is associated with conditions of pathologic β-hCG elevation, multiple gestations, and abnormal pregnancy states.

Gross features
Luteomas are usually 6–12 cm in diameter but may exceed 20 cm. They are circumscribed, multinodular solid masses with a soft gray-brown to tan cut surface. Small cystic spaces may be present. Those removed in the puerperium may be softer and paler or even frankly necrotic.

Microscopic features
Luteomas display sheets of large eosinophilic cells that are broken up into alveolar groups by numerous delicate blood vessels (Figures 22.15–22.20). An organoid pattern (Figure 22.16) is common. A trabecular arrangement is less frequently seen and a solitary case has displayed sertoliform tubular structures.[56] The cell size is intermediate between that of granulosa and theca–lutein cells. The reticulin pattern of fibers around groups rather than individual cells is also intermediate between the abundant pericellular distribution of reticulin fibers in the

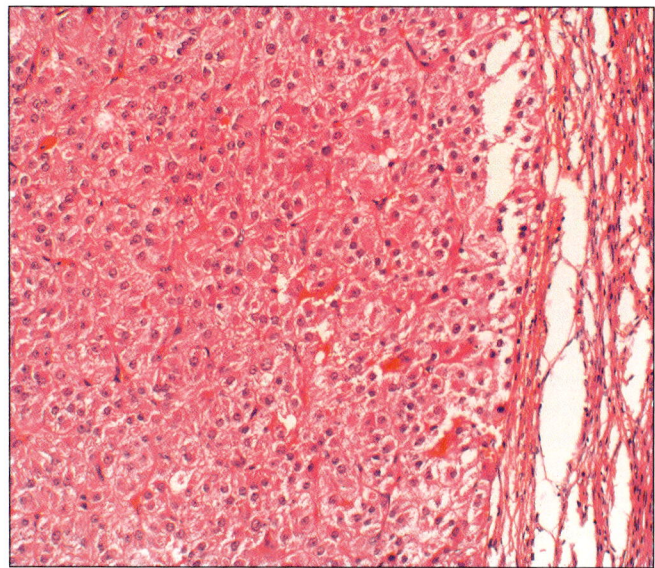

Fig. 22.15 Luteoma of pregnancy. A 4 cm solitary nodule excised at cesarean section. Well-defined 'tumor' margin is present at right.

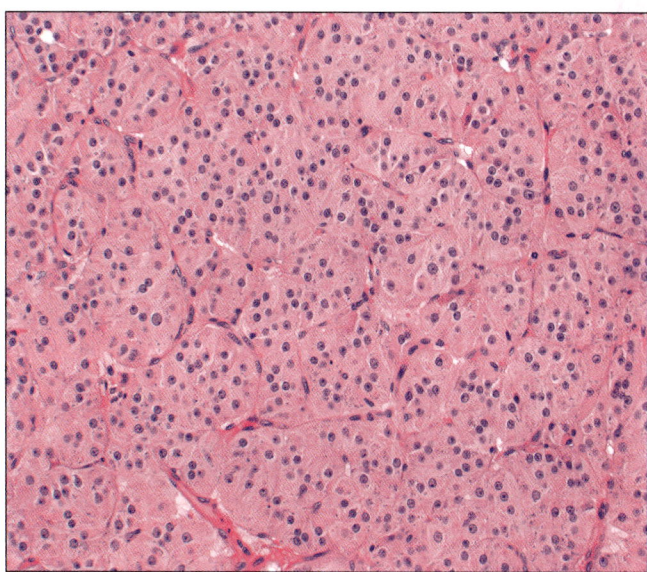

Fig. 22.16 Luteoma of pregnancy. Distinctly organoid pattern with cell groups separated by delicate vessels. Note mild nuclear variation.

theca interna and the paucity of fibers in the granulosa layer. Follicular spaces containing colloid-like material may be present (Figures 22.17 and 22.18) but the intracellular hyaline droplets ('colloid bodies') typical of corpora lutea of pregnancy are rarely identified. The cytoplasm is eosinophilic and sometimes finely vacuolated but contains little stainable lipid. The round central nuclei have a prominent nucleolus and abundant euchromatin. There may be mild nuclear pleomorphism and some mitotic figures – under 3 per 10 high-power fields (HPFs) (Figures 22.16 and 22.19). The remainder of the ovary shows the physiologic changes of pregnancy but small theca–lutein cysts may be evident as well. Early involutional changes include nuclear pyknosis and increased cytoplasmic vacuolation. Eventually the luteoma is reduced to sheets of necrotic cells (Figure 22.20). Even at this late stage, the typical reticulin pattern may still be useful diagnostically.

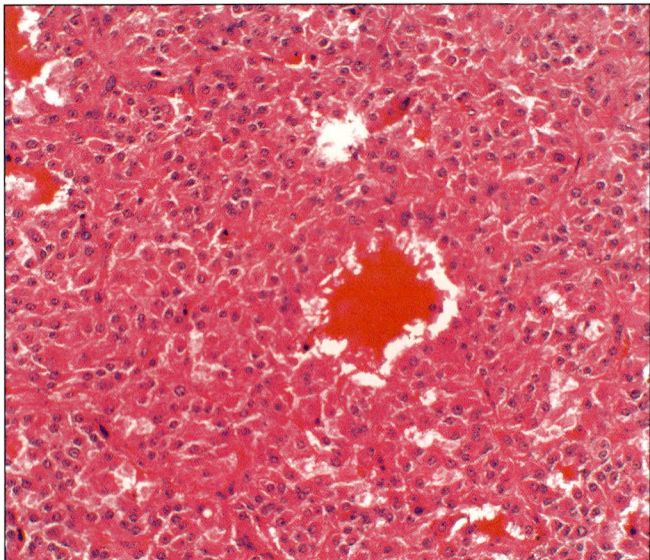

Fig. 22.17 Luteoma of pregnancy. Uniform cells in alveolar groups, and follicular spaces containing colloid-like material.

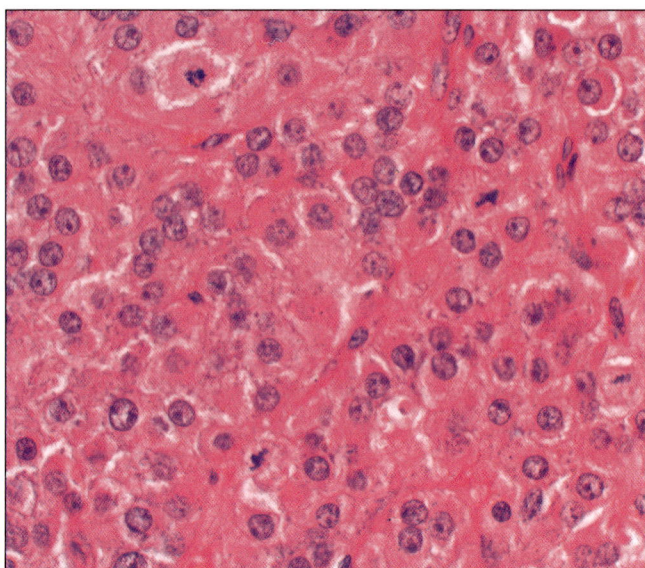

Fig. 22.19 Luteoma of pregnancy. Luteoma cells with abundant cytoplasm, mildly pleomorphic nucleim and mitoses.

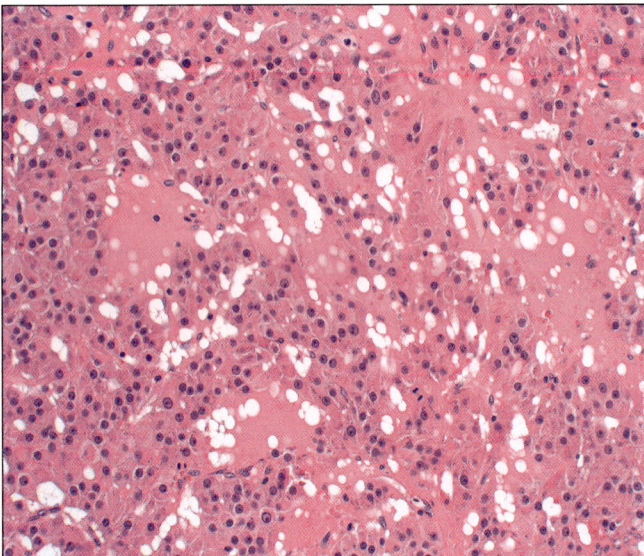

Fig. 22.18 Luteoma of pregnancy. The alveolar groups and follicular spaces are less well defined in this example, but nevertheless present.

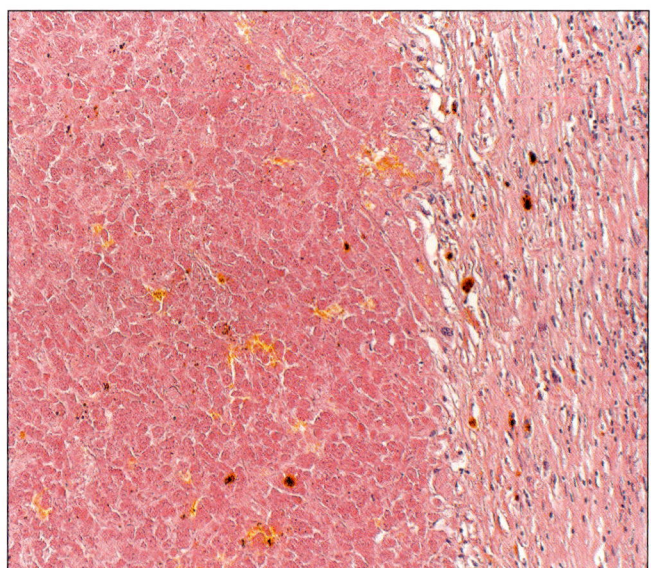

Fig. 22.20 Luteoma of pregnancy. Involuted luteoma 5 months postpartum; sheets of ghost cells with some organization (granulation tissue) at margin.

Differential diagnosis

Non-cystic aggregates of large lutein-like cells include a plethora of entities in the differential diagnosis, some neoplastic, some not. While these are listed in Figure 22.21, the clinical context and gross features of the lesions all contribute materially to their separation.

Nodular stromal hyperthecosis may occur in pregnancy. The ovaries are uniformly enlarged and display multiple microscopic nodules of spindle-shaped luteinized stromal cells, arranged in bundles rather than alveoli. Reticulin fibers invest individual cells that have pale or finely vacuolated cytoplasm containing abundant lipid.

Lipid cell tumors are almost always unilateral (with the exception of stromal luteomas) and sometimes arise in the ovarian hilus. They are solid lobulated tumors composed of eosinophilic or finely vacuolated cells arranged in a diffuse or, less commonly, a trabecular pattern – not dissimilar to that of luteomas. Reticulin surrounds single cells or small groups. Mitotic activity is variable but rarely as prominent as in luteomas of pregnancy. The most helpful distinguishing microscopic features are the abundant stainable intracytoplasmic lipid in all lipid cell tumors and the presence of crystalloids of Reinke in Leydig cell tumors (Table 22.2).

Thecomas are usually unilateral. They may be focally luteinized in pregnancy and resemble luteomas. However, the basic spindle shape of the cells is still evident. Sclerosing stromal tumors, closely related to thecomas, display a striking lobulated pattern that is due to bands of edematous immature or mature collagenous stroma (absent in luteomas). Within the lobules there is abundant pericellular reticulin as seen in thecomas. Another helpful distinguishing feature is the mixed

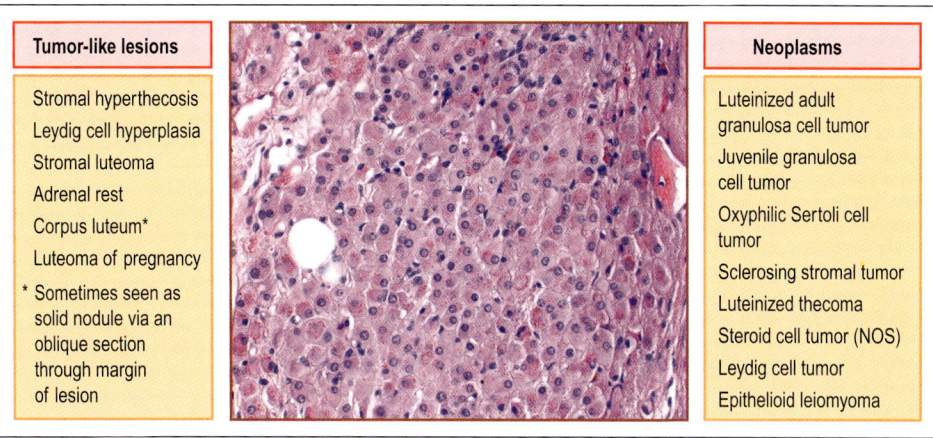

Tumor-like lesions	Neoplasms
Stromal hyperthecosis Leydig cell hyperplasia Stromal luteoma Adrenal rest Corpus luteum* Luteoma of pregnancy * Sometimes seen as solid nodule via an oblique section through margin of lesion	Luteinized adult granulosa cell tumor Juvenile granulosa cell tumor Oxyphilic Sertoli cell tumor Sclerosing stromal tumor Luteinized thecoma Steroid cell tumor (NOS) Leydig cell tumor Epithelioid leiomyoma

Fig. 22.21 Non-cystic aggregates of lutein-like cells: differential diagnosis.

Table 22.2 Steroid cell tumor versus pregnancy luteoma: differential diagnosis

	Steroid cell tumor	Pregnancy luteoma
Clinical		
Mean age:	47 years	26 years
Relationship to pregnancy	None	Diagnosed at or near term or in puerperium
Racial tendency	None	80% in black women
Laterality	Almost always unilateral	Often bilateral and multicentric
Endocrine features	75% of women virilized	25% develop hirsutism during pregnancy; female newborn sometimes with hermaphroditic signs
Histologic		
Intracellular lipid	Abundant	Relatively little or none
Necrosis	If present, only focal	Diffuse acute regressive changes if removed postpartum
Adjacent uninvolved ovary	No pregnancy changes	Pregnancy changes (deciduosis, hyperthecosis)

population of spindle and polyhedral eosinophilic cells (mostly the latter). Granulosa cell tumors are rare in pregnancy but, when they occur, are usually of the juvenile type, which may closely resemble luteomas.

MULTIPLE THECA–LUTEIN CYSTS (HYPERREACTIO LUTEINALIS)

Etiology and clinical features
While theca–lutein cysts (luteinized follicular cysts) can occur at any age and in many different clinical situations, multiple bilateral theca–lutein cysts are classically associated with molar pregnancies or choriocarcinoma, occurring in 25% of such cases. They also occur in association with Rhesus isoimmunization, non-immune hydrops, chronic renal failure,[17] multiple pregnancies,[72] and even apparently normal singleton pregnan-

cies.[19,42] Rarely, a similar clinicopathologic picture results from ovarian hyperstimulation, provoked by ovulation-induction agents (see below). This condition is occasionally associated with clinical evidence of hyperglycemia or virilization.[69]

Although multiple bilateral theca–lutein cysts are usually associated with abnormally elevated β-hCG levels, additional factors may be necessary for their genesis. The cysts may persist into, or appear first in, the puerperium when β-hCG levels have fallen. In the latter situation the cysts probably initially developed during pregnancy under the influence of β-hCG but were then maintained by the FSH and LH levels that rose soon after parturition if lactation was not established. The condition almost always regresses within a few weeks after parturition. For this reason surgery during pregnancy, which is often required for diagnostic purposes or for management of acute abdomen or shock, should be as conservative as possible. Intraoperative frozen-section examination of an incisional ovarian biopsy may obviate unnecessarily extensive surgery based on the erroneous presumption of malignant disease.

Gross and microscopic features
Both ovaries are involved and measure up to 15 cm across. Sectioning shows multiple cysts 1–4 cm in diameter that contain yellowish fluid or blood, separated by edematous stroma (Figure 22.22). The follicular cysts show hyperplasia and prominent luteinization of the theca interna layer; the granulosa is often luteinized as well (Figures 22.23 and 22.24). The edematous stroma may also contain large clusters of luteinized stromal cells.

Differential diagnosis
Solitary luteinized follicular cysts of pregnancy and the puerperium (see below) are large, unilateral and unilocular. Hemorrhage and edema are usually absent. There is no distinct separation of granulosa and theca layers.

SOLITARY LUTEINIZED FOLLICULAR CYSTS OF PREGNANCY AND PUERPERIUM

Definition
A large, distinctive follicular cyst of the ovary may occur during pregnancy.[31,77] Such cysts present as adnexal masses in the third to fourth months of pregnancy or postpartum, or are incidental

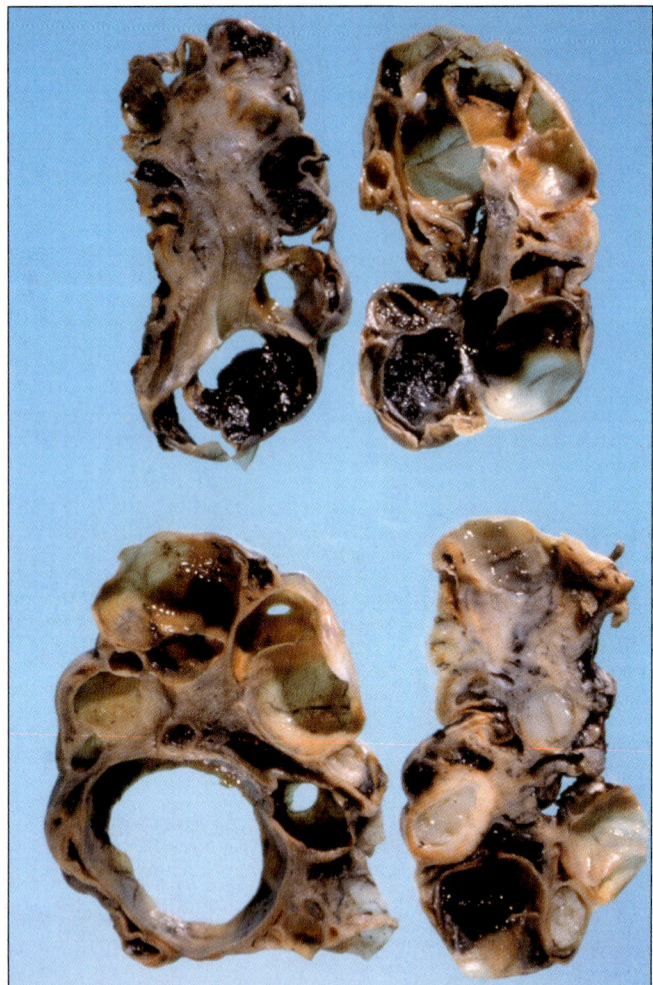

Fig. 22.22 Multiple theca–lutein cysts in pregnancy. Multiple cysts and intervening hemorrhagic edematous stroma.

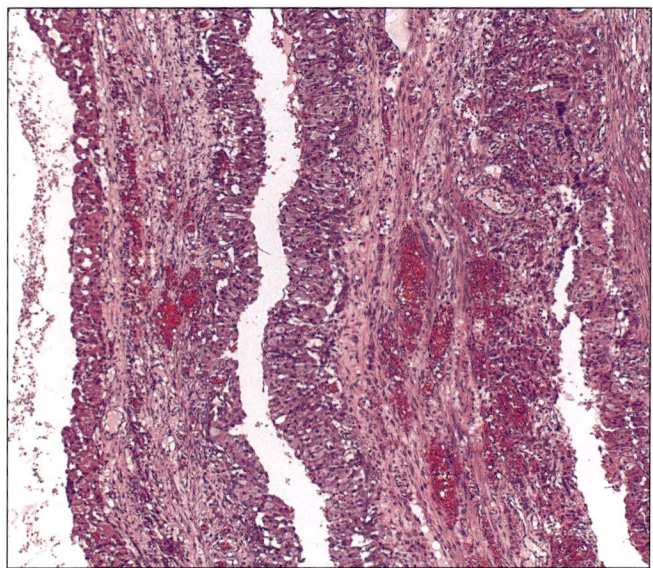

Fig. 22.24 Detail of Figure 22.23. Luteinization of both theca and granulosa with some early necrosis (cytoplasmic eosinophilia) of the lining (at left).

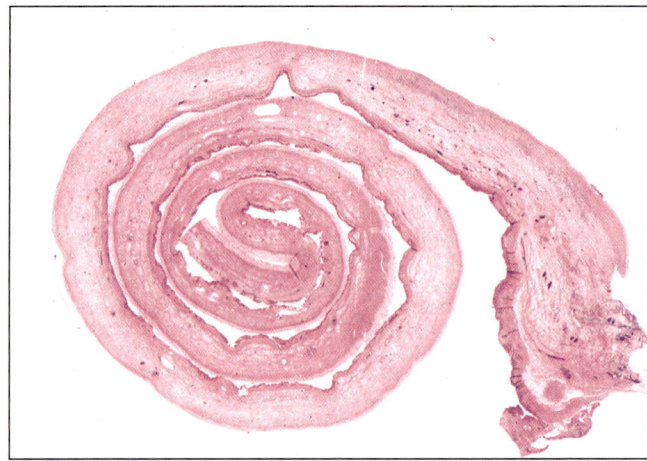

Fig. 22.25 Solitary 23 cm luteinized follicular cyst ('jam roll' preparation). Removed 2 months postpartum following torsion.

findings at cesarean section. The involved ovaries exhibit large (average diameter 25 cm), unilocular, thin-walled cysts (Figure 22.25) that contain clear or mucoid fluid. The pathogenesis is unknown, but β-hCG stimulation is probably important.

Microscopic features

Microscopically, a single layer or multiple layers of large luteinized cells line the cysts, with only a sparse reticulin network. Similar cells are sometimes also present in the fibrous wall of the cysts but these cells are not obviously thecal in type, i.e., there is no clear definition of the granulosa and theca elements of the cyst wall usually seen in cysts of follicular origin. A striking feature is the focal presence of large pleomorphic hyperchromatic nuclei in the luteinized cells (Figure 22.26). This feature, together with the remarkably large cyst size and lack of recognizable separation of lining cells into granulosa and theca layers, distinguish this entity morphologically from the follicular cysts of non-pregnant women.

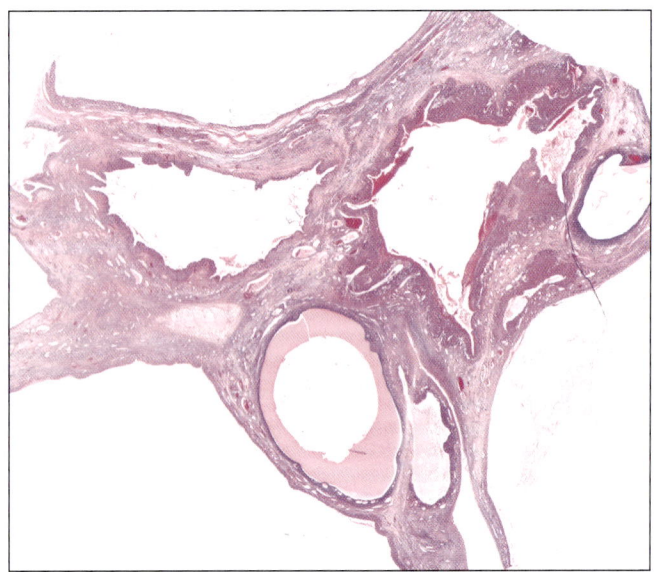

Fig. 22.23 Multiple theca–lutein cysts in pregnancy. Ribbons of luteinized cells line cysts.

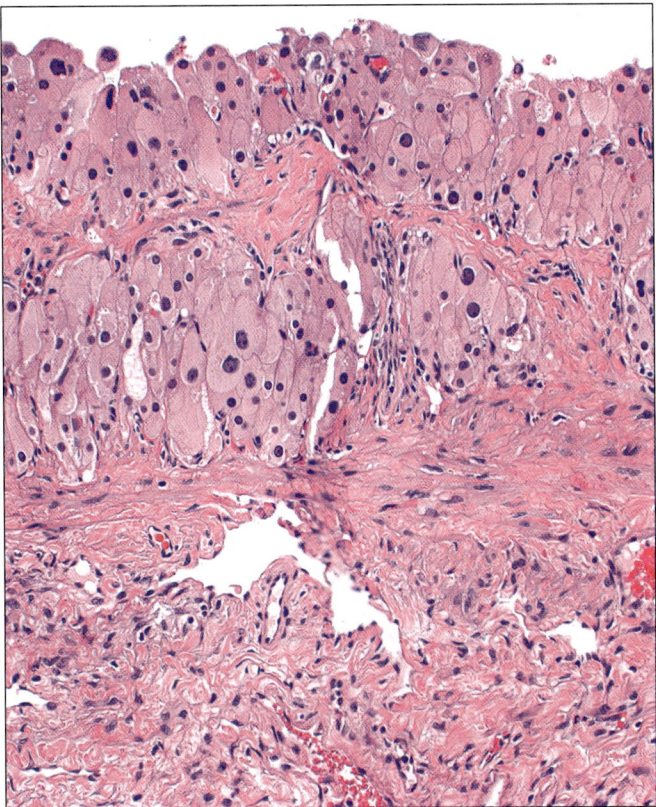

Fig. 22.26   Theca–lutein cyst. Detail of cyst wall showing luteinized cells with pleomorphic hyperchromatic nuclei (same case as Figure 22.25).

LEYDIG (HILUS) CELL HYPERPLASIA

This condition has a close association with pregnancy. It is asymptomatic but may be found incidentally in ovaries biopsied or excised for indications such as tumor. For greater detail, see below.

DECIDUOSIS

Etiology

Deciduosis (extrauterine decidual change) is a quasi-physiologic process that arises in the subcelomic mesenchyme as a result of the progesterone stimulus of pregnancy. It is thus an expression of müllerianosis (see Chapter 33). It can be identified, if carefully sought, in most ovaries from term or near-term pregnancies. It is found with greater difficulty in the first and second trimesters.

Deciduosis also develops on the peritoneal surfaces of other pelvic and abdominal structures and may be exaggerated in patients with trophoblastic disease. This decidual change is also regularly observed in the stroma of ovarian endometriotic deposits during pregnancy.

Gross and microscopic features

Deciduosis appears as serosal macules 1–5 mm across, which are flat or slightly raised in contour. Decidual foci consist of superficial discrete collections of cells cytologically similar to the decidual cells of gestational endometrium, i.e., distinct cell margins, abundant, slightly eosinophilic, finely granular cytoplasm and central, small round pale nuclei with conspicuous

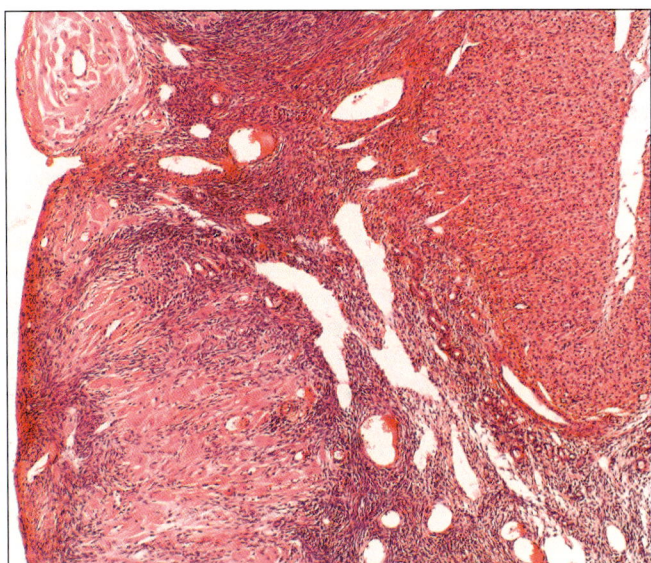

Fig. 22.27   Ovarian deciduosis. Subserosal plaque, with central capillary, plus clustered decidual cells in adjacent cortex. Note stromal luteinization at right.

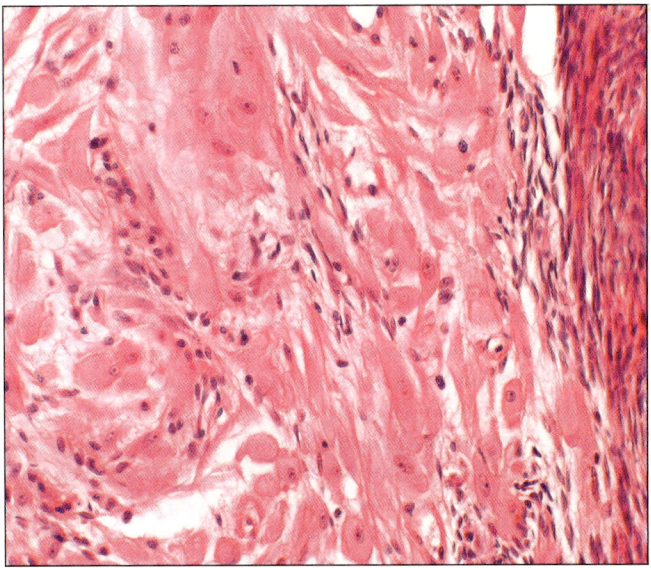

Fig. 22.28   Detail of deciduosis (same case as Figure 22.27). Decidual cells showing abundant cytoplasm, round to oval nuclei with prominent nucleoli. Occasional lymphocytes present.

nucleoli. Capillaries are prominent and the decidual cells sometimes appear to sheath them. A sprinkling of lymphocytes may be present (Figures 22.27 and 22.28). Most commonly the foci are nodular or plaque-like but some lie just beneath the serosal surface and are surrounded by edematous stroma. Decidual foci may become confluent. Individual decidual cells may also be seen, usually adjacent to the larger foci described above.

OVARIAN GRANULOSA CELL PROLIFERATIONS OF PREGNANCY

Definition

Proliferations of granulosa cells occur rarely as incidental findings in pregnant women. The lesions are usually multiple and are present within atretic follicles.[65]

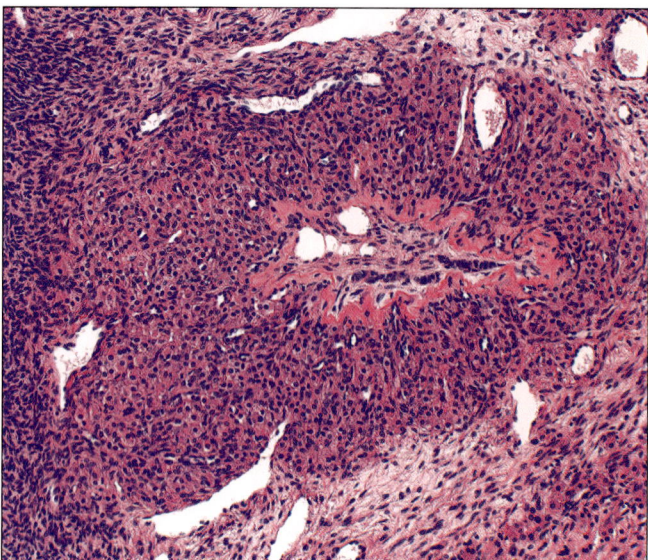

Fig. 22.29 Re-emergence of granulosa cells within an atretic follicular remnant in pregnancy. Small trabecular arrangements are seen centrally. The residual perifollicular theca cells are luteinized as are scattered stromal cells nearby.

Microscopic features

The arrangement of the granulosa cells mimics similar patterns seen with granulosa cell tumors, i.e., solid, microfollicular, trabecular or insular (Figure 22.29). Usually, the granulosa cells contain scanty cytoplasm and grooved nuclei resembling the cells of the adult-type granulosa cell tumor. Less commonly, the cells are luteinized with non-grooved nuclei of variable size, or sertoliform with vacuolated cytoplasm suggestive of lipid.

OVARIAN PREGNANCY

Definition

Definitive diagnosis of ovarian pregnancy requires proof of ovarian nidation and exclusion of tubal nidation with secondary ovarian involvement, and the following criteria are applicable:

- The tube must be intact and clearly separate from the ovary.
- The fetal sac should occupy the normal position of the ovary and be connected to the uterus by the utero-ovarian ligament.
- Definite ovarian tissue must be present in the sac wall. (These criteria become more difficult to establish in more advanced gestations. In these cases confirmation of ovarian pregnancy requires the demonstration of ovarian tissue at several places in the fetal sac wall.)
- The serum β-hCG should fall to non-pregnant levels upon removal of the ovarian lesion.

Etiology

Ovarian nidation occurs about once in every 10 000 pregnancies and accounts for approximately 0.5–3% of ectopic gestations.[23,59,60] Exceptionally rarely, the ovarian nidation may be multiple,[45] or occur with an isochronous intrauterine pregnancy.[48,68] A strong relationship exists between ovarian ectopic pregnancies and use of intrauterine contraceptive devices

(IUDs), but the nature of this relationship remains unclear.[59] In marked contrast to patients with tubal ectopics, patients with ovarian pregnancies are highly fertile and have a lower than average incidence of pelvic inflammatory disease and endometriosis. The pathogenesis is best explained by chance fertilization of an unexpectedly mature ovum within the fimbria, or on the ovarian surface, and subsequent implantation in the ovarian parenchyma. Intrafollicular implantation and development of the conceptus within the corpus luteum itself is considered highly unlikely. This is not only because the ovum would not have completed its first meiotic division and matured to the point of being able to accept fertilization, but also because of the inhospitable environment in the hemorrhagic corpus luteum. Ovarian endometriosis is thought to play no role in local nidation.

Microscopic features

Histologic examination is necessary to confirm that trophoblastic tissue is present in juxtaposition to unequivocal ovarian structures. A corpus luteum of pregnancy can often be identified close to the hemorrhagic implantation site (Figures 22.30 and 22.31). Deciduosis and other pregnancy-associated alterations may be noted in the adjacent parenchyma. If a partial rather than a complete oophorectomy has been performed, it may be difficult to confirm the diagnosis solely by pathologic examination of the material submitted.

PRIMARY OVARIAN TROPHOBLASTIC DISEASE

Ovarian hydatidiform mole is an extremely rare lesion that develops subsequent to ovarian pregnancy. The ovary is grossly enlarged and replaced by an encapsulated hemorrhagic mass of vesicles. Confirmation of primary ovarian origin requires exclusion of extension from a molar pregnancy arising within the uterus or fallopian tube as well as demonstration that the molar tissue is intraovarian. Gestational choriocarcinoma in the ovary may be either metastatic from the uterus or a primary tumor developing subsequent to ovarian pregnancy.[20,51] Exclusion of the former beyond reasonable doubt is implicit in confirming the latter possibility, something that is extraordinarily difficult to do. It has been suggested that a useful term would be 'choriocarcinoma occurring solely in the ovary' rather than forcing a particular case into the primary or metastatic category. Ovarian choriocarcinoma can also coexist with an apparently normal uterogestation, further confounding the issue. The morphology of choriocarcinoma and the problems in diagnosis of non-gestational choriocarcinoma (germ cell tumor)[3] are discussed in Chapter 27.

OTHER OVARIAN LESIONS

TORSION

Between 10 and 20% of all cases of torsion of both tumorous and non-tumorous ovaries occurs during pregnancy[7] and is thought to be due to physiologic dislocation of the ovaries in pregnancy and the softening and edema of the pelvic tissues, especially ligaments. Torsion involves all forms of cysts and neoplasms that occur during the reproductive years (see below) and rarely may even involve a primary ovarian pregnancy itself.[54]

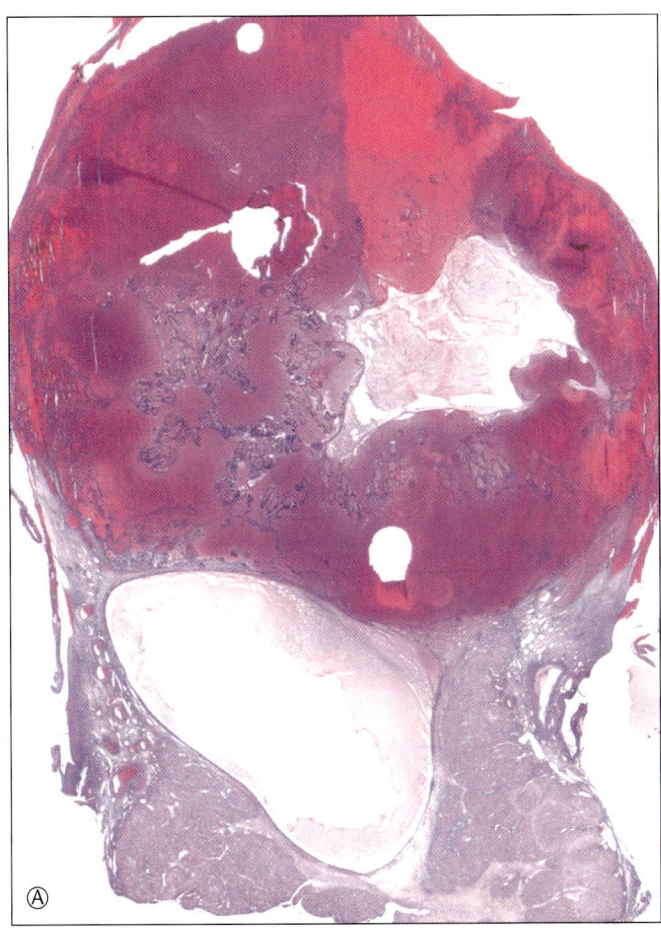

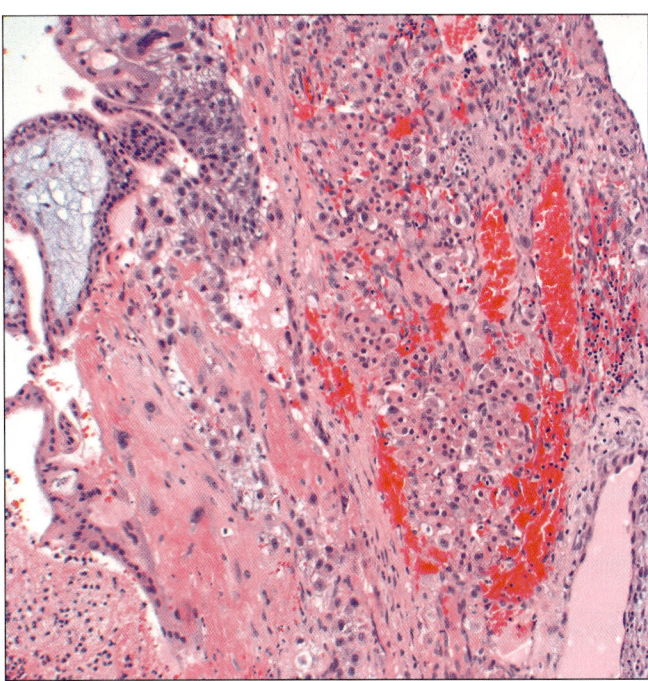

Fig. 22.31 Ectopic ovarian pregnancy. Note immature villi and villous trophoblast to the left and scattered extravillous trophoblastic cells infiltrating the granulosa lutein cells of the corpus luteum to the right.

DISSEMINATED PERITONEAL LEIOMYOMATOSIS

Disseminated peritoneal leiomyomatosis displays innumerable nodules, 2–3 mm in diameter, scattered throughout the peritoneal cavity but particularly conspicuous in the pelvis and omentum. Ovarian involvement occurs in 25% of cases. The nodules are superficial, discrete and well circumscribed, and composed of whorled smooth muscle, similar to the familiar uterine leiomyomas; they may also contain some fibroblasts and decidual cells. The condition usually presents in association with pregnancy or use of the oral contraceptive pill. Resolution may be spontaneous after parturition but can also be accelerated by progesterone (see Chapters 25 and 33).

OVARIAN NEOPLASMS

The true incidence of ovarian neoplasms in pregnancy is difficult to assess from the literature and to a great extent depends on the method of diagnosis (clinical or surgical) and whether non-neoplastic lesions have been included.[9,58,66] A reasonable figure based on multiple series is one tumor per 1000 live births, of which 2–5% are malignant (contrasted with 20% of ovarian tumors in general) (Table 22.3).

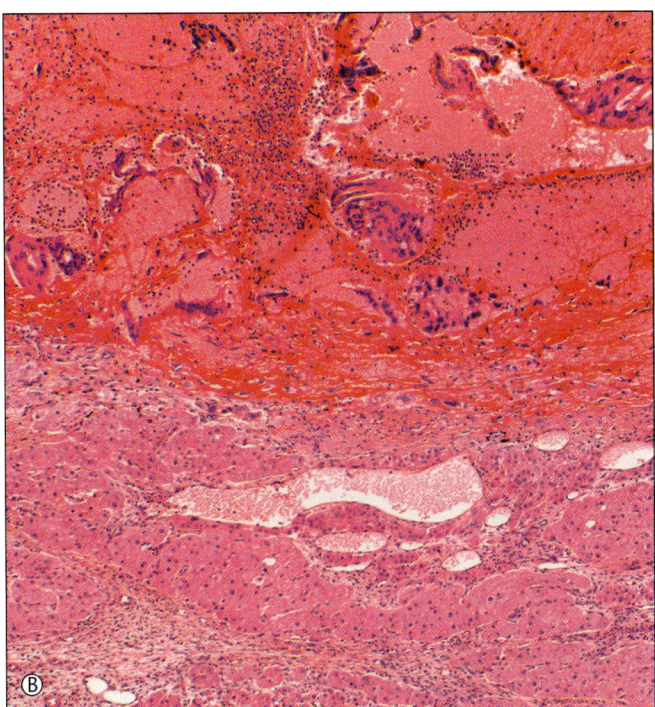

Fig. 22.30 Ectopic ovarian pregnancy. **(A)** Chorionic vesicle and immature villi surrounded by blood clot. Corpus luteum at bottom. **(B)** Higher power showing juxtaposition of immature villous tissue and corpus luteum.

REACTIVE STROMAL TUMOR-LIKE LESIONS

POLYCYSTIC OVARY SYNDROME

Definition

Polycystic ovary syndrome (PCOS) is the prototypic form of chronic hyperandrogenic anovulation. It is a common heterogeneous metabolic disorder that is often familial, affecting at least 10% of reproductive women. By definition, the syndrome

Table 22.3 Primary ovarian tumors diagnosed or removed during pregnancy*

Surface epithelial–stromal tumors	
Serous	
Benign	13
Proliferating	1
Mucinous	
Benign	24
Proliferating	1
Malignant	1
Sex cord–stromal tumors	
Thecoma	1
Sclerosing stromal tumor	1
Fibroma	1
Germ cell tumors (teratomas)	
Immature	1
Mature (dermoid cysts)	67
Monodermal (struma)	2
Total	133

*119 157 livebirths King George V Hospital 1950–1975.

Table 22.4 Criteria for diagnosing polycystic ovary syndrome and related disorders

Criteria of the US National Institutes of Health

Polycystic ovary syndrome
  Presence of menstrual abnormalities and anovulation
  Presence of clinical and/or biochemical hyperandrogenemia
  Absence of hyperprolactinemia or thyroid disease
  Absence of late-onset congenital adrenal hyperplasia
  Absence of Cushings syndrome

Polycystic ovaries
  Presence of polycystic ovaries on ultrasound examination
  Absence of menstrual or cosmetic symptoms
  Absence of biochemical hyperandrogenemia

Idiopathic hirsutism
  Presence of excess hair growth
  Absence of biochemical hyperandrogenemia

Proposed criteria (European Society of Human Reproduction and Embryology and American Society of Reproductive Medicine)*

Polycystic ovary syndrome is diagnosed if any two of the following are present:
  Presence of polycystic ovaries on ultrasound examination
  Clinical or biochemical hyperandrogenism
  Menstrual dysfunction with anovulation

* Symposium on PCOS, Rotterdam, The Netherlands, 1 May 2003.

is unassociated with any underlying adrenal or pituitary disorders or ovarian tumors. It may manifest hyperinsulinemia, hyperlipidemia, diabetes mellitus, and cardiac disease, as well as the better recognized hyperandrogenism, hirsutism, infertility, and chronic anovulation.

Presenting features are, to some extent, age dependent, from precocious puberty in childhood, through hirsutism and menstrual irregularities in teenagers, infertility and glucose intolerance in adulthood, to frank diabetes and cardiovascular disease in older patients.

The term 'polycystic ovaries' as used by some applies to many (possibly up to 25%) asymptomatic women with typical ultrasound features,[39] the term 'polycystic ovary syndrome' being reserved for those women who have morphologic features of polycystic ovaries associated with typical clinical symptoms. Indeed, some recent publications exclude polycystic ovaries as a key diagnostic criterion for PCOS (Table 22.4). Polycystic ovaries may simply reflect the pathology of that subset of women who seem to ovulate best when thin, unlike their 'normal' counterparts who need a certain amount of body fat to ovulate regularly and would thus become amenorrheic when pathologically thin. Some believe that 'polyfollicular' should replace the term 'polycystic' and that 'functional hyperandrogenism' should replace 'PCOS'.[28]

Etiology

The disorder is probably the most common hormonal abnormality in women of reproductive age and certainly is a leading cause of infertility. In young women, precocious puberty and hyperinsulinemia are early manifestations of PCOS. It is frequently associated with insulin resistance and type 2 diabetes, possibly on the basis of pancreatic β-cell dysfunction,[55] and management with insulin sensitizers such as metformin is currently popular for the induction of ovulation.[25] Obesity exacerbates the insulin resistance and favors the progression from impaired glucose tolerance to clinical diabetes in these patients.[64] Whether obesity is a cause or an effect of PCOS is unclear, but the latter is more likely. A valid distinction is possible between

the 'lean' and 'obese' PCOS patient. The typical obesity of PCOS is abdominal, rather than in the thighs and hips – the type associated with greater risk of hypertension, diabetes, and lipid abnormalities. A key to the way the body uses energy is insulin, which promotes the storage of fat to ensure a constant source of fuel, calories, ensuring the body's most efficient operation.

Insulin also, in turn, signals the body to release testosterone, with somatic as well as skin and hair manifestations. Skin symptoms, such as acne or hirsutism, are not only determined by serum androgen levels but also by the activity of the skin's hormone receptors and the activity of enzymes such as 5-α reductase. Women who exhibit amenorrhea, hirsutism, and enlarged polycystic ovaries represent the severe end of the disease spectrum.

One significant study suggests that an increase of antimüllerian hormone (AMH) serum level in PCOS is the consequence of the androgen-induced excess in small developing antral follicles and that each follicle produces a normal amount of AMH.[57] Possibly an increased AMH tone within the cohort affects follicular arrest so characteristic of PCOS by interacting negatively with FSH at the time of selection.

A distinct familial clustering of women with PCOS suggests that hereditary factors are also etiologically important. Indeed, PCOS is currently thought to be related to interactions of susceptibility and protective genomic variants, modified by environmental factors. Candidate genes for PCOS include those related to androgenic pathways and metabolic associations of the syndrome. More recently, genes encoding inflammatory cytokines have been identified as target genes for PCOS, as proinflammatory genotypes and phenotypes are also associated with obesity, insulin resistance, type 2 diabetes, PCOS, and increased cardiovascular risk.[62] From a series of linkage and association studies using affected sibling-pair analysis and the transmission/disequilibrium test to explore candidate genes, evidence is mounting for a susceptibility gene that maps near D19S884 on chromosome 19p13.3.

Existing data suggest that the putative PCOS gene lying in this region is probably involved in signal transduction mechanisms leading to altered expression of a suite of genes that affect theca cell steroidogenesis as well as the metabolic phenotype of other cell types, including muscle and fat.[71] Nevertheless, despite much detailed investigation, no one gene seems to play a pivotal role in the genesis of PCOS. It remains probable that PCOS is the final outcome of different, interrelated genetic anomalies that influence each other and perpetuate the syndrome.[26]

Investigational profile

Nearly all patients with PCOS have at least subtle laboratory abnormalities. Often, they are at the upper limits of 'normal', showing only a tendency, rather than a discrete abnormality. By contrast, serious pathology may be more evident by a marked elevation, or suppression, of a single test. Glucose (fasting insulin levels and a glucose tolerance test) and lipid testing should be in the morning after fasting (no food or drink after midnight the night before).

Many have sustained high LH levels due to an increase in LH pulse size and frequency. These high LH levels (usually above 20 IU/L) are involved in the excessive theca cell growth and consequent androgen production. Amongst women with PCOS, this subgroup with high serum LH levels is at highest risk for infertility and miscarriage.[33] Most patients have normal or slightly lower levels of FSH, and an LH:FSH ratio greater than 2. Provided the LH level is not lower than 8 IU/L, this may be used to suggest the diagnosis in women with clinical features of PCOS.

Hyperinsulinemia or abnormalities of the insulin-like growth factor axis are frequently found. Although the women are often obese, their hyperinsulinemia appears independent of their obesity. Insulin inhibits sex hormone-binding globulin production and stimulates ovarian androgen production.[63] Most have demonstrable androgen excess with raised levels of total testosterone (usually 2.4–4.2 nmol/L), androstenedione (usually 10.5–17.5 nmol/L), DHEA, and DHEA sulfate (about 40% of women with PCOS will have at least one of these androgens elevated). Obese and anovulatory women with PCOS usually have low levels of sex hormone-binding globulin, resulting in high free testosterone levels. The presence or absence of hirsutism depends on whether or not these androgens are converted peripherally by 5-α reductase to the more potent androgen DHT (dihydrotestosterone) and 3-α-diol-G as reflected by increased levels of 3-α-diol-G.

About 20% of women with PCOS also have mildly elevated levels of prolactin (20–30 ng/mL), possibly related to increased pulsatility of gonadotrophin-releasing hormone (GnRH) or to a relative dopamine deficiency, or both.

The most consistent ultrasound feature is the presence of more than 10 peripherally placed symmetrical small follicles (2–8 mm in diameter – the so-called 'string of pearls') in association with increased stroma and often an ovarian volume greater than 12 cm³. In some cases the ovary is virtually filled with small cysts. In other cases, it is heterogeneously dense with barely detectable microcystic changes (some women with characteristic clinical features of PCOS have normal-sized ovaries). It must be remembered that any hyperandrogenic state may be manifested by these appearances in the ovaries. Diffusely

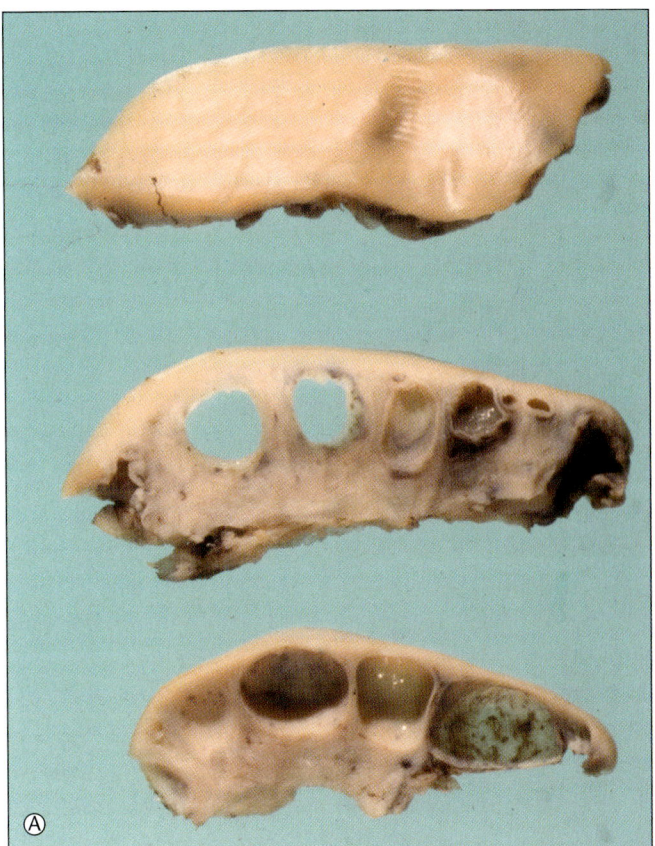

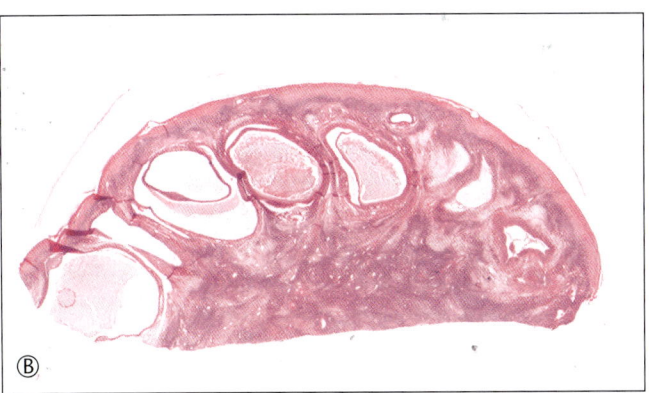

Fig. 22.32 Polycystic ovary syndrome. **(A)** Cut surface showing thickened capsule and relatively uniform development of antral follicles. **(B)** Whole mount of same case highlighting above features as well as absence of stigmata of ovulation.

enlarged ovaries without a discrete mass on ultrasound, in the absence of adrenal findings, are consistent with the diagnosis of hyperthecosis, which is probably a less common variant in the PCOS spectrum.

Gross features

Both ovaries are ovoid or globular and usually symmetrically enlarged to twice their normal size or more, with a thickened glistening white capsule. The cut surfaces typically show a somewhat thickened capsule with a linear subcapsular aggregation of multiple small follicles up to about 8 mm in diameter and containing clear fluid, and an absence of stigmata of previous ovulation (Figure 22.32).

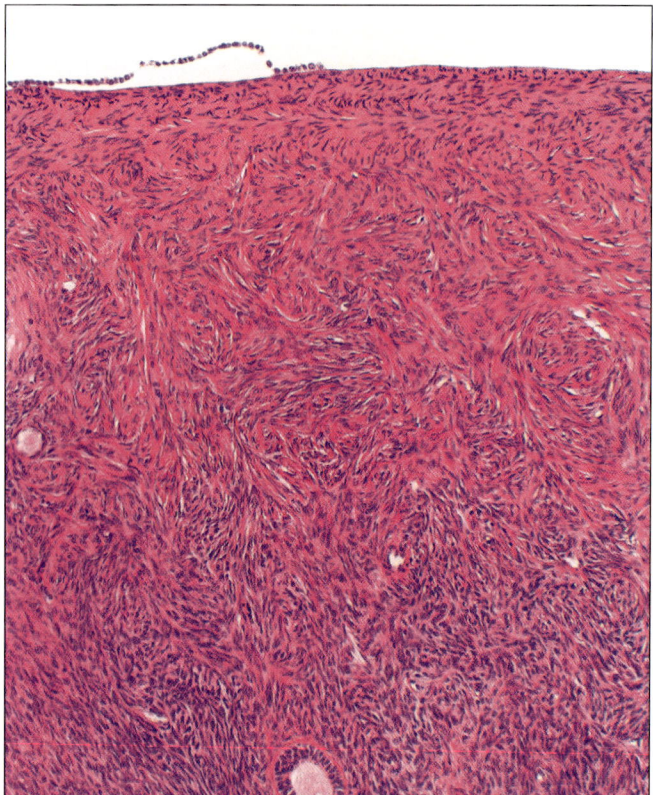

Fig. 22.33 Low power of thickened and somewhat fibrotic tunica delimited by the serosa and subjacent primordial and primary follicles.

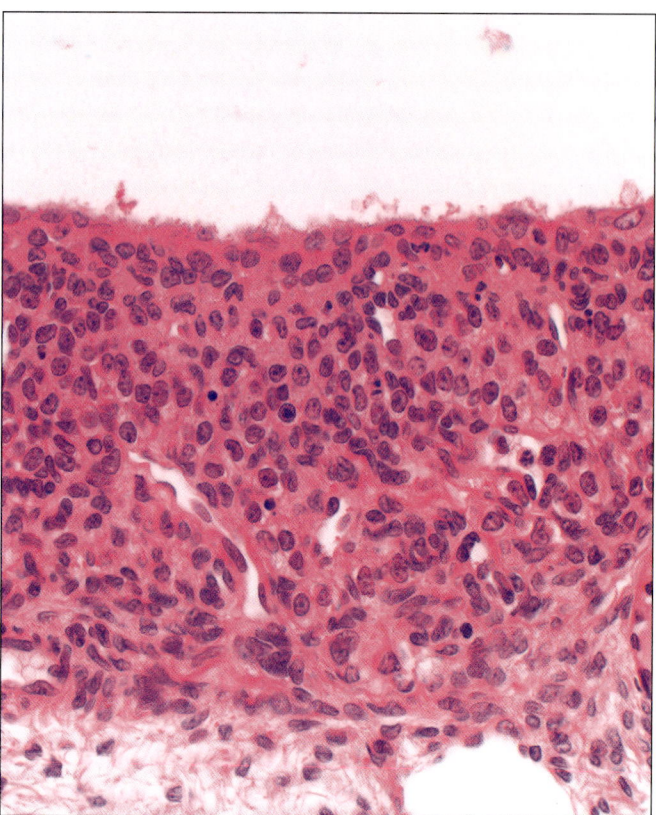

Fig. 22.34 Polycystic ovary syndrome. Hyperplastic and partly luteinized theca interna and an attenuated, effete granulosa (top) are typical changes in many of the follicles.

Microscopic features

The tunica albuginea is usually but not always thickened, often three-fold, but occasionally up to 10-fold, with an accentuation of the layered interlacing bundles of acellular fibrocollagenous connective tissue (Figure 22.33). This finding is not specific for PCOS and is found in many anovulatory states. Follicular development deviates markedly from normal in many ways. Primordial follicles are present in appropriate or slightly reduced numbers and there are many cystic follicles at about the 4–8 mm stage of development (Figure 22.32B). The relatively uniform size of the cystic follicles is a typical feature of PCOS. Anovulatory women will have a conspicuous absence of residua of ovulation. Follicular atresia is prominent. Apart from aberrant follicular development, theca cell hyperplasia occurs in all cases. The theca interna layer is often two to three times thicker than normal. The theca cells may be larger than normal with more obvious eosinophilic cytoplasm or appear frankly luteinized. The granulosa of these follicles is either indistinguishable from normal or exhibits early regressive changes with disaggregation and lack of mitotic activity.

Atretic follicles may also show persistence of the prominent theca cell layer (Figure 22.34). The persistence of these theca cells, often to the point where other components of the atretic follicles have completely disappeared, offers a possible explanation for the infrequent, isolated aggregates or clusters of such cells in the deep cortical and medullary stroma (Figure 22.35). These clusters are occasionally seen in normal ovaries but are much more prominent in, and typical of, hyperthecosis.

Differential diagnosis

The morphologic changes described above have been found in other clinical settings such as 92% of women with idiopathic hirsutism, 87% of women with oligomenorrhea, 82% of women with congenital adrenal hyperplasia, and almost 25% of 'normal women'. They should, therefore, be regarded as typical but not diagnostic of polycystic ovary syndrome. Using pelvic ultrasound, polycystic ovaries and multicystic ovaries may be difficult to distinguish, although the main characteristic feature of polycystic ovaries is the presence of more than 10 peripheral small follicles in association with increased stroma. Clinically, late onset congenital adrenal hyperplasia and other virilizing disorders may mimic polycystic ovaries.

For the pathologist, other conditions that may resemble polycystic ovary syndrome include the ovarian hyperstimulation syndrome, the swollen ovary syndrome, and hyperreactio luteinalis with multiple theca–lutein cysts and prominence of luteinized stromal cells in enlarged ovaries. The clinical context of this latter condition associated with a pregnancy episode or trophoblastic disease hardly lends itself to ready confusion.

STROMAL HYPERPLASIA AND HYPERTHECOSIS

Definitions and clinical features

Stromal hyperplasia is the exaggerated presence of cortical stroma that is characteristically ovarian. Mild hyperplasia of the cortical and medullary stroma is found in the ovaries of about one-third of perimenopausal and postmenopausal women. It is

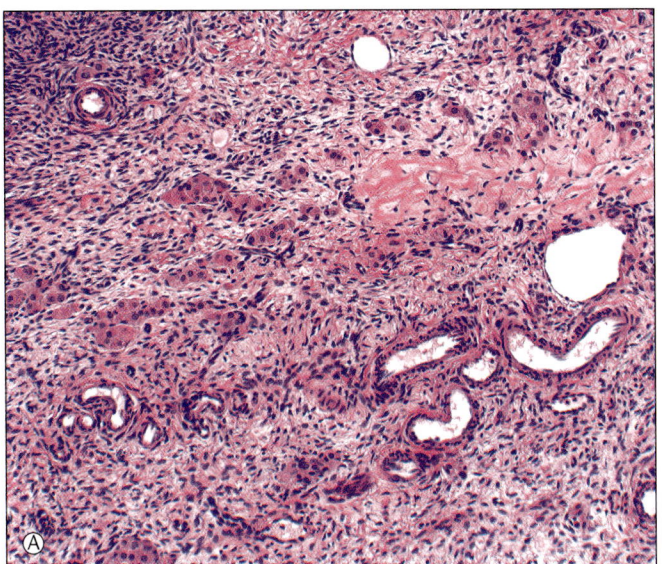

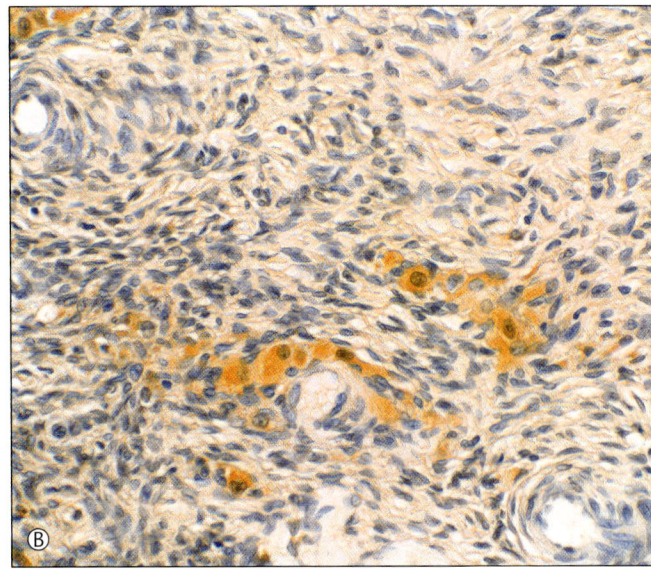

Fig. 22.35 Polycystic ovary syndrome. **(A)** Clusters of prominent stromal lutein cells with rounded nuclei and eosinophilic slightly granular cytoplasm, around an old follicular remnant. **(B)** The prominence of these cells is enhanced through immunostaining for estradiol.

nearly always diffusely bilateral. As the apparent severity of the changes does not correlate well with clinical symptomatology, some suggest that the term 'stromal hyperplasia' should be reserved for definite and florid cases. Minimum criteria should be an obliterated normal distinction between cortex and medulla or at least some nodularity to the proliferating stroma. Most women are older and many are postmenopausal. Clinical symptoms result from excess androgen (androstenedione) production by the hyperplastic stroma,[43,70] with or without dominant peripheral aromatization to estrone.[35]

Hyperthecosis is the presence of luteinized cells of thecal origin located in the stroma distant from the follicles. They may be single or in groups, clustered or scattered diffusely. Hyperthecosis occurs regularly in association with ovarian stromal hyperplasia on the one hand and merges imperceptibly with the polycystic ovary syndrome on the other. Like stromal hyperplasia, it may on occasion be asymptomatic, but is more usually accompanied by marked defeminization and virilization[44] and only occasionally by estrogenic signs. Although isolated luteinized stromal cells are common in postmenopausal ovaries, clinical hyperthecosis occurs mostly in women of reproductive age and may rarely present as virilization in pregnancy that ameliorates spontaneously after delivery, or as endometrial hyperplasia. Not rarely, these changes are seen in association with endometrial hyperplasias and cancer.

Gross features

Both ovaries are enlarged, up to twice normal size. The capsule is thickened and the cut surface is uniformly pale yellow to fawn in color, often with blurring of the division into cortex and medulla (Figure 22.36). In severe cases, nodularity will be present.

Microscopic features

Stromal hyperplasia shows a variable but marked proliferation of plump but otherwise undistinguished spindled stromal cells, each invested by reticulin fibrils, recapitulating the storiform swathes and whorls of normal ovarian stroma (Figure 22.37).

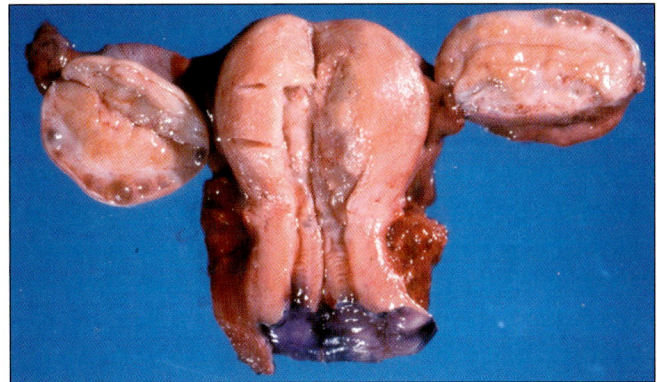

Fig. 22.36 Cortical stromal hyperplasia. Extrafascial hysterectomy for endometrial carcinoma (note tumor in right fundus). Ovaries are uniformly enlarged and the soft, fawn cut surface shows blurring of usual distinction between cortex and medulla.

The medulla is most affected by this proliferation and the usually obvious corticomedullary interface may be obliterated. Stromal hyperplasia may be entirely diffuse (Figure 22.38), but rather more commonly exhibits a focal or widespread nodular pattern, particularly in the cortex. Fat stains usually reveal widespread intracytoplasmic lipid. Small foci of hyalinization are quite frequently encountered in the superficial cortex (Figure 22.39). Some lesions include histiocytes, which impart an overall 'granulomatous' character microscopically, suggesting an end stage regression of the luteinized stromal cells.

Stromal hyperthecosis is typified by isolated or aggregated lutein-like cells throughout each ovary. These cells generally are more numerous in the medulla (Figure 22.40) than the cortex (Figure 22.41), and they are large and polyhedral with abundant eosinophilic granular or finely vacuolated cytoplasm and rounded central nuclei, each with a single, small to sometimes prominent nucleolus (Figure 22.40). Focal regression is sometimes seen with hyalinization and a mild lymphohistiocytic infiltrate (Figure 22.42). A continuum exists between such diffuse cases and those in which the lutein cells form multiple

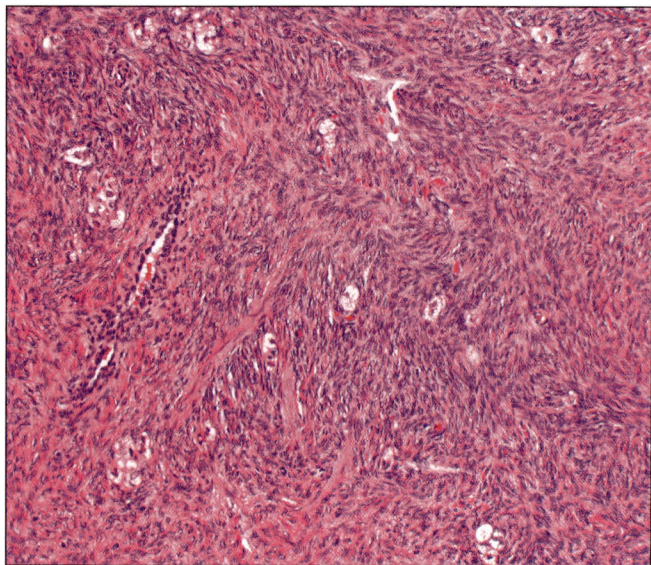

Fig. 22.37 Cortical stromal hyperplasia. Characterized by swirls and bands of small spindle cells, more cellular but otherwise indistinguishable from normal ovarian cortex. It is a moot point as to how prominent isolated luteinized cells with foamy cytoplasm can be without reclassifying a lesion as hyperthecosis (see Figure 22.41).

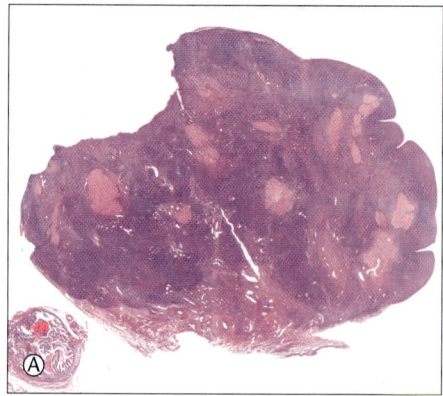

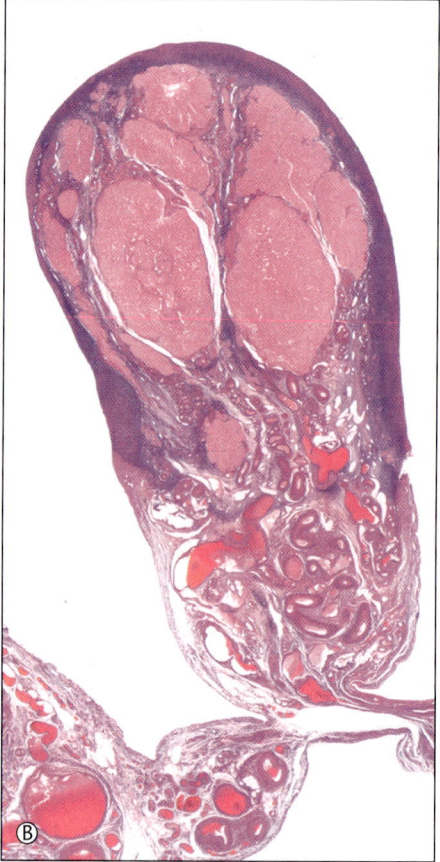

Fig. 22.38 **(A)** Section of diffusely hyperplastic postmenopausal ovary. Note obliteration of normal corticomedullary junction. **(B)** Normal postmenopausal ovary for comparison.

discrete small nodules (Figure 22.43 – nodular stromal hyperthecosis). The cortex frequently contains small cystic follicles, each with a prominent luteinized theca interna layer. Stigmata of recent ovulation are absent, but follicular atresia is sometimes increased.

Differential diagnosis

In occasional cases, one or more of these nodules becomes dominant, suggesting a neoplasm graced by a specific name – stromal luteoma. In accord with similar pathologic processes in other endocrine glands (e.g., thyroid, parathyroid), the diagnosis of stromal luteoma should be made with caution in the presence of multiple hyperplastic nodules of theca-like cells, and the term is best reserved for those lipid cell tumors of stromal origin that arise in the absence of such diffuse or nodular ovarian stromal hyperplasia or hyperthecosis. These tumor-like nodules are comprised entirely of large rounded lutein cells (Figure 22.44), and average about 1 cm in diameter. Reinke crystalloids are absent, distinguishing them from Leydig cell tumors of stromal (or non-hilar) origin. Paradoxically, Leydig cell hyperplasia and Leydig cell tumors may also occur in association with hyperthecosis. The spindled non-luteinized theca-like cells of partly luteinized thecomas (see Chapter 26) are also absent, as are the perivascular hyaline plaques typical of thecomas.

Behavior and treatment

Virilizing hyperthecosis, unlike polycystic ovary syndrome, tends not to respond to clomiphene treatment, but a measure of success has been achieved with the use of GnRH agonists.[40]

LEYDIG (HILUS) CELL HYPERPLASIA

Definition

Leydig cells are rounded to polygonal cells with moderately sized, vesicular, central nuclei and eosinophilic, granular to

finely vacuolated cytoplasm that are infrequently observed in routine sections of the ovaries unless specifically sought, despite their documented presence in at least 80% of cases. Their casual observation, therefore, usually indicates some degree of hyperplasia.

Etiology

Prominent Leydig cells are most regularly seen in response to raised gonadotrophin levels during pregnancy or at the menopause. Occasionally the pregnancy-associated Leydig cell hyperplasia is severe, sufficient to produce visible mitotic activity in these cells (an otherwise extremely rare occurrence). In non-pregnant women, Leydig cell hyperplasia most frequently occurs against a background of stromal hyperplasia and hyperthecosis.

Clinical features

Leydig cell hyperplasia is generally of a mild degree and unassociated with clinical endocrine disturbance. Although the endocrine profile is not consistent or specific for Leydig cell hyperplasia, there may be increased serum testosterone levels.

Microscopic features

The hyperplasia appears as clusters and nodules of typical rounded or polygonal Leydig cells with moderately sized, vesicular, central nuclei and eosinophilic, granular to finely vacuolated cytoplasm (Figure 22.45). Yellow-brown intracytoplasmic lipochrome (lipofuscin) pigment is often focally observed, and Reinke crystalloids are sometimes found in occasional cells although they may be sparse. Their prominence does not cor-

relate with the severity of the hyperplasia. Nuclear pleomorphism is not common, although bizarre hyperchromatic nuclei may be encountered in the hyperplastic Leydig cells of postmenopausal women.

The nodules or clusters of Leydig cells vary greatly from area to area and, although most prominent in the ovarian hilus, may extend into the mesovarium. Small capillary vessels are identifiable amongst the Leydig cells, and non-myelinated nerves can be disclosed in apposition to many of the cell clusters (Figure 22.46). Cells immunostain strongly for α-inhibin and calretinin.

Leydig cells (with typical Reinke crystalloids) may also be found in a limited range of hyperplastic and neoplastic conditions, derived from the ovarian stroma and distinct from the ovarian hilus cells. These non-neoplastic stromal Leydig cells may be seen in simple stromal hyperplasias or stromal proliferations reactive to metastatic carcinomas or primary epithe-

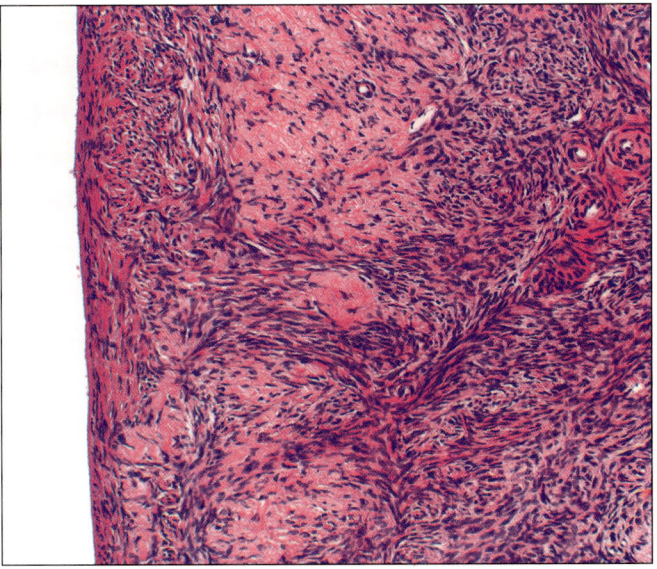

Fig. 22.39   Cortical stromal hyperplasia. Focal hyalinization but no 'granulomas'.

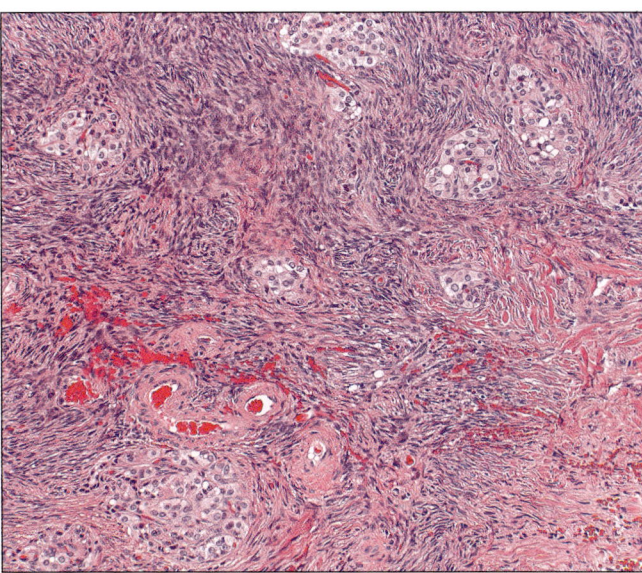

Fig. 22.41   Stromal hyperthecosis. Discrete clusters of luteinized stromal cells in hyperplastic cortical stroma.

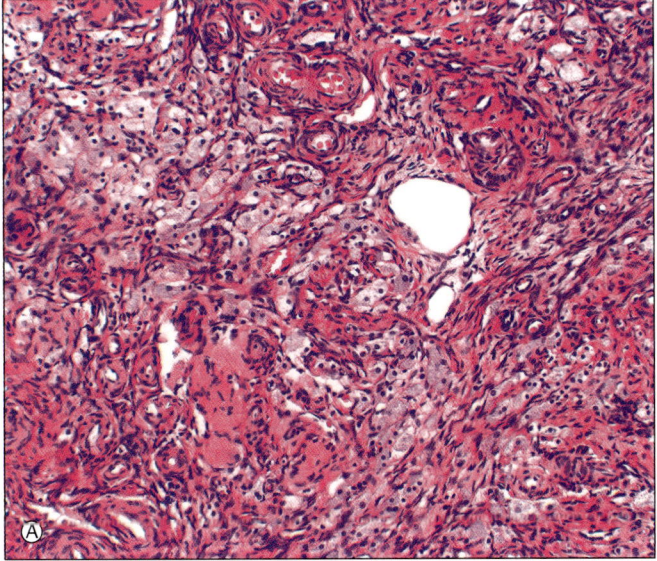

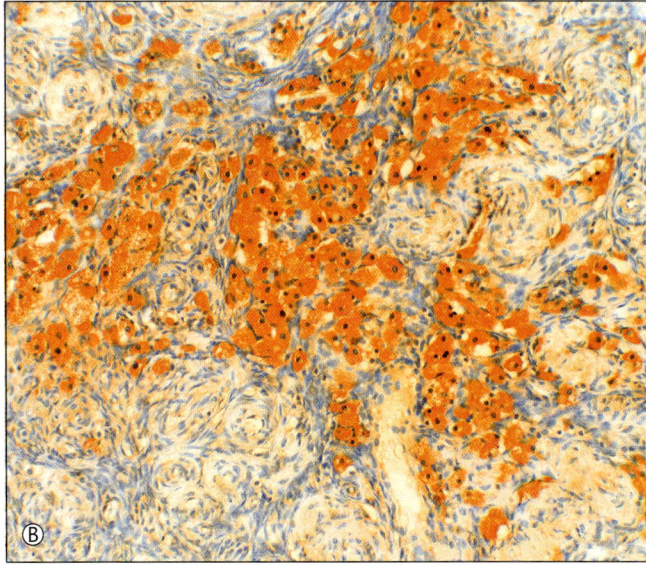

Fig. 22.40   Stromal hyperthecosis. Medullary clusters of luteinized stromal cells. **(A)** H&E; **(B)** immunostain for estradiol.

lial ovarian neoplasms (see Chapter 24). Rarely, typical Leydig cells are noted in benign ovarian stromal tumors, the so-called 'stromal-Leydig cell tumors' and 'pure Leydig cell tumors of non-hilar type'. Unlike Leydig cell tumors of hilus cell origin, these lesions are characteristically multinodular, bilateral, and found in ovaries with stromal hyperplasia and hyperthecosis.

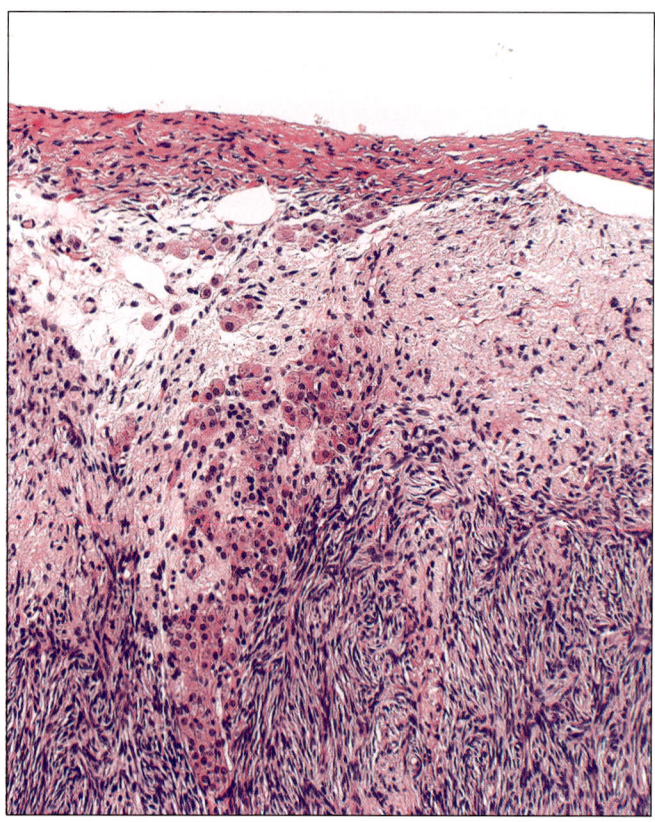

Fig. 22.42 Hyperthecosis. A small collection of residual luteinized stromal cells is noted, while the remainder of the focus has undergone hyalinization.

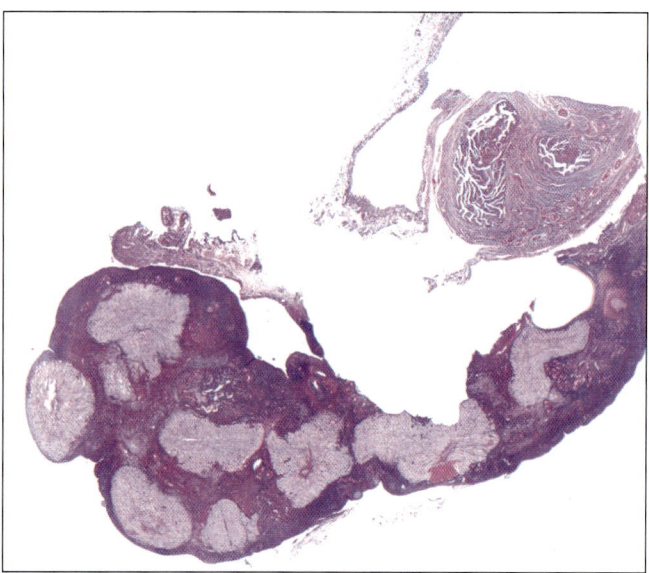

Fig. 22.43 Nodular stromal hyperthecosis from a virilized woman. Multiple discrete nodules of large pale lutein cells against a background of stromal hyperplasia.

MASSIVE OVARIAN EDEMA AND FIBROMATOSIS

MASSIVE OVARIAN EDEMA

Definition
This rare tumor-like entity exhibits gross enlargement of one or both ovaries by an accumulation of edema fluid in the stroma that separates normal follicular structures.

Etiology
Massive ovarian edema is thought to result from partial or intermittent torsion of an otherwise normal ovary (observed at operation in one-half of cases), compromising venous and lymphatic drainage but not causing ischemic necrosis.[12,27,50,53]

Clinical features
Most examples occur in women in their second and third decades, although rarely in prepubertal girls.[27,36,50,52,53] These women present with acute abdominal pain and/or a palpable adnexal mass, and less commonly with menstrual disturbances. Masculinization of varying degrees is sometimes present, clinically suggestive of the polycystic ovary syndrome in some cases, a pathologic condition that may coexist with massive ovarian edema.[30] Possibly, both the edema and the abnormal hormone production result from a local paraendocrine factor.

Gross and microscopic features
The enlarged ovary may be up to 35 cm in diameter (average, 11 cm) with a soft pearly external surface. The cut surface is almost featureless and myxoid, from which regularly exudes protein-rich edema fluid (Figure 22.47). The typical histologic features are diffuse edema of the medulla and inner cortex with relative sparing of the superficial cortex and tunica albuginea, which are often thick and fibrotic. Cystic follicles beneath the tunica (Figure 22.48) and other normal cortical and medullary structures such as corpora albicantia are normal if seen, but separated by loose myxoid tissue. Small fields of normal-appearing ovarian stroma may be present in less edematous

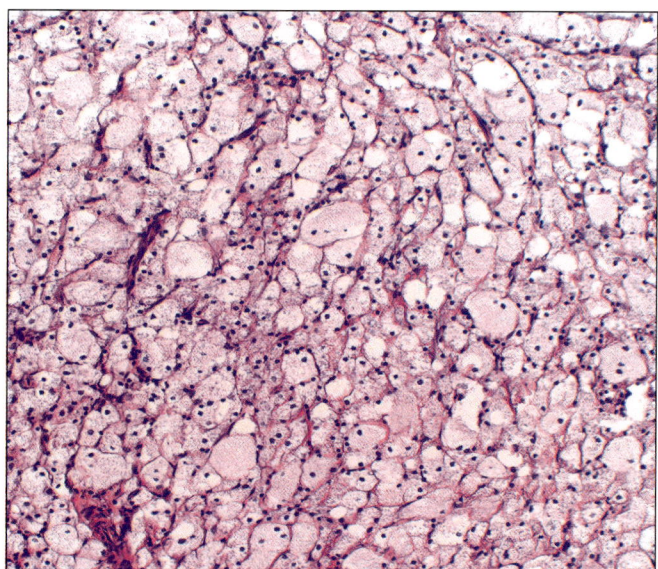

Fig. 22.44 Stromal luteoma. Large vacuolated lutein cells from a solitary 9 mm nodule.

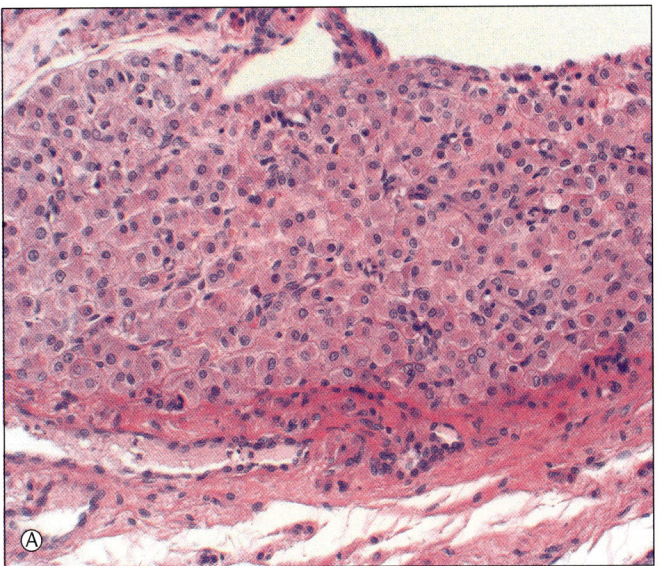
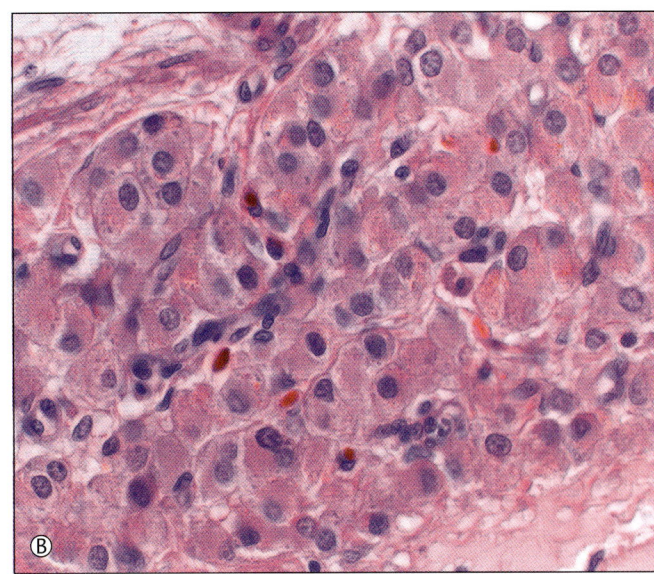

Fig. 22.45 Leydig cell hyperplasia. **(A)** Large nodule of typical polygonal Leydig cells associated with a number of small vessels. **(B)** Leydig cells with uniform, rounded, central, vesicular nuclei and eosinophilic, slightly granular cytoplasm containing abundant cytochrome pigment and occasional refractile Reinke crystals.

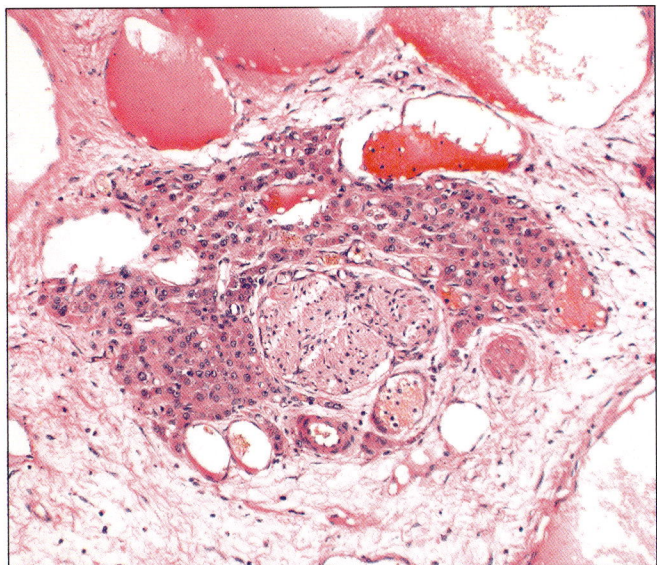

Fig. 22.46 Leydig cell hyperplasia. Small nodule of Leydig cells adjacent to a number of small vessels and sheathing a small nerve.

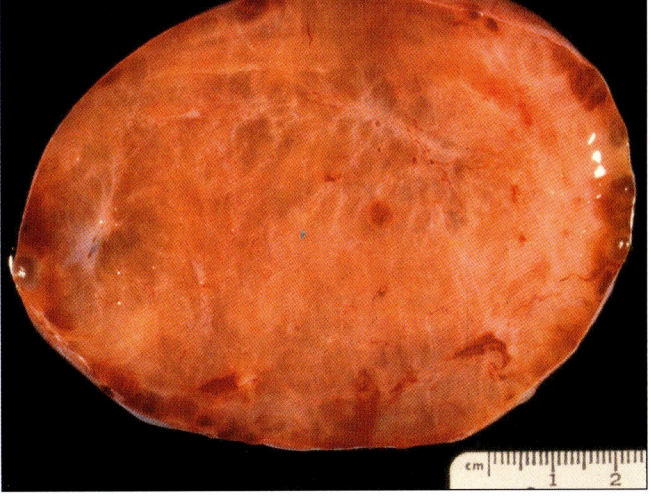

Fig. 22.47 Massive ovarian edema. Featureless cut surface of an ovary with massive edema. Follicles are apparent beneath the capsule.

areas. The marked edema widely separates stellate stromal cells and scanty intervening collagen (Figure 22.49), making vascular and lymphatic channels abnormally prominent. There may be some congestion and foci of red cell extravasation. Small numbers of lymphocytes, mast cells, and macrophages may be observed rarely. Focal necrosis is uncommon. Over 40% of examples show isolated or clustered luteinized stromal cells, thought to be the source of excess steroid hormone production in those patients presenting with virilization. The luteinization is usually confined to edematous areas, but may also be seen in the contralateral edematous or non-edematous ovary. It appears to be related directly to the duration of symptoms.

Differential diagnosis
Other ovarian lesions that may show marked focal or generalized edema include ovarian fibromas and thecofibromas

(see Chapter 26). The relationship between massive ovarian edema and fibromatosis is yet to be settled but is more likely to represent disparate responses to the same pathologic stimulus rather than one (fibromatosis) being a precursor of the other (massive edema). Sclerosing stromal tumors (see Chapter 26) tend to compress the surrounding normal ovarian tissue and have a pseudolobular pattern with focal hyalinization. Metastatic carcinomas and malignant lymphomas may be sufficiently edematous as to grossly resemble massive ovarian edema. This applies particularly to Krukenberg tumors, in which the diagnostic signet-ring cells may be quite sparse indeed. In cases of patchy edema and focal condensation of plump cortical stromal cells, either a stain for mucin, such as with alcian blue, or an immunostain for cytokeratins, is helpful to identify the metastatic signet-ring cells.

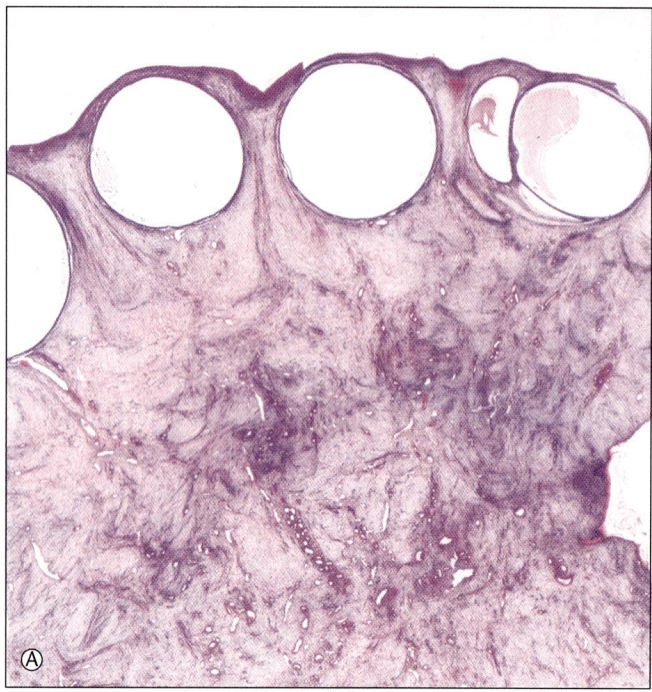

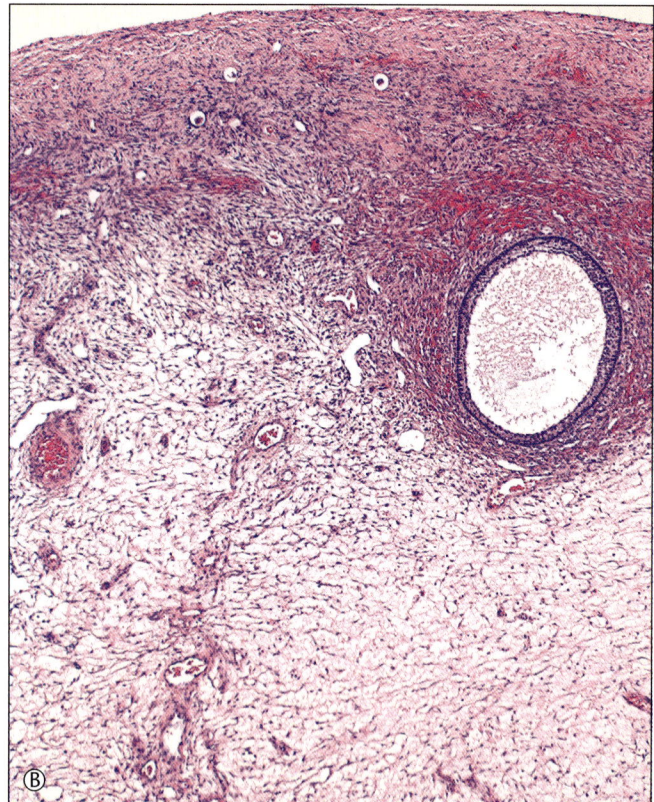

Fig. 22.48 Massive ovarian edema. **(A)** Edema maximal in the deeper cortex and medulla, with relative sparing of the superficial cortex. **(B)** Higher power showing preservation of follicular structures in the superficial cortex.

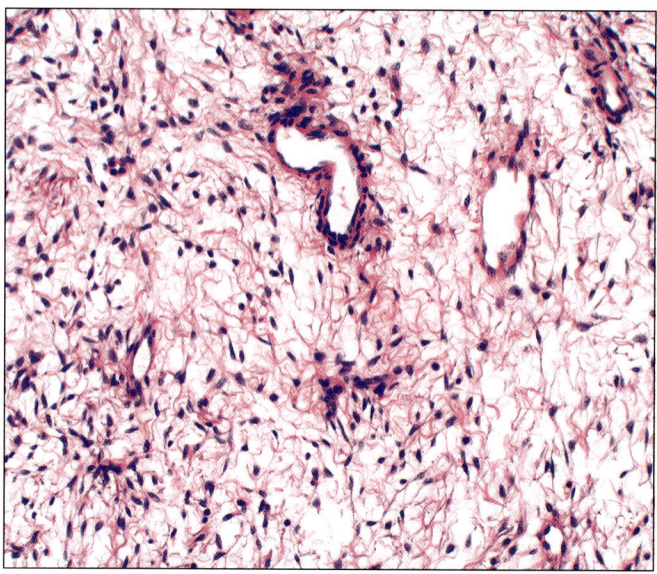

Fig. 22.49 Massive ovarian edema. Stellate stromal cells widely separated by gross interstitial edema. Same case as Figure 22.48A.

is mostly unilateral and furthermore, it is argued, exclusion of an underlying neoplastic process that may have predisposed to the partial torsion in an individual case cannot be achieved without microscopic examination of the enlarged ovary. The young age of the patients, a small but significant risk of bilaterality or of 'recurrence' in the contralateral ovary,[21,61,76] and the consequent importance of retention of reproductive capacity, however, suggest a more conservative approach. Preoperative ultrasound or MRI may be helpful.[74,75] An intraoperative frozen section examination of a large wedge biopsy of the affected ovary to exclude underlying neoplasia and to confirm viability of the edematous ovary can be followed by surgical tethering of the ovary to the uterus or side wall of the pelvis.[38] This course of action is usually, although not always, clinically successful.[32] An alternative conservative approach has involved use of oral contraceptive agents.

FIBROMATOSIS

Definition

The various manifestations of non-neoplastic proliferations of the 'undifferentiated' ovarian stroma collectively may be described as 'fibromatosis'. The term was first applied to a tumor-like condition of unknown cause, characterized by florid overgrowth of collagen-producing spindle cells that enveloped normal follicular structures and led to thickening of the superficial cortex.

Etiology

The strong clinical overlap with massive edema – young age, clinical manifestations of menstrual irregularities, abdominal pain and less commonly virilization, and identification of torsion in some cases at operation – as well as transitional appearances between the two entities, suggest a common pathogenesis. We believe that they represent different parts of a single pathologic spectrum. In our view, many examples in the earlier reports[78] represent the chronic, 'burnt-out' end stage of this florid reactive proliferative process. At the 'immature' or acute end of this pathologic process, the usually large

Behavior and treatment

Unilateral salpingo-oophorectomy has been the traditional surgical procedure for massive ovarian edema, largely driven by a failure to consider the diagnosis preoperatively, or when faced, at laparotomy, with a unilateral solid ovarian 'mass'. It

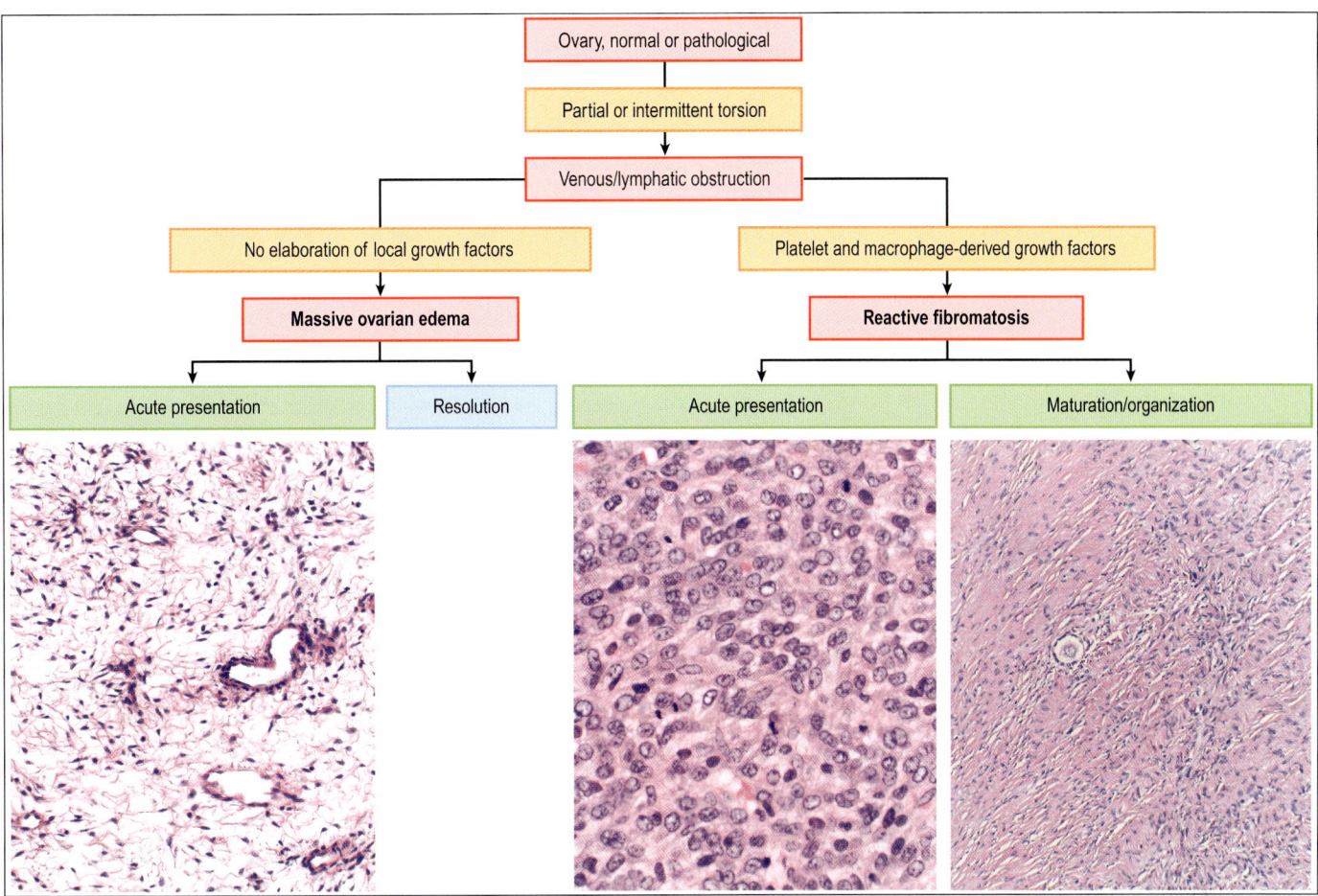

Fig. 22.50 Ovarian fibromatosis and massive edema. Notional relationships within this group of pathologic entities.

ovarian masses are either 'acellular' lesions (typical massive ovarian edema – see above) or, rarely, highly cellular fibroblastic tumor-like lesions that have been variously reported as 'thecomas', 'secondary massive edema', 'sarcoma-like ovarian nodules', 'malignant luteinized thecoma', 'fibromatosis',[67] and 'luteinized thecoma with sclerosing peritonitis'.[15] The characteristics of this combined group are:

- young age (mean age 24 years, range 4–76 years);
- abdominal pain and swelling associated with pelvic masses and ascites/pleural effusions in many cases;
- frequent association between abdominal fibromatosis/sclerosing peritonitis and ovarian fibromatosis/massive ovarian edema;
- occasional exposure to antiepileptic drugs or to β-adrenergic blocking agents (particularly in patients under 10 years of age); and
- personally observed cases of massive edema in one ovary and florid 'immature' fibromatosis in the contralateral ovary.

Although the underlying mechanism for ovarian fibromatosis is unknown, it is speculated that local tissue injury (e.g., surgery, incomplete or intermittent ovarian torsion) stimulates platelets and macrophages to secrete locally acting growth factors that in turn induce massive fibroblastic proliferation and/or edema. Possibly, patients who present in the acute phase exhibit either massive ovarian edema or florid mitotically active 'immature' fibromatosis with/without associated peritoneal pathology,

and those who present in a subacute or resolving phase exhibit the better documented 'mature' form of acellular sclerotic fibromatosis (Figure 22.50).

Gross features

The ovaries are enlarged but sometimes only marginally so. The cut surface of the 'mature' forms is densely sclerotic and pale. The 'immature' or cellular variants are usually large solid masses, averaging about 15 cm in diameter with fibrinous adhesions on the external surface, with tan-white and smooth cut surfaces, frequently focally hemorrhagic (Figure 22.51).

Microscopic features

The mature variant of fibromatosis exhibits collagen-producing spindle cells that proliferate around and between normal follicles (Figure 22.52) and produce a thickened fibrotic cortex. The proliferative process varies from densely acellular bands of collagen to intersecting bundles of spindle cells with a storiform pattern resembling ovarian cortex. Minor foci of uninvolved cortex and edema may be present (Figure 22.53), as may rare luteinized cells in the fibromatous zones or adjacent normal cortex. Microscopic foci of sex-cord differentiation may appear as isolated epithelial-like structures (Figure 22.54), or may be aggregated around areas of hypercellularity suggesting development from old follicular remnants.

'Immature' ovarian fibromatosis shows densely cellular swathes and intersecting bundles of spindle-shaped fibroblasts or myofibroblasts (Figure 22.55). Areas of apparent maturation of the myofibroblastic stroma (Figure 22.56) suggest a transition from 'immature' fibromatosis towards more typical or familiar examples of fibromatosis (Figures 22.52 and 22.53). In most instances, this process totally obliterates the normal architecture of the ovary, but in ovaries that are only slightly enlarged, it may be confined to the cortex. The proliferating myofibroblastic cells, which are immunoreactive for vimentin and smooth muscle actin, have scanty cytoplasm and round to oval, vesicular, but remarkably bland nuclei. Nucleoli are small or inapparent. Mitoses are numerous, regularly exceeding 20 mitotic figures per 10 HPFs; atypical mitoses are not seen (Figure 22.57). Reticulin stains show a fine pericellular meshwork of fibrils. Hemorrhage is seen focally but no necrosis.

This architectural pattern merges into areas more typical of massive ovarian edema with conspicuous intercellular edema fluid, microcyst formation, dilated lymphatics, and sinusoidal blood vessels and interstitial hemorrhages. At the interfaces,

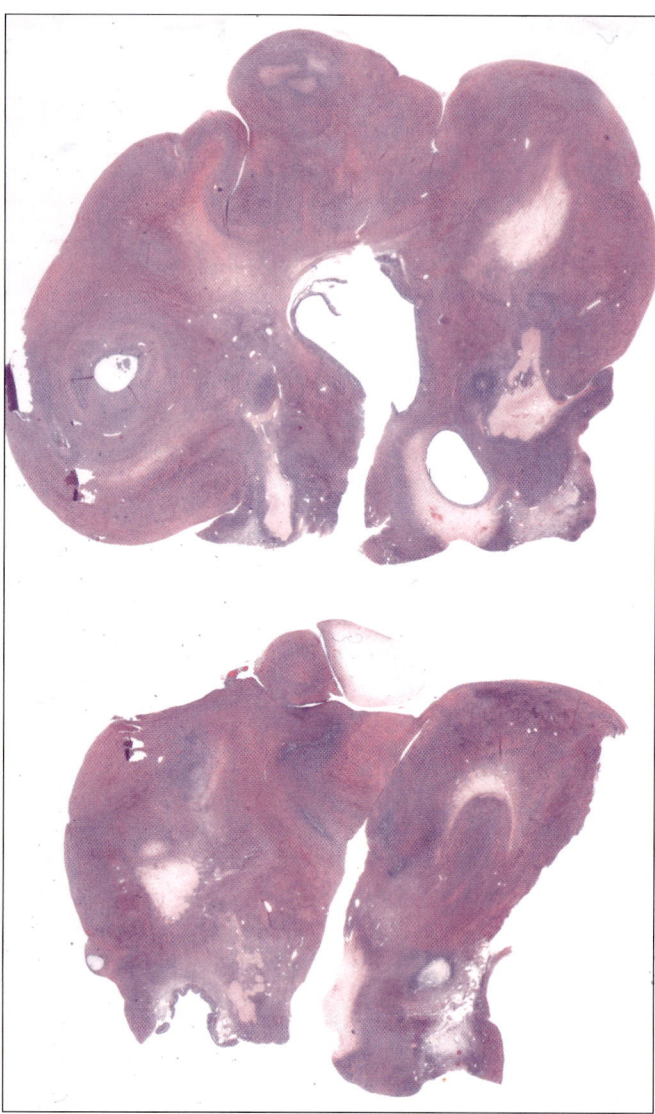

Fig. 22.53 Low power survey of ovarian fibromatosis. Irregular replacement by dense sclerotic fibrous tissue is seen with focal edema, entrapped follicular remnants and small areas of uninvolved cortex.

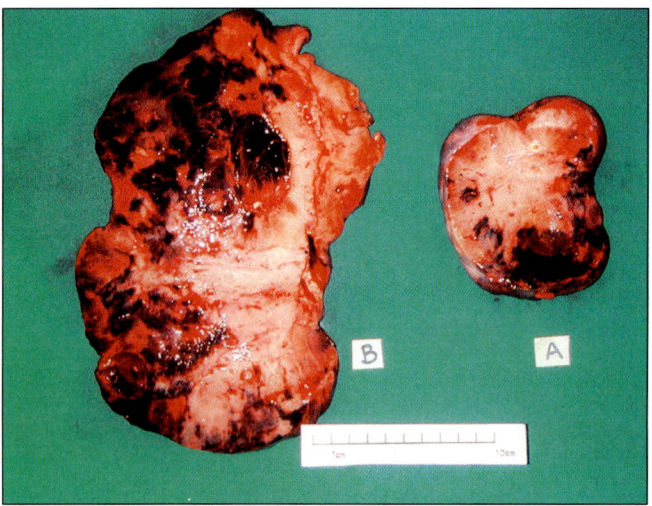

Fig. 22.51 'Immature' ovarian fibromatosis. Bilateral, large, soft, hemorrhagic masses, with otherwise featureless cut surfaces. An entrapped primordial follicle is present.

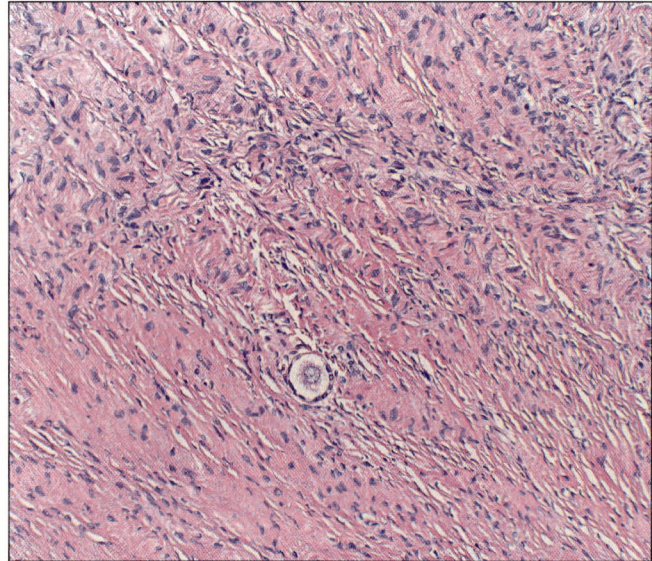

Fig. 22.52 Ovarian fibromatosis. Characterized by uniform, dense fibrocollagenous connective tissue. An entrapped primordial follicle is present.

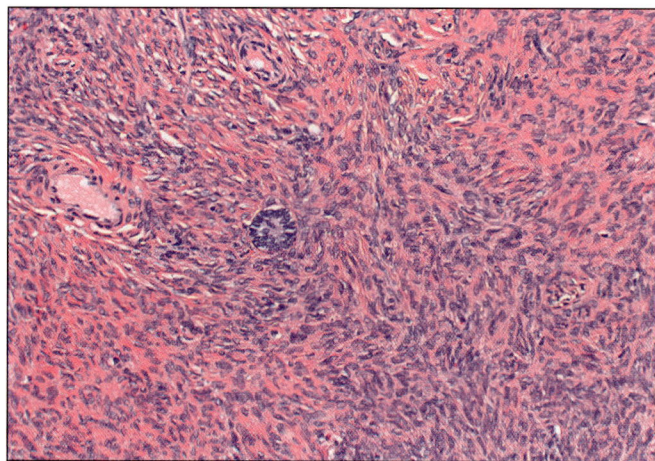

Fig. 22.54 Ovarian fibromatosis. Showing rare sex cord-like structure, deep within the fibroblastic nodule.

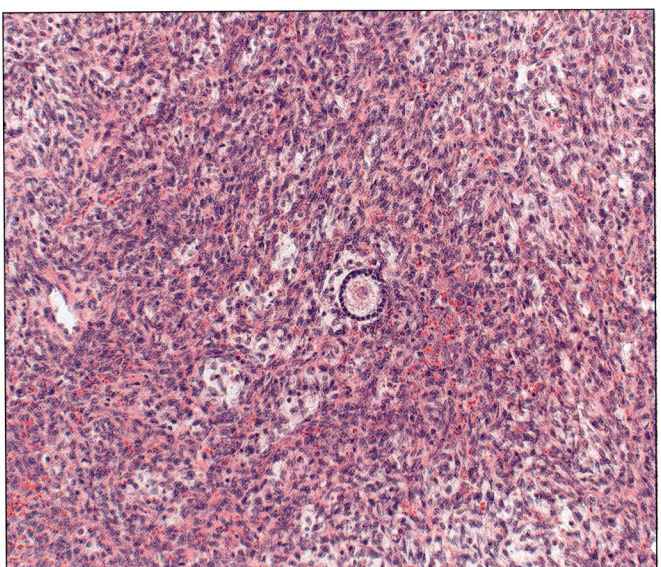

Fig. 22.55 'Immature' fibromatosis. Plump, spindle-shaped myofibroblastic cells enveloping residual primordial follicle.

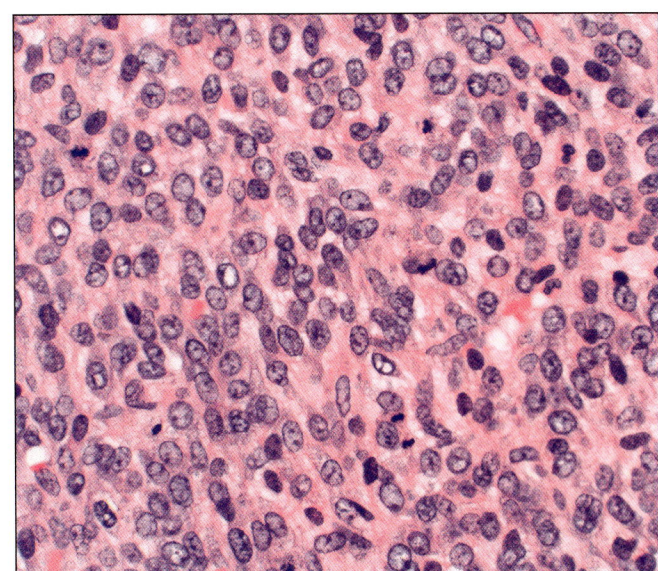

Fig. 22.57 'Immature' fibromatosis. Higher power of proliferating myofibroblastic cells seen in Figure 22.55. Note bland oval nuclei, but numerous mitoses.

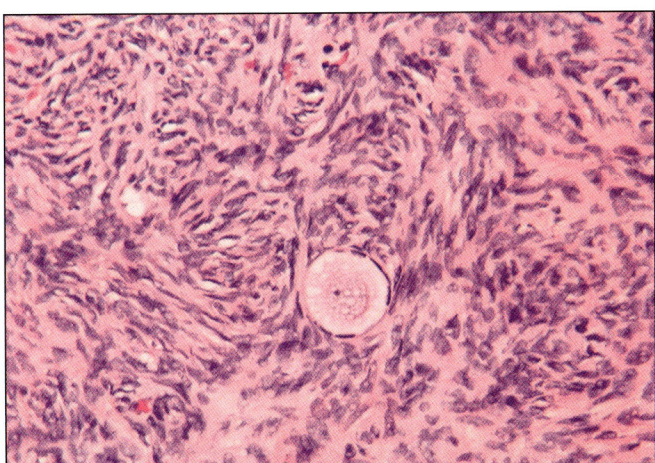

Fig. 22.56 Ovarian fibromatosis. Stromal cellularity intermediate between that seen in Figure 22.55 and that of 'end-stage' disease seen in Figure 22.52.

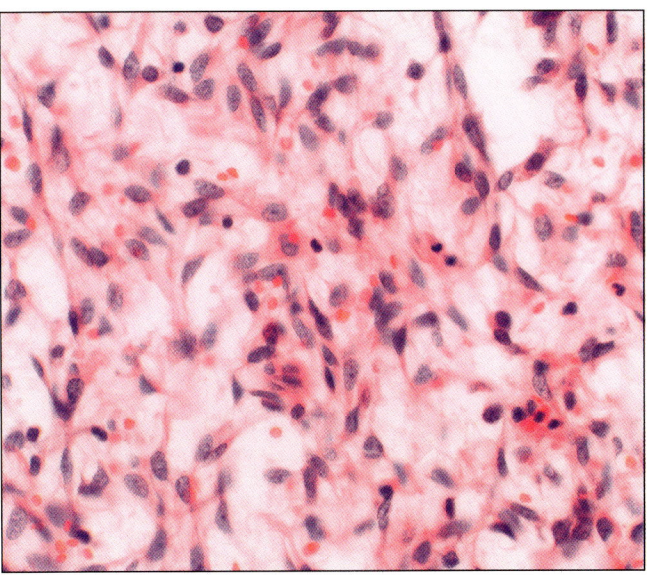

Fig. 22.58 'Immature' fibromatosis. Intercellular edema imparts a 'tissue culture' appearance to proliferating mesenchymal cells, and a morphologic pattern that overlaps that of massive ovarian edema.

the proliferating fibroblasts assume a 'tissue-culture' appearance (Figure 22.58).

Scattered in both the cellular fibroblastic and edematous areas are single or nested lutein-like cells. These cells exhibit small to moderate amounts of eosinophilic cytoplasm and rounded central nuclei, often with an obvious central nucleolus (Figure 22.59). Cells intermediate between the lutein-like cells and fibroblasts are seen.

Another important morphologic feature, reported occasionally, is the identification of entrapped follicular structures, crucial because (as with massive ovarian edema) it represents strong evidence that the process is not neoplastic. These are usually unremarkable primordial follicles (Figures 22.52, 22.55 and 22.56), but may be 'dysplastic' (see above).

Differential diagnosis

Stromal hyperthecosis (see above), like many cases of 'immature' fibromatosis, is commonly bilateral and occurs in young women. It is not associated, however, with ascites or an acute presentation, does not cause massive enlargement of the

ovaries, does not obliterate ovarian architecture, and is not associated with either collagen production or proliferating mitotically active fibroblastic cells.

Luteinized thecomas, the neoplasms that most closely resemble 'immature' fibromatosis, may occur in young women, but with vanishing rarity under the age of 20 years. In contrast, one half of patients with fibromatosis in which the ovary shows florid proliferative features are younger than 20 years of age; some are under 10 years. Most luteinized thecomas are estrogenic (>50%), unilateral (>90%), and unassociated with ascites or peritoneal pathology, while fibromatosis is endocrinologically inactive or occasionally androgenic, commonly bilateral, and may present in association with similar fibroblastic peritoneal lesions. Histologically, luteinized thecomas are not edematous and do not incorporate native ovarian follicles.

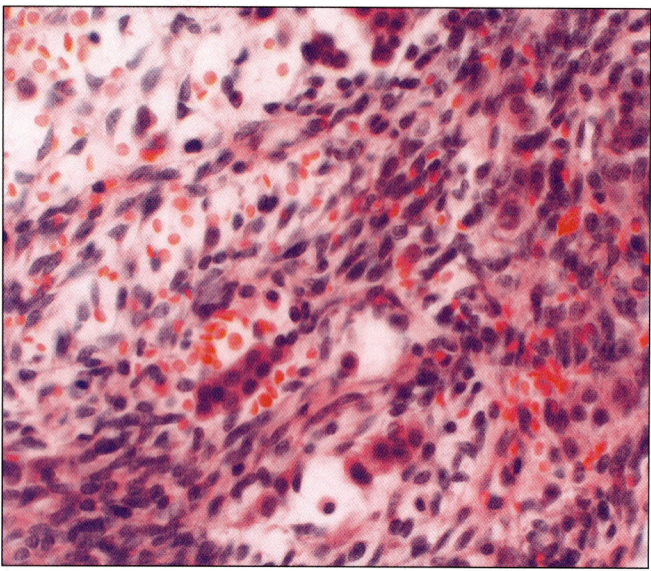

Fig. 22.59 Nests of small to medium sized lutein cells with eosinophilic granular cytoplasm, rounded nuclei each with a central nucleolus.

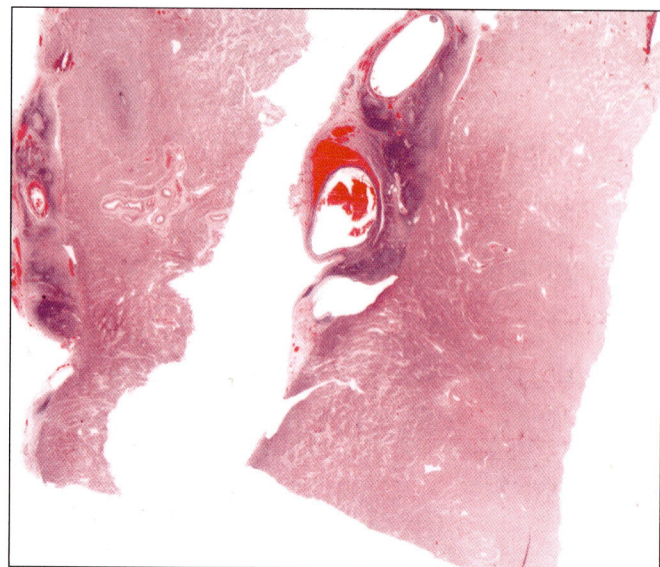

Fig. 22.60 Ovarian remnant. An island of identifiable ovarian cortical tissue containing developing follicles, densely adherent to the uterine wall.

SEQUELAE OF SURGERY OR TRAUMA

OVARIAN REMNANT SYNDROME (RESIDUAL OVARY SYNDROME)

Definition
This condition exists if a patient, who has had a 'total bilateral oophorectomy', later develops a palpable mass or experiences pelvic pain or other symptoms referable to ovarian tissue that has been left behind.[10,11]

Etiology
Residual ovarian tissue should not be confused with accessory or supernumerary ovaries (see above). The incomplete oophorectomy is usually the consequence of difficult surgical dissection secondary to adhesions caused by endometriosis or pelvic inflammatory disease, which has often been complicated further by previous surgery.

Clinical features
In a premenopausal patient, climacteric symptoms fail to develop and, if the uterus has been left behind, continuing cyclic vaginal bleeding may occur. In these patients clinical suspicions of the syndrome will be confirmed if the serum FSH and LH remain within the premenopausal range.

Pathology
At re-exploration, ovarian remnants may be found attached by usually dense adhesions to any of the residual pelvic structures, including the uterus (Figure 22.60) or the pelvic wall. Remnants may be grossly enlarged by the presence of endometriotic or dysfunctional cysts,[11] but some consist simply of normal functional ovarian parenchyma. Obstruction or compression of the ureter, the colon or bladder may occur.[73]

Ovarian 'drilling' for polycystic ovary syndrome
One form of surgical therapy for patients resistant to medical management of polycystic ovary syndrome is so-called laparo- scopic 'drilling'. This has largely replaced the older forms of corticomedullary stromal reduction such as wedge resection[4] and produces a peculiar pattern of tissue necrosis (Figure 22.61). Although pathognomonic and instantly identifiable with prior experience, this appearance would be utterly mysterious to the pathologist without relevant clinical information.

SPLENOSIS (AUTOTRANSPLANTANTION OF SPLENIC TISSUE)

Etiology
This most often follows trauma, usually a motor vehicle accident, which has resulted in splenic rupture necessitating splenectomy, or rupture of a diseased spleen.[37] Nodules of splenic tissue, usually less than 1 cm in diameter, are randomly distributed in the peritoneal cavity and may be found adherent to the ovaries (Figure 22.62). Splenosis is generally asymptomatic but may cause abdominal or pelvic pain simulating endometriosis, or produce intestinal obstruction due to the development of adhesions. The gynecologic surgeon may encounter splenosis as an incidental finding or mistakenly interpret the widespread fleshy reddish-brown or purplish peritoneal nodules as endometriotic deposits.

Microscopic features
The implants are encased by fibrous tissue that simulates a splenic capsule, but lack smooth muscle and elastic fibers. Larger nodules usually show all the histologic components of normally sited splenic parenchyma (Figure 22.62) but, in smaller lesions, red pulp only may be evident.

IATROGENIC DISORDERS OF THE OVARIES

RADIOTHERAPY DAMAGE

Etiology
The ovaries may be exposed to external high-dose ionizing radiation for various reasons, most commonly for the treat-

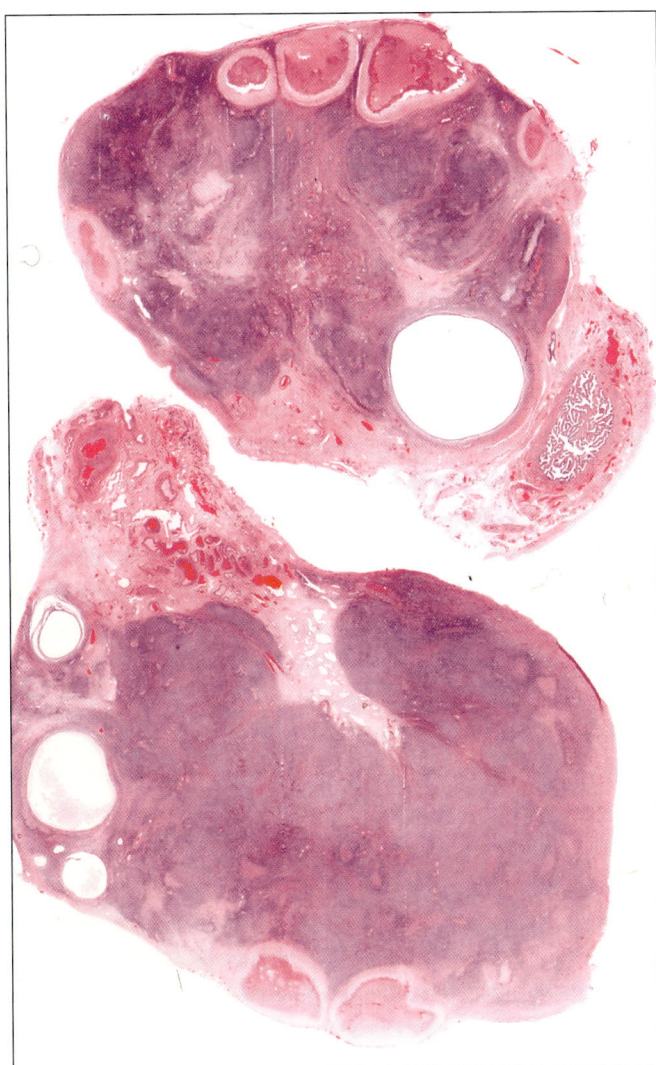

Fig. 22.61 Ovarian 'drilling.' A distinct pattern of acute focal tissue necrosis induced by laparoscopic diathermy to the ovarian cortex and superficial medulla of an ovary in a patient with polycystic ovary syndrome.

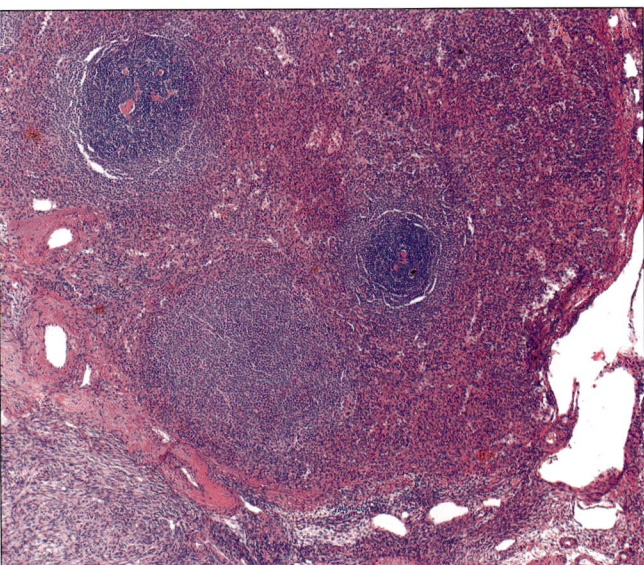

Fig. 22.62 Ovarian splenosis. Ovarian splenotic nodules thought to represent endometriosis at laparotomy in a 28-year-old woman with infertility. History of motor vehicle accident followed by splenectomy 17 years previously. Note ovarian cortical stroma at bottom left.

ment of malignant disease, either in children or in adults. In the past, radiotherapy was used to induce an artificial menopause and to treat some non-malignant conditions such as endometriosis. Apart from achieving the desired radiotherapeutic effect on tumor growth, the most important issue at stake for young patients undergoing treatment for malignant disease is that of subsequent fertility. In contrast to gametogenesis in males, proliferation of oogonia ceases *in utero* and the number of oocytes is then fixed and cannot be replenished. Destruction of these germ cells *in utero* may lead to ovarian dysgenesis and postnatally to premature ovarian failure. The mitotically active oogonia are much more sensitive to radiation than oocytes that are in a resting phase (prophase of their first meiotic division) until just before ovulation. Ovarian follicles also vary in their sensitivity. Actively growing follicles are most vulnerable, possibly because their rapidly proliferating granulosa cells are radiosensitive, and their destruction may lead to death of the oocyte that they invest. Doses of less than 150 rads are not harmful to the ovaries of young women whereas 400 rads will render most women over 40 years permanently amenorrheic. Doses of 800 rads (acute or fractionated) sterilize vir-

tually all women. Intermediate doses will cause a variable number of younger women to have temporary or permanent amenorrhea. Children display a greater resistance to radiation-induced ovarian failure. However, high doses (2000–3000 rads), as used in the treatment of abdominal malignancies, will produce permanent ovarian failure. Oophoropexy and lead shielding are only partially successful in preserving fertility. As with chemotherapy, return of regular menses or even pregnancy after treatment does not necessarily mean that the ovaries have not been damaged. It may be years before a reduced oocyte pool becomes evident as premature ovarian failure.[47]

Microscopic features

The first observable light-microscopic change in radiated oocytes is nuclear pyknosis. Condensation of chromatin and damage to the nuclear envelope are evident ultrastructurally. The cytoplasmic damage that follows is manifest as eosinophilia. Granulosa cells exhibit pyknosis and karyolysis very soon after a radiation insult and, if a sufficient number of these cells are destroyed and regeneration is inadequate, the oocyte will die and the follicle will undergo atresia. Granulosa lutein cells show cytoplasmic vacuolation. The chronic effect on the follicular apparatus is a decrease in follicular activity, demonstrated by a progressive reduction in the numbers of growing and involuting follicles and corpora lutea, culminating in primordial follicle depletion.

The acute and chronic radiation effects in the non-specialized ovarian structures are similar to those documented more often in other organs. Stromal edema and fibrin exudation progress to stromal hyalinization, fibrosis, and capsular adhesions (Figure 22.63). Vascular changes are most conspicuous in arteries, which show fibrinoid necrosis, thrombosis, hyalinized media, foam cell accumulation, and myointimal proliferation. However, damage to the microvasculature is considered to be the prime mediator of delayed radiation injury, particularly ischemic necrosis and fibrosis.

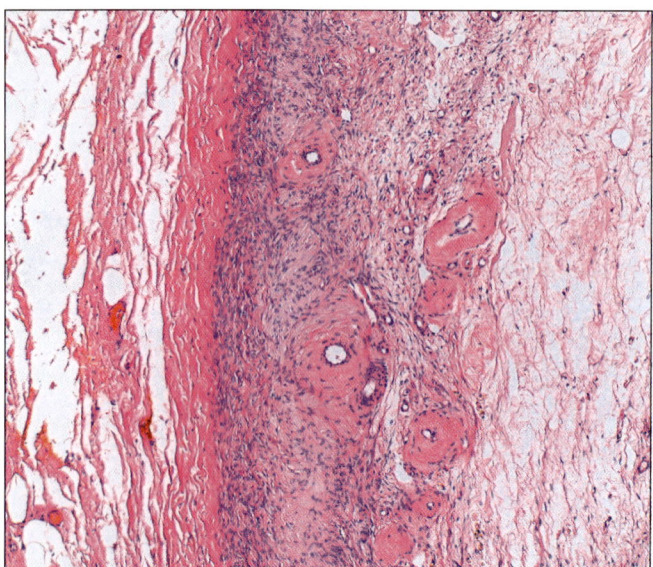

Fig. 22.63 Chronic radiation damage. Dense periovarian adhesions are subtended by atrophic, hyalinized cortex displaying vessels with hyalinized media and some fibrinoid change.

CHEMOTHERAPEUTIC AND IMMUNOSUPPRESSIVE DRUGS

Etiology

From limited morphologic studies, antineoplastic drugs have a similar general effect on the ovary as ionizing radiation, i.e., death of selected cells, especially those that are proliferating at the time of the insult. Individual drugs have a variable ovarian toxicity, and factors that influence the response of patients to radiotherapy also operate with respect to chemotherapy.[47] Adult women are more likely to develop temporary or permanent amenorrhea due to oocyte destruction than prepubertal children treated for cancer with cytotoxics alone, due to the low level of ovarian follicular activity before puberty. Attempts to simulate a quiescent state, and thus mitigate the damaging effect of chemotherapy in adults, have been made by giving oral contraceptives during therapy.

Microscopic features

Biopsies show capsular thickening, peri-oophoritis, stromal fibrohyalinization, necrotizing vasculitis, hemorrhage, and disintegrating follicles.

ORAL CONTRACEPTIVES

Etiology

Combined estrogen–progestogen contraceptive pills inhibit ovulation chiefly by suppressing the release of pituitary gonadotrophins (see also Chapter 13). With 20 µg dosages of ethinyl estradiol, follicular activity is more common so that contraception depends on suppression of the LH surge or disruption of the endometrial cycle.[24]

Microscopic features

Morphologic effects on the ovaries depend on the type of preparation administered. High-dose formulas suppress all func-

tional activity, and the ovaries shrink to postmenopausal size. Follicular growth is inhibited, no corpora lutea are formed, and the ovarian stroma becomes dense and fibrous. The basement membrane around primordial follicles thickens but oocytes are unaffected. After several months of therapy, corpora albicantia may be the only evidence of previous follicular activity. With low-dose preparations, there may be continuing folliculogenesis, including the development of mature (Graafian) follicles. Ovulation is still inhibited; the follicles undergo atresia and corpora lutea do not form. Randomized controlled trials indicate that modern oral contraceptives are unlikely to prevent the development of functional cysts or to hasten their disappearance.[24]

Differential diagnosis

Although practical problems in differential diagnosis are unlikely to arise, similar morphologic ovarian changes that correlate with functional arrest are also seen in women with (see above) hypogonadotrophic hypogonadism, resistant ovary syndrome, and prolonged hyperprolactinemia.

PROGESTERONE

Etiology

Short-term, high-dose progestogen therapy is used to manage various gynecologic disorders, including endometriosis and abnormal uterine bleeding, especially that due to anovulation. Low-dose progestogens are used in the contraceptive 'mini-pill'.

Microscopic features

High-dose progesterone suppresses follicular activity and ovulation can be inhibited. Foci of deciduosis may occur in the ovarian cortex and beneath the pelvic peritoneum (Figure 22.64). Ovarian (and extraovarian) endometriotic lesions may exhibit a progestogenic effect similar to that more commonly encountered in the endometrium. The endometriotic glands are small, poorly developed, and relatively inactive, while the stroma shows a decidual reaction. Low-dose progestogens do not cause such conspicuous morphologic alterations. Follicular activity usually continues and ovulation, with formation of a normal corpus luteum, occurs in about 40% of cases. There is defective ovulation in a further 30%. Follicular cysts have been noted occasionally.

DANAZOL

Etiology

This is an isoxazol derivative of a synthetic steroid 17-α ethinyltestosterone, used in the treatment of endometriosis, dysfunctional uterine bleeding, benign breast disease, and angioneurotic edema, and causes profound ovarian suppression and inhibits ovulation. It has a complex action, interfering with cyclic FSH and LH production, directly inhibiting follicular development and steroidogenesis, and also having a weak impeded androgenic effect.

Microscopic features

The ovaries become small and follicular activity is arrested. Endometriotic lesions shrink and may be difficult to identify,

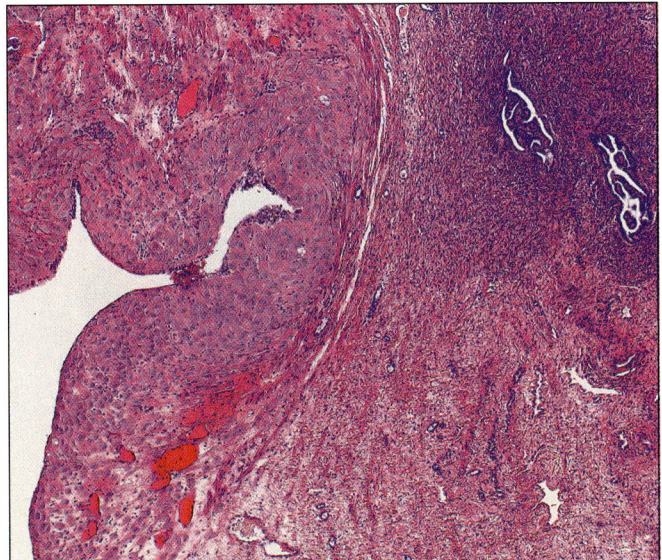

Fig. 22.64 Pseudodeciduosis beneath the mesothelium of the ovarian hilus. From a woman recently treated with progesterone.

even microscopically. The endometriotic glands become very small and are lined by atrophic cuboidal cells that display characteristic ultrastructural changes. The endometriotic stroma is compact and similarly inactive, and may be difficult to differentiate from cortical stroma.

GONADOTROPHIN-RELEASING HORMONE (GnRH) ANALOGUES

The most widely studied GnRH analogue is goserelin. It acts on the hypothalamic–pituitary axis to suppress ovarian function, decreasing LH and estradiol levels to postmenopausal values. By virtue of its mode of action, goserelin causes the ovaries to become small and follicular activity ceases. Unlike tamoxifen (see below), there is no estrogen agonist-like effect.[34]

OVULATION-INDUCTION AGENTS

Ovulation-induction agents (especially clomiphene citrate), pulsatile GnRH therapy, and human menopausal gonadotrophins produce an iatrogenic form of hyperreactio luteinalis (see above) known as the 'ovarian hyperstimulation syndrome' (OHSS). This complication develops only after β-hCG is given at the time of ovulation, and is particularly prone to occur in women with the polycystic ovary syndrome. Pathology is localized to the ovaries at the time the condition is triggered. The syndrome is unpredictable and potentially life-threatening when organs different from the ovaries become involved, causing ascites, hydrothorax or coagulation disturbances resulting in thromboembolic phenomena. The different clinical signs are the basis of a proposal for a local and systemic classification.[16]

Pathology
In severe cases the ovaries become massively enlarged and although surgical intervention is usually not required, patho-

logic examination shows changes identical to multiple theca–lutein cysts as well as one or more corpora lutea.

TAMOXIFEN

Tamoxifen is increasingly used as adjuvant therapy in premenopausal women with breast cancer. The hormonal effects of tamoxifen in premenopausal women are associated with increased levels of estradiol and progesterone whereas FSH and LH remain normal or increase slightly. Tamoxifen is structurally similar to clomiphene and is equivalent for induction of ovulation. The elevated serum levels of estrogen and progesterone may result from maturation of multiple ovarian follicles. There is no evidence that tamoxifen exposure is associated with an increase in benign or malignant primary or metastatic ovarian neoplasms. Further study is necessary to better define any association between tamoxifen and endometriosis and the effect of tamoxifen on ovarian cancer risk.[46]

Microscopic features
Multiple and single ovarian follicular cysts have been reported in premenopausal women treated with tamoxifen but it is debatable whether their incidence is increased. Necrosis and torsion are recognized but rare complications.

OVARIAN HEMORRHAGE AND ADNEXAL TORSION

OVARIAN HEMORRHAGE

Etiology
Small hemorrhages are common in normally functioning ovaries. The well-vascularized theca interna of developing follicles is prone to hemorrhage but usually only a small intrafollicular or perifollicular hematoma is formed. Slight bleeding occurs with follicular rupture at ovulation. Bleeding also occurs regularly in the vascularization stage of the corpus luteum. This is usually slight but, if excessive, may lead to the formation of a corpus luteum cyst (see below).

On occasion, profuse hemorrhage from the above sources (mostly corpora lutea) causes ovarian rupture and bleeding into the peritoneal cavity. Hemoperitoneum from a corpus luteum may occur at any time during the reproductive years but especially during pregnancy. The risk is increased in patients receiving anticoagulants of any type,[13,18] and, rarely, spontaneous thrombocytopenia.[14] Rupture occurs most often on day 20–26 of the menstrual cycle, and two-thirds of cases involve the right ovary.

Microscopic features
Pathologic examination of the excised tissues (oophorectomy, wedge excision or cystectomy) will readily identify the source of the bleeding, except when extensive interstitial hemorrhage has obscured morphologic detail. In these cases, the operative findings and clinical features should provide a presumptive diagnosis. Sometimes examination of the blood clot evacuated from the peritoneal cavity may yield diagnostic material such as groups of lutein cells, chorionic villi or tumor fragments (Figure 22.65).

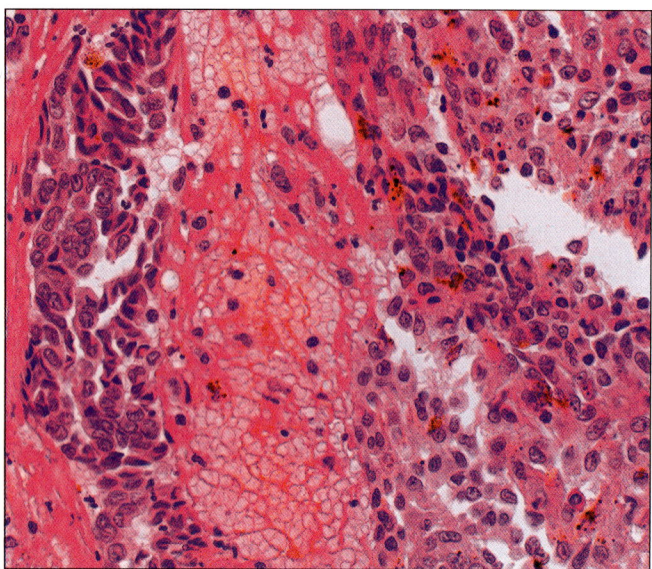

Fig. 22.65 Peritoneal blood clot, containing granulosa cells, retrieved at laparotomy from a young woman with a ruptured follicular cyst.

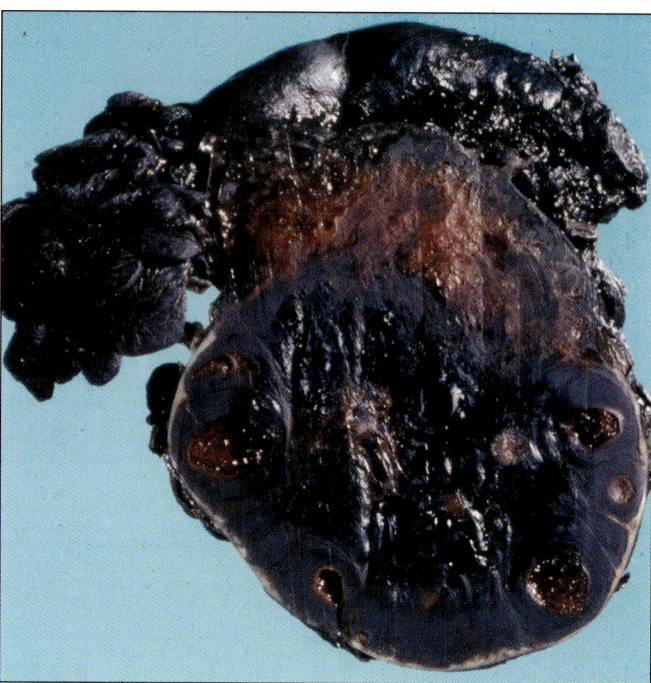

Fig. 22.66 Idiopathic torsion of ovary and tube in a young woman. Several follicles are evident in the hemorrhagic infarcted ovary, but no cyst or neoplasm could be identified.

ADNEXAL TORSION

Etiology

Torsion involving the ovary may occur in isolation (see above) or together with the fallopian tube. It is an uncommon but not rare gynecologic occurrence.[8] It presents most frequently during the reproductive years, but about 25% of cases involve children and, of these, a significant minority occurs in neonates and infants less than 8 months of age. Otherwise, unexplained absence of an ovary has been attributed to subclinical torsion and consequent 'autoamputation' occurring in childhood or, perhaps, even *in utero*. Massive ovarian edema may be a variation on the theme, the clinicopathologic differences being dictated by the degree and speed of torsion and the stage at which the condition is diagnosed.

The tube and ovary usually undergo torsion as a single unit, rotating around the broad ligament as an axis (Figure 22.66). Less commonly, the ovary twists alone, around the mesovarium and even more rarely the tube alone undergoes torsion.[2] The right side is more commonly affected, the left ovary being less freely mobile because of the presence of the sigmoid colon.

In adults, most cases are secondary to pathologic ovarian enlargements. Ovaries, once exceeding a diameter of 6 cm, are lifted out of the pelvic confines and become more freely mobile. A wide range of cystic and neoplastic diseases have been identified in twisted ovaries, the most common lesions being cystic teratomas (Figure 22.67A) or cystadenomas. There is an increased risk of torsion of normal fallopian tube and ovary in pregnancy because of increased ovarian mobility within the abdomen during this period, most usually in the first half of pregnancy.[7,54] Torsion also occurs in association with ovarian hyperstimulation syndrome (see above).[6]

In children, torsion of apparently normal ovaries accounts for approximately one-third of cases, and occasionally may be bilateral.[1,5]

Microscopic features

Microscopy confirms hemorrhage, edema, and ischemic change and often, frank necrosis. Normal structures may be difficult to identify. Multiple blocks of more solid or apparently viable areas, especially cyst walls, should be examined to determine the nature of any underlying pathologic condition and to exclude the possibility of a malignant neoplasm (Figure 22.67A). We have found that staining for reticulin fibres, which regularly survive prolonged *in vivo* infarction, is particularly helpful in giving a 'skeletal' picture of the underlying vascular, stromal, and epithelial architecture long after all cellular detail is lost or obscured by hemorrhage. Complex cystic or papillary patterns are suspicious of underlying neoplasms and may even give the experienced observer hints of histologic type (Figure 22.67B,C). Organoid structures may represent the infarcted tissues of a dermoid cyst. The accompanying fallopian tube, if torted, may show similar ischemic changes and, less frequently, the apparent cause of adnexal torsion, such as a hydrosalpinx.

MÜLLERIANOSIS AND REACTIVE MESOTHELIAL LESIONS

'Müllerianosis' is a generic term applied to that group of epithelial and mesenchymal 'metaplasias' and proliferations that are frequent in the female peritoneal cavity, commonly around the pelvic viscera and especially the ovaries. In many ways, they exhibit the same morphologic features as their cellular analogues lining or forming the müllerian duct derivatives, such as endosalpinx (the fallopian tube mucosal lining), endometrium, smooth muscle and so forth.

Their origin is far from agreed on in the literature, and their relationships to either clinical symptoms or various forms of

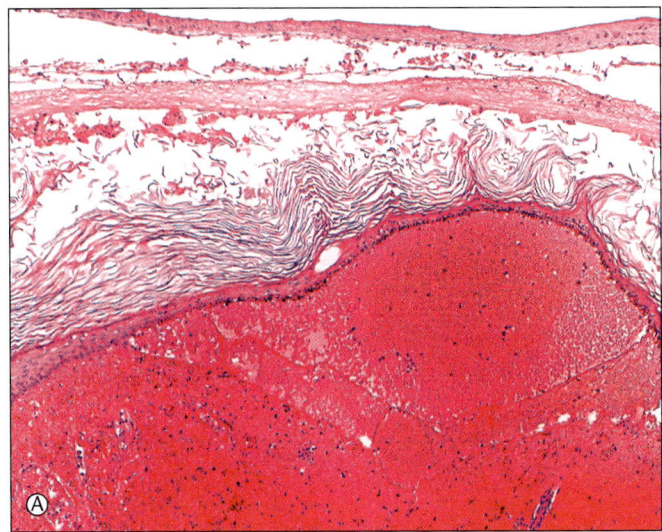

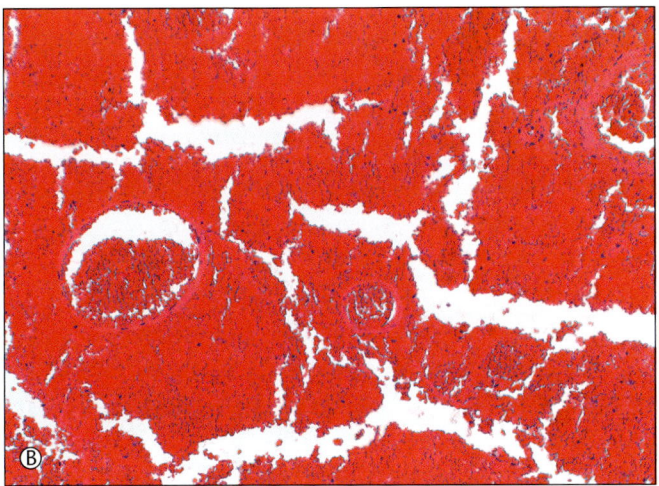

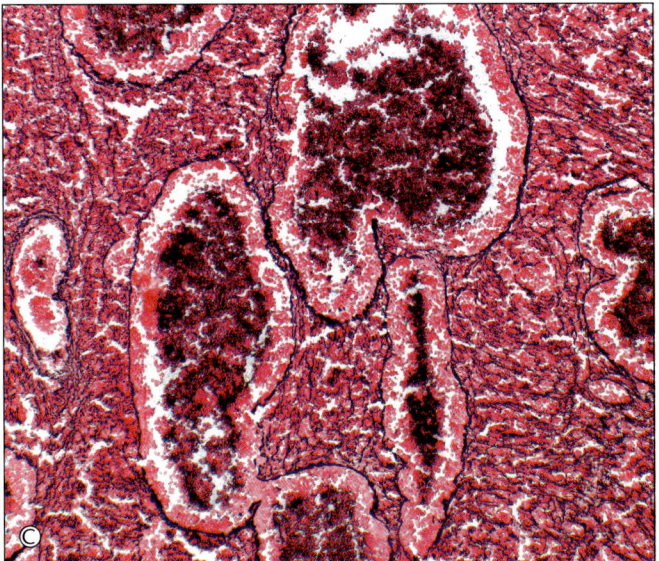

Fig. 22.67 Torsion due to benign tumor. **(A)** Diffuse hemorrhage into the wall of a mature cystic teratoma with surviving squamous lining at left. **(B)** Torsion of benign mucinous tumor, showing a featureless hemorrhagic necrotic area. **(C)** Similar area with glandular morphology highlighted by reticulin stain.

neoplastic transformation are also controversial. Their various, and apparently quite tissue-specific, anatomic distributions and pathologic correlates are outlined in greater detail in Chapter 33, while the relationship of endosalpingeal or serous type to serous ovarian neoplasms is explored in Chapter 24.

The epithelial metaplasias that fall loosely into this group of lesions would, therefore, include 'endosalpingiosis' (also called 'serous change' by some) and 'endocervicosis'. Extension by common usage rather than rational argument might also include transitional cell metaplasia as occurs in Walthard cell rests. The mesenchymal or stromal lesions in this group include 'deciduosis' (regularly encountered in pregnant patients) and 'disseminated peritoneal leiomyomatosis'. Mixed lesions would include endometriosis. Non-specific peritoneal inclusions and proliferations are to one side of this morphologic spectrum, but clearly are to be considered in their pathogenesis.

REFERENCES

1. Abes M, Sarihan H. Oophoropexy in children with ovarian torsion. Eur J Pediatr Surg 2004;14:168–71.
2. Antoniou N, Varras M, Akrivis C, Kitsiou E, Stefanaki S, Salamalekis E. Isolated torsion of the fallopian tube: a case report and review of the literature. Clin Exp Obstet Gynecol 2004;31:235–8.
3. Balat O, Kutlar I, Ozkur A, Bakir K, Aksoy F, Ugur MG. Primary pure ovarian choriocarcinoma mimicking ectopic pregnancy: a report of fulminant progression. Tumori 2004;90:136–8.
4. Balen A. Surgical treatment of polycystic ovary syndrome. Best Pract Res Clin Endocrinol Metab 2006;20:271–80.
5. Beaunoyer M, Chapdelaine J, Bouchard S, Ouimet A. Asynchronous bilateral ovarian torsion. J Pediatr Surg 2004;39:746–9.
6. Bellver J, Escudero E, Pellicer A. Bilateral partial oophorectomy in the management of severe ovarian hyperstimulation syndrome (OHSS): ovarian mutilating surgery is not an option in the management of severe OHSS. Hum Reprod 2003;18:1363–7.
7. Born C, Wirth S, Stabler A, Reiser M. Diagnosis of adnexal torsion in the third trimester of pregnancy: a case report. Abdom Imaging 2004;29:123–7.
8. Bouguizane S, Bibi H, Farhat Y, et al. [Adnexal torsion: a report of 135 cases]. J Gynecol Obstet Biol Reprod (Paris) 2003;32:535–40.
9. Bromley B, Benacerraf B. Adnexal masses during pregnancy: accuracy of sonographic diagnosis and outcome. J Ultrasound Med 1997;16:447–52; quiz 53–4.
10. Bryce GM. Ovarian remnant syndrome. J R Soc Med 1995;88:60.
11. Burke M, Talerman A, Carlson JA, Bibbo M. Residual ovarian tissue mimicking malignancy in a patient with mucinous carcinoid tumor of the ovary. A case report. Acta Cytol 1997;41(4 Suppl):1377–80.
12. Carvalho JP, Diegoli MS, Carvalho FM, Diegoli CA. Adnexal torsion following gonadotropin-releasing hormone analog therapy: a case report. Rev Hosp Clin Fac Med Sao Paulo 2004;59:128–30.
13. Castellino G, Cuadrado MJ, Godfrey T, Khamashta MA, Hughes GR. Characteristics of patients with antiphospholipid syndrome with major bleeding after oral anticoagulant treatment. Ann Rheum Dis 2001;60:527–30.
14. Castro-Lizano N, Calleja C, Galindo-Rodriguez G, Avina-Zubieta JA. Ovarian haemorrhage, rupture and haemoperitoneum secondary to thrombocytopenia in a patient with SLE. Lupus 2003;12:648–50.
15. Clement PB, Young RH, Hanna W, Scully RE. Sclerosing peritonitis associated with luteinized thecomas of the ovary. A clinicopathological analysis of six cases. Am J Surg Pathol 1994;18:1–13.
16. Cobellis L, Pecori E, Stradella L, De Lucia E, Messalli EM, Cobellis G. Ovarian hyperstimulation syndrome: distinction between local and systemic disease. Gynecol Endocrinol 2003;17:95–9.
17. Coccia ME, Pasquini L, Comparetto C, Scarselli G. Hyperreactio luteinalis in a woman with high-risk factors. A case report. J Reprod Med 2003;48:127–9.
18. Cretel E, Cacoub P, Huong DL, Gompel A, Amoura Z, Piette JC. Massive ovarian haemorrhage complicating oral anticoagulation in the antiphospholipid syndrome: a report of three cases. Lupus 1999;8:482–5.
19. Csapo Z, Szabo I, Toth M, Devenyi N, Papp Z. Hyperreactio luteinalis in a normal singleton pregnancy. A case report. J Reprod Med 1999;44:53–6.
20. Danihel L, Sokol L, Breitenecker G, et al. [Extrauterine choriocarcinoma – a rare form of gestational trophoblastic disease]. Bratisl Lek Listy 1996;97:279–83.
21. de la Cruz SI, Llanos Arriaga V, Narro Tristan H, Andrade Manzano A, Fernandez Martinez RL. [Bilateral ovary massive edema. Unusual gynecologic pathology. Report of 2 cases]. Ginecol Obstet Mex 2001;69:72–6.
22. de Sanctis C, Lala R, Matarazzo P, Andreo M, de Sanctis L. Pubertal development in patients with McCune–Albright syndrome or

pseudohypoparathyroidism. J Pediatr Endocrinol Metab 2003;16(Suppl 2):293–6.

23. Ercal T, Cinar O, Mumcu A, Lacin S, Ozer E. Ovarian pregnancy: relationship to an intrauterine device. Aust N Z J Obstet Gynaecol 1997;37:362–4.

24. ESHRE Capri Workshop Group. Ovarian and endometrial function during hormonal contraception. Hum Reprod 2001;16:1527–35.

25. Fleming R. The use of insulin sensitising agents in ovulation induction in women with polycystic ovary syndrome. Hormones (Athens) 2006;5:171–8.

26. Fratantonio E, Vicari E, Pafumi C, Calogero AE. Genetics of polycystic ovarian syndrome. Reprod Biomed Online 2005;10:713–20.

27. Friedrich M, Ertan AK, Axt-Fliedner R, Hollander M, Schmidt W. Unilateral massive ovarian edema (MOE): a case report. Clin Exp Obstet Gynecol 2002;29:65–6.

28. Geisthovel F. A comment on the European Society of Human Reproduction and Embryology/American Society for Reproductive Medicine consensus of the polycystic ovarian syndrome. Reprod Biomed Online 2003;7:602–5.

29. Grimes DA, Jones LB, Lopez LM, Schulz KF. Oral contraceptives for functional ovarian cysts. Cochrane Database Syst Rev 2006:CD006134.

30. Guvenal T, Cetin A, Tasyurt A. Unilateral massive ovarian edema and polycystic ovaries. A case report. Eur J Obstet Gynecol Reprod Biol 2001;97:258–9.

31. Haddad A, Mulvany N, Billson V, Arnstein M. Solitary luteinized follicle cyst of pregnancy. Report of a case with cytologic findings. Acta Cytol 2000;44:454–8.

32. Hill LM, Pelekanos M, Kanbour A. Massive edema of an ovary previously fixed to the pelvic side wall. J Ultrasound Med 1993;12:629–32.

33. Homburg R. Adverse effects of luteinizing hormone on fertility: fact or fantasy. Baillieres Clin Obstet Gynaecol 1998;12:555–63.

34. Jonat W. Luteinizing hormone-releasing hormone analogues – the rationale for adjuvant use in premenopausal women with early breast cancer. Br J Cancer 1998;78(Suppl 4):5–8.

35. Jongen VH, Hollema H, van der Zee AG, Santema JG, Heineman MJ. Ovarian stromal hyperplasia and ovarian vein steroid levels in relation to endometrioid endometrial cancer. BJOG 2003;110:690–5.

36. Kanumakala S, Warne GL, Stokes KB, Chan YF, Grover S. Massive ovarian edema causing early puberty. J Pediatr Endocrinol Metab 2002;15:861–4.

37. Khosravi MR, Margulies DR, Alsabeh R, Nissen N, Phillips EH, Morgenstern L. Consider the diagnosis of splenosis for soft tissue masses long after any splenic injury. Am Surg 2004;70:967–70.

38. Kocak M, Caliskan E, Haberal A. Laparoscopic conservation of the ovaries in cases with massive ovarian oedema. Gynecol Obstet Invest 2002;53:129–32.

39. Koivunen R, Laatikainen T, Tomas C, Huhtaniemi I, Tapanainen J, Martikainen H. The prevalence of polycystic ovaries in healthy women. Acta Obstet Gynecol Scand 1999;78:137–41.

40. Krug E, Berga SL. Postmenopausal hyperthecosis: functional dysregulation of androgenesis in climacteric ovary. Obstet Gynecol 2002;99(5 Pt 2):893–7.

41. Kuroiwa M, Hatakeyama SI, Suzuki N, Murai H, Toki I, Tsuchida Y. Neonatal ovarian cysts: management with reference to magnetic resonance imaging. Asian J Surg 2004;27:43–8.

42. Le Vaillant C, Tremouilhac C, Boog G. [Luteinized cystic ovarian hyperplasia during a normal pregnancy]. J Gynecol Obstet Biol Reprod (Paris) 2003;32:368–74.

43. Leong S, Trivedi AN. A case of ovarian stromal hyperplasia causing hirsutism in a post-menopausal woman. Aust N Z J Obstet Gynaecol 2001;41:102–3.

44. Manieri C, Di Bisceglie C, Fornengo R, et al. Postmenopausal virilization in a woman with gonadotropin dependent ovarian hyperthecosis. J Endocrinol Invest 1998;21:128–32.

45. Marret H, Hamamah S, Alonso AM, Pierre F. Case report and review of the literature: primary twin ovarian pregnancy. Hum Reprod 1997;12:1813–5.

46. McGonigle KF, Vasilev SA, Odom-Maryon T, Simpson JF. Ovarian histopathology in breast cancer patients receiving tamoxifen. Gynecol Oncol 1999;73:402–6.

47. Meirow D, Nugent D. The effects of radiotherapy and chemotherapy on female reproduction. Hum Reprod Update 2001;7:535–43.

48. Melilli GA, Avantario C, Farnelli C, Papeo R, Savona A. Combined intrauterine and ovarian pregnancy after in vitro fertilization and embryo transfer: a case report. Clin Exp Obstet Gynecol 2001;28:100–1.

49. Mittermayer C, Blaicher W, Grassauer D, et al. Fetal ovarian cysts: development and neonatal outcome. Ultraschall Med 2003;24:21–6.

50. Mohan H, Mohan P, Bal A, Tahlan A. Massive ovarian oedema: report of two cases. Arch Gynecol Obstet 2004;270:199–200.

51. Namba A, Nakagawa S, Nakamura N, et al. Ovarian choriocarcinoma arising from partial mole as evidenced by deoxyribonucleic acid microsatellite analysis. Obstet Gynecol 2003;102(5 Pt 1):991–4.

52. Natarajan A, Wales JK, Marven SS, Wright NP. Precocious puberty secondary to massive ovarian oedema in a 6-month-old girl. Eur J Endocrinol 2004;150:119–23.

53. Nogales FF, Martin-Sances L, Mendoza-Garcia E, Salamanca A, Gonzalez-Nunez MA, Pardo Mindan FJ. Massive ovarian oedema. Histopathology 1996;28:229–34.

54. Pan HS, Huang LW, Lee CY, Hwang JL, Chang JZ. Ovarian pregnancy torsion. Arch Gynecol Obstet 2004;270:119–21.

55. Pelusi B, Gambineri A, Pasquali R. Type 2 diabetes and the polycystic ovary syndrome. Minerva Ginecol 2004;56:41–51.

56. Piana S, Nogales FF, Corrado S, Cardinale L, Gusolfino D, Rivasi F. Pregnancy luteoma with granulosa cell proliferation: an unusual hyperplastic lesion arising in pregnancy and mimicking an ovarian neoplasia. Pathol Res Pract 1999;195:859–63.

57. Pigny P, Merlen E, Robert Y, et al. Elevated serum level of anti-müllerian hormone in patients with polycystic ovary syndrome: relationship to the ovarian follicle excess and to the follicular arrest. J Clin Endocrinol Metab 2003;88:5957–62.

58. Pitynski K, Basta A, Szczudrawa A, Oplawski M. [Ovarian tumors in pregnancy in the material of the Department of Gynecology and Oncology Collegium Medicum of Jagiellonian University in Cracow]. Ginekol Pol 2002;73:371–5.

59. Raziel A, Schachter M, Mordechai E, Friedler S, Panski M, Ron-El R. Ovarian pregnancy – a 12-year experience of 19 cases in one institution. Eur J Obstet Gynecol Reprod Biol 2004;114:92–6.

60. Raziel A, Mordechai E, Schachter M, Friedler S, Pansky M, Ron-El R. A comparison of the incidence, presentation, and management of ovarian pregnancies between two periods of time. J Am Assoc Gynecol Laparosc 2004;11:191–4.

61. Roberts CL, Weston MJ. Bilateral massive ovarian edema: a case report. Ultrasound Obstet Gynecol 1998;11:65–7.

62. Roldan B, San Millan JL, Escobar-Morreale HF. Genetic basis of metabolic abnormalities in polycystic ovary syndrome: implications for therapy. Am J Pharmacogenomics 2004;4:93–107.

63. Sabuncu T, Harma M, Harma M, Nazligul Y, Kilic F. Sibutramine has a positive effect on clinical and metabolic parameters in obese patients with polycystic ovary syndrome. Fertil Steril 2003;80:1199–204.

64. Salehi M, Bravo-Vera R, Sheikh A, Gouller A, Poretsky L. Pathogenesis of polycystic ovary syndrome: what is the role of obesity? Metabolism 2004;53:358–76.

65. Satyanarayana S, Bohre JK. Ovarian granulosa cell 'tumorlet' and mature follicles with ectopic decidua in pregnancy – a case report. Indian J Pathol Microbiol 2001;44:149–50.

66. Sayedur Rahman M, Al-Sibai MH, Rahman J, et al. Ovarian carcinoma associated with pregnancy. A review of 9 cases. Acta Obstet Gynecol Scand 2002;81:260–4.

67. Scurry J, Allen D, Dobson P. Ovarian fibromatosis, ascites and omental fibrosis. Histopathology 1996;28:81–4.

68. Selo-Ojeme DO, GoodFellow CF. Simultaneous intrauterine and ovarian pregnancy following treatment with clomiphene citrate. Arch Gynecol Obstet 2002;266:232–4.

69. Sherer DM, Dalloul M, Khoury-Collado F, et al. Hyperreactio luteinalis presenting with marked hyperglycemia and bilateral multicystic adnexal masses at 21 weeks gestation. Am J Perinatol 2006;23:85–8.

70. Sluijmer AV, Heineman MJ, Koudstaal J, Theunissen PH, de Jong FH, Evers JL. Relationship between ovarian production of estrone, estradiol, testosterone, and androstenedione and the ovarian degree of stromal hyperplasia in postmenopausal women. Menopause 1998;5:207–10.

71. Strauss JF, 3rd. Some new thoughts on the pathophysiology and genetics of polycystic ovary syndrome. Ann N Y Acad Sci 2003;997:42–8.

72. Tanaka Y, Yanagihara T, Ueta M, et al. Naturally conceived twin pregnancy with hyperreactio luteinalis, causing hyperandrogenism and maternal virilization. Acta Obstet Gynecol Scand 2001;80:277–8.

73. Terzibachian JJ, Gay C, Bertrand V, Bouvard M, Knoepffler F. [Value of ureteral catheterization in laparoscopy]. Gynecol Obstet Fertil 2001;29:427–32.

74. Umesaki N, Tanaka T, Miyama M, Kawamura N. Sonographic characteristics of massive ovarian edema. Ultrasound Obstet Gynecol 2000;16:479–81.

75. Umesaki N, Tanaka T, Miyama M, Nishimura S, Kawamura N, Ogita S. Successful preoperative diagnosis of massive ovarian edema aided by comparative imaging study using magnetic resonance and ultrasound. Eur J Obstet Gynecol Reprod Biol 2000;89:97–9.

76. Valenzuela P, Dominguez P. Bilateral massive ovarian edema of the ovary. Zentralbl Gynakol 1999;121:258–9.

77. Wang XY, Vinta MK, Myers S, Fan F. Solitary luteinized follicle cyst of pregnancy and puerperium. Pathol Res Pract 2006;202:471–3.

78. Young RH, Scully RE. Fibromatosis and massive edema of the ovary, possibly related entities: a report of 14 cases of fibromatosis and 11 cases of massive edema. Int J Gynecol Pathol 1984;3:153–78.

Ovarian neoplasia: epidemiology and etiology

23

James V. Lacey Jr   Mark E. Sherman

Malignant ovarian tumors are divisible largely into three histopathologic tumor categories that differ in etiology, biology, and clinical behavior: (1) surface epithelial–stromal tumors; (2) sex cord-stromal tumors; and (3) germ cell tumors. Surface epithelial–stromal tumors, which generally are called simply 'ovarian carcinomas', account for 95% of all ovarian cancers and are the focus of this chapter. (The term 'surface epithelial tumors' is problematic because growing evidence suggests that similar-appearing tumors may arise from several different histologic structures.) The epidemiology and etiology of ovarian carcinomas have been extensively studied. Considerably less is known about gonadal–stromal and germ cell tumors. This chapter reviews current knowledge about the epidemiology and etiology of ovarian carcinomas and discusses the implications for understanding ovarian carcinogenesis. Sex cord-stromal tumors and germ cell tumors are discussed elsewhere (see Chapters 26 and 27).

DESCRIPTIVE EPIDEMIOLOGY

Approximately 20 180 women were diagnosed with ovarian cancer in the United States in 2006. Among US women, ovarian cancer accounts for approximately 3% of incident cancers and is the second most frequently diagnosed gynecologic cancer.[72] The average annual age-adjusted incidence ovarian cancer rate is 16 per 100 000 US women.[149] Roughly one of every 70 American women will be diagnosed during her lifetime.[150] Since the mid-1970s, overall ovarian cancer incidence rates have slightly declined.[71]

Stage at presentation is the most important prognostic factor in ovarian carcinoma. Stage-specific relative survival rates for ovarian cancer are comparable to other gynecologic cancers – 5-year survival for localized ovarian cancer is over 90%.[72] However, in contrast to other gynecologic cancers, about 70% of ovarian cancers present with disseminated disease, and only 19% of tumors are organ confined at diagnosis. Not surprisingly, given the advanced presentation of most tumors, the overall 5-year relative survival rate for ovarian cancer was only 45% between 1995 and 2001.[72] That statistic underscores the need to improve ovarian cancer detection, prevention, and treatment.

The average annual age-adjusted ovarian cancer mortality rate is 7.6 per 100 000 women,[150] and an estimated 15 310 US women died of ovarian cancer in 2006.[72] Ovarian cancer causes more deaths than uterine cervical and uterine corpus cancers combined. In contrast with cervical cancer, screening strategies that have been tested to date have not proven successful.[68]

However, introduction of platinum-based therapies in the 1980s has produced better rates of complete and overall remission and improved 5-year survival.[30]

Incidence rates are higher in developed than developing countries.[133] Age-standardized incidence rates vary 4.5-fold by region: North American, Scandinavian, and Northern European countries have the highest incidence rates, while African and some Asian nations, such as China, have lower rates.[133] Mortality data show a similar, but less dramatic, pattern. The estimated age-standardized mortality rates are 6.2 per 100 000 in developed countries and 2.8 per 100 000 in developing countries.[139]

Rates for invasive ovarian cancer are approximately twice as high among white as among black women in the US.[105] Although incidence rates are higher among white than black women, mortality rates in these two groups are nearly identical.[105] Reasons for the racial disparities in incidence rates are not clear.

Despite the consistent picture that emerges from incidence and mortality rates, important questions remain. Ovarian cancer rates are usually not corrected for oophorectomy status. Not only is oophorectomy prevalence difficult to estimate, but so are variations introduced by racial or ethnic groups and geography. In addition, different histopathologic types of ovarian carcinoma might differ in etiology and pathogenesis, and therefore histology-specific rates might prove more informative than overall ovarian cancer rates. Data from the National Cancer Institute's Surveillance, Epidemiology and End Results (SEER) program for the period 1978–1998 showed increasing rates among white women for serous, endometrioid, and clear cell carcinoma histologies but declining rates among blacks for mucinous and serous carcinoma histologies. Shifting pathologic classification, compounded by poor reproducibility of histologic typing and a tendency for ovarian carcinomas to demonstrate multiple patterns of differentiation or minimal differentiation, could influence these trends. More research is needed to define subsets of tumors with distinctive etiology or pathogenesis to facilitate targeted detection, prevention, and surveillance.

RISK AND PROTECTIVE FACTORS FOR SPORADIC OVARIAN CARCINOMA

Environmental, genetic, and lifestyle factors all influence ovarian cancer risk (Figure 23.1). Many determinants of this disease are established at young ages – in the second and third decades – and appear to produce long-lasting effects.

601

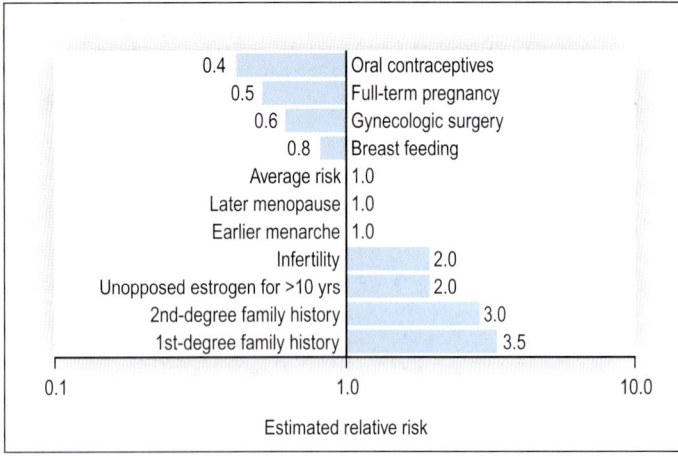

Fig. 23.1 Relative importance of factors associated with the development of ovarian cancer.

REPRODUCTIVE VARIABLES

Parity is strongly associated with decreased risk for ovarian carcinoma.[9,54,73,156,212,216] A single pregnancy reduces risk by approximately 40–60%, and each additional pregnancy decreases the relative risk another 10–15%. Despite these consistent data, potential protection associated with highly correlated factors, such as timing of births or fertility, is unresolved.

Most studies concluded that age at first or last birth was not related to risk after accounting for parity,[73,116,201] but some authors argue that both number and timing of births matter.[118] A recent study reported that older compared with younger age at last birth increased the risk,[210] but the strong correlations between age, parity, and ages at first and last birth raise questions about the potential independence of such associations. Some studies observed decreased risks associated with increasing number of incomplete pregnancies,[15,52,117] but others showed no such association.[45]

Nulligravid women are at higher risk than gravid women, but nulligravidity can be due to infertility (i.e., an absence of conception after 12 continuous months of contraceptive-free sexual intercourse), subfertility, or reproductive choice.[80] Higher risks among infertile women support some role for abnormal endocrine factors.[73,116,212,214] Two studies[9,214] reported higher (up to six-fold) relative risks among sexually active women who were not using contraceptives and had not conceived over long intervals compared with other women. More recent data highlight the importance of the potential causes of infertility. In a large cohort of US women evaluated for infertility, higher ovarian cancer risks were found among patients with primary infertility than secondary infertility, and especially among patients with primary infertility and endometriosis.[13]

Assisted reproductive technologies, such as ovulation-stimulating infertility medications, may also affect risk.[167,212] Some,[108,167] but not all,[141,200] cohort studies have reported increased risks with particular medications, whereas few of the published case-control studies observed associations with fertility drug use or specific medications.[40,113,132,179] However, a recent analysis of a large US cohort with lengthy follow-up

found that women who had used clomiphene citrate or gonadotrophins were not at increased risk for ovarian carcinoma.[12,13] These studies face several particular challenges: potential detection bias due to clinical workups in infertile women, recall bias associated with fertility treatments, and difficulties controlling for causes of infertility. Nonetheless, current evidence suggests that causes of subfertility and infertility, rather than the associated treatments, appear as more important predictors of ovarian cancer risk.[75,80,123] Additional studies of infertility treatments and ovarian carcinoma risk are needed, especially given that lengthy follow-up may be required to identify associations for rare outcomes.

In several studies, women who breastfed their children had lower ovarian carcinoma risks than women who did not.[9,156,164,180,193] However, in contrast with breast carcinoma, risk does not seem to progressively decrease with increasing duration of breastfeeding.

Age at menopause has a debatable effect on ovarian cancer risk.[9,38,171,216] Similarly, earlier age at menarche has not been associated with risk in most analyses, although some studies have reported weak positive associations.[9,38,216]

These variables may coalesce as the total number of lifetime menstrual cycles. The interval between menarche and menopause, accounting for periods of oral contraceptive use, parity, or breastfeeding, can approximate lifetime number of cycles, which has been positively associated with ovarian cancer.[138,144] A recently constructed mathematical model of ovarian cancer incidence incorporating time since menopause, duration of ovulation (duration of premenopause minus parity and years of oral contraceptive use), and tubal ligation best predicts the observed incidence in two large US cohort studies.[166] Accurately estimating lifetime cycles is difficult and at present does not fully capture other ovarian changes.[112]

GYNECOLOGIC SURGERY

Simple hysterectomy or tubal ligation consistently decreases the risk of subsequent ovarian cancer.[9,49,55,82,106,156,165,212,214] After gynecologic surgery, a woman's relative risk of developing ovarian cancer falls by 30–40%.

How and why these surgeries reduce risk is unknown. One possibility involves reduced blood flow to the ovaries, which might alter the hormonal milieu, although evidence for both explanations is lacking.[207] Gynecologic surgery potentially facilitates preferential removal of ovaries that appear grossly abnormal at laparotomy. However, gross examination seems unlikely to identify high-risk ovaries because proven methods for detecting preclinical ovarian cancer are lacking,[29,69] and therefore unaided clinical examination would also seem unlikely to detect early abnormalities. Tubal ligation has been linked to reduced risk for endometrioid and clear cell carcinomas. If these specific histopathologic tumor types arise from endometriosis, then tubal ligation might reduce risk by preventing expelled endometrial tissue from reaching the ovaries, where it might create endometriotic implants.

EXOGENOUS HORMONES

Oral contraceptive use has been consistently demonstrated to reduce risk for ovarian carcinoma. Long-term use generates substantial protection,[9,41,156,163,209,216] but even a few months of use produces long-term protective effects. Long-term users (≥10 years) were 80% less likely than non-users to develop ovarian carcinoma in one study,[1] and protection persisted for years after last use.[9,41,163,216] Despite some uncertainty about changing formulations, recent data indicate that newer lower-dose oral contraceptives reduce risk to the same extent as their higher-dose predecessors.[51,124,168,170]

Exogenous hormones used in menopausal hormone therapy, in contrast, appear to increase risk. Early studies produced diverse results – null,[212] inverse,[61] and positive[208] associations – that were difficult to reconcile.[18,43] Questions still remain,[125,153,181] but recent studies, including three large cohorts,[37,88,159] point to an increased risk among women who used menopausal estrogens (i.e., 'estrogen replacement therapy') for long durations.[46,111,119,143,151]

Based on limited data for hysterectomized women with intact ovaries, it appears that unopposed estrogen may increase ovarian carcinoma risk in this group,[88,111,138] although not all studies agree.[181] Among women with intact uteri, questions remain about whether combined estrogen and progestin therapy increases ovarian carcinoma risk. Interpretation of these data is often complex because women may have used unopposed estrogen before using estrogen plus progestin.[88,103,111,151] Limited data suggest that this formulation does not increase risk overall;[88,111,138,151,181] however, data are insufficient to estimate risk associated with long-term or recent use of either sequential or continuous estrogen plus progestin regimens.

ENDOGENOUS HORMONES

Associations with endogenous hormone levels have received less attention than associations with exogenous hormones. The ovary is itself a source of hormones, and hormone levels within the ovarian parenchyma, clefts, or cysts formed from invaginations of surface epithelium could differ from circulating hormone levels. One study found that women who developed ovarian cancer had higher levels of androgens and lower levels of gonadotrophins than controls.[65] In pooled data from three studies, ovarian cancer was not associated with circulating estrogens, androgens, sex hormone binding globulin (SHBG), insulin-like growth factor-1 (IGF-1), insulin-like growth factor binding proteins (IGFBPs), or follicle-stimulating hormone (FSH).[94,95] As existing cohort studies mature, additional opportunities to revisit this hypothesis will arise. Testing this hypothesis in premenopausal women may prove especially informative but would require large studies with sufficient numbers of ovarian carcinoma patients and accurate measurements of hormone levels in cycling women.

ENERGY BALANCE

Obesity is receiving increasing attention as a potential risk factor for ovarian cancer. Some studies reported increased risks among heavier women only for serous or endometrioid tumors.[35] Attempts to replicate those data instead raised more uncertainty by reporting increased risks only among women who are clinically obese,[174] whose body mass index (BMI; kg/m^2) is higher at age 18,[93] who are diagnosed before menopause,[34] who never used menopausal estrogens,[158] or who were physically inactive.[145] Other studies concluded that obese women had decreased ovarian cancer risk.[96,131] These diverse results could reflect statistical chance or other systematic biases specific to analyzing obesity as a risk factor for ovarian cancer.

Data on ovarian cancer and physical activity are not consistent. Case-control studies in China,[218,219] Canada,[129] and the US[17] have reported potential inverse associations with increasing activity, but two cohort analyses[3,7,104] observed that increasing activity might put women at increased, rather than decreased, risk. Another US cohort study of primarily postmenopausal women found a null association between ovarian cancer and increasing activity.[56] In the absence of strong inverse associations from prospective studies, the inverse associations that tend to occur in retrospective studies with hospital-based controls warrant careful scrutiny and await definitive replication.[129]

Correlations between ovarian cancer incidence and per capita fat availability (i.e., increased incidence rates among migrants who moved to areas with higher per-capita fat availability) have stimulated interest in dietary risk factors.[4] Mixed results followed. Initial studies in unique populations, such as ovolactovegetarians[137] or meat abstainers[79] provided conflicting results. Since then, studies have primarily focused on a few classes of foods: lactose and dairy foods, fats, vitamins, fiber, and fruits and vegetables.

Higher consumption of yogurt, cottage cheese, and other lactose-rich dairy products was linked with increased risk in an early case-control study.[20] Galactose-related enzymes can influence gonadotrophin levels, which are hypothesized to be crucial ovarian cancer risk determinants. A meta-analysis of 22 published studies concluded that the association between ovarian cancer and milk or dairy product consumption was null.[146] However, two large cohort studies – one from the US[32] and one from Sweden[91] – reported increased risks associated with dairy and milk consumption.

Fat intake can be closely correlated with dairy consumption, and most case-control studies produced positive associations between increasing fat consumption and ovarian cancer.[22,86,155,178] Certain fatty foods (e.g., eggs, butter, and meats) have received substantial attention, but recent data are less supportive of the hypothesis that higher intake of fat increases ovarian cancer risk.[6,85,100,130]

A heterogeneous group of related exposures – fiber, fruits, vegetables, and vitamins – has yielded surprisingly consistent inverse associations with ovarian cancer. In several studies, total vegetable intake,[10,85,130,178] different types of fiber,[99,135] or particular vitamins (e.g., beta-carotene, vitamin A, or vitamin B[14,130,182,195]) were associated with reduced risks of ovarian cancer. Some studies, however, reported null associations.[31,100]

Several early studies linked coffee consumption to an elevated risk of ovarian cancer,[87,194,213] but few studies replicated that association.[62,83,102,140,183] Recent studies are equally inconclusive.[74,92] Before 1990, most reports showed no association with alcohol use.[14,53,86,213] Recent studies generally replicated those findings.[48,83] However, one case-control study reported an inverse association with two or more drinks per week,[48,205] and a Swedish analysis of a cohort of women diagnosed with alcoholism over 30 years identified marginally fewer than expected ovarian cancers: standardized incidence ratio (SIR) of 0.86, 95% confidence interval, 0.68–1.08. Alcohol's ability to suppress gonadotrophin levels might possibly account for the apparent reduced risk.[90] A Swedish cohort study found no association with wine, beer, or spirits consumption,[101] but an Australian case-control study reported strong inverse associations. Compared with women who never consumed alcohol, women who consumed two or more drinks per week had a 50% reduced odds ratio, and even women who consumed less than one drink per week had a reduced risk of ovarian cancer.[205] The prospective Iowa Women's Health Study published a similar inverse association that, on further exploration, was limited to women with both high alcohol and high folate intake.[78]

OTHER RISK FACTORS

Potential associations between ovarian cancer and diabetes, hypertension and thyroid diseases have not been confirmed.[131,206] Pelvic inflammatory disease has been linked with ovarian cancer,[154] but this hypothesis requires further testing. Polycystic ovaries do not seem to be more likely than normal ovaries to develop ovarian cancer.[42]

Case-control studies generally report positive associations between ovarian cancer and perineal talc exposure. A lack of consistent statistical significance and inconsistent associations with different types of talc use raise questions about the validity of this association.[16,23,59,213] One large cohort study reported no such association.[44]

Smoking is not considered a major risk factor for ovarian cancer. Some recent investigations argued that smoking increases the risk for tumors of mucinous histology only. Cohort[190] and case-control studies[50,98,110] have found increased risks for mucinous tumors after reporting null or weak positive associations based on all tumor histologies. The potential for smoking-related mucinous adenocarcinoma primary cancers (such as those of gastrointestinal origin) to metastasize to the ovary and be misclassified as primary mucinous ovarian carcinoma might contribute to these discrepancies, but improved histopathology- and immunohistochemistry-based diagnoses should avoid this problem. Future studies that address this question would ideally possess adequate statistical power for *a priori* histology-specific analyses and employ standardized histologic review of the original pathology data. Recent attempts to address passive smoking[47] signal a reasonable direction for future research.

Certain occupations came under scrutiny when studies linked hair dyes and triazine herbicides to ovarian cancer.[8,27] Linkage studies in Finland,[198] Sweden,[176] and the US[169] suggested a pattern of increased risks among certain professions (e.g., healthcare workers) or with particular occupational exposures (e.g., solvents). Until additional data address the potential for inconsistent or chance findings and the challenge of finding large populations with sufficient data on other potential confounding variables, occupation will likely not be considered a major risk factor for ovarian cancer.[175]

After initial studies reported suggestive inverse associations among women who used anti-inflammatory or analgesic medications,[19,157,196] later studies showed, at most, a weak and inconsistent association.[33,114,162] However, if anti-inflammatory drugs are protective, they may only have an effect during the premenopause by reducing damaging effects of postovulatory inflammatory reactions. Assessing premenopausal drug use is difficult, especially for medications that can be purchased without a prescription. In contrast, psychotropic medications, particularly those operating through dopaminergic mechanisms, appeared to increase ovarian cancer risk.[57,58] Here, too, subsequent studies that employed cohort designs or improved exposure assessment reported null associations.[26,28,76,89]

HOST FACTORS

Although only 5–10% of ovarian cancer patients have a first-degree relative with ovarian cancer,[66] a family history of ovarian cancer is a strong risk factor for developing ovarian cancer. Women whose first-degree relatives have ovarian cancer are three times as likely to develop the disease as women with unaffected relatives.[81,172,187] Higher numbers of affected relatives or relatives affected at earlier ages appear to be more important than which family member had ovarian cancer.[66] Women with two or more affected relatives or whose relative was diagnosed before age 50 experience a particularly increased risk.[136]

Compared with the 1–2% absolute risk in the general population, women whose relatives have ovarian cancer have a 9.4% absolute risk of developing ovarian cancer in their lifetime.[63] Women who inherit a mutation in autosomal dominant breast cancer susceptibility gene 1 (*BRCA1*) or breast cancer susceptibility gene 2 (*BRCA2*) have a 15–40% absolute risk of developing ovarian cancer.[188,199,204,215] Despite these increases, *BRCA1/2* mutations explain less than one-third of the elevated risk in women with familial ovarian cancer.[136] Other candidate high-risk genes have not been identified but likely exist.[66]

Both *BRCA1* and *BRCA2* are tumor-suppressor genes that appear to preserve cells' ability to efficiently repair double-stranded DNA breaks.[184] Although these genes are expressed in many tissues throughout the body, mutations in *BRCA1* and *BRCA2* are highly associated with particular cancer sites: ovaries, fallopian tubes, peritoneum, and breasts. Compared with ovarian cancers in women with wild-type *BRCA1* and *BRCA2*, ovarian cancers in mutation carriers are more often serous adenocarcinomas and display TP53 (tumor protein p53) dysregulation.[72,184,192] Mutation carriers tend to be diagnosed at younger ages than women without mutations, but their risk remains elevated at later ages, too.[11] However, both disease-free and overall survival rates for *BRCA1/2*-linked ovarian cancer do not appear to be lower than survival rates for sporadic ovarian cancer.[11]

Three *BRCA* founder mutations in Ashkenazi Jewish women – 185delAG and 5382insC in *BRCA1* and 6174delT in *BRCA2* – account for much of the increased risk reported in North American data. The 6174delT *BRCA2* mutation is located within the 'ovarian cancer cluster region' (OCCR), which covers approximately 3300 nucleotides whose mutations are associated with higher risks of ovarian cancer than are mutations in other regions of the gene.[191] A substantial portion of *BRCA1* and *BRCA2* mutations in women with ovarian cancer are not founder mutations and fall outside the OCCR, but the clinical significance of these reported and novel mutations is uncertain.[128] Particular mutations might be especially important in certain populations. For example, Icelandic investigators have reported one founder mutation each in *BRCA1* and *BRCA2*, but a survey of all ovarian cancer patients diagnosed between 1999 and 2003 revealed the *BRCA1* mutation in only one mother–daughter pair. In contrast, the 999del5 *BRCA2* mutation was detected in 6% of invasive cancer patients compared with only 0.3% of a non-affected population sample.[147]

Although one-third of US women report a family history of breast or ovarian cancer,[67] the prevalence of a *BRCA1* or *BRCA2* mutation in the general population is estimated to be much lower – perhaps 1 in 300 to 1 in 500 women.[120] For women at elevated risk due to a confirmed *BRCA* mutation or a strong family history, bilateral salpingo-oophorectomy can dramatically reduce the risk of ovarian cancer. Ovarian, peritoneal or fallopian tube cancer is occasionally detected at the time of surgery,[77,148] but the subsequent risk of developing ovarian cancer falls by at least 85%.[2] (Although risk might be expected to fall to zero after bilateral salpingo-oophorectomy, carcinoma can arise in residual ovarian tissue or in the peritoneal cavity.) Referral for genetic counseling is currently recommended for women with clinically significant *BRCA* mutations and for women whose family history is associated with an increased risk of carrying a *BRCA1* or *BRCA2* mutation.[2] For other women at elevated risk of ovarian cancer, key questions remain unanswered; referral for genetic counseling and evaluation for *BRCA* testing is not currently recommended.

Whether oral contraceptives might effectively reduce risk in women at highly elevated lifetime risk due to a *BRCA1* or *BRCA2* mutation has generated substantial interest. To date, data are not clear. Studies in high-risk clinics have reported similar protection among oral contraceptive users with and without confirmed mutations,[101,115,211] although some have argued that those study settings are particularly prone to potential biases.[202] A case-control study in Israel reported that oral contraceptive use reduced ovarian cancer risk only among non-carriers. Oral contraceptive use was not associated with ovarian cancer in women with confirmed mutations, but this analysis was limited by the low prevalence of mutations among the disease-free control group.[107]

BRCA mutations are associated with the vast majority of hereditary ovarian cancer. Hereditary non-polyposis colorectal cancer (HNPCC) syndrome appears to be responsible for the rest, which represent perhaps 10% of hereditary ovarian cancers and 1–2% of all ovarian cancers.[142] Defective mismatch repair is the genetic hallmark of HNPCC, and mutations in three genes – *hMLH1*, *hMSH2*, and *hMSH6* – are present in approximately 95% of all HNPCC-associated cancers.[97] The lifetime risk of ovarian cancer in women with HNPCC is between 8 and 15%.[97] Although ovarian cancer risks are lower than lifetime risks of developing colorectal cancer or endometrial cancer for HNPCC families, some authors have argued that a family history suggestive of HNPCC should prompt the same consideration of genetic counseling and potential prophylactic surgery as would a family history of hereditary breast and ovarian cancer.[97] In one study of women with HNPCC-associated germ-line mutations, prophylactic oophorectomy was associated with sharply reduced risks of ovarian cancer,[173] although the study design likely introduced bias that would overestimate the efficacy of surgery.[127] With the increasing recognition of HNPCC-associated ovarian cancer, future studies will surely evaluate risk assessment, screening, and prophylactic surgery in this high-risk group.

Low-penetrance genetic factors, such as single-nucleotide polymorphisms or haplotypes, might be expected theoretically to influence ovarian cancer risk, although to date, there have been no conclusive reports. In one study, the CAG repeat length in the androgen receptor (AR) gene was not associated

with ovarian cancer in studies of primarily sporadic[185] or *BRCA1/2* mutation carriers.[25] After initial null results for progesterone receptor (PR) polymorphisms and ovarian cancer,[109] recent papers suggest specific polymorphisms[189] or related haplotypes[134] might be associated with ovarian cancer. This route of exploration, although promising, is particularly prone to false-positive results,[203] and even larger studies would be required to assess potential differences by histologic type or other molecular features. Replication in sufficiently large population-based studies and consortia of well-conducted studies will be required. Ongoing analyses of pooled data from multiple large studies should clarify these associations.

SCREENING

By one estimate, effective ovarian cancer screening could extend survival by 3 years.[197] Screening could reduce mortality, but clinical trials have not yet demonstrated a benefit to screening; ongoing studies should provide informative data in the near future.[68] Current screening studies use elevated cancer antigen 125 (CA125) levels in serum or ovarian abnormalities detected via transvaginal ultrasonography. New work suggests that the rate of change rather than the absolute level of CA125 may be diagnostically useful.

One challenge facing screening is the low prevalence of ovarian cancer in the population. Targeted efforts in high-risk women could improve the performance of screening by focusing on populations at higher baseline risk. Even in these groups, however, results have been equivocal. In one recent study, intensive surveillance via pelvic examination, CA125, and transvaginal ultrasonography did not identify ovarian cancers at early stages, leading to the conclusion that prophylactic surgery was likely to be more efficient at reducing ovarian cancer risk than such a resource-intense screening.[126]

HISTOLOGY-SPECIFIC ASSOCIATIONS

Many epidemiologic studies consider ovarian cancer to be an etiologically homogeneous disease that is associated with a common set of causes. However, differences in histologic characteristics or molecular alterations could reflect divergent etiologies. Understanding these differences might identify factors that are more strongly associated with certain tumor types than with ovarian cancer as a whole, which would suggest different public health strategies for prevention. Alternatively, identifying essential exposures or mechanisms that are common to all types of ovarian carcinoma might permit the identification of single strategies with broad potential for detecting or preventing most types of ovarian cancer. Understanding factors that are necessary for carcinogenesis among women at high risk due to family history or high-penetrance genetic mutations could improve decision-making regarding the risks and benefits of prophylactic oophorectomy in this setting.

A recent pooled analysis of data from 10 case-control studies of US white women, including 1834 invasive epithelial ovarian cancers and 7484 controls, investigated whether potential ovarian cancer risk factors varied by histologic type.[84] Differences in the frequencies of epidemiologic factors among women with specific histologic tumors were generally small, but interesting patterns emerged. The strong reproductive protective factors, oral contraceptive use and parity, were associated with reduced risks of each histologic type. Non-reproductive factors, such as BMI and smoking, showed potentially different associations with mucinous or endometrioid tumor types, but the results were not consistent. Such differences could have emerged by chance or been due to biases, but the data raise questions about whether stratification of tumors by other characteristics, such as molecular markers, would reveal larger differences.

ORIGINS OF OVARIAN CARCINOMA AND MODELS OF CARCINOGENESIS

Despite the generally consistent epidemiologic data linking ovarian cancer to specific risk factors, little is known about ovarian carcinoma natural history, precursors, or early stages of carcinogenesis. By the time most carcinomas are surgically removed for diagnosis and treatment, their obliteration of the surrounding, once-normal ovarian tissue often obscures clues related to their origins from precursor lesions. However, there is substantial evidence[177] that ovarian carcinomas can develop from different types of distinct tissue structures, including ovarian surface epithelium, the epithelial lining of surface inclusion cysts, foci of endometriosis, and borderline tumors (i.e., tumors of low malignant potential). In addition to the (albeit inconclusive) risk factor differences by histopathologic type, studies have suggested that ovarian carcinomas can be classified into subsets based on gene expression profiles, cytogenetic abnormalities, and similar mechanisms of pathogenesis.[70]

From an etiologic perspective, models of ovarian carcinogenesis have focused on the consistent observation that repeated ovulation provides a unifying explanation for several risk factors and protective factors. Conditions associated with reduced ovulation, e.g., pregnancy and oral contraceptives, consistently reduce risk. Combining these and other menstrual factors into single 'ovulatory age' or 'lifetime ovulatory cycles' indices have generally produced the expected associations with ovarian cancer risk, i.e., older ovulatory ages[39] or higher cycle counts[144] increase risk. However, the imprecision inherent in developing these indices leads to different risk estimates depending on the method of calculation.[112] In addition, the magnitude of risk reduction for short-term oral contraceptive use or a single pregnancy is unexpectedly large for the associated reduction in lifetime number of ovulatory cycles. This observation underscores the need to understand the mechanism that underlies the risk associated with ovulation.

One possible mechanism that could account for the risk associated with repeated ovulation is that repeated epithelial trauma and re-epithelialization increase the risk for random mutations to develop and persist. Ovulation prompts a cascade of epithelial events, including minor trauma and increased local concentrations of estrogen-rich follicular fluid. These 'incessant ovulation' events may lie on the causal path to ovarian cancer.[36,217] This is consistent with most of the endocrine-related risk factors except for the risks associated with clinical infertility.

However, this explanation would not account for the disproportionate protection from a single pregnancy or short-term oral contraceptive use. Exposure to high levels of progesterone or reduced levels of androgen during pregnancy,

or to oral contraceptives, seems to produce disproportionately large effects compared with the absolute decrease in number of ovulatory cycles.[152] In animal models, progesterone promotes apoptosis of surface epithelium, a process that could potentially eliminate damaged cells and reduce the risk of carcinogenesis.[160]

Re-epithelialization after ovulation might also increase the formation of cysts lined by ovarian surface epithelium. Increased ovulation might increase the formation of epithelial inclusion cysts, thus providing a microenvironment that is prone to malignant transformation yet protected from mechanical dislodgement. However, this perspective is challenged by the comparatively weak associations between lifetime number of cycles and prevalence of inclusion cysts.[64] Furthermore, cross-sectional studies have found inconsistent relationships between the presence of inclusion cysts and carcinoma,[60] and ultrasound-based screening to detect and surgically remove cysts has not been shown to reduce the mortality from ovarian cancer.[24]

A second commonly considered unifying hypothesis makes ovarian cancer the result of accumulated exposure to circulating pituitary gonadotrophins.[21,186] Although this hypothesis is consistent with the protective effects of parity and oral contraceptive use and the increased risk associated with cumulative number of lifetime ovulations, serum gonadotrophin levels were unrelated to risk in the two epidemiologic studies that have directly compared serum levels in specimens obtained before the diagnosis of cancer.[5,65,94] According to this hypothesis, early menopause should increase risk because of the earlier rise in luteinizing hormone (LH) and follicle-stimulating hormone (FSH) levels, and menopausal estrogen therapy should decrease risk because it reduces circulating gonadotrophins, but neither association has been observed in epidemiologic studies. Some have argued that this hypothesis is based on experimental data that are related to the development of stromal cancers in animals, and therefore may not apply to the development of ovarian carcinomas in humans.[5]

Other models help account for specific subsets of tumors that arise from surface epithelium. For example, one model invokes two pathways for serous ovarian carcinoma.[177] One form arises from pre-existing neoplasms, such as serous borderline tumors. These tumors develop via a multistage model of carcinogenesis and display generally indolent clinical behavior. Low-grade serous carcinoma is representative of this group. In contrast, this model postulates a second high-grade form thought to develop rapidly *de novo* from non-neoplastic surface epithelium either on the ovarian surface or lining cyst. In support of this theory, nearly 70% of borderline tumors and low-grade serous carcinomas exhibit mutations in *braf* and *ras* in contrast with none of the high-grade serous carcinomas. Furthermore, 50–80% of borderline and low-grade serous tumors show upregulated expression of wild-type *p53*, and 67% of high-grade serous carcinomas demonstrate *p53* mutations.

Each theory accommodates some, but not all, of the available data. A unifying hypothesis may lie in a combination of ovulation, hormones, and local effects. Additional factors, such as genetic alterations; androgens, progestogens, and other hormones;[152,161] inflammation;[122] and endometriosis,[121] also appear to be important. By the time a woman reaches menopause, two apparent *bona fide* protective factors – oral contraceptive use and parity – are essentially static. Against a backdrop of risk set by a woman's cumulative number of ovulatory cycles, these other factors might sufficiently stimulate tumor promotion or capably keep carcinogenesis in check. How these theories intertwine is likely to be complex, but the intersections of the available hypotheses are also likely to be the most fruitful areas for future hypothesis-driven research.

CONCLUSION

Ovarian cancer epidemiology includes relative extremes. Some risk factor data are entirely consistent, such as the inverse associations with oral contraceptives and parity and the positive associations with family history. Other data are highly uncertain, such as the data on lifestyle factors like smoking and obesity. Histology-specific associations, which could reflect histology-specific etiologies, might account for some of these differences, but other unknown differences at the molecular or population level could be important. Incorporating these knowns and unknowns into existing models of ovarian cancer etiology will be the major challenge for current and future research.

REFERENCES

1. The reduction in risk of ovarian cancer associated with oral-contraceptive use. The Cancer and Steroid Hormone Study of the Centers for Disease Control and the National Institute of Child Health and Human Development. N Engl J Med 1987;316:650–5.
2. Genetic risk assessment and BRCA mutation testing for breast and ovarian cancer susceptibility: recommendation statement. Ann Intern Med 2005;143:355–61.
3. Anderson JP, Ross JA, Folsom AR. Anthropometric variables, physical activity, and incidence of ovarian cancer: The Iowa Women's Health Study. Cancer 2004;100:1515–21.
4. Armstrong B, Doll R. Environmental factors and cancer incidence and mortality in different countries, with special reference to dietary practices. Int J Cancer 1975;15:617–31.
5. Arslan AA, Zeleniuch-Jacquotte A, Lundin E, et al. Serum follicle-stimulating hormone and risk of epithelial ovarian cancer in postmenopausal women. Cancer Epidemiol Biomarkers Prev 2003;12:1531–5.
6. Bertone ER, Rosner BA, Hunter DJ, et al. Dietary fat intake and ovarian cancer in a cohort of US women. Am J Epidemiol 2002;156:22–31.
7. Bertone ER, Willett WC, Rosner BA, et al. Prospective study of recreational physical activity and ovarian cancer. J Natl Cancer Inst 2001;93:942–8.
8. Boffetta P, Andersen A, Lynge E, Barlow L, Pukkala E. Employment as hairdresser and risk of ovarian cancer and non-Hodgkin's lymphomas among women. J Occup Med 1994;36:61–5.
9. Booth M, Beral V, Smith P. Risk factors for ovarian cancer: a case-control study. Br J Cancer 1989;60:592–8.
10. Bosetti C, Negri E, Franceschi S, et al. Diet and ovarian cancer risk: a case-control study in Italy. Int J Cancer 2001;93:911–5.
11. Boyd J, Sonoda Y, Federici MG, et al. Clinicopathologic features of BRCA-linked and sporadic ovarian cancer. JAMA 2000;283:2260–5.
12. Brinton LA, Lamb EJ, Moghissi KS, et al. Ovarian cancer risk after the use of ovulation-stimulating drugs. Obstet Gynecol 2004;103:1194–203.
13. Brinton LA, Lamb EJ, Moghissi KS, et al. Ovarian cancer risk associated with varying causes of infertility. Fertil Steril 2004;82:405–14.
14. Byers T, Marshall J, Graham S, Mettlin C, Swanson M. A case-control study of dietary and nondietary factors in ovarian cancer. J Natl Cancer Inst 1983;71:681–6.
15. Chen MT, Cook LS, Daling JR, Weiss NS. Incomplete pregnancies and risk of ovarian cancer (Washington, United States). Cancer Causes Control 1996;7:415–20.
16. Cook LS, Kamb ML, Weiss NS. Perineal powder exposure and the risk of ovarian cancer. Am J Epidemiol 1997;146:459–65.
17. Cottreau CM, Ness RB, Kriska AM. Physical activity and reduced risk of ovarian cancer. Obstet Gynecol 2000;96:609–14.
18. Coughlin SS, Giustozzi A, Smith SJ, Lee NC. A meta-analysis of estrogen replacement therapy and risk of epithelial ovarian cancer. J Clin Epidemiol 2000;53:367–75.
19. Cramer DW, Harlow BL, Titus-Ernstoff L, Bohlke K, Welch WR, Greenberg ER. Over-the-counter analgesics and risk of ovarian cancer. Lancet 1998;351:104–7.
20. Cramer DW, Harlow BL, Willett WC, et al. Galactose consumption and metabolism in relation to the risk of ovarian cancer. Lancet 1989;2:66–71.
21. Cramer DW, Welch WR. Determinants of ovarian cancer risk. II. Inferences regarding pathogenesis. J Natl Cancer Inst 1983;71:717–21.
22. Cramer DW, Welch WR, Hutchison GB, Willett W, Scully RE. Dietary animal fat in relation to ovarian cancer risk. Obstet Gynecol 1984;63:833–8.
23. Cramer DW, Welch WR, Scully RE, Wojciechowski CA. Ovarian cancer and talc: a case-control study. Cancer 1982;50:372–6.
24. Crayford TJ, Campbell S, Bourne TH, Rawson HJ, Collins WP. Benign ovarian cysts and ovarian cancer: a cohort study with implications for screening. Lancet 2000;355:1060–3.
25. Dagan E, Friedman E, Paperna T, Carmi N, Gershoni-Baruch R. Androgen receptor CAG repeat length in Jewish Israeli women who are BRCA1/2 mutation carriers: association with breast/ovarian cancer phenotype. Eur J Hum Genet 2002;10:724–8.
26. Dalton SO, Johansen C, Mellemkjaer L, et al. Antidepressant medications and risk for cancer. Epidemiology 1999;11:171–6.
27. Donna A, Crosignani P, Robutti F, et al. Triazine herbicides and ovarian epithelial neoplasms. Scand J Work Environ Health 1989;15:47–53.
28. Dublin S, Rossing MA, Heckbert SR, Goff BA, Weiss NS. Risk of epithelial ovarian cancer in relation to use of antidepressants, benzodiazepines, and other centrally acting medications. Cancer Causes Control 2002;13:35–45.
29. Ellsworth LR, Allen HH, Nisker JA. Ovarian function after radical hysterectomy for stage IB carcinoma of cervix. Am J Obstet Gynecol 1983;145:185–8.
30. Eltabbakh GH, Awtrey CS. Current treatment for ovarian cancer. Expert Opin Pharmacother 2001;2:109–24.
31. Fairfield KM, Hankinson SE, Rosner BA, Hunter DJ, Colditz GA, Willett WC. Risk of ovarian carcinoma and consumption of vitamins A, C, and E and specific carotenoids: a prospective analysis. Cancer 2001;92:2318–26.
32. Fairfield KM, Hunter DJ, Colditz GA, et al. A prospective study of dietary lactose and ovarian cancer. Int J Cancer 2004;110:271–7.
33. Fairfield KM, Hunter DJ, Fuchs CS, Colditz GA, Hankinson SE. Aspirin, other NSAIDs, and ovarian cancer risk (United States). Cancer Causes Control 2002;13:535–42.
34. Fairfield KM, Willett WC, Rosner BA, Manson JE, Speizer FE, Hankinson SE. Obesity, weight gain, and ovarian cancer. Obstet Gynecol 2002;100:288–96.
35. Farrow DC, Weiss NS, Lyon JL, Daling JR. Association of obesity and ovarian cancer in a case-control study. Am J Epidemiol 1989;129:1300–4.
36. Fathalla MF. Incessant ovulation – a factor in ovarian neoplasia? Lancet 1971;2:163.
37. Folsom AR, Anderson JP, Ross JA. Estrogen replacement therapy and ovarian cancer. Epidemiology 2004;15:100–4.
38. Franceschi S, La Vecchia C, Booth M, et al. Pooled analysis of 3 European case-control studies of ovarian cancer: II. Age at menarche and at menopause. Int J Cancer 1991;49:57–60.
39. Franceschi S, La Vecchia C, Helmrich SP, Mangioni C, Tognoni G. Risk factors for epithelial ovarian cancer in Italy. Am J Epidemiol 1982;115:714–9.
40. Franceschi S, La Vecchia C, Negri E, et al. Fertility drugs and risk of epithelial ovarian cancer in Italy. Hum Reprod 1994;9:1673–5.
41. Franceschi S, Parazzini F, Negri E, et al. Pooled analysis of 3 European case-control studies of epithelial ovarian cancer: III. Oral contraceptive use. Int J Cancer 1991;49:61–5.
42. Gadducci A, Gargini A, Palla E, Fanucchi A, Genazzani AR. Polycystic ovary syndrome and gynecological cancers: is there a link? Gynecol Endocrinol 2005;20:200–8.
43. Garg PP, Kerlikowske K, Subak L, Grady D. Hormone replacement therapy and the risk of epithelial ovarian carcinoma: a meta-analysis [see comments]. Obstet Gynecol 1998;92:472–9.
44. Gertig DM, Hunter DJ, Cramer DW, et al. Prospective study of talc use and ovarian cancer. J Natl Cancer Inst 2000;92:249–52.
45. Gierach GL, Modugno F, Ness RB. Relations of gestational length and timing and type of incomplete pregnancy to ovarian cancer risk. Am J Epidemiol 2005;161:452–61.
46. Glud E, Kjaer SK, Thomsen BL, et al. Hormone therapy and the impact of estrogen intake on the risk of ovarian cancer. Arch Intern Med 2004;164:2253–9.
47. Goodman MT, Tung K-H. Active and passive smoking and the risk of borderline and invasive ovarian cancer (United States). Cancer Causes Control 2003;14:569–77.
48. Goodman MT, Tung KH. Alcohol consumption and the risk of borderline and invasive ovarian cancer. Obstet Gynecol 2003;101:1221–8.
49. Green A, Purdie D, Bain C, et al. Tubal sterilisation, hysterectomy and decreased risk of ovarian cancer. Survey of Women's Health Study Group. Int J Cancer 1997;71:948–51.
50. Green A, Purdie D, Bain C, Siskind V, Webb PM. Cigarette smoking and risk of epithelial ovarian cancer (Australia). Cancer Causes Control 2001;12:713–9.
51. Greer JB, Modugno F, Allen GO, Ness RB. Androgenic progestins in oral contraceptives and the risk of epithelial ovarian cancer. Obstet Gynecol 2005;105:731–40.
52. Greggi S, Parazzini F, Paratore MP, et al. Risk factors for ovarian cancer in central Italy. Gynecol Oncol 2000;79:50–4.
53. Gwinn ML, Webster LA, Lee NC, Layde PM, Rubin GL. Alcohol consumption and ovarian cancer risk. Am J Epidemiol 1986;123:759–66.

54. Hankinson SE, Colditz GA, Hunter DJ, et al. A prospective study of reproductive factors and risk of epithelial ovarian cancer. Cancer 1995;76:284–90.

55. Hankinson SE, Hunter DJ, Colditz GA, et al. Tubal ligation, hysterectomy, and risk of ovarian cancer. A prospective study. JAMA 1993;270:2813–8.

56. Hannan LM, Leitzmann MF, Lacey JV, Jr, et al. Physical activity and risk of ovarian cancer: a prospective cohort study in the United States. Cancer Epidemiol Biomarkers Prev 2004;13:765–70.

57. Harlow BL, Cramer DW. Self-reported use of antidepressants or benzodiazepine tranquilizers and risk of epithelial ovarian cancer: evidence from two combined case-control studies (Massachusetts, United States). Cancer Causes Control 1995;6:130–4.

58. Harlow BL, Cramer DW, Baron JA, Titus-Ernstoff L, Greenberg ER. Psychotropic medication use and risk of epithelial ovarian cancer. Cancer Epidemiol Biomarkers Prev 1998;7:697–702.

59. Harlow BL, Weiss NS. A case-control study of borderline ovarian tumors: the influence of perineal exposure to talc. Am J Epidemiol 1989;130:390–4.

60. Hartge P, Hayes R, Reding D, et al. Complex ovarian cysts in postmenopausal women are not associated with ovarian cancer risk factors: preliminary data from the prostate, lung, colon, and ovarian cancer screening trial. Am J Obstet Gynecol 2000;183:1232–7.

61. Hartge P, Hoover R, McGowan L, Lesher L, Norris HJ. Menopause and ovarian cancer. Am J Epidemiol 1988;127:990–8.

62. Hartge P, Lesher LP, McGowan L, Hoover R. Coffee and ovarian cancer. Int J Cancer 1982;30:531–2.

63. Hartge P, Whittemore AS, Itnyre J, McGowan L, Cramer D. Rates and risks of ovarian cancer in subgroups of white women in the United States. The Collaborative Ovarian Cancer Group. Obstet Gynecol 1994;84:760–4.

64. Heller DS, Murphy P, Westhoff C. Are germinal inclusion cysts markers of ovulation? Gynecol Oncol 2005;96:496–9.

65. Helzlsouer KJ, Alberg AJ, Gordon GB, et al. Serum gonadotropins and steroid hormones and the development of ovarian cancer. JAMA 1995;274:1926–30.

66. Hemminki K, Granstrom C. Familial invasive and borderline ovarian tumors by proband status, age and histology. Int J Cancer 2003;105:701–5.

67. Hughes KS, Roche C, Campbell CT, et al. Prevalence of family history of breast and ovarian cancer in a single primary care practice using a self-administered questionnaire. Breast J 2003;9:19–25.

68. Jacobs I. Screening for familial ovarian cancer: the need for well-designed prospective studies. J Clin Oncol 2005;23:5443–5.

69. Jacobs IJ, Skates SJ, MacDonald N, et al. Screening for ovarian cancer: a pilot randomised controlled trial [see comments]. Lancet 1999;353:1207–10.

70. Jazaeri AA, Yee CJ, Sotiriou C, Brantley KR, Boyd J, Liu ET. Gene expression profiles of BRCA1-linked, BRCA2-linked, and sporadic ovarian cancers. J Natl Cancer Inst 2002;94:990–1000.

71. Jemal A, Murray T, Ward E, et al. Cancer statistics, 2005. CA Cancer J Clin 2005;55:10–30.

72. Jemal A, Siegel R, Ward E, et al. Cancer statistics, 2006. CA Cancer J Clin 2006;56:106–30.

73. Joly DJ, Lilienfeld AM, Diamond EL, Bross ID. An epidemiologic study of the relationship of reproductive experience to cancer of the ovary. Am J Epidemiol 1974;99:190–209.

74. Jordan SJ, Purdie DM, Green AC, Webb PM. Coffee, tea and caffeine and risk of epithelial ovarian cancer. Cancer Causes Control 2004;15:359–65.

75. Kashyap S, Moher D, Fung MF, Rosenwaks Z. Assisted reproductive technology and the incidence of ovarian cancer: a meta-analysis. Obstet Gynecol 2004;103:785–94.

76. Kato I, Zeleniuch-Jacquotte A, Toniolo PG, Akhmedkhanov A, Koenig K, Shore RE. Psychotropic medication use and risk of hormone-related cancers: the New York University Women's Health Study. J Public Health Med 2000;22:155–60.

77. Kauff ND, Barakat RR. Surgical risk-reduction in carriers of BRCA mutations: where do we go from here? Gynecol Oncol 2004;93:277–9.

78. Kelemen LE, Sellers TA, Vierkant RA, Harnack L, Cerhan JR. Association of folate and alcohol with risk of ovarian cancer in a prospective study of postmenopausal women. Cancer Causes Control 2004;15:1085–93.

79. Kinlen LJ. Meat and fat consumption and cancer mortality: a study of strict religious orders in Britain. Lancet 1982;1:946–9.

80. Klip H, Burger CW, Kenemans P, van Leeuwen FE. Cancer risk associated with subfertility and ovulation induction: a review. Cancer Causes Control 2000;11:319–44.

81. Koch M, Gaedke H, Jenkins H. Family history of ovarian cancer patients: a case-control study. Int J Epidemiol 1989;18:782–5.

82. Kreiger N, Sloan M, Cotterchio M, Parsons P. Surgical procedures associated with risk of ovarian cancer. Int J Epidemiol 1997;26:710–5.

83. Kuper H, Titus-Ernstoff L, Harlow BL, Cramer DW. Population based study of coffee, alcohol and tobacco use and risk of ovarian cancer. Int J Cancer 2000;88:313–8.

84. Kurian AW, Balise RR, McGuire V, Whittemore AS. Histologic types of epithelial ovarian cancer: have they different risk factors? Gynecol Oncol 2005;96:520–30.

85. Kushi LH, Mink PJ, Folsom AR, et al. Prospective study of diet and ovarian cancer. Am J Epidemiol 1999;149:21–31.

86. La Vecchia C, Decarli A, Negri E, et al. Dietary factors and the risk of epithelial ovarian cancer. J Natl Cancer Inst 1987;79:663–9.

87. La Vecchia C, Franceschi S, Decarli A, et al. Coffee drinking and the risk of epithelial ovarian cancer. Int J Cancer 1984;33:559–62.

88. Lacey JV, Jr, Mink PJ, Lubin JH, et al. Menopausal hormone replacement therapy and risk of ovarian cancer. JAMA 2002;288:334–41.

89. Lacey JV, Jr, Sherman ME, Hartge P, Schatzkin A, Schairer C. Medication use and risk of ovarian carcinoma: a prospective study. Int J Cancer 2004;108:281–6.

90. Lagiou P, Ye W, Wedren S, et al. Incidence of ovarian cancer among alcoholic women: a cohort study in Sweden. Int J Cancer 2001;91:264–6.

91. Larsson SC, Bergkvist L, Wolk A. Milk and lactose intakes and ovarian cancer risk in the Swedish Mammography Cohort. Am J Clin Nutr 2004;80:1353–7.

92. Larsson SC, Wolk A. Coffee consumption is not associated with ovarian cancer incidence. Cancer Epidemiol Biomarkers Prev 2005;14:2273–4.

93. Lubin F, Chetrit A, Freedman LS, et al. Body mass index at age 18 years and during adult life and ovarian cancer risk. Am J Epidemiol 2003;157:113–20.

94. Lukanova A, Lundin E, Akhmedkhanov A, et al. Circulating levels of sex steroid hormones and risk of ovarian cancer. Int J Cancer 2003;104:636–42.

95. Lukanova A, Lundin E, Toniolo P, et al. Circulating levels of insulin-like growth factor-I and risk of ovarian cancer. Int J Cancer 2002;101:549–54.

96. Lukanova A, Toniolo P, Lundin E, et al. Body mass index in relation to ovarian cancer: a multi-centre nested case-control study. Int J Cancer 2002;99:603–8.

97. Malander S, Rambech E, Kristoffersson U, et al. The contribution of the hereditary nonpolyposis colorectal cancer syndrome to the development of ovarian cancer. Gynecol Oncol 2006;101:238–43.

98. Marchbanks PA, Wilson H, Bastos E, Cramer DW, Schildkraut JM, Peterson HB. Cigarette smoking and epithelial ovarian cancer by histologic type. Obstet Gynecol 2000;95:255–60.

99. McCann SE, Freudenheim JL, Marshall JR, Graham S. Risk of human ovarian cancer is related to dietary intake of selected nutrients, phytochemicals and food groups. J Nutr 2003;133:1937–42.

100. McCann SE, Moysich KB, Mettlin C. Intakes of selected nutrients and food groups and risk of ovarian cancer. Nutr Cancer 2001;39:19–28.

101. McGuire V, Felber GA, Mills M, et al. Relation of contraceptive and reproductive history to ovarian cancer risk in carriers and noncarriers of BRCA1 gene mutations. Am J Epidemiol 2004;160:613–8.

102. Miller DR, Rosenberg L, Kaufman DW, et al. Epithelial ovarian cancer and coffee drinking. Int J Epidemiol 1987;16:13–17.

103. Mills PK, Riordan DG, Cress RD. Epithelial ovarian cancer risk by invasiveness and cell type in the Central Valley of California. Gynecol Oncol 2004;95:215–25.

104. Mink PJ, Folsom AR, Sellers TA, Kushi LH. Physical activity, waist-to-hip ratio, and other risk factors for ovarian cancer: a follow-up study of older women. Epidemiology 1996;7:38–45.

105. Mink PJ, Sherman ME, Devesa SS. Incidence patterns of invasive and borderline ovarian tumors among white women and black women in the United States. Results from the SEER Program, 1978–1998. Cancer 2002;95:2380–9.

106. Miracle-McMahill HL, Calle EE, Kosinski AS, et al. Tubal ligation and fatal ovarian cancer in a large prospective cohort study. Am J Epidemiol 1997;145:349–57.

107. Modan B, Hartge P, Hirsh-Yechezkel G, et al. Parity, oral contraceptives, and the risk of ovarian cancer among carriers and noncarriers of a BRCA1 or BRCA2 mutation. N Engl J Med 2001;345:235–40.

108. Modan B, Ron E, Lerner-Geva L, et al. Cancer incidence in a cohort of infertile women. Am J Epidemiol 1998;147:1038–42.

109. Modugno F. Ovarian cancer and polymorphisms in the androgen and progesterone receptor genes: a HuGE review. Am J Epidemiol 2004;159:319–35.

110. Modugno F, Ness RB, Cottreau CM. Cigarette smoking and the risk of mucinous and nonmucinous epithelial ovarian cancer. Epidemiology 2002;13:467–71.

111. Moorman PG, Schildkraut JM, Calingaert B, Halabi S, Berchuck A. Menopausal hormones and risk of ovarian cancer. Am J Obstet Gynecol 2005;193:76–82.

112. Moorman PG, Schildkraut JM, Calingaert B, Halabi S, Vine MF, Berchuck A. Ovulation and ovarian cancer: a comparison of two methods for calculating lifetime ovulatory cycles (United States). Cancer Causes Control 2002;13:807–11.

113. Mosgaard BJ, Lidegaard O, Kjaer SK, Schou G, Andersen AN. Infertility, fertility drugs, and invasive ovarian cancer: a case-control study. Fertil Steril 1997;67:1005–12.

114. Moysich KB, Mettlin C, Piver MS, Natarajan N, Menezes RJ, Swede H. Regular use of analgesic drugs and ovarian cancer risk. Cancer Epidemiol Biomarkers Prev 2001;10:903–6.

115. Narod SA, Risch H, Moslehi R, et al. Oral contraceptives and the risk of hereditary ovarian cancer. Hereditary Ovarian Cancer Clinical Study Group. N Engl J Med 1998;339:424–8.

116. Nasca PC, Greenwald P, Chorost S, Richart R, Caputo T. An epidemiologic case-control study of ovarian cancer and reproductive factors. Am J Epidemiol 1984;119:705–13.

117. Negri E, Franceschi S, La Vecchia C, Parazzini F. Incomplete pregnancies and ovarian cancer risk. Gynecol Oncol 1992;47:234–8.

118. Negri E, Franceschi S, Tzonou A, et al. Pooled analysis of 3 European case-control studies: I. Reproductive factors and risk of epithelial ovarian cancer. Int J Cancer 1991;49:50–6.

119. Negri E, Tzonou A, Beral V, et al. Hormonal therapy for menopause and ovarian cancer in a collaborative re-analysis of European studies. Int J Cancer 1999;80:848–51.

120. Nelson HD, Huffman LH, Fu R, Harris EL. Genetic risk assessment and BRCA mutation testing for breast and ovarian cancer susceptibility: systematic evidence review for the U.S. Preventive Services Task Force. Ann Intern Med 2005;143:362–79.

121. Ness RB. Endometriosis and ovarian cancer: thoughts on shared pathophysiology. Am J Obstet Gynecol 2003;189:289–94.

122. Ness RB, Cottreau C. Possible role of ovarian epithelial inflammation in ovarian cancer. J Natl Cancer Inst 1999;91:1459–67.

123. Ness RB, Cramer DW, Goodman MT, et al. Infertility, fertility drugs, and ovarian cancer: a pooled analysis of case-control studies. Am J Epidemiol 2002;155:217–24.

124. Ness RB, Grisso JA, Klapper J, et al. Risk of ovarian cancer in relation to estrogen and progestin dose and use characteristics of oral contraceptives. SHARE Study Group. Steroid Hormones and Reproductions. Am J Epidemiol 2000;152:233–41.

125. Noller K L. Estrogen replacement therapy and risk of ovarian cancer. JAMA 2002;288:368–9.

126. Oei AL, Massuger LF, Bulten J, Ligtenberg MJ, Hoogerbrugge N, de Hullu JA. Surveillance of women at high risk for hereditary ovarian cancer is inefficient. Br J Cancer 2006;94:814–9.

127. Offit K, Kauff ND. Reducing the risk of gynecologic cancer in the Lynch syndrome. N Engl J Med 2006;354:293–5.

128. Pal T, Permuth-Wey J, Betts JA, et al. BRCA1 and BRCA2 mutations account for a large proportion of ovarian carcinoma cases. Cancer 2005;104:2807–16.

129. Pan SY, Ugnat AM, Mao Y. Physical activity and the risk of ovarian cancer: a case-control study in Canada. Int J Cancer 2005;117:300–7.

130. Pan SY, Ugnat AM, Mao Y, Wen SW, Johnson KC. A case-control study of diet and the risk of ovarian cancer. Cancer Epidemiol Biomarkers Prev 2004;13:1521–7.

131. Parazzini F, Moroni S, La Vecchia C, Negri E, dal Pino D, Bolis G. Ovarian cancer risk and history of selected medical conditions linked with female hormones. Eur J Cancer 1997;33:1634–7.

132. Parazzini F, Negri E, La Vecchia C, Moroni S, Franceschi S, Crosignani PG. Treatment for infertility and risk of invasive epithelial ovarian cancer. Hum Reprod 1997;12:2159–61.

133. Parkin DM, Bray F, Ferlay J, Pisani P. Global cancer statistics, 2002. CA Cancer J Clin 2005;55:74–108.

134. Pearce CL, Hirschhorn JN, Wu AH, et al. Clarifying the PROGINS allele association in ovarian and breast cancer risk: a haplotype-based analysis. J Natl Cancer Inst 2005;97:51–9.

135. Pelucchi C, La Vecchia C, Chatenoud L, et al. Dietary fibres and ovarian cancer risk. Eur J Cancer 2001;37:2235–9.

136. Pharoah PD, Ponder BA. The genetics of ovarian cancer. Best Pract Res Clin Obstet Gynaecol 2002;16:449–68.

137. Phillips RL, Garfinkel L, Kuzma JW, Beeson WL, Lotz T, Brin B. Mortality among California Seventh-Day Adventists for selected cancer sites. J Natl Cancer Inst 1980;65:1097–107.

138. Pike MC, Pearce CL, Peters R, Cozen W, Wan P, Wu AH. Hormonal factors and the risk of invasive ovarian cancer: a population-based case-control study. Fertil Steril 2004;82:186–95.

139. Pisani P, Parkin DM, Bray F, Ferlay J. Estimates of the worldwide mortality from 25 cancers in 1990. Int J Cancer 1999;83:870–3.

140. Polychronopoulou A, Tzonou A, Hsieh CC, et al. Reproductive variables, tobacco, ethanol, coffee and somatometry as risk factors for ovarian cancer. Int J Cancer 1993;55:402–7.

141. Potashnik G, Lerner-Geva L, Genkin L, Chetrit A, Lunenfeld E, Porath A. Fertility drugs and the risk of breast and ovarian cancers: results of a long-term follow-up study. Fertil Steril 1999;71:853–9.

142. Prat J, Ribe A, Gallardo A. Hereditary ovarian cancer. Hum Pathol 2005;36:861–70.

143. Purdie DM, Bain CJ, Siskind V, et al. Hormone replacement therapy and risk of epithelial ovarian cancer. Br J Cancer 1999;81:559–63.

144. Purdie DM, Bain CJ, Siskind V, Webb PM, Green AC. Ovulation and risk of epithelial ovarian cancer. Int J Cancer 2003;104:228–32.

145. Purdie DM, Bain CJ, Webb PM, Whiteman DC, Pirozzo S, Green AC. Body size and ovarian cancer: case-control study and systematic review (Australia). Cancer Causes Control 2001;12:855–63.

146. Qin LQ, Xu JY, Wang PY, Hashi A, Hoshi K, Sato A. Milk/dairy products consumption, galactose metabolism and ovarian cancer: meta-analysis of epidemiological studies. Eur J Cancer Prev 2005;14:13–19.

147. Rafnar T, Benediktsdottir KR, Eldon BJ, et al. BRCA2, but not BRCA1, mutations account for familial ovarian cancer in Iceland: a population-based study. Eur J Cancer 2004;40:2788–93.

148. Rebbeck TR, Lynch HT, Neuhausen SL, et al. Prophylactic oophorectomy in carriers of BRCA1 or BRCA2 mutations. N Engl J Med 2002;346:1616–22.

149. Ries LAG, Eisner MP, Kosary CL, et al. SEER Cancer Statistics Review 1975–2000. Bethesda, MD: National Cancer Institute; 2003. Online. Available: http://seer.cancer.gov/csr/1975_2000.

150. Ries LAG, Kossary CL, Hankey BF. SEER Cancer Statistics Review, 1973–1995. Bethesda, MD: National Cancer Institute; 1998.

151. Riman T, Dickman PW, Nilsson S, et al. Hormone replacement therapy and the risk of invasive epithelial ovarian cancer in Swedish women. J Natl Cancer Inst 2002;94:497–504.

152. Risch HA. Hormonal etiology of epithelial ovarian cancer, with a hypothesis concerning the role of androgens and progesterone. J Natl Cancer Inst 1998;90:1774–86.

153. Risch HA. Hormone replacement therapy and the risk of ovarian cancer. Gynecol Oncol 2002;86:115–7.

154. Risch HA, Howe GR. Pelvic inflammatory disease and the risk of epithelial ovarian cancer. Cancer Epidemiol Biomarkers Prev 1995;4:447–51.

155. Risch HA, Jain M, Marrett LD, Howe GR. Dietary fat intake and risk of epithelial ovarian cancer. J Natl Cancer Inst 1994;86:1409–15.

156. Risch HA, Marrett LD, Howe GR. Parity, contraception, infertility, and the risk of epithelial ovarian cancer. Am J Epidemiol 1994;140:585–97.

157. Rodriguez C, Henley SJ, Calle EE, Thun MJ. Paracetamol and risk of ovarian cancer mortality in a prospective study of women in the USA. Lancet 1998;352:1354–5.

158. Rodriguez C, Calle EE, Fakhrabadi-Shokoohi D, Jacobs EJ, Thun MJ. Body mass index, height, and the risk of ovarian cancer mortality in a prospective cohort of postmenopausal women. Cancer Epidemiol Biomarkers Prev 2002;11:822–8.

159. Rodriguez C, Patel AV, Calle EE, Jacob EJ, Thun MJ. Estrogen replacement therapy and ovarian cancer mortality in a large prospective study of US women. JAMA 2001;285:1460–5.

160. Rodriguez GC, Nagarsheth NP, Lee KL, et al. Progestin-induced apoptosis in the Macaque ovarian epithelium: differential regulation of transforming growth factor-beta. J Natl Cancer Inst 2002;94:50–60.

161. Rodriguez GC, Nagarsheth NP, Lee KL, et al. Progestin-induced apoptosis in the Macaque ovarian epithelium: differential regulation of transforming growth factor-beta. J Natl Cancer Inst 2002;94:50–60.

162. Rosenberg L, Palmer JR, Rao RS, et al. A case-control study of analgesic use and ovarian cancer. Cancer Epidemiol Biomarkers Prev 2000;9:933–7.

163. Rosenberg L, Palmer JR, Zauber AG, et al. A case-control study of oral contraceptive use and invasive epithelial ovarian cancer. Am J Epidemiol 1994;139:654–61.

164. Rosenblatt KA, Thomas DB. Lactation and the risk of epithelial ovarian cancer. The WHO Collaborative Study of Neoplasia and Steroid Contraceptives. Int J Epidemiol 1993;22:192–7.

165. Rosenblatt KA, Thomas DB. Reduced risk of ovarian cancer in women with a tubal ligation or hysterectomy. The World Health Organization Collaborative Study of Neoplasia and Steroid Contraceptives. Cancer Epidemiol Biomarkers Prev 1996;5:933–5.

166. Rosner BA, Colditz GA, Webb PM, Hankinson SE. Mathematical models of ovarian cancer incidence. Epidemiology 2005;16:508–15.

167. Rossing MA, Daling JR, Weiss NS, Moore DE, Self SG. Ovarian tumors in a cohort of infertile women. N Engl J Med 1994;331:771–6.

168. Royar J, Becher H, Chang-Claude J. Low-dose oral contraceptives: protective effect on ovarian cancer risk. Int J Cancer 2001;95:370–4.

169. Sala M, Dosemeci M, Zahm SH. A death certificate-based study of occupation and mortality from reproductive cancers among women in 24 US states. J Occup Environ Med 1998;40:632–9.

170. Schildkraut JM, Calingaert B, Marchbanks PA, Moorman PG, Rodriguez GC. Impact of progestin and estrogen potency in oral contraceptives on ovarian cancer risk. J Natl Cancer Inst 2002;94:32–8.

171. Schildkraut JM, Cooper GS, Halabi S, Calingaert B, Hartge P, Whittemore AS. Age at natural menopause and the risk of epithelial ovarian cancer. Obstet Gynecol 2001;98:85–90.

172. Schildkraut JM, Thompson WD. Familial ovarian cancer: a population-based case-control study. Am J Epidemiol 1988;128:456–66.

173. Schmeler KM, Lynch HT, Chen LM, et al. Prophylactic surgery to reduce the risk of gynecologic cancers in the Lynch syndrome. N Engl J Med 2006;354:261–9.

174. Schouten LJ, Goldbohm RA, van den Brandt PA. Height, weight, weight change, and ovarian cancer risk in the Netherlands cohort study on diet and cancer. Am J Epidemiol 2003;157:424–33.

175. Shen N, Weiderpass E, Antilla A, et al. Epidemiology of occupational and environmental risk factors related to ovarian cancer. Scand J Work Environ Health 1998;24:175–82.

176. Shields T, Gridley G, Moradi T, Adami J, Plato N, Dosemeci M. Occupational exposures and the risk of ovarian cancer in Sweden. Am J Ind Med 2002;42:200–13.

177. Shih I, Kurman RJ. Molecular pathogenesis of ovarian borderline tumors: new insights and old challenges. Clin Cancer Res 2005;11:7273–9.

178. Shu XO, Gao YT, Yuan JM, Ziegler RG, Brinton LA. Dietary factors and epithelial ovarian cancer. Br J Cancer 1989;59:92–6.

179. Shushan A, Paltiel O, Iscovich J, Elchalal U, Peretz T, Schenker JG. Human menopausal gonadotropin and the risk of epithelial ovarian cancer. Fertil Steril 1996;65:13–18.

180. Siskind V, Green A, Bain C, Purdie D. Breastfeeding, menopause, and epithelial ovarian cancer. Epidemiology 1997;8:188–91.

181. Sit AS, Modugno F, Weissfeld JL, Berga SL, Ness RB. Hormone replacement therapy formulations and risk of epithelial ovarian carcinoma. Gynecol Oncol 2002;86:118–23.

182. Slattery ML, Schuman KL, West DW, French TK, Robison LM. Nutrient intake and ovarian cancer. Am J Epidemiol 1989;130:497–502.

183. Snowdon DA, Phillips RL. Coffee consumption and risk of fatal cancers. Am J Public Health 1984;74:820–3.

184. Sowter HM, Ashworth A. BRCA1 and BRCA2 as ovarian cancer susceptibility genes. Carcinogenesis 2005;26:1651–6.

185. Spurdle AB, Webb PM, Chen X, et al. Androgen receptor exon 1 CAG repeat length and risk of ovarian cancer. Int J Cancer 2000;87:637–43.

186. Stadel BV. The etiology and prevention of ovarian cancer [letter]. Am J Obstet Gynecol 1975;123:772–4.

187. Stratton JF, Pharoah P, Smith SK, Easton D, Ponder BA. A systematic review and meta-analysis of family history and risk of ovarian cancer. Br J Obstet Gynaecol 1998;105:493–9.

188. Struewing JP, Hartge P, Wacholder S, et al. The risk of cancer associated with specific mutations of BRCA1 and BRCA2 among Ashkenazi Jews. N Engl J Med 1997;336:1401–8.

189. Terry KL, De Vivo I, Titus-Ernstoff L, Sluss PM, Cramer DW. Genetic variation in the progesterone receptor gene and ovarian cancer risk. Am J Epidemiol 2005;161:442–51.

190. Terry PD, Miller AB, Jones JG, Rohan TE. Cigarette smoking and the risk of invasive epithelial ovarian cancer in a prospective cohort study. Eur J Cancer 2003;39:1157–64.

191. Thompson D, Easton D. Variation in cancer risks, by mutation position, in BRCA2 mutation carriers. Am J Hum Genet 2001;68:410–9.

192. Thompson D, Easton DF. Cancer incidence in BRCA1 mutation carriers. J Natl Cancer Inst 2002;94:1358–65.

193. Titus-Ernstoff L, Perez K, Cramer DW, Harlow BL, Baron JA, Greenberg ER. Menstrual and reproductive factors in relation to ovarian cancer risk. Br J Cancer 2001;84:714–21.

194. Trichopoulos D, Papapostolou M, Polychronopoulou A. Coffee and ovarian cancer. Int J Cancer 1981;28:691–3.

195. Tung KH, Wilkens LR, Wu AH, et al. Association of dietary vitamin A, carotenoids, and other antioxidants with the risk of ovarian cancer. Cancer Epidemiol Biomarkers Prev 2005;14:669–76.

196. Tzonou A, Polychronopoulou A, Hsieh CC, Rebelakos A, Karakatsani A, Trichopoulos D. Hair dyes, analgesics, tranquilizers and perineal talc application as risk factors for ovarian cancer. Int J Cancer 1993;55:408–10.

197. Urban N. Screening for ovarian cancer. We now need a definitive randomised trial. BMJ 1999;319:1317–8.

198. Vasama-Neuvonen K, Pukkala E, Paakkulainen H, et al. Ovarian cancer and occupational exposures in Finland. Am J Ind Med 1999;36:83–9.

199. Venkitaraman AR. Cancer susceptibility and the functions of BRCA1 and BRCA2. Cell 2002;108:171–82.

200. Venn A, Watson L, Bruinsma F, Giles G, Healy D. Risk of cancer after use of fertility drugs with in-vitro fertilisation. Lancet 1999;354:1586–90.

201. Voigt LF, Harlow BL, Weiss NS. The influence of age at first birth and parity on ovarian cancer risk. Am J Epidemiol 1986;124:490–1.

202. Wacholder S. Bias in intervention studies that enroll patients from high-risk clinics. J Natl Cancer Inst 2004;96:1204–7.

203. Wacholder S, Chanock S, Garcia-Closas M, El Ghormli L, Rothman N. Assessing the probability that a positive report is false: an approach for molecular epidemiology studies. J Natl Cancer Inst 2004;96:434–42.

204. Wacholder S, Struewing JP, Hartge P, Greene MH, Tucker MA. Breast cancer risks for BRCA1/2 carriers. Science 2004;306:2187–91.

205. Webb PM, Purdie DM, Bain CJ, Green AC. Alcohol, wine, and risk of epithelial ovarian cancer. Cancer Epidemiol Biomarkers Prev 2004;13:592–9.

206. Weiderpass E, Ye W, Vainio H, Kaaks R, Adami HO. Diabetes mellitus and ovarian cancer (Sweden). Cancer Causes Control 2002;13:759–64.

207. Weiss NS, Harlow BL. Why does hysterectomy without bilateral oophorectomy influence the subsequent incidence of ovarian cancer? Am J Epidemiol 1986;124:856–8.

208. Weiss NS, Lyon JL, Krishnamurthy S, Dietert SE, Liff JM, Daling JR. Noncontraceptive estrogen use and the occurrence of ovarian cancer. J Natl Cancer Inst 1982;68:95–8.

209. Weiss NS, Lyon JL, Liff JM, Vollmer WM, Daling JR. Incidence of ovarian cancer in relation to the use of oral contraceptives. Int J Cancer 1981;28:669–71.

210. Whiteman DC, Siskind V, Purdie DM, Green AC. Timing of pregnancy and the risk of epithelial ovarian cancer. Cancer Epidemiol Biomarkers Prev 2003;12:42–6.

211. Whittemore AS, Balise RR, Pharoah PD, et al. Oral contraceptive use and ovarian cancer risk among carriers of BRCA1 or BRCA2 mutations. Br J Cancer 2004;91:1911–5.

212. Whittemore AS, Harris R, Itnyre J. Characteristics relating to ovarian cancer risk: collaborative analysis of 12 US case-control studies. II. Invasive epithelial ovarian cancers in white women. Collaborative Ovarian Cancer Group. Am J Epidemiol 1992;136:1184–203.

213. Whittemore AS, Wu ML, Paffenbarger RS, Jr, et al. Personal and environmental characteristics related to epithelial ovarian cancer. II. Exposures to talcum powder, tobacco, alcohol, and coffee. Am J Epidemiol 1988;128:1228–40.

214. Whittemore AS, Wu ML, Paffenbarger RS, Jr, et al. Epithelial ovarian cancer and the ability to conceive. Cancer Res 1989;49:4047–52.

215. Wooster R, Weber BL. Breast and ovarian cancer. N Engl J Med 2003;348:2339–47.

216. Wu ML, Whittemore AS, Paffenbarger RS, Jr, et al. Personal and environmental characteristics related to epithelial ovarian cancer. I. Reproductive and menstrual events and oral contraceptive use. Am J Epidemiol 1988;128:1216–27.

217. Zajicek J. Ovarian cystomas and ovulation, a histogenetic concept. Tumori 1977;63:429–35.

218. Zhang M, Lee AH, Binns CW. Physical activity and epithelial ovarian cancer risk: a case-control study in China. Int J Cancer 2003;105:838–43.

219. Zhang M, Xie X, Lee AH, Binns CW. Sedentary behaviours and epithelial ovarian cancer risk. Cancer Causes Control 2004;15:83–9.

Ovarian serous and mucinous epithelial–stromal tumors

Jaime Prat

SURFACE EPITHELIAL–STROMAL TUMORS

The tumors in this category account for approximately two-thirds of all ovarian tumors and for about 90% of all ovarian cancers in the Western world.[96,113] They are thought to arise either directly or indirectly from the ovarian surface epithelium (modified mesothelium) and the underlying ovarian stroma. The epithelial–stromal tumors are primarily subclassified according to their epithelial component into serous, mucinous, endometrioid, clear, transitional, and squamous cell types.

Some tumors, particularly those in the serous subtype, may be exophytic or intracystic (endophytic), or both. The presence of exophytic growth is indicated by the word 'surface', which is added to the designation, i.e., 'serous surface papillary adenocarcinoma'. In contrast, cystic tumors with intracystic growth are variably called 'serous adenocarcinoma' or described by the prefix cyst- before their name, i.e., 'serous cystadenocarcinoma'. Most surface epithelial–stromal neoplasms are predominantly epithelial, with only a minor component derived from the ovarian stroma. When gland-forming tumors have a predominant stromal component, the terms 'adenofibroma' and 'cystadenofibroma' (if grossly visible cysts are present) are used. However, the subdivision of epithelial–stromal tumors that is most important from a clinical viewpoint is their classification into benign, borderline, and carcinoma forms, because it generally correlates with prognosis. This is done according to the amount of tumor cell proliferation, the degree of nuclear atypia, and the presence or absence of stromal invasion.[96,113] Only serous and mucinous borderline tumors have been clearly defined clinicopathologically.

BORDERLINE TUMORS

Borderline tumors (also designated as tumors of low malignant potential) show histologic and cytologic features that are intermediate between those of clearly benign and clearly malignant tumors of the same cell type(s). They exhibit epithelial proliferation greater than that seen in their benign counterparts but an absence of *destructive invasion* of the stroma or confluent growth, and are associated with a much better prognosis, stage for stage, than that of ovarian carcinomas.[63,95,113] Even in the absence of invasiveness within the ovary, borderline tumors of serous type can either implant on peritoneal surfaces or be associated with independent foci of primary serous peritoneal neoplasia; rarely, invasion of the underlying tissues occurs in both circumstances.[11,34–36,53,69,97,116] Exceptionally, tumors of borderline malignancy spread via lymphatics and blood vessels. In addition, a small number of these tumors are combined with

or transform over time into obviously invasive carcinomas.[53,69,97] Although favorable in most cases, the biologic behavior of borderline tumors differs from that of the obviously benign tumors of the same cell type(s). Therefore, the designation 'tumors of borderline malignancy' should be kept. Alternative terms such as *proliferating, atypical,* and *atypical proliferating*[117] are misleading because they do not imply the malignant potential of a small but significant number of these tumors and discourage complete surgical staging and follow-up of the patients.[63,95–97,113] Although the word 'borderline' may suggest uncertainty, it accurately describes the ambiguous histologic and biologic features of these neoplasms and remains the most appropriate term.

The distinction between borderline tumors and carcinomas is one of the most common problems in ovarian tumor pathology, yet the literature on borderline tumors is confusing, particularly with regard to their diagnostic features and treatment. Although the World Health Organization (WHO)[63] has recommended the presence or absence of 'obvious invasion' of the stroma, most practitioners do not require obvious stromal invasion for the diagnosis of carcinoma if the epithelial cells are malignant cytologically. To promote terminology agreement, the WHO has proposed essential diagnostic criteria for distinguishing borderline tumors from carcinomas,[113] and also incorporated a variant designated as borderline tumor *with intraepithelial carcinoma*. The extent of the carcinomatous epithelium should be noted in the pathology report.[113]

SEROUS TUMORS

Definition

Serous tumors in both their benign and borderline forms show ciliated epithelial cells and other cell types resembling those of the fallopian tube. Although the less differentiated tumors lose the cytologic features of tubal epithelium, they usually exhibit distinctive patterns of growth, including fine and complex papillary structures with prominent cellular budding, glands with irregular slit-like lumens, and solid sheets. Psammoma bodies and larger calcific deposits are usually found. Serous tumors, whether benign, borderline or malignant, tend to be uniform throughout a given specimen, usually lacking the admixtures of these three subtypes so common in mucinous tumors. The Systematized Nomenclature of Medicine (SNOMED) classification of serous tumors is as follows:

- Benign serous tumors
  - serous adenofibroma, cystadenofibroma
  - serous surface papilloma

– serous cystadenoma
– serous papillary cystadenoma
- Serous borderline tumor
- Serous carcinoma.

Epidemiology

In the Western world, serous tumors account for 30–40% of all ovarian tumors. Of these, approximately 70% are benign, 5–10% borderline, and 20–25% carcinomas.[113] Borderline and invasive serous tumors together account for about 30% of all ovarian cancers.

BENIGN SEROUS TUMORS

Clinical features

Benign serous tumors may occur at any age but are most common during the fifth decade. Usually, the tumors are asymptomatic and discovered incidentally during ultrasound investigation of another gynecologic disorder.

Macroscopic features

Benign serous tumors are usually endophytic (cystadenomas), but may be exophytic (surface papillomas), or both. Serous cystadenomas are usually unilocular (Figure 24.1) but may be multilocular, and have thin-walled cyst(s) (Figure 24.2) filled with watery or occasionally thin-mucinous fluid. They average about 10 cm in size. The cyst(s) may have a smooth inner surface or one with polypoid excrescences (Figure 24.3), which are firm if their stroma is fibrous and soft if it is edematous (Figure 24.4). Serous cystadenomas are bilateral in approximately 10–20% of cases (Figure 24.2).

Serous surface papillomas appear as polypoid excrescences on the outer surface of the ovary. The surface tumors are often accompanied by underlying cystic components. Serous adenofibromas are hard, white, predominantly fibromatous tumors with small glands or cysts that contain clear fluid. When bilateral, their firm consistency may suggest the diagnosis of cancer.

Microscopic features

The cysts and polypoid excrescences of benign serous tumors are typically lined by a single epithelium similar to that of the fallopian tube, which is frequently ciliated (Figure 24.5). Tumors lined entirely by non-ciliated cuboidal or columnar

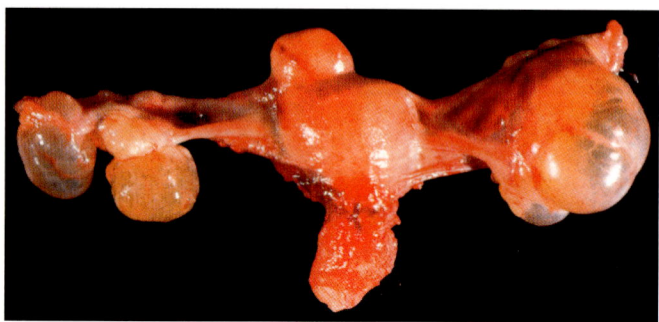
Fig. 24.2 Serous cystadenoma, bilateral.

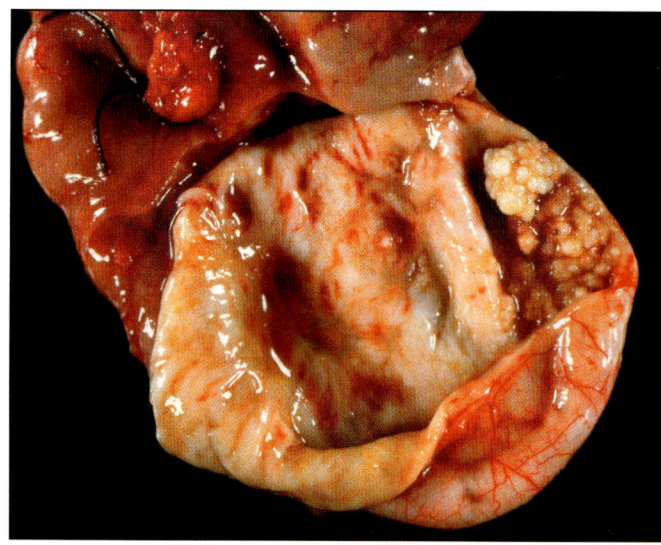
Fig. 24.3 Serous cystadenoma. A papillary growth is present in the lumen of the cyst.

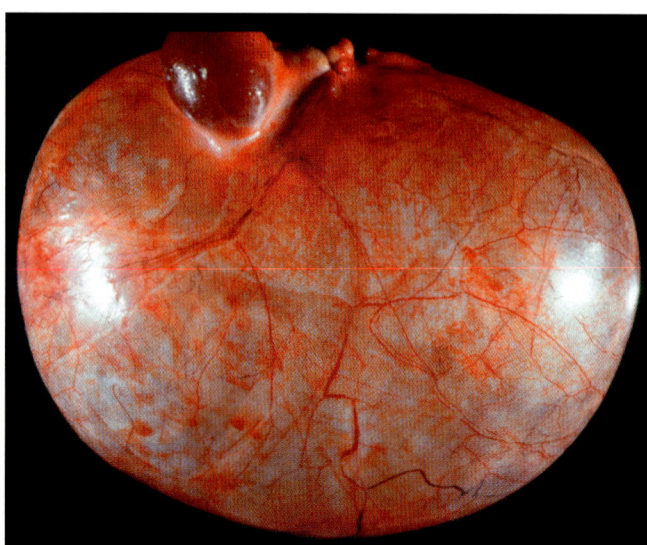

Fig. 24.1 Serous cystadenoma. Unilocular, thin-walled cyst.

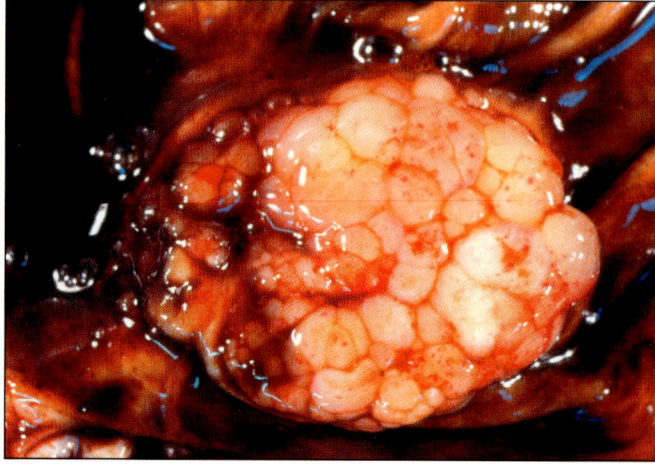
Fig. 24.4 Serous papillary cystadenoma. Intracystic polyp with confluent papillae which were soft and edematous.

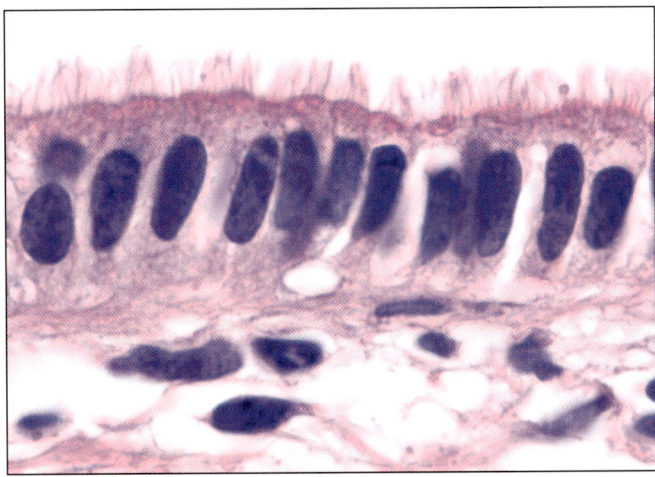

Fig. 24.5 Serous cystadenoma. Ciliated epithelium similar to that of the fallopian tube. Reproduced with permission from Prat.[96]

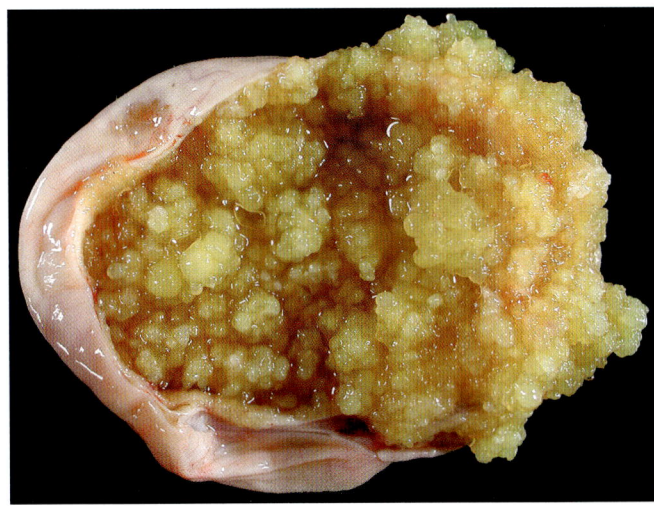

Fig. 24.7 Serous borderline tumor. Intracystic growth of soft papillary excrescences. Courtesy of Dr J Forteza, Santiago, Spain.

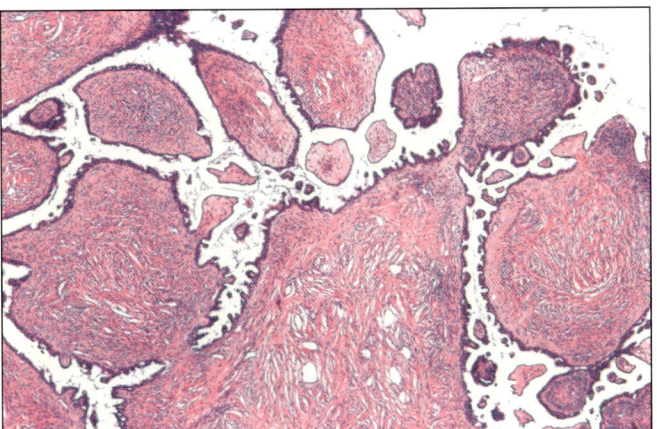

Fig. 24.6 Serous papillary cystadenoma. The polypoid excrescences are composed predominantly of dense fibrous tissue. Reproduced with permission from Prat.[96]

epithelium that resembles ovarian surface epithelium are also generally included in the serous category despite their indifferent appearance. The epithelial cells of benign serous tumors may secrete mucin, but when it is present, it is usually confined to the lumens of cysts and apical portion of the cytoplasm of the epithelial cells. Mitoses are rare. There is no nuclear atypia. Psammoma bodies are infrequent. Papillae when found are composed almost entirely of stroma (Figure 24.6), which may be collagenous or markedly edematous. In adenofibromas and cystadenofibromas, glands and cysts are scattered within a predominantly fibromatous stroma. Otherwise typical benign cystic or surface serous tumors containing minor foci consistent with borderline neoplasia (cell stratification and nuclear atypia) are kept in the benign category for clinical purposes.[113]

Differential diagnosis

Serous cystadenomas may be confused with rare examples of cystic struma ovarii (Chapter 27), but the latter exhibits at least minor foci of identifiable thyroid follicles in the cyst's outer wall. Rare rete cystadenomas may simulate serous cystadenomas but, in addition to their hilar location, often show a thick

layer of smooth muscle and are lined by cells lacking cilia. Serous surface papillary adenofibromas should be distinguished from the common small surface stromal proliferations sometimes seen in adult women. The latter lesions are typically multifocal, have a simple cuboidal epithelial lining, and do not form a mass lesion.

SEROUS BORDERLINE TUMORS

Clinical features

Serous borderline tumors (SBTs) account for from one-fourth to one-third of malignant serous tumors.[57,92] According to most publications, they are most common in the fourth and fifth decades, with an average patient age of 42 years.[69] Although often asymptomatic, the tumor may sometimes present with abdominal enlargement and pain due to rupture or torsion. Approximately 70% are confined to one or both ovaries (stage 1) at the time of diagnosis; the remaining tumors have spread within the pelvis (stage 2) or upper abdomen (stage 3). Only rare cases have extended beyond the abdomen (stage 4) at the time of presentation.[92,97] One-third of the stage 1 tumors are bilateral.[92]

Macroscopic features

Serous borderline tumors have one or more cysts that are lined to varying extents by polypoid excrescences and closely packed finer papillae (endophytic growth) (Figure 24.7). The cysts contain thick mucinous fluid, which does not necessarily indicate the mucinous nature of the tumor. The polypoid excrescences contain fibrous or edematous stroma (Figure 24.7). Serous cystadenofibromas of borderline malignancy are firm, white, fibromatous tumors with a cystic component of variable size. In almost 50% of SBTs the papillary growth covers the outer surface of the ovary (serous surface papillary borderline tumor) (Figure 24.8).[114] Frequently both exophytic and endophytic papillary components are present (Figure 24.9). The typical gross features of serous carcinomas, such as friability, hemorrhage, and necrosis, are not seen in SBTs.

PRIMARY TUMORS

Serous borderline tumors show stromal polypoid excrescences, glands, and papillae lined by stratified cuboidal to columnar epithelial cells and ciliated cells resembling those of the fallopian tube (Figures 24.10–24.14). Larger hobnail cells with ample eosinophilic cytoplasm (Figure 24.15) and mesothelial-like cells may also be present. Eosinophilic cells are increased when microinvasion has occurred. The degree to which the lining epithelial cells show nuclear atypia varies from mild to moderate (rarely severe) within an individual tumor, and mitoses are rare; therefore, the histologic pattern usually differs from that of carcinoma *in situ* (CIS) of other organs. Psammoma bodies are found in about one-fourth of cases. The three most important diagnostic features are: (1) arborizing papillae that form increasingly smaller branches ending in clusters of epithelial cells that appear to be detached from the stroma (hierarchical pattern of branching); (2) varying degree of nuclear atypia; and (3) absence of 'frank' stromal invasion or solid sheets of tumor with a cribriform pattern.[113]

Several changes within SBTs may result in overdiagnosis of carcinoma. The pathologist's main diagnostic problems while dealing with SBTs are as follows:

- Pseudoinvasion
- Self-implantation
- Mesothelial cell hyperplasia
- Micropapillary pattern
- Microinvasion
- Peritoneal implants
- SBT in lymph nodes
- SBT of the peritoneum

PSEUDOINVASION, AUTOIMPLANTS, AND MESOTHELIAL CELL HYPERPLASIA

Serous borderline tumors often show a relatively complex proliferation of glands and papillae (Figure 24.16). The glands often invaginate into the stroma and, particularly when sectioned tangentially, may appear as if they have invaded the stroma.[113] This *pseudoinvasion* differs, however, from the destructive stromal invasion of a carcinoma. The stroma about the pseudoinvasion is similar to the stroma elsewhere and the glands have an orderly distribution. In carcinoma, it forms a desmoplastic stroma typically and the neoplastic glands have a more disorderly arrangement. Exceptionally, an SBT implants on itself and may exhibit focal desmoplastic stroma.

Autoimplants are sharply circumscribed desmoplastic plaques usually on the outer surface but occasionally on the inner (cystic) surface of the tumor, resembling non-invasive

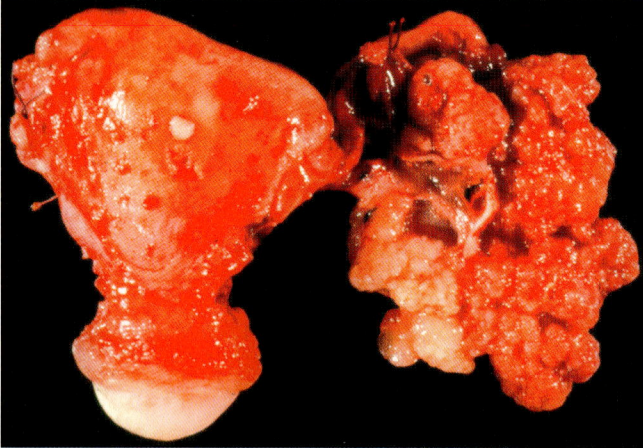

Fig. 24.8 Serous surface papillary borderline tumor. Exophytic papillary growth. Reproduced with permission from Prat.[96]

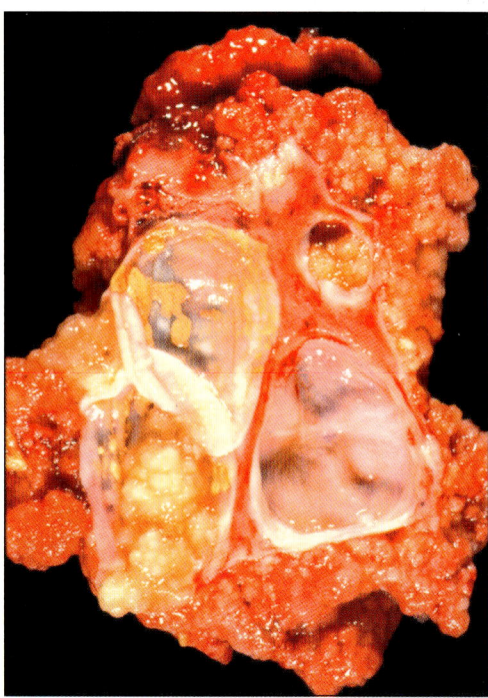
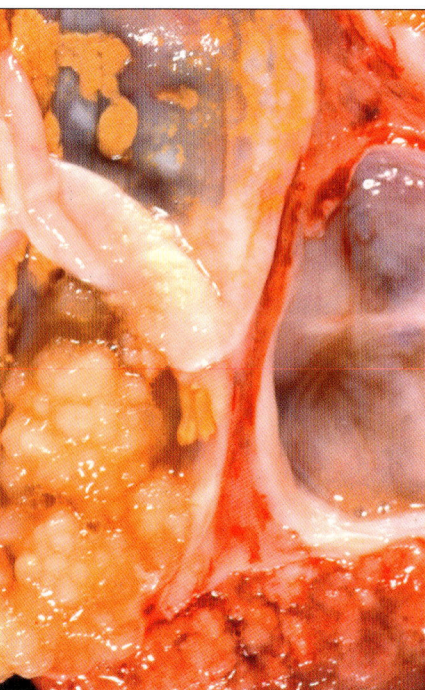

Fig. 24.9 Serous borderline tumor. Left: The external surface is covered by confluent polypoid excrescences and closely packed small papillae (exophytic growth). The sectioned surface shows a solid and cystic tumor with intracystic papillary growth. Right: Closer view of the intracystic papillae which were soft and edematous. Reproduced with permission from Prat.[96]

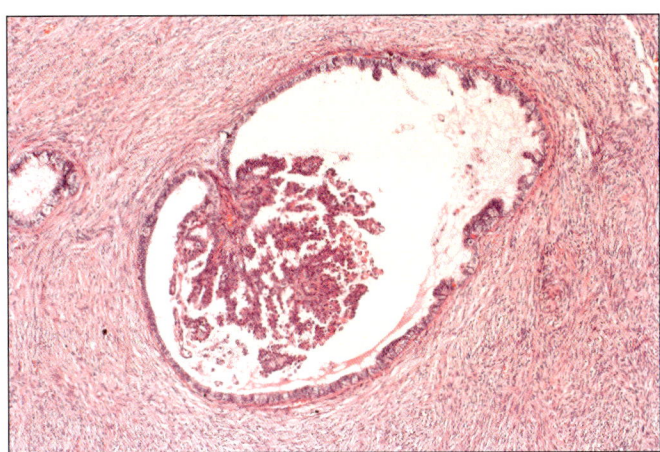

Fig. 24.10 Incipient serous borderline tumor arising within a surface epithelial inclusion cyst. Reproduced with permission from Prat.[96]

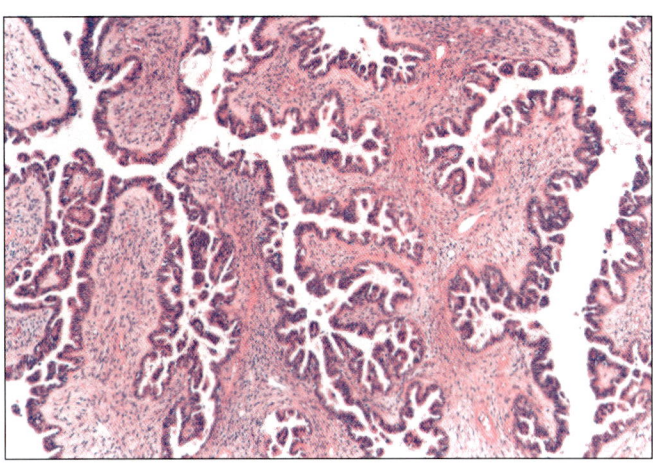

Fig. 24.13 Serous borderline tumor, typical pattern. The papillae are lined by stratified cuboidal-to-columnar epithelial cells with hyperchromatic nuclei.

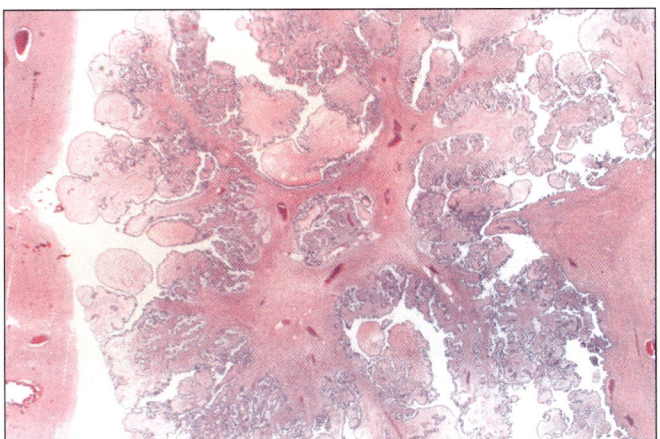

Fig. 24.11 Serous borderline tumor, typical pattern. The epithelial papillae show hierarchical and complex branching without stromal invasion. Some papillae have fibroedematous stalks.

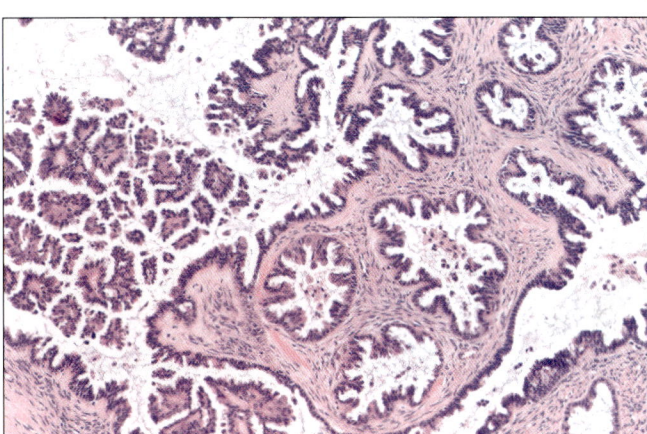

Fig. 24.14 Serous borderline tumor, typical pattern. Detachment of small cell nests from the stratified lining epithelium. The nuclei are slightly atypical. The lumen of the cyst contains basophilic mucin.

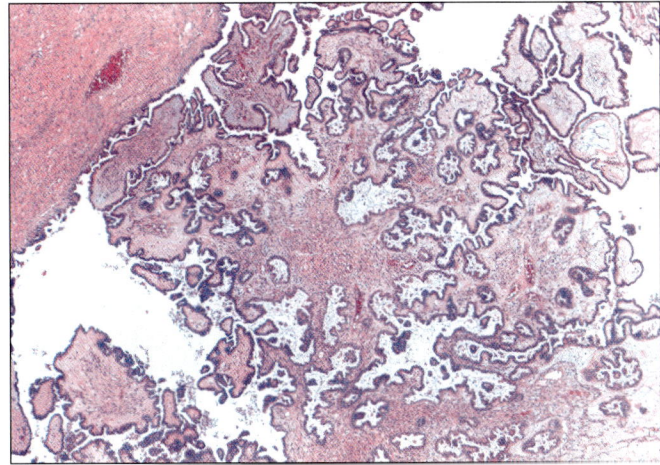

Fig. 24.12 Serous borderline tumor, typical pattern. Orderly penetration of the stroma by glands and microcysts with papillae, without stromal reaction.

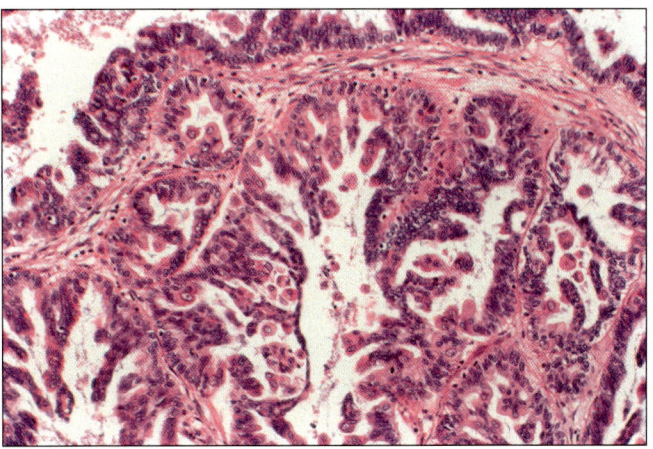

Fig. 24.15 Serous borderline tumor. The lining cells are stratified with cellular budding and show moderate atypia. Larger hobnail cells with abundant eosinophilic cytoplasm are seen. Reproduced with permission from Prat.[96]

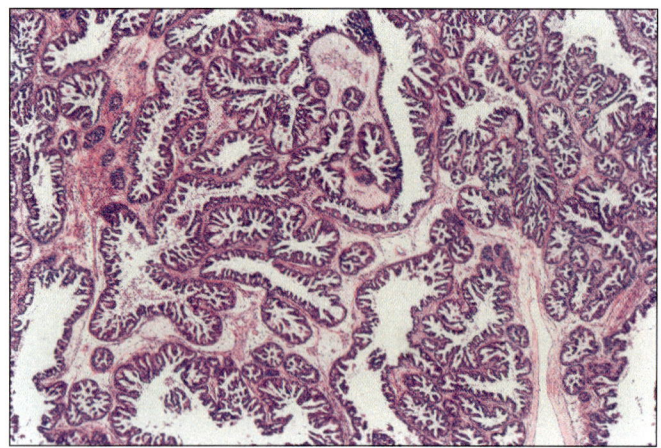

Fig. 24.16 Serous borderline tumor. Complex proliferation of glands and papillae not to be interpreted as stromal invasion. No stromal reaction is seen. Reproduced with permission from Prat.[96]

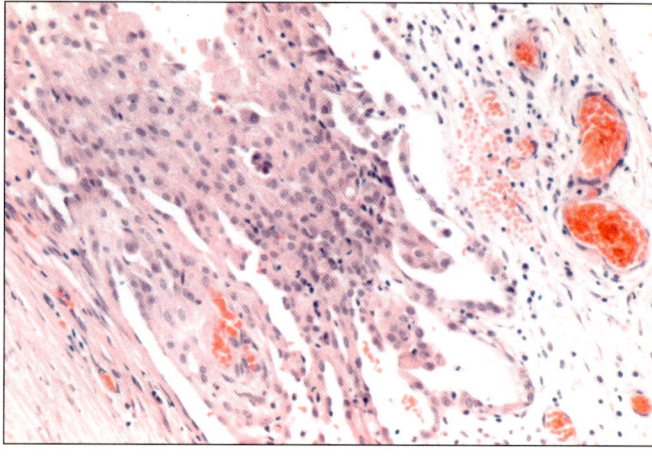

Fig. 24.18 Mesothelial hyperplasia on the surface of a serous borderline tumor. The mesothelial cells lack nuclear atypia and are typically arranged in a linear fashion. Reproduced with permission from Prat.[96]

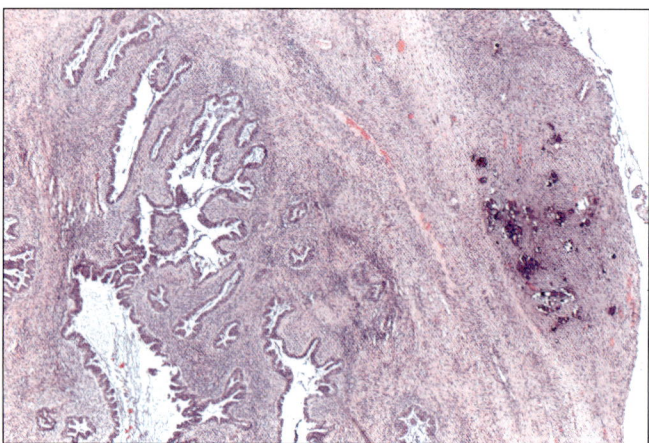

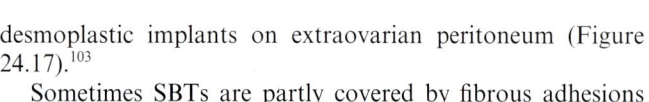

Fig. 24.17 Serous borderline tumor with autoimplantation. The upper right corner of the figure shows desmoplastic tissue with numerous psammoma bodies creating an image similar to that of a desmoplastic peritoneal implant. Note the sharp demarcation with the ovarian stroma. Reproduced with permission from Prat.[96]

desmoplastic implants on extraovarian peritoneum (Figure 24.17).[103]

Sometimes SBTs are partly covered by fibrous adhesions associated with *mesothelial hyperplasia*, which may be erroneously interpreted as surface borderline tumor or even carcinoma. The mesothelial cells, however, lack nuclear atypia and are typically arranged in a linear fashion (Figure 24.18).

MICROPAPILLARY PATTERN

Rarely, an exuberant and delicate 'micropapillary' (or focal cribriform) proliferation without destructive stromal invasion is found in SBTs (Figure 24.19). Some designate this growth pattern as 'micropapillary serous carcinoma' because, according to the proponents,[17] it is frequently associated with aggressive behavior. Most investigators[28,31,36,69,97,128] do not share this viewpoint and prefer the designation SBT with micropapillary pattern (or micropapillary SBT). The microscopic features include a filigree pattern of highly complex micropapillae growing in a non-hierarchical fashion from fibrous stalks

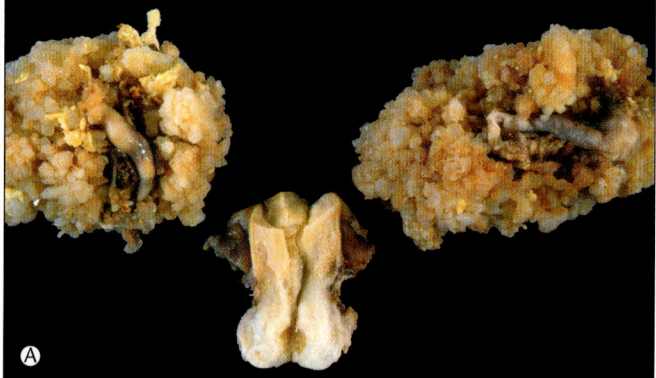

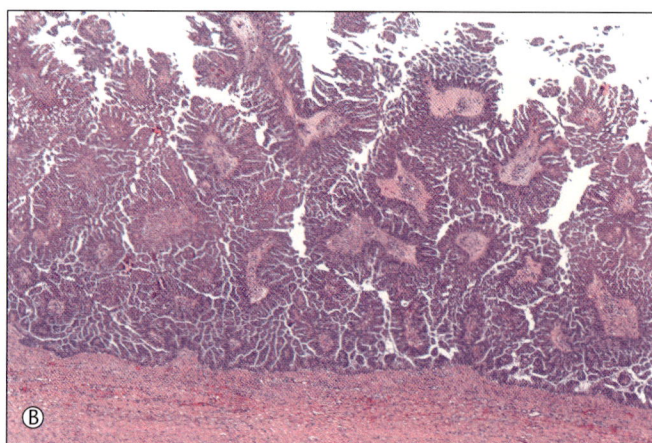

Fig. 24.19 **(A)** Bilateral serous borderline tumor with micropapillary proliferation. Both tumors show prominent exophytic papillary growth. **(B)** Serous borderline tumor with micropapillary pattern. The highly complex micropapillae grow in a non-hierarchical fashion from fibrovascular stalks. Stromal invasion is not present. Reproduced with permission from Prat.[96]

(Figure 24.20) and composed of stratified non-ciliated cuboidal cells with a high nuclear:cytoplasmic ratio. Nuclear atypia is only mild with occasional higher grade nuclei present (Figure 24.21). Mitotic figures are rare and no abnormal forms are seen.[17]

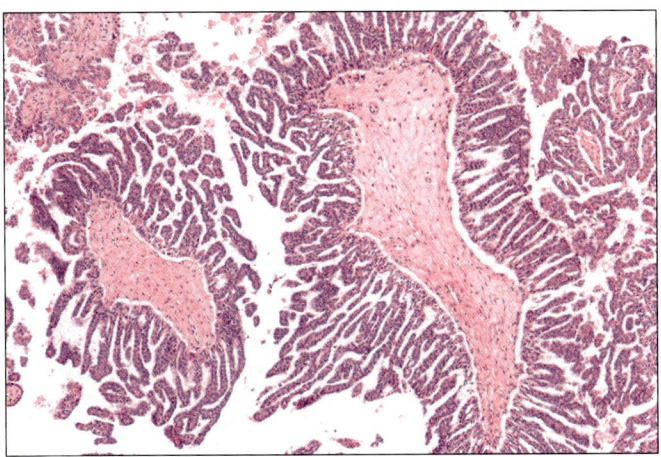

Fig. 24.20 Serous borderline tumor with micropapillary pattern ('Medusa head-like appearance'). Filigree network of small micropapillae – at least five times as long as wide – arising directly from papillary stalks.

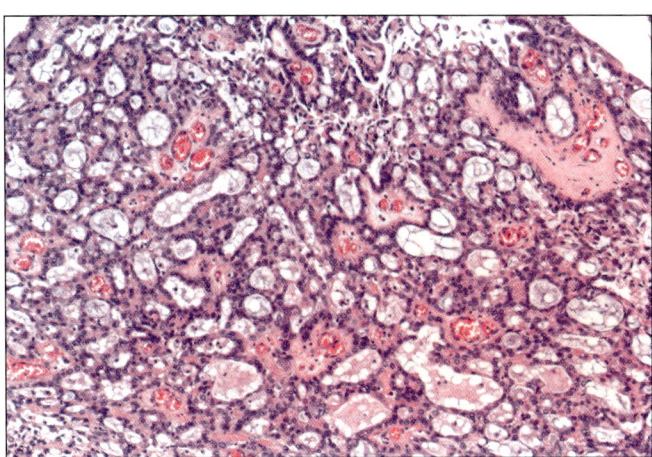

Fig. 24.22 Serous borderline tumor with cribriform architecture.

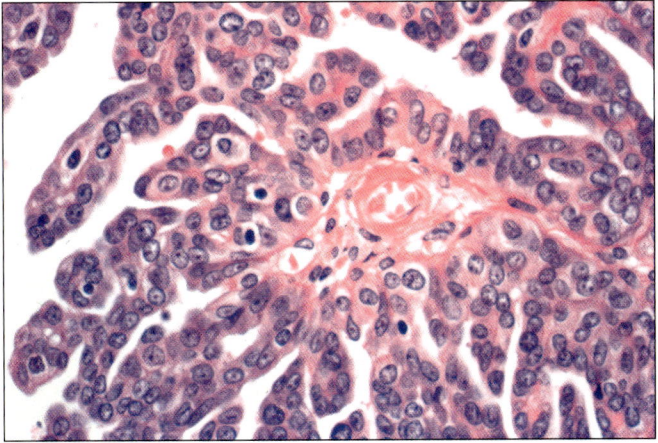

Fig. 24.21 Serous borderline tumor with micropapillary pattern. Nuclear atypia is uniform and only moderate (grade 2). Reproduced with permission from Prat.[96]

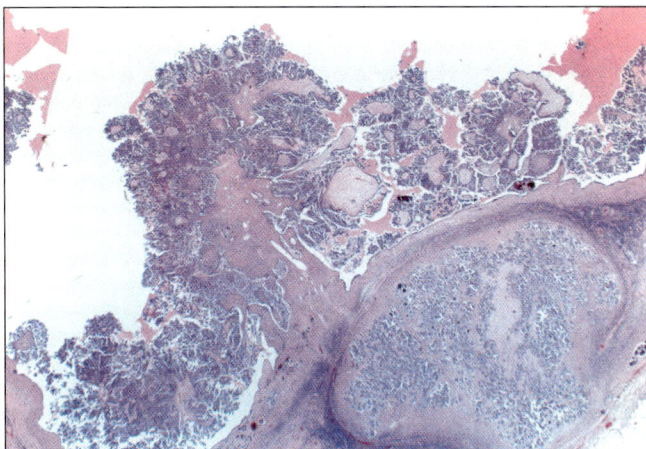

Fig. 24.23 Serous micropapillary adenocarcinoma. Note the presence of destructive stromal invasion (larger than 10 mm²). Reproduced with permission from Prat.[96]

In contrast to the typical SBT, which usually shows variable degrees of cell proliferation and nuclear atypia, the micropapillary or cribriform tumor (Figure 24.22) exhibits a homogeneous and marked degree of cell proliferation and uniform nuclear atypia. Most micropapillary tumors contain areas of typical SBT, indicating the former's probable origin.[17] When the micropapillary architecture exceeds 5 mm in greatest dimension, the original proponents[17] recommended segregating these tumors from the less proliferative SBTs, claiming that they are likely to progress to invasive carcinoma, particularly as invasive peritoneal implants. Subsequently, another group of investigators[31] required that the 'micropapillae' should be five times as long as wide (Figure 24.20).

At least six recent investigations have failed to demonstrate that the overall survival of patients with advanced stage micropapillary SBTs differs from that of patients with typical SBTs.[28,31,36,69,97,128] They have shown that bilaterality, ovarian surface growth, and advanced stage (non-invasive implants) are more common features of micropapillary SBTs than of typical SBTs, but a strong association of the former tumors with invasive implants and poor outcome has been inconsis-

tent. Although in three of these studies[28,31,69] micropapillary SBTs were more frequently associated with invasive implants, micropapillary architecture did not have a significant adverse effect on survival when controlled for implant type. The findings of these studies reinforce the view that micropapillary SBTs have a prognosis much closer to typical SBTs than to carcinomas.

Although largely non-invasive, serous tumors with prominent micropapillary architecture may contain areas of frank stromal invasion (Figure 24.23); therefore, extensive sampling is indicated in such cases. However, acceptance of the micropapillary pattern as synonymous with invasive carcinoma in not obviously invasive tumors is unjustified, for several reasons: (1) all patients with stage 1 tumors survived; (2) stage 2–3 micropapillary tumors with non-invasive peritoneal implants had the same good prognosis as typical SBTs (Table 24.1); (3) as indicated above, a clear association with invasive implants has not been demonstrated in the general population; and (4) patients who died of recurrent tumor almost all had invasive peritoneal implants which, *per se*, is the key feature associated with a poor prognosis.

The micropapillary pattern (Figures 24.20 and 24.21), almost always associated with typical SBT, most likely repre-

Table 24.1 Literature comparison: advanced stage serous borderline tumors with micropapillary pattern

	Burks et al.[17]	Seidman & Kurman[116]	Eichhorn et al.[31]	Prat & de Nictolis[97]	Longacre et al.[69]
Total cases	10	11	19	13	23
Cases with invasive implants	6[b]	10[b]	3	1	5
Chemotherapy[a]	8/10 (80%)	5/9 (56%)	5/17 (29%)	9/12 (75%)	ND
Five-year follow-up	5	10	10	9	23
Alive, no tumor	0	3	6	8	17
Alive, recurrent tumor in contralateral oophorectomy	0	0	2	1	0
Alive, progressive residual/recurrent tumor	2[b]	3[b]	0	1[c]	0
Died of tumor	2	4	2	0	5
Died of unrelated causes	1	0	0	0	1
Follow-up <5years	5	1	5	3	0
Lost to follow-up	0	0	3	1	0
Recent cases	0	0	1	0	0

[a]Number of patients/number of patients with postoperative treatment information (%).
[b]Including 'implants with micropapillary' pattern but without recognizable invasion of underlying tissue.
[c]Patient died of tumor subsequent to her report.
ND, no data available.

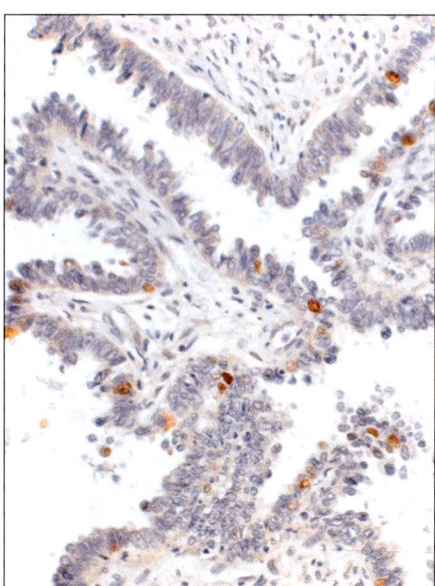
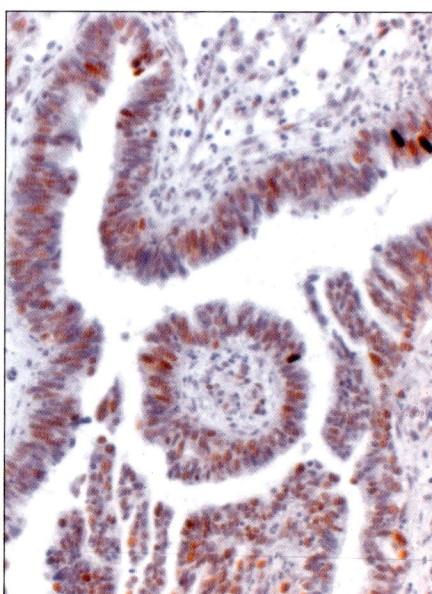

Fig. 24.24 Serous borderline tumor with multiple pelvic recurrences. P53 immunostaining was stronger in the third (right) than in the first (left) recurrent tumor. Reproduced with permission from Prat.[96]

sents a degree of epithelial proliferation closer to invasive carcinoma than SBT.[113] Immunohistochemical and mutational studies have demonstrated differences among SBTs, micropapillary SBTs, and conventional serous carcinomas of the ovary.[52] Immunostaining for p53 is weak and focal in SBTs, moderate and diffuse in micropapillary SBTs (Figure 24.24), and intense in most serous carcinomas. Both ordinary SBTs and micropapillary SBTs lack *p53* mutations, which are detected in two-thirds of the serous carcinomas.[52] Similarly, comparative genomic hybridization studies revealed greater chromosomal imbalances in micropapillary SBTs than in SBTs and fewer than in serous carcinomas.[131] These findings suggest that micropapillary SBTs represents a neoplastic epithelial proliferation intermediate between SBT and serous carcinoma. By analogy

with cervical neoplasia, the difference between typical SBT and micropapillary SBT is like that between CIN 2 and CIN 3. Although the micropapillary pattern in combination with other clinical and pathologic features (i.e., advanced stage, invasive implants, and microinvasion) may be associated with increased risk of disease progression, taken individually, micropapillarity is not a specific predictor of adverse prognosis.[69]

MICROINVASION

Approximately 10% of otherwise typical SBTs contain one or more discrete foci of stromal microinvasion,[8,53,69,78,84,97,134] which are made up of single epithelial cells or small clusters of such cells with abundant eosinophilic cytoplasm (Figures 24.25 and

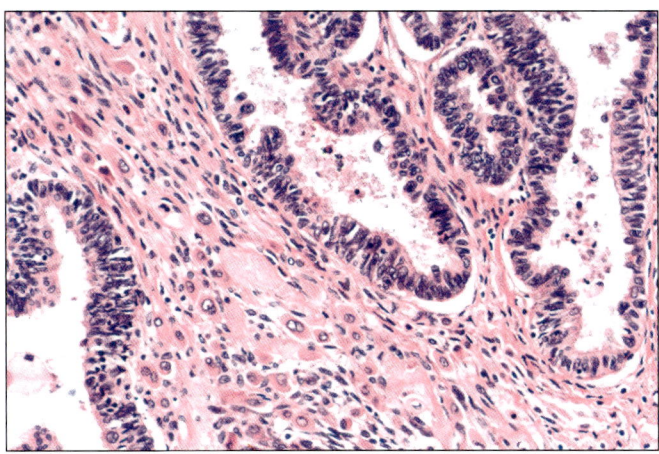

Fig. 24.25 Serous borderline tumor with microinvasion. Stromal microinvasion by single epithelial cells and small clusters of such cells with abundant eosinophilic cytoplasm. Reproduced with permission from Prat.[96]

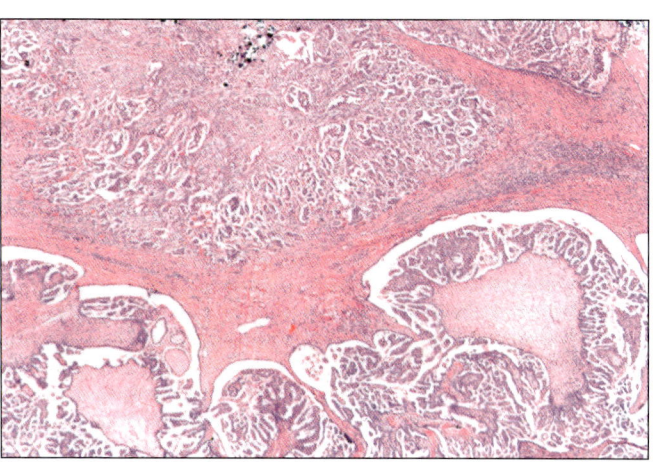

Fig. 24.27 Serous borderline tumor showing both a micropapillary pattern (bottom) and microinvasion (top).

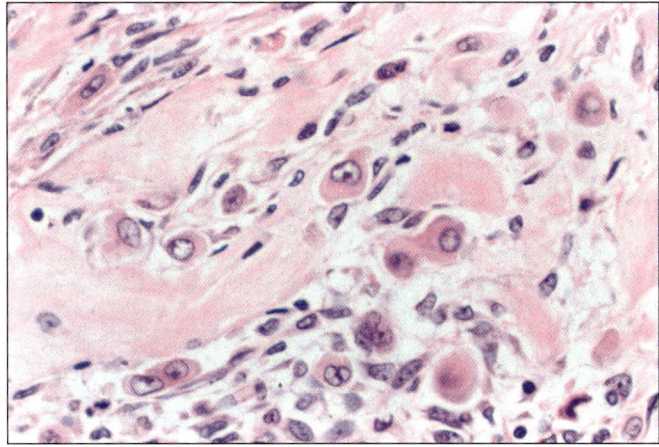

Fig. 24.26 Serous borderline tumor with microinvasion. The invasive cells show ample eosinophilic cytoplasm and vesicular nuclei with prominent nucleoli. Reproduced with permission from Prat.[96]

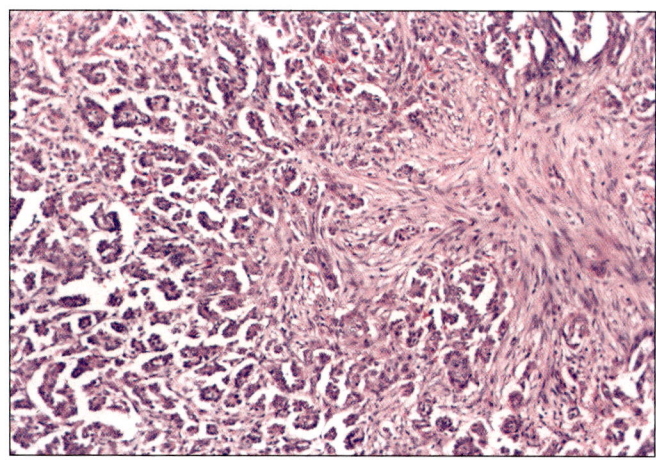

Fig. 24.28 Serous borderline tumor with microinvasion. The stroma contains numerous small papillae and clusters of tumor cells surrounded by clefts.

24.26). Often, the cell nests appear surrounded by clefts that separate the epithelium from the stroma (Figures 24.27–24.29). These microscopic foci (arbitrarily defined as not exceeding 10 mm^2 in area, or 3 mm maximum linear dimension) are typically unassociated with a significant stromal reaction and are easily overlooked on routinely stained sections.[113] Cytokeratin stains help to visualize the invasive epithelial cells (Figure 24.30). Occasionally, foci of lymphatic invasion may be present.[8] Several patients with these tumors have been pregnant at the time of diagnosis.[78]

Serous borderline tumors with microinvasion are associated with a higher frequency of bilaterality, exophytic ovarian surface growth, and advanced stage than typical SBTs lacking microinvasion, yet the rate of invasive implants is similar in both tumor groups.[97] At least five studies (Table 24.2)[8,53,84,97,134] have confirmed that SBTs with or without microinvasion have a similar prognosis. However, a recent report suggests that microinvasion may represent a risk factor for disease progression that is independent of stage and implant status.[69,78] SBTs with microinvasion should be distinguished from SBTs with *microinvasive carcinoma*. The latter shows 'destructive'

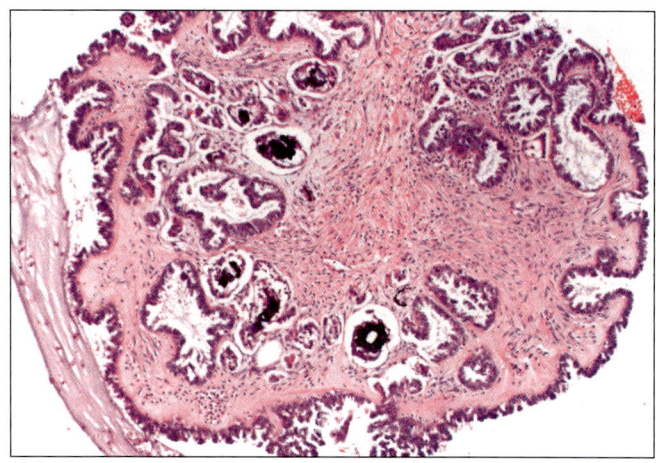

Fig. 24.29 Serous borderline tumor with microinvasion. Rounded epithelial cell aggregates lying in clear stromal spaces.

Table 24.2 Literature comparison: serous borderline tumors with microinvasion

	Tavassoli[134]	Bell & Scully[8]	Nayar et al.[84]	Kennedy & Hart[53]	Prat & de Nictolis[97]	McKenney et al.[78]
Total cases	18	21	7	4	20	60
Advanced stage	6	2	ND	1	9	26
Invasive implants/distant metastasis	1	1	0	0	1	2
Lymph node metastasis	1	1	0	0	2	7
Chemotherapy	4	3	ND	3	4	9
Radiotherapy	1	0	ND	0	1	4
Five-year follow-up (or until death)	5	ND	6	3	11	ND
Alive, no tumor	4	ND	6	3	9	41
Alive, progressive residual/recurrent tumor	0	1	0	0	1	2
Died of tumor	1	0	0	0	1*	7
Follow-up <5 years	13	ND	1	1	5	ND
Lost to follow-up	0	4	0	0	4	10

*Incomplete surgical staging.
ND, no data available.

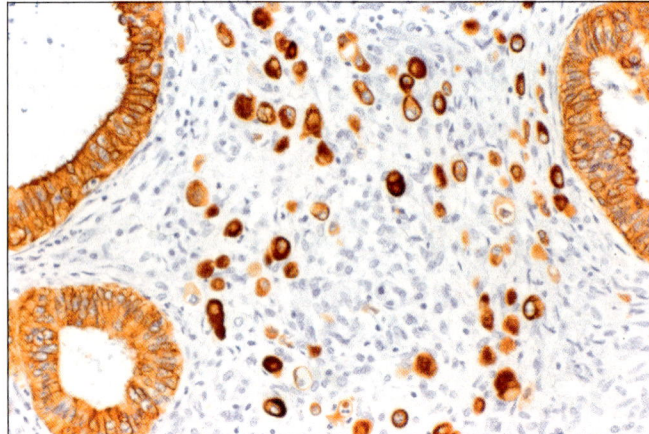

Fig. 24.30 Serous borderline tumor with microinvasion. The invasive cells are strongly reactive for cytokeratin. Reproduced with permission from Prat.[96]

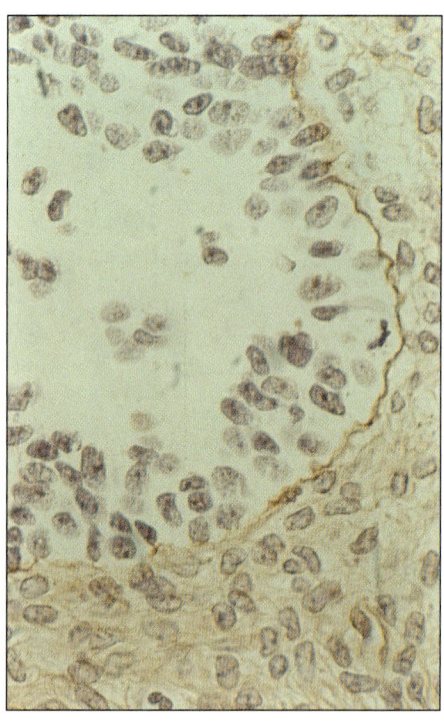

Fig. 24.31 Serous adenocarcinoma. The basement membrane appears focally interrupted (bottom). Type IV collagen immunostaining. Reproduced with permission from Prat.[96]

invasion of the stroma by malignant-appearing cells and its desmoplastic stromal response.[7]

Immunohistochemistry

Whereas all benign serous cystadenomas show a continuous basement membrane and weak or negative type IV collagenase expression, serous carcinomas exhibit frequent disruptions or complete absence of the basement membrane (Figure 24.31) and moderate to intense type IV collagenase immunostaining. SBTs with microinvasion also show focal absence of type IV collagen around the clusters of invasive cells that reacted strongly for type IV collagenase. This enzyme is also identified in the non-invasive cells with abundant eosinophilic cytoplasm.[25]

PERITONEAL IMPLANTS

One controversial aspect of SBTs is their association in about 30 to 40% of cases with peritoneal implants.[11,34–36,53,69,97,116]

Implants are found more frequently in patients with tumors that have an exophytic component than in those which do not.[114] They rarely present as bulky disease (Figure 24.32A), and, in most cases, are either microscopic or small macroscopic (≤1–2 cm) lesions. Their histologic appearance may vary greatly, ranging from foci of benign glandular epithelium resembling endosalpingiosis (an accepted, but suboptimal term, in common usage – see Chapter 33), to non-invasive papillae, plaques or nodules of borderline epithelium and

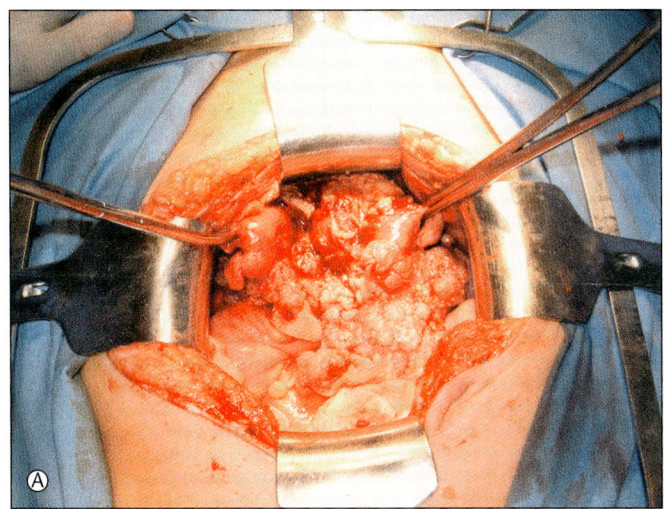

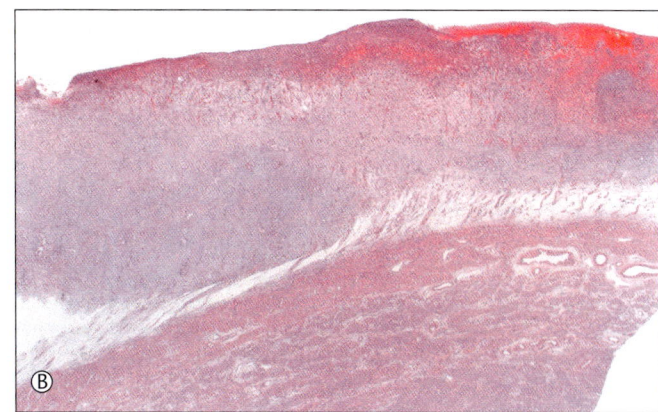

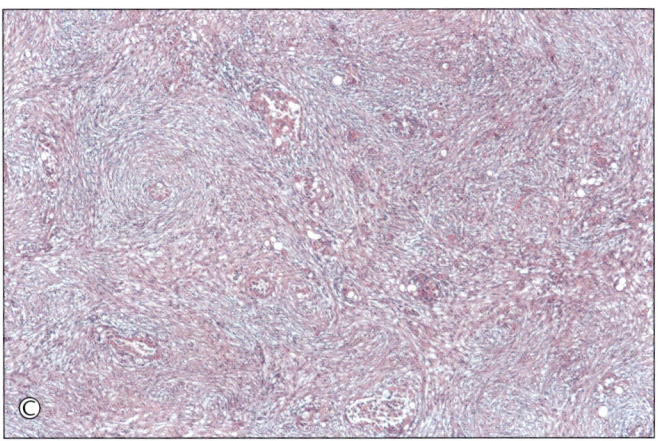

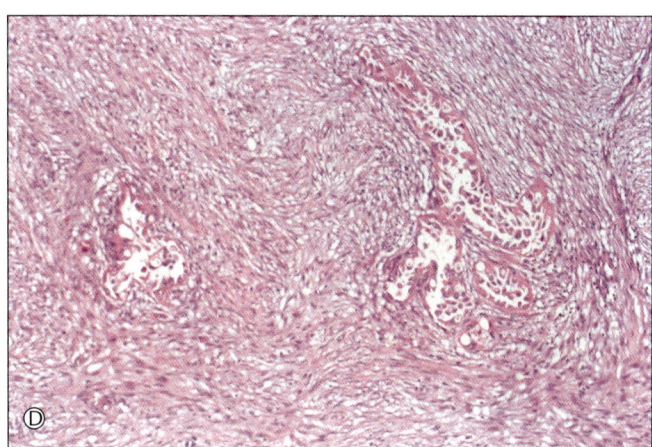

Fig. 24.32 **(A)** Serous borderline tumor with non-invasive implants. At laparotomy, the uterus was covered by a soft gray-white and hemorrhagic mass (400 g). Courtesy of Dr I Boguna, Barcelona, Spain. **(B)** Non-invasive desmoplastic implant of serous borderline tumor. The implant appears plastered upon the uterine serosa without invading the underlying myometrium. The surface of the implant shows hemorrhage and necrosis. **(C)** The implant is largely composed of a fibroblastic proliferation which surpasses quantitatively the glandular epithelial component. **(D)** Two epithelial glands containing hobnail cells with moderately atypical nuclei are surrounded by dense fibroblastic stroma.

stroma, to invasive implants resembling a low-grade serous carcinoma.[11] Endosalpingiosis – typified by glands, cysts, and occasionally papillae with psammoma bodies – is a benign peritoneal lesion frequently associated with ovarian SBTs (Figure 24.33). It may rarely be the substrate for the development of peritoneal SBTs or carcinomas, but its presence should not change the stage of a synchronous ovarian SBT.

The peritoneal implants of SBTs have been classified histologically into *non-invasive* and *invasive* types, with the former being further subdivided into *epithelial* and *desmoplastic* subtypes.[11]

- The *epithelial* subtype of non-invasive implants shows papillary proliferations of atypical epithelial cells resembling those of the ovarian SBT (Figure 24.34); they are typically present on the surface of the peritoneum (Figure 24.35) or in smoothly contoured subperitoneal invaginations, and exhibit little or no stromal reaction.[11]
- In contrast, the *desmoplastic* subtype of non-invasive implant is largely composed of a stromal proliferation, which is plastered upon serosal surfaces or invaginations

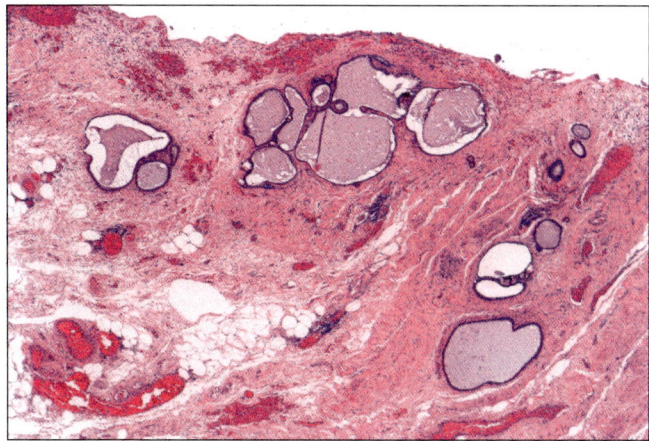

Fig. 24.33 Endosalpingiosis. Glands lined by flattened tubal-like epithelium lie in the parametrium.

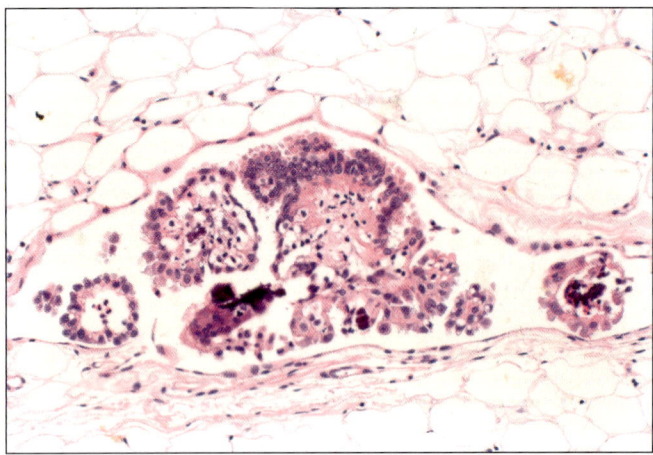

Fig. 24.34 Non-invasive epithelial implant of serous borderline tumor within a smoothly contoured invagination of the omental fat. The epithelial proliferation contains psammoma bodies and resembles that of the primary ovarian tumor.

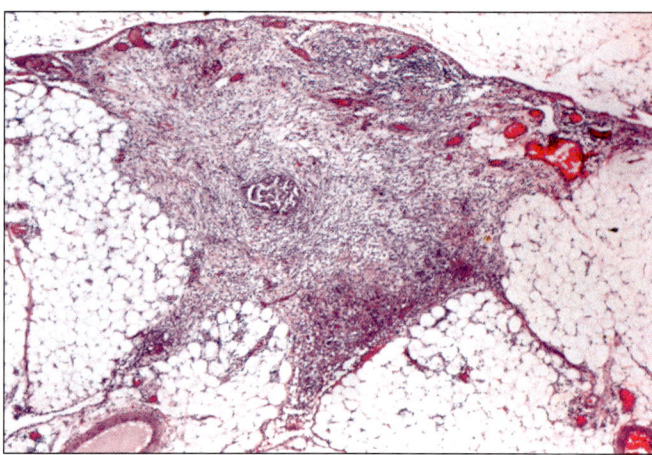

Fig. 24.36 Non-invasive desmoplastic implant of serous borderline tumor. The implant invaginates between adjacent lobules of omental fat. Scattered nests of tumor cells are present within a loose fibroblastic stroma. Reproduced with permission from Prat.[95]

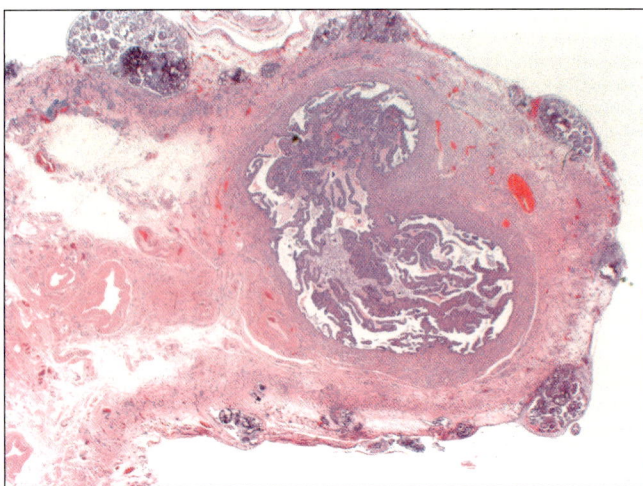

Fig. 24.35 Non-invasive epithelial implants of serous borderline tumor on the serosa of the fallopian tube. Reproduced with permission from Prat and de Nictolis.[97]

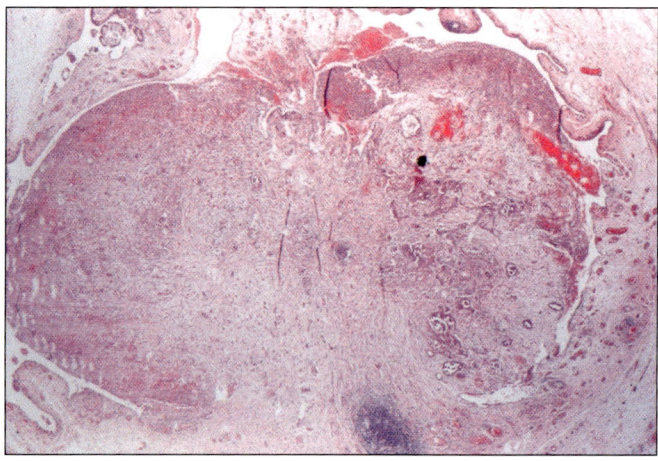

Fig. 24.37 Non-invasive desmoplastic implant of serous borderline tumor. The sharply circumscribed nodule is composed predominantly of granulation tissue-like stroma and contains only scattered nests of tumor cells. Foci of hemorrhage and necrosis are seen at the periphery. Reproduced with permission from De Nictolis et al.[26]

between lobules of omental fat (Figure 24.32B–D, 24.36 and 24.37). The stromal reaction surpasses quantitatively the epithelial component of the implant. In late lesions, small glands and papillae lined by atypical serous cells as well as psammoma bodies are entrapped by dense fibroblastic tissue that is often infiltrated by acute and chronic inflammatory cells. Early implants show necrosis with surface fibrin deposition and hemorrhage (Figure 24.37).[11]

• *Invasive* implants, which represent approximately 12% of the cases,[11,31,36,69,97] manifest a disorderly infiltration of normal tissues, such as the omentum; in contrast to the well-defined limits of the desmoplastic implants, the invasive implants exhibit irregular borders (Figure 24.38). They usually show a greater epithelial cell population (Figure 24.39) and resemble histologically a low-grade serous adenocarcinoma (Figure 24.40); marked cytologic atypia may be present.[11]

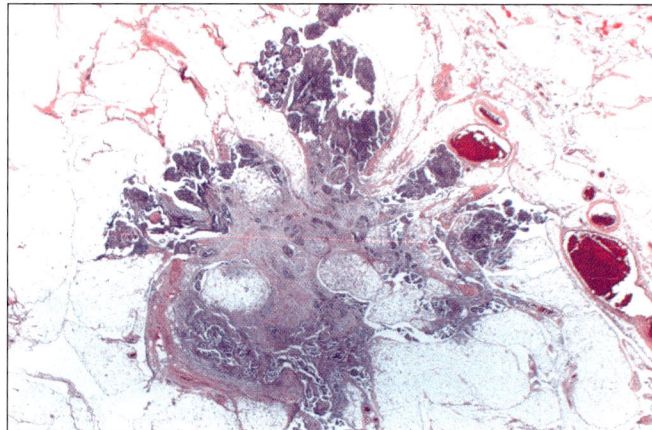

Fig. 24.38 Invasive omental implant of serous borderline tumor. The implant is composed predominantly of epithelial cells which invade the adipose tissue in an irregular fashion. Reproduced with permission from Prat.[96]

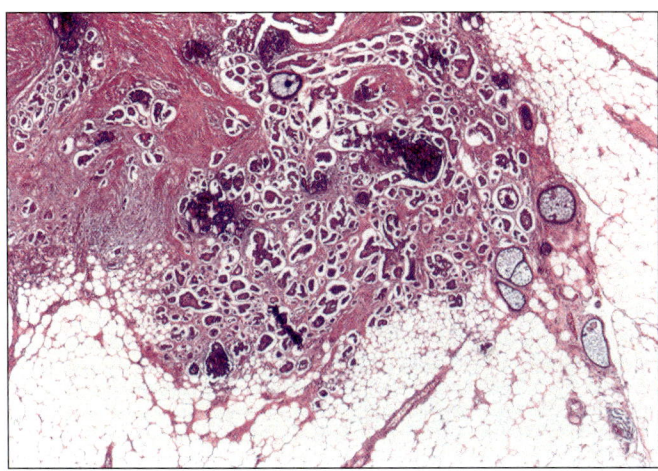

Fig. 24.39 Invasive omental implant of serous borderline tumor. The tumor glands and papillae appear disorderly distributed within a desmoplastic ('collagenized') stroma and many of them are surrounded by clefts. Reproduced with permission from Prat and de Nictolis.[97]

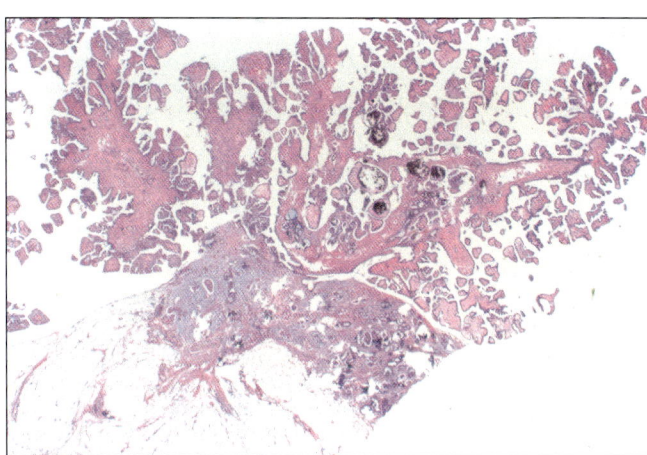

Fig. 24.41 Mixed non-invasive and invasive omental implant of serous borderline tumor. The non-invasive component shows exophytic growth with hierarchical branching papillae (top) whereas the invasive tumor infiltrates the adipose tissue (bottom). Reproduced with permission from Prat.[96]

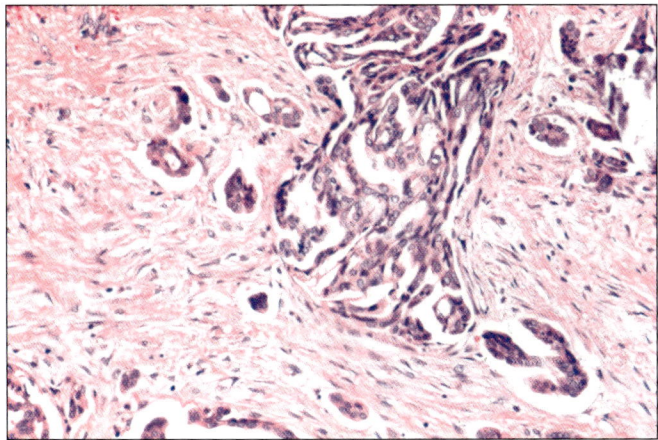

Fig. 24.40 Invasive omental implant of serous borderline tumor. The tumor resembles a low-grade serous adenocarcinoma. Reproduced with permission from De Nictolis et al.[26]

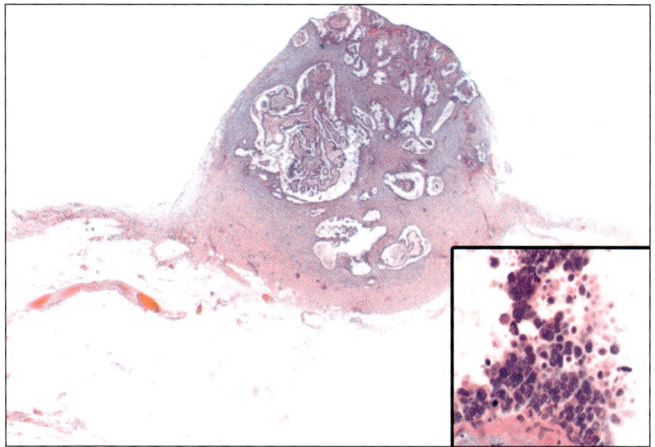

Fig. 24.42 Desmoplastic non-invasive omental implant of serous carcinoma. Numerous glands and papillae are present. The tumor cells exhibit an unusually high nuclear atypia for the ordinary serous borderline tumor. Reproduced with permission from Prat.[96]

Implants should be sampled extensively since non-invasive and invasive implants may coexist (Figure 24.41). Also, some implants of serous carcinomas may be non-invasive and simulate the desmoplastic non-invasive implants of SBTs. The former implants, however, usually contain highly atypical epithelial cells (Figure 24.42).[113]

At least 10 studies of SBTs with peritoneal implants (Table 24.3)[11,12,26,31,34,35,53,69,76,97,116] have clearly demonstrated that separation of the implants into invasive and non-invasive subtypes carries important prognostic implications. The rare tumors that were fatal were mostly those with *invasive* peritoneal implants.

Despite the poor prognosis associated with invasive implants when they actually invade the underlying tissues, their diagnostic criteria remain problematic. Truly invasive implants are rare lesions; i.e., from a population exceeding 3 million people, only six patients with stage 3 SBTs with invasive implants were encountered during a 17-year period.[36] Some investigators, however, have reported higher rates of invasive implants (up to 35% in one series) but a lack of correlation between their

presence and adverse prognosis.[34] Such a discrepancy could be explained by the inclusion of desmoplastic non-invasive implants in the category of invasive implants.[11]

Although the use of more liberal histologic criteria (i.e., solid epithelial nests surrounded by clefts and micropapillary architecture) increased the proportion of invasive implants in a recently reported series to more than 50%,[12] association with death due to progressive disease was less significant than by three other groups using more stringent diagnostic rules.[31,36,97] In fact, one of the latter studies confirmed that solid epithelial nests surrounded by clefts and micropapillary architecture are found more often in invasive than non-invasive implants;[97] in that series, obvious destructive invasion was the only feature of the peritoneal implants specifically associated with poor outcome.[97] As stated earlier, the presence of epithelial cell clusters surrounded by clefts or halos is a characteristic feature of stromal microinvasion (which is associated with a favorable prognosis) (Figure 24.29). In contrast, an abundant epithelial component (Figures 24.38 and 24.39), whether micropapillary

Table 24.3 Death from tumor among patients with ovarian serous borderline tumors associated with peritoneal implants (literature review, 1984–2005)

	Non-invasive implants	Invasive implants
McCaughey et al.[76]	2/13	4/5
Bell et al.[11]	3/50	5/6[a]
De Nictolis et al.[26]	0/10	4/9
Kennedy & Hart[53]	1/25[b]	0/1[c]
Seidman & Kurman[116]	1/51	2/3
Gershenson et al.[34,35]	6/73	6/39
Eichhorn et al.[31]	0/30	2/3
Bell et al.[12]	2/29[d]	6/31[e]
Prat & De Nictolis[97]	0/34	3/6[f]
Longacre et al.[69]	2/85	5/14[g]
Total	17/400	37/117

[a] One patient died of tumor subsequent to her report.
[b] Transformation into serous carcinoma.
[c] Follow-up 23 months.
[d] One patient was alive with progressive disease (AWPD).
[e] 13 patients were AWPD.
[f] The other three patients were AWPD.
[g] One patient was AWPD and one died of leukemia but had persistent tumor.

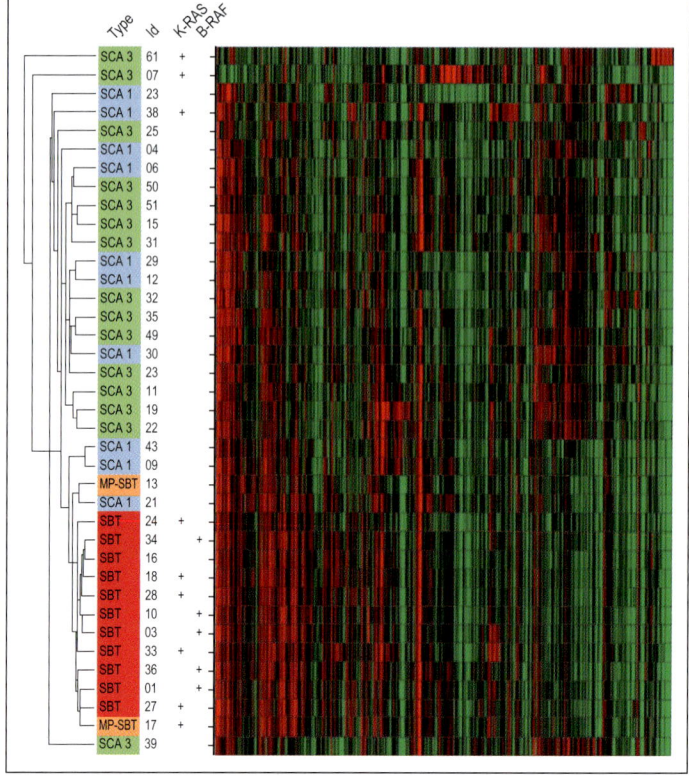

Fig. 24.43 Unsupervised hierarchical cluster analysis of 38 ovarian neoplasms and *B-Raf/K-ras* mutation status. In the heat map each row represents a tumor and each column a single gene. Red indicates higher-than-average expression and green indicates lower-than-average expression. *K-ras* and *B-raf* mutations are indicated by + in two columns. Tumor types have been colored to facilitate identification of groups, whereas the dendrogram shows the proximity of samples. MP-SBT, micropapillary pattern SBT; SBT, serous borderline tumor, SCA, serous carcinoma. Reproduced with permission from Sieben et al.[122]

or not, favors the diagnosis of invasion. Non-invasive desmoplastic implants typically contain an excess of granulation tissue-like stroma and minimal epithelial component in the form of small cellular nests or glands (Figures 24.32B–D, 24.36 and 24.37).[11] The finding of single isolated cells in the stroma is not enough histologic evidence to diagnose the implant as invasive; such isolated cells can also be found in approximately one-third of non-invasive desmoplastic implants.[12]

The characteristics of non-invasive epithelial, non-invasive desmoplastic, and invasive implants can be summarized as follows:

- Non-invasive epithelial implants:
  - Papillary proliferations resembling ovarian SBT
  - On peritoneal surface or in smoothly contoured invaginations
  - Well-defined margins
  - Little or no stromal reaction
  - Psammoma bodies.
- Non-invasive desmoplastic implants:
  - Stromal proliferation plastered on serosal surfaces or between lobules of omental fat
  - Well-defined margins
  - Excess of granulation tissue-like stroma (>50%) and minimal epithelial component
  - Hemorrhage, necrosis (early changes), fibrosis, and calcification (late changes).
- Invasive implants:
  - Disorderly distributed glands destructively invading normal tissue
  - Poorly defined irregular margins
  - Abundant epithelial component

- Dense collagenous stroma without significant inflammation
- Resemble low-grade serous carcinomas
- Aneuploidy.

Because the ovarian and peritoneal lesions in stage 2–3 SBTs may have various histologic appearances, and as the extraovarian peritoneal mesothelium has the potential to give rise to müllerian epithelial lesions, i.e., endosalpingiosis and serous neoplasms, some investigators have postulated that some of the peritoneal implants associated with ovarian SBTs are independent foci of primary peritoneal neoplasia rather than true implants.[109] Others, however, favor the 'implantation' explanation based on the fact that two-thirds of SBTs with an exophytic component are associated with implants (in contrast to less than 5% of those that are exclusively endophytic).[114]

Somatic genetics

Recent molecular genetic studies indicate that SBTs and conventional serous carcinomas represent separate pathogenetic entities. SBTs with and without micropapillary pattern frequently display *B-Raf/K-ras* mutations (Figure 24.43) but rarely mutant *p53*. In contrast, *B-Raf/K-ras* mutations are rare in conventional high-grade serous carcinomas (Figure 24.43), but *p53* mutations occur in approximately 60% of cases (see below[18,125]). *B-Raf/K-ras* mutations also occur in the epithelium of cystadenomas adjacent to SBTs, suggesting that they precede the development of the latter tumors.[45] *K-ras* mutations are also present in the glandular inclusions (endosalpingiosis) in the peritoneum and lymph nodes of patients with ovarian SBT.[2] RNA expression profiles of ovarian serous tumors have recently disclosed that the mitogenic (RAS-RAF-MEK-ERK-MAP) kinase pathway is activated in SBTs; however, activation of downstream genes involved in extracellular matrix degradation is absent, suggesting an uncoupling of both events.[122] Two genes involved in regulating this uncoupling – ERK-inhibitor *Dusp-4* and uPA-inhibitor *Serpina 5* – are downregulated in serous carcinomas in contrast to SBTs. In serous carcinomas, this also involves downstream activation of matrix metalloprotease-9.[122] Gene expression profiling has also shown prominent expression of *p53*, cyclin-dependent kinase inhibitor *p21*, and other *p53*-modulated genes in SBTs, suggesting that this signaling pathway may play an important role in the distinct phenotype associated with this lesion.[14] Although the profiles for invasive low-grade serous carcinomas did not contain the enhanced p53 signaling activity observed in SBTs, the former tumors were aligned with the SBTs instead of high-grade serous tumors.[14] These findings provide additional proof that typical SBT, SBT with micropapillary pattern, and invasive low-grade serous carcinoma are closely related neoplasms, which are different from usual invasive serous carcinomas. The rare cases of invasive low-grade serous carcinomas with micropapillary pattern (Figure 24.44) (which also have *B-Raf/K-ras* mutations) probably represent SBTs with infiltrative stromal invasion greater than microinvasion.

Clonality studies have examined whether multiple, synchronous or metachronous SBTs (found at different sites in the abdominal cavity) arise as a result of spread from a single ovarian site, or whether such deposits are polyclonal, representing independent primary tumors. Two studies based on X chromosome inactivation analysis support a multifocal origin of bilateral and advanced SBTs.[39,71] However, tumor-related changes may interfere with X chromosome inactivation and this method poorly assesses clonality. In contrast, loss of heterozygosity (LOH) is an irreversible genetic event acquired during tumorigenesis. Its weakness, however, is that the absence of informative markers and the failure to detect LOH underestimates the frequency of clonality. In a study for evaluating LOH on chromosome 17p13, genetic concordance was found between the non-invasive peritoneal implants and the primary ovarian SBTs in all three cases studied.[142] Subsequently, clonality has been assessed by a genome-wide allelotyping in 47 synchronous and/or metachronous bilateral ovarian SBTs and a single non-invasive peritoneal implant from 22 patients using 59 microsatellite markers.[121] Concordant results were obtained in seven of nine SBTs with LOH in informative markers and identical chromosomal breakpoints in six of seven cases. Although the subsequent involvement of the contralateral ovary in a patient who had a previously resected unilateral SBT (Figure 24.45) is usually interpreted as development of second and independent serous borderline tumor, these molecular genetic findings lend further support to the implantation theory. More recently, clonality of invasive and non-invasive peritoneal implants and lymph node deposits has been investigated by genome-wide allelotyping and *B-Raf/K-ras* mutation analysis in 10 patients using 23 microsatellite markers. Concordant LOH for 1–5 microsatellite markers was found in all five informative cases in all tumor sites. In addition, identical *K-ras* and *B-Raf* mutations were detected in four and two cases, respectively (Figure 24.46).[123] These findings strongly support the metastatic nature of non-invasive and invasive peritoneal implants and lymph node deposits.

Differential diagnosis

SBTs are only rarely confused with other neoplasms. Their distinction from serous carcinomas has already been discussed. SBTs differ from endocervical-like mucinous borderline tumors by the lack of both intracellular mucin and a neutrophilic infiltrate (see below). SBTs may also occur as a component of mixed müllerian borderline tumors. Retiform Sertoli–Leydig cell tumors (Chapter 26) can have areas indistinguishable from SBTs on routine staining, but occur in a younger age group, have other distinctive features such as long ribbons of sex cord-type cells, and other patterns of Sertoli–Leydig cell tumors.

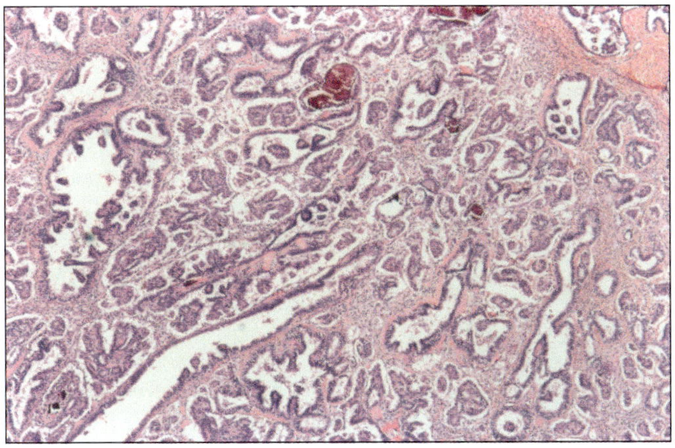

Fig. 24.44 Serous papillary adenocarcinoma, well differentiated. The tumor, which also had an extensive borderline component, shows stromal invasion by glands and papillae with only mild to moderate nuclear atypia. Psammoma bodies and larger calcific deposits are seen. Reproduced with permission from Prat.[96]

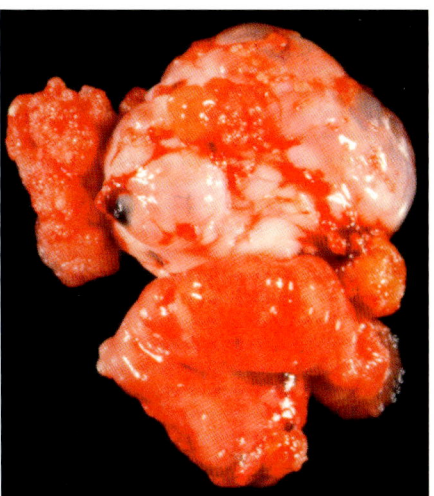

Fig. 24.45 Recurrent cystic and surface papillary serous borderline tumor. The patient had undergone unilateral salpingo-oophorectomy for a similar tumor of the contralateral ovary 2 years before. Reproduced with permission from Prat.[96]

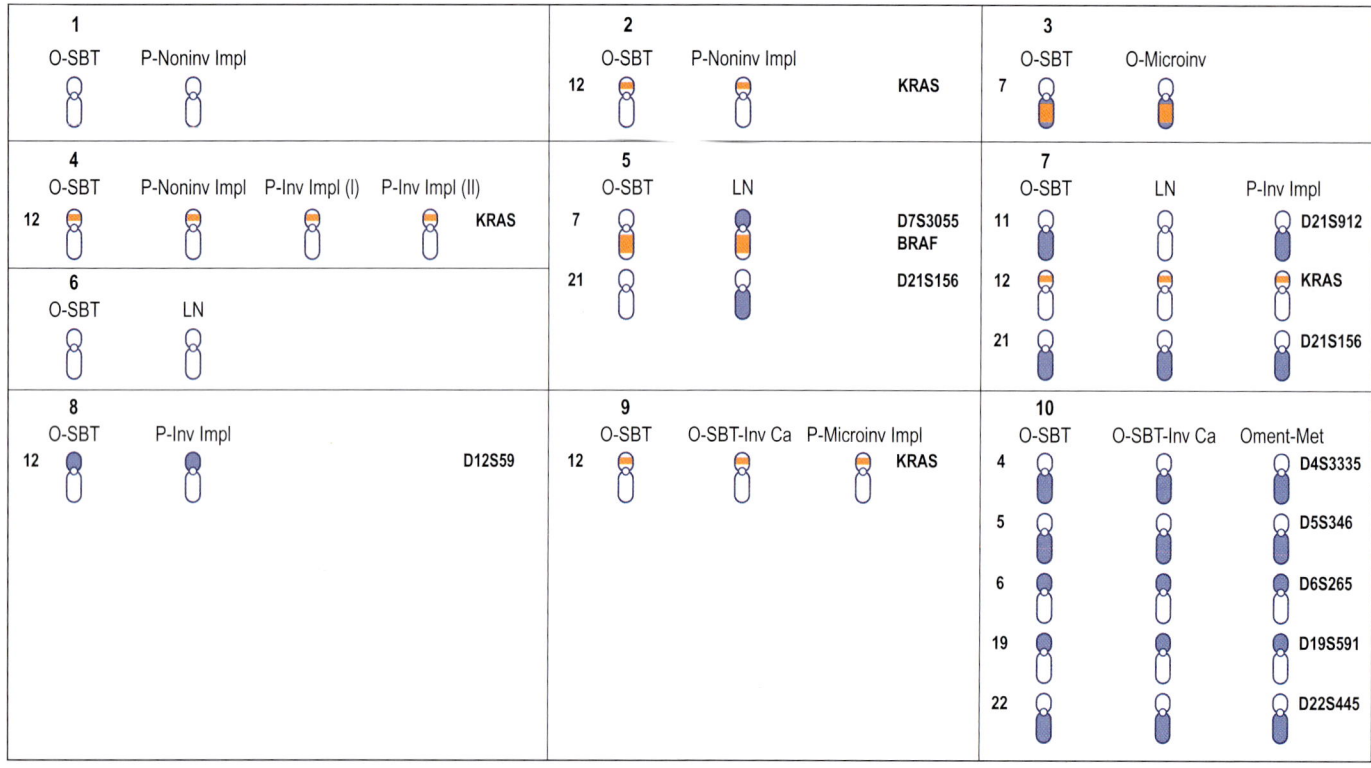

Fig. 24.46 Clonal analysis of 10 serous borderline tumors with peritoneal implants and/or lymph node involvement. O-SBT, ovarian serous borderline tumor; P-Noninv Impl, non-invasive peritoneal implant; O-Microinv, ovarian SBT with focus of microinvasion, too small to warrant the diagnosis of serous carcinoma; P-Inv Impl, invasive peritoneal implant; LN, SBT with lymph node involvement; O-SBT-Inv Ca, ovarian SBT with invasive foci allowing the diagnosis of low-grade serous carcinoma; P-Microinv Impl, non-invasive peritoneal implant with foci of microinvasion; Oment-Met, omental metastasis of serous carcinoma. Loss of heterozygosity (LOH) is indicated in blue; *B-RAF/K-RAS* mutation is indicated in red; microsatellite markers for which the LOH was found are indicated on the right. Chromosome numbers where LOH and mutations were found are on the left. Reproduced with permission from Sieben et al.[123]

These tumors, like most sex-cord tumors, are often reactive for α-inhibin.

Biologic behavior

The overall outcome of SBTs is extremely favorable. For patients with stage 1 tumors, the risk of recurrence or the development of a second SBT has been estimated to be only 5–10%.[53,69,97] The tumors rarely recur beyond 10 years.

Most SBTs maintain their microscopic features and indolent clinical behavior, and usually do not progress over the years to frankly invasive carcinoma.[53] Some of the rare cases in which transformation into carcinoma has been described[124] have been reinterpreted as examples of insufficiently sampled or misdiagnosed serous carcinomas from the beginning. It is possible that some of these cases represent independent serous carcinomas of the peritoneum. In a recent study, however, transformation of SBT to low-grade serous carcinoma occurred in 6–7% of patients late in the course of the disease and was associated with poor prognosis. Almost 80% occurred in patients without prior history of invasive implants.[69] Of eight cases of SBT with malignant behavior, all had ovarian surface involvement, three exhibited focal stromal invasion greater than microinvasion, and only two were micropapillary SBT (SBT-MP).[60] Malignant transformation of SBT to high-grade carcinoma may also occur early[91] or following multiple recurrences[97] (Figure 24.47).

Although exophytic SBTs are more often associated with synchronous peritoneal implants than intracystic SBTs, the presence of ovarian surface involvement (Figure 24.8) does not necessarily predict progression of disease.[53,114] As previously stated, most fatal SBTs have had invasive implants.[11,12,26,31,53,69,76,97,116]

SEROUS BORDERLINE TUMORS IN LYMPH NODES

The frequency of lymph node involvement by SBTs is unknown. The pelvic or para-aortic lymph nodes, or both, were involved in 23% of the cases in one study.[59] This high frequency of regional lymph node 'metastasis' may be artificial. Glandular inclusions lined by benign serous epithelium may be encountered in pelvic and para-aortic lymph nodes (Figure 24.48) of women who have had a lymphadenectomy as part of the treatment of squamous cell carcinoma of the cervix.[51] Thus, it is not surprising that occasionally proliferative changes, including SBTs, develop in this epithelium. When this occurs in a patient with an SBT of the ovary, the distinction between primary nodal and metastatic tumor can be difficult.[30] If the SBT in the nodes is a focal finding confined to the parenchyma or capsule of the lymph node, and appears associated with numerous benign inclusions, it is logical to interpret the nodal proliferation in these cases as synchronous neoplasia.[113] In other cases there is involvement of vascular sinuses at the periphery of the

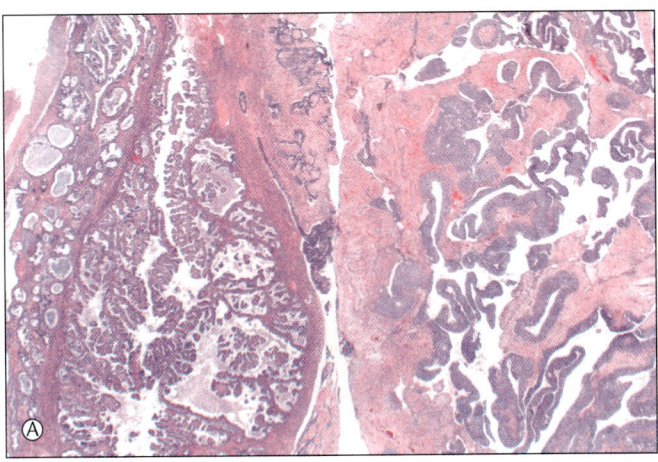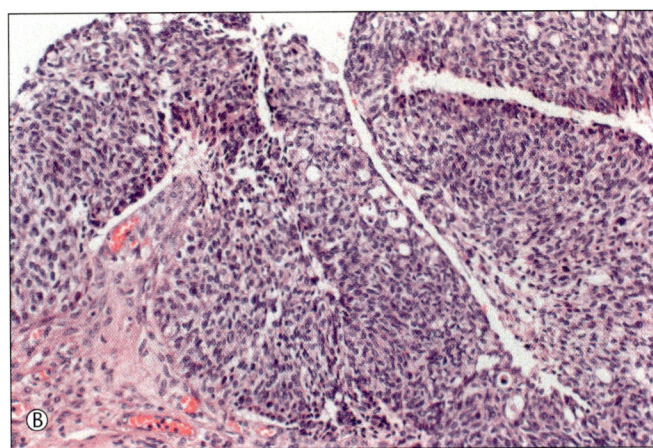

Fig. 24.47 **(A)** Serous borderline tumor with malignant transformation. The sixth recurrent pelvic tumor shows a component of transitional cell carcinoma (right) which had not been identified in previous specimens. The patient had 12 recurrent tumors resected over a period of 11 years. **(B)** Higher magnification of the transitional cell carcinoma. Reproduced with permission from Prat.[96]

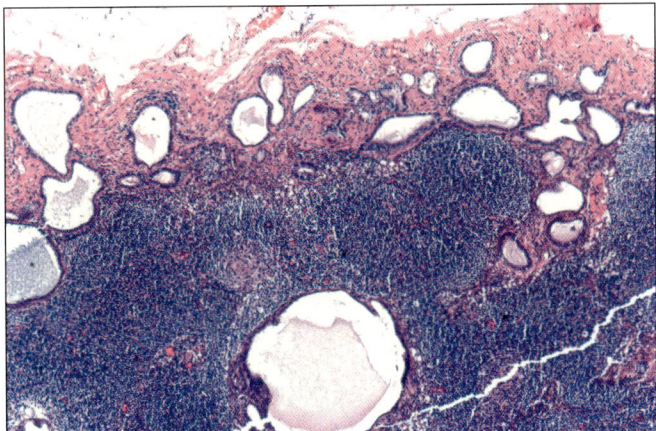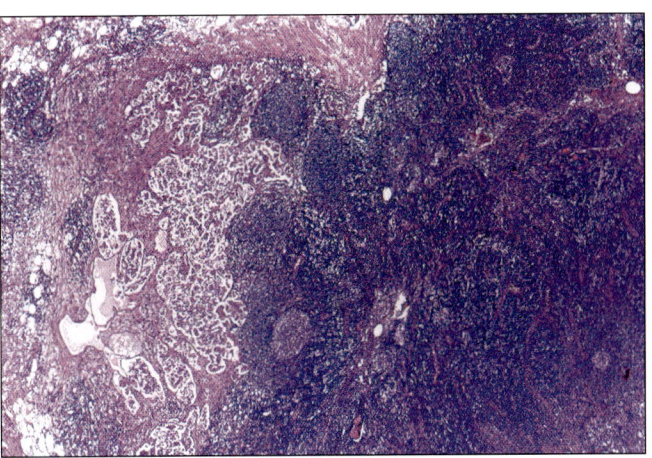

Fig. 24.48 Benign müllerian inclusion glands in a pelvic lymph node. Reproduced with permission from Prat.[96]

Fig. 24.49 Serous borderline tumor within the marginal sinus of a pelvic lymph node. The patient had a similar ovarian tumor.

node (Figures 24.49 and 24.50) suggesting metastatic spread to the node.[113] Recently, molecular genetic evidence has shown that some glandular inclusions may represent bland-appearing forms of metastatic SBT.[82]

Whether the lymph node involvement represents synchronous neoplasia or true metastatic SBT does not change the favorable prognosis of these patients and should not influence their treatment. A recent report, however, has suggested that nodular epithelial aggregates (Figure 24.51) (1–8 mm), often accompanied by desmoplastic stromal reaction (Figure 24.52) and micropapillary architecture, are associated with decreased disease-free survival.[77] Rarely, SBTs extend to extra-abdominal lymph nodes including cervical lymph nodes.[97,133] Occasionally, extensive lymph node metastases occur in patients with invasive peritoneal implants and are associated with poor prognosis.[97]

Another nodal lesion that may cause confusion in identifying metastatic tumor is cytokeratin-positive mesothelial cells,

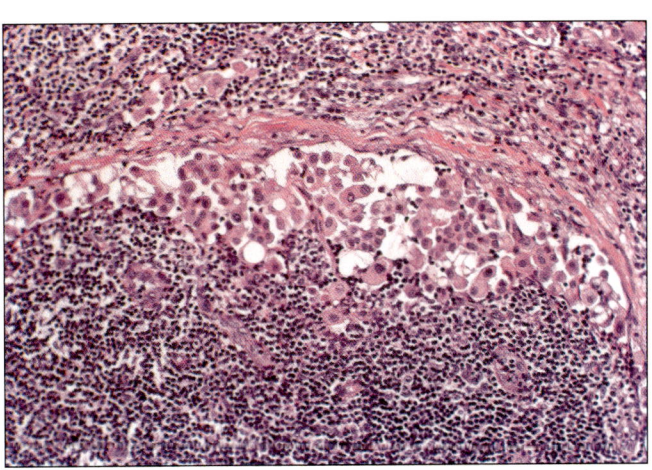

Fig. 24.50 Serous borderline tumor within a lymphatic of a lymph node.

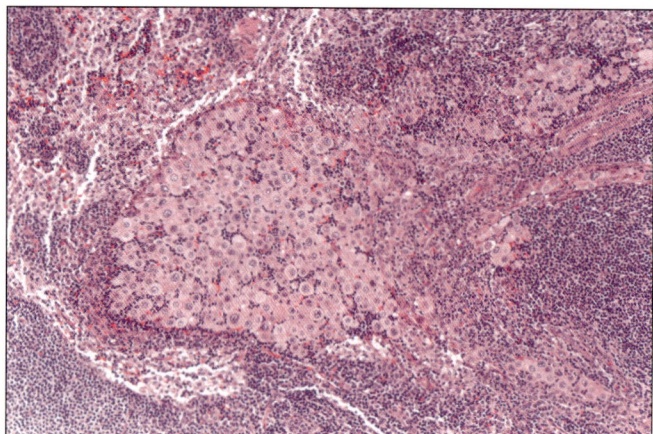

Fig. 24.51 Serous borderline tumor with lymph node involvement by nodular epithelial aggregates.

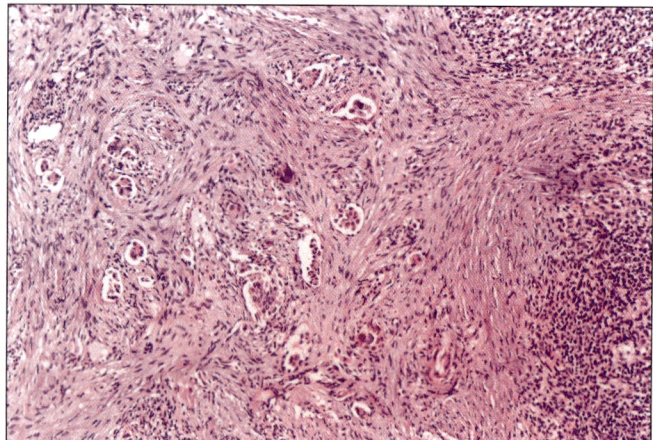

Fig. 24.52 Serous borderline tumor with lymph node involvement and desmoplastic stromal reaction.

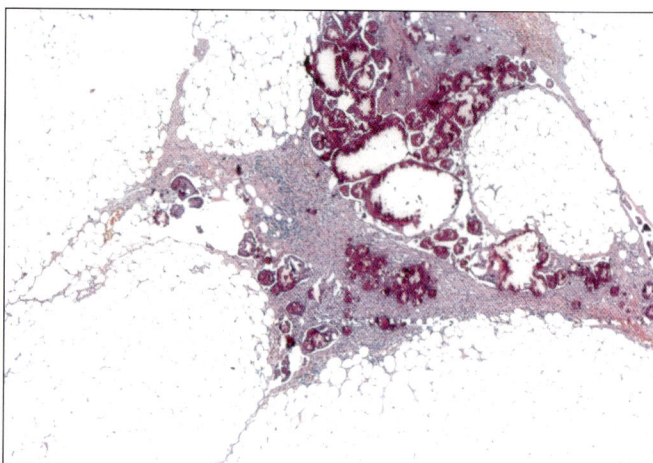

Fig. 24.53 Serous borderline tumor of the peritoneum. The tumor is well circumscribed and resembles a non-invasive desmoplastic implant. Psammoma bodies and larger calcific deposits are seen. Reproduced with permission from Prat.[96]

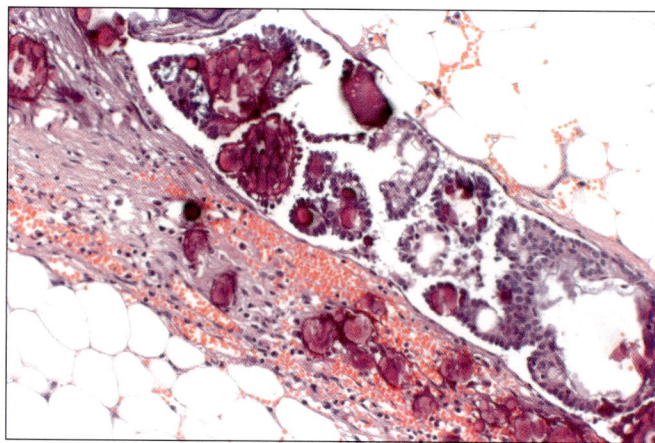

Fig. 24.54 Serous borderline tumor of the peritoneum. The tumor extends between lobules of adipose tissue. The ovaries were free of tumor. Reproduced with permission from Prat.[96]

singly or in groups, occupying either the subcapsular sinuses or the lymph node parenchyma.[22] This phenomenon is due to marked proliferation of mesothelial cells as a result of peritoneal involvement by tumor; the mesothelial cells are subsequently filtered ('deportation') from the peritoneal fluid by regional lymph nodes.[3] Immunostaining with a panel of antibodies may be of help. The most useful markers are Ber-EP4, which reacts with serous tumors but not with mesothelioma. In contrast, calretinin, cytokeratin 5 (CK5), and thrombomodulin all react with mesothelioma but not with serous carcinomas.[88,139]

SEROUS BORDERLINE TUMORS OF THE PERITONEUM

Tumors histologically identical to SBTs may arise as primary neoplasms of the peritoneum with minimal or no ovarian surface involvement.[9,13] The ages of the patients range from 16 to 67 years (mean age, 32 years). Infertility and abdominal pain are the most frequent presenting symptoms but one-third of the lesions are incidental findings at laparotomy performed for various other reasons.[9] At operation, the peritoneal lesions may be focal or diffuse. They typically appear as fibrous adhe-

sions or granular lesions of the peritoneal surfaces (up to 6 mm in diameter) and may be mistaken for peritoneal carcinomatosis. They are found mainly in the pelvic peritoneum, but can involve the upper abdominal peritoneum including omentum.[9] In these patients, the ovaries are typically of normal size, and frequently exhibit adhesions and focal granularity similar to that seen in the extraovarian peritoneum. Microscopically, the tumors may resemble either the epithelial or desmoplastic subtypes of non-invasive implants of ovarian SBTs (Figures 24.53 and 24.54).[9] Endosalpingiosis and chronic salpingitis are common associated findings in these patients.[9]

The standard treatment is total abdominal hysterectomy and bilateral salpingo-oophorectomy (TAH-BSO) and omentectomy. Younger patients who desire to maintain fertility may be treated conservatively.[13] The prognosis is excellent, although rarely, invasive low-grade serous carcinoma of the peritoneum may develop and occasional death due to tumor may occur.[9]

Treatment

Surgery is the cornerstone of treatment for patients with SBTs. In menopausal and postmenopausal women and in those who have completed their childbearing, the standard treatment is TAH-BSO. Abdominal exploration, careful staging, and removal of all grossly identifiable tumor should be done. In young women with unilateral tumors and normal-appearing contralateral ovaries who wish to preserve their reproductive capacity, unilateral oophorectomy, or even an ovarian cystectomy, can be safely performed.[5,53,67] Although a staging procedure for SBTs is often thought to be too radical, comprehensive surgical staging is recommended in patients with apparent stage 1 SBTs to exclude the presence of peritoneal implants.[68] Between 16 and 30% of patients with stage 1 and 75% with stage 2 have been upgraded to stage 3 after a restaging operation.[68] Follow-up examination is mandatory. After the patient's family is complete, hysterectomy with residual salpingo-oophorectomy has been advocated, but its value has been questioned.[89] If a similar tumor develops in the contralateral ovary (5–10% of the cases), the patient can be successfully treated in most cases by reoperation alone.[53,97]

For patients with advanced stage SBTs, postoperative treatment has varied from no additional therapy to various forms of chemotherapy and radiation therapy. The literature presents no clear evidence that adjuvant therapy alters the course of the disease and, unfortunately, many patients have died as a result of adverse complications of such treatments.[53] The current treatment approach is to recommend postoperative chemotherapy (carboplatin plus paclitaxel) to those patients with invasive peritoneal implants, or non-invasive implants with macroscopic residual disease.[33,53] For patients with recurrent SBTs, secondary cytoreductive surgery and optimal resection has been associated with high overall survival.[16]

Prognosis

Survival of patients with SBTs is much higher than that of serous carcinomas (see below). According to the most recent 'annual' report (2003) of the International Federation of Gynecology and Obstetrics (FIGO),[44] the 5-year survival rates for patients with disease that is stages 1–3B are roughly between 88 and >95% and about 60% for disease that is stage 3C or 4. Estimates of 20-year survival are about 80%. Other than the adverse effect of invasive implants, there is no agreement in the literature as to which prognostic factors are important. Although positive peritoneal cytology is predictive for survival in cases of ovarian carcinoma, this is not the case in SBTs.[143] According to most investigators, SBTs with micropapillary pattern or SBTs with microinvasion have a prognosis similar to that of tumors lacking these features. Likewise, focal lymph node involvement has not demonstrated any effect on survival. The vast majority of SBTs display a diploid DNA histogram. Aneuploid SBTs are thought to be associated with poorer prognosis.[143]

SEROUS CARCINOMAS

Clinical features

The average age of women with serous carcinomas is 56 years (age range, 45–65 years).[113] Although most patients have symptoms, these are often subtle and easily confused with those of benign conditions of the gastrointestinal tract. As a result,

about 70% of patients present when the tumor is in advanced stage, i.e., it has metastasized to the upper abdomen. The tumors spread mainly by local extension, intra-abdominal dissemination, and through lymphatics. Rarely, they also spread through the bloodstream. In early stage (stage 1), a mobile but irregular pelvic mass can often be palpated by pelvic examination, especially if the tumor is more than about 5–6 cm in size and has not protruded above the pelvic brim. As the disease spreads into the pelvic cavity, nodules may be found in the cul-de-sac, particularly on bimanual rectovaginal examination (stage 2). Ascites may occur in all stages, but becomes more evident when the tumor involves the upper abdomen (stage 3). Metastatic disease is commonly found in the omentum. Pelvic and para-aortic lymph nodes are involved in approximately 40–70% of stage 3 tumors. Finally, the disease may spread to the supraclavicular lymph nodes and into the pleura, causing malignant effusion (stage 4). Advanced intra-abdominal tumor is often associated with signs of intestinal obstruction, including nausea, vomiting, and abdominal pain. Ultrasound, magnetic resonance imaging, and computed tomography have no clearly established role in preoperative tumor staging. Laparotomy and surgical exploration of the abdominal cavity remain the standard approach for staging.

In approximately 10% of stage 3 serous carcinomas, the ovaries are small and show only minimal superficial involvement; these findings warrant a diagnosis of peritoneal serous carcinoma (see 'Differential diagnosis' and Chapter 23).[108,112] Malignant serous tumors may be found in all anatomic regions of the adult female genital tract.

Macroscopic features

Serous carcinomas range in size from microscopic to over 20 cm in diameter and are bilateral in two-thirds of all cases (one-third of stage 1 cases).[113] Well-differentiated tumors are typically solid and cystic with soft papillae within the cysts or on the surface (Figures 24.55 and 24.56). The papillae tend to be softer and more confluent than those of SBTs. Rare serous

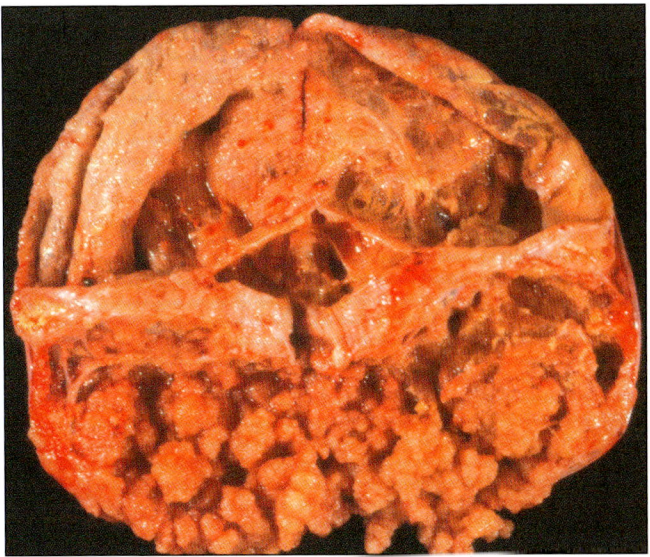

Fig. 24.55 Serous papillary cystadenocarcinoma, well differentiated. The tumor is solid and cystic and shows confluent papillae within the cysts. Reproduced with permission from Prat.[96]

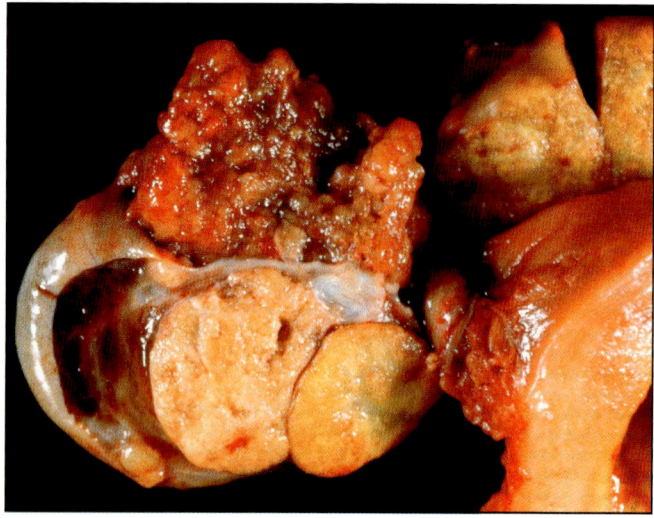

Fig. 24.56 Serous papillary cystadenocarcinoma, well differentiated. Solid and cystic tumor with an exophytic borderline component (top).

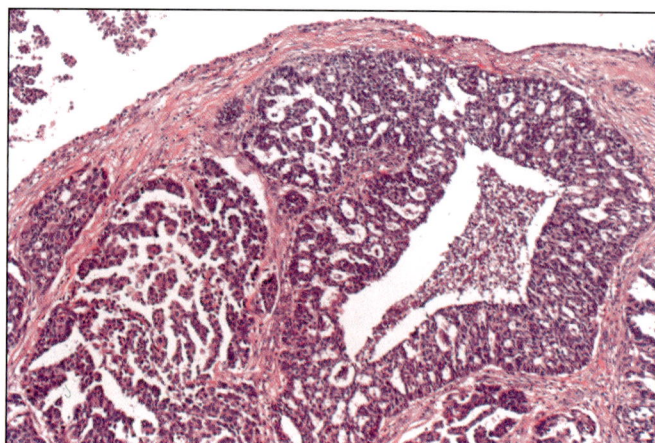

Fig. 24.58 Serous papillary adenocarcinoma, high grade. The tumor is characterized by small cellular papillae without fibrous cores and solid areas with slit-like spaces.

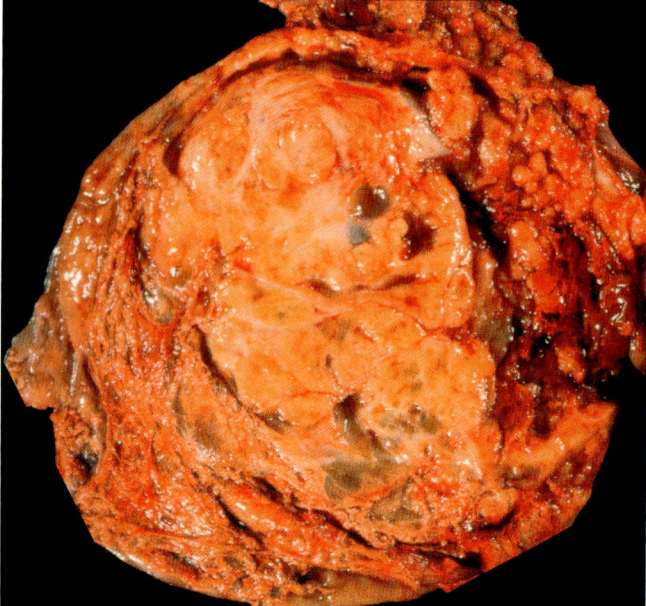

Fig. 24.57 Serous papillary cystadenocarcinoma, high grade. The tumor is solid and cystic with extensive hemorrhage and necrosis.

carcinomas appear as closely packed soft surface papillae, requiring microscopic examination for their distinction from SBTs. Poorly differentiated tumors are predominantly solid, multinodular masses with necrosis and hemorrhage (Figure 24.57). Omental metastases are usually firm tumor masses with grayish-white cut surfaces. Grossly normal omentum contains microscopic tumor in 20% of cases.

Microscopic features

Most serous carcinomas are high-grade tumors and frequently show obvious stromal invasion. Architecturally, they show irregularly branching and highly cellular papillae with little or no stromal support (Figures 24.58–24.60), and slit-like glandular lumens within more solid areas (Figure 24.61). The slit-like spaces tend to be uniform in size and oriented radially (Figure 24.62). The tumor cells are small and uniform, but scattered bizarre mononuclear giant cells are frequently seen (Figure 24.63). Mitoses are numerous and tumor necrosis is often extensive. The stroma may be scanty or desmoplastic (Figure 24.64). Psammoma bodies are often present in varying numbers (30–40%). Serous carcinomas tend to be uniform throughout. Rarely do high- and low-grade forms coexist.

Low-grade serous carcinomas are rare. They show irregular infiltration of small, tight nests and papillae of tumor cells within variable amounts of desmoplastic or hyaline stroma, which often contains psammoma bodies or larger calcific deposits (Figures 24.44 and 24.65). In contrast to high-grade carcinomas, the tumor cells contain small grade 1 nuclei and rare mitoses (Figure 24.66).[129]

Psammocarcinoma is a very rare form of low-grade serous carcinoma with a favorable prognosis.[37] This tumor, which behaves clinically more like an SBT than a serous carcinoma, differs in its microscopic features from the former by infiltrating the ovarian stroma (Figures 24.67 and 24.68). Four criteria recommended for the diagnosis of psammocarcinoma include: (1) invasion of the ovarian stroma (or, in extraovarian sites, invasion of any intraperitoneal tissue); (2) only mild to moderate nuclear atypia; (3) epithelial nests <15 cells in their largest dimension; and (4) the presence of psammoma bodies in at least 75% of papillae or nests.[37] Although all 18 reported tumors were stage 3 at presentation, there has been only one death, turning out a survival rate of 94%.

Another pattern of well-differentiated serous carcinoma shows the presence within fibrous stroma of broad papillae lined by tumor cells lying in non-lymphatic spaces (Figure 24.69); the spaces probably result from secretion of serous fluid by the neoplastic cells.[113] Serous carcinomas may contain various other cell types as a minor component (<10%), but do not influence the outcome. Rare serous carcinomas undergo focal squamous differentiation.

Immunohistochemistry

Serous carcinomas are reactive for CK7, but not CK20. They are also reactive for CAM 5.2, AE1/AE3, epithelial membrane antigen (EMA), B72.3, Ber-EP4, Leu-M1, and CA125 (85%),

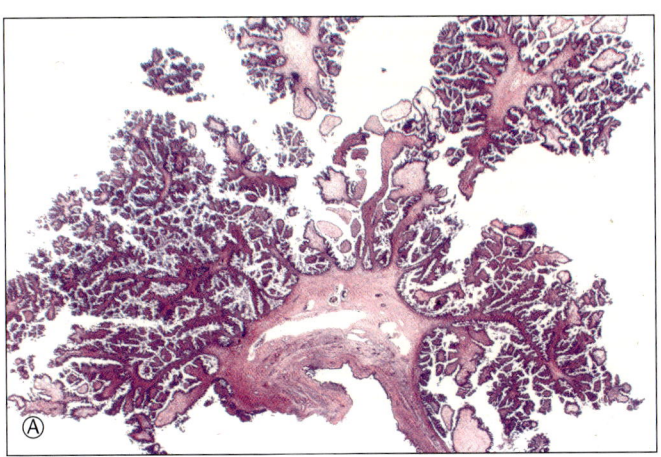
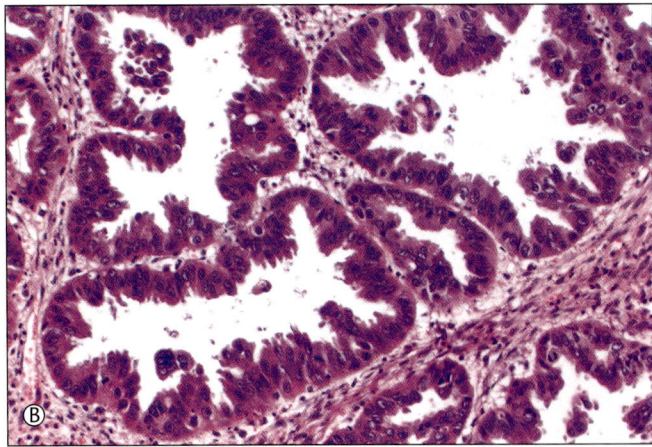

Fig. 24.59 Serous papillary adenocarcinoma, moderately differentiated. **(A)** Hierarchical and complex branching without obvious stromal invasion. **(B)** The tumor cells show moderate nuclear atypia, prominent nucleoli, and mitotic activity.

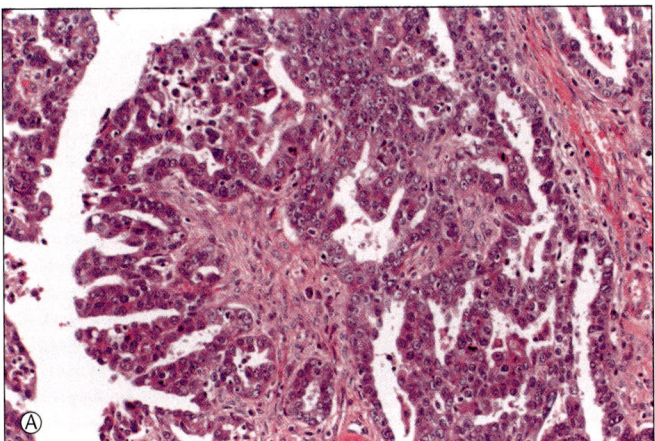
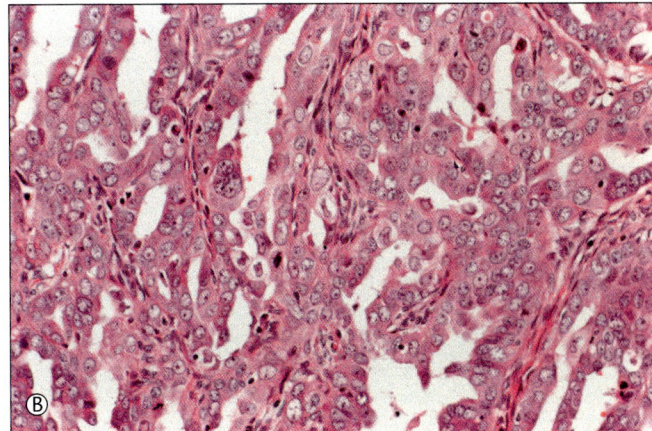

Fig. 24.60 Serous papillary adenocarcinoma, poorly differentiated. **(A)** Closely packed papillae lacking fibrous cores. **(B)** Papillae are lined by cells with atypical nuclei and high nuclear:cytoplasmic ratios.

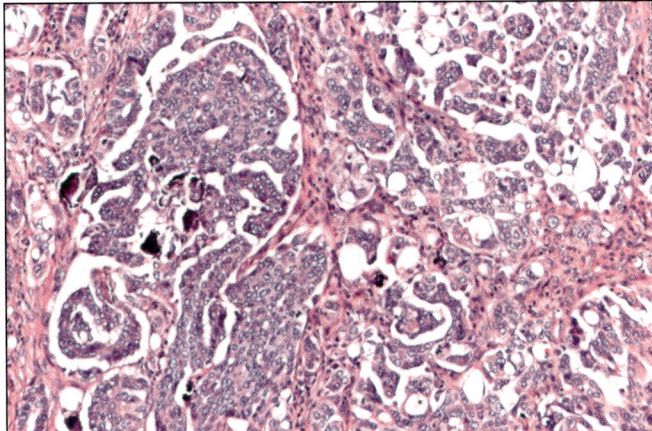
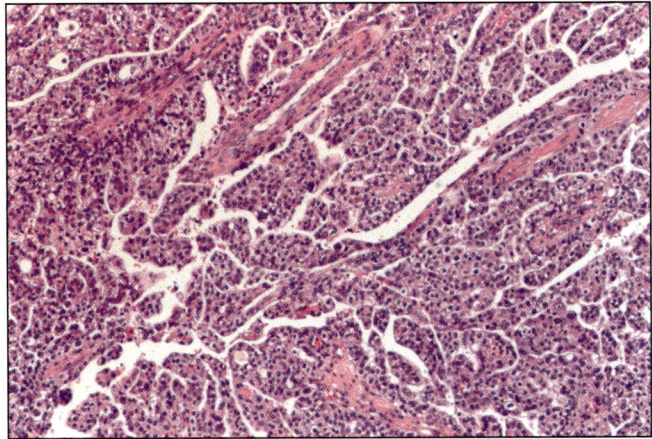

Fig. 24.61 Serous papillary adenocarcinoma, poorly differentiated. The tumor shows closely packed papillae and solid proliferation of tumor cells (left). Reproduced with permission from Prat.[96]

Fig. 24.62 Serous papillary adenocarcinoma, poorly differentiated. The regular slit-like spaces are radially oriented.

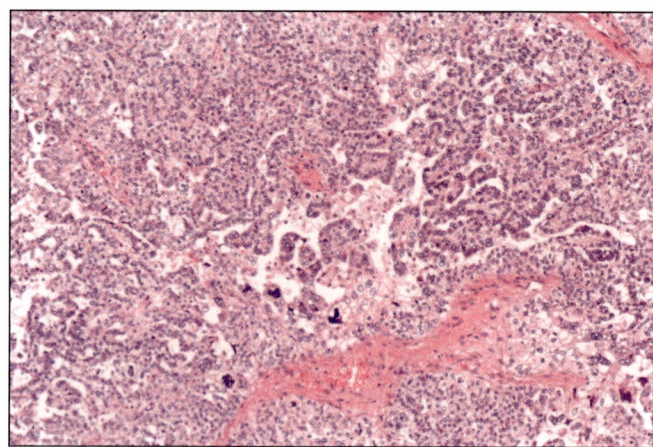

Fig. 24.63 Serous papillary adenocarcinoma, poorly differentiated. Although tumor cells are predominantly small and uniform, a few bizarre mononuclear giant cells are seen.

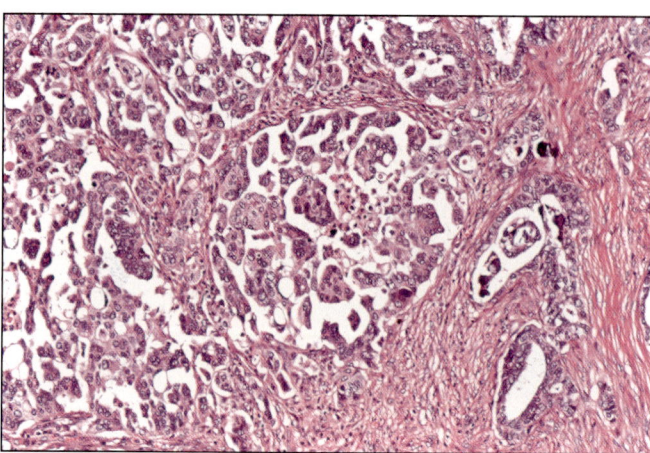

Fig. 24.64 Serous papillary adenocarcinoma, poorly differentiated. Lace-like architecture.

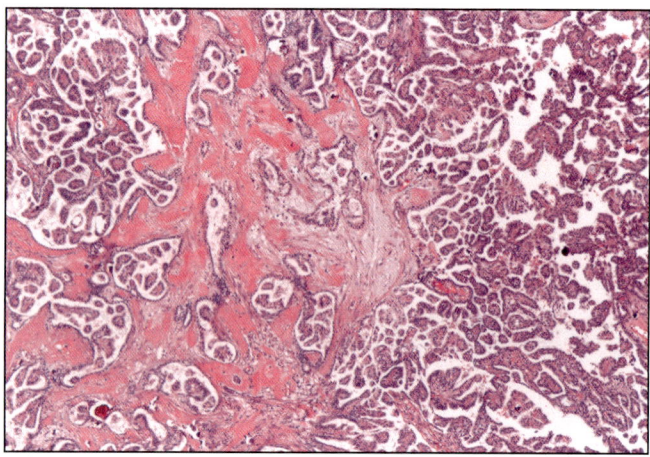

Fig. 24.65 Serous papillary adenocarcinoma, well differentiated. The tumor shows invasive (left) and non-invasive (right) components.

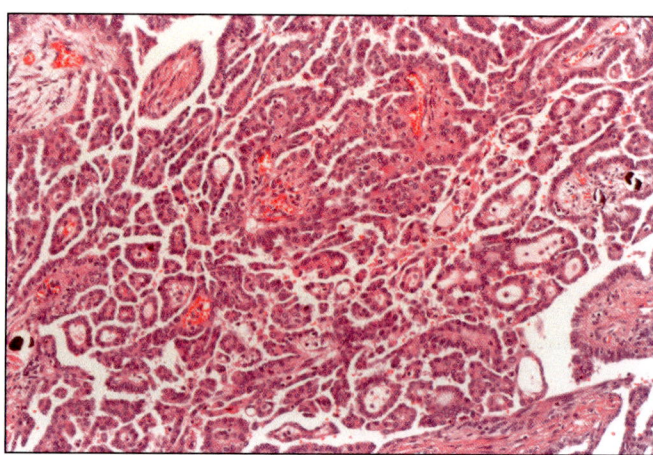

Fig. 24.66 Serous papillary adenocarcinoma, well differentiated. The tumor shows slender papillae with fibrovascular cores lined by small cells with grade 1 nuclei. Occasional psammoma bodies are seen.

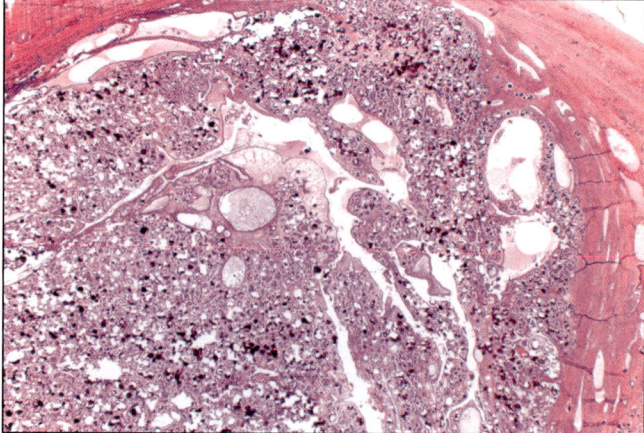

Fig. 24.67 Serous psammocarcinoma. The invasive and well-differentiated epithelial component is partly covered by psammoma bodies. Reproduced with permission from Prat.[96]

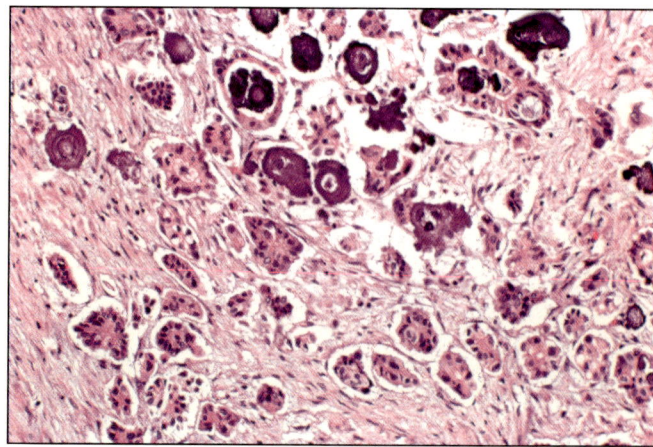

Fig. 24.68 Serous psammocarcinoma. Well-differentiated epithelial cells lying in a fibrous stroma with psammoma bodies. Reproduced with permission from Prat.[96]

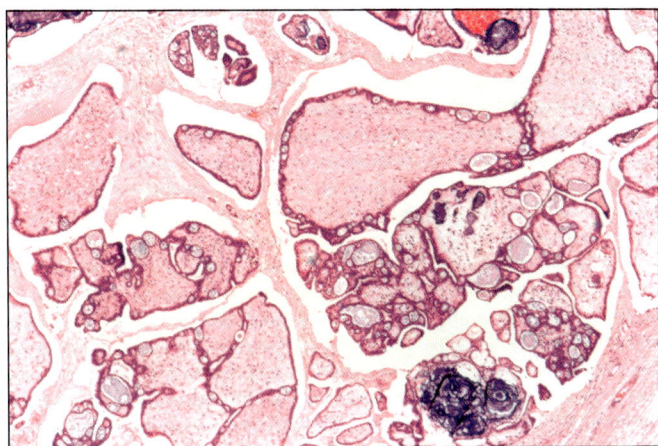

Fig. 24.69 Serous papillary adenocarcinoma, low grade. Broad papillae lined by tumor cells appear in non-lymphatic spaces within fibrous stroma. Reproduced with permission from Prat.[96]

but not for calretinin, CK5, and other mesothelial markers. Alpha-inhibin may be rarely reactive.

Histogenesis and somatic genetics

Most high-grade serous carcinomas are thought to arise *de novo* from the surface epithelium or its inclusion cysts and spread rapidly early in their course.[10] Early on, microscopic foci of carcinoma can be seen on the surface of the ovaries, within clefts or in cortical inclusions cysts.[10] In contrast, low-grade serous carcinomas typically arise within borderline tumors and only occasionally *de novo* from the surface epithelium.[93] Early serous carcinomas of the conventional type are already high-grade tumors that morphologically resemble their advanced stage counterparts. The histologic similarities correlate with recent molecular genetic findings demonstrating *p53* mutations in small stage 1 serous carcinomas.[66] Approximately 60% of advanced stage ovarian serous carcinomas have mutant *p53*.[126] In contrast, SBTs with and without micropapillary pattern, as well as the uncommon low-grade serous carcinomas, frequently display *K-ras* mutations but rarely mutant *p53*.[18,125] *K-ras* mutations are very rarely found in conventional high-grade serous carcinomas.[18,125] Accordingly, a dualistic model for ovarian serous carcinogenesis has recently been proposed.[125] One pathway involves a stepwise progression from SBT to non-invasive (SBT-MP) and then invasive low-grade ('micropapillary') serous carcinoma. The other pathway has rapid transformation of the ovarian surface epithelium into a high-grade serous carcinoma. Gene expression profiling has shown that, in contrast to SBTs and low-grade invasive serous carcinomas, high-grade serous cancers have enhanced expression of genes linked to cell cycle control (S and G_2–M checkpoint regulation), chromosomal instability (*STK6*, *E2F3*), and epigenetic silencing.[14] These alterations are absent in SBTs and low-grade invasive carcinomas. The latter tumors, however, do not contain the enhanced *p53* signaling activity encountered in SBTs.[14]

Differential diagnosis

Serous carcinomas of the ovary should be distinguished from serous carcinomas that are primary in the peritoneum. Clonality studies in cases of the latter tumors show polyclonality[83] in contrast to the monoclonality of peritoneal carcinomatosis associated with ovarian serous carcinomas.[135] According to the Gynecologic Oncology Group, if the carcinoma is confined to the ovarian surface and is the only intraperitoneal tumor, it is considered to be of ovarian origin; if the ovarian tumor is invasive, it is considered primary if the depth of invasion of the ovarian parenchyma is at least 5 mm, even though peritoneal tumor masses may be much larger. From a clinical viewpoint, the distinction is not critical because the prognosis and treatment are similar.

Although serous carcinoma is the epithelial cancer most often associated with papillae, other carcinomas, particularly endometrioid, clear cell, and transitional cell carcinomas (TCCs), may be papillary as well, and enter the differential diagnosis. The papillae in endometrioid carcinomas are typically larger and villous, as in uterine villoglandular carcinomas. Squamous differentiation is common in endometrioid carcinomas but rare in serous carcinomas. Endometrioid carcinomas are more likely associated with coexistent adenocarcinoma of the uterine endometrium (in 15–20% of cases)[49] and with non-neoplastic endometriosis in the ovaries or elsewhere in the pelvis (about 30%) than their serous counterparts. The papillae in clear cell carcinomas are lined by hobnail or clear cells and typically have hyalinized cores; other distinctive features of clear cell carcinoma are almost always present. Hobnail cells may be seen in otherwise typical serous carcinomas but are almost always present in small foci. A coarsely papillary configuration with multilayered epithelium is seen uncommonly and should not be misinterpreted as evidence of transitional differentiation. A further useful marker is the presence of occasional bizarre mononuclear giant cells (Figure 24.63) among sheets of small uniform cells. These may be the only feature suggestive of serous neoplasia in otherwise undifferentiated carcinomas.

Some serous carcinomas contain cells with abundant eosinophilic cytoplasm and may mimic malignant mesotheliomas (see Chapter 25) but are usually distinguished by their intra-ovarian location, distinctive glandular pattern, and nuclear features. The typical tubular and papillary patterns of mesotheliomas differ from the more disorderly patterns of serous carcinomas. Malignant mesothelioma cells are typically less pleomorphic than those of serous carcinoma and their papillae are less cellular. Psammoma bodies are much less common in mesotheliomas than in serous carcinomas. Immunohistochemical staining may be helpful (see Chapter 25).[88,139]

Primary serous carcinoma of the ovary must be distinguished from metastatic serous carcinoma of the fallopian tube and endometrium. In cases exhibiting myometrial vascular invasion, bilateral and surface ovarian involvement, and tumor present in the ovarian hilus within vascular spaces, the diagnosis of secondary involvement by the endometrial carcinoma is obvious. In other cases, either the ovarian tumor is an independent primary neoplasm or is the only primary tumor that has spread to the endometrium (see Chapter 25).

Occasionally, metastatic poorly differentiated carcinoma from the breast may closely simulate serous carcinoma both microscopically and in its pattern of spread within the abdomen. In such cases, a history of breast cancer and comparison of both tumors in terms of their grades, patterns, and cell types facilitates the diagnosis. In mammary carcinomas, nucleoli tend to be less prominent, and chromatin less coarse, than in serous carcinomas. The 'single-file' infiltrative pattern typical of lobular breast carcinoma is rarely seen in serous carcinomas. Demonstration of intracellular mucin is useful. Immunohistochemistry may be helpful in difficult cases. Reactivity for gross cystic disease fluid protein-15 favors metastatic breast carcinoma whereas CA125 reactivity favors primary ovarian carcinoma; however, neither stain is entirely specific.

Treatment and prognosis

The initial treatment includes abdominal exploration, meticulous staging, and resection of all grossly identifiable disease (bulk resection).[19] Stage 1 serous carcinoma is treated by bilateral salpingo-oophorectomy with total hysterectomy. Alternatively, unilateral salpingo-oophorectomy can be performed on a young woman when the tumor is of low-grade malignancy. Close follow-up is essential in those cases; residual adnexa and uterus may be removed after childbearing is completed. Postoperatively, patients with grade 3 serous carcinomas receive combination chemotherapy. The chemotherapeutic agents most commonly used for epithelial ovarian cancers are platinum compounds (cisplatin and carboplatin), alkylating agents, and taxol.

Various grading systems have been proposed for serous carcinomas. A three-tiered grading system modeled after the widely accepted criteria for grading of breast carcinomas has been recently proposed.[120] FIGO 5-year survival figures for patients with serous carcinoma are: stage 1, 76%; stage 2, 56%; and stage 3, 25%.[92] Patients with high-grade serous carcinomas that contain large nuclei have a shorter overall survival than women with high-grade serous carcinomas that contain smaller nuclei.[47]

MUCINOUS TUMORS

Definition and general features

Mucinous tumors show cysts and glands lined by epithelial cells containing intracytoplasmic mucin. The tumor cells may resemble those of the endocervix, gastric pylorus, or intestine. They are typically diastase resistant, periodic acid-Schiff (PAS) positive and mucicarmine positive. Mucinous tumors account for 10–15% of all primary ovarian tumors.[57] Approximately 80% are benign and the remainder are borderline tumors, non-invasive carcinomas, and invasive carcinomas.[57] Although they generally occur in older women (mean age, 51–54 years), mucinous borderline tumors and carcinomas are more common in the first two decades than their serous counterparts.[113] Mucinous tumors, especially the borderline tumors, tend to be the largest of all ovarian tumors. Many of them are 15–30 cm in diameter and weigh up to 4000 g or more.[113]

Mucinous ovarian tumors are difficult to interpret. Over the past 50 years, their classification has changed considerably as a result of : (1) the establishment of a mucinous borderline subcategory separately from mucinous adenocarcinomas; (2) the recognition of mucinous borderline tumors *with intraepithelial carcinoma*; (3) the recent recognition that most ovarian mucinous cystic tumors associated with pseudomyxoma peritonei are metastases (secondary tumors) as almost all are of appendiceal origin; and (4) the increasing recognition of metastatic adenocarcinomas of intestinal and pancreatic origin that closely resemble primary ovarian mucinous tumors.

Although mucinous ovarian tumors are currently classified as surface epithelial tumors, their origin is unclear in most cases. Some mucinous tumors are of germ cell origin (monodermal teratomas), but neometaplasia of the ovarian surface epithelium is an alternative explanation for their development.[113] In fact, transitions between mucinous tumors and serous and endometrioid tumors are occasionally seen. Also, serous and endometrioid tumors may secrete mucin from the apical pole of the epithelial cells, resulting in abundant intracystic mucus, but not generally intracytoplasmic. Mucinous tumors may be associated with dermoid cysts (3–5%), Brenner tumors, and mucinous tumors of other organs such as uterine cervix and appendix.[113] In patients with the Peutz–Jeghers syndrome, well-differentiated mucinous ovarian tumors may be accompanied by minimal deviation adenocarcinomas ('adenoma malignum') of the cervix. Occasionally, mucinous cystic ovarian tumors may develop from heterologous gastrointestinal elements in a Sertoli–Leydig cell tumor.

Mucinous ovarian tumors are among the most common non-endocrine neoplasms presenting hormonal manifestations. Most times, the endocrine symptoms are due to the secretion of steroid hormones, produced by the ovarian stroma adjacent to the tumor.[75,113] The serum level of inhibin (a hormone produced by ovarian granulosa and lutein cells that inhibits the secretion of follicle-stimulating hormone by the anterior pituitary gland) is considered to be a tumor marker for mucinous borderline tumors and carcinomas, possibly due to the reactive luteinized cells that develop in the adjacent stroma.[43] Less frequently, patients present the Zollinger–Ellison syndrome, secondary to gastrin secretion by neuroendocrine cells in the gastrointestinal mucinous epithelium, and rarely, the carcinoid syndrome (see Chapter 27). CA125, carcinoembryonic antigen (CEA), and CA19–9 are often elevated in mucinous carcinomas.

Ovarian mucinous tumors are subdivided into benign, borderline, and malignant categories depending on their degree of cell proliferation, nuclear atypia, and the presence or absence of stromal invasion. In contrast to serous tumors, which are characteristically homogeneous in their degree of differentiation, mucinous tumors are often heterogeneous. Benign-appearing, borderline, and invasive patterns may coexist within an individual neoplasm; also, not infrequently, the degree of malignancy of the carcinomatous component varies from non-invasive to invasive, and from well-differentiated to poorly differentiated or even undifferentiated (anaplastic) carcinoma. Such a morphologic continuum suggests that tumor progression occurs from cystadenoma and borderline tumor to non-invasive, microinvasive, and invasive carcinoma. This hypothesis is supported by studies of *K-ras* mutations which are common in mucinous ovarian tumors and represent an early event in mucinous ovarian tumorigenesis. Mucinous borderline tumors have a higher frequency of *K-ras* mutations than that of mucinous cystadenomas but a lower rate than that of mucinous carcinomas.[24,48,73,81] Using microdissection, the same *K-ras* mutation has been detected in benign-appearing, borderline, and malignant areas of the same tumor.[24] From a practical viewpoint, the prognostic evaluation of mucinous ovarian tumors other than benign cystadenomas is difficult because of their typical large size, and the great variation in the degree of differentiation of individual tumors, often requiring extensive microscopic sampling. For this reason, extensive sampling is important, especially of areas that appear nodular or solid. The SNOMED classification of mucinous tumors is as follows:

- Benign mucinous tumors
  - mucinous adenofibroma
  - mucinous cystadenoma
- Mucinous borderline tumor
- Mucinous adenocarcinoma.

BENIGN MUCINOUS TUMORS

Clinical profile

Benign mucinous cystadenomas comprise approximately 80% of ovarian mucinous tumors. They occur most frequently during the third to sixth decades, although they may also be encountered in younger women. This age distribution accounts for their frequent occurrence during pregnancy.

Macroscopic features

Mucinous cystadenomas are often large, unilateral, multilocular, but sometimes unilocular cystic tumors containing mucoid material (Figures 24.70 and 24.71). The outer cyst wall is often thick with a smooth or bosselated surface. The rare mucinous cystadenofibromas and adenofibromas are partly to almost completely solid with small cysts (Figure 24.72). Benign mucinous tumors are bilateral in 2–5% of cases, and are associated with a dermoid cyst or a Brenner tumor in about 5% of cases.[113]

Microscopic features

Mucinous cystadenomas are composed of glands and cysts lined by a single layer of columnar cells with abundant intracellular mucin. Cellular stratification is minimal, and nuclei are basally located with only mild atypia (Figures 24.73 and 24.74).[6] Papillae are unusual, except in cases of mucinous cystadenomas of endocervical-like type which are conspicuously papillary. Goblet cells, neuroendocrine cells and, rarely, Paneth cells may be encountered in mucinous cystadenomas of gastrointes-

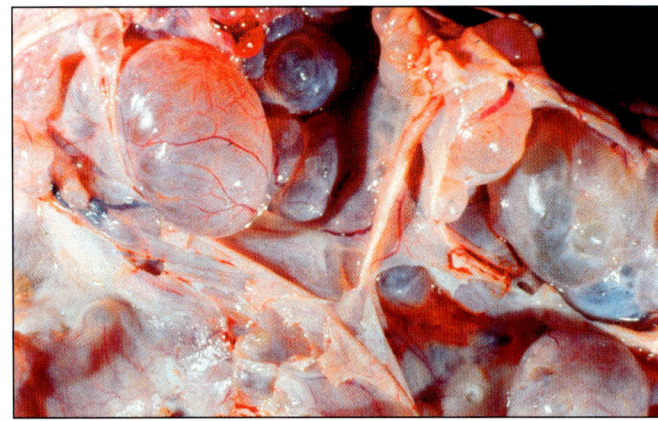

Fig. 24.71 Mucinous cystadenoma. The section surface shows a multiloculated tumor with large cysts.

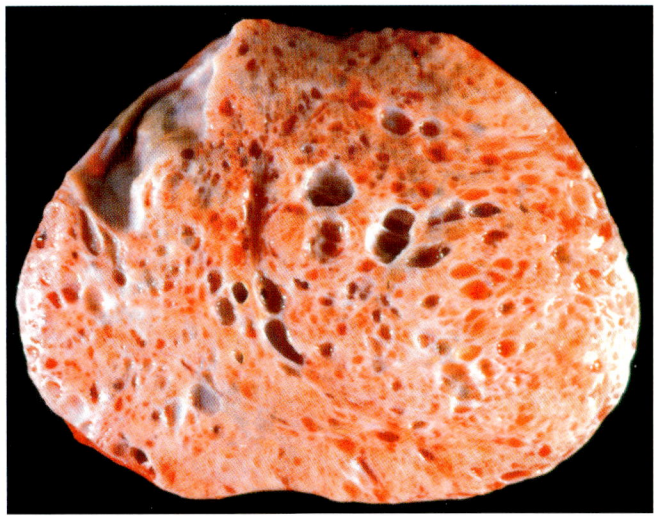

Fig. 24.72 Mucinous cystadenofibroma. The sectioned surface appears partly solid with numerous small cysts.

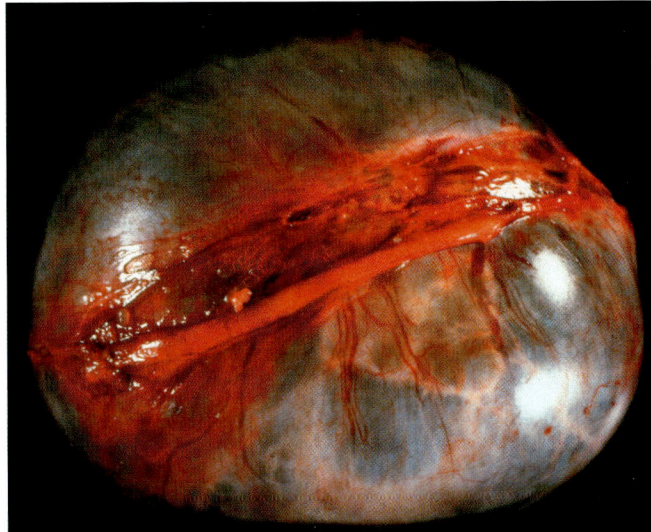

Fig. 24.70 Mucinous cystadenoma.

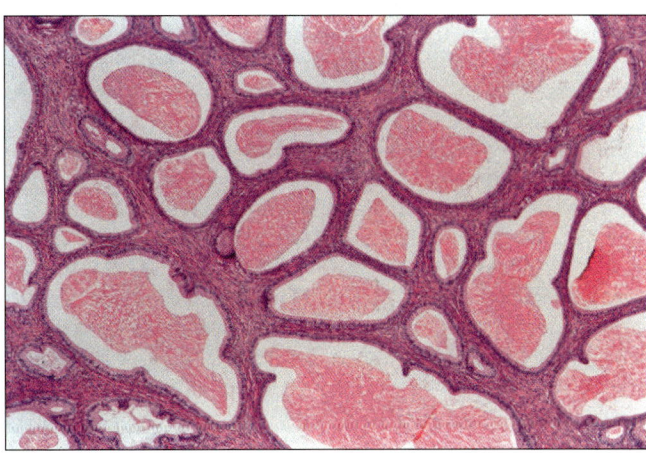

Fig. 24.73 Mucinous cystadenoma. Cystic glands lined by mucin-filled columnar cells with basal nuclei.

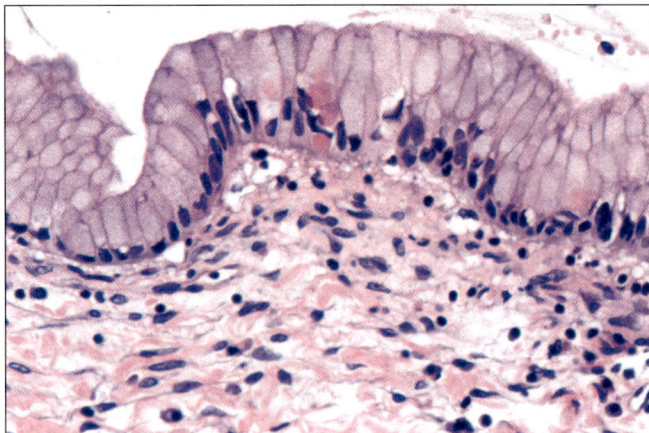

Fig. 24.74 Mucinous cystadenoma. The cytoplasm is mucin-rich and the nuclei are small and basal. Reproduced with permission from Prat.[96]

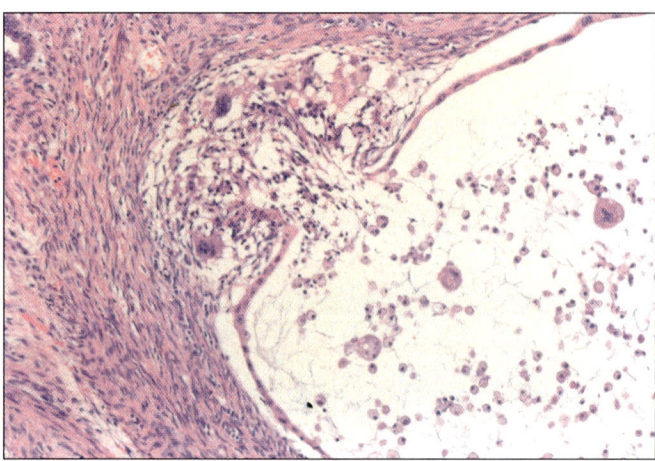

Fig. 24.76 Mucinous cystadenofibroma. Ruptured gland with mucin granuloma.

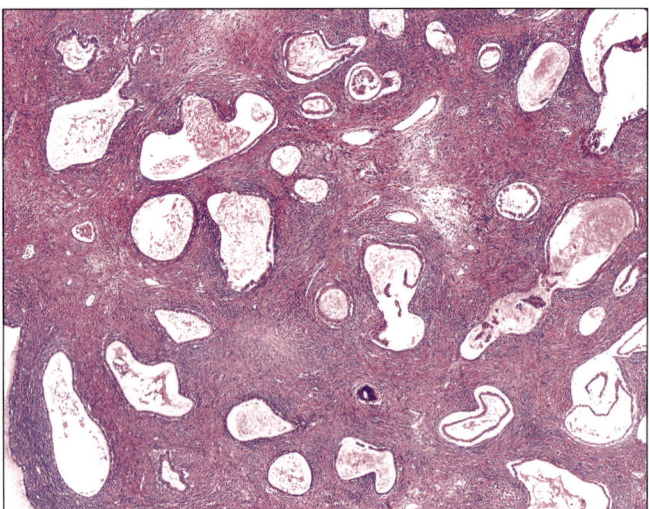

Fig. 24.75 Mucinous cystadenofibroma. Benign mucinous cystic glands lie in dense fibrous stroma.

tinal nature. Gastrointestinal differentiation, however, is found more often in borderline tumors and carcinomas. The stroma is fibrocollagenous and the cellularity, although variable, rarely approaches that of the serous tumors. Occasionally, marked prominence of the stroma exists between locules, giving rise to patterns of adenofibroma (Figure 24.75). Stromal cellularity may be increased in the vicinity of the epithelium and in this zone lutein-like cells are seen in 25% of cases. Rare benign tumors may show definite Leydig cells (with crystals) in the adjacent stroma. Smooth muscle may develop sometimes in the stroma running parallel to the cyst linings.

Rupture of mucinous glands and cysts is common, resulting in extravasation of mucin into the stroma, and often a marked inflammatory response. Such a finding must be distinguished from large pools of dissecting mucin (pseudomyxoma ovarii), which is a characteristic feature of mucinous ovarian tumors associated with pseudomyxoma peritonei (see below). In about 5% of mucinous cystadenomas, the mucin in the stroma typically elicits a histiocytic and foreign body giant cell response (mucin granuloma) (Figure 24.76). Extruded neoplastic epithelium from an adjacent ruptured gland, particularly if accompanied by a mucin granuloma, should be distinguished from stromal microinvasion (see below).

MUCINOUS BORDERLINE TUMORS

Mucinous borderline tumors (MBTs) exhibit an epithelial proliferation of mucinous-type cells greater than that seen in their benign counterparts, but without destructive stromal invasion. In the Western world, they are less common than SBTs. Of the 20% of primary mucinous tumors that are not cystadenomas, MBTs outnumber the invasive carcinomas.[41] MBTs have been subclassified into two different clinicopathologic forms: the most common form is composed of intestinal-type epithelium and has been designated MBT of *intestinal type*. A second and less common variant of MBT contains endocervical-type epithelium and has been named MBT *endocervical-like* (Figure 24.77).[110]

MUCINOUS BORDERLINE TUMORS ENDOCERVICAL-LIKE

Endocervical MBTs,[110] also designated as müllerian mucinous borderline tumors, account for 10–15% of MBTs. About 140 cases have been reported.[29,101,110,119] These tumors differ in many respects from intestinal MBTs as shown in Table 24.4. The average age of patients with endocervical MBTs is 40 years, with a range of 15–84 years.[29,101,110,119] An association with endometriosis is frequent. About 20% of the tumors have spread to the peritoneum or lymph nodes at the time of diagnosis.[110] No association with pseudomyxoma peritonei has been described.

Macroscopic features

The tumors average 8–10 cm in diameter, with a range from 2 to 36 cm. About 80% are unilocular or contain three or fewer locules. Most of them show grossly visible intracystic papillae (Figure 24.78). From 12 to 40% are bilateral at presentation[29,101,110,119] and the contralateral ovary is subsequently involved by an endocervical-type MBT in an additional 7% of cases.[110]

Microscopic features

The tumors contain complex papillae architecturally similar to those of SBTs (Figure 24.79). The epithelial lining is composed

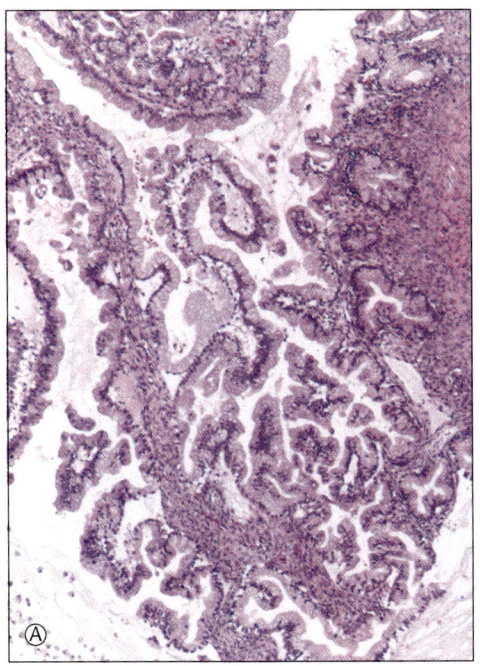
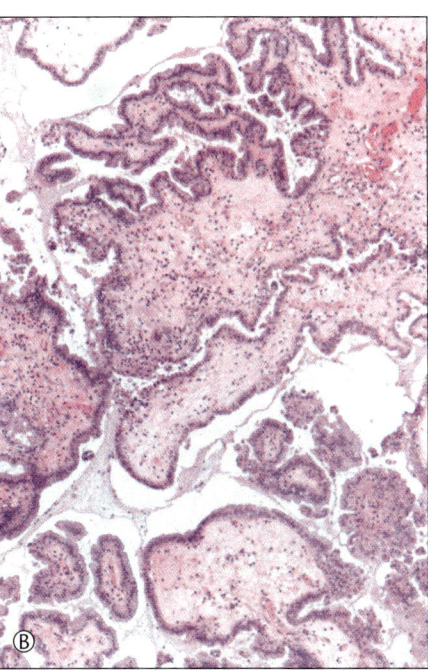

Fig. 24.77 Mucinous borderline tumors. **(A)** The intestinal-type tumor resembles a colonic polyp and contains goblet cells. **(B)** The endocervical-like tumor shows mucinous epithelial cells resembling endocervical epithelium. None of the tumors shows stromal invasion.

Table 24.4 Mucinous borderline tumors (MBT)

	Endocervical-like MBT (%)	Intestinal type MBT (%)
Frequency	15	85
Average age (years)	34	41
Bilaterality	40	6
Diameter (cm)	8	19
Multilocular	20	72
Goblet cells	0	100
Grimelius +ve cell	3	86
Acute inflammation	100	0
Endometriosis	30	6
Stage 2–3	24	10
Implants and/or lymph node metastases	20	0
Pseudomyxoma peritonei	0	17

Data from Rutgers and Scully.[110]

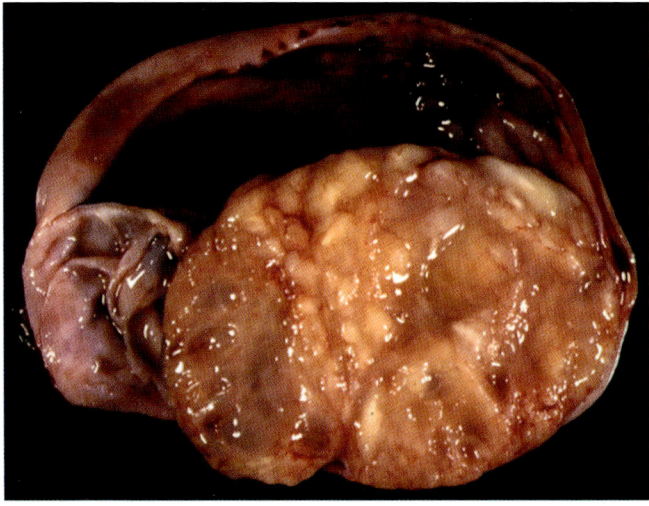

Fig. 24.78 Mucinous borderline tumor, endocervical-like. The sectioned surface shows solid and cystic mucinous papillae arising in an endometriotic cyst.

of columnar, mucin-containing cells that resemble endocervical cells as well as indifferent polygonal cells with abundant eosinophilic cytoplasm that are usually located at the tips of papillae (Figure 24.80).[110] The nuclei exhibit mild to focally severe atypia. Mitotic figures are infrequent. No destructive invasion of the stroma is observed. Nuclear stratification in the absence of recognizable stromal invasion cannot be used as a diagnostic criterion of carcinoma in endocervical-type MBTs as the polygonal eosinophilic cells may be stratified up to 20 μm or more in height (Figure 24.81).[110] Rare tumors exhibit foci of micropapillary growth similar to the micropapillary pattern seen in

SBTs.[119] Other müllerian-like epithelial cell types may be present, including ciliated serous cells, endometrioid cells, and squamous epithelium. From 30 to 50% of the tumors show a transition from mucinous neoplasia to endometriosis.[101,110,111] No areas of intestinal differentiation are usually seen. Typically, polymorphonuclear leukocytes infiltrate the stroma of the papillae, the neoplastic epithelium, and the intraluminal mucin in almost all cases (Figure 24.82).

Endocervical-type MBTs with intraepithelial carcinoma have been recently described.[29,101,119] Morphologic features of the intraepithelial carcinoma include foci showing a cribriform pattern of growth and stroma-free cellular papillae, or nuclear features of malignancy (Figure 24.83). In most cases, the intraepithelial carcinoma in endocervical-type MBT consists of

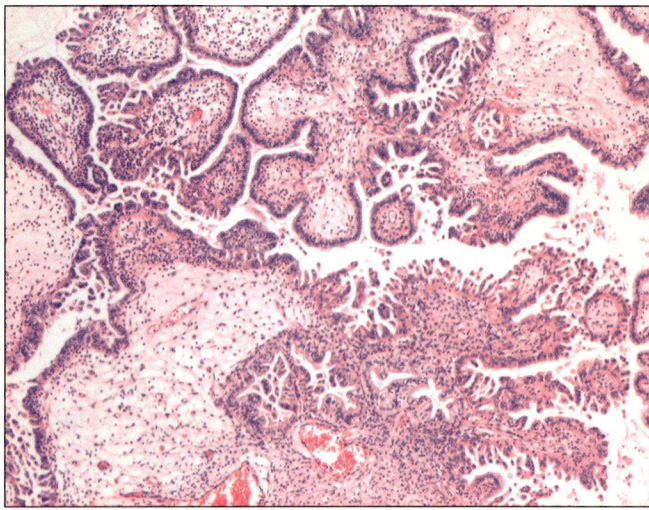

Fig. 24.79 Mucinous borderline tumor, endocervical-like. Typical low-power papillary architecture. The papillae show edematous stromal cores and are lined by endocervical-type mucinous cells.

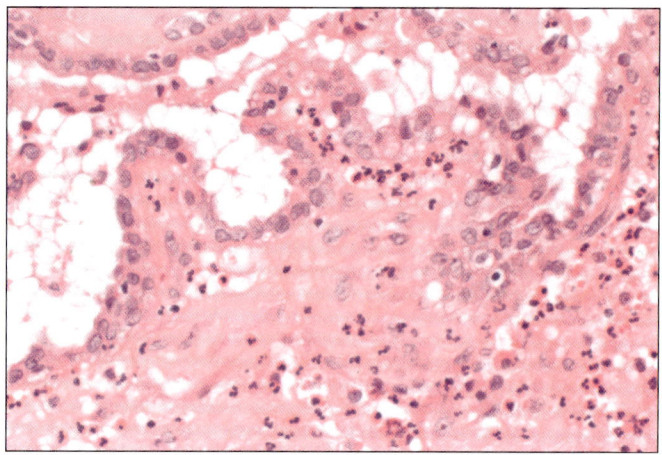

Fig. 24.82 Mucinous borderline tumor, endocervical-like. Note the characteristic intraepithelial neutrophil infiltration. Reproduced with permission from Prat.[96]

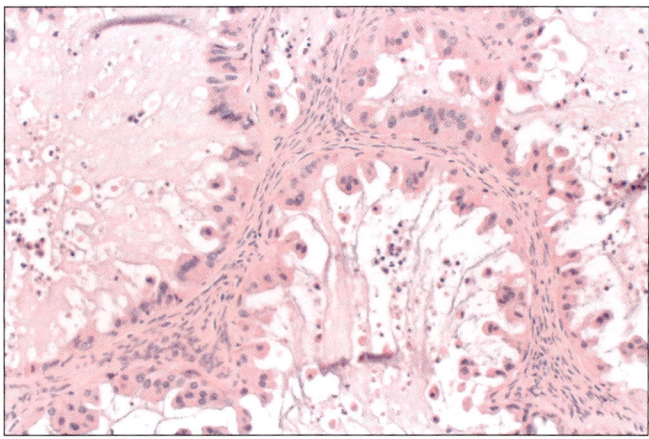

Fig. 24.80 Mucinous borderline tumor, endocervical-like. Indifferent cells with eosinophilic cytoplasm and tufting. Reproduced with permission from Prat.[96]

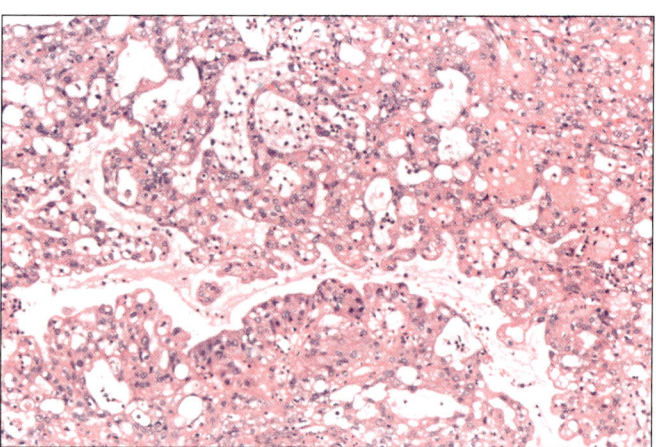

Fig. 24.83 Mucinous borderline tumor, endocervical-like. Microglandular hyperplasia with cell stratification and moderate nuclear atypia ('intraepithelial carcinoma'). Numerous polymorphonuclear leukocytes are seen. Reproduced with permission from Prat.[96]

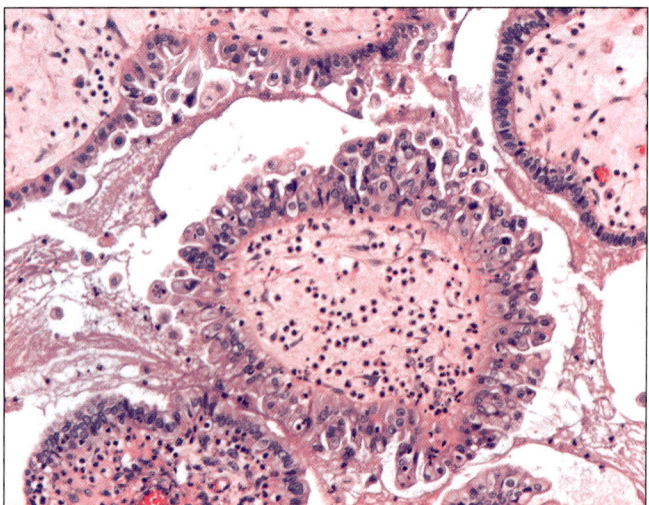

Fig. 24.81 Mucinous borderline tumor, endocervical-like. Stratification with cellular budding is evident. Neutrophils are seen in the stroma and epithelium. Reproduced with permission from Rodriguez et al.[101]

multiple foci usually measuring less than 1 or 2 mm in linear dimension. Classification of these tumors as intraepithelial carcinoma seems justified by the mean 7-year disease-free follow-up interval for 10 patients with this diagnosis.[29,101,119] Since few cases have been reported and the follow-up intervals relatively short, the favorable behavior of these tumors needs confirmation by additional investigations.

Microinvasion has been described in 24 endocervical-type MBTs (19%) from five different series.[29,54,84,101,119] The microinvasive foci ranged from <2 to 5 mm in greatest diameter, and were similar to those found more commonly in SBTs (Figures 24.84 and 24.85). Twelve patients with prolonged follow-up were without evidence of disease at an average of 8 years.[29,54,84,101]

Endocervical-type MBTs may be associated with pelvic or abdominal implants (3–20%) which are characteristically discrete and contain mucinous glands in a fibrous stroma (desmoplastic implants) (Figure 24.86).[101,110] In some cases the peritoneal implants may arise from independent foci of endometriosis. Some implants may appear invasive.

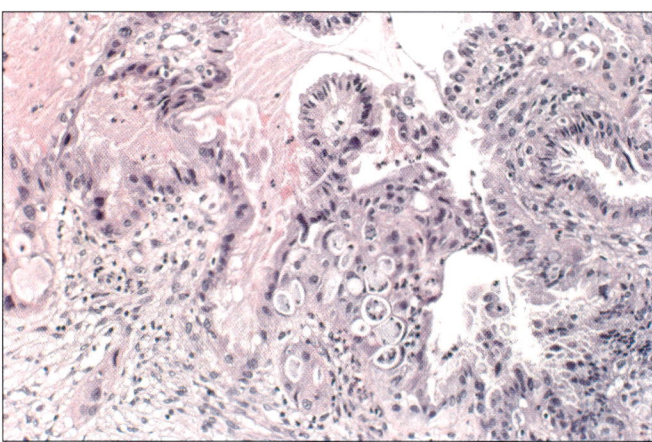

Fig. 24.84 Mucinous endocervical-like borderline tumor with intraepithelial carcinoma and microinvasion. The lining epithelium shows cell stratification, cribriform pattern, and marked nuclear atypia. A nest of invasive cells is seen at the lower left corner of the figure. Reproduced with permission from Prat.[96]

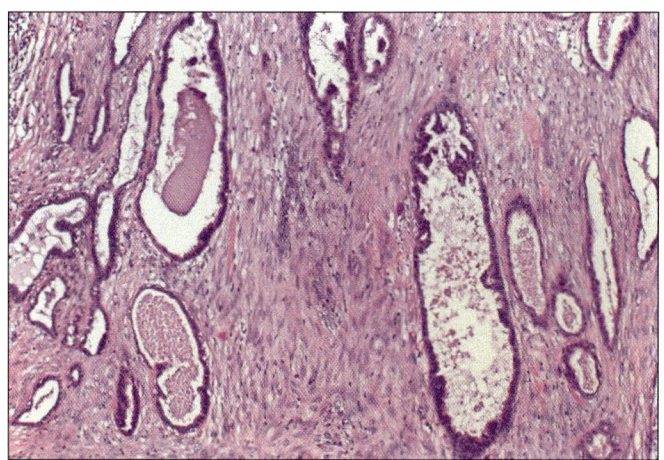

Fig. 24.85 Mucinous endocervical-like borderline tumor with microinvasion. Tubular glands with desmoplastic stromal response.

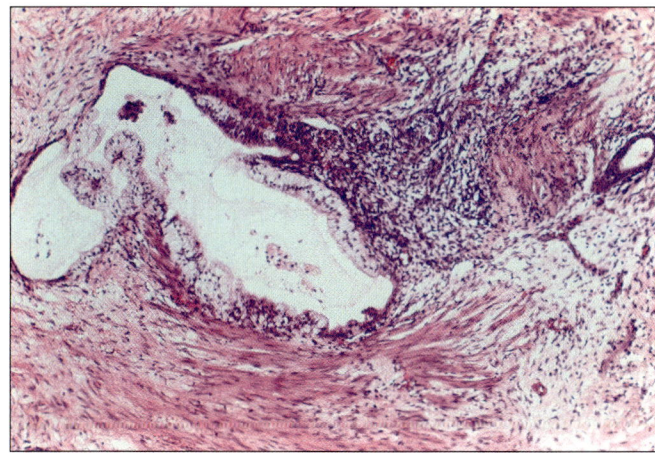

Fig. 24.86 Isolated peritoneal implant of mucinous endocervical-like borderline tumor.

Treatment and prognosis

Stage 1 endocervical-type MBTs are generally treated like SBTs (see above). If the contralateral normal-appearing ovary is conserved, the patient should be followed closely for possible development of a similar tumor in it. The prognosis of endocervical-type MBT is excellent and approximates that of SBTs. Recent studies report that foci of intraepithelial carcinoma (IEC) or microinvasion have not affected the prognosis.[29,101,119] No deaths from these tumors have been well documented, although most reported follow-up has been under 5 years.[40,86,101,110,119,127] There is no evidence that chemotherapy is necessary or helpful, even for patients with higher-stage disease.[110,113]

MUCINOUS BORDERLINE TUMORS OF INTESTINAL TYPE

Intestinal-type MBTs account for 85% of MBTs and occur most frequently in the fourth to seventh decades (average age, 52 years).[113] About 80–90% are stage 1 and only 5% are bilateral.[113] Of note, metastatic mucinous tumors in the ovary often mimic primary ovarian mucinous neoplasms, particularly adenocarcinomas of the pancreas and large intestine (see Chapter 29).[141] Microscopically, the metastatic tumor may appear deceptively 'benign', 'borderline' or malignant. It has recently been established that most, if not all, ovarian mucinous tumors associated with pseudomyxoma peritonei are metastatic tumors, frequently from low-grade appendiceal mucinous neoplasms (see below).[140] Bilaterality is exceptional in stage 1 ovarian mucinous tumors; therefore, tumor involvement of both ovaries should raise the suspicion of metastatic carcinoma.

Macroscopic features

On gross examination, the tumors average 19 cm in diameter, are usually cystic and multilocular, and contain mucinous fluid (Figure 24.87).[113] Papillae and polypoid excrescences may line

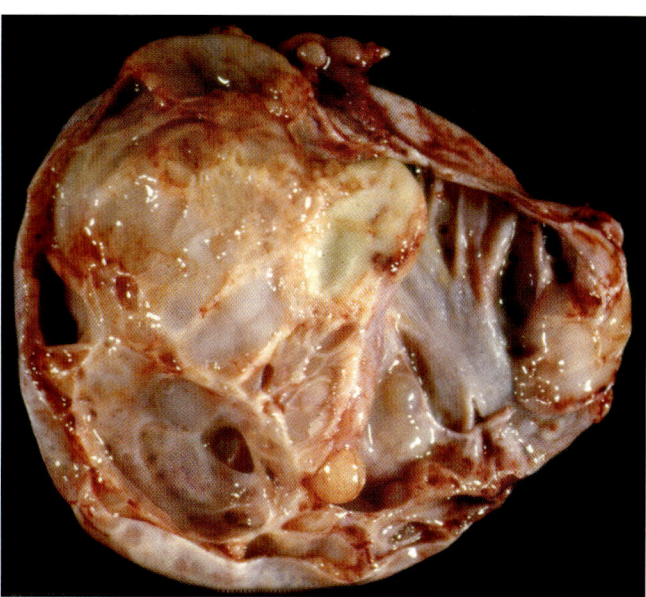

Fig. 24.87 Mucinous cystic borderline tumor of intestinal type. The sectioned surface shows a multiloculated cystic tumor with largely smooth cyst walls. Reproduced with permission from Prat.[96]

the cysts. Intestinal-type MBTs cannot be distinguished grossly from mucinous cystadenoma and cystadenocarcinoma. These tumors should be sampled extensively, particularly the solid portions, since variable degrees of epithelial proliferation and nuclear atypia (from benign to borderline, and to carcinoma) are frequent within an individual neoplasm.[41]

Microscopic features

Microscopically, intestinal-type MBTs consist of cysts and glands lined by atypical epithelium of gastrointestinal type (Figure 24.88). The cysts may contain papillae that are typically thin and branching. The lining epithelium almost always contains goblet cells and may have argyrophil cells and occasional Paneth cells. The epithelial cells are usually stratified to two or three layers, nuclear atypia is mild to moderate, and mitotic figures vary from few to numerous. Stromal invasion

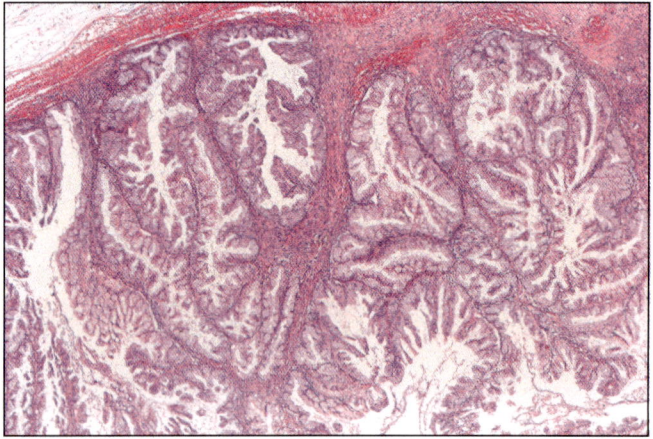

Fig. 24.88 Mucinous cystic borderline tumors of intestinal type. Packed intraglandular proliferation of mucinous epithelium with filiform branching papillae. There is no stromal invasion. Reproduced with permission from Rodriguez and Prat.[102]

is not seen (Figure 24.89). The overall appearance resembles that of a hyperplastic or adenomatous colonic polyp. Most tumors also contain foci of benign mucinous epithelium, which resembles endocervical or gastric epithelium. Occasionally, pools of extravasated mucin dissect into the stroma and may be associated with a histiocytic and foreign-body giant-cell reaction (mucin granuloma) or may lack an inflammatory cell response (pseudomyxoma ovarii). Focal necrosis and acute inflammation are not uncommon.

Non-invasive intestinal-type MBTs may exhibit areas of epithelial cell proliferation of four or more layers, scattered foci of cribriform or stroma-free papillary architecture, and moderate (grade 2) or severe atypical (grade 3) nuclei (Figure 24.90 and 24.91). Whether tumors with such areas should be classified as non-invasive carcinomas or as borderline tumors has remained controversial for many years.[41] Recent studies,[27,46,62,100,102] however, have shown these tumors to be almost always clinically benign. We recommend they be classified as mucinous borderline tumors *with intraepithelial carcinoma*.[63,113] The latter diagnosis is mainly based on cytologic features. No minimum quantity of malignant-appearing epithelium is required for inclusion into this histologic category. The upper limit, however, merges imperceptibly with invasive carcinoma with an expansile growth pattern (see below) and has been arbitrarily established as 10 mm^2. Because of their *in situ* malignant change, an MBT with intraepithelial carcinoma requires more extensive sampling than pure intestinal-type MBTs to exclude stromal invasion. Cell pseudostratification and cribriform-like pattern caused by tangential sectioning should not be interpreted as intraepithelial carcinoma, which characteristically lacks high-grade nuclear atypia.[41]

Ten per cent of intestinal-type MBTs contain one or more foci of stromal microinvasion (also arbitrarily defined as not exceeding 10 mm^2). Individual microinvasive foci usually are <1 or 2 mm in greatest dimension. Their histologic appearances vary from small nests of tumor cells admixed with extracellular mucin in a normal ovarian stroma to irregular glands associated with a fibroblastic or edematous stroma, or tiny

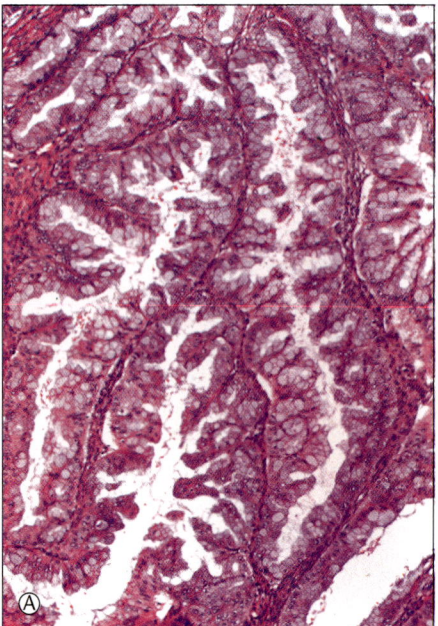

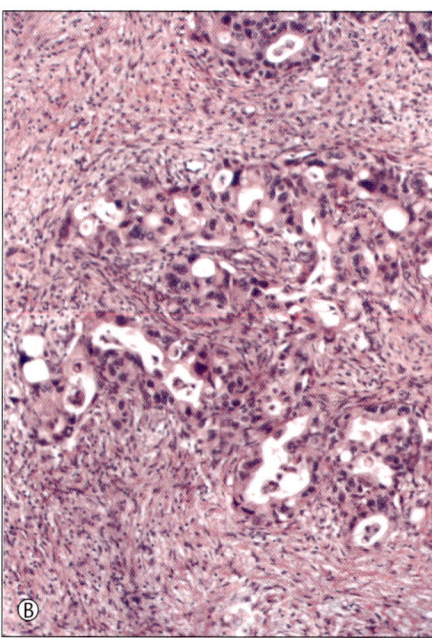

Fig. 24.89 Mucinous borderline tumor **(A)** and mucinous carcinoma **(B)**. The borderline tumor shows branching papillae with minimal stromal support, stratification into two or three cell layers, and mild nuclear atypia without stromal invasion. In contrast, the carcinoma exhibits severe nuclear atypia and obvious stromal invasion.

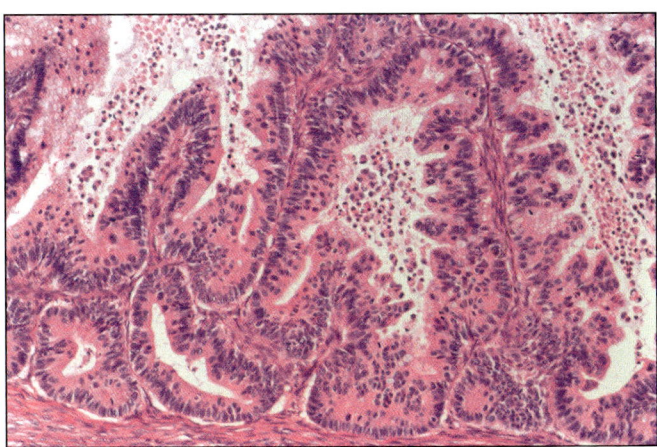

Fig. 24.90 Mucinous borderline tumor with intraepithelial carcinoma. There is cell proliferation with glandular architectural complexity. The glands are lined by grade 2 malignant nuclei with mitotic figures.

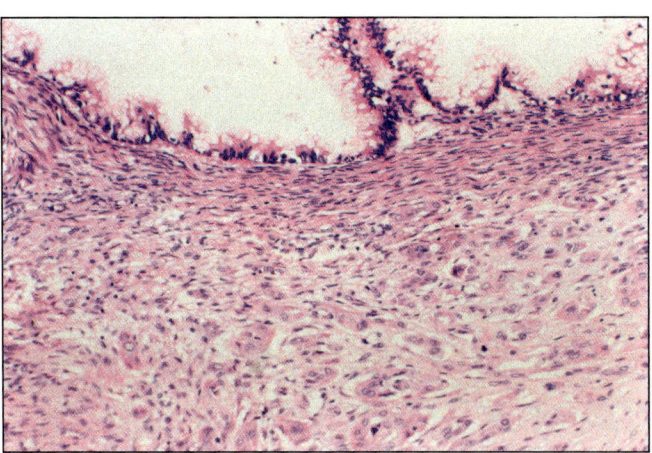

Fig. 24.92 Mucinous borderline tumor with microinvasion. Stromal microinvasion by single epithelial cells and small clusters of such cells with abundant eosinophilic cytoplasm and minimal nuclear atypia.

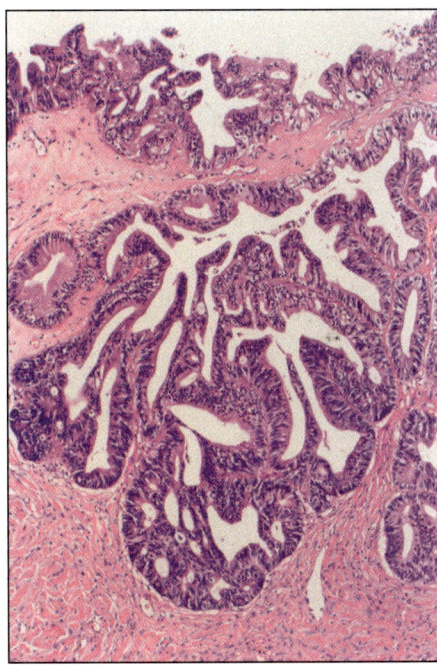

Fig. 24.91 Mucinous borderline tumor with intraepithelial carcinoma. Architectural complexity with cribriform pattern.

nests or isolated tumor cells within clear spaces. On the basis of less than 40 reported cases,[54,62,84,100,102] the presence of these foci does not alter the favorable prognosis of intestinal-type MBT. Nevertheless, MBT with microinvasion should be distinguished from microinvasive carcinoma. Whereas the microinvasive component and the adjacent glands of the former tumors exhibit only low-grade (borderline) nuclear atypia (Figure 24.92), the cells of microinvasive carcinomas usually contain grade 3 nuclei (Figure 24.93). Recently, a case of MBT with intraepithelial carcinoma with microinvasive carcinoma associated with aggressive behavior has been reported.[72] Stromal microinvasion may be difficult to distinguish from extruded neoplastic epithelium from an adjacent ruptured gland, particularly if accompanied by a mucin granuloma (Figure 24.76). Cytokeratin immunostaining reveals that mucin

granulomas contain tumor cells more often than suspected on H&E.[56]

Immunohistochemistry

The immunophenotype of endocervical MBT differs from intestinal MBT. Both types of mucinous borderline tumors are reactive for cytokeratin 7 (CK7) (Figure 24.94), but only the intestinal type immunoreacts for cytokeratin 20 (CK20)[79] and CEA. The endocervical-type but not the intestinal-type MBT is reactive for estrogen and progesterone receptors, CA125, mesothelin, and WT1.[136]

Treatment and prognosis

Stage 1 intestinal-type MBTs are treated similarly to SBTs. In a young woman who wishes to preserve her reproductive function, unilateral oophorectomy can be safely performed. Prolonged follow-up is recommended to exclude development of a similar tumor in the contralateral ovary. When performing a consultation in the operating theater (frozen section), the pathologist should be mindful that additional postoperative sampling may disclose that a carcinomatous component may be present in the permanent sections. When this is done, the surgeon is more likely to undertake appropriate staging. If there is gross evidence of pseudomyxoma peritonei or the patient has bilateral ovarian tumors, removal of the appendix as well as exploration of the abdomen for a possible source of metastasis are recommended.

According to the FIGO annual report,[92] MBTs are confined to one or both ovaries (stage 1) in 82% of the cases, stage 2 in 6%, stage 3 in 10%, and stage 4 in 2%. Almost all stage 2–3 intestinal MBTs are associated with pseudomyxoma peritonei. Excluding this group of patients in which the ovarian tumor is virtually always secondary (metastatic) from a primary appendiceal tumor (see below), some have questioned whether the non-invasive intestinal-type MBT has any malignant potential as the 5-year survival nears 100% in these women. Some investigators[100] have proposed abandoning the borderline denomination for these tumors and replacing it with 'atypical proliferative mucinous tumors'. Others,[62,102] however, believe that the term 'borderline' should be retained because it better reflects the view that these tumors represent intermediate stages of mucinous tumorigenesis and may be accompanied by

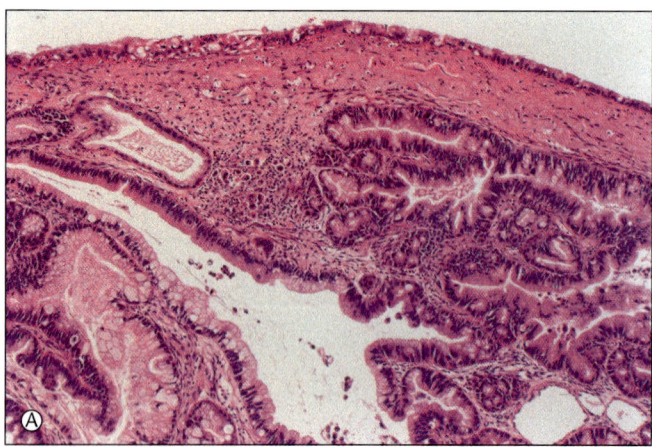
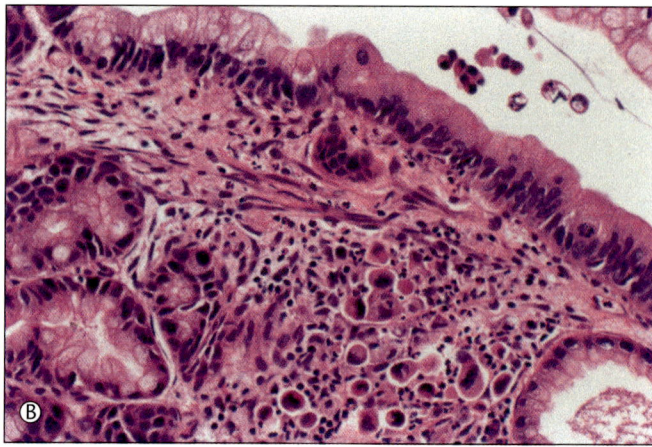

Fig. 24.93 Mucinous borderline tumor with intraepithelial and microinvasive carcinoma. **(A)** Stromal microinvasion by single epithelial cells with severe nuclear atypia. **(B)** Detail of microinvasive single epithelial cells.

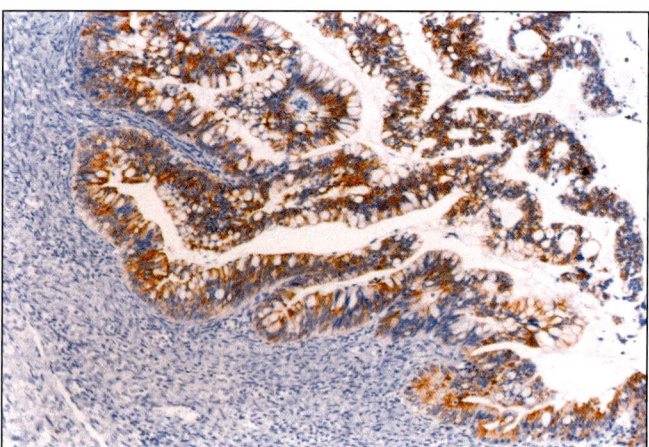

Fig. 24.94 Mucinous borderline tumor. Immunoreaction for cytokeratin 7.

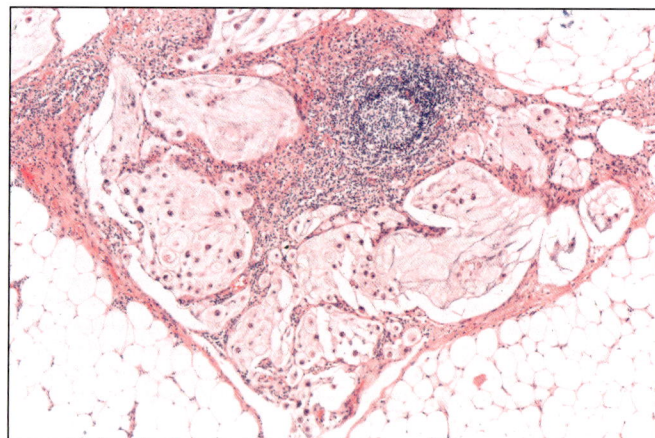

Fig. 24.95 Pseudomyxoma peritonei associated with mucinous tumors of the appendix and ovaries. Note the presence of tumor cells floating in pools of mucin dissecting through the fat. Reproduced with permission from Prat.[96]

intraepithelial and frankly invasive carcinomas. Also, some intestinal-type MBTs may account for the rare cases of pseudomyxoma peritonei in which the appendix does not contain a mucinous tumor.[62]

In advanced stage intestinal-type MBTs not associated with pseudomyxoma peritonei, the metastases appear as invasive peritoneal implants and the prognosis is similar to that of ovarian mucinous carcinomas with metastases. In these cases, it is likely that areas of invasion within the ovarian tumor were not sampled.[41,62,102] In fact, in a recent large study, the only ruptured stage 1 intestinal-type MBT that recurred contained intraepithelial carcinoma.[62]

MUCINOUS CYSTIC TUMORS ASSOCIATED WITH PSEUDOMYXOMA PERITONEI

Pseudomyxoma peritonei, a disease of MUC2-expressing goblet cells,[87] is a clinical term for localized or widespread intraperitoneal deposits of extracellular mucin ('gelatinous ascites') caused by rupture or leakage of an intra-abdominal tumor (Figure 24.95). Unlike MUC5AC, which is not specific

for pseudomyxoma peritonei, the MUC2 goblet cells secrete voluminous quantities of extracellular mucin in a ratio of mucin:cells exceeding 10:1. The mucus may be acellular or may contain mucinous epithelial cells. The gelatinous material should be thoroughly sampled and examined microscopically. The degree of cellular atypia (variously described as low grade or high grade, or alternatively as benign, borderline, or malignant) should be indicated in the report, as well as whether the mucin dissects into tissues with a fibrous response or is merely on the surface. Patients in whom the tumor appears benign or borderline usually have a more favorable clinical course than those where the tumor appears histologically malignant (peritoneal carcinomatosis).[62,107] Nevertheless, the former tumors may lead to significant morbidity and mortality (10-year survival rate of 45%)[80] and their designation as low-grade mucinous carcinomas has recently been proposed.[15] While there is general agreement today that most tumors arise in the appendix,[62,63,98,104,140] it is still open to question whether some of these neoplasms are ovarian in origin. One explanation, albeit rare, is an origin in a mature ovarian teratoma where the appendix is proven to be normal.[62,74,94,105] In most reported cases, the mucinous tumors were of borderline malignancy and not reac-

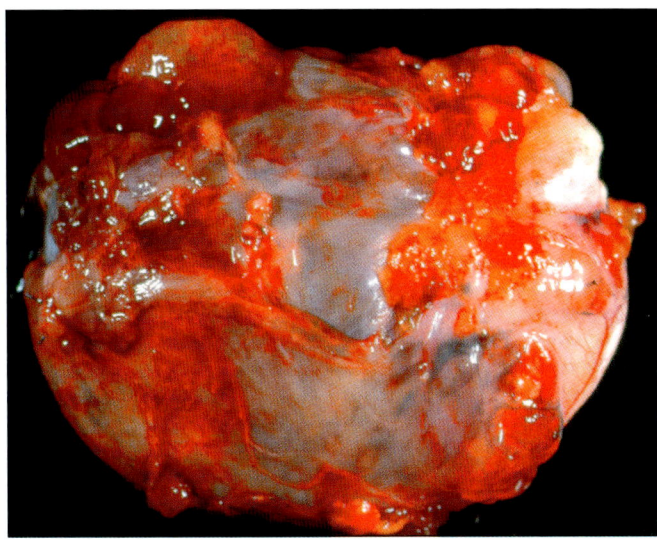

Fig. 24.96 Mucinous cystic ovarian tumor associated with pseudomyxoma peritonei and a similar appendiceal tumor. Note the presence of mucin deposits on the surface of the cyst. Reproduced with permission from Prat.[96]

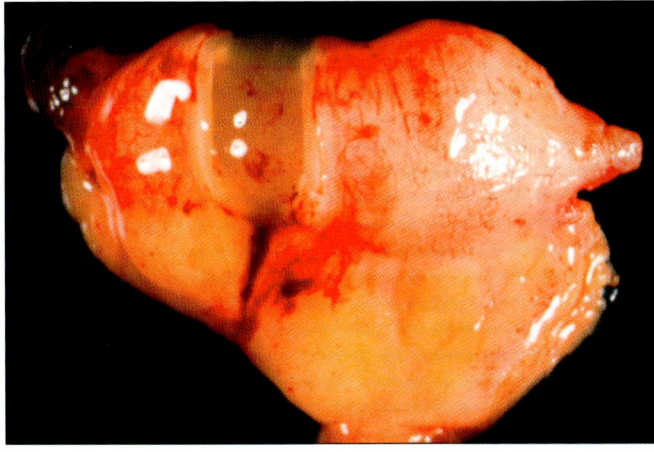

Fig. 24.97 Mucinous appendiceal tumor (mucocele) associated with pseudomyxoma peritonei and bilateral ovarian mucinous tumors. Reproduced with permission from Prat.[96]

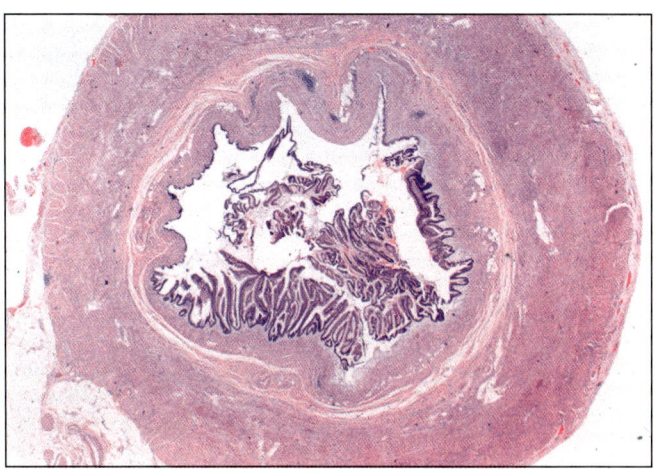

Fig. 24.98 Mucinous appendiceal tumor associated with pseudomyxoma peritonei and bilateral ovarian mucinous tumors. Reproduced with permission from Prat.[95]

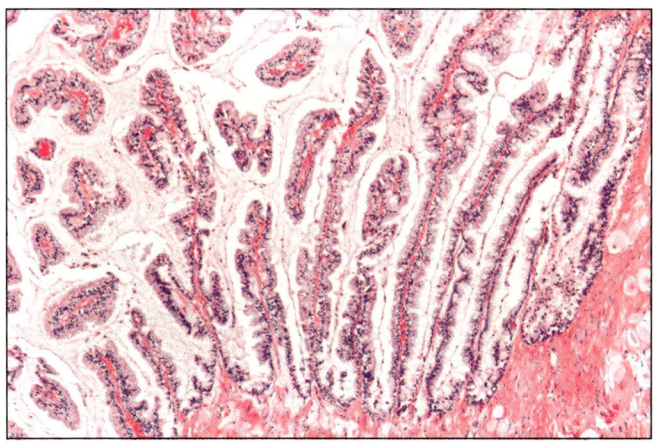

Fig. 24.99 Mucinous ovarian tumor associated with pseudomyxoma peritonei and a similar appendiceal tumor. The tumor resembles a mucinous borderline tumor of the ovary. Reproduced with permission from Cuatrecasas et al.[23]

tive for CK7. Reactivity for CK20 supported their gastrointestinal-type teratomatous origin.[62,105] Some studies of 'ovarian' borderline and low-grade mucinous tumors associated with peritoneal spread recognize deficiencies in establishing their origin since the appendix had not been removed in these cases.[62] In our experience, and that of others, removal of the appendix not uncommonly reveals either gross enlargement or a small primary tumor, which is found after blocking the entire organ. The synchronous ovarian and appendiceal tumors were traditionally considered as independent primary neoplasms, but there is now convincing evidence that in most cases the ovarian tumors (Figure 24.96) represent metastases from the appendiceal lesions (Figures 24.97 and 24.98).[41,98,104,140]

The gross and microscopic evidence includes:

(1) simultaneous presentation of the ovarian and appendiceal tumors in cases of pseudomyxoma peritonei; (2) their histologic similarity (Figure 24.99); (3) high frequency of bilaterality of the ovarian tumors (ovarian intestinal-type MBTs are usually unilateral and only occasionally associated with pseudomyxoma peritonei); (4) right-sided predominance of unilateral ovarian tumors; (5) ovarian surface involvement (Figure 24.100) and/or presence of pools of mucin dissecting through the ovarian stroma (pseudomyxoma ovarii) (Figure 24.101), a rare finding in primary mucinous ovarian tumors; (6) unusually tall mucinous epithelium of the ovarian tumors in the presence of appendiceal and peritoneal involvement; and (7) appendiceal tumors always showing the histologic features of a primary tumor, being either adenomas or adenocarcinomas.[41,98,104,140]

Features against the secondary nature of the ovarian tumors are: (1) large size and presence of a benign-appearing epithelial component in the ovarian tumors; (2) small size, low grade or benign microscopic appearance of the appendiceal tumors with intact appendiceal wall on gross inspection or even microscopic examination; (3) occasional presentation of the appendiceal tumor months to years after the discovery of the ovarian tumor;

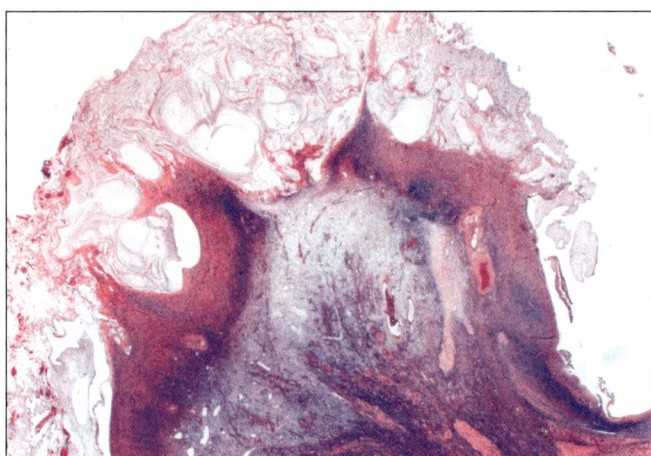

Fig. 24.100 Mucinous ovarian tumor associated with a similar mucinous tumor of the appendix and pseudomyxoma peritonei. Ovarian surface involvement. Reproduced with permission from Prat.[96]

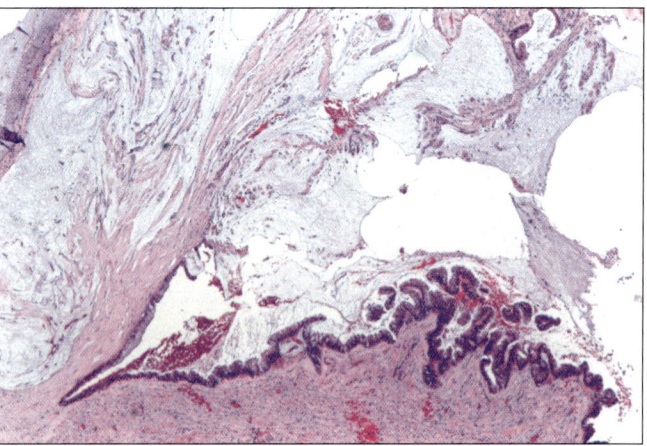

Fig. 24.101 Mucinous ovarian tumor associated with a mucinous tumor of the appendix and pseudomyxoma peritonei. Pools of mucin dissecting through the ovarian stroma (pseudomyxoma ovarii). Reproduced with permission from Prat.[96]

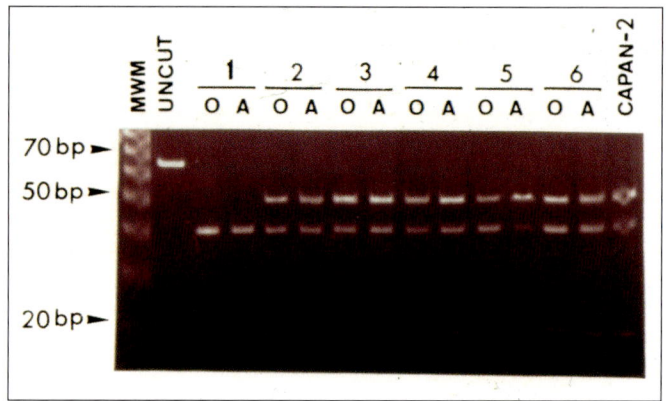

Fig. 24.102 Mucinous ovarian tumors associated with mucinous tumors of the appendix and pseudomyxoma peritonei. Mutational pattern studied by RFLP-PCR. MWM, molecular weight marker, 10 bp DNA Ladder (Life Technologies Inc., Gaithersburg, MD); UNCUT, undigested 65 bp DNA amplified PCR product. Lane 15, CAPAN 2: positive control (CAPAN 2 cell line). Cases 1–6 are underlined. The mutational band (52 bp) for codon 12 *c-K-ras* point mutation is present in both (O, Ovary; A, Appendix) samples in five of the six cases (Cases 2–6). The 40 bp fragment represents the normal allele. Reproduced with permission from Cuatrecasas et al.[23]

Molecular genetic studies have also addressed this problem.[21,23,132] Loss of heterozygosity (LOH) on chromosomes 17q (nm23), 3p (VHL), and 5q has disclosed divergent findings in the ovarian and appendiceal tumors in some cases (supporting two separate primaries) and similar findings in others (supporting a single primary tumor with metastatic spread).[21] Using a different approach, *K-ras* mutations were studied in synchronous ovarian and appendiceal tumors.[23,132] The clinicopathologic features (simultaneous presentation, bilaterality or right-sided predominance, similar histopathologic findings, and presence of pseudomyxoma peritonei) suggested that they were primary appendiceal tumors metastatic to the ovaries. Moreover, the concordance of a *K-ras* mutational pattern in both tumors in each patient (Figure 24.102) also suggested their clonal nature and supported the hypothesis that they had originated from the same clone, which – in the light of the clinicopathologic data – was most likely of appendiceal origin.

Prognosis and treatment

Patients with pseudomyxoma peritonei containing epithelial cells that are benign or borderline appearing usually have a protracted clinical course. The 5- and 10-year survival rates are 75% and 68%, respectively. In contrast, when the epithelial cells of the pseudomyxoma peritonei appear malignant (peritoneal carcinomatosis), the clinical course is more aggressive and approximately 90% of patients die within 3 years. Cytoreductive surgery at initial presentation and repeated palliative debulking, mucolytic agents, chemotherapy and/or radiotherapy have done relatively little to modify the natural history of this disease.[38,70,138]

MUCINOUS CARCINOMAS

The establishment of the borderline subcategory of mucinous tumors, as well as the increasing recognition of metastatic adenocarcinomas that resemble primary ovarian mucinous

(4) differences in the histologic grade of the ovarian and appendiceal tumors; (5) discordant epithelial immunohistochemical staining in the ovarian and appendiceal tumors; and (6) more favorable clinical behavior in these patients than that expected for patients with metastatic carcinomas.[115] Authors in favor of the metastatic nature of ovarian tumors have contended all the above points and stated that the appendiceal source of the pseudomyxoma peritonei can only be excluded after adequate sampling and microscopic examination of the appendix.[41,98,104,140] The appendiceal tumors may be small and rupture sites can be sealed after evacuation of mucus and retraction of the appendiceal wall.[140] Differences in the histologic appearance and immunohistochemical staining between appendiceal and ovarian tumors may reflect tumor heterogeneity or incomplete sampling of the neoplasms.[113] Moreover, mucinous tumors metastatic to the ovary typically show a much higher degree of differentiation than the primary neoplasms and may appear deceptively 'benign' in some areas.[113,140] Concordant negative immunostaining reactions for human alveolar macrophage 56 (HAM-56) and CK7 in both tumors also support their appendiceal origin.[106]

tumors, have narrowed significantly the number of mucinous ovarian tumors currently diagnosed as carcinoma (Figure 24.103). Of 688 primary mucinous tumors confined to the ovary at diagnosis in the first modern study, only 22 (3%) were obviously invasive carcinomas.[42] Thus, the reported frequency of 15% for mucinous adenocarcinomas primary in the ovary may be overestimated, and most contemporary studies have been based on a relatively small number of cases.[46,62,102] According to a recent report, mucinous carcinomas comprise <3% of ovarian carcinomas.[118] In contrast to borderline mucinous tumors, mucinous adenocarcinomas have not usually been subclassified into intestinal and endocervical-like (see below).

Macroscopic features

Mucinous carcinomas are usually large (8–40 cm; mean 16–19 cm in greatest dimension),[46] unilateral, multilocular or unilocular cystic masses containing mucinous fluid (Figure 24.104). They often exhibit papillary and solid areas that may be soft and mucoid, or firm, hemorrhagic, and necrotic. Extensive sampling of mucinous ovarian tumors, especially the more solid areas, is critical, as benign, borderline, and malignant components may coexist within a single specimen and the malignant areas may involve only a small portion of the tumor. The tumors are bilateral in only 5% of the cases. Bilateral mucinous carcinomas or unilateral carcinomas under 10 cm in greatest dimension should raise the suspicion of metastases.

Microscopic features

Over 80% of frankly invasive mucinous carcinomas have components of intestinal-type MBT or mucinous cystadenoma, or both, suggesting a progression from benign to malignant neoplasia. The remaining 20% of the carcinomas appear exclusively malignant. Recently, the proposal has been made to divide mucinous carcinomas into two categories: an *expansile* type without demonstrable destructive stromal invasion, but exhibiting back-to-back or complex malignant glands without or with minimal intervening stroma and exceeding 10 mm² in area (>3 mm in each of two linear dimensions) (Figures 24.105–24.107); and an *infiltrative* type, showing obvious stromal invasion in the form of glands, cell clusters, or individual cells, disorderly infiltrating the stroma and frequently associated with a desmoplastic stromal reaction (Figures 24.108 and 24.109).[62] The expansile pattern of growth has also been referred to as the 'non-invasive', 'intraglandular'[46] or 'confluent glandular'[100] pattern.

Rare mucinous carcinomas of the endocervical-like or mixed müllerian type have been described;[61,119] three cases were associated with endometriosis and one with an endocervical-type MBT of the contralateral ovary.[61]

Differential diagnosis

The most important differential diagnosis of mucinous ovarian carcinoma is with metastatic mucinous carcinoma that may

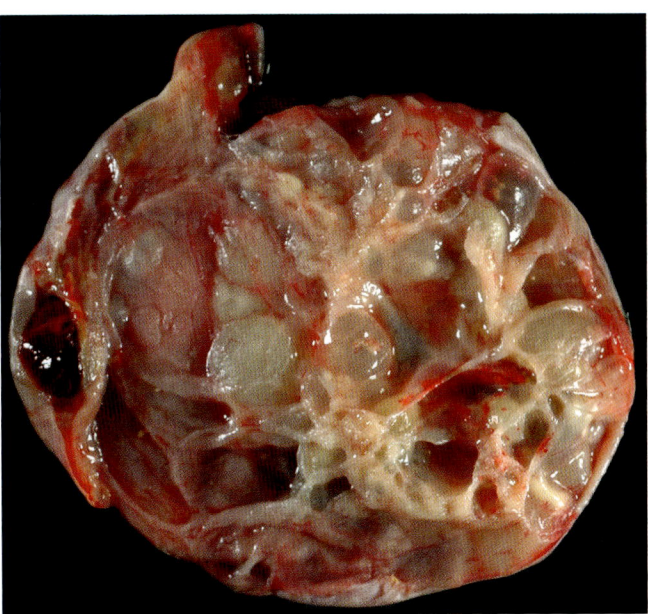

Fig. 24.104 Mucinous cystadenocarcinoma. The sectioned surface shows a multiloculated tumor.

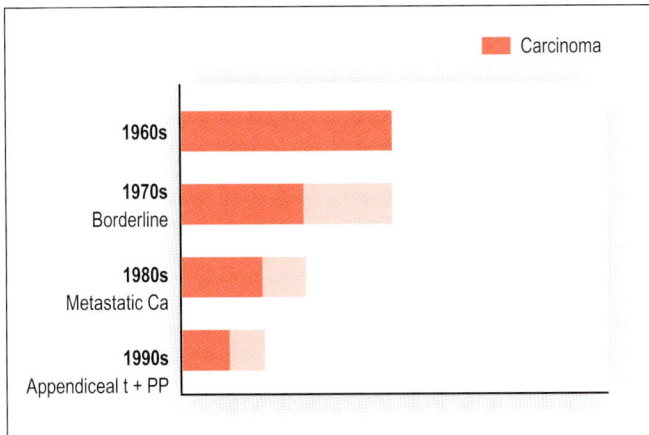

Fig. 24.103 Mucinous tumors of the ovary. Over the last 40 years, the percentage of primary mucinous carcinomas (Ca) of the ovary has progressively reduced because of the introduction of the borderline category of tumors (1970s); the realization that metastatic adenocarcinomas, particularly of the large intestine and pancreas, can simulate primary ovarian tumors (1980s); and, lastly, the finding that most mucinous ovarian tumors associated with 'pseudomyxoma peritonei' (PP) are secondary neoplasms, often from the appendix. Reproduced with permission from Prat.[96]

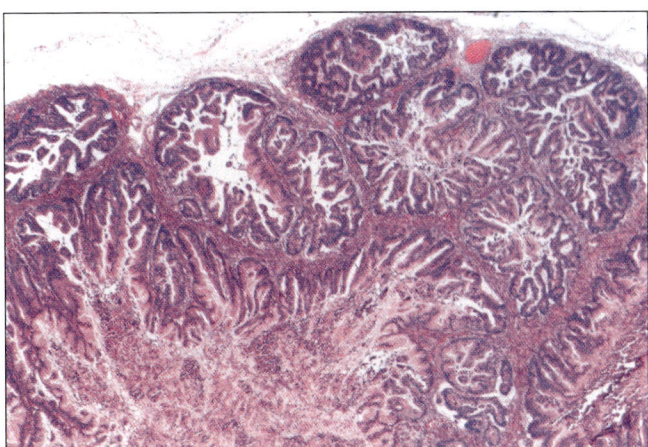

Fig. 24.105 Mucinous carcinoma with expansile invasion. Confluent, complex glandular proliferation without obvious stromal invasion. Reproduced with permission from Prat.[96]

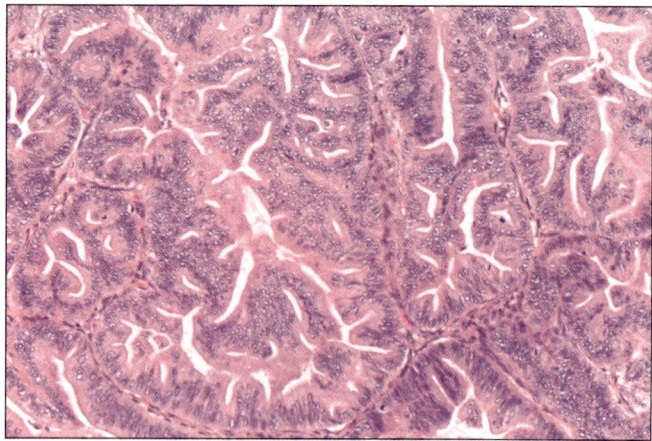

Fig. 24.106 Mucinous carcinoma with expansile invasion. Closely packed (back-to-back) malignant glands with little to no stromal support. Stromal invasion is not obvious. Mitotic figures are seen. Reproduced with permission from Prat.[96]

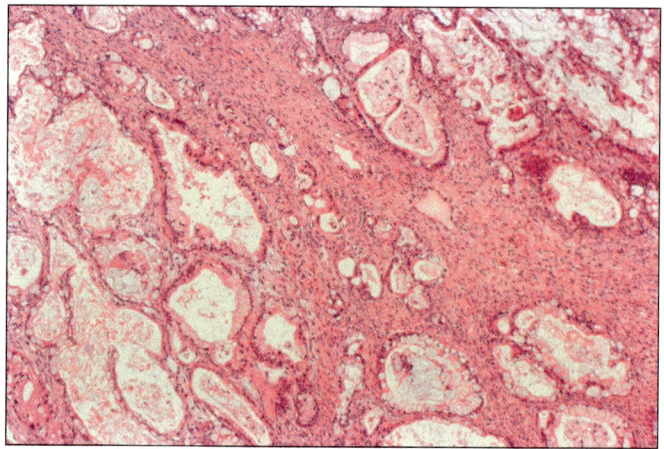

Fig. 24.109 Mucinous carcinoma with infiltrative invasion. Mucinous glands infiltrate a desmoplastic stroma.

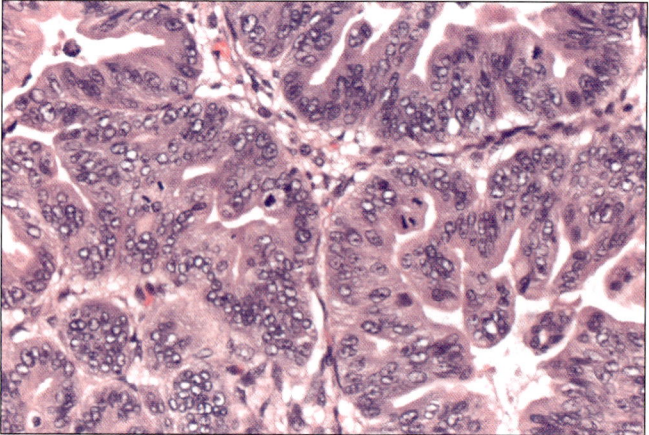

Fig. 24.107 Mucinous carcinoma with expansile invasion. Papillary glands lined by cells with grade 2–3 malignant nuclei. Mitotic figures are seen. Reproduced with permission from Prat.[96]

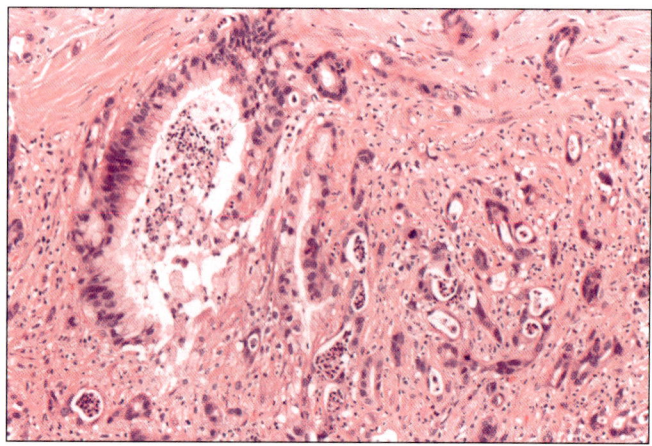

Fig. 24.108 Mucinous carcinoma with infiltrative invasion. Mucinous glands and individual nests of tumor cells infiltrate a desmoplastic stroma in a disorderly fashion. Reproduced with permission from Prat.[96]

present clinically as a primary ovarian tumor. Most of these originate in the large intestine, appendix, pancreas, biliary tract, stomach, or cervix (see Chapter 28).[50,64,90,140,141] Common features that favor a primary mucinous carcinoma are an expansile pattern of invasion and a complex papillary architecture; a borderline or benign-appearing component is commonly found.[64] Features favoring a metastatic mucinous carcinoma are bilaterality, small size (<10 cm), a multinodular growth pattern, ovarian surface involvement by epithelial cells (surface implants), hilar involvement, signet-ring cell component, vascular space invasion, and presence of extraovarian disease.[64] The finding of abundant extracellular mucin (pseudomyxoma ovarii) should always raise the suspicion of metastatic carcinoma. Most primary mucinous carcinomas of the ovary are unilateral and stage 1.[46,62,100,102] Nevertheless, metastatic mucinous adenocarcinomas, particularly colorectal carcinomas, may be large (≥10 cm) and unilateral in approximately 40% of cases.[55]

Well-differentiated endometrioid carcinomas containing foci of benign-appearing endocervical-like cells are best interpreted as endometrioid adenocarcinomas, grade 1, with areas of mucinous metaplasia. Some endometrioid adenocarcinomas secrete large amounts of mucin into the lumens of their glands and cysts, but the mucin is present only in the glycocalyx of the tumor cells. These tumors are considered to be mucin-rich endometrioid carcinomas rather than mucinous carcinomas.[113]

Sertoli–Leydig cell tumors with heterologous mucinous elements may appear on gross examination as mucinous cystic tumors. The problem may be accentuated if a mucinous tumor is producing androgens and virilizing the patient because of its luteinized stroma. Microscopically, there is Sertoli–Leydig cell tumor, typically of the intermediate type with abundant sex cord-like structures, between the cyst locules, rather than stroma or lutein cells. Other heterologous elements such as carcinoid or mesenchymal tissues (skeletal muscle or cartilage) may also be present in heterologous Sertoli–Leydig cell tumors to aid in the differential diagnosis.[113]

Immunohistochemistry

Although selected immunostains help to distinguish primary from secondary ovarian tumors, immunohistochemistry is considerably less useful when the ovarian neoplasm is of mucinous type. Most ovarian mucinous borderline tumors and carcinomas are of intestinal type and, therefore, their immunophenotype frequently overlaps with that of metastatic gastrointestinal tumors. Cytokeratin immunostains are the most commonly used.[137] Primary ovarian mucinous tumors are almost always (up to 80%) immunoreactive for CK7 whereas colorectal adenocarcinomas are usually CK7 negative.[79,90] However, CK7 is usually positive in metastatic carcinomas of the pancreas, notorious for masquerading as primary ovarian tumors, and it is also focally expressed by many other carcinomas, including those of stomach, gall bladder, small bowel, appendix, lung, breast, thyroid, uterus, and bladder.[20,50,65,130] Ovarian mucinous borderline tumors and carcinomas are immunoreactive for CK20 in 65% and 75% of cases, respectively, but the reaction is typically weak and focal.[20,50] In contrast, colorectal adenocarcinomas are diffusely and strongly reactive for CK20.[50,65,90] Therefore, a CK7-negative/CK20-positive immunoprofile suggests metastatic adenocarcinoma.[50,137] Although the vast majority of colorectal adenocarcinomas express CK20, poorly differentiated and right-sided tumors can be CK20 negative.[90] Thus, immunostains for CK7 and CK20 should be interpreted with caution, always in the light of all clinical information, and with the understanding that no tumor shows absolute consistency in its staining with these markers.

Other immunohistochemical stains have greater overlap in their expressions and should not be used individually in this differential diagnosis. Nevertheless, after taking into account the clinicopathologic findings and the results of the CK immunostains, a lack of reactivity for vimentin, CA125, B72.3, and gastric mucin gene MUC5AC,[1,58] and strong reactivity for carcinoembryonic antigen (CEA) and MUC2,[1,58] favors metastatic colorectal cancer over primary ovarian adenocarcinoma. Loss of Dpc4 immunoreactivity occurs in almost 50% of metastatic carcinomas of the pancreas, whereas most primary ovarian mucinous carcinomas are focally or diffusely positive.[50]

Human papillomavirus (HPV) DNA assessment may be helpful for distinguishing mucinous adenocarcinoma of the cervix metastatic to the ovary from a primary ovarian mucinous carcinoma; p16 expression is also a reliable surrogate marker for HPV.[32]

Somatic genetics

As indicated above, tumor heterogeneity is common and probably reflects progression from benign to malignant neoplasia that occurs in mucinous carcinogenesis (Figures 24.110 and 24.111). Recent studies strongly suggest that in the sequence of malignant transformation from benign and borderline mucinous tumors to infiltrative carcinoma, intraepithelial (non-invasive) carcinomas and carcinomas with purely expansile (not obvious) invasion represent transitional stages of mucinous carcinogenesis.[62,102] Recent molecular studies support this hypothesis of genetic alterations in mucinous tumors.[24,73] An increasing frequency of codon 12/13 *K-ras* mutations in benign, borderline, and carcinomatous mucinous ovarian tumors favors the viewpoint that *K-ras* mutational activation is an early event in mucinous ovarian tumorigenesis (Figure 24.112–24.115).[24,73]

Treatment and prognosis

Treatment of mucinous carcinomas is similar to that of serous carcinomas (see above). FIGO stage is the single most impor-

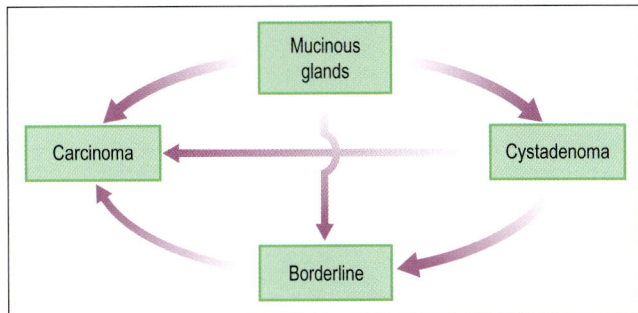

Fig. 24.110 Mucinous carcinomas: histogenesis. In contrast to serous carcinomas, which are thought to arise *de novo* from the surface epithelium and its inclusion cysts, malignant mucinous intestinal tumors frequently exhibit a transition from benign, to borderline, and to carcinoma. Reproduced with permission from Prat.[96]

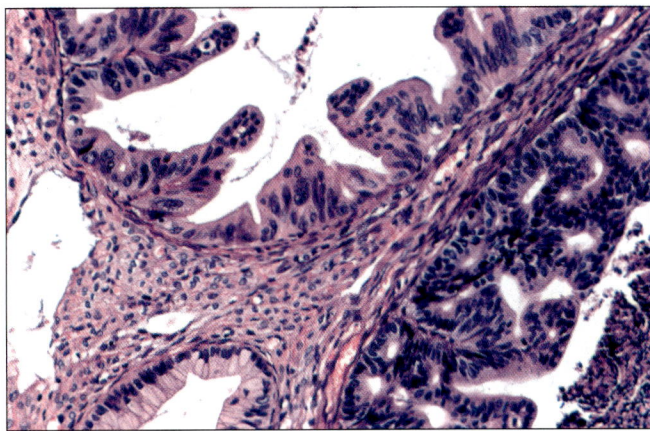

Fig. 24.111 Mucinous tumor of intestinal type. Three neoplastic components appear next to each other: benign (bottom left), borderline with marked proliferation and nuclear atypia (top), and carcinoma with cribriform pattern and central necrosis (bottom right). Reproduced with permission from Prat.[95]

tant prognostic factor, and stage 1 carcinomas have an excellent prognosis. However, the prognosis in cases with extraovarian spread is poor.[46,62,85,100,102] According to the FIGO annual report,[92] mucinous carcinomas are confined to one or both ovaries in 49% of the cases, are stage 2 in 11%, stage 3 in 29%, and stage 4 in 10%. The 5-year survival for patients with stage 1 mucinous carcinomas is 83%; stage 2, 55%; stage 3, 21%; and stage 4, 9%.[92] After excluding cases of metastatic tumor from non-ovarian sites and cases of pseudomyxoma peritonei of intestinal origin, more than 80% of mucinous carcinomas are stage 1 (confined to ovary) at the time of diagnosis.[46,62,102]

Prognosis within and across FIGO stage also reflects specifics of histologic features. Infiltrative stromal invasion is biologically more aggressive than expansile invasion. Among 59 cases of invasive carcinoma in two recent series,[62,102] all 20 cases with expansile invasion were stage 1 and none experienced recurrent disease. Of the 25 infiltrative carcinomas with follow-up data, only 9 of 13 patients with stage 1 disease and 1 of 12 with higher stage disease (stage 2A) had favorable outcomes. Furthermore, in contrast to previous reports,[46,62,100] one series[102]

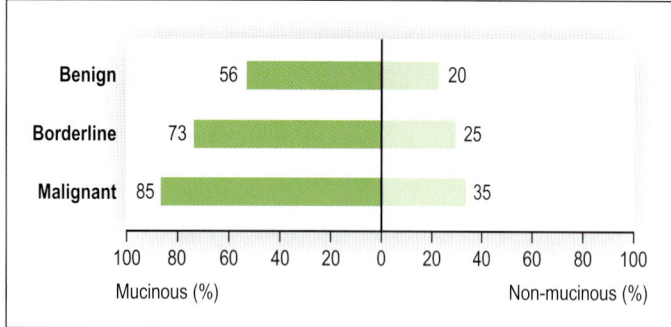

Fig. 24.112 K-*ras* investigation in two large series of mucinous and non-mucinous epithelial ovarian tumors. K-*ras* mutations were encountered more frequently in mucinous (68%) than in non-mucinous (30%) tumors. They occurred in benign, borderline, and fully malignant tumors, but their presence increased significantly with the degree of malignancy.[24] Reproduced with permission from Prat.[96]

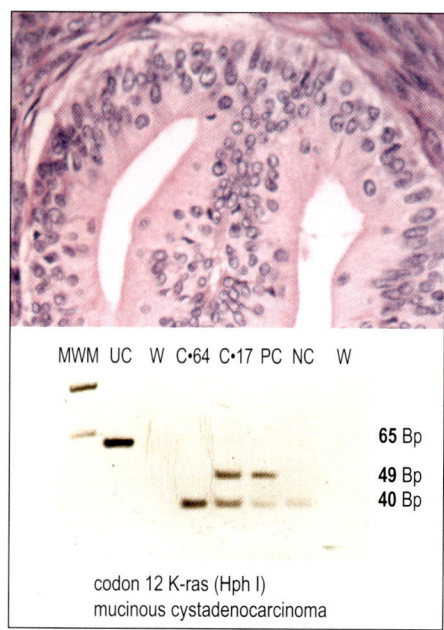

Fig. 24.114 Well-differentiated mucinous carcinoma. Restriction fragment length polymorphism-polymerase chain reaction (RFLP-PCR) analysis shows a point mutation at codon 12 of *K-ras* (Case 17). The 49 and 40 bp bands correspond to the mutant and normal alleles, respectively. Note that both the positive control (PC) and the investigated tumor (C-17) are heterozygous and show two bands. Reproduced with permission from Prat.[96]

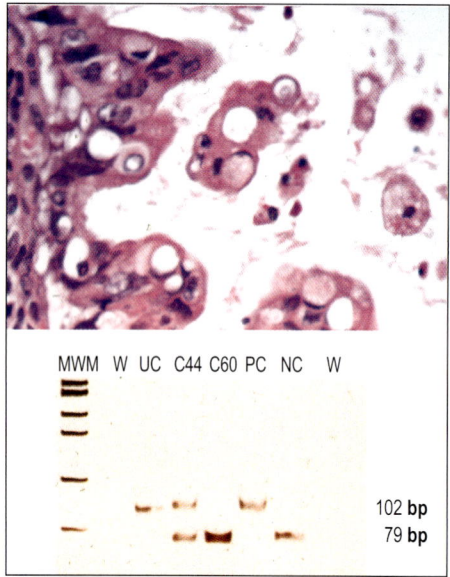

Fig. 24.113 Mucinous borderline tumor of intestinal type. Restriction fragment length polymorphism-polymerase chain reaction (RFLP-PCR) analysis reveals a point mutation at codon 12 of *K-ras*. (Case 44). The 102 and 79 bp bands correspond to the mutant and normal alleles, respectively. Note that the positive control (PC) is homozygous and the investigated tumor (C44) is heterozygous. Reproduced with permission from Prat.[96]

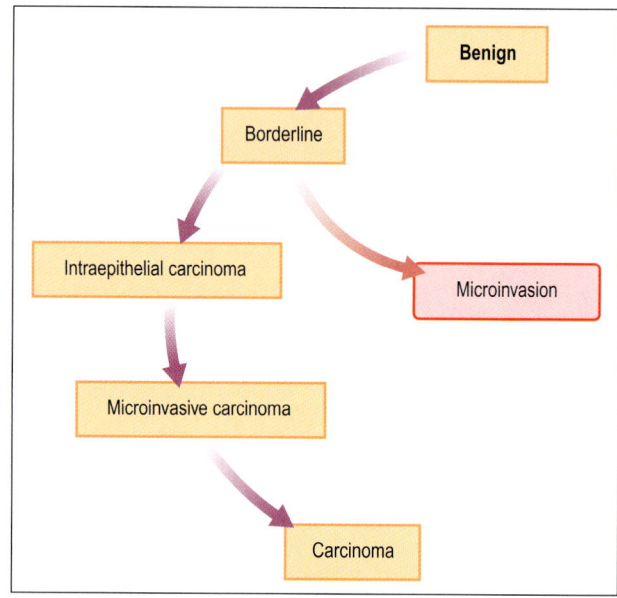

Fig. 24.115 Progression of mucinous tumors. Reproduced with permission from Prat.[96]

showed that high nuclear grade (grade 3) was predictive of behavior independent of the surgical stage.

The combination of extensive and infiltrative stromal invasion, high nuclear grade, and tumor rupture should be considered a strong predictor of recurrence for stage 1 mucinous carcinomas (Table 24.5).[102]

Foci of stromal invasion <10 mm² have been designated 'microinvasive', and cases with this finding have had a favorable outcome.[54,62,84,86,102,127] However, experience with these tumors is still scarce, and occasional carcinomas with stromal invasion barely beyond the limit accepted for microinvasion have produced metastases (Figures 24.116 and 24.117).[85]

Table 24.5 Stage 1 mucinous carcinomas: prognosis

Favorable	Unfavorable	
Expansile	Infiltrative	(P = 0.005)
Nuclear G1–2	Nuclear G3	(P = 0.021)
Intact	Ruptured	

Data from Rodriguez and Prat.[102]

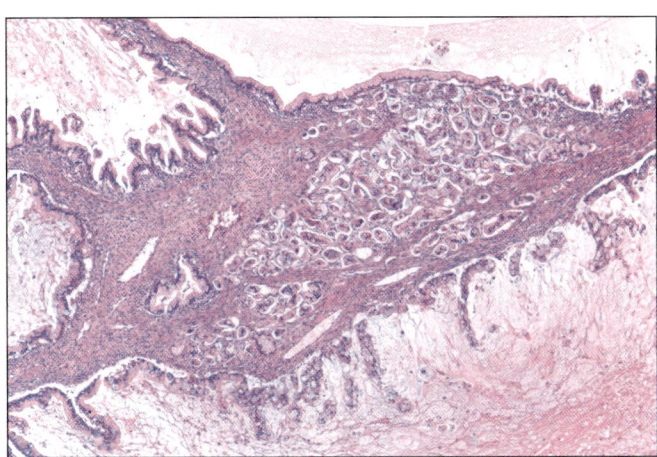

Fig. 24.116 Invasive mucinous carcinoma. Small focus (1.5 mm²) of microinvasion. The adjacent glandular epithelium appears benign or borderline. This stage 3B ruptured cystic tumor contained several additional foci of stromal invasion, the largest 10.2 mm² in area. Reproduced with permission from Prat.[96]

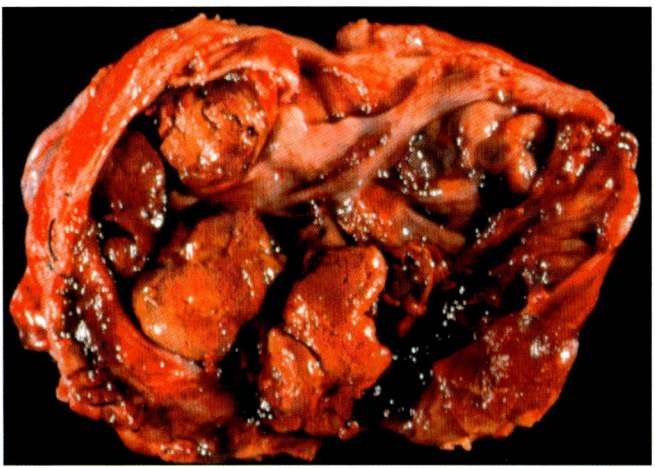

Fig. 24.118 Sarcoma-like mural nodules in a mucinous cystic tumor. Four red to brown nodules protrude into the lumen of the cyst. Reproduced with permission from Prat.[96]

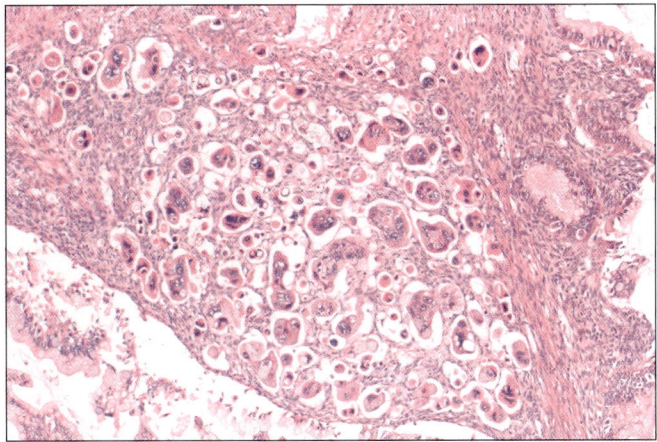

Fig. 24.117 Invasive mucinous carcinoma. Small focus (1.3 mm²) of microinvasion. Notice the presence of highly malignant (nuclear grade 3) carcinomatous cells. Reproduced with permission from Prat.[96]

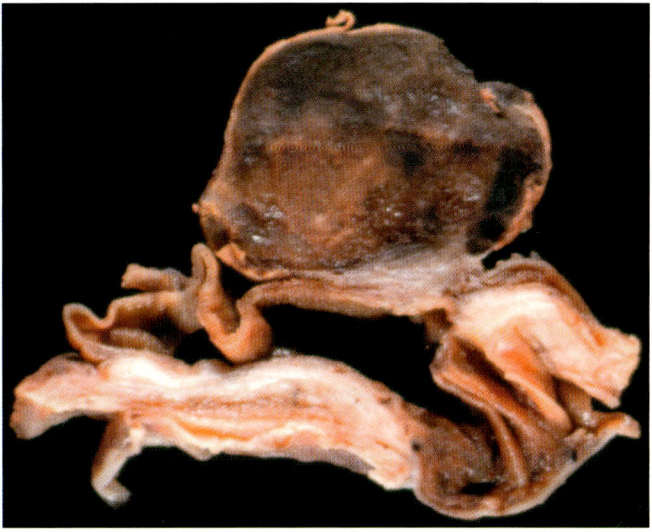

Fig. 24.119 Sarcoma-like mural nodules in a mucinous cystic tumor. The sectioned surface shows a hemorrhagic nodule which appears well circumscribed. Reproduced with permission from Prat.[95]

MURAL NODULES

Mucinous cystic tumors of the ovary, whether benign, borderline, or malignant, may contain one or more mural nodules that differ notably in their microscopic features from those of the underlying mucinous neoplasm. The nodules have been classified into three major subtypes: sarcoma-like mural nodules, nodules of anaplastic carcinoma, and sarcoma.[4] Mixed nodules have also been described.

Sarcoma-like mural nodules occur predominantly in middle-aged women (mean age, 39 years) as red-brown nodules (0.6–6 cm in diameter) (Figure 24.118) that appear sharply demarcated from the adjacent mucinous epithelium (Figures 24.119 and 24.120). They are associated with mucinous carcinomas in about half the cases and with benign and MBTs in the remainder (Figure 24.121). The nodules are almost always multiple. They exhibit a heterogeneous cell population with numerous multinucleated cells of the epulis type (Figure 24.122), atypical spindle cells (Figure 24.123), and inflammatory cells. In some nodules the predominant elements are spindle-shaped cells of moderate size containing hyperchromatic nuclei and pleomorphic mononucleated or binucleated giant cells. The mitotic index in the most cellular areas is 5–10 mitoses per 10 high-power fields (HPFs). Immunohistochemical staining shows reactivity with histiocytic markers and vimentin, and weak and focal staining for cytokeratin (Figure 24.124), suggesting a possible origin from submesothelial mesenchymal cells,[4] possibly stimulated to proliferate due to spillage of mucin or hemorrhage into aggregates of these cells within the ovary. All lesions so far described have had a benign clinical course.[4]

Nodules of anaplastic carcinoma exhibit either a diffuse collection of: (1) large rhabdoid cells with abundant eosinophilic cytoplasm (Figure 24.125), eccentric nuclei, and one or more prominent nucleoli; (2) sarcomatoid spindle cells with atypical and vesicular nuclei often exhibiting a herringbone pattern; or (3) pleomorphic cells.[99] The cells react strongly for cytokeratin (Figure 24.126). These lesions occur almost always

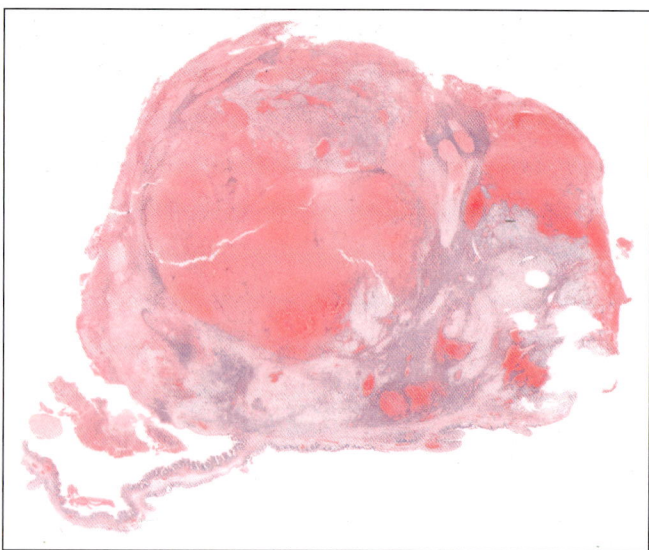

Fig. 24.120 *Sarcoma-like mural nodule in a mucinous cystic tumor. The nodule shows extensive hemorrhage and is well demarcated from the mucinous epithelial component (bottom). Reproduced with permission from Prat.[96]*

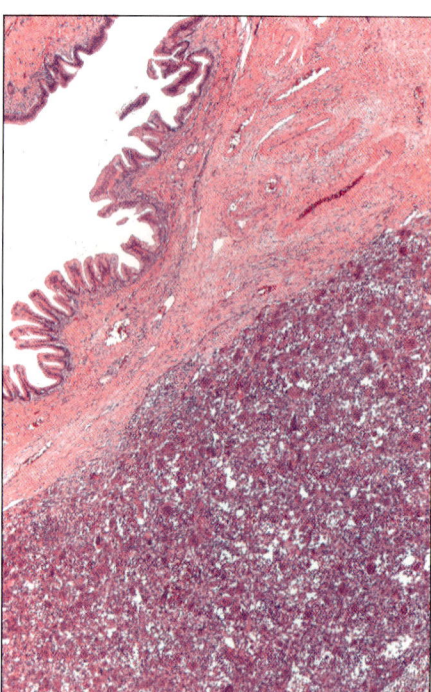

Fig. 24.121 *Sarcoma-like nodule in wall of mucinous cystic tumor. The nodule exhibits a heterogeneous cell population with numerous multinucleated cells of the epulis type. Reproduced with permission from Prat.[95]*

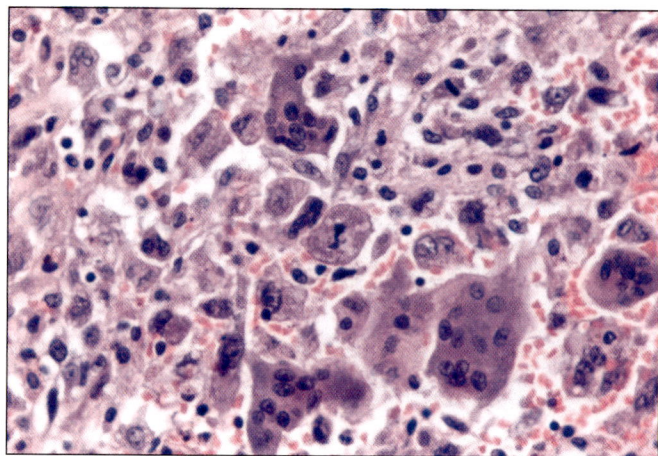

Fig. 24.122 *Sarcoma-like mural nodule in a mucinous cystic tumor. The cells of the nodule include osteoclast-like giant cells and smaller mononuclear cells. Two atypical mitotic figures are present. Reproduced with permission from Prat.[96]*

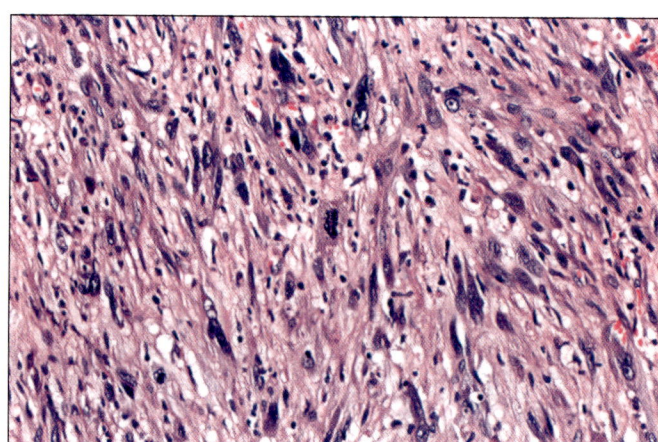

Fig. 24.123 *Sarcoma-like mural nodule in a mucinous cystic tumor. The cells of the nodule appear pleomorphic and spindle. An atypical mitosis is seen in the center. Reproduced with permission from Prat.[96]*

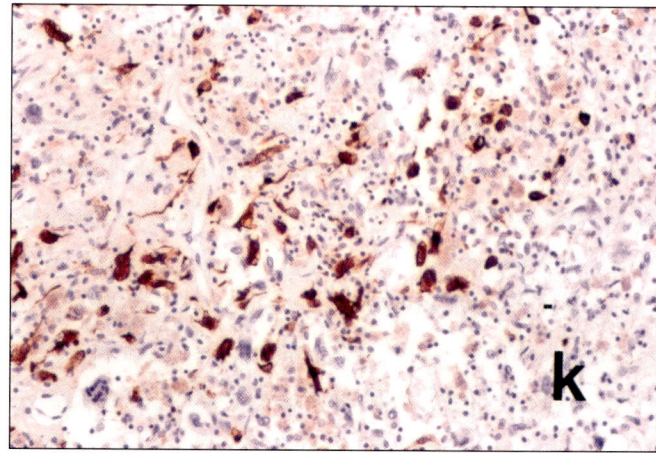

Fig. 24.124 *Sarcoma-like mural nodule in a mucinous cystic tumor. The pleomorphic and spindle cells are weakly immunoreactive for cytokeratin. Reproduced with permission from Prat.[96]*

in malignant or borderline mucinous tumors, and only rarely in cystadenomas. Their sizes range from microscopic to about 10 cm and they may be single or multiple. Frequently, the surrounding tissue is invaded, and in a minority of cases, the vascular space may show invasion as well.[99,102] Although initially thought to carry an invariably unfavorable prognosis, newer data indicate that these nodules, when found within unruptured stage 1 mucinous cystic tumors, may also be associated with a favorable prognosis.[99,102]

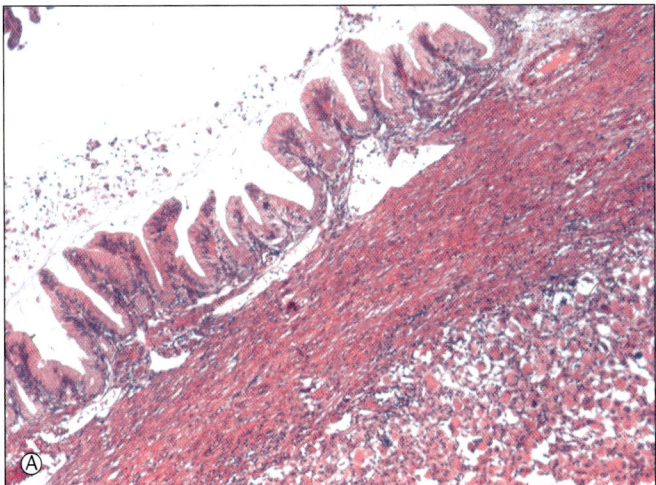

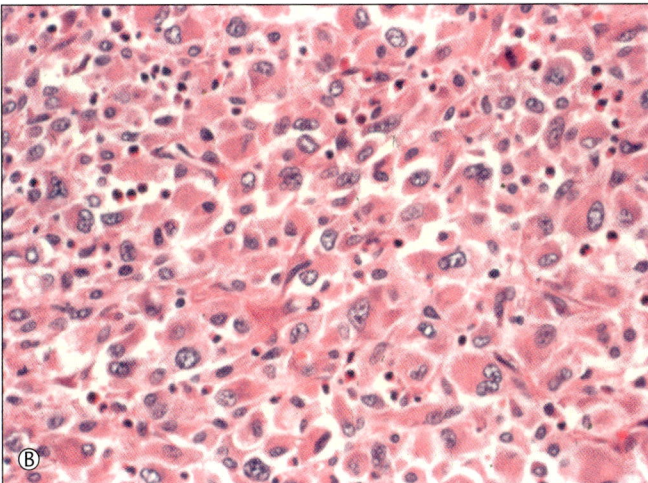

Fig. 24.125 Anaplastic carcinoma in mucinous cystic tumor. The epithelial lining of the cyst appears of borderline malignancy **(A)**. The undifferentiated component is characterized by a diffuse arrangement of cells with abundant eosinophilic cytoplasm and grade 3 nuclei **(B)**. Reproduced with permission from Prat.[96]

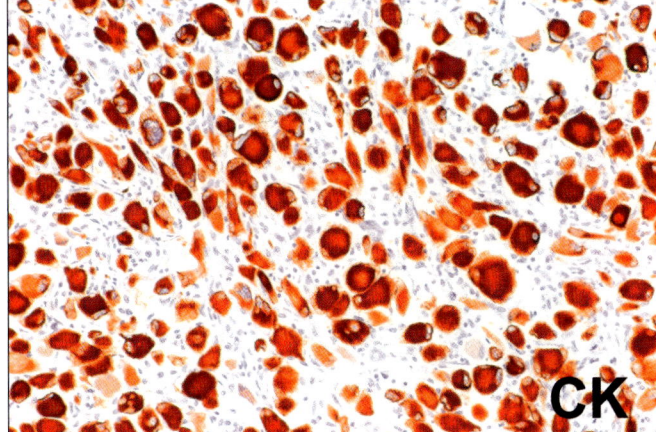

Fig. 24.126 Anaplastic carcinoma in mucinous cystic tumor. Strongly positive cytokeratin immunostain. Reproduced with permission from Prat.[96]

Various types of true sarcomatous nodules have been reported, such as fibrosarcoma, rhabdomyosarcoma, and undifferentiated sarcoma. These tumors carry a poor prognosis. Mixed nodules usually consist of small foci of anaplastic carcinoma within what appears to be a sarcoma-like nodule. Also, in tumors containing multiple nodules, some may be of one type and others of another type.

REFERENCES

1. Albarracin CT, Jafri J, Montag AG, Hart J, Kuan SF. Differential expression of MUC2 and MUC5AC mucin genes in primary ovarian and metastatic colonic carcinoma. Hum Pathol 2000;31:672–7.
2. Alvarez AA, Moore WF, Robboy SJ, et al. K-ras mutations in mullerian inclusion cysts associated with serous borderline tumors of the ovary. Gynecol Oncol 2001;80:201–6.
3. Argani P, Rosai J. Hyperplastic mesothelial cells in lymph nodes: report of six cases of a benign process that can simulate metastatic involvement by mesothelioma or carcinoma. Hum Pathol 1998;29:339–46.
4. Bagué S, Rodríguez IM, Prat J. Sarcoma-like mural nodules in mucinous cystic tumors of the ovary revisited: a clinicopathologic analysis of 10 additional cases. Am J Surg Pathol 2002;26:1467–76.
5. Barnhill DR, Kurman RJ, Brady MF, et al. Preliminary analysis of the behavior of stage I ovarian serous tumors of low malignant potential: a Gynecologic Oncology Group study. J Clin Oncol 1995;13:2752–6.
6. Bell DA. Mucinous adenofibromas of the ovary. A report of 10 cases. Am J Surg Pathol 1991;15:227–32.
7. Bell DA, Longacre TA, Prat J, et al. Serous borderline (low malignant potential, atypical proliferative) ovarian tumors. Workshop perspectives. Hum Pathol 2004;35:934–48.
8. Bell DA, Scully RE. Ovarian serous borderline tumors with stromal microinvasion: a report of 21 cases. Hum Pathol 1990;21:397–403.
9. Bell DA, Scully RE. Serous borderline tumors of the peritoneum. Am J Surg Pathol 1990;14:230–9.
10. Bell DA, Scully RE. Early *de novo* ovarian carcinoma. A study of fourteen cases. Cancer 1994;73:1859–64.
11. Bell DA, Weinstock MA, Scully RE. Peritoneal implants of ovarian serous borderline tumors. Histologic features and prognosis. Cancer 1988;62:2212–22.
12. Bell KA, Smith Sehdev AE, Kurman RJ. Refined diagnostic criteria for implants associated with ovarian atypical proliferative serous tumors (borderline) and micropapillary serous carcinomas. Am J Surg Pathol 2001;25:419–32.
13. Biscotti CV, Hart WR. Peritoneal serous papillomatosis of low malignant potential (serous borderline tumors of the peritoneum). A clinicopathologic study of 17 cases. Am J Surg Pathol 1992;16:467–75.
14. Bonome T, Lee JY, Park DC, et al. Expression profiling of serous low malignant potential, low-grade, and high-grade tumors of the ovary. Cancer Res 2005;65:10602–12.
15. Bradley RF, Stewart JH, Russell GB, Levine EA, Geisinger KR. Pseudomyxoma peritonei of appendiceal origin: a clinicopathologic analysis of 101 patients uniformly treated at a single institution, with literature review. Am J Surg Pathol 2006;30:551–9.
16. Bristow RE, Gossett DR, Shook DR, et al. Recurrent micropapillary serous ovarian carcinoma: the role of secondary cytoreductive surgery. Cancer 2002;95:791–800.
17. Burks RT, Sherman ME, Kurman RJ. Micropapillary serous carcinoma of the ovary. A distinctive low-grade carcinoma related to serous borderline tumors. Am J Surg Pathol 1996;20:1319–30.
18. Caduff RF, Svoboda-Newman SM, Ferguson AW, Johnston CM, Frank TS. Comparison of mutations of Ki-ras and p53 immunoreactivity in borderline and malignant epithelial ovarian tumors. Am J Surg Pathol 1999;23:323–8.
19. Cannistra SA. Cancer of the ovary. N Engl J Med 2004;351:2519–29.
20. Chu PG, Weiss LM. Keratin expression in human tissues and neoplasms. Histopathology 2002;40:403–39.
21. Chuaqui RF, Zhuang Z, Emmert-Buck MR, et al. Genetic analysis of synchronous mucinous tumors of the ovary and appendix. Hum Pathol 1996;27:165–71.
22. Clement PB, Young RH, Oliva E, Sumner HW, Scully RE. Hyperplastic mesothelial cells within abdominal lymph nodes: mimic of metastatic ovarian carcinoma and serous borderline tumor – a report of two cases associated with ovarian neoplasms. Mod Pathol 1996;9:879–86.
23. Cuatrecasas M, Matias-Guiu X, Prat J. Synchronous mucinous tumors of the appendix and the ovary associated with pseudomyxoma peritonei: a clinicopathologic study of six cases with comparative analysis of c-Ki-ras mutations. Am J Surg Pathol 1996;20:739–46.
24. Cuatrecasas M, Villanueva A, Matias-Guiu X, Prat J. K-ras mutations in mucinous ovarian tumors: a clinicopathologic and molecular study of 95 cases. Cancer 1997;79:1581–6.

25. De Nictolis M, Garbisa S, Lucarini G, et al. 72-KiloDalton type IV collagenase, type IV collagen, and Ki67 antigen in serous tumors of the ovary: a clinicopathologic, immunohistochemical and serological study. Int J Gynecol Pathol 1996;15:102–9.

26. De Nictolis M, Montironi R, Tommasoni S, et al. Serous borderline tumors of the ovary: a clinicopathologic, immunohistochemical and quantitative study of 44 cases. Cancer 1992;70:152–60.

27. De Nictolis M, Montironi R, Tommasoni S, et al. Benign, borderline and well-differentiated malignant intestinal mucinous tumors of the ovary: a clinicopathologic, histochemical, immunohistochemical and nuclear quantitative study of 57 cases. Int J Gynecol Pathol 1994;13:10–21.

28. Deavers MT, Gershenson DM, Tortolero-Luna G, Malpica A, Lu KH, Silva EG. Micropapillary and cribriform patterns in ovarian serous tumors of low malignant potential. A study of 99 advanced stage cases. Am J Surg Pathol 2002;26:1129–41.

29. Dubé V, Roy M, Plante M, Renaud MC, Tetu B. Mucinous ovarian tumors of Mullerian-type: an analysis of 17 cases including borderline tumors and intraepithelial, microinvasive, and invasive carcinomas. Int J Gynecol Pathol 2005;24:138–46.

30. Ehrmann RL, Federschneider JM, Knapp RC. Distinguishing lymph node metastases from benign glandular inclusions in low-grade ovarian carcinoma. Am J Obst Gynecol 1980;136:737–46.

31. Eichhorn JH, Bell DA, Young RH, Scully RE. Ovarian serous borderline tumors with micropapillary and cribriform patterns: a study of 40 cases and comparison with 44 cases without these patterns. Am J Surg Pathol 1999;23:397–409.

32. Elishaev E, Gilks CB, Miller D, Srodon M, Kurman RJ, Ronnett BM. Synchronous and metachronous endocervical and ovarian neoplasms: evidence supporting interpretation of the ovarian neoplasms as metastatic endocervical adenocarcinomas simulating primary ovarian surface epithelial neoplasms. Am J Surg Pathol 2005;29:281–94.

33. Gershenson DM. Contemporary treatment of borderline ovarian tumors. Cancer Invest 1999;17:206–10.

34. Gershenson DM, Silva EG, Levy L, Burke TW, Wolf JK, Tornos C. Ovarian serous borderline tumors with invasive peritoneal implants. Cancer 1998;82:1096–103.

35. Gershenson DM, Silva EG, Tortolero-Luna G, Levenback C, Morris M, Tornos C. Serous borderline tumors of the ovary with noninvasive peritoneal implants. Cancer 1998;83:2157–63.

36. Gilks CB, Alkushi A, Yue JJ, Lanvin D, Ehlen TG, Miller DM. Advanced-stage serous borderline tumors of the ovary: a clinicopathological study of 49 cases. Int J Gynecol Pathol 2003;22:29–36.

37. Gilks CB, Bell DA, Scully RE. Serous psammocarcinoma of the ovary and peritoneum. Int J Gynecol Pathol 1990;9:110–21.

38. Gough DB, Donohue JH, Schutt AJ, et al. Pseudomyxoma peritonei. Long-term patient survival with an aggressive regional approach. Ann Surg 1994;219:112–19.

39. Gu J, Roth LM, Younger C, et al. Molecular evidence for the independent origin of extra-ovarian papillary serous tumors of low malignant potential. J Natl Cancer Inst 2001;93:1147–52.

40. Guerrieri C, Hogberg T, Wingren S, Fristedt S, Simonsen E, Boeryd B. Mucinous borderline and malignant tumors of the ovary. A clinicopathologic and DNA ploidy study of 92 cases. Cancer 1994;74:2329–40.

41. Hart WR. Mucinous tumors of the ovary: A review. Int J Gynecol Pathol 2005;24:4–25.

42. Hart WR, Norris HJ. Borderline and malignant mucinous tumors of the ovary. Histologic criteria and clinical behavior. Cancer 1973;31:1031–45.

43. Healy DL, Burger HG, Mamers P, et al. Elevated serum inhibin concentrations in postmenopausal women with ovarian tumors. N Engl J Med 1993;329:1539–42.

44. Heintz AP, Odicino F, Maisonneuve P, et al. Carcinoma of the ovary. Int J Gynecol Obstet 2003;83S:133–66.

45. Ho CL, Kurman RJ, Dehari R, Wang TL, Shi Ie M. Mutations of BRAF and RAS precede the development of ovarian serous borderline tumors. Cancer Res 2004;64:6915–18.

46. Hoerl HD, Hart WR. Primary ovarian mucinous cystadenocarcinomas. A clinicopathologic study of 49 cases with long term follow-up. Am J Surg Pathol 1998;22:1449–62.

47. Hsu CY, Kurman RJ, Vang R, et al. Nuclear size distinguishes low- from high-grade ovarian serous carcinoma and predicts outcome. Hum Pathol 2005;36:1049–54.

48. Ichikawa Y, Nishida M, Suzuki H, et al. Mutation of K-ras proto-oncogene is associated with histological subtypes in human mucinous ovarian tumors. Cancer Res 1994;54:33–5.

49. Irving JA, Catasus L, Gallardo A, et al. Synchronous endometrioid carcinomas of the uterine corpus and ovary: Alterations in the beta-catenin (CTNNB1) pathway are associated with independent primary tumors and favorable prognosis. Hum Pathol 2005;36:605–19.

50. Ji H, Isacson C, Seidman J, Kurman RJ, Ronnett BM. Cytokeratins 7 and 20, Dpc4, and MUC5AC in the distinction of metastatic mucinous carcinomas in the ovary from primary ovarian mucinous tumors: Dpc4 assists in identifying metastatic pancreatic carcinomas. Int J Gynecol Pathol 2002;21:391–400.

51. Karp LA, Czernobilsky B. Glandular inclusions in pelvic and abdominal para-aortic lymph nodes. A study of autopsy and surgical material in males and females. Am J Clin Pathol 1969;52:212–18.

52. Katabuchi H, Tashiro H, Cho KR, Kurman RJ, Hedrick Ellenson L. Micropapillary serous carcinoma of the ovary: an immunohistochemical and mutational analysis of p53. Int J Gynecol Pathol 1998;17:54–60.

53. Kennedy AW, Hart WR. Ovarian papillary serous tumors of low malignant potential (serous borderline tumors). A long term follow-up study, including patients with microinvasion, lymph node metastasis, and transformation to invasive serous carcinoma. Cancer 1996;78:278–86.

54. Khunamornpong S, Russell P, Dalrymple JC. Proliferating (LMP) mucinous tumors of the ovaries with microinvasion: morphologic assessment of 13 cases. Int J Gynecol Pathol 1999;18:238–46.

55. Khunamornpong S, Suprasert P, Pojchamarnwiputh S, Na Chiangmai W, Settakorn J, Siriaungkul S. Primary and metastatic mucinous adenocarcinomas of the ovary: evaluation of the diagnostic approach using tumor size and laterality. Gynecol Oncol 2006;101:152–7.

56. Kim K-R, Lee H-I, Lee S-K, Ro JY, Robboy SJ. Is stromal microinvasion in primary mucinous ovarian tumors with 'mucin granuloma' true invasion? Am J Surg Pathol 2007;31:546–54.

57. Koonings PP, Campbell K, Mishell DR, Jr, Grimes DA. Relative frequency of primary ovarian neoplasms: a ten year review. Obstet Gynecol 1989;74:921–6.

58. Lau SK, Weiss LM, Chu PG. Differential expression of MUC1, MUC2 and MUC5AC in carcinomas of various sites: an immunohistochemical study. Am J Clinl Pathol 2004;122:61–9.

59. Leake JF, Rader JS, Woodruff JD, Rosenshein NB. Retroperitoneal lymphatic involvement with epithelial ovarian tumors of low malignant potential. Gynecol Oncol 1991;42:124–30.

60. Lee KR, Castrillon DH, Nucci MR. Pathologic findings in eight cases of ovarian serous borderline tumors, three with foci of serous carcinoma, that preceded death or morbidity from invasive carcinoma. Int J Gynecol Pathol 2001;20:329–34.

61. Lee KR, Nucci MR. Ovarian mucinous and mixed epithelial carcinomas of mullerian (endocervical-like) type: a clinicopathologic analysis of four cases of an uncommon variant associated with endometriosis. Int J Gynecol Pathol 2003;22:42–51.

62. Lee KR, Scully RE. Mucinous tumors of the ovary. A clinicopathologic study of 196 borderline tumors (of intestinal type) and carcinomas, including an evaluation of 11 cases with 'pseudomyxoma peritonei'. Am J Surg Pathol 2000;24:1447–64.

63. Lee KR, Tavassoli FA, Prat J, et al. Tumours of the ovary and peritoneum: surface epithelial–stromal tumours. In: Tavassoli FA, Devilee P, eds. World Health Organization Classification of Tumours. Pathology and Genetics of Tumours of the Breast and Female Genital Organs. Lyon: IARC Press; 2003.

64. Lee KR, Young RH. The distinction between primary and metastatic mucinous carcinomas of the ovary: gross and histologic findings in 50 cases. Am J Surg Pathol 2003;27:281–92.

65. Lee MJ, Lee HS, Kim WH, Choi Y, Yang M. Expression of mucins and cytokeratins in primary carcinomas of the digestive system. Mod Pathol 2003;16:403–10.

66. Leitao MM, Soslow RA, Baergen RN, Olvera N, Arroyo C, Boyd J. Mutation and expression of the TP53 gene in early stage epithelial ovarian carcinoma. Gynecol Oncol 2004;93:301–6.

67. Lim-Tan SK, Cajigas HE, Scully RE. Ovarian cystectomy for serous borderline tumors: a follow-up study of 35 cases. Obstet Gynecol 1988;72:775–81.

68. Lin PS, Gershenson DM, Bevers MW, Lucas KR, Burke TW, Silva EG. The current status of surgical staging of ovarian serous borderline tumors. Cancer 1999;85:905–11.

69. Longacre TA, McKenney JK, Tazelaar HD, Kempson RL, Hendrickson MR. Ovarian serous tumors of low malignant potential (borderline tumors). Outcome-based study of 276 patients with long-term (≥ 5-year) follow-up. Am J Surg Pathol 2005;29:707–23.

70. Look KY, Stehman FB, Moore DH, Sutton GP. Intraperitoneal 5-fluorouracil for pseudomyxoma peritonei. Int J Gynecol Cancer 1995;5:361–5.

71. Lu KH, Bell DA, Welch WR, Berkowitz PS, Mok SC. Evidence for the multifocal origin of bilateral and advanced human serous borderline ovarian tumors. Cancer Res 1998;58:2328–30.

72. Ludwick C, Gilks CB, Miller D, Yaziji H, Clement PB. Aggressive behavior of stage I ovarian mucinous tumors lacking extensive infiltrative invasion: a report of four cases and review of the literature. Int J Gynecol Pathol 2005;24:205–17.

73. Mandai M, Konishi I, Kuroda H, et al. Heterogeneous distribution of K-ras-mutated epithelia in mucinous ovarian tumors with special reference to histopathology. Hum Pathol 1998;28:34–40.

74. Marquette S, Amant F, Vergote I, Moerman P. Pseudomyxoma peritonei associated with a mucinous ovarian tumor arising from a mature cystic teratoma. A case report. Int J Gynecol Pathol 2006;25:340–3.

75. Matias-Guiu X, Prat J. Ovarian tumors with functioning stroma: an immunohistochemical study with hCG mono and polyclonal antibodies. Cancer 1990;65:2001–5.

76. McCaughey WTE, Kirk ME, Lester W, Dardick I. Peritoneal epithelial lesions associated with proliferative serous tumors of ovary. Histopathology 1984;8:195–208.

77. McKenney JK, Balzer BL, Longacre TA. Lymph node involvement in ovarian serous tumors of low malignant potential (borderline tumors): pathology, prognosis, and proposed classification. Am J Surg Pathol 2006;30:614–24.

78. McKenney JK, Balzer BL, Longacre TA. Patterns of stromal invasion in ovarian serous tumors of low malignant potential (borderline tumors): a reevaluation of the concept of stromal microinvasion. Am J Surg Pathol 2006;30:1209–21.
79. Miettinen M. Keratin 20: immunohistochemical marker for gastrointestinal, urothelial, and Merkel cell carcinomas. Mod Pathol 1995;8:384–8.
80. Misdraji J, Yantiss RK, Graeme-Cook FM, Balis UJ, Young RH. Appendiceal mucinous neoplasms. A clinicopathologic analysis of 107 cases. Am J Surg Pathol 2003;27:1089–103.
81. Mok SC, Bell DA, Knapp RC, et al. Mutation of K-ras protooncogene in human ovarian epithelial tumors of borderline malignancy. Cancer Research 1993;53:1489–92.
82. Moore WF, Bentley RC, Berchuck A, Robboy SJ. Some mullerian inclusion cysts in lymph nodes and peritoneum are metastases from serous borderline tumors of the ovary. Am J Surg Pathol 2000;24:710–18.
83. Muto MG, Welch WR, Mok SC, et al. Evidence for a multifocal origin of papillary serous carcinoma of the peritoneum. Cancer Res 1995;55:490–2.
84. Nayar R, Siriaunkgul S, Robbins KM, McGowan L, Ginzan S, Silverber SG. Microinvasion in low malignant potential tumors of the ovary. Hum Pathol 1996;27:521–7.
85. Nomura K, Aizawa S. Noninvasive, microinvasive, and invasive mucinous carcinomas of the ovary. A clinicopathologic analysis of 40 cases. Cancer 2000;89:1541–6.
86. Nomura K, Aizawa S. Clinicopathologic and mucin histochemical analyses of 90 cases of ovarian mucinous borderline tumors of intestinal and mullerian types. Pathol Int 1996;46:575–80.
87. O'Connell JT, Tomlinson JS, Roberts AA, McGonigle KF, Barsky SH. Pseudomyxoma peritonei is a disease of MUC2-expressing goblet cells. Am J Pathol 2002;161:551–64.
88. Ordonez NG. Role of immunohistochemistry in distinguishing epithelial peritoneal mesotheliomas from peritoneal and ovarian serous carcinomas. Am J Surg Pathol 1998;22:1203–14.
89. Papadimitriou DS, Martin-Hirsch P, Kitchener HC, Lolis DE, Dalkalitsis N, Paraskevaidis E. Recurrent borderline tumors after conservative treatment management in women wishing to retain their fertility. Eur J Gynecol Oncol 1999;20:94–7.
90. Park SY, Kim HS, Hong EK, Kim WH. Expression of cytokeratins 7 and 20 in primary carcinomas of the stomach and colorectum and their value in the differential diagnosis of metastatic carcinomas to the ovary. Hum Pathol 2002;33:1078–85.
91. Parker RL, Clement PB, Chercover DJ, et al. Early recurrence of ovarian serous borderline tumor as high-grade carcinoma: a report of two cases. Int J Gynecol Pathol 2004;23:265–72.
92. Pettersson F. Annual report of the results of treatment in gynecological cancer. Stockholm: International Federation of Gynecology and Obstetrics; 1991.
93. Powell DE, Puls L, van Nagell I. Current concepts in epithelial ovarian tumors: does benign to malignant transformation occur? Hum Pathol 1992;23:846–7.
94. Pranesh N, Menasce LP, Wilson MS, O'Dwyer ST. Pseudomyxoma peritonei: unusual origin from an ovarian mature cystic teratoma. J Clin Pathol 2005;58:1115–17.
95. Prat J. Ovarian tumors of borderline malignancy (tumors of low malignant potential): a critical appraisal. Adv Anat Pathol 1999;6:247–74.
96. Prat J. Pathology of the Ovary. Philadelphia: Saunders; 2004:83–109.
97. Prat J, de Nictolis M. Serous borderline tumors of the ovary. A long-term follow-up study of 137 cases, including 18 with micropapillary pattern and 20 with microinvasion. Am J Surg Pathol 2002;26:1111–28.
98. Prayson RA, Hart WR, Petras RE. Pseudomyxoma peritonei. A clinicopathologic study of 19 cases with emphasis on site of origin and nature of associated ovarian tumors. Am J Surg Pathol 1994;18:591–603.
99. Provenza C, Young RH, Prat J. Anaplastic carcinoma in mucinous ovarian tumors: A clinicopathologic study of 34 cases emphasizing the crucial impact of stage on prognosis, their histologic spectrum, and overlap with sarcoma-like mural nodules. Am J Surg Pathol 2008;32:383–9.
100. Riopel MA, Ronnett BM, Kurman RJ. Evaluation of diagnostic criteria and behavior of ovarian intestinal-type mucinous tumors. Atypical proliferative (borderline) tumors and intraepithelial, microinvasive, invasive and metastatic carcinomas. Am J Surg Pathol 1999;23:617–35.
101. Rodriguez IM, Irving JA, Prat J. Endocervical-like mucinous tumors of the ovary. A clinicopathologic analysis of 31 cases. Am J Surg Pathol 2004;28:1311–18.
102. Rodriguez IM, Prat J. Mucinous tumors of the ovary. A clinicopathologic analysis of 75 borderline tumors (of intestinal type) and carcinomas. Am J Surg Pathol 2002;26:139–52.
103. Rollins SE, Young RH, Bell DA. Autoimplants in serous borderline tumors of the ovary: a clinicopathologic study of 30 cases of a process to be distinguished from serous adenocarcinoma. Am J Surg Pathol 2006;30:457–62.
104. Ronnett BM, Kurman RJ, Zahn CM, et al. Pseudomyxoma peritonei in women: a clinicopathologic analysis of 30 cases with emphasis on site of origin, prognosis, and relationship to ovarian mucinous tumors of low malignant potential. Hum Pathol 1995;26:509–24.
105. Ronnett BM, Seidman JD. Mucinous tumors arising in ovarian mature cystic teratomas: relationship to the clinical syndrome of pseudomyxoma peritonei. Am J Surg Pathol 2003;27:650–7.

106. Ronnett BM, Shmookler BM, Diener-West M, Sugarbaker PH, Kurman RJ. Immunohistochemical evidence supporting the appendiceal origin of pseudomyxoma peritonei in women. Int J Gynecol Pathol 1997;16:1–9.
107. Ronnett BM, Yan H, Kurman RJ, et al. Patients with pseudomyxoma peritonei associated with disseminated peritoneal adenomucinosis have a significantly more favorable prognosis than patients with peritoneal mucinous carcinomatosis. Cancer 2001;92:85–91.
108. Rothacker D, Mobius G. Varieties of serous surface papillary carcinoma of the peritoneum in northern Germany: A thirty-year autopsy study. Int J Gynecol Pathol 1995;14:310–18.
109. Russell P. Borderline epithelial tumors of the ovary: a conceptual dilemma. Clin Obstet Gynecol 1984;11:259–77.
110. Rutgers JL, Scully RE. Ovarian müllerian mucinous papillary cystadenomas of borderline malignancy. A clinicopathologic analysis. Cancer 1988;61:340–8.
111. Rutgers JL, Scully RE. Ovarian mixed-epithelial papillary cystadenomas of borderline malignancy of müllerian type. A clinicopathologic analysis. Cancer 1988;61:546–54.
112. Schorge JO, Muto MG, Lee SJ, et al. BRCA1-related papillary serous carcinoma of the peritoneum has a unique molecular pathogenesis. Cancer Res 2000;60:1361–64.
113. Scully RE, Young RH, Clement PB. Tumors of the ovary, maldeveloped gonads, fallopian tube, and broad ligament. In: Rosai J, Sobin LH, eds. Atlas of Tumor Pathology, 3rd edn., Vol. 23. Washington, DC: Armed Forces Institute of Pathology; 1998.
114. Segal GH, Hart WR. Ovarian serous tumors of low malignant potential (serous borderline tumors). The relationship of exophytic surface tumor to peritoneal 'implants'. Am J Surg Pathol 1992;16:577–83.
115. Seidman JD, Elsayed AM, Sobin LH, Tavassoli FA. Association of mucinous tumors of the ovary and appendix. A clinicopathologic study of 25 cases. Am J Surg Pathol 1993;17:22–34.
116. Seidman JD, Kurman RJ. Subclassification of serous borderline tumors of the ovary into benign and malignant types. A clinicopathologic study of 65 advanced stage cases. Am J Surg Pathol 1996;20:1331–45.
117. Seidman JD, Kurman RJ. Ovarian serous borderline tumors: a critical review of the literature with emphasis on prognostic factors. Hum Pathol 2000;31:539–57.
118. Seidman JD, Kurman RJ, Ronnett BM. Primary and metastatic mucinous adenocarcinomas in the ovaries. Incidence in routine practice with a new approach to improve intraoperative diagnosis. Am J Surg Pathol 2003;27:985–93.
119. Shappell HW, Riopel MA, Smith Sehdev AE, Ronnett BM, Kurman RJ. Diagnostic criteria and behavior of ovarian seromucinous (endocervical-type mucinous and mixed cell-type) tumors: atypical proliferative (borderline) tumors, intraepithelial, microinvasive, and invasive carcinomas. Am J Surg Pathol 2002;26:1529–41.
120. Shimizu Y, Kamoi S, Amada S, Akiyama F, Silverberg SG. Toward the development of a universal grading system for ovarian epithelial carcinoma: testing of a proposed system in a series of 461 patients with uniform treatment and follow-up. Cancer 1998;82:893–901.
121. Sieben NLG, Kolkman-Uljee SM, Flanagan AM, et al. Molecular genetic evidence for monoclonal origin of bilateral ovarian serous borderline tumors. Am J Pathol 2003;162:1095–101.
122. Sieben NLG, Oosting J, Flanagan AM, et al. Differential gene expression in ovarian tumors reveals *Dusp-4* and *Serpina-5* as key regulators for benign behavior of serous borderline tumors. J Clin Oncol 2005;23:7257–64.
123. Sieben NLG, Roemen GMJM, Oosting J, Fleuren GJ, Engeland Mv, Prat J. Clonal analysis favours a monoclonal origin for serous borderline tumours with peritoneal implants. J Pathol 2006;210:405–11.
124. Silva EG, Tornos C, Zhuang Z, Merino MJ, Gershenson DM. Tumor recurrence in stage I ovarian serous neoplasms of low malignant potential. Int J Gynecol Pathol 1998;17:1–6.
125. Singer G, Kurman RJ, Chang H-W, Cho SKR, Shih I-M. Diverse tumorigenic pathways in ovarian serous carcinoma. Am J Pathol 2002;160:1223–28.
126. Singer G, Stöhr R, Cope L, et al. Patterns of p53 mutations separate ovarian serous borderline tumors and low- and high-grade carcinomas and provide support for a new model of ovarian carcinogenesis. A mutational analysis with immunohistochemical correlation. Am J Surg Pathol 2005;29:218–24.
127. Siriaunkgul S, Robbins KM, McGowan L, Silverberg SG. Ovarian mucinous tumors of low malignant potential: a clinicopathologic study of 54 tumors of intestinal and müllerian type. Int J Gynecol Pathol 1995;14:198–208.
128. Slomovitz BM, Caputo TA, Gretz HF, et al. A comparative analysis of 57 serous borderline tumors with and without a noninvasive micropapillary component. Am J Surg Pathol 2002;26:592–600.
129. Smith Sehdev AE, Sehdev PS, Kurman RJ. Noninvasive and invasive micropapillary (low-grade) serous carcinoma of the ovary. A clinicopathologic analysis of 135 cases. Am J Surg Pathol 2003;27:725–36.
130. Soslow RA, Rouse RV, Hendrickson MR, Silva EG, Longacre TA. Transitional cell neoplasms of the ovary and urinary bladder: a comparative immunohistochemical analysis. Int J Gynecol Pathol 1996;15:257–65.
131. Staebler A, Heselmeyer-Haddad K, Bell K, et al. Micropapillary serous carcinoma of the ovary has distinct patterns of chromosomal imbalances by comparative genomic hybridization compared with atypical proliferative serous tumors and serous carcinomas. Hum Pathol 2002;33:47–59.

132. Szych C, Staebler A, Connolly DC, Wu R, Cho KR, Ronnett BM. Molecular genetic evidence supporting the clonality and appendiceal origin of pseudomyxoma peritonei in women. Am J Pathol 1999;154:1849–55.
133. Tan LK, Flynn SD, Carcangiu ML. Ovarian serous borderline tumors with lymph node involvement. Clinicopathologic and DNA content study of seven cases and review of the literature. Am J Surg Pathol 1994;18:904–12.
134. Tavassoli FA. Serous tumor of low malignant potential with early stromal invasion (serous LMP with microinvasion). Mod Pathol 1988;1:407–13.
135. Tsao SW, Mok CH, Knapp RC, et al. Molecular genetic evidence of a unifocal origin for human serous ovarian carcinomas. Gynecol Oncol 1993;48:5–10.
136. Vang R, Gown AM, Barry TS, Wheeler DT, Ronnett BM. Ovarian atypical proliferative (borderline) mucinous tumors: gastrointestinal and seromucinous (endocervical-like) types are immunophenotypically distinctive. Int J Gynecol Pathol 2006;25:83–9.
137. Wauters CC, Smedts F, Gerrits LGM, Bosman FT, Ramaekers FC. Keratins 7 and 20 as diagnostic markers of carcinomas metastatic to the ovary. Hum Pathol 1995;26:852–5.
138. Wertheim I, Fleischhacker D, McLachlin CM, et al. Pseudomyxoma peritonei: a review of 23 cases. Obstet Gynecol 1994;84:17–21.
139. Yaziji H, Gown AM. Immunohistochemical analysis of gynecologic tumors. Int J Gynecol Pathol 2001;20:64–78.
140. Young RH, Gilks CB, Scully RE. Mucinous tumors of the appendix associated with mucinous tumors of the ovary and pseudomyxoma peritonei. A clinicopathological analysis of 22 cases supporting an origin in the appendix. Am J Surg Pathol 1991;15:415–29.
141. Young RH, Hart WR. Metastases from carcinomas of the pancreas simulating primary mucinous tumors of the ovary: a report of seven cases. Am J Surg Pathol 1989;13:748–56.
142. Zanotti KM, Hart WR, Kennedy AW, Belinson JL, Casey G. Allelic imbalance on chromosome 17p13 in borderline (low malignant potential) ovarian epithelial tumors. Int J Gynecol Pathol 1999;18:247–53.
143. Zuna RE, Behrens A. Peritoneal washing cytology in gynecologic cancers. J Natl Cancer Inst 1996;88:980–7.

Ovarian endometrioid, clear cell, Brenner, and rare epithelial–stromal tumors

25

Jaime Prat

ENDOMETRIOID TUMORS

Definition

Endometrioid tumors of the ovary resemble those encountered more frequently in the endometrium.[41,78] They include endometrioid carcinomas, endometrioid stromal sarcomas, adenosarcomas, and malignant müllerian mixed tumors (carcinosarcomas). Endometrioid carcinomas are the most common. Although an origin from endometriosis can be demonstrated in some cases, it is not required for the diagnosis (almost all müllerian tumors can originate from endometriosis).[41,78] Recent molecular genetic studies, however, suggest that most endometrioid cancers arise by the malignant transformation of endometriosis and not the ovarian surface epithelium.[33,56,77]

The epithelial cells of endometrioid tumors resemble those of proliferative endometrium. Diastase-periodic acid-Schiff (PAS), and mucicarmine staining reveal some extracellular mucin plus staining of the luminal glycocalyx. Ten per cent of tumors contain Grimelius-positive argyrophil cells. Secretory changes similar to those seen in postovulatory endometrium are frequently seen in well-differentiated tumors and squamous elements are common. Most endometrioid ovarian carcinomas are moderately or well differentiated since, when poorly differentiated, they are often classified as serous carcinomas. The Systematized Nomenclature of Medicine (SNOMED) classification of endometrioid tumors is as follows:

- Adenofibroma
  - cystadenofibroma
- Cystadenoma
- Endometrioid borderline tumor
- Endometrioid adenocarcinoma, not otherwise specified
  - malignant adenofibroma (adenocarcinofibroma)
  - variant with squamous differentiation
  - ciliated variant
  - oxyphilic variant
  - secretory variant
  - sertoliform variant
- Malignant mesodermal (müllerian) mixed tumor (carcinosarcoma)
- Adenosarcoma
- Endometrioid stromal and undifferentiated sarcoma.

EPITHELIAL TUMORS

Clinical features

Endometrioid epithelial tumors represent 2–4% of all ovarian tumors.[78] Benign endometrioid tumors (mostly adenofibromas) are rare and account for <1% of benign ovarian tumors. Only 2–3% of borderline ovarian tumors are endometrioid. Endometrioid carcinomas account for 10–20% of ovarian carcinomas, representing the second most common form of ovarian epithelial malignancy.[78]

Benign, borderline, and malignant endometrioid epithelial tumors occur most commonly in women in the perimenopausal or postmenopausal age groups, with mean ages of 56, 51, and 56 years, respectively.[78] About 40% of endometrioid carcinomas are associated with documented ipsilateral ovarian or pelvic endometriosis.[27,78] Patients whose tumors occur in association with endometriosis are, on average, 5–10 years younger than patients without associated ovarian endometriosis.[53,76,78] Endometriosis-related ovarian carcinomas are more frequently low grade and low stage and have a more favorable prognosis than carcinomas unrelated to endometriosis.[10] Endometrioid carcinomas are confined to the ovaries and adjacent pelvic structures in 70% of cases. They are bilateral in 28% of all cases and in 13% of those in FIGO stages 1–2.

Endometrioid carcinoma of the ovary is associated in 15–20% of cases with carcinoma of the endometrium.[31,78] The favorable outcome in those cases in which the tumor is limited to both organs suggests that these neoplasms are mostly independent primary tumors arising as a result of a müllerian field effect.[23,31] The criteria for distinguishing ovarian endometrioid carcinoma with spread to the corpus, the opposite situation, and independent primary tumors of both organs are presented below.

Like most ovarian carcinomas, many endometrioid carcinomas are asymptomatic. Some present as a pelvic mass with or without pain, and may be associated with endocrine symptoms secondary to steroid hormone secretion by the specialized ovarian stroma.[50] Serum CA125 is elevated in over 80% of the cases.[40]

Pathogenesis

The frequent association of ovarian endometrioid carcinomas with endometriosis (Figure 25.1), endometrial carcinoma, or both, suggests that some ovarian endometrioid carcinomas may have the same risk factors for their development as endo-

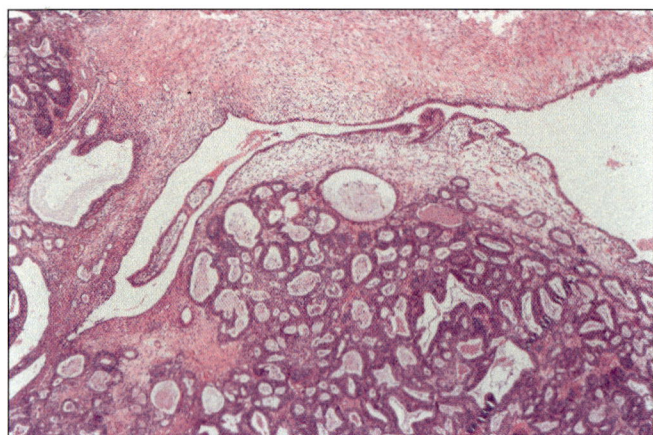

Fig. 25.1   Well-differentiated endometrioid adenocarcinoma arising from an endometriotic cyst.

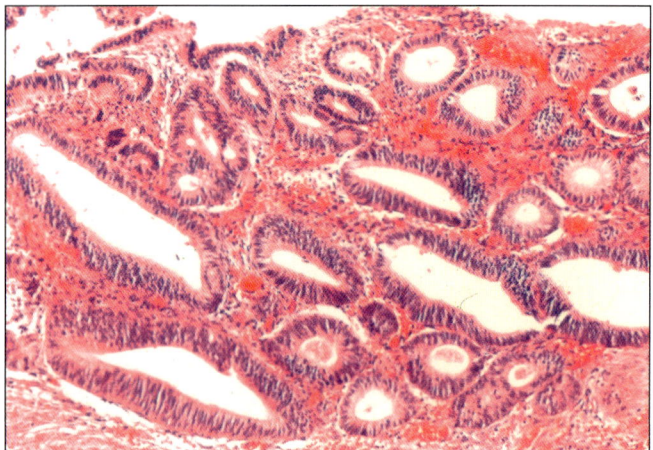

Fig. 25.2   Endometrial hyperplasia in endometriotic cyst.

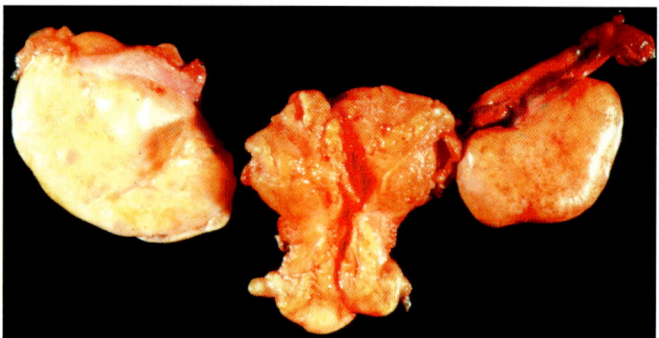

Fig. 25.3   Bilateral endometrioid adenofibroma.

The rare endometrioid cystadenomas are similar to endometriotic cysts but lack endometrial stroma, hemosiderin-laden macrophages, and a myofibroblastic wall. Nevertheless, their frequent merging with endometriotic cysts suggests that a pure endometrioid cystadenoma may not even exist. Adenofibromas have non-mucinous glands lying within an abundant fibromatous stroma. Tall columnar epithelium resembles that of proliferative endometrium, with basophilic to deeply eosinophilic cytoplasm and elongate nuclei with relatively coarse chromatin and small but obvious nucleoli, or inactive endometrium with uniform dark nuclei and scanty cytoplasm. Mitoses are rarely seen. Squamous differentiation in the form of morules is a common finding.[41,78]

BORDERLINE ENDOMETRIOID TUMORS

Pathology

Borderline endometrioid tumors may appear as either multilocular cystadenofibromas similar to benign tumors or cystic tumors with solid but friable mural nodules.

There is no agreement on the criteria for the diagnosis of endometrioid tumors of borderline malignancy. Most are adenofibromatous and show crowded endometrial-like glands and cystic spaces embedded in stroma that varies from ovarian to hyaline or collagenous (Figure 25.4). By WHO criteria, these tumors exhibit glands or cysts lined by atypical or cytologically malignant endometrioid-type cells without obvious stromal invasion (Figure 25.5).[41] Mitoses range up to 4 mitotic figures per 10 high-power fields (HPFs) but are rarely atypical. Squamous metaplasia, present in one-third to one-half of cases, may occasionally be both florid and keratinizing (Figure 25.6). It may give rise to a foreign-body, giant cell reaction. Stromal luteinization occasionally occurs. An uncommon stromal change is focal metaplastic benign bone formation. When the epithelial component is carcinomatous the term borderline endometrioid tumor with *intraepithelial carcinoma* is used and the tumor is graded 1–3 (Figure 25.5). Microinvasion is arbitrarily defined as the presence of one or more foci of epithelial cells haphazardly infiltrating the stroma, 10 mm² or less in area.[78] Tumors exhibiting confluent glandular growth (5 mm or more in maximum diameter) and destructive stromal invasion greater than microinvasion are diagnosed as invasive carcinomas. Cytologic atypia and microinvasion do not appear to affect the favorable prognosis of borderline endometrioid tumors and conservative treatment, i.e., unilateral salpingo-oophorectomy, appears to be curative. However, only a few cases have been reported and clinical follow-up data are limited.[6]

metrial carcinomas. Up to 42% of endometrioid carcinomas are associated with ipsilateral ovarian or pelvic endometriosis,[53] an entity in which the entire spectrum of endometrial hyperplasia can be seen (Figure 25.2)[27] (see Chapter 20). Several epidemiologic studies have shown that ovarian endometriosis is associated with an increased risk of developing ovarian endometrioid and clear cell carcinomas.[9,10,22,84] Atypical ipsilateral endometriosis occurs in up to 23% of endometrioid carcinomas and may have a role in the process of transformation to malignancy.[27] Not infrequently, the lining epithelium of endometriotic cysts shows large cells with abundant eosinophilic cytoplasm and large, hyperchromatic, smudgy nuclei. This cytologic change is often seen in the absence of carcinoma and its malignant potential is unknown.[80]

BENIGN ENDOMETRIOID TUMORS

Most benign endometrioid tumors are unilateral endometrioid adenofibromas. These rare tumors have a mean size of about 10 cm in diameter, and about one-sixth are bilateral (Figure 25.3). The external surface is smooth and the cut surface is firm and densely fibrous displaying variably sized cystic spaces. The cysts contain clear or yellowish fluid. Occasionally, the tumors are predominantly cystic.

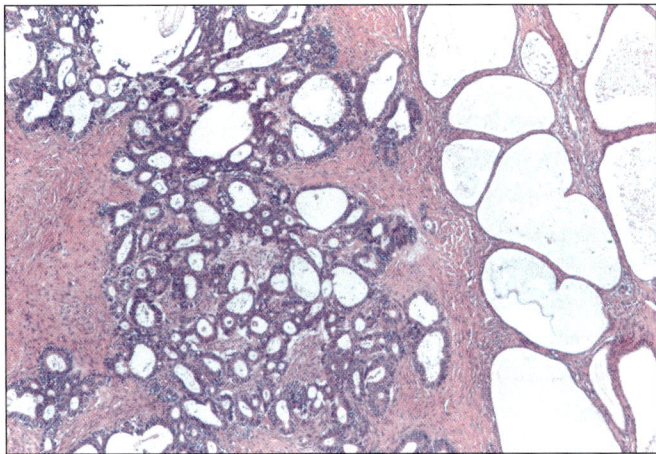

Fig. 25.4 Borderline endometrioid adenofibroma. Crowded endometrial-like glands and cystic spaces are embedded in dense fibrous stroma.

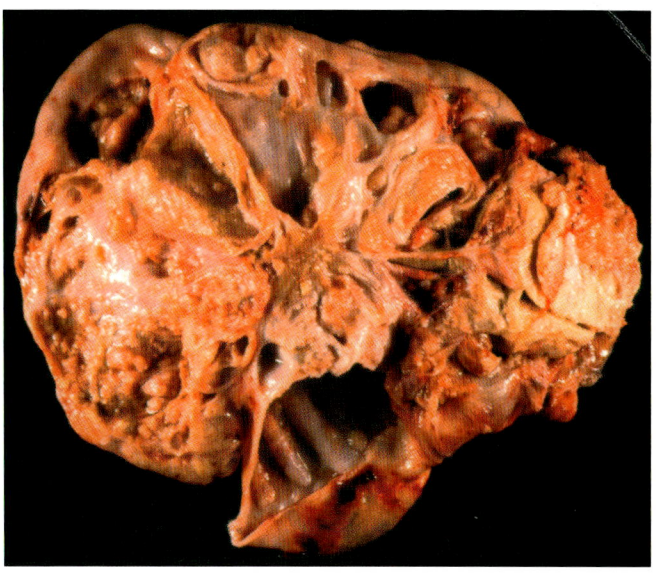

Fig. 25.7 Endometrioid adenocarcinoma. The solid and cystic tumor shows polypoid masses with focal necrosis.

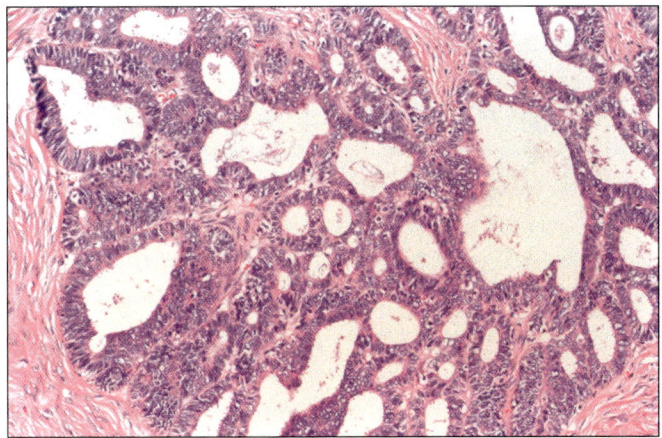

Fig. 25.5 Borderline endometrioid adenofibroma with well-differentiated (grade 1) intraepithelial carcinoma. Well-demarcated cribriform islands without obvious stromal invasion.

Immunohistochemistry and somatic genetics

The immunohistochemical profile of borderline endometrioid tumors resembles that of endometrioid carcinomas (see below). In both, β-catenin gene mutation appears to be an early event in tumorigenesis.[59] In a study of eight borderline endometrioid tumors, a strong nuclear β-catenin immunoreaction (both in the glandular and squamous components) was obtained in all cases, and seven (90%) had β-catenin gene (*CTNNB1*) mutations. This slight discrepancy could be attributed to technical problems, limiting the mutational analysis to exon 3, or alterations in other genes that may interfere with β-catenin levels. Only one tumor had a *PTEN* mutation. Neither *K-ras* mutations nor microsatellite instability (MI) were encountered.

ENDOMETRIOID CARCINOMAS

Macroscopic features

Endometrioid carcinomas are predominantly cystic, measuring 12–20 cm in diameter, with usually smooth outer surfaces. The cut surfaces reveal friable soft masses or papillae partly filling cystic spaces that may contain bloodstained fluid (Figure 25.7). Rarely, they are completely solid, exhibiting hemorrhage or necrosis. Mucus may sometimes fill the cystic spaces. The tumor, if it has arisen in an endometriotic cyst, tends to be a polypoid nodule projecting into the lumen of a thick-walled, blood-filled cyst (Figure 25.8).

Microscopic features

Ovarian endometrioid carcinomas closely resemble endometrioid carcinomas of the uterine corpus. Most are well differentiated – particularly those arising from endometriotic cysts – and show round, oval, or tubular glands lined by stratified non-mucin-containing epithelium (Figures 25.9 and 25.10). Mitoses range up to about 5 per 10 HPFs. Cribriform or villoglandular patterns may be present (Figure 25.11). The broad blunt papillae with obvious connective tissue cores differ from the usually fine micropapillae of serous carcinomas. Squamous differentiation occurs in 30–50% of the cases, often in the form of morules

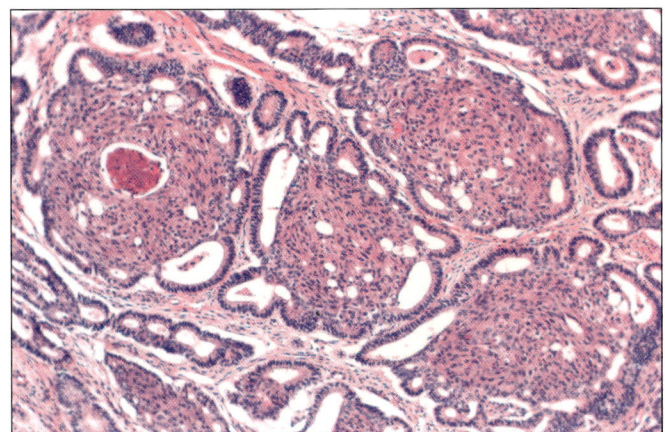

Fig. 25.6 Borderline endometrioid adenofibroma. Squamous morules with occasional central necrosis partly replace endometrioid glands. Reproduced from Prat,[68] with permission from Lippincott Williams & Wilkins.

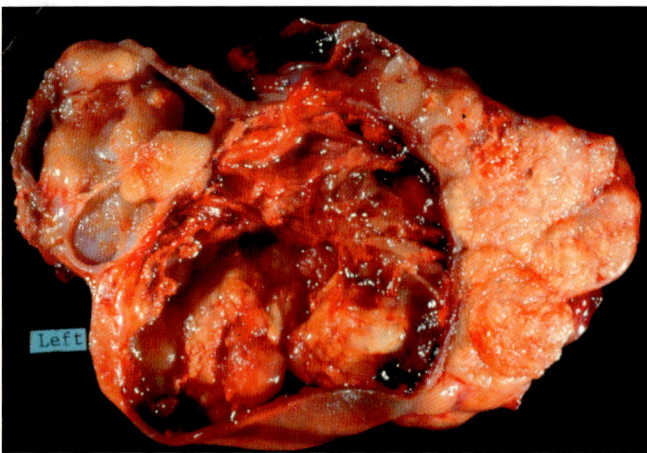

Fig. 25.8 Endometrioid adenocarcinoma arising from an endometriotic cyst. The polypoid tumor protrudes from the inner surface of the sectioned cyst and has extended through the capsule.

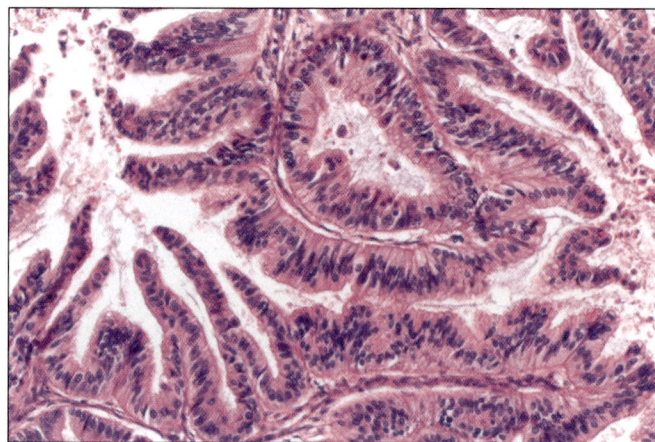

Fig. 25.11 Well-differentiated endometrioid adenocarcinoma with villoglandular architecture. Reproduced with permission from Prat.[69]

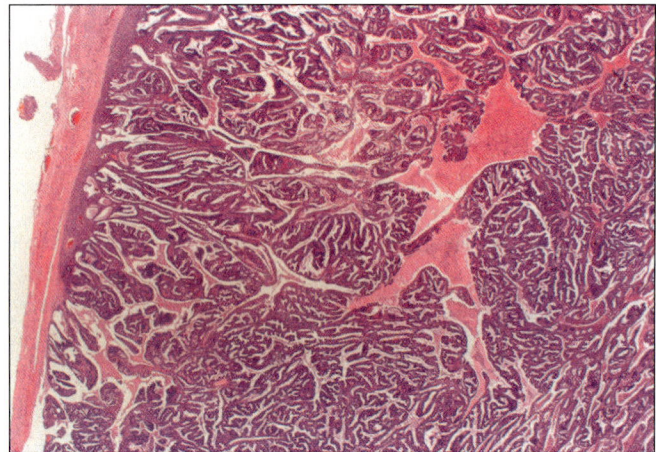

Fig. 25.9 Well-differentiated endometrioid adenocarcinoma (grade 1). The tumor shows a villoglandular pattern.

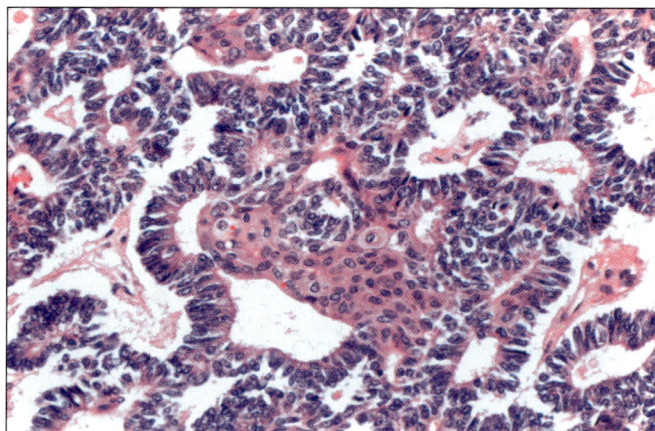

Fig. 25.12 Well-differentiated endometrioid adenocarcinoma. There is squamous differentiation in the form of squamous morules.

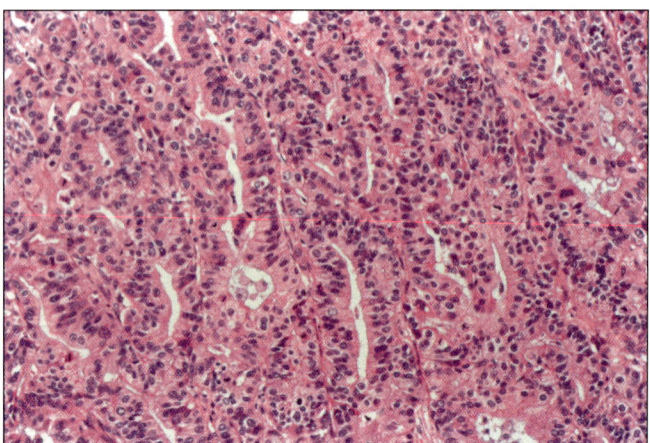

Fig. 25.10 Endometrioid adenocarcinoma. The crowded neoplastic glands are lined by stratified non-mucin-containing epithelium. Nuclear atypia is moderate.

(cytologically benign-appearing squamous cells) (Figure 25.12).[78] Occasionally, the squamous elements appear malignant and are then intimately admixed with or separated from the glandular component. The current designation 'endometrioid carcinoma with squamous differentiation' is generally preferable to adenoacanthoma or adenosquamous carcinoma, even though the latter terms in many cases more succinctly convey the degree of histologic differentiation of the squamous epithelium.[41,78] Aggregates of spindle-shaped epithelial cells are an occasional finding in endometrioid carcinoma (Figure 25.13).[86] Rarely, the spindle cell nests undergo a transition to clearly recognizable squamous cells suggesting that the former may represent abortive squamous differentiation.[89] Some well-differentiated endometrioid carcinomas, almost always with a squamous component, may have a prominent fibrous stroma (malignant adenofibromas). Stromal invasion in such tumors is difficult to document and inferred only by the extent and complexity of the glandular component and the presence of a desmoplastic stroma.

Rare examples of mucin-rich (Figure 25.14), secretory, ciliated cell, and oxyphilic types have been described.[17,67] In the mucin-rich variant, glandular lumens and apex of the cell cytoplasm are occupied by mucin.[2] The secretory type contains vacuolated cells with supranuclear and/or subnuclear vacuoles

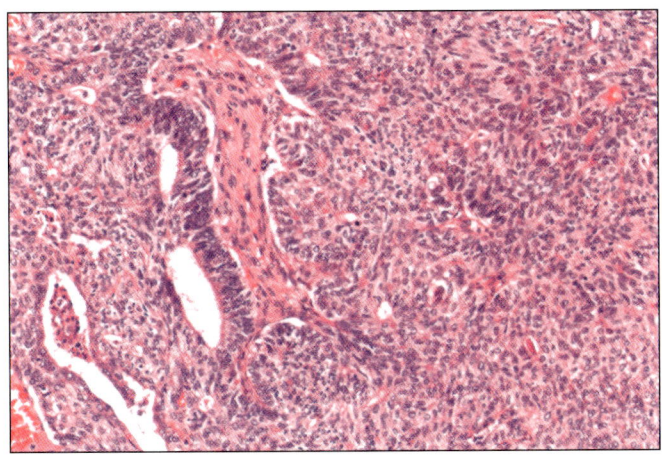

Fig. 25.13 Endometrioid adenocarcinoma with spindle-shaped epithelial cells. The spindle-shaped cells merge almost imperceptibly with the glandular epithelium (abortive squamous differentiation). Reproduced with permission from Prat.[69]

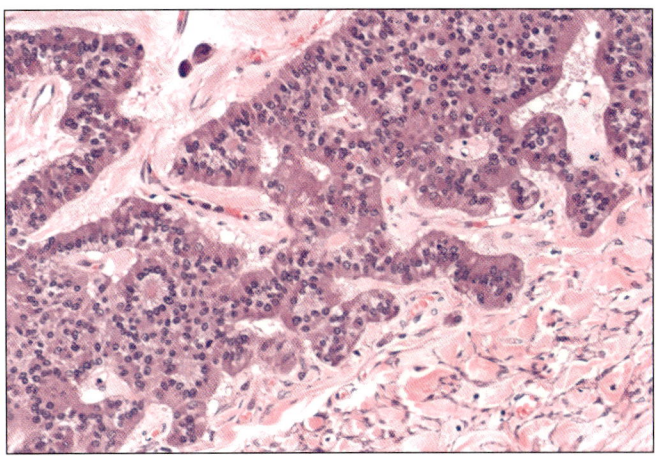

Fig. 25.15 Endometrioid adenocarcinoma resembling a granulosa cell tumor. The tumor cells are arranged in islands and line small glands simulating Call–Exner bodies. The microglands contain eosinophilic secretion. The nuclei are round and hyperchromatic. Reproduced with permission from Prat.[69]

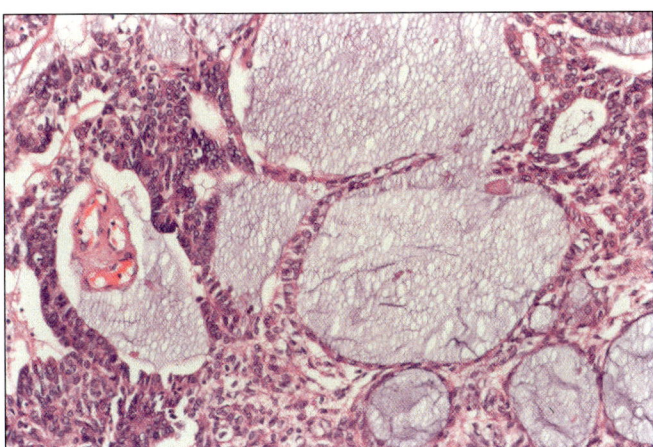

Fig. 25.14 Endometrioid adenocarcinoma, mucin-rich form. The glands are filled with mucin.

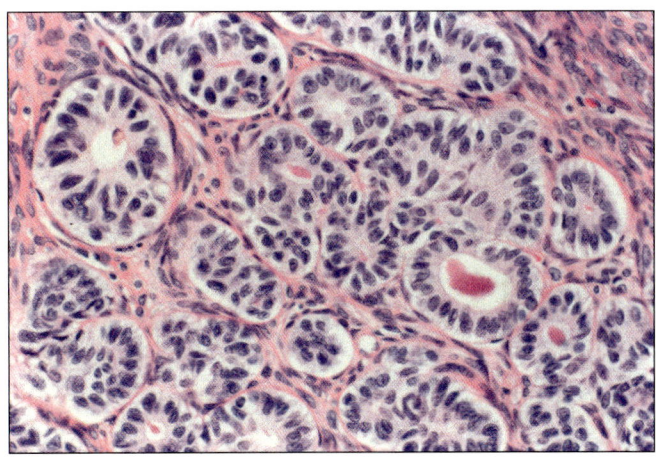

Fig. 25.16 Endometrioid adenocarcinoma resembling a Sertoli cell tumor. Tubular glands lined by cells with oval nuclei and clear cytoplasm, resembling the tubules of a Sertoli cell tumor.

resembling those of an early secretory endometrium.[78] Hobnail cells are not seen. The oxyphilic variant has a prominent component of large polygonal tumor cells with abundant eosinophilic cytoplasm and round central nuclei with prominent nucleoli.[67]

Occasional tumors contain solid areas punctuated by tubular or round glands or small rosette-like glands (microglandular pattern) simulating an adult granulosa cell tumor (Figure 25.15).[95] Unlike the Call–Exner bodies found in granulosa cell tumors, the microglands in endometrioid carcinomas contain intraluminal mucin. The nuclei of endometrioid carcinomas are usually round and hyperchromatic, whereas those of granulosa cell tumors are round, oval, or angular, pale and grooved[95] (see Chapter 26). Rare cases of endometrioid carcinomas of the ovary show focal to extensive areas resembling Sertoli and Sertoli–Leydig cell tumors (Figures 25.16 and 25.17).[60,75,95] They contain small, well-differentiated hollow tubules, solid tubules or, rarely, thin cords resembling sex cords. When the stroma is luteinized (Figure 25.18), this variant may be mistaken for a Sertoli–Leydig cell tumor, particularly if the patient is virilized. Nevertheless, typical glands of endometrioid carci-

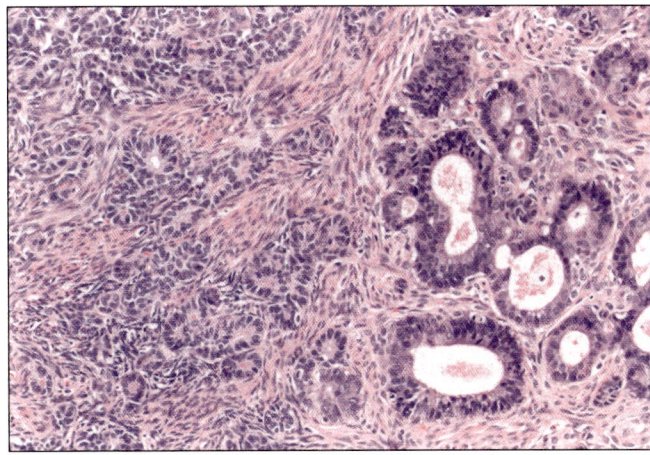

Fig. 25.17 Endometrioid adenocarcinoma resembling a Sertoli cell tumor. The small tubular glands, resembling the tubules of a Sertoli cell tumor (left), appear adjacent to typical glands of endometrioid carcinoma (right).

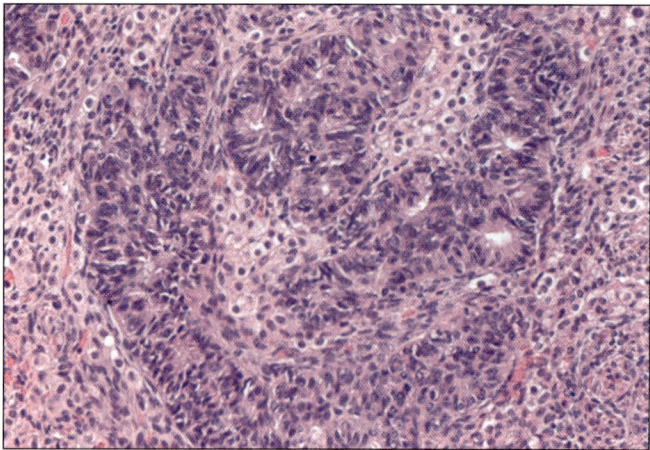

Fig. 25.18 Endometrioid adenocarcinoma resembling a Sertoli–Leydig cell tumor. The tubular glands contain high-grade nuclei. The luteinized ovarian stromal cells resemble Leydig cells.

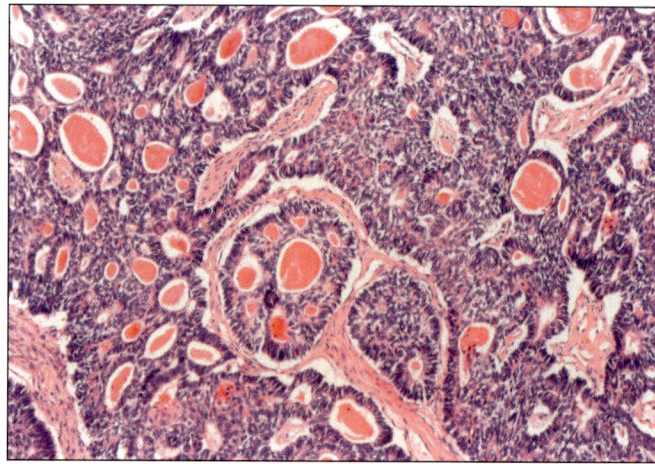

Fig. 25.20 Endometrioid carcinoma. The tumor exhibits an adenoid basal carcinoma component.

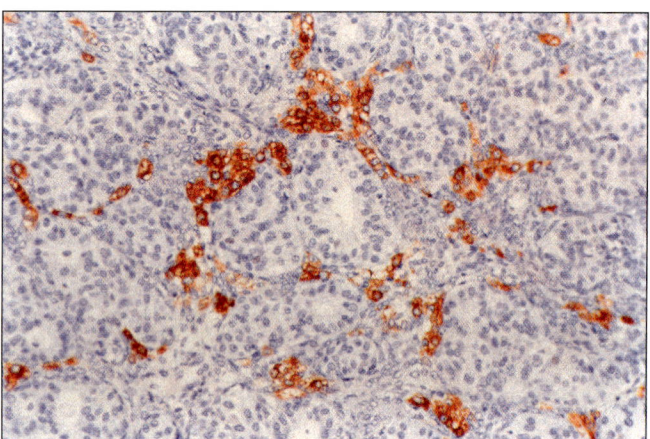

Fig. 25.19 Endometrioid adenocarcinoma resembling a Sertoli–Leydig cell tumor. Immunoreaction for α-inhibin is positive in the luteinized stromal cells and negative in the epithelial cells.

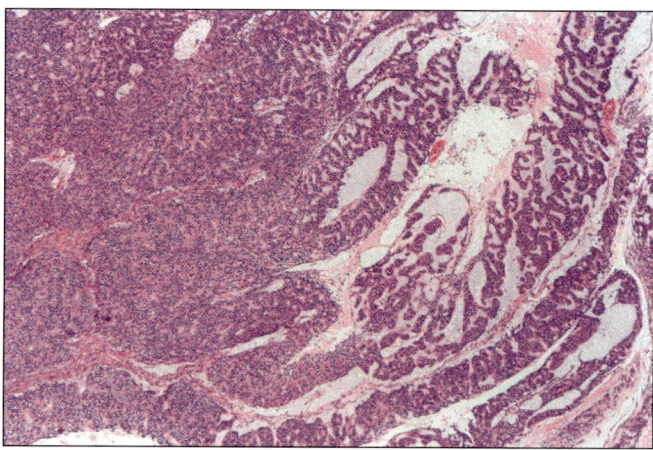

Fig. 25.21 Adenoid cystic-like component in endometrioid carcinoma.

noma and squamous differentiation are each present in 75% of the tumors, facilitating their recognition as an endometrioid carcinoma.[95] Furthermore, immunostains for α-inhibin (Figure 25.19) and calretinin show reactivity in Sertoli cells but not in the cells of endometrioid carcinoma.[49]

Poorly differentiated endometrioid carcinomas have a predominantly solid pattern with focal microglandular areas. Mitotic activity is high (up to 5 or more mitoses per HPF) and squamous or secretory change is rare. Hemorrhage and/or necrosis are prominent.

Approximately one-third of ovarian carcinomas with a predominantly endometrioid component are mixed with other epithelial types such as clear cell and serous carcinoma. Generally, a mixed epithelial tumor is diagnosed when 10% or more of a second or third type of epithelium is present.[41] Rarely, endometrioid carcinomas may exhibit an adenoid basal (Figure 25.20) or adenoid cystic-like component (Figure 25.21). About 10% of endometrioid carcinomas contain argyrophilic cells of neuroendocrine type. Occasionally, bone metaplasia can be found.

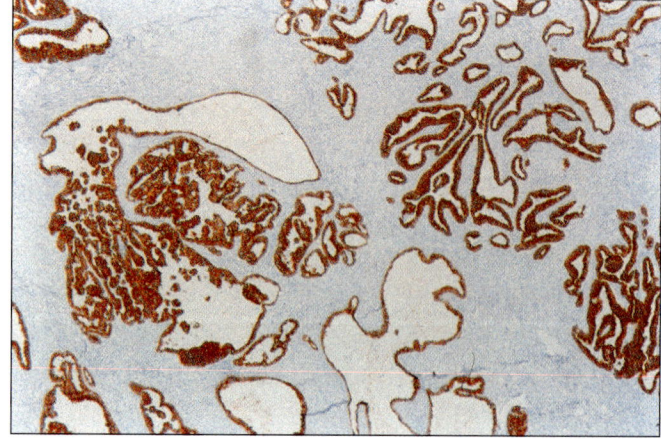

Fig. 25.22 Endometrioid adenocarcinoma with reactivity for cytokeratin 7.

Immunohistochemistry

Endometrioid carcinomas are immunoreactive for cytokeratins (CK7, 97%; CK20, 13%) (Figures 25.22 and 25.23), epithelial membrane antigen (EMA), B72.3, CA125 (76%), and estrogen and progesterone receptors. Some are also reactive for carcino-

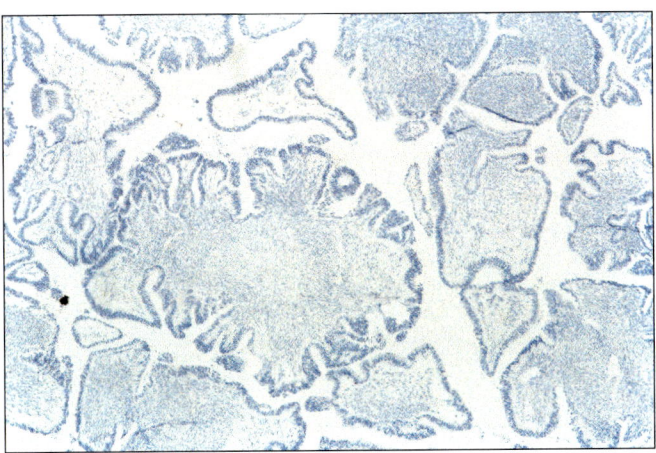

Fig. 25.23 Endometrioid adenocarcinoma with no reactivity for cytokeratin 20.

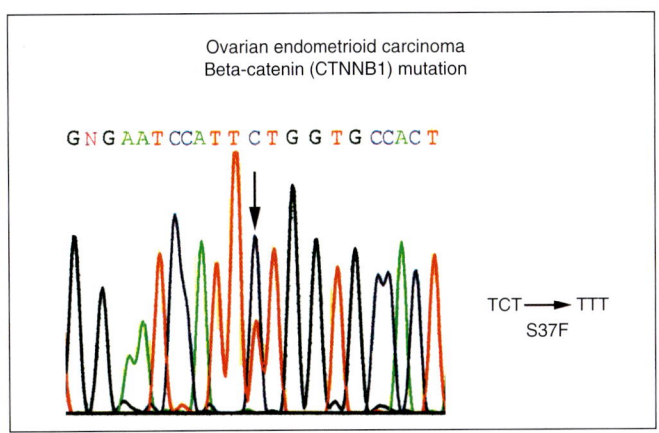

Fig. 25.25 Endometrioid adenocarcinoma. DNA sequencing of exon 3 of the β-catenin (*CTNNB1*) gene discloses a TCT to TTT point mutation at codon 37 (S37F). Reproduced with permision from Prat.[69]

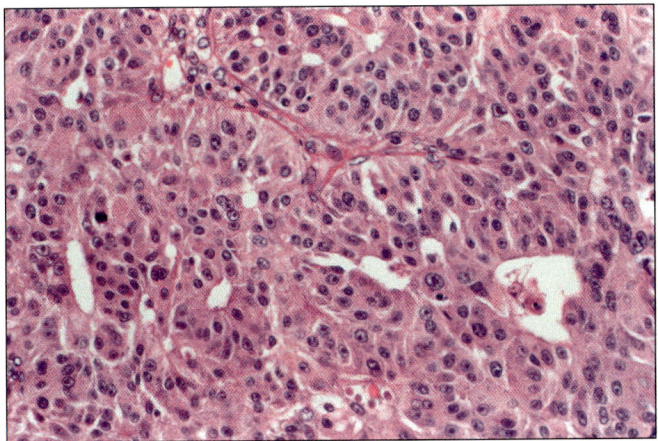

Fig. 25.24 Endometrioid carcinoma, predominantly solid, with grade 3 nuclei.

embryonic antigen (CEA) (30%) and vimentin. Alpha-inhibin is usually negative.[3,49]

Grading

Grading of endometrioid carcinoma of the ovary uses the same criteria as for endometrial adenocarcinoma.[96] Grade 1 tumors are glandular or papillary neoplasms exhibiting <5% of solid tumor growth (Figure 25.10). Grade 2 tumors show 5–50% solid growth, and grade 3 tumors show >50% solid tumor growth (Figure 25.24). Areas of squamous or spindle cell differentiation are not counted as solid growth. When the nuclei are highly atypical and the architectural glandular pattern is grade 1 or 2, the overall tumor grade is increased by one.

Spread and metastasis

Stage 1 carcinomas are bilateral in 17% of cases. The stage distribution of endometrioid carcinomas differs from that of serous carcinomas. According to the FIGO annual report, 31% of the tumors are stage 1, 20% stage 2, 38% stage 3, and 11% stage 4.[65] However, in a recent review of 874 cases from 19 series, 43% of the tumors were stage 1.[6]

Genetic susceptibility

Most endometrioid carcinomas occur sporadically but occasional cases develop in families with germline mutations in DNA mismatch repair genes, mainly *MSH-2* and *MLH-1* (Muir–Torre syndrome).[45] This syndrome, a variant of the hereditary non-polyposis colorectal cancer syndrome, reflects an inherited autosomal dominant susceptibility to develop cutaneous and visceral neoplasms.[83]

Somatic genetics

Somatic mutations of the β-catenin (*CTNNB1*) and *PTEN* genes are the most common genetic abnormalities identified in sporadic ovarian endometrioid carcinomas. Compared with uterine endometrioid carcinomas, the ovarian tumors have similar frequency of β-catenin abnormalities but a lower rate of MI and *PTEN* alterations.[11] Beta-catenin protein, encoded by the *CTNNB1* gene located in 3p21, maintains cell polarity by interacting with E-cadherin at the cell membrane. In the cytoplasm, free β-catenin interacts with APC (adenomatous polyposis coli) protein and may function as a transcription factor. Abnormal nuclear β-catenin accumulation resulting from mutations in *CTNNB1* and related genes produces transcriptional activation through the LEF/Tcf pathway. The APC protein downregulates β-catenin by cooperating with the glycogen synthase kinase 3-beta (GSK3-β), inducing phosphorylation of the serine–threonine residues coded in exon 3 of the *CTNNB1* gene and its degradation through the ubiquitin–proteasome pathway. *CTNNB1* mutations alter recognition sequences and inhibit phosphorylation, resulting in cytoplasmic and nuclear accumulation of β-catenin, signal transduction, and transcriptional activation. Increased β-catenin immunoexpression caused by *CTNNB1* or *APC* mutations results in uncontrolled activation of target gene expression such as matrix metalloproteinase-7 (*MMP-7*), and cyclin D1 (*CD1*). The frequencies of *CTNNB1* mutations range from 38 to 50% (Figure 25.25).[11,54,64] Beta-catenin is immunohistochemically detectable in carcinoma cells in more than 80% of the cases. Endometrioid carcinomas with β-catenin mutations usually are early stage tumors associated with good prognosis.[11,28]

PTEN/MMAC1/TEP1 tumor suppressor gene is located in chromosome 10q23.3, a genomic region undergoing loss of

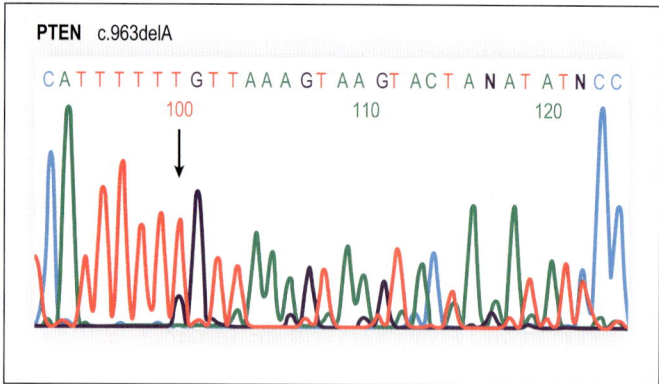

Fig. 25.26 Endometrioid adenocarcinoma. Partial representative nucleotide sequencing of antisense strand around the (A)₆ tract in exon 8 of *PTEN*. Sequence analysis of the polymerase chain reaction product of tumor DNA showed the deletion of one nucleotide in the polyA tract. Reproduced with permission from Irving et al.[31]

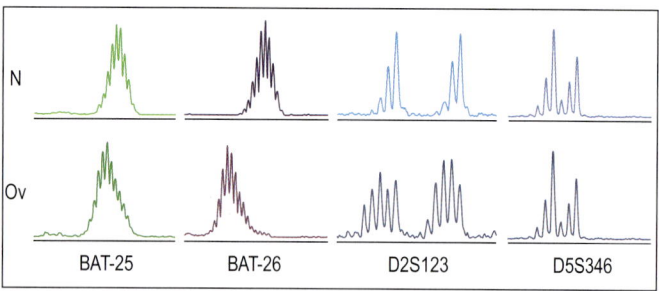

Fig. 25.27 Endometrioid adenocarcinoma. Microsatellite instability for the loci BAT-25, BAT-26, D2S123, and D5S346 (capillary electrophoresis).

heterozygosity (LOH) in a wide variety of human cancers. *PTEN* encodes a phosphatase that antagonizes the PI3K/AKT pathway by dephosphorylating PIP₃, the product of PI3K. Decreased *PTEN* activity causes increased cell proliferation and survival through modulation of signal transduction pathways. *PTEN* may be inactivated by several mechanisms such as mutation, LOH at 10q23, and promoter hypermethylation. Loss of function of the two alleles is needed for *PTEN* inactivation and, usually, mutation and LOH coexist. *PTEN* is mutated in approximately 20% of endometrioid ovarian tumors (Figure 25.26) and in 46% of those with 10q23 LOH.[11,56] *PTEN* mutations occur between exons 3 and 8. The majority of endometrioid carcinomas with *PTEN* mutations are well differentiated and stage 1 tumors, suggesting that *PTEN* inactivation is an early event in this subset of ovarian tumors.[11,56] The finding of 10q23 LOH and *PTEN* mutations in endometriotic cysts that are adjacent to endometrioid carcinomas with similar genetic alterations provides additional evidence for the precursor role of endometriosis in ovarian carcinogenesis.[77]

Microsatellite instability also occurs in sporadic endometrioid carcinomas of the ovary (Figure 25.27) although less frequently than in uterine endometrioid carcinomas. The reported frequency in the ovary ranges from 12.5 to 19%.[11,30,54] Like endometrial carcinomas, many ovarian carcinomas with MI follow the same process of *MLH-1* promoter methylation and frameshift mutations at coding mononucleotide repeat microsatellites.[11,30] For a fuller description, see Reference 11.

Differential diagnosis

The distinction of endometrioid tumors from serous and mucinous neoplasms has been discussed in Chapter 24.

1. *Endometrioid adenofibroma vs Brenner tumor*: Both tumors exhibit a prominent fibrous stromal component. Endometrioid tumors generally have an epithelial component in the form of glands with lumens, whereas in Brenner tumors the epithelial component typically consists of branching nests and trabeculae of transitional cells; a glandular component, if present in the Brenner tumor, is frequently mucinous. Nuclear grooves, characteristic of the transitional cells of Brenner tumors, are not found in squamous morules.

2. Endometrioid adenocarcinoma, secretory type, vs clear cell adenocarcinoma: The secretory form of endometrioid adenocarcinoma displays glands lined by well-differentiated cells with basal and supranuclear vacuoles. The tubulocystic pattern of clear cell carcinoma exhibits glands lined by hobnail cells with high-grade nuclei. In addition, the clear cell carcinoma, unlike secretory carcinoma, usually contains areas where the tumor is composed of sheets of tumor cells with clear cytoplasm.

3. *Endometrioid adenocarcinoma vs ovarian tumor of wolffian origin*: The glands of endometrioid carcinoma commonly contain intraluminal mucin, which is absent in wolffian tumors. Wolffian tumors are also rarely reactive for EMA and B72.3.51.[78]

4. *Endometrioid carcinoma vs yolk sac tumor (glandular variant)*: Yolk sac tumors typically occur in young women, show other more common patterns, and exhibit reactivity for α-fetoprotein (see Chapter 27). Occasionally, yolk sac differentiation is encountered in endometrioid carcinomas.[55]

5. *Endometrioid carcinomas vs granulosa cell tumor (insular, trabecular, or microfollicular)*: Endometrioid carcinomas may contain microglands with basally oriented nuclei, luminal cytoplasm, and intraluminal mucin (Figure 25.15) which differ from Call–Exner bodies where the nuclei are haphazardly oriented about the central cavity. In addition, the nuclei of endometrioid carcinomas are usually round and hyperchromatic, whereas those of granulosa cell tumors are round or oval, or angular, pale and grooved.[95] Carcinomas are reactive for EMA, whereas granulosa cell tumors are reactive for α-inhibin (Figure 25.19) and calretinin.

6. *Endometrioid carcinomas vs Sertoli-stromal cell tumors*: Sertoli-stromal cell tumors generally occur in young women (average age, 25 years) and almost always are unilateral (98%), whereas endometrioid carcinomas are not uncommonly bilateral (28%). Typical glands of endometrioid carcinomas (Figure 25.17) with intraluminal mucin and squamous differentiation are each found in three-fourths of tumors resembling Sertoli-stromal cell tumors.[95] Nearly all Sertoli-stromal tumors are reactive for α-inhibin (Figure 25.19) and calretinin.[3,49]

7. *Identical patterns of endometrioid carcinoma involving both the ovary and uterine corpus (independent primaries vs metastatic tumors)*: This problem is discussed below. The good prognosis experienced when the tumor is limited to both organs is one piece of evidence that the neoplasms are usually independent primaries.[23,31] Using FIGO rules

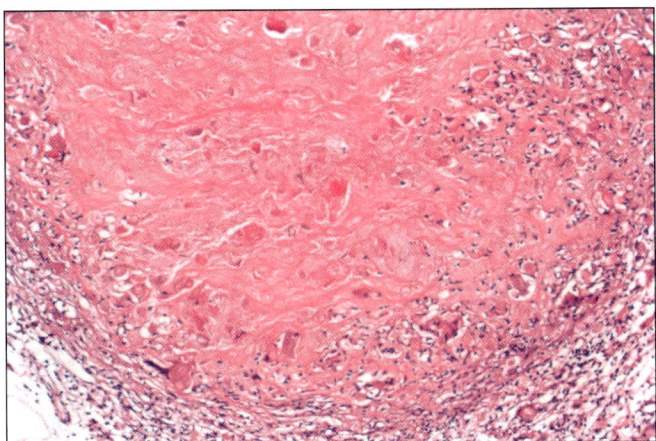

Fig. 25.28 Peritoneal foreign body granuloma to keratin. The patient had an ovarian endometrioid carcinoma with squamous differentiation. No viable tumor cells are seen. Reproduced with permission from Prat.[69]

for staging, the primary site is determined by the initial clinical manifestations.[65]

8. *Endometrioid carcinoma vs metastatic colonic adenocarcinoma*: This differential diagnosis is covered more fully in Chapter 29. Bilaterality, 'dirty' necrosis, amputated glands, desmoplastic stroma, vascular invasion, and 'too high grade' nuclei all favor metastatic carcinoma. In addition, metastatic colonic carcinoma is usually reactive for CK20, whereas endometrioid carcinoma is reactive for CK7 (Figure 25.22).

Treatment and prognosis

The treatment of endometrioid carcinomas is similar to that of ovarian cancers in general. The 5-year survival rate of patients with stage 1 carcinoma is 78%; stage 2, 63%; stage 3, 24%; and stage 4, 6%.[65] Patients with grade 1 and 2 tumors have a higher survival rate than those with grade 3 tumors. Peritoneal foreign-body granulomas to keratin found in cases of endometrioid carcinoma with squamous differentiation do not seem to affect the prognosis adversely in the absence of viable-appearing tumor cells (Figure 25.28).[78] Endometrioid carcinomas with a mixed clear cell, serous, or undifferentiated carcinoma component are reported to have a worse prognosis.[88]

SIMULTANEOUS ENDOMETRIOID CARCINOMAS OF THE OVARY AND ENDOMETRIUM

Simultaneous carcinomas of the ovary and uterine corpus, usually detected as synchronous and less frequently as metachronous tumors, occur in 15–20% of ovarian tumors and in approximately 5% of uterine tumors.[41] Both tumors are of endometrioid type in the majority of cases. Accurate diagnosis as separate independent primary tumors, or as primary tumor in one site with metastasis to the other site, has important prognostic implications and is necessary for appropriate staging and treatment. Independent primary tumors of low histologic grade, usually of endometrioid type, and with involvement limited to the endometrium and ovary, are associated with favorable outcome and often require no additional treatment other than oophorectomy and hysterectomy. In contrast, tumors that are metastatic from the uterus to ovary, or from

the ovary to uterus, usually carry an adverse prognosis and adjuvant therapy is generally indicated.

The criteria for distinguishing metastatic from independent primary carcinomas rely mainly upon conventional clinico-pathologic findings. The presence of a precancerous process is strong evidence of *in situ* genesis. In the endometrium, these processes include endometrial hyperplasia, especially if atypical, or endometrial intraepithelial neoplasia (EIN). Similarly, the presence of potentially precancerous processes in the ovary, such as endometriosis or a pre-existing benign or borderline tumor of similar histologic type, suggest *de novo* development of the cancer also in the ovary. Certain features reliably favor metastatic disease. The most important of these is the presence of a multinodular growth pattern or implants of tumor onto the ovarian surface, a feature not seen with primary ovarian tumors. Rapid patient demise also favors metastatic disease. Tumor in the lumen of the fallopian tubes suggests metastasis. This is most often associated with serous tumors arising in the endometrium that implant on the ovary by retrograde transmission. Synchronous tumors that are regarded as metastases are usually of high histologic grade, e.g., adenosquamous carcinomas, mixed müllerian tumors, and non-endometrioid carcinomas (serous and clear cell). Some cases of metastases to the endometrium show small tumor nodules perched on the superficial endometrium as might be expected of an implant. Other features include the presence and extent of blood vessel and myometrial invasion. By paying attention to these findings, the precise diagnosis can be established in most cases. Occasionally, however, the differential diagnosis can be difficult or impossible as the tumors may show overlapping features.[41]

Application of molecular pathology

In difficult cases, comparative analysis of the immunohistochemical and DNA flow cytometric features of the two neoplasms may be of some help.[23,70] The presence of identical aneuploid DNA indices in two separate carcinomas suggests metastasis from one to the other.[70] Differing indices, while suggesting the possibility of two independent primaries, still does not completely exclude the metastatic nature of one, since a changing DNA index sometimes reflects tumor progression.

Clonality analysis using various molecular methods can also be helpful.[47] These include LOH,[21,24,31,43,81] gene mutation,[24,31,43,54] and clonal X-inactivation analysis.[26] Although LOH pattern concordance in two separate carcinomas is highly suggestive of a common clonal origin (i.e., one tumor is a metastasis from the other), the finding of different LOH patterns does not necessarily mean that they represent independent tumors since different areas of the same tumor may be heterogeneous.[8] Similarly, while discordant *PTEN* mutations and different MI in the two neoplasms usually suggest independent primaries, metastatic carcinomas may also exhibit gene mutations that differ from those of the corresponding primary tumors as a result of tumor progression.[24,31] Alternatively, two independent primary carcinomas may exhibit identical gene mutations reflecting induction of the same genetic alterations by a common carcinogenic agent acting in two separate sites of a single anatomic region (Figure 25.29).[31,47] In other words, the genetic profile can be identical in independent tumors and different in metastatic carcinomas.[31] Therefore, clonality analysis is useful in the distinction of independent primary carcinomas from

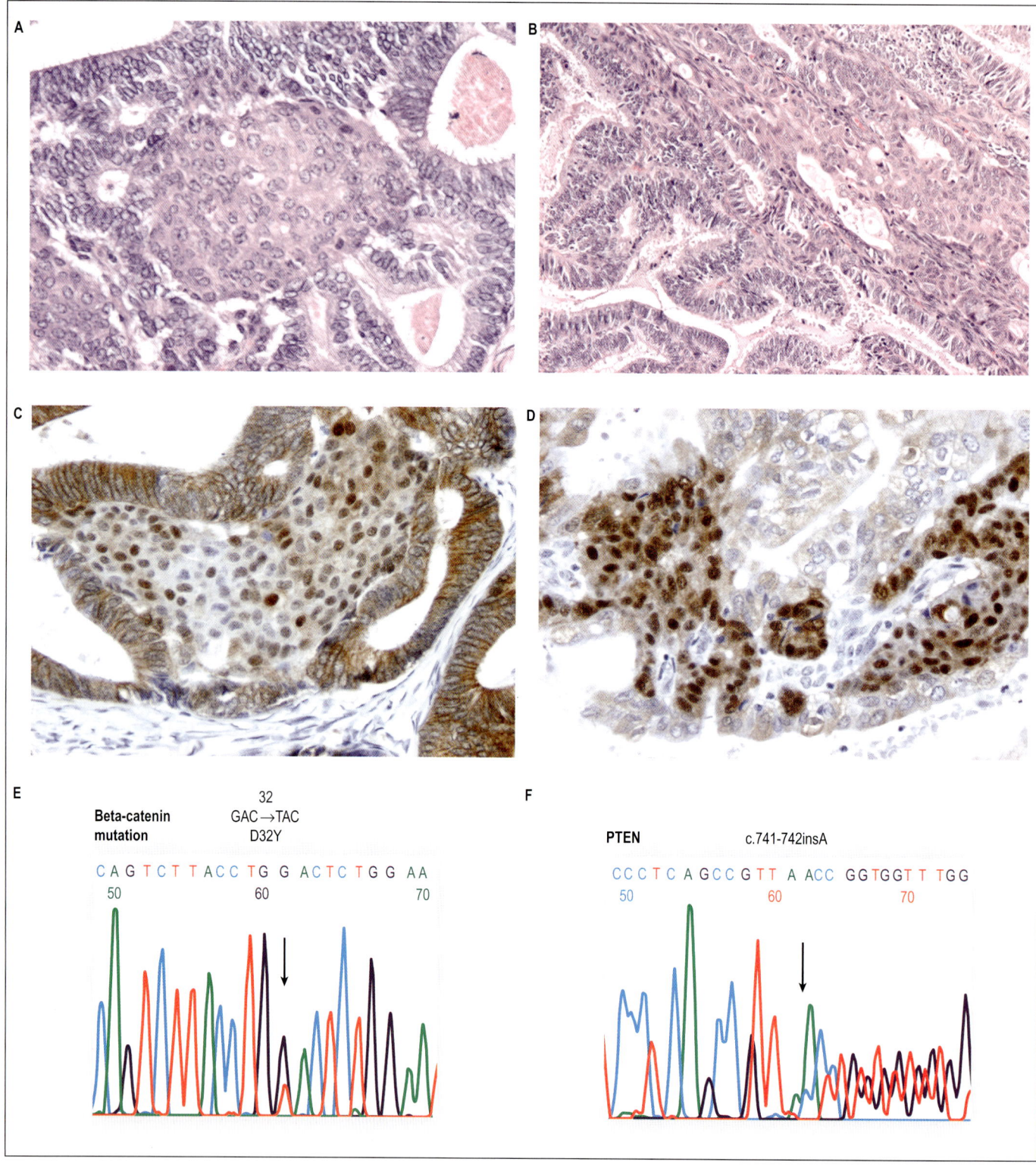

Fig. 25.29 Synchronous, independent, primary endometrioid carcinomas of the uterus (left panel) and ovary (right panel). Both tumors were grade 1 with squamous differentiation as shown in **(A)** (uterus) and **(B)** (ovary). Nuclear accumulation of β-catenin was most prominent in squamous morules **(C**, uterus; **D**, ovary). Sequence analysis of exon 3 of *CTNNB1* revealed an identical GAC→TAC point mutation (D32Y) in both uterine and ovarian tumors **(E)**. Sequencing histogram of *PTEN* frameshift mutation **(F)**. An identical bp insertion in exon 7 was detected in both tumors. Reproduced with permission from Irving et al.[31]

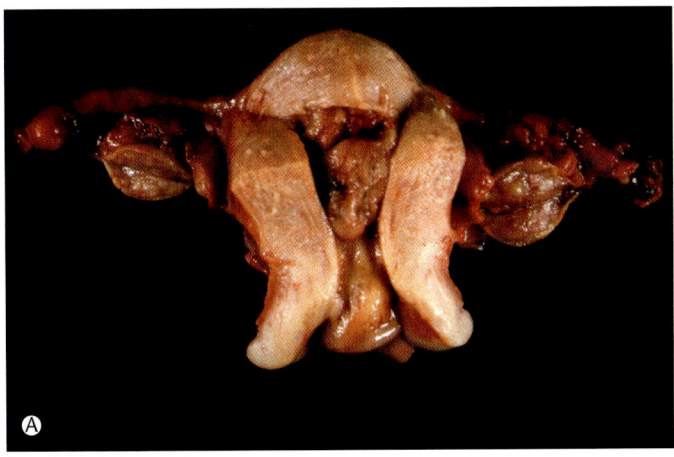
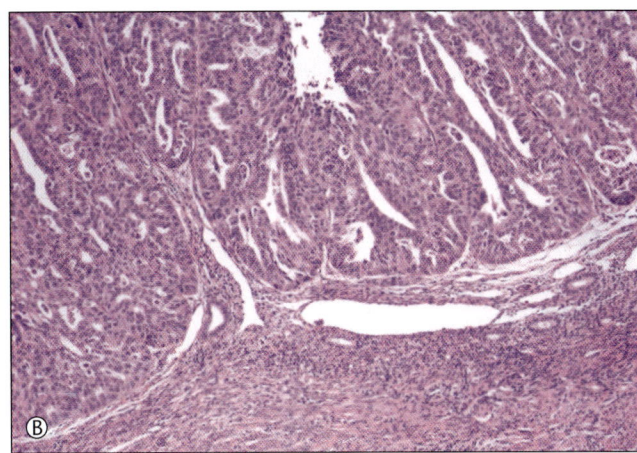
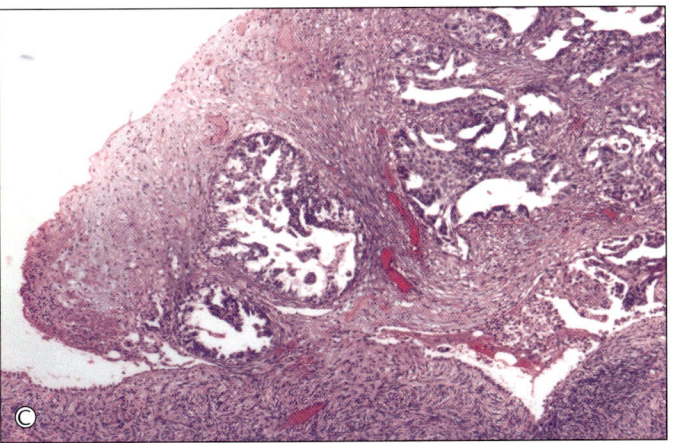
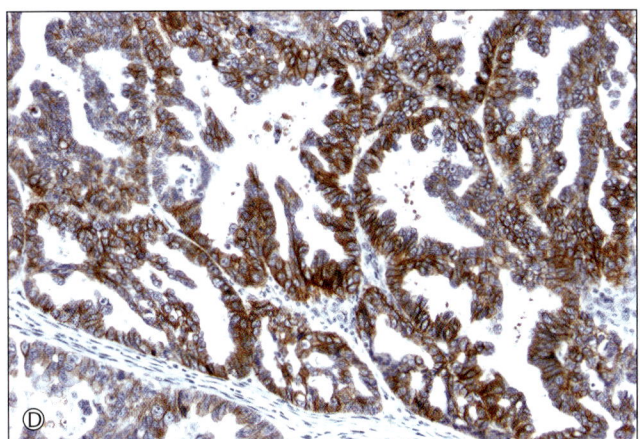

Fig. 25.30 Primary endometrioid carcinoma of the uterine corpus with bilateral ovarian metastases. **(A)** Polypoid tumor filling the endometrial cavity, with surface involvement of both ovaries. **(B)** The uterine tumor was a minimally invasive (<1 mm), grade 3 endometrioid carcinoma. **(C)** The ovarian surfaces were extensively involved by metastatic grade 3 endometrioid carcinoma. **(D)** Membranous pattern of β-catenin immunoreactivity was observed in the uterine tumor (shown) as well as both ovaries and omental metastases. Reproduced with permission from Irving et al.[31]

metastatic carcinomas provided the diagnosis does not rely exclusively on a single molecular result and the molecular data are interpreted in the light of appropriate clinical and pathologic findings.[31]

A recent study has revealed a frequency of molecular alterations in both independent and metastatic tumors, including MI and *PTEN* mutations, which is higher than that observed in single sporadic tumors. Nuclear immunoreactivities for β-catenin and *CTNNB1* mutations were restricted to independent uterine and ovarian tumors and were absent in metastatic tumors (Figure 25.30). These findings correlated with the clinical outcome.[31]

TUMORS WITH A SARCOMATOUS COMPONENT

These tumors are uncommon in the ovary and display neoplastic stromal or mesenchymal cells exhibiting varying degrees of proliferation as well as many patterns of mesenchymal differentiation. Many also contain neoplastic epithelial elements that may be benign or malignant. Similar tumors occur more frequently in the uterus and, rarely, in the pelvic and abdominal peritoneum or the omentum.

MALIGNANT MESODERMAL MIXED TUMORS (CARCINOSARCOMAS)

Definition
This class of tumors is composed of both carcinomatous and sarcomatous elements. The former may be of differing müllerian types, usually as serous or endometrioid, while the latter component may be homologous (tissue types native to the müllerian tract, i.e., endometrial stroma, fibrous tissue, and smooth muscle) or heterologous (foreign tissue, such as skeletal muscle, adipose tissue, cartilage, and bone). Any of these various components may be widespread or limited to small foci.[41] Approximately one-third fall into the homologous group. Occasionally, these complex neoplasms arise in ovarian endometriosis.

General features
Malignant mesodermal (müllerian) mixed tumors (MMMTs) account for <1% of all ovarian cancers.[41,78] They occur in the sixth to eighth decades, and are rare below the age of 40 years.[78] Recent immunohistochemical and molecular genetic studies[1,25,86] support a clonal origin of both tumor components (epithelial and mesenchymal-like elements) and, accordingly, a proposal to designate these tumors 'undifferentiated or metaplastic car-

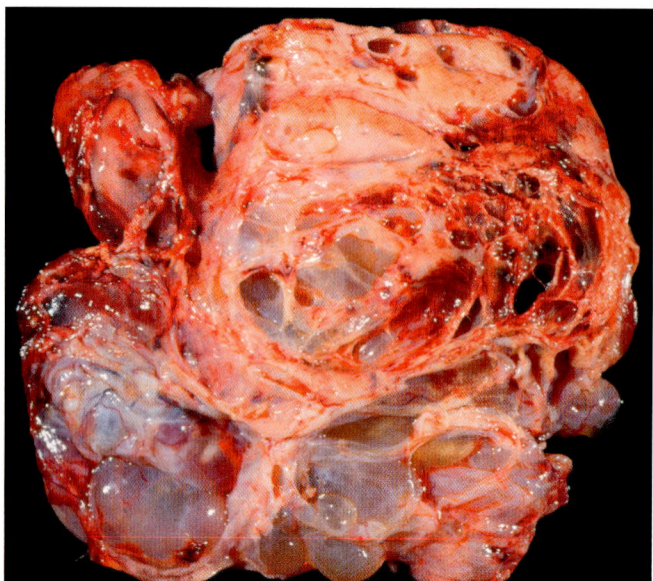

Fig. 25.31 Malignant mesodermal mixed tumor (carcinosarcoma). The sectioned surface reveals a solid and cystic tumor with areas of hemorrhage.

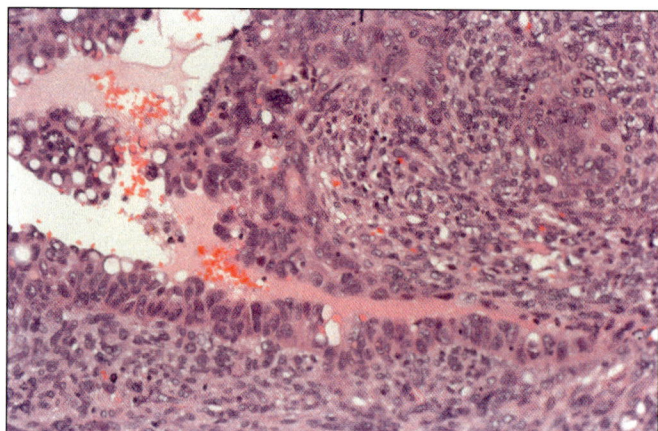

Fig. 25.33 Malignant mesodermal mixed tumor (carcinosarcoma). Biphasic growth of high-grade carcinoma and sarcoma. Hyaline globules are seen.

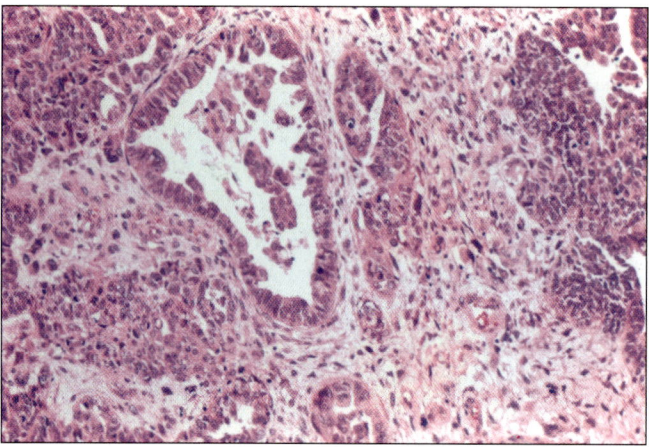

Fig. 25.32 Malignant mesodermal mixed tumor (carcinosarcoma). Poorly differentiated glands are surrounded by spindle-shaped and pleomorphic cells. Reproduced with permission from Prat.[69]

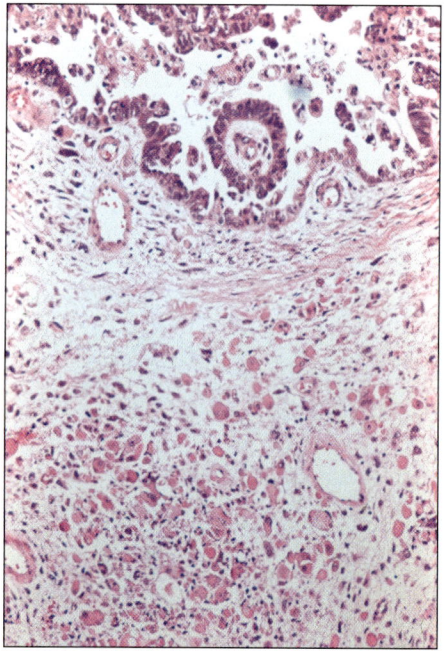

Fig. 25.34 Malignant mesodermal mixed tumor, heterologous. Rhabdomyosarcomatous component (bottom). Reproduced with permission from Prat.[69]

cinoma' has been made.[52] However, preserving the currently accepted term MMMT, which indicates the type(s) of neoplastic differentiation, is recommended because of the unique clinicopathologic features of this tumor.

Macroscopic features
The tumors are bilateral in one-third of the cases.[78] They are usually large (15–20 cm mean diameter), friable, solid and/or cystic with areas of necrosis and hemorrhage (Figure 25.31). Occasionally, bone or cartilage can be palpated.

Microscopic features
Most tumors display a complex admixture of epithelial and malignant stromal elements and transitions are uncommon. The epithelial component is most frequently high-grade serous (Figure 25.32), endometrioid, or undifferentiated carcinoma. Occasionally, squamous, mucinous, or clear cell carcinoma is found. If the epithelium is mucinous, care should be taken to differentiate such tumors from mucinous cystic tumors with mural nodules (see below and Chapter 24). The sarcomatous elements are usually hypercellular sheets of small, hyperchromatic, round to spindle-shaped cells with a high mitotic rate and lacking apparent differentiation. In the homologous type, the sarcoma-like component resembles fibrosarcoma, malignant fibrous histiocytoma, or high-grade endometrial stromal sarcoma (Figure 25.33). The heterologous tumor most often contains chondrosarcoma, rhabdomyosarcoma (Figure 25.34), or both. Rarely, osteosarcoma or liposarcoma is present. PAS-positive, diastase-resistant hyaline bodies (Figure 25.33) are common in the sarcomatous component. Glial, neuronal, and trophoblastic differentiation may be encountered.

Immunohistochemistry

As a general rule, reactivity for EMA and cytokeratins (AE1/AE3 and CAM 5.2) but not for vimentin helps distinguish poorly differentiated carcinoma from sarcoma. However, in MMMTs, the sarcoma-like component may also react for cytokeratins and EMA,[7] and reactivity with vimentin is not uncommon in the epithelial component. Reactivity with chromogranin, neuron-specific enolase, and synaptophysin is found in one-sixth of the cases.

Somatic genetics

MMMTs are probably monoclonal as the histologically different components share similar allelic losses and retentions.[1,25,86] A cell line developed from an MMMT has expressed both epithelial and mesenchymal antigens.[5] Tumor progression (clonal evolution) could explain the heterogeneous pattern of LOH in either the carcinomatous or sarcoma-like components of the neoplasm.[25]

Differential diagnosis

1. *MMMT vs immature teratoma*: Immature teratoma occurs predominantly in children and adolescents and typically contains elements derived from all three germ layers. Neuroectodermal tissue, which is rarely found in MMMT, is almost always the predominant malignant component. In addition, the malignant epithelial component of immature teratoma has an embryonal appearance and the cartilaginous component resembles fetal cartilage with uniform nuclei, in contrast to the cartilage found in MMMT in which the cells are bizarre and appear clearly malignant (chondrosarcoma) (see Chapter 27).

2. *MMMT vs poorly differentiated Sertoli–Leydig cell tumor with heterologous elements:* The latter tumor nearly always occurs in young women, many of whom present because of virilization. Usually, some area is better differentiated and readily diagnosable as Sertoli–Leydig tumors. Reactivity for α-inhibin and calretinin (Sertoli–Leydig) and EMA (in MMMT) also facilitates the diagnosis (see Chapter 26).

3. *MMMT vs endometrioid stromal sarcomas with sex cord-like differentiation*: The latter tumors are better differentiated than MMMTs and often exhibit sex cord differentiation (see below).

4. *MMMT vs sarcoma-like mural nodules in mucinous cystic tumor*: The mural nodules may be reactive, composed of anaplastic carcinoma or truly sarcomatous (see Chapter 24).

Tumor spread and prognosis

Over 75% of MMMTs have spread beyond the ovary at the time of diagnosis, 60% being stage 3 and 10% stage 4.[41] The metastases commonly contain both carcinomatous and sarcomatous components. The prognosis is very poor. After cytoreductive surgery and platinum-based chemotherapy, the overall 5-year survival is under 30%. Only 25% of patients survive 2 years (median survival, 10 months).[41]

MÜLLERIAN ADENOSARCOMAS

Ovarian adenosarcomas are usually unilateral and predominantly solid tumors containing numerous small cysts. Over 50 cases have been reported.[19] They occur in older women (mean

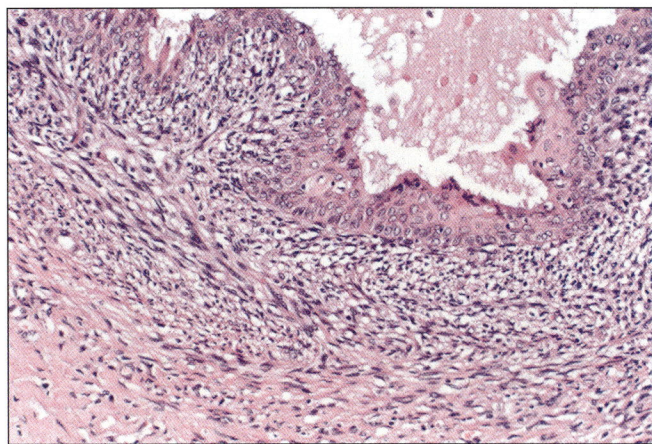

Fig. 25.35 Adenosarcoma. Squamous differentiation and cuff of cellular stroma. Reproduced with permision from Prat.[69]

age, 54 years) and have a much worse prognosis than their more common uterine counterparts. Fifty per cent die within 5 years.

Microscopically, the tumors exhibit both a malignant stromal and a glandular component. The glandular epithelium, which is usually of endometrioid type (Figure 25.35), appears benign or less frequently atypical. The stroma resembles a cellular fibroma, low-grade fibrosarcoma, or low-grade endometrial-stromal sarcoma. Typically, it is most cellular adjacent to the glands forming cuffs around them ('periglandular cuffing'). The glands become cystic and polypoid projections of stroma into the lumens are often present. Mitoses in the stromal cells range from 2 to over 40 per 10 HPFs.[19] Heterologous elements, sex cord-like structures, and sarcomatous overgrowth are occasionally found.

Adenosarcomas should be distinguished from adenofibromas, polypoid endometriosis, sex cord-stromal tumors, and endometrial stromal sarcomas.

Adenosarcoma of the ovary is a far more aggressive tumor than its counterpart in the endometrium. About half will have spread beyond the ovary by the time of diagnosis. Treatment is primarily surgical, although radiation therapy and chemotherapy have also been used. For stage 1 cancer, tumor rupture, high-grade, and sarcomatous overgrowth are associated with a higher rate of recurrence.[19]

ENDOMETRIOID STROMAL SARCOMAS

Definition

These tumors consist of cells resembling the stromal cells of normal proliferative endometrium. They may derive from foci of ovarian endometriosis (coexistent endometriosis is present in almost half the cases), from foci of gland-free endometrial stroma in the ovary (stromal endometriosis) or, possibly, may arise directly from the ovarian stromal cells following metaplasia into endometrial stromal-type cells.[92]

Clinical features

Endometrioid stromal sarcoma (ESS) of the ovary is not a common tumor.[12,92] Patients are 11–76 years of age. The majority of tumors occur during the fifth and sixth decades. The presenting symptoms, which are non-specific, are related to the

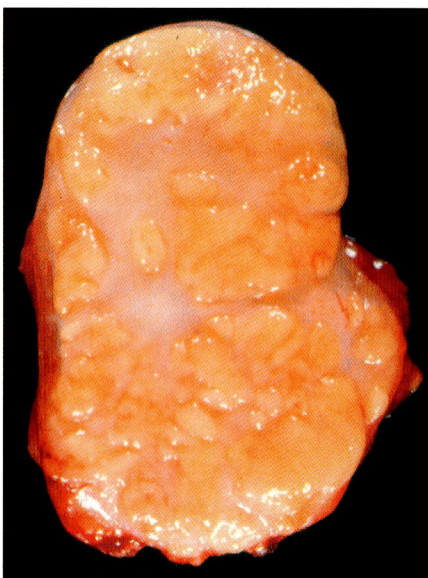

Fig. 25.36 Endometrioid stromal sarcoma. The sectioned surface of the tumor is solid and multinodular.

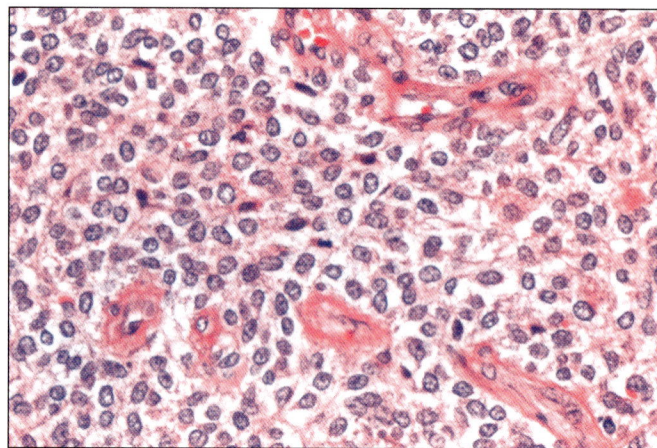

Fig. 25.37 Endometrioid stromal sarcoma, low grade. The tumor is composed of a monotonous collection of small cells resembling endometrial stromal cells. Note the presence of small arterioles resembling the spiral arterioles of the normal late secretory endometrium.

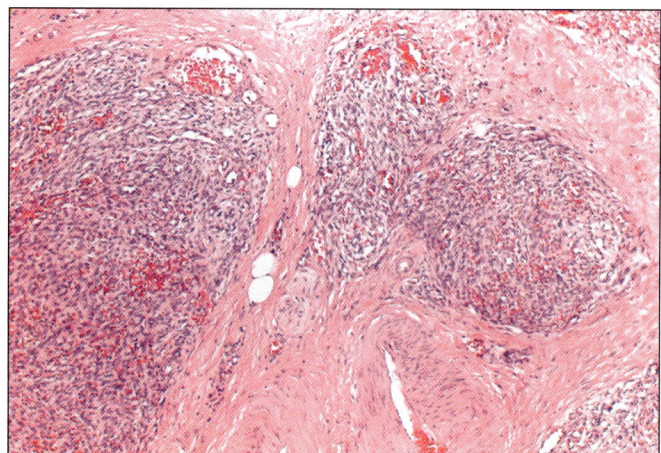

Fig. 25.38 Endometrioid stromal sarcoma, low grade. Cellular nodules intersected by dense fibrous bands. Reproduced with permission from Prat.[69]

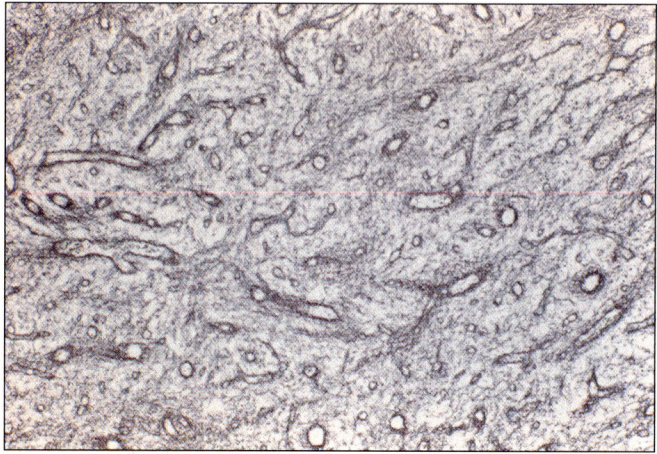

Fig. 25.39 Endometrioid stromal sarcoma, low grade. Reticulin staining discloses a prominent vascular pattern.

presence of a pelvic mass. In one of the larger series,[92] the tumor was, at the time of operation, confined to the ovary in only one-sixth of patients; it involved other pelvic structures or had spread into the abdomen in over one-third for each group and had metastasized to the lungs in the remaining. About 30% of the patients had a similar tumor in the uterus for which reason a metastasis to the ovary was strongly considered in some.[92]

Macroscopic features

The tumors generally are up to 15 cm in diameter and unilateral in 75% of cases.[92] They are predominantly solid, though foci of cystic change are present in over half. On section they usually have a yellow-white homogeneous appearance (Figure 25.36), with foci of necrosis being relatively uncommon.

Microscopic features

Histologically, ovarian ESSs, like their more common uterine counterparts, exhibit sheets of uniform cells resembling the stromal cells of normal proliferative endometrium (Figure 25.37). In contrast to the uterine tumors, fibromatous areas are frequently present (Figure 25.38).[92] An important diagnostic feature is the presence of a prominent network of small arterioles (Figure 25.37), closely resembling the spiral vessels seen in normal late secretory endometrium. This network is most clearly seen in reticulin-stained sections (Figure 25.39).[92] The tumor cells are small and oval to spindle-shaped, and usually have scanty cytoplasm. The intravascular growth characteristic of uterine ESSs of low-grade malignancy is not seen within the ovarian tumors but is typically present when the neoplasm extends beyond the ovary (Figure 25.40).[92] The tumor cells may contain abundant intracellular lipid (Figure 25.41) and, although usually growing in uniform sheets, can, like similar uterine tumors, show an epithelial or sex cord-like pattern. In almost half the cases, endometriosis is identified adjacent to the tumor (Figure 25.42), or a few glands of endometrioid type are found within it.[92]

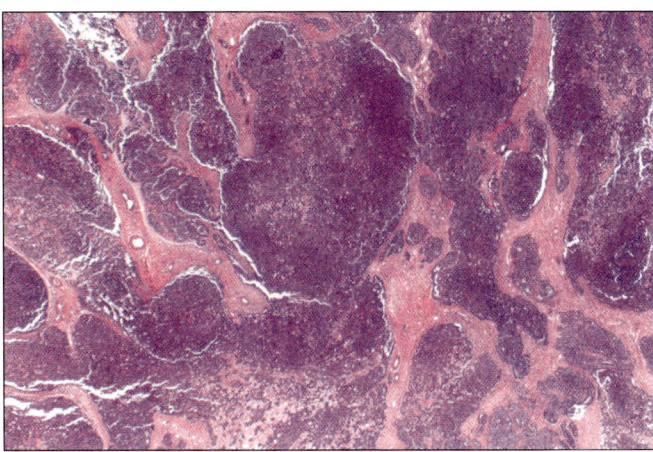

Fig. 25.40 Endometrioid stromal sarcoma, low grade, metastatic to the omentum. Densely cellular tumor nodules.

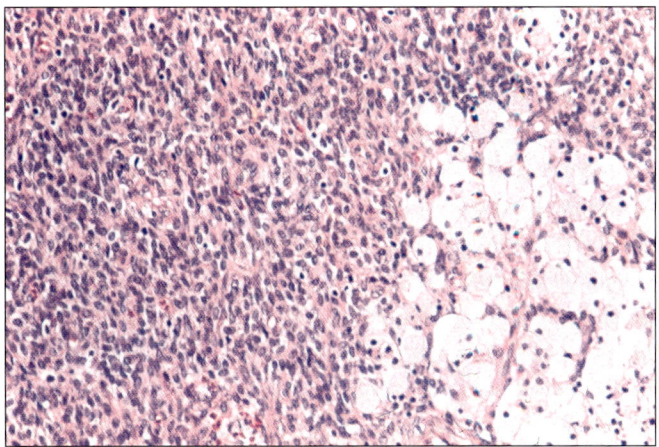

Fig. 25.41 Endometrioid stromal sarcoma, low grade. Clusters of foam cells (right). Reproduced with permission from Young et al.[92]

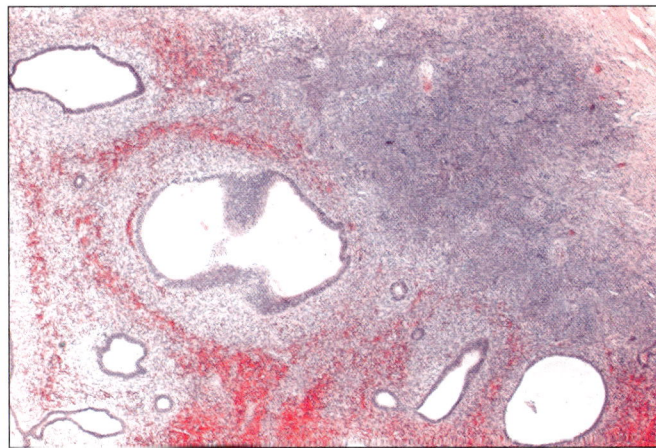

Fig. 25.42 Endometrioid stromal sarcoma, low grade, arising from endometriosis. Reproduced with permission from Young et al.[92]

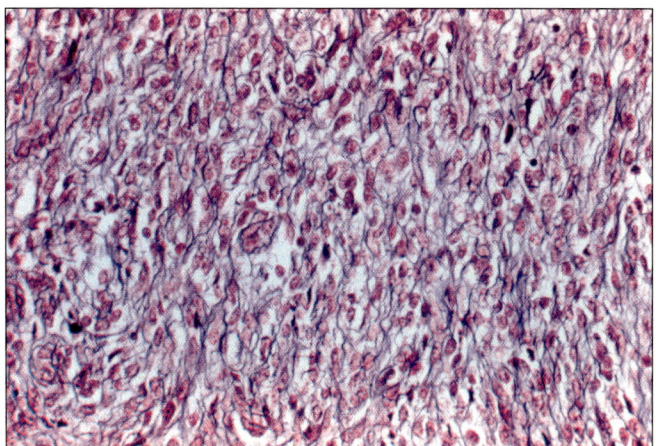

Fig. 25.43 Endometrioid stromal sarcoma, low grade. Reticulin staining discloses individual investment of the tumor cells by fibrils.

Immunohistochemistry

ESSs immunoreact for vimentin and CD10. Muscle-associated proteins and low-molecular weight cytokeratins are only focally expressed. Calretinin and α-inhibin are not expressed.

Differential diagnosis

The cytologic features and the presence of a rich vascular network allow for the differentiation of ESSs from other types of ovarian sarcoma. An adenosarcoma may, however, be mimicked if endometriotic glands are trapped within the tumor. Nevertheless, the focal presence of the glands, as opposed to their uniform distribution throughout an adenosarcoma, together with the absence of any stromal condensation around the glands (periglandular cuffing), usually indicates the correct diagnosis. A sex cord-like pattern, if a prominent feature of an ESS, may lead to confusion with a granulosa cell tumor; the epithelial-like cells, however, lack the nuclear features of granulosa cells. Furthermore, granulosa cell tumors lack the individual cellular investment by reticulin fibrils (Figure 25.43) so characteristic of ESS. The usual advanced stage and the frequent bilaterality of ESS argue against a diagnosis of any tumor in the sex cord-stromal category. A lack of reactivity for calretinin and/or α-inhibin also helps to identify the tumor as a stromal sarcoma.[15,98]

Nearly one-third of ovarian ESSs are associated with a prior, synchronous, or subsequent uterine ESS.[92] When the uterine lesions precede the ovarian neoplasms by many years, the tumors most likely represent independent primary neoplasms of each organ. In synchronous cases, however, it may be impossible to exclude metastasis from one organ to the other, especially if other pelvic structures are involved. Some[12] regard the tumor as an ovarian primary only if both the tumor is confined to the ovary and the uterus has been shown to be disease free on pathologic examination. Others[78] also accept ovarian endometriosis as evidence of an ovarian origin. Obviously, it is important to review any prior hysterectomy specimen in a patient with an ovarian ESS. If the uterus has not been removed at the time of operation, it is more than a remote possibility that a uterine ESS may have been left behind or will subsequently develop.[78]

Tumors that lack endometrial stromal differentiation and are composed of pleomorphic mesenchymal cells with highly atypical nuclei and prominent nucleoli should be diagnosed as undifferentiated ovarian sarcoma.[12]

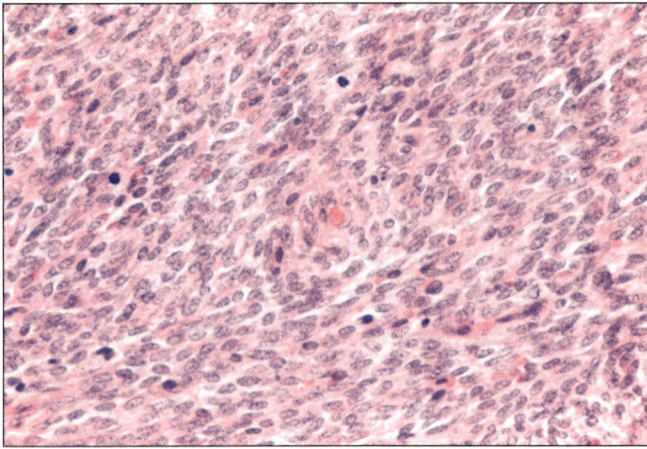

Fig. 25.44 Endometrioid stromal sarcoma, high grade with several mitotic figures. Reproduced with permission from Prat.[69]

Prognosis

Ovarian ESSs behave similarly to uterine ESSs, with mitotic activity being of major prognostic significance. Tumors with <10 mitoses per 10 HPFs are associated with a good prognosis, even if there is extrauterine spread. In the largest series reported,[92] only 10% of patients whose neoplasms contained <10 mitoses per 10 HPFs died of their disease. While patients with extraovarian spread survived over the short term, longer term follow-up studies indicate that the disease may nonetheless be fatal even after 10 years.[78] The prognosis associated with tumors containing more than 10 mitoses per 10 HPFs (Figure 25.44) was comparable to that of other ovarian sarcomas, and three-fourths of women die within 4 years.[92]

Treatment

The primary treatment of ovarian ESS is surgical. In menopausal or postmenopausal patients, hysterectomy with bilateral salpingo-oophorectomy is the treatment of choice. Because of the high frequency of bilateral ovarian involvement and the possibility of synchronous or subsequent uterine ESS, a similar approach may be optimal even for younger women. Both progesterone and radiotherapy have been used for residual or recurrent disease. Tumors of low-grade malignancy (<10 mitoses per 10 HPFs) typically run an indolent course and patients with untreated residual disease may remain free of symptoms for many years.

TUMORS OF SMOOTH MUSCLE

LEIOMYOMAS

Ovarian leiomyomas are rare.[42] The mean age at presentation is 43 years, but they have been encountered in females as young as age 3 and as old as 103 years. Most are asymptomatic but about a third complained of non-specific pelvic mass symptoms such as abdominal pain or swelling. Rarely, torsion occurs. Ascites has developed in a few patients.

The tumors are usually unilateral, and range in size from 1 to 24 cm in diameter. Although lacking a true capsule, leiomyomas tend to be sharply circumscribed, which helps distinguish them from the far more common ovarian fibromas, which are solid and firm and on section have a white, gray or

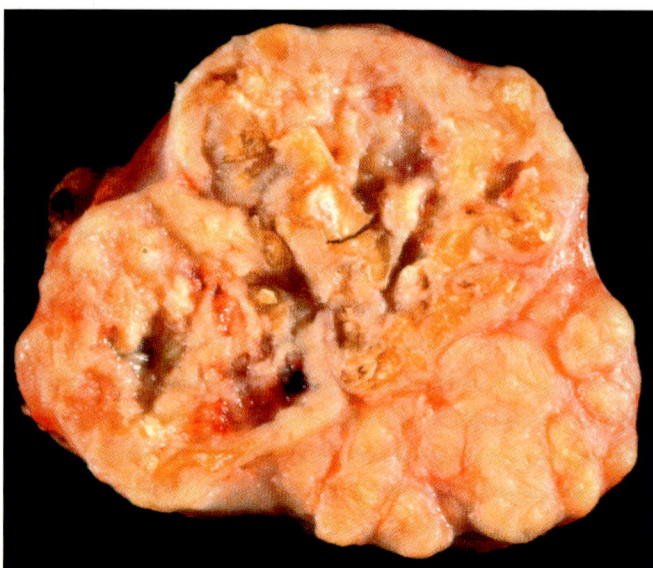

Fig. 25.45 Ovarian leiomyoma with calcification and cystic degeneration on cut section.

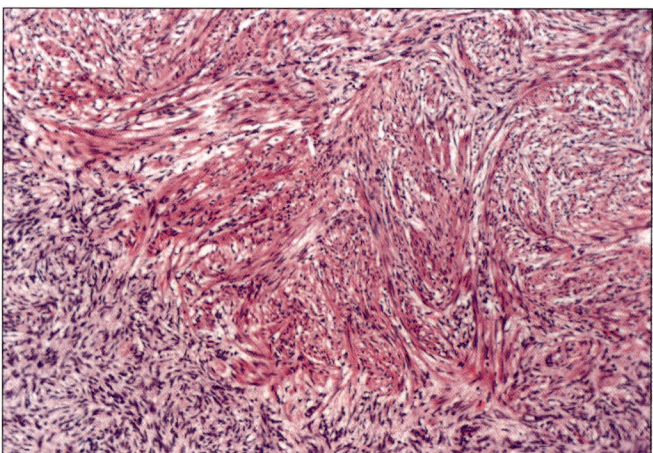

Fig. 25.46 Ovarian leiomyoma with spindle cells arranged in intersecting bundles.

brown cut surface. Leiomyomas have a whorled or multinodular structure and although commonly solid may show areas of myxoid or pseudocystic change (Figure 25.45). Foci of hemorrhage, necrosis, or calcification are common.

Histologically, the ovarian leiomyoma has the typical features of that associated with the uterus (Figure 25.46), i.e., interlacing bundles of smooth muscle fibers, sometimes admixed with collagenous septa. The muscle cells have elongated blunt-ended or cigar-shaped nuclei. Occasional multinucleated giant cells may be present, but there is otherwise no pleomorphism. Mitotic figures are either absent or extremely sparse. Like the uterine counterpart, cellular and mitotically active ovarian leiomyomas exist.[42] Both lack significant nuclear atypia. Mitotically active ovarian leiomyomas may contain up to 15 mitoses per 10 HPFs, but should not have atypical mitotic figures. Leiomyomas with extensive hyalinization and epithelioid cells (Figure 25.47) may be confused with sex cord-stromal tumors (see Chapter 26) and those exhibiting myxoid change may resemble yolk sac tumors (see Chapter 27).[42] Immunostains for

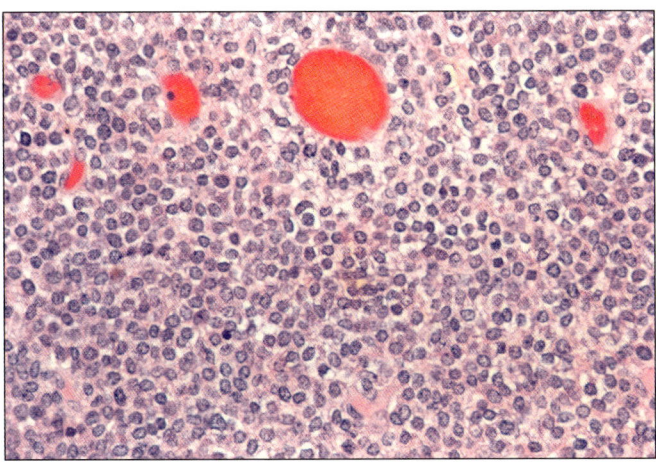

Fig. 25.47 Epithelioid leiomyoma. Courtesy of Dr S Carinelli, Milan, Italy.

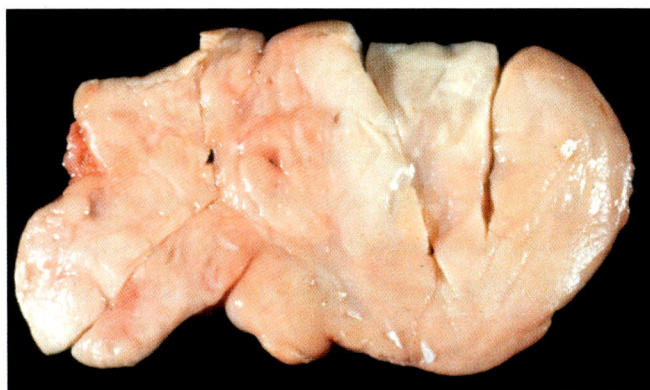

Fig. 25.48 Ovarian leiomyosarcoma. Fleshy nodular tumor showing a solid sectioned surface. Reproduced with permission from Prat.[69]

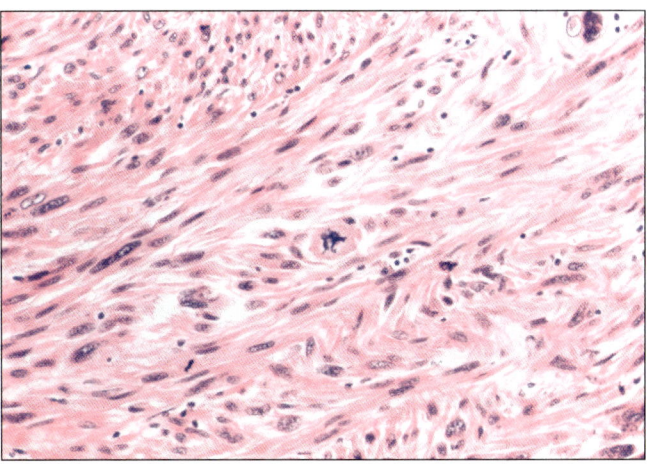

Fig. 25.49 Well-differentiated ovarian leiomyosarcoma. Interlacing fascicles of smooth muscle fibers. An atypical mitotic figure is present. Reproduced with permission from Prat.[69]

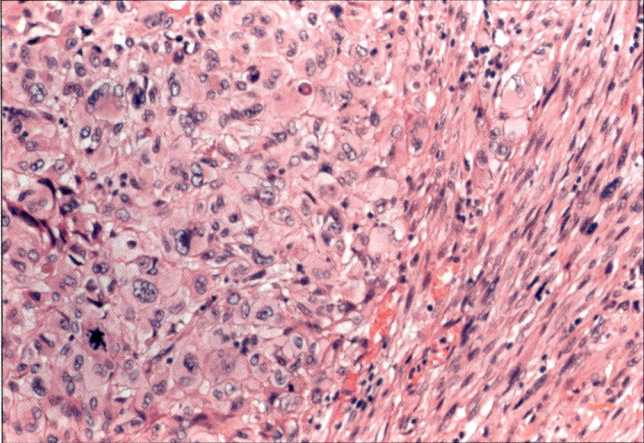

Fig. 25.50 Epithelioid leiomyosarcoma. Typical leiomyosarcoma is seen to the right and epithelioid cells with abundant eosinophilic cytoplasm on the left. An atypical mitotic figure is seen. Reproduced with permission from Prat.[69]

desmin, α-inhibin, calretinin, and α-fetoprotein may facilitate the diagnosis.

The histogenesis of ovarian leiomyomas is uncertain. Possible origins are from the smooth muscle fibers of the ovarian ligaments, ovarian blood vessels, or smooth muscle fibers of the cortical stroma.

Ovarian leiomyomas, including those considered as cellular or 'mitotically active', are benign and can be treated conservatively. Criteria for distinguishing between benign and malignant smooth muscle tumors of the ovary are similar to those used for uterine smooth muscle tumors. Moderate to severe nuclear atypia, tumor cell necrosis, and infiltrative margins correlated with malignant behavior.[42] Cytologically atypical leiomyomas with less than 5 mitoses per 10 HPFs that lack tumor cell necrosis may be considered of 'uncertain malignant potential'.[42] A mitotic count of greater than 5 mitoses per 10 HPFs in a cytologically atypical ovarian smooth muscle tumor should be regarded as an adverse sign, especially if any other adverse histologic features are present.

LEIOMYOSARCOMAS

Ovarian leiomyosarcomas are extremely uncommon and fewer than 50 examples have been reported.[42] The tumors usually occur in elderly women (mean age, 58 years). The presenting symptoms are abdominal pain or an awareness of an abdominal mass. The tumors are almost always unilateral and are generally large with a mean of 14 cm; some are as large as 30 cm.[42] Grossly the tumors have a nodular outer surface and on section most are predominantly solid (Figure 25.48), often with extensive hemorrhage and necrosis. The cut surface tends to be gray-white and usually has a more fleshy texture than that of a leiomyoma. The histologic appearances are variable and range from very well-differentiated tumors (Figure 25.49) that resemble atypical leiomyomas to highly pleomorphic sarcomas (Figures 25.50 and 25.51) with only a few areas of a recognizably smooth muscle nature. As in the uterus, the diagnosis rests on the presence of at least two of the following three histologic features: moderate or severe cytologic atypia, a mitotic count of ≥10 mitoses per 10 HPFs, and geographic tumor cell necrosis. The mitotic count may range from 4 to 25 mitoses per 10 HPFs and atypical mitoses are frequently seen.

However, in the absence of tumor cell necrosis, a mitotic count of ≥5 mitoses per 10 HPFs in a cytologically atypical ovarian tumor warrants a diagnosis of leiomyosarcoma.[42]

Ovarian leiomyosarcomas are aggressive neoplasms and have commonly spread beyond the ovary at the time of initial

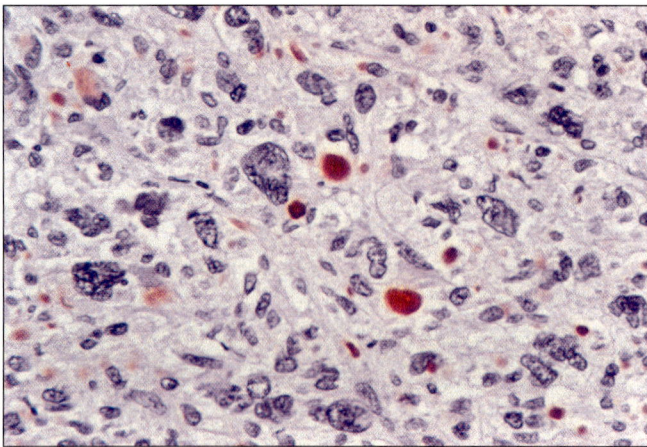

Fig. 25.51 Pleomorphic leiomyosarcoma, focally reactive for desmin.

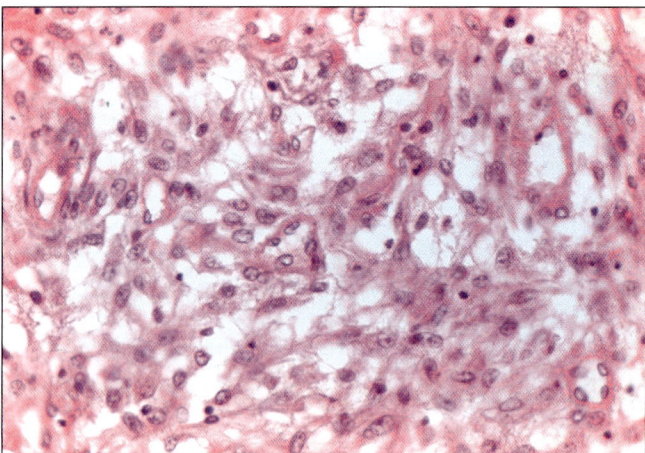

Fig. 25.52 Myxoid leiomyosarcoma with a loose reticular meshwork of elongated cells without significant atypicality or mitotic activity. Reproduced with permission from Prat.[69]

diagnosis. The treatment of choice is probably radical surgery, although radiotherapy or chemotherapy may prolong survival in some instances. Approximately 70% of patients develop recurrent disease at a mean of 20 months and 62% died of tumor within a year.[42]

MYXOID LEIOMYOSARCOMA

Myxoid leiomyosarcoma of the ovary is an extremely rare tumor.[42] Unlike the usual leiomyosarcoma, the myxoid variant is a large gelatinous mass sowing cystic change, necrosis, and hemorrhage. Microscopically, the tumors exhibit a reticular meshwork of elongated cells surrounded by abundant basophilic myxoid material (Figure 25.52). The differential diagnosis includes massive edema, ovarian myxoma, yolk sac tumor (see Chapter 27), and myxoid sarcomatous component of MMMT (see above). Positive immunoreactions for smooth muscle markers (Figure 25.51) may be helpful in establishing the nature of the tissue and hence the diagnosis. Due to the decreased cellular density the myxoid change causes, mitotic counts are usually low and therefore deceptive. Clinical stage seems to be the most reliable prognostic indicator, but unfortunately, this feature is of no use if the tumor is stage 1A. Like

its uterine counterpart, myxoid leiomyosarcoma of the ovary is highly aggressive, with most patients dying within 2 years of diagnosis.[42]

CLEAR CELL TUMORS

General features

Clear cell tumors are composed of the following types of epithelial cells: clear cells (containing glycogen) similar to those of renal cell carcinoma, 'hobnail' cells (with large nuclei that protrude the apparent cytoplasmic limits into a lumen) that line cysts and tubules, and less frequently flat, cuboidal, oxyphilic, or mucin-containing signet-ring cells.[41] Mucicarmine and diastase-resistant PAS-stained material is sometimes present at the luminal border of the cells and commonly in the luminal secretions, whereas abundant, particulate, diastase-digestible, PAS-positive glycogen is usually readily demonstrable in the cytoplasm.

Benign clear cell tumors are exceptional, and the borderline forms account for less than 1% of ovarian borderline tumors.[78] Clear cell adenocarcinomas (CCCs) represent 6% of surface epithelial–stromal cancers.[65,78] Most are diagnosed during the fifth to seventh decades.[35] Among the epithelial–stromal cancers, they have the highest association with ovarian and pelvic endometriosis and paraendocrine hypercalcemia.[90] CCC occurs not only in the ovary, but also in the endometrium, fallopian tube, cervix, and vagina.

Historically, the origin of CCC was considered to be from mesonephric remnants, for which reason the designations 'mesonephroma' and 'mesonephric carcinoma' were used. It is now accepted that these tumors are müllerian in nature.[78] Most occur along the course of müllerian duct derivatives or within the ovary, which is covered by a surface epithelium capable of differentiating into neoplastic müllerian cell types, or involved by endometriosis commonly associated with CCC (up to 40% of cases). CCC also arises from the bed of tissue where müllerian-derived vaginal adenosis is found in girls and young women exposed prenatally to diethylstilbestrol (DES),[78] but to date no cases of CCC in the endometrium or ovary has ever been associated with the drug.[78] Lastly, CCC recapitulates the hypersecretory endometrium of pregnancy.[78]

The SNOMED classification of clear cell tumors is as follows:

- Clear cell cystadenoma
- Clear cell cystadenofibroma
- Clear cell tumor of borderline malignancy
- Clear cell adenofibroma of borderline malignancy
- Clear cell adenocarcinoma
- Clear cell adenocarcinofibroma.

Macroscopic features

Benign or borderline CCCs have a non-specific gross appearance and an average diameter of about 10–12 cm.[78] CCCs may be predominantly solid (Figure 25.53) but are more often predominantly cystic (unilocular or multilocular) containing one or more white, yellow, or brown polypoid masses that protrude into the lumens (Figure 25.54).[35,41,78] Occasionally, the cystic glands may be so extensive as to render the tumor's sectioned surface as sponge-like (parvilocular cystoma) (Figure 25.55).

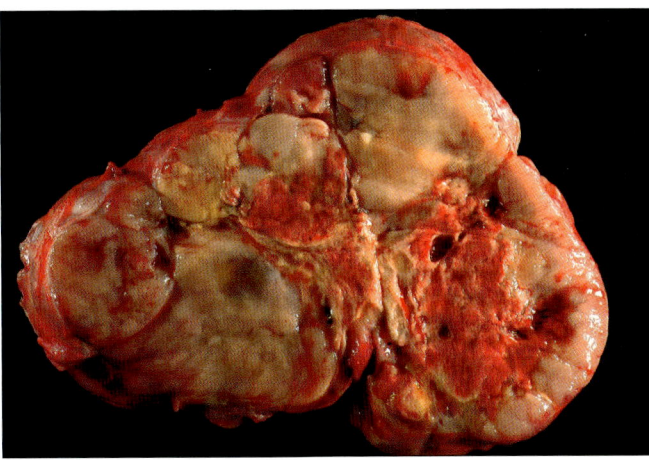

Fig. 25.53 Clear cell adenocarcinoma with a predominantly solid and fleshy sectioned surface with areas of necrosis.

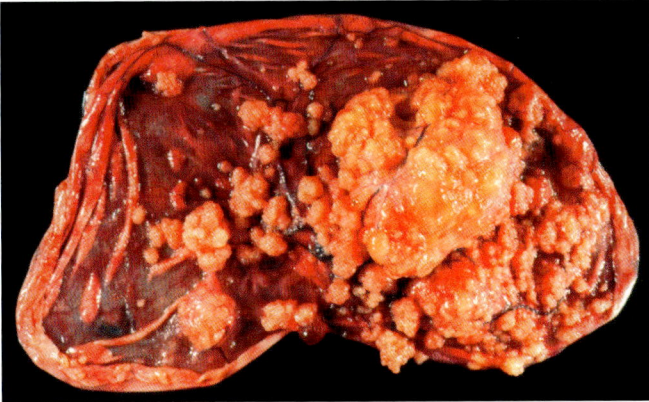

Fig. 25.54 Clear cell adenocarcinoma. The predominantly cystic tumor contains multiple yellow-brown polypoid masses that protrude into the lumen of the cyst.

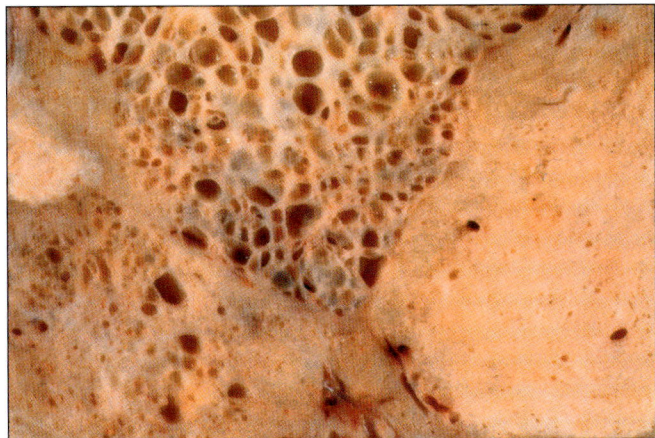

Fig. 25.55 Borderline clear cell adenofibroma, showing numerous small cysts (parvilocular cystoma) on cross-section.

The cyst lumens contain serous or mucinous fluid, or chocolate-colored material when the tumor has arisen in an endometriotic cyst (Figure 25.56). Benign and borderline clear cell tumors are almost always unilateral; stage 1 carcinomas are bilateral in 2% of the cases.[65]

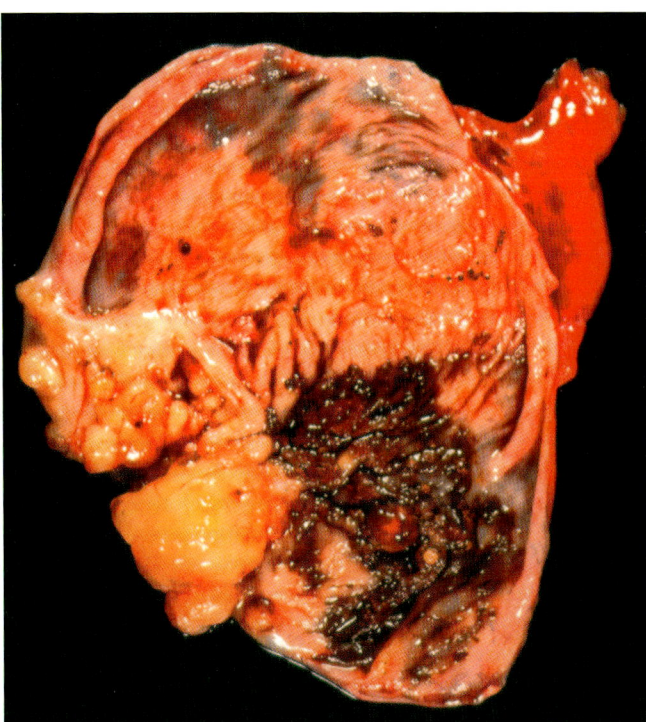

Fig. 25.56 Clear cell adenocarcinoma arising in endometriotic cyst. The polypoid yellow tumor protrudes into the lumen of a unilocular endometriotic (chocolate) cyst. Reproduced with permission from Matias-Guiu et al.[48]

BENIGN CLEAR CELL TUMORS

Nearly all benign clear cell tumors are adenofibromas. The tubular spaces are lined by a single layer of hobnail cells, clear cells or, less commonly, 'indifferent' cuboidal cells. The nuclei are regular in size and shape. Cellular atypia, if present, is only mild and focal. Solid sheets of clear cells and luminal tufting are absent. Mitoses are rarely encountered. The intervening stroma is compact and fibrocollagenous, often being more cellular adjacent to the epithelial elements.

BORDERLINE CLEAR CELL TUMORS

Borderline clear cell tumors (Figure 25.57) show atypical epithelium without invasion (one or more foci each under 10 mm² do not alter the designation) (Figure 25.58).[41,78] Nuclear atypia, epithelial budding, and mitoses (up to 3 per 10 HPFs) are present. True papillae are rarely seen. Before a diagnosis of a benign or a borderline clear cell adenofibroma is rendered, the specimen should be extensively sampled for occult CCC in as much as these tumor subtypes occur far more often in the company of CCC than in pure form (Figure 25.59).[78]

CLEAR CELL ADENOCARCINOMAS

Clear cell adenocarcinomas (CCCs) exhibit a variety of patterns and cell types that are often admixed.[78] The most common patterns are tubulocystic (Figure 25.60) and papillary (Figure 25.61). A predominantly solid pattern is less frequent (Figure 25.62). The papillae are often complex. Rarely, CCC has a reticular pattern, simulating a yolk sac tumor (Figure 25.63).

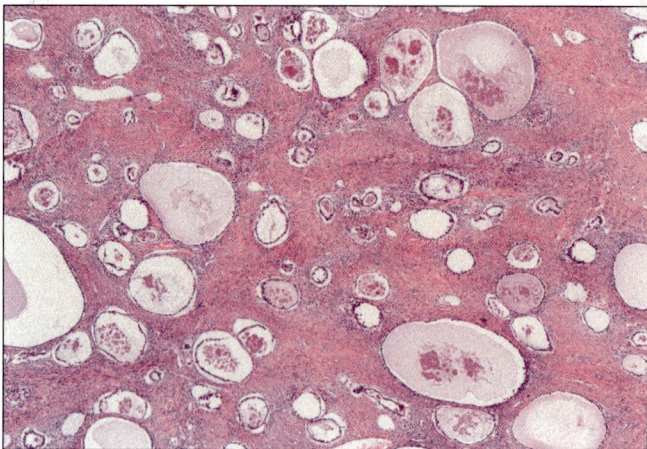

Fig. 25.57 Borderline clear cell adenofibroma with microinvasion. Cystic glands lined by flat and hobnail cells lie in an abundant fibromatous stroma.

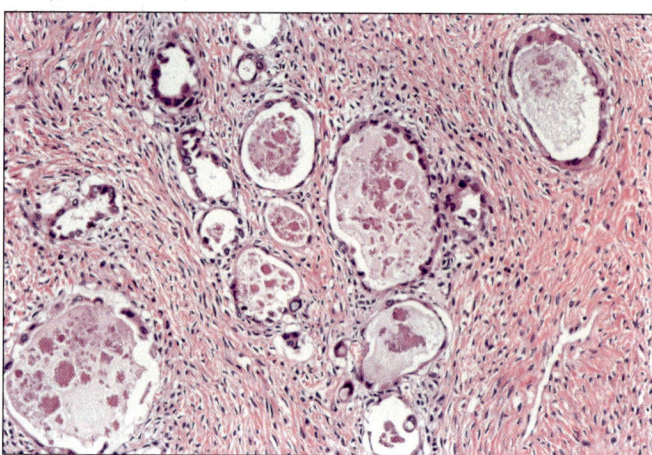

Fig. 25.58 Borderline clear cell adenofibroma with microinvasion. Small glands and single tumor cells have invaded the stroma.

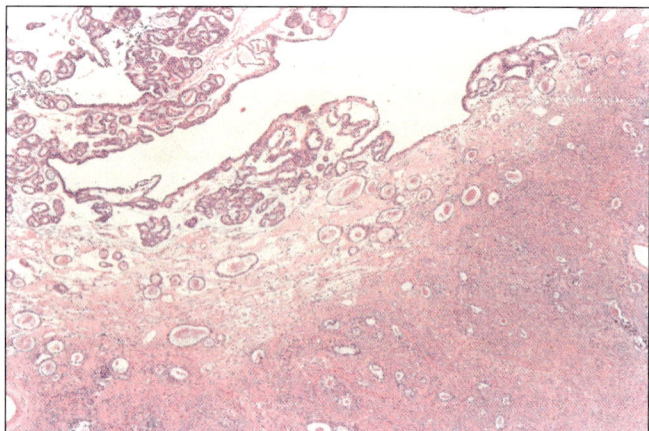

Fig. 25.59 Clear cell adenocarcinoma in borderline adenofibroma. The invasive carcinoma, composed of oxyphilic cells, appears on the upper left corner of the figure. Reproduced with permission from Prat.[69]

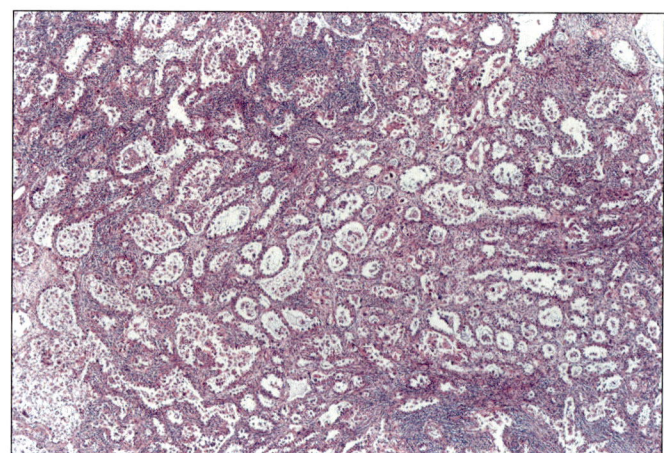

Fig. 25.60 Clear cell adenocarcinoma, tubulocystic pattern.

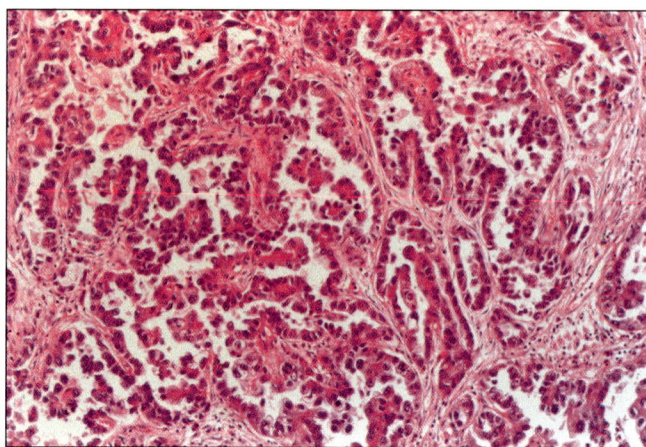

Fig. 25.61 Clear cell adenocarcinoma, papillary pattern. The papillae are lined by hobnail cells and have hyalinized cores.

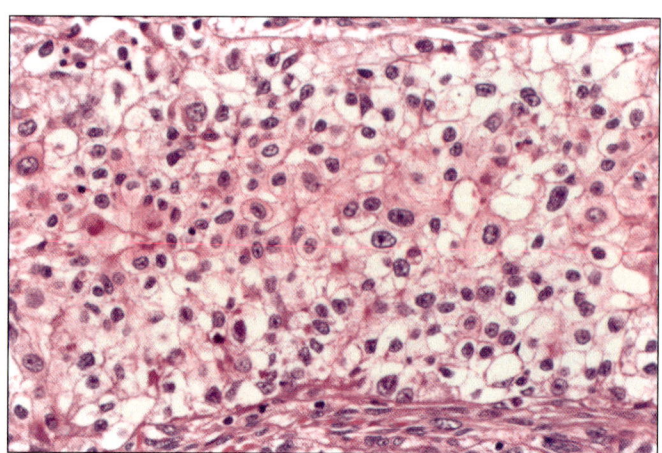

Fig. 25.62 Clear cell adenocarcinoma, solid pattern. The clear cells are polyhedral and have eccentric hyperchromatic nuclei. Reproduced with permission from Prat.[69]

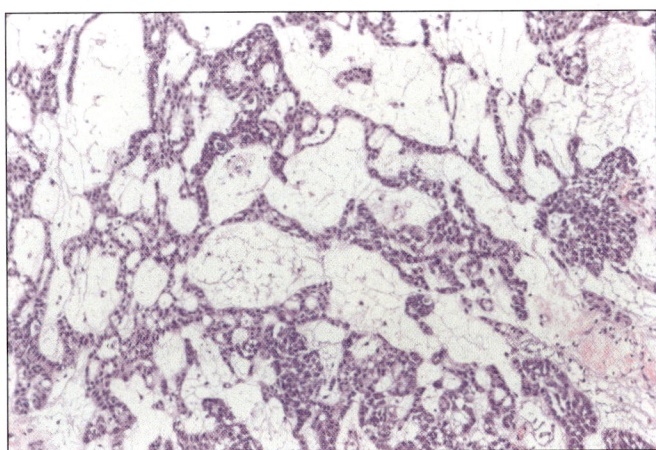

Fig. 25.63 Clear cell adenocarcinoma, reticular pattern. The edematous stroma simulates a yolk sac tumor. Reproduced with permission from Prat.[69]

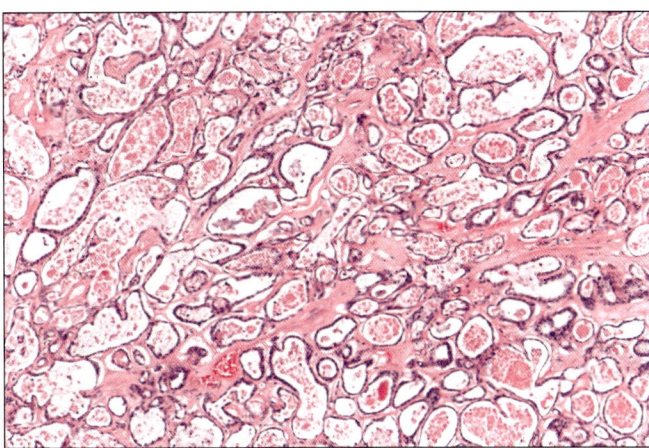

Fig. 25.66 Clear cell adenocarcinoma with tubulocystic pattern. The dilated cysts are lined by flat cells which have a deceptively benign appearance. Note the presence of inspissated eosinophilic secretion within the cystic glands. Reproduced with permission from Prat.[69]

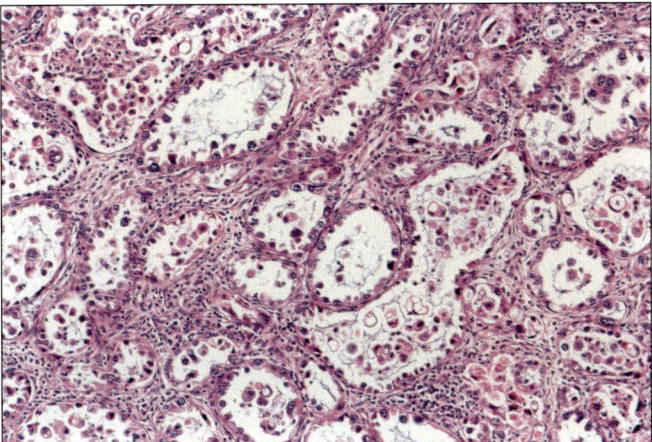

Fig. 25.64 Clear cell adenocarcinoma with tubulocystic pattern and markedly atypical hobnail cells.

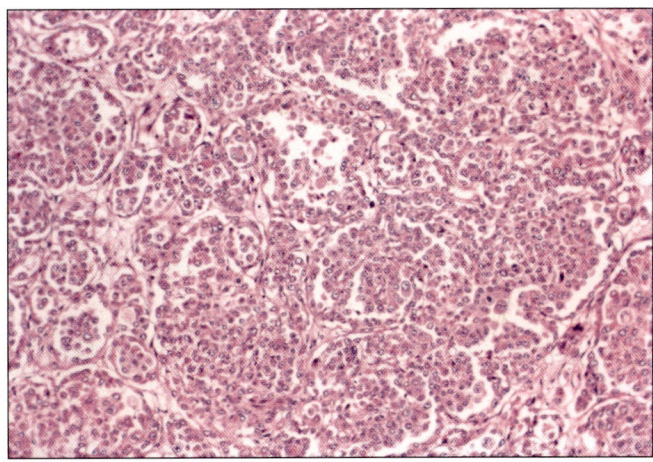

Fig. 25.67 Clear cell adenocarcinoma, oxyphilic type. The tumor cells have abundant eosinophilic cytoplasm and form solid aggregates.

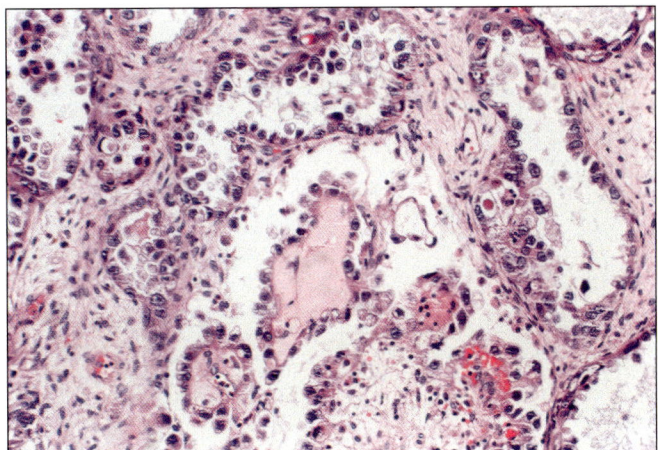

Fig. 25.65 Clear cell adenocarcinoma with tubulocystic and papillary features, and occasional signet-ring cells.

The most common cell types are the clear and the hobnail cells. Clear cells are clustered in solid nests or masses (Figure 25.62) whereas hobnail cells line lumens and papillae (Figure 25.64). Clear cells are rounded or polyhedral, have distinct cell borders, and contain eccentric rounded nuclei with prominent

nucleoli. The hobnail cells contain bulbous dark nuclei that protrude into lumens beyond their apparent cytoplasmic limits (Figure 25.65). Less common cell types are flat cells (deceptively benign looking) (Figure 25.66), cuboidal cells, oxyphilic cells with abundant eosinophilic cytoplasm (Figure 25.67),[78] and signet-ring cells containing mucin, typically in the form of inspissated eosinophilic material in the center of the vacuole (bull's-eye appearance) (Figures 25.68–25.70). Rarely, the latter cells predominate in CCC. The various patterns are often admixed (Figure 25.71). Mitoses are less frequent than in other types of ovarian carcinomas and usually number <2 per 10 HPFs. Indeed, a mitotic rate of ≥6 per 10 HPFs is regarded as an adverse prognostic variable.[34]

Three characteristic microscopic features help in the diagnosis of CCC: (1) multiple complex papillae (Figure 25.61); (2) dense hyaline basement membrane material expanding the cores of the papillae (Figure 25.72);[78] and (3) hyaline bodies, which are present in approximately 25% of cases (Figure 25.73). In exceptional cases, extensive amounts of basement membrane material, which characteristically stains for type IV col-

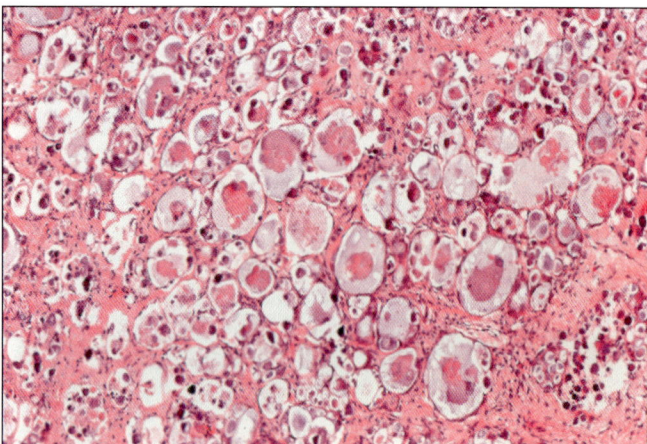

Fig. 25.68 Clear cell adenocarcinoma with small cystic glands and signet-ring cells. The glands contain inspissated eosinophilic secretion.

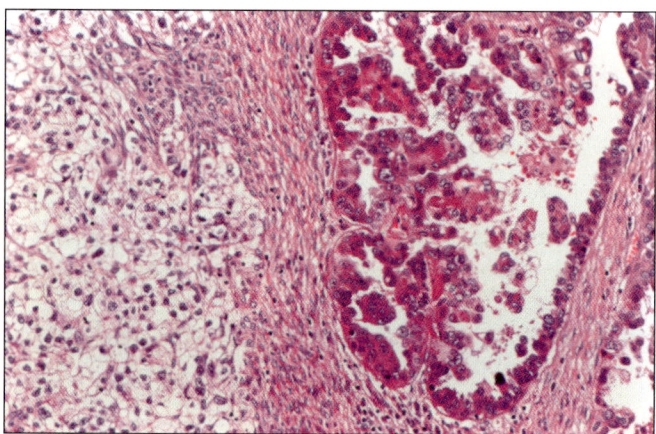

Fig. 25.71 Clear cell adenocarcinoma, mixed papillary and solid patterns. Reproduced with permission from Prat.[69]

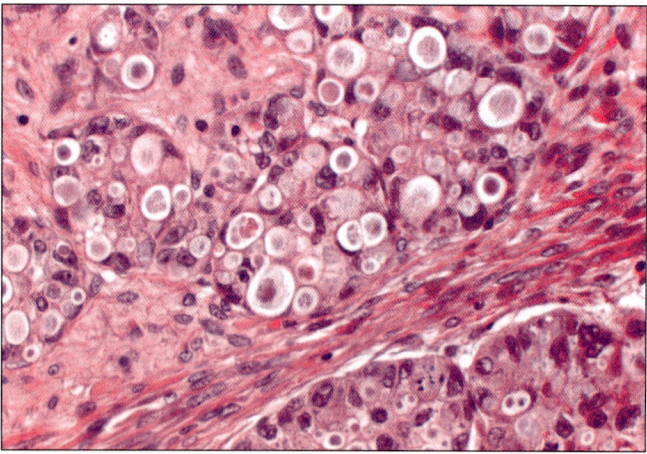

Fig. 25.69 Clear cell adenocarcinoma, signet-ring type. The vacuolated tumor cells resemble those of a Krukenberg tumor.

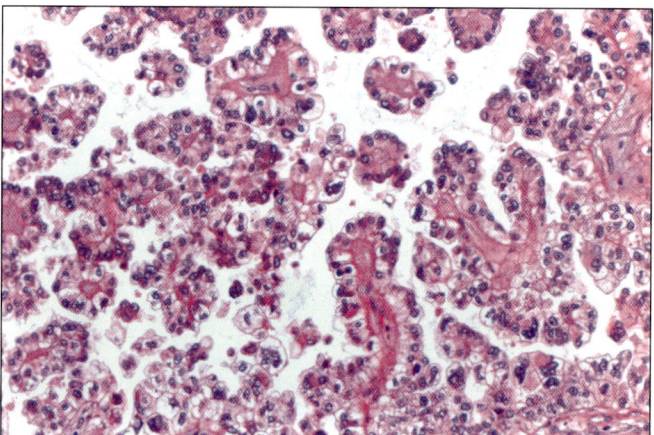

Fig. 25.72 Clear cell adenocarcinoma. The papillae are lined by clear cells and have hyalinized cores.

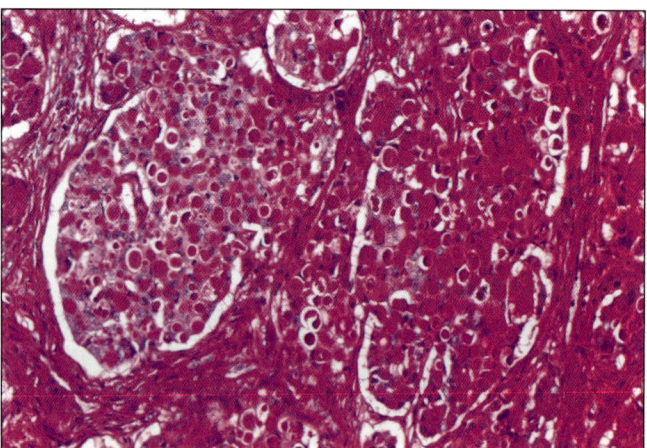

Fig. 25.70 Clear cell adenocarcinoma, signet-ring type. The inspissated secretion was stained by PAS and was diastase resistant.

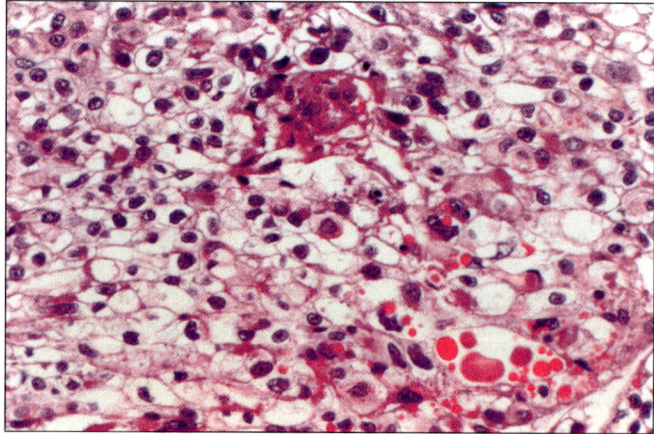

Fig. 25.73 Clear cell adenocarcinoma. Numerous intracytoplasmic hyaline globules are seen on the lower right corner of the figure. Reproduced with permission from Prat.[69]

lagen and laminin, occupy the stroma. Clear cell carcinoma is occasionally admixed with endometrioid carcinoma, to which it is closely related.

The clear cells contain glycogen (Figure 25.74). Except in the mucin-containing signet-ring cells, mucinous secretion (dia-stase-resistant, PAS-positive), if present, is found in the lumens and along the cytoplasmic apex of the lining cells. Electron microscopy reveals short, irregular, blunt microvilli on the surface of the luminal cells, glycogen, and rough endoplasmic reticulum within the cytoplasm (Figure 25.75).

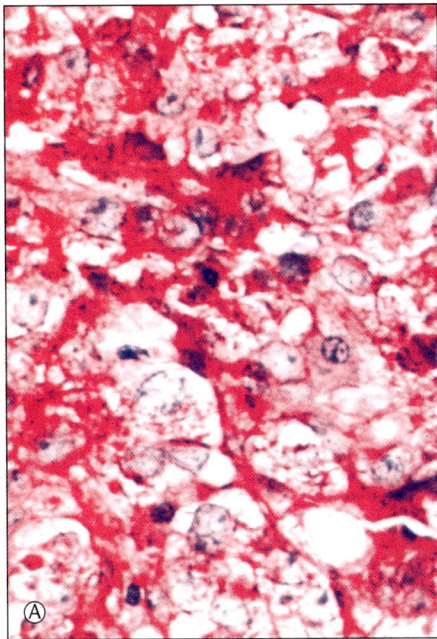
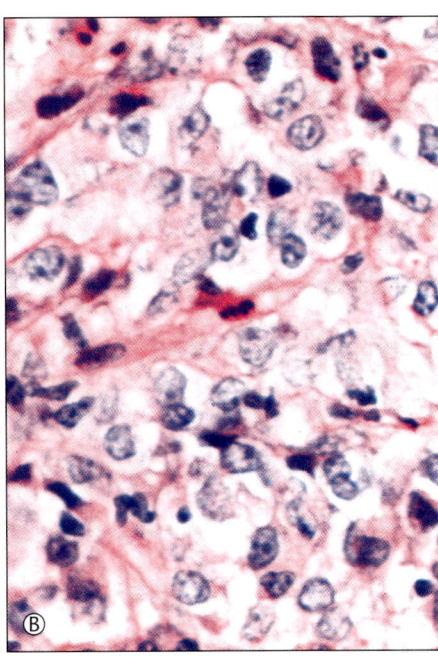

Fig. 25.74 Clear cell adenocarcinoma. The tumor cells contain glycogen which is stained by PAS (**A**) and digested by diastase (**B**). Reproduced with permission from Prat.[69]

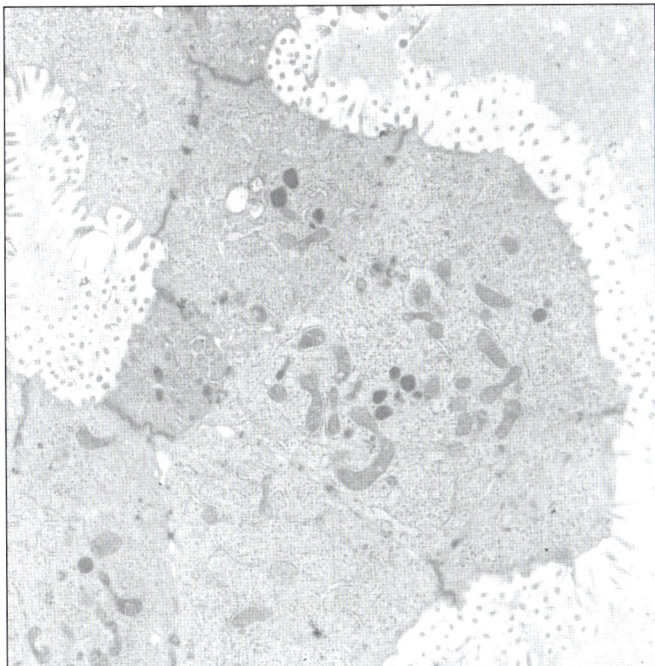

Fig. 25.75 Clear cell adenocarcinoma. Electron microscopy reveals short, irregular, blunt microvilli on the cell surface, glycogen, and rough endoplasmic reticulum within the cytoplasm. Courtesy of Dr J Lloreta, Barcelona, Spain.

Immunohistochemistry

CCCs stain diffusely and strongly for keratins, EMA, Leu-M1, and B72.3. Stains for CA125 are positive in 50% of cases and for CEA in 38%. Rarely is CCC immunoreactive for α-feto-protein (AFP).

Somatic genetics

The genetic alterations encountered in CCC resemble those of endometrioid carcinomas (see above).

Differential diagnosis

1. *Dysgerminoma*: A CCC may simulate a dysgerminoma when it has a diffuse pattern composed entirely of clear cells (Figure 25.62). The dysgerminoma cell is rounded with flattened edges in contrast to the polyhedral cell of CCC, and the nuclei of dysgerminoma, unlike those of the CCC, are central and contain one to several prominent nucleoli. Lymphocytes are almost always seen in dysgerminoma, especially in fibrous septa, which are lacking in CCC. Granulomas are also often seen in dysgerminoma, but rarely, if ever, in CCC. Immunoreactions for placental-like alkaline phosphatase (PLAP) are more commonly positive in dysgerminoma than in CCC. Contrariwise, CCC shows reactivity for cytokeratins and EMA, as expected in an epithelial tumor. Finally, the older age of patients with CCC would be unusual in germ cell tumors.

2. *Yolk sac tumor*: CCC may display a loose, edematous appearance (Figure 25.63) simulating the reticular pattern of a yolk sac tumor and both tumors may be papillary and contain hyaline bodies. The nuclei in yolk sac tumors, however, almost always appear more primitive than in CCC and their papillae may occasionally contain a central vessel (Schiller–Duval body) and lack a hyalinized eosinophilic core. The presence of other types of germ cell neoplasia within the neoplasm excludes a diagnosis of CCC. Of note, hyaline bodies are seen in one-fourth of CCCs as well as commonly in yolk sac tumors. AFP is demonstrable in almost all yolk sac tumors but in only 10% of CCCs.

3. *Juvenile granulosa cell tumor*: The young age of the patient, the associated estrogenic symptoms, α-inhibin reactivity, and the presence of more typical tumor patterns facilitate the diagnosis.

4. *Krukenberg tumor*: Rare cases of CCC that are predominantly composed of mucin-containing signet-ring cells (Figures 25.69 and 25.70) may be difficult to distinguish from a Krukenberg tumor. However,

Krukenberg tumors occur in patients who are known to have a primary mucinous carcinoma elsewhere, and are bilateral in 80% of the cases. Additional sections usually show the typical microscopic features of CCC, i.e., hyalinized papillae, hobnail cells, and tubulocystic pattern.

5. *Metastatic renal cell carcinoma*: The very rare metastatic renal cell carcinoma may be indistinguishable from the rare primary ovarian CCC that is composed exclusively of clear cells (Figure 25.62). In most cases of ovarian CCC, however, the additional presence of other patterns (e.g., tubulocystic) and cell types and conspicuous extracellular luminal mucin permits microscopic differentiation. Clinical data, including radiologic studies, may be necessary in some cases to exclude metastatic renal cell carcinoma.

6. *Steroid cell tumor/hepatoid yolk sac tumor/hepatoid carcinoma*: CCC composed predominantly or exclusively of oxyphilic cells (Figure 25.67) may closely resemble steroid cell tumors or other ovarian tumors exhibiting abundant eosinophilic cytoplasm such as the hepatoid yolk sac tumor and hepatoid carcinoma. However, typical foci of CCC are usually present in the oxyphilic variant of the tumor. In addition, the nuclei in oxyphilic CCC are typically eccentric in contrast to the central nuclei of steroid cell tumors. The degree of cytologic atypia in CCC generally exceeds that of steroid cell tumors. The hepatoid yolk sac tumor generally occurs in young females and, in addition, often contains other foci of more typical yolk sac neoplasia. Hepatoid carcinoma occurs in an age group that is generally similar to that of CCC but lacks the typical foci of CCC usually present in the oxyphilic form of the tumor. In contrast to oxyphilic CCC, hepatoid yolk sac tumor and hepatoid carcinoma are reactive for AFP.

7. *Arias-Stella change*: The glands of CCC resemble the hypersecretory glands of the Arias-Stella phenomenon, which occasionally may be encountered in ovarian endometriosis associated with either intrauterine or extrauterine pregnancy or trophoblastic disease. The Arias-Stella phenomenon usually involves a focus of closely packed glands. The epithelial cells exhibit marked nuclear pleomorphism and hyperchromatism; of importance, however, the nuclear material has a smudged appearance. The cytoplasm is vacuolated and clear or may be densely eosinophilic. Unlike CCC, the Arias-Stella phenomenon is associated with decidua and typically shows nuclear polyploidy. CCC develops predominantly in postmenopausal women, and usually contains near diploid or aneuploid nuclear DNA.

Tumor spread and staging
Patients with CCC present as stage 1 disease in 43% of cases, stage 2 in 19%, stage 3 in 29%, and stage 4 in 9%.[65]

Treatment and prognosis
Treatment is similar to that applied to other ovarian carcinomas. Most patients with clear cell borderline tumors, including those with microinvasion, have a favorable prognosis. CCC is currently considered as an unfavorable histologic type with a worse prognosis in advanced stages than other malignant epithelial–stromal tumors, and a poor response to platinum-based

chemotherapy.[29] The prognosis of CCC resembles that of undifferentiated carcinoma.[29] The 5-year survival rate for patients with stage 1 carcinoma is 69%; stage 2, 55%; stage 3, 14%; and stage 4, 4%.[41]

TRANSITIONAL CELL TUMORS

Definition
Ovarian tumors composed of epithelial cells histologically resembling those of the urothelium are grouped in the transitional cell category of tumors. This group of neoplasms constitutes 1–2% of all ovarian tumors and includes: (1) benign Brenner tumors, exhibiting a prominent stromal component and transitional cell nests; (2) borderline (non-invasive) and malignant (invasive) Brenner tumors, both of which are associated with a benign Brenner tumor component; and (3) transitional cell carcinomas (TCCs) not associated with a benign or borderline Brenner component.[41]

The SNOMED classification of transitional cell tumors is as follows:

- Brenner tumor
- Borderline Brenner tumor
- Malignant Brenner tumor
- Transitional cell carcinoma (non-Brenner).

Pathogenesis
Transitional cell tumors appear to derive directly from the ovarian surface epithelium that undergoes metaplasia to form urothelial-like epithelium. Although transitional cell differentiation in the form of Walthard rests occurs frequently in the pelvic peritoneum (perisalpinx and ovarian hilus), it represents the least common type of ovarian surface epithelial differentiation.[78] Walthard rests and small Brenner tumors have been found to arise occasionally from the rete ovarii, which is also of celomic or mesonephric derivation.[78] In rare cases, Brenner nests lie adjacent to or within a dermoid cyst, a struma ovarii, or a carcinoid tumor, suggesting a possible germ cell origin for at least some cases.[78] The similarity of Walthard rests and transitional cell tumors to urothelium is evident at both histologic and ultrastructural levels. However, the cytokeratin (CK) immunohistochemical profile of the ovarian transitional cell tumors parallels that of müllerian (negative CK20) rather than urothelial (positive CK20) tumors.[44,62,82] CK7, CEA, EMA, and CA19-9 may be expressed by both ovarian and urinary tract neoplasms. Urothelial markers such as uroplakin III (Uro-III) and thrombomodulin are consistently positive in Brenner tumors but rarely positive in TCC of the ovary.[44,57] Additionally, the ovarian tumors are CA125 positive. These findings, along with a frequent mixture of other müllerian epithelial elements (mucinous, serous) in the tumors, have prompted grouping of transitional cell tumors with the other 'epithelial–stromal tumors'.

BENIGN BRENNER TUMOR
Clinical features
Benign Brenner tumors represent less than 5% of benign epithelial–stromal tumors.[41] They are found in women of both reproductive and postmenopausal years, usually between the ages of 30 and 60 years.[78] Most are asymptomatic and

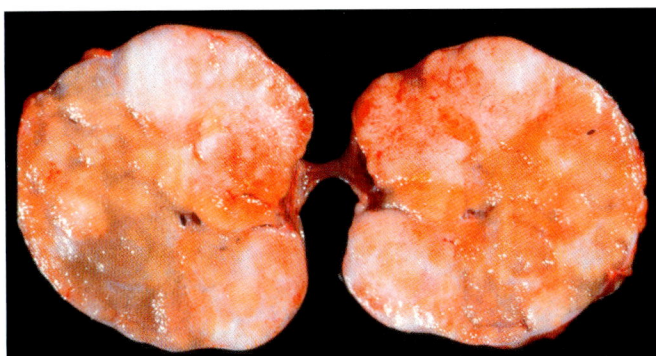

Fig. 25.76 Brenner tumor. On section, the tumor appears solid, yellowish-brown, and multinodular. The gray areas correspond to the fibromatous stroma. Reproduced with permission from Prat.[69]

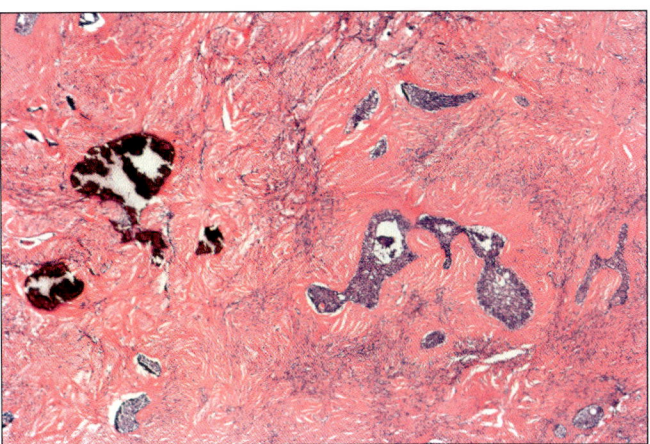

Fig. 25.77 Brenner tumor. Several nests of transitional cells lie in a fibromatous stroma showing focal calcification.

are typically found incidentally in ovaries removed for some other reason. Brenner tumors with functioning stroma are associated with endocrine symptoms of estrogenic or androgenic type.

Macroscopic features

Approximately half of the benign Brenner tumors are grossly visible. Many are under 2 cm in size and only a few exceed 10 cm in diameter. Less than 10% are bilateral. The sectioned surface of the typical Brenner tumor shows a nodular, sharply circumscribed (but unencapsulated), and lobulated fibrous mass that has a brownish tinge (Figure 25.76). Small cysts are common, and a rare tumor is predominantly cystic. Focal calcification may be seen. About one-fourth exhibit a cystic component, but this usually represents mixed (mucinous) epithelial differentiation.

Microscopic features

Benign Brenner tumors show round to oval nests or trabeculae of mature transitional cells within a prominent fibromatous stroma (Figure 25.77). The apparent islands are in reality branches of a tree-like structure that in cortical tumors is in continuity with the ovarian surface epithelium. The epithelial cells are round to polygonal with distinct cell membranes and eosinophilic to clear cytoplasm. The oval nuclei have fine, evenly dispersed chromatin, obvious nucleoli, and often longitudinal grooving (so-called 'coffee-bean' appearance). This latter feature is not always prominent and, moreover, it is non-specific. It can be found in other ovarian tumors such as the adult granulosa cell tumor. Epithelial atypia is rare, as are mitoses (<1 per 10 HPFs). The nests may be solid or have a central cavity containing densely eosinophilic, mucin-positive material. The lumina may be lined by mucinous (Figure 25.78), sometimes ciliated-serous, or indifferent epithelium. Occasionally, squamous differentiation is found within the Brenner nests. Often the cell nests become cystic and these microcysts (containing eosinophilic debris or mucin) are mostly lined by otherwise unremarkable transitional cells. Cystic change may be more prominent – to the point of having macroscopically visible cysts forming a significant portion of the tumor. Typical transitional cell epithelium commonly lines these cysts but, sometimes, it is a mucinous epithelium that gives rise to one-sided overgrowth. The extreme of this spectrum is for a small nodule of transitional cell tumor to be found in the wall of an

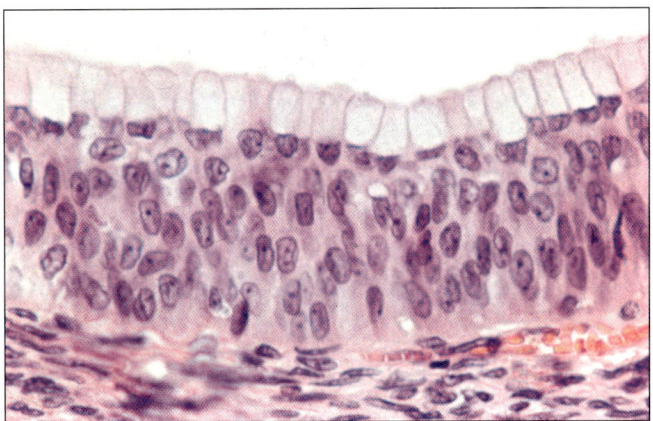

Fig. 25.78 Brenner tumor. Cavitated nest of transitional cells lined by mucinous columnar epithelium. Reproduced with permission from Prat.[69]

otherwise typical benign mucinous cystadenoma (see 'Mixed epithelial tumors' below).

The Brenner epithelial nests are scattered throughout a stromal component that has the microscopic features of an ovarian fibroma or more rarely a thecoma, and may contain luteinized cells. There is much variation in cellularity, which is inversely proportional to collagen formation and hyalinization, the latter most often prominent around, or in juxtaposition to, epithelial nests. Dystrophic spiculate calcification is frequently present in such sites (Figure 25.77). New bone formation and marked stromal edema may occur.

Immunohistochemistry and somatic genetics

As evidence of some urothelial differentiation, benign Brenner tumors express Uro-III and thrombomodulin in three-fourths of cases, but they do not immunoreact for CK20.[44,57,62,63,73,82] One-third of the tumors contain intracytoplasmic neuroendocrine granules, which are reactive for serotonin, but not for peptide hormones. K-ras mutations at codon 12 have been identified in three of five benign Brenner tumors in one study.[14] This finding supports the hypothesis that, in ovarian tumors, K-ras mutations are genetic events closely related to the mucinous phenotype.

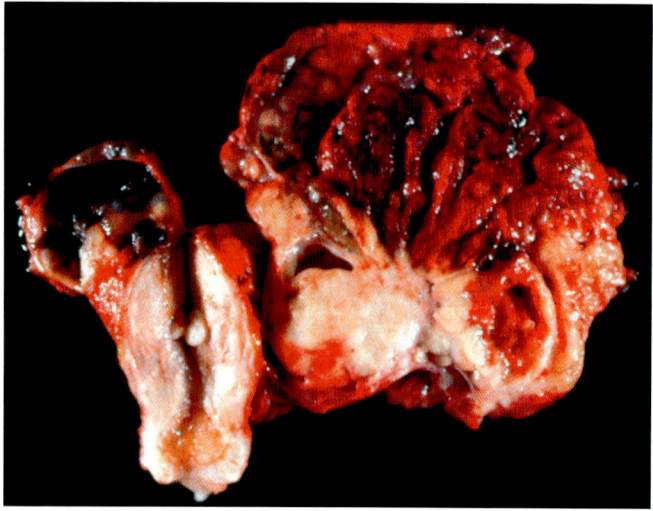

Fig. 25.79 Malignant Brenner tumor. A large solid and cystic tumor with polypoid masses composed of fleshy, partly hemorrhagic, tumor tissue. A fibroma-like component (benign Brenner tumor) is seen at the bottom. The contralateral ovary shows a mucinous cystadenoma.

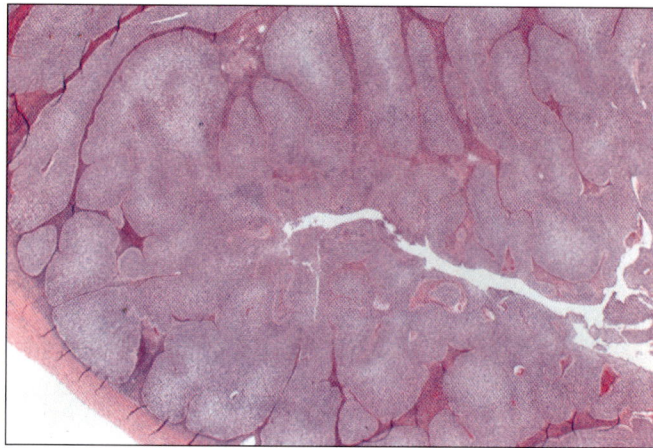

Fig. 25.80 Borderline Brenner tumor. Confluent papillae lined by transitional cells protrude into a cystic space. Reproduced with permission from Prat.[69]

BORDERLINE AND MALIGNANT BRENNER TUMORS

Clinical features

Only 5% of Brenner tumors are borderline or malignant and, unlike their benign counterparts, the great majority occur in women over 50 years of age.[41,78] The patients present with an abdominal mass or pain. Some may have abnormal vaginal bleeding. Most tumors are confined to the ovary at the time of diagnosis. While borderline tumors are almost always unilateral, 10% of malignant Brenner tumors are bilateral.[78]

Macroscopic features

Borderline Brenner tumors are typically large with a median size of 16–20 cm. Although they are usually cystic and unilocular or multilocular, with papillomatous masses protruding into one or more of the locules, occasional tumors are solid. Malignant Brenner tumors may be solid or cystic with mural nodules; they have no distinctive features except that, in contrast to transitional cell carcinomas, they may exhibit a benign Brenner tumor component which may be fibromatous and calcified (Figure 25.79).[41,78]

Microscopic features

Microscopically, the polyps of the borderline tumors resemble urothelial papillary neoplasms (Figure 25.80) and exhibit the same spectrum of architectural and cytologic features. By definition, there is no stromal invasion (Figure 25.81). A benign Brenner tumor component is typically present (Figure 25.82) but may be small and easily overlooked. The mitotic rate is highly variable and focal necrosis is common. Mucinous metaplasia may be extensive. The criteria for the diagnosis of borderline and frankly malignant Brenner tumors and the designations used for these neoplasms are somewhat controversial. Since there are no reported cases of borderline tumors of any grade that have spread beyond the ovary or have followed an aggressive behavior, some investigators have desig-

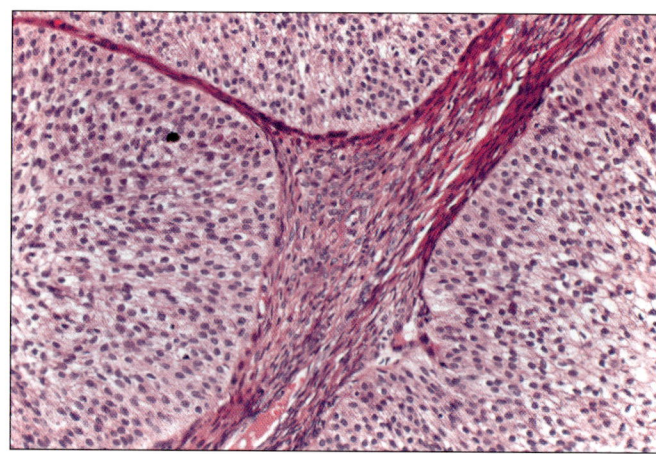

Fig. 25.81 Borderline Brenner tumor. The lining of the papillae is composed of low-grade transitional cells resembling that of a grade 1 papillary transitional cell carcinoma of the bladder. Reproduced with permission from Prat.[69]

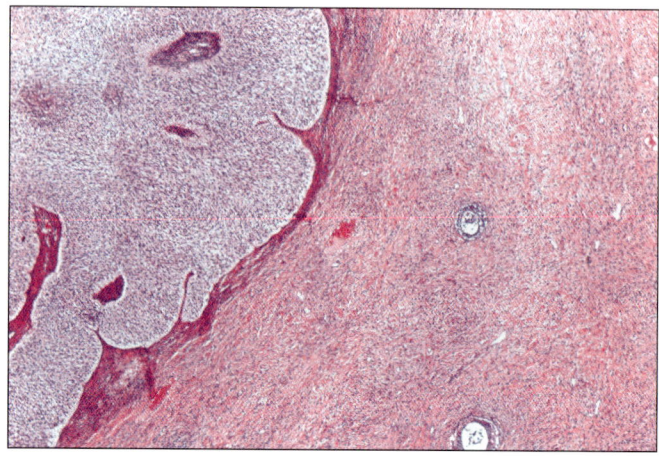

Fig. 25.82 Borderline Brenner tumor. Two benign Brenner nests with central cavities lie in the adjacent fibromatous stroma. Reproduced with permission from Prat.[69]

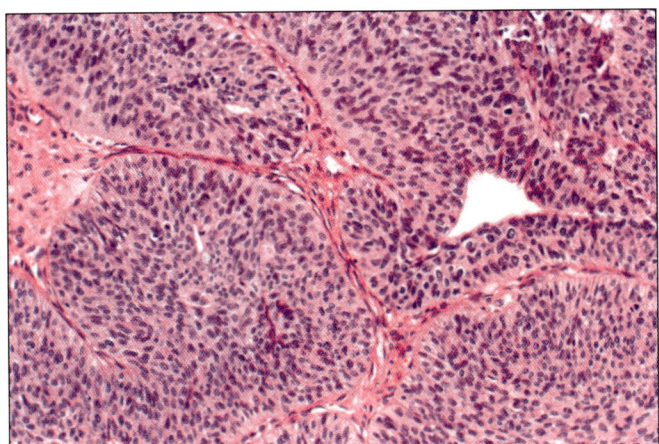

Fig. 25.83 Malignant Brenner tumor. Large, closely-packed, solid aggregates of transitional cells.

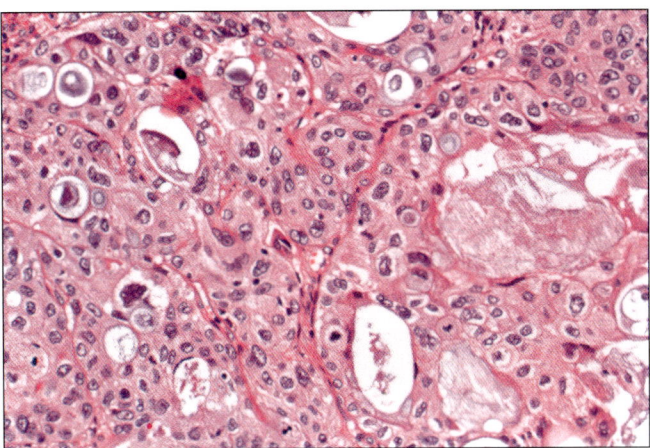

Fig. 25.85 Malignant Brenner tumor. The irregular masses of transitional cell carcinoma contain many small pools filled with mucin.

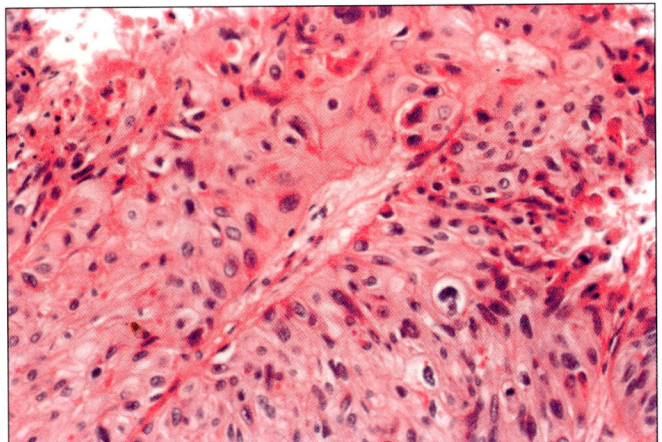

Fig. 25.84 Malignant Brenner tumor. Early squamous differentiation.

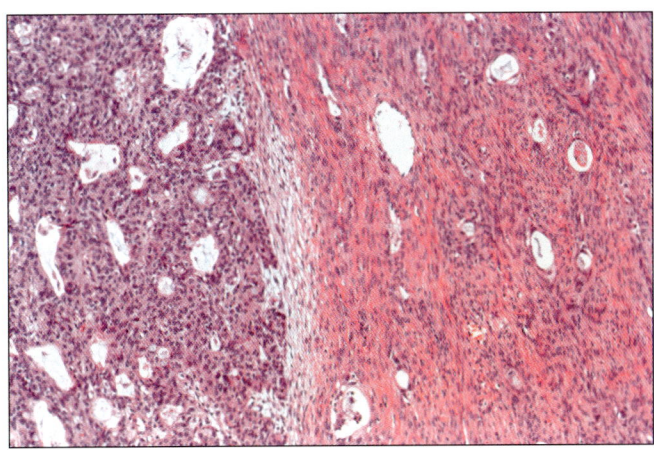

Fig. 25.86 Malignant Brenner tumor. Several cavitated nests of benign Brenner component are seen in the vicinity.

nated these tumors as 'proliferating' rather than borderline. Others, however, designate those resembling grade 2 or 3 transitional cell carcinoma of the urinary tract as borderline 'with intraepithelial carcinoma'.[78] The finding of severe atypia should suggest further sampling in order to exclude the presence of an invasive component.

Malignant Brenner tumors are usually suspected on sectioning when solid cancerous masses are found. Microscopically, invasive transitional or squamous cell carcinoma (Figures 25.83–25.85), alone or mixed with each other, is evident together with a benign or borderline Brenner component (Figure 25.86).[41,78] Cysts are lined by multilayered epithelium featuring hyperchromatic and pleomorphic nuclei and prominent mitotic activity. With the exception of a few reported cases in which cellular atypia has been described as mild, the malignancy of the tumor cells is usually quite obvious. Discrete nests of carcinoma cells may undergo central necrosis producing a 'comedo carcinoma' pattern and occasional bizarre tumor giant cells are seen. However, as in other malignant epithelial adenofibromas, the demonstration of unequivocal stromal invasion is subjective and may necessitate extensive sampling. Irregularity, branching and confluent epithelial nests, depletion of stroma by crowded epithelial masses, and desmoplastic stromal reac-

tions are useful diagnostic features. Mucinous elements and, more rarely, mucinous adenocarcinoma may coexist with the transitional component. A recent case of a stage 1A malignant Brenner tumor containing a prominent signet-ring mucinous component, which closely simulates a Krukenberg tumor, is shown in Figure 25.87.

Immunohistochemistry

The immunoprofile resembles that of benign Brenner tumors (see above) with a variable pattern of antigen expression in the invasive component of the frankly malignant counterpart (Figures 25.88 and 25.89). Loss of expression of pRb and p16, associated with overexpression of p21 and cyclin D, has recently been found in six borderline and one malignant Brenner tumors. These findings suggest that dysregulation of the cell cycle G_1–S phase transition plays a pathogenetic role.[72]

Differential diagnosis

In the absence of a benign or proliferating transitional cell component, the distinction between malignant Brenner tumors and other poorly differentiated ovarian carcinomas may be difficult. Identification of a mucin-secreting adenocarcinoma

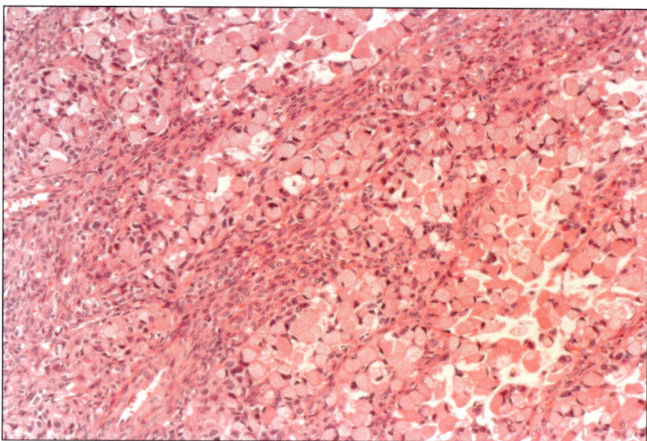

Fig. 25.87 Malignant Brenner tumor with a prominent signet-ring mucinous epithelial component.

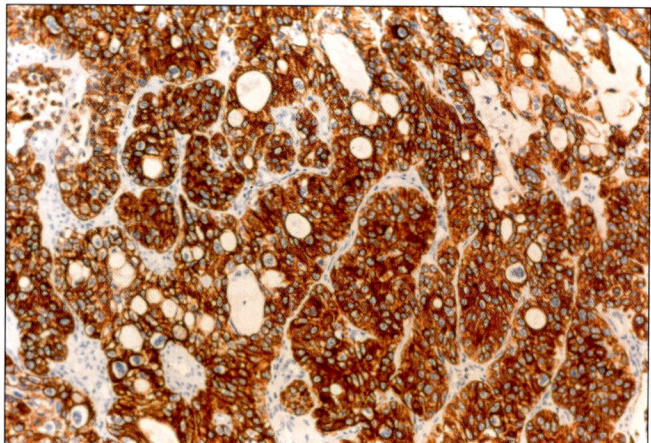

Fig. 25.88 Malignant Brenner tumor. Positive immunoreaction for cytokeratin 7.

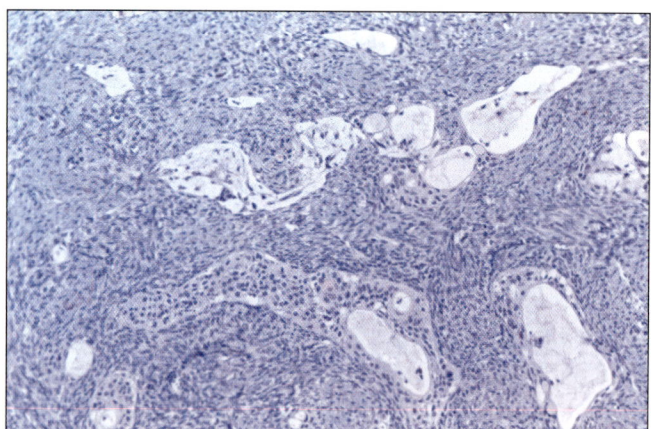

Fig. 25.89 Malignant Brenner tumor. Negative immunoreaction for cytokeratin 20.

component, if present, would strongly favor malignant Brenner tumor, while origin from, or juxtaposition to, an endometriotic cyst would favor a tumor of endometrioid type. Differentiating between transitional cell carcinoma primary in the ovary versus metastases to the ovaries from the urinary tract often requires clinical information.

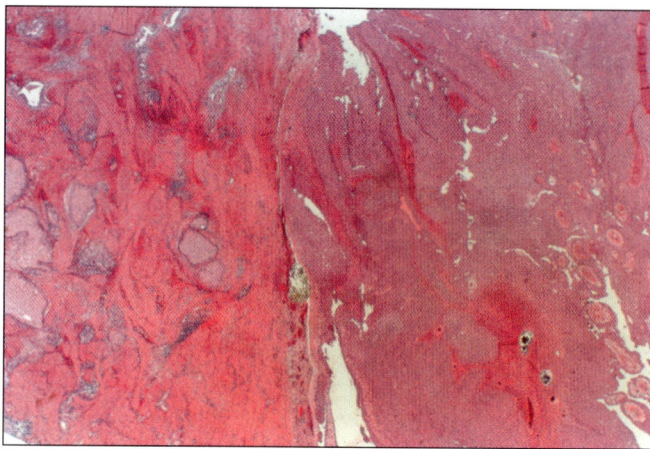

Fig. 25.90 Recurrent borderline Brenner tumor. The recurrent tumor forms confluent papillae on the uterine serosa (right) and infiltrates the underlying myometrium (left).

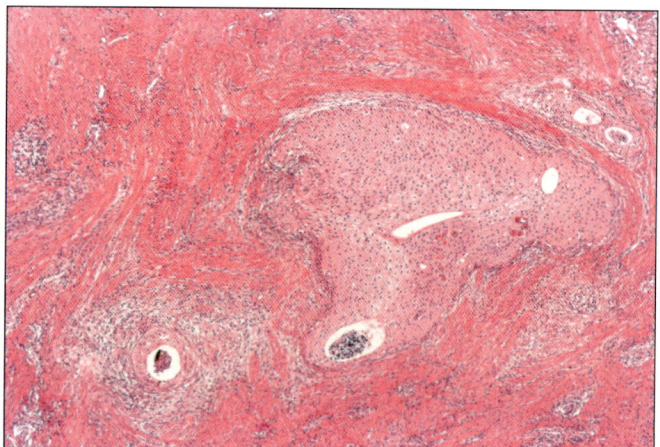

Fig. 25.91 Recurrent borderline Brenner tumor. Myometrial invasion by partly cavitated masses of transitional tumor cells.

Treatment and prognosis

Borderline Brenner tumors can be treated by conservative surgery when they occur in young women. Malignant Brenner tumors are treated like other epithelial cancers. Although none of more than 50 reported borderline Brenner tumors is known to have spread beyond the ovary,[78] we have recently seen a borderline Brenner tumor that recurred in the uterus after incomplete laparoscopic resection (Figures 25.90 and 25.91). Most malignant Brenner tumors are stage 1 and have an excellent prognosis (88% 5-year survival). About one-fifth, however, present with extraovarian spread and behave similarly to other ovarian cancers.[4] Nevertheless, the prognosis of advanced stage malignant Brenner tumors has been reported to exceed that of transitional cell carcinomas.[4]

TRANSITIONAL CELL CARCINOMAS

Clinical features

Transitional cell carcinoma (TCC) is the pure or predominant element in 6% of ovarian carcinomas. The mean age of patients is 60 years. Abdominal pain and swelling are the most common

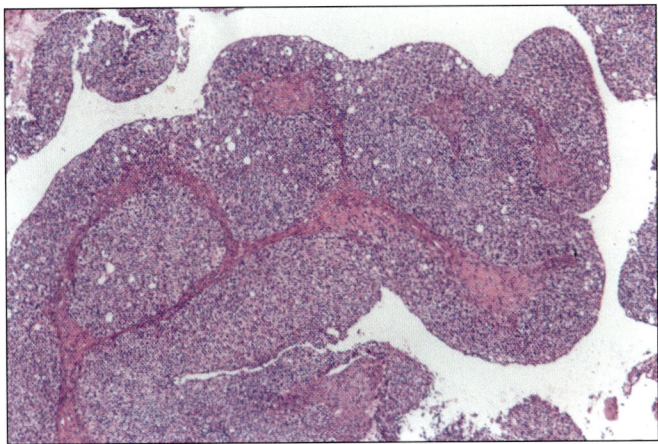

Fig. 25.92 Transitional cell carcinoma. Multilayered papilla with smooth luminal borders protruding into an empty space. Reproduced with permission from Prat.[69]

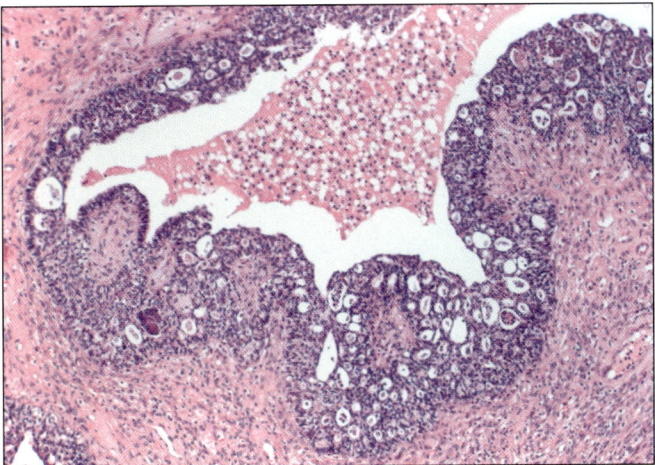

Fig. 25.93 Transitional cell carcinoma. Intraepithelial microspaces containing eosinophilic or amphophilic material. Reproduced with permission from Prat.[69]

presenting symptoms. Bladder or bowel disturbances are also common. TCC does not differ from other high-grade ovarian carcinomas regarding stage (often high) and bilaterality (15% of cases).[18]

Microscopic features

TCCs resemble those occurring in the urinary tract and lack a benign or borderline Brenner tumor component. The tumor cells characteristically form undulating thick bands lining cysts (93%) or large papillae that protrude into empty spaces (63%) (Figure 25.92). The cysts, which are often compressed, appear empty or contain cellular necrotic debris. The papillae have cores of fibrovascular tissue and show a smooth luminal border ('papillary type'). The bands of epithelium are multilayered, have a relative uniform width of at least a dozen cells, and typically contain microspaces (Figure 25.93) of the size of or slightly larger than Call–Exner bodies (87%).[18] Diffuse (solid), insular, and trabecular patterns are found in half of cases. Slit-like fenestrations or filiform papillae are seen focally in a minority of tumors. Tumor cell necrosis occurs in the majority of cases.[18] At low magnification, the tumor cells are usually monomorphic and evenly spaced. The nuclei are round and often exhibit large eosinophilic nucleoli or longitudinal grooves. The cytoplasm is moderately abundant and frequently pale and granular. Generally, the nuclear atypicality is moderate or marked and mitotic activity high. As in urothelial carcinoma, glandular and/or squamous differentiation may occur. Unlike malignant Brenner tumors, TCCs are frequently associated or mixed with carcinomas of other types, usually poorly differentiated serous or endometrioid carcinomas.

Immunohistochemistry

Ovarian TCCs have an immunoprofile that differs from TCCs of the urinary tract, resembling ovarian epithelial stromal tumors.[44,62,82] Ovarian TCCs are unreactive for CK20 and Uro-III, and sometimes reactive for thrombomodulin (30% of cases). Unlike bladder cancer, ovarian TCC is reactive for vimentin and CA125. Unlike Brenner tumors (see above), TCC overexpresses p53 and preserves pRb, and p16 expression.[72]

Differential diagnosis

TCC is distinguished from undifferentiated carcinoma by the presence of thick, undulating papillae with smooth luminal borders in contrast to the pseudopapillae secondary to tumor cell necrosis that may be present in undifferentiated carcinoma. Microspaces are also more frequent in TCC than in undifferentiated carcinomas. The tumor cells in TCC have moderate cytoplasm, and in well-differentiated areas the nuclei have a distinctive 'urothelial' appearance with low cytoplasmic to nuclear ratios and nuclear grooves.

The adult granulosa cell tumor (adult GCT) with a diffuse pattern may also be considered in the differential diagnosis. However, the microspaces of TCC differ from Call–Exner bodies. The former are larger and more variable in size and, in contrast to the latter, their lumens are sharply demarcated from the surrounding epithelial cells. Also, TCC nuclei often have prominent nucleoli and high mitotic activity. Finally, the clinical and operative findings can be helpful. Adult GCTs are often associated with estrogenic manifestations, are unilateral in 95% of cases, and confined to the ovary (stage 1) in 90% of the cases.

Treatment and prognosis

TCCs are treated like other epithelial cancers. At the time of diagnosis, TCC has spread beyond the ovary in over two-thirds of cases. Some believe that carcinomas with metastatic transitional cell differentiation behave more favorably than poorly differentiated carcinomas of the other types, apparently due to their better response to chemotherapy.[36] A propensity for micronodular spread and better surgical resectability might contribute to the survival benefit.[36] The overall 5-year survival rate for TCC is 35%.

SQUAMOUS CELL LESIONS

EPIDERMOID (SQUAMOUS CELL) CYSTS

These rare lesions are usually incidental findings. Epidermoid cysts not associated with teratomatous elements may originate from the surface epithelium of the ovary or from the rete ovarii. They are lined by keratinizing squamous epithelium and

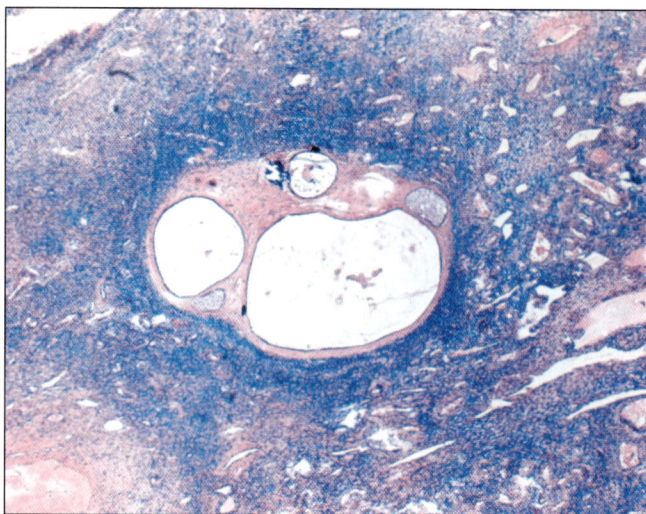

Fig. 25.94 Epidermoid cyst. The lining epithelium is flat. Two Walthard rests are seen within the wall of the cyst. Reproduced with permission from Prat.[69]

contain a creamy material that is usually seen on gross examination (Figure 25.94). Multiple sections are required to rule out a dermoid cyst.

SQUAMOUS CELL CARCINOMAS

Ovarian squamous cell carcinomas may have several histogenetic origins. Most seem to be of germ cell origin, as they arise from the walls of dermoid cysts. Less frequently, they occur in association with endometriosis, as a component of a malignant Brenner tumor, or in pure form where they are considered to be of epithelial–stromal origin.[66] Rare cases are associated with squamous cell carcinoma of the cervix (*in situ* or invasive), raising the question of their metastatic nature.[46,85] The finding of a benign epithelial lesion, such as endometriosis, mucinous cystadenoma, Brenner tumor, or epidermoid cysts within the same ovary suggests a primary epithelial neoplasm. The presence of these associated lesions may have prognostic implications, as pure squamous cell carcinomas generally behave more aggressively than those arising in endometriosis. Also, a malignant squamous cell component can be extensive in ovarian carcinomas of other types, particularly endometrioid carcinomas and malignant Brenner tumors. Most ovarian squamous cell carcinomas have spread beyond the ovary at the time of presentation, and the prognosis is poor.[66]

MIXED EPITHELIAL TUMORS

Definition

Most ovarian epithelial–stromal tumors are pure and easily classified into one of the five major categories (i.e., serous, mucinous, endometrioid, clear cell, and transitional). In some cases, however, two or more histologic types reside within the same tumor, or the tumor type cannot be identified by available criteria. Sampling of the tumor should be extensive enough to include all different components. Using WHO convention, mixed epithelial ovarian tumors are those in which the minor components are grossly recognizable, or account for at least

10% of the tumor on microscopic examination.[41] Mixed epithelial tumors represent less than 4% of epithelial–stromal tumors. Endometrioid tumors with squamous differentiation and neuroendocrine tumors associated with an epithelial–stromal tumor are excluded from this definition.

The SNOMED classification of mixed epithelial tumors is as follows:

- Benign mixed epithelial tumor
- Borderline mixed epithelial tumor
- Malignant mixed epithelial tumor.

The association of different types of epithelial–stromal tumors is not surprising in view of their common origin. Almost all combinations of mixed epithelial tumors have been described. Among the best known are: Brenner tumor with a mucinous cystic component; endocervical-like mucinous cystadenoma of borderline malignancy exhibiting other epithelial cell types of müllerian derivation;[78] endometrioid carcinoma admixed with clear cell carcinoma (Figure 25.95);[88] endometrioid carcinoma with a serous (Figure 25.96) or undifferentiated component; and transitional cell carcinoma with another type of carcinoma. In fact, transitional cell differentiation is commonly found in endometrioid and serous carcinomas.

Whereas in benign and borderline tumors the mixture of different cell types is not prognostically relevant, the presence of a serous or undifferentiated component in a carcinoma has long been known to have a negative effect on prognosis, particularly for stage 3 and 4 tumors. The 5-year survival rate for stage 3 tumors falls from 63 to 8%.[88] Prognostic data regarding transitional cell differentiation in carcinomas are still controversial and, similarly, there is no statistical evidence that mixed endometrioid and clear cell carcinomas behave differently from either of the two pure types.

UNDIFFERENTIATED CARCINOMAS

Definition

Undifferentiated carcinomas are tumors of epithelial–stromal origin that lack significant differentiation, or contain only minor (< 5%) areas of differentiation.[41,78] They probably account for less than 5% of ovarian cancers of epithelial type. The SNOMED classification is undifferentiated carcinoma.

Clinical features

The patients generally are older (mean age, 54 years) with a range of ages from 39 to 72 years. The clinical presentation resembles that of other ovarian cancers: abdominal pain, swelling, weight loss, and urinary or intestinal symptoms. At laparotomy, 90% of the tumors show extraovarian spread, and half are stage 3 (Figure 25.97).[41,78]

Pathology

Undifferentiated carcinomas are bilateral in 15% of cases (Figure 25.98). They are predominantly solid with extensive hemorrhage and necrosis. Surface adhesions and capsular rupture are common. Microscopically, they show a uniform population of large to medium-sized cells arranged in solid groups with high-grade nuclei and numerous mitotic figures (Figures 25.99 and 25.100). Foci of high-grade serous or transitional cell carcinoma may be present. Rare undifferentiated

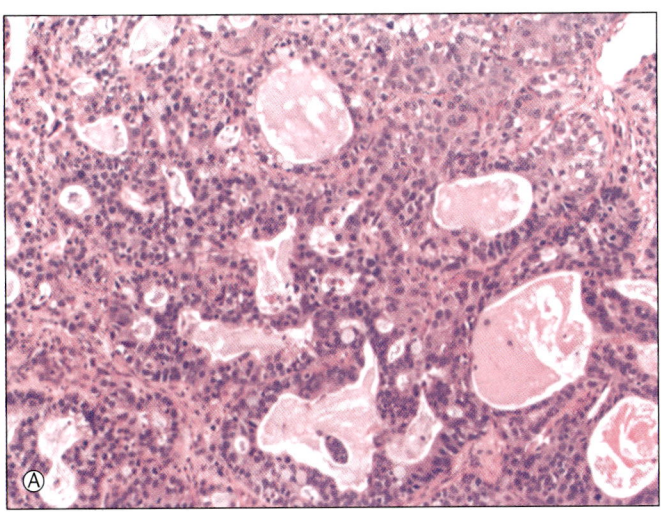 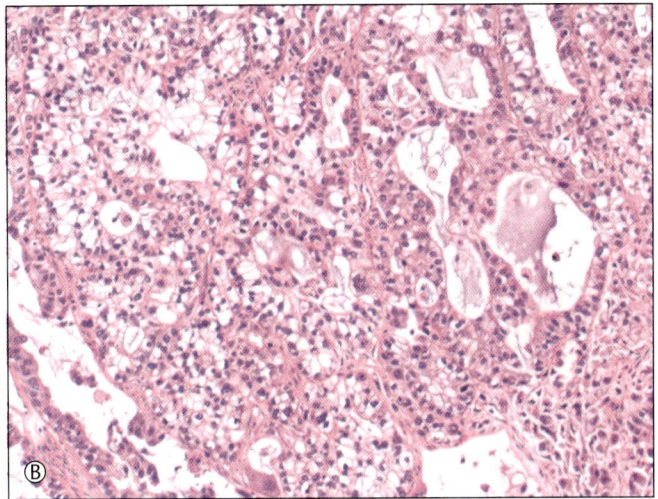

Fig. 25.95 Mixed epithelial tumor. Endometrioid adenocarcinoma **(A)** was admixed with clear cell adenocarcinoma **(B)**. Reproduced with permission from Prat.[69]

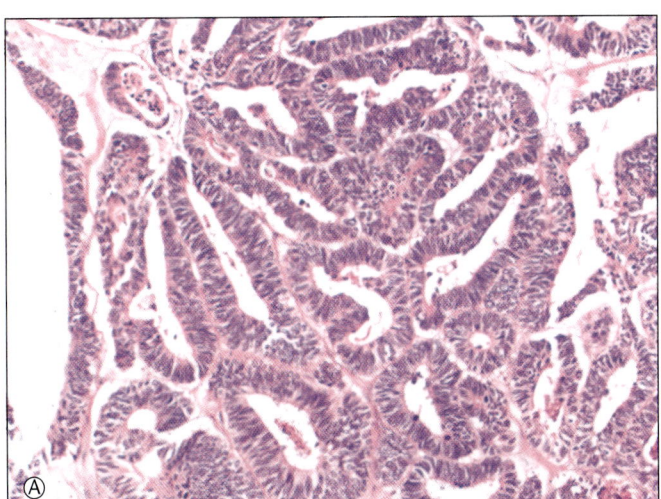 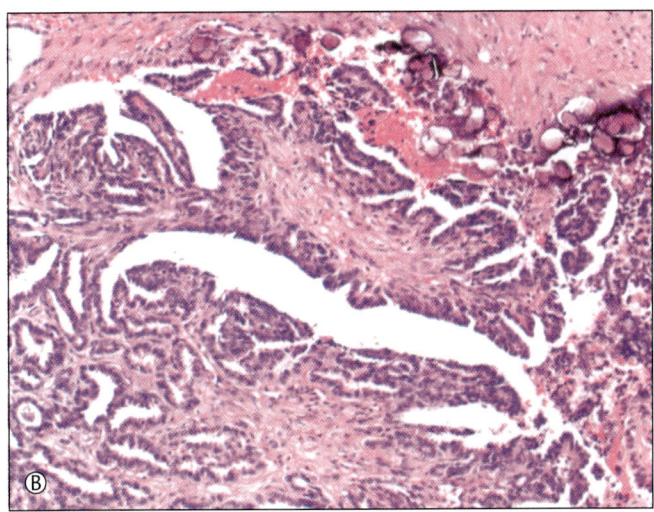

Fig. 25.96 Mixed epithelial tumor. The tumor was composed of endometrioid carcinoma **(A)** and serous papillary carcinoma **(B)**. Reproduced with permission from Prat.[69]

carcinomas are of small cell type or show neuroendocrine features (see below).[16,20] Undifferentiated carcinomas may occasionally exhibit focal choriocarcinoma with human chorionic gonadotrophin (hCG) secretion.[58]

Immunohistochemistry
Undifferentiated carcinoma is reactive for EMA and cytokeratin, and unreactive for vimentin. Occasionally it is CA125 reactive.[38]

Differential diagnosis
Undifferentiated carcinomas may be confused with diffuse granulosa cell tumors of the adult type, which have much

better prognosis, and with transitional cell carcinomas. Most granulosa cell tumors have a low-grade nuclear appearance and lack both the frequency of mitotic activity and abnormal mitotic figures so characteristic of undifferentiated carcinomas. Moreover, granulosa cell tumors fail to react with EMA but typically react with vimentin and α-inhibin. Undifferentiated carcinomas of small cell type show the same immunoprofile as the large cell type.[74] Estrogenic and androgenic endocrine manifestations so commonly associated with granulosa cell tumors are not seen in patients with undifferentiated carcinomas. The distinctions between undifferentiated and transitional cell carcinomas are discussed above.

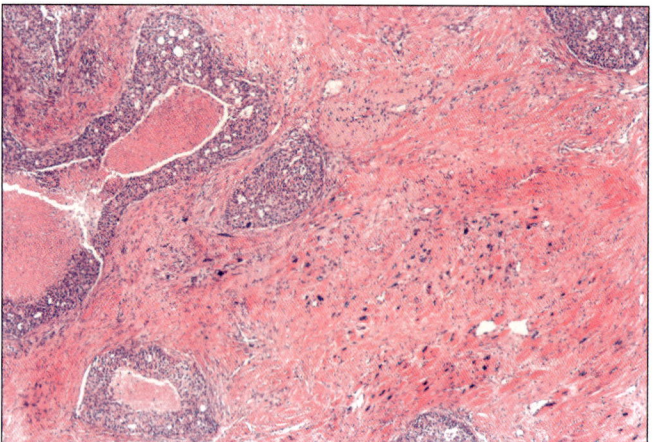

Fig. 25.97 Metastatic undifferentiated carcinoma to the right undersurface of the diaphragm.

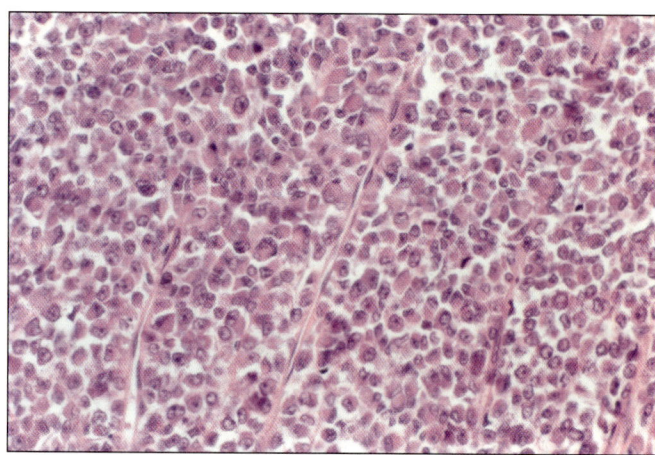

Fig. 25.100 Undifferentiated carcinoma with rhabdoid features. The tumor cells have eccentric atypical nuclei with single prominent nucleoli and abundant eosinophilic cytoplasm.

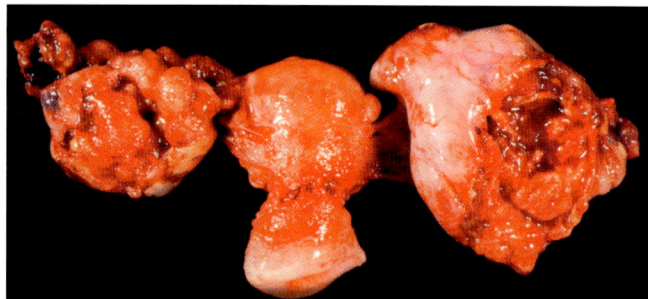

Fig. 25.98 Undifferentiated carcinoma, bilateral. Predominantly solid tumors which have extended through the capsule.

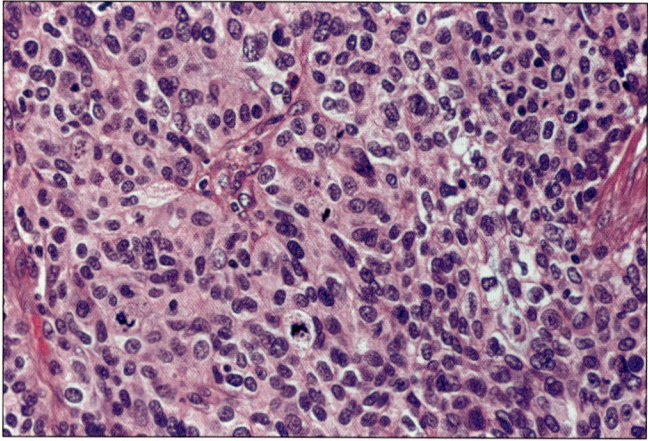

Fig. 25.99 Undifferentiated carcinoma. The tumor cells have atypical nuclei with abnormal mitoses and moderate amount of cytoplasm.

Undifferentiated carcinomas of epithelial–stromal origin should also be distinguished from poorly differentiated ovarian tumors of other types, particularly small cell carcinoma with hypercalcemia (see below) which typically occurs in the first three decades of life, neuroendocrine carcinomas (see below), and lymphomas. Rarely, undifferentiated carcinomas from other organs metastasize to the ovary (Chapter 28).

Prognosis

The 5-year survival rate of patients with undifferentiated carcinoma ranges from 17% (stage 3) to 68% (stage 1).

MISCELLANEOUS AND UNCLASSIFIED TUMORS

SMALL CELL UNDIFFERENTIATED CARCINOMA, HYPERCALCEMIC TYPE

Clinical features

This tumor typically develops in females between 2 and 46 years of age (average age, 24 years) and is associated with hypercalcemia in two-thirds of cases.[94] The mechanism by which hypercalcemia develops, and spontaneously regresses after the tumor is extirpated, relates to 'parathyroid hormone-related protein' (PTHrp) in many cases.[51] The tumor is occasionally familial.[94] Most patients present with abdominal swelling and pain related to the tumor. Even though the neoplasm is almost always unilateral, half will already be extra-ovarian at the time of laparotomy.[94]

Pathology

Grossly, the small cell carcinoma of hypercalcemic type is usually large (15–20 cm) and predominantly solid, resembling a lymphoma or dysgerminoma because of its cream-colored and uniform cut surface (Figure 25.101). Hemorrhage, necrosis, and cystic degeneration are common. Two patterns are found microscopically.[94] The more common shows tumor cells that are small, closely packed, and frequently arranged in diffuse sheets (Figures 25.102–25.104), and cords resembling a lymphoma or a juvenile granulosa cell tumor. Follicle-like structures lined by tumor cells are present in 80% of the cases (Figure 25.105). These spaces typically contain eosinophilic fluid, but sometimes it is basophilic. The nuclei may display a single prominent nucleolus and mitoses are numerous. The second form consists of larger cells exhibiting epithelioid or rhabdoid features (Figure 25.106), such as abundant eosino-philic cytoplasm and prominent nucleoli. Mixed patterns often

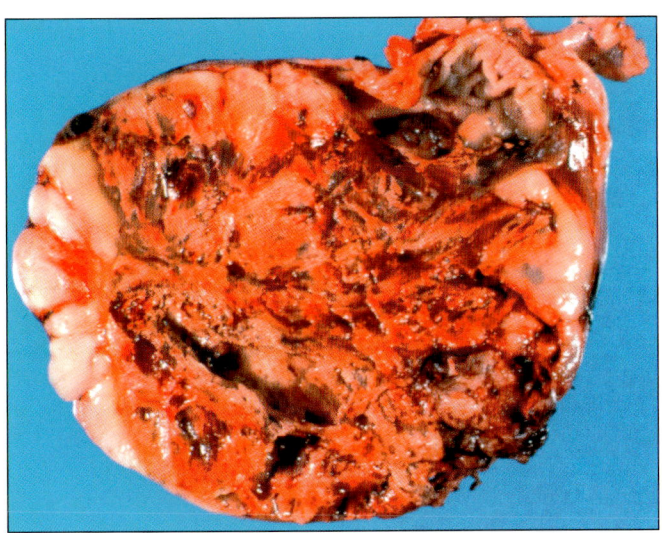

Fig. 25.101 Small cell carcinoma, hypercalcemic type. The sectioned surface appears lobulated and composed of fleshy tissue resembling that of a dysgerminoma or lymphoma. There is extensive hemorrhage and necrosis. Courtesy of Dr R E Scully, Boston, MA.

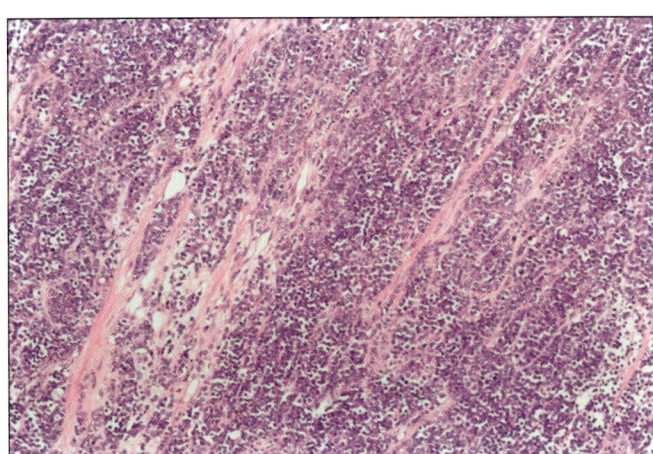

Fig. 25.102 Small cell carcinoma, hypercalcemic type. The tumor cells grow in nests.

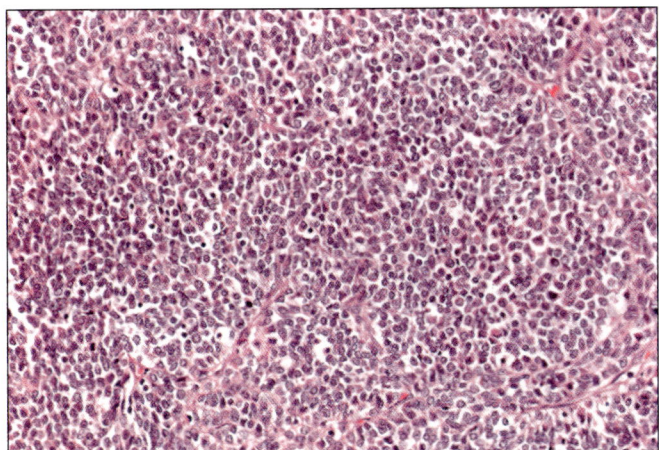

Fig. 25.103 Small cell carcinoma, hypercalcemic type. Diffuse arrangement of small tumor cells with scanty cytoplasm.

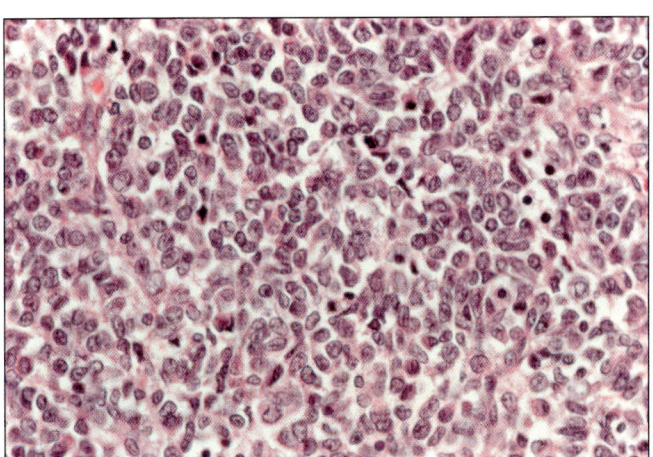

Fig. 25.104 Small cell carcinoma, hypercalcemic type. Closely packed epithelial cells exhibiting hyperchromatic nuclei and scanty cytoplasm.

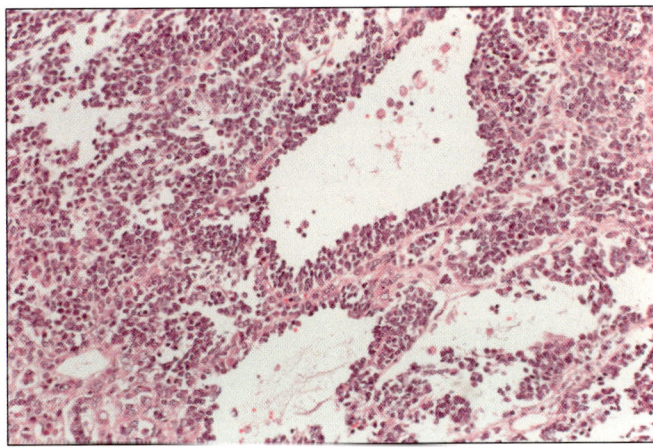

Fig. 25.105 Small cell carcinoma, hypercalcemic type. Follicle-like structures.

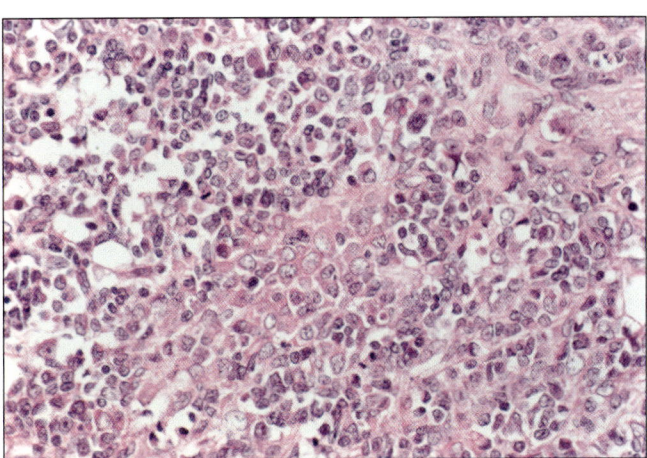

Fig. 25.106 Small cell carcinoma, hypercalcemic type. Large cells with abundant eosinophilic cytoplasm and round clear nuclei with prominent nucleoli appear admixed with smaller cells.

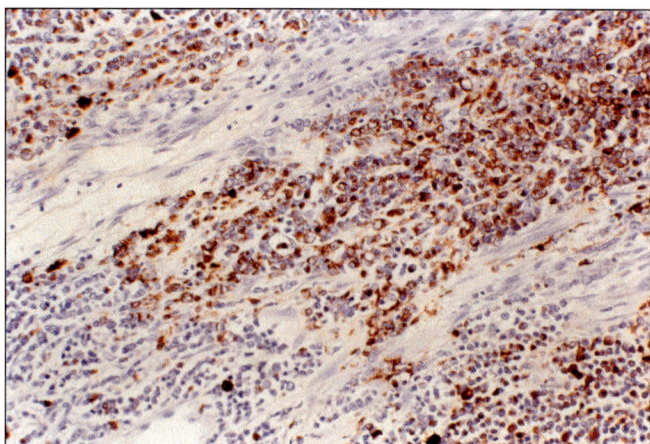

Fig. 25.107 Small cell carcinoma, hypercalcemic type. Cytokeratin immunoreaction.

occur. The tumor stroma may be edematous or myxoid. Interestingly, mucinous glands, atypical mucinous cells, or signet-ring cells are present in 10% of the tumors.[94]

Immunohistochemistry, DNA cytometry, and ultrastructure
The tumor cells are diploid[94] and typically reactive for cytokeratins (CAM 5.2) (Figure 25.107), EMA, and also vimentin, but unreactive for α-inhibin.[2] It is variable for neuron-specific enolase, chromogranin, parathyroid hormone, and parathyroid hormone-related protein.[2,51] Immunohistochemistry is useful in order to exclude lymphoma, primitive neuroectodermal tumor, metastatic melanoma, and desmoplastic small round cell tumor. Ultrastructural analysis shows the tumor to be of epithelial appearance with small desmosomes and tight junctions. The cytoplasm contains dilated granular endoplasmic reticulum with amorphous material. Some neurosecretory granules have been found.[94]

Differential diagnosis
Small cell carcinomas are most often misinterpreted as granulosa cell tumors of either the adult or the juvenile type. These differential diagnoses are discussed in Chapter 26. The absence of membrane immunostaining for MIC2 protein (CD99) distinguishes small cell carcinomas from primitive neuroectodermal tumors. Small cell carcinomas can also be confused with malignant lymphomas and sometimes with metastatic malignant melanoma and metastatic alveolar rhabdomyosarcoma (see Chapters 28 and 29). Clinicopathologic features and immunohistochemistry usually clarify these differential diagnoses.

Prognosis
The prognosis is poor even for stage 1 tumors, with only one-third of patients surviving 5 years. Most patients with higher stage tumors will die of disease within 2 years.[94]

SMALL CELL CARCINOMA, PULMONARY TYPE
These highly malignant tumors are histologically similar to small cell carcinomas of the lung and should be distinguished from metastases of the latter. Patients are generally older than those with small cell carcinomas of the hypercalcemic type and most of them present with high stage disease.[20] Microscopically, most

cells have scanty cytoplasm, nuclei with stippled chromatin, and inconspicuous nucleoli that are typically molded by adjacent nuclei. Although the histogenesis of these tumors is unclear, the concurrence of some with endometrioid carcinomas or its variants, or with Brenner tumor, suggests a surface epithelial derivation. Most tumors are aneuploid.[20]

UNDIFFERENTIATED CARCINOMA OF NON-SMALL CELL (NEUROENDOCRINE) TYPE
These tumors, which are highly malignant and occur in older women (average age, 60 years), are recognized because of their trabecular and insular growth pattern. The tumor cells are of medium to large size and contain large nuclei which may exhibit central macronucleoli. Each of the eight reported cases was admixed with surface epithelial tumors (seven mucinous and one endometrioid). The diagnosis is established by the presence of argyrophilic granules and reactivity for chromogranin, serotonin, and neuron-specific enolase. The associated surface epithelial components confirm the primary nature of the tumor.[16]

CYSTS AND ADENOMAS OF THE RETE OVARII
Rete ovarii tubules may become dilated to form cysts. These are usually only small hilar lesions but larger cysts, up to 12 cm in diameter, also occur. Some have been associated with virilization in postmenopausal women. The cysts are lined by non-ciliated cuboidal or, less commonly, ciliated columnar epithelium, and their fibrous walls exhibit bundles of smooth muscle and often peripheral Leydig cell hyperplasia. The epithelial lining may undergo squamous metaplasia, representing one possible origin of ovarian epidermoid cysts (see above). Adenomas disclose cords and tubules lined by cells similar to those seen in the normal rete.

ADENOMATOID TUMORS
These tumors are more frequently encountered, as incidental findings, subserosally in the uterus and fallopian tubes. They may also occur rarely in the hilar region where they form well-circumscribed white to yellow nodules 1–1.5 cm in diameter. The cut surface shows a honeycomb pattern of small cystic spaces. Microscopically, vascular-like spaces are lined by flattened or cuboidal cells, in turn surrounded by stroma. The tumor cells have eosinophilic or vacuolated cytoplasm that is alcian blue-positive at pH 2.5; this reaction, including the non-specific stromal staining, can be eliminated by prior incubation with hyaluronidase. Adenomatoid tumors are reactive for anti-mesothelial antibodies such as HBME1 and calretinin but not for Ber-EP4.

OVARIAN MESOTHELIOMAS
Secondary ovarian involvement by malignant mesothelioma is common and is usually limited to the ovarian surface or superficial stroma (Figure 25.108). Occasionally, the ovary is extensively involved and the clinical picture simulates that of ovarian cancer.[13] Microscopically, malignant mesotheliomas show tubular, papillary, and solid patterns and relatively uniform cells with abundant eosinophilic cytoplasm (Figure 25.109). Rare tumors with an exclusive sheet-like pattern containing polygonal cells may be confused with ectopic decidual reaction.

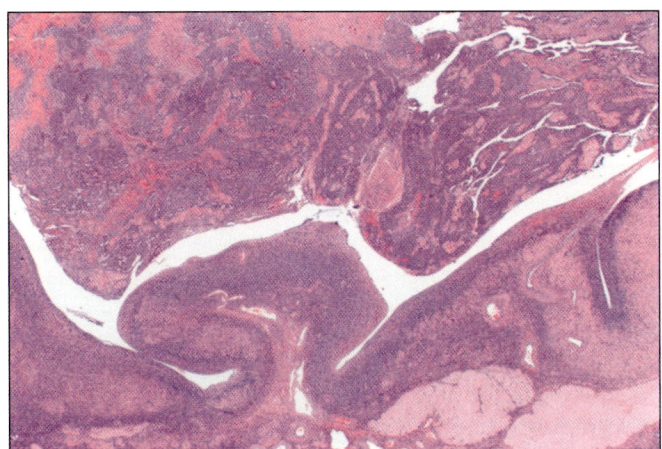

Fig. 25.108 Malignant mesothelioma involving the ovary. The tumor (top) covers the surface of the ovary (bottom).

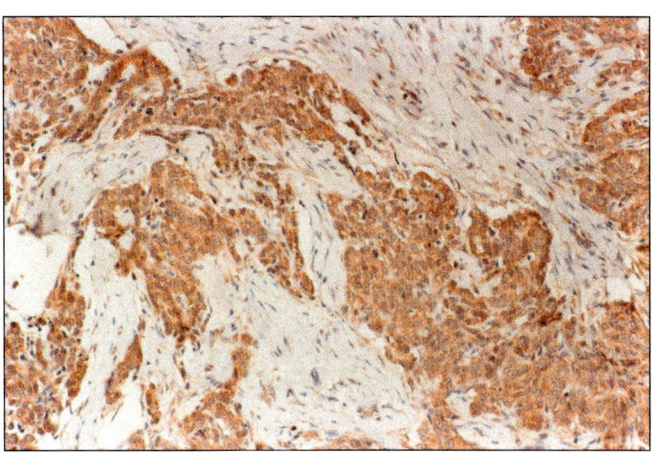

Fig. 25.110 Malignant epithelial mesothelioma involving the ovary. The tumor cells are immunoreactive for calretinin.

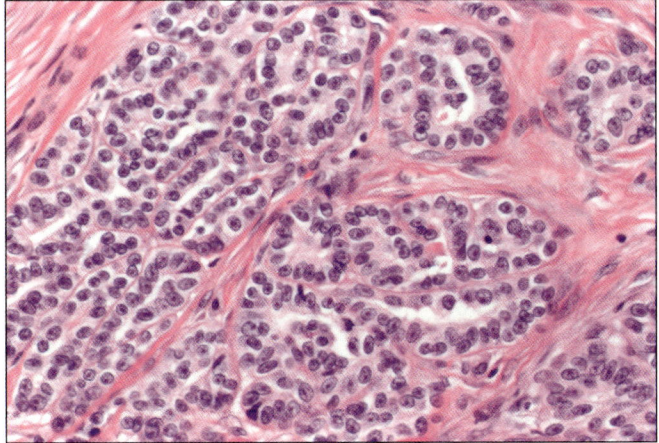

Fig. 25.109 Malignant epithelial mesothelioma involving the ovary. The tumor cells have a uniform appearance and are separated by slit-like spaces.

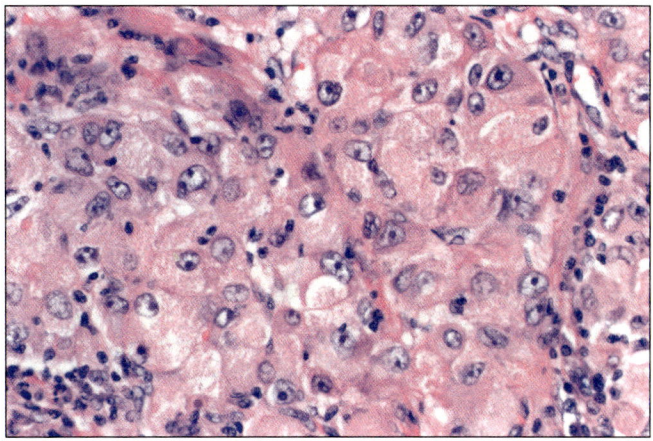

Fig. 25.111 Hepatoid carcinoma. The polygonal tumor cells have abundant eosinophilic cytoplasm and round nuclei with prominent nucleoli.

In routinely stained H&E sections, mesotheliomas are usually readily distinguishable from serous carcinoma by their pattern of growth and cytologic features, although immunohistochemical stains are sometimes necessary to confirm the diagnosis. In contrast to adenocarcinomas, mesotheliomas lack neutral mucins (digested PAS-negative) and contain hyaluronic acid within vacuoles (alcian blue-positive, hyaluronidase-sensitive). Hyaluronic acid, however, may leach from formalin-fixed tumors, resulting in false-negative staining. The most useful immunohistochemical markers are the Ber-EP4-defined surface glycoprotein which shows reactivity in serous carcinomas but not in mesothelioma, and calretinin (Figure 25.110), CK5, and thrombomodulin, all three of which are reactive in mesothelioma but not in serous carcinomas.[61,91] Additionally, no reactivity for CEA, B72.3, Leu-M1, and CA125 favors a diagnosis of mesothelioma over carcinoma.

HEPATOID CARCINOMAS

This rare subtype of ovarian carcinoma resembles hepatocellular carcinoma (Figure 25.111) and gastric hepatoid carci-

noma, and shows reactivity for AFP and α_1-antitrypsin (Figure 25.112).[32] Most women are postmenopausal and by the time of diagnosis, most tumors will have spread beyond the ovary.[32] Sheets, trabeculae, and cords of cells with moderate to large amounts of eosinophilic cytoplasm and round to oval central nuclei are characteristic. Hyaline bodies may be numerous. These tumors are commonly admixed with serous or, less frequently, with mucinous or endometrioid carcinomas, strongly suggesting a surface epithelial origin.[32,79,87]

Hepatoid carcinoma must be distinguished from the rare hepatocellular carcinoma metastatic to the ovary and other ovarian tumors that have cells with abundant eosinophilic cytoplasm, particularly the hepatoid yolk sac tumor (see Chapter 27), steroid cell tumors (see Chapter 26), and oxyphilic clear cell carcinomas (see above). Clinicopathologic features must be considered in making the distinction between hepatoid carcinoma and metastatic hepatocellular carcinoma. A hepatic mass suggestive of a primary neoplasm is strong evidence in favor of metastasis to the ovary.

The presence of bile pigment cannot be considered diagnostic of hepatic origin as it is found sometimes in hepatoid carci-

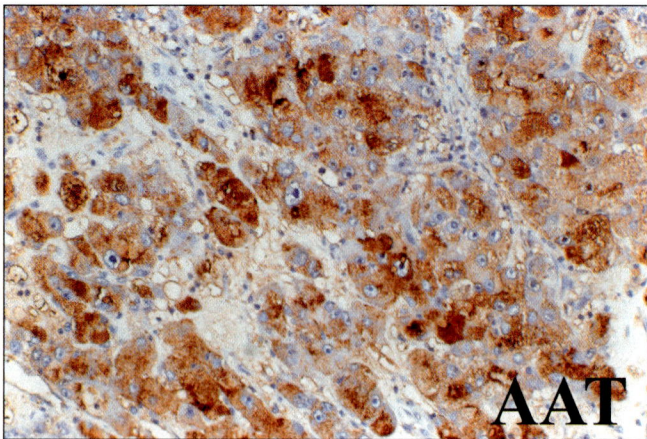

Fig. 25.112 Hepatoid carcinoma. Immunoreaction for α_1-antitrypsin.

nomas arising at other sites. Hepatoid yolk sac tumor almost always develops in young women and usually shows additional typical patterns of yolk sac/germ cell neoplasia. Steroid cell tumors are often associated with endocrine manifestations and generally are not reactive for AFP. Similarly, hepatoid carcinoma is not reactive for α-inhibin.

DESMOPLASTIC SMALL CELL TUMORS OF CHILDHOOD

See Chapter 33.

FEMALE ADNEXAL TUMORS OF WOLFFIAN ORIGIN

See Chapter 33.

REFERENCES

1. Abeln EC, Smit VT, Wessels JW, de Lee UW, Cornelisse CJ, Fleuren GJ. Molecular genetic evidence for the conversion hypothesis of the origin of malignant mixed müllerian tumours. J Pathol 1997;183:424–31.
2. Aguirre P, Thor AD, Scully RE. Ovarian small cell carcinoma: histogenetic considerations based on immunohistochemical and other findings. Am J Clin Pathol 1989;92:140–9.
3. Aguirre P, Thor AD, Scully RE. Ovarian endometrioid carcinomas resembling sex cord-stromal tumors. An immunohistochemical study. Int J Gynecol Pathol 1989;8:364–73.
4. Austin RM, Norris HJ. Malignant Brenner tumor and transitional cell carcinoma of the ovary: a comparison. Int J Gynecol Pathol 1987;6:29–39.
5. Becker JL, Papenhausen PR, Widen RH. Cytogenetic, morphologic and oncogene analysis of a cell line derived from a heterologous mixed müllerian tumor of the ovary. In Vitro Cell Dev Biol Anim 1997;33:325–31.
6. Bell KA, Kurman RJ. A clinicopathologic analysis of atypical proliferative (borderline) tumors and well-differentiated endometrioid adenocarcinomas of the ovary. Am J Surg Pathol 2000;24:1465–79.
7. Bitterman P, Chun B, Kurman RJ. The significance of epithelial differentiation in mixed mesodermal tumors of the uterus. A clinicopathologic and immunohistochemical study. Am J Surg Pathol 1990;14:317–28.
8. Blaker H, Graf M, Rieker RJ, Otto HF. Comparison of losses of heterozygosity and replication errors in primary colorectal carcinomas and corresponding liver metastases. J Pathol 1999;188:258–62.
9. Borgfeldt C, Andolf E. Cancer risk after hospital discharge diagnosis of benign ovarian cysts and endometriosis. Acta Obstet Gynecol Scand 2004;83:395–400.
10. Brinton LA, Gridley G, Persson I, Bergqvist A. Cancer risk after a hospital discharge diagnosis of endometriosis. Am J Obstet Gynecol 1997;176:572–9.
11. Catasús L, Bussaglia E, Rodríguez IM, et al. Molecular genetic alterations in endometrioid carcinomas of the ovary: similar frequency of beta-catenin

abnormalities but lower rate of microsatellite instability and PTEN alterations than in uterine endometrioid carcinomas. Hum Pathol 2004;35:1360–8.
12. Chang KL, Crabtree GS, Lim Tan SK, Kempson RL, Hendrickson MR. Primary extrauterine endometrial stromal neoplasms: a clinicopathologic study of 20 cases and a review of the literature. Int J Gynecol Pathol 1993;12:282–96.
13. Clement PB, Young RH, Scully RE. Malignant mesotheliomas presenting as ovarian masses. A report of nine cases, including two primary ovarian mesotheliomas. Am J Surg Pathol 1996;20:1067–80.
14. Cuatrecasas M, Erill N, Musulen E, Costa I, Matias-Guiu X, Prat J. K–ras mutations in nonmucinous ovarian epithelial tumors: a molecular analysis and clinicopathological study of 144 patients. Cancer 1998;82:1088–95.
15. Deavers MT, Malpica A, Liu J, Broaddus R, Silva G. Ovarian sex cord-stromal tumors: an immunohistochemical study including a comparison of calretinin and inhibin. Mod Pathol 2003;16:584–90.
16. Eichhorn JH, Lawrence WD, Young RH, Scully RE. Ovarian neuroendocrine carcinomas of non small cell type associated with surface epithelial adenocarcinomas. A study of five cases and a review of the literature. Int J Gynecol Pathol 1996;15:303–14.
17. Eichhorn JH, Scully RE. Endometrioid ciliated-cell tumors of the ovary: a report of five cases. Int J Gynecol Pathol 1996;15:248–56.
18. Eichhorn JH, Young RH. Transitional cell carcinoma of the ovary. A morphologic study of 100 cases with emphasis on differential diagnosis. Am J Surg Pathol 2004;28:453–63.
19. Eichhorn JH, Young RH, Clement PB, Scully RE. Mesodermal (Müllerian) adenosarcoma of the ovary: a clinicopathologic analysis of 40 cases and review of the literature. Am J Surg Pathol 2002;26:1243–58.
20. Eichhorn JH, Young RH, Scully RE. Primary ovarian small cell carcinoma of pulmonary type. A clinicopathologic, immunohistologic, and flow cytometric analysis of 11 cases. Am J Surg Pathol 1992;16:926–38.
21. Emmert-Buck MR, Chuaqui R, Zhuang Z, Nogales F, Liotta LA, Merino MJ. Molecular analysis of synchronous uterine and ovarian endometrioid tumors. Int J Gynecol Pathol 1997;16:143–8.
22. Erzen M, Rakar S, Klancnik B, Syrjanen K. Endometriosis-associated ovarian carcinoma (EAOC): an entity distinct from other ovarian carcinomas as suggested by a nested case-control study. Gynecol Oncol 2001;83:100–8.
23. Falkenberry SS, Steinhoff MM, Gordinier M, Rappoport S, Gajewski W, Granai CO. Synchronous endometrioid tumors of the ovary and endometrium. A clinicopathologic study of 22 cases. J Reprod Med 1996;41:713–18.
24. Fujii H, Matsumoto T, Yoshida M, et al. Genetics of synchronous uterine and ovarian endometrioid carcinoma: combined analyses of loss of heterozygosity, PTEN mutation, and microsatellite instability. Hum Pathol 2002;33:421–8.
25. Fujii H, Yoshida M, Gong ZX, et al. Frequent genetic heterogeneity in the clonal evolution of gynecological carcinosarcoma and its influence on phenotypic diversity. Cancer Res 2000;60:114–20.
26. Fujita M, Enomoto T, Wada H, Inoue M, Okudaira Y, Shroyer KR. Application of clonal analysis. Differential diagnosis for synchronous primary ovarian and endometrial cancers and metastatic cancer. Am J Clin Pathol 1996;105:350–9.
27. Fukunaga M, Nomura K, Ishikawa E, Ushigome S. Ovarian atypical endometriosis: its close association with malignant epithelial tumors. Histopathology 1997;30:249–55.
28. Gamallo C, Palacios J, Moreno G, Calvo de Mora J, Suarez A, Armas A. Beta-catenin expression pattern in stage I and II ovarian carcinomas: relationship with beta-catenin gene mutations, clinicopathological features, and clinical outcome. Am J Pathol 1999;155:527–36.
29. Goff BA, Sainz de la Cuesta R, Muntz HG, et al. Clear cell carcinoma of the ovary: a distinct histologic type with poor prognosis and resistance to platinum-based chemotherapy in stage III disease. Gynecol Oncol 1996;60:412–17.
30. Gras E, Catasus LL, Arguelles R, et al. Microsatellite instability, MLH-1 promoter hypermethylation, and frameshift mutations at coding mononucleotide repeat microsatellites in ovarian tumors. Cancer 2001;92:2829–36.
31. Irving JA, Catasus L, Gallardo A, et al. Synchronous endometrioid carcinomas of the uterine corpus and ovary: alterations in the beta-catenin (CTNNB1) pathway are associated with independent primary tumors and favorable prognosis. Hum Pathol 2005;36:605–19.
32. Ishikura H, Scully RE. Hepatoid carcinoma of the ovary. A newly described tumor. Cancer 1987;60:2775–84.
33. Jiang X, Hitchcock A, Bryan EJ, et al. Microsatellite analysis of endometriosis reveals loss of heterozygosity at candidate ovarian tumor suppressor gene loci. Cancer Res 1996;56:3534–9.
34. Kennedy AW, Biscotti CV, Hart WR, Tuason LJ. Histologic correlates of progression-free interval and survival in ovarian clear cell adenocarcinoma. Gynecol Oncol 1993;50:334–8.
35. Komiyama S, Aoki D, Tominaga E, Susumu N, Udagawa Y, Nozawa S. Prognosis of Japanese patients with ovarian clear cell carcinoma associated with pelvic endometriosis: clinicopathologic evaluation. Gynecol Oncol 1999;72:342–6.
36. Kommoss F, Kommoss S, Schimdt D, et al. Survival benefits for patients with advanced-stage transitional cell carcinomas vs. other subtypes of ovarian carcinoma after chemotherapy with platinum and paclitaxel. Gynecol Oncol 2005;97:195–9.

37. Kommoss F, Oliva E, Bahn AK, Young RH, Scully RE. Inhibin expression in ovarian tumors and tumor-like lesions: an immunohistochemical study. Mod Pathol 1998;11:656–64.
38. Kuwashima Y, Takayama S. Immunohistochemical characterization of undifferentiated carcinomas of the ovary. J Cancer Res Clin 1994;120:672–7.
39. Ladanyi M, Gerald W. Fusion of the EWS and WT1 genes in the desmoplastic small round cell tumor. Cancer Res 1994;54:2837–40.
40. Leake J, Woolas RP, Daniel J, Oram DH, Brown CL. Immunocytochemical and serological expression of CA 125: a clinicopathological study of 40 malignant ovarian epithelial tumours. Histopathology 1994;24:57–64.
41. Lee KR, Tavassoli FA, Prat J, et al. Tumours of the ovary and peritoneum: surface epithelial–stromal tumours. In: Tavassoli FA, Devilee P, eds. World Health Organization Classification of Tumours. Pathology and Genetics of Tumours of the Breast and Female Genital Organs. Lyon: IARC Press; 2003.
42. Lerwill MF, Sung R, Oliva E, Prat J, Young RH. Smooth muscle tumors of the ovary. A clinicopathologic study of 54 cases emphasizing prognostic criteria, histologic variants, and differential diagnosis. Am J Clin Pathol 2004;28:1436–51.
43. Lin WM, Forgacs E, Warshal DP, et al. Loss of heterozygosity and mutational analysis of the PTEN/MMAC1 gene in synchronous endometrial and ovarian carcinomas. Clin Cancer Res 1998;4:2577–83.
44. Logani S, Oliva E, Amin MB, Folpe AL, Cohen C, Young RH. Immunoprofile of ovarian tumors with putative transitional cell (urothelial) differentiation using novel urothelial markers: histogenetic and diagnostic implications. Am J Surg Pathol 2003;27:1434–41.
45. Machin P, Catasus L, Pons C, et al. Microsatellite instability and immunostaining for MSH-2 and MLH-1 in cutaneous and internal tumors from patients with the Muir–Torre syndrome. J Cutan Pathol 2002;29:415–20.
46. Mai KT, Yazdi HM, Bertrand MA, Le Saux N, Cathcart LL. Bilateral primary ovarian squamous cell carcinoma associated with human papillomavirus infection and vulvar and cervical intraepithelial neoplasia. Am J Surg Pathol 1996;20:767–72.
47. Matias-Guiu X, Lagarda H, Catasus LI, et al. Clonality analysis in synchronous or metachronous tumors of the female genital tract. Int J Gynecol Pathol 2002;21:205–11.
48. Matias-Guiu X, Lerma E, Prat J. Clear cell tumors of the female genital tract. Semin Diagn Pathol 1997;14:233–9.
49. Matias-Guiu X, Pons C, Prat J. Müllerian inhibiting substance, alpha-inhibin, and CD99 expression in sex cord-stromal tumors and endometrioid ovarian carcinomas resembling sex cord-stromal tumors. Hum Pathol 1998;29:840–5.
50. Matias-Guiu X, Prat J. Ovarian tumors with functioning stroma. An immunohistochemical study of 100 cases with human chorionic gonadotropin monoclonal and polyclonal antibodies. Cancer 1990;65:2001–5.
51. Matias-Guiu X, Prat J, Young RH, et al. Human parathyroid hormone-related protein in ovarian small cell carcinoma. An immunohistochemical study. Cancer 1994;73:1878–81.
52. McCluggage WG. Uterine carcinosarcomas (malignant mixed Müllerian tumors) are metaplastic carcinomas. Int J Gynecol Cancer 2002;12:687–90.
53. McMeekin DS, Burger RA, Manetta A, et al. Endometrioid adenocarcinoma of the ovary and its relationship to endometriosis. Gynecol Oncol 1995;59:81–6.
54. Moreno-Bueno G, Gamallo C, Perez-Gallego L, Calvo de Mora J, Suarez A, Palacios J. Beta-catenin expression pattern, beta-catenin gene mutations, and microsatellite instability in endometrioid ovarian carcinomas and synchronous endometrial carcinomas. Diagn Mol Pathol 2001;10:116–22.
55. Nogales FF, Bergeron C, Carvia RE, Alvaro T, Fulwood HR. Ovarian endometrioid tumors with yolk sac tumor component, an unusual form of ovarian neoplasm. Analysis of six cases. Am J Surg Pathol 1996;20:1056–66.
56. Obata K, Morland SJ, Watson RH, et al. Frequent PTEN/MMAC mutations in endometrioid but not serous or mucinous epithelial ovarian tumors. Cancer Res 1998;58:2095–7.
57. Ogawa K, Johansson SL, Cohen SM. Immunohistochemical analysis of uroplakins, urothelial specific proteins, in ovarian Brenner tumors, normal tissues, and benign and neoplastic lesions of the female genital tract. Am J Pathol 1999;155:1047–50.
58. Oliva E, Andrada E, Pezzica E, Prat J. Ovarian carcinomas with choriocarcinomatous differentiation. Cancer 1993;72:2441–6.
59. Oliva E, Sarrio D, Brachtel EF, et al. High frequency of beta-catenin mutations in borderline endometrioid tumors of the ovary. J Pathol 2006;208:708–13.
60. Ordi J, Schammel DP, Rasekh L, Tavassoli FA. Sertoliform endometrioid carcinomas of the ovary: a clinicopathologic and immunohistochemical study of 13 cases. Mod Pathol 1999;12:933–40.
61. Ordonez NG. Role of immunohistochemistry in distinguishing epithelial peritoneal mesotheliomas from peritoneal and ovarian serous carcinomas. Am J Surg Pathol 1998;22:1203–14.
62. Ordonez NG. Transitional cell carcinomas of the ovary and bladder are immunophenotypically different. Histopathology 2000;36:433–8.
63. Ordonez NG, Mackay B. Brenner tumor of the ovary: a comparative immunohistochemical and ultrastructural study with transitional cell carcinoma of the bladder. Ultrastruct Pathol 2000;24:157–67.
64. Palacios J, Gamallo C. Mutations in the beta-catenin gene (CTNNBI) in endometrioid ovarian carcinomas. Cancer Res 1998;58:1344–7.
65. Pettersson F. Annual report of the results of treatment in gynecological cancer. Stockholm: International Federation of Gynecology and Obstetrics; 1991.
66. Pins MR, Young RH, Daly WJ, Scully RE. Primary squamous cell carcinoma of the ovary. A report of 37 cases. Am J Surg Pathol 1996;20:823–33.
67. Pitman MB, Young RH, Clement PB, Dickersin GR, Scully RE. Endometrioid carcinoma of the ovary and endometrium, oxyphilic cell type: a report of nine cases. Int J Gynecol Pathol 1994;13:290–301.
68. Prat J. Ovarian tumors of borderline malignancy (tumors of low malignant potential): a critical appraisal. Adv Anat Pathol 1999;6:247–74.
69. Prat J. Pathology of the ovary. Philadelphia: Saunders; 2004.
70. Prat J, Matias-Guiu X, Barreto J. Simultaneous carcinoma involving the endometrium and the ovary. A clinicopathologic, immunohistochemical, and DNA flow cytometric study of 18 cases. Cancer 1991;68:2455–9.
71. Rahilly MA, Williams ARW, Krausz T, al Nafussi A. Female adnexal tumor of probable Wolffian origin: a clinicopathologic and immunohistochemical study of three cases. Histopathology 1995;26:69–74.
72. Ribe A, Larrosa CV, Catasus L, Palacios J, Prat J. Brenner tumors but not transitional cell carcinomas of the ovary show dysregulation of cell cycle G_1–S phase transition [abstract]. Mod Pathol 2006;19S1:194A.
73. Riedel I, Czernobilsky B, Lifschitz-Mercer B, et al. Brenner tumors but not transitional cell carcinomas of the ovary show urothelial differentiation: immunohistochemical staining of urothelial markers, including cytokeratins and uroplakins. Virchows Arch 2001;438:181–91.
74. Riopel MA, Perlman EJ, Seidman JD, Kurman RJ, Sherman ME. Inhibin and epithelial membrane antigen immunohistochemistry assist in the diagnosis of sex cord-stromal tumors and provide clues to the histogenesis of hypercalcemic small cell carcinomas. Int J Gynecol Pathol 1998;17:46–53.
75. Roth LM, Liban E, Czernobilsky B. Ovarian endometrioid tumors mimicking Sertoli and Sertoli–Leydig cell tumors. Sertoliform variant of endometrioid carcinoma. Cancer 1982;50:1322–31.
76. Sainz de la Cuesta R, Eichhorn JH, Rice LW, Fuller AF, Jr, Nikrui N, Goff BA. Histologic transformation of benign endometriosis to early epithelial ovarian cancer. Gynecol Oncol 1996;60:238–44.
77. Sato N, Tsunoda H, Nishida M, et al. Loss of heterozygosity on 10q23.3 and mutation of the tumor suppressor gene PTEN in benign endometrial cyst of the ovary: possible sequence progression from benign endometrial cyst to endometrioid carcinoma and clear cell carcinoma of the ovary. Cancer Res 2000;60:7052–6.
78. Scully RE, Young RH, Clement PB. Tumors of the ovary, maldeveloped gonads, fallopian tube, and broad ligament. In: Atlas of Tumor Pathology: third series. Fascicle 23. Washington, DC: Armed Forces Institute of Pathology; 1998:153–64.
79. Scurry JP, Brown RW, Jobling T. Combined ovarian serous papillary and hepatoid carcinoma. Gynecol Oncol 1996;63:138–42.
80. Seidman JD. Prognostic importance of hyperplasia and atypia in endometriosis. Int J Gynecol Pathol 1996;15:1–9.
81. Shenson DL, Gallion HH, Powell DE, Pieretti M. Loss of heterozygosity and genomic instability in synchronous endometrioid tumors of the ovary and endometrium. Cancer 1995;76:650–7.
82. Soslow RA, Rouse RV, Hendrickson MR, Silva EG, Longacre TA. Transitional cell neoplasms of the ovary and urinary bladder: a comparative immunohistochemical analysis. Int J Gynecol Pathol 1996;15:257–65.
83. Southey MC, Young M-A, Whitty J, et al. Molecular pathologic analysis enhances the diagnosis and management of Muir–Torre syndrome and gives insight into its underlying molecular pathogenesis. Am J Surg Pathol 2001;25:936–41.
84. Stern RC, Dash R, Bentley RC, Snyder MJ, Haney AF, Robboy SJ. Malignancy in endometriosis: frequency and comparison of ovarian and extraovarian types. Int J Gynecol Pathol 2001;20:133–9.
85. Sworn MJ, Jones H, Letchworth AT, Herrington CS, McGee JO. Squamous intraepithelial neoplasia in an ovarian cyst, cervical intraepithelial neoplasia and human papillomavirus. Hum Pathol 1995;26:344–7.
86. Thompson L, Chang B, Barsky SH. Monoclonal origins of malignant mixed tumors (carcinosarcomas). Evidence for a divergent histogenesis. Am J Surg Pathol 1996;20:277–85.
87. Tochigi N, Kishimoto T, Supriatna Y, et al. Hepatoid carcinoma of the ovary: a report of three cases admixed with common surface epithelial carcinoma. Int J Gynecol Pathol 2003;22:266–71.
88. Tornos C, Silva EG, Khorana SM, Burke TW. High–stage endometrioid carcinoma of the ovary. Prognostic significance of pure versus mixed histologic types. Am J Surg Pathol 1994;18:687–93.
89. Tornos C, Silva EG, Ordonez NG, Gershenson DM, Young RH, Scully RE. Endometrioid carcinoma of the ovary with a prominent spindle-cell component, a source of diagnostic confusion. A report of 14 cases. Am J Surg Pathol 1995;19:1343–53.
90. Tsunematsu R, Saito T, Iguchi H, Fukuda T, Tsukamoto N. Hypercalcemia due to parathyroid hormone-related protein produced by primary ovarian clear cell adenocarcinoma: case report. Gynecol Oncol 2000;76:218–22.
91. Yazili H, Gown AM. Immunohistochemical analysis of gynecologic tumors. Int J Gynecol Pathol 2001;20:64–78.
92. Young RH, Prat J, Scully RE. Endometrioid stromal sarcomas of the ovary: a clinicopathologic analysis of 23 cases. Cancer 1984;53:1143–55.
93. Young RH, Eichhorn JH, Dickersin GR, Scully RE. Ovarian involvement by the intra-abdominal desmoplastic small round cell tumor with divergent differentiation: a report of three cases. Hum Pathol 1992;23:454–64.

94. Young RH, Oliva E, Scully RE. Small cell carcinoma of the ovary, hypercalcemic type. A clinicopathologic analysis of 150 cases. Am J Surg Pathol 1994;18:1102–16.

95. Young RH, Prat J, Scully RE. Ovarian endometrioid carcinomas resembling sex cord-stromal tumors. A clinicopathologic analysis of 13 cases. Am J Surg Pathol 1982;6:513–22.

96. Zaino RJ, Kurman RJ, Diana KL, Morrow CP. The utility of the revised International Federation of Gynecology and Obstetrics histologic grading of endometrial adenocarcinoma using a defined nuclear grading system: a Gynecologic Oncology Group study. Cancer 1995;75:81–6.

97. Zaloudek C, Miller TR, Stern JR. Desmoplastic small cell tumor of the ovary: a unique polyphenotypic tumor with an unfavorable prognosis. Int J Gynecol Pathol 1995;14:260–5.

98. Zheng W, Sung CJ, Hanna I, et al. Alpha and beta subunits of inhibin/activin as sex cord-stromal differentiation markers. Int J Gynecol Pathol 1997;16:263–71.

Ovarian sex cord-stromal and steroid cell tumors

26

Peter Russell   Stanley J. Robboy   Jaime Prat

GRANULOSA CELL TUMORS

Definition and cell types

Granulosa cell tumors are the archetypal feminizing sex cord-stromal tumors and their hallmark is the conspicuous presence of cells (at least a 10% representation in the material examined) that resemble those of the follicular granulosa or their luteinized variants. Other cells (of ovarian stromal origin and similar to those in the theca interna or externa of the developing follicle or their luteinized variants) commonly accompany them, and these latter cells may indeed be a dominant component without negating the diagnosis. Tumors with a small granulosa cell component may be designated as 'fibromas with minor sex-cord elements'. It is not known whether the variable ovarian stromal element is reactive to the presence of the neoplastic granulosa cells or is an integral part of the tumor.

Granulosa cells are small, usually round to polygonal, but may be spindle shaped with scanty amphophilic cytoplasm, usually containing only occasional small lipid droplets, and having indistinct cell borders. Their bland round, oval or angular nuclei often show a deep longitudinal groove and may exhibit a small, variably prominent nucleolus (Figure 26.1A,B). Nuclear chromatin may be compact and dense or loose and vesicular. Luteinized granulosa cells, seen particularly in the diffuse, multicystic, and 'juvenile' types of granulosa cell tumors, have larger, more rounded, and generally non-grooved nuclei of similar general appearance and abundant pale eosinophilic lipid-laden cytoplasm. Granulosa cells regularly express α-inhibin, calretinin, and WT1.[11] They contain vimentin and smooth muscle actin intermediate filaments (Figure 26.1C) and, less commonly, juxtanuclear aggregates of cytokeratins (Figure 26.1D, Table 26.1). While the better differentiated tumors show a clear demarcation between sex cord and stromal elements, this distinction is blurred in poorly differentiated lesions, particularly those with a diffuse or so-called 'sarcomatoid' pattern. A reticulin stain is often of use, showing only sparse fibrils in the granulosa cell component except around small blood vessels, while the theca cells are individually invested by reticulin fibrils (Figure 26.2). Intermediate reticulin patterns occasionally are encountered.

The perimenopausal clustering of cases of granulosa cell tumor suggests a role for pituitary trophins in their genesis. The evidence for the genesis in women who have been subjected to clomiphene citrate or gonadotrophin therapy for ovarian stimulation remains controversial.[100,104]

GRANULOSA CELL TUMOR, ADULT TYPE

Clinical profile

Most granulosa cell tumors occur in adult women (peak incidence, 45–55 years) and rather more than half occur after the menopause. Patients present with non-specific abdominal symptoms (20%), complaints suggesting an endocrinologic disturbance (50%), or both (30%). Abdominal pain and swelling, backache, dysuria or dyspareunia occur in one-third of patients. Abdominal distension is due to either tumor mass or ascites that accompanies nearly 10% of lesions. Rarely, Meigs syndrome is diagnosed. Occasional patients complain of acute abdominal pain due to hemorrhage into the tumor or rupture of a cystic neoplasm with hemoperitoneum, particularly in young women who are pregnant. Elevated serum levels of estradiol and estrone are often found. In premenopausal women, the most common 'endocrine' symptoms are irregular menstruation or menorrhagia, less frequently prolonged amenorrhea, or painfully enlarged breasts. Postmenopausal women usually complain of vaginal bleeding and sometimes breast enlargement. A high proportion of tumors have concomitant endometrial hyperplasias (about 50%) and carcinoma (about 10%). Occasional tumors, especially those that are unilocular cysts, present with signs of virilization.[81] Granulosa cell tumors occurring in pregnancy may produce large amounts of estrogen without clinical effect, whereas occasionally they are associated with signs of virilization. Serum inhibin, a polypeptide secreted by granulosa cells to regulate follicle stimulating hormone (FSH) secretion from the pituitary, is a useful tumor marker.[75] Antimüllerian hormone, produced by normal and neoplastic granulosa cells, has also been investigated in the same context.[44]

Macroscopic features

These tumors vary from tiny subclinical lesions to quite extraordinary masses filling the abdomen, with a mean diameter of about 13 cm. The external surface may be smooth or bosselated. The cut surface is typically partly solid and partly cystic (over half of cases). Solid areas may be hard and rubbery or soft in consistency and somewhat yellowish to gray in color (Figure 26.3), while cystic spaces contain proteinaceous fluid or old altered blood. Thin-walled parvilocular cystic granulosa

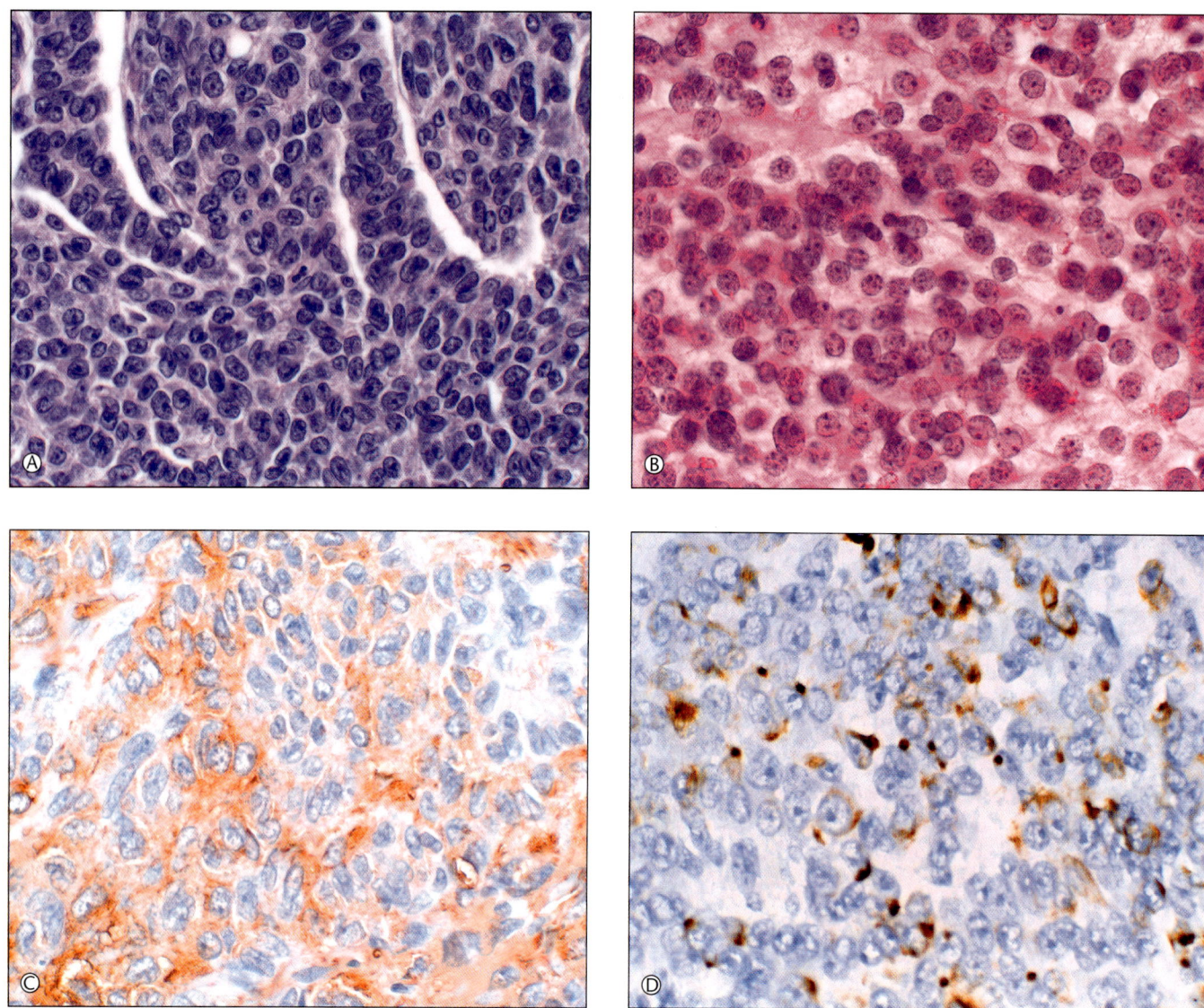

Fig. 26.1 Well-differentiated granulosa cell tumor. **(A)** Cells are typically crowded with scanty cytoplasm and bland, elongate, often longitudinally grooved nuclei. **(B)** Non-cohesive sheets of uniform granulosa cells from an intraoperative scalpel scraping of a solid tumor. Nuclear grooves are less apparent in such preparations. **(C)** Scattered cells displaying cytoplasmic staining for smooth muscle actin. **(D)** Patchy, focally 'punctate', cytoplasmic staining for cytokeratins (AE1/AE3).

cell tumors may be mistaken grossly for benign serous cysts. Hemorrhage and necrosis are common. At laparotomy, the tumors are confined to the ovaries in 90% of patients and are bilateral in only 2%.

Microscopic features

Any one particular pattern of growth may dominate, but variation in the histologic appearance from area to area in any given tumor is much more common.

Well-differentiated granulosa cell tumors exhibit one or more of so-called 'microfollicular', 'macrofollicular', 'trabecular' or 'insular' patterns. The microfollicular variant (Figure 26.4), the most easily recognized, shows multiple small rounded spaces formed by cystic degeneration in small aggregates of granulosa cells, and containing eosinophilic periodic acid-Schiff (PAS)-positive material (chondroitin 6-sulphate) and often fragments of nuclear debris or pyknotic nuclei. These

spaces, known as Call–Exner bodies, are found in only 30–50% of tumors. The granulosa cell nuclei are oriented somewhat radially, but haphazardly, around these cavitated structures (Figure 26.5), and lack the cellular precision of adenocarcinoma cells around an acinus. The macrofollicular variant (Figure 26.6) comprises cysts of differing sizes lined by multilayered well-differentiated granulosa cells, often cuffed by a layer of theca-like cells, and apparently also formed by cystic degeneration in large masses of granulosa cells. Either or both of these cell layers may be luteinized. In the uncommon totally cystic granulosa cell tumors, the lining cells of the cysts may so closely resemble those of non-neoplastic ovarian follicle cysts that differentiation on purely histologic criteria is problematic.

The trabecular variant exhibits cells arranged as anastomosing ribbons or cords one (Figure 26.7) to several (Figure 26.8) cells wide. The granulosa cell cords are set in a background of

Table 26.1 Immunophenotype of granulosa cell tumors	
Antibody	**Frequency**
Calretinin	100%
Vimentin	100%
α- and β-Inhibin	100%
Smooth muscle actin	90%
CD 99	80%
WT1	60%
S-100 protein	50%
35BH11	40%
AE1/AE3	40%
CAM 5.2	35%
Desmin	20%
CA-125	–
Epithelial membrane antigen	–
B72.3	–
Carcinoembryonic antigen	–
Chromogranin	–

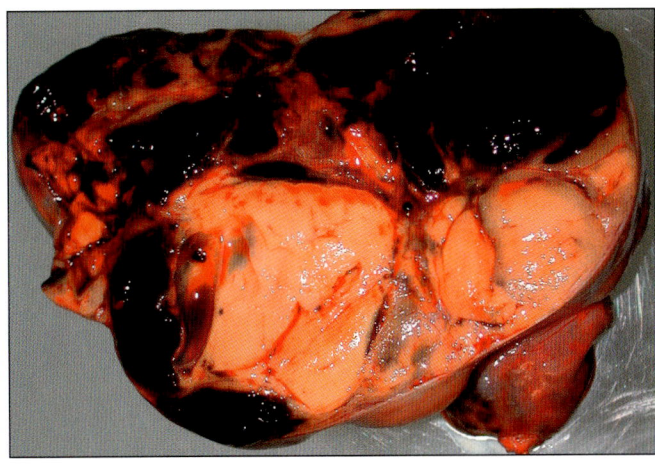

Fig. 26.3 Cut surface of a typical granulosa cell tumor. Solid areas are pale yellow/fawn and featureless, but with focal necrosis. Cystic spaces are filled with blood.

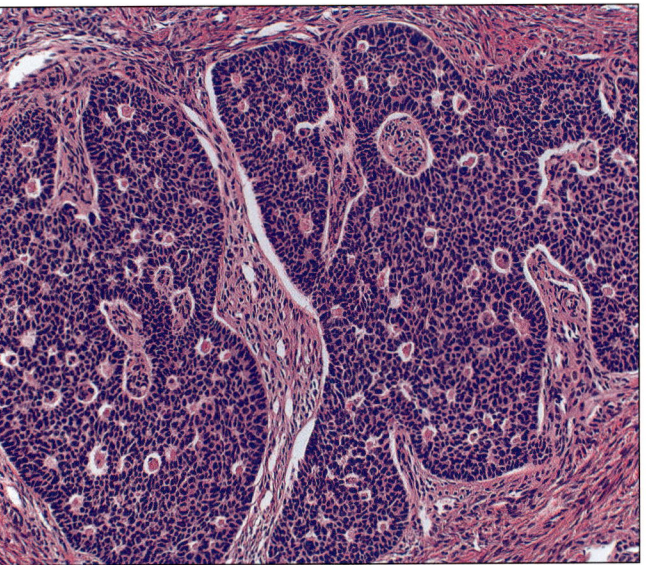

Fig. 26.4 Well-differentiated granulosa cell tumor with a microfollicular pattern. Cells show some palisading around the periphery of cell masses but rarely more pronounced than illustrated here. Call–Exner bodies are numerous.

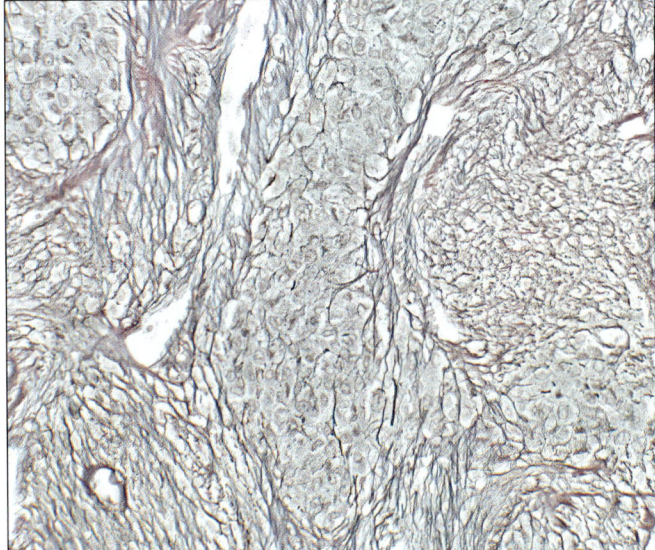

Fig. 26.2 Granulosa – theca cell tumor. Reticulin-poor granulosa cell areas with intervening zones of theca cells densely enmeshed by reticulin fibers. Reticulin stain.

stromal cells and show variable peripheral nuclear palisading. They may rarely produce true tubules, but any significant presence of these strongly suggests Sertoli cell differentiation. A trabecular pattern with hyaline or mucoid change in the stroma gives rise to the so-called 'cylindromatous' form of granulosa cell tumor (Figure 26.9), which at times may merge into the tumorous sex-cord tumor with annular tubules (SCTAT) (see below).

Insular variants exhibit masses or islands of polyhedral granulosa cells with peripherally palisaded nuclei separated by a fibroma-like or thecoma-like stroma (Figure 26.10). Call–Exner bodies are more common in this variant, but still are found in only a minority of cases. The insular pattern also shows overlap with the microfollicular pattern described above. Occasional, otherwise unremarkable, well-differentiated granulosa cell tumors exhibit small foci where cells have enlarged bizarre nuclei (Figures 26.11 and 26.12) and/or multinucleated giant cells. These foci are degenerative in nature and in no way alter the classification, typing or grading of the tumor in which they are found. Another unusual degenerative phenomenon is central sclerosis within islands or masses of granulosa cells, again probably ischemic in nature (Figure 26.13). Rare cases of granulosa cell tumor have scattered eosinophilic polygonal cells in the stroma that show an immunophenotype of true hepatic cell differentiation.[1]

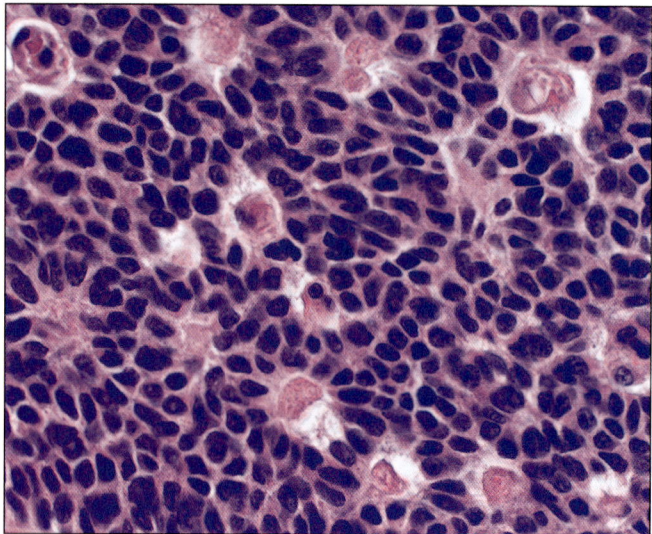

Fig. 26.5 Well-differentiated granulosa cell tumor, microfollicular pattern. Numerous Call–Exner bodies containing hyaline material and cellular debris.

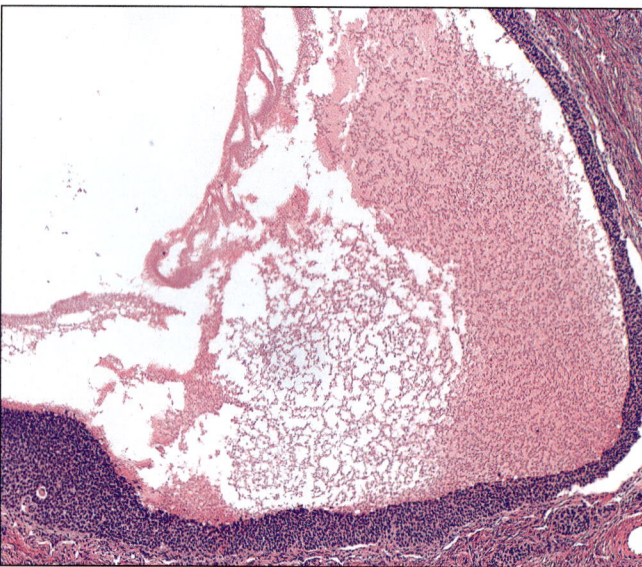

Fig. 26.6 Well-differentiated granulosa cell tumor, macrofollicular pattern. Lining cells closely resemble those of normal preovulatory follicles. No thecal layer is present in this example.

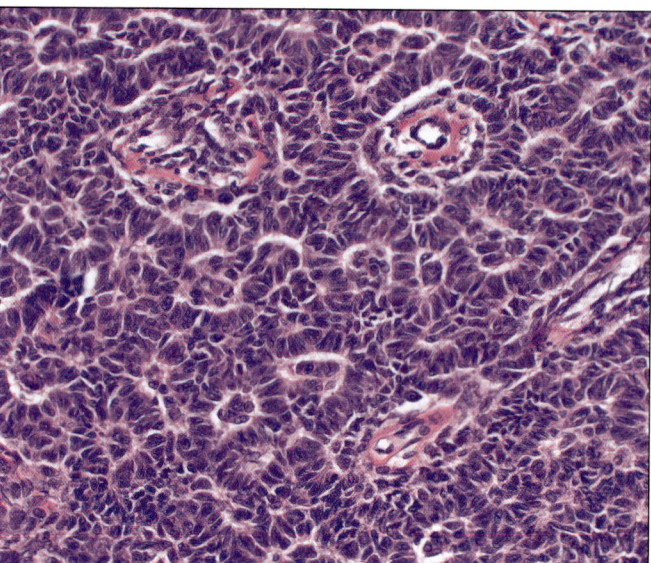

Fig. 26.7 Well-differentiated granulosa cell tumor, trabecular pattern. Cords of cells vary from one to two cells thick with oval nuclei oriented perpendicularly.

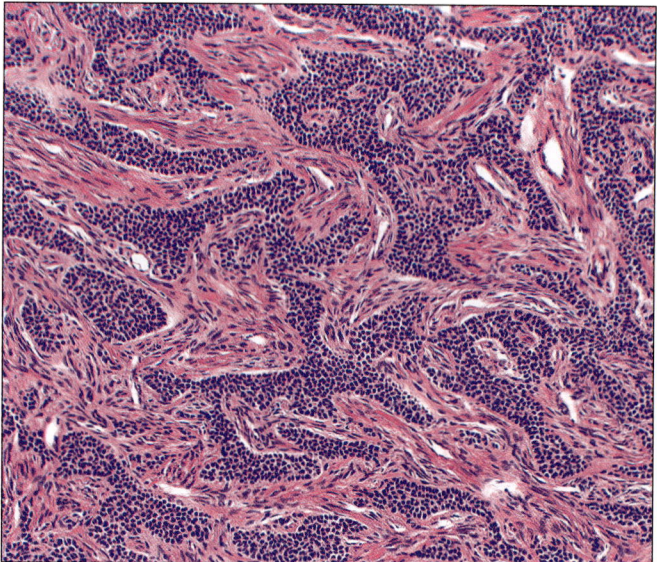

Fig. 26.8 Well-differentiated granulosa cell tumor, trabecular pattern. Cords of cells are much thicker than in the previous variant (Figure 26.7) and are separated by prominent fibrothecoma-like stroma.

In moderately differentiated forms, the trabecular pattern is more complex and is composed of fine narrow undulating cords of granulosa cells with little intervening stroma, producing so-called 'watered-silk' ('moiré-silk') or gyriform appearances (Figure 26.14). Insular patterns also become increasingly complex with diminution of the intervening stroma.

Poorly differentiated diffuse or 'sarcomatoid' forms produce monotonous cellular growth resembling a low-grade round cell (Figure 26.15A) or spindle cell sarcoma (Figure 26.15B). The uniform cells are closely packed and arranged in poorly circumscribed sheets that often appear to merge at their periphery with nearby acellular areas or the surrounding normal ovarian stroma. Luteinization further effaces the architecture (Figure 26.16). The cells contain regular and relatively bland nuclei and, although mitoses may at times be numerous, they lack the

high counts observed in the undifferentiated carcinomas or sarcomas forming the differential diagnosis of this variant of granulosa cell tumors. Fewer than 10% of granulosa cell tumors exhibit over 5 mitoses per 10 high-power fields (HPFs). Diffuse granulosa cell tumors contain variable amounts of reticulin fibrils, depending on the relative presence of a stromal (theca cell) component, and such reticulin as is present tends to outline groups rather than individual cells, this being of some help in differentiating them from low-grade endometrioid sarcomas, in which individual cells are ensheathed.

Isolated case reports detail combined granulosa cell tumor and benign mucinous tumor (Figures 26.17 and 26.18) that appear analogous to the Sertoli–Leydig cell tumors with heterologous elements.[13,59,69]

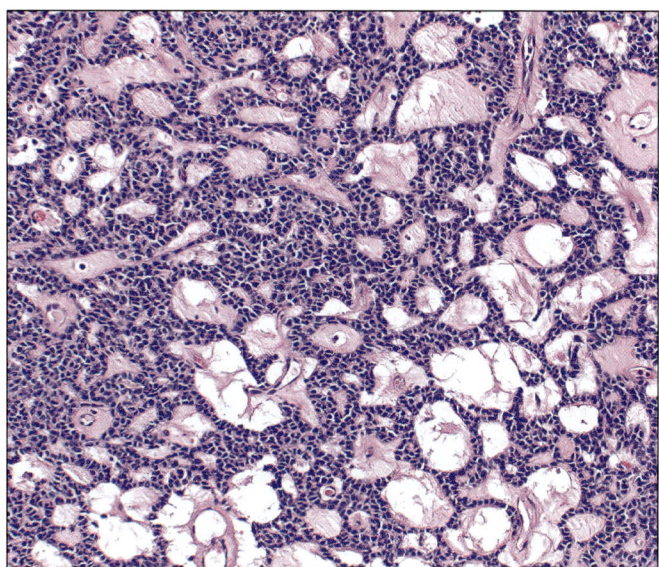

Fig. 26.9 Well-differentiated granulosa cell tumor. With the addition of hyaline change to the stroma, the tumor acquires a 'cylindromatous' appearance.

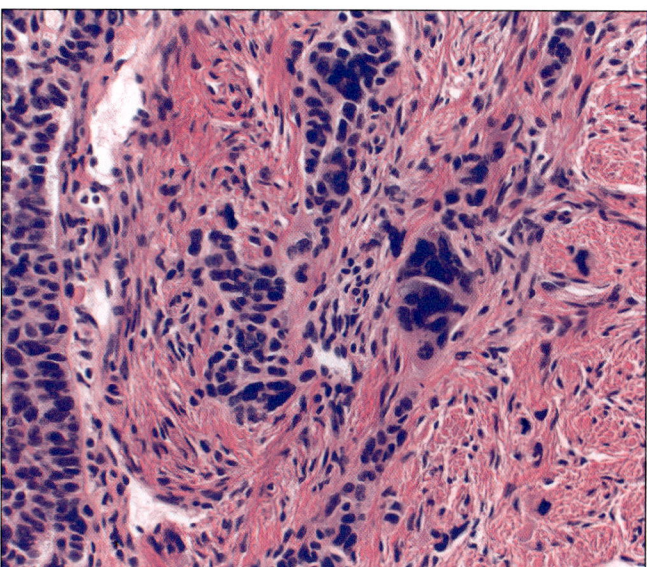

Fig. 26.11 Well-differentiated granulosa cell tumor with focally bizarre nuclei. They may occur in any of the histologic variants of this tumor. Isolated bizarre nuclei seen here in small trabecular of granulosa cells.

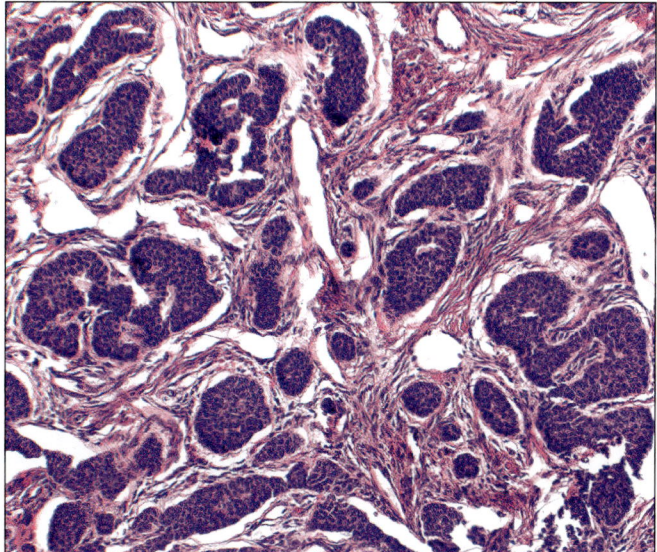

Fig. 26.10 'Insular' variant of microfollicular granulosa cell tumor. This pattern is important only in the difficulty it may present in being distinguished from ovarian carcinoid tumors.

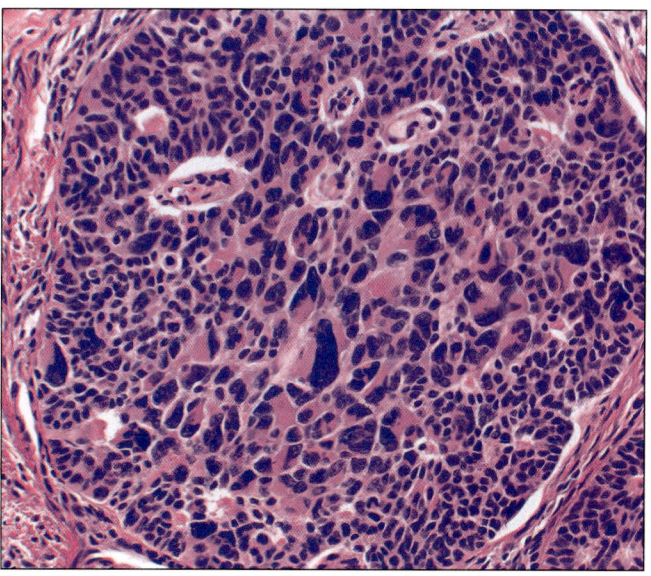

Fig. 26.12 Well-differentiated granulosa cell tumor with focally bizarre nuclei. Bizarre nuclei seen within cell nest of microfollicular tumor.

Differential diagnosis

The discrimination between an undifferentiated small cell carcinoma of the ovary of hypercalcemic type (see Chapter 25) and a granulosa cell tumor is important. If a tumor behaves in an unexpectedly aggressive fashion for one originally diagnosed as granulosa cell tumor, particularly in a younger woman, the possibility of such a misdiagnosis must be considered. The growth patterns, including the presence of follicle-like spaces and the monotonous uniformity of the constituent cells, can be similar in both entities. The most readily appreciable discriminatory criterion is the appearance of the nuclei. The nuclei are typically bland and often grooved in granulosa cell tumors and have few mitoses, but show variation in size and shape, marked hyperchromasia, and are rarely grooved in undifferentiated small cell carcinomas. Numerous mitoses, frequently atypical, and apop-

totic bodies are often also found in the latter. Immunohistochemistry regularly distinguishes inhibin and calretinin reactivity in the granulosa cell tumor, but not in small cell carcinoma.[54] Reactivity for epithelial membrane antigen (EMA) is less reliable, being regularly reactive in small cell carcinomas and only occasionally reactive in adult granulosa cell tumors, but not infrequently positive in juvenile granulosa cell tumors.[55]

Granulosa cell tumors may be readily confused with carcinoid tumors, particularly those that have an insular pattern. The cells in an insular carcinoid tumor, however, usually have well-defined cell margins, eosinophilic granular cytoplasm peripherally, and more regular and rounded nuclei than those in granulosa cell tumors. Acini of insular carcinoids show well-formed circular lumens and columnar cells lining the tumor in which the cytoplasm is luminal and the nuclei basal. Call–Exner

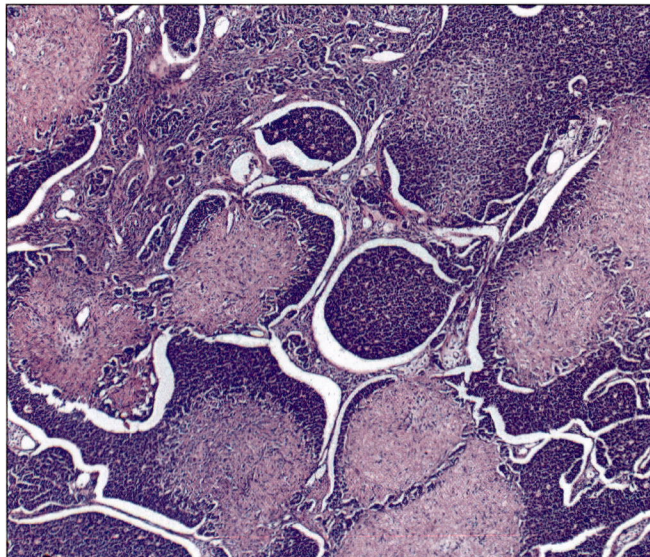

Fig. 26.13 Microfollicular granulosa cell tumor. This example displays pronounced central sclerosis in large islands of granulosa cells.

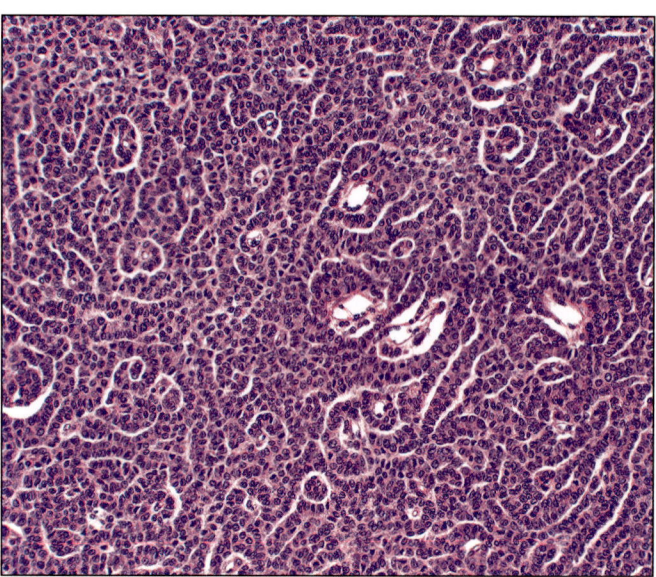

Fig. 26.14 Moderately differentiated granulosa cell tumor, gyriform or 'moiré-silk' pattern. Nuclei are still uniform and bland with few mitoses.

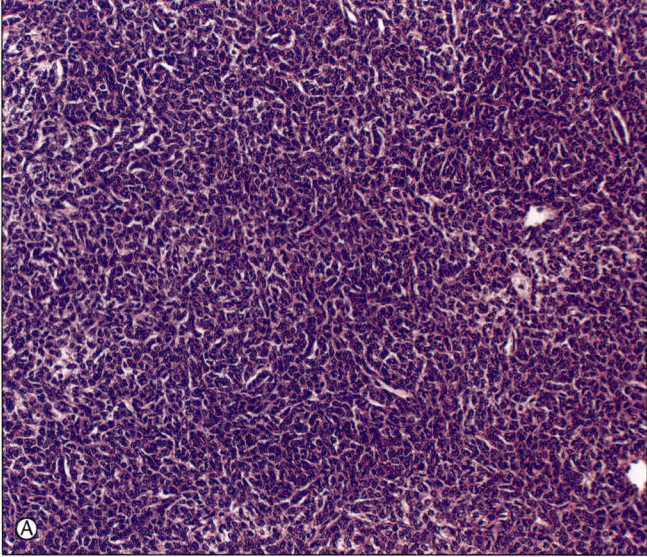

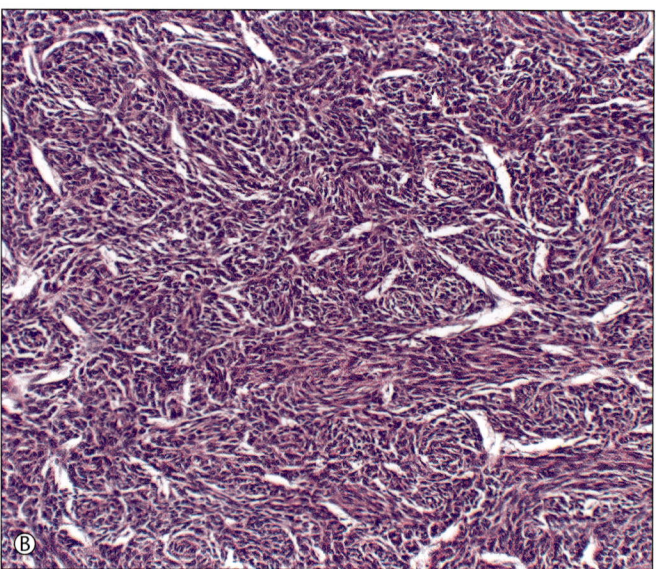

Fig. 26.15 Poorly differentiated diffuse granulosa cell tumor. Solid sheets and fascicles of **(A)** small round cells or **(B)** small spindled cells. Vascular spaces are infrequent compared to low-grade endometrioid stromal sarcoma.

body nuclei usually haphazardly line the degenerative central space. Large numbers of argyrophil cells and chromogranin-reactive cells are demonstrable in carcinoid tumors.

Call–Exner bodies should not be confused with the glands of adenocarcinomas and the hyaline bodies of similar size observed in gonadoblastomas and sex-cord tumors with annular tubules. The acini of adenocarcinomas are often filled with thick mucin and the nuclei are usually more pleomorphic than those of the granulosa cell tumor. The hyaline bodies in gonadoblastoma and sex-cord tumor with annular tubules are denser than Call–Exner bodies and are sometimes continuous with hyaline basement membrane material around the periphery of the tumor cell nests. These bodies may also be calcified.

Most granulosa cell tumors are easily distinguished from androblastomas (Sertoli–Leydig cell tumors), but this distinction may be impossible in very poorly differentiated cases and,

of course, mixed tumors do occur (see 'Gynandroblastomas' below). In difficult cases, we categorize the sex cord-stromal tumor as of indeterminate differentiation. As stated above, the granulosa cell component of a granulosa cell tumor may be minor. The watershed between such tumors and the so-called 'fibromas with minor sex-cord elements' is arbitrarily set at 10% representation by the sex-cord (granulosa cell) components (Figure 26.19).

Prognosis and treatment

Recurrent disease sometimes presents within 5 years of removal of the primary tumor, but more commonly it is evident only later (average of 8–9 years). Many recur even after 10 years, thus leading to corrected death rates of 87–94% at 5 years, 76–82% at 10 years, and 50–62% at 20 years.[47,83] Celomic spread is the commonest route of dissemination when meta-

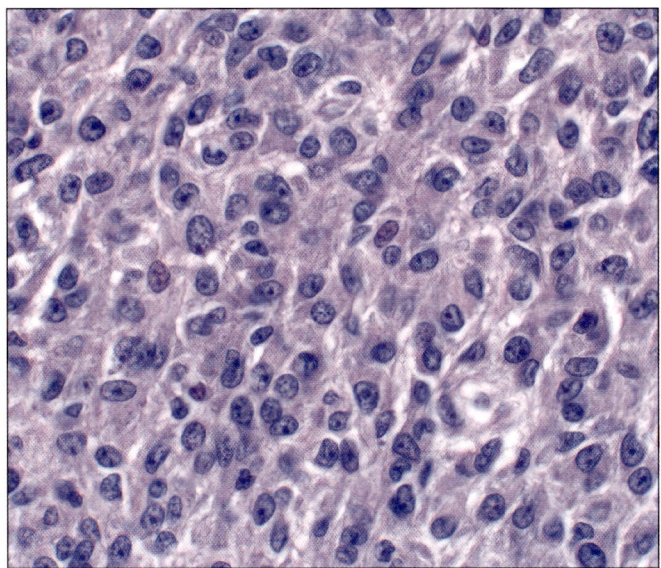

Fig. 26.16 Poorly differentiated and luteinized granulosa cell tumor. Nuclei are bland and uniform. Longitudinal grooves tend to disappear in such variants.

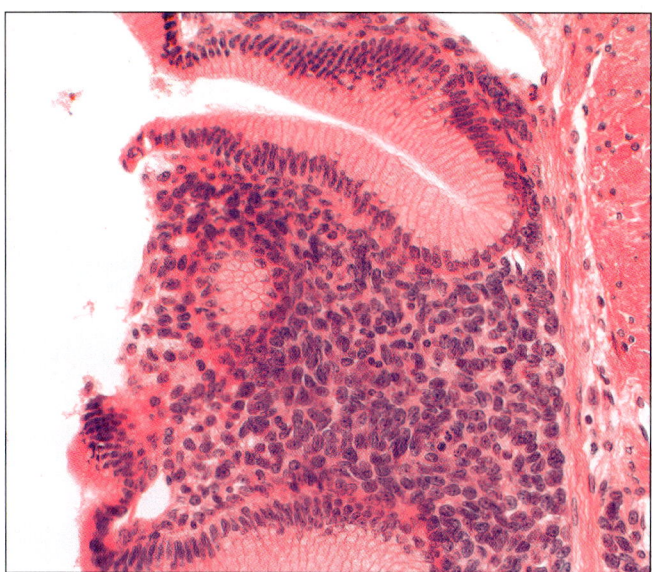

Fig. 26.18 Combined granulosa cell/benign mucinous tumor. Benign müllerian (endocervical) mucinous glands intimately mixed with typical granulosa cells.

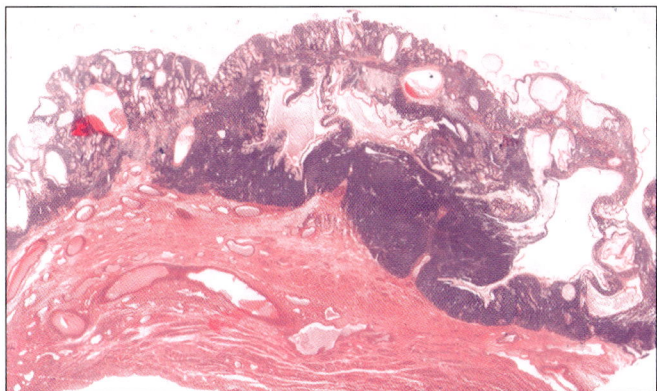

Fig. 26.17 Combined granulosa cell/benign mucinous tumor. Survey showing broad band of dense hypercellular tumor lining the cyst with included gland-like spaces.

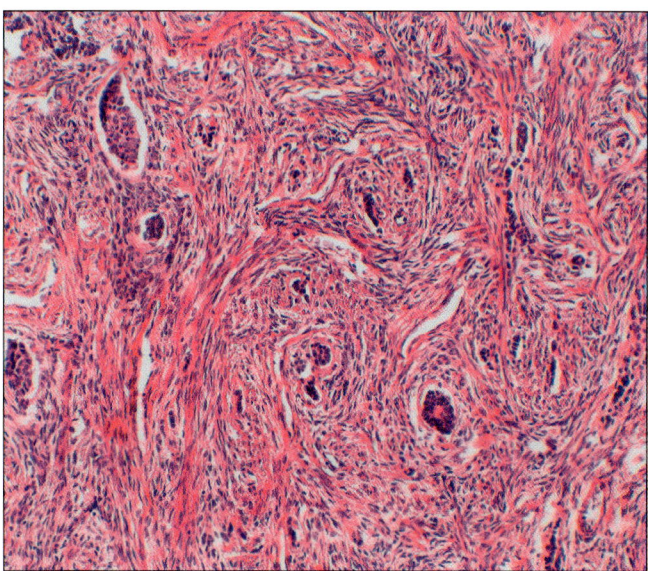

Fig. 26.19 Trabecular granulosa cell tumor with only minor sex-cord components.

static disease is present. Spread occurs mostly within the pelvis or lower abdominal cavities. Metastasis to retroperitoneal nodes is uncommon. Distant metastases are rare, but have been reported in lungs, brain, bones, and liver. The surgical approach employed with epithelial–stromal ovarian tumors is also used to treat granulosa cell tumors. Where fertility is an issue in management, unilateral salpingo-oophorectomy and peritoneal biopsies with an ipsilateral pelvic and para-aortic lymph node dissection is the recommended surgical treatment. The cornerstone of a sustained progression-free interval for advanced disease appears to be radical cytoreductive surgery. The role of chemotherapy and radiotherapy in cases of advanced disease remains controversial, although response to cisplatin, etoposide, and bleomycin has been noted.[79]

Regardless of the particular microscopic pattern observed, all granulosa cell tumors are considered as low-grade malignancies. In our present state of knowledge, clinical factors are as important as pathologic features in identifying those adult granulosa cell tumors likely to progress or recur. Adverse fea-

tures include age over 50 years,[110] extraovarian spread at laparotomy (stages 2–4), and residual tumor after primary surgery,[91,101] while for stage 1A cases, spontaneous rupture of tumor, tumor diameter >5 cm and numerous mitotic figures (≥5 mitoses per 10 HPFs) appear significant.[82]

GRANULOSA CELL TUMOR, JUVENILE TYPE

Clinical profile

A small but definable subset of granulosa cell tumors – which includes 90% of examples in prepubertal girls, many in adolescents, and only infrequently in adult women – has a distinctive histologic appearance designated as 'juvenile' granulosa cell tumor. A disproportionate number of granulosa cell tumors removed or diagnosed during pregnancy belong to this histologic group.[33,97] Over 80% of juvenile granulosa cell tumors that occur in prepubertal girls present with an anovulatory form of isosexual precocious pseudopuberty, including galactorrhea.[41,78] Rarely, they present with secondary amenorrhea and biochemical evidence of androgen secretion.[45] More acute thoracoabdominal symptoms may be present in some. There has also been documented an infrequent association with multiple enchondromatosis (Ollier disease), enchondromatosis with hemangiomas (Maffucci syndrome),[66] and rarely with leprechaunism, tuberous sclerosis,[30] and hypercalcemia.[19] They may occur rarely in dysgenetic gonads. Cytogenetics on juvenile granulosa cell tumors regularly reveals trisomy 12, trisomy 14 or monosomy 22,[53] a pattern similar but not identical to that found in adult granulosa cell tumors.[48]

Pathology

The macroscopic features resemble those of the adult tumor. Microscopically, the juvenile granulosa cell tumor shows partially coalescing solid nodules of proliferating granulosa cells arranged randomly in sheets or around irregular follicle-like spaces in which the secretory fluids in the follicles are amphophilic. Intersecting fibrous bands accentuate this nodularity (Figure 26.20), occasionally (when marked) producing a superficial resemblance to sclerosing stromal tumors (see below).

Intercellular edema may be quite pronounced, particularly if the patient is pregnant. The thick-walled follicles and cavities (Figure 26.21) are smaller than those seen in adult macrofollicular granulosa cell tumors and may contain mucicarmine-positive material in over one-half of cases. Solid tubular patterns are sometimes seen. Theca cells are often prominent, particularly at the periphery of the nodules, but may be intimately admixed with the granulosa cells. Reticulin stains can be employed to highlight the relative proportions of these two cellular elements.

Cytologically, both cell types appear less 'mature' than their equivalents in other types of granulosa cell tumors. The nuclei are larger and more hyperchromatic and the granulosa cells

rarely show nuclear grooving (Figure 26.22). Mitoses, occasionally atypical, are often prominent, and average about 7 mitotic figures per 10 HPFs. Luteinization is also a common feature of both granulosa and theca cell elements. Rare and isolated examples of juvenile granulosa cell tumors showing focal specific mesenchymal differentiation towards skeletal muscle[71] or Wilms tumor[64] have been reported.

Prognosis

Juvenile granulosa cell tumors, although appearing poorly differentiated and pleomorphic, typically have a high cure rate, except in high stage cases that recur early and progress rapidly.[25]

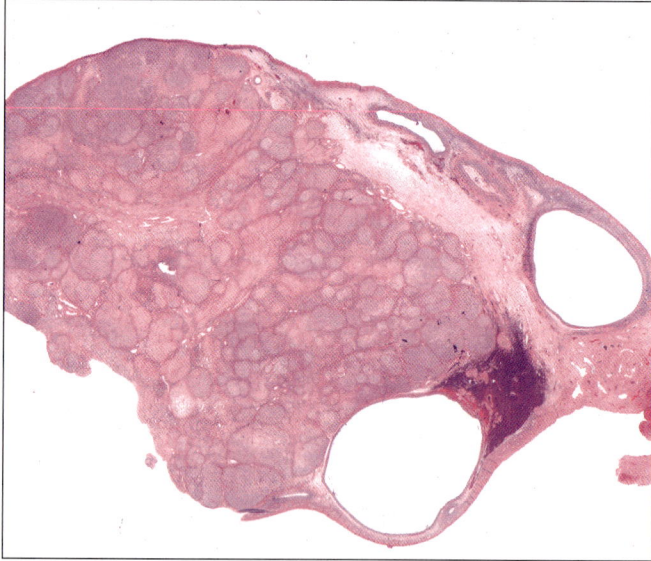

Fig. 26.20 Juvenile granulosa cell tumor. Survey of small tumor from 7-year-old girl presenting with precocious pseudopuberty. Note solid lobular growth pattern. (See also juvenile granulosa cell component of gynandroblastoma, Figure 26.74A.)

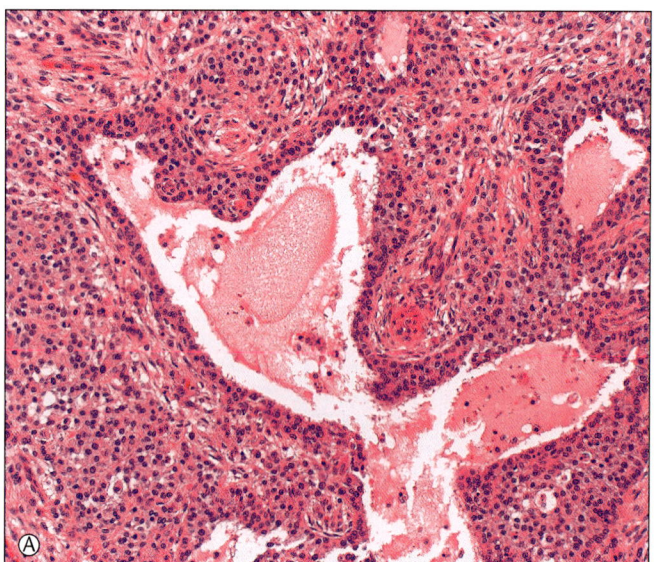
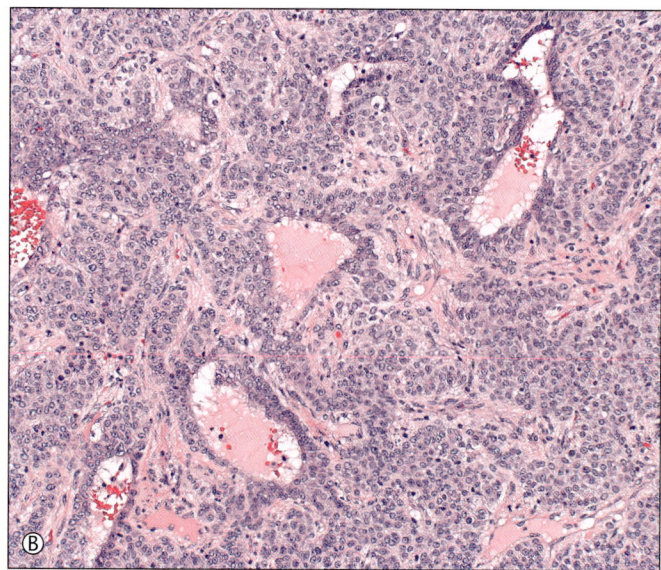

Fig. 26.21 Juvenile granulosa cell tumor. **(A, B)** Irregular follicle-like structures lined by a variably thickened polyhedral granulosa cell layer with adjacent, less well-organized aggregates of cells with pale cytoplasm and rounded, 'immature', non-grooved nuclei. (See also juvenile granulosa cell component of gynandroblastoma, Figure 26.74B.)

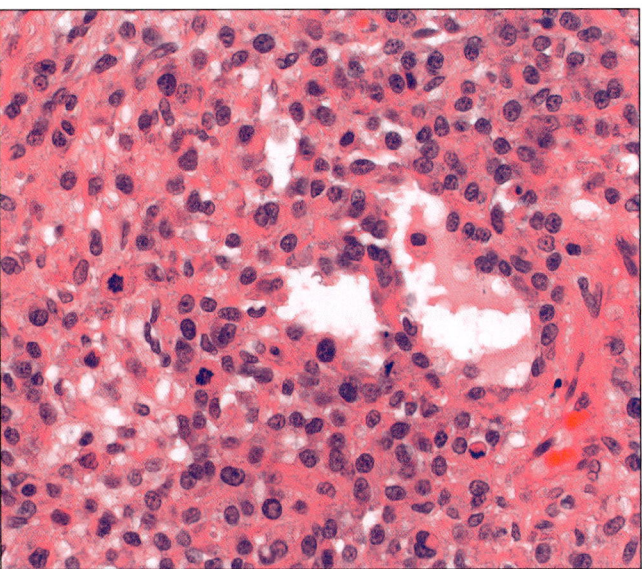

Fig. 26.22 Juvenile granulosa cell tumor. Solid nodule of 'immature' granulosa cells with hyperchromatic nuclei and obvious mitoses.

THECOMA–FIBROMA GROUP OF TUMORS

Definition
These neoplasms arise from the ovarian stroma and exhibit a spectrum of histologic appearances that includes, at one end, simple fibromas and, at the other end, tumors showing distinct differentiation to specialized perifollicular or follicular theca cells or their luteinized variants. Tumors in the thecoma–fibroma group vary from microscopic to very large and fibromas, particularly, are frequently quite small and incidental findings at operation. We have chosen 1 cm diameter, widely adopted for the benign surface epithelial–stromal tumors, as the lower limit for size. The presence of occasional small aggregates of cells of sex-cord type is acceptable without altering the primary diagnosis. Applying these general guidelines, ovarian fibromas are by far the commonest ovarian neoplasms of sex cord-stromal origin and account for 6% of all primary ovarian tumors. Typical thecomas, on the other hand, are uncommon lesions while tumors with features intermediate between these histologic extremes are only somewhat more frequently encountered.

THECOMAS

Definition
Thecomas are benign tumors composed of plump spindled cells with obvious lipid-containing cytoplasm and resembling cells of the ovarian theca interna.

Clinical profile
Thecoma occurs at any age but is most common after age 40 years. They rarely develop in children. The mean age at presentation is about 55 years, and 75% occur after the menopause. Luteinized variants are more likely to occur in younger women. Estrogenic manifestations are by far the commonest mode of clinical presentation and usually take the form of menstrual irregularities or postmenopausal bleeding. Androgenic theco-

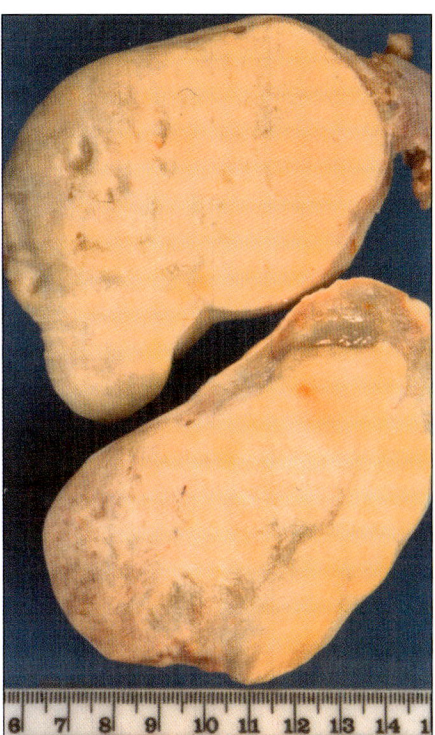

Fig. 26.23 Thecoma. Solid, well-circumscribed tumor with pale, variably yellow cut surface.

mas are rare, although luteinized thecomas may cause virilization in pregnancy.[40] Non-specific abdominal symptoms relating to the tumor itself are less common, although abdominal pain and swelling and even Meigs syndrome occur.[105] Rare associated pathologic entities include pancreatic cysts[16] and a steroid cell tumor (see below) in the contralateral ovary.[18]

Macroscopic features
The size range varies from small subclinical nodules to large, firm, solid, rubbery tumors several centimeters in diameter. The cut surface characteristically is bright yellow to orange, although many appear paler in hue (Figure 26.23). They are almost always unilateral. The remainder of the ovary and, indeed, the contralateral ovary may show diffuse or nodular hyperplasia.

Microscopic features
Most tumors conform to one of two patterns. Typical thecomas consist of large, often ill-defined, somewhat nodular masses (Figure 26.24) of eosinophilic or vacuolated cells interspersed by relatively less conspicuous bands of fibrous connective tissue. The fibrous bands are composed mostly of tight bundles of elongated fibroblastic cells but often exhibit hyalinized plaques (Figure 26.25). The theca cells are uniformly plump and spindle shaped, with small, pale, round or ovoid, central, non-grooved nuclei (Figure 26.26A). The immunoprofile of the tumor cells includes reactivity for calretinin and α-inhibin (Figure 26.26B).[8,56] Reticulin stains show a fine meshwork of fibrils about individual cells. Mitoses are rare (<1 per 10 HPFs in most tumors). Edema or myxoid change is often prominent and some tumors show an occasional focus of dystrophic calcification (i.e., ragged spicules of mineralization in areas of stromal degeneration/hyalinization) or even ossification.[62] A particular subtype showing extensive calcification is occasionally noted in

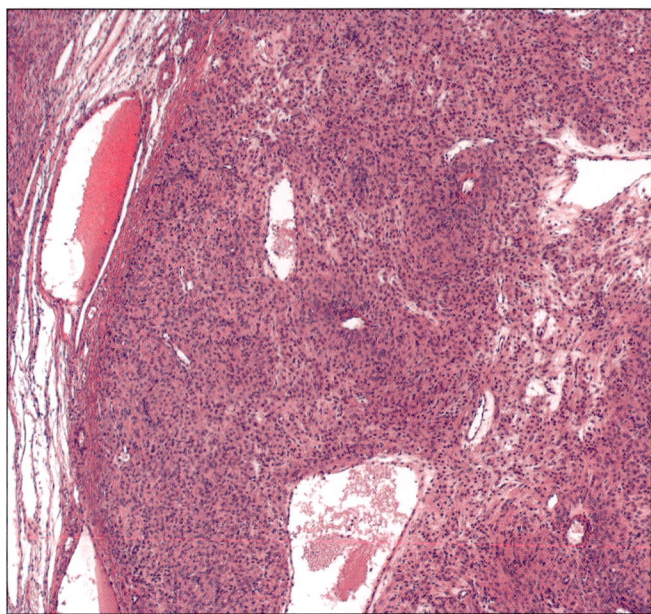

Fig. 26.24 Ovarian thecoma. Circumscribed nodule, showing featureless masses of plump spindle cells.

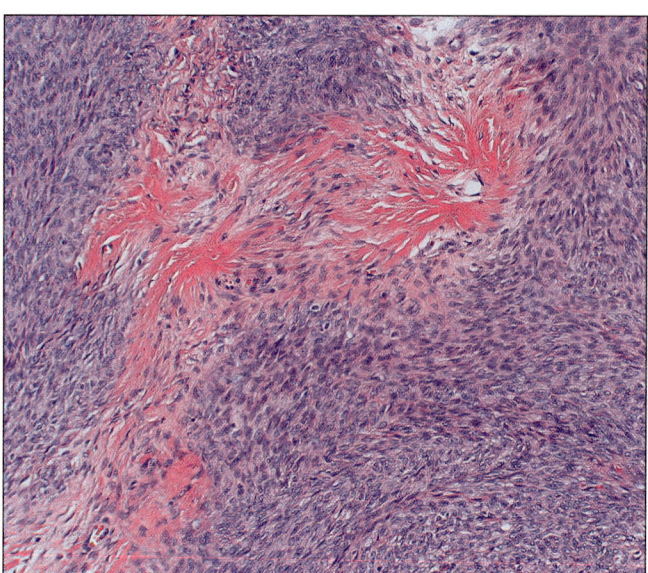

Fig. 26.25 Ovarian thecoma. Plump theca-like cells with eosinophilic cytoplasm. Hyalinization of the stroma is prominent.

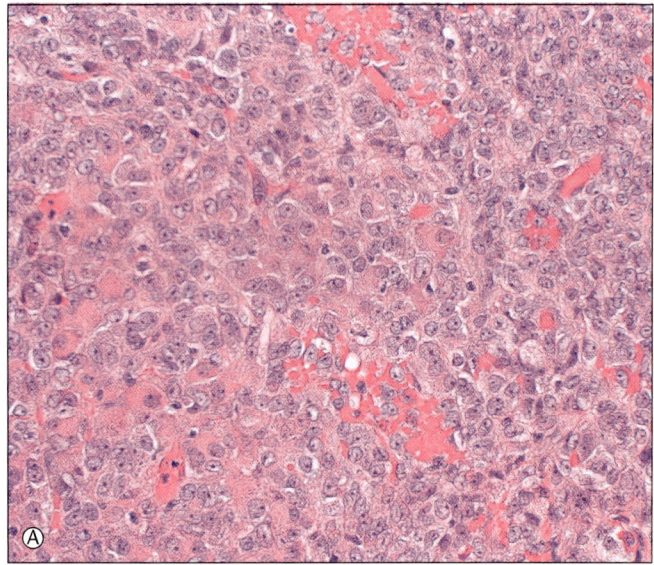

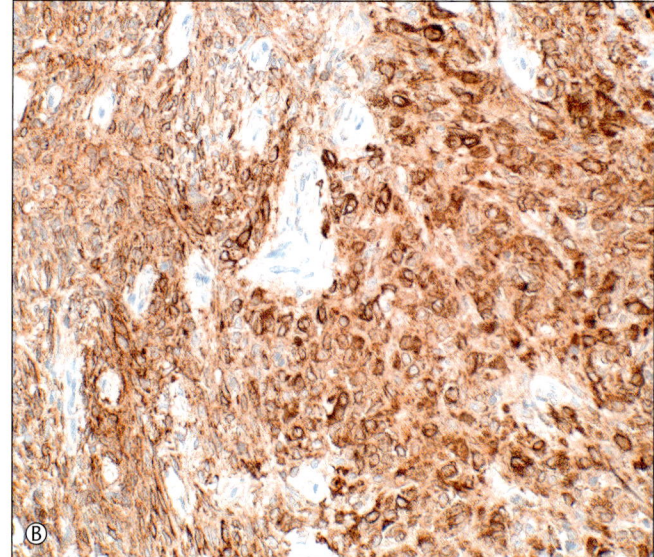

Fig. 26.26 Ovarian thecoma. **(A)** Plump theca-like cells with eosinophilic cytoplasm and uniform, round-to-oval central nuclei. **(B)** Prominent cytoplasmic staining for α-inhibin.

young women, although this needs to be distinguished from extensively calcified sclerosing stromal tumors.[98]

Occasional small nests of granulosa-like cells are found; such tumors are called 'thecomas with minor sex-cord elements'. Over 50% of thecomas are associated with stromal hyperplasia in the same and/or contralateral ovary that may be diffuse or nodular (including nodular thecal hyperplasia).

The second defined histologic pattern, designated 'luteinized thecoma', is an otherwise typical thecoma or perhaps a more fibromatous tumor throughout which clusters of large eosinophilic lipid-laden lutein cells are scattered (Figure 26.27). Over 10% of such luteinized thecomas are androgenic. Luteinized thecomas tend to be solitary lesions and occur more frequently in younger women. They are unassociated with a background

of stromal hyperplasia and therefore distinguishable from stromal luteomas. Stromal luteomas are almost always seen as dominant nodules in a background of nodular thecal hyperplasia (stromal hyperplasia with focal luteinization) and we regard them as hyperplastic or tumor-like in nature (see Chapter 22). The term 'luteinized thecoma' has also been applied, erroneously in our view, to an acutely presenting ovarian mass, sometimes associated with sclerosing peritonitis[6,63] and forming part of the spectrum of fibromatosis (see Chapter 22).

Malignant thecoma, the existence of which some challenge, is accepted in principle by us and by others, based on calretinin or inhibin reactivity in frankly malignant spindle cell tumors.[58] In our experience, however, is important to concede that, like fibromas (see below), otherwise typical thecomas occasionally

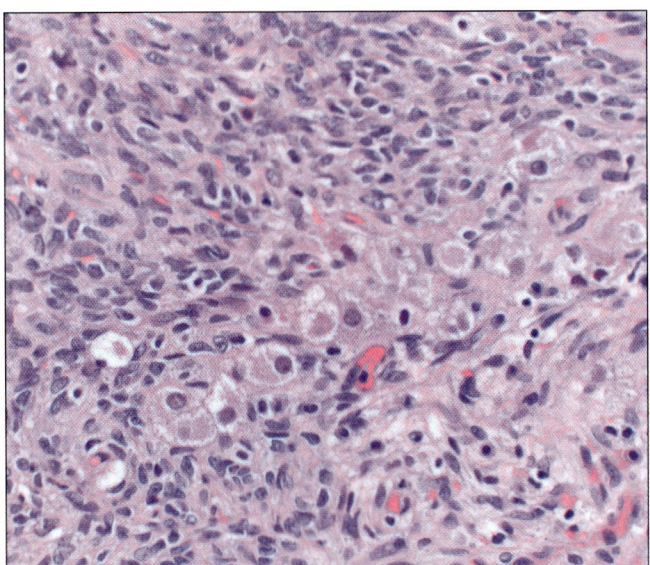

Fig. 26.27 Luteinized thecoma. Isolated clusters of large, clearly luteinized theca cells (abundant eosinophilic cytoplasm, round, slightly hyperchromatic, vesicular nuclei) in a background of smaller spindled cells.

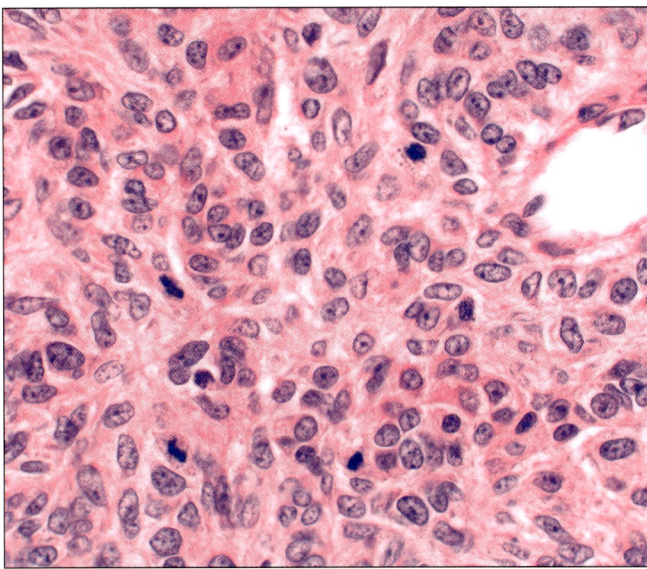

Fig. 26.28 Mitotically active ovarian thecoma. Otherwise typical thecomas occasionally display numerous mitoses.

display numerous mitoses (Figure 26.28). The explanation for this is not clear but may be low-grade ischemia (partial torsion). In the absence of established criteria, thecomatous tumors confined to the ovary and exhibiting both hypercellularity and ≥4 mitotic figures per 10 HPFs should be regarded with suspicion and the patient followed clinically.[105] Nuclear atypia *per se* is not an indication of malignancy and rare thecomas or luteinized thecomas may contain focal aggregates of bizarre nuclei without compromising the patient's prognosis.

THECAFIBROMAS

Clinical profile
These tumors exhibit a much lower frequency of associated endometrial pathology and evidence of endocrine disturbance than do the 'pure' thecomas and in this respect more closely resemble the largely hormonally inactive fibromas and sclerosing stromal tumors. The general age at presentation and clinical findings also resemble those for ovarian fibromas. The existence of tumors intermediate between thecomas and fibromas is evidence of the specialized ovarian stromal origin of most if not all ovarian fibromas. For all practical purposes, these tumors are benign, although a solitary reported case (with positive inhibin reactivity)[58] blurs the distinction with fibrosarcoma (see below).

Pathology
Thecafibromas are solid rubbery tumors showing gross feature indistinguishable from those of ovarian fibromas. The basic architecture of these tumors is that of a cellular fibroma with variably interlaced bundles of thin spindle cells producing collagen in some areas quite prominently (Figure 26.29). Edema is present in half and often pronounced. The collagenous component is usually fibrillary in appearance but hyalinization is sometimes seen. The latter is often accentuated perivascularly. These elements are well represented in scalpel scrapes of the fresh tumor (Figure 26.30).

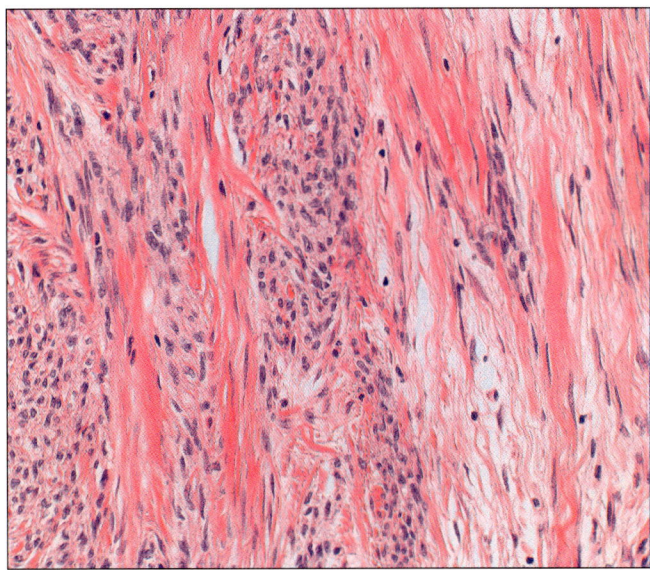

Fig. 26.29 Thecofibroma. Sheets of plump theca cells (top) and attenuated fibroblastic cells (right) interspersed by hyalinized bands of collagen.

Theca cells are present in variable numbers but are usually seen in small clusters, often observed only on close examination of several sections, or as larger but isolated fields in fibrous tumors (Figure 26.29). By convention, luteinized theca cells are not seen, as their presence alters the diagnosis to luteinized thecoma (see above).

SCLEROSING STROMAL TUMORS

Clinical profile
Sclerosing stromal tumors are separated from other sex cord-stromal tumors due to their unusual clinical setting (80% occur under 30 years of age and rarely in childhood[23]) and a surprising lack (given the histologic features) of hormonally related

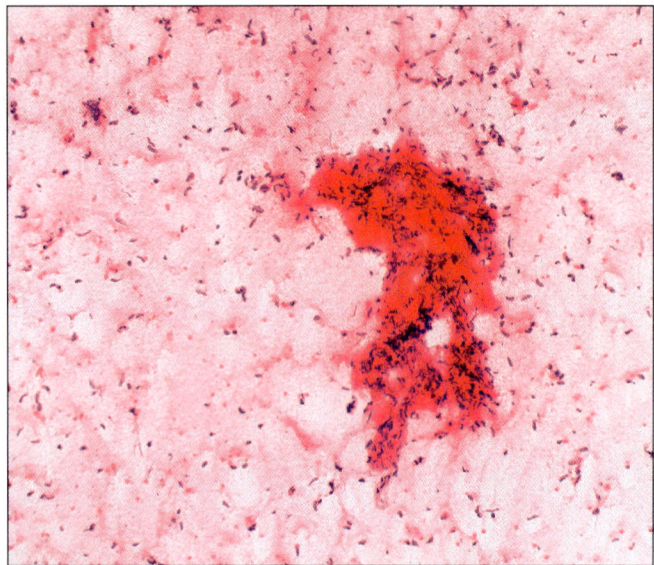

Fig. 26.30 Thecofibroma – scalpel scrape from fresh tumor. Densely eosinophilic collagen containing distorted spindle cells and a background of predominantly 'stripped' small bipolar nuclei (same tumor as Figure 26.29).

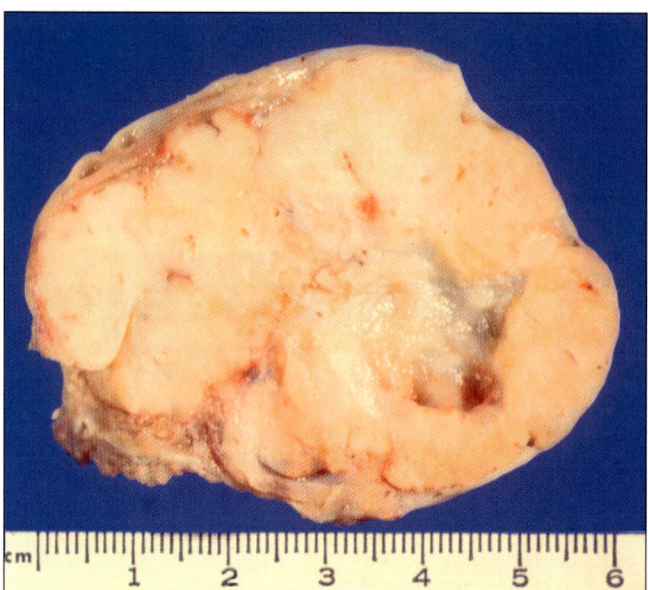

Fig. 26.31 Sclerosing stromal tumor. Cystic degeneration and vague pseudolobulation are apparent in the cut surface.

abnormalities.[92] They arise from perifollicular myoid stromal cells – a population of muscle-specific actin-positive cells in the theca externa. Some patients have presented with anovulation, due to the secretion of estrogen, progesterone, and testosterone, or masculinization, particularly in pregnancy,[21,31] which resolved spontaneously once the tumor was removed. Ascites and abnormal uterine bleeding in elderly patients are rare presenting symptoms. All sclerosing stromal tumors have, to date, pursued a benign course. Cytogenetics commonly reveals trisomy 12 in these tumors.[39]

Macroscopic features

They are unilateral (with a solitary exception[14]), solid, distinctly lobulated, firm tumors, averaging 3–5 cm in diameter, that are sharply circumscribed from the adjacent ovarian parenchyma. The cut surface is pale, 'fleshy' and variegated with focal yellowish areas and sometimes patchy cystic degeneration (Figure 26.31). Occasionally, they form a single large cyst. Extensive calcification is seen in rare cases.[98,109] A solitary case is known to have arisen in an accessory ovary.[2]

Microscopic features

They exhibit a characteristic pseudolobular pattern of cellular zones separated by broad swathes of acellular sclerotic or edematous connective tissue (Figures 26.32 and 26.33). Within the cellular nodules, fine strands of this sclerotic stroma also interdigitate randomly between individual cells and small groups of cells (Figure 26.34). Numerous branching vascular spaces of various sizes are present in the cellular areas. The cells are typically rounded to polyhedral with vacuolated (Figure 26.34) or eosinophilic cytoplasm (Figure 26.35), or are spindle-shaped fibroblasts. It is this variety of cell types that is distinctive. Component cells have small, dark, non-grooved nuclei, sometimes with a prominent nucleolus. Mitoses are rare. Individual cells are surrounded by a fine meshwork of reticulin fibers. Isolated spindle cells in the cellular areas are reactive for smooth muscle actin (Figure 26.36),[92,98] but not for estrogen

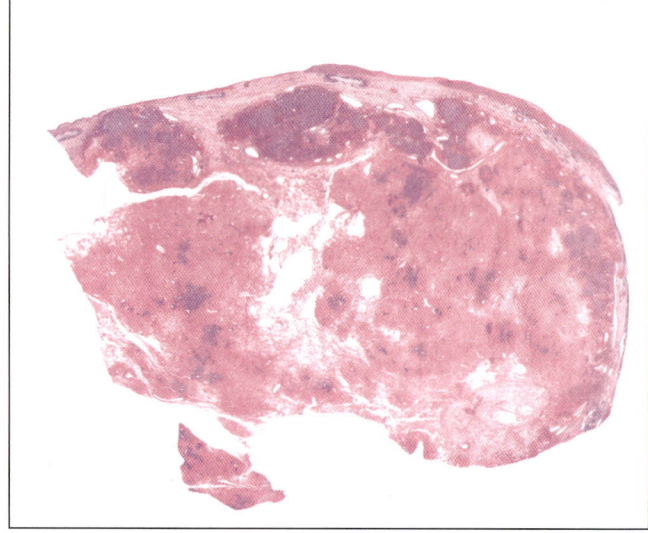

Fig. 26.32 Sclerosing stromal tumor. Survey of tumor in which pseudolobulation is marked with clear division into cellular and fibrous zones.

and progesterone receptors.[36,92] Mast cells may be prominent in the stroma. Occasional vacuolated cells have crescentic nuclei resembling signet-ring cells and, when embedded in dense stroma, may erroneously suggest a diagnosis of Krukenberg tumor. These cells are mucin negative.

The vascular, sclerotic, and edematous stromal changes are constant features of these tumors (Figure 26.37) and relate to the local elaboration of vascular permeability and vascular endothelial growth factors.[36,39] The edema is zonal in contrast to that seen in massive ovarian edema (see Chapter 22) or an edematous fibroma (see Figure 26.41). Dystrophic spiculate stromal calcification is rarely present, but may be extreme.[98,109]

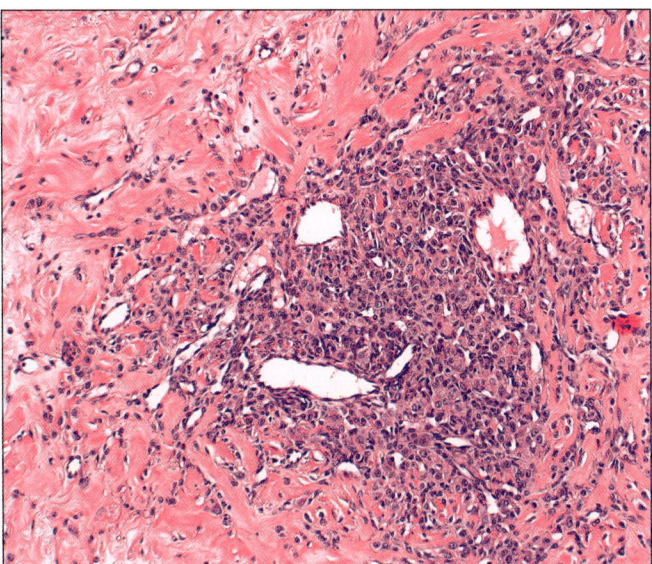

Fig. 26.33 Sclerosing stromal tumor. A key diagnostic feature is the nature of the interface between cellular and stromal zones.

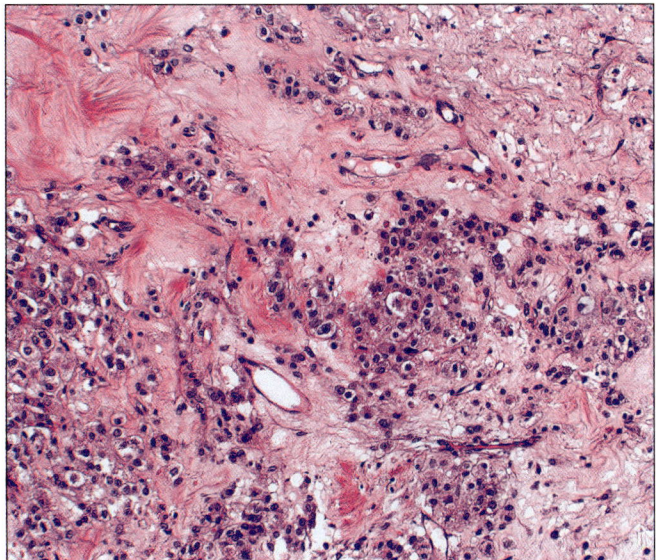

Fig. 26.34 Sclerosing stromal tumor. Periphery of cellular area showing encroachment of hyalinized connective tissue between nests and individual polyhedral lutein-like tumor cells.

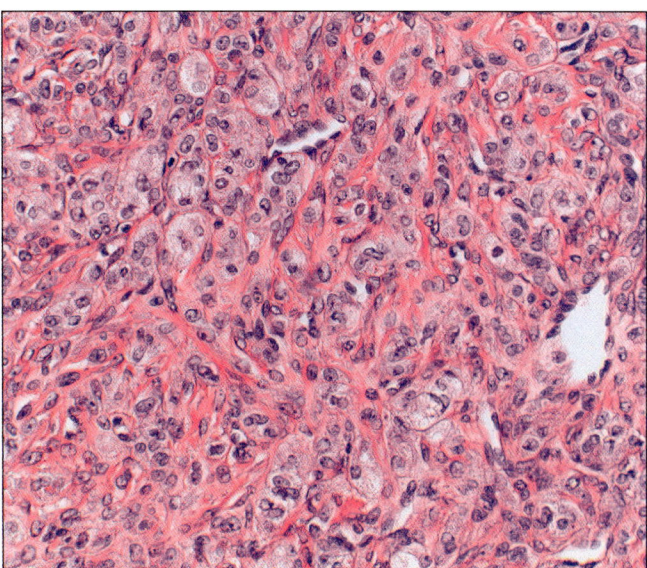

Fig. 26.35 Sclerosing stromal tumor. Cellular area with an admixture of large polyhedral and spindled tumor cells. Polyhedral cells have rather more vesicular nuclei and obvious nucleoli. Compare with area of benign thecoma seen in Figure 26.26A.

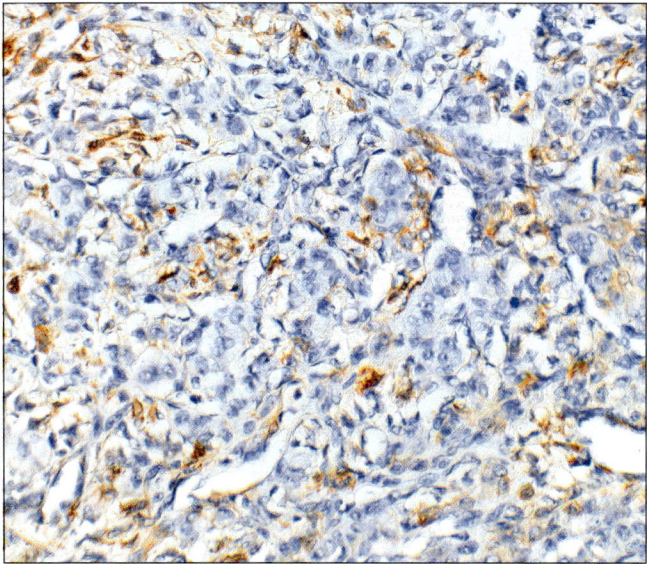

Fig. 26.36 Sclerosing stromal tumor. Cellular area in same case as Figure 26.35 in which spindled cells stain strongly for smooth muscle actin, but not the polyhedral cells.

Differential diagnosis

It is the histologic pattern of stromal sclerosis (particularly the transition from dense acellular hyaline connective tissue, through broad bands of similar stroma to fine tentacles interposed between the theca-like cells in the cellular nodules) that allows differentiation of sclerosing stromal tumors from 'luteinized thecoma' (Table 26.2) and from various other forms of thecofibroma.

Sclerosing stromal tumors are only one of several ovarian neoplasms that may contain signet-ring-like cells. Some such cells are thought to be stromal, while others are apparently of sex cord or even epithelial origin.[10,20] The association of signet-ring-like cells and edematous stroma may raise the possibility of Krukenberg tumor, but the signet-ring cells of Krukenberg tumors contain mucin rather than lipid and are immunoreac-

tive for cytokeratins. Krukenberg tumors also occur typically in women in the sixth and seventh decades, are mostly bilateral, and lack the pseudolobulated pattern of sclerosing stromal tumors on cut surfaces.

FIBROMAS

Clinical profile

Fibromas are, by far, the most commonly encountered subtype of the sex cord-stromal tumors, accounting for almost two-thirds of neoplasms in this group. The mean age of occurrence is 48 years and 90% or more occur in women over the age of 30 years. Ascites is the most frequent general abdominal

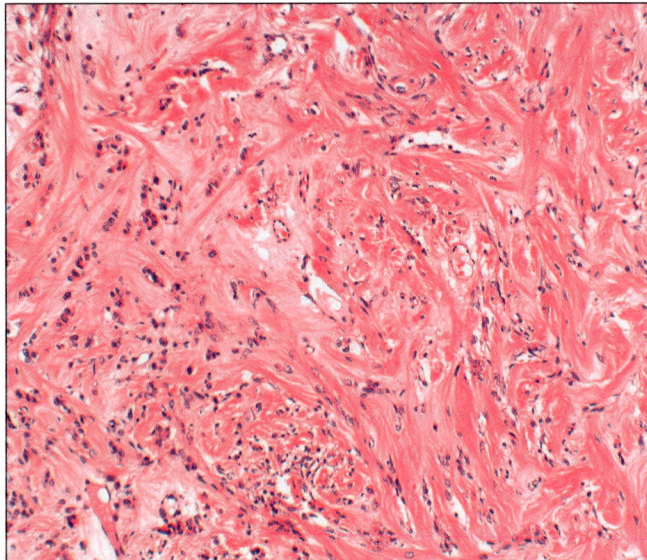

Fig. 26.37 Sclerosing stromal tumor. Margin between cellular and acellular zones, the latter showing profound hyaline change in collagenous connective tissue.

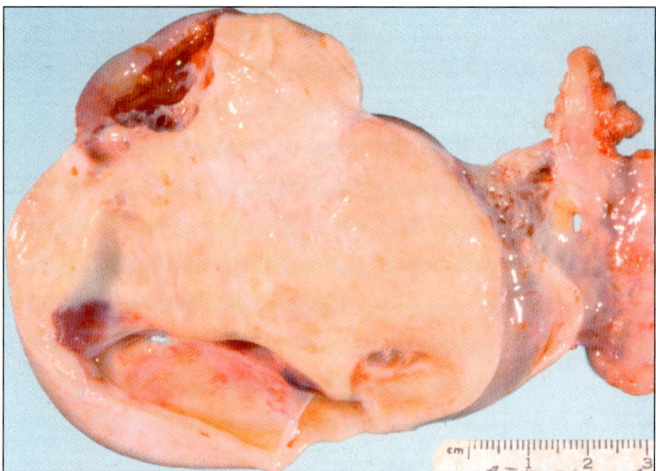

Fig. 26.38 Ovarian fibroma. Gray/white cut surface, featureless apart from areas of cystic degeneration.

Table 26.2 Differential diagnosis: sclerosing stromal tumor versus luteinized thecoma of ovary

Sclerosing stromal tumor	Luteinized thecoma
Clinical diagnosis	
75% aged <30 years (mean 25 years)	90% aged >30 years (mean 48 years)
Mostly hormonally inactive	Typically estrogenic
Histologic diagnosis	
Marked pseudolobulation	Uniform architecture
Prominent sclerosis around clusters and individual cells	No sclerosis
Prominent vasculature	Inapparent vasculature
No perivascular hyaline plaques	Perivascular hyaline plaques
Adjacent ovary normal	Adjacent ovary may be hyperplastic

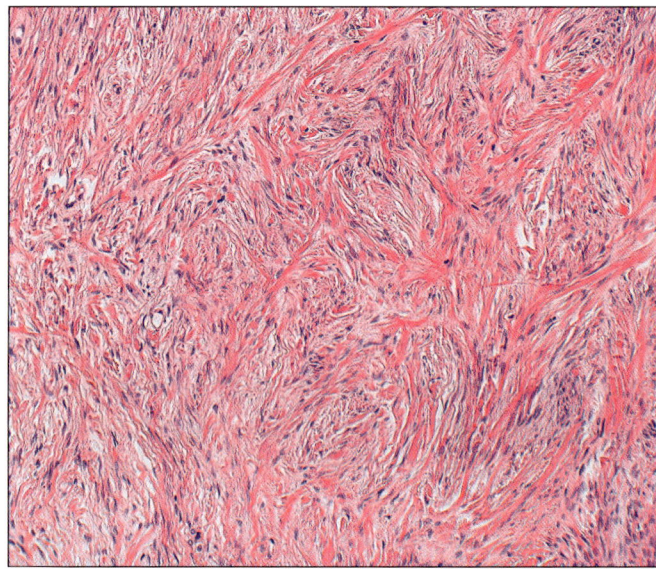

Fig. 26.39 Ovarian fibroma. Typical lesion showing woven bundles of relatively hypocellular collagenous connective tissue.

symptom associated with ovarian fibromas,[88] being present in over 10% of cases. Tumor size is the most important (though not sole) determinant (fibromas over 10 cm in diameter are associated with ascites in 40% of cases). Edematous fibromas are more likely to be associated with ascites than those with sclerotic or cellular stroma. The only clinical condition statistically associated with an increased risk of ovarian fibroma is the hereditary 'basal cell nevus syndrome',[34] although one has been found in a patient with Maffucci syndrome.[15] Trisomy 12 is a constant finding in benign and cellular fibromas, as with many other stromal tumors, while trisomy 8 has been identified in cases of clinically malignant fibrosarcomas.[99]

Macroscopic features
Fibromas are bilateral in about 5% of instances. One-third are 3 cm in diameter or smaller, but they commonly exceed 15 cm. Larger tumors have a smooth or slightly bosselated serosal surface. They are solid and vary from rubbery to 'rock-hard' in consistency. Smaller lesions may appear as polypoid nodules on the ovarian surface or poorly circumscribed nodules within the ovary. The cut surface is white and faintly whorled, often with areas of cystic degeneration (Figure 26.38). In extreme cases, this gives rise to large ragged-walled cysts filled with protein-rich serous fluid. Other degenerative phenomena such as calcification (that may be extreme) are occasionally present, particularly in fibromas occurring as part of the rare basal cell nevus syndrome. The rare cellular fibromas and fibrosarcomas tend to be large and friable, attached to pelvic structures, and to exhibit hemorrhage and necrosis.

Microscopic features
The basic architectural pattern of fibromas comprises variably cellular bundles and intersecting swathes of collagenous fibrous tissue (Figure 26.39), occasionally with a striking storiform pattern resembling ovarian cortex (Figure 26.40). The elongate fibroblastic tumor cells have spindle-shaped nuclei and may

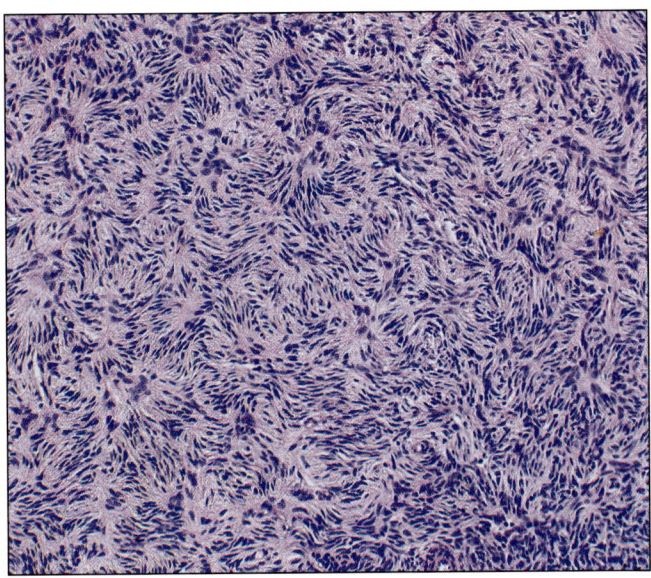

Fig. 26.40 Ovarian fibroma. Tightly whorled 'storiform' pattern of small spindled cells more closely resembling normal ovarian cortical stroma.

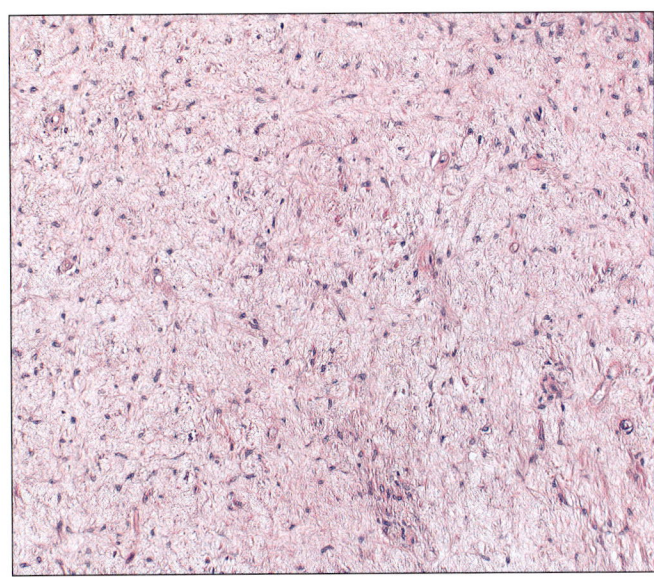

Fig. 26.41 Edematous ovarian fibroma. Relatively acellular collagenous connective tissue dispersed by intercellular edema fluid.

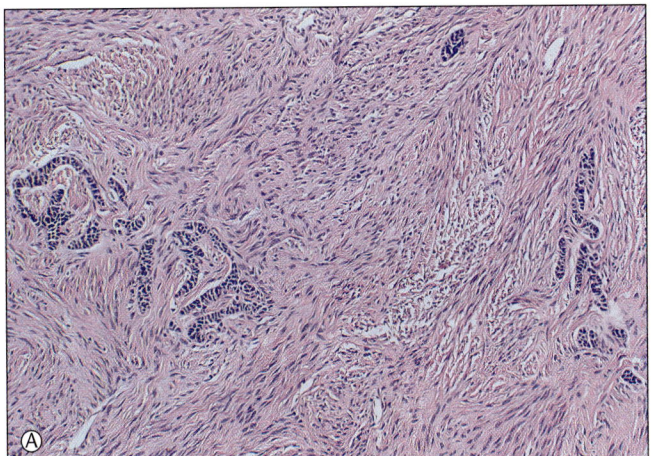

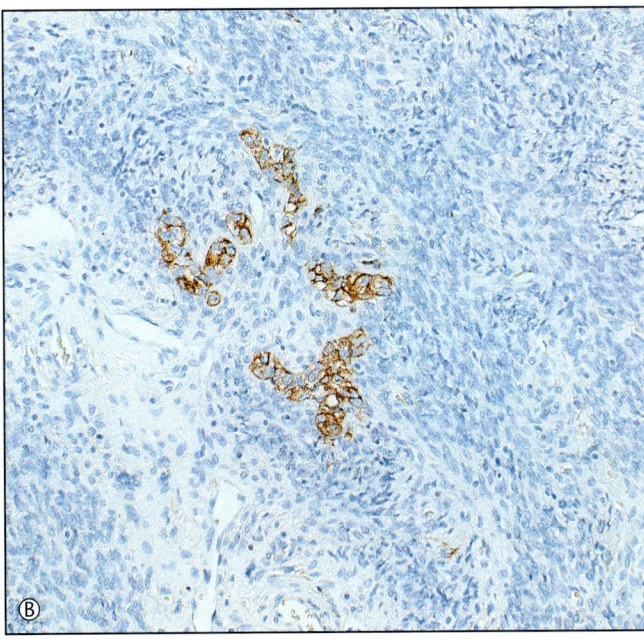

Fig. 26.42 Fibroma with minor sex-cord element. **(A)** Occasional small cords or tubule-like structures of ill-defined sex-cord cells set in an otherwise unremarkable fibroma. Contrast with Figure 26.22. **(B)** Immunostains for cytokeratins are useful to confirm the 'epithelial' nature of poorly defined sex cords.

contain small amounts of lipid in their otherwise inapparent cytoplasm. The immunoprofile of the tumor cells includes reactivity for vimentin and often, but not always, scattered α-inhibin and calretinin reactivity.[11] The collagen usually appears hyaline or somewhat wavy. The cellularity varies inversely with both collagen production and stromal edema, both of which may be quite marked (Figure 26.41). Dystrophic spiculate calcification is occasionally seen as are focal necrosis and hemorrhage. Nuclear atypia and mitoses are rarely encountered in the average case except in the presence of partial torsion and low-grade ischemia. The uninvolved portion of the ovary and/or the contralateral ovary sometimes shows nodular or diffuse stromal hyperplasia.

Rare, otherwise typical, fibromas contain sparse, poorly formed tubular structures composed of Sertoli-like cells or nests of cells resembling granulosa cells. These have been called fibromas with minor sex-cord elements as, by definition, the sex-cord elements must amount to less than 10% of the tumor in the tissue reviewed (Figure 26.42). Fibromas that exhibit aggregates of lipid-laden lutein-like cells are termed 'luteinized thecomas' (see above).

Occasional fibromatous tumors are hypercellular and/or show appreciable mitotic activity. Based on follow-up studies, cellular fibromas (Figure 26.43) displaying bland nuclei can be expected to behave in a benign fashion, although they may

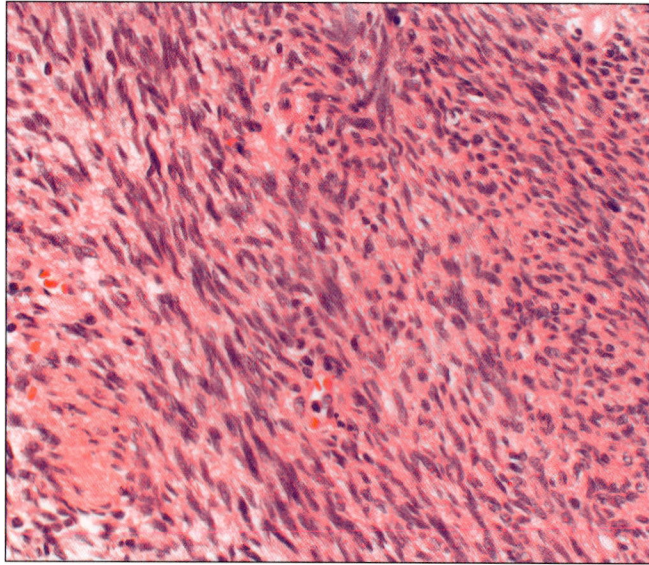

Fig. 26.43 Benign cellular fibroma. Woven bundles and fascicles of ill-defined spindle cells separated by wavy collagen. Cells have thin, elongate, tapered nuclei and few, or patchy, mitoses.

Table 26.3 Differential diagnosis: edematous ovarian fibroma versus massive edema of ovary

Edematous fibroma	Massive edema
Clinical diagnosis	
90% aged >30 years (mean 48 years)	Almost all aged <30 years (mean 20 years)
Abdominal mass and ascites	Abdominal pain
Hormonally inactive	Often masculinizing (clinical background of polycystic ovary syndrome frequently present)
Histologic diagnosis	
Displaces ovarian structures	Incorporates ovarian structures
Circumscribed/nodular lesion	Involves ovary uniformly
No luteinized cells	Luteinized stromal cells
Adjacent ovary may be hyperplastic	

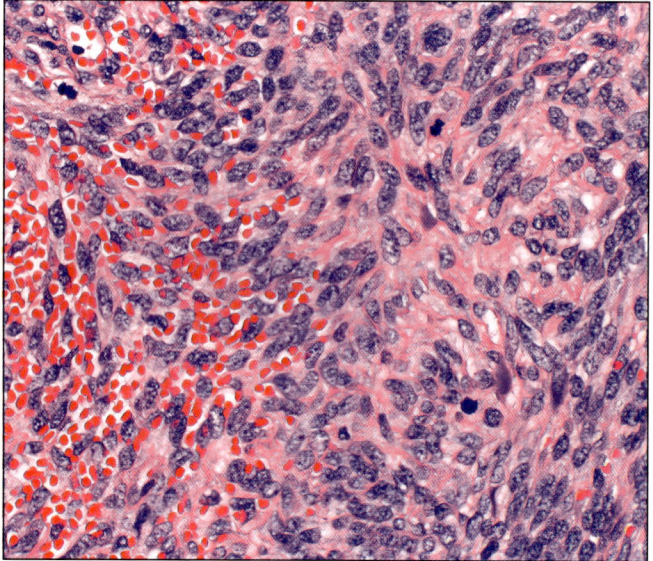

Fig. 26.44 Ovarian fibrosarcoma. Marked hypercellularity, nuclear hyperchromatism, and obvious mitotic activity are characteristic of this lesion.

occasionally recur locally. It has been suggested that those with a mitotic count >4 per 10 HPFs, yet bland nuclear features, be designated as 'mitotically active cellular fibromas'.[35] Fibrosarcomas have a mitotic rate of ≥4 per 10 HPFs over a minimum of 40 HPFs counted and, in our experience, all display diffuse nuclear hyperchromasia (Figure 26.44) and regularly pursue a frankly malignant course. An alternative approach to highly cellular, mitotically active, spindle cell tumors of the ovary is to consider them as *ovarian stromal sarcomas* (Figure 26.45), supported with an appropriate immunoprofile of α-inhibin and/or calretinin reactivity.

Differential diagnosis

A sometimes difficult histologic distinction is between an edematous ovarian fibroma and massive ovarian edema (Table 26.3).

Discrimination of fibrosarcomas from poorly differentiated sex cord-stromal tumors, particularly Sertoli–Leydig cell tumors, is on the basis of total absence of even poorly formed epithelial-like structures or identifiable intracytoplasmic lipid. It is arguable whether or not the presence of scattered α-inhibin and calretinin immunostaining is a valid basis for separation.

ANDROBLASTOMAS (SERTOLI–LEYDIG CELL TUMORS)

Definition and cell types

Androblastomas are extremely uncommon neoplasms, accounting for only about 1% of all sex cord-stromal tumors (0.1–0.5% of all primary ovarian neoplasms) and exhibiting Sertoli cells resembling those of the developing or adult testis, Leydig cells and/or fibroblastic cells in differing relative proportions and at various levels of differentiation. Synonyms include Sertoli–Leydig cell tumor and the quaintly archaic arrhenoblastoma. Detailed studies have not conclusively established the origin of the Sertoli cells in these ovarian neoplasms, although their 'pseudo-male' differentiation is not due to any perturbation at a molecular level of the sex-determining region Y (*SRY*) gene or the X chromosome activation state.[38] Definitive evidence shows that the Leydig cell component is an integral part of the neoplastic process in these tumors (unlike the theca cells in granulosa cell tumors – see above). This takes the form of Leydig cells being found in the metastatic deposits (Figure 26.46) and is the justification for discussing Leydig cell tumors in this section, separately from other 'steroid cell' tumors with which they share many common features, particularly as classification is based principally on the finding of Reinke crystalloids – ephemeral structures at best, and even seen in typical testicular Leydig cell tumors in only 40% of cases. In the ovaries, Sertoli–Leydig cell tumors outnumber both pure Sertoli cell tumors and pure Leydig cell tumors, the reverse of their relative frequencies in the testes.[107]

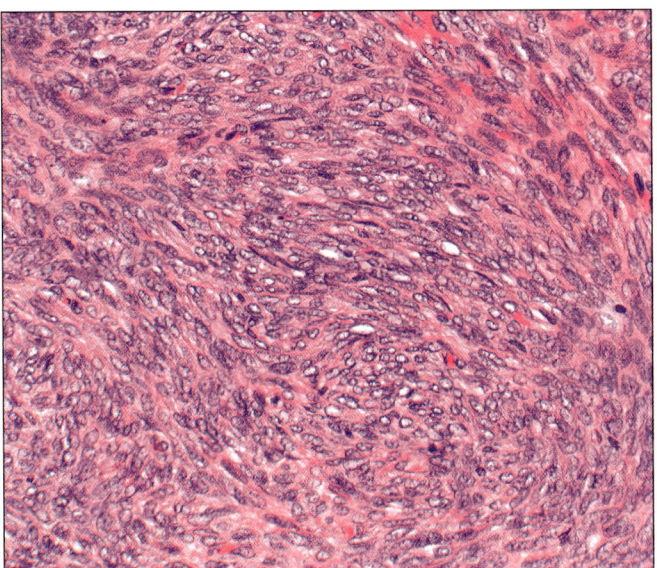

Fig. 26.45 'Ovarian stromal sarcoma'. An alternative concept for the high-grade malignant end of the 'fibroma' spectrum. Tumor cells have elongate but blunt-ended or oval nuclei and an ill-defined storiform architectural pattern.

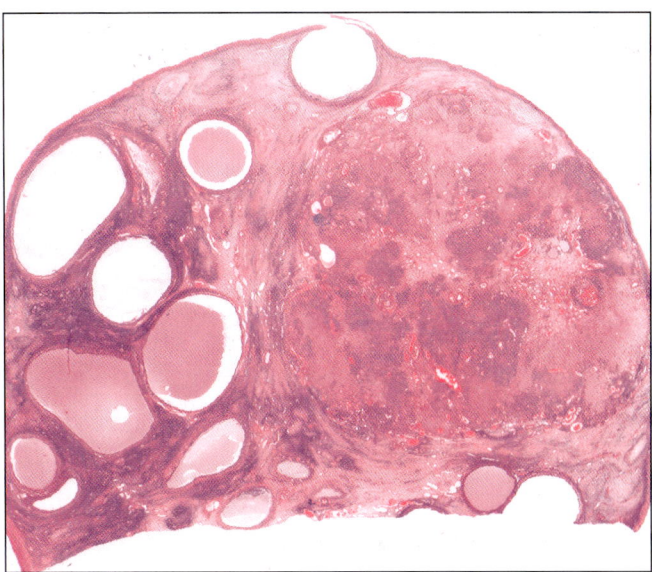

Fig. 26.47 Small, poorly differentiated Sertoli–Leydig cell tumor. Tumor found incidentally in the left ovary of a patient undergoing hysterectomy.

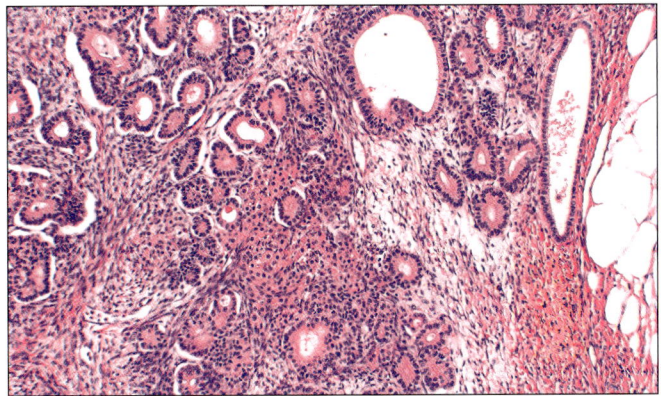

Fig. 26.46 Metastatic deposit of well-differentiated Sertoli–Leydig cell tumor in omentum. Note omental fat at bottom and central aggregates of typical Leydig cells.

Clinical profile

As a group, androblastomas occur predominantly in the second and third decades (mean age about 25 years), rarely before puberty and fewer than 10% after the menopause.[9] They are bilateral in less than 2% and confined to the ovaries in over 95% of cases. Individual subtypes deviate little from this general pattern. Pure Sertoli cell tumors and, to a lesser extent, pure Leydig cell tumors have bimodal age distributions with incidence peaks in the third and seventh decades. In 40–50% of patients, the presenting symptoms relate to clinical signs of androgenic activity while most of the remainder are non-specific abdominal symptoms referable to the physical presence of a tumor mass. Endocrinologically, Sertoli–Leydig cell tumors produce a mixture of C-19 steroids (mostly dehydro-epiandrosterone and androstenedione, with small amounts of testosterone)[80] while pure Leydig cell tumors tend to produce only the far more potent testosterone[18] and thus will present clinically when much smaller in size. Occasionally, they are incidental findings at hysterectomy for unrelated pathology (Figure 26.47).

Pure well-differentiated Sertoli cell tumors are mostly estrogenic and, in prepubertal girls, they may even be associated with isosexual precocious pseudopuberty or Peutz–Jeghers syndrome. Well-differentiated Sertoli–Leydig cell tumors are often endocrinologically inactive but may be androgenic or sometimes feminizing. By contrast, while pure Leydig cell tumors and poorly differentiated Sertoli–Leydig cell tumors may also be feminizing, at least half are clinically androgenic. Virilizing signs may persist after removal of the tumor, but not the symptoms. Estrogenic manifestations may be explained either by direct estrogen production by the tumor or, more probably, by peripheral conversion of androgenic secretions from the tumor to estrogens.

Sertoli–Leydig cell tumors may be associated with raised serum levels of α-fetoprotein, but rarely to the levels seen with yolk sac tumors. Immunohistochemical studies indicate that the origin of this oncoprotein is in the Leydig cells,[22] the Sertoli cells, and/or heterologous hepatocytes.[46] Androblastomas presenting during pregnancy less often exhibit androgenic manifestations than equivalent tumors occurring in non-pregnant women, presumably as the placenta can aromatize androgens into estrogens.

WELL-DIFFERENTIATED SERTOLI CELL TUMORS

Clinical profile

Well-differentiated ovarian Sertoli cell tumors ('tubular androblastomas') are histologically indistinguishable from their more commonly encountered homologues within the testis. Indeed, in patients who are genetic males but phenotypic females (intersex) with the testicular feminization syndrome, the 'tumor' that most commonly develops is the Sertoli cell adenoma. They are mostly estrogenic, regardless of the presence or absence of intracellular lipid storage. They are associated unduly frequently with anomalies of the internal genitalia. Many of these Sertoli cell tumors, but certainly not all, are probably hamartomas rather than true benign neoplasms.

Macroscopic features

Sertoli cell tumors vary markedly in size, but most are smaller than 10 cm in diameter. They tend to be solid, firm, encapsulated and lobulated masses, typically yellow or tan in color. Small cystic areas are infrequently present. They are unilateral in normal women and more often bilateral in phenotypic females with testicular feminization.

Microscopic features

Well-differentiated Sertoli cell tumors are composed of lobules of uniform, tortuous, solid or hollow tubules, filled with or lined by one or more layers of cuboidal to columnar benign-appearing cells with eosinophilic or vacuolated cytoplasm and dark, oval, basal nuclei (Figure 26.48A). The immunoprofile of these cells includes focal reactivity for CD99[28], antimüllerian hormone,[51,73] α-inhibin, calretinin, low molecular weight cytokeratins, and a lack of reactivity for EMA. Mitoses are rare and nucleoli are not prominent. The Sertoli cells, in some tumors, have well-defined cell borders and apical surfaces. More frequently, the apical margins of the cells are indistinct and the lateral cell boundaries poorly defined. The Sertoli cells usually contain lipid droplets but, in some tumors, they are grossly vacuolated (Figure 26.48B) and distended by fat, giving rise to the so-called 'Sertoli cell tumor with lipid storage' or 'lipid-rich Sertoli cell tumor'. The tubules in this tumor generally are solid and in larger discrete masses. Nodules of the polyhedral vacuolated cells are also noted. Luminal mucin (stained by mucicarmine) is occasionally present. Occasional Sertoli cell tumors may have abundant eosinophilic cytoplasm.[24]

Intervening stroma is usually represented by a few bands of acellular connective tissue that are either edematous or hyalinized and, by definition, contain few or no Leydig cells. Less commonly, the hyalinized stroma is more prominent, and rarely, the stroma is the dominant component with the tumors then resembling ovarian fibromas with only a minor tubular element. Such lesions have been reclassified as 'fibromas with minor sex-cord elements'. Pure Sertoli cell tumors with marked nuclear atypia and mitotic activity have been reported as Sertoli cell carcinomas (see below).

WELL-DIFFERENTIATED SERTOLI–LEYDIG CELL TUMORS

Clinical profile

These very uncommon benign tumors, occurring in women with a mean age in the mid thirties, differ from the well-differentiated Sertoli cell tumors described above only in the presence of an obvious Leydig cell component. They account for 10% of all Sertoli–Leydig cell tumors. As with pure Sertoli cell tumors, there is a statistical association with either congenital anomalies of the internal genitalia in otherwise normal women or with the testicular feminization syndrome.

Macroscopic features

Well-differentiated Sertoli–Leydig cell tumors are almost always unilateral and appear as well circumscribed, solitary, firm tumor masses in the ovary. They range in size up to 20 cm in diameter, measuring, on average, 5–6 cm across. The hilar location may still be apparent in the occasional small lesion. The cut surface is yellow and characteristically lobulated (Figure 26.49). Small cysts may be present and there is often focal hemorrhage. Rare cases may be extensively calcified or even ossified.[61]

Microscopic features

Histologically, tumors consist of uniform solid or hollow tubular structures lined by Sertoli-type cells (Figures 26.50 and 26.51) and show the features outlined in the previous section. Tubules may contain eosinophilic secretion but are more frequently empty. The intervening stroma contains variable numbers of Leydig cells. These tend to be packed in ribbons or

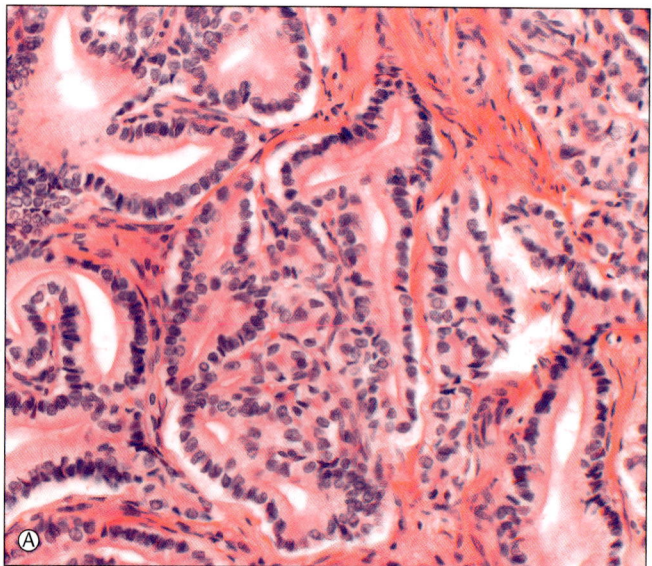
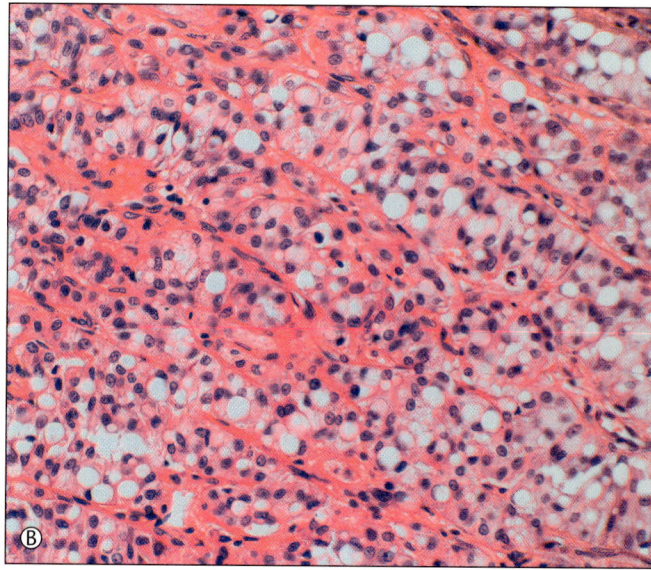

Fig. 26.48 Well-differentiated Sertoli cell tumor (tubular androblastoma). **(A)** With characteristic hollow tubules lined by tall columnar cells with basal nuclei and clear or vacuolated cytoplasm. **(B)** With lipid storage in the tumor cells, obscuring to some extent the tubular architecture.

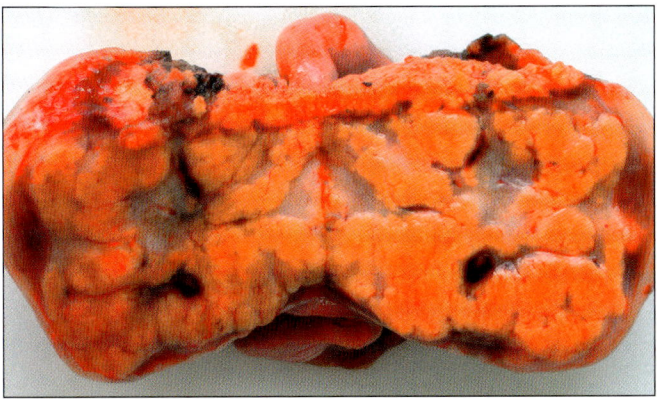

Fig. 26.49 Well-differentiated Sertoli–Leydig cell tumor. The cut surface is typically yellow, firm and lobulated.

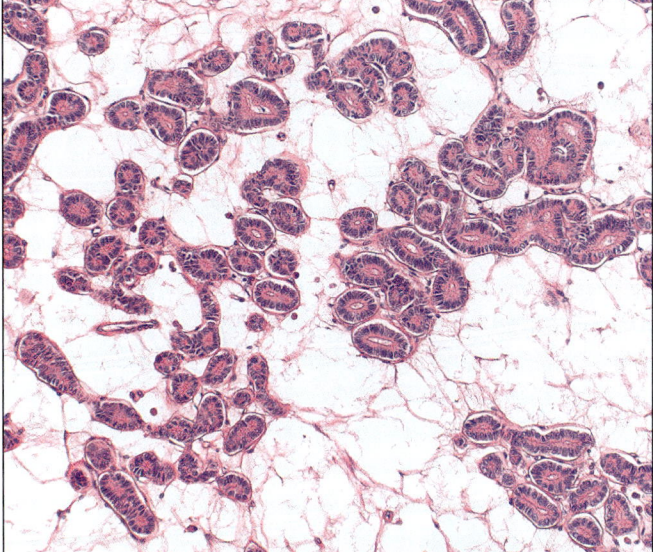

Fig. 26.50 Well-differentiated Sertoli–Leydig cell tumor. Edematous areas with widely separated Sertoli cell tubules. Leydig cells were present only at the periphery of such areas.

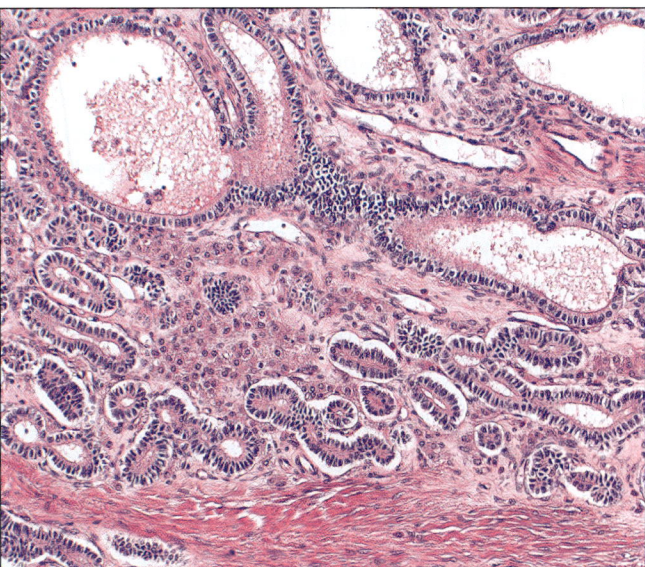

Fig. 26.51 Well-differentiated Sertoli–Leydig cell tumor. Tubular and cystic spaces lined by Sertoli cells, separated by sheets of uniform eosinophilic Leydig cells with regular rounded nuclei.

nests between the Sertoli cell tubules but may form more solid sheets in some tumors (Figure 26.51). The cytologic details of these cells are given below (pure Leydig cell tumors). Mitoses are rare in these tumors.

An interesting histologic feature of some tumors in this group is the coarse architectural arrangement into cellular and acellular areas, reminiscent of the nodular or pseudolobular pattern of sclerosing stromal tumors (Figure 26.52). The acellular areas have the same dense hyaline and collagenous tissue background, also with prominent dilated sinusoidal vessels.

A further unusual variant is the large unilocular fibrous-walled cyst, in which are scattered tubules and cystic spaces lined by typical Sertoli cells as well as clusters of Leydig-like cells.

LEYDIG (HILUS) CELL TUMORS

Leydig cell neoplasms of the ovary are formed exclusively of large eosinophilic cells similar to those usually present in the ovarian hilus. They are most uncommon. They are thought to

derive directly from hilus cells, or as a one-sided development of a Sertoli–Leydig cell tumor, or rarely from the ovarian stromal cells. For all practical purposes they are benign (see the discussion on steroid cell tumors below), although rare cases of metastasizing Leydig cell tumor are known. Most are masculinizing,[72] but about 10–20% have some estrogenic effect, most readily recognized in the endometrium (hyperplasia or carcinoma). The very rare 'stromal Leydig cell tumors' are either estrogenic or androgenic in approximately equal numbers.[94]

Macroscopic features
Leydig cell tumors are unilateral (only a handful of bilateral hilus cell or stromal Leydig cell tumors have been described) and vary in size. Most exceed 5 cm in diameter, but rarely are sufficiently large to produce symptoms relating to their mass alone. They usually occupy the hilar region of the ovary (Figure 26.53A) and adjacent mesovarium. They are well-circumscribed, soft, fleshy, yellow-to-brown nodules in which focal hemorrhage is common (Figure 26.53B).

Microscopic features
Leydig cell tumors are composed of closely packed sheets (Figure 26.54A), nests (Figure 26.54B) or solid cords of uniform, polyhedral, eosinophilic cells measuring about 20 μm across. Nuclei are round, central, and vary somewhat in size. They have relatively sparse chromatin and one or more intensely basophilic nucleoli. Cytoplasmic pseudoinclusions may be noted. They frequently give an appearance of being unevenly distributed in the tumor with 'nuclear-rich' and 'nuclear-poor' zones a feature we regard as almost pathognomonic of Leydig cell differentiation, even in the absence of Reinke crystalloids. Mitoses are rare. Leydig cell cytoplasm is densely eosinophilic and finely granular with small sudanophilic lipid-containing cytoplasmic vacuoles. PAS-positive yellow-brown lipochrome pigment is seen in many cells. The immunoprofile of these cells includes consistently strong reactivity for calretinin,[49] α-

inhibin,[111] relaxin-like factor[3] and vimentin, but not cytokeratins and EMA.

Reinke crystalloids are slender birefringent rods with square or tapered ends, within an incomplete 'halo', and best seen when stained bright red with Mallory trichrome stain. They are found in just over 50% of these tumors, but are irregularly

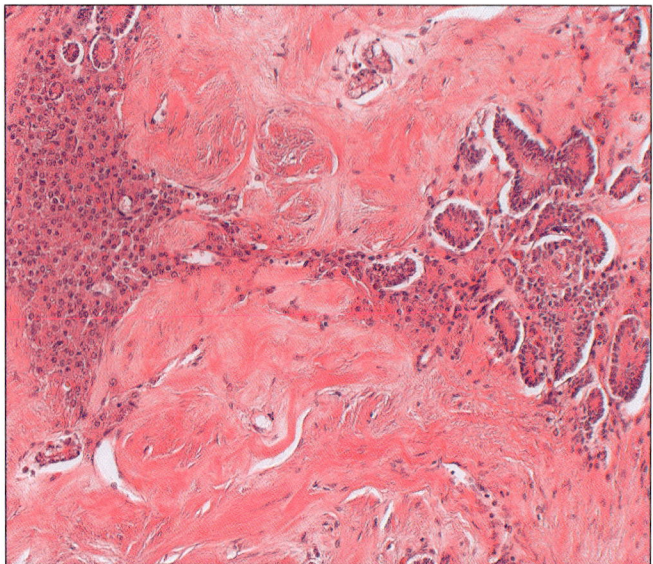

Fig. 26.52 Well-differentiated Sertoli–Leydig cell tumor. This field shows an interface between acellular sclerotic zones with dilated vascular spaces and more cellular zones. Aggregates of Leydig cells are seen at left and Sertoli cell tubules at right.

distributed in the tumor and thus may require extensive searching to locate. While generally regarded as pathognomonic of Leydig cell differentiation, Reinke crystalloids may rarely be found in tumors of adrenal origin.[77] Variably sized rounded colloid bodies may be seen in some cells, thought to be precursors of Reinke crystalloids.

At the tumor margins, the Leydig cells sometimes become more spindle shaped (Figure 26.55), tending to merge with the adjacent stromal cells. Reticulin stains show a fine meshwork of fibrils and accentuate the marked vascularity that, in an H&E stained section, often imparts an 'organoid' appearance. Collagen is rarely conspicuous (Figure 26.56). The walls of moderately sized vessels show fibrinoid change in about 40% of tumors. The adjacent compressed ovarian tissue shows stromal hyperplasia, focal luteinization or occasional hilus cell hyperplasia. Rare cases have minor sex-cord elements.

Differential diagnosis

Differentiation between Leydig cell tumors and Leydig cell hyperplasias may, on occasions, be difficult. Many Leydig cell tumors display a conspicuous admixture of large vacuolated cells similar to those in the adrenal cortex. A diagnosis of mixed Leydig cell/adrenal cell tumor suggests itself in some of these tumors, but has little to commend other than the morphologic variability of the component cells. However, there is definite histologic and histogenetic justification to support the rare 'stromal Leydig cell tumors' as discrete and valid variants.[94] In these tumors, nondescript ovarian stromal cells comprise the bulk, with focal single or clustered Leydig-like cells. These cells contain Reinke crystalloids by definition, their presence being the only distinguishing feature between stromal Leydig cell

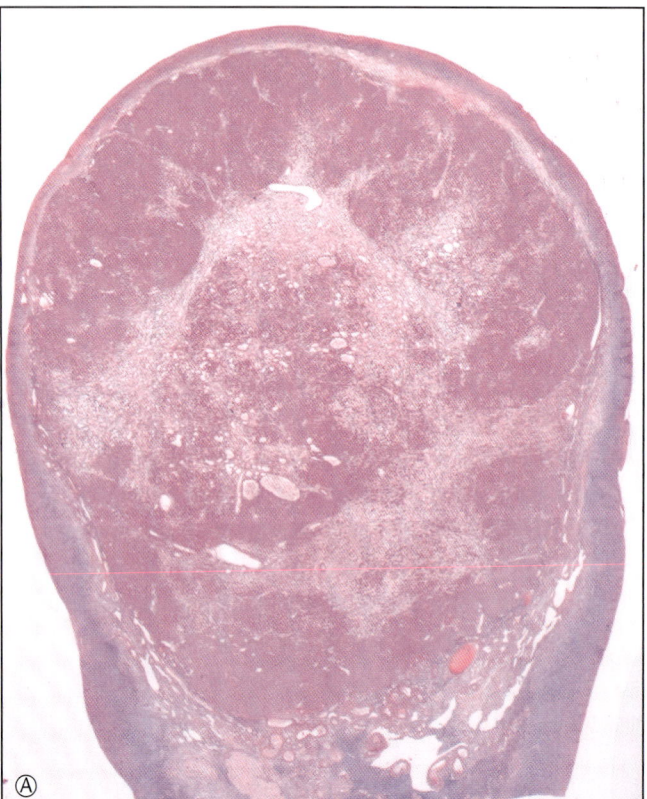

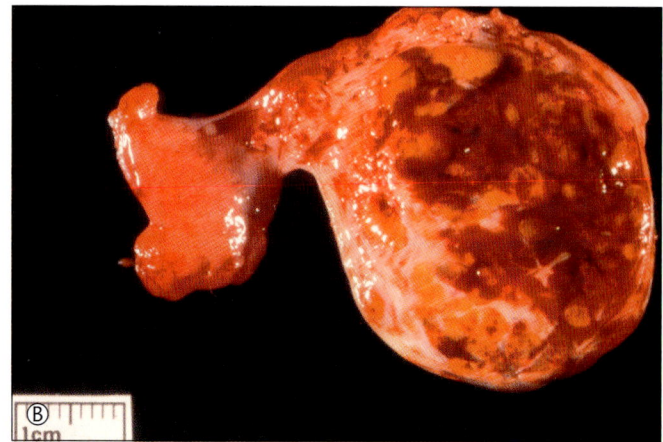

Fig. 26.53 Leydig (hilus) cell tumor. **(A)** Whole section demonstrating the clearly defined margins and the hilar position. **(B)** Small Leydig (hilus) cell tumor, the cut surface of which demonstrated nodules of orange-brown tissue separated by hemorrhage.

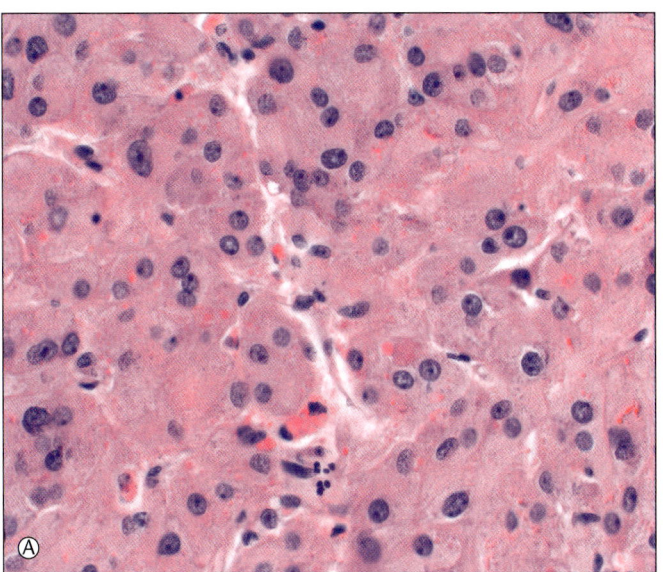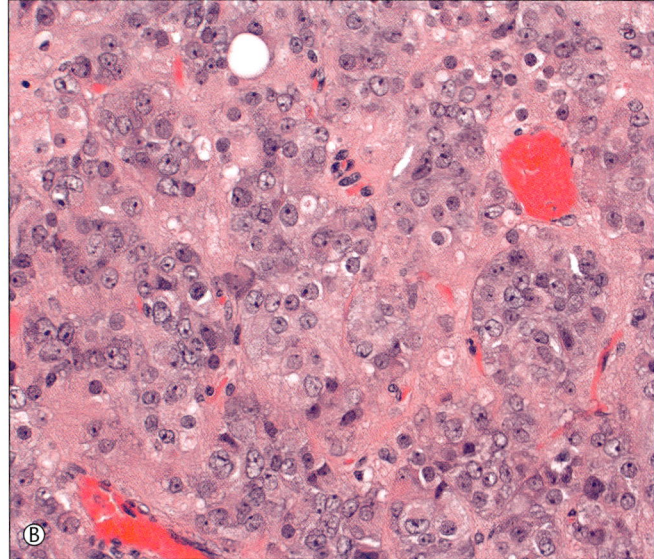

Fig. 26.54 Leydig cell tumor. **(A)** Irregularity of distribution of nuclei is due to cellular orientation to the fine network of capillary vessels. Nuclei are round with one or more prominent nucleoli. **(B)** Nested Leydig cells.

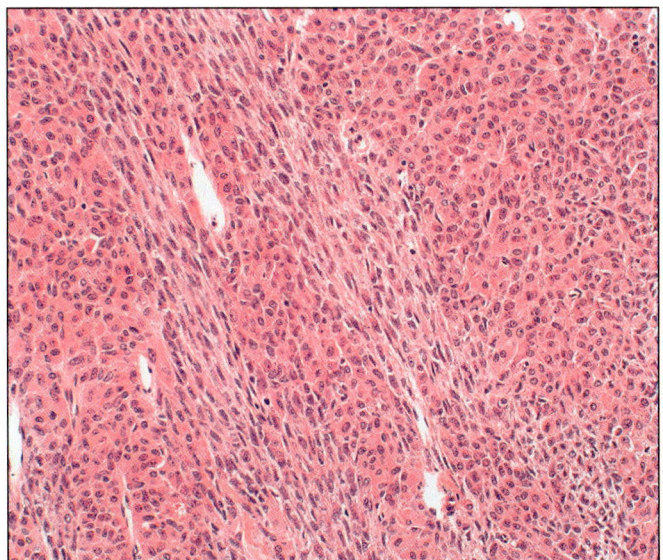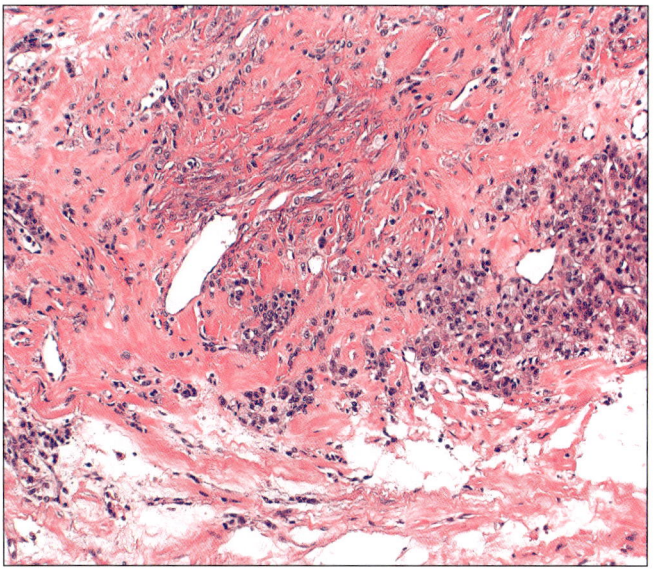

Fig. 26.55 Leydig cell tumor. Alternating zones of spindle-shaped and polyhedral cells.

Fig. 26.56 Leydig cell tumor with pronounced stromal hyalinization, resembling sclerosing stromal tumor (compare with Figure 26.34).

tumors and the much less rare luteinized thecomas (see above). This single criterion may not be absolute in confirming or excluding a diagnosis of Leydig (hilus) cell tumor, and such an argument is germane to this pair of non-hilar tumors as well.

MODERATELY AND POORLY DIFFERENTIATED SERTOLI–LEYDIG CELL TUMORS

Together, these form the most common subtype of androblastomas, and account for two-thirds of all ovarian Sertoli–Leydig cell tumors. Moderately and poorly differentiated Sertoli–Leydig cell tumors are part of a histologic continuum, and frequently particular tumors will show poor differentiation in

one area and moderate differentiation in another. The Sertoli and Leydig cells may vary independently in their degree of maturity or differentiation.

Macroscopic features

These tumors are bilateral in less than 2% of cases. The mean diameter is 15 cm. They are usually well circumscribed and have bosselated outer surfaces. The cut surfaces are typically partly solid and partly cystic. Smooth-walled cysts, in general, are more frequently present in larger neoplasms and those with a 'retiform' pattern (see below). Cysts most often contain clear yellow fluid and, unlike granulosa cell tumors, only occasionally contain altered blood clot. Polypoid masses may project into the cystic spaces. Solid portions of the tumor are lobulated, firm or fleshy in consistency (Figure 26.57) and usually

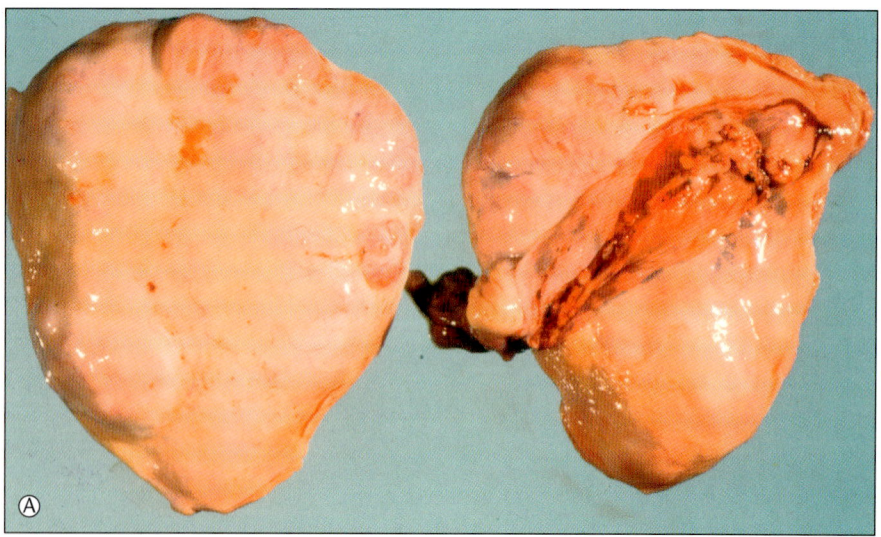

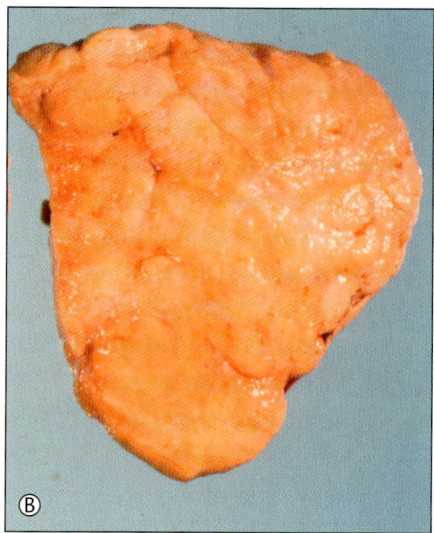

Fig. 26.57 Solid, poorly differentiated Sertoli–Leydig cell tumor, 15 cm in diameter. The external surface **(A)** is slightly bosselated; the cut surface **(B)** is lobulated and fleshy in appearance.

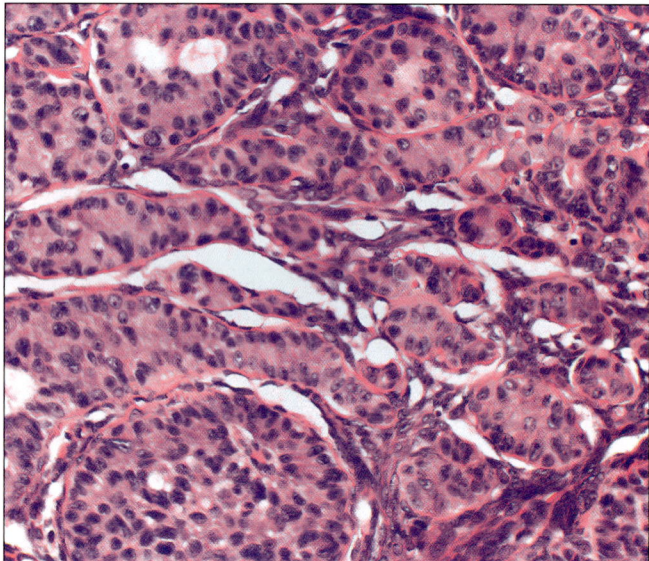

Fig. 26.58 Moderately differentiated Sertoli–Leydig cell tumor. Tubules are predominantly solid and occasionally complex.

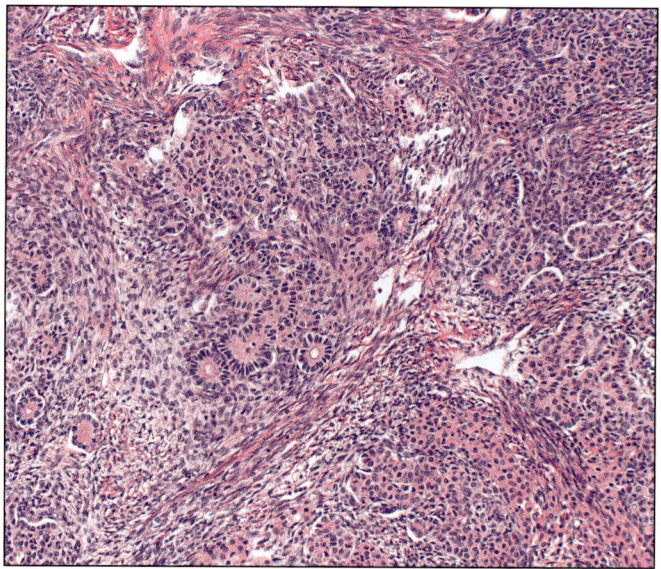

Fig. 26.59 Moderately differentiated Sertoli–Leydig cell tumor. Some Sertoli cell tubules have lumens; some are solid. Leydig cells are obvious in the stromal background.

yellow-gray in color. Necrosis and hemorrhage are frequently prominent.

Microscopic features

Moderately differentiated Sertoli–Leydig cell tumors exhibit cellular nodules or 'lobules' of readily apparent epithelial cells separated by zones of loose fibrous or fibromyxoid mesenchymal stroma. Immature Sertoli-type cells, with small oval or angular nuclei and either scanty, or rather more obvious pale cytoplasm, are arranged in short, thin cords (resembling the sex cords of the immature testes and having double rows of cells with nuclei arranged antipodally – Figure 26.58), true hollow tubules (Figure 26.59) or poorly circumscribed cell nests and sheets. Such cells form the major components of the

cellular lobules while tubules or cords extend irregularly into the surrounding fibrous or fibromyxoid zones. Nuclei are relatively bland and mitoses infrequent (average 5 per 10 HPFs). Rarely, thin-walled cysts lined by flattened Sertoli cells (Figure 26.60) create a sieve-like pattern. The indifferent fibrous mesenchyme is relatively abundant and consists of closely packed spindle-shaped cells (Figure 26.61) associated with a very variable amount of collagen that may be hyalinized. Mature Leydig cells are usually apparent in this stroma, particularly around the perimeter of the tumor or at the margins of cellular nodules, as sheets, clusters or single cells, and less commonly within the cellular zones. In some instances the stromal (Leydig cell) component may also appear densely cellular. Sertoli and/or Leydig cell elements may contain varying

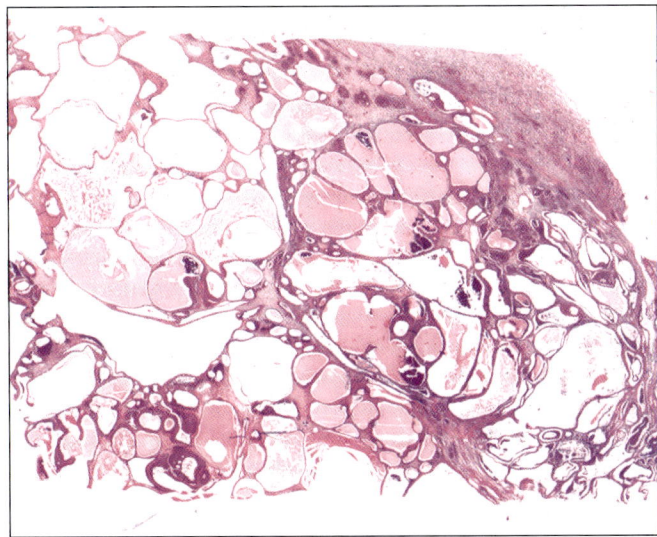

Fig. 26.60 Moderately differentiated Sertoli–Leydig cell tumor. Survey showing a sieve-like pattern of thin-walled cysts lined by Sertoli cells.

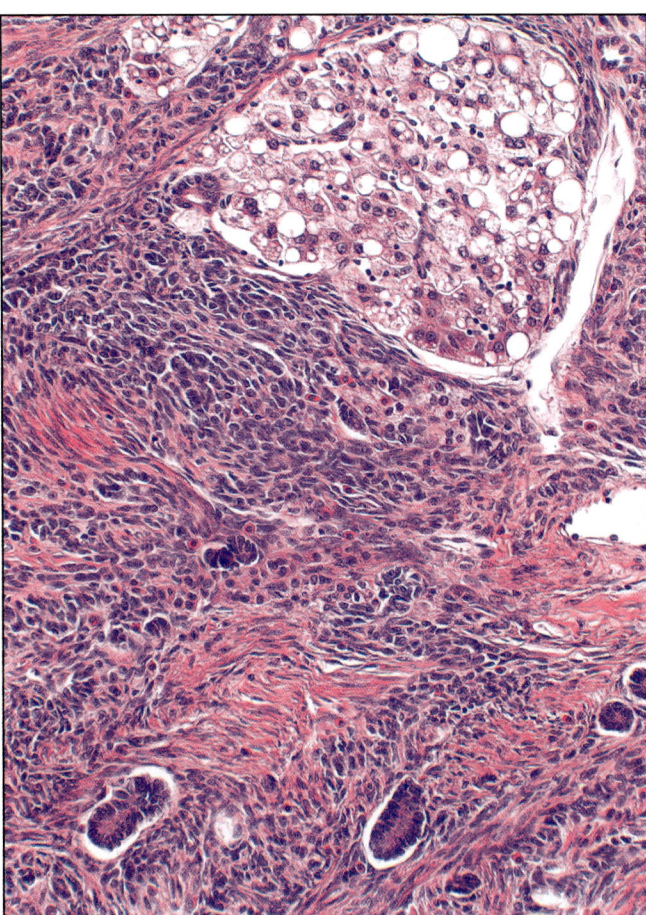

Fig. 26.61 Moderately differentiated Sertoli–Leydig cell tumor. Tumor composed predominantly of indifferent mesenchyme with occasional solid Sertoli cell tubules and nests of lipid-laden Leydig cells (upper right).

amounts of lipid in the form of cytoplasmic vacuolation (Figure 26.61) and, on rare occasions, show foci of bizarre nuclei as an isolated phenomenon.

Poorly differentiated Sertoli–Leydig cell tumors consist largely of sheets of spindle-shaped cells in which there may be occasional thin cord-like structures or trabeculae (Figure 26.62). These sarcoma-like areas (Figure 26.63) may contain numerous mitoses (nearly always exceeding 1 per HPF). Cribriform, trabecular (Figure 26.64) and 'moiré-silk' areas simulating granulosa cell tumors may rarely be seen, and thought must be given to applying rigid criteria before diagnosing gynandroblastoma (see below). Focal variations in otherwise typical tumors may lead to 'organoid' or solid trabecular patterns (Figure 26.65). Leydig cells may also be seen, but these are usually infrequent and require extensive searching to locate. As in moderately differentiated Sertoli–Leydig cell tumors, they are most readily found in loose mesenchyme adjacent to cellular nodules, and may have eosinophilic or foamy amphophilic cytoplasm (Figure 26.66). The very rare pure Sertoli cell carcinoma[67,103] with hollow or solid tubular architecture (Figure 26.67) also belongs in the poorly differentiated group.

RETIFORM VARIANTS OF SERTOLI–LEYDIG CELL TUMOR

Fourteen per cent of moderately and 30% of poorly differentiated ovarian Sertoli–Leydig cell tumors exhibit 'retiform' foci, so-called because of a resemblance to the rete testis. Tumors with this pattern occur at a slightly younger age (mean age, 17 years) than those without and are also less likely to produce clinical signs of virilization.[107] The retiform pattern, represented by minor foci (Figure 26.68) or large fields (Figure 26.69), shows an irregular network of slit-like spaces and cysts, often containing papillae of various shapes. The cystic and compressed tubular spaces and the papillae are lined by flattened or cuboidal cells with the same general cytologic features as the immature Sertoli cells described above. Papillae may be short and rounded with hyalinized cores, large and bulbous with edematous cores,

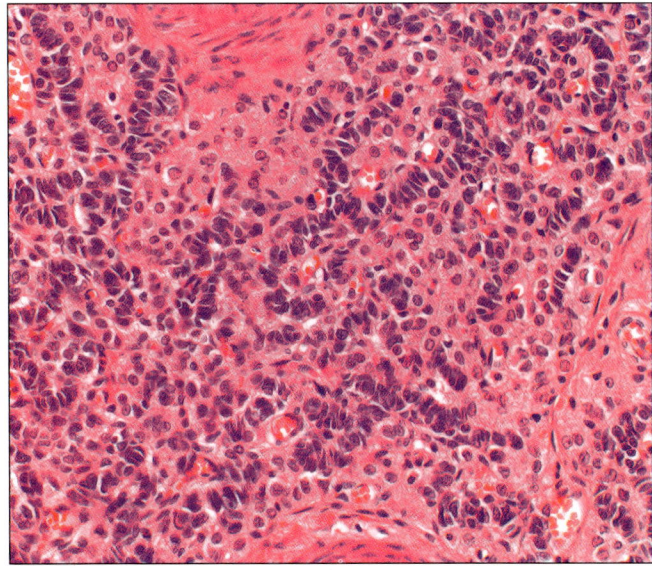

Fig. 26.62 Poorly differentiated Sertoli–Leydig cell tumor. An area showing primitive solid cords and trabeculae of cells with oval nuclei, scanty cytoplasm, and mitoses. Leydig cells are dispersed between the sex-cord elements (same case as Figure 26.47).

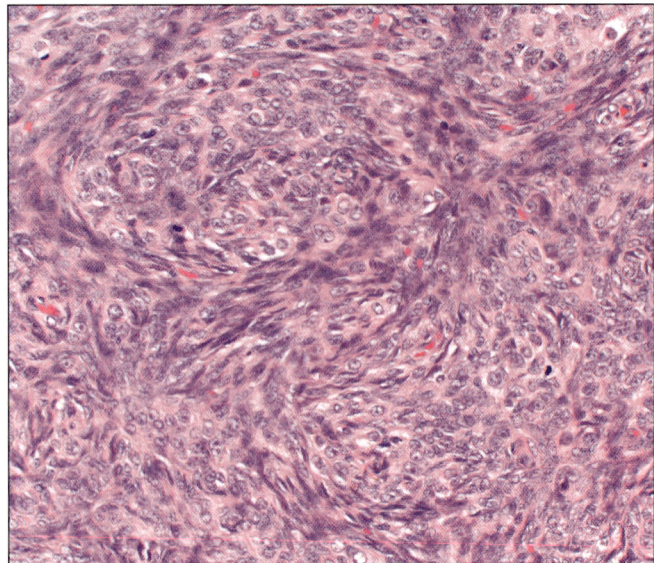

Fig. 26.63 Poorly differentiated Sertoli–Leydig cell tumor. Sarcoma-like area of indifferent spindle cells showing conspicuous mitotic activity and some vague suggestion of 'biphasic' cell differentiation.

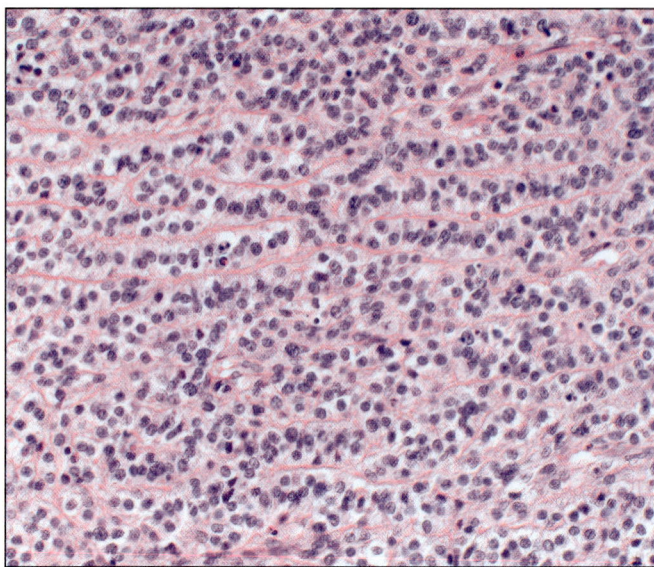

Fig. 26.65 Poorly differentiated Sertoli–Leydig cell tumor. Solid area of cords of immature Sertoli cells with rounded nuclei and clear or vacuolated cytoplasm.

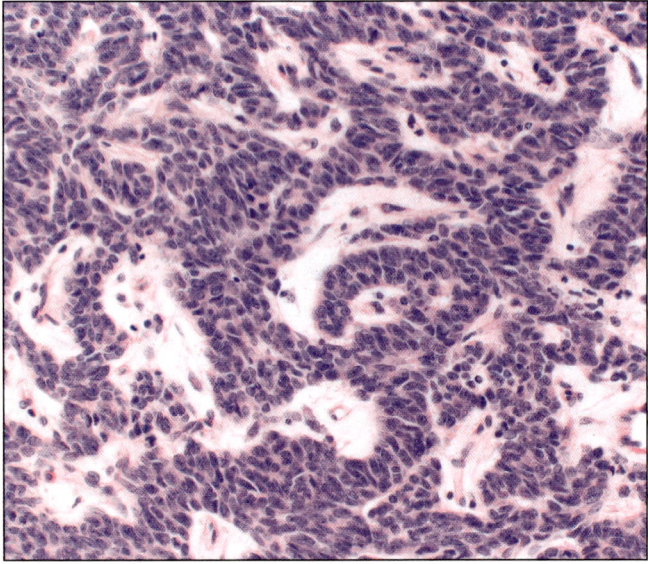

Fig. 26.64 Poorly differentiated Sertoli–Leydig cell tumor. Fine trabecular area simulating patterns seen in granulosa cell tumor.

or more complex and branched, occasionally simulating those of serous or endometrioid epithelial carcinomas.

Heterologous elements, such as intestinal-type mucinous epithelium, fat, cartilage, skeletal muscle, bone, etc. are found in over 20% of moderately differentiated and a smaller proportion of poorly differentiated Sertoli–Leydig cell tumors (in 40% of those with a retiform pattern – see below).

The adjacent ovarian tissue is usually unremarkable, although it may be distinctly edematous if removed during pregnancy. Rarely, moderately and poorly differentiated Sertoli–Leydig cell tumors are associated with the morphologic changes of the polycystic ovary syndrome in the affected or contralateral ovary.[89] There are reports but probably an incidental association with coexisting discrete benign adult cystic

teratoma (4%) and benign mucinous cysts (3%) in either the same or contralateral ovary.

Differential diagnosis

Carcinomas, primary or metastatic, with imperfectly formed acini may be mistaken for a moderately well-differentiated Sertoli–Leydig cell tumor, especially if the stromal cells undergo luteinization and thus come to resemble Leydig cells. This is particularly so for moderately differentiated ovarian endometrioid carcinomas, some of which show marked superficial resemblances to either granulosa cell tumors or Sertoli–Leydig cell tumors (so-called 'sertoliform' variants).[65] The age ranges and clinical settings of these tumors should facilitate their differentiation, as should squamous metaplasia or luminal mucins when found in the endometrioid tumors. An immunoprofile of 'epithelial' elements also facilitates diagnosis. Broad spectrum and low molecular weight cytokeratins (AE1/AE3 and CAM 5.2) are usually only focally reactive in epithelial-like areas of Sertoli–Leydig cell tumors, but will be diffusely and strongly positive in the glandular epithelium of the endometrioid carcinomas. Similarly, these elements will be consistently unreactive for EMA and estrogen and/or progesterone receptors (ER/PR) in the Sertoli–Leydig cell tumors, but consistently reactive (EMA) or often reactive (ER/PR) in the carcinomas. The Sertoli cells are frequently reactive for α-inhibin and calretinin while the carcinomas are not. Though heterologous mucinous epithelium is found in 20% of all androblastomas, such epithelium will show intracellular as well as luminal mucin, differentiating it from the non-mucin-secreting epithelium of 'sertoliform' endometrioid adenocarcinoma. The so-called tubular Krukenberg tumors (see Chapter 29) may be mistaken for moderately differentiated Sertoli–Leydig cell tumors, particularly if there is prominent stromal response to individual tumor cells, prominent stromal luteinization, and clinical masculinization. The majority of these former tumors, however, are bilateral and a mucicarmine stain reveals typical signet-ring cells in all cases. The reti-

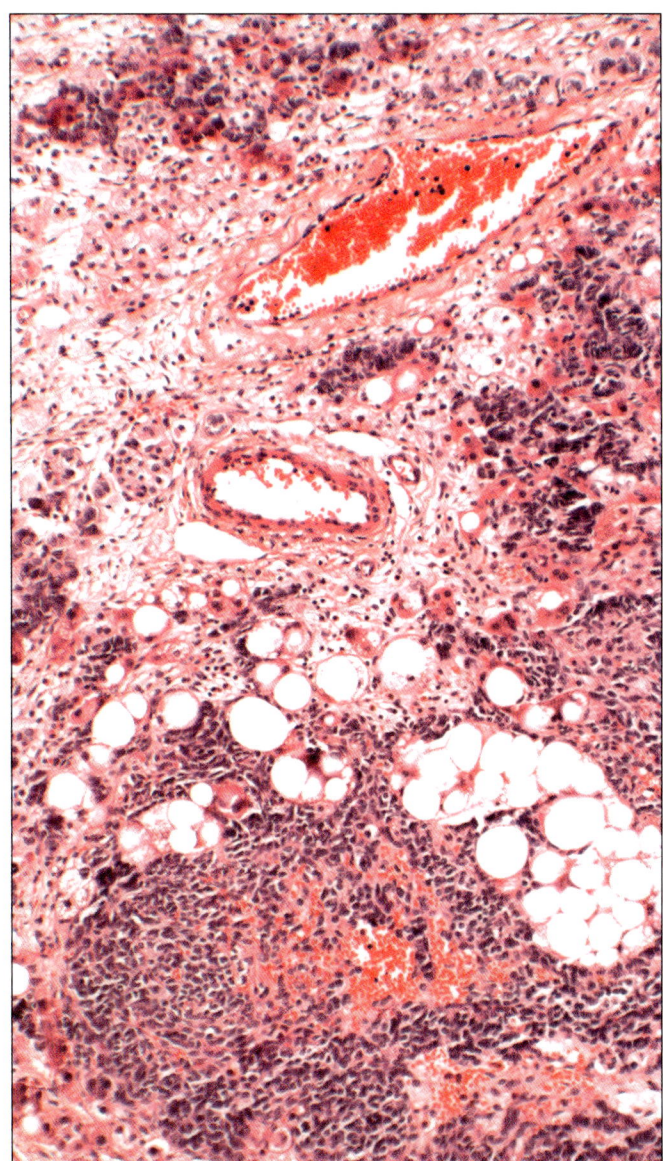

Fig. 26.66 Poorly differentiated Sertoli–Leydig cell tumor. Edge of cellular area with obvious Leydig cells. Those scattered near the center and top have dense eosinophilic cytoplasm, while those aggregated below center have grossly vacuolated cytoplasm.

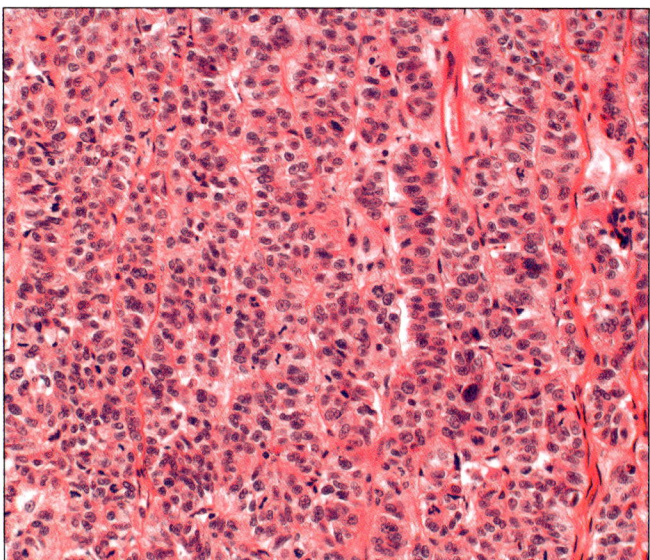

Fig. 26.67 Malignant, pure Sertoli cell tumor. Tumor composed of solid gyriform tubules and cords of cells with ovoid nuclei and numerous mitoses.

Prognosis and treatment

The incidence of clinical malignancy in these tumors is 10–30%. The most reliable indication of malignancy is evidence of local extraovarian spread or metastases at the time of staging laparotomy, all such tumors pursuing an aggressive and usually fatal course, regardless of therapy. Histologic grade correlates to some extent with the likely clinical outcome; 11% of 'moderately' well-differentiated tumors are clinically malignant while 20% of those with heterologous mesenchymal elements (see below) and 60% of poorly differentiated tumors are also likely to progress clinically. Recurrences or metastases in apparently early stage disease are usually apparent within 12 months – often before 6 months – and are commonly preceded by an exacerbation of the patient's virilization. Metastases occur in the omentum, abdominal lymph nodes or the liver, but have also been reported in lungs, bones, intestine, kidney, mediastinum, and brain.

Patients with early stage disease and well-differentiated tumors rarely experience recurrences. Unilateral salpingo-oophorectomy is the recommended surgical procedure when fertility is a management issue, and may be performed laparoscopically in suitable cases,[43,110] otherwise total hysterectomy and bilateral salpingo-oophorectomy is performed.

ANDROBLASTOMAS WITH HETEROLOGOUS ELEMENTS

These tumors are separable from other moderately and poorly differentiated Sertoli–Leydig cell tumors on purely histologic grounds – namely the presence of heterologous elements, the most common of which is gastrointestinal mucin-secreting epithelium.[50] It is seen in about 20% of Sertoli–Leydig cell tumors. About 5% contain immature skeletal muscle[42] and/or cartilage.[107] Rarely they exhibit neuroblastoma, fat, carcinoid, smooth muscle, bone, hepatocytes giving rise to elevated serum α-fetoprotein,[60] endometrium or endometrioid adenofibroma.

form variant may be confused with endodermal sinus tumors (see Chapter 27), serous epithelial carcinomas (see Chapter 24) or carcinosarcomas – either homologous or heterologous (see Chapter 25).

The differentiation between granulosa and Sertoli–Leydig cell tumors may be impossible in the least differentiated forms and a history of virilization is insufficient to justify attaching this diagnostic label to a neoplasm that would be better categorized as a sex cord-stromal tumor of indeterminate type. Differential immunoprofiles[102] may be utilized, more for academic than pragmatic reasons. However, in relatively mature tumors, the Sertoli cells do show appreciable differences from granulosa cells, even though the basic histologic architecture may be similar in some cases. Call Exner bodies are not found in androblastomas, while true tubules and Leydig cells (containing Reinke crystalloids) are not present in granulosa cell tumors.

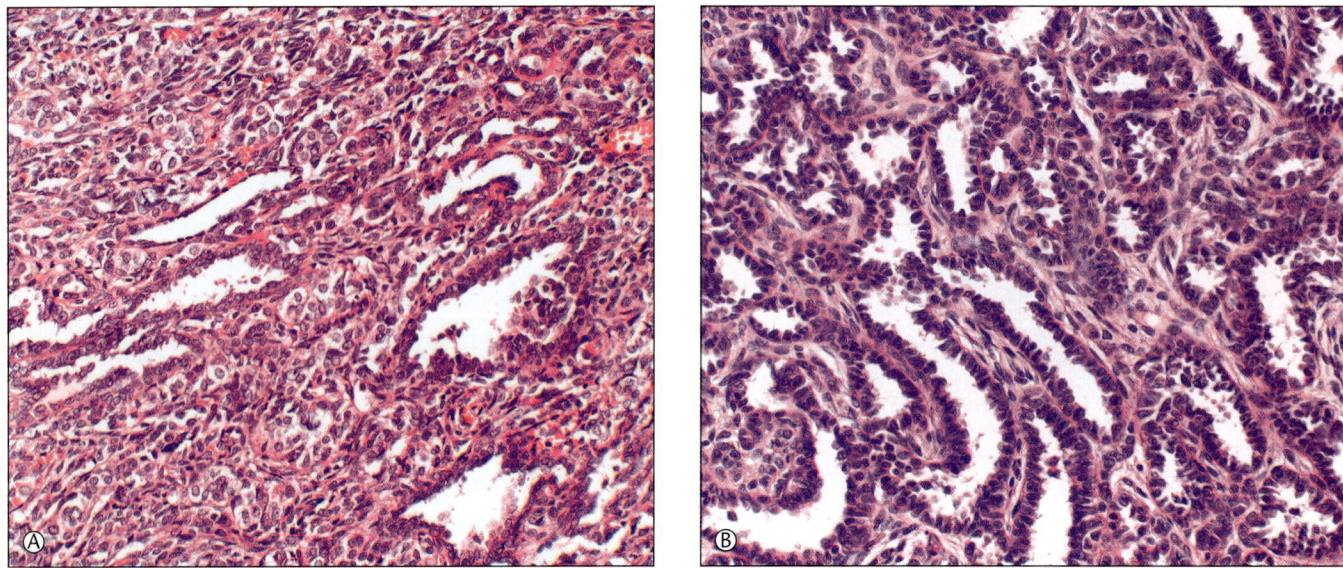

Fig. 26.68 Small 'retiform' foci in poorly differentiated Sertoli–Leydig cell tumors. **(A)** Angular, branching, slit-like spaces lined by cuboidal epithelial cells are noted centrally. **(B)** Better defined cuboidal epithelial cells ('hobnail-like') lining the irregularly shaped retiform spaces.

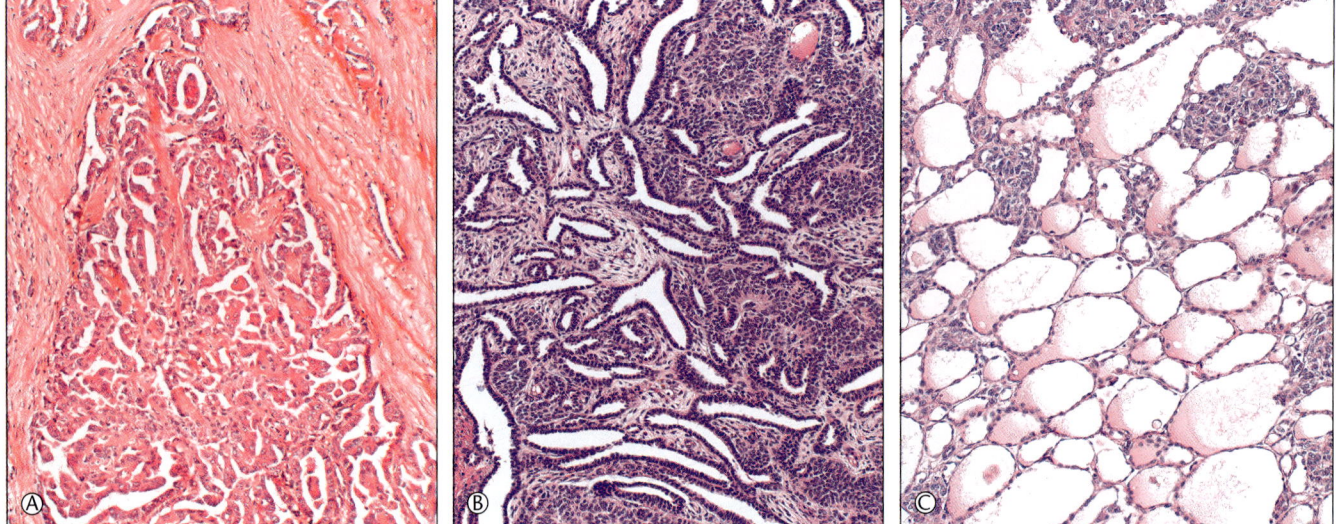

Fig. 26.69 Poorly differentiated Sertoli–Leydig cell tumors. Large fields with 'retiform' patterns in otherwise typical neoplasms. **(A)** Branching, slit-like tubular spaces contain small papillary processes with hyalinized connective tissue cores. Epithelial cells are cuboidal. **(B)** The retiform character of the slit-like spaces is particularly striking in this field. **(C)** Sieve-like area with cystic spaces lined by flattened or cuboidal ('hobnail-like') cells.

Clinical profile

The clinical and endocrinologic profiles of these neoplasms are the same as those of Sertoli–Leydig cell tumors without heterologous elements. About 20% behave aggressively.

Macroscopic features

Sertoli–Leydig cell tumors with heterologous elements tend to be larger than those without such elements. The tumors are bosselated, with some showing grossly visible mucin-filled cysts on the cut surfaces. Solid areas of friable yellow-gray tissue are comparable to solid areas in 'pure' Sertoli–Leydig cell tumors, and extensive hemorrhage and necrosis may be observed here.

Microscopic features

The mucinous epithelium in these tumors (Figure 26.70A) is usually benign (but may be malignant) and is clearly enteric in type. The columnar cells are identical to those of normal small intestine, being commonly interspersed with goblet cells, Paneth cells, and basally situated argentaffin cells or other cells immunoreactive for neuron-specific enolase. The latter may give rise to carcinoid or adenocarcinoid foci. The mucinous component varies from a minor element up to and including almost pure mucinous cystadenomas with only microscopic evidence of Sertoli–Leydig cell differentiation. Similarly, mesenchymal elements vary enormously in their relative prominence and their degree of differentiation.

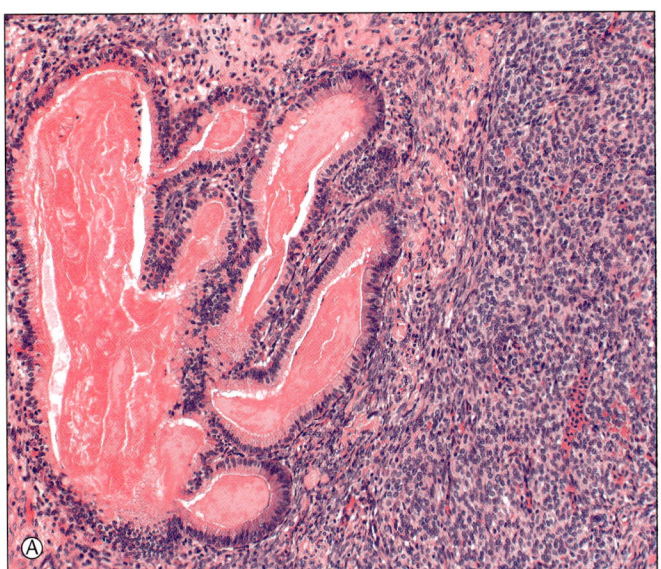

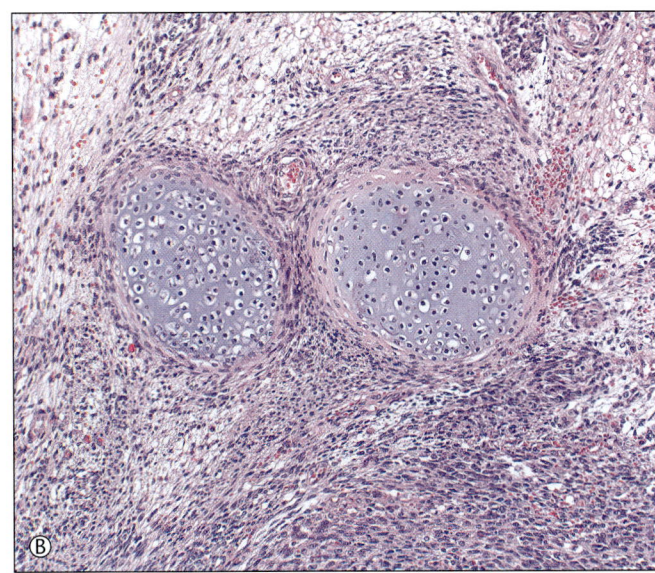

Fig. 26.70 Poorly differentiated androblastoma with heterologous elements. **(A)** Cystic spaces containing eosinophilic mucinous material and lined by enteric-type epithelium. Goblet cells are a prominent feature of such epithelium. Poorly differentiated spindle cell tumor at right. **(B)** Two circumscribed nodules of cartilage adjacent to a sarcoma-like area (bottom).

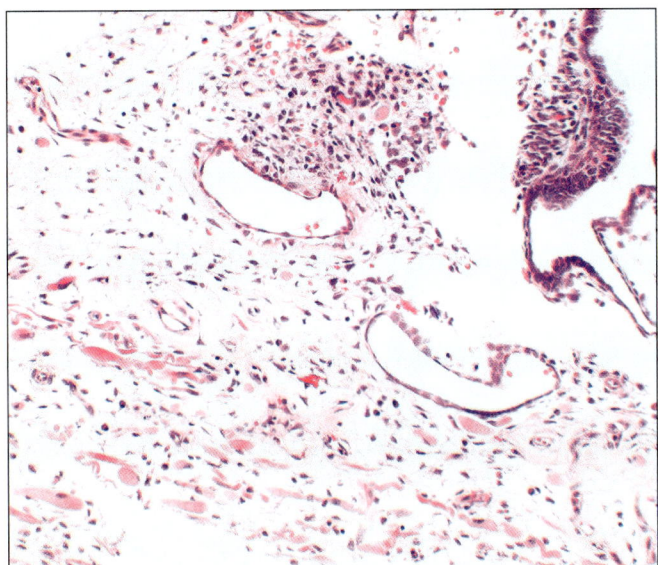

Fig. 26.71 Poorly differentiated retiform Sertoli–Leydig cell tumor with heterologous elements. Rhabdomyoblasts, with strap-like eosinophilic cytoplasm, are seen at bottom with an irregular retiform glandular structure at top right.

Relatively banal immature cartilaginous islands (Figure 26.70B) are readily apparent, but skeletal muscular components (Figure 26.71) are frequently admixed with densely cellular spindle-cell tissue and easily missed. The wide range of tissue types seen in immature teratomas is characteristically absent, thus distinguishing these two entities. If the Sertoli–Leydig cell component is small and overlooked, the tumor may be mistyped as a pure sarcoma. This has been proposed as an alternative explanation for the genesis of some pure chondrosarcomas and rhabdomyosarcomas of the ovary rather than monophasic carcinosarcoma.

The androblastomatous components of these tumors are indistinguishable morphologically from those of Sertoli–Leydig cell tumors without heterologous elements. They are predominantly moderately differentiated in association with mucinous cysts and almost always poorly differentiated when mesenchymal elements or sarcoma are present.

GYNANDROBLASTOMAS

The term 'gynandroblastoma' defines those tumors that show intermingling of prominent well-differentiated ovarian and testicular elements – the importance of the 'intermingling' being to exclude theoretical cases of collision tumor. These extremely rare neoplasms have been capriciously overdiagnosed in the past and few acceptable examples are known.[26,37,96] The amount required of each component necessary to establish the diagnosis remains controversial. We prefer to ignore small foci in making the diagnosis, but some will nonetheless diagnose gynandroblastomas occasionally if the tumor exhibits small focal areas simulating granulosa cell differentiation. Alternatively, rare hollow tubules lined by typical Sertoli cells may also be encountered in otherwise unremarkable granulosa cell tumors. Occasional cases have been reported in which the ovarian elements have been of juvenile rather than adult granulosa cell type,[7,12,95] and in which the testicular or Sertoli–Leydig cell areas exhibited heterologous elements.[57]

Most well-documented cases have been virilizing and have presented in women with a mean age of 31 years (age range, 15–65 years), although a rare patient may be postmenopausal.[106] To date, no case has pursued a malignant course, but follow-up prior to case reporting is traditionally short.

Macroscopic features

The few cases reported have been unilateral, small (2–6 cm in diameter), solid, pale tumors; occasionally as small, incidentally found lesions (Figure 26.72). The cut surfaces often show

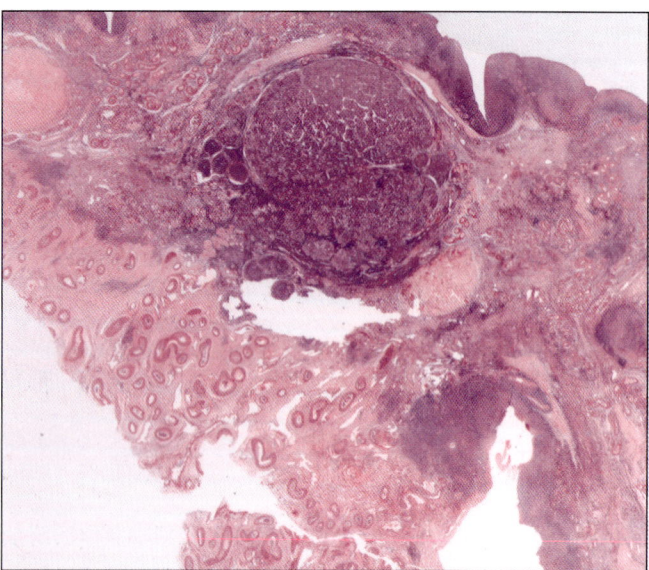

Fig. 26.72 Gynandroblastoma. A very small neoplasm identified in the medulla of an ovary removed from a 45-year-old woman with uterine fibroids. The rounded nodule at the top showed Sertoli cell differentiation only. The adjacent scattered small micronodules showed granulosa cell differentiation.

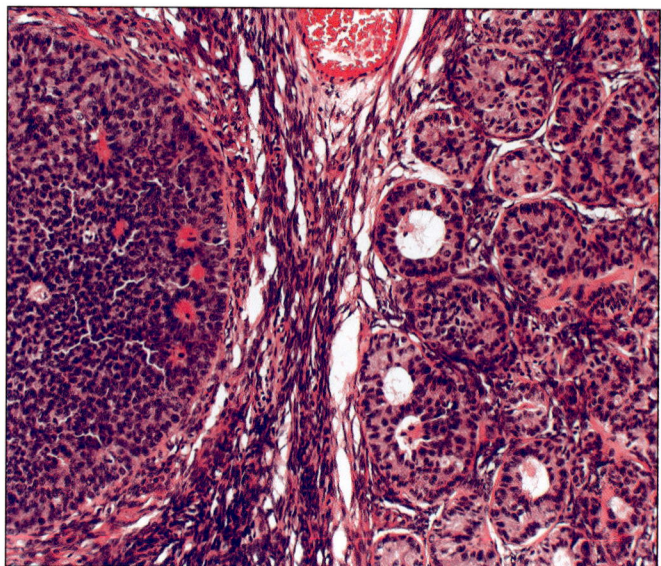

Fig. 26.73 Gynandroblastoma (same case as Figure 26.72). The interface between the Sertoli cell nodule (right) with hollow tubules lined by tall columnar cells and an adjacent granulosa cell nest with a microfollicular pattern and typical Call–Exner bodies.

pink-to-yellow fleshy nodules with coarse intervening fibrous septa.

Microscopic features

Ovarian elements are seen as nests of mature granulosa cells in which Call–Exner bodies may be found (Figure 26.73). Rarely, the granulosa component is of juvenile type (Figure 26.74). Male or testicular components may be tubules lined by typical Sertoli cells and/or Leydig cells containing Reinke crystalloids (described in four cases only). The residual rims of ovarian tissue and the contralateral ovaries have shown no noteworthy abnormalities. At the ultrastructural level, the tubular elements of gynandroblastomas more closely resemble the 'retiform' variant of Sertoli–Leydig cell tumors, while the Call–Exner bodies tend to be of the 'hyaline' rather than 'spongiform' type more commonly identified in granulosa cell tumors. Poorly differentiated sex cord-stromal tumors in which less than definite granulosa and Sertoli cell differentiation is seen are excluded from this diagnosis and should be categorized as sex cord-stromal tumors of indeterminate type.

SEX-CORD TUMORS WITH ANNULAR TUBULES (SCTAT)

Divergent histogenetic views continue to be promoted, particularly concerning those SCTAT unassociated with Peutz–Jeghers syndrome, claiming granulosa cell or Sertoli cell origin, the latter principally on ultrastructural evidence. This has led, in the past, to 'Sertoli cell tumor, annular tubular type' being suggested as an alternative name for SCTAT.

Clinical profile

Separation of SCTAT from otherwise unclassified sex cord-stromal tumors appears warranted on both morphologic and clinical grounds. They occur in two clinical settings.

- Firstly, nearly all female patients with Peutz–Jeghers syndrome (generalized hamartomatous intestinal polyposis and melanin spots of the oral mucosa, lips, and digits) develop SCTAT tumors. Such cases account for one-third of reported examples of ovarian SCTAT. Germline-inactivating mutations in one allele of the *STK11/LKB1* tumor suppressor gene at chromosome 19p13.3 have been found in most patients with Peutz–Jeghers syndrome, but not in patients lacking the phenotypic changes of Peutz–Jeghers syndrome.[17] In this setting, the tumors occur at almost any age but the mean is 27 years, and are associated with menstrual irregularities in about 40% of instances. The tumors are typically bilateral, multifocal, calcified and very small (frequently microscopic), and are probably hamartomatous tumorlets rather than neoplasms. This concept is supported by the finding of similar structures of dysgenetic follicular origin in the ovaries of normal fetuses, infants, children and adults, and in ovarian dysgenesis and failure[27] (see Chapter 22). All SCTAT associated with Peutz–Jeghers syndrome have been clinically benign, although they may rarely be associated with so-called 'adenoma malignum of the uterine cervix' and other genital tract neoplasms and metaplasias.[52,68,87] This small risk should always be borne in mind in the postoperative management and follow-up of these women.
- Secondly, unassociated with Peutz–Jeghers syndrome, SCTAT have almost always been large and unilateral, and should be regarded as true neoplasms, with at least 20% pursuing a malignant course.[85] Serum inhibin, müllerian-inhibiting substance (MIS), and progesterone levels may all be used as tumor markers in such patients.[70] The mean age at presentation for these patients, unassociated with Peutz–Jeghers syndrome, is 34 years. Over half of patients present with postmenopausal bleeding, menstrual irregularities or isosexual pseudopuberty suggesting hyperestrogenism. Rare cases of SCTAT have been

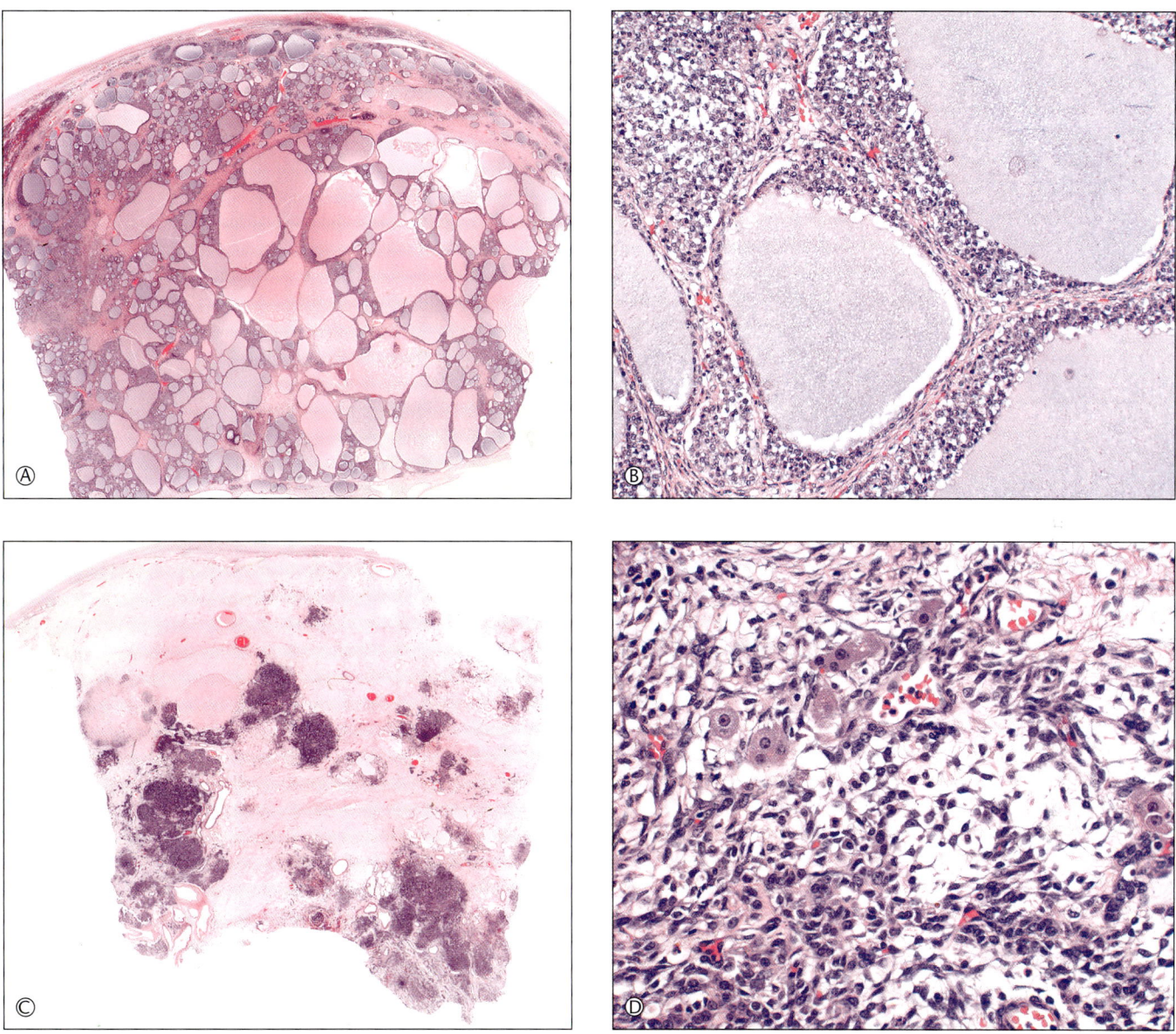

Fig. 26.74 Gynandroblastoma with juvenile granulosa cell tumor and poorly differentiated Sertoli–Leydig cell tumor. **(A)** Survey of sieve-like juvenile granulosa cell tumor zone. **(B)** High power of juvenile granulosa cell area. **(C)** Survey of adjacent poorly differentiated Sertoli–Leydig cell tumor zone. **(D)** High power of Sertoli–Leydig cell area.

associated with a gestagen-like effect on the endometrium.[85] Solitary extraovarian examples have been reported in the fallopian tube[29] and umbilicus.[4]

Macroscopic features

The examples occurring in conjunction with Peutz–Jeghers syndrome are usually multifocal, bilateral, and almost always very small tumorlets found incidentally in ovaries. The tumorlets frequently have a yellow cut surface. Focal calcification is occasionally obvious.

SCTAT, in patients lacking the syndrome, are almost always unilateral and present as a solitary, large solid mass up to 20 cm in diameter (although in rare cases the tumor is microscopic and multifocal SCTAT).[108] They are commonly described as having nodules of firm yellow to tan tissue, occasionally with cysts and areas of hemorrhage and necrosis. Adhesions to adja-

cent pelvic organs, when present, are usually reactive to local capsular infiltration by tumor.

Microscopic features

SCTAT typically exhibit well-circumscribed, rounded or oval, epithelial islands made up of ring-shaped, lumenless tubules encircling glassy, acidophilic, PAS-positive, basement membrane-like material. The rings themselves are set in fibrous ovarian stroma (Figure 26.75), which may contain foci of luteinized cells and show focal hyalinization that, in some lesions, is pronounced (Figure 26.76). The stroma regularly condenses around the perimeter of cell nests to form thick hyaline basement membranes (showing immunoreactivity for type IV collagen[95]) and is continuous with the blunt-ended ellipsoid deposits of hyaline material within the cell nests. Sometimes simple annular cords envelop single deposits of

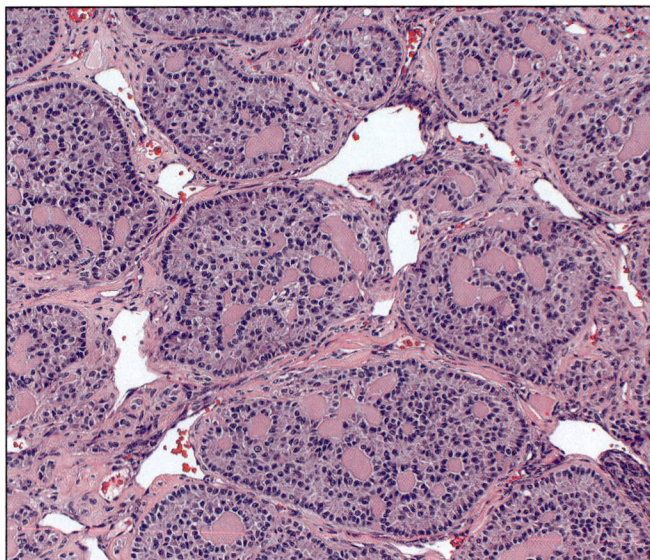

Fig. 26.75 Sex-cord tumor with annular tubules. Clustered nests of columnar cells arranged in a complex ring-like or annular fashion around hyaline deposits.

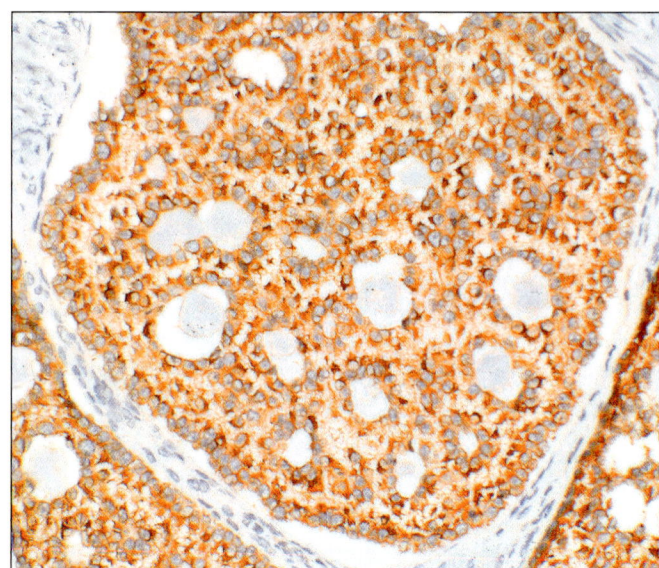

Fig. 26.77 Sex-cord tumor with annular tubules. Small typical cell nest displaying strong cytoplasmic immunostaining for α-inhibin.

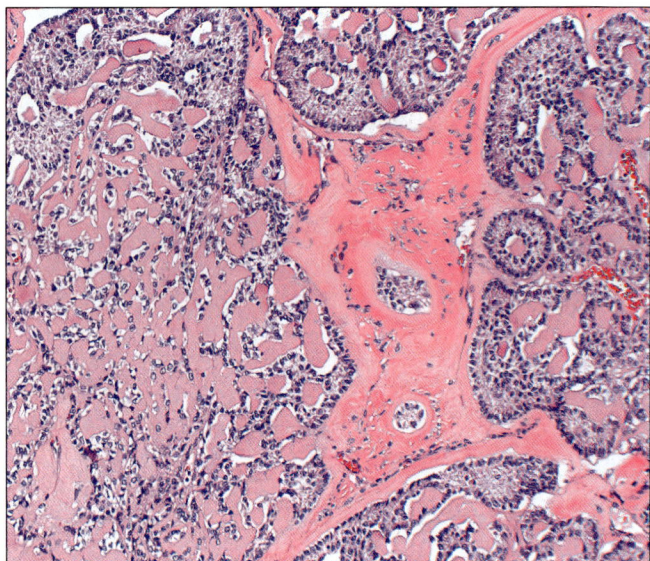

Fig. 26.76 Sex-cord tumor with annular tubules. Tumor featuring exaggerated deposition of hyaline material that, in places, may almost totally efface the tumor architecture.

hyaline material, but, more commonly, a network of complex tubules encompasses and interdigitates with many such deposits. The tubular cell cytoplasm is abundant, pale, and vacuolated or slightly granular. Regular, rounded, occasionally grooved nuclei, often with a single small nucleolus, are generally arranged in a double row – one row at the periphery of the cell nests and the second around the hyaline deposits. They may also proliferate towards the centers of the tubules to a variable degree. Microscopic focal calcification is observed in over half of the cases. Mitoses are rare.

Tumors occurring in patients without Peutz–Jeghers syndrome differ somewhat from those in women with this syndrome inasmuch as there is focal differentiation towards microfollicular or cylindroma-like granulosa cell tumor and/or

areas indistinguishable from Sertoli cell tumor with elongated solid tubules (ultrastructurally confirmed by finding Charcot–Bottcher crystalloids in the neoplastic cells). Calcification is rare. The immunophenotype of the tumor cells includes strong reactivity for α-inhibin (Figure 26.77) and vimentin intermediate filaments.[111] Hyalinized stroma may occasionally be profound and associated with degenerative changes in the tubular epithelial cells. Coagulative necrosis may be present. Mitoses are uncommon (<1 per 10 HPFs) and vascular permeation and destructive stromal invasion are not obvious, even in clinically malignant examples. Transition from typical SCTAT, through sertoliform tubular areas, to foci resembling well-differentiated endometrioid carcinoma may rarely be present, and is probably analogous to the equally rare occurrence of so-called 'endometrioid' areas in otherwise typical Sertoli–Leydig cell tumors.

Differential diagnosis

SCTAT must be discriminated from microfollicular granulosa cell tumors, well-differentiated Sertoli cell tumors, and gonadoblastomas. The cells of SCTAT are larger with more obvious and paler (or clear) cytoplasm than in granulosa cell tumors. The hyaline acidophilic deposits in the center of the cell nests are larger than the Call–Exner bodies of granulosa cell tumors, are frequently complex, and lack cellular debris. Nuclear palisading, prominent in SCTAT, is not a feature of granulosa cell tumors.

The cell morphology of SCTAT is similar to that of well-differentiated Sertoli cell tumors. The latter tumors, however, are composed predominantly of hollow, simple tubules not seen in SCTAT.

SCTAT may superficially resemble gonadoblastomas in the patterns of cell nests, stromal calcification, and stromal Leydig cells. Gonadoblastomas are composed of two cell types – large germ cells and smaller dark cells of sex-cord origin. These smaller cells may produce rosettes resembling Call–Exner bodies or be radially oriented around individual germ cells. They do not, however, produce annular tubules or cords with antipodally disposed nuclei as seen in SCTAT.

UNCLASSIFIED SEX CORD-STROMAL TUMORS

Occasional ovarian neoplasms are associated with clinical or histologic features that suggest sex cord or gonadal stromal origin, yet do not conveniently conform to any of the previously described tumor types. This is largely a function of their rarity and the precision with which established subgroups of tumors are defined. Our approach is to restrict this category of tumors largely to those very uncommon poorly differentiated, diffuse or spindle cell tumors with occasional tubular or cord-like structures that are impossible to further categorize (Figures 26.78 and 26.79).

Well-differentiated stromal tumors (fibromas) with minor sex-cord elements (Figures 26.42 and 26.80) represent another rare category of tumors that, until recently, we would have placed within this unclassified group (see above). Tumors that are intermediate between thecomas and fibromas (and these, by contrast, are frequently observed) are placed in an 'unclassified' subgroup of the thecoma–fibroma group in the WHO classification, but are termed 'thecafibromas' in our schema.

STEROID CELL TUMORS

Steroid (lipid or lipoid) cell tumors, not otherwise specified, are infrequently encountered ovarian neoplasms that exhibit an organoid or diffuse arrangement of large, rounded or

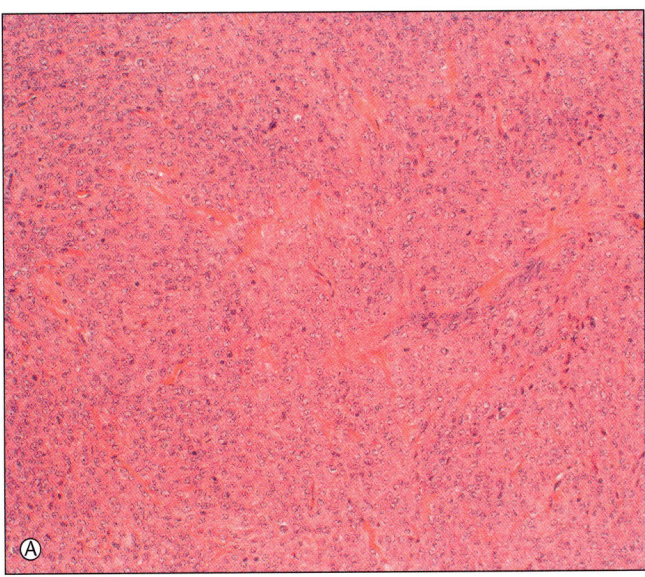
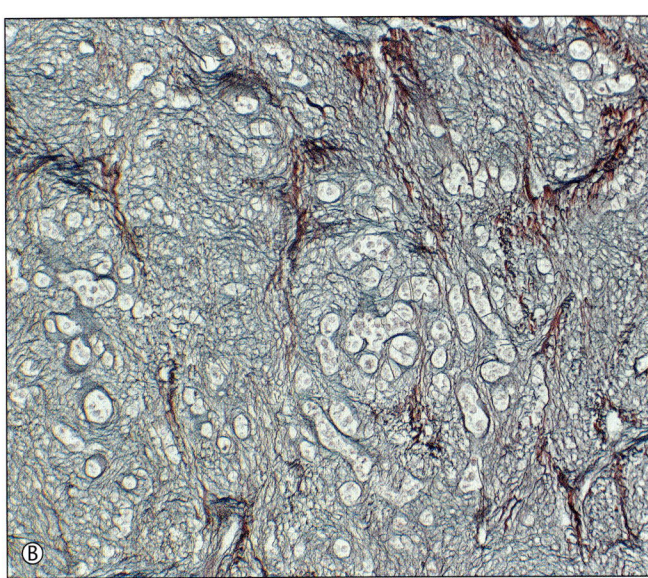

Fig. 26.78 Poorly differentiated sex cord-stromal tumor, not otherwise classifiable. **(A)** Mass composed of patternless sheets of uniform round to slightly spindled cells (compare with Figure 26.63). The 'sex-cord' elements are not discernible in the routine H&E sections. **(B)** Same field as (A). The distinction between sex-cord and stromal elements is highlighted by staining for reticulin fibers, but further classification according to the nature of the sex-cord elements is not possible.

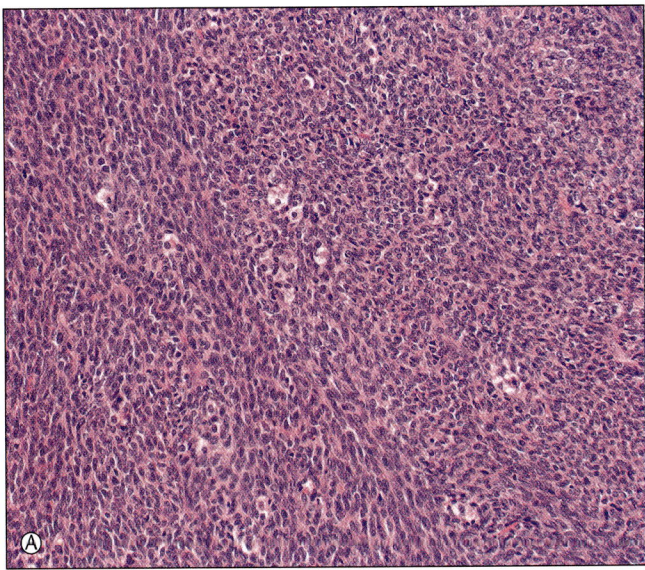
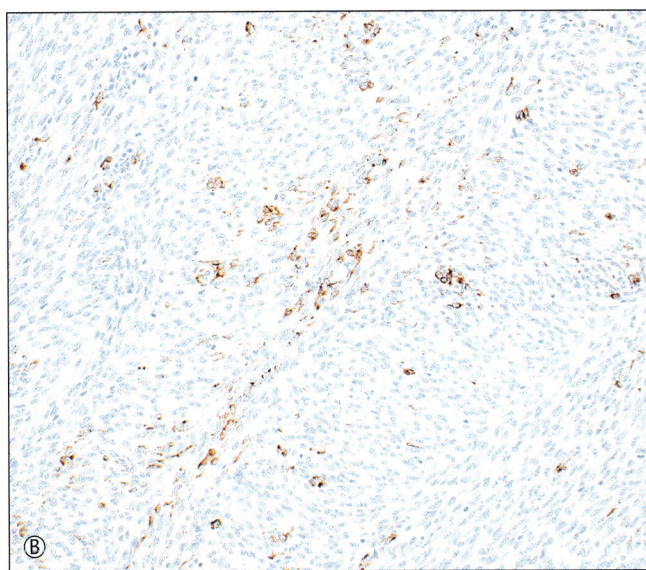

Fig. 26.79 Poorly differentiated sex cord-stromal tumor, not otherwise classifiable. **(A)** Patternless and densely cellular sheets of small uniform spindle cells with sparsely scattered single cells suggestive of lutein differentiation. **(B)** These cells are highlighted by immunostaining for α-inhibin.

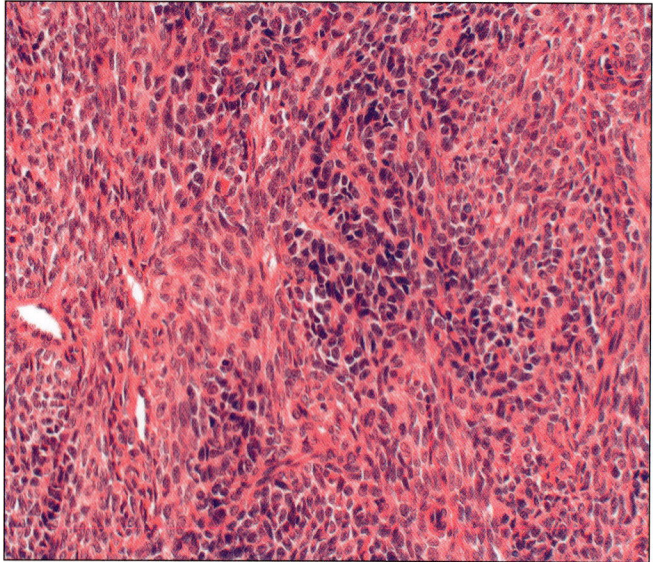

Fig. 26.80 Cellular fibroma with minor and poorly formed sex-cord elements. Cellular anaplasia and nuclear atypia are absent and this tumor behaved in a benign fashion.

Table 26.4 Differential diagnosis: steroid cell tumor versus pregnancy luteoma

Steroid cell tumor	Pregnancy luteoma
Clinical diagnosis	
Mean age 47 years	Mean age 26 years
No relationship to pregnancy	Diagnosed near term, or in puerperium
No racial tendency	80% in black women
Almost always unilateral	Often bilateral and multicentric
75% of women virilized	Asymptomatic
Histologic diagnosis	
Abundant intracellular lipid	Relatively little or no lipid
Necrosis, if present, only focal	Diffuse acute regressive changes if removed in puerperium
No pregnancy changes in adjacent uninvolved ovary	Pregnancy changes in adjacent ovary (deciduosis, hyperthecosis)

polygonal cells that resemble Leydig, stromal lutein or adrenal cortical cells. By convention, neoplasms with cellular features pathognomonic of a particular tumor type are excluded. Hilus or Leydig cells derived from the ovarian stroma, indeed, are a suggested source for some steroid cell tumors. As Leydig cells can only be identified positively by finding Reinke crystalloids, and these structures are often sparse in typical Leydig cell tumors of the ovary (see above), it is highly likely that some steroid cell tumors are unidentifiable Leydig cell tumors, where either size, or lack of differentiation, precludes the tumor from forming Reinke crystalloids.

Other likely cells of origin of these tumors are theca–lutein or stromal lutein cells. Evidence supporting this includes a marked resemblance of tumor cells to stromal lutein cells and the demonstrable origin of occasional small discrete lesions, indistinguishable from typical steroid cell tumors, within the ovarian stroma. These nodules, associated often with stromal hyperthecosis (nodules of lutein cells in the neighboring stroma), have been designated as stromal luteomas, although in our view it is debatable whether such lesions are true neoplasms. Pregnancy luteomas, or nodular theca–lutein hyperplasia of pregnancy (see Chapter 22), are histologically very similar to the steroid cell group of tumors and demonstrate the proliferative potential of the ovarian stroma. The differentiation of pregnancy luteomas from steroid cell tumors, not otherwise specified, is given in Table 26.4.

Although the lipid-rich cells of many of these tumors closely resemble adrenocortical cells, this similarity cannot, of itself, be regarded as a serious basis for tumor classification. Adrenal cortical rests in the vicinity of the ovary have also been proposed as a possible origin for some lesions. However, while such rests are common, they occur in the broad ligament, mesosalpinx, fallopian tube wall, and mesovarium rather than within the ovarian stroma. Steroid cell tumors, by contrast, occur in the cortical and medullary stroma of the ovaries and only isolated reports exist of steroid cell tumors located outside the normally sited ovaries.[76,86]

Clinical profile

Most often they occur in women of reproductive age, particularly during the third and fourth decades, and rarely in postmenopausal women or children.[32] They are clinically androgenic in 40% of cases[5] and regularly secrete androstenedione, α-hydroxyprogesterone, testosterone, and dehydroepiandrosterone. The onset of virilization tends to be gradual rather than abrupt and is usually preceded by amenorrhea and defeminization. Also, a further 7% of cases develop Cushing-like syndromes, with elevated serum cortisol levels. Non-specific symptoms referable to the physical presence of the tumor, abdominal pain and swelling, occur in relatively few patients.

Macroscopic features

These tumors are almost always well circumscribed, solid and unilateral without predilection for either ovary. Cystic variants, due to focal degeneration and secondary intracystic hemorrhage, occur. They vary greatly in size from 0.5 to 45 cm in diameter. The cut surface, which bulges in the fresh state, is frequently lobulated and ranges in color from bright yellow through reddish-brown to dark green-brown. The smaller tumors tend to occupy the medulla or hilus of the ovary. Necrosis and hemorrhage may be present in larger tumors.

Microscopic features

Steroid cell tumors are well demarcated from the surrounding compressed ovarian stroma. They usually have an organoid pattern common to many steroid-producing tumors, consisting of rounded or polygonal vacuolated cells arranged in nests or columns (Figure 26.81) and separated by a rich network of capillaries and vascular sinusoids. The columns may be arranged centripetally from the capsule, simulating the adrenal cortex. Less commonly there is a diffuse arrangement of cells (Figure 26.82). The tumor cell cytoplasm is moderate to abundant in amount and varies correspondingly from granular and eosinophilic (as seen in the adrenal zona reticularis – Figure 26.81) to foamy and lipid-rich (as seen in the zona fasciculata – Figure 26.82). Stains for neutral lipid are strongly positive in 75% of tumors. Lipochrome pigment granules vary from very

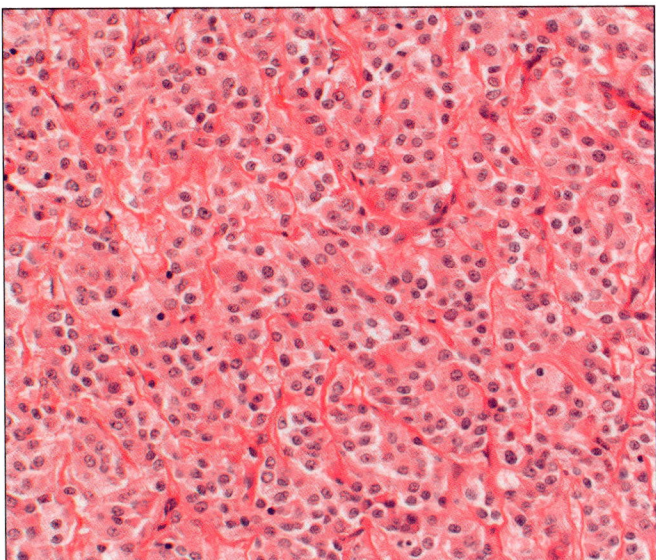

Fig. 26.81 Steroid cell tumor. A solid tumor, presenting with omental metastases, in a 37-year-old woman. A fascicular pattern due to the cord-like arrangement of tumor cells and the intervening vascular stroma.

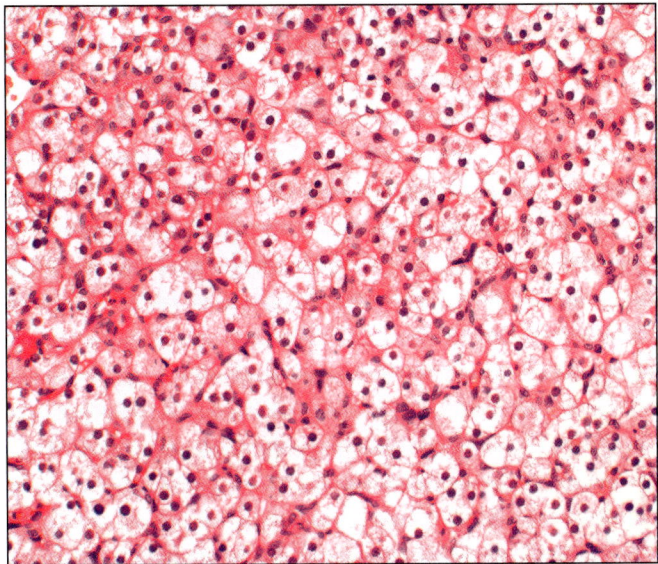

Fig. 26.82 Steroid cell tumor. A solid pattern of growth of large polyhedral cells with vacuolated lipid-rich cytoplasm.

sparse to numerous. Cytoplasmic glycogen may be present in some cases. Reticulin fibers invest individual or small groups of cells, but interstitial fibrosis and hyalinization are rarely prominent. Nuclei tend to be small and central with effaced chromatin and, while varying degrees of nuclear pleomorphism and mitotic activity (usually more than in ovarian Leydig cell tumors) have been observed, a diagnosis of malignancy can only really be made morphologically in the presence of local invasion. Necrosis, hemorrhage, and hyaline fibrosis (that may be calcified) are sometimes present, as are broad areas of myxoid-like connective tissue containing clusters or cords of tumor cells.

Immunohistochemically, these tumors are reactive regularly for α-inhibin,[74,90] 75% for vimentin, 40% focally for various cytokeratins, and 30% for smooth muscle actin.[84] Steroid cell

tumors are unreactive for chromogranin, Leu-M1, α-fetoprotein, carcinoembryonic antigen (CEA), and HMB45.

Differential diagnosis
From the group of solid tumors composed of lipid-rich, steroid-producing cells, the diagnosis of steroid cell tumor is basically one of exclusion. The specific histologic features that enable identification of Leydig cell tumors are discussed in that section, and those that clinically distinguish pregnancy luteomas (rare large nodules of lutein cells that develop during pregnancy and regress spontaneously postpartum) from steroid cell tumors are outlined in Table 26.4. Luteinized thecomas (see above) exhibit clusters of lutein cells that are similar to those of steroid cell tumors, but these cells are found in a background of spindled fibroblastic or theca-type cells. Primary clear cell carcinomas of müllerian epithelial type may have a uniform solid pattern of clear cells, although other patterns are usually present. These latter cells, however, are rich in glycogen and contain scanty lipid, in direct contrast to those of typical steroid cell tumors. They are only occasionally virilizing and are associated with pelvic endometriosis in 40% or more of cases.

Prognosis and treatment
Over 30% of steroid cell tumors pursue a malignant clinical course with spread within the abdomen and occasional distant metastases. Tumor size (8 cm in diameter or larger), 2 or more mitoses per 10 HPFs, necrosis and hemorrhage, and marked nuclear atypia are adverse correlates of prognosis. Unilateral salpingo-oophorectomy appears adequate management for small ovarian tumors apparently encapsulated and therefore confined to one ovary at thorough staging laparotomy. Tumors greater than 8 cm in diameter or that show evidence of extra-ovarian extension should be treated by more extensive surgery. Inadequate experience with adjuvant therapy precludes sensible evaluation of its efficacy.

REFERENCES

1. Ahmed E, Young RH, Scully RE. Adult granulosa cell tumor of the ovary with foci of hepatic cell differentiation: a report of four cases and comparison with two cases of granulosa cell tumor with Leydig cells. Am J Surg Pathol 1999;23:1089–93.
2. Andrade LA, Gentilli AL, Polli G. Sclerosing stromal tumor in an accessory ovary. Gynecol Oncol 2001;81:318–19.
3. Bamberger AM, Ivell R, Balvers M, et al. Relaxin-like factor (RLF): a new specific marker for Leydig cells in the ovary. Int J Gynecol Pathol 1999;18:163–8.
4. Baron BW, Schraut WH, Azizi F, Talerman A. Extragonadal sex cord tumor with annular tubules in an umbilical hernia sac: a unique presentation with implications for histogenesis. Gynecol Oncol 1988;30:71–5.
5. Bernasconi D, Del Monte P, Marinaro E, Marugo A, Marugo M. [Severe postmenopausal hyperandrogenism due to an ovarian lipoid cell tumor: a case report]. Minerva Endocrinol 2004;29:25–9.
6. Bianco R, de Rosa G, Staibano S, Somma P, Bianco AR. Ovarian luteinized thecoma with sclerosing peritonitis in an adult woman treated with leuprolide and toremifene in complete remission at 5 years. Gynecol Oncol 2005;96:846–9.
7. Broshears JR, Roth LM. Gynandroblastoma with elements resembling juvenile granulosa cell tumor. Int J Gynecol Pathol 1997;16:387–91.
8. Cao QJ, Jones JG, Li M. Expression of calretinin in human ovary, testis, and ovarian sex cord-stromal tumors. Int J Gynecol Pathol 2001;20:346–52.
9. Caringella A, Loizzi V, Resta L, Ferreri R, Loverro G. A case of Sertoli–Leydig cell tumor in a postmenopausal woman. Int J Gynecol Cancer 2006;16:435–8.
10. Cashell AW, Jerome WG, Flores E. Signet ring stromal tumor of the ovary occurring in conjunction with Brenner tumor. Gynecol Oncol 2000;77:323–6.
11. Cathro HP, Stoler MH. The utility of calretinin, inhibin, and WT1 immunohistochemical staining in the differential diagnosis of ovarian tumors. Hum Pathol 2005;36:195–201.

12. Chan JK, Zhang M, Kaleb V, et al. Prognostic factors responsible for survival in sex cord stromal tumors of the ovary – a multivariate analysis. Gynecol Oncol 2005;96:204–9.

13. Chandran R, Rahman H, Gebbie D. Composite mucinous and granulosa-theca-cell tumour of the ovary: an unusual neoplasm. Aust N Z J Obstet Gynaecol 1993;33:437–9.

14. Chang W, Oiseth SJ, Orentlicher R, Agarwal G, Yahr LJ, Cayten CG. Bilateral sclerosing stromal tumor of the ovaries in a premenarchal girl. Gynecol Oncol 2006;101:342–5.

15. Christman JE, Ballon SC. Ovarian fibrosarcoma associated with Maffucci's syndrome. Gynecol Oncol 1990;37:290–1.

16. Colovic R, Barisic G, Colovic N, Markovic V, Nadj G. Double mucinous cystadenoma of the pancreas associated with thecoma of the ovary. Acta Chir Iugosl 2002;49:95–7.

17. Connolly DC, Katabuchi H, Cliby WA, Cho KR. Somatic mutations in the STK11/LKB1 gene are uncommon in rare gynecological tumor types associated with Peutz–Jeghers syndrome. Am J Pathol 2000;156:339–45.

18. Cserepes E, Szucs N, Patkos P, et al. Ovarian steroid cell tumor and a contralateral ovarian thecoma in a postmenopausal woman with severe hyperandrogenism. Gynecol Endocrinol 2002;16:213–16.

19. Daubenton JD, Sinclair-Smith C. Severe hypercalcemia in association with a juvenile granulosa cell tumor of the ovary. Med Pediatr Oncol 2000;34:301–3.

20. Dickersin GR. The role of electron microscopy in gynecological pathology. Int J Gynecol Pathol 2000;19:56–66.

21. Duska LR, Flynn C, Goodman A. Masculinizing sclerosing stromal cell tumor in pregnancy: report of a case and review of the literature. Eur J Gynaecol Oncol 1998;19:441–3.

22. Farley JH, Taylor RR, Bosscher JR. Late presentation of an alpha-fetoprotein secreting isolated large upper abdominal retroperitoneal Sertoli–Leydig cell tumor recurrence. Gynecol Oncol 1995;56:319–22.

23. Fefferman NR, Pinkney LP, Rivera R, Popiolek D, Hummel-Levine P, Cosme J. Sclerosing stromal tumor of the ovary in a premenarchal female. Pediatr Radiol 2003;33:56–8.

24. Ferry JA, Young RH, Engel G, Scully RE. Oxyphilic Sertoli cell tumor of the ovary: a report of three cases, two in patients with the Peutz–Jeghers syndrome. Int J Gynecol Pathol 1994;13:259–66.

25. Frausto SD, Geisler JP, Fletcher MS, Sood AK. Late recurrence of juvenile granulosa cell tumor of the ovary. Am J Obstet Gynecol 2004;191:366–7.

26. Fukunaga M, Endo Y, Ushigome S. Gynandroblastoma of the ovary: a case report with an immunohistochemical and ultrastructural study. Virchows Arch 1997;430:77–82.

27. Garcia-Galiana S, Monteagudo C, Tortajada M, Llombart A, Cano A. Ovarian sex cord tumor with annular tubules in a woman with premature ovarian failure. Fertil Steril 2001;76:1264–6.

28. Gordon MD, Corless C, Renshaw AA, Beckstead J. CD99, keratin, and vimentin staining of sex cord-stromal tumors, normal ovary, and testis. Mod Pathol 1998;11:769–73.

29. Griffith LM, Carcangiu ML. Sex cord tumor with annular tubules associated with endometriosis of the fallopian tube. Am J Clin Pathol 1991;96:259–62.

30. Guo H, Keefe KA, Kohler MF, Chan JK. Juvenile granulosa cell tumor of the ovary associated with tuberous sclerosis. Gynecol Oncol 2006;102:118–20.

31. Gurbuz A, Karateke A, Kabaca C, Gaziyiz GO, Kir G. Sclerosing stromal cell tumor of the ovary in pregnancy: a case report. Eur J Gynaecol Oncol 2004;25:534–5.

32. Harris AC, Wakely PE, Jr, Kaplowitz PB, Lovinger RD. Steroid cell tumor of the ovary in a child. Arch Pathol Lab Med 1991;115:150–4.

33. Hasiakos D, Papakonstantinou K, Goula K, Karvouni E, Fotiou S. Juvenile granulosa cell tumor associated with pregnancy: report of a case and review of the literature. Gynecol Oncol 2006;100:426–9.

34. Howell CG, Jr, Rogers DA, Gable DS, Falls GD. Bilateral ovarian fibromas in children. J Pediatr Surg 1990;25:690–1.

35. Irving JA, Alkushi A, Young RH, Clement PB. Cellular fibromas of the ovary: a study of 75 cases including 40 mitotically active tumors emphasizing their distinction from fibrosarcoma. Am J Surg Pathol 2006;30:929–38.

36. Ishioka S, Sagae S, Saito T, et al. A case of a sclerosing stromal ovarian tumor that expresses VEGF. J Obstet Gynaecol Res 2000;26:35–8.

37. Kalir T, Friedman F, Jr. Gynandroblastoma in pregnancy: case report and review of literature. Mt Sinai J Med 1998;65:292–5.

38. Kato N, Fukase M, Ono I, Matsumoto K, Okazaki E, Motoyama T. Sertoli-stromal cell tumor of the ovary: immunohistochemical, ultrastructural, and genetic studies. Hum Pathol 2001;32:796–802.

39. Kawauchi S, Tsuji T, Kaku T, Kamura T, Nakano H, Tsuneyoshi M. Sclerosing stromal tumor of the ovary: a clinicopathologic, immunohistochemical, ultrastructural, and cytogenetic analysis with special reference to its vasculature. Am J Surg Pathol 1998;22:83–92.

40. Khiari K, Ben Abdallah N, Cheikhrouhou H, et al. [Virilism during pregnancy]. J Gynecol Obstet Biol Reprod (Paris) 2003;32(3 Pt 1):261–5.

41. Koksal Y, Reisli I, Gunel E, Caliskan U, Bulun A, Kale G. Galactorrhea-associated granulosa cell tumor in a child. Pediatr Hematol Oncol 2004;21:101–6.

42. Kostopoulou E, Talerman A. Ovarian Sertoli–Leydig cell tumor of intermediate differentiation with immature skeletal muscle heterologous elements. Acta Obstet Gynecol Scand 2003;82:197–8.

43. Kriplani A, Agarwal N, Roy KK, Manchanda R, Singh MK. Laparoscopic management of Sertoli–Leydig cell tumors of the ovary. A report of two cases. J Reprod Med 2001;46:493–6.

44. La Marca A, Volpe A. Anti-Mullerian hormone (AMH) in female reproduction: is measurement of circulating AMH a useful tool? Clin Endocrinol 2006;64:603–10.

45. Larizza D, Calcaterra V, Sampaolo P, et al. Unusual presentation of juvenile granulosa cell tumor of the ovary. J Endocrinol Invest 2006;29:653–6.

46. Larsen WG, Felmar EA, Wallace ME, Frieder R. Sertoli–Leydig cell tumor of the ovary: a rare cause of amenorrhea. Obstet Gynecol 1992;79(5 Pt 2):831–3.

47. Lauszus FF, Petersen AC, Greisen J, Jakobsen A. Granulosa cell tumor of the ovary: a population-based study of 37 women with stage I disease. Gynecol Oncol 2001;81:456–60.

48. Lin YS, Eng HL, Jan YJ, et al. Molecular cytogenetics of ovarian granulosa cell tumors by comparative genomic hybridization. Gynecol Oncol 2005;97:68–73.

49. Lugli A, Forster Y, Haas P, et al. Calretinin expression in human normal and neoplastic tissues: a tissue microarray analysis on 5233 tissue samples. Hum Pathol 2003;34:994–1000.

50. Mathur SR, Bhatla N, Rao IS, Singh MK. Sertoli–Leydig cell tumor with heterologous gastrointestinal epithelium: a case report. Indian J Pathol Microbiol 2003;46:91–3.

51. Matias-Guiu X, Pons C, Prat J. Mullerian inhibiting substance, alpha-inhibin, and CD99 expression in sex cord-stromal tumors and endometrioid ovarian carcinomas resembling sex cord-stromal tumors. Hum Pathol 1998;29:840–5.

52. Matseoane S, Moscovic E, Williams S, Huang JC. Mucinous neoplasm in the cervix associated with a mucinous neoplasm in the ovary and concurrent bilateral sex cord tumors with annular tubules: immunohistochemical study. Gynecol Oncol 1991;43:300–4.

53. Mayr D, Kaltz-Wittmer C, Arbogast S, Amann G, Aust DE, Diebold J. Characteristic pattern of genetic aberrations in ovarian granulosa cell tumors. Mod Pathol 2002;15:951–7.

54. McCluggage WG. Ovarian neoplasms composed of small round cells: a review. Adv Anat Pathol 2004;11:288–96.

55. McCluggage WG. Immunoreactivity of ovarian juvenile granulosa cell tumours with epithelial membrane antigen. Histopathology 2005;46:235–6.

56. McCluggage WG, Maxwell P. Immunohistochemical staining for calretinin is useful in the diagnosis of ovarian sex cord-stromal tumours. Histopathology 2001;38:403–8.

57. McCluggage WG, Sloan JM, Murnaghan M, White R. Gynandroblastoma of ovary with juvenile granulosa cell component and heterologous intestinal type glands. Histopathology 1996;29:253–7.

58. McCluggage WG, Sloan JM, Boyle DD, Toner PG. Malignant fibrothecomatous tumour of the ovary: diagnostic value of anti-inhibin immunostaining. J Clin Pathol 1998;51:868–71.

59. McKenna M, Kenny B, Dorman G, McCluggage WG. Combined adult granulosa cell tumor and mucinous cystadenoma of the ovary: granulosa cell tumor with heterologous mucinous elements. Int J Gynecol Pathol 2005;24:224–7.

60. Mooney EE, Nogales FF, Tavassoli FA. Hepatocytic differentiation in retiform Sertoli–Leydig cell tumors: distinguishing a heterologous element from Leydig cells. Hum Pathol 1999;30:611–7.

61. Mooney EE, Vaidya KP, Tavassoli FA. Ossifying well-differentiated Sertoli–Leydig cell tumor of the ovary. Ann Diagn Pathol 2000;4:34–8.

62. Morizane M, Ohara N, Mori T, Murao S. Ossifying luteinized thecoma of the ovary. Arch Gynecol Obstet 2003;267:167–9.

63. Nishida T, Ushijima K, Watanabe J, Kage M, Nagaoka S. Sclerosing peritonitis associated with luteinized thecoma of the ovary. Gynecol Oncol 1999;73:167–9.

64. O'Dowd J, Ismail SM. Juvenile granulosa cell tumour of the ovary containing a nodule of Wilms' tumour. Histopathology 1990;17:468–70.

65. Ordi J, Schammel DP, Rasekh L, Tavassoli FA. Sertoliform endometrioid carcinomas of the ovary: a clinicopathologic and immunohistochemical study of 13 cases. Mod Pathol 1999;12:933–40.

66. Outwater EK, Wagner BJ, Mannion C, McLarney JK, Kim B. Sex cord-stromal and steroid cell tumors of the ovary. Radiographics 1998;18:1523–46.

67. Phadke DM, Weisenberg E, Engel G, Rhone DP. Malignant Sertoli cell tumor of the ovary metastatic to the lung mimicking neuroendocrine carcinoma: report of a case. Ann Diagn Pathol 1999;3:213–19.

68. Podczaski E, Kaminski PF, Pees RC, Singapuri K, Sorosky JI. Peutz–Jeghers syndrome with ovarian sex cord tumor with annular tubules and cervical adenoma malignum. Gynecol Oncol 1991;42:74–8.

69. Price A, Russell P, Elliott P, Bannatyne P. Composite mucinous and granulosa-cell tumor of ovary: case report of a unique neoplasm. Int J Gynecol Pathol 1990;9:372–8.

70. Puls LE, Hamous J, Morrow MS, Schneyer A, MacLaughlin DT, Castracane VD. Recurrent ovarian sex cord tumor with annular tubules: tumor marker and chemotherapy experience. Gynecol Oncol 1994;54:396–401.

71. Raafat F, Klys H, Rylance G. Juvenile granulosa cell tumor. Pediatr Pathol 1990;10:617–23.

72. Regnier C, Bennet A, Malet D, et al. Intraoperative testosterone assay for virilizing ovarian tumor topographic assessment: report of a Leydig cell tumor of the ovary in a premenopausal woman with an adrenal incidentaloma. J Clin Endocrinol Metab 2002;87:3074–7.

73. Rey R, Sabourin JC, Venara M, et al. Anti-Mullerian hormone is a specific marker of sertoli- and granulosa-cell origin in gonadal tumors. Hum Pathol 2000;31:1202–8.
74. Rishi M, Howard LN, Bratthauer GL, Tavassoli FA. Use of monoclonal antibody against human inhibin as a marker for sex cord-stromal tumors of the ovary. Am J Surg Pathol 1997;21:583–9.
75. Robertson DM, Burger HG, Fuller PJ. Inhibin/activin and ovarian cancer. Endocr Relat Cancer 2004;11:35–49.
76. Roth LM, Davis MM, Sutton GP. Steroid cell tumor of the broad ligament arising in an accessory ovary. Arch Pathol Lab Med 1996;120:405–9.
77. Ryan JJ, Rezkalla MA, Rizk SN, Peterson KG, Wiebe RH. Testosterone-secreting adrenal adenoma that contained crystalloids of Reinke in an adult female patient. Mayo Clin Proc 1995;70:380–3.
78. Santala M, Suvanto-Luukkonen E, Kyllonen A, Ruokonen A, Puistola U. Hyperprolactinemia complicating juvenile granulosa cell tumor of the ovary. Gynecol Oncol 2001;82:389–91.
79. Savage P, Constenla D, Fisher C, et al. Granulosa cell tumours of the ovary: demographics, survival and the management of advanced disease. Clin Oncol (R Coll Radiol) 1998;10:242–5.
80. Sawetawan C, Rainey WE, Word RA, Carr BR. Immunohistochemical and biochemical analysis of a human Sertoli–Leydig cell tumor: autonomous steroid production characteristic of ovarian theca cells. J Soc Gynecol Investig 1995;2:30–7.
81. Sayegh RA, DeLellis R, Alroy J, Lechan R, Ball HG. Masculinizing granulosa cell tumor of the ovary in a postmenopausal woman. A case report. J Reprod Med 1999;44:821–5.
82. Schumer ST, Cannistra SA. Granulosa cell tumor of the ovary. J Clin Oncol 2003;21:1180–9.
83. Sehouli J, Drescher FS, Mustea A, et al. Granulosa cell tumor of the ovary: 10 years follow-up data of 65 patients. Anticancer Res 2004;24(2C):1223–9.
84. Seidman JD, Abbondanzo SL, Bratthauer GL. Lipid cell (steroid cell) tumor of the ovary: immunophenotype with analysis of potential pitfall due to endogenous biotin-like activity. Int J Gynecol Pathol 1995;14:331–8.
85. Shen K, Wu PC, Lang JH, Huang RL, Tang MT, Lian LJ. Ovarian sex cord tumor with annular tubules: a report of six cases. Gynecol Oncol 1993;48:180–4.
86. Smith D, Crotty TB, Murphy JF, Crofton ME, Franks S, McKenna TJ. A steroid cell tumor outside the ovary is a rare cause of virilization. Fertil Steril 2006;85:227.
87. Song SH, Lee JK, Saw HS, et al. Peutz–Jeghers syndrome with multiple genital tract tumors and breast cancer: a case report with a review of literature. J Korean Med Sci 2006;21:752–7.
88. Spinelli C, Gadducci A, Bonadio AG, Berti P, Miccoli P. Benign ovarian fibroma associated with free peritoneal fluid and elevated serum CA 125 levels. Minerva Ginecol 1999;51:403–7.
89. Spremovic-Radjenovic S, Radosavljevic A, Petkovic S, et al. [The polycystic ovary syndrome associated with ovarian tumor]. Srp Arh Celok Lek 1997;125:375–7.
90. Stewart CJ, Jeffers MD, Kennedy A. Diagnostic value of inhibin immunoreactivity in ovarian gonadal stromal tumours and their histological mimics. Histopathology 1997;31:67–74.
91. Stuart GC, Dawson LM. Update on granulosa cell tumours of the ovary. Curr Opin Obstet Gynecol 2003;15:33–7.
92. Stylianidou A, Varras M, Akrivis C, Fylaktidou A, Stefanaki S, Antoniou N. Sclerosing stromal tumor of the ovary: a case report and review of the literature. Eur J Gynaecol Oncol 2001;22:300–4.
93. Takeshima Y, Inai K. Ovarian sex cord tumor with annular tubules – a case report and review of the literature in Japanese. Hiroshima J Med Sci 1992;41:37–42.
94. Takeuchi S, Ishihara N, Ohbayashi C, Itoh H, Maruo T. Stromal Leydig cell tumor of the ovary. Case report and literature review. Int J Gynecol Pathol 1999;18:178–82.
95. Talerman A. Gynandroblastoma with elements of juvenile granulosa cell tumor. Int J Gynecol Pathol 1998;17:190.
96. Talmon GA, Persidskii I, Gulizia JA. A cystic mass in a young woman with presumed polycystic ovarian syndrome. Gynandroblastoma. Arch Pathol Lab Med 2006;130:225–6.
97. Tanyi J, Rigo J, Jr, Csapo Z, Szentirmay Z. Trisomy 12 in juvenile granulosa cell tumor of the ovary during pregnancy. A report of two cases. J Reprod Med 1999;44:826–32.
98. Tiltman AJ, Haffajee Z. Sclerosing stromal tumors, thecomas, and fibromas of the ovary: an immunohistochemical profile. Int J Gynecol Pathol 1999;18:254–8.
99. Tsuji T, Kawauchi S, Utsunomiya T, Nagata Y, Tsuneyoshi M. Fibrosarcoma versus cellular fibroma of the ovary: a comparative study of their proliferative activity and chromosome aberrations using MIB-1 immunostaining, DNA flow cytometry, and fluorescence in situ hybridization. Am J Surg Pathol 1997;21:52–9.
100. Unkila-Kallio L, Leminen A, Tiitinen A, Ylikorkala O. Nationwide data on falling incidence of ovarian granulosa cell tumours concomitant with increasing use of ovulation inducers. Hum Reprod 1998;13:2828–30.
101. Uygun K, Aydiner A, Saip P, et al. Granulosa cell tumor of the ovary: retrospective analysis of 45 cases. Am J Clin Oncol 2003;26:517–21.
102. Vang R, Herrmann ME, Tavassoli FA. Comparative immunohistochemical analysis of granulosa and sertoli components in ovarian sex cord-stromal tumors with mixed differentiation: potential implications for derivation of sertoli differentiation in ovarian tumors. Int J Gynecol Pathol 2004;23:151–61.
103. Watson B, Siegel CL, Ylagan LR. Metastatic ovarian Sertoli-cell tumor: FNA findings with immunohistochemistry. Diagn Cytopathol 2003;29:283–6.
104. Willemsen W, Kruitwagen R, Bastiaans B, Hanselaar T, Rolland R. Ovarian stimulation and granulosa-cell tumour. Lancet 1993;341:986–8.
105. Wu L, Zhang W, Li H, Li L, Kong W, Liu L. [Clinical analysis of 74 cases with ovarian thecoma]. Zhonghua Fu Chan Ke Za Zhi 2002;37:101–3.
106. Yamada Y, Ohmi K, Tsunematu R, et al. Gynandroblastoma of the ovary having a typical morphological appearance: a case study. Jpn J Clin Oncol 1991;21:62–8.
107. Young RH. Sex cord-stromal tumors of the ovary and testis: their similarities and differences with consideration of selected problems. Mod Pathol 2005;18(Suppl 2):S81–98.
108. Young RH, Welch WR, Dickersin GR, Scully RE. Ovarian sex cord tumor with annular tubules: review of 74 cases including 27 with Peutz–Jeghers syndrome and four with adenoma malignum of the cervix. Cancer 1982;50:1384–402.
109. Zamecnik M. Calcifying sclerosing tumor of the ovary: a late stage of sclerosing stromal tumor? Cesk Patol 2002;38:121–4.
110. Zhang M, Cheung MK, Shin JY, et al. Prognostic factors responsible for survival in sex cord stromal tumors of the ovary – an analysis of 376 women. Gynecol Oncol 2007;104:396–400.
111. Zheng W, Sung CJ, Hanna I, et al. Alpha and beta subunits of inhibin/activin as sex cord-stromal differentiation markers. Int J Gynecol Pathol 1997;16:263–71.

Ovarian germ cell tumors

Peter Russell   Stanley J. Robboy   Jaime Prat

27

DYSGERMINOMAS

Definition and cell types

Dysgerminomas, thought to arise from premeiotic oogonia, consist entirely of sheets of large uniform pale cells that have the phenotype of primordial germ cells and can be activated to express pluripotential capacity. While once thought to be terminally differentiated, dysgerminoma cells are now believed to be pluripotential, as recently evidenced by their consistent elaboration of OCT4, a POU-domain transcription factor (also known as OCT3, OTF3, and POU5F1). This factor, encoded by the *POU5F1* gene, located on chromosome 6p21.3, helps regulate pluripotential capacity during normal development and is detectable in embryonic stem and germ cells. Of ovarian germ cell neoplasms, it is detected in dysgerminomas and embryonal carcinomas only.[14,29,69,104]

Tumor cells have abundant pale, slightly granular eosinophilic to clear cytoplasm, and exhibit well-delineated cell boundaries and a large central vesicular nucleus. The cytoplasm contains variable amounts of glycogen demonstrable by the periodic acid-Schiff (PAS) reaction; cytoplasmic lipid can also be demonstrated in frozen sections. Nuclei are oval to round with finely granular chromatin and usually a single prominent eosinophilic nucleolus (Figure 27.1).

Clinical profile

Dysgerminomas are infrequently encountered neoplasms and, when pure, comprise only about 1% of all primary ovarian malignant tumors, about 1–2% of all ovarian germ cell tumors, and something over 25% of malignant ovarian germ cell tumors.[85] They may present at any age from infancy to old age but are rare under 5 years of age and after the menopause. Most cases occur in the second and third decades with 80–85% of patients aged under 30 years. Familial clustering is rarely documented.[3,61] Rare cases have been associated with Downs syndrome and a genetic relationship suggested.[158] Molecular studies of sporadic cases commonly reveals a chromosome 12p abnormality.[39]

The presenting symptoms resemble those observed in patients with other ovarian neoplasms, though often of shorter duration. If they complicate pregnancy, the association compromises neither tumor prognosis nor fetal outcome.[16] Some have bizarre presentations, such as with paraneoplastic granulomatous nephritis.[79]

Infrequently, they are found incidentally, such as during investigation for primary amenorrhea. In these latter 3–5% of cases, some form of gonadal dysgenesis is often found associated with a karyotype containing a Y chromosome. In such patients, the resulting dysgerminoma is commonly a small tumor and almost invariably supervenes upon a gonadoblastoma.

Dysgerminomas are fast growing tumors, but metastases do not commonly occur early in the clinical course. They are confined to the ovaries (FIGO stage 1) in two-thirds of cases,[12] of which bilateral examples account for 15%. This latter figure includes 6% in which contralateral ovarian involvement is only microscopic and may be a second primary lesion, underpinning the importance of biopsy examination of both ovaries in patients for whom conservative surgery is planned (see below). Unilateral tumors show a slight tendency to be right-sided. Lymphatic spread affects first the common iliac and lowermost para-aortic groups of nodes, and subsequently the mediastinal and supraclavicular nodes. Blood-borne spread to distant organs typically occurs late, with liver, lungs, kidneys, and bones the most common sites for secondary deposits.

Macroscopic features

Dysgerminomas are almost always firm solid tumors with rounded or bosselated contours (Figure 27.2) and smooth gray-white external surfaces featuring prominent vessels. They vary in size up to large masses weighing over 5 kg, with a median diameter of 15 cm. Large lesions particularly may be associated with inflammatory adhesions to the surrounding structures due to torsion, or the tumor capsule may be ruptured or invaded, leading to local tumor adhesions and intraperitoneal spread. The cut surface is characteristically featureless (Figure 27.2) and, in the fresh state, is gray-pink to cream in color. Hemorrhage or necrosis may be seen, especially in large tumors, and may occasionally produce cysts. Grossly visible calcification is only seen in dysgerminomas arising from a gonadoblastoma. Our examination of dysgerminomas routinely includes a specimen radiograph as an aid to location of focal calcification.

Microscopic features

Typical dysgerminomas consist of aggregates, islands or cords of large (15–25 μm in diameter), uniform, polyhedral cells separated by varying numbers of delicate connective tissue septa containing lymphocytes (Figure 27.3). Mitotic activity varies from area to area within individual tumors. Conspicuous uniformity of cell and nuclear size and appearance is a hallmark of dysgerminomas (Figure 27.4), although isolated large or giant cells may be seen – either histiocytic or, in 3% of cases, single or small aggregates of syncytiotrophoblastic cells. These latter cells (Figure 27.5A), while secreting beta-human chorionic gonadotrophin (β-hCG) and human placental lactogen (hPL), are not foci of choriocarcinoma, differing in both the

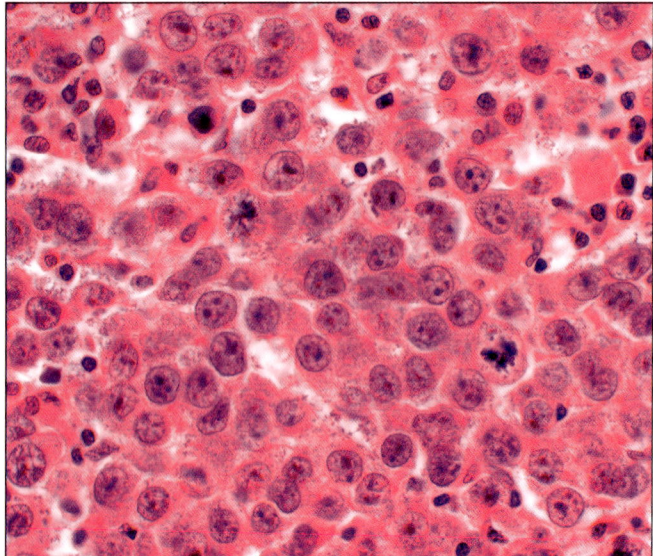

Fig. 27.1 Cellular detail of dysgerminomas. Tumor cells are large (note plasma cell at top right for comparison) with round-to-slightly angular vesicular nuclei, prominent nucleoli, granular cytoplasm with often indistinct cell borders.

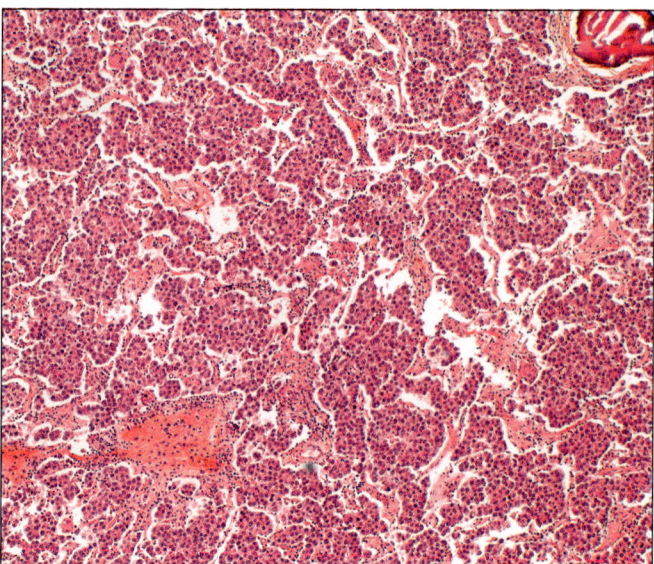

Fig. 27.3 Architectural arrangement of dysgerminomas. Cords, nests or nodules of uniform tumor cells are separated by fine connective tissue septa containing lymphocytes. Rare circumscribed foci of calcification (top right) may be seen in the absence of a pre-existing gonadoblastoma.

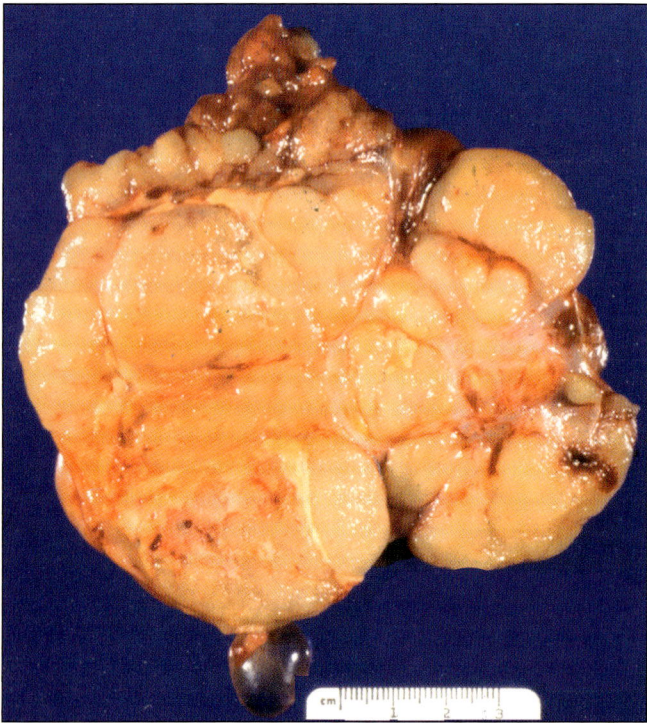

Fig. 27.2 Dysgerminoma. A typical, solid, bosselated tumor with a uniform, pale, cut surface. Focal necrosis is noted in the lower left of the tumor.

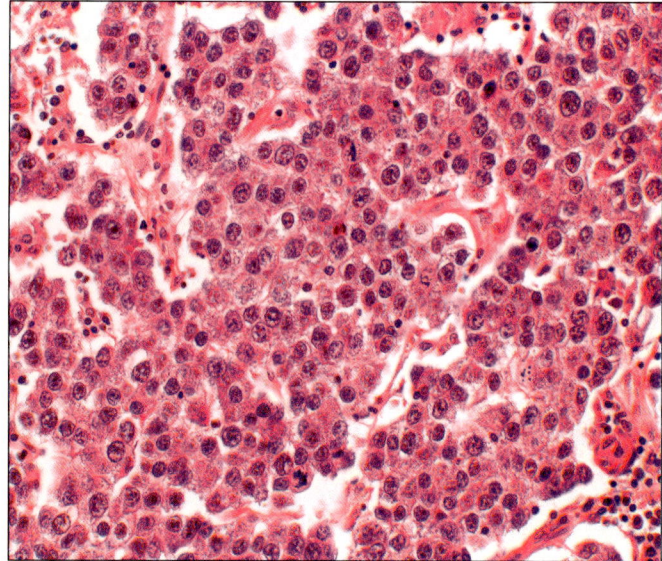

Fig. 27.4 Cellular uniformity is a cardinal histologic feature of dysgerminomas.

complete absence of any cytotrophoblastic element and the poor prognosis of a choriocarcinoma. The immunophenotype of ovarian dysgerminomas is seen in Table 27.1. Clusters of luteinized stromal cells (Figure 27.5B) and luteinized follicles may sometimes be found in the ovarian parenchyma adjacent to the tumor nodules. Rarely, pure dysgerminomas are associated with raised β-hCG levels in the absence of demonstrable syncytiotrophoblast-like cells.

The stromal network usually consists of loose edematous connective tissue in delicate strands but may be quite dense and hyalinized (Figure 27.6A). It may be a dominant component, leading to the wide separation of islands of dysgerminoma cells (Figure 27.6B). It is almost always infiltrated by lymphocytes (Figure 27.3) that are predominantly of T-cell lineage.[48,167] Less commonly histiocytes, eosinophils, and plasma cells (Figure 27.1) may be identified. The lymphocytic infiltration varies from slight to dense and may include lymphoid follicles with germinal centers. The histiocytic component, when prominent, has a granulomatous appearance, ranging from ill-defined aggregates of histiocytes (Figure 27.7A) to well-formed palisaded granulomas (Figure 27.7B) with histiocytic giant cells and a cuff of small lymphocytes (20% of lesions).

Focal necrosis and hemorrhage are common and, in large tumors, may be prominent. Small deposits of dystrophic spiculate calcification (Figure 27.3) are occasionally seen in dysgerminomas in association with necrosis, hemorrhage, fibrosis, or hyalinization. More obvious and more rounded foci of calcification are found in dysgerminomas that arise from gonadoblastoma. Aberrant or dysgenetic follicles may be found at the periphery of dysgerminomas in karyotypically normal females (Figure 27.8) and these should not be mistaken for gonadoblastoma nests. Other uncommonly encountered phenomena include the invasion by dysgerminoma cells of entrapped developing follicles (Figure 27.9).

Cellular tumors with minimal stroma, vascular invasion, only slight lymphocytic infiltration, marked nuclear pleomorphism, and a high mitotic rate (>3 mitotic figures per high-power field) generally are termed 'anaplastic dysgerminomas' and are more aggressive. However, in view of the inconstancy of these findings and the marked histologic variations within

the same tumor, there is no general agreement that the behavior of individual tumors can be assessed from their histologic appearances. Vascular invasion and capsular penetration may adversely alter prognosis, but it is uncertain whether these variables are independent of stage (see below).

Metastatic deposits generally exhibit the same histologic features as the primary tumors (Figure 27.10). Occasionally, apparently pure dysgerminomas are associated with metastases composed of other neoplastic germ cell elements, stressing the importance of adequate sampling of such tumors (see Chapter 35). In contralateral ovaries, microscopic 'metastases' usually take the form of small cords or individual dysgerminoma cells infiltrating between normal ovarian cortical structures (Figure 27.11).

Differential diagnosis

About 15% of ovarian 'dysgerminomas' contain obvious malignant germ cell elements of other types (e.g., choriocarcinoma, yolk sac tumor, immature teratoma). These tumors are classified as malignant mixed germ cell tumors and are discussed later in this chapter.

Few tumors are mistaken for typical dysgerminomas, particularly in young patients in whom there is a raised level of suspicion of malignant germ cell tumor. However, other malignant germ cell tumors (especially embryonal carcinoma), malignant stromal tumors (juvenile granulosa cell tumor), and metastatic neoplasms (diffuse large cell lymphoma and malignant melanoma) may cause problems.

Embryonal carcinomas are rare and biologically aggressive tumors that occur in young females. Unlike dysgerminomas, most present with hormonal manifestations (precocious puberty, abnormal vaginal bleeding). Microscopically, the large tumor cells have large vesicular nuclei containing one or more prominent nucleoli. These nuclei tend to be more pleomorphic and hyperchromatic than those of dysgerminoma cells, and the cell cytoplasm is copious and amphophilic to eosinophilic rather than clear (Table 27.2). Transitional patterns between dysgerminomas and embryonal carcinoma have been observed.[137] Embryonal carcinoma cells may be orien-

Table 27.1 Immunoprofile of dysgerminomas

Antibody against	Expression
Lactate dehydrogenase	100%
Placental alkaline phosphatase	100%
OCT4 (POU5F1)	100%
CD117 (c-kit)	87%
Neuron-specific enolase (NSE)	75%
AE1/AE3	10%
β-Human chorionic gonadotrophin	5%
Epithelial membrane antigen (EMA)	–
S-100 protein	–
Leukocyte common antigen (LCA)	–
Vimentin	–
α-Fetoprotein	–

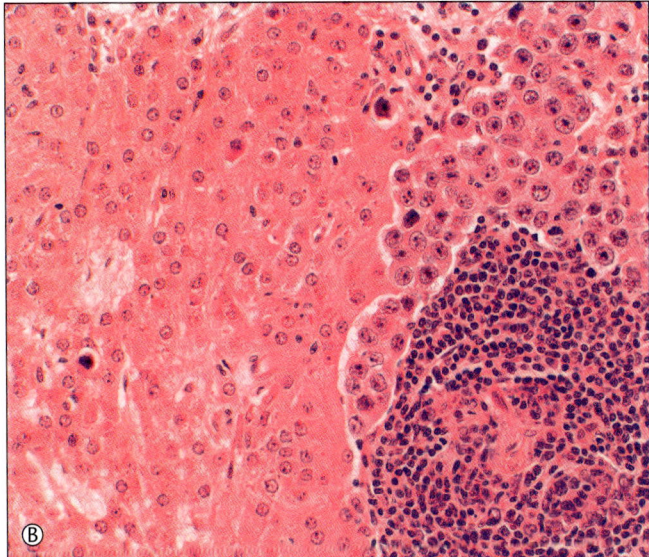

Fig. 27.5 Dysgerminoma. **(A)** Large multinucleated syncytiotrophoblast-like cell (center) in an otherwise typical dysgerminoma. **(B)** Same tumor showing an irregular island of well-luteinized stromal cells (left half). Contrast with dysgerminoma cells in right half.

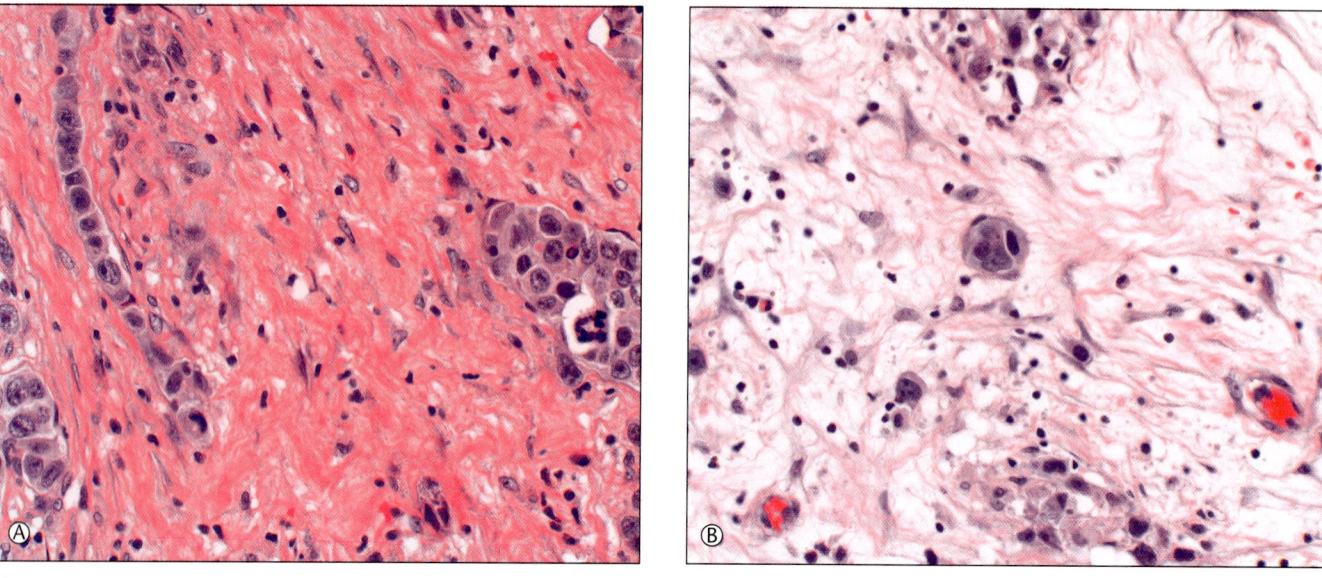

Fig. 27.6 Dysgerminoma. **(A)** Dense fibrocollagenous or **(B)** loose myxoid stroma separates cords of dysgerminoma cells with large hyperchromatic nuclei.

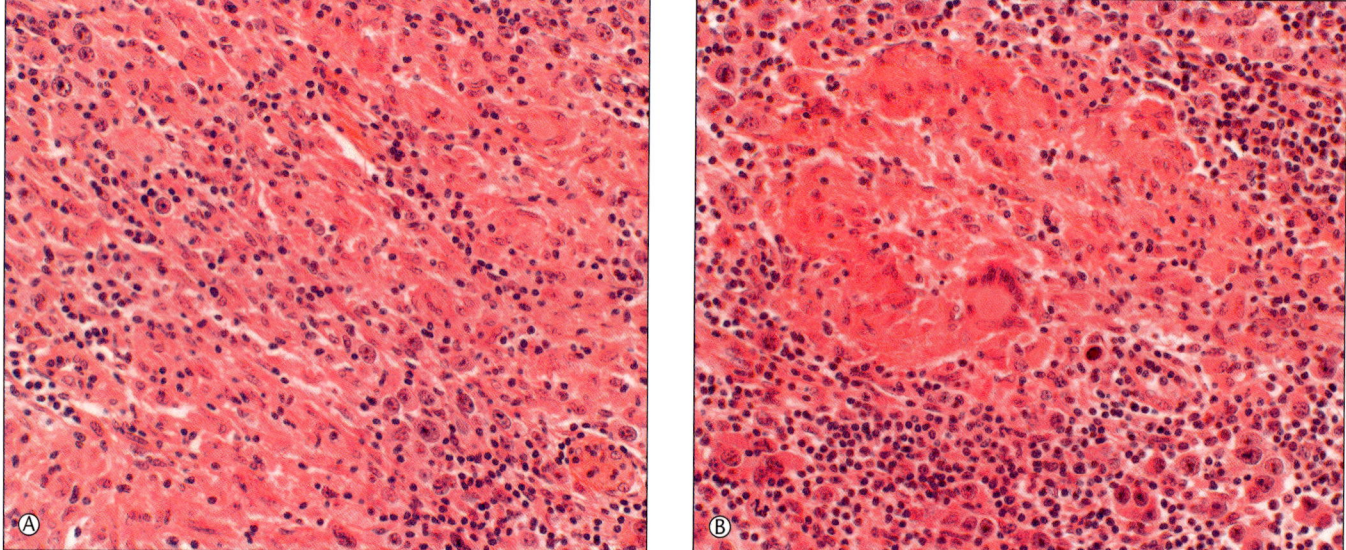

Fig. 27.7 Dysgerminoma. Histiocytic stromal infiltrates ranging from **(A)** marked and diffuse with a few residual tumor cells to **(B)** focal and granuloma-like aggregates with a cuff of lymphocytes.

tated around gland-like clefts, giving them an epithelioid appearance (many such cells produce α-fetoprotein, AFP), or may produce areas more closely resembling primitive mesenchyme. Both features are absent from dysgerminomas. Syncytiotrophoblastic giant cells that produce β-hCG (demonstrated immunohistochemically) are also often seen, whilst these are only rarely seen in dysgerminomas. Strong reactivity to cytokeratins in tumor cells of embryonal carcinomas is in contrast to the weak, scanty staining in 10% of dysgerminomas.

Juvenile granulosa cell tumors also occur at this age and histologically have a predominantly diffuse pattern of large polyhedral cells with rounded vesicular nuclei containing a relative prominent nucleolus. However, there are usually poorly formed follicular structures not seen in dysgerminomas, and the cells have eosinophilic granular cytoplasm (often luteinized) rather than clear cytoplasm containing abundant glycogen. Neither the connective tissue septa containing lymphocytes

nor histiocytic granulomas are present in juvenile granulosa cell tumors and these features aid in distinguishing between these two entities.

Malignant diffuse large cell lymphomas (see Chapter 28) may present as ovarian tumors, although rarely in young women, and, in their monotonous architecture, give rise to some uncertainty. One particular subtype that causes difficulty is the immunoblastic sarcoma, where the lymphoma cells have pale-to-clear cytoplasm and a large nucleolus. However, ovarian lymphomas are commonly (50%) bilateral (see Table 28.5). The lymphoma cells lack glycogen and have indistinct cell borders. Lymphoma cells of large B-cell type may show cytoplasmic positivity with methyl green pyronin (not seen in dysgerminoma cells). On closer examination, there may also be an admixture of smaller lymphoid cells, and the large lymphoma cells may have reniform or convoluted nuclei quite different from the rounded pale vesicular nuclei of uniform

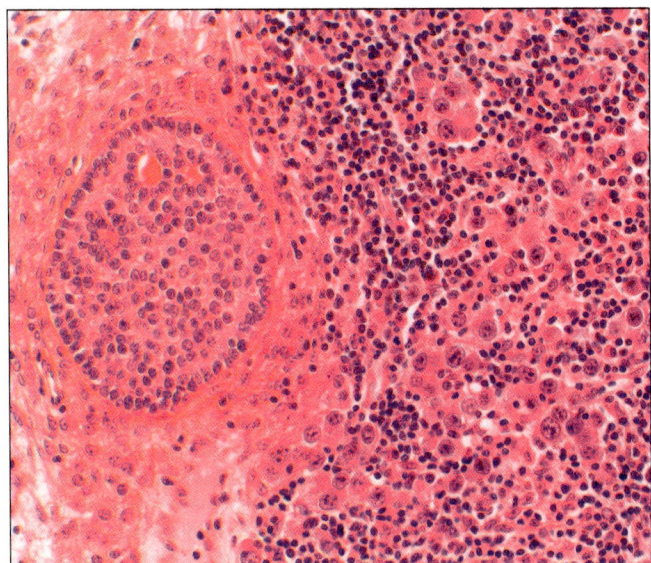

Fig. 27.8 A dysplastic or dysgenetic follicle at the margin of a dysgerminoma. The patient was a karyotypically normal female.

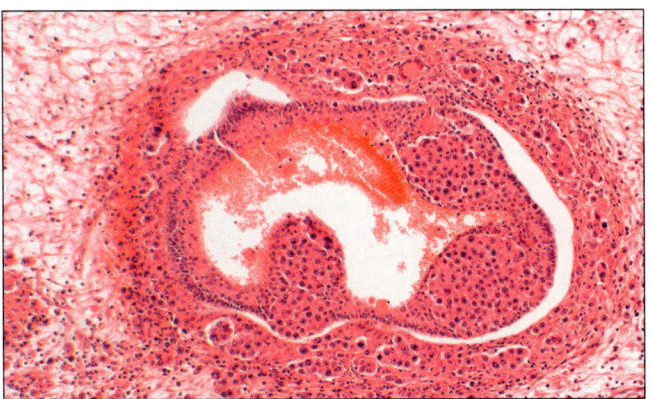

Fig. 27.9 Unusual pattern of infiltration by dysgerminoma cells. The granulosa of a developing follicle has been invaded from without.

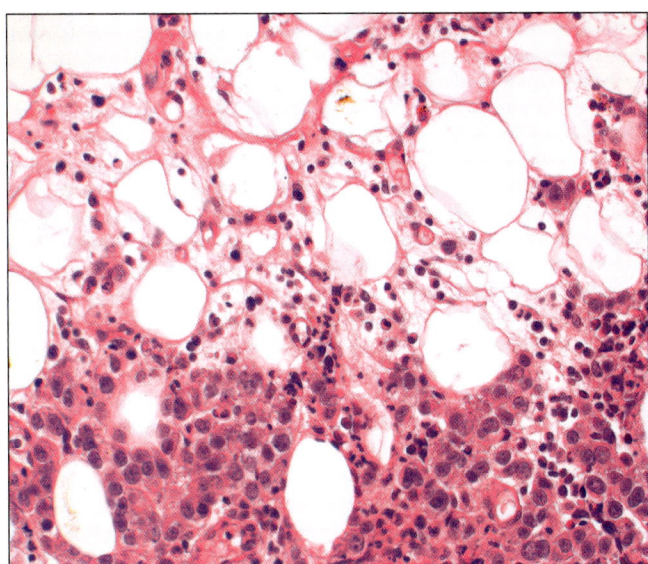

Fig. 27.10 Metastatic dysgerminoma in omentum. The character of the primary tumor, including the lymphocytic infiltrate, is recapitulated in the secondary deposit.

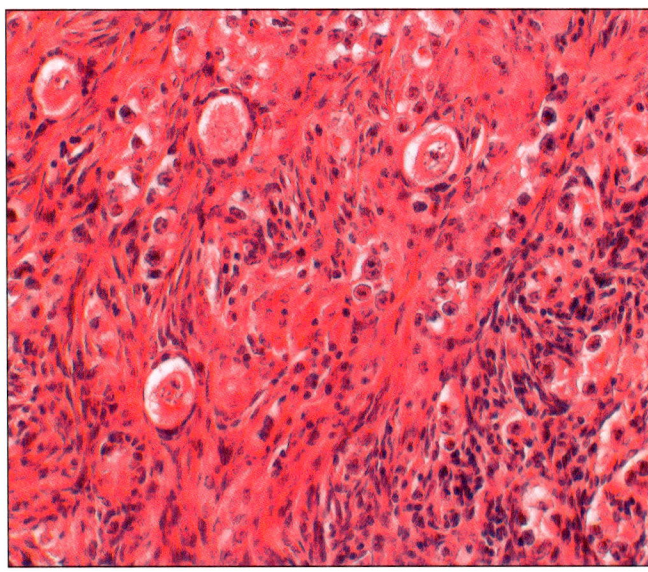

Fig. 27.11 Dysgerminoma. Microscopic tumor in a normal-sized ovary from a patient with a large contralateral ovarian mass. Note residual primordial follicles.

Table 27.2 Dysgerminoma versus embryonal carcinoma: differential diagnosis

Dysgerminoma	Embryonal carcinoma
Clinical	
Bilateral in 15% of cases	Essentially always unilateral
Hormonal manifestations rare	Hormonal manifestations in 60%
Histologic	
Uniformity of cell type and architecture	Variability from area to area; epithelial and mesenchyme-like areas
Stroma contains lymphocytes and often histiocytic granulomas	Scattered lymphocytes; no granulomas
Syncytiotrophoblast-like giant cells in 3%	Syncytiotrophoblast-like giant cells common
Immunohistochemical	
α-Fetoprotein negative, mostly cytokeratin negative	α-Fetoprotein positive, cytokeratin positive

sized dysgerminoma cells. Reactivity to leukocyte common antigen (LCA) and either T-cell or B-cell surface markers, as well as the absence of POU5F1 in the lymphoma cells should complete the differentiation.

Finally, metastatic amelanotic malignant melanomas may masquerade as primary ovarian cancer in young women and, in one of its many guises, can be readily mistaken for dysgerminoma. Melanoma cells, however, tend to have eosinophilic rather than pale or clear cytoplasm, indistinct cell borders and usually an 'acantholytic' appearance. The diagnosis can almost always be confirmed by reactivity to S-100 protein, HMB45 and tyrosinase, and by an appeal for relevant clinical information.

Treatment and prognosis

Rigorously defined FIGO stage at laparotomy and size of tumor are the most important prognostic indicators. Dysger-

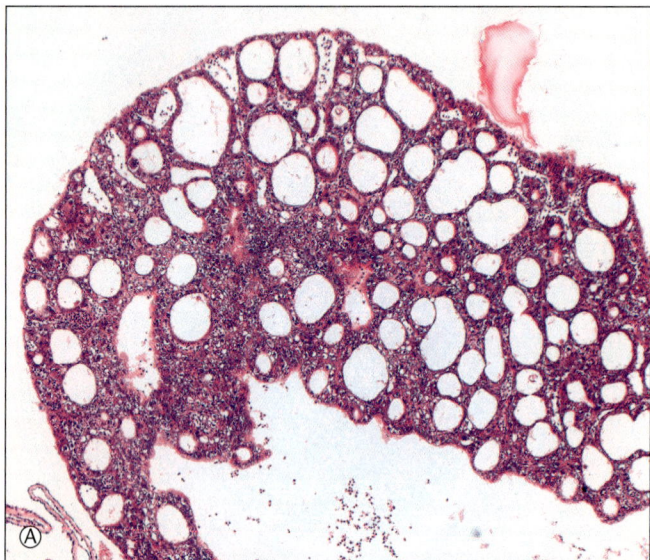
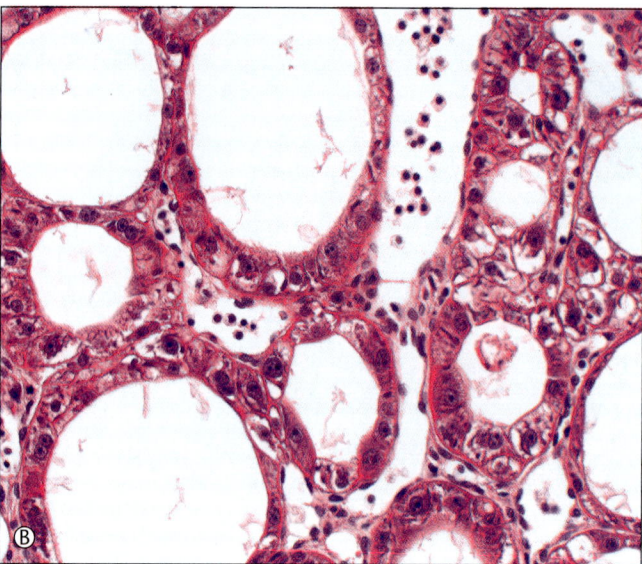

Fig. 27.12 Well-developed yolk sac of an early human embryo (9 weeks amenorrhea). **(A)** Low power showing coarse cribriform arrangement of endodermal spaces. **(B)** High power of large cuboidal endodermal cells lining variably sized spaces. Note the nucleated red blood cells in the rich vascular network between these spaces.

minomas are associated with an overall 5-year survival rate of 80–90%,[12,85] while survival of patients with 'encapsulated' stage 1A tumors (i.e., the tumor capsules are not invaded by dysgerminoma cells) is over 95%, despite a significant (about 25%) recurrence rate, and 60% for patients with spread beyond the ovaries. Over 75% of recurrences occur in the first year after diagnosis. Age below 20 years or above 40 years is also an adverse prognostic sign.

Conservative therapy (unilateral salpingo-oophorectomy) is appropriate for the two-thirds of patients who are karyotypically normal young women with an encapsulated unilateral tumor, for whom retention of fertility is important, and in whom a thorough staging laparotomy reveals no other evidence of tumor.[25,109] This staging procedure includes washings of the peritoneal cavity and biopsy of retroperitoneal nodes and particularly the contralateral ovary (as 10% will show occult involvement). Sustained remission following conservative surgery alone for stage 1A disease is high,[110] and careful follow-up of the patients – utilizing serum lactic dehydrogenase and its isoenzymes, placental-like alkaline phosphatase (PLAP), and β-hCG as tumor markers – allows BEP (bleomycin, etoposide and cisplatin) chemotherapy of any metastases or recurrences with near 100% survival.[20] Other patients with bilateral or extraovarian disease or for whom fertility is not an issue are treated by hysterectomy and bilateral salpingo-oophorectomy followed by chemotherapy with cure rates approaching 90%.

YOLK SAC TUMORS (ENDODERMAL SINUS TUMORS)

Definition

Yolk sac tumors show preferential differentiation toward yolk sac or vitelline structures. Given that the human yolk sac (Figure 27.12) is directly contiguous with the primitive gut in early embryonic development, these two structures are frequently referred to as primary and secondary yolk sac vesicles, respectively. The 'polyvesicular vitelline tumor' (see below) is

thought to represent structurally the transition from the larger primary to the smaller secondary yolk sac and is thus included amongst variants of yolk sac or endodermal sinus tumor. This relationship with primordial gut structures is supported by the ultrastructural demonstration in yolk sac tumors of cells resembling gut epithelium with Paneth cells, gastric parietal cells and hepatocytes. More pronounced hepatic differentiation may lead to the so-called 'hepatoid yolk sac tumor' in which densely eosinophilic tumor cells resemble those seen in hepatocellular carcinoma.

During fetal life, AFP is produced by the yolk sac, liver, and upper gastrointestinal tract. In addition, the human yolk sac produces other proteins (e.g., α_1-antitrypsin), the focal presence of which has been shown by immunohistochemical techniques within many, but not all, yolk sac tumors (Table 27.3).

Clinical profile

Pure yolk sac tumors are uncommon ovarian neoplasms, their frequency being half that of dysgerminomas. They may rarely arise outside the normally sited gonads.[44,59] The age distribution of patients at presentation ranges from infancy to the seventh decade,[90] but almost all occur before 30 years of age (median age 18 years). Isolated ovarian examples have been found in elderly patients associated with ovarian epithelial–stromal tumors and presumably arise from the latter by genetic de-repression and tumor transformation.[106,131]

The presenting symptoms are usually abdominal enlargement and pain of short duration (1 week or less in half of cases). Torsion or rupture of the tumor with acute pain may cause the patient to present as an abdominal emergency. Raised serum levels of AFP (>20 ng/mL) are routinely found and this is a useful, although not pathognomonic, serologic marker for the presence of yolk sac tumor elements in a primary ovarian neoplasm, its metastases and/or recurrences.

As AFP has a biologic half-life of about 5 days, blood levels assayed in the immediate postoperative period (i.e., after diagnosis has been made histologically) may still be useful in estab-

Table 27.3 Immunoprofile of yolk sac tumors	
Antibody against	**Expression**
AE1/AE3	100%
CAM 5.2	100%
CD10	100%
α-Fetoprotein	80%
Leu-M1 (CD15)	60%
Placental alkaline phosphatase	45%
α₁-Antitrypsin	45%
Vimentin	25%
CD117 (c-kit)	20%
OCT4 (POU5F1)	–
β-Human chorionic gonadotrophin	–
Epithelial membrane antigen (EMA)	–
S-100 protein	–
CK7	–

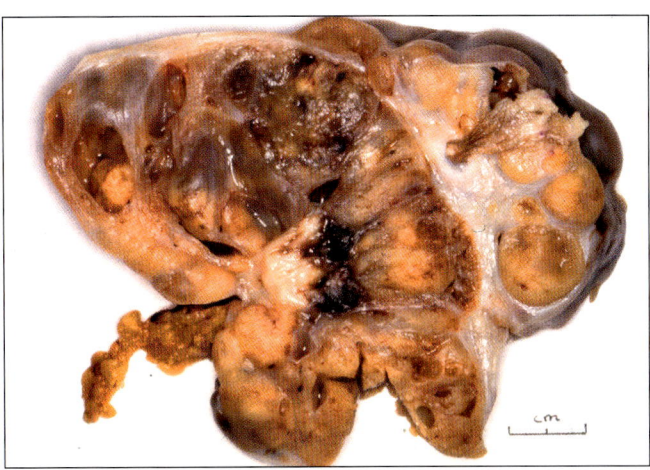

Fig. 27.13 Variegated cut surface of a large, partly solid yolk sac tumor.

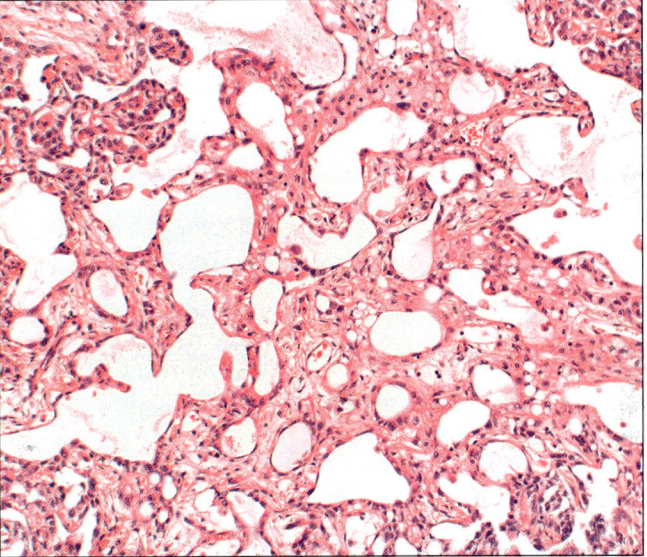

Fig. 27.14 Yolk sac tumor. Reticular pattern with variably sized cystic spaces lined by attenuated epithelial cells.

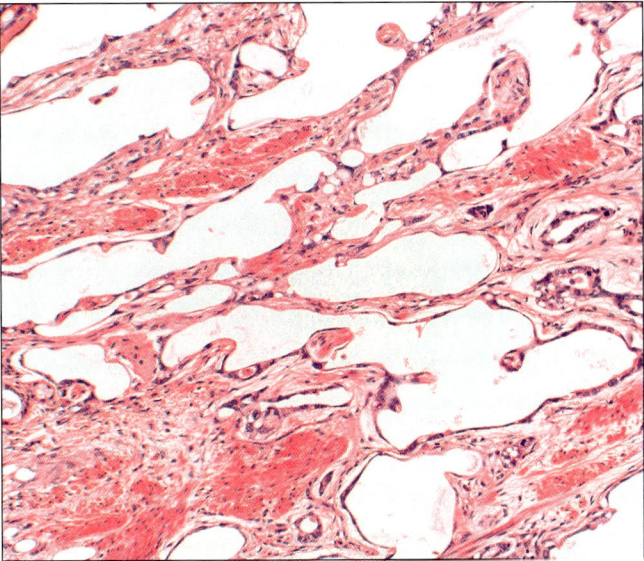

Fig. 27.15 Yolk sac tumor. Reticular pattern with branching and anastomosing channels lined by attenuated and cuboidal epithelial cells. Transitions between these and polyvesicular vitelline patterns may be seen.

lishing baseline values. In the absence of residual disease, the postoperative serum AFP level falls to normal in 4–6 weeks. An increase in serum AFP heralds the onset of recurrent disease, often prior to other clinical evidence.[83] Occasional cases also present during pregnancy, with attendant difficulties in determining the contributions to the serum AFP levels attributable to the pregnancy and to the tumor.[7] Serum β-hCG is not elevated in patients with pure yolk sac tumors.

Macroscopic features

Pure yolk sac tumors are virtually always unilateral, showing a slight predilection for the right ovary. They are usually large, friable, bosselated masses, with the majority being over 15 cm in diameter and occasionally weighing up to 5 kg. Rupture before or during operation occurs in a third of cases. A solid, variegated, gray-yellow cut surface with areas of hemorrhage, necrosis, and cystic or 'myxoid' degeneration is characteristic (Figure 27.13). The fluid present in these cystic areas tends to be clear and gelatinous in consistency.

Microscopic features

Yolk sac tumors exhibit several distinctive patterns and, although all or most can be readily identified in most tumors (if sufficient blocks are taken), one or two usually predominate.

The 'reticular', microcystic or myxomatous pattern is the most frequently encountered. In this, loose vacuolated honeycombed networks of variably sized cystic spaces (Figure 27.14) or channels (Figure 27.15) are lined by flattened, pleomorphic cells, with large hyperchromatic or vesicular nuclei (with one or more prominent nucleoli), the size of the cystic spaces seeming to increase with progressive distance from the dilated nutrient vessels of the tumor. Mitoses, although obvious, are less numerous than in areas of yolk sac tumor showing other histologic patterns. Extramedullary erythropoiesis may be noted in the reticular areas of some tumors, possibly reflecting this role of the yolk sac in early embryonic life. The cystic spaces and channels may contain pale, proteinaceous, PAS-positive material, or small, rounded, brightly eosinophilic hyaline droplets that are PAS positive and diastase resistant. These hyaline bodies, found also within the cytoplasm of many tumor cells, may be numerous and prominent in some yolk sac tumors and are found in areas exhibiting any of the histologic patterns described below. They are thought to be elaborated by tumor cells and accumulate intracytoplasmically, and are thence discharged into the surrounding tissue upon rupture of the cells. These droplets contain AFP and α_1-antitrypsin.

Focal areas of loose myxoid tissue containing alveolar spaces and occasional glandular structures lined by cuboidal epithelium may be seen together with reticular areas. This loose myxoid pattern is considered to be analogous to the magma reticulare of the exocelomic extraembryonic mesoderm. These mesenchymal elements coexpress vimentin and keratin intermediate filaments, suggesting derivation from the epithelial cells[117] and may, rarely, exhibit definitive mesenchymal differentiation such as skeletal muscle (or extramedullary erythropoiesis as noted above).

The endodermal sinus, pseudopapillary or 'festoon' pattern (Figure 27.16) is the most distinctive. It includes the pathognomonic Schiller–Duval bodies, yet present in only 20% of all cases. These bodies are thought to recapitulate the endodermal sinuses in the rat placenta. They consist of narrow cords of loose connective tissue, each with a longitudinal capillary blood vessel in the center and covered by a monolayer mantle of primitive cuboidal or low columnar, mitotically active epithelial cells (Figure 27.16). The cytoplasm of these cells is typically clear, containing glycogen and occasionally small amounts of lipid. In cross-section they appear as epithelial papillae projecting into the surrounding, poorly formed, capsular sinusoid space which, in turn, is lined by a single layer of flat cells with prominent hyperchromatic nuclei (Figure 27.17). In most yolk sac tumors, these Schiller–Duval bodies are poorly formed or absent. The general background pattern in festoon areas consists of a complex labyrinth of branching and communicating spaces and channels, with papillary processes resembling abortive Schiller–Duval bodies radiating into the surrounding stroma. The stroma may contain scat-

tered lymphocytes and, rarely, histiocytic granulomas. Hyaline PAS-positive material, forming bands or connective tissue cores surrounded by tumor cells, is frequently seen in festoon areas.

The 'solid' pattern is usually less conspicuous, occurring principally at the margins of the tumor deposits. It is composed of rounded aggregates (Figure 27.18) or solid masses (Figure 27.19) of small primitive epithelial cells with slightly vacuolated cytoplasm, large vesicular or hyperchromatic nuclei with prominent nucleoli. They often exhibit marked mitotic activity.

The 'alveolar–glandular' pattern consists of gland-like spaces and cavities lined by flattened or cuboidal epithelial cells (Figure 27.20) and surrounded by myxoid stroma. Some of these spaces may have a multilayered cell lining and occasionally these lining cells give rise to small papillary luminal projections. A probably related variant reported as showing 'endometrioid-like' glands, and composed of tall columnar or cuboidal cells with vacuolated cytoplasm resembling secretory endometrium[34] (Figures 27.21 and 27.22), is equally interpretable, in our view, as showing true yolk sac differentiation (compare with Figure 27.12). It consists of nests of primitive endodermal glands within loose or hyalinized stroma. One such 'endometrioid-like' yolk sac tumor coexisted with a Sertoli–Leydig cell tumor in the same ovary. This patient had Y heterochromatin inserted into the 1qh region of chromosome 1.[155]

The 'polyvesicular vitelline' pattern is encountered only occasionally and consists of many 'pear-shaped' vesicles surrounded by loose cellular mesenchyme (Figure 27.23). These vesicles are lined at the narrow ends by cuboidal epithelial cells, often with basal or supranuclear vacuoles that may stain for neutral mucins, and at the broader ends by flattened mesothelial-like cells. These lining cells are also reactive for AFP. Individual vesicles vary in size and shape and the division into broad and narrow segments which are thought to represent primary and secondary yolk sac vesicles, respectively, is often accentuated by a slight luminal constriction at this epithelial interface. Occasional glandular or cystic spaces are encoun-

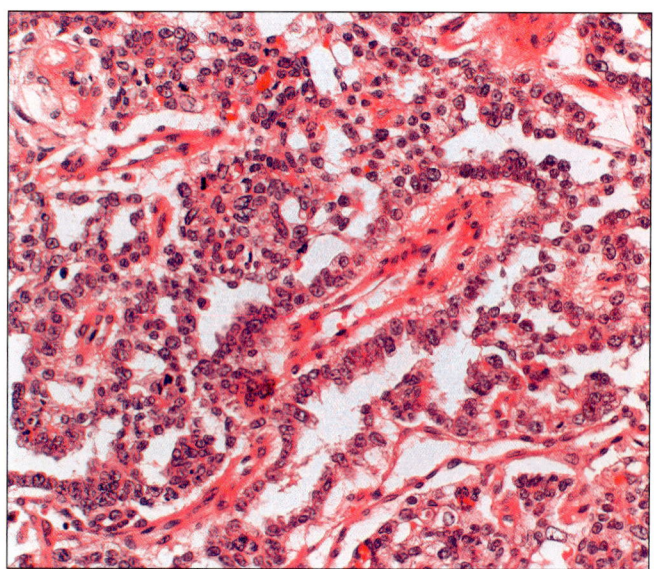

Fig. 27.16 Festoon pattern of yolk sac tumor. Endodermal sinus structures are seen in longitudinal section (center).

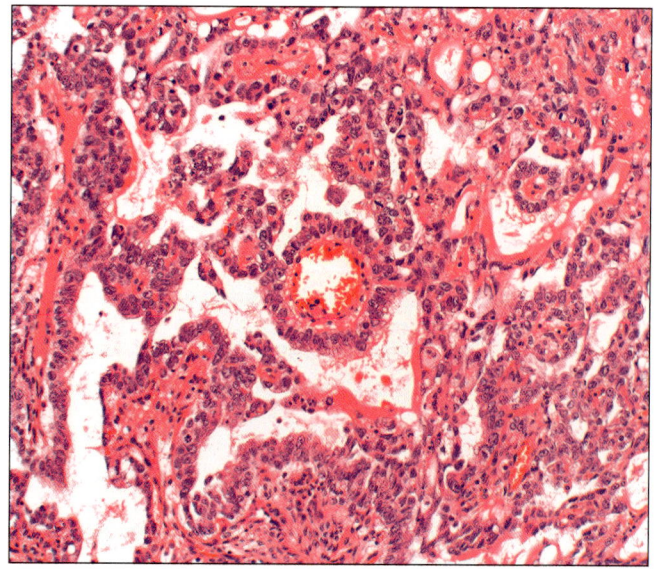

Fig. 27.17 Festoon pattern of yolk sac tumor. Well-formed Schiller–Duval body (center).

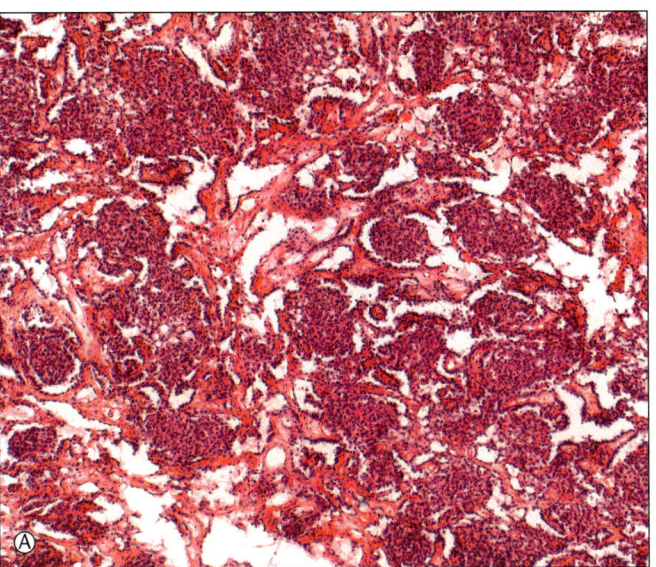 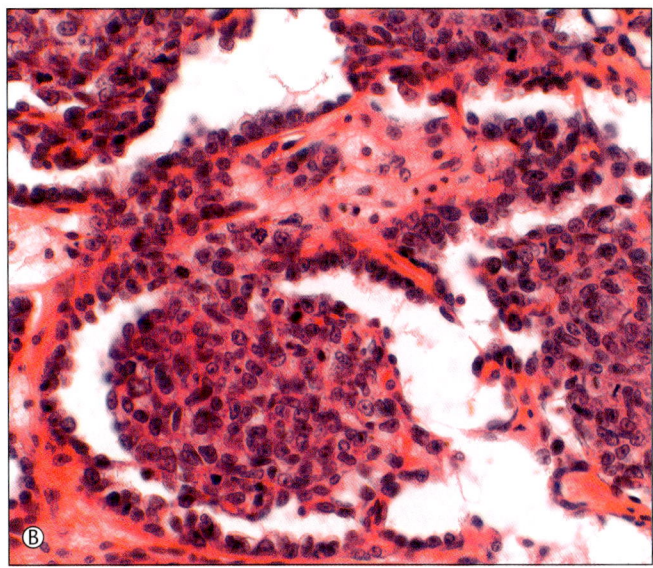

Fig. 27.18 Solid pattern of yolk sac tumor. **(A)** Several small cellular morules at the margin of a typical festoon area. **(B)** Primitive, mitotically active cells with crowded hyperchromatic nuclei.

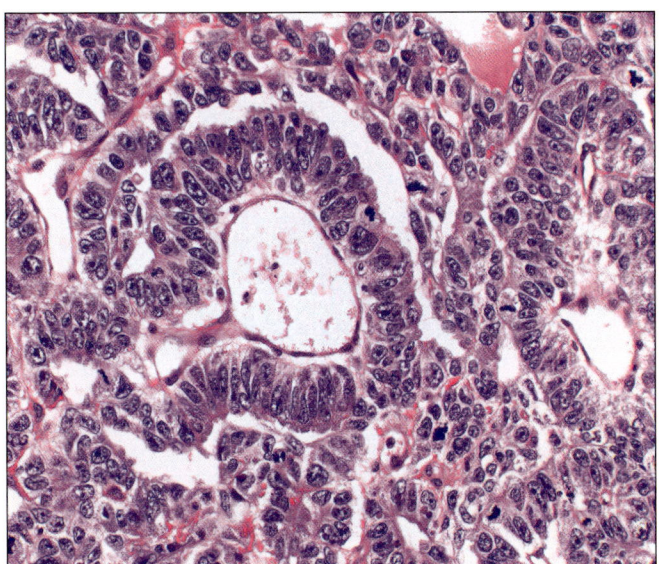 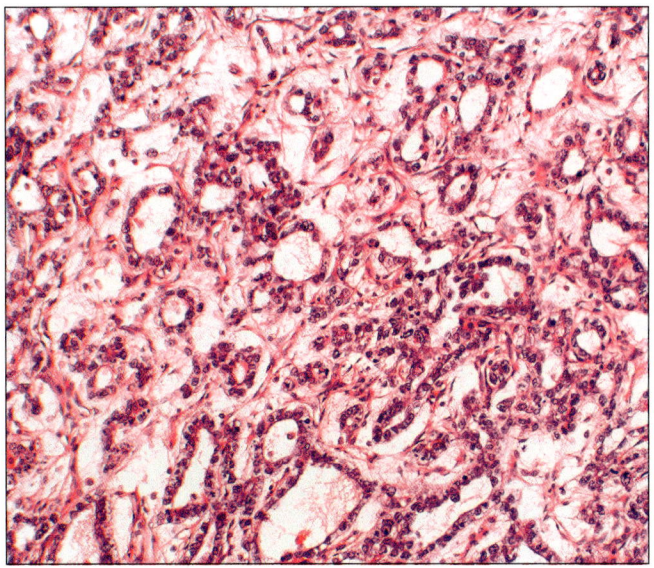

Fig. 27.19 Solid pattern of yolk sac tumor. An area of complex solid epithelial growth composed of primitive cells and suggesting differentiation towards embryonal endodermal structures.

Fig. 27.20 So-called 'alveolar–glandular' pattern of yolk sac tumor.

tered in which the epithelium exhibits more definite intestinal differentiation. Extremely rarely, entire tumors exhibit the polyvesicular vitelline pattern and such neoplasms are termed 'polyvesicular vitelline tumors'.

In addition to these well-defined patterns, further variants termed 'yolk sac tumors with hepatoid differentiation' ('hepatoid yolk sac carcinomas') have a mostly solid pattern typified by sheets and nests of eosinophilic, mitotically active cells in a cellular fibrous stroma (Figure 27.24) and resembling hepatocellular carcinoma.[180] Small foci of hepatoid differentiation are seen in 16–48% of otherwise unremarkable yolk sac tumors, thus strengthening this association (Figure 27.25). How much of this 'somatic' or 'embryonal' differentiation is required to reclassify such tumors as mixed malignant germ cell in type (see below) has not been determined. Rarely these tumors produce bile. Tumor cells in these areas may be reactive for hepatocyte

paraffin-1 antibody.[140] Variably sized cystic spaces filled with mucicarmine-positive material may be present, giving a honeycomb appearance, and this tumor pattern occasionally merges with adjacent areas showing the polyvesicular vitelline variant described above. The tumor cells are polygonal with distinct cell borders, eosinophilic cytoplasm, and large rounded central nuclei, each containing a single prominent nucleolus. PAS-positive, diastase-resistant hyaline droplets as described above are prominent. AFP and α_1-antitrypsin are demonstrable in tumor cell cytoplasm and, to a lesser extent, in the hyaline droplets. Rare foci of respiratory epithelial differentiation may also be encountered (Figure 27.26).

Differential diagnosis
Müllerian clear cell and, to a lesser extent, endometrioid carcinomas (see Chapter 25) and embryonal carcinomas (see

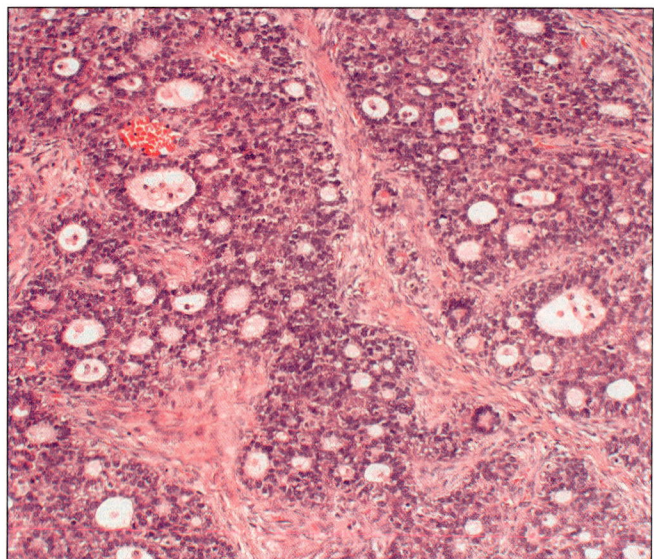

Fig. 27.21 So-called 'endodermal sinus tumor with intestinal differentiation'. Architecturally, this variant resembles normal early human yolk sac (Figure 27.12). Courtesy of Dr J Molnar, San Francisco, CA.

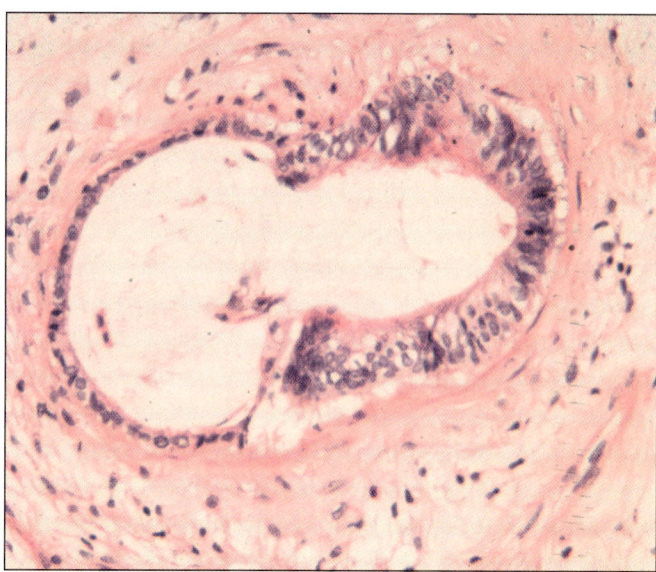

Fig. 27.23 Yolk sac tumor. Polyvesicular vitelline area shows pear-shaped vesicle lined partly by attenuated and partly by cuboidal epithelium.

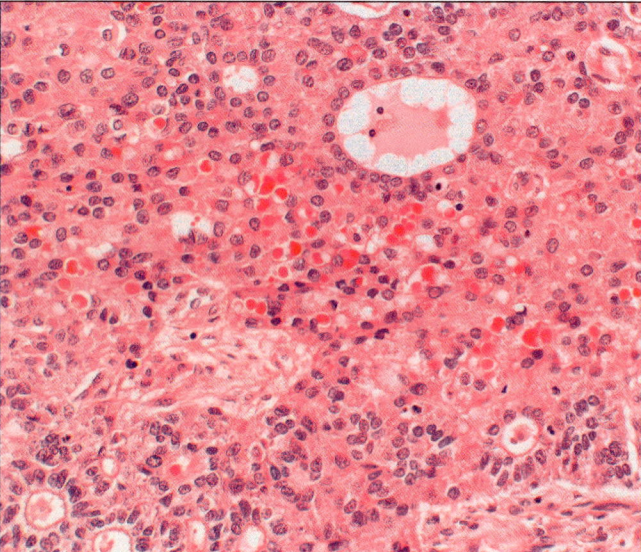

Fig. 27.22 Higher power of tumor shown in Figure 27.25, with occasional gland-like spaces. Glands interspersed amongst polygonal cells with prominent cell borders and eosinophilic cytoplasm, some containing PAS-positive, diastase-resistant, eosinophilic hyaline bodies. Courtesy of Dr J Molnar, San Francisco, CA.

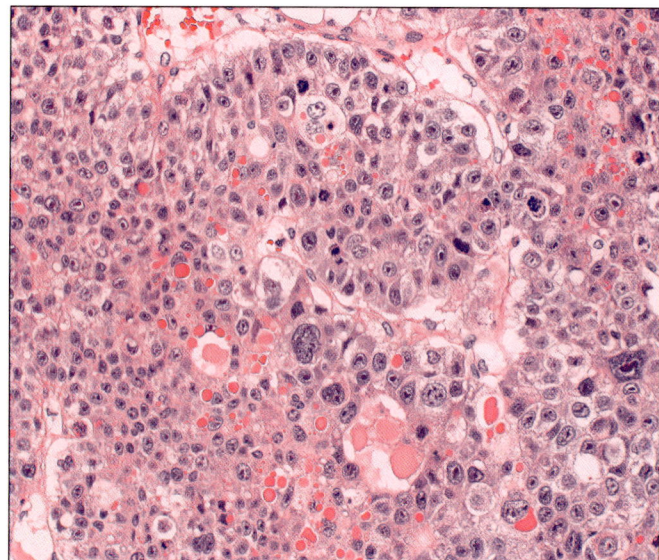

Fig. 27.24 Hepatoid yolk sac tumor. Sheets of uniform polyhedral cells with irregular angulated nuclei and abundant cytoplasm containing eosinophilic inclusions.

below) of the ovaries are the three neoplasms with which yolk sac tumors might be confused pathologically.

Clear cell and endometrioid carcinomas, which usually occur in the fifth to seventh decades, typically are large thick-walled cystic tumors with numerous yellow-fawn, fleshy nodules projecting into the lumen (Table 27.4). Histologically, clear cell carcinomas show much more regular tubulopapillary patterns and lack the honeycomb meshwork of cystic spaces and channels of yolk sac tumors. The tubular lining cells either have abundant clear cytoplasm or are hobnailed with nuclei that bulge into the lumen, in contrast to the rather pleomorphic primitive cells of yolk sac tumors. Large bulbous hobnail cells are rarely seen in yolk sac tumors. In clear cell carcinomas the papillary processes are finer and more frond-like and are also

lined by polyhedral clear cells. Typical Schiller–Duval bodies are absent. Sheets of large pavement-like cells with clear cytoplasm containing small, dark, uniform, eccentric nuclei, typical of the solid pattern of clear cell carcinoma, are not seen in yolk sac tumors. Benign (parvilocular) clear cell tumors, composed entirely of cystic spaces, may resemble superficially the reticular (Figure 27.15) or polyvesicular vitelline (Figure 27.23) patterns of yolk sac tumor. However, the epithelial linings in the former are either typical hobnail cells or large clear cells rather than the two types of epithelia (mesothelial-like cells in the broader portion and columnar mucus-secreting cells in the narrow portion) seen in the different segments of the pear-shaped vesicles characteristic of polyvesicular vitelline tumors. Similarly, the frequently associated architectural features of

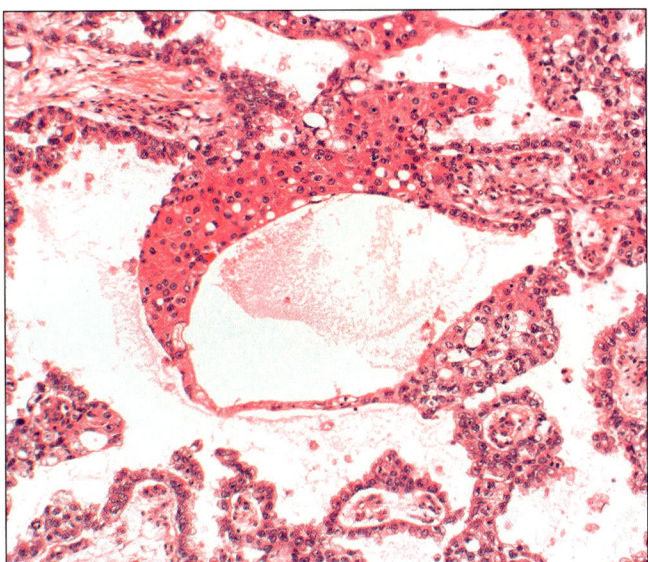

Fig. 27.25 Yolk sac tumor. Small focal aggregate of polyhedral eosinophilic hepatoid cells in an otherwise typical lesion.

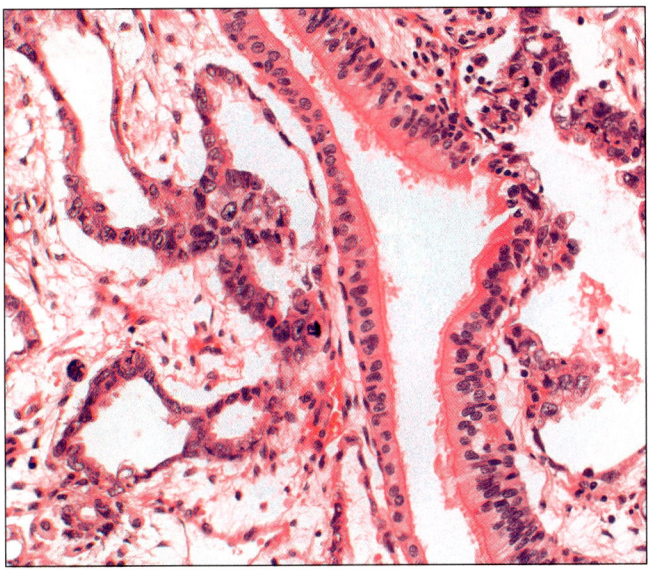

Fig. 27.26 Yolk sac tumor. An isolated strip of ciliated respiratory epithelium in an otherwise typical yolk sac tumor with a reticular pattern.

Table 27.4 Yolk sac tumor versus clear cell carcinoma: differential diagnosis

Yolk sac tumor	Clear cell carcinoma
Clinical profile	
Almost always <30 years	Occur in the fifth to seventh decades, peak incidence 50 years
Macroscopic features	
Solid, friable, with hemorrhage, necrosis and soft myxoid or gelatinous areas	Thick-walled, unilocular cysts with fleshy, yellow-fawn mural nodules
Microscopic features	
Festoon areas:	Tubulopapillary areas:
Schiller–Duval bodies	Regular frond-like papillae
Typical hobnail-like cells extremely rare	Hobnail cells common
Solid areas:	
Composed mostly of small primitive cells	Pavement-like clear cells with regular nuclei
Mitoses very numerous	Mitoses rare
Polyvesicular vitelline areas:	Parvilocular areas:
Vesicles lined by either polyhedral cuboidal mucus-secreting cells or mesothelial-like cells	Cysts lined by clear cells or hobnail cells
Immunoprofile	
EMA and CK7 negative. Only focally positive for Leu-M1 in 60%	Diffusely positive for EMA, CK7 and Leu-M1

CK7, cytokeratin 7; EMA, epithelial membrane antigen.

endometrioid carcinomas, such as squamous differentiation, mucinous or ciliated cell metaplasia and nearby endometriosis, assist in differentiating these neoplasms from the exceptionally rare glandular or 'endometrioid-like' yolk sac tumors. The immunoprofile of yolk sac tumors includes almost uniform lack of reactivity for cytokeratin 7 (CK7) and epithelial membrane antigen (EMA), both of which müllerian clear cell and endometrioid carcinomas strongly express.[143]

Pure embryonal carcinomas, rare in the ovaries, are regularly associated with hormonal manifestations of β-hCG and lack the specific histologic patterns observed in yolk sac tumors, as described above. Poorly differentiated embryonal carcinomas consist of cell masses with more granular amphophilic cytoplasm, greater nuclear pleomorphism, and even more prominent nucleoli. Syncytiotrophoblastic giant cells are regularly seen and these elaborate immunoreactive chorionic gonadotrophin. Better differentiated embryonal carcinomas exhibit cords, tubules or cleft spaces lined by primitive epithelial cells, and somewhat more closely resemble poorly differentiated adult-type adenocarcinomas rather than particular patterns of yolk sac tumors. Primitive mesenchymal elements such as islands of cartilage may also be present. Tumor cells are reactive for POU5F1, whilst those of yolk sac tumors are not.[14,104]

Treatment and prognosis

These neoplasms grow rapidly and metastasize early to the retroperitoneal nodes, liver, lungs, and bowel. Local invasion and intraperitoneal spread leads to extensive disease in 30% of cases by the time of diagnosis. The remaining 70% of patients with tumor apparently confined to one ovary at laparotomy (stage 1A) usually have occult metastases. The 5-year survival rates in stages 1, 2, 3, and 4 are approximately 95%, 90%, 30%, and 25%, respectively.[40,127] There is some evidence that yolk sac tumors displaying a diversity of histologic patterns behave less aggressively than those exhibiting only one or two of the patterns described above,[157] but no evidence that the presence of other malignant germ cell tumor elements, preoperative serum AFP levels or p53 status of the tumor have any effect on survival.[127] Most current regimes use tumor-reductive surgery (wherever practicable) followed by combination cisplatin-based chemotherapy. Patients who do not respond to chemotherapy tend to die within 3 years of first treatment.

EMBRYONAL CARCINOMAS

Definition

Embryonal carcinomas are the least differentiated of all ovarian germ cell tumors and are considered to be homologues of embryonal carcinomas of adult testes. Individual examples display the capacity to differentiate towards either embryonic (teratoid elements) or extraembryonic (yolk sac or trophoblast) structures but, by definition, this is minimal. Tumors exhibiting obvious differentiation in either direction are termed 'mixed malignant germ cell tumors' and are discussed below, and this is the more pedestrian setting in which embryonal carcinoma as a distinct histologic pattern is identified. The pluripotential nature of these neoplasms is evidenced by their consistent elaboration of OCT4, a POU-domain transcription factor (also known as OCT3, OTF3, and POU5F1). This factor, encoded by the *POU5F1* gene and located on chromosome 6p21.3, helps regulate pluripotential capacity during normal development and is detectable in embryonic stem and germ cells. Of ovarian germ cell neoplasms, it is detected in dysgerminomas and embryonal carcinomas only.[14,29,69,104]

Pure ovarian embryonal carcinomas are extremely rare. The reason for their apparent rarity in the ovaries, while their histologic homologues in the testes are relatively more common, is unknown.[180] Embryonal carcinomas occasionally arise from pre-existing gonadoblastomas.

Clinical profile

As with other malignant germ cell tumors, the majority present in patients in their second and third decades (median age, 15 years), but exceptionally can occur in women as old as 50 years.[81,122] Most patients present with an abdominal or pelvic mass and, unlike yolk sac tumors and dysgerminomas, about two-thirds have hormonal manifestations (precocious pseudo-puberty or abnormal uterine bleeding). Serum β-hCG levels are usually elevated. Familial clustering of malignant germ cell tumors involving both sexes and including embryonal carcinomas may occur.[3,61,112]

Macroscopic features

Pure embryonal carcinomas are large, soft, solid, unilateral masses with smooth external surfaces. The cut surfaces show yellow-gray tissue with widespread hemorrhage and necrosis and usually a minor cystic component.

Microscopic features

The least differentiated variants are composed of sheets and masses of pleomorphic primitive cells, superficially resembling cytotrophoblastic cells, and showing little or no architectural organization (Figure 27.27). Tumor cells are medium to large in size, polyhedral in shape, and have obvious pale amphophilic granular cytoplasm but ill-defined cell borders. They often form syncytial cell masses with central necrosis. Nuclei are central and pleomorphic, with vesicular chromatin, and may contain one or more large nucleoli. Mitoses are frequent and abnormal mitotic figures are regularly seen. Giant multinucleated syncytiotrophoblastic cells elaborating β-hCG are common (see Figure 27.28). These cells may be clustered at the periphery of tumor nodules or scattered randomly throughout. Intervening mononuclear tumor cells, however, lack β-hCG but stain irregularly for AFP in 85% of cases. Hyaline droplets

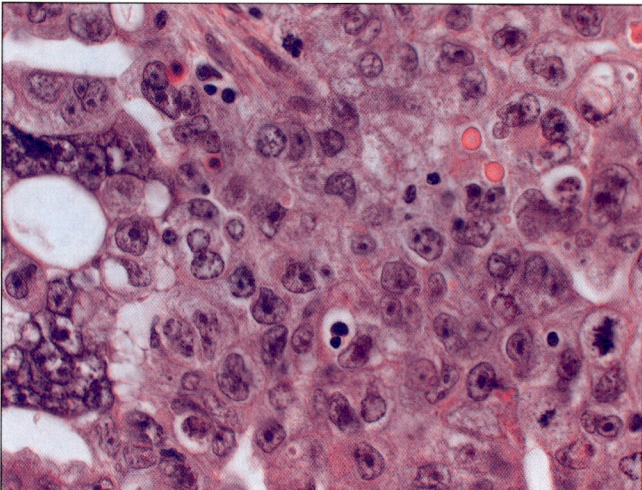

Fig. 27.27 Embryonal carcinoma. Solid sheets of primitive cells with characteristic large vesicular nuclei and prominent nucleoli.

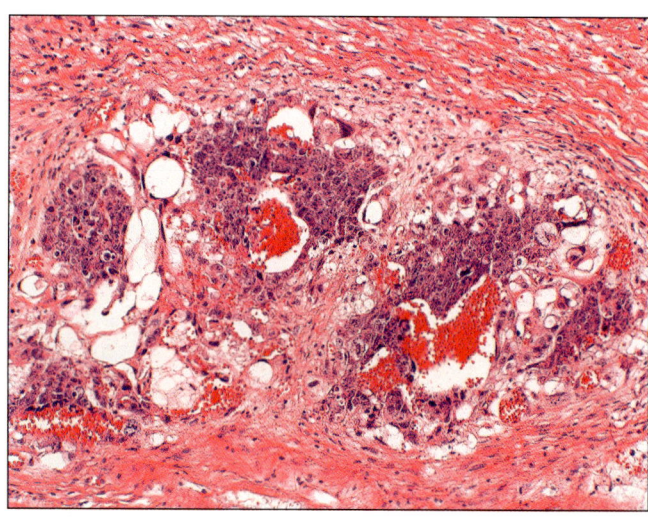

Fig. 27.28 Embryonal carcinoma. A rare focus showing two amorphous embryoid bodies and multinucleated syncytiotrophoblastic cells.

similar to those described in yolk sac tumors (also reactive for AFP) are seen within and between the mononuclear tumor cells. Stromal and epithelial elements consistent with truncated somatic differentiation (minute foci of cartilage and islands of squamous epithelium) are rarely found. More obvious differentiation is absent (particularly neuroepithelium), thus distinguishing these tumors from immature teratomas.

In the somewhat better differentiated examples, tumor cells tend to line cleft-like glandular spaces (Figure 27.29) and appear a little more epithelial and less pleomorphic, thus superficially resembling poorly differentiated adult-type carcinomas. True glands are uncommon but, when present, they may be lined by cells elaborating cytoplasmic mucin. Papillary structures, if present, are composed of solid aggregates of cells and must be differentiated from the typical Schiller–Duval bodies of yolk sac tumors. Occasional abortive embryoid bodies may be seen (Figure 27.28). Mesenchymal differentiation manifests as zones of either loose and edematous or dense fibrosarcoma-like tissue containing spindle cells. Focal necrosis and hemorrhage are common. Vascular invasion is more obvious than in

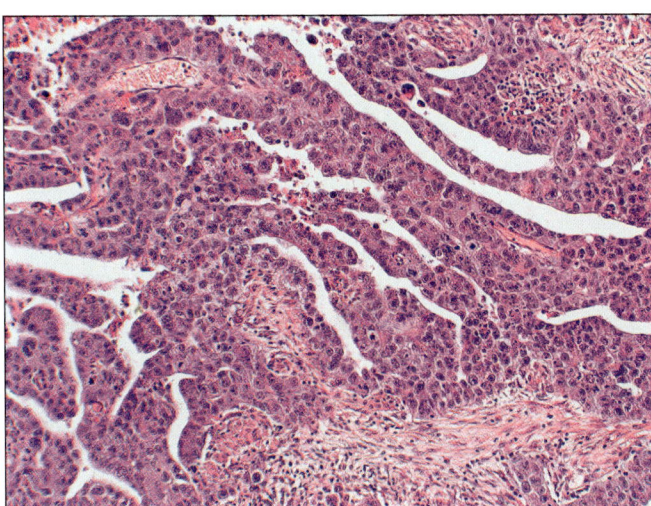

Fig. 27.29 Embryonal carcinoma. Area showing more obvious 'epithelial' differentiation with irregular slit-like spaces lined by primitive cells.

other malignant germ cells tumors (with the exception of choriocarcinoma).

The contralateral ovary in many instances shows the changes of hyperreactio luteinalis (see Chapter 22) due to the raised β-hCG levels in these patients.

Differential diagnosis

The solid undifferentiated forms of embryonal carcinoma may occasionally be confused with anaplastic dysgerminomas (Table 27.2), an important discrimination to make because of the markedly different prognoses and therapies of these tumors. The presence of clefts, alveoli, or any cell-lined spaces precludes the diagnosis of dysgerminoma. Embryonal carcinoma cells are usually larger and more pleomorphic and, in contrast to dysgerminoma cells, are strongly reactive for cytokeratins. AFP is readily demonstrated in the mononuclear tumor cells, and syncytiotrophoblastic cells are much more numerous and more frequently seen in embryonal carcinomas than in dysgerminomas.

A more difficult pathologic differentiation, though rarely a clinical conundrum, is between embryonal carcinomas and undifferentiated carcinomas of common epithelial origin. The latter neoplasms, as a general rule, occur in much older women and are commonly bilateral. Although, histologically, both may show large sheets of pleomorphic cells, the large primitive vesicular nuclei, each with one or more prominent central nucleoli, of the embryonal carcinoma cells should be readily distinguishable from the variable hyperchromatic, angular nuclei seen in undifferentiated epithelial malignant tumors. An absence of primitive mesenchyme (except in carcinosarcomas) and syncytiotrophoblast-like giant cells in the latter are also important discriminatory elements, as are the relevant immunophenotypes.

Treatment and prognosis

They are highly malignant, locally aggressive, and spread widely throughout the peritoneal cavity, although extra-abdominal metastases occur somewhat later than with yolk sac tumors. Lungs, liver, and retroperitoneal lymph nodes are documented sites for metastases. Sixty per cent of patients present with stage 1A tumors at laparotomy. Half of stage 1A

cases treated by simple surgical excision alone have a fatal outcome, indicating the high rate of occult metastases at the time of diagnosis and the need for postoperative adjuvant chemotherapy in all cases. Patients with residual extraovarian disease at surgery do poorly. The primary treatment of embryonal carcinomas is surgery (unilateral salpingo-oophorectomy is adequate for stage 1A cases) followed by chemotherapy (usually a combination of cisplatin, vinblastine, and bleomycin). Embryonal carcinomas are not radiosensitive. Monitoring the progress of these tumors is facilitated by the serial assessment of both serum β-hCG and AFP.

POLYEMBRYOMAS (POLYEMBRYONIC EMBRYOMAS)

Definition

Polyembryomas are vanishingly rare ovarian germ cell tumors containing myriads of variably formed 'embryoid bodies' that resemble normal presomite human embryos of approximately days 15–16 of development, although occasional embryoid bodies are more readily encountered in ovarian malignant mixed germ cell tumors made up predominantly of other neoplastic elements such as immature teratoma or embryonal carcinoma. Embryoid bodies are subtyped as complete, imperfect or amorphous depending upon the closeness with which they resemble normal presomite embryos, but this morphologic subtyping has no pathologic significance. Although theories vary on the origin of embryoid bodies, they most likely form after initiation of teratogenesis from multipotential embryonal cells in the tumors rather than directly from germ cells. Embryoid bodies should not be regarded as intermediate stages in transformation of embryonal cells towards immature teratomatous structures or tissues but rather as intransitive endpoints of differentiation or maturation in their own right.

Clinical profile

Fewer than 20 cases of ovarian polyembryoma have been reported,[129] almost all being malignant mixed germ cell tumors with a major component of polyembryoma associated with other germ cell elements, mainly immature teratoma or choriocarcinoma. Most have occurred in young patients, the oldest being 43 years of age.[28] Clinical findings are those of patients with other ovarian malignant germ cell tumors. Most cases have shown invasion of adjacent structures and organs and intraperitoneal metastases, and behaved in an aggressive fashion.

Macroscopic features

Polyembryomas are solid, unilateral tumors that grossly resemble other malignant germ cell tumors. They range in size from about 10 cm in diameter to giant masses filling the whole abdominal cavity. Hemorrhagic and necrotic areas are prominent. The cut surface of the tumor may exhibit a fine granularity, which represents the presence of the myriad small embryoid bodies (Figure 27.30).

Microscopic features

The hallmark of polyembryomas is the presence of embryoid bodies, the better differentiated of which include an embryonic disc, amniotic cavity, and yolk sac surrounded by a variable cuff of primitive extraembryonic mesenchyme (Figures 27.31

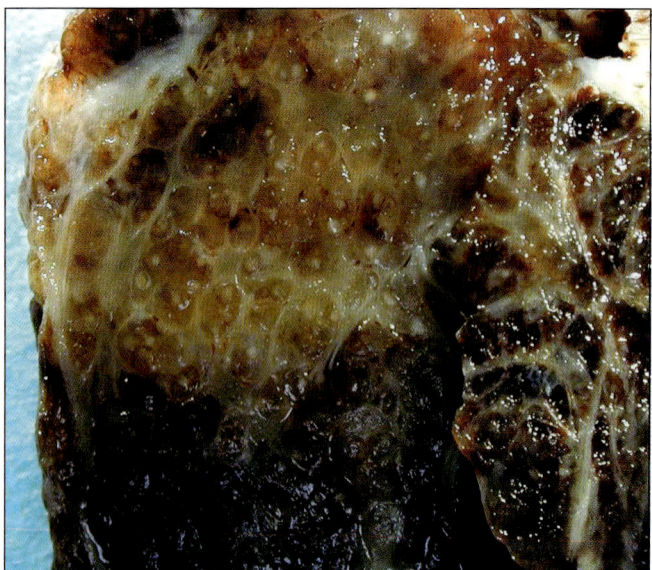

Fig. 27.30 Ovarian polyembryoma. Cut surface of tumor showing innumerable but circumscribed zones of myxoid connective tissue each containing a central embryoid body. Courtesy of Dr C Camaris, Sydney, Australia.

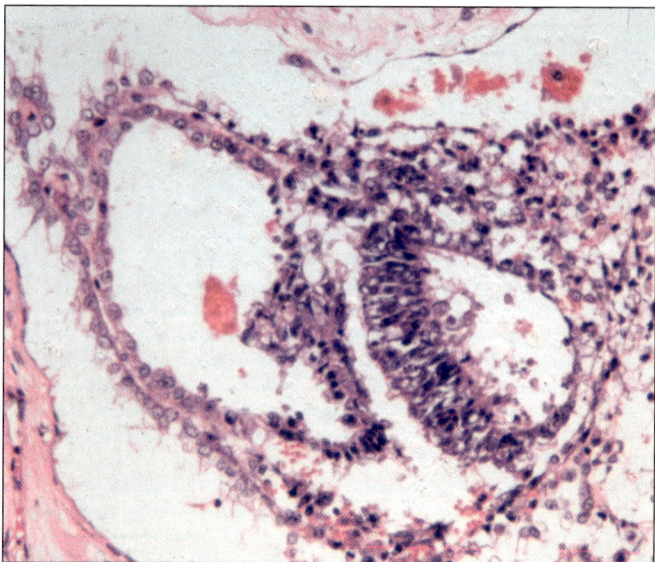

Fig. 27.31 Ovarian polyembryoma. Slightly distorted embryoid body lying in loose myxoid connective tissue. Courtesy of Dr A Takeda, Nagoya, Japan.

and 27.32). In well-formed bodies, the embryonic trilaminar disc is lined on one side by uniform cuboidal epithelial cells, resembling endoderm and continuous with the yolk sac. The epithelium lining the yolk sac reacts strongly for AFP, while the primitive 'endodermal' epithelium of the embryonic disc reacts weakly. The other side of the embryonic disc exhibits tall columnar 'ectodermal' epithelium that merges with amniotic epithelium lining the rest of the cavity. The cuff of immature extraembryonic mesenchyme consists of regular, loosely packed, mitotically active, spindle-shaped cells.

Teratomatous structures such as neuroglia, epidermis and skin appendages, cords of liver cells (Figure 27.33), respiratory and intestinal epithelium, in various stages of differentiation may be seen among the embryoid bodies. Transitions between the 'amniotic cavity' and intestinal or squamous elements, and between the 'yolk sac' and hepatic elements, may be seen but not between embryoid bodies and other teratomatous elements derived from the embryonic disc. Syncytiotrophoblastic giant cells that stain for β-hCG and hPL are sometimes present at the periphery of the embryoid bodies.

When less well-formed, embryoid bodies contain a medullary plate and amnion associated with a blastocystic space or with a cuff of extraembryonic mesenchyme. They may have two or more amniotic cavities and share a single yolk sac cavity or vice versa. There may be disproportion between the two cavities, and the cavities may be malformed. In any one tumor, embryoid bodies may vary in size and their degree of maturation (but not beyond the 18-day stage of embryonic development). Some examples may be severely malformed and bizarre examples (Figure 27.34).

Treatment and prognosis

There is no merit in discriminating at a prognostic or therapeutic level between these and other malignant mixed germ cell tumors on the basis of so few reported cases, although one patient surgically staged and confined to one ovary has been treated successfully by salpingo-oophorectomy alone.[28]

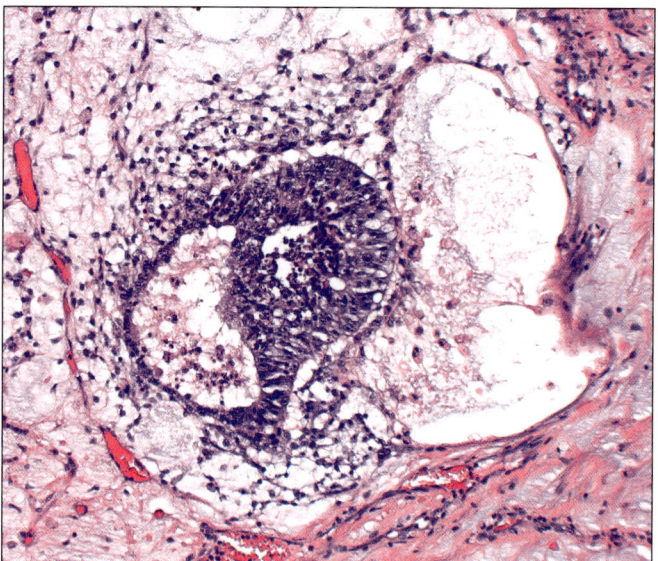

Fig. 27.32 Ovarian polyembryoma. Well-formed but somewhat degenerate embryoid body lying in loose myxoid extraembryonic mesenchyme. Courtesy of Dr C Camaris, Sydney, Australia.

CHORIOCARCINOMAS

Definition

Trophoblastic differentiation in malignant ovarian tumors is found in various entities. They may be a metastasis from primary gestational choriocarcinoma in the uterus, much less commonly primary gestational choriocarcinoma from an ovarian pregnancy,[107] a 'non-gestational choriocarcinoma' (a malignant germ cell tumor showing partial or occasionally complete trophoblastic differentiation[18,38,65,94,142,183]) or choriocarcinoma arising by dedifferentiation from within a surface epithelial–stromal tumor.[71,134,136] For the purposes of this discussion, a fifth possibility – namely that of widespread chorio-

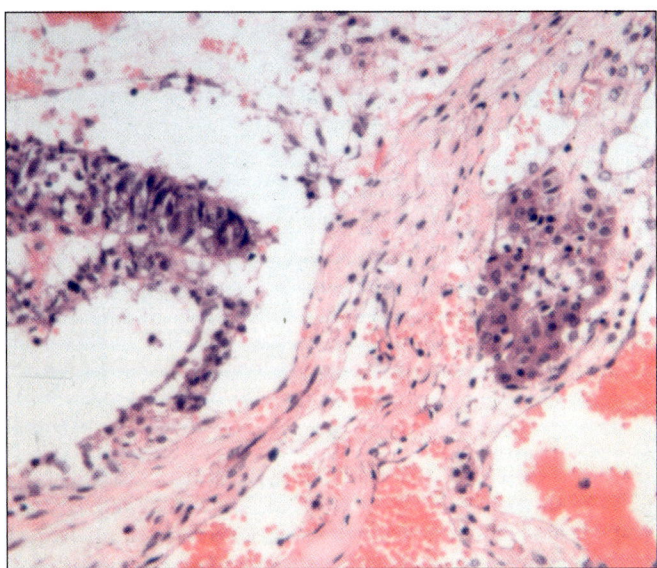

Fig. 27.33 Ovarian polyembryoma. Island of primitive hepatic cells adjacent to an embryoid body. Courtesy of Dr A Takeda, Nagoya, Japan.

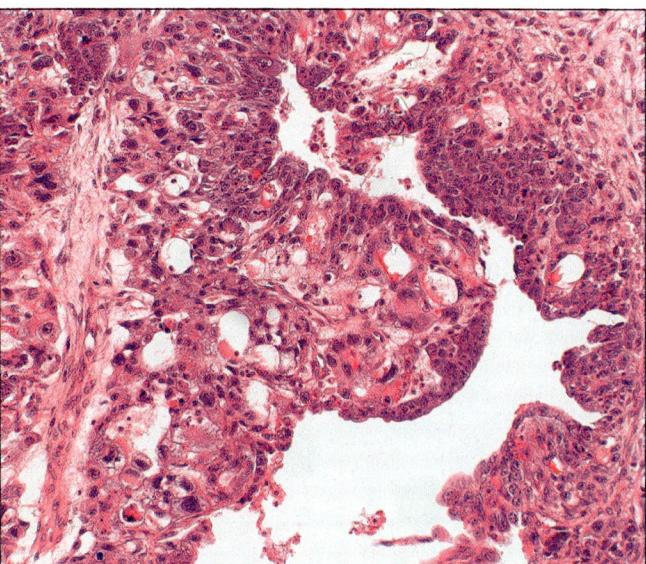

Fig. 27.35 Non-gestational ovarian choriocarcinoma. A ragged cystic space lined by a complex mixture of cytotrophoblast (small dark cells) and large bizarre syncytiotrophoblast.

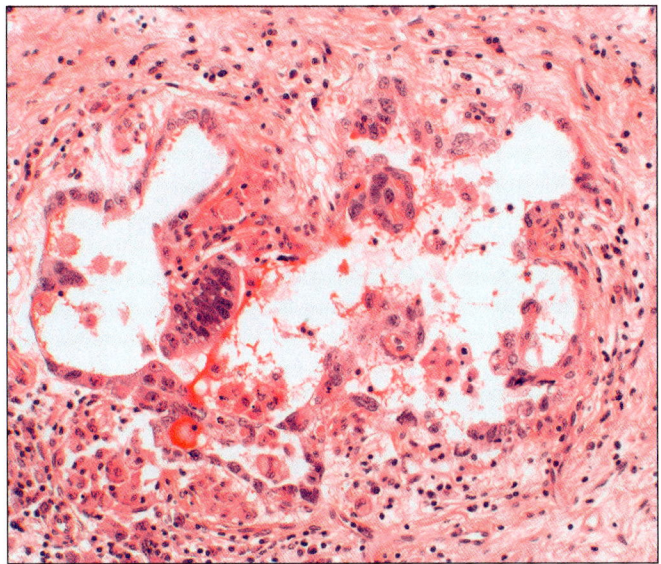

Fig. 27.34 Ovarian polyembryoma. Amorphous embryoid body with bizarre development of amnionic and yolk sac vesicles.

carcinoma in the neonate from a primary tumor arising in its placenta – is not considered relevant.

Choriocarcinomas are characterized by an intimate admixture of cytotrophoblast and its derivative cell, syncytiotrophoblast. Along with yolk sac tumors, they thus represent extraembryonic differentiation within the spectrum of malignant germ cell neoplasia. Pure non-gestational ovarian choriocarcinomas are extremely rare and highly malignant.[18,38,62,142,183]

Other reported so-called ovarian choriocarcinomas have trophoblast mixed with other malignant germ cell elements. This latter feature is valuable in discriminating gestational from non-gestational origin of choriocarcinomas in women in the reproductive age group. Without access to DNA polymorphism analysis,[177] non-gestational ovarian choriocarcinomas were formerly only diagnosed with confidence in prepubertal

girls. This has no doubt influenced the age profile of the cases in the literature, most being under the age of 20 years. This point is of clinical relevance as the adolescent years of 15–19 also include one of the periods of highest risk for gestational trophoblastic neoplasia.

Clinical profile

The clinical findings overlap those observed in patients with other ovarian malignant germ cell tumors, with the addition of hormonal manifestations occasioned by the elaboration of β-hCG and overt bleeding from metastatic deposits. Bilateral spontaneous pneumothorax has also been reported. Prepubertal girls show signs of isosexual pseudoprecocity, while adult patients may present with signs clinically suggestive of 'ectopic pregnancy'. Quantitative assay of serum be β-hCG assists in diagnosing choriocarcinoma and monitoring the progress of the disease and its therapeutic response.

These tumors invade the adjacent pelvic structures, spread widely in the peritoneal cavity, and metastasize via both lymphatics and, to a lesser extent, blood vessels.

Pathology

These tumors are usually large, unilateral, solid masses. The cut surfaces are hemorrhagic, and focal necrosis is seen. On microscopic examination, they display an intimate admixture of two types of cells, cytotrophoblast and syncytiotrophoblast, both of which are essential for a definite diagnosis, although occasional fields may be encountered in which one or the other cell type is present exclusively (Figure 27.35). Cytotrophoblastic cells are medium-sized polygonal or round cells with clear or amphophilic cytoplasm, well-defined cell borders, and either small, round, hyperchromatic central nuclei or larger vesicular nuclei, each containing a conspicuous nucleolus.

Mitoses are numerous within cytotrophoblastic cells, which do not elaborate β-hCG, but react strongly for cytokeratins. Syncytiotrophoblastic cells, by contrast, are giant irregular symplastic cells with abundant dense amphophilic and fre-

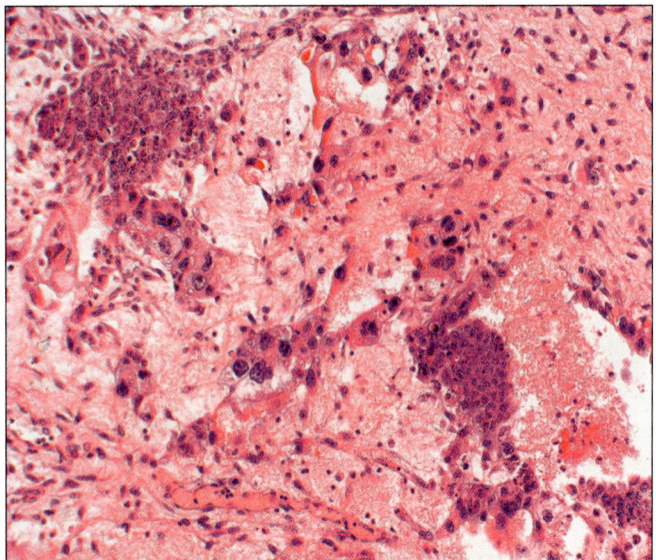

Fig. 27.36 Non-gestational ovarian choriocarcinoma. Nests of cytotrophoblastic cells and syncytiotrophoblastic cells in loose myxoid connective tissue.

quently vacuolated cytoplasm, and multiple hyperchromatic nuclei which vary in shape and size Mitoses are not seen in these cells. Syncytiotrophoblastic cells are reactive for cyto-keratins, CD10, HLA-G, inhibin, and β-hCG and commonly for other pregnancy-associated proteins such as hPL and preg-nancy-specific β-glycoprotein (SPI). Large mononuclear or 'intermediate' trophoblastic cells have been demonstrated by these techniques in ovarian germ cell tumors, including choriocarcinomas.

Variability from area to area in both relative proportions and architectural relationships of the cytotrophoblast and syn-cytiotrophoblast (Figure 27.36) is a hallmark of non-gestational choriocarcinoma and, when the tumor cells form solid aggregates, the cytotrophoblastic cells are usually dis-posed centrally with a partial or complete peripheral collection of syncytiotrophoblast cells. Hemorrhage and necrosis may be extensive with a thin rim of tumor tissue that is often barely discernible.

Differential diagnosis

Diagnosis of choriocarcinoma is not difficult if the strict con-vention of identifying both cyto- and syncytiotrophoblast is observed. The presence of syncytiotrophoblastic cells alone does not constitute choriocarcinoma, and their isolated pres-ence in malignant germ cell tumors of other types (e.g., dysger-minomas, embryonal carcinomas, polyembryomas), or indeed non-germ cell tumors, alters neither their diagnosis nor prog-nosis and management.

The challenge to establish whether or not a pure ovarian choriocarcinoma is gestational or non-gestational cannot be met by histologic means alone, and DNA polymorphism analy-sis[177] is required for this purpose. The presence of other neoplas-tic elements, a clear indication of non-gestational or germ cell tumor origin, may vary from isolated islands of primitive mes-enchyme-like stroma (without negating the diagnosis) to con-spicuous fields of tumor showing dysgerminomatous, embryonic or extraembryonic differentiation. In this latter case the tumor is reclassified as a mixed malignant germ cell tumor.

TREATMENT AND PROGNOSIS

The clinical outcome for patients with non-gestational chorio-carcinomas has been regarded traditionally as less favorable than for those with the gestation-related choriocarcinomas, although more recent studies suggest that the surgical stage of pure ovarian choriocarcinomas may be more important in clinical outcome than the determination of gestational or non-gestational origin. Since the presence of other malignant germ cell elements cannot be entirely excluded in any given case, even with extensive histologic assessment, current treatment is similar to that recommended for other malignant germ cell tumors. Thus, cytoreductive surgery (unilateral salpingo-oophorectomy in apparent stage 1A cases) is followed by meth-otrexate-based chemotherapy, this having achieved some success.[38,65]

TERATOMAS

IMMATURE TERATOMAS

Definition

These teratomas, thought to arise from post-meiotic germ cells, contain immature (embryonal) structures, as well as mature elements in most cases. By analogy with normal fetal tissues studied at various stages of development, the ontogeny of immature teratomas corresponds to an embryonic stage of between 2 and 8 weeks (fertilization age).[30] Pure immature tera-tomas comprise about 1% of ovarian teratomas[176] overall with only 10–20% of the latter occurring in the first two decades of life. Most immature teratomas include elements from all three germ layers but a small number are predominantly or exclu-sively monodermal. The presence of mitotically active embry-onic-type neuroepithelium or, less commonly, cellular and mitotically glial tissue is thought to be definitional by some.[180] The additional presence of other malignant germ cell tumor elements (a not uncommon occurrence) places the tumor in the malignant mixed germ cell tumor group (see below).

Clinical profile

Immature teratomas occur predominantly in the first two decades of life with a peak incidence at 14–19 years of age. Rare examples occur in women over the age of 40 years.[51] Patients usually present with abdominal enlargement, pain, and a readily palpable tumor. Ascites is not uncommon. Nausea, vomiting, and fever may also occur. Raised serum β-hCG and AFP levels signal the possibility of a mixed malignant germ cell tumor, although elevated serum AFP levels are found in up to 60% of patients with immature teratomas, including some that have been exhaustively sampled for the presence of other germ cell components. This may be explained by the immunohisto-chemical detection of AFP in a wide variety of both endoder-mally and ectodermally derived tissues of an immature teratoma, suggesting that endodermal sinus tissue is not the only possible source of this substance or, alternatively, that yolk sac tumor forms part of the background stroma of many germ cell tumors. Other tumor markers used in follow-up and management of these neoplasms include CA19–9, CA125 and carcinoembryonic antigen (CEA).[101]

The tumors grow rapidly, and extraovarian spread is present at initial laparotomy in about one-third of cases. As a result of rupture or capsular penetration, the tumor seeds throughout the peritoneal cavity. Direct local spread with formation of adhesions also occurs. In addition, tumors may metastasize to retroperitoneal and para-aortic lymph nodes, as well as to liver, lungs, and brain, but these distant deposits are rarely found even at autopsy.

Peritoneal metastatic deposits of mature teratomatous tissue, sometimes called 'implants', are often composed almost entirely or exclusively of mature glial tissue – 'gliomatosis peritonei' (see Chapter 33). This phenomenon occurs in association with approximately 10% of patients with immature teratomas and is biologically benign so long as the implants are histologically mature. In some instances, gliomatosis peritonei is not evident until 'second-look' laparotomy. Gliomatosis peritonei does not develop in association with immature teratoma exclusively; in fact, the majority of cases are associated with mature solid or cystic teratomas (see below)[60] or primary extraovarian teratomas and even, bizarrely, from non-neoplastic intracranial glial tissue via a ventriculoperitoneal shunt.[70] At laparotomy the small peritoneal nodules may be mistaken for carcinomatosis or miliary tuberculosis. The lesions are thought to result from release of mature neural tissue through a ruptured capsule (a common finding in these tumors, if specifically sought) or from the maturation of peritoneal deposits of immature neural tissue. An intriguing alternative possibility, which raises more questions than it answers, is that these lesions arise *in situ* by metaplasia from pluripotential cells beneath the peritoneum,[56,159] a concept supported by molecular genetic evidence. Lymphatic spread has also been suggested and this would account for the rare concurrent presence of glial tissue in lymph nodes. Long-term follow-up of patients with untreated gliomatosis peritonei shows that most lesions persist unchanged, undergo fibrous replacement or disappear entirely.

Macroscopic features

Immature teratomas are almost always unilateral, but a second, mature cystic teratoma is present in 5–10% of the contralateral ovaries. Their size is generally in the range of 14–18 cm, but may be up to 35 cm. The tumors form round, oval or lobulated masses that may display capsular adhesions and/or rupture but elsewhere have smooth surfaces. The consistency may be soft or firm depending on the nature of the teratomatous components. The tumors are predominantly solid but usually show multiple small cysts (Figure 27.37), generally less than 1 cm in diameter, but occasionally one or more large ones are present. Some contain sebaceous material or hair but most are degenerative in type and filled with clear, mucoid or bloodstained fluid. The solid areas are variable in appearance. Important areas to sample are those with a white or gray soft 'encephaloid' appearance. Hemorrhage and necrosis are relatively common and these foci should also be examined because they are likely to include the less well-differentiated tissues. Bone, cartilage or gritty calcified areas are often noted.

Gliomatosis peritonei consists of multiple tiny firm gray-white superficial peritoneal nodules resembling miliary tubercles. They generally are localized to the pelvic peritoneum, may be limited to the immediate vicinity of the ovarian tumor, and sometimes appear to be spatially related to the point of tumor rupture. Widespread plaque-like involvement of both abdominal and pelvic peritoneum may also occur. The implants are not generally associated with adhesions. The nodules range in size from 0.1 to 1.1 cm with an average of 0.3 cm. By contrast,

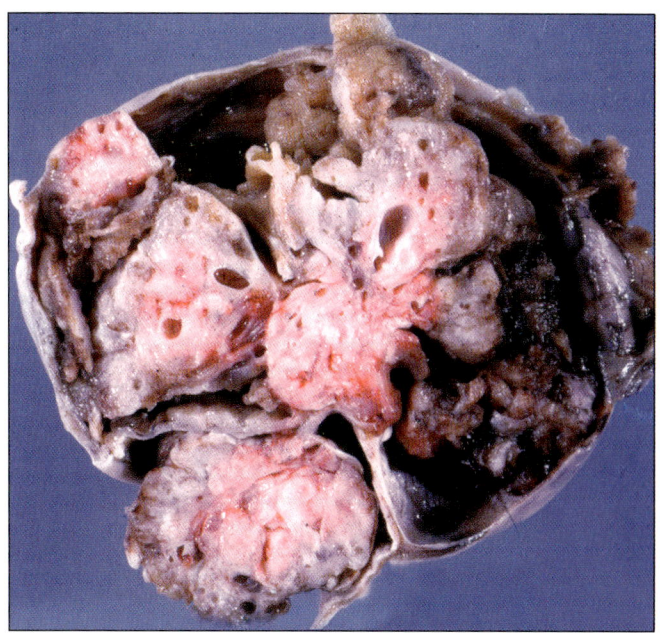

Fig. 27.37 Immature teratoma (high grade). Large cystic spaces are present at top and right. The 'solid' areas contain multiple tiny cysts. Dark areas are foci of hemorrhage and necrosis (right).

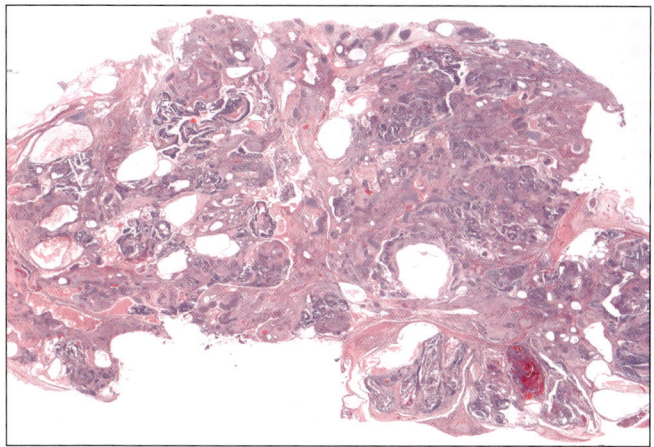

Fig. 27.38 Immature teratoma (high grade). Same case as Figure 27.37. Tissue components are randomly arranged. Large dark areas are predominantly neuroglia.

immature teratomatous metastatic deposits tend to be fewer in number, larger in size, and associated with adhesions.

Microscopic features

All three germ cell layers are generally evident and the range of tissues includes all those that may be identified in benign cystic teratomas. There is a marked predominance of ectodermal and mesodermal components and it is in these that the immaturity is also most clearly evident. The various tissues are admixed in a haphazard arrangement throughout the tumor and this contrasts sharply with benign cystic teratomas in which there is some semblance of organization (Figure 27.38). A striking feature on low-power examination may be the proliferation of neural tissues to form nodular masses mimicking some of the familiar intracranial tumors such as glioblastomas, neuroblastomas, medulloblastomas, and ependymomas.

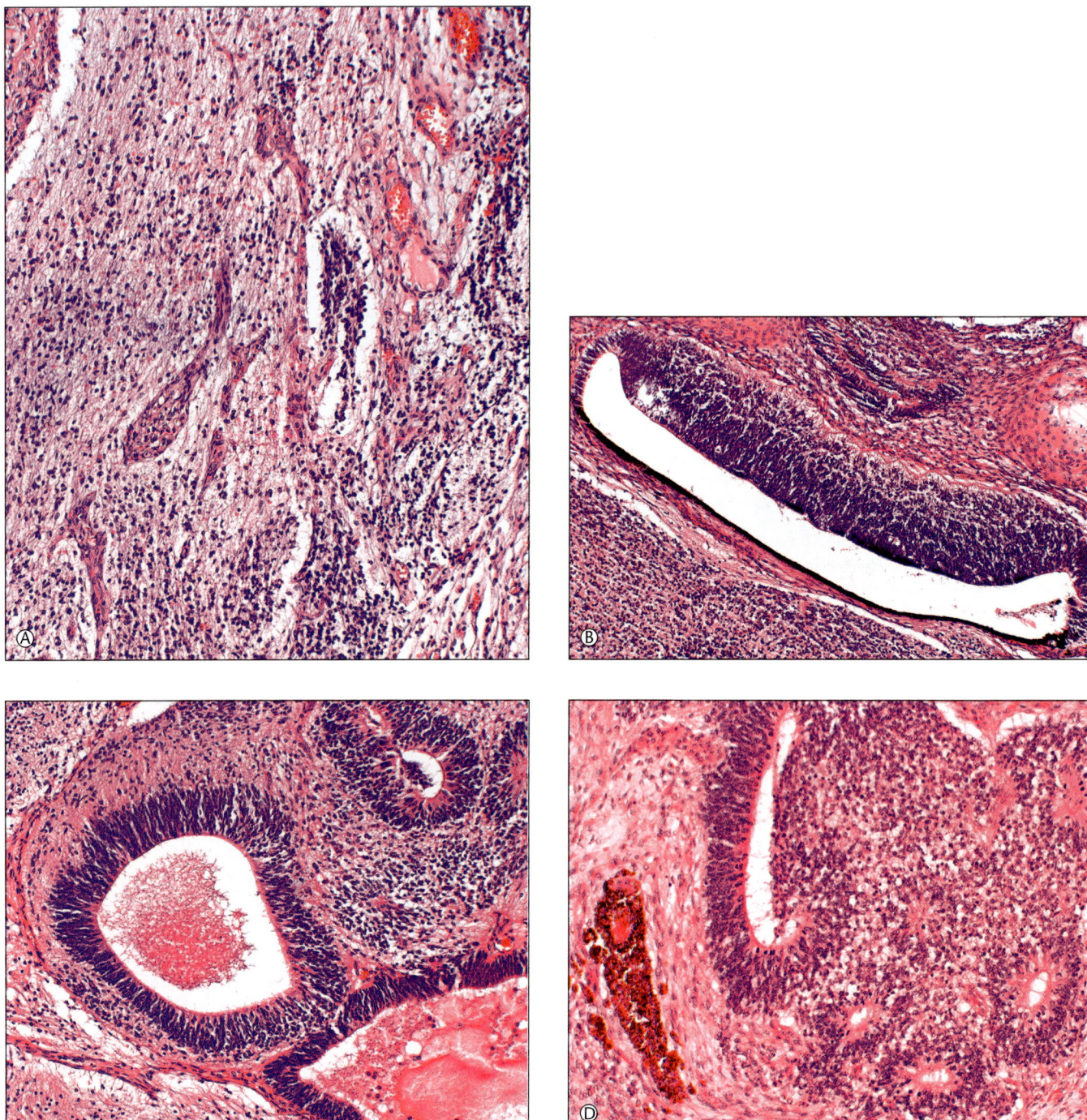

Fig. 27.39 Neural elements in high-grade immature teratomas. **(A)** Cellular neuroglia resembling glioblastoma. **(B)** Immature neuroglia and adjacent pigmented neuroepithelium resembling embryonic optic cup. **(C)** Neuroglia with neuroepithelial tubes showing well-defined luminal margin and elongate nuclei. **(D)** Highly cellular neuroglia forming neuroepithelial rosettes. At left is some densely pigmented neuroepithelium.

Ectoderm is chiefly represented by neural tissue (Figure 27.39) in the form of (roughly in decreasing order of frequency) glia, neuroepithelium, neuroblastic tissue, choroid plexus, nerve fibers, microglia, ganglia, cerebellar tissue, and pigmented neuroepithelium. Gliomatous tissue is present in varying degrees of immaturity and atypicality and may exhibit the vascular proliferative changes characteristic of astrocytomas (Figure 27.39A; see also Figure 27.42). An expected immunoprofile of reactivity to glial fibrillary acid protein (GFAP),

sulfoglucuronyl carbohydrate (HNK-1), neuron-specific enolase (NSE), and S-100 protein is seen, with about 50% of tumors also showing expression of vimentin filaments and infrequently showing reactivity for neurofilaments. Mitotic activity and atypicality increase in proportion to the degree of immaturity. Neuroepithelium is most readily recognizable where it forms tubules, simulating embryonic neural tubes (Figure 27.39C,D). These have a well-defined luminal margin lined by tall columnar cells, sometimes ciliated, with elongate

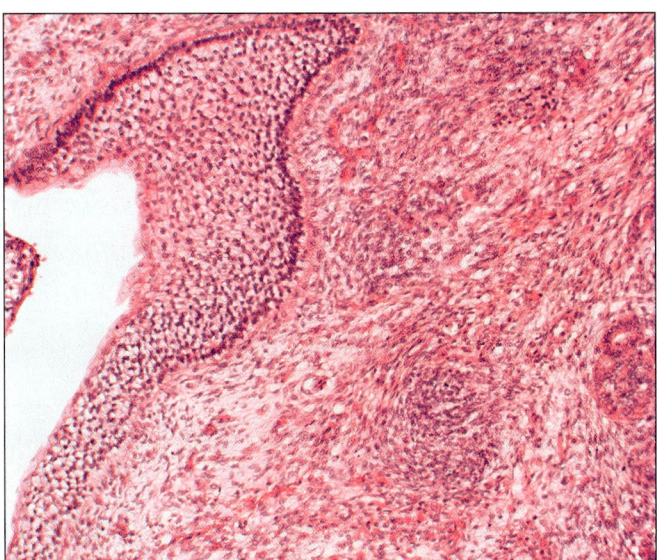

Fig. 27.40 Low-grade immature teratomas. Cyst lined by immature squamous epithelium. Note cellularity of underlying mesenchyme.

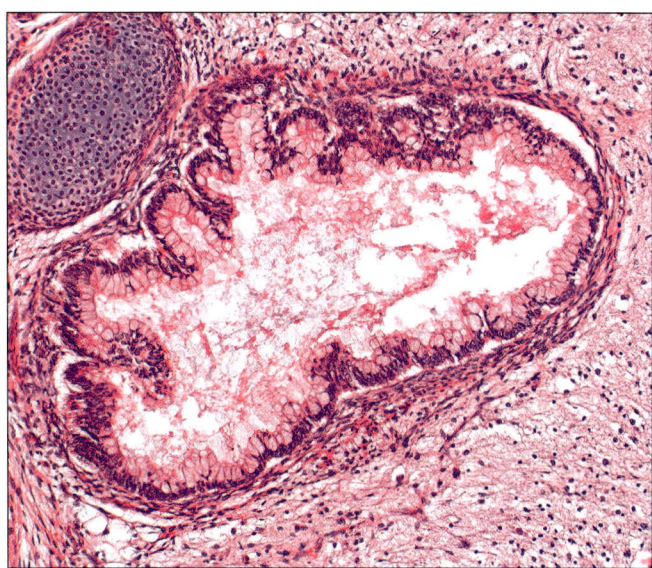

Fig. 27.42 High-grade immature teratoma. Small nodule of immature cartilage and adjacent gastrointestinal epithelium. Neuroglial tissue surrounding this resembles fibrillary astrocytoma.

tumor immaturity, resembles more closely undifferentiated myxoid embryonic mesenchyme and exhibits increased mitotic activity (Figure 27.40). Immature cartilage characteristically also shows immunoreactivity of chondrocytes for CD34 and bcl-2.[30] Tooth anlagen may be prominent in low-grade tumors. Smooth, but not striated, muscle is quite commonly observed.

Endoderm is less well represented than the above elements in most tumors, and only rarely predominates.[130] It is usually manifest as tubules lined by non-specific columnar epithelium, sometimes with subnuclear glycogen vacuoles. Gastrointestinal (Figure 27.42) or bronchial epithelium (Figure 27.41) is found less often, as are isolated groups of hepatic cells.

Histologic grading of all tumors is recommended and presupposes adequate tumor sampling. The presently used semi-quantitative system, based on the overall proportion of neuroepithelium,[133] advocates a two-tiered system:

- *Low grade*: Neoplasms containing less than one low-power field of immature neuroepithelium on any one microscope section.
- *High grade*: Immature neuroepithelium is common and exceeds one low-power field on one or more tumor sections in the tissue available for review (Figure 27.38).

Gliomatosis peritonei usually consists of nodules, sometimes aggregated, of mature glial tissue with no cytologic atypia and scarce or absent mitotic activity (Figure 27.43). The individual lesions may be surrounded by loose fibrous connective tissue and a light mixed inflammatory infiltrate in which lymphocytes predominate. A small proportion of lesions include neurons or non-neural teratomatous components such as mature cartilage or squamous elements, the latter sometimes consisting only of some keratinous debris. Reactivity for GFAP aids in the localization and identification of gliomatous foci.

Deposits of metastatic immature teratoma may show a wide variety of tissue components (both neural and other) and degree of immaturity within a single patient (Figure 27.44). The nearby peritoneum may display a florid inflammatory reaction making identification of the small metastatic lesions problematic (Figure 27.45).

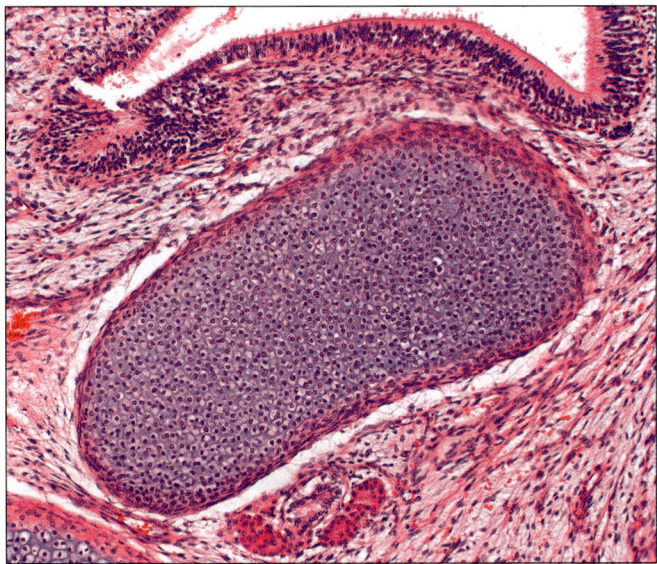

Fig. 27.41 Low-grade immature teratoma. Nodules of immature (fetal) cartilage and respiratory epithelium.

hyperchromatic nuclei. Spindle-shaped cells with similar nuclei stream out towards the surrounding tissues. With increasing tumor grade, nuclear atypicality and mitotic activity become more conspicuous and the thickness of rosette epithelium increases from one cell to many cells. Pigmented neuroepithelium is quite common and foci may resemble embryonic optic discs (Figure 27.39B), pigmented medulloblastoma or retinal anlage tumor. Neuroblastomatous areas exhibit sheets of small cells with hyperchromatic nuclei forming rosettes, as seen in neuroblastomas of the adrenal glands.

Squamous epithelium is usually present, disposed in small islands, and generally lacks cytologic malignancy. Skin adnexal structures are also common (Figure 27.40).

Small islands of cartilage and bone are usually present and these often express immaturity and resemble their embryonic counterparts (Figures 27.41 and 27.42). Mesoderm shows widely distributed loose fibrous connective tissue, that, with increasing

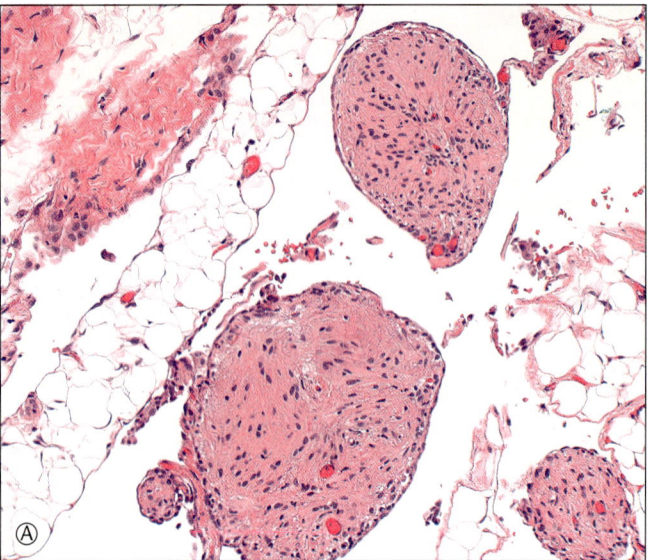 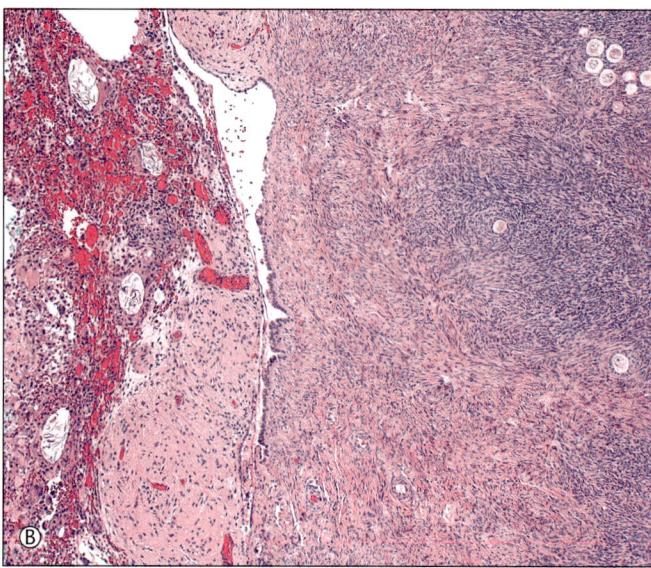

Fig. 27.43 Gliomatosis peritonei associated with ruptured immature teratoma. **(A)** Clustered omental nodules of mature glial tissue. The lesions are well circumscribed, and lack any cellular atypia. **(B)** Glial nodules on surface of contralateral ovary. Note inflammatory reaction to groups of anucleate squames.

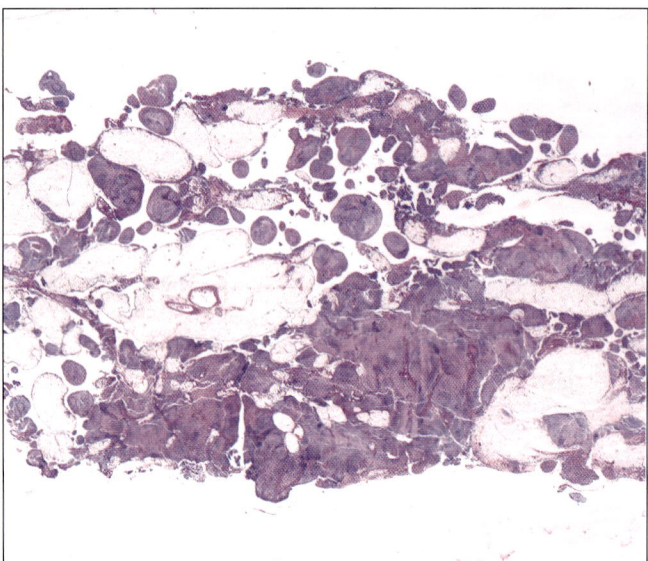

Fig. 27.44 Peritoneal metastases of immature teratoma. Florid deposition of variably mature and variably circumscribed neuroglia.

Fig. 27.45 Peritoneal metastases of immature teratoma. Deposits of immature neuroglia have induced, and are obscured by, a florid peritoneal reaction.

Differential diagnosis

Immature teratomas must be differentiated from benign mature cystic teratomas, since even the low-grade tumors have the potential to recur and kill the patient. This diagnostic pitfall can be avoided by adequately sampling all apparently straightforward, predominantly cystic, teratomas, concentrating on solid areas, particularly any that are unusually soft (encephaloid), hemorrhagic or necrotic. Reactivity for GFAP helps identify mature and immature glial tissue, and similarly, HNK-1 (CD57) for other neuroectodermal tissue. In immature teratomas the various tissues are admixed haphazardly throughout the tumor, contrasting sharply with benign cystic teratomas in which there is some semblance of organization.

Immature teratoma is a common component of malignant mixed germ cell tumors, and the possibility of a mixed tumor should be explored by extensive histologic sampling. If more than one low-power field of other malignant germ cell tumor elements is found, such tumors must be excluded from the pure immature teratoma category. Elevated preoperative β-hCG or AFP levels should lead to a careful search for the corresponding histologic components.

Carcinosarcomas (see Chapter 25) exhibit a variety of tissue types and may be a source of confusion. However, they are derived from mesoderm only and therefore neural elements are virtually never present. The adenocarcinomatous components are usually readily distinguishable from the tubular neuroepithelial elements of immature teratoma but, if in doubt, reactivity for cytokeratin and lack of reactivity for GFAP and HNK-1 (CD57) are confirmatory. Chondroid elements are frequently present in müllerian tumors but they are highly pleomorphic, contrasting with the common chondroid components of immature teratomas that have an embryonal rather than a chondrosarcomatous appearance. Rhabdomyoblasts are not uncommon in müllerian tumors but are rare in immature teratomas.[188] A clinical feature helpful in differential diagnosis is that carcinosarcomas occur predominantly in postmenopausal women, whereas immature teratomas have never been reported in this age group.

The monodermal variants of immature teratoma, e.g., malignant neuroectodermal tumors, should be clearly identified as such in the final diagnosis since some have a significantly worse prognosis.

Treatment and prognosis

The prognosis of immature teratomas depends principally on the histologic grade of the ovarian tumor (in stage 1 cases) or that of its metastases (in higher stage cases). The grading system for these tumors is unique in ovarian tumor pathology, being based on the degree of tissue immaturity in the neuroepithelium. The grade of the primary tumor appears to determine the likelihood of extraovarian spread whereas the grade of the metastases in addition correlates with the likelihood of recurrence and possible death from uncontrolled tumor growth. Large size of tumor (>1500 g), rupture (spontaneous or operative), and increasing age are further adverse factors. Recurrences, if they occur, usually develop within the first postoperative year so that the published 2- and 5-year survival rates are similar. Refinement in modern combination chemotherapy has seen a remarkable improvement in long-term clinical outcome with overall disease-free survival rates of over 95%.[101,110] Only very large grade 1, stage 1 solid teratomas (greater than 1500 g) progress and warrant consideration of adjuvant chemotherapy. Clinical tumor staging does not correlate with prognosis as well as might be expected from experience with ovarian tumors in general, since the presence of metastases that are histologically mature may presage maturation of the primary tumor and therefore confers a paradoxically good prognosis on some high stage tumors.

There is general agreement on management. Conservative, fertility-sparing surgery is recommended, with careful follow-up, for patients with stage 1–2, low-grade tumors. This is reasonable in view of the rarity of bilateral immature teratomas and the possibility of future fertility that it offers young patients. However, the surgeon must be aware that about one-sixth of contralateral ovaries will contain a dermoid cyst. Patients with high-grade, stage 1–2 tumors, or with stage 3 tumors of any grade of immaturity, or those with tumor recurrence, have benefited from combination chemotherapy. All the excised metastatic tumor tissue should be examined histologically since the deposits may vary in their degree of maturation. If all are mature (gliomatosis peritonei) and the underlying ovarian teratoma is mature, no further immediate treatment is required, although rare malignant transformation of mature peritoneal glial deposits may be encountered.[161] Radiotherapy has not proved useful in controlling the disease.

MATURE TERATOMAS

MATURE SOLID TERATOMAS

Definition

These solid teratomas consist exclusively of mature or adult tissues and are rare compared with the cystic form (dermoid cyst). The age distribution at presentation is comparable to that of immature teratomas but the clinical features are otherwise similar to those of the common cystic form. Gliomatosis peritonei (peritoneal implantation of mature glial tissue) occurs in about one-third of cases but does not indicate malignancy.[60,126] A confident diagnosis of mature solid teratoma can only be made after thorough sampling to exclude immature areas or other malignant germ cell tumor components.

Pathology

The macroscopic features are similar to those of immature teratomas, although hemorrhage and necrosis are uncommon unless torsion has occurred. Histologic examination reveals a wide variety of mature tissues from all three germ cell layers. These are more finely intermingled than in the cystic variants but still retain some degree of organization. Neural elements often predominate and these must be carefully scrutinized for evidence of immaturity or mitotic activity.

Treatment and prognosis

The clinical course is always benign, and the recommended treatment is unilateral salpingo-oophorectomy with excision of peritoneal lesions, if present, as thoroughly as is practicable.

MATURE CYSTIC TERATOMAS

Definition

These tumors, derived from postmeiotic germ cells,[185] display predominantly one or more cysts lined by epidermis, accompanied by its appendages, and usually one or more other adult-type tissues. The component tissues correspond to those of a developing fetus of over 8 weeks development (fertilization age).[30] Another speculative pathogenetic mechanism is the fusion or coalescence of primordial follicles to give binovular forms.[125] Rare examples of familial incidence suggest genetic predisposition in some patients.[77]

Mature cystic teratomas are by far the most common form of germ cell tumor and constitute 15–25% of ovarian tumors overall. The proportion is greater in children, 40–50%.[43] The term 'dermoid cyst', while only appropriate for those examples composed exclusively of epidermal and adnexal structures, is in such common use for mature cystic teratomas that there is no realistic expectation that it will be changed.

Clinical profile

Mature cystic teratomas occur at all ages, but are rare in infancy. Most cases are diagnosed in the reproductive years (mean age, 35 years).[13] Although many patients present with non-specific signs and symptoms of an ovarian tumor, a considerable proportion (up to 60% of all cases) are asymptomatic and discovered only as incidental findings during pelvic examination, caesarean section or surgery for other indications. Some are detected during laparotomy for the removal of a contralateral germ cell tumor. Menstrual disturbances are unusual and rarely related to the presence of the tumor. However, mature cystic teratomas have, on occasions, been associated with symptomatic excessive production of estrogen or androgen.[105]

Complications that have often been associated with mature cystic teratomas include torsion (in 5% of cases),[13] spontaneous rupture (in 2% of cases), infection (<1% of cases), malignant transformation (in 1.5% of cases),[36] and autoimmune hemolytic anemia.[64] One case was accompanied by sclerosing peritoni-

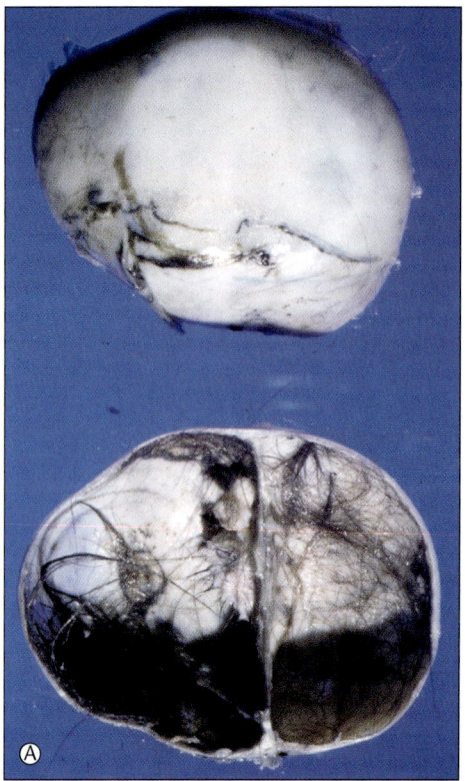

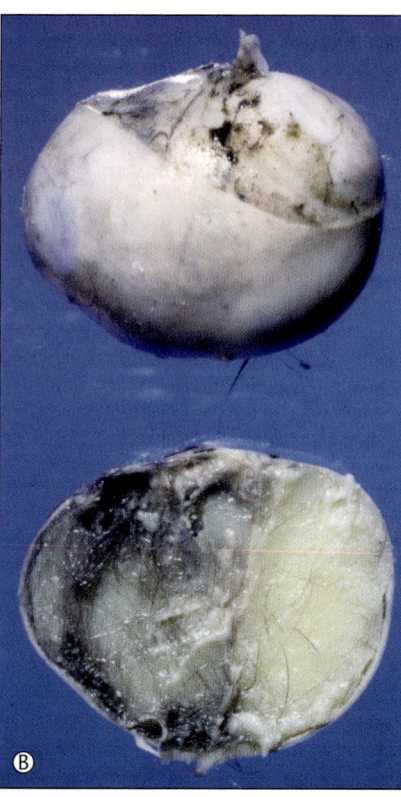

Fig. 27.46 Bilateral mature cystic teratomas in pregnancy. **(A)** Left ovarian cyst is bilocular; dermal papilla (Rokitansky tubercle) and teeth are present in left locule. **(B)** Right ovarian cyst shows typical content of thick greasy sebaceous material and hairs; note thick capsule.

tis,[166] an entity more usually seen with ovarian fibromatosis (see Chapter 22).

With spontaneous rupture, there is usually an insidious leakage of contents into the peritoneal cavity, which may cause a widespread peritoneal granulomatous reaction that mimics carcinomatosis or tuberculosis (see Chapter 33) or result in gliomatosis peritonei (a complication much more commonly associated with solid mature or immature teratomas). Rarely, rupture and intraperitoneal spillage is followed, many years later, by recurrence of discrete intraperitoneal tumor masses,[92] a phenomenon that must be distinguished from the so-called 'growing teratoma syndrome' – a result of previous chemotherapy for non-dysgerminomatous malignant germ cell tumors.[128,146,174] Other rare complications relate to hormonal function of endocrine tissues present in the tumor such as thyroid tissue[5,52] or trophin-producing pituitary tissue,[24] or to the subsequent development of malignant germ cell tumors in the residual ovarian tissue of patients whose mature cystic teratomas were removed by cystectomy alone.[6]

Macroscopic features
Mature cystic teratomas are bilateral in 9–16% of cases (Figure 27.46). In 1% of cases, multiple, apparently discrete tumors are found within the ovary. Some patients harbor an additional cyst in an extraovarian site such as omentum, retroperitoneum, spinal canal, lung or round ligament.[80] Omental lesions most probably represent parasitic ovarian cysts that have detached following torsion.[181]

The tumors are round or ovoid and range in size from 1 cm to over 30 cm, but most are 5–10 cm in maximum diameter when excised. They have thick white capsules, generally free of adhesions, which display prominent blood vessels. Their consistency is doughy, and palpation results in a pitting indentation. On incision, the tumors are usually unilocular cysts filled with thick greasy sebaceous material and matted hair (Figure 27.46) which sometimes round up to form sebum and hair balls.[4] Once cooled or refrigerated, sebum solidifies. Washing under hot water dissolves this material, facilitating the further examination of the tumour and its component parts (see Chapter 35). Less commonly, cysts contain only mucoid material or clear fluid, which has the biochemical characteristics of cerebrospinal fluid. This latter phenomenon is more common in childhood and, if pronounced, has been dubbed 'ovarian hydrocephalus'. About 5–10% of tumors are multilocular.

After emptying the cyst contents, a polypoid nodule (or occasionally nodules) called the dermal papilla or Rokitansky tubercle can almost always be identified protruding into the lumen (Figure 27.46). The cyst lining is generally white and smooth, resembling skin. The hairs usually emanate from the tubercle, and their color in most instances matches that of the host. Teeth have been identified in up to one-third of cases. They are usually found in the soft tissue of the cyst wall but may be loose in the cavity or embedded in bone (Figure 27.46). Incisors, molars and less commonly canines at various stages of development have been identified. Other tissues that are frequently present and readily recognized macroscopically are bone, cartilage, adipose tissue, and brain tissue. Rarely, pigmented foci may be present. Older lesions may exhibit marked dystrophic calcification. Prominent vascular components may simulate cavernous hemangiomas. Sometimes organized structures resembling portions of intestines, skeletal structures or eyes may be recognized. Rare, bizarre cases demonstrate feti-

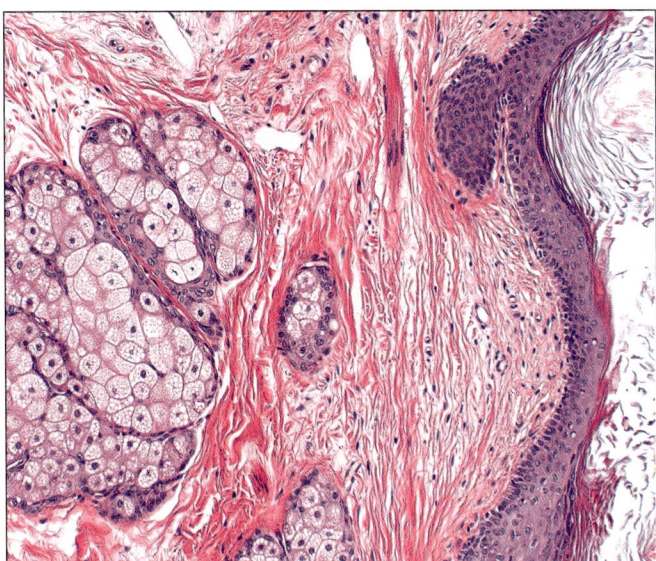

Fig. 27.47 Mature cystic teratoma. This cyst is lined by mature epidermis and subtended by connective tissue containing exuberant dermal appendages (pilosebaceous follicles).

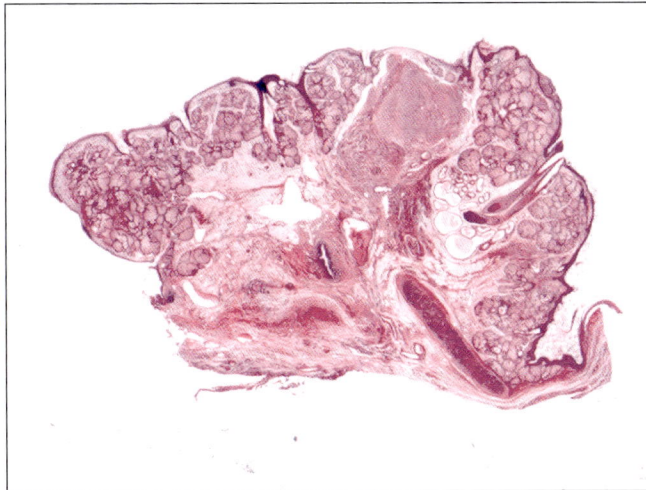

Fig. 27.48 Survey view of dermal papilla from mature cystic teratoma. Cyst is lined chiefly by squamous epithelium with underlying adnexal structures.

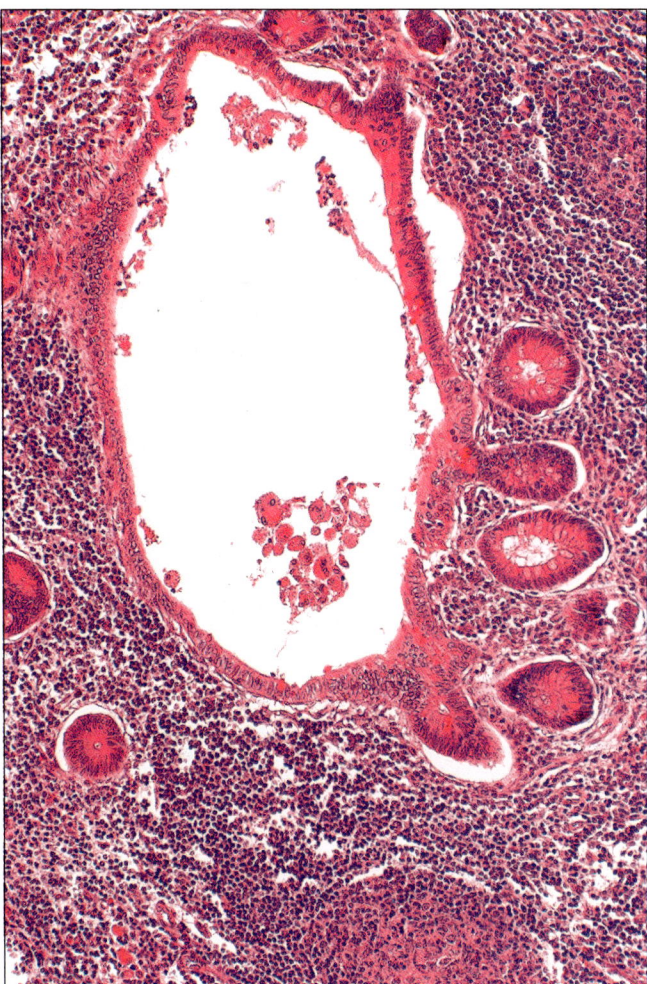

Fig. 27.49 Mature cystic teratoma. Colonic mucosa with lymphoid aggregates mimicking the appendix.

form structures (homunculi)[96] attached to the inner lining of the cyst; these show a predominance of lower extremity and distal parts.

Microscopic features

Various mature tissues are usually present, derived from two or all three germ cell layers. Ectodermal tissues are present almost universally (Figures 27.47 and 27.48) while mesodermal and endodermal tissues are identified in at least half of all cases.

Keratinized squamous epithelium and occasionally respiratory epithelium or neuroglia commonly line the cysts (Figures 27.51 and 27.52). Skin adnexal structures (i.e., hair follicles, sebaceous and sweat glands) are common and are most prolific in the dermal papilla (Figure 27.48). It is here also that the majority of other tissues are most often identified, while adipose tissue, neural tissue, and smooth muscle are more widely dis-

tributed. 'Supradiaphragmatic' tissues predominate. There is always some degree of organization of different tissues following the rules of normal embryogenesis. Skin appendages bear their usual relationship to the epidermis (Figure 27.48) and intestinal epithelium includes argyrophil cells and may be subtended by lymphoid aggregates (Figure 27.49) and smooth muscle, even containing interstitial cells of Cajal.[1] The rare presence of male tissues, e.g., prostatic glands (Figure 27.50), in cystic teratomas is difficult to explain, unless induction by locally produced androgens is invoked. The immunophenotype is identical to that of normal prostate.[68,184]

A summary is presented below, of tissues found in such tumors.

- *Tissues very commonly present* (>66% of cases): epidermis, hair follicles, sebaceous glands, smooth muscle, adipose tissue, cerebrum (children).
- *Tissues commonly present* (33–66% of cases): sweat glands, cerebrum (adults), peripheral nerve, cartilage, bone, respiratory epithelium (Figure 27.52).
- *Tissues occasionally present* (5–33% of cases): teeth, gastrointestinal epithelium (Figure 27.49), thyroid tissue (Figure 27.53), salivary glands, ependyma.

- *Tissues rarely present (<5% of cases)*: prostate (Figure 27.50), retina, breast, pituitary, choroid plexus (Figure 27.51B), ganglia (Figure 27.54A), lung (Figure 27.55), kidney, liver, cardiac muscle, adrenal, thymus, cerebellum (Figure 27.54B), striated muscle (Figure 27.56) or erectile tissue (Figure 27.57).

One-fourth of tumors show focal loss of the squamous epithelial lining, and consequent florid granulomatous reaction to the exposed hair fragments and keratinous debris (Figure 27.58). The response to exposed lipid, keratinous debris, and hair may rarely, however, be extremely florid, even to the extent of simulating a neoplastic process (Figure 27.59). Another common finding is a lattice or sieve-like pattern of spaces outlined by attenuated foreign-body giant cells (Figure 27.58B), also referred to as a 'pneumatosis cystoides-like' appearance, which represents a granulomatous lipophagic reaction to interstitial

oily sebaceous material. Rarely there is reactive new bone formation in response to organized connective tissue around hair shafts (Figure 27.58C).

Individual tissues retain their functional potential and may respond 'appropriately' to an altered hormonal milieu, e.g., secretory activity in mammary tissue of a pregnant host. Degenerative and inflammatory changes that occur in normally sited tissues have also been reported in teratomas, e.g., neuronal degeneration (see Figure 27.62), reactive astrocytic changes, odontogenic structures showing caries or variants of fibrous dysplasia (Figure 27.60), graying of hair, gastric mucosa showing peptic ulceration[154] or ischemic ulceration (Figure 27.61), and thyroiditis.[49] Epidermal melanocytes have been observed in 40–75% of negroid and 7–12% of Caucasian patients. Intradermal, compound, and blue nevi have been found in association with the epidermal lining of the cysts,[97]

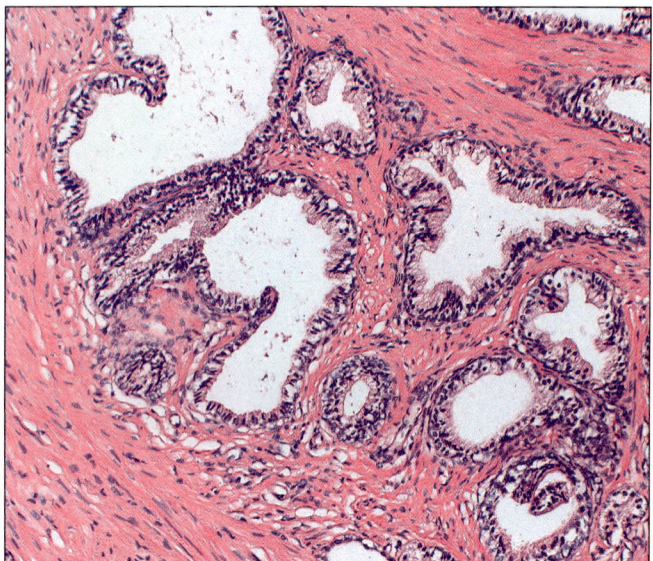

Fig. 27.50 Mature cystic teratoma. Typical prostatic glands.

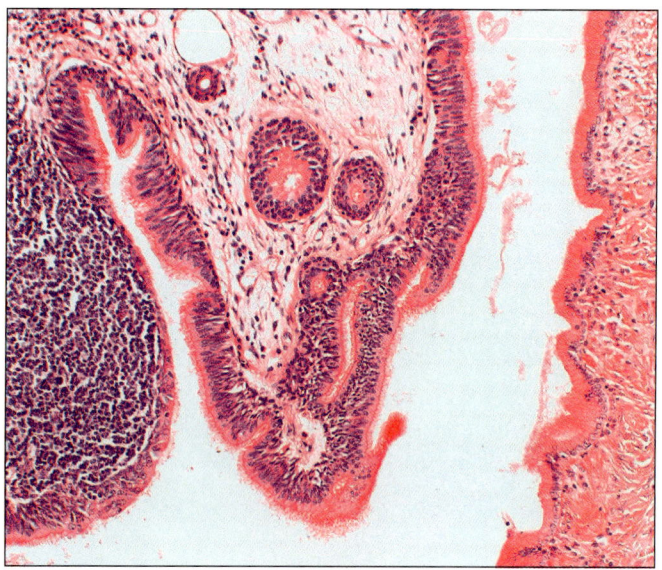

Fig. 27.52 Mature cystic teratoma. Small cystic space lined by an endocervical-like simple mucinous epithelium at left and respiratory mucosa at right.

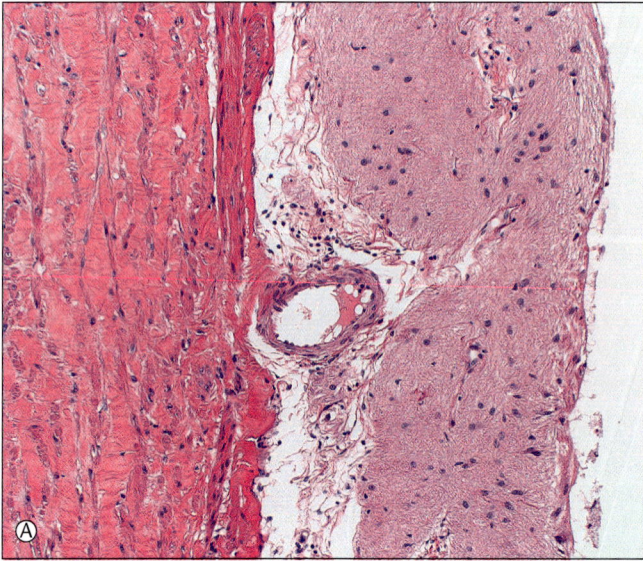

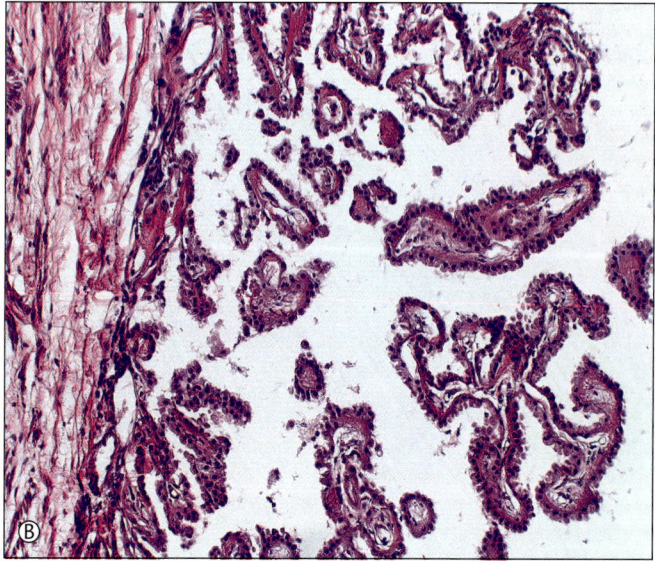

Fig. 27.51 Mature cystic teratoma. Cysts are occasionally lined by **(A)** mature neuroglia or **(B)** ependyma with choroid plexus formation.

and their existence is of interest when considering the origin of primary ovarian malignant melanomas (see below).

Differential diagnosis

The pathologic features of mature cystic teratomas are so well known that problems in differential diagnosis rarely arise. Despite the classic macroscopic appearance, the solid portions of the tumor should be well sampled to exclude the possibility of immature teratoma, other germ cell tumor elements or secondary malignant transformation, all of which carry important prognostic implications. Conversely, a not uncommon diagnostic error that we have seen in consultation is to mistake mature cerebellar tissue for immature neuroglia or, indeed, for small cell carcinoma.

Mixed müllerian tumors may include a variety of tissues, both mesenchymal and epithelial, but all are of mesodermal origin and one or more components usually show malignant characteristics (see Chapter 25).

Treatment and prognosis

Growth of the tumors is slow. However, surgical removal is generally recommended in order to confirm the nature of the neoplasm and to avert the development of complications, including malignant transformation. In women who wish to preserve optimal childbearing potential, cystectomy rather than total oophorectomy may be attempted, and the recurrence rate after this procedure appears to be very low. Up to one-sixth of contralateral ovaries will contain or subsequently develop a mature cystic teratoma. Clinical and morphologic characteristics said to be risk factors for recurrence are young age and a greater diversity of tissues including those of central nervous system type.[191]

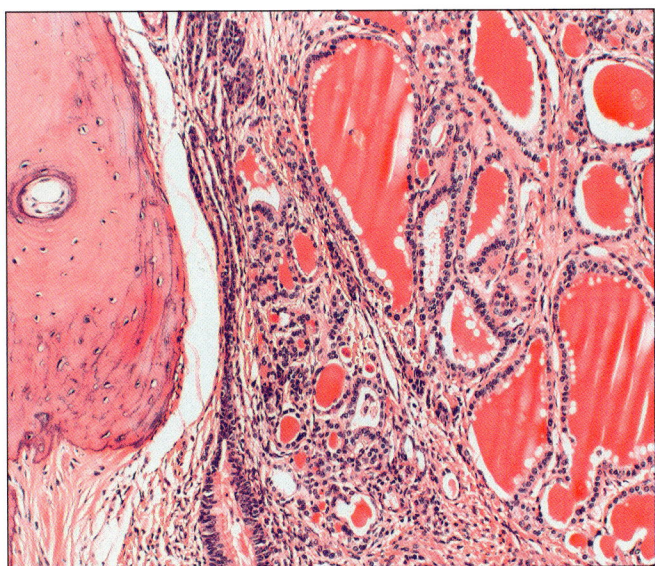

Fig. 27.53 Mature cystic teratoma. Small focus of thyroid tissue, adjacent to a bony nodule, in cyst wall.

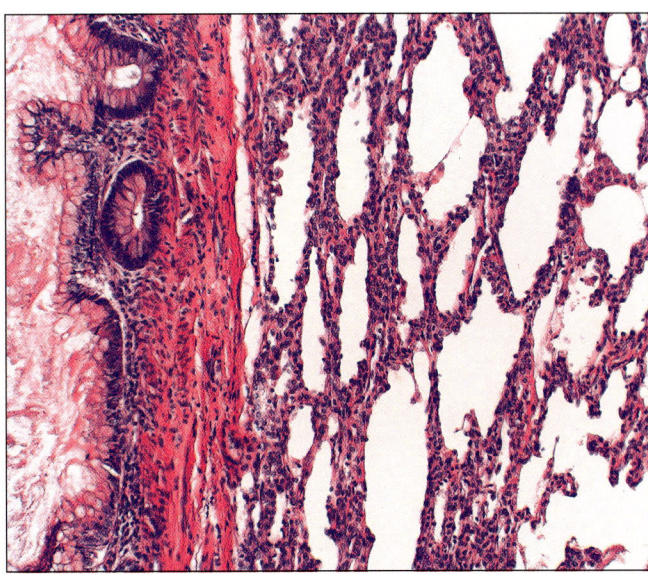

Fig. 27.55 Pulmonary tissue is a rare finding in mature cystic teratomas. Here it is subtended by gastrointestinal epithelium (left).

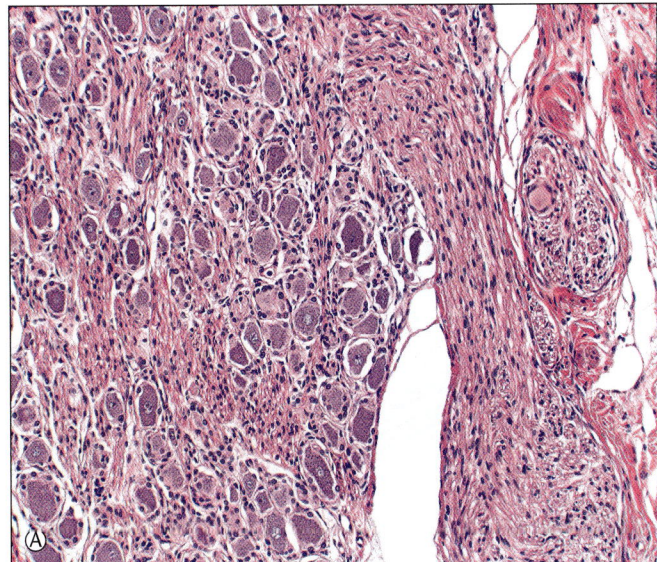

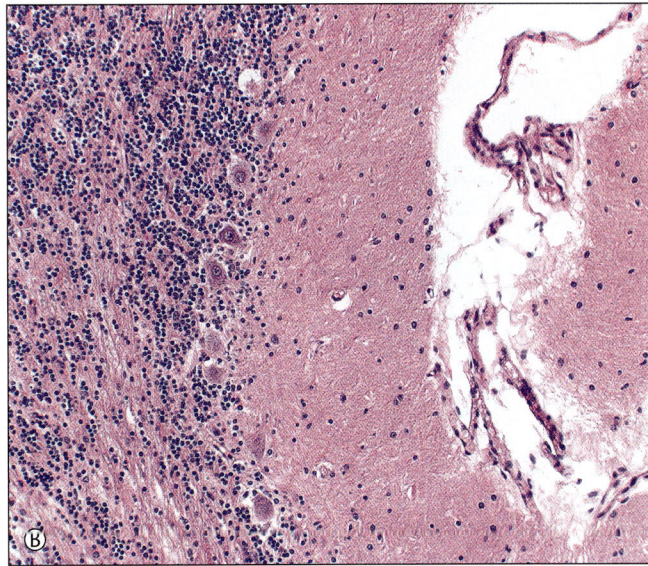

Fig. 27.54 Neural tissues in mature cystic teratomas. **(A)** Ganglion and large nerve bundle. **(B)** Nodule of cerebellar tissue; the cyst was lined by ependyma.

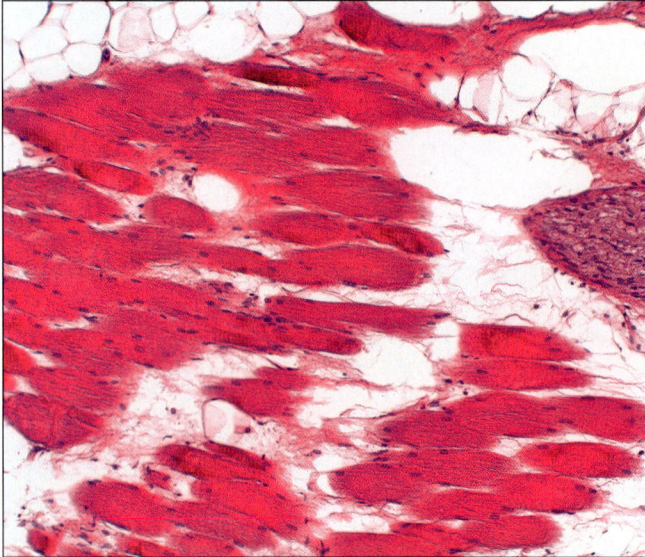

Fig. 27.56 Striated muscle is unusually identified in mature cystic teratomas. Here it is surrounded by adipose tissue.

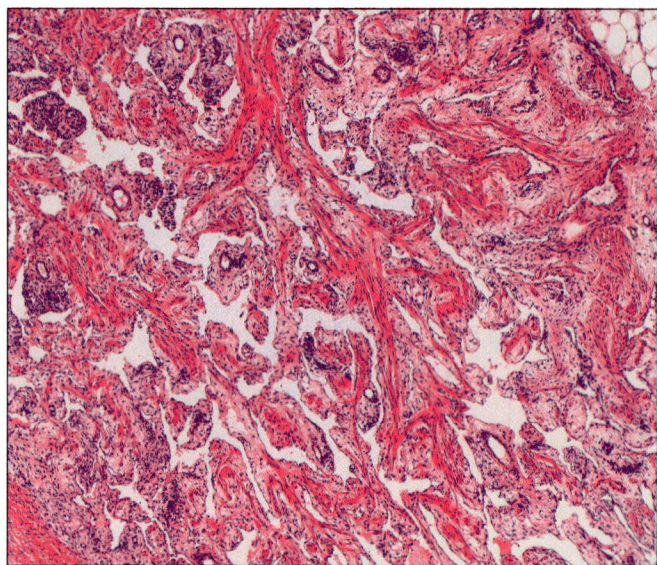

Fig. 27.57 Small discrete and partly organoid focus of vascular erectile tissue. Adipose tissue is seen at bottom left.

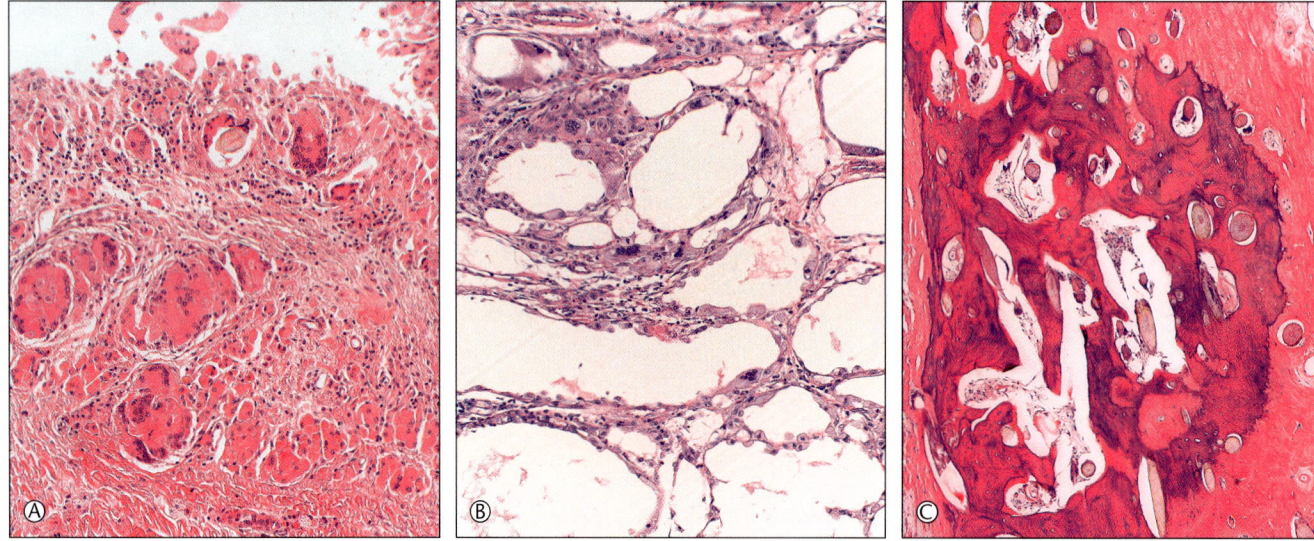

Fig. 27.58 Mature cystic teratoma. Reactive changes in walls of cystic teratomas where cyst lining has broken down. **(A)** Sheets of foamy macrophages, some multinucleated, surround hair fragments. **(B)** Sieve-like (so-called 'lattice') pattern in wall of cyst. Some of the fat spaces are lined by large macrophages. **(C)** Reactive new bone formation around extruded cyst contents and hair.

TERATOMAS WITH SECONDARY MALIGNANT TRANSFORMATION

Definition

This category does not include all malignant neoplasms arising from, or in association with, benign cystic teratomas. By convention, malignancies associated with monodermal teratomas are excluded. Thyroid carcinomas and carcinoids are therefore discussed separately. Tumors that include malignant germ cell tumor elements, such as choriocarcinoma, as well as teratomatous elements are also excluded as these form part of the malignant mixed germ cell tumor group. Malignant transformation, as thus defined, develops in approximately 1.5% of mature cystic teratomas. This complication occurs most often in postmenopausal women but is also, albeit rarely, seen in younger women (including those who are pregnant) and girls as young as 9 years. Exceptional cases may disclose more than one malignant component (Figure 27.62).[178,189] The validity of malignant neural tumors arising in mature cystic teratomas is questioned and those reported in young women usually but not always represent immature teratomas that characteristically contain neural elements.

Clinical profile

There are no distinctive clinical features, although as a group they are more likely than uncomplicated teratomas to be associated with abdominal swelling (sometimes due to ascites), pain, and systemic symptoms.

At laparotomy, malignancy can be suspected when there is capsular tumor penetration and adhesions, infiltration of adjacent structures or peritoneal metastases. In others the diagnosis is suspected on incising the excised ovarian mass, but in about

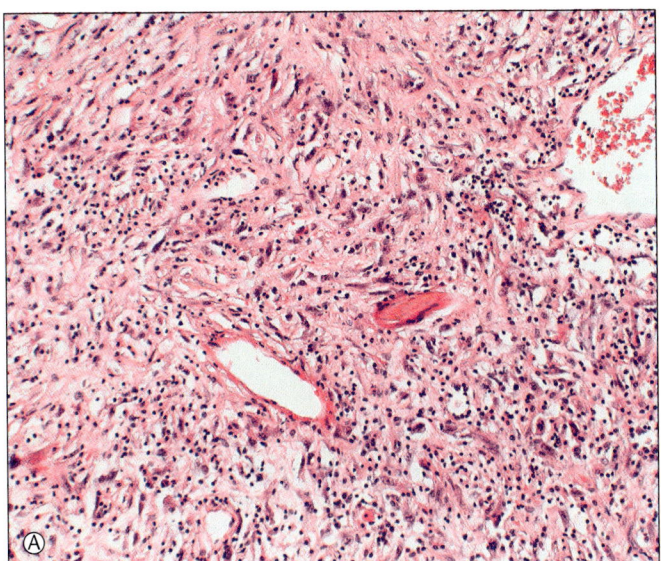

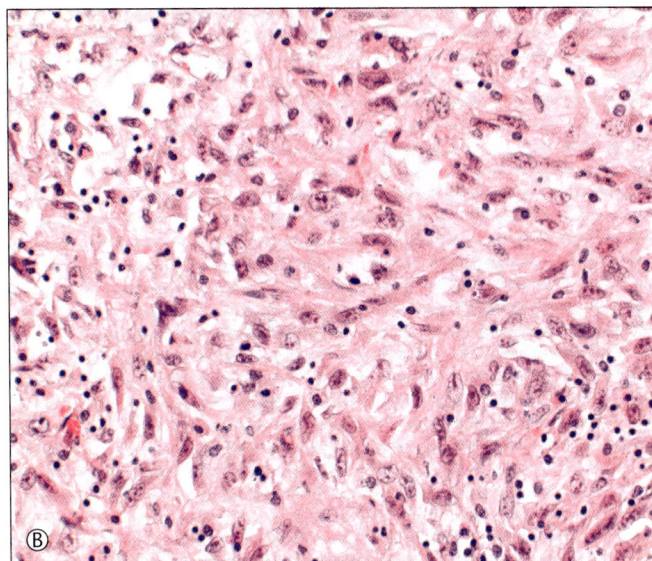

Fig. 27.59 Mature cystic teratoma. A 10 cm soft hemorrhagic tumor-like mass occupying much of the lumen displayed **(A)** an intense fibroxanthomatous response to exposed lipid, keratinous debris, and hair fragments and **(B)** a vigorous proliferation of atypical fibrohistiocytic cells with a somewhat storiform pattern and a patchy mixed inflammatory infiltrate in the background.

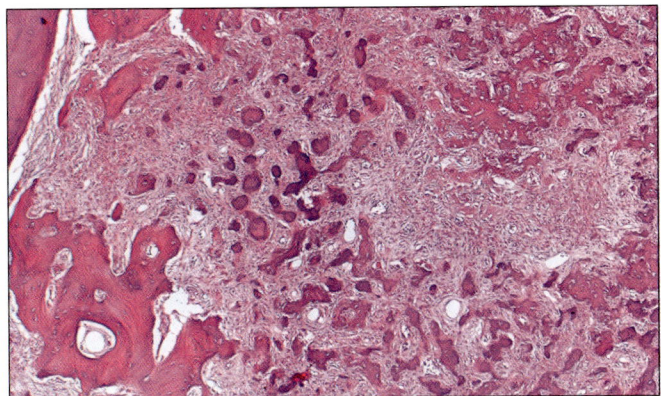

Fig. 27.60 Mature cystic teratoma. A focus, between an island of cortical bone (left) and a nearby tooth, showing 'cemento-osseous' dysplasia. Florid metaplastic bone formation includes some islands resembling cementum.

one-fourth the diagnosis is made only after the tumor is examined histologically. Tumors spread predominantly by local direct infiltration and subsequent intraperitoneal dissemination. Distant lymphatic and blood-borne metastases are distinctly unusual except in sarcomas.

Macroscopic features

Malignant transformation is always unilateral, but an uncomplicated mature cystic teratoma may be present in the contralateral ovary in one-sixth of cases. They mostly are larger than their benign counterparts, generally in the range of 15–20 cm in diameter. At least half display tumor-associated adhesions and capsular penetration. In these more advanced cases, malignant tumor is generally obvious on bisecting the ovaries, presenting as necrotic crumbly masses projecting into the cavity and/or infiltrating the cyst wall. Carcinomas often develop in or close to the dermal papilla. Malignant melanomas form pigmented mural nodules (Figure 27.63). Sarcomas are generally hemorrhagic. However, in many cases tumor growth is

more subtle and may only be represented by a plaque-like focus in the cyst lining or an area of induration in the wall. It is imperative, therefore, that all mature cystic teratomas should be examined histologically with particular attention to any unusual or solid areas. Even if there is an overgrowth of malignant tumor tissue, the presence of an underlying mature cystic teratoma usually declares itself by the presence of hair and/or sebaceous material in the cyst cavity.

Microscopic features

A wide variety of malignant tumors may arise within previously benign mature cystic teratomas, but by far the most common are squamous cell carcinomas.[50,87] They account for over 75% of cases (Figure 27.64). The remainder comprises various adenocarcinomas (7%),[36,57,68,89,98,100,120,168] undifferentiated carcinomas, melanomas,[67,102,193] basal cell carcinomas (<1%), and various sarcomas (7%). Malignant tumors documented to have arisen in mature cystic teratomas of the ovary are listed below with recent or key references to the rarer of these entities.

- Squamous cell carcinoma
- Malignant melanoma
- Thyroid carcinoma (Figure 27.65)
- Adenocarcinoma (Figure 27.66)
- Carcinoid tumor
- Sebaceous carcinoma[182]
- Eccrine adnexal carcinoma[189]
- Apocrine adenocarcinoma[124]
- Adenosquamous carcinoma[76]
- Extramammary Pagets disease[123]
- Clear cell carcinoma[160]
- Undifferentiated carcinoma[27]
- Small cell carcinoma of pulmonary type[103]
- Basal cell carcinoma[31]
- Carcinosarcoma[9]
- Fibrosarcoma[95]
- Osteogenic sarcoma[2,11,55]

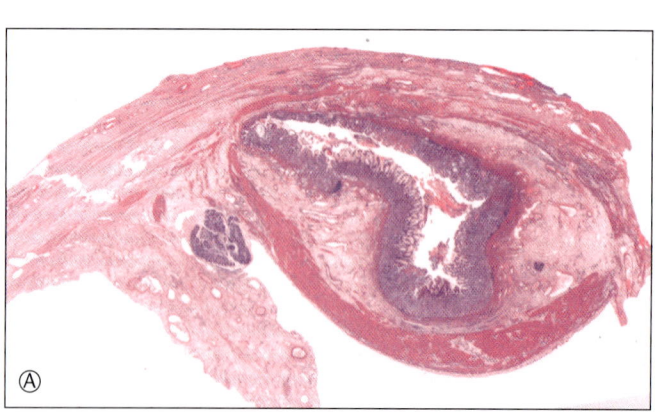

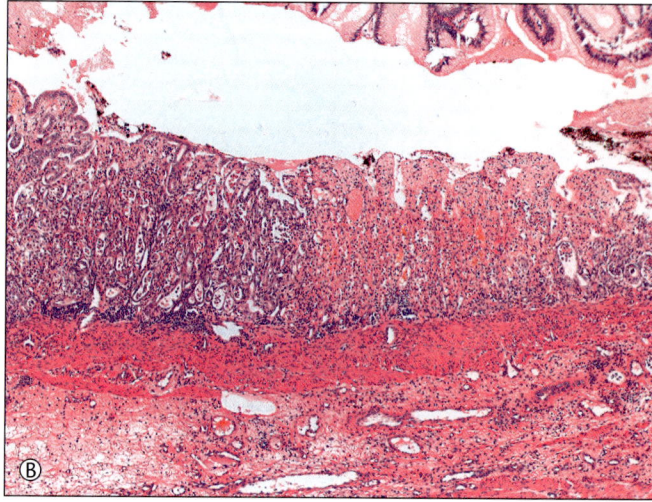

Fig. 27.61 Gastric differentiation in mature cystic teratoma. **(A)** Survey showing transverse section with mixed body-type and antral mucosa, and small central, extramural nodule of exocrine pancreas. **(B)** One of several small punched-out ischemic ulcers with mucosal hemorrhage and necrosis and submucosal inflammation.

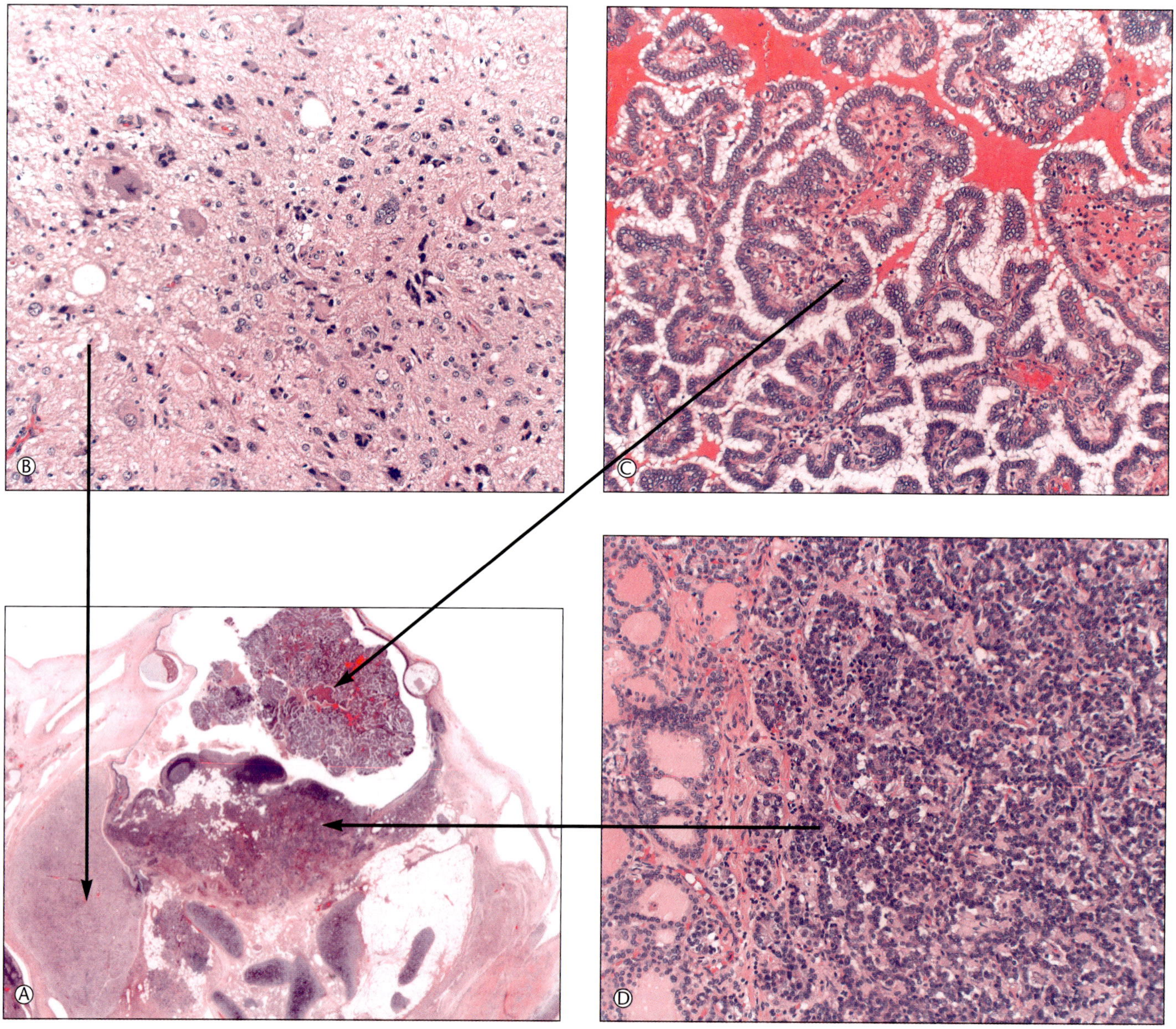

Fig. 27.62 Mature cystic teratoma with multiple malignancies. **(A)** Large mature teratoma with substantial focus of adenocarcinoma (top of field). **(B)** Neural tissue displaying degenerative and dysmorphic changes. **(C)** Papillary carcinoma of thyroid (malignant stroma). **(D)** Trabecular carcinoid.

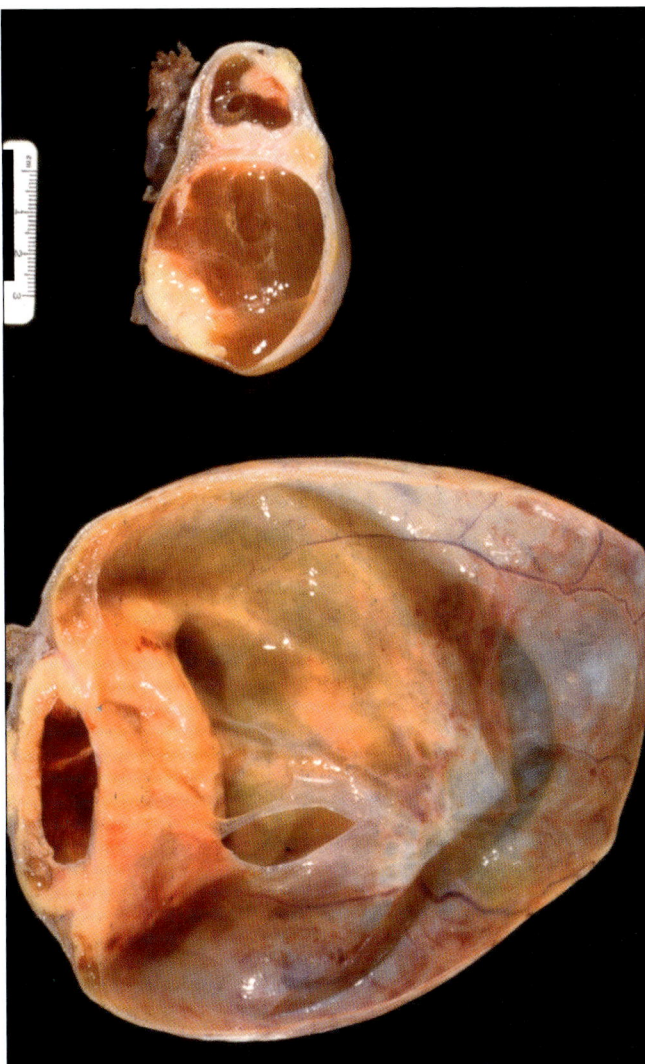

Fig. 27.63 Malignant melanoma arising in a benign cystic teratoma. Discrete, poorly pigmented polypoid projections are seen projecting into the lumen of a somewhat crenated, thin-walled cyst, lined predominantly by neuroglia. Sebaceous and gelatinous debris has been removed to demonstrate the solid tumor masses.

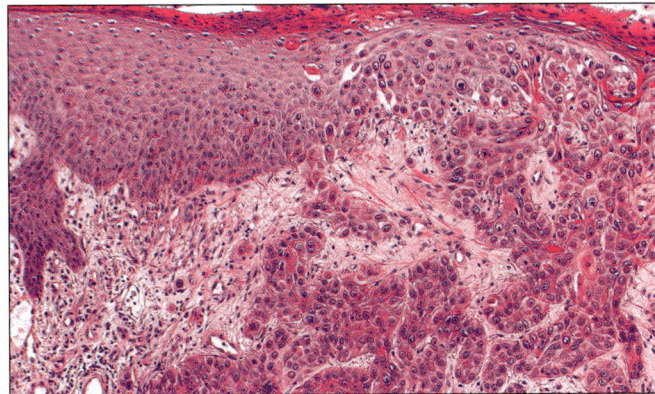

Fig. 27.64 Squamous cell carcinoma arising in the mature cystic teratoma of a 61-year-old woman. The carcinoma formed an 11 cm nodule in the cyst wall.

- Chondrosarcoma[35]
- Leiomyosarcoma[26]
- Malignant mixed mesodermal tumor[54]
- Malignant fibrous histiocytoma[179]
- Angiosarcoma[42,45,78,132]
- Neuroblastoma[145]
- Primitive neuroectodermal tumor[82]
- Glioblastoma[46]
- Paraganglioma[115]

The histologic appearances are diverse, reflecting the wide range of malignancies that may arise within teratomas. Squamous cell carcinomas can often be seen to arise from metaplastic squamous epithelium lining the cyst (Figure. 27.64), sometimes within a zone of dysplastic or *in situ* carcinomatous epithelium or from a focus of ciliated or non-ciliated columnar mucosa. Invading squamous cell carcinoma may also exhibit a pseudosarcomatous stromal reaction.

Adenocarcinomas may arise from a variety of tissues but a specific histogenesis is usually difficult to confirm except in tumors of distinctive histology such as sebaceous carcinoma.[182] Tumors suggestive of mammary, sweat gland or salivary gland origin have been described. Mucinous carcinoma of respiratory type may occasionally develop adjacent to respiratory type tissues.[36,98]

Ovarian malignant melanomas are usually pigmented and show all the histologic patterns seen at other sites.[102,116] Some have junctional activity in the adjacent epidermis-lined cyst.

Differential diagnosis

The teratomatous origin of these tumors may be overlooked if histologic sampling is inadequate; the lesion is then likely to be misdiagnosed as a metastasis. However, there is the possibility that growth of the malignant component may have obliterated the pre-existing teratoma. The clinical presentation should always be taken into account and the pattern of extraovarian spread, if present, should be consistent with a primary ovarian neoplasm.

The most frequent misdiagnosis is immature teratoma, a clinically malignant neoplasm found in girls and young women. This tumor, almost always a predominantly solid lesion, has abundant immature neural components. In addition, other tissue components often show immaturity and malignant cytologic features, unlike mature cystic teratomas with malignant transformation in which only one cancerous component (rarely neural) is demonstrable.

Carcinosarcomas (see Chapter 25) occur in the same age group as the tumors under discussion and exhibit a variety of tissue components. However, they are generally solid and lack the characteristic squamous epithelium-lined cyst and associated adnexal structures. Malignancy is commonly expressed in both the epithelial component (generally resembling serous carcinoma) and the mesenchymal component (usually resembling endometrial stromal sarcoma, at least in part). Endodermally and ectodermally derived structures are, for all practical purposes, absent, but islands of malignant squamous epithelium (of müllerian mesodermal origin) are occasionally present, and rare examples have included malignant neuroectodermal tissues. Such neoplasms have been termed teratoid carcinosarcomas.[53,172]

Some Sertoli–Leydig cell tumors include heterologous elements and these variants (see Chapter 26) may mimic adeno-

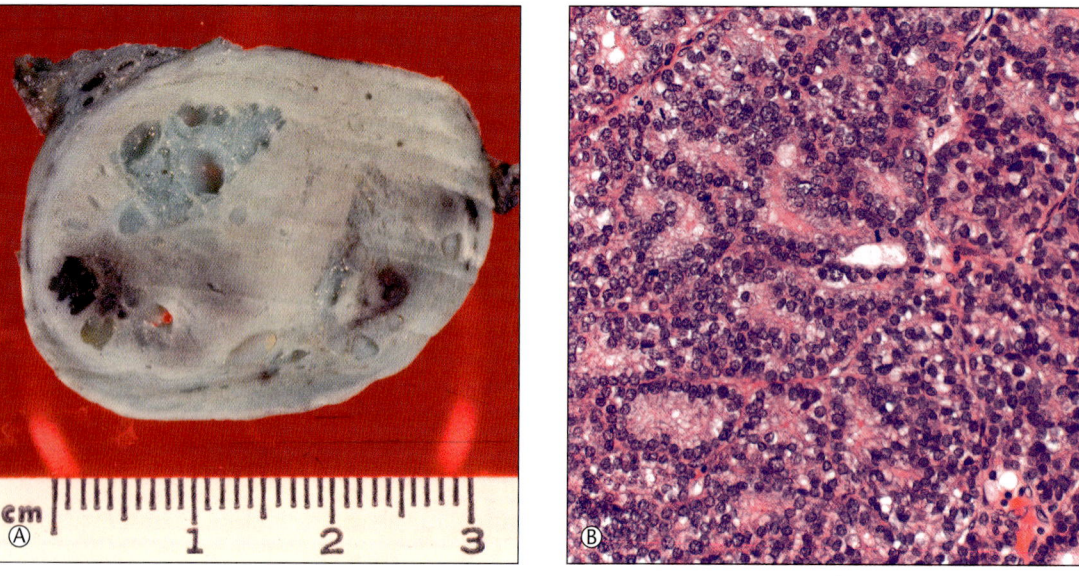

Fig. 27.65 Malignant struma in a 48-year-old woman. **(A)** Ovarian mass. The subsequent clinical course (alive with local disease at 10 years) supported a diagnosis of malignancy. **(B)** Circumscribed but unencapsulated nodule of cellular well-differentiated follicular carcinoma with overlapping nuclei and mitoses.

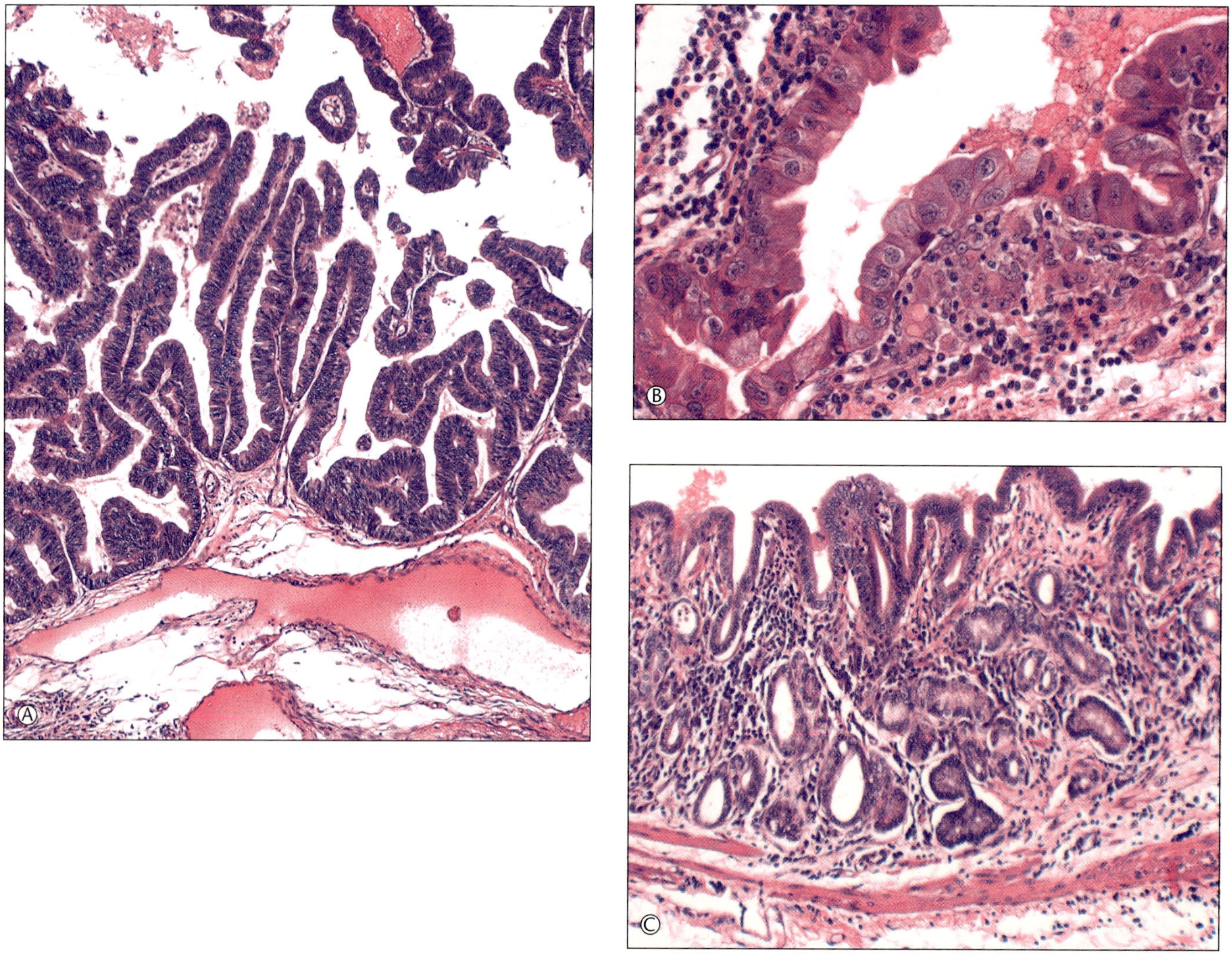

Fig. 27.66 Adenocarcinoma arising from a dermoid cyst in a 62-year-old woman. **(A)** Papillary adenocarcinoma. **(B)** Field of adenocarcinoma *in situ* between carcinoma seen in (a) and benign gastric antral type mucosa seen in **(C)**.

carcinomas or sarcomas arising in mature cystic teratomas. Mucinous epithelium of colonic type is the most common heterologous element but squamous epithelium, almost universal in mature cystic teratomas, is not seen. Sertoli cell tubules tend to be admixed with other heterologous tissues rather than forming a discrete mass as would carcinoma arising in a mature cystic teratoma. When the heterologous elements are malignant and form the major element of the tumor, exhaustive sampling may be the only means to establish the androblastomatous, as opposed to teratomatous, origin of the malignancy. Leydig cells may be scattered within groups throughout the stroma. They are rarely present in the parenchyma of teratomas even though they are common at the peripheral margins. A clinical point of distinction is the occurrence of androblastomas predominantly in young women whereas teratomas with secondary malignant transformation develop typically in postmenopausal women.

The difficulties in distinguishing primary ovarian malignant melanomas from the more common metastatic lesions[67] are also discussed in Chapter 29.

Treatment and prognosis

The prognosis for patients with malignant transformation in teratomas is very poor, with most women dying within a year. Extraovarian spread, if present at the time of diagnosis, carries a dismal outlook. Outcome is less gloomy for patients with squamous cell carcinomas confined to the ovary at the time of surgical treatment,[87] with a 5-year survival rate of 63% compared with 15% for the remainder. Poor prognostic factors include dissemination, cyst wall invasion, ascites, spontaneous or accidental rupture, adhesions, and tumor type other than squamous carcinoma.

The mainstay of treatment is surgery, with pelvic clearance being indicated in most cases. Unilateral oophorectomy may represent sufficient treatment in younger women in whom the ovarian capsule is not breached and the diagnosis is made only on pathologic examination.

MONODERMAL AND HIGHLY SPECIALIZED TERATOMAS

These teratomas consist predominantly or exclusively of one adult tissue and are presumed to result either from teratomatous development involving only one germ cell layer or overgrowth of one tissue at the expense of others originally present. Examples include struma ovarii, carcinoid tumors, epidermoid cysts, and neuroectodermal tumors.

STRUMA OVARII

In this teratoma, thyroid tissue is exclusively present or constitutes a major or grossly recognizable component of a more complex teratoma. Since 5–13% of mature cystic teratomas of the ovary include some thyroid tissue histologically, the diagnosis usually requires that more than 50% of the tumor is made up of thyroid tissue or that the thyroid tissue, regardless of size, is functionally active. By convention, thyroid tissue that is histologically or biologically malignant is also classified as struma. Strumas are generally considered to account for less than 5% of mature teratomas. Conversely, while 50–60% of strumas are associated with, or part of, mature cystic teratomas, most of

the remainder are pure, and a very small percentage are associated with carcinoid tumors (strumal carcinoids) or mucinous cystadenomas in the same ovary. Rare examples also occur in the neighboring tissues of the female genital tract, e.g., the fallopian tube.[73]

Clinical profile

The age range for struma ovarii is narrower than for mature cystic teratomas in general, most cases occurring in the reproductive years with a peak in the early forties. Like mature cystic teratomas of the ovary, most present with non-specific abdominal symptoms or are incidental findings. Rarely, patients develop symptoms or signs indicating estrogen excess, considered to be due to the activity of luteinized stromal cells surrounding the tumor. Up to one-third develop ascites, which can be quite marked but does not signify malignancy. It settles rapidly after tumor removal. Some of these patients also develop a hydrothorax (Meigs syndrome).

Hyperthyroidism is a much discussed complication of struma ovarii[52] but, using biochemical criteria to confirm the clinical impression (not available in most early studies), less than 5% of strumas have this association. In order to attribute biochemically established hyperthyroidism to struma ovarii, thyroid activity should be demonstrated in the ovary by means of a ^{131}I scan[19] and, preferably, a radionucleotide angiogram. The pathogenesis of hyperthyroidism associated with struma ovarii is of interest. The ectopic thyroid tissue appears to act autonomously in a manner analogous to toxic nodular goiter and the thyroid gland itself may be suppressed.

Occasional examples of strumas are clinically malignant, i.e., associated with metastatic disease.[41,152] Genuine metastases occur up to 26 years after oophorectomy, to peritoneum, mesentery, contralateral ovary, liver, bones, mediastinum, lung, and brain.[194] The well-known difficulties in diagnosing malignancy in the thyroid gland are exaggerated in ectopically sited tissue where criteria such as capsular invasion cannot be readily applied. Extraovarian spread appears to be the only valid criterion, so that many cases from the older literature have been discredited by modern reviewers; the original diagnoses were sometimes based on morphology alone (anaplasia and mitotic activity) or on a misinterpretation of what we now know to be strumal carcinoid tumors.[150] Spread of banal thyroid tissue to the peritoneal cavity, peritoneal strumosis (see below), while sometimes described as a benign condition,[21] can in our experience recur.

Macroscopic features

Struma ovarii is almost always unilateral. The contralateral ovary rarely harbors an additional struma, but is more likely to contain an uncomplicated mature cystic teratoma. The tumors vary greatly in size but typical lesions are about 10 cm in diameter (but somewhat larger if cystic in nature or if associated with mature cystic teratomas). Strumas associated with hyperthyroidism are generally more than 6 cm in diameter. They are most often found as circumscribed nodules in the walls of mature cystic teratomas but, if pure, form encapsulated lobulated masses with smooth surfaces, often displaying prominent blood vessels. Sectioning of the tumors reveals soft or firm red-brown or yellowish tissue with a glistening surface. Tumors are mostly solid but usually include multiple small cystic spaces containing colloid or mucoid material. Cystic variants contain clear to green-brown fluid. Hemorrhage, necrosis, and fibrosis may be apparent and, in fact, the gross appearance may closely resemble that of nodular colloid or adenomatous goiters (Figure 27.67).

Microscopic features

The thyroid tissue of struma ovarii exhibits morphologic and biochemical identity with thyroid tissue in the neck (Figure 27.68A). It may appear histologically 'normal' but more commonly shows a range of minor abnormalities. There is generally a great variability in follicular size and maturity, with macrofollicular, microfollicular, and solid (embryonal) patterns being commonly observed. Small numbers of oxyphil cells may also be encountered, as rarely may clear cell variants (Figure 27.68B).[108] The colloid is PAS positive and contains birefringent oxalate crystals. The identity of the tissue can be

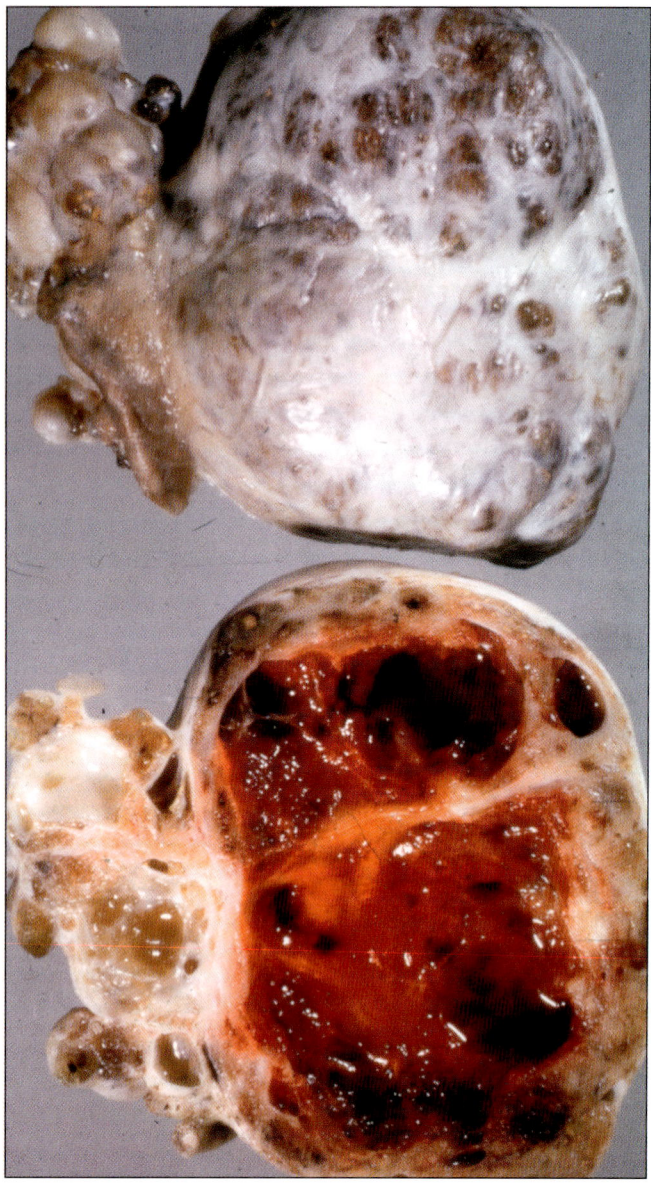

Fig. 27.67 Struma ovarii. Encapsulated mass of glistening thyroid tissue with foci of cystic degeneration and fibrosis. No other heterologous elements were present in this tumor.

readily confirmed by immunohistochemical stain for thyroglobulin. All the microscopic features associated with nodular colloid or adenomatous goiters may be encountered, e.g., fibrosis, hemorrhage, and cystic degeneration. This latter feature may lead to a paucity of thyroid follicles in the cyst wall with an accompanying danger of the diagnosis being overlooked.[169]

Follicular adenoma-like areas are not infrequently seen but their significance is unknown. One group[47] has subcategorized the largest series of such cases as 'proliferative struma' to indicate tumor-like architectural and cellular features but separable from 'malignant struma' by the lack of 'ground glass', overlapping nuclei, vascular space invasion or mitotic activity. All their 'proliferative struma' cases pursued a benign clinical course. In our own experience, excessive cellularity is sometimes a marker of progressive clinical course, albeit manifesting many years after removal of the primary ovarian mass.[151,152] No capsule normally separates thyroid tissue from adjacent teratomatous elements, if present, or residual ovarian parenchyma, and capsular invasion, an important parameter in the assessment of follicular tumors in the thyroid gland of the neck, is not available in equivalent ovarian thyroid masses.

Stromal luteinization or, rarely, Leydig cell hyperplasia, may be seen at the margins of the tumor (Figure 27.69), much like any teratoma. In patients with hyperthyroidism, and some without, histologic features of hyperplasia may be evident, i.e., diminution in colloid with scalloping of its margin and tall columnar epithelium with focal intraluminal tufting. Florid diffuse hyperplasia is rarely seen and correlates poorly with toxicity. As in the thyroid gland, mild nuclear atypia and mitotic activity can be present without generating suspicions of malignancy. Vascular invasion should be regarded as indicating a tumor of uncertain malignant potential. Indisputable malignant strumas, i.e., with documented extraovarian spread, have manifested primarily papillary patterns,[135] rarely follicular variants,[148] and commonly a hypercellular pattern as seen in adenomas.

More frequently than might be expected by chance, struma ovarii is seen associated with benign Brenner tumors,[22,171,190] with intermediate immunoprofiles in some of the transitional cell nests.

Benign thyroid tissue outside the ovaries (strumosis peritonei) is seen as variably sized colloid-like nodules on or just beneath the visceral peritoneum (Figure 27.70).

Differential diagnosis

Colloid-like follicles or microfollicular foci may be encountered in some clear cell carcinomas, androblastomas, endometrioid carcinomas, granulosa cell tumors, and pregnancy luteomas. These areas, however, constitute only minor components of these tumors, and other characteristic patterns will be seen elsewhere. Teratomatous elements are not present. If still in doubt, the demonstration of birefringent oxalate crystals in the acini or reactivity for thyroglobulin in the lining epithelium will be conclusive.

Metastatic thyroid carcinoma should not be seriously considered except in a patient with a known primary since, even in this situation, ovarian metastases are exceedingly rare.[192]

Care must be taken not to overlook a strumal carcinoid (see below). The carcinoid component of these tumors is usually trabecular in type and is either intimately admixed with the thyroid follicles or occurs as a discrete focus. The cellular char-

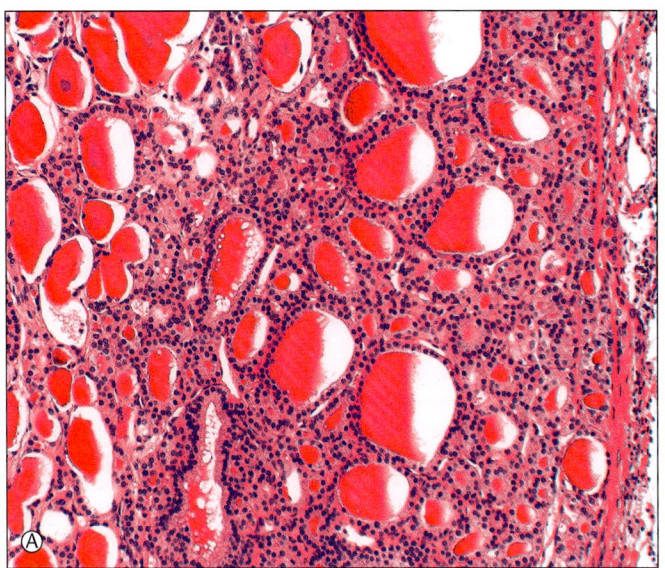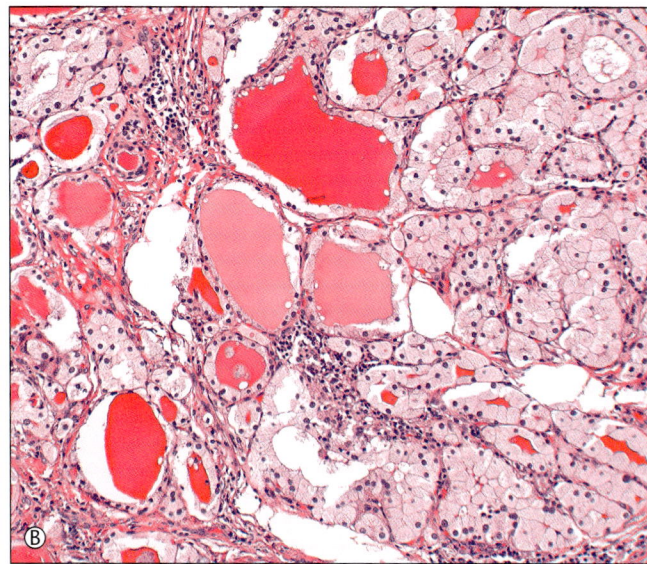

Fig. 27.68 Struma ovarii. **(A)** Variably sized banal thyroid follicles (contrast with Figure 27.65B). **(B)** Rare clear cell struma.

acteristics are the same as in pure carcinoid tumors and most are argyrophilic (see below). Mitotic activity is minimal.

Treatment and prognosis

Oophorectomy is adequate treatment for straightforward struma ovarii. Pelvic clearance is recommended for malignant tumors, with additional thyroidectomy and adjunctive therapy, e.g., ^{131}I, for those with extraovarian spread.[41,194]

CARCINOID AND STRUMAL CARCINOID TUMORS

Primary carcinoid tumors constitute less than 5% of ovarian teratomas and are rarer than struma ovarii, yet are four times as common as carcinoids metastatic to the ovaries. Approximately half are insular, one-third trabecular, and one-sixth strumal in type. A few are mucinous carcinoids (goblet cell or adenocarcinoids),[15,23] or rarely both mucinous and stromal.[113]

A slight majority of primary ovarian carcinoids are associated with other obvious teratomatous elements.[164] Some arise in close proximity to gastrointestinal or respiratory epithelium that includes APUD cells, a possible source of the neoplastic proliferation, or directly from teratomatous primitive neuroectodermal cells or uncommitted endodermal epithelial cells that have the potential for APUD cell differentiation. Rarely, they occur with Sertoli–Leydig cell tumors. Neuroendocrine cells are identified in 6% of non-neoplastic ovaries and these may be the origin of carcinoids not associated with teratomas.

Biochemical, histochemical and morphologic (including ultrastructural) studies indicate that ovarian insular carcinoids are analogous to midgut carcinoids whereas trabecular carcinoids are analogous to foregut or hindgut carcinoids. Strumal carcinoids are composed of carcinoid (mostly trabecular and analogous to hindgut carcinoid) and thyroid elements, both considered to be of endodermal teratomatous origin. Mucinous carcinoids are analogous to the more familiar appendiceal tumors and show biphasic differentiation along mucinous and argentaffin cell lines.

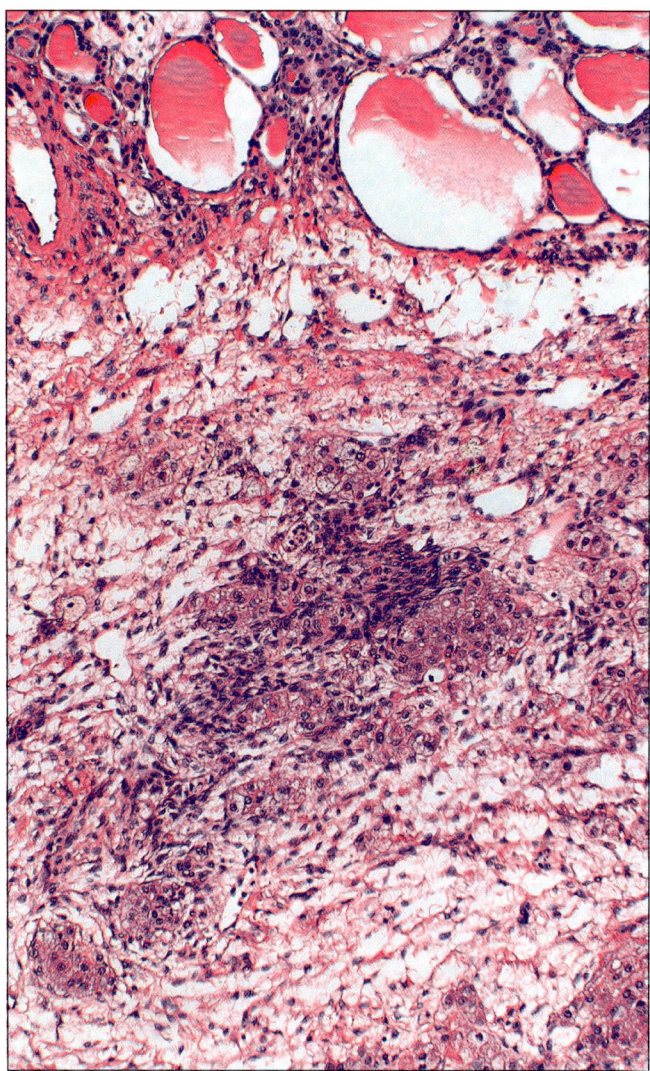

Fig. 27.69 Margin of a struma ovarii showing peripheral Leydig cell hyperplasia. Such Leydig cell clusters were prominently situated around much of the perimeter of the struma.

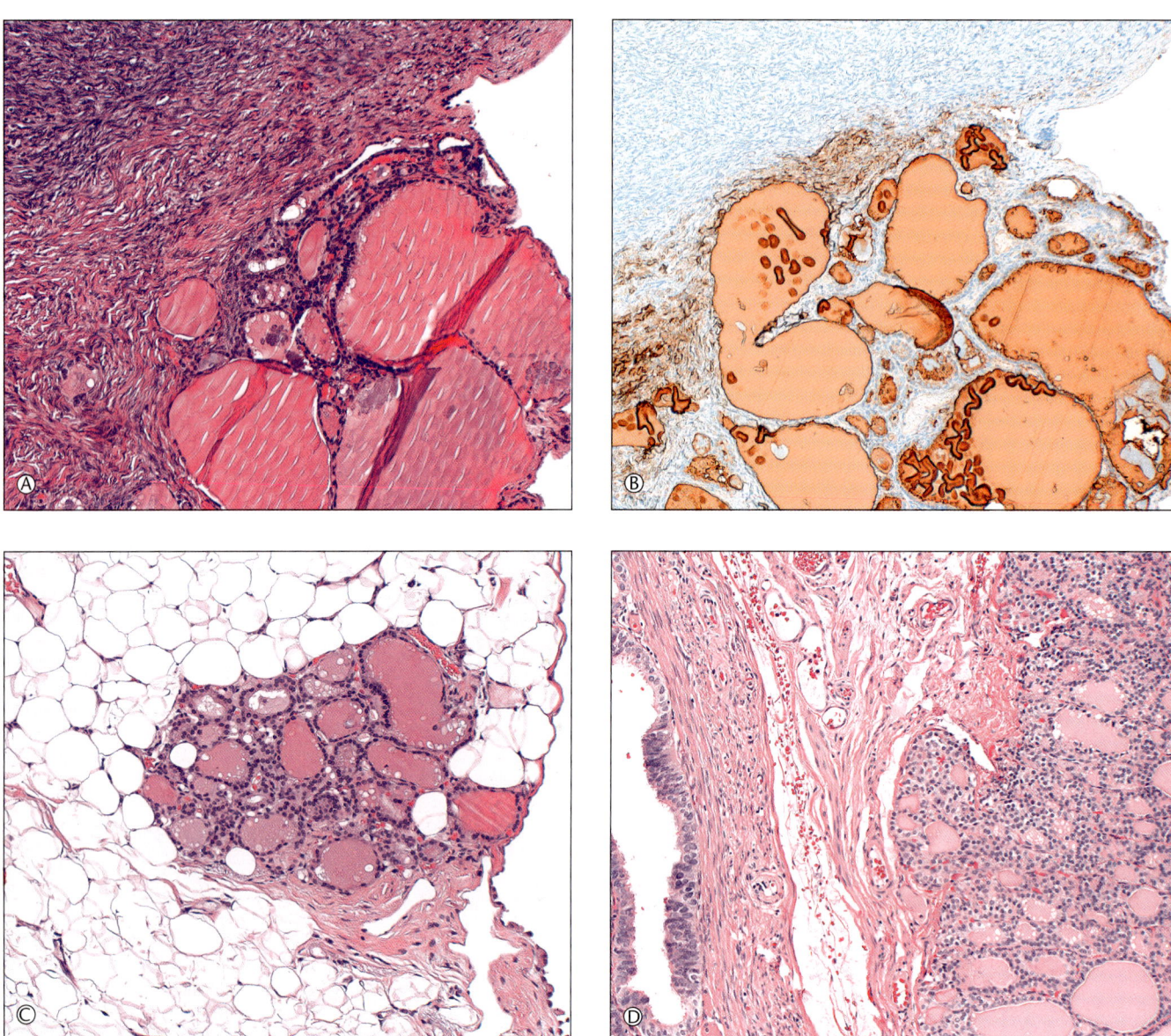

Fig. 27.70 Peritoneal strumosis. A contralateral ovarian dermoid cyst had been removed 25 years previously. **(A)** Strumal tissue is seen on the surface of the residual ovary which, in **(B)**, immunostains for thyroglobulin. Strumal deposits were seen **(C)** in omentum and **(D)** on the serosal surface of the fallopian tube.

Clinical profile

The age range of patients with ovarian carcinoids is wide but most tumors are seen in peri- or postmenopausal women. Mucinous carcinoids occur in somewhat younger women. Most patients present with symptoms relating to an enlarging ovarian mass, or the lesion is an incidental finding. A small percentage of patients present with manifestations of estrogen or androgen excess (abnormal uterine bleeding or virilization) or features of hyperthyroidism.

One-third of patients with insular carcinoids (usually those with a carcinoid tumor >4 cm across) and a very much smaller proportion of patients with trabecular carcinoids[164] display symptoms or signs of the carcinoid syndrome. The flushing attacks must be carefully distinguished from menopausal symptoms that are encountered in the age group in which these tumors most commonly occur. It is a more common complication of ovarian, contrasted with gastrointestinal, carcinoids since the secretory products of the tumor, particularly 5-hydroxytryptamine (serotonin), can reach the systemic circulation without passing through the liver where otherwise they would be detoxified. If the syndrome is suspected preoperatively, it may be confirmed by measuring serum serotonin or urinary 5-hydroxyindoleacetic acid (5-HIAA) levels that are always raised in these patients. Alternatively, constipation may accompany ovarian trabecular carcinoid tumors, due to the elaboration of peptide-YY.[187]

Macroscopic features

Primary ovarian carcinoids are virtually always unilateral, but up to 15% of cases exhibit a mature cystic teratoma or mucinous tumor in the contralateral ovary. Most (60%) are components of mature cystic teratomas or, less commonly, mucinous cystadenomas. In these cases, the mucinous tumor is usually a one-sided overgrowth of the teratoma and the carcinoid tumor, in turn, a one-sided overgrowth of the mucinous tumor. Mucinous carcinoids tend to be pure tumors.

Carcinoid tumors most commonly appear as firm circumscribed nodules in the walls of mature cystic teratomas (or mucinous cystadenomas). The size of the carcinoid component ranges from small to massive, but the maximum dimension is generally about 10 cm. Unlike struma ovarii there is as yet no minimum size criterion for the diagnosis of carcinoid tumors, but a 1 cm nodular proliferation would seem to be a reasonable lower limit. On sectioning, the tumor tissue is grayish-yellow or tan colored (Figure 27.71A). Hemorrhage and necrosis are generally not apparent but may occasionally be seen in strumal and mucinous carcinoids. Cystic spaces containing clear or mucoid fluid are usually present in addition to the cystic teratomatous components. The thyroid component of strumal carcinoids may sometimes be recognized macroscopically, especially if it forms a discrete mass. These areas are soft to very firm and the cut surface is red-brown and glistening contrasted with the yellow-gray of carcinoid tissue. Pure tumors form firm nodular masses with smooth bosselated surfaces.

Microscopic features

In ovarian insular carcinoids (Figure 27.72), tumor cells are arranged in round, oval or angular islands with some peripheral palisading. Small acini are present, typically at the margins of the islands but sometimes diffusely. They contain eosinophilic secretions that stain positively for mucin and may become inspissated and calcified resembling psammoma bodies. The tumor cells are remarkably uniform in appearance. Cytoplasm is abundant and may exhibit myriads of tiny eosinophilic granules, particularly at the periphery of the islands. The nuclei are central and round, with evenly distributed clumped chromatin. Mitotic activity is rarely observed. The proportion of stroma is variable; it is dense and fibroma-like and is occasionally focally luteinized. Minor trabecular areas are seen in less than 5% of cases (Figure 27.72B). All tumors are argentaffinic and this is most readily appreciated in the granular cells described above. The argyrophilic reaction (Grimelius and Bodian protargol stain) is usually weakly positive. Reactivity for low molecular weight cytokeratins, NSE, chromogranin B and various neuronal peptides, including calcitonin, can be demonstrated, as well as prostatic acid phosphatase,[162] this latter interpreted as a further similarity between such tumors in the ovaries and rectal carcinoids. Microscopic features that best correlate with the presence of the carcinoid syndrome are an insular pattern with a volume greater than a 40 mm diameter sphere, abundance of acini, and prominence of argentaffin granules. The associated teratomatous components are chiefly of endodermal derivation.

The histologic features of ovarian trabecular carcinoids resemble those of hindgut, e.g., rectal, carcinoids. The most characteristic pattern is that of orderly long wavy ribbons, one or two cells thick, interspersed with a small amount of loose fibrous connective tissue. Where the ribbons appear shorter, the stroma tends to be denser. The elongate cells are orientated perpendicularly to the long axes of the ribbons (Figure 27.73A). Wide bands and trabeculae are also present, as well as scattered small cell nests (Figure 27.73B). This latter feature should not be misinterpreted as vascular permeation or evidence of aggressive local invasion. A minor but definite insular component is seen in 20% of cases. The tumor often includes multiple small cystic spaces lined by mucinous epithelium that appear to form an intrinsic part of the tumor. The cytologic characteristics are similar to insular carcinoids as described above. The tumor cells are argyrophilic, but argentaffinic in only two-thirds. Neuronal peptides, including calcitonin, have been identified immunohistochemically. Stromal luteinization is common.

The diagnostic feature of strumal carcinoids is the admixture of carcinoid and thyroid elements. These vary in their relative proportions and may be intimately admixed throughout the mass or merge only at the interface between separate masses of thyroid and carcinoid tissue (Figure 27.74). The carcinoid component is purely trabecular in half the cases and, in the remainder, is a mixture of trabecular and insular patterns or, uncommonly, mucinous carcinoid.[113] Rarely, it is entirely insular in type. The thyroid component is both macro- and microfollicular and includes typical colloid. Where the tissues are admixed, follicular epithelium appears to stream into the ribbons of carcinoid cells, or carcinoid cells seem to replace

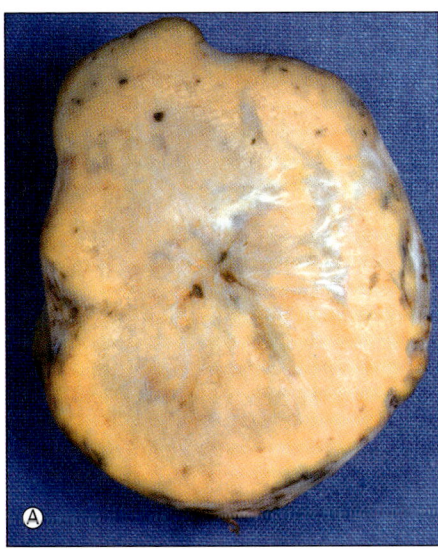
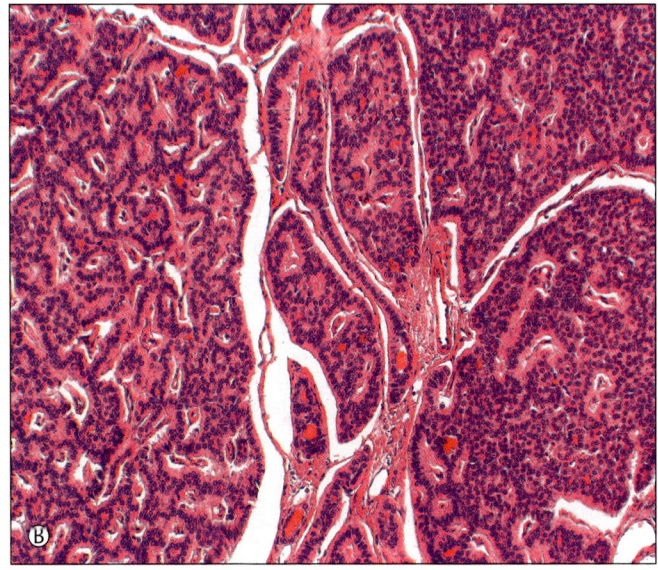

Fig. 27.71 Ovarian carcinoid tumor. **(A)** Cut surface of 4 cm solid tan tumor. **(B)** Low power showing insular pattern above and trabecular area below.

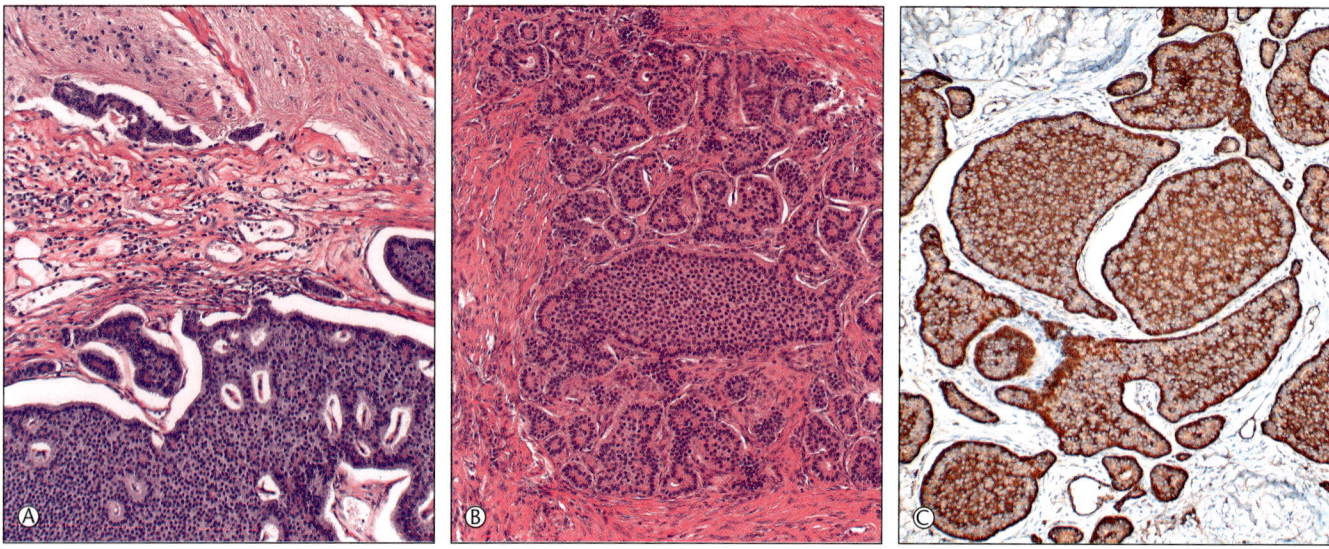

Fig. 27.72 Ovarian insular carcinoid tumor. **(A)** Interface between carcinoid tumor displaying numerous small acini below and benign teratomatous neuroglial tissue at top. **(B)** Typical insular pattern. **(C)** Immunostain for synaptophysin.

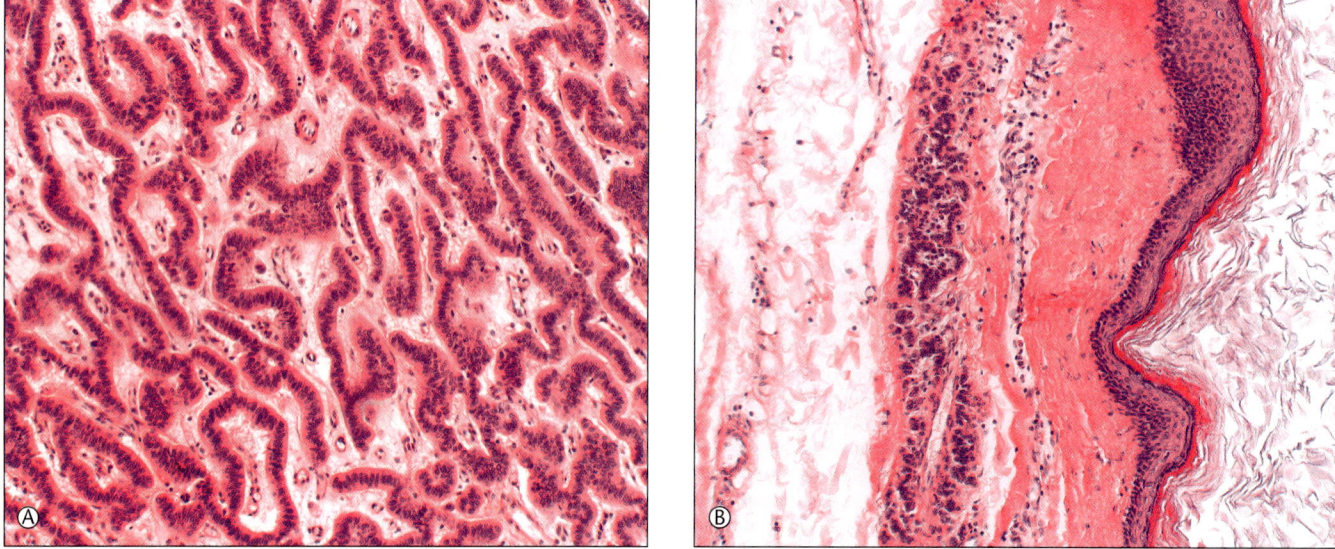

Fig. 27.73 Detail of trabecular carcinoid tumor. **(A)** Neat sinuous ribbons of elongate cells are orientated at right angles to the long axes of the ribbons. The small nuclei are round or ovoid with dense but regular chromatin. **(B)** One of a myriad of small, scattered cell nests around the perimeter of the main tumor mass, this one beneath the squamous lining of the teratomatous cyst.

part of the follicular lining (Figure 27.74). The individual components retain their innate cytologic and immunohistochemical characteristics; the follicular epithelium is thyroglobulin-reactive while the carcinoid component contains various neuropeptides, including calcitonin in a small number of cases. Some workers have identified, in the transitional zones, an intermediate cell population (resembling thyroid 'C' cells) showing both follicular thyroid and neuroendocrine differentiation. Mucinous epithelium may be evident as a few or many cysts or as individual cells within the carcinoid component. The stroma is variable in quantity and character and may contain amyloid – a property that enhances the morphologic similarity of some lesions to medullary carcinomas of the thyroid gland. Stromal luteinization has been observed in one-third of cases.

There are no histologic features that are reliably predictive of a malignant clinical course in non-mucinous carcinoids, although those associated with obvious teratomas are less likely to metastasize than 'pure' carcinoids.[164] Other unusual features observed in metastasizing tumors have included prominent mitotic activity (>3 mitotic figures per high-power field), conspicuous nucleoli, necrosis, paucity of acini, and 'anaplasia'. The histologic descriptions of these tumors (often limited) suggest that some of them are more in keeping with 'atypical' or malignant carcinoid tumors as documented in extraovarian sites.

Mucinous carcinoids consist of small and large acini containing mucin surrounded by cuboidal or columnar cells. Interstitial mucin and signet-ring cells may be observed occasionally to the point of resembling Krukenberg tumors. The small round or oval nuclei resemble more closely those of carcinoid tumors rather than colonic adenocarcinomas, but show more nuclear atypia and mitotic activity than other varieties of

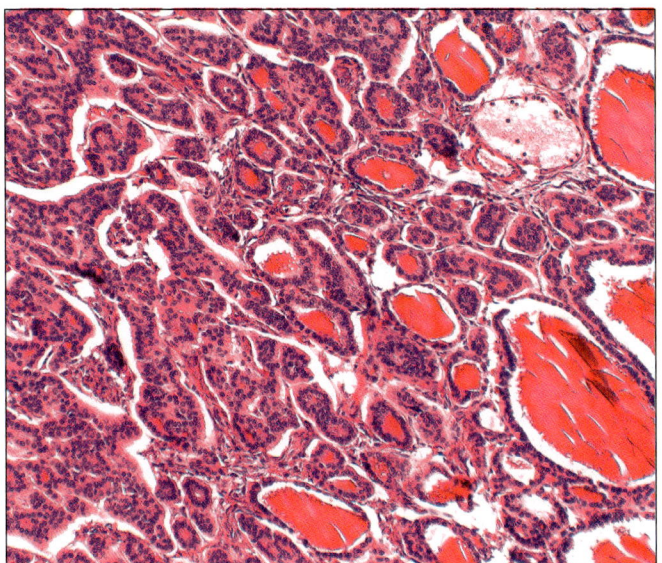

Fig. 27.74 Strumal carcinoid tumor. Low power view of a transitional area between thyroid follicles and carcinoid ribbons.

Table 27.5 Trabecular carcinoid versus androblastoma: differential diagnosis

Trabecular carcinoid	Androblastoma
Clinical profile	
Virilization very rare	Virilization common
Microscopic features	
Ribbons of uniform width throughout tumor	Narrower ribbons, other patterns present
Stroma fibromatous	Stroma often contains Leydig cells
Cytoplasm copious, often granular	Less cytoplasm, sometimes vacuolated
Argyrophilic, usually argentaffinic	Both reactions negative
Teratomatous elements mostly present	Mucinous cysts may be present

primary ovarian carcinoids. The cytoplasm of some cells is argyrophilic and sometimes argentaffinic as well, corresponding to the presence of immunoreactive neuropeptides, e.g., serotonin and chromogranin A. The stroma is not abundant and may be loose or dense.

Differential diagnosis

Metastatic carcinoids (see Chapter 29), which are usually insular in type, can be histologically indistinguishable from primary 'pure' ovarian lesions but there are usually discriminating clinical and surgical features. Metastatic tumors are almost always bilateral and extraovarian metastases may be evident. The tumors are multinodular and not associated with teratomatous elements. Identification of a primary tumor, usually in the ileum, clinches the diagnosis (see Table 29.2).

Granulosa cell tumors (see Chapter 26) are the neoplasms that are most likely to be confused with insular carcinoids. Call–Exner bodies may resemble carcinoid acini but their margins are less regular and the lumens may contain nuclear debris as well as eosinophilic material. The 'lumens' in Call–Exner bodies are degenerative and the nuclei lie randomly around them, in contrast to carcinoids where the glands form true acini. The nuclei are arranged basally and separated from the lumens by obvious cytoplasm. The granulosa cells have grooved nuclei and the scanty cytoplasm is neither argyrophilic nor argentaffinic. Teratomatous elements are not present.

Poorly differentiated primary or metastatic adenocarcinomas may superficially resemble insular carcinoid tumors but the nuclei are never as uniform and there is always obvious mitotic activity. Argentaffin and argyrophil reactions are usually negative as are immunohistochemical reactions (e.g., chromogranin) for neurosecretory granules.

Brenner tumors (see Chapter 25) display epithelial islands but these are broken up by large amounts of fibromatous stroma. The epithelial component is composed of transitional cells without acinus formation. The nuclei are often grooved and the cytoplasm is not argyrophilic or argentaffinic.

Androblastomas (see Chapter 26) may be confused with trabecular carcinoids, particularly those with luteinized stroma.

The Sertoli cell ribbons are, however, thinner and shorter, and the constituent cells have sparser cytoplasm that is sometimes vacuolated and lacks granularity or argyrophilia. Examination of further sections will usually reveal other typical growth patterns and clumps of Leydig cells. Teratomatous elements are absent but cysts lined by mucinous epithelium, including occasional argentaffin cells, may be present in both (Table 27.5).

Malignant strumas need to be distinguished from strumal carcinoids, with which they have often been confused in the past. Thyroid carcinomas sometimes show a fair degree of anaplasia and mitotic activity. Ribbon-like growth is not apparent and the cells are not argyrophilic or argentaffinic.

Treatment and prognosis

Insular and 'mixed' carcinoids are best considered as tumors of low malignant potential. The tumors grow slowly and recurrences or metastases are rare. Trabecular carcinoids are very infrequently associated with metastases. The metastases of strumal carcinoids may be either thyroidal or carcinoid in type.[8,86] Approximately 5% of cases have proved fatal, with extensive peritoneal, liver, and abdominal lymph node deposits and, rarely, widespread systemic dissemination.

Treatment of uncomplicated carcinoid tumors is bilateral salpingo-oophorectomy and hysterectomy. In the rare young patient desirous of retaining her fertility, or in cases with trabecular carcinoid tumors, unilateral salpingo-oophorectomy is acceptable. Close clinical follow-up is mandatory in all patients. In cases of extraovarian spread, excision of metastases, as far as is practicable, is recommended, followed by chemotherapy. Serum serotonin or urinary 5-HIAA levels can be used to monitor the progress of the disease. Most symptoms and signs of the carcinoid syndrome regress quickly postoperatively. However, carcinoid heart disease (pulmonary stenosis, tricuspid stenosis/incompetence, and right-sided heart failure) can continue to progress without obvious recurrence of tumor.

The clinical course of mucinous carcinoids is more aggressive and in this respect they are comparable with their homologues in the appendix. Metastases may be present at the time of laparotomy. Treatment therefore needs to be radical, more in keeping with that employed in patients with ovarian müllerian carcinomas.

OTHER (RARE) MONODERMAL AND HIGHLY SPECIALIZED TERATOMAS

Pituitary adenomas

Rare pituitary corticotrophin adenomas,[186] forming discrete nodules in the wall of otherwise typical mature cystic teratomas, can cause Cushings syndrome.[24]

Epidermoid cysts

These cysts are most often considered to be of teratomatous origin but there are other histogenetic possibilities (see other miscellaneous epithelial lesions, Chapter 25).

Endodermal variants of mature cystic teratomas

A mature monodermal teratoma, consisting of a 9 cm cyst lined by respiratory epithelium (with focal squamous metaplasia), developed in a 5-year-old girl.[33]

Giant sebaceous tumors

Rare ovarian tumors consist almost exclusively of benign sebaceous glandular tissue.[32] Only slightly less rarely, are malignant variants (sebaceous carcinoma) observed to arise from mature cystic teratomas.[149,182]

Salivary tumors

We have encountered in a 26-year-old patient a benign monomorphic (basal cell) salivary adenoma (Figure 27.75) that consisted of mixed adenoid cystic and cribriform patterns of growth.[153] Small discrete cribriform nests of basaloid cells showed peripheral palisading and cuffing with hyalinized basal lamina material (Figure 27.76). Centrally, epithelial islands showed a sponge-like arrangement with deposits of sialomucins. The cells were reactive for cytokeratins, S-100 protein, and salivary amylase.

Neuroectodermal tumors and gliomas

Although rare, there are a wide variety of ovarian tumors of neuroectodermal origin. Some are dominant components of otherwise typical mature or immature teratomas, while others are apparently pure and may, indeed, produce cystic lesions composed exclusively of mature brain tissue.[58] Some may result from secondary malignant transformation in pre-existing mature cystic teratomas, but most probably represent monodermal teratomatous development. In the ovary these resemble their counterparts of the same names occurring in the brains of children and are of three main histologic subtypes: differentiated (usually ependymomas), primitive,[84,88] and anaplastic (glioblastoma multiforme). Some investigators attempt to distinguish between immaturity and 'intrinsic malignancy' in this group of tumors but both qualities have similar clinical implications. Most occur in young women (rarely in postmenopausal women) and many poorly differentiated examples are clinically aggressive.[84,91,99,144]

Primitive neuroectodermal tumors (PNET) The average age of patients is about 19 years and there is a high mortality rate. The tumors are unilateral, large, partly solid and partly cystic. They consist chiefly of patternless sheets of undifferentiated small pleomorphic cells (Figure 27.77A) resembling neuroblasts. There are also foci of glial differentiation, and some tumors include ependymal rosettes, medulloepitheliomatous or medulloblastomatous patterns (Figure 27.77B), and primitive

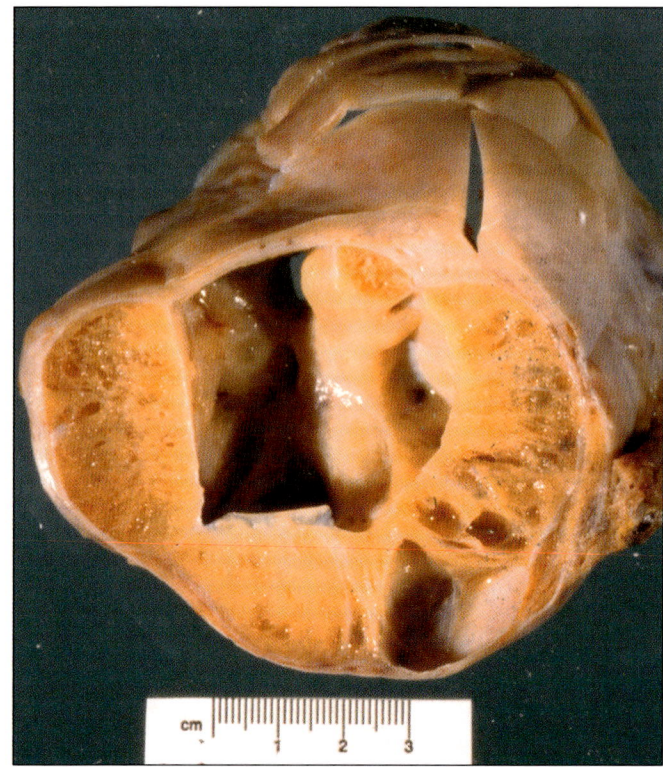

Fig. 27.75 Monomorphic (basal cell) salivary adenoma. Slice through tumor to reveal various-sized cystic spaces, fine 'honeycomb' areas, and solid nodules.

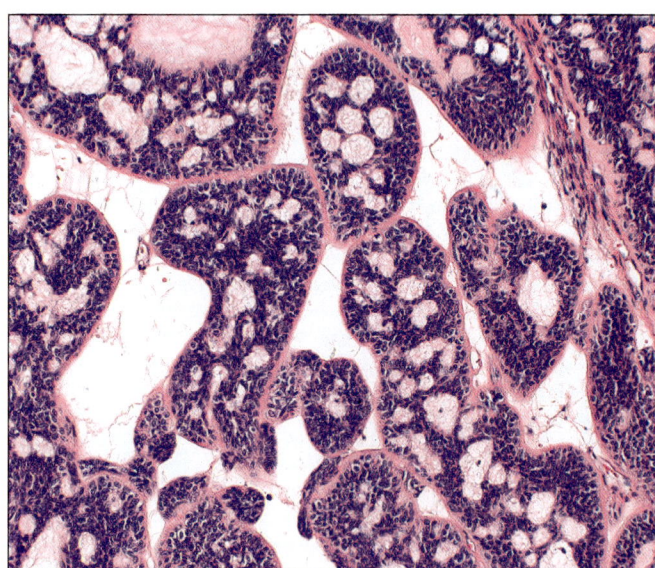

Fig. 27.76 Monomorphic (basal cell) salivary adenoma. Cribriform nest of small basaloid cells with peripheral palisading and cuffing with hyalinized basal lamina material.

neural tube-like structures. Some show foci of mature teratoma, including typical dermoid cysts (Figure 27.78). Those that lack these components may be confused with other types of ovarian neoplasms such as granulosa cell tumors, undifferentiated small cell carcinomas of hypercalcemic type or desmoplastic small cell tumors (see Chapter 25). The background of small, undifferentiated pleomorphic cells distinguishes these tumors from the other ovarian neuroectodermal tumors mentioned above. The immunophenotype of the cells generally includes focal reactivity for GFAP, synaptophysin, neurofilaments, and MIC2 (CD99) but not for cytokeratins,[82,91,99] while some exhibit the characteristic balanced t(11;22)(q24;q12) chromosomal translocation specific for the PNET/Ewing sarcoma family of neoplasms.[84,88]

Anaplastic neuroectodermal tumors These tumors resemble high-grade gliomas (glioblastoma). Focal squamous differentiation is an indication of their teratomatous origin. Anaplastic tumor cells are arranged in sheets and contain variable amounts of cytoplasm with eosinophilic processes. Bizarre nuclei and mitoses are common. Cells are reactive for GFAP.

Melanotic neuroectodermal tumors of the ovary These are similar to the retinal anlage tumors or pigmented progonomas of infancy. They are generally cystic and show sheets of small dark cells with scant cytoplasm, among which are tubules lined by larger cells containing abundant melanin. Structures resembling primitive optic vesicles may be found.

Ependymomas These occur in women aged 16–68 years.[63,66,91,93,119] Over half of cases are confined to one ovary and the remainder have intraperitoneal metastases. The primary tumor is usually at least partly cystic. Microscopically, ependymomas are indistinguishable from those of the central nervous system (contrasting with those of the sacrococcygeal

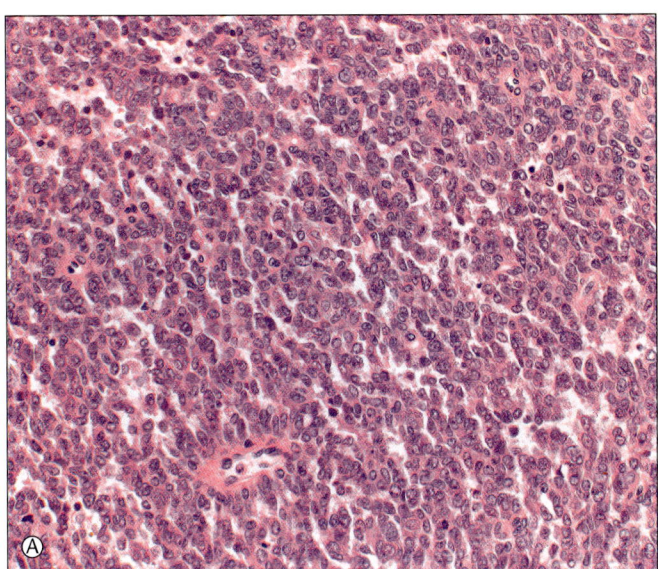
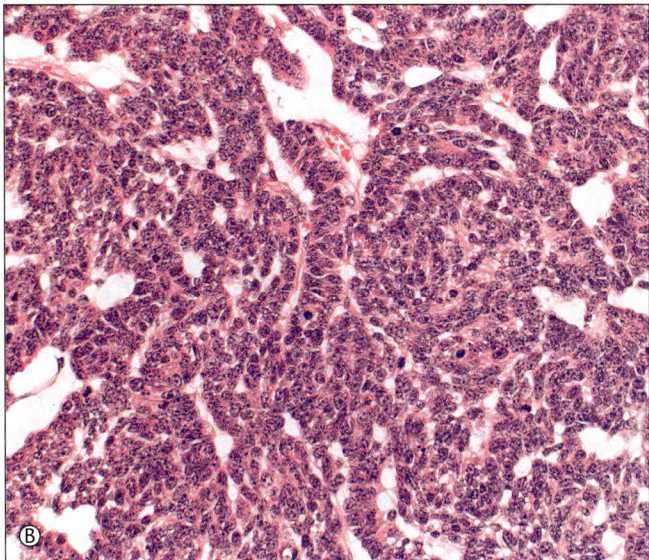

Fig. 27.77 Primitive neuroectodermal tumor (PNET). **(A)** Patternless sheets of small pleomorphic cells. In a patient of this age, differentiation is required from undifferentiated small cell tumor of hypercalcemic type and from desmoplastic small cell tumor of peritoneum (see Chapter 33). **(B)** Some focal suggestion of medulloblastomatous differentiation.

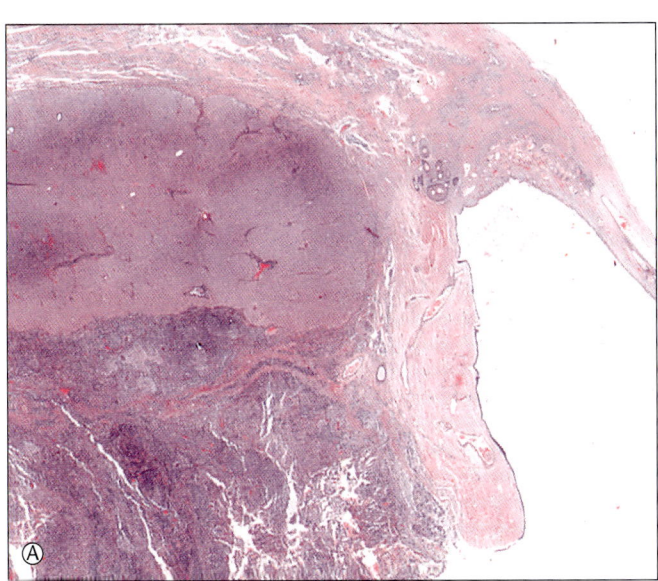
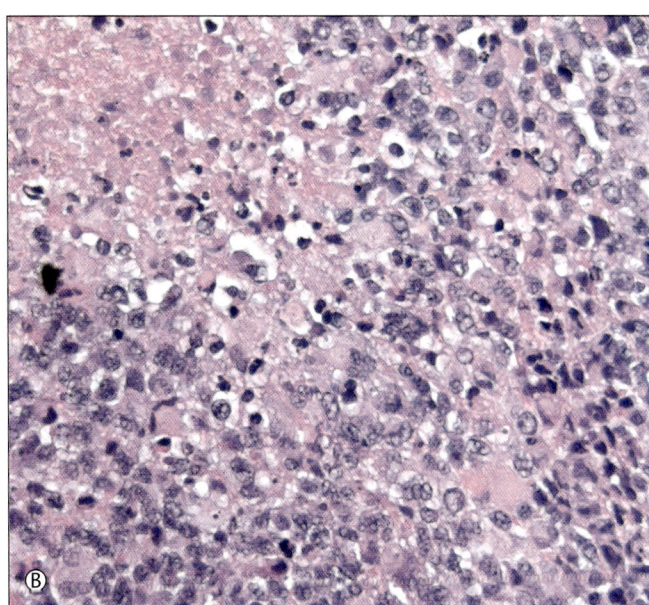

Fig. 27.78 PNET arising from a glioma within a mature cystic teratoma. **(A)** Scan of tumor showing cystic teratoma at left, anaplastic astrocytoma at center bottom, and densely cellular PNET at top. **(B)** High power of central type PNET with small dark cells and necrosis (bottom right).

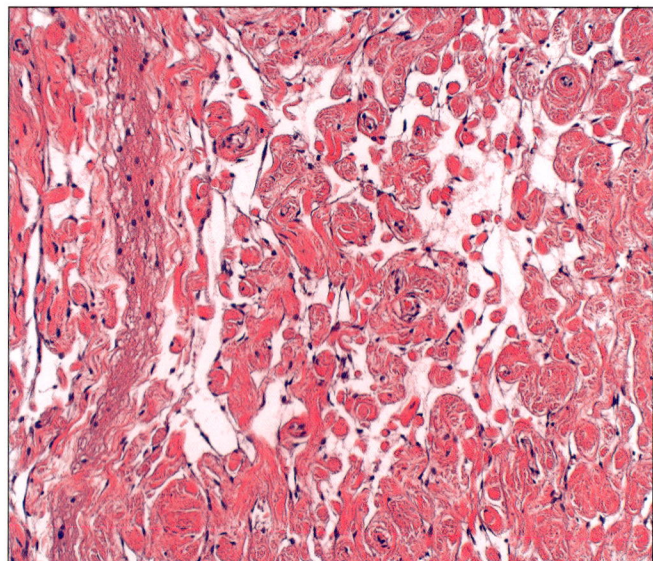

Fig. 27.79 Angioblastic (angiomatous) meningioma arising from a mature cystic teratoma. Note strip of glial tissue traversing meningioma near right of field.

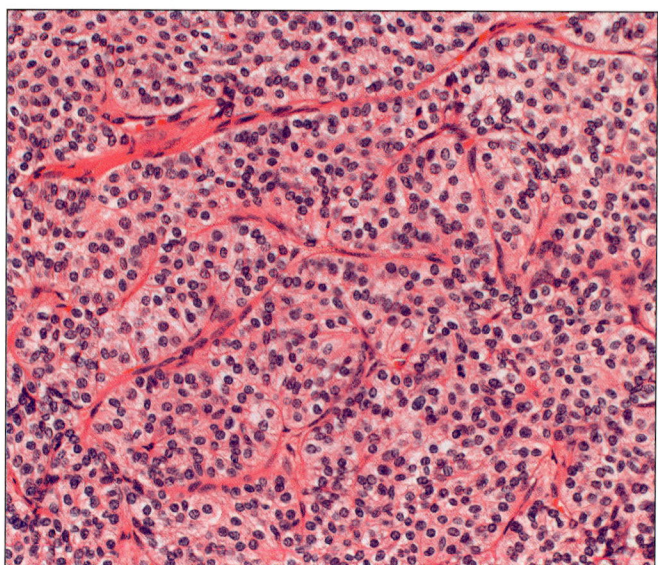

Fig. 27.80 A 13 cm non-chromaffin paraganglioma. Other teratomatous elements were sought and not found and the origin of the tumor is unclear. Organoid pattern of small cells with rounded central nuclei and pale, slightly granular cytoplasm.

region) and show predominantly a diffuse or lobular pattern of cells separated by relatively acellular stroma. Perivascular pseudorosettes are prominent, as are fibrillary cytoplasmic processes. Occasional true rosettes can be found. The nature of the cells is confirmed by immunostaining showing reactivity for vimentin, MDM-2, GFAP, and S-100 protein (in 50% of cases) but not for many cytokeratins (e.g., CAM 5.2) and EMA. The tumors may superficially resemble endometrioid (with large gland-like spaces) or serous carcinomas (with complex papillary patterns and psammoma bodies). Although other obvious heterologous tissues are absent, the teratomatous origin of these tumors is supported by the known occurrence of ependymal tissue in ovarian mature cystic teratomas, and of focal ependymal differentiation in immature teratomas. A suggested alternative histogenesis is neometaplasia of müllerian duct-derived tissue.[66] The identification of progesterone receptors in a bilateral ovarian ependymoma suggests the possibility of hormone responsiveness that may be of value in management.

Gliomas Rare examples of central neurocytoma,[72] meningioma[170] (Figure 27.79) and glioblastoma[46] arising in teratomas have all been reported.

Other differentiated neuroectodermal tumors (e.g., non-chromaffin paragangliomas) These are occasionally encountered[111,115] and some are presumably of teratomatous origin (Figure 27.80). Morphologically, they exhibit the typical organoid pattern of 'Zellballen' or nests of uniform rounded cells with small central nuclei, showing delicate stippled chromatin, and pale or granular cytoplasm. Reticulin fibers separate cell nests from the vascular network of the stroma. Immunostaining of the main tumor cells ('chief cells') for neuroendocrine markers (NSE and chromogranin A) shows reactivity, as may inhibin and calretinin.[115] Peripheral sustentacular cells are highlighted by strong immunostaining for S-100 protein. Other possible origins are from hilar neural elements.

MALIGNANT MIXED GERM CELL TUMORS

Definition
Malignant mixed germ cell tumors are composed of two or more of the neoplastic germ cell elements already described in this chapter and, collectively, they comprise <10% of all *malignant* ovarian germ cell tumors.[17,197] By convention, benign mature cystic teratomas with secondary malignant change (most commonly squamous carcinoma and occurring in much older women) are excluded from this category. Gonadoblastomas and other mixed germ cell-sex cord-stromal tumors are also excluded (tumors containing sex cord-stromal derivatives as well as germ cells or germ cell tumors).

Clinical profile
Mixed germ cell tumors occur in young women, almost all under 30 years of age (median, 12 years),[197] but rarely in perimenopausal women.[81] About one-third of prepubertal girls with malignant mixed germ cell tumors present with isosexual pseudoprecocity and occasionally lesions of female intersex.[147] Serum levels of either β-hCG or AFP, or both, may be raised, depending on the composition of the individual tumor. However, a raised serum β-hCG does not necessarily indicate choriocarcinoma, since isolated syncytiotrophoblastic cells as part of embryonal carcinoma, polyembryoma or dysgerminoma (and, rarely, non-germ cell tumors) may elaborate this hormone. As with mediastinal germ cell tumors, rare examples occur with hematologic disorders.[121,173] An association has been observed with membranoproliferative glomerulonephritis.[156] Molecular genetic studies commonly reveal isochromosome 12p.[141]

Macroscopic features
Mixed germ cell tumors usually are large, averaging about 15 cm in diameter, with smooth or bosselated external surfaces and cut surfaces that vary markedly depending on the histo-

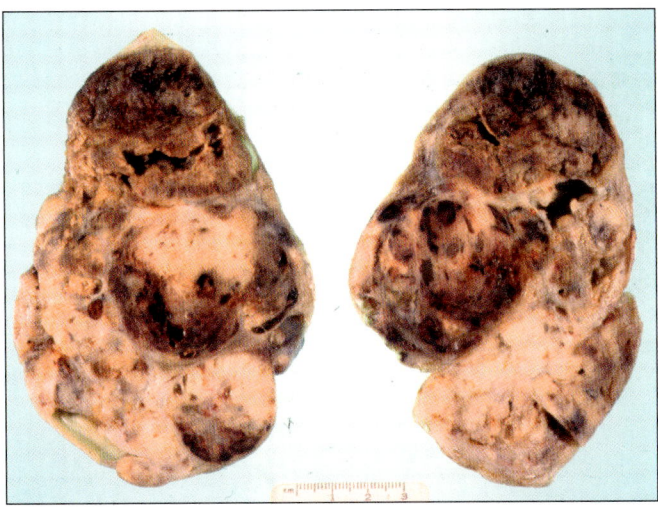

Fig. 27.81 Solid malignant mixed germ cell tumor. The cut surface showing variation from area to area is characteristic of such neoplasms.

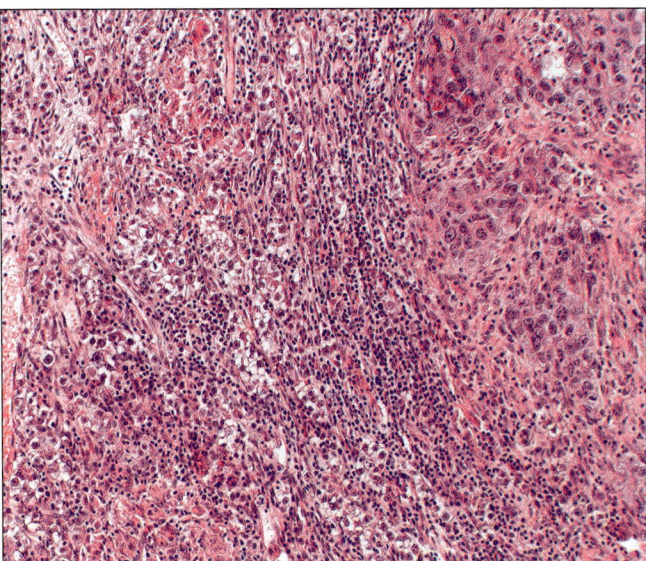

Fig. 27.83 Malignant mixed germ cell tumor. Dysgerminoma (left) and embryonal carcinoma (right).

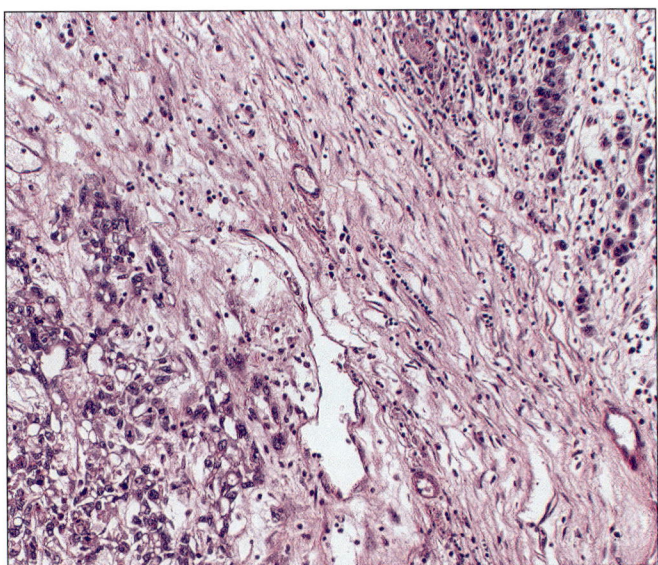

Fig. 27.82 Malignant mixed germ cell tumor. Dysgerminoma (left) and reticular pattern of yolk sac tumor (right).

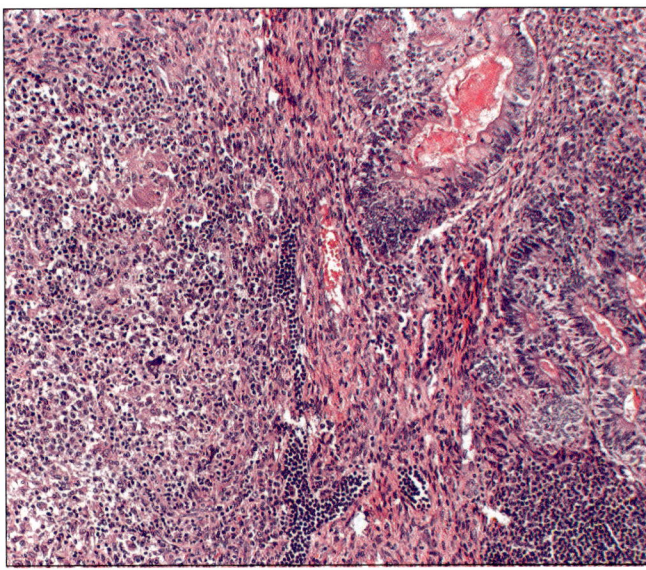

Fig. 27.84 Malignant mixed germ cell tumor. High-grade immature teratoma (left) and dysgerminoma (right).

logic components present (Figure 27.81). Microcystic or 'honeycomb' areas suggest immature teratoma. Solid, soft fleshy areas usually indicate dysgerminoma. Hemorrhage, although often non-specific, may point to choriocarcinoma, and the margins of such areas must be adequately sampled. Necrosis is almost always obvious.

Microscopic features

The various elements in these tumors may be extensively admixed or may form separate areas in juxtaposition or separated by fibrous tissue septa. Malignant neoplasms in this group are classified according to component elements listed in decreasing order of prominence, but this depends on all areas of varying appearance being thoroughly sampled and examined histologically. Dysgerminoma is the commonest component of malignant mixed germ cell tumors, being present in over 75% of reported cases (Figures 27.82–27.84). Only slightly less frequent are the various patterns of yolk sac tumor (Figures 27.82 and 27.85). Immature teratoma occurs in half of these

tumors (Figures 27.84 and 27.85) while embryonal carcinoma (Figure 27.83) and choriocarcinoma are relatively less common (20% of cases).

Treatment and prognosis

Sixty per cent of malignant mixed germ cell tumors are apparently confined to one ovary (stage 1A) at presentation but, prior to the advent of modern chemotherapy, 50% of these patients died from tumor, indicating a considerable proclivity for occult metastases. If dysgerminoma is a component of the tumor, there is about a 5–10% likelihood of contralateral involvement. Inspection of the second ovary, and exclusion of bilaterality, should thus precede any decision to employ conservative surgery. Tumor size (>10 cm in diameter) and histologic composition (more than one-third of choriocarcinoma, yolk sac tumor, and/or high-grade teratoma) are the two major pathologic correlates of poor clinical outcome for stage 1 malignant mixed germ cell tumors. Postoperative multiple-agent chemotherapy (usually vincristine or platinum based[175]), an integral component of management based partly on the microscopic composition of the individual tumor, has dramatically improved the survival rates for these patients, which are now close to 100% regardless of clinical stage.

MIXED GERM CELL AND SEX CORD-STROMAL TUMORS (GONADAL ANLAGE TUMORS)

Tumors composed of germ cells and stromal elements pose a problem in pathogenesis and hence nomenclature. By general

usage the term 'mixed germ cell-sex cord-stromal tumor'[10,165] is reserved for those few otherwise unclassified neoplasms composed of these cell types which exhibit distinctive histologic appearances and clinicopathologic features differing from those of gonadoblastomas. An alternative proposed terminology is 'gonadal anlage tumor with male differentiation' ('gonadoblastoma') and 'gonadal anlage tumor with female differentiation' ('pflugeroma' or 'mixed germ cell-sex cord-stromal tumor').

As a group, these mixed tumors are composed of two and commonly three cell types. The two cellular elements common to all are germ cells and cells of sex-cord origin resembling immature granulosa or Sertoli cells. Theca-lutein or Leydig-like cells are also present in most examples of gonadoblastoma type.

Over 80% of acceptable examples of gonadoblastoma have occurred in phenotypic females. However, over 95% of 'females' with gonadal tumors of this type have abnormal karyotypes that include 46,XY or numerical and structural aberrations of the sex chromosomes. The additional evidence of electron microscopic similarities between the sex-cord elements of gonadoblastomas and those of normal testes supports the hypothesis that many represent disordered or abortive attempts at testicular differentiation, and the likelihood of neoplasms is related more to the severity of the disturbed gonadal organogenesis.[163] These lesions are briefly included in this text as they mostly present to the surgical pathologist as 'ovarian tumors' but are covered more fully in the discussion of intersex (see Chapter 34). Also, rare cases genuinely arise in essentially normal ovaries (Figure 27.86).

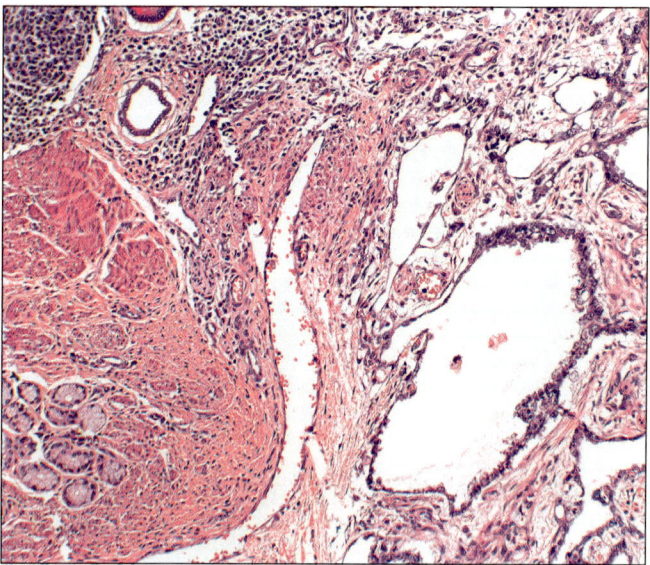

Fig. 27.85 Malignant mixed germ cell tumor. Yolk sac tumor with reticular pattern (left) and adjacent mature teratoma (immature elsewhere).

GONADOBLASTOMAS

The component germ cells in gonadoblastomas closely resemble dysgerminoma cells while the intermixed cells are similar to immature granulosa/Sertoli-type cells. Isolated nests of cells resembling those of gonadoblastoma are occasionally seen in

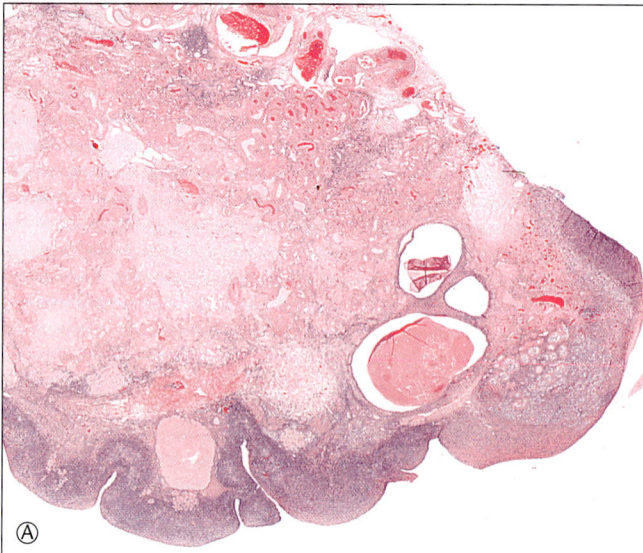

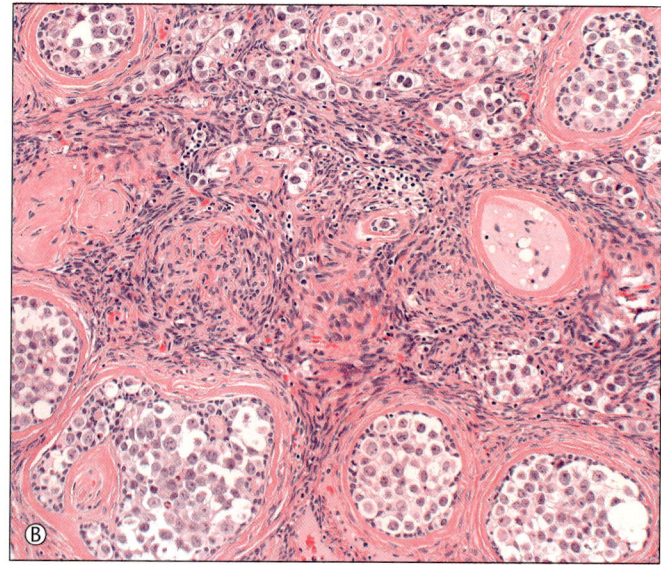

Fig. 27.86 Gonadoblastoma. Rare lesion arising in normal ovary of a 55-year-old multiparous woman with a 46,XX karyotype. **(A)** Scan of the ovarian section, showing small tumor centered at the corticomedullary junction at left pole of ovary and presence of normal follicular and luteal remnants. **(B)** Circumscribed gonadoblastoma nests with both germ cells and peripheral small sex cord-like cells to the top and left, and surrounded by hyalinized basement membrane material, and progressing to dysgerminoma at the bottom.

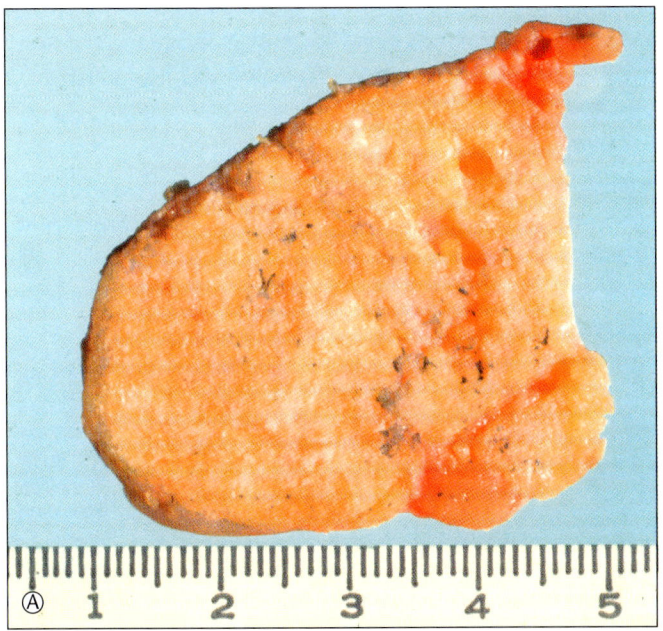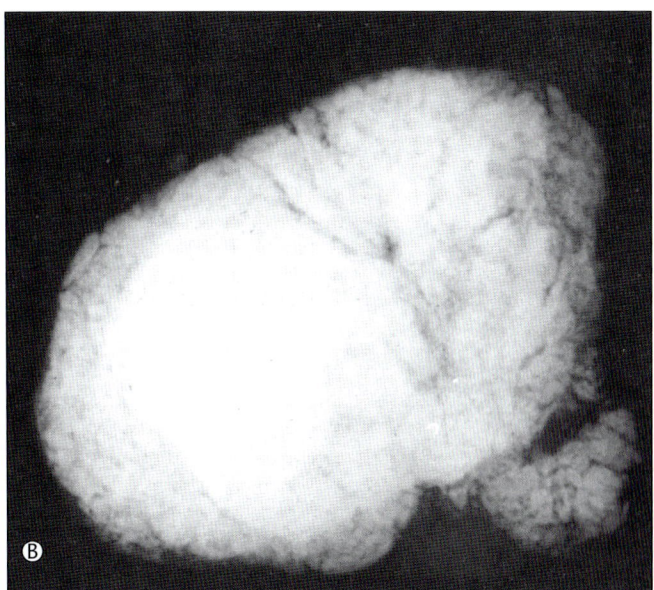

Fig. 27.87 Heavily calcified gonadoblastoma. **(A)** Pale, gritty cut surface with a small soft tissue nodule in the lower right corner which was histologically dysgerminoma. **(B)** Specimen radiograph (Faxitron®) of the same tumor.

abnormal gonads and malformed seminiferous tubules and have been variously termed 'gonadoblastosis', 'intersexual formations' or 'ring tubules'. This continuous morphologic spectrum has also been interpreted as suggesting a hamartomatous nature for gonadoblastomas. No case of pure gonadoblastoma has been associated with documented metastases. Where a superimposed malignant germ cell tumor has led to metastases, the secondary deposits have not recapitulated the patterns of gonadoblastoma. This suggests that these tumors should be regarded, at most, as *in situ* malignant germ cell neoplasms.

Clinical profile

Over 80% of patients with gonadoblastomas are phenotypically female, while the remainder are cryptorchid males. Of these 'females', 60% are virilized and over 95% of them have an abnormal karyotype that includes a Y chromosome (46,XY in 50%, 45,X/46,XY in 25%) and underlying anomalies of gonadal development (see Chapter 34). Rare patients have stigmata of pure gonadal dysgenesis syndrome but have Y chromosomal fragments.[75,114] Gonadoblastomas have also been seen in true hermaphrodites, with a 46,XX karyotype or a 46,XY karyotype, also generally with Y chromosomal fragments. Rarely, these tumors have occurred in siblings.

Patient age at diagnosis ranges from birth to 38 years, with most presenting in the second and third decades. Detection shortly after birth occurs during surgical evaluation of ambiguous genitalia. The majority of phenotypic females with gonadoblastomas present with primary amenorrhea or early-onset secondary amenorrhea, during the investigation of which the lesions are identified. Much less commonly, they may present as unilateral or bilateral gonadal masses – radiographic examination frequently shows fine stippled calcification in such pelvic masses – presumptive evidence of gonadoblastoma. Occasional patients have exhibited isosexual pseudoprecocity, while very rare women have cycled spontaneously and become pregnant.[195] We have encountered one example in a 55-year-old multiparous woman, an incidental finding at hysterectomy for prolapse.[37]

Macroscopic features

These tumors are bilateral in over one-third of cases. Unilateral cases show a slight right-sided predominance. About one-fourth are diagnosed only after microscopic examination. The macroscopic appearances of the obvious gonadoblastomas vary with size (usually 2–3 cm across, but from microscopic to 10 cm in diameter), the presence or absence of a supervening malignant germ cell tumor, and whether or not calcification is prominent (in 45% of cases). Pure gonadoblastomas are almost always solid tumors (although cystic variants have been encountered) with smooth or slightly lobulated external surfaces. They vary in consistency from soft and fleshy to firm and densely calcified. The cut surface is gray-yellow or white and granular, if calcified (Figure 27.87).

Microscopic features

The basic architecture of gonadoblastomas depends on the presence of numerous well-circumscribed cell nests, each invested by a thick basal lamina and embedded in fibrous connective tissue stroma (Figure 27.88). The nests are small, oval to round, and solid (only rarely cystic; Figure 27.89). They contain an intimate mixture of germ cells and other cells of sex-cord type that resemble immature granulosa or Sertoli cells. Lymphocytes and even granulomas (Figure 27.90) are occasionally seen within the discrete nests.

The germ cells are large and polyhedral, with pale, slightly granular cytoplasm and large round vesicular nuclei, often with a prominent nucleolus. The cells sometimes exhibit appreciable mitotic activity, and are reactive for PLAP and for OCT4 (POU5F1).[29,104] The small ovoid sex-cord cells have dark, slightly elongated nuclei (Figure 27.91). Mitoses are not seen in these cells. They are considered to be Sertoli cells or their precursors, or primitive sex-cord stromal cells defying further categorization, and are reactive for CK18, vimentin, and α-

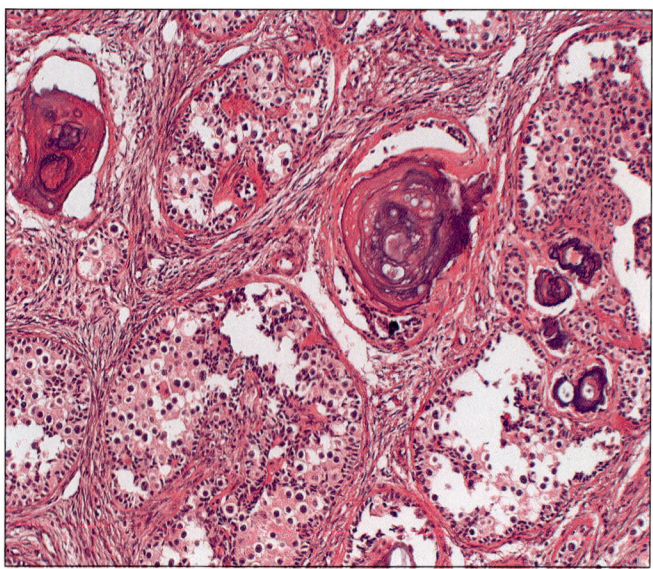

Fig. 27.88 Well-circumscribed nests of a gonadoblastoma with central dystrophic calcification. Small rounded calcified bodies resembling psammoma bodies coalesce to form larger irregular masses.

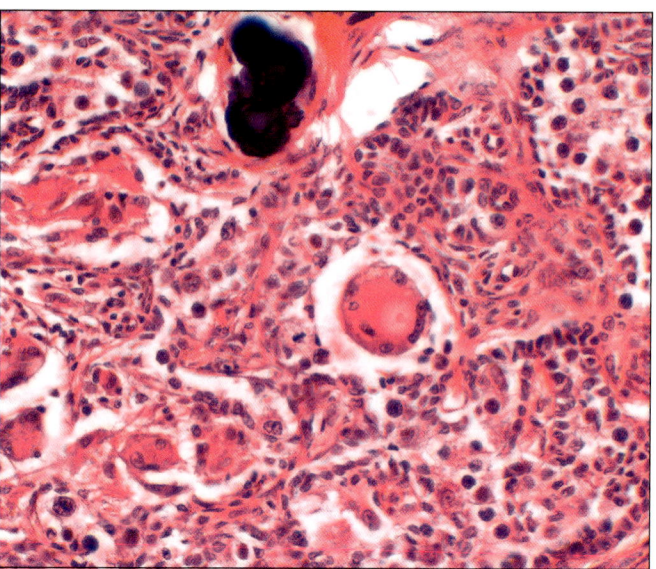

Fig. 27.90 Gonadoblastoma. Histiocytic giant cells included within the gonadoblastoma cell nests.

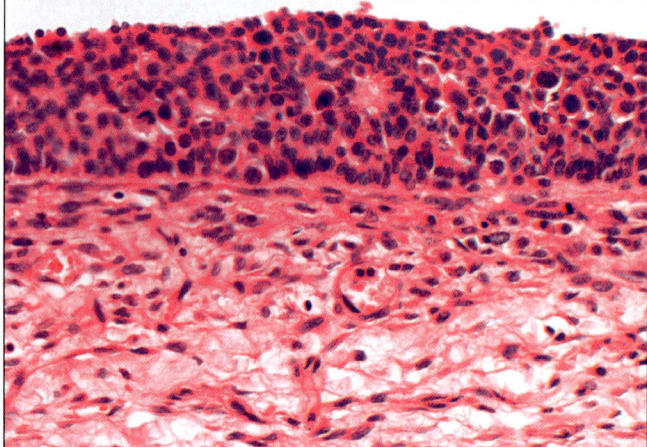

Fig. 27.89 Gonadoblastoma. Rare cystic tumor showing the same intimate mixture of large germ cells and smaller 'supportive' or sex cord-stromal cells.

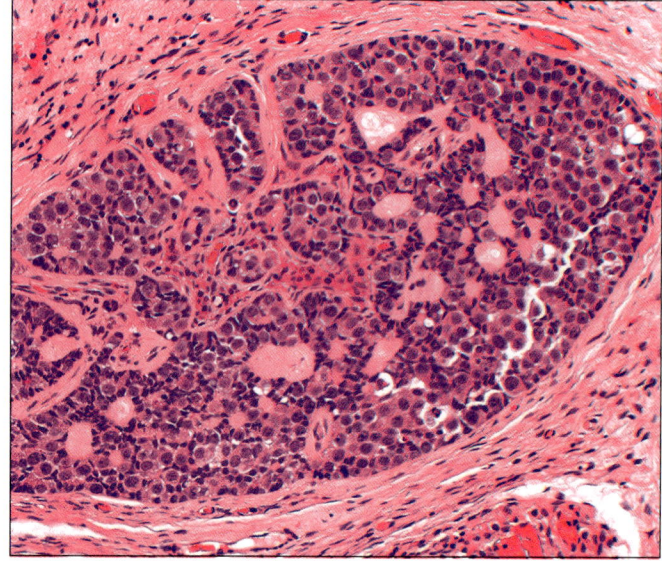

Fig. 27.91 Gonadoblastoma. A typical cell nest showing 'supportive' Sertoli-like cells arranged radially around individual germ cells and around hyaline deposits.

inhibin.[138] They are organized within the cell nests in three different patterns:

- To form a peripheral palisade around aggregates of germ cells (Figures 27.88 and 27.89).
- To form a corona around individual or groups of germ cells in a microfollicular pattern similar to the granulosa of primary follicles.
- To radially surround small deposits of hyaline, eosinophilic PAS-positive material (Figure 27.91) similar to Call–Exner bodies or the laminations of sex-cord tumors with annular tubules.

These rounded, hyaline deposits, composed of aggregated basal lamina material (laminin), are sometimes continuous with linear hyaline deposits around the periphery of the cell nests. Similarities with the hyaline bodies of the sex-cord tumor

with annular tubules (see Chapter 26), and differences from typical Call–Exner bodies, have been noted ultrastructurally.

The fibrous connective tissue stroma that separates the cellular nests contains lutein or Leydig-like cells in 66–75% of cases overall, but significantly more commonly in postpubertal teenagers than in younger children, possibly in response to gonadotrophin stimulation. They vary considerably in their numbers from case to case and, although they usually contain lipochrome pigment, Reinke crystals are rarely observed. This intervening fibrous stroma also varies greatly in amount and in cellularity, from dense and hyalinized to tissue more closely resembling ovarian cortex, the latter particularly so in tumors that have arisen in a gonadal streak. In some gonadoblastomas, the stroma is loose and edematous.

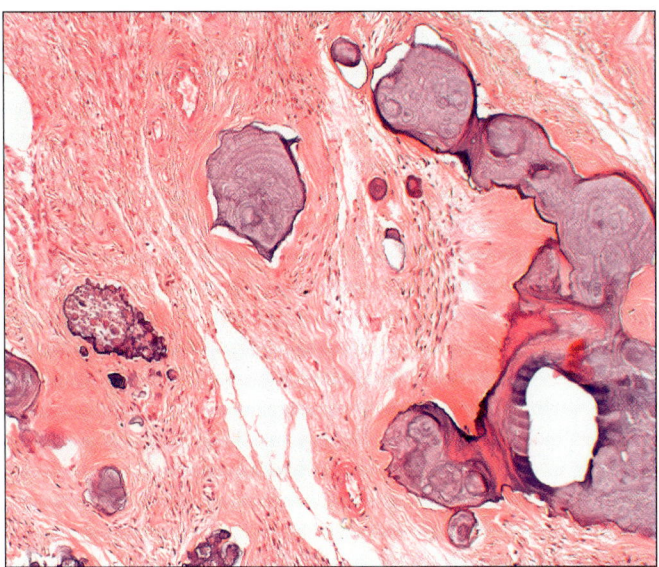

Fig. 27.92 So-called 'burnt-out' gonadoblastoma. A streak gonad characterized by the pattern of calcification set in fibrous gonadal stroma.

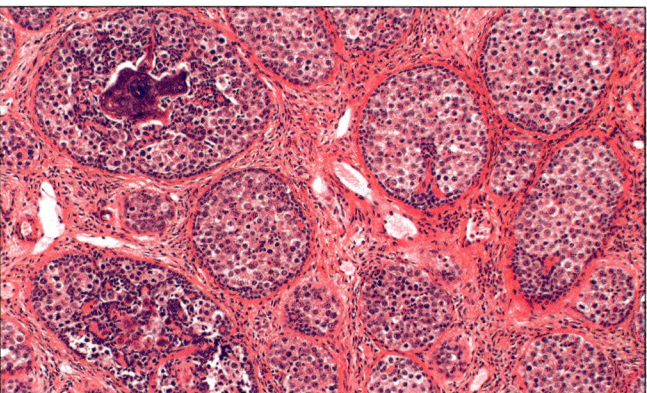

Fig. 27.93 Gonadoblastoma exhibiting progression to dysgerminoma. Typical gonadoblastoma nests (left) are seen in which germ cell proliferation is active but still confined to the cell nests (so-called 'dysgerminoma *in situ*'). Gradual obliteration of the 'supportive' cells (right) ultimately leads to infiltrative dysgerminoma.

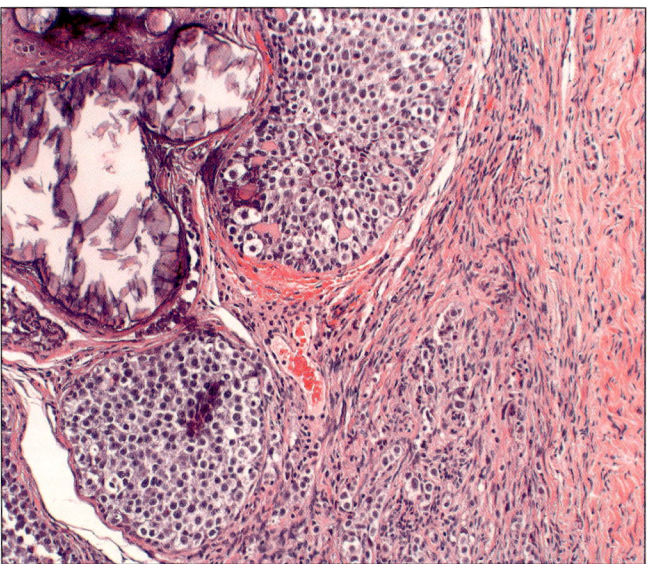

Fig. 27.94 Gonadoblastoma progressing to infiltrating dysgerminoma. Calcified remnants of gonadoblastoma to right with *in situ* dysgerminoma to the immediate left and progressing to invasive dysgerminoma to the centre top.

Gonadoblastomas usually obliterate most or all of the gonads in which they arise. These in turn, in the case of smaller tumors, can be shown to be gonadal streaks or abnormal abdominal testes of pure gonadal dysgenesis or mixed gonadal dysgenesis types.

The appearances of gonadoblastomas may be considerably modified by hyalinization, calcification, and the overgrowth by dysgerminoma or other malignant germ cell tumor. Hyalinization occurs by coalescence and extension of the amorphous, hyaline bodies and the peripheral basal lamina-like band. The hyaline material replaces tumor cells, sometimes entirely. Calcification, seen microscopically in 80% of lesions, usually begins in the hyaline bodies with formation of small laminated calcispherules resembling psammoma bodies (Figure 27.88). The process continues with enlargement and fusion of the calcified bodies and spiculate dystrophic calcification of the hyaline material, finally forming a calcified mass around the whole nest. The process may extend to the stroma between the cellular nests. In such cases, the tumor cells are sparse or even absent, and the pattern of calcification (Figure 27.92) and the presence of lutein or Leydig-like cells may be the only indication of gonadoblastoma. Although this appearance is not considered pathognomonic of gonadoblastoma – it has been graced with the term 'burnt-out' gonadoblastoma – it is highly suggestive and, in such circumstances, a careful search for more typical areas of tumor should be undertaken.

Otherwise typical dysgerminoma overgrows gonadoblastoma in 30% of cases.[139] This progression can be demonstrated by an *in situ* phase (Figures 27.93 and 27.94). This overgrowth may vary from a small focus of germ cells in the stroma outside the gonadoblastoma nests to gross tumor growth that obliterates the antecedent tumor. The only clue to the presence of the original lesion may be tiny foci of calcification (the detection of which is facilitated by radiographic examination of the specimen) and the patient's genotype. In a further 10% of cases, a more malignant type of germ cell tumor, i.e., immature teratoma, yolk sac tumor, embryonal carcinoma or choriocarcinoma, is found.

Differential diagnosis

Gonadoblastomas, because of their distinctive histologic appearances and cellular composition, are readily distinguished from the more frequently encountered gonadal neoplasms. Those from which differentiation may be problematical are the mixed germ cell-sex cord-stromal tumors (see below), and the ovarian sex-cord tumors with annular tubules (SCTAT) that are usually found in patients with Peutz–Jeghers syndrome. These latter lesions are composed of tubules lined by Sertoli and granulosa-like cells arranged in nests, contain similar round, eosinophilic, hyaline deposits, and tend to calcify in the same manner as gonadoblastomas. They are, however, completely devoid of germ cells.

Treatment and prognosis

Female patients with dysgenetic gonads whose genotype includes Y chromosomal material have an approximately 25% likelihood of harboring a gonadoblastoma or malignant germ

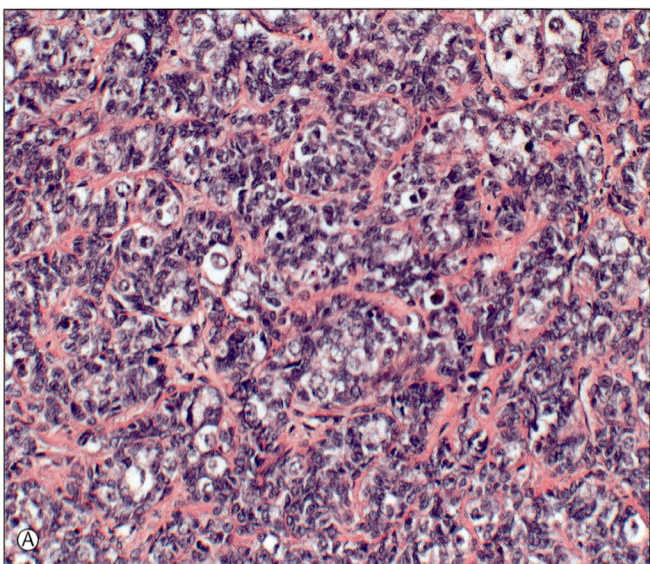 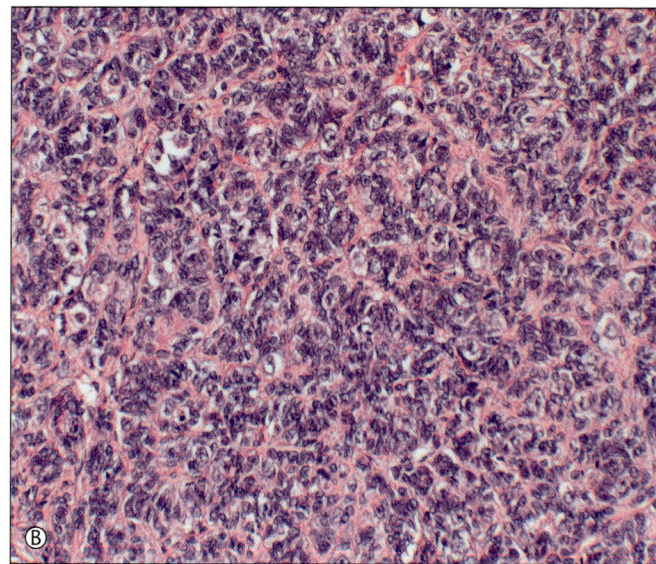

Fig. 27.95   A mixed germ cell and sex cord-stromal tumor. In **(A)** and **(B)** the presence of large germ cells and smaller 'supportive' or sex cord-stromal cells is universal, although their proportions vary from field to field. Courtesy of Dr A Talerman, Philadelphia, PA.

cell tumor – a risk that argues strongly in favor of prophylactic bilateral salpingo-oophorectomy, especially as these dysgenetic gonads are incapable of normal function and retention of reproductive capability is not an issue.[74] Furthermore, the dysgenetic gonads may be virilizing influences even if a malignant tumor does not supervene.

Of those patients with proven gonadoblastoma that has progressed to invasive dysgerminoma, the clinical outcome is still good. Metastases occur later and less frequently than in dysgerminomas unassociated with gonadoblastoma and are rarely fatal. By contrast, the more malignant forms of germ cell tumor behave in a fashion similar to those unassociated with gonadoblastoma.

UNCLASSIFIED MIXED GERM CELL AND SEX CORD-STROMAL TUMORS

Clinical profile

Only rare examples have been adequately documented of this category that includes all neoplasms containing variable mixtures of germ cells and sex-cord elements,[10,118,163,165] but lack the characteristic cellular arrangements of gonadoblastomas. Occasionally theca-lutein and Leydig-like cells are encountered. They arise from normally developed ovaries in karyotypically and phenotypically normal children under 10 years of age, although one case has displayed monosomy 22.[165]

The most frequent presenting symptoms are an abdominal mass and acute abdominal pain due to torsion. Some children exhibit signs of isosexual pseudoprecocity.[196]

Macroscopic features

These tumors are almost always unilateral and vary in size up to 18 cm in diameter and 1 kg in weight. They are usually round to oval and of firm consistency with a smooth, glistening capsule and a gray-pink to pale fawn solid cut surface. Cysts are occasionally present. Necrosis and macroscopic calcification have not been observed.

Microscopic features

The germ cells are similar to those in dysgerminomas/seminomas. They show brisk mitotic activity and are immunoreactive for PLAP, POU5F1 (OCT4) and c-kit protein.[118] Some of the germ cells occasionally appear to be more mature than those seen in gonadoblastomas or dysgerminomas, with large round nuclei lacking a prominent nucleolus. They tend to resemble 'primordial cells' or 'clear cells of another type'. The cells of sex-cord origin resemble Sertoli cells rather more closely than granulosa cells, but may be very immature, and also show variable mitotic activity. While the relative proportion of germ cells to sex-cord cells varies from area to area within individual tumors, their intimate admixture is universal (Figure 27.95). Tumors are predominantly solid in pattern, but with occasional small cleft-like or cystic spaces, the latter resembling the follicle-like spaces of granulosa cell tumors or the retiform patterns of moderately or poorly differentiated Sertoli–Leydig cell tumors. Heterologous elements have been rarely encountered.

There are three discernible architectural arrangements of the component cells. The first shows long, branching cords of variable thickness surrounded by moderate amounts of loose, edematous or dense, fibrous connective tissue. There is some similarity between these trabeculae and the primitive sex cords of the developing ovary. The second pattern shows pseudotubular structures surrounded by a fine network of similar fibrous connective tissue. They resemble the gonadal Sertoli cell congeries of the androgen insensitivity syndrome (testicular feminization syndrome). There may be merging of this pseudotubular pattern, via small clusters of larger round or oval cellular masses, with the third pattern that exhibits germ cell aggregates surrounded by variable, but usually prominent, sex-cord elements. The nest-like pattern of gonadoblastomas is not observed in these tumors. Hyaline bodies and focal stromal dystrophic calcification are very rare or absent.

Normal ovarian stroma with primordial or developing follicles is present at the periphery in all cases. A pure dysgerminoma has been reported as supervening upon the germ cell

27

Table 27.6 Gonadoblastoma versus unclassified mixed germ cell-sex cord-stromal tumor: differential diagnosis

Gonadoblastoma	Unclassified mixed germ cell-sex cord-stromal tumor
Clinical profile	
Most common in second and third decades	Almost all under the age of 10 years
Most have abnormal karyotype (including Y chromosome)	All have 46,XX karyotype
Tumors hormonally inert or associated with masculinization and primary amenorrhea	Phenotypically normal females, isosexual pseudoprecocity in occasional cases
Macroscopic features	
Small tumors	Large tumors
Bilateral in 38%	Always unilateral
Calcified in 45%	Not calcified grossly
Microscopic features	
Typical nest-like pattern	Multiplicity of patterns
Hyaline bodies/microcalcification common	Hyaline bodies/microcalcification absent
Stromal lutein cells common	Stromal lutein cells rare
Dysgerminoma or other germ cell tumor in 60%	Other germ cell tumor types very rare

element in this type of tumor. Intermediate patterns between typical gonadoblastomas and tumors in this category have also been encountered. An apparently unique case demonstrated a sex-cord stromal element reminiscent of SCTAT.[10]

Differential diagnosis

The neoplasms with which mixed germ cell-sex cord-stromal tumors may be most easily confused are, of course, gonadoblastomas (Table 27.6). These girls have a normal female 46,XX karyotype, while those patients with gonadoblastomas are mostly chromosomally abnormal, the karyotype containing a Y chromosome. There is no evidence of virilization. Signs of hormonal activity, if present, are usually estrogenic (isosexual pseudoprecocity). Macroscopically, these tumors are generally larger than uncomplicated gonadoblastomas and they arise in normal ovaries, without evidence of gonadal dysgenesis or phenotypic abnormality. They differ microscopically from gonadoblastomas by the presence of multiple histologic patterns (described above) and greater proliferative activity, particularly in the sex-cord elements. Calcification and stromal hyalinization are absent in these tumors, while the vast majority of cases lack theca-lutein and Leydig cells.

Confusion between mixed germ cell-sex cord-stromal tumors and pure sex cord-stromal tumors should be countered by sampling sufficiently to find the germ cell element and, conversely, they can be differentiated from dysgerminomas by correctly identifying the sex-cord component that may be scanty but is always present.

Treatment and prognosis

The true malignant potential of these tumors has not been firmly determined but, to date, recurrences and/or metastases

after unilateral salpingo-oophorectomy have been recorded only occasionally,[10] and this therefore remains the recommended therapy. Furthermore, in the case of the 31-year-old woman, a dysgerminoma had supervened upon the mixed germ cell-sex cord-stromal tumor, yet the patient was free of disease 4 years after local excision and radiotherapy.

REFERENCES

1. Agaimy A, Lindner M, Wuensch PH. Interstitial cells of Cajal (ICC) in mature cystic teratoma of the ovary. Histopathology 2006;48:208–9.
2. Ajithkumar TV, Abraham EK, Nair MK. Osteosarcoma arising in a mature cystic teratoma of the ovary. J Exp Clin Cancer Res 1999;18:89–91.
3. Akyuz C, Koseoglu V, Gogus S, Balci S, Buyukpamukcu M. Germ cell tumours in a brother and sister. Acta Paediatr 1997;86:668–9.
4. Al Hilli F, Ansari N. Pathogenesis of balls in mature ovarian cystic teratoma. Report of 3 cases and review of literature. Int J Gynecol Pathol 2006;25:347–53.
5. Amareen VN, Haddad FH, Al-Kaisi NS. Hypothyroidism due to Hashimoto thyroiditis post struma ovarii excision. Saudi Med J 2004;25:948–50.
6. Anteby EY, Ron M, Revel A, Shimonovitz S, Ariel I, Hurwitz A. Germ cell tumors of the ovary arising after dermoid cyst resection: a long-term follow-up study. Obstet Gynecol 1994;83:605–8.
7. Aoki Y, Higashino M, Ishii S, Tanaka K. Yolk sac tumor of the ovary during pregnancy: a case report. Gynecol Oncol 2005;99:497–9.
8. Armes JE, Ostor AG. A case of malignant strumal carcinoid. Gynecol Oncol 1993;51:419–23.
9. Arora DS, Haldane S. Carcinosarcoma arising in a dermoid cyst of the ovary. J Clin Pathol 1996;49:519–21.
10. Arroyo JG, Harris W, Laden SA. Recurrent mixed germ cell-sex cord-stromal tumor of the ovary in an adult. Int J Gynecol Pathol 1998;17:281–3.
11. Aygun B, Kimpo M, Lee T, Valderrama E, Leonidas J, Karayalcin G. An adolescent with ovarian osteosarcoma arising in a cystic teratoma. J Pediatr Hematol Oncol 2003;25:410–3.
12. Ayhan A, Bildirici I, Gunalp S, Yuce K. Pure dysgerminoma of the ovary: a review of 45 well staged cases. Eur J Gynaecol Oncol 2000;21:98–101.
13. Ayhan A, Bukulmez O, Genc C, Karamursel BS, Ayhan A. Mature cystic teratomas of the ovary: case series from one institution over 34 years. Eur J Obstet Gynecol Reprod Biol 2000;88:153–7.
14. Baker PM, Oliva E. Immunohistochemistry as a tool in the differential diagnosis of ovarian tumors: an update. Int J Gynecol Pathol 2005;24:39–55.
15. Baker PM, Oliva E, Young RH, Talerman A, Scully RE. Ovarian mucinous carcinoids including some with a carcinomatous component: a report of 17 cases. Am J Surg Pathol 2001;25:557–68.
16. Bakri YN, Ezzat A, Akhtar, Dohami, Zahrani. Malignant germ cell tumors of the ovary. Pregnancy considerations. Eur J Obstet Gynecol Reprod Biol 2000;90:87–91.
17. Balat O, Kudelka AP, Edwards CL, Verschraegen C, Kavanagh JJ. Remission of recurrent mixed germ cell tumor of the ovary after treatment with vincristine, carboplatin, fluorouracil, and ifosfamide: a case report and review of the literature. Eur J Gynaecol Oncol 1996;17:342–4.
18. Balat O, Kutlar I, Ozkur A, Bakir K, Aksoy F, Ugur MG. Primary pure ovarian choriocarcinoma mimicking ectopic pregnancy: a report of fulminant progression. Tumori 2004;90:136–8.
19. Bartel TB, Juweid ME, O'Dorisio T, Sivitz W, Kirby P. Scintigraphic detection of benign struma ovarii in a hyperthyroid patient. J Clin Endocrinol Metab 2005;90:3771–2.
20. Brewer M, Gershenson DM, Herzog CE, Mitchell MF, Silva EG, Wharton JT. Outcome and reproductive function after chemotherapy for ovarian dysgerminoma. J Clin Oncol 1999;17:2670–5.
21. Brogsitter C, Wonsak A, Wurl K, Kotzerke J. Peritoneal strumosis. Eur J Nucl Med Mol Imaging 2004;31:1057.
22. Burg J, Kommoss F, Bittinger F, Moll R, Kirkpatrick CJ. Mature cystic teratoma of the ovary with struma and benign Brenner tumor: a case report with immunohistochemical characterization. Int J Gynecol Pathol 2002;21:74–7.
23. Burke M, Talerman A, Carlson JA, Bibbo M. Residual ovarian tissue mimicking malignancy in a patient with mucinous carcinoid tumor of the ovary. A case report. Acta Cytol 1997;41(4 Suppl):1377–80.
24. Candrina R, Sleiman I, Zorzi F. ACTH-secreting pituitary adenoma within an ovarian teratoma. Eur J Intern Med 2005;16:359–60.
25. Casey AC, Bhodauria S, Shapter A, Nieberg R, Berek JS, Farias-Eisner R. Dysgerminoma: the role of conservative surgery. Gynecol Oncol 1996;63:352–7.
26. Chang A, Schuetze SM, Conrad EU, 3rd, Swisshelm KL, Norwood TH, Rubin BP. So-called 'inflammatory leiomyosarcoma': a series of 3 cases providing additional insights into a rare entity. Int J Surg Pathol 2005;13:185–95.
27. Chang DH, Hsueh S, Soong YK. Small cell carcinoma with neurosecretory granules arising in an ovarian dermoid cyst. Gynecol Oncol 1992;46:246–50.

28. Chapman DC, Grover R, Schwartz PE. Conservative management of an ovarian polyembryoma. Obstet Gynecol 1994;83(5 Pt 2):879–82.

29. Cheng L, Thomas A, Roth LM, Zheng W, Michael H, Karim FW. OCT4: a novel biomarker for dysgerminoma of the ovary. Am J Surg Pathol 2004;28:1341–6.

30. Cho NH, Kim YT, Lee JH, et al. Diagnostic challenge of fetal ontogeny and its application on the ovarian teratomas. Int J Gynecol Pathol 2005;24:173–82.

31. Chumas JC, Scully RE. Sebaceous tumors arising in ovarian dermoid cysts. Int J Gynecol Pathol 1991;10:356–63.

32. Cicchini C, Larcinese A, Ricci F, Aurello P, Mingazzini PL, Indinnimeo M. Monodermal highly specialized teratoma of the ovary: a sebaceous gland tumor. Eur J Gynaecol Oncol 2002;23:442–4.

33. Clement PB, Dimmick JE. Endodermal variant of mature cystic teratoma of the ovary: report of a case. Cancer 1979;43:383–5.

34. Clement PB, Young RH, Scully RE. Endometrioid-like variant of ovarian yolk sac tumor. A clinicopathological analysis of eight cases. Am J Surg Pathol 1987;11:767–78.

35. Climie AR, Heath LP. Malignant degeneration of benign cystic teratomas of the ovary. Review of the literature and report of a chondrosarcoma and carcinoid tumor. Cancer 1968;22:824–32.

36. Cobellis L, Schurfeld K, Ignacchiti E, Santopietro R, Petraglia F. An ovarian mucinous adenocarcinoma arising from mature cystic teratoma associated with respiratory type tissue: a case report. Tumori 2004;90:521–4.

37. Cooper C, Cooper M, Carter J, Russell P. Gonadoblastoma progressing to dysgerminoma in a 55-yr-old woman with normal karyotype. Pathology 2007;39:284–5.

38. Corakci A, Ozeren S, Ozkan S, Gurbuz Y, Ustun H, Yucesoy I. Pure nongestational choriocarcinoma of ovary. Arch Gynecol Obstet 2005;271:176–7.

39. Cossu-Rocca P, Zhang S, Roth LM, et al. Chromosome 12p abnormalities in dysgerminoma of the ovary: a FISH analysis. Mod Pathol 2006;19: 611–5.

40. Dallenbach P, Bonnefoi H, Pelte MF, Vlastos G. Yolk sac tumours of the ovary: an update. Eur J Surg Oncol 2006;32:1063–75.

41. Dardik RB, Dardik M, Westra W, Montz FJ. Malignant struma ovarii: two case reports and a review of the literature. Gynecol Oncol 1999;73:447–51.

42. Davidson B, Abeler VM. Primary ovarian angiosarcoma presenting as malignant cells in ascites: case report and review of the literature. Diagn Cytopathol 2005;32:307–9.

43. De Backer A, Madern GC, Oosterhuis JW, Hakvoort-Cammel FG, Hazebroek FW. Ovarian germ cell tumors in children: a clinical study of 66 patients. Pediatr Blood Cancer 2006;46:459–64.

44. Dede M, Pabuccu R, Yagci G, Yenen MC, Goktolga U, Gunhan O. Extragonadal yolk sac tumor in pelvic localization. A case report and literature review. Gynecol Oncol 2004;92:989–91.

45. den Bakker MA, Ansink AC, Ewing-Graham PC. 'Cutaneous-type' angiosarcoma arising in a mature cystic teratoma of the ovary. J Clin Pathol 2006;59:658–60.

46. den Boon J, van Dijk CM, Helfferich M, Peterse HL. Glioblastoma multiforme in a dermoid cyst of the ovary. A case report. Eur J Gynaecol Oncol 1999;20:187–8.

47. Devaney K, Snyder R, Norris HJ, Tavassoli FA. Proliferative and histologically malignant struma ovarii: a clinicopathologic study of 54 cases. Int J Gynecol Pathol 1993;12:333–43.

48. Dietl J, Horny HP, Ruck P, Kaiserling E. Dysgerminoma of the ovary. An immunohistochemical study of tumor-infiltrating lymphoreticular cells and tumor cells. Cancer 1993;71:2562–8.

49. Doldi N, Taccagni GL, Bassan M, et al. Hashimoto's disease in a papillary carcinoma of the thyroid originating in a teratoma of the ovary (malignant struma ovarii). Gynecol Endocrinol 1998;12:41–2.

50. Dos Santos L, Mok E, Iasonos A, et al. Squamous cell carcinoma arising in mature cystic teratoma of the ovary: a case series and review of the literature. Gynecol Oncol 2007;105:321–4.

51. Doss BJ, Jacques SM, Qureshi F, et al. Immature teratomas of the genital tract in older women. Gynecol Oncol 1999;73:433–8.

52. Dunzendorfer T, deLas Morenas A, Kalir T, Levin RM. Struma ovarii and hyperthyroidism. Thyroid 1999;9:499–502.

53. Ehrmann RL, Weidner N, Welch WR, Gleiberman I. Malignant mixed mullerian tumor of the ovary with prominent neuroectodermal differentiation (teratoid carcinosarcoma). Int J Gynecol Pathol 1990;9:272–82.

54. Ergeneli MH, Demirhan B, Duran EH, Coskun M. Malignant mixed mesodermal tumor arising in a benign cystic teratoma. Eur J Obstet Gynecol Reprod Biol 1999;83:191–4.

55. Fadare O, Bossuyt V, Martel M, Parkash V. Primary osteosarcoma of the ovary: a case report and literature review. Int J Gynecol Pathol 2007;26:21–5.

56. Ferguson AW, Katabuchi H, Ronnett BM, Cho KR. Glial implants in gliomatosis peritonei arise from normal tissue, not from the associated teratoma. Am J Pathol 2001;159:51–5.

57. Fishman A, Edelstein E, Altaras M, Beyth Y, Bernheim J. Adenocarcinoma arising from the gastrointestinal epithelium in benign cystic teratoma of the ovary. Gynecol Oncol 1998;70:418–20.

58. Fogt F, Vortmeyer AO, Ahn G, et al. Neural cyst of the ovary with central nervous system microvasculature. Histopathology 1994;24:477–80.

59. Fujiwara K, Shirotani T, Kohno I. Supernumerary ovary found by ultrasonogram and FSH measurement after an extensive operation for a yolk sac tumor of the ovary. Gynecol Obstet Invest 1999;48:138–40.

60. Gabrys M, Blok K, Rabczynski J, et al. Gliomatosis peritonei with mature teratoma of the ovary. Ginekol Pol 2002;73:1224–7.

61. Galani E, Alamanis C, Dimopoulos MA. Familial female and male germ cell cancer. A new syndrome? Gynecol Oncol 2005;96:254–5.

62. Gangadharan VP, Mathew BS, Kumar KS, Chitrathara K. Primary choriocarcinoma of the ovary. Report of two cases. Indian J Cancer 1999;36:213–5.

63. Garcia-Barriola V, De Gomez MN, Suarez JA, Lara C, Gonzalez JE, Garcia-Tamayo J. Ovarian ependymoma. A case report. Pathol Res Pract 2000;196:595–9.

64. Glorieux I, Chabbert V, Rubie H, et al. [Autoimmune hemolytic anemia associated with a mature ovarian teratoma]. Arch Pediatr 1998;5:41–4.

65. Goswami D, Sharma K, Zutshi V, Tempe A, Nigam S. Nongestational pure ovarian choriocarcinoma with contralateral teratoma. Gynecol Oncol 2001;80:262–6.

66. Guerrieri C, Jarlsfelt I. Ependymoma of the ovary. A case report with immunohistochemical, ultrastructural, and DNA cytometric findings, as well as histogenetic considerations. Am J Surg Pathol 1993;17:623–32.

67. Gupta D, Deavers MT, Silva EG, Malpica A. Malignant melanoma involving the ovary: a clinicopathologic and immunohistochemical study of 23 cases. Am J Surg Pathol 2004;28:771–80.

68. Halabi M, Oliva E, Mazal PR, Breitenecker G, Young RH. Prostatic tissue in mature cystic teratomas of the ovary: a report of four cases, including one with features of prostatic adenocarcinoma, and cytogenetic studies. Int J Gynecol Pathol 2002;21:261–7.

69. Hattab EM, Tu PH, Wilson JD, Cheng L. OCT4 immunohistochemistry is superior to placental alkaline phosphatase (PLAP) in the diagnosis of central nervous system germinoma. Am J Surg Pathol 2005;29:368–71.

70. Hill DA, Dehner LP, White FV, Langer JC. Gliomatosis peritonei as a complication of a ventriculoperitoneal shunt: case report and review of the literature. J Pediatr Surg 2000;35:497–9.

71. Hirabayashi K, Yasuda M, Osamura RY, Hirasawa T, Murakami M. Ovarian nongestational choriocarcinoma mixed with various epithelial malignancies in association with endometriosis. Gynecol Oncol 2006;102:111–7.

72. Hirschowitz L, Ansari A, Cahill DJ, Bamford DS, Love S. Central neurocytoma arising within a mature cystic teratoma of the ovary. Int J Gynecol Pathol 1997;16:176–9.

73. Hoda SA, Huvos AG. Struma salpingis associated with struma ovarii. Am J Surg Pathol 1993;17:1187–9.

74. Hoepffner W, Horn LC, Simon E, et al. Gonadoblastomas in 5 patients with 46,XY gonadal dysgenesis. Exp Clin Endocrinol Diabetes 2005;113:231–5.

75. Horn LC, Limbach A, Hoepffner W, et al. Histologic analysis of gonadal tissue in patients with Ullrich–Turner syndrome and derivative Y chromosomes. Pediatr Dev Pathol 2005;8:197–203.

76. Hsu CY, Yang CF, Chen WY, Chiang H. Adenosquamous carcinoma and schneiderian papilloma-like lesion in a mature cystic teratoma of the ovary: a case report. Zhonghua Yi Xue Za Zhi (Taipei) 1996;57:375–9.

77. Indinnimeo M, Cicchini C, Larcinese A, Kanakaki S, Ricci F, Mingazzini PL. Two twins with teratoma of the ovary. An unusual association: case report. Eur J Gynaecol Oncol 2003;24:199–201.

78. Jha S, Chan KK, Poole CJ, Rollason TP. Pregnancy following recurrent angiosarcoma of the ovary – a case report and review of literature. Gynecol Oncol 2005;97:935–7.

79. Kakarla N, Boswell HB, Zurawin RK. A large pelvic mass in an adolescent patient with granulomatous nephritis: case report and discussion of treatment challenges. J Pediatr Adolesc Gynecol 2006;19:223–9.

80. Kaleli B, Aktan E, Bayramoglu H, Alatas E. Mature cystic teratoma in round ligament: case report. Eur J Obstet Gynecol Reprod Biol 1997;74:195–6.

81. Kammerer-Doak D, Baurick K, Black W, Barbo DM, Smith HO. Endodermal sinus tumor and embryonal carcinoma of the ovary in a 53-year-old woman. Gynecol Oncol 1996;63:133–7.

82. Kanbour-Shakir A, Sawaday J, Kanbour AI, Kunschner A, Stock RJ. Primitive neuroectodermal tumor arising in an ovarian mature cystic teratoma: immunohistochemical and electron microscopic studies. Int J Gynecol Pathol 1993;12:270–5.

83. Kawai M, Kano T, Furuhashi Y, et al. Prognostic factors in yolk sac tumors of the ovary. A clinicopathological analysis of 29 cases. Cancer 1991;67:184–92.

84. Kawauchi S, Fukuda T, Miyamoto S, et al. Peripheral primitive neuroectodermal tumor of the ovary confirmed by CD99 immunostaining, karyotypic analysis, and RT-PCR for EWS/FLI-1 chimeric mRNA. Am J Surg Pathol 1998;22:1417–22.

85. Kdous M, Hachicha R, Gamoudi A, Boussen H, Benna F, Rahal K. [Pure dysgerminoma of the ovary. 12 case reports]. Tunis Med 2003;81:937–43.

86. Khadilkar UN, Pai RR, Lahiri R, Kumar P. Ovarian strumal carcinoid – report of a case that metastasized. Indian J Pathol Microbiol 2000;43:459–61.

87. Kikkawa F, Ishikawa H, Tamakoshi K, Nawa A, Suganuma N, Tomoda Y. Squamous cell carcinoma arising from mature cystic teratoma of the ovary: a clinicopathologic analysis. Obstet Gynecol 1997;89:1017–22.

88. Kim KJ, Jang BW, Lee SK, Kim BK, Nam SL. A case of peripheral primitive neuroectodermal tumor of the ovary. Int J Gynecol Cancer 2004;14:370–2.

89. Kim SM, Choi HS, Byun JS, et al. Mucinous adenocarcinoma and strumal carcinoid tumor arising in one mature cystic teratoma of the ovary with synchronous cervical cancer. J Obstet Gynaecol Res 2003;29:28–32.

90. Kinoshita K. A 62-year-old woman with endodermal sinus tumor of the ovary. Am J Obstet Gynecol 1990;162:760–2.

91. Kleinman GM, Young RH, Scully RE. Primary neuroectodermal tumors of the ovary. A report of 25 cases. Am J Surg Pathol 1993;17:764–78.

92. Kommoss F, Emond J, Hast J, Talerman A. Ruptured mature cystic teratoma of the ovary with recurrence in the liver and colon 17 years later. A case report. J Reprod Med 1990;35:827–31.

93. Komuro Y, Mikami M, Sakaiya N, et al. Tumor imprint cytology of ovarian ependymoma. A case report. Cancer 2001;92:3165–9.

94. Koo HL, Choi J, Kim KR, Kim JH. Pure non-gestational choriocarcinoma of the ovary diagnosed by DNA polymorphism analysis. Pathol Int 2006;56:613–6.

95. Kruger S, Schmidt H, Kupker W, Rath FW, Feller AC. Fibrosarcoma associated with a benign cystic teratoma of the ovary. Gynecol Oncol 2002;84:150–4.

96. Kuno N, Kadomatsu K, Nakamura M, Miwa-Fukuchi T, Hirabayashi N, Ishizuka T. Mature ovarian cystic teratoma with a highly differentiated homunculus: a case report. Birth Defects Res A Clin Mol Teratol 2004;70:40–6.

97. Kuroda N, Hirano K, Inui Y, et al. Compound melanocytic nevus arising in a mature cystic teratoma of the ovary. Pathol Int 2001;51:902–4.

98. Kushima M. Adenocarcinoma arising from mature cystic teratoma of the ovary. Pathol Int 2004;54:139–43.

99. Lawlor ER, Murphy JI, Sorensen PH, Fryer CJ. Metastatic primitive neuroectodermal tumour of the ovary: successful treatment with mega-dose chemotherapy followed by peripheral blood progenitor cell rescue. Med Pediatr Oncol 1997;29:308–12.

100. Levine DA, Villella JA, Poynor EA, Soslow RA. Gastrointestinal adenocarcinoma arising in a mature cystic teratoma of the ovary. Gynecol Oncol 2004;94:597–9.

101. Li H, Hong W, Zhang R, Wu L, Liu L, Zhang W. Retrospective analysis of 67 consecutive cases of pure ovarian immature teratoma. Chin Med J (Engl) 2002;115:1496–500.

102. Liberati F, Maccio T, Ascani S, et al. Primary malignant melanoma arising in an ovarian cystic teratoma. Acta Oncol 1998;37:381–3.

103. Lim SC, Choi SJ, Suh CH. A case of small cell carcinoma arising in a mature cystic teratoma of the ovary. Pathol Int 1998;48:834–9.

104. Looijenga LH, Stoop H, de Leeuw HP, et al. POU5F1 (OCT3/4) identifies cells with pluripotent potential in human germ cell tumors. Cancer Res 2003;63:2244–50.

105. Lopez-Beltran A, Calanas AS, Jimena P, et al. Virilizing mature ovarian cystic teratomas. Virchows Arch 1997;431:149–51.

106. Lopez JM, Malpica A, Deavers MT, Ayala AG. Ovarian yolk sac tumor associated with endometrioid carcinoma and mucinous cystadenoma of the ovary. Ann Diagn Pathol 2003;7:300–5.

107. Lorigan PC, Grierson AJ, Goepel JR, Coleman RE, Goyns MH. Gestational choriocarcinoma of the ovary diagnosed by analysis of tumour DNA. Cancer Lett 1996;104:27–30.

108. Loughrey MB, McCusker G, Heasley RN, Alkalbani M, McCluggage WG. Clear cell struma ovarii. Histopathology 2003;43:495–7.

109. Low JJ, Perrin LC, Crandon AJ, Hacker NF. Conservative surgery to preserve ovarian function in patients with malignant ovarian germ cell tumors. A review of 74 cases. Cancer 2000;89:391–8.

110. Lu KH, Gershenson DM. Update on the management of ovarian germ cell tumors. J Reprod Med 2005;50:417–25.

111. Mahdavi A, Silberberg B, Malviya VK, Braunstein AH, Shapiro J. Gangliocytic paraganglioma arising from mature cystic teratoma of the ovary. Gynecol Oncol 2003;90:482–5.

112. Mandel M, Toren A, Kende G, Neuman Y, Kenet G, Rechavi G. Familial clustering of malignant germ cell tumors and Langerhans' histiocytosis. Cancer 1994;73:1980–3.

113. Matias-Guiu X, Forteza J, Prat J. Mixed strumal and mucinous carcinoid tumor of the ovary. Int J Gynecol Pathol 1995;14:179–83.

114. Mazzanti L, Cicognani A, Baldazzi L, et al. Gonadoblastoma in Turner syndrome and Y-chromosome-derived material. Am J Med Genet A 2005;135:150–4.

115. McCluggage WG, Young RH. Paraganglioma of the ovary: report of three cases of a rare neoplasm, including two exhibiting inhibin positivity. Am J Surg Pathol 2006;30:600–5.

116. McCluggage WG, Bissonnette JP, Young RH. Primary malignant melanoma of the ovary: a report of 9 definite or probable cases with emphasis on their morphologic diversity and mimicry of other primary and secondary ovarian neoplasms. Int J Gynecol Pathol 2006;25:321–9.

117. Michael H, Ulbright TM, Brodhecker CA. The pluripotential nature of the mesenchyme-like component of yolk sac tumor. Arch Pathol Lab Med 1989;113:1115–9.

118. Michal M, Vanecek T, Sima R, et al. Mixed germ cell sex cord-stromal tumors of the testis and ovary. Morphological, immunohistochemical, and molecular genetic study of seven cases. Virchows Arch 2006;449:612–22.

119. Mikami M, Komuro Y, Sakaiya N, et al. Primary ependymoma of the ovary, in which long-term oral etoposide (VP-16) was effective in prolonging disease-free survival. Gynecol Oncol 2001;83:149–52.

120. Min KJ, Jee BC, Lee HS, Kim YB. Intestinal adenocarcinoma arising in a mature cystic teratoma of the ovary: a case report. Pathol Res Pract 2006;202:531–5.

121. Miyagawa S, Hirota S, Park YD, et al. Cutaneous mastocytosis associated with a mixed germ cell tumour of the ovary: report of a case and review of the literature. Br J Dermatol 2001;145:309–12.

122. Miyazaki C, Kato R, Nishimura N, Nagamatsu M, Kodama S, Honma S. [A case of embryonal carcinoma of the ovary occurred in a 50-year-old woman]. Nippon Sanka Fujinka Gakkai Zasshi 1992;44:483–6.

123. Monteagudo C, Torres JV, Llombart-Bosch A. Extramammary Paget's disease arising in a mature cystic teratoma of the ovary. Histopathology 1999;35:582–4.

124. Morimitsu Y, Nakashima O, Nakashima Y, Kojiro M, Shimokobe T. Apocrine adenocarcinoma arising in cystic teratoma of the ovary. Arch Pathol Lab Med 1993;117:647–9.

125. Muretto P, Chilosi M, Rabitti C, Tommasoni S, Colato C. Biovularity and 'coalescence of primary follicles' in ovaries with mature teratomas. Int J Surg Pathol 2001;9:121–5.

126. Nanda S, Kalra B, Arora B, Singh S. Massive mature solid teratoma of the ovary with gliomatosis peritonei. Aust N Z J Obstet Gynaecol 1998;38:329–31.

127. Nawa A, Obata N, Kikkawa F, et al. Prognostic factors of patients with yolk sac tumors of the ovary. Am J Obstet Gynecol 2001;184:1182–8.

128. Nimkin K, Gupta P, McCauley R, Gilchrist BF, Lessin MS. The growing teratoma syndrome. Pediatr Radiol 2004;34:259–62.

129. Nishida T, Oda T, Sugiyama T, Kataoka A, Honda S, Yakushiji M. Ovarian mixed germ cell tumor comprising polyembryoma and choriocarcinoma. Eur J Obstet Gynecol Reprod Biol 1998;78:95–7.

130. Nogales FF, Ruiz Avila I, Concha A, del Moral E. Immature endodermal teratoma of the ovary: embryologic correlations and immunohistochemistry. Hum Pathol 1993;24:364–70.

131. Nogales FF, Bergeron C, Carvia RE, Alvaro T, Fulwood HR. Ovarian endometrioid tumors with yolk sac tumor component, an unusual form of ovarian neoplasm. Analysis of six cases. Am J Surg Pathol 1996;20:1056–66.

132. Nucci MR, Krausz T, Lifschitz-Mercer B, Chan JK, Fletcher CD. Angiosarcoma of the ovary: clinicopathologic and immunohistochemical analysis of four cases with a broad morphologic spectrum. Am J Surg Pathol 1998;22:620–30.

133. O'Connor DM, Norris HJ. The influence of grade on the outcome of stage I ovarian immature (malignant) teratomas and the reproducibility of grading. Int J Gynecol Pathol 1994;13:283–9.

134. Oliva E, Andrada E, Pezzica E, Prat J. Ovarian carcinomas with choriocarcinomatous differentiation. Cancer 1993;72:2441–6.

135. Osmanagaoglu M, Bozkaya H, Reis A. Malignant struma ovarii: a case report and review of the literature. Indian J Med Sci 2004;58:206–10.

136. Ozaki Y, Shindoh N, Sumi Y, Kubota T, Katayama H. Choriocarcinoma of the ovary associated with mucinous cystadenoma. Radiat Med 2001;19:55–9.

137. Parkash V, Carcangiu ML. Transformation of ovarian dysgerminoma to yolk sac tumor: evidence for a histogenetic continuum. Mod Pathol 1995;8:881–7.

138. Pauls K, Franke FE, Buttner R, Zhou H. Gonadoblastoma: evidence for a stepwise progression to dysgerminoma in a dysgenetic ovary. Virchows Arch 2005;447:603–9.

139. Pena-Alonso R, Nieto K, Alvarez R, et al. Distribution of Y-chromosome-bearing cells in gonadoblastoma and dysgenetic testis in 45,X/46,XY infants. Mod Pathol 2005;18:439–45.

140. Pitman MB, Triratanachat S, Young RH, Oliva E. Hepatocyte paraffin 1 antibody does not distinguish primary ovarian tumors with hepatoid differentiation from metastatic hepatocellular carcinoma. Int J Gynecol Pathol 2004;23:58–64.

141. Poulos C, Cheng L, Zhang S, Gersell DJ, Ulbright TM. Analysis of ovarian teratomas for isochromosome 12p: evidence supporting a dual histogenetic pathway for teratomatous elements. Mod Pathol 2006;19:766–71.

142. Radotra BD. Pure non-gestational choriocarcinoma of ovary: a case report with autopsy findings. Indian J Pathol Microbiol 2001;44:503–5.

143. Ramalingam P, Malpica A, Silva EG, Gershenson DM, Liu JL, Deavers MT. The use of cytokeratin 7 and EMA in differentiating ovarian yolk sac tumors from endometrioid and clear cell carcinomas. Am J Surg Pathol 2004;28:1499–505.

144. Rangan A, Lobo FD, Rao AA. Primary primitive neuroectodermal tumor of the ovary: a case report. Indian J Pathol Microbiol 2003;46:58–9.

145. Reid HA, van der Walt JD, Fox H. Neuroblastoma arising in a mature cystic teratoma of the ovary. J Clin Pathol 1983;36:68–73.

146. Rekha W, Amita M, Sudeep G, Shubhada K, Hemant T. Growing teratoma syndrome in germ cell tumour of the ovary: a case report. Aust N Z J Obstet Gynaecol 2005;45:170–1.

147. Reyes Rivera ML, Wong Sanchez E, Casas Santisrebe AL, de Leon RA, Castillo Menchaca F. [Female pseudohermaphroditism. Mixed germ cell tumor of the ovary. A case report]. Ginecol Obstet Mex 1998;66:24–8.

148. Ribeiro-Silva A, Bezerra AM, Serafini LN. Malignant struma ovarii: an autopsy report of a clinically unsuspected tumor. Gynecol Oncol 2002;87:213–5.

149. Ribeiro-Silva A, Chang D, Bisson FW, Re LO. Clinicopathological and immunohistochemical features of a sebaceous carcinoma arising within a benign dermoid cyst of the ovary. Virchows Arch 2003;443:574–8.

150. Robboy SJ, Scully RE. Strumal carcinoid of the ovary: an analysis of 50 cases of a distinctive tumor composed of thyroid tissue and carcinoid. Cancer 1980;46:2019–34.

151. Robboy SJ, Krigman HR, Donohue J. Prognostic indexes in malignant struma ovarii – clinicopathological analysis of 36 patients with 20+-year follow-up. Lab Invest 1995;72:A95.

152. Robboy SJ, Szyfelbein WM, Peng RY, et al. Malignant struma ovarii: an analysis of 82 cases, including 23 with extraovarian spread [unpublished data]. 2008.

153. Russell P, Wills EJ, Watson G, Lee J, Geraghty T. Monomorphic (basal cell) salivary adenoma of ovary: report of a case. Ultrastruct Pathol 1995;19: 431–8.

154. Sahin AA, Ro JY, Chen J, Ayala AG. Spindle cell nodule and peptic ulcer arising in a fully developed gastric wall in a mature cystic teratoma. Arch Pathol Lab Med 1990;114:529–31.

155. Sala E, Villa N, Crosti F, et al. Endometrioid-like yolk sac and Sertoli–Leydig cell tumors in a carrier of a Y heterochromatin insertion into 1qh region: a causal association? Cancer Genet Cytogenet 2007;173:164–9.

156. Salazar-Exaire D, Rodriguez A, Galindo-Rujana ME, et al. Membranoproliferative glomerulonephritis associated with a mixed-cell germinal ovary tumor. Am J Nephrol 2001;21:51–4.

157. Sasaki H, Furusato M, Teshima S, et al. Prognostic significance of histopathological subtypes in stage I pure yolk sac tumour of the ovary. Br J Cancer 1994;69:529–36.

158. Satge D, Honore L, Sasco AJ, Vekemans M, Chompret A, Rethore MO. An ovarian dysgerminoma in Down syndrome. Hypothesis about the association. Int J Gynecol Cancer 2006;16(Suppl 1):375–9.

159. Schmidt D, Kommoss F. [Teratoma of the ovary: clinical and pathological differences between mature and immature teratomas]. Pathologe 2007;28:203–8.

160. Sekiya S, Iwasawa H, Morikawa S, Takamizawa H. Malignant change of dermoid cysts of the ovary. Report on an adenosquamous cell carcinoma and a clear cell carcinoma. Eur J Gynaecol Oncol 1984;5:16–20.

161. Shefren G, Collin J, Soriero O. Gliomatosis peritonei with malignant transformation: a case report and review of the literature. Am J Obstet Gynecol 1991;164(6 Pt 1):1617–20; discussion 20–1.

162. Sidhu J, Sanchez RL. Prostatic acid phosphatase in strumal carcinoids of the ovary. An immunohistochemical study. Cancer 1993;72:1673–8.

163. Slowikowska-Hilczer J, Romer TE, Kula K. Neoplastic potential of germ cells in relation to disturbances of gonadal organogenesis and changes in karyotype. J Androl 2003;24:270–8.

164. Soga J, Osaka M, Yakuwa Y. Carcinoids of the ovary: an analysis of 329 reported cases. J Exp Clin Cancer Res 2000;19:271–80.

165. Speleman F, Dermaut B, De Potter CR, et al. Monosomy 22 in a mixed germ cell-sex cord-stromal tumor of the ovary. Genes Chromosomes Cancer 1997;19:192–4.

166. Stenram U. Sclerosing peritonitis in a case of benign cystic ovarian teratoma. A case report. Apmis 1997;105:414–6.

167. Stewart CJ, Farquharson MA, Foulis AK. Characterization of the inflammatory infiltrate in ovarian dysgerminoma: an immunocytochemical study. Histopathology 1992;20:491–7.

168. Sumi T, Ishiko O, Maeda K, Haba T, Wakasa K, Ogita S. Adenocarcinoma arising from respiratory ciliated epithelium in mature ovarian cystic teratoma. Arch Gynecol Obstet 2002;267:107–9.

169. Szyfelbein WM, Young RH, Scully RE. Cystic struma ovarii: a frequently unrecognized tumor. A report of 20 cases. Am J Surg Pathol 1994;18:785–8.

170. Takeshima Y, Kaneko M, Furonaka O, Jeet AV, Inai K. Meningioma in mature cystic teratoma of the ovary. Pathol Int 2004;54:543–8.

171. Takeuchi K, Ohbayashi C, Kitazawa S, Ohara N, Maruo T. Coexistence of Brenner tumor and struma ovarii: case report. Eur J Gynaecol Oncol 2005;26:109–10.

172. Tanimoto A, Arima N, Hayashi R, Hamada T, Matsuki Y, Sasaguri Y. Teratoid carcinosarcoma of the ovary with prominent neuroectodermal differentiation. Pathol Int 2001;51:829–32.

173. Teitell M, Rowland JM. Systemic mast cell disease associated with primary ovarian mixed malignant germ cell tumor. Hum Pathol 1998;29:1546–7.

174. Tejura H, O'Leary A. Growing teratoma syndrome after chemotherapy for germ cell tumour of the ovary. J Obstet Gynaecol 2005;25:296–7.

175. Tewari K, Cappuccini F, Disaia PJ, Berman ML, Manetta A, Kohler MF. Malignant germ cell tumors of the ovary. Obstet Gynecol 2000;95:128–33.

176. Trabelsi A, Conan-Charlet V, Lhomme C, Morice P, Duvillard P, Sabourin JC. [Peritoneal glioblastoma: recurrence of ovarian immature teratoma (report of a case)]. Ann Pathol 2002;22:130–3.

177. Tsujioka H, Hamada H, Miyakawa T, Hachisuga T, Kawarabayashi T. A pure nongestational choriocarcinoma of the ovary diagnosed with DNA polymorphism analysis. Gynecol Oncol 2003;89:540–2.

178. Tyagi SP, Maheshwari V, Tyagi N, Tewari K. Double malignancy in a benign cystic teratoma of the ovary (a case report). Indian J Cancer 1993;30:140–2.

179. Ueda G, Sato Y, Yamasaki M, et al. Malignant fibrous histiocytoma arising in a benign cystic teratoma of the ovary. Gynecol Oncol 1977;5:313–22.

180. Ulbright TM. Germ cell tumors of the gonads: a selective review emphasizing problems in differential diagnosis, newly appreciated, and controversial issues. Mod Pathol 2005;18(Suppl 2):S61–79.

181. Ushakov FB, Meirow D, Prus D, Libson E, BenShushan A, Rojansky N. Parasitic ovarian dermoid tumor of the omentum – a review of the literature and report of two new cases. Eur J Obstet Gynecol Reprod Biol 1998;81:77–82.

182. Vartanian RK, McRae B, Hessler RB. Sebaceous carcinoma arising in a mature cystic teratoma of the ovary. Int J Gynecol Pathol 2002;21:418–21.

183. Vautier-Rit S, Ducarme G, Devisme L, Vinatier D, Leroy JL. [Primary choriocarcinoma of the ovary: a case report]. Gynecol Obstet Fertil 2004;32:620–3.

184. Vlodavsky E, Kerner H. Prostatic tissue in a benign cystic teratoma of the ovary. Report of two cases. Isr Med Assoc J 2000;2:783–4.

185. Vortmeyer AO, Devouassoux-Shisheboran M, Li G, Mohr V, Tavassoli F, Zhuang Z. Microdissection-based analysis of mature ovarian teratoma. Am J Pathol 1999;154:987–91.

186. Waugh MS, Soler AP, Robboy SJ. Silent corticotroph cell pituitary adenoma in a struma ovarii. Int J Gynecol Pathol 2007;26:26–9.

187. Yaegashi N, Tsuiki A, Shimizu T, et al. Ovarian carcinoid with severe constipation due to peptide YY production. Gynecol Oncol 1995;56:302–6.

188. Yanai H, Matsuura H, Kawasaki M, Takada Y, Tabuchi Y, Yoshino T. Immature teratoma of the ovary with a minor rhabdomyosarcomatous component and fatal rhabdomyosarcomatous metastases: the first case in a child. Int J Gynecol Pathol 2002;21:82–5.

189. Yoon HK, Park SM, Joo JE. Combined microcystic adnexal carcinoma and squamous cell carcinoma arising in the ovarian cystic teratoma – a brief case report. J Korean Med Sci 1994;9:432–5.

190. Yoshida M, Obayashi C, Tachibana M, Minami R. Coexisting Brenner tumor and struma ovarii in the right ovary: case report and review of the literature. Pathol Int 2004;54:793–7.

191. Yoshikata R, Yamamoto T, Kobayashi M, Ota H. Immunohistochemical characteristics of mature ovarian cystic teratomas in patients with postoperative recurrence. Int J Gynecol Pathol 2006;25:95–100.

192. Young RH, Jackson A, Wells M. Ovarian metastasis from thyroid carcinoma 12 years after partial thyroidectomy mimicking struma ovarii: report of a case. Int J Gynecol Pathol 1994;13:181–5.

193. Zarbo R, Scibilia G, Conoscenti G, Scollo P. Ovarian cystic teratoma with primary epithelial cell melanoma. Eur J Gynaecol Oncol 2005;26:71–4.

194. Zekri JM, Manifold IH, Wadsley JC. Metastatic struma ovarii: late presentation, unusual features and multiple radioactive iodine treatments. Clin Oncol (R Coll Radiol) 2006;18:768–72.

195. Zhao S, Kato N, Endoh Y, Jin Z, Ajioka Y, Motoyama T. Ovarian gonadoblastoma with mixed germ cell tumor in a woman with 46,XX karyotype and successful pregnancies. Pathol Int 2000;50:332–5.

196. Zuntova A, Motlik K, Horejsi J, Eckschlager T. Mixed germ cell-sex cord stromal tumor with heterologous structures. Int J Gynecol Pathol 1992;11:227–33.

197. Zuntova A, Sumerauer D, Teslik L, Kabickova E, Koutecky J. [Mixed germ cell tumours of the ovary in childhood and adolescence]. Cesk Patol 2004;40:92–101.

Ovarian lymphoid and hematopoietic neoplasms

28

Anand S. Lagoo   Peter Russell   Stanley J. Robboy

The ovaries can be involved by lymphomas and leukemias. Although presentation of these diseases as ovarian masses is a rare event, their highly specialized, and often curative, treatment regimens differ completely from those of the more common epithelial and germ cell tumors and it is crucial that these neoplasms be correctly identified and appropriately classified. Most lymphoid neoplasms can manifest either as a mass lesion (lymphoma) or as circulating cells (lymphocytic or lymphoblastic leukemia) in different patients or in the same patient over the course of the disease, although the former is initially more usual for many of these neoplasms. Hematopoietic cell neoplasms more commonly present as leukemias, either acute or chronic myelogenous leukemia. Occasionally, a primary extramedullary presentation, referred to as granulocytic sarcoma, can affect various sites including the ovaries.

In addition to the vanishingly rare primary involvement of ovaries in lymphomas or granulocytic sarcoma, they are somewhat more often involved as part of disseminated lymphomas and leukemias.

LYMPHOMA

Our understanding has changed greatly in recent decades regarding the pathogenesis and pathology of lymphomas with the realization that the various lymphomas constitute different diseases, each with distinct clinicopathologic features and prognoses.[3] The current World Health Organization (WHO) classification[19] and its predecessor, the Revised European and American Lymphoma (REAL) classification,[14] best exemplify this paradigm as it departs from most previous classifications, including the popular working formulation,[1] which considered most non-Hodgkins lymphomas as morphologic variants of the same basic disease process. The new WHO classification defines lymphomas as separate diseases based on morphologic, immunophenotypic, cytogenetic and clinical features. As the various lymphomas differ widely in their rates of progression, overall life expectancy after diagnosis, and the response to individual forms of treatment, accurate subtyping has become imperative.[2] As new therapies are being introduced that target specific antigens expressed on the surface of the lymphoma cells (e.g., rituximab, an anti-CD20 antibody) or to abnormal proteins these cells produce (e.g., imatinib against the BCR/ABL product of the Philadelphia chromosome, t(9;22)), it is critical that all lymphomas be completely characterized by immunophenotype, cytogenetic features, and even molecular abnormalities.[15,36] Moreover, specific immunophenotypic, cytogenetic or molecular features of the more commonly occurring lymphomas and leukemias provide prognostic information about subsets of these diseases, which may be used for making treatment decisions in an individual patient.

A standardized workup for all specimens suspected of harboring lymphomas is necessary for optimal management of these patients and should include flow cytometry and cytogenetic testing when possible. Even if lymphoma is not suspected prior to surgery, as occurs frequently with ovarian lymphoma, some of the same information may be salvaged through immunohistochemistry, polymerase chain reaction-based methods applied to DNA retrieved from paraffin-embedded tissue, and interphase fluorescent *in situ* hybridization (FISH) on paraffin sections. Experience is required to interpret the results of these studies. Some general features of practical significance in the modern lymphoma classification are discussed below.

Classification

This section presents general principles. For a ready reference, Table 28.1 lists the commonly encountered antigenic markers in leukemia/lymphoma diagnosis and their significance. Like all earlier classifications, the newest WHO classification[19] also recognizes the fundamental distinction between Hodgkin and non-Hodgkin lymphomas. Hodgkin lymphomas are further classified into classic and nodular lymphocyte-predominant types. The immunophenotype of the Reed–Sternberg (R-S) cell in classic Hodgkin lymphoma (CD15+, CD30+, CD20–, CD45–) differs from the lymphocyte and histiocyte (L&H) or 'popcorn' cell in nodular lymphocyte-predominant Hodgkin lymphoma (CD15–, CD30–, CD20+, CD45+). However, the malignant cells (R-S cells or L&H cells) in both types of Hodgkin lymphoma are scarce, most cells in the involved organ being reactive cells including lymphocytes, histiocytes, plasma cells, and eosinophils.[31]

Non-Hodgkin lymphomas comprise several entities which are first broadly classified as B-cell or T-cell processes, with each group being further subclassified as precursor cell or mature cell neoplasm. B-cell lymphomas constitute the vast majority of lymphomas in Western countries (>80%) and generally respond better to current chemotherapy than do T-cell lymphomas and therefore have a better prognosis.[11,24] The precursor cell diseases, which manifest with a blast morphology and high proliferation rate, are aggressive, but potentially curable with modern chemotherapy. Burkitt lymphoma, a tumor of mature B-cell origin, also grows very rapidly due to a specific chromosomal translocation resulting in an activated c-*myc* oncogene.

Mature B-cell lymphomas with large cells are aggressive and more proliferative, whereas those with small cells are generally indolent. There are, however, important exceptions. Mantle

Table 28.1 Significance of immunophenotypic markers commonly used in lymphoma/leukemia diagnosis

Antigen	Primary cellular distribution	Significance in lymphoma/leukemia diagnosis
CD1a	Thymocytes, immature T-cells	Expressed in precursor T-cell neoplasms
CD2	All T-cells, NK cells	May be lost in T-cell lymphoma
CD4	1. Helper T-cells 2. Monocytes (lower expression)	1. Coexpression with CD8 or absence of both CD4 and CD8 in precursor T-cell neoplasms 2. Acute monoblastic or monocytic leukemia and granulocytic sarcoma
CD3	All T-cells	Most specific for T-cell lineage Only cytoplasmic expression may be seen
CD5	All T-cells, some naïve B-cells	1. When expressed in B-cells, indicates either CLL or MCL 2. May be lost in T-cell lymphoma
CD7	All T-cells	1. Most commonly lost in T-cell lymphomas 2. Most commonly expressed in AML
CD10 (CALLA)	Follicular B-cells, hematogones	1. Expressed in precursor B-cell lymphoblastic lymphoma, Burkitts lymphoma, and follicular lymphoma 2. Expressed in AILD-type T-cell lymphoma
CD14	Monocytes	Acute myelomonocytic, monoblastic, and monocytic leukemia and granulocytic sarcoma
CD15	Monocytes, granulocytes	Reed–Sternberg (R-S) cells in classic Hodgkin lymphoma
CD20	B-cells	Loss on B-cells indicates precursor B-cells or plasma cells
CD23	Follicular dendritic cells	Used to differentiate CD5+ B-cell lymphomas: CLL, CD23+, and MCL, CD23–
CD30	Immunoblasts (B and T)	R-S cells in classic Hodgkin lymphoma, ALCL
CD34	Hematopoietic stem cells	Acute leukemias
CD38	Plasma cells, many other lymphoid cells	Expression on CLL/SLL cells is a poor prognostic indicator
CD45 (LCA)	Leukocytes	Absent in erythroid precursors, plasma cells, and R-S cells
CD56	NK cells, some T-cells	Abnormal plasma cells and monocytes
CD57	NK cells, T-cell subset	Increased in lymphocyte-predominant Hodgkin lymphoma
CD68	Histiocytes, monocytes	Some cases of acute monocytic leukemia
CD79a	B-cells (expressed before CD20), plasma cells	Precursor B-cell, mature B-cell, and plasma cell neoplasms
CD99	MIC2 gene product	25–80% lymphomas, especially precursor cell and T-cell lymphomas, Ewings sarcoma/PNET
CD117	Promyelocytes, mast cells	Acute promyelocytic leukemia, other acute myeloid leukemias
CD138	Plasma cells	Plasmacytoma, plasma cell myeloma
Alk-1	Not detected in normal cells	Anaplastic large cell lymphoma with t(2;5)
Bcl-2	Many lymphocytes, but *not* in reactive follicle centers	Expressed in follicle in follicular lymphoma
Bcl-6	Follicle center cells	Indicates origin from follicle center cells in DLBCL
Cyclin D1	Only cytoplasmic staining in normal lymphoid cells	Nuclear expression characteristic for MCL and some cases of plasma cell myeloma
EBNA2	EBV-infected cells	Endemic Burkitt, some Hodgkin lymphomas, nasal type NK/T-cell lymphoma
EBV-LMP	EBV-infected cells	Same as EBNA2
EMA	Epithelial tissue	'Popcorn' cells in lymphocyte-predominant Hodgkin lymphoma, ALCL
Ki-67 (MIB1)	Proliferating cells	Burkitt-like lymphoma and Burkitt lymphoma have >99% nuclear staining
MPO	Promyelocytes and more mature myeloid cells	Distinction between monocytic and myeloid type of granulocytic sarcoma
TdT	Thymocytes, immature T-, B-, and myeloid blasts	1. Distinction between Burkitt lymphoma (TdT–) and precursor B-cell lymphoblastic lymphoma (TdT+). 2. Distinction between peripheral T-cell and lymphoblastic lymphomas (TdT+)
TIA-1	Cytotoxic T-cells and NK cells	Lymphomas arising from these cells

AILD, angioimmunoblastic lymphadenopathy with dysproteinemia; ALCL, anaplastic large cell lymphoma; AML, acute myeloid leukemia; CLL, chronic lymphocytic leukemia; DLBCL, diffuse large B-cell lymphoma; EBV, Epstein–Barr virus; EBV-LMP, Epstein–Barr virus latent membrane protein; EMA, epithelial membrane antigen; MCL, mantle cell lymphoma; NK, natural killer; PNET, primitive neuroectodermal tumor; SLL, small lymphocytic lymphoma.

cell lymphoma (MCL) is a diffuse small cell lymphoma which superficially resembles the indolent B-cell small lymphocytic lymphoma (SLL), but responds poorly to therapy and has an aggressive course. This behavior is predicated on the specific cytogenetic abnormality, t(11;14), which causes overexpression of the cell cycle controlling enzyme, cyclin D1. Reactivity to cyclin D1 in the nuclei of the lymphoma cells provides a specific test for MCL.[42] Another fundamental concept to emerge in the past two decades is that of lymphomas arising from the mucosa-associated lymphoid tissue (MALT).[5] Interestingly, these so-called 'MALT lymphomas' can occur as a result of long-standing chronic inflammation and can affect virtually any organ, e.g., stomach, skin, conjunctiva, thyroid, lung, kidney, genital tract, etc.

The T-cells and natural killer (NK) cells are linked developmentally and biologically. Lymphomas arising from these two cell types have many similarities and are grouped together in the WHO classification. The clinical behavior of T/NK cell lymphomas, unlike B-cell lymphomas, lacks correlation with cell size (Table 28.2). Because the infiltrate in these lymphomas is often polymorphous and shows many histiocytes, it may be confused with reactive conditions or Hodgkin lymphoma. Specific immunophenotypes or cytogenetic abnormalities are usually not identified in T/NK cell lymphomas with the notable exception of anaplastic large T-cell lymphoma, which expresses CD30 and the protein product of the *Alk-1* gene due to a t(2;5)

cytogenetic abnormality.[38] Many T/NK cell lymphomas have characteristic extranodal involvement patterns which, together with other clinical features, form the basis of diagnosis in many cases.

Table 28.2 lists the salient diagnostic and clinical features of the more common non-Hodgkin lymphomas (NHL).

Incidence

Worldwide, the incidence of lymphoma has nearly doubled in the past three decades.[27] While the overall incidence of lymphomas is about 11.5 per 100 000 person years,[11] primary extranodal lymphomas constitute about a fifth to a third of these.[22] Primary ovarian lymphomas are rare, constituting only 0.1–0.2% of all lymphomas. Even in patients aged below 20 years, in whom epithelial ovarian tumors are uncommon, primary ovarian lymphoma still remains a relatively rare form of ovarian malignancy, estimated at about 0.6% of all ovarian tumors. A prominent exception occurs in areas with endemic Burkitt lymphoma, where it accounts for over half the ovarian tumors in young patients. Worldwide, ovarian involvement by disseminated lymphoma is much less rare.

Ovarian involvement by malignant lymphomas takes three forms:

1. Incidental involvement of ovaries in disseminated lymphoma: This is the most common form and is seen in

Table 28.2 Important clinicopathologic features of common lymphomas

Lymphoma	Immunophenotype	Cytogenetic abnormality	Clinical behavior
B-cell non-Hodgkins lymphomas			
Precursor B-cell lymphoblastic lymphoma/acute lymphoblastic leukemia	CD45+/–, CD19+, CD22+, CD20–/+, CD10+, TdT+/–, sIg–	Hyperdiploidy or other numeric t(9;22)	Aggressive, curable (80%) *Bad prognostic indicator*
Burkitt lymphoma/leukemia	CD45+/–, CD19+, CD22+, CD20+, CD10+, TdT–, sIg+	t(8;14) or less commonly t(2;14) or t(14;22)	Aggressive, curable (90%)
Follicular lymphoma	CD45+/–, CD19+, CD22+, CD20+, CD10+, TdT–, sIg+, bcl-2+, bcl-6+	t(14;18)	Indolent (grades 1 and 2), incurable *Moderately aggressive (grade 3), incurable*
Diffuse large B-cell lymphoma	CD45+/–, CD19+, CD22+, CD20+, CD10–/+, TdT–, sIg+, bcl-2–/+, bcl-6+/–		Aggressive, curable (50%)
Small cell lymphoma	Pan-B antigens+, CD5+, CD23+	Abnormal chromosomes 11,12, or 13	Indolent, incurable
Mantle cell lymphoma	Pan-B antigens+, CD5+, CD23–/+, cyclin D1+	t(11;14)	Moderately aggressive, bulky disease, incurable
Marginal zone lymphoma	Pan-B antigens+, CD5–, CD10–	t(11;18)	Localized; curable *Bad prognostic indicator*
T-cell lymphomas			
Precursor T-cell lymphoblastic lymphoma/acute lymphoblastic Leukemia	CD3–/+, CD5+, CD7+, CD1a+, TdT+	Involving chromosome 14q11 or 7p14 (T-cell receptor genes) in about 33%, not specific for the disease	Aggressive, curable (50%)
Peripheral T-cell lymphoma, NOS	CD3+, CD5+/–, CD7–/+, CD1a–, TdT–	Multiple abnormalities described, none is specific	Variable, incurable
Anaplastic large cell lymphoma	CD3+, CD5+/–, CD7–/+, CD1a–, TdT–, CD30+, ALK1+/–	t(2;5)	Good if t(2;5) present

about 20% patients with widespread lymphoma. Many B-cell lymphomas spread widely, whereas T-cell lymphomas frequently remain localized to a particular tissue (e.g., skin) until late in the course. B-cell lymphomas are much more common than T-cell lymphomas in the Western world. Both factors contribute to most ovarian lymphomas being of B-cell type.[26] Occasionally there may be bilateral ovarian enlargement due to massive edema secondary to vascular compromise occurring in patients with retroperitoneal lymphoma.[6]

2. Presentation as an ovarian mass in patients with undisclosed disseminated lymphoma, occurring in 0.3% of patients with lymphoma: Most of these patients also have occult nodal involvement, and overt generalized disease usually develops within a short time. Indeed it has been suggested that all primary ovarian lymphomas should be treated as a local manifestation of systemic disease.[10] Diffuse large B-cell lymphoma and follicular lymphoma constitute the most common NHLs in the Western world and ovarian involvement occurs more commonly than with other forms. The non-endemic form of Burkitt lymphoma is primarily an abdominal disease and involves the ovaries in a disproportionately large number of cases.

3. Ovarian lymphoma as a primary extranodal lymphoma: This diagnosis requires staging and follow-up studies showing no evidence of any systemic disease. Although many are skeptical about this entity given the lack of a normal B-lymphocyte population in the ovaries,[37] rare but well-documented reports support the existence of primary ovarian lymphoma.[7,16,17] A case of a collision tumor with a proliferating serous ovarian cystadenoma[35] and primary ovarian lymphoma in an HIV-positive patient has been described.[23] The definition of primary and secondary ovarian lymphoma also revolves around the staging system used and the stage assigned to bilateral ovarian involvement.[21,40] Some investigators have considered any involvement of non-ovarian structures, even when contiguous with the involved ovary, as evidence of secondary involvement of ovary while others consider these as primary ovarian lymphomas. This is more fully discussed in the section on staging of ovarian lymphomas.

Clinical features

The ages at which malignant lymphomas initially manifest in the ovaries parallel those of patients with equivalent nodal disease.[11] Variations relate more to histologic type than to the anatomic site affected. Diffuse large B-cell lymphoma is most common in the 35–45 years age group while follicular lymphoma and small lymphocytic lymphoma are more often found in older women. Although endemic Burkitt lymphoma typically affects children in the 5–10 years age group, ovaries in adult patients can be involved as well.[20] The sporadic variant usually occurs in young adults, occasionally complicating pregnancy.[25,29]

Presentation is similar to that of other ovarian tumors, namely an abdominal or pelvic mass, often accompanied by pain which is sometimes severe.[41] Ascites occasionally occurs. Less commonly, the tumors are incidental findings at routine pelvic examination or surgery for other indications. In patients

with apparent gonadal disease only, staging procedures reveal more advanced disease (FIGO stages 2–4) in half of cases, for which reason systemic therapy is routinely recommended. While some patients enjoyed long survival after surgery alone,[30] before the advent of modern chemotherapy, the outcome of ovarian lymphoma treated with radical surgery was usually dismal, and only limited success occurred in cases treated with radiotherapy following surgery.[32] Localized ovarian lymphomas treated with modern combination chemotherapy have a favorable prognosis, with 75% experiencing long-term survival.[26] It appears that the failure-free survival in ovarian NHL treated with chemotherapy is similar to that of nodal NHL.[8] In cases of systemic lymphoma involving the ovary, survival is influenced by the type of lymphoma and possibly also by the other accepted prognostic factors including age, tumor stage, number of extranodal sites, performance status, and serum lactate dehydrogenase (LDH) levels. Aggressive chemotherapy now achieves cures in numerous cases in precursor B-cell and T-cell lymphomas, Burkitts lymphoma, diffuse large B-cell lymphoma (DLBCL), and anaplastic large cell lymphoma (ALCL). It is still relatively ineffective with small lymphocytic lymphoma (SLL), follicular lymphoma (FCL), and mantle cell lymphoma (MCL); myeloablative and non-myeloablative stem cell transplantation have shown some success in MCL. Patients with primary ovarian lymphoma have shown a good prognosis in some studies,[41] while others report prognosis similar to nodal lymphomas of the same type.[8]

Staging

A staging system for a group of tumors is clinically most useful if it can accurately assess the anatomic extent of disease that allows uniform reporting of treatment results and pooling of data from various institutions. The Ann Arbor staging system of Hodgkins lymphoma was introduced in 1971 and in 1973 was adopted as the principal staging system for most non-Hodgkins lymphomas (Table 28.3). In a disease like Hodgkins lymphoma, which has a tendency to spread by continuity and contiguity, this system was particularly suitable. However, with the rare exception of marginal zone lymphoma of MALT type, most non-Hodgkins lymphomas spread by bloodstream or

Table 28.3 Ann Arbor staging systems with designations appropriate for involvement of the female genital tract

Stage	Definition
I	Involvement of a single lymph node region (I) or of a single extralymphatic organ or site (IE)
II	Involvement of two or more lymph node regions on the same side of the diaphragm (II) or localized involvement of an extralymphatic organ site and of one or more lymph node regions on the same side of the diaphragm (IIE)
III	Involvement of lymph node regions on both sides of the diaphragm (III), which may also be accompanied by localized involvement of the spleen (IIS), extralymphatic site (IIIE) or both (IIISE)
IV	Diffuse or disseminated involvement of one or more extralymphatic organs or tissues with or without associated lymph node enlargement

lymphatics and the Ann Arbor system has proved less accurate in predicting prognostic groups. Thus, an international prognostic index (IPI) has been developed to take into account the patient's age, stage (Ann Arbor system), number of extranodal sites involved, performance status, and serum LDH level. The IPI appears to provide more accurate prognostic information for lymphomas than staging alone. With the advent of antibody-based therapies, a revised index has been proposed.[33] Whether this is applicable to primary extranodal lymphomas is not clear.

The International Federation of Gynecology and Obstetrics (FIGO) has developed staging systems for malignant tumors of various female reproductive organs (see Appendix A). In its most simple form, stage 1 restricts the tumor to the lining and deeper tissue of the involved organ (including bilateral ovarian involvement), stage 2 with spread by contiguity or immediately adjacent to contiguous tissues, stage 3 with involved regional lymph nodes or for ovary with peritoneal involvement, and stage 4 with distant metastasis. While many studies on genital tract lymphoma have used this schema, many have found the Ann Arbor system[8,10,26] to be more satisfactory. Some studies have not used any staging information.[41]

The relative lack of consistency in staging ovarian lymphomas has previously been a subject of some discussion.[40] Only rare studies have directly compared the two staging systems,[10,13] finding that the Ann Arbor system is prognostically more sensitive. This apparent insensitivity of the FIGO system may in part stem from reports that inadequately subclassify each stage.[30] An additional reason may relate to the biology of these tumors. Ovarian lymphomas tend to show bilateral involvement and extensive peritoneal involvement more frequently than involvement of supradiaphragmatic lymph nodes.[8] In a study where both FIGO and Ann Arbor stage are recorded,[10] there are many Ann Arbor stage II and IV patients, but none with stage III disease. Of note, bilateral ovarian disease or even microscopic peritoneal seeding would be assigned stage IV in the Ann Arbor system, while these would not affect the main stage in the FIGO system. Previous studies have found that unilateral ovarian disease has a better prognosis regardless of stage,[10,30] but the FIGO system does not stratify patients according to this parameter. On the other hand, the FIGO system records the local extent of disease in the other female genital organs more accurately than the Ann Arbor system. We believe lymphomas of the female genital tract merit staging by both systems.

Pathology

Lymphomas presenting as ovarian disease are bilateral in half of cases, regardless of stage. Burkitt lymphoma is almost always bilateral (Figure 28.1). The ovarian tumors vary greatly in size, with most measuring 8–15 cm in diameter. Ovaries incidentally involved by disseminated lymphoma may be of normal size or only slightly enlarged. The ovaries are usually free of adhesions and show a nodular or bosselated surface. The cut surface is uniformly pale or gray-white to tan with a rubbery or fleshy consistency. Interaction of the infiltrating cells with ovarian stroma may obscure the typical 'fish-flesh' appearance seen in involved lymph nodes. Gross edema, small foci of necrosis, cystic degeneration, and hemorrhage may all be present in the cut surface (Figure 28.2), but rarely are conspicuous features. Although the ovaries seem preferentially infiltrated relative to the remainder of the female genital tract,

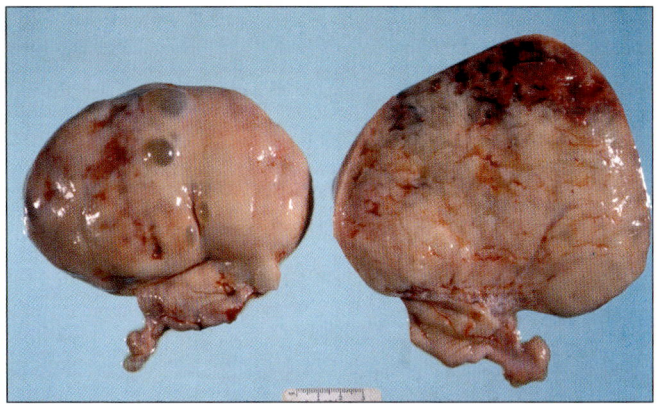

Fig. 28.1 Burkitt lymphoma presenting as bilateral ovarian masses in a 16-year-old girl. The external surfaces (left side) are smooth without adhesions. The cut surface (right side) shows fleshy tumor with focal degenerative changes and hemorrhage.

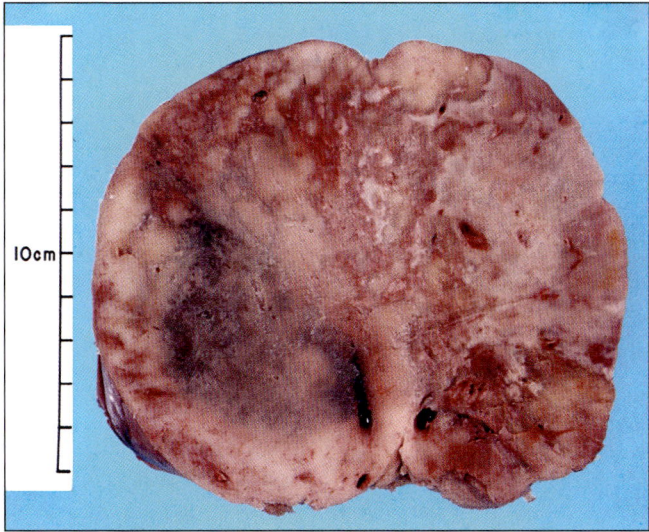

Fig. 28.2 Ovarian lymphoma. The interaction of the ovarian stroma with the tumor may obscure the typical fish-flesh appearance seen in lymph nodes involved by lymphoma. Degenerative and cystic changes and hemorrhage are not uncommon in aggressive lymphomas such as diffuse large B-cell lymphoma.

other organs, especially the adjacent fallopian tubes, may also appear swollen and edematous owing to peritoneal or interstitial infiltration.

A careful morphologic assessment of 4–5 μm H&E sections are necessary to formulate a short differential diagnosis (Figure 28.3), even though the final diagnosis almost always requires ancillary studies (Figure 28.4). The sections should be examined initially at low power, with the illumination turned down, to assess if the lymphomatous infiltrate is diffuse (Figure 28.3A), sometimes with a 'starry-sky' pattern produced by large macrophages interspersed amongst small uniform lymphoma cells (Figure 28.3B), or nodular (Figure 28.5B1). The nodularity of the infiltrate may be focal or quite subtle. Presence or absence of fibrosis, necrosis, tingible body macrophages (histiocytes containing nuclear and cellular debris) (Figure

28.3C, arrows), granulomas, and variation in cell morphology should also be noted. The size of the lymphoma cells is assessed at high (40–50×) magnification. All cells smaller than or equal to a histiocyte (or endothelial cell) nucleus are defined as 'small' (Figure 28.3D) and those larger than the histiocyte nucleus are defined as 'large' (Figure 28.3E). In Burkitt lymphoma, the cells are usually medium in size (Figure 28.3C, arrows). In small cells, the nucleus can be round with condensed chromatin (in small lymphocytic lymphoma or chronic lymphocytic leukemia) resembling small lymphocytes seen in peripheral blood, or round with open chromatin and small nucleoli (in lymphoblastic and Burkitt or Burkitt-like lymphomas) (Figure 28.3D), or irregularly oval, cleaved or crinkled like a raisin with moderately condensed chromatin (in follicular lymphoma and

mantle cell lymphoma) (Figure 28.3F). Large cell nuclei may have prominent central nucleoli (immunoblastic DLBCL), smaller nucleoli (centroblastic DLBCL) (Figure 28.3G) or may be anaplastic (Figure 28.3E). The presence of Reed–Sternberg cells (Figure 28.5F1) or mononuclear variants of these cells should be noted.

The infiltrate of diffuse lymphoma often forms cords, sometimes only one cell thick. The malignant cells may infiltrate and surround structures, e.g., pre-existing follicles, corpora lutea and corpora albicantes, without destroying them. The tumor cells also invade blood vessel walls in this way. Follicular lymphoma and some cases of DLBCL may demonstrate bands of fibrous tissue or even dense sclerotic areas. Microscopic focal necrosis may be found in addition to those foci evident mac-

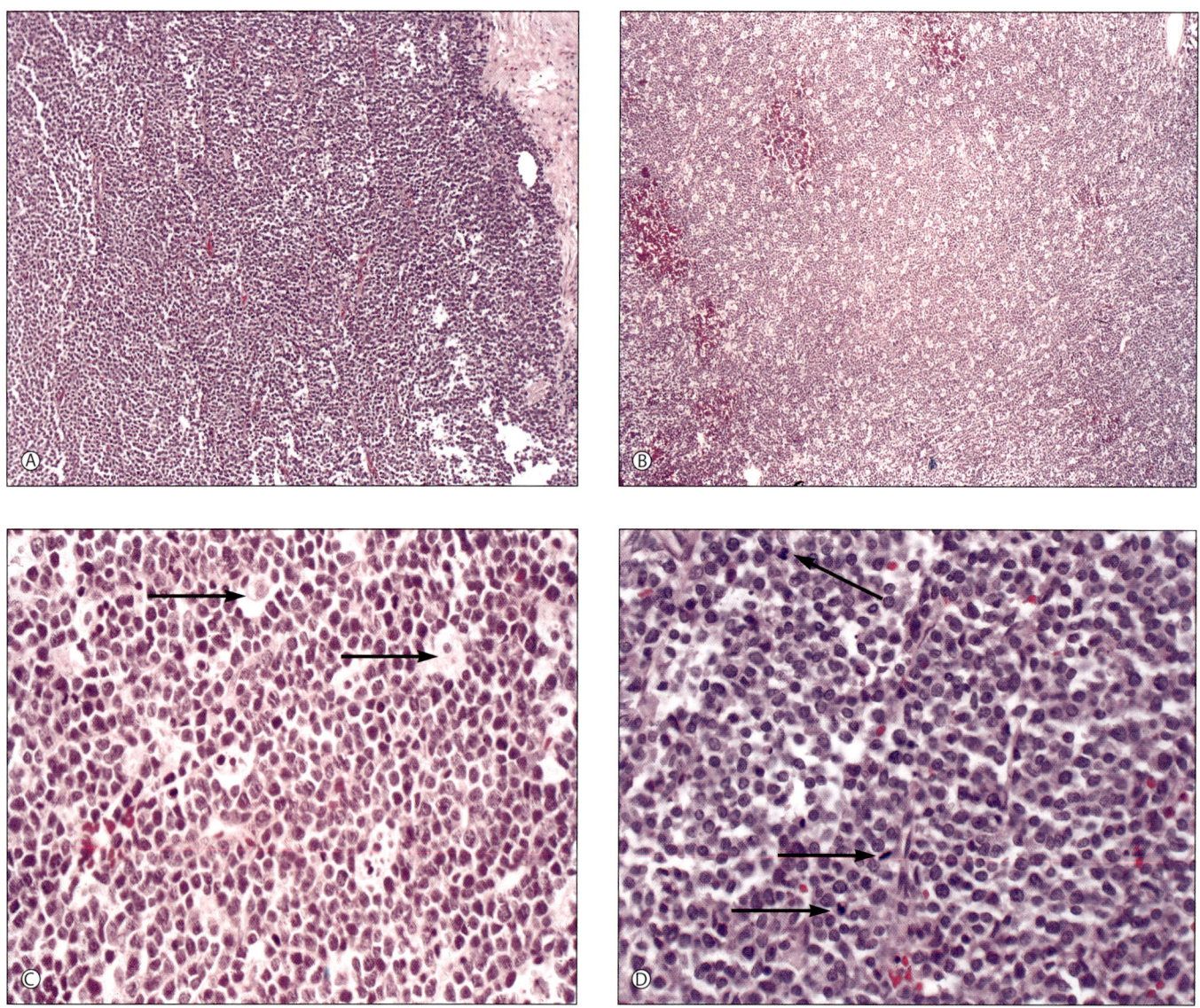

Fig. 28.3 General histologic characteristics of lymphomas with H&E staining. **(A)** Low power magnification shows a diffuse pattern of involvement (100×) (contrast with the follicular or nodular involvement in Figure 28.5B). **(B)** Starry-sky pattern of *Burkitts lymphoma* (40×). **(C)** At higher magnification the uniform cells of *Burkitt lymphoma* are about the same size as the nuclei of histiocytes (arrows). The latter contain cellular debris in their cytoplasm and are referred to as 'tingible body macrophages'. The lymphoma cells have round nuclei with fine chromatin and small nucleoli (400×). **(D)** *Lymphoblastic lymphoma* consists of small cells with a high nuclear:cytoplasmic ratio, fine chromatin, and small nucleoli. Mitoses are present (arrows) (400×).

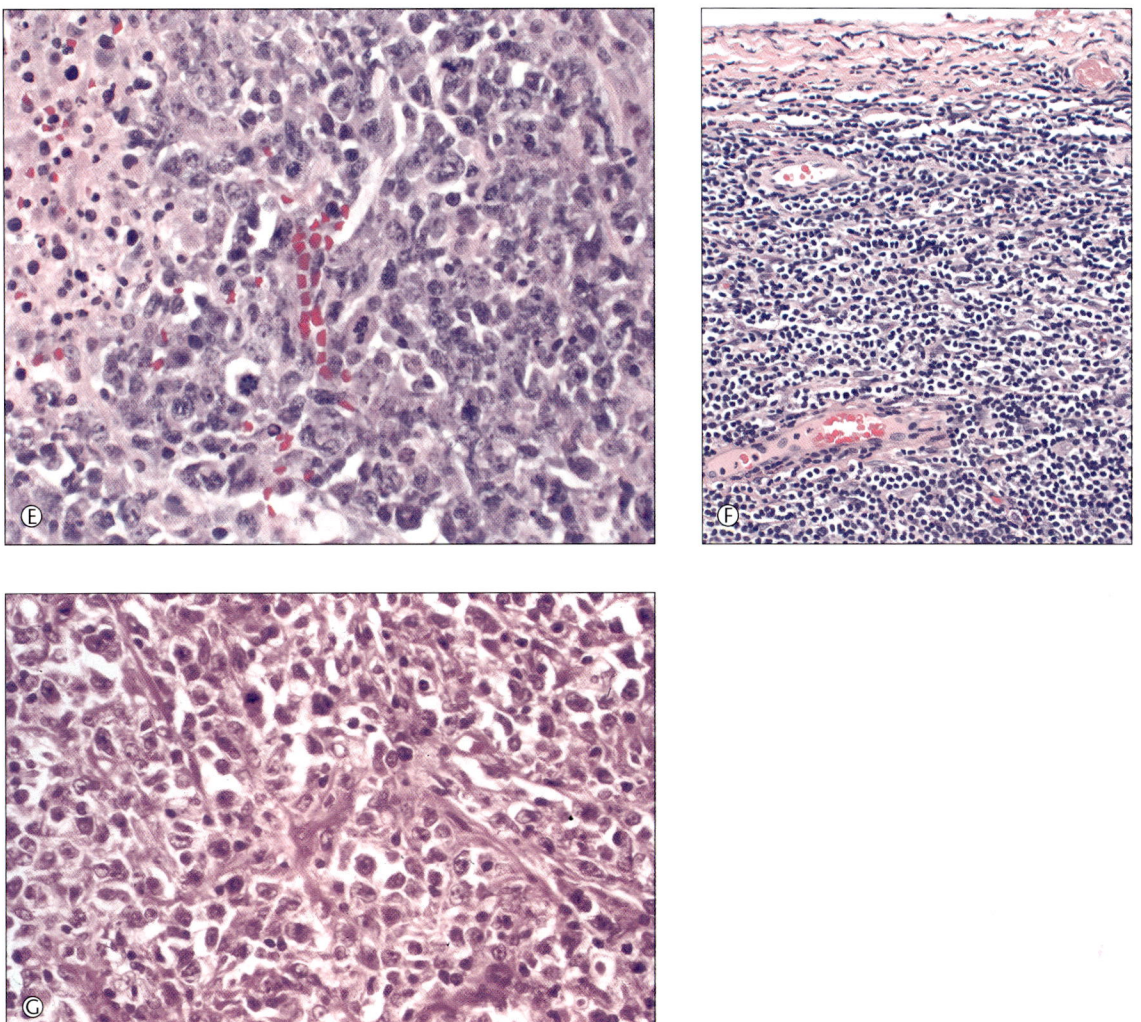

Fig. 28.3, Continued **(E)** The cells and their nuclei in *large cell lymphoma* vary moderately in size and shape. Nucleoli are variably prominent. Necrosis with acute inflammatory infiltrate is seen in upper left corner. This proved to be a T-cell lymphoma (see Figure 28.4C) (400×). **(F)** A low-grade *follicular lymphoma* with oval, cleaved nuclei with condensed chromatin. Note that follicular lymphoma involving ovary may lack a follicular pattern (200×). **(G)** So-called centroblastic morphology of *diffuse large B-cell lymphoma* (DLBCL). The biologic significance of the various morphologic subtypes of DLBCL is uncertain (400×).

roscopically. In high-grade tumors with rapid cell turnover, e.g., DLBCL, lymphoblastic and especially Burkitt lymphoma, a starry-sky appearance is typical (Figure 28.3B).

When microscopic examination suggests a diagnosis of lymphoma, the following immunohistochemical panel should be performed, starting with the screening panel. In a large cell lymphoma, identifying the lymphoma as a B-cell (CD20+) process may be sufficient. Small cell lymphomas, on the other hand, usually require additional workup for accurate classification. For prognostic purposes, additional immunostains may be performed in DLBCL, in which some experience is required to properly interpret the results.

1. Screening panel: CD45, CD20, CD3, cytokeratin.
2. Small B-cell lymphomas (CD20+): CD5, CD10, cyclin D1, CD23, bcl-2, bcl-6.
3. Blasts or DLBCLs: CD10, CD79a, cyclin D1, bcl-6, Ki-67, TdT, EBV-LMP, EBNA2.
4. T-cell neoplasms (usually CD3+): CD1a, CD2, CD5, CD7, TdT, CD30, Alk-1, TIA-1.
5. Hodgkins lymphoma: CD15, CD30, CD57, EMA.
6. Leukemic infiltration (CD45+, CD3−, CD20−): CD4, CD34, CD68, CD117, MPO.

Nearly all primary lymphomas (80–95%) of the ovary are B-cell neoplasms[8,26,41] and, as such, are reactive for the pan-B cell antigen, CD20 (Figure 28.4A). Staining for CD10 (Figure 28.4B) and CD5 is helpful in determining the further classification of small B-cell lymphomas. When a lesion suspected to be a lymphoma is not reactive for CD20, four possibilities should be considered: (1) a T-cell lymphoma; (2) a granulocytic sarcoma; (3) a precursor B-cell neoplasm such as precursor B-cell lymphoblastic leukemia/lymphoma; or (4) the patient has previously received treatment with anti-CD20 antibody. CD20 may be undetectable for several months following such therapy on normal as well as abnormal (lymphoma) B-cells.[34] In such

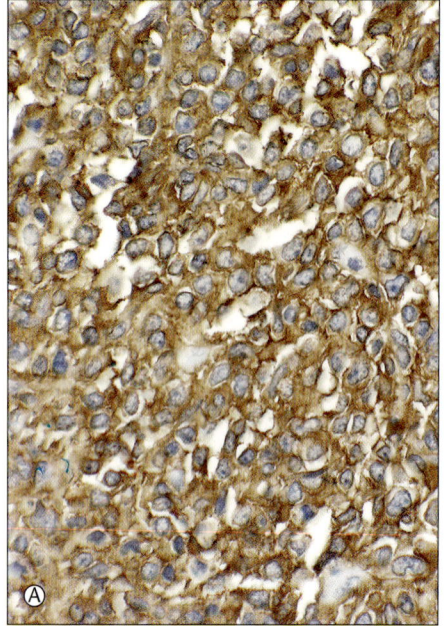

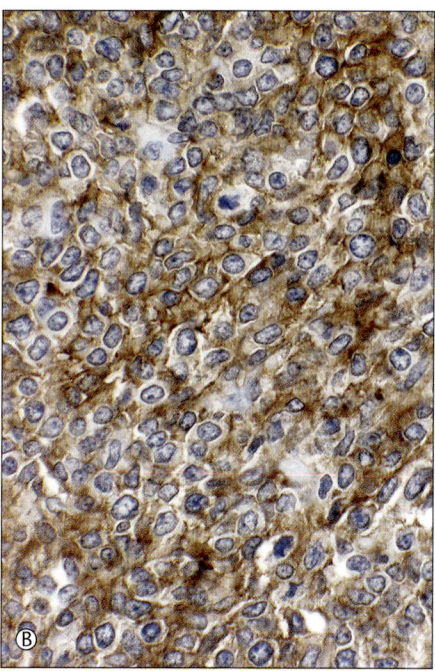

Fig. 28.4 Some typical immunohistochemical staining patterns of lymphomas. **(A)** CD20 reactivity in lymphoblastic lymphoma. **(B)** CD10 reactivity in the same tumor is reactive for CD10. Follicular lymphomas and some large cell lymphomas are also reactive for CD10 and the cell morphology is used to make the correct diagnosis. Additional immunostains such as TdT may also be employed. **(C)** CD3 reactivity in the large cell lymphoma of Figure 28.3E. **(D)** The same tumor shows a loss of a pan-T-cell marker, CD5. The small reactive T-cells on the right are reactive for CD5. Such reactivity is useful as internal quality control (all 400×).

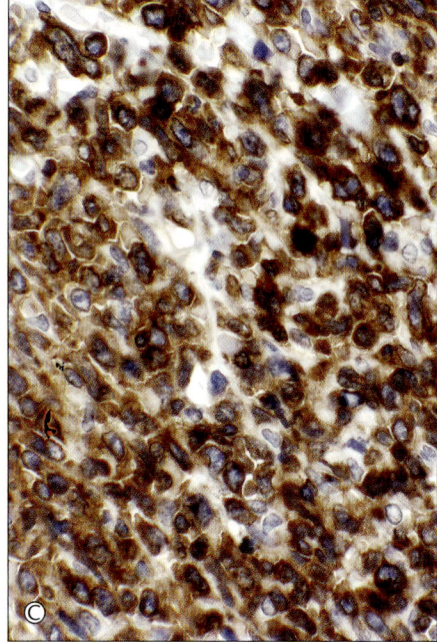

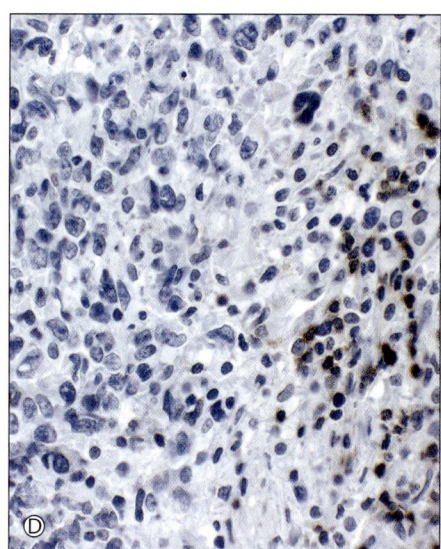

cases, other B-cell markers like CD79a or PAX5 may be useful. The existence of a T-cell lymphoma is evident when the cells are reactive for CD3 (Figure 28.4C). However, many T-cell lymphomas show loss of one or more pan-T-cell antigens, CD2, CD5 (Figure 28.4D) or CD7, and some may not express CD3 itself. Anaplastic T-cell lymphomas, which are typically reactive for CD30, may not express many of the T-cell antigens, and even the common leukocyte antigen CD45 is usually not expressed. To confuse the issue further, these cells may express the epithelial membrane antigen (EMA), suggesting the possibility of a carcinoma. Cytokeratin is not expressed by these cells, however. The lymphomas encountered most often in the ovary are diffuse large B-cell lymphoma (Figure 28.3G)

and Burkitts lymphoma (Figure 28.3C), each type being reported at a frequency of 30–65% of all ovarian lymphomas in various series.[8,10,26,30,41]

The proportion of these two tumors reflects the age of the patient population in the study: Burkitt lymphoma is common in patients under 20 years of age and diffuse large B-cell lymphoma in older patients.[30] Ovarian follicular lymphomas (Figures 28.3F and 28.5B1) constitute about 15% of ovarian lymphomas, can be associated with significant diffuse areas (containing either small cleaved cells or large cells; Figure 28.3F), and occur almost exclusively in older patients.[4,10,26,30] Lymphoblastic lymphoma (usually of T-cell origin, but also of B-cell origin; Figures 28.3D and 28.4A) occurs in younger

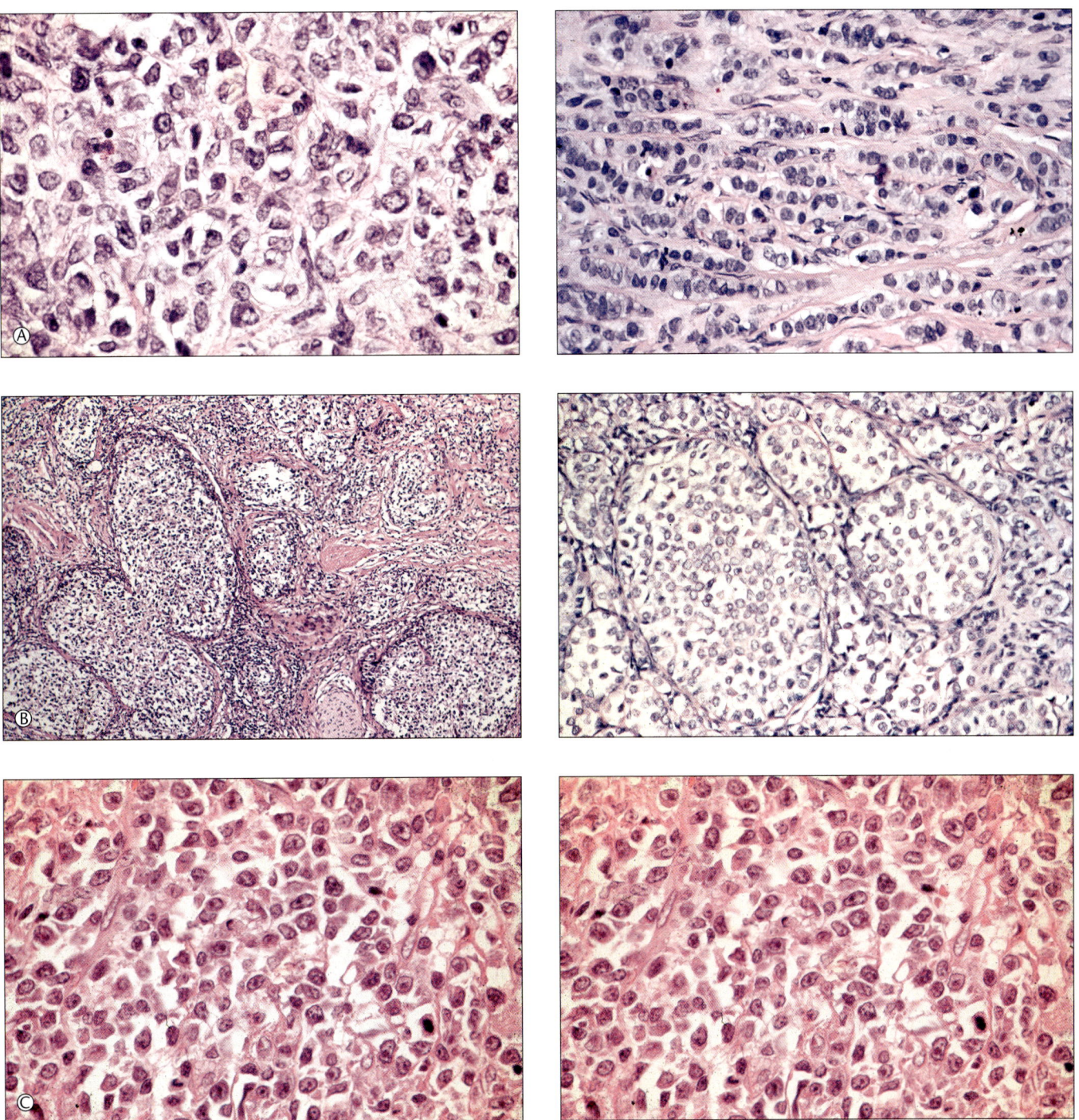

Fig. 28.5 Differential diagnosis of ovarian lymphoma. **(A)** Indian file pattern: (A1) Diffuse large B-cell lymphoma: the lymphoma cells may infiltrate ovarian stroma in a cord-like fashion. (A2) Metastatic lobular carcinoma of breast showing 'Indian file' arrangement of malignant cells. **(B)** Nodules: (B1) Follicular lymphoma, grade 3: large cells in nodules separated by variable amount of stroma. (B2) Metastatic breast carcinoma with solid nests of cells resembles the back-to-back arrangement of follicles in follicular lymphoma. **(C)** Prominent nucleoli: (C1) Diffuse large B-cell lymphoma: the cells in the immunoblastic variant of this lymphoma have a single prominent nucleolus dysgerminoma. (C2) Cytologic features mimic lymphoma.

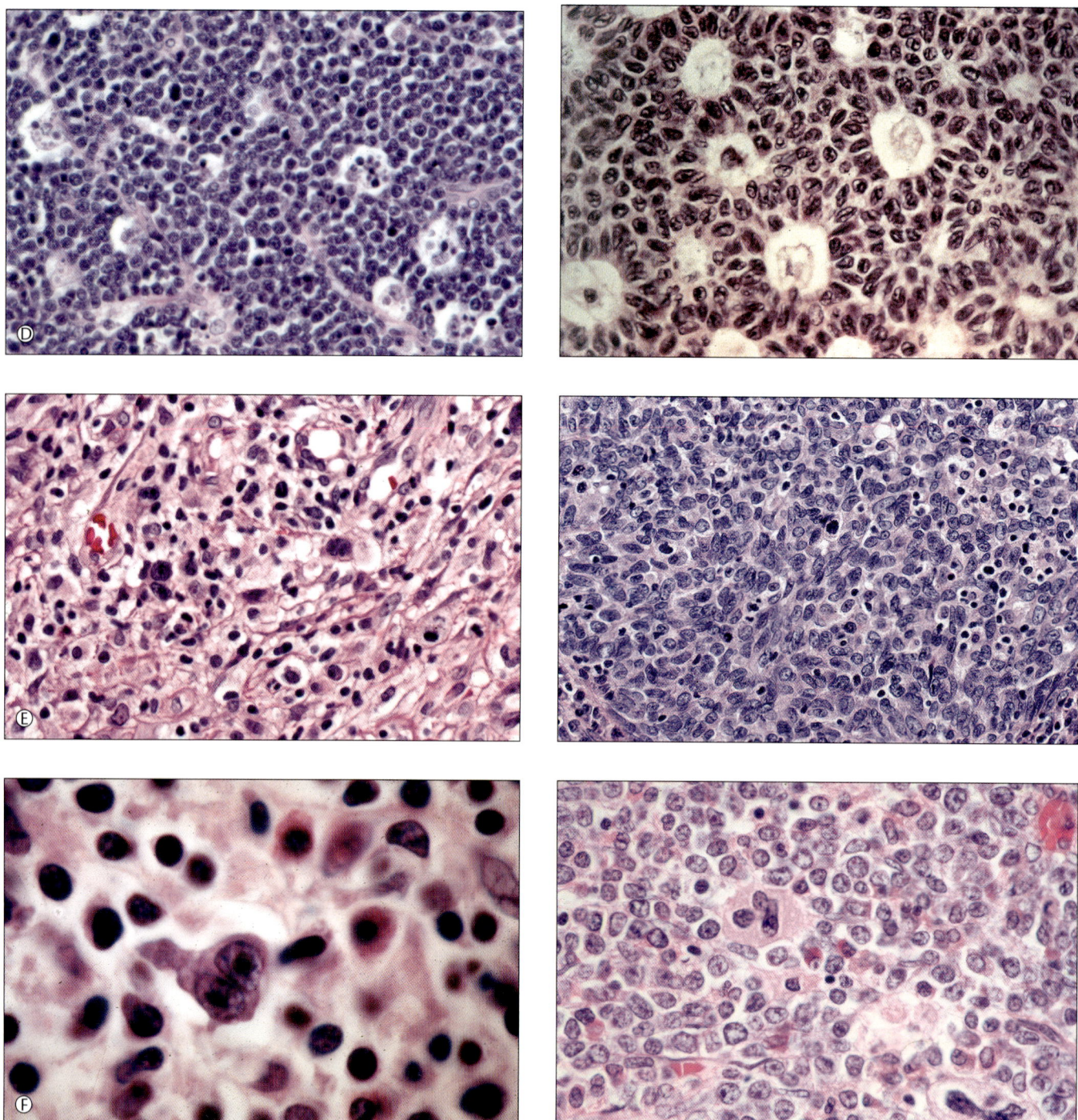

Fig. 28.5, Continued **(D)** Starry-sky pattern Burkitts lymphoma: (D1) The tingible body macrophages produce clear spaces in a background of small blue cells. (D2) Granulosa cell tumor: the Call–Exner bodies produce a starry-sky pattern in this tumor. **(E)** Anaplasia: (E1) Anaplastic large cell lymphoma: large atypical cells with abnormally shaped nuclei and variation in nuclear size. The lack of lymphoid markers, including CD45, makes diagnosis difficult. These tumors are typically CD30+. (E2) Anaplastic carcinoma: the sheet-like arrangement of large abnormal cells resembles anaplastic large cell lymphoma. Immunohistochemical staining is required for diagnosis. **(F)** Reed–Sternberg cell: (F1) Hodgkins lymphoma with Reed–Sternberg cell. The cells show reactivity for CD15 and CD30. Note also the reactive background containing lymphocytes, plasma cells, eosinophils, and histiocytes. (F2) Granulocytic sarcoma (extramedullary myeloid leukemia) with megakaryocyte: most of the background cells have the morphology of immature blasts. However, eosinophilic metamyelocytes are characteristically present.

patients, even infants.[18,39] Other T-cell lymphomas are rarely seen and include anaplastic large cell lymphoma (Figure 28.5E1) or peripheral T-cell lymphoma, not otherwise specified (Figure 28.3E).[41] T-cell lymphomas appear to occur more frequently in east Asia,[28] mirroring the relatively higher frequency of these neoplasms in this region. Primary Hodgkins lymphoma (Figure 28.5F1) is not unknown, being reported mostly as case reports and in some larger series as well.[32] Multiple myeloma has been observed to involve ovaries at autopsy and even primary plasmacytoma of the ovary has been reported.[9]

Differential diagnosis

The key to diagnosing lymphoma in the ovary is to suspect it! Fortunately, many ancillary studies are now available to confirm the diagnosis and subtype the lymphoma/leukemia.

Leukemias may present macroscopic and microscopic features indistinguishable from those of lymphomas. The histologic and immunohistochemical properties of myeloid leukemias are discussed in the next section. The distinction between lymphoid leukemias and lymphomas is often arbitrary, as many of these conditions can present either as mass lesions (lymphoma) or as lymphocytosis and bone marrow involvement (leukemia). CD45 is generally reactive in most leukemias as well as in lymphomas. Plasma cell neoplasms (plasmacytomas), some acute lymphoblastic leukemias, and anaplastic large cell lymphomas are usually negative for CD45. CD138 is positive in plasma cell neoplasms and CD30 in anaplastic large cell lymphomas. In cases of acute lymphoblastic leukemia other B-cell and T-cell markers known to be expressed in immature cells must be used. For B-cells CD79a and for T-cells CD7, CD2, and CD1a are useful, while TdT (terminal deoxynucleotidyl transferase) staining may be present in either type. Imprints from fresh tumor tissue stained by a Romanowsky technique can facilitate the identification of any cytoplasmic granulation in myeloid leukemic cells as well as the characteristic cytoplasmic vacuoles in Burkitts lymphoma. Eosinophilic metamyelocytes can usually be identified easily on H&E-stained sections or touch preparations and are a clue to the myeloid nature of the infiltrate. Similarly, megakaryocytes (Figure 28.5F2) may sometimes be present in these infiltrates.

The non-hemopoietic tumors most commonly confused with lymphomas are granulosa cell tumors and dysgerminomas; others are metastatic carcinomas and primary undifferentiated small cell carcinomas. In children, embryonal rhabdomyosarcoma and neuroblastoma remain possibilities.

Granulosa cell tumor (see Chapter 26) occurs over a wide age range, but many patients also exhibit clinical or pathologic evidence of endocrine dysfunction such as abnormal uterine bleeding or endometrial hyperplasia. The tumors are rarely bilateral (5%) and are often hemorrhagic with prominent cystic areas, features unusual in lymphoma. Although the diffuse or sarcomatoid variants of granulosa cell tumor may closely resemble ovarian lymphoma, some sections will almost always reveal other more specific patterns, e.g., follicular and trabecular. Call–Exner bodies should not be confused with the starry-sky pattern of Burkitts and some other lymphomas (Figure 28.5D2). Nuclear clefts occur in both tumors, but deep longitudinal grooves are found only in granulosa cell tumor. Nucleoli are not prominent and the mitotic rate is usually low. The relevant immunoprofile of granulosa cell tumor includes non-

Table 28.4 Lymphoma versus granulosa cell tumor: differential diagnosis

Lymphoma	Granulosa cell tumor
Clinical profile	
50% bilateral	5% bilateral
No endocrine function	Often estrogenic
Usually rapidly progressive	Indolent course
Microscopic features	
Nuclei pleomorphic, sometimes clefted	Nuclei bland, uniform; deep groove in half the cases
Nucleoli often prominent	Nucleoli inconspicuous
Mitoses variable, but usually conspicuous	Mitoses variable but usually infrequent
Starry-sky pattern in some cases	Call–Exner bodies sometimes present
Immunophenotype	
Reactivity for CD45 and B- or T-cell markers	Non-reactive for CD45, reactive for vimentin and inhibin

reactivity for CD45 and reactivity for vimentin, calretinin, and inhibin. Electron microscopy can also readily distinguish granulosa cell tumor from lymphoma but is rarely used (Table 28.4).

Dysgerminoma (see Chapter 27) is unusual in patients older than 30 years and is uncommonly bilateral (14%). Although it exhibits a diffuse pattern as in lymphomas, fine septa will contain mature lymphocytes and plasma cells (Figure 28.5C2) and, sometimes, small epithelioid granulomas. Dysgerminoma cells are large and have distinct cell membranes; the nuclei are central, large, and vesicular with a prominent central nucleolus and a moderate amount of clear cytoplasm containing periodic acid-Schiff (PAS) positive material (glycogen). The nuclei in dysgerminoma are not convoluted. Dysgerminoma may resemble immunoblastic lymphomas, but the latter demonstrate poor cellular cohesion, nuclei that are often eccentric, and strongly pyroninophilic cytoplasm. Dysgerminoma cells are non-reactive for CD45 and reactive for placental alkaline phosphatase (Table 28.5).

Metastatic carcinomas (see Chapter 29) are found most often in middle-aged or older women, and sometimes in the absence of a history of carcinoma elsewhere. They are frequently bilateral. Metastatic tumors are often composed of multiple nodules rather than a diffuse infiltration, and central necrotic foci are frequently found. Metastatic poorly differentiated carcinoma (especially mammary) may be arranged in sheets or cords (Figure 28.5A2), as in lymphoma, but a desmoplastic stromal reaction favors the former diagnosis. Metastasis of lobular carcinoma of the breast may superficially resemble a high-grade follicular lymphoma (Figure 28.5B2). The cells in lobular carcinoma are more monotonous and show fine chromatin and inconspicuous nucleoli. Infiltrating carcinomas destroy and obliterate pre-existing structures, whereas these are often preserved in lymphomas. Carcinoma cells are usually more cohesive than those of lymphoma and a small amount of

Table 28.5 Lymphoma versus dysgerminoma: differential diagnosis

Lymphoma	Dysgerminoma
Clinical profile	
50% bilateral	10% bilateral (plus 5% microscopic)
Most >35 years	Most <35 years
Microscopic features	
Nuclei pleomorphic, sometimes clefted	Nuclei regular, round to oval
Cells non-cohesive	Cell borders distinct
Cytoplasm scanty, sometimes basophilic	Cytoplasm moderate, poorly stained with H&E, but PAS positive
Immunophenotype	
Reactive for CD45	Non-reactive for CD45, reactive for placental alkaline phosphatase

Table 28.6 Lymphoma versus metastatic carcinoma: differential diagnosis

Lymphoma	Metastatic carcinoma
Macroscopic features	
Single mass	Multiple nodules
Fleshy or rubbery texture	Granular and friable
Necrosis inconspicuous	Necrosis common
Microscopic features	
Cytoplasm usually scanty, sometimes basophilic	Cytoplasm moderate amount, often acidophilic
Fibrous septa sometimes	Desmoplasia frequent
Reticulin sparse or around single cells	Reticulin around cell groups
Occasional necrotic cells	Obvious necrotic foci
Immunoprofile	
Reactive for CD45, non-reactive for EMA	Non-reactive for CD45, reactive for EMA and cytokeratin

EMA, epithelial membrane antigen.

mucin may be demonstrable either in the cytoplasm or in the rare acini. Reticulin stains demonstrate fibers around groups of cells, whereas in lymphomas, reticulin fibers are either present around individual cells or are sparse throughout. Carcinoma cells are reactive for cytokeratins and non-reactive for CD45 (Table 28.6).

Metastatic undifferentiated small cell carcinoma of pulmonary or other origin rarely presents as a clinical diagnostic problem but can simulate lymphomas histologically (Figure 28.5E2), with their diffuse pattern of small cells displaying scanty cytoplasm and dense hyperchromatic nuclei with a high mitotic rate. Necrosis is more conspicuous than in lymphoma and includes the characteristic zones of smudgy hematoxylino-

philic debris. The cytoplasm is often reactive for neuron-specific enolase and electron microscopy often shows neuro-secretory granules.

Primary small cell carcinoma of 'hypercalcemic type' (see Chapter 25) occurs in young women (mean age 22 years). All reported cases have been unilateral. Their growth pattern is diffuse, insular or trabecular. The closely packed cells have scanty cytoplasm and small round to oval nuclei with solitary nucleoli. There is usually prominent necrosis and a high mitotic rate that exceeds that usually associated with lymphomas. Tumor cells are non-reactive for CD45 and EMA.

LEUKEMIA

Leukemias are broadly classified as lymphoid and non-lymphoid (i.e., myeloid) with acute and chronic subtypes in each category. Lymphoid leukemias usually have a counterpart in a lymphoma, and the two entities are considered to be the same disease presenting primarily as a disseminated involvement of blood and bone marrow (leukemia) or localized disease presenting as a tumor mass (lymphoma). Thus chronic lymphocytic leukemia (CLL) and small lymphocytic lymphoma (SLL) are the same disease and are designated as CLL/SLL in the WHO classification. When acute myeloid leukemias present as solitary masses, these are called granulocytic sarcomas or chloromas (because of their greenish hue) and can pose a diagnostic challenge. The cells in these tumors, particularly those with monocytoid differentiation, closely resemble a diffuse large cell lymphoma. Judicious use of immunohistochemical stains is necessary for correct interpretation of these lesions.

The WHO classification[19] of acute myeloid leukemias differs from the French–American–British (FAB) classification in that certain recurrent cytogenetic abnormalities, namely t(15;17), inv(16), t(8;21) and those involving 11q23 are used to define distinct subtypes as they appear to determine prognosis in these conditions. In addition, most other subtypes identified on the basis of morphology of the leukemic blasts (designated as M0 through M7 in the FAB classification) are also retained, albeit with more descriptive names such as acute myeloid leukemia, minimally differentiated or acute monoblastic leukemia, etc. The WHO classification also emphasizes the adverse prognostic implications of acute leukemia arising from a myelodysplastic syndrome or from a chronic myeloproliferative condition (chronic myelogenous leukemia, CML and others) or following chemotherapy for another malignancy.

Ovarian infiltration occurs more commonly in patients with leukemias than with lymphomas and is seen more often in children than in adults. Ovarian infiltrates have been detected in two-thirds of leukemic patients at autopsy, but clinically enlarged ovaries are rare. An acute abdomen-like presentation can occur following excessive bleeding from a corpus luteum in acute myeloid leukemia.[12] Distinction between acute lymphoblastic and acute myeloid leukemias is critical since the two groups are treated differently. Acute lymphoblastic leukemias, like the lymphomas, are primarily divided according to their B-cell or T-cell origin. The acute myeloid leukemias are classified in the WHO scheme first according to the presence of specific cytogenetic abnormalities. In the absence of these well-

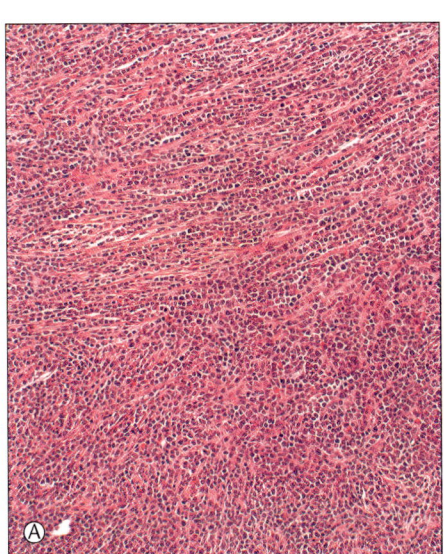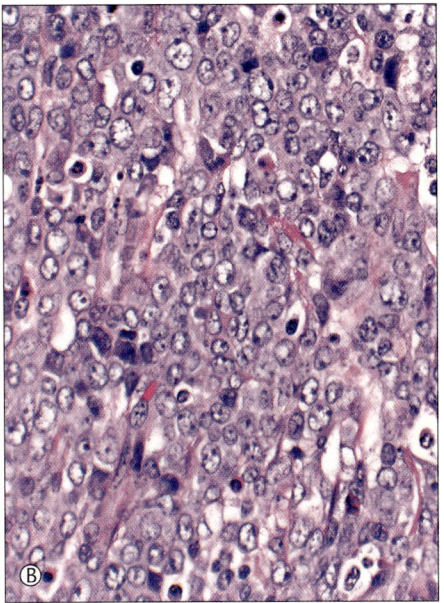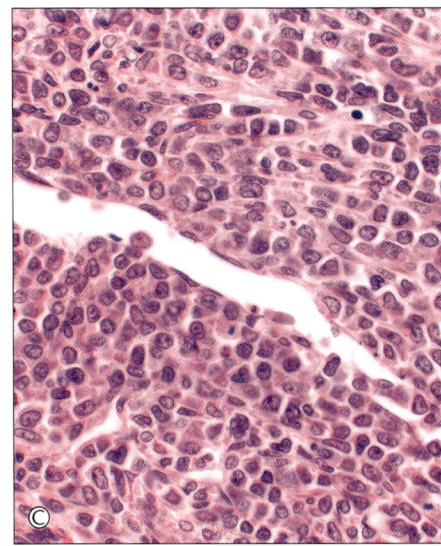

Fig. 28.6 Leukemic infiltrate of ovary by acute myeloid leukemia. **(A)** The cells are uniform and show minimal variation in nuclear size or shape. There is a very fine trabecular pattern, with ribbons only one cell thick, at the top, merging with a more diffuse pattern at the bottom (100×). **(B)** This acute myeloid leukemia with monocytoid differentiation shows moderate variation in cellular and nuclear detail and closely mimics a large cell lymphoma (400×). **(C)** Ill-defined granular cytoplasm is present in this case, but the granularity is not demonstrable without recourse to naphthol AS-D chloroacetate esterase or Giemsa staining.

defined cytogenetic abnormalities the presence of dysplasia in the hematopoietic cells is used to define the next group. The level of differentiation and primary direction of differentiation (granulocytic, monocytic, erythroid, or megakaryocytic) help define the remaining cases, which constitute over 60% of all cases.[19]

Since the cytogenetic abnormalities correlate with prognosis, cytogenetic studies are critical for proper evaluation. FISH studies on paraffin-embedded tissue provide a valuable alternative when fresh tissue is no longer available. Myeloid leukemias are encountered more frequently than the lymphoblastic types, but ovarian involvement in relapses of acute lymphoblastic leukemia is not uncommon. Hematologic investigations usually reveal leukemia, but rarely a leukemic picture may not develop for some time and even be absent at the time of death, despite the bone marrow showing infiltration.

Microscopic features

The histologic features of leukemias can closely mimic those of ovarian lymphomas. If the possibility of extramedullary acute leukemia is ignored, the results of the common immunohistochemical stains used to analyze gynecologic malignancies will be perplexing (see below). Diffuse cellular infiltrates are present, sometimes with cord-like formations as in the diffuse lymphomas (Figure 28.6A). While the infiltrate is generally more monotonous in acute leukemia than in lymphoma, this is by no means invariable and some granulocytic sarcomas show moderate variation in cellular and nuclear size to closely resemble large cell lymphomas (Figure 28.6B). Leukemic infiltrates may also surround and invade follicular structures without destroying them. The nuclear features are those of the corresponding blast cells in the leukemic bone marrow. The folded nuclei of myeloid leukemic cells may mimic the cleft or irregularly shaped nuclei of some lymphomas (Figure 28.6C). In myeloid leukemias, cytoplasmic granulation may be apparent in the H&E-stained sections, and the presence of eosinophil metamyelocytes is considered characteristic. PAS or Giemsa stains highlight neutrophilic and eosinophilic precursors, respectively, but differentiation may be completely lacking. The Leder stain for naphthol AS-D chloroacetate esterase activity also shows myeloid differentiation.

Imprints of fresh tumor tissue stained by a Romanowsky technique can aid in identifying cytoplasmic granules and provide clear nuclear cytologic detail. More commonly, a screening immunohistochemical panel is used (Figure 28.7). A result showing CD45+, CD20–, CD3– cytokeratin reactivity patterns should raise the possibility of acute leukemic involvement, but some cases of lymphoblastic leukemia may even be non-reactive for CD45. Many blasts are reactive for CD34, which can be helpful in suggesting the presence of acute leukemic infiltrate. Additional immunohistochemical stains for myeloperoxidase and CD117 (myeloid cells); lysozyme, CD4, and CD68 (monocytic differentiation); CD79a and CD10 (precursor B-cells); and CD1a, TdT, CD2, or CD7 (precursor T-cells), are required to fully characterize the leukemic infiltrate. Among the acute myeloid leukemias, those with monocytic or myelomonocytic differentiation have a higher propensity for extramedullary involvement. These cells may be reactive for CD68 and other monocytic markers. Other cell types that may be difficult to identify unless specifically sought are blastoid or anaplastic plasma cells (CD45–, CD138+) and cells of anaplastic large cell lymphoma (CD45–, CD20–, CD3–, CD30+).

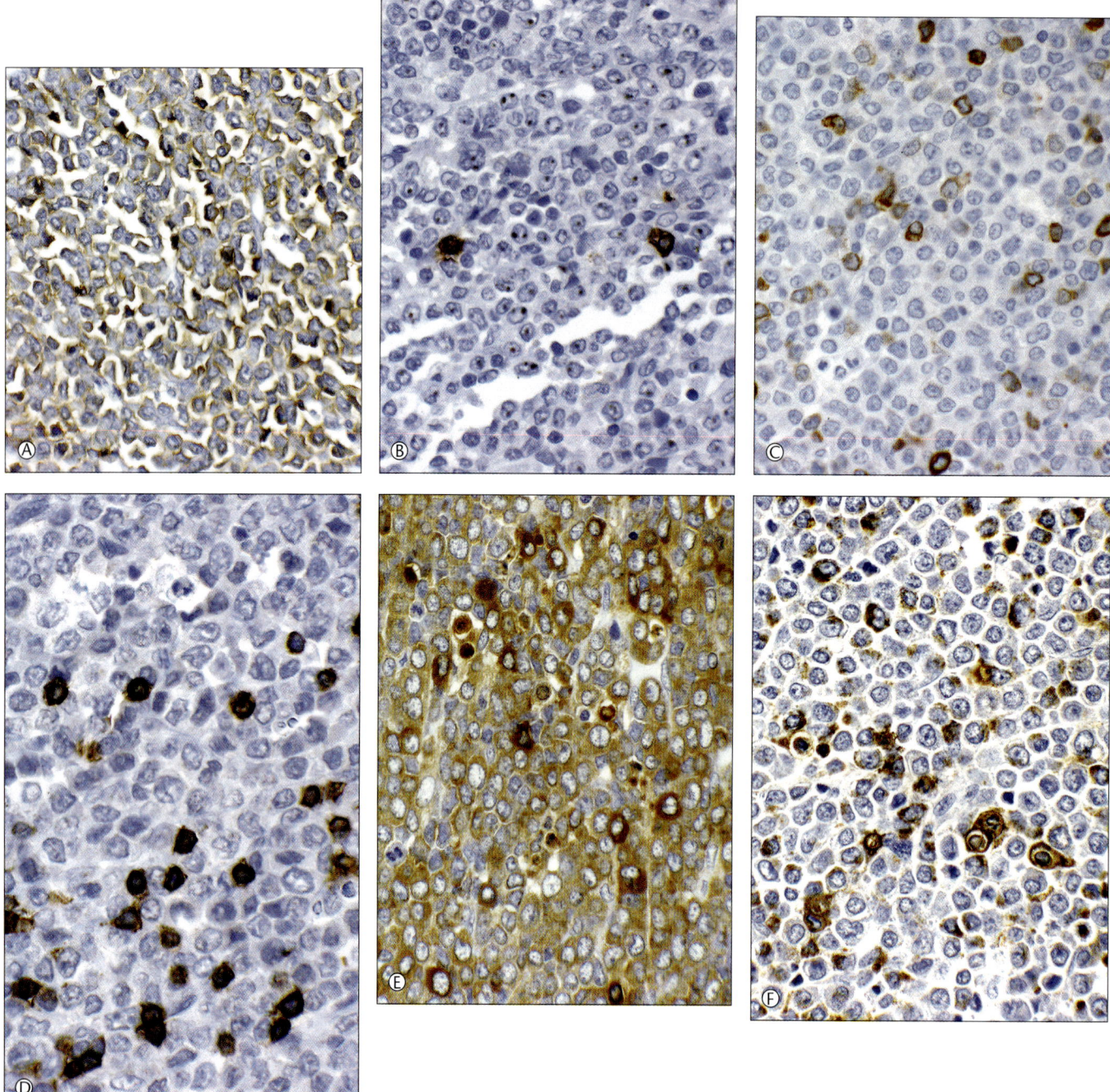

Fig. 28.7 Immunophenotypic profile in extramedullary acute myeloid leukemia (granulocytic sarcomas) of ovary. **(A)** The cells are reactive for CD45, but not for B-cell markers CD20 **(B)** or CD79a **(C)** or T-cell marker CD3 **(D)**. Myeloid maturation is evident from the strong reactivity for myeloperoxidase **(E)**. **(F)** Monocytic differentiation in some cells is reflected by the reactivity for CD68 in some cells. (All 400×.)

Differential diagnosis

Leukemias share many clinical and pathologic features with lymphoma and the differential diagnosis for the latter, therefore, is applicable. Discrimination of lymphoma from leukemia is discussed above.

Treatment and prognosis

The specific subtype and the cytogenetic abnormality present generally govern the prognosis of acute leukemias. Precursor B-cell acute lymphoblastic leukemias have the best overall cure rate, but acute myeloid leukemia is the type most commonly encountered in primary ovarian disease. Even when systemic disease is absent, these patients need chemotherapy. Complete remission now occurs in over half of cases with current chemotherapy, but many patients relapse within 5 years, particularly if they lack a favorable cytogenetic abnormality such as t(15;17), inv(16), or t(8;21). Acute myeloid leukemias arising from a myelodysplastic syndrome or as blast transformation of chronic myelogenous leukemia generally carry a poor prognosis. Acute leukemia arising after chemotherapy for other malignancies including lymphomas similarly carries a poor prognosis. Stem cell transplantation offers hope of cure in some cases.

REFERENCES

1. National Cancer Institute sponsored study of classifications of non-Hodgkin's lymphomas: summary and description of a working formulation for clinical usage. The Non-Hodgkin's Lymphoma Pathologic Classification Project. Cancer 1982;49:2112–35.
2. A clinical evaluation of the International Lymphoma Study Group classification of non-Hodgkin's lymphoma. The Non-Hodgkin's Lymphoma Classification Project. Blood 1997;89:3909–18.
3. Armitage JO, Weisenburger DD. New approach to classifying non-Hodgkin's lymphomas: clinical features of the major histologic subtypes. Non-Hodgkin's Lymphoma Classification Project. J Clin Oncol 1998;16:2780–95.
4. Boyle FM, Taylor KM, Bell JR. Ovarian follicular non-Hodgkins lymphoma. Pathology 1991;23:164–6.
5. Cavalli F, Isaacson PG, Gascoyne RD, Zucca E. MALT lymphomas. In: Schechter GP, Broudy VC, Williams ME, eds. Hematology 2001. Washington, DC: American Society of Hematology; 2001:241–58.
6. Dalloul M, Sherer DM, Gorelick C, et al. Transient bilateral ovarian enlargement associated with large retroperitoneal lymphoma. Ultrasound Obstet Gynecol 2007;29:236–8.
7. Dao AH. Malignant lymphoma of the ovary: report of a case successfully managed with surgery and chemotherapy. Gynecol Oncol 1998;70:137–40.
8. Dimopoulos MA, Daliani D, Pugh W, Gershenson D, Cabanillas F, Sarris AH. Primary ovarian non-Hodgkin's lymphoma: outcome after treatment with combination chemotherapy. Gynecol Oncol 1997;64:446–50.
9. Emery JD, Kennedy AW, Tubbs RR, Castellani WJ, Hussein MA. Plasmacytoma of the ovary: a case report and literature review. Gynecol Oncol 1999;73:151–4.
10. Fox H, Langley FA, Govan AD, Hill AS, Bennett MH. Malignant lymphoma presenting as an ovarian tumour: a clinicopathological analysis of 34 cases. Br J Obstet Gynaecol 1988;95:386–90.
11. Groves FD, Linet MS, Travis LB, Devesa SS. Cancer surveillance series: non-Hodgkin's lymphoma incidence by histologic subtype in the United States from 1978 through 1995. J Natl Cancer Inst 2000;92:1240–51.
12. Habek D, Cerkez Habek J, Galic J, Goll-Baric S. Acute abdomen as first symptom of acute leukemia. Arch Gynecol Obstet 2004;270:122–3.
13. Harris NL, Scully RE. Malignant lymphoma and granulocytic sarcoma of the uterus and vagina. A clinicopathologic analysis of 27 cases. Cancer 1984;53:2530–45.
14. Harris NL, Jaffe ES, Stein H, et al. A revised European–American classification of lymphoid neoplasms: a proposal from the International Lymphoma Study Group. Blood 1994;84:1361–92.
15. Hennessy BT, Hanrahan EO, Daly PA. Non-Hodgkin lymphoma: an update. Lancet Oncol 2004;5:341–53.
16. Iaffaioli RV, Frasci G, Di Tuoro AS, et al. Malignant lymphoma of the ovary: report on two cases and review of the literature. Eur J Gynaecol Oncol 1990;11:205–4.
17. Imaizumi E, Seki K, Kikuchi Y, et al. Primary ovarian lymphoma. A case report. Arch Gynecol Obstet 1993;252:209–13.
18. Iyengar P, Ismiil N, Deodhare S. Precursor B-cell lymphoblastic lymphoma of the ovaries: an immunohistochemical study and review of the literature. Int J Gynecol Pathol 2004;23:193–7.
19. Jaffe ES, Harris NL, Stein H, Vardiman JW, eds. Pathology and Genetics of Tumours of Haematopoietic and Lymphoid Tissues. WHO Classification of Tumours series. Lyon: IARC Press; 2001.
20. Konje JC, Otolorin EO, Odukoya OA, Ladipo OA, Ogunniyi J. Burkitts lymphoma of the ovary in Nigerian adults – a 27-year review. Afr J Med Sci 1989;18:301–5.
21. Kosari F, Daneshbod Y, Parwaresch R, Krams M, Wacker HH. Lymphomas of the female genital tract: a study of 186 cases and review of the literature. Am J Surg Pathol 2005;29:1512–20.
22. Krol AD, le Cessie S, Snijder S, Kluin-Nelemans JC, Kluin PM, Noordijk EM. Primary extranodal non-Hodgkin's lymphoma (NHL): the impact of alternative definitions tested in the Comprehensive Cancer Centre West population-based NHL registry. Ann Oncol 2003;14:131–9.
23. Lanjewar DN, Dongaonkar DD. HIV-associated primary non-Hodgkin's lymphoma of ovary: a case report. Gynecol Oncol 2006;102:590–2.
24. Lopez-Guillermo A, Cid J, Salar A, et al. Peripheral T-cell lymphomas: initial features, natural history, and prognostic factors in a series of 174 patients diagnosed according to the R.E.A.L. classification. Ann Oncol 1998;9:849–55.
25. Magloire LK, Pettker CM, Buhimschi CS, Funai EF. Burkitt's lymphoma of the ovary in pregnancy. Obstet Gynecol 2006;108(3 Pt 2):743–5.
26. Monterroso V, Jaffe ES, Merino MJ, Medeiros LJ. Malignant lymphomas involving the ovary. A clinicopathologic analysis of 39 cases. Am J Surg Pathol 1993;17:154–70.
27. Muller AM, Ihorst G, Mertelsmann R, Engelhardt M. Epidemiology of non-Hodgkin's lymphoma (NHL): trends, geographic distribution, and etiology. Ann Hematol 2005;84:1–12.
28. Nakamura S, Kato M, Ichimura K, et al. Peripheral T/natural killer-cell lymphoma involving the female genital tract: a clinicopathologic study of 5 cases. Int J Hematol 2001;73:108–14.
29. Ng SP, Leong CF, Nurismah MI, Shahila T, Jamil MA. Primary Burkitt lymphoma of the ovary. Med J Malaysia 2006;61:363–5.
30. Osborne BM, Robboy SJ. Lymphomas or leukemia presenting as ovarian tumors. An analysis of 42 cases. Cancer 1983;52:1933–43.
31. Papadaki T, Stamatopoulos K. Hodgkin disease immunopathogenesis: long-standing questions, recent answers, further directions. Trends Immunol 2003;24:508–11.
32. Rotmensch J, Woodruff JD. Lymphoma of the ovary: report of twenty new cases and update of previous series. Am J Obstet Gynecol 1982;143:870–5.
33. Sehn LH, Berry B, Chhanabhai M, et al. The revised International Prognostic Index (R-IPI) is a better predictor of outcome than the standard IPI for patients with diffuse large B-cell lymphoma treated with R-CHOP. Blood 2007;109:1857–61.
34. Seliem RM, Freeman JK, Steingart RH, Hasserjian RP. Immunophenotypic changes and clinical outcome in B-cell lymphomas treated with rituximab. Appl Immunohistochem Mol Morphol 2006;14:18–23.
35. Skodras G, Fields V, Kragel PJ. Ovarian lymphoma and serous carcinoma of low malignant potential arising in the same ovary. A case report with literature review of 14 primary ovarian lymphomas. Arch Pathol Lab Med 1994;118:647–50.
36. Smith JK, Mamoon NM, Duhe RJ. Emerging roles of targeted small molecule protein-tyrosine kinase inhibitors in cancer therapy. Oncol Res 2004;14:175–225.
37. Suzuki T, Sasano H, Takaya R, et al. Leukocytes in normal-cycling human ovaries: immunohistochemical distribution and characterization. Hum Reprod 1998;13:2186–91.
38. ten Berge RL, Oudejans JJ, Ossenkoppele GJ, et al. ALK expression in extranodal anaplastic large cell lymphoma favours systemic disease with (primary) nodal involvement and a good prognosis and occurs before dissemination. J Clin Pathol 2000;53:445–50.
39. Turken A, Ciftci AO, Akcoren Z, Koseoglu V, Akata D, Senocak ME. Primary ovarian lymphoma in an infant: report of a case. Surg Today 2000;30:305–7.
40. Vang R, Medeiros LJ, Deavers MT. Current problems with staging lymphomas involving the ovary. Am J Surg Pathol 2006;30:1202–3.
41. Vang R, Medeiros LJ, Warnke RA, Higgins JP, Deavers MT. Ovarian non-Hodgkin's lymphoma: a clinicopathologic study of eight primary cases. Mod Pathol 2001;14:1093–9.
42. Yatabe Y, Nakamura S, Seto M, et al. Clinicopathologic study of PRAD1/cyclin D1 overexpressing lymphoma with special reference to mantle cell lymphoma. A distinct molecular pathologic entity. Am J Surg Pathol 1996;20:1110–22.

Ovarian tumors: miscellaneous and metastatic

Peter Russell   Jennifer M. Roberts   Stanley J. Robboy

UNCLASSIFIED AND MISCELLANEOUS 'EPITHELIAL' TUMORS

OVARIAN MESOTHELIOMAS

Tumors arise on the ovarian surface that morphologically, histochemically, and ultrastructurally resemble mesotheliomas originating elsewhere in the serous cavities. Such cases may include a variety of benign lesions and rare primary ovarian malignant mesotheliomas.[4] This class of tumor is discussed more fully in Chapter 33.

ADENOMATOID TUMORS

Adenomatoid tumors constitute one form of mesothelial neoplasms, and are discussed more fully in Chapter 19. They are not uncommonly encountered, as incidental findings, in the uterus and fallopian tubes but rarely in the ovaries[69,168,221] and even more rarely in both uterus and ovaries in the same patient.[61] They occur in the hilar region where they form well-circumscribed white to yellow nodules 1–1.5 cm in diameter. Typically, the cut surface reveals a honeycomb pattern of small cystic spaces, although a solitary lesion has been described with transitions to so-called benign multicystic mesothelioma.[220]

Microscopic features
Vascular-like spaces are lined by flattened or cuboidal cells, characteristically with thin thread-like cytoplasmic processes that bridge these spaces.[69] The spaces are, in turn, surrounded by stroma rich in elastic, collagen, and smooth muscle fibers. Cords and small clusters of vacuolated cells may also be present. The tumor cells have eosinophilic or vacuolated cytoplasm that is alcian blue positive at pH 2.5, a reaction, including the non-specific stromal staining, that prior incubation with hyaluronidase eliminates. Tumors regularly react with vimentin, calretinin, mesothelin, WT1, and cytokeratin 5/6.[107,137,168,221]

EPIDERMOID CYSTS

These uncommon cysts are lined by epidermis unaccompanied by skin appendages or other teratomatous elements (Figure 29.1). The small cysts are usually incidental findings but the larger examples reported to date have been associated with abdominal pain and swelling. They are located in the hilus, medulla or cortex and are filled with yellowish creamy material. Generally, they are considered to be of teratomatous origin (ectodermal or endodermal), but other histogenetic possibili-

ties include squamous metaplasia of endometriotic cysts, rete ovarii, mesonephric tubules or epithelium of celomic derivation. Some cysts have exhibited mural nests of epithelial cells resembling those of Walthard rests or Brenner tumors – a finding that supports the theory of celomic origin. Possibly, not all cysts share the same origin; rather, the histogenesis may vary according to location.[6,9,138,143,173]

SQUAMOUS CELL CARCINOMAS

In addition to the benign squamous or epidermoid ovarian cysts, examples of 'pure' (i.e., non-teratomatous) squamous carcinoma *in situ* (CIN)[141] and invasive carcinoma[25,110,136,144] have been reported. Often, it is particularly difficult to exclude a coexisting teratoma that an expanding carcinoma has overrun. Other possible origins should be explored histologically, which may require extensive sampling of the ovarian mass.

Focal glandular differentiation might be evidence for an endometrioid (adenosquamous) carcinoma, and sampling of cyst walls, if present, may reveal evidence of a pre-existing endometriotic cyst (see Chapters 20 and 25).[18,144] Glandular differentiation or areas resembling transitional cell carcinoma also raise the possibility of malignant Brenner tumor, which requires (by convention) confirmation by finding areas of typical benign (solid fibrous areas) or proliferating Brenner tumor (see Chapter 25). Squamous carcinoma metastatic to the ovaries is rare[121,127] (see below). Although we have encountered such cases – for example, originating from the cervix – we have not seen one presenting as an adnexal tumor. Occasional examples of pure ovarian squamous carcinomas that coexist with squamous CIN of the uterine cervix have raised the potential that such lesions may be caused by high-risk human papillomavirus infection.[110,112,141,145]

Microscopic features
Histologically, ovarian squamous CIN is usually identified as atypical squamous epithelium lining a cyst (Figure 29.2) or, rarely, as an extension onto the ovarian serosa of widespread squamous CIN involving the müllerian duct derivatives. Infiltrating squamous carcinoma (well-differentiated keratinizing squamous carcinoma in the only examples we have encountered – Figure 29.3) occurs as mural nodules in epidermoid cysts or, less commonly, as solid masses.

HEPATOID CARCINOMAS

Rare examples have been reported of primary, poorly differentiated ovarian adenocarcinomas composed mainly of cells with phenotypic features similar to those of hepatocellular

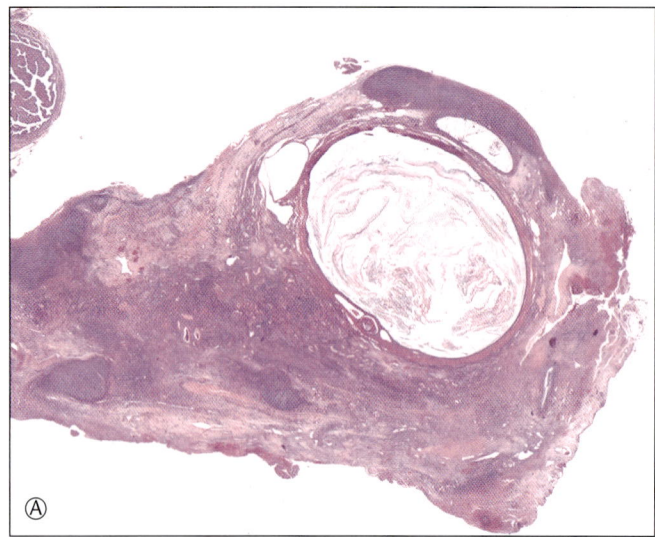

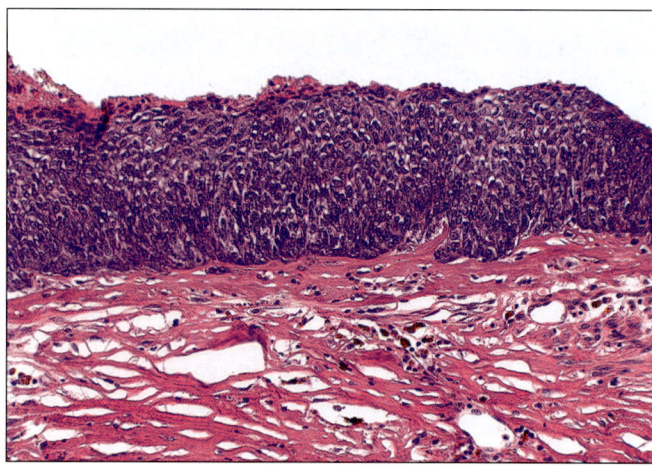

Fig. 29.2 Epidermoid cyst of the ovary. Lined by markedly atypical squamous epithelium (squamous carcinoma *in situ*).

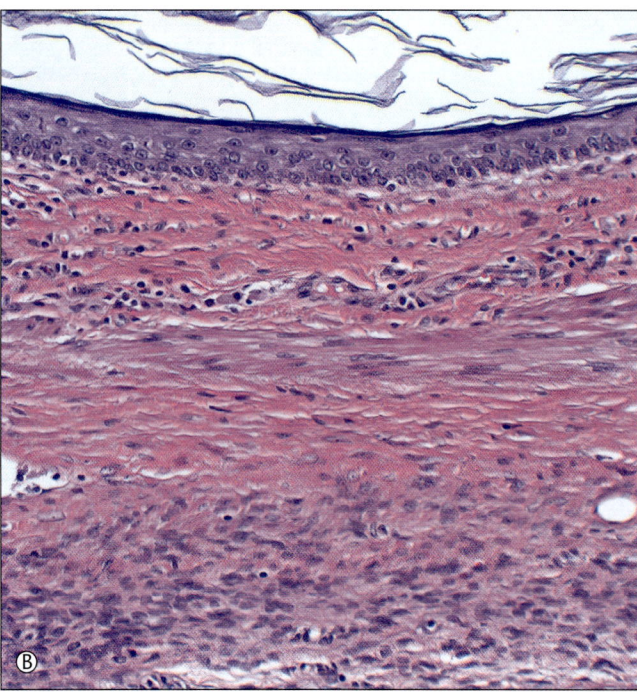

Fig. 29.1 Epidermoid cyst of ovary. **(A)** Survey of lesion indicating its medullary position and showing thick keratinous debris in the lumen. **(B)** High power of benign squamous epithelial lining of the cyst wall.

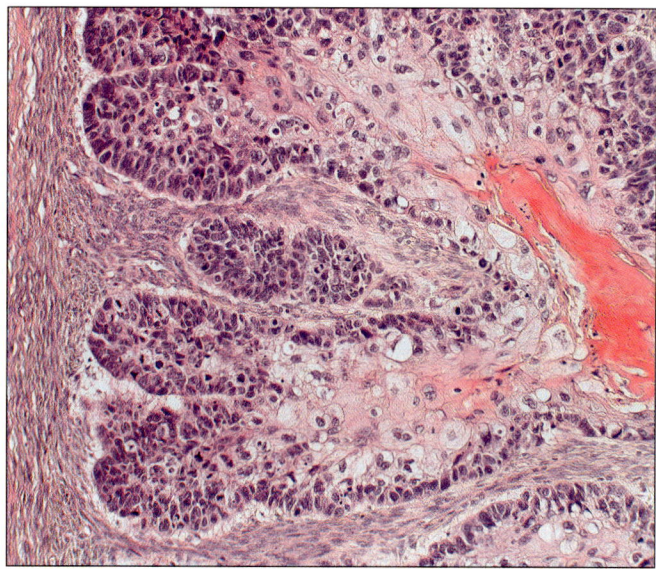

Fig. 29.3 Primary well-differentiated keratinizing squamous cell carcinoma of the ovary. Tumor tissue abutting normal ovarian stroma at the right margin.

carcinomas.[97,113,147,169,171,191,193,202] The patients are aged from 36 to 77 years. The large polygonal component cells have abundant eosinophilic cytoplasm and central nuclei (Figure 29.4), and resemble those of hepatocellular carcinomas, with focal positive immunostaining for α-fetoprotein, frequent but not universal staining with hepatocyte paraffin 1 (Hep Par 1), a canalicular pattern of staining for polyclonal carcinoembryonic antigen (CEA) and staining for cytokeratin 7 (CK7).[147,195] By definition, the tumors do not show any patterns suggestive of endodermal sinus tumor, and several reported examples exhibit areas of surface epithelial–stromal carcinoma of the usual types.[169,171,191] Nevertheless, opinions are divided as to whether the origin of these tumors is germ cell or surface epithelial.[191,202]

Hepatoid yolk sac tumor is the most important entity in the differential diagnosis (see Chapter 27). Features in favor of this diagnosis are the young age of the patient (predominantly below 30 years) and the presence, if found, of other yolk sac tumor patterns or other malignant germ cell tumor elements.

OVARIAN TUMORS OF PROBABLE MESONEPHRIC (WOLFFIAN) ORIGIN

The basis for considering these ovarian and broad ligament tumors[90,175] to be of mesonephric (wolffian) origin, derived from vestigial embryonic remnants in the broad ligaments or ovarian hilus, is the similarity, especially the presence of conspicuous basement membranes, to normal mesonephric duct remnants (see Chapters 5 and 6). This class of tumor is discussed more fully in Chapter 19.

CYSTS AND ADENOMAS OF THE RETE OVARII

Rete ovarii tubules may dilate to form cysts. These are usually only small hilar lesions but substantial cysts also occur. Some have been associated with virilization in postmenopausal women, while rare lesions have been reported in children.[1] The cysts are lined by non-ciliated cuboidal or, less commonly, ciliated columnar epithelium, and their fibrous wall includes bundles of smooth muscle, which may 'crenate' the cyst lining after fixation (Figure 29.5A). The wall often also discloses peripheral Leydig cell hyperplasia (Figure 29.5B). The epithelial lining may undergo squamous metaplasia, which may represent one possible origin of ovarian epidermoid cysts (see above). Adenomatous hyperplasia of the rete ovarii[66] shows poorly circumscribed proliferation of both tubular structures, which blends with the existing rete ductal architecture, and fibromuscular stroma. These features as well as the lack of papillary structures are thought to differentiate hyperplasia from true adenomas.[130] These latter lesions display a complex tubulopapillary pattern with epithelial structures,

lined by regular columnar with clear cytoplasm, similar to those seen in the normal rete. A conspicuous papillary pattern begs differentiation from a serous epithelial neoplasm, while those neoplasms that display prominent Leydig cells in the stroma require distinction from retiform Sertoli–Leydig cell tumors. Immunohistochemically, rete tumors are diffusely reactive for epithelial membrane antigen (EMA), CAM 5.2, vimentin, and CA125.[130]

MISCELLANEOUS MESENCHYMAL TUMORS

Ovarian mesenchymal tumors are of diverse origin. Fibromas are discussed with the tumors of gonadal stromal origin (see Chapter 26) and smooth muscle tumors are included in the group of müllerian mesenchymal tumors (see Chapter 25). The remaining tumors discussed below arise from those connective tissue elements of the ovaries not committed to its specific gonadal function, e.g., vessels and nerves. They may also arise from monophyletic teratomas, secondary malignant transformation in mature cystic teratomas or be the predominant sarcomatous component in mixed müllerian tumors[84,166] or Sertoli–Leydig cell tumors. With exceptional rarity, they may arise as benign mesenchymal components of surface epithelial–stromal tumors.[71] In view of their diverse nature, the neoplasms should be sampled extensively for evidence of a specific origin since this may influence prognosis.

VASCULAR AND RELATED TUMORS

HEMANGIOMAS

Some controversy exists as to whether these represent malformations, hamartomas or true tumors. Among the 40 some reported cases,[20,27,28,53,58,83,85,119,167,196,203] most were found in children or young adults as incidental findings at surgery or autopsy. Some patients present with abdominal masses or ascites[53,85] or pain due to torsion.[109] Some patients also have

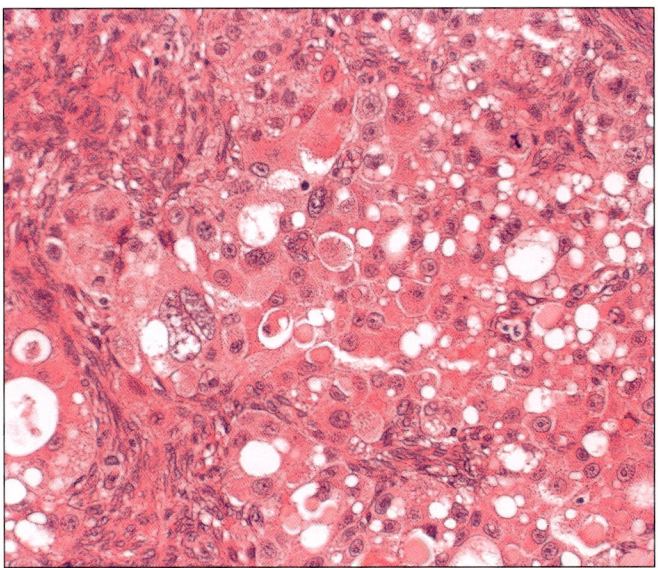

Fig. 29.4 Hepatoid carcinoma of ovary. Courtesy of Dr R Brown, Melbourne, Australia.

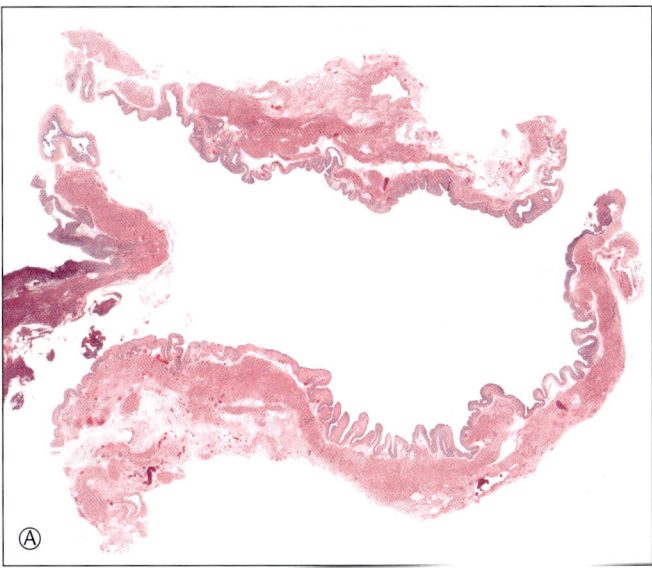

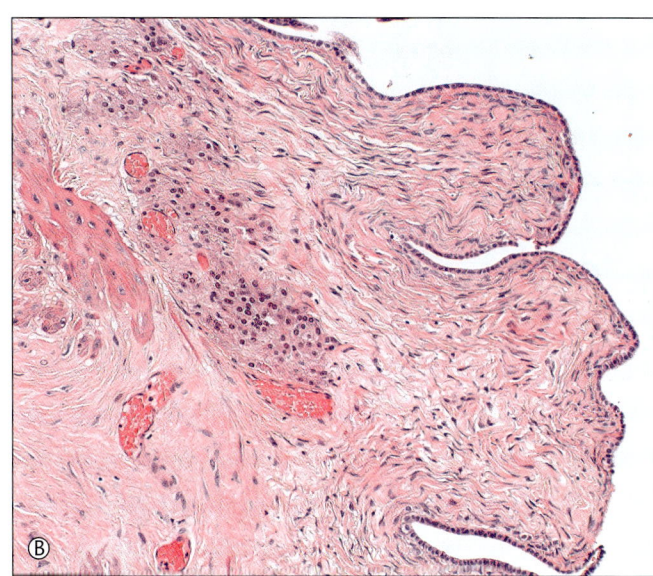

Fig. 29.5 Cyst of rete ovarii. **(A)** Survey of lesion showing crenation of the lining due to the smooth muscle in the cyst wall. **(B)** Non-ciliated cuboidal epithelium lines cyst with Leydig cells (center) and smooth muscle in cyst wall.

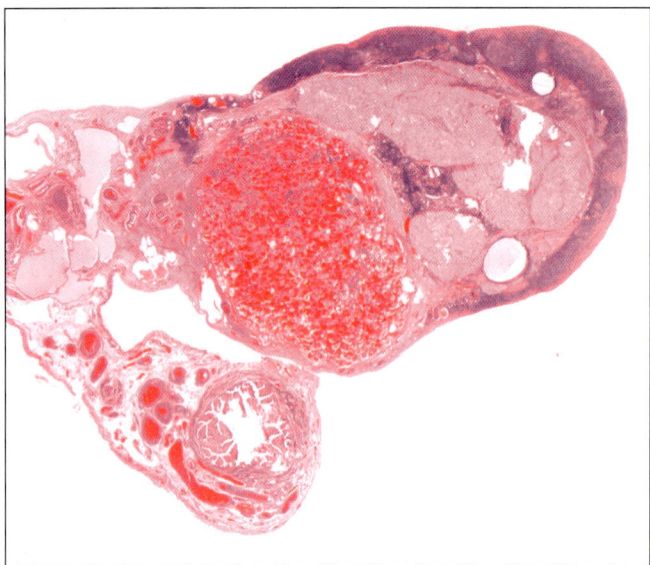

Fig. 29.6 Benign ovarian hemangioma. Incidental finding at hysterectomy for endometrial carcinoma in 57-year-old woman.

generalized or abdominopelvic hemangiomatosis or hemangiomas elsewhere in the genital tract.

Most tumors are unilateral, bilaterality being associated with some cases of generalized or abdominopelvic hemangiomatosis. Most are under 1.5 cm in diameter, in the hilus or medulla, and clearly demarcated from the surrounding tissues, a feature distinguishing them from the prominent coils of blood vessels normally present in this region. The capsule is smooth and the cut surface shows spongy red or purplish tissue.

Most tumors are of the cavernous or mixed cavernous–capillary type (Figure 29.6). The vascular channels are lined by a single layer of endothelial cells, and focal thrombosis may be present. Investigators have specifically reported the presence[119] or absence[58,83] of estrogen and progesterone receptors in the endothelial cells. The intervening scanty fibrous tissue may show some hyalinization or calcification and occasionally luteinization.[20,58,119,167,203]

The differential diagnosis includes normal medullary vasculature, lymphangiomas (see below), and cystic teratomas with prominent vascular components.[78] A solitary example of an infantile hemangioendothelioma (cellular hemangioma of infancy) has been reported in the ovary of a newborn.[153]

HEMANGIOENDOTHELIOMAS (ANGIOSARCOMAS)

These exceptionally rare tumors have been reported only in adults (age range, 19–77 years) and have presented as abdominal pain or masses. Torsion and rupture are not uncommon complications. The tumors are large, soft, friable, spongy, unilateral masses with areas of hemorrhage and necrosis.[33,81,128,132,150,154] The vascular spaces are lined by endothelial cells showing nuclear pleomorphism and mitotic activity that, although sometimes only focal, may be the only features that distinguish them from hemangiomas. The presence of solid cores of endothelial cells helps to confirm the diagnosis. The tumors are reactive for CD31, CD34 and, less reliably, factor VIII-related antigen.[81,132] They pursue a malignant course with local infiltration, peritoneal seeding, and vascular dissemination. The differential diagnosis also includes teratomas with prominent vascular components, lymphangiosarcomas, hemangiopericytomas, and metastatic angiosarcomas (see below), and even exceptionally an epithelioid angiosarcoma arising in a leiomyoma.[37]

HEMANGIOPERICYTOMAS

Ovarian hemangiopericytomas have only been reported since the early 1990s and it is doubtful that any but the best documented of these represents genuine examples.[201] Tumors that may, in whole or in part, resemble hemangiopericytomas are endometrial stromal tumors, sclerosing stromal tumors, granulosa cell tumors, and leiomyomas, and these probably account for most of the tumors previously designated as 'hemangiopericytomas'. These lesions have a complex vascular network composed of gaping thin-walled channels that often show a staghorn pattern of branching. The tumor cells that surround the vessels are regular ovoid fibroblast-like cells, each surrounded by abundant reticulin fibers. Fibrosis and myxoid change may be present.

In endometrial stromal tumors, abundant, regularly distributed, small blood vessels are present but they lack the branching pattern characteristic of hemangiopericytomas. Collagenization and myxoid change are rarely present.

GLOMUS TUMORS

Benign glomus tumor are vanishingly rare, one having been reported as an apparently pure lesion[55] and one having arisen in a mature cystic teratoma.[177] They exhibited the typical gross appearances of glomus tumors elsewhere (circumscribed solid yellow/gray masses) with vaguely organoid growth patterns histologically. Two cells types were present: small epithelioid cells arranged in nests and around large vessels, and larger spindle cells arranged in fascicles that merged with the vessel walls. Oncocytic change was also observed. Tumor cells were reactive for smooth muscle actin and vimentin. A small proportion of cells were reactive for estrogen and progesterone receptors.[55]

LYMPHANGIOMAS

Lymphangiomas are even rarer than hemangiomas.[3,41,100] The tumors are usually unilateral, up to 6 cm in diameter, and with smooth gray capsules. The cut surfaces show cystic spaces containing clear yellowish fluid. The microscopic features are typical of extraovarian lymphangiomas and differ from hemangiomas only by the absence of red cells in the anastomosing channels and the frequent presence of lymphocytes in their walls. The differential diagnosis includes adenomatoid tumors, cystic mesotheliomas (see Chapter 33), and cystic teratomas with sieve-like foci (see Chapter 27). One occurred after local irradiation for a childhood Wilms tumor.[68]

TUMORS OF MUSCULOSKELETAL TYPE SUPPORTIVE TISSUE

TUMORS OF STRIATED MUSCLE ORIGIN

Ovarian rhabdomyomas are extraordinarily rare, either pure[72] or in association with a benign serous tumor.[71] By contrast, rhabdomyosarcoma is the most common of the pure hetero-logous ovarian sarcomas.[129,148,166] Although striated muscle tumors possibly arise from undifferentiated ovarian mesen-chyme, they may also represent one-sided development of mixed müllerian tumors (in which rhabdomyosarcoma is a relatively frequent component) or Sertoli–Leydig cell tumors (see Chapter 26). Diagnosis of pure primary rhabdomyosar-coma requires the examination of multiple blocks to exclude these other diagnostic possibilities. The age at presentation ranges from early childhood to old age, usually with an initial complaint of a rapidly enlarging abdominal mass and pain.

The tumors are unilateral and usually greater than 10 cm in diameter. The cut surfaces show soft gray-white tissue with areas of hemorrhage, necrosis, and cystic degeneration. The histologic subtypes are comparable with extraovarian rhabdo-myosarcomas. Embryonal and alveolar types are most common in young patients and pleomorphic in the elderly. Microcystic areas may resemble small cell carcinoma of hypercalcemic type and other small round cell tumors such as malignant lym-phoma, leukemia, and primitive neuroectodermal tumors and, of course, metastatic rhabdomyosarcoma. Although metasta-ses are often apparent at initial presentation and death usually occurs within a year, there have been some good responses to surgery, chemotherapy, and radiotherapy.

CHONDROGENIC TUMORS

Only one case of an ovarian chondroma[156] and isolated cases of pure ovarian chondrosarcoma[172,188] are known. Ovarian tumors with conspicuous benign cartilaginous components are most likely to be fibromas with cartilaginous metaplasia or teratomas with prominent cartilage formation. Malignant car-tilaginous tumors are most often carcinosarcomas or, rarely, metastatic neoplasms.[186]

BONE TUMORS

The rare reports of ovarian osteomas[59] probably represent examples of osseous metaplasia in fibromas, leiomyomas or non-neoplastic lesions.

Pure osteogenic sarcomas, i.e., with no evidence of associ-ated teratoma or carcinosarcoma, have been described rarely.[44,70] Patients range from 24 to 75 years of age, and have a poor prognosis, many dying within months of diagnosis. The large tumors have histologic features similar to those of skele-tal osteogenic sarcomas. Some cases[165] are associated with a cyst lined by ciliated epithelium.

GIANT CELL TUMORS

Benign giant cell tumors, histologically similar to the familiar skeletal lesions, form mural nodules in ovarian cysts of muci-nous (see Chapter 24),[105] serous[36,47] or uncertain type. Pure giant cell tumors are exceedingly rare.[43] One we have seen in an older woman was unilateral, large (10 cm), cytologically malignant (Figure 29.7), and lacked epithelial components.

SYNOVIAL SARCOMA

We have reported the first case of primary synovial sarcoma arising as a 500 g mass in the left ovary of a 90-year-old woman.[178] The tumor displayed the characteristic biphasic

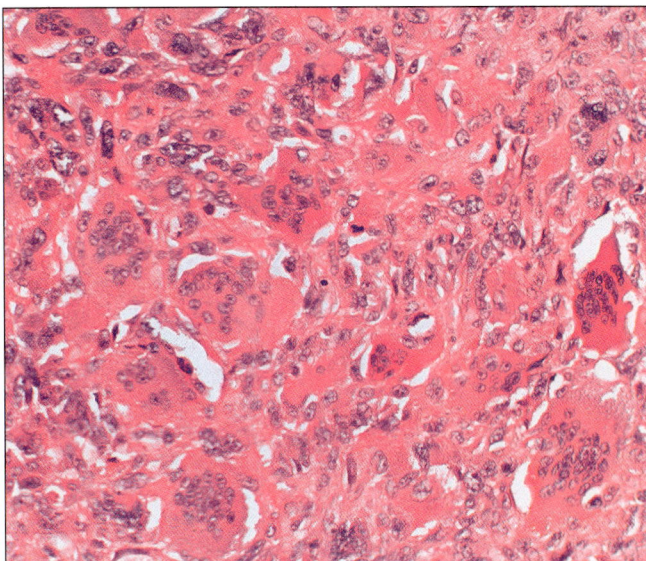

Fig. 29.7 Malignant giant cell tumor of ovary. Lesion composed of multinucleated giant cells and background of mononuclear cells that show more marked nuclear pleomorphism. Courtesy of Dr D Buntine, Brisbane, Australia.

pattern (Figure 29.8A), with the 'epithelial' component high-lighted by cytokeratin reactivity (Figure 29.8B).

NEURAL AND RELATED TUMORS

These are very rare and their histogenesis is that proposed for other mesenchymal ovarian tumors. Some are associated with von Recklinghausens disease. Neuroectodermal tumors (epen-dymomas, neuroblastomas, glioblastomas), even if apparently pure, are considered to be of teratomatous origin and are discussed with immature and monodermal teratomas (see Chapter 27).

NEUROFIBROMAS, NEUROFIBROSARCOMAS

All have been associated with von Recklinghausens disease.[56,67] These neoplasms may cause ovarian enlargement with worri-some features at laparotomy that simulate a malignant tumor (even when benign).

NEURILEMMOMAS (SCHWANNOMAS)

There have been rare cases, all with symptoms of a pelvic mass and an uneventful postoperative course. Tumors are solid and histologically similar to non-ovarian neurilemmomas (Figure 29.9). Two malignant schwannomas have been reported in elderly women who died with metastatic disease 5–18 months after initial surgery,[174,184] and a third woman, aged 58 years, who presented with metastatic disease in the axilla but remains well 17 months after definitive surgery.[96]

GANGLIONEUROMAS

Small ganglioneuromas in the ovarian hilus have to be distin-gushed from the non-neoplastic proliferations of ganglion cells sometimes seen in this region. Larger examples have been described.

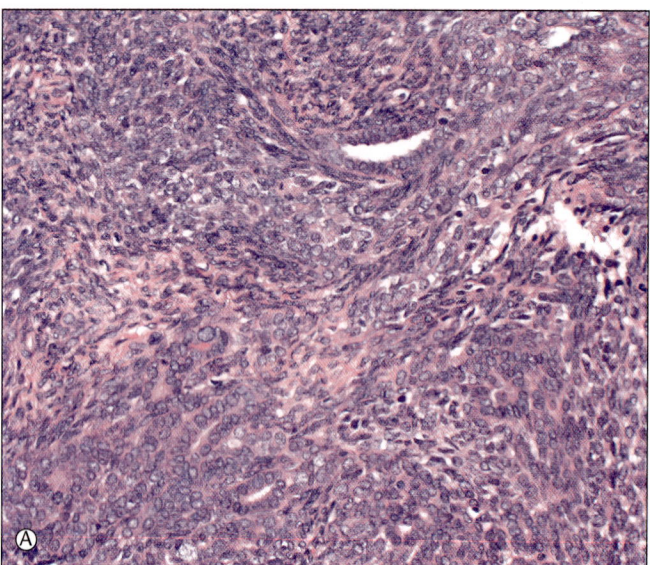
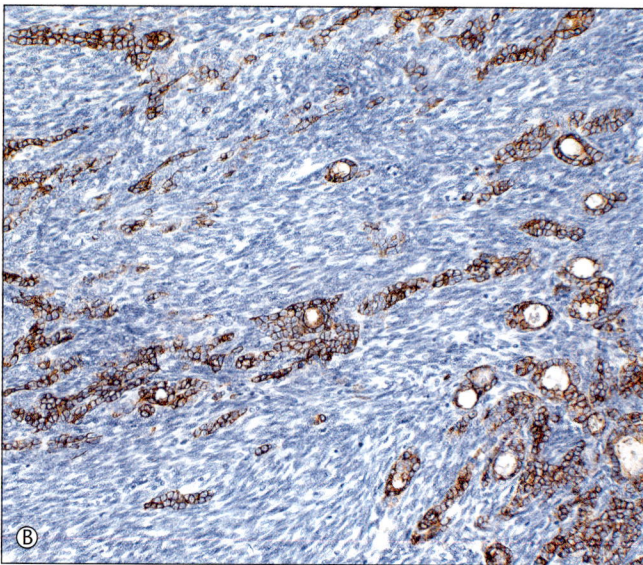

Fig. 29.8 Primary synovial sarcoma of ovary. **(A)** The tumor displayed a subtle biphasic pattern. **(B)** The 'epithelial' component is highlighted by immunostaining for cytokeratin 7.

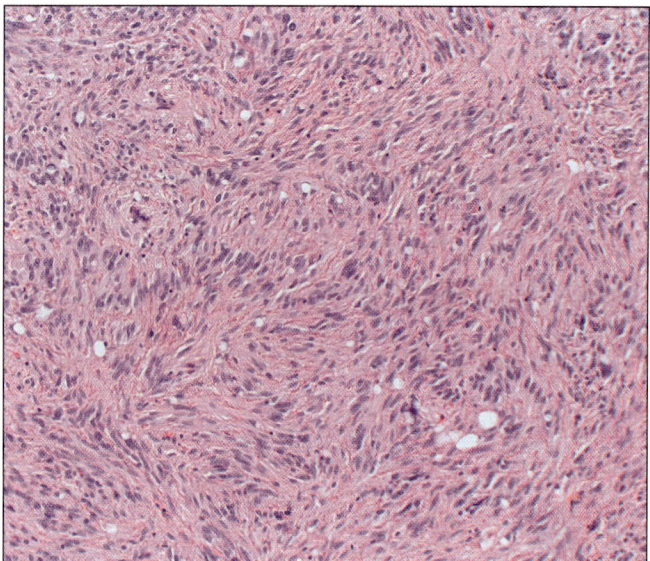

Fig. 29.9 Ovarian schwannoma. Typical Antoni-A area in solid tumor removed from patient with neurofibromatosis.

PHEOCHROMOCYTOMAS

Ovarian pheochromocytoma is exceeding rare. We have encountered one, 1.5 cm in size, which was an incidental finding in a 59-year-old woman. Another older case was in a 15-year-old girl who presented with hypertension, fits, and a left-sided abdominal mass. Catecholamines were extracted from the 970 g tumor. The symptoms disappeared rapidly postoperatively.

MISCELLANEOUS SOFT TISSUE TUMORS

MYXOMAS

Ovarian myxomas are rare.[30,38,161,190] The ages of the patients range from 13 to 65 years. Presentation is usually with an asymptomatic unilateral adnexal mass.

The tumors show stellate and spindle cells in a pale blue to pink myxoid stroma containing mucopolysaccharides stainable by alcian blue and colloidal iron. Hyaluronic acid is present. Tumors are well vascularized and the vessels are capillary-like. The overall picture is typically uniform and fibrosis, if present, is limited and focal. Immunohistochemically, myofibroblastic tumor cells are reactive for vimentin and smooth muscle actin, but only rarely for desmin, features shared with some tumors of the thecoma–fibroma group and raised as evidence for myxomas being part of this neoplastic spectrum.[31]

The tumors most frequently encountered that are likely to cause difficulties in differential diagnosis are edematous fibromas. However, these consist predominantly of fibrous tissue with only focal edematous or myxoid areas, similar to the patterns seen in uterine leiomyomas.

More important distinctions are from myxoid liposarcomas (distinguished by their characteristic plexiform vascular patterns and lipoblasts), pseudomyxoma ovarii (strips and clusters of mucin-secreting epithelial cells in pools of extracellular mucin), and sarcoma botryoides (pleomorphic cells, including rhabdomyoblasts). They also should not be confused with massive edema.

Myxomas, even when treated by conservative surgery, rarely recur.[38,190] In the one study with a recurrence, DNA flow cytometry showed an aneuploid cell population. The tumor cells are immunoreactive for vimentin and usually actin, focally for desmin, but not for S-100 protein, neuron-specific enolase (NSE), neurofilament, Leu-M7, EMA, cytokeratins or factor VIII-related antigen.

LIPOGENIC TUMORS

There are no well-documented cases of pure ovarian lipomas. Lesions that simulate lipomas are benign cystic teratomas with prominent adipose tissue,[52] adherent adipose tissue or auto-amputated infarcted appendices epiploicae and adipocytic prosoplasia. In the last condition, most often observed in perimenopausal obese women, small accumulations of fat cells are found in the ovarian cortex. No pure primary ovarian liposarcoma has been reported but liposarcoma may be identified in the ovary as a component of a carcinosarcoma or as a metastasis.

MYOFIBROBLASTOMA

A solitary example of a benign solid ovarian tumor has been reported, arising in a 22-year-old woman, with histologic and electron microscopic features of a myofibroblastoma.[160] The neoplasm was encapsulated and composed of fascicles of bland spindled cells with architectural patterns similar to those seen in solitary fibrous tumor. The immunoprofile included strong reactivity for smooth muscle actin and muscle specific actin, and weak focal reactivity for CD34.

SARCOMAS NOT OTHERWISE DIFFERENTIATED

Rarely, a malignant mesenchymal tumor is encountered that lacks apparent specific differentiation or evidence of underlying lesions known to be associated with, or complicated by, sarcomas. Multiple blocks should be examined closely for evidence of müllerian epithelial components or teratomatous elements. Immunohistochemical stains for epithelial markers help exclude undifferentiated carcinoma. The possibility of a metastasis should also be considered; the clinical history and operative findings should be reviewed. If the patient is a young woman with hypercalcemia, primary small cell 'carcinoma' enters the differential diagnosis (see Chapter 25).

MALIGNANT TUMORS METASTATIC TO THE OVARIES

The ovaries provide fertile soil for metastases and are the most commonly involved organs in the female genital tract, regardless of the location of the primary tumor. Overall, in cancer-associated deaths, ovarian metastases are likely to be macroscopically evident in approximately 6% and histologically identifiable in an additional 6%. For individual tumors this figure rises to a peak of 50% for gastric carcinoma. Since primary ovarian carcinomas account for only 6% of cancer deaths in women, malignant ovarian tumors identified at autopsy are more likely to be secondary than primary lesions. By contrast, the probability that a malignant ovarian tumor encountered at laparotomy is metastatic varies from about 6 to 22%, reflecting the incidence of different types of cancer in different populations.[64]

Mechanisms of spread

There are several routes of tumor spread to the ovaries, one or more of which can often be inferred from careful histologic examination in a given case. The lymphatic route is probably the most important and accounts for many metastases from the genitourinary tract as well as from the colon, stomach, and breast.[21] Lymphatic permeation is most readily recognized in the ovarian hilus (Figure 29.10) and may also be conspicuous in tubal submucosal lymphatics (Figure 29.11).

Evidence of hematogenous dissemination is most often seen in patients with advanced disease, and other blood-borne metastases are usually apparent. The well-vascularized ovaries of premenopausal women are particularly receptive to seeding in this way.

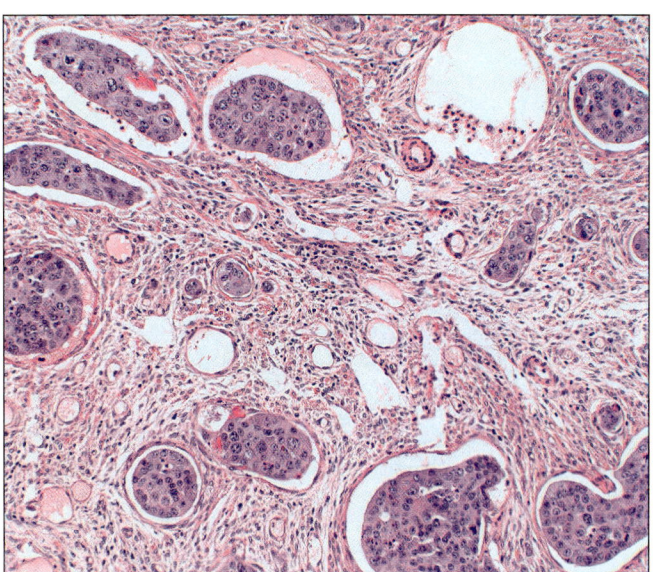

Fig. 29.10 Metastatic pulmonary squamous carcinoma in lymphatics of ovarian medulla.

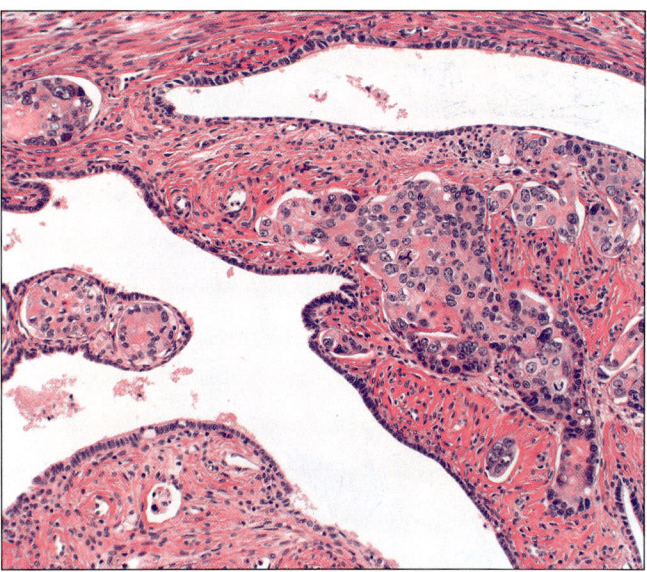

Fig. 29.11 Metastatic colonic adenocarcinoma. Extensive infiltration of mucosal and mural lymphatics of fallopian tube.

Transcelomic spread is associated principally with primary tumors of the abdominal viscera. Viable malignant cells are exfoliated into the peritoneal cavity and may establish themselves on the ovarian serosa, as well as other pelvic and abdominal organs (Figure 29.12).

A transluminal route may be utilized by endometrial and tubal carcinomas. Clusters of carcinoma cells can regularly be identified in the tubal lumen in these cases (Figure 29.13) and it is likely that cells, shed from the ostia, implant on the ovaries (Figure 29.14). The route of transtubal spread appears to be the primary method by which serous carcinomas of the endometrium spread to the peritoneal cavity.[179]

Direct infiltration by tumors arising in pelvic organs is also important, especially in advanced disease. Uterine, tubal,

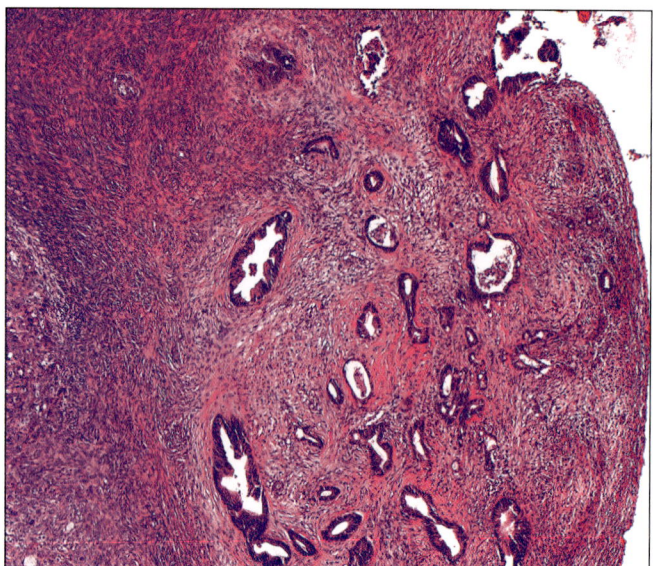

Fig. 29.12 Metastatic colonic adenocarcinoma. Capsular nodule of carcinoma with adjacent loosely adherent clusters of tumor cells (top right). Carcinoma also infiltrates cortical stroma below.

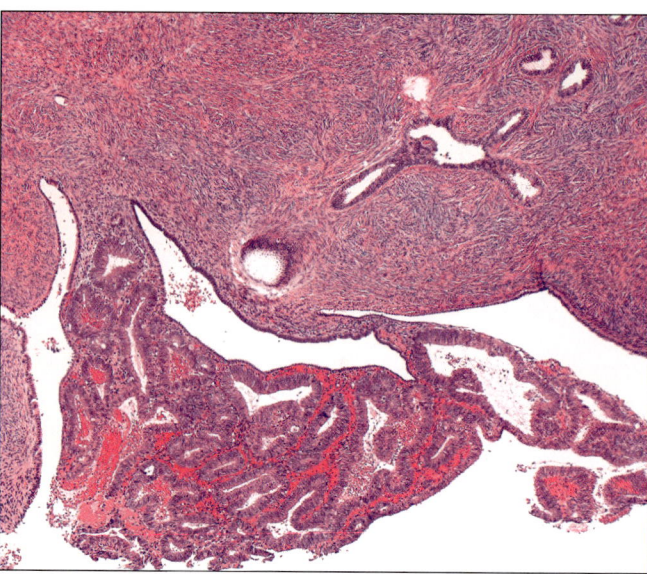

Fig. 29.14 Well-differentiated endometrial adenocarcinoma which has implanted, via transtubal spread, on to the surface of the ovary.

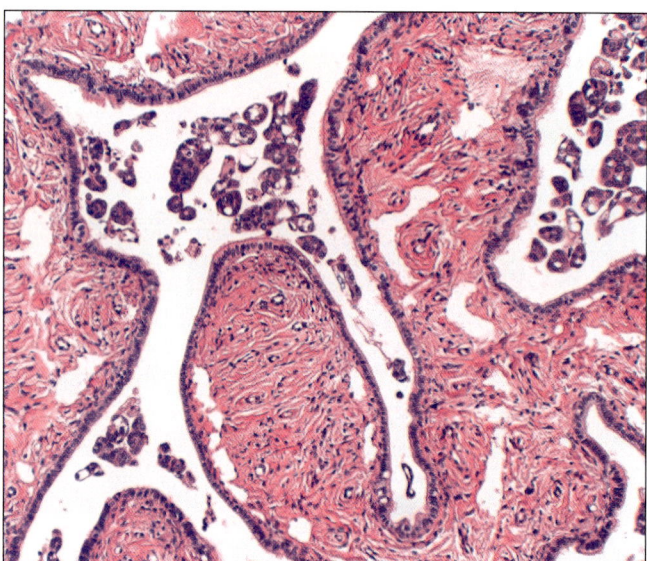

Fig. 29.13 Clusters of carcinoma cells in the lumen of the fallopian tube.

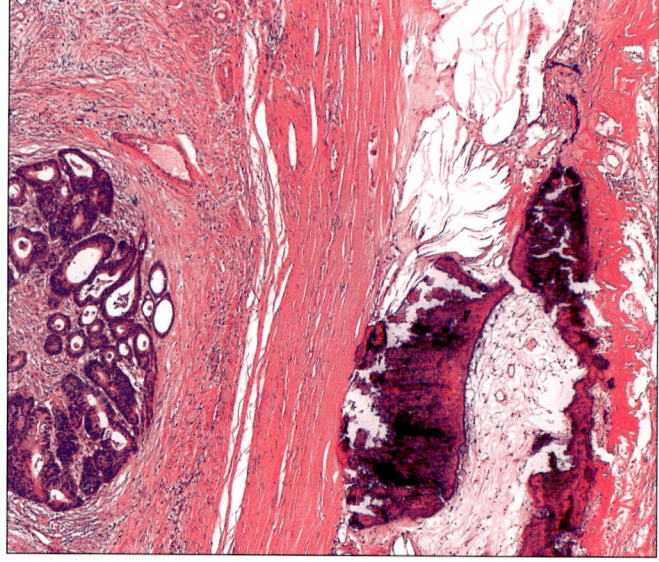

Fig. 29.15 Colonic adenocarcinoma (Dukes stage C) metastatic to a mature cystic teratoma. The 15 cm cyst was filled with necrotic tumor tissue, sebaceous material, and hair fragments (left). The thick fibrous, calcified, and partly ossified wall was infiltrated by metastatic carcinoma (right).

colonic, bladder, mesothelial, and retroperitoneal tumors may involve the ovaries in this way.

As well as metastasizing to the ovarian parenchyma, spread to a pre-existing primary ovarian neoplasm is also well known. For example, breast carcinoma has metastasized to a Brenner tumor, and melanoma and colonic adenocarcinoma to mature cystic teratomas (Figure 29.15).

Clinical profile

Ovarian metastases are usually a manifestation of advanced disease, developing within a few years of diagnosis of the

primary neoplasm. Sometimes they simulate primary ovarian carcinomas clinically, and the source of the metastases may remain obscure for some months or even years after oophorectomy. In these circumstances, a high index of suspicion is necessary and a multidisciplinary approach should be adopted, incorporating clinical, radiologic, serologic, and pathologic features.[116,207,208] Patients with metastases to the ovaries tend to be younger than those with primary ovarian neoplasms. This partly reflects the propensity of tumors to seed to the well-vascularized premenopausal ovaries and partly that tumors commonly metastasizing to the ovaries, especially gastric and mammary carcinomas, occur commonly in younger women.

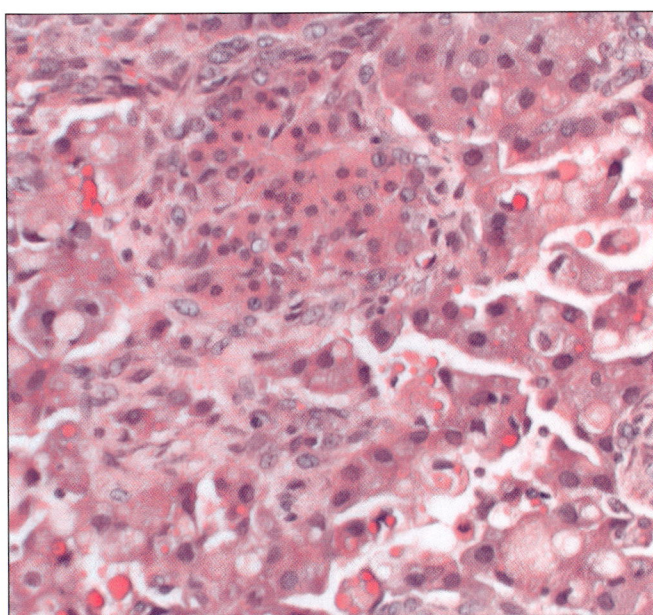

Fig. 29.16 Metastatic hepatocellular carcinoma. Large ovarian mass from a woman with a history of a primary hepatic tumor resected a few months previously. Trabeculae of tumor cells, some vacuolated, and some containing hyaline globules that are α-fetoprotein positive. There is marked stromal luteinization, manifest as compact groups of smaller cells with dense cytoplasm.

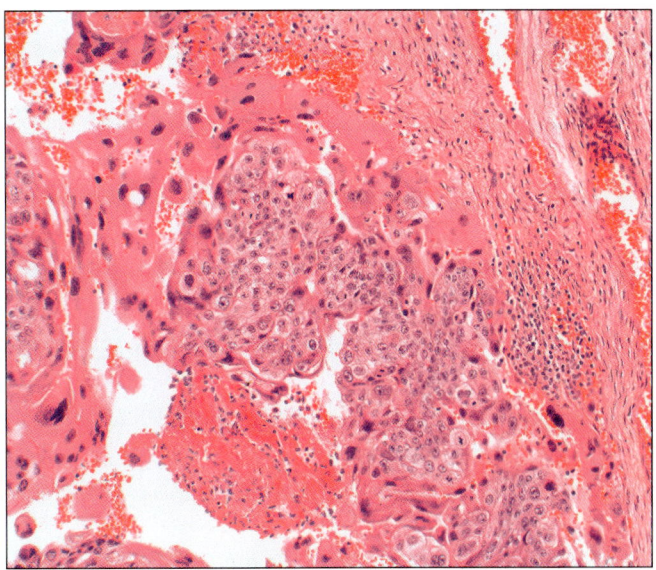

Fig. 29.17 Metastatic choriocarcinoma. The hemorrhagic tumor, adjacent to medullary stroma, displays both syncytio- and cytotrophoblastic proliferation. From a 53-year-old woman with irregular vaginal bleeding; no history of gestational trophoblastic disease or germ cell tumor.

For example, most women with Krukenberg tumors are premenopausal. The prognosis for most patients with ovarian metastases is poor, with an overall 5-year survival rate of 12%.

A small percentage of women with metastatic ovarian neoplasms may suffer from menstrual abnormalities, postmenopausal bleeding, virilization, or the delivery of a masculinized female fetus. These manifestations result from hormonally active luteinized stromal cells (Figure 29.16; see also Figure 29.36) that have been identified in approximately one-third of metastatic neoplasms. This phenomenon occurs particularly often where the metastatic carcinoma is mucinous in type, e.g., of colorectal origin. The ovarian masses of postmenopausal women commonly produce estrogen and progesterone. Stromal luteinization is gonadotrophin responsive, explaining its relative frequency in pregnancy and the postmenopausal period. Additionally, tumors such as choriocarcinoma metastatic to the ovaries may produce beta-human chorionic gonadotrophin (β-hCG) (Figure 29.17).

If there is a known primary malignant tumor outside the ovaries, the presence of an ovarian mass or masses should ensure that appropriate assessment can take place. Ninety per cent of ovarian metastases are from the gastrointestinal and female genital tract. Unusual patterns of spread for a primary ovarian tumor and even the presence of any extraovarian tumor, e.g., lung, liver, and peritoneum, should alert the pathologist that ovarian metastasis rather than primary neoplasm must be considered, and confirmed or excluded. An extraovarian primary neoplasm should be sought if the pathologic features of the ovarian mass indicate this likelihood. The following general features may help to make such a decision.

Macroscopic features

The appearances of ovaries containing metastases vary greatly. Features most helpful are bilaterality and the presence of multiple large nodules either within the substance of the ovaries or on the surface (Figures 29.18 and 29.19). The tumors may be solid or cystic. Cyst formation, while favoring primary neoplasia, does not exclude a metastasis. Metastases may be cystic even when the primary tumor is solid.[64]

Metastases are grossly bilateral in approximately 75% of all cases.[64] Primary ovarian serous and undifferentiated carcinomas are also commonly bilateral, but primary tumors showing mucinous, endometrioid or clear cell features (the types with which metastatic tumors are most likely to be confused) are bilateral in less than 15% of cases. When bilateral tumors are mucinous or endometrioid they are likely to be metastatic.

The bilateral ovarian metastatic masses are commonly of different sizes. In one older series, the larger metastasis was on average 14 cm in diameter, while the other was 6 cm smaller, or 8 cm in diameter. Not uncommonly, the textures of the two may also be quite different. The larger may show areas of hemorrhage and necrosis, due to the out-stripped blood supply, whereas the smaller ovary may appear firm without such changes. Sometimes, especially if less than about 5 cm in diameter, the smaller ovary may appear superficially normal. An important macroscopic clue to occult metastasis in these cases is that the normal architecture in the smaller gonad is often obliterated, such that corpora lutea, corpora albicantia, follicles, and all other structures that are expected to be present are absent. Another clue is the presence of high stage disease, involving peritoneum, liver, omentum, and retroperitoneal lymph nodes.

A recently proposed algorithm to differentiate primary and metastatic carcinomas involving the ovaries has proved useful with mucinous and low-grade adenocarcinomas,[87,170,183,204a] correctly classifying neoplasms in 81–90% of cases. The algorithm, which when used intraoperatively can enhance the accuracy of

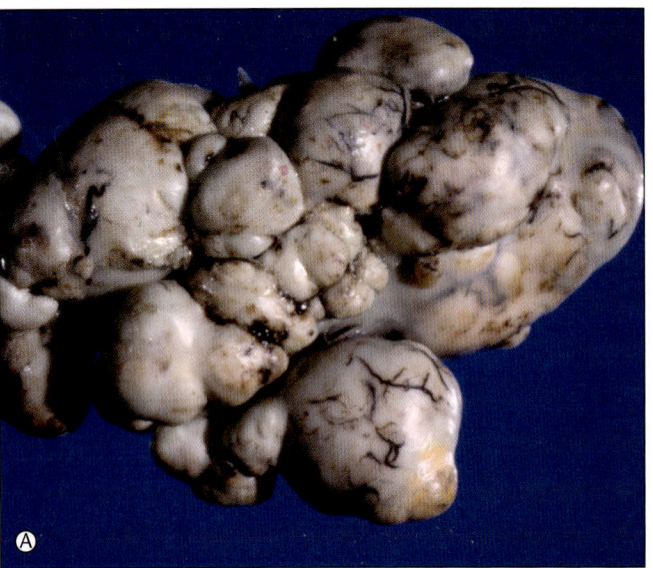
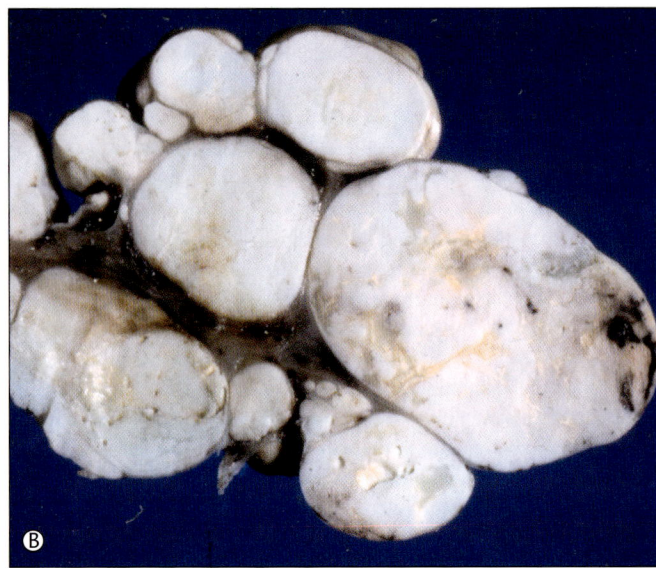

Fig. 29.18 Metastatic colonic adenocarcinoma. Such a multinodular mass would be quite uncharacteristic of a primary ovarian carcinoma. **(A)** External surface. **(B)** Cut surface.

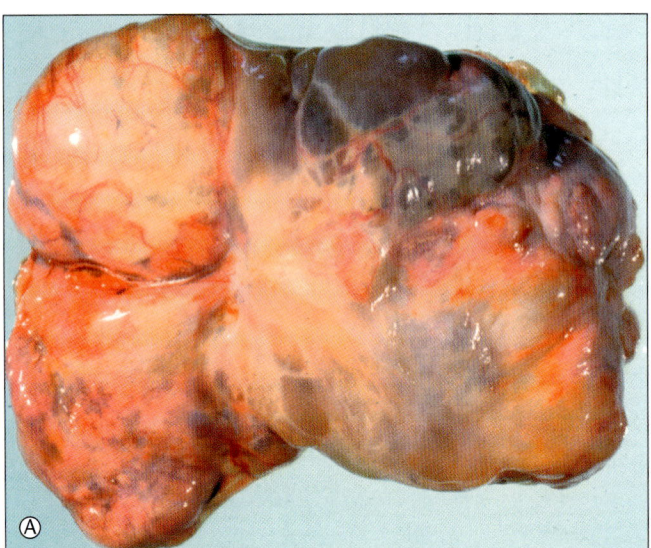
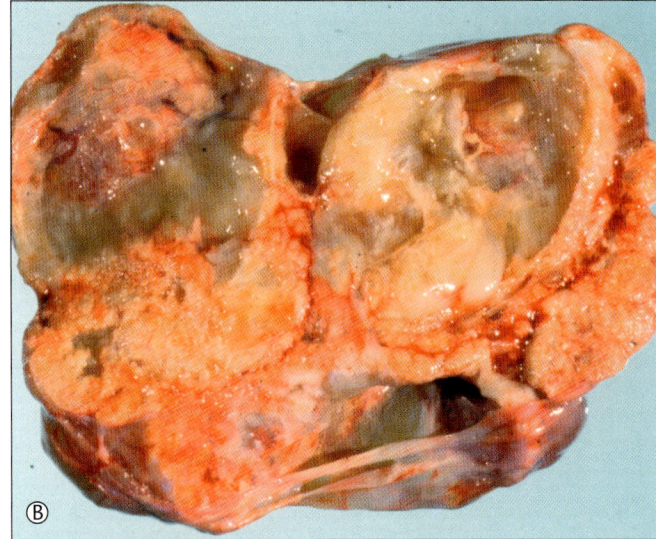

Fig. 29.19 Intestinal carcinoma metastatic to the ovary. **(A)** External surface is bosselated with coarse vessels and cysts visible. **(B)** Cut surface shows ragged friable necrotic tissue and mucin-filled cysts.

frozen sections, classifies all bilateral carcinomas as metastatic, unilateral tumors less than 10 cm in diameter as metastatic, and unilateral tumors 10 cm or greater in diameter as primary.

Microscopic features

Metastatic tumors display various appearances largely depending on their site of origin. The text that follows is organized by the site of origin. In approaching the differential diagnosis, it is important also to think of the pattern presented, from which the type of lesions that can be present, either as metastases or primary, can be considered. This approach is developed in Table 29.1.

Features more commonly observed in metastatic lesions include growth in multiple nodules and the presence of disease on the serosa (that may have been visible macroscopically). Lymphatic or blood vessel invasion is useful also, as lymphatic permeation is only extremely infrequently seen at the periphery of primary ovarian carcinomas. The tumors may form both small and large cysts.

Other features more likely to predict metastasis are small tumors confined to the medulla, tumors with an infiltrative pattern of stromal invasion that spares or infiltrates rather than obliterates follicular structures (Figure 29.20; see also Figures 29.22 and 29.23), single cell infiltration and signet-ring forms, cells floating in mucin, and variation in growth pattern from one nodule to another.[116] Follicle-like spaces are not uncommon in ovarian metastases and may arise due to inadequate lymphatic drainage.[74,214] Metastases with mucinous differentia-

Table 29.1 Differential diagnosis of metastatic tumors to the ovary

Pattern	Metastasis to ovary	Differential diagnosis (primary tumors)	Useful immunostains
Endometrioid	GI tract	Endometrioid Ca, endometriosis, yolk sac, serous	CK7, CK20, CEA, CDX2, villin, CD10, AFP, WT1, Ber-EP4
Mucinous	GI tract, cervix	Mucinous tumors, clear cell, mucinous carcinoid	CK7, CK20 CDX2, villin, CEA, chromogranin, synaptophysin, PAS
Signet ring (Krukenberg)	GI tract, bladder, breast	Fibroma, carcinoid, S-L, mucinous, clear cell, sclerosing stromal, signet-ring stromal, lymphoma	Wide range
Clear cell	Renal cell, colon	Clear cell, yolk sac, secretory variant of endometrioid	Vimentin, CD10, RCC, CDX2, AFP
Transitional	Carcinoid, urinary TCC	Brenner, transitional, undifferentiated Ca	CK7, CK18, chromogranin, synaptophysin
Serous	Fallopian tube, serous endometrium, breast, mesothelioma, mesothelial proliferation	Serous, yolk sac, retiform S-L	CK7, CK20, calretinin, inhibin, Ber-EP4, EMA, AFP
Small acini	Insular carcinoid, breast, microadenocarcinoma of pancreas	Granulosa, carcinoid mucinous, yolk sac, struma, adenomatoid tumor	Chromogranin, GCDFP, CK7, CK20, CA19–9, inhibin, AFP, TTF-1, thyroglobulin, calretinin
Tubular	Krukenberg, carcinoid	Sertoli, S-L, granulosa, SCTAT, endometrioid Ca, carcinoid	CK7, Ber-EP4, vimentin, inhibin, calretinin, chromogranin, synaptophysin, EMA
Cords and columns	Breast (especially lobular), lymphoma, carcinoid, small cell lung	Granulosa, S-L, carcinoid	CK7, CD45, inhibin, calretinin, vimentin, chromogranin, synaptophysin, Ber-EP4, GCDFP-15, TTF-1
Follicle-like spaces	Carcinoid, melanoma, oat cell, thymus, adenoid cystic salivary, alveolar rhabdomyosarcoma, desmoplastic round cell tumor, lymphoma	Small cell with high calcium, granulosa cell, endometrioid, undifferentiated Ca, embryonal, struma, adenomatoid, ovarian tumor of probable wolffian origin	Wide range
Small cell	Oat cell, thymus, neuroblastoma, alveolar rhabdomyosarcoma, melanoma, Merkel cell, lymphoma, Ewings, desmoplastic round cell tumor	Small cell with high calcium, PNET, neuroblastoma, small cell neuroendocrine, dysgerminoma	Wide range

Table 29.1 *Continued*

Pattern	Metastasis to ovary	Differential diagnosis (primary tumors)	Useful immunostains
Abundant eosinophilic cytoplasm	Melanoma, hepatocellular, large cell of lung, adrenal, carcinoid	Steroid cell tumor, luteinized granulosa, oxyphil clear cell, hepatoid yolk sac, hepatoid, primary melanoma, Leydig cell, undifferentiated Ca, luteinized thecoma, Leydig cell hyperplasia, decidua, pregnancy luteoma, large solitary luteinized follicle cyst, exuberant corpus luteum	HMB-45, MART-1, Hep Par, inhibin, calretinin, TTF-1, chromogranin, synaptophysin, AFP, CK7, EMA
Insular (nesting)	Breast, carcinoid, microadenocarcinoma of pancreas, oat cell, melanoma	Brenner, gonadoblastoma, undifferentiated Ca, granulosa, dysgerminoma, carcinoid	CK7, CK20, EMA, PLAP, GCDFP-15, TTF-1, chromogranin, synaptophysin, CA19–9, S-100, MART-1, HMB-45, inhibin
Sarcomatoid	Endometrial–stromal sarcoma, leiomyosarcoma, melanoma	Mucinous, serous, fibrosarcoma, rare sarcomas	CD10, desmin, actin, h-caldesmon, HMB-45, CK7, inhibin, calretinin, progesterone receptor
Diffuse	Breast, endometrial stromal	Granulosa, gonadoblastoma, dysgerminoma, undifferentiated Ca, yolk sac, embryonal Ca	Wide range
Fibroma/thecoma	Endometrial–stromal sarcoma, Krukenberg	Fibroma/thecoma, fibromatosis, stromal hyperplasia, stromal hyperthecosis, sclerosing stromal tumor, leiomyoma	CD10, alcian blue, h-caldesmon, actin, desmin, inhibin, calretinin, cytokeratin
Mixed epithelial–stromal	Krukenberg, carcinoid	Adenofibroma, MMMT, adenosarcoma	Alcian blue, chromogranin, CD10, vimentin, Ber-EP4
Myxoid tumors	Krukenberg	Yolk sac, massive edema, torsion, fibroma, sclerosing stromal tumor, myxoma	Cytokeratin, AFP, calretinin, EMA
Heterologous elements	Rare sarcomas	Teratoma, S–L, rare sarcomas	Wide range, depending on element seen
Eosinophilic hyaline globules	Solid pseudopapillary neoplasm of pancreas (numerous)	Yolk sac, clear cell (few)	AFP, vimentin, CD10, CD56, cytokeratin

AFP, a-fetoprotein; Ca, carcinoma; CDX2, caudal-related homeobox 2; CEA, carcinoembryonic antigen; CK, cytokeratin; EMA, epithelial membrane antigen; GCDFP, gross cystic disease fluid protein; GI, gastrointestinal; Hep Par, hepatocyte paraffin; MART-1, melanoma antigen recognized by T cells 1; MMMT, mesodermal (müllerian) mixed tumor; PAS, periodic acid-Schiff; PLAP, placental-like alkaline phosphatase; PNET, primitive neuroectodermal tumor; RCC, renal cell carcinoma; SCTAT, sex-cord tumors with annular tubules; S-L, Sertoli–Leydig; TCC, transitional cell carcinoma; TTF-1, thyroid transcription factor-1; WT1, Wilms tumor 1.

Modified adaptation from James Small MD PhD and Robert Young MD.

tion not uncommonly display a maturation phenomenon, with a spectrum of appearances, simulating benign and borderline (proliferating) cystadenoma.[65,116] Other (non-mucinous) metastases usually lack such transitional appearances. Prominent stromal luteinization around the tumor nodules is also suspicious for metastasis (Figure 29.16; see also Figure 29.36).

METASTASES FROM THE FEMALE GENITAL TRACT

METASTASES FROM CERVIX

Ovarian metastases from cervical carcinoma are considered rare. Usually the metastatic nature of the ovarian lesion is evident clinically but occasionally the cervical tumor is occult and the ovarian mass causes the presenting symptoms.[40,116,151] Both squamous carcinoma and adenocarcinoma may metastasize to the ovaries, with the latter occurring significantly more often than the former.[125,185,187] Increasing clinical stage correlates with an increased frequency of ovarian metastases for both types of carcinoma[125,126,176] and tumor size of greater than 30 mm for adenocarcinoma.[125] Metastases in apparent stage 1 disease are rare.

While we have not encountered occult cervical squamous cell carcinoma presenting as an adnexal tumor, primary squamous cell carcinoma of the ovary should not be diagnosed until metastasis from the cervix or elsewhere is excluded. Squamous cell carcinoma of the cervix has been reported as a metastasis to an ovarian Brenner tumor.[82]

The assessment of synchronous and metachronous endocervical and ovarian adenocarcinomas can be difficult because metastases can share gross and microscopic features with primary ovarian epithelial neoplasms, both mucinous and endometrioid, and both proliferating tumors and well-differentiated carcinoma.[40,116] A microscopic clue to the metastatic nature of an ovarian tumor is a 'hybrid' epithelium with features of both endometrioid and mucinous differentiation or very atypical mucinous epithelium as well as many apical mitoses and numerous apoptotic bodies. These features are more typical of endocervical than primary ovarian adenocarcinoma.[40] Utilizing in situ hybridization and polymerase chain reaction (PCR) for detection of human papillomavirus (HPV) and reactivity for p16 and hormone receptors, these authors showed the metastatic nature of 10 ovarian neoplasms originally thought to be primary. The ovarian and endocervical tumors contained identical HPV genotypes, were diffusely reactive for p16, and generally lacked reactivity for estrogen and progesterone receptors. In two cases, the discovery that the ovarian lesions were metastases led to reinterpretation of cervical adenocarcinoma in situ (AIS) lesions as invasive, and in two further cases, patients without known cervical disease were then found to have occult endocervical adenocarcinoma.

Cervical adenoma malignum may be associated with synchronous ovarian mucinous tumors, sometimes in the setting of Peutz–Jeghers syndrome. In this instance, as adenoma malignum is not HPV related, assessing their HPV DNA status is not useful.[40,46,146,192] Assessing cytokeratin reactivity is also of little help as both primary cervical and ovarian tumors should be reactive for CK7 and unreactive for CK20.

Massive ovarian edema may occur as a result of lymphatic permeation by metastatic squamous cell carcinoma and adeno-

carcinoma of the cervix.[93] Metastatic endocervical adenocarcinoma may also present as a virilizing ovarian mass simulating a primary endometrioid carcinoma.[151]

Small cell cervical carcinomas metastasize to the ovaries, as have mixed, transitional cell, and undifferentiated carcinomas.[218]

METASTASES FROM FALLOPIAN TUBES

Metastases from fallopian tube carcinoma are rarely reported. This reflects both the perceived rarity of these tubal carcinomas and the difficulty in establishing the temporal primacy of coexisting tubal and ovarian lesions.[162] Given that most tubal carcinomas show similar microscopic features to serous or undifferentiated tumors of the ovaries, rarely is it possible when both organs are involved to say where the tumor originated. Although cases of mucinous, endometrioid or clear cell carcinoma are uncommon primary malignancies in the tubes, when specifically studied they may reveal evidence of primary tubal disease and spread to the adjacent ovaries.[155]

METASTASES FROM ENDOMETRIUM AND MYOMETRIUM

When carcinomas are found in one or both ovaries and the endometrial cavity, they are usually of similar histologic type, raising the question as to whether they are synchronous primary or metastatic lesions. The principles used in distinguishing primary independent ovarian carcinomas from metastatic endometrial carcinoma (Figure 29.20) are discussed in Chapter 25.

In a series of sarcomas metastatic to the ovaries,[210] slightly more than half were from uterine primaries (two-thirds endometrial stromal sarcomas and one-third leiomyosarcomas). Leiomyosarcomas usually involve the ovaries when there is evidence of widespread disease. The ovaries may be enlarged but microscopic metastases can occur. Secondary stromal

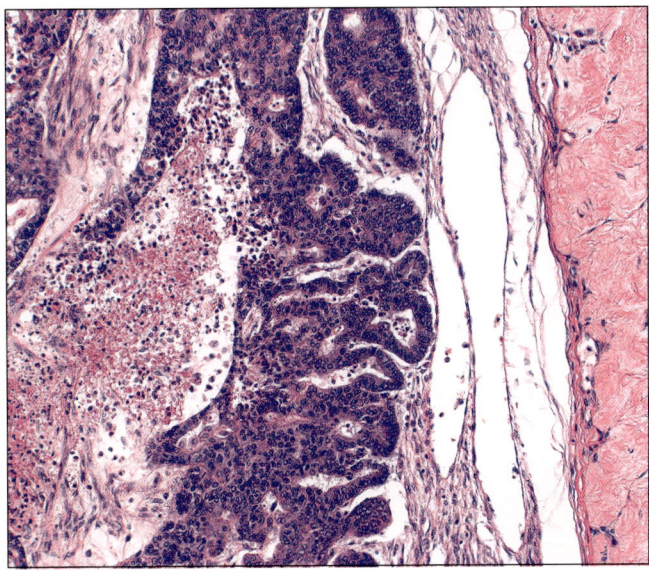

Fig. 29.20 Moderately differentiated endometrioid adenocarcinoma, metastatic from a large primary uterine tumor, and forming a small medullary deposit adjacent to an old corpus albicans. Such a site is virtually pathognomonic of metastatic epithelial malignancy

sarcomas also must be distinguished from primary ovarian endometrioid stromal sarcoma, which usually is unilateral and associated with endometriosis. Stromal sarcoma may also mimic thecoma[219] and other sex cord-stromal tumors, including granulosa cell tumor. The metastases are usually bilateral and extraovarian disease is regularly present.

METASTATIC TROPHOBLASTIC DISEASE

Primary choriocarcinoma of the ovary of either gestational or germ cell origin is often impossible to distinguish from a metastasis of an intrauterine choriocarcinoma that has regressed, on purely morphologic grounds (Figure 29.17). Patient age helps only in prepubertal girls. Thorough sampling of the ovarian tumor is necessary to identify other germ cell elements.

Placental site trophoblast tumors metastatic to the ovaries have been described, as has invasive hydatidiform mole with ovarian involvement.

METASTASES FROM BREAST

Breast carcinoma accounts for a considerable percentage of lesions metastatic to the ovaries and is probably the most common of all silent metastases. Ovarian secondaries have been found at autopsy in up to 40% of women dying with widespread breast cancer. The frequency of ovarian involvement in patients undergoing therapeutic oophorectomy for advanced disease is 30%[123] and <10% when the oophorectomy is 'prophylactic'. Ovarian metastases are usually silent clinically, only rarely producing endocrine symptoms. They present exceptionally as 'primary' ovarian neoplasms, prior to the discovery of the breast tumor. Conversely, they may present decades after the primary tumor was successfully treated.[120]

Patients with breast cancer are at increased risk of developing primary ovarian carcinoma, especially if they have a hereditary predisposition to breast and ovarian cancer due to *BRCA1* or *BRCA2* mutations.[116] It is not surprising then that patients with known breast cancer who present with 'new' findings of an adnexal or pelvic mass are more likely to have independent ovarian or tubal malignancy than metastases from the breast cancer by a 3:1 ratio.[32]

Diagnosis

Multiple small nodules or a confluent mass may be evident (Figure 29.21). The ovaries are usually only mildly enlarged, with a smooth surface and a bosselated nodular appearance. Ductal carcinoma is more common as an ovarian metastasis but a higher proportion of lobular carcinomas metastasize to the ovaries. Any of the various histologic patterns of primary breast carcinomas may be recapitulated in ovarian metastases, such as trabeculae, acini, cribriform glands, sheets, and Indian files. Not uncommonly, several different patterns will be evident in a single tumor (Figure 29.22). Infiltration of follicular structures is frequently observed and lymphatic permeation is usually readily apparent (Figures 29.21, 29.23 and 29.24). Small lesions may merge imperceptibly with the adjacent stroma and simulate foci of nodular stromal hyperplasia, especially if the interspersed stromal cells are luteinized (Figure 29.25). Lobular carcinoma in particular may be subtle at low power. However, the malignant cytologic characteristics of the infiltrate are readily apparent on closer inspection. Krukenberg-type metastases from the breast have also been reported, though rarely. An unusual case is breast carcinoma metastasizing to a benign ovarian fibroma.[142]

Differential diagnosis

Diffuse and Indian file patterns are often found in lymphomas and leukemias (see below). The ovarian lesions most commonly mimicked by metastatic breast carcinomas are sex cord-stromal tumors, dysgerminomas, granulosa cell tumors, and carcinoid tumors.[50]

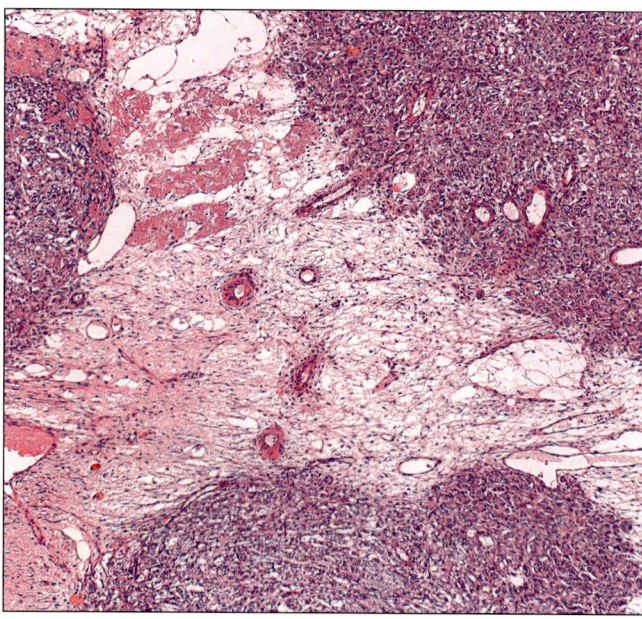

Fig. 29.21 Metastatic breast carcinoma. Multiple discrete nodules are present in the ovarian stroma and there is invasion of a corpus fibrosum at top left.

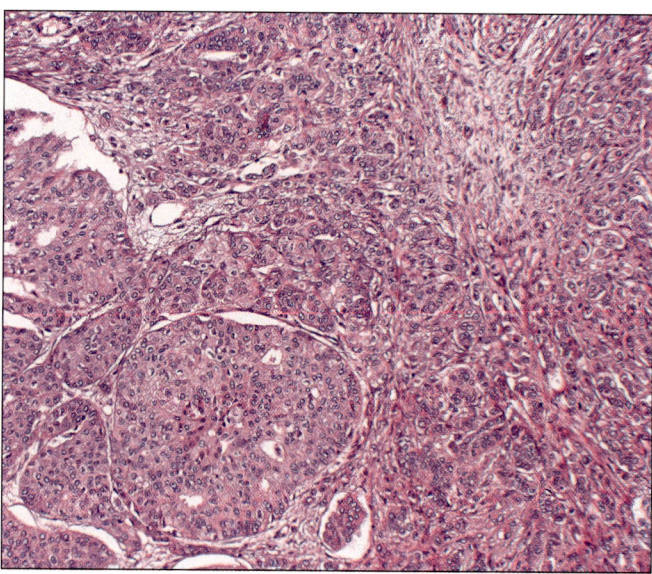

Fig. 29.22 Patterns of breast carcinoma metastatic to the ovary – trabecular (left) and cribriform (right).

Carcinoid and sex cord-stromal tumors, especially Sertoli cell tumors, may simulate the cord-like and trabecular patterns of metastatic breast carcinomas. However, these tumors have regular round to elongate nuclei and lack the obvious malignant cytologic features of metastatic breast carcinomas. Breast carcinoma cells are reactive for EMA, but are not argyrophilic, and are unreactive for NSE and chromogranin. The cells often exhibit luminal or cytoplasmic mucin.

Metastases from intestinal carcinomas, while forming pseudocystic necrotic masses with obvious mucinous glandular differentiation, may occasionally form small acini and cords with only scanty mucin production and thus resemble metastases from breast. The clinical history and surgical findings should provide the necessary information to establish the site of the primary tumor. Immunohistochemical analysis shows the breast carcinoma typically to be reactive for CK7 but not CK20, while the pattern with colorectal carcinoma is usually reversed.[116]

Metastatic breast carcinomas may need to be distinguished from primary ovarian adenocarcinomas. Ductal carcinoma may mimic a primary ovarian endometrioid carcinoma with small acini but differentiation from poorly differentiated serous carcinoma is more often a diagnostic challenge. Foci of a feathery papillary pattern should suggest an ovarian primary. Reactivity with CA125 and WT1 favors serous carcinoma, whereas reactivity with gross cystic disease fluid protein-15 (GCDFP-15, also known as BRST-2) suggests a breast origin[7] (see Chapter 24). If a panel of four antibodies is used, a decision tree effectively discriminates among primary ovarian carcinoma and metastases of breast and colonic origin in 86% of cases.[95] Estrogen receptors are commonly found in breast and ovarian primary tumors, but not in colonic carcinomas.

METASTASES FROM GASTROINTESTINAL TRACT

In recent decades the incidence of gastric carcinoma has fallen and, in most Western countries, colonic carcinomas are now encountered more frequently by a factor of at least three. Both carcinomas spread readily to the ovaries and together they form the bulk of clinically apparent tumors metastatic to these organs. Ovarian secondaries are identified at autopsy in 15–50% of women with gastric carcinoma and in 15–30% of those with colorectal carcinoma. Yet, in clinical series, ovarian metastases are diagnosed in only 3–8% of cases.

A very small percentage of gastrointestinal tumors metastatic to the ovaries originate in the appendix, pancreas, gall bladder, small intestine or esophagus (squamous cell carcinoma). Recognition that the ovarian tumor is mucinous and possibly intestinal in origin (commonly, a partial garland of mucin-poor intestinal type glands surrounds necrosis showing extensive cellular debris, so-called 'dirty' necrosis) can play an

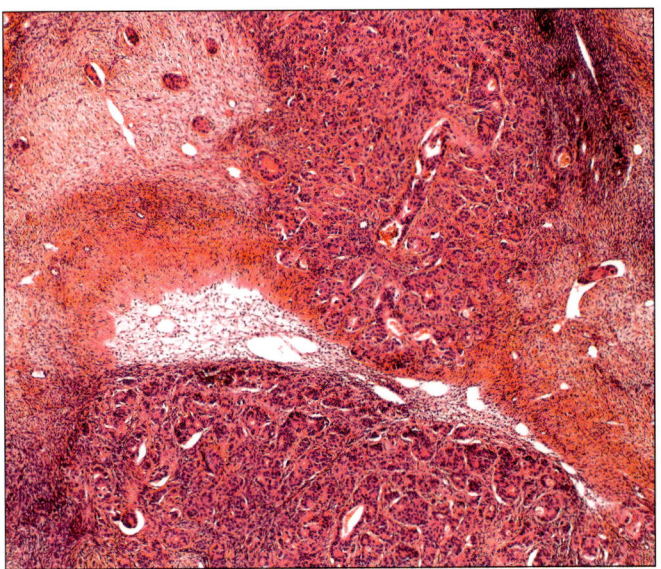

Fig. 29.23 Metastatic breast carcinoma invading the wall of an atretic follicle. Lymphatic permeation is seen at bottom right.

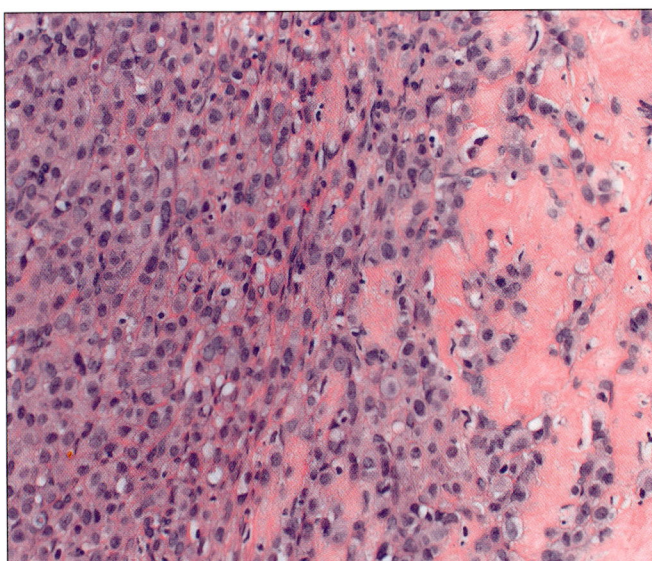

Fig. 29.24 Metastatic breast carcinoma infiltrating a corpus albicans. Tumor cells have a moderate amount of cytoplasm. Nuclei are pleomorphic and hyperchromatic.

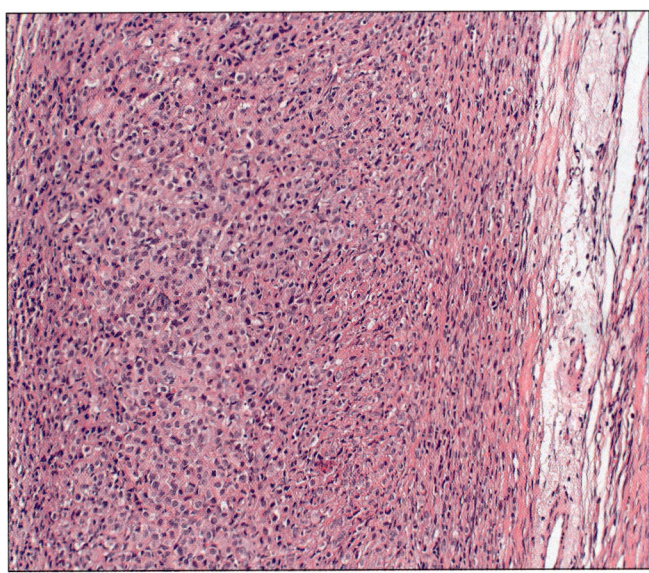

Fig. 29.25 Metastatic breast carcinoma. Nodule that merges imperceptibly with adjacent stroma, simulating a focus of stromal hyperplasia.

important role in patient management. If the mucinous tumor is diagnosed by frozen section during the operative procedure and the possibility of metastasis entertained, the surgeon can carefully examine the bowel for the true primary lesion. It is our experience that intestinal obstruction will usually occur within 3 months of detection of the ovarian metastasis. Therefore, recognition of the primary tumor and its removal at the initial operation will almost surely save the patient a second, and often emergency, operation.

KRUKENBERG TUMORS

The term 'Krukenberg tumor' denotes an ovarian adenocarcinoma with a distinctive histologic pattern showing pleomorphic mucin-filled signet-ring cells, commonly invested in a cellular sarcoma-like proliferation of ovarian stroma. This latter feature, however, is not definitional as some variants have the classic signet-ring cells without the cellular stroma.[152] Krukenberg tumors account for 3–8% of all carcinomas metastatic to the ovaries. Gastric carcinomas account for 40–95% of all cases (depending on the population studied) and colorectal carcinomas less than 20%. Indeed most, if not all, metastases to the ovaries from the stomach are of the Krukenberg type. The historical development and characterization of Krukenberg tumors, as well as related metastases to the ovaries, has been masterfully reviewed by Young.[207,208]

Breast carcinomas uncommonly produce metastases of Krukenberg type. Rare sources are the gall bladder, ampulla of Vater, and small intestine, appendix, cervix, and bladder.[152]

Clinical profile

The average age of patients with Krukenberg tumors is approximately 45 years (range, 13–84 years),[91] which is younger than most patients with metastatic carcinoma. Common presenting symptoms are abdominal pain and swelling that relate to the usually bilateral and often large ovarian masses. Gastrointestinal disturbances are less common, and endocrine symptoms are rare and generally restricted to pregnant patients who may become virilized or deliver a masculinized female fetus.[49,200] Interestingly, metastatic gastric carcinoma has a proclivity for involving the ovaries during pregnancy.[54,116] Ascites is present in more than 50% of the cases. Only 25% of patients have a history of prior tumor with an average elapsed interval, before the appearance of ovarian lesions, of less than 6 months. The primary carcinoma is sometimes occult, even at laparotomy, and may not be detected until the postoperative period (and, rarely, not at all). Peritoneal involvement is usually inconspicuous at laparotomy, an observation that supports the theory of retrograde lymphatic spread as the pathogenesis of some tumors. The prognosis is poor, with death usually occurring within a year. However, bilateral oophorectomy in patients with no other obvious metastases may confer a survival benefit, increasing the median survival time from 3 to 17 months.[24] In addition, prophylactic oophorectomy has been suggested as a strategy to improve survival in women under 50 years with more than six positive nodes at gastrectomy.[89]

Macroscopic features

The tumors are bilateral in about 80% of cases. The ovaries are asymmetrically enlarged (Figure 29.26), with one usually greater than 10 cm in maximum diameter and sometimes as large as 30 cm. The ovaries are transformed into rounded or

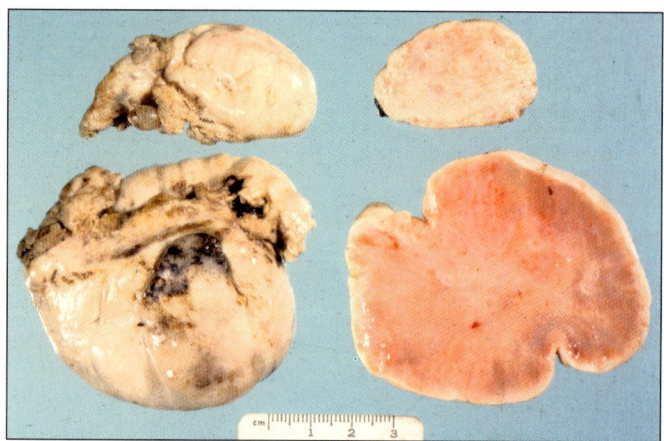

Fig. 29.26 Krukenberg tumors from a 61-year-old woman with primary gastric carcinoma. Capsular surfaces of the asymmetrically enlarged left and right ovaries are bosselated. Cut surfaces show uniform edematous gelatinous tumor tissue.

lobulated masses of firm white or yellowish tissue with brown or purple foci of degeneration. In smaller tumors the overall ovarian contours may be preserved. The capsular surface is typically free of adhesions or peritoneal deposits. Parts of the tumors may be gelatinous, spongy or edematous. Cystic degeneration is common in larger masses. Frank necrosis is generally not conspicuous.

Microscopic features

Krukenberg tumors typically exhibit multiple, ill-defined nodules displaying an intimate admixture of pleomorphic signet-ring cells and crowded, plump, spindled stromal cells, the latter presenting a sarcoma-like appearance (Figures 29.27A and 29.28A). Compact cellular areas and pale edematous areas often alternate, with occasional pools of basophilic mucin prominent in the latter. A pseudocapsule of compact tumor may be seen between the central edematous zone and the ovarian surface epithelium. The epithelial component consists chiefly of single or clustered signet-ring cells, but trabeculae, tubules, acini, and small cysts may also be present. The signet-ring cells are identical to those seen in gastric carcinomas, with vacuolated cytoplasm and eccentric hyperchromatic nuclei. Mitotic activity is sparse. The carcinoma cells may also display granular eosinophilic cytoplasm, particularly when located within tubules (Figure 29.27). Neutral mucin is the predominant secretion and the diastase-periodic acid-Schiff (PAS) or mucicarmine stains inexpensively demonstrate the nature and arrangement of the cells (Figure 29.28B). Immunohistochemical markers of epithelial differentiation, such as cytokeratins (CK7 and CK20) and EMA, also successfully highlight the carcinoma cells. It is germane to recall that metastatic gastric carcinomas in the ovaries, unlike intestinal metastases, are commonly unreactive or only focally reactive for CK20.[139] By contrast, gastric carcinomas are usually reactive for CK7, while intestinal metastases are usually unreactive. Lymphatic invasion is conspicuous in over one half of cases, and although best observed in the hilus, it can also be readily demonstrated in the mesosalpinx and mesovarium if these tissues are available for review.

The mesenchymal component varies considerably in amount. Of ovarian stromal origin, it is composed of bundles of spindle

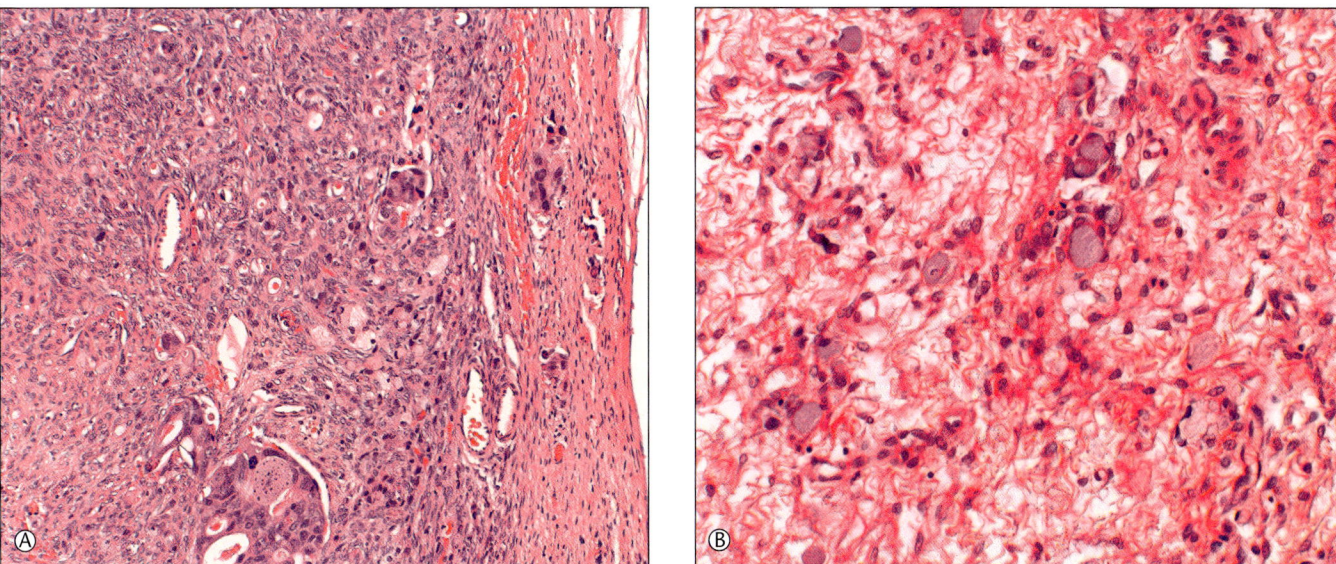

Fig. 29.27 Krukenberg tumors. Single and clustered vacuolated carcinoma cells, including signet-ring forms with abundant granular eosinophilic cytoplasm and pleomorphic nuclei, infiltrate between hyperplastic stromal cells **(A)** and in edematous stroma **(B)**.

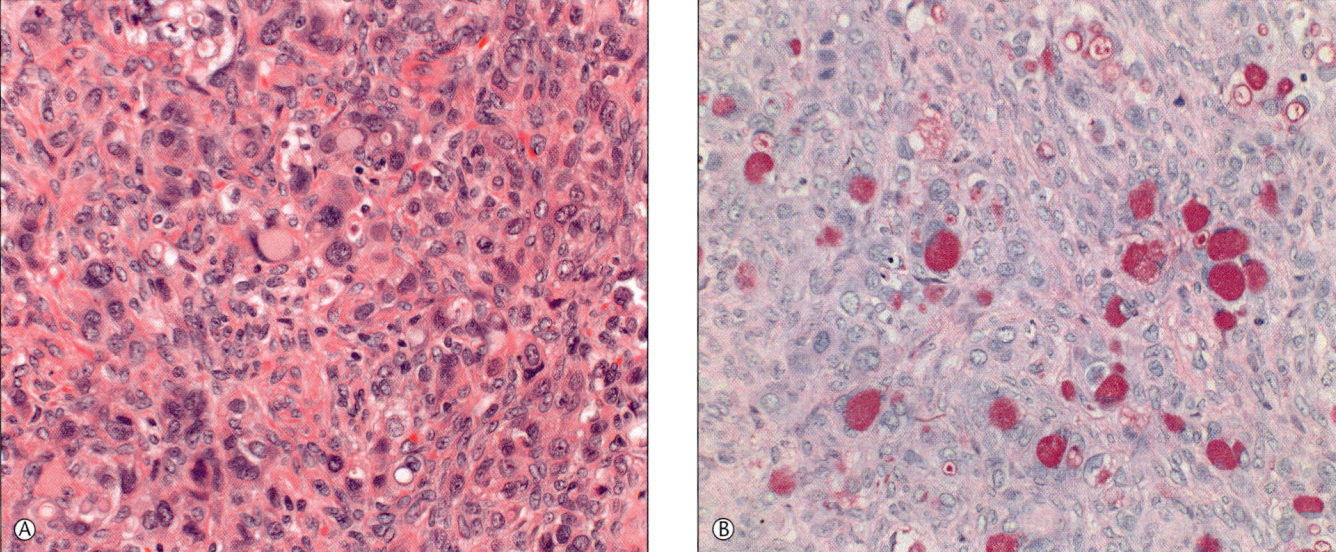

Fig. 29.28 Krukenberg tumor. The ovarian stroma is hyperplastic and luteinized. **(A)** The infiltrate of carcinoma cells is difficult to appreciate in this H&E-stained section. **(B)** Same area with carcinoma cells highlighted by mucicarmine stain.

cells resembling those seen in stromal hyperplasia (Figures 29.27A and 29.28A). There is minimal cytologic atypia or mitotic activity. The stroma may become collagenized and may also show a storiform pattern, resembling a fibroma, particularly in the superficial portions of the tumors. The deeper portions of the tumors are generally more cellular and the stromal cells plumper. Edema is present focally (Figure 29.27B), especially in the medulla, but is sometimes diffuse and marked, to the extent of forming pseudocysts or simulating 'massive edema'.[10] Uncommonly, pools of interstitial mucin are present (Figure 29.29). Although the stroma is hypercellular, luteinized stromal cells are only identified in about 20% of tumors[91] and are far less common than in metastatic colorectal carcinomas.

Some Krukenberg tumors display a predominant tubular pattern and have been subclassified as 'tubular Krukenberg tumors', as distinct from the classic type.[49,159] They constitute up to 20% of all Krukenberg tumors and may represent a somewhat better differentiated group (Figure 29.30). Signet-ring cells are present both in tubules and intermingled with stromal cells. Scattered argentaffinic and argyrophilic cells may be identified. Luteinized stromal cells are relatively more frequent than in the classic variant.

A difficult pattern to recognize in Krukenberg tumors is when the signet-ring cells are few and the stromal response extensive. In these cases, the relatively banal stroma will simulate the stroma of a Sertoli–Leydig tumor. The

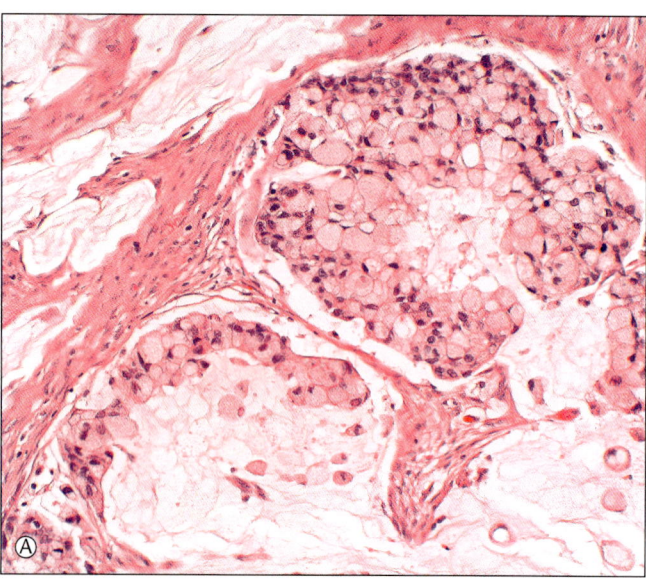
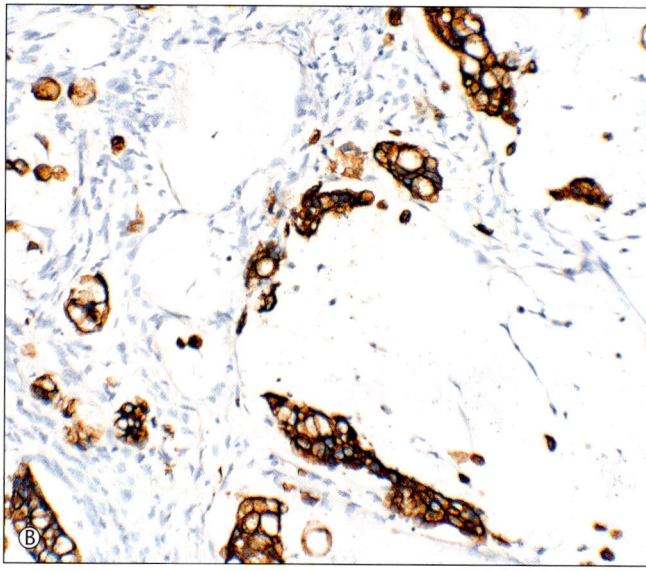

Fig. 29.29 Krukenberg tumor. **(A)** Focal areas of prominent extracellular mucin production are present, containing aggregates of typical signet-ring cells. **(B)** Tumor cells are strongly immunoreactive for cytokeratin 7.

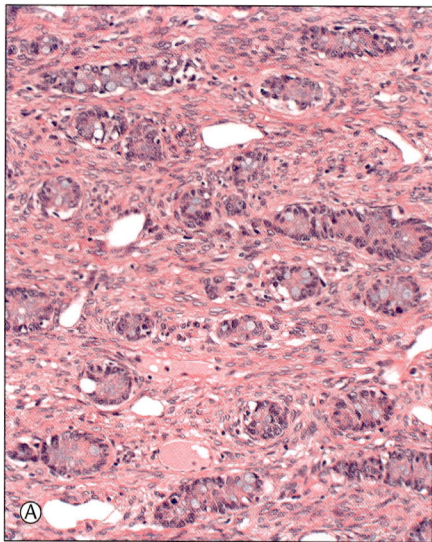
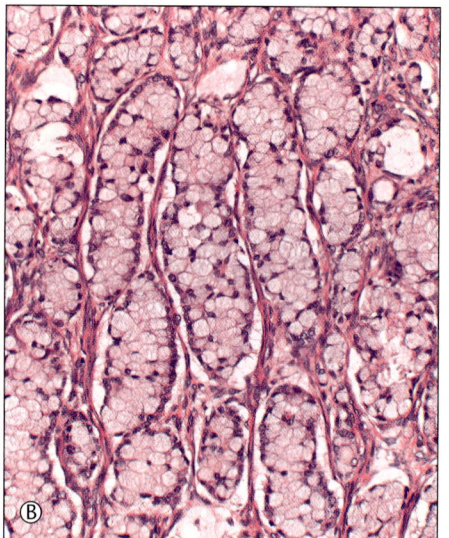

Fig. 29.30 Tubular Krukenberg tumors. **(A)** Tubules are composed of mucin-secreting cells with high-grade nuclei and set in dense cellular stroma. **(B)** Crowding of tubules to the exclusion of intervening stroma may yield a sertoliform pattern.

nodularity of the stroma may provide the only clue in routine sections.

Differential diagnosis

Fibromas may resemble Krukenberg tumors macroscopically, although the former are usually unilateral. The erroneous impression may be reinforced microscopically if the Krukenberg tumor has abundant fibromatous stroma with only sparse carcinoma cells. The correct diagnosis will not be missed if tumors are well sampled and sections showing vacuolated cells are stained for mucin.

Sertoli–Leydig cell tumors may simulate tubular Krukenberg tumors. Although vacuolated cells are sometimes present in Sertoli cell tubules, they lack mucin and the cells lack significant cytologic atypia. The stromal components of Sertoli–

Leydig cell tumors lack signet-ring cells but contain Leydig cells that may be difficult to distinguish from the luteinized stromal cells of Krukenberg tumors. The accompanying stromal cells in Krukenberg tumors may be reactive for α-inhibin and calretinin (as are sex cord-stromal tumors), so it is vital to carefully identify which cells are reactive.[116]

Vacuolated cells are present in sclerosing stromal tumors and in its apparently unique variant 'signet-ring stromal tumor of ovary' (see Chapter 26) but neither of these contains mucin. Vacuolated cells have also been described in gastrointestinal stromal tumors metastatic to the ovaries; mucin is absent and the signet-ring cells merge with adjacent spindle cells.[75]

Mucinous (goblet cell) carcinoids may have large numbers of mucin-rich signetring cells but will stain with Grimelius stain as well as for chromogranin and synaptophysin.[152] Primary

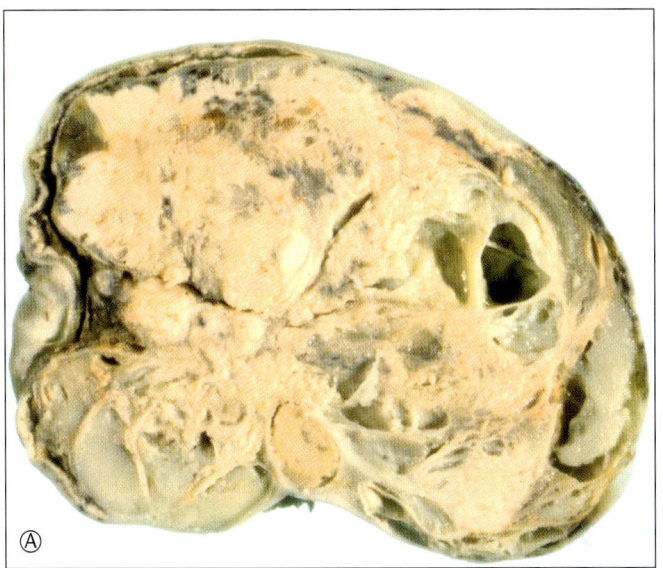
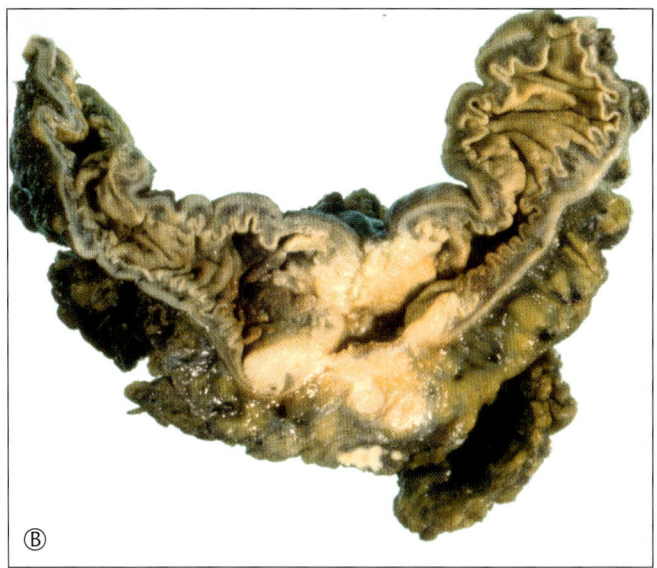

Fig. 29.31 Metastatic colonic adenocarcinoma. Large solid/cystic ovarian metastasis (**A**), from Dukes stage D carcinoma (**B**).

mucinous carcinoids would be expected to have associated teratomatous components in most cases.[198]

Krukenberg tumors may exhibit numerous small cysts lined by flattened cells and suggestive of clear cell carcinoma. Conversely, clear cell adenocarcinomas may also have signet-ring areas, but distinctive more typical clear cell areas should be present (see Chapter 25).

Rarely, 'primary' Krukenberg tumors have been reported. It is vital that, before this diagnosis is made, extensive investigations (which may involve a thorough autopsy) and/or prolonged follow-up (at least 10 years after oophorectomy) occur, in order to exclude a primary elsewhere.[91,116,152]

Prognosis
Krukenberg tumors are associated with an average survival of a little over 1 year, irrespective of whether or not there is a known or declared primary site.[91] Krukenberg tumors presenting in pregnancy are associated with a particularly aggressive clinical course.[54]

METASTASES FROM COLON AND RECTUM
Clinical profile
The most commonly occurring metastatic carcinoma to mimic primary ovarian carcinoma is that of large bowel origin.[34,64] Patients with such metastases are generally older (peri- or postmenopausal) than those with metastases from gastric carcinoma. The ovarian metastases in over half of patients are part of diffuse intraperitoneal disease. A few have abnormal uterine bleeding or virilization resulting from the endocrine activity of luteinized ovarian stromal cells. This phenomenon may occur with any secondary tumor but is most common with colorectal malignancies. About 75% have had an intestinal carcinoma removed, in most cases less than 3 years previously. However, clinicians may not provide this information or even consider it relevant in the workup of a gynecologic cancer. The remainder present as an apparent primary ovarian neoplasm. Women with colorectal carcinomas have an increased risk of developing primary ovarian carcinomas, particularly those with hered-

itary non-polyposis colon cancer.[108] For this reason, as well as to avoid the possibility of subsequent bulky ovarian metastases and the need for further surgery, some have recommended prophylactic bilateral oophorectomy at the time of initial colorectal surgery, especially for peri- or postmenopausal women. The issue, however, remains controversial.[62] Certainly, removal of ovarian metastases as part of radical cytoreductive surgery improves survival in some women.[62,118,157]

Pseudo-Meigs syndrome occasionally occurs in association with ovarian metastases from colorectal carcinoma.[45,124,135] In these cases, the non-malignant ascites and/or pleural effusion resolve after resection of the primary and metastatic tumors. Women with colorectal carcinoma metastatic to the ovaries have raised serum CA125 levels in one-third of cases, prior to oophorectomy.[99]

Macroscopic features
Approximately 70% of colorectal metastases are bilateral and, like those of gastric origin, may be large (Figure 29.31). Capsular adhesions, associated with peritoneal metastases or direct tumor infiltration, are sometimes present. The lobulated or multinodular masses frequently have a cystic component with spaces filled with necrotic debris (Figure 29.32) or, less often, clear or mucinous fluid, and they may thus simulate primary ovarian mucinous carcinomas. Other intra-abdominal metastases are commonly present. Lymph nodes and liver parenchyma are often involved.

Microscopic features
Metastases typically resemble the corresponding primary colorectal carcinoma. In most cases, this means that the tumor mimics a primary ovarian endometrioid carcinoma. Glandular spaces of varying sizes are present and cribriform foci are common (Figures 29.33 and 29.34). A characteristic feature is pseudocyst formation that results from central necrosis of tumor nodules, leaving a rim of viable epithelium, the so-called 'garland-like' growth pattern (Figure 29.32). The presence of karyorrhectic material and inflammatory cells in the densely eosinophilic coarsely granular necrotic debris has led to the

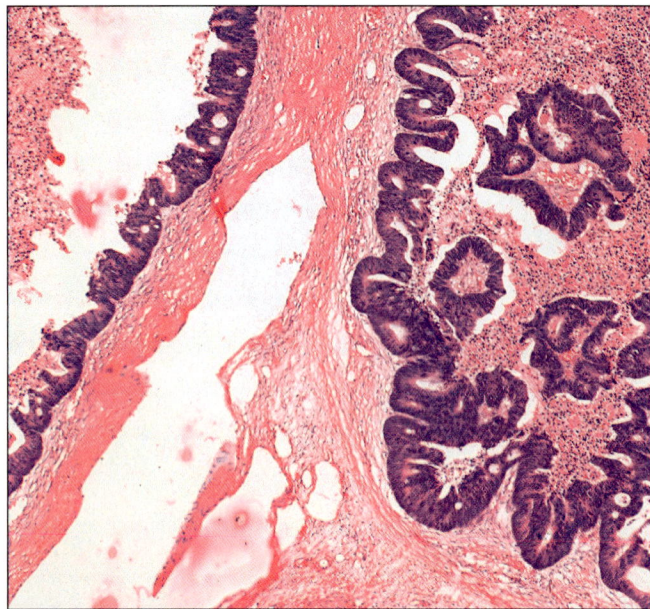

Fig. 29.32 Pseudocystic change in metastatic colonic carcinoma. Necrosis in center of tumor nodules leaves a rim of viable epithelium – the so-called 'garland' pattern – responsible for specific cytologic features (so-called 'dirty' necrosis).

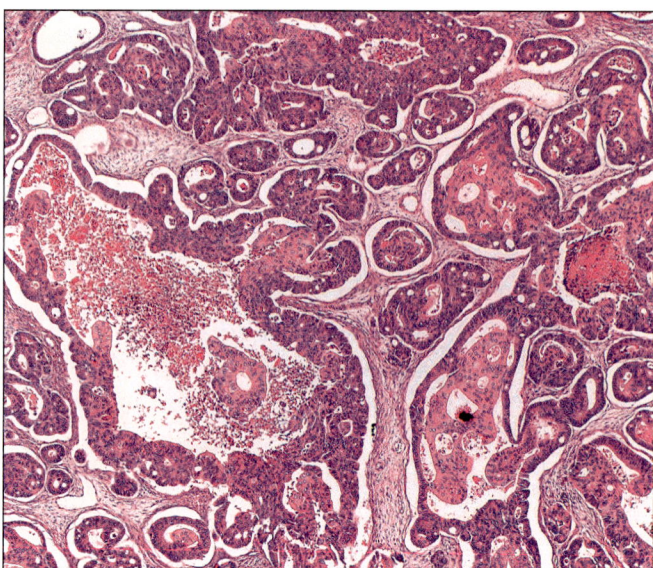

Fig. 29.34 Ovarian metastasis from colonic adenocarcinoma. Cellular arrangement is cribriform (pseudoendometrioid) with garland pattern at bottom. Note the intraluminal cellular aggregates where the cells have enlarged to resemble squamous morules (left center).

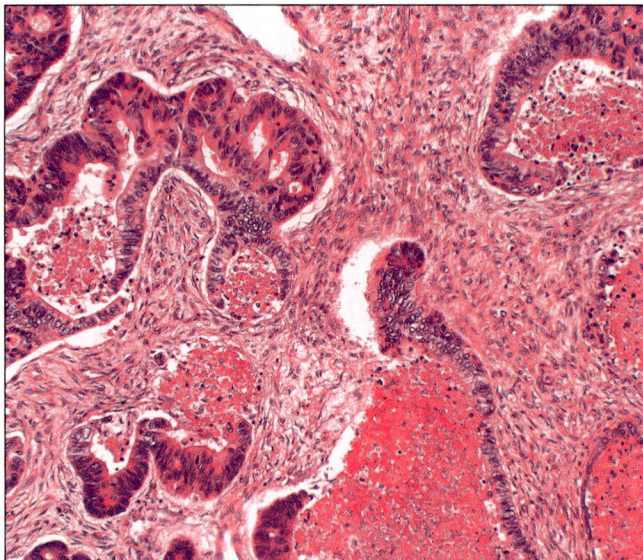

Fig. 29.33 Metastatic colonic adenocarcinoma showing a cribriform pattern resembling endometrioid carcinoma. The glandular epithelium is focally necrotic (center and left) producing a characteristic crescent of viable tumor. Contrast with Figure 29.35 (mucinous type).

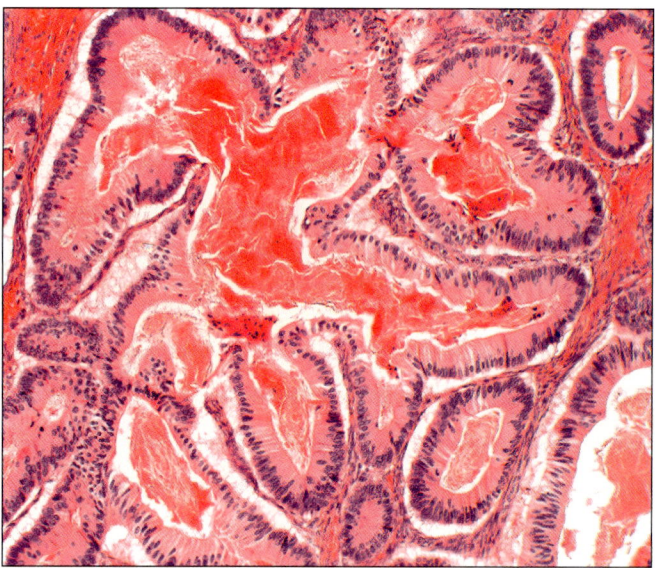

Fig. 29.35 Metastatic colonic carcinoma of mucinous type. Epithelium lining glands appears deceptively bland at this magnification. Contrast with Figure 29.33 (pseudoendometrioid pattern).

term 'dirty' necrosis for this appearance.[64] Individual glands may also show segmental necrosis of their epithelial lining (Figure 29.33). Mucin production is almost always demonstrable but is generally limited to the apical cytoplasm and gland lumens. Occasional goblet cells may be seen. A metastatic colorectal adenocarcinoma would be expected to show more cellular pleomorphism with more hyperchromatic nuclei than a primary ovarian lesion.

In a smaller proportion of cases, the tumor may mimic a primary ovarian mucinous neoplasm. There may be areas resembling benign (Figure 29.35) and borderline (proliferating) mucinous cystadenoma, as well as areas with destructive stromal invasion. Trabecular patterns and foci of Krukenberg-type infiltration are occasionally encountered.

The stroma is very variable in amount and may show collagenization, edema or myxoid change. The stroma in half of tumors is thecoma-like, being composed of plump spindle cells. About one-third of all colorectal metastases contain foci of frank stromal cell luteinization. Luteinized cells have abundant vacuolated or granular eosinophilic cytoplasm. They are arranged in small clusters or appear to ensheath groups of carcinoma cells and are often most conspicuous at the margins of the tumor (Figure 29.36). In pregnancy, luteinized cells may

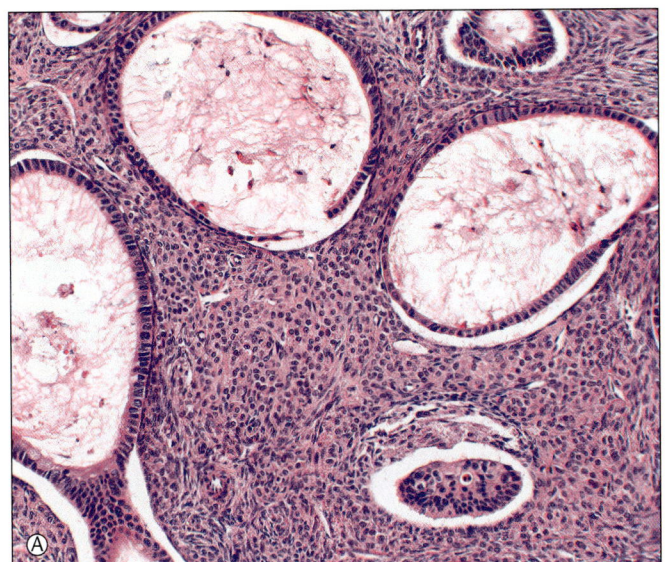 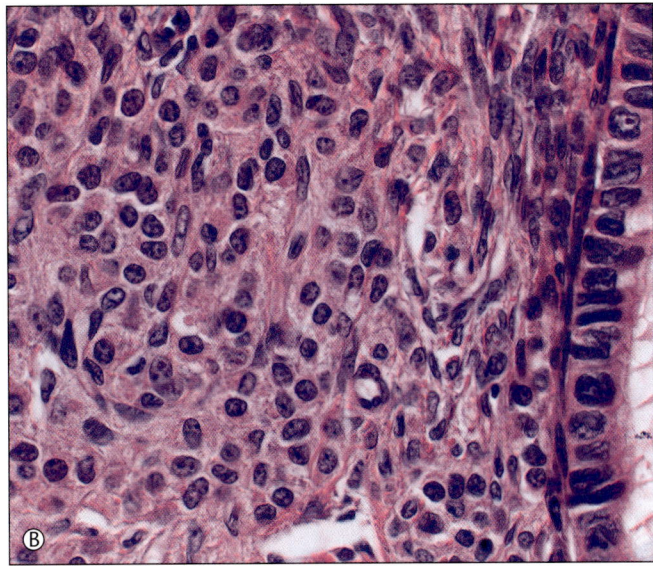

Fig. 29.36 Stromal luteinization associated with metastatic colonic carcinoma. **(A)** Hyperplastic stroma separates the malignant glands. **(B)** Detail of stromal cells showing abundant eosinophilic cytoplasm. The nuclei are round to oval and cytologically benign.

become confluent and fill the spaces between the epithelial components.

Less than 10% of colorectal metastases have the pathologic characteristics of Krukenberg tumors (see above). Rare colorectal metastases have a clear cell morphology[213] and mimic either a primary ovarian clear cell carcinoma or the secretory variant of endometrioid carcinoma. A thorough search should be made for more typical areas of metastatic colorectal carcinoma.

Sections of capsular adhesions may reveal direct tumor infiltration or small discrete peritoneal metastases (Figure 29.12). Lymphatic permeation is often present in the ovarian hilus and accompanying fallopian tube (Figure 29.11).

Differential diagnosis

In women without a prior history of intestinal carcinoma and in whom no other abdominal neoplasm is readily apparent at the time of oophorectomy, the often difficult problem arises of distinguishing a primary ovarian adenocarcinoma (mucinous or endometrioid) from a colorectal metastasis. Features favoring metastatic carcinoma are bilaterality, multinodular pattern, surface tumor deposits, extensive lymphovascular permeation (especially in hilar and para-ovarian vessels), extensive necrosis, lack of a fibrous capsule or a true cystic component, an infiltrative pattern of stromal invasion, and prominent stromal luteinization (Table 29.2).[98] The 'garland' pattern with cribriform areas and 'dirty' necrosis seem to be the most useful microscopic features to allow differentiation from primary endometrioid carcinoma although this is not always a reliable criterion.[116] The presence of squamous differentiation strongly favors endometrioid adenocarcinoma, but rare primary adenosquamous carcinomas of the large intestine do occur.[63] Additionally, the presence of an adenofibromatous area or coexisting endometriosis favor an ovarian primary.

Confusingly, about one-third of metastatic mucinous tumors will display areas simulating benign and/or proliferating mucinous cystadenoma and non-invasive carcinoma, known as the 'maturation phenomenon'.[64,208] Single cell invasion, signet-ring cells, and microscopic surface mucin point towards a metasta-

Table 29.2 Primary mucinous adenocarcinoma of ovary versus metastatic colonic carcinoma: differential diagnosis

Primary mucinous carcinoma	Metastatic colonic carcinoma
Clinical profile	
Bilateral in <20%	Bilateral in 70%
Metastases, if present, are peritoneal and superficial	Other metastases common, in lymph nodes and liver parenchyma
Macroscopic features	
Cystic component prominent	Multinodular solid tumors
Necrosis mild to moderate	Necrosis usually marked, producing pseudocysts
Microscopic features	
Thick acellular fibrous capsule around periphery in many	No peripheral capsule
Epithelial transitions common	Epithelial transitions uncommon ('maturation' phenomenon)
Stromal luteinization uncommon	Stromal luteinization common
Immunoprofile	
Mostly CK-7 positive, CK-20 negative	Mostly CK-7 negative, CK-20 positive

sis. Features favoring a primary mucinous tumor include size >10 cm, an expansile pattern of invasion, a complex papillary pattern, a smooth external surface, and the presence of a coexisting Brenner tumor, teratoma or mural nodule.[64,98]

Specific immunohistochemical panels have proven useful in distinguishing ovarian tumors from gastrointestinal tumors in many instances. Endometrioid and clear cell carcinomas of müllerian origin are reactive for CA125 and CK7, but not CK20 and CEA (except in foci of squamous differentiation) while tumors of gastrointestinal origin with an endometrioid

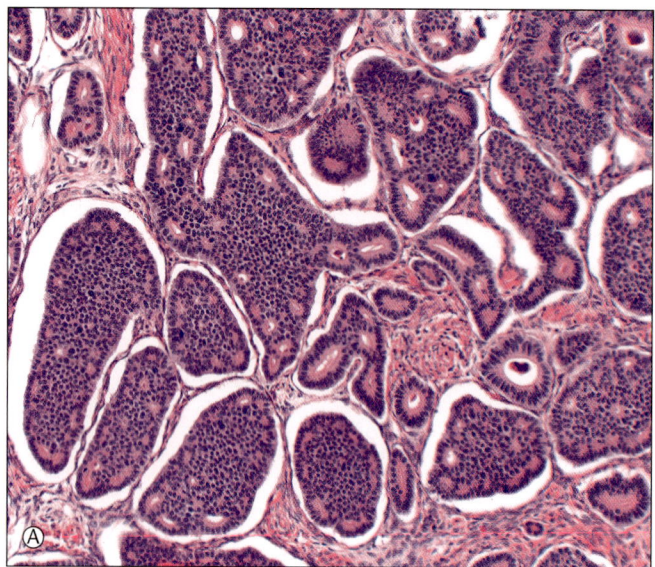
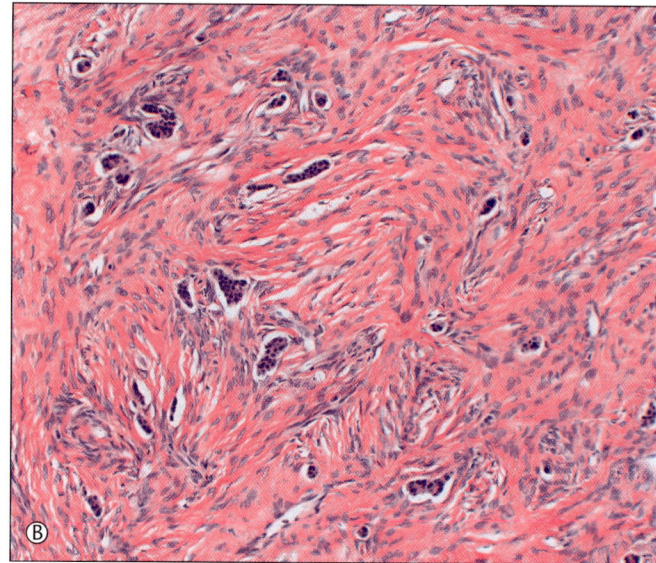

Fig. 29.37 Metastatic carcinoid tumor, insular type. From a 71-year-old woman with widespread intraperitoneal disease; a primary ileal tumor had been resected 2 years previously. **(A)** Uniform closely packed groups of cells with peripheral palisading. Retraction artifact is prominent. A few acini are present. **(B)** In this area, the cell groups are separated by abundant sclerotic stroma.

or clear cell appearance have findings that generally are reversed.[64,116,199]

Differentiation between primary and metastatic mucinous carcinomas can be more difficult. Immunohistochemical overlap is sufficient to reduce its value, while complex rules apply and with many exceptions. Primary ovarian mucinous carcinomas are reactive for CK7 (unless they are teratomatous in origin) but, in contrast to the endometrioid tumors, many show focal or even widespread reactivity for CK20 (see Chapter 25), reflecting intestinal differentiation.[64] Conversely, colorectal carcinomas of mucinous type are usually strongly and diffusely reactive for CK20 and, at most, exhibit only focal CK7 reactivity. Poorly differentiated and right-sided colonic carcinomas, by contrast, can have a reactive CK7/unreactive CK20 immunophenotype.[64,152]

MUC5AC is said to identify ovarian mucinous tumors but is also positive in some colorectal mucinous tumors. MUC2 is reactive in 90% of metastatic colonic carcinomas but also stains a variable proportion of ovarian mucinous primaries, and we have not found it particularly useful. Cdx2 and β-catenin typically show nuclear reactivity in colorectal carcinomas.[115] Ovarian mucinous primaries show wide variation in reported reactivity to Cdx2.[7,64,116] Nuclear reactivity of primary ovarian mucinous tumors for β-catenin is infrequent.[26]

Alpha-methylacyl-coenzyme A racemase, also known as P504S, is a recently described cytoplasmic protein that has been utilized in a panel with Cdx2 and β-catenin. Reactivity with all three markers is diagnostic of a colorectal origin.[102] Human alveolar macrophage 56 (HAM-56) reactivity favors an ovarian primary while the opposite is true for strong immunoreactivity for p53.[152] CEA is a poor discriminator. In view of these immunohistochemical inconsistencies, it is vital that the final diagnosis of any mucinous neoplasm in the ovaries be made only after taking into account all morphologic and immunohistochemical features, as well as clinical and operative information.

METASTATIC CARCINOID TUMORS

Carcinoid tumors account for less than 2% of tumors metastatic to the ovaries but it is important to distinguish them from primary ovarian carcinoid tumors and from other ovarian tumors that share some histologic characteristics but carry disparate prognoses.

Clinical profile
Most patients with metastatic carcinoid are over 40 years of age. Symptoms of pelvic or abdominal masses are commonly present and the carcinoid syndrome is present preoperatively in 40% of surgical cases. The ileum is the most common site of the primary tumor. Cecum, appendix, jejunum, and pancreas are less common sites. Metastasis from a bronchial carcinoid is quite rare.[74]

At operation, both ovaries are invariably involved, sometimes only apparent on microscopic examination. Abdominal metastases (mesenteric, omental, and peritoneal) are usually also evident, but liver involvement is often only minimal or absent (except in patients with the carcinoid syndrome).

Diagnosis
Any or all of the typical histologic patterns of carcinoid tumors may be present, but the most common is the insular pattern typical of midgut carcinoids, which reflects the most frequent source of these tumors. The cell groups often show peripheral palisading of nuclei, and small acini may be present in the center or more prominently at the margins of the islands (Figures 29.37A and 29.38), especially in those tumors that are functional. An unusual variant has shown central spindling within the islands of metastatic carcinoid cells (Figure 29.39). Large follicle-like spaces have been described, probably due to lymphatic obstruction as the tumor grows.[214] The nuclei are central with coarse but evenly clumped chromatin. Mitoses are

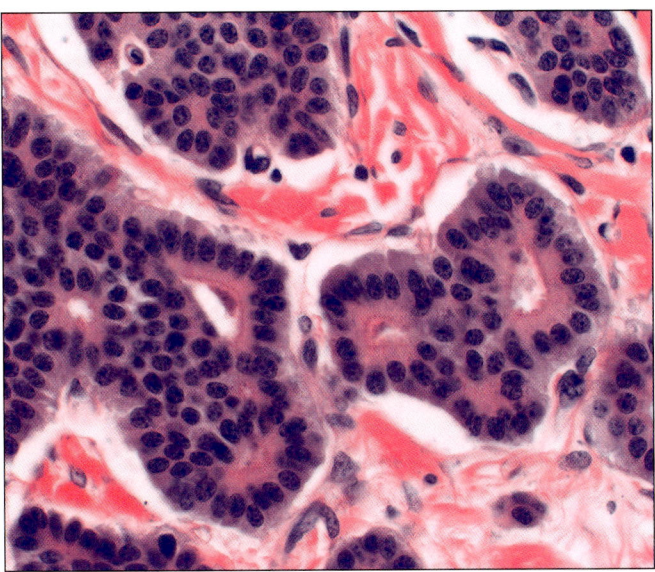

Fig. 29.38 Metastatic carcinoid tumor. Some cell groups form acini; central lumens are well defined and surrounded by radially orientated low columnar cells, in contrast to the Call–Exner bodies of granulosa cell tumors.

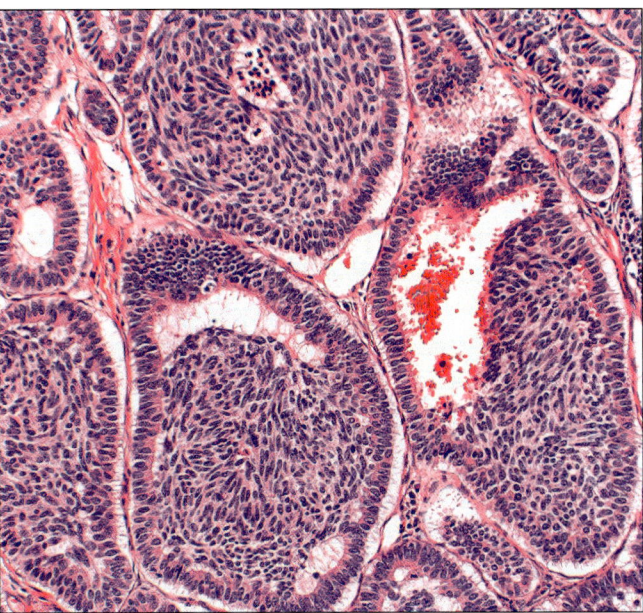

Fig. 29.39 Metastatic carcinoid tumor in an 89-year-old woman. The large solid right ovarian mass was characterized by islands of small central spindled cells with distinct peripheral palisading by tall columnar cells with eosinophilic cytoplasm. Immunostains were strongly positive for chromogranin and synaptophysin. Courtesy of Dr J Ferguson, Canberra, Australia.

usually sparse. The eosinophilic, sometimes granular, cytoplasm is usually argentaffinic.

The cells' neuroendocrine nature can be confirmed simply by demonstrating immunohistochemical reactivity for NSE, chromogranin, synaptophysin or specific secretory products such as serotonin. The abundant fibromatous stroma, thought to be at least partly induced by fibroblast growth factors elaborated by the enterochromaffin cells,[42] may become hypocellular and hyalinized (Figure 29.37B) or, less commonly, luteinized. Calcification of the stroma or intraluminal secretions may be present. Vascular invasion is sometimes observed. The microscopic pattern of mucinous or goblet cell carcinoid should also be recognized. These are almost always of appendiceal origin (see below). They contain goblet cells as well as argentaffin or argyrophil cells.

Differential diagnosis

Distinction from a primary ovarian carcinoid tumor may be difficult except when there is evidence of coexisting cystic teratoma on the one hand, or an intestinal tumor on the other. Without these strong clues, bilaterality is the most useful discriminator (Table 29.3) and bilateral tumors should be considered as metastatic cancer until proven otherwise. Primary tumors rarely have peritoneal deposits at initial presentation. The above observations mandate that if an ovarian carcinoid tumor is diagnosed at frozen section, the contralateral ovary and abdominal contents should be carefully examined for evidence of further tumor. Sometimes the contralateral ovary will be normal in size, but involved, emphasizing the importance of microscopic examination of even normal-appearing ovaries (Figure 29.40). On macroscopic examination, primary tumors present a more homogeneous and less nodular appearance than that of secondary tumors. Postoperative radiologic examination of the abdomen and urinary 5-hydroxyindoleacetic acid (5-HIAA) estimations may be helpful. If the ovarian tumors are metastatic, abdominal recurrences usually become apparent within a few months.

Table 29.3 Primary versus secondary carcinoid tumor: differential diagnosis

Metastatic carcinoid	Primary carcinoid
Clinical profile	
Primary site apparent in 80%	No intestinal tumor
Peritoneal seeding and abdominal metastases frequent	Extraovarian spread uncommon
Early recurrence and progression	Low rate of recurrence
Macroscopic features	
Bilateral almost always	Unilateral always
Cut surface nodular and variegated	Cut surface homogeneous
Microscopic features	
Teratomatous elements absesnt	Teratomatous elements usually present

Granulosa cell tumors display insular and trabecular patterns and have true macrofollicles; however, other patterns, e.g., diffuse and follicular, not found in carcinoids, are also present. Call–Exner bodies are distinguished from the true acinar spaces with luminal cytoplasm of carcinoid tumors by the haphazard rather than radial arrangement of cells and peripheral nuclei that border them (Figure 29.38). Granulosa cells have grooved oval rather than round nuclei. The scanty cytoplasm of granulosa cell tumors is reactive for inhibin and calretinin, but is not argyrophilic, and is unreactive for cytokeratins and neuroendocrine markers.

Transitional cell tumors have abundant fibromatous stroma surrounding islands of multilayered cells with elongate grooved

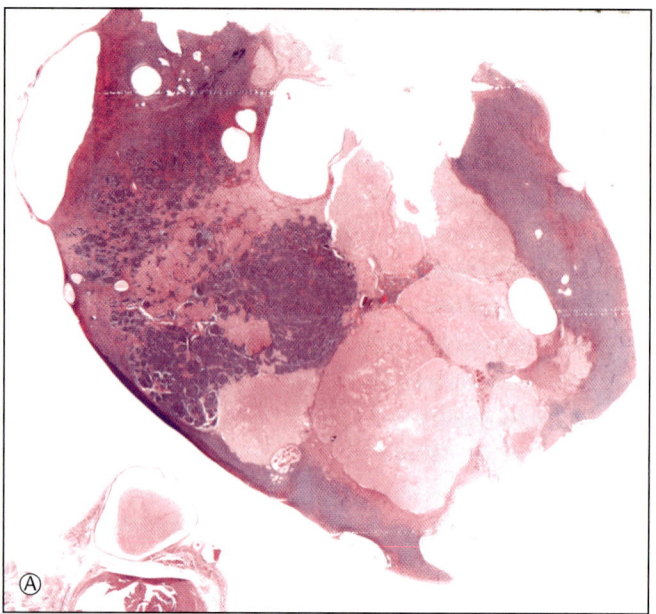

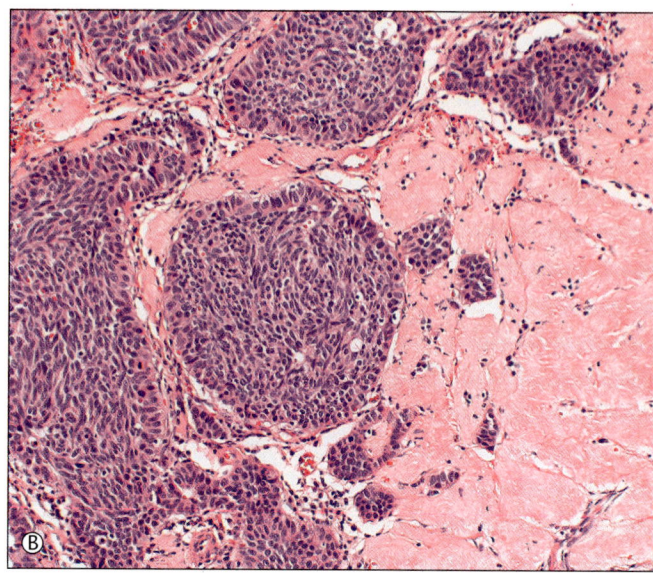

Fig. 29.40 Metastatic carcinoid tumor. Small atrophic contralateral ovary from same patient as Figure 29.39. **(A)** Survey of ovary. **(B)** Carcinoid tumor infiltrating the margin of an old corpus albicans. Courtesy of Dr J Ferguson, Canberra, Australia.

nuclei. The cytoplasm is only focally argyrophilic. The islands often include central mucinous epithelial cells and there may also be separate simple mucinous cysts.

Adenofibromas very occasionally resemble carcinoid tumors microscopically and on low-power microscopic examination. However higher magnification will reveal that the cystic spaces are lined by typical müllerian epithelia.

Poorly differentiated primary or metastatic adenocarcinomas, including small cell neuroendocrine carcinomas,[48] may superficially resemble metastatic carcinoid tumors, but closer inspection reveals focal necrosis, obvious nuclear pleomorphism and numerous mitoses. The neat organoid patterns of carcinoids are absent.

Metastatic mucinous carcinoids[92] need to be distinguished from metastatic adenocarcinomas. Mucinous carcinoids may contain foci of pure adenocarcinoma; conversely, metastatic gastric carcinoma may contain scattered argentaffin or argyrophil cells. The diagnosis of a mucinous carcinoid (apart from finding the appendiceal primary tumor) should be made in the presence of the typical pattern of nests containing an admixture of signet-ring cells and cells containing argentaffin granules.

Treatment and prognosis

As discussed above, recognition in the operating theater that a carcinoid tumor is metastatic to the ovary can prompt an immediate search for the intestinal primary. This will almost certainly thwart an obstructive episode that otherwise usually occurs within months. The prognosis for patients with ovarian metastases from a carcinoid tumor is poor. One-third of patients die within 1 year and two-thirds within 4 years. At autopsy, there is usually extensive peritoneal and nodal disease as well as hepatic and other visceral metastases. Morphologic evidence of carcinoid heart disease is present in 70%.

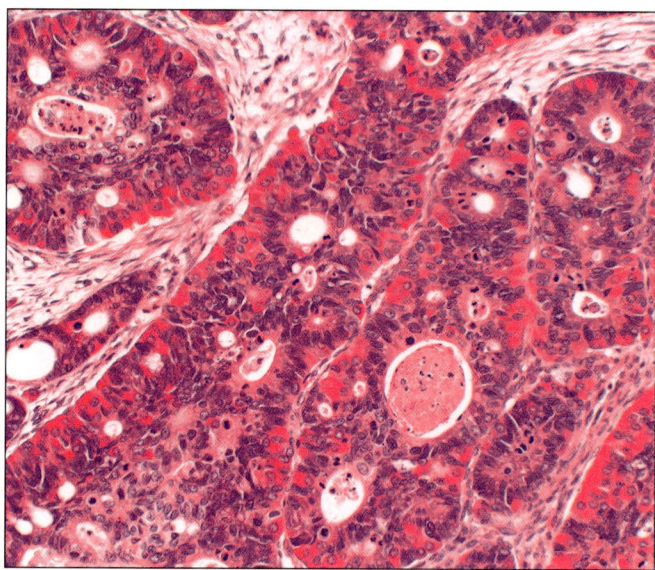

Fig. 29.41 Metastatic adenocarcinoma from jejunum. A prominent cribriform pattern is complemented by extreme prominence of brightly eosinophilic Paneth cells.

METASTASES FROM SMALL INTESTINE

Ovarian metastases from other tumors of the small intestine are rare. A handful of metastatic adenocarcinomas from duodenum and jejunum (Figure 29.41) is known.[88,103,163,164] Of the few reported cases, most have been glandular and a solitary one was a Krukenberg tumor. The potential for misdiagnosis as primary ovarian carcinoma exists and, once again, a high index of suspicion is warranted. Although these gastrointesti-

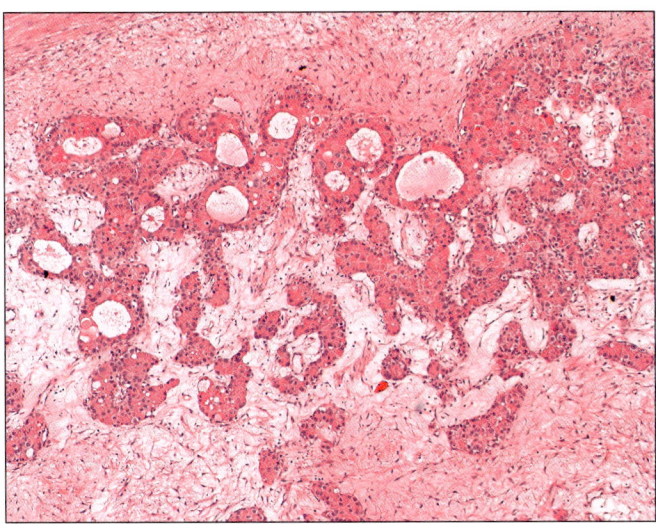

Fig. 29.42 Metastatic adenocarcinoid (mucinous carcinoid) tumor of appendiceal origin.

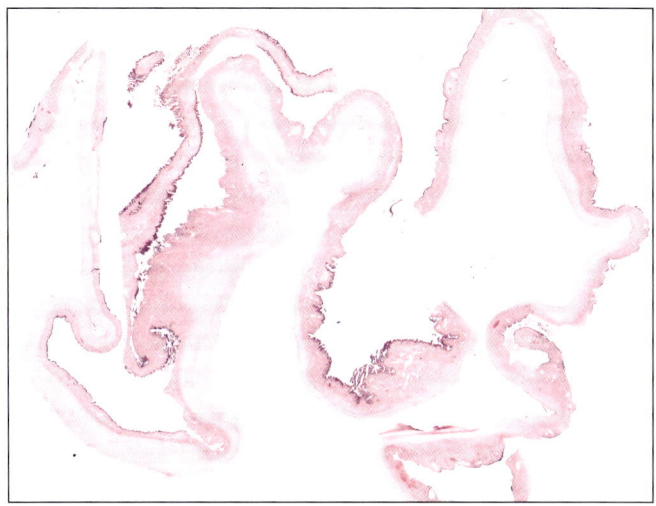

Fig. 29.43 Metastatic pancreatic carcinoma. Scan of section displaying parvilocular cystic pattern.

nal tumors were reactive for CK20 and CEA, but not CK7 or CA125,[88,163] variations in their immunoprofile may occur. In one study, most primary small intestinal carcinomas were reactive for CK7 and one-third not for CK20.[23]

Gastrointestinal stromal tumor can also metastasize to the ovaries.[75] In one case bilateral ovarian tumors manifested 27 years after the bowel primary and, in another, the intestinal tumor was not evident until autopsy 18 months later. The differential diagnosis in such cases is broad, encompassing leiomyosarcoma (primary or metastatic), endometrial stromal neoplasm (primary or metastatic), other mesenchymal neoplasms (benign or malignant), sarcomatoid sex cord-stromal tumor, and melanoma. Reactivity with c-kit (CD117) and CD34, but not desmin, is expected.

Primary jejunal leiomyosarcoma has also been described with metastasis to the ovaries.[104]

METASTASES FROM THE APPENDIX

Appendiceal metastases are of three main types: frankly invasive adenocarcinoma, carcinoid (usually mucinous), and low-grade mucinous epithelial tumors. Adenocarcinomas metastasize to the ovaries in about 10% of cases. They can present, however, as an ovarian mass. They may resemble primary mucinous or endometrioid carcinoma or may have a signet-ring morphology.[64] A similar approach as for metastatic large bowel tumors should be taken.[29]

The least common appendiceal carcinomas to metastasize to the ovary are adenocarcinoids, also known as mucinous or goblet cell carcinoids (Figure 29.42). Metastases of these rare tumors occur at a rate that warrants bilateral oophorectomy at the time the primary tumor is resected. Furthermore, close inspection of the appendix should be done routinely whenever any mucinous tumor of the ovaries is removed. Microscopically, both the appendiceal and ovarian lesions show rounded nests containing goblet cells and argentaffin or argyrophil cells. They may also have foci resembling Krukenberg tumor[111] or mucinous cystadenocarcinoma.[22,73] Immunohistochemical studies for neuroendocrine markers may be necessary to confirm the tumor's nature.[111,116] The differential diagnosis

includes the vanishingly rare primary ovarian goblet cell carcinoids, which display other neoplastic associations suggesting primary ovarian tumorigenesis (e.g., teratomatous elements in about one half of cases, other patterns of carcinoid tumor, proliferating mucinous tumors, etc.) and are usually confined to one ovary.[64,116]

The frequency with which patients with low-grade mucinous tumors of the appendix also have similar tumors in one or both ovaries and pseudomyxoma peritonei is high. The origin and nature of these tumors were and still remain somewhat controversial, although studies of mucin gene expression, cytokeratin profiles, and molecular genetics have strongly favored a metastatic nature to the vast majority of ovarian tumors.[64] This is discussed further in Chapters 24 and 33.

METASTASES FROM PANCREAS

Metastases from the exocrine pancreas are particularly rare but are noteworthy for the frequency with which they simulate primary ovarian cancer. This is particularly likely if the pancreatic neoplasm is in the body or tail of the pancreas, as symptoms from these tumors may not appear until late in the course of the disease.[116] The ovarian secondaries are often large multicystic masses (Figure 29.43) that show a range of microscopic appearances mimicking mucinous cystadenoma, proliferating mucinous tumor (i.e., 'of borderline malignancy') (Figure 29.44), and well-differentiated mucinous cystadenocarcinoma. The tumor may require extensive sampling to reveal destructive stromal invasion.[116]

Differential diagnosis

As in other metastatic lesions, features suggesting an extraovarian primary include bilaterality, nodular growth pattern, surface desmoplastic implants, lymphovascular invasion, and extensive intra-abdominal spread. Cytokeratin immunohistochemistry is unproductive for differentiating these from primary ovarian mucinous carcinoma. Both are regularly reactive for CK7, and while the primary ovarian carcinoma may be unreactive for CK20, so may the pancreatic metastases (Figure 29.45). Loss of the nuclear transcription factor DPC4, which occurs

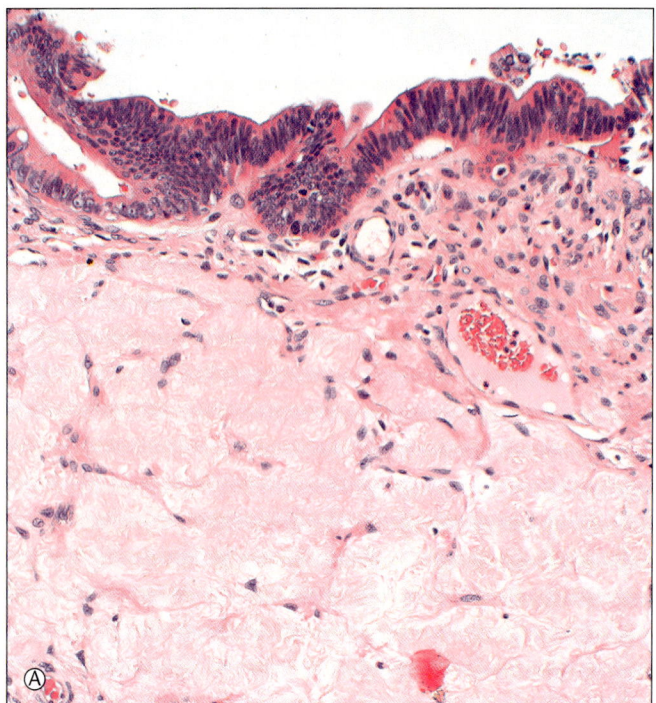

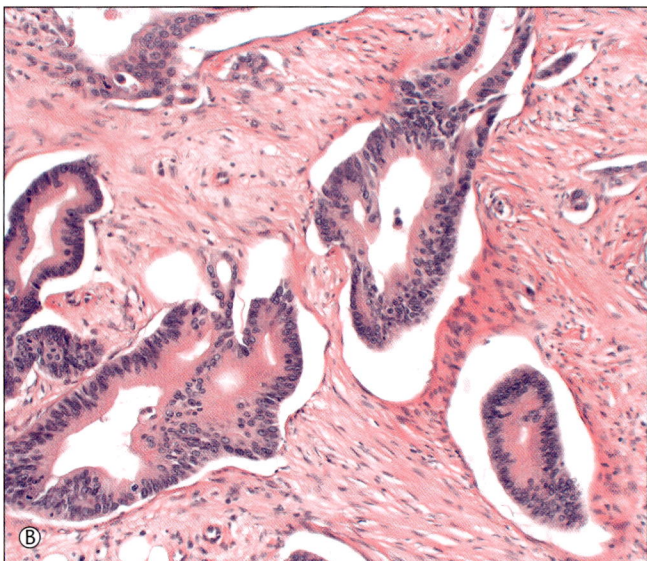

Fig. 29.44 Metastatic pancreatic adenocarcinoma (same case as Figure 29.43). **(A)** While the epithelium is clearly atypical, its lack of variability differs from the usual pattern of a primary mucinous carcinoma. Note also the predominantly mid-cellular position of the vertically oriented cigar-shaped nuclei. **(B)** The primary pancreatic neoplasm in this case, for comparison.

in 50% of pancreatic carcinomas, indicates a pancreatic primary as most ovarian mucinous tumors are reactive.[116] Other recently described markers may also prove useful. Mesothelin, fascin, and prostate stem cell antigen (PSCA) more often all show reactivity in metastatic pancreatic carcinoma (73%, 73%, and 82%, respectively), unlike primary ovarian mucinous carcinoma (17%, 26%, and 43%, respectively) where reactivity is much less common.[19]

Pancreatic carcinomas can give rise to Krukenberg tumors and also to tumors resembling insular carcinoid.[64] If there is extensive omental or peritoneal disease, the differential diagnosis may include ovarian or primary peritoneal serous carcinoma. Reactivity for WT1 will confirm a müllerian serous malignancy as pancreatic neoplasms are unreactive.[116]

METASTASES FROM GALL BLADDER AND BILE DUCTS

Carcinomas of the gall bladder or bile ducts (Figure 29.46) sporadically metastasize to the ovary.[5,51,79,189] Patients' ages range from 33 to 73 years. Like other primaries, the presentation may be that of an ovarian mass, be discovered synchronously or appear up to 2 years later.

The tumors may vary in their appearances, resembling endometrioid or mucinous carcinoma, a Krukenberg tumor or even a Sertoli–Leydig cell tumor. As with other metastases, diagnosis depends on an awareness of a possible extraovarian origin as well as on the usual features of bilaterality, multinodularity (macroscopically and/or microscopically), and implants on the ovarian surface.

METASTASES FROM LIVER

METASTATIC HEPATOCELLULAR CARCINOMA

Hepatocellular carcinoma metastatic to the ovaries is exceptionally rare (Figure 29.16) but must be included in the differential diagnosis of ovarian oxyphil cell tumors. In the handful of known cases,[13,35,86,147,217] the patients' ages were 17–67 years. The ovarian masses were identified synchronously with the liver tumor or occurred some later time. In one case, the ovarian metastasis presented 2 years after orthotopic liver transplantation for hepatocellular carcinoma.[35]

Macroscopically, the ovarian tumors are usually bilateral, range from 4 to 11 cm in diameter, and may be solid or cystic. Microscopically, they consist of cells with moderate-to-abundant eosinophilic cytoplasm, either diffusely or arranged in nodules, nests and trabeculae. Cysts or glands and bile may be present. The lesion should be differentiated from primary hepatoid carcinoma of the ovaries[205,217] (see above), hepatoid variant of yolk sac tumor (see above), metastatic hepatoid tumors from other organs, eosinophilic variants of endometrioid and clear cell carcinoma, and steroid cell tumor.[116] Extensive sampling usually reveals the diagnosis. Immunohistochemical analysis for α-fetoprotein and Hep Par 1 does not distinguish among any of these entities as all are reactive.[116] B72.3, an oncofetal glycoprotein, is more useful as hepatoid carcinomas are reactive, unlike hepatocellular carcinoma.[106]

METASTATIC HEPATOBLASTOMA

One hepatoblastoma occurred in a 19-year-old woman with bilateral ovarian metastases.[57]

METASTATIC MALIGNANT MELANOMA

Ovarian metastases are present in about 15% of women who die of malignant melanoma, but only occasionally do they present as surgical biopsy specimens. The metastases usually

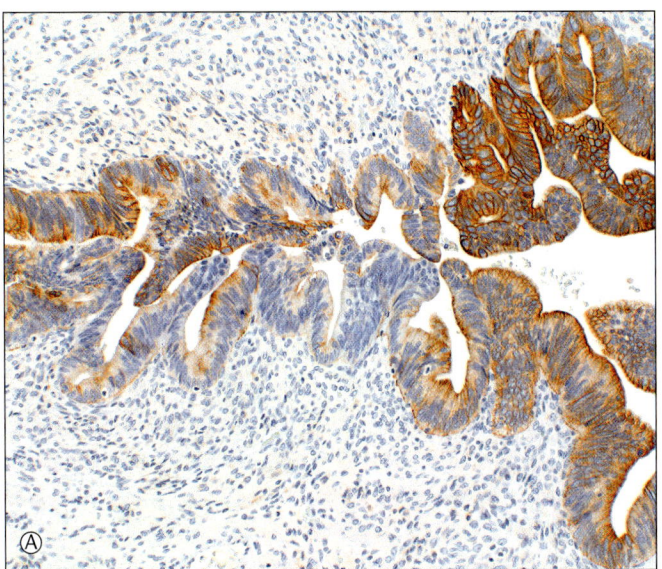
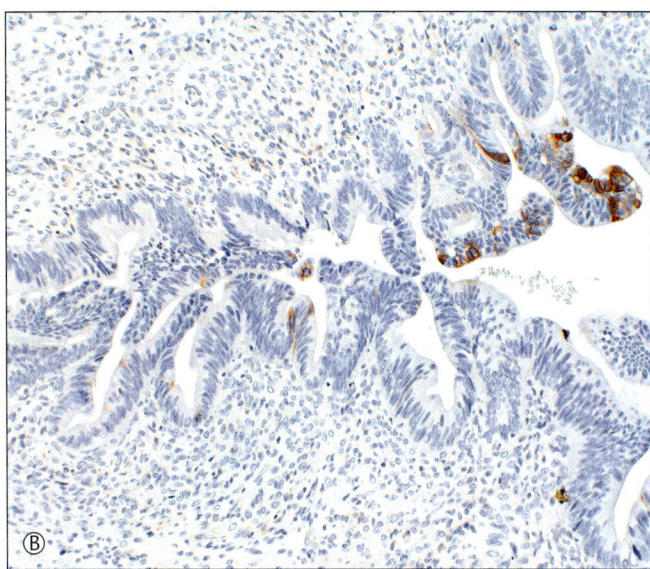

Fig. 29.45 Metastatic pancreatic adenocarcinoma (same case as Figure 29.43). The epithelium shows **(A)** strong immunostaining for CK7 and **(B)** focal immunostaining for CK20.

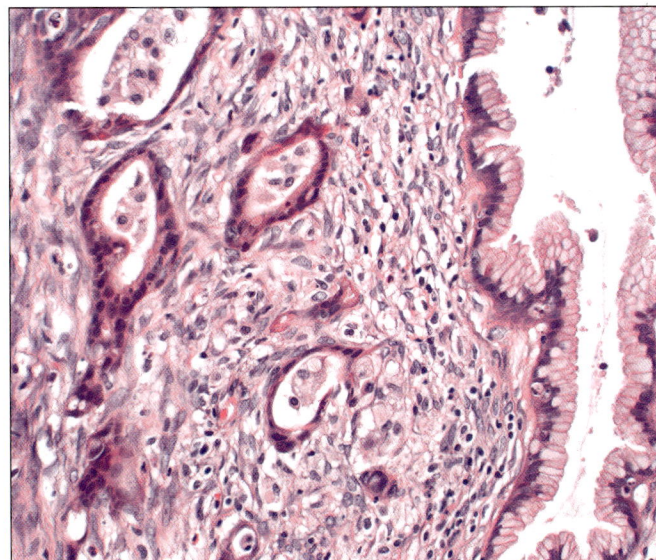

Fig. 29.46 Metastatic cholangiocarcinoma, from a tumor arising in the extrahepatic bile ducts. Epithelium at the left is deceptively bland, while infiltrating carcinoma is noted to the right.

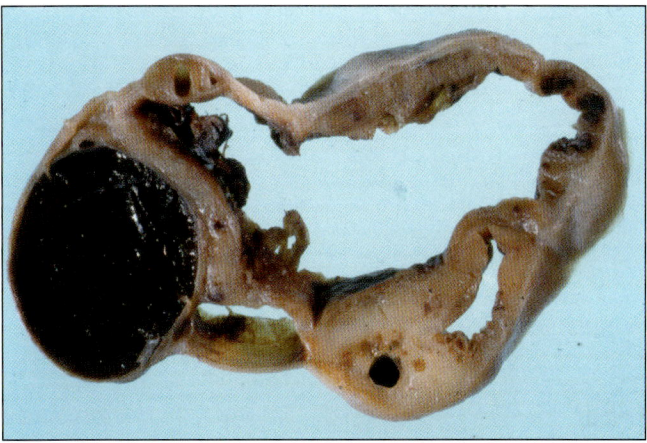

Fig. 29.47 Malignant melanoma metastatic to the ovary of an 18-year-old girl. A skin lesion had been excised a few weeks previously. The large mass is hemorrhagic, cystic, and focally pigmented.

result from hematogenous spread and occur in a setting of disseminated disease, though rarely may prove to be solitary.[80] They outnumber primary ovarian malignant melanomas by a ratio of at least 2:1. The ovarian lesions only occasionally clinically manifest as apparent primary neoplasm.[149,158,211] In countries with high frequencies of cutaneous melanomas, such as Australia, these tumors may constitute up to 10% of surgically resected ovarian metastases. They may present up to 25 years after the primary lesion has been excised. Sometimes the primary lesion undergoes regression or is clinically occult (adrenal gland, eye, mucosal sites) and is not identified during life or even by thorough autopsy examination. Rare ovarian

melanomas are true primary neoplasms – generally considered to be of teratomatous origin[14] (see Chapter 27).

Pathology

Ovarian metastases of malignant melanoma usually form soft, multinodular masses. Importantly, in one recent series, over 90% of definitively metastatic lesions were unilateral.[60] The involved ovaries are enlarged, averaging 11 cm in diameter. Hemorrhage, cystic degeneration, and necrosis are usually conspicuous but pigmentation is variable (Figure 29.47). The microscopic features are those of metastatic melanoma elsewhere, but can be extremely variable and can simulate a variety of primary ovarian neoplasms (Figure 29.48).

Differential diagnosis

Pigmented metastases generally cause no problem in differential diagnosis, particularly if there is a known extraovarian

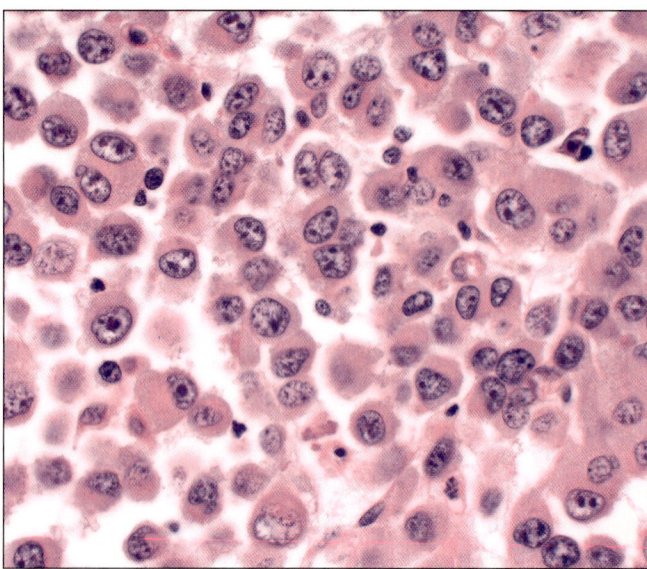

Fig. 29.48 Metastatic malignant melanoma. Diffuse pattern of large, non-cohesive polyhedral cells, with oval irregular nuclei containing single prominent nucleoli and abundant eosinophilic cytoplasm.

primary lesion. Amelanotic melanomas can be confused with primary or metastatic undifferentiated carcinomas, oxyphilic variants of clear cell and endometrioid carcinoma, sex cord-stromal tumors, endometrial stromal sarcomas, primary ovarian small cell carcinomas of hypercalcemic type (see above), large cell lymphoma (e.g., Ki-1 lymphoma; see Chapter 28), and dysgerminomas (see Chapter 27). Follicle-like structures have been described, leading to confusion with juvenile granulosa cell tumor and ovarian small cell carcinomas of hypercalcemic type.[60,116] An immunoprofile of reactivity for S-100 protein, melan-A, and HMB45, but not cytokeratin, usually confirms the diagnosis. However, sex cord-stromal tumors may be reactive for S-100 and melan-A and some steroid cell tumors are reactive for HMB45. Occasional melanomas are also reactive for α-inhibin, potentially confounding differentiation from sex cord-stromal tumors.[60, 116] Electron microscopy may prove useful in some cases.

An admittedly rare and difficult differential diagnosis is between primary and metastatic ovarian melanoma, a distinction of importance since the former is associated with a much better prognosis. Tumors associated with teratomatous elements suggest primary ovarian origin, although a solitary older case has been reported of bilateral metastases to dermoid cysts. Conversely, lack of teratomatous elements does not exclude primary ovarian origin since such evidence may have been obliterated by tumor growth or missed as a result of inadequate sampling. Evidence of primary origin is most convincing if lesions can be demonstrated to arise from a focus of preinvasive melanocytic proliferation such as junctional activity in the cyst lining of a teratoma, and prolonged follow-up during which no alternative primary site of melanoma declares itself, even including a regressed cutaneous melanoma.[117] Common sense dictates that, without specific evidence, an ovarian melanoma should be considered metastatic until proven otherwise.

METASTATIC NON-GENITAL CARCINOMAS AND SARCOMAS

METASTASES FROM KIDNEYS

Ovarian metastases are found at autopsy in <1% of women with renal adenocarcinomas. They rarely present clinical problems but they can be the initial manifestation of the disease[116,131,181] or present as isolated secondary lesions many years after nephrectomy.[2,197] Coexistent primary carcinomas of kidney and ovary may also occur.[8,194]

Differential diagnosis

On the rare occasion that clear cell adenocarcinoma of the kidney metastasizes to the ovaries, it must be distinguished from primary ovarian clear cell carcinoma.[212] Many features that usually suggest metastatic disease, e.g., bilaterality and macroscopic appearance of multiple nodules, are absent in these cases. The microscopic features that suggest metastatic renal cell carcinoma are a characteristic sinusoidal vascular pattern, the absence of hobnail cells lining the tubules and glands, the absence of intraluminal mucin, and hyaline basement membrane-like material. Primary ovarian clear cell carcinomas are more likely to have an admixture of patterns, such as tubulocystic, solid, and papillary, but morphologic overlap may occur.[116] The presence of endometriosis in the same ovary favors an ovarian primary.[182] A panel of antibodies can assist in distinguishing the two entities. An ovarian primary will display reactivity for CK7 and 34βE12 (a high molecular weight keratin cocktail including cytokeratins 1, 5, 10, and 14), and often estrogen and progesterone receptors and CA125, while renal clear cell carcinoma will be unreactive for these. In addition, renal cell carcinoma shows reactivity for CD10 and renal cell carcinoma (RCC) marker.[7,116,131]

The only other tumor that could enter the differential diagnosis is a steroid cell tumor but such neoplasms rarely have a tubular pattern. Reactivity for α-inhibin supports a diagnosis of steroid cell tumor.[116]

METASTASES FROM BLADDER

Metastatic transitional cell carcinoma (TCC) from the bladder or elsewhere in the urinary tract, to the ovaries, is also a rare occurrence. While bilaterality favors metastatic disease, primary ovarian TCC may also be bilateral. Extensive sampling is required to identify or exclude a component of benign or proliferating Brenner tumor or other ovarian surface epithelial–stromal tumor, which – if identified – would confirm a primary lesion. Immunohistochemical markers may contribute. Ovarian TCC is reactive for CK7 and CA125, may show nuclear reactivity with an antibody against the N-terminal of WT1 (analogous to ovarian serous carcinomas), and is unreactive for CK20. Bladder TCC is reactive for both CK7 and CK20 as well as uroplakin III and thrombomodulin.[7,77,116]

METASTASES FROM OTHER URINARY TRACT TUMORS

Bilateral Krukenberg tumors were found in a patient with primary renal pelvic TCC that had a prominent signet-ring cell component.[76] Occasionally, metastases from other tumors of the urinary tract such as a Wilms tumor or a rhabdoid tumor

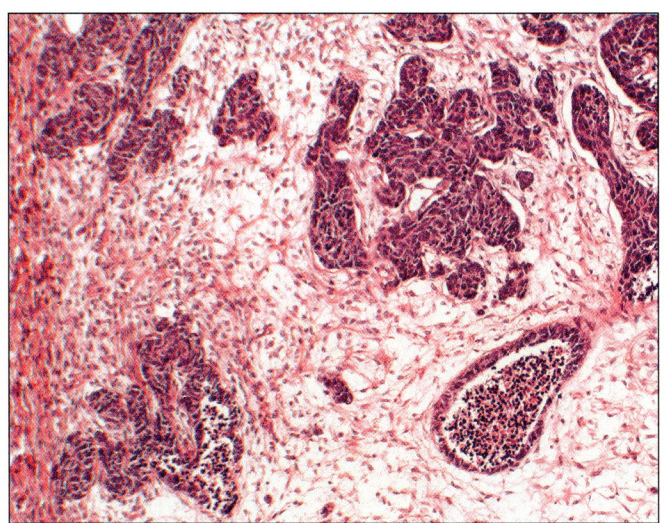

Fig. 29.49 Metastatic small cell undifferentiated carcinoma of the lung, previously treated. The cell groups show central necrosis. Nuclei are hyperchromatic and cytoplasm is scanty.

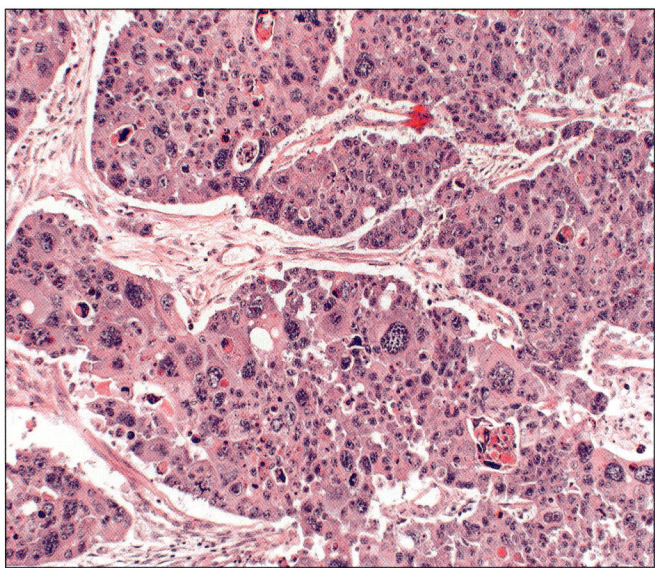

Fig. 29.50 Keratinizing squamous carcinoma of lung metastatic to the ovaries. Lesion in a 44-year-old woman (same case as Figure 29.10).

present as primary ovarian carcinoma.[114,215] Bladder adenocarcinoma has presented initially as a Krukenberg tumor[16,209] and a urachal adenocarcinoma has simulated primary ovarian mucinous adenocarcinoma.[134,206]

METASTASES FROM LUNGS AND MEDIASTINUM

Ovarian metastases from lung carcinomas account for only 0.4% of ovarian metastases but are increasing in frequency as the disease becomes more common in women[74] (Figures 29.49 and 29.50). Most women present with symptoms of the lung lesion and are subsequently found to have a pelvic tumor. However, if the ovarian lesions manifest earlier, they invariably pose a considerable diagnostic challenge. All major histologic types of lung cancer can spread to the ovaries and potentially mimic a primary carcinoma. Squamous cell carcinomas, the most common form of lung cancer, rarely metastasize to ovaries (one-sixth of metastases).[74] The metastases from primary lung adenocarcinomas are slightly more frequent (one-third of metastases). Thyroid transcription factor-1 (TTF-1) reactivity helps identify lungs as a potential primary site in cases of metastatic adenocarcinoma of unknown origin, being reactive in 60–75% of primary lung adenocarcinomas, but not reactive in primary ovarian adenocarcinomas. Undifferentiated small cell (oat cell) carcinomas of the lung, the most common type of tumor to metastasize (nearly half), should not be confused with primary small cell carcinomas of ovary of either 'hypercalcemic type' or 'pulmonary type' (see Chapter 25) although all of the tumors have a poor prognosis. Ovarian small cell carcinomas of hypercalcemic type occur in young women and, like other ovarian tumors, are negative for TTF-1, while more than half of small cell lung carcinomas are reactive.[7,74] Primary ovarian small cell carcinoma of pulmonary type typically differs from metastatic small cell lung carcinoma in its proclivity for peritoneal spread and its association with surface epithelial–stromal neoplasia, in particular endometrioid carcinoma. It may also be associated with Brenner tumor or mature cystic teratoma.[74] Interestingly, however, small cell carcinoma of the lung has been reported to metastasize to pre-existing ovarian tumors, including benign Brenner tumors, a fibroma, a Sertoli–Leydig cell tumor, and a mucinous carcinoma.[12,74]

Metastatic large cell carcinomas must be distinguished from morphologically similar oxyphilic tumors, both primary and secondary, including melanoma. Bronchioloalveolar carcinomas rarely are metastatic to the ovaries.[204]

Small cell carcinomas arising in sites other than lung, such as mediastinum, uterine cervix, and gastrointestinal tract, may also metastasize to the ovaries.[39,218] Isolated cases with metastases include posterior mediastinal neuroblastoma[215] and mediastinal thymoma.[15,17]

METASTASES FROM ENDOCRINE TUMORS

Carcinomas of the endocrine glands rarely feature in series of metastatic ovarian tumors. Rarely, ovarian metastasis from thyroid carcinoma may mimic struma ovarii.[101,216] This is discussed more fully in Chapter 27.

Neuroblastoma of the adrenal gland does metastasize to the ovaries but this is usually an autopsy finding. Rarely, the metastasis can present clinically.[114,180,215] The typical histologic features of neuroblastoma are present. The clinical context is a reliable discriminator between such lesions and the even rarer neuroblastomas primary in the ovaries (see Chapter 27).

Exceedingly rare instances include an oncocytic adrenocortical carcinoma[94] and an adrenocorticotropic hormone (ACTH)-secreting islet cell tumor of the endocrine pancreas, causing Cushings syndrome and bilateral ovarian metastases. The mechanism of spread in this latter case was thought to be peritoneal seeding as there were several peritoneal nodules at laparotomy. The lack of hepatic metastases was considered to have excluded vascular spread.[133]

METASTASES FROM EXTRAGENITAL SARCOMAS

Sarcomas rarely metastasize to the ovaries and are more likely to be primary tumors at that site. Leiomyosarcomas (from

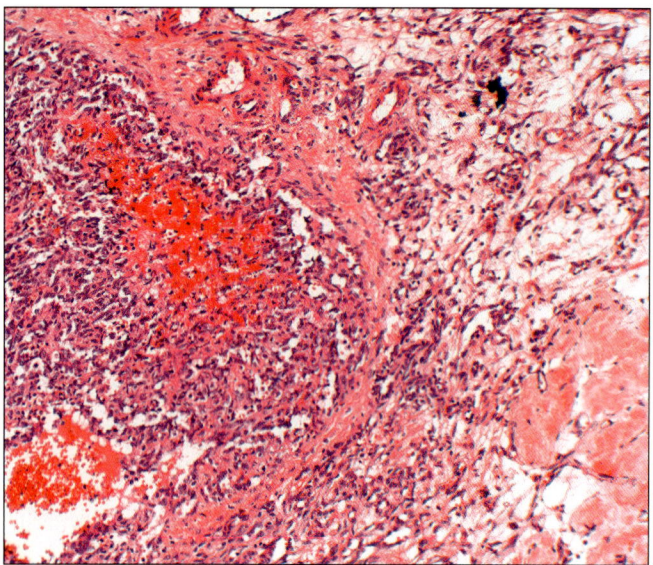

Fig. 29.51 Metastatic angiosarcoma from the breast in a 42-year-old woman. The tumor, which impinges on a corpus albicans (top left), consists of a network of small vascular spaces.

stomach, small bowel, and retrovesical tissue) are the least rare.[210] Isolated examples include fibrosarcoma of the anterior abdominal wall, sarcoma of the mesentery of smooth muscle of neural type, hemangiosarcoma of the heart, osteosarcoma of the maxilla, chondrosarcoma of the rib, Ewings sarcoma of a pubic bone, angiosarcoma[140] (Figure 29.51), alveolar rhabdomyosarcoma,[114,215] Ewings sarcoma of the fibula,[215] chordoma,[222] and malignant hemangiopericytoma.[11] In children, rhabdomyosarcoma is said to be the most common sarcoma to spread to ovary.[215] Metastatic retinoblastoma is also known.[114,122]

REFERENCES

1. Acikalin MF, Tokar B. Giant cyst of the rete ovarii in a child. J Pediatr Surg 2005;40:e17–19.
2. Adachi Y, Sasagawa I, Nakada T, et al. Bilateral ovarian metastasis from left renal cell carcinoma. Urol Int 1994;52:169–71.
3. Ahluwalia J, Girish V, Saha S, Dey P. Lymphangioma of the ovary. Acta Obstet Gynecol Scand 2000;79:894–5.
4. Attanoos RL, Gibbs AR. Primary malignant gonadal mesotheliomas and asbestos. Histopathology 2000;37:150–9.
5. Ayhan A, Guney I, Saygan-Karamursel B, Taskiran C. Ovarian metastasis of primary biliary and gallbladder carcinomas. Eur J Gynaecol Oncol 2001;22:377–8.
6. Azzena A, Zannol M, Bertezzolo M, Zen T, Chiarelli S. Epidermoid cyst and primary trabecular carcinoid of the ovary: case report. Eur J Gynaecol Oncol 2002;23:317–9.
7. Baker PM, Oliva E. Immunohistochemistry as a tool in the differential diagnosis of ovarian tumors: an update. Int J Gynecol Pathol 2005;24:39–55.
8. Balat O, Kudelka AP, Ro JY, et al. Two synchronous primary tumors of the ovary and kidney: a case report. Eur J Gynaecol Oncol 1996;17:257–9.
9. Bateman AC, Sworn MJ, Theaker JM, Buckingham MS. Pure epidermoid cysts of the ovary. J Obstet Gynaecol 1997;17:96–7.
10. Bazot M, Detchev R, Cortez A, Uzan S, Darai E. Massive ovarian edema revealing gastric carcinoma: a case report. Gynecol Oncol 2003;91:648–50.
11. Begum M, Katabuchi H, Tashiro H, Suenaga Y, Okamura H. A case of metastatic malignant hemangiopericytoma of the ovary: recurrence after a period of 17 years from intracranial tumor. Int J Gynecol Cancer 2002;12:510–4.
12. Bing Z, Adegboyega PA. Metastasis of small cell carcinoma of lung into an ovarian mucinous neoplasm: immunohistochemistry as a useful ancillary technique for diagnosis and classification of rare tumors. Appl Immunohistochem Mol Morphol 2005;13:104–7.
13. Bocher WO, Lohr HF, Steegmuller KW, et al. Detection of hepatitis C virus replication in ovarian metastases of a patient with hepatocellular carcinoma. J Hepatol 1994;21:47–51.
14. Boscaino A, D'Antonio A, Orabona P, Tornillo L, Staibano S, De Rosa G. Primary malignant melanoma of the ovary. Pathologica 1995;87:685–8.
15. Bott-Kothari T, Aron BS, Bejarano P. Malignant thymoma with metastases to the gastrointestinal tract and ovary: a case report and literature review. Am J Clin Oncol 2000;23:140–2.
16. Bowlby LS, Smith ML. Signet-ring cell carcinoma of the urinary bladder primary presentation as a Krukenberg tumor. Gynecol Oncol 1986;25:376–81.
17. Briese V, Rohde E. [Ovarian metastasis of a thymoma]. Zentralbl Gynakol 1984;106:473–6.
18. Campagnutta E, Sopracordevole F, Spolaor L, Doglioni C, Parin A, Scarabelli C. Squamous cell carcinoma in ovarian endometriosis. A case report. J Reprod Med 1994;39:557–60.
19. Cao D, Ji H, Ronnett BM. Expression of mesothelin, fascin, and prostate stem cell antigen in primary ovarian mucinous tumors and their utility in differentiating primary ovarian mucinous tumors from metastatic pancreatic mucinous carcinomas in the ovary. Int J Gynecol Pathol 2005;24:67–72.
20. Carder PJ, Gouldesbrough DR. Ovarian haemangiomas and stromal luteinization. Histopathology 1995;26:585–6.
21. Chang TC, Changchien CC, Tseng CW, et al. Retrograde lymphatic spread: a likely route for metastatic ovarian cancers of gastrointestinal origin. Gynecol Oncol 1997;66:372–7.
22. Chen KT. Appendiceal adenocarcinoid with ovarian metastasis. Gynecol Oncol 1990;38:286–8.
23. Chen ZM, Wang HL. Alteration of cytokeratin 7 and cytokeratin 20 expression profile is uniquely associated with tumorigenesis of primary adenocarcinoma of the small intestine. Am J Surg Pathol 2004;28:1352–9.
24. Cheong JH, Hyung WJ, Chen J, Kim J, Choi SH, Noh SH. Survival benefit of metastasectomy for Krukenberg tumors from gastric cancer. Gynecol Oncol 2004;94:477–82.
25. Chien SC, Sheu BC, Chang WC, Wu MZ, Huang SC. Pure primary squamous cell carcinoma of the ovary: a case report and review of the literature. Acta Obstet Gynecol Scand 2005;84:706–8.
26. Chou YY, Jeng YM, Kao HL, Chen T, Mao TL, Lin MC. Differentiation of ovarian mucinous carcinoma and metastatic colorectal adenocarcinoma by immunostaining with beta-catenin. Histopathology 2003;43:151–6.
27. Cormio G, Loverro G, Iacobellis M, Mei L, Selvaggi L. Hemangioma of the ovary. A case report. J Reprod Med 1998;43:459–61.
28. Correa-Rivas MS, Colon-Gonzalez G, Lugo-Vicente H. Cavernous hemangioma presenting as a right adnexal mass in a child. P R Health Sci J 2003;22:311–13.
29. Cortina R, McCormick J, Kolm P, Perry RR. Management and prognosis of adenocarcinoma of the appendix. Dis Colon Rectum 1995;38:848–52.
30. Costa MJ, Thomas W, Majmudar B, Hewan-Lowe K. Ovarian myxoma: ultrastructural and immunohistochemical findings. Ultrastruct Pathol 1992;16:429–38.
31. Costa MJ, Morris R, DeRose PB, Cohen C. Histologic and immunohistochemical evidence for considering ovarian myxoma as a variant of the thecoma-fibroma group of ovarian stromal tumors. Arch Pathol Lab Med 1993;117:802–8.
32. Curtin JP, Barakat RR, Hoskins WJ. Ovarian disease in women with breast cancer. Obstet Gynecol 1994;84:449–52.
33. Davidson B, Abeler VM. Primary ovarian angiosarcoma presenting as malignant cells in ascites: case report and review of the literature. Diagn Cytopathol 2005;32:307–9.
34. Daya D, Nazerali L, Frank GL. Metastatic ovarian carcinoma of large intestinal origin simulating primary ovarian carcinoma. A clinicopathologic study of 25 cases. Am J Clin Pathol 1992;97:751–8.
35. de Groot ME, Dukel L, Chadha-Ajwani S, Metselaar HJ, Tilanus HW, Huikeshoven FJ. Massive solitary metastasis of hepatocellular carcinoma in the ovary two years after liver transplantation. Eur J Obstet Gynecol Reprod Biol 2000;90:109–11.
36. De Rosa G, Donofrio V, De Rosa N, Fulciniti F, Zeppa P. Ovarian serous tumor with mural nodules of carcinomatous derivation (sarcomatoid carcinoma): report of a case. Int J Gynecol Pathol 1991;10:311–18.
37. Drachenberg CB, Faust FJ, Borkowski A, Papadimitriou JC. Epithelioid angiosarcoma of the uterus arising in a leiomyoma with associated ovarian and tubal angiomatosis. Am J Clin Pathol 1994;102:388–9.
38. Eichhorn JH, Scully RE. Ovarian myxoma: clinicopathologic and immunocytologic analysis of five cases and a review of the literature. Int J Gynecol Pathol 1991;10:156–69.
39. Eichhorn JH, Young RH, Scully RE. Nonpulmonary small cell carcinomas of extragenital origin metastatic to the ovary. Cancer 1993;71:177–86.
40. Elishaev E, Gilks CB, Miller D, Srodon M, Kurman RJ, Ronnett BM. Synchronous and metachronous endocervical and ovarian neoplasms: evidence supporting interpretation of the ovarian neoplasms as metastatic endocervical adenocarcinomas simulating primary ovarian surface epithelial neoplasms. Am J Surg Pathol 2005;29:281–94.
41. Evans A, Lytwyn A, Urbach G, Chapman W. Bilateral lymphangiomas of the ovary: an immunohistochemical characterization and review of the literature. Int J Gynecol Pathol 1999;18:87–90.

42. Facco C, La Rosa S, Dionigi A, Uccella S, Riva C, Capella C. High expression of growth factors and growth factor receptors in ovarian metastases from ileal carcinoids: an immunohistochemical study of 2 cases. Arch Pathol Lab Med 1998;122:828–32.

43. Fadare O, Mariappan MR, Ocal IT, Parkash V. A malignant ovarian tumor with osteoclast-like giant cells. Am J Surg Pathol 2003;27:854–60.

44. Fadare O, Bossuyt V, Martel M, Parkash V. Primary osteosarcoma of the ovary: a case report and literature review. Int J Gynecol Pathol 2007;26:21–5.

45. Feldman ED, Hughes MS, Stratton P, Schrump DS, Alexander HR, Jr. Pseudo-Meigs' syndrome secondary to isolated colorectal metastasis to ovary: a case report and review of the literature. Gynecol Oncol 2004;93:248–51.

46. Ferguson AW, Svoboda-Newman SM, Frank TS. Analysis of human papillomavirus infection and molecular alterations in adenocarcinoma of the cervix. Mod Pathol 1998;11:11–18.

47. Franco V, Florena AM, Orlando E, Becchina G. Giant cell tumor of the ovary. Immunohistochemical evidence of origin from stromal ovarian cells. Histol Histopathol 1995;10:55–60.

48. Fukunaga M, Endo Y, Miyazawa Y, Ushigome S. Small cell neuroendocrine carcinoma of the ovary. Virchows Arch 1997;430:343–8.

49. Fung MF, Vadas G, Lotocki R, Heywood M, Krepart G. Tubular Krukenberg tumor in pregnancy with virilization. Gynecol Oncol 1991;41:81–4.

50. Gagnon Y, Tetu B. Ovarian metastases of breast carcinoma. A clinicopathologic study of 59 cases. Cancer 1989;64:892–8.

51. Garcia A, De la Torre J, Castellvi J, Gil A, Lopez M. Ovarian metastases caused by cholangiocarcinoma: a rare Krukenberg's tumour simulating a primary neoplasm of the ovary: a two-case study. Arch Gynecol Obstet 2004;270:281–4.

52. Gardella C, Chumas JC, Pearl ML. Ovarian lipoma of teratomatous origin. Obstet Gynecol 1996;87(5 Pt 2):874–5.

53. Gehrig PA, Fowler WC, Jr, Lininger RA. Ovarian capillary hemangioma presenting as an adnexal mass with massive ascites and elevated CA-125. Gynecol Oncol 2000;76:130–2.

54. Glisic A, Atanackovic J. Krukenberg tumor in pregnancy. The lethal outcome. Pathol Oncol Res 2006;12:108–10.

55. Gokden N, Peterdy G, Philpott T, Maluf HM. Glomus tumor of the ovary: report of a case with immunohistochemical and ultrastructural observations. Int J Gynecol Pathol 2001;20:390–4.

56. Gordon MD, Weilert M, Ireland K. Plexiform neurofibromatosis involving the uterine cervix, endometrium, myometrium, and ovary. Obstet Gynecol 1996;88(4 Pt 2):699–701.

57. Green LK, Silva EG. Hepatoblastoma in an adult with metastasis to the ovaries. Am J Clin Pathol 1989;92:110–5.

58. Gucer F, Ozyilmaz F, Balkanli-Kaplan P, Mulayim N, Aydin O. Ovarian hemangioma presenting with hyperandrogenism and endometrial cancer: a case report. Gynecol Oncol 2004;94:821–4.

59. Gupta B, Sehgal A, Punia RP, Bakshi P, Malhotra S. Osteoma of the ovary causing obstructed labour. Aust N Z J Obstet Gynaecol 2001;41:230–1.

60. Gupta D, Deavers MT, Silva EG, Malpica A. Malignant melanoma involving the ovary: a clinicopathologic and immunohistochemical study of 23 cases. Am J Surg Pathol 2004;28:771–80.

61. Hanada S, Okumura Y, Kaida K. Multicentric adenomatoid tumors involving uterus, ovary, and appendix. J Obstet Gynaecol Res 2003;29:234–8.

62. Hanna NN, Cohen AM. Ovarian neoplasms in patients with colorectal cancer: understanding the role of prophylactic oophorectomy. Clin Colorectal Cancer 2004;3:215–22.

63. Harpaz N, Saxena R. Large intestine. In: Weidner N, Cote RJ, Suster S, Weiss LM, eds. Modern Surgical Pathology. Philadelphia: Saunders; 2003:749–852.

64. Hart WR. Diagnostic challenge of secondary (metastatic) ovarian tumors simulating primary endometrioid and mucinous neoplasms. Pathol Int 2005;55:231–43.

65. Hart WR. Mucinous tumors of the ovary: a review. Int J Gynecol Pathol 2005;24:4–25.

66. Heatley MK. Adenomatous hyperplasia of the rete ovarii. Histopathology 2000;36:383–4.

67. Hegg CA, Flint A. Neurofibroma of the ovary. Gynecol Oncol 1990;37:437–8.

68. Heinig J, Beckmann V, Bialas T, Diallo R. Lymphangioma of the ovary after radiation due to Wilms' tumor in childhood. Eur J Obstet Gynecol Reprod Biol 2002;103:191–4.

69. Hes O, Perez-Montiel DM, Alvarado Cabrero I, et al. Thread-like bridging strands: a morphologic feature present in all adenomatoid tumors. Ann Diagn Pathol 2003;7:273–7.

70. Hines JF, Compton DM, Stacy CC, Potter ME. Pure primary osteosarcoma of the ovary presenting as an extensively calcified adnexal mass: a case report and review of the literature. Gynecol Oncol 1990;39:259–63.

71. Huang TY, Chen JT, Ho WL. Ovarian serous cystadenoma with mural nodules of genital rhabdomyoma. Hum Pathol 2005;36:433–5.

72. Iizuka S, Nagata J, Fukuo S, Kosaka J. [A case of rhabdomyoma arising from the ovary]. Nippon Sanka Fujinka Gakkai Zasshi 1992;44:1197–200.

73. Ikeda E, Tsutsumi Y, Yoshida H, Yanagi K. Goblet cell carcinoid of the vermiform appendix with ovarian metastasis mimicking mucinous cystadenocarcinoma. Acta Pathol Jpn 1991;41:455–60.

74. Irving JA, Young RH. Lung carcinoma metastatic to the ovary: a clinicopathologic study of 32 cases emphasizing their morphologic spectrum and problems in differential diagnosis. Am J Surg Pathol 2005;29:997–1006.

75. Irving JA, Lerwill MF, Young RH. Gastrointestinal stromal tumors metastatic to the ovary: a report of five cases. Am J Surg Pathol 2005;29:920–6.

76. Irving JA, Vasques DR, McGuinness TB, Young RH. Krukenberg tumor of renal pelvic origin: report of a case with selected comments on ovarian tumors metastatic from the urinary tract. Int J Gynecol Pathol 2006;25:147–50.

77. Ishii Y, Itoh N, Takahashi A, Masumori N, Ikeda T, Tsukamoto T. Bladder cancer discovered by ovarian metastasis: cytokeratin expression is useful when making differential diagnosis. Int J Urol 2005;12:104–7.

78. Itoh H, Wada T, Michikata K, et al. Ovarian teratoma showing a predominant hemangiomatous element with stromal luteinization: report of a case and review of the literature. Pathol Int 2004;54:279–83.

79. Jain V, Gupta K, Kudva R, Rodrigues GS. A case of ovarian metastasis of gall bladder carcinoma simulating primary ovarian neoplasm: diagnostic pitfalls and review of literature. Int J Gynecol Cancer 2006;16(Suppl 1):319–21.

80. Jeremic K, Berisavac M, Argirovic R, et al. Solitary ovarian metastasis from cutaneous melanoma – case report. Eur J Gynaecol Oncol 2006;27:443–4.

81. Jha S, Chan KK, Poole CJ, Rollason TP. Pregnancy following recurrent angiosarcoma of the ovary – a case report and review of literature. Gynecol Oncol 2005;97:935–7.

82. Johnson TL, Keohane ME, Danzey TJ, Hicks ML. Squamous cell carcinoma of the cervix metastatic to an ovarian Brenner tumor. Mod Pathol 1995;8:307–11.

83. Jurkovic I, Dudrikova K, Boor A. Ovarian hemangioma. Cesk Patol 1999;35:133–5.

84. Jylling AM, Jorgensen L, Holund B. Mucinous cystadenocarcinoma in combination with hemangiosarcoma in the ovary. Pathol Oncol Res 1999;5:318–9.

85. Kaneta Y, Nishino R, Asaoka K, Toyoshima K, Ito K, Kitai H. Ovarian hemangioma presenting as pseudo-Meigs' syndrome with elevated CA125. J Obstet Gynaecol Res 2003;29:132–5.

86. Khunamornpong S, Siriaunkgul S, Chunduan A. Metastatic hepatocellular carcinoma of the ovary. Int J Gynaecol Obstet 1999;64:189–91.

87. Khunamornpong S, Suprasert P, Pojchamarnwiputh S, Na Chiangmai W, Settakorn J, Siriaunkgul S. Primary and metastatic mucinous adenocarcinomas of the ovary: evaluation of the diagnostic approach using tumor size and laterality. Gynecol Oncol 2006;101:152–7.

88. Kilic G, Abadi M. Jejunal adenocarcinoma presenting as a primary ovarian carcinoma. Gynecol Oncol 2000;78:255–8.

89. Kim NK, Kim HK, Park BJ, et al. Risk factors for ovarian metastasis following curative resection of gastric adenocarcinoma. Cancer 1999;85:1490–9.

90. Kinkor Z, Michal M. [Female adnexal tumor of probable Wolffian origin (Wolffian adenoma) – 2 case reports and literature review]. Ceska Gynekol 2003;68:280–3.

91. Kiyokawa T, Young RH, Scully RE. Krukenberg tumors of the ovary: a clinicopathologic analysis of 120 cases with emphasis on their variable pathologic manifestations. Am J Surg Pathol 2006;30:277–99.

92. Klein EA, Rosen MH. Bilateral Krukenberg tumors due to appendiceal mucinous carcinoid. Int J Gynecol Pathol 1996;15:85–8.

93. Krasevic M, Haller H, Rupcic S, Behrem S. Massive edema of the ovary: a report of two cases due to lymphatic permeation by metastatic carcinoma from the uterine cervix. Gynecol Oncol 2004;93:564–7.

94. Kurek R, Von Knobloch R, Feek U, Heidenreich A, Hofmann R. Local recurrence of an oncocytic adrenocortical carcinoma with ovary metastasis. J Urol 2001;166:985.

95. Lagendijk JH, Mullink H, van Diest PJ, Meijer GA, Meijer CJ. Immunohistochemical differentiation between primary adenocarcinomas of the ovary and ovarian metastases of colonic and breast origin. Comparison between a statistical and an intuitive approach. J Clin Pathol 1999;52:283–90.

96. Laszlo A, Ivaskevics K, Sapi Z. Malignant epithelioid ovarian schwannoma: a case report. Int J Gynecol Cancer 2006;16(Suppl 1):360–2.

97. Lee CH, Huang KG, Ueng SH, Swei H, Chueh HY, Lai CH. A hepatoid carcinoma of the ovary. Acta Obstet Gynecol Scand 2002;81:1080–2.

98. Lee KR, Young RH. The distinction between primary and metastatic mucinous carcinomas of the ovary: gross and histologic findings in 50 cases. Am J Surg Pathol 2003;27:281–92.

99. Lewis MR, Euscher ED, Deavers MT, Silva EG, Malpica A. Metastatic colorectal adenocarcinoma involving the ovary with elevated serum CA125: a potential diagnostic pitfall. Gynecol Oncol 2007;105:395–8.

100. Logani KB, Agarwal K. Lymphangioma of the ovary. J Indian Med Assoc 1997;95:146, 152.

101. Logani S, Baloch ZW, Snyder PJ, Weinstein R, LiVolsi VA. Cystic ovarian metastasis from papillary thyroid carcinoma: a case report. Thyroid 2001;11:1073–5.

102. Logani S, Oliva E, Arnell PM, Amin MB, Young RH. Use of novel immunohistochemical markers expressed in colonic adenocarcinoma to distinguish primary ovarian tumors from metastatic colorectal carcinoma. Mod Pathol 2005;18:19–25.

103. Loke TK, Lo SS, Chan CS. Case report: Krukenberg tumours arising from a primary duodenojejunal adenocarcinoma. Clin Radiol 1997;52:154–5.

104. Long CY, Lee YM, Tsai KB, Su JH, Hsu SC. Primary jejunal leiomyosarcoma mimicking a gynecologic tumor. Gynecol Obstet Invest 2002;54:180–2.

105. Lorentzen M. Giant cell tumor of the ovary. Virchows Arch A Pathol Anat Histol 1980;388:113–22.

106. Loy TS, Nashelsky MB. Reactivity of B72.3 with adenocarcinomas. An immunohistochemical study of 476 cases. Cancer 1993;72:2495–8.

107. Lugli A, Forster Y, Haas P, et al. Calretinin expression in human normal and neoplastic tissues: a tissue microarray analysis on 5233 tissue samples. Hum Pathol 2003;34:994–1000.

108. Lynch HT, Lynch JF. 25 years of HNPCC. Anticancer Res 1994;14(4B):1617–24.

109. M'Pemba Loufoua-Lemay AB, Peko JF, Mbongo JA, Mokoko JC, Nzingoula S. [Ovarian torsion revealing an ovarian cavernous hemangioma in a child]. Arch Pediatr 2003;10:986–8.

110. Mai KT, Yazdi HM, Bertrand MA, LeSaux N, Cathcart LL. Bilateral primary ovarian squamous cell carcinoma associated with human papilloma virus infection and vulvar and cervical intraepithelial neoplasia. A case report with review of the literature. Am J Surg Pathol 1996;20:767–72.

111. Mandai M, Konishi I, Tsuruta Y, et al. Krukenberg tumor from an occult appendiceal adenocarcinoid: a case report and review of the literature. Eur J Obstet Gynecol Reprod Biol 2001;97:90–5.

112. Manolitsas TP, Lanham SA, Hitchcock A, Watson RH. Synchronous ovarian and cervical squamous intraepithelial neoplasia: an analysis of HPV status. Gynecol Oncol 1998;70:428–31.

113. Maymon E, Piura B, Mazor M, Bashiri A, Silberstein T, Yanai-Inbar I. Primary hepatoid carcinoma of ovary in pregnancy. Am J Obstet Gynecol 1998;179(3 Pt 1):820–2.

114. McCarville MB, Hill DA, Miller BE, Pratt CB. Secondary ovarian neoplasms in children: imaging features with histopathologic correlation. Pediatr Radiol 2001;31:358–64.

115. McCluggage WG. Immunohistochemical and functional biomarkers of value in female genital tract lesions. Int J Gynecol Pathol 2006;25:101–20.

116. McCluggage WG, Wilkinson N. Metastatic neoplasms involving the ovary: a review with an emphasis on morphological and immunohistochemical features. Histopathology 2005;47:231–47.

117. McCluggage WG, Bissonnette JP, Young RH. Primary malignant melanoma of the ovary: a report of 9 definite or probable cases with emphasis on their morphologic diversity and mimicry of other primary and secondary ovarian neoplasms. Int J Gynecol Pathol 2006;25:321–9.

118. McCormick CC, Giuntoli RL, 2nd, Gardner GJ, et al. The role of cytoreductive surgery for colon cancer metastatic to the ovary. Gynecol Oncol 2007;105:791–5.

119. Miliaras D, Papaemmanouil S, Blatzas G. Ovarian capillary hemangioma and stromal luteinization: a case study with hormonal receptor evaluation. Eur J Gynaecol Oncol 2001;22:369–71.

120. Mohseni H, Truong P, Hadjseyd M, et al. [Uterine and ovarian metastases 28 years after the discovery of breast cancer]. Presse Med 2003;32:67–9.

121. Morice P, Haie-Meder C, Pautier P, Lhomme C, Castaigne D. Ovarian metastasis on transposed ovary in patients treated for squamous cell carcinoma of the uterine cervix: report of two cases and surgical implications. Gynecol Oncol 2001;83:605–7.

122. Moshfeghi DM, Wilson MW, Haik BG, Hill DA, Rodriguez-Galindo C, Pratt CB. Retinoblastoma metastatic to the ovary in a patient with Waardenburg syndrome. Am J Ophthalmol 2002;133:716–8.

123. Mueller MD, Dreher E, Eggimann T, Linder H, Altermatt H, Hanggi W. Is laparoscopic oophorectomy rational in patients with breast cancer? Surg Endosc 1998;12:1390–2.

124. Nagakura S, Shirai Y, Hatakeyama K. Pseudo-Meigs' syndrome caused by secondary ovarian tumors from gastrointestinal cancer. A case report and review of the literature. Dig Surg 2000;17:418–9.

125. Nakanishi T, Wakai K, Ishikawa H, et al. A comparison of ovarian metastasis between squamous cell carcinoma and adenocarcinoma of the uterine cervix. Gynecol Oncol 2001;82:504–9.

126. Natsume N, Aoki Y, Kase H, Kashima K, Sugaya S, Tanaka K. Ovarian metastasis in stage IB and II cervical adenocarcinoma. Gynecol Oncol 1999;74:255–8.

127. Nguyen L, Brewer CA, DiSaia PJ. Ovarian metastasis of stage IB1 squamous cell cancer of the cervix after radical parametrectomy and oophoropexy. Gynecol Oncol 1998;68:198–200.

128. Nielsen GP, Young RH, Prat J, Scully RE. Primary angiosarcoma of the ovary: a report of seven cases and review of the literature. Int J Gynecol Pathol 1997;16:378–82.

129. Nielsen GP, Oliva E, Young RH, Rosenberg AE, Prat J, Scully RE. Primary ovarian rhabdomyosarcoma: a report of 13 cases. Int J Gynecol Pathol 1998;17:113–9.

130. Nogales FF, Carvia RE, Donne C, Campello TR, Vidal M, Martin A. Adenomas of the rete ovarii. Hum Pathol 1997;28:1428–33.

131. Nolan LP, Heatley MK. The value of immunocytochemistry in distinguishing between clear cell carcinoma of the kidney and ovary. Int J Gynecol Pathol 2001;20:155–9.

132. Nucci MR, Krausz T, Lifschitz-Mercer B, Chan JK, Fletcher CD. Angiosarcoma of the ovary: clinicopathologic and immunohistochemical analysis of four cases with a broad morphologic spectrum. Am J Surg Pathol 1998;22:620–30.

133. Oberg KC, Wells K, Seraj IM, Garberoglio CA, Akin MR. ACTH-secreting islet cell tumor of the pancreas presenting as bilateral ovarian tumors and Cushing's syndrome. Int J Gynecol Pathol 2002;21:276–80.

134. Ohira S, Shiohara S, Itoh K, Ashida T, Fukushima M, Konishi I. Urachal adenocarcinoma metastatic to the ovaries: case report and literature review. Int J Gynecol Pathol 2003;22:189–93.

135. Ohsawa T, Ishida H, Nakada H, et al. Pseudo-Meigs' syndrome caused by ovarian metastasis from colon cancer: report of a case. Surg Today 2003;33:387–91.

136. Ohtani K, Sakamoto H, Masaoka N, et al. A case of rapidly growing ovarian squamous cell carcinoma successfully controlled by weekly paclitaxel–carboplatin administration. Gynecol Oncol 2000;79:515–8.

137. Ordonez NG. Application of mesothelin immunostaining in tumor diagnosis. Am J Surg Pathol 2003;27:1418–28.

138. Ozercan IH, Cobanoglu B, Simsek M, Dogan C, Ozercan MR. Epidermoid cyst of the ovary: a case report. Pathologica 2000;92:284–5.

139. Park SY, Kim HS, Hong EK, Kim WH. Expression of cytokeratins 7 and 20 in primary carcinomas of the stomach and colorectum and their value in the differential diagnosis of metastatic carcinomas to the ovary. Hum Pathol 2002;33:1078–85.

140. Patel T, Ohri SK, Sundaresan M, et al. Metastatic angiosarcoma of the ovary. Eur J Surg Oncol 1991;17:295–9.

141. Pellegrino A, Cormio G, Cappellini A, Perego P, Rossi R. Squamous carcinoma in situ of the ovary. Gynecol Obstet Invest 1997;44:278–80.

142. Perry LJ, Lewis JC, Ball RY. Adenocarcinoma of the breast metastatic to benign ovarian fibroma. Gynecol Oncol 1996;62:408–10.

143. Peters K, Gassel AM, Muller T, Dietl J. [Ovarian epidermoid cyst and endometrioid carcinoma: do they share their origin?]. Zentralbl Gynakol 2002;12:443–5.

144. Pins MR, Young RH, Daly WJ, Scully RE. Primary squamous cell carcinoma of the ovary. Report of 37 cases. Am J Surg Pathol 1996;20:823–33.

145. Pins MR, Young RH, Crum CP, Leach IH, Scully RE. Cervical squamous cell carcinoma in situ with intraepithelial extension to the upper genital tract and invasion of tubes and ovaries: report of a case with human papilloma virus analysis. Int J Gynecol Pathol 1997;16:272–8.

146. Pirog EC, Kleter B, Olgac S, et al. Prevalence of human papillomavirus DNA in different histological subtypes of cervical adenocarcinoma. Am J Pathol 2000;157:1055–62.

147. Pitman MB, Triratanachat S, Young RH, Oliva E. Hepatocyte paraffin 1 antibody does not distinguish primary ovarian tumors with hepatoid differentiation from metastatic hepatocellular carcinoma. Int J Gynecol Pathol 2004;23:58–64.

148. Piura B, Rabinovich A, Yanai-Inbar I, Cohen Y, Glezerman M. Primary sarcoma of the ovary: report of five cases and review of the literature. Eur J Gynaecol Oncol 1998;19:257–61.

149. Piura B, Kedar I, Ariad S, Meirovitz M, Yanai-Inbar I. Malignant melanoma metastatic to the ovary. Gynecol Oncol 1998;68:201–5.

150. Platt JS, Rogers SJ, Flynn EA, Taylor RR. Primary angiosarcoma of the ovary: a case report and review of the literature. Gynecol Oncol 1999;73:443–6.

151. Powell JL, Bock KA, Gentry JK, White WC, Ronnett BM. Metastatic endocervical adenocarcinoma presenting as a virilizing ovarian mass during pregnancy. Obstet Gynecol 2002;100(5 Pt 2):1129–33.

152. Prat J. Ovarian carcinomas, including secondary tumors: diagnostically challenging areas. Mod Pathol 2005;18(Suppl 2):S99–111.

153. Prus D, Rosenberg AE, Blumenfeld A, et al. Infantile hemangioendothelioma of the ovary: a monodermal teratoma or a neoplasm of ovarian somatic cells? Am J Surg Pathol 1997;21:1231–5.

154. Quesenberry CD, Li C, Chen AH, Zweizig SL, Ball HG, 3rd. Primary angiosarcoma of the ovary: a case report of stage I disease. Gynecol Oncol 2005;99:218–21.

155. Rabczynski J, Ziolkowski P. Primary endometrioid carcinoma of fallopian tube. Clinicomorphologic study. Pathol Oncol Res 1999;5:61–6.

156. Ramos Martinez E, Rodriguez Moguel L, Quijano Narezo M, Santiago Payan H. [Primary chondroma of the ovary. Report of a case]. Ginecol Obstet Mex 1983;51:95–8.

157. Rayson D, Bouttell E, Whiston F, Stitt L. Outcome after ovarian/adnexal metastectomy in metastatic colorectal carcinoma. J Surg Oncol 2000;75:186–92.

158. Remadi S, McGee W, Egger JF, Ismail A. Ovarian metastatic melanoma. A diagnostic pitfall in histopathologic examination. Arch Anat Cytol Pathol 1997;45:43–6.

159. Resta L, De Benedictis G, Colucci GA, et al. Secondary tumors of the ovary. III. Tumors of the gastrointestinal tract and other sites. Eur J Gynaecol Oncol 1990;11:289–98.

160. Rhoades CP, McMahon JT, Goldblum JR. Myofibroblastoma of the ovary: report of a case. Mod Pathol 1999;12:907–11.

161. Rix GH, Perez-Clemente MP, Spencer PJ, Al-Rufaie HK. Myxoma of the ovary. J Obstet Gynaecol 1998;18:295–6.

162. Rose PG, Piver MS, Tsukada Y. Fallopian tube cancer. The Roswell Park experience. Cancer 1990;66:2661–7.

163. Sakai Y, Hatano B. Metastatic duodenal carcinoma simulating primary mucinous tumor of the ovary. Arch Gynecol Obstet 2005;272:84–6.

164. Sakakura C, Hagiwara A, Yoshikawa T, Hamada T, Yamagishi H. Huge ovarian metastasis from jejunal cancer occurring immediately after initial operation. Hepatogastroenterology 2005;52:425–8.

165. Sakata H, Hirahara T, Ryu A, Sawada T, Yamamoto M, Sakurai I. Primary osteosarcoma of the ovary. A case report. Acta Pathol Jpn 1991;41:311–7.

166. Sant'Ambrogio S, Malpica A, Schroeder B, Silva EG. Primary ovarian rhabdomyosarcoma associated with clear cell carcinoma of the ovary: a case report and review of the literature. Int J Gynecol Pathol 2000;19:169–73.

167. Savargaonkar PR, Wells S, Graham I, Buckley CH. Ovarian haemangiomas and stromal luteinization. Histopathology 1994;25:185–8.

168. Schwartz EJ, Longacre TA. Adenomatoid tumors of the female and male genital tracts express WT1. Int J Gynecol Pathol 2004;23:123–8.

169. Scurry JP, Brown RW, Jobling T. Combined ovarian serous papillary and hepatoid carcinoma. Gynecol Oncol 1996;63:138–42.

170. Seidman JD, Kurman RJ, Ronnett BM. Primary and metastatic mucinous adenocarcinomas in the ovaries: incidence in routine practice with a new approach to improve intraoperative diagnosis. Am J Surg Pathol 2003;27:985–93.

171. Senzaki H, Kiyozuka Y, Mizuoka H, et al. An autopsy case of hepatoid carcinoma of the ovary with PIVKA-II production: immunohistochemical study and literature review. Pathol Int 1999;49:164–9.

172. Shakfeh SM, Woodruff JD. Primary ovarian sarcomas: report of 46 cases and review of the literature. Obstet Gynecol Surv 1987;42:331–49.

173. Sheikh SS, Amr SS. Epidermoid cyst of the ovary. J Obstet Gynaecol 2003;23:213.

174. Shetty MR, Boghossian HM, Duffell D, Freel R, Gonzales JC. Tumor-induced hypoglycemia: a result of ectopic insulin production. Cancer 1982;49:1920–3.

175. Sheyn I, Mira JL, Bejarano PA, Husseinzadeh N. Metastatic female adnexal tumor of probable Wolffian origin: a case report and review of the literature. Arch Pathol Lab Med 2000;124:431–4.

176. Shimada M, Kigawa J, Nishimura R, et al. Ovarian metastasis in carcinoma of the uterine cervix. Gynecol Oncol 2006;101:234–7.

177. Silver SA, Tavassoli FA. Glomus tumor arising in a mature teratoma of the ovary: report of a case simulating a metastasis from cervical squamous carcinoma. Arch Pathol Lab Med 2000;124:1373–5.

178. Smith CJ, Ferrier AJ, Russell P, Danieletto S. Primary synovial sarcoma of the ovary: first reported case. Pathology 2005;37:385–7.

179. Snyder MJ, Bentley R, Robboy SJ. Transtubal spread of serous adenocarcinoma of the endometrium: an underrecognized mechanism of metastasis. Int J Gynecol Pathol 2006;25:155–60.

180. Somjee S, Kurkure PA, Chinoy RF, Deshpande RK, Advani SH. Metastatic ovarian neuroblastoma: a case report. Pediatr Hematol Oncol 1999;16:459–62.

181. Spencer JR, Eriksen B, Garnett JE. Metastatic renal tumor presenting as ovarian clear cell carcinoma. Urology 1993;41:582–4.

182. Stern RC, Dash R, Bentley RC, Snyder MJ, Haney AF, Robboy SJ. Malignancy in endometriosis: frequency and comparison of ovarian and extraovarian types. Int J Gynecol Pathol 2001;20:133–9.

183. Stewart CJ, Brennan BA, Hammond IG, Leung YC, McCartney AJ. Accuracy of frozen section in distinguishing primary ovarian neoplasia from tumors metastatic to the ovary. Int J Gynecol Pathol 2005;24:356–62.

184. Stone GC, Bell DA, Fuller A, Dickersin GR, Scully RE. Malignant schwannoma of the ovary. Report of a case. Cancer 1986;58:1575–82.

185. Sutton GP, Bundy BN, Delgado G, et al. Ovarian metastases in stage IB carcinoma of the cervix: a Gynecologic Oncology Group study. Am J Obstet Gynecol 1992;166(1 Pt 1):50–3.

186. Swift R, Jalleh R, Patel A, Hutton K, Gaer J, Wood C. Chondrosarcoma from a rib metastasizing to the ovary. Acta Orthop Scand 1991;62:76.

187. Tabata M, Ichinoe K, Sakuragi N, Shiina Y, Yamaguchi T, Mabuchi Y. Incidence of ovarian metastasis in patients with cancer of the uterine cervix. Gynecol Oncol 1987;28:255–61.

188. Talerman A, Auerbach WM, van Meurs AJ. Primary chondrosarcoma of the ovary. Histopathology 1981;5:319–24.

189. Taranto AJ, Lourie R, Lau WF. Ovarian vascular pedicle sign in ovarian metastasis arising from gall bladder carcinoma. Australas Radiol 2006;50:504–6.

190. Tetu B, Bonenfant JL. Ovarian myxoma. A study of two cases with long-term follow-up. Am J Clin Pathol 1991;95:340–6.

191. Tochigi N, Kishimoto T, Supriatna Y, Nagai Y, Nikaido T, Ishikura H. Hepatoid carcinoma of the ovary: a report of three cases admixed with a common surface epithelial carcinoma. Int J Gynecol Pathol 2003;22:266–71.

192. Toki T, Zhai YL, Park JS, Fujii S. Infrequent occurrence of high-risk human papillomavirus and of p53 mutation in minimal deviation adenocarcinoma of the cervix. Int J Gynecol Pathol 1999;18:215–9.

193. Trivedi P, Dave K, Shah M, Karelia N, Patel D, Wadhwa M. Hepatoid carcinoma of the ovary – a case report. Eur J Gynaecol Oncol 1998;19:167–9.

194. Tsekeris P, Mavreas S, Zioga A, Paizi P, Kalef-Ezra J. A case report on two primary malignancies of the ovary and kidney. Eur J Gynaecol Oncol 1999;20:38–9.

195. Tsung JS, Yang PS. Hepatoid carcinoma of the ovary: characteristics of its immunoreactivity. A case report. Eur J Gynaecol Oncol 2004;25:745–8.

196. Uppal S, Heller DS, Majmudar B. Ovarian hemangioma – report of three cases and review of the literature. Arch Gynecol Obstet 2004;270:1–5.

197. Valappil SV, Toon PG, Anandaram PS. Ovarian metastasis from primary renal cell carcinoma: report of a case and review of literature. Gynecol Oncol 2004;94:846–9.

198. Vang R, Bague S, Tavassoli FA, Prat J. Signet-ring stromal tumor of the ovary: clinicopathologic analysis and comparison with Krukenberg tumor. Int J Gynecol Pathol 2004;23:45–51.

199. Vang R, Gown AM, Barry TS, Wheeler DT, Ronnett BM. Immunohistochemistry for estrogen and progesterone receptors in the distinction of primary and metastatic mucinous tumors in the ovary: an analysis of 124 cases. Mod Pathol 2006;19:97–105.

200. Vauthier-Brouzes D, Vanna Lim-You K, Sebagh E, Lefebvre G, Darbois Y. [Krukenberg tumor during pregnancy with maternal and fetal virilization: a difficult diagnosis. A case report]. J Gynecol Obstet Biol Reprod (Paris) 1997;26:831–3.

201. Verswijvel G, Termote B, Sannen G, Ombelet W, Palmers Y. Hemangiopericytoma of the ovary. JBR-BTR 2004;87:229–30.

202. Watanabe Y, Umemoto M, Ueda H, Nakai H, Hoshiai H, Noda K. Cytopathologic and clinicopathologic features of ovarian hepatoid carcinoma. A case report. Acta Cytol 2003;47:78–82.

203. Yamawaki T, Hirai Y, Takeshima N, Hasumi K. Ovarian hemangioma associated with concomitant stromal luteinization and ascites. Gynecol Oncol 1996;61:438–41.

204. Yeh KY, Chang JW, Hsueh S, Chang TC, Lin MC. Ovarian metastasis originating from bronchioloalveolar carcinoma: a rare presentation of lung cancer. Jpn J Clin Oncol 2003;33:404–7.

204a. Yemelyanova AV, Vang R, Judson K, Wu LS, Ronnett BM. Distinction of primary and metastatic mucinous tumors involving the ovary: analysis of size and laterality data by primary site with reevaluation of an algorithm for tumor classification. Am J Surg Pathol 2008;32:128–38.

205. Young RH. New and unusual aspects of ovarian germ cell tumors. Am J Surg Pathol 1993;17:1210–24.

206. Young RH. Urachal adenocarcinoma metastatic to the ovary simulating primary mucinous cystadenocarcinoma of the ovary: report of a case. Virchows Arch 1995;426:529–32.

207. Young RH. From Krukenberg to today: the ever present problems posed by metastatic tumors in the ovary. Part I: Historical perspective, general principles, mucinous tumors including the Krukenberg tumor. Adv Anat Pathol 2006;13:205–27.

208. Young RH. From Krukenberg to today: the ever present problems posed by metastatic tumors in the ovary. Part II. Adv Anat Pathol 2007;14:149–77.

209. Young RH, Scully RE. Urothelial and ovarian carcinomas of identical cell types: problems in interpretation. A report of three cases and review of the literature. Int J Gynecol Pathol 1988;7:197–211.

210. Young RH, Scully RE. Sarcomas metastatic to the ovary: a report of 21 cases. Int J Gynecol Pathol 1990;9:231–52.

211. Young RH, Scully RE. Malignant melanoma metastatic to the ovary. A clinicopathologic analysis of 20 cases. Am J Surg Pathol 1991;15:849–60.

212. Young RH, Hart WR. Renal cell carcinoma metastatic to the ovary: a report of three cases emphasizing possible confusion with ovarian clear cell adenocarcinoma. Int J Gynecol Pathol 1992;11:96–104.

213. Young RH, Hart WR. Metastatic intestinal carcinomas simulating primary ovarian clear cell carcinoma and secretory endometrioid carcinoma: a clinicopathologic and immunohistochemical study of five cases. Am J Surg Pathol 1998;22:805–15.

214. Young RH, Scully RE. Differential diagnosis of ovarian tumors based primarily on their patterns and cell types. Semin Diagn Pathol 2001;18:161–235.

215. Young RH, Kozakewich HP, Scully RE. Metastatic ovarian tumors in children: a report of 14 cases and review of the literature. Int J Gynecol Pathol 1993;12:8–19.

216. Young RH, Jackson A, Wells M. Ovarian metastasis from thyroid carcinoma 12 years after partial thyroidectomy mimicking struma ovarii: report of a case. Int J Gynecol Pathol 1994;13:181–5.

217. Young RH, Gersell DJ, Clement PB, Scully RE. Hepatocellular carcinoma metastatic to the ovary: a report of three cases discovered during life with discussion of the differential diagnosis of hepatoid tumors of the ovary. Hum Pathol 1992;23:574–80.

218. Young RH, Gersell DJ, Roth LM, Scully RE. Ovarian metastases from cervical carcinomas other than pure adenocarcinomas. A report of 12 cases. Cancer 1993;71:407–18.

219. Yu TJ, Iwasaki I, Horie H, Tamaru J, Takahashi A. Endolymphatic stromal myosis of the uterus with metastasis to ovary and recurrence in vagina. Acta Pathol Jpn 1986;36:301–8.

220. Zamecnik M, Gomolcak P. Composite multicystic mesothelioma and adenomatoid tumor of the ovary: additional observation suggesting common histogenesis of both lesions. Cesk Patol 2000;36:160–2.

221. Zhu L, Li B. [Clinical pathological analysis of adenomatoid tumor in uterus and ovaries]. Zhonghua Bing Li Xue Za Zhi 2001;30:43–5.

222. Zukerberg LR, Young RH. Chordoma metastatic to the ovary. Arch Pathol Lab Med 1990;114:208–10.

Nidation and placenta

Eoghan E. Mooney Stanley J. Robboy

30

INTRODUCTION

Placental pathology has historically received little attention by obstetricians and pathologists alike. The old midwifery term, 'afterbirth', reflects the attitude of many clinicians that placental examination was at best an afterthought. This has changed with the recognition that many adverse pregnancy outcomes reflect prepartum rather than intrapartum events. It is not necessary to examine all placentas in the laboratory.[120] Indications for examination are essentially any disease of the mother, the infant or any clinically accepted placental abnormality (funny mother, funny infant or funny disease). In most institutions, this constitutes approximately 15% of deliveries.

Placental examination is an integral part of the fetal or perinatal autopsy and adds conclusive or important information in over a third of such cases.[76] Within these parameters, the extent of the examination will vary with different healthcare systems. While the delivery suite may be the ideal place to initiate ancillary investigations such as microbiology and cytogenetics,[75] many pathologists prefer a laboratory-based grossing station with adequate photographic and other facilities. Even though the value of many ancillary investigations has been questioned,[56] a careful gross examination with retention of formalin-fixed tissue can permit subsequent histologic examination in cases where an abnormality becomes apparent in neonatal life, rather than at birth. The litigious climate of most Western countries has spurred placental examination with clinical correlation, and indeed some insurance companies have offered a reduction in obstetric insurance based on routine placental examination.

In examining the placenta, the pathologist has the advantage of having the entire organ. Even so, many other variables must be taken into account to correctly interpret the morphologic findings. The gestational age may not be entirely accurate. Important data such as infant's weight, changes in growth patterns, and other biophysical parameters are not always provided. Even with these, the variable villous patterns can make clinical correlation difficult. Proper sampling when taking sections for histology is also important in order to avoid false conclusions.

This chapter aims to provide the pathologist with a structured approach to the placental features most commonly encountered in routine practice. Background information on morphogenesis is provided to assist in interpretation. Indeed, an appreciation of morphogenesis is important, for the placenta is unique to the body in that its entire life is only 9 months long. It continually undergoes elaborate change during this time, and at the end is discarded.

ANATOMY AND EMBRYOLOGY

EARLY PREGNANCY

Fertilization, cell division, formation of the morula, and later formation of blastocyst are independent of maternal contact. The blastocyst reaches the uterus on day 3 after fertilization and implants by the end of day 7. While our understanding of implantation, especially its molecular basis,[8] is still evolving, implantation involves a highly choreographed expression of adhesion and antiadhesion molecules both in the embryo and endometrium, together with alterations in the endometrial extracellular matrix.

The process of implantation has three phases: muscular, adhesive, and invasive. The muscular phase concerns transport of the conceptus to the optimal site for implantation, which in humans is the mid-to-high posterior wall of the uterus in the mid-sagittal plane (Figure 30.1). This phase is probably more important in animals where multiple births are the norm and even spacing for adequate nidation is advantageous. During the adhesive phase, the normally repulsive interactions between two epithelial surfaces (endometrium and trophoblast) are reversed.[26]

In the invasive phase, irregular projections of syncytiotrophoblast invade into the endometrium (Figure 30.2). This phase lasts until approximately day 8 postconception and is called the prelacunar phase, based on the appearance of the blastocyst. At day 8, vacuoles appear in the syncytiotrophoblast, which become confluent to form lacunae. This change commences at the implantation pole and becomes confluent over the blastocyst by day 13. At this stage, the earliest forms of chorionic villi begin to form (Figure 30.3) and the primary chorionic plate consists of a continuous layer of cytotrophoblast on the embryoblast side of the lacunae. Infiltration of the pillars of syncytiotrophoblast surrounding the lacunae by cytotrophoblast from the chorionic plate is followed by expansion of these pillars as extraembryonic mesenchyme follows cytotrophoblast. The outermost layer of trophoblast (the trophoblast shell) is formed by syncytiotrophoblast, and later by cytotrophoblast as well. Cytotrophoblast continues to invade endometrium and is seen as clusters of extratrophoblast ('X' cells) and trophoblastic giant cells in what will become the basal plate. The lacunar space becomes the intervillous space, and the embryologic development of villi proceeds during gestation. These developments are maximal at the deep aspect of the blastocyst and normally only this persists to form the true placenta (chorion frondosum). The remainder atrophies (chorion laeve) (Figure 30.4).

829

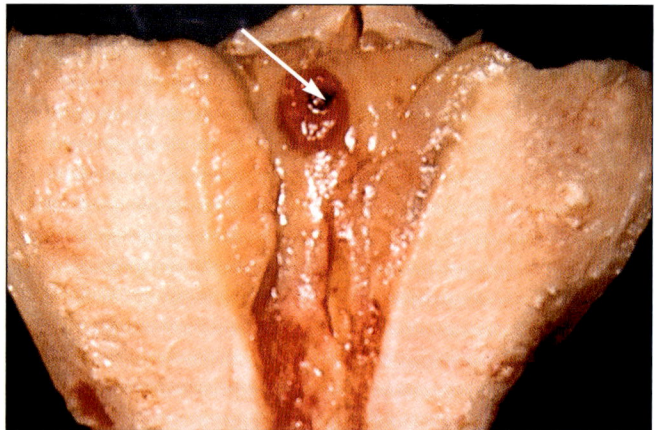

Fig. 30.1 Implantation (arrow) in early pregnancy.

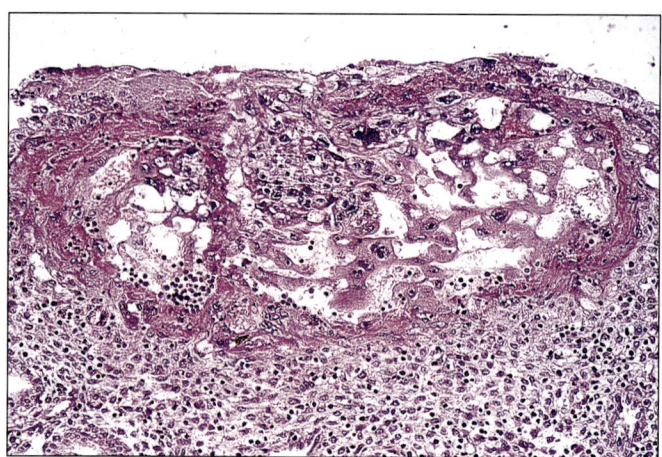

Fig. 30.2 Primitive trophoblast. Chorionic villi have not yet formed in the pregnancy of about 1-week duration.

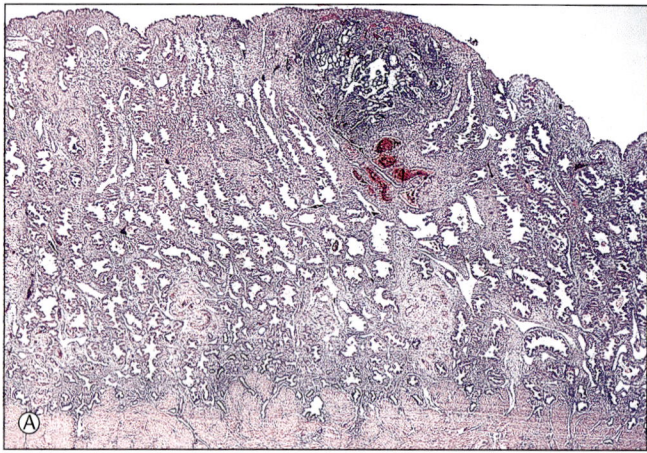

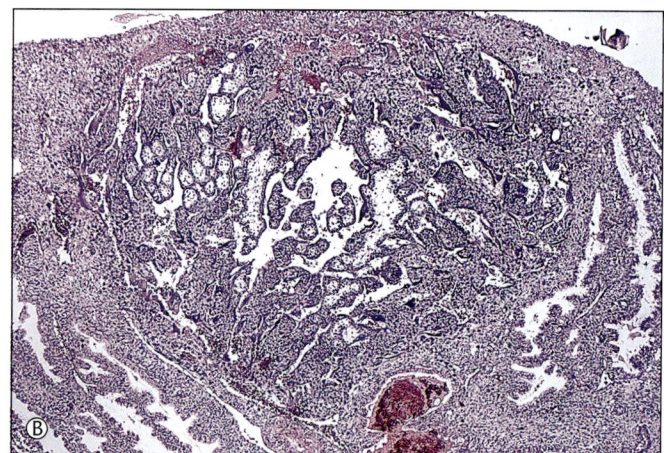

Fig. 30.3 **(A)** Day 14 conceptus as tiny implant in superficial endometrium. **(B)** Detail of earliest stage of chorionic villi formation.

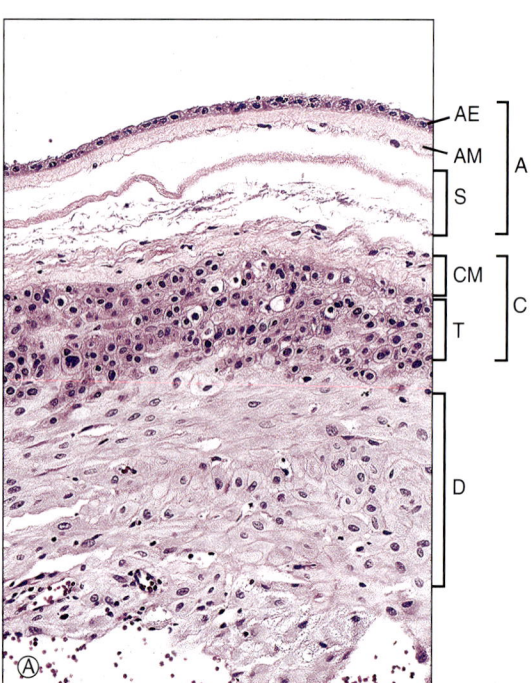

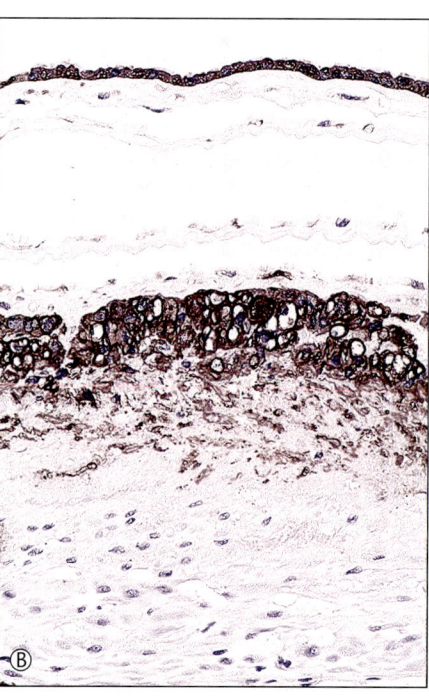

Fig. 30.4 Normal membrane in a third-trimester placenta. **(A)** Amnion (A), parts of which include amnionic epithelium (AE), amnionic mesoderm (AM) and spongy level (S). The chorionic plate (C) is composed of chorionic mesoderm (CM) and trophoblast (T). Beneath that is the maternal decidua (D). **(B)** Both the trophoblasts and amnionic epithelium are markedly reactive for cytokeratin (CAM 5.2).

The cytotrophoblastic shell thins and is replaced by Nitabuchs fibrin layer, which is composed of matrix-type fibrinoid and lies between the shell and the decidual boundaries. The fibrinoid between the shell and the intervillous space is called Rohrs fibrinoid and is fibrin-type fibrinoid. The two are indistinguishable by routine H&E sections, but may be differentiated immunohistochemically using antibodies directed against oncofetal fibronectin for matrix-type fibrinoid and fibrin for fibrin-type fibrinoid.[17]

PLACENTAL MORPHOLOGY

Villous development takes place during gestation and results both in growth of the placenta and the morphologic alterations necessary to meet increasing fetal demands. Protrusions of trophoblast (trophoblast sprouts) into the lacunae are the forerunners of villi.[21] Initially, the sprouts consist of syncytiotrophoblast, which are followed by cytotrophoblast and by connective tissue containing fetal capillaries. The villi thus formed are termed mesenchymal villi and are the precursors of all other villous types. While they are the dominant type in the first trimester, some trophoblast sprouting and mesenchymal villous development probably occurs up to term.

The immature intermediate villi are formed from the mesenchymal villi and are primarily responsible for placental growth (Figure 30.5). They have a complete trophoblastic mantle with many cytotrophoblastic cells present, but lack vasculosyncytial membranes. The syncytial nuclei are evenly dispersed without knots. They have a loose (reticular) stroma with abundant stromal channels containing Hofbauer cells. They are the dominant villous type seen in the second trimester and are transformed into stem villi when their production from mesenchymal villi decreases.

Stem villi are defined by 50% or more of their stroma being compact and containing vessels with media or adventitia identifiable on light microscopy (Figure 30.6) They range in size from 80 to 5000 µm and connect the chorionic plate to the remaining distal villous tree. Some stem villi connect to the basal plate (anchoring villi). They have both an arterial and a venous circulation, which (depending on size) consist of either arteries and veins or arterioles and venules. The trophoblastic cover is predominantly syncytiotrophoblast and may be replaced with fibrinoid in the mature placenta. A perivascular capillary network is more prominent in less mature stem villi and reflects their origin from immature intermediate villi. The localization of myofibroblasts and smooth muscle cells in stem villi has been defined immunohistochemically and these cells may play a role in villous vascular regulation.[31]

The mature intermediate villi (Figure 30.7) are formed from the mesenchymal villi in the third trimester and give rise to the majority of terminal villi. They are 60–150 µm in diameter and contain capillaries, arterioles, and venules. The stroma is loose and the vessels comprise less than half the villous cross-sectional area. The syncytiotrophoblast has a uniform structure without vasculosyncytial membranes or knots. At term, mature intermediate villi make up one-fourth of the parenchyma.

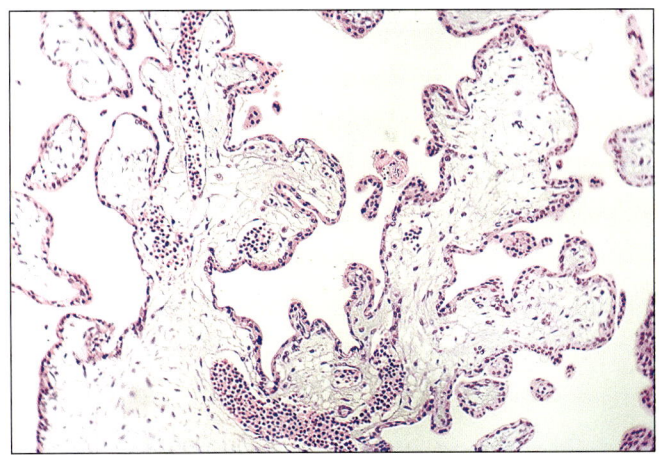
Fig. 30.6 Stem villus.

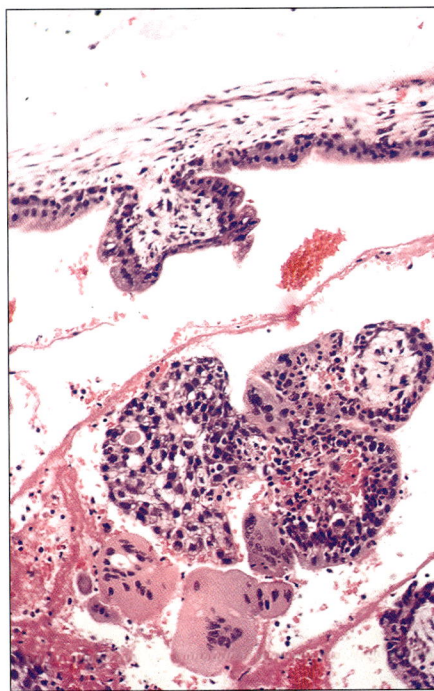
Fig. 30.5 Mesenchymal villus.

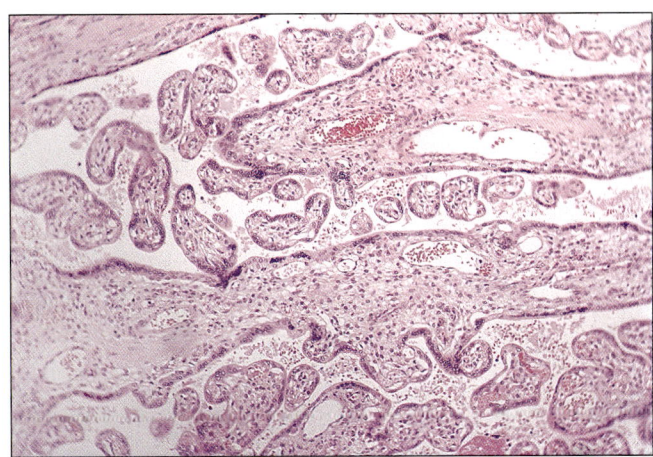
Fig. 30.7 Mature intermediate villus.

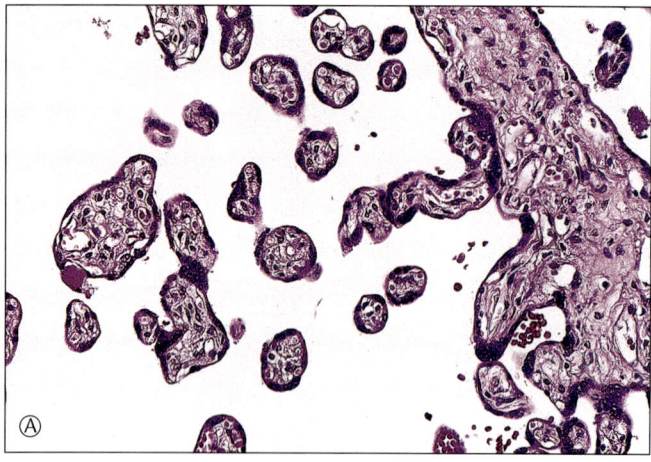 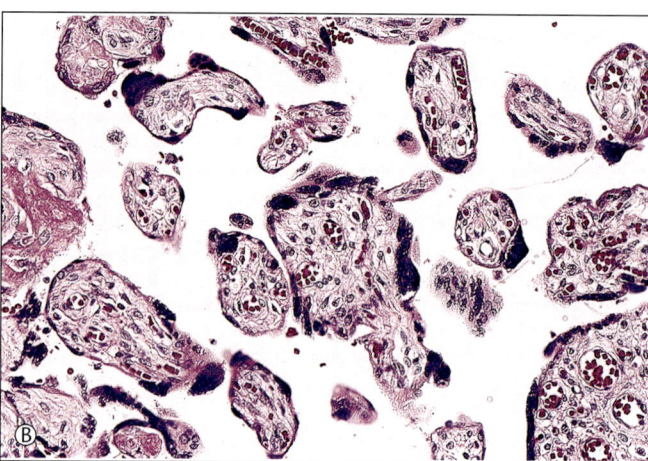

Fig. 30.8 **(A)** Terminal villi. **(B)** Detail.

The terminal villi (Figure 30.8) are the site of gaseous exchange and derive from the mature intermediate villi. They arise as capillary growths which, in exceeding that of parent mature intermediate villi, result in trophoblastic protrusions. The capillaries are dilated and comprise over 50% of the villus cross-sectional area. Optimal gas exchange requires the formation of vasculosyncytial membranes. The syncytiotrophoblast nuclei become pushed to one side so that only a very thin attenuated layer of syncytiotrophoblastic cytoplasm remains applied to its basement membrane, which is itself applied to the capillary's basement membrane. The capillaries are 3–5 mm long and each maintains its own non-branching structure. They do not form a capillary network, but remain as long capillaries. In addition, the capillaries have varicosities where their diameters enlarge considerably. The exact functional significance of these varicosities is unknown, although a rheologic function from vascular deformation and altered flow has been proposed. These villi appear at 27 weeks of gestation and increase in number until term.

The placenta's maternal surface divides into partitions and is caused by placental septum formation. As collections of cytotrophoblast, the so-called 'cell columns', anchor the decidua to the villi, their growth rates differ so that slow-growing ones tend to pull up the decidual basal plate, buckling it into the placental septa. These septa are incomplete and rarely reach the chorionic plate. Therefore, they have no precise anatomic relationship to the functional units of the placenta.

INTERVILLOUS (MATERNAL) CIRCULATION

The labyrinthine space ultimately becomes the intervillous space into which maternal blood flows through the altered spiral arteries. The timing of this development is uncertain. The circulation through lacunae and subsequent intervillous space has been shown to be indirect in animal models.[37] This may be the normal pattern in the first trimester in the human, with intervillous circulation gradually establishing itself rather than commencing abruptly at the end of the first trimester.[73]

The advantage to the embryo of such a delay is protection against the teratogenic effects of high ambient oxygen concentration, and elevated pressure from spiral arteries. Abnormal

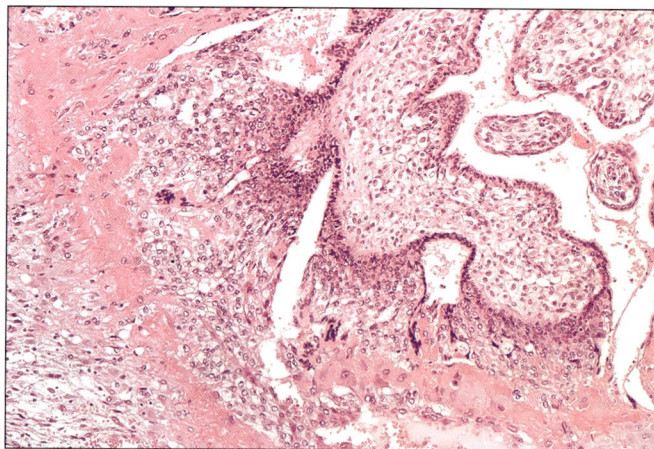

Fig. 30.9 Anchoring cytotrophoblastic cell columns.

implantation may alter this sequence and result in pregnancy loss. Plugs of trophoblast in the lumen of spiral arteries are a feature of normal pregnancies[59] and are less commonly seen in spontaneous abortions in contrast with therapeutic or elective abortions.[55] Their absence correlates with the more frequent presence of blood clot in the intervillous space and other features that may reflect defective implantation. Thus, the untimely development of the intervillous circulation may result from defective implantation and is one mechanism by which early pregnancy loss occurs.

DEVELOPMENT OF THE UTEROPLACENTAL VESSELS

Early in gestation, the cytotrophoblastic cells stream out from the tips of the anchoring villi (Figure 30.9), penetrate the trophoblastic shell, and colonize the decidua and adjacent myometrium of the placental bed. These cells, which are reactive for human placental lactogen (hPL) and cytokeratins (Figure 30.10), are called the 'interstitial extravillous trophoblast'. They are responsible for the placental site reaction.

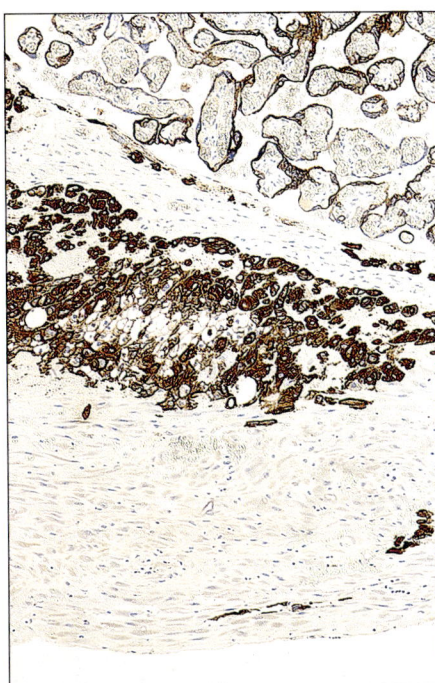

Fig. 30.10 Cytokeratin staining of extravillous interstitial trophoblast (CAM 5.2).

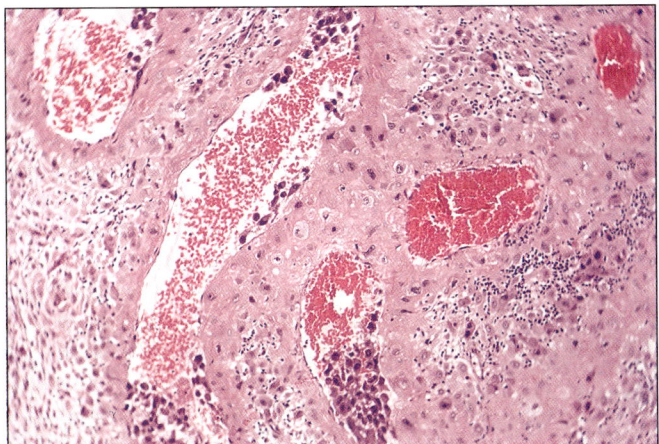

Fig. 30.11 A transforming spiral artery. Intravascular trophoblast and extravillous interstitial trophoblast are present.

In addition, cytotrophoblast called the 'intravascular extravillous cytotrophoblast' invades and plugs the lumens of the decidual spiral arteries. The cells destroy the endothelium and the elastic and muscular tissues of the media, which are then replaced by fibrinoid material derived from fibrin and trophoblastic secretions (Figures 30.11 and 30.12). This produces large diameter vessels lacking intrinsic tone that allow a high-flow, low-pressure system to develop. The first wave of transformation continues until the decidual–myometrial junction is completed at approximately 12 weeks' gestation. After a pause, intravascular trophoblast activity commences again at 14–16 weeks and transforms the myometrial segment of the spiral arteries to as far as the junction with the radial arteries. This process completes by the end of week 20.

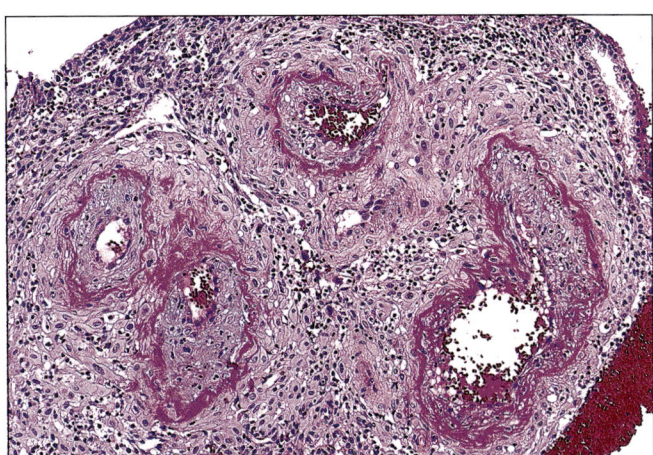

Fig. 30.12 A transforming spiral artery. There is extensive intravascular trophoblast and extravillous interstitial trophoblast filling the maternal vessels.

The mechanisms that control trophoblast invasion are complex and poorly understood. Low oxygen tension may help control entry of cytotrophoblast into the S phase of the cell cycle, while proliferation and high ambient oxygen tension may lead to an invasive phenotype.[44] The higher oxygen tensions in the non-transformed spiral arteries may induce the expression of invasive integrins, a vascular adhesion molecule phenotype, and cessation of mitotic activity. This may explain why trophoblast only superficially invades the uterine veins. Their oxygen tensions are low, so a differentiated adhesive phenotype is not expected.

FUNCTIONAL UNIT OF THE PLACENTA

The placenta's functional unit is variously known as the fetal lobule, fetal cotyledon, or fetal villous tree.[78] At term, the normal placenta contains 40–60 lobules, each 2–4 cm in diameter. The central area receives the oxygenated blood from the maternal spiral arteries and shows an increased number of immature intermediate villi. The surrounding, more densely packed villi show a predominance of mature intermediate and terminal villi. This is the area where gas exchange is maximal, as the blood slowly percolates around small villi that have vasculosyncytial membranes. At the lobule's periphery is the venous outflow area through which blood drains to the 50–200 maternal venous outlets. Despite the apparent continuity of the intervillous space, each lobule relies upon its own spiral artery. Thrombosis of that artery results in infarction in that lobule.

EXAMINATION OF THE PLACENTA

The average term placenta measures about $18 \times 16 \times 2.3$ cm (Figure 30.13).

UMBILICAL CORD

The cord should be measured, but the pathologist must remember that sections of the cord may have been removed shortly

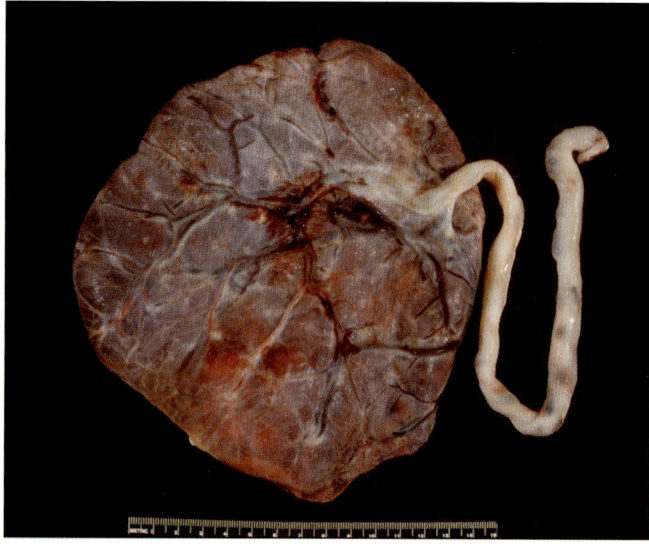

Fig. 30.13   Normal term placenta.

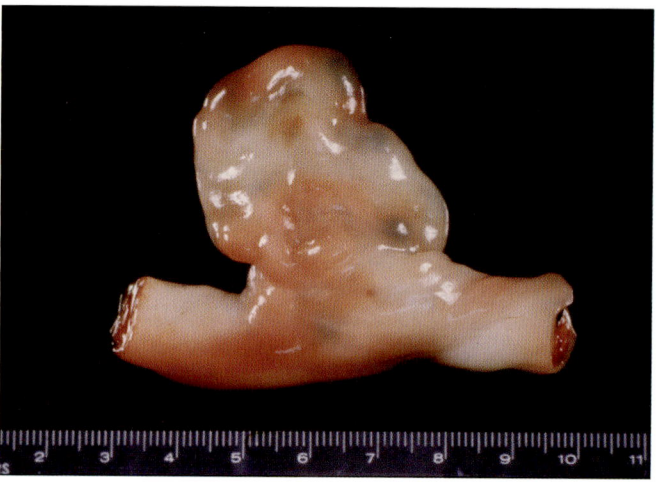

Fig. 30.15   Umbilical cord with false knots (vascular loops).

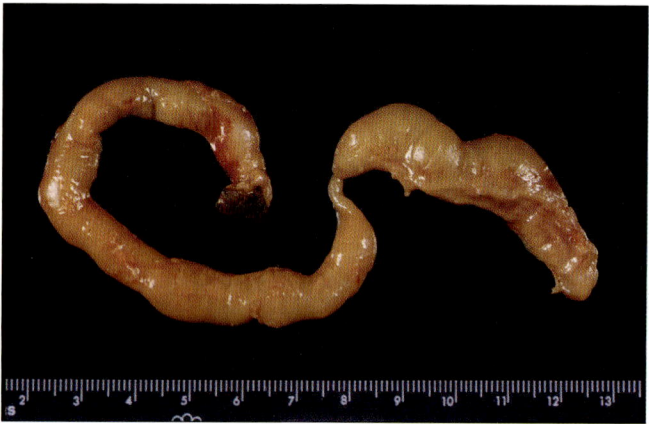

Fig. 30.14   Stricture in umbilical cord.

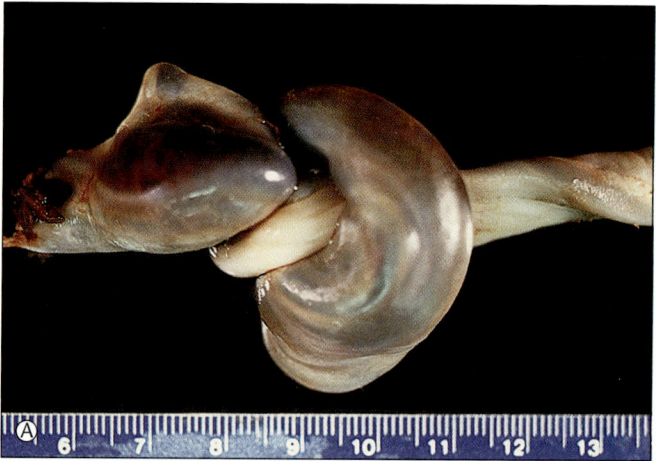

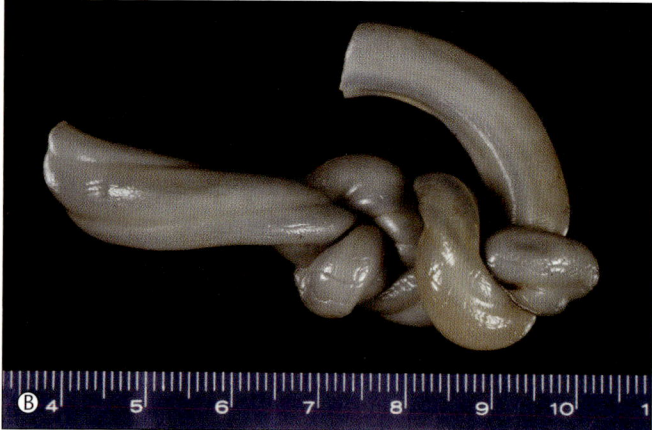

Fig. 30.16   Umbilical cord with **(A)** a single true knot and **(B)** multiple true knots.

after delivery for blood gas analysis. This possibility should be excluded before a short cord is reported. The average cord length is 60 cm. Longer cords are associated with hypermotility and shorter ones with hypomotility. Neural tube defects and chromosomal abnormalities are sometimes the underlying cause of the latter. In an 18-year retrospective review, excessively long cords (≥70 cm) were associated with a range of gross and microscopic features, and with abnormal neurologic status in infants.[11] Clinical or pathologic abnormalities of the cord were found in 70% of infants with fetal thrombotic vasculopathy.[106] Rarely does the cord show a stricture (Figure 30.14). False knots (vascular loops) may be present (Figure 30.15), but usually are of no clinical significance. The cross-sectional area of the cord and the size of the vessels should be noted. In routine practice maximum diameter is easier to measure. An association between adverse neonatal outcome and an umbilical vein area ≤10th percentile on sonography has been noted[46] and a reduction in vascular profiles has been found in cases of intrauterine growth restriction (IUGR) with abnormal Doppler waveforms.[19]

The significance of true knots is unclear. They are more likely to occur with a long cord, with hydramnios, and with male fetuses. The knots many be single (Figure 30.16A) or multiple (Figure 30.16B). The fetus with a long cord is less able to exert traction on the knot *in utero*. The effects of a knot are mediated by its tightening with traction, causing vascular compromise. This may happen at delivery, but then the chronic

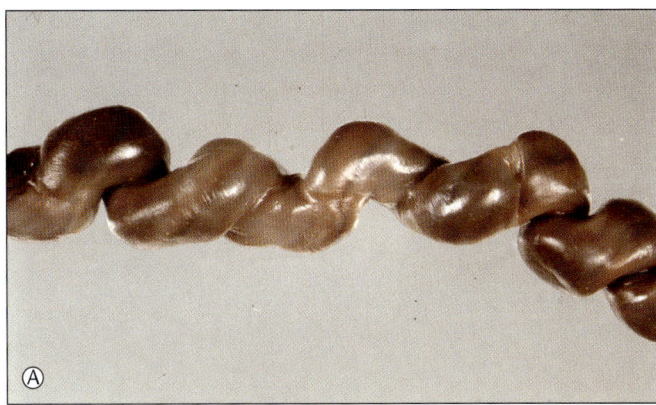

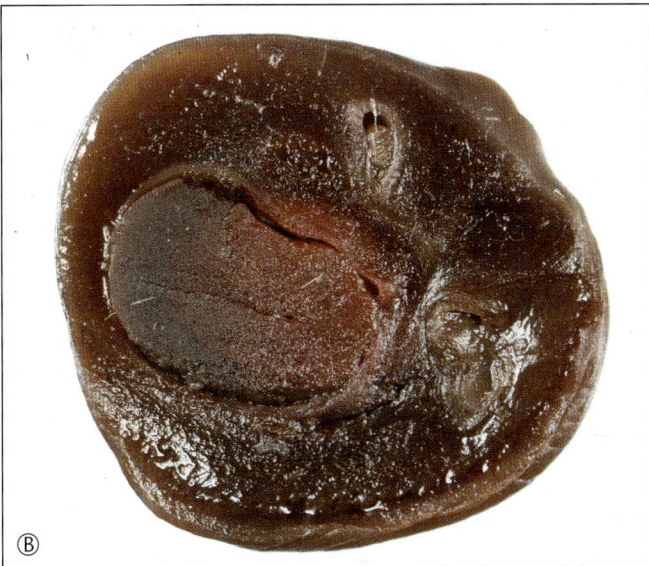

Fig. 30.17 **(A)** Torsed umbilical cord that has thrombosed. **(B)** Cross-section.

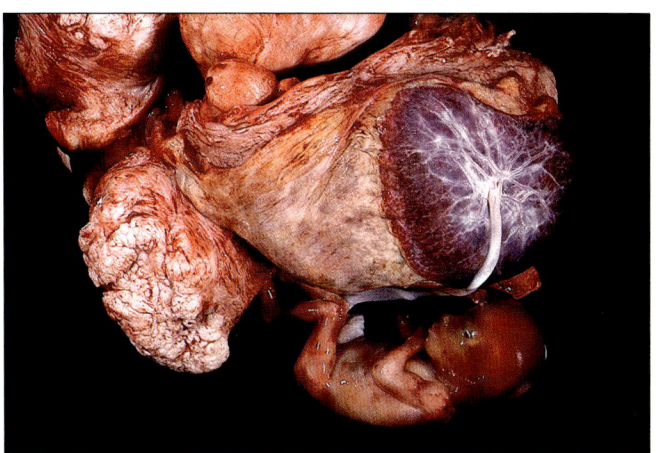

Fig. 30.18 Normal fetus and placenta showing implantation of the placenta as it is in the uterus.

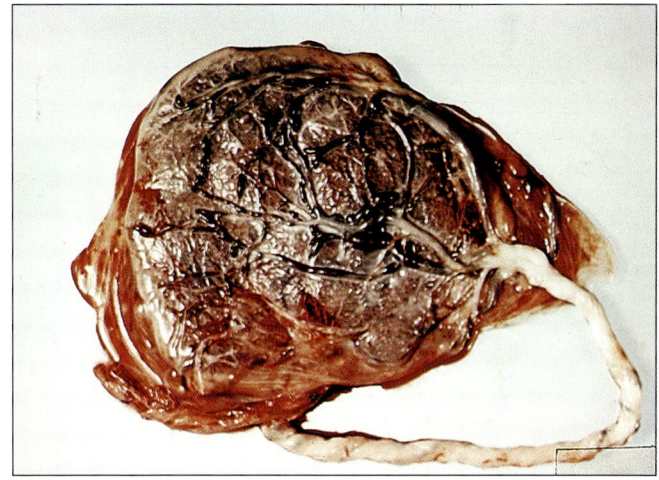

Fig. 30.19 Marginal insertion of umbilical cord ('battledore' placenta).

changes (fixed grooving of the cord, edema, vascular congestion, and thrombosis) induced by tightening will be absent. When these features are absent, the pathologist should be cautious in attributing fetal death to a true knot, remembering that a loose knot may be formed after intrauterine death. The lack of a difference in blood gas values between neonates with true knots and those without supports the interpretation that most knots are clinically insignificant.[82] However, a true knot is more commonly associated with other cord problems including nuchal cord and cord prolapse, either of which may contribute to the observed increase in antepartum (but not intrapartum) stillbirths.[53]

Coiling of the cord is normal. The normal range is one coil per 5 cm.[81] A literature review has indicated 0.17 ± 0.009 spirals completed per centimeter.[29] The 10th to 90th percentile range is one per 3 cm to one per 14 cm on this basis. Hypo- and hypercoiling of the cord is associated with a range of adverse pregnancy outcomes, including pregnancy loss and IUGR.[29,81] Occasionally the cord will torse and thrombose (Figure 30.17).

The cord may insert centrally (Figure 30.18), eccentrically, marginally or have a velamentous insertion. The latter two are the most significant. In marginal insertion, the cord joins the disc at its edge. This is sometimes called a 'battledore' placenta, because of the fancied resemblance to the racquet (racket) used in battledore, a precursor to badminton (Figure 30.19). Cord insertion directly onto the membranes (velamentous insertion) occurs in approximately 1% of singleton deliveries. The vessels are at risk of compression and thrombosis.[120] Rupture of these vessels can lead to significant fetal blood loss and hypoxia. In addition to intrapartum events, velamentous insertion is associated with an increased risk of preterm delivery, low birth weight, and abnormalities of fetal heart rate.[52] Vessels may be present in the membranes in up to 7% of placentas, but vasa previa (vessels in the membranes in advance of the presenting part) are less common (1:2500 deliveries). Prenatal diagnosis reduces the mortality rate in such cases from 56 to 3%.[98]

In the third stage of labor, avulsion of the cord may occur due to traction and this may cause subamniotic hemorrhage. However, this form of hemorrhage may also occur where a central or eccentric insertion is furcate (Figure 30.20), i.e., where cord vessels have lost their cover of Whartons jelly and have splayed out prior to inserting into the disc. In most cases fresh subamniotic hemorrhage is of no clinical significance. In some cases there may be hematomas of the cord without apparent explanation (Figure 30.21).

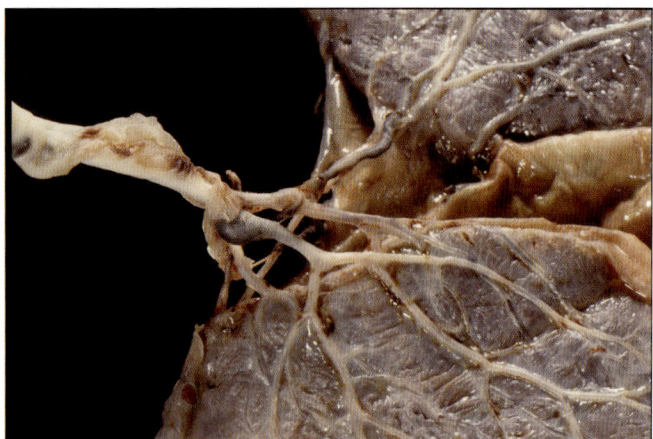

Fig. 30.20 Furcate insertion of umbilical cord.

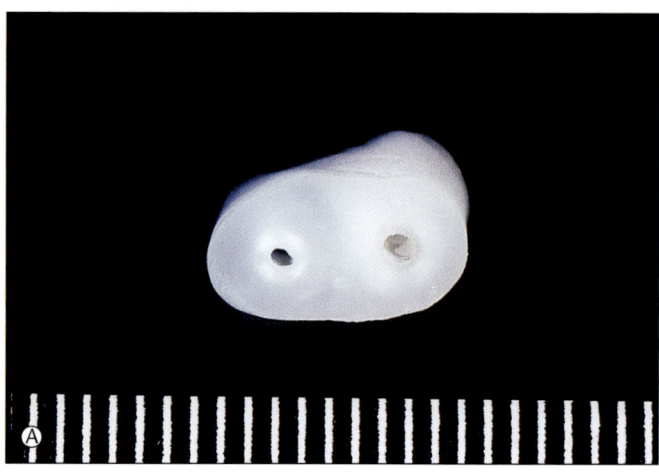

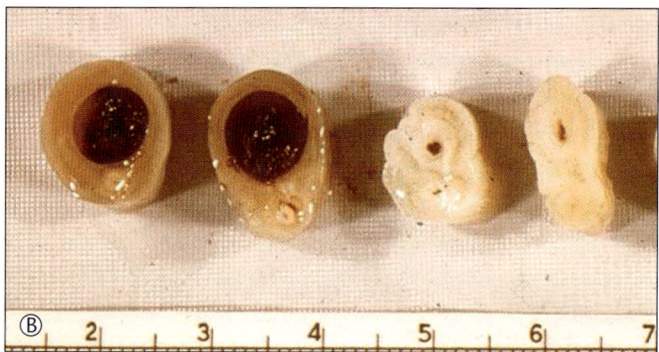

Fig. 30.22 **(A)** Two-vessel umbilical cord. **(B)** One vessel is thrombosed.

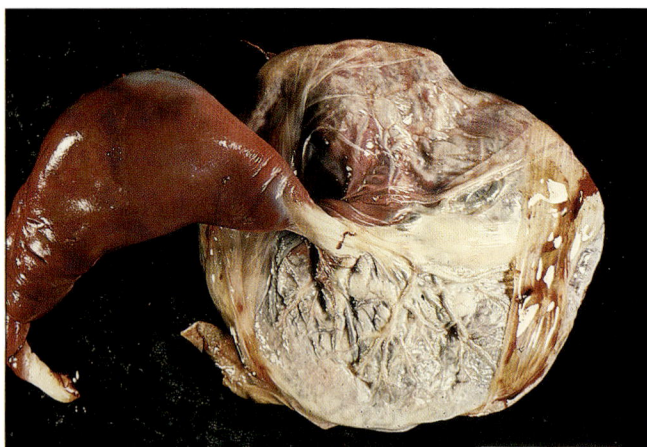

Fig. 30.21 Hematoma of umbilical cord.

The normal cord has three vessels – two umbilical arteries and one umbilical vein. Their presence should be confirmed in every cord examined, as 0.5–1.0% have only a single umbilical artery, i.e., a two-vessel cord (Figure 30.22). This abnormality, in one-third of cases, is associated with other congenital abnormalities, including those of the heart, gastrointestinal and urinary tracts, and central nervous system.[24] It also occurs in association with recognized syndromes, such as trisomy 18.[65] As some renal abnormalities may be minor and of little clinical significance, the extent to which the finding of a single umbilical artery requires further investigation is controversial. A meta-analysis of 37 studies concluded that, in the absence of other risk factors for malformation, intensive investigation of asymptomatic neonates with a single umbilical artery is not justified.[132]

Supernumerary vessels are rare and may be either arterial or venous. Tumors of the cord are also rare. Most are hemangiomas,[126,128] but rare angiomyxomas[131] and teratomas[71] have been reported. Thinned media of cord vessels may occur rarely. Confirmation of a possible association with congenital malformations is needed, given the small numbers of cases reported.[102] Grossly or sonographically visible cysts may develop from the vestigial remnants that are usually found as incidental microscopic findings. These remnants may be of the allantoic duct (possessing a flattened or transition cell-type epithelium; Figure 30.23A) or omphalomesenteric duct (cuboidal epithelium with mucinous component; Figure 30.23B).

The surface of the cord may appear edematous in some cases with acute inflammation. Traction and/or clamping should be excluded. An edematous cord with a reddish discoloration typically occurs with maceration.

MEMBRANES

Examination of the membranes for evidence of acute inflammation is of considerable importance. Acute chorioamnionitis is mainly caused by bacteria. It has been associated with bacterial vaginosis, a condition in which the vaginal pH rises above 4.5 and where a polymicrobial population containing *Bacteroides* sp., *Gardnerella vaginalis*, *Mycoplasma hominis*, *Ureaplasma urealyticum*, and *Peptostreptococcus* sp. replaces the lactobacilli normally present in the vagina.[119] It seems that *G. vaginalis* may interact with other organisms, such as *M. hominis*, to cause clinically significant infection.[48] Group B hemolytic *Streptococcus* is responsible for two neonatal syndromes: one, an infection in the first week, causes neonatal sepsis with a mortality of 15–20%; the second causes meningitis of later onset. Intrapartum infection can lead to early neonatal sepsis and the neonate may present almost immediately with respiratory distress syndrome. Although chorioamnionitis occurs with streptococcal infection, the organism is also known for its

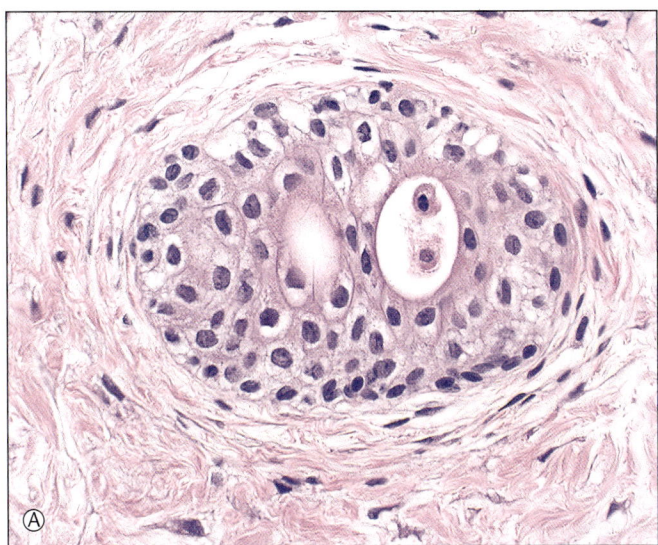

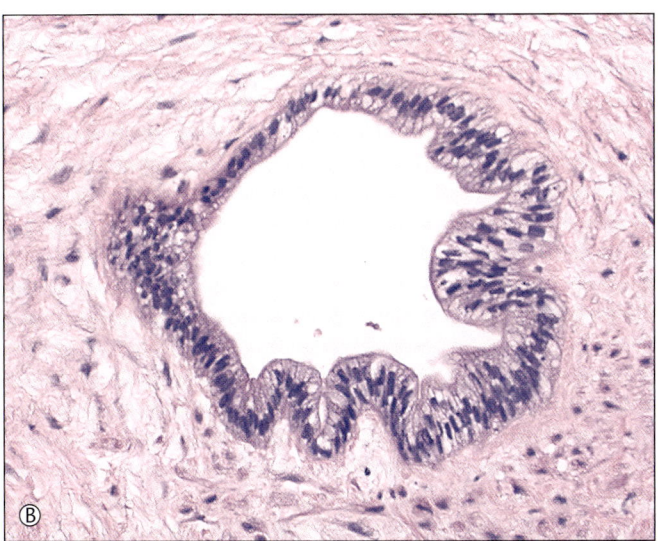

Fig. 30.23 Normal findings in umbilical cord. **(A)** Allantoic duct (possessing a flattened or transition cell-type epithelium), residual urinary tract system. **(B)** Omphalomesenteric duct (cuboidal epithelium with mucinous component), residual digestive system.

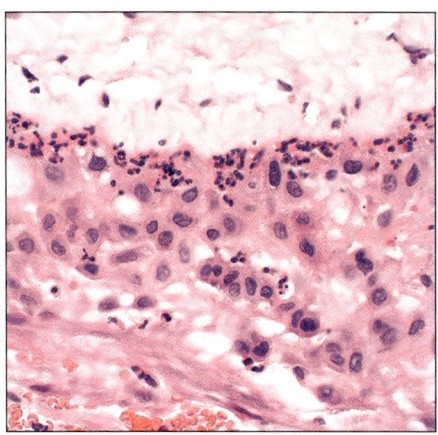

Fig. 30.24 Acute chorioamnionitis, stage 1. The inflammation involves the trophoblast, but not the spongy layer of the amnion.

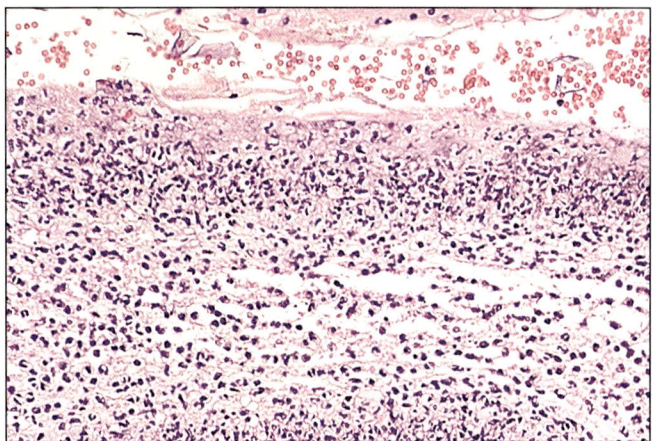

Fig. 30.25 Acute chorioamnionitis, stage 3 (Society of Pediatric Pathology). The inflammation pervades all structures and destroys the amnionic epithelium.

ability to infect the fetus even though the membranes remain intact and show little if any maternal response.

With early, mild acute inflammation, regardless of the type of organism, the membranes may be grossly normal. More advanced inflammation produces a milky opacity, altering the normal gray purple color of the disc. There may be frank pus with an offensive odor. Meconium may obscure the alterations of the acute inflammatory infiltrate.

The easiest method to assess inflammation is from a section of membranes cut from the rupture site to the margin of the disc and prepared for histologic examination as a roll, variously known as a 'Swiss roll', 'jam roll', and 'jelly roll'. One method used to report the severity of the inflammation is histologic staging.[38,113,134] In stage 1 the neutrophils permeate the trophoblastic layers, but not into the spongy layer of the amnion (Figure 30.24). The next more advanced stage (stage 2) is where neutrophils have infiltrated into the spongy layer of the amnion. In stage 3, all layers of the amnion are involved,

but the epithelium is preserved. Newer systems have collapsed stages 2 and 3 into a single stage 2. In stage 4 (stage 3 by the newer system of the Society of Pediatric Pathology) necrotizing inflammation has destroyed the amnion (Figure 30.25). Even though the histologic stages have shown some correlation with stages of microbial infection,[118] there is frequently a discrepancy between the clinical and histologic diagnosis of chorioamnionitis.[127]

The neutrophils in chorioamnionitis are maternal in origin, as examination of the chorionic plate reveals. In contrast, the inflammatory response in the wall of cord vessels (funisitis) (most commonly the vein, but in severe cases, the arteries as well) represents the response of a live fetus to infected amniotic fluid. The inflammatory pattern and the time taken to mount an inflammatory response may primarily reflect the virulence of the infecting organism. Organisms of low virulence (e.g., *Ureaplasma*, *Mycoplasma*, and anaerobes) may cause preterm labor, but not bacteremia in the neonate. They probably take days rather than hours to reach the placenta. Virulent organisms e.g., Group B *Streptococcus*, *Escherichia coli*, and *Listeria* can cause bacteremia and may reach the placenta in hours rather than days. However, membrane integrity, maternal immune status, and cytokine gene polymorphisms play a role,

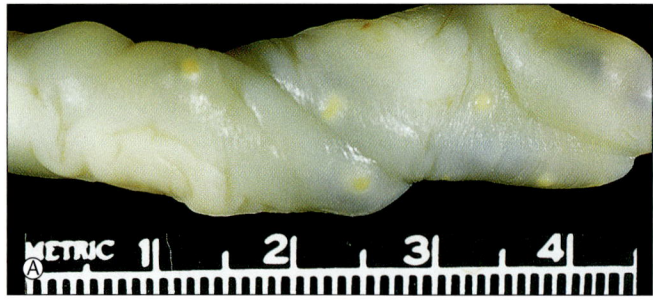

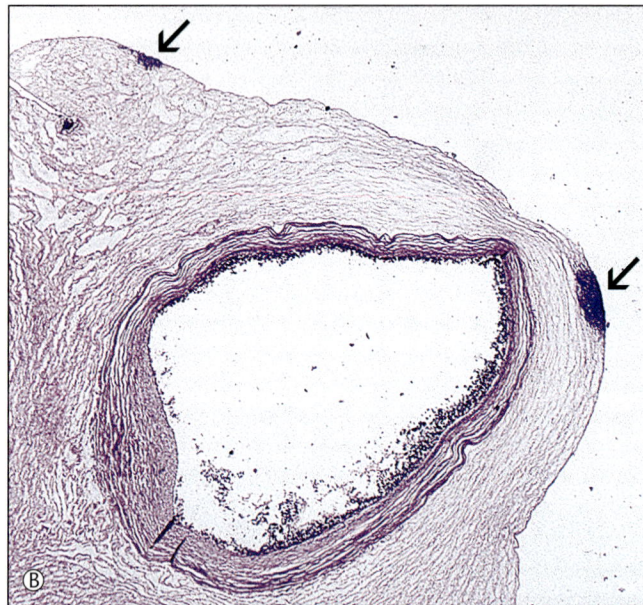

Fig. 30.26 *Candida* funisitis. **(A)** Small white flecks are on the surface, which **(B)** microscopically are *Candida* organisms (arrows).

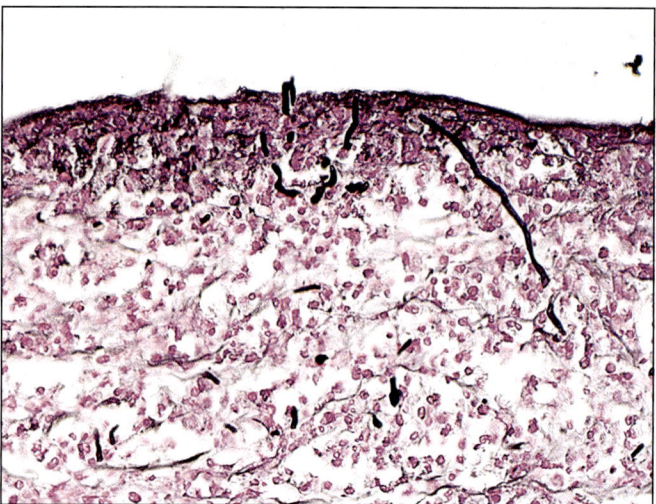

Fig. 30.27 Pseudohyphae (black) of *Candida* infecting the umbilical cord. (Methenamine silver stain.)

and assessment of timing in an individual case may be difficult. Gestational age is also of importance – chorionic vasculitis is less prevalent with increased gestational age.[28] In addition to bacteria, fungi and viruses may also cause infection via the ascending pathway. In *Candida* chorioamnionitis, numerous yellow-white spongy flecks stud the membranes and umbilical cord (Figures 30.26 and 30.27). Some feel these are pathognomonic of *Candida* infection.[62]

The clinical significance of chorioamnionitis and funisitis depends on gestational age and severity. Ascending infection is a major cause of preterm premature rupture of the membranes, which accounts for 30–40% of preterm births.[9] Increasing stages of chorioamnionitis show a significant association with funisitis, preterm birth and perinatal death.[134] Funisitis has been directly linked with development of fetal germinal matrix hemorrhages, choroiditis with intraventricular hemorrhage, and periventricular leukomalacia.[49,94,135,136] For term infants, there is an increased risk of sepsis following chorioamnionitis, but neurologic morbidity may be related to other complications of labor.[3] In one study of very low birth weight infants,[112] vascular thrombi in placentas that were associated with chorioamnionitis were felt to account for neurologic impairment. An association between chorioamnionitis and adverse developmental outcome has not been demonstrated in other studies on similar groups.[32] The presence of acutely inflamed membranes should prompt a search for associated lesions such as thrombi, and exclusion of coexistent pathology, such as retroplacental hemorrhage, where chorioamnionitis is more common.[104] There is a correlation between increased interleukin 6 (IL-6) levels and increasing extent of fetal vessel vasculitis. Morphologic patterns differ with gestational age, with earlier elevation of IL-6 in term infants.[117] Decidual necrosis manifests as a shaggy, cream-yellow area, usually present near the margin of the placental disc. Nodularity of the amnion may be due either to amnion nodosum (Figure 30.28) or squamous metaplasia (Figure 30.29). The two can usually be distinguished on gross examination. Amnion nodosum is a consequence of oligohydramnios and presents as approximately 3 mm nodules, which may be relatively easily detached by running a finger over the involved area. Microscopy shows aggregates of amorphous and cellular debris, and even occasionally detached hair (Figure 30.28B). With squamous metaplasia, which has no known clinical associations, the nodules are only detached with difficulty.

Abnormalities of the placenta may cause fetal malformation.[25] Some may be fatal such as body stalk anomaly. Amniotic bands should be sought in the context of more restricted fetal abnormalities, including amputation, acral deformities, or even craniofacial abnormalities that may resemble neural tube defect. These bands are delicate strands of amnion and mesoderm whose effects may be predominantly or exclusively mechanical. They may be focal or extensive, and histologic examination of carefully selected areas will confirm absence of the amnion from its normal location.

MECONIUM ON CORD AND MEMBRANES

We regard the presence of scanty macrophages with non-hemosiderin pigments as normal and physiologic: indeed, fetal defecation has been documented sonographically.[103] More extensive meconium staining produces a green discoloration grossly. Its passage is generally felt to reflect hypoxic stress in the fetus. Meconium acts as a vasoconstrictor on the

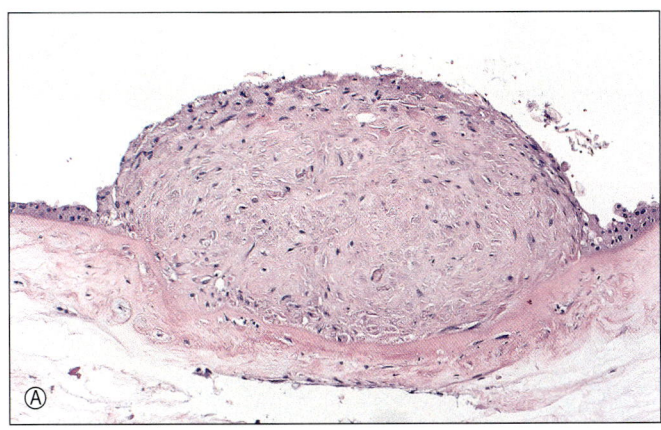

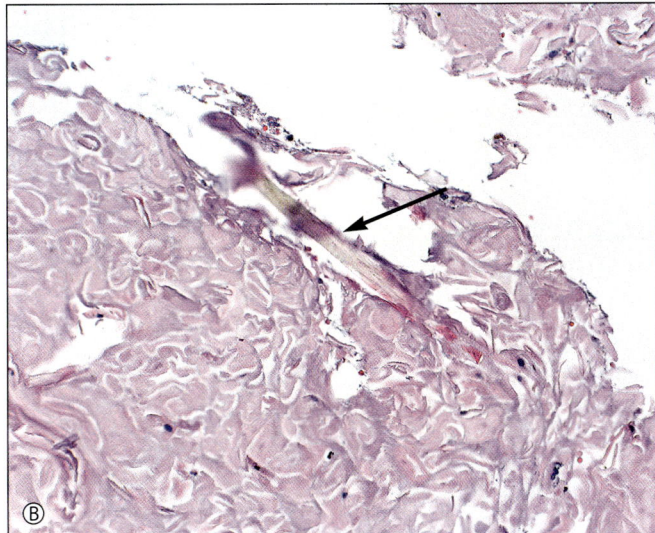

Fig. 30.28 **(A)** Amnion nodosum. **(B)** Embedded hair shaft (arrow).

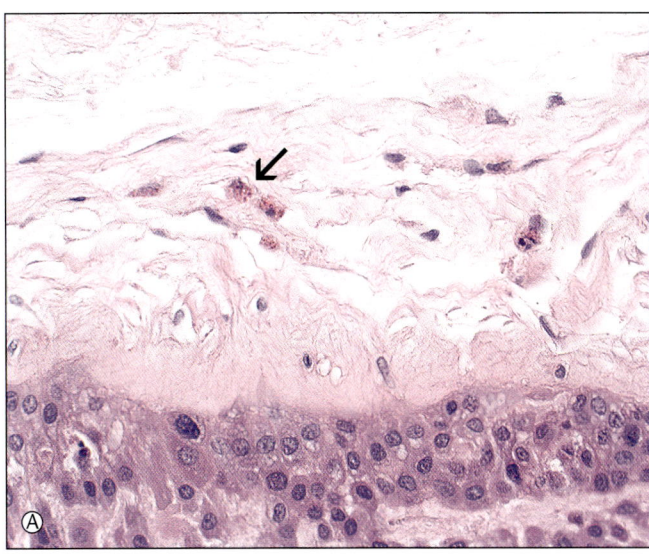

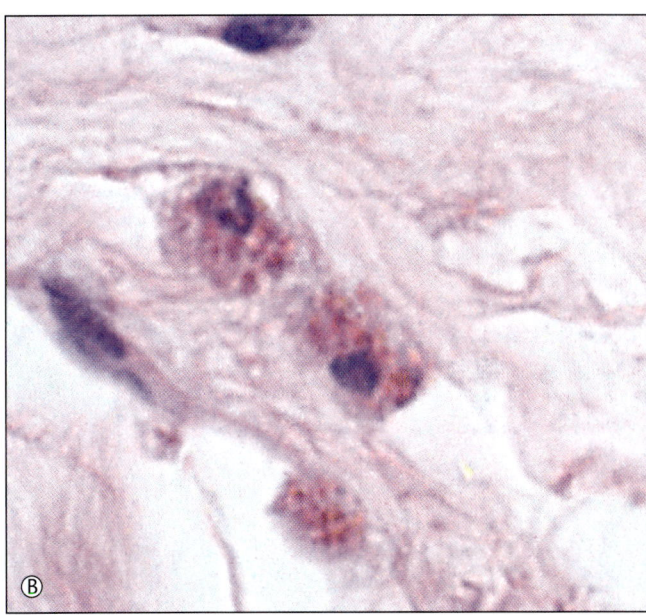

Fig. 30.30 Meconium. **(A)** A light green-brown pigment barely visible at low magnification fills the macrophage (arrow). **(B)** Detail (inset)

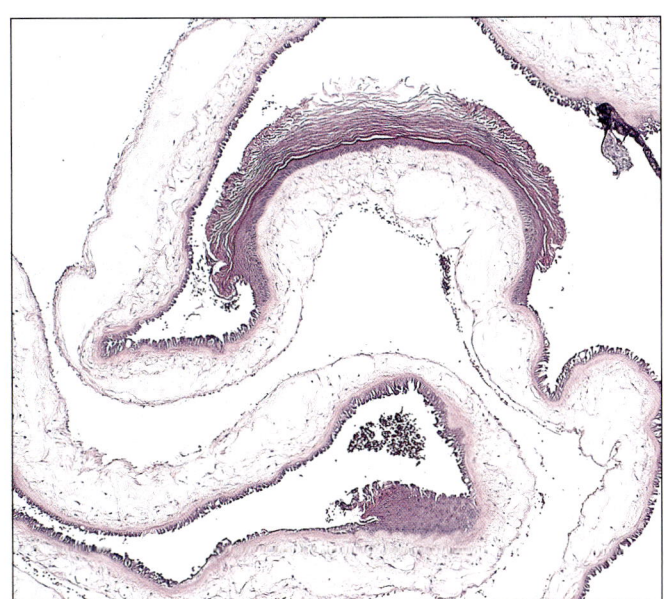

Fig. 30.29 Squamous metaplasia.

fetoplacental vasculature[54] and the vascular spasm that ensues has been suggested as a cause of adverse pregnancy outcome.[4] Morphologically, meconium may result in necrosis of smooth muscle cells of umbilical cord vessels or cause ulceration of the cord.[20] The changes in muscle cells may mimic a vasculitis.[45]

The presence of meconium in amnionic macrophages (Figure 30.30) indicates its presence on the membranes for at least 3 hours.[93] Macrophages with meconium can remain in the amnion or chorion for a week after the meconium is no longer visible in the amniotic fluid.[93] If aspirated, meconium produces significant pneumonitis. The inflammation that the meconium induces is maximal in the cord, but is less intense and more focal than that due to the vasculitis of chorioamnionitis.[20]

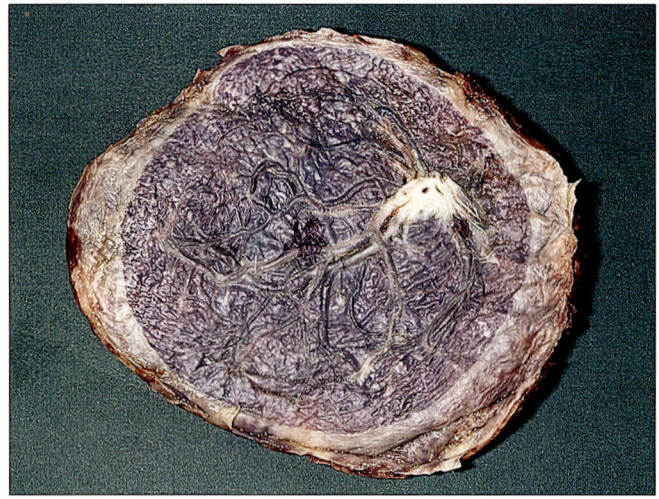

Fig. 30.31 Circummarginate placenta.

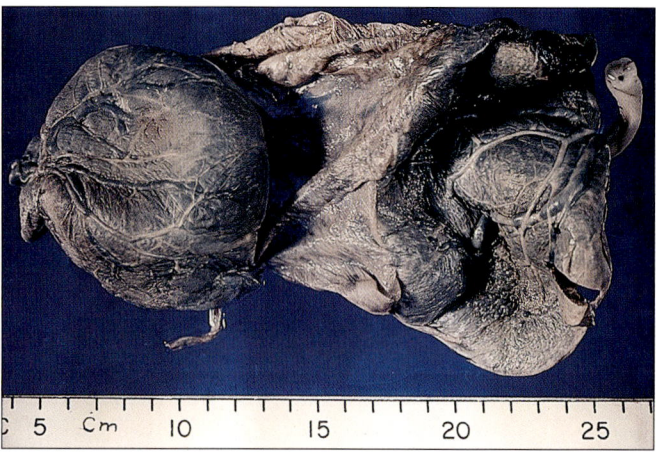

Fig. 30.33 Bilobate placenta.

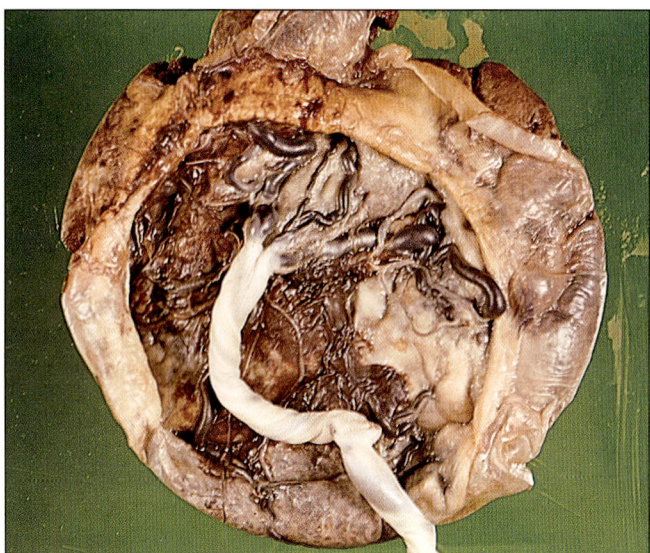

Fig. 30.32 Circumvallate placenta. The membranes fold back upon themselves on the surface of the placenta.

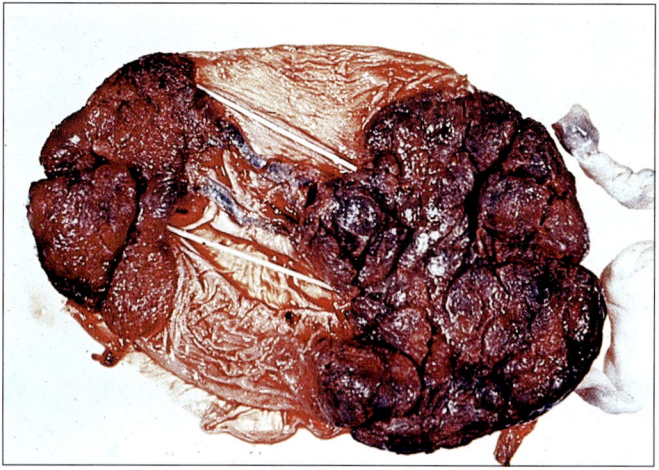

Fig. 30.34 Succenturiate lobe of placenta.

ARCHITECTURAL AND DEVELOPMENTAL ABNORMALITIES

Extrachorial placentas have the chorion laeve inserting at some distance inside rather than at the rim of the placenta. The term 'extrachorial' implies that the edge of the placenta is uncovered except for fibrin and, sometimes, old clotted blood. Thus, the edge of the placental villous tissue protrudes from under the chorion laeve/membranes. Vaginal bleeding may occasionally originate from this site. If the transition is flat, the placenta is called 'circummarginate'; if the edge is rolled up and folded over itself ('plicated'), the placenta is then called 'circumvallate'.

The circummarginate form (Figure 30.31) has no known clinical associations. The circumvallate form (Figure 30.32), however, is associated with threatened abortion, membrane rupture, and antepartum hemorrhage leading to prematurity,

but not to an increase in perinatal mortality. Circumvallation is significantly associated with iron-laden macrophages in the membranes, termed 'diffuse chorioamnionic hemosiderosis',[111] suggesting circumvallation may be caused by chronic peripheral separation of the placenta. Both types of extrachorial placentation are rarely total and mixtures between the two and normal placentation are more frequently encountered.

The bilobed placenta has two nearly equal sized discs with the umbilical cord inserting between the two either velamentously or marginally in the larger half (Figure 30.33). An initial lateral implantation in the endometrium that is relatively avascular leads to trophotropism and placentation on both the anterior and posterior endometrial surfaces. These placentas are associated with multiparity, older maternal age, previous history of infertility, assisted reproduction, retention, and abnormal adherence. The vessels between the two may thrombose or present as vasa previa. Higher orders of lobation are extremely rare.

Accessory (succenturiate) lobes are found in 6% of placentas and are small areas of placental tissue joined by either an isthmus or velamentous vessels to the main disc (Figure 30.34). If symptomatic, they may present as placenta previa with or without fetal hemorrhage or be retained *in utero* postpartum. Placenta membranacea arises when there is failure of villous regression to form a chorion laeve. Thus, an abnormally thin placenta comes to cover an unusually large area of the uterine lining. The entire conceptual sac is covered with villi and the placenta becomes, in addition, a placenta previa. The placenta on cut section is thinned from the normal 2.5 or 3 cm to perhaps 1 cm or less in the fixed state. This condition is sometimes associated with mid-trimester antepartum hemorrhage. It may also sometimes show undue adherence, but normal third-stage delivery usually occurs.

A fenestrate placenta is one where a placental lobule appears missing. Careful inspection of the maternal aspect shows that the lobules surrounding the expected location of the missing lobule are smooth, and the featureless overlying chorion is smooth. A girdle or ring placenta is one with the membranes above and below the placental ring. They are rare in humans.

PLACENTAL WEIGHT

Opinions vary on the utility of placental weight.[17,40,93] As the placenta varies considerably in length, breadth, and depth, we feel that this single metric parameter conveys information, despite the variables impinging on it. It is especially useful when combined with a description, e.g., in cases of hydrops, where a severely affected placenta is pale and heavy. The placenta should be weighed trimmed of cord and membranes, with any adherent clot removed and weighed separately.

Placental weight depends on the *in utero* environment, timing of cord clamping, storage interval, and fixation.[39] The timing of umbilical cord clamping at delivery will either trap a considerable quantity of blood within the placenta if early, or lead to a relatively bloodless organ if delayed. The practice of placental examination in the unfixed state will be associated with fluid loss of variable extent, but it tends to increase with storage time. Formalin fixation of the placenta will result in a gain in weight of often 8–10%, and occasionally up to 15%. The relatively few studies published all show a trend for increasing placental weight during this past century, which is most likely due to improved nutritional status and environmental factors. Twin placental weights have a ratio of 1.69 above that of the same gestational age singletons.[101] Singleton placental weight gain was more than that in twins, but waned after 37 weeks. Placental weight in isolation is of limited use because there is a large spread of acceptable weights for gestational age. However, the figures of 190 g ± 45 at 24 weeks, 320 g ± 70 at 30 weeks, and 540 g ± 100 at 40 weeks provide a general indication of normality or otherwise. The ratio of normal placental to fetal weight at term is 0.14, with a range of 0.1–0.2.

Lesions found with IUGR, especially when more than a single lesion, are often associated with a decreased placental weight.[109] Pre-eclamptic placentas tend to be small, as do those with fetal congenital anomalies, infection, and chromosomal errors. Large placentas are found in women living at high altitude. They are often large in women with diabetes mellitus, rhesus incompatibility, fetal hydrops, maternal and fetal anemia, and some chronic intrauterine infections, e.g., syphilis.

FETAL SURFACE OF PLACENTA

The normal color of the fetal surface is a gray purple and is due to the presence of blood in the parenchyma as seen through clear membranes. Small (usually <3 cm) subamniotic cysts and

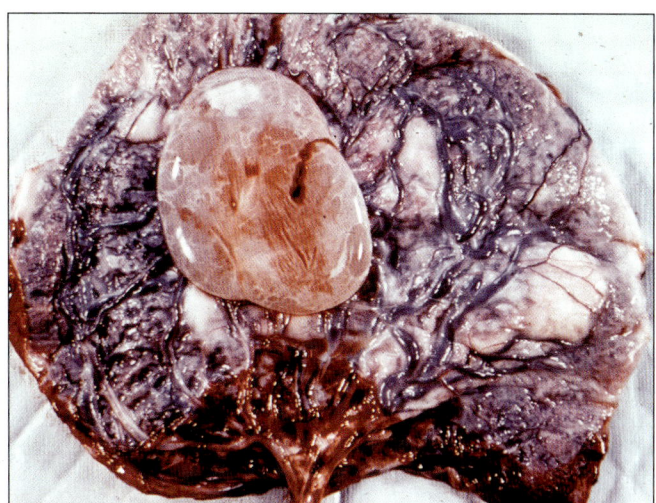

Fig. 30.35 Subamniotic cyst.

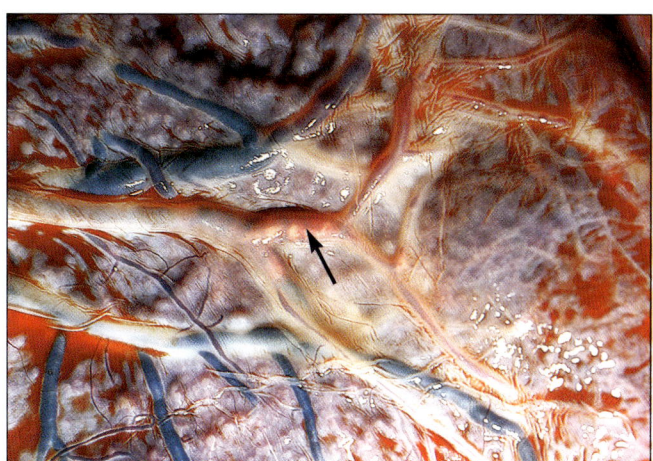

Fig. 30.36 Arterial thrombus (arrow), visible on the fetal surface.

rarely large (Figure 30.35) may be present as incidental findings. Stripping the amnion allows more detailed inspection of the chorionic plate vessels. Normally, fetal arteries run over (i.e., uppermost) veins. This is valuable as the arteries may be difficult to distinguish histologically. Thrombi, which may appear grossly as thickened white areas of the vessel wall, may be subtle and only appreciated on close examination. Thrombi may be seen in arteries (Figure 30.36), but more often are in veins (Figure 30.37).[69] Barium gelatin injection of the umbilical arteries is one definitive method to identify arteries (Figure 30.38).

Mesenchymal dysplasia can manifest as malformed surface chorionic vessels and proximal portions of the stem villous vessels (Figure 30.39).[77,123] The placentas have aneurysmally dilated chorionic plate vessels and focally cystic stem villi with myxomatous stroma and cistern formation, but lack the trophoblastic features of partial mole. Furthermore, cell lines derived from placentas with mesenchymal dysplasia have a diploid genome. Some cases have been associated with Beckwith–Wiedemann syndrome,[60,74] placental chorangiomas, and fetal hemangiomas.[23]

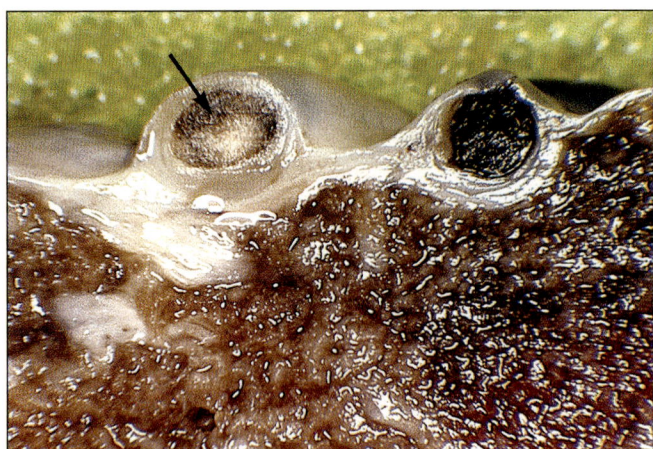

Fig. 30.37 Thrombus in a chorionic plate vessel (arrow). The vessel is probably a vein (left).

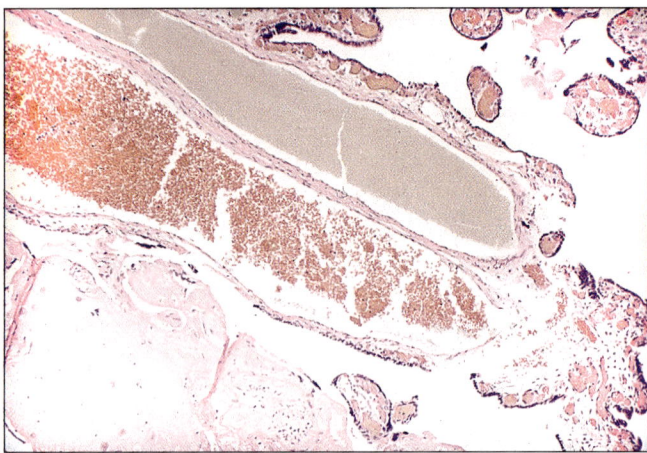

Fig. 30.38 Intra-arterial injection of barium gelatin distinguishes artery from vein. Courtesy of Dr Peter Kelehan, National Maternity Hospital, Dublin.

MATERNAL SURFACE OF THE PLACENTA

The cotyledons of the placenta should be examined to ensure that the placenta is intact. Evidence of old hemorrhage, manifest as foci of tan-colored granularity, should be sought, especially where there is a clinical history of pre-eclampsia or extensive or central infarction. The presence of hemorrhage and the percentage of the surface affected, its location (central or peripheral), and the presence or absence of cavitation should be noted. A wrinkled gyriform pattern is characteristic of maternal floor infarction. The basal plate should be examined to detect thrombosed spiral arteries.[70,105]

CUT SURFACE

The placenta should be serially sectioned and examined at intervals of 1–2 cm. The parenchyma varies in color depending on the amount of maternal and fetal blood present. A degree of pallor is normal where the disc has been drained. A dramatic color change in an intact placenta, i.e., a 'two-tone' effect, may be seen in cases of retroplacental hemorrhage.[89] Any lesions should be described and the percentage of the parenchyma affected estimated and recorded.

INFARCTION

The placenta requires both maternal and fetal blood flow for normal function. Acute cessation of maternal blood flow in the presence of a live fetus results in a placental infarct. The placenta can withstand loss of a variable percentage, often given as one-third, of its functional tissue before this become clinically manifest. However, this may be influenced by how rapidly infarction develops and by the quality of the remaining parenchyma.

On cut section, an acute infarct is red and as it ages the color changes through brown, to tan, to off-white (Figures 30.40–30.42). The consistency changes from firm to hard. Central

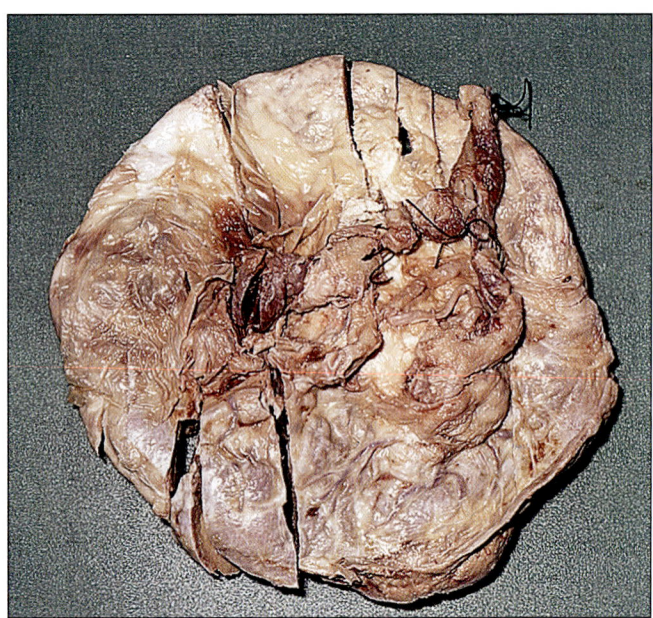

Fig. 30.39 Mesenchymal dysplasia. The fetal surface shows a mass of large caliber vessels.

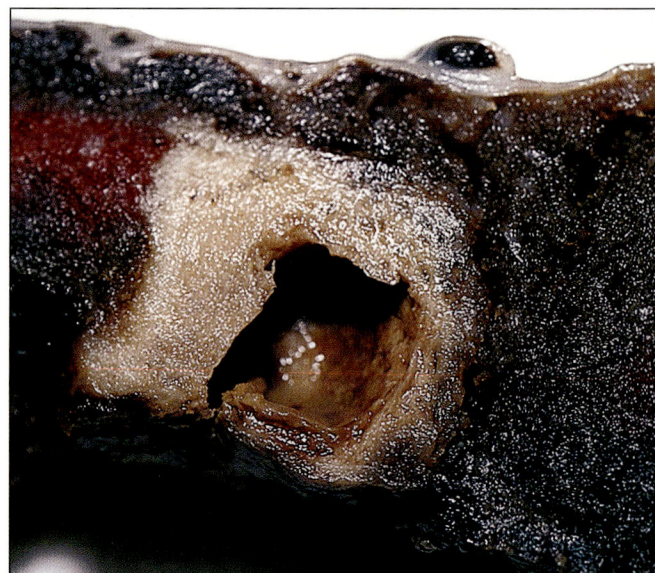

Fig. 30.40 Old infarction. The cavity was due to a hematoma that caused compression. The retroplacental nature of the hematoma cannot be appreciated from this section.

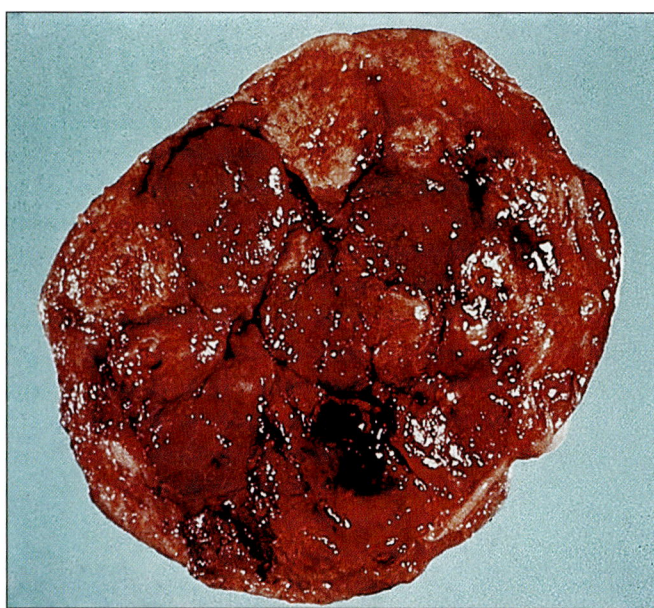

Fig. 30.41 Old infarcts. The infarcts appear as off-white, triangular-shaped, inverted pyramids.

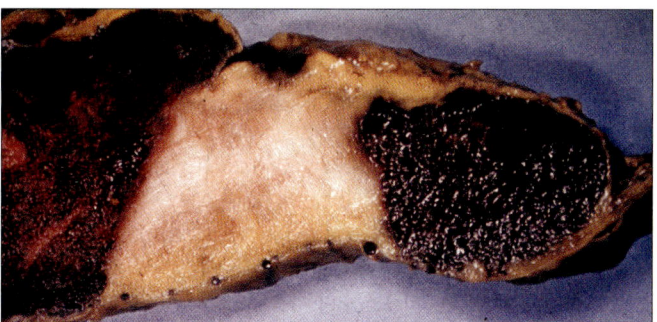

Fig. 30.42 Old infarct, transmural. The infarct is off-white to yellow, and triangular shaped.

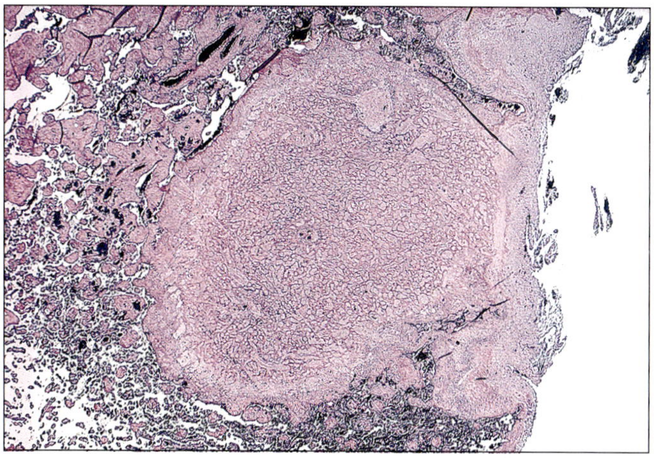

Fig. 30.43 Infarct. The chorionic villi are ghost-like. No viable cells are present either in them or the surrounding fibrin.

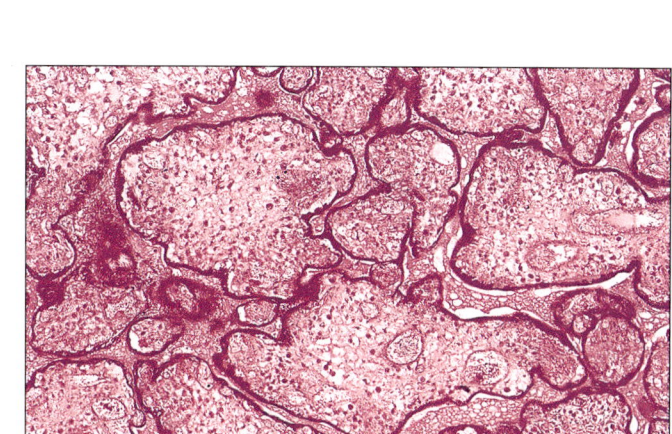

Fig. 30.44 Infarct with ghost outlines of villi. As time passes, the outlines become less pronounced.

infarcts and those occurring earlier in gestation are more likely to be significant, whereas peripheral infarction of even 5% at term is considered physiologic. The age of the infarct(s), location, percentage at parenchymal involvement, and presence of associated retroplacental hemorrhage should be noted.

Histologically, the acute infarct is composed of non-viable villi with erythrocyte extravasation and areas of syncytiotrophoblastic nuclear pyknosis. The intervillous space is narrowed and later obliterated by fibrin deposition. Aging lesions have ghost-like villi surrounded by fibrin (Figures 30.43 and 30.44). Infarction is associated with IUGR fetal hypoxia and intrauterine fetal death. Infarction is the morphologic expression of a severely compromised uteromaternal vascular supply. A reduction in fetal blood flow may sometimes precede infarction.[84]

PERIVILLOUS FIBRIN DEPOSITION AND MATERNAL FLOOR 'INFARCTION'

Perivillous fibrin deposition is seen macroscopically as areas of firm gray-white waxy material, usually peripherally, but some-

times throughout the placenta (Figure 30.45). Larger lesions show eosinophilic fibrin that separates villi (Figure 30.46). The syncytiotrophoblast is degenerate and cytotrophoblast prominent. The villi become atrophic and non-functional. Perivillous fibrin deposition is seen increasingly from 30 weeks gestational age, but is not unduly increased in post-term deliveries. It is less prominent where maternal blood flow is reduced, i.e., with pre-eclampsia, essential hypertension, and diabetes. With maternal floor infarction there is an increase in basal plate fibrin over the entire maternal floor that exceeds 3 mm thickness. Fibrin encroaches on the intervillous space and causes the maternal surface to develop a gyriform pattern macroscopically (Figure 30.47). Histologically, the fibrin layer of the basal plate thickens, with perivillous fibrin extending to surround adjacent villi, sometimes through the thickness of the placenta.

Another pattern, massive perivillous fibrin deposition (≥25% of villi encased by fibrin), is strongly associated with IUGR.[63] Some believe that the increase in fibrin only occurs after fetal death as a protection against postmortem hemorrhage, but it can occur with live births.[7] It is associated with an increase in

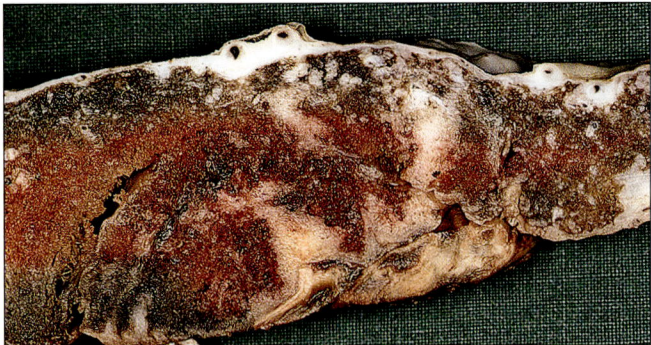

Fig. 30.45 Perivillous fibrin deposition showing large waxy plaques.

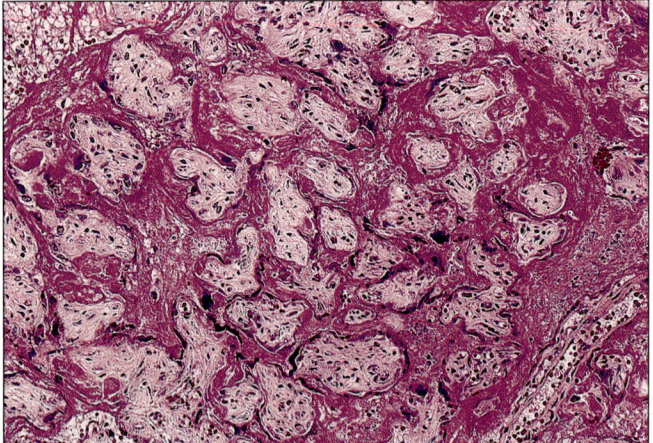

Fig. 30.46 Extensive perivillous fibrin around villi.

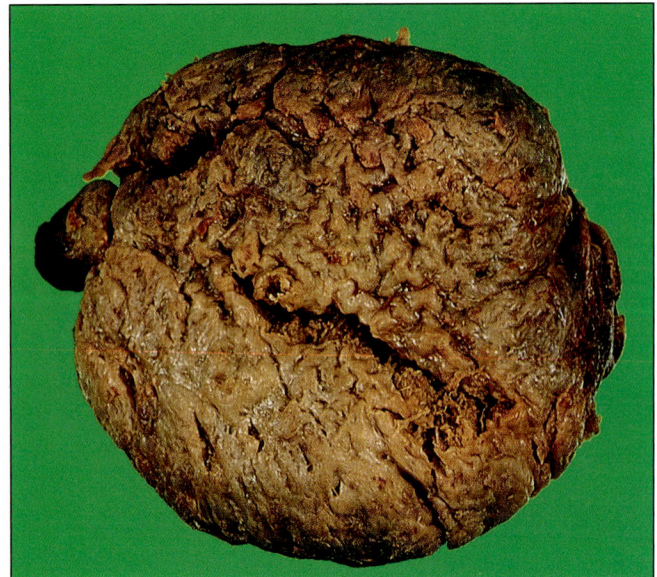

Fig. 30.47 Maternal floor infarction with gyriform fibrin deposition. Courtesy of Dr D.G. Fagan, University Hospital, Queen's Medical Centre, Nottingham.

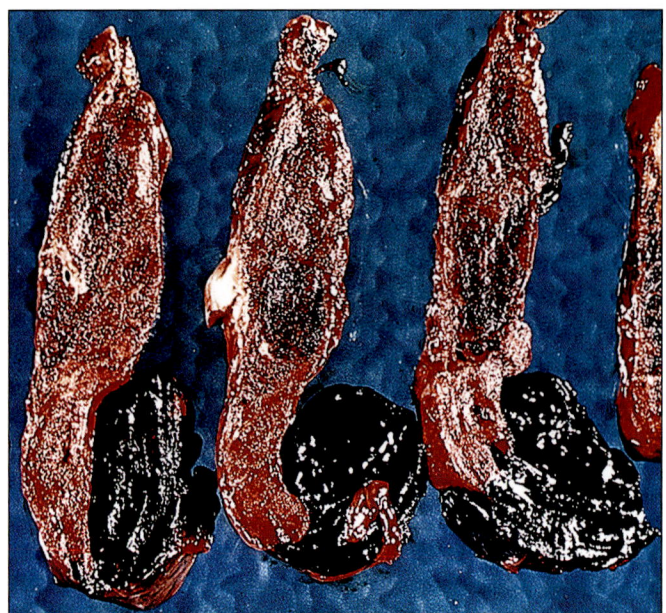

Fig. 30.48 Abruptio placenta with adherent retroplacental clot.

perinatal mortality and fetal growth restriction.[13] It may cause a rise in maternal serum α-fetoprotein and cases may be recognized prospectively by the combination of IUGR, oligohydramnios, and increased placental echogenicity.[83] This condition is important to recognize in the delivered placenta since it may recur in subsequent pregnancies.[13,43] Subchorionic fibrin deposition results from changes in blood flow and eddy currents. It is usually laminated and roughly pyramidal in shape with its base at the chorionic plate. As it lacks (or has very few) enmeshed villi, placental function is not lost. The observations of an absence of subchorionic fibrin deposition in fetuses with movement disorders, short umbilical cords, and later neurologic handicap has prompted the opinion, now questioned, that the fetus normally damages the subchorionic plate fibrin layer, which may then lead to thrombosis.[92] Against this view, the subchorionic trophoblastic layer is already partially degenerate and replaced by fibrin by the time that fetal movements are sufficiently robust to cause damage.[41]

HEMATOMA

Retroplacental hematomas separate the placenta's basal plate from the uterine wall, causing fetal anoxia and maternal hemorrhage (Figure 30.48).[41] Retroplacental hemorrhage is found in 5% of placentas, occurring considerably more commonly than the clinical diagnosis would suggest. Many small hemorrhages are clinically silent. Conversely, a dramatic abruption with rapid cesarean section may have no placental manifestations. A more slowly developing retroplacental hematoma will indent the parenchyma and cause compression infarction of the overlying parenchyma (Figure 30.49). Small yellow flecks of decidua may be seen on the outer and inner surface of the hematoma. Acute lesions consist almost entirely of red blood cells, but with aging these degenerate and are replaced by fibrin. The overlying decidua is frequently necrotic and infiltrated by neutrophils and macrophages. Long-standing lesions may contain hemosiderin-laden macrophages.

The following have been associated with retroplacental hematoma and abruption: pre-eclampsia, essential hypertension, obstruction of the inferior vena cava, folic acid deficiency, cigarette smoking, anticardiolipin antibodies, blunt abdominal trauma, and chorioamnionitis. An association with cocaine use may be overstated.[90] A pregnancy with abruption carries a much higher risk for adverse perinatal outcome such as stillbirth and preterm delivery and increases the risk for recurrence in a subsequent pregnancy.[5] Vascular malformations in placental bed biopsies in cases of abruption have been described in addition to failure of physiologic transformation.[34] The cause is therefore likely to be multifactorial.[88] The extent of the hematoma, the speed of onset, and the status of the uteroplacental vasculature all interact to determine outcome.

A marginal hematoma is a collection of blood adjacent to the margin of the placenta with stripping of the chorion laeve, usually seen as a crescent around the placental periphery. It may be associated with antepartum hemorrhage.

SUBCHORIAL THROMBOSIS (BREUS MOLE)

Subchorial thromboses are found both with abortions and live term pregnancies (Figure 30.50). The fetal surface shows numerous bosselations while the cut surface discloses a laminated thrombus between the chorionic plate and the underlying villous tissue. Strands of stem villi may be found within the thrombus. The subchorial thrombosis should be at least 2 cm thick. The pathogenesis is not fully understood, but may be caused by sudden slowing of blood flow in the subchorionic region.[41]

INTERVILLOUS THROMBOSIS

Intervillous thrombi mark the site of fetal–maternal hemorrhage and consist of laminated blood clot comprising both fetal and maternal red cells. A rim of compressed and infarcted villi, which may be numerous, is found in about a third of term placentas. Occasionally, these thrombi are found in cases of maternal–fetal rhesus incompatibility. A fresh thrombus, sometimes called a Kline's hemorrhage, may appear on section as a hole in the villous parenchyma in which the blood is easily washed out.[42] The pathogenesis probably lies in small disruptions in the villous capillaries.

OTHER CONDITIONS

Calcifications in the placenta are common in primigravidas, especially in those who deliver in the summer and autumn months. It is not more common in post-term placentas and is of no clinical significance.

Septal cysts are collections of gelatinous gray fluid seen at the apex of placental septa. The fluid is probably derived from the surrounding mantle of X cells or intermediate trophoblast. They are more common in edematous than normal placentas, but have no apparent clinical significance.

MULTIPLE GESTATION

Multiple births occur normally in slightly under 1% of spontaneously conceived pregnancies and may be dizygotic or monozygotic (Figure 30.51). Dizygotic twinning has a strong

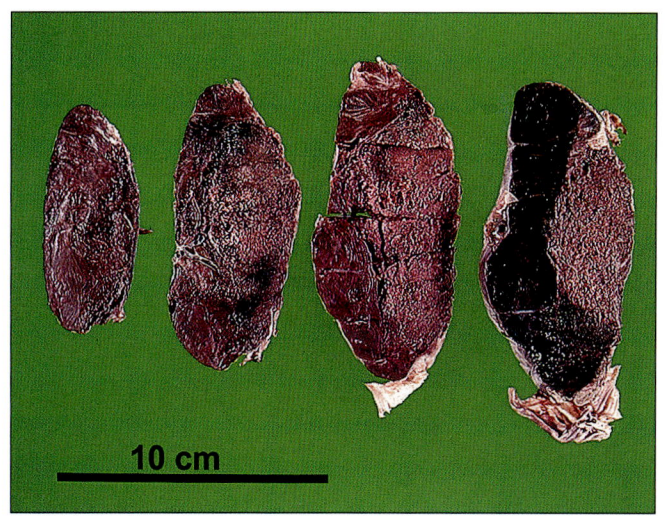

Fig. 30.50 A 2 cm subchorionic hemorrhage. There was also abruption at time of delivery of the premature infant.

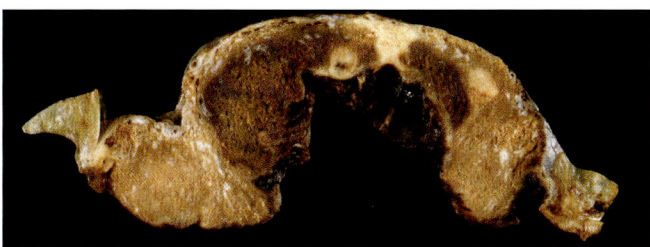

Fig. 30.49 Abruptio placenta with dramatic indentation of the parenchyma. The parenchyma is infarcted between the hemorrhage and the chorionic plate.

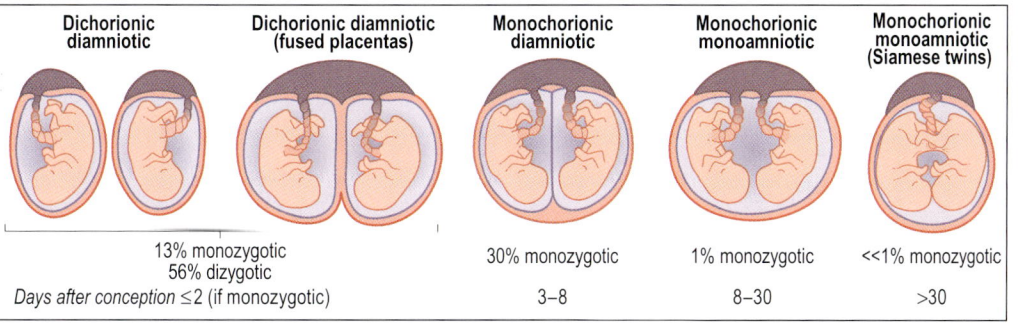

Fig. 30.51 Placental structure in twin pregnancy. The listed percentages are for each variant and total 100%. After Robboy et al.[115]

Dichorionic diamniotic	Dichorionic diamniotic (fused placentas)	Monochorionic diamniotic	Monochorionic monoamniotic	Monochorionic monoamniotic (Siamese twins)
13% monozygotic 56% dizygotic		30% monozygotic	1% monozygotic	<<1% monozygotic
Days after conception ≤2 (if monozygotic)		3–8	8–30	>30

hereditary component, which is confined to the maternal side. The frequency of dizygotic twinning and multiple gestations is substantially increased in women who have undergone artificial induction of ovulation with hormones.

Separate placentas develop when two fertilized ova implant apart from one another. If the ova implant near one another, the two placentas show varying degrees of fusion and may appear as one (Figure 30.52). When the ova implant apart, there are discrete conceptuses, each placenta having its own amniotic sac. In the case of placental fusion, microscopic examination of the intervening membranes between the two fetuses discloses two chorions and two amnions, i.e., a dichorionic diamniotic gestation (Figure 30.53).

The early division of a single fertilized ovum results in twins that are genetically identical and therefore of the same sex. If a single fertilized ovum divides within two days of fertilization, before the trophoblast has differentiated, two separate embryos develop, each with its own placenta and amniotic sac (dichorionic diamniotic twinning). Hence, scrutiny of the placenta cannot always distinguish between monozygotic and dizygotic twinning. If division occurs between days 3 and 8 after conception, the trophoblast but not the amniotic cavity has already differentiated, and a single placenta with two amniotic sacs develops (monochorionic diamniotic twinning) (Figure 30.54). A monochorionic monoamniotic placenta forms if division occurs between days 8 and 30 after conception, because the

amniotic cavity has already developed (Figure 30.55). Division at later periods results in conjoint (Siamese) twins (Figure 30.56).

Because monochorionic twins are at an increased risk of complications and adverse perinatal outcome compared with dichorionic twins,[87] it is important that each placenta be

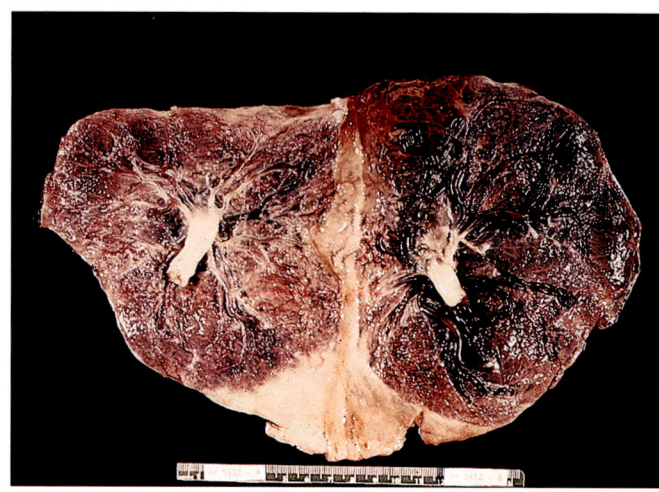

Fig. 30.52 Fused placenta.

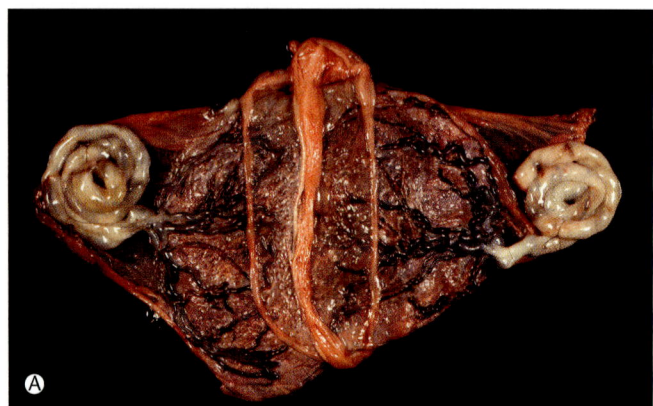

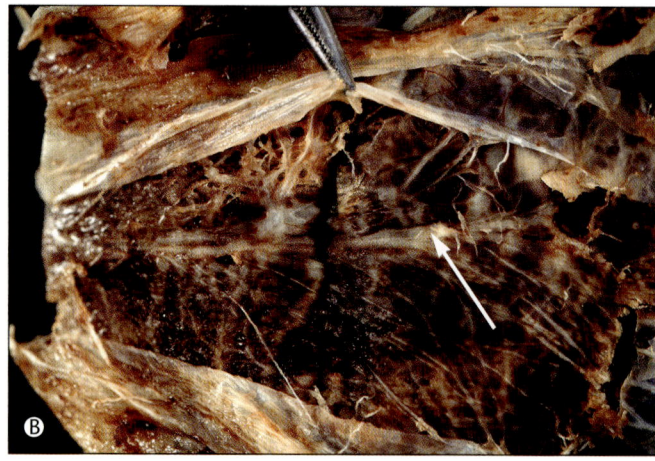

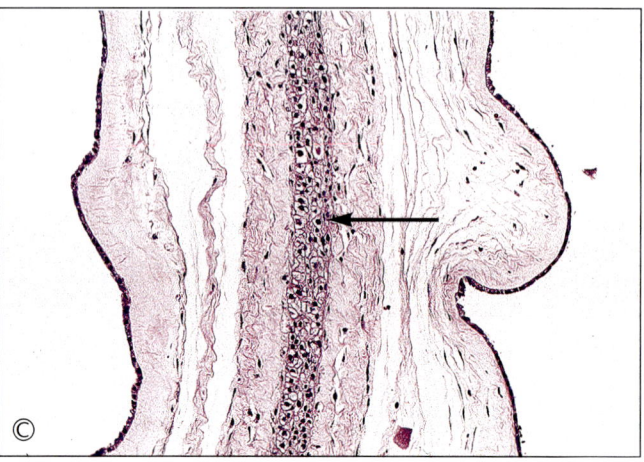

Fig. 30.53 Dichorionic diamniotic placenta. **(A)** Grossly, a low ridge (arrow) is present at the junction of the two chorions; attempts to remove it expose the underlying villous parenchyma **(B)**. **(C)** Microscopically, a chorionic membrane separates two diamniotic fetuses, shown by the presence of trophoblast (arrow) between the two amnions.

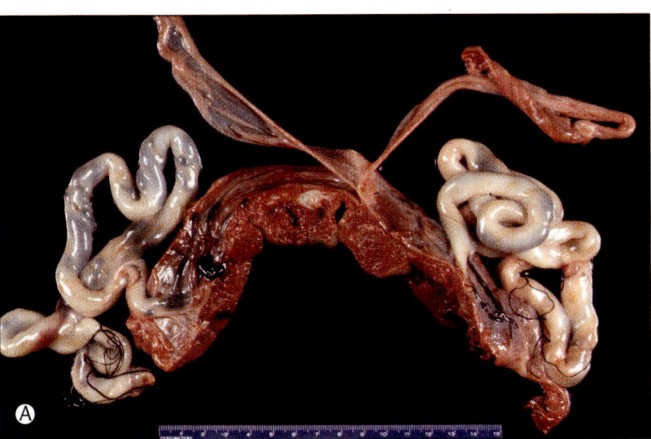

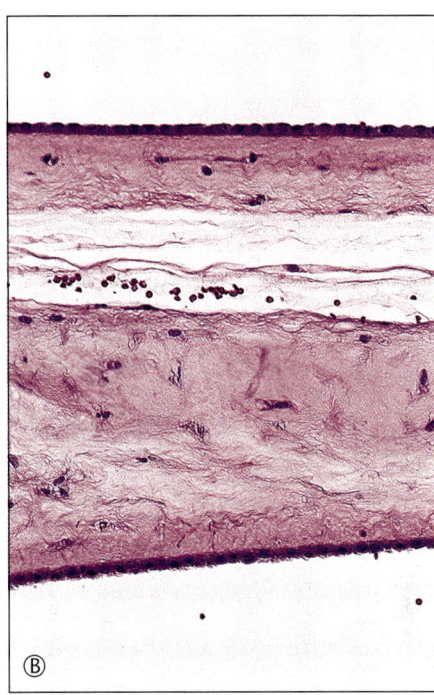

Fig. 30.54 Monochorionic diamniotic placenta. **(A)** Grossly, both amnions can be separated and pulled towards their respective cords, leaving a clear chorionic surface below. **(B)** Microscopically, no trophoblastic layer is present between the two amnions.

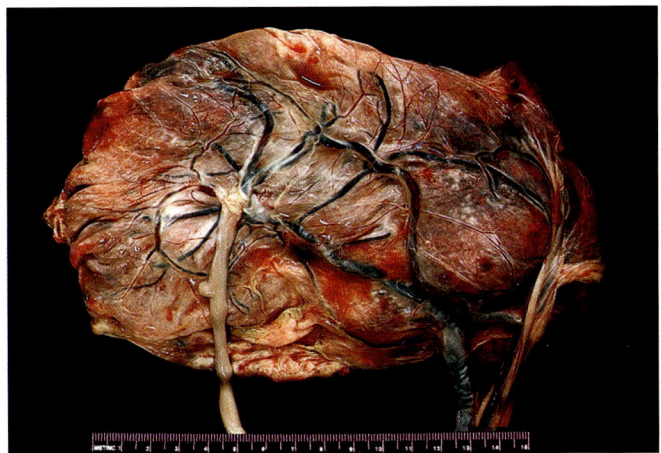

Fig. 30.55 Monochorionic monoamniotic placenta.

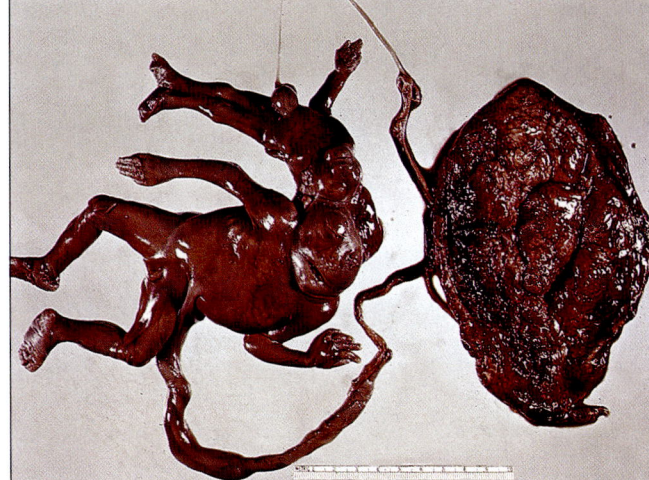

Fig. 30.56 Siamese twin.

examined separately. To facilitate this examination and permit information about each placenta to link to the proper child, each placenta should be clearly designated in the delivery ward (e.g., by one clamp on the cord of twin 1, two on that of twin 2, etc.).

On examination of the placenta, the chorionicity should be established prior to the removal of the cords and membranes. For practical purposes, a monochorionic placenta means the twins are monozygotic, or, in common parlance, 'identical'. In view of postzygotic events, the former term is preferable,[80] especially as discordance for sex[100,129] and karyotype[95] can occur on occasion in monochorionic twins. However, it is still important to recognize that almost all monochorionic placentas are from monozygotic twins. Dichorionic placentas mean that

there is a chance (approximately 10–15%) that the twins are monozygotic.

To establish chorionicity, the dividing membrane should be examined. If both amnions can be separated and pulled towards their respective cords, leaving a clear chorionic surface below, the placenta is monochorionic (Figure 30.54A). In dichorionic placentation, a low ridge formed by the junction of the two chorions is present at this point (Figure 30.53B), and attempts to remove it will expose the underlying villous parenchyma. The contents of the membranes forming this ridge can be confirmed histologically, but this is usually unnecessary.

An important consequence of monochorionic placentation is that vascular anastomoses may be present and twin–twin

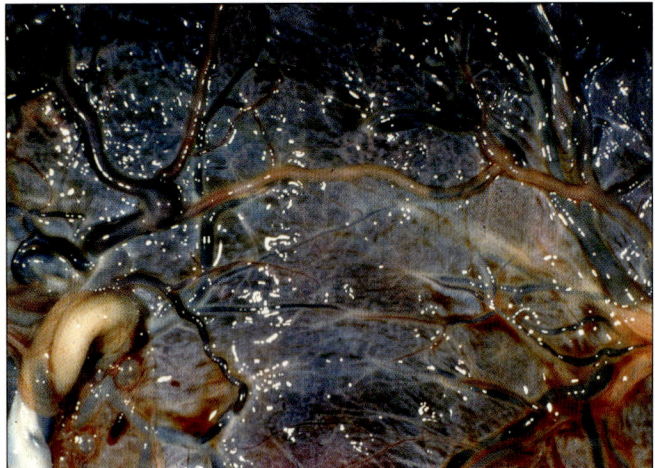

Fig. 30.57 Twin–twin superficial anastomosis.

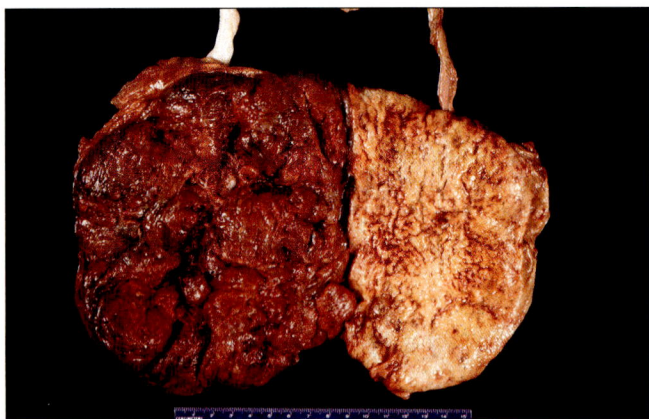

Fig. 30.58 Twin–twin transfusion syndrome with pale donor placenta and congested recipient placenta.

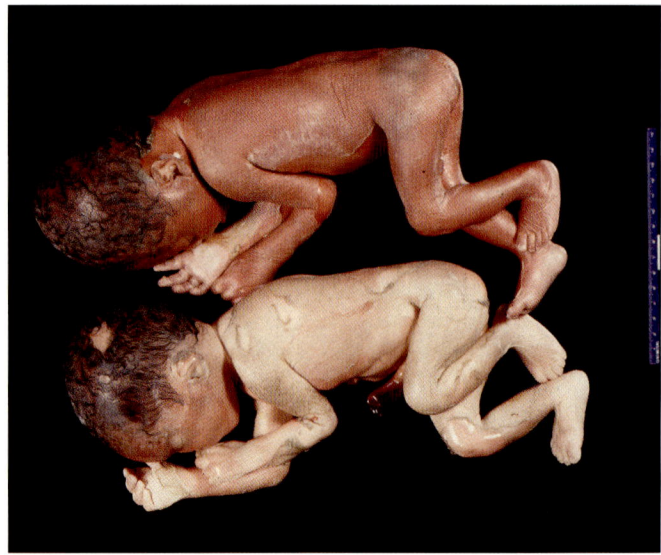

Fig. 30.59 Twin–twin transfusion syndrome.

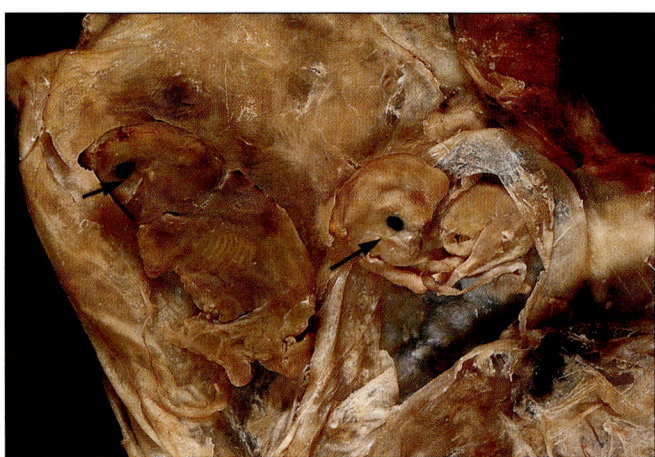

Fig. 30.60 Fetus papyraceus. Two macerated fetuses (arrows) are each about 2 cm in length. This mother delivered three normal triplets.

transfusion syndrome (TTTS) may occur. Surface vessels may cross from one placenta to the other and form anastomoses (Figure 30.57). These may be demonstrated by injection of air or gelatin, but their absence does not mean that significant vascular shunting did not occur in the parenchyma during intrauterine life. The rarity of TTTS in monochorionic monoamniotic twins has been related to arterial–arterial anastomoses in almost 100% of these cases, in contrast to the greater frequency of venoarterial anastomoses in dichorionic monoamniotic twins.[133] Diagnosis of TTTS may be difficult and the entity may be under-recognized in monoamniotic twins if oligohydramnios in the donor and polyhydramnios in the recipient is a criterion.[133] The placenta of the donor twin may be pale and bulky, with edematous villi and inconspicuous vessels, whereas that of the recipient may be congested (Figure 30.58). TTTS may be acute, but is usually chronic and the donor and the recipient may change with time. Even where both fetuses are available for autopsy, it may be difficult to be certain of the pattern of the condition (Figure 30.59).[15] TTTS rarely occurs in dichorionic twins.[27] Endoscopic laser coagulation of anastomoses is used increasingly in the treatment of severe TTTS.[124]

Other complications of twin pregnancy are acardia and fetus papyraceus. Acardia occurs where one twin lacks or has only rudimentary cardiac structures, but receives its blood supply from the other twin via vascular anastomoses. The term 'twin-reversed arterial perfusion' (TRAP) is sometimes used for this condition. The acardiac twin usually shows a variable degree of somatic organization, sometimes with only rudimentary structures, and the donor or 'pump twin' may develop cardiac failure and hydrops. The cord of the acardiac twin usually has a single umbilical artery. The placenta is most commonly monochorionic diamniotic.[25]

Fetus papyraceus occurs when one twin dies and becomes compressed, occasionally to the extent as appearing as thickened membranes. This occurs most commonly with triplets or more (Figure 30.60). There are various etiologies, including twin–twin transfusion, cord accidents, and, less commonly, maternal trauma.[99] Complications of twin pregnancy where the placental findings are minor or negligible are discussed elsewhere.[27]

MICROSCOPIC LESIONS OF THE PLACENTA

PLACENTAL INFLAMMATION AND INFECTION

The placenta, its membranes and umbilical cord may become infected by numerous routes, but the two most common and clinically important are ascending infection and hematogenous spread. Maternal infection may be subclinical. Other routes include the fallopian tube itself, foci of abdominal infection using the fallopian tube as a conduit, chronic endometritis, and invasive procedures such as amniocentesis and cordocentesis (transabdominal blood sampling of the fetal umbilical cord performed under ultrasound guidance, i.e., funipuncture additionally). Intrauterine transfusion of infected blood can lead to placental infection via the fetus. Chronic endometritis is associated with reduced fertility and as such is an uncommon source of placental infection.

VILLITIS

Villitis has a frequency of about 10% (Figure 30.61) as well as number of blocks prepared for microscopic examination. In most (95–98%) cases, no etiologic agent is found and the term 'villitis of unknown etiology' (VUE) is used. In some cases, the etiology is viral or protozoal in origin and spread hematogenously, unlike ascending infections, which are usually bacterial. The inflammatory reaction that develops in the villous stroma has been variously described as 'proliferative', 'necrotizing', 'granulomatous' or 'reparative'. The end result is a sclerotic functionless villus.

Many cases are associated with a prior maternal history of abortion or stillbirth, sometimes multiple. Some cases may be due to varicella or *Toxoplasma*, overlooked in the absence of clinically relevant information.[18] Many cases yield etiologic agents if modern diagnostic techniques such as immunohistochemistry, *in situ* hybridization, and polymerase chain reaction are used. The demonstration that a substantial fraction of the inflammatory cells is maternal in origin[108] supports the hypothesis that villitis is frequently a maternal immunologic response to fetal tissue.

Macroscopically, placentas with villitis may be small and pale or normal. On microscopic examination of four parenchymal sections, villitis may be divided into four grades:[41]

- Grade 1 (very mild villitis): 1–2 foci with few villi involved.
- Grade 2 (mild villitis): up to <6 foci of villous inflammation, each focus containing maximally 20 villi.
- Grade 3 (moderate villitis): Multiple inflammatory foci present, each occupying up to half a low-power field.
- Grade 4 (severe villitis): Large areas of most sections inflamed.

On low power magnification the villi tend to be swollen, and exhibit some sclerosis, an increase in perivillous fibrin, and adhesions among villi (Figure 30.62). On higher power magnification, the villi disclose an infiltrate of lymphocytic, histiocytic or both cell types (Figure 30.63), all of which are readily distinguished from the normal stromal cells that are more generally elongate and bland. Some villi, although enlarged and exhibiting increased numbers of stromal cells, lack inflammatory cells and therefore are not villitis (Figure 30.64). Additional signs of villitis include some disruption of the villi, destruction of the normal vasculature, and spillover of inflammatory cells into the adjacent perivillous space (Figure 30.63). The infiltrate usually consists of either or both lymphocytes (CD45 reactive) (Figure 30.65A), which are predominantly, but not exclusively, T-cells of maternal origin, or macrophages, which are intravillous, CD68 reactive (Figure 30.65B), and of fetal origin.[91] The presence of plasma cells should lead to a thorough search for a specific infection such as cytomegalovirus (CMV) (see Chapter 31, Figures 31.20–31.23).

Villitis and infarction frequently coexist in cases of pre-eclampsia and overdiagnosis of villitis adjacent to infarcts may be a problem.[66] Similarly, a mild increase in stromal mononuclear cells should be distinguished from a true inflammatory infiltrate. Villitis of grades 2–4 is associated with IUGR.[121] Vil-

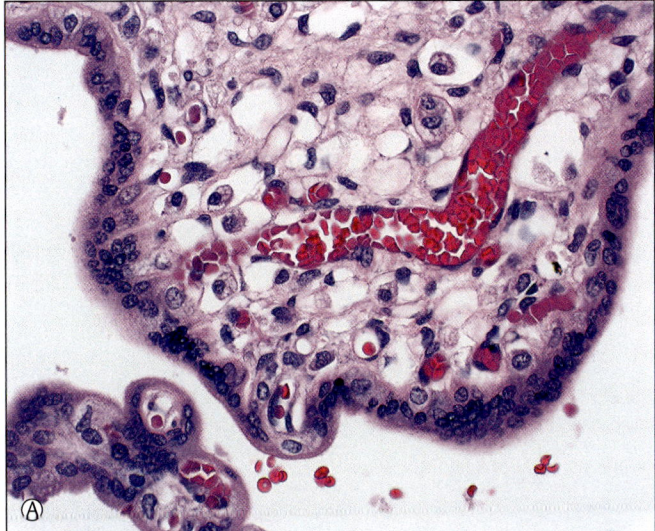
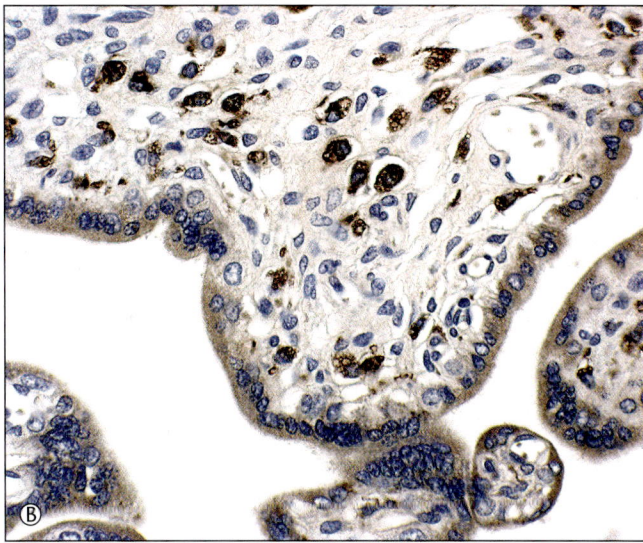

Fig. 30.61 Villus: **(A)** normal with **(B)** some CD68 reactive (Hofbauer) macrophages (fetal origin).

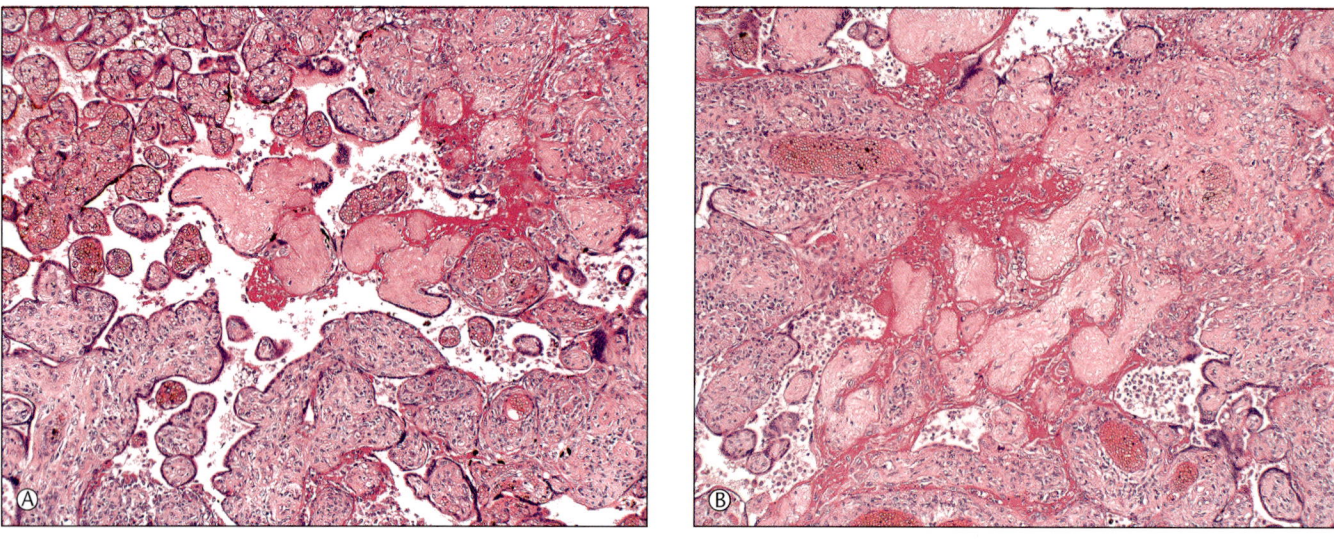

Fig. 30.62 Villitis: **(A)** low magnification; **(B)** with swollen villi, some sclerotic, and an increase in perivillous fibrin, with adhesions among villi.

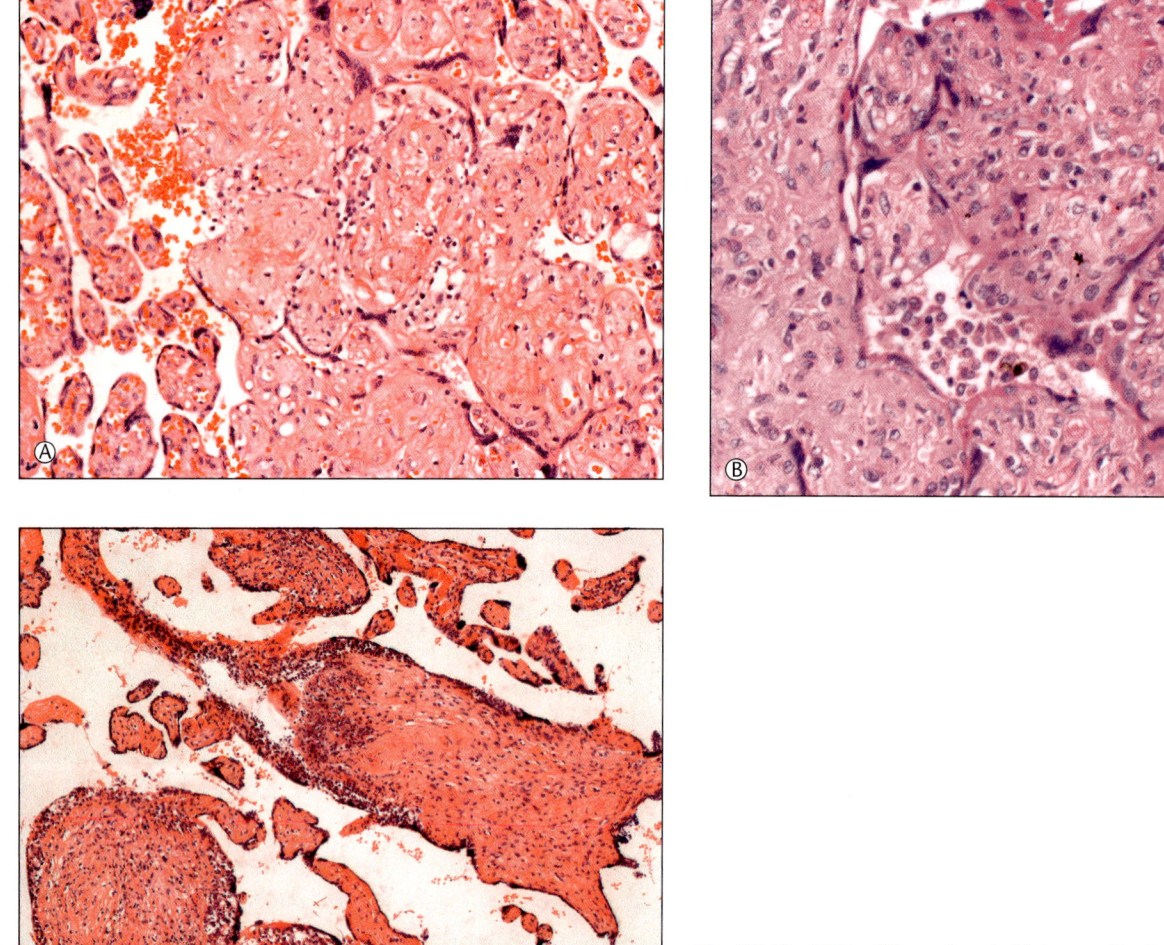

Fig. 30.63 Villitis: **(A)** medium to high magnification, with an inflammatory infiltrate. Additionally some villi are disrupted, show **(B)** spillover of inflammatory cells into the adjacent perivillous space, and **(C)** in a stem villus, show destruction of the normal vasculature.

litis with obliterative fetal vessel vasculopathy is one of the placental findings associated with neurologic impairment in term infants.[107] This feature is usually seen in grades 3 and 4 villitis, although we comment on its presence or absence in addition to allocating a grade. As with other entities in placental pathology, recognition of cofactors, e.g., maternal hypertension, is increasingly important.[14] There is no relationship between villitis and the presence of rubella antibodies.

The specific viruses and bacterial infections that give rise to villitis are described more fully in Chapter 31.

DECIDUITIS

Acute inflammation of the decidua alone is insufficient to diagnose ascending infection reliably, particularly in the absence of funisitis. Foci of necrosis and acute inflammation are commonly seen in placentas of stillbirths, and may be associated with fresh retroplacental hemorrhage. A well-demarcated area of acute inflammation in the decidua from term membranes may represent the cervical mucus plug – a barrier to, rather than a source of, infection. Scattered lymphocytes are commonly found in the decidua, but a heavy infiltrate of chronic inflammatory cells may be associated with increased perinatal mortality. Not unexpectedly, pathologists more confidently make the histologic diagnosis of chronic inflammation involving the decidua rather than villi.[68] Basal plate inflammation was more common in placentas from males in one study of severely premature infants.[47] In reporting deciduitis, we comment on the intensity of inflammation and the presence or absence of an associated basal villitis. What its contribution is, if any, to perinatal outcome or preceding or subsequent endometrial pathologic status is unknown.

CHRONIC INTERVILLOSITIS

Chronic intervillositis, an inflammatory infiltrate in the intervillous space unrelated to the villi and usually without effect on the villi (i.e., without villitis),[57] discloses mainly mononuclear cells (histiocytes and lymphocytes) with rare neutrophils (Figure 30.66). Most cells are reactive for the macrophage marker CD68. There is also intervillous and perivillous fibrin deposition. Fetal outcome is poor.

Intervillositis is associated with pregnancy-induced hypertension, lupus erythematosus, maternal drug use, and diabetes. Chronic intervillositis has also been associated with recurrent abortions[36] and may be identified at any stage of pregnancy. Chronic intervillositis is also found in nearly 20% of cases of malaria.[97] Over half of neonates with malaria and chronic intervillositis have low birth weights, but show no neonatal morbidity.

VASCULAR LESIONS

FETAL VESSEL THROMBI

Vascular occlusions may occur in vessels at various levels in the fetal circulation, from the umbilical cord to the villous capillaries, and their detection is a function not only of their extent, but also of sampling[110] and interpretation.[105]

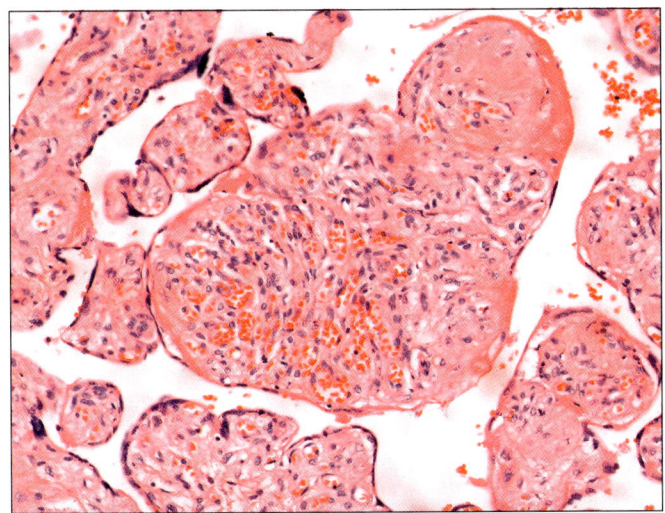

Fig. 30.64 Hypercellular villus without an increase in inflammatory cells.

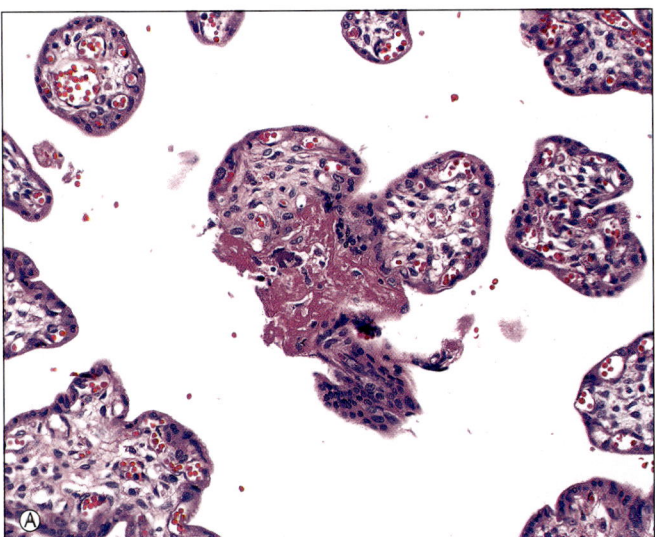
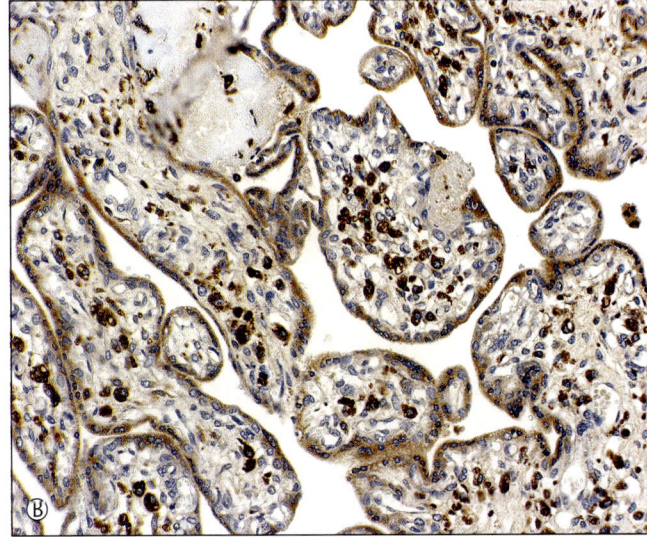

Fig. 30.65 Villitis, with **(A)** fibrinous adhesions among villi and **(B)** CD68 reactive infiltrate.

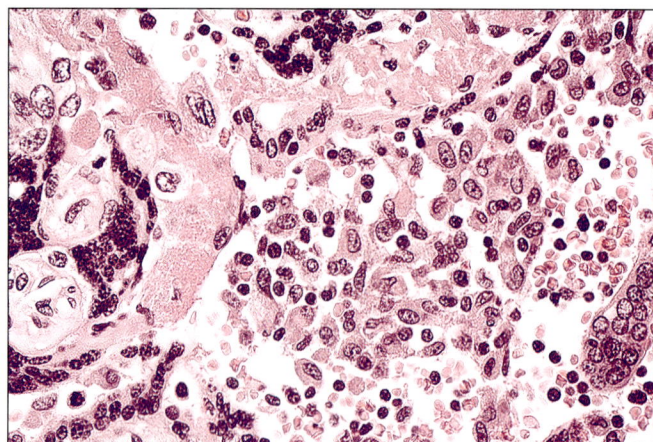

Fig. 30.66 Intervillositis from an infant with IUGR. The cells in the maternal space show a histiocytic morphology.

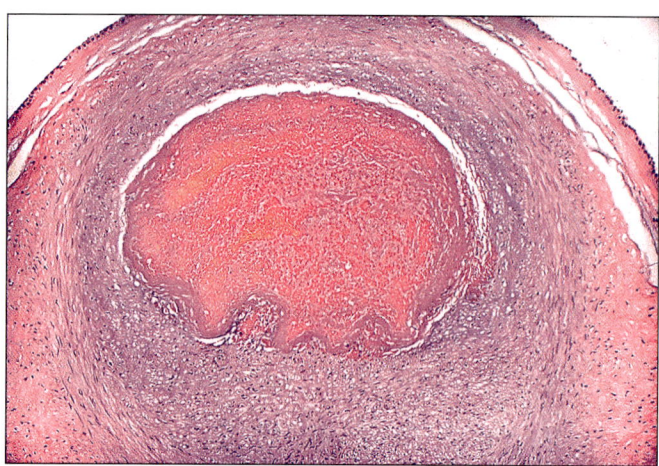

Fig. 30.67 Thrombus in large surface vessels. The lumen is completely occluded, and because of its age shows peripheral organization.

The umbrella term 'fetal thrombotic vasculopathy' (FTV)[110] encompasses fetal surface or stem vessel thrombi or occlusion, clusters of avascular sclerotic villi, and hemorrhagic endovasculitis. FTV occurs in approximately 3% of placentas from term deliveries.[86]

The components of FTV are now described individually. Thrombi may be seen grossly (Figure 30.37) or may only be apparent microscopically (Figure 30.67), completely occluding blood flow. Following cessation of blood flow, the vessels fibrose (Figure 30.68). Hemorrhagic endovasculitis shows vascular fibrosis with entrapment, fragmentation, and exocytosis of red blood cells through the vessel walls. Medial myocyte necrosis is also present.[122] There is no associated inflammation. We regard hemorrhagic endovasculitis (and hemorrhagic villitis) in livebirths as part of FTV. Many of these changes are also seen in placentas of stillbirths.

Occasional sclerotic villi are found in many placentas. The term 'extensive' is used when clusters of fibrotic villi constitute more than 2.5% of the parenchyma in multiple sections, or constitute a single lesion greater than 0.25 cm^2.[110] Avascular villi are sharply demarcated from the surrounding normal villi (Figure 30.69) and characteristically show an increase in trophoblast basement membrane hemosiderin deposition,[85] reflecting the inability of the fetal circulation to remove iron absorbed by the trophoblast. In some cases, often with hemorrhagic endovasculitis in the stem vessels, distal villi are bulbous and normocellular with karyorrhectic debris in vessels, rather than being small, sclerotic, and avascular. This may represent an earlier stage in the evolution of avascular villi, or in some cases where the picture persists, a 'sublethal hit' on these villi. Extensive avascular villi are the most common manifestation of FTV.

Our understanding of the causes and significance of FTV continues to evolve and emphasizes the need for detailed placental examination. Thrombi in the cord or in chorionic plate vessels may also be secondary to compression, acute inflammation or true knots. Obliterated distal stem vessels are frequently seen with severe villitis. Lesions of the cord, both clinical and pathologic, were seen in two-thirds of cases with FTV.[106] FTV is found four times more commonly in placentas of infants with neonatal encephalopathy[86] and it undoubtedly reflects chronic and sometimes acute disturbance in the fetoplacental circula-

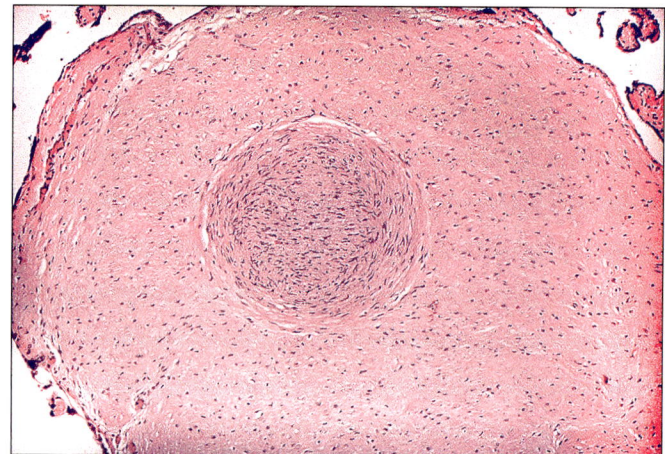

Fig. 30.68 Total fibrous obliteration of stem vessel.

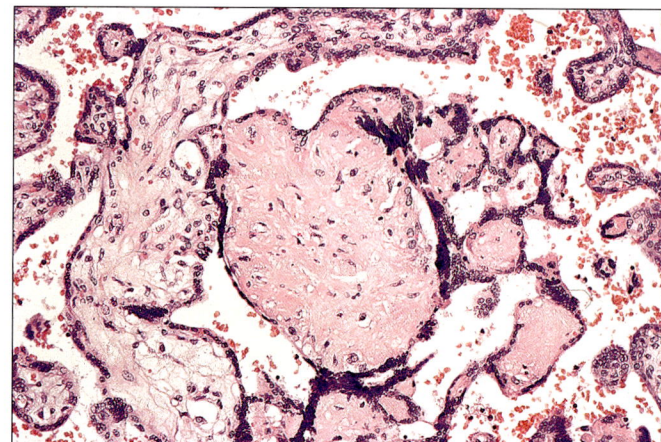

Fig. 30.69 Avascular villi. The presence of hemosiderin deposits in villi such as these should alert the pathologist to the possibility of previous CMV infection.

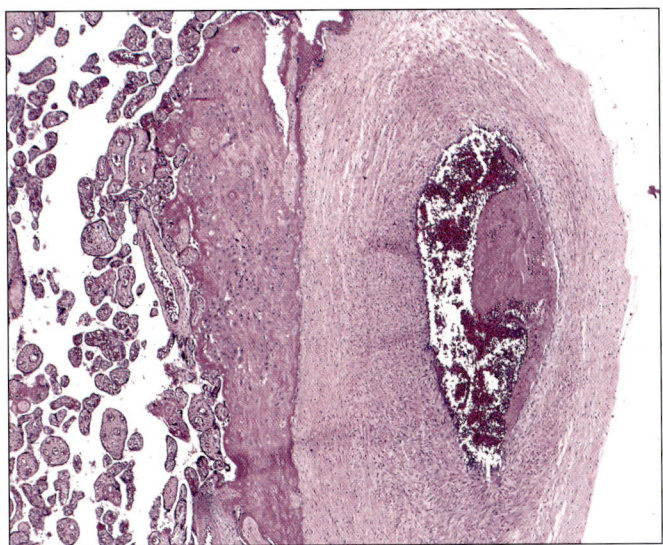

Fig. 30.70 Mural thrombus atop endothelial 'cushion' with peripheral recanalization.

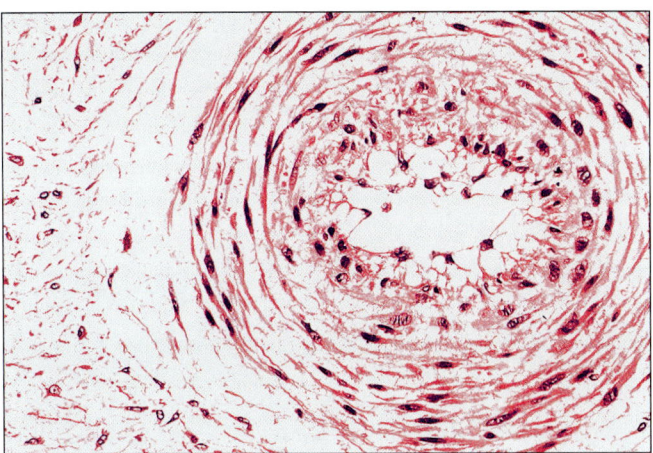

Fig. 30.71 So-called 'obliterative endarteritis'. Partial luminal obliteration by ballooned endothelial cells is artifactual.

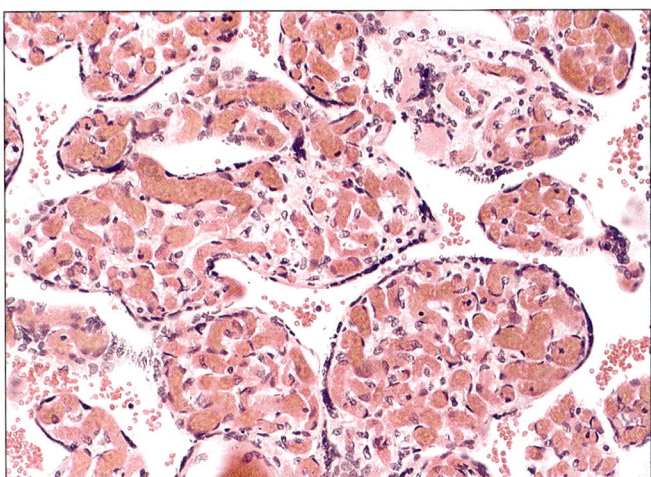

Fig. 30.72 Chorangiosis. Multiple (more than 10) vascular profiles are present.

tion. The predictive value of FTV is uncertain, and the problem has been likened to the finding of a deep vein thrombus in the leg vein of an adult.[70] An as yet unknown number of cases of cerebral palsy may have their etiology in antepartum vascular events rather than reflecting an intrapartum hypoxia. FTV was found in 40% of placentas from infants in neonatal intensive care that had thrombosis.[79] Over half of the placentas of infants with neurologic impairment showed one or more of findings of FTV, villitis with vascular obliteration, chorioamnionitis with severe fetal vessel vasculitis, and meconium-induced vascular necrosis.[107]

Fibrin deposition may be seen in about 10% of placentas focally in an exophytic area of the vessel wall (Figure 30.70). This protrusion consists of loose connective tissue that blends with the cap of fibrin. These protrusions have been referred to as endothelial 'cushions' and held by some to be normal features of vascular bifurcations.[17] These mural fibrin thrombi are seen in 8–10% of placentas[86] and may be single or multiple. These overlap with the entity termed 'fibrinous vasculosis' and may be seen in placentas with fetal thrombotic vasculopathy. However, the clinical significance of isolated lesions is unclear.

The spectrum of thrombotic lesions and its correlation with inherited defects of coagulation continues as a subject of intense investigation. A high proportion of women with obstetric complications, including pre-eclampsia, abruption, stillbirth, and IUGR, have a thrombophilic mutation (52% vs 17% in women without complications).[72] Among women with an adverse pregnancy outcome whose placentas have thrombotic lesions, mutated Factor V Leiden (54%) and protein S deficiency (23%) are common.[10] Further studies are necessary to establish the relevance and implications for treatment of isolated placental thrombi.[69]

Spontaneously aborted fetuses have a higher frequency of mutated Factor V Leiden than the general population (8.6% vs 4.2%). The carrier frequency for mothers with a miscarriage has been reported at 6.8%.[33] However, there is no consensus yet to the relative importance of thrombophilic mutations and no evidence base for treating women with such abnormalities.[12]

So-called 'obliterative endarteritis' (Figure 30.71) is manifest by muscular arteries in the villi having markedly reduced luminal areas in which the intimal cells feature clear cytoplasm. Ultrastructurally contracted smooth muscle cells show cytoplasm herniated into the intima. It also demonstrates that the apparently clear-appearing endothelial cells are actually a fixation artifact.

CHORANGIOSIS

Chorangiosis (which differs from chorangioma and chorangiomatosis, see below) may be an important and possibly unrecognized entity of increased villous capillaries that occurs with chronic fetal hypoxia (Figure 30.72).[6] It involves terminal villi, generally is not seen before 32 weeks, and is most common after 37 weeks. This condition is defined using a ×10 objective. There should be at least 10 villi with 10 or more vessels on cross-section in 10 different areas on one slide and should be seen in at least three different locations within the placenta. One villus should have more than 15 vascular profiles. It may be overdiagnosed in cases where the placenta is congested, and underdiagnosed (due to collapse of the villous vessels) when umbilical cord clamping has been delayed. This condition of excessive fetal capillary growth occurs over a few weeks. It occurs in placentas with extensive avascular villi[110] and is associated with IUGR. However, as it is frequently only focal, some believe it has little importance as a diagnostic entity.[41] We have encountered it in 4% of all placentas, often where many villi are non-functional due to villitis.

ABNORMALITIES OF THE UTEROPLACENTAL VESSELS

The endovascular trophoblast invades in two waves during fetal life. The first completes by 12 weeks and the second by 20 weeks. In this way, the decidual portions of the spiral arteries are converted to uteroplacental vessels by the end of the first trimester. The intramyometrial portions of the spiral arteries are converted during the second trimester.

Uteroplacental vascular perfusion defects are associated with a failure of the second wave of endovascular trophoblast. With patience and a good magnifying light, it is possible to see the attached fragments of the non-transformed uteromaternal vessels as well as their potential site of entry into the decidua. The findings of completely muscularized vessels in the basal decidua or in the decidua capsularis after 14 weeks should be considered abnormal (Figure 30.73). These arteries may subsequently undergo acute atherosis (Figure 30.74), which appears as acute fibrinoid necrosis of the vessel wall with subintimal accumulations of lipophages. There may later be a transmural chronic inflammatory infiltrate. Acute atherosis is pathognomonic of uteromaternal perfusion defect. It is not specific for pre-eclampsia as it occurs in systemic lupus erythematosus with the lupus anticoagulant, diabetes, hypertension, and idiopathic IUGR. Only half of cases of pre-eclampsia will show atherosis of basal plate vessels. Acute fibrinoid necrosis of the maternal uteroplacental vessels, either marked (Figure 30.75) or slight, may also be the only histologic manifestation of maternal vascular disease.

VILLOUS LESIONS

VILLOUS MATURITY

Villous maturation may be disturbed chronologically by either being delayed or accelerated. Its recognition demands adequate and appropriate placental sampling, and awareness of the normal variation of the villi within the functional unit. Assessing villous maturity and/or maldevelopment is difficult. While it is tempting to state that this assessment should be performed only by pathologists who report large numbers of placentas, even experienced placental pathologists are unable to date pregnancies more accurately than within 6 weeks.[67]

We avoid the term 'dysmaturity', preferring to characterize an abnormal pattern as either more advanced or delayed than expected. While recognizing the teleologic nature of this argument, it does provide a relatively simple and descriptive starting point in composing a report that is intelligible to the clinician. We assess villi in the center of the disc on a number of sections, avoiding peripheral and subchorionic areas, areas near infarcts, and the center of placental lobules.

Delayed villous maturation is classically associated with maternal diabetes mellitus, rhesus isoimmunization, syphilis, and Downs syndrome. The villi appear less developed than would be expected for the gestational age. The cross-sectional profile is more bulbous, and tertiary villi are reduced in number.

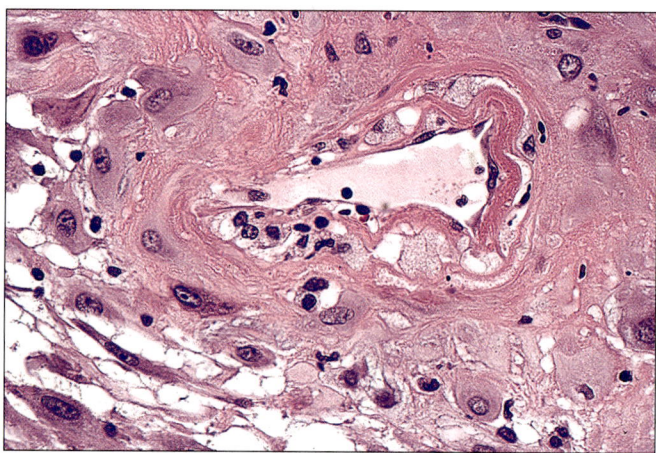

Fig. 30.74 Vessel with acute atherosis. The vessels show fibrinoid mural change, lipid-laden macrophages (arrows) and scattered chronic inflammatory cells in the wall.

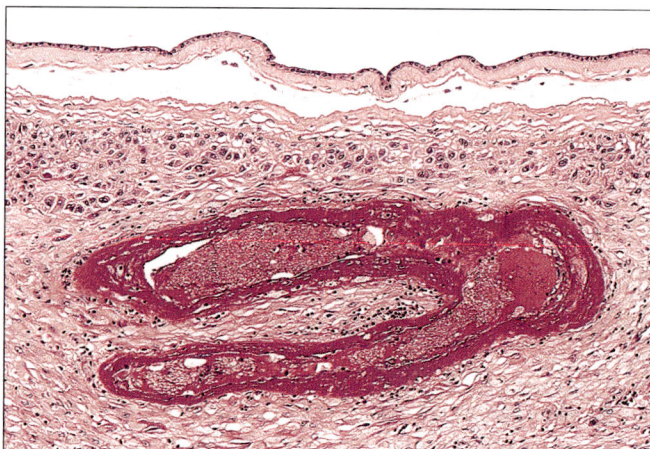

Fig. 30.75 Maternal vascular disease. This is an extreme example of fibrinoid necrosis in a maternal vessel found in the decidua beneath the chorion in a woman with severe pre-eclampsia.

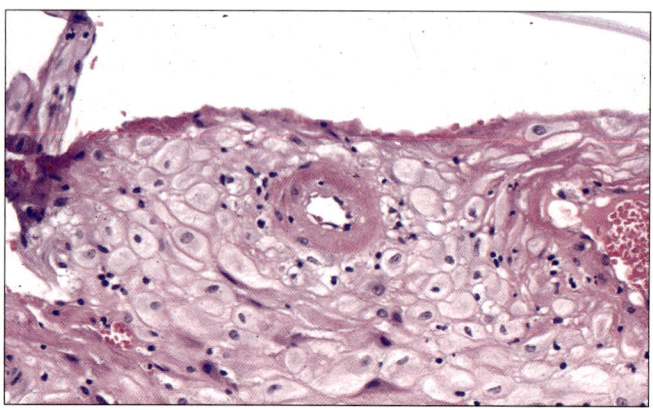

Fig. 30.73 Muscularized vessel in decidua capsularis.

Also, there may be persistence of stromal channels, which are a characteristic feature of immature intermediate villi. Vasculosyncytial membrane formation is decreased. With this approach, approximately 5% of placentas in our practice receive a histologic diagnosis of delayed maturation. It is seen with congenital abnormalities, including trisomies and gastroschisis. In some cases there may be IUGR. It is the only abnormality seen in some patients with neonatal encephalopathy. One review of over 17 000 placentas found delayed maturation in 5.7%. Only a minority of fetuses whose placenta showed this pattern died, but a 70-fold risk of death was claimed compared with those with a normal placenta.[130]

Accelerated villous maturation, in contrast, shows a markedly increased number of small, sclerotic villi, with an increase in syncytiotrophoblast knots. It has also been referred to as distal villous hypoplasia. The extreme is the Tenney–Parker effect (Figure 30.76). The placental response to chronic hypoxia is the basis for the morphologic changes seen in accelerated villous maturation.

Sometimes a mixed pattern is seen, with areas of delayed maturation alternating with areas of accelerated maturation. Such a pattern may occur in diabetes, where changes of uteroplacental ischemia are superimposed on a delayed maturation pattern. Occasional cases of pre-eclampsia show delayed maturation, instead of the advanced pattern more usually seen.

VILLOUS EDEMA

Severe villous edema is easily recognized. The placenta is pale and hydropic and the villi show stromal edema and persistent stromal channels. It may be associated with fetal hydrops. The diagnosis and significance of milder forms are contentious. Second trimester villi show prominent stromal channels and some pathologists feel villous edema is a normal feature of the second trimester, whereas others maintain that villous edema is a major cause of fetal mortality and neonatal morbidity. Possibly the increased villus size effectively reduces the size of the intervillous space and hence perfusion. Villous edema is found in immune and non-immune hydrops and in some infections, including CMV. The mechanism of its production outside these scenarios remains unknown. Less mature villi in the center of the fetal lobule should not be used to diagnose edema.

MISCELLANEOUS VILLOUS CHANGES

The villous response to reduced oxygen concentration in the maternal blood includes cytotrophoblastic hyperplasia (Figure 30.77). This is best appreciated on a periodic acid-Schiff (PAS) stain. Cytotrophoblast cells are relatively clear staining compared to the overlying syncytiotrophoblastic cells, which are slightly basophilic. As the cytotrophoblast produces basement membrane, focal thickenings become apparent. Those are thought to be errors in production of basement membrane proteins.

The villi also may be subject to fibrinoid necrosis. In this condition, the cytotrophoblast undergoes degeneration and then is replaced by matrix-type fibrinoid. The fibrinoid then gradually replaces the entire villus such that the overlying syncytiotrophoblast eventually degenerates. *Mycoplasma* bodies have been found within villi that show fibrinoid necrosis, but it is not certain whether these are entrapped innocent bystand-

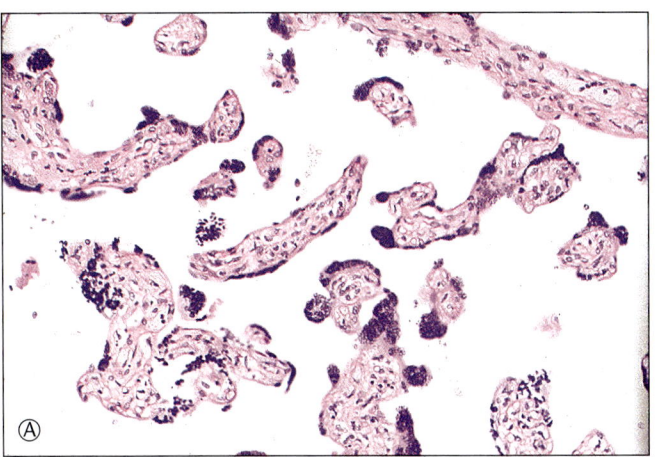

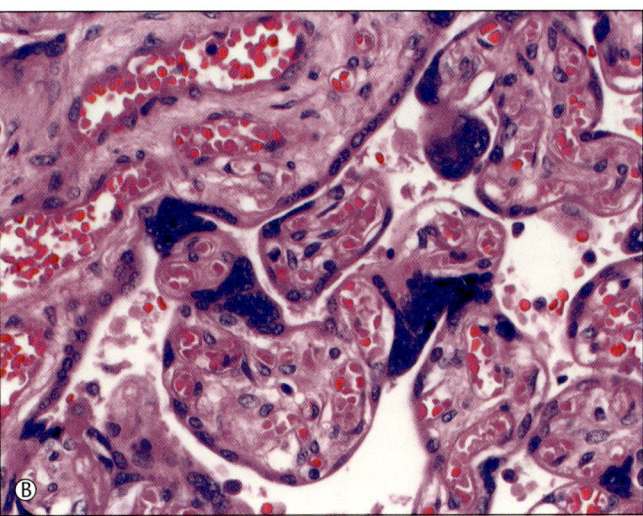

Fig. 30.76 Syncytial knots (Tenney–Parker effect). **(A)** Three-dimensional reconstructions have shown that the abundant syncytiotrophoblast knots are an artifact of tangential cuts through terminal villi. **(B)** Detail of knots.

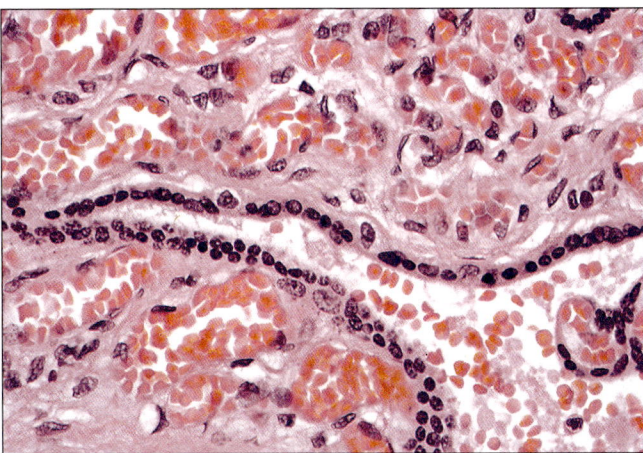

Fig. 30.77 Cytotrophoblast nuclei. They can be distinguished from syncytiotrophoblast by their paler nuclei and their proximity to the basement membrane.

ers or have etiologic significance. Villous calcifications should be distinguished from the more common calcifications of the basal plate, as they may be a sequel of previous villitis.

Vacuolated cells in multiple tissues, including syncytiotrophoblast, intermediate trophoblast, and Hofbauer cells, should raise the suspicion of storage disease. A known family history can be helpful in planning the needed investigations. These might include, for instance, electron microscopy, fibroblast culture, and enzyme analysis. Congenital abnormalities may accompany some cases,[51] but in others, placental examination may provide the first clue to the diagnosis.[116] Of course, metabolic products of the various storage diseases may not always accumulate to any significant degree in the immature placenta.[61]

NON-TROPHOBLASTIC TUMORS OF THE PLACENTA

There are relatively few non-trophoblastic tumors of the placenta.

CHORANGIOMA

The chorangioma or placental hemangioma is the most common placental tumor with a frequency of 0.6%.[16] They are more common with increased maternal age (>30 years) and in pregnancies with hypertension and diabetes.[50] Macroscopically, the tumor may protrude from the fetal surface or less frequently the maternal surface, replacing a lobule. It may be located in the membranes, but more commonly is contained within the substance of the placenta and is only visible on the cut surface. They may be single or multiple, varying from incidental microscopic findings to over 5 cm in size (Figures 30.78 and 30.79). They can also be microscopic in size (Figure 30.80A), even to being small obliterative tangles of vessels (Figure 30.80B). The color of chorangiomas varies from purple-red through tan to off-white. They appear encapsulated and are firmer than the surrounding placental parenchyma.

Histologically, the chorangioma consists of multiple vessels, usually of capillary size, although they can be cavernous, arising from a stem villus. The villus is expanded by the blood vessels (Figure 30.81A), demonstrated well with both CD34 (Figure 30.81B) and desmin, and variable amounts of mesenchymal stroma, and shows an attenuated trophoblastic cover-

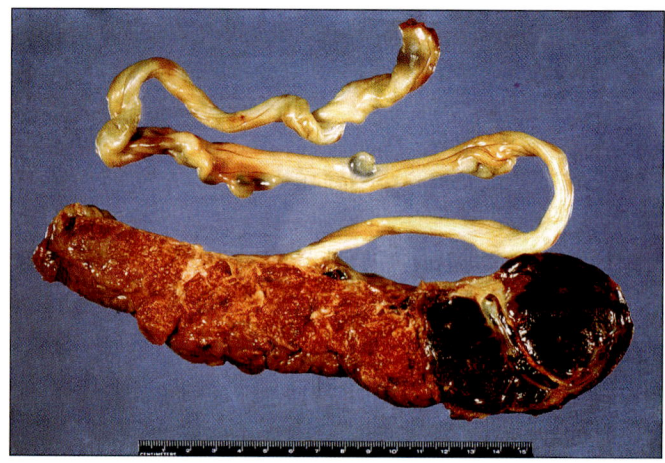

Fig. 30.79 Chorangioma, cross-section, large, panmural.

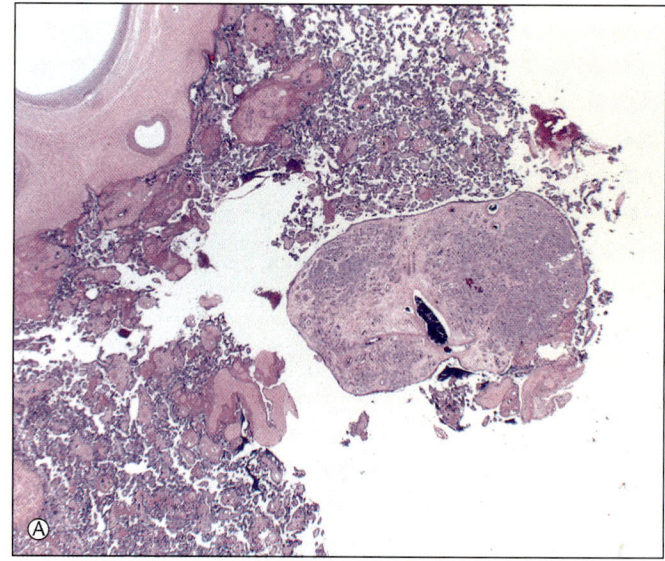

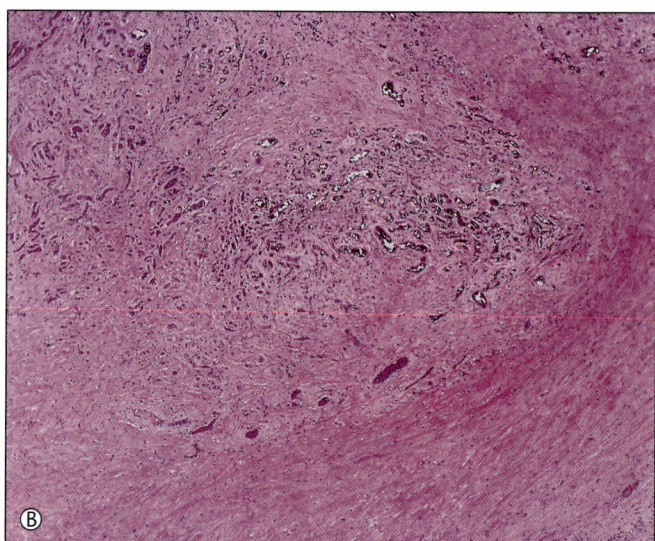

Fig. 30.80 Chorangioma, H&E. **(A)** Low magnification of usual nodule. **(B)** Obliterative nodule.

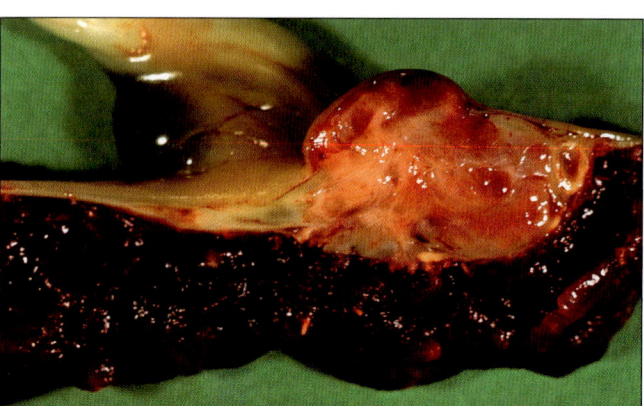

Fig. 30.78 Chorangioma, subchorial.

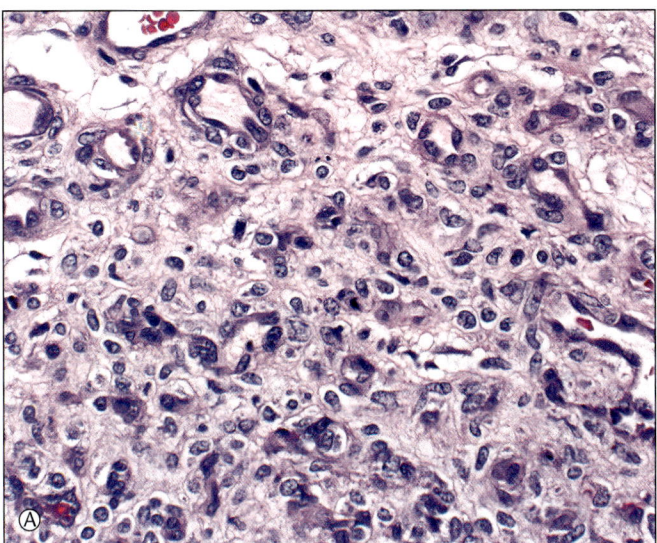

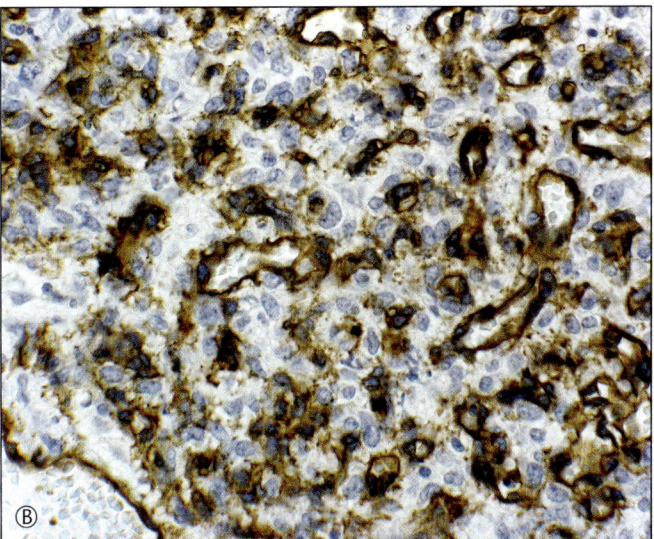

Fig. 30.81 Chorangioma showing vascular channels: **(A)** H&E; **(B)** CD34.

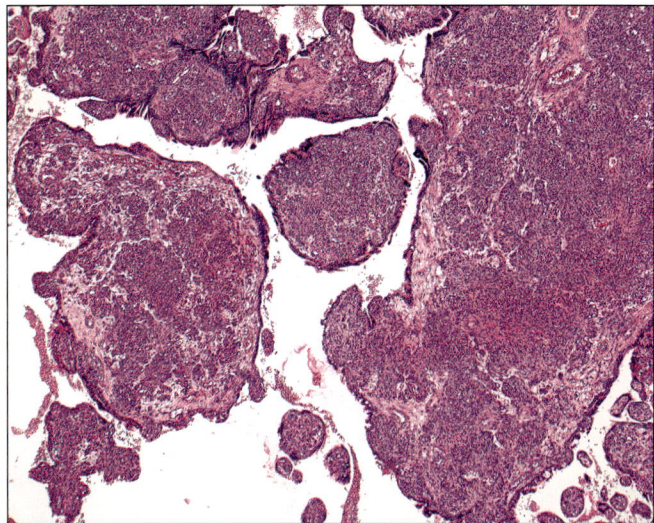

Fig. 30.82 Chorangiomatosis involving multiple villi.

ing. Degenerative changes include myxoid, hyalinized, necrotic, and calcified areas. Mitoses are occasionally seen, but even allowing for endothelial and stromal atypia, there is no evidence that these tumors are malignant.[41]

Chorangiomatosis is a rare microscopic finding. In contrast to chorangiosis, where the changes are confined to terminal villi, the vascular proliferation is also seen at the periphery of stem vessels – the proliferation 'permeates normal villous structures' (Figure 30.82). It may be found in placentas that also contain chorangiomas.

Complications of larger tumors include polyhydramnios with subsequent premature rupture of membranes, antepartum hemorrhage, and dystocia. The fetus may suffer intrauterine death, IUGR, transient cardiomegaly, bleeding disorders, hypoalbuminemia, anemia, and hydrops fetalis, the last being the highest risk of death.[125] The hematologic disorders may be due to entrapped red blood cells and/or platelets in the tumorous capillaries resulting in disseminated intravascular coagulation. In addition, chorangiomas have been found with fetal

angiomas, Beckwith–Wiedemann syndrome, mesenchymal dysplasia, and high altitude.[74,114] The etiology is still debated. Chorangiomas have not been found in first-trimester aborted gestations so it seems unlikely that they result from defective villous angiogenesis.[41] They must therefore be acquired later in pregnancy. There have been instances where chorangiomas have partially infarcted with subsequent alleviation of symptoms of patchy hydramnios.[22]

CHORANGIOCARCINOMA (CHORANGIOMAS WITH TROPHOBLASTIC PROLIFERATION)

So-called chorangiocarcinoma exhibits a mantle of atypical trophoblast around a chorangioma. Among the few reported cases, all mothers and infants were well during the short periods of follow-up available. When routinely diagnosed chorangiomas were reviewed and assessed with proliferation markers, 65% could be called chorangiocarcinoma, suggesting that a better term for this group is 'chorangiomas with trophoblastic proliferation'.[64] While given a name of malignancy, there is no indication that any of these lesions are biologically malignant.

INTRAPLACENTAL CHORIOCARCINOMA

This is also known as choriocarcinoma *in situ*, and grossly resembles an infarct in a term placenta. As such, it may be under-reported (Figure 30.83). Microscopically, there is central necrosis and a rim of abnormal trophoblast with choriocarcinomatous features (Figure 30.84). Systemic metastases are seen in some mothers, but other patients appear free of disease on follow-up.[58]

TERATOMAS

Teratomas may arise in the placenta, or more accurately between the amnion and chorion, either on the placental disc or within the membranes. They are composed of mature elements containing skin, brain, gut, and cartilage. They probably arise from faulty migration of germ cells from the mesentery

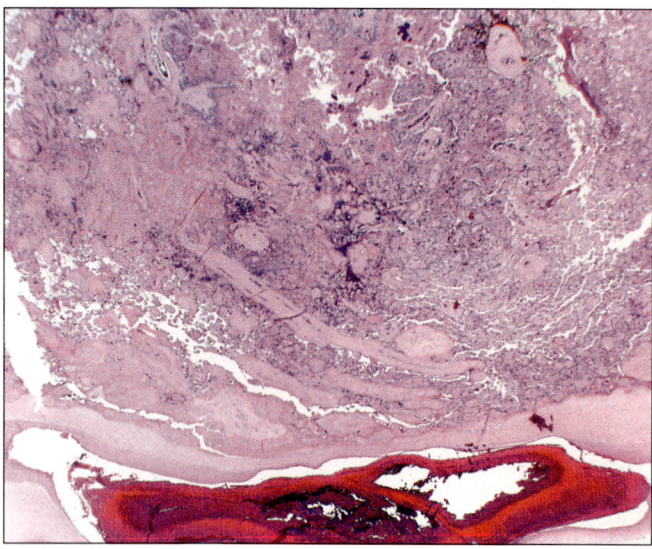

Fig. 30.83 Choriocarcinoma *in situ*. Grossly, the small nodule appeared yellow as in infarct.

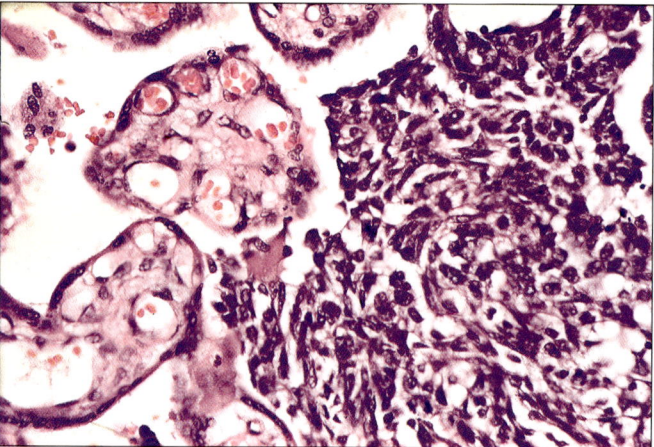

Fig. 30.85 Metastatic breast carcinoma. Aggregates of poorly differentiated malignant cells lie in the intervillous space.

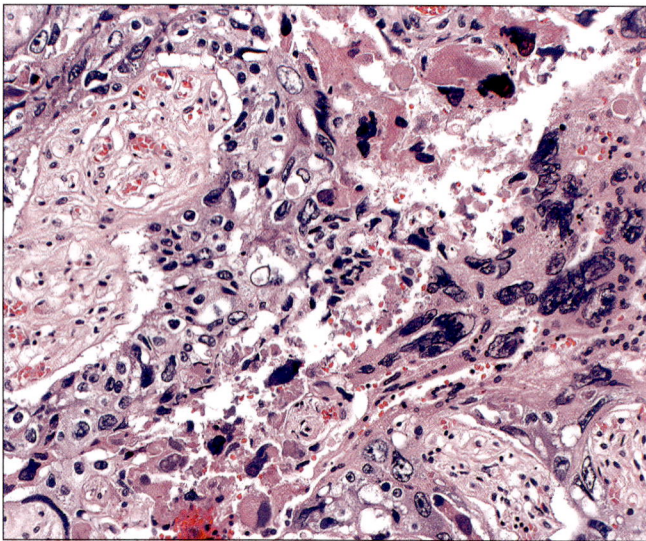

Fig. 30.84 Choriocarcinoma *in situ*. The trophoblasts growing about the residual villi are in the typical pattern of choriocarcinoma.

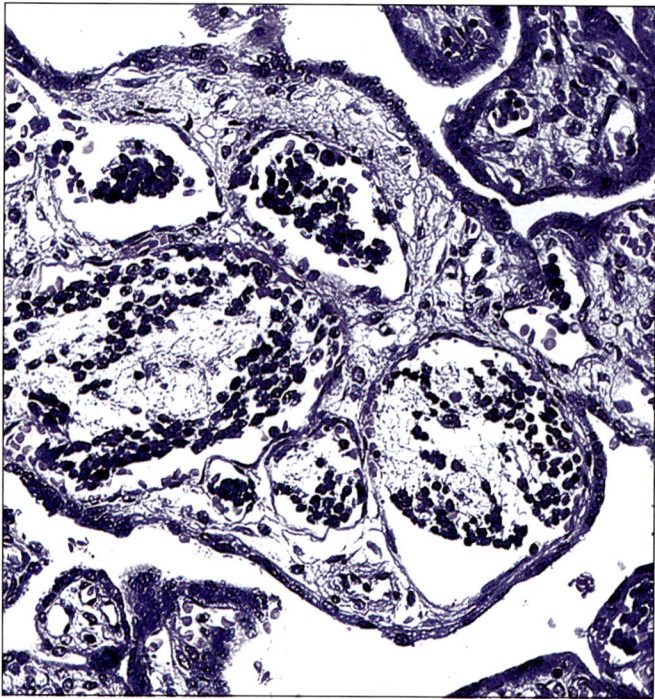

Fig. 30.86 Metastatic neuroblastoma within villous blood vessels.

of the bowel when it is within the umbilical cord and hence may give rise to teratomas of the cord. This is the same site as the calcified yolk sac vestige that may be found, implying another possible mechanism for germ cell sequestration. Hepatocellular adenoma and an adrenal heterotopia have also been described.

METASTATIC TUMOR

The placenta may rarely harbor maternal and even more exceptionally congenital fetal tumor metastases.[1] Metastatic tumors may be seen macroscopically in 60% of involved placentas, especially in cases of pigmented melanomas. Melanomas comprise 30%, breast carcinomas 18% (Figure 30.85), and hematopoietic malignancies 13% of the cases. Metastatic sarcomas, lung carcinoma, Hodgkins and non-Hodgkins lymphoma have

all been described. Melanoma most regularly invades the villous stroma. In one series, the fetus was affected in 22% of cases.[2] Other tumors tend to remain in the intervillous space. Some suggest that all placental metastases be reported,[1] the minimum data set required being maternal age, race, prior malignancy and treatment, maternal and fetal outcome, gross features, and histology of placenta. The chronologic relationship among diagnosis, pregnancy, and tumor behavior throughout pregnancy should also be recorded.

Neuroblastoma may present with intraplacental metastases with tumor cells being seen in villous vessels (Figure 30.86). The fetus is usually hydropic due to the large abdominal tumor load that restricts the venous return. Most fetuses are stillborn.

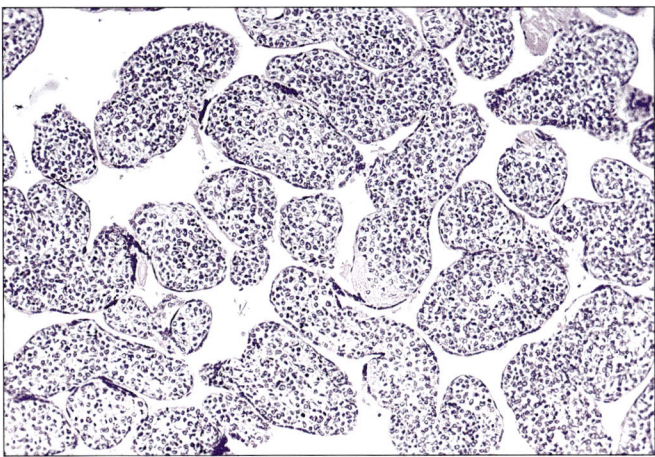

Fig. 30.87 Congenital leukemia.

Other malignancies that may be diagnosed primarily on placental examination include hepatoblastoma[35] and primitive epithelial tumor of the liver.[96] Congenital leukemias may also occasionally be seen in villous vessels (Figure 30.87). Transient myeloproliferative disease, which mimics congenital leukemia, may show numerous blast cells in fetal vessels with early vessel wall infiltration.[30]

REFERENCES

1. Ackerman J, Gilbert-Barness E. Malignancy metastatic to the products of conception: a case report with literature review. Pediatr Pathol Lab Med 1997;17:577–86.
2. Alexander A, Samlowski WE, Grossman D, et al. Metastatic melanoma in pregnancy: risk of transplacental metastases in the infant. J Clin Oncol 2003;21:2179–86.
3. Alexander JM, McIntire DM, Leveno KJ. Chorioamnionitis and the prognosis for term infants. Obstet Gynecol 1999;94:274–8.
4. Altshuler G, Arizawa M, Molnar-Nadasdy G. Meconium-induced umbilical cord vascular necrosis and ulceration: a potential link between the placenta and poor pregnancy outcome. Obstet Gynecol 1992;79(5 Pt 1):760–6.
5. Ananth CV, Savitz DA, Williams MA. Placental abruption and its association with hypertension and prolonged rupture of membranes: a methodologic review and meta-analysis. Obstet Gynecol 1996;88:309–18.
6. Ananth CV, Berkowitz GS, Savitz DA, Lapinski RH. Placental abruption and adverse perinatal outcomes. JAMA 1999;282:1646–51.
7. Andres RL, Kuyper W, Resnik R, Piacquadio KM, Benirschke K. The association of maternal floor infarction of the placenta with adverse perinatal outcome. Am J Obstet Gynecol 1990;163:935–8.
8. Aplin JD. The cell biology of human implantation. Placenta 1996;17:269–75.
9. Arias F, Gonzalez-Ruiz AR, Jacobson RL. Recent advances in the pathophysiology and management of preterm premature rupture of the fetal membranes. Curr Opin Obstet Gynecol 1999;11:141–7.
10. Arias F, Romero R, Joist H, Kraus FT. Thrombophilia: a mechanism of disease in women with adverse pregnancy outcome and thrombotic lesions in the placenta. J Matern Fetal Med 1998;7:277–86.
11. Baergen RN, Malicki D, Behling C, Benirschke K. Morbidity, mortality, and placental pathology in excessively long umbilical cords: retrospective study. Pediatr Dev Pathol 2001;4:144–53.
12. Baglin T. Thrombophilia testing: what do we think the tests mean and what should we do with the results? J Clin Pathol 2000;53:167–70.
13. Bane AL, Gillan JE. Massive perivillous fibrinoid causing recurrent placental failure. BJOG 2003;110:292–5.
14. Becroft DM, Thompson JM, Mitchell EA. Placental villitis of unknown origin: epidemiologic associations. Am J Obstet Gynecol 2005;192:264–71.
15. Bendon RW. Twin transfusion: pathological studies of the monochorionic placenta in liveborn twins and of the perinatal autopsy in monochorionic twin pairs. Pediatr Pathol Lab Med 1995;15:363–76.
16. Benirschke K. Recent trends in chorangiomas, especially those of multiple and recurrent chorangiomas. Pediatr Dev Pathol 1999;2:264–9.
17. Benirschke K, Kaufmann P, Baergen R. Pathology of the Human Placenta, 5th edn. New York: Springer; 2006.
18. Benirschke K, Coen R, Patterson B, Key T. Villitis of known origin: varicella and toxoplasma. Placenta 1999;20:395–9.
19. Bruch JF, Sibony O, Benali K, Challier JC, Blot P, Nessmann C. Computerized microscope morphometry of umbilical vessels from pregnancies with intrauterine growth retardation and abnormal umbilical artery Doppler. Hum Pathol 1997;28:1139–45.
20. Burgess AM, Hutchins GM. Inflammation of the lungs, umbilical cord and placenta associated with meconium passage in utero. Review of 123 autopsied cases. Pathol Res Pract 1996;192:1121–8.
21. Castellucci M, Scheper M, Scheffen I, Celona A, Kaufmann P. The development of the human placental villous tree. Anat Embryol (Berl) 1990;181:117–28.
22. Chazotte C, Girz B, Koenigsberg M, Cohen WR. Spontaneous infarction of placental chorioangioma and associated regression of hydrops fetalis. Am J Obstet Gynecol 1990;163(4 Pt 1):1180–1.
23. Chen CP, Chern SR, Wang TY, Huang ZD, Huang MC, Chuang CY. Pregnancy with concomitant chorangioma and placental vascular malformation with mesenchymal hyperplasia. Hum Reprod 1997;12:2553–6.
24. Chow JS, Benson CB, Doubilet PM. Frequency and nature of structural anomalies in fetuses with single umbilical arteries. J Ultrasound Med 1998;17:765–8.
25. Craven C, Ward K. Placental causes of fetal malformation. Clin Obstet Gynecol 1996;39:588–606.
26. Cross JC, Werb Z, Fisher SJ. Implantation and the placenta: key pieces of the development puzzle. Science 1994;266:1508–18.
27. D'Alton ME, Simpson LL. Syndromes in twins. Semin Perinatol 1995;19:375–86.
28. Dammann O, Allred EN, Leviton A, et al. Fetal vasculitis in preterm newborns: interrelationships, modifiers, and antecedents. Placenta 2004;25:788–96.
29. de Laat MW, Franx A, van Alderen ED, Nikkels PG, Visser GH. The umbilical coiling index, a review of the literature. J Matern Fetal Neonatal Med 2005;17:93–100.
30. de Tar MW, Dittman W, Gilbert J. Transient myeloproliferative disease of the newborn: case report with placental, cytogenetic, and flow cytometric findings. Hum Pathol 2000;31:396–8.
31. Demir R, Kosanke G, Kohnen G, Kertschanska S, Kaufmann P. Classification of human placental stem villi: review of structural and functional aspects. Microsc Res Tech 1997;38:29–41.
32. Dexter SC, Malee MP, Pinar H, Hogan JW, Carpenter MW, Vohr BR. Influence of chorioamnionitis on developmental outcome in very low birth weight infants. Obstet Gynecol 1999;94:267–73.
33. Dizon-Townson DS, Meline L, Nelson LM, Varner M, Ward K. Fetal carriers of the factor V Leiden mutation are prone to miscarriage and placental infarction. Am J Obstet Gynecol 1997;177:402–5.
34. Dommisse J, Tiltman AJ. Placental bed biopsies in placental abruption. Br J Obstet Gynaecol 1992;99:651–4.
35. Doss BJ, Vicari J, Jacques SM, Qureshi F. Placental involvement in congenital hepatoblastoma. Pediatr Dev Pathol 1998;1:538–42.
36. Doss BJ, Greene MF, Hill J, Heffner LJ, Bieber FR, Genest DR. Massive chronic intervillositis associated with recurrent abortions. Hum Pathol 1995;26:1245–51.
37. Enders AC, King BF. Early stages of trophoblastic invasion of the maternal vascular system during implantation in the macaque and baboon. Am J Anat 1991;192:329–46.
38. Faye-Petersen OM, Heller DS, Joshi VJ. Handbook of Placental Pathology, 2nd edn. London: Taylor and Francis; 2006.
39. Fox GE, Van Wesep R, Resau JH, Sun CC. The effect of immersion formaldehyde fixation on human placental weight. Arch Pathol Lab Med 1991;115:726–8.
40. Fox H. Aging of the placenta. Arch Dis Child Fetal Neonatal Ed 1997;77:F171–5.
41. Fox H. Pathology of the Placenta, 2nd edn. London: W.B. Saunders; 1997.
42. Fujikura T, Sho S. Placental cavities. Obstet Gynecol 1997;90:112–6.
43. Fuke Y, Aono T, Imai S, Suehara N, Fujita T, Nakayama M. Clinical significance and treatment of massive intervillous fibrin deposition associated with recurrent fetal growth retardation. Gynecol Obstet Invest 1994;38:5–9.
44. Genbacev O, Zhou Y, Ludlow JW, Fisher SJ. Regulation of human placental development by oxygen tension. Science 1997;277:1669–72.
45. Genest DR, Granter S, Pinkus GS. Umbilical cord 'pseudo-vasculitis' following second trimester fetal death: a clinicopathological and immunohistochemical study of 13 cases. Histopathology 1997;30:563–9.
46. Ghezzi F, Raio L, Gunter Duwe D, Cromi A, Karousou E, Durig P. Sonographic umbilical vessel morphometry and perinatal outcome of fetuses with a lean umbilical cord. J Clin Ultrasound 2005;33:18–23.
47. Ghidini A, Salafia CM. Gender differences of placental dysfunction in severe prematurity. BJOG 2005;112:140–4.
48. Gibbs RS. Chorioamnionitis and bacterial vaginosis. Am J Obstet Gynecol 1993;169(2 Pt 2):460–2.
49. Grafe MR. The correlation of prenatal brain damage with placental pathology. J Neuropathol Exp Neurol 1994;53:407–15.
50. Guschmann M, Henrich W, Entezami M, Dudenhausen JW. Chorioangioma – new insights into a well-known problem I. Results of a clinical and morphological study of 136 cases. J Perinat Med 2003;31:163–9.

51. Hale LP, van de Ven CJ, Wenger DA, Bradford WD, Kahler SG. Infantile sialic acid storage disease: a rare cause of cytoplasmic vacuolation in pediatric patients. Pediatr Pathol Lab Med 1995;15:443–53.
52. Heinonen S, Ryynanen M, Kirkinen P, Saarikoski S. Perinatal diagnostic evaluation of velamentous umbilical cord insertion: clinical, Doppler, and ultrasonic findings. Obstet Gynecol 1996;87:112–7.
53. Hershkovitz R, Silberstein T, Sheiner E, et al. Risk factors associated with true knots of the umbilical cord. Eur J Obstet Gynecol Reprod Biol 2001;98:36–9.
54. Holcberg G, Huleihel M, Katz M, et al. Vasoconstrictive activity of meconium stained amniotic fluid in the human placental vasculature. Eur J Obstet Gynecol Reprod Biol 1999;87:147–50.
55. Hustin J, Jauniaux E, Schaaps JP. Histological study of the materno-embryonic interface in spontaneous abortion. Placenta 1990;11:477–86.
56. Incerpi MH, Miller DA, Samadi R, Settlage RH, Goodwin TM. Stillbirth evaluation: what tests are needed? Am J Obstet Gynecol 1998;178:1121–5.
57. Jacques SM, Qureshi F. Chronic intervillositis of the placenta. Arch Pathol Lab Med 1993;117:1032–5.
58. Jacques SM, Qureshi F, Doss BJ, Munkarah A. Intraplacental choriocarcinoma associated with viable pregnancy: pathologic features and implications for the mother and infant. Pediatr Dev Pathol 1998;1:380–7.
59. Jaffe R, Jauniaux E, Hustin J. Maternal circulation in the first-trimester human placenta – myth or reality? Am J Obstet Gynecol 1997;176:695–705.
60. Jauniaux E, Nicolaides KH, Hustin J. Perinatal features associated with placental mesenchymal dysplasia. Placenta 1997;18:701–6.
61. Jones CJ, Lendon M, Chawner LE, Jauniaux E. Ultrastructure of the human placenta in metabolic storage disease. Placenta 1990;11:395–411.
62. Kaplan C. Placental pathology for the nineties. Pathol Annu 1993; 28(Pt 1):15–72.
63. Katzman PJ, Genest DR. Maternal floor infarction and massive perivillous fibrin deposition: histological definitions, association with intrauterine fetal growth restriction, and risk of recurrence. Pediatr Dev Pathol 2002;5:159–64.
64. Khong TY. Chorangioma with trophoblastic proliferation. Virchows Arch 2000;436:167–71.
65. Khong TY, George K. Chromosomal abnormalities associated with a single umbilical artery. Prenat Diagn 1992;12:965–8.
66. Khong TY, Staples A, Moore L, Byard RW. Observer reliability in assessing villitis of unknown aetiology. J Clin Pathol 1993;46:208–10.
67. Khong TY, Staples A, Bendon RW, et al. Observer reliability in assessing placental maturity by histology. J Clin Pathol 1995;48:420–3.
68. Khong TY, Bendon RW, Qureshi F, et al. Chronic deciduitis in the placental basal plate: definition and interobserver reliability. Hum Pathol 2000;31:292–5.
69. Kraus FT. Placental thrombi and related problems. Semin Diagn Pathol 1993;10:275–83.
70. Kraus FT. Cerebral palsy and thrombi in placental vessels of the fetus: insights from litigation. Hum Pathol 1997;28:246–8.
71. Kreczy A, Alge A, Menardi G, Gassner I, Gschwendtner A, Mikuz G. Teratoma of the umbilical cord. Case report with review of the literature. Arch Pathol Lab Med 1994;118:934–7.
72. Kupferminc MJ, Eldor A, Steinman N, et al. Increased frequency of genetic thrombophilia in women with complications of pregnancy. N Engl J Med 1999;340:9–13.
73. Kurjak A, Kupesic S. Doppler assessment of the intervillous blood flow in normal and abnormal early pregnancy. Obstet Gynecol 1997;89:252–6.
74. Lage JM. Placentomegaly with massive hydrops of placental stem villi, diploid DNA content, and fetal omphaloceles: possible association with Beckwith–Wiedemann syndrome. Hum Pathol 1991;22:591–7.
75. Langston C, Kaplan C, Macpherson T, et al. Practice guideline for examination of the placenta: developed by the Placental Pathology Practice Guideline Development Task Force of the College of American Pathologists. Arch Pathol Lab Med 1997;121:449–76.
76. Larsen LG, Graem N. Morphological findings and value of placental examination at fetal and perinatal autopsy. APMIS 1999;107:337–45.
77. Lee GK, Chi JG, Cha KS. An unusual venous anomaly of the placenta. Am J Clin Pathol 1991;95:48–51.
78. Leiser R, Kosanke G, Kaufmann P. Human placental vascularization. Structural and quantitative aspects. In: Soma H, ed. Placenta: Basic Research for Clinical Application. Basel: Karger; 1991:32–45.
79. Leistra-Leistra MJ, Timmer A, van Spronsen FJ, Geven WB, van der Meer J, Erwich JJ. Fetal thrombotic vasculopathy in the placenta: a thrombophilic connection between pregnancy complications and neonatal thrombosis? Placenta 2004;25(Suppl A):S102–5.
80. Machin GA. Some causes of genotypic and phenotypic discordance in monozygotic twin pairs. Am J Med Genet 1996;61:216–28.
81. Machin GA, Ackerman J, Gilbert-Barness E. Abnormal umbilical cord coiling is associated with adverse perinatal outcomes. Pediatr Dev Pathol 2000;3:462–71.
82. Maher JT, Conti JA. A comparison of umbilical cord blood gas values between newborns with and without true knots. Obstet Gynecol 1996;88:863–6.
83. Mandsager NT, Bendon R, Mostello D, Rosenn B, Miodovnik M, Siddiqi TA. Maternal floor infarction of the placenta: prenatal diagnosis and clinical significance. Obstet Gynecol 1994;83(5 Pt 1):750–4.
84. McDermott M, Gillan JE. Chronic reduction in fetal blood flow is associated with placental infarction. Placenta 1995;16:165–70.
85. McDermott M, Gillan JE. Trophoblast basement membrane haemosiderosis in the placental lesion of fetal artery thrombosis: a marker for disturbance of maternofetal transfer? Placenta 1995;16:171–8.
86. McDonald DG, Kelehan P, McMenamin JB, et al. Placental fetal thrombotic vasculopathy is associated with neonatal encephalopathy. Hum Pathol 2004;35:875–80.
87. Minakami H, Honma Y, Matsubara S, Uchida A, Shiraishi H, Sato I. Effects of placental chorionicity on outcome in twin pregnancies. A cohort study. J Reprod Med 1999;44:595–600.
88. Misra DP, Ananth CV. Risk factor profiles of placental abruption in first and second pregnancies: heterogeneous etiologies. J Clin Epidemiol 1999;52:453–61.
89. Mooney EE, al Shunnar A, O'Regan M, Gillan JE. Chorionic villous haemorrhage is associated with retroplacental haemorrhage. Br J Obstet Gynaecol 1994;101:965–9.
90. Mooney EE, Boggess KA, Herbert WN, Layfield LJ. Placental pathology in patients using cocaine: an observational study. Obstet Gynecol 1998;91:925–9.
91. Myerson D, Parkin RK, Benirschke K, Tschetter CN, Hyde SR. The pathogenesis of villitis of unknown etiology: analysis with a new conjoint immunohistochemistry-in situ hybridization procedure to identify specific maternal and fetal cells. Pediatr Dev Pathol 2006;9:257–65.
92. Naeye RL. The clinical significance of absent subchorionic fibrin in the placenta. Am J Clin Pathol 1990;94:196–8.
93. Naeye RL. Disorders of the Placenta, Fetus and Neonate. Diagnosis and Clinical Significance. St Louis: Mosby; 1992.
94. Nelson KB, Dambrosia JM, Grether JK, Phillips TM. Neonatal cytokines and coagulation factors in children with cerebral palsy. Ann Neurol 1998;44:665–75.
95. Nieuwint A, Van Zalen-Sprock R, Hummel P, et al. 'Identical' twins with discordant karyotypes. Prenat Diagn 1999;19:72–6.
96. Ohyama M, Ijiri R, Tanaka Y, et al. Congenital primitive epithelial tumor of the liver showing focal rhabdoid features, placental involvement, and clinical features mimicking multifocal hemangioma or stage 4S neuroblastoma. Hum Pathol 2000;31:259–63.
97. Ordi J, Ismail MR, Ventura PJ, et al. Massive chronic intervillositis of the placenta associated with malaria infection. Am J Surg Pathol 1998;22:1006–11.
98. Oyelese Y, Catanzarite V, Prefumo F, et al. Vasa previa: the impact of prenatal diagnosis on outcomes. Obstet Gynecol 2004;103(5 Pt 1):937–42.
99. Peleg D, Ferber A, Orvieto R, Bar-Hava I, Ben-Rafael Z. Single intrauterine fetal death (fetus papyraceus) due to uterine trauma in a twin pregnancy. Eur J Obstet Gynecol Reprod Biol 1998;80:175–6.
100. Perlman EJ, Stetten G, Tuck-Muller CM, et al. Sexual discordance in monozygotic twins. Am J Med Genet 1990;37:551–7.
101. Pinar H, Sung CJ, Oyer CE, Singer DB. Reference values for singleton and twin placental weights. Pediatr Pathol Lab Med 1996;16:901–7.
102. Qureshi F, Jacques SM. Marked segmental thinning of the umbilical cord vessels. Arch Pathol Lab Med 1994;118:826–30.
103. Ramon y Cajal CL, Martinez RO. Defecation in utero: a physiologic fetal function. Am J Obstet Gynecol 2003;188:153–6.
104. Rana A, Sawhney H, Gopalan S, Panigrahi D, Nijhawan R. Abruptio placentae and chorioamnionitis – microbiological and histologic correlation. Acta Obstet Gynecol Scand 1999;78:363–6.
105. Rayne SC, Kraus FT. Placental thrombi and other vascular lesions. Classification, morphology, and clinical correlations. Pathol Res Pract 1993;189:2–17.
106. Redline RW. Clinical and pathological umbilical cord abnormalities in fetal thrombotic vasculopathy. Hum Pathol 2004;35:1494–8.
107. Redline RW. Severe fetal placental vascular lesions in term infants with neurologic impairment. Am J Obstet Gynecol 2005;192:452–7.
108. Redline RW, Patterson P. Villitis of unknown etiology is associated with major infiltration of fetal tissue by maternal inflammatory cells. Am J Pathol 1993;143:473–9.
109. Redline RW, Patterson P. Patterns of placental injury. Correlations with gestational age, placental weight, and clinical diagnoses. Arch Pathol Lab Med 1994;118:698–701.
110. Redline RW, Patterson P. Pre-eclampsia is associated with an excess of proliferative immature intermediate trophoblast. Hum Pathol 1995;26:594–600.
111. Redline RW, Wilson-Costello D. Chronic peripheral separation of placenta. The significance of diffuse chorioamnionic hemosiderosis. Am J Clin Pathol 1999;111:804–10.
112. Redline RW, Wilson-Costello D, Borawski E, Fanaroff AA, Hack M. Placental lesions associated with neurologic impairment and cerebral palsy in very low-birth-weight infants. Arch Pathol Lab Med 1998;122:1091–8.
113. Redline RW, Faye-Petersen O, Heller D, Qureshi F, Savell V, Vogler C. Amniotic infection syndrome: nosology and reproducibility of placental reaction patterns. Pediatr Dev Pathol 2003;6:435–48.
114. Reshetnikova OS, Burton GJ, Milovanov AP, Fokin EI. Increased incidence of placental chorioangioma in high-altitude pregnancies: hypobaric hypoxia as a possible etiologic factor. Am J Obstet Gynecol 1996;174:557–61.

115. Robboy SJ, Duggan M, Kurman RT. The female reproductive system. In: Rubin E, Farber J, eds. Pathology, 3rd edn. Philadelphia: Lippincott; 1999:962–1028.

116. Roberts DJ, Ampola MG, Lage JM. Diagnosis of unsuspected fetal metabolic storage disease by routine placental examination. Pediatr Pathol 1991;11:647–56.

117. Rogers BB, Alexander JM, Head J, McIntire D, Leveno KJ. Umbilical vein interleukin-6 levels correlate with the severity of placental inflammation and gestational age. Hum Pathol 2002;33:335–40.

118. Romero R, Salafia CM, Athanassiadis AP, et al. The relationship between acute inflammatory lesions of the preterm placenta and amniotic fluid microbiology. Am J Obstet Gynecol 1992;166:1382–8.

119. Romero R, Mazor M, Morrotti R, et al. Infection and labor. VII. Microbial invasion of the amniotic cavity in spontaneous rupture of membranes at term. Am J Obstet Gynecol 1992;166(1 Pt 1):129–33.

120. Salafia CM, Vintzileos AM. Why all placentas should be examined by a pathologist in 1990. Am J Obstet Gynecol 1990;163(4 Pt 1):1282–93.

121. Salafia CM, Vogel CA, Bantham KF, Vintzileos AM, Pezzullo J, Silberman L. Preterm delivery: correlations of fetal growth and placental pathology. Am J Perinatol 1992;9:190–3.

122. Sander CH, Kinnane L, Stevens NG, Echt R. Haemorrhagic endovasculitis of the placenta: a review with clinical correlation. Placenta 1986;7:551–74.

123. Sander CM. Angiomatous malformation of placental chorionic stem vessels and pseudo-partial molar placentas: report of five cases. Pediatr Pathol 1993;13:621–33.

124. Senat MV, Deprest J, Boulvain M, Paupe A, Winer N, Ville Y. Endoscopic laser surgery versus serial amnioreduction for severe twin-to-twin transfusion syndrome. N Engl J Med 2004;351:136–44.

125. Sepulveda W, Alcalde JL, Schnapp C, Bravo M. Perinatal outcome after prenatal diagnosis of placental chorioangioma. Obstet Gynecol 2003;102(5 Pt 1):1028–33.

126. Shipp TD, Bromley B, Benacerraf BR. Sonographically detected abnormalities of the umbilical cord. Int J Gynaecol Obstet 1995;48:179–85.

127. Smulian JC, Shen-Schwarz S, Vintzileos AM, Lake MF, Ananth CV. Clinical chorioamnionitis and histologic placental inflammation. Obstet Gynecol 1999;94:1000–5.

128. Sondergaard G. Hemangioma of the umbilical cord. Acta Obstet Gynecol Scand 1994;73:434–6.

129. Souter VL, Kapur RP, Nyholt DR, et al. A report of dizygous monochorionic twins. N Engl J Med 2003;349:154–8.

130. Stallmach T, Hebisch G, Meier K, Dudenhausen JW, Vogel M. Rescue by birth: defective placental maturation and late fetal mortality. Obstet Gynecol 2001;97:505–9.

131. Tennstedt C, Chaoui R, Bollmann R, Dietel M. Angiomyxoma of the umbilical cord in one twin with cystic degeneration of Wharton's jelly. A case report. Pathol Res Pract 1998;194:55–8.

132. Thummala MR, Raju TN, Langenberg P. Isolated single umbilical artery anomaly and the risk for congenital malformations: a meta-analysis. J Pediatr Surg 1998;33:580–5.

133. Umur A, van Gemert MJ, Nikkels PG. Monoamniotic-versus diamniotic-monochorionic twin placentas: anastomoses and twin-twin transfusion syndrome. Am J Obstet Gynecol 2003;189:1325–9.

134. van Hoeven KH, Anyaegbunam A, Hochster H, et al. Clinical significance of increasing histologic severity of acute inflammation in the fetal membranes and umbilical cord. Pediatr Pathol Lab Med 1996;16:731–44.

135. Verma U, Tejani N, Klein S, et al. Obstetric antecedents of intraventricular hemorrhage and periventricular leukomalacia in the low-birth-weight neonate. Am J Obstet Gynecol 1997;176:275–81.

136. Wharton KN, Pinar H, Stonestreet BS, et al. Severe umbilical cord inflammation – a predictor of periventricular leukomalacia in very low birth weight infants. Early Hum Dev 2004;77:77–87.

Placenta – clinical scenarios

31

Eoghan E. Mooney   Emma Doyle   Peter Gearhart   Stanley J. Robboy

Gross examination of the placenta by the obstetrician is a routine practice at the time of delivery. Inspection of the membranes, umbilical cord, and cotyledons can help determine if there is any retained tissue that may result in postpartum hemorrhage, or in any gross abnormalities that might prompt a closer evaluation of the newborn baby. In most institutions the decision to request a pathologic evaluation of the placenta is made by the delivering clinician.

The discussion of diseases involving placental pathology has been divided for ease of presentation. Despite much overlap, the prior chapter emphasizes entities where the pathology is the central feature and this chapter good clinical–pathologic correlation of placental abnormalities and the pregnancy itself which may be useful in understanding antenatal events that may have contributed to the adverse pregnancy outcome.

This chapter focuses on the placental findings in common clinical scenarios. Points of particular relevance in the gross examination of the placenta are highlighted. While substantial overlap exists for some entities, e.g., intrauterine growth restriction (IUGR) and uteroplacental insufficiency, the scenarios are presented separately for ease of discussion. A constant theme throughout this chapter is the relevance of placental examination to diagnosis of disease in the offspring. Often chronic conditions can be demonstrated as the cause of cerebral palsy, and identification of disease in the placenta can reduce or negate the medico-legal charge of birth-related injury.

ECTOPIC PREGNANCY

Ectopic pregnancy (see also Chapter 19) is a conceptus implanted outside the uterine cavity. Nearly all (98%) ectopics occur in the fallopian tube. The remaining 2% are found in the uterine cornua or cervix (Figure 31.1),[125] abdomen, or ovary.[124]

The consequences of ectopic pregnancy are severe. It is one of the important causes of maternal death in the USA during the first trimester.[20] It is substantially more dangerous (38 deaths/100 000 events) than either childbirth or legal abortion (9:<1 death, respectively).[41]

Ectopic pregnancy is uncommon, but has increased in some areas to 2% of pregnancies.[71] In one large catchment area in Ireland, the rates rose more than two-fold in a 10-year period. As the risk factors seemed stable over that time period, the increase was attributed to the more widespread availability of serum beta-human chorionic gonadotrophin (β-hCG) testing and a corresponding earlier time in pregnancy when the diagnosis could be established (falling from 8 to 6 weeks).[90] Several factors, however, influence the rates. Women who have achieved pregnancy with the use of assisted reproductive tech-

nology have seen rates increase dramatically to 1:100.[77,99] Women exposed in utero to diethylstilbestrol have also experienced significantly higher rates of ectopic pregnancy.

The risk of tubal ectopic pregnancy is strongly associated with prior tubal surgery, tubal ligation,[140] previous ectopic pregnancies, intrauterine contraceptive devices, infertility, and other tubal pathology such as salpingitis isthmica nodosa, endometriosis, and pelvic inflammatory disease. Intrauterine contraceptive devices prevent uterine pregnancy more effectively than they prevent tubal pregnancy, and so there is a relative increase in the latter. Ectopic pregnancies can result from complications of infertility treatment (e.g., functional motility problems following ovarian stimulation and placement procedures for gametes, zygotes, and embryos).

Macroscopically, the tube with an ectopic pregnancy expands. Half of cases disclose a rupture, with chorionic villi present on the serosal surface or protruding through the ostium at the fimbrial end. Implantation is most commonly ampullary (80%), followed by isthmic (12%), fimbrial (6%), and interstitial (2%), with ampullary and isthmic implantation increased following assisted reproduction.[99]

Ectopic pregnancies usually rupture, but may be expelled via the uterus or abort through the fimbrial end of the tube. The ruptured ectopic may secondarily implant in the abdomen, within the broad ligament or less commonly the ovary. The implantation site in the fallopian tube is of the accreta type because there is no decidua and extravillous trophoblast widely infiltrates the muscle layers leading to rupture. Microscopically, trophoblast can be seen within vascular lumens. There may also be foci of acute and chronic inflammation, necrosis and sometimes obvious chorionic villi. Frequently, eosinophils are prominent in the wall of the tube. If chorionic villi are not grossly obvious, which is the usual situation, all blood clot should be processed for it is in the clot that both chorionic villi and extravillous trophoblast are most easily found. Fetal abnormalities and gestational trophoblastic disease may also occur. The interstitial ectopic is the most threatening to the mother with an associated maternal mortality rate of 2% following uterine rupture.[73]

The endometrium in ectopic pregnancies decidualizes to the degree expected in a normal intrauterine pregnancy, but without inflammation or placental site trophoblastic reaction. In an intrauterine pregnancy, on the other hand, small amounts of inflammation are present throughout the decidua. While not pathognomonic, the absence of inflammation is a useful feature to help lead the pathologist to consider that an ectopic pregnancy might be present. Regardless, tissues of fetal origin should be identified to exclude the presence of an ectopic pregnancy so as to safeguard the patient.

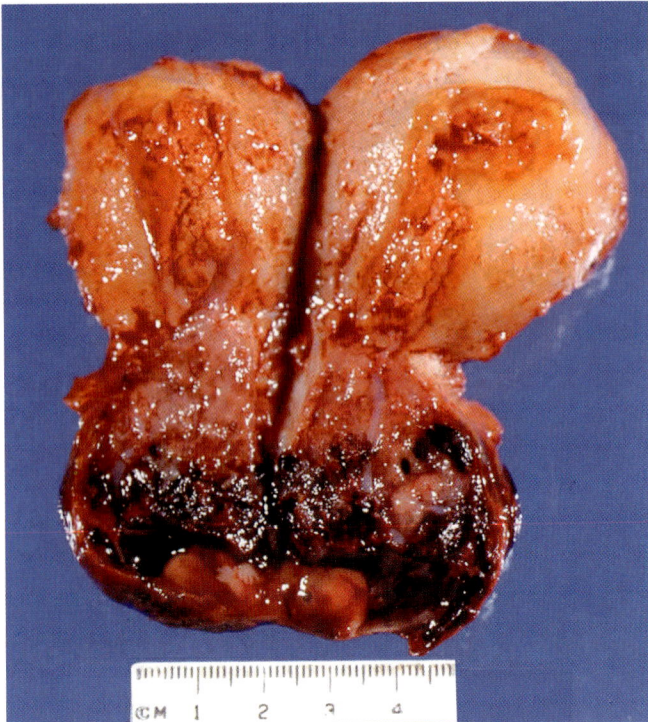

Fig. 31.1 Ectopic pregnancy of cervix. Courtesy of Dr Stephen Ruby, Palo Heights, IL, USA.

Ovarian ectopic pregnancies are rare. They are associated with young maternal age, multiparity, and intrauterine contraceptive devices. Four criteria should be met to diagnose an ovarian pregnancy with certainty:[103] (1) the fallopian tube should be normal and separate from the ovary; (2) the conceptus should be in the normal anatomic location of the ovary; (3) the conceptus should be connected to the uterus by the ovarian ligament; and (4) ovarian tissue should be histologically demonstrated within the placental tissue. All of these criteria are rarely met.

Abdominal ectopic pregnancies are quite rare with incidence estimates ranging from 1 in 7000 to 1 in 40 000 deliveries.[86] They are associated with a high maternal and fetal mortality. There is no decidual reaction, and vascular invasion with subsequent separation and hemorrhage is the usual mode of fetal loss.

Heterotopic (i.e. synchronous intrauterine and ectopic) pregnancy is rare with an estimate of 1 in 30,000 deliveres.[77,99]

EARLY PREGNANCY LOSS (SPONTANEOUS MISCARRIAGE)

The term 'abortion' is often replaced by the term 'miscarriage' in clinical practice. The World Health Organization defines abortion as the expulsion from its mother of a fetus weighing less than 500 g before weeks 20–22. It also includes 'an otherwise product of conception' of any age to include gestational trophoblastic disease.[138] In practice, the definition includes all fetal losses before the legal age of viability, which in the United Kingdom is 24 weeks. However, in many US institutions viability can be sustained at 23 weeks and sometimes even at 22 weeks. With advances in medical technology, and thereby with increased numbers of survivors of earlier gestations, this legal definition may soon require revision. The incidence of miscarriage is difficult to ascertain as many women miscarry before they are aware of the pregnancy. Approximately 15–25% of pregnancies will end in a miscarriage, and recurrent miscarriage (loss of three or more consecutive pregnancies) will affect approximately 1% of fertile couples. In the majority of cases, the exact etiology is unknown.

There are three basic duties the histopathologist has in reporting the findings from miscarriages. These are:

- To show that a pregnancy has in fact occurred (presence of tissues of fetal origin, i.e., embryonic parts, chorionic villi or trophoblast).
- To confirm the location of the pregnancy (i.e., intrauterine or ectopic).
- To identify or exclude a serious disease process, especially gestational trophoblastic disease.

We believe selected tissue from all miscarriages should be examined microscopically. The extreme position of only examining products macroscopically is faulty, as tissues thought to be present macroscopically are sometimes absent histologically. The converse is also true.[44] In the case of evacuated retained products or elective terminations, the finding of villous or fetal tissues confirms the procedure was successful, whereas the finding of decidua only should lead to further clinical intervention. The finding where the specimen is composed solely of decidua free of inflammation is also a clue that the pregnancy may not be intrauterine or that the evacuation procedure was faulty, leading to further investigative procedures and/or repeat curettage.

Fetal parts, when present, may be examined in accordance with parental wishes. Suction termination disrupts the fetus, but measurements of a hand or foot permit comparison against tables of growth rates. Whole fetuses and large embryos may be examined according to published protocols.

In general, the appearances from early pregnancies are as follows:

- At the mean age of 9.4 weeks, gelatinous sacs that may be empty or contain a disorganized embryo or umbilical cord stump. Macroscopically, the villi are edematous. Some may show fibrosis and vascular obliteration. Nucleated red blood cells, commonly present during the 2 weeks before (Figure 31.2), are now being replaced by red blood cells produced by the bone marrow, and if present, often appear partially pyknotic. The highest incidence of karyotypic abnormalities occurs in this group.
- At the mean age of 14.1 weeks, placental or decidual tissue with or without a macerated embryo. Microscopically, the villi are collapsed with or without nucleated red blood cells, have stromal fibrosis, and feature obliterative changes of the vessels together with some syncytial knotting and mineralization.
- At the mean age of 18.6 weeks, placental tissue or decidua associated with or without a fresh embryo. Microscopically, the villi are normal for gestational age with no degenerative changes.

Chromosomal abnormalities in the conceptus are more frequently identified in earlier than in later fetal losses, with up to 75% of first trimester miscarriages having an abnormal karyotype.[97] Most will be sporadic events, but a small minority result from balanced translocations in one of the parents and hence

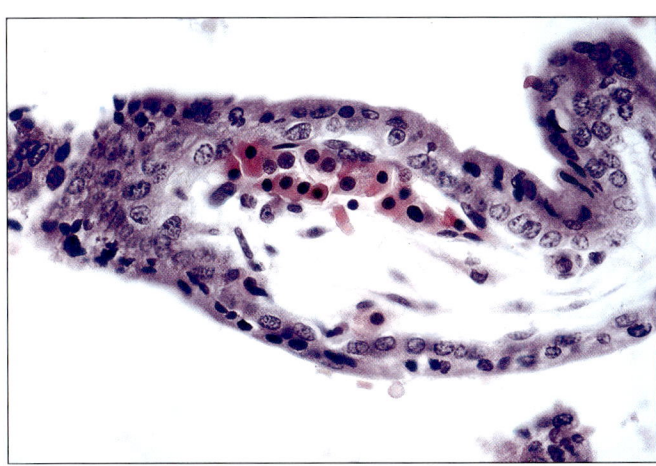

Fig. 31.2 First trimester normal chorionic villus from a normal fetus. There is a uniform inner layer of cytotrophoblasts and outer layer of syncytiotrophoblasts. At 8 weeks, the red cells are nucleated and hepatic in origin. Hofbauer cells are present in the stroma.

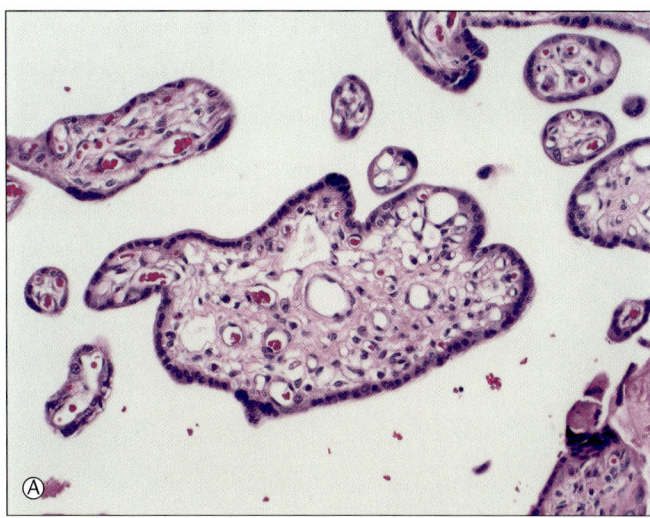

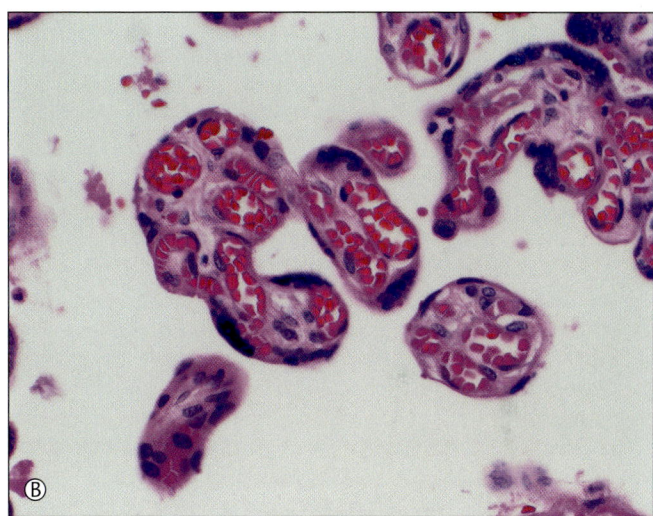

Fig. 31.3 **(A)** Second trimester normal chorionic villus. The syncytiotrophoblast layer is now discontinuous. **(B)** Third trimester normal chorionic villus. The residual trophoblasts have largely coalesced into knots and the perimeter of each villus is large a cytoplasmic membrane.

may recur. Some of the more commonly encountered karyotypic abnormalities are trisomies, especially 16 and 13, and monosomy X (45,X). There is a clear association between congenital abnormality (with a normal karyotype) and miscarriage. The incidence of neural tube defects and other minor abnormalities, such as cleft lip and palate or polydactyly, is strikingly higher in abortuses than in live births.

Frequently, the placenta is the only tissue available when examining the early conceptus. As the extraembryonic mesoderm is derived from the embryo, the embryo must survive until day 12–15 postfertilization, after which the placenta may continue to grow on its own, having obtained the mesenchyme it requires from the embryo. In most first trimester miscarriages, chorionic villi are the only tissues of fetal origin identified. As a rule of thumb, the fetus is within the first trimester if the outer layer of syncytiotrophoblast and inner layer of cytotrophoblast are distinct, uniform, and continuous around all of the villi (Figure 31.2). The fetus can be assessed as 'normal' if the stroma is loose and nucleated red blood cells are plentiful. Only in the second trimester does the syncytiotrophoblast layer become discontinuous (Figure 31.3a). By the third trimester the residual trophoblasts have coalesced largely into knots and the perimeter of each villus is largely a cytoplasmic membrane (Figure 31.3b). Finally, the condition of the villi provides a clue to the time of fetal death. If the villi are extensively fibrotic, a vascular tree is not seen, and virtually all of the vessels are atrophic, it can be assumed that fetal death occurred some time before (Figure 31.4).

The presence or absence and the quantity of nucleated red blood cells also provides a clue to the health of the specimen as well as to duration of the pregnancy. Nucleated fetal red blood cells derived from the yolk sac are seen at 6.5 weeks' menstrual age (4.5 weeks postconception). The switch from nucleated yolk sac-derived red blood cells to anucleate liver-derived red blood cells starts at week 9. By week 11, the nucleated red blood cells make up only 10–15% of the cells. They disappear completely at approximately 12 weeks.[129] In this way, the timing of a lethal event can be assessed.

There have been several attempts to determine the etiology of early fetal loss by morphologic examination. Villous features

thought to represent karyotypic abnormalities include vesicular change, irregular villous contour, presence of trophoblastic pseudoinclusions, trophoblastic hyperplasia, abnormal stromal cells and, in the case of 45,XO monosomy, villous fibrosis and hypoplasia. By including analysis of pathologic features of the maternal–embryonic interface (i.e., absence of interstitial trophoblast columns, absence of intravascular trophoblast plugs, and absence of physiologic changes in spiral arteries), the sensitivity of histology for chromosomal abnormalities may be increased.[55] Examination of material from recurrent miscarriage cannot distinguish recurrent from sporadic cases, or ascertain the cause in the majority of cases.[58] Elegant light and electron microscopic studies support the concept that many early pregnancy losses result from premature onset of the maternal–placental circulation secondary to inadequate trophoblast invasion.[57]

Uterine abnormalities such as leiomyomas, cervical incompetence, and congenital abnormalities of müllerian duct fusion may all contribute to early pregnancy loss. Infection becomes

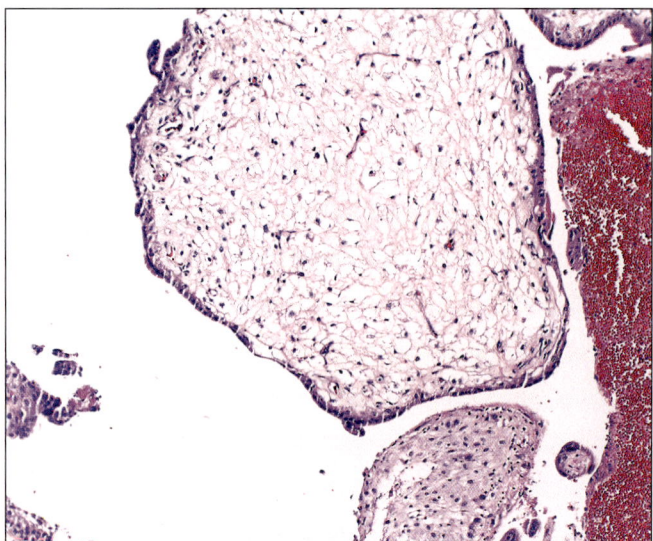

Fig. 31.4 Early miscarriage in which vascular channels have largely disappeared. Several single nucleated red blood cells are partially pyknotic in withered vessels.

increasingly important later in gestation as the influence of abnormal karyotype wanes. Early on, *Campylobacter* sp., *Listeria monocytogenes*, *Toxoplasma gondii*, rubella, cytomegalovirus, and syphilis are important.

The finding of a placental site trophoblastic reaction is important as it generally excludes that the pregnancy was ectopic in the fallopian tube and merely became displaced into the uterus following miscarriage. The presence of chorionic villi and decidua by themselves theoretically do not achieve this according to some reports in the literature,[42] but none of the authors or editors has ever encountered an example of chorionic villi in the uterus where the origin proved to be an ectopic pregnancy. Similarly, wording of the diagnosis can be important because of its use as a guide to management. In our practices, we avoid the term 'products of conception' (POC), but rather describe the findings, if intrauterine, as 'intrauterine contents', followed by a morphologic description, usually consisting of 'chorionic villi and decidua present'. Avoidance of the term POC eliminates the possibility that the clinician can incorrectly interpret a report of decidua only as an indication of an intrauterine pregnancy.

In the absence of easily identified chorionic villi, immunohistochemical stains for cytokeratins and human placental lactogen (see Chapter 30, Figures 30.4 and 30.13) are useful for facilitating the identification of extravillous trophoblast in decidual fragments.

In summary, examination of the early pregnancy loss will:

- confirm intrauterine gestation in most cases
- exclude hydatidiform mole in the vast majority of cases
- identify an occasional case of chronic intervillositis
- not identify the etiology in most cases.

MID TO LATE PREGNANCY LOSS

Analysis of second trimester losses may only show changes of intrauterine death in the placenta. If the miscarriage is fresh,

infection is a likely cause and examination should focus on the membranes. A small placenta is frequently found in trisomies and should prompt cytogenetic analysis – a success rate exceeding 85% can be expected from placental cultures even when maceration is present.[27] Early onset pre-eclampsia will show changes as described below.

Late losses are more likely to reveal placental pathology. The infant is frequently macerated. In this context, we are cautious in applying the term 'fetoplacental thrombotic vasculopathy' unless there is unequivocal evidence of antemortem vascular pathology, such as clearly defined avascular villi. However, other pathologies such as villitis and delayed villous maturation can still be discerned.

The contribution of uteroplacental vascular insufficiency to growth restriction has been discussed below. Placental infarction is associated with cerebral ischemia in the fetus, particularly in growth-restricted infants.[12,13,15] In cases of intrauterine fetal death, intrauterine infection and intrauterine ischemia (the latter possibly due to cord pathology) are also major contributors.[14] However, most of the observations on the cord were clinical, i.e., nuchal cord, and only one of five cords in this group had any structural abnormality (single umbilical artery). Examination of the parenchyma may show villous congestion, stromal hemorrhage, and raised nucleated red cells in cases of cord compression. Abnormal cord coiling, assessed as both under- and overcoiled cords, is associated with fetal death.[23–25,96] Cord coiling is frequently presented as an explanation for fetal death. However, as many of these fetuses are macerated, it is also possible that the passive fetal movement around a cord whose turgor has vanished may account for overcoiling in some of the cases. In the absence of associated pathology such as calcification or thrombosis, we keep an open mind on its role in fetal loss.

ABRUPTION

Abruption, a condition in which the placenta detaches if not tears away from the uterine wall, can be a dramatic obstetric event. Although abruption and retroplacental hemorrhage are sometimes used interchangeably, abruption signifies a clinical event with signs and symptoms, whereas retroplacental hemorrhage is a pathologic finding, often with no clinical correlation (see Chapter 30). Occurring in 1% of pregnancies, abruption is a leading cause of vaginal bleeding in the latter half of pregnancy, and an important cause of perinatal morbidity. It also accounts for 12% of perinatal deaths.[1] The effect on the mother depends primarily on the severity of the abruption, whereas the effect on the fetus depends both on the severity of the abruption as well as the fetus's gestational age. Risk factors include prior abruption, smoking, trauma, multifetal gestation, hypertension, pre-eclampsia, thrombophilias, advanced maternal age, preterm premature rupture of the membranes, intrauterine infections, and hydramnios.[93] Cocaine abuse may also be a cause.[50,93,121] From the pathologist's viewpoint, chorionic villus hemorrhage and villus edema are more frequent in cocaine users.[83]

Questions frequently posed to the pathologist are: does an abruption exist, how extensive is it, and is it recent, old or ongoing? More often than not, none of these questions can be answered based solely on the pathologic examination, leading the pathologist to come away disappointed at not being able

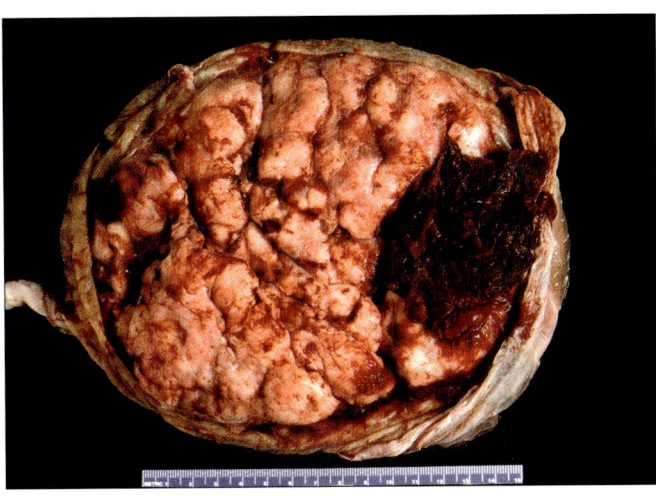

Fig. 31.5 Peripheral and probably clinically insignificant abruption/retroplacental hemorrhage.

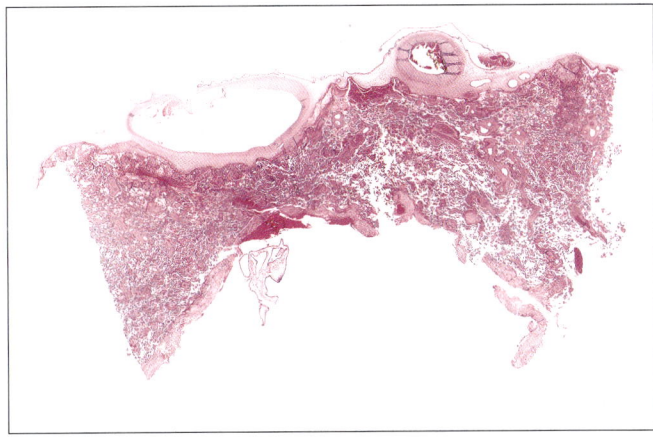

Fig. 31.7 Abruptio placenta with marked compression of the overlying parenchyma.

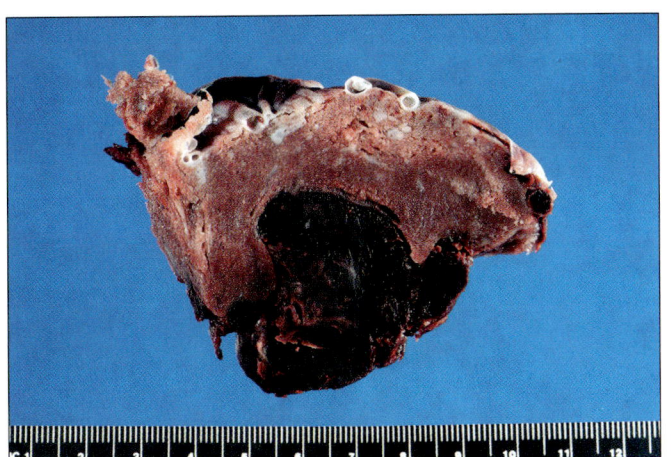

Fig. 31.6 Abruption with parenchymal compression nearly half the placental thickness.

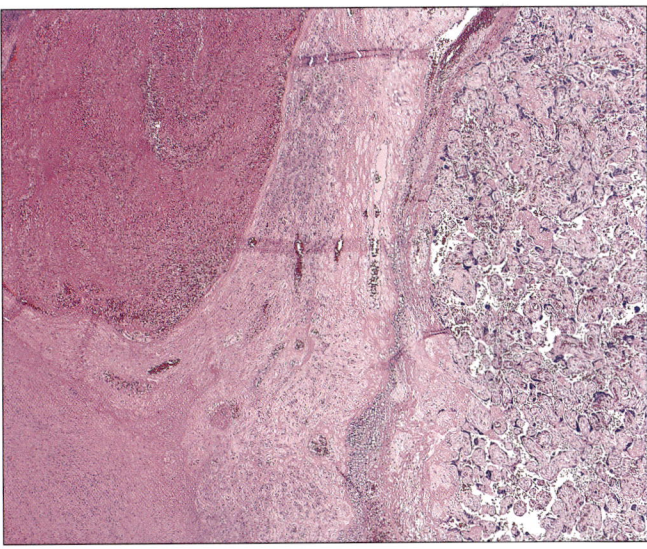

Fig. 31.8 Abruption, clinically of 1 day's duration. An acute inflammatory infiltrate has developed at the interphase of the bleeding and parenchyma.

to add much of clinical use. Most are peripheral (Figure 31.5) and, if recent, will not be detected by pathologic examination, since the hemorrhage will most likely have escaped peripherally and presented as vaginal bleeding. Retroplacental hemorrhage towards the center is far more significant, since the displaced placenta can no longer support fetal functions (Figure 31.6) (see also Chapter 30, Figures 30.48 and 30.49). In a study of over 53 000 pregnancies,[2] the extent of the placental separation profoundly affected the chance of stillbirth. With a 75% separation, the relative risk of fetal death was 31. Even a 50% separation showed profound effects. The risk for preterm delivery was also substantially increased when the separation was mild (with a separation of 25%, the relative risk was 5). The clinical correlate as to the amount of bleeding is best gauged by the volume of retroplacental clot found at cesarean section, or secondarily by the amount of blood clot that accompanies the placenta to the pathology laboratory. The duration of the bleeding is best gauged by whether the parenchyma has been displaced by the blood, whether the junction of the blood and parenchyma shows discoloration from pigment breakdown, and whether the parenchyma near the abruption is infarcted.

Macroscopically, the location, diameter of the involved area, depth of the concave depression (indentation) (Figure 31.7), and thickness of the normal placenta above should be recorded, measurements that will help determine the significance of the abruption. Microscopic sections should be taken at several areas of the junction between the blood and viable placenta, for the presence of tissue reactions can help date the minimum amount of time that the abruption was present. From our experience, nearly a day will have ensued before the villi degenerate and an inflammatory response will be evident at the villus–hemorrhage junction (Figure 31.8). Within several days hemoglobin breakdown will show. Some placentas will show different changes at different areas, for while placental abruption is generally regarded as an acute event, accumulating data indicate that it is often an end result of chronic processes that have begun earlier in pregnancy, even possibly extending to near the time of conception.[4]

HYPERTENSIVE DISORDERS

PRE-ECLAMPSIA

Pre-eclampsia, a disorder only of pregnancy, occurs in about 5–8% of pregnant women and appears during the last trimester, especially in the first pregnancy. Risk factors include nulliparity, women who are at the extremes of reproductive age, multiple gestation, and chronic diseases such as diabetes mellitus, kidney disease, and chronic hypertension. It usually begins insidiously after week 20 of pregnancy with excessive weight gain, marked fluid retention, increase in maternal systemic blood pressure, and the appearance of proteinuria. The essential diagnostic criteria consist of only three elements: pregnancy, proteinuria, and hypertension. Mild pre-eclampsia is declared when the blood pressure is sustained at or above 140 mm Hg systolic or 90 mm Hg diastolic and the urinary protein excretion exceeds 300 mg/day (3+ protein on the urine dipstick).[136]

Progression of mild pre-eclampsia can be slow or rapid and can manifest in many different ways. With increasing blood pressure and declining renal function the resulting fluid retention may result in pulmonary edema. The systemic vasospasm that occurs is particularly noticeable in organs with microvasculature. Hence the classic signs and symptoms of pre-eclampsia, including: visual disturbances from retinopathy; headache from cerebral vasculature changes; chest pain and shortness of breath from cardiopulmonary changes; right upper quadrant discomfort from hepatic dysfunction; proteinuria and glomerulopathy from decreased renal blood flow; systemic edema from peripheral vasospasm; and oligohydramnios and non-reassuring fetal testing from decreased placental perfusion.

Pre-eclampsia can eventually progress further to include grave complications for the mother and the fetus. Maternal complications include eclamptic seizure, the syndrome of *h*emolysis, *e*levated *l*iver enzymes, and *l*ow *p*latelets (HELLP syndrome), subcapsular liver hematoma, pulmonary edema, acute renal failure, intracerebral hemorrhage, and death. The disseminated intravascular coagulation (DIC) that sometimes develops is not part of the pre-eclampsia itself as much as a consequence of the developing HELLP syndrome, abruption or hematoma. Fetal complications include non-reassuring fetal testing, placental abruption, oligohydramnios, intrauterine growth retardation, and death.

Pre-eclampsia is treated with magnesium sulfate and antihypertensive agents, but the definitive therapy is the removal of the placenta, usually by induction of labor or by cesarean delivery.

Much is known about the pathophysiology of pre-eclampsia and eclampsia (Figure 31.9), yet the etiology remains obscure. Immunologic and genetic factors have been invoked,[111] as well as altered vascular reactivity, endothelial injury, and coagulation abnormalities,[108,133] nitric oxide,[87] and oxidative stress.[52] An elevation in circulating angiogenic factors such as sFlt-1 is seen in pregnancies where pre-eclampsia develops[75,126,131] and in trisomy 13,[8] where there is an increased risk of pre-eclampsia. Pre-eclampsia sometimes occurs with hydatidiform mole, which suggests that the trophoblast is the most likely responsible tissue and that pre-eclampsia may be a trophoblastic disease. Recent work has also shown that women with pre-eclampsia have increased expression of specific placental

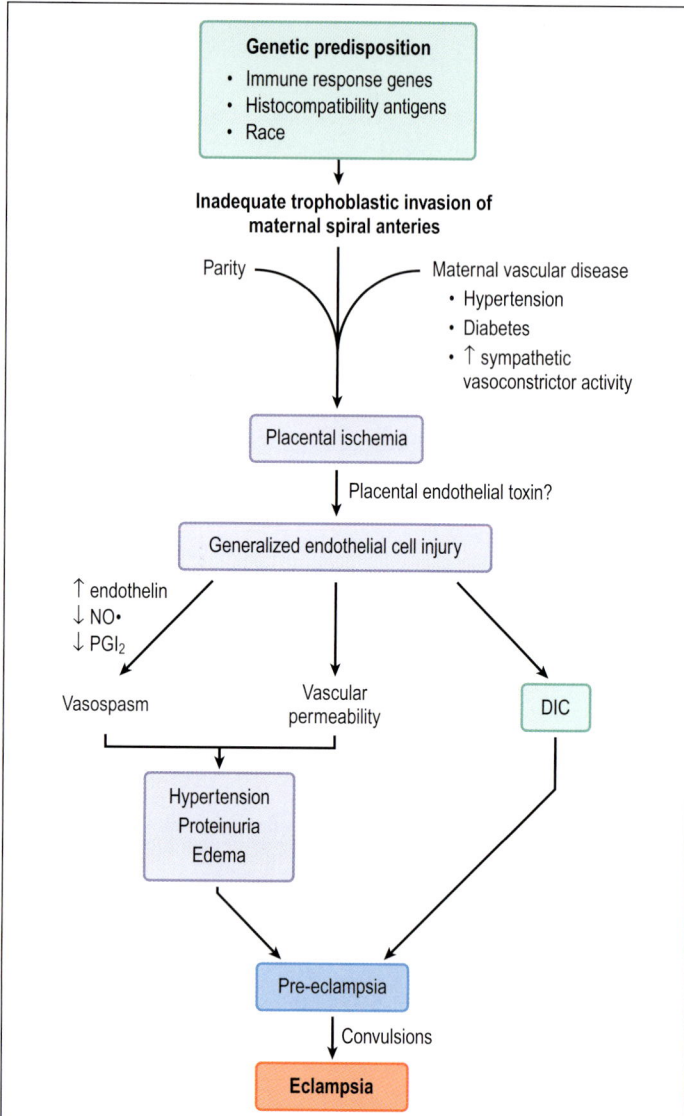

Fig. 31.9 Pathogenesis of pre-eclampsia and eclampsia. From Robboy et al.[109] Reprinted by permission of Lippincott.

miRNAs,[98] furthering that the placenta is a significant factor in pre-eclampsia.

The combination of increased placental bulk combined with decreased perfusion seems to be of particular importance.[84] Even though the hemodynamic, renal, and endothelial systems are essential to the pathophysiology of this disorder, pre-eclampsia is not a primary disease of any of these systems. Early onset pre-eclampsia and IUGR share many placental pathologic findings. Some believe a predisposition to endothelial dysfunction exists in both, with the metabolic syndrome (obesity, insulin resistance, hyperlipidemia, hyperglycemia) being a key link with pre-eclampsia.[85] The abnormal implantation common to both is variably influenced by maternal factors and by habits such as diet and smoking.[17,115,123]

The pathologic changes in the placenta reflect reduced maternal blood flow to the uteroplacental unit. The key factor resides in the arteries of the placental bed. Normally, extravillous trophoblast invades these arteries and these vessels become high-volume, low-pressure conduits of blood from the mother

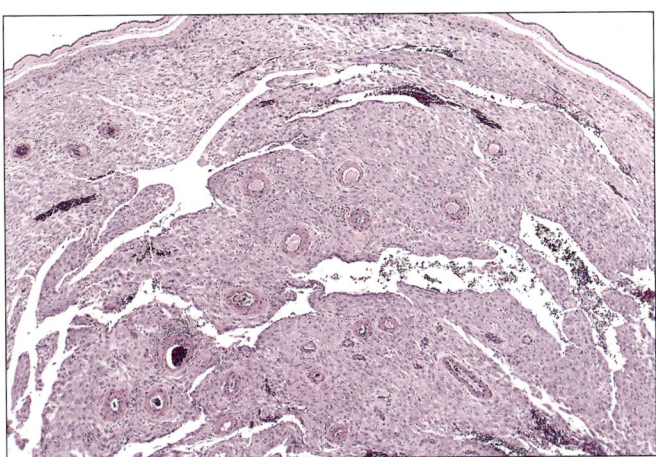

Fig. 31.10 Maternal hypertension with a serpiginous spiral artery with a thickened, untransformed wall.

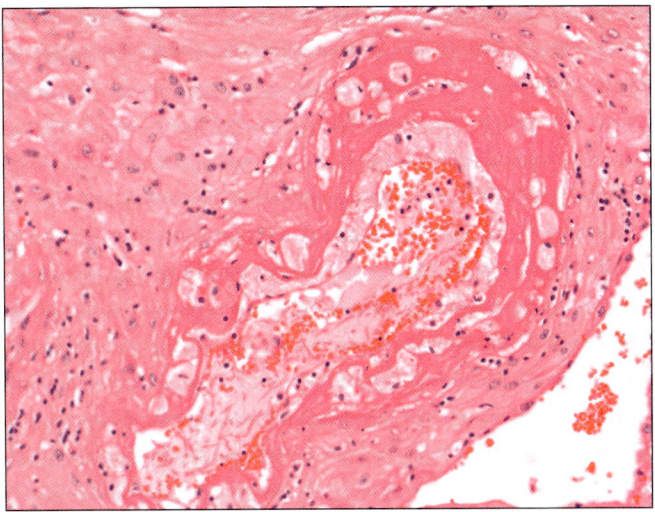

Fig. 31.12 Maternal hypertension. Untransformed wall, but with atherosis.

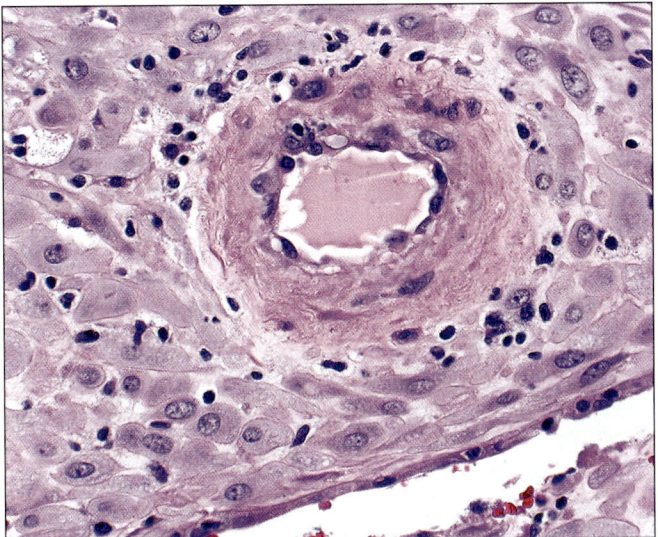

Fig. 31.11 Maternal hypertension with untransformed vessel wall.

to the uteroplacental unit. In pre-eclampsia, these arteries never fully dilate, secondary to inadequate colonization by endovascular trophoblast. The arteries are smaller than normal in absolute size and retain their musculoelastic wall (Figures 31.10 and 31.11). Spiral arteries commonly exhibit acute atherosis (Figure 31.12), a lesion of the vessel wall consisting of fibrinoid necrosis with the accumulation of lipid-laden macrophages and chronic inflammatory cells. Thrombosis of these vessels is frequent and results in placental infarcts. The combination of vasoconstriction and structural changes in the spiral arteries contributes to inadequate blood flow and placental ischemia that are the physiologic hallmarks of the disease. Turnover of villous trophoblast is increased in pre-eclampsia, with necrosis superimposed on cells undergoing apoptosis (aponecrosis). These fragments may contribute to local placental damage and to the systemic features of pre-eclampsia.[53]

Pathology

The principal pathologic changes in pre-eclampsia are decidual vasculopathy, infarcts, villous maldevelopment, and abruption.[101,110] In assessing the placenta, the pathologist

should make a distinction between early onset pre-eclampsia (i.e., before 34 weeks' gestation), a condition with fetal implications, and late-onset pre-eclampsia, essentially a maternal condition. The classic early onset pre-eclamptic placenta is small. Extensive infarction of the placenta (exceeds 10% of parenchyma) occurs in nearly a third of patients with severe pre-eclampsia, although it may be negligible in mild cases. A strong association exists between women with early onset severe pre-eclampsia and antiphospholipid syndrome,[82] which can result in the formation of arterial and venous thromboses. Microscopically, the contrast with normal placental development can be appreciated at low power. The chorionic villi show signs of underperfusion, with only a few remaining immature intermediate villi, and Tenney–Parker changes of increased syncytial knotting in fibrotic, deformed terminal villi. Cytotrophoblasts are increased, with focal basement membrane thickenings best appreciated on the periodic acid-Schiff (PAS) stain. Decidual vessels in the decidua capsularis (best found in the membrane roll) may show acute atherosis and failed transformation of the spiral arteries.

INTRAUTERINE GROWTH RESTRICTION (IUGR)

IUGR, formerly known as intrauterine growth retardation, overlaps with small for gestational age (SGA).[95] Both entities are commonly defined as fetal weight below the 10th percentile for gestational age, although debate continues as to what is the best percentile and whether or not to include abdominal circumference to help identify abnormal infants. Approximately 70% of infants in this group are constitutionally small and have no pathology. Nevertheless, compared to a population of normal size, the perinatal mortality rate is six to eight times higher. Outside of prematurity, IUGR is the second leading cause of perinatal mortality. Of the different growth parameters associated with an increased risk of perinatal mortality, a decreased abdominal circumference relative to the head circumference is a highly sensitive marker.

IUGR in reality is a late stage manifestation of a collection of diseases of many causes. The etiologies can be divided into two broad categories: maternal causes and fetoplacental factors. In mothers, these include chronic disease, particularly diabetes, together with vasculopathy, hypertension, systemic lupus erythematosus, antiphospholipid syndrome, anemia, hemoglobinopathies, multiple gestation, substance abuse, poor weight gain, and malnutrition. Fetoplacental factors include fetal genetic disorders, chromosomal abnormalities, congenital malformations, and problems of placentation including the syndrome of unexplained elevated maternal serum α-fetoprotein (MSAFP). Antenatal identification of a growth restricted fetus is important in order to intervene with delivery before stillbirth or hypoxic ischemic encephalopathy occurs. Mothers who have a history of IUGR with a prior pregnancy are also at risk for recurrence in subsequent pregnancies, including an increased risk of subsequent stillbirth.[128]

Separation of IUGR from those infants who are small but have achieved their full growth potential can be problematic. For the purposes of placental analysis, we request that all placentas of small infants (<10% of normal for age body weight) be sent for examination. While practical, this is less than ideal, as it does not incorporate data on race, birth order, and parental body characteristics that can help improve identification of true growth restriction.[19] Agreement between customized standards and a population standard on growth restriction can be expected in approximately two-thirds of births.

In IUGR, the placenta is not uncommonly small. The fetal surface should be examined for vascular thrombosis and the maternal surface for infarcts. The cut surface may show infarcts or increased perivillous fibrin. However, many diseases responsible for causing IUGR can only be diagnosed microscopically, such as villitis. Among 104 IUGR cases seen in our practice over a recent 2-year period (2004/5), nearly 30% of the placentas were microscopically normal. Of these, one-third were grossly small for the expected gestational age, consistent with the observation that fetal growth depends on placental weight.[45] Changes of uteroplacental insufficiency were the most common finding, being observed in 25% of cases. Of these, one-third had manifestations of early onset pre-eclampsia. Villitis was seen as the primary pathology in one-fifth of cases, with severe grades disproportionately represented. Secondary pathology was seen in 22% of cases.

OTHER PATHOLOGIC CONDITIONS EVALUATED IN THE CONTEXT OF IUGR

CONFINED PLACENTAL MOSAICISM

Confined placental mosaicism occurs where the placenta's karyotype differs from that of the fetus.[61] This may cause both IUGR and fetal loss. The mechanism by which this occurs is unknown but may be confined to specific chromosomes. In one study of IUGR with matched controls, confined placental mosaicism was significantly higher (15.7% vs 1.4% in controls).[139] While these placentas often showed decidual vasculopathy and infarction, there are no diagnostic criteria on light microscopy. Rather the diagnosis rests with awareness of the condition and use of appropriate further investigations such as fluorescent *in situ* hybridization or comparative genomic hybridization.[74]

ABSENCE OR REVERSAL OF END-DIASTOLIC FLOW (ARED FLOW)

Umbilical artery Doppler velocimetry, an antenatal ultrasound technique that examines placental resistance, is useful to determine ARED flow, abnormalities of which are associated with prominent placental histologic lesions, namely infarction and massive perivillous fibrin deposition. The testing is usually done in the third trimester. The affected fetus is usually growth restricted, and the ultrasonic abnormalities reflect attempts to maximize perfusion of vital organs. These are high-risk pregnancies, with a perinatal mortality reaching about 30%[63–65] if the baby is not delivered electively.

The placentas are usually small, but the fetal:placental weight ratio is often maintained. Microscopically, the tertiary villi are thin and poorly vascularized in contrast to the branching vessels seen in IUGR where end-diastolic flow is maintained.[132] Reduction, absence, and reversal seem not to constitute a spectrum of morphologic abnormality and the entire villous tree may be underdeveloped in absent end-diastolic flow. A combination of Doppler velocimetry studies, placental assessment by ultrasound, and serum assessment for raised α-fetoprotein and β-hCG levels in the second trimester is useful diagnostically.

ARED flow is more common in males, with males also showing a higher birth weight:placental weight ratio, suggesting impaired placentation may be causal.[29] Similarly, more severe chronic inflammation is found at the implantation site, which is the site where the fetus's trophoblast invades into the maternal decidua and maternal endovasculature. The risk of pre-eclampsia, preterm delivery, and abruption are also all increased in males.[33] Collectively, these findings may suggest an immunologic component to abnormal placentation in some males, which reflects an abnormal maternal immune response. This subject requires further investigation for resolution.

ADVERSE NEUROLOGIC OUTCOME: NEONATAL ENCEPHALOPATHY AND CEREBRAL PALSY

The area of neonatal neurologic disability is a contentious one, especially in the courtroom, and the erroneous attribution of such damage to 'birth asphyxia' has led to obstetricians becoming uninsurable in many Western jurisdictions. The incidence of cerebral palsy has remained between 2 and 3 per 1000 live births over the last three decades, with similar figures from many centers.[18] Few cases of cerebral palsy are related to birth asphyxia, determined in one center to be 4% (2 of 46) of cases when the objective American College of Obstetricians and Gynecologists (ACOG)/American Academy of Pediatrics criteria are used.[127]

Placental examination, when combined with relevant clinical information, can add much to the understanding of events in many cases that sequentially have taken place and led to a bad outcome. Any center wishing to examine such placentas must first have in place a mechanism for identifying, retrieving, and processing them, without producing an impossibly large workload. A diagnosis of cerebral palsy may often not be made until the non-progressive nature of the impairment is clear, and, as such, placental analysis may have to proceed with a less definitive label. For term infants, neonatal encephalopathy is the best predictor of long-term neurologic disability.

Macroscopic examination should focus on the cord, membranous vessels, fetal surface vessels, and, if present, on maternal blood clots or areas of compression. At a minimum, a section of parenchyma, cord, and membranes should be available for microscopy. The key lesions to be sought, graded, and reported are those of inflammation and thrombosis.[51,67,81,105,106,135] The presence of both, with lesions of different age and duration, appears to increase the risk of cerebral palsy. The coexistence of subacute and chronic pathology is significantly more likely to be identified in a cohort of medico-legal cases than in controls (24% vs 2%, respectively).[104] The placental findings in cerebral palsy can be expected to overlap with those in IUGR, as in fetuses beyond 33 weeks, the two conditions are associated.[31]

In as much as infection appears to play an important role in the genesis of cerebral palsy, it is important to try to identify the infection's cause. Not uncommonly, the infectious agents may exist in the placenta without apparent histologic findings. Nearly three-fourths of neonates with poor outcomes in one study had viral or bacterial disease (Coxsackie virus 46%, bacteria 38%, herpes 8%, parvovirus 4%, and picornavirus 4%) when tested with *in situ* hybridization or reverse transcriptase polymerase chain reaction (RT-PCR), compared with none of the controls.[32] In a population-based study, perinatal exposure to neurotropic viruses, in particular herpes B viruses, showed an association with cerebral palsy.[34] Given the prevalence of viral nucleic acids in the control population (almost 40%), the need for a cofactor or trigger might be necessary to result in damage.

In summary, to maximize the benefit of placental examination, pathologists must integrate and use clinical, morphologic, and molecular techniques.

DIABETES MELLITUS

Assessment of the placenta from a diabetic requires knowledge of glucose control in pregnancy and details regarding hypertension. With good control and without macrosomia, placental weight may be normal and there may be no discernable changes by routine light microscopy.[80] Both placental weight and macrosomia increase with poor control. Changes include delayed villous maturation (villous immaturity), villous edema, and chorangiosis. Maternal hypertensive disorders also impact on the placental morphology.[56] With stereologic assessment, more subtle changes may be detected, even in type 1 diabetics with good glycemic control, with enhanced angiogenesis.[79]

HYDROPS FETALIS (MATERNAL RHESUS ISOIMMUNIZATION)

Maternal rhesus (Rh) isoimmunization and to a lesser extent anti-Kell, Duffy and other minor antibodies and ABO incompatibility produce similar placental changes. However, with modern obstetric practice, full-blown cases of immune hydrops fetalis are uncommon. The Rh-negative mother may be sensitized in her first pregnancy, either before birth from fetal–maternal hemorrhage, or during birth. The risk of sensitization increases in cases of operative removal of the placenta.

Macroscopically, the placenta ranges from normal to enlarged and bulky. The villi may show appropriate or delayed maturity, with an increase in immature intermediate villi. Generally, the placental changes are inconstant in any given placenta, appearing as a mosaic of normal areas admixed with others that are edematous. The cytotrophoblasts are mildly increased and there is focal basement membrane thickening. Focal syncytiotrophoblast necrosis can be appreciated on electron microscopy. Up to 30% of cases show increased numbers of intervillous thromboses and fibrinoid necrosis of villi. The villous capillaries (which tend to be sparser than normal) contain nucleated fetal red blood cells. The villous stroma is edematous and macrophages (Hofbauer cells) are easily identified. The cause of the edema is believed to be a consequence of fetal anemia leading to high-output cardiac failure. These changes are not pathognomonic for rhesus isoimmunization.

PLACENTA ACCRETA (INCLUDING INCRETA AND PERCRETA)

Placenta accreta, which occurs in about 0.9% of deliveries,[38] substantially increases the risk of preterm delivery and SGA babies.[39] The disorder is associated with prior manual removal of the placenta, cornual implantation, leiomyomas, and prior endometrial scarring. It is frequently diagnosed clinically when there is a difficult delivery of the placenta and relates to undue adherence of the placenta to the uterine myometrium. Although ultrasound with Doppler imaging of the placental vasculature can also suggest this finding, particularly in the case of a complete placenta previa in a patient with history of prior uterine scar, ultrasonography and MRI of the placenta can confirm these suspicions,[137] thus helping to guide management of the delivery. Nevertheless, despite predelivery preparations, significant blood loss may occur.

The primary defect is thought to be a lack of decidual response in the endometrium, with the consequent apposition of chorionic villi and myometrium. There is little fibrin deposition and extravillous trophoblast (X cells) may be mistaken for decidua if immunohistologic evaluation is neglected. Increta implies a moderate degree of myometrial penetration and percreta means penetration by chorionic villi through the entire wall to the level of the serosa, or more. In the extreme, not only is the wall breached, but there is contiguous invasion of adjacent pelvic organs. In practice, all types are sometimes referred to as placenta accreta, although more often this term is used to mean attached placenta without myometrial invasion. Accreta is the most common (75% of cases), increta (20% of cases), and percreta (5% of cases).

Placenta accreta is one of the most common indications for postpartum hysterectomy[66] and this scenario is most likely where there is a prior cesarean section and current placenta previa. The placenta will have a markedly disrupted maternal surface and careful dissection is needed to identify chorionic villi adjacent to or admixed with myometrial fibers. The finding of only trophoblast admixed with superficial myometrial fibers is insufficient for the diagnosis, as this occurs normally in the uncomplicated state. In a hysterectomy specimen the chorionic villi are found lying directly on the surface of the myometrium (Figure 31.13) or in the uterine wall with placenta increta

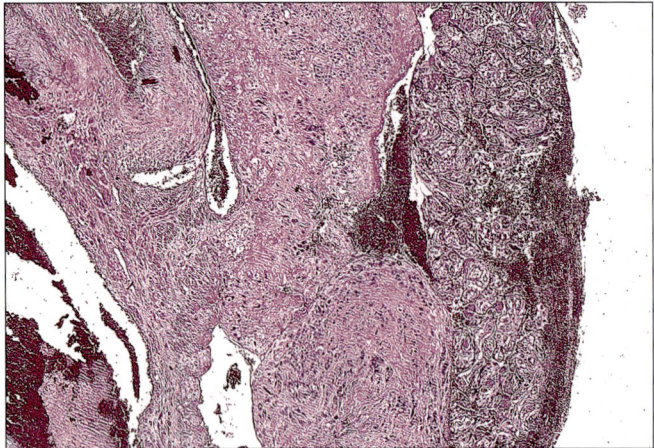

Fig. 31.13 Placenta accreta. The placenta is adherent to the superficial-most myometrium requiring postpartum hysterectomy.

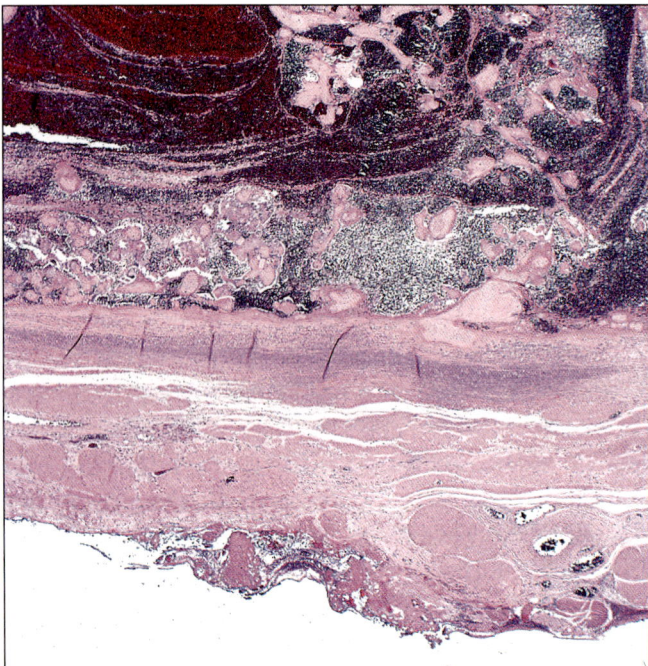

Fig. 31.14 Placenta increta. The placenta penetrates deep into the myometrial wall.

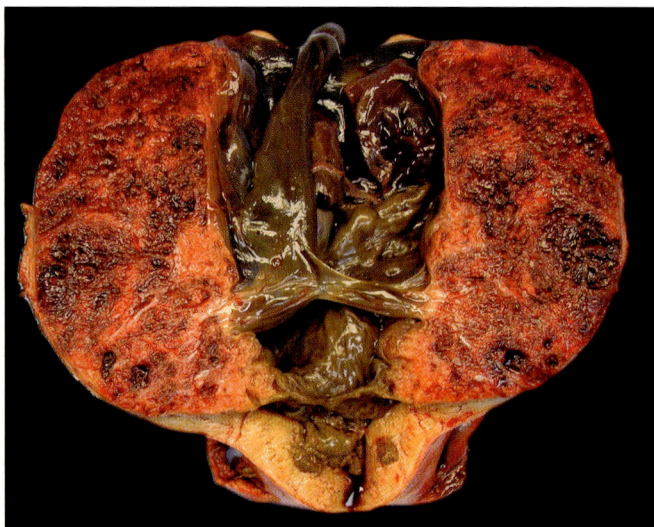

Fig. 31.15 Placenta percreta. The placenta penetrates the myometrium to the level of the serosal covering.

sac that will further enlarge and progress with growth of the placenta.

THROMBOPHILIA

Thrombophilia is a laboratory definition for factors, inherited or acquired, that predispose to the development of thrombosis,[102] which is a major threat for the mother and fetus during pregnancy. Some relatively common mutations, such as Factor V Leiden, an autosomal dominant condition in which the coagulation factor cannot be destroyed by activated protein C (aPC), are relatively weakly thrombogenic, whereas other rarer mutations such as protein C or protein S deficiency are strongly thrombogenic. The fetal genotype is important, as seen from cases of discordant twins.[68] In one large Caucasian Australian population, inherited thrombophilic polymorphisms were commonly found within 64% and 25% of the birth population homozygous and heterozygous, respectively, for at least one of four polymorphisms (Factor V Leiden 9.5% and 0.7%, prothrombin gene 4.1% and 0.2%, gene A1298C 38.3% and 11.8%, and methylenetetrahydrofolate reductase (MTHFR) gene C677T 37.3% and 12.4%).[36]

Correlative studies as to the diseases associated with thrombophilia are conflicting.[72] Some have shown that fetal thrombophilic polymorphisms may be related to adverse pregnancy outcomes, such as SGA[37] and, if preterm, for cerebral palsy.[35] Infarcts and a decreased placental weight are more common in women with complicated pregnancies and thrombophilia than in those without thrombophilia. However, when placentas from 64 infants with IUGR, pre-eclampsia or abruption were correlated with fetal and maternal thrombophilic status, no increase in the prevalence of fetal thrombotic lesions was seen.[5]

Antiphospholipid antibodies, which also give rise to thrombophilia, are a heterogeneous group of autoantibodies that may be unassociated with other diseases (primary) or found in the context of autoimmune disease (secondary). They are associated with recurrent pregnancy loss and defective endovascular trophoblast invasion.[120] Placentas from affected gestations

(Figure 31.14). Occasionally, the placenta pervades and destroys nearly the entire thickness of the uterine wall (placenta percreta) (Figure 31.15).

Previous cesarean section is also a risk factor for placenta previa, where implantation on the lower uterine segment scar mimics placenta accreta clinically. Cesarean section is also associated with an increased frequency of abruption in the next pregnancy.[46] Alterations in the myometrial wall seen following cesarean section include distortion and widening, inflammation and adenomyosis. A grossly visible defect may be present in the anterior wall. Implantation on either a normally healed or a diseased scar will not have the protective effect provided by the presence of decidua, and so postpartum separation is less likely to occur. Implantation in the lower segment (adjacent to the defect) can cause expansion of the defect, dehiscence of the wall, and the formation of a

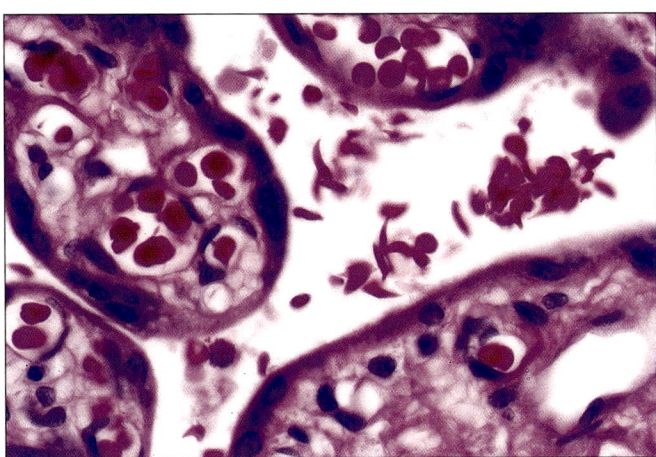

Fig. 31.16 Sickled red cells. Compare the sickled red cells in the perivillous space with the perfectly round and smooth fetal red cells in chorionic villi.

do not show specific features. Most pregnancies are uncomplicated, but features of uteroplacental vascular insufficiency, such as placental infarction and pre-eclampsia, are more commonly seen.[119] A small subgroup will show massive perivillous fibrin deposition.[119]

SICKLE CELL TRAIT AND DISEASE

The heterozygous trait (sickle cell trait) appears not to be associated with placental pathology. In the homozygous form, maternal anemia and veno-occlusive disease result in a preplacental type of fetal hypoxia. Alterations in the endothelium of the umbilical vein, demonstrable by scanning and transmission electron microscopy, may also be due to hypoxia.[26] Of import to the mother, the initial clue that the disease exists may be from the finding of the sickled cells in the intervillous space of the placenta (Figure 31.16).

TWIN PREGNANCY

As discussed in Chapter 30, establishing chorionicity (e.g., monochorionic or dichorionic) is critical in assessing the pathology that may be present in a twin pregnancy. Twins have a higher incidence of perinatal morbidity and mortality than singleton pregnancies, and monochorionic twins are at higher risk than dichorionic. Ten per cent of twins with dichorionic placentae are monozygotic, and fetal outcome is related to chorionicity rather than to zygosity.[16] Monoamniotic monochorionic twins (MoMo) have a 20% fetal mortality rate.[48] This is usually attributed to prematurity, congenital abnormalities, and rarely twin–twin transfusion syndrome (TTTS). Cord entanglement is seen in 40% of MoMo twins, but its contribution to mortality may be lower than previously anticipated.[21] Monochorionic twins weigh less than twins from dichorionic gestations.[3] Severe growth discordance between the twins (>25%) has an overall prevalence of approximately 9% in twin pregnancies,[130] but is more common in MoMo twins[134] where it is associated with an increased perinatal mortality. MoMo placentas have significantly greater numbers of both superficial

and deep anastomoses than do uncomplicated monochorionic diamniotic pregnancies, which may provide a vascular basis for the twin–twin transfusion syndrome that occurs on rare occasions in monoamniotic pregnancies.[7] Monochorionic twins have a 3% mortality.[134]

Assessing growth restriction in twins may be problematic, and use of a twin nomogram with allowance for chorionicity has been advised. Peripheral cord insertion reflective of a spatially limited intrauterine compartment and avascular villi indicative of occluded fetal vessels in the placenta are associated with moderate growth discordance (>15% of birth weight) or abnormal birth weight (SGA, <10th percentile).[107] Decreased placental weight, velamentous insertions, and single umbilical artery have also been associated with severe growth discordance.[134] Other findings such as thrombotic lesions differ according to chorionicity; non-occlusive mural thrombi in fetal vessels are more common in monochorionic than dichorionic twins or in singletons, and are associated with avascular villi in the latter two groups.[116]

A systematic review of observational studies over a 15-year period has shown that following death of one twin, monochorionic and dichorionic twins have a death risk of 12% and 4%, respectively, with a risk of neurologic disability of 18% and 1%.[91] The survival of the co-twin following intrauterine death is inversely related to the time of the first fetal death, with mortality being higher for same-sex twins.[59]

PROLONGED PREGNANCY

Prolonged pregnancy is generally defined as a gestation, based on menstrual age, exceeding 42 weeks.[78] With the estimated date of confinement (EDC), or due date, for normal pregnancies calculated as 38 weeks after conception, or 40 weeks from the first day of the last normal menstrual period, about 18% of pregnancies in the US extend 1 week beyond the normal due date and 7% beyond 2 weeks. (Some differences between statistics in the US and Canada seem to relate to whether menstrual or clinical dates are used.[60,69]) Truly prolonged pregnancy probably occurs in 1–1.5% in most Western countries due to increased accuracy of dating techniques and intervention with induction of labor specifically to avoid risks of post-term pregnancy, which are significant both in terms of perinatal death and maternal morbidity.[88,89] Compared to ongoing pregnancies at 37 weeks' gestation, there is an eight-fold increased risk of mortality (stillbirths plus infant mortality) for pregnancies that are ongoing at 43 weeks' gestation.[49] One explanation widely advanced in the past is that the placenta can fail because of age, but this concept has been challenged.[30] That a placenta can show such weight increase seems incompatible with the concept of failure. Oligohydramnios is another factor in the controversy of what defines 'postmaturity'. There is normally a reduction in amniotic fluid volume as term approaches and the term placenta is not directly responsible for amniotic fluid production. Postmature placentas may be normal, without increased infarctions, calcifications or perivillous fibrin deposition. Features suggestive of reduced fetal blood flow occur in one-fifth of cases, and those of mild ischemia in up to one-sixth. Delayed villous maturation may be more important to recognize in this cohort. It typically permits normal growth, but in a manner as yet unknown fails, with a resultant normally formed macerated term stillbirth.

MATERNAL INFECTIONS AND THE PLACENTA

The possible effects of exposure to infections during pregnancy are a cause of great anxiety. In addition to serologic evaluation during pregnancy, examination of the placenta may help to confirm or refute the effects of many organisms.

TOXOPLASMOSIS

Toxoplasmosis, an infection caused by the protozoan parasite *Toxoplasma gondii,* may begin by the eating of contaminated meat or from exposure to contaminated soil or cat litter. Immunocompetent individuals are usually asymptomatic. Acute infections in pregnant women can be transmitted to the fetus, although approximately 75% of congenitally infected newborns are asymptomatic.[114] Consequences include mental retardation, blindness, and epilepsy, but today, the classic triad of chorioretinitis, hydrocephalus, and cerebral calcifications is relatively rare. The risk of maternal–fetal transmission increases with gestational age at the time of exposure, whereas the incidence of severe disease decreases. If infection occurs just before or during the first trimester, it may cause miscarriage, intrauterine death or severe neurologic lesions, whereas fetal infection occurring late in pregnancy may result in either congenital disease or a subclinical state. The classic finding in the placenta is villitis (Figure 31.17), but manifestations range from no sign of inflammation to necrotizing inflammation. Toxoplasma cysts may be seen in the cord and membranes (Figures 31.18 and 31.19), and fetal vessel calcification may be found.[9] Toxoplasmosis is a rare cause of granulomatous villitis.[141]

RUBELLA

Rubella is transmitted via droplet spread from respiratory tract secretions of infected individuals. Clinical disease exhibits a generalized maculopapular rash, lymphadenopathy, and fever, although nearly one-half of those infected are asymptomatic. The virus can be transmitted to the fetus through the placenta and is capable of causing serious congenital defects, miscarriages, and stillbirths. With immunization, rubella infection

and congenital rubella syndrome are rarely seen today. The risk of fetal infection varies according to the time of onset of maternal infection. It is about 80% if the fetal infection occurs in the first trimester, 67% in the second, and 35% in the third. Serologic tests and viral cultures are useful in confirming the diagnosis. Serious complications, such as deafness, ocular, cardiovascular, and CNS damage, result almost exclusively from infection in the first 16 weeks of gestation.

Placental changes reflect the time of the infection. Early on, there is a focal necrotizing villitis with endarteritis, focal trophoblastic necrosis with or without neutrophilic infiltration, and perivillous fibrin deposition. Rarely, eosinophil inclusions may be seen in trophoblast or endothelial cells. Hofbauer cells are increased and there may be a perivasculitis. Infection during later pregnancy causes chronic inflammatory infiltrates in the placental membranes, cord, and deciduas. These features are non-specific and may be caused by herpes viruses or cytomegalovirus (CMV). The end stage is stromal fibrosis, although both acute and chronic features may be present simultaneously.

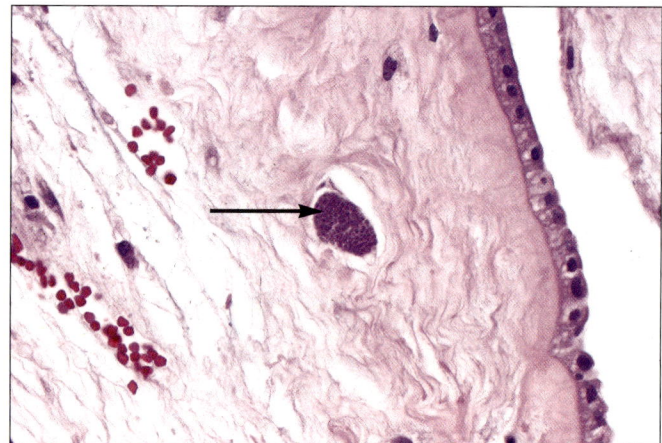

Fig. 31.18 Toxoplasma cysts in amniotic membrane (arrow).

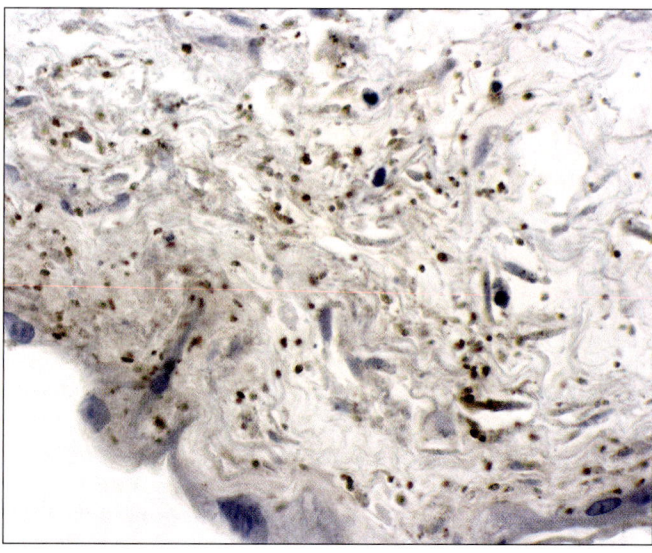

Fig. 31.19 Toxoplasma (immunoperoxidase stain).

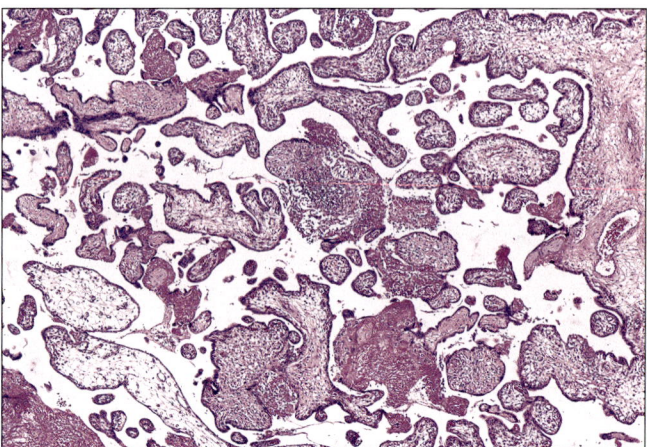

Fig. 31.17 Toxoplasmosis manifest on low power as villitis.

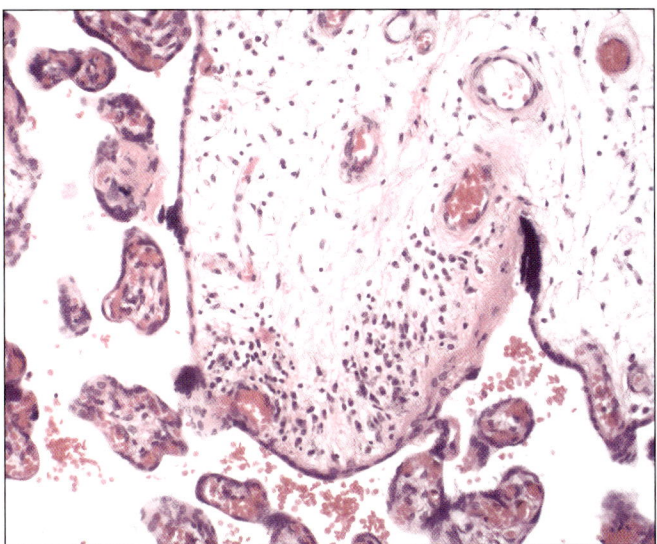

Fig. 31.20 CMV villous edema and chronic inflammatory cells.

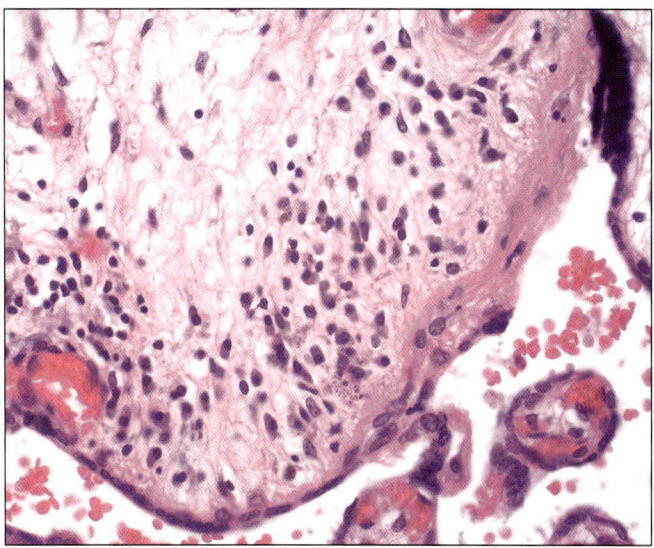

Fig. 31.21 CMV plasma cells and hemosiderin prominent in villus.

CYTOMEGALOVIRUS

CMV is considered one of the most common and important congenital infections in developed nations with approximately 1% of pregnant women acquiring a primary infection.[28] It is also the most common agent of the TORCH (acronym for *t*oxoplasmosis, *o*ther infections, *r*ubella, *c*ytomegalovirus infection and *h*erpes simplex) group to infect the placenta and fetus.

With 40% of the women transmitting the infection to their fetuses, the risk of serious fetal injury is great. While the risk of transmission is greatest if the infection is acquired during the third trimester, the risk of serious fetal injury is greatest if acquired during the first or early part of the second trimester. The virus is transmitted in blood and body fluids, including saliva. Infection in a pregnant woman is usually asymptomatic. The virus can be transmitted following a primary infection in the mother during pregnancy or a recrudescence of a latent infection acquired at a time before pregnancy. Most (75–85%) infants suffer no adverse effects. Those that do may suffer from IUGR and serious neurologic impairment, including deafness and ocular damage. Coinfection with HIV in AIDS patients may enhance CMV transmission and lead to more severe tissue damage.

The combination of a lymphoplasmacytic villitis (Figure 31.20), villous sclerosis, and hemosiderin deposition (Figure 31.21) is commonly found. The characteristic deposition of hemosiderin pigment in sclerotic villi reflects the virus's endotheliotropic nature. Intranuclear inclusions (Figure 31.22) may be seen adjacent to necrotic debris in the villous stroma, although these may be few or absent, even with immunohistochemistry (Figure 31.23).

The diagnosis can be otherwise confirmed by serologic testing, viral culture, and PCR assay to detect CMV DNA in fetal and placental tissues, especially in endothelial cells and Hofbauer cells in the villi.[117] Of import, however, only about one-fourth of pregnant women with positive screening tests for CMV in one large study actually had primary infections once confirmatory testing was completed.[43]

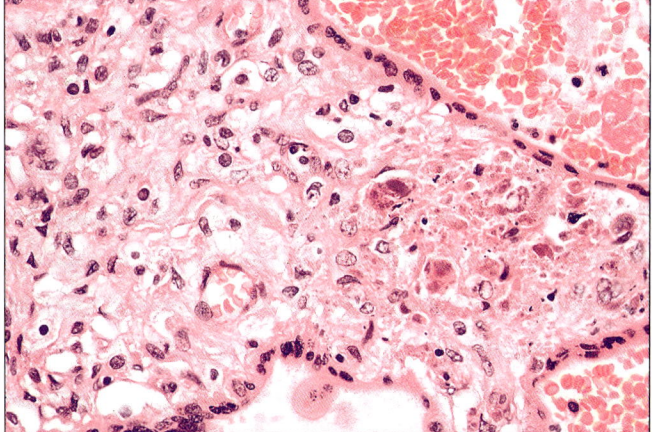

Fig. 31.22 CMV inclusions.

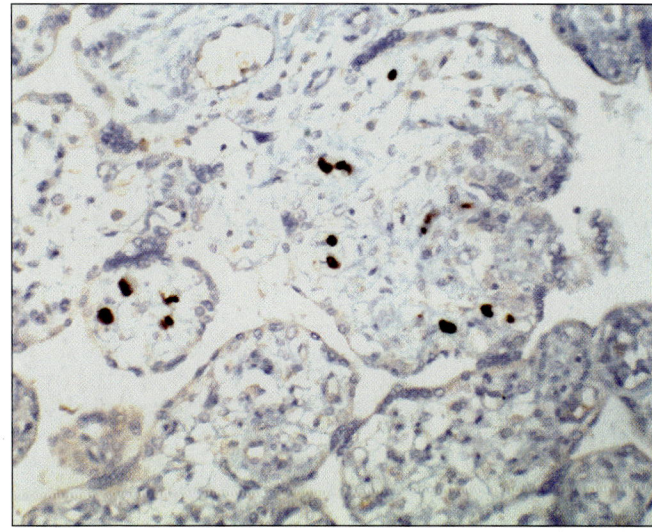

Fig. 31.23 CMV (immunoperoxidase stain).

HERPES SIMPLEX

Herpes simplex viruses (HSV) types 1 and 2 cause genital herpes. Direct contact with infected maternal secretions can lead to neonatal herpetic infection. The risks are greatest when a woman acquires a new infection (primary genital herpes) during late pregnancy, before the development of protective maternal antibodies. Most maternal infections are asymptomatic or go unrecognized and it may be difficult to distinguish clinically between primary and recurrent HSV infection. If primary genital herpes is present at the time of delivery and the baby is delivered vaginally, the risk of neonatal herpes is about 40%.[11] Recurrent genital herpes does not pose a significant risk for the development of neonatal herpes infection. Occasionally, *in utero* infection of the fetus and placenta does occur, and morphologic placental features include giant cell change, usually in the decidua and extravillous trophoblast.[6] There is often marked immaturity of the placenta with inflammatory changes in all placental areas. A heavy plasma cell infiltrate in the chorion should raise the suspicion of herpes, and there may be a chronic villitis with necrosis. Diagnosis is confirmed by immunohistochemistry for type 1 and type 2 in conjunction with viral culture and PCR.

VARICELLA ZOSTER

Primary infection with varicella zoster virus causes chickenpox. The virus remains dormant in the dorsal root ganglion and may reactivate as shingles at a later time. Chickenpox is highly contagious and is spread by droplet transmission or by direct personal contact with vesicular fluid. Primary infection in pregnancy is associated with an increased risk of complications, including maternal death and the fetal varicella syndrome. Women from tropical and subtropical areas are more likely to be seronegative for varicella zoster virus IgG and therefore are more susceptible to developing chickenpox. The risks to the fetus are greatest when the primary infection occurs prior to the 20th week of gestation or after 36 weeks. Fetal varicella syndrome does not occur at the time of the initial fetal infection, but is believed to result from subsequent herpes zoster reactivation *in utero* and only occurs in a minority of infected fetuses. It occurs in 1–2% of maternal varicella infections that take place prior to 20 weeks' gestation. Placental histologic findings include chronic villitis with multinucleated giant cells, granulomatous inflammation, and fetal vessel occlusion.[9] The diagnosis can be confirmed by immunohistochemistry.

HIV

Before the era of highly active antiretroviral therapy, the risk of mother to child transmission of HIV neared 20% in non-breastfeeding women in Europe and up to 40% in breastfeeding African populations. The principal obstetric risk factors for mother–child transmission are maternal plasma viral load, vaginal delivery, duration of membrane rupture, chorioamnionitis, preterm delivery, and breastfeeding.[70] Mother–child transmission is largely preventable with universal antenatal screening, antiretroviral therapy, delivery by cesarean section in certain circumstances, and artificial formula feeding. In women who do not breastfeed and lacking intervention, over

80% of HIV transmissions from mother to child occur late in the third trimester (from 36 weeks) and during labor and at delivery. Fewer than 2% of transmissions occur during the first and second trimesters.

Placentas from cases with fetal transmission of HIV-1 subtype E (the type most frequently seen in South-east Asia) show chorioamnionitis, chronic deciduitis, and decidual necrosis.[10] No specific features are seen.[40] HIV-infected women have an increased risk of chorioamnionitis, but less frequent villitis.[118] Chorioamnionitis and funisitis are almost always associated with ascending maternal infection and therefore their prevalence among HIV-infected women may result from HIV-associated factors (e.g., sexual exposure, vaginitis, sexually transmitted infections).

HUMAN PAPILLOMAVIRUS (HPV)

HPV is a DNA virus tropic for squamous epithelium, but may be found in the placenta. Syncytiotrophoblasts are the cells most likely to be infected.[47,76] There are no specific histologic features in the placenta and its role in the pathogenesis of early pregnancy loss is uncertain.

PARVOVIRUS B19

Parvovirus B19 virus causes erythema infectiosum, also called 'slapped cheek syndrome'. Approximately 50–75% of adult women are immune. Primary infection in adults is usually subclinical or causes non-specific flu-like symptoms and arthralgia. Maternal infection with parvovirus B19 occurs in <1–6% of susceptible pregnancies. Transplacental transmission occurs in 25–50% of cases and appears to increase in later gestations. The virus is a recognized cause of first trimester miscarriage and hydrops fetalis. It is frequently diagnosed by detection of maternal IgM as part of a workup for an ultrasound diagnosis of hydrops.

The primary site of parvovirus B19 infections is within erythroid precursor cells and it has an affinity for the late normoblast stage (Figure 31.24). Cardiac myocytes are also infected. Hydrops is due to fetal anemia, myocarditis, and resulting cardiac failure.

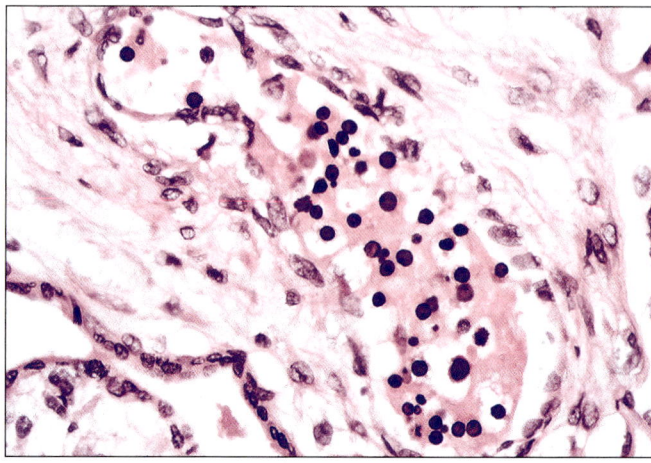

Fig. 31.24 Nucleated red blood cells with parvovirus inclusions.

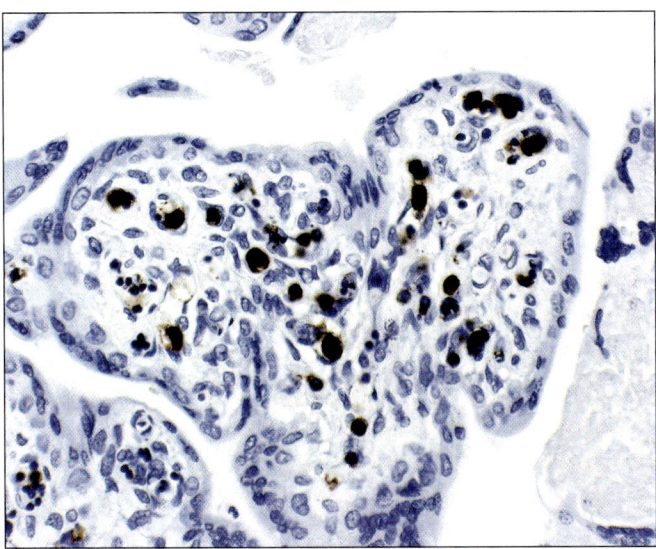

Fig. 31.25 Parvovirus in nucleated red blood cells (immunohistochemical stain).

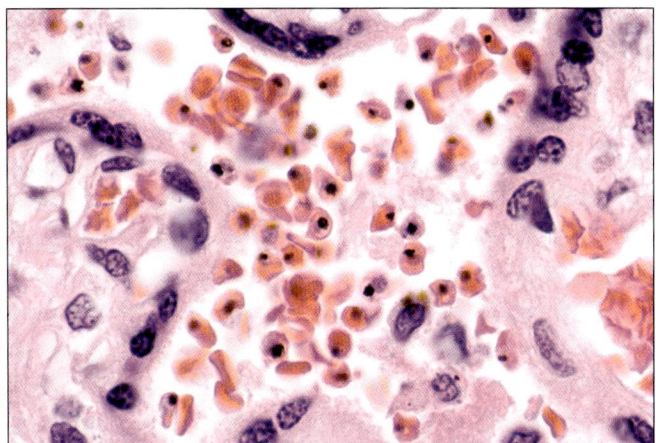

Fig. 31.26 Malaria parasitic in red blood cells.

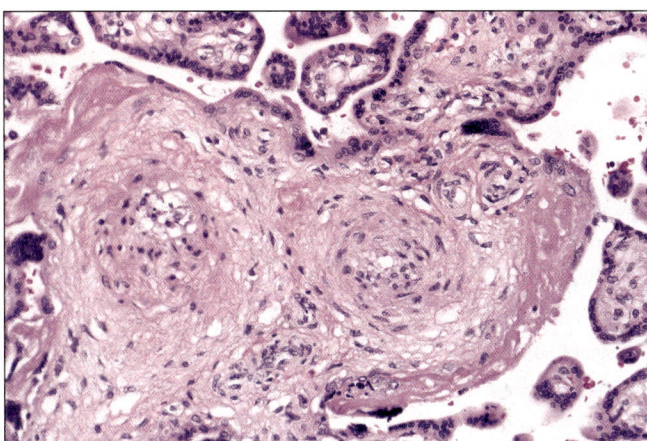

Fig. 31.27 Syphilis with proliferative vascular changes (obliterative endarteritis).

The placenta is usually bulky, pale, and edematous. Histologically, there is villous edema with villous tissue dysmaturity, villitis, and intervillitis. A fetal nucleated red cell response (erythroblastosis) is seen in capillaries. Some nucleated red blood cells show a characteristic appearance of marginated chromatin with central nuclear clearing.[112] Diagnosis can also be made by immunohistochemistry (Figure 31.25) and by detection of B19 DNA by PCR in both placental and fetal tissue.[100]

MALARIA

Pregnant women from endemic areas (especially primiparous women, who have more severe disease and significantly higher prevalence rates of malarial infection) are more prone to develop malaria than non-pregnant women. Infection in pregnancy is associated with extensive parasitic infection of the placenta, maternal anemia, and a reduction in birth weight. In the non-immune population traveling to malaria regions, severe disease is more common in pregnancy and is associated with miscarriage, preterm birth, and neonatal and maternal death.

The villi, *per se*, are not involved by parasites. Rather they parasitize red blood cells (Figure 31.26). In active infection, the parasitized cells attach to villi in areas of syncytiotrophoblast damage.[22] A mononuclear inflammatory infiltrate (intervillositis), malarial pigment, and an increase in perivillous fibrin are also seen. Fibrinoid necrosis, basal membrane thickening, and increased numbers of syncytial knots are features also associated with malarial infection.[54,92,113] Chronic infections show the most severe changes whereas placentas with acute infections exhibit a mild increase in inflammatory cells only and those with past infections show only minimal differences compared with non-infected placentas.

SYPHILIS

Congenital syphilis is caused by transplacental transmission of the spirochete *Treponema pallidum*. Congenital syphilis remains a major cause of stillbirth and long-term morbidity globally. If untreated, the sequelae of congenital syphilis can be lifelong, including neurologic abnormalities, bone and joint malformations, and deafness secondary to eighth nerve involvement. The transmission rate from mother to fetus approaches 100% if the primary or secondary syphilis in the mother remains untreated during pregnancy. Perinatal death may result from congenital infection in more than 40% of untreated pregnancies. A pregnant woman with syphilis who has not received therapy or who has received inadequate therapy may transmit the infection to the fetus at any clinical stage of the disease, although this more frequently occurs following early syphilis.

Grossly, the placenta may be pale and bulky, and necrotizing funisitis lends a 'barber's pole' appearance to the cord. Classic gummas are rare today. The syphilitic 'triad' includes enlarged hypercellular (immature) villi, proliferative vascular changes (obliterative endarteritis) (Figure 31.27), and acute or chronic villitis with plasma cells. Other features may be present, such as granulomatous, proliferative, and necrotizing villitis (Figure 31.28) with multinucleated giant cells. The decidua may also disclose a plasma cell infiltrate. These findings are present to varying degrees in an affected placenta and are not specific for syphilis. Necrotizing funisitis may also occur and is also a non-specific finding. In one cohort, necrotizing funisitis, villous enlargement, and acute villitis were significantly

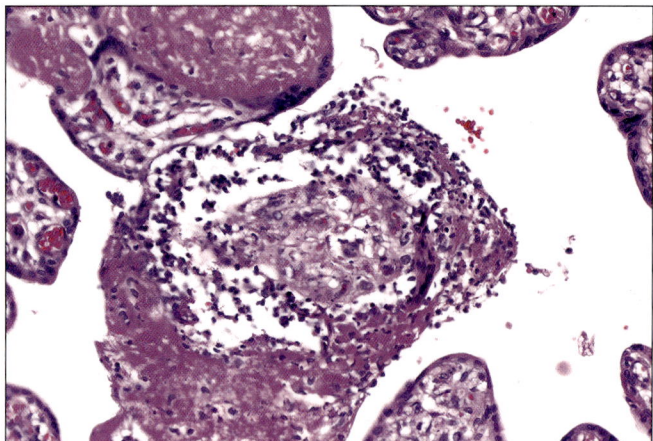

Fig. 31.28 Syphilis with necrotizing villitis.

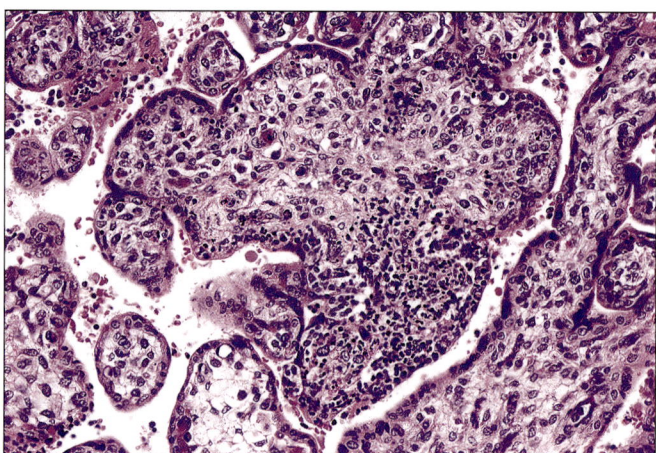

Fig. 31.30 *Listeria* villitis. Inflamed villi show disrupted trophoblast lining, fibrin accumulation, and adhesion to adjacent villi.

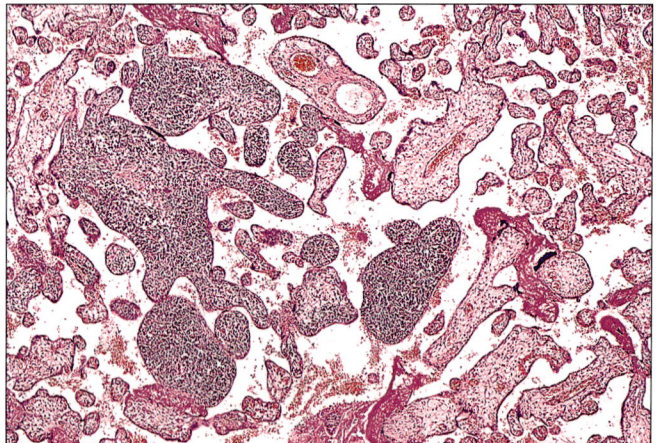

Fig. 31.29 *Listeria* villitis. A low-power view shows hypercellular villi.

more common in both stillborn and liveborn infants with congenital syphilis. Placental examination improved the detection rate in both liveborn and stillborn infants.[122]

Diagnosis may be confirmed by PCR for treponemal DNA. In untreated cases, Warthin–Starry silver stain, or more recently introduced immunohistochemical methods for tissue in paraffin, may demonstrate spirochetes in placental and umbilical cord tissue. As with villitis of unknown etiology, the predominant inflammatory cells are maternal in origin and are CD8-positive T lymphocytes.[62]

LISTERIA MONOCYTOGENES

A commonly encountered bacterial infection is due to *Listeria monocytogenes*. The placentas are frequently studded with microabscesses on their maternal and cut surfaces and usually have an associated chorioamnionitis. Histologically, there are multiple microabscesses with associated necrosis within the intervillous space and villi (Figures 31.29 and 31.30). *Listeria* may infect the placenta via the hematogenous and ascending routes. Although maternal infection produces little systemic upset, it causes devastating fetal sepsis with congenital pneumonia, gastritis, and esophagitis. Immunohistochemistry

detection of *Listeria* antigens may be useful in cases where culture has not been possible.[94]

OTHER ORGANISMS

Mycobacterium tuberculosis may infect the placenta, and produces the classic granulomatous inflammation in the placenta and decidua.

Other parasitic infections include trypanosomiasis and schistosomiasis.

REFERENCES

1. Ananth CV, Wilcox AJ. Placental abruption and perinatal mortality in the United States. Am J Epidemiol 2001;153:332–7.
2. Ananth CV, Berkowitz GS, Savitz DA, Lapinski RH. Placental abruption and adverse perinatal outcomes. JAMA 1999;282:1646–51.
3. Ananth CV, Vintzileos AM, Shen-Schwarz S, Smulian JC, Lai YL. Standards of birth weight in twin gestations stratified by placental chorionicity. Obstet Gynecol 1998;91:917–24.
4. Ananth CV, Oyelese Y, Prasad V, Getahun D, Smulian JC. Evidence of placental abruption as a chronic process: associations with vaginal bleeding early in pregnancy and placental lesions. Eur J Obstet Gynecol Reprod Biol 2006;128:15–21.
5. Ariel I, Anteby E, Hamani Y, Redline RW. Placental pathology in fetal thrombophilia. Hum Pathol 2004;35:729–33.
6. Avgil M, Ornoy A. Herpes simplex virus and Epstein–Barr virus infections in pregnancy: consequences of neonatal or intrauterine infection. Reprod Toxicol 2006;21:436–45.
7. Bajoria R. Abundant vascular anastomoses in monoamniotic versus diamniotic monochorionic placentas. Am J Obstet Gynecol 1998; 179(3 Pt 1):788–93.
8. Bdolah Y, Palomaki GE, Yaron Y, et al. Circulating angiogenic proteins in trisomy 13. Am J Obstet Gynecol 2006;194:239–45.
9. Benirschke K, Coen R, Patterson B, Key T. Villitis of known origin: varicella and toxoplasma. Placenta 1999;20:395–9.
10. Bhoopat L, Khunamornpong S, Sirivatanapa P, et al. Chorioamnionitis is associated with placental transmission of human immunodeficiency virus-1 subtype E in the early gestational period. Mod Pathol 2005;18:1357–64.
11. Brown ZA, Selke S, Zeh J, et al. The acquisition of herpes simplex virus during pregnancy. N Engl J Med 1997;337:509–15.
12. Burke C, Gobe G. Pontosubicular apoptosis ('necrosis') in human neonates with intrauterine growth retardation and placental infarction. Virchows Arch 2005;446:640–5.
13. Burke C, Sinclair K, Cowin G, et al. Intrauterine growth restriction due to uteroplacental vascular insufficiency leads to increased hypoxia-induced cerebral apoptosis in newborn piglets. Brain Res 2006;1098:19–25.
14. Burke CJ, Tannenberg AE. Intrapartum stillbirths in hospital unrelated to uteroplacental vascular insufficiency. Pediatr Dev Pathol 2007;10:35–40.

15. Burke CJ, Tannenberg AE, Payton DJ. Ischaemic cerebral injury, intrauterine growth retardation, and placental infarction. Dev Med Child Neurol 1997;39:726–30.
16. Carroll SG, Tyfield L, Reeve L, Porter H, Soothill P, Kyle PM. Is zygosity or chorionicity the main determinant of fetal outcome in twin pregnancies? Am J Obstet Gynecol 2005;193(3 Pt 1):757–61.
17. Chappell LC, Seed PT, Briley AL, et al. Effect of antioxidants on the occurrence of pre-eclampsia in women at increased risk: a randomised trial. Lancet 1999;354:810–6.
18. Clark SL, Hankins GD. Temporal and demographic trends in cerebral palsy – fact and fiction. Am J Obstet Gynecol 2003;188:628–33.
19. Clausson B, Gardosi J, Francis A, Cnattingius S. Perinatal outcome in SGA births defined by customised versus population-based birthweight standards. BJOG 2001;108:830–4.
20. Condous G. Ectopic pregnancy – risk factors and diagnosis. Aust Fam Physician 2006;35:854–7.
21. Cordero L, Franco A, Joy SD. Monochorionic monoamniotic twins: neonatal outcome. J Perinatol 2006;26:170–5.
22. Crocker IP, Tanner OM, Myers JE, Bulmer JN, Walraven G, Baker PN. Syncytiotrophoblast degradation and the pathophysiology of the malaria-infected placenta. Placenta 2004;25:273–82.
23. de Laat MW, van der Meij JJ, Visser GH, Franx A, Nikkels PG. Hypercoiling of the umbilical cord and placental maturation defect: associated pathology? Pediatr Dev Pathol 2007;10:293–9.
24. de Laat MW, Nikkels PG, Franx A, Visser GH. The Roach muscle bundle and umbilical cord coiling. Early Hum Dev 2007;83:571–4.
25. de Laat MW, van Alderen ED, Franx A, Visser GH, Bots ML, Nikkels PG. The umbilical coiling index in complicated pregnancy. Eur J Obstet Gynecol Reprod Biol 2007;130:66–72.
26. Decastel M, Leborgne-Samuel Y, Alexandre L, Merault G, Berchel C. Morphological features of the human umbilical vein in normal, sickle cell trait, and sickle cell disease pregnancies. Hum Pathol 1999;30:13–20.
27. Doyle EM, McParland P, Carroll S, Kelehan P, Mooney EE. The role of placental cytogenetic cultures in intrauterine and neonatal deaths. J Obstet Gynaecol 2004;24:878–80.
28. Duff P. A thoughtful algorithm for the accurate diagnosis of primary CMV infection in pregnancy. Am J Obstet Gynecol 2007;196:196–7.
29. Edwards A, Megens A, Peek M, Wallace EM. Sexual origins of placental dysfunction. Lancet 2000;355:203–4.
30. Fox H. Aging of the placenta. Arch Dis Child Fetal Neonatal Ed 1997;77:F171–5.
31. Gaffney G. Etiology of fetal and neonatal brain damage. In: Squier W, ed. Acquired Damage to the Developing Brain – Timing and Causation. London: Arnold; 2002:39–55.
32. Genen L, Nuovo GJ, Krilov L, Davis JM. Correlation of in situ detection of infectious agents in the placenta with neonatal outcome. J Pediatr 2004;144:316–20.
33. Ghidini A, Salafia CM. Gender differences of placental dysfunction in severe prematurity. BJOG 2005;112:140–4.
34. Gibson CS, MacLennan AH, Goldwater PN, Haan EA, Priest K, Dekker GA. Neurotropic viruses and cerebral palsy: population based case-control study. BMJ 2006;332:76–80.
35. Gibson CS, MacLennan AH, Hague WM, et al. Associations between inherited thrombophilias, gestational age, and cerebral palsy. Am J Obstet Gynecol 2005;193:1437.
36. Gibson CS, MacLennan AH, Rudzki Z, et al. The prevalence of inherited thrombophilias in a Caucasian Australian population. Pathology 2005;37:160–3.
37. Gibson CS, MacLennan AH, Janssen NG, et al. Associations between fetal inherited thrombophilia and adverse pregnancy outcomes. Am J Obstet Gynecol 2006;194:947 e1–10.
38. Gielchinsky Y, Rojansky N, Fasouliotis SJ, Ezra Y. Placenta accreta – summary of 10 years: a survey of 310 cases. Placenta 2002;23:210–4.
39. Gielchinsky Y, Mankuta D, Rojansky N, Laufer N, Gielchinsky I, Ezra Y. Perinatal outcome of pregnancies complicated by placenta accreta. Obstet Gynecol 2004;104:527–30.
40. Goldenberg RL, Mudenda V, Read JS, et al. HPTN 024 study: histologic chorioamnionitis, antibiotics and adverse infant outcomes in a predominantly HIV-1-infected African population. Am J Obstet Gynecol 2006;195:1065–74.
41. Grimes DA. The morbidity and mortality of pregnancy: still risky business. Am J Obstet Gynecol 1994;170(5 Pt 2):1489–94.
42. Gruber K, Gelven PL, Austin RM. Chorionic villi or trophoblastic tissue in uterine samples of four women with ectopic pregnancies. Int J Gynecol Pathol 1997;16:28–32.
43. Guerra B, Simonazzi G, Banfi A, et al. Impact of diagnostic and confirmatory tests and prenatal counseling on the rate of pregnancy termination among women with positive cytomegalovirus immunoglobulin M antibody titers. Am J Obstet Gynecol 2007;196:221 e1–6.
44. Heatley MK, Clark J. The value of histopathological examination of conceptual products. Br J Obstet Gynaecol 1995;102:256–8.
45. Heinonen S, Taipale P, Saarikoski S. Weights of placentae from small-for-gestational age infants revisited. Placenta 2001;22:399–404.
46. Hendricks MS, Chow YH, Bhagavath B, Singh K. Previous cesarean section and abortion as risk factors for developing placenta previa. J Obstet Gynaecol Res 1999;25:137–42.
47. Hermonat PL, Kechelava S, Lowery CL, Korourian S. Trophoblasts are the preferential target for human papilloma virus infection in spontaneously aborted products of conception. Hum Pathol 1998;29:170–4.
48. Heyborne KD, Porreco RP, Garite TJ, Phair K, Abril D. Improved perinatal survival of monoamniotic twins with intensive inpatient monitoring. Am J Obstet Gynecol 2005;192:96–101.
49. Hilder L, Costeloe K, Thilaganathan B. Prolonged pregnancy: evaluating gestation-specific risks of fetal and infant mortality. Br J Obstet Gynaecol 1998;105:169–73.
50. Hladky K, Yankowitz J, Hansen WF. Placental abruption. Obstet Gynecol Surv 2002;57:299–305.
51. Horvath B, Grasselly M, Turay A, Hegedus A, Oreg Z. Histologic chorioamnionitis is associated with cerebral palsy. Orv Hetil 2006;147:211–6.
52. Hubel CA. Oxidative stress in the pathogenesis of preeclampsia. Proc Soc Exp Biol Med 1999;222:222–35.
53. Huppertz B, Kadyrov M, Kingdom JC. Apoptosis and its role in the trophoblast. Am J Obstet Gynecol 2006;195:29–39.
54. Ismail MR, Ordi J, Menendez C, et al. Placental pathology in malaria: a histological, immunohistochemical, and quantitative study. Hum Pathol 2000;31:85–93.
55. Jauniaux E, Hustin J. Histological examination of first trimester spontaneous abortions: the impact of materno-embryonic interface features. Histopathology 1992;21:409–14.
56. Jauniaux E, Burton GJ. Villous histomorphometry and placental bed biopsy investigation in type I diabetic pregnancies. Placenta 2006;27:468–74.
57. Jauniaux E, Hempstock J, Greenwold N, Burton GJ. Trophoblastic oxidative stress in relation to temporal and regional differences in maternal placental blood flow in normal and abnormal early pregnancies. Am J Pathol 2003;162:115–25.
58. Jindal P, Regan L, Fourkala EO, et al. Placental pathology of recurrent spontaneous abortion: the role of histopathological examination of products of conception in routine clinical practice: a mini review. Hum Reprod 2007;22:313–6.
59. Johnson CD, Zhang J. Survival of other fetuses after a fetal death in twin or triplet pregnancies. Obstet Gynecol 2002;99(5 Pt 1):698–703.
60. Joseph KS, Huang L, Liu S, et al. Reconciling the high rates of preterm and postterm birth in the United States. Obstet Gynecol 2007;109:813–22.
61. Kalousek DK. Current topic: confined placental mosaicism and intrauterine fetal development. Placenta 1994;15:219–30.
62. Kapur P, Rakheja D, Gomez AM, Sheffield J, Sanchez P, Rogers BB. Characterization of inflammation in syphilitic villitis and in villitis of unknown etiology. Pediatr Dev Pathol 2004;7:453–8; discussion 421.
63. Karsdorp VH. Abnormal Doppler velocities in the umbilical artery. Eur J Obstet Gynecol Reprod Biol 1998;80:129–31.
64. Karsdorp VH, Dirks BK, van der Linden JC, van Vugt JM, Baak JP, van Geijn HP. Placenta morphology and absent or reversed end diastolic flow velocities in the umbilical artery: a clinical and morphometrical study. Placenta 1996;17:393–9.
65. Karsdorp VH, van Vugt JM, van Geijn HP, et al. Clinical significance of absent or reversed end diastolic velocity waveforms in umbilical artery. Lancet 1994;344:1664–8.
66. Kelehan P, Mooney EE. Pathology of the uterus. In: Lynch C, Keith L, Lalonde A, Karoshi M, eds. A Textbook of Postpartum Hemorrhage. Kirkmahoe, Dumfriesshire: Sapiens; 2006:326–39.
67. Keogh JM, Badawi N. The origins of cerebral palsy. Curr Opin Neurol 2006;19:129–34.
68. Khong TY, Hague WM. Biparental contribution to fetal thrombophilia in discordant twin intrauterine growth restriction. Am J Obstet Gynecol 2001;185:244–5.
69. Klebanoff MA. Gestational age: not always it seems. Obstet Gynecol 2007;109:798–9.
70. Kourtis AP, Bulterys M, Nesheim SR, Lee FK. Understanding the timing of HIV transmission from mother to infant. JAMA 2001;285:709–12.
71. Kriebs JM, Fahey JO. Ectopic pregnancy. J Midwifery Womens Health 2006;51:431–9.
72. Kujovich JL. Thrombophilia and pregnancy complications. Am J Obstet Gynecol 2004;191:412–24.
73. Lau S, Tulandi T. Conservative medical and surgical management of interstitial ectopic pregnancy. Fertil Steril 1999;72:207–15.
74. Lestou VS, Lomax BL, Barrett IJ, Kalousek DK. Screening of human placentas for chromosomal mosaicism using comparative genomic hybridization. Teratology 1999;59:325–30.
75. Levine RJ, Maynard SE, Qian C, et al. Circulating angiogenic factors and the risk of preeclampsia. N Engl J Med 2004;350:672–83.
76. Liu Y, You H, Hermonat PL. Studying the HPV life cycle in 3A trophoblasts and resulting pathophysiology. Methods Mol Med 2005;119:237–45.
77. Ludwig M, Kaisi M, Bauer O, Diedrich K. Heterotopic pregnancy in a spontaneous cycle: do not forget about it! Eur J Obstet Gynecol Reprod Biol 1999;87:91–3.
78. Management of Prolonged Pregnancy. Rockville, MD: Agency for Healthcare Research and Quality. Online. Available: www.ahrq.gov/downloads/pub/evidence/pdf/prolpreg/prolpreg.pdf.
79. Mayhew TM. Enhanced fetoplacental angiogenesis in pre-gestational diabetes mellitus: the extra growth is exclusively longitudinal and not accompanied by microvascular remodelling. Diabetologia 2002;45:1434–9.

80. Mayhew TM, Jairam IC. Stereological comparison of 3D spatial relationships involving villi and intervillous pores in human placentas from control and diabetic pregnancies. J Anat 2000;197(Pt 2):263–74.

81. McDonald DG, Kelehan P, McMenamin JB, et al. Placental fetal thrombotic vasculopathy is associated with neonatal encephalopathy. Hum Pathol 2004;35:875–80.

82. Moodley J, Bhoola V, Duursma J, Pudifin D, Byrne S, Kenoyer DG. The association of antiphospholipid antibodies with severe early-onset pre-eclampsia. S Afr Med J 1995;85:105–7.

83. Mooney EE, Boggess KA, Herbert WN, Layfield LJ. Placental pathology in patients using cocaine: an observational study. Obstet Gynecol 1998;91:925–9.

84. Morgan T, Ward K. New insights into the genetics of preeclampsia. Semin Perinatol 1999;23:14–23.

85. Ness RB, Sibai BM. Shared and disparate components of the pathophysiologies of fetal growth restriction and preeclampsia. Am J Obstet Gynecol 2006;195:40–9.

86. Nisenblat V, Leibovitz Z, Tal J, et al. Primary ovarian ectopic pregnancy misdiagnosed as first-trimester missed abortion. J Ultrasound Med 2005;24:539–43, quiz 544–5.

87. Norris LA, Higgins JR, Darling MR, Walshe JJ, Bonnar J. Nitric oxide in the uteroplacental, fetoplacental, and peripheral circulations in preeclampsia. Obstet Gynecol 1999;93:958–63.

88. Olesen AW, Basso O, Olsen J. Risk of recurrence of prolonged pregnancy. BMJ 2003;326:476.

89. Olesen AW, Westergaard JG, Olsen J. Perinatal and maternal complications related to postterm delivery: a national register-based study, 1978–1993. Am J Obstet Gynecol 2003;189:222–7.

90. Ong S, Wingfield M. Increasing incidence of ectopic pregnancy: is it iatrogenic? Ir Med J 1999;92:364–5.

91. Ong SS, Zamora J, Khan KS, Kilby MD. Prognosis for the co-twin following single-twin death: a systematic review. BJOG 2006;113:992–8.

92. Ordi J, Ismail MR, Ventura PJ, et al. Massive chronic intervillositis of the placenta associated with malaria infection. Am J Surg Pathol 1998;22:1006–11.

93. Oyelese Y, Ananth CV. Placental abruption. Obstet Gynecol 2006;108:1005–16.

94. Parkash V, Morotti RA, Joshi V, Cartun R, Rauch CA, West AB. Immunohistochemical detection of Listeria antigens in the placenta in perinatal listeriosis. Int J Gynecol Pathol 1998;17:343–50.

95. Peleg D, Kennedy CM, Hunter SK. Intrauterine growth restriction: identification and management. Am Fam Physician 1998;58:453–60, 66–7.

96. Peng HQ, Levitin-Smith M, Rochelson B, Kahn E. Umbilical cord stricture and overcoiling are common causes of fetal demise. Pediatr Dev Pathol 2006;9:14–19.

97. Philipp T, Philipp K, Reiner A, Beer F, Kalousek DK. Embryoscopic and cytogenetic analysis of 233 missed abortions: factors involved in the pathogenesis of developmental defects of early failed pregnancies. Hum Reprod 2003;18:1724–32.

98. Pineles BL, Romero R, Montenegro D, et al. Distinct subsets of microRNAs are expressed differentially in the human placentas of patients with preeclampsia. Am J Obstet Gynecol 2007;196:261 e1–6.

99. Pisarska MD, Carson SA. Incidence and risk factors for ectopic pregnancy. Clin Obstet Gynecol 1999;42:2–8, quiz 55–6.

100. Quemelo PR, Lima DM, da Fonseca BA, Peres LC. Detection of parvovirus B19 infection in formalin-fixed and paraffin-embedded placenta and fetal tissues. Rev Inst Med Trop Sao Paulo 2007;49:103–7.

101. Raspollini MR, Taddei GL. Histologic features of maternal vasculopathy and clinical manifestations of preeclampsia: still the correlation to be demonstrated. Am J Obstet Gynecol 2007;196:e14, author reply e14.

102. Raspollini MR, Oliva E, Roberts DJ. Placental histopathologic features in patients with thrombophilic mutations. J Matern Fetal Neonatal Med 2007;20:113–23.

103. Raziel A, Golan A, Pansky M, Ron-El R, Bukovsky I, Caspi E. Ovarian pregnancy: a report of twenty cases in one institution. Am J Obstet Gynecol 1990;163(4 Pt 1):1182–5.

104. Redline R. Placental lesions and neurologic outcome. In: Baker P, Sibley C, eds. Clinics in Developmental Medicine. London: McKeith Press; 2006:58–69.

105. Redline RW. Placental pathology and cerebral palsy. Clin Perinatol 2006;33:503–16.

106. Redline RW, O'Riordan MA. Placental lesions associated with cerebral palsy and neurologic impairment following term birth. Arch Pathol Lab Med 2000;124:1785–91.

107. Redline RW, Shah D, Sakar H, Schluchter M, Salvator A. Placental lesions associated with abnormal growth in twins. Pediatr Dev Pathol 2001;4:473–81.

108. Redman CW, Sacks GP, Sargent IL. Preeclampsia: an excessive maternal inflammatory response to pregnancy. Am J Obstet Gynecol 1999;180(2 Pt 1):499–506.

109. Robboy SJ, Duggan M, Kurman RT. The female reproductive system. In: Rubin E, Farber J, eds. Pathology, 3rd edn. Philadelphia: Lippincott; 1999:962–1028.

110. Roberts DJ, Oliva E. Clinical significance of placental examination in perinatal medicine. J Matern Fetal Neonatal Med 2006;19:255–64.

111. Roberts JM, Cooper DW. Pathogenesis and genetics of pre-eclampsia. Lancet 2001;357:53–6.

112. Rogers BB, Over CE. Parvovirus B19 in fetal hydrops. Hum Pathol 1999;30:247.

113. Rogerson SJ, Beeson JG. The placenta in malaria: mechanisms of infection, disease and foetal morbidity. Ann Trop Med Parasitol 1999;93(Suppl 1):S35–42.

114. Rorman E, Zamir CS, Rilkis I, Ben-David H. Congenital toxoplasmosis – prenatal aspects of Toxoplasma gondii infection. Reprod Toxicol 2006;21:458–72.

115. Salafia C, Shiverick K. Cigarette smoking and pregnancy II: vascular effects. Placenta 1999;20:273–9.

116. Sato Y, Benirschke K. Increased prevalence of fetal thrombi in monochorionic-twin placentas. Pediatrics 2006;117:e113–17.

117. Satosar A, Ramirez NC, Bartholomew D, Davis J, Nuovo GJ. Histologic correlates of viral and bacterial infection of the placenta associated with severe morbidity and mortality in the newborn. Hum Pathol 2004;35:536–45.

118. Schwartz DA, Sungkarat S, Shaffer N, et al. Placental abnormalities associated with human immunodeficiency virus type 1 infection and perinatal transmission in Bangkok, Thailand. J Infect Dis 2000;182:1652–7.

119. Sebire NJ, Backos M, El Gaddal S, Goldin RD, Regan L. Placental pathology, antiphospholipid antibodies, and pregnancy outcome in recurrent miscarriage patients. Obstet Gynecol 2003;101:258–63.

120. Sebire NJ, Fox H, Backos M, Rai R, Paterson C, Regan L. Defective endovascular trophoblast invasion in primary antiphospholipid antibody syndrome-associated early pregnancy failure. Hum Reprod 2002;17:1067–71.

121. Shankaran S, Lester BM, Das A, et al. Impact of maternal substance use during pregnancy on childhood outcome. Semin Fetal Neonatal Med 2007;12:143–50.

122. Sheffield JS, Sanchez PJ, Wendel GD, Jr, et al. Placental histopathology of congenital syphilis. Obstet Gynecol 2002;100:126–33.

123. Shiverick KT, Salafia C. Cigarette smoking and pregnancy I: ovarian, uterine and placental effects. Placenta 1999;20:265–72.

124. Sowter MC, Farquhar CM. Ectopic pregnancy: an update. Curr Opin Obstet Gynecol 2004;16:289–93.

125. Starita A, Di Miscia A, Evangelista S, Donadio F, Starita A. Cervical ectopic pregnancy: clinical review. Clin Exp Obstet Gynecol 2006;33:47–9.

126. Stepan H, Faber R, Dornhofer N, Huppertz B, Robitzki A, Walther T. New insights into the biology of preeclampsia. Biol Reprod 2006;74:772–6.

127. Strijbis EM, Oudman I, van Essen P, MacLennan AH. Cerebral palsy and the application of the international criteria for acute intrapartum hypoxia. Obstet Gynecol 2006;107:1357–65.

128. Surkan PJ, Stephansson O, Dickman PW, Cnattingius S. Previous preterm and small-for-gestational-age births and the subsequent risk of stillbirth. N Engl J Med 2004;350:777–85.

129. Szulman AE. Examination of the early conceptus. Arch Pathol Lab Med 1991;115:696–700.

130. Tan H, Wen SW, Fung Kee Fung K, Walker M, Demissie K. The distribution of intra-twin birth weight discordance and its association with total twin birth weight, gestational age, and neonatal mortality. Eur J Obstet Gynecol Reprod Biol 2005;121:27–33.

131. Tjoa ML, Levine RJ, Karumanchi SA. Angiogenic factors and preeclampsia. Front Biosci 2007;12:2395–402.

132. Todros T, Ronco G, Fianchino O, et al. Accuracy of the umbilical arteries Doppler flow velocity waveforms in detecting adverse perinatal outcomes in a high-risk population. Acta Obstet Gynecol Scand 1996;75:113–19.

133. van Beck E, Peeters LL. Pathogenesis of preeclampsia: a comprehensive model. Obstet Gynecol Surv 1998;53:233–9.

134. Victoria A, Mora G, Arias F. Perinatal outcome, placental pathology, and severity of discordance in monochorionic and dichorionic twins. Obstet Gynecol 2001;97:310–5.

135. Vogler C, Petterchak J, Sotelo-Avila C, Thorpe C. Placental pathology for the surgical pathologist. Adv Anat Pathol 2000;7:214–29.

136. Wagner LK. Diagnosis and management of preeclampsia. Am Fam Physician 2004;70:2317–24.

137. Warshak CR, Eskander R, Hull AD, et al. Accuracy of ultrasonography and magnetic resonance imaging in the diagnosis of placenta accreta. Obstet Gynecol 2006;108(3 Pt 1):573–81.

138. WHO97. WHO: Recommendation, definitions, terminology and format for statistical tables related to the perinatal period and the use of a new certificate for cause of perinatal deaths. Acta Obstet Gynecol Scand 1997;56:247–53.

139. Wilkins-Haug L, Quade B, Morton CC. Confined placental mosaicism as a risk factor among newborns with fetal growth restriction. Prenat Diagn 2006;26:428–32.

140. Wittich AC. Primary ovarian pregnancy after postpartum bilateral tubal ligation – a case report. J Reprod Med 2004;49:759–61.

141. Yavuz E, Aydin F, Seyhan A, et al. Granulomatous villitis formed by inflammatory cells with maternal origin: a rare manifestation type of placental toxoplasmosis. Placenta 2006;27:780–2.

Gestational trophoblastic disease

32

Annie N-Y Cheung

WHAT IS GESTATIONAL TROPHOBLASTIC DISEASE?

The trophoblast is an integral component of the human placenta responsible for mediating the implantation of the embryo, protecting the fetus from the maternal immune system, delivering nutrients, and removing waste products, as well as producing vital pregnancy hormones. The trophoblast is subclassified into several distinct types to serve such diverse functions. Even in a normal pregnancy, placental trophoblast cells possess the ability to proliferate, invade host tissue, evade the host's immune control and even metastasize, features that ironically typify malignant tumor.[137]

Occasionally, placental trophoblast gives rise to a heterogeneous group of diseases, each with specific clinical, histopathologic, and cytogenetic features. This collective family of 'gestational trophoblastic disease' (GTD)[14,95] encompasses partial and complete hydatidiform moles, invasive mole, choriocarcinoma, placental site trophoblastic tumor (PSTT), and epithelioid trophoblastic tumor (ETT) (Table 32.1). Several non-neoplastic trophoblastic lesions are often also included for comparison and differential diagnosis.

TROPHOBLAST TYPES

In the normal placenta, each type of trophoblast may be classified according to its location and morphologic features. Regarding the locations, villous trophoblast grows with chorionic villi while the extravillous trophoblast usually infiltrates the decidua, chorion, myometrium, and blood vessels of the placental site. The trophoblastic populations are further differentiated into three discrete types: cytotrophoblast, syncytiotrophoblast, and intermediate trophoblast, each based on different morphologic, biologic, and immunohistochemical features.[110,133]

The cytotrophoblast is the mononuclear germinal trophoblastic cell responsible for proliferation, while the syncytiotrophoblast is the multinucleated differentiated cell that produces most placental hormones such as human chorionic gonadotrophin (hCG) and human placental lactogen (hPL). Intermediate trophoblast shows overlapping histologic features of both cytotrophoblast and syncytiotrophoblast[81] and depending on their locations, can be further divided, into villous intermediate trophoblast located in the trophoblastic columns, implantation site intermediate trophoblast in the placental site, and chorionic-type intermediate trophoblast in the chorion laeve of the fetal membranes.[134] Villous trophoblast consists predominantly of cytotrophoblast and syncytiotrophoblast as well as intermediate trophoblast which forms trophoblastic columns that anchor the placenta to the implantation site (Figures 32.1 and 32.2). The extravillous trophoblast consists mainly of intermediate trophoblast (Figures 32.3 and 32.4).[131,134]

While hydatidiform mole and choriocarcinoma arise from villous cytotrophoblast, syncytiotrophoblast, and intermediate trophoblast, a range of neoplastic and non-neoplastic lesions have been described in the past two decades that derive from intermediate trophoblast at various sites (Table 32.2).[131] Exaggerated placental site and placental site trophoblastic tumor (PSTT) are lesions of intermediate trophoblast in the implantation site (implantation site intermediate trophoblast), while placental site nodule and ETT relate to the intermediate trophoblast of the chorion laeve (chorionic-type intermediate trophoblast). Exaggerated placental site and placental site nodule are non-neoplastic lesions, whereas PSTT and ETT are neoplasms with a potential for local invasion and metastasis.

TROPHOBLAST MARKERS

IMPORTANCE OF IDENTIFYING TROPHOBLAST IN HISTOLOGY SECTIONS

The confirmation or exclusion of gestational products in surgical pathology samples, especially those of uterine curettings, is important to the diagnosis of recent intrauterine or ectopic pregnancy. This is critical if trophoblastic cells are detected on conventional histologic sections, especially when they are few in number or when chorionic villi are not found. Cytokeratin immunostaining, which is both highly sensitive and specific for trophoblast, is particularly fruitful in the setting of chorionic villi-negative specimens without obvious extravillous trophoblast (Figure 32.5).[79]

In addition to documenting the presence of trophoblast, trophoblast markers may also help as adjunct tools to distinguish trophoblastic lesions from non-trophoblastic lesions occurring in the female genital tract. Moreover, the distinctive expression patterns of various trophoblast markers may help improve our understanding of trophoblast biology. For example, p53 is expressed mainly in the nuclei of cytotrophoblast,[19] while c-fms, p21, and bcl-2 are expressed predominantly in syncytiotrophoblast.[17,20,21] The difference in the localization of oncogene expression may indicate that different genes operate at different stages in the proliferation and differentiation cascade of the trophoblast system.

Table 32.1 Classification of gestational trophoblastic disease[14,110,133,135]

Hydatidiform mole	Complete (classic) / Partial
Invasive mole	
Choriocarcinoma	
Placental site trophoblastic tumor	
Epithelioid trophoblastic tumor	
Trophoblastic lesions, miscellaneous	Exaggerated placental site / Placental site nodule or plaque
Unclassified trophoblastic lesions	

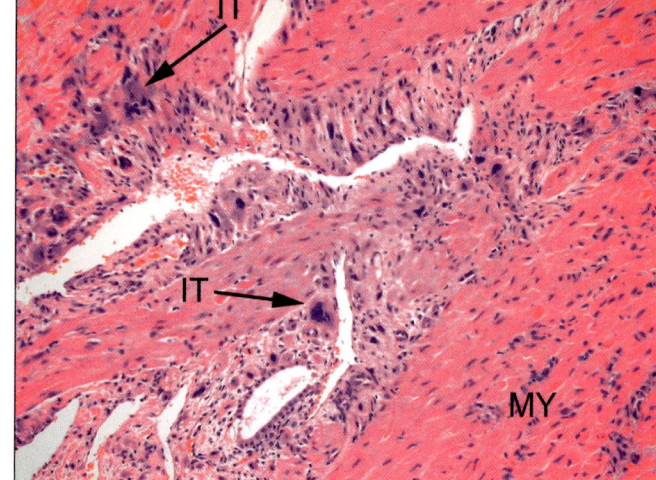

Fig. 32.3 Infiltrative intermediate trophoblast (IT) in the myometrium (MY).

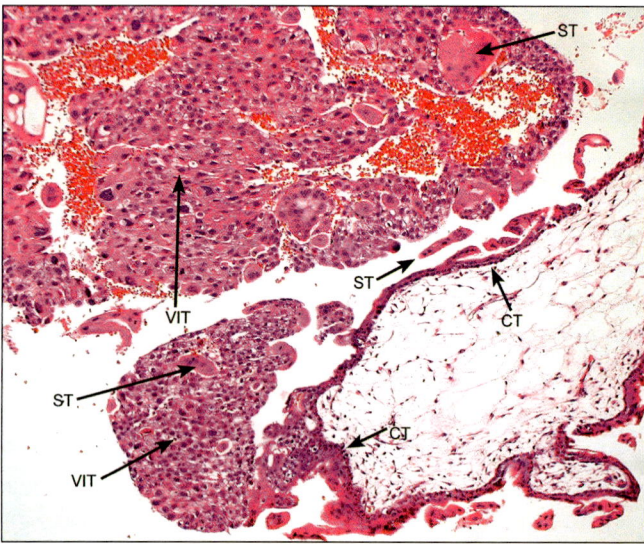

Fig. 32.1 The villous trophoblasts are composed of villous cytotrophoblast (CT), syncytiotrophoblast (ST) and intermediate trophoblast (VIT).

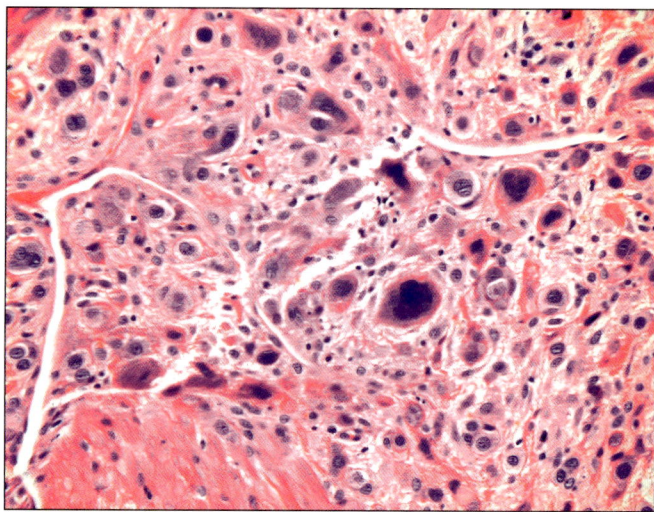

Fig. 32.4 Intermediate trophoblast infiltrating the decidua.

EXAMPLES OF TROPHOBLAST MARKERS

Besides the traditional markers involving pregnancy-associated hormones, such as *hCG* or *hPL*, several trophoblast biomarkers have been identified recently.

- *Alpha-inhibin* is found in nearly all populations of trophoblast except cytotrophoblast.[130] It is found in choriocarcinoma mainly localized within syncytiotrophoblast[96] and in the intermediate trophoblast population of PSTT.[112] It is essentially expressed in all categories of GTD, but not in carcinomas or smooth muscle tumors of the female genital tract. Immunohistochemical detection of α-inhibin is therefore helpful in the differential diagnosis of gestational trophoblastic lesions.

- *Melanoma cell adhesion molecule (Mel-CAM)*, also known as MUC18, is a cell adhesion molecule belonging to the immunoglobulin supergene family. Mel-CAM is a specific

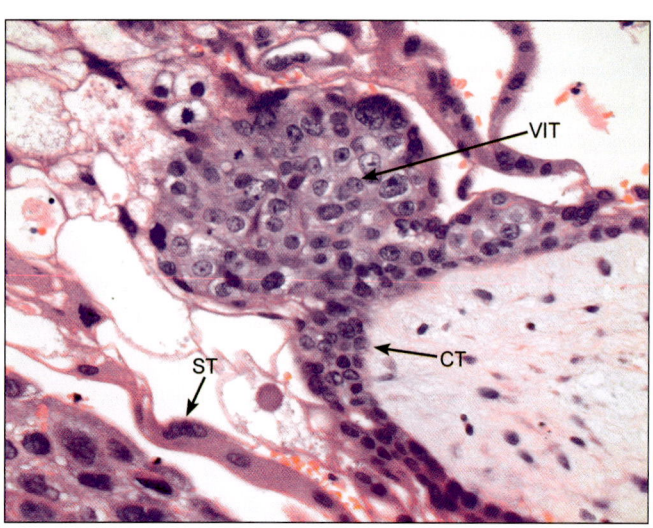

Fig. 32.2 Detail of proliferating cytotrophoblasts and syncytiotrophoblasts.

Table 32.2 Trophoblast types and related lesions

Trophoblast origin	Trophoblast subtype	Location subtype	Lesions	Presence of chorionic villi	Reactive vs neoplastic nature	Hormones
Villous	Cytotrophoblast		Hydatidiform mole	Yes	Potential of malignant transformation	hCG
	Syncytiotrophoblast					
	Intermediate	Anchoring type located in trophoblastic columns	Choriocarcinoma	No	Malignant	hCG
Extravillous	Intermediate	Implantation site	PSTT	No	Malignant	hPL
			Exaggerated placental site	No	Non-neoplastic	hPL
	Intermediate	Chorion laeve type	Epithelioid trophoblastic tumor	No	Malignant	hPL
			Placental site nodule	No	Non-neoplastic	hPL

hCG, human chorionic gonadotrophin; hPL, human placental lactogen, PSTT, placental site trophoblastic tumor.

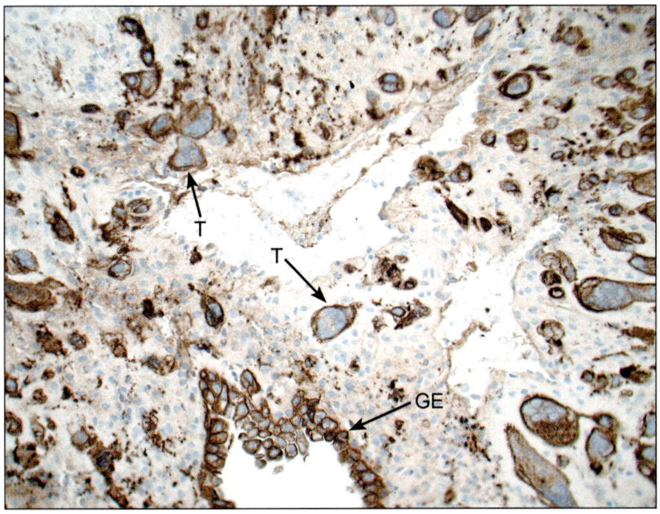

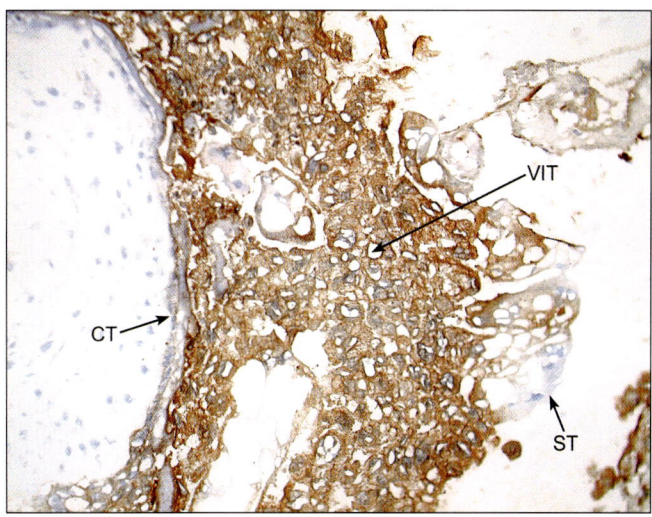

Fig. 32.5 Decidua with infiltrating intermediate trophoblasts (T) highlighted by immunoreactivity for cytokeratin AE1/3. GE, glandular epithelium.

Fig. 32.6 HLA-G immunoreactivity in villous intermediate trophoblast column of villi (VIT). CT, cytotrophoblast; ST, syncytiotrophoblast.

and sensitive marker for intermediate trophoblast differentiation in normal placentas, implantation sites, and in gestational trophoblastic lesions.[127]

- *HLA-G* is a non-classic major histocompatibility complex (MHC) class I antigen with immunoreactivity reported in choriocarcinoma, PSTT, ETT, placental site nodules, and exaggerated placental sites (Figure 32.6).[136] It has not been detected in non-trophoblastic uterine neoplasms. This specificity for trophoblast fosters its role as a useful marker in the differential diagnosis of these lesions.

- Immunoreactivity for *c-mos*, a proto-oncogene involved in the mitogen-activating protein kinase pathway in both normal placenta and GTD, is strongly expressed in syncytiotrophoblast, moderately in villous intermediate trophoblast (Figure 32.7), but not in implantation site intermediate trophoblast, chorionic-type intermediate trophoblast or villous cytotrophoblast. Non-trophoblastic

tumors, including carcinomas, sarcomas, and germ cell tumors, lack *c-mos* expression.[158] Immunohistochemical detection of *c-mos* thus helps differentiate choriocarcinoma from PSTT and non-trophoblastic tumors of the female genital tract that may sometimes cause problems in differential diagnosis.

- The *p63* gene is a transcription factor belonging to the *p53* family and has several isoforms classified in two groups designated TA-p63 and δN-p63 isoforms, which display *p53*-like tumor suppressor function and oncogenic effects, respectively. Cytotrophoblast expresses the δN-p63 isoform (Figure 32.8)[132] while the chorionic-type intermediate trophoblast in the fetal membranes, placental site nodules, and epithelioid trophoblastic tumors expresses the TA-p63 isoform. Intermediate trophoblast in the implantation site and placental site trophoblastic tumors do not express *p63*.

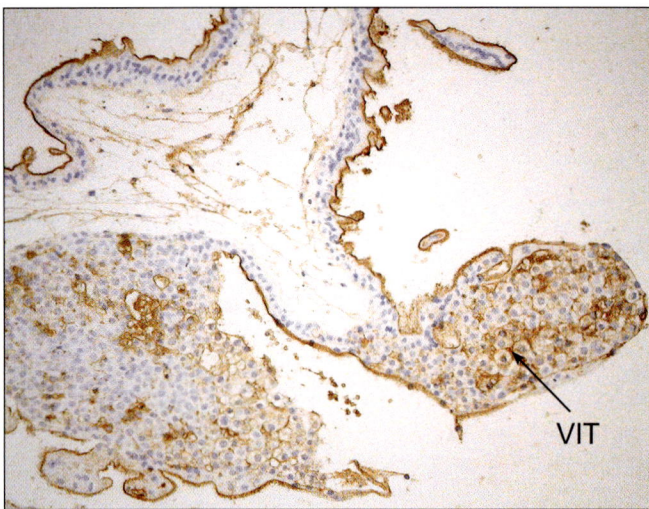

Fig. 32.7 *c-mos* immunoreactivity found at syncytiotrophoblast and villous intermediate trophoblast (VIT) but not cytotrophoblast or implantation intermediate trophoblast.

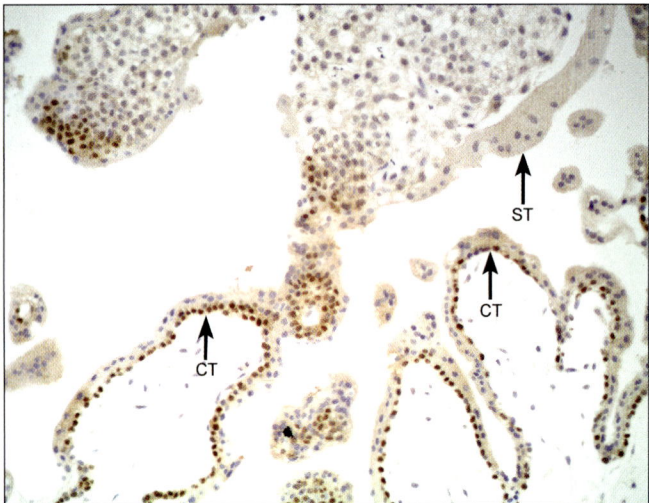

Fig. 32.8 δN-p63 isoform of *p63* gene localized to cytotrophoblast (CT). ST, syncytiotrophoblast.

FEATURES OF GESTATIONAL TROPHOBLASTIC DISEASES

GTD includes a heterogeneous family encompassing various neoplastic and non-neoplastic lesions arising from different types of villous and non-villous trophoblast (Tables 32.1 and 32.2).[53,110,133,135] Lesions included under GTD are unique because they can be considered as allografts arising from a conceptus that has invaded the maternal tissues. They have unusual genetic composition with usually unbalanced dominance in paternal contribution. Some lesions, like choriocarcinoma, PSTT, and ETT, are definitely neoplastic. Others, like hydatidiform mole, are abnormal placentas that are prone to malignant transformation. Each has distinct clinical, morphologic, pathologic, and genetic features.

EPIDEMIOLOGY

There are wide variations in the reported incidence of hydatidiform mole and choriocarcinoma throughout the world. The former ranges from 11.5 per 1000 deliveries in Indonesia to less than 1 per 1000 deliveries in the United States.[13,107] The frequency of choriocarcinoma varies from 2 per 1000 pregnancies in Taiwan to 1 in 40 000 pregnancies in the United States and Europe. The incidence rates are higher in Asia, Africa, and Latin America than in Europe, Australia, and North America.

The incidence rates are difficult to compare because of various limitations in the methodologies of these studies. Common limitations include lack of clear definition of the disease entities and inconsistencies in diagnostic criteria. Moreover, many studies are biased as only hospital populations are analyzed, disregarding uncomplicated births and unreported spontaneous or induced abortions in the community. Ideally, the incidence rate should be based on the total number of all pregnancies, which would be the best denominator to evaluate the risk of GTD in a population. Since such data are extremely difficult to ascertain, other denominators, such as the total number of deliveries or live births, have been used to determine incidence rates.

To accurately assess the frequency of partial mole is even more difficult and this is reflected by the wide variation of published data. The figures vary from 3 to 35% of all hydatidiform moles. Some partial moles may have been overlooked in cases considered to be missed abortions.

RISK FACTORS

The reasons for the geographical variation in the frequency of gestational trophoblastic disease are also unclear.

Age All women with hydatidiform mole are in the reproductive years. It is well recognized that hydatidiform mole is most frequent at the extremes of the reproductive age. The tendency to continue having pregnancies in late reproductive life in high incidence areas may be one of the underlying reasons. For instance, studies of the incidence of mole in a Chinese population in Hong Kong showed that women aged over 39 and who already had five or more children had a significantly higher risk of having a molar pregnancy.[13]

Past obstetric history A history of previous spontaneous abortions is more common in patients with hydatidiform mole or choriocarcinoma. Furthermore, women with a previous history of hydatidiform mole are at greater risk of having another molar pregnancy.[9,109] In contrast, live births and term pregnancies seem to be related to a decreased possibility. Such observations support the hypothesis that hydatidiform mole is basically a pregnancy with chromosomal abnormalities.

Gestational choriocarcinoma may arise in association with any type of pregnancy: 50% arise in association with hydatidiform mole, 25% follow abortion or tubal pregnancy, and 25% follow term gestation. About 2–3% of hydatidiform moles progress to choriocarcinoma.

Diet The geographical variation in the incidence rates of hydatidiform mole and choriocarcinoma also lead to the belief that socioeconomic environment or dietary factors may be of significance in the development of GTD. One case-control study suggested that dietary deficiency of carotene, a vitamin A precursor, may predispose to molar pregnancy.[9]

Blood group Studies on the ABO blood group system have suggested its potential role in trophoblastic disease, affecting both risk and prognosis. However, the risk association seems to be weaker compared with maternal age and a previous history of hydatidiform mole.[107]

TYPES OF GESTATIONAL TROPHOBLASTIC DISEASE

HYDATIDIFORM MOLE

Hydatidiform moles are subclassified into two distinct entities – complete and partial. Both classically exhibit hydropic swelling and trophoblastic proliferation of some or all chorionic villi (Table 32.3).[139,140,145,146] Traditionally, complete hydatidiform mole is a hydatidiform mole without an embryo/fetus. There is pronounced hydropic swelling of the majority of placental villi and variable degrees of trophoblastic hyperplasia. Partial hydatidiform mole is a molar pregnancy with a mixture of enlarged edematous villi and normal sized villi. There may be evidence of fetal development.

The genetic basis of hydatidiform mole is one of the most fascinating issues in human diseases. Moreover, few parameters have been found useful in predicting the clinical progress of hydatidiform mole. Last but not least, the difficulty in diagnosis and classification of hydatidiform mole at early gestational age has been increasingly recognized in recent years.

Pathogenesis and genetic basis
The pathogenesis of hydatidiform mole remains controversial. Historical thoughts attributed the primary etiology to overgrown villous trophoblast that 'oversecreted' leading to hydropically swollen villi and thus vascular obliteration and fetal death. In contrast, others proposed that early death of the embryo was causative and failure of the fetal circulation development lead to hydropic swelling.[59,117] It has recently been suggested that the proper vasculogenic differentiation is significantly retarded in early complete mole due to increased apoptosis in the precursor cells of blood vessels, leading to progressive accumulation of vesicular fluid and subsequent formation of cistern.[75]

Thus, hydatidiform mole has been considered essentially as a form of pregnancy with chromosomal abnormalities that are prone to malignant transformation, but are not, strictly speaking, neoplastic.[43,110,133] As discussed in earlier paragraphs, studies on risk factors, especially regarding age and past obstetric history, support such hypotheses.[9,13,109]

Karyotyping of hydatidiform mole
Karyotypic and genetic analysis of hydatidiform mole has helped to subclassify molar pregnancies into complete or partial moles. Nearly all complete moles are diploid (46,XX; 46,XY) and most partial moles are triploid (69,XXY; 69,XXX; 69,XYY) (Figure 32.9).[65,92,120,139,140,150] Recent genetic analysis on hydatidiform moles using comparative genomic hybridiza-

tion (CGH) revealed balanced profiles without detectable chromosomal gains or deletions.[1] These findings may be limited by the resolution power of the CGH technique.

Genetic origin of hydatidiform mole
Complete moles The vast majority of diploid complete moles are of pure androgenetic origin since their entire nuclear DNA is paternally derived[65,92,120,139,140,150] and transmitted from the sperm to an anuclear ovum devoid of nuclear DNA. The cytoplasmic structures, including mitochondrial DNA, are maternally derived.[22] Most complete moles are monospermic arising from fertilization of an anucleate egg by a haploid sperm which undergoes endoreduplication (Figure 32.9B).[121] Around one-fifth of complete moles are dispermic, formed after fertilization of an anucleate egg by two sperms (Figure 32.9C).

Occasional triploid or tetraploid complete moles as well as tetraploid partial moles have been reported.[46] These also have an excess of paternal contributions. Triploid or tetraploid complete moles remain androgenetic while tetraploid partial moles have one maternal and three paternal haploid contributions to the genome.

Under rare situations, there are complete moles that are diploid but biparental, rather than purely androgenetic. These unusual biparental complete moles tend to be recurrent in a patient or affect several members of a family. Familial recurrent hydatidiform mole is characterized by recurrent complete hydatidiform moles of biparental, rather than the more usual androgenetic, origin. In most such families, genetic mapping has shown that the responsible gene is located in a 1.1 Mb region on chromosome 19q13.4.[37,38] Mutations in this gene result in dysregulation of imprinting in the female germline with abnormal development of both embryonic and extraembryonic tissue. About 75% of the subsequent pregnancies in women diagnosed with this condition are likely to be complete moles. The others may suffer from miscarriages and partial moles. Women with familial recurrent hydatidiform mole have a similar risk of progressing to persistent trophoblastic disease similar to that of androgenetic complete mole.

Partial moles Most partial moles are triploid gestations carrying 69 chromosomes,[90] with an extra chromosomal haploid set from the father (Figure 32.9D).[64,91] Partial moles thus usually arise as a result of fertilization of an ovum by two sperms although fertilization of an egg by a single diploid sperm cannot be excluded.

Partial moles with such diandric composition constitute 80–90% of triploid gestations.[24,88,162] On the other hand, the digynic triploid placentas, which have two maternal contributions to the nuclear genome (46 maternal chromosomes and 23 paternal chromosomes), do not fulfill the criteria for diagnosis of partial mole.[116] Instead, the digynic triploid conceptions have abnormally small placentas and growth-retarded fetuses.[97] Mild villous abnormalities with preservation of fetal tissues and fetal red blood cells in the villi may be found.

Repetitive partial molar pregnancy may occur, just as with complete molar pregnancy.[78,118]

Genetic aberrations in hydatidiform mole
Similar to other human neoplasms, malignant transformation in GTD most likely involves multiple genetic alterations, including activation of oncogenes and inactivation of tumor suppressor genes, aberrant expression of telomerase and apop-

Table 32.3 Comparison among hydropic abortus and complete and partial hydatidiform moles[61,87,109,121]

	Hydropic abortus	Partial hydatidiform mole		Complete hydatidiform mole	
Karyotype	Diploid, often with abnormal karyotype	Triploid (69)		Diploid (46,XX; 46,XY) or tetraploid (92)	
Gestational age at diagnosis when aborted or evacuated	Earliest (mean = 11 weeks)	Mean = 12 weeks		Latest (mean = 15 weeks)	
Embryo/fetus/amnion	May be present	May be present		Absent, generally	
		<12 weeks	>12 weeks	<12 weeks	>12 weeks
Villous size	Uniform	Varied	Varied	Varied	Varied
Villous enlargement	May be marked	Varied	Some enlarged, but often not prominent	Minimal	Marked
Villous outline	Smooth, round to ovoid (balloon-shaped)	Irregular	Scalloped with pseudoinclusions and frond-like invaginations	Club-shaped budding	Round to ovoid (balloon-shaped)
Villous cisterns	Absent	Varied	Variable, but usually not prominent	Uncommon	Prominent
Villous stroma	Hydropic	Fibrotic	Hydropic	Mucoid/myxoid	Hydropic
Karyorrhexis in stromal cells of well-preserved villi[109]	Inconspicuous; karyorrhexis within fetal vessels may be present	Inconspicuous	Inconspicuous	Present and increasing	Common and intense
Trophoblastic proliferation	Polar	May be focal. Lace-like pattern around the villus	Focal	Multifocal	Circumferential
Trophoblastic atypia	None	Absent to minimal	Absent to minimal	Minimal	Often present
Trophoblast pseudoinclusions	Rare	Present	Present	Present	Present
Normal villi present	Sometimes	Present	Present	Some	None to few
Nucleated red blood cell	Present	Present	Present	Occasionally	Absent
Blood vessels	Absent, collapsed	Present	Present	Sometimes	Absent, generally
Implantation site	Normal	Normal	Normal	Florid	Florid
Relative level of serum β-hCG	Variable; relatively low (around 8000 IU)	Moderately elevated; around 66 000 IU		Moderately elevated; around 184 000 IU	
Return of serum β-hCG to normal (without chemotherapy)	Mean = 47 days	Mean = 63 days		Mean = 78 days	

β-hCG, beta-human chorionic gonadotrophin.

totic activity, and altered dynamics of cell–cell and cell–matrix dynamics, leading to a dysregulation of cellular processes including proliferation, differentiation, apoptosis, and invasion.[50,94]

Because of the predominant androgenetic origin of hydatidiform mole, it is believed that the malignancy following a hydatidiform mole results from recessive mutational genetic factors that control cell growth dynamics. Some believe that if the mutation is homozygous, the normal control mechanism of cell growth is lost.[70,101]

Imprinting genes may be involved.[27,37] The preferential expression of genes based on the gamete of origin, defined as genomic imprinting, has emerged as a fundamental mechanism in mammalian biology and appears to be of pathogenetic importance in GTD. For example, in androgenetic complete mole, expression of H19 from the paternal allele is seen in the villous cytotrophoblast cell layer surrounding the villous stroma, whereas the normal placenta expresses H19 only from the maternal allele. This represents relaxation of imprinting.[37] As discussed earlier, women with recurrent hydatidiform moles may carry an autosomal recessive mutation, provisionally mapped to 19q13.3–13.4, which may be important in regulating the maternal imprint in the ovum.[37] Such mutations may involve dysregulated imprinting marks in the maternal germline or for their maintenance in the embryo, and may be responsible for development of recurrent molar pregancies.[144]

Clinicopathologic features
Complete hydatidiform mole
Clinical presentation In the past, complete mole usually presented between 11 and 25 weeks of pregnancy with vaginal bleeding or excessive uterine enlargement for gestational age.

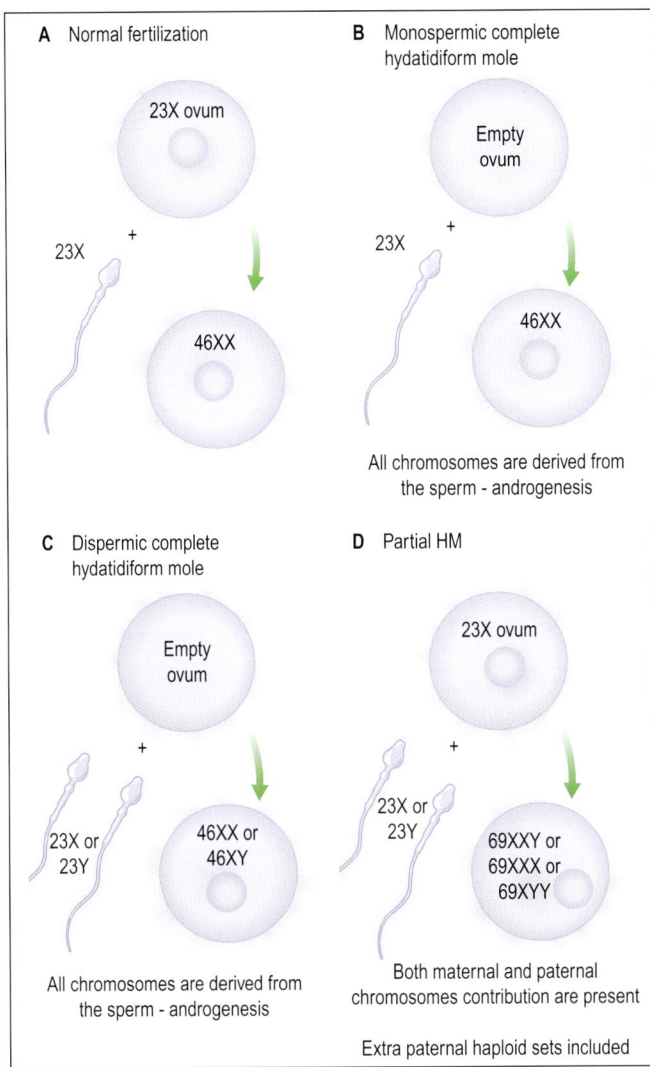

A Normal fertilization

23X ovum

23X

+

46XX

B Monospermic complete hydatidiform mole

Empty ovum

23X

+

46XX

All chromosomes are derived from the sperm - androgenesis

C Dispermic complete hydatidiform mole

Empty ovum

+

23X or 23Y

46XX or 46XY

All chromosomes are derived from the sperm - androgenesis

D Partial HM

23X ovum

+

23X or 23Y

69XXY or 69XXX or 69XYY

Both maternal and paternal chromosomes contribution are present

Extra paternal haploid sets included

Fig. 32.9 Normal fertilization involves one paternal and one maternal haploid chromosome sets (**A**). In monospermic complete mole (**B**), one sperm fertilizes an empty ovum with no nuclear chromosome followed by duplication. In dispermic complete mole (**C**), two sperms fusing in an empty ovum also result in diploid chromosome composition. In a partial mole (**D**), extra haploid set(s) of paternal genome fuse with the ovum, with retained maternal haplotype producing a triploid genome.

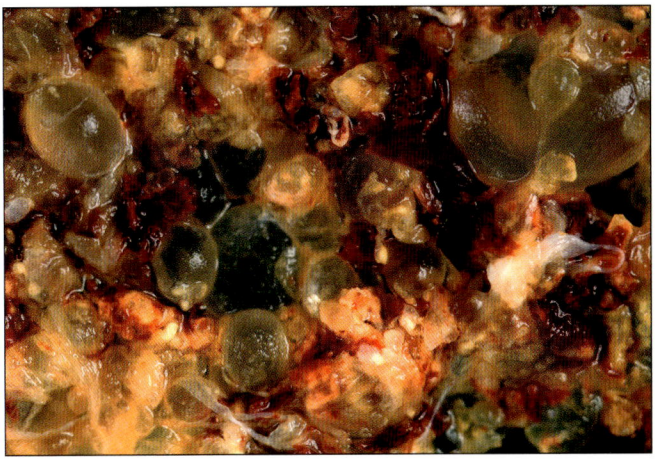

Fig. 32.10 Complete hydatidiform mole with 5–15 mm grossly visible vesicles. The specimen was floated in water for photography.

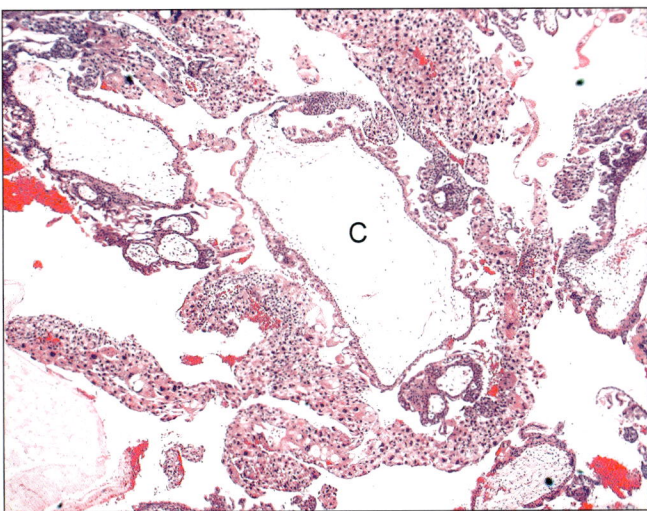

Fig. 32.11 A complete mole with well-formed cistern (C) and circumferential trophoblastic hyperplasia.

Pelvic ultrasound examination often revealed a characteristic 'snowstorm appearance' suggestive of molar pregnancy. Common application of pelvic ultrasound now enables the diagnosis at earlier gestational ages with complete moles not uncommonly being diagnosed as early as 6–8 weeks. The hCG level is usually markedly raised, although in recent decades the levels are less pronounced as the disease is being discovered at earlier gestational ages. Some complete moles may be incidentally diagnosed by histologic study of spontaneously passed or surgically evacuated tissue from patients with missed abortion or undergoing elective abortion. The diagnosis is not suspected before histologic examination and such findings emphasize the importance of sending all such aborted material for histologic examination.[141]

Pathology Macroscopically, a complete mole in the second trimester exhibits clusters of vesicles with variable dimensions developed from transformation of chorionic villi (Figure 32.10). Although the vesicles are usually at least 1 mm in size, many will exceed 5 mm or even 1 cm. Indeed, the term 'hydatidiform mole' derives from this remarkable 'bunch of grapes' appearance. An embryo/fetus is almost always absent in complete hydatidiform mole.[119]

Microscopically, a complete mole exhibits markedly distended chorionic villi due to the accumulation of abundant stromal fluid with central cistern formation. A substantial degree of multifocal to circumferential proliferation of both cytotrophoblast and syncytiotrophoblast is usually obvious in contrast to bipolar proliferation in normal early placenta (Figures 32.11 and 32.12). Fetal stromal blood vessels are almost always absent, often in association with obvious karyorrhexis of stromal cells[23,154] (Figures 32.13 and 32.14).

The availability of high-resolution ultrasonography has recently made possible the diagnosis of complete mole before

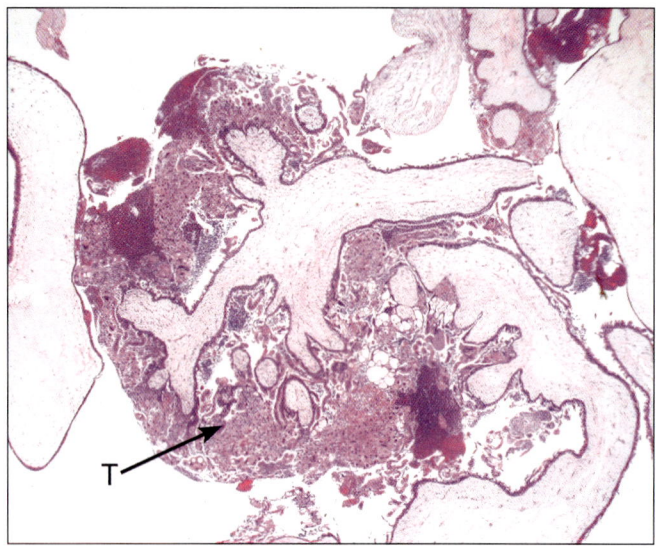

Fig. 32.12 Early complete hydatidiform mole. The villus ends are club shaped and diffusely surrounded by atypical trophoblastic (T) cells. Cistern formation is not conspicuous.

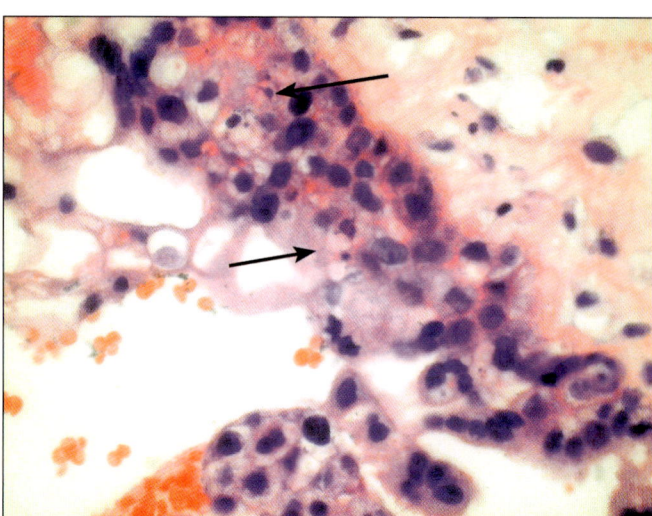

Fig. 32.14 Increased karyorrhexis in the trophoblast mantle.

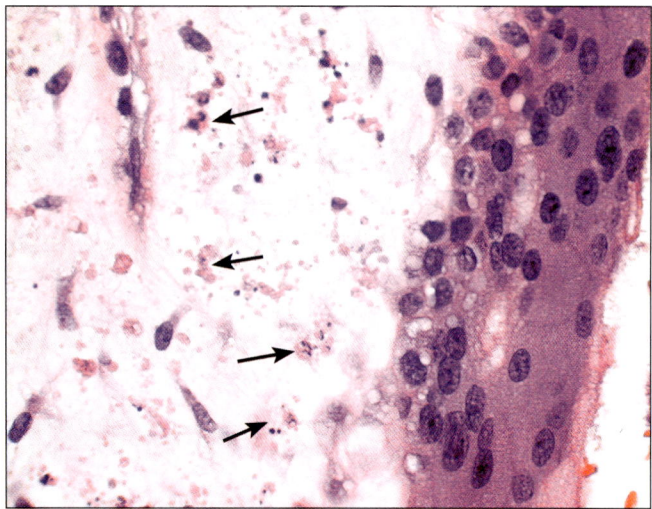

Fig. 32.13 Increased karyorrhexis in stromal cells of a hydropic villus of a complete mole.

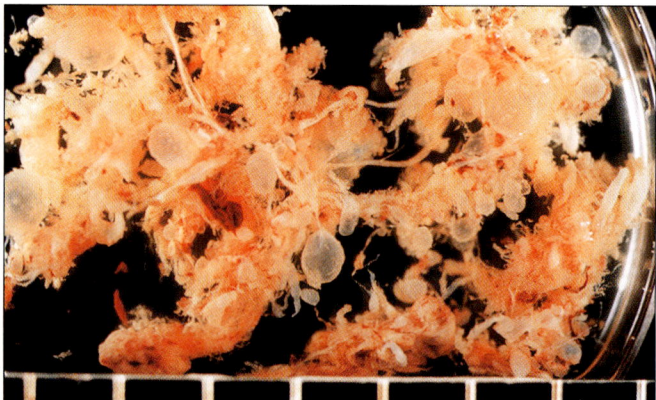

Fig. 32.15 Partial mole. Vesicles were identified in the uterine curettings macroscopically.

12 weeks' gestation. These early complete moles may show previously unfamiliar histologic features such as numerous club-shaped secondary villous sprouts from a larger villus and non-hydropic myxoid or mucoid hypercellular stroma.[72,110] Poorly demarcated central cisterns may be seen in early complete moles. While there is reduction in mature blood vessels with distinct lumen, immature vascular networks without lumen and CD31-positive primitive stromal cells may be abundant.[75] There is, however, increased apoptosis in the precursor cells of blood vessels.

Partial hydatidiform mole

Clinical presentation Patients with partial mole are less likely to present with frank symptoms and signs as seen in complete mole. They are clinically more commonly diagnosed as a missed abortion.

Pathology The macroscopic appearances are variable. The placental tissue is usually less bulky with variable proportions of vesicles (Figures 32.15 and 32.16). There may be an identifiable fetus, or fetal parts. The fetus may be well-formed or carry multiple congenital anomalies including syndactyly of the fingers and toes.

Microscopically, an admixture of hydropic and normal sized villi may be present (Figure 32.17), although the presence of non-hydropic villi cannot reliably discriminate between partial and early complete mole.[109] The hydropic villi show variable degrees of swelling with central cistern formation, usually less extensive than that found in complete mole (Figures 32.18 and 32.19). They often have irregular scalloped outlines (Figure 32.20) and trophoblastic inclusions (Figures 32.21 and 32.22). The cisterns are usually not well formed, with development of an irregular maze-like pattern. Normal sized degenerated villi are also found. Fetal development may be suspected by rudimentary blood vessels that contain fetal red blood cells (Figure 32.23).

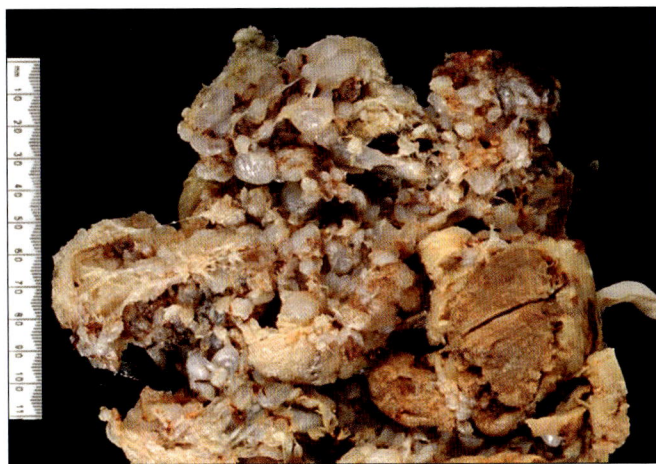

Fig. 32.16 A partial mole with vesicles found in the placenta focally.

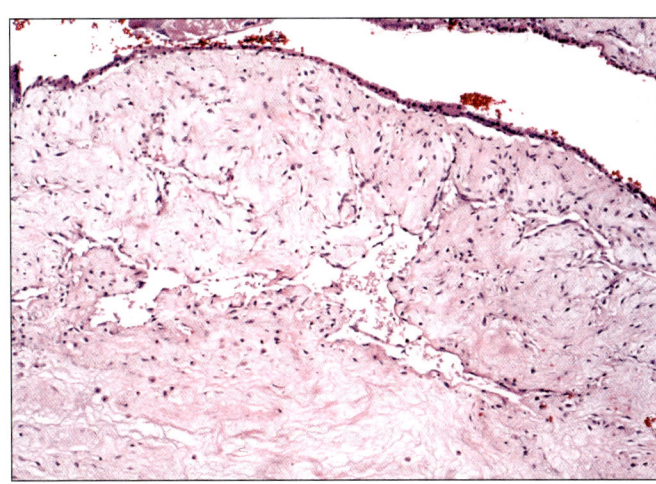

Fig. 32.19 Irregular ill-formed cistern is found within hydropic chorionic villi of a partial mole.

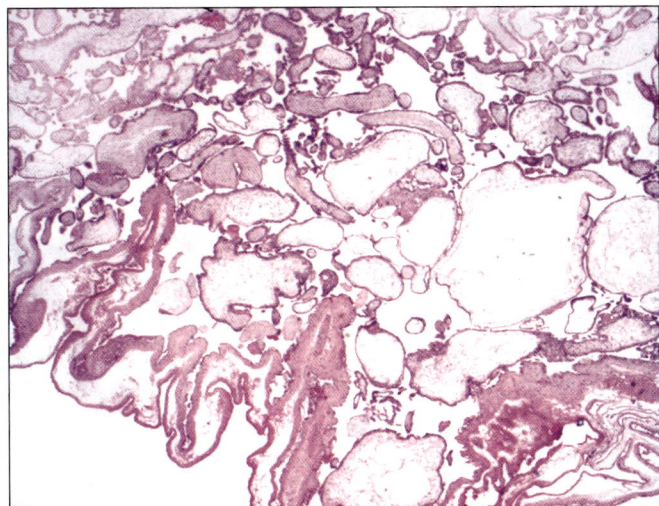

Fig. 32.17 Partial mole with discernable cisterns and hydropic chorionic villi of heterogeneous sizes.

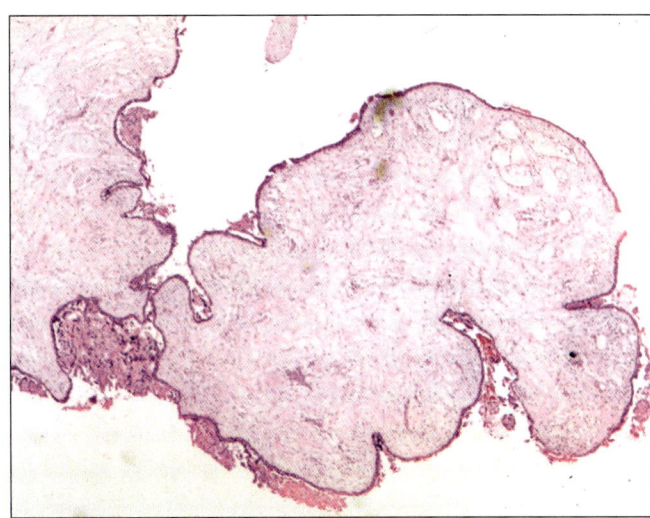

Fig. 32.20 Hydropic chorionic villi in partial mole with irregular indentations.

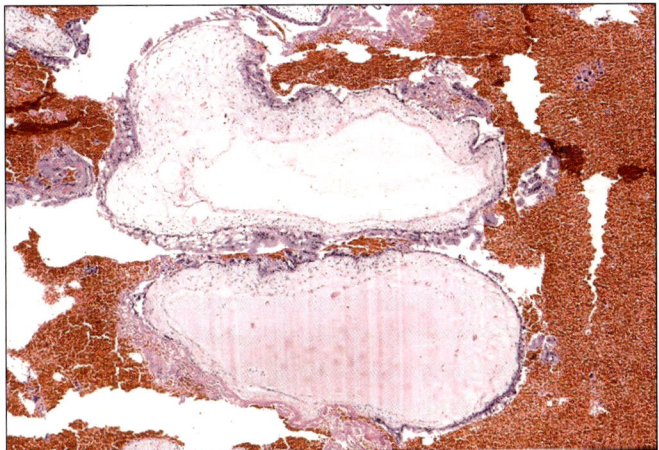

Fig. 32.18 Well-formed cistern in hydropic villi of a partial mole.

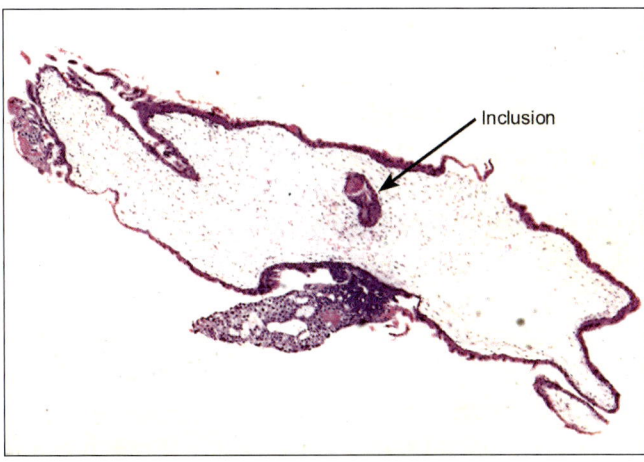

Fig. 32.21 Partial mole with trophoblastic indentation and inclusion in hydropic villi.

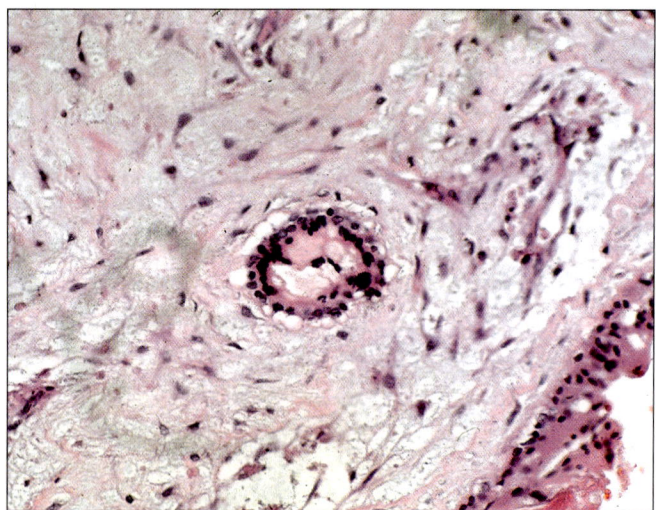

Fig. 32.22 Trophoblastic inclusions in hydropic chorionic villi of a partial mole.

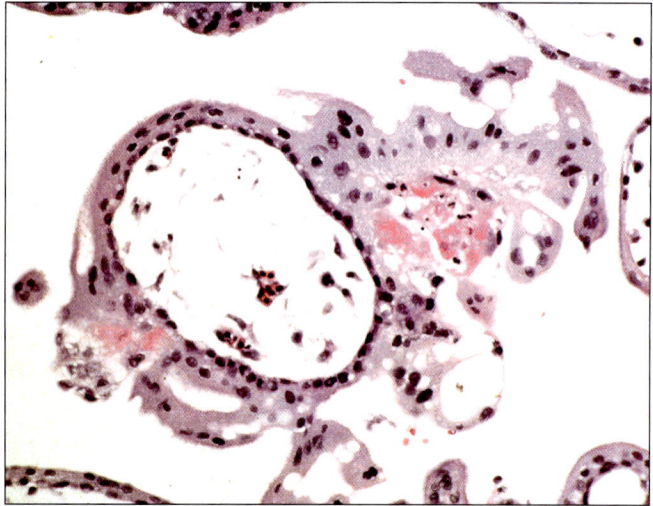

Fig. 32.23 Nucleated red blood cells in villi may provide evidence of fetal development in a partial mole.

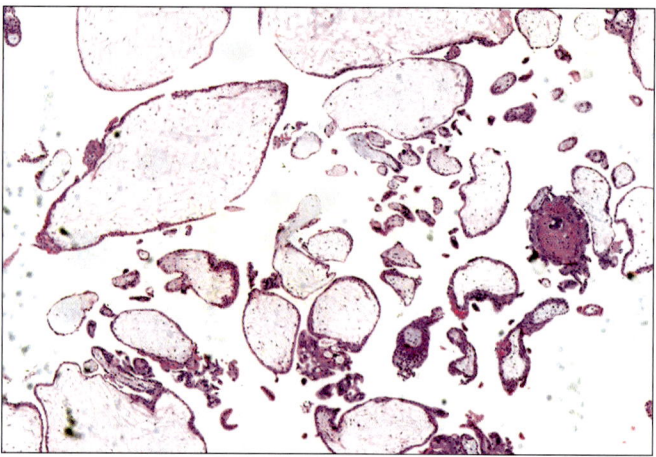

Fig. 32.24 Chorionic villi with hydropic change in a hydropic abortion.

Problems in diagnosis of hydatidiform mole

Flow of evaluation Histologic evaluation of products of gestation is a common daily task of anatomic pathologists. In evaluating whether disease is present, it is important initially to decide whether the chorionic villi show morphologic abnormalities such as hydropic change. If present, the pathologist must decide whether the changes are consistent with hydatidiform mole or with non-molar placental abnormalities, including digynic hydropic abnormalities or placental mesenchymal dysplasia. If hydatidiform mole is the preferred diagnosis, then assessment must be made as to whether it is a complete or partial mole.

It is worth noting that histologic diagnosis and classification of hydatidiform mole is subject to substantial intra- and interobserver variations even among expert placental pathologists.[47,60,67] Discordance most frequently occurs in the differential diagnosis between partial mole and hydropic abortion.

Practical approach Of import, all material should be processed and examined so that all evacuated villi can be assessed. It may be impossible to make a firm diagnosis based purely on histopathologic evaluation if only relatively few villi with well-developed histologic features are available. Ancillary laboratory investigations such as ploidy, imprinting gene marker or other molecular studies may be necessary. If such techniques are not routinely available, a report may be issued stating the most likely diagnosis and the reasons for uncertainty.[108] The patient may need to be registered for brief hCG monitoring. In cases of non-molar hydropic abortion, the hCG level usually falls rapidly, with an average of less than 7 weeks. Follow-up can be stopped. This course of action will result in a small number of non-molar hydropic abortions receiving a brief hCG follow-up. However, this can reduce the chance of missing hydatidiform moles leading to the otherwise preventable gestational trophoblastic neoplasia.

Differentiation of a hydatidiform mole from abortion with hydropic villi Distinguishing a hydatidiform mole, in particular an early complete mole or a partial mole, from an abortion with hydropic villi may be diagnostically challenging (Table 32.3). Hydropic abortion shows edema with mesenchymal swelling of chorionic villi and absence of villous blood vessels (Figures 32.24 and 32.25), features also found in hydatidiform mole.

Traditionally, an abortion specimen is not a molar pregnancy that shows villous edema only microscopically and has minimal or no cistern formation.[133] However, it is becoming progressively more difficult to distinguish hydropic abortion from hydatidiform mole of early gestational age, a time by which cistern formation is not usually established.[28,30,85,99] Some clues help in the distinction. A hydropic abortus usually has far less tissue at the time of evacuation with no macroscopically recognizable embryo. Microscopy of the hydropic abortus shows a diffuse spectrum of villous sizes ranging from small, to medium sized, to large. In particular, two distinct populations of villi are not found (Figures 32.24 and 32.25). The pattern of trophoblastic hyperplasia often helps to distinguish a partial mole from a simple hydropic abortion. In partial moles, the villous trophoblast may be focal, multifocal or circumferentially proliferated, whereas in first trimester abortions the proliferation is polar (Figure 32.26). Moreover, the trophoblast is

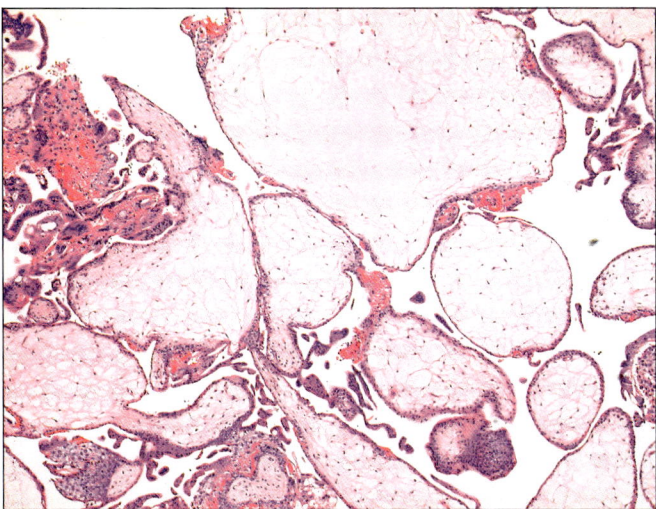

Fig. 32.25 Conspicuous hydropic change in a spontaneous abortion that is difficult to distinguish from early partial or even complete mole.

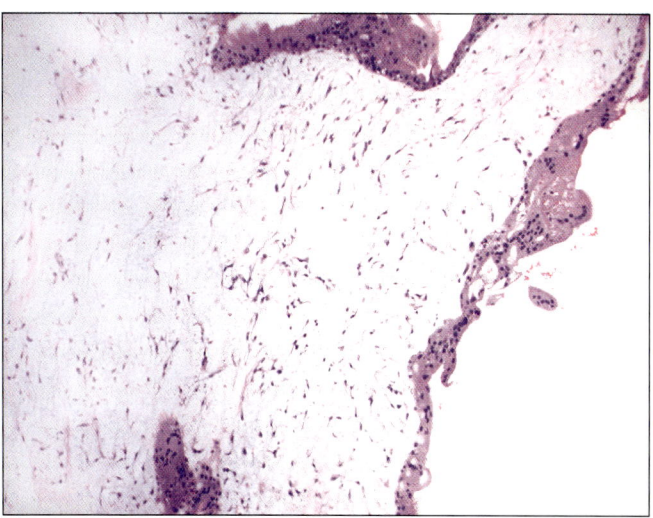

Fig. 32.27 Early complete mole with a conspicuous myxoid villous stroma.

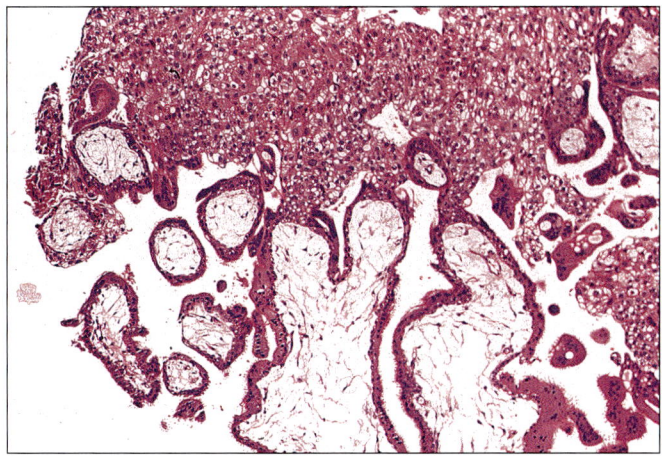

Fig. 32.26 Polar anchoring trophoblast. The first trimester placenta normally has anchoring villi that show localized proliferations of trophoblast at one edge of the villi.

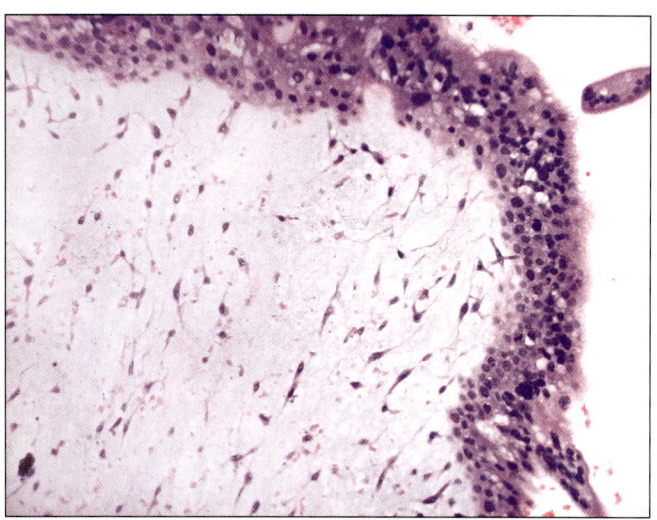

Fig. 32.28 A myxoid stroma is often seen in early complete mole.

attenuated and thin, and tightly covers the villous surface, rather than projecting as little clubs of syncytiotrophoblast (trophoblastic knuckles) or as lacy mounds of trophoblast.

Diagnosis of early hydatidiform mole In recent decades, pathologists have been obliged to histologically evaluate products of conception evacuated as early as 6 weeks' gestational age due to early diagnosis of spontaneous miscarriage or therapeutic termination of pregnancy.[52,125] In such early gestations, the conventional histologic features of complete or partial hydatidiform mole are not well developed and may produce diagnostic problems.[72] To make the problems more difficult, about two-thirds of such first-trimester pregnancies eventually diagnosed histologically as hydatidiform mole lack the typical clinical presentation or classic ultrasound appearance. The risk of subsequent development of persistent trophoblastic disease is independent of gestational age at evacuation.[61,109,121,124] Correct diagnosis of an early hydatidiform mole has become a significant and important challenge to pathologists.

New histologic criteria more relevant to the diagnosis of early hydatidiform mole have been described in recent years. Characteristically, the villi of very early complete mole may not demonstrate significant cistern formation and trophoblast proliferation, and the diagnostic histologic hallmarks of a hydatidiform mole are thus absent. There is, however, a distinctive villous stroma, which is typically myxoid and hypercellular, with a phylloides-like configuration (Figures 32.27–32.30). Conspicuous karyorrhexis of the stromal cells is usually observed (Figures 32.13 and 32.14). This is often associated with markedly atypical intermediate trophoblasts at the placental implantation site. Also, features traditionally thought to be associated with partial moles, such as vessels and nucleated red blood cells, may also be seen in early complete moles.[52,53]

Differentiation of a partial mole from a complete mole This can also be difficult. Identification of fetal tissues within a mole, such as embryonic tissue, amnion or fetal red blood cells in villous vessels, is insufficient to classify a hydatidiform mole as a partial mole. It can be a complete mole developed from a twin placenta or genuine preservation of fetal development in a complete mole.[84,109] Similarly, the presence of chorionic villi of relatively normal morphology or of villous blood vessels does not reliably differentiate between partial mole and early complete mole.

Some histologic features, however, have been found useful in distinction. Complete mole, even very early in gestation, usually displays more florid trophoblastic hyperplasia (Figures 32.11 and 32.12) whereas the trophoblastic hyperplasia of partial mole is normally only focal and is usually lacy or club-like (Figure 32.21). The villous outlines of the complete mole are outwardly projecting, finger-like in early gestations (Figure 32.30), and smooth and balloon-like in later gestations, in contrast to the scalloped 'fjord-like' outline of the partial mole with its stromal trophoblastic inclusions (Figures 32.20 and 32.21).[74,87,119,142] On the other hand, stromal karyorrhexis is a common feature in complete mole.[75] Moreover, most complete moles display conspicuous trophoblast invasion and destruction of blood vessels with interstitial hemorrhage. These features help discriminate between complete and partial mole.

Distinguishing a partial molar pregnancy from a twin pregnancy with one normal twin and one complete mole Both conditions may display embryonic/fetal tissues, some hydropic villi, and some relatively normal villi. The hallmarks of twin pregnancy with coexisting complete mole include: (1) marked trophoblastic hyperplasia on the surface of some villi (Figures 32.11 and 32.12); (2) distended, outwardly clubbed villi (Figure 32.31); and (3) trophoblast with striking atypia (markedly enlarged intermediate trophoblast with large, hyperchromatic nuclei) at the implantation site (Figure 32.32). In contrast, partial molar pregnancy has: (1) focal trophoblastic atypia; (2) scalloped villi; and (3) focal hyperplasia with less atypia at the implantation site.

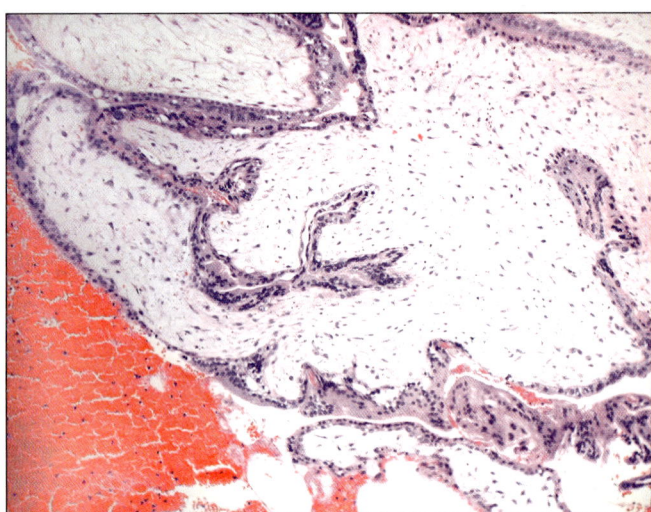

Fig. 32.29 Phylloides-like configuration may be noted in an early complete mole.

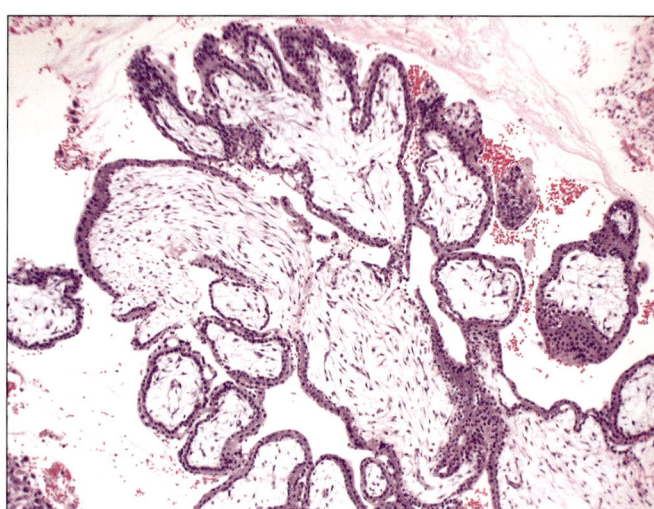

Fig. 32.31 Club-shaped villi are more commonly found in complete mole.

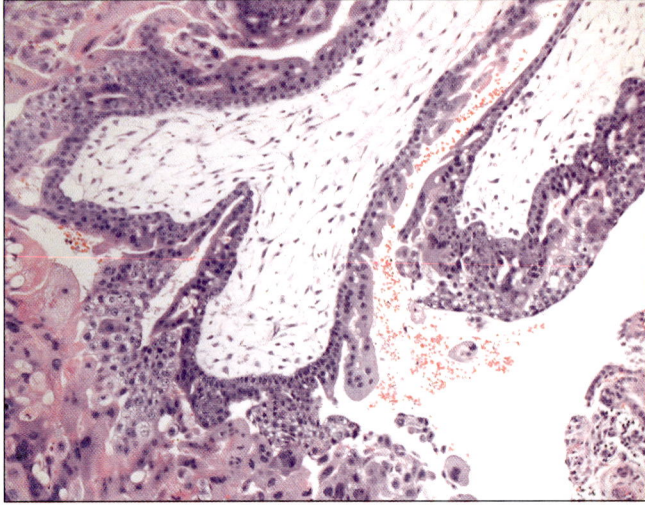

Fig. 32.30 Polypoid, sprout-like villi are often seen in early complete mole.

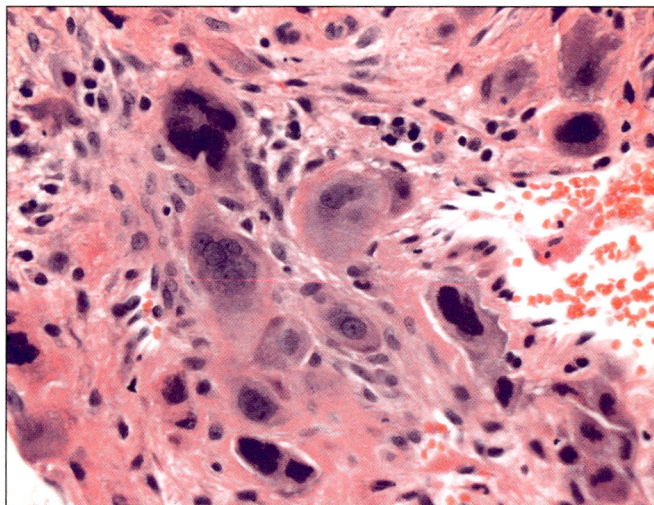

Fig. 32.32 Cytologic atypia of intermediate trophoblast in a complete mole.

Diagnosis of ectopic hydatidiform mole Ectopic GTD, including hydatidiform mole and choriocarcinoma, is uncommon, with a UK incidence of approximately 1.5 per 1 000 000 births.[54] Initial management is usually surgical removal of the conceptus. Referral to a specialist center is recommended. Expert review indicates that overdiagnosis of definite complete or partial hydatidiform mole was significantly less in ectopic pregnancy (6%) than in uterine curettage specimens (90%),[122] even though it is easy to overdiagnose hydatidiform mole in *early tubal ectopic pregnancy*.[11] Polar trophoblastic proliferation and hydropic villi may be found normally in early placentation, or in cases of hydropic abortion. Sheets of extravillous trophoblast may be particularly prominent in tubal ectopic gestation. The absence of circumferential trophoblastic proliferation, scalloped outline or stromal karyorrhexis should caution against the diagnosis of hydatidiform mole.

When large aggregates of proliferating trophoblast are found without villi, the *differential diagnosis of choriocarcinoma or PSTT* should be considered. If extensive sheets of trophoblast occur in the presence of villi, which are not molar, the rare possibility of intraplacental choriocarcinoma should be considered regardless of gestational age (see below).

Rarely, *placental mesenchymal dysplasia*, with or without Beckwith-Wiedemann syndrome, may be misdiagnosed as partial mole (Figure 32.33).[111] These cases often display cyst

formation, terminal villous hydropic change, and marked aneurysmal dilatation of stem villous vessels. There may be focal chorioangiomatoid change and extramedullary hematopoiesis, but not excessive trophoblast proliferation and trophoblastic inclusions, which are typical of partial mole.

Chorangiocarcinoma is a rare placental tumor in which there is a proliferation of both the vascular and epithelial (trophoblast) components of the chorionic villi. It is usually found in term placentas in association with infarction and fibrin deposition as discrete yellowish white nodules. It may involve the stem villi. Scattered chorionic villi with florid stromal vascular proliferation resembling chorangioma as well as hyperplastic villous trophoblast are found (Figures 32.34 and 32.35). The trophoblast may display marked cytologic atypia and increased

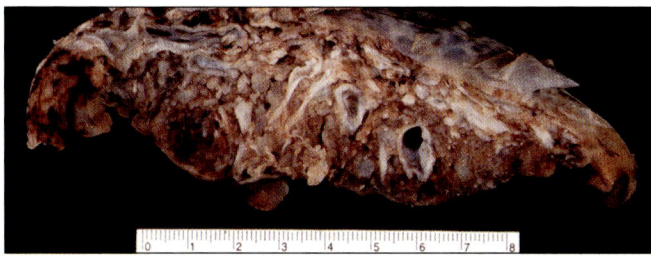

Fig. 32.33 Remarkable cystic spaces found in serial sections of a nonmolar condition of placental mesenchymal dysplasia. When the cystic spaces are detected in an antenatal ultrasound, hydatidiform mole must be suspected.

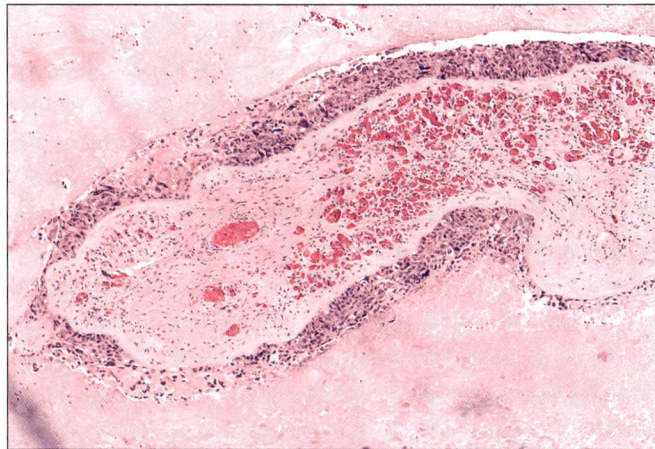

Fig. 32.34 Chorangiocarcinoma. An abnormal villus shows intense vascularity, a thin rim of hyperplastic villous trophoblast, and adjacent tumor infarction.

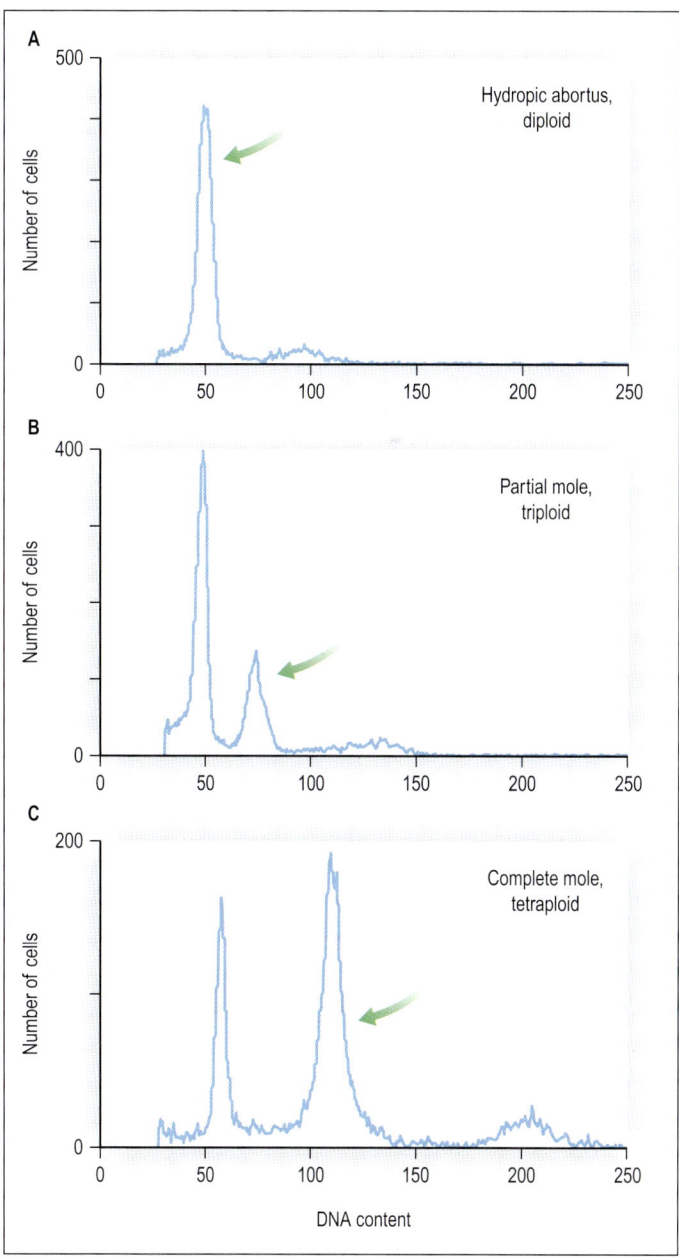

Fig. 32.35 Chorangiocarcinoma. Detail of abnormal villus with intense vascularity, a thin rim of atypical, mitotically active villous trophoblast, and adjacent necrosis.

mitotic activity. There is no invasion of the maternal intervillous space or the villous stroma. The trophoblast is strongly reactive for cytokeratin while only focally reactive for hCG and hPL.[142] Some chorangiocarcinomas may bear resemblance to ETT. Despite the atypia and proliferative activity of the villous trophoblast, no significant malignant sequelae have been experienced in the small number of cases reported.[73,87,119,142] One patient with chorangiocarcinoma had previous hydatidiform molar pregnancies. There is current uncertainty as to whether this lesion should be classified as high reactive, benign, borderline or malignant.

Ancillary techniques to assist histologic diagnosis and classification

During recent years, several immunohistochemical markers and molecular techniques (Table 32.4) have been developed that are particularly helpful in distinguishing hydropic abortion from hydatidiform mole as well as partial from complete hydatidiform moles. Such applications are particularly useful in early pregnancy.

These tests are based on genetic knowledge that a complete mole is diploid without maternal contribution, whereas a partial mole is triploid with one maternal chromosome haploid set. But the diagnosis of partial mole cannot be assumed for every triploid gestation, as only about two-thirds of triploidies show diagnostic features of partial moles.[61] A triploid gestation can derive from a paternal and two maternal genomes giving rise to a fetus with intrauterine growth retardation and dysmorphic features with a small placenta.

p57 is a paternally imprinted inhibitor gene and, if expressed, implies a maternal contribution to the gestational products. Absence of p57 expression thus supports the diagnosis of complete mole, which is of pure androgenetic origin.[45,46,68] However, for reasons not yet understood, the trophoblast in these cases still shows p57 reactivity. p57 immunostaining cannot distinguish partial mole from hydropic abortion since both involve a maternal genome contribution and both will be immunoreactive. Other ancillary diagnostic methods that detect ploidy of the gestational products, such as flow or image cytometry[48,86] and chromosome *in situ* hybridization[89] (see below), may be helpful in such situations, especially if applied in a combined approach. A p57 positive hydropic conception that is diploid would favor a hydropic abortion while a triploid one would support a diagnosis of partial mole.

The *proliferative index* of a hydropic conceptus may also be helpful in differential diagnosis. A relatively new marker now in use is MCM7, which is a member of the multicopy maintenance (MCM) protein family that regulates DNA replication during the S phase. In quiescent cells, human MCM7 mRNA is almost undetectable. It increases during the late G_1 to S phase as the cells enter the cell cycle, making it a good marker for proliferation. This novel proliferation marker demonstrates less variability than more well-established markers, such as proliferating cell nuclear antigen (PCNA) and MIB1 (Ki-67), and therefore may be a better proliferation marker (Figure 32.36). The MCM7 index is significantly higher in partial and complete moles than in spontaneous abortion. MCM7 may be useful in differentiating molar and non-molar gestations although it does not discriminate partial from complete mole or in predicting the development of persistent disease.[157] The trophoblast of hydatidiform moles is more likely to show overexpression of *p53, p21*, cyclin E or apoptotic

Table 32.4 Molecular markers in trophoblastic lesions

Genetic and molecular events	Relative level when compared with normal placentas		Relative level in HM in relation to subsequent development of GTN
	HM	CCA	
Oncogenes, tumor suppressor genes, and cell-cycle regulators			
p53[17,19,51,115]	↑	↑	
p21[17,51]	↑	↑	
Mdm-2[17,51]	↑	↑	
Rb[51]	↑	↑	
DOC-2/hDab2[49]		↑	
c-erb B-2[12,159]	↑	↑	
c-fms[20]	↑		
Cyclin E[76,106]	↑	↑	
Promoter hypermethylation of p16[155]	↑	↑	↑
Cell death and senescence			
Telomerase[3,21]	↑	↑	↑
Apoptosis[23,115,154]	↑	↑	↑
bcl-2[115,154]	↓	↓	
Mcl-1[41]	↑		↑
Ki-67[17,106,129]	↑	↑	
MCM7[157]	↑	↑	
Id1[156]	↑	↑	
Caspase[42]	↓	↓	
Cell adhesion, motility, and invasion			
E-cadherin/β-catenin[93]	↓	↓	
MMPs[113,147]		↑	
TIMPs[34]		↓	
Promoter methylation of TIMP3[34,155]		↑	
Promoter hypermethylation of E-cadherin[155]	↑	↑	
Insulin-like growth factor binding protein 1[36]			↓
KIAA1200[35]	↑		
Osteopontin[8,10,35]	↓		
Immunomodulation			
Ferritin light polypeptide[36]			↓
Human chorionic gonadotrophin, beta subunit (CGB)[35]	↑		

↑, increased expression; ↓, decreased expression; CCA, choriocarcinoma; GTN, gestational trophoblastic neoplasia; HM, hydatidiform mole.

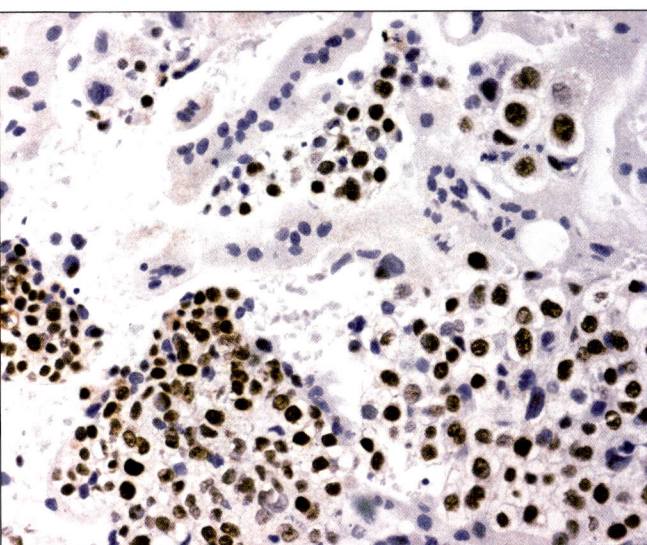

Fig. 32.36 MCM7, a proliferation marker, shown in cytotrophoblast nuclei in choriocarcinoma.

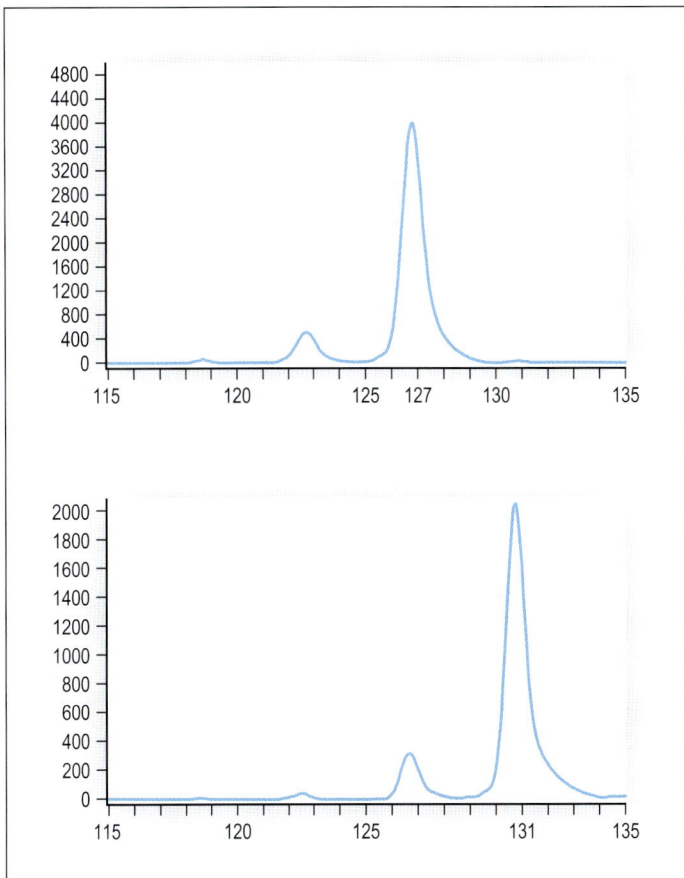

Fig. 32.38 Microsatellite polymorphisms of the patient and the diploid hydatidiform mole (HM). The patient was homozygous for the marker D3S1358, generating an allele of 127 bp. The HM was also homozygous for D3S1358, giving rise to an allele of 131 bp.

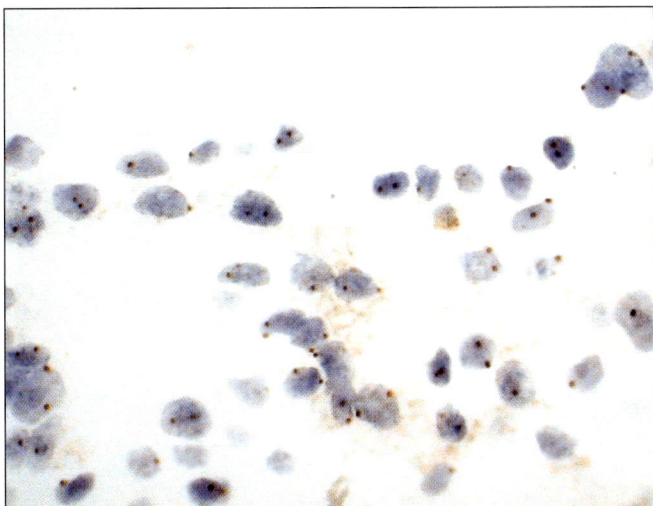

Fig. 32.37 Two hybridization signals for DNA probes (arrows) for chromosome 16 found in most nuclei of complete hydatidiform mole, confirmed by genotyping.

markers,[16,17,19,23,76,106,154] but it is unclear if such differences can be used for routine surgical diagnosis.

Detection of the *chromosome composition* of hydropic products of conception by flow cytometry, chromosome *in situ* hybridization, and DNA genotyping after microdissection have proven useful in differentiating hydropic abortion, complete mole, and partial mole.[15,40,89,109,143] Genotyping results correlate with the histologic evaluation in nearly 90% of hydatidiform moles and with chromosome *in situ* hybridization findings in virtually all cases. In other words, triploid hydatidiform moles possess maternal-derived alleles, while diploid hydatidiform moles (Figure 32.37) are purely androgenetic (Figure 32.38). The former favors a partial mole while the latter supports a diagnosis of complete mole. Genotyping and chromosome *in situ* hybridization are thus reliable adjuncts to histology, especially when the histologic evaluation is not clear and the specimen is of an early gestational age.[89] Using the

same approach in a recent study, most cases originally histologically diagnosed as partial moles that subsequently developed metastatic diseases were found to be complete moles. This study recapitulates the difficulty in histologically distinguishing partial from complete moles. It is worth emphasizing that a small number of partial moles progressed to metastatic disease or even choriocarcinoma. Thus, all patients with hydatidiform mole should be followed closely regardless of histologic subclassification.[15]

Progress of hydatidiform mole

Most hydatidiform moles regress after suction evacuation, the serum and urine hCG levels returning rapidly to normal. About 5–15%[2,114,121,153] of patients with hydatidiform mole require chemotherapy due to development of gestational trophoblastic neoplasia (GTN). GTN refers to evidence of trophoblastic activity after evacuation as shown by a stationary or rising hCG level. There may or may not be evidence of metastases. The frequency with which GTN is diagnosed after a hydatidiform mole depends on the mode of primary therapy, sensitivity of the follow-up hCG assay, duration of follow-up, and the diagnostic definitions. The wide ranges may reflect inconsistency in criteria used by various centers in managing GTD, rendering conclusive observations from epidemiologic studies difficult.[138]

The natural history for partial molar pregnancy is much more benign than that of complete molar pregnancy. For instance, in a recent study including over 1000 patients with complete hydatidiform mole, 15% of patients developed persistent GTN.[153] In contrast, only 1–5% of all partial mole pregnancy patients needed chemotherapy for persistent trophoblastic disease.[98,103,151] Nevertheless, women with partial molar pregnancy should still be followed up with serial β-hCG determinations for variable periods of time.

Few indices predict the progression of hydatidiform mole to GTN. To date, the *hCG regression pattern* remains the most specific prognostic indicator.[103,114,152] Controversies exist regarding potential *histopathologic parameters* useful in identifying high-risk patients. While earlier reports suggested that histopathologic grading based on the degree of trophoblastic hyperplasia and atypia facilitated prediction of the clinical outcome in cases of hydatidiform mole, most studies disagreed.[13,100,110] Thus, studies involving various clinicopathologic, biologic, and molecular markers have been conducted to explore alternative prognostic indices (Table 32.4).

Ancillary techniques to assist prediction of clinical outcome

Whether the *heterozygous (dispermic)* complete mole has a higher malignant potential than its *homozygous (monospermic)* counterpart remains controversial. Some studies have found that heterozygous moles, which include both 46,XX or 46,XY genotype, have greater malignant potential than their homozygous counterparts,[26,69,148,149] but this has been rejected by others.[18,39,102,143] Also, there is no correlation between the presence of a Y chromosome and the development of persistent GTN with or without metastasis.[18,102]

More recent approaches have achieved better success. Studies on the *apoptotic index* of hydatidiform mole using the terminal deoxynucleotidyl transferase (TdT)-mediated deoxyuridine triphosphate (dUTP) nick end labeling (TUNEL) approach and the caspase-sensitive M30 cytodeath immunohistochemistry method have found greater agreement with subsequent development of GTN chemotherapy (Figure 32.39).[23,154]

The apoptotic index of those hydatidiform moles that spontaneously regressed was significantly higher than the cases that developed persistent disease requiring chemotherapy. Similarly, high *telomerase activity* in hydatidiform mole was more likely associated with future aggressive disease that would require chemotherapy.[21] From differential expression microarray analysis, aberrant expression of Mcl-1, insulin-like growth factor binding protein 1 (IGFBP1), and ferritin light polypeptide also appear to be useful markers for predicting clinical behavior.[36,41]

In a recent study investigating the distribution of the alleles in the short tandem repeat sequences at loci D16S539, D7S820, and D13S317 in genetically complete hydatidiform moles, there were significant differences in allele frequencies between the complete moles and the local population.[163] Significant difference in specific allele frequency also existed among those cases that developed persistent disease.

INVASIVE MOLE

Clinicopathologic features

Invasive moles, which are defined by the finding of hydropic villi from a hydatidiform mole invading into the myometrium, blood vessels or even extrauterine sites, are found in about one-sixth of patients with complete moles. The patients usually have persistently high hCG levels and may in some cases present with uterine rupture. Chemotherapy and sometimes hysterectomy may be indicated. The diagnosis is usually made on a hysterectomy specimen.

The macroscopic appearance of an invasive mole varies with the extent of invasion. Variable numbers of molar vesicles may be seen in the endometrial cavity, myometrium, and adjacent extrauterine tissue (Figure 32.40). Significant hemorrhage is usually present. Microscopically, invasive moles exhibit molar villi within the myometrium or the blood vessels (Figure 32.41).

Diagnostic problems

Trophoblast has the capacity to invade or even metastasize, even in normal non-molar pregnancy. This phenomenon is sometime referred to as 'pseudo-malignancy'. In *placenta accreta*, for instance, non-molar villi invade directly into the

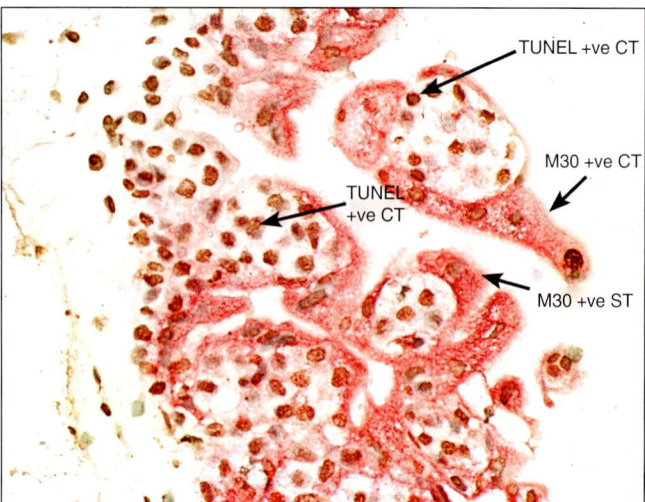

Fig. 32.39 Immunoreactivity for TUNEL and M30 cytodeath antibody: markers for different stages of apoptosis were found at the nuclei of cytotrophoblast (CT) and cytoplasm of syncytiotrophoblast (ST), respectively.

TUNEL +ve CT

M30 +ve CT

TUNEL +ve CT

M30 +ve ST

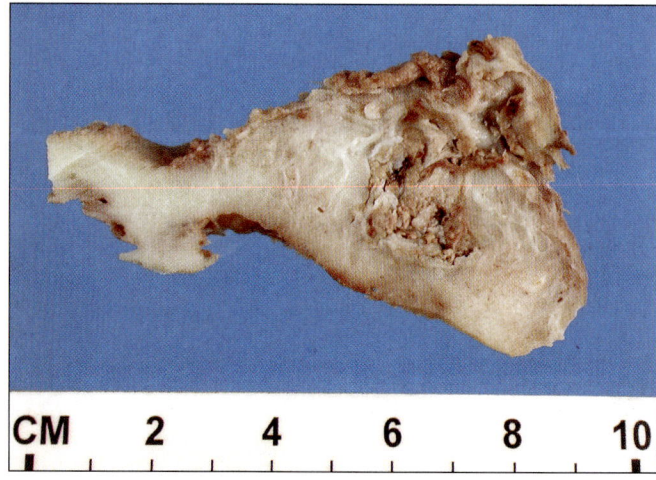

Fig. 32.40 Longitudinal section of a uterus showing an invasive mole.

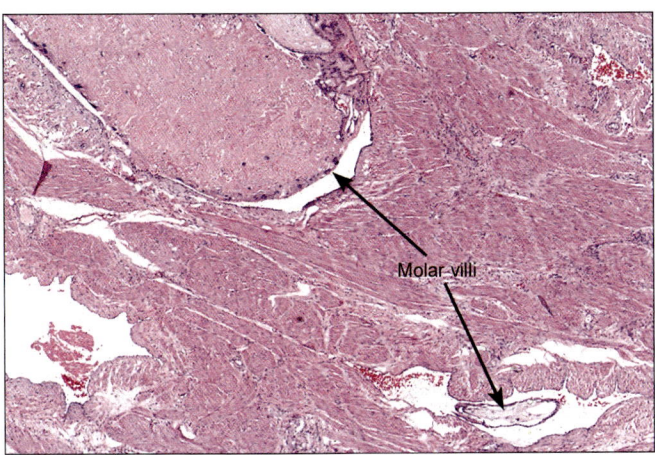

Fig. 32.41 Molar villi infiltrating myometrium and blood vessels in invasive mole.

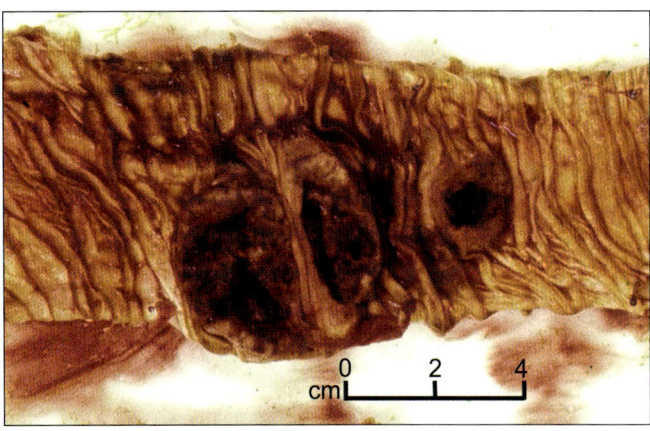

Fig. 32.42 Metastatic choriocarcinoma in intestine. The chief complaint was massive melena.

uterine myometrium in the absence of decidua formation. Clinically this may pose problems in obstetric management.

Invasive mole also needs to be distinguished from *choriocarcinoma*. Chorionic villi are absent in the latter while invasive moles exhibit chorionic villi, even in metastatic foci.

CHORIOCARCINOMA

Clinical presentation

Choriocarcinoma is a malignant tumor of admixed proliferating cytotrophoblast, intermediate trophoblast and syncytiotrophoblast. Depending on the extent of involvement, patients with choriocarcinoma may present with vaginal bleeding or symptoms related to extrauterine metastases. There may be hemorrhagic events in the central nervous system, liver, and gastrointestinal tract. Approximately half of the cases of choriocarcinoma present following a complete mole, but some may be preceded by non-molar abortions or even an unremarkable term delivery. Only rare cases of choriocarcinoma develop either *in situ* or in a partial hydatidiform mole.[58]

Pathology

Macroscopically, choriocarcinoma usually appears as single or multiple well-circumscribed hemorrhagic nodular lesions. The primary uterine tumor may extend deeply into the myometrium. The lungs, brain, and liver are the most common metastatic sites (Figure 32.42), suggesting a predominantly hematogenous route of dissemination. Lymph node metastasis is rare in gestational choriocarcinoma, in contrast with choriocarcinoma of non-gestational (germ cell) origin.

Microscopically, choriocarcinoma exhibits a biphasic pattern with a central core of mononuclear cytotrophoblast surrounded by a peripheral rim of multinucleated syncytiotrophoblast (Figure 32.43). The viable and better preserved tumor cells are found mainly at the lesion's periphery while extensive hemorrhage and necrosis are more often central. As a general rule, choriocarcinoma should not be diagnosed in the presence of chorionic villi. A few mitotic figures may be found in the cytotrophoblast, but there is no apparent correlation between mitotic activity and prognosis. The syncytiotrophoblast is reactive for hCG and α-inhibin. Occasionally, a small biopsy of choriocarcinoma may reveal only scanty syncytiotropho-

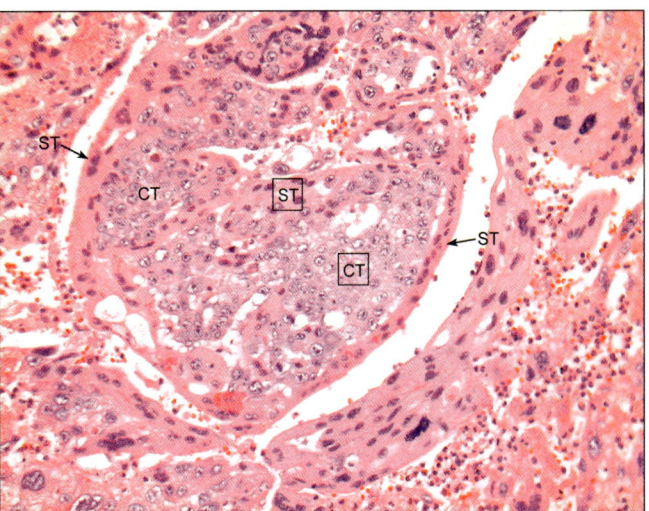

Fig. 32.43 Typical biphasic pattern of admixed cytotrophoblast (CT) and syncytiotrophoblast (ST) in choriocarcinoma.

blast and the morphologic features may mimic a poorly differentiated carcinoma. The diagnosis may then become difficult, especially in extrauterine sites. Immunohistochemical biomarkers for trophoblast help confirm the diagnosis (Figures 32.44–32.47).

Human chorionic gonadotrophin-related changes may be found in the genital tract of patients suffering from choriocarcinoma, including Arias-Stella phenomenon, decidual reaction mimicking progestogen-induced effect, cervical microglandular hyperplasia, and bilateral ovarian theca-lutein cysts. Such ovarian cysts have been considered a sign of recurrent or persistent choriocarcinoma despite treatment.

Pathogenesis

The pathogenesis of choriocarcinoma is also unclear. About half of gestational choriocarcinomas are preceded by a complete mole, the others by abortions, normal or even ectopic pregnancies.[31,107] Choriocarcinoma occurring after a normal pregnancy might be an intramyometrial metastasis from a small intraplacental choriocarcinoma.[44,53]

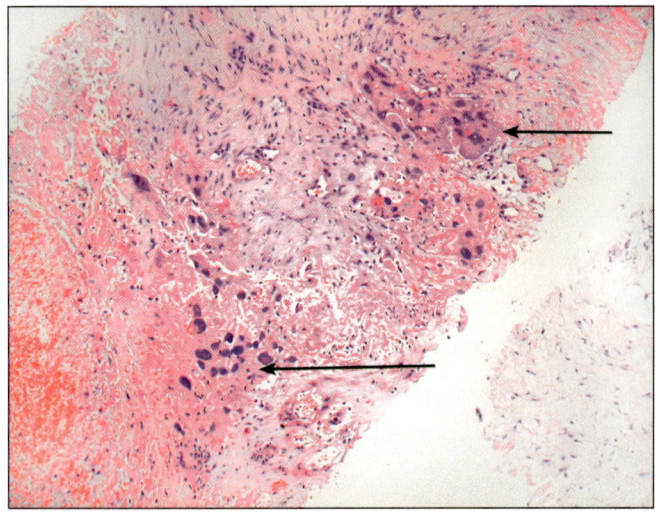

Fig. 32.44 An extensive pelvic tumor with extensive hemorrhage and necrosis. Only small foci of viable tumor cells (arrows) can be identified.

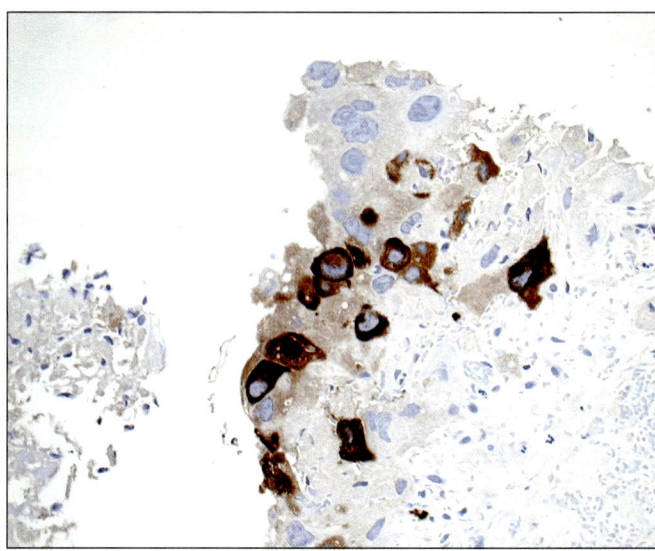

Fig. 32.46 Occasional tumor cells are positive for hPL.

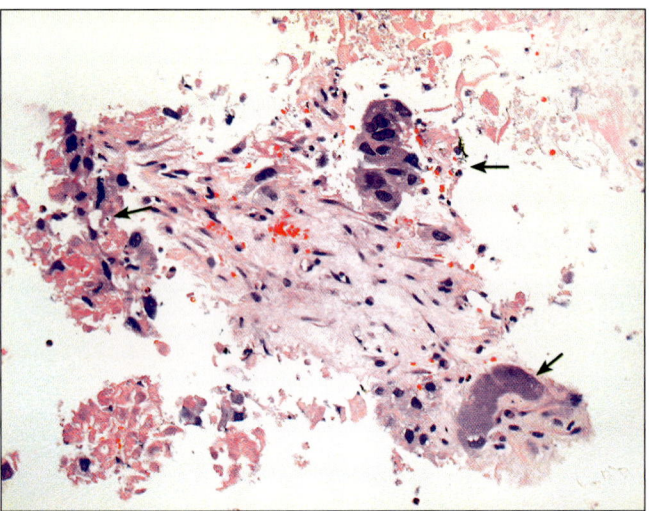

Fig. 32.45 Fragments of choriocarcinomatous cells (arrows) spread throughout abdomen.

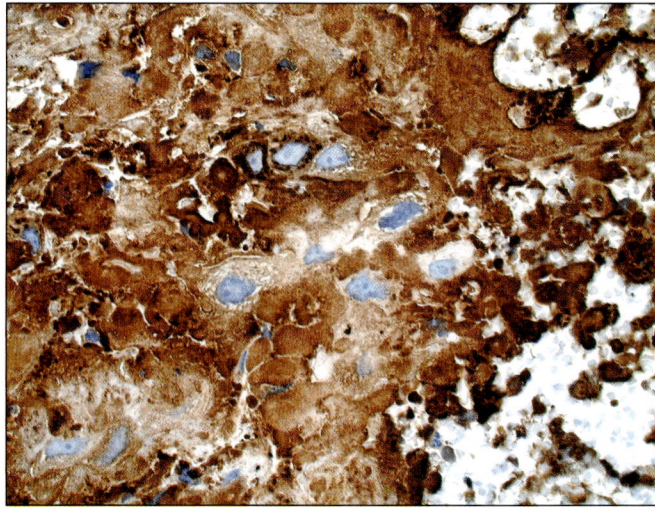

Fig. 32.47 The tumor cells are extensively positive for hCG.

Comparative genomic hybridization studies show similar chromosomal imbalances in three-fourths of choriocarcinomas with consistent amplification of 7q21–q31 and loss of 8p12–p21 detected.[1] Recently, a suppressor gene, identified as NECC1 (not expressed in choriocarcinoma clone 1), has been found.[4,95] Normal placental villi abundantly express it, but not choriocarcinoma cell lines and most surgically removed choriocarcinoma tissue samples. When transfected into choriocarcinoma cell lines, remarkable alterations occur in cell morphology and suppression of *in vivo* tumorigenesis. Induction of chorionic hormones by transfection of this gene showed differentiation of choriocarcinoma cells to syncytiotrophoblast-like cells, suggesting that loss of NECC1 expression is involved in malignant conversion of placental trophoblasts.[95]

Significant chromosomal gains or deletions have been detected in the majority of choriocarcinomas by CGH analysis.[1]

Diagnostic problems

Choriocarcinoma should be distinguished from invasive mole, PSTT, ETT, and non-gestational choriocarcinoma (germ cell tumor). Moreover, ectopic hCG production may also be found in carcinomas of the lung, kidney, and breast, melanomas and lymphoma.[110,133]

Postpartum choriocarcinoma probably originates from asymptomatic intraplacental choriocarcinomas (Figure 32.48).[14,44] When small, it may appear as an incidental finding as a hemorrhagic nodule in an otherwise normal third trimester placenta with no adverse effects on mother or baby. About half of the cases may present as metastatic maternal disease.[123] Occasionally, disseminated fatal infantile choriocarcinoma may occur. Macroscopic examination of the placenta appears unremarkable or may resemble a placental infarct or 'blood clot'.[7,66] Histologically, some villi adjacent to the choriocarcinoma may be covered focally or completely by neoplastic tro-

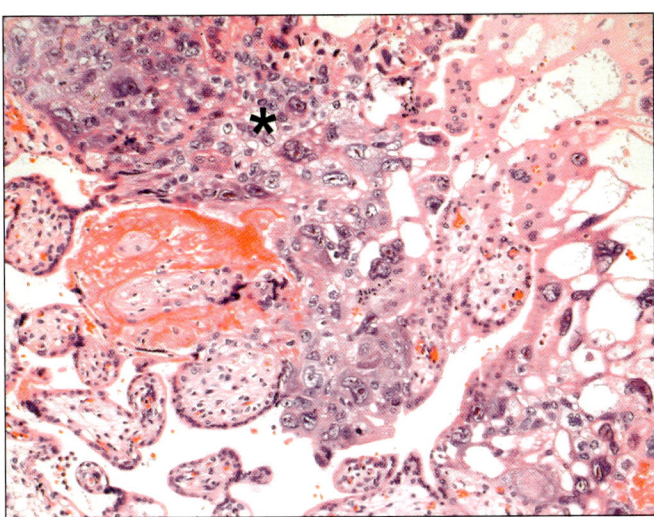

Fig. 32.48 Tiny intraplacental choriocarcinoma (asterisk) found in retrospective examination of macroscopically normal placenta after diagnosis of postpartum choriocarcinoma established.

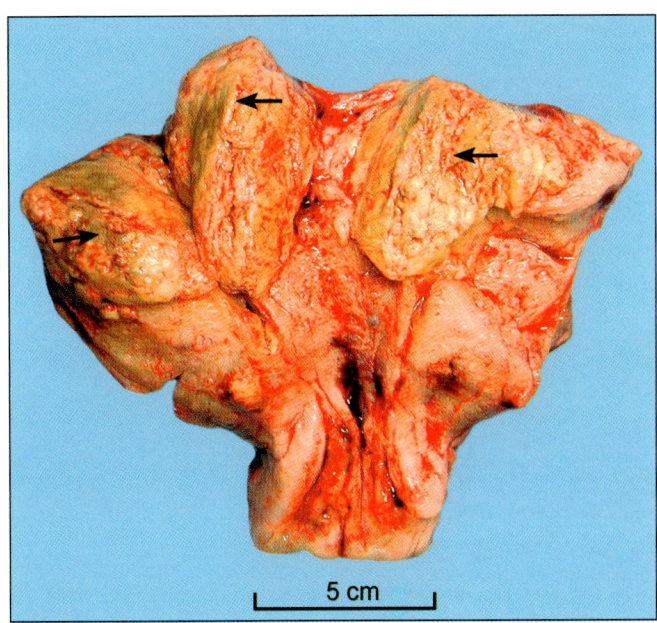

5 cm

Fig. 32.49 Multiple intramyometrial nodules (arrows) in a case of PSTT.

phoblast, but are not neoplastic. The presence of chorionic villi is only acceptable at such an early stage of choriocarcinoma without violating the diagnosis. On the other hand, most intraplacental choriocarcinomas support the view that the tumor arises from villous trophoblast.

It is essential that thorough microscopic examination be performed on all curetted specimens of all gestational ages.[48] Timely diagnosis is prognostically important since intraplacental choriocarcinomas can give rise to both maternal and fetal metastases during pregnancy. A patient with an incidentally discovered intraplacental choriocarcinoma should be extensively investigated for evidence of metastases with serial hCG measurements in both mother and child.

PLACENTAL SITE TROPHOBLASTIC TUMOR

Clinical presentation

Placental site trophoblastic tumor (PSTT) is a neoplasm composed predominantly of intermediate trophoblast. The patients are usually in the reproductive age group, their ages ranging from 20 to 62 (average 32) years.[6] There may be a clinical history of amenorrhea or abnormal bleeding.[29,55,82] In a recent review involving a large number of patients, about 80% of the tumors were diagnosed at stage 1, occurring on an average of 34 months after the last known gestation.

Macroscopic features

The macroscopic features of PSTT are variable. The tumors are on average 5 cm in greatest dimension. The tumor may appear as an ill-defined or well-circumscribed nodule in the myometrium with or without endometrial protrusion (Figure 32.49). It may be tan or yellow with foci of necrosis, but rarely shows conspicuous hemorrhage.

Microscopic features

Microscopically, the tumor consists of a diffuse monomorphic population of mononuclear trophoblast as solid aggregates, sheets, and irregular cords (Figures 32.50 and 32.51). The tumor cells have irregular nuclear membranes, hyperchromatic

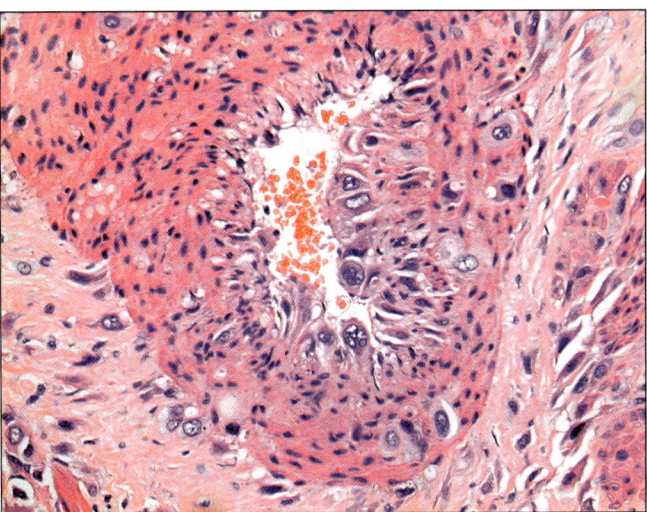

Fig. 32.50 Neoplastic intermediate trophoblast of placental site type replacing endothelium in PSTT.

nuclei, and dense eosinophilic to amphophilic cytoplasm (Figure 32.52). The biphasic pattern of choriocarcinoma is absent although occasional multinucleated cells may be found. Chorionic villi are absent. The tumor cells infiltrate between myometrial bundles typically without destroying the myometrial cells. They also frequently permeate the vascular endothelium, and exhibit abundant extracellular eosinophilic fibrinoid material (Figure 32.53). The tumor cells are strongly and extensively reactive for hPL (Figure 32.54) while hCG reactivity is focal and relatively weak (Figure 32.55). Like other trophoblastic tumors, PSTT cells are usually immunoreactive for inhibin (Figure 32.56). The cytologic appearance and immunophenotype of the PSTT tumor cells are compatible with intermediate trophoblast of placental site type.[83] The Ki-67 index in PSTT (mean 14%) is significantly higher than that in the

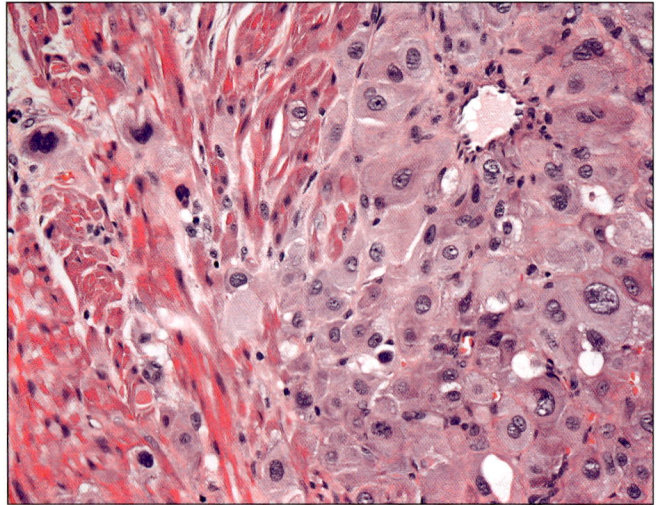

Fig. 32.51 Confluent mass of neoplastic intermediate trophoblast replaces myometrium in PSTT.

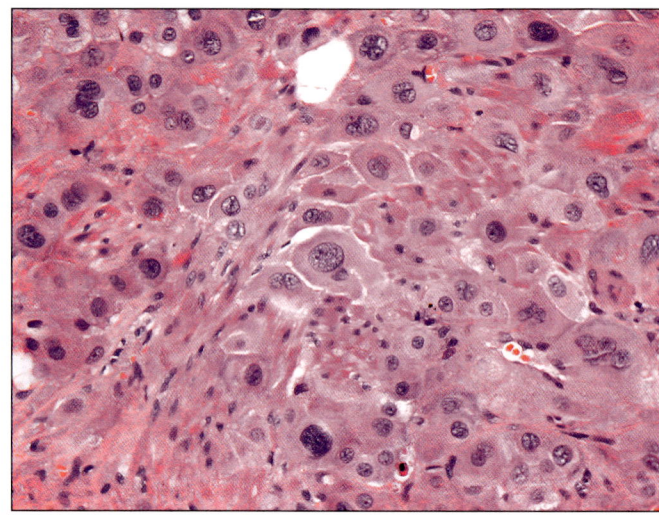

Fig. 32.52 Some PSTT cells had relatively eosinophilic cytoplasm.

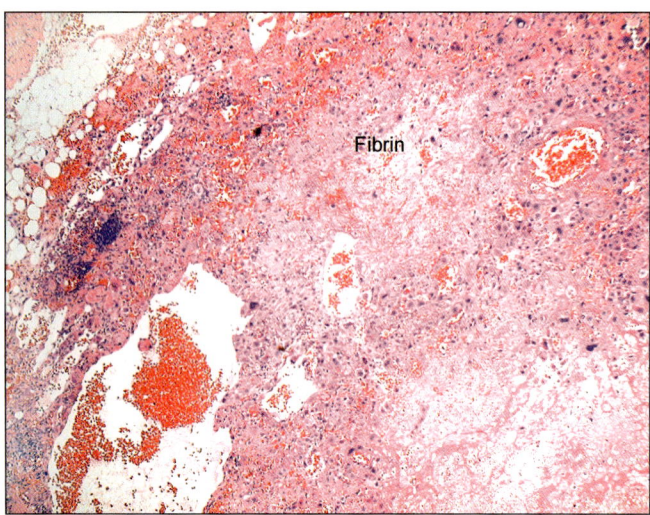

Fig. 32.53 Abundant fibrinoid deposit in metastatic foci of PSTT in lymph nodes.

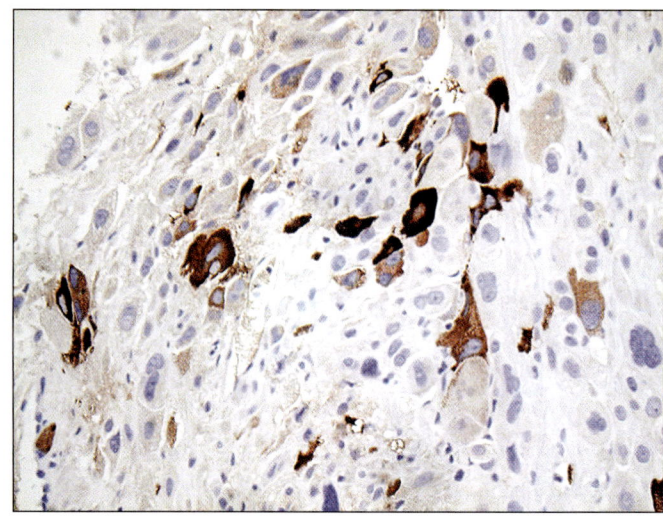

Fig. 32.54 Trophoblastic tumor cells in PSTT immunoreactive for hPL.

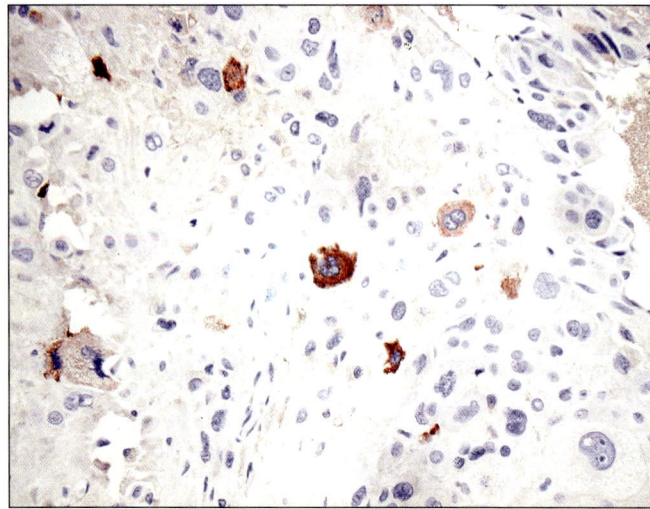

Fig. 32.55 Few PSTT cells immunoreactive for hCG.

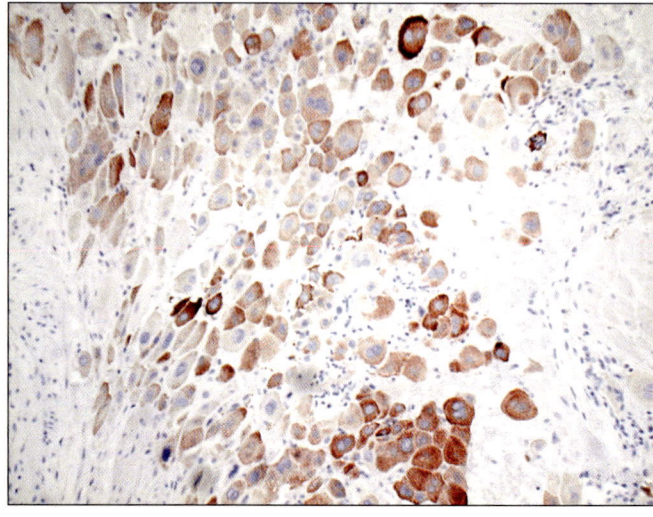

Fig. 32.56 Trophoblastic tumor cells in PSTT cells immunoreactive for inhibin.

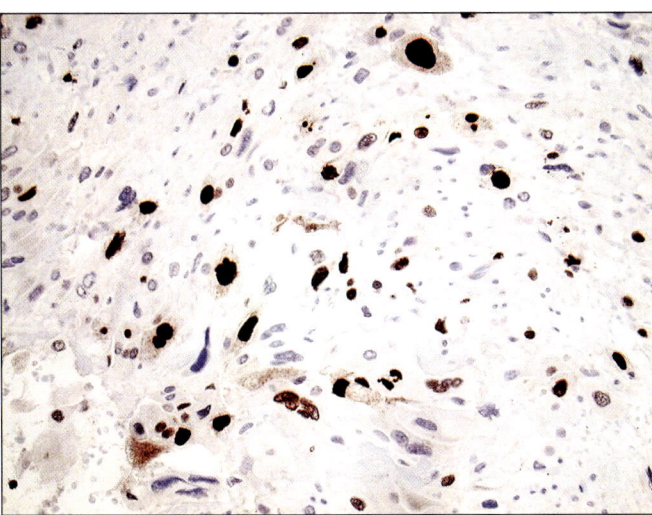

Fig. 32.57 Numerous trophoblastic tumor cells in PSTT immunoreactive for MIB1 (Ki-67), a proliferation marker.

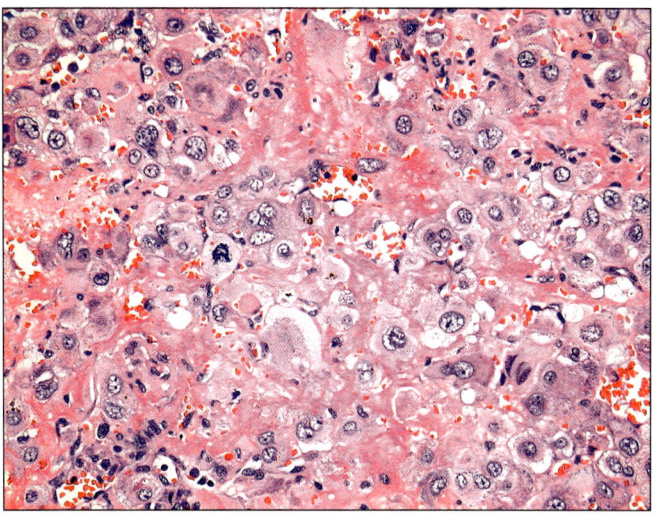

Fig. 32.59 PSTT: detail showing monomorphic cells with copious cytoplasm.

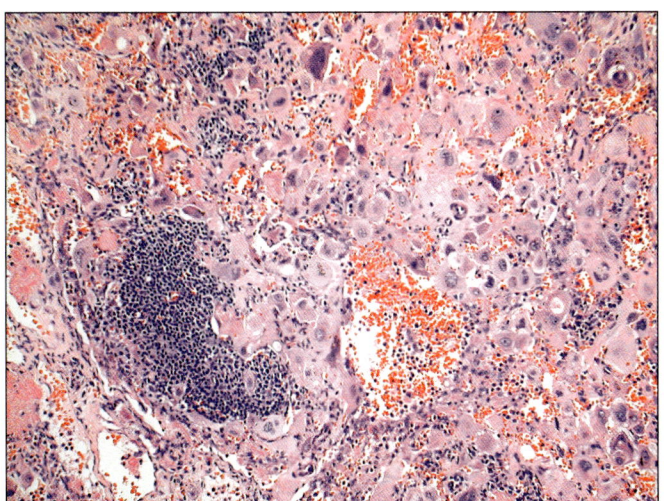

Fig. 32.58 Metastatic PSTT in lymph nodes may poise diagnostic difficulty for pathologists not suspecting the diagnosis.

exaggerated placental site reaction (mean <5%) (Figure 32.57).[129]

Clinical behavior

PSTT is often a self-limiting disease, even for cases with deep myometrial invasion. Some patients are cured by curettage only. However, some PSTT are aggressive with widespread metastasis. The most common metastatic sites are lungs, liver, and vagina (Figures 32.58 and 32.59). Lymph nodes may also be involved. Histologic identification may be a problem for the unwary, especially in cases where the histologic features are masked by extensive fibrin deposit. Hysterectomy is the primary mode of treatment in most cases. However, chemotherapy can still play a major role when curative surgery is not feasible.

Significant factors associated with adverse survival are age over 35 years, interval since the last pregnancy of over 2 years, deep myometrial invasion, stage 3 or 4, maximum hCG level >1000 mIU/mL, extensive coagulative necrosis, high mitotic rate (>5 mitoses per 10 high-power fields), and the presence of cells with clear cytoplasm.[6,33,57]

PSTT is occasionally associated with glomerular disease[29,161] and the patients may develop proteinuria. Renal biopsies show eosinophilic deposits in the capillary lumens immunoreactive for fibrinogen and immunoglobulin M (IgM).

Pathogenesis

By demonstrating alleles in PSTT and ETT that are not present in adjacent normal uterine tissue, Oldt et al. have demonstrated molecular evidence that placental site trophoblastic tumors and epithelioid trophoblastic tumors are of fetal (trophoblastic) origin.[105] PSTT and ETT seem to be more common after female gestations.[62] Since the male has only one X chromosome of maternal origin, it is possible that the paternal X chromosome may play a role in development of such tumors. Most reports on genetic studies on PSTT using comparative genomic hybridization reported the absence of detectable chromosomal gain or loss.[63,157] This is probably related to the resolution power of this genetic analysis approach. In occasional cases, regional gains have been found at 21q11–q21.[63]

Diagnostic problems

Pathologists often need to distinguish PSTT from exaggerated placental site reaction. Histologic features in favor of the latter include absence of a mass-forming lesion, the presence of normal chorionic villi, and proliferating mononuclear intermediate trophoblasts admixed evenly with multinucleated trophoblasts. In difficult cases, Ki-67 immunostaining can be helpful: a low level of Ki-67 labeling (1%) is seen in an exaggerated placental site, whereas PSTT generally shows a higher index (>10%) (Figure 32.57).[61]

PSTT may be difficult to distinguish from poorly differentiated carcinoma and sarcomas, especially epithelioid leiomyosarcomas, choriocarcinoma, melanoma, and even exaggerated placental site reaction. This may be particularly problematic in the clinical situation when frozen section diagnosis of an unknown intrauterine lesion is necessary. Helpful clues to the diagnosis are the characteristic pattern of blood vessel invasion and preserved bundles of myometrial cells split apart by invasive tumor cells, as well as extensive fibroid deposition of fibrinoid material. Chorionic villi are absent. Rarely, a trophoblastic tumor with histologic features of both choriocarcinoma and PSTT occurs.[133]

Separation of PSTT from the epithelioid smooth muscle tumor, although rare, can be difficult. Immunohistochemical studies for hPL, HLA-G, α-inhibin, cytokeratin 18, and various smooth muscle markers can be helpful.

EPITHELIOID TROPHOBLASTIC TUMOR

Definition
Epithelioid trophoblastic tumor (ETT) is a neoplastic growth composed of a relatively uniform population of mononucleate intermediate trophoblastic cells of the type found in the chorion laeve.

Clinical presentation
Patients are usually of reproductive age and present with abnormal vaginal bleeding. Occasionally, ETT may first present at extrauterine sites, such as the lungs, following a hydatidiform mole, invasive mole, or even term pregnancy.[56] Serum hCG levels are usually mildly elevated. Occasionally, ETT may coexist with choriocarcinoma or PSTT.[126]

Macroscopic features
Epithelioid trophoblastic tumor in the uterus usually appears as a discrete, hemorrhagic, solid, and cystic lesion (Figure 32.60). It may be found in the fundus, lower uterine segment, or endocervix. It can also be found in unusual sites such as the broad ligament.[80]

Microscopic features
Microscopically, a relatively uniform population of mononuclear trophoblastic cells appears in the form of nests and solid masses surrounded by extensive necrosis and a hyaline-like matrix (Figure 32.61), the resulting 'geographic' pattern being characteristic. The tumor cells have eosinophilic or clear cytoplasm and round nuclei (Figure 32.62) and are focally immunoreactive for hPL, hCG, cytokeratin, and α-inhibin (Figure 32.63), features of intermediate trophoblastic cells in the chorion laeve. The Ki-67 index in ETT is usually lower than that in choriocarcinoma but higher than that in the placental site nodule.

Diagnostic problems
The monomorphic growth pattern of ETT can distinguish it from choriocarcinoma, which exhibits a biphasic pattern of syncytiotrophoblast and cytotrophoblast. Compared with PSTT that grows with an infiltrative pattern, ETT grows in a nodular fashion. Moreover, ETT cells are relatively smaller and display less nuclear pleomorphism.

In some cases, ETT may replace the endocervical tissue, mimicking a primary cervical cancer. The hyaline-like material in ETT resembles keratin and the tumor can be erroneously diagnosed as a keratinizing squamous cell carcinoma of the cervix. It may even mimic high-grade squamous intraepithelial lesions if the neoplastic cells focally replace the endocervical surface and glandular epithelium.[32]

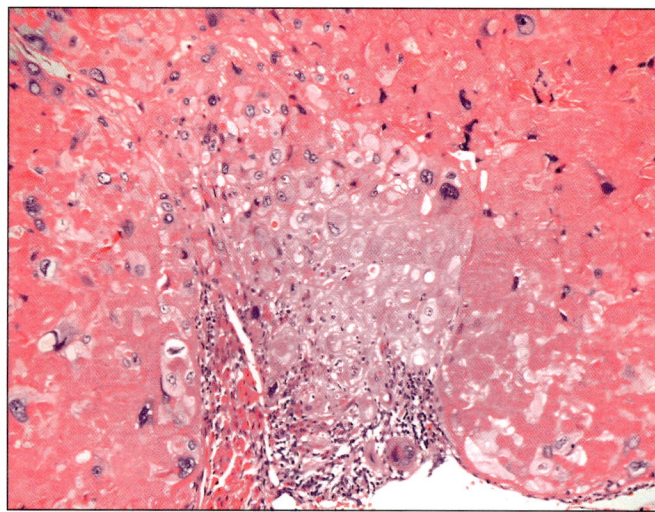

Fig. 32.61 An epithelioid trophoblastic tumor with abundant fibrin deposit.

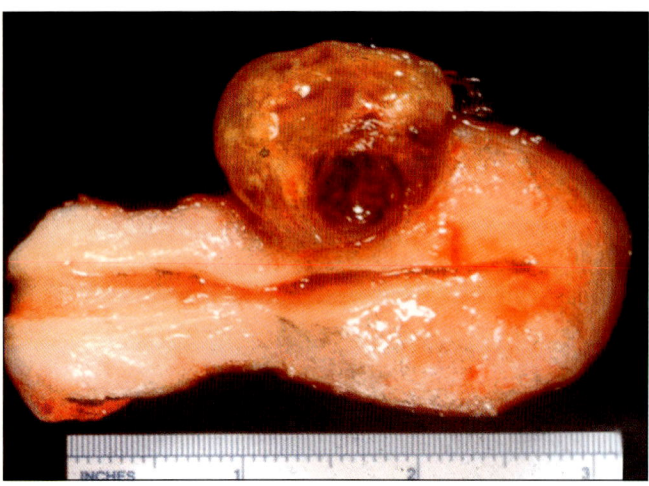

Fig. 32.60 Epithelioid trophoblastic tumor, localized in the lower uterine segment, invading the myometrium. Courtesy of Dr M Martel, Department of Pathology, Yale University, New Haven, CT.

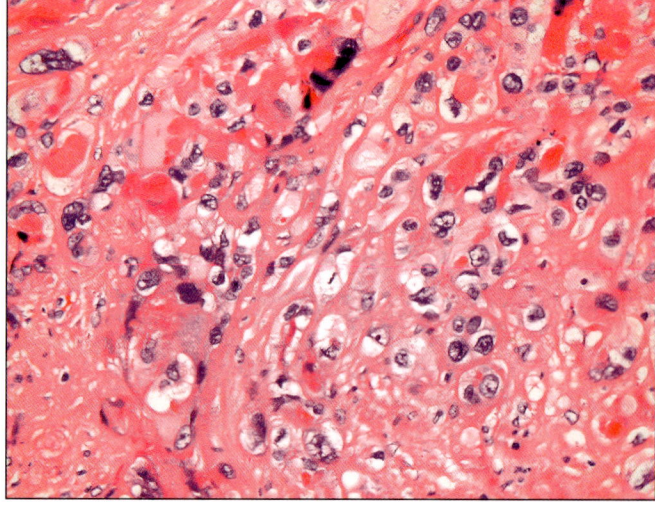

Fig. 32.62 Epithelioid trophoblastic tumor cells with bland cytology, resembling intermediate trophoblast of chorion type.

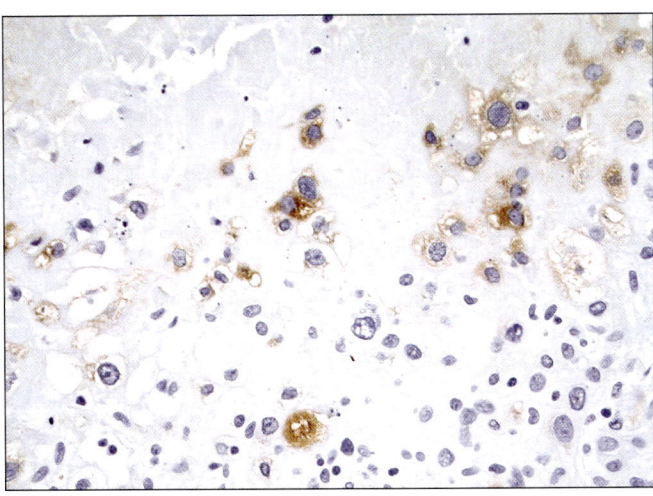

Fig. 32.63 Epithelioid trophoblastic tumor cells immunoreactive for inhibin.

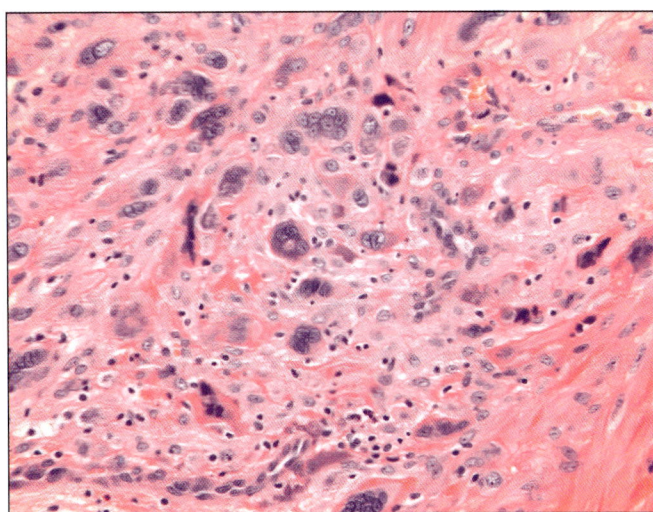

Fig. 32.64 Aggregates of intermediate trophoblast in a placental site with occasional multinucleated cells.

Epithelioid trophoblastic tumor should also be distinguished from non-neoplastic lesions of intermediate trophoblast including exaggerated placental site reaction and placental site nodule. While such non-neoplastic lesions of intermediate trophoblast are considered benign, rare cases will show extrauterine spread.[5]

Clinical behavior
Epithelioid trophoblastic tumor is a rare, though distinctive, gestational trophoblastic tumor.[25,56,71,77,104,126,128] It can behave in a malignant fashion, although it is less aggressive than choriocarcinoma and resembles more closely PSTT behavior.

TROPHOBLASTIC LESIONS, MISCELLANEOUS

EXAGGERATED PLACENTAL SITE

In this reactive lesion, there is florid infiltration of the endometrium and myometrium at the implantation site by populations of intermediate trophoblast and sometimes syncytiotrophoblast.[131] Its former name, syncytial endometritis, is no longer used since the lesion is not inflammatory, not confined to the endometrium or composed mainly of syncytiotrophoblast.[66] It can be found in association with normal pregnancy, abortion or hydatidiform mole. Despite the extensive infiltration by trophoblastic cells, endometrial and myometrial architecture are preserved. Histologic elements associated with pregnancy such as decidua or villi may be found, but confluent masses and necrosis are not (Figure 32.64). Trophoblast may occasionally permeate the blood vessels (Figure 32.65). Mitotic activity is rare or absent in the trophoblastic cells and the Ki-67 index is low. The histologic distinction between PSTT and an exaggerated placental site can be difficult. The low Ki-67 labeling index in the latter supports the diagnosis of exaggerated placental site.[129]

PLACENTAL SITE NODULES OR PLAQUES

Placental site nodules or plaques are occasionally found in patients of the reproductive age group. The patients may have

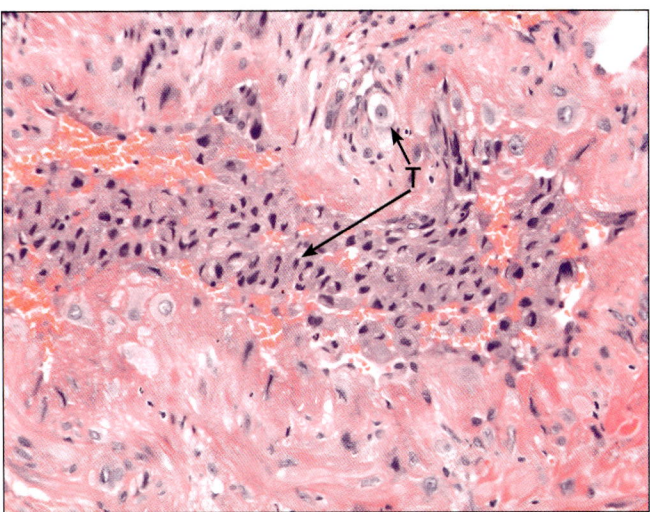

Fig. 32.65 Embolic trophoblast in a blood vessel in a placental site.

endometrial curettage or aspirate due to menorrhagia or irregular uterine bleeding when the lesion is discovered in the endometrial sample. Sometimes, it is an incidental finding in a hysterectomy specimen. The nodules are single or multiple, well-circumscribed plaques that are extensively hyalinized (Figures 32.66 and 32.67).[67] Cellularity varies and the lesional cells have abundant cytoplasm that is amphophilic, eosinophilic or occasionally vacuolated. The nuclei have irregular outlines. Mitotic figures are usually absent or rare.[135,160] The trophoblastic cells are reactive for cytokeratin, placental-like alkaline phosphatase (PLAP), hPL, and pregnancy-specific beta-1 glycoprotein (SP1). Occasional cells may be reactive for hCG and epithelial membrane antigen (EMA).

Differential diagnosis of lesions derived from intermediate trophoblast
More than one subpopulation of intermediate trophoblast with distinctive morphologic and immunohistochemical features give rise to different neoplastic and non-neoplastic lesions.[131]

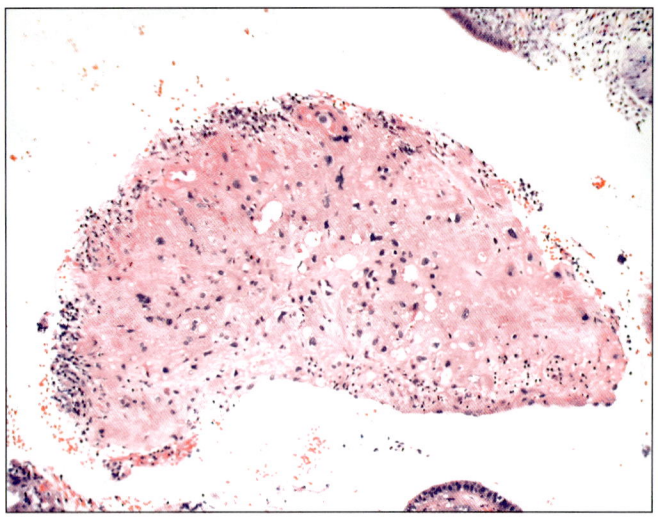

Fig. 32.66 Placental site nodule. A small hyalinized nodule with trophoblast lies adjacent to non-diagnostic endometrium. The patient's last pregnancy was 3 years before.

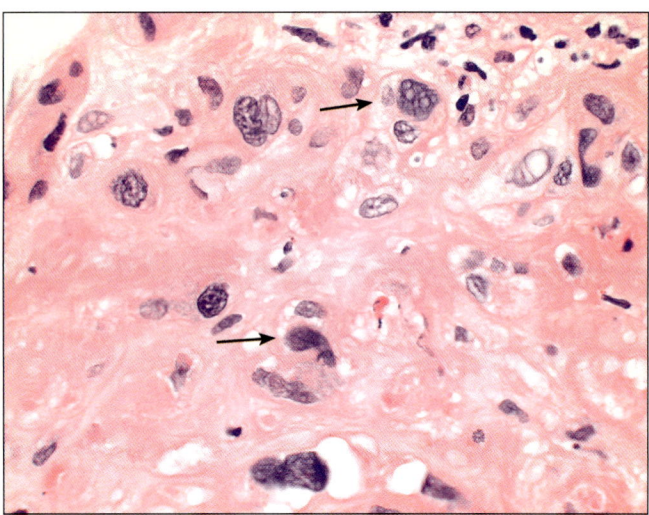

Fig. 32.67 Placental site nodule. Higher magnification showing intermediate trophoblasts (arrows) in the nodule.

Implantation site intermediate trophoblast accounts for exaggerated placental site and its neoplastic counterpart, PSTT, while chorionic-type intermediate trophoblast is related to placental site nodule and its neoplastic counterpart, ETT. Villous intermediate trophoblast may contribute to choriocarcinoma.

UNCLASSIFIED TROPHOBLASTIC LESIONS

Unclassified trophoblastic lesions refer to unusual cases of gestational trophoblastic lesions that cannot be specifically placed in well-established subgroups of GTD. For instance, some lesions with macroscopic features of a hydatidiform mole lack abnormal trophoblastic proliferation. Other lesions exhibit abnormal trophoblastic activity but only non-molar villi are found.

Diagnostic problems

A difficult diagnostic dilemma is the presence of trophoblastic proliferation in the absence of detectable villi or characteristic features of choriocarcinoma or PSTT.

If trophoblasts, whether cytotrophoblast or syncytiotrophoblast, are found in the absence of discernable chorionic villi in the uterine curettage from a patient with a recent diagnosis of hydatidiform mole, residual trophoblastic disease should be diagnosed. In contrast, if found in a curettage obtained after a normal pregnancy or non-molar abortion, a better diagnosis is 'trophoblast suspicious for but not diagnostic of choriocarcinoma'. Careful clinical follow-up with serum hCG assays should resolve the problem.

Occasionally, trophoblast, predominantly intermediate trophoblast, with or without associated chorionic villi, may be found at extrauterine sites, especially the lungs, vagina or pelvic wall. While villous 'metastasis' occurs almost exclusively in association with invasive mole, non-molar villi may occasionally deport, although these extrauterine lesions usually regress.

SUMMARY

GTD is a heterogeneous group of diseases with different clinical, morphologic, and biologic characteristics. Recent advances have been in the discovery of the epithelioid trophoblastic tumor and recognition that intermediate trophoblast gives rise to various categories of neoplastic and non-neoplastic lesions. With advances in ultrasound investigation and alertness of patients, histologic distinction between hydropic abortion and partial mole, and between complete and partial moles, especially at early gestational age, may be difficult. Moreover, histopathology has a limited role in predicting prognosis of GTD, in particular hydatidiform mole. New immunohistochemical markers and molecular techniques are now available to facilitate the diagnosis of cases with histopathologic dilemma. Such adjunct laboratory investigations may also help predict the progress of GTD and enhance better patient management.

REFERENCES

1. Ahmed MN, Kim K, Haddad B, Berchuck A, Qumsiyeh MB. Comparative genomic hybridization studies in hydatidiform moles and choriocarcinoma: amplification of 7q21–q31 and loss of 8p12–p21 in choriocarcinoma. Cancer Genet Cytogenet 2000;116:10–15.
2. Allen JE, King MR, Farrar DF, Miller DS, Schorge JO. Postmolar surveillance at a trophoblastic disease center that serves indigent women. Am J Obstet Gynecol 2003;188:1151–3.
3. Amezcua CA, Bahador A, Naidu YM, Felix JC. Expression of human telomerase reverse transcriptase, the catalytic subunit of telomerase, is associated with the development of persistent disease in complete hydatidiform moles. Am J Obstet Gynecol 2001;184:1441–6.
4. Asanoma K, Kato H, Inoue T, Matsuda T, Wake N. Analysis of a candidate gene associated with growth suppression of choriocarcinoma and differentiation of trophoblasts. J Reprod Med 2004;49:617–26.
5. Baergen RN, Rutgers J, Young RH. Extrauterine lesions of intermediate trophoblast. Int J Gynecol Pathol 2003;22:362–7.
6. Baergen RN, Rutgers JL, Young RH, Osann K, Scully RE. Placental site trophoblastic tumor: a study of 55 cases and review of the literature emphasizing factors of prognostic significance. Gynecol Oncol 2006;100:511–20.
7. Barghorn A, Bannwart F, Stallmach T. Incidental choriocarcinoma confined to a near-term placenta. Virchows Arch 1998;433:89–91.
8. Batorfi J, Fulop V, Kim JH, et al. Osteopontin is down-regulated in hydatidiform mole. Gynecol Oncol 2003;89:134–9.

9. Berkowitz RS, Cramer DW, Bernstein MR, et al. Risk factors for complete molar pregnancy from a case-control study. Am J Obstet Gynecol 1985;152:1016–20.
10. Briese J, Oberndorfer M, Schulte HM, Loning T, Bamberger AM. Osteopontin expression in gestational trophoblastic diseases: correlation with expression of the adhesion molecule, CEACAM1. Int J Gynecol Pathol 2005;24:271–6.
11. Burton JL, Lidbury EA, Gillespie AM, et al. Over-diagnosis of hydatidiform mole in early tubal ectopic pregnancy. Histopathology 2001;38:409–17.
12. Cameron B, Gown AM, Tamimi HK. Expression of c-erb B-2 oncogene product in persistent gestational trophoblastic disease. Am J Obstet Gynecol 1994;170:1616–21.
13. Cheung AN. Gestational trophoblastic diseases. In: Ho FCS, Wu PC, eds. Topics in Pathology for Hong Kong. Hong Kong: Hong Kong University Press; 1995:147–63.
14. Cheung AN. Pathology of gestational trophoblastic diseases. Best Pract Res Clin Obstet Gynaecol 2003;17:849–68.
15. Cheung AN, Khoo US, Lai CY, et al. Metastatic trophoblastic disease after an initial diagnosis of partial hydatidiform mole: genotyping and chromosome in situ hybridization analysis. Cancer 2004;100:1411–17.
16. Cheung AN, Ngan HY, Collins RJ, Wong YL. Assessment of cell proliferation in hydatidiform mole using monoclonal antibody MIB1 to Ki-67 antigen. J Clin Pathol 1994;47:601–4.
17. Cheung AN, Shen DH, Khoo US, Wong LC, Ngan HY. p21WAF1/CIP1 expression in gestational trophoblastic disease: correlation with clinicopathological parameters, and Ki67 and p53 gene expression. J Clin Pathol 1998;51:159–62.
18. Cheung AN, Sit AS, Chung LP, et al. Detection of heterozygous XY complete hydatidiform mole by chromosome in situ hybridization. Gynecol Oncol 1994;55:386–92.
19. Cheung AN, Srivastava G, Chung LP, et al. Expression of the p53 gene in trophoblastic cells in hydatidiform moles and normal human placentas. J Reprod Med 1994;39:223–7.
20. Cheung AN, Srivastava G, Pittaluga S, et al. Expression of c-myc and c-fms oncogenes in trophoblastic cells in hydatidiform mole and normal human placenta. J Clin Pathol 1993;46:204–7.
21. Cheung AN, Zhang DK, Liu Y, et al. Telomerase activity in gestational trophoblastic disease. J Clin Pathol 1999;52:588–92.
22. Chiu PM, Liu VW, Ngan HY, Khoo US, Cheung AN. Detection of mitochondrial DNA mutations in gestational trophoblastic disease. Hum Mutat 2003;22:177.
23. Chiu PM, Ngan YS, Khoo US, Cheung AN. Apoptotic activity in gestational trophoblastic disease correlates with clinical outcome: assessment by the caspase-related M30 CytoDeath antibody. Histopathology 2001;38:243–9.
24. Conran RM, Hitchcock CL, Popek EJ, et al. Diagnostic considerations in molar gestations. Hum Pathol 1993;24:41–8.
25. Coulson LE, Kong CS, Zaloudek C. Epithelioid trophoblastic tumor of the uterus in a postmenopausal woman: a case report and review of the literature. Am J Surg Pathol 2000;24:1558–62.
26. Davis JR, Surwit EA, Garay JP, Fortier KJ. Sex assignment in gestational trophoblastic neoplasia. Am J Obstet Gynecol 1984;148:722–5.
27. Devriendt K. Hydatidiform mole and triploidy: the role of genomic imprinting in placental development. Hum Reprod Update 2005;11:137–42.
28. Driscoll SG. Problems and pitfalls in the histopathologic diagnosis of gestational trophoblastic lesions. J Reprod Med 1987;32:623–8.
29. Eckstein RP, Paradinas FJ, Bagshawe KD. Placental site trophoblastic tumor (trophoblastic pseudotumor): a study of four cases requiring hysterectomy including one fatal case. Histopathology 1982;6:211–26.
30. Elston CW. The histopathology of trophoblastic tumors. J Clin Pathol Suppl (R Coll Pathol) 1976;10:111–31.
31. Elston CW. Trophoblastic tumors of the placenta. In: Fox H, ed. Pathology of the Placenta. London: Saunders; 1976:368–425.
32. Fadare O, Parkash V, Carcangiu ML, Hui P. Epithelioid trophoblastic tumor: clinicopathologic features with an emphasis on uterine cervical involvement. Mod Pathol 2006;19:75–82.
33. Feltmate CM, Genest DR, Wise L, et al. Placental site trophoblastic tumor: a 17-year experience at the New England Trophoblastic Disease Center. Gynecol Oncol 2001;82:415–19.
34. Feng H, Cheung AN, Xue WC, et al. Down-regulation and promoter methylation of tissue inhibitor of metalloproteinase 3 in choriocarcinoma. Gynecol Oncol 2004;94:375–82.
35. Feng HC, Tsao SW, Ngan HY, et al. Differential gene expression identified in complete hydatidiform mole by combining suppression subtractive hybridization and cDNA microarray. Placenta 2006;27:521–6.
36. Feng HC, Tsao SW, Ngan HY, et al. Differential expression of insulin-like growth factor binding protein 1 and ferritin light polypeptide in gestational trophoblastic neoplasia: combined cDNA suppression subtractive hybridization and microarray study. Cancer 2005;104:2409–16.
37. Fisher RA, Hodges MD. Genomic imprinting in gestational trophoblastic disease – a review. Placenta 2003;24(Suppl A):S111–S118.
38. Fisher RA, Hodges MD, Newlands ES. Familial recurrent hydatidiform mole: a review. J Reprod Med 2004;49:595–601.
39. Fisher RA, Lawler SD. Heterozygous complete hydatidiform moles: do they have a worse prognosis than homozygous complete moles? Lancet 1984;2:51.
40. Fisher RA, Newlands ES. Rapid diagnosis and classification of hydatidiform moles with polymerase chain reaction. Am J Obstet Gynecol 1993;168:563–9.
41. Fong PY, Xue WC, Ngan HY, et al. Mcl-1 expression in gestational trophoblastic disease correlates with clinical outcome: a differential expression study. Cancer 2005;103:268–76.
42. Fong PY, Xue WC, Ngan HY, et al. Caspase activity is downregulated in choriocarcinoma: a cDNA array differential expression study. J Clin Pathol 2006;59:179–83.
43. Fox H. Gestational trophoblastic disease. BMJ 1997;314:1363–4.
44. Fox H, Laurini RN. Intraplacental choriocarcinoma: a report of two cases. J Clin Pathol 1988;41:1085–8.
45. Fukunaga M. Immunohistochemical characterization of p57 (KIP2) expression in early hydatidiform moles. Hum Pathol 2002;33:1188–92.
46. Fukunaga M. Immunohistochemical characterization of p57 Kip2 expression in tetraploid hydropic placentas. Arch Pathol Lab Med 2004;128:897–900.
47. Fukunaga M, Katabuchi H, Nagasaka T, et al. Interobserver and intraobserver variability in the diagnosis of hydatidiform mole. Am J Surg Pathol 2005;29:942–7.
48. Fukunaga M, Ushigome S, Fukunaga M, Sugishita M. Application of flow cytometry in diagnosis of hydatidiform moles. Mod Pathol 1993;6:353–9.
49. Fulop V, Colitti CV, Genest D, et al. DOC-2/hDab2, a candidate tumor suppressor gene involved in the development of gestational trophoblastic diseases. Oncogene 1998;17:419–24.
50. Fulop V, Mok SC, Gati I, Berkowitz RS. Recent advances in molecular biology of gestational trophoblastic diseases. A review. J Reprod Med 2002;47:369–79.
51. Fulop V, Mok SC, Genest DR, et al. p53, p21, Rb and mdm2 oncoproteins. Expression in normal placenta, partial and complete mole, and choriocarcinoma. J Reprod Med 1998;43:119–27.
52. Gemer O, Segal S, Kopmar A, Sassoon E. The current clinical presentation of complete molar pregnancy. Arch Gynecol Obstet 2000;264:33–4.
53. Genest DR, Berkowitz RS, Fisher R, et al. Gestational trophoblastic disease. In: Tavassoli FA, Devilee P, eds. World Health Organization Classification of Tumours. Pathology and Genetics. Tumours of Breast and Female Genital Organs. Lyon: IARC Press; 2003:250–6.
54. Gillespie AM, Lidbury EA, Tidy JA, Hancock BW. The clinical presentation, treatment, and outcome of patients diagnosed with possible ectopic molar gestation. Int J Gynecol Cancer 2004;14:366–9.
55. Gloor E, Hurlimann J. Trophoblastic pseudotumor of the uterus: clinicopathologic report with immunohistochemical and ultrastructural studies. Am J Surg Pathol 1981;5:5–13.
56. Hamazaki S, Nakamoto S, Okino T, et al. Epithelioid trophoblastic tumor: morphological and immunohistochemical study of three lung lesions. Hum Pathol 1999;30:1321–7.
57. Hassadia A, Gillespie A, Tidy J, et al. Placental site trophoblastic tumor: clinical features and management. Gynecol Oncol 2005;99:603–7.
58. Heifetz SA, Czaja J. In situ choriocarcinoma arising in partial hydatidiform mole: implications for the risk of persistent trophoblastic disease. Pediatr Pathol 1992;12:601–11.
59. Hertig AT, Edmonds HW. Genesis of hydatidiform mole. Arch Pathol 1940;30:260.
60. Howat AJ, Beck S, Fox H, et al. Can histopathologists reliably diagnose molar pregnancy? J Clin Pathol 1993;46:599–602.
61. Hui P, Martel M, Parkash V. Gestational trophoblastic diseases: recent advances in histopathologic diagnosis and related genetic aspects. Adv Anat Pathol 2005;12:116–25.
62. Hui P, Parkash V, Perkins AS, Carcangiu ML. Pathogenesis of placental site trophoblastic tumor may require the presence of a paternally derived X chromosome. Lab Invest 2000;80:965–72.
63. Hui P, Riba A, Pejovic T, et al. Comparative genomic hybridization study of placental site trophoblastic tumor: a report of four cases. Mod Pathol 2004;17:248–51.
64. Jacobs PA, Szulman AE, Funkhouser J, Matsuura JS, Wilson CC. Human triploidy: relationship between parental origin of the additional haploid complement and development of partial hydatidiform mole. Ann Hum Genet 1982;46:223–31.
65. Jacobs PA, Wilson CM, Sprenkle JA, Rosenshein NB, Migeon BR. Mechanism of origin of complete hydatidiform moles. Nature 1980;286:714–16.
66. Jacques SM, Qureshi F, Doss BJ, Munkarah A. Intraplacental choriocarcinoma associated with viable pregnancy: pathologic features and implications for the mother and infant. Pediatr Dev Pathol 1998;1:380–7.
67. Javey H, Borazjani G, Behmard S, Langley FA. Discrepancies in the histological diagnosis of hydatidiform mole. Br J Obstet Gynaecol 1979;86:480–3.
68. Jun SY, Ro JY, Kim KR. p57kip2 is useful in the classification and differential diagnosis of complete and partial hydatidiform moles. Histopathology 2003;43:17–25.
69. Kajii T, Kurashige H, Ohama K, Uchino F. XY and XX complete moles: clinical and morphologic correlations. Am J Obstet Gynecol 1984;150:57–64.
70. Kajii T, Ohama K. Androgenetic origin of hydatidiform mole. Nature 1977;268:633–4.
71. Kamoi S, Ohaki Y, Mori O, et al. Epithelioid trophoblastic tumor of the uterus: cytological and immunohistochemical observation of a case. Pathol Int 2002;52:75–81.

72. Keep D, Zaragoza MV, Hassold T, Redline RW. Very early complete hydatidiform mole. Hum Pathol 1996;27:708–13.

73. Khong TY. Chorangioma with trophoblastic proliferation. Virchows Arch 2000;436:167–71.

74. Khong TY. Chorangioma with trophoblastic proliferation. Virchows Arch 2000;436:167–71.

75. Kim MJ, Kim KR, Ro JY, Lage JM, Lee HI. Diagnostic and pathogenetic significance of increased stromal apoptosis and incomplete vasculogenesis in complete hydatidiform moles in very early pregnancy periods. Am J Surg Pathol 2006;30:362–9.

76. Kim YT, Cho NH, Ko JH, et al. Expression of cyclin E in placentas with hydropic change and gestational trophoblastic diseases: implications for the malignant transformation of trophoblasts. Cancer 2000;89:673–9.

77. Knox S, Brooks SE, Wong-You-Cheong J, et al. Choriocarcinoma and epithelial trophoblastic tumor: successful treatment of relapse with hysterectomy and high-dose chemotherapy with peripheral stem cell support: a case report. Gynecol Oncol 2002;85:204–8.

78. Koc S, Ozdegirmenci O, Tulunay G, et al. Recurrent partial hydatidiform mole: a report of a patient with three consecutive molar pregnancies. Int J Gynecol Cancer 2006;16:940–3.

79. Konoplev SN, Dimashkieh HH, Stanek J. Cytokeratin immunohistochemistry: a procedure for exclusion of pregnancy in chorionic villi-negative specimen. Placenta 2004;25:146–52.

80. Kuo KT, Chen MJ, Lin MC. Epithelioid trophoblastic tumor of the broad ligament: a case report and review of the literature. Am J Surg Pathol 2004;28:405–9.

81. Kurman RJ, Main CS, Chen HC. Intermediate trophoblast: a distinctive form of trophoblast with specific morphological, biochemical and functional features. Placenta 1984;5:349–69.

82. Kurman RJ, Scully RE, Norris HJ. Trophoblastic pseudotumor of the uterus: an exaggerated form of 'syncytial endometritis' simulating a malignant tumor. Cancer 1976;38:1214–26.

83. Kurman RJ, Young RH, Norris HJ, et al. Immunocytochemical localization of placental lactogen and chorionic gonadotropin in the normal placenta and trophoblastic tumors, with emphasis on intermediate trophoblast and the placental site trophoblastic tumor. Int J Gynecol Pathol 1984;3:101–21.

84. Lage JM, Young RH. Pathology of trophoblastic disease. In: Clement RB, Young RH, eds. Tumors and tumor-like lesions of the uterine corpus and cervix. New York: Churchill Livingstone; 1993:426.

85. Lage JM. Diagnostic dilemmas in gynecologic and obstetric pathology. Semin Diagn Pathol 1990;7:146–55.

86. Lage JM. Gestational trophoblastic tumors: refining histologic diagnoses by using DNA flow and image cytometry. Curr Opin Obstet Gynecol 1994;6:359–63.

87. Lage JM. Gestational trophoblastic diseases. In: Robboy SJ, Anderson MC, Russell P, eds. Pathology of the Female Reproductive Tract. Edinburgh: Churchill Livingstone; 2001:759–81.

88. Lage JM, Mark SD, Roberts DJ, et al. A flow cytometric study of 137 fresh hydropic placentas: correlation between types of hydatidiform moles and nuclear DNA ploidy. Obstet Gynecol 1992;79:403–10.

89. Lai CY, Chan KY, Khoo US, et al. Analysis of gestational trophoblastic disease by genotyping and chromosome in situ hybridization. Mod Pathol 2004;17:40–8.

90. Lane SA, Taylor GR, Quirke P. The diagnosis of molar disease. In: Lowe D, Fox H, eds. Advances in Gynaecological Pathology. Edinburgh: Churchill Livingstone; 1992:235–60.

91. Lawler SD, Fisher RA, Pickthall VJ, Povey S, Evans MW. Genetic studies on hydatidiform moles. I. The origin of partial moles. Cancer Genet Cytogenet 1982;5:309–20.

92. Lawler SD, Povey S, Fisher RA, Pickthall VJ. Genetic studies on hydatidiform moles. II. The origin of complete moles. Ann Hum Genet 1982;46:209–22.

93. Li HW, Cheung AN, Tsao SW, Cheung AL, O WS. Expression of e-cadherin and beta-catenin in trophoblastic tissue in normal and pathological pregnancies. Int J Gynecol Pathol 2003;22:63–70.

94. Li HW, Tsao SW, Cheung AN. Current understandings of the molecular genetics of gestational trophoblastic diseases. Placenta 2002;23:20–31.

95. Matsuda T, Wake N. Genetics and molecular markers in gestational trophoblastic disease with special reference to their clinical application. Best Pract Res Clin Obstet Gynaecol 2003;17:827–36.

96. McCluggage WG, Ashe P, McBride H, Maxwell P, Sloan JM. Localization of the cellular expression of inhibin in trophoblastic tissue. Histopathology 1998;32:252–6.

97. McFadden DE, Kwong LC, Yam IY, Langlois S. Parental origin of triploidy in human fetuses: evidence for genomic imprinting. Hum Genet 1993;92:465–9.

98. Menczer J, Girtler O, Zajdel L, Glezerman M. Metastatic trophoblastic disease following partial hydatidiform mole: case report and literature review. Gynecol Oncol 1999;74:304–7.

99. Messerli ML, Parmley T, Woodruff JD, et al. Inter- and intra-pathologist variability in the diagnosis of gestational trophoblastic neoplasia. Obstet Gynecol 1987;69:622–6.

100. Montes M, Roberts D, Berkowitz RS, Genest DR. Prevalence and significance of implantation site trophoblastic atypia in hydatidiform moles and spontaneous abortions. Am J Clin Pathol 1996;105:411–16.

101. Murdoch S, Djuric U, Mazhar B, et al. Mutations in NALP7 cause recurrent hydatidiform moles and reproductive wastage in humans. Nat Genet 2006;38:300–2.

102. Mutter GL, Pomponio RJ, Berkowitz RS, Genest DR. Sex chromosome composition of complete hydatidiform moles: relationship to metastasis. Am J Obstet Gynecol 1993;168:1547–51.

103. Niemann I, Petersen LK, Hansen ES, Sunde L. Predictors of low risk of persistent trophoblastic disease in molar pregnancies. Obstet Gynecol 2006;107:1006–11.

104. Ohira S, Yamazaki T, Hatano H, et al. Epithelioid trophoblastic tumor metastatic to the vagina: an immunohistochemical and ultrastructural study. Int J Gynecol Pathol 2000;19:381–6.

105. Oldt RJ, III, Kurman RJ, Shih I. Molecular genetic analysis of placental site trophoblastic tumors and epithelioid trophoblastic tumors confirms their trophoblastic origin. Am J Pathol 2002;161:1033–7.

106. Olvera M, Harris S, Amezcua CA, et al. Immunohistochemical expression of cell cycle proteins E2F-1, Cdk-2, Cyclin E, p27(kip1), and Ki-67 in normal placenta and gestational trophoblastic disease. Mod Pathol 2001;14:1036–42.

107. Palmer JR. Advances in the epidemiology of gestational trophoblastic disease. J Reprod Med 1994;39:155–62.

108. Paradinas FJ. The diagnosis and prognosis of molar pregnancy: the experience of the National Referral Centre in London. Int J Gynaecol Obstet 1998;60(Suppl 1):S57–S64.

109. Paradinas FJ, Browne P, Fisher RA, et al. A clinical, histopathological and flow cytometric study of 149 complete moles, 146 partial moles and 107 non-molar hydropic abortions. Histopathology 1996;28:101–10.

110. Paradinas FJ, Elston CW. Gestational trophoblastic diseases. In: Fox H, Wells M, eds. Haines and Taylor Obstetrical and Gynaecological Pathology. Edinburgh: Churchill Livingstone; 2003:1359–1430.

111. Paradinas FJ, Sebire NJ, Fisher RA, et al. Pseudo-partial moles: placental stem vessel hydrops and the association with Beckwith–Wiedemann syndrome and complete moles. Histopathology 2001;39:447–54.

112. Pelkey TJ, Frierson HF, Jr, Mills SE, Stoler MH. Detection of the alpha-subunit of inhibin in trophoblastic neoplasia. Hum Pathol 1999;30:26–31.

113. Petignat P, Laurini R, Goffin F, Bruchim I, Bischof P. Expression of matrix metalloproteinase-2 and mutant p53 is increased in hydatidiform mole as compared with normal placenta. Int J Gynecol Cancer 2006;16:1679–84.

114. Pisal N, Tidy J, Hancock B. Gestational trophoblastic disease: is intensive follow up essential in all women? BJOG 2004;111:1449–51.

115. Qiao S, Nagasaka T, Harada T, Nakashima N. p53, Bax and Bcl-2 expression, and apoptosis in gestational trophoblast of complete hydatidiform mole. Placenta 1998;19:361–9.

116. Redline RW, Hassold T, Zaragoza MV. Prevalence of the partial molar phenotype in triploidy of maternal and paternal origin. Hum Pathol 1998;29:505–11.

117. Reynolds SR. Hydatidiform mole: a vascular congenital anomaly. Obstet Gynecol 1976;47:244–50.

118. Rice LW, Lage JM, Berkowitz RS, Goldstein DP, Bernstein MR. Repetitive complete and partial hydatidiform mole. Obstet Gynecol 1989;74:217–19.

119. Rosai J. Ackerman's Surgical Pathology. St. Louis: Mosby; 1989.

120. Saji F, Tokugawa Y, Kimura T, et al. A new approach using DNA fingerprinting for the determination of androgenesis as a cause of hydatidiform mole. Placenta 1989;10:399–405.

121. Sebire NJ, Fisher RA, Rees HC. Histopathological diagnosis of partial and complete hydatidiform mole in the first trimester of pregnancy. Pediatr Dev Pathol 2003;6:69–77.

122. Sebire NJ, Lindsay I, Fisher RA, Savage P, Seckl MJ. Overdiagnosis of complete and partial hydatidiform mole in tubal ectopic pregnancies. Int J Gynecol Pathol 2005;24:260–4.

123. Sebire NJ, Lindsay I, Fisher RA, Seckl MJ. Intraplacental choriocarcinoma: experience from a tertiary referral center and relationship with infantile choriocarcinoma. Fetal Pediatr Pathol 2005;24:21–9.

124. Sebire NJ, Makrydimas G, Agnantis NJ, et al. Updated diagnostic criteria for partial and complete hydatidiform moles in early pregnancy. Anticancer Res 2003;23:1723–8.

125. Sebire NJ, Rees H, Paradinas F, Seckl M, Newlands E. The diagnostic implications of routine ultrasound examination in histologically confirmed early molar pregnancies. Ultrasound Obstet Gynecol 2001;18:662–5.

126. Shen DH, Khoo US, Ngan HY, et al. Coexisting epithelioid trophoblastic tumor and choriocarcinoma of the uterus following a chemoresistant hydatidiform mole. Arch Pathol Lab Med 2003;127:e291–e293.

127. Shih IM, Kurman RJ. Expression of melanoma cell adhesion molecule in intermediate trophoblast. Lab Invest 1996;75:377–88.

128. Shih IM, Kurman RJ. Epithelioid trophoblastic tumor: a neoplasm distinct from choriocarcinoma and placental site trophoblastic tumor simulating carcinoma. Am J Surg Pathol 1998;22:1393–1403.

129. Shih IM, Kurman RJ. Ki-67 labeling index in the differential diagnosis of exaggerated placental site, placental site trophoblastic tumor, and choriocarcinoma: a double immunohistochemical staining technique using Ki-67 and Mel-CAM antibodies. Hum Pathol 1998;29:27–33.

130. Shih IM, Kurman RJ. Immunohistochemical localization of inhibin-alpha in the placenta and gestational trophoblastic lesions. Int J Gynecol Pathol 1999;18:144–50.

131. Shih IM, Kurman RJ. The pathology of intermediate trophoblastic tumors and tumor-like lesions. Int J Gynecol Pathol 2001;20:31–47.

132. Shih IM, Kurman RJ. p63 expression is useful in the distinction of epithelioid trophoblastic and placental site trophoblastic tumors by profiling trophoblastic subpopulations. Am J Surg Pathol 2004;28:1177–83.

133. Shih IM, Mazur MT, Kurman RJ. Gestational trophoblastic disease and related lesions. In: Kurman RJ, ed. Blaustein's pathology of the female genital tract. New York: Springer Verlag; 2002:1193–224.

134. Shih IM, Seidman JD, Kurman RJ. Placental site nodule and characterization of distinctive types of intermediate trophoblast. Hum Pathol 1999;30:687–94.

135. Silverberg SG, Kurman RJ. Tumors of the uterine corpus and gestational trophoblastic disease. In: Atlas of Tumor Pathology, third series. Fascicle 3. Washington, DC: Armed Force Institute of Pathology; 1992.

136. Singer G, Kurman RJ, McMaster MT, Shih I. HLA-G immunoreactivity is specific for intermediate trophoblast in gestational trophoblastic disease and can serve as a useful marker in differential diagnosis. Am J Surg Pathol 2002;26:914–20.

137. Soundararajan R, Rao AJ. Trophoblast 'pseudo-tumorigenesis': significance and contributory factors. Reprod Biol Endocrinol 2004;2:15.

138. Steigrad SJ. Epidemiology of gestational trophoblastic diseases. Best Pract Res Clin Obstet Gynaecol 2003;17:837–47.

139. Szulman AE, Surti U. The syndromes of hydatidiform mole. I. Cytogenetic and morphologic correlations. Am J Obstet Gynecol 1978;131:665–71.

140. Szulman AE, Surti U. The syndromes of hydatidiform mole. II. Morphologic evolution of the complete and partial mole. Am J Obstet Gynecol 1978;132:20–7.

141. Tasci Y, Dilbaz S, Secilmis O, et al. Routine histopathologic analysis of product of conception following first-trimester spontaneous miscarriages. J Obstet Gynaecol Res 2005;31:579–82.

142. Trask C, Lage JM, Roberts DJ. A second case of 'chorangiocarcinoma' presenting in a term asymptomatic twin pregnancy: choriocarcinoma in situ with associated villous vascular proliferation. Int J Gynecol Pathol 1994;13:87–91.

143. van de Kaa CA, Schijf CP, de Wilde PC, et al. Persistent gestational trophoblastic disease: DNA image cytometry and interphase cytogenetics have limited predictive value. Mod Pathol 1996;9:1007–14.

144. Van den Veyver IB, Al-Hussaini TK. Biparental hydatidiform moles: a maternal effect mutation affecting imprinting in the offspring. Hum Reprod Update 2006;12:233–42.

145. Vassilakos P, Kajii T. Hydatidiform mole: two entities [letter]. Lancet 1976;1:259.

146. Vassilakos P, Riotton G, Kajii T. Hydatidiform mole: two entities. A morphologic and cytogenetic study with some clinical consideration. Am J Obstet Gynecol 1977;127:167–70.

147. Vegh GL, Selcuk TZ, Fulop V, et al. Matrix metalloproteinases and their inhibitors in gestational trophoblastic diseases and normal placenta. Gynecol Oncol 1999;75:248–53.

148. Wake N, Fujino T, Hoshi S, et al. The propensity to malignancy of dispermic heterozygous moles. Placenta 1987;8:319–26.

149. Wake N, Seki T, Fujita H, et al. Malignant potential of homozygous and heterozygous complete moles. Cancer Res 1984;44:1226–30.

150. Wake N, Takagi N, Sasaki M. Androgenesis as a cause of hydatidiform mole. J Natl Cancer Inst 1978;60:51–7.

151. Wielsma S, Kerkmeijer L, Bekkers R, et al. Persistent trophoblast disease following partial molar pregnancy. Aust N Z J Obstet Gynaecol 2006;46:119–23.

152. Wolfberg AJ, Berkowitz RS, Goldstein DP, Feltmate C, Lieberman E. Postevacuation hCG levels and risk of gestational trophoblastic neoplasia in women with complete molar pregnancy. Obstet Gynecol 2005;106:548–52.

153. Wolfberg AJ, Feltmate C, Goldstein DP, Berkowitz RS, Lieberman E. Low risk of relapse after achieving undetectable HCG levels in women with complete molar pregnancy. Obstet Gynecol 2004;104:551–4.

154. Wong SY, Ngan HY, Chan CC, Cheung AN. Apoptosis in gestational trophoblastic disease is correlated with clinical outcome and Bcl-2 expression but not Bax expression. Mod Pathol 1999;12:1025–33.

155. Xue WC, Chan KY, Feng HC, et al. Promoter hypermethylation of multiple genes in hydatidiform mole and choriocarcinoma. J Mol Diagn 2004;6:326–34.

156. Xue WC, Feng HC, Chan KY, et al. Id helix–loop–helix proteins are differentially expressed in gestational trophoblastic disease. Histopathology 2005;47:303–9.

157. Xue WC, Khoo US, Ngan HY, et al. Minichromosome maintenance protein 7 expression in gestational trophoblastic disease: correlation with Ki67, PCNA and clinicopathological parameters. Histopathology 2003;43:485–90.

158. Xue WC, Khoo US, Ngan HY, et al. c-mos immunoreactivity aids in the diagnosis of gestational trophoblastic lesions. Int J Gynecol Pathol 2004;23:145–50.

159. Yazaki-Sun S, Daher S, de Souza Ishigai MM, et al. Correlation of c-erbB-2 oncogene and p53 tumor suppressor gene with malignant transformation of hydatidiform mole. J Obstet Gynaecol Res 2006;32:265–72.

160. Young RH, Kurman RJ, Scully RE. Placental site nodules and plaques. A clinicopathologic analysis of 20 cases. Am J Surg Pathol 1990;14:1001–9.

161. Young RH, Scully RE, McCluskey RT. A distinctive glomerular lesion complicating placental site trophoblastic tumor: report of two cases. Hum Pathol 1985;16:35–42.

162. Zaragoza MV, Surti U, Redline RW, et al. Parental origin and phenotype of triploidy in spontaneous abortions: predominance of diandry and association with the partial hydatidiform mole. Am J Hum Genet 2000;66:1807–20.

163. Zhang XW, Zhu HB, Wu SY, et al. Distribution of the alleles at loci D16S539, D7S820, and D13S317 in hydatidiform mole genome from Chinese women and its relationship with clinical prognosis. Cancer Genet Cytogenet 2006;164:133–6.

The peritoneum

John H. Eichhorn   Stanley J. Robboy   Rex C. Bentley   Maria Merino   Peter Russell

33

NORMAL PERITONEUM

Knowledge of the peritoneum is important in understanding the pathology of the female genital tract. Its epithelial covering, the mesothelium, shares many features with the progenitor epithelium of tumors arising from the müllerian system. It is also the site of many important diseases in women.

The peritoneum is a nearly continuous membrane that lines the abdominal cavity, thus allowing free movement between the viscera and the abdominal wall. In males, the peritoneal cavity forms a closed system. In females, the peritoneum is an 'open system' in that it is interrupted in the pelvis by the fallopian tubes. The fallopian tubes are potential final conduits for the transmission of pathogens, chemical and biologic, that have ascended through the genital tract from the external environment.

Parietal peritoneum covers the abdominal wall, diaphragm, and anterior surface of the retroperitoneal viscera and pelvis, while the visceral peritoneum ensheaths the intestines and intra-abdominal organs. Mesothelial cells in the peritoneum are morphologically, histochemically, immunocytochemically, and ultrastructurally similar to those found in the pleura and pericardium.[33]

The cells that line the peritoneal cavity and those that form the serosa of the ovary are both of celomic epithelial origin. This has led to discussion of whether tumors and tumor-like lesions of the peritoneum and ovary, i.e., the müllerian epithelial lesions, are the same entity in both locations. It has also led to the introduction of the concept of the so-called 'secondary müllerian system' as a mechanism by which tumors of müllerian histology might arise from the peritoneum.[125] While noteworthy differences exist between the cells lining the peritoneal cavity and those covering the ovary, each is capable of giving rise to müllerian epithelial inclusions, particularly of the serous type.

Normal mesothelium is a single layer of small cells with small central nuclei. Cytoplasm is minimal with crisp, well-defined cell borders. Nucleoli are not apparent.

Immunocytochemistry has proven valuable in characterizing the normal mesothelial cell and features that distinguish it from cells generally considered to be müllerian in origin. This subject is covered in detail below.

On an ultrastructural basis, mesothelial cells show prominent and numerous long microvilli. This is in contrast to many müllerian epithelia, especially serous epithelia, where cilia are obvious by light microscopy and greatly overshadow the slender microvilli. Whereas the microvilli in typical adenocarcinomas tend to be shorter, stubbier and are fewer in number

than those of mesothelial cells, microvilli in adenocarcinomas related to müllerian epithelium may be exceptional in terms of length and complexity. As ultrastructural examination is rarely used today to distinguish between lesions of mesothelial and ovarian origin, this aspect is not discussed further.

Submesothelial mesenchyme anchors the mesothelium to the underlying tissue. A subject that has long been controversial is the role of the submesothelial stromal cell. While early works suggested that these stromal cells contribute to re-epithelialize denuded mesothelium, more recent work indicates that healing of injured serosa progresses by replication and inward migration of the mesothelial cells at the periphery of the wound.[33] This would suggest that the adjacent mesothelial cells actively orchestrate the regeneration of new mesothelial cells and that the subjacent cells do not play an active role in repair. These stromal cells may, however, be important in the development of deciduosis, endometriosis, and disseminated peritoneal leiomyomatosis (see below).

INFLAMMATORY AND REACTIVE LESIONS

Since the introduction of antibiotic use over a half century ago, the problem of peritoneal infection, usually bacterial infection, has diminished greatly. In adult females, most infections are ascending, usually in the form of pelvic inflammatory disease. Peritoneal inflammations that occur in both sexes, such as those caused by appendicitis or diverticulitis, although common, are not covered here. In addition to the acute inflammatory reaction itself, chronic changes may occur, such as are seen in granulomatous and histiocytic reactions. In some cases, the inflammatory process leads to reactive changes.

GRANULOMATOUS PERITONITIS

Granulomas are generally induced by foreign material including keratin, by vernix caseosa or meconium, in the form of necrotic pseudoxanthomatous nodules or as a postcautery reaction.[36]

SUTURE MATERIALS

Foreign-body granulomas are most commonly associated with suture material retained from surgery performed at an earlier time. The sutures may consist of dense hyaline material in varying degrees of disintegration, or translucent threads. The foreign-body component of the granulomas can be highlighted

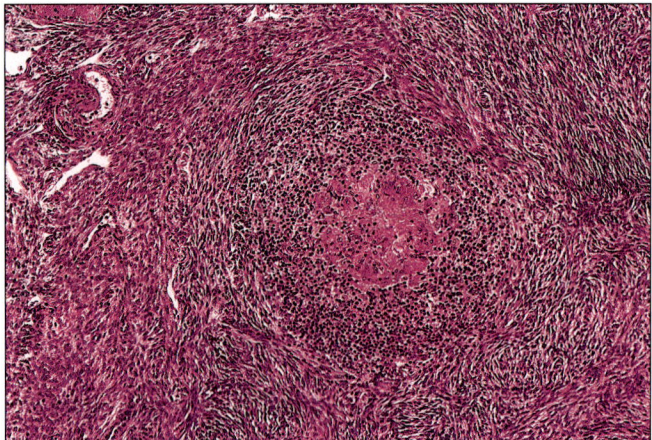

Fig. 33.1 Sarcoidal granuloma. These granulomas lack necrosis.

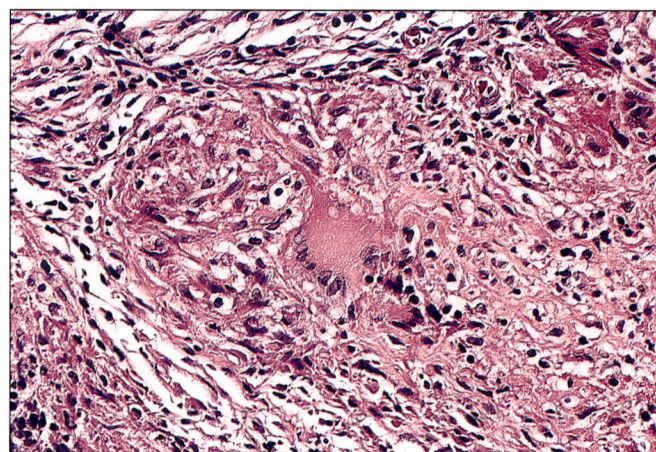

Fig. 33.2 Tuberculous granuloma. Langhans giant cells are present in this biopsy specimen but necrosis is absent.

with polarizing filters. Cellular reaction consists of macrophages, some multinucleated, and lymphocytes. There is both local fibrosis and serosal adhesions.

SURGICAL GLOVE POWDER

Surgical glove powder, either talc or starch-based, is a common cause of granulomas. The widespread peritoneal granulomas may simulate carcinomatosis or tuberculosis at subsequent laparotomy. Usually the starch granulomas resolve within a few months, leaving no residua or only adhesions. Although generally lacking clinical significance, some patients develop chronic fibrosing peritonitis while others suffer an acute illness (abdominal pain and fever) 2–4 weeks postoperatively. Talc, while now carefully modified for surgical use and no longer contaminated with asbestos,[96] is a greater irritant than starch, and is poorly absorbed by some patients. A hypersensitivity reaction may be involved. As well as being surgically introduced, talc and starch may enter the peritoneal cavity by ascending the genital tract, the most usual sources being powder in contraceptives, deodorants, and gloves used for vaginal examination.

Talc granulomas are of the typical foreign-body type. Multinucleated giant cells are usually numerous and contain pleomorphic crystal spicules readily seen with polarized light.

Starch granulomas exhibit several histologic patterns. The most common is a typical foreign-body reaction. Some lesions include prominent polymorphonuclear leukocytes, especially eosinophils, to the extent of forming microabscesses. An uncommon pattern is sarcoid granulomas (Figure 33.1),[19,24] which lack necrosis, or tuberculoid granulomas (Figures 33.2 and 33.3), which variably show necrotic foci. The latter appearance may be misinterpreted as tuberculosis. The presence of starch can usually be suspected with careful focusing in H&E sections by finding 10 µm polyhedral translucent blue-green bodies. Examination with polarized light reveals the pathognomonic Maltese cross. Starch particles can also be stained with periodic acid-Schiff, methenamine silver or Lugols iodine. Since starch is readily introduced by the pathologist during the gross examination of the tissue, its presence exclusively on the surface should be disregarded. Rarely, fat necrosis and rheumatoid-type necrotizing foci are identified as reactions to starch.

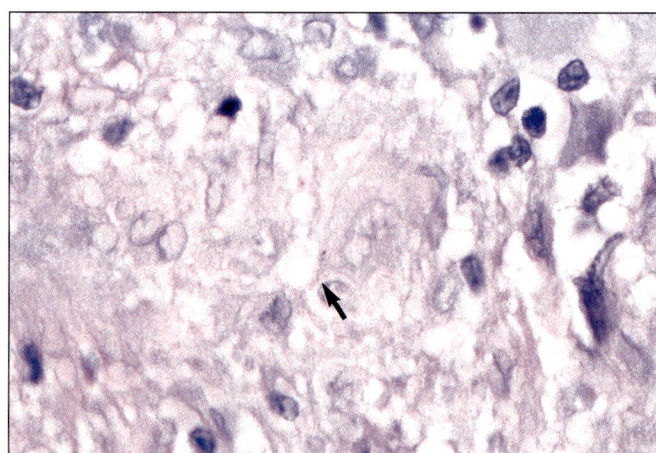

Fig. 33.3 *Mycobacterium tuberculosis.* Only a single rod-shaped organism (arrow) is demonstrable, despite an extensive search (Ziehl–Neelsen).

CONTRAST MEDIA

Peritoneal granulomas may result from exposure to hysterosalpingographic contrast media. Oil-based contrast media absorb slowly from the peritoneal cavity, and lipogranulomas sometimes form. These appear as foreign-body giant cell reactions orientated around clear spherical vacuoles from which lipid has been removed during processing (similar to the pattern seen in lymph nodes following lymphangiograms or cholecystograms). Lipogranulomas may become confluent, and focal necrosis may occur. If uterine or tubal tissue is available for examination, lipogranulomas and foamy macrophages may be evident in the endometrial stroma and tubal lamina propria. Peritoneal granulomas have also been reported, but less frequently, after the use of water-based contrast media.

INTESTINAL CONTENTS

Foreign-body granulomas to intestinal contents may be seen following perforation such as in Crohns disease, diverticulitis or malignant fistulae. These granulomas are generally confined to the serosa, but plant material and barium from a perforated colon may be identified in the wall or subserosal fat.

CYSTIC TERATOMA (DERMOID CYST) RUPTURE

Widespread peritoneal granulomas and adhesions frequently develop if a mature cystic teratoma (dermoid cyst) ruptures. When extruded, the squamous cells, hairs, and sebum typically trigger a local foreign-body reaction in the adjacent ovarian parenchyma. In the peritoneum, however, the incited inflammatory response is often pervasive due to more extensive spread. This phenomenon occurs especially when the teratoma is removed by cystectomy during laparoscopic surgery.[184] On occasion the reaction may also appear as a sclerosing peritonitis (see below).[176]

KERATIN

Peritoneal foreign-body granulomas to keratin may be found in association with endometrial or ovarian adenoacanthomas.[232] Uterine examples are thought to result from retrograde transmission of acellular keratinous debris through the fallopian tubes (Figure 33.4). Occasionally this follows radiotherapy, indicative that the viable glandular component of the tumor has been destroyed with only the non-viable keratin debris or ghost cells remaining. Granulomas have been seen on the serosa of the adnexa, uterus, colon, and appendix. These granulomas are easily misinterpreted as deposits of metastatic carcinoma, and care must be taken to determine whether tumor cells are or are not present. While it would seem that cell-free granulomas should not carry any adverse connotations for the patient, we have seen occasional cases where recurrence followed.

CAUTERIZED TISSUE

Florid foreign-body granulomatous reactions to cauterized tissue in pelvic peritoneal and ovarian biopsies are occasionally encountered in patients who have had endometriotic or other lesions treated in the weeks prior to biopsy. The lesions show central eosinophilic, focally refractile, amorphous material (representing the coagulated tissue and carbonaceous debris), palisaded by large numbers of multinucleated foreign-body giant cells and a peripheral lymphocytic infiltrate (Figure 33.5). Lesions tend to hyalinize with age and may persist for many years.

CESAREAN DELIVERY

Complicating cesarean delivery and occasionally found during a spontaneous vaginal delivery, the amniotic fluid contents may spill into the peritoneal cavity causing a syndrome clinically similar to bowel perforation.[48,221] Amniotic fluid contains squamous cells, keratin, and sometimes lanugo hair. It may also contain meconium, which itself is composed of bile, pancreatic, and intestinal secretions.[75] Grossly, the amniotic fluid contents appear as cheese-like yellow patches limited to the serosal layer of visceral organs.[134] Squamous cells appear as large, relatively solid collections of flattened squamous cells lying one upon another, but without nuclei. The hallmark of meconium peritonitis is calcification, which presumably results from the action of pancreatic enzymes.

TUBERCULOSIS

Tuberculosis, the disease that must always be considered in the differential diagnosis whenever granulomas are found with Langerhans giant cells, is still encountered in the peritoneum, usually in underdeveloped countries or in recent migrants to Western countries.[118,165,212,213,222] It also may occur as a complication of chronic peritoneal dialysis.[1] Clinically, it may manifest non-specifically as any of various abdominal pathologies, not uncommonly as widespread carcinomatosis.[86] The presence of ascites, a pelvic mass, and marked elevation of serum levels of CA125 may lead to a false clinical suspicion of ovarian cancer.[118,165]

HISTIOCYTIC, NON-GRANULOMATOUS PERITONEAL LESIONS

Histiocytic infiltrates rather than discrete granulomas are occasionally found in the peritoneum.[184] Melanin-rich histiocytes are sometimes found in cases where an ovarian dermoid cyst has ruptured. The spillage contains melanin, which the peritoneal histiocytes phagocytose. Grossly, the peritoneum may appear to be stained black or display small tumor-like nodules on its surface. Microscopically, the histiocytes are usually present in a fibrous stroma. The melanin-rich histio-

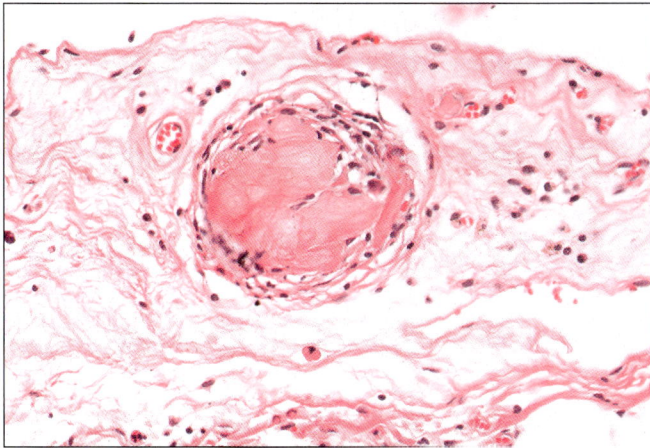

Fig. 33.4 Keratin nodule in omentum. Radiotherapy was used to treat the endometrial adenoacanthoma.

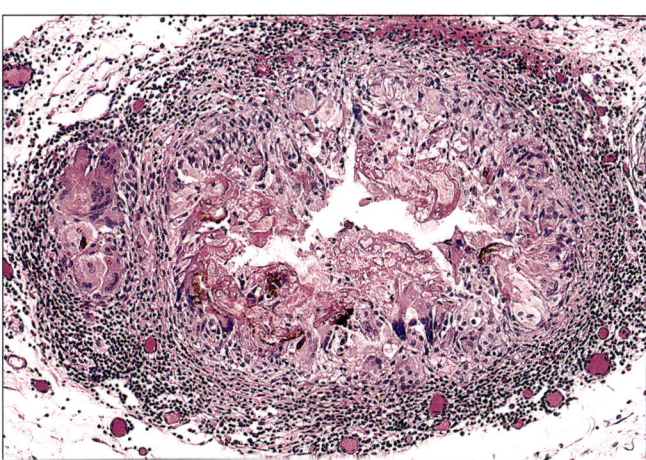

Fig. 33.5 Florid foreign-body granulomatous reactions to cauterized tissue.

cytes lack atypia. Appropriate immunohistochemical stains can further indicate that the cells are histiocytes resembling the dark pigmentation of melanin[109] and not atypical melanocytes.

Occasionally, foci of endometriosis may disclose an abundance of histiocytes filled with ceroid, a wax-like, finely granular, golden to yellow-brown pigment that is a form of lipofuscin, a lipid-containing residue of lysosomal digestion that is considered an aging or 'wear and tear' pigment. Ceroid is believed to be the end result of the breakdown of blood products after removal of iron. These histiocytic foci are sometimes called 'necrotic pseudoxanthomatous nodules'.[32,36,200]

spared. Nodules contain bland, slender, and stellate cells with long tapering cytoplasmic processes throughout. In addition to cytokeratin reactivity, the cells also disclose immunoreactivity for vimentin and smooth muscle actin. The interpretation given to this finding is that the nodules have features of myofibroblasts.[41,214]

Occasionally, sclerosing lesions may be difficult to differentiate from desmoplastic mesothelioma, especially when the biopsy specimen is small. Features that favor a diagnosis of mesothelioma include nuclear atypia, necrosis, organized patterns of collagen deposition (fascicular or storiform), and destructive infiltration into adjacent tissues.

FIBROSING LESIONS

Sclerosing peritonitis is a reactive process in which a thickened fibrous or myofibromatous stroma develops on the peritoneal serosa. It is often idiopathic,[50,68] although in some cases the cause is identified, such as in association with a ruptured ovarian dermoid and spillage of the contents (see granulomatous reactions, above),[176,215] chronic dialysis,[3,31,52,74,119] or after surgical procedures. These are rarely diagnostic problems.

In some cases, the sclerosing peritonitis has been described as part of a syndrome, often in association with so-called 'luteinized thecoma of the ovary'.[41,105,152,214,228] We believe many if not all of these ovarian lesions are actually a form of reactive fibromatosis (see Chapter 22). Clinically, most of the women are young, usually under 30 years of age. Common presenting signs include abdominal enlargement and sometimes small bowel obstruction. Ascites may be present. Even when the patients have a luteinized thecoma, none has endocrine symptoms. Only the occasional person presents with signs of acute abdominal pain. A significant number of patients have been exposed to propranolol-type beta-blocking agents or antiepileptics.

Grossly, opaque to light brown 1–3 mm granules or nodules appear matted together on the peritoneum or on the serosa of the involved organs. The omentum is usually indurated. Microscopic examination discloses a fibrotic process, with various chronic inflammatory cells (Figure 33.6). There is usually some degree of mesothelial hyperplasia. Deeper tissues are relatively

REACTIVE MESOTHELIAL PROLIFERATIONS

MESOTHELIAL HYPERPLASIA

The mesothelium covering the pelvic and abdominal organs and omentum and lining the peritoneal cavity is a highly active tissue that participates in the surface proliferations accompanying inflammatory adhesions.[90] As used commonly in the literature, mesothelial hyperplasia refers to a slight increase in the number of mesothelial cells, and signifies a reactive phenomenon. The term also refers less commonly to where the cells are substantially increased in number and have an altered cytologic appearance such that a preneoplastic process must be contemplated.

With the slightest irritation, such as occurs with injury, ascites or inflammation, the mesothelial cells can undergo remarkable change. Grossly, the cellular proliferation cannot be appreciated until the surface layer, with its accompanying inflammatory exudate, becomes opaque. Microscopically, the changes range from a mild (Figure 33.7) to a substantial increase in the number of mesothelial cells (Figure 33.8), most of which have transformed from being flat and relatively inconspicuous to cuboidal or even columnar. Even though the cell borders may begin to blur, the cytoplasm remains substantial. With pronounced hyperplasia, the mesothelial proliferations may appear as sheets, clusters, ribbons, tubules, and sometimes as papillary formations that can be misinterpreted as metastatic adenocarcinoma (Figure 33.9).

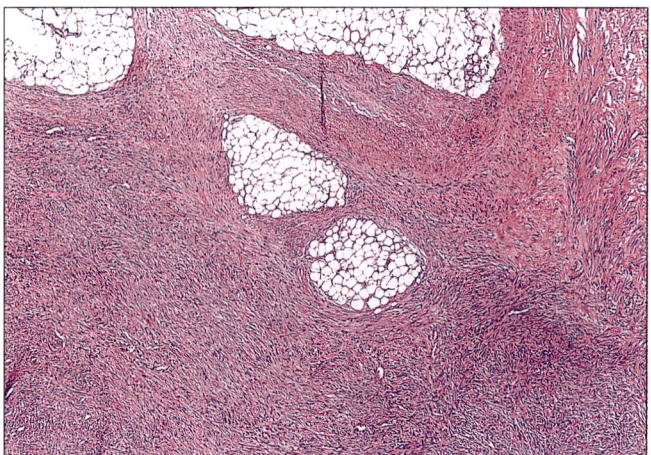

Fig. 33.6 Sclerosing peritonitis.

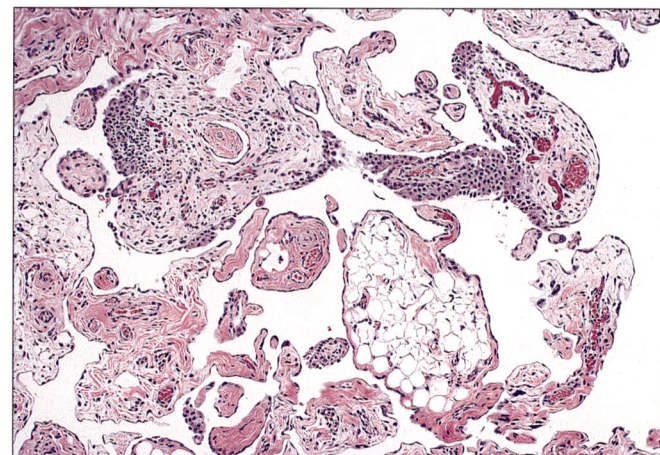

Fig. 33.7 Slight mesothelial hyperplasia of peritoneum.

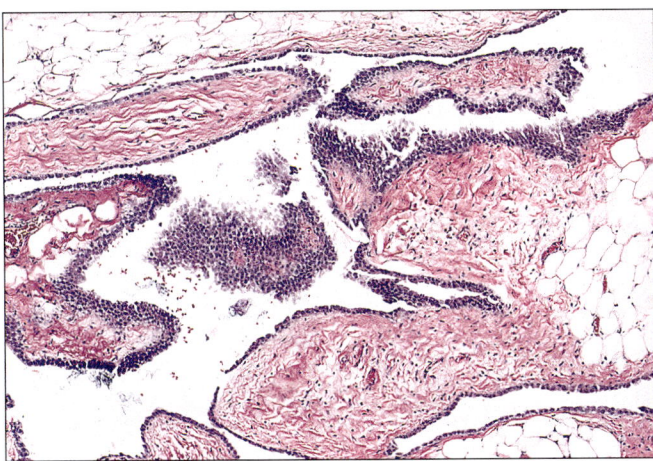

Fig. 33.8 Thin layer of moderately reactive mesothelium.

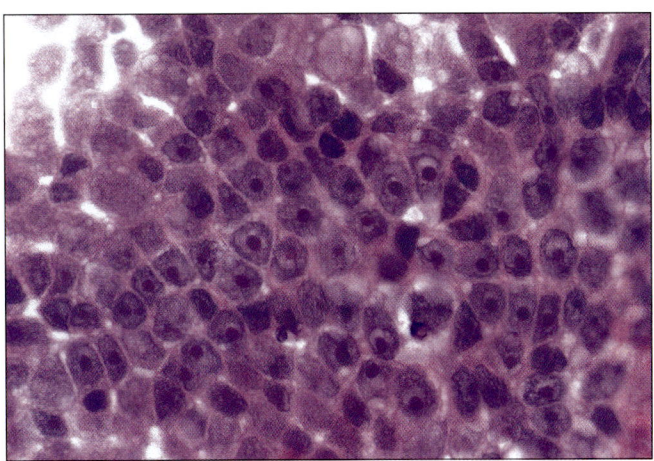

Fig. 33.10 Markedly reactive mesothelial cells with prominent nucleoli. The cytologic washing from this patient was strongly considered as adenocarcinoma.

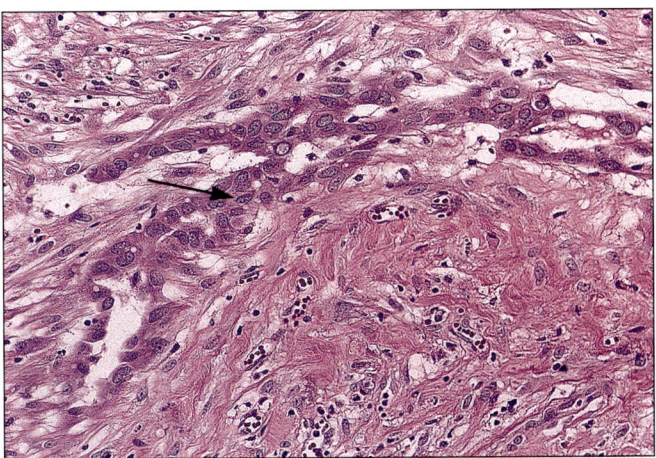

Fig. 33.9 Reactive mesothelium. The enlarged mesothelial cells (arrow) that cover a focus of fibrous reaction superficially resemble metastatic adenocarcinoma.

Reactive mesothelial cells tend to be uniform in appearance. With minor degrees of reactivity, the nuclei are small, regular, and round or oval. Nucleoli are central and the cytoplasm is eosinophilic or sometimes vacuolated. With increasing degrees of reactivity, the nuclei enlarge and the chromatin increases. Nucleoli become more apparent and, in the extreme case, may become quite large and singularly prominent (Figure 33.10). Cells may become bi- or multinucleated. Cytologic preparations especially show the dramatic change from normal to reparative to markedly hyperplastic mesothelium, even to the point where, on occasion, the large macronucleoli may be mistaken as evidence for malignancy.

The immunoprofile of normal mesothelium differs from that expected of an 'epithelial' covering. As anticipated, it expresses cytokeratin intermediate filaments typical of epithelial cells. But it also expresses vimentin and desmin, which are indicative, respectively, of mesenchymal differentiation and specialization into muscle. This includes cases where the reactive mesothelium is on the surface of the peritoneum as well as where cuboidal cells are entrapped in clefts below the basal lamina and in sheets. In contrast, ovarian serosa is immunoreactive for vimentin and desmin in fewer than half of cases.

Ovarian inclusion cysts are non-reactive for vimentin and desmin, as are benign and borderline (proliferating) ovarian tumors. The differential reactivity of mesothelium (and mesothelioma) and müllerian tissue (and ovarian tumors) is explored more fully below.

With greater degrees of injury, a layer of spindle-shaped mesenchymal cells may sometimes appear below the mesothelial cells. In the resting state, this layer is inconspicuous, but when stimulated, the cells may proliferate and produce a highly cellular desmoplastic tissue. Cells also express cytokeratin, vimentin, and desmin. These cells simulate myofibroblasts, and are thought to give rise occasionally to the muscular cells in the condition 'disseminated peritoneal leiomyomatosis'.

The exuberant and sometimes pseudoinfiltrative growth that mesothelium can show, together with the increased mitotic activity that is frequently observed, may lead to a false impression of primary or metastatic carcinoma, despite the benign cytologic appearance of the cells.[38] Carcinoma cells generally demonstrate greater nuclear pleomorphism and more conspicuous mitotic activity. Clusters of mesothelial cells are easily mistaken for metastatic carcinoma. This is true especially when mesothelial cells extensively involve sinusoids in pelvic lymph nodes either as small papillary clusters or as sheets of somewhat dishesive cells.[42] Exuberant surface proliferations, sometimes forming sessile or polypoid nodules, can also simulate mesothelioma, a problem also encountered in the walls of hernia sacs. A useful morphologic feature that can help distinguish reactive mesothelial cell aggregates from metastatic carcinoma is their orientation at low-power magnification to one another (often in a line that can be traced for some considerable distance) (Figure 33.9) and their relation to the position of the original peritoneal surface (as demonstrated by the presence of the peritoneal elastic lamina).[117]

Organization of surface proliferative lesions and inflammatory exudates may leave adhesions of variable density, ranging from delicate strands of loose connective tissue to broad bands of dense well-vascularized collagenous fibrous tissue. Entrapped inflammatory exudate within granulation tissue and proliferating sheets of mesothelial cells may lead to mesothelial (peritoneal) cyst formation. These may not become clinically apparent until months or years after the precipitating event.

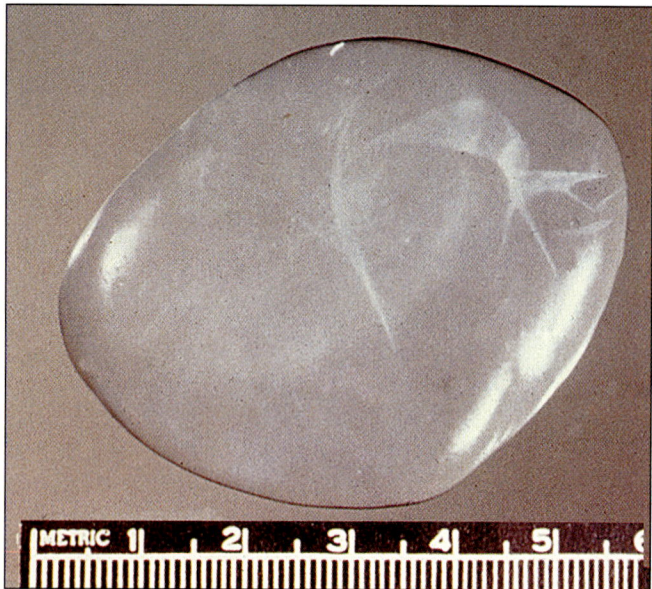

Fig. 33.11 Mesothelial cystic proliferation.

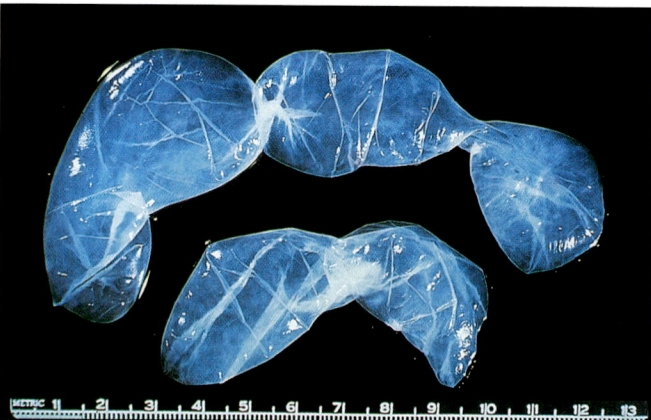

Fig. 33.13 Multiple large mesothelial cysts.

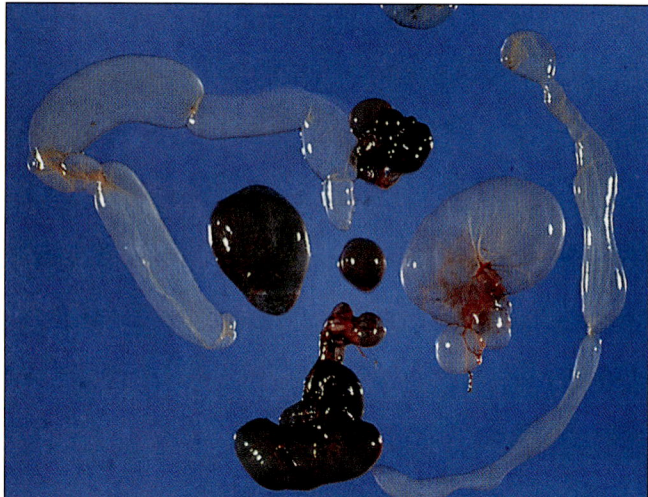

Fig. 33.12 Multiple small mesothelial cysts.

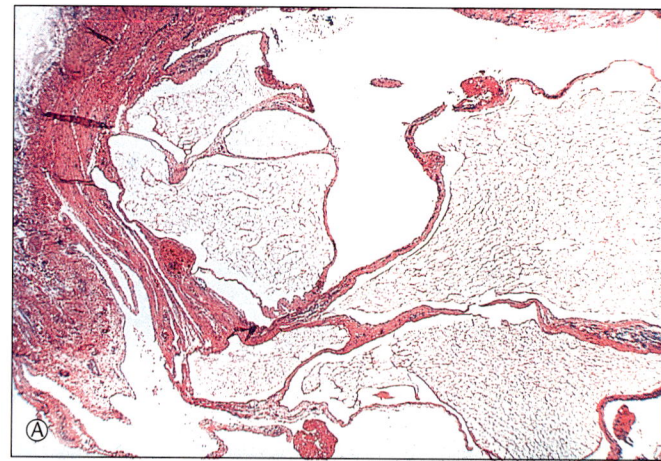

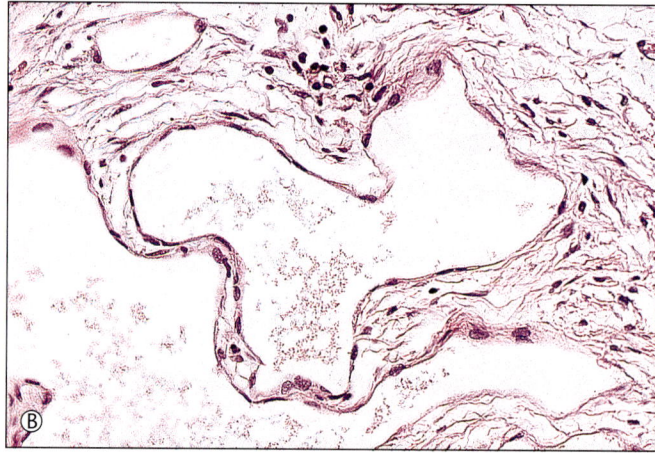

Fig. 33.14 **(A)** Thin-walled mesothelial cysts in peritoneum. **(B)** Normal mesothelium covered by fibrous adhesions, not to be confused with lymphatic vessels.

PERITONEAL MESOTHELIAL INCLUSION CYSTS AND CYSTIC PROLIFERATION

Peritoneal inclusion cysts are of several types. Those that appear as a clinical entity occur most often in young women and are frequently associated with prior abdominal surgery.[123] The cysts are generally considered reactive, although some believe the larger lesions are neoplastic. Benign multicystic mesothelioma is an alternative epithet for this condition that reflects this notion.

Inclusion cysts are usually several millimeters in diameter and multiple. Cystic proliferations are larger (Figures 33.11–33.13). Some may reach 20 cm diameter and form multilocular masses simulating an ovarian cystadenoma. Cysts are usually thin walled, contain clear proteinaceous fluid, and are lined by attenuated mesothelial cells (Figure 33.14). Metaplasia of the mesothelial lining sometimes occurs and is tubal in type. This

may be one way that serous change (also called 'endosalpingiosis', see below) develops. Inflammatory infiltrates, if present at all, are limited to sparse lymphocytic collections.

A more common form of cyst is one that is actually normal, but in a location that can be mistaken for carcinoma. In patients where there has been peritonitis, layers of fibrinous adhesions

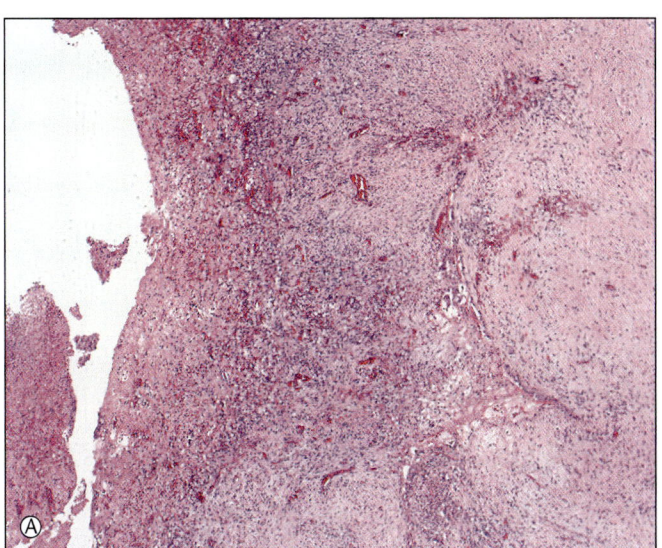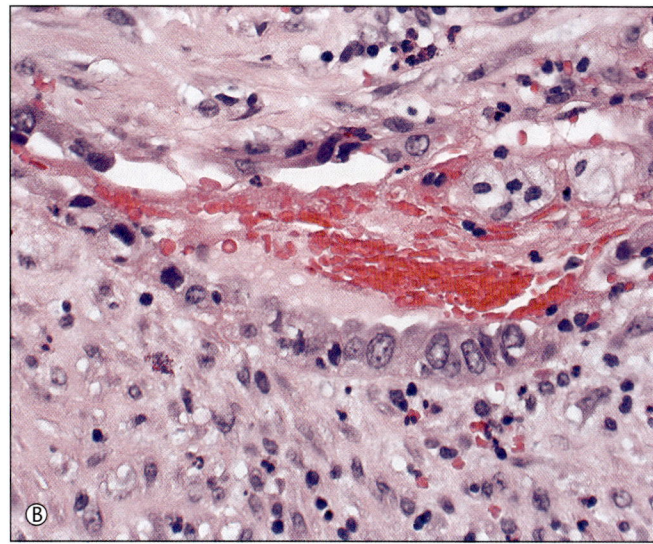

Fig. 33.15 (A) Serosa covered by adhesions. It is easy to mistake the normal mesothelium for serous adenocarcinoma due to its location within the peritoneal wall. **(B)** Detail of mesothelial inclusion.

develop that then are superficial to the deeper lining of normal mesothelium. The epithelium may appear cystic and not uncommonly is misconstrued for invasive serous adenocarcinomas until attention is paid to its regularity and benign histology (Figure 33.15).

MÜLLERIANOSIS (MÜLLERIAN TUMOR-LIKE CONDITIONS)

There is no widely accepted generic term for the various manifestations of müllerian-directed changes, whether they are benign, metaplastic or neoplastic, or epithelial or mesenchymal, that develop in the omentum, pelvic peritoneum, pelvic walls, and beneath the ovarian serosa. Endosalpingiosis, a term in common usage, describes lesions composed of benign, tubal-like epithelium. Yet whenever such lesions show signs of neoplasia, the nomenclature reflects the more standard terminology associated with neoplasms, e.g., serous adenocarcinoma. 'Endocervicosis' has been used to indicate the rare but analogous mucinous epithelial lesions. Again, if a tumor develops, the name shifts to the more usual terminology associated with neoplasms, e.g., mucinous adenocarcinoma. 'Müllerian or paramesonephric metaplasia', 'benign glandular inclusions', 'inclusion cysts', 'benign tubular lesions', and 'implants' (if associated with ovarian carcinoma) are other terms found in the recent literature. However, all these terms may be criticized as they lack precision. Since there is widespread agreement that these various lesions are of müllerian origin, the term 'müllerianosis' has been proposed as a simple 'umbrella' term that is sufficiently descriptive of the spectrum to justify wider use.[186]

The pathogenesis of müllerian lesions is unclear. Metaplasia is an appropriate term only if it is accepted that, in the development of these lesions, one adult tissue, e.g., serous epithelium, replaces another, such as ovarian serosa (or pelvic mesothelium). Acknowledging that this transformation may proceed through intermediate undifferentiated or stem cells, 'metaplasia' is probably the best term available. The undifferentiated

cells involved in the genesis of müllerianosis are thought to be those of the subcelomic mesenchyme, which is inapparent in postnatal life but contributes substantially during embryonic development to the genesis of the müllerian ducts. Thus, the pelvic and abdominal peritonea retain a potential for müllerian differentiation conditioned by its embryonic origin. This potential is greatest in the ovaries and decreases with increasing distance from them.[125] The difficulty with this proposed theory is the lack of any experimental data.

The factors that stimulate müllerian derivatives to develop are unknown. A few believe the tissues are embryologic rests that remain in place for years and then later proliferate, but such rests have not been observed. Some consider müllerianosis to be acquired and induced by changes in the hormonal milieu that follows puberty. Some instances of peritoneal disease may represent implanted disease from the ovary, especially in terms of serous tumors of borderline malignancy in the peritoneum, and others may derive from müllerian inclusion cysts in the peritoneal cavity or retroperitoneal lymph nodes (see below). Some lesions described as müllerianosis are in fact endometriosis, which may not be a disease that develops *de novo* from the peritoneum, but rather from retrograde transmission of endometrium from the uterine corpus (see Chapter 20). In short, the etiologic factors leading to the development of müllerian epithelium in the peritoneum remain a mystery.

What is clear, however, is that each of the entities described here has a characteristic anatomic distribution and set of clinicopathologic correlates that are far from random and seem to be type specific. For example, the presence of serous epithelium, also called endosalpingiosis or müllerian inclusion cysts (see below), when present, commonly involves the pelvic visceral serosa, omentum, and pelvic lymph nodes and is seen with increased frequency in women who also have serous ovarian neoplasms (and may actually represent extremely well-differentiated metastases to the peritoneum from the ovarian tumor). Endometriosis, should this be included, has a very different anatomic distribution, but almost never includes the omentum or pelvic lymph nodes. Endocervicosis usually involves the posterior peritoneal surface of the bladder in the midline. Transitional cell rests are seen typically on the superior and posterior surfaces of the fallopian tubes – and they can and do occur together in the same patient and can show transitions from one pattern to another in individual lesions – and that doesn't take into account the 'stromal' variants.

The most common form of epithelial differentiation is of the serous ('tubal') type, perhaps reflecting the hypothesis that it may be the prototypic müllerian epithelium.[177,187] Endometrioid epithelium unaccompanied by endometrioid stroma, and mucinous and clear cell forms are rare.

ENDOSALPINGIOSIS (SEROUS CHANGE)

Endosalpingiosis is the presence of a lining epithelium that resembles the lining of the normal fallopian tube. The term was coined in the 1930s to reflect the proposed mechanism whereby the cells lining the fallopian tube were believed to have sloughed and implanted onto the peritoneum. No data exist to support this hypothesis, however. To avoid this potential association, some of us have adopted a synonym, 'serous change'. Some cases accompany endometriosis in laparoscopic biopsies of women being investigated for infertility.[108] Many examples, as discussed below, may not be primary at all, but rather exceedingly well-differentiated metastases from borderline serous tumors of the ovary.[145]

Endosalpingiosis, if seen macroscopically, may appear as a focal granularity, with a single to few tiny bumps, or a single to few tiny cysts. In its most simple histologic form it appears as individual small, round-to-oval glands with an obvious lumen and devoid of any architectural disorder (Figure 33.16). Occasionally, the gland may be larger, but shows neither cytologic nor architectural abnormalities (Figure 33.17). A peripheral basement membrane is present and cilia are often prominent. Psammoma bodies (calcospherites) are commonly present and usually in continuity with the epithelium. If the epithelium is destroyed, the psammoma bodies may be found free in the stroma. The epithelium is usually only one cell layer thick, but there may be stratification or occasionally mild papillary infoldings. Nuclei are basally situated, mitotic activity is

absent, and there is no nuclear atypia. Serous change is not associated with mesothelial reactions, adhesions or inflammation, apart from occasional lymphocytes.

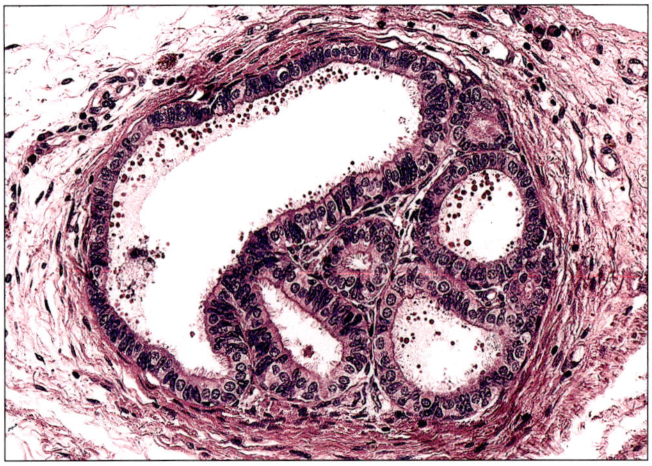

Not uncommonly, the serous foci exhibit more epithelial proliferation than would be expected in benign lesions. The criteria used for assessing whether the excessive growth reflects neoplasms of borderline malignancy are identical to those for serous tumors in general and are summarized in Table 33.1.

Several important questions, yet to be answered definitively, have sparked substantial controversy and discussion. These include:

- How frequently does serous change represent implants of serous epithelium from an ovarian tumor of a similar histology?
- Are there diagnostic tools, either by ordinary histology or molecular biology, capable of distinguishing between primary lesions in the peritoneum and metastases to the peritoneum?
- Should endosalpingiosis in which the cells are atypical and proliferative be designated at least as a borderline tumor?

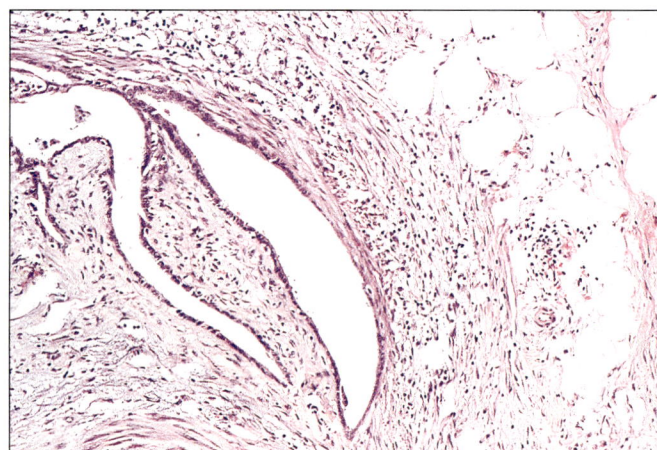

Fig. 33.17 'Endosalpingiosis' (serous change). The serous epithelium is unremarkable without any observable cytologic or architectural atypia.

Fig. 33.16 Endosalpingiosis. Several serous glands lack architectural and cytologic atypia. This lesion has been also called 'serous change' by some, or a form of müllerian inclusion cyst, which reflects the bias toward pathogenesis.

Table 33.1 Features distinguishing endosalpingiosis (serous change) from serous borderline tumor of the peritoneum		
	Endosalpingiosis (serous change)	**Serous borderline tumor (primary and implanted)**
Location	Surface and subperitoneal	Surface and subperitoneal
Architecture	Simple round or oval gland	Simple glands, often with focal or complex papillary epithelial tufts, detached cell clusters and psammoma bodies
Cytology	No atypia	Mild-to-severe atypia and often cellular stratification
Stromal reaction	None to focal hyalinization	None to, in one form, exuberant desmoplasia

Modified from a presentation by D.A. Bell, Boston, MA.

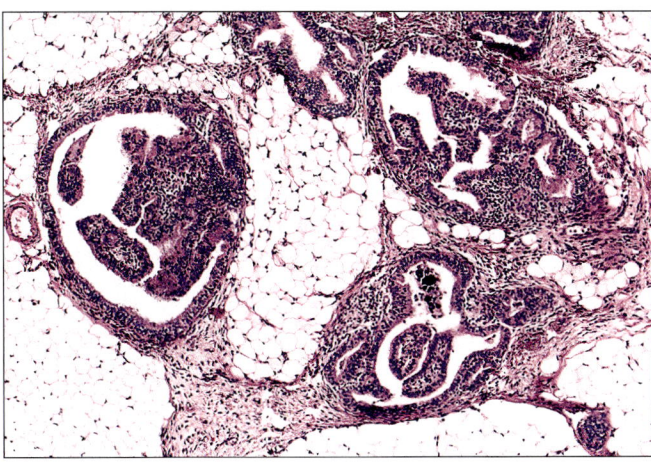

Fig. 33.18 Florid endosalpingiosis or serous borderline tumor? The photograph shown has been called florid endosalpingiosis by some and serous borderline tumor by others.

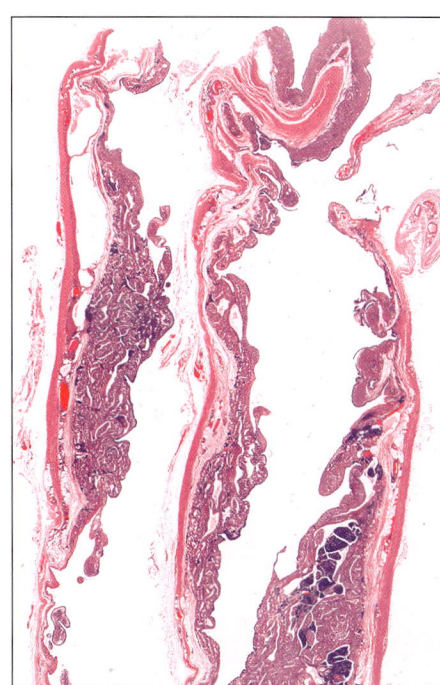

Fig. 33.19 Cystic endosalpingiosis displaying mural smooth muscle proliferation typical of lymphangioleiomyomatosis and with similar lymph node changes.

Can the serous change behave as a malignancy and still be designated by a term that implies a relatively mild disease process, i.e., 'endosalpingiosis with tumor-like manifestations'?

The literature contains many references to serous change that is considered to have arisen from the peritoneum. Yet in these same references, most patients have synchronous ovarian tumors of generally the similar histologic type. In one series, 25 of the 40 patients with serous change in the omentum had ovarian tumors.[172] In another study that dealt with ovarian serous neoplasms of borderline malignancy that later recurred, 8 of 11 patients had 'endosalpingiosis' found in the peritoneum at the time of the initial operation.[211] As endosalpingiosis in the peritoneum is commonly found together with implants of serous borderline tumor of ovary that has metastasized to the peritoneum,[22] it may well be that the foci of 'endosalpingiosis' in many of these cases were implants in the first place. Conversely, whatever the underlying pathogeneses of peritoneal endosalpingiosis and ovarian serous neoplasia, it is not improbable that they are related and that the presence of one might correlate positively with the presence of the other. The critical issue is that there is insufficient information available at this time to definitively answer this query.

A recent report describes florid cystic serous change with tumor-like manifestations in four patients, all of whom had cysts transmurally in the uterine wall.[39] Most of the glands were lined by a single layer of unremarkable serous-type epithelium. Some photographs, however, show intraglandular papillae with various degrees of pseudostratification that might equally be considered as tumors of borderline malignancy (Figure 33.18). By contrast, we have seen rare examples of cystic endosalpingiosis displaying the sort of mural smooth muscle proliferation typical of lymphangioleiomyomatosis and with similar lymph node changes (Figure 33.19).

ENDOCERVICOSIS (MUCINOUS CHANGE)

Lesions composed of mucinous columnar epithelium have been described and given the name 'endocervicosis'. This is a controversial condition and if it should exist as an entity, the question is then raised as to its pathogenesis and significance as well as the best nomenclature. No investigators have suggested they derive, by retrograde menstruation, from the lining epithelium of the endocervical canal. Does its occurrence in various sites represent the same or different lesions? Nearly all reported cases involve the peritoneum overlying the bladder.[37,151] Since this organ is lined by transitional epithelium, which is well known to show mucinous metaplasia, might not many of the examples reflect an innate property of urothelium to undergo mucinous change rather than invoking müllerian metaplasia of the peritoneum? Unanswered is how and why the change manifests on the outside of the bladder. Paraurethral glands develop mucinous cysts and mucinous cysts develop in the vulva, yet these would not be considered as endocervicosis.

Another possible explanation is that the lesions on the posterior peritoneal surface of the bladder derive from urachal remnants, in which case they should best not be thought of as müllerian in origin or type.

Yet, the cases described as endocervicosis that overlie the bladder can present as microscopic foci or they can be large, and they are composed of mucinous epithelium alone, or occasionally mucinous together with serous or endometrioid-type epithelium. In the latter situation, the lesions have been called 'müllerianosis of the urinary bladder'.[37,234] One case, reported as an example of a retroperitoneal cyst, was 8 cm in diameter.[49] Another case has been reported in the vagina,[136] an area where mucinous adenosis is well known to develop, even in the absence of diethylstilbestrol exposure.[179] The occurrence of mucinous cysts in the peritoneum is, in our experience, exceedingly rare.

ENDOMETRIOID, CLEAR CELL, AND TRANSITIONAL CELL CHANGES

Occasional cysts have been seen lined by endometrioid epithelium, but it is often unclear whether these may represent endometriosis in which the stroma is absent or atrophic. Rare cases with clear cells, usually in the form of clear cell adenocarcinoma, also appear in the older literature. These are so uncommon that it is difficult to assess today whether these truly have arisen from peritoneal mesothelium or are manifestations of clear cell adenocarcinoma, which itself has arisen from peritoneal endometriosis. Walthard rests, which are rests of transitional (urothelial-like) epithelium, are common occurrences on the tubal serosa, particularly the superior and posterior surfaces, and throughout the broad ligament. They occasionally occur beneath the ovarian serosa but, in any other peritoneal location, are exceedingly rare.

MÜLLERIAN INCLUSION CYSTS

Müllerian inclusion cysts (MIC) are small glandular cysts lined by 'normal' müllerian-type epithelium. Although reported to occur in lymph nodes in up to 20% of women, the more realistic frequency is quite low, ranging in two large series of women with cervical cancer treated with Wertheim hysterectomy from 3.5%[102] to under 1%.[145] Including cases where the pathogenesis of the cysts may include an exceedingly well-differentiated form of metastases from borderline serous tumors of ovary, müllerian inclusion cysts may be found in decreasing order in lymph nodes, pelvic peritoneum and omentum, bowel and uterine serosa, and parametrial connective tissues.[145] Men are not affected. The pathologic features below relate to their presence in pelvic lymph nodes only.

Pathology

Inclusion cysts are not grossly identifiable as such. Occasionally, cysts that are on the surface may appear as bumps, but we are not aware of any instance in which the surgeon suspected their nature. About three-fourths of cases will have 2–5 lymph nodes with inclusions, while most of the rest have only a single node with an inclusion. Similarly, most involved nodes

will contain only 1 or 2 inclusions (Figure 33.20). A minority will contain 3–10 inclusions. Rarely, a node may contain 20 or more inclusions (Figure 33.21).

Microscopically, the inclusions consist of small glands with a simple architecture (Figures 33.22 and 33.23). They are round to slightly bosselated. A single layer of müllerian-type epithelium, generally with prominent cilia, lines the glands. Epithelium is usually a mixture of ciliated, secretory, and intercalated cells. Lumens are usually clear, but occasionally contain a thin, amphophilic secretion. Cells are cytologically bland and cuboidal to columnar. Nuclear contours are regular, the chromatin is even, and nucleoli are rarely seen. Mitoses should not be identified. Neither we[145] nor others[219] have encountered inclusion cysts in lymph nodes lined by mucinous columnar cells.

Pathogenesis

Names given to this condition in the past reflect the various hypothetical pathogeneses.[66,102,110,167,188,207,234] For example, some have considered this condition to be a form of endosalpingiosis, reasoning that the cells lining the fallopian tube sloughed and reimplanted onto the peritoneum and then drained to the

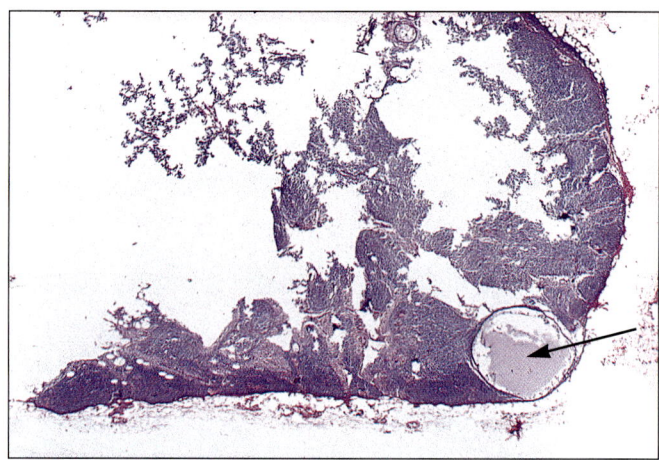

Fig. 33.20 Müllerian inclusion cyst in lymph nodes (arrow). A small metastasis cannot be seen at this low-power magnification. This patient had a borderline serous tumor of the ovary.

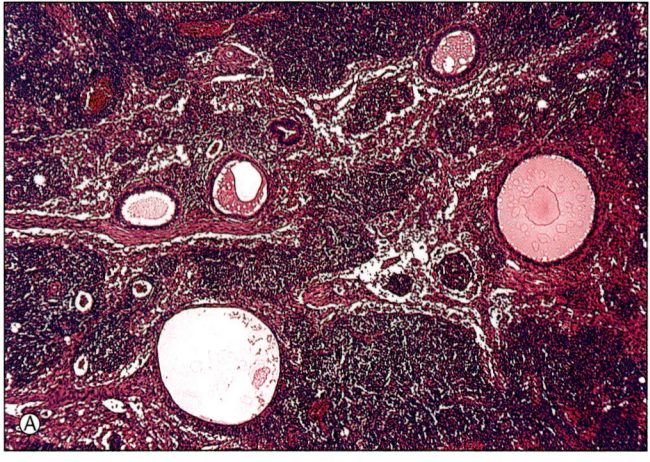
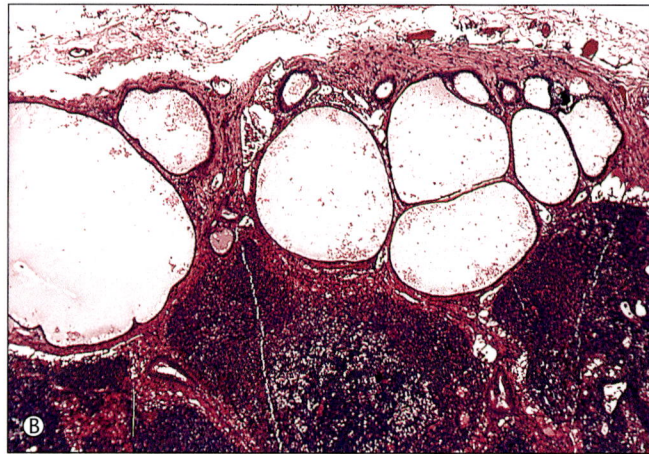

Fig. 33.21 (A, B) Multiple müllerian inclusion cysts in lymph node.

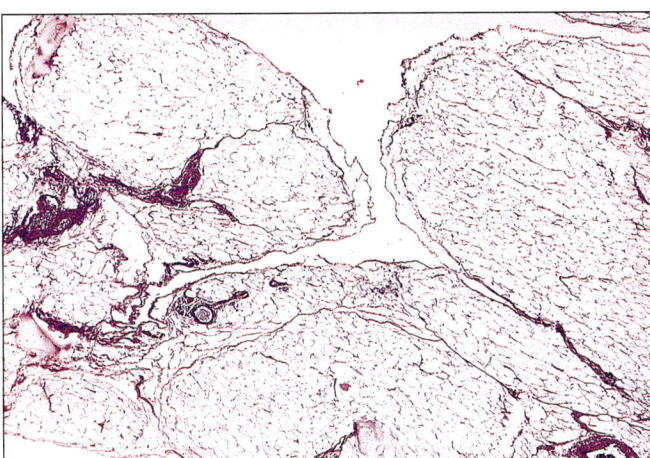

Fig. 33.22 Müllerian inclusion cyst in peritoneum. This patient had a borderline serous tumor of the ovary.

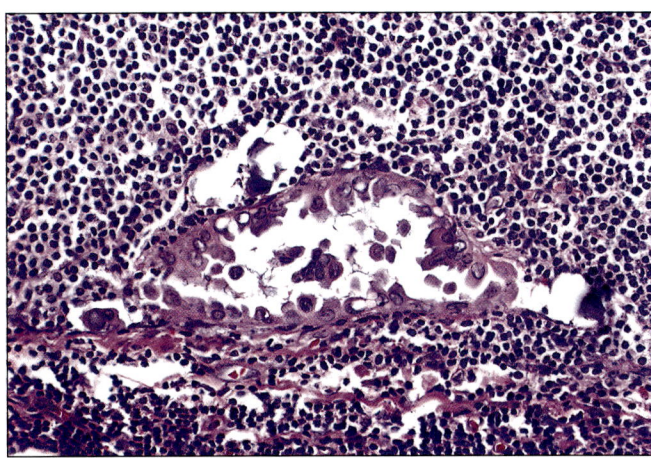

Fig. 33.24 Lymph node metastasis from ovarian borderline serous tumor. The tumor is adjacent to a müllerian inclusion cyst.

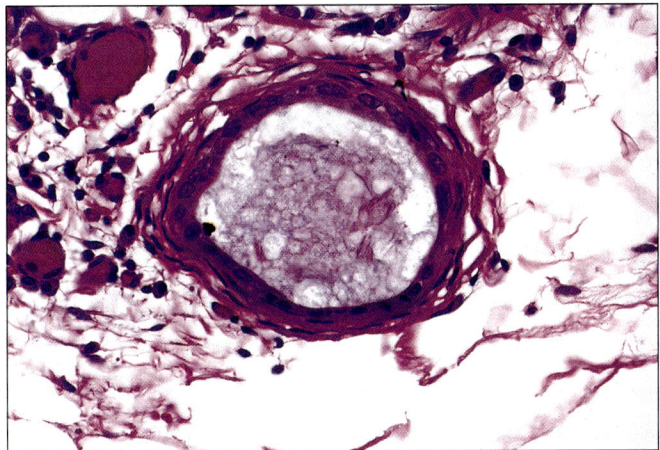

Fig. 33.23 Müllerian inclusion cyst in the peritoneum, high magnification. This patient had a borderline serous tumor of the ovary.

regional lymph nodes. Others have classified such bland glandular inclusions as derivatives of endometriosis, whether or not a stromal component could be identified.[104,174] Another explanation proposes that these inclusions are a metaplastic phenomenon involving the conceptual secondary müllerian system of celom-derived peritoneum.[125]

Several investigators have also shown that MIC can resemble and in many cases are probably extremely well-differentiated nodal metastases.[145] In the setting of gynecologic tumors, some have considered these inclusions as definite nodal metastases. However, some consider MIC as incidental and benign, even when the inclusions are papillary and could be easily considered to be borderline serous tumors on morphologic grounds alone.[44]

These theories have both a theoretical and a practical importance. If the cysts arise *in situ* and are benign, they might provide an explanation for how borderline or cancerous müllerian-type tumors might arise as primary tumors of the peritoneum.[167] On the other hand, if the inclusions represent metastases, then their presence will change the staging of the patient, which could alter subsequent therapy.

A comprehensive series reporting MIC in multiple sites including peritoneum showed that these lesions were most common in women with borderline and grade 1 malignant serous ovarian tumors, and substantially more so than in women with high-grade invasive ovarian cancers.[145] This assumes even greater relevance today with new observations that borderline and grade 1 malignant serous ovarian cancers have a different mode of pathogenesis from high-grade serous carcinomas.[204,205] This association with borderline tumors has been seen by others. (In another recent study,[173] 48% of all cases of peritoneal MIC – called 'endosalpingiosis' by the authors – were associated with borderline serous tumor or adenofibroma of the ovary.) Moreover, when focusing only on lymph nodes, the inclusions were present in lymph nodes in 45% of cases of borderline serous tumor, 2% of invasive serous cancers, and 2.6% of all other conditions for which staging laparotomy was done. Providing additional evidence for the concept that the glands might represent metastases from the primary ovarian tumor in many cases, one study showed K-*ras* mutations in three of six (50%) glands in lymph nodes as well as the associated borderline tumors. All mutations were in codon 12 (Gly to Val in two cases, Gly to Asp in one case).[8] Others have arrived at similar conclusions.[61] Additional molecular studies are required to decipher the relation between borderline ovarian tumors and MIC and to examine the prognostic significance of the latter.

Differential diagnosis

In considering the dilemma of correctly classifying MIC and understanding their malignant potential in the spectrum of müllerian proliferative lesions, it is useful to examine the significance of *bona fide* metastatic borderline lesions, especially of those identified in lymph node dissections. An example is illustrated where lymph nodes with typical MIC had tiny foci of tumor found in the same node (Figure 33.24). In a study of retroperitoneal nodes involved with epithelial ovarian tumors of low malignant potential, patients with involved lymph nodes had a significantly higher rate of recurrence, but without any substantial impact on survival.[126] A more recent study of 74 patients found that cases can be stratified into two risk categories by the histologic pattern of nodal involvement.[138] Patients with nodular aggregates of intranodal epithelium exceeding

1 mm have significantly decreased *disease-free* survival rates when compared with patients with other patterns of nodal involvement.

Available survival data for women with resected ovarian serous tumors of borderline malignancy concur with these findings. It is known that stage 1 and even stage 2A borderline tumors have an excellent prognosis with a nearly 100% 5-year survival and 95% 10-year survival. Even when borderline serous tumors of all stages are considered, the expected 5-year survival rate is about 80–95%.[211] In a recent study of 80 patients with high stage tumors with only non-invasive implants, however, the *disease-free* survival rates fell steadily as observation intervals are extended to 10, 15, and 20 years.[210] These data are pertinent in considering the biologic significance of MIC. If low malignant potential tumors metastatic to nodes do not affect short-term mortality, MIC should be even less likely to show adverse effects.

When a bland lesion that appears to be glandular is encountered in lymph nodes or in the peritoneum or omentum, several entities that simulate MIC need to be excluded. The 'prime suspect' must be a borderline serous tumor, especially if psammoma bodies or slightly more irregular calcifications are found.

Mesothelial inclusions and hyperplasia can sometimes closely resemble MIC.[218] Generally, mesothelium may be recognized by its flat to cuboidal cells with central, vesicular nuclei, moderate to large amounts of eosinophilic, vacuolated cytoplasm and possibly enlarged nucleoli. Extensive cilia and intercalated cells are absent. In cases with florid mesothelial hyperplasia, significant solid and papillary growth may be found, far beyond that consistent with MIC. Commonly, immunohistochemistry has been used to distinguish mesothelial lesions, and is discussed below (Table 33.2).

Endometriosis is also a potential pitfall in the diagnosis of glandular lesions, particularly in the setting of concomitant gynecologic carcinomas. However, the distinction between MIC and endometriosis should usually be easily made, especially in lymph nodes where endometriosis is exceedingly rare. While it has been postulated that MIC are endometriosis in a form without observable stroma, the majority of the literature requires observable stroma to diagnose endometriosis. Immunostains for CD10 and vimentin can also be useful to help identify the presence of stroma. Also, the composition of the epithelium in endometriosis can be helpful, although not always diagnostic. Epithelium of endometriosis is usually endometrioid and lacks cilia, whereas the epithelium in MIC often has a tubal morphology with either cilia or intercalated cells. In our experience, endometriosis is virtually never encountered in lymph nodes.

The issue of distinction (if it exists at all) between MIC and what has been considered as 'endosalpingiosis' is discussed below in this chapter under the topic of serous borderline tumors.

TUMOR-LIKE CONDITIONS

ENDOMETRIOSIS

Endometriosis is a disease principally involving the peritoneal cavity (see Chapter 20).

Table 33.2 Immunohistochemical panel to differentiate mesothelioma from serous carcinoma[a]

	Percentage positive	
	Mesothelioma	Serous
h-Caldesmon	>90%	5%
Calretinin	>90%	10%[b]
Cytokeratin panel (AE1/AE3 and CAM 5.2)	>90%	100%
Cytokeratin (CK) 5/6	>90%	25%[b]
D2–40	>90%	20%
Epithelial membrane antigen (EMA)	>80%	100%
Thrombomodulin	50–75%	5%[b]
Desmin	40%	Negative
Vimentin	25%	35%
CA125	15–30%	95%
MOC-31	5%[b]	95%
S-100	0–10%	33–85%
Ber-EP4	0–10%[b]	100%
Leu-M1 (CD15)	0–10%	65%
Carcinoembryonic antigen (CEA)	<5%	15%
Placental-like alkaline phosphatase (PLAP)	<5%	65%
B72.3	<5%	85%
CA19.9	<5%	67%
Estrogen receptor	<5%	95%
Progesterone receptor	<5%	65%

Note: Mesothelial cells showing reactive atypia show an identical immunophenotype to malignant mesothelioma (with the exception of EMA immunoreactivity).

[a]The percentages for serous carcinoma of ovary and serous carcinoma primary in the peritoneum are essentially identical.

[b]Trace to focally positive. Ber-EP4 is derived from a membrane-enriched fraction derived from the MDF7 breast carcinoma cell line and reacts with an epitope present in two glycoproteins that are not covalently bound. CA125 is an antibody to ovarian carcinoma antigen 125. MOC-31 is an antibody that recognizes a glycoprotein of unknown function present in epithelial cells. B72.3, a monoclonal antibody generated using a membrane-enriched fraction derived from human breast cancer cells, recognizes a tumor-associated glycoprotein called TAG-72. CA19.9 is a sialylated lacto-N-fucopentaose II related to the Lewis blood group.

OVARIAN REMNANT SYNDROME

This condition exists if a patient who has had a 'total bilateral oophorectomy' later develops a palpable mass or experiences pelvic pain or other symptoms referable to ovarian tissue that has been left behind (Figure 33.25). This condition is described more fully elsewhere (see Chapter 22).

SUPERNUMERARY OR ACCESSORY OVARIES

Supernumerary ovaries are ectopic ovaries located at some distance from the eutopic ovary. It is rare but occasional cases

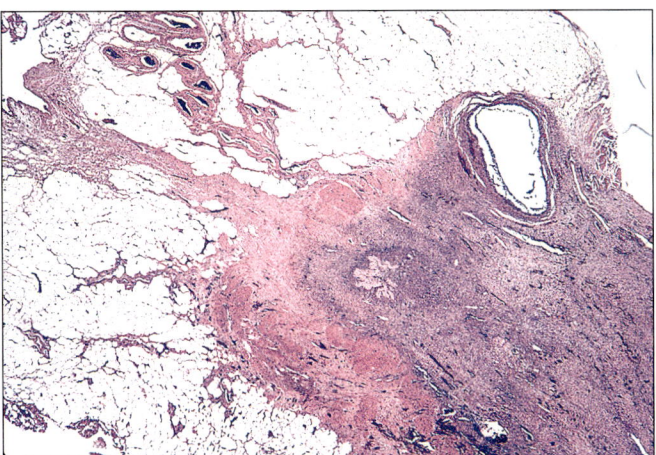

Fig. 33.25 Ovarian remnant syndrome. Ovarian tissue that was left behind at the time of oophorectomy has regrown and is functional.

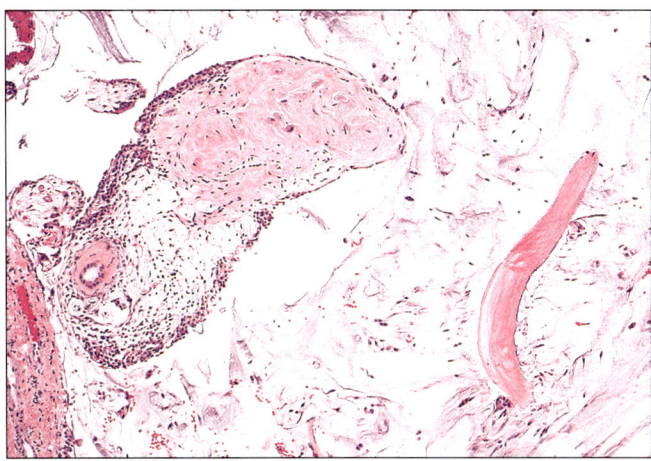

Fig. 33.26 Trophoblastic implant in peritoneum. The patient had a ruptured ectopic pregnancy.

have been reported in the peritoneal cavity.[120] This condition is described more fully elsewhere (see Chapter 21).

SPLENOSIS (AUTOTRANSPLANTATION OF SPLENIC TISSUE)

Nodules of splenic tissue, usually less than 1 cm in diameter, are randomly distributed in the peritoneal cavity. The etiology is trauma, most commonly a motor vehicle accident, which has resulted in splenic rupture.[189] Splenosis is generally asymptomatic but may cause abdominal or pelvic pain simulating endometriosis, or produce intestinal obstruction due to the development of adhesions. Splenosis may be encountered as an incidental finding or mistakenly interpreted as endometriosis because the nodules are widespread, fleshy, and reddish-brown or purplish.[129,162,226]

Implants are encased by fibrous tissue that simulates a splenic capsule, but lacks smooth muscle and elastic fibers. Larger nodules usually disclose all of the histologic components of normally sited splenic parenchyma. In smaller lesions, only the red pulp may be evident.

Splenunculi (supernumerary spleens) can be distinguished from splenotic foci by their restricted distribution, limited numbers, regular shapes, presence of a capsule and miniature hilus, and lack of associated adhesions.

TROPHOBLASTIC IMPLANTS

Finding disseminated trophoblastic implants in the peritoneum is uncommon (Figure 33.26). They may occur on occasion with peritoneal pregnancy, or following laparoscopic treatment of tubal pregnancy, where the frequency has been estimated at 3.6%.[175,223] Viability is suggested by rising human chorionic gonadotrophin concentrations following surgery. The condition is best avoided by meticulous inspection of the abdomen after resection of the tubal pregnancy.

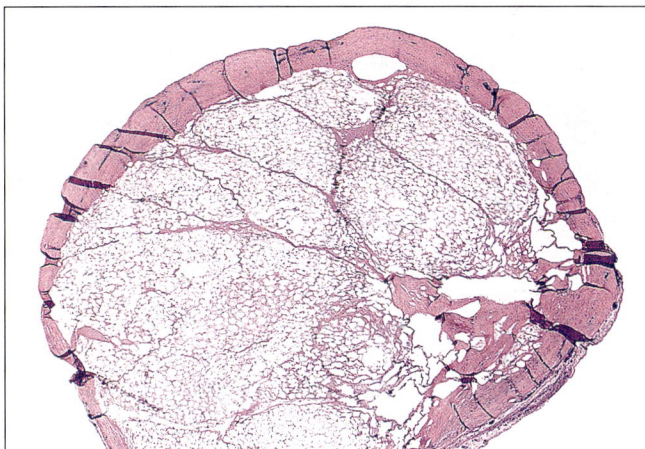

Fig. 33.27 Infarcted appendix epiploica.

INFARCTED APPENDIX EPIPLOICA

Appendices epiploicae, also known as 'epiploic tags', are small polypoid processes of adipose tissue that project from the serosa of the large intestine, especially the transverse and sigmoid colon. Occasionally, they undergo torsion, infarction, and later detachment and can be found lying free within the peritoneal cavity.[80,225] Typically in these cases, the center contains hyalinized fibrous tissue and often some residual adipose tissue that is mummified. The outer rim and variable portions of the core may calcify (Figure 33.27).

DECIDUOSIS

Deciduosis, a form of 'stromal müllerianosis' disclosing foci of ectopic decidualized stromal cells, is commonly observed in association with pregnancy. Groups of decidual cells, indistinguishable from those found in gestational endometrium, occasionally appear in the pelvic and lower abdominal peritoneum, beneath the ovarian surface epithelium, and in the plicae of the fallopian tubes. It is also rarely seen in lymph nodes. Patients

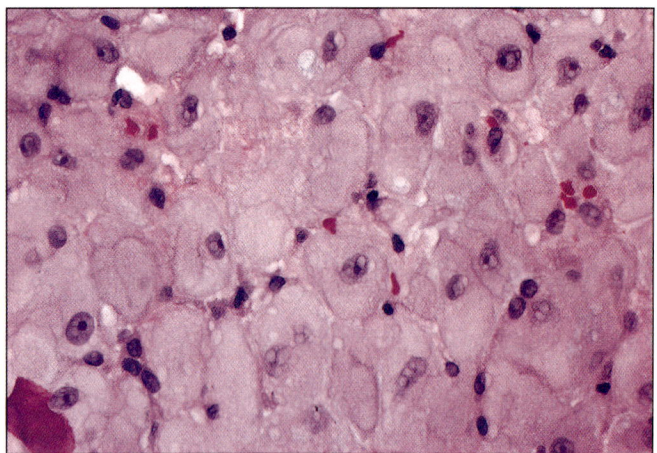

Fig. 33.28 Decidual reaction of pregnancy.

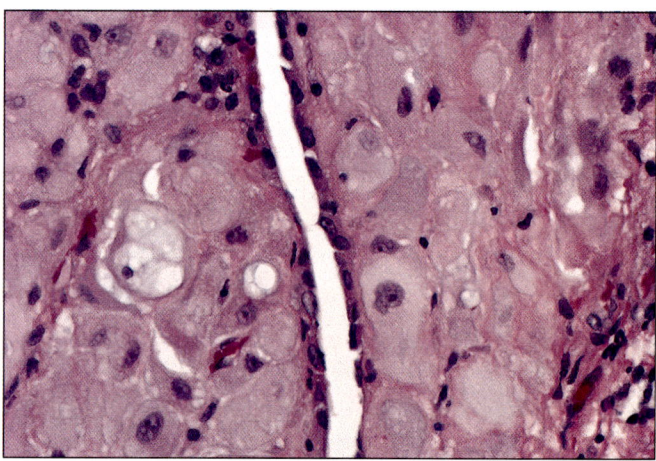

Fig. 33.29 Decidual reaction of pregnancy. Several cells show signs of degeneration.

with trophoblastic disease also regularly exhibit deciduosis, mediated, as in a normal pregnancy, by high plasma levels of chorionic gonadotrophins. Ectopic pseudodecidual reactions also occur with exogenous progesterone administration. These changes occur rarely in the absence of such histories and have mostly been identified in premenopausal women. Most lesions are incidental findings.

If seen grossly, the nodules are tan to pale brown, slightly gelatinous, and rarely more than several millimeters. Occasionally, it may reach several centimeters in size and consist of multiple, tiny, soft nodules separated by thin, white, rubbery septa.[14]

In many locations, such as in fallopian tube plicae or adjacent to a corpus luteum, the decidua-like cells are pure. In the peritoneum, the decidualized cells are often admixed with smooth muscle cells, giving rise to the condition 'disseminated peritoneal leiomyomatosis', also known as 'leiomyomatosis peritonealis disseminata'. Although the presence of the decidua in such cases has been used to argue that this condition develops by differentiation of the subcelomic mesenchyme with the formation of multiple tumor-like nodules (see below), there is no consensus that this is the true mechanism.

The decidual reaction most often appears as solid clusters of cohesive, decidualized cells with sharp cell borders (Figures 33.28 and 33.29). Cytoplasm may be abundant and glass-like or may show some degrees of degeneration (Figure 33.30). Some cells have a clear vacuolated cytoplasm that superficially resembles the soap-bubble-like physaliferous cell of chordoma (Figure 33.30). Some nodules may also show transitions between a more solid and a more myxoid pattern of decidual reaction (Figure 33.31).

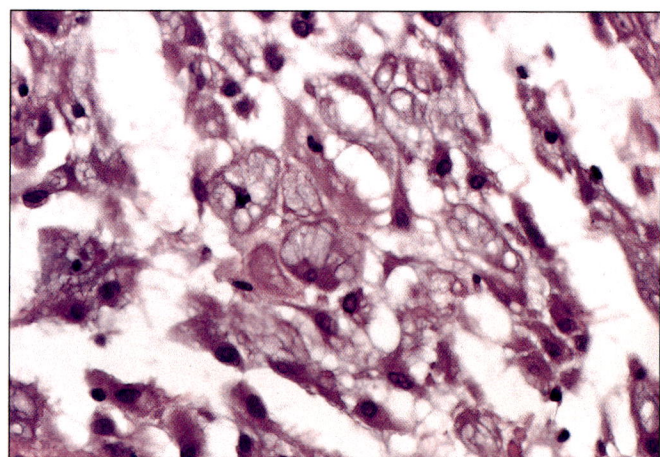

Fig. 33.30 Decidual reaction of pregnancy. Numerous decidual cells are degenerative.

DISSEMINATED PERITONEAL LEIOMYOMATOSIS

Multiple nodules of proliferating smooth muscle found throughout the peritoneum characterize leiomyomatosis peritonealis disseminata (see Chapter 18). This rare condition is usually observed in women of reproductive age,[7,95,124] although it occurs occasionally in postmenopausal women. It develops on a background of an altered hormonal milieu, such as with pregnancy, oral contraceptive use,[191] hormonal therapy, or

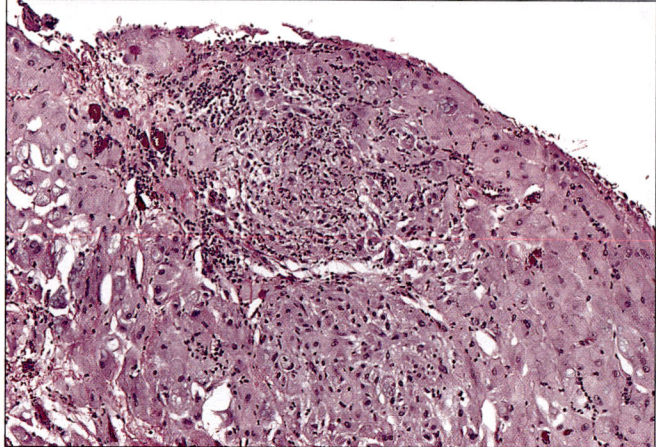

Fig. 33.31 Nodules intermediate between decidua and smooth muscle proliferation. Shows features of both deciduosis and disseminated peritoneal leiomyomatosis.

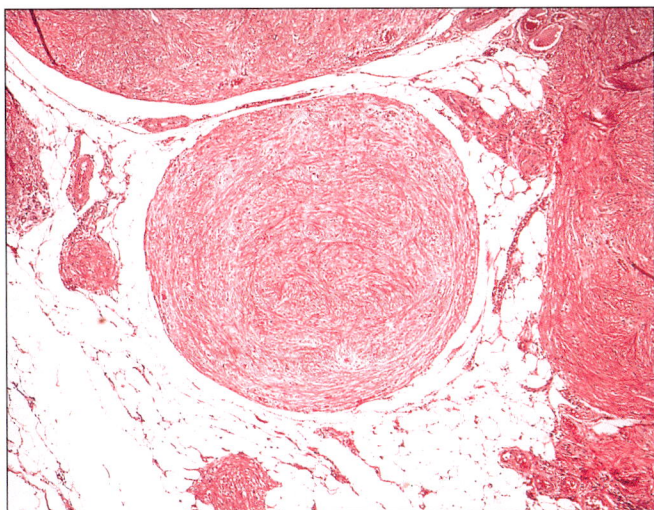

Fig. 33.32 Disseminated peritoneal leiomyomatosis.

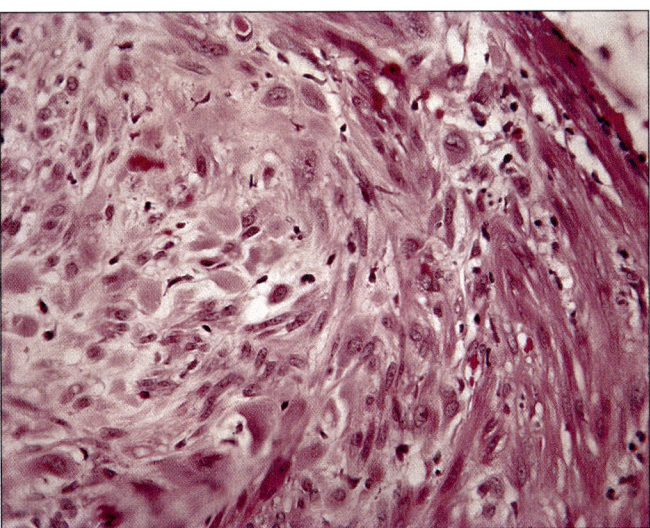

Fig. 33.33 Disseminated peritoneal leiomyomatosis. There is both extensive smooth muscle and decidua.

steroid-producing ovarian tumors.[92] While this condition is often classified as a tumor-like condition, since it commonly regresses, the lesions in some cases persist, suggesting a neoplastic process. On rare occasions, some have shown malignant transformation.[15,73,99]

Pathology

Grossly, multiple gray-white nodules that may be granular to several millimeters in diameter are found covering the peritoneal surfaces of the pelvis, pelvic organs, intestines, and omentum. Microscopically, the nodules consist of smooth muscle arranged like leiomyomas (Figure 33.32). Cells usually lack atypia and mitotic activity, and only rarely have features of malignancy. In many cases, the tumor is admixed with stromal cells resembling decidua (Figure 33.33). Smooth muscle cells are markedly reactive for desmin and muscle-specific antigens, but without reactivity for keratin. This pattern of staining has been used to argue in support of the hypothesis that the

condition arises from multicentric differentiation of submesothelial stem cells.[131] Ultrastructural examination discloses myofilamentous bundles with focal electron-dense bodies typical of smooth muscle cell differentiation.

Pathogenesis

Progesterone stimulation appears to be critical in the development of these tumors in nearly all cases. They are virtually always strongly reactive for progesterone receptors and usually reactive for estrogen receptors although with less intensity.[27] In postpartum women, estrogen receptor reactivity in decidualized nodules is either weak or absent.[29] Such an immunohistochemical staining pattern might be expected, since ovarian and placentally derived progesterone is critical in transforming endometrial stromal cells into decidua during pregnancy and since foci of decidual cells are found with the smooth muscle cells.

Regression has been documented in cases where excess hormonal stimulation has been removed, e.g., with the cessation of oral contraceptives, oophorectomy, or following childbirth.[92] A hormonal stimulus is thus believed to facilitate the development of the smooth muscle nodules, as suggested by older animal models where peritoneal and omental nodular spindle cell proliferations developed in guinea pigs exposed to large doses of progesterone and estrogen.

Based on the above observations, the general view has been that disseminated peritoneal leiomyomas are metaplastic in origin and hormonally responsive. Yet, rather than this lesion being polyclonal, one study in which 42 leiomyomatous lesions from four patients were studied found that the leiomyomas were monoclonal, which strongly suggests that the lesions are neoplastic and from the same precursor lesion.[171]

Other conditions also give rise to one or more peritoneal leiomyomas. Uterine subserosal leiomyomas may become detached and implant elsewhere on the peritoneum (parasitic leiomyomas). Leiomyomas arising in the deep retroperitoneal–abdominal soft tissue can involve the peritoneum.[20,161] Like uterine leiomyomas, they can be hormonally reactive, which is unlike leiomyomas of deep somatic soft tissue, e.g., extremities, which are hormonally unreactive.[21]

MESOTHELIAL NEOPLASMS

Tumors of mesothelial origin form an array of conditions that range from those that are neoplastic but benign, through those that are extremely well differentiated and rarely act in a malignant fashion, to those that are multicentric, moderately to poorly differentiated, and aggressive. Some of these tumors are also easily confused with tumors of müllerian lineage and especially serous carcinoma, which itself usually arises from the ovary but on occasion arises *de novo* in the peritoneal cavity. Immunohistochemistry is particularly important to confirm that the tissue identified is mesothelial in type or to differentiate mesotheliomas from serous tumors (see Table 33.2).

ADENOMATOID TUMOR

Adenomatoid tumors are benign neoplasms of mesothelial origin, encountered most often in the fallopian tubes where frequently they are sieve-like or multicystic. In contrast, they

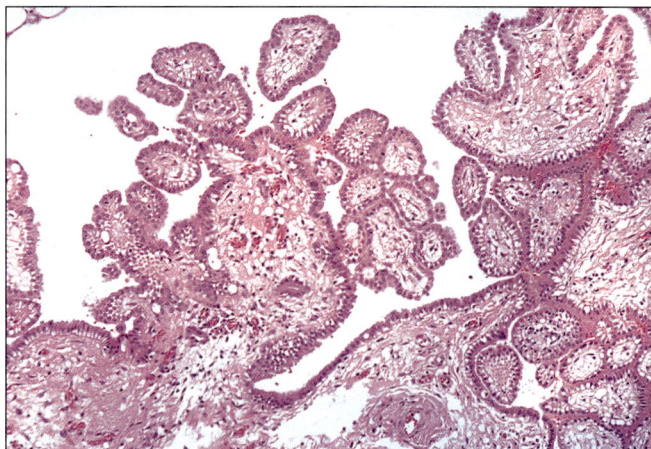

Fig. 33.34 Well-differentiated peritoneal mesothelioma.

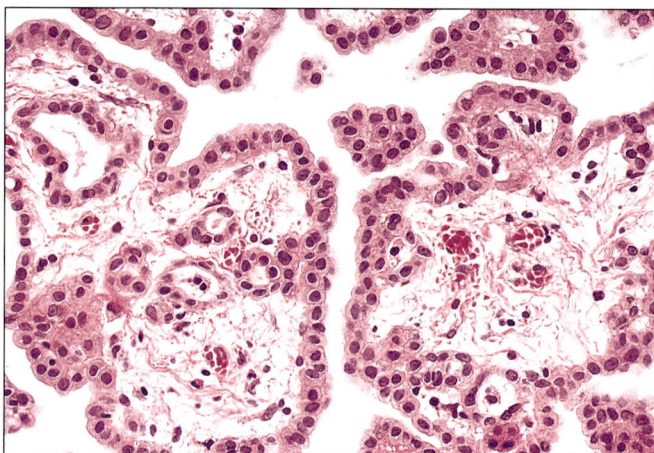

Fig. 33.35 Detail of well-differentiated peritoneal mesothelioma.

are also found subserosally in the uterine corpus near the fallopian tube, where they more usually simulate leiomyomas. They are seldom encountered elsewhere in the peritoneal cavity (see Chapter 19).

WELL-DIFFERENTIATED PAPILLARY MESOTHELIOMA

An extremely rare form of peritoneal mesothelioma is the well-differentiated papillary mesothelioma. Most women are of reproductive age, although an occasional patient has been postmenopausal. Also encountered in males, less common sites include the tunica vaginalis testis, pericardium, and pleura. Lesions typically cause no symptoms, and usually are found incidentally at operation. Tumors grossly are typically solitary, broad based, wart-like excrescences that are polypoid or slightly nodular. Color and texture are similar to ovarian cortical tissue but sometimes firmer. They are generally small, usually measuring from 8 mm to <2 cm in diameter.[84] An occasional tumor is multicentric.[217]

On microscopic examination, the neoplasm consists of relatively thick papillae composed of dense fibrous or hyalinized tissue covered by a single layer of cytologically benign, small cuboidal cells (Figure 33.34). Nuclei are bland, with a low nuclear grade (Figure 33.35). Mitoses are rare, usually under 1, but may be as high as 3 mitotic figures per 10 high-power fields (HPFs). The diagnosis should be made with caution, as malignant mesotheliomas may have foci that, viewed in isolation, resemble this tumor.[10] These lesions can usually be reliably distinguished from serous epithelial tumors, since the architecture of the latter usually discloses feathery irregular clusters of cells in which the nuclei are far more atypical and higher grade. Psammoma bodies may be encountered in rare cases. These tumors are nearly always benign, but rare tumors have acted aggressively.[28,101]

MULTICYSTIC MESOTHELIOMA

Multicystic mesotheliomas are rare indolent forms of mesothelial tumor. They occur in young women (average age 35 years, range 23–74 years), and most often are found in the pelvis.

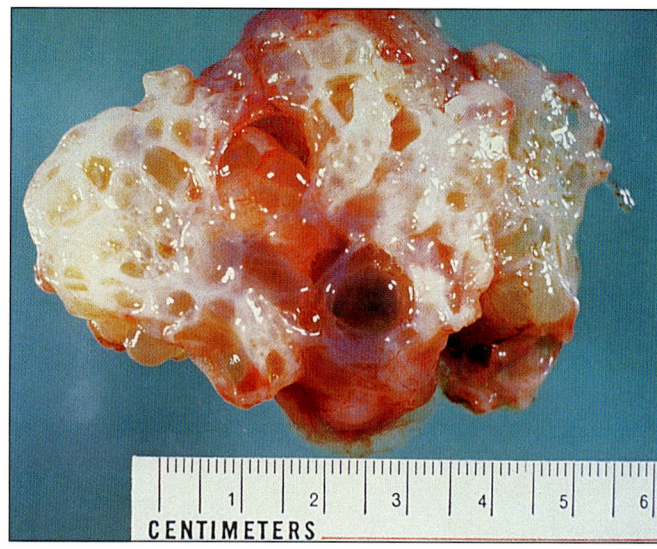

Fig. 33.36 Multicystic mesothelioma.

While some may be reactive in origin and may well represent variants of mesothelial hyperplasia or multiloculated peritoneal inclusion cyst (see above), the fact that some can be substantial in size and have atypical nuclei suggests that the latter examples may be neoplastic. Grossly, the tumors are multicystic with thin-walled cysts separated by thin fibrous septa (Figure 33.36). Cells lining the cysts may be flat to 'hobnail' in shape (Figures 33.37–33.39). While most cells are bland, the nuclei in some cases may be atypical. At the other end of a wide morphologic spectrum, some lesions may be virtually indistinguishable from adenomatoid tumors. Occasional tumors have recurred.[190]

DIFFUSE MALIGNANT MESOTHELIOMA

Peritoneal diffuse malignant mesotheliomas, tumors arising from the mesothelium covering the peritoneum, are much less common than their pleural counterparts, accounting for about 10% of all malignant mesotheliomas.[47] It is important that

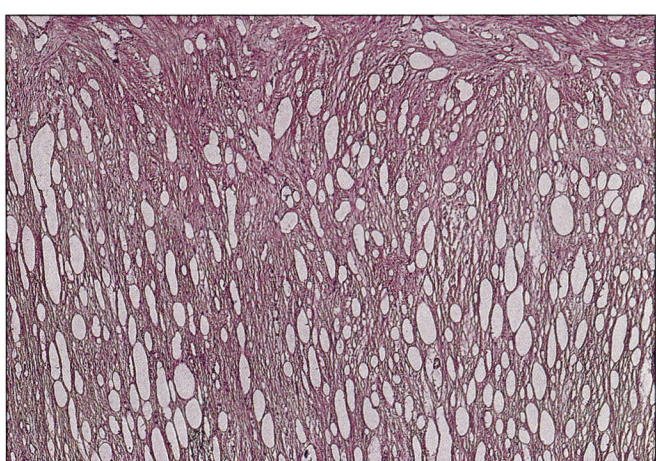

Fig. 33.37 Multicystic mesothelioma. On low power, the tumor resembles an adenomatoid tumor.

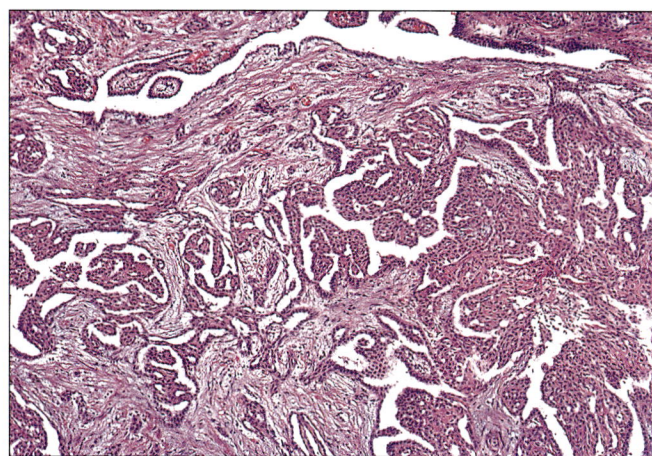

Fig. 33.40 Diffuse malignant mesothelioma.

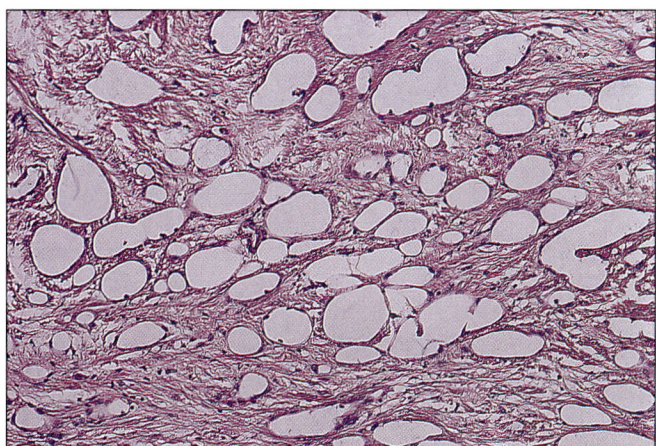

Fig. 33.38 Detail of multicystic mesothelioma.

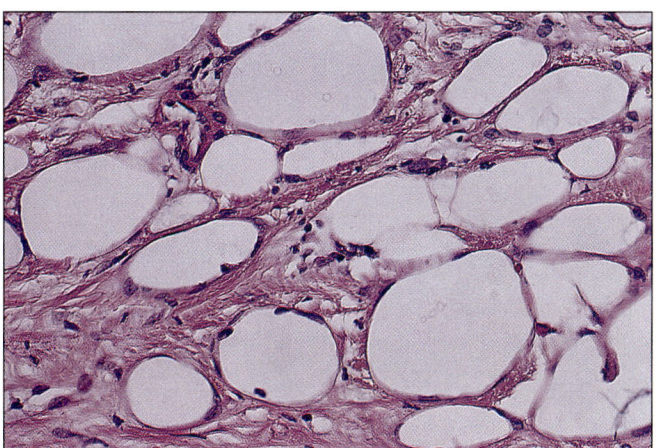

Fig. 33.39 Multicystic mesothelioma, high-power magnification.

these tumors be distinguished from serous adenocarcinomas, including those arising from the peritoneal surface itself and those metastatic from an ovarian primary, because the survival rate for women with malignant mesothelioma is worse than that for women with serous adenocarcinoma, and the treat-

ment of the two diseases currently differs. In our experience, this is less of a diagnostic problem than is generally inferred in the literature. Peritoneal diffuse malignant mesotheliomas occasionally develop in young women, but most patients are middle-aged or postmenopausal, and the tumor frequency increases with age.

Clinical manifestations usually are non-specific and include ascites, abdominal discomfort, digestive disturbances, and weight loss. Presentation with acute appendicitis, acute chole-cystitis, incarcerated hernia or 'Sister Mary Joseph nodule' (deep subcutaneous nodule in the umbilical area) has been reported in exceptional cases.[113,156] In contrast to malignant mesotheliomas of the pleura, there is no gender disparity in the prevalence of peritoneal malignant mesotheliomas. Moreover, while most tumors are highly aggressive, some peritoneal malignant mesotheliomas pursue a more indolent course.[114] Finally, the evidence for a causal link between asbestos exposure and peritoneal mesothelioma is weaker for women than for men. It is generally stated in the literature that asbestos exposure is uncommon in women with peritoneal mesothelioma. In one recent population-based study of peritoneal malignant mesotheliomas, 29% of 96 men had asbestos-related jobs whereas none of 113 women had occupational or environmental risk factors.[98] One study has shown asbestos burdens of 56 738 to 1 963 250 fibers per gram of wet weight tissue in six of seven women examined.[97] In contrast, men with peritoneal mesotheliomas typically have had an even heavier burden and more prolonged exposure to asbestos than men with pleural mesotheliomas.

Pathology

Tumors may extensively involve and diffusely thicken the peritoneum and the serosa of the various abdominal and pelvic organs. On microscopic examination, most tumors have only an epithelial component, which usually has a tubulopapillary to focally solid pattern. Unlike pleural mesotheliomas, sarcomatoid or fibrous variants are extremely rare.[10,23,114,153] The epithelial variant of malignant mesothelioma has polygonal or cuboidal cells with moderately abundant eosinophilic cytoplasm (Figures 33.40–33.42). Cells tend to have a more or less constant nuclear:cytoplasmic ratio and only mild to moderate nuclear atypia (Figures 33.43 and 33.44), although in some cases the nuclei become larger and more bizarre as the cyto-

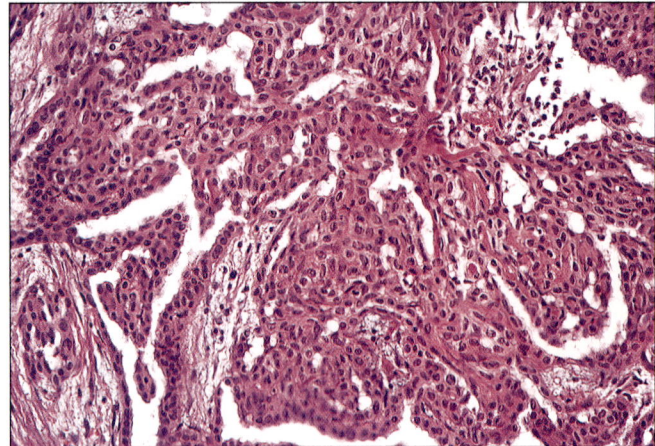

Fig. 33.41 Diffuse malignant mesothelioma, detail.

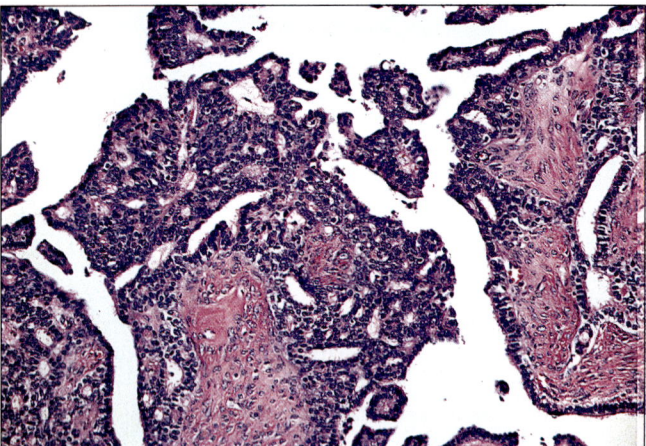

Fig. 33.42 Diffuse malignant mesothelioma with a somewhat glandular pattern.

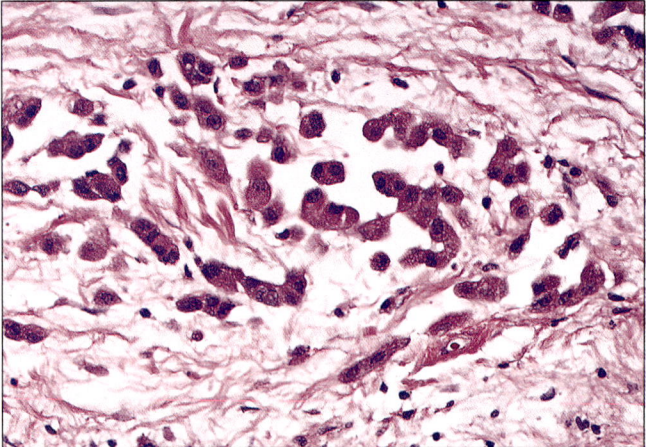

Fig. 33.43 Diffuse malignant mesothelioma. Individual cells have central banal nuclei and copious eosinophilic cytoplasm.

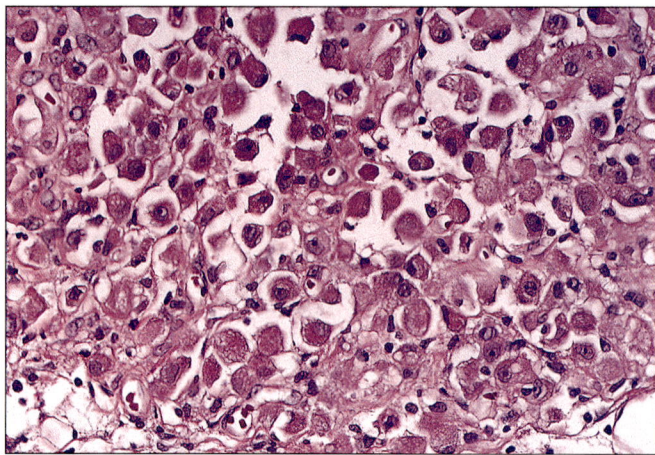

Fig. 33.44 Diffuse malignant mesothelioma in which the cells display a more or less constant nuclear:cytoplasmic ratio and only mild to moderate nuclear atypia.

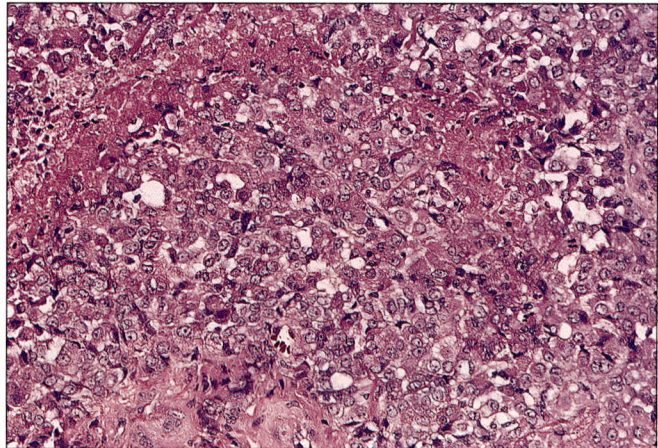

Fig. 33.45 Diffuse malignant mesothelioma in which the compact cells display a more or less constant nuclear:cytoplasmic ratio.

plasmic volume increases (Figure 33.45).[137] In rare cases, the cytoplasm is abundant, amphophilic, and glassy, mimicking decidual change (so-called 'deciduoid mesothelioma').[10,201] Biphasic histology, increased mitotic index, and p16 loss also independently correlate with increased risk of death according to one study,[23] while another failed to identify any morphologic features that differentiated those cases with a highly aggressive course from indolent ones.[114]

Differential diagnosis

The two types of lesion that are most difficult to distinguish from diffuse malignant mesothelioma are florid mesothelial hyperplasia and serous adenocarcinoma, whether the latter is primary in the peritoneum or metastatic from the ovary or another site. In contrast to hyperplasia, malignant mesothelioma often has grossly visible nodules, necrosis, and conspicuous large cytoplasmic vacuoles, and may have severe nuclear pleomorphism. Destructive tissue invasion should be sought as an important pointer to biologic malignancy. Reactive mesothelial cells generally have smaller nuclei than those of malignant mesothelioma. In some cases the reactive mesothelial proliferations may be indolent and remain for years.

The diagnosis that results in substantially differing treatment plans is the high-grade serous adenocarcinoma (Table 33.3). Psammocarcinoma and low-grade serous carcinoma with abundant psammoma bodies are readily distinguished from mesothelioma, in which psammoma bodies are few when

Table 33.3 Malignant mesothelioma versus serous carcinoma: differential diagnosis

Feature	Malignant mesothelioma	Serous carcinoma
Clinical		
History of asbestos exposure	Often positive	None
Diffuse peritoneal tumor mass	Yes	Usually dominant ovarian
Responsive to therapy	Rapidly fatal and unresponsive	Some respond
Histologic		
Sarcomatoid and adenomatoid foci	Present	Absent
Columnar cells	Rare	Numerous
Psammoma bodies	Rare	Often present
Nuclei	Round	Oval or elongate
Mucins (scanty)	Cytoplasmic acid mucin	Apical neutral mucin
Ultrastructural		
Tonofilaments	Abundant	Usually sparse
Cilia	Never numerous	Often numerous
Intracytoplasmic lumina	Common	Uncommon
Apical 'snouts'	Rare	Common

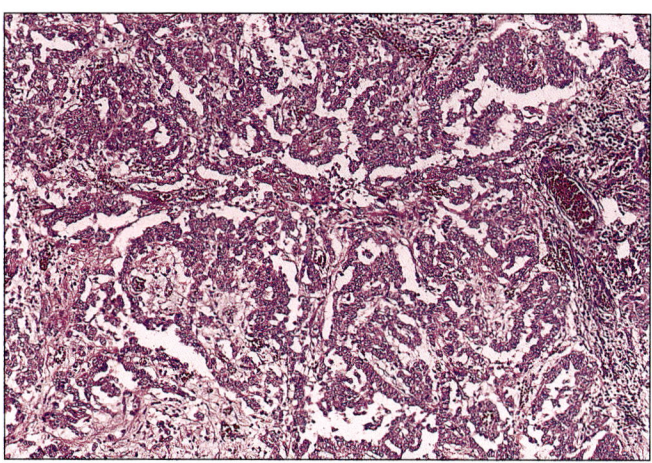

Fig. 33.46 Diffuse malignant mesothelioma in which tumor cells lie on the surface.

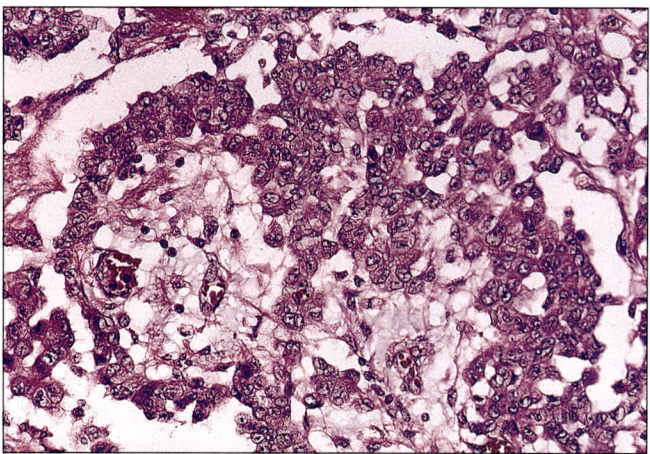

Fig. 33.47 Diffuse malignant mesothelioma, high-power magnification.

they are present. Mesothelial cells tend to be uniform, polygonal, and have moderate-to-extensive amounts of eosinophilic cytoplasm. Adenocarcinomas, in contrast, tend to have columnar cells, occasional cells with bizarre nuclear features, and variable numbers of psammoma bodies. Complicating the distinction, it is now recognized that malignant mesotheliomas can on rare occasion arise within the ovary.[40]

Often, immunohistochemistry is critically important in establishing the proper diagnosis. Many investigations have explored the differential staining patterns of the two conditions.[9,43,85,139] A summary of their findings is presented in Table 33.2. Calretinin, a 29 kDa calcium-binding protein, is present in nearly all epithelial mesotheliomas (Figures 33.46–33.48), but rare in adenocarcinomas. The exact function of this protein is unknown, although it seems to be involved in the metabolic process that regulates the maintenance of tumor cells in the cell cycle, prohibiting their entrance into the apoptotic pathway.[158] A cytokeratin cocktail made up of low-weight cytokeratins is usually positive in both mesothelioma and adenocarcinoma. Cytokeratin 5/6 is usually expressed by mesotheliomas, but seldom by adenocarcinomas. Vimentin and desmin are commonly detected in mesotheliomas. Once, it was believed that vimentin expression favored a diagnosis of mesothelioma, but it is now known that this intermediate filament is seen in normal and neoplastic cells of both epithelial and mesenchymal origin. Moreover, keratins and vimentin are commonly coexpressed by adenocarcinomas of müllerian type. CA125, an antigen initially identified in cell lines of ovarian serous adenocarcinomas, can be expressed by mesotheliomas.

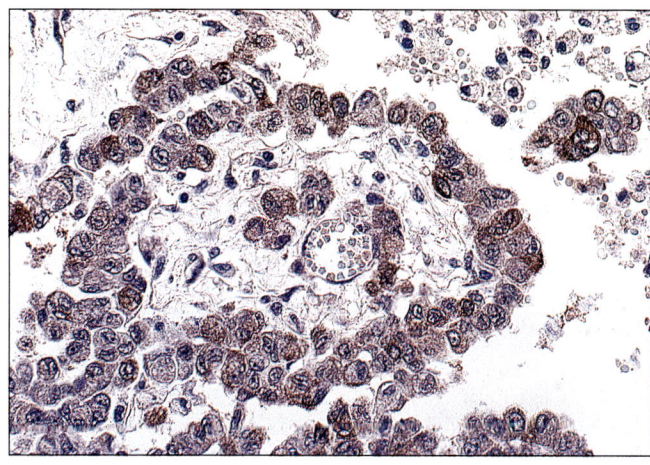

Fig. 33.48 Diffuse malignant mesothelioma, calretinin immunoreaction.

SEROUS TUMORS (PRIMARY AND METASTATIC)

In the ovary, the most frequently encountered tumors are in the class of surface epithelial–stromal neoplasms. They account for nearly 60% of all ovarian tumors.[178] The most common subtype is the serous neoplasm, accounting for 45% of the common epithelial tumors. Other frequently occurring types are the mucinous, endometrioid, and clear cell tumors.

In the peritoneum, the serous tumor is the only müllerian-type tumor encountered with a notable frequency. The rare occurrence of endometrioid or clear cell tumors and müllerian-type sarcomas and malignant mixed mesodermal tumors is usually associated with development from endometriosis. Mucinous tumors that are primary in the peritoneum, i.e., not retroperitoneal in location, are so rare as to be reportable. Most mucinous tumors in the peritoneum are metastatic from a gastrointestinal or rarely an ovarian primary.

SEROUS TUMOR OF BORDERLINE MALIGNANCY (PROLIFERATING TUMORS, TUMORS OF LOW MALIGNANT POTENTIAL)

Peritoneal tumors that are histologically identical to serous borderline tumors of the ovary, but where the patient is free of ovarian disease, are well known.[103,227] The age range is wide (mean, 32 years, range 16–77 years) and in two-thirds of cases only the pelvic peritoneum is involved. Many patients given limited treatment so as to preserve fertility had no evidence of persistent tumor years later. Invasive low-grade peritoneal serous carcinoma developed in 8% of them.

Considerably more common are cases in which these peritoneal lesions are accompanied by an ovarian serous tumor of borderline malignancy, and, in such cases, many or all of these peritoneal proliferations are regarded as 'implants' from the ovarian neoplasm. The origin and significance of serous borderline tumors arising in the peritoneum or implanting onto it are two very controversial subjects in gynecologic pathology.[208] Some of the numerous issues include the following:

- What is an appropriate microscopic definition of peritoneal serous borderline tumor? Is it biologically or functionally equivalent to implants (metastases) from an ovarian neoplasm? As stated above, we feel that many cases listed as showing endosalpingiosis are actually metastases.
- What is atypical endosalpingiosis, and indeed, is there such a thing? If so, does this condition give rise to borderline serous tumor?
- What features distinguish peritoneal implants of ovarian serous borderline tumor from a primary peritoneal invasive carcinoma (sometimes elastic stains) when a marked desmoplastic stromal response develops?
- What features help to distinguish between invasive and non-invasive implants, especially when the tumor has elicited a marked desmoplastic stromal response?
- What histologic features permit the pathologist to distinguish reliably among the various conditions listed below?

Some of these controversial issues are also addressed in Chapter 24.

Pathology

Papillary processes, small clusters of cells, cell stratification, detached cellular clusters, nuclear atypia, and mitotic activity in the absence of invasion identify a serous tumor as being of borderline malignancy, whether it is in the ovary or in the peritoneum. Grossly, the implants of serous borderline tumors appear as fine granularities ('miliary granularities') or small nodules several millimeters in diameter that are present on the surface or just beneath it (Figure 33.49) Low-power microscopic examination discloses extensive clusters of blunt papillae or glandular structures, often with complex cellular tufts (Figures 33.50 and 33.51). Psammoma bodies are common and may fill the core of the papilla (Figure 33.52). Commonly the papillae and even the psammoma bodies overshadow the epithelial component (Figure 33.53). Some clusters of cells may be detached. There is usually mild-to-severe cytologic atypia with some stratification, but substantially less than that with typical adenocarcinoma (Figure 33.54). These features, except for the prominence of the psammoma bodies, are all typical of serous borderline tumor as described for the ovary.[22] When in

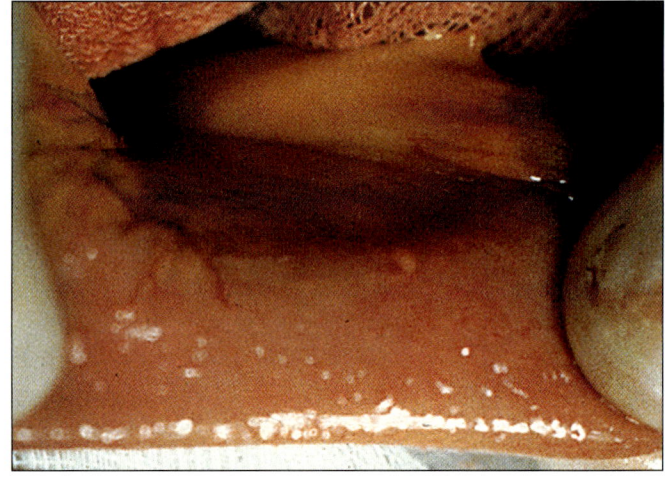

Fig. 33.49 Miliary peritoneal implants of serous borderline tumor of ovary.

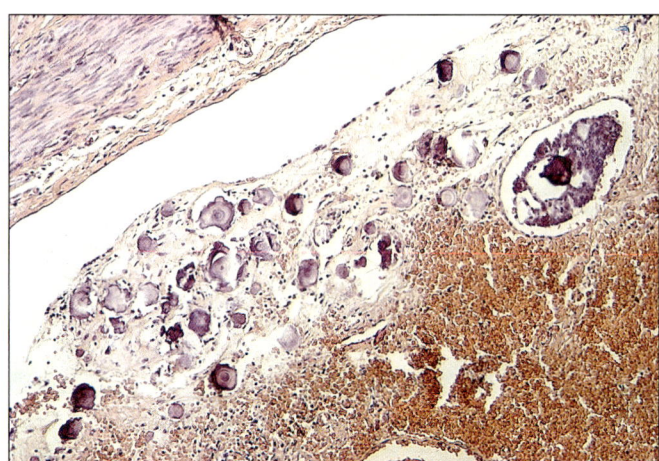

Fig. 33.50 Non-invasive implants. The peritoneal tumor from the borderline serous tumor of ovary shows numerous blunt glands and papillae with extensive psammoma bodies.

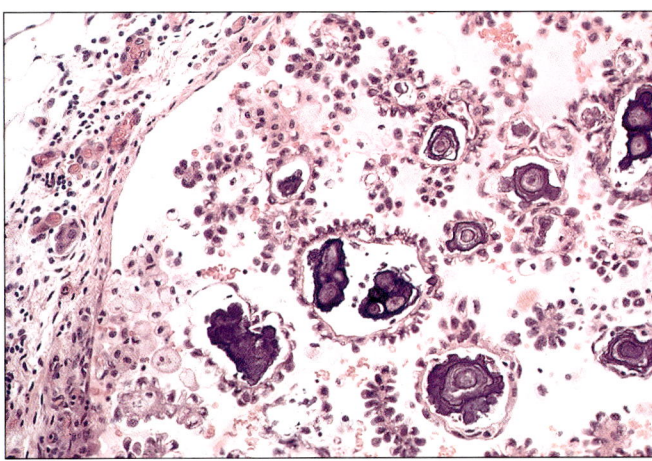

Fig. 33.51 Non-invasive implants with epithelial tufts and psammoma bodies.

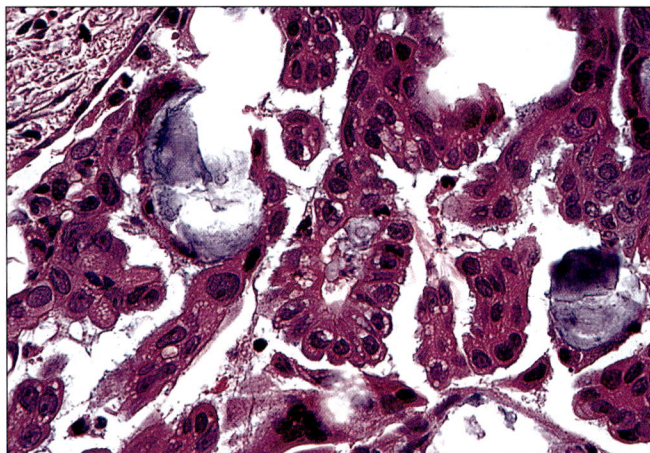

Fig. 33.54 Peritoneal implants with slightly atypical epithelial cells and prominent calcifications.

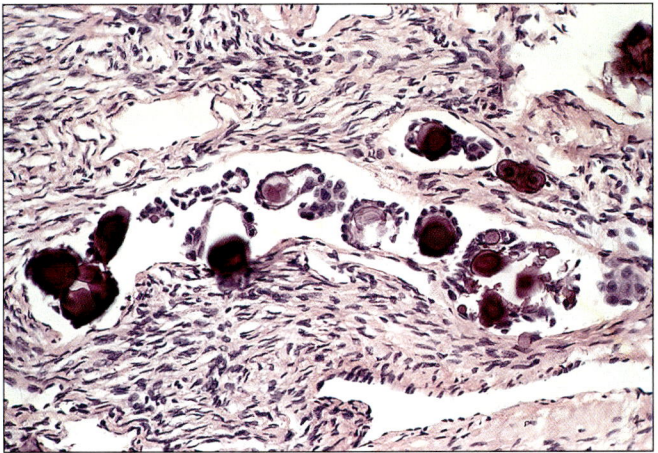

Fig. 33.52 Non-invasive implants with prominent psammoma bodies.

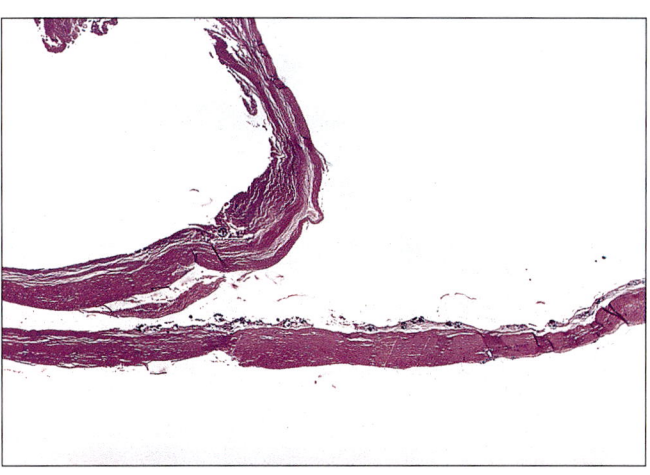

Fig. 33.55 Extensive numbers of psammoma bodies in peritoneal deposits. Clinically, the surface was gritty to touch.

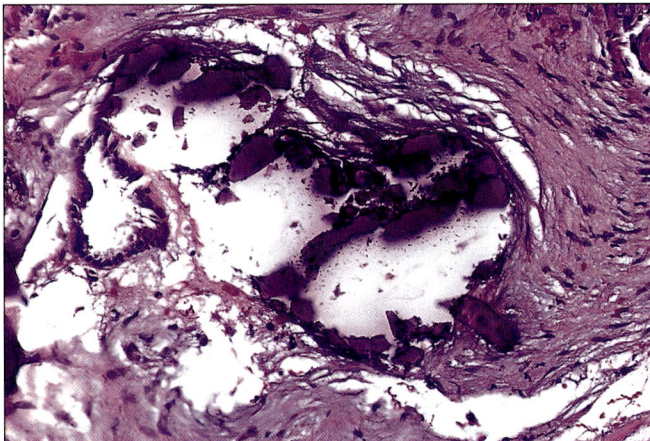

Fig. 33.53 Peritoneal deposits of borderline serous tumor. Few foci of slightly atypical epithelial cells are seen among the extensive psammomatous calcifications. (Note: each subsequent photomicrograph denoted by an asterisk (*) is from the same patient who had a serous borderline tumor of the ovary and various forms of implants in the peritoneum. She is well after 25 years.)

the omentum, and especially when found in crevices between lobules of omentum, borderline tumors may occasionally elicit a marked desmoplastic stromal response. Not uncommonly, biopsies of the peritoneum will disclose the presence of only psammoma bodies (Figures 33.55 and 33.56). In a rare case, these have even been encountered in routine cervical smears (Figure 33.57). It has been our experience that where extensive biopsies have been performed, for example in a staging laparotomy, some foci will show the more typical epithelial changes of borderline serous tumor.

The presence of only psammoma bodies on the peritoneum poses a special problem. They may reflect serous epithelium, often as borderline serous tumor, where the epithelium has undergone degeneration leaving only the residua of psammoma bodies. They may also represent intraperitoneal shedding to dependent regions from tumor growing on the ovarian serosa. In the absence of an epithelial component, we prefer to note the causes of psammoma bodies in the differential diagnosis, but refrain from considering them as definitive evidence of tumor, either primary or metastatic implants to the peritoneum.

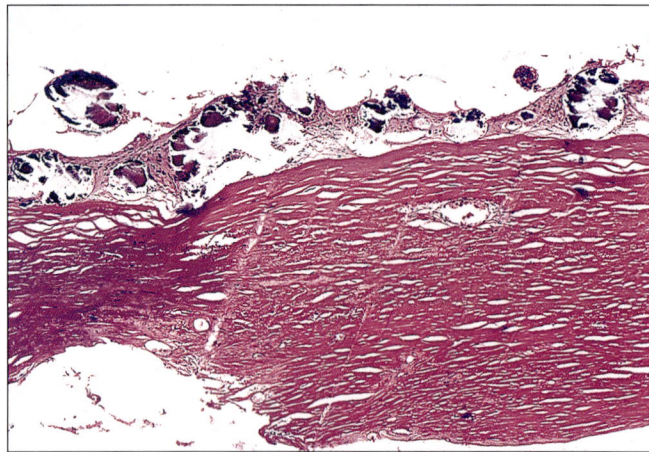

Fig. 33.56 Peritoneal deposits of borderline serous tumor. Medium–low magnification showing almost exclusive psammomatous calcifications*.

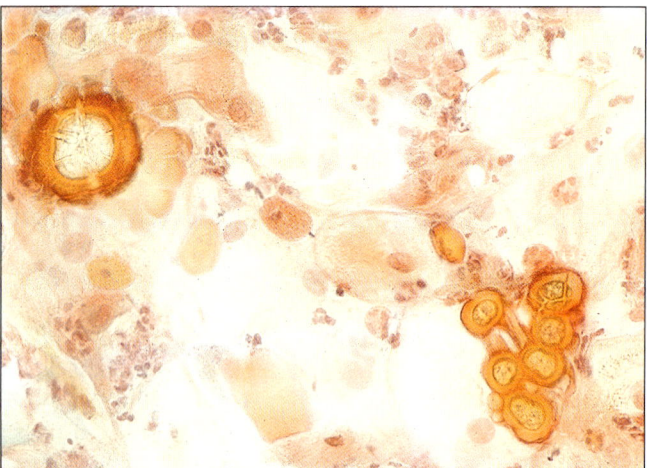

Fig. 33.57 Extensive psammoma bodies in a Papanicolaou smear. The patient had a serous borderline tumor of the ovary and extensive implants in the peritoneum.

Types of implant

Regardless of whether peritoneal serous lesions arise in that location or implant onto it, they fall into several relatively well-characterized groups. More than one of these types of implant may be encountered in any given patient, at either the initial procedure or a subsequent operation. The presence of one of these implant types (invasive implant), and maybe others, portends progression of the disease to a low-grade carcinoma.

Implant types include the following (Figure 33.58).

* Categories well accepted:
  – non-invasive epithelial implants
  – non-invasive desmoplastic implants
  – invasive implants
* Categories about which ambiguity exists:
  – non-invasive implants with atypical features
  – implants, indeterminate for invasion.

All of the types of non-invasive implant may show marked cytologic atypia, variable mitoses, single cell infarction, and calcifications.[130] Key features helpful in distinguishing non-invasive and invasive implants are summarized in Table 33.4.

Non-invasive epithelial implants These implants demonstrate no invasion into the underlying normal tissue (Figures 33.59–33.61). Epithelium shows papillary proliferations lined by typical serous cells and it resides on the peritoneal surfaces or just beneath it. If embedded in subperitoneal stroma, the implants are in smoothly lined locules. In the omentum these may lie between lobules (Figure 33.61). A stromal reaction, if present, is rarely more than minimal. Implants usually show minimal cytologic atypia.

Non-invasive desmoplastic implants These show small clusters of tumor cells (and rarely single cells or large broad papillae) that lie in a dense, markedly reactive, fibrotic stroma that is layered upon the serosal surfaces, frequently in the septa between omental fatty lobules (Figures 33.62–33.66). They may also be found on the peritoneum in dependent areas. Well-developed examples appear as plaques in which the desmoplastic stroma is more abundant than the epithelium, the entrapped epithelial cells are somewhat evenly distributed within the stroma, and inflamed granulation tissue covers the surface. Other than in the omentum, they are usually separated from the underlying tissue by the peritoneal elastic membrane, which can be stained for by routine elastic stains. As the tumor cells or papillary fragments die, or are entrapped and compressed by the fibroblastic proliferation, they may undergo dystrophic calcification, forming psammoma bodies. In most areas of pathology, desmoplasia is considered as a warning sign that invasive tumor cells may be nearby. In the peritoneum, reactive or desmoplastic stroma may occur in response to displaced or degenerated cells or cellular debris (see above), including implants from a borderline or frank ovarian carcinoma. Inflammation probably also helps to embed peritoneal metaplastic epithelial inclusions, giving the appearance of invasion. Also, ovarian carcinomas do not always elicit a stromal response when they metastasize to peritoneal surfaces, and in such cases they must be recognized by other attributes.

Invasive implants These show any of the following patterns (Figures 33.67–33.69).

* Destructive infiltration of underlying tissue.
* Abundant single cell infiltration.
* Irregular or angulated margins of clustered tumor cells. This reflects tumor cells dissecting along stromal cell planes. When papillae or small clusters of tumor cells invade into the stroma, the stromal margins may appear retracted (an artifact), and display sharp angulations and pointed contours.
* Small clusters of cells irregularly clumped in a pale, loose stroma. These may appear as small, irregular tongues of tumor cells that extend from the base of glands in a pattern similar to microinvasive cancer of the cervix.
* Solid clusters of cells, especially with a cribriform pattern (intraglandular bridging).

Non-invasive implants with atypical features The literature during the past decades is replete with conflicting interpretations of various histologic harbingers of adverse outcome. Some implants, in the absence of frank invasion into adjacent tissue, exhibit features that some investigators associate with a worse behavior, and thus warranting more aggressive therapy. The 'micropapillary' pattern is the most notorious of these.

Serous peritoneal implants

Fig. 33.58 Types of serous peritoneal implants associated with serous borderline tumor of ovary.

Non-invasive

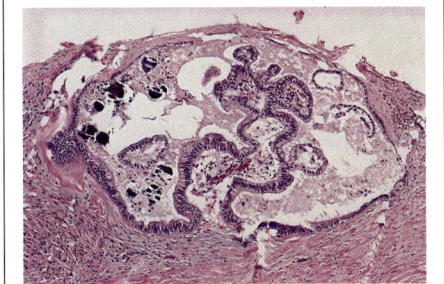

Surface implant

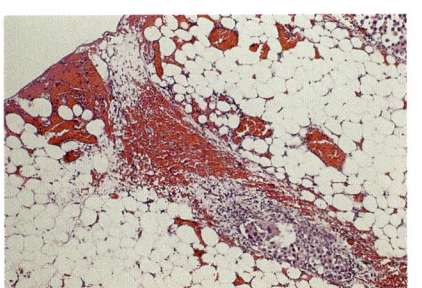

Implant between fat lobules

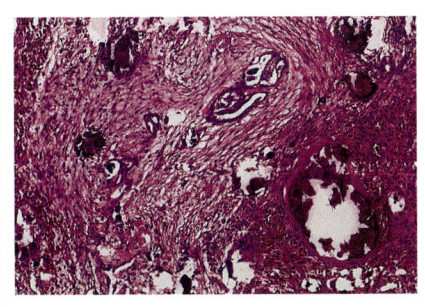

Desmoplastic implant

Invasive

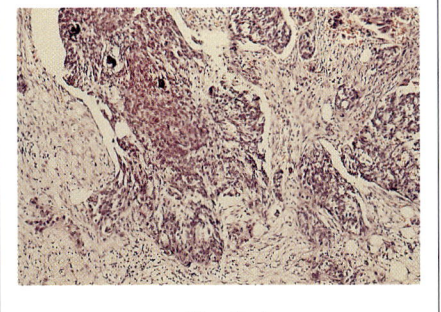

Solid angulated margins

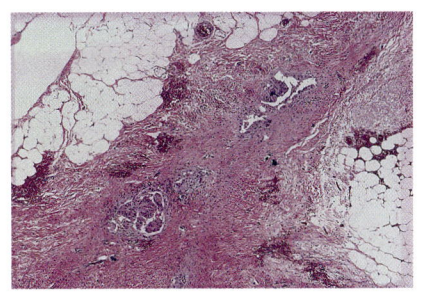

Single cell infiltration

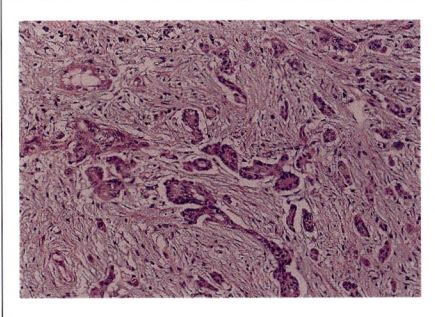

Clustered cell infiltration with retraction

Since this feature was first introduced[26,196] and later reviewed[16] as an adverse feature, others have shown that the feature is associated with more extensive abdominal spread and hence higher stage, but not with a worse prognosis.[82,168,169] Only invasive implants are associated with fatality.

Another pattern described as atypical is the conspicuous presence of small, solid or cribriform epithelial nests. While these features are generally regarded as signs of histologic malignancy, they do not influence prognosis if microscopically small in quantity. Finally, tiny clusters of tumor cells sur-rounded by cleft-like spaces are presently considered malignant. While these patterns have sometimes been considered as covariants,[16] others provided evidence that this pronouncement might be premature.[82,130]

Implants, indeterminate for invasion It is important to separate, wherever possible, invasive from non-invasive implants. Sometimes this cannot be done with certainty. Examples might include biopsies that are tiny, heavily calcified, or suboptimally preserved or processed. We recommend that small superficial

Table 33.4 Features distinguishing non-invasive and invasive implants in serous tumor involving the peritoneum

	Non-invasive	Invasive
Architectural features	Sharp plane demarcating tumor and underlying normal tissue	Irregular infiltration of parietal, visceral or omental fat ('destructive growth')
	Well-defined involvement of omental crevices, preserving normal lobular architecture of surrounding tissue	Bulky expansion of crevices between omental fat lobules, obliterating normal architecture and incorporating fat cells into the reactive process
	Solid and cribriform pattern generally absent. Small compact nests and single cells may be present, but with few cleft-like spaces around them	Sheets of tumor, with or without cribriform pattern, that sometimes extends radially beyond the desmoplastic stromal response; peritumoral cleft-like spaces and single cells may be abundant
	Papillae and small nests sometimes in a desmoplastic stromal reaction, but lacking features of dissection	Papillae and small nests with dissection, and sometimes with desmoplastic stromal reaction and retraction
Cytologic features	Usually nil-to-moderate nuclear atypia with no more than rare mitoses	May show marked nuclear atypia with multiple mitoses, sometimes atypical
Ancillary techniques	DNA diploid (euploid)	DNA diploid or aneuploid

Modified from a presentation by D.A. Bell, Boston, MA.

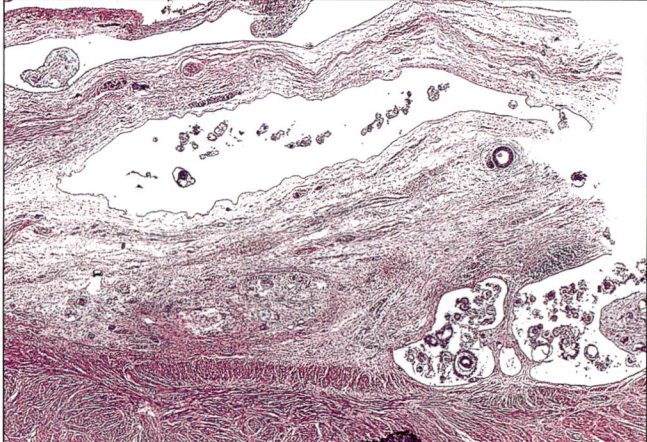

Fig. 33.59 Non-invasive implants.

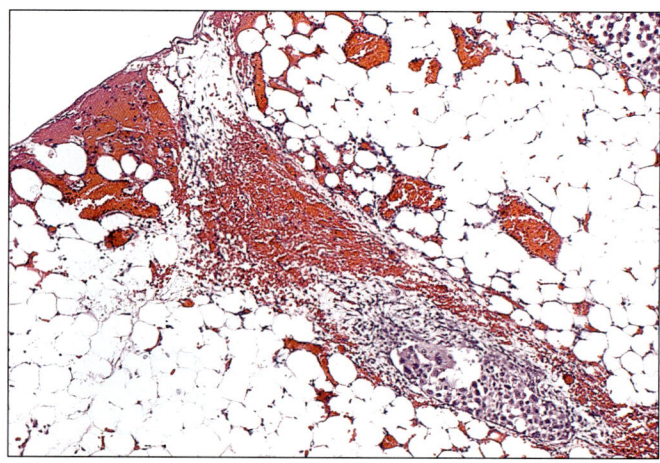

Fig. 33.61 Non-invasive implant between fat lobules in omentum.

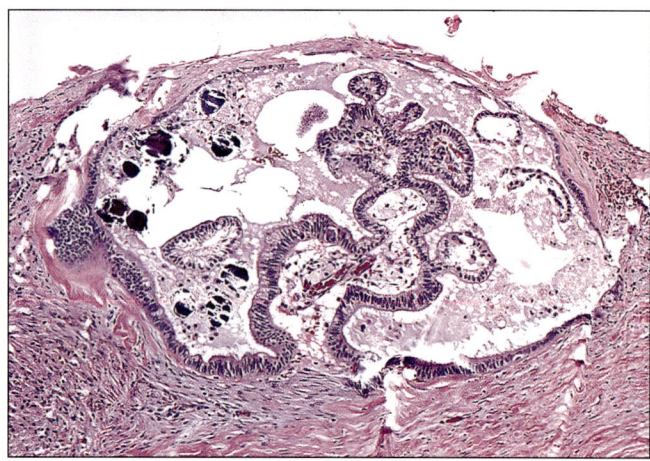

Fig. 33.60 Non-invasive surface implant. The exuberant epithelial proliferation and obvious calcifications lie distant from the extensive pure psammomatous calcifications seen in several preceding photomicrographs from this series*.

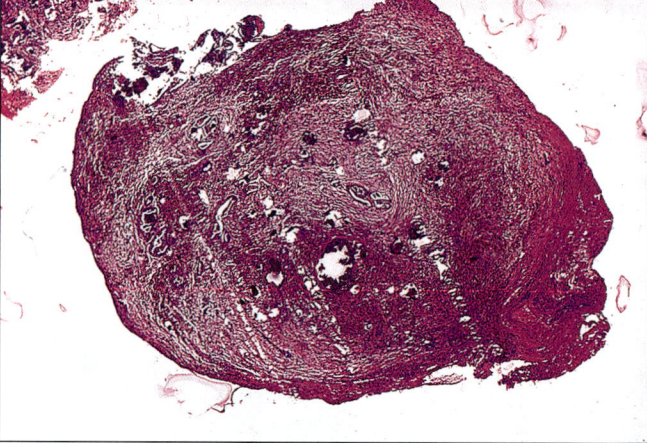

Fig. 33.62 Desmoplastic implant in pelvis*.

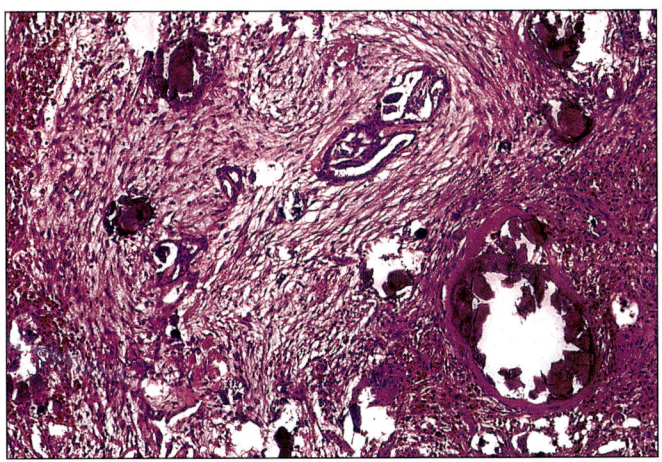

Fig. 33.63 Desmoplastic implant in pelvis, medium magnification*.

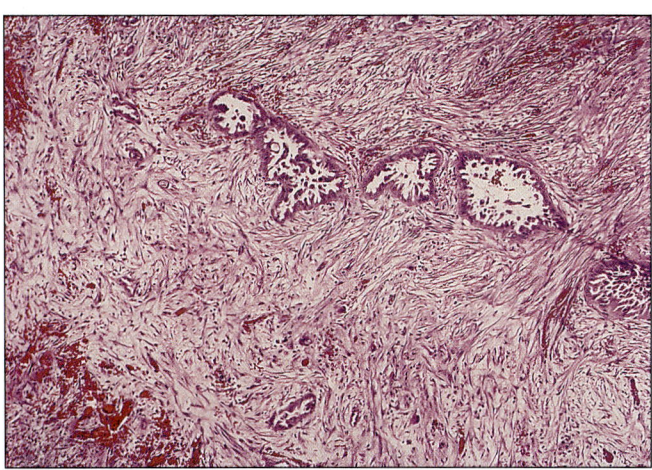

Fig. 33.64 Desmoplastic implant. The borderline serous tumor is entrapped in the marked fibrous reaction.

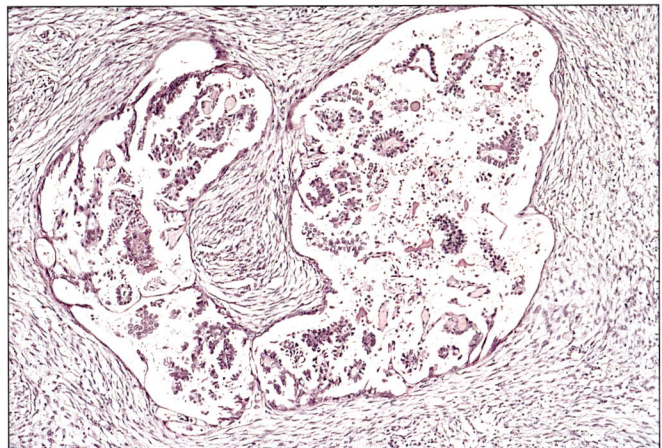

Fig. 33.65 Desmoplastic implant. Borderline serous tumor is entrapped in the marked fibrous reaction.

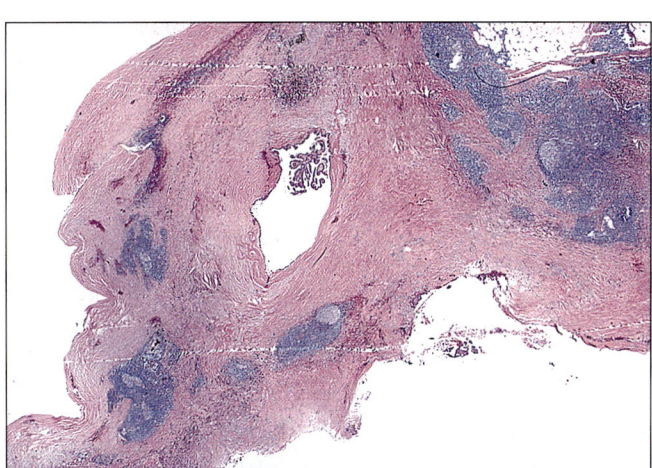

Fig. 33.66 Massive fibrous nodule in liver. The core contains an obvious focus of borderline serous tumor*.

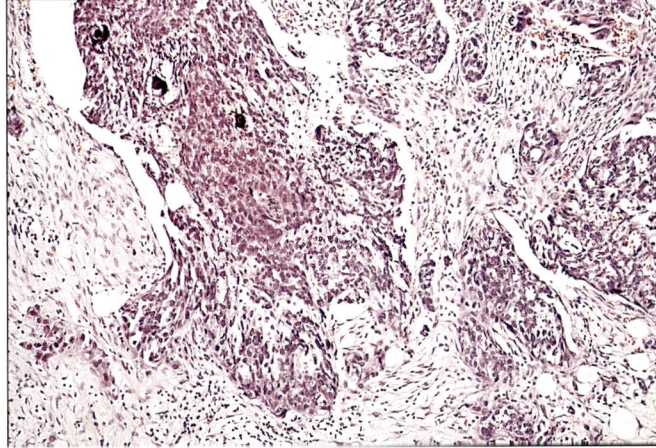

Fig. 33.67 Invasive implant. Solid clusters of tumor cells have irregular, angulated margins.

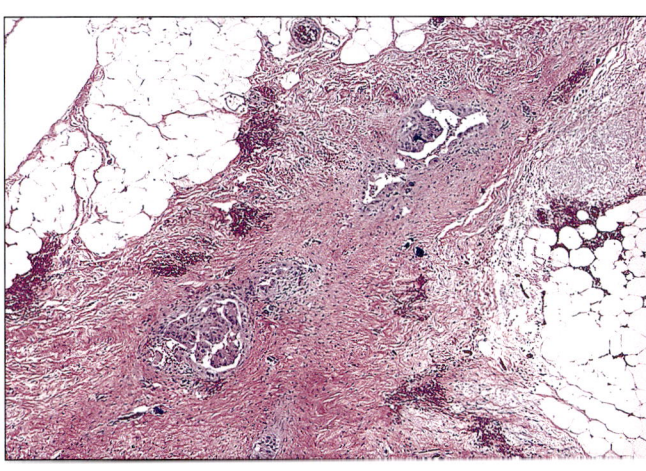

Fig. 33.68 Invasive implant with single cells irregularly dissecting into desmoplastic stroma.

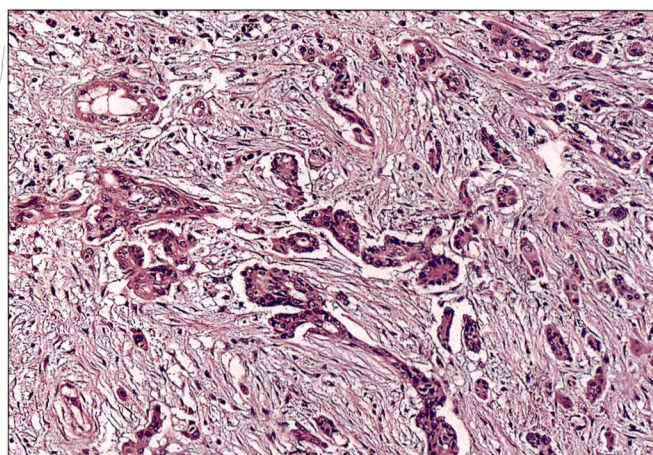

Fig. 33.69 Invasive implant. Small clusters of cells infiltrate into the desmoplastic stroma. The stroma about the tumor cells shows artifactual retraction.

biopsies of desmoplastic implants in which subjacent normal tissue is not present be classified as non-invasive implants, on the assumption that they would have been stripped away with ease by the surgeon.

Prognostic features
Patients with serous borderline tumors confined to the ovaries have an excellent prognosis and in these cases it is accepted practice that surgical resection alone is sufficient treatment. Prognosis and treatment for patients with extraovarian implants (accounting for about 40% of cases) and primary peritoneal tumors are less certain. In a comprehensive review, 16% of patients with extraovarian disease had recurrence or died of tumor.[197] From a practical point of view, three features have been identified to date that indicate a higher risk for aggressive biologic behavior:

- FIGO stage of disease
- invasive implants
- residual tumor after primary surgery.

These are findings that identify a small subgroup of patients with a more guarded prognosis.

The heterogeneous appearances of peritoneal implants and the adverse prognostic impact of invasive ones have been known for several decades. Unfortunately, various institutions have differing definitions of what constitutes an invasive implant and what is destructive infiltration.[54] Additionally, when strictly defined, other lesions associated with an adverse prognosis are sometimes missed. In a recent population-based study of 49 advanced stage serous borderline tumors, invasive implants were identified in only 12% of cases.[82] Use of more liberal definitions, however, has diminished the prognostic value of this feature.

Not uncommonly, clinicians are unclear as to how to treat patients with serous borderline tumors with non-invasive peritoneal implants, which promotes the tumor, if of ovarian origin, to at least FIGO stage 2 and more commonly to FIGO stage 3. Should the patient be re-explored to debulk the existing tumor and perform a staging laparotomy, or treated postoperatively with chemotherapy? Increasingly, it is becoming recognized that non-invasive implants carry some long-term risk

to the patient. While of a relatively low malignant potential, they nevertheless are prognostically adverse, leading to tumor recurrence in 44% of patients, with 10% of recurrences occurring within 5 years, 19% between 5 and 10 years, 10% between 10 and 15 years, and 5% after 15 years.[209] In another study of patients with only non-invasive implants, with a median follow-up time of over 10 years, 15% of patients with macroscopic residual disease at completion of initial surgery who subsequently underwent second-look surgery had responded to chemotherapy.[78] Thirty per cent developed progressive disease or had a relapse with a median time of 7 years from the date of diagnosis to relapse. In two-thirds of these patients, the tumor had transformed histologically to an invasive low-grade serous adenocarcinoma. These findings were interpreted to indicate that the presence of macroscopic residual disease is an adverse predictor of subsequent disease. However, other series have experienced no such malignant transformation, even with equally long follow-up periods.[22]

The presence of residual macroscopic disease also appeared to be a major predictor of recurrence and survival in a study of patients with invasive implants.[79] The median time from date of diagnosis to recurrence in this study was about 2 years, and of these patients most had invasive low-grade serous adenocarcinoma diagnosed in the recurrence. Although slightly more than half of the few patients who were able to be evaluated with second-look operations showed a response to chemotherapy, it was unclear prospectively which patients should be selected for such forms of therapy.

SEROUS CARCINOMA (OF PERITONEAL ORIGIN)

Ever since primary peritoneal serous carcinoma was first recognized a half century ago as an entity, there has been considerable debate about its nomenclature, biologic behavior, and differentiation from serous carcinoma metastatic to the peritoneum from the ovary (or elsewhere).[56] It has only one-tenth the frequency of serous carcinoma arising in the ovary,[69,185] which assumes that none of these cancers are actually metastases from small ovarian cancers where the peritoneum has provided a more hospitable site for growth than the ovary.[195] The mean age of women with this tumor is 50–65 years.[58,112] Abdominal pain and ascites are frequent primary symptoms and signs.[12] Like ovarian cancer in general, serous carcinoma primary in the peritoneum may have a familial basis.[11,112,166] Like ovarian cancer, it can also metastasize to distant locations.[57]

Definition of primary disease
The most widely accepted definition of primary peritoneal serous carcinoma uses the criteria advocated by the Gynecologic Oncology Group. These are:

- Ovaries are normal in size or enlarged by a benign process.
- The extraovarian sites of carcinoma are of significantly greater volume than the tumor present on either ovary.
- The ovarian tumor component is non-existent, confined to the ovarian surface with or without stromal invasion measuring in aggregate less than 5×5 mm, or within the ovarian substance and measuring less than 5×5 mm.
- The histologic characteristics indicate serous carcinoma of any grade.

While these criteria do not assure that each individual case in the peritoneum is truly primary, they certainly minimize the chance that any significant numbers are metastases from the ovary to the peritoneum.

Pathology

The peritoneal tumor is generally bulky and widespread, showing extensive peritoneal carcinomatosis, and almost always involves the omentum. Occasionally, smaller tumors may appear as discrete nodules arising from multiple peritoneal surfaces. Microscopically, the tumor primary in the peritoneum is morphologically identical to serous adenocarcinoma arising in the ovary (see Chapter 24). Tumor cells have a typical feathery low-power appearance with extensive papillae and a variable scattering of psammoma bodies. Tumor grade spans the same range as is seen in the ovarian analogues but, in our experience, a disproportionate number are high-grade carcinomas.

Pathogenesis

Molecular studies suggest that some but not all peritoneal cancers may be polyclonal and multifocal in origin.[55,112,143,149,193] This differs from ovarian carcinoma, which is almost always monoclonal.[121,143,149,193,194] In one study, seven cases of primary peritoneal carcinoma were diagnosed among more than 1200 women in the Gilda Radner Ovarian Cancer Detection Program, a program established for women at known high risk for developing ovarian or peritoneal cancer based on a familial history.[112] Tumors in these women were identified in different ways, including elevated levels of CA125, abnormal ultrasonographs or abdominal symptoms. Five of the tumors studied for clonality demonstrated differing patterns of gene expression in differing tumor sites. Markers included p53, bcl-2, HER-2/neu and nm-23. While these findings indicated polyclonality and were suggestive of multifocal origin, an origin from a single site could not be excluded for several reasons.[77] One possibility was that the cancer originated at one site, but that in metastasizing acquired additional genetic aberrations or genetic instability. In addition, gene expression may be under different control mechanisms at differing sites. These observations do, however, support the hypothesis that serous carcinoma of the peritoneum has a molecular pathogenesis distinct from that of analogous ovarian neoplasms. In another report, the polyclonal nature was defined more thoroughly. Using tumor cells microdissected from paraffin-embedded samples, loss of heterozygosity, a molecular genetic approach used to identify tumor suppressor genes, was found commonly in sporadic peritoneal carcinoma. At least two foci were affected, both on chromosome 17: the *p53* gene on the short arm and the *BRCA1* gene on the long arm.

Clinicopathologic correlation

Clinicopathologic studies generally have not shown significant epidemiologic differences between cancers arising within the peritoneum and in the ovary.[59,88,106]

Currently there is no accepted staging system for peritoneal carcinoma, complicating analysis of this tumor type as well as comparisons with ovarian serous carcinoma. One study, attempting to segregate the cases of serous carcinoma of the peritoneum, compared cases of ovarian serous carcinoma where the involvement was largely on the surface and divided these into groups where the involvement was small versus more extensive.[147] No differences in survival were found. Several studies have compared the survival of women who had tumor arising from the peritoneum with those who had tumors metastatic to the peritoneum from the ovary. Again no differences in biologic behavior and survival were observed.[17,164] As with primary ovarian carcinoma, debulking surgery with little residual tumor is a critical factor in subsequent survival.[220]

Lymph nodes are involved in 10–30% of cases with primary peritoneal carcinoma,[60] with a pattern of spread not unlike that of ovarian carcinoma. Whether lymph nodes are involved or not does not appear to separately affect prognosis.[60]

Recently the fallopian tube, particularly the fimbrial end, has been proposed as a potential site of origin of some ovarian or peritoneal serous cancers.[116,163] Woman with germline *BRCA* mutations have an increased risk of cancers in all of these sites.[4,127,128] One difficulty in evaluating those studies that propose a tubal origin for ovarian and peritoneal cancers is that they rely heavily on cases in which 'intraepithelial carcinoma' is the only tubal lesion. How can such lesions be defined with certainty in this location? Cannot a 'drop metastasis' to the tubal mucosa from another site mimic perfectly an *in situ* carcinoma, using the existing basement membrane as a scaffold for its expansion (something we have observed on a number of occasions). One feature that may be useful to identify metastatic origin from endometrium is non-reactivity of WT1, in contrast to expression of WT1 for serous carcinomas of the ovary, fallopian tube, and peritoneum.[2,6,62,94]

PSAMMOCARCINOMA

Psammocarcinoma, a rare form of serous carcinoma,[81] may arise as a primary tumor in the peritoneum or as an ovarian cancer that has metastasized to the peritoneum. For a tumor to be called 'psammocarcinoma' rather than 'serous carcinoma', psammoma bodies need to involve more than 75% of all papillae and there needs to be destructive invasion of tissue. The neoplastic epithelium should show only mild cytologic atypia, and epithelial sheets of tumor should not be present (see Chapter 24). This quantitative threshold, however, is arbitrary as the tumor may just be a subset of well-differentiated serous carcinomas. We suspect that some of the cases described in the peritoneum[144,148] are actually examples of serous borderline tumors (see above). Peritoneal implants in borderline serous tumors show many variations and psammoma body formation can be substantial, especially in areas where there is a marked desmoplastic stromal response or massive infarction. The overall prognosis of the psammocarcinoma, described as excellent, is the same as that of the borderline serous tumor,[229] but bad outcomes have been reported.[5]

MISCELLANEOUS PRIMARY TUMORS

INTRA-ABDOMINAL DESMOPLASTIC SMALL ROUND CELL TUMOR

Desmoplastic small round cell tumor is the descriptive designation for a rare, undifferentiated, and highly aggressive tumor that with few exceptions involves the peritoneal serosa[122] and contiguous organs such as the kidney and ovary.[236] It usually appears during adolescence and early adulthood, with a mean age of 25 years, but occasionally may be found in older women.[71,231] It is far more common in men than in women. The prognosis is poor.

Grossly, most tumors are bulky abdominal masses that have spread diffusely over the peritoneal surface. The characteristic microscopic pattern is nests of 'small, blue cells' embedded in a dense to massive and reactive fibrous stroma. About one-third of tumors exhibit a wider range of morphologic features, principally as spindle-shaped cells with epithelioid to focally sarcomatoid arrangements.

Virtually all tumors are cytokeratin (CK) positive (cytokeratin 'cocktail' monoclonal antibodies CAM 5.2, AE1/AE3), but lack CK20 expression, indicative that they are not of large intestinal origin.[76,159,160] Roughly four-fifths are also reactive with antibodies to epithelial membrane antigen (EMA), neuron-specific enolase (NSE), desmin (with paranuclear dot-like reactivity), and vimentin, suggestive that there is both epithelial and mesenchymal differentiation. Between two-fifths and two-thirds of tumors express Ber-EP4, CD57 (Leu-7), CD15 (Leu-M1), and CA125, suggestive that the tumor is not mesothelial in origin. Wilms tumor (WT1) protein is detected immunohistochemically in 90% of cases.[13] Most other common immunohistochemical stains lack reactivity in most cases. Electron microscopic examination shows the tumor cells have mesenchymal–fibroblastic features.

Coexpression of epithelial and mesenchymal antigens distinguishes the desmoplastic small round cell tumor from other small round and blue cell tumors occurring in this age group. These antigenic properties have challenged the popular notion that the intra-abdominal desmoplastic small round cell tumor is a 'blastomatous' tumor derived exclusively from the primitive mesothelium.

Several members of the undifferentiated small round cell tumor family share specific cytogenetic alterations.[51] A translocation involves the Ewing sarcoma gene (*EWS1*) on chromosome 22 and the Wilms tumor gene (*WT1*) on chromosome 11. The translocation, t(11;22)(p13;q12), resulting in a loss of three specific amino acids,[115] appears to have an oncogenic effect. Other translocation patterns have also been described.[157,206] The fusion protein that is produced seems to function as a potent activator of transcription, suggesting that the Wilms tumor gene gains function as a result of the fusion. Thus, the fusion gene seems to function as a dominant oncogene in this disease.[18]

SOLITARY FIBROUS TUMOR OF PERITONEUM ('FIBROUS MESOTHELIOMA')

Solitary fibrous tumors, previously called 'fibrous mesotheliomas', are primitive tumors composed of fibroblasts and primitive mesenchymal cells that can manifest multidirectional differentiation. They are rare tumors found most often in the pleura,[91] but do occur occasionally in the peritoneum.[70,72] Most patients remain well after tumor excision, although occasional neoplasms have acted aggressively.

Grossly, the tumors vary in size from 1 cm to over 20 cm in diameter (Figure 33.70). They are usually solitary and appear encapsulated by fibrous tissue. Microscopically, tumors are composed of spindle cells in a markedly collagenized stroma,

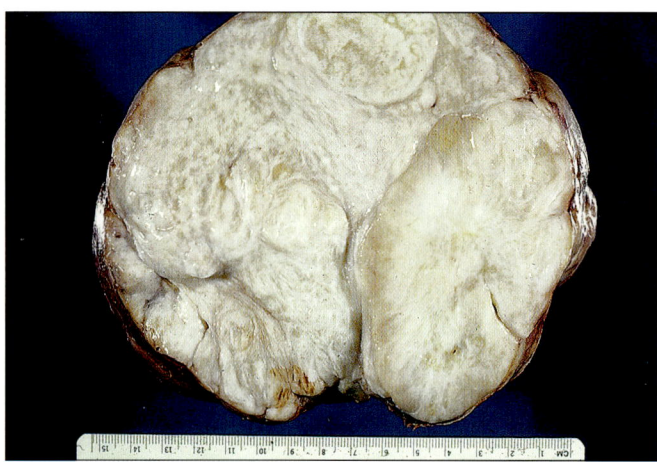

Fig. 33.70 Solitary benign fibrous mesothelioma. Courtesy of Dr Victor Roggli, Durham, NC.

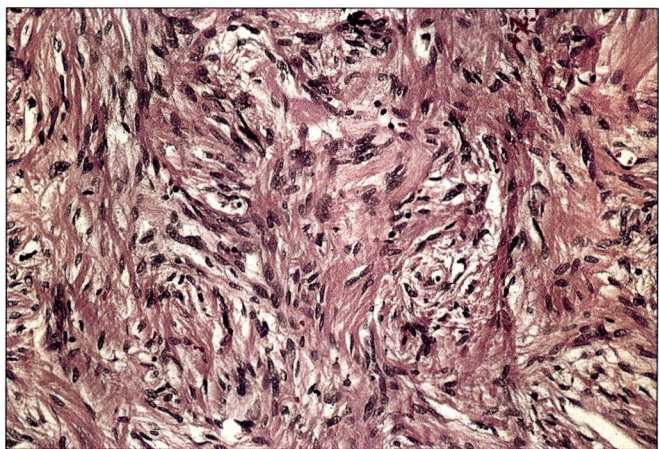

Fig. 33.71 Solitary benign mesothelioma. The tumor is composed of spindle cells in a markedly collagenized stroma. Courtesy of Dr Victor Roggli, Durham, NC.

often with abundant blood vessels, in a hemangiopericytoma-like pattern (Figure 33.71). Tumor cells may have fascicular, cord-like, and irregular arrangements and are found interspersed in strands in between thick collagen bundles. Nuclei are often vesicular and the nucleoli inconspicuous. Mitoses are rare.

Tumor cells are reactive for vimentin but not for cytokeratin. CD34, a sialylated transmembrane glycoprotein found initially in endothelial cells and myeloid progenitor cells, is usually demonstrable.[91] CD31, a platelet endothelial cell adhesion molecule, is not. By contrast, desmoplastic mesotheliomas, tumors in the differential diagnosis, are reactive for cytokeratin but not for CD34.[64]

OTHER TUMORS

A variety of tumors arise rarely in the peritoneum. Their histogenesis is not always certain. Of the less rare tumors, adenosarcomas are often associated with endometriosis.[216] Carcinosarcomas have also been described,[203] as have the stromal sarcomas[34] and rhabdomyosarcomas.[111] Pure epithelial tumors, such as clear cell adenocarcinoma, have been described, also in association with endometriosis.[216] It would seem likely that any tumor usually associated with an endometrial origin could well have arisen in extrauterine endometriosis, as have some of the above cited cases. This subject is discussed more fully in Chapter 20.

METASTATIC TUMORS

PSEUDOMYXOMA PERITONEI

Pseudomyxoma peritonei refers to the accumulation of jelly-like mucus in the pelvic or peritoneal cavity. The earlier interpretation that this condition represented a stage 3 spread from mucinous tumors of the ovaries was challenged more than a decade ago, with the recognition that most, but not all, of these tumors arose from the appendix.[67]

Pathology
Grossly, pools of gelatinous material are present in the peritoneal cavity. The volume encountered may vary greatly. Pseudomyxoma peritonei may be extensive and appear as semisolid gelatin covering all of the pelvic and abdominal structures or, in contrast, it may appear as little more than a slightly thickened gelatinous coat over a focal area of bowel or omentum. It is critical during the operation for the surgeon to inspect, and remove, the appendix in each case. Usually, the appendix will be enlarged or adherent to an omentum that is covered with the gelatinous material. In several cases where re-exploration was performed, the appendiceal tumor was not readily apparent and was identified only because the surgeon palpated a slight swelling. We have seen cases of pseudomyxoma peritonei where the appendix that was removed at operation appeared grossly normal, but a primary tumor was found within it on thorough histologic evaluation.

On microscopic examination, the mucinous deposits may have several histologic appearances,[25,107,140,233] some engendering differing names. The neoplastic epithelium in one subset appears banal. The gelatin may be devoid of all tumor cells (mucinous ascites) (Figure 33.72). The mucinous material often contains inflammatory cells, mesothelial cells, and, if present for some time, may display capillaries and fibroblasts indicating that organization has occurred. More commonly, strips of extremely well-differentiated intestinal-type mucinous epithelium are found in the gelatinous material (Figures 33.73–33.75). If only isolated foci are present, the epithelium may be so well differentiated as to resemble that of a mucinous adenoma, a term we prefer to the 'disseminated peritoneal adenomucinosis' of others.[25]

When there is sufficient neoplastic tissue, the finding of occasional mitoses or cytoplasm that has largely lost its intra-cytoplasmic mucin suggests that the tumor is of at least borderline malignancy. Alternatively, cribriform patterns or other histologic features of malignancy such as signet-ring cells are found that warrant a diagnosis of adenocarcinoma.[25] One report indicates cytologic washings are sufficient to distinguish histologically benign from malignant specimens.[107]

Pathogenesis
The origin of pseudomyxoma peritonei has been a matter of active investigation and debate.[233] Historically, most of these tumors were thought to be ovarian in origin, especially when

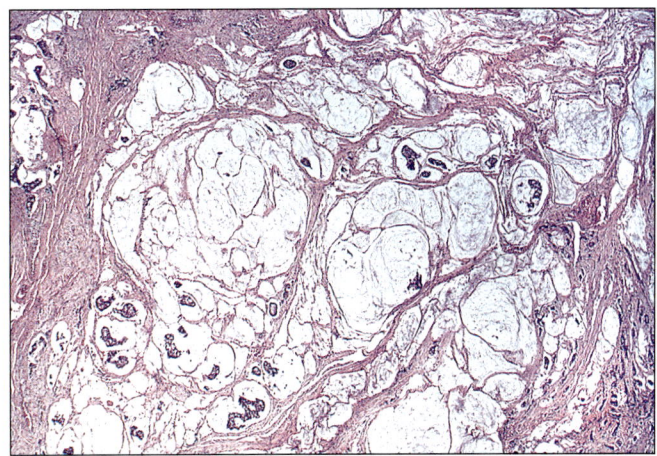

Fig. 33.73 Pseudomyxoma peritonei. Multiple clusters of tumor cells are present in the mucinous material.

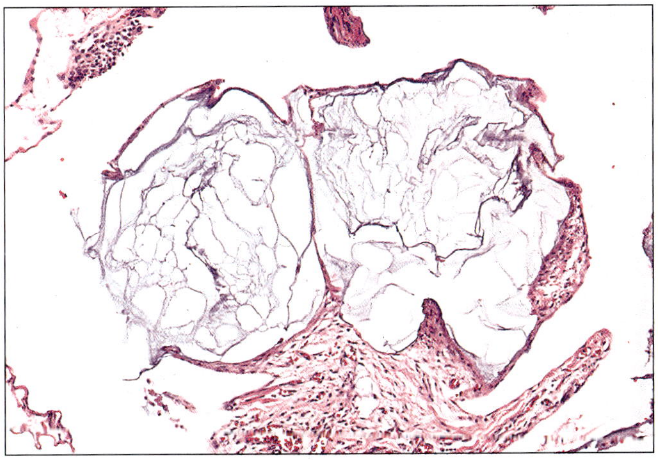

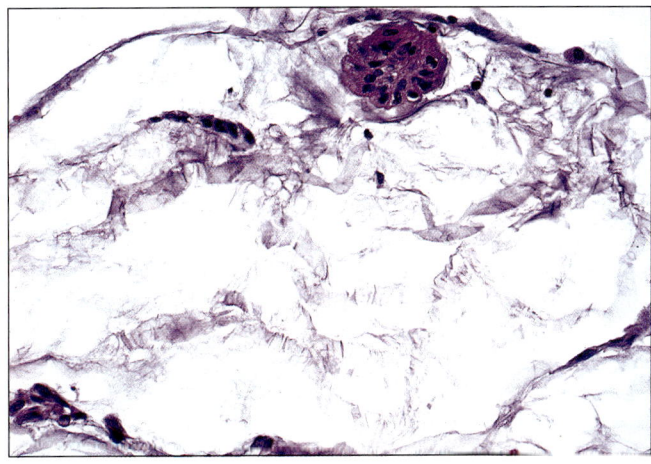

Fig. 33.74 Pseudomyxoma peritonei, high magnification. Clusters of tumor cells are present in the mucin.

Fig. 33.72 Pseudomyxoma peritonei. Only mucin is present in this photograph.

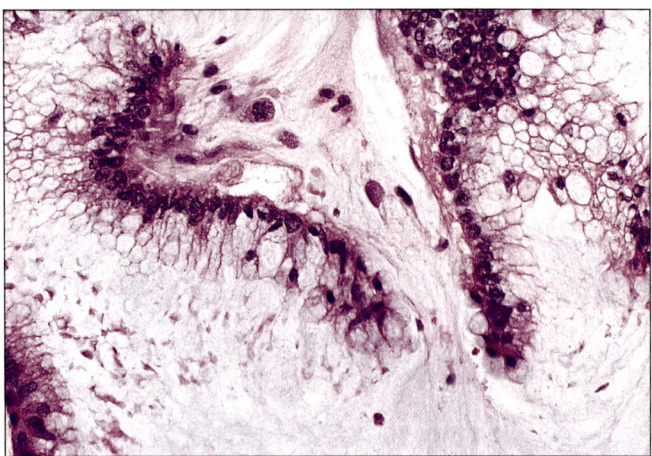

Fig. 33.75 Cluster of intestinal-type epithelium in pseudomyxoma peritonei.

the ovarian neoplasm was substantial in size or had the appearance of a mucinous tumor of borderline malignancy. Almost two decades ago[235] the opinions began to shift towards the appendix as the site of origin in most cases,[170,181–183] although some have provided evidence implicating the ovary to be the source in many cases.[35,198,199,202] Based on genetic analyses, most cases are now believed to be of appendiceal origin,[45] and more specifically from goblet cells expressing MUC2.[155] A minority of cases then became thought due to ovarian origin.[35] A recent review has gone so far as to state, 'pseudomyxoma peritonei almost never results from a ruptured primary ovarian neoplasm, but often produces secondary borderline-like ovarian tumors'.[93] In an exceptional case, however, pseudomyxoma peritonei can arise from the rupture of a mucinous tumor of intestinal type that has arisen in ovarian teratomas.[135] Other exceptions, such as personally observed cases in which the appendix had been removed more than 20 years previously in childhood, may be encountered, but these only serve to reinforce the general rule.

Mucinous cysts of the spleen in some cases are associated with pseudomyxoma peritonei. Splenomegaly due to cystic intrasplenic mucinous epithelial lesions may occasionally be the presenting feature of pseudomyxoma peritonei or herald tumor recurrence.[53] The clinicopathologic profile of these cases has conformed to that of neoplastic pseudomyxoma peritonei, with similar ages of onset, outcomes, and histologic features. A confirmed or suspected appendiceal primary has been found in most cases. By immunohistochemical methods, the epithelium within the splenic cysts was reactive for CK20, but not CK7 (see below).

A second and related issue, and the subject of burgeoning literature, revolves about the genetic[35,154] and immunocytochemical differences between mucinous tumors arising in the gastrointestinal tract and those that have originated in the ovary, with spread to the peritoneal cavity. Multiple immunohistochemical panels have been introduced with varying degrees of success. Several antigens, namely Leu-M1, B72.3, milk fat globule protein, and carcinoembryonic antigen (CEA), have proven unsuccessful in distinguishing these conditions.[198] HAM-56, an antibody to human alveolar macrophages, has shown some promise as a tool for diagnosing tumors of intes-

tinal origin in one study,[65] but not in another.[132] The topic is also addressed in Chapter 29.

Most recently, specific cytokeratin panels have been employed to distinguish ovarian mucinous tumors from gastrointestinal mucinous tumors. Cytokeratins are a complex family of proteins composed of 20 members in humans.[141,142] They have a specific distribution pattern in normal epithelia, a feature retained in neoplasms derived from them. Tumors of müllerian origin are usually reactive for CK7 but not CK20, whereas tumors of lower intestinal origin have findings that generally are reversed, i.e., CK20 reactivity but generally not for CK7.[87,133,180,181,224] In a small percentage of cases, the ovarian neoplasm is reactive for CK20 but not CK7. Most cases of pseudomyxoma peritonei show reaction patterns consistent with an appendiceal origin.[182,183]

New and bizarre manifestations of pseudomyxoma peritonei continue to be recognized that without cytokeratin immunostains might otherwise have resisted confirmation. Several cases have been reported in which abnormal mucinous epithelium was seen in the endometrium and the cervix that was of the intestinal type and resembled what is often seen in a tumor of borderline malignancy. Findings in these cases led ultimately to the discovery of a primary tumor in the appendix, which was confirmed by the immunoprofile of an intestinal-type tumor.[146]

Treatment and prognosis

Low-grade tumors are usually treated for cure, which consists of aggressive surgical debulking and intraperitoneal chemotherapy.[230] With the recognition that some cases are histologically a high-grade malignancy, the patients are treated symptomatically to avoid the high morbidity rates associated with aggressive therapy and the lack of improved long-term survival.

GLIOMATOSIS PERITONEI

Gliomatosis peritonei is a rare condition in which peritoneal implants composed largely or exclusively of fully mature glial tissue are found in the abdominal cavity, usually in association with a solid ovarian teratoma,[83,89,150] which can be mature or immature.[192] Tears in the capsule of the ovarian tumor have been identified, suggesting a mechanism by which the gliomatous tissue leaks into the abdominal cavity (Figure 33.76). One recent study, however, provides evidence from molecular studies that glial implants arise by metaplasia of pluripotent peritoneal stem cells,[63] which is indeed strange in that some are part of teratomatous explants and nearly all are associated with dermoid cysts that show evidence of rupture.

At the time of laparotomy, either when the ovarian tumor is discovered or at some subsequent period, implants in the peritoneum usually are found to be composed of glial tissue only (Figures 33.77 and 33.78). Occasionally, other teratomatous elements are identified. Microscopic implants should be graded separately from the ovarian tumor, and this will determine whether subsequent therapy is needed. Usually, the implants are grade 0 or 1 (Figure 33.78). In some cases, they are grade 2 or 3. Most patients with this condition do well, although recurrences have been recorded[30] as well as later malignant transformation.[46] This condition is described more fully in the section on ovarian teratomas (see Chapter 27).

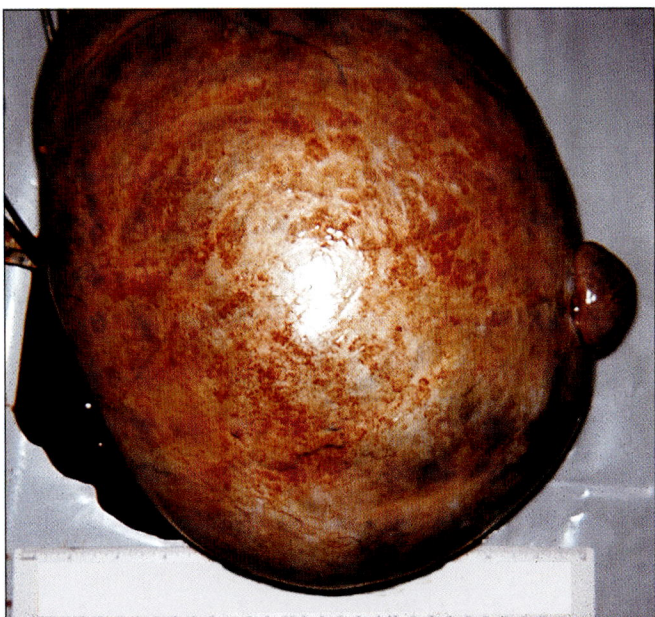

Fig. 33.76 Solid teratoma of ovary with capsular rent. Glial tissue protrudes through a large rent in the capsule.

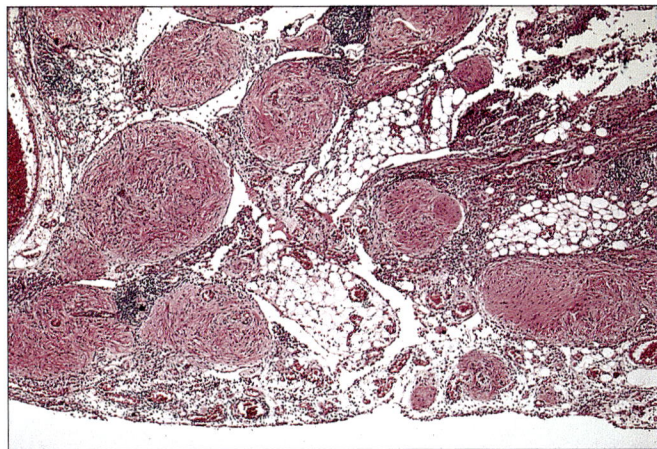

Fig. 33.77 Gliomatosis peritonei. Multiple nodules of mature glial tissue are implanted within omental adipose tissue.

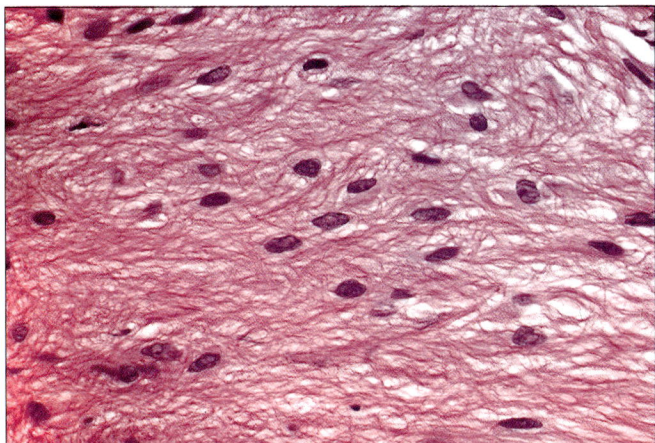

Fig. 33.78 Gliomatosis peritonei. Uniform glial cells, all highly differentiated (grade 0), show an extensive neurofibrillary background.

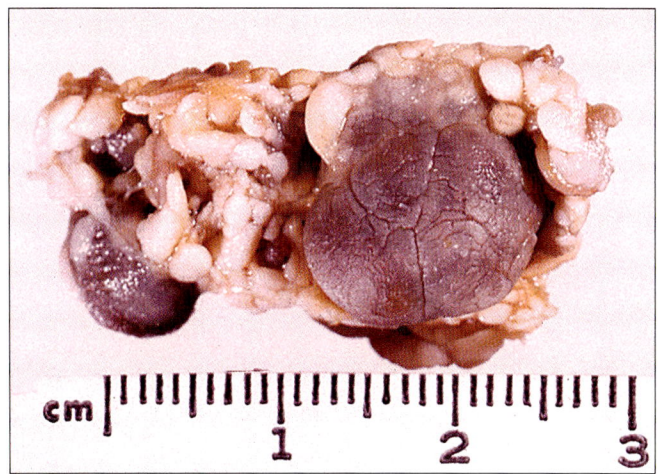

Fig. 33.79 Strumosis peritonei.

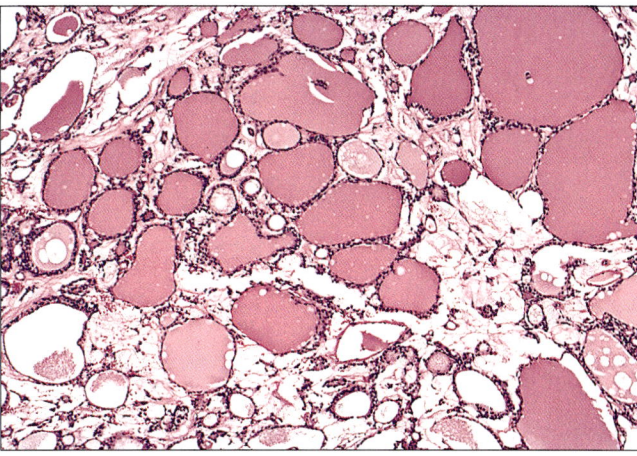

Fig. 33.80 Strumosis peritonei with macrofollicular appearance.

Gliomatosis peritonei has also been reported in a patient with a ventriculoperitoneal shunt.[100]

STRUMOSIS PERITONEI

Strumosis peritonei is a rare condition in which nodules found singly or throughout the omentum are composed largely of well-differentiated thyroid tissue. While rare, and reported as if it were some specialized entity, we have seen several in our consultation practices and believe it to represent a metastatic or implanted form of malignant struma ovarii. Most cases occur in association with a solid ovarian teratoma or a struma ovarii. Nodules may be several millimeters to centimeters in size and grossly, on cut section, resemble colloid (Figure 33.79). Microscopically, the thyroid may resemble a macrofollicular adenoma (Figure 33.80). Like gliomatosis peritonei, a defective capsule has been found in most cases with 'implants' from the ovary, suggesting a mechanism of spread into the abdominal cavity. While some patients with the condition do well, recurrence is unpredictable. We have seen patients survive for more than 20 years and at autopsy show atrophic scarred tumor. Some patients have had a clinically more aggressive course. This condition is described more fully on ovarian teratomas (see Chapter 27).

REFERENCES

1. Abraham G, Mathews M, Sekar L, Srikanth A, Sekar U. Tuberculous peritonitis in a cohort of continuous ambulatory peritoneal dialysis patients. Peritoneal Dialysis Int 2001;21(Suppl):S202–4.
2. Acs G, Pasha T, Zhang PJ. WT1 is differentially expressed in serous, endometrioid, clear cell, and mucinous carcinomas of the peritoneum, fallopian tube, ovary, and endometrium. Int J Gynecol Cancer 2004;23:110–18.
3. Afthentopoulos IE, Passadakis P, Oreopoulos DG. Sclerosing peritonitis in continuous ambulatory peritoneal dialysis patients: one center's experience and review of the literature. Adv Ren Replace Ther 1998;5:157–67.
4. Agoff SN, Mendelin JE, Grieco VS, Garcia RL. Unexpected gynecologic neoplasms in patients with proven or suspected BRCA-1 or -2 mutations: implications for gross examination, cytology, and clinical follow-up. Am J Surg Pathol 2002;26:171–8.
5. Akbulut M, Kelten C, Bir F, Soysal ME, Duzcan SE. Primary peritoneal serous psammocarcinoma with recurrent disease and metastasis: a case report and review of the literature. Gynecol Oncol 2007;105:248–51.
6. Al-Hussaini M, Stockman A, Foster H, McCluggage WG. WT-1 assists in distinguishing ovarian from uterine serous carcinoma and in distinguishing between serous and endometrioid ovarian carcinoma. Histopathology 2004;44:109–15.
7. Altinok G, Usubutun A, Kucukali T, Gunalp S, Ayhan A. Disseminated peritoneal leiomyomatosis – a benign entity mimicking carcinomatosis. Arch Gynecol Obstet 2000;264:54–5.
8. Alvarez AA, Moore WF, Robboy SJ, et al. K-ras mutations in Mullerian inclusion cysts associated with serous borderline tumors of the ovary. Gynecol Oncol 2001;80:201–6.
9. Attanoos RL, Webb R, Dojcinov SD, Gibbs AR. Value of mesothelial and epithelial antibodies in distinguishing diffuse peritoneal mesothelioma in females from serous papillary carcinoma of the ovary and peritoneum. Histopathology 2002;40:237–44.
10. Baker PM, Clement PB, Young RH. Malignant peritoneal mesothelioma in women – a study of 75 cases with emphasis on their morphologic spectrum and differential diagnosis. Am J Clin Pathol 2005;123:724–37.
11. Bandera CA, Muto MG, Schorge JO, Berkowitz RS, Rubin SC, Mok SC. BRCA1 gene mutations in women with papillary serous carcinoma of the peritoneum. Obstet Gynecol 1998;92:596–600.
12. Barda G, Menczer J, Chetrit A, et al. Comparison between primary peritoneal and epithelial ovarian carcinoma: a population-based study. Am J Obstet Gynecol 2004;190:1039–45.
13. Barnoud R, Delattre O, Peoc'h M, et al. Desmoplastic small round cell tumor: RT-PCR analysis and immunohistochemical detection of the Wilm's tumor gene WT1. Pathol Res Pract 1998;194:693–700.
14. Begin LR. Florid soft-tissue decidual reaction – a potential mimic of neoplasia. Am J Surg Pathol 1997;21:348–53.
15. Bekkers RLM, Willemsen WNP, Schijf CPT, Massuger LFAG, Bulten J, Merkus JMWM. Leiomyomatosis peritonealis disseminata: does malignant transformation occur? A literature review. Gynecol Oncol 1999;75:158–63.
16. Bell KA, Sehdev AES, Kurman RJ. Refined diagnostic criteria for implants associated with ovarian atypical proliferative serous tumors (borderline) and micropapillary serous carcinomas. Am J Surg Pathol 2001;25:419–32.
17. BenBaruch G, Sivan E, Moran O, Rizel S, Menczer J, Seidman DS. Primary peritoneal serous papillary carcinoma: a study of 25 cases and comparison with stage III–IV ovarian papillary serous carcinoma. Gynecol Oncol 1996;60:393–6.
18. Benjamin LE, Fredericks WJ, Barr FG, Rauscher FJ, 3rd. Fusion of the EWS1 and WT1 genes as a result of the t(11;22)(p13;q12) translocation in desmoplastic small round cell tumors. Mod Pediatr Oncol 1996;27:434–9.
19. Bernaciak J, Spina JC, Curros ML, Maya G, Venditti J, Chacon C. Case report: peritoneal sarcoidosis in an unusual location. Semin Resp Crit Care Med 2002;23:597–600.
20. Billings SD, Folpe AL, Weiss SW. Do leiomyomas of deep soft tissue exist? An analysis of highly differentiated smooth muscle tumors of deep soft tissue supporting two distinct subtypes. Am J Surg Pathol 2001;25:1134–42.
21. Billings SD, Folpe AL, Weiss SW. Do leiomyomas of deep soft tissue exist? An analysis of highly differentiated smooth muscle tumors of deep soft tissue supporting two distinct subtypes. Am J Surg Pathol 2001;25:1134–42.
22. Biscotti CV, Hart WR. Peritoneal serous micropapillomatosis of low malignant potential (serous borderline tumors of the peritoneum). A clinicopathologic study of 17 cases. Am J Surg Pathol 1992;16:467–75.
23. Borczuk AC, Taub RN, Hesdorffer M, et al. P16 loss and mitotic activity predict poor survival in patients with peritoneal malignant mesothelioma. Clin Cancer Res 2005;11:3303–8.
24. Bourdillon L, Lanier-Gachon E, Stankovic K, et al. Lofgren syndrome and peritoneal involvement by sarcoidosis – case report. Chest 2007;132:310–2.
25. Bradley RF, Stewart JH, Russell GB, Levine EA, Geisinger KR. Pseudomyxoma peritonei of appendiceal origin: a clinicopathologic analysis of 101 patients uniformly treated at a single institution, with literature review. Am J Surg Pathol 2006;30:551–9.
26. Burks RT, Sherman ME, Kurman RJ. Micropapillary serous carcinoma of the ovary: a distinctive low-grade carcinoma related to serous borderline tumors. Am J Surg Pathol 1996;20:1319–30.
27. Butnor KJ, Burchette JL, Robboy SJ. Progesterone receptor activity in leiomyomatosis peritonealis disseminata. Int J Gynecol Pathol 1999;18:259–64.
28. Butnor KJ, Sporn TA, Hammar SP, Roggli VL. Well-differentiated papillary mesothelioma. Am J Surg Pathol 2001;25:1304–9.
29. Buttner A, Bassler R, Theele C. Pregnancy-associated ectopic decidua (deciduosis) of the greater omentum. An analysis of 60 biopsies with cases of fibrosing deciduosis and leiomyomatosis peritonealis disseminata. Pathol Res Pract 1993;189:352–9.
30. Calder CJ, Light AM, Rollason TP. Immature ovarian teratoma with mature peritoneal metastatic deposits showing glial, epithelial, and endometrioid differentiation – a case report and review of the literature. Int J Gynecol Pathol 1994;13:279–82.
31. Cancarini GC, Sandrini M, Vizzardi V, Bertoli S, Buzzi L, Maiorca R. Clinical aspects of peritoneal sclerosis. J Nephrol 2001;14(Suppl):S39–S47.
32. Carey M, Kirk ME. Necrotic pseudoxanthomatous nodules of the omentum and peritoneum – a peculiar reaction to endometriotic cyst contents. Obstet Gynecol 1993;82(4 Part 2):650–2.
33. Carter D, True L, Otis CN. Serous membranes. In: Sternberg SS, ed. Histology for Pathologists, 2nd edn. Philadelphia: Lippincott; 1997:223–42.
34. Chang KL, Crabtree GS, Limtan SK, Kempson RL, Hendrickson MR. Primary extrauterine endometrial stromal neoplasms – a clinicopathologic study of 20 cases and a review of the literature. Int J Gynecol Pathol 1993;12:282–96.
35. Chuaqui RF, Zhuang ZP, Emmertbuck MR, et al. Genetic analysis of synchronous mucinous tumors of the ovary and appendix. Hum Pathol 1996;27:165–71.
36. Clement PB. Reactive tumor-like lesions of the peritoneum. Am J Clin Pathol 1995;103:673–6.
37. Clement PB, Young RH. Endocervicosis of the urinary bladder. A report of six cases of a benign mullerian lesion that may mimic adenocarcinoma. Am J Surg Pathol 1992;16:533–42.
38. Clement PB, Young RH. Florid mesothelial hyperplasia associated with ovarian tumors – a potential source of error in tumor diagnosis and staging. Int J Gynecol Pathol 1993;12:51–8.
39. Clement PB, Young RH. Florid cystic endosalpingiosis with tumor-like manifestations – a report of four cases including the first reported cases of transmural endosalpingiosis of the uterus. Am J Surg Pathol 1999;23:166–75.
40. Clement PB, Young RH, Scully RE. Malignant mesotheliomas presenting as ovarian masses – a report of nine cases, including two primary ovarian mesotheliomas. Am J Surg Pathol 1996;20:1067–80.
41. Clement PB, Young RH, Hanna W, Scully RE. Sclerosing peritonitis associated with luteinized thecomas of the ovary. A clinicopathological analysis of six cases. Am J Surg Pathol 1994;18:1–13.
42. Clement PB, Young RH, Oliva E, Sumner HW, Scully RE. Hyperplastic mesothelial cells within abdominal lymph nodes: mimic of metastatic ovarian carcinoma and serous borderline tumor – a report of two cases associated with ovarian neoplasms. Mod Pathol 1996;9:879–86.
43. Comin CE, Saieva C, Messerini L. h-Caldesmon, calretinin, estrogen receptor, and Ber-EP4: a useful combination of immunohistochemical markers for differentiating epithelioid peritoneal mesothelioma from serous papillary carcinoma of the ovary. Am J Surg Pathol 2007;31:1139–48.
44. Copeland LJ, Silva EG, Gershenson DM, Sneige N, Atkinson EN, Wharton JT. The significance of mullerian inclusions found at second-look laparotomy in patients with epithelial ovarian neoplasms. Obstet Gynecol 1988;71:763–70.
45. Cuatrecasas M, Matias-Guiu X, Prat J. Synchronous mucinous tumors of the appendix and the ovary associated with pseudomyxoma peritonei: a clinicopathologic study of six cases with comparative analysis of c-Ki-ras mutations. Am J Surg Pathol 1996;20:739–46.
46. Dadmanesh F, Miller DM, Swenerton KD, Clement PB. Gliomatosis peritonei with malignant transformation. Mod Pathol 1997;10:597–601.
47. Davidson B, Risberg B, Berner A, Bedrossian CW, Reich R. The biological differences between ovarian serous carcinoma and diffuse peritoneal malignant mesothelioma. Semin Diagn Pathol 2006;23:35–43.
48. Davis JR, Miller HS, Feng JD. Vernix caseosa peritonitis: report of two cases with antenatal onset. Am J Clin Pathol 1998;109:320–3.
49. de Peralta MN, Delahoussaye PM, Tornos CS, Silva EG. Benign retroperitoneal cysts of mullerian type: a clinicopathologic study of three cases and review of the literature. Int J Pathol 1994;13:273–8.
50. Dehner LP, Coffin CM. Idiopathic fibrosclerotic disorders and other inflammatory pseudotumors. Semin Diagn Pathol 1998;15:161–73.
51. Dei Tos AP, Dal Cin P. The role of cytogenetics in the classification of soft tissue tumours. Virchows Arch 1997;431:83–94.
52. Di Paolo N, Garosi G. Peritoneal sclerosis. J Nephrol 1999;12:347–61.
53. du Plessis DG, Louw JA, Wranz PA. Mucinous epithelial cysts of the spleen associated with pseudomyxoma peritonei. Histopathology 1999;35:551–7.
54. Eichhorn JH, Bell DA, Young RH, Scully RE. Ovarian serous borderline tumors with micropapillary and cribriform patterns – a study of 40 cases and comparison with 44 cases without these patterns. Am J Surg Pathol 1999;23:397–409.
55. Eisen A, Weber BL. Primary peritoneal carcinoma can have multifocal origins: implications for prophylactic oophorectomy. J Natl Cancer Inst 1998;90:797–9.
56. Eltabbakh GH, Piver MS. Extraovarian primary peritoneal carcinoma. Oncology (Williston Park) 1998;12:813–9.

57. Eltabbakh GH, Piver MS, Werness BA. Primary peritoneal adenocarcinoma metastatic to the brain. Gynecol Oncol 1997;66:160–3.
58. Eltabbakh GH, Werness BA, Piver S, Blumenson LE. Prognostic factors in extraovarian primary peritoneal carcinoma. Gynecol Oncol 1998;71:230–9.
59. Eltabbakh GH, Piver MS, Natarajan N, Mettlin CJ. Epidemiologic differences between women with extraovarian primary peritoneal carcinoma and women with epithelial ovarian cancer. Obstet Gynecol 1998;91:254–9.
60. Eltabbakh GH, Piver MS, Hempling RE, Werness BA, Blumenson LE. Importance of lymph node metastases in primary peritoneal carcinoma. J Surg Oncol 1998;68:144–8.
61. Emerson RE, Wang M, Liu F, Lawrence WD, Abdul-Karim FW, Cheng L. Molecular genetic evidence of an independent origin of serous low malignant potential implants and lymph node inclusions. Int J Gynecol Pathol 2007;26:387–94.
62. Euscher ED, Malpica A, Deavers MT, Silva EG. Differential expression of WT-1 in serous carcinomas in the peritoneum with or without associated serous carcinoma in endometrial polyps. Am J Surg Pathol 2005;29:1074–8.
63. Ferguson AW, Katabuchi H, Ronnett BM, Cho KR. Glial implants in gliomatosis peritonei arise from normal tissue, not from the associated teratoma. Am J Pathol 2001;159:51–5.
64. Flint A, Weiss SW. CD-34 and keratin expression distinguishes solitary fibrous tumor (fibrous mesothelioma) of pleura from desmoplastic mesothelioma. Hum Pathol 1995;26:428–31.
65. Fowler LJ, Maygarden SJ, Novotny DB. Human alveolar macrophage-56 and carcinoembryonic antigen monoclonal antibodies in the differential diagnosis between primary ovarian and metastatic gastrointestinal carcinomas. Hum Pathol 1994;25:666–70.
66. Fox H. Primary neoplasia of the female peritoneum. Histopathology 1993;23:103–10.
67. Fox H. Pseudomyxoma peritonei. Br J Obstet Gynaecol 1996;103:197–8.
68. Frigerio L, Taccagni GL, Mariani A, Mangili G, Ferrari A. Idiopathic sclerosing peritonitis associated with florid mesothelial hyperplasia, ovarian fibromatosis, and endometriosis: a new disorder of abdominal mass. Am J Obstet Gynecol 1997;176:721–2.
69. Fromm GL, Gershenson DM, Silva EG. Papillary serous carcinoma of the peritoneum. Obstet Gynecol 1990;75:89–95.
70. Fukunaga M, Naganuma H, Ushigome S, Endo Y, Ishikawa E. Malignant solitary fibrous tumour of the peritoneum. Histopathology 1996;28:463–6.
71. Fukunaga M, Endo Y, Takaki K, Ishikawa E, Ushigome S. Postmenopausal intra-abdominal desmoplastic small cell tumor. Pathol Int 1996;46:281–5.
72. Fukunaga M, Naganuma H, Nikaido T, Harada T, Ushigome S. Extrapleural solitary fibrous tumor: a report of seven cases. Mod Pathol 1997;10:443–50.
73. Fulcher AS, Szucs RA. Leiomyomatosis peritonealis disseminata complicated by sarcomatous transformation and ovarian torsion: presentation of two cases and review of the literature. Abdom Imaging 1998;23:640–4.
74. Garosi G, Di Paolo N, Sacchi G, Gaggiotti E. Sclerosing peritonitis: a nosological entity. Perit Dial Int 2005;25(Suppl):S110.
75. George E, Leyser S, Zimmer HL, Simonowitz DA, Agress RL, Nordin DD. Vernix caseosa peritonitis. An infrequent complication of cesarean section with distinctive histopathologic features. Am J Clin Pathol 1995;103:681–4.
76. Gerald WL, Ladanyi M, de Alava E, et al. Clinical, pathologic, and molecular spectrum of tumors associated with t(11;22)(p13;q12): desmoplastic small round-cell tumor and its variants. J Clin Oncol 1998;16:3028–36.
77. Gershenson DM. Peritoneal serous papillary carcinoma, a phenotypic variant of familial ovarian cancer: implications for ovarian cancer screening – discussion. Am J Obstet Gynecol 1999;180:925–7.
78. Gershenson DM, Silva EG, Tortolero-Luna G, Levenback C, Morris M, Tornos G. Serous borderline tumors of the ovary with noninvasive peritoneal implants. Cancer 1998;83:2157–63.
79. Gershenson DM, Silva EG, Levy L, Burke TW, Wolf JK, Tornos C. Ovarian serous borderline tumors with invasive peritoneal implants. Cancer 1998;82:1096–103.
80. Ghosh P, Strong C, Naugler W, Haghighi P, Carethers JM. Peritoneal mice implicated in intestinal obstruction – report of a case and review of the literature. J Clin Gastroenterol 2006;40:427–30.
81. Gilks CB, Bell DA, Scully RE. Serous psammocarcinoma of the ovary and peritoneum. Int J Gynecol Pathol 1990;9:110–21.
82. Gilks CB, Alkushi A, Yue JJW, Lanvin D, Ehlen TG, Miller DM. Advanced-stage serous borderline tumors of the ovary: a clinicopathological study of 49 cases. Int J Gynecol Pathol 2003;22:29–36.
83. Gocht A, Lohler J, Scheidel P, Stegner H-E. Gliomatosis peritonei combined with mature ovarian teratoma. Pathol Res Pract 1995;191:1029–35.
84. Goldblum J, Hart WR. Localized and diffuse mesotheliomas of the genital tract and peritoneum in women – a clinicopathologic study of nineteen true mesothelial neoplasms, other than adenomatoid tumors, multicystic mesotheliomas, and localized fibrous tumors. Am J Surg Pathol 1995;19:1124–37.
85. Gown AM. Uses of antibody panels in the analysis of metastatic carcinomas of unknown primary. Acta Histochem Cytochem 1999;32:153–9.
86. Groutz A, Carmon E, Gat A. Peritoneal tuberculosis versus advanced ovarian cancer: a diagnostic dilemma. Obstet Gynecol 1998; 91(5 Pt 2):868.
87. Guerrieri C, Franlund B, Fristedt S, Gillooley JF, Boeryd B. Mucinous tumors of the vermiform appendix and ovary, and pseudomyxoma peritonei: histogenetic implications of cytokeratin 7 expression. Hum Pathol 1997;28:1039–45.
88. Halperin R, Zehavi S, Hadas E, Habler L, Bukovsky I, Schneider D. Immunohistochemical comparison of primary peritoneal and primary ovarian serous papillary carcinoma. Int J Gynecol Pathol 2001;20:341–5.
89. Hamada Y, Tanano A, Sato M, et al. Ovarian teratoma with gliomatosis peritonei: report of two cases. Surg Today 1998;28:223–6.
90. Hammar SP. Critical commentary to 'Malignant peritoneal mesothelioma mimicking mesenteric inflamatory disease'. Pathol Res Pract 1994;190:623–4.
91. Hanau CA, Miettinen M. Solitary fibrous tumor: histological and immunohistochemical spectrum of benign and malignant variants presenting at different sites. Hum Pathol 1995;26:440–9.
92. Hardman IWJ, Majmudar B. Leiomyomatosis peritonealis disseminata: clinicopathologic analysis of five cases. South Med J 1996;89:291–4.
93. Hart WR. Mucinous tumors of the ovary: a review. Int J Gynecol Pathol 2005;24:4–25.
94. Hashi A, Yuminamochi T, Murata SI, Iwamoto H, Honda T, Hoshi K. Wilms tumor gene immunoreactivity in primary serous carcinomas of the fallopian tube, ovary, endometrium, and peritoneum. Int J Gynecol Pathol 2003;22:374–7.
95. Heinig J, Neff A, Cirkel U, Klockenbusch W. Recurrent leiomyomatosis peritonealis disseminata after hysterectomy and bilateral salpingo-oophorectomy during combined hormone replacement therapy. Eur J Obstet Gynecol Reprod Biol 2003;111:216–8.
96. Heller DS, Gordon RE, Katz N. Correlation of asbestos fiber burdens in fallopian tubes and ovarian tissue. Am J Obstet Gynecol 1999;181:346–7.
97. Heller DS, Gordon RE, Clement PB, Turnnir R, Katz N. Presence of asbestos in peritoneal malignant mesotheliomas in women. Int J Gynecol Cancer 1999;9:452–5.
98. Hemminki K, Li XJ. Time, trends and occupational risk factors for peritoneal mesothelioma in Sweden. J Occup Environ Med 2003;45:451–5.
99. Herrero J, Kamali P, Kirschbaum M. Leiomyomatosis peritonealis disseminata associated with endometriosis: a case report and literature review. Eur J Obstet Gynecol Reprod Biol 1998;76:189–91.
100. Hill DA, Dehner LP, White FV, Langer JC. Gliomatosis peritonei as a complication of a ventriculoperitoneal shunt: case report and review of the literature. J Pediatr Surg 2000;35:497–9.
101. Hoekstra AV, Riben MW, Frumovitz M, Liu JS, Ramirez PT. Well-differentiated papillary mesothelioma of the peritoneum: a pathological analysis and review of the literature. Gynecol Oncol 2005;98:161–7.
102. Horn LC, Bilek K. Frequency and histogenesis of pelvic retroperitoneal lymph node inclusions of the female genital tract. An immunohistochemical study of 34 cases. Pathol Res Pract 1995;191:991–6.
103. Hutton RL, Dalton SR. Primary peritoneal serous borderline tumors. Arch Pathol Lab Med 2007;131:138–44.
104. Hwang HC, Gown AM. Benign glandular inclusions in pelvic lymph nodes: endosalpingiosis or endometriosis? Lab Invest 1997;76:102A.
105. Iwasa Y, Minamiguchi S, Konishi I, Onodera H, Zhou J, Yamabe H. Sclerosing peritonitis associated with luteinized thecoma of the ovary. Pathol Int 1996;46:510–14.
106. Jaaback KS, Ludeman L, Clayton NL, Hirschowitz L. Primary peritoneal carcinoma in a UK cancer center: comparison with advanced ovarian carcinoma over a 5-year period. Int J Gynecol Cancer 2006;16(Suppl):123–8.
107. Jackson SL, Fleming RA, Loggie BW, Geisinger KR. Gelatinous ascites: a cytohistologic study of pseudomyxoma peritonei in 67 patients. Mod Pathol 2001;14:664–71.
108. Jansen RP, Russell P. Nonpigmented endometriosis: clinical, laparoscopic, and pathologic definition. Am J Obstet Gynecol 1986;155:1154–9.
109. Jaworski RC, Boadle R, Greg J, Cocks P. Peritoneal 'melanosis' associated with a ruptured ovarian dermoid cyst: report of a case with electron-probe energy dispersive x-ray analysis. Int J Gynecol Pathol 2001;20:386–9.
110. Kadar N, Krumerman M. Possible metaplastic origin of lymph node 'metastases' in serous ovarian tumor of low malignant potential (borderline serous tumor). Gynecol Oncol 1995;59:394–7.
111. Kaplan AM, Creager AJ, Livasy CA, Dent GA, Boggess JF. Intra-abdominal embryonal rhabdomyosarcoma in an adult. Gynecol Oncol 1999;74:282–5.
112. Karlan BY, Baldwin RL, Lopez-Luevanos E, et al. Peritoneal serous papillary carcinoma, a phenotypic variant of familial ovarian cancer: implications for ovarian cancer screening. Am J Obstet Gynecol 1999;180:917–25.
113. Kerrigan SAJ, Cagle P, Churg A. Malignant mesothelioma of the peritoneum presenting as an inflammatory lesion – a report of four cases. Am J Surg Pathol 2003;27:248–53.
114. Kerrigan SAJ, Turnnir RT, Clement PB, Young RH, Churg A. Diffuse malignant epithelial mesotheliomas of the peritoneum in women – a clinicopathologic study of 25 patients. Cancer 2002;94:378–85.
115. Kim J, Lee K, Pelletier J. The desmoplastic small round cell tumor t(11;22) translocation produces EWS/WT1 isoforms with differing oncogenic properties. Oncogene 1998;16:1973–9.
116. Kindelberger DW, Lee Y, Miron A, et al. Intraepithelial carcinoma of the fimbria and pelvic serous carcinoma: evidence for a causal relationship. Am J Surg Pathol 2007;31:161–9.
117. Knudsen PI. The peritoneal elastic lamina. J Anat 1991;177:41–6.
118. Koc S, Beydilli G, Tulunay G, et al. Peritoneal tuberculosis mimicking advanced ovarian cancer: a retrospective review of 22 cases. Gynecol Oncol 2006;103:565–9.

119. Krediet RT, Zweers MM, van Westrhenen R, Ho-dac-Pannekeet MM, Struijk DG. What can we do to preserve the peritoneum? Perit Dial Int 2003;23(Suppl):S14–S19.

120. Kuga T, Esato K, Takeda K, Sase M, Hoshii Y, Takahashi M. A supernumerary ovary of the omentum with cystic change: report of two cases and review of the literature. Pathol Int 1999;49:566–70.

121. Kupryjanczyk J, Thor AD, Beauchamp R, Poremba C, Scully RE, Yandell DW. Ovarian, peritoneal, and endometrial serous carcinoma: clonal origin of multifocal disease. Mod Pathol 1996;9:166–73.

122. Lae ME, Roche PC, Jin L, Lloyd RV, Nascimento AG. Desmoplastic small round cell tumor – a clinicopathologic, immunohistochemical, and molecular study of 32 tumors. Am J Surg Pathol 2002;26:823–35.

123. Lamovec J, Sinkovec J. Multilocular peritoneal inclusion cyst (multicystic mesothelioma) with hyaline globules. Histopathology 1996;28:466–9.

124. Langenberg R, Wojdat R, Volz-Koster S, Volz J. Disseminated intraperitoneal leiomyomatosis – case report of a rare differential diagnosis of metastasizing ovarian malignancy. Geburt Frauenheil 2005;65:1074–6.

125. Lauchlan SC. The secondary mullerian system revisited. Int J Gynecol Pathol 1994;13:73–9.

126. Leake JF, Rader JS, Woodruff JD, Rosenshein NB. Retroperitoneal lymphatic involvement with epithelial ovarian tumors of low malignant potential. Gynecol Oncol 1991;42:124–30.

127. Leeper K, Garcia R, Swisher E, Goff B, Greer B, Paley P. Pathologic findings in prophylactic oophorectomy specimens in high-risk women. Gynecol Oncol 2002;87:52–6.

128. Levine DA, Argenta PA, Yee CJ, et al. Fallopian tube and primary peritoneal carcinomas associated with BRCA mutations. J Clin Oncol 2003;21:4222–7.

129. Lim C, McIlroy K, Briggs G, Tan L. Splenosis mimicking lymphoma. Pathology 2007;39:183–5.

130. Longacre TA, McKenney JK, Tazelaar HD, Kempson RL, Hendrickson MR. Ovarian serous tumors of low malignant potential (borderline tumors) – outcome-based study of 276 patients with long-term (≥5-year) follow-up. Am J Surg Pathol 2005;29:707–23.

131. Losch A, Kainz C, Gitsch G, Breitenecker G. Leiomyomatosis peritonealis disseminata – a case report. Wien Klin Wochenschr 1996;108:153–6.

132. Loy TS, Abshier J. Immunostaining with HAM56 in the diagnosis of adenocarcinomas. Mod Pathol 1993;6:473–5.

133. Loy TS, Calaluce RD, Keeney GL. Cytokeratin immunostaining in differentiating primary ovarian carcinoma from metastatic colonic adenocarcinoma. Mod Pathol 1996;9:1040–4.

134. Mahmoud A, Silapaswan S, Lin K, Penney D. Vernix caseosa: an unusual cause of post-cesarean section peritonitis. Am Surg 1997;63:382–5.

135. Marquette S, Amant F, Vergote I, Moerman P. Pseudomyxoma peritonei associated with a mucinous ovarian tumor arising from a mature cystic teratoma. A case report. Int J Gynecol Pathol 2006;25:340–3.

136. Martinka M, Allaire C, Clement PB. Endocervicosis presenting as a painful vaginal mass: a case report. Int J Gynecol Pathol 1999;18:274–6.

137. McCaughey WT, Colby TV, Battifora H, et al. Diagnosis of diffuse malignant mesothelioma: experience of a US/Canadian Mesothelioma Panel. Mod Pathol 1991;4:342–53.

138. McKenney JK, Balzer BL, Longacre TA. Lymph node involvement in ovarian serous tumors of low malignant potential (borderline tumors): pathology, prognosis, and proposed classification. Am J Surg Pathol 2006;30:614–24.

139. Miller RT. Immunocytochemistry of epithelial tumors. In: ASCP National Meeting; 1999; New Orleans, LA: American Society of Clinical Pathology; 1999:1–47.

140. Misdraji J, Yantiss RK, Graeme-Cook FM, Balis UJ, Young RH. Appendiceal mucinous neoplasms – a clinicopathologic analysis of 107 cases. Am J Surg Pathol 2003;27:1089–103.

141. Moll R. Molecular diversity of cytokeratins: significance for cell and tumor differentiation. Acta Histochem Suppl 1991;41:117–27.

142. Moll R, Lowe A, Laufer J, Franke WW. Cytokeratin 20 in human carcinomas. A new histodiagnostic marker detected by monoclonal antibodies. Am J Pathol 1992;140:427–47.

143. Moll UM, Valea F, Chumas J. Role of p53 alteration in primary peritoneal carcinoma. Int J Gynecol Pathol 1997;16:156–62.

144. Molpus KL, Wu H, Fuller AF. Recurrent psammocarcinoma of the peritoneum with complete response to tamoxifen therapy. Gynecol Oncol 1998;68:206–9.

145. Moore WF, Bentley RC, Berchuck A, Robboy SJ. Some mullerian inclusion cysts in lymph nodes may sometimes be metastases from serous borderline tumors of the ovary. Am J Surg Pathol 2000;24:710–18.

146. Moore WF, Bentley RC, Kim KR, Olatidoye B, Gray SR, Robboy SJ. Goblet-cell mucinous epithelium lining the endometrium and endocervix: evidence of metastasis from an appendiceal primary tumor through the use of cytokeratin-7 and -20 immunostains. Int J Gynecol Pathol 1998; 17:363–7.

147. Mulhollan TJ, Silva EG, Tornos C, Guerrieri C, Fromm GL, Gershenson D. Ovarian involvement by serous surface papillary carcinoma. Int J Gynecol Pathol 1994;13:120–6.

148. Munkarah AR, Jacques SM, Qureshi F, Deppe G. Conservative surgery in a young patient with peritoneal psammocarcinoma. Gynecol Oncol 1999;73:312–14.

149. Muto MG, Welch WR, Mok SCH, et al. Evidence for a multifocal origin of papillary serous carcinoma of the peritoneum. Cancer Res 1995;55:490–2.

150. Nanda S, Kalra B, Arora B, Singh S. Massive mature solid teratoma of the ovary with gliomatosis peritonei. Aust N Z J Obstet Gynaecol 1998;38:329–31.

151. Nazeer T, Ro JY, Tornos C, Ordonez NG, Ayala AG. Endocervical type glands in urinary bladder: a clinicopathologic study of six cases. Hum Pathol 1996;27:816–20.

152. Nishida T, Ushijima K, Watanabe J, Kage M, Nagaoka S. Sclerosing peritonitis associated with luteinized thecoma of the ovary. Gynecol Oncol 1999;73:167–9.

153. Nonaka D, Kusamura S, Baratti D, et al. Diffuse malignant mesothelioma of the peritoneum – a clinicopathologic study of 35 patients treated locoregionally at a single institution. Cancer 2005;104:2181–8.

154. Noumoff J, Livolsi V, Mikuta J, Faruqi S. An insight into the etiology of pseudomyxoma peritonei by chromosomal and immunohistochemical analysis. Gynecol Oncol 1993;29:136.

155. O'Connell JT, Tomlinson JS, Roberts AA, McGonigle KF, Barsky SH. Pseudomyxoma peritonei is a disease of MUC2-expressing goblet cells. Am J Pathol 2002;161:551–64.

156. Odashiro D, Miiji L, Odashiro M, et al. Peritoneal malignant mesothelioma first presenting as Sister Mary Joseph's nodule. Mod Pathol 2006;19(Suppl):184–5.

157. Ordi J, de Alava E, Torne A, et al. Intraabdominal desmoplastic small round cell tumor with EWS/ERG fusion transcript. Am J Surg Pathol 1998;22:1026–32.

158. Ordonez NG. Value of calretinin immunostaining in differentiating epithelial mesothelioma from lung adenocarcinoma. Mod Pathol 1998;11:929–33.

159. Ordonez NG. Desmoplastic small round cell tumor: I: a histopathologic study of 39 cases with emphasis on unusual histological patterns. Am J Surg Pathol 1998;22:1303–13.

160. Ordonez NG. Desmoplastic small round cell tumor: II: an ultrastructural and immunohistochemical study with emphasis on new immunohistochemical markers. Am J Surg Pathol 1998;22:1314–27.

161. Paal E, Miettinen M. Retroperitoneal leiomyomas: a clinicopathologic and immunohistochemical study of 56 cases with a comparison to retroperitoneal leiomyosarcomas. Am J Surg Pathol 2001;25:1355–63.

162. Peitsidis P, Akrivos T, Vecchini G, Rodolakis A, Akrivos N, Markaki S. Splenosis of the peritoneal cavity resembling an adnexal tumor: case report. Clin Exp Obstet Gynecol 2007;34:120–2.

163. Piek JMJ, Kenemans P, Verheijen RHM. Intraperitoneal serous adenocarcinoma: a critical appraisal of three hypotheses on its cause. Am J Obstet Gynecol 2004;191:718–32.

164. Piura B, Meirovitz M, Bartfeld M, YanaiInbar I, Cohen Y. Peritoneal papillary serous carcinoma: study of 15 cases and comparison with stage III–IV ovarian papillary serous carcinoma. J Surg Oncol 1998;68:173–8.

165. Piura B, Rabinovich A, Leron E, Yanai-Inbar I, Mazor M. Peritoneal tuberculosis – an uncommon disease that may deceive the gynecologist. Eur J Obstet Gynecol Reprod Biol 2003;110:230–4.

166. Piver MS, Jishi MF, Tsukada Y, Nava G. Primary peritoneal carcinoma after prophylactic oophorectomy in women with a family history of ovarian cancer – a report of the Gilda Radner Familial Ovarian Cancer Registry. Cancer 1993;71:2751–5.

167. Prade M, Spatz A, Bentley R, Duvillard P, Bognel C, Robboy SJ. Borderline and malignant serous tumor arising in pelvic lymph nodes: evidence of origin in benign glandular inclusions. Int J Gynecol Pathol 1995;14:87–91.

168. Prat J. Serous tumors of the ovary (borderline tumors and carcinomas) with and without micropapillary features. Int J Gynecol Pathol 2003;22:25–8.

169. Prat J, de Nictolis M. Serous borderline tumors of the ovary – a long-term follow-up study of 137 cases, including 18 with a micropapillary pattern and 20 with microinvasion. Am J Surg Pathol 2002;26:1111–28.

170. Prayson RA, Hart WR, Petras RE. Pseudomyxoma peritonei. A clinicopathologic study of 19 cases with emphasis on site of origin and nature of associated ovarian tumors. Am J Surg Pathol 1994;18:591–603.

171. Quade BJ, McLachlin CM, Soto-Wright V, Zuckerman J, Mutter GL, Morton CC. Disseminated peritoneal leiomyomatosis: clonality analysis by X chromosome inactivation and cytogenetics of a clinically benign smooth muscle proliferation. Am J Pathol 1997;150:2153–66.

172. Quddus MR, Sung CJ, Lauchlan SC. A comparison of omental endosalpingiosis and endometriosis. Mod Pathol 1998;11:112A.

173. Quddus MR, Sung CJ, Lauchlan SC. Benign and malignant serous and endometrioid epithelium in the omentum. Gynecol Oncol 1999;75:227–32.

174. Regidorbrandau PA, Pfaffenbach B, Metz KA, Schindler AE. Endometriosis in retroperitoneal lymphatic nodes. Geburt Frauenheil 1994;54:372–4.

175. Rehbock J, Dimpfl T, Assemi C. Disseminated peritoneal trophoblastic implants after surgery of tubal pregnancies – a typical complication of the laparoscopic technique? Geburt Frauenheil 1997;57:155–7.

176. Reich O, Kometter R, Pickel H. Chronic sclerosing peritonitis after spontaneous rupture of a cystic teratoma: a pitfall in surgical staging of ovarian tumours. Geburt Frauenheil 1999;59:94–5.

177. Robboy SJ. A hypothetic mechanism of diethylstilbestrol (DES)-induced anomalies in exposed progeny. Hum Pathol 1983;14:831–3.

178. Robboy SJ, Duggan M, Kurman RT. The female reproductive system. In: Rubin E, Farber J, eds. Pathology, 3rd edn. Philadephia: Lippincott; 1999:962–1028.

179. Robboy SJ, Hill EC, Sandberg EC, Czernobilsky B. Vaginal adenosis in women born prior to the diethylstilbestrol era. Hum Pathol 1986;17:488–92.

180. Ronnett BM, Kurman RJ, Shmookler BM, Sugarbaker PH, Young RH. The morphologic spectrum of ovarian metastases of appendiceal adenocarcinomas: a clinicopathologic and immunohistochemical analysis of tumors often misinterpreted as primary ovarian tumors or metastatic tumors from other gastrointestinal sites. Am J Surg Pathol 1997;21:1144–55.

181. Ronnett BM, Shmookler B, Diener-West M, Sugarbaker PH, Kurman RJ. Immunohistochemical evidence supporting the appendiceal origin of pseudomyxoma peritonei in women. Int J Gynecol Pathol 1997;16:1–9.

182. Ronnett BM, Zahn CM, Kurman RJ, Kass ME, Sugarbaker PH, Shmookler BM. Disseminated peritoneal adenomucinosis and peritoneal mucinous carcinomatosis: a clinicopathologic analysis of 109 cases with emphasis on distinguishing pathologic features, site of origin, prognosis, and relationship to 'pseudomyxoma peritonei'. Am J Surg Pathol 1995;19:1390–408.

183. Ronnett BM, Kurman RJ, Zahn CM, et al. Pseudomyxoma peritonei in women: a clinicopathologic analysis of 30 cases with emphasis on site of origin, prognosis, and relationship to ovarian mucinous tumors of low malignant potential. Hum Pathol 1995;26:509–24.

184. Rosen DMB, Lam AM, Carlton MA, Cario GM. The safety of laparoscopic treatment for ovarian dermoid tumours. Aust N Z J Obstet Gynaecol 1998;38:77–9.

185. Rothacker D, Mobius G. Varieties of serous surface papillary carcinoma of the peritoneum in northern Germany: a thirty-year autopsy study. Int J Gynecol Pathol 1995;14:310–8.

186. Russell P, Farnsworth A. Surgical Pathology of the Ovaries, 2nd edn. New York: Churchill Livingstone; 1997.

187. Russell P, Bannatyne PM, Solomon HJ, Stoddard LD, Tattersall MH. Multifocal tumorigenesis in the upper female genital tract – implications for staging and management. Int J Gynecol Pathol 1985;4:192–210.

188. Ryuko K, Miura H, Abu-Musa A, Iwanari O, Kitao M. Endosalpingiosis in association with ovarian surface papillary tumor of borderline malignancy. Gynecol Oncol 1992;46:107–10.

189. Sarraf KM, Abdalla M, Al-Omari O, Sarraf MG. Diagnostic difficulties of pelvic splenosis: case report. Ultrasound Obstet Gynecol 2006;27:220–1.

190. Sawh RN, Malpica A, Deavers MT, Liu JS, Silva EG. Benign cystic mesothelioma of the peritoneum: a clinicopathologic study of 17 cases and immunohistochemical analysis of estrogen and progesterone receptor status. Hum Pathol 2003;34:369–74.

191. Scharlau LL, Scharlau J, Mathuis C, Schremmer CN. Diffuse peritoneal leiomyomatosis: a case report. Geburt Frauenheil 2000;60:225–8.

192. Schmidt D, Kommoss F. Teratoma of the ovary. Clinical and pathological differences between mature and immature teratomas. Pathologe 2007;28:203–8.

193. Schorge JO, Mok SC. Understanding the pathogenesis of primary peritoneal carcinoma: involvement of the BRCA1 and p53 genes. Hum Pathol 1999;30:115–6.

194. Schorge JO, Muto MG, Welch WR, et al. Molecular evidence for multifocal papillary serous carcinoma of the peritoneum in patients with germline BRCA1 mutations. J Natl Cancer Inst 1998;90:841–5.

195. Scully RE. Extraovarian primary peritoneal carcinoma. Oncology (Williston Park) 1998;12:820.

196. Seidman JD, Kurman RJ. Subclassification of serous borderline tumors of the ovary into benign and malignant types: a clinicopathologic study of 65 advanced stage cases. Am J Surg Pathol 1996;20:1331–45.

197. Seidman JD, Kurman RJ. Ovarian serous borderline tumors: a critical review of the literature with emphasis on prognostic indicators. Hum Pathol 2000;31:539–57.

198. Seidman JD, Elsayed AM, Sobin LH, Tavassoli FA. Association of mucinous tumors of the ovary and appendix – a clinicopathologic study of 25 cases. Am J Surg Pathol 1993;17:22–34.

199. Seidman JD, Elsayed AM, Sobin LH, Tavassoli FA. Pseudomyxoma peritonei. Am J Surg Pathol 1993;17:1070–1.

200. Seidman JD, Oberer S, Bitterman P, Aisner SC. Pathogenesis of pseudoxanthomatous salpingiosis. Mod Pathol 1993;6:53–5.

201. Shanks JH, Harris M, Banerjee SS, et al. Mesotheliomas with deciduoid morphology – a morphologic spectrum and a variant not confined to young females. Am J Surg Pathol 2000;24:285–94.

202. Shen DH, Ng TY, Us K, Xue WC, Cheung ANY. Pseudomyxoma peritonei – a heterogenous disease. Int J Gynecol Pathol 1998;62:173–82.

203. Shen DH, Khoo US, Xue WC, et al. Primary peritoneal malignant mixed mullerian tumors – a clinicopathologic, immunohistochemical, and genetic study. Cancer 2001;91:1052–60.

204. Shih IM, Kurman RJ. Ovarian tumorigenesis – a proposed model based on morphological and molecular genetic analysis. Am J Pathol 2004;164:1511–18.

205. Shih IM, Kurman RJ. Molecular pathogenesis of ovarian borderline tumors: new insights and old challenges. Clin Cancer Res 2005;11:7273–9.

206. Shimizu Y, Mitsui T, Kawakami T, et al. Novel breakpoints of the EWS gene and the WT1 gene in a desmoplastic small round cell tumor. Cancer Genet Cytogenet 1998;106:156–8.

207. Shiraki M, Otis CN, Donovan JT, Powell JL. Ovarian serous borderline epithelial tumors with multiple retroperitoneal nodal involvement: metastasis or malignant transformation of epithelial glandular inclusions? Gynecol Oncol 1992;46:255–8.

208. Silva EG, Kurman RJ, Russell P, Scully RE. Symposium: Ovarian tumors of borderline malignancy. Int J Gynecol Pathol 1996;15:281–302.

209. Silva EG, Gershenson DM, Malpica A, Deavers M. The recurrence and the overall survival rates of ovarian serous borderline neoplasms with noninvasive implants is time dependent. Am J Surg Pathol 2006;30:1367–71.

210. Silva EG, Gershenson DM, Malpica A, Deavers M. The recurrence and the overall survival rates of ovarian serous borderline neoplasms with noninvasive implants is time dependent. Am J Surg Pathol 2006;30:1367–71.

211. Silva EG, Tornos C, Zhuang ZP, Mcrino MJ, Gershenson DM. Tumor recurrence in stage I ovarian serous neoplasms of low malignant potential. Int J Gynecol Pathol 1998;17:1–6.

212. Sinha P, Johnson AN, Chidamberan-Pillai S. Pelvic tuberculosis: an uncommon gynaecological problem presenting as ovarian mass. Br J Obstet Gynaecol 2000;107:139–40.

213. Sinha R, Gupta D, Tuli N. Genital tract tuberculosis with myometrial involvement. Int J Gynecol Oncol 1997;57:191–2.

214. Spiegel GW, Swiger FK. Luteinized thecoma with sclerosing peritonitis presenting as an acute abdomen. Gynecol Oncol 1996;61:275–81.

215. Stenram U. Sclerosing peritonitis in a case of benign cystic ovarian teratoma. A case report. APMIS 1997;105:414–6.

216. Stern RC, Dash R, Bentley RC, Snyder MJ, Haney AF, Robboy SJ. Malignancy in endometriosis: frequency and comparison of ovarian and extraovarian types. Int J Gynecol Pathol 2001;20:133–9.

217. Swan N. Peritoneal mesothelioma. Am J Surg Pathol 1997;21:122–3.

218. Sykes PH, Mulvaney NJ. Mesothelial cell hyperplasia in laparoscopy sites may cause difficulties in the diagnosis, staging, and management of ovarian tumors: a case report. Int J Gynecol Cancer 1998;8:345–8.

219. Sykes PH, Quinn MA, Rome RM. Ovarian tumors of low malignant potential: a retrospective study of 234 patients. Int J Gynecol Cancer 1997;7:218–26.

220. Taus P, Petru E, Gucer F, Pickel H, Lahousen M. Primary serous papillary carcinoma of the peritoneum: a report of 18 patients. Eur J Gynaecol Oncol 1997;18:171–2.

221. Tawfik O, Prather J, Bhatia P, Woodroof J, Gunter J, Webb P. Vernix caseosa peritonitis as a rare complication of cesarean section. A case report. J Reprod Med 1998;43:547–50.

222. Thoreau N, Fain O, Babinet P, et al. Peritoneal tuberculosis: 27 cases in the northeastern suburbs of Paris. Int J Tuberc Lung Dis 2002;6:253–8.

223. Tsutsumi O, Ando K, Momoeda M. Ruptured isthmal pregnancy following laparoscopic salpingostomy in the ipsilateral tube. Int J Gynecol Obstet 1997;57:187–9.

224. Vang R, Gown AM, Barry TS, et al. Cytokeratins 7 and 20 in primary and secondary mucinous tumors of the ovary: analysis of coordinate immunohistochemical expression profiles and staining distribution in 179 cases. Am J Surg Pathol 2006;30:1130–9.

225. Vuong PN, Guyot H, Moulin G, Houissa-Vuong S, Berrod JL. Pseudotumoral organization of a twisted epiploic fringe or 'hard-boiled egg' in the peritoneal cavity. Arch Pathol Lab Med 1990;114:531–2.

226. Vydianath B, Gurumurthy M, Crocker J. Solitary ovarian splenosis. J Clin Pathol 2005;58:1224–5.

227. Weir MM, Bell DA, Young RH. Grade 1 peritoneal serous carcinomas: a report of 14 cases and comparison with 7 peritoneal serous psammocarcinomas and 19 peritoneal serous borderline tumors. Am J Surg Pathol 1998;22:849–62.

228. Werness BA. Luteinized thecoma with sclerosing peritonitis. Arch Pathol Lab Med 1996;120:303–6.

229. Whitcomb BP, Kost ER, Hines JF, Zahn CM, Hall KL. Primary peritoneal psammocarcinoma: a case presenting with an upper abdominal mass and elevated CA-125. Gynecol Oncol 1999;73:331–4.

230. Wirtzfeld DA, Rodriguez-Bigas M, Weber T, Petrelli NJ. Disseminated peritoneal adenomucinosis: a critical review. Ann Surg Oncol 1999;6:797–801.

231. Wolf AN, Ladanyi M, Paull G, Blaugrund JE, Westra WH. The expanding clinical spectrum of desmoplastic small round-cell tumor: a report of two cases with molecular confirmation. Hum Pathol 1999;30:430–5.

232. Wu TI, Chang TC, Hsueh S, Lai CH. Ovarian endometrioid carcinoma with diffuse pigmented peritoneal keratin granulomas: a case report and review of the literature. Int J Gynecol Cancer 2006;16:426–9.

233. Young RH. Pseudomyxoma peritonei and selected other aspects of the spread of appendiceal neoplasms. Semin Diagn Pathol 2004;21:134–50.

234. Young RH, Clement PB. Mullerianosis of the urinary bladder. Mod Pathol 1996;9:731–7.

235. Young RH, Gilks CB, Scully RE. Mucinous tumors of the appendix associated with mucinous tumors of the ovary and pseudomyxoma peritonei. A clinicopathological analysis of 22 cases supporting an origin in the appendix. Am J Surg Pathol 1991;15:415–29.

236. Young RH, Eichhorn JH, Dickersin GR, Scully RE. Ovarian involvement by the intra-abdominal desmoplastic small round cell tumor with divergent differentiation: a report of three cases. Hum Pathol 1992;23:454–64.

Disorders of sexual development

34

Stanley J. Robboy   Francis Jaubert

Continuing new insights into the biology of sexual development (see Chapter 1) and advances in chromosome analysis are leading to earlier identification and more prompt treatment of the intersexual patient, the results of which facilitate a more normal life for affected individuals. With more sophisticated abilities to diagnose earlier and with greater precision have come many implications and opportunities. The families as well as the healthcare team can better understand the nature of the condition. It becomes easier to offer more appropriate counseling for gender assignment, hormone treatment, and fertility options and information about the risk of future gonadal malignancy that might develop either in the youngster or later in life. Based on these various advances, a classification of abnormal sexual development has been developed and refined that correlates the gonadal and genital anatomy with the chromosomal findings and specific genetic or metabolic defects (Tables 34.1 and 34.2).

In a shift from a classification anchored about whether the intersex revolves about a specific gene or whole chromosomal abnormality, the current classification is organized by broader categories into which the intersexual disorders are divided into 'abnormalities of genital differentiation', due largely to the abnormal production or sensitivity of a single hormone, or 'abnormalities in sex determination', due to abnormal gonadal differentiation, usually testicular, with or without chromosomal aberration.[60,95,118]

That the subject is complex is evident from collaborative studies where precise assignment of the etiologic cause cannot be determined in nearly half of cases, despite the synergistic cooperative endeavor of clinicians, biochemists, molecular biologists, and pathologists. The current classification is an integrated approach to this complex group of disorders and is organized according to the manner by which patients present as well as on the pathophysiologic basis of the defect. The classification also groups patients who are at high risk for development of gonadal neoplasia (Table 34.3).

DISORDERS OF GENITAL DIFFERENTIATION (DISORDERS GENERALLY ASSOCIATED WITH A NORMAL CHROMOSOME CONSTITUTION AND NORMAL GONAD)

FEMALE PSEUDOHERMAPHRODITISM (FEMALE INTERSEX)

Female pseudohermaphroditism occurs as a result of relative androgen excess *in utero* in an individual with two ovaries and two X chromosomes (46,XX). The elevated levels of androgen present during embryogenesis usually result in genital ambiguity and may result in a male phenotype.

FETAL DEFECTS

Adrenogenital syndrome

Congenital adrenal hyperplasia, unlike all other conditions responsible for the appearance of ambiguous genitalia in the newborn, may be life threatening because of a lack of synthesis of specific adrenal steroids. Prompt diagnosis and appropriate therapy are essential. With early treatment, normal external genitalia and fertility can be achieved. The manifestations of the adrenogenital syndrome in the XX individual are most easily understood by examining the simplified biosynthetic pathways of mineralocorticoid, glucocorticoid, and sex steroids (Figure 34.1).[26,98,99] Two enzymes, 21-hydroxylase and 11β-hydroxylase, participate in the formation of the glucocorticoids, desoxycorticosterone and cortisol, and the mineralocorticoid, aldosterone, but neither in testosterone nor the estrogens, estrone or estradiol. Deficiency of either enzyme in the 46,XX female leads to elevated adrenocorticotropic hormone (ACTH) products and hence elevated levels of testosterone and other strongly androgenic intermediates, which may result in sexual ambiguity or marked virilization of the newborn's external genitalia (Table 34.4).[29,38]

3β-Hydroxysteroid dehydrogenase is required for testosterone formation. In its absence, the principal androgen to form is the weak androgen, dehydroepiandrosterone (DHEA), which has one-twentieth the potency of testosterone. Patients with deficiency of this enzyme, therefore, show signs of no more than mild virilization, usually with clitoral hypertrophy but not with labial fusion or anterior displacement of the urethral orifice.[90]

21-Hydroxylase deficiency is inherited as an autosomal recessive trait caused by an abnormal gene on chromosome 6 that encodes for cytochrome P450c21 (i.e., *CYP21*) (see footnote in Table 34.2 for origin of cytochrome nomenclature). It accounts for more than 95% of cases of congenital adrenal hyperplasia, occurring once in 15 000 births. It is especially high in Ashkenazi Jews (1:27 live births). The genetic aberrations responsible for expression of the disease are complicated. This gene exists in tandem with a pseudogene, *CYP21P*, which is believed to be non-transcribable as it contains a high number of documented mutations.[94] The clinical manifestation depends upon the absence of the single active gene (*CYP21*, formerly called *CYP21B*) that actively expresses the 21-hydroxylase enzyme, or of the rearrangements, deletions or point mutations transferred from the pseudogene present.[26,77,94] Approximately

Table 34.1 Classification of intersexual disorders*

Disorders of genital differentiation (disorders generally associated with a normal chromosome constitution and normal gonad)

FEMALE PSEUDOHERMAPHRODITISM (FEMALE INTERSEX)

Fetal defect
  Adrenogenital syndrome (testosterone overproduction due to adrenocorticoid insufficiency)
    21α-Hydroxylase deficiency
    11β-Hydroxylase deficiency
  Placental aromatase defect

Maternal influence
  Maternal ingestion of progestins or androgens
  Maternal virilizing tumor

MALE PSEUDOHERMAPHRODITISM (MALE INTERSEX)

Primary gonadal defects
  Testicular regression syndrome (gonadal destruction)
  Leydig cell agenesis
    Defective hCG-LH receptor
  Defects in testosterone synthesis
    Testosterone and adrenocorticoid insufficiency
      Defect in cholesterol synthesis (Smith–Lemli–Opitz syndrome)
      20,22-Desmolase deficiency (StAR deficiency)
      3β-Hydroxylase dehydrogenase deficiency
      17α-Hydroxylase deficiency
    Testosterone insufficiency only
      17,20-Desmolase deficiency
      17β-Hydroxysteroid (17-ketosteroid reductase) dehydrogenase deficiency
      Persistent müllerian duct syndrome (defect in müllerian inhibiting substance system)

End-organ defects
  Androgen receptor binding deficiency
    Androgen insensitivity syndrome (testicular feminization)
    Incomplete androgen insensitivity syndrome (Reifenstein syndrome)
  Peripheral androgen transformation deficiency
    5α-Reductase deficiency

Disorders of sex determination (disorders generally associated with an abnormal sex chromosome constitution leading to abnormal gonadal formation)

SEXUAL AMBIGUITY INFREQUENT

Klinefelter syndrome (XXY)

Turner syndrome and Turner-like (XO and X mosaicism)

XX male (sex reversal)

Pure gonadal dysgenesis, bilateral

Disorders of Wilms tumor gene (*WT1*)
  Denys–Drash syndrome
  Frasier syndrome

SEXUAL AMBIGUITY INFREQUENT

XY disorder of sex development (DSD) (mixed gonadal dysgenesis (MGD)), including
  Turner-like (some forms)
  Dysgenetic male pseudohermaphroditism

XY male to female sex reversal
  Steroidogenic Factor 1 (SF1) abnormality
  Deleted chromosome 9p

True hermaphroditism

*'Idiopathic' or 'unclassified' conditions exist within each major category. We assume that each category of male pseudohermaphroditism with defects in specific protein products or receptors has forms where the abnormality is total or partial, or where the defect results from a qualitatively abnormal structure.

Table 34.2 Genes involved in disorders of intersex

Gene	Name	Location	Cells affected	Function	Abnormality
AMH (MIS)	Antimüllerian hormone (müllerian inhibiting substance, type 1)	19q13	Sertoli cells	Causes regression of fetal müllerian ducts, inhibits Leydig cells	Persistent müllerian duct syndrome
AMHR2 MISR II	Antimüllerian hormone type 2 receptor Müllerian inhibiting substance II	12q12–13	Primary sex cords	Serine threonine kinase receptor	Persistent müllerian duct syndrome
AR	Androgen receptor	Xq11–12	Target cell depends on cofactor specifics	Androgen receptor, a ligand transcription factor	Male pseudohermaphroditism, complete or partial androgen insensitivity syndrome
StAR	Steroidogenic acute regulatory protein	8p11.2	Mitochondria of adrenal, testis, ovary	Steroidogenic acute regulatory protein	Congenital lipoid adrenal hyperplasia
HSD3B2	3β-Hydroxysteroid dehydrogenase type II	1p13.1	Microsome of adrenal, testis, ovary	3β-Hydroxysteroid dehydrogenase type II	Congenital adrenal hyperplasia
HSD17B3	17β-Hydroxysteroid dehydrogenase III	9q22	Microsome of adrenal, testis, ovary	17β-Hydroxysteroid dehydrogenase, 17-ketosteroid reductase 3	Male pseudohermaphroditism
Cytochrome P450C17	See footnote (previously CYP17)	10q24–25	Microsome of adrenal, testis, ovary	17-Hydroxylase: 20–22 lyase	Male pseudohermaphroditism
Cytochrome P450C21	See footnote (previously CYP21)	6q21.3	Microsome of adrenal, testis, ovary	21-Hydroxylase	Congenital adrenal hyperplasia, female pseudohermaphroditism
Cytochrome P450C11B1	See footnote (previously CYP11)	8q24	Microsome of adrenal, testis, ovary	11β-Hydroxylase	Congenital adrenal hyperplasia
SRD5A2	Steroid 5α-reductase 2	2p23	Fetal genital skin and male accessory organs	5α-Reductase type 2	Male pseudohermaphroditism*
TSPY	Testis-specific protein Y (one component of GBY)	Ypter-p11.2	Spermatogonia	Spermatogonial proliferation in a phosphorylation-dependent manner	Gonadoblastoma
GBY	Gonadoblastoma Y	Y, near centromere	Spermatogonia	Undefined physiologic function in normal males	Gonadoblastoma
DMRT1	DM-Domain gene expressed in testis	9p24.3	? Spermatogenesis	Human testis differentiation	XY male to female sex reversal
SF1	Steroidogenic factor-1	9q33	? Sertoli cell	Gonadal differentiation and steroidogenesis	XY male to female sex reversal; male pseudohermaphroditism

'CYP' is a host of enzymes that use iron to oxidize things, largely as a strategy by which the body disposes of potentially harmful substances by making them more water soluble. CYP in humans is found in the *liver*, the main organ involved in drug and toxin removal and small intestine. CYP resides in the endoplasmic reticulum. In the adrenal and gonads, CYP is vital to the formation of *cholesterol and steroid* metabolites. Of the 1000 plus known CYPs in nature, humans have only about 50 (49 genes and 15 pseudogenes have been sequenced). It is thought that the massive heterogeneity of these oxidases in nature reflects the complex interdependence (read: 'ongoing battle') between plants and animals: plants develop new alkaloids to limit their consumption by animals; animals develop new enzymes to metabolize the plant toxins, and so it goes on. From an evolutionary viewpoint, the number of CYP genes exploded when organisms moved from the oceans to dry land – around 400 million years ago! The name cytochrome P450 comes from CY (cytochrome) and P (pigment) when a solution exposed to carbon monoxide absorbs light at a wavelength of 450 nm. See http://www.anaesthetist.com/physiol/basics/metabol/cyp/cyp.htm for a more detailed explanation.

one-fourth of cases of classic congenital adrenogenital syndrome result from the deleted *CYP21* gene. The remainder are due to non-deleted mutant gene sequences that have been transferred from the pseudogene, rendering the active gene non-functional.[26] If the allele carries a defect encoding for a mild defect, then the child will develop a non-classic form of adrenal hyperplasia, which by definition occurs after birth and

is never associated with genital ambiguity.[94] This latter syndrome is common, occurring in 1% of all women, and is thought to be a major cause of adult-onset virilism.

In the congenital form of the adrenogenital syndrome, the extent of virilization depends upon the timing in fetal life when the disease begins. If the onset begins after week 16 of gestation, the clitoris may be enlarged. If androgen excess occurs

Table 34.3 Gonadal tumors of abnormal sexual development

Leydig cell hyperplasia (pseudotumor)	Adrenogenital syndrome
Luteoma of pregnancy	Maternal virilizing tumor
Intratubular germ cell neoplasia	Congenital lipoid adrenal hyperplasia (defect in steroidogenic acute regulatory (*StAR*) gene)
Sertoli cell hamartomas; Leydig cell nodules; seminoma	Androgen insensitivity syndrome (testicular feminization)
Mediastinal germ cell tumors; Leydig cell tumors (rare) Breast cancer; hematologic malignancies	Klinefelter syndrome (XXY)
Non-germ cell (serous carcinoma of ovary; endometrial carcinoma); stromal luteoma or hilus cell hyperplasia; extragonadal tumor of neurogenic origin	Turner syndrome and Turner-like (XO and X mosaicism)
Wilms tumor; gonadoblastoma	Denys–Drash syndrome
Gonadoblastoma	Frasier syndrome
Gonadoblastoma	46,XY disorder of sex development
Germinoma; gonadoblastoma rare	True hermaphroditism

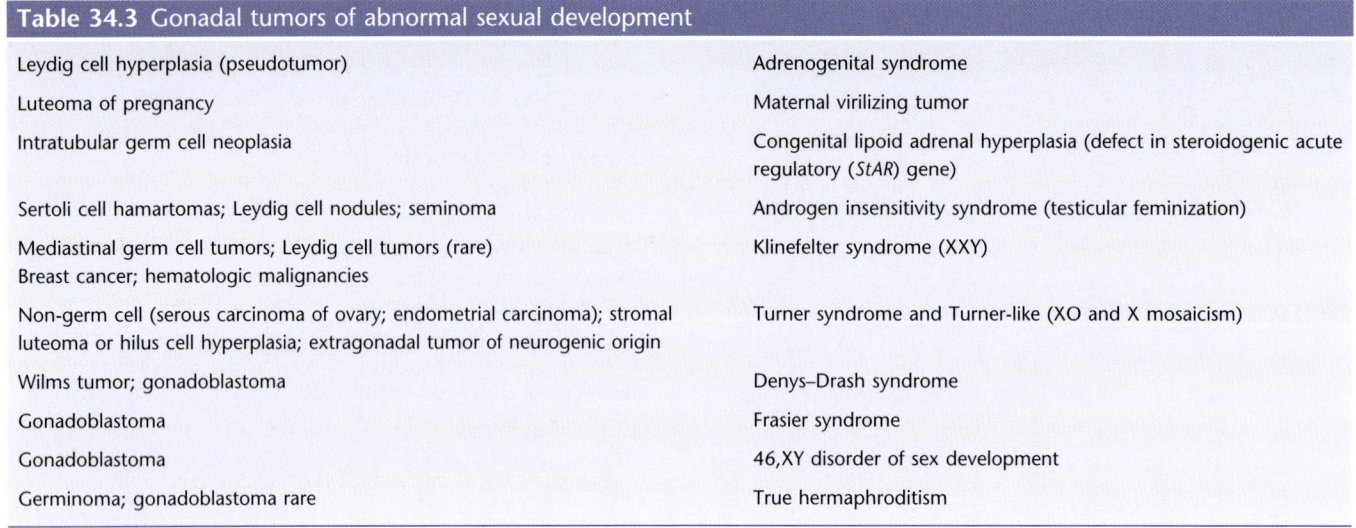

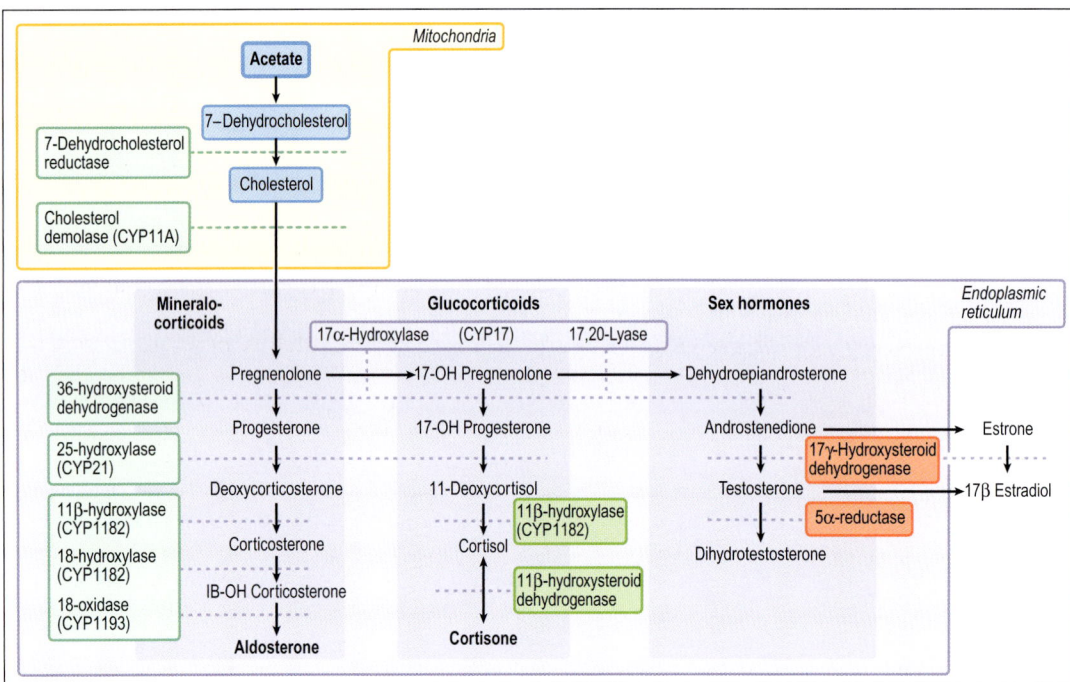

Fig. 34.1 Biosynthesis of mineralocorticoids, glucocorticoids, and sex steroids.

earlier, the vagina and urethra may open into a common urogenital sinus. More marked clitoral enlargement and an opening of the urogenital sinus at the clitoral base may mimic penile hypospadias and suggest an even earlier temporal effect. On occasion, the changes have been of such severity that the female infants have been misdiagnosed as cryptorchid males with or without hypospadias.

Tumor development in genetic females with this condition is rare. In one unusual case, prostatic adenocarcinoma developed with osteoblastic skeletal metastases. Presumably, the initial development of the prostate itself was based on excessive testosterone formation during embryogenesis, which itself was reflective of 21-hydroxylase deficiency.[154] In addition, the patient subsequently developed clear cell carcinoma of the endometrium.

Males who have the adrenogenital syndrome show no evidence of genital ambiguity, but may have an enlarged phallus and a hyperpigmented rugated scrotum. Clinically detectable bilateral testicular nodules occasionally develop during childhood or young adulthood and must be distinguished from true Leydig cell tumors (Figures 34.2 and 34.3).[116] Usually the cells are composed of interstitial cells larger than Leydig cells, secrete cortisol and respond to treatment with the adrenolytic agent o,p'-DDD (mitotane), indicative that these cells are adrenal or adrenal-like in origin. Bilaterality and decreasing tumor size after corticosteroid therapy are features indicative that the testicular 'tumor' of the adrenogenital syndrome is hyperplastic rather than neoplastic.[122] Screening examinations with ultrasonography and magnetic resonance imaging have shown that intratesticular masses are far more common than

Table 34.4 Forms of adrenal hyperplasia affecting the external genitalia

Deficiency	Syndrome	Ambiguous genitalia	Postnatal virilization
Steroidogenic acute regulatory protein (StAR)	–	Males	
3β-Hydroxysteroid dehydrogenase	Classic	Males	Yes
	Non-classic	No	Yes
17α-Hydroxylase	–	Males	No
21-Hydroxylase	Salt-wasting	Females	Yes
	Simple virilizing	Females	Yes
	Non-classic	No	Yes
11β-Hydroxylase	Classic	Females	Yes
	Non-classic	No	Yes

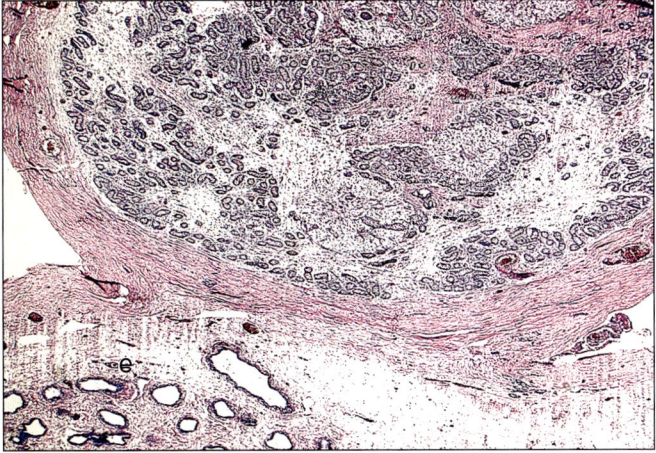

Fig. 34.2 Interstitial cell tumor of testis in child with adrenogenital syndrome. The epididymis (e) is adjacent to the testis.

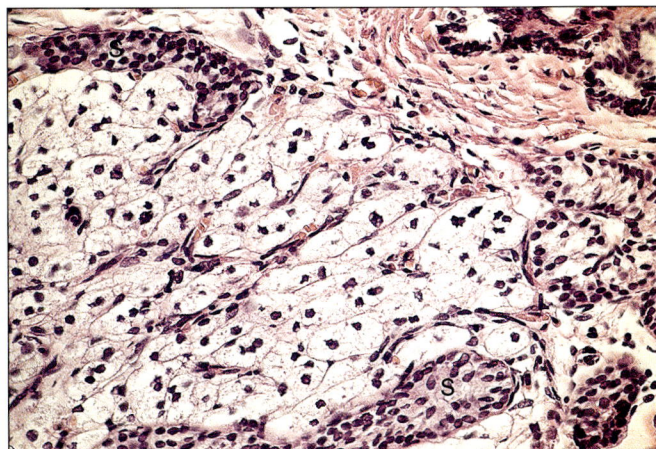

Fig. 34.3 Interstitial cell tumor of adrenogenital syndrome. The tumor cells (t), which lie adjacent to immature seminiferous tubules (s), resemble adrenocortical cells more closely than Leydig cells.

expected, being present in 40% of affected males.[12] Rare cases have also been reported of ovarian tumors associated with severe virilizing symptoms.[4,15] The tumors, like those which arise in the testes, are bilateral, and are composed of cells with abundant cytoplasm, cytoplasmic lipochrome pigment, and some nuclear pleomorphism.

Placental aromatase defect

Placental aromatase deficiency is a rare cause of maternal virilization during pregnancy and pseudohermaphroditism of the female fetus.[63,79] Mutations in the aromatase gene, *CYP19*, which causes abnormally low conversion of androstenedione to 17β-estradiol and estrone, result in virilization of the mother and her female fetus because of the accumulation of potent androgens that are not converted to estrogens. The mothers usually show the onset of progressive virilization during the third trimester. The male fetus has normal genitalia.

MATERNAL INFLUENCE

Maternal ingestion of progestins or androgens

Maternal ingestion of synthetic progestins was implicated as a cause of female pseudohermaphroditism in the late 1950s when such treatment was employed for threatened or habitual abortion. Subsequently, progestins have also been implicated in the development of hypospadias in male offspring. Most cases of female pseudohermaphroditism in this category developed after maternal ingestion of Norlutin (17α-ethinyl-19-nortestosterone), less often with ethisterone (17α-ethinyltestosterone), and occasionally after the ingestion of Enovid, diethylstilbestrol, androgens or the intramuscular administration of progesterone.

Masculinization usually consists of phallic enlargement and variable degrees of labioscrotal fusion, depending on the time during gestation when the therapy was administered. Although the degree of masculinization is usually less than that associated with the adrenogenital syndrome, the sexual ambiguity in female infants has been of such severity in some instances as to result in male sex assignment. The degree of virilization does not progress with age. The gonads and internal genital organs are unaffected, and ovulation, menstruation, and normal secondary female characteristics appear at puberty.

Maternal virilizing lesions

A variety of benign and malignant tumors and tumor-like conditions, primary as well as metastatic to the ovary, have been associated with virilization of the mother and/or her female offspring.[42,143] The luteoma of pregnancy and the probably related hyperreactio luteinalis are the most common lesions that cause maternal virilization during pregnancy.[142] This is a benign hyperplastic lesion of the ovaries that is encountered most often as an incidental finding at the time of cesarean section or postpartum sterilization, usually in women who are multiparous. Occasional cases have been detected prenatally.[84] Elevated levels of human chorionic gonadotropin (hCG) are thought to induce hyperplasia of theca–lutein or stroma–lutein cells, which are responsible for the production of androgen (principally androstenedione). A small percentage of the female infants become masculinized, with mild enlargement of the clitoris and occasionally minimal degrees of labioscrotal fusion or rugate, hyperpigmented ('scrotal') labia. The nature of these changes indicates that the ovarian nodules do not function until the second half of gestation, which agrees with the occasional onset of masculinization in the mother during the third trimester.

Elevated plasma and tissue levels of testosterone, dihydrotestosterone, androstenedione, and DHEA have been detected in virilized patients. The plasma levels return to normal once the tumor is extirpated. Even without treatment, the nodules regress and disappear soon after delivery. Rarely, a functional luteoma may reoccur during a subsequent pregnancy.

Other primary functioning lesions of the ovary that may lead to virilized female offspring as well as metastatic tumors to the ovary that induce the stroma to function during pregnancy are discussed elsewhere in this book.

MALE PSEUDOHERMAPHRODITISM (MALE INTERSEX)

Male pseudohermaphroditism defines a heterogeneous group of intersex conditions that are characterized by an intrauterine state of relative functional androgen deficiency, an apparently normal 46,XY karyotype, and either identifiable testes or evidence that testes were present during fetal development. The external genitalia are usually female or ambiguous, although in certain categories (e.g., testicular regression syndrome) they may appear as phenotypically male. The responsible defect may be in the gonad, leading to deficiency in androgens, deficiency in müllerian inhibiting substance (MIS), or both. Alternatively, end-organ defects in which developing tissues are unresponsive to androgens or MIS may lead to the abnormal phenotype.

PRIMARY GONADAL DEFECTS

A primary defect of the gonad in an XY karyotype individual may lead to male pseudohermaphroditism by any one of the following mechanisms: regression (destruction) of the gonads or their anlage during intrauterine life; agenesis of the Leydig cells; a specific enzymatic defect in testosterone, dihydrotestosterone synthesis or receptors to these hormones; or a defect in elaboration or action of MIS.

Testicular regression syndrome

Testicular regression follows the irreparable destruction of both testes at a critical stage of fetal development in an XY individual, with resulting endocrine/hormonal disturbances. Unilateral testicular destruction does not result in the testicular regression syndrome, as the causative mechanisms and manifestations differ.

The phenotype of an affected individual with testicular regression syndrome reflects the specific stage of fetal development during which the testes were damaged. In general, gonadal regression that occurs during embryonic life, before the elaboration of MIS and/or androgenic steroids by the testes, leads to a female phenotype. Regression of the testes during late embryonic through mid-fetal life permits a masculine phenotype (Figure 34.4). The testicular regression syndrome has a variety of etiologies, some possibly as diverse as inherited genetic defect, intrauterine infection, or infarction. The heterogeneity in the presentation of this syndrome and its relative rarity has led to numerous and sometimes confusing terms for this disorder, including: true agonadism, testicular dysgenesis, rudimentary testis, vanishing testis, and complete bilateral anorchia. Pure gonadal dysgenesis (Swyer syndrome) has been used to designate some forms of the testicular regression syndrome, but this term is better avoided so as not to confuse it with other conditions similarly named and discussed below.

At one end of the spectrum of the testicular regression syndrome, the internal genitalia and gonads are absent and the external genitalia are female. Presumably, the urogenital ridge was destroyed in its entirety during early embryonic life, even before the müllerian ducts began to differentiate (prior to day 42).

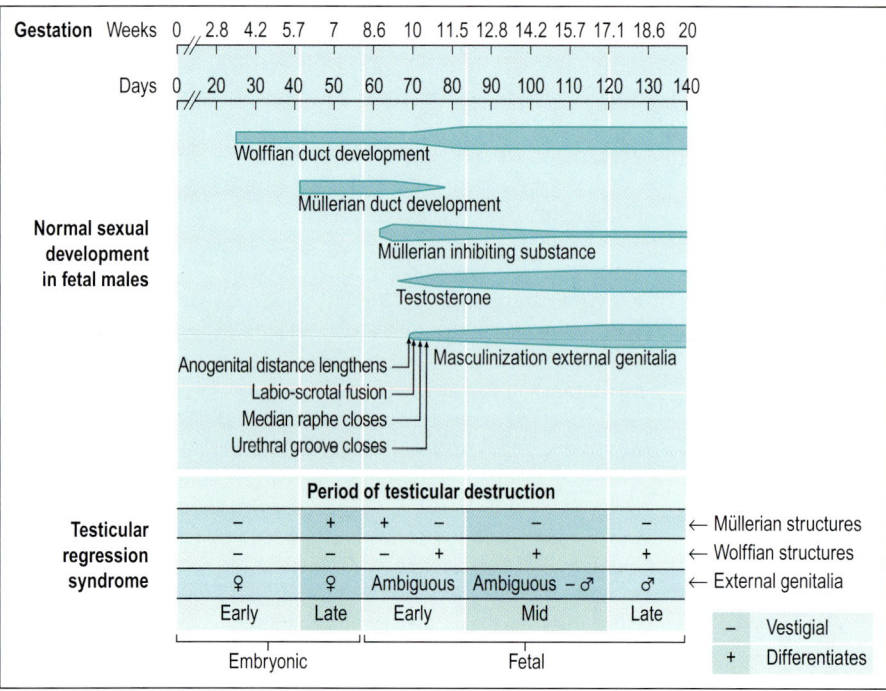

Fig. 34.4 Testicular regression syndrome. The phenotypic appearance of the internal genitalia abnormalities relates to the time during embryogenesis when the normal development of the genital tract was damaged.

At the other end of the spectrum, which approximates the endpoint of normal genital development, the patients are phenotypic males with infantile to nearly normal male external genitalia, normally differentiated wolffian duct structures and completely inhibited müllerian duct development. Often in these cases, no gonadal tissue is identified. However, there is sometimes a focus of vascularized fibrosis (85%), hemorrhage or hemosiderin deposition (70%), calcification (60%) or giant cells at the expected site of the gonad, which is near the residual vas deferens or epididymis (Figures 34.5 and 34.6).[28,92,132] Occasionally, atrophic seminiferous tubules may be found amidst the fibrous stroma. Testicular regression presumably develops during the late fetal period (after 120 days) when müllerian structures have already atrophied under the influences of MIS, and testosterone and dihydrotestosterone have exerted a major influence on the normal development of internal and external genitalia, respectively. Torsion and infarction of improperly descended testes have been suggested.[131]

Intermediate in the spectrum of this disorder are patients with ambiguous genitalia and various combinations of wolffian and/or müllerian duct development. Testes that regress during

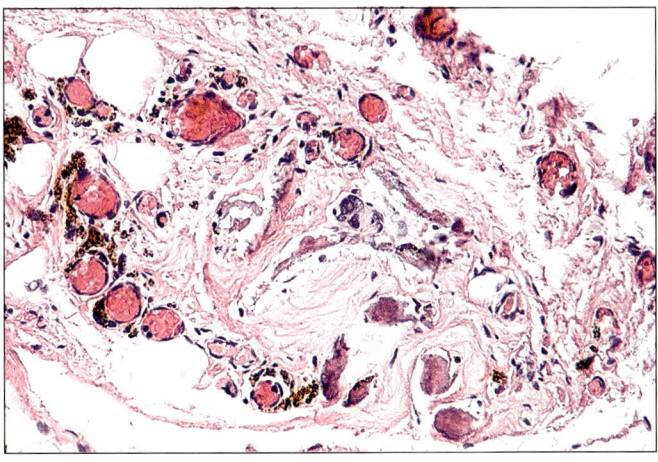

Fig. 34.5 Testicular regression syndrome. Vascularized fibrosis, hemosiderin deposition, and calcification are seen at the expected site of both gonads.

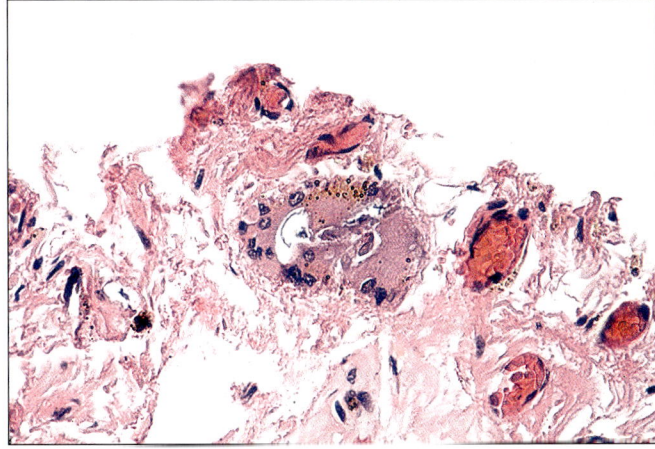

Fig. 34.6 Testicular regression syndrome. Foreign-body giant cells are seen at the expected site of the gonad.

the late embryonic period (day 43–59) usually secrete insufficient testosterone to affect the wolffian duct. The production of MIS is variable, resulting in poorly differentiated or rudimentary müllerian structures (incomplete inhibition). In the absence of systemic androgens, the external genitalia appear female.

Regression of the testes during the early fetal period (day 59–84), which is after Sertoli cell (MIS) and Lcydig cell (testosterone) function have begun or are about to begin, results in an individual with ambiguous external genitalia. Various combinations of wolffian and müllerian structures develop depending on the duration of androgen secretion and müllerian inhibition.

Regression of the testes during the mid-fetal period (day 84–120) results in more advanced masculinization of the external genitalia, although degrees of ambiguity are usually present. Since müllerian duct inhibition is normally completed by day 80, the müllerian structures will have been suppressed and wolffian structures develop.

Leydig cell deficiency

Leydig cell deficiency is a rare cause of male pseudohermaphroditism that may have more than one cause. Some cases may lack Leydig cells altogether, while in others the presence of enzymatic machinery can be seen in fibroblast-like cells by appropriate antibodies, but some other dysfunction leads to the Leydig cell dysfunction.[10] Affected individuals have a 46,XY karyotype and testes with interstitial fibrosis, but lack mature Leydig cells and testosterone production. Tubules with Sertoli cells and, sometimes, immature spermatogonia are found. The müllerian structures are absent, indicating appropriate testicular production of MIS by Sertoli cells during fetal life. The wolffian duct system is developed either partially or fully such that identifiable vasa deferentia and epididymides are present. The phenotype varies and is usually female with unremarkable or ambiguous external genitalia, although unambiguous males with evidence of primary hypogonadism have been reported. The presence of wolffian duct development and the variable degrees of masculinized external genitalia indicate that some Leydig cells must have differentiated and functioned during early fetal life. Luteinizing hormone levels are elevated in affected individuals. Because this condition is so rare, it is uncertain whether the underlying defect is an absence or a defect of the luteinizing hormone (LH)-hCG receptor on the Leydig cell or with some other, unknown, factor arresting Leydig cell development.

Defects in testosterone synthesis

Congenital deficiency of any enzyme involved in testosterone production in the testis or adrenal gland results in a state of androgen deficiency (relative estrogen excess). The histologic appearance of the testicular tissue is variable. Although described occasionally as 'normal', the photomicrographs in some reports have disclosed large clusters of Leydig cells surrounding tubules lined only by Sertoli cells. Spermatogonia are often normal in children, but disappear by puberty.[13] In general, the number of gonads studied for any of the conditions and the ranges of ages studied (infancy, childhood, adulthood) have been limited. Müllerian structures are absent, but wolffian duct structures may be present. The degree to which the external genitalia develop depends upon the type and severity of the defect.

Defect in cholesterol synthesis (Smith–Lemli–Opitz syndrome) Cholesterol synthesis is required for testosterone and all other hormones that the gonads and adrenal glands produce. The Smith–Lemli–Opitz syndrome, inherited as an autosomal recessive trait, results from an enzymatic defect in the last step of cholesterol metabolism (reduction of 7-dehydrocholesterol (7-DCH) due to mutations in the 7-dehydrocholesterol reductase gene).[39,102,104] These patients variably show ambiguous genitalia with hypospadias, and more constantly a wide range of other somatic abnormalities including a distinctive facial appearance (microcephaly, ptosis, small upturned nose, micrognathia), cleft palate and limb anomalies (proximally placed thumbs, polydactyly, and 2–3 toe syndactyly).[109] This entity is considered as the first known true metabolic syndrome of multiple congenital malformations.

Several 46,XY infants with female external genitalia and intra-abdominal testes with epididymides and deferent ducts had a normally shaped uterus and vagina.[18,41] One biochemical study using probes for 26 'loci' including *SRY* found that the Y chromosome was entirely normal.[41] Studies of testicular function both *in vivo* and *in vitro* in a 46,XY patient with ambiguous genitalia and raised as a girl suggested that the fetal testes might have failed to respond to placental hCG at the time of male external genital differentiation.[17] Testicular histology in this patient was normal for age.

Congenital lipoid adrenal hyperplasia Congenital lipoid adrenal hyperplasia (lipoid CAH), the most severe form of CAH, results from mutations in the steroidogenic acute regulatory (*StAR*) gene as the primary defect (Table 34.2).[69,73] The *StAR* gene, located on chromosome 8, encodes a protein that helps transport cholesterol into the mitochondria.[27] The principal effect is the absence of cholesterol intermediates capable of converting to pregnenolone. Additional damage occurs from the subsequent steroidogenic loss independent of *StAR*, and results from the effects of the cholesterol esters that accumulate in the adrenal cortex. This leads to cellular damage in the form of salt wasting, hyponatremia, hypovolemia, hyperkalemia, acidosis, and death in infancy. This state of hypergonadotrophic hypogonadism shows markedly elevated levels of gonadotrophic hormones (LH, follicle-stimulating hormone, ACTH), but markedly impaired synthesis of all gonadal and adrenal cortical steroids, even with trophic stimulation tests.

In the 46,XY male, the external genitalia may be ambiguous to female, but sufficient testosterone must have been secreted during embryogenesis since the internal genitalia are male. Some of these patients may have a palpable gonad in the inguinal canal. These testes disclose immature seminiferous tubules with spermatogonia. Occasional Leydig cells are present. The germ cells may disappear over time, resulting in a Sertoli-only syndrome, although this is not inevitable. Germ cells can persist and rarely develop into intratubular germ cell neoplasia.[73]

Congenital adrenal hyperplasia Several inherited enzymatic defects, which cause the syndrome of congenital adrenal hyperplasia, involve both the synthesis of adrenal mineralocorticoid and glucocorticoid hormones as well as the adrenal and testicular sex hormones. Due to these genetic defects, one or more adrenal cortical enzymes fail to be synthesized or are defective.

The deficiency of 3β-hydroxylase dehydrogenase, like the 20,22-desmolase deficiency, results in decreased synthesis of mineralocorticoid and glucocorticoid hormones as well as adrenal and testicular sex hormones, and may lead to life-threatening salt wasting in infancy. DHEA, a weak androgen secreted in high amounts, results in slight clitoral enlargement in the female, but rarely completely masculinizes the external genitalia in males. Hence, the male may be born with ambiguous genitalia and may resemble a virilized female. Males in whom the defect is partial may be born with hypospadias, but at puberty develop gynecomastia. Over time, the Sertoli cells, which may initially appear normal, undergo atrophy and the spermatogonia change from abundant to rare to absent. The number of Leydig cells may increase with age, but it is unclear whether the hyperplasia is absolute or relative to the atrophy of other elements.[91]

In contrast to the early age of diagnosis in the above two syndromes, the diagnosis in most patients with 17β-hydroxylase deficiency is not suspected until the anticipated time of puberty or later. Occasionally, detailed steroid analysis of the urine of a newborn male presenting with ambiguous genitalia has been performed, indicating that the correct diagnosis can be made in the young.

Deficiency of two enzymes, 17,20-desmolase and 17-hydroxysteroid dehydrogenase (formerly 17-ketosteroid reductase), results in deficient testosterone synthesis but does not affect the production of either mineralocorticoids or glucocorticoids. The former defect (conversion of 17-hydroxypregnenolone to DHEA) is extremely rare. The patients reported presented with ambiguous external genitalia and inguinal or intra-abdominal testes. Spermatogonia were present in the testes of infants but were absent in the biopsies of their older teenage relatives. All had third-degree hypospadias, but normal male internal ductal differentiation.

Genetic males with 17β-hydroxysteroid dehydrogenase (17β-HSD) deficiency have uniformly been raised as females and have unambiguous female external genitalia. Most are diagnosed at or after puberty when they fail to menstruate and instead show signs of virilization such as clitoromegaly (enlarged phallus) and hirsutism.[156] Breast development may or may not take place. At surgery, müllerian duct derivatives are absent, consistent with normal antimüllerian hormone action. Wolffian duct differentiation, indicative of testosterone secretion during embryogenesis, is normal.[9] The testes present in the inguinal canal or labia majora contain rare to no spermatogonia, and may exhibit numerous Leydig cells. Detailed endocrine studies have shown that testicular 17β-HSD is under a different genetic control from that in extragonadal tissues, and while affected males lack testicular 17β-HSD, the extragonadal activity is normal or enhanced. More than 15 mutations have been identified in the responsible gene.[9,20,90]

Defect in müllerian inhibiting system

The persistent müllerian duct syndrome, also known as 'hernia uteri inguinalis', is a rare form of male pseudohermaphroditism where müllerian duct structures persist in 46,XY phenotypic males (Figure 34.7). Most patients present when young with unilateral or bilateral cryptorchid testes, normal or almost normal male external genitalia, and an inguinal hernia into which prolapses an infantile uterus and fallopian tubes.[24,117] Some patients may be older.[37] The testes are histologically normal, wolffian duct structures are developed, the pubertal development is normal, and a rare patient has been fertile.

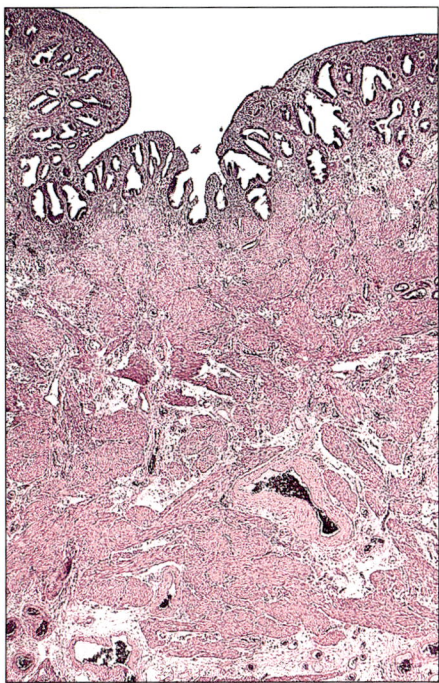

Fig. 34.7 Uterus in persistent müllerian duct syndrome.

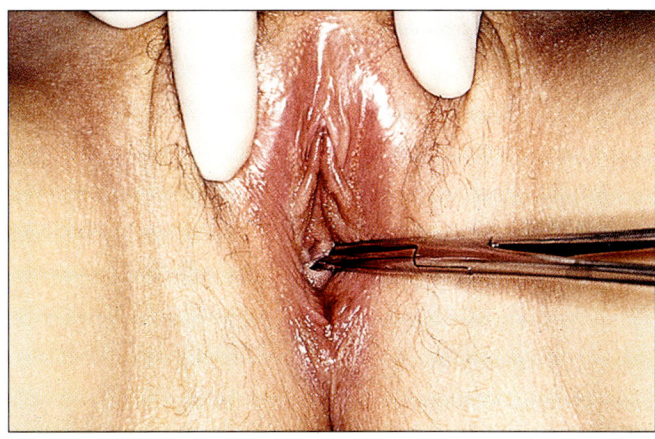

Fig. 34.8 'Normal' phenotypic feminine genitalia in androgen insensitivity syndrome.

Treatment is surgical, consisting of orchiopexy and herniorrhaphy with hysterectomy and bilateral salpingectomy.

If at operation any patient has a streak gonad or a tumor rather than bilateral testes, the diagnosis of mixed gonadal dysgenesis should be considered. In most cases of persistent müllerian duct syndrome, the vas deferens is embedded in the wall of the upper vagina and sometimes the müllerian structures must be left intact to preserve the vas deferens. Malignant testicular tumors have been reported in the very rare cases of adult patients with persistent müllerian duct syndrome and uncorrected cryptorchid testes.

Persistent müllerian duct syndrome is a heterogeneous group of disorders caused by at least two different defects in the müllerian inhibiting system. The most common is a defect in the müllerian inhibiting substance (*MIS*) gene, also known as the antimüllerian hormone (*AMH*) gene. The next most common is a defective AMH receptor (type II).[16,65] The effect of these abnormalities is that some patients produce no biologically functional MIS, whereas others that produce normal amounts of biologically active MIS have end-organ insensitivity to MIS or an abnormality of the timing of MIS secretion.

On a rare occasion, a germ cell tumor may develop in the gonad, and, exceptionally, a müllerian-type tumor may develop in the genital tract.[127]

END-ORGAN DEFECTS

The normal development of the wolffian duct derivatives and the external genitalia requires that these structures be responsive to androgen and that the enzyme 5α-reductase be present in the anlage of the prostate and external genitalia to convert testosterone to dihydrotestosterone. A molecular defect of the androgen receptor system (e.g., unstable androgen receptor or lack of androgen receptor) leads to impaired development of both wolffian duct structures and external genitalia in 46,XY

individuals. If only 5α-reductase is absent or defective, the abnormalities in the reproductive tract are confined to the external genitalia and prostate.

Androgen receptor disorders (androgen insensitivity syndromes)

Disordered androgen receptor function results in various phenotypes ranging from phenotypic women with intra-abdominal testes to individuals with ambiguous genitalia to phenotypic men with minimal clinical abnormalities. One classification scheme[87] lists four categories, which are, in order of increasing virilization (decreasing feminization):

- complete testicular feminization
- incomplete testicular feminization
- Reifenstein phenotype
- infertile and/or undervirilized man.

About 70% of cases share an X-linked recessive inheritance through the carrier mothers, the result of mutational defects in the androgen receptor gene, which has been localized to the long arm of the X chromosome. In another 30%, the mutation arises *de novo*.[71] A variety of different genetic mutations have been characterized,[51,110] many of which are limited to individual families.[66] These mutations may lead to functional absence of the androgen receptor because the primary sequences of the gene are affected. These patients generally present as complete testicular feminization. The more common defect results from single amino acid substitutions and is associated with the various other forms of the disease as described below. In rare patients the androgen receptor disorder has occurred in combination with other unusual karyotypes, e.g., 47,XXY[139] and 47,XYY.[97]

Complete androgen receptor insufficiency (complete testicular feminization) Complete testicular feminization, the most common form of male pseudohermaphroditism, occurs in 1:20000 newborns. The external genitalia are phenotypically female (Figure 34.8) and, for this reason, the condition is rarely diagnosed before puberty unless an inguinal hernia or labial mass is encountered or unless the disease is known to be familial.[6,130] Primary amenorrhea is the most common complaint leading to evaluation and subsequent diagnosis. The medical history usually reveals that breast development occurred as

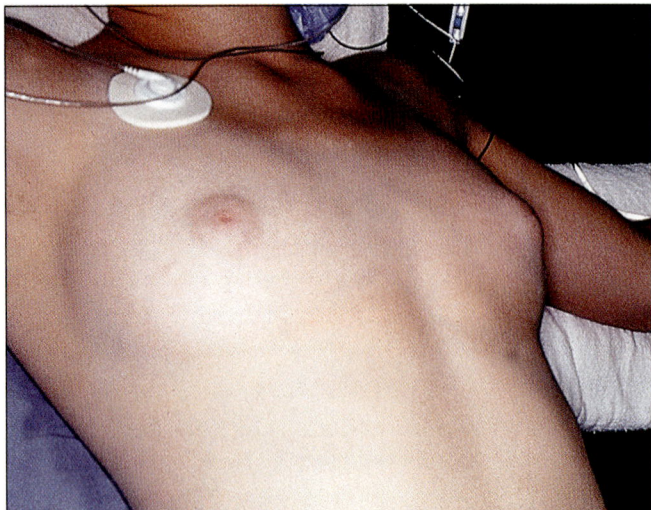

Fig. 34.9 Immature breast development and lack of axillary hair in androgen insensitivity syndrome.

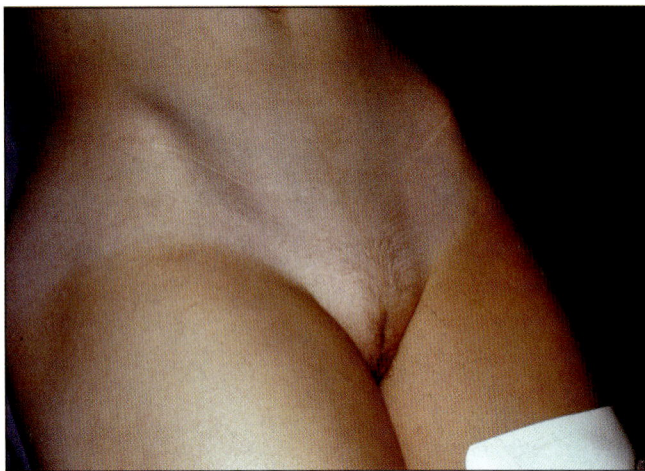

Fig. 34.10 Lack of pubic hair in androgen insensitivity syndrome.

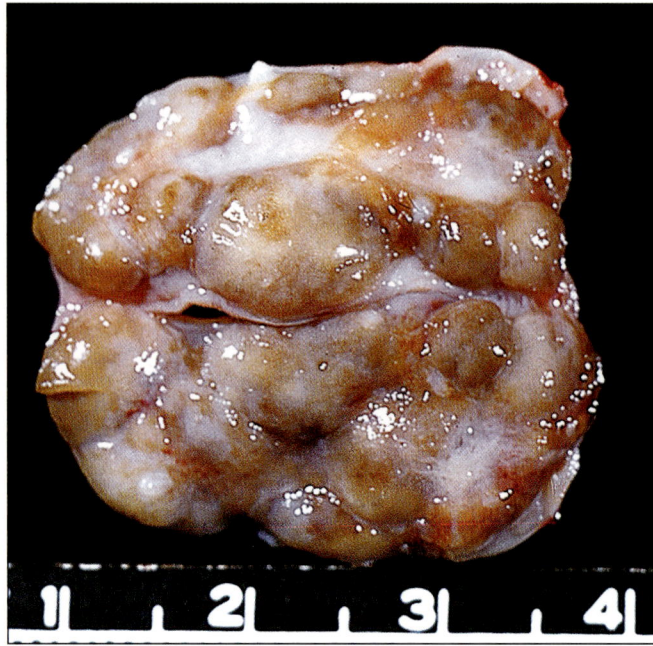

Fig. 34.11 Testis in androgen insensitivity syndrome without tumor.

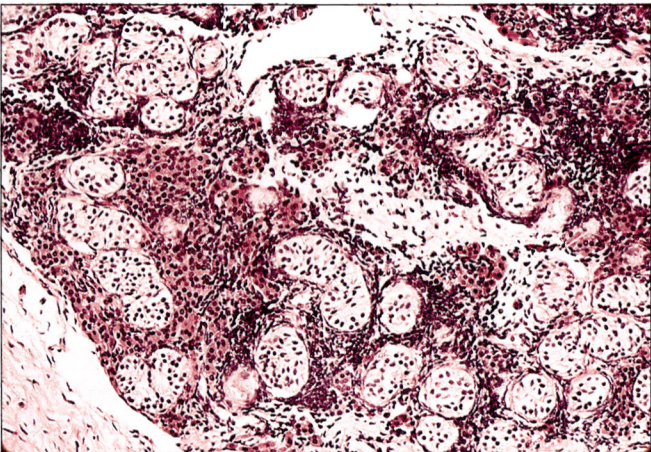

Fig. 34.12 Androgen insensitivity syndrome. Immature seminiferous tubules, numerous Leydig cells, and rare foci of immature ovarian-type stroma comprise the testis.

expected at puberty, but remains in the pubertal state (Figure 34.9). Pubic and axillary hair is scant (Figure 34.10) and the vagina is shortened. The epididymides are usually cystic and not connected to the testes. The vasa differentia, seminal vesicles, and prostate are absent. As a rule, both the cervix and the uterine corpus are absent. A fragment of fallopian tube may be found in up to one-third of cases.[121] The testes are cryptorchid and may be located in the inguinal canal, the pelvis or rarely the labia. In the complete or almost complete form of the syndrome, the individual exhibits a truly female consciousness gender identity with normal extragenital erotogenic sensitivity and normal maternal attitude, emphasizing the need to support the patient as a woman, even with reconstructive surgery.[145] This condition should be differentiated from defects in SF1 mutations (XY, sex reversal with androgen insensitivity-like features) with which it can be confused.

The gonads in infants and young children are relatively normal but by age 5 years, they show abnormalities. By young adulthood, the gonad is often involved with benign or malignant tumors as described below. If tumors are not present by this age, the gonad is usually small and on section is tan to brown and traversed by thin white bands (Figure 34.11). Microscopic examination of the testicular parenchyma discloses immature seminiferous tubules. At earlier ages, the tubules may be clustered in small aggregates (Figure 34.12), but with time they become more sparsely distributed (Figure 34.13). Spermatogonia may be present, but spermatogenesis is absent. The number of spermatogonia found is also age dependent, diminishing as the patient ages. The interstitium, which resembles ovarian stroma, is usually abundant at an early age and over time often becomes more fibrous (Figure 34.14). Fetal-type Leydig cells may be abundant. The physical findings indicate that Leydig cells are active hormone producers. The Leydig cells in individuals with testicular feminization have an ultrastructure typical of cells involved in active hormone syn-

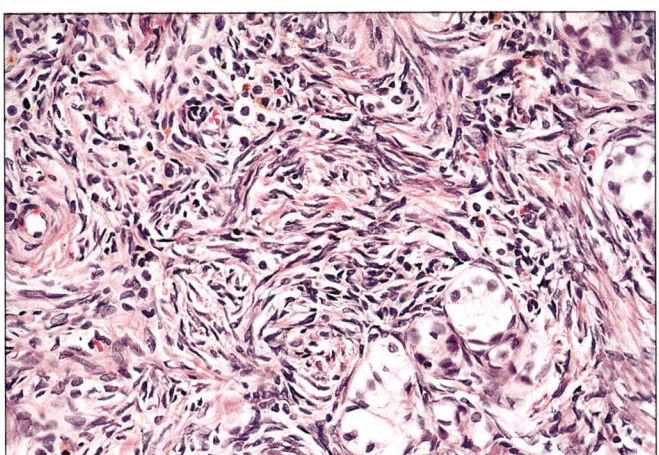

Fig. 34.13 Androgen insensitivity syndrome. Scattered immature seminiferous tubules are embedded in the dense ovarian-type cortical stroma present in the testis.

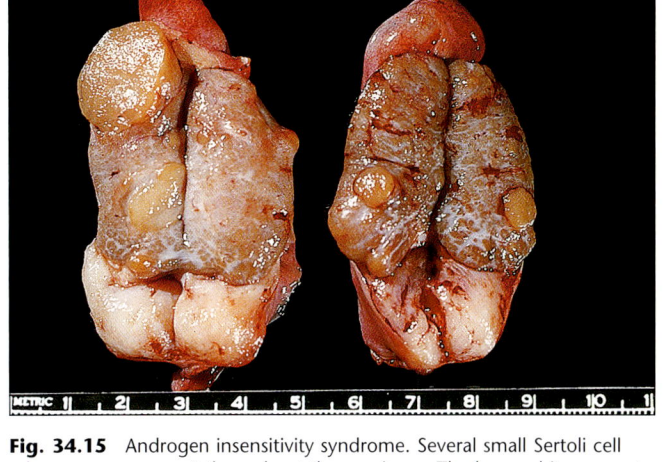

Fig. 34.15 Androgen insensitivity syndrome. Several small Sertoli cell adenomas are present throughout the specimen. The large white mass at the inferior pole may represent a hypertrophied gubernaculum testis or a leiomyoma present since birth.

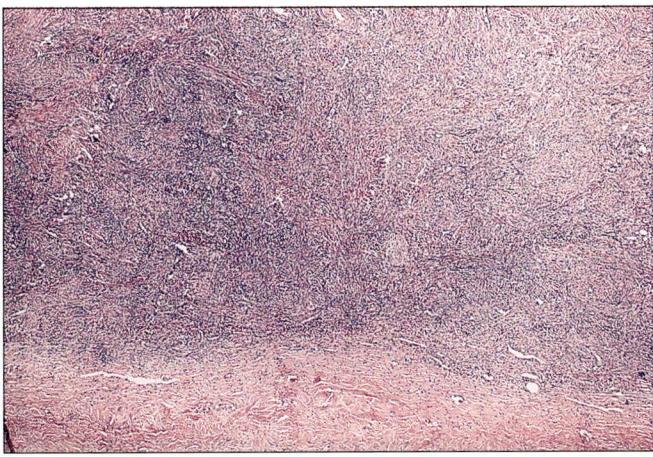

Fig. 34.14 Androgen insensitivity syndrome in an older gonad. Dense ovarian-type cortical stroma with extremely rare scattered immature seminiferous tubules comprise the testis.

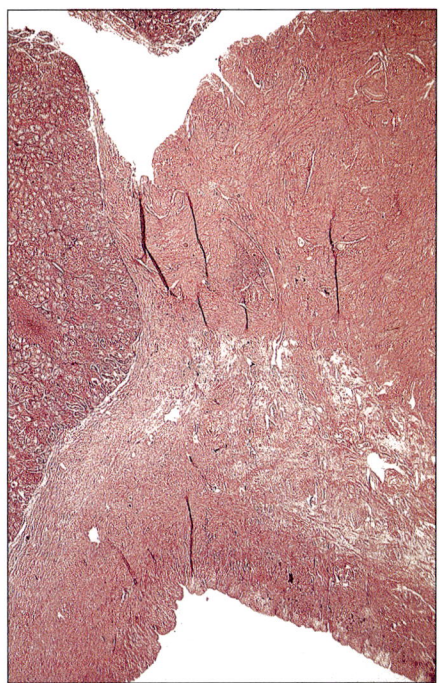

Fig. 34.16 Nodule of hypertrophied gubernaculum in androgen insensitivity syndrome.

thesis and the systemic androgen levels in these individuals are characteristically elevated. These findings indicate that the pathologic defect in the testicular feminization syndrome is an end-organ defect and not lack of hormone production by the testes.

More often than not, the testis macroscopically discloses nodules that are hamartomatous (e.g., Sertoli cell adenoma) or neoplastic (e.g., dysgerminoma or gonadoblastoma-like). One finding we have seen characteristically is a 1–2 cm firm white nodule of hyalinized smooth muscle leiomyoma-like tissue that is usually present at one pole of the testis (Figure 34.15). Theories regarding what this nodule might represent include an abnormally hypertrophied gubernaculum (Figures 34.16 and 34.17) or paratesticular leiomyoma. That it is reactive for smooth muscle actin (Figure 34.17C) confirms its smooth muscle origin. It is unlikely that this represents a rudimentary uterine structure.

Most testes of affected individuals contain multiple benign nodules that are discrete, firm, yellow to brown and bulge above the sectioned surface (Figure 34.15). These hamartoma-

tous nodules are present, usually bilaterally, in virtually every case we have examined personally. The typical size varies from 1 mm to 1 cm, but occasionally up to 4 cm.[121] The bulk of the nodule consists of seminiferous tubules lacking lumina (Figure 34.18). Spermatogonia may be present (Figure 34.19). The seminiferous tubules that have a diffuse distribution and are located outside the nodules have a lamina propria that is of normal thickness in prepubertal testes, but thickened and hyalinized in the adult.[112] Sertoli cell adenomas, which average 3 cm in diameter, but range to 25 cm (Figure 34.20), are hamartomas composed predominantly or exclusively of closely packed immature seminiferous tubules lacking lumina and lined by immature, uniform Sertoli cells (Figure 34.21), some with germ cells (Figure 34.22).[50,121]

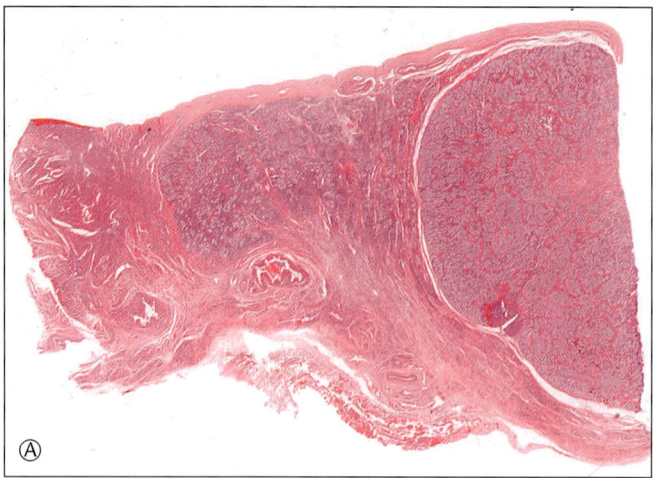

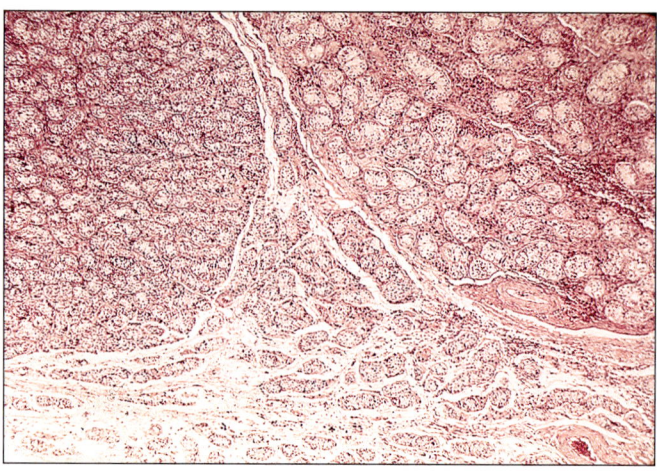

Fig. 34.18 Sertoli cell adenoma in which tubules lack lumens in androgen insensitivity syndrome.

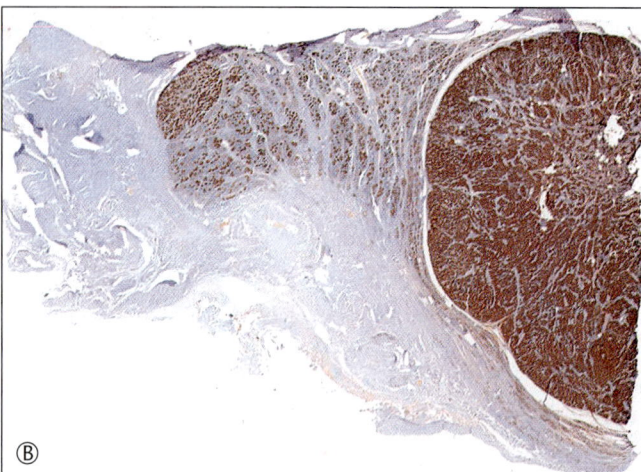

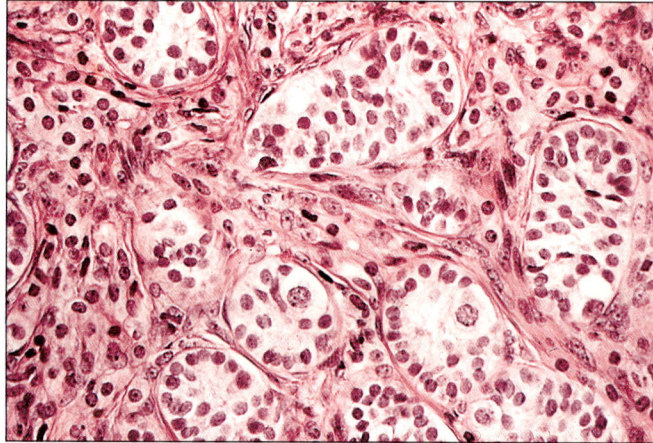

Fig. 34.19 Seminiferous tubules with occasional spermatogonia in androgen insensitivity syndrome.

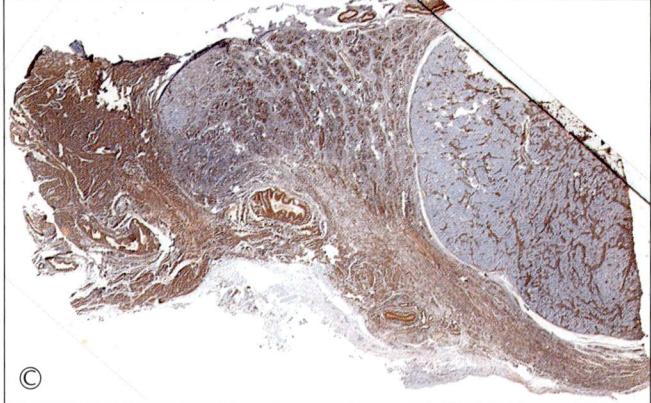

Fig. 34.17 Androgen insensitivity syndrome with **(A)** Sertoli adenoma (right) and hypertrophied gubernaculum (left). **(B)** Antimüllerian hormone. **(C)** Smooth muscle actin.

The interstitium in the testes of affected patients often resembles ovarian stroma, and frequently contains Leydig cells (Figure 34.12). On rare occasion, Leydig cell nodules form, and have been considered benign tumors (Figures 34.23 and 34.24). Even though tumors have been reported occasionally as malignant, none has shown evidence of invasion or dissemination grossly or microscopically.[58] In summary, the name applied to

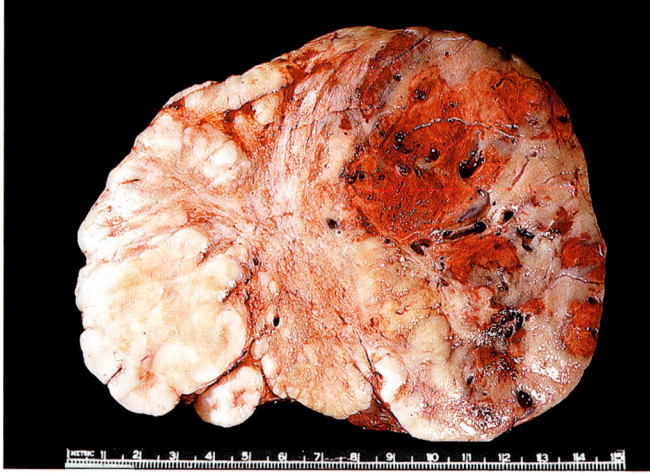

Fig. 34.20 Giant Sertoli cell adenoma.

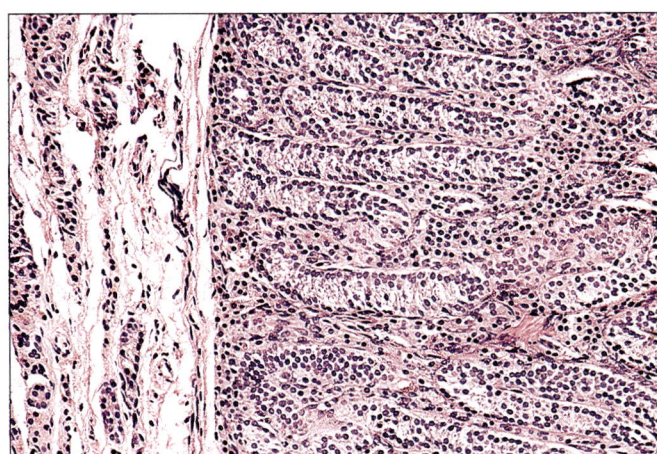

Fig. 34.21 Interface of Sertoli cell adenoma and adjacent seminiferous tubules in androgen insensitivity syndrome.

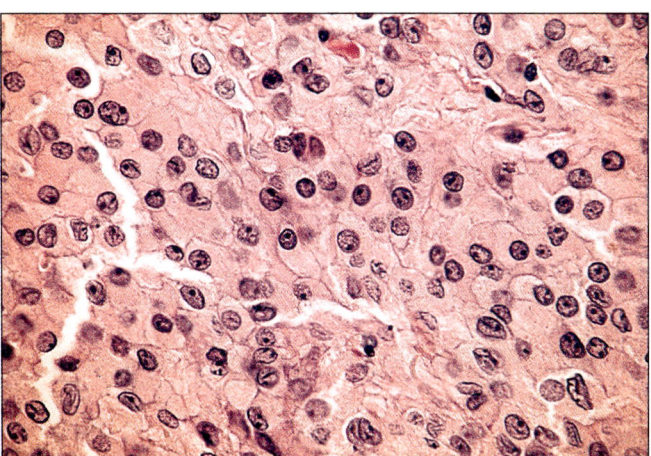

Fig. 34.24 Leydig cell tumor in androgen insensitivity syndrome. Detail of cells with large central nucleus and copious cytoplasm.

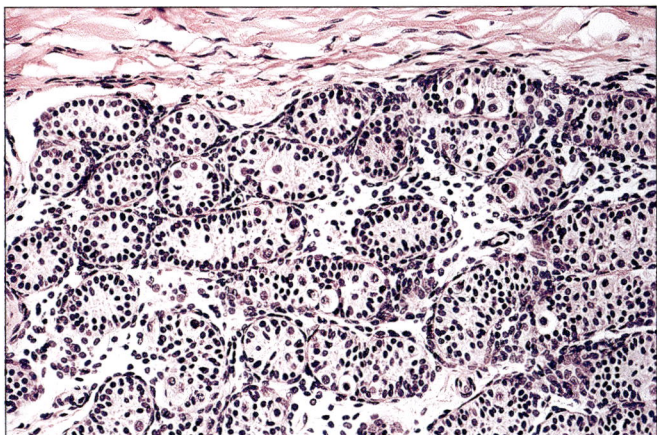

Fig. 34.22 Germ cells in Sertoli cell adenoma.

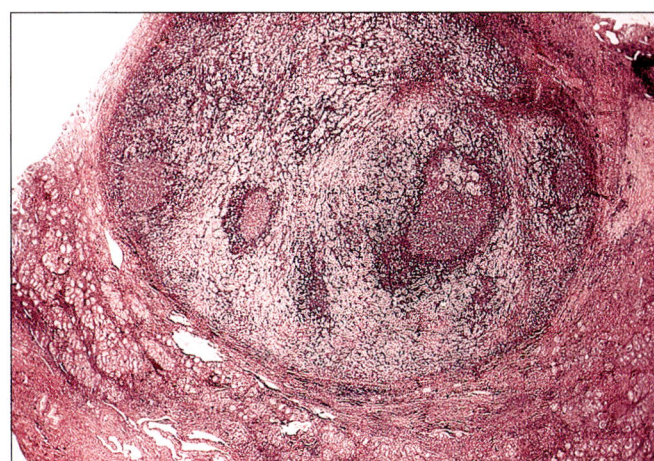

Fig. 34.25 Seminoma in androgen insensitivity syndrome.

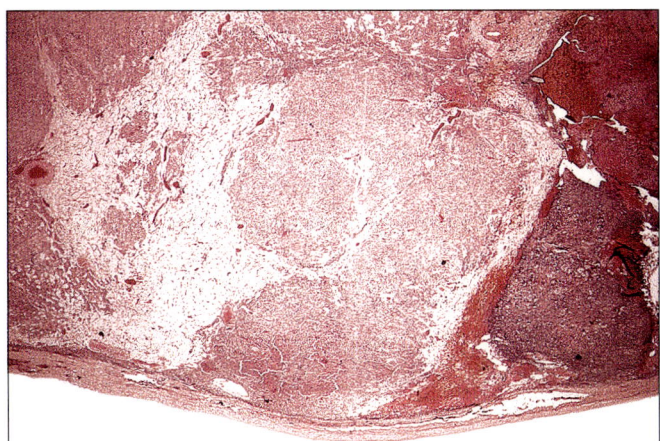

Fig. 34.23 Leydig cell tumor in androgen insensitivity syndrome.

each type of nodule is somewhat arbitrary and depends largely upon the types of component present as well as their number and size. Most nodules are classified as hamartomas, Sertoli cell adenomas, or rarely as Leydig cell tumors.

Malignant gonadal tumors develop with increasing frequency with age in patients with testicular feminization. Semi-

noma is the most commonly encountered gonadal malignancy in this syndrome. Intratubular germ cell neoplasia is sometimes seen, either independently or in association with seminoma (Figures 34.25 and 34.26). Other malignant germ cell tumors and malignant sex-cord tumors are also encountered rarely. One malignant sex-cord stromal tumor that was estrogen secreting has been reported.[86] Unlike mixed gonadal dysgenesis in which tumors develop in young individuals, the risk of malignancy in patients with testicular feminization is only 4% by the age of 25 years, but reaches 33% by 50 years.[81] Since malignant tumors rarely develop before completion of puberty, castration can usually be delayed until after adolescence, thus permitting the patient to undergo normal pubertal development with spontaneous female secondary sex characteristics.

Partial androgen receptor insufficiency (incomplete testicular feminization) About 10–50% of patients with the androgen insensitivity syndrome have an incomplete variant.[52,150] The clinical manifestations vary depending on the classification system used. If restricted, it resembles complete testicular feminization except that there is partial fusion of the labioscrotal folds and usually some clitoromegaly at birth. If inclusive of all forms of the androgen insensitivity syndrome that are not

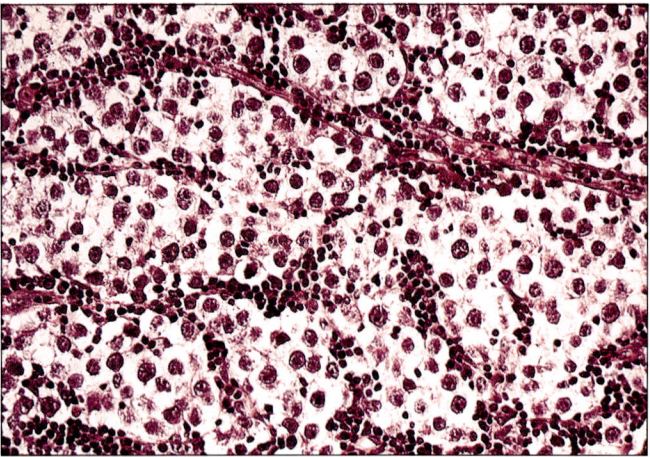

Fig. 34.26 Seminoma in androgen insensitivity syndrome. Detail of neoplastic germ cells surrounded by fibrous stroma invested with numerous lymphocytes.

considered *complete* testicular feminization, then greater percentages of patients will look and be raised as males.[52,150] Viewed broadly, patients with partial androgen receptor insufficiency form one of the largest groups of intersex patients born with male sex ambiguity.[95] Like the complete form, underdeveloped wolffian duct derivatives are often present. If the diagnosis is established during childhood, gonadectomy should be performed before puberty, since disfiguring virilization may accompany breast development at puberty. Estrogen therapy should be given at the appropriate time to initiate feminization. The pathologic findings are those described for the complete form of testicular feminization.[112]

Other forms Reifenstein syndrome, infertile male syndrome, and undervirilized male syndrome are other forms of incomplete androgen insensitivity in which the phenotype is male. There are few reports describing the microscopic findings of the gonads.

- Patients with Reifenstein syndrome usually present with gynecomastia and severe hypospadias, as children or teenagers with perineoscrotal hypospadias. However, the phenotypic spectrum is wide, even within the same affected family with a single androgen receptor abnormality in all affected family members. The usual abnormalities include hypospadias, breast development at puberty, female habitus, azoospermia, cryptorchism, and hypoplasia or absence of wolffian duct structures.
- Infertile male syndrome is a rare androgen receptor defect characterized by a phenotypically normal man with infertility caused by azoospermia.
- In the undervirilized male syndrome, the individual is a male with gynecomastia, a small penis, decreased beard and body hair, a normal male urethra, a normal sperm density, and an identifiable androgen receptor defect. Most affected individuals are infertile.

5α-Reductase type 2 deficiency

This is a disorder of testosterone metabolism. Functional deficiency from the mutated enzyme, 5α-reductase 2, impairs the conversion of testosterone to dihydrotestosterone, the hormone that masculinizes the indifferent urogenital sinus and induces development of the prostate.[56] The disorder, formerly known as 'pseudovaginal perineoscrotal hypospadias', has an autosomal recessive inheritance and is rare. The majority of reported cases have come from family clusters found in a number of relatively isolated geographic locations.[5] Several unrelated patients have been found to have an identical mutation, suggesting a common ancestral founder.[129] The type 2 isoenzyme develops in the fetus and is detectable in the genital skin and the male accessory sex organs. The type 1 isoenzyme is not detectable in the fetus; its activation in skin at the time of puberty is responsible for the clinical virilization these patients later express.

Affected males are usually phenotypically female with female to ambiguous external genitalia at birth.[128] The small clitoris-like phallus lacks a urethral orifice. In most affected individuals the urogenital sinus opens on the perineum and within the sinus an anterior orifice leads to the urethra and a posterior orifice to a blind vaginal pouch. The testes are in the inguinal canals or labia. The müllerian-derived structures are absent whereas wolffian-derived structures (vas deferens, epididymis, and seminal vesicle), the anlagen of which respond to testosterone, are normal.

At puberty, virilization occurs due to type 1 isoenzyme activation, but the breasts fail to develop. The penis lengthens, the bifid scrotum grows and becomes rugated and hyperpigmented, and the testes enlarge and descend. Testicular biopsy specimens reveal spermatogenesis and tubular atrophy in some individuals, complete spermatogenic arrest and Leydig cell hyperplasia in others. The prostate remains rudimentary and the seminal vesicles underdeveloped, which results in affected adults having highly viscous semen and extremely low ejaculate volume. Erection and ejaculation are possible in some affected individuals, but few of these individuals are fertile.

Neonates with this disorder frequently go unrecognized and are raised as females. After the virilization that accompanies puberty, individuals raised as girls sometimes reverse their sex roles and function as men, often with a stormy period of adjustment. Interestingly, the syndrome was known in New Guinea as 'penis at 12' where a familial clustering of the disorder was predictably seen among a group of pubescent children. Individuals with a male gender identity benefit from surgical correction of hypospadias and cryptorchism. High doses of testosterone enhance virilization. Persons raised as females who elect to continue to function as females into adulthood benefit from orchiectomy before the onset of puberty to avoid the accompanying virilization. Estrogen therapy is useful to promote feminization. No patients are known to have developed testicular germ cell tumors, although there has been a single case report of a vaginal squamous cell carcinoma occurring at age 50 years.[1]

DISORDERS OF SEX DETERMINATION (DISORDERS GENERALLY ASSOCIATED WITH AN ABNORMAL SEX CHROMOSOME CONSTITUTION LEADING TO ABNORMAL GONADAL FORMATION)

Additions, deletions, and mosaicism of the sex chromosomes characterize individuals in this category. The appearance of the gonads is variable and ranges from the presence of a streak

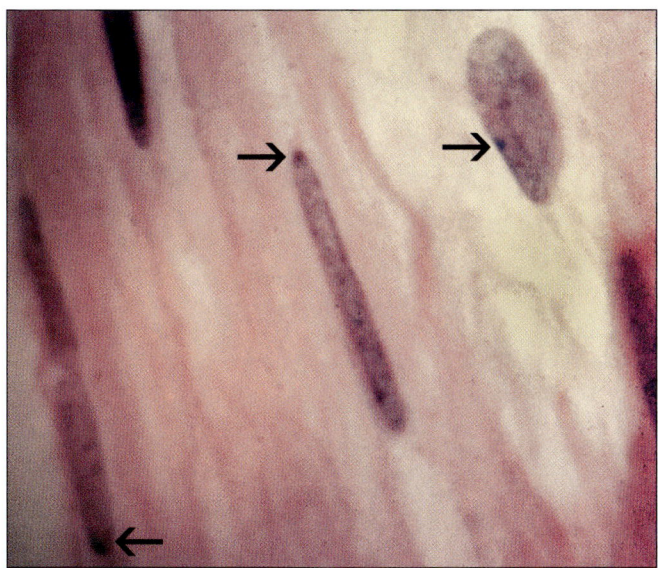

Fig. 34.27 Single Barr body. A single mass of densely staining chromatin material (arrow) is present at the periphery of the nucleus. As the number of sex chromatin masses is one less than the actual number of X chromosomes, this patient has two X chromosomes.

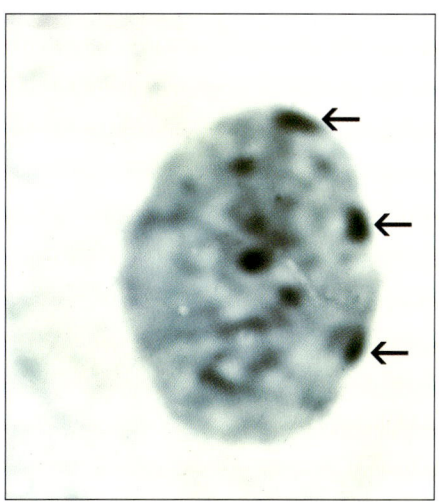

Fig. 34.28 Three Barr bodies. Three masses of densely staining chromatin material (arrows) are present at the periphery of the nucleus. As the number of sex chromatin masses is one less than the actual number of X chromosomes, this patient has four X chromosomes.

gonad to a nearly normal female or male gonad on both gross and microscopic examination. These disorders are subdivided into two broad categories depending on the frequency with which sexual ambiguity occurs.

While this chapter does not deal extensively with laboratory manifestations, the pathologist can sometimes suspect that a specimen is from a patient with abnormal sexual development by determining whether a sex chromatin body is present. The Barr body, as it is often called, refers to the mass of densely staining chromatin material found at the periphery of the nucleus in patients with more than one X chromosome. The nuclei in smooth muscle cells in arteries are particularly useful for this examination. The number of Barr bodies is one less than the number of 'X' chromosomes present so that a single Barr body signifies an XX karyotype and three Barr bodies, for example, represent an XXXX karyotype. This simple technique is often useful in helping to determine whether the patient is a genetic male (XY = zero Barr bodies), genetic female (XX = 1 Barr body) (Figure 34.27), or has some unusual manifestation of multiple X chromosomes (Figures 34.28 and 34.29).

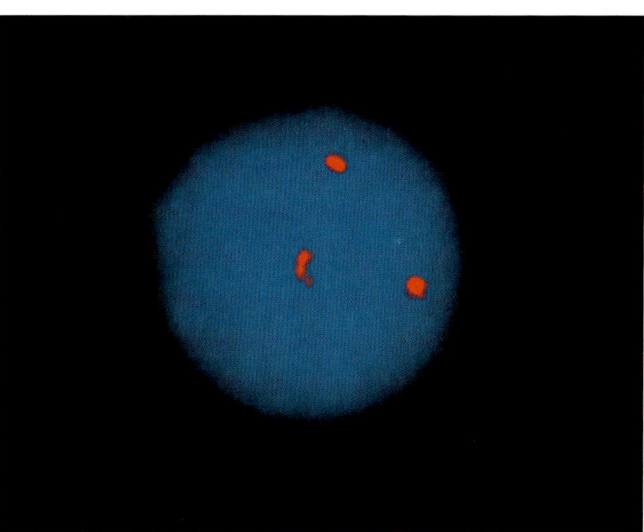

Fig. 34.29 Three Barr bodies by fluorescent *in situ* hybridization.

SEXUAL AMBIGUITY INFREQUENT

KLINEFELTER SYNDROME

Klinefelter syndrome, one of the most common causes of prepubertal delay and primary hypogonadism in males, occurs in about one of every 1000 live newborn males and accounts for about 3% of infertile males. The karyotype is usually 47,XXY in four-fifths of cases, which usually results from non-disjunction occurring during meiosis of either paternal or maternal gametes.[75] The remainder have a higher grade chromosomal aneuploidy (48,XXXY, 49,XXXXY, 48,XXYY) or mosaicism (47,XXY/46,XY) caused by non-disjunction during mitosis of the developing zygote. Molecular probe studies have shown that both parents contribute the extra chromosome in about half of the incidences. In the father they result as an error in the first paternal meiotic division, but in the mother over one-fourth occur (28%) at the second maternal meiotic division.[54] Unlike trisomy 21, which occurs as a failure of the first maternal meiotic division, the likelihood of Klinefelter syndrome is not increased with advancing maternal age.

The clinical picture varies depending on the age at which the diagnosis is first suspected. Some estimate that upwards of two-thirds of persons with Klinefelter syndrome remain undiagnosed; about 10% are diagnosed prenatally with genetic screening programs and one-fourth at adolescence or during adult life when the patient presents with gynecomastia, obesity, and signs of infertility, or is evaluated for malignancy[75] (Figures 34.30 and 34.31). Although infants with Klinefelters syndrome usually have normal external male genitalia at birth, the syndrome is sometimes discovered during evaluations of newborns

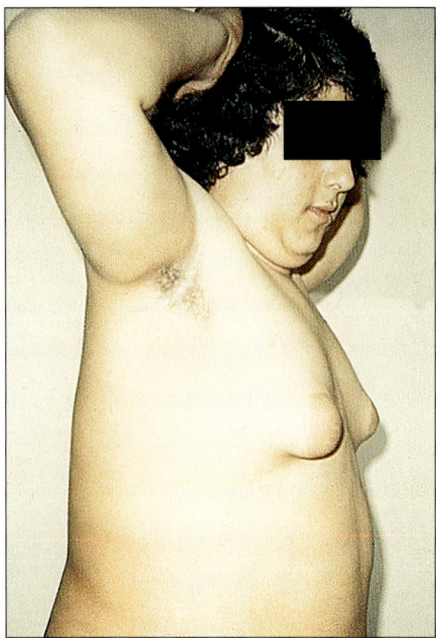

Fig. 34.30 Klinefelter syndrome. Gynecomastia is present and axillary hair is absent.

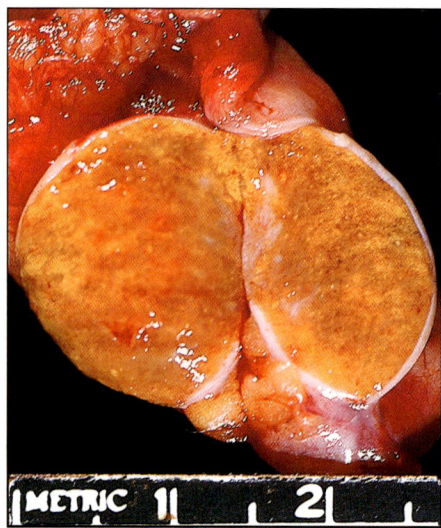

Fig. 34.32 Testis in Klinefelter syndrome. The parenchyma is golden-yellow to slightly brown.

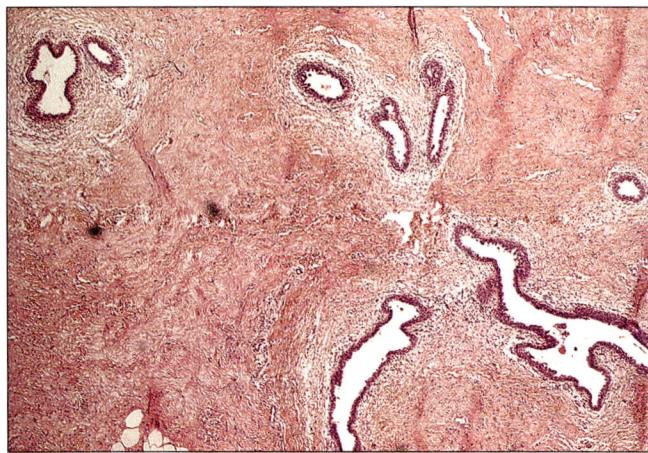

Fig. 34.31 Gynecomastia in Klinefelter syndrome. The breast tissue is composed solely of ducts; no lobular tissue is present.

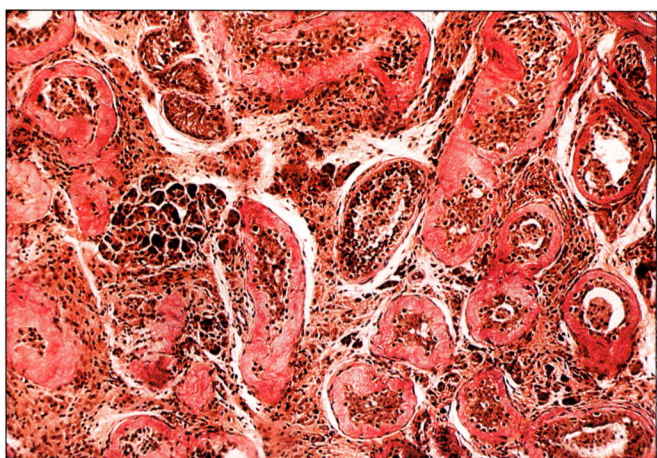

Fig. 34.33 Postpubertal end-stage testis in Klinefelter syndrome. Elastic tissue is present in the hyalinized sclerotic wall of seminiferous tubules.

with hypospadias, micropenis, and small, soft testes or crypt-orchism. Before puberty, the only physical signs may be small testes or long-leggedness resulting in a diminished upper to lower body segment ratio. After puberty, signs of androgen deficiency become apparent. The beard and body hairs are frequently sparse. Half of the patients develop gynecomastia. By the age of 25 years, two-thirds of patients complain of decreased libido. Frequently associated clinical findings include learning disabilities, behavioral disorders, reduced economic striving, and limited sexual drive. Laboratory tests reveal elevated gonadotrophin levels (postpuberty), low testosterone levels, and azoospermia.

The Klinefelter testes in adult 47,XXY individuals are small and rarely exceed 2 cm in maximal dimension (Figure 34.32). The seminiferous tubules may show some degenerative changes during fetal life, and by late childhood the primary spermatogonia are already greatly reduced in number. Shortly before the expected time of puberty, the progressive degenerative changes dramatically accelerate.[3] The absence or presence of elastic fibers in the tubular wall indicates whether the process of atrophy began prepubertally or postpubertally (Figure 34.33), respectively. On microscopic examination, the testes in adults are largely atrophic, have hyalinized seminiferous tubules, and a relative increase in the number of Leydig cells (Figure 34.34). Some tubules may be preserved, but lined only by Sertoli cells. Rarely, an occasional seminiferous tubule of the adult testis contains germ cells in varying stages of maturation. In these cases it is unusual for development to extend beyond the stage of first spermatocyte.[54] If sperm are detected, mosaicism, most likely of the 46,XY/47,XXY pattern, should be suspected. Patients with this mosaic karyotype are sometimes fertile.

The Leydig cells become pronounced in number some time after puberty. Although they appear hyperplastic relative to the

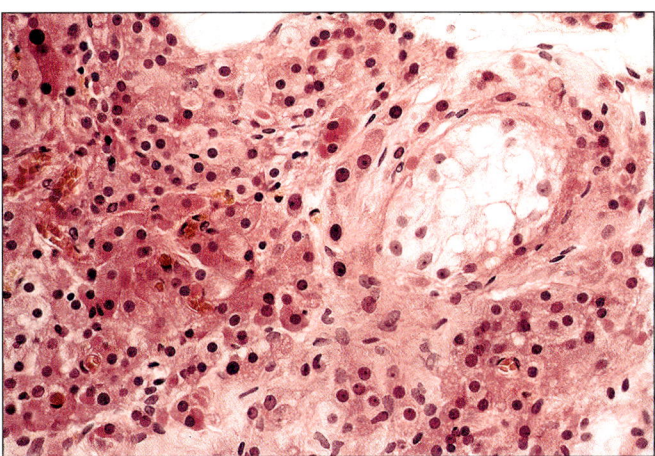

Fig. 34.34 Leydig cells surrounding a seminiferous tubule composed of only Sertoli cells in Klinefelters syndrome.

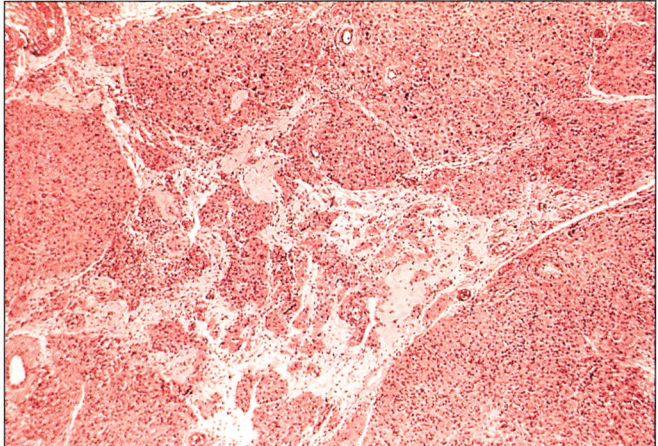

Fig. 34.35 Leydig cell neoplasm in Klinefelters syndrome.

atrophic appearance of the other elements, it is uncertain whether the absolute volume is greater than in normal testes. Functionally, the Leydig cells are abnormal, evidenced by the low levels of serum testosterone in the setting of elevated serum LH and follicle-stimulating hormone levels and subnormal increase in response to an hCG challenge.

Various neoplasms have been associated with Klinefelter syndrome. Both gonadal and extragonadal germ cell tumors develop with increased frequency. Most extragonadal tumors occur in the mediastinum as teratoma and embryonal cell carcinoma (teratocarcinoma) or choriocarcinoma.[2,151] In the testis, seminoma, teratoma, and embryonal cell carcinoma have been encountered.[83] Leydig cell tumors are rare (Figure 34.35).[103] The risk of breast carcinoma in men with Klinefelter syndrome may be 20% higher than in normal men. Hematologic malignancies have also been reported, including acute leukemia, Hodgkin disease, malignant lymphoma, and chronic myeloid leukemia.[68]

TURNER SYNDROME

In the classic form, Turner syndrome is a disorder in which sexually immature phenotypic females of short stature have various congenital anomalies and streak gonads. The cytogenetic hallmark is the 45,X karyotype with a sporadic, nonfamilial pattern of inheritance. A critical region is the short arm of the X chromosome (Xp11.2–p22).[157] Other karyotypes identified less frequently in this syndrome include mosaic 45,X/46,XX and 45,X/47,XXX/46,XX, or additional anomalies of the X chromosome. The X chromosome in 75% of cases is maternal in origin.[59,82] Patients with a 45,X/46,XY mosaic karyotype (considered in mixed gonadal dysgenesis) usually present with obvious sexual ambiguity, but sometimes present as phenotypic females with the clinical stigmata of Turner syndrome. Depending upon the definition used for Turner syndrome, some studies have identified a small number of patients with a Y chromosome.[46] In cases where conventional cytogenetic analysis disclosed pure X monosomy, additional studies also found hidden 'Y' mosaicism or cryptic Y chromosomal material present in 3–10%[23,25,78,85,126] of the patients. The complex nature of karyotyping is expressed in a study where the blood from a single adult with Turners syndrome was examined in 287 cytogenetic laboratories with many differing results.[106]

A significant difference between patients with a 45,X/46,XY mosaic karyotype and those with classic 45,X Turner syndrome is that gonadoblastoma and malignant germ cell tumors are common in patients with the former and rare in the latter. Currently, it is common practice to actively exclude Y mosaicism in individuals with Turner syndrome if virilization or a small marker chromosome is seen.[30] Some have recommended that Y chromosomal exclusion should be carried out in all Turner patients.[78] In an occasional instance, microscopic gonadoblastoma or other germ cell tumor has been found in some of these Turner-like patients with a cryptic Y chromosome.[23]

At a molecular level, a specific deficiency has been proposed to help explain the syndrome's development.[153] The gene *RPS4* (ribosomal protein S4) is necessary for ribosomal function. This gene is normally located on the X and Y chromosomes near the pseudoautosomal region and are both interchangeable. It is speculated that normal human development requires at least two *RPS4* genes in each cell, and that the Turner phenotype may be due, in part at least, to the presence of only one.

About 98% of fetuses with a 45,X karyotype abort. This accounts for the frequency of Turners syndrome being about 1 in 100 conceptions, but only about 1 in 3000–10 000 liveborn females. In the newborn, the overt findings relate to lymph stasis, which manifests as edema of the dorsum of the hands or feet or, less frequently, as a swelled nape of the neck (cystic hygroma) (Figure 34.36). Later in childhood and in adult life, a webbed neck and elevated distal portion of the nails are residua of more marked swellings present during fetal life and may still provide a clue to the correct diagnosis. A rare, but important, major presentation is hydronephrosis due to ureteropelvic stenosis. All female neonates with a ureteropelvic obstruction should have chromosomal analysis. Congenital anomalies of other organ systems associated with Turner syndrome include a short fourth metacarpal, hypoplastic nails, multiple pigmented nevi, and coarcted aorta. Growth retardation (short stature) is common.[44] More than 40 somatic anomalies are associated with this condition.

Spontaneous puberty occurs in 5–10% of women with Turner syndrome.[53] While most patients will have been diag-

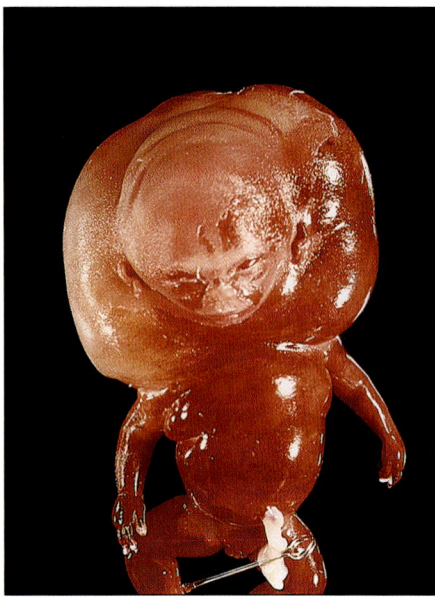

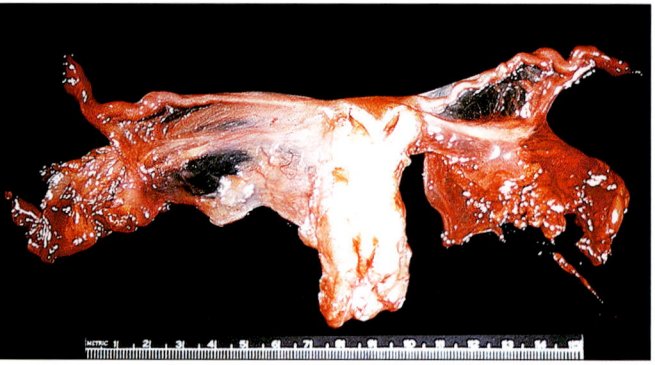

Fig. 34.37 Streak ovary in Turner syndrome. The adult gonads appear as white fibrous streaks, 2–3 cm long and 0.5 cm in diameter, located in the position normally occupied by the ovary.

Fig. 34.36 Fetus with Turner syndrome. The overt finding related to lymph stasis manifests as swellings of the nape of the neck (cystic hygroma).

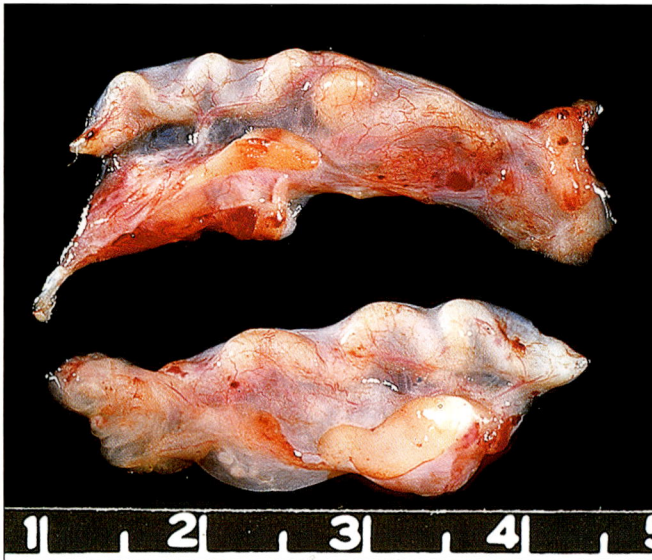

Fig. 34.38 Streak ovary in Turner syndrome. Macroscopic view of adult gonads, which are white fibrous streaks located adjacent to the fallopian tube.

nosed earlier, those who reach adolescence undiagnosed often present with primary amenorrhea. Examination reveals underdeveloped secondary sex characteristics and a small uterus. Urinary gonadotrophins are always elevated and the vaginal smear lacks cornified cells. The buccal smear in a 45,X individual reveals few if any Barr bodies; in those 20% of patients with a mosaic karyotype (usually 45,X/46,XX or 45,X/47,XXX) the smear discloses a subnormal number of chromatin-positive cells (about 5–15% for a female). Only rare patients with Turner syndrome have become pregnant and most of these have been mosaics with a 46,XX cell line. Some of these women have mosaic patterns that are found only after extensive search.[80] Oocyte donation programs have recently proven effective with one center recording 20 clinical pregnancies in 18 women, the majority of whom achieved a liveborn via cesarean section.[40]

At laparotomy, the internal genitalia are female and, although small, are in normal relation to one another. The adult gonads appear as white fibrous streaks, 2–3 cm long and 0.5 cm in diameter, and are located in the position normally occupied by the ovary (Figures 34.37 and 34.38). On microscopic examination a streak consists of an attenuated cortex, a medulla, and a hilus (Figures 34.39 and 34.40). The cortex consists of characteristic ovarian stroma in which the cells are elongated, wavy and have a conspicuous nucleus with scant cytoplasm. Rete tubules (rete ovarii) and hilar cells are typically present in the hilus region. Oocytes are almost always absent in adults with Turner syndrome. Comparative analyses have shown that in the normal ovary numerous oogonia are visible and organized in cord-like structures within mesenchymal cells by the 18th week, whereas the gonads of Turners patients have increased small oogonia, with the few large oogonia showing signs of degeneration.[115] In normal gonads primordial follicles are found by the 20th week, and preantral and antral follicles by the 26th week. These finding are absent in the Turner gonads.

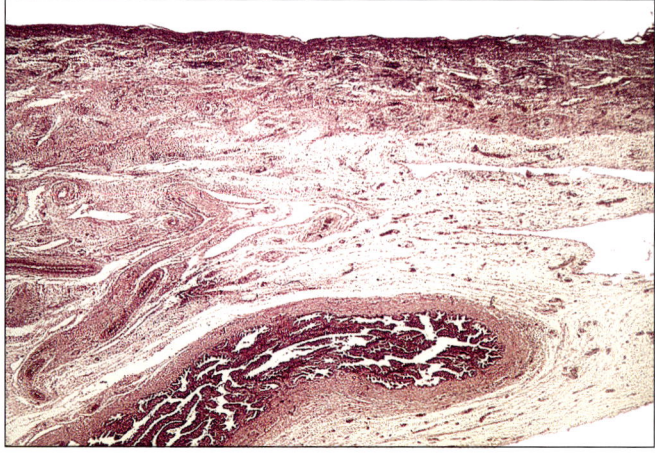

Fig. 34.39 Streak ovary in Turner syndrome with adjacent fallopian tube.

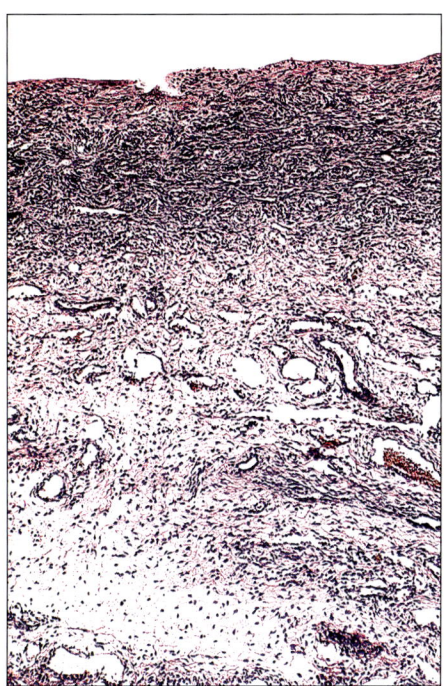

Fig. 34.40 Streak ovary in Turner syndrome. The streak consists of an attenuated cortex, a medulla, and a hilus. The cortex consists of characteristic ovarian stroma with cells that have elongated, wavy conspicuous nuclei and scant cytoplasm.

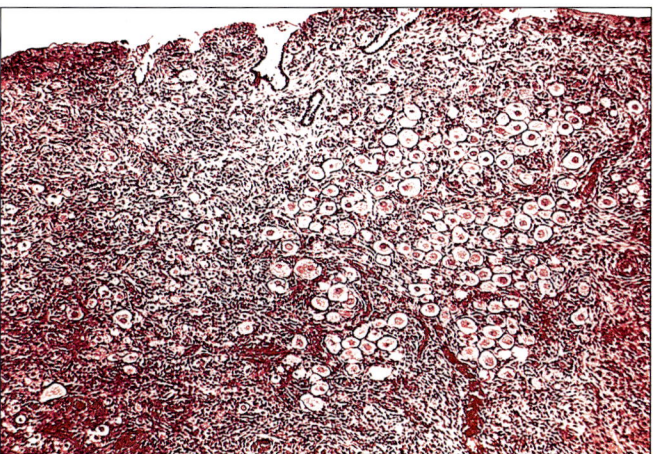

Fig. 34.41 Embryonic ovary in Turner syndrome. Oocytes are present in normal numbers before week 12 of gestation.

Oocytes are present in normal numbers in 45,X embryos before week 12 of gestation (Figure 34.41), but older fetuses and young children show accelerated rates of oocyte depletion relative to the normal number for the age. Usually before the time of menarche in the normal girl, Turners women will have no oocytes, thus leading to primary amenorrhea. These findings are interpreted to suggest that the second X chromosome is necessary for granulosa cell development and primary follicle formation. Without this X chromosome, granulosa cells fail to differentiate and, as a result, the oocytes degenerate. Gonadal tumors are exceedingly rare. Tumors of germ cell origin are undoubtedly rare because of the paucity of germ cells. While occasional germ cell tumors have been reported,[108] more sophis-

ticated chromosomal testing, especially with newer molecular biologic techniques, has found cryptic Y chromosomal fragments associated with the tumor tissue.[57,88] Most reported cases with a gonadoblastoma component have had a mosaic pattern with a Y chromosome,[88,141] and more appropriately are considered as mixed gonadal dysgenesis.

Non-germ cell tumors occur. Some patients also have had virilization with stromal luteoma or hilus cell hyperplasia.[88] Development of neoplasms of the so-called 'surface epithelial type' suggest that the celomic epithelium encapsulating the gonad can undergo malignant change even if the gonad is a streak. Endometrial carcinoma occurred occasionally in those patients who had received long-term high-dose exogenous estrogen therapy to foster the appearance of the female secondary sex characteristics. Both natural estrogens and synthetic non-steroidal estrogens have been implicated and the duration of usage usually exceeded 3 years. Today, this is so rare that it is not even recognized to occur, although there have been several cases described where the tumor developed even in the absence of hormone replacement therapy.[70] Extragonadal tumors, most often of neurogenic origin, have also been reported in children and young adults.

XX MALE (SEX REVERSAL)

The XX male syndrome is a disorder exhibiting a nearly normal but infertile phenotypic male with a 46,XX karyotype. This syndrome, one of the rarest of all sex chromosome anomalies, occurs in about 1 of 24 000 newborn males.[135] XX males share many characteristics of men with Klinefelters syndrome. Both have a generally masculine appearance, normal or near normal external genitalia, male psychosexual orientation, normal-to-weak secondary sexual characteristics, normal-to-low androgen levels, and azoospermia. The testes are small with prominent Leydig cells and tubules lined only by Sertoli cells. Like Klinefelters patients, the most common reasons for adult evaluation are infertility and abnormal secondary sexual characteristics. But they also differ. XX males are generally shorter in height, and the frequency of hypospadias and gynecomastia is higher. The frequency of impaired intelligence is not increased in XX males relative to the general population. Increasingly, with ultrasonography and genetic analyses being performed during the gestation, the XX male syndrome is now being discovered prenatally.[45]

The XX male syndrome results potentially from at least three distinctly different mechanisms. About 70% of these patients have a small portion of paternally derived Y chromosome that contains the *SRY* gene present abnormally on the X chromosome. The *SRY* gene is normally found on the short arm of the Y chromosome adjacent to the pseudoautosomal pairing region. During meiosis in the father, an abnormal exchange sometimes leads to the transfer onto the X chromosome of the entire pseudoautosomal region plus the adjacent portion of the Y chromosome with the *SRY* gene. Inheritance of such an X chromosome from the father leads to the Y(+) XX male syndrome. The inheritance pattern of this syndromic form is sporadic. These patients have normal male external genitalia. Hypospadias and ambiguous genitalia are virtually never found. Apparently, the presence of the *SRY* gene is adequate to lead to normal male phenotype. Azoospermia in these patients results from the lack of other genes normally found on the Y chromosome necessary for sperm development.

Some patients with the XX male syndrome lack Y-derived DNA. Such Y(–) XX males might result by two different mechanisms. The first accounts for the familial transmission of an autosomal dominant or X-linked inheritance of XX maleness. These patients usually have ambiguous genitalia. This indicates that genes exist, which can trigger testis determination when mutated.[72] A second potential mechanism that might lead to the Y(–) condition is chromosomal mosaicism with a prevalent XX lineage. In such patients, the Y-containing cell line might simply be technically too difficult to identify because of the small number of such cells. Alternatively, a 47,XXY zygote might lose its Y chromosome by non-disjunction early in ontogeny, thus allowing a 46,XX cell line to persist. The 47,XXY cell line may have persisted only long enough to induce male gonadal development. Such patients, just as patients with familial Y(–) XX maleness, often present with sexual ambiguity suggesting that patients with Y(–) XX male syndrome are closely related both phenotypically and etiologically to XX true hermaphrodites, who present with both testicular and ovarian tissue.

PURE GONADAL DYSGENESIS

Usual form

Pure gonadal dysgenesis, and its eponym, Swyer syndrome, are terms that historically have encompassed diverse conditions, including testicular regression syndrome at one end of the spectrum and mixed gonadal dysgenesis (now 46,XY disorder of sex development) at the other. As used in this chapter, 'pure gonadal dysgenesis' refers to a phenotypic female where the internal genitalia include müllerian structures (uterus and fallopian tubes) and generally streak gonads, the constellation of which probably still encompasses a multitude of diverse conditions. The patients may appear phenotypically normal or have hypoplastic external genitalia. The pure gonadal dysgenesis syndrome occurs with both 46,XX and 46,XY karyotypes and has both familial and sporadic patterns of inheritance.

The 46,XX type pure gonadal dysgenesis is usually an autosomal recessive disorder, but, less frequently, may be due to an abnormality of the X chromosome, possibly as a mosaic 45,X cell line confined to the gonad.[93] Deletions of the short or long arm of an X chromosome have been identified in some cases. Such patients have greater ovarian development than those with 46,XY pure gonadal dysgenesis or Turner syndrome and present more often with signs of ovarian dysfunction (secondary amenorrhea or infertility) rather than primary gonadal failure (primary amenorrhea). Some patients may also have mosaic cell lines with the *SRY* gene absent in some tissues (peripheral leukocytes), but present in others (testicular tissue).[33]

The 46,XY type pure gonadal dysgenesis is more common than the 46,XX form of the disorder. The syndrome of pure gonadal dysgenesis may be sporadic or familial with either X-linked recessive or autosomal recessive patterns of inheritance.[19,120] Some patients have a mosaic 45,X/46,XY karyotype. The 46,XY type may also involve deletion of the *SRY* gene, a mutated inactive *SRY* gene or a defective promoter cofactor.[124,137,138] One gene believed crucial for regulating the *SRY* gene is *DAX* (see Table 34.2) located on the X chromosomal short arm.[144] The gene is unusual in that only one copy, which is normal, is insufficient to negate the effects of the *SRY* gene. A double dosage, i.e., the presence of two active copies in tandem, results in sex reversal from male to female. (It seems that the *DAX* locus is normally subject to X inactivation as patients with Klinefelter syndrome have two copies of the affected X chromosome locus.)[148] In one series of 14 XY females with pure gonadal dysgenesis, patients who had normal *SRY* had gonads composed of undifferentiated stroma in which were tubules or a rete structure suggesting some differentiation towards testis. In those cases where there were mutations in *SRY*-orf (*SRY*-opening reading frames), no tubules were observed; the gonads were composed exclusively of ovarian-like stroma with sclerohyaline nodules in some areas. These data also suggested that *SRY* may play a role in rete testis formation.[149]

Patients with 46,XX pure gonadal dysgenesis, as those with Turner syndrome, only rarely have gonadal tumors. Some have had hilus cell hyperplasia and hilus cell tumors with the usual associated virilizing effects. Epithelial tumors are extremely rare, but of these mucinous tumors occur more frequently than serous.[74] Rare examples of germ cell tumors have been reported,[96] and even though no identifiable Y chromosome component could be detected in some, the possibility of a cryptic Y fragment cannot be excluded. Patients with 46,XY pure gonadal dysgenesis are at high risk for gonadoblastoma and other germ cell tumors, as is true of all patients with streak gonads and a Y chromosome.[138] In one series, 11 of 20 patients had gonadal neoplasms; eight were gonadoblastomas, half of which were bilateral, and eight were dysgerminoma, all unilateral.[111] On this basis, patients with 46,XY pure gonadal dysgenesis might be considered a subset of the broader condition of mixed gonadal dysgenesis.

DEFECT IN THE WILMS TUMOR SUPPRESSOR (*WT1*) GENE

Denys–Drash syndrome

Denys–Drash syndrome is a rare disorder that, like Frasiers syndrome, results from a mutated Wilms tumor suppressor (*WT1*) gene, which is located on chromosome band 11p13. The two entities, however, have differing mutations, the heterozygous point mutations altering the zinc finger encoding exons in the former, and mutations in intron 9 of the same gene in the latter.[14] Denys–Drash syndrome consists of congenital nephropathy, Wilms tumor, and intersex disorders, sometimes with the development of gonadoblastoma. Most children present with renal disease in the form of proteinuria. Most develop Wilms tumor and nearly all die from renal failure by 3 years of age. Males with ambiguous genitalia are more commonly diagnosed earlier than females in whom the genitalia are normal.[60,61]

Multiple gonadal abnormalities described to date include normal ovaries with signs of early ovarian failures, normal müllerian and wolffian ducts, and normal to dysgenetic testes. Early prophylactic nephrectomy is important to prevent the development of the malignant renal tumors.[11]

Frasier syndrome

Frasier syndrome, like Denys–Drash syndrome, is rare and results from a mutated *WT1* gene, specifically mutation of intron 9.[14] The syndrome is defined by male pseudohermaphroditism and progressive glomerulopathy. Patients usually present because of the glomerulopathy, usually with proteinuria as the initial manifestation. During the ensuing workup, they are found to have normal female external genitalia, streak gonads, XY karyotype, and sometimes gonadoblastoma.[123,152] When raised as a female, a presenting sign may be absence of anticipated pubertal sexual development.[22] The nephropathy is usually focal segmental glomerulosclerosis, which differs from the diffuse mesangial sclerosis seen in Denys–Drash. The renal disease is relentless, but end-stage renal disease may not occur until late childhood.

Mutations in the *WT1* gene occur in a region different from that in Denys–Drash. Abnormal splicing at intron 9 leads to an unbalanced ratio of the WT1 isoforms needed for normal glomerular and gonadal development.[34] Patients with Frasier syndrome have no increased risk for Wilms tumor because the KTS-negative isoform of the WT1 protein retains its tumor suppressor function.[100] The elevated risk of gonadoblastoma reflects the overall high risk of tumorigenesis in dysgenetic gonads. Molecular mechanisms that underlie the intersex state and nephropathy in Frasier syndrome are poorly understood.

SEXUAL AMBIGUITY FREQUENT

Patients in this category exhibit a wide range of phenotypic appearances and internal genitalia. A 'Y' chromosome is often present, usually as part of a mosaic complement. Sexual ambiguity is a common finding. This is an area currently undergoing rapid change as detailed genetic analyses at the molecular level are just beginning to identify an ever-expanding group of conditions that given rise to the phenotype described below. These are described in a broader sense as 46,XY disorders of sex development followed by one condition where the specific genotypes (steroidogenic factor 1 abnormality or deletion of chromosome 9p) are known.

46,XY DISORDERS OF SEX DEVELOPMENT (MIXED GONADAL DYSGENESIS)

Mixed gonadal dysgenesis (MGD) is a heterogeneous syndrome with a 45,X/46,XY or 46,XY karyotype, persistent müllerian duct structures, a dysgenetic testis, and a contralateral streak gonad.[7] It is one of the most frequent causes of male sexual ambiguity.[95] The functional deficit imposed by the abnormal testis is expressed as incomplete inhibition of müllerian development, incomplete differentiation of wolffian duct structures, and incomplete male development of the external genitalia. Often, incomplete mediation of testicular descent occurs, resulting in both internal and external asymmetry of the genitalia and a mixture of male and female features in an individual in whom neither gonad is normal. About two-thirds of affected individuals are raised as females and the remainder as males, in part for psychological and cultural reasons and so as to prevent the future development of cancer, which is not uncommon. The subject of gender assignment is many faceted.[95,113]

Given the overlap, we believe that the syndrome of MGD should be enlarged to incorporate some patients with bilateral streak gonads, streak-like areas but with tubules (described above as 46,XY type pure gonadal dysgenesis) or bilateral abnormal testes with a mosaic 45,X/46,XY karyotype (dysgenetic male pseudohermaphroditism) because the clinical, pathologic, and chromosomal features of these syndromes closely resemble each other. In turn, some patients with MGD exhibit the phenotypic features of a Turner-like syndrome.[8,136]

A variety of different genetic abnormalities appear to result in MGD, thus leading to its phenotypic heterogeneity. Partial deletions of both the short and long arms of chromosome Y have been detected in these individuals. Most cases where no detectable Y chromosomal anomaly is observed by conventional chromosome analysis have a Y fragment found when additional testing is performed.[43]

Clinically, MGD is usually detected in the neonate because of ambiguous external genitalia (Figures 34.42 and 34.43). Frequently, a palpable testis bulges through an indirect inguinal hernia or descends completely into the labioscrotal fold, resulting in asymmetry of the genital swellings. This clinical appearance prompted some earlier investigators to name the syndrome 'asymmetric gonadal dysgenesis'. If the gonads are intraabdominal, the labioscrotal folds may appear as normal labia or as empty scrotal sacs. The condition is likely to go unrecognized unless the clitoris is sufficiently enlarged to mandate investigation, which is common. The gonad that descends is

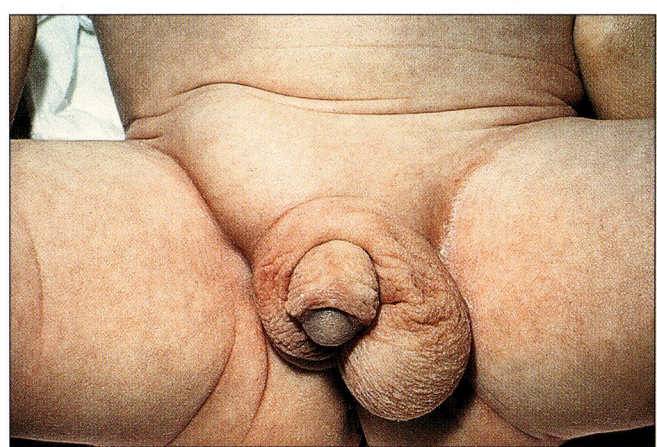

Fig. 34.42 External genitalia in mixed gonadal dysgenesis. The left testis had descended into the scrotum; the right streak was in the abdominal cavity. Because of this characteristic appearance, some investigators prefer the name 'asymmetric gonadal dysgenesis' rather than 'mixed gonadal dysgenesis'.

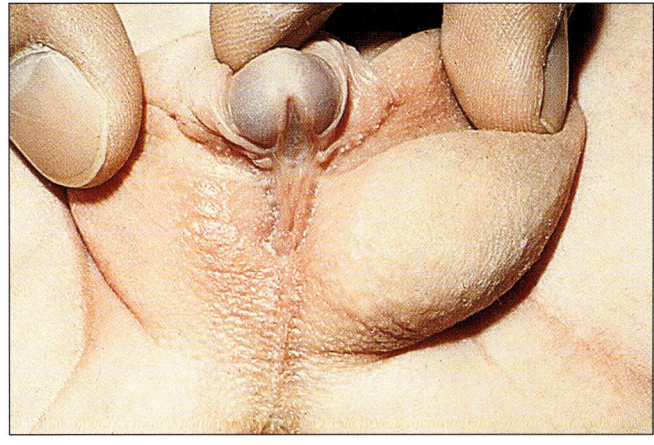

Fig. 34.43 External genitalia in mixed gonadal dysgenesis. Only the left testis had descended into the scrotum.

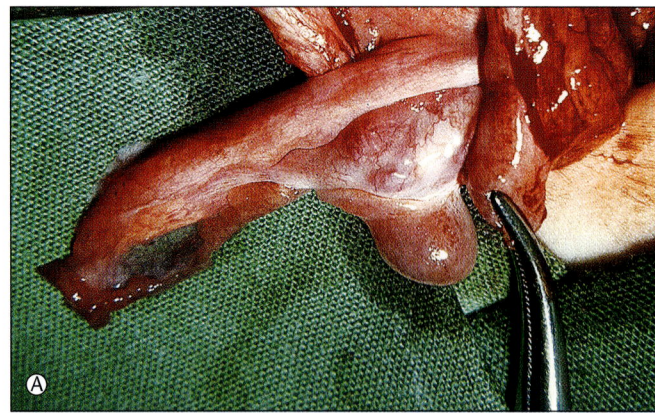

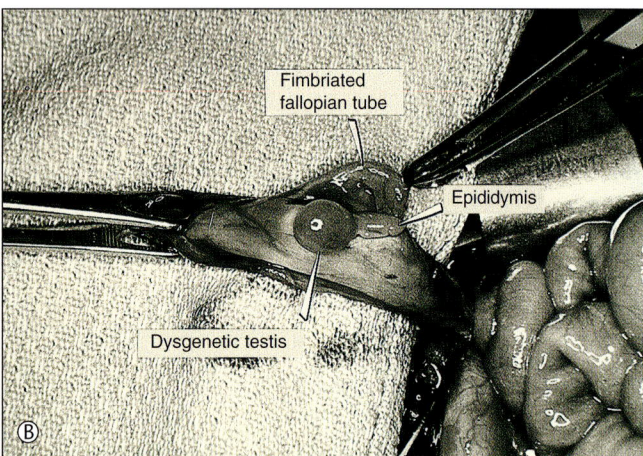

Fig. 34.44 Internal genitalia in mixed gonadal dysgenesis. **(A)** At operation. **(B)** Labeled.

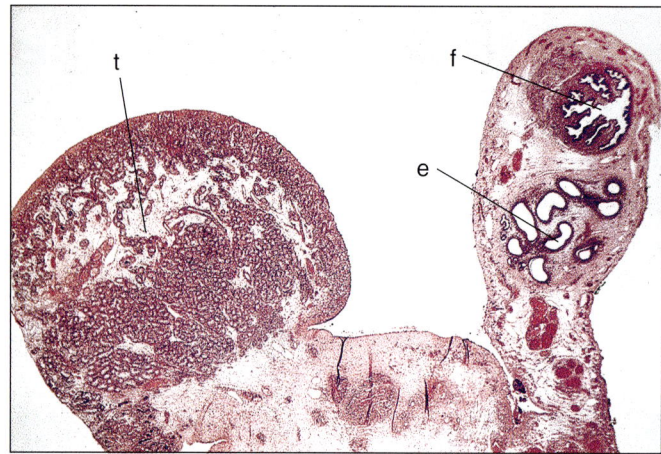

Fig. 34.45 Organs in mixed gonadal dysgenesis. Testis (t), fallopian tube (f), and epididymis (e).

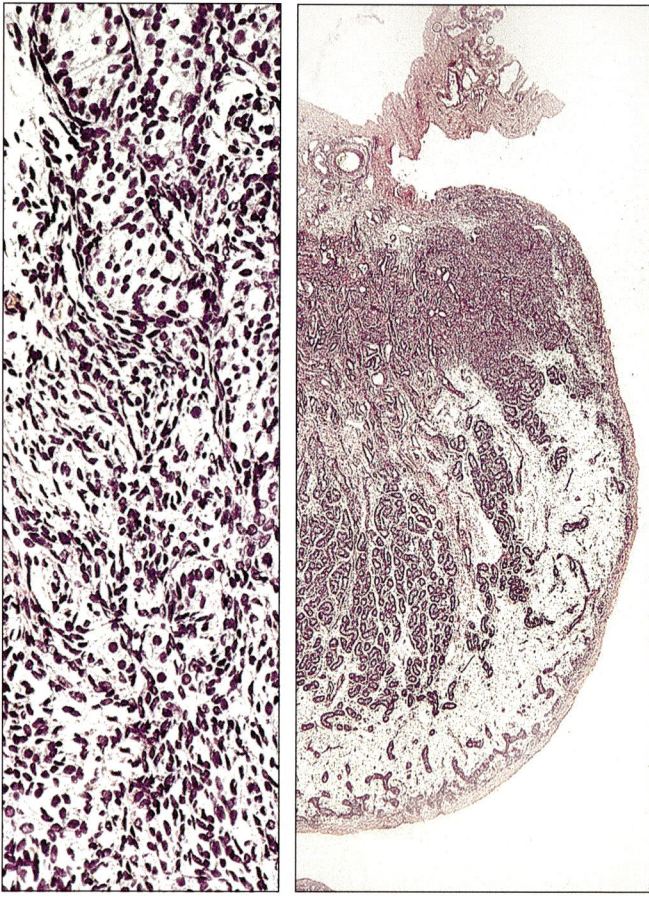

Fig. 34.46 Testis in mixed gonadal dysgenesis. The dysgenetic testis has a thin rim of cortex (right bottom), relatively normal medulla (right middle), and hilus (right top), which in detail (left) shows the various tissue components blending together such that they are indistinguishable.

usually a testis, and the streak gonads are always intra-abdominal unless dragged into a 'hernia uteri inguinale'.

Organs derived from the müllerian duct persist in 95% of cases (Figures 34.44 and 34.45).[89,119] The uterus is usually infantile or rudimentary, but occasionally may be normal. The fallopian tubes are frequently bilateral. If a testis is grossly near normal size and well differentiated, the fimbria of the ipsilateral tube may be absent, but in only one-third of cases is the ipsilateral tube entirely absent. Organs of wolffian duct derivation may also be present, but the frequency is variable. An epididymis is identified in two-thirds of cases and is usually present on the side where there is a testis. The vas deferens is encountered less frequently. The seminal vesicle is identified only rarely, probably because tissue near the bladder/prostate region is not usually removed.

The gonad may be a testis or a streak. Streak gonads may be partially differentiated toward testis, or suggestion of differentiation toward ovary with gonadal-type stroma and even a very rare primordial follicle, but not ovary which requires the presence of differentiation with follicles in at least the antral stage. Bilateral gross testes, frequently of an asynchronous degree of maturity, are found in about 15% of cases whereas a unilateral gross testis is found in 60%. The testis is consistently abnormal architecturally, its organization being divided into three zones, each of which reflects the quantity and type of cellular components present (Figure 34.46). The three zones, which are described below in detail, include: (1) the region of the tunica albuginea or cortex, which exhibits a range of findings from widely spaced seminiferous tubules (Figure 34.47) or differentiation toward streak, usually with ovarian-like stroma to immature zones indeterminate between female and male

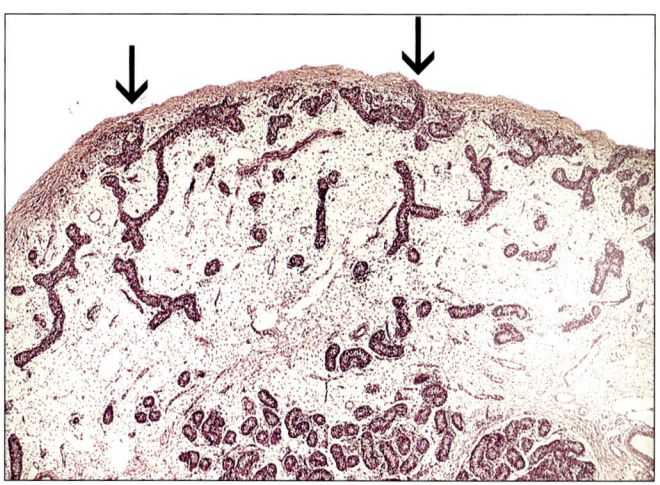

Fig. 34.47 Cortex of testis in mixed gonadal dysgenesis. The seminiferous tubules are scattered and penetrate the tunica albuginea to open onto the surface (arrows).

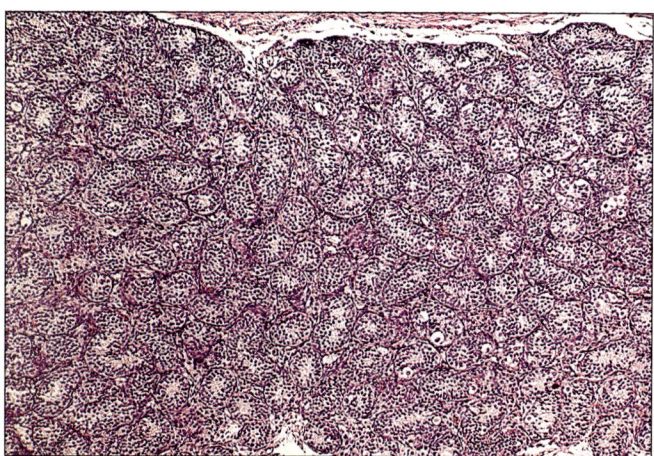

Fig. 34.49 Medulla of testis in mixed gonadal dysgenesis. The testicular tissue looks relatively normal.

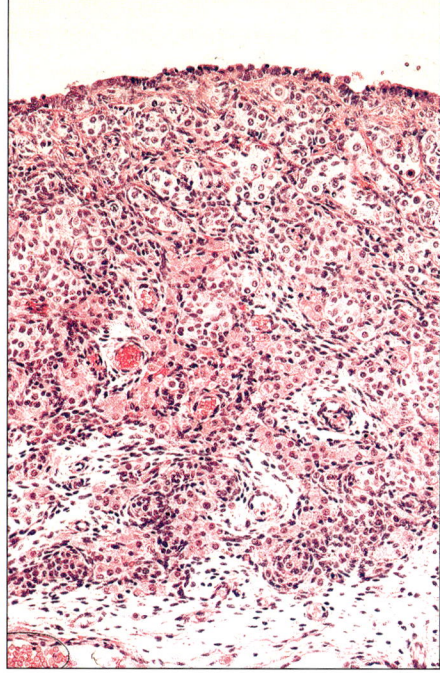

Fig. 34.48 Rim of gonadal cortex in mixed gonadal dysgenesis with persistent primary sex cords. It is difficult to determine whether the organ is testis or ovary.

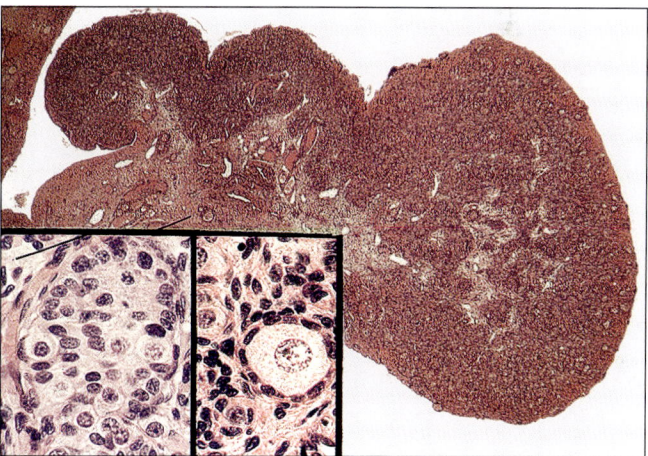

Fig. 34.50 Gonad in mixed gonadal dysgenesis. In an unusual finding, some areas show early formation of seminiferous tubules while rare foci disclose primordial follicles, but nothing more advanced in development. Over time, the entire organ will atrophy and appear as a streak gonad.

structures with primary sex cords (Figure 34.48); (2) the medulla, which is composed of normal or near-normal seminiferous tubules and interstitium (Figure 34.49); and (3) a hilar region with poorly differentiated seminiferous tubules that are only partly differentiated toward testis (Figure 34.46). It is uncertain whether this zone may represent hypertrophied rete testis.

The superficial cortex may contain seminiferous tubules that are often widely separated by edematous, undifferentiated stroma. Sometimes the tubules penetrate the incompletely formed tunica albuginea and open onto the serosa. Occasionally, broad zones of cortex differentiate slightly toward streak-

like ovary, even displaying rare primordial follicles, but as mentioned above, without more fully developed follicles would still be called a streak (or, as some prefer, a 'streak-testis') (Figure 34.50). In some cases it is difficult to distinguish between female and male structures.

The central zone (medulla) of the macroscopic infant testis is usually architecturally and cytologically normal (Figure 34.49). Narrow closed seminiferous tubules are lined by Sertoli cells with abundant cytoplasm. The numbers of spermatogonia vary. Advanced forms of spermatogenic maturation are not observed. Occasionally, the germ cells are seen to lie directly on the basement membrane of the seminiferous tubule rather than being surrounded normally by Sertoli cells (Figure 34.51). Leydig cells are present in small clusters of varying size. The nuclei of the Leydig cells contain finely dispersed chromatin, and the cytoplasm varies from minimal and amphophilic or slightly basophilic to abundant and eosinophilic. In older patients, the medulla is atrophic and the tubules are lined only by Sertoli cells (Figure 34.52). The basement membranes are often thickened. Prominent clusters of Leydig cells fill the inter-

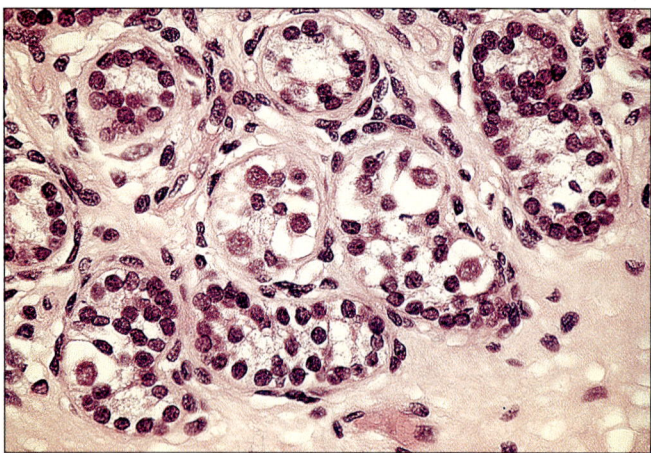

Fig. 34.51 Abnormally located germ cells in mixed gonadal dysgenesis. Numerous germ cells lie directly on the basement membrane of the seminiferous tubule rather than being surrounded normally by Sertoli cells.

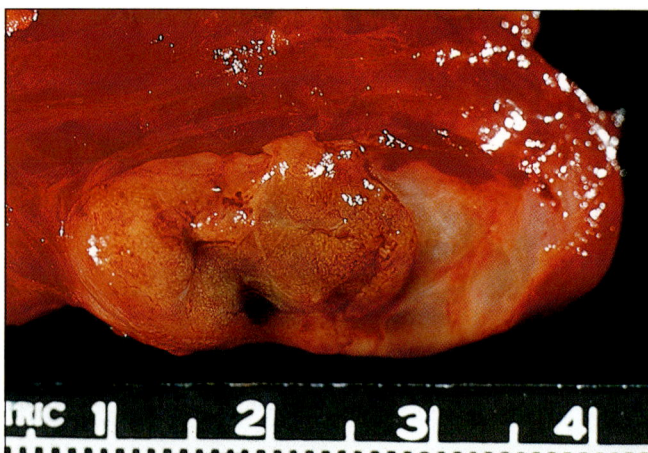

Fig. 34.53 Testis in a 35-year-old phenotypic male with mixed gonadal dysgenesis. The tunica albuginea is tan and maximally 1 mm thick. The parenchyma is golden yellow.

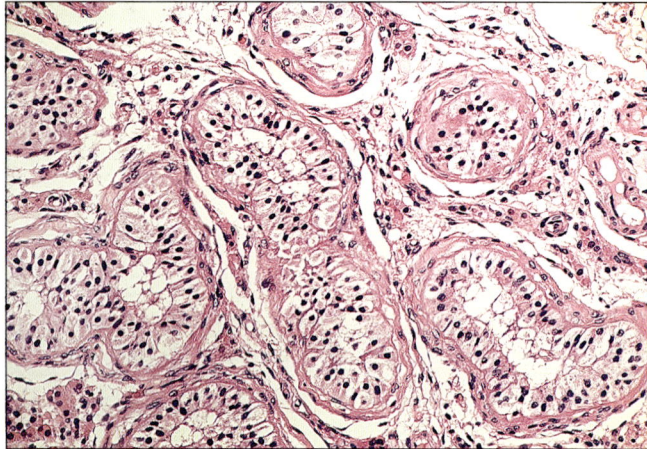

Fig. 34.52 Seminiferous tubules lined by only Sertoli cells in mixed gonadal dysgenesis. The interstitium is filled with Leydig cells.

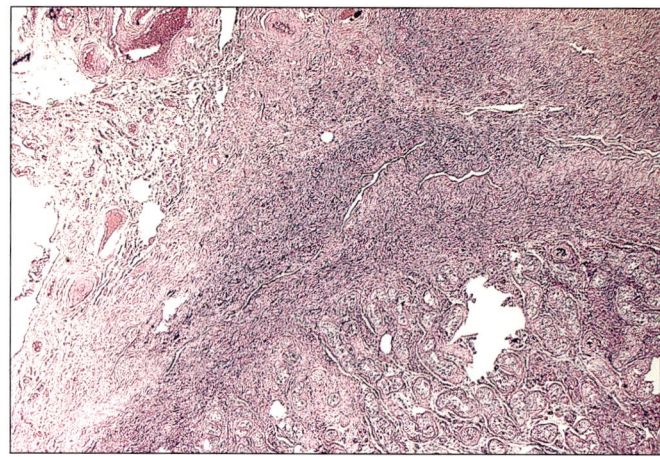

Fig. 34.54 Cross-section of tunica albuginea in mixed gonadal dysgenesis. The testicular stroma resembles the stroma of ovarian cortex. The medulla contains seminiferous tubules.

stitium. (In the specimen shown in Figures 34.52–34.54 the patient was a 35-year-old phenotypic male, with a small gonad, which was golden brown on cut section.) The tunica albuginea is composed of stroma resembling the stroma of ovarian cortex (Figure 34.54).

The architecturally disorganized hilar region discloses seminiferous tubules that are swollen by increased numbers of Sertoli cells and are lined by indistinct basement membranes. These tubules also merge with the surrounding stroma, imparting the appearance of a homogeneous blend of Leydig cells, germ cells, Sertoli cells, and an indeterminate type of interstitial stroma. The region resembles neither fetal ovary nor testis (Figure 34.46). It is uncertain whether some of this region may represent rete testis.

The streak gonads appear similar to those found in Turner syndrome. We have not observed a gonad that has been identifiable grossly as an ovary or has been shown microscopically to contain Graafian follicles, corpora lutea or corpora albicantia. However, the presence of rare primordial follicles or, especially as in the fetal ovary, aggregates of germ cells partially surrounded by immature granulosa cells are evidence that a streak gonad can differentiate toward ovary. Morphologic changes may occur over time in the streak gonads. Myriads of germ cells present in a streak of an infant may degenerate and disappear by puberty (Figure 34.55), resulting in a gonad composed exclusively of fibrous tissue and a few rete tubules. Similar changes occur in the streak gonads of Turner syndrome (45,X karyotype).

Tumors develop in about 10% of patients with mixed gonadal dysgenesis.[119] The most common, the gonadoblastoma, is discussed below. Approximately 30% of gonadoblastomas are overgrown by a malignant germ cell tumor, usually the germinoma (Figures 34.56 and 34.57); 8% are overgrown by yolk sac tumor, immature teratoma, embryonal carcinoma or choriocarcinoma. An occasional gonad may also show proliferative sex-cord elements and resemble a Sertoli cell tumor[101] or disclose nodules suggestive of a juvenile granulosa cell tumor.[107] Although the gonadoblastoma itself does not metastasize and therefore can be considered as a precancer or an *in situ* malignancy, the typically malignant behavior of the other tumors makes early prophylactic removal of the gonads in all patients advisable. Also, to avoid the consequences of onset of

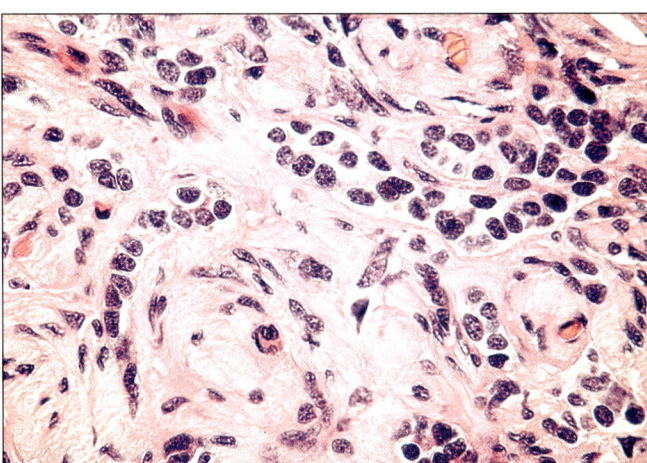

Fig. 34.55 Changes over time in mixed gonadal dysgenesis. When the patient was an infant, the streak gonad resembled a fetal ovary with germ cells and immature sex cords or tubules. When the streak gonad was removed in entirety 13 years later, it existed only as several microscopic areas of wispy ovarian-type cortical stroma and rete ovarii.

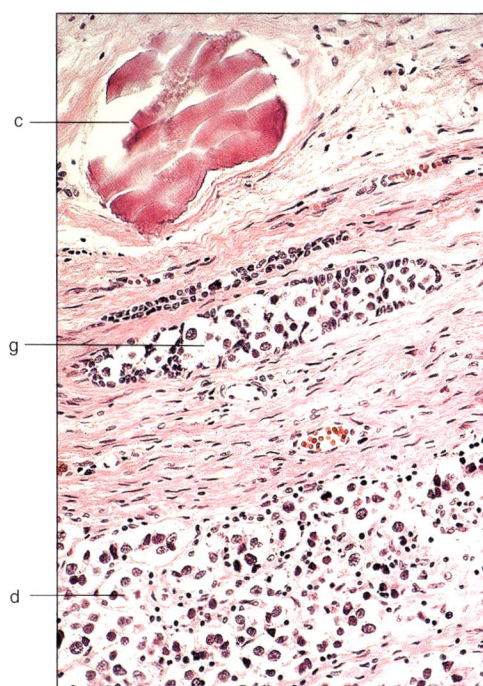

Fig. 34.57 Gonadoblastoma with superimposed dysgerminoma. A small focus of calcification (c) lies adjacent to the gonadoblastoma (g) in which malignant germ cells are surrounded by immature granulosa/Sertoli cells. Adjacent is typical dysgerminoma (d), which by definition lacks surrounding supporting sex-cord supporting elements.

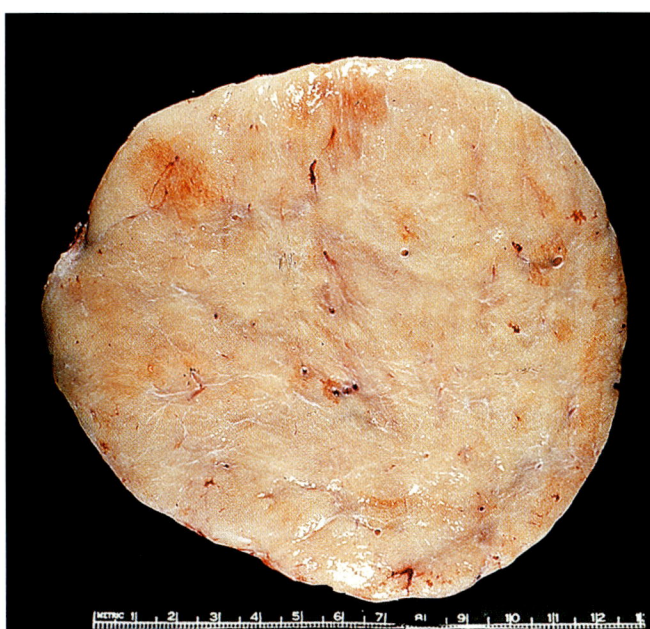

Fig. 34.56 A 15 cm dysgerminoma in mixed gonadal dysgenesis arising from gonadoblastoma.

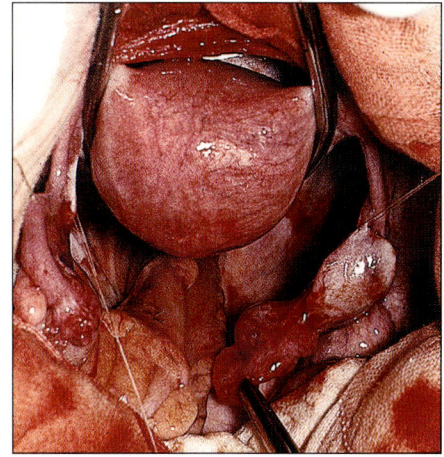

Fig. 34.58 Mixed gonadal dysgenesis with ovary, streak gonads, and endometrial adenocarcinoma. The patient had been treated with long-term estrogen therapy.

virilization if the patient is to be raised as a female, it is important that gonadectomy be performed before the patient reaches puberty. The ultimate gender identity that a patient may desire is an area of controversy.[21] Patients who have been treated with long-term administration of estrogen may on occasion develop endometrial carcinoma (Figure 34.58). Congenital cardiovascular anomalies have also been reported in patients with MGD.

Gonadoblastoma
Definition
Gonadoblastoma is a precancerous or *in situ* form of germ cell cancer unique to patients with abnormal sexual development.

It consists of malignant germ cells that are surrounded individually or in groups or by immature cells that are of sex-cord derivation (immature Sertoli/granulosa-like cells). The tumor nearly always occurs in association with a whole or component of a 'Y' chromosome,[125] although cases are known that have arisen in tumors with a 46,XX karyotype and even where the patient has given birth.[155] Although most cases are detected in children or young adults, the tumor may develop prenatally.[64]

Clinical features

Most gonadoblastomas occur in phenotypic females with abnormal gonads.[125] Some occur in phenotypic males, almost all of whom have cryptorchism or abnormal external or abnormal internal genitalia. Only the rare patient is a normal phenotypic male without apparent abnormal genitals.[49] Nearly all gonadoblastomas occur in patients with MGD. Gonadoblastoma accounts for three-fourths of the gonadal tumors arising in dysgenetic gonads and is usually discovered during the first to fourth decades of life. Many of the isolated reports of gonadoblastoma associated with other forms of hermaphroditism described clinically and pathologically may in actuality be examples of MGD.

Genetic changes

The role of the Y chromosome in the development of cancer is controversial. Since much of the Y chromosome (except for the pseudoautosomal regions at both ends of the chromosomes, initialed PAR) neither pairs with nor recombines with the X chromosome during meiosis, it has been difficult to study this chromosome and identify its oncogenic genes and tumor-suppressor genes. The gonadoblastoma Y gene locus (*GBY*) appears to be located on the short or long arm of the Y chromosome near the centromere. It may be that more than one gene is involved. Possibly the gonadoblastoma gene functions as an oncogene only in the dysgenetic gonad, and otherwise has a normal function in the normally developing testis. A multicopy gene, called *TSPY* (testis specific protein Y), which is an oncogene located in the GBY critical region, has emerged as the most likely GBY candidate.[35,76] This oncogene is expressed in spermatogonial cells in normal testis, suggesting a function early in spermatogenesis, and is drastically reduced in the gonads of patients with androgen insensitivity, a syndrome not associated with gonadoblastoma. Currently, it is not yet clear how and why the oncogenic function of *TSPY* predisposes the abnormal gonad to cancer development. In gonadoblastoma, the Y chromosome signal is significantly higher in the tumor cells than in adjacent non-tumor cells.[55]

Pathology

The gross appearance of the gonad with gonadoblastoma varies according to the size of the neoplasm, the presence of calcification (Figure 34.59), and whether the gonadoblastoma has been overgrown by a malignant form of germ cell tumor (usually germinoma) (Figure 34.57). The immunoprofile of the tumor cells shows reactivity with placental alkaline phosphatase (PLAP) (Figure 34.60A), c-kit (Figure 34.60B), and FOXL2 (Figure 34.60C). Most gonadoblastomas, if macroscopically visible, are small. About 20% of gonadoblastomas arise in a streak gonad (Figure 34.61) and another 20% arise in a dysgenetic testis. A very rare case is found with ovarian tissue or at least dysgenetic gonads with rare primordial follicles (Figure 34.62). In the remaining cases, the nature of the underlying gonad cannot be determined with certainty because tumor replaces it. Abut a fifth of gonadoblastomas are discovered solely because a streak gonad was examined microscopically. The contralateral gonad also contains a gonadoblastoma in more than one-third of patients.

On microscopic examination, the gonadoblastoma appears as circumscribed nests of neoplastic germ cells having the cytologic properties of germinoma (dysgerminoma and seminoma) and are encompassed individually or in groups by sex-cord

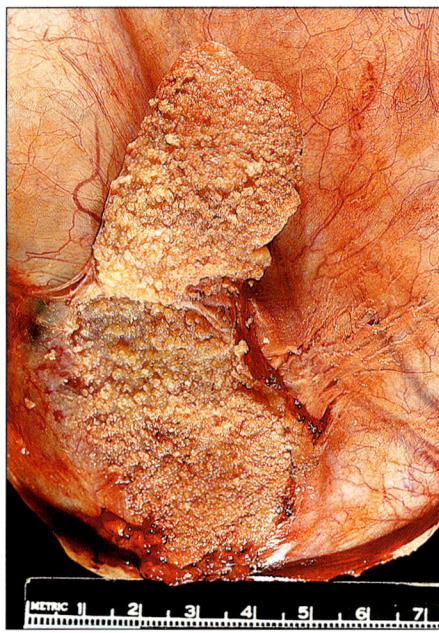

Fig. 34.59 Calcified gonadoblastoma. The 5 × 2 × 0.5 cm calcified focus was apparent radiographically.

derivatives with inconspicuous cytoplasm and small round to oval nuclei resembling immature Sertoli cells (Figures 34.62 and 34.63). The germ cells are of two forms, one of which is an immature small cell form with a high nuclear:cytoplasmic ratio resembling gonocytes/oogonia and believed to be the cell that can progress to dysgerminoma.[67] The small cell also gives rise to the larger and mature form of germ cells which resemble prespermatogonia/oocytes and have copious amounts of light to clear cytoplasm, usually with a distinct cytoplasmic membrane. The mature large cell is not precancerous. Both types of germ cell have centrally placed nuclei in the cell and obvious macronucleoli that are one to several in number. Histologically, these precancerous germ cells resemble the carcinoma *in situ* (CIS) germ cells often found in seminiferous tubules that are adjacent to seminomas which develop in genetically normal 46,XY men.

Recent immunohistochemical studies provide some insight into the progression of precancerous germ cells into invasive malignancy, especially in the form of seminoma/dysgerminoma.[67] OCT 3/4, an octamer binding transcription factor, is present diffusely and strongly in the immature form of precancerous germ cell, in malignant germ cells at the junction of gonadoblastoma and seminoma/dysgerminoma, and in the seminoma/dysgerminoma distant from the gonadoblastoma. It is not present in the mature form of gonadoblastoma germ cell. TSPY, the testis Y specific protein,[76] is present in the larger mature gonadoblastoma germ cell, but minimally noticeable to absent in the precancerous immature form. While it is variably present in the early invasive component of seminoma/dysgerminoma, it is absent from the malignant germ cells deep within the invasive cancer. These data suggest that TSPY may be involved in the initial selection of tumorigenic cells, but once the process has begun and the malignant germ cells are duplicating as a seminoma/dysgerminoma, TSPY dependency is lost. Neither PLAP nor c-kit (CD117) (Figure 34.60), both markers of germ cells, reliably demonstrates the malig-

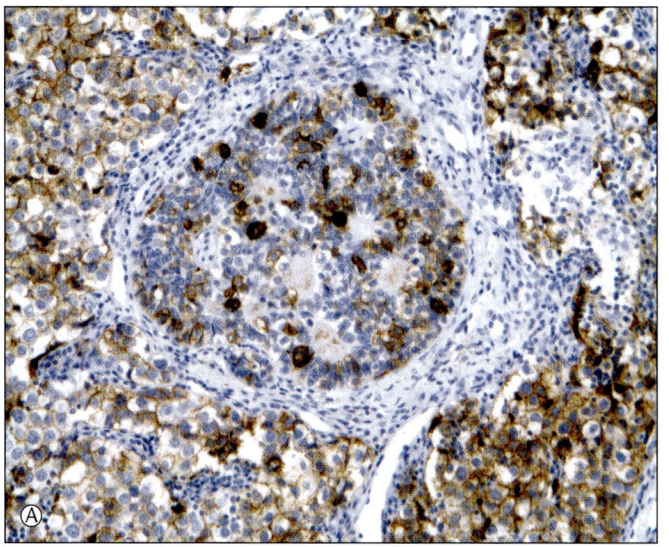

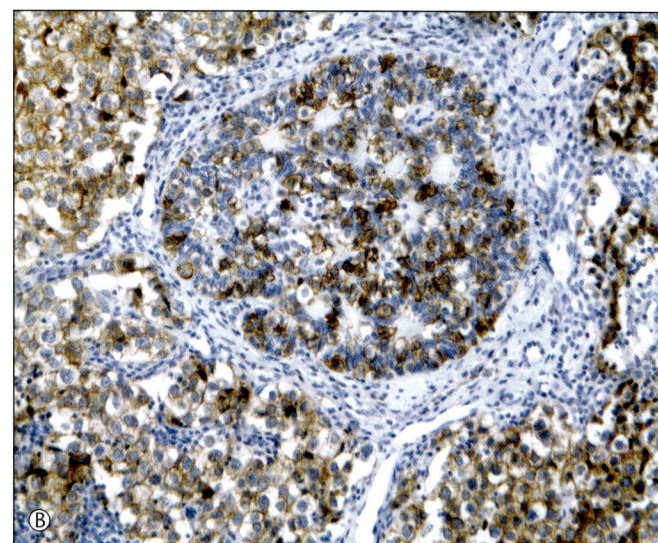

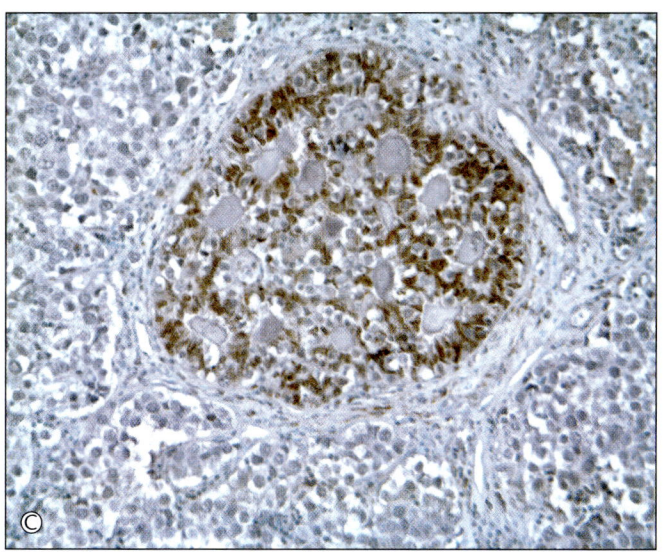

Fig. 34.60 Gonadoblastoma showing reactivity with placental alkaline phosphatase (PLAP) **(A)**, c-kit **(B)** and FOXL2 **(C)**.

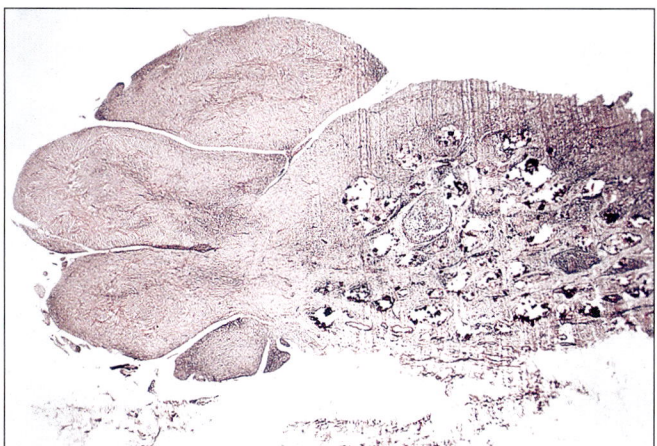

Fig. 34.61 Gonadoblastoma occupying a gonadal streak.

nant germ cells, nor do they help explain the pathogenetic process.

Inhibin reactivity and AMH[114] are commonly demonstrable in the surrounding cells, which is in keeping with the sex-cord cells (immature Sertoli/granulosa cells) being an integral part of the tumor. Hyaline, composed of basement membrane material, is found along the margin or as nodules within the nests of gonadoblastoma. In four-fifths of cases, the hyaline material is calcified, initially appearing as small, laminated spheres (Figures 34.57 and 34.64), which eventually fuse and coalesce into large mulberry-like masses. Not infrequently, the only evidence that a dysgerminoma originated in a gonadoblastoma is the presence focally of mulberry-like calcifications. Hormonally active cells that resemble lutein and Leydig cells are found interspersed among the nests of tumor in about two-thirds of cases. These hormonally active cells are found least frequently in non-virilized phenotypic females, more often in virilized females, and most frequently in phenotypic males. To some degree, their appearance may reflect the postpubertal age of the patient when the gonad is examined.

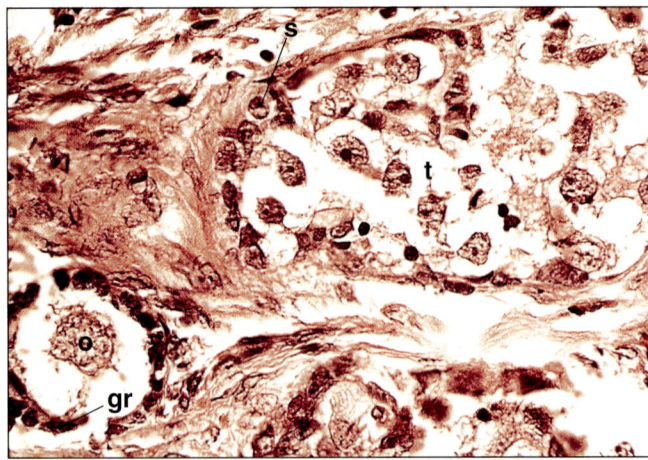

Fig. 34.62 Gonadoblastoma adjacent to primordial follicle. The gonadoblastoma (t) shows malignant nuclei with large central nucleoli and a zone of immature stromal elements (s) around the entire nest. Adjacent to it is a normal primordial follicle. The single central oocyte (o), which has a large central nucleus, fine nuclear chromatin, and copious cytoplasm, is surrounded by a rim of immature granulosa cells (gr). The rarity of primordial follicles, the absence of any of other structures showing more advanced development, and this history that such lesions will atrophy and fibrose over time suggest this is not an ovotestis.

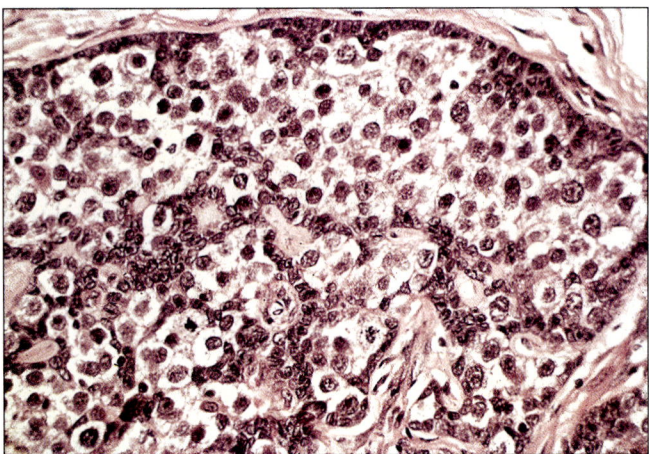

Fig. 34.63 Gonadoblastoma with immature granulosa/Sertoli cells surrounding nests of tumor.

XY FEMALE (SEX REVERSAL)

Steroidogenic factor 1 (SF1) is an orphan nuclear receptor (i. e., no identified natural ligand) that regulates the transcription of multiple genes implicated in reproduction, steroidogenesis, and male sexual differentiation, including *AMH*, *DAX1*, *CYP11A1*, steroidogenic acute regulatory protein (STAR), and those encoding steroid hydroxylases, gonadotrophins, and aromatase. Some of the heterozygous SF1 mutations result in a spectrum of end-organ defects similar to that of androgen receptor mutations and are discussed above. In rare instances, mutations in SF1 can lead to a testicular regression-like syndrome with 46,XY sex reversal but without adrenal insufficiency. One patient described had an eunuchoid habitus, no breast development and ambiguous genitalia with an enlarged clitoris, single perineal opening, and without palpable gonads

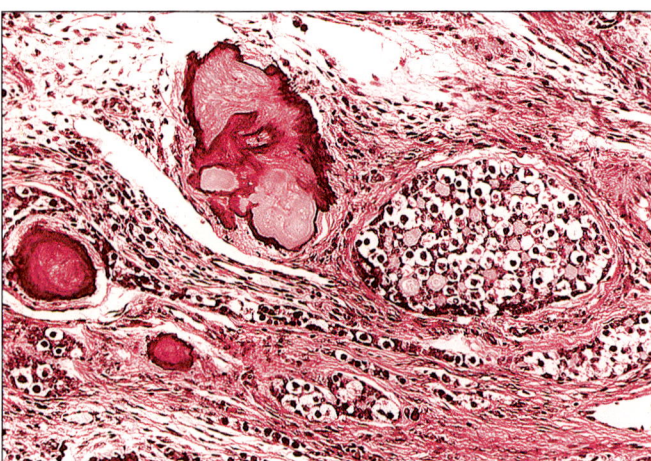

Fig. 34.64 Gonadoblastoma with multifocal calcification.

(absence histologically confirmed).[31,36] The rarity of identifying this form of XY sex reversal has suggested that other genes participate in the sex determination cascade.

Deletion of a gene on chromosome 9p is a newly described cause of sex reversal in the genetic XY male.[147] The gene, *DMRT*, located at 9p24.3 and transcribed only in the embryonic gonads of both sexes and in fetal and adult testis, is required for postnatal differentiation of both somatic and germ cells in the mouse testis. One patient,[147] born with sexually ambiguous genitalia, had a 46,XY,del(9)(p22-pter) karyotype. The gonads appeared like that of a postnatal testis. The müllerian ducts had regressed and the wolffian derivatives had developed normally. One of the two pelvic testes had a poorly developed albuginea. One-third of the gonad at one pole was maldeveloped with ill-defined, large trabeculae rich in germ cells with non-centered nuclei and vacuolated cytoplasm. The cells were cohesive, thus differing from primitive cords. There was no follicle differentiation in the deeper part. Another patient had no uterus, but a fallopian tube on the right and bilateral ovotestes.[105] The locus on 9p apparently maintains testis differentiation in the male rather than determining the primary sex, since the dysgenetic testes exhibit WT1, SRY, and MIS.

Several 46,XX females, including some of postpubertal age, with deletions at 9p or other abnormalities, showed normal ovarian development, suggesting that the 9p22–p24 deletion does not contain a locus required for early ovarian differentiation.[105,147]

TRUE HERMAPHRODITISM

True hermaphroditism is defined as the presence of both testicular and ovarian tissue in a patient. Affected individuals may have either a female or a male phenotype with variable degrees of sexual ambiguity (Figure 34.65). Because the wavy, cortical-type stroma typically seen in the female gonad can be found in both female and male gonads and therefore is non-specific, follicular structures must be identified to classify gonadal tissue as ovarian and seminiferous tubules to classify the tissue as testicular. In true hermaphrodites, the gonads may be ovary and testis separately or combined in an ovotestis.

True hermaphroditism is a rare condition both in North American and Europe,[48] but one of the more common etiologies of male sexual ambiguity.[95] It is, in contrast, common in Africa, especially in South Africa.[140] Clusters in other geographic locations are known,[32,47] some with data differing from the summary given below.

The ovotestis is the most frequently encountered type of gonad in true hermaphroditism (Figures 34.66–34.68).[146] In four-fifths of cases the ovarian and testicular tissues are arranged in an end-to-end fashion. The ovarian portion of an ovotestis has a convoluted surface while the testicular portion is smooth and glistening. Frequently, a distinct line demarcates the two tissues. The firm nature of the palpable ovarian tissue and the soft texture of the testis are valuable clinical signs when evaluating the nature of a gonad in an infant with ambisexual external genitalia.

An ovary, which preferentially develops on the left side, is the second most common gonad in true hermaphrodites. Every patient over 15 years of age in one series had either a corpus

luteum or a corpus albicans.[140] The testis, which is the gonad least often encountered, develops preferentially on the right.

The location of the gonad is influenced by the type and quantity of gonadal tissue present. Increasing amounts of

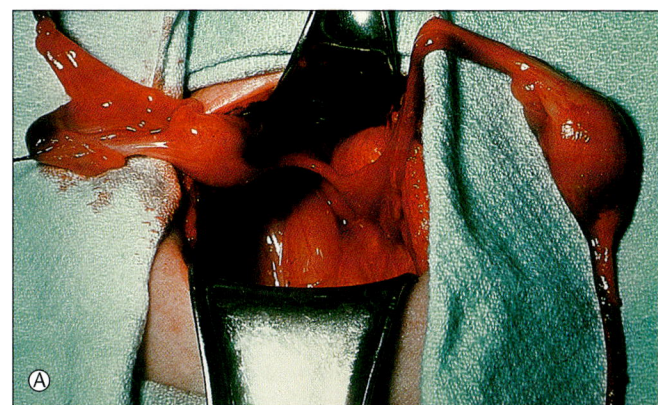
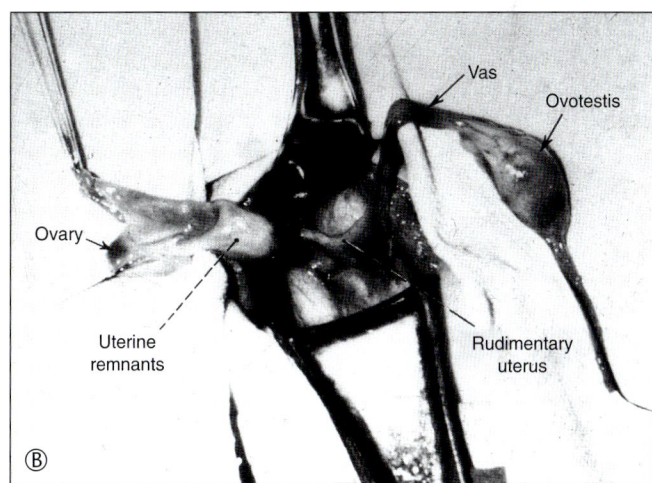

Fig. 34.66 True hermaphroditism. **(A)** Gonads as seen during the operation. **(B)** Labeled.

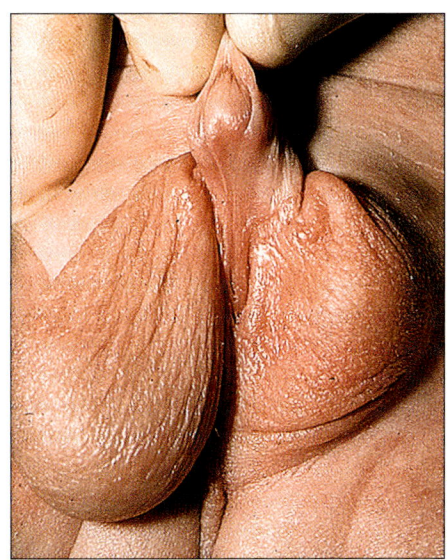

Fig. 34.65 True hermaphroditism with bifid scrotum.

Fig. 34.67 Ovotestis. Seminiferous tubules are at one pole and a solid cluster of primordial follicles at the other.

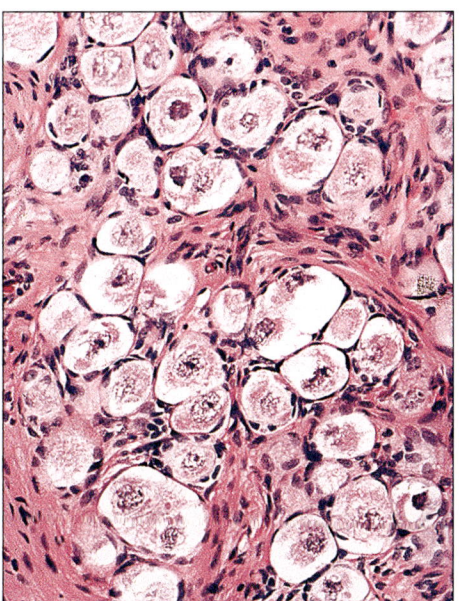
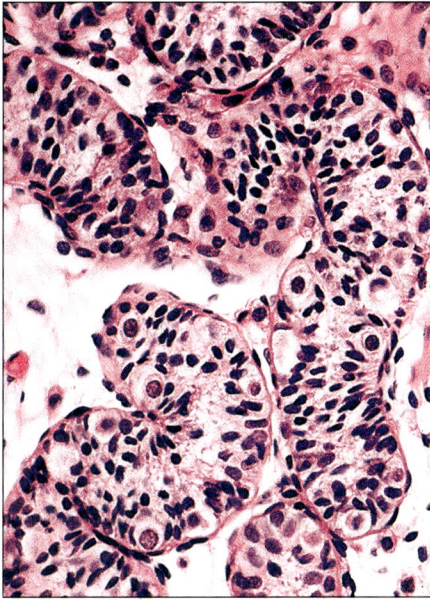

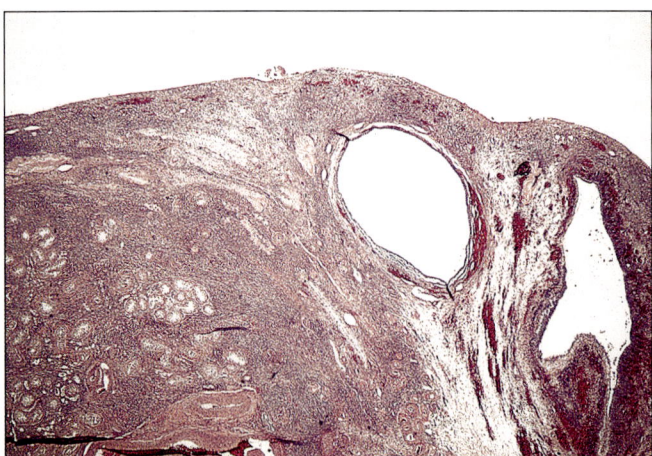

Fig. 34.68 Ovotestis in true hermaphrodite. The gonad showed Graafian follicle formation indicative of ovary in one half of the gonad and seminiferous tubules in the other indicative of testicular formation.

ovarian tissue increase the probability that the gonad will be in an ovarian position. It is felt that this may be due to deficient or absent MIS, which is needed for the initial descent of the testis to occur. When a gonad with the macroscopic features of an ovary is situated in the inguinal canal or in the labioscrotal fold, the possibility of it being an ovotestis should be seriously considered. The position of the testis is less constant. Most (63%) reside in the scrotum, 14% in the inguinal region, 1% in the internal inguinal ring, and 22% in a normal ovarian position.

The nature of the genital structure adjacent to a gonad in true hermaphroditism depends upon the nature of the gonad, which is in contrast to MGD in which a fallopian tube is often adjacent to the gonad, regardless of whether it is a testis or a streak. In true hermaphroditism a fallopian tube is adjacent to an ovary and an epididymis or vas deferens is adjacent to a testis. Either a müllerian or wolffian structure, but not both, is adjacent to an ovotestis. MIS appears to be functional. Ninety-five per cent of fallopian tubes adjacent to ovotestes have closed ostia. Only 10% of uteri are normal; the other patients have absent uteri (13%), unicornuate uteri (10%), absent cervix (14%) or uterine hypoplasia (46%).

The most common karyotypes in true hermaphroditism are 46,XX (60%), 46,XY (12%), and mosaic (28%), usually 46,XX/46,XY, 46,XY/47,XXY, or least frequently 45,X/46,XY. Patients with a 'Y' chromosome have a two- to three-fold increased frequency of having a testis as opposed to an ovotestis. Nearly 75% of true hermaphrodites with an ovary and an ovotestis have a 46,XX karyotype.

As in other disorders of intersex, genetic aberrations appear to play a key role in the development of true hermaphroditism. For example, chromosome Y-specific genes (e.g., *SRY*) have been detected in some 46,XX true hermaphrodites, suggesting one potential mechanism for the development of XX true hermaphroditism, similar to individuals with XX male syndrome.[48] In some series, *SRY* was undetected in the 46,XX patients,[47] indicating that other mechanisms may also be important. But such data must be read with care as other case reports identify examples where the patient may be 46,XX and lack the *SRY*

gene in usual cells examined (leukocytes). Yet cells from the gonad itself demonstrate *SRY*.[62] Mutations that mimic the *SRY* gene have been suggested as one possibility where the *SRY* gene was absent.[130] One explanation proposed for patients with an XY chromosome constitution is the possibility that the *SRY* gene, if present, may act at a time too late to stimulate the development of a testis, hence permitting ovarian tissue to develop.

The clinical presentations of true hermaphrodites vary to some extent depending upon their ages at the time of diagnosis. Until recently, the condition often went undetected until adolescence when phenotypic male patients were evaluated for gynecomastia, or for cysts in the testis and treated surgically, and phenotypic female patients were evaluated for amenorrhea or failure to develop secondary sex changes. Thus, in one series,[140] three-fourths of patients were raised as males and one-fourth as females. Many patients, however, menstruated and a few became pregnant. Phenotypic males may experience monthly hematuria because of menstruation into a persistent urogenital sinus. With an increased awareness of intersex states, the condition is recognized more often in infants because of ambiguous genitalia, usually in the form of a small phallus (enlarged clitoris).[32,48] Like MGD, the scrotum may be asymmetric, with the larger, more normal-appearing hemiscrotum containing a testis. Among 160 patients the external genitalia were asymmetric in three-fourths (labioscrotal folds in 63% and hemiscrota in 13%).

On microscopic examination, the gonadal tissue often appears normal if the patient is young. In infants, the ovarian tissue contains numerous follicles, whereas the testicular parenchyma discloses normal-appearing seminiferous tubules with spermatogonia. Patients in the reproductive years may have ovarian tissue with structures indicative of ovulation, e.g., follicles, corpora lutea, and corpora albicantia, but spermatogenesis is rare in the testicular portion. The testicular portion of an ovotestis is usually abnormal with incomplete development, loss of germ cells, and tubular sclerosis. Scrotal testes in these patients show less severe changes, sometimes showing faulty spermatogenesis.

At times, distinction between true hermaphroditism and MGD can be difficult, if not impossible. In the newborn, asymmetric ambiguous genitalia may be observed in both conditions. If a streak gonad from a patient with MGD is serially sectioned, a rare primordial follicle may be encountered in what otherwise appears to be a testis with well-developed seminiferous tubules. If the gonad is not removed, over time the gonad will progress to a streak gonad. If the term 'true hermaphroditism' is restricted to those patients in whom the ovarian and testicular tissue are both apparent grossly and the definition of an ovary requires development of at least the antral stage of follicular development, it should usually be possible to segregate more clearly those individuals in whom the ovarian tissue may be functional.

Gonadal tumors occur in less than 3% of affected individuals, and in one large series with long-term follow-up, not at all.[146] Germinoma is the most common type of tumor, but gonadoblastomas and a variety of other tumors have been reported.[133] One case has been reported where the primitive sex-cord cellular elements adjacent to seminiferous tubules in a testis gave rise to cancer in the form of a juvenile granulosa cell tumor.[134]

REFERENCES

1. Aartsen EJ, Snethlage RAI, Vangeel AN, Gallee MPW. Squamous cell carcinoma of the vagina in a male pseudohermaphrodite with 5 alpha-reductase deficiency. Int J Gynecol Cancer 1994;4:283–7.
2. Aguirre D, Nieto K, Lazos M, et al. Extragonadal germ cell tumors are often associated with Klinefelter syndrome. Hum Pathol 2006;37:477–80.
3. Aksglaede L, Wikstrom AM, Rajpert-De Meyts E, Dunkel L, Skakkebaek NE, Juul A. Natural history of seminiferous tubule degeneration in Klinefelter syndrome. Hum Reprod Update 2006;12:39–48.
4. Al-Ahmadie HA, Stanek J, Liu J, Mangu PN, Niemann T, Young RH. Ovarian 'tumor' of the adrenogenital syndrome – the first reported case. Am J Surg Pathol 2001;25:1443–50.
5. Al-Attia HM. Male pseudohermaphroditism due to 5 alpha-reductase-2 deficiency in an Arab kindred. Postgrad Med J 1997;73:802–7.
6. Alvarez-Nava F, Gonzalez S, Soto M, Martinez C, Prieto M. Complete androgen insensitivity syndrome: clinical and anatomopathological findings in 23 patients. Genet Couns 1997;8:7–12.
7. Alvarez-Nava F, Gonzalez S, Soto M, Pineda L, Morales-Machin A. Mixed gonadal dysgenesis: a syndrome of broad clinical cytogenetic and histopathologic spectrum. Genet Couns 1999;10:233–43.
8. Alvarez-Nava F, Martinez MC, Gonzalez S, Soto M, Borjas L, Rojas A. FISH and PCR analysis of the presence of Y-chromosome sequences in a patient with Xq-isochromosome and testicular tissue. Clin Genet 1999;55:356–61.
9. Andersson S, Moghrabi N. Physiology and molecular genetics of 17 beta-hydroxysteroid dehydrogenases. Steroids 1997;62:143–7.
10. Arnhold IJ, Latronico AC, Batista MC, Mendonca BB. Menstrual disorders and infertility caused by inactivating mutations of the luteinizing hormone receptor gene. Fertil Steril 1999;71:597–601.
11. Auber F, Lortat-Jacob S, Sarnacki S, et al. Surgical management and genotype/phenotype correlations in WT1 gene-related diseases (Drash, Frasier syndromes). J Pediatr Surg 2003;38:124–9.
12. Avila NA, Premkumar A, Merke DP. Testicular adrenal rest tissue in congenital adrenal hyperplasia: comparison of MR imaging and sonographic findings. Am J Roentgenol 1999;172:1003–6.
13. Bale PM, Howard NJ, Wright JE. Male pseudohermaphroditism in XY children with female phenotype. Pediatr Pathol 1992;12:29–49.
14. Barbosa AS, Hadjiathanasiou CG, Theodoridis C, et al. The same mutation affecting the splicing of WT1 gene is present on Frasier syndrome patients with or without Wilms' tumor. Hum Mutat 1999;13:146–53.
15. Bas F, Saka N, Darendeliler F, et al. Bilateral ovarian steroid cell tumor in congenital adrenal hyperplasia due to classic 11beta-hydroxylase deficiency. J Pediatr Endocrinol Metab 2000;13:663–7.
16. Belville C, Josso N, Picard JY. Persistence of Mullerian derivatives in males. Am J Med Genet 1999;89:218–23.
17. Berenzstein E, Torrado M, Belgorosky A, Rivarola M. Smith–Lemli–Opitz syndrome: in vivo and in vitro study of testicular function in a prepubertal patient with ambiguous genitalia. Acta Paediatr 1999;88:1229–32.
18. Bialer MG, Penchaszadeh VB, Kahn E, Libes R, Krigsman G, Lesser ML. Female external genitalia and mullerian duct derivatives in a 46,XY infant with the Smith–Lemli–Opitz syndrome. Am J Med Genet 1987;28:723–31.
19. Bilbao JR, Loridan L, Castano L. A novel postzygotic nonsense mutation in SRY in familial XY gonadal dysgenesis. Hum Genet 1996;97:537–9.
20. Bilbao JR, Loridan L, Audi L, Gonzalo E, Castano L. A novel missense (R80W) mutation in 17-beta-hydroxysteroid dehydrogenase type 3 gene associated with male pseudohermaphroditism. Eur J Endocrinol 1998;139:330–3.
21. Birnbacher R, Marberger M, Weissenbacher G, Schober E, Frisch H. Gender identity reversal in an adolescent with mixed gonadal dysgenesis. J Pediatr Endocrinol Metab 1999;12(5 Suppl):687–90.
22. Bonte A, Schroder W, Denamur E, Querfeld U. Absent pubertal development in a child with chronic renal failure: the case of Frasier syndrome. Nephrol Dial Transplant 2000;15:1688–90.
23. Brant WO, Rajimwale A, Lovell MA, et al. Gonadoblastoma and Turner syndrome. J Urol 2006;175:1858–60.
24. Buchholz NP, Biyabani R, Herzig MJU, et al. Persistent mullerian duct syndrome. Eur Urol 1998;34:230–2.
25. Canto P, Kofman-Alfaro S, Jimenez AL, et al. Gonadoblastoma in Turner syndrome patients with nonmosaic 45,X karyotype and Y chromosome sequences. Cancer Genet Cytogenet 2004;150:70–2.
26. Carlson AD, Obeid JS, Kanellopoulou N, Wilson RC, New MI. Congenital adrenal hyperplasia: update on prenatal diagnosis and treatment. J Steroid Biochem Mol Biol 1999;69:19–29.
27. Caron KM, Soo SC, Wetsel WC, Stocco DM, Clark BJ, Parker KL. Targeted disruption of the mouse gene encoding steroidogenic acute regulatory protein provides insights into congenital lipoid adrenal hyperplasia. Proc Natl Acad Sci U S A 1997;94:11540–5.
28. Cendron M, Schned AR, Ellsworth PI. Histological evaluation of the testicular nubbin in the vanishing testis syndrome. J Urol 1998;160(3 Pt 2):1161 3.
29. Cerame BI, Newfield RS, Pascoe L, et al. Prenatal diagnosis and treatment of 11beta-hydroxylase deficiency congenital adrenal hyperplasia resulting in normal female genitalia. J Clin Endocrinol Metab 1999;84:3129–34.
30. Chu C. Y-chromosome mosaicism in girls with Turner's syndrome. Clin Endocrinol 1999;50:17–18.
31. Correa RV, Domenice S, Bingham NC, et al. A microdeletion in the ligand binding domain of human steroidogenic factor 1 causes XY sex reversal without adrenal insufficiency. J Clin Endocrinol Metab 2004;89:1767–72.
32. Damiani D, Fellous M, McElreavey K, et al. True hermaphroditism: clinical aspects and molecular studies in 16 cases. Eur J Endocrinol 1997;136:201–4.
33. Dardis A, Saraco N, Mendilaharzu H, Rivarola M, Belgorosky A. Report of an XX male with hypospadias and pubertal gynecomastia, SRY gene negative in blood leukocytes but SRY gene positive in testicular cells. Hormone Res 1997;47:85–8.
34. de Nanclares GP, Castano L, Bilbao JR, et al. Molecular analysis of Frasier syndrome: mutation in the WT1 gene in a girl with gonadal dysgenesis and nephronophthisis. J Pediatr Endocrinol Metab 2002;15:1047–50.
35. Delbridge ML, Longepied G, Depetris D, et al. TSPY, the candidate gonadoblastoma gene on the human Y chromosome, has a widely expressed homologue on the X – implications for Y chromosome evolution. Chromosome Res 2004;12:345–56.
36. Domenice S, Correa RV, Costa EM, et al. Mutations in the SRY, DAX1, SF1 and WNT4 genes in Brazilian sex-reversed patients. Braz J Med Biol Res 2004;37:145–50.
37. Erk A, Ozeren S, Ozbay O, Vural B, Elcioglu N. Persistent mullerian duct syndrome – a case report. J Reprod Med 1999;44:135–8.
38. Ferrari P, Obeyesekere VR, Li K, et al. Point mutations abolish 11 beta-hydroxysteroid dehydrogenase type II activity in three families with the congenital syndrome of apparent mineralocorticoid excess. Mol Cell Endocrinol 1996;119:21–4.
39. Fitzky BU, Glossmann H, Utermann G, Moebius FF. Molecular genetics of the Smith–Lemli–Opitz syndrome and postsqualene sterol metabolism. Curr Opin Lipidol 1999;10:123–31.
40. Foudila T, Soderstrom-Anttila V, Hovatta O. Turner's syndrome and pregnancies after oocyte donation. Hum Reprod 1999;14:532–5.
41. Fukazawa R, Nakahori Y, Kogo T, et al. Normal Y sequences in Smith–Lemli–Opitz syndrome with total failure of masculinization. Acta Paediatr 1992;81:570–2.
42. Fung MF, Vadas G, Lotocki R, Heywood M, Krepart G. Tubular Krukenberg tumor in pregnancy with virilization. Gynecol Oncol 1991;41:81–4.
43. Gibbons B, Tan SY, Yu CC, Cheah E, Tan HL. Risk of gonadoblastoma in female patients with Y chromosome abnormalities and dysgenetic gonads. J Paediatr Child Health 1999;35:210–3.
44. Gicquel C, Gaston V, Cabrol S, Le Bouc Y. Assessment of Turner's syndrome by molecular analysis of the X chromosome in growth-retarded girls. J Clin Endocrinol Metab 1998;83:1472–6.
45. Ginsberg NA, Cadkin A, Strom C, Bauer-Marsh E, Verlinsky Y. Prenatal diagnosis of 46,XX male fetuses. Am J Obstet Gynecol 1999;180:1006–7.
46. Gravholt CH, Fedder J, Naeraa RW, Muller J. Occurrence of gonadoblastoma in females with Turner syndrome and Y chromosome material: a population study. J Clin Endocrinol Metab 2000;85:3199–202.
47. Guerra Junior G, de Mello MP, Assumpcao JG, et al. True hermaphrodites in the southeastern region of Brazil: a different cytogenetic and gonadal profile. J Pediatr Endocrinol Metab 1998;11:519–24.
48. Hadjiathanasiou CG, Brauner R, Lortat-Jacob S, et al. True hermaphroditism: genetic variants and clinical management. J Pediatr 1994;125(5 Pt 1):738–44.
49. Hatano T, Yoshino Y, Kawashima Y, et al. Case of gonadoblastoma in a 9-year-old boy without physical abnormalities. Int J Urol 1999;6:164–6.
50. Hawkyard S, Poon P, Morgan DR. Sertoli tumour presenting with stress incontinence in a patient with testicular feminization. Br J Urol Int 1999;84:382–3.
51. Hiort O, Holterhus PM, Nitsche EM. Physiology and pathophysiology of androgen action. Baillieres Clin Endocrinol Metab 1998;12:115–32.
52. Hiort O, Sinnecker GH, Holterhus PM, Nitsche EM, Kruse K. The clinical and molecular spectrum of androgen insensitivity syndromes. Am J Med Genet 1996;63:218–22.
53. Hovatta O. Pregnancies in women with Turner's syndrome. Ann Med 1999;31:106–10.
54. Hunter RHF. Abnormal sexual development in man. In: Hunter RHF, ed. Sex Determination, Differentiation and Intersexuality in Placental Mammals. Cambridge: Cambridge University Press; 1995:204–38.
55. Iezzoni JC, von Kap-Herr C, Golden WL, Gaffey MJ. Gonadoblastomas in 45,X/46,XY mosaicism – analysis of Y chromosome distribution by fluorescence in situ hybridization. Am J Clin Pathol 1997;108:197–201.
56. Imperato-McGinley J. 5 alpha-reductase-2 deficiency. Curr Ther Endocrinol Metab 1997;6:384–7.
57. Ito K, Kawamata Y, Osada H, Ijichi M, Takano E, Sekiya S. Pure yolk sac tumor of the ovary with mosaic 45X/46X+mar Turner's syndrome with a Y-chromosomal fragment. Arch Gynecol Obstet 1998;262:87–90.
58. Iwamoto I, Yanazume S, Fujino T, Yoshioka T, Douchi T. Leydig cell tumor in an elderly patient with complete androgen insensitivity syndrome. Gynecol Oncol 2005;96:870–2.
59. Jacobs P, Dalton P, James R, et al. Turner syndrome: a cytogenetic and molecular study. Ann Hum Genet 1997;61(Pt 6):471–83.
60. Jaubert F, Nihoul-Fekete C, Lortat-Jacob S, Josso N, Fellous M. Hermaphroditism pathology. Ann Pathol (Fr) 2004;24:499–509.

61. Jaubert F, Vasiliu V, Patey-Mariaud de Serre N, et al. Gonad development in Drash and Frasier syndromes depends on WT1 mutations. Arkh Patol 2003;65:40–4.

62. Jimenez AL, Kofman-Alfaro S, Berumen J, et al. Partially deleted SRY gene confined to testicular tissue in a 46,XX true hermaphrodite without SRY in leukocytic DNA. Am J Med Genet 2000;93:417–20.

63. Jones MEE, Boon WC, McInnes K, Maffei L, Carani C, Simpson ER. Recognizing rare disorders: aromatase deficiency. Nat Clin Prac Endocrinol Metab 2007;3:414–21.

64. Jorgensen N, Muller J, Jaubert F, Clausen OP, Skakkebaek NE. Heterogeneity of gonadoblastoma germ cells: similarities with immature germ cells, spermatogonia and testicular carcinoma in situ cells. Histopathology 1997;30:177–86.

65. Josso N, Belville C, di Clemente N, Picard JY. AMH and AMH receptor defects in persistent Mullerian duct syndrome. Hum Reprod Update 2005;11:351–6.

66. Kanayama H, Naroda T, Inoue Y, Kurokawa Y, Kagawa S. A case of complete testicular feminization: laparoscopic orchiectomy and analysis of androgen receptor gene mutation. Int J Urol 1999;6:327–30.

67. Kersemaekers AM, Honecker F, Stoop H, et al. Identification of germ cells at risk for neoplastic transformation in gonadoblastoma: an immunohistochemical study for OCT3/4 and TSPY. Hum Pathol 2005;36:512–21.

68. Keung YK, Buss D, Chauvenet A, Pettenati M. Hematologic malignancies and Klinefelter syndrome: a chance association? Cancer Genet Cytogenet 2002;139:9–13.

69. Khoury K, Ducharme L, LeHoux JG. Family of two patients with congenital lipoid adrenal hyperplasia due to StAR mutation. Endocrinol Res 2004;30:925–9.

70. Kocova M, Basheska N, Papazovska A, Jankova R, Toncheva D, Popovska S. Girls with Turner's syndrome with spontaneous menarche have an increased risk of endometrial carcinoma: a case report and review from the literature. Gynecol Oncol 2005;96:840–5.

71. Kohler B, Lumbroso S, Leger J, et al. Androgen insensitivity syndrome: somatic mosaicism of the androgen receptor in seven families and consequences for sex assignment and genetic counseling. J Clin Endocrinol Metab 2005;90:106–11.

72. Kolon TF, Ferrer FA, McKenna PH. Clinical and molecular analysis of XX sex reversed patients. J Urol 1998;160(3 Pt 2):1169–72.

73. Korsch E, Peter M, Hiort O, et al. Gonadal histology with testicular carcinoma in situ in a 15-year-old 46,XY female patient with a premature termination in the steroidogenic acute regulatory protein causing congenital lipoid adrenal hyperplasia. J Clin Endocrinol Metab 1999;84:1628–32.

74. Lam SK, Yu MY, To KF, Chan MKM, Chun TKH. Ovarian epithelial tumour in gonadal dysgenesis: a case report and literature review. Aust N Z J Obstet Gynaecol 1996;36:106–9.

75. Lanfranco F, Kamischke A, Zitzmann M, Nieschlag E. Klinefelter's syndrome. Lancet 2004;364:273–83.

76. Li Y, Vilain E, Conte F, Rajpert-De Meyts E, Lau YF. Testis-specific protein Y-encoded gene is expressed in early and late stages of gonadoblastoma and testicular carcinoma in situ. Urol Oncol 2007;25:141–6.

77. Ludwig M, Beck A, Wickert L, et al. Female pseudohermaphroditism associated with a novel homozygous G-to-A (V370-to-M) substitution in the P-450 aromatase gene. J Pediatr Endocrinol Metab 1998;11:657–64.

78. Lvarez-Nava AF, Soto M, Sanchez MA, Fernandez E, Lanes R. Molecular analysis in Turner syndrome. J Pediatr 2003;142:336–40.

79. MacGillivray MH, Morishima A, Conte F, Grumbach M, Smith EP. Pediatric endocrinology update: an overview. The essential roles of estrogens in pubertal growth, epiphyseal fusion and bone turnover: lessons from mutations in the genes for aromatase and the estrogen receptor. Hormone Res 1998;49(Suppl 1):2–8.

80. Magee AC, Nevin NC, Armstrong MJ, McGibbon D, Nevin J. Ullrich–Turner syndrome: seven pregnancies in an apparent 45,X woman. Am J Med Genet 1998;75:1–3.

81. Manuel M, Katayama PK, Jones HW, Jr. The age of occurrence of gonadal tumors in intersex patients with a Y chromosome. Am J Obstet Gynecol 1976;124:293–300.

82. Martinez-Pasarell O, Nogues C, Bosch M, Egozcue J, Templado C. Analysis of sex chromosome aneuploidy in sperm from fathers of Turner syndrome patients. Hum Genet 1999;104:345–9.

83. Matsuki S, Sasagawa I, Kakizaki H, Suzuki Y, Nakada T. Testicular teratoma in a man with XX/XXY mosaic Klinefelter's syndrome. J Urol 1999;161:1573–4.

84. Mazza V, Di Monte I, Ceccarelli PL, et al. Prenatal diagnosis of female pseudohermaphroditism associated with bilateral luteoma of pregnancy. Hum Reprod 2002;17:821–4.

85. Mazzanti L, Cicognani A, Baldazzi L, et al. Gonadoblastoma in Turner syndrome and Y-chromosome-derived material. Am J Med Genet A 2005;135:150–4.

86. McNeill SA, O'Donnell M, Donat R, Lessells A, Hargreave TB. Estrogen secretion from a malignant sex cord stromal tumor in a patient with complete androgen insensitivity. Am J Obstet Gynecol 1997;177:1541–2.

87. McPhaul MJ, Griffin JE. Male pseudohermaphroditism caused by mutations of the human androgen receptor. J Clin Endocrinol Metab 1999;84:3435–41.

88. Mendes JRT, Strufaldi MWL, Delcelo R, et al. Y-chromosome identification by PCR and gonadal histopathology in Turner's syndrome without overt Y-mosaicism. Clin Endocrinol 1999;50:19–26.

89. Mendez JP, Ulloa-Aguirre A, Kofman-Alfaro S, et al. Mixed gonadal dysgenesis: clinical, cytogenetic, endocrinological, and histopathological findings in 16 patients. Am J Med Genet 1993;46:263–7.

90. Mendonca BB, Arnhold IJ, Bloise W, Andersson S, Russell DW, Wilson JD. 17 Beta-hydroxysteroid dehydrogenase 3 deficiency in women. J Clin Endocrinol Metab 1999;84:802–4.

91. Mendonca BB, Inacio M, Arnhold IJP, et al. Male pseudohermaphroditism due to 17 beta-hydroxysteroid dehydrogenase 3 deficiency – diagnosis, psychological evaluation, and management. Medicine (Baltimore) 2000;79:299–309.

92. Merry C, Sweeney B, Puri P. The vanishing testis: anatomical and histological findings. Eur Urol 1997;31:65–6.

93. Meyers CM, Boughman JA, Rivas M, Wilroy RS, Simpson JL. Gonadal (ovarian) dysgenesis in 46,XX individuals: frequency of the autosomal recessive form. Am J Med Genet 1996;63:518–24.

94. Moran C, Knochenhauer ES, Azziz R. Non-classic adrenal hyperplasia in hyperandrogenism: a reappraisal. J Endocrinol Invest 1998;21:707–20.

95. Morel Y, Rey R, Teinturier C, et al. Aetiological diagnosis of male sex ambiguity: a collaborative study. Eur J Pediatr 2002;161:49–59.

96. Morimura Y, Nishiyama H, Yanagida K, Sato A. Dysgerminoma with syncytiotrophoblastic giant cells arising from 46,XX pure gonadal dysgenesis. Obstet Gynecol 1998;92(4 Pt 2 Suppl):654–6.

97. Naguib KK, Al-Etreibi NN, Al-Awadi SA, El-Harbi MK, Kamal AS. Complete testicular feminization syndrome with 47,XYY karyotype: a double hit phenomenon. Med Princ Pract 1997;6:216–21.

98. New MI. Diagnosis and management of congenital adrenal hyperplasia. Annu Rev Med 1998;49:311–28.

99. Newfield RS, New MI. 21-hydroxylase deficiency. Ann N Y Acad Sci 1997;816:219–29.

100. Niaudet P, Gubler MC. WT1 and glomerular diseases. Pediatr Nephrol 2006;21:1653–60.

101. Nomura K, Matsui T, Aizawa S. Gonadoblastoma with proliferation resembling Sertoli cell tumor. Int J Gynecol Pathol 1999;18:91–3.

102. Nowaczyk MJ, Whelan DT, Heshka TW, Hill RE. Smith–Lemli–Opitz syndrome: a treatable inherited error of metabolism causing mental retardation. Can Med Assoc J 1999;161:165–70.

103. Okada H, Gotoh A, Takechi Y, Kamidono S. Leydig cell tumour of the testis associated with Klinefelter's syndrome and Osgood–Schlatter disease. Br J Urol 1994;73:457.

104. Opitz JM. RSH (so-called Smith–Lemli–Opitz) syndrome. Curr Opin Pediatr 1999;11:353–62.

105. Ounap K, Uibo O, Zordania R, et al. Three patients with 9p deletions including DMRT1 and DMRT2: a girl with XY complement, bilateral ovotestes, and extreme growth retardation, and two XX females with normal pubertal development. Am J Med Genet 2004;130:415–23.

106. Park JP, Brothman AR, Butler MG, et al. Extensive analysis of mosaicism in a case of Turner syndrome: the experience of 287 cytogenetic laboratories. College of American Pathologists/American College of Medical Genetics Cytogenetics Resource Committee. Arch Pathol Lab Med 1999;123:381–5.

107. Pena-Alonso R, Nieto K, Alvarez R, et al. Distribution of Y-chromosome-bearing cells in gonadoblastoma and dysgenetic testis in 45,X/46,XY infants. Mod Pathol 2005;18:439–45.

108. Pierga JY, Giacchetti S, Vilain E, et al. Dysgerminoma in a pure 45,X Turner syndrome: report of a case and review of the literature. Gynecol Oncol 1994;55(3 Part 1):459–64.

109. Porter FD. Human malformation syndromes due to inborn errors of cholesterol synthesis. Curr Opin Pediatr 2003;15:607–13.

110. Quigley CA, DeBellis A, Marschke KB, El-Awady MF, Wilson EM, French FS. Androgen receptor defects: historical, clinical, and molecular perspectives. Endocrinol Rev 1995;16:271–321.

111. Radakovic B, Jukic S, Bukovic D, Ljubojevic N, Cima I. Morphology of gonads in pure XY gonadal dysgenesis. Coll Antropol 1999;23:203–11.

112. Regadera J, Martinez-Garcia F, Paniagua R, Nistal M. Androgen insensitivity syndrome – an immunohistochemical, ultrastructural, and morphometric study. Arch Pathol Lab Med 1999;123:225–34.

113. Reiner WG. Assignment of sex in neonates with ambiguous genitalia. Curr Opin Pediatr 1999;11:363–5.

114. Rey R, Sabourin JC, Venara M, et al. Anti-Mullerian hormone is a specific marker of sertoli- and granulosa-cell origin in gonadal tumors. Hum Pathol 2000;31:1202–8.

115. Reynaud K, Cortvrindt R, Verlinde F, De Schepper J, Bourgain C, Smitz J. Number of ovarian follicles in human fetuses with the 45,X karyotype. Fertil Steril 2004;81:1112–9.

116. Rich MA, Keating MA, Levin HS, Kay R. Tumors of the adrenogenital syndrome: an aggressive conservative approach. J Urol 1998;160:1838–41.

117. Rizk DEE, Ezimokhai M, Hussein AS, Gerami S, Deb P. Persistent Mullerian duct syndrome. Arch Gynecol Obstet 1998;261:105–7.

118. Robboy SJ, Jaubert F. Neoplasms and pathology of sexual developmental disorders (intersex). Pathology 2007;39:147–63.

119. Robboy SJ, Miller T, Donahoe PK, et al. Dysgenesis of testicular and streak gonads in the syndrome of mixed gonadal dysgenesis: perspective derived

from a clinicopathologic analysis of twenty-one cases. Hum Pathol 1982;13:700–16.

120. Rutgers JL. Advances in the pathology of intersex conditions. Hum Pathol 1991;22:884–91.

121. Rutgers JL, Scully RE. The androgen insensitivity syndrome (testicular feminization): a clinicopathologic study of 43 cases. Int J Gynecol Pathol 1991;10:126–44.

122. Rutgers JL, Young RH, Scully RE. The testicular 'tumor' of the adrenogenital syndrome. A report of six cases and review of the literature on testicular masses in patients with adrenocortical disorders. Am J Surg Pathol 1988;12:503–13.

123. Saxena AK, van Tuil C, Schultze-Everding A. Frasier syndrome in a pre-menarchal girl: laparoscopic resection of gonadoblastoma. Eur J Pediatr 2006;165:917–9.

124. Scherer G, Held M, Erdel M, et al. Three novel SRY mutations in XY gonadal dysgenesis and the enigma of XY gonadal dysgenesis cases without SRY mutations. Cytogenet Cell Genet 1998;80:188–92.

125. Scully RE, Young RH, Clement RB. Tumors of the Ovary, Maldeveloped Gonads, Fallopian Tube, and Broad Ligament, 3rd edn. Washington, DC: Armed Forces Institute of Pathology; 1998.

126. Semerci CN, Satiroglu-Tufan NL, Turan S, et al. Detection of Y chromosomal material in patients with a 45,X karyotype by PCR method. Tohoku J Exp Med 2007;211:243–9.

127. Shinmura Y, Yokoi T, Tsutsui Y. A case of clear cell adenocarcinoma of the mullerian duct in persistent mullerian duct syndrome: the first reported case. Am J Surg Pathol 2002;26:1231–4.

128. Sinnecker GH, Hiort O, Dibbelt L, et al. Phenotypic classification of male pseudohermaphroditism due to steroid 5 alpha-reductase 2 deficiency. Am J Med Genet 1996;63:223–30.

129. Skordis N, Patsalis PC, Bacopoulou L, Sismani C, Sultan C, Lumbroso S. 5 alpha-reductase 2 gene mutations in three unrelated patients of Greek Cypriot origin: identification of an ancestral founder effect. J Pediatr Endocrinol Metab 2005;18:241–6.

130. Slaney SF, Chalmers IJ, Affara NA, Chitty LS. An autosomal or X linked mutation results in true hermaphrodites and 46,XX males in the same family. J Med Genet 1998;35:17–22.

131. Smith NM, Byard RW, Bourne AJ. Testicular regression syndrome – a pathological study of 77 cases. Histopathology 1991;19:269–72.

132. Spires SE, Woolums CS, Pulito AR, Spires SM. Testicular regression syndrome – a clinical and pathologic study of 11 cases. Arch Pathol Lab Med 2000;124:694–8.

133. Talerman A, Verp MS, Senekjian E, Gilewski T, Vogelzang N. True hermaphrodite with bilateral ovotestes, bilateral gonadoblastomas and dysgerminomas, 46,XX/46,XY karyotype, and a successful pregnancy. Cancer 1990;66:2668–72.

134. Tanaka Y, Sasaki Y, Tachibana K, Suwa S, Terashima K, Nakatani Y. Testicular juvenile granulosa cell tumor in an infant with X/XY mosaicism clinically diagnosed as true hermaphroditism. Am J Surg Pathol 1994;18:316–22.

135. Tateno T, Sasagawa I, Ashida J, Nakada T. Deletion of Y chromosome involving the DAZ (deleted in azoospermia) gene in XX males. Arch Androl 1999;42:179–83.

136. Telvi L, Lebbar A, Del Pino O, Barbet JP, Chaussain JL. 45,X/46,XY mosaicism: report of 27 cases. Pediatrics 1999;104(2 Pt 1):304–8.

137. Tsutsumi O, Iida T, Nakahori Y, Taketani Y. Analysis of the testis-determining gene SRY in patients with XY gonadal dysgenesis. Horm Res 1996;46(Suppl 1):6–10.

138. Uehara S, Funato T, Yaegashi N, et al. SRY mutation and tumor formation on the gonads of XY pure gonadal dysgenesis patients. Cancer Genet Cytogenet 1999;113:78–84.

139. Uehara S, Tamura M, Nata M, et al. Complete androgen insensitivity in a 47,XXY patient with uniparental disomy for the X chromosome. Am J Med Genet 1999;86:107–11.

140. van Niekerk WA, Retief AE. The gonads of human true hermaphrodites. Hum Genet 1981;58:117–22.

141. Vanderbijl AE, Fleuren GJ, Kenter GG, Dejong D. Unique combination of an ovarian gonadoblastoma, dysgerminoma, and mucinous cystadenoma in a patient with Turners syndrome – a cytogenetic and molecular analysis. Int J Gynecol Pathol 1994;13:267–72.

142. Vanslooten AJ, Rechner SF, Dodds WG. Recurrent maternal virilization during pregnancy caused by benign androgen-producing ovarian lesions. Am J Obstet Gynecol 1992;167:1342–3.

143. Vauthier-Brouzes D, Vanna Lim-You K, Sebagh E, Lefebvre G, Darbois Y. Krukenberg tumor during pregnancy with maternal and fetal virilization: a difficult diagnosis. A case report. J Gynecol Obstet Biol Reprod (Paris) 1997;26:831–3.

144. Veitia R, Ion A, Barbaux S, et al. Mutations and sequence variants in the testis-determining region of the Y chromosome in individuals with a 46,XY female phenotype. Hum Genet 1997;99:648–52.

145. Velidedeoglu HV, Coskunfirat OK, Bozdogan MN, Sahin U, Turkguven Y. The surgical management of incomplete testicular feminization syndrome in three sisters. Br J Plastic Surg 1997;50:212–6.

146. Verkauskas G, Jaubert F, Lortat-Jacob S, Malan V, Thibaud E, Nihoul-Fekete C. The long-term followup of 33 cases of true hermaphroditism: a 40-year experience with conservative gonadal surgery. J Urol 2007;177:726–31; discussion 731.

147. Vialard F, Ottolenghi C, Gonzales M, et al. Deletion of 9p associated with gonadal dysfunction in 46,XY but not in 46,XX human fetuses. J Med Genet 2002;39:514–8.

148. Vilain E, McCabe ERB. Mammalian sex determination: from gonads to brain. Mol Genet Metab 1998;65:74–84.

149. Vilain E, Jaubert F, Fellous M, McElreavey K. Pathology of 46,XY pure gonadal dysgenesis: absence of testis differentiation associated with mutations in the testis-determining factor. Differentiation 1993; 52:151–9.

150. Viner RM, Teoh Y, Williams DM, Patterson MN, Hughes IA. Androgen insensitivity syndrome: a survey of diagnostic procedures and management in the UK. Arch Dis Child 1997;77:305–9.

151. Volkl TM, Langer T, Aigner T, et al. Klinefelter syndrome and mediastinal germ cell tumors. Am J Med Genet 2006;140:471–81.

152. Wang NJ, Song HR, Schanen NC, Litman NL, Frasier SD. Frasier syndrome comes full circle: genetic studies performed in an original patient. J Pediatr 2005;146:843–4.

153. Watanabe M, Zinn AR, Page DC, Nishimoto T. Functional equivalence of human X- and Y-encoded isoforms of ribosomal protein S4 consistent with a role in Turner syndrome. Nat Genet 1993;4:268–71.

154. Winters JL, Chapman PH, Powell DE, Banks ER, Allen WR, Wood DP. Female pseudohermaphroditism due to congenital adrenal hyperplasia complicated by adenocarcinoma of the prostate and clear cell carcinoma of the endometrium. Am J Clin Pathol 1996;106:660–4.

155. Zhao S, Kato N, Endoh Y, Jin Z, Ajioka Y, Motoyama T. Ovarian gonadoblastoma with mixed germ cell tumor in a woman with 46,XX karyotype and successful pregnancies. Pathol Int 2000;50: 332–5.

156. Zhu YS, Katz MD, Imperato-McGinley J. Natural potent androgens: lessons from human genetic models. Baillieres Clin Endocrinol Metab 1998;12:83–113.

157. Zinn AR, Tonk VS, Chen Z, et al. Evidence for a Turner syndrome locus or loci at Xp11.2–p22.1. Am J Hum Genet 1998;63:1757–66.

Cutup – gross description and processing of specimens

35

Stanley J. Robboy   George L. Mutter   Ruthy Shako-Levy   Sarah M. Bean
Jaime Prat   Rex C. Bentley   Peter Russell

GENERAL ASPECTS

The surgical pathologist reports the histopathologic diagnosis and specific information relating to prognosis and treatment, and, therefore, must have sufficient familiarity with the management of gynecologic and obstetric disorders to assure that the report, as its major focus, communicates the clinically relevant information. This chapter provides an approach to the processing of gynecologic and obstetric tissue specimens. The techniques of gross examination and the method of reporting the pathologic findings are guided by the clinical principles on which patient management is based. Several textbooks are now devoted entirely to this topic.[8,12,14]

In general, most tissue specimens submitted to the surgical pathology laboratory fall into one of two categories:

- biopsy specimens, or
- therapeutic resections.

The philosophies differ in the techniques used in the examination of each, although some specimens such as cervical cone/loop electrosurgical excision procedure (LEEP) biopsies and lymph node resections serve both purposes.

The main purpose of a biopsy is to provide a histologic diagnosis that will guide management. Since biopsy specimens tend to be small and without specific gross diagnostic features, the major pathology resides in the tissue slides. The gross description plays a relatively unimportant role other than to ensure that what is received in the pathology laboratory and submitted for microscopic examination matches the slides returned from the histology laboratory for the pathologist to examine. Any apparent disparity between the findings on a slide and that expected based on the gross description is often the only clue that a slide or block may have been mislabeled. A good gross description should be therefore precise and brief. Examples of good descriptions are '3 ovoid fragments 2 to 4 mm in diameter', 'multiple shreds of tissue 5 cm in aggregate' or the exact size given in three dimensions. For some specimens, it is also useful to note whether it is largely blood, mucin or tissue. When the case may need review later, only the tissue slides themselves are used. Generally, the gross description will be of little utility at that later time.

In therapeutic resections in contrast, the gross description that the pathologist provides is often the most important aspect of the entire report. These are usually larger operative specimens, and the pathologist is the only person who has the specimen available for examination. Once the specimen is examined in the gross state and dissected, it is normally discarded after several weeks; after that time, the gross specimen is no longer available for any other physician to examine. There is no way at later times to return to the specimen and determine the position and size of any lesion, its margins, its relations to neighboring organs, or any other facets about its growth pattern.

For operative specimens, particularly those containing a malignancy, information in the surgical pathology report should describe the extent of the tumor and specific features that relate to prognosis and staging. The adequacy of the surgical treatment as well as the need for additional therapy depends on these findings. Since the gynecologic surgeon has seen the pathology in vivo, it is important that the surgeon communicate the operative findings, since these will bear directly on how the pathologist processes the specimen. For example, adequacy of resection margins requires an appreciation of the orientation of the specimen to certain anatomic landmarks that are obvious to the surgeon, but which the pathologist cannot always reconstruct in the laboratory.

A good gross description enables the reader to reconstruct an image that corresponds to the specimen and its lesion. Since the histologic diagnosis for many tumors has been made by biopsy before the operative procedure, the gross description of the specimen should focus on the site and extent of the lesion and its relationship to adjacent structures. Key findings should be suggested from the gross examination of the specimen. Microscopic findings should be complementary to those identified grossly, and it should be uncommon for them to be in conflict. A careful gross examination is mandatory to ensure that the appropriate microscopic sections are obtained. Conversely, an inattentive gross examination often leads to preparation of needless 'representative' slides (read: 'haphazard' or 'taken without thinking'), or worse yet, an incorrect diagnosis.

Inclusion or absence of microscopic descriptions within the report varies by custom in differing countries and even to individual pathologists within a single department; if absent, they should not alter the effectiveness of the report. If present, they should be brief and add information not already apparent from the final diagnosis. For example, there is no need to describe tubules and cysts lined by cells with bulbous nuclei protruding into the lumen when the final diagnosis is 'clear cell adenocarcinoma, tubulocystic type'. Conversely, in cases lacking a microscopic description, often pertinent microscopic findings germane to the clinician can be added to a comment following the diagnosis. In the US, where payment requires proof that a procedure was performed, every stain, whether with positive or non-contributory findings, needs to be mentioned somewhere in the report.

The final diagnosis of a tumor should include its cell type, grade, dimensions, location, and extent, as well as the adequacy of the resection margins, presence of lymphatic or vascular invasion, and status of the regional lymph nodes. It is one thing to report an 'endometrial adenocarcinoma' but far better to report 'serous carcinoma of the endometrium extensive throughout the corpus with vascular invasion, penetrating to within 0.2 mm of the 1.2 cm thick myometrium, with metastases to 2 of 24 lymph nodes' with a detailed listing to follow of which lymph nodes, and how many in each group, are involved. The former merely reaffirms what was known before the operation, whereas the latter presents information that helps to predict prognosis and plan further treatment. Since 2004, all hospitals wishing to achieve certification/designation as a cancer institute by the American College of Surgeons must issue reports listing all of the data points deemed mandatory by the College of American Pathologists. Appendix C addresses the details of reporting, but suffice it to say here that an appropriate gross description and selection of blocks for microscopy requires a full understanding of what should be in the final report for each specimen type, and why.

SECTION CODES AND THE REPORT

Many operations result in two or more separate specimens being submitted to the pathology department. Cervical examinations often produce two or three colposcopically directed biopsies plus an endocervical curettage. Twenty or more specimens from a staging laparotomy are also common. As a first step, each container received should be numbered and checked against the clinical manifest to ensure that all specimens removed have in fact reached the pathologist. This information is usually listed on the requisition sheet ('specimens submitted'). Each specimen should be uniquely labeled (see below). Payment issues also require that each container be given an identifiable diagnosis.

TYPES OF SECTION CODE

It is important that every department settle on a numbering system that is clear and used consistently throughout the specimen. The most common systems in use today are computer generated, providing the accession number for the overall case, the container number for each portion of the specimen when it is received in multiple parts, an identifier for each paraffin block, the level within each paraffin block, and the type of stain used with any given slide.

Most systems use a one- or two-letter prefix to identify the general type of case received (S = surgical, C or P = cytology, and A = autopsy), followed by a two-digit number designating the year (00 = 2000), followed by a sequential five- or six-digit number. One system, in common use worldwide, then assigns a unique letter to each container received, starting at the beginning of the alphabet, i.e., 'A'. Each block sampled from that specimen/container then receives a sequential number, e.g., A1, A2, . . . An. Each subsequent specimen/container receives the next available letter, e.g., B, with multiple blocks from the container having sequential numbers, B1 . . . Bn. If multiple levels of a single paraffin block are made, a practice for cervical biopsies in many institutions, the letter 'L' is appended with the designation of the slide level, e.g., -L2 for the second level of the block. Thus a typical specimen number might be SG-00-02167 B4-L2, which translates to 'Surgical specimen of a gynecologic nature, received in year 2000, accession number 2167, container B, fourth block taken from specimen B, and second slide prepared from that paraffin block'. Variants of the above system typically utilize letters in upper and lower case, Roman numerals, and Arabic numbers, usually in some combination and defined sequence. (Of course, multiple numbering systems exist, and it is not the purpose of this chapter to pick which is best; the purpose is rather to help ensure that whatever system used is clear, such that any other person not associated with the case can determine solely from the slide number exactly what area of the specimen was sampled.)

In departments where numbers are assigned manually, some systems label all blocks consecutively regardless of the parent container. The block number may be in alphabetical order, e.g., A, B, C . . . Z, proceeding thereafter to AA. After AZ, proceed to BA and so forth. Another method common in manual systems is to label organs with letters, e.g., RO and LO for right and left ovaries. Although this method has the advantage of providing an intuitive link to the organ sampled, it may lead to ambiguities when dealing with margins and relations with other organs, and sometimes leads to overly complex lettering schemes. This method is usually only practical in a group of one or two pathologists who can agree on the abbreviations chosen. Use of idiosyncratic labeling systems can cause significant difficulty for other pathologists attempting to review these cases.

LOCATION OF SECTION CODES IN THE REPORT

Most pathologists prefer a section code summary at the end of the gross while some prefer entering block codes within the gross text. In either case, the report must be clear, both to the pathologist and to any person who at a later time will need to utilize the report. Block summaries, if used, by necessity duplicate substantial parts of the gross, but cannot be used in its place. In general, inclusion within the gross offers greater clarity and brevity when describing a lesion that has some unusual feature, e.g., a probable leiomyosarcoma. 'The borders in one region are sharp and distinct from the surrounding myometrium (Block B10) while elsewhere it blends into the adjacent myometrium (Block B11).' Integration within the gross is clearer and easier to write than repeating the verbiage in detail in the block summary. If the codes are listed sequentially at the end of the report, the site and feature identified require presentation in sufficient detail so that the reader can link the gross description with the slide. Using the example above, it would be inappropriate for the coding block at the end to state B10 and B11 are myometrium as it is unclear which sample has the sharp borders and is probably a leiomyomatous tumor and which has blurred borders and may potentially be sarcomatous. A section code at the end might better read, 'B10 Myometrium, sharply circumscribed medial border'.

SPECIMEN AND SITE IDENTIFICATION

Regardless of the section code method used, it is critical that the reader can link the tissues received to the sections processed and both to the final diagnoses. For example, four cervical biopsies from the same patient are received in separate containers, but from the same operation. Information on the requisition slip indicates the colposcopically directed specimens are from 3, 6, 9, and 12 o'clock, respectively. In this example, the accession number might be SG-00-02167, and the containers are labeled A, B, C, and D, respectively. Since the paraffin block usually is identified solely by the code, then this same code should appear throughout. Thus, the gross might read 'A. 3:00 bx' (the wording exactly replicating what the clinician wrote on the container itself) while the final diagnosis would include 'A. Cervix, Biopsy at 3 o'clock: Diagnostic finding'. Obviously, the label on the slide must provide all of the necessary identifiers.

A most perplexing problem we encounter in referred specimens is where the label assigned to the container in the gross description differs in some significant manner from that given in the microscopic description to that given in the final diagnosis. For example, the container might be 'A' in the gross description which refers to a specimen consisting of uterus, ovaries, and fallopian tubes, whereas the final diagnosis is '1. Endometriosis of the ovary'. Such cases require substantial effort on the part of the consultant pathologist to determine (and sometimes guess) which gross description truly belongs to which slide and both to the listed final diagnosis.

GROSS DESCRIPTION

If possible, describe specimens received in the fresh state before fixation. Formalin alters natural color and consistency of tissue. The opening sentence of the gross description should indicate how the tissue is received (fresh or fixed) and labeled. Does the specimen received correspond with its label? For example, the container received states 'Uterus, tubes, and ovaries', yet the left adnexa is absent. Such a gross description might read, 'Received fresh is a uterus and right ovary and fallopian tube. The left ovary and fallopian tube are absent.' Give measurements and weights of the individual diseased organs (e.g., 'the 710 g, 18 × 15 × 8 cm uterus'). Conglomerate measurements and weights are meaningless (uterus, tubes, and ovaries which together weigh 710 g and measure 18 × 15 × 8 cm) since they are ambiguous as to the role played by each organ and where the pathology resides. Rather than removing and weighing each organ, estimate by subtracting the estimated weight of the uninvolved organs.

The gross description should proceed in an orderly fashion, focusing on the primary lesion. Several common methods are in use. In one, the pathology in any given container/specimen is emphasized first. This highlights the pathology and de-emphasizes the normal. In practice, descriptions are full but economical in words and space. The second method is to follow a routine pattern whereby the same order is followed in every case, e.g., ovary, fallopian tube, uterine corpus, cervix, etc. This method, while usually easier for the novice, lends itself to loquacious reports filled with tedious description. All too often the true pathology is treated least well or even inadequately, as it is buried deep in the description if it is even described. At times the pathology is virtually omitted. Not uncommonly, such travelogues lead to reports several pages long, but with a description of the tumor under several lines in toto. With the novice, detailed descriptions force careful examination, but with experience, can be refined to a more concise and readable form.

Avoid elaborate descriptions of normal incidental anatomy. In a radical hysterectomy for cervical cancer, there is no need for an overly elaborate description of a normal fallopian tube.

The following is excessive, '7 cm long, elongate structure with a 1 mm internal diameter and 4 mm external diameter with a tan, smooth, glistening serosa, a 2 mm thick wall, and a lumen without identifiable abnormality'. Simply 'the fallopian tube is 7 cm long, 4 mm in diameter and unremarkable' will do.

Similarly, we believe experience should allow the pathologist to describe grossly obvious lesions in diagnostic terms rather than non-specific and frequently long-winded descriptions, a practice with which many also disagree. Leiomyoma, or where useful, the diagnostic term with one or two adjectives ('well circumscribed, whorled leiomyoma'), is far more useful than the excessive description ('numerous, discrete, circumscribed, rounded lesions with a bulging whorled cut surface, white in color, and compressing the adjacent myometrium') which is tedious to read. At worst the description is vague ('rounded lesions'). Purposeful uncertainty, where it exists, can also be introduced with adjectives ('5 cm soft, focally necrotic leiomyomatous nodule with irregular borders suspicious for sarcomatous change').

The gross description, especially of small specimens, should conclude stating how much of the tissue has been processed for microscopic examination. This is especially important in the case of endometrial curettings removed for a suspected intra-uterine pregnancy where neither chorionic villi nor other tissues of fetal origin are found and all of the tissue has been submitted. Specify the number of each type of block sampled and from where each was obtained. An example of a useful gross description is: 'The endometrium, which is 2 mm thick, discloses no obvious tumor. The entire endometrium including the superficial myometrium is blocked and submitted *in toto*.'

INKING

Application of ink, often in multiple colors, can be useful to identify margins that lack natural boundaries (e.g., various surgical margins) or to determine if the lesion present truly involves the margin or is present only where the tissue has been cut on a bias, thus simulating a margin. If used, apply sparingly and blot dry the applied ink to prevent spill-over or running. Acetone or distilled white vinegar can be used to set the ink. As inking is a procedure all too often done indiscriminately, determine first whether it is even useful. There is no need to ink a uterine serosa in cases of cervical intraepithelial neoplasia (CIN) or in cases where the endometrial cancer is small and non-invasive and the serosa is obviously normal and uninvolved. Ink sometimes is helpful (and sometimes the only clue) in determining the serosa of the ovary replaced by tumor. Determine also that the ink does not inadvertently cover disease, e.g., endometriosis or a metastasis on the serosa.

Sections parallel to margins often are taken to evaluate the excision lines, a method that sometimes can use fewer sections than those taken perpendicular to the line of resection. One difficulty commonly encountered is if tumor is found by the histopathologist to be in the parallel margin. The section may have been taken from the outside of the block or it may have been inadvertently taken from the inside. If tangential margins are used, then the inner face should be inked telling the histology technologist to sample the other (non-inked) side when preparing the histology slides.

DRAWINGS AND PHOTOGRAPHS

Include drawings and/or photographs if this simplifies portrayal of complicated relationships or permits better orientation, especially of surgical resection margins. Today, most photographs use digital technology. Document scanners can also be used for this purpose and can create surprisingly high-quality images. Block diagrams can be made from digital photographs or Xerox copies and are particularly useful in complex cases.

FIXATIVES

Formalin-based fixatives are generally the most practical and commonly used today. A specimen submitted for tissue processing should be less than 3 mm thick. Thicker specimens are difficult to dehydrate and inhibit paraffin infiltration, thus leading to inadequate slides. Sometimes, it is much easier and more efficient to cut blocks from tissue that has been fixed for several hours instead of attempting to cut 3 mm thick slices directly from the fresh specimen. Large specimens should be cross-sectioned and cut at intervals 1 cm thick. This permits adequate penetration by formalin, after which the tissue can be trimmed into 3 mm thick blocks. For large specimens, e.g., uteri removed for leiomyomata, placing the tissue blocks into cassettes (with all labeling complete) and retaining them in the fluid fixative for an extra day facilitates better sections.

With the advent of a rapidly increasing library of immunocytochemical techniques that will work with paraffin-embedded tissue, two common practices of the past are less common today. One has been to fix some tissue from tumors in glutaraldehyde for possible electron microscopy or examination with 1 μm thick sections. This is now largely confined to sarcomas, lymphomas, pediatric tumors, and pituitary tumors. The other is to snap freeze tissues for immunocytochemical analyses where formalin fixation destroys the ability of the antibodies to bind to the sought antigens.

NUMBER OF SECTIONS REQUIRED

Judging what number of blocks must be sampled to optimally examine a specimen is one of the more controversial subjects not only in gynecologic pathology, but in all branches of surgical pathology. In general, the authors believe that far too many blocks are taken, adding expense but not furthering the diagnostic information gained. A useful exercise is to determine what single slide would be taken if the entire prosection permitted were limited to the single slide. This forces thinking about which single slide would demonstrate the lesion as well as pertinent margins or neighboring relations. Such forethought often has a major influence on how a specimen is opened and/or sampled. For example, an excisional biopsy of vulvar tumor might be best sampled by six equidistant perpendicular blocks sampling the central tumor, deep margin, and lateral margins rather than eight tangential lateral margins, shave margins of the base, and several of only the tumor. Leiomyomas/equivocal leiomyosarcomas should include not only the tumor but also the neighboring tissue and margins if possible. Endometrial tumors can easily be sampled to include the adjacent 'normal' endometrium.

SYNOPTIC CHECKLISTS

As the complexity of information contained in reports increases and tumor cases are accessioned into trials with specific entry criteria, checklists are being used with increasing frequency to record and evaluate the details of operative and pathologic findings. Appendix C covers this topic fully.

VULVA[2]

EXCISIONAL BIOPSIES

Biopsies of the vulva should be handled like skin biopsies. Assess the deep and lateral resection margins. Have the surgeon place a suture for orientation. Ink (often in several colors for orientation) facilitates recognition on microscopic examination.

WIDE LOCAL EXCISION

These specimens are usually highly variable in their composition. In general, wide local excisions are performed for non-invasive neoplasms such as VIN 3 or Pagets disease of the vulva, as well as superficially invasive (less than 1 mm) stage 1 carcinomas. Lymph node dissections are added for stage 1B carcinomas (greater than 1 mm invasive). Orientation is critical in these specimens and if not clearly indicated, consultation with the surgeon may be required prior to fixation and examination. Operative specimens often include labia minora and majora, clitoris, perineal body, and perianal tissue (Figure 35.1). Describe and measure the lesions, distances to resection margins, and the anatomic structures involved. Examine the coloration and surface texture carefully as intraepithelial lesions are subtle, being typically red-brown to white and roughened.

As lesions are often multifocal and difficult to discern macroscopically, examine all surgical resection margins microscopically. This requires sections through all obvious lesions to exclude the presence of invasive carcinoma, and sections from all the peripheral resection margins. Sections parallel to margins ('tangential') are often taken to evaluate the excision lines, a method that sometimes can use fewer sections than those taken perpendicular to the line of resection. This method is particularly useful for tumors such as Pagets disease that are notorious for being extensive and cannot be seen grossly at the margin. One difficulty commonly encountered is to determine if tumor found in the slide truly involves the margin or was from the inner face, and therefore not a true representation of the margin. This is discussed more fully in the section above on 'Inking'.

For tumors that are discreet and can be seen, such as squamous cell carcinoma, we feel that multiple radial sections are more advantageous as the central lesion, margins, and intervening areas can be included in one slide and tumor close to the margin is easier to evaluate (Figure 35.2). Facilitate sectioning by pinning the specimen on a corkboard or a block of paraffin and fix first for several hours or overnight. When pinned to a corkboard, the specimen can then be floated upside down in a tub of formalin, which avoids compression that gravity

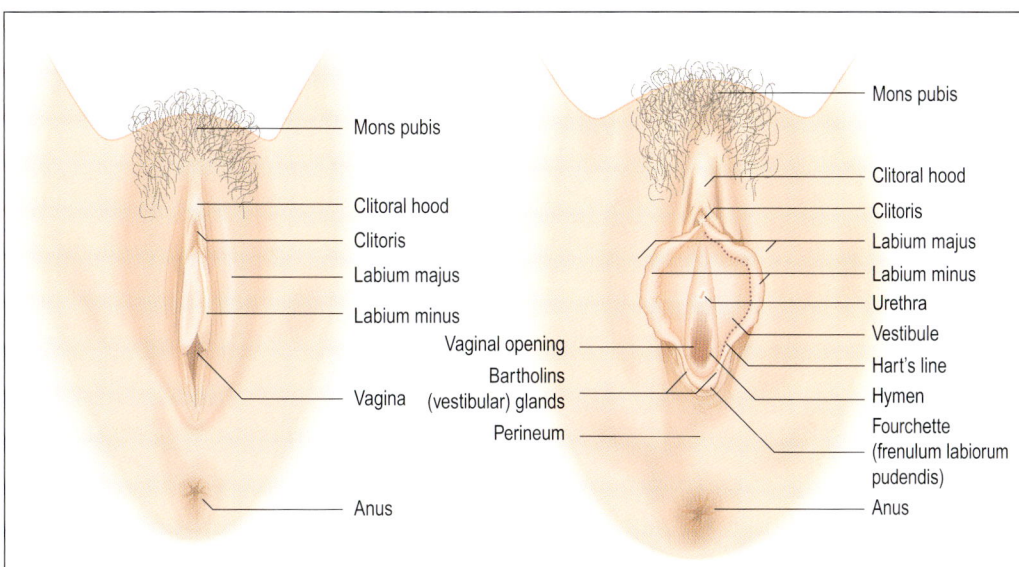

Fig. 35.1 External genitalia.

Mons pubis

Clitoral hood
Clitoris
Labium majus
Labium minus
Vaginal opening
Bartholins (vestibular) glands
Vagina
Perineum
Anus

Mons pubis

Clitoral hood
Clitoris
Labium majus
Labium minus
Urethra
Vestibule
Hart's line
Hymen
Fourchette (frenulum labiorum pudendis)
Anus

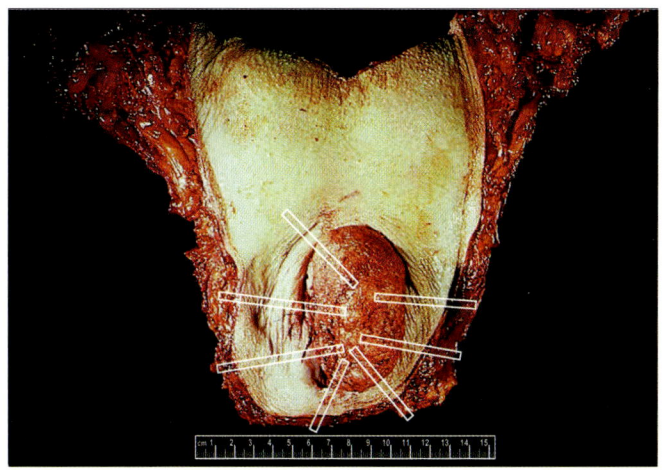

Fig. 35.2 Radial sections for examination of vulvar cancer. Sections, which are full thickness, include tumor and all margins.

otherwise introduces. Diagrams or photographs are often useful if the number of sections taken is substantial or relations are complicated.

SKINNING VULVECTOMY

A skinning vulvectomy removes the superficial vulvar skin at the level of the dermis, preserving the clitoris, and replacing it with a split thickness skin graft. Because this preserves the underlying vulvar soft tissue, the vulvar contour is retained, and there is improved cosmetic outcome and sexual function. This is by definition a superficial excision, meaning it is performed almost entirely for non-invasive neoplasms (VIN 3 and Pagets disease). The gross description will be similar to that of wide local excision.

SIMPLE (OR TOTAL) VULVECTOMY

This includes the entire vulva and subcutaneous fat (dissection to deep fascia). It is typically performed for non-invasive neoplasms that widely involve the vulva. Pin, fix, and section the specimen at 0.5 cm intervals to evaluate for invasive carcinoma. For Pagets disease, palpate the underlying dermis for associated carcinoma. Typically, the extent of Pagets disease exceeds that visible macroscopically as occult foci are often present within normal-appearing skin. The resection margins must be thoroughly evaluated, but use discretion for the number of sections submitted! As Pagets disease frequently recurs even with pathologically 'negative' margins, some recent studies suggest that margin status may be of little or no value in predicting recurrence.[1,13]

RADICAL VULVECTOMY

Radical vulvectomy consists of vulva excised to the deep fascia of the thigh, the periosteum of the pubis, and the inferior fascia of the urogenital diaphragm. It is most commonly performed together with at least an inguinal lymph node dissection, which may be included en bloc with the vulvectomy. Total radical vulvectomies have largely been replaced in favor of more limited excisions, with the surgery designed to completely excise the primary tumor with a minimum 2 cm margin, and dissection to the deep fascia and periosteum of the pubic symphysis. True radical total vulvectomies are now performed primarily in the setting of large and/or aggressive tumors. The gross description should include the size, location, and depth the primary lesion penetrates, and all resection margins, including perianal and vaginal margins. Sectioning may be aided if the specimen is fixed for several hours or overnight. The technique of pinning and flotation as described above is also useful. Sections should include the tumor, showing the maximum depth of invasion, labia majora and minora, clitoris, distal urethra, resection margins including the vaginal margin, and all lymph nodes. Sections should evaluate the status of the skin immediately adjacent to the primary lesion, as preinvasive disease is often present. Separate lymph nodes into superficial and deep groups (Figure 35.3). Invasive vulvar neoplasms are solitary in contrast to intraepithelial lesions, which are often multifocal. Consequently, evaluation of resection margins can be largely limited to the margins near the tumor. Lymph nodes are best identified in the fresh state. Adequate palpation is crucial. The report should include microscopic diagnosis, tumor grade, dimensions, location and maximum depth of invasion, presence of lymphatic invasion, number and location of involved lymph nodes, and distance to resection margins. Diagrams and/or photographs may be useful aids.

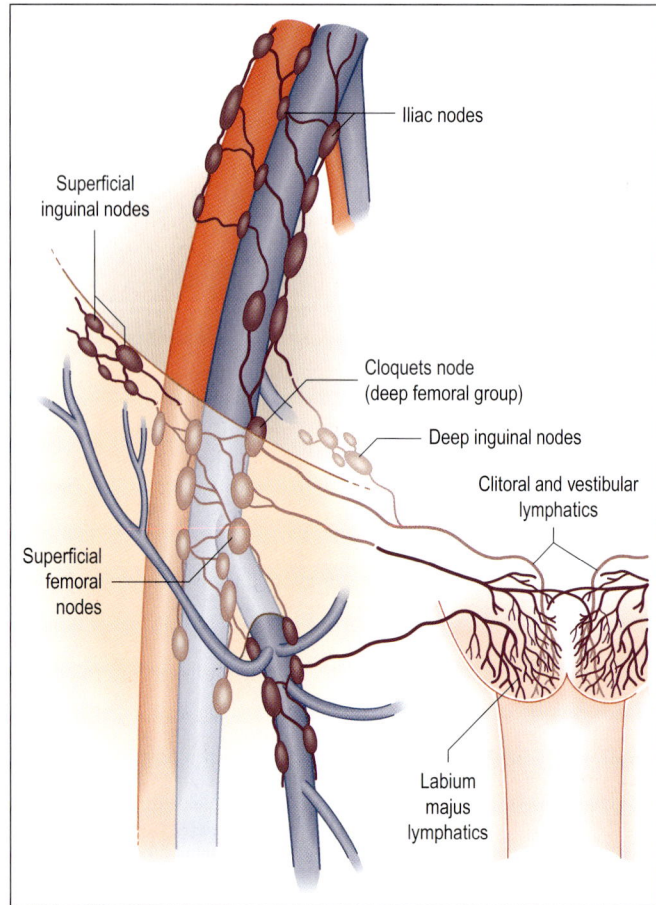

Fig. 35.3 Lymphatics of the vulva. (Modified from Schmidt).[13]

CERVIX[3]

Specimens from the cervix include punch biopsies, endocervical curettages, cone biopsies (various methods), total hysterectomy specimens, and radical hysterectomy specimens.

PUNCH BIOPSIES

Biopsies are usually colposcopically directed. The best specimens are at least several millimeters long with underlying stroma to a depth of 2–4 mm. We do not request that the biopsy be attached to filter paper or any such medium because even if the specimen curls, the presence of epithelium in relation to stroma nearly always permits the correct orientation to be established. It is important to search the container in which the specimen was received, especially the underside of the lid, for any stray fragments of tissue. If the fragments are tiny, they can be placed in a mesh bag for processing. Record the number of pieces received. The fixed, curled biopsy may be bisected transversally to produce two pieces that are approximately pyramidal in shape. These are then embedded with the flat, cut surface downwards so that this surface is cut by the microtome. We cut each biopsy at three levels. This degree of sampling is generally adequate for most purposes and saves substantial

time, effort, and overall cost in reducing the number of time recuts at deeper levels are needed. Step-serial sectioning is not necessary routinely.

Common problems we have encountered in interpreting biopsies are where stroma is absent or the highly dysplastic epithelium is so extensive as to raise the concern that invasion may possibly be present. In both cases the diagnostic impression is given, together with the warning that the possibility of invasion cannot be excluded. When invasion of squamous cells into underlying stroma is seen, the definition of microinvasive carcinoma often precludes that the diagnosis can be made reliably on a colposcopic biopsy. We report the diagnosis in terms such as 'stromal invasion is seen'. Based on the findings, we sometimes attempt to identify whether the lesion is microinvasive or whether the extent of the invasion cannot be determined without a more definitive procedure, e.g., a cone biopsy. Often, it is possible to diagnose clinical cancer (stage 1B or greater) on a colposcopic biopsy definitively if tumor diffusely pervades the entire biopsy specimen. Telephone calls and a close working relation with the gynecologist are important.

ENDOCERVICAL CURETTAGE

Endocervical curettage is performed to evaluate the presence of endocervical neoplasms, cervical neoplasia in the endocervical canal, or to determine whether endometrial carcinoma has spread into the cervix. As subsequent clinical management depends upon whether disease is present in the curettings, considerable care must be exercised in handling specimens, which typically are scant and composed mostly of blood and mucus. Endocervical scrapings should be submitted as a separate specimen in a mesh bag (e.g., a Shandon mesh bag or tea bag) before being placed into the cassette. This avoids small fragments of tissue from becoming lost during processing. Most cancers, when present in the curettage specimen, are generally easy to diagnose.

Several problems we have encountered with some frequency create an element of uncertainty in the validity of diagnosis. All revolve about detached fragments of intraepithelial neoplasia. The question arises whether the fragment with slightly atypical nuclei represents a tangential cut of normal epithelium or CIN. The presence of any dysplastic tissue in the endocervical specimen will often lead the gynecologist to consider additional therapy, or at least additional diagnostic workup. The second situation occurs with the finding of atypical glandular nuclei bathed in mucin. We have seen this represent small endocervical carcinomas. A third situation is where the endocervical curettage has been performed in conjunction with a cone biopsy/loop procedure. Any disease present in the curettage can be considered endocervical in origin if the curettage has been performed after the cone/loop procedure. If the curettage precedes the cone/loop procedure, it must be questioned whether the lesion is truly endocervical or simply removed *en passant* as the curettage instrument passes over the neoplastic region on the ectocervix.

CONE BIOPSY

Cone biopsy and its variants are the standard procedures performed for women with CIN. The cone biopsy can be a diagnostic or a therapeutic procedure. Commonly, it is both simultaneously. The conventional cone biopsy is obtained using a scalpel ('cold knife') but more commonly today, is done with laser or low-voltage, large-loop diathermy methods (LEEP). Variant names are also used. Excision with loop diathermy has the advantage that there is usually less bleeding and the cervix heals with better preservation of anatomy. It can also be performed as an outpatient procedure without the need for general anesthetic. One disadvantage, especially if the instrument is used at suboptimal power levels, is thermal damage that may make diagnosis and, in particular, the examination of the edges of the specimen, difficult. Some suggest loop electrosurgical excision procedures should not be used for glandular lesions, as evaluation of the margins in these cases is also particularly difficult.

The cone biopsy is a roughly cone-shaped excision of the uterine cervix to include a portion of exocervix, external os, and endocervical canal with varying amounts of deep tissues. We ask the surgeon to note the 12 o'clock position with a black suture.

The surgical pathologist can limit the gross description to the measurements of the specimen and any obvious lesion. Care should be given to a clear statement (or a uniform procedure used) as to what is being measured. The measurements should include the cranial–caudal distance (which is not the same as the diameter), the diameter if the specimen is not

opened or circumference if opened, and the thickness if opened.

Cone biopsy specimens can be processed in several ways. Radial sectioning from the center is the preferred method (Figure 35.4), but parallel cuts (anteroposterior) (Figure 35.5) can be taken from one side to the other (left to right or vice versa). With the latter, the specimen must be opened longitudinally with a sharp scissors, fixed, and then blocked in entirety from one end to the other. Both the ectocervical and endocervical edges of the specimen need to be assessed, which can prove to be problematic if a specimen is bowed and cut tangentially or on a bias (Figure 35.6).

Application of differential ink is useful to determine endocervical and ectocervical margins and whether neoplasm involves the margin. Multiple color inks (alcian blue ink, India ink, and yellow ink) often aid in identifying the various margins. Blot dry the tissue and apply ink sparingly. Then pin the tissue on a corkboard with the mucosa facing up. Inking is easier to perform generally before the specimen is opened. Fixation for 3 hours before cutting is usually adequate, but longer times sometimes may be required. Assure the correct face of each block is prepared for cutting. Place one face down in the cassette and mark the opposite side with a dot of India ink, if necessary. Most laboratories will embed the side opposite ink down (the side that will be cut).

Serially cut blocks should be submitted in separate cassettes numbered consecutively. Submit the entire specimen in a clockwise direction (Block A1 = 1 o'clock, etc.). If there are many sections, and especially if they are small, convenience and economy dictate placing two or three sections per cassette. In usual practice, cold knife cones usually lead to 12 blocks and loop procedures to six.

The report on a cone biopsy specimen should include an assessment of the degree of CIN, if present, together with any other incidental pathology, and whether or not the abnormal

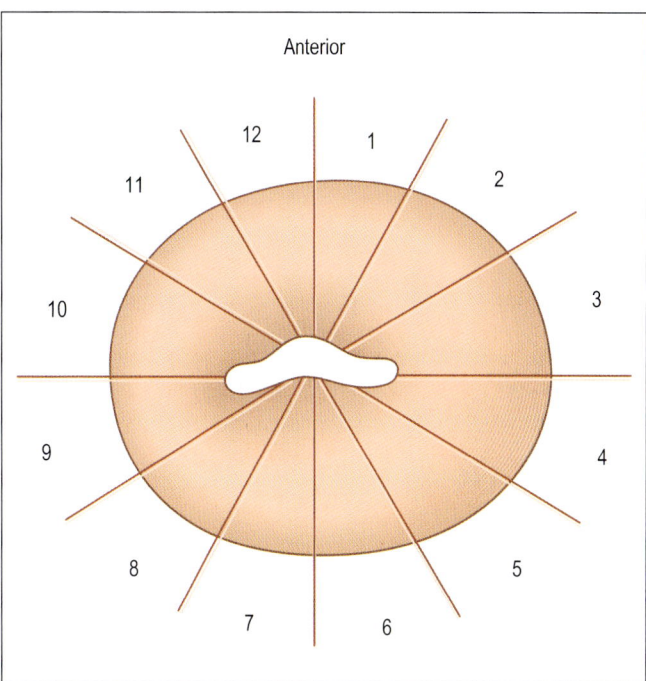

Fig. 35.4 Radial sectioning of a cone biopsy.

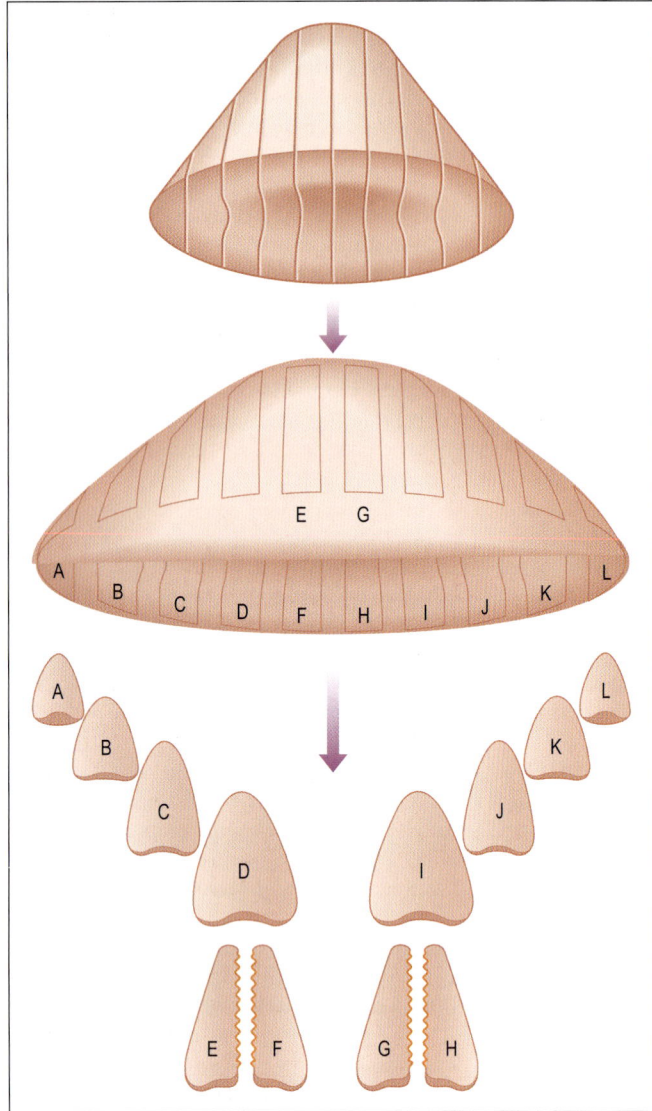

Fig. 35.5 Cone biopsy of cervix blocked with serial parallel cuts. This technique in general offers less information than in Figure 35.4.

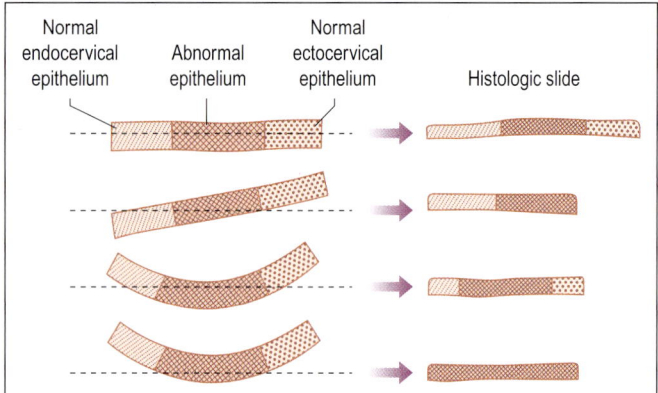

Fig. 35.6 Examples of potential errors introduced if paraffin blocks are embedded and cut tangentially or on a bias. (Modified from Schmidt).[13]

epithelium extends to the excision margins of the specimen. It is usual practice to record if the crypts are involved, as this sometimes has a bearing on additional therapy. It is often useful to note the distribution of the lesions. Invasion, if present, needs to be described in detail, including measurements of the maximum depth of invasion, the maximum width of the lesion, whether lymphatic channels are involved, whether the growth pattern is confluent, and a statement on the completeness of excision of both intraepithelial and invasive elements.

MALIGNANT CERVICAL DISEASE

Simple hysterectomy is commonly performed for high-grade intraepithelial neoplasms and many microinvasive cancers. Radical hysterectomy, which refers to the removal of paracervical soft tissue, is common for stage 1 squamous carcinomas, depending on size and configuration of the tumor in the endocervical canal, and for some stage 2A tumors. The word 'radical' has nothing to do with whether the ovaries or pelvic lymph nodes are removed, or whether there is a vaginal cuff, although commonly radical hysterectomies will include these additional tissues.

For uteri removed for the treatment of CIN, the extent of the workup depends upon what question is to be answered. Is there the need to document the fullest topographical extent of the disease, or is the purpose simply to document the disease diagnosed preoperatively? One method is to amputate the cervix at least 0.5 cm above the level of the external os and process similarly to a cone biopsy. Unless there is some compelling reason, usually four cassettes (one for each quadrant) will suffice. If the clinical history dictates a more detailed analysis, the cervix should be serially blocked in the way that has been described above for a cone biopsy.

Pin the amputated cervix and fix it in formalin for at least 3 hours before cutting. Include the maximum amount of endocervix that will fit into the cassette. Each section should be full thickness to include the endocervical mucosa, squamocolumnar junction, exocervix, and outer adventitia. If a vaginal cuff has been submitted, measure the distance from the exocervix to the line of resection. Sections may be circumferential or perpendicular as long as the blocking process is thorough. We prefer sections perpendicular to the line of resection as they permit assessment of the cervical lesion together with the margins in context.

The gross description from a radical hysterectomy needs to include the tumor dimensions, tumor location – especially with respect to the vaginal fornix and the vaginal margin – depth of invasion, and an impression of whether the lymph nodes contain metastases. Sections of the cervix need to demonstrate both the maximum depth of invasion and the relationship of the tumor to the surgical margins. One or more blocks should contain a complete section from the mucosal surface of uterus through to the serosa. If the wall is too thick for one cassette, divide the section in two and identify both appropriately. Additional sections of the tumor's interface to non-neoplastic mucosa will often demonstrate the CIN from which the invasive tumor arose. These sections need only sample the mucosa and inner wall. Also sample the region of the internal os – lower uterine segment. Evaluate the vaginal resection margin as described above. Since the cervical lymphatics drain laterally toward the parametrium, these areas are especially important in defining the spread of disease. Submit all of the parametrial tissue since this represents the lateral and most significant resection margin. Inking the parametrium is sometimes useful if definition of the true surgical margins is necessary. The surgeon will usually group lymph nodes by areas. Separate and group as right and left, further by location (internal iliac, external iliac, obturator, etc.).

UTERINE CORPUS[4]

ENDOMETRIAL BIOPSIES AND CURETTINGS

All tissues should be submitted from diagnostic procedures, whereas selected samples can be submitted from therapeutic procedures in which large volumes of tissue are received, e.g., curettage performed for termination of pregnancy. The gross description should estimate the aggregate volume. The cassettes should be packed loosely to permit proper fixation and dehydration. Wrap specimens in fine Shandon mesh/tea bags or equivalent and submit in entirety, documenting in the dictation that this was done.

Fat in curettings should be reported immediately to the clinician, as this almost certainly indicates uterine perforation.

For specimens with obvious aborted products of conception (POC), evaluate completeness of fetal and placental removal when possible. Therapeutic abortions, if performed after week 8, will more often show fetal fragments than spontaneous abortions. Single small samples of fetal parts and placenta suffice for sectioning. When fetal parts are absent, pay particular attention to finding chorionic villi. Chorionic villi are soft grey-white tissue fragments that arborize when submerged in fluid such as formalin. Soft, tan, solid and often shiny gray tissue is decidua and, in itself, does not diagnose the presence of an intrauterine pregnancy. For this reason our reports avoid the words 'products of conception'; rather we report: 'Intrauterine contents: Chorionic villi (and any other diagnostic tissues) present'.

At times, the specimen may consist of a uterine cast. Look for an intact or ruptured gestational sac in spontaneous abortions especially. Embedding a portion of the sac with the embryo in agar may improve the chances of observing it microscopically. When a fetus or fetal parts are identified grossly, usually one section is sufficient for documentation, unless there is a gross abnormality. Note crown–rump length and head circumference of the fetus, if possible, and obtain the weight. Since the fetus is often disrupted in therapeutic abortions, another measurement useful to assess fetal age is the toe–heel (foot) length. Only if microscopic examination fails to reveal tissues of fetal origin should additional tissue be processed. Avoid blood clots. In contrast to ectopic pregnancy in the fallopian tube where blood clots typically contain chorionic villi, uterine blood clots almost always lack chorionic villi, even when villi are flagrantly present elsewhere.

If no tissues of fetal origin are found after examination of all tissues, notify the clinician about the possibility of an ectopic pregnancy. Occasionally, this warning informs the clinician that a therapeutic abortion has failed and must be repeated.

Rarely, this may provide the sole indication of an undiagnosed bicornuate uterus. In the appropriate clinical setting, for example, habitual abortion or a previous newborn with multiple congenital malformations, cytogenetic analysis should be considered. As the tissue must be sterile, this type of examination is best instigated and effected by the obstetric service in the delivery room.

Curettings from hydatidiform moles often come in two parts: suction curettage and sharp curettage. Examine carefully for fetal parts. Use common sense regarding the amount of tissue that should be submitted. Three blocks are usually ample. Tissue from the sharp curettage should be processed entirely, since it must be evaluated for myometrial invasion. It should also be remembered that with suction curettage, most vesicles will have been forcibly disrupted and the classic gross appearance will not be present.

SAMPLING CONSIDERATIONS

Precancerous changes of the endometrium are usually of sufficient bulk to present a substantial target for random sampling devices such as a curette or biopsy apparatus. In the premenopausal and perimenopausal years, a bulky persistent proliferative or polyp-bearing endometrium usually presents plenty of material for histologic examination. Less consistent is the postmenopausal patient with an atrophic endometrium which may be highly fragmented due to its fragile and thin nature. In that setting, the precancerous lesion itself usually comprises the largest tissue fragments and stands out from the background.

The extent of random sampling will determine the likelihood of missing a precancerous lesion using transcervical devices, now the preferred endometrial sampling method in the United States. Sharp curettage by a rigid device requires anesthesia and cervical dilatation, and samples less than half of the uterine cavity in about 60% of cases. Pipelle biopsies using a 3.2 mm diameter flexible cannula that removes a tissue core as it spirals across the endometrial surface are small enough that cervical dilatation and anesthesia are unnecessary. Barring some specific exceptions, tissue adequacy and interpretive ease are as good as or better for the Pipelle compared to curettage. Intraluminal mass lesions such as polyps or leiomyomas may deflect the Pipelle instrument, making some areas inaccessible. If one of these conditions is known through examination or ultrasonographic studies, a rigid sampling device may have benefits. Previous studies of atypical hyperplasia diagnostic performance can provide some estimate of these devices to find precancer. Sensitivity of atypical hyperplasia detection is 82% and 67%, respectively, for Pipelle and Vabra devices. Respective specificity is 100% and >99%.

Visually directed hysteroscopic biopsies for precancer detection require operator skill and some common sense. The hysteroscope permits access to areas of an abnormally shaped cavity that may be otherwise inaccessible. While this is an advantage, the hysteroscopist should never assume that precancerous lesions can be reliably targeted by visual appearance alone. Sampling of hysteroscopically evident lesions must always be accompanied by a broader and representative sampling of the remaining otherwise unremarkable endometrial lining. The hysteroscopist should choose an appropriate biopsy device that minimizes artifactual distortion and provides a sufficiently large sample that includes lesion as well as its interface with adjacent tissues. 'Hot' biopsy devices, such as cautery loops, and very small crushing jaw devices should be avoided.

UTERUS REMOVED FOR BENIGN FUNCTIONAL DISEASE

This includes hysterectomy for leiomyomas, endometrial hyperplasia, persistent abnormal bleeding, uterine prolapse, or intractable pelvic pain, the last due sometimes to unrecognized organic causes, e.g., adenomyosis or endometriosis on the serosa.

List specimens received, including whether the adnexae are attached or separate. Several methods are available for orientation. One easy method to determine laterality is to lift the specimen by the two ovaries, which will be posterior to the fallopian tubes (Figure 35.7). Another method is to observe the peritoneum. The uterine posterior surface covers a larger area and extends farther down toward the cervix than anteriorly, where it is reflected high over the bladder.

Weigh the specimen without adnexae (i.e., subtract the estimated adnexal weight). Nomenclature is given in Figure 35.8.

Normal weights
Nulliparous: 30–40 g
Parous: 75–100 g
After eight pregnancies: 240 g
Postmenopausal: 20–40 g

Normal measurements
Top of fundus to exocervix: 5–8 cm
Cornu to cornu: 3–5 cm
Anterior to posterior surface: 2–4 cm
Cervical length and diameter: 3 cm each

Examine the uterine serosa, particularly the posterior surface, for adhesions and brown hemosiderin deposits, so-

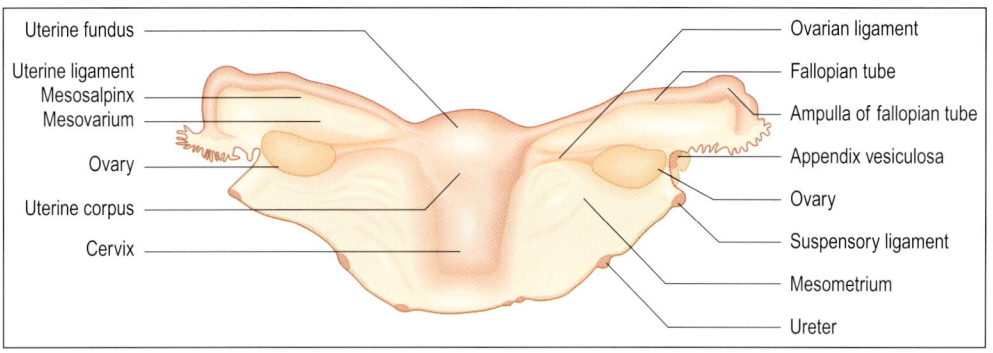

Labels (left): Uterine fundus, Uterine ligament, Mesosalpinx, Mesovarium, Ovary, Uterine corpus, Cervix

Labels (right): Ovarian ligament, Fallopian tube, Ampulla of fallopian tube, Appendix vesiculosa, Ovary, Suspensory ligament, Mesometrium, Ureter

Fig. 35.7 The uterus and adnexa. One easy method for determining laterality is to suspend the two ovarian ligaments, which are posterior to the fallopian tube and therefore define right from left.

Fig. 35.8 Components of the human female uterus.

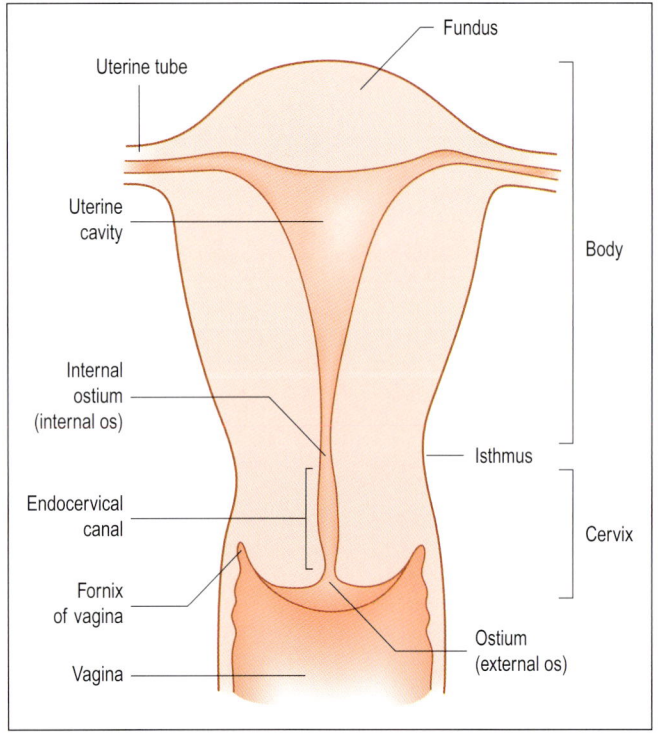

Labels: Uterine tube, Uterine cavity, Internal ostium (internal os), Endocervical canal, Fornix of vagina, Vagina, Fundus, Body, Isthmus, Cervix, Ostium (external os)

called 'powder burns', if endometriosis is suspected, and small vesicles or gritty implanted foci of borderline serous tumor or endosalpingiosis (these of often the same lesion, an issued debated by some), ovarian cancer implants, and psammoma bodies. Examine the exocervix for lacerations, scarring, ulcerations, and nabothian cysts.

Before opening the uterus, probe the cervical canal and endometrial cavity to establish the canal's patency; this also facilitates opening the uterus. With a scalpel incise the outer wall from the cervical os to the cornu along one lateral margin, and then along the fundal top and opposite side. Complete the opening with a scissors. Note that scissors blunt rapidly or even fail if the muscular wall is not cut initially with the scalpel. Another useful trick is to pass a pair of long fine forceps through the cervical os all the way to the fundus and cut the uterus open by a scalpel run between the forceps blades. Cut half way through to open the cavity or cut all the way through if wished.

Measure the average thickness of the endometrium and assess whether it is atrophic, polypoid, lush or hemorrhagic, smooth or rough surfaced. Record polyp measurements and locations. Evaluate the myometrium and state its average and maximum thicknesses. A focally or asymmetrically thickened myometrium with or without small cysts or focal hemorrhage suggests adenomyosis. For a normal cervix, usually one section is adequate if it includes the entire wall to involve the endocervix, squamocolumnar junction, exocervix, and paracervical soft tissue. Some pathologists prefer one section each of the anterior and posterior lips. The section through the endometrium, if the lesion is benign, should be 2 cm long and include the full endometrial thickness and a wedge of myometrium with serosa if not too thick. Generally, two sections, one each from the anterior and posterior corpus, usually in the fundus, suffice if the woman is in reproductive years and one if the uterus is atrophic and the woman in the postmenopausal years. If there is no apparent pathology and the preoperative diagnosis is pain or dysfunctional uterine bleeding, then increase the number of sections to at least four that are full thickness through the left and right sides of both the anterior and posterior walls near the fundus (Figure 35.9). It is surprising how frequently adenomyosis is confined to only a single area in a single slide. Longitudinal or oblique rather than horizontal sections more commonly provide representative endometrium for review with few sections.

Uteri removed for endometrial hyperplasia require multiple sections of the endomyometrium to exclude carcinoma. For example, six sections, each 2 cm long and cut as wedges can usually fit into two to three cassettes (Figure 35.10). If the uterus is not enlarged, this number of sections often samples 75% of the endometrium. Some pathologists prefer to block in the entire endometrium with sections through to the serosa so as not to miss the possibility of invasive cancer and be able to measure the depth of invasion.

If removed for leiomyomas, record the number present, their location (submucosal, intramural, subserosal) and size (e.g., 'ten <1 cm and two measuring 13 and 18 cm in diameter'). If submucosal, state whether the tumor distorts the endometrial cavity or protrudes into the lower uterine canal or cervix. Each leiomyoma should be sectioned and examined grossly, but not necessarily microscopically. If all are white, firm, and whorled, have well-circumscribed margins, are small and lack areas that are soft, necrotic, or hemorrhagic, even one

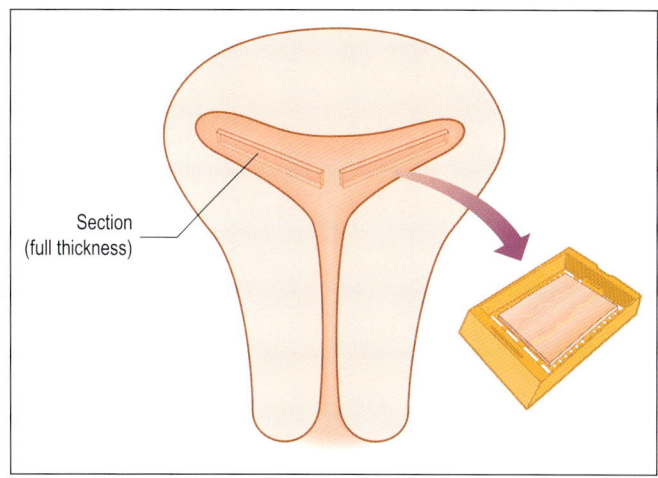

Fig. 35.9 Sampling of uterine body for complaint of bleeding where no obvious gross disease is present (e.g., occult adenomyosis). Two full thickness sections anteriorly and two posteriorly extensively and efficiently sample the endometrium and myometrial wall.

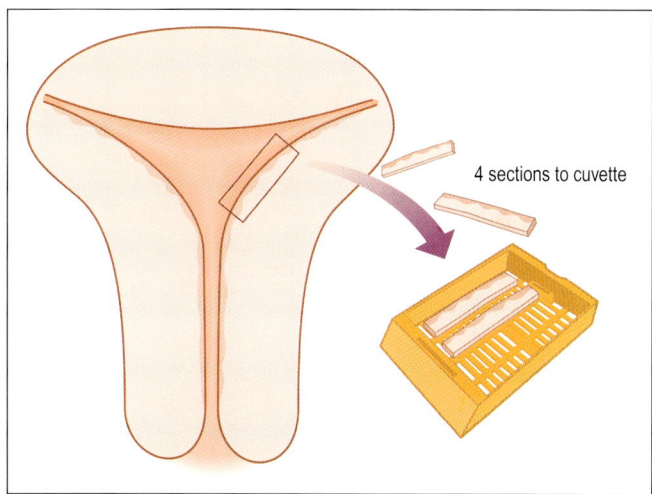

Fig. 35.10 Efficient but extensive sampling of uterine body for endometrial hyperplasia.

block can be sufficient. As leiomyosarcomas less than 5 cm virtually never metastasize regardless of microscopic appearance, routine microscopic examination of every typical leiomyoma is unnecessary. Conversely, as leiomyosarcomas generally grow as a single nodule or mass and exhibit soft and degenerative areas, all suspicious areas should be thoroughly sampled. As a rule, take one microscopic section per 1–2 cm of the suspicious regions, for these areas usually yield more useful information. The transition between smooth muscle tumors and surrounding myometrium is the preferred site for histologic sampling. 'Random' sections of grossly typical leiomyomas generally are of little use! For myomectomy specimens, transect each leiomyoma and take one section of each if the number is not excessive, or more if any areas are suspicious.

UTERUS REMOVED DURING OBSTETRIC PROCEDURES

Hysterectomy during delivery is performed for intractable hemorrhage, placenta accreta, uterine rupture or cervical neoplasia. For the last, process the specimen as described previously. For the other conditions, focus the gross description and sectioning on the relation of the placenta and membranes to the uterus. Describe lacerations, usually lateral, carefully as to location, extent, and depth of penetration. Uterine rupture may have occurred at the site of a previous lower segment cesarean section scar and sections across the site of rupture should be oriented to optimize its identification as a predisposing factor. Also, placenta previa, placenta accreta, and previous cesarean section in the lower segment not infrequently go together. Obtain sections from these sites. For placenta previa, sample carefully the zone of the internal os to identify associated placenta accreta. Full-thickness sections at the site of suspected placental retention are useful in defining placenta accreta, increta, and percreta.

MALIGNANT UTERINE DISEASE

Evaluate all specimens with a preoperative diagnosis of malignancy for residual tumor. If present, determine the maximum depth of myometrial invasion and cervical involvement (mucosal or stromal) and take sections to document these findings.

The gross description must include the overall size, location, distribution (focal or diffuse), and shape (sessile or polypoid). For example, a 6 × 5 cm sessile tumor wall extends to involve the anterior lower uterine segment, but not the endocervix. The tumor penetrates largely 5 mm and maximally 10 mm into a 23 mm thick wall. If the tumor is polypoid and protrudes into the endometrial cavity, identify the borders of the adjacent normal endometrium, draw an imaginary line between, and then report measurements above and below the line. Thus the 1 cm thick tumor, which protrudes 7 mm into the endometrial cavity, penetrates 3 mm into the superficial myometrium (Figure 35.11). Describe and sample the uninvolved endometrium, including the lowermost margin of the neoplasm (Figures 35.11 and 35.12). The gross depth of myometrial invasion should be recorded. At least one microscopic section should permit measurement of the greatest depth of tumor invasion. For intramural tumors, describe the interface between the tumor and myometrium (circumscribed, irregular, or infiltrative) and note any worm-like extrusions of tumor in surrounding tissues that could represent grossly involved lymphatic/vascular channels (seen most commonly in endometrial stromal sarcomas and intravenous leiomyomatosis).

When the interface between the neoplastic endometrium and the myometrium is wavy and disconcerting for invasion, an important clue is to determine whether any residual normal endometrial glands are present deep at the junction and deep

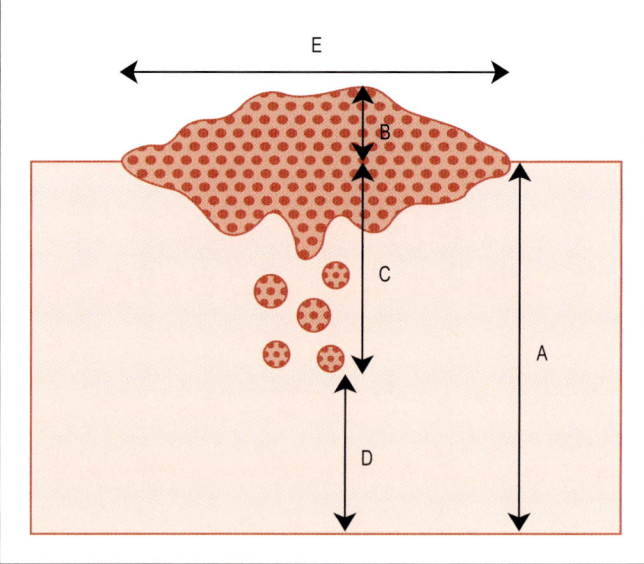

Fig. 35.11 Measurements of depth to which tumor invades. A, full thickness of myometrial wall, measured from where endometrium adjacent to tumor is normal (or hyperplasic). B, component of tumor exophytic and rising above imaginary line drawn between adjacent normal endometrium. C, depth of invasion. D, tumor-free zone. E, width of tumor. We generally report a tumor as measuring $n \times n \times n$ and 'C' cm invasive into a wall 'A' cm thick.

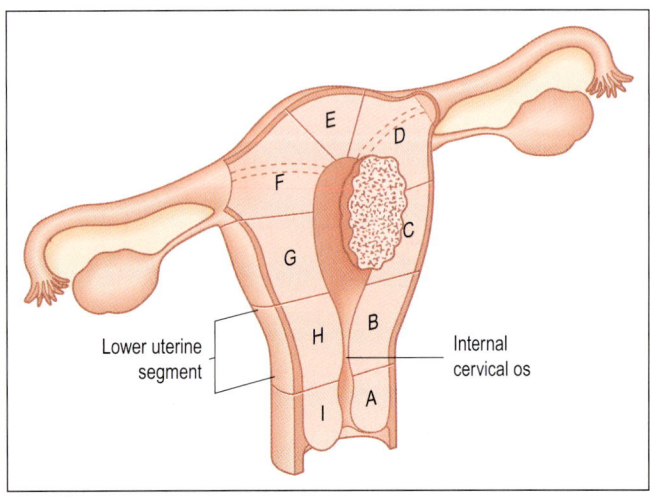

Fig. 35.12 Technique for sectioning the uterus. Sampling includes cervix (e.g., A, I), margins adjacent and deep to a cancer (e.g., C, D), lower uterine segment and uppermost endocervix – for example, to determine whether an endometrial cancer involves the cervix, thus upstaging it (e.g., B, H), the wall for adenomyosis (e.g., D, F), and endometrium with areas partially or totally seemingly free of tumor (e.g., C, G).

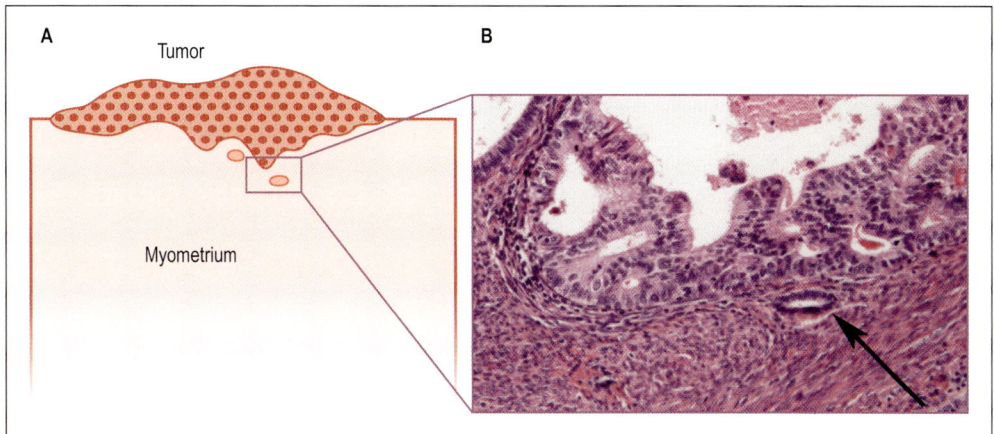

Fig. 35.13 Intraendometrial tumor in which normal endometrial glands (arrow) lie deep to the tumor and on the interface between endometrium and myometrium. Without this point of normal demarcation, the tumor would appear invasive.

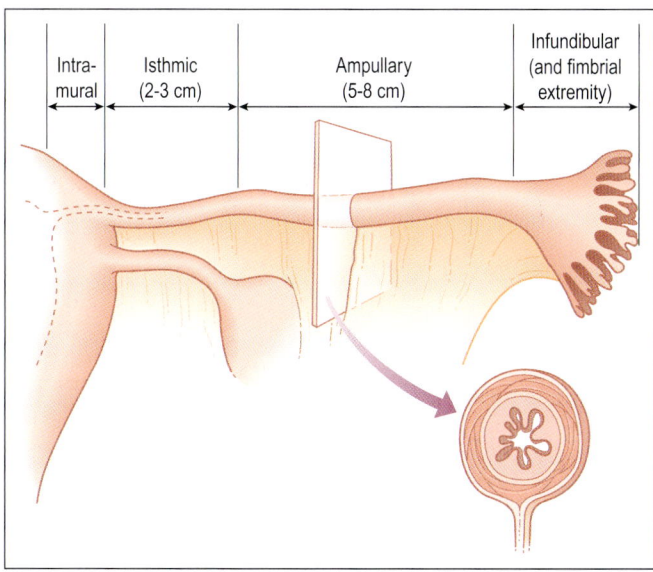

Fig. 35.14 Technique for sectioning fallopian tube free of abnormalities. Transverse sections are obtained from the isthmic, ampullary, and infundibular regions. Modified from Schmidt.[13]

to the neoplasm (Figure 35.13). Many a seemingly invasive tumor is actually confined entirely to the endometrium.

Lymph nodes removed for staging of endometrial carcinoma present a particular challenge. Because studies have shown that the higher numbers of removed pelvic and para-aortic lymph nodes (12 or greater) are more prognostically powerful, particularly when negative,[9] substantial pressure may be placed on the pathologist to produce high lymph node counts. Careful dissection of lymphadenectomy specimens, with submission of any possible lymph node is all that is necessary, however. Pathologists should resist the temptation to artificially elevate the node count. If the gross lymph node count is small and if the remnant soft tissue is small, it may be worthwhile to entirely submit the remaining soft tissue for histologic examination. This can reassure the surgeon that a thorough examination of the tissue has been performed.

FALLOPIAN TUBE[10]

Most fallopian tube specimens (salpingectomy) are performed in conjunction with oophorectomy and hysterectomy, especially in older women in whom it is no longer necessary to preserve fertility. In these cases, there is typically no pathologic condition in the fallopian tubes. The overall length and diameter of the tube should be measured, and if there is no apparent pathology, usually a single section from each suffices. For convenience, each tube is usually submitted for histologic examination together with the corresponding section of ovary.

STERILIZATION

When removed for ligation, the single most important finding is that indeed the tube has been ligated. This requires that a complete cross-section of the tube, which includes the lumen, be identified and differentiated from round ligament. Measure the length and the diameter of each tube (Figure 35.14). One method for sampling is to slice the tube into sections 1–3 mm long and to submit all for microscopic examination, each piece being cut on end. This is particularly important for serous tumors of the endometrium or for women who are *BRCA* carriers. Even if per chance some sections are cut tangentially, usually at least some will be intact to document that the lumen is present. This saves substantial time and effort by not having to request additional recuts. Another technique that saves effort is to place the specimens into agar to preclude incorrect embedding. The procedure for examining a failed ligation is discussed elsewhere (see Chapter 20).

TUBAL ECTOPIC PREGNANCY

Record the site and location of the pregnancy. A rupture site, if present, should be described and sampled. If the ectopic pregnancy is not obvious, a focal enlargement or swelling should be sought. Blood distending the lumen should be documented as it is unlikely to result from any other cause. Sometimes the area must be sectioned extensively. A tubal abortion leaves foci of trophoblast at the implantation site. Blood clot in the tube, sometimes submitted as a separate specimen, should be examined carefully for gray-white tissue and sampled microscopically for trophoblast or chorionic villi. Multiple cross-sections of the fallopian tube at the site of swelling or bleeding demonstrate chorionic villi efficiently. Sections of fallopian tube, even slightly away from the swelling, may be normal, but should be sampled to confirm or exclude pre-existing pathology such as agglutinated plicae in healed salpingitis.

NEOPLASM

Tubal cancer is uncommon. Its behavior is similar to ovarian carcinoma and frequently appears as a solid mass in the wall of a grossly dilated tube. Describe its size, location, and extent, with reference to other pelvic structures. Transverse sections through the full tubal wall permit determination of the depth of penetration. Include this information plus the grade of the tumor in the pathology report.

OVARY[11]

The pathologist may receive ovarian tissue from patients in a variety of clinical circumstances, each of which determines different manners in which the specimen is handled. If oophorectomy is performed in association with a hysterectomy with no expectation or realization of ovarian pathology, a simple 'routine' pathologic examination will usually suffice. By contrast, ovaries excised for suspected or proven neoplasms may

require several different specialized analyses in addition to histologic assessment. In some circumstances, e.g., ovarian failure, it may be appropriate to have a preoperative consultation to discuss the appropriate site and size of the biopsy and its immediate handling in the operating theater in order to optimize analysis of the clinical problem.

GENERAL RULES

Several general rules can be applied when the specimen is small, and either incidental or where no substantial pathology is anticipated.

- The specimen should be examined fresh or at most fixed for a short period.
- It should be weighed and measured.
- The external surface should be inspected for adhesions, excrescences, hemorrhage or hemosiderin (powder burns) indicative of possible endometriosis.
- Sections should be taken perpendicularly through the adhesions to include the capsule and parenchyma to determine whether or not the adhesions are due to inflammation or neoplasm. Note the presence of a corpus luteum, cystic follicles (if excessive in number), or cysts. Their combined absence may indicate an otherwise unexpected diffuse metastasis.
- Residual uninvolved ovary in a neoplastic mass is sometimes found immediately adjacent to the fallopian tube. The ovary should be incised by parallel transverse cuts (Figure 35.15). Take cross-sections through the tube to include a wedge of ovary.
- One block is sufficient from a macroscopically normal ovary, but this should include cortex, medulla, and hilus, conveniently sampled by a single section through the middle of the ovary. Additional blocks of possible pathologic structures will be required.

LARGE CYSTIC OR NEOPLASTIC OVARIES

Ovaries should be measured in three dimensions. Weighing large ovarian tumors may provide a more readily appreciable assessment of the size of the lesion. Document whether the ovarian tumor is received intact or ruptured (intraoperative rupture can upstage the patient). If a tubo-ovarian mass is submitted, careful dissection may be necessary to identify its components. In pelvic inflammatory disease the ovary is

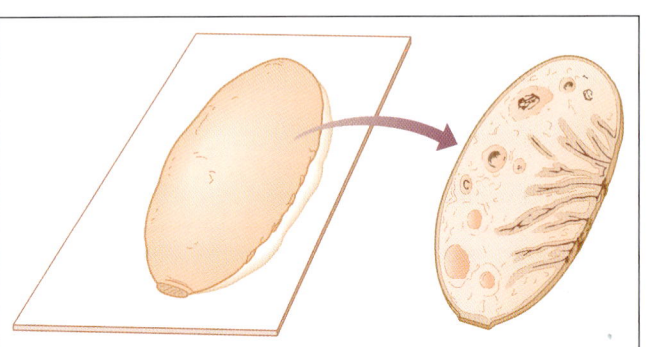

Fig. 35.15 Technique for sectioning ovary in the absence of abnormalities. The cross-section shows cortex, medulla, and hilum. Modified from Schmidt.[13]

relatively spared and should be readily recognized once the surrounding adhesions have been teased away. The course of the fallopian tubes should be identified and the condition of the fimbriae noted. A hydrosalpinx or paraovarian cyst, especially if associated with adhesions, may cause confusion if diligent efforts are not made to establish the anatomic relationships.

Pay attention to the capsule as indicated above and then slice the ovary at 1 cm intervals. Many ovarian tumors are cystic and all locules should be opened with scissors or sliced through with a sharp long-bladed knife. Note the character of the cyst contents (serous (i.e., watery), mucoid, bloodstained, oily, gelatinous, pultaceous) and the smoothness of its lining. A smooth shiny lining usually indicates a benign lesion. Large thin-walled cysts can be sampled effectively by making a 'membrane-roll' from a strip of cyst wall (Figure 35.16). Ragged hemorrhagic cyst linings suggest endometriosis, but several blocks may be necessary in order to identify the diagnostic portion of the lining. In about 5% of mucinous adenomas, one of the hundreds of cysts will contain hair, indicative that the mucinous component is a cystic teratoma with a monodermal overgrowth of mucinous tissue.

If the ovary has undergone torsion, the tissues may be extremely edematous, hemorrhagic or even necrotic. Slice the ovary finely, looking for any viable tissue or residua of a cyst or solid tumor that may have undergone torsion. Reticulin stains on suspicious areas may help to highlight the underlying pathology. The accompanying fallopian tube, if also involved, should be closely examined because it may be, albeit rarely, the site of the inciting lesion. However, in children, torsion of normal adnexa is not uncommon.

Mature cystic teratomas (dermoid cysts) should be emptied as completely as possible of the trapped hair and sebaceous material. Remove sebum by washing with hot water (liquefies the sebum). Short exposures do not destroy the epithelial lining. Block any knobby protuberance (Rokitansky tubercle) or where the wall is thickened. This will be the most rewarding source of diagnostic material. Granularity, fine friable papillary excrescences, or soft fleshy nodules arising from cyst walls should arouse suspicions of malignancy and be thoroughly sampled. If the tumor has a variegated appearance, then sample as many apparently different areas as possible. Take blocks

from areas where the tumor comes closest to the capsule or resection margin and particularly from the surface adhesions if tumor is close to the capsule at these points. In addition, look for and sample residual non-tumorous ovarian tissue. Look for the fallopian tube, which may be incorporated in or stretched over the tumor mass/cyst. It may contain coexistent mucosal neoplasia.

For neoplasms, the gross examination is critical. Carefully examine the capsule for rents, adhesions, implants, or extension and penetration of the underlying tumor. For small tumors, identify location as cortical, medullary, or hilar. Cut larger tumors into slabs at 1 cm intervals. If cystic, examine for papillary excrescences and small solid foci, since these may reveal areas of low malignant potential or cancer. If mucinous, find the most solid regions and sample extensively. The cystic areas will be benign or microscopically disclose little more than borderline tumor. Only the solid areas generally show areas definable as adenocarcinoma.

MICROSCOPIC SECTIONS

Document if adhesions, inflammatory or true tumor, involve the external surface. This is important in staging. Request that the surgeons place a stitch in adhesions noted during operative procedure. Ink can be useful to document the tumor's serosal surface.

The best blocks of tumor are where the tissue is viable. Include the capsule and tumor, and include tumor with adjacent normal parenchyma.

Use discretion in the number of blocks obtained. Generally, about one block per 2 cm of greatest tumor dimension will suffice to document the tumor process. Serous tumors tend to be relatively uniform throughout, and need fewer blocks. Often, three slides of serous tumors are sufficient. Mucinous tumors, in contrast, often vary greatly. It is common for any single tumor to have large areas that are benign or borderline, with only few areas that are unequivocally malignant. Commonly, areas with multilocular thin-walled cysts are benign, or at most of borderline malignancy. Areas that are more solid are usually borderline and sometimes frankly malignant. Quite commonly, only 10% of solid areas may show unequivocal malignancy, which in a 10 cm tumor translates to only two slides with malignancy out of 20 sampled. Search for solid areas and sample them thoroughly. Unilocular cysts with a smooth inner-wall lining may be large, but require few sections.

Germ cell tumors, especially if associated with gonadoblastoma, should be sampled extensively, especially at various different areas. Not uncommonly, the tumor may seem pure, even after microscopic examination has been completed, yet the recurrence is of a different type. These tumors should initially be X-rayed for calcifications, which might indicate the area of gonadoblastoma. These regions should be sampled thoroughly for gonadoblastoma and any other tumor type present; a useful technique is to identify the fallopian tube, hold it, and take sections perpendicular through it to include the ovarian surface. Finally, all variations in the gross appearance, e.g., foci of hemorrhage, etc. should be specifically sampled as they may represent different tumor types, e.g., foci of embryonal cell carcinoma or endodermal sinus tumor arising in association with a dysgerminoma.

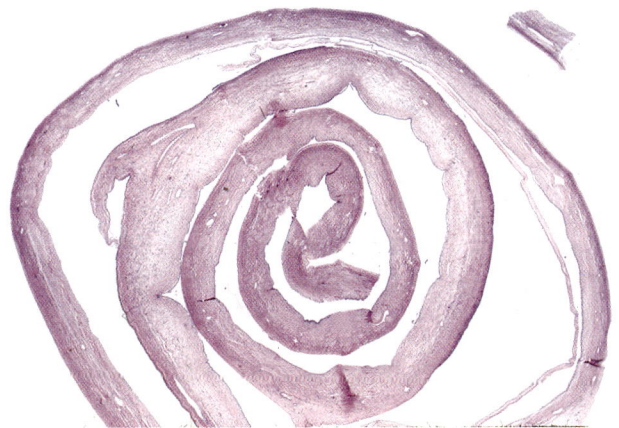

Fig. 35.16   'Membrane-roll' made from thin-walled ovarian cyst.

Dermoid cysts should be washed with hot water to remove the sebum and hair, and microscopic sections taken from the solid tissue. It is of little use to sample the wall that grossly shows only skin and hair as microscopic sections will disclose only the same. Sample solid nodules. These are the business components, and the ones that will disclose the carcinoid, strumas, etc.

Membrane rolls composed of extensive quantities of cyst wall tissue can be examined if the wall is made into a membrane roll and a cross-section slide prepared (Figure 35.16).

STAGING OPERATIONS

There is need for close cooperation between surgeon and pathologist in the staging operations for assessment of both primary ovarian carcinoma and for second-look of previously treated cancer. These may involve intraoperative assessment of excised tissues, including frozen section, as well as the histo-logic examination of multiple specimens and cytologic assessment of peritoneal washings and ascitic fluid. General guidelines for the surgeon include:

1. Evaluate the ovarian mass to exclude metastasis from colon, stomach, or elsewhere. Note penetration through capsule and biopsy areas of adherence.
2. Obtain ascitic fluid or saline washings for cytology.
3. Inspect all peritoneal surfaces. Prove that apparent implants are malignant by frozen section, or submit multiple samples for permanent section, or both. Inspect the diaphragm, with biopsy of visible lesions or scrapings for cytology.
4. Confirm accuracy of apparent stage 1 or 2 disease by generous omental biopsy and biopsy of palpable pelvic and para-aortic nodes.
5. After excision, mark the specimen indicating for the pathologist the site(s) of rupture and/or area(s) of adherence. Record residual disease location and estimate extent.

Specimens submitted for pathologic examination are likely to include:

- Uterus with attached or separately submitted adnexa, preferably delivered fresh to the pathologist immediately after excision. Before taking fresh tissue samples for DNA flow cytometry, etc., carefully examine the whole specimen noting the excisional margins if necessary. Complete the assessment of the ovaries as recommended above. Before fixation, open the uterine cavity, keeping in mind the possibility of a coexisting endometrial carcinoma or hyperplasia. Scrutinize the uterine serosal surface for tumor deposits and section any adhesions to exclude microscopic metastases (since these will raise the FIGO stage from at least stage 1 to at least stage 2A).
- Omentum. Slice finely, looking for tumor deposits and block these. If none is found, sample any unusually firm areas (usually fibrous adhesions which may or may not be associated with microscopic tumor deposits). If none is found, one to two blocks of normal tissue should be sufficient. In over 20% of cases, the grossly normal omentum will disclose microscopic foci of tumor.
- Pelvic and/or para-aortic lymph nodes. Block all lymphoid tissue.

- Peritoneal biopsies. These are often very small and should be handled accordingly, using a mesh bag if necessary.
- Peritoneal washings. The surgeon collects these by saline irrigation from the left and right paracolic gutters, subdiaphragmatic region, and pouch of Douglas. The fluids are cytocentrifuged and the spun deposits are used to make direct smears. When available, examination of the fluid using modern liquid based cytology techniques (e.g. ThinPrep) can also be helpful. Process the remainder of the deposit as a cell block. Ascitic fluid is treated similarly.

FETUS AND PLACENTA[5]

SECOND TRIMESTER FETUS

In many institutions, special permission is required to examine a fetus nearing viability. Statutes variously define the cut-off as a fetus older than 20 weeks' gestation, greater than 15 cm crown–rump length or greater than 300 g weight. Regardless, the placenta can be submitted as a surgical pathology specimen.

Measure and record the fetal weight, crown–heel length, crown–rump length, and head circumference. Other common measurements include femur length, arm span, thorax and abdominal circumferences. Foot length may be recorded as well. Sex can usually be determined by external examination. If the genitalia are ambiguous, then describe them as such, but never give a 'best guess' for sex assignments. Look for obvious external anomalies. More subtle ones are difficult to observe in early gestation. Measure cord length and state the number of blood vessels. Describe the skin surface and, after the body is opened, observe the organs *in situ*. Determine situs and note any obvious abnormalities. Retrieve the gonads and place them in a mesh bag at this point. Take sections of various organs. We find that weighing organs that are part of a surgical specimen is often a futile exercise. Include each lobe of lung, both gonads, and small sections of every other organ including various parts of gastrointestinal tract and skin. Macerated fetuses are difficult to sample adequately because of the usually severe softening of the tissues; submit sections of more solid tissue (lungs, heart, kidneys). Often the entire examination consists of no more than three cassettes filled with tissue.

PLACENTA

Abnormalities of the placenta are frequently associated with adverse outcomes in either the fetus or the mother.[5,6] However, examination of the placenta is not routinely performed in most institutions unless specific indications are present. The College of American Pathologists practice guidelines[7] include recommendations of indications for placental examination (Table 35.1). To determine which placentas should be examined, remember the three funnies: funny mother, funny infant, funny disease. This should lead to the examination of about one in three placentas, although in practice fewer are examined (about one in five).[5]

Table 35.1 Examination of the placenta

Recommended maternal indications (general agreement)

Systemic disorders with clinical concerns for mother or infant (e.g., severe diabetes, impaired glucose metabolism, hypertensive disorders, collagen disease, seizures, severe anemia (<9 g))

Premature delivery ≤34 weeks' gestation

Peripartum fever and/or infection

Unexplained third trimester bleeding or excessive bleeding >500 cm³

Clinical concern for infection during this pregnancy (e.g., human immunodeficiency virus, syphilis, cytomegalovirus, primary herpes, toxoplasma, rubella)

Severe oligohydramnios

Unexplained or recurrent pregnancy complication (e.g., intrauterine growth retardation, stillbirth, spontaneous abortion, premature birth)

Invasive procedures with suspected placental injury

Abruption

Non-elective pregnancy termination

Thick and/or viscid meconium

Other maternal indications (less general agreement)

Premature delivery >34–37 weeks' gestation

Severe unexplained polyhydramnios

History of substance abuse

Gestational age ≥42 weeks

Severe maternal trauma

Prolonged (>24 hours) rupture of membranes

Recommended fetal/neonatal indications

Admission or transfer to other than a level 1 nursery

Stillbirth or perinatal death

Compromised clinical condition defined as any of the following: cord blood pH, <7.0; Apgar score, ≤6 at 5 minutes; ventilatory assistance, >10 minutes; or severe anemia, hematocrit <35%

Hydrops fetalis

Birthweight <10th percentile

Seizures

Infection or sepsis

Major congenial anomalies, dysmorphic phenotype, or abnormal karyotype

Discordant twin growth >20% weight difference

Multiple gestation with same-sex infants and fused placentas

Other fetal/neonatal indications (less general agreement)

Birthweight >95th percentile

Asymmetric growth

Multiple gestation without other indication

Vanishing twin beyond the first trimester

Recommended placental indications

Physical abnormality (e.g., infarct, mass, vascular thrombosis, retroplacental hematoma, amnion nodosum, abnormal coloration or opacification, malodor)

Small or large placental size or weight for gestational age

Umbilical cord lesions (e.g., thrombosis, torsion, true knot, single artery, absence of Whartons jelly)

Total umbilical cord length <32 cm at term

Other placental indications (less general agreement)

Abnormalities of placental shape

Long cord (>100 cm)

Marginal or velamentous cord insertion

Due to the not infrequent occurrence of AIDS and AIDS-related diseases in the general population, many routinely fix all placentas for 24 hours before examination. If indicated, sterile samples for cytogenetics or culture should be taken prior to fixation. Fresh samples should also be taken for metabolic/biochemical studies and/or electron microscopy if the history is suggestive.

Identify the site of membrane rupture. If far from the placenta proper, consider it to be unremarkable and make no comment. Record the presence or absence of hemorrhage in the membranes, and the approximate distance of it to the margin of the placenta.

Remove the membranes and cord and weigh the placenta. Measure the overall length and width and comment on shape (discoid, ovoid, irregular). Systematically describe all parts (Figure 35.17).

- *Fetal surface*: Describe the color, surface characteristics (smooth, roughened, opaque, etc.), vascularity. Note the margins. Are the membranes inserted in the usual manner? Is there thickening, circummarginate or circumvallate insertion, etc.? If present, estimate the percentage of circumference affected.
- *Umbilical cord*: Describe insertion (central, eccentric, marginal, velamentous); measure length and cross-sectional diameter (state as average or range); state number of blood vessels. Look for varicosities, excessive coiling, false knots, true knots, edema, discoloration, thrombosis, hemorrhage, etc.
- *Membranes*: The amnion is the layer adjacent to the fetus. Usually the chorion and amnion are loosely fused (easily separated), but may be completely separate. Look for thickening, opacity and adherent blood clot. Describe color, clarity, edema, etc. Make a membrane roll to include the area of rupture. Membrane rolls can be made on fixed tissue provided the membranes are neither edematous nor covered with meconium. There are several methods of membrane rolling, of which one is:
  1. Remove the membranes from the placenta.
  2. Cut a 10 cm wide strip to include both chorion and amnion extending from the edge that was attached to the placenta to the edge where the rupture occurred.
  3. Gently blot the membranes with gauze. Grasp one cut edge with non-toothed forceps and while maintaining a grip on the membranes, roll the membranes around the forceps with the amnion (which is smoother) on the outside of the roll.
  4. Relax the grip on the forceps slightly and use the blunt side of a knife blade to remove the roll from the forceps.
  5. Carefully slice the roll (use the sharp edge of the blade for this!) into 2–3 mm thick slices, and place into the cassette; alternatively, pin the membrane roll onto cork and cut sections or fix the membrane roll overnight and cut transverse sections the next day.
- *Maternal surface*: Is the surface intact or disrupted? If disrupted, estimate whether all tissue is present. Describe the cotyledon pattern, fibrin, calcification, and blood clot. Describe well-defined depressions. Estimate the percentage of surface affected. Give the average thickness. Describe any succenturiate lobes. Cross-section the

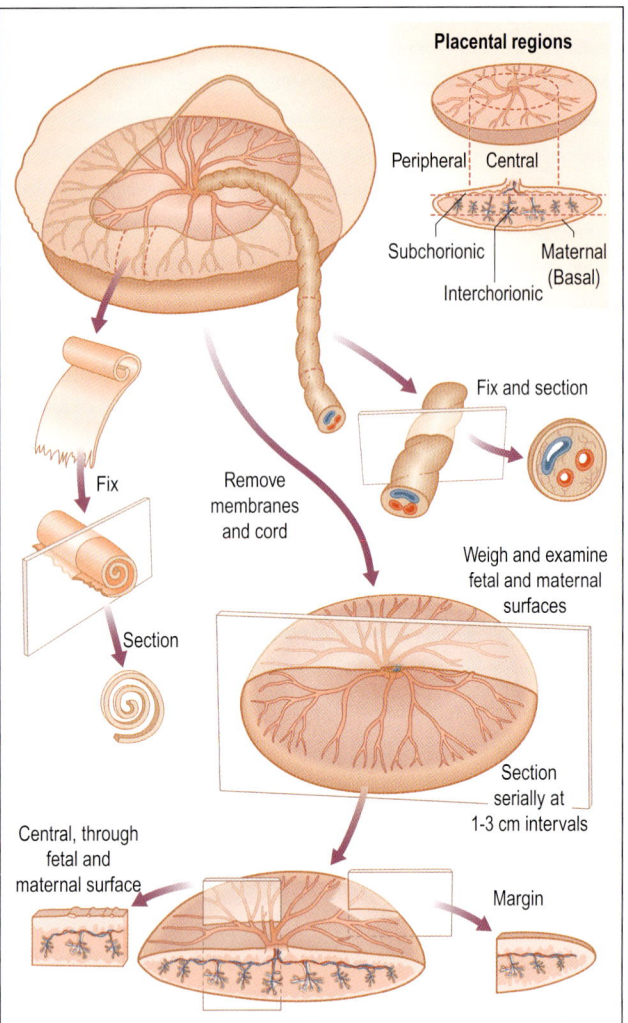

Placental regions

Peripheral | Central

Subchorionic | Maternal (Basal)

Interchorionic

Fix and section

Fix

Remove membranes and cord

Section

Weigh and examine fetal and maternal surfaces

Section serially at 1-3 cm intervals

Central, through fetal and maternal surface

Margin

Fig. 35.17 Placental examination. Adequate sampling for histologic study includes membrane roll, cross-section of cord, and specific placental regions, specifically cut to display fetal and maternal surfaces. Modified from Schmidt.[13]

specimen and look for and describe lesions, infarcts, blood clots, masses, etc. Estimate the percentage of the area involved.

- *Tissue sections*: It is our preference to submit at least three sections for microscopic examination: (1) cross-section of the umbilical cord; (2) membrane roll; and (3) cross-section of normal parenchyma somewhere centrally. Other sections should be taken as appropriate.

TWINS

Determine the type of twin placenta, i.e., dichorionic diamniotic, monochorionic diamniotic, monochorionic monoamniotic. Unless it is a monochorionic monoamniotic placenta, take a strip of the dividing membranes (T-zone), roll it, fix, and then section (Figure 35.18). Sections of membrane other than T-zone should also be rolled, fixed, and submitted. Examine, weigh, and cut the placenta (or placentas if not fused) as for a singleton placenta. If the placentas are fused, estimate the percentage each placenta comprises of the total, and note any differences in color between each placenta.

Monoamniotic twin placentas are uncommon and result in a high rate of fetal morbidity and mortality. These twins are always identical (monozygotic).

Monochorionic diamniotic placentas have two layers of amnion separating the two fetal sacs (see Figure 30.54). These membranes are thin and can be easily stripped from the fetal surface leaving no trace. Careful examination of the fetal surface often reveals vascular anastomoses between the two fetal circulations. Injection of colored dye is a useful way to demonstrate vascular anastomoses before fixation. These twins are also always identical.

Fused dichorionic diamniotic or separate twin placentas have amnion–chorion–amnion layers which can be divided into three or sometimes four layers and are more opaque/white, often with visible blood vessels in the membranous position. The two amnion layers can be easily stripped away, but the chorion is firmly attached and cannot easily be pulled away from the placental surface. Removal leaves a thin low ridge of firm tan tissue. Vascular anastomoses are absent. These twins may be identical or fraternal (dizygotic). If of the same sex, approximately 75% will be fraternal and 25% monozygotic or identical.

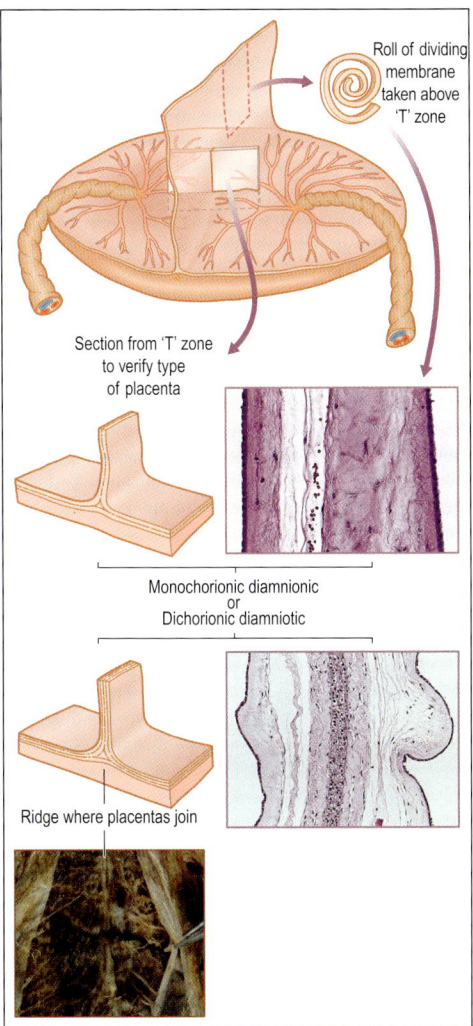

Fig. 35.18 Examination of placenta of twins. Sampling of a twin placenta includes a section of septal membrane dividing the amniotic cavities, cut to display the T-zone, where the septal membrane attaches to the placental surface. Modified from Schmidt.[13]

Similar principles apply to the examination of placentas from gestations greater than two (triplets, etc.).

REFERENCES

1. Black D, Tornos C, Soslow RA, Awtrey CS, Barakat RR, Chi DS. The outcomes of patients with positive margins after excision for intraepithelial Paget's disease of the vulva. Gynecol Oncol 2007;104:547–50.
2. Branton PA. Vulva. 2005. Online. Available: www.cap.org/apps/docs/cancer_protocols/2005/vulva05_pw.pdf
3. Branton PA. Uterine cervix. 2005. Online. Available: www.cap.org/apps/docs/cancer_protocols/2005/uterinecervix05_pw.pdf
4. Branton PA, Moore WF. Endometrium. 2005. Online. Available: www.cap.org/apps/docs/cancer_protocols/2005/endometrium05_pw.pdf
5. Curtin WM, Krauss S, Metlay LA, Katzman PJ. Pathologic examination of the placenta and observed practice. Obstet Gynecol 2007;109:35–41.
6. Kraus FT. Introduction: the importance of timely and complete placental and autopsy reports. Semin Diagn Pathol 2007;24:1–4.
7. Langston C, Kaplan C, Macpherson T, et al. Practice guideline for examination of the placenta: developed by the Placental Pathology Practice Guideline Development Task Force of the College of American Pathologists. Arch Pathol Lab Med 1997;121:449–76.
8. Lester SC. Manual of Surgical Pathology. Edinburgh: Churchill Livingstone; 2006.
9. Lutman CV, Havrilesky LJ, Cragun JM, et al. Pelvic lymph node count is an important prognostic variable for FIGO stage I and II endometrial carcinoma with high-risk histology. Gynecol Oncol 2006;102:92–7.
10. Oliva E, Branton PA, Scully RE. Fallopian tube. 2005. Online. Available: www.cap.org/apps/docs/cancer_protocols/2005/fallopian05_pw.pdf
11. Oliva E, Branton PA, Scully RE. Ovary. 2005. Online. Available: www.cap.org/apps/docs/cancer_protocols/2005/ovary05_pw.pdf
12. Tebes S, Cardosi R, Hoffman M. Paget's disease of the vulva. Am J Obstet Gynecol 2002;187:281–3; discussion 283–4.
13. Schmidt WA. Principles and Techniques of Surgical Pathology. Menlo Park, Addison-Westley, 1983.
14. Westra WH, Hruban RH, Phelps TH, Isacson C. Surgical Pathology Dissection: An Illustrated Guide. New York: Springer; 2003.

Immunohistochemical and functional biomarkers of value in female genital tract lesions

36

W. Glenn McCluggage

INTRODUCTION

Recent years have witnessed a veritable explosion in the use of immunohistochemical markers in gynecologic pathology.[91,102,107,134,202] Most relate to their use in the diagnosis of gynecologic neoplasms but some have prognostic or predictive value. In general, panels of markers provide better information than a single antibody. Predictably, most antibodies, although initially thought specific for a given tumor, later have proven to have a broader range of reactivity with a more diverse set of tumor types. As an example, calretinin, an excellent marker for mesothelium, is also remarkably sensitive for ovarian sex-cord tumors. The focus of this chapter is to provide a survey of the antibodies commonly used in the diagnosis of gynecologic lesions grouped as to function or type. Markers of prognostic or predictive value, such as Ki-67, a marker of nuclear proliferation, are discussed where appropriate, understanding that only a handful are sufficiently informative to be used in routine practice.

BROAD SPECTRUM DIFFERENTIATION MARKERS

The following biomarkers are expressed commonly in many cell types. They are useful in a wide variety of settings and in differential diagnoses. In some cases, their combinations may be unique to a particular entity.

EPITHELIAL MARKERS

CYTOKERATINS

Cytokeratins (CKs) belong to the group of filament proteins that are intermediate between microfilaments and microtubules. They constitute the cytoskeleton of virtually all epithelial cells, both benign and malignant. Some non-epithelial cell types and tumors derived from these may also express CKs. The cytokeratin family of proteins, coded by different genes, have been classified and numbered (numbers 1 to 20).[127] The expression of the various CKs in cells and tumors depends on their embryonic origin and also the degree of cellular differentiation.[64] One broad group of CKs, type I (CK9–20), has an acidic isoelectric point. The other group, type II (CK1–8), has a basic-neutral isoelectric point. Antibodies against CKs help confirm the epithelial lineage of a neoplasm. In this regard monoclonal antibodies, such as AE1/3 and CAM 5.2, are available that recognize multiple members of the CK family, e.g., AE1/3 reacts against almost all of the CK family of proteins (AE1 recognizes most type I CKs whereas AE3 reacts against most type II CKs). CAM 5.2 reacts against CK8 and CK18. Additionally, antibodies are available that react against specific CKs, e.g., CK7 or CK20. The following sections detail the use of various anti-CK antibodies in the diagnosis of female genital tract lesions.

Broad spectrum CKs

Broad spectrum anti-CK antibodies, such as AE1/3, often prove of value in confirming the epithelial lineage of a neoplasm. For example, in distinguishing a poorly differentiated carcinoma from sarcoma, melanoma or lymphoma, reactivity with AE1/3, especially if widespread, favors a diagnosis of carcinoma, i.e., a malignant epithelial tumor. However, the anti-CK antibodies, such as AE1/3, occasionally react with tumors of melanocytic,[11] mesenchymal, and lymphoid origin.[98] Even smooth muscle tumors may react with anti-CK antibodies.[15,132] This may result in diagnostic difficulties, especially if dealing with an epithelioid smooth muscle neoplasm. Such common experiences underscore the necessity to use panels of antibodies.

Endometrial stromal neoplasms may also be CK positive on occasion.[42] Broad spectrum anti-CK antibodies are reactive with trophoblastic cells and often are useful in distinguishing intermediate trophoblast from decidua, thus confirming the presence of a placental site.

CAM 5.2

CAM 5.2 does not react against normal squamous epithelium but is reactive against most glandular epithelia. Besides its utility in diagnosing an epithelial neoplasm, its differential staining of squamous and glandular epithelia often helps in the diagnosis of vulvar Pagets disease. The Paget cells usually react (the residual squamous cells do not) and this may be of value in diagnosis and helping to exclude mimics such as melanocytic tumors, pagetoid Bowens disease, and mycosis fungoides.

Cytokeratins 7 and 20

In recent years a combination of antibodies against CK7 and CK20 (differential CK staining) has been widely used in ovarian and peritoneal pathology to distinguish between a primary ovarian or peritoneal adenocarcinoma and a metastatic adenocarcinoma, especially of colorectal origin.[12,69,81,145,197] In general, primary ovarian carcinomas exhibit diffuse CK7 reactivity and are unreactive with CK20. Primary ovarian adenocarcinomas of serous, endometrioid, and clear cell type also usually exhibit this same immunophenotype. Primary ovarian mucinous neoplasms are more variable. In general, they are diffusely reactive with CK7 and unreactive or at most focally reactive with CK20. However, there are many exceptions with occasional primary ovarian mucinous neoplasms, especially those which exhibit intestinal differentiation, being diffusely CK20 positive. In the distinction between a primary ovarian endometrioid adenocarcinoma and a metastatic colorectal adenocarcinoma with an endometrioid appearance, differential CK staining is very useful, the former usually being diffusely CK7 reactive and CK20 unreactive, while the latter generally exhibits diffuse CK20 reactivity and is CK7 unreactive. In the case of an ovarian mucinous neoplasm, differential CK staining is not uncommonly difficult to interpret when distinguishing a primary ovarian tumor from a secondary colorectal neoplasm since many primary ovarian mucinous neoplasms may be CK20 reactive and, conversely, colorectal adenocarcinoma with a mucinous appearance may be focally CK7 positive. In addition, mucinous tumors arising in a teratoma often have staining patterns of the gastrointestinal component of the teratoma. In this regard, other antibodies (discussed below) are sometimes of value (Table 36.1).

Differential CK staining is of limited value in distinguishing between a primary ovarian carcinoma and a metastatic adenocarcinoma from other organs, since many of these tumors exhibit a CK7 positive/CK20 unreactive or focally positive immunophenotype. However, dual CK7 and CK20 reactivity raises the possibility of a primary neoplasm in the stomach, pancreas, biliary tree or urinary bladder (Table 36.2).[26,74,145,195] Breast, pulmonary, endometrial, and endocervical adenocarcinomas are most commonly CK7 positive and CK20 unreactive.

CK7 and CK20 staining also helps to confirm that most cases of pseudomyxoma peritonei in women are of appendiceal (or more rarely colorectal) origin rather than originating from a ruptured ovarian mucinous neoplasm.[58,162] In cases of pseudomyxoma peritonei with coexistent appendiceal and ovarian mucinous neoplasms, the epithelial elements in all locations, i.e., the appendix, ovary, and peritoneum, are usually diffusely CK20 positive and unreactive or focally positive with CK7, in keeping with an intestinal origin.

CK7 may be of value in the vulva in confirming a diagnosis of Pagets disease and excluding mimics such as malignant melanoma and mycosis fungoides, since the cells of primary vulvar Pagets disease are usually intensely CK7 positive.[54,55] In addition to its diagnostic value in Pagets disease, CK7 may assist in assessing the margins. With H&E-stained slides, it is often exceedingly difficult to identify that single isolated tumor cell located at the margin. CK20, while usually unreactive, may sometimes be focally reactive in vulvar Pagets disease.[16,54,55] Strong CK20 reactivity should result in consideration of secondary Pagets disease, either from the colorectum or urinary tract. Positive reactivity with uroplakin III is also suggestive of secondary Pagets disease from the urinary tract.[16]

Cytokeratin 5/6

CK5/6 is often reactive in mesothelial cells, be they normal, reactive or neoplastic, and therefore is helpful, as part of a panel, to distinguish mesothelial proliferations from epithelial.[32] This is often problematic in ovarian and peritoneal pathology, the main differential diagnosis usually being between a serous epithelial proliferation (benign, borderline or malignant) and a mesothelial proliferation (benign or malignant). Mesothelial proliferations generally react with CK5/6 while epithelial lesions often, although not always, do not. In this regard, CK5/6 should be used as part of a panel that may include Ber-EP4 (an epithelial membrane marker reactive in most epithelial lesions and generally unreactive in mesothelial lesions). Other antibodies generally reactive in mesothelial lesions are calretinin, HBME1, thrombomodulin, and CD44H (generally unreactive in epithelial lesions).[7]

Other cytokeratins

Although the remaining specific CKs have found little place in diagnostic gynecologic pathology, assessment of the qualitative changes in the cells expressing various CKs plus other non-CKs are proving helpful in assessing the progression from

Table 36.1 Typical reaction patterns in primary ovarian and metastatic colorectal adenocarcinoma

Antibody	Endometrioid ovarian adenocarcinoma	Mucinous ovarian adenocarcinoma	Colorectal adenocarcinoma
CK7	Diffuse +	Diffuse or focal +	–
CK20	–	Negative, focal or diffuse +	Diffuse +
CA125	Diffuse +	–	–
CEA	–	Negative, focal or diffuse +	Diffuse +
β-Catenin	Negative, focal or diffuse +	–	Focal or diffuse +
Cdx2	–	Negative, focal or diffuse +	Diffuse +
Villin	–	Negative, focal or diffuse +	Diffuse +
MUC5AC	Diffuse +	Diffuse +	–

Table 36.2 Typical differential cytokeratin reaction patterns in tumors

	CK7	CK20
Mucinous ovarian adenocarcinoma	+	– or +
Non-mucinous ovarian adenocarcinoma	+	–
Colorectal adenocarcinoma	–	+
Cervical adenocarcinoma	+	–
Endometrial adenocarcinoma	+	–
Pancreatic/biliary adenocarcinoma	+	+ or –
Gastric adenocarcinoma	+	+ or –
Renal cell carcinoma	–	–
Bladder adenocarcinoma	+	+ or –
Breast adenocarcinoma	+	–
Pulmonary adenocarcinoma	+	–
Mesothelioma	+	–

normal cervical squamous epithelium to low- and high-grade cervical intraepithelial neoplasia (CIN) to invasive squamous carcinoma. In brief, reactivity with CK14, 18, and 19 in the basal cell compartment increases while the expression of CK13 decreases.[130] Functional expression of these biomarkers is explored more fully in Chapter 8. Staining with the high molecular weight CK 34βE12 may assist in highlighting the basal cell layer in ectopic prostatic tissue within the cervix.[120]

EPITHELIAL MEMBRANE ANTIGEN (EMA) AND BER-EP4

EMA (a glycoprotein found in human milk fat globule membranes) and Ber-EP4 (an epithelial specific antigen to a membrane-bound glycoprotein) are both similar and help to confirm that a neoplasm has an epithelial lineage. Trophoblast and trophoblastic neoplasms are also reactive. Both are used commonly in panels to distinguish an ovarian adenocarcinoma such as a serous or endometrioid carcinoma (reactive) from a sex cord-stromal tumor (unreactive).[29,160] Ber-EP4 is useful in distinguishing a serous adenocarcinoma of the ovary or peritoneum and implants in the peritoneum (reactive) from mesothelial-derived lesions (unreactive). Although EMA reactivity is rare in ovarian sex cord-stromal tumors (even though reactivity with anti-CK antibodies is not uncommon), focal immunoreactivity inexplicably is common (50% of a small series) in ovarian juvenile granulosa cell tumors.[119] EMA is generally unreactive in the female adnexal tumor of probable wolffian origin (FATWO).[37] This is diagnostically useful since FATWO may be confused with an epithelial neoplasm, which is usually EMA reactive.

MESENCHYMAL CELL MARKERS

VIMENTIN

Vimentin is the most widely distributed of the intermediate filament proteins and is expressed in virtually all mesenchymal cells and in most mesenchymal neoplasms in the female genital tract. Occasionally there is a need to determine whether a tumor is mesenchymal or epithelial, in which case vimentin staining may be important, but in most cases the distinction is apparent from the H&E-stained slide.

By contrast, there are selected circumstances where vimentin staining may be of value. In the cervix, vimentin may be used as an aid to distinguish between tuboendometrioid metaplasia and endometriosis (usually vimentin reactive) and adenocarcinoma *in situ* (AIS) (usually vimentin unreactive).[92] Vimentin may also be useful in differentiating between an endometrial adenocarcinoma of endometrioid type and an endocervical adenocarcinoma.[22,72,110,203] The former usually exhibits diffuse vimentin reactivity whereas endocervical adenocarcinomas generally do not. The situation is less clear with a mucinous adenocarcinoma of the endometrium and an endometrioid adenocarcinoma of the cervix, although some believe that vimentin reactivity depends more on the pattern of differentiation (endometrioid versus mucinous) than the site of origin (endometrial versus cervical).[72]

Vimentin helps distinguish between a microglandular variant of endometrioid or mucinous adenocarcinoma of the endometrium (usually vimentin reactive) and cervical microglandular

hyperplasia (vimentin unreactive).[152] Reactivity may help confirm that a primary cervical adenocarcinoma is of mesonephric derivation.[177]

SMOOTH MUSCLE MARKERS

Multiple biomarkers reactive against smooth muscle antigens include alpha-smooth muscle actin (α-SMA), desmin, and h-caldesmon. These markers are helpful in several diagnostic scenarios, especially in confirming smooth muscle differentiation within a neoplasm, such tumors potentially occurring at any site within the female genital tract. However, some smooth muscle neoplasms, especially malignant and epithelioid variants, are unreactive or only focally reactive.[137] Of the three most commonly used antibodies, h-caldesmon is the most specific, but is less sensitive than desmin. Desmin is not a specific smooth muscle marker, as it also stains skeletal muscle.

In the uterine corpus, the main value of smooth muscle markers is in establishing a diagnosis of a smooth muscle neoplasm, either benign or malignant. An antibody panel composed of desmin, h-caldesmon, and CD10 (discussed later) helps distinguish cellular leiomyomatous neoplasms from endometrial stromal neoplasms (Table 36.3). In general, leiomyomatous neoplasms are diffusely reactive with desmin and h-caldesmon.[133,137,163] CD10 is usually unreactive or focally reactive, although some cellular leiomyomatous neoplasms and leiomyosarcomas may also be diffusely reactive.[27,106,184] Endometrial stromal neoplasms are usually diffusely CD10 reactive, and unreactive (most cases) or maximally focally positive to desmin and h-caldesmon.[27,106,184] α-SMA is of limited value since many endometrial stromal neoplasms are diffusely reactive, an indication that considerable immunophenotypic overlap exists between uterine smooth muscle and endometrial stromal neoplasms. This is perhaps not unexpected since these two cell types develop from a common progenitor within the uterus. Uterine tumor resembling ovarian sex-cord tumor, sex cord-like areas within endometrial stromal neoplasms, and uterine perivascular epithelioid cell tumor (PEComa) are also variably reactive with smooth muscle markers.[191]

In the cervix, α-SMA distinguishes normal endocervical glands or non-neoplastic endocervical glandular lesions from the banal glands of adenoma malignum. The presence of many α-SMA reactive stromal cells suggests a desmoplastic response to tumor.[122] This is usually accompanied by loss of estrogen receptor (ER) expression in the stromal cells.

Table 36.3 Typical reaction patterns in endometrial stromal and smooth muscle neoplasm

Antibody	Smooth muscle neoplasm	Endometrial stromal neoplasm
Desmin	Diffuse +	– or focal +
α-Smooth muscle actin	Diffuse +	Negative, focal or diffuse +
h-Caldesmon	Diffuse +	–
CD10	Negative, focal or diffuse +	Diffuse +
Oxytocin receptor	Diffuse +	–

In the vulvovaginal region, many of the wide range of relatively site-specific mesenchymal neoplasms such as angiomyofibroblastoma, aggressive angiomyxoma, and superficial cervicovaginal myofibroblastoma react with smooth muscle markers, especially desmin.[113] Thus, none of these markers is of value in confirming that a mesenchymal lesion represents a leiomyomatous neoplasm. However, non-reactivity with smooth muscle antibodies is of value in diagnosing cellular angiofibroma, which in contrast to most other neoplasms in the differential diagnosis does not usually react.[68,113,116] Some believe that cellular angiofibroma exhibits fibroblastic differentiation while most of the other neoplasms mentioned are myofibroblastic in origin.

Another tumor that commonly shows reactivity with desmin is intra-abdominal desmoplastic small round cell tumor (in females this may present as a primary ovarian neoplasm), usually with paranuclear dot-like immunoreactivity.[143] This is useful in diagnosis, especially in differentiating this neoplasm from the wide range of 'small blue cell tumors' that may involve the ovary and peritoneum. Desmin sometimes assists in the distinction between benign and malignant mesothelial proliferations. Benign mesothelial cells are usually desmin reactive while the cells of malignant mesothelioma are generally unreactive, although there is significant overlap.

SKELETAL MUSCLE MARKERS

A variety of skeletal muscle markers are available, including myoglobin, myoD1, and sarcomeric actin. These markers assist in confirming the presence of rhabdomyosarcoma.[108] Embryonal rhabdomyosarcomas generally are rare in the female genital tract, being most common in the vagina where the differential diagnosis usually includes the 'small blue cell tumors of childhood'. Rhabdomyosarcomas rarely arise in the cervix, uterus or ovary. Skeletal muscle markers may also assist in establishing a diagnosis of a pleomorphic rhabdomyosarcoma in the uterus or ovary and in confirming rhabdomyoblastic differentiation in a uterine or ovarian carcinosarcoma.

ENDOMETRIAL STROMAL MARKERS

CD10

CD10 – also known as the common acute lymphoblastic leukemia antigen (CALLA) – is a cell-surface neutral endopeptidase expressed by lymphoid precursor cells and B lymphoid cells of germinal center origin. Antibodies against CD10 are widely used in lymphoma panels.

CD10 is important in diagnosing an endometrial stromal neoplasm, since most endometrial stromal nodules and endometrial stromal sarcomas (formerly low-grade endometrial stromal sarcomas) exhibit diffuse intense reactivity, although fibrous variants may be unreactive.[13,27,106,184] In the distinction between an endometrial stromal and a smooth muscle neoplasm, CD10 should be used as part of a panel, since conventional uterine smooth muscle tumors may be focally reactive and it is common for cellular and highly cellular leiomyomas (which are frequently mistaken for endometrial stromal neoplasms) and leiomyosarcomas to be diffusely reactive.

CD10 is also characteristically reactive in mesonephric lesions within the female genital tract. Cervical mesonephric remnants and mesonephric remnants elsewhere within the female genital tract usually exhibit luminal CD10 reactivity.[112,141,142] CD10 reactivity in a benign cervical glandular lesion is good evidence of a mesonephric origin,[112] although prostatic metaplasia may also be reactive.[120] However, CD10 is of limited value in confirming a mesonephric origin for an adenocarcinoma since many usual endocervical and endometrial adenocarcinomas are also reactive.[112] FATWO may be CD10 reactive as this neoplasm most likely has a mesonephric origin.[141]

Other uses of CD10 staining in gynecologic pathology include the distinction between a metastatic renal clear cell carcinoma involving the ovary (CD10 reactive)[19] and a primary ovarian clear cell carcinoma (CD10 unreactive). In addition, most trophoblastic cell populations and trophoblastic neoplasms are reactive.[142] CD10 also help confirm the presence of endometrial stroma and in establishing a diagnosis of endometriosis.[183] However, this is of limited value in the cervix since a rim of CD10 reactive stromal cells surrounds normal endocervical glands.[112] Other gynecologic neoplasms that may be CD10 reactive include leiomyosarcoma, carcinosarcoma, undifferentiated uterine sarcoma, ovarian sex cord-stromal tumors, uterine tumors resembling ovarian sex-cord tumors, and mixed tumors of the vagina.[138,139,193] However, CD10 immunoreactivity in these neoplasms is inconsistent and unlikely to be of diagnostic value. In summary, CD10 is expressed in a much wider range of gynecologic neoplasms than was originally appreciated. When used as an aid to diagnosis, CD10 should always be part of a panel, the makeup of which will depend on the differential diagnoses under consideration.

MESOTHELIAL MARKERS

Calretinin

Calretinin is a 29 kDa calcium-binding protein, best known for its role in the diagnosis of mesothelioma. In the distinction between a mesothelioma and an adenocarcinoma, calretinin should be used as part of a panel. Calretinin and Ber-EP4, an epithelial membrane antigen marker, are the two most useful antibodies to distinguish between a serous epithelial and a mesothelial proliferation.[7] Most serous proliferations are Ber-EP4 reactive and calretinin unreactive, the converse being the rule for mesothelial lesions. Nuclear reactivity with calretinin is more specific than cytoplasmic staining for mesothelial cells.[7]

Calretinin is also found in most ovarian sex cord-stromal tumors.[20,105,128,169] In comparison to α-inhibin, calretinin is a slightly more sensitive but less specific marker of ovarian sex cord-stromal tumors. Calretinin is more likely to be reactive in an ovarian fibroma than α-inhibin. However, ovarian adenocarcinomas are more likely to be reactive with calretinin than α-inhibin.

In general, neoplasms reactive for α-inhibin also show reactivity with calretinin. Other gynecologic neoplasms that may show calretinin reactivity include FATWO, uterine tumor resembling ovarian sex-cord tumors, sex cord-like areas within endometrial stromal neoplasms, and adenomatoid tumors. Mesonephric lesions, both benign and malignant, within the cervix and elsewhere in the female genital tract may show reactivity.[112]

BLOOD VESSEL MARKERS

CD34

CD34, a single chain transmembrane glycoprotein, leukocyte differentiation antigen, is expressed by hematopoietic progenitor cells (decreases with maturation), endothelial cells, and fixed connective tissue cells (e.g., fibroblasts in skin). CD34 is inconsistently expressed in several vulvovaginal mesenchymal lesions, including aggressive angiomyxoma, cellular angiofibroma, and superficial myofibroblastoma.[49,68,113,116] Solitary fibrous tumors rarely occur at various sites within the female genital tract and are CD34 reactive.[194] Endometrial stromal neoplasms are CD34 unreactive, which may be of use in differential diagnosis in that many mimics, especially those in an extrauterine location, are reactive.[13] Metastatic gastrointestinal stromal tumor (GIST) to the ovary or elsewhere in the female genital tract usually expresses CD34,[67] as do the rare primary GISTs arising in the vulvovaginal region or rectovaginal septum.[82]

NARROW SPECTRUM DIFFERENTIATION MARKERS

These are cell type specific (pathognomonic) markers that are often useful to rule in or exclude a targeted question.

TROPHOBLASTIC MARKERS

A major application of broad-spectrum cytokeratins, as discussed above, is simple confirmation of presence or absence of an implantation site. Because trophoblast cells are reactive for keratin and decidual stroma is not, keratin reactivity is an easy method to identify trophoblast in uterine products of conception or the implantation site when trying to exclude the presence of an ectopic pregnancy. Although cytokeratin is more robust than beta-human chorionic gonadotrophin (β-hCG) or human placental lactogen (hPL), and the intensity is uniform throughout gestation, it is not useful in the evaluation of trophoblastic disease. The value of α-inhibin and CD10 as trophoblastic markers has already been discussed.

BETA-HUMAN CHORIONIC GONADOTROPHIN (β-HCG)

Human chorionic gonadotrophin (hCG) is a glycoprotein comprising a protein core and a carbohydrate side chain, and composed of two dissimilar subunits – α and β. The α subunits are indistinguishable from the α subunits of luteinizing hormone, follicle-stimulating hormone, and thyroid-stimulating hormone. The β subunits differ and confer specificity.

β-hCG reacts against syncytiotrophoblast but not cytotrophoblast. All trophoblastic neoplasms express reactivity. Choriocarcinoma shows the strongest and most diffuse reactivity. The placental site trophoblastic tumor (PSTT) and epithelioid trophoblastic tumor (ETT) are less reactive. Trophoblastic elements in mixed germ cell tumors show reactivity, as does syncytiotrophoblast when it sporadically occurs in neoplasms such as dysgerminoma and endometrial carcinoma. β-hCG may be found on occasion in a variety of non-trophoblastic neoplasms, including cervical squamous carcinoma.[61]

PLACENTAL-LIKE ALKALINE PHOSPHATASE (PLAP)

The alkaline phosphatases are a heterogeneous group of glycoproteins that are usually confined to the cell surface. PLAP is a dimer of 65 kD subunits and is synthesized during the G_1

phase of the cell cycle. PLAP is expressed in syncytiotrophoblast and in some intermediate trophoblastic populations, reactivity being stronger in lesions derived from chorion-type intermediate trophoblast, such as placental site nodule, than in lesions of implantation site intermediate trophoblast which are usually only focally positive. Ovarian dysgerminoma is also reactive.

HUMAN PLACENTAL LACTOGEN (HPL)

Human placental lactogen, a member of the gene family that includes human growth hormone and human prolactin, is expressed in intermediate trophoblast and is useful in panels to diagnose trophoblastic neoplasms. In general, expression is stronger and more diffuse in placental site trophoblastic tumor than in choriocarcinoma.

MEL-CAM (CD146)

Mel-CAM is expressed in implantation site intermediate trophoblastic cells.[170,172] Chorion-type intermediate trophoblastic cells are usually unreactive or focally reactive. Placental site trophoblastic tumor and exaggerated placental site, being lesions of implantation site intermediate trophoblast, express Mel-CAM, whereas placental site nodules and epithelioid trophoblastic tumor, which are lesions of chorion-type intermediate trophoblast, are usually Mel-CAM unreactive. In distinguishing placental site trophoblastic tumor from exaggerated placental site, double immunohistochemical staining with Mel-CAM and MIB1 has proven of value.[170] In exaggerated placental site, the MIB1 index in intermediate trophoblastic cells is close to zero whereas it is significantly elevated (14 ± 6.9%) in placental site trophoblastic tumor.[170]

HLA-G (HUMAN LEUKOCYTE ANTIGEN) (CYTOTROPHOBLAST)

HLA-G, present in all implantation-types and chorion-types of intermediate trophoblast, is expressed in all known trophoblastic tumors, including choriocarcinoma, placental site trophoblastic tumor, and epithelioid trophoblastic tumor, as well as in benign trophoblastic lesions, such as placental site nodule and exaggerated placental site.[178] HLA-G is generally unreactive in non-trophoblastic uterine neoplasms.[178] HLA-G reactivity has been found in ovarian carcinomas.[33]

MELANOCYTIC MARKERS

HMB45

HMB45 is probably the most specific marker of malignant melanoma, being melanosome associated. HMB45 reactivity is useful to confirm the diagnosis of malignant melanoma at any site within the female genital tract, most commonly found in the vulva or vagina. Metastatic melanoma in the ovary can assume an unusual array of morphologic appearances and easily fool the pathologist if there is no history of melanoma. HMB45 may assist in this regard.[60] However, occasional ovarian steroid cell tumors, which may mimic melanoma, are HMB45 reactive.[35] This is true also for melan-A (MART-1), which is discussed below. Another neoplasm characteristically reactive with HMB45 is perivascular epithelioid cell tumor (PEComa).[191] This is an extremely rare neoplasm, which in the female genital tract most commonly involves the uterine myometrium.[191] Clusters of epithelioid cells with clear cytoplasm coexpress both HMB45 and smooth muscle markers. In addition, uterine epithelioid leiomyosarcomas with a clear cell appearance may also express HMB45.[66,176]

MELAN-A (MART-1)

Melan-A, also known as MART-1, is another melanocytic marker of value in the diagnosis of malignant melanoma. Ovarian sex cord-stromal tumors are also commonly reactive.[182,201]

S-100 PROTEIN

S-100 protein is useful in the diagnosis of malignant melanoma, either primary or metastatic, at various sites within the female genital tract. Other neoplasms in the female genital tract that may be S-100 protein reactive include ovarian sex cord-stromal tumors and cartilaginous areas within carcinosarcomas.[186]

NEUROENDOCRINE MARKERS

There are various commercially available neuroendocrine markers, including chromogranin, CD56, synaptophysin, and PGP9.5. These vary in their specificity and sensitivity. For example, chromogranin is a highly specific but poorly sensitive marker while CD56 is sensitive but lacks specificity. Neuroendocrine markers may be used to confirm neuroendocrine differentiation within a neoplasm and establish a diagnosis of a small cell or large cell neuroendocrine carcinoma. Reactivity with neuroendocrine markers is not necessary to establish a diagnosis of a small cell neuroendocrine carcinoma since many of these are sparsely granulated and unreactive with neuroendocrine markers. In contrast, reactivity with neuroendocrine markers is a prerequisite for a diagnosis of large cell neuroendocrine carcinoma. Rare paraganglioma and typical and atypical carcinoid occur within the female genital tract and are reactive.[63] CD56 is a sensitive marker of ovarian sex cord-stromal tumors with most morphological subtypes being reactive.

LYMPHOID ANTIBODIES

Markers against lymphoid cells are of value in diagnosing rare hematopoietic malignancies, either lymphoma or leukemia, within the female genital tract. This complex area is discussed in detail in Chapter 29.

Several markers may assist in the diagnosis of a low-grade endometritis, usually resting on the morphologic identification of plasma cells that may be difficult to visualize with H&E when few in number. Both B and T lymphoid markers help. In the normal endometrium, most lymphoid cells are of T cell or natural killer (NK) cell lineage. B lymphocytes account for less than 1% of endometrial leukocytes, being mainly located in lymphoid aggregates. The use of B lymphoid markers, such as CD20 and CD79a, reveals substantially increased numbers of B cells in unusual locations such as beneath the surface epithelium and intraepithelially.[38] *In situ* hybridization for kappa and lambda light chains helps in diagnosing endometritis,[41] as may antibodies against plasma cells, such as syndecan and VS38.[10,85]

Aberrant reactivity to the following markers usually indicates a disease state and therefore helps in distinguishing it from normal. The pattern of expression may be pathognomonic for a particular disease state, and thus useful in resolving a differential diagnosis.

TUMOR MARKERS

CA19.9

CA19.9, an antigen of sialyl Lewis(a) containing glycoprotein, is usually reactive in pancreatic, biliary or colorectal adenocarcinoma metastatic to the ovary. This antigen commonly shows reactivity, whereas most primary ovarian adenocarcinomas are unreactive,[81] although mucinous neoplasms may be focally reactive.

CARCINOEMBRYONIC ANTIGEN (CEA)

CEA consists of a heterogeneous family of related oncofetal glycoproteins secreted into the glycocalyceal surface of gastrointestinal cells. The monoclonal antibody to CEA was raised against tumor cells derived from a hepatic metastasis of colorectal carcinoma.

Monoclonal CEA helps distinguish non-mucinous ovarian adenocarcinomas (usually unreactive) from colorectal adenocarcinoma (usually reactive), when used as part of a panel (Table 36.1).[12,81] Primary ovarian mucinous adenocarcinomas are also often reactive. Adenocarcinomas from other organs, such as pancreas and stomach, are variably reactive.

CEA often forms part of a panel to help distinguish endometrioid endometrial adenocarcinoma from endocervical adenocarcinoma.[22,72,110,203] Endocervical adenocarcinomas are usually, but not always, diffusely reactive with CEA. Primary endometrioid adenocarcinomas of the corpus are unreactive or focally reactive, although the associated squamous elements may be diffusely reactive. CEA staining patterns of primary mucinous carcinomas of the endometrium are not well studied but at least a proportion are reactive. CEA is usually reactive in cervical AIS and unreactive in benign endocervical glandular lesions.[28]

CEA is usually reactive in primary vulvar Pagets disease and, like CK7 and CAM 5.2, helps exclude mimics or assess margins.

CA125 (OC125)

CA125, a mucin-like glycoprotein, is an antibody to an ovarian carcinoma antigen. Serum CA125 levels are commonly elevated in patients with ovarian cancer, especially of the serous type. Although elevated levels are not specific for an ovarian cancer, serum CA125 measurements may be useful in diagnosis and especially in the follow-up of patients with ovarian cancer.

Immunohistochemical staining with CA125 helps to distinguish between a primary and a metastatic ovarian adenocarcinoma and in the evaluation of a disseminated peritoneal tumor in women.[102,107] In general, primary ovarian (or peritoneal) adenocarcinomas of serous, endometrioid, and clear cell types exhibit diffuse CA125 reactivity. Primary ovarian mucinous carcinomas are usually unreactive as are colorectal adenocarcinomas. In distinguishing primary ovarian adenocarcinoma from a metastatic colorectal adenocarcinoma, CA125 should be used in a panel including CK7, CK20, and CEA, as well as other markers of colorectal adenocarcinoma, which are discussed later. CA125 reactivity is not specific for an ovarian adenocarcinoma, as primary adenocarcinomas of many other organs, including breast, lung, cervix, and uterine corpus, exhibit reactivity in a proportion of cases. Mesotheliomas are commonly reactive as are benign mesothelial cells.[9]

INHIBIN

Inhibin is a dimeric 32 kDa peptide hormone composed of an α and a β subunit produced by the ovarian granulosa and theca cells. Individual antibodies are available against each subunit. Most ovarian sex cord-stromal tumors show focal to diffuse cytoplasmic reactivity with α-inhibin, although fibroma, poorly differentiated Sertoli–Leydig and sarcomatoid granulosa cell tumor are sometimes unreactive.[30,34,59,77,93,96,118,146,160,161,181,201] Small numbers of other ovarian sex cord-stromal tumors are also unreactive. Since ovarian sex cord-stromal tumors, such as granulosa and Sertoli cell tumors, may be morphologically confused with a wide range of neoplasms, especially endometrioid carcinomas, immunohistochemical evaluation with α-inhibin (and other sex cord-stromal markers such as calretinin) may be extremely useful in primary diagnosis and also when confirming a metastatic neoplasm, which may occur years or decades later.[45] In distinguishing between a sex cord-stromal tumor and an endometrioid carcinoma, the former is almost always unreactive with EMA[29,59,160] and Ber-EP4 (Table 36.4). Ovarian sex cord-stromal tumors are unreactive with CK7, but may be focally reactive with a broad spectrum anti-CK antibody.[44] Most carcinomas are unreactive with α-inhibin, although a rare tumor is focally reactive. Of import, activated ovarian stromal cells that occur in association with and at the periphery of any ovarian neoplasm may be reactive with sex cord-stromal markers, so that close attention must be paid to the cellular morphology of the particular clusters that are immunohistochemically reactive.

With the advent of fine needle aspiration cytology (FNAC), α-inhibin staining has assumed greater importance in the evaluation of ovarian cysts.[99,104] Reactivity of the cells in an aspirate with α-inhibin and unreactive staining with EMA helps confirm the presence of granulosa cells, indicating a follicular rather than an epithelial lined cyst. α-Inhibin may also help to demonstrate luteinized stromal cells in cases of ovarian stromal hyperthecosis, or in association with ovarian neoplasms of non-sex cord-stromal type that have resulted in androgenic or estrogenic manifestations.[104]

Other gynecologic neoplasms that are variably reactive with α-inhibin include FATWO, cervical mesonephric adenocarcinoma, uterine tumor resembling ovarian sex-cord tumor, and sex cord-like areas within endometrial stromal neoplasms.[8,37,78,100,188] α-Inhibin also stains some trophoblastic cell populations, syncytiotrophoblast and some intermediate trophoblastic cells showing reactivity while cytotrophoblast is unreactive.[97,171] Choriocarcinoma and other trophoblastic neoplasms, especially PSTT and ETT, may be α-inhibin reactive. β-inhibin is less useful diagnostically than α-inhibin since many ovarian and extraovarian carcinomas are reactive.[101]

OCT4

OCT4 (also called POU5F1) is an octamer binding transcription factor expressed in both mouse and human embryonic stem and germ cells. Nuclear reactivity is expressed in ovarian dysgerminoma and embryonal carcinoma and in the germ cell component of gonadoblastoma.[24] Most ovarian epithelial and sex cord-stromal tumors are unreactive, although occasional clear cell carcinomas have expressed reactivity.[24] As clear cell carcinoma and dysgerminoma often superficially resemble each other and in some areas may appear almost identical, the information about OCT4 reactivity must be assessed with great caution. Testicular seminomas and embryonal carcinomas are also OCT4 reactive.

HIK1083

HIK1083, a monoclonal antibody against gastric gland mucous cell mucin, is reactive in cervical minimal deviation adenocarcinoma of mucinous type (adenoma malignum).[121,190] This may be diagnostically useful as normal endocervical glands are consistently unreactive. Focal reactivity may be present in ordinary endocervical adenocarcinomas and less well differentiated areas in adenoma malignum may be unreactive.

The benign endocervical glandular lesion, lobular endocervical glandular hyperplasia, which can mimic adenoma malignum, may also be reactive with HIK1083.[121] This may be due, if believed, to lobular endocervical glandular hyperplasia being a precursor of adenoma malignum as rare cases with transitional features have been described.

CDx2

Cdx2 is a gene that encodes for a transcription factor involved in the development and differentiation of the small and large intestines. Colorectal adenocarcinomas usually exhibit diffuse nuclear reactivity with antibodies against *Cdx2*[57,156,189,198] and this may be useful, as part of a panel (Table 36.1), in distinguishing between a primary ovarian adenocarcinoma and a metastatic colorectal adenocarcinoma. To complicate this interpretation, the percentages vary widely among studies stating that the primary ovarian endometrioid adenocarcino-

Table 36.4 Antibodies of value in distinguishing between ovarian endometrioid adenocarcinoma and sex cord-stromal tumor

Antibody	Endometrioid adenocarcinoma	Sex cord-stromal tumor
Cytokeratin 7	+	−
Epithelial membrane antigen	+	−
α-Inhibin	−	+
Calretinin	− or +	+
Broad spectrum cytokeratins	Diffuse +	− or focal +

mas rarely exhibit *Cdx2* reactivity whereas some primary ovarian mucinous tumors do.[57,156,189,198] This reinforces the caution that markers of intestinal differentiation may on occasion be expressed in primary ovarian mucinous neoplasms and that a panel of antibodies should always be used to distinguish between a primary ovarian and metastatic colorectal carcinoma. In summary, *Cdx2* is a relatively sensitive marker of colorectal cancer, but is of limited specificity. Intestinal type AIS and adenocarcinoma in the cervix may be Cdx2 reactive.

ALPHA-FETOPROTEIN (AFP)

AFP is a glycoprotein composed of 590 amino acid residues present in yolk sac tumors and some cases of hepatocellular carcinoma. In the female genital tract, AFP helps to establish a diagnosis of yolk sac tumor of ovarian or extraovarian origin. Primary hepatoid carcinomas of the ovary, metastatic hepatocellular carcinoma, and metastatic hepatoid carcinomas from other organs may also be reactive. Some Sertoli–Leydig cell tumors in the ovary express AFP and are associated with an elevated AFP serum level.[48]

HEP PAR 1

Hep Par 1 (hepatocyte paraffin 1) is expressed in most hepatocellular carcinomas, ovarian hepatoid yolk sac tumors, primary ovarian hepatoid carcinomas, and hepatoid carcinomas metastatic to the ovary from organs in addition to the liver.[151] Hep Par 1 is of no value in distinguishing any of these tumors from each other. Occasional cervical carcinomas, either of glandular or squamous type, may also express Hep Par 1.[187]

MUC ANTIBODIES

Mucins are high molecular weight glycoproteins. Several mucin genes have been identified or cloned (*MUC1–MUC12*) and monoclonal antibodies to these are available.[51] Expression of the mucin gene *MUC5AC* helps distinguish colonic adenocarcinoma metastatic to the ovary (unreactive) from a primary ovarian adenocarcinoma (reactive).[2,69] Appendiceal and pancreatic adenocarcinomas typically express *MUC5AC*;[69] colorectal adenocarcinomas express *MUC2*. *MUC2* expression in vulvar Pagets disease favors an underlying colorectal adenocarcinoma.[80] *MUC2* reactivity is also useful to confirm that pseudomyxoma peritonei is of appendiceal origin.[135,136] *MUC5AC* is expressed in endocervical glands.

CD99

The CD99 antigen, or MIC2 gene product, is a cell surface glycoprotein involved in cell adhesion processes. CD99 is important in antibody panels used to diagnose small round blue cell tumors.

In the female genital tract, CD99 helps establish the diagnosis of peripheral primitive neuroectodermal tumor (PNET) which has rarely been described in the ovary, uterus, cervix, and vulva.[73] The reactivity should be membranous. Cytoplasmic reactivity is less specific. Ovarian sex cord-stromal tumors also commonly exhibit membranous CD99 reactivity, as may uterine tumors resembling ovarian sex-cord tumors and sex cord-like areas within endometrial stromal neoplasms.[8,78,90]

TUMOR SUPPRESSOR GENES

WT1

The *WT1* gene is a tumor suppressor gene located on the short arm of chromosome 11 at p13. Although first reported as a candidate for the main gene implicated in Wilms tumor development, *WT1* immunohistochemical expression is found but restricted to the normal tissues of ovary, kidney, testis, spleen, and mesothelium. *WT1* is expressed in a number of malignancies, including malignant mesothelioma and intra-abdominal desmoplastic small round cell tumor (IADSRCT).

Antibodies are available against both the C-terminal and the N-terminal of *WT1* and nuclear staining is regarded as positive. IADSRCT is reactive with antibodies against the C-terminal.[143] This may be useful in diagnosis and in the distinction of IADSRCT from the other small blue cell tumors, such as rhabdomyosarcoma and neuroblastoma, which rarely may involve the ovary and peritoneum.[114]

Primary ovarian, peritoneal, and tubal serous carcinomas are usually *WT1* positive (antibody against N-terminal).[3,39,56,62,115,175] In a poorly differentiated ovarian carcinoma, nuclear *WT1* reactivity favors a serous neoplasm since most endometrioid, clear cell, and mucinous carcinomas are unreactive. Transitional cell carcinomas of the ovary are also commonly *WT1* reactive.[88] With a disseminated serous carcinoma involving more than one site, diffuse reactivity with *WT1* favors an ovarian, peritoneal or tubal primary. Most uterine serous carcinomas are unreactive or only focally reactive, although the literature is somewhat contradictory.[3,39,56,62,115,175] When dealing with such cases, correlation among clinical, pathologic, radiologic, and serologic parameters is critical.

When disseminated adenocarcinoma involves the abdomen and peritoneal cavity in a female, diffuse nuclear *WT1* reactivity strongly favors a serous carcinoma arising from the ovary, peritoneum or fallopian tube. Most pancreatic, biliary, gastric, breast, and colorectal carcinomas are *WT1* unreactive. In this regard *WT1* should be employed as one element of a panel of markers.

Ovarian small cell carcinoma of hypercalcemic type is usually reactive with an antibody against the N-terminal of *WT1*.[114,117] As this small cell tumor often morphologically resembles juvenile granulosa cell tumor (JGCT), a panel of antibodies to *WT1*, α-inhibin, and EMA may be of value (Table 36.5).

Other neoplasms involving the female genital tract that may be *WT1* reactive include malignant mesothelioma, adenoma-

Table 36.5 Antibodies of value in distinguishing between ovarian small cell carcinoma of hypercalcemic type and juvenile granulosa cell tumor

Antibody	Ovarian small cell carcinoma of hypercalcemic type	Juvenile granulosa cell tumor
WT1 (N-terminal)	Diffuse + (intense)	– or focal + (weak)
α-Inhibin	–	Diffuse or focal +
Epithelial membrane antigen	Focal +	– or focal +

toid tumor (not surprising since these are of mesothelial derivation), endometrial stromal neoplasms, leiomyomatous tumors, and ovarian sex cord-stromal tumors.[167,184]

DPC4

DPC4 (for deleted in pancreatic cancer, locus 4) is a tumor suppressor gene that is inactivated by allelic loss in approximately 50% of pancreatic cancers. Such cases lack immunohistochemical staining.[69] In contrast, ovarian, colorectal, and appendiceal carcinomas are usually *DPC4* reactive[69] since there is no allelic loss. Since pancreatic adenocarcinoma metastatic to ovary may closely mimic a primary ovarian mucinous adenocarcinoma histologically (or even a benign or borderline mucinous cystadenoma), evaluation of *DPC4* reactivity is helpful diagnostically.

p53

p53 is a tumor suppressor gene, located on the short arm of chromosome 17, which encodes a 35 kDa nuclear protein involved in regulating cell growth. *p53* mutations are among the most commonly detected genetic abnormalities in human neoplasia. Mutations result in a conformational change of the protein, which becomes stabilized, thus allowing for immunohistochemical detection. The most widely used anti-*p53* antibody is D07. Usually, but not always, a diffuse intense nuclear reactivity is found whenever *p53* mutation occurs. However, lower levels of *p53* reactivity may occur without mutation, resulting from stabilized wild-type *p53* by non-mutational events.

Diffuse intense nuclear *p53* reactivity is characteristic of uterine serous carcinoma and *p53* is of value in distinguishing this carcinoma (especially those glandular variants without papillary formation) from an endometrioid carcinoma that usually exhibits much lower levels.[5,83,205] Diffuse *p53* staining in a papillary endometrial carcinoma is more in keeping with a serous adenocarcinoma than an endometrioid adenocarcinoma with papillary folds. However, there are many exceptions. An occasional serous adenocarcinoma may be *p53* unreactive and some endometrioid adenocarcinomas show significant nuclear reactivity. *p53* helps identify the precursor lesion of serous carcinoma, namely endometrial intraepithelial carcinoma (EIC). This is often a subtle lesion that not uncommonly involves an endometrial polyp. In this situation, *p53* immunohistochemistry may be combined with ER and PR, as discussed below. In some studies, the *p53* labeling index has proven to be an independent prognostic factor in endometrial carcinoma[4] but in others it is dependent on cell type and other pathologic parameters. Some believe that the *p53* labeling index is an independent prognostic factor only in endometrioid type endometrial adenocarcinomas.[4] Regardless, *p53* helps distinguish serous adenocarcinoma, EIC, and clear cell carcinoma from benign papillary endometrial proliferations and metaplasias, including the Arias-Stella effect,[154,192] a problem most likely to be encountered in small endometrial biopsies. Endometrial metaplasias may exhibit a weak heterogeneous pattern of *p53* reactivity.[154] Diffuse *p53* reactivity is much more common in uterine leiomyosarcomas than benign leiomyomatous neoplasms, including symplastic or atypical leiomyoma.[124]

In ovarian carcinoma, diffuse *p53* reactivity is more common in serous and undifferentiated carcinomas than in other mor-

phologic subtypes.[53] Recently, a dualistic pathway of ovarian serous carcinogenesis has been proposed.[164,173] Diffuse *p53* staining is far more common in high-grade compared to low-grade ovarian serous carcinoma.[140] *p53* mutation is likely to occur early in the evolution of high-grade ovarian serous carcinoma, since diffuse reactivity has been identified in small microscopic high-grade serous carcinomas, especially in prophylactic oophorectomy in patients with *BRCA1* and *BRCA2* mutations. It is generally absent or focally reactive in low-grade tumors and borderline serous tumors, which is one of several pieces of evidence that the borderline tumor pathogenetically is entirely different from the ordinary high-grade serous adenocarcinoma. *p53* reactivity has also been found in atypical epithelium in ovarian cortical inclusion cysts adjacent to serous carcinomas, so-called ovarian dysplasia or ovarian intraepithelial neoplasia.[43]

In the vulva, *p53* helps distinguish undifferentiated vulvar intraepithelial neoplasia (VIN) (unreactive) from simplex VIN (reactive). Strong *p53* reactivity confined to the basal cell layer favors differentiated VIN,[200] although *p53* reactivity may also be seen in lichen sclerosis in the absence of differentiated VIN. *p53* reactivity in vulvar Pagets disease helps predict cases in which there is associated dermal invasion.[204]

p63

The *p63* gene is a transcription factor which belongs to the *p53* family. The p63 protein has six isoforms, three each classified into two groups, designated TA-p63 and δN-p63.[174] Cytotrophoblast expresses the δN-p63 isoform whereas chorion-type intermediate trophoblast in the fetal membranes, placental site nodules, and epithelioid trophoblastic tumors express the TA-p63 isoform.[174] Intermediate trophoblast in the implantation site and placental site trophoblastic tumor do not express *p63*.

p63 helps distinguish cervical small cell neuroendocrine carcinoma from small cell non-keratinizing squamous carcinoma.[196] Most squamous carcinomas diffusely react while neuroendocrine carcinomas, including small cell neuroendocrine carcinoma, are unreactive or focally reactive.[196] In the cervix, *p63* is preferentially expressed in immature cells of squamous lineage, including basal and reserve cells.[153]

PTEN

PTEN (phosphatase and tensin homolog deleted on chromosome 10) is a tumor suppressor gene mutated in a high percentage of endometrioid adenocarcinomas of the endometrium.[17] *PTEN* mutation is generally associated with loss of *PTEN* immunohistochemical staining.[129] *PTEN* is also mutated in some endometrioid adenocarcinomas of the ovary.[23] *PTEN* mutation occurs early in the development of endometrioid-type endometrial adenocarcinoma since mutation with associated absence of immunohistochemical reactivity has been found in over half of the cases of the precursor lesion, called endometrial intraepithelial neoplasia (EIN) in one classification scheme and atypical endometrial hyperplasia in another. Of note, EIN is different from EIC, the precursor lesion to serous adenocarcinoma of the endometrium.

PTEN-null glands also occur not uncommonly in normal cyclical endometrium,[129] especially normal secretory endometrium, and therefore a lack of reactivity cannot be used to diagnose EIN or atypical endometrial hyperplasia. Further-more, not all cases of EIN exhibit an absence of *PTEN* reactivity and in other cases loss of expression precedes the development of morphologic features of EIN.

The most widely used anti-*PTEN* antibody is 6H2.1. The PTEN-null rate in endometrial adenocarcinoma varies by tumor subtype, ranging from a low of 13% of serous cancers to almost 60% of all endometrioid cancers.[129] *PTEN* inactivation is highest for those tumors preceded by an EIN lesion, in which case 66% of EIN and 83% of their associated adenocarcinomas are PTEN-null.[129]

PROTO-ONCOGENES

bcl-2

Located on chromosome 18, the proto-oncogene *bcl-2* encodes a 25 kDa protein mainly localized to the inner mitochondrial membrane. This extends cell survival by blocking apoptosis.

In proliferative endometrium, *bcl-2* is diffusely expressed in the gland cell cytoplasm. The activity is reduced in the glands of both atypical hyperplasia and endometrioid-type adenocarcinomas.[65] Furthermore, endometrioid adenocarcinomas of the corpus express *bcl-2* more commonly than non-endometrioid tumors. In the cervix, *bcl-2* is normally expressed in the basal cell layer of the squamous epithelium. Normal fallopian tube epithelium is *bcl-2* reactive,[109] as are foci of ciliated metaplasia involving the ovarian surface epithelium and the epithelium of cortical inclusion cysts.[147]

Tuboendometrial metaplasia and endometriosis in the cervix generally exhibit diffuse cytoplasmic reactivity, which helps distinguish them from AIS, which is generally unreactive.[18,94] Endometrial stromal neoplasms are also commonly *bcl-2* reactive but this is of limited value since many other tumors included in the differential diagnosis are also reactive.[13]

CD117 (C-KIT)

CD117, a transmembrane tyrosine kinase receptor, is expressed in metastatic GIST within the ovary or elsewhere in the female genital tract[67] and in rare primary GISTs arising in the vulvo-vaginal region or rectovaginal septum.[82] Some gynecologic sarcomas, including leiomyosarcoma,[157,158] may express CD117, as occasionally do other tumors, including uterine carcinosarcoma, ovarian serous carcinoma, and germ cell tumors such as dysgerminoma and gonadoblastoma.[140,199]

CELL CYCLE AND NUCLEAR PROLIFERATION

KI-67 (MIB1)

The best known markers of cell proliferation are MIB1 (reactive against the Ki-67 antigen) and proliferating cell nuclear antigen (PCNA). MIB1 identifies all cells in non-G_0 phases of the cell cycle, i.e., all proliferating cells. PCNA expression is highest during the S phase of the cell cycle but due to a relatively long half-life persists in cells that are no longer cycling and are in G_0.

Cervical squamous lesions exhibit an increased MIB1 proliferation index from normal through CIN 3.[79,95,123,149] In normal

squamous epithelium, MIB1 reactivity is largely confined to the basal and parabasal layers. While MIB1 reactivity helps somewhat to distinguish among the spectrum of CIN lesions, its major use is to distinguish between CIN and benign mimics such as atrophic squamous epithelium, transitional metaplasia and immature squamous metaplasia, the benign mimics exhibiting a low MIB1 proliferation index while there is usually substantial to nearly full thickness reactivity (>90%) in CIN 3. MIB1 also helps to evaluate cauterized cervical resection margins, i.e., cauterized CIN 3 from cauterized non-dysplastic squamous epithelium.[123]

Similarly in the endocervix, MIB1 helps to distinguish endocervical AIS and benign mimics such as tuboendometrial metaplasia, endometriosis, and microglandular hyperplasia (MGH).[18,28,84,94,150] Benign mimics usually exhibit a low MIB1 proliferation index of <10% while in AIS the proliferation index is in excess of 30% and usually much greater. In general, only scattered nuclei react in benign mimics while most nuclei react in AIS and a semi-quantitative assessment is all that is necessary. Problematically, there may be overlap at the lower end of the high-grade AIS spectrum and the upper end of the benign spectrum (especially in cases of tuboendometrial metaplasia and endometriosis). MIB1 should form part of a panel including bcl-2 and p16 (Table 36.6). MIB1 may also assist in evaluating cauterized cervical resection margins, differentiating precancer from normal.

In the vulva, MIB1 has some utility in evaluating squamous lesions.[87,148] Koilocytotic changes there may be less well developed than in the cervix. True human papillomavirus (HPV) infection of the vulva is associated with clusters of MIB1-reactive cells in the middle and upper thirds of the epithelium,[148] which helps to definitively categorize the lesion in which an equivocal diagnosis of condyloma might be made. The cells of high-grade VIN express MIB1 throughout much of the full epithelial thickness, which helps distinguish high-grade VIN from atrophic squamous epithelium.

MIB1, together with hormone receptors and p53, helps to distinguish endometrioid endometrial cancer from primary clear cell or serous carcinoma. The former generally exhibits a much lower MIB1 proliferation index than serous and clear cell tumors where almost every nucleus is reactive. This also assists in identifying small foci of EIC, the putative precursor lesion to serous carcinoma. Proliferation indices in endometrial cancers are an independent prognostic factor in some, but not all, studies.[50,165,180]

Proliferation markers have been used when assessing trophoblastic lesions.[85] There is no significant difference in the proliferation index in chorionic villi between hydatidiform mole and hydropic abortion.[185] Reactivity with proliferation

Table 36.6 Antibodies of value in distinction between cervical tuboendometrial metaplasia and endometriosis and adenocarcinoma *in situ* (AIS)

Antibody	Tuboendometrial metaplasia/endometriosis	Cervical AIS
MIB1	<30%	>50%
bcl-2	Diffuse +	–
p16	– or focal +	Diffuse +

markers is largely confined to villous cytotrophoblast. Proliferation markers do not predict progression of hydatidiform moles to persistent trophoblastic disease. MIB1 also aids in distinguishing PSTT and an exaggerated placental site.[170] In the former, the MIB1 index is significantly elevated ($14 \pm 7\%$) whereas it is nearly zero in the latter.[170] Care should be taken to exclude reactivity in small lymphocytes in the latter. MIB1 also helps distinguish PSTT from choriocarcinoma, since the latter exhibits a much higher proliferation index.[170]

p16

p16, also known as cyclin-dependent kinase 4 inhibitor (CDK4I), is the product of the *INK4A* gene and binds specifically to cyclin D:CDK4/6 complexes to control the cell cycle at the G_1–S interphase (see Chapter 8 for a fuller discussion of the entire pathway). In the cervix, diffuse p16 staining usually correlates with the presence of high-risk HPV.[71,75,76] Thus, there is diffuse p16 expression (usually a combination of nuclear and cytoplasmic staining) in high-grade CIN. A proportion of cells in low-grade CIN may also show reactivity.[71] In cervical squamous lesions, p16 may help identify small focal areas of high-grade CIN and distinguish atypical immature squamous metaplasia from high-grade CIN involving immature metaplastic squamous epithelium.[1,75]

Most neoplastic and preneoplastic endocervical glandular lesions exhibit diffuse p16 reactivity since these are generally associated with high-risk HPV.[18,131,159] p16 may also be useful in diagnosing endocervical AIS (also known as high-grade cervical glandular intraepithelial neoplasia; HCGIN), which is usually diffusely reactive, and distinguishing this from mimics such as tuboendometrial metaplasia (TEM) and endometriosis which are either unreactive or focally reactive.[18] In this regard, p16, MIB1, and bcl-2 can be used as part of a panel[18] (Table 36.6). As discussed above, p16 helps distinguish endocervical adenocarcinoma, which exhibits diffuse reactivity, from endometrial adenocarcinoma of endometrioid type, which is unreactive or focally reactive.[6,111] The squamous areas in endometrial adenocarcinomas may be strongly reactive. Rare cases of uterine corpus endometrioid adenocarcinoma will exhibit diffuse reactivity but this is exceptional. Some endometrial serous carcinomas also react diffusely with p16.[6]

p16 is useful to distinguish metastatic cervical adenocarcinoma in the ovary (p16 reactive) from primary ovarian endometrioid or mucinous adenocarcinoma (p16 unreactive).[40] In the vulva, p16 reactivity is characteristic of bowenoid, warty or undifferentiated VIN,[155,166] since this disease in all stages of its development is associated with HPV infection. Differentiated or simplex VIN is usually p16 unreactive since there is no association with HPV.[155,166] Similarly, HPV-associated vulvar squamous carcinomas are p16 reactive while those not associated with HPV are unreactive.

p57

p57, also known as Kip2, is a cell cycle inhibitor of cell proliferation and tumor suppressor encoded by a strongly paternally imprinted, maternally expressed gene. p57 is only expressed when maternal DNA is present. A particular use is in the distinction of complete hydatidiform mole from partial hydatidiform mole and hydropic abortion. p57 is expressed in the nuclei of cytotrophoblast and villous mesenchyme in the normal pla-

centa, hydropic villi, and villi of partial mole since all have a maternal component.[21,31,47,52,70] In contrast, p57 is absent in the villous cytotrophoblastic cell nuclei in the complete mole, since these villi are paternally derived and lack maternal DNA. Positive reactivity in decidua and extravillous trophoblast (it is not known why extravillous trophoblast reacts) acts as an internal positive control. p57 cannot determine whether a trophoblastic neoplasm has arisen from a pre-existing partial or complete mole or non-molar pregnancy.[168]

HORMONE RECEPTORS

ESTROGEN RECEPTOR (ER) AND PROGESTERONE RECEPTOR (PR)

Many native normal tissues and tumors arising within the female genital tract exhibit reactivity with antibodies against ER and PR. There are several situations in which these markers have diagnostic value.

Most of the vulvovaginal mesenchymal lesions react with ER and PR, including aggressive angiomyxoma, angiomyofibroblastoma, cellular angiofibroma, superficial cervicovaginal myofibroblastoma, and smooth muscle neoplasms.[49,68,103,113,116,] Therefore, assessing ER and PR reactivity does not assist in distinguishing between these neoplasms, most of which are thought to arise from the zone of hormone receptor-positive subepithelial cells that extend from the cervix to the vulva. That aggressive angiomyxoma is often hormone receptor positive is the rationale for treating these neoplasms with gonadotrophin-releasing hormone agonists, especially recurrent neoplasms and those tumors not amenable to surgical resection.[44]

Endometrial cancers of endometrioid type, often referred to as type I cancers, are commonly ER and PR reactive, whereas serous and clear cell tumors, the so-called type II cancers, are not.[36] Pathogenetically, endometrioid cancers often arise on a background of EIN and in some as yet undefined mechanism are often related to abnormal estrogen exposure or abnormal estrogen receptivity. All EIN lesions are reactive for both ER and PR. All anovulatory endometria (this encompasses the balance of 'hyperplasias') are also all essentially positive.

The serous and clear cell tumors occur in an older population of women, have an adjacent endometrium that is atrophic, and are unrelated pathogenetically to estrogen. In practice there may be immunohistochemical overlap, with some type I cancers being ER and PR unreactive while some type II cancers are reactive, albeit usually focally so. In spite of this, immunohistochemical staining with ER and PR may assist in distinguishing between types of neoplastic classes. For example, a papillary endometrioid carcinoma may be mistaken for a serous carcinoma whereas a glandular variant of serous carcinoma without papillary formation may be mistaken for an endometrioid adenocarcinoma. Diffuse strong nuclear reactivity with ER and PR favors an endometrioid adenocarcinoma whereas negativity or focal reactivity suggests a serous carcinoma. In practice it is useful to combine ER and PR with p53, the latter usually being diffusely reactive in serous carcinomas and unreactive or only focally reactive in endometrioid cancers. Similarly, a combination of ER, PR, and p53 may help distinguish problematic endometrial metaplasias and benign papillary proliferations from a small uterine serous carcinoma or its presumed precursor lesion endometrial intraepithelial

Table 36.7 Typical reaction patterns of endometrial adenocarcinoma of endometrioid type and endocervical adenocarcinoma

Antibody	Endometrioid-type endometrial adenocarcinoma	Endocervical adenocarcinoma
Estrogen receptor	Diffuse +	–
Vimentin	Diffuse +	–
Monoclonal carcinoembryonic antigen	– or focal +	Diffuse or focal +
p16	– or focal +	Diffuse +

carcinoma (EIC). Endometrial metaplasias usually exhibit a weak heterogeneous pattern of p53 staining whereas EIC generally exhibits diffuse intense reactivity.[154] Quantitative ER and PR are also of prognostic value in endometrial cancers in that hormone receptor-positive neoplasms have a better prognosis than those that are unreactive. However, the prognostic value of ER and PR staining is not independent of other parameters, such as tumor type and grade. Many other uterine neoplasms may be ER and PR positive, including endometrial stromal sarcoma and smooth muscle neoplasms, both benign and malignant.

ER assessment as part of a panel helps differentiate endometrioid adenocarcinoma of the endometrium and an endocervical adenocarcinoma (Table 36.7).[6,22,72,110,203] This may be a difficult distinction to make when tumor is present in both endometrial and cervical biopsies or in a hysterectomy specimen where tumor involves both the corpus and cervix. Endometrial adenocarcinomas of endometrioid type are generally diffusely ER reactive while endocervical adenocarcinomas are unreactive or at most focally reactive.[22,110] In a panel with vimentin, monoclonal CEA, and p16,[6,111] endometrioid-type endometrial adenocarcinomas are usually vimentin reactive, CEA unreactive or focally reactive, and p16 unreactive or focally reactive. In contrast, endocervical adenocarcinomas are usually vimentin unreactive and diffusely reactive with CEA and p16. Squamoid elements in endometrioid adenocarcinomas of the uterus may be both CEA and p16 reactive. Techniques such as in situ hybridization that demonstrate HPV may also be of value. Endometrioid adenocarcinoma in the corpus is unreactive, whereas endocervical adenocarcinoma often is reactive.[179]

Other situations in which ER and PR may be of diagnostic value are the distinction between a primary ovarian adenocarcinoma and a secondary adenocarcinoma from outside the female genital tract. In general, ER and/or PR reactivity suggests an ovarian primary, although many primary ovarian adenocarcinomas are unreactive. However, ER and PR are of no value in the distinction between a primary ovarian adenocarcinoma and a metastasis from the breast or from elsewhere within the female genital tract.

ANDROGEN RECEPTOR

In both the cervix and vagina, androgen receptor (AR) is reactive in mesonephric remnants and ectopic prostatic tissue.[120] Normal endocervical glands are usually unreactive, although the expression of AR in the wide range of benign endocervical

glandular lesions has not been extensively studied. Normal cervical and vaginal stromal fibroblasts are AR positive.[120] Other neoplasms in the female genital tract found to express AR in a variable percentage of cases include endometrial adenocarcinoma, endometrial stromal sarcoma, cervical mesonephric adenocarcinoma, and female adnexal tumor of probable wolffian origin.[14,37,126]

OXYTOCIN RECEPTOR

Oxytocin is produced by the posterior pituitary and is released into the systemic circulation in response to stimuli such as parturition and suckling. Oxytocin receptor is present in the non-pregnant uterus, in both the endometrium and myometrium.[46] An antibody against oxytocin receptor helps to distinguish uterine smooth muscle tumor (oxytocin receptor reactive) from an endometrial stromal neoplasm (oxytocin receptor unreactive).[86]

CELL ADHESION MARKERS

BETA-CATENIN

Beta-catenin (β-catenin) and adenomatous polyposis coli gene mutations are common in colorectal carcinoma.[125] As a result of these mutations, β-catenin is localized to the nucleus of colorectal carcinomas where it may be detected immunohistochemically. β-Catenin may be a useful addition to the panel of antibodies employed to distinguish between a primary ovarian adenocarcinoma and a metastatic colorectal adenocarcinoma (Table 36.1).[25] Most, but not all, colorectal adenocarcinomas exhibit nuclear reactivity while the majority of primary ovarian mucinous neoplasms are unreactive. Primary ovarian endometrioid adenocarcinomas may exhibit nuclear reactivity since they can be associated with β-catenin gene mutation[25] and the squamoid elements are often intensely positive.[89] Membranous β-catenin staining is the norm in epithelial cells and only nuclear reactivity is of diagnostic value.

REFERENCES

1. Agoff SN, Lin P, Morihara J, Mao C, Kiviat NB, Koutsky LA. p16 INK4A expression correlates with degree of cervical neoplasia: a comparison with Ki-67 expression and detection of high-risk HPV types. Mod Pathol 2003;16:665–73.
2. Albarracin CT, Jafri J, Montag AG, Hart J, Kuan S. Differential expression of MUC2 and MUC5AC mucin genes in primary ovarian and metastatic colonic carcinoma. Hum Pathol 2000;31:672–7.
3. Al-Hussaini M, Stockman A, Foster H, McCluggage WG. WT-1 assists in distinguishing ovarian from uterine serous carcinoma and in distinguishing serous and ovarian endometrioid carcinoma. Histopathology 2004;44: 109–15.
4. Alkushi A, Lim P, Coldman A, Huntsman D, Miller D, Gilks CB. Interpretation of p53 immunoreactivity in endometrial carcinoma: establishing a clinically relevant cut-off level. Int J Gynecol Pathol 2004;23:129–37.
5. Ambros RA, Sheehan CE, Kallakury BV, et al. MDM2 and p53 protein expression in the histologic subtypes of endometrial carcinoma. Mod Pathol 1996;9:1165–9.
6. Ansari-Lari MA, Staebler A, Zaino RJ, Shah KV, Ronnett BM. Distinction of endocervical and endometrial adenocarcinomas: immunohistochemical p16 expression correlated with human papillomavirus (HPV) DNA detection. Am J Surg Pathol 2004;28:160–7.
7. Attanoos RL, Webb R, Dojcinov SD, Gibbs AR. Value of mesothelial and epithelial antibodies in distinguishing diffuse peritoneal mesothelioma in females from serous papillary carcinoma of the ovary and peritoneum. Histopathology 2002;40:237–44.

8. Baker RJ, Hildebrandt RH, Rouse RV, Hendrickson MR, Longacre TA. Inhibin and CD99 (MIC2) expression in uterine stromal neoplasms with sex cord-like elements. Hum Pathol 1999;30:671–9.

9. Bateman AC, al-Talib RK, Newman T, Williams JH, Herbert A. Immunohistochemical phenotype of malignant mesothelioma: predictive value of CA125 and HBME-1 expression. Histopathology 1997;30:49–56.

10. Bayer-Garner IB, Korourian S. Plasma cells in chronic endometritis are easily identified when stained with syndecan-1. Mod Pathol 2001;14:877–9.

11. Ben-Izhak O, Stark P, Levy R, Bergman R, Lichtig C. Epithelial markers in malignant melanoma. A study of primary lesions and their metastases. Am J Dermatopathol 1994;16:241–6.

12. Berezowski K, Stasny JF, Kornstein MJ. Cytokeratins 7 and 20 and carcinoembryonic antigen in ovarian and colonic carcinoma. Mod Pathol 1996;9:426–9.

13. Bhargava R, Shia J, Hummer AJ, et al. Distinction of endometrial stromal sarcomas from 'hemangiopericytomatous' tumors using a panel of immunohistochemical stains. Mod Pathol 2005;18:40–7.

14. Bozdogan O, Atasoy P, Erekul S, Bozdogan N, Bayram M. Apoptosis-related proteins and steroid hormone receptors in normal, hyperplastic, and neoplastic endometrium. Int J Gynecol Pathol 2002;21:375–82.

15. Brown DC, Theaker JM, Banks PM, Gatter KC, Mason DY. Cytokeratin expression in smooth muscle and smooth muscle tumours. Histopathology 1987;11:477–86.

16. Brown HM, Wilkinson EJ. Uroplakin-III to distinguish primary vulvar Paget disease from Paget disease secondary to urothelial carcinoma. Hum Pathol 2002;33:545–8.

17. Bussaglia E, del Rio E, Matias-Guiu X, Prat J. PTEN mutations in endometrial carcinomas: a molecular and clinicopathologic analysis of 38 cases. Hum Pathol 2000;31:312–17.

18. Cameron RI, Maxwell P, Jenkins D, McCluggage WG. Immunohistochemical staining with MIB-1, bcl2 and p16 assists in the distinction of cervical glandular intraepithelial neoplasia from tubo-endometrial metaplasia, endometriosis and microglandular hyperplasia. Histopathology 2002;41:313–21.

19. Cameron RI, Ashe P, O'Rourke DM, Foster H, McCluggage WG. A panel of immunohistochemical stains assists in the distinction between ovarian and renal clear cell carcinoma. Int J Gynecol Pathol 2003;22:272–6.

20. Cao QJ, Jones JG, Li M. Expression of calretinin in human ovary, testis and ovarian sex cord-stromal tumors. Int J Gynecol Pathol 2001;20:346–52.

21. Castrillon DH, Sun DQ, Weremowicz S, Fisher RA, Crum CP, Genest DR. Discrimination of complete hydatidiform mole from its mimics by immunohistochemistry of the paternally imprinted gene product p57 (KIP2). Am J Surg Pathol 2001;25:1225–30.

22. Castrillon DH, Lee KR, Nucci MR. Distinction between endometrial and endocervical adenocarcinoma: an immunohistochemical study. Int J Gynecol Pathol 2002;21:4–10.

23. Catasus L, Bussaglia E, Rodrguez I, et al. Molecular genetic alterations in endometrioid carcinomas of the ovary: similar frequency of beta-catenin abnormalities but lower rate of microsatellite instability and PTEN alterations than in uterine endometrioid carcinomas. Hum Pathol 2004;35:1360–8.

24. Cheng L, Thomas A, Roth CM, et al. OCT4. A novel biomarker for dysgerminoma of the ovary. Am J Surg Pathol 2004;18:1341–6.

25. Chou YY, Jeng YM, Kao HL, Chen TJ, Mao TL, Lin MC. Differentiation of ovarian mucinous carcinoma and metastatic colorectal adenocarcinoma by immunostaining with β-catenin. Histopathology 2003;43:151–6.

26. Chu P, Wu E, Weiss LM. Cytokeratin 7 and cytokeratin 20 expression in epithelial neoplasms: a survey of 435 cases. Mod Pathol 2000;13:962–72.

27. Chu PG, Arber PA, Weiss LM, et al. Utility of CD10 in distinguishing between endometrial stromal sarcoma and uterine smooth muscle tumors: an immunohistochemical comparison of 34 cases. Mod Pathol 2001;14:465–71.

28. Cina SJ, Richardson MS, Austin RM, Kurman RJ. Immunohistochemical staining for Ki-67 antigen, carcinoembryonic antigen, and p53 in the differential diagnosis of glandular lesions of the cervix. Mod Pathol 1997;10:176–80.

29. Costa MJ, De Rose PB, Roth LM, et al. Immunohistochemical phenotype of ovarian granulosa cell tumors: absence of epithelial membrane antigen has diagnostic value. Hum Pathol 1994;25:60–6.

30. Costa MJ, Ames PF, Walls J, Roth CM. Inhibin immunohistochemistry applied to ovarian neoplasms: a novel, effective diagnostic tool. Hum Pathol 1997;28:1247–54.

31. Crisp H, Burton JL, Stewart R, Wells M. Refining the diagnosis of hydatidiform mole: image ploidy analysis and p57 KIP2 immunohistochemistry. Histopathology 2003;43:363–73.

32. Cury PM, Butcher DN, Fisher C, Corrin B, Nicholson AG. Value of the mesothelium-associated antibodies thrombomodulin, cytokeratin 5/6, calretinin, and CD44H in distinguishing epithelioid pleural mesothelioma from adenocarcinoma metastatic to the pleura. Mod Pathol 2000;13:107–12.

33. Davidson B, Elstrand MB, McMaster MT, et al. HLA-G expression in effusions is a possible marker of tumor susceptibility to chemotherapy in ovarian carcinoma. Gynecol Oncol 2005;96:42–7.

34. Deavers MT, Malpica A, Liu J, Broaddus R, Silva EG. Ovarian sex cord-stromal tumors: an immunohistochemical study including a comparison of calretinin and inhibin. Mod Pathol 2003;16:584–90.

35. Deavers MT, Malpica A, Ordonez NG, Silva EG. Ovarian steroid cell tumors: an immunohistochemical study including a comparison of calretinin with inhibin. Int J Gynecol Pathol 2003;22:162–7.

36. Demopoulos RL, Mesia AF, Mittal K, Vamvakas E. Immunohistochemical comparison of uterine papillary serous and papillary endometrioid carcinoma: clues to pathogenesis. Int J Gynecol Pathol 1999;18:233–7.

37. Devouassoux-Shisheboran M, Silver SA, Tavassoli FA. Wolffian adnexal tumor, so-called female adnexal tumor of probable Wolffian origin (FATWO): immunohistochemical evidence in support of a Wolffian origin. Hum Pathol 1999;30:85–63.

38. Disep B, Innes BA, Cochrane HR, Tijani S, Bulmer JN. Immunohistochemical characterization of endometrial leucocytes in endometritis. Histopathology 2004;45:625–32.

39. Egan JA, Ionescu ML, Eapen E, Jones JG, Marshall DS. Differential expression of WT1 and p53 in serous and endometrioid carcinoma of the endometrium. Int J Gynecol Pathol 2004;23:119–22.

40. Elishaev E, Gilks CB, Miller D, Srodon M, Kurman RJ, Ronnett BM. Synchronous and metachronous endocervical and ovarian neoplasms: evidence supporting interpretation of the ovarian neoplasms as metastatic endocervical adenocarcinomas simulating primary ovarian surface epithelial neoplasms. Am J Surg Pathol 2005;29:281–94.

41. Euscher E, Nuovo GJ. Detection of kappa- and lambda-expressing cells in the endometrium by in situ hybridization. Int J Gynecol Pathol 2002;21:383–90.

42. Farhood AI, Abrams J. Immunohistochemistry of endometrial stromal sarcoma. Hum Pathol 1991;22:224–30.

43. Feeley KM, Wells M. Precursor lesions of ovarian epithelial malignancy. Histopathology 2001;38:87–95.

44. Fine BA, Munoz AK, Litz CE, Gershenson DM. Primary medical management of recurrent aggressive angiomyxoma of the vulva with a gonadotropin-releasing hormone agonist. Gynecol Oncol 2001;81:120–2.

45. Flemming P, Wellmann A, Maschek H, Lang H, Georgii A. Monoclonal antibodies against inhibin represent key markers of adult granulosa cell tumors of the ovary even in their metastases. A report of three cases with late metastasis, being previously misinterpreted as hemangiopericytoma. Am J Surg Pathol 1995;19:927–33.

46. Fuchs AR, Fuchs F, Soloff MS. Oxytocin receptors in nonpregnant human uterus. J Clin Endocrinol Metab 1985;60:37–41.

47. Fukunaga M. Immunohistochemical characterization of p57 KIP2 expression in early hydatidiform moles. Hum Pathol 2002;33:1188–92.

48. Gagnon S, Tetu B, Silva EG, McCaughey WT. Frequency of alpha-fetoprotein production by Sertoli–Leydig cell tumors of the ovary: an immunohistochemical study of eight cases. Mod Pathol 1989;2:63–7.

49. Ganesan R, McCluggage WG, Hirschowitz L, Rollason TP. Superficial myofibroblastoma of the lower female genital tract: report of a series including tumours with a vulval location. Histopathology 2005;46:137–43.

50. Geisler JP, Geisler HE, Miller GA, Wiemann MC, Zhou Z, Crabtree W. MIB-1 in endometrial carcinoma: prognostic significance with 5–year follow-up. Gynecol Oncol 1999;75:432–6.

51. Gendler SJ, Spicer AP. Epithelial mucin genes. Annu Rev Physiol 1995;57:607–34.

52. Genest DR, Dorfman DM, Castrillon DH. Ploidy and imprinting in hydatidiform moles. Complementary use of flow cytometry and immunohistochemistry of the imprinted gene product p57 KIP2 to assist molar classification. J Reprod Med 2002;47:342–6.

53. Gilks CB. Subclassification of ovarian surface epithelial tumors based on correlation of histologic and molecular pathologic data. Int J Gynecol Pathol 2004;23:200–5.

54. Goldblum JR, Hart WR. Vulvar Paget's disease: a clinicopathologic and immunohistochemical study of 19 cases. Am J Surg Pathol 1997;21:1178–87.

55. Goldblum JR, Hart WR. Perianal Paget's disease – a histologic and immunohistochemical study of 11 cases with and without associated rectal adenocarcinoma. Am J Surg Pathol 1998;2:170–1.

56. Goldstein NS, Uzieblo A. WT-1 immunoreactivity in uterine papillary serous carcinoma is different from ovarian serous carcinomas. Am J Clin Pathol 2002;117:541–5.

57. Groisman GM, Meir A, Sabo E. The value of Cdx2 immunostaining in differentiating primary ovarian carcinomas from colonic carcinomas metastatic to the ovaries. Int J Gynecol Pathol 2004;23:52–7.

58. Guerrieri C, Franlund B, Fristedt S, Gillooley JF, Boeryd B. Mucinous tumors of the vermiform appendix and ovary, and pseudomyxoma peritonei: histogenetic implications of cytokeratin 7 expression. Hum Pathol 1997;28:1039–45.

59. Guerrieri C, Franlund B, Malmstrom H, Boeryd B. Ovarian endometrioid carcinomas simulating sex cord-stromal tumors; a study using inhibin and cytokeratin 7. Int J Gynecol Pathol 1998;17:266–71.

60. Gupta D, Deavers MT, Silva EG, Malpica A. Malignant melanoma involving the ovary: a clinicopathologic and immunohistochemical study of 23 cases. Am J Surg Pathol 2004;28:771–80.

61. Hameed A, Miller DS, Muller CY, Coleman RL, Albores-Saavedra J. Frequent expression of beta-human chorionic gonadotropin (β-hCG) in squamous cell carcinoma of the cervix. Int J Gynecol Pathol 1999;18:381–6.

62. Hashi A, Yuminamochi T, Murata S-I, Iwamoto H, Honda T, Hoshi K. Wilms tumor gene immunoreactivity in primary serous carcinomas of the fallopian tube, ovary, endometrium and peritoneum. Int J Gynecol Pathol 2003;22:374–7.

63. Hassan A, Bennet A, Bhalla S, Ylagan LR, Mutch D, Dehner LP. Paraganglioma of the vagina: report of a case, including immunohistochemical and ultrastructural findings. Int J Gynecol Pathol 2003;22:404–6.

64. Heatley MK. Cytokeratins and cytokeratin staining in diagnostic histopathology. Histopathology 1996;28:479–83.

65. Henderson GS, Brown KA, Perkins SL, Abbott TM, Clayton F. bcl-2 is down-regulated in atypical endometrial hyperplasia and adenocarcinoma. Mod Pathol 1996;9:430–8.

66. Hurrell DP, McCluggage WG. Uterine leiomyosarcoma with HMB45 positive clear cell areas: report of two cases. Histopathology 2005;47:540–2.

67. Irving JA, Lerwill MF, Young RH. Gastrointestinal stromal tumors metastatic to the ovary: a report of five cases. Am J Surg Pathol 2005;29:920–6.

68. Iwasa Y, Fletcher CD. Cellular angiofibroma: clinicopathologic and immunohistochemical analysis of 51 cases. Am J Surg Pathol 2004;28:1426–35.

69. Ji H, Isacson C, Seidman JD, Kurman RJ, Ronnett BM. Cytokeratins 7 and 20, Dpc4, and MUC5AC in the distinction of metastatic mucinous carcinomas in the ovary from primary ovarian mucinous tumors: Dpc4 assists in identifying metastatic pancreatic carcinomas. Int J Gynecol Pathol 2002;21:391–400.

70. Jun S-Y, Ro JY, Kim K-R. p57 KIP2 is useful in the classification and differential diagnosis of complete and partial hydatidiform moles. Histopathology 2003;43:17–25.

71. Kalof AN, Evans MF, Simmons-Arnold L, Beatty BG, Cooper K. p16INK4A immunoexpression and HPV in situ hybridization signal patterns: potential markers of high-grade cervical intraepithelial neoplasia. Am J Surg Pathol 2005;29:674–9.

72. Kamoi S, Al Juboury ML, Akin MR, et al. Immunohistochemical staining in the distinction between endometrial and endocervical adenocarcinomas: another viewpoint. Int J Gynecol Pathol 2002;21:217–23.

73. Kawrachi S, Fukuda T, Miyamoto S, et al. Peripheral primitive neuroectodermal tumor of the ovary confirmed by CD99 immunostaining, karyotypic analysis and RT-PCR for EWS/FLI-1 chimeric mRNA. Am J Surg Pathol 1998;22:1417–22.

74. Kim MA, Lee HS, Yang HK, Kim WH. Cytokeratin expression profile in gastric carcinomas. Hum Pathol 2004;35:576–81.

75. Klaes R, Benner A, Friedrich T, et al. p16INK4a immunohistochemistry improves interobserver agreement in the diagnosis of cervical intraepithelial neoplasia. Am J Surg Pathol 2002;26:1389–99.

76. Klaes R, Friedrich T, Spitkovsky D, et al. Overexpression of p16 (INK4A) as a specific marker for dysplastic and neoplastic epithelial cells of the cervix uteri. Int J Cancer 2002;92:276–84.

77. Kommoss F, Oliva E, Bhan AK, Young RH, Scully RE. Inhibin expression in ovarian tumors and tumor-like lesions: an immunohistochemical study. Mod Pathol 1998;11:656–64.

78. Krishnamurthy S, Jungbloth AA, Busam KJ, Rosai J. Uterine tumors resembling ovarian sex cord tumors have an immunophenotype consistent with true sex cord differentiation. Am J Surg Pathol 1998;22:1078–82.

79. Kruse A-J, Baak JPA, Helliesen T, et al. Evaluation of MIB-1 positive cell clusters as a diagnostic marker for cervical intraepithelial neoplasia. Am J Surg Pathol 2002;26:1501–7.

80. Kuan SF, Montag AG, Hart J, Krausz T, Recant W. Differential expression of mucin genes in mammary and extramammary Paget's disease. Am J Surg Pathol 2001;25:1469–77.

81. Ladendijk JA, Mullink EH, van Diest PJ, et al. Tracing the origin of adenocarcinomas with unknown primary using immunohistochemistry. Differential diagnosis between colonic and ovarian carcinomas as primary sites. Hum Pathol 1998;29:491–7.

82. Lam MM, Corless CL, Goldblum JR, et al. Extragastrointestinal stromal tumours (EGISTs) presenting as vulvovaginal/rectovaginal septal masses: a diagnostic pitfall. Mod Pathol 2003;18:885A.

83. Lax SF, Kendall B, Tashiro H, Slebos RJ, Hedrick L. The frequency of p53, K-ras mutations, and microsatellite instability differs in uterine endometrioid and serous carcinoma: evidence of distinct molecular genetic pathways. Cancer 2000;88:814–25.

84. Lee KR, Sun D, Crum CP. Endocervical intraepithelial glandular atypia (dysplasia): a histopathologic, human papillomavirus, and MIB-1 analysis of 25 cases. Hum Pathol 2000;1:656–64.

85. Leong ASY, Vinyuvat S, Leong FJWM, et al. Anti-CD38 and VS38 antibodies for detection of plasma cells in the diagnosis of chronic endometritis. Appl Immunohistochem 1997;5:189–93.

86. Loddenkemper C, Mechsner S, Foss H-D, et al. Use of oxytocin receptor expression in distinguishing between uterine smooth muscle tumors and endometrial stromal sarcoma. Am J Surg Pathol 2003;27:1458–62.

87. Logani S, Cu D, Quint WGV, Ellenson LH, Pirog EC. Low-grade vulvar and vaginal intraepithelial neoplasia: correlation of histologic features with human papillomavirus DNA detection and MIB1 immunostaining. Mod Pathol 2003;16:735–41.

88. Logani S, Oliva E, Amin MB, Folpe AL, Cohen C, Young RH. Immunoprofile of ovarian tumors with putative transitional cell (urothelial) differentiation using novel urothelial markers: histogenetic and diagnostic implications. Am J Surg Pathol 2003;27:1434–41.

89. Logani S, Oliva E, Arnell PM, Amin MB, Young RH. Use of novel immunohistochemical markers expressed in colonic adenocarcinoma to distinguish primary ovarian tumors from metastatic colorectal carcinoma. Mod Pathol 2005;18:19–25.

90. Loo KT, Leung AKF, Chan JKC. Immunohistochemical staining of ovarian granulosa cell tumours with MIC2 antibody. Histopathology 1995;27:388–90.

91. Marjoniemi VM. Immunohistochemistry in gynaecological pathology: a review. Pathology 2004;36:109–19.

92. Marques T, Andrade LA, Vassallo J. Endocervical tubal metaplasia and adenocarcinoma in situ: role of immunohistochemistry for carcinoembryonic antigen and vimentin in differential diagnosis. Histopathology 1996;28:549–50.

93. Matias-Guiu X, Pons C, Prat J. Mullerian inhibiting substance, alpha-inhibin, and CD99 expression in sex cord-stromal tumors and endometrioid ovarian carcinomas resembling sex cord-stromal tumors. Hum Pathol 1998;29:840–5.

94. McCluggage WG, Maxwell P, McBride HA, Hamilton PW, Bharucha H. Monoclonal antibodies Ki-67 and MIB1 in the distinction of tuboendometrial metaplasia from endocervical adenocarcinoma and adenocarcinoma in situ in formalin fixed material. Int J Gynecol Pathol 1995;14:209–16.

95. McCluggage WG, Tang L, Maxwell P, Bharucha H. Monoclonal antibody MIB1 in the assessment of cervical squamous intraepithelial lesions. Int J Gynecol Pathol 1996;15:131–6.

96. McCluggage WG, Maxwell P, Sloan JM. Immunohistochemical staining of ovarian granulosa cell tumors with monoclonal antibody against inhibin. Hum Pathol 1997;28:1034–8.

97. McCluggage WG, Ashe P, McBride H, Maxwell P, Sloan JM. Localization of the cellular expression of inhibin in trophoblastic tissue. Histopathology 1998;32:252–6.

98. McCluggage WG, el-Agnaff M, O'Hara MD. Cytokeratin positive T cell malignant lymphoma. J Clin Pathol 1998;51:404–6.

99. McCluggage WG, Patterson A, White J, Anderson NH. Immunocytochemical staining of ovarian cyst aspirates with monoclonal antibody against inhibin. Cytopathology 1998;9:336–42.

100. McCluggage WG. Uterine tumours resembling ovarian sex cord tumours: immunohistochemical evidence for true sex cord differentiation. Histopathology 1999;34:373–80.

101. McCluggage WG, Maxwell P. Adenocarcinomas of various sites may exhibit immunoreactivity with anti-inhibin antibodies. Histopathology 1999;35:216–20.

102. McCluggage WG. Recent advances in immunohistochemistry in the diagnosis of ovarian neoplasms. J Clin Pathol 2000;53:327–34.

103. McCluggage WG, Patterson A, Maxwell P. Aggressive angiomyxoma of pelvic parts exhibits oestrogen and progesterone receptor positivity. J Clin Pathol 2000;53:603–5.

104. McCluggage WG. The value of inhibin staining in gynecological pathology. Int J Gynecol Pathol 2001;20:79–85.

105. McCluggage WG, Maxwell P. Immunohistochemical staining for calretinin is useful in the diagnosis of ovarian sex cord-stromal tumours. Histopathology 2001;38:403–8.

106. McCluggage WG, Sumathi VP, Maxwell P. CD10 is a sensitive and diagnostically useful immunohistochemical marker of normal endometrial stroma and of endometrial stromal neoplasms. Histopathology 2001;39:273–8.

107. McCluggage WG. Recent advances in immunohistochemistry in gynaecological pathology. Histopathology 2002;40:309–26.

108. McCluggage WG, Lioe TF, McClelland HR, et al. Rhabdomyosarcoma of the uterus: report of two cases, including one of the spindle cell variant. Int J Gynecol Cancer 2002;12:128–32.

109. McCluggage WG, Maxwell P. Bcl-2 and p21 staining of cervical tuboendometrial metaplasia. Histopathology 2002;40:107.

110. McCluggage WG, Sumathi VP, McBride HA, et al. A panel of immunohistochemical stains, including carcinoembryonic antigen, vimentin and estrogen receptor aids the distinction between primary endometrial and endocervical adenocarcinomas. Int J Gynecol Pathol 2002;21:11–15.

111. McCluggage WG, Jenkins D. Immunohistochemical staining with p16 may assist in the distinction between endometrial and endocervical adenocarcinoma. Int J Gynecol Pathol 2003;22:231–5.

112. McCluggage WG, Oliva E, Herrington CS, McBride H, Young RH. CD10 and calretinin staining of endocervical glandular lesions, endocervical stroma and endometrioid adenocarcinoma of the uterine corpus: CD10 positivity is characteristic of, but not specific for, mesonephric lesions and is not specific for endometrioid stroma. Histopathology 2003;43:144–50.

113. McCluggage WG. A review and update of morphologically bland vulvovaginal mesenchymal lesions. Int J Gynecol Pathol 2004;24:26–38.

114. McCluggage WG. Ovarian neoplasms composed of small round cells. A review. Adv Anat Pathol 2004;11:288–96.

115. McCluggage WG. WT1 is of value in ascertaining the site of origin of serous carcinomas within the female genital tract. Int J Gynecol Pathol 2004;23:97–9.

116. McCluggage WG, Ganesan R, Hirschowitz L, Rollason TP. Cellular angiofibroma and related fibromatous lesions of the vulva: report of a series of cases with a morphological spectrum wider than previously described. Histopathology 2004;45:360–8.

117. McCluggage WG, Oliva E, Connolly LE, McBride HA, Young RH. An immunohistochemical analysis of ovarian small cell carcinoma of hypercalcemic type. Int J Gynecol Pathol 2004;23:330–6.

118. McCluggage WG, Young RH. Non-neoplastic granulosa cells within ovarian vascular channels: a rare potential diagnostic pitfall. J Clin Pathol 2004;57:151–4.

119. McCluggage WG. Immunoreactivity of ovarian juvenile granulosa cell tumours with epithelial membrane antigen. Histopathology 2005;46:235–6.

120. McCluggage WG, Ganesan R, Hirschowitz L, et al. Ectopic prostatic tissue in the uterine cervix and vagina: report of a series with a detailed immunohistochemical analysis. Am J Surg Pathol 2006;30:209–15.

121. Mikami Y, Kiyokawa T, Hata S, et al. Gastrointestinal immunophenotype in adenocarcinomas of the uterine cervix and related glandular lesions: a possible link between lobular endocervical glandular hyperplasia/pyloric gland metaplasia and adenoma malignum. Mod Pathol 2004;17:962–72.

122. Mikami Y, Kiyokawa T, Moriya T, Sasano H. Immunophenotypic alteration of the stromal component in minimal deviation adenocarcinoma ('adenoma malignum') and endocervical glandular hyperplasia: a study using oestrogen receptor and alpha-smooth muscle actin double immunostaining. Histopathology 2005;46:130–6.

123. Mittal K. Utility of MIB1 in evaluating cauterised cervical cone biopsy margins. Int J Gynecol Pathol 1999;18:211–14.

124. Mittal K, Demopoulos RI. MIB-1 (Ki-67), p53, estrogen receptor, and progesterone receptor expression in uterine smooth muscle tumors. Hum Pathol 2001;32:984–7.

125. Miyoshi Y, Nagase H, Ando H, et al. Somatic mutations of the APC gene in colorectal tumors: mutation cluster region in the APC gene. Hum Mol Genet 1992;1:229–33.

126. Moinfar F, Regitnig P, Tabrizi AD, Denk H, Tavassoli FA. Expression of androgen receptors in benign and malignant endometrial stromal neoplasms. Virchows Arch 2004;444:410–14.

127. Moll R, Franke WW, Schiller DL, Geiger B, Krepler R. The catalog of human cytokeratins: patterns of expression in normal epithelia, tumors and cultured cells. Cell 1982;31:11–24.

128. Movahedi-Lankarani S, Kurman RJ. Calretinin, a more sensitive but less specific marker than α-inhibin for ovarian sex cord-stromal neoplasms. An immunohistochemical study of 215 cases. Am J Surg Pathol 2002;26:1477–83.

129. Mutter GL, Ince TA, Baak JP, Kust GA, Zhou XP, Eng C. Molecular identification of latent precancers in histologically normal endometrium. Cancer Res 2001;61:4311–14.

130. Nair SA, Nair MB, Jayaprakash PG, Rajalekshmy TN, Nair MK, Pillai MR. Increased expression of cytokeratins 14, 18 and 19 correlates with tumor progression in the uterine cervix. Pathobiology 1997;65:100–7.

131. Negri G, Egarter-Vigl E, Kasal A, et al. p16 (INK4a) is a useful marker for the diagnosis of adenocarcinoma of the cervix uteri and its precursors. Am J Surg Pathol 2003;27:187–93.

132. Norton AJ, Thomas JA, Isaacson PG. Cytokeratin-specific monoclonal antibodies are reactive with tumours of smooth muscle derivation. An immunocytochemical and biochemical study using antibodies to intermediate filament cytoskeletal proteins. Histopathology 1987;11:487–99.

133. Nucci MR, O'Connell JT, Huettner PC, et al. h-Caldesmon expression effectively distinguishes endometrial stromal tumors from uterine smooth muscle tumors. Am J Surg Pathol 2001;25:253–8.

134. Nucci MR, Castillon DH, Bai H, et al. Biomarkers in diagnostic obstetric and gynecologic pathology: a review. Adv Anat Pathol 2003;10:55–68.

135. O'Connell JT, Hacker CM, Barsky SH. MUC2 is a molecular marker for pseudomyxoma peritonei. Mod Pathol 2002;15:958–72.

136. O'Connell JT, Tomlinson JS, Roberts AA, McGonigle KF, Barsky SH. Pseudomyxoma peritonei is a disease of MUC2-expressing goblet cells. Am J Pathol 2002;161:551–64.

137. Oliva E, Young RH, Amin MB, Clement PB. An immunohistochemical analysis of endometrial stromal and smooth muscle tumors of the uterus: a study of 54 cases emphasizing the importance of using a panel because of overlap in immunoreactivity for individual antibodies. Am J Surg Pathol 2002;26:403–12.

138. Oliva E. CD10 expression in the female genital tract: does it have useful diagnostic applications? Adv Anat Pathol 2004;11:310–15.

139. Oliva E, Gonzalez L, Dionigi A, Young RH. Mixed tumors of the vagina: an immunohistochemical study of 13 cases with emphasis on the cell of origin and potential aid in differential diagnosis. Mod Pathol 2004;17:1243–50.

140. O'Neill CJ, Deavers MT, Malpica A, et al. An immunohistochemical comparison between low grade and high grade ovarian serous carcinomas: significantly higher expression of p53, MIB1, bcl2, HER-2/neu and C-KIT in high grade neoplasms. Am J Surg Pathol 2005;29:1034–41.

141. Ordi J, Nogales FF, Palacia A, et al. Mesonephric adenocarcinoma of the uterine corpus: CD10 expression as evidence of mesonephric differentiation. Am J Surg Pathol 2001;25:1540–5.

142. Ordi J, Romagosa C, Tavassoli FA, et al. CD10 expression in epithelial tissues and tumors of the gynecologic tract: a useful marker in the diagnosis of mesonephric, trophoblastic and clear cell tumors. Am J Surg Pathol 2003;27:178–86.

143. Ordonez NG. Desmoplastic small round cell tumour, II. An ultrastructural and immunohistochemical study with emphasis on new immunohistochemical markers. Am J Surg Pathol 1998:22:1314–27.

144. Otis CN, Powell JC, Barbuto D, et al. Intermediate filamentous proteins in adult granulosa cell tumors. An immunohistochemical study of 25 cases. Am J Surg Pathol 1992;16:962–8.

145. Park SY, Kim HS, Hong EK, Kim WH. Expression of cytokeratins 7 and 20 in primary carcinomas of the stomach and colorectum and their value in the differential diagnosis of metastatic carcinomas to the ovary. Hum Pathol 2002;33:1078–85.

146. Pelkey TJ, Frierson HF Jr, Mills SE, Stoler MH. The diagnostic value of inhibin staining in ovarian neoplasms. Int J Gynecol Pathol 1998;17:97–105.

147. Piek JM, Verheijen RH, Menko FH, et al. Expression of differentiation and proliferation related proteins in epithelium of prophylactically removed ovaries from women with a hereditary female adnexal cancer predisposition. Histopathology 2003;43:26–32.

148. Pirog EC, Chen Y-T, Isacson C. MIB1 immunostaining is a beneficial adjunct test for accurate diagnosis of vulvar condyloma acuminatum. Am J Surg Pathol 2000;24:1393–9.

149. Pirog EC, Baergen RN, Soslow RA, et al. Diagnostic accuracy of cervical low-grade squamous intraepithelial lesions is improved with MIB1 immunostaining. Am J Surg Pathol 2002;26:70–5.

150. Pirog EC, Isacson C, Szabolcs MJ, et al. Proliferative activity of benign and neoplastic endocervical epithelium and correlation with HPV DNA detection. Int J Gynecol Pathol 2002;21:22–6.

151. Pitman MB, Triratanachat S, Young RH, Oliva E. Hepatocyte paraffin 1 antibody does not distinguish primary ovarian tumors with hepatoid differentiation from metastatic hepatocellular carcinoma. Int J Gynecol Pathol 2004;23:58–64.

152. Qiu W, Mittal K. Comparison of morphologic and immunohistochemical features of cervical microglandular hyperplasia with low-grade mucinous adenocarcinoma of the endometrium. Int J Gynecol Pathol 2003;22:261–5.

153. Quade BJ, Yang A, Wang Y, et al. Expression of the p53 homologue p63 in early cervical neoplasia. Gynecol Oncol 2001;80:24–9.

154. Quddus MR, Sung CJ, Zheng W, Lauchlan SC. p53 immunoreactivity in endometrial metaplasia with dysfunctional uterine bleeding. Histopathology 1999;35:44–9.

155. Quddus MR, Xu C, Steinhoff MM, Zhang C, Lawrence WD, Sung CJ. Simplex (differentiated) type VIN: absence of p16INK4 supports its weak association with HPV and its probable precursor role in non-HPV related vulvar squamous cancers. Histopathology 2005;46:718–20.

156. Raspollini MR, Amunni G, Villanucci A, Baroni G, Taddei A, Taddei GL. Utility of CDX-2 in distinguishing between primary and secondary (intestinal) mucinous ovarian carcinoma. Appl Immunohistochem Mol Morphol 2004;12:127–31.

157. Raspollini MR, Amunni G, Villanucci A, et al. c-Kit expression in patients with uterine leiomyosarcomas: a potential alternative therapeutic treatment. Clin Cancer Res 2004;10:3500–3.

158. Raspollini MR, Paglierani M, Taddei GL, Villanucci A, Amunni G, Taddei A. The protooncogene c-KIT is expressed in leiomyosarcomas of the uterus. Gynecol Oncol 2004;93:718.

159. Riethdorf L, Riethdorf S, Lee KR, Cviko A, Loning T, Crum CP. Human papillomaviruses, expression of p16 INK4A, and early endocervical glandular neoplasia. Hum Pathol 2002;33:899–904.

160. Riopel MA, Perlman EJ, Seidman JD, Kurman RJ, Sherman ME. Inhibin and epithelial membrane antigen immunohistochemistry assist in the diagnosis of sex cord-stromal tumors and provide clues to the histogenesis of hypercalcemic small cell carcinoma. Int J Gynecol Pathol 1998;17:46–53.

161. Rishi M, Howard LN, Bratthauer GL, Tavassoli FA. Use of monoclonal antibody against human inhibin as a marker for sex cord-stromal tumors of the ovary. Am J Surg Pathol 1997;21:583–9.

162. Ronnett BM, Shmookler BM, Diener-West M, Sugarbaker PH, Kurman RJ. Immunohistochemical evidence supporting the appendiceal origin of pseudomyxoma peritonei in women. Int J Gynecol Pathol 1997;16:1–9.

163. Rush DS, Tan JY, Baergen RN, et al. h-Caldesmon, a novel smooth muscle-specific antibody, distinguishes between cellular leiomyoma and endometrial stromal sarcoma. Am J Surg Pathol 2001;25:253–8.

164. Russell SE, McCluggage WG. A multistep model for ovarian tumorigenesis: the value of mutation analysis in the KRAS and BRAF genes. J Pathol 2004;203:617–19.

165. Salvesen HB, Iversen OE, Akslen LA. Prognostic significance of angiogenesis and Ki-67, p53, and p21 expression: a population-based endometrial carcinoma study. J Clin Oncol 1999;17:1382–90.

166. Santos M, Montagut C, Mellado B, et al. Immunohistochemical staining for p16 and p53 in premalignant and malignant epithelial lesions of the vulva. Int J Gynecol Pathol 2004;23:206–14.

167. Schwartz EJ, Longacre TA. Adenomatoid tumors of the female and male genital tract express WT1. Int J Gynecol Pathol 2004;23:123–8.

168. Sebire NJ, Rees HC, Peston D, Seckl MJ, Newlands ES, Fisher RA. p57(KIP2) immunohistochemical staining of gestational trophoblastic tumours does not identify the type of the causative pregnancy. Histopathology 2004;45:135–41.

169. Shah VI, Freites ON, Maxwell P, McCluggage WG. Inhibin is more specific than calretinin as an immunohistochemical marker for differentiating sarcomatoid granulosa cell tumor of the ovary from other spindle cell neoplasms. J Clin Pathol 2003;56:221–4.

170. Shih IM, Kurman RJ. Ki-67 labelling index in the differential diagnosis of exaggerated placental site, placental site trophoblastic tumor and choriocarcinoma. A double immunohistochemical staining technique using Ki-67 and Mel-CAM antibodies. Hum Pathol 1998;29:27–33.

171. Shih IM, Kurman RJ. Immunohistochemical localization of inhibin-alpha in the placenta and gestational trophoblastic lesions. Int J Gynecol Pathol 1999;18:144–50.

172. Shih IM, Kurman RJ. The pathology of intermediate trophoblastic tumors and tumor-like lesions. Int J Gynecol Pathol 2001;20:31–47.

173. Shih IM, Kurman RJ. Ovarian tumorigenesis: a proposed model based on morphological and molecular genetic analysis. Am J Pathol 2004;164:1511–18.
174. Shih IM, Kurman RJ. p63 expression is useful in the distinction of epithelioid trophoblastic and placental site trophoblastic tumors by profiling trophoblastic subpopulations. Am J Surg Pathol 2004;28:1177–83.
175. Shimizu M, Toki T, Takagi Y, et al. Immunohistochemical detection of the Wilms' tumor gene (WT1) in epithelial ovarian tumors. Int J Gynecol Pathol 2000;19:158–63.
176. Silva EG, Deavers MT, Bodurka DC, Malpica A. Uterine epithelioid leiomyosarcomas with clear cells: reactivity with HMB-45 and the concept of PEComa. Am J Surg Pathol 2004;28:244–9.
177. Silver SA, Devouassoux-Shisheboran M, Mezzetti TP, Tavassoli FA. Mesonephric adenocarcinomas of the uterine cervix: a study of 11 cases with immunohistochemical findings. Am J Surg Pathol 2001;25:379–87.
178. Singer G, Kurman RJ, McMaster MT, Shih IM. HLA-G immunoreactivity is specific for intermediate trophoblast in gestational trophoblastic disease and can serve as a useful marker in differential diagnosis. Am J Surg Pathol 2002;26:914–20.
179. Staebler A, Sherman ME, Zaino RJ, et al. Hormone receptor immunohistochemistry and human papillomavirus in situ hybridization are useful for distinguishing endocervical and endometrial adenocarcinomas. Am J Surg Pathol 2002;26:998–1006.
180. Stefansson IM, Salvesen HB, Immervoll H, Akslen LA. Prognostic impact of histological grade and vascular invasion compared with tumour cell proliferation in endometrial carcinoma of endometrioid type. Histopathology 2004;44:472–9.
181. Stewart CJR, Jeffers MD, Kennedy A. Diagnostic value of inhibin immunoreactivity in ovarian gonadal stromal tumours and their histological mimics. Histopathology 1997;31:67–74.
182. Stewart CJR, Nandini CL, Richmond JA. Value of A103 (melan-A) immunostaining in the differential diagnosis of ovarian sex cord tumours. J Clin Pathol 2000;53:206–11.
183. Sumathi VP, McCluggage WG. CD10 is useful in demonstrating endometrial stroma at ectopic sites and in confirming a diagnosis of endometriosis. J Clin Pathol 2002;55:391–2.
184. Sumathi VP, Al-Hussaini M, Connolly LE, Fullerton L, McCluggage WG. Endometrial stromal neoplasms are immunoreactive with WT-1 antibody. Int J Gynecol Pathol 2004;23:241–7.
185. Suresh UR, Hale RJ, Fox H, Buckley CH. Use of proliferation cell nuclear antigen immunoreactivity for distinguishing hydropic abortions from partial hydatidiform moles. J Clin Pathol 1993;46:48–50.
186. Tanaka Y, Carney JA, Ijiri R, Kato K, Miyake T, Nakatani Y, Misugi K. Utility of immunostaining for S-100 protein subunits in gonadal sex cord-stromal tumors, with emphasis on the large-cell calcifying Sertoli cell tumor of the testis. Hum Pathol 2002;33:285–9.
187. Thamboo TP, Wee A. Hep Par 1 expression in carcinoma of the cervix: implications for diagnosis and prognosis. J Clin Pathol 2004;57:48–53.
188. Tiltman AJ, Allard U. Female adnexal tumours of probable Wolffian origin: an immunohistochemical study comparing tumours, mesonephric remnants and para-mesonephric derivatives. Histopathology 2001;38:237–42.
189. Tornillo L, Moch H, Diener PA, Lugli A, Singer G. CDX-2 immunostaining in primary and secondary ovarian carcinomas. J Clin Pathol 2004;57:641–3.
190. Utsugi K, Hira Y, Takeshima N, Akiyama F, Sakurai S, Hasumi K. Utility of the monoclonal antibody HIK1083 in the diagnosis of adenoma malignum of the uterine cervix. Gynecol Oncol 1999;75:345–8.
191. Vang R, Kempson RL. Perivascular epithelioid cell tumour (PEComa) of the uterus: a subset of HMB-45 positive epithelioid mesenchymal neoplasms with an uncertain relationship to pure smooth muscle tumors. Am J Surg Pathol 2002;26:1–13.
192. Vang R, Barner R, Wheeler DT, Strauss BL. Immunohistochemical staining for Ki-67 and p53 helps distinguish endometrial Arias-Stella reaction from high grade carcinoma, including clear cell carcinoma. Int J Gynecol Pathol 2004;23:223–33.
193. Vang R, Herrmann ME, Tavassoli FA. Comparative immunohistochemical analysis of granulosa and Sertoli components in ovarian sex cord-stromal tumors with mixed differentiation: potential implications for derivation of Sertoli differentiation in ovarian tumors. Int J Gynecol Pathol 2004;23:151–61.
194. Wakami K, Tateyama H, Kawashima H, et al. Solitary fibrous tumor of the uterus producing high-molecular-weight insulin-like growth factor II and associated with hypoglycemia. Int J Gynecol Pathol 2005;24:79–84.
195. Wang HL, Lu DW, Yerian LM, et al. Immunohistochemical distinction between primary adenocarcinoma of the bladder and secondary colorectal adenocarcinoma. Am J Surg Pathol 2001;25:1380–7.
196. Wang TY, Chen BF, Yang YC, et al. Histologic and immunophenotypic classification of cervical carcinomas by expression of the p53 homologue p63: a study of 250 cases. Hum Pathol 2001;32:479–86.
197. Wauters CCAP, Smedts F, Gerrits LGM, et al. Keratins 7 and 20 as diagnostic markers of carcinomas metastatic to the ovary. Hum Pathol 1995;26:852–5.
198. Werling RW, Yaziji H, Bacchi CE, Gown AM. CDX2, a highly sensitive and specific marker of adenocarcinomas of intestinal origin: an immunohistochemical survey of 476 primary and metastatic carcinomas. Am J Surg Pathol 2003;27:303–10.
199. Winter WE 3rd, Seidman JD, Krivak TC, et al. Clinicopathological analysis of c-kit expression in carcinosarcomas and leiomyosarcomas of the uterine corpus. Gynecol Oncol 2003;91:3–8.
200. Yang B, Hart WR. Vulvular intraepithelial neoplasia of the simplex (differentiated) type: a clinicopathologic study including analysis of HPV and p53 expression. Am J Surg Pathol 2000;24:429–41.
201. Yao DX, Soslow RA, Hedvat CV, Leitao M, Baergen RN. Melan-A (A103) and inhibin expression in ovarian neoplasms. Appl Immunohistochem Mol Morphol 2003;11:244–9.
202. Yaziji H, Gown AM. Immunohistochemical analysis of gynecologic tumors. Int J Gynecol Pathol 2001;20:64–78.
203. Zaino RJ. The fruits of our labours: distinguishing endometrial from endocervical adenocarcinoma. Int J Gynecol Pathol 2002;21:1–3.
204. Zhang C, Zhang P, Sung J, Lawrence WD. Overexpression of p53 is correlated with stromal invasion in extramammary Paget's disease of the vulva. Hum Pathol 2003;34:880–5.
205. Zheng W, Cao P, Zheng M, Kramer EE, Godwin TA. p53 overexpression and bcl-2 persistence in endometrial carcinoma: comparison of papillary serous and endometrioid subtypes. Gynecol Oncol 1996;61:167–74.

Appendix A:
FIGO staging rules of cancers of the female genital tract

Modified without altered meaning from Pecorelli S, Ngan HYS, Hacker NF, 26th Annual Report on the Results of Treatment in Gynecologic Cancer. Int J Gynecol Obstet 2006;95: S1–S257. In addition, the UICC staging pertinent for pathology is given, together with the FIGO stage equivalent. In 2008, shortly after this book appears in print, the FIGO Committee on Gynecologic Oncology will recommend multiple changes to FIGO staging rules. For the convenience of our readers and to keep our text 'cutting edge', the appropriate new rules are being reprinted. We ask the reader to verify the new rules have become sanctioned. All anticipated changes in the current (old) classifications are marked with a '*'.

APPENDIX A1: CARCINOMA OF THE VULVA[1]

FIGO SURGICAL STAGING SYSTEM

Stage 0*   Intraepithelial neoplasia grade 3 (CIS, VIN 3)

Stage 1*   Lesions ≤ 2 cm in size, confined to vulva or perineum, no nodal metastasis
    1A   Stromal invasion[2] ≤ 1.0 mm
    1B*   Stromal invasion[2] >1.0 mm

Stage 2   Tumor confined to vulva and/or perineum; >2 cm in dimension, no nodal metastasis

Stage 3*   Tumor any size with adjacent spread to the lower urethra and/or vagina, or anus, and/or unilateral regional lymph node metastasis[3]

Stage 4
    4A*   Tumor invades any of: upper urethra, bladder mucosa, rectal mucosa, pelvic bone, and/or bilateral regional node metastases
    4B   Any distant metastasis including pelvic lymph nodes

---

1. Melanomas use a separate system.

2. Depth of invasion: the tumor is measured from the epithelial–stromal junction of the adjacent most superficial dermal papilla to the deepest point of invasion.

3. Regional nodes are femoral and inguinal nodes. Distal nodes include the pelvic lymph nodes (external iliac, internal iliac, and common iliac).

UICC STAGING SYSTEM

FIGO Stage	UICC T	N	M
0	Tis	N0	M0
IA	T1a	N0	M0
IB	T1b	N0	M0
II	T2	N0	M0
III	T1	N1	M0
	T2	N1	M0
	T3	N1	M0
IVA	T1	N2	M0
	T2	N2	M0
	T3	N2	M0
	T4	Any N	M0
IVB	Any T	Any N	M1

Where

Regional lymph nodes (N)

- NX – Regional lymph nodes cannot be assessed
- N0 – No regional lymph node metastasis
- N1 – Unilateral regional lymph node metastasis
- N2 – Bilateral regional lymph node metastases

Distant metastasis (M)

- MX – Distant metastasis cannot be assessed
- M0 – No distant metastasis
- M1 – Distant metastasis

PROPOSED CHANGES IN STAGING OF CARCINOMA OF VULVA (FIGO 2008)

Stage 0   Deleted

Stage 1   Tumor confined to vulva

    1A   Tumor ≤ 2 cm in size, and stromal invasion ≤1.0 mm

    1B   Tumor > 2 cm in size or stromal invasion >1.0 mm

Stage 2   Tumor any size with extension to adjacent perineal structures ($\frac{1}{3}$ lower urethra, $\frac{1}{3}$ lower vagina, anus) with negative nodes.

Stage 3   As Stage 2 with positive nodes.

    3A   (i)   With 1 lymph node metastasis (≥5 mm), or

            (ii)   1–2 lymph node metastasis(es) (<5 mm)

    3B   (i)   With ≥2 lymph node metastases (≥5 mm), or

            (ii)   ≥3 lymph nodal metastases (<5 mm)

    3C   With positive nodes with extracapsular spread.

Stage 4   Tumor invades other regional ($\frac{2}{3}$ upper urethra, $\frac{2}{3}$ upper vagina), or distant structures.

    4A   Tumor invades:

            (i)   upper urethral and/or vaginal mucosa, bladder mucosa, rectal mucosa, or fixed to pelvic bone, or

            (ii)   fixed or ulcerated femoral-inguinal lymph nodes.

APPENDIX A2: CARCINOMA OF THE VAGINA[1]

FIGO SURGICAL STAGING SYSTEM

Stage 0   Intraepithelial neoplasia grade 3 (VaIN, CIS)

Stage 1   Carcinoma limited to vaginal wall

Stage 2   Carcinoma involves subvaginal tissue but has not extended to pelvic wall

Stage 3   Carcinoma extends to pelvic wall

Stage 4   Carcinoma extends beyond the true pelvis or involves the mucosa of the bladder or rectum; bullous edema as such does not allot the case to stage 4

    4A   Tumor invades bladder and/or rectal mucosa and/or direct extension beyond the true pelvis

    4B   Spread to distant organs

UICC STAGING SYSTEM

FIGO Stage	UICC T	N	M
0	Tis	N0	M0
I	T1	N0	M0
II	T2	N0	M0
III	T1	N1	M0
	T2	N1	M0
	T3	N0	M0
	T3	N1	M0
IVA	T4	Any N	M0
IVB	Any T	Any N	M1

Where

Regional lymph nodes (N)

- NX – Regional lymph nodes cannot be assessed
- N0 – No regional lymph node metastasis
- N1 – Pelvic or inguinal lymph node metastasis

Distant metastasis (M)

- MX – Distant metastasis cannot be assessed
- M0 – No distant metastasis
- M1 – Distant metastasis

---

1. Classify as 'cervical' if the cervical os is involved, even if most of the tumor is in the vagina. Classify as 'vulvar' if any portion of the vulva is involved.

APPENDIX A3: CARCINOMA OF THE CERVIX[1]

CURRENT FIGO CLINICAL STAGING SYSTEM (MONTREAL 1994)

Stage 0*   Preinvasive carcinoma (CIN 3, CIS)

Stage 1   Carcinoma strictly confined to cervix (disregard extension to corpus)

1A   Invasive cancer identified only microscopically. Depth[2] <5.0 mm; Width[2] <7.0 mm

1A1*   Depth ≤3.0 mm

1A2   Depth >3.0 mm

1B   Cancer > stage 1A and confined to cervix

1B1   Clinical size ≤4.0 cm

1B2   Clinical size >4.0 cm

Stage 2   Invasive carcinoma that extends beyond cervix but not reached either lateral pelvic wall. Vaginal involvement limited to upper two-thirds

2A*   No obvious parametrial involvement

2B   Obvious parametrial involvement

Stage 3   Invasive carcinoma that extends to either lateral pelvic wall and/or lower third of vagina. On rectal examination, no cancer-free space exits between tumor and pelvic wall. All cases with hydronephrosis or non-functioning kidney are included, unless due to other cause

3A   Involves lower third of vagina

3B   Extension to pelvic wall and/or hydronephrosis or non-functioning kidney

Stage 4   Invasive carcinoma that involves the mucosa of the urinary bladder and/or rectum (biopsy proven) or extends beyond the true pelvis

4A   Spread of growth to adjacent organs

4B   Spread to distant organs

---

1. The tumor is classified as cervical once the external os is involved, even if the cancer originates in the vagina.
2. Measured from the base of the diseased epithelium – superficial or glandular.

UICC STAGING SYSTEM

FIGO Stage	UICC T	N	M
0	Tis	N0	M0
IA1	T1a1	N0	M0
IA2	T1a2	N0	M0
IB1	T1b1	N0	M0
IB2	T1b2	N0	M0
IIA	T2a	N0	M0
IIB	T2b	N0	M0
IIIA	T3a	N0	M0
IIIB	T1	N1	M0
	T2	N1	M0
	T3a	N1	M0
	T3b	Any N	M0
IVA	T4	Any N	M0
IVB	Any T	Any N	M1

Where

Regional lymph nodes (N)

- NX – Regional lymph nodes cannot be assessed
- N0 – No regional lymph node metastasis
- N1 – Regional lymph node metastasis

Distant metastasis (M)

- MX – Distant metastasis cannot be assessed
- M0 – No distant metastasis
- M1– Distant metastasis

PROPOSED CHANGES IN STAGING OF CARCINOMA OF CERVIX (FIGO 2008)

Stage 0   Deleted

Stage 1A1   Depth ≤ 3 mm

1A1   Exclude microscopic epithelial buds from this category and report them separately in a note.

2A   Without parametrial invasion.

2A1   Clinically visible lesion ≤ 4.0 cm in greatest dimension.

2A2   Clinically visible lesion > 4 cm in greatest dimension.

APPENDIX A4: CARCINOMA OF THE ENDOMETRIUM

CURRENT FIGO SURGICAL STAGING SYSTEM (RIO DE JANERRO, 1988)

Stage 0*   Preinvasive carcinoma

Stage 1   Tumor confined to uterine corpus
1A*   Limited to endometrium
1B*   Invasion less than half of myometrium
1C*   Invasion more than half of myometrium

Stage 2   Tumor involves cervix
2A*   Endocervical glands involved only
2B*   Invasion into cervical stroma

Stage 3
3A*   Tumor invades serosa of corpus uteri and/or adnexae and/or positive cytologic findings
3B   Vaginal metastases
3C*   Metastases to pelvic/para-aortic lymph nodes

Stage 4
4A   Tumor invades bladder mucosa and/or bowel mucosa
4B   Distant metastases, including intra-abdominal metastasis and/or inguinal lymph nodes

Grading Notes:

Endometrioid tumors are graded 1–3; serous, clear cell and carcinosarcomas are graded 3.

Architectural degree of gland formation:

G1: ≤5% of the non-squamous or non-morular solid-growth pattern is solid.
G2: 6–50% of the non-squamous or non-morular solid-growth pattern is solid.
G3: >50% of the non-squamous or non morular solid-growth pattern is solid.

On nuclear grading

1. Notable nuclear atypia, inappropriate for the architectural grade, raises the grade of a grade 1 or 2 tumor by 1.
2. Adenocarcinomas with squamous differentiation are graded by the nuclear grade of the glandular component.

UICC STAGING SYSTEM

FIGO Stage	UICC T	N	M
0	Tis	N0	M0
IA	T1a	N0	M0
IB	T1b	N0	M0
IC	T1c	N0	M0
IIA	T2a	N0	M0
IIB	T2b	N0	M0
IIIA	T3a	N0	M0
IIIB	T3b	N0	M0
IIIC	T1	N1	M0
	T2	N1	M0
	T3a	N1	M0
	T3b	N1	M0
IVA	T4	Any N	M0
IVB	Any T	Any N	M1

Where

Regional lymph nodes (N)

- NX – Regional lymph nodes cannot be assessed
- N0 – No regional lymph node metastasis
- N1 – Regional lymph node metastasis

Distant metastasis (M)

- MX – Distant metastasis cannot be assessed
- M0 – No distant metastasis
- M1 – Distant metastasis

PROPOSED CHANGES IN STAGING OF CARCINOMA OF UTERINE CORPUS (FIGO 2008)

Stage 0   Deleted
Stage 1   Tumor confined to uterine corpus.
1A   Invasion less than half of myometrium
1B   Invasion more than half of myometrium
Stage 2   Tumor invades cervical stroma
Stage 3   Local and/or regional spread.
3A   Tumor invades serosa of corpus uteri and/or adnexae[#].
3C   Metastases to pelvic and/or para-aortic lymph nodes[#].
3C1   Positive pelvic nodes
3C2   Positive para-aortic lymph nodes

Either G1, G2, or G3
[#]Positive cytology is to be reported separately, but does not change the stage.

PROPOSED NEW STAGING OF UTERINE SARCOMAS (FIGO 2008)

(Stage Carcinosarcoma as Endometrial Carcinoma; Stage Adenosarcoma separately as below)

UTERINE SARCOMA NOS

Stage 1	Tumor limited to uterus
1A	≤5 cm
1B	>5 cm
Stage 2	Tumor extends to the pelvis
2A	Adnexa involved
2B	Tumor extends to extrauterine pelvic tissue
Stage 3	Tumor invades abdominal tissues (not just protruding into the abdomen).
3A	1 site
3B	>1 site
3C	Metastasis to pelvic and/or para-aortic lymph nodes
Stage 4	Tumor invades bladder and/or rectum and/or distant metastasis
4A	Tumor invades bladder and/or rectum
4B	Distant metastasis

ADENOSARCOMA

Stage 1	Tumor limited to uterus
1A	Tumor limited to endometrium/endocervix (without myometrial invasion)
1B	Tumor invades < half of myometrium
1C	Tumor invades > half of myometrium
Stage 2	Tumor extends to the pelvis
2A	Adnexa involved
2B	Tumor extends to extrauterine pelvic tissue
Stage 3	Tumor invades abdominal tissues (not just protruding into the abdomen).
3A	1 site
3B	>1 site
3C	Metastasis to pelvic and/or para-aortic lymph nodes
Stage 4	Tumor invades bladder and/or rectum and/or distant metastasis
4A	Tumor invades bladder and/or rectum
4B	Distant metastasis

APPENDIX A5: CARCINOMA OF THE FALLOPIAN TUBE

FIGO SURGICAL STAGING SYSTEM

Stage 0   Carcinoma *in situ*

Stage 1   Tumor limited to the fallopian tubes
  1A   One tube involved; serosa not involved; no ascites
  1B   Both tubes involved; other features as above
  1C   Tumor either stage 1A or 1B, tubal serosa involved, or malignant cells present in ascites or peritoneal washings

Stage 2   Tumor involves one or both fallopian tubes with pelvic extension
  2A   Extension and/or metastasis to the uterus and/or ovaries
  2B   Extension to other pelvic tissues
  2C   Tumor either stage 2A or 2B, tubal serosa involved, or malignant cells present in ascites or peritoneal washings

Stage 3   Tumor involves one or both fallopian tubes, with peritoneal implants outside the pelvis and/or positive regional nodes
  3A   Microscopic metastases to abdominal peritoneal surfaces
  3B   Macroscopic metastases to abdominal peritoneal surfaces, none >2 cm
  3C   Abdominal implants >2 cm in diameter and/or positive regional nodes

Stage 4   Distant metastases beyond peritoneal cavity Pleural effusions, if present, require positive cytology

UICC STAGING SYSTEM

FIGO Stage	UICC T	N	M
IA	T1a	N0	M0
IB	T1b	N0	M0
IC	T1c	N0	M0
IIA	T2a	N0	M0
IIB	T2b	N0	M0
IIC	T2c	N0	M0
IIIA	T3a	N0	M0
IIIB	T3b	N0	M0
IIIC	T3c	N0	M0
Any T	N1	M0	
IV	Any T	Any N	M1

Where

Regional lymph nodes (N)

- NX – Regional lymph nodes cannot be assessed
- N0 – No regional lymph node metastasis
- N1 – Regional lymph node metastasis

Distant metastasis (M)

- MX – Distant metastasis cannot be assessed
- M0 – No distant metastasis
- M1 – Distant metastasis

APPENDIX A6: CARCINOMA OF THE OVARY

FIGO SURGICAL STAGING SYSTEM

Stage 1   Tumor confined to the ovaries
  1A   Tumor limited to one ovary; capsule intact; no tumor on external surface; washings and ascites free of malignant cells
  1B   Tumor limited to both ovaries; other features identical
  1C   Stage 1A or 1B, but with tumor on serosa, or capsule ruptured (spontaneous or iatrogenic), or malignant cells in ascites or peritoneal washings

Stage 2   Tumor involves one or both ovaries with pelvic extension
  2A   Extension and/or metastases to the uterus and/or tubes; washings and ascites free of malignant cells
  2B   Extension to other pelvic tissues; washings and ascites free of malignant cells
  2C   Tumor either stage 2A or 2B, but other features of stage 1C

Stage 3   Tumor involving one or both ovaries with microscopically confirmed peritoneal implants outside pelvis and/or positive regional lymph nodes
  3A   Microscopic peritoneal metastases beyond pelvis
  3B   Macroscopic peritoneal metastases beyond pelvis ≤ 2 cm
  3C   Peritoneal metastasis beyond the pelvis >2 cm, or positive regional lymph nodes

Stage 4   Distant metastases beyond peritoneal cavity

Note: Liver capsule metastasis is T3/Stage III, liver parenchymal metastasis is M1/Stage IV. Pleural effusion must have positive cytology.

UICC STAGING SYSTEM

FIGO Stage	UICC T	N	M
IA	T1a	N0	M0
IB	T1b	N0	M0
IC	T1c	N0	M0
IIA	T2a	N0	M0
IIB	T2b	N0	M0
IIC	T2c	N0	M0
IIIA	T3a	N0	M0
IIIB	T3b	N0	M0
IIIC	T3c	N0	M0
	Any T	N1	M0
IV	Any T	Any N	M1

Where

Regional lymph nodes (N)

- NX – Regional lymph nodes cannot be assessed
- N0 – No regional lymph node metastasis
- N1 – Regional lymph node metastasis

Distant metastasis (M)

- MX – Distant metastasis cannot be assessed
- M0 – No distant metastasis
- M1 – Distant metastasis (excludes peritoneal metastasis)

APPENDIX A7: CARCINOMA OF THE GESTATIONAL TROPHOBLASTIC DISEASES (GTD)

FIGO SURGICAL STAGING SYSTEM

Stage 1   Disease confined to uterus

Stage 2   GTD extends outside uterus, but limited to genital structures (adnexa, vagina, broad ligament)

Stage 3   GTD extends to lungs, with or without known genital tract involvement

Stage 4   All other metastatic sites

MODIFIED WHO SCORING SYSTEM COMBINED WITH FIGO STAGING

FIGO (WHO) risk factor scoring with FIGO staging	0	1	2	4
Age	<40	$\geqq$40	–	–
Antecedent pregnancy	Hydatidiform mole	Abortion	Term	–
Interval months from index pregnancy	<4	4–6	7–12	>12
Pretreatment hCG mIU/mL	<10^3	10^3–10^4	>10^4–10^5	>10^5
Largest tumor size including uterus	–	3–4 cm	$\geqq$5 cm	–
Metastatic sites including uterus	Lung	Spleen Kidney	GI tract	Brain Liver
Number of metastases identified	–	1–4	5–8	>8
Previous failed chemotherapy	–	–	Single drug	Two or more drugs

Appendix B:
Histologic classification of tumors and precursor conditions of the female genital tract

(Modified from WHO Classification, AFIP Fascicles, and International Society of Gynecologic Pathologists' Classification)

SNOMED-RT CODE*

T-81000 D7-70060	**VULVA**
M-801F9	**Epithelial Tumors and Related Lesions**
T-00261 M-01100	*Squamous lesions*
M-80520	Epithelial papillomas and polyps
T-81290 M-80520	Vestibular squamous papilloma (vestibular papilloma)
M-76810	Fibroepithelial polyp
DE-32A20	Condyloma acuminatum
M-72750	Seborrheic keratosis
M-72680	Keratoacanthoma
M-67015	Squamous intraepithelial lesions
T-81000 + M-code	(dysplasia, carcinoma in situ, vulvar intraepithelial neoplasia (VIN))
M-74001	Mild dysplasia (VIN 1)
M-74002	Moderate dysplasia (VIN 2)
M-74003	Severe dysplasia (VIN 3)
M-80712	Carcinoma *in situ* (VIN 3)
M-80703	Squamous cell carcinoma
M-80713	Keratinizing
M-80723	Non-keratinizing
M-81233	Basaloid
M-80513	Verrucous
M-76700 M-80703	Warty (condylomatous)
M-80903	Basal cell carcinoma
T-1A310 M-01100	*Glandular lesions*
M-84050	Papillary hidradenoma
M-84020	Clear cell hidradenoma
M-84070	Syringoma
M-81000	Trichoepithelioma
M-81020	Trichilemmoma
T-81520 M-81400	Adenoma of minor vestibular glands
M-85423	Pagets disease
T-81510 M-80103	*Bartholin gland carcinomas*
M-81403	Adenocarcinoma
M-80703	Squamous cell carcinoma
M-82003	Adenoid cystic carcinoma
M-85603	Adenosquamous carcinoma
M-81203	Transitional cell carcinoma
M-8FFFF D4–48014	*Tumors arising from ectopic breast tissue*
T-01380 M-80103	*Carcinomas of sweat gland origin*
M-880F9	**Soft Tissue Tumors**
M-88000	*Benign*
M-88500/M-88510	Lipoma and fibrolipoma

M-91200	Hemangiomas
M-91310	Capillary
M-91210	Cavernous
M-91200 DF-00260	Acquired
M-91410	Angiokeratoma
M-44020	Pyogenic granuloma
M-91700	Lymphangioma
M-88100	Fibroma
M-88900	Leiomyoma
M-95800	Granular cell tumor
M-95400	Neurofibroma
M-95600	Schwannoma (neurilemmoma)
M-87110	Glomus tumor
M-88300 G-A249	Benign fibrous histiocytoma
M-89000	Rhabdomyoma
M-88003	*Malignant*
M-89103	Embryonal rhabdomyosarcoma (sarcoma botryoides)
M-88411 F-93032	Aggressive angiomyxoma
M-88903	Leiomyosarcoma
M-88323	Dermatofibrosarcoma protuberans
M-88303	Malignant fibrous histiocytoma
M-88043	Epithelioid sarcoma
M-89633	Malignant rhabdoid tumor
M-954F9 G-A425	Malignant nerve sheath tumors
M-91203	Angiosarcoma
M-91403	Kaposi sarcoma
M-91501	Hemangiopericytoma
M-88503	Liposarcoma
M-95813	Alveolar soft part sarcoma

	Miscellaneous Tumors
M-872F9	*Melanocytic tumors*
D4-40370	Congenital melanocytic nevus
M-87200	Acquired melanocytic nevus
M-87800	Blue nevus
M-87270	Dysplastic melanocytic nevus
M-87203	Malignant melanoma
M-95903/M-98003	Lymphoma and leukemia
M-90713	Yolk sac tumor (endodermal sinus tumor)
M-82473	Merkel cell tumor
M-80006	**Secondary Tumors**
T-82000	**VAGINA**
M-801F9	**Epithelial Tumors and Related Lesions**
T-00261 M-01100	*Squamous lesions*
M-80520	Squamous papilloma
DE-32A20	Condyloma acuminatum
M-67015	Squamous intraepithelial lesions (dysplasia, carcinoma *in situ*; VaIN)
M-74001	Mild dysplasia (VaIN 1)
M-74002	Moderate dysplasia (VaIN 2)
M-74003	Severe dysplasia (VaIN 3)
M-80712	Carcinoma *in situ* (VaIN 3)
M-80703	Squamous cell carcinoma
M-80713	Keratinizing
M-80733	Non-keratinizing
M-80513	Verrucous
M-76700 M-80703	Warty (condylomatous)

1024

T-1A310 M-01100	*Glandular lesions*
T-F6490 M-80500	Müllerian papilloma

M-74200	Adenosis
M-74200 G-A248	Atypical adenosis
M-81403	Adenocarcinoma
M-83103	Clear cell adenocarcinoma
M-83803	Endometrioid adenocarcinoma
M-84803	Mucinous adenocarcinoma
T-83231	Endocervical type
M-81443	Intestinal type

Other epithelial tumors

M-91103	Mesonephric adenocarcinoma
M-85603	Adenosquamous carcinoma
M-82003	Adenoid cystic carcinoma
M-80753 G-A123	Adenoid basal carcinoma
M-82403	Carcinoid tumor
M-80413	Small cell carcinoma
M-80103 G-F504	Undifferentiated carcinoma

T-11061 M-8FFFF	**Mesenchymal Tumors**
M-88900	Leiomyoma
M-89000	Rhabdomyoma
M-88903	Leiomyosarcoma
M-89103	Sarcoma botryoides (embryonal rhabdomyosarcoma)
M-89303	Endometrioid stromal sarcoma

M-89901	**Mixed Epithelial and Mesenchymal Tumors**
M-89400	Mixed tumor
M-89333	Adenosarcoma
M-89803	Carcinosarcoma (malignant mesodermal mixed tumor, malignant müllerian mixed tumor)
M-89400 M-90403	Mixed tumor resembling synovial sarcoma

	Miscellaneous Tumors
M-872F9	*Melanocytic lesions*
M-87200	Melanocytic nevus
M-87800	Blue nevus
M-87203	Malignant melanoma

M-90643	*Tumors of germ cell type*
M-90713	Yolk sac tumor (endodermal sinus tumor)
M-90840	Dermoid cyst (mature cystic teratoma)
M-90540	Adenomatoid tumor
M-82611	Villous adenoma
M-95903/M-98003	Lymphoma and leukemia

M-80006	**Secondary Tumors**

T-83200	**UTERINE CERVIX**

M-801F9	**Epithelial Tumors and Related Lesions**
T-00261 M-01100	*Squamous lesions*
DE-32A20	Condyloma acuminatum
M-80772	Squamous cell (cervical) intraepithelial neoplasia (CIN)
M-74001	CIN 1 (Mild dysplasia)
M-74002	CIN 2 (Moderate dysplasia)
M-74003	CIN 3 (Severe dysplasia and carcinoma *in situ*)
M-80763	Microinvasive squamous cell carcinoma
M-80703	Squamous cell carcinoma
M-80713	Non-keratinizing
M-80723	Keratinizing
M-80413	Small cell (non-endocrine)
G-A643	Variants
M-80513	Verrucous carcinoma

1025

M-76700 M-80703	Warty
M-80503	Papillary
M-80823 M-80103	Lymphoepithelioma-like carcinoma
T-1A310 M-01100	*Glandular lesions*
T-83200 T-1A310	Cervical glandular intraepithelial neoplasia (CGIN)
T-1A310 M-74000/M-81402	(glandular dysplasia and adenocarcinoma *in situ*)
G-A001	Low grade
G-A003	High grade
M-81403	Adenocarcinoma
M-84803	Mucinous adenocarcinoma
T-83231	Endocervical type
M-81443	Intestinal type
M-83803	Endometrioid adenocarcinoma
M-83103	Clear cell adenocarcinoma
M-84413	Serous adenocarcinoma
	Villoglandular adenocarcinoma
	Adenoma malignum (minimal deviation adenocarcinoma)
	Other epithelial tumors
M-85603 (M-84303)	Adenosquamous carcinoma (mucoepidermoid carcinoma)
None	Glassy cell carcinoma
M-82003	Adenoid cystic carcinoma
M-80753 G-A123	Adenoid basal carcinoma
T-B0000 M-8FFFF	Endocrine tumor
M-82403	Carcinoid tumor (small cell/neuroendocrine carcinoma)
M-82403 G-A248	Atypical carcinoid tumor
M-80123 M-82463	Large cell neuroendocrine carcinoma
M-80413 (M-80423)	Small (oat) cell carcinoma
T-F6460 M-91103	Mesonephric duct adenocarcinoma
M-80103 G-F504	Undifferentiated carcinoma
T-11061 M-8FFFF	**Mesenchymal Tumors**
M-88900	Leiomyoma
M-88903	Leiomyosarcoma
T-83240 M-89303	Endocervical stromal sarcoma
M-89103	Embryonal rhabdomyosarcoma (sarcoma botryoides)
M-89303	Endometrioid stromal sarcoma
M-95813	Alveolar soft part sarcoma
M-89901	**Mixed Epithelial and Mesenchymal Tumors**
M-89320	Adenomyoma
M-89320 G-A248 M-76800	Atypical polypoid adenomyoma (variant)
M-89333	Adenosarcoma
M-89803	Carcinosarcoma (malignant mesodermal mixed tumor, malignant müllerian mixed tumor)
M-89603	Wilms tumor
	Miscellaneous Tumors
M-872F9	*Melanocytic lesions*
M-87200	Melanocytic nevus
M-87800	Blue nevus
M-87203	Malignant melanoma
M-91103	Mesonephric adenocarcinoma
M-95903/M-98003	Lymphoma and leukemia
M-90643	*Tumors of germ cell type*
M-90713	Yolk sac tumor (endodermal sinus tumor)
M-90840	Dermoid cyst (mature cystic teratoma)
M-80006	**Secondary Tumors**

M-801F9 **Epithelial Tumors and Related Lesions**
D7-75620 *Endometrial hyperplasia* (with cytologic atypia)
G-A537   Simple
G-A540 (M-72420)   Complex (adenomatous)

M-72005 *Atypical endometrial hyperplasia*
G-A537   Simple
G-A540 (M-72420 G-A248)   Complex (adenomatous with atypia)

T-83400 M-80103 *Endometrial carcinoma*
M-83803   Endometrioid adenocarcinoma
G-A643 G-A308   Common variant
M-83803   Endometrioid adenocarcinoma with squamous differentiation
M-85703/M-85603   (adenoacanthoma and adenosquamous carcinoma)
G-A643 G-7156   Rare variants
        Villoglandular adenocarcinoma
        Secretory adenocarcinoma
T-E0460 T-E0000 M-81403   Ciliated cell adenocarcinoma
M-84413   Serous adenocarcinoma
M-83103   Clear cell adenocarcinoma
M-84803   Mucinous adenocarcinoma
M-80703   Squamous cell carcinoma
M-80103 G-A660   Mixed types of carcinoma
M-80103 G-F504   Undifferentiated carcinoma

T-11061 M-8FFFF **Mesenchymal Tumors and Related Lesions**
M-A9301 *Endometrial stromal tumors*
M-89300   Endometrial stromal nodule
M-89303   Endometrial stromal sarcoma
M-89303 M-85901   Endometrial stromal tumor resembling ovarian sex-cord tumors
M-A9301 T-83426   Endometrial stromal neoplasms with endometrial glands

T-83000 M-88003 G-F504 *Undifferentiated uterine sarcoma*

M-88971 *Smooth muscle tumors*
M-88900   Leiomyoma
G-A643   Variants of leiomyoma
M-88920   Cellular leiomyoma
(/M-88910/T-AB787)   Epithelioid (plexiform, leiomyoblastoma, clear cell)
M-88920 M-37000   Hemorrhagic cellular leiomyoma
        Lipoleiomyoma
M-88930   Symplastic (atypical or bizarre)
M-88903   Leiomyosarcoma
G-A643   Variants of leiomyosarcoma
M-88913   Epithelioid
M-88963   Myxoid
    Other smooth muscle neoplasms
M-88900 M-80006 G-A249   Benign metastasizing leiomyoma
M-88901   Diffuse leiomyomatosis
(T-D4400 G-A324) M-88901   Disseminated peritoneal leiomyomatosis
M-88901   Intravenous leiomyomatosis

Mixed endometrial stromal and smooth muscle tumors
M-90540 *Adenomatoid tumor*

Other mesenchymal tumors
F-C0280   Homologous
F-C0290   Heterologous

M-89901 **Mixed Epithelial and Mesenchymal Tumors**
M-88000 *Benign*
    Adenofibroma

M-89320	Adenomyoma
M-89320 G-A248 M-76800	Atypical polypoid adenomyoma (variant)
M-89403	*Malignant*
M-89333	Adenosarcoma
F-C0280	Homologous
F-C0290	Heterologous
	Carcinofibroma
M-89803	Carcinosarcoma (malignant mesodermal mixed tumor; malignant müllerian mixed tumor)
F-C0280	Homologous
F-C0290	Heterologous
M-90643	Tumors of germ cell type
M-93643	Neuroectodermal tumors
M-95903/M-98003	Lymphoma and leukemia
M-80006	**Secondary Tumors**
T-88000	**FALLOPIAN TUBE**
M-801F9	**Epithelial Tumors**
M-88000	*Benign*
M-76800	Endometrioid polyp
M-80500	Papilloma
M-8FFFF G-A469 M-73000	Metaplastic papillary tumor
M-80103	*Malignant*
M-81403	Adenocarcinoma *in situ*
M-84413	Serous adenocarcinoma
M-84803	Mucinous adenocarcinoma
M-83803	Endometrioid adenocarcinoma
M-83103	Clear cell adenocarcinoma
M-81203	Transitional cell carcinoma
M-80703	Squamous cell carcinoma
M-82813	Mixed carcinoma
M-80103 G-F504	Undifferentiated carcinoma
M-89901	**Mixed Epithelial–Mesenchymal Tumors**
M-89403	*Malignant*
M-89333	Adenosarcoma
M-89803	Carcinosarcoma
M-880F9	**Soft Tissue Tumors**
M-88000	*Benign*
M-88900	Leiomyoma
M-88003	*Malignant*
M-88903	Leiomyosarcoma
M-905F9	**Mesothelial Tumors**
M-90503 G-A224	Solitary mesothelioma
M-90540	Adenomatoid tumor
M-90643	**Germ Cell Tumors**
M-90801	*Teratoma*
M-90801	Mature
M-90840	Dermoid cyst
M-90801	Solid
M-90803	Immature
	Struma
M-82403	Carcinoid

M-80006   **Secondary Tumors**

T-87000	**OVARY**
(T-00250 M-8FFFF/ **M-85901) G-A168**	**Surface Epithelial-Stromal Tumors**
M-01120	*Tumor-like conditions*
D7–72050	Serous inclusion cyst
	Serous tumors
M-88000	Benign
M-84410/M-84600	Cystadenoma and papillary cystadenoma
M-84610	Surface papilloma
M-90140/M-90140	Adenofibroma and cystadenofibroma
M-84423	Of borderline malignancy (of low malignant potential; proliferating)
M-844F9/M-84521	Cystic tumor and papillary cystic tumor
M-84613	Surface papillary tumor
M-90140/M-90140	Adenofibroma and cystadenofibroma
M-80103	Malignant
	Adenocarcinoma, papillary adenocarcinoma, and papillary cystadenocarcinoma
M-84613	Surface papillary adenocarcinoma
M-90130 G-A425/M-90130 G-A425	Malignant adenofibroma and cystadenofibroma
	Mucinous tumors, endocervical-like and intestinal types
M-01120	Tumor-like lesions
M-33410 M-33440	Mucinous inclusion cysts
M-88000	Benign
M-84700	Cystadenoma
M-90140/M-90140	Adenofibroma and cystadenofibroma
M-84723	Of borderline malignancy (of low malignant potential; proliferating)
M-844F9	Cystic tumor
M-90140/M-90140	Adenofibroma and cystadenofibroma
M-84806	Pseudomyxoma ovarii
M-80103	Malignant
M-81403/M-84403	Adenocarcinoma and cystadenocarcinoma
M-90130 G-A425/M-90130 G-A425	Malignant adenofibroma and cystadenofibroma
M-84803	Colloid adenocarcinoma
M-84903 (M-84906)	Primary signet cell 'Krukenberg' adenocarcinoma
M-83803 M-8FFFF	*Endometrioid tumors*
M-01120	Tumor-like lesions
M-76500	Endometriosis
M-88000	Benign
M-83800	Cystadenoma
M-83800 T-00261 G-F5F8	Cystadenoma with squamous differentiation
M-90140/M-90140	Adenofibroma and cystadenofibroma
M-90140/M-90140 T-00261 G-F5F8	Adenofibroma and cystadenofibroma with squamous differentiation
M-83801	Of borderline malignancy (of low malignant potential; proliferating)
M-844F9	Cystic tumor
T-00261 G-F5F8	With squamous differentiation
M-90140/M-90140	Adenofibroma and cystadenofibroma
T-00261 G-F5F8	With squamous differentiation
M-80103	Malignant
M-81403/M-84403	Adenocarcinoma and cystadenocarcinoma
	Secretory type
T-00261 G-F5F8	With squamous differentiation
M-90130 G-A425/M-90130 G-A425	Malignant adenofibroma and cystadenofibroma
T-00261 G-F5F8	With squamous differentiation
T-AB787 M-8FFFF	*Clear cell tumors*
M-01120	Tumor-like conditions
M-88000	Benign
M-84400	Cystadenoma
M-90140/M-90140	Adenofibroma and cystadenofibroma

G-A425	Of borderline malignancy (of low malignant potential; proliferating)
M-844F9	Cystic tumor
M-90140/M-90140	Adenofibroma and cystadenofibroma
M-80103	Malignant
M-81403	Adenocarcinoma
M-90130 G-A425/M-90130	Malignant adenofibroma and cystadenofibroma
G-A425	
T-1A151 M-8FFFF	*Transitional cell tumors*
M-01120	Tumor-like conditions
M-90000	Brenner tumor
M-90001	Brenner tumor of borderline malignancy (proliferating)
M-90003	Malignant Brenner tumor
M-81203	Transitional cell carcinoma (non-Brenner type)
M-805F9	*Squamous cell tumors*
	Epithelial–stromal and stromal
M-80000/M-01120	Benign tumors and tumor-like conditions
(T-D4400 G-A324) M-8890	Disseminated peritoneal leiomyomatosis
M-88900 G-A643 G-B003	Leiomyoma and histologic variants
M-76500/None	Endometriosis, deciduosis
M-80003	Malignant tumors
M-88003	Pure sarcomas
F-C0280	Homologous
M-88903	Leiomyosarcoma
M-89303 G-A001	Low-grade stromal sarcomas (endolymphatic stromal myosis stromatosis)
M-89303 G-A003	High-grade endometrioid stromal sarcomas
F-C0290	Heterologous
M-89003	Rhabdomyosarcoma
M-92203	Chondrosarcoma
M-91803	Osteogenic sarcoma
M-89901	Mixed epithelial and stromal tumors
M-89333 G-A001	Low grade (adenosarcoma)
F-C0280	Homologous
F-C0290	Heterologous
G-A003/M-89803	High grade (carcinosarcoma)
M-89901	*Mixed epithelial tumors (specify types)*
M-88000	Benign
G-A425	Of borderline malignancy (of low malignant potential; proliferating)
M-80103	Malignant
M-80103 G-F504	*Undifferentiated carcinoma*
M-85901	**Sex Cord-Stromal Tumors**
M-01120	*Tumor-like conditions*
T-87000 M-36300 M-78800	Massive ovarian edema and fibromatosis
M-72430 G-A321/M-73040	Diffuse stromal hyperplasia and hyperthecosis
M-33400/DB-21500	Dysfunctional cysts and polycystic ovary syndrome
	Hyperreactio luteinalis (multiple luteinized follicle cysts)
M-86201 M-85901 M-89400	*Granulosa-stromal cell tumors*
M-86201	Granulosa cell tumor
DF-00230	Adult
M-86221	Juvenile
M-8FFFF M-86000 M-8810	Tumors in thecoma–fibroma group
M-86000	Thecoma
M-86000	Typical
M-86010	Luteinized
M-86003	Malignant thecoma
M-86000	Fibrothecoma
M-88100	Fibroma
M-88100	Typical

T-E0000 M-88100	Cellular fibroma
M-88100 M-85901 G-A217	Fibroma with minor sex-cord elements
M-88103	Fibrosarcoma
M-86020	Sclerosing stromal tumor
M-86100	(Stromal luteoma)
M-86400 M-85901/M-86301	*Sertoli-stromal cell tumors; androblastomas*
G-F501	Well differentiated
M-86400	Sertoli cell tumor (tubular androblastoma)
M-86310	Sertoli–Leydig cell tumor
M-86310 G-F502	Sertoli–Leydig cell tumor of intermediate differentiation
F-C0290 G-A643	Variant – with heterologous elements (specify type)
M-86310 G-F503	Sertoli–Leydig cell tumor, poorly differentiated (sarcomatoid)
F-C0290 G-A643	Variant – with heterologous elements (specify type)
	Retiform
F-C0290 G-A643	Variant – with heterologous elements (specify type)
M-86231	Sex-cord tumor with annular tubules
M-86321	Gynandroblastoma
M-86700	**Steroid (Lipid) Cell Tumors**
M-01120	*Tumor-like conditions*
D7-55195	Leydig cell hyperplasia
M-73040 M-03010	Nodular hyperthecosis
M-86100	Stromal luteoma
M-79680	Luteoma of pregnancy
M-8FFFF	*Tumors*
M-86501	Leydig cell tumor, hilus and stromal variants
M-86710	Adrenal rest tumor
M-86700	Steroid cell tumor, unclassified (not otherwise specified)
M-90643	**Germ Cell Tumors**
M-90603	Dysgerminoma
With G-A643	Variant – with syncytiotrophoblast cells
M-90713	Yolk sac tumor (endodermal sinus tumor)
M-90713	Variants – polyvesicular vitelline tumor
	Hepatoid
T-1A310	Glandular (also called 'endometrioid-like')
M-90703	Embryonal carcinoma
M-90723	Polyembryoma
M-91003 F-84200	Choriocarcinoma, non-gestational
M-90801	*Teratoma*
M-90803	Immature
M-90801	Mature
M-90801	Solid
M-90840	Cystic (dermoid cyst)
M-8FFFF G-A570	With secondary tumor (specify type)
	Fetiform (homunculus)
	Monodermal
M-90900	Struma ovarii
(M-8FFFF G-A570) G-A643	Variant – with secondary tumor (specify type)
M-82403	Carcinoid tumor
	Insular
	Trabecular
M-90911	Strumal carcinoid tumor
M-82433	Mucinous carcinoid tumor
M-93643	Neuroectodermal tumors (specify type)
T-01310 M-8FFFF	Sebaceous tumors
M-90853	Mixed germ cell tumors (specify types)
M-90853	**Mixed Germ Cell and Sex Cord-Stromal Tumors**

M-90731	Gonadoblastoma
M-90603 G-A643	Variant – with dysgerminoma or other germ cell tumor
M-90643/M-85901/M-85901	**Germ cell-sex cord-stromal tumor of non-gonadoblastoma type**
(M-90731 G-0042)	
M-9060 G-A643	Variant – with dysgerminoma or other germ cell tumor
T-87410 M-8FFFF	**Tumors of Rete Ovarii**
M-81400/M-84400	Adenoma and cystadenoma
M-81403	Adenocarcinoma
M-905F9	**Mesothelial Tumors**
M-90540	Adenomatoid tumor
M-90503	Mesothelioma
M-8FFFF	**Tumors of Uncertain Origin and Miscellaneous Tumors**
M-80413	Small cell carcinomas
(T-F6460 G-2002) M-8FFFF	Tumor of probable wolffian origin
	Hepatoid carcinoma
M-88400	Myxoma
D8-00180	**Gestational Trophoblastic Diseases**
M-880F9	**Soft Tissue Tumors Not Specific to Ovary**
M-95903/M-98003	**Malignant Lymphomas and Leukemias**
M-80006	**Secondary (metastatic) Tumors**
D8-00180	**GESTATIONAL TROPHOBLASTIC-DISEASE**
M-91000	**Hydatidiform Mole**
M-91000	Complete
M-91030	Partial
M-91001	**Invasive Hydatidiform Mole**
M-91001	(Chorioadenoma destruens)
M-91003	**Choriocarcinoma**
M-91041	**Placental Site Trophoblastic Tumor**
	Miscellaneous Trophoblastic Lesions
T-F1900	Exaggerated placental site
T-F1900 M-03010/M-01470	Placental site nodule and plaque
D8-00180 G-A650	**Unclassified Trophoblastic Lesions**

* SNOMED RT is a Registered Trademark and is copyrighted by SNOMED International of the College of American Pathologists.

Appendix C:
Synoptic reports/checklists

Stanley J. Robboy   Rex C. Bentley

INTRODUCTION

The use of synoptic reports has been advocated for many years, both to include the necessary data points a clinician finds useful for treatment and to better standardize the method in which the information is presented. Edition 1 of this book presented a complete set of synoptic reports for gynecologic pathology that had been developed some years before by a group of senior gynecologic pathologists.[1] More recently, the College of American Pathologists developed a set of synoptic reports for the entire body, the data items for which have been deemed required for inclusion in pathology reports if the pathologist's hospital is to achieve accreditation as a tumor registry certified by the American College of Surgeons. The templates listed below are abstracted from the CAP website (www.CAP.org → Reference resources → Practice Resources, subheading Cancer Protocols). Two examples for each organ are then presented, one where the details of primary cancer are given first, followed by the sites and details of the metastases. The final section lists findings in the non-involved organs. The second example, a form more common to most pathologists, lists the findings for each container in order for any given patient accession. In the authors' department, the mandated information on pathologic staging and the procedure the clinician performed are listed in a section separate from the diagnosis, as the true procedure and the final clinical and even some of the information useful for pathologic staging are not always available to the pathologist.

SECTION ON STAGING IN THE REPORT

PROCEDURE:
PATHOLOGIC STAGE: PT_pN_pM_
NOTE: Information on pathology staging and the operative procedure is being transmitted to this Institution's Cancer Registry as required for accreditation purposes by the Commission on Cancer. Pathology staging is based solely upon the current tissue specimen being evaluated, and does not incorporate information on any specimens submitted separately to our Cytology section, past pathology information, imaging studies, or clinical or operative findings. Anatomic pathology staging is a component to be considered only in determining the clinical stage, but should not be confused with nor substituted for it. The exact operative procedure is available in the surgeon's operative report.

VULVAR CARCINOMA

GENERIC TEMPLATE LISTING CRITICAL FEATURES

Specimen type: ____ [expand]
VULVA (location of submitted specimen)
   Histologic type: ____ carcinoma.
   Tumor grade: ____ [FIGO 1, 2, or 3, if applicable].
   Location of tumor: ____
   Tumor size: ____ × ____ × ____ cm.
   Depth of invasion: ____ cm, in a specimen ____ cm thick (including subq tissue).
   Lymphatic/vascular invasion: ____ [present, absent].
   Margins: ____
      Vaginal cuff: ____ [involved, not involved].
      Anal: ____ [involved, not involved].
      Closest disease-free margin: ____ cm.
   Epidermis adjacent to tumor: ____
   Additional findings: ____

(*Omit what is not relevant*)
The following contain tumor:
The following are free of tumor:
Left superficial inguinal lymph nodes: ____ [findings].
Right superficial inguinal lymph nodes ____ [findings].

EXAMPLE: KEY DIAGNOSIS FIRST AND CLUSTERED

C. 'Vulva':
   Histologic type: Squamous cell carcinoma, invasive.
   Tumor grade: Moderately differentiated.
   Location of tumor: Left vulva.
   Tumor size: 6.0 × 4.5 cm.
   Depth of invasion: 0.5 cm, in a specimen 1.0 cm thick, including subcutaneous tissue.
   Lymphatic/vascular invasion: Absent.
   Margins: Completely excised.
      Vaginal cuff: N/A.
      Closest disease-free margin: 0.5 cm.
   Epidermis adjacent to tumor: Atrophic.
   Additional findings: None.

The following contain metastatic tumor:
B. Left inguinal lymph nodes: three of nine nodes contain tumor (3/9).

The following specimens are free of tumor:
A. Right inguinal lymph nodes: no tumor in eight lymph nodes (0/8).

EXAMPLE: DIAGNOSIS LISTED IN ORDER OF RECEIPT IN PATHOLOGY LAB

A. Right inguinal lymph nodes: no tumor in eight lymph nodes (0/8).
B. Left inguinal lymph nodes: three of nine nodes contain tumor (3/9).
C. 'Vulva':
　　Histologic type: Squamous cell carcinoma, invasive.
　　Tumor grade: Moderately differentiated.
　　Location of tumor: Left vulva.
　　Tumor size: 6.0 × 4.5 cm.
　　Depth of invasion: 0.5 cm, in a specimen 1.0 cm thick, including subcutaneous tissue.
　　Lymphatic/vascular invasion: Absent.
　　Margins: Completely excised.
　　　　Vaginal cuff: N/A.
　　　　Closest disease-free margin: 0.5 cm.
　　Epidermis adjacent to tumor: Atrophic.
　　Additional findings: None.

VAGINAL CARCINOMA

GENERIC TEMPLATE LISTING CRITICAL FEATURES

VAGINA
　　Histologic type: ____ carcinoma, invasive.
　　Tumor grade: ____ [FIGO 1, 2, or 3, if applicable].
　　Tumor size: ____ × ____ × ____ cm.
　　Location: ____ [upper, middle, lower thirds and ant/post and laterality R/L].
　　Depth of invasion: ____ cm, in a wall ____ cm thick.
　　Margins: ____ [present, where].
　　　　Tumor-free distance to closest margin: ____ cm.
　　Additional findings: ____

CERVICAL MICROINVASIVE AND CARCINOMA

GENERIC TEMPLATE LISTING CRITICAL FEATURES

MICROINVASIVE SQUAMOUS CELL CARCINOMA [of cervix]
　　Depth of invasion: ____ mm.
　　Horizontal size of invasive tumor: ____ mm.
　　Lymphatic/vascular invasion: ____ [yes/no].
　　Endocervical glands involved: ____ [yes/no].
　　Margins of resection:
　　　　Ectocervical: ____
　　　　Endocervical: ____
　　　　Deep: ____

EXAMPLE:

Microinvasive squamous cell carcinoma [of cervix]
　　Depth of invasion: 0.5 mm.
　　Horizontal size of invasive tumor: 2 mm.
　　Lymphatic/vascular invasion: No.
　　Additional finding: Extensive CIN3 with involvement of endocervical gland crypts.

Margins of resection:
　　Ectocervical: Negative.
　　Endocervical: Involved.
　　Deep: Negative.

NOTE: The microinvasive component is of the 'spray bud' type and consists of two microscopic foci, each miniscule and much smaller than ½ millimeter in size. These are completely excised. However, the extensive CIN3 does involve the endocervical margin. These findings have been discussed with Dr. James Johnson (11/9/07, 2:20pm).

GENERIC TEMPLATE LISTING CRITICAL FEATURES

UTERUS: ____ grams.
　　Cervix:
　　　　Location: ____ [o'clock boundaries].
　　　　Histologic type: ____ carcinoma, invasive.
　　　　Tumor grade: ____ [FIGO 1, 2, or 3, if applicable].
　　　　Tumor size: ____ × ____ × ____ cm.
　　　　Depth of invasion: ____ cm, in a wall ____ cm thick.
　　　　Lymphatic/vascular invasion: ____ no tumor seen [present, supfl or deep].
　　　　Vaginal cuff: ____ [tumor present, absent].
　　　　Parametria: ____ [tumor present (which side), absent].
　　　　Margins: ____ [present, where].
　　　　　　Tumor-free distance to closest margin: ____ [cm].
　　Endometrium: ____ [involved by carcinoma; or benign dx if no cancer].
　　Myometrium: ____ [involved by carcinoma; or benign dx if no cancer].
　　Serosa: ____

EXAMPLE: KEY DIAGNOSIS FIRST AND CLUSTERED

A. 'Uterus': 159 grams.
　　Cervix:
　　　　Location: Endocervix, diffuse, circumferential.
　　　　Histologic type: Squamous cell carcinoma, non-keratinizing type, invasive.
　　　　Tumor grade: N/A.
　　　　Tumor size: 5 × 4 × 3 cm (estimate).
　　　　Depth of invasion: 1.5 cm, in a wall 1.5 cm thick.
　　　　Lymphatic/vascular invasion: Perivascular and major vascular venous invasion.
　　　　Vaginal cuff: Unremarkable.
　　　　Parametria: Involved.
　　　　Margins: Uninvolved.
　　　　　　Tumor-free distance to closest margin: 0.2 mm.
　　Endometrium: Quiescent.
　　Myometrium: Involved with tumor.
　　Serosa: No pathologic diagnosis.

The following specimens disclose metastatic/implanted tumor:
B. Right pelvic lymph node: microscopic (≪ 1 mm) focus in one of nine lymph nodes (1/9).

The following specimens are free of tumor:
A. Ovaries and fallopian tubes, bilateral: no pathologic diagnosis.
C. Left pelvic lymph nodes: no tumor in six lymph nodes (0/6).

EXAMPLE: DIAGNOSIS LISTED IN ORDER OF RECEIPT IN PATHOLOGY LAB

A. 'Uterus': 159 grams.
  Cervix:
    Location: Endocervix, diffuse, circumferential.
    Histologic type: Squamous cell carcinoma, non-keratinizing type, invasive.
    Tumor grade: N/A.
    Tumor size: 5 × 4 × 3 cm (estimate).
    Depth of invasion: 1.5 cm, in a wall 1.5 cm thick.
    Lymphatic/vascular invasion: Perivascular and major vascular venous invasion.
    Vaginal cuff: Unremarkable.
    Parametria: Involved.
    Margins: Uninvolved.
      Tumor-free distance to closest margin: 0.2 mm.
  Endometrium: Quiescent.
  Myometrium: Involved with tumor.
  Serosa: No pathologic diagnosis.
  Ovaries and fallopian tubes, bilateral: no pathologic diagnosis.
B. Right pelvic lymph node: microscopic (≪1 mm) focus in one of nine lymph nodes (1/9).
C. Left pelvic lymph nodes: no tumor in six lymph nodes (0/6).

ENDOMETRIAL CANCER (EXCLUDES STROMAL TUMORS)

GENERIC TEMPLATE LISTING CRITICAL FEATURES

UTERUS: ____ grams.
  Endometrium:
    Tumor site: ____ [diffuse, fundus, corpus, LUS, R/L cornu].
    Histologic type: ____ adenocarcinoma [histo type, or N/A].
    FIGO grade: ____ [FIGO 1, 2, or 3, if applicable]
    Tumor size: ____ × ____ × ____ cm.
    Maximum depth of myometrial invasion: ____ cm, in a ____ cm thick wall.
    Lymphatic/vascular invasion: ____ [pos, neg].
    Adjacent non-neoplastic endometrium: ____ [nl, atrophic, hyperplasia, absent].
    Remaining myometrium: ____ [leiomyoma, adenomyosis].
  Cervix: ____ [if involved, note mucosal vs stromal invasion; list other benign dx].
  Serosa: ____ [free of tumor, other findings].
  Specimen margins: ____

EXAMPLE: KEY DIAGNOSIS FIRST AND CLUSTERED

A. 'Uterus': 56 grams.
  Endometrium:
    Tumor site: Fundus.
    Histologic type: Carcinosarcoma (malignant mixed müllerian tumor).
    FIGO grade: 2.
    Tumor size: 2.5 × 1.5 × 1.3 cm.
    Maximum depth of myometrial invasion: 0.6 cm, in a 1.4 cm thick wall.
    Lymphatic/vascular invasion: Negative.
    Adjacent non-neoplastic endometrium: Atrophy.
    Remaining myometrium: No pathologic diagnosis.

Cervix: Negative for malignancy.
Serosa: Negative for malignancy.
Specimen margins: negative for malignancy.

The following specimens disclose metastatic/implanted tumor:
B. Left ovary.
C. Right ovary.
D. Left pelvic sidewall (biopsy).

The following specimens are free of tumor:
B. Left fallopian tube.
C. Right fallopian tube.
E. Left pelvic lymph node (biopsy): eight lymph nodes, negative for malignancy (0/8).
F. Right aortic node (biopsy): five lymph nodes, negative for malignancy (0/5).
G. Left aortic node (biopsy): three lymph nodes, negative for malignancy (0/3).
H. Right highest periaortic node (biopsy): two lymph nodes, negative for malignancy (0/2).
I. Right pelvic nodes (biopsy): twenty lymph nodes, negative for malignancy (0/20).

EXAMPLE: DIAGNOSIS LISTED IN ORDER OF RECEIPT IN PATHOLOGY LAB

A. 'Uterus': 56 grams.
  Endometrium:
    Tumor site: Fundus.
    Histologic type: Carcinosarcoma (malignant mixed müllerian tumor).
    FIGO grade: 2.
    Tumor size: 2.5 × 1.5 × 1.3 cm.
    Maximum depth of myometrial invasion: 0.6 cm, in a 1.4 cm thick wall.
    Lymphatic/vascular invasion: Negative.
    Adjacent non-neoplastic endometrium: Atrophy.
    Remaining myometrium: No pathologic diagnosis.
  Cervix: Negative for malignancy.
  Serosa: Negative for malignancy.
  Specimen margins: negative for malignancy.
B. 'Left tube and ovary' (left salpingo-oophorectomy):
    Ovary with metastatic carcinosarcoma.
    Fallopian tube: no pathologic diagnosis.
    See comment.
C. 'Right tube and ovary' (right salpingo-oophorectomy):
    Ovary with metastatic carcinosarcoma.
    Fallopian tube: no pathologic diagnosis.
    See comment.
D. 'Left pelvic sidewall' (biopsy):
    Metastatic carcinosarcoma.
    See comment.
E. 'Left pelvic lymph node' (biopsy):
    Eight lymph nodes, negative for malignancy (0/8).
F. 'Right aortic node' (biopsy):
    Five lymph nodes, negative for malignancy (0/5).
    Granulomatous inflammation.
G. 'Left aortic node' (biopsy):
    Three lymph nodes, negative for malignancy (0/3).
H. 'Right highest periaortic node' (biopsy):
    Two lymph nodes, negative for malignancy (0/2).
I. 'Right pelvic nodes' (biopsy):
    Twenty lymph nodes, negative for malignancy (0/20).
    Granulomatous inflammation.

FALLOPIAN TUBE CARCINOMA

GENERIC TEMPLATE LISTING CRITICAL FEATURES

'____ FALLOPIAN TUBE' [side]
   ____ Adenocarcinoma [histologic type, or as applicable].
   FIGO grade: ____ [FIGO 1, 2, or 3, if applicable].
   Tumor size: ____ × ____ × ____ cm.
   Weight: ____ grams.
   Tumor site: ____ [fimbria, ampulla, infundibulum, isthmus].
   Relation to ovary: ____ [fused].
   Status of fimbriated end: ____ [open, closed].
   Specimen integrity: ____ [intact, ruptured, fragmented].
   Lymphatic/vascular invasion: ____ [yes/no].
   Additional findings: ____ [salpingitis].

OVARIAN CARCINOMA (EXCLUDING GERM CELL TUMORS)

GENERIC TEMPLATE LISTING CRITICAL FEATURES

'____ OVARY': [side]
   ____ Adenocarcinoma [histologic type, or as applicable].
   FIGO grade: ____ [FIGO 1, 2, or 3, if applicable].
   Tumor size: ____ × ____ × ____ cm.
   Weight: ____ grams.
   Serosa: ____ [growth on surface, rupture].
   Additional findings: ____ [endometriosis].
Specimens with metastatic/implanted tumor.
Specimens free of tumor.

EXAMPLE: KEY DIAGNOSIS FIRST AND CLUSTERED

A,B. 'Right ovary':
   Type: Serous borderline tumor.
   FIGO grade: N/A.
   Tumor size: 14.5 × 9.5 × 4 cm.
   Weight: 129 grams.
   Serosa: Involved.
   Additional findings: None.

Specimens with metastatic/implanted tumor:
C. Appendix.
D. Right gutter peritoneum.
E. Omentum.

Specimens free of tumor:
F. Left ovary and bilateral fallopian tubes.

NOTE: The various extragonadal specimens disclose numerous tumor implants, many with foci of desmoplastic stromal responses, but no definitive invasive implants.

EXAMPLE: DIAGNOSIS LISTED IN ORDER OF RECEIPT IN PATHOLOGY LAB

A. 'Right ovary' biopsy: serous borderline tumor.
B. 'Right ovary':
   Type: Serous borderline tumor.
   FIGO grade: N/A.
   Tumor size: 14.5 × 9.5 × 4 cm.
   Weight: 129 grams.
   Serosa: Involved.
   Additional findings: None.
C. Appendix: Implants of borderline serous tumor.
D. Right gutter peritoneum: Implants of borderline serous tumor
E. Omentum: Implants of borderline serous tumor.
F. Left ovary and bilateral fallopian tubes: No pathologic diagnosis.

NOTE: The various extragonadal specimens disclose numerous tumor implants, many with foci of desmoplastic stromal responses, but no definitive invasive implants.

GESTATIONAL TROPHOBLASTIC TUMOR

GENERIC TEMPLATE LISTING CRITICAL FEATURES

Specimen type: ____ [partial or radical vaginectomy]
   GESTATIONAL TROPHOBLASTIC DISEASE
   Histologic type: ____
   Tumor size: ____ × ____ × ____ cm.
   Location: ____ depth of invasion: ____ cm, in a wall ____ cm thick.
   Margins: ____ [present, where].
   Tumor-free distance to closest margin: ____ cm.
   Lymphatic/vascular invasion: ____ [yes/no].
   Additional findings: ____
   Fetal tissue: ____ [present, absent].

REFERENCE

1. Robboy SJ, Bentley RC, Krigman H, Silverberg SG, Norris HJ, Zaino RJ. Synoptic reports in gynecologic pathology. Int J Gynecol Pathol 1994;13:161–74.

Appendix D:
Coding with SNOMED CT (Systematized Nomenclature of Medicine-Clinical Terminology)

Christopher B. Hubbard   John F. Madden   Rajesh Dash   Stanley J. Robboy

This textbook, largely descriptive, aims to help the user achieve dexterity in rendering a correct diagnosis based on the histologic and immunocytochemical features present. Once rendered, the more pressing issue pertinent in today's perspective of global health care is to more effectively allow information exchange, such that the diagnosis can easily be shared wherever a patient's record is stored, used for statistical purposes or quality assurance, or even compared with institutions around the world. Free text is difficult to compare. Structured coding, in contrast, is realistic and preferred.

For more than 40 years, the US College of American Pathologists (CAP) has been developing a standard medical nomenclature and coding language, SNOMED (Systematized Nomenclature of Medicine). In the early 2000s, the CAP's then current version SNOMED RT (for Reference Terminology) joined with the United Kingdom's Clinical Terms Version 3 (CTV3) to form SNOMED CT® (Clinical Terminology). SNOMED CT® is a scientifically validated, comprehensive clinical healthcare terminology that today is the most complete multilingual clinical terminology now existing in the world.

SNOMED CT® is now the US standard for electronic health information exchange in interoperability specifications defined by the Healthcare Information Technology Standards Panel (HITSP), an arm of the US Government. It has also been adopted for electronic information interchange by the US Departments of Health and Human Services, Defense, and Veterans Affairs, through the Consolidated Health Informatics (CHI) initiative. In May 2004, the US National Library of Medicine adopted SNOMED CT® and integrated it into its Unified Medical Language System (UMLS) Metathesaurus. Through the UMLS Metathesaurus, SNOMED CT® is free for use by anyone in the United States. As of April 2007 the intellectual property rights to SNOMED CT® were transferred to the International Health Terminology Standards Organization (IHTSDO) in a move aimed at making SNOMED CT® a truly international standard with worldwide adoption. At the time of this writing, the following charter member countries support SNOMED CT®: Australia, Canada, Denmark, Lithuania, The Netherlands, New Zealand, Sweden, the United Kingdom, and the United States.

SNOMED CT® is commonly used for coding, retrieval, and analysis of clinical data. In its basic form, SNOMED CT® has a core set of over 376 000 'concepts' that represent granular clinical terms across the spectrum of health care. All SNOMED CT® concepts fall into one of the following 19 *root concept* categories:

- *Clinical finding*
- *Procedure*
- *Observable entity*
- *Body structure*
- *Organism*
- *Substance*
- *Pharmaceutical/biologic product*
- *Specimen*
- *Special concept*
- *Physical force*
- *Event*
- *Environments/geographical locations*
- *Social context*
- *Situation with explicit context*
- *Staging and scales*
- *Linkage concept*
- *Qualifier value*
- *Record artifact*
- *Physical object*

SNOMED CT® includes a number of data tables (Figure D.1). The core data tables include concepts, descriptions, and relationships. In addition to these tables, SNOMED CT® also includes tables to manage historical changes, indicate subsets of concepts, cross maps to different terminologies such as ICD-9 and LOINC, and others.

Medical concepts can be expressed accurately by a number of terms and abbreviations. For example, endometrial intraepithelial neoplasia may also be referred to as simply 'EIN'. To accommodate widely diverse terminology for the same clinical concept, SNOMED CT® provides for potentially an unlimited number of synonyms know as *descriptions*. Descriptions can be one of several description 'types' including *Fully Specified Name*, *Preferred Term*, or *Synonym*. All concepts have at least a *Fully Specified Name* and a *Preferred Term* description.

To express complex medical concepts and relationships, SNOMED CT® allows concepts to be combined in what are known as *relationships*. Relationships are formed through the use of *Linkage Concepts*. Related concepts maybe be expressed as concept A '*is a*' concept B, or concept A '*has a finding site*' of concept B, for example. These relationships form an ontology that represents the true power of SNOMED CT®.

Other than the core tables, there are several other noteworthy features. SNOMED CT® has cross mappings to other coding systems like ICD-9-CM, ICD-10, and LOINC. Cross mappings correlate SNOMED CT® concepts with codes in these other coding systems. The mappings can be one to one, many to one, or many to many. Cross mappings even contain information regarding the accuracy of the mapping.

Subsets are another important feature of SNOMED CT® (Figure D.1). A subset is lists of concepts, descriptions or relationships that are an index to relevant concepts for a specific topic. Subsets contain concepts for only part of SNOMED CT® but do not limit the full use of SNOMED CT®. Subsets

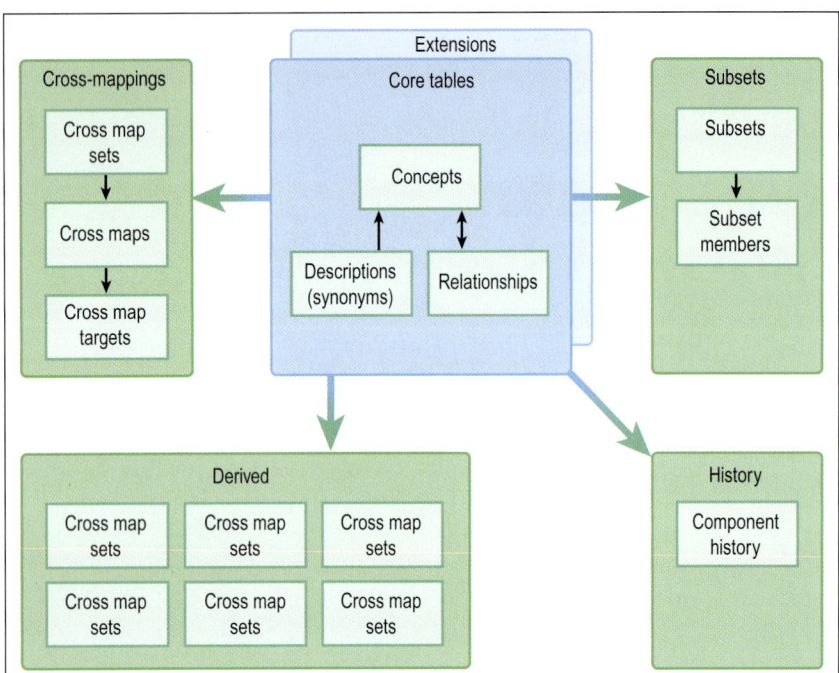

Fig. D.1 Overview of SNOMED CT Data Table.

Table D.1 Potential issues with free text

Accuracy	Text processing generally relies on 'rules' to evaluate freely entered text. These rules can be broken relatively easily (e.g., through misspelling or poor grammar) causing false positives or omissions during term retrieval of codes to match the free text.
Event propagation	Without further processing, trigger alarms, audits, safety alerts, reflex orders, care maps, billing, etc. Example: *In a uterine scraping for intrauterine pregnancy that discloses no chorionic villi, a trigger alert as an e-mail or telephone call to the clinician would be quite useful, stating that in the absence of any definite signs of intrauterine pregnancy, an ectopic pregnancy should be considered quickly.*
Cannot be processed efficiently by computers	Codes that represent granular concepts are much more efficiently processed by computers.

can help reduce the number of concepts one is looking for by filtering out irrelevant terms. This can improve coding accuracy for medical data of a specific context (e.g., anesthesiology, gynecology, pathology, etc.).

SNOMED CT® comes with a useful freeware software tool known as CliniClue.[1] CliniClue provides an easy to use tool for finding SNOMED CT® concepts and visualizing built-in concept relationships (Figure D.2).

WHY CODE? WHY SNOMED?

Health care is rapidly moving towards digitized records. The US Federal Government has called for this movement and even mandates it in certain cases. The digital promise is an increased ease of use on many levels and the portability of information. However, much healthcare information is free text which has proven problematic for reliable digital use (Table D.1). To fully utilize digital healthcare information safely and efficiently, coded terminology is a requirement.

The coding of healthcare information is certainly not new. Many aspects of health care have been coded for years with systems such as ICD-9, ICD-10, and CPT. So why not just use one of these systems? The reason is these systems are more generalized in nature, were not designed for clinical notation coding, and the data collected are to a different standard. Additionally, these systems have no facility to combine expressions to clarify meaning and the updates from gatekeepers are too slow to respond to rapidly evolving areas of clinical practice. Using coded information for patient care requires a degree of precision for which these systems were simply not made.

SNOMED CT® was specifically designed to address clinical coding issues. Through the use of the many SNOMED CT® features one can precisely and accurately convey clinical information (Table D.2).

Some of the benefits to health care coding with SNOMED CT® include the following:

- Common national, international, and multilingual terminology that allows direct correlation.
- Concise, legible data.
- Computer friendly data for quick and efficient processing.
- Ability to search for information not actually present through relationships (e.g., substances in drugs).
- Improved patient safety (alerts, reflexive processing, drug interactions, auditing, etc.).
- Improves interoperability between systems by providing a common terminology.

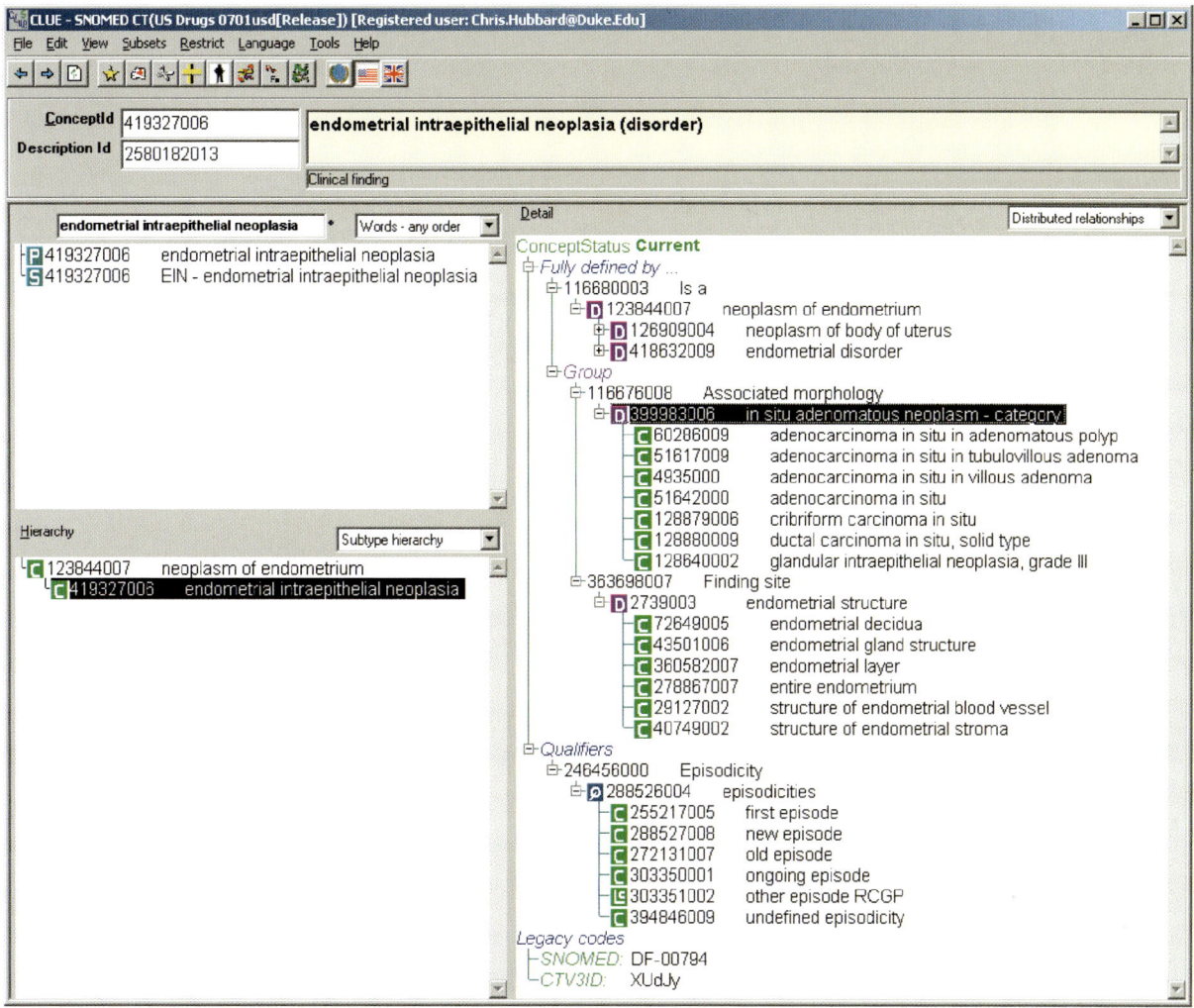

Fig. D.2 Example of clinical features associated with a SNOMED concept.

Table D.2 Examples of SNOMED CT® coded diagnosis

Sample diagnosis	SNOMED CT code – concept
Mild dysplasia	(43185009) Mild dysplasia (morphologic abnormality)

Endometrial intraepithelial neoplasia of endometrium	(419327006) Endometrial intraepithelial neoplasia (disorder)
	   (363698007) Finding site (attribute)
	     (2739003) Endometrial structure (body structure)

Pseudomyxoma peritonei arising in the appendix metastatic to ovary	(112679004) Pseudomyxoma peritonei (morphologic abnormality)
	   (114158018) Arising in (attribute)
	     (181255000) Entire appendix (body structure)
	     (77879006) Metastatic to (attribute)
	       (181464007) Entire ovary (body structure)

- Improved intraorganizational continuity of care (e.g., allergies gathered at admission can be automatically used by a pharmacist).
- Improved information flow between public/private and primary/secondary/tertiary care providers.
- Improved local, national, and international disease monitoring and epidemiology.
- Improved auditing.
- Improved research and other use services.
- Improved care mapping and disease management.

- Improved billing and reimbursement.
- Improved decision support.
- Improved aggregate, administrative, performance, and resource reporting.

REFERENCE

1. CLUE and CliniClue are available as freeware from The Clinical Information Consultancy Ltd. Online. Available: www.cliniclue.com.

Appendix E: Abbreviations

5-HIAA	5-hydroxyindoleacetic acid
ACOG	American College of Obstetricians and Gynecologists
ACTH	adrenocorticotropic hormone
AFP	α-fetoprotein
AGUS	atypical glandular cells of undetermined significance
AHC	adrenal hypoplasia congenita [gene]
AILD	angioimmunoblastic lymphadenopathy with dysproteinemia
AIS	adenocarcinoma *in situ*
ALCL	anaplastic large T-cell lymphoma
AMH	antimüllerian hormone (see MIS)
AML	acute myeloid leukemia
aPC	activated protein C
APC	adenomatous polyposis coli
APUD	amine precursor uptake and decarboxylation
AR	androgen receptor
AREDF	absence or reverse of end-diastolic flow
ASC-H	atypical squamous cells – HSIL cannot be excluded
ASCUS	atypical squamous cells of undetermined significance
BCC	basal cell carcinoma
BEP	bleomycin, etoposide and cisplatin [chemotherapy]
BMI	body mass index
BPES	blepharophimosis ptosis epicanthus inversus syndrome
BRCA1	breast cancer gene 1
CAH	congenital adrenal hyperplasia
CALLA	common acute lymphoblastic leukemia antigen
CAP	College of American Pathologists
CCC	clear cell adenocarcinoma
CDK4I	cyclin-dependent kinase 4 inhibitor
CDKN2A	cyclin-dependent kinase inhibitor 2A
CD*nn*	cluster designation number, e.g., CD31
Cdx2	caudal-related homeobox 2 [gene/protein]
CEA	carcinoembryonic antigen
CGH	comparative genomic hybridization
CGIN	cervical glandular intraepithelial neoplasia
CHI	Consolidated Health Informatics
CIN	cervical intraepithelial neoplasia
CIS	carcinoma *in situ*
CK	cytokeratin
CLL	chronic lymphocytic leukemia
CML	chronic myelogenous leukemia
CMV	cytomegalovirus
CTZ	congenital transformation zone
CYP	cytochrome pseudogene
D&C	dilatation and curettage
DAX1	DSS-AHC on the X chromosome, where DSS = dosage sensitive sex reversal gene and AHC = adrenal hypoplasia congenita gene
DAZ	deleted in azoospermia
DCH	dehydrocholesterol
DES	diethylstilbestrol (Stilbestrol)
DESAD	Diethylstilbestrol Adenosis [project]
DHEA	dehydroepiandrosterone
DHT	dihydrotestosterone
DIC	disseminated intravascular coagulation
DLBCL	diffuse large B-cell lymphoma
DMPA	depot-medroxyprogesterone acetate
DPC	deleted in pancreatic cancer
DSD	disorder of sex development
DSS	dosage sensitive sex reversal [gene]
dUTP	deoxyuridine triphosphate
EBV	Epstein–Barr virus
EBV-LMP	Epstein–Barr virus latent membrane protein
ECC	endocervical curettage
EDC	estimated date of confinement
EGD	endocervical glandular dysplasia
EGF	epidermal growth factor
EGFR	epidermal growth factor receptor
EIA	enzyme immunoassay
EIC	endometrial intraepithelial carcinoma
EIN	endometrial intraepithelial neoplasia
EMA	epithelial membrane antigen
EmGD	endometrial glandular dysplasia
ER	estrogen receptor
ESA	epithelial specific antigen
ESN	endometrial stromal nodule
ESS	endometrial (endometrioid) stromal sarcoma
ETT	epithelioid trophoblastic tumor
FATWO	female adnexal tumor of (probable) wolffian origin
FCL	follicular lymphoma
FDA	Food and Drug Administration
FIGO	Federation International of Gynecologists and Obstetricians
FISH	fluorescent *in situ* hybridization
FNAC	fine needle aspiration cytology
FSH	follicle-stimulating hormone
FTV	fetal thrombotic vasculopathy
FUS	focused ultrasound
GBY	gonadoblastoma Y [gene]
GCDFP	gross cystic disease fluid protein
GCT	granulosa cell tumor

GFAP	glial fibrillary acid protein		LUF	luteinized unruptured follicle [syndrome]
GIST	gastrointestinal stromal tumor		LVSI	lymphovascular involvement
GMS	Gomori methenamine silver [stain]		MALT	mucosa-associated lymphoid tissue
GnRH	gonadotrophin-releasing hormone		MART-1	melanoma antigen recognized by T cells-1
GOG	Gynecologic Oncology Group		MBT	mucinous borderline tumor
GTD	gestational trophoblastic disease		mCEA	monoclonal carcinoembryonic antigen
GTN	gestational trophoblastic neoplasia		MCL	mantle cell lymphoma
HAM-56	human alveolar macrophage-56		MCM	multicopy maintenance [protein family]
hCG	human chorionic gonadotrophin		MEA	microwave energy
HCGIN	high-grade cervical glandular intraepithelial neoplasia		Mel-CAM	melanoma cell adhesion molecule
			MGD	mixed gonadal dysgenesis
HELLP	hemolysis, elevated liver enzymes, low platelets [syndrome]		MGH	microglandular hyperplasia
			MHA-TP	microhemagglutination assay for antibodies to *T. pallidum*
Hep Par 1	hepatocyte paraffin 1			
HGSIL	high-grade squamous intraepithelial lesion		MHC	major histocompatibility complex
HITSP	Healthcare Information Technology Standards Panel		MI	microsatellite instability; myocardial infarction
			MIC	müllerian inclusion cysts
HLA	human leukocyte antigen		MIS	müllerian inhibiting substance (see AMH)
HMG	high motility gene		Mitf	microphthalmia-associated transcription factor
HNPCC	hereditary non-polyposis colorectal cancer		MMMT	mesodermal (müllerian) mixed tumor/ malignant mixed müllerian tumor
HPF	high power field			
hPL	human placental lactogen		MoMo	monochorionic monoamniotic [twins]
HPV	human papillomavirus		MRgFUS	magnetic resonance guided focused ultrasound
HRT	hormone replacement therapy		MSAFP	maternal serum α-fetoprotein
HSD	hydroxysteroid dehydrogenase		MTHFR	methylenetetrahydrofolate reductase [gene]
HSIL	high-grade squamous intraepithelial lesion		NCAM	neural cell adhesion molecule
HSV	herpes simplex virus		NCBD	nuclear changes bordering on dyskaryosis
IADSRCT	intra-abdominal desmoplastic small round cell tumor		NCR	non-coding region
			NECC1	not expressed in choriocarcinoma clone 1 [gene]
IEC	intraepithelial carcinoma			
IFN	interferon		NHL	non-Hodgkin lymphoma
Ig	immunoglobulin		NK	natural killer
IGF	insulin-like growth factor		NSE	neuron-specific enolase
IGFBP	insulin-like growth factor binding protein		o,p′-DDD	chemical name for mitotane
IHTSDO	International Health Terminology Standards Organization		OC	oral contraceptive
			OCCR	ovarian cancer cluster region
IL	interleukin		OHSS	ovarian hyperstimulation syndrome
IPI	international prognostic index		ORF	open reading frame
ISGP	International Society of Gynecological Pathologists		PAR	pseudoautosomal [pairing] region
			PAS	periodic acid-Schiff
ISVVD	International Society for the Study of Vulvovaginal Disease		PCNA	proliferating cell nuclear antigen
			PCOS	polycystic ovary syndrome
IUD	intrauterine contraceptive device		PCR	polymerase chain reaction
IUGR	intrauterine growth restriction		PDGF	platelet-derived growth factor
JGCT	juvenile granulosa cell tumor		PDGFB	platelet-derived growth factor beta
KPI	karyopyknotic index		PEComa	perivascular epithelioid cell tumor
LBC	liquid-based cytology		PEPI	Postmenopausal Estrogen/Progestin Interventions (PEPI) Trial
LCA	leukocyte common antigen			
LCGIN	low-grade cervical glandular intraepithelial neoplasia		PID	pelvic inflammatory disease
			PLAP	placental-like alkaline phosphatase
LCH	Langerhan cell histiocytosis		PNET	primitive neuroectodermal tumor
LCR	long control region		POC	products of conception
LDH	lactate dehydrogenase		PPV	positive predictive values
LEEP	loop electrosurgical excision procedure		PR	progesterone receptor
LGSIL	low-grade squamous intraepithelial lesion		PRb	retinoblastoma protein
LH	luteinizing hormone		PSCA	prostate stem cell antigen
LHRH	luteinizing hormone-releasing hormone		PSTT	placental site trophoblastic tumor
LMP	latent membrane protein		PTAH	phosphotungstic acid hematoxylin [stain]
LOH	loss of heterozygosity		PTEN	phosphatase and tensin homolog deleted on chromosome 10 [gene]
LOINC	Logical Observation Identifiers Names and Codes			
			PTHrp	parathyroid hormone-related protein
LSIL	low-grade squamous intraepithelial lesion		Rb	retinoblastoma [gene]

RCC	renal cell carcinoma
RFLP	restriction fragment length polymorphism
Rh	maternal rhesus
RPR	rapid plasma reagin
RT-PCR	reverse transcriptase polymerase chain reaction
SBT	serous borderline tumor
SBT-MP	micropapillary serous borderline tumor
SCC	squamous cell carcinoma
SCCA	squamous cell carcinoma antigen
SCTAT	sex-cord tumors with annular tubules
SEER	Surveillance, Epidemiology and End Results [database]
SERM	selective estrogen receptor modulator
SF1	steroidogenic factor 1
SGA	small for gestational age
SGO	Society of Gynecologic Oncologists
SHBG	sex hormone binding globulin
SI	stratification index
SIL	squamous intraepithelial lesion
SIN	salpingitis isthmica nodosa
SIR	standardized incidence ratio
SLL	small lymphocytic lymphoma
SMA	smooth muscle actin
SMILE	stratified mucin-producing intraepithelial lesion
SNOMED	Systematized Nomenclature of Medicine (© College of American Pathologists)
SOX9	SRY-related high motility gene box group
SRY	sex determining region Y
StAR	steroidogenic acute regulatory protein
STI	sexually transmitted infection
STUMP	smooth muscle tumor of uncertain malignant potential

TAH-BSO	total abdominal hysterectomy and bilateral salpingo-oophorectomy
TCC	transitional cell carcinoma
TDF	testis determining factor
TdT	terminal deoxynucleotidyl transferase
TEM	transmission electron microscopy; tuboendometrial metaplasia
TGF	transforming growth factor
TIS	ThinPrep Imaging System
TNF	tumor necrosis factor
TORCH	toxoplasmosis, other infections, rubella, cytomegalovirus infection and herpes simplex [syndrome]
TP53	tumor protein p53
TPHA	*T. pallidum* hemabsorption [test]
TRAP	twin-reversed arterial perfusion
TSPY	testis-specific protein Y
TTF-1	thyroid transcription factor-1
TTTS	twin–twin transfusion syndrome
TUNEL	terminal dUTP nick end labeling
UICC	International Union Against Cancer
UMLS	Unified Medical Language System
URR	upstream regulatory region
UTROSCT	uterine tumor resembling ovarian sex-cord tumor
VaIN	vaginal intraepithelial neoplasia
VDRL	venereal disease research laboratory
VIN	vulvar intraepithelial neoplasia
VLP	virus-like particle
VUE	villitis of unknown etiology
WHO	World Health Organization
WT	Wilms tumor

Index

Page numbers in *italics* represent figures or tables.